VETERINARY MEDICINE

A Textbook of the Diseases of
Cattle, Sheep, Pigs, Goats and Horses

D.C. BLOOD, OBE, BVSc, MVSc, FACVS, HonLLD(Sask),
HonARCVS, HonDVSc, HonLLD(Guelph)
Professor Emeritus,
School of Veterinary Science, University of Melbourne, Australia

O.M. RADOSTITS, DVM, MSc
Professor of Veterinary Medicine,
Department of Veterinary Internal Medicine, University of Saskatchewan,
Saskatoon, Canada
Diplomate of the American College of Veterinary Internal Medicine

J.H. ARUNDEL, BVSc, MVSc
Reader in Veterinary Parasitology,
School of Veterinary Science, University of Melbourne, Australia

C.C. GAY, DVM, MVSc, FACVS
Professor of Veterinary Medicine,
Department of Veterinary Clinical Medicine and Surgery,
Washington State University, Pullman, Washington, USA

VETERINARY MEDICINE

A Textbook of the Diseases of Cattle, Sheep, Pigs, Goats and Horses

by

D.C. BLOOD

and

O.M. RADOSTITS

with contributions by

J.H. Arundel and C.C. Gay

SEVENTH EDITION

Baillière Tindall

London Philadelphia Sydney Tokyo Toronto

Baillière Tindall
W.B. Saunders

24–28 Oval Road
London NW1 7DX

The Curtis Center
Independence Square West
Philadelphia, PA 19106–3399, USA

55 Horner Avenue
Toronto, Ontario M8Z 4X6, Canada

Harcourt Brace Jovanovich Group (Australia) Pty Limited
30–52 Smidmore Street
Marrickville, NSW 2204, Australia

Harcourt Brace Jovanavich (Japan) Inc.
Ichibancho Central Building, 22–1 Ichibancho
Chiyoda-Ku, Tokyo 102, Japan

First published 1960
Fourth edition 1974
Fifth edition 1979
Sixth edition 1983
Reprinted 1985 and 1988
Seventh edition 1989
Reprinted 1990

English Language Book Society Edition of Sixth Edition 1983
French edition (Vigot Frères, Paris) 1976
Italian edition (Editoriale Grasso, Bologna) 1980
Japanese edition (Buneido, Tokyo) 1981
Portuguese edition (Guanabara Koogan, Rio de Janeiro) 1978
Spanish edition (Editorial Interamericana, Mexico) 1982
English Language Book Society Edition of Seventh Edition 1989

This book is printed on acid-free paper ∞

British Library Cataloguing in Publication Data

Blood, D.C. (Douglas Charles),
Veterinary medicine.—7th ed.
1. Livestock. Diseases
I. Title II. Radostits, O.M.
636.089′6

ISBN 0–7020–1286–6

Typeset by Setrite Typesetters Ltd.
Printed and bound in Great Britain by
Mackays of Chatham PLC, Chatham, Kent

Contents

PART ONE GENERAL MEDICINE

PART TWO SPECIAL MEDICINE

List of Tables

List of Illustrations

Preface to the Seventh Edition

WE have undertaken the writing of this new edition because there have been sufficient changes in all sections of the book to warrant an updating of the text. It has been a much bigger task than ever before because of the tremendous increase in volume of veterinary literature which has occurred in the last 5 years. There are many more journals, with many more very good papers by more writers, due in no small part to the increase in number of veterinary schools and therefore in academic staff. Our task of reading, abstracting, collating and annotating has therefore been more time-consuming and also more onerous because of the need to again keep the size of the text similar to that of the last edition, which is close to maximum in our view.

We have found it necessary to rewrite some of the more complex diseases to which much additional information has been added. This list includes bovine virus diarrhea, chronic obstructive pulmonary disease, sarcoidosis, cryptosporidiosis, monensin poisoning, caprine arthritis-encephalitis, equine ehrlichial colitis, swamp cancer and acute interstitial pneumonia. We have also bowed to many requests from Asian and African colleagues and included trypanosomiasis, theileriosis, East Coast fever, surra, sweating sickness and heartwater and assume that we now have a completely international coverage of the medicine of food animals and horses. There are a number of additional poisons and poisonous plants and inherited diseases and many new minor diseases including wool slip, summer slump, cold cow syndrome and watery mouth of lambs; Nairobi sheep disease, giardiasis and yersiniosis have also been added. There are some new findings about rye grass staggers and summer fescue toxicosis. The chapters on therapeutics, nutritional deficiency diseases and helminth and arthropod parasites have had major overhauls, and there have been additions to the sections on chronic renal disease and chronic laminitis.

The major change in the book's format has been the inclusion of an introductory essay on the principles and objectives of food animal medicine. We are of the opinion that these principles and objectives are now so different from those of companion animal medicine that they need to be set down clearly and unequivocally. We hope we have done that and perhaps clarified the views of undergraduates with respect to the expectations that the profession and clients have of them.

We have continued to purge our reference list but they continue to grow in spite of that. Computer-assisted diagnosis has not expanded as much as we expected and the sections on decision analysis and the making of a diagnosis have been expanded proportionally to their importance to medicine at this time.

Since the last edition, the textbook list for food animal veterinarians has been augmented by some significant additions including *Herd Health* by O.M. Radostits and D.C. Blood; *Veterinary Epidemiology* by M. Thrusfield and *Veterinary Virology* by F. Fenner *et al.*

It is again our great pleasure to record our indebtedness to C.C. Gay for Chapters 4 and 8 and some other items and to J.H. Arundel for Chapters 26 and 27. Heather Pearce has been an exemplary typist and translated our less than elegant hand-writing into perfect manuscript with great speed, efficiency and dedication.

D.C. BLOOD
Saskatoon, 1987 O.M. RADOSTITS

DEDICATED
TO THE MEMORY OF
H.B. PARRY
WHO FIRST BASED THE TEACHING OF
VETERINARY INTERNAL MEDICINE
ON PHYSIOLOGY AND PATHOLOGY

AND

TO
J.A. HENDERSON
WHO ALWAYS EXAMINED THE SICK COW FIRST
AND THEN SAID
"NOW LETS LOOK AT THE REST OF THE HERD"

Introduction

OBJECTIVES AND PRINCIPLES OF FOOD-PRODUCING ANIMAL PRACTICE

THE primary objective of this book is to provide the veterinary student and the practitioner with the knowledge and information necessary to provide animal health management for food-producing animals. This is an essay on the objectives and principles of veterinary practice related to the production of cattle, sheep, goats and swine.

Food-producing animal veterinary practice provides service primarily to the owners of the meat-, milk- and fiber-producing animals such as dairy and beef cattle, swine, sheep and goats. In recent years, veterinarians have begun to provide service to owners of wildlife species such red deer, elk and moose which are being raised under farm conditions for the production of meat and byproducts such as hides. While some commercially processed horsemeat is consumed by humans, the market is small compared to beef and pork, and horses are not usually included in discussions about food-producing animal veterinary practice. Poultry, fish and rabbits are also important sources of human food.

For the past 40 years the major activity in food-producing animal practice, and a major source of income, was the provision of emergency veterinary service to the owners of herds or flocks in which a single animal or a few animals were affected with one of the common diseases. Occasionally, outbreaks of disease affecting several animals occurred. In addition, routine elective veterinary services such as castration, vaccination, dehorning, deworming, the testing for diseases such as brucellosis and tuberculosis, and the dispensing of veterinary drugs, pharmaceuticals and biologics accounted for a significant source of revenue for the veterinarian. In the last 10 years there has been a shift from emphasis and dependence on emergency veterinary medicine and routine procedures to more attention being paid by the veterinarian and the producer to planned animal health and production management using the whole farm approach. Livestock producers are now much more knowledgeable and articulate about animal agriculture than they used to be and they are concerned about the cost-effectiveness and the scientific basis of the recommendations made by veterinarians and agricultural advisors. More and more producers are doing the routine elective procedures themselves. From first-hand experience and extension courses provided for them, they have also learned how to diagnose and treat many of the common diseases of farm livestock. Many veterinary pharmaceuticals, antimicrobials and biologics can now be purchased by producers from either veterinary or non-veterinary sources.

The intensification of animal agriculture has created complex animal health and production problems for which there are no simple and reliable therapeutic and preventive procedures, and this has made the task of the veterinarian much more difficult. For example, acute undifferentiated respiratory disease of feedlot cattle is a major problem which is difficult to treat and control effectively because the etiology and epidemiology are complex. Acute diarrhea of newborn calves can be caused by many different enteropathogens but a knowledge of the risk factors or epidemiological determinants such as colostral immunity and population density is probably more important for effective clinical management and control of the disease. The rearing of pigs intensively and in complete confinement has exaggerated problems such as neonatal mortality due to crushing by the sow, suboptimal reproductive performance due to a variety of management and environmental factors, and pneumonia in growing and finishing pigs which may be almost impossible to eradicate unless the herd is depopulated and repopulated with minimal disease breeding stock. The solutions to these complex problems are not readily available, in part, because insufficient research on their etiology and epidemiology has been done in the herds where the problems are occurring. As a result, the veterinarian must become knowledgeable and skillful in the principles of epidemiology, applied nutrition and animal housing, in the education and training of animal attendants, the analysis of production indices and profit and loss, which includes the use of computers, in addition to being skillful in the traditional veterinary disciplines of medicine, reproduction, pharmacology, pathology and the like. In summary, the food-producing animal practitioner must become more skilled in the simultaneous management of animal health and production; the modern livestock producer is cost conscious and anything veterinarians do or recommend must be cost-effective.

In contrast, the developments in companion animal medicine have followed in the footsteps of human medicine with an ever increasing emphasis and reliance on extensive use of clinical pathology for the in-depth evaluation of the hematology, clinical chemistry, enzymology, immune status and many other body functions of clinical cases. Several diagnostic techniques such as ultrasonography, endoscopy, nuclear imaging and computerized axial tomography, in addition to the traditional radiographic techniques commonly used in small animal practice, are now also being introduced primarily in veterinary teaching hospitals but also in specialty referral private practices. These in-depth "diagnostic workups" presumably lead to a greater understanding of the etiology and pathophysiology of disease with the ultimate aim of a more accurate and early diagnosis which allows much more effective medical and surgical therapy than is economically possible or necessary in food-producing animals. There is not the same emphasis on the efficiency of production, epidemiology and cost effectiveness which constantly face the food-producing animal practitioner. Instead, pet-owners, because of the sentimental value of their animals, and the growing importance of the human–companion animal bond, are willing to pay for the costs associated with extensive laboratory and sophisticated diagnostic tests and the intensive and prolonged veterinary hospital care. Palliative care for dogs and cats which are affected with diseases which may not be curable over the long term is now a recognized fact in small animal practice.

In many ways, equine practice has evolved along similar lines to small animal practice. Some aspects of it, such as reproduction, intensive clinical care of the newborn foal, and the treatment of medical and surgical diseases of valuable athletic and competitive horses have advanced a great deal. The great strides which have been made in our understanding of the diagnosis, prognosis and medical and surgical therapy of colic in the horse must be attributed to the in-depth diagnostic laboratory work and the medical and surgical expertise which have been used. Understanding the prognosis of equine colic has in part been due to discriminant analysis of the clinical and laboratory findings which is a triumph for analytical epidemiology. In addition to the advanced diagnostic and therapeutic procedures being conducted on valuable horses at veterinary teaching hospitals there are now many privately-owned equine veterinary centers which provide the same service. Undoubtedly the high financial value of some horses has provided the impetus to the development of these services.

It appears that there are major differences between the objectives and principles of companion animal practice and those of food-producing animal practice. In companion animal practice the objective is the restoration of the clinically ill animal to a normal state if possible, or in some cases a less than normal state is acceptable providing it is a quality life, using all of the readily available diagnostic and therapeutic techniques which can be afforded by the client. While in food-producing animal practice the objective is to improve the efficiency of animal production using the most economical methods of diagnosis, treatment and control including the disposal by culling or slaughter of animals which are difficult to treat and are economic losses.

This growing dichotomy in the delivery of veterinary services to the food-producing animal owner and to the companion animal owner prompted us to present a short introductory essay on the objectives and principles of food-producing animal practice.

THE OBJECTIVES OF FOOD ANIMAL PRODUCING PRACTICE

The most important objective is the continuous improvement of the efficiency of livestock production by the management of animal health. This involves several different but related activities and responsibilities which include the following:

- Providing the most economical method of diagnosis and treatment of sick and injured animals and returning them to an economically productive status, or to a point where slaughter for salvage is possible in the shortest possible time. The financially conscious producer wants to know the probability of success following treatment of a disease in an animal and to minimize the costs of prolonged convalescence and repetitive therapy
- Monitoring animal health and production of the herd on a regular basis so that actual performance can be compared with targets and the reasons for the shortfalls in production or increases in the incidence of disease can be identified as soon as possible so that appropriate and cost-effective action can be taken. The number of pigs weaned per litter, preweaning piglet milk yield, annual wool cut per sheep are examples of criteria of performance and disease prevalence
- Recommending of specific preventive veterinary programs against diseases which are risks in the particular environment, e.g. vaccination of cattle against blackleg and sheep against footrot, the strategic use anthelmintics
- Setting up planned herd and flock health programs for individual farms with the objective of maintaining optimum productivity through animal health management. This subject is presented in the companion volume to this book, *Herd Health* by O.M. Radostits and D.C. Blood (published in 1985 by W.B. Saunders)
- Advising on nutrition, breeding and general management practices. Food-producing animal practitioners must be interested in these matters when they affect animal health, it is a large part of preventive veterinary medicine to do so, and it is now common for veterinarians to expand their health-oriented animal husbandry advisory service to include an animal production advisory service. To do so is a matter of individual preference, an option

which some veterinarians take up and others do not. Those who do not may form a loose collaborative association with agricultural scientists. However, veterinarians still require a working knowledge of the relevant subjects; at least enough to know when to call in the collaborating advisor for advice. Members of both groups should be aware of the extensive list of subjects and species-oriented textbooks on these subjects which should be used to support this kind of service

- Encouraging livestock producers to maintain standards of animal welfare which comply with the views of the community is emerging as a major responsibility of the veterinarian. The production of food-producing animals under intensified conditions has now become an animal welfare concern which practitioners must face
- Promoting management practices which ensure that the meat and milk are free of biological and chemical agents which are capable of causing disease in man must also become a preoccupation for food-producing animal veterinarians. This is because the general public is concerned about the safety of the meat and milk products it consumes and the most effective way to minimize hazards presented by certain infectious agents and chemical residues in meat and milk is to control these agents at their point of entry into the food-chain, namely, during the production phase on the farm. Veterinarians will undoubtedly become involved in the surveillance of the use of antimicrobial compounds and other chemicals which are added to feed supplies to promote growth or prevent infections.

MODERN TECHNIQUES IN FOOD-PRODUCING ANIMAL PRACTICE

A unique feature of a food-producing animal veterinary practice is that most of the service is provided by the veterinarian who makes visits to the farm. In some areas of the world where veterinarians had to travel long distances to farms, an alternative strategy grew up. Large animal clinics were established and producers brought their animals which needed veterinary attention to the clinic. For the past 25 years these clinics have provided excellent facilities in which, for example, surgical procedures such as caesarean sections could be done and intensive fluid therapy for dehydrated diarrheic calves could be administered much more effectively and at a higher standard than on the farm. However, much less veterinary service is being provided in these clinics now because of the high operating costs of providing hospital care and the limited economic returns which are possible for the treatment of food-producing animals which have a fixed economic value. Producers have also become less enthusiastic about transporting animals to and from a veterinary clinic because of the time and expense involved.

Another feature is that the diagnosis, treatment and control of diseases of food-producing animals is heavily dependent on the results of the clinical examination of animals on the farm and the intensive examination of the environment and management techniques. This means that the veterinarian must become highly skilled in obtaining an accurate and useful history on the first visit to an animal or group of animals and in conducting an adequate clinical examination in order to make the best diagnosis possible quickly and economically so that treatment and control measures can be instituted as soon as possible. For example, the veterinarian must be able to recognize peracute coliform mastitis in a recently calved dairy cow and differentiate it clinically from parturient hypocalcemia because the administration of calcium salts to a cow with peracute mastitis but which is diagnosed incorrectly as parturient hypocalcemia can cause sudden death. On the farm, during the day, or in the middle of the night, the veterinarian will not have ready access to a laboratory for the rapid determination of a cow's serum calcium level. The practitioner must therefore become an astute diagnostician and a skillful user of the physical diagnostic skills of visual observation, auscultation, palpation, percussion, succussion, ballottement and olfactory perception. On the farm the clinical findings, including the events of the recent disease history of an animal, are often much more powerful, diagnostically, than laboratory data. It therefore becomes increasingly important that clinicans' examination should be repeated until the clinician is assured that all of the clinically significant abnormalities have been detected. An outline of the clinical examination of an animal and the different methods for making a diagnosis are presented in Chapter 1. Becoming efficient in clinical examination requires the diligent application of a systematic approach to the task and, most importantly, evaluation of the outcome. A very rewarding method of becoming a skillful diagnostician is to retrospectively correlate the clinical findings with the pathology of those cases which die and are submitted for necropsy. A great deal of clinical medicine can be learned at the time of necropsy. The correlation of the clinical findings with the clinical pathology data, if available, is also an excellent method of evaluation but is not routinely available in most private practices. The food-producing animal practitioner must also be a competent field pathologist and be able to carry out a necropsy in the field, usually under less than desirable conditions, and to make a tentative etiological diagnosis so that additional cases in the herd can be properly handled or prevented. Doing necropsies on the farm or having them done by a local diagnostic laboratory can be a major activity in a specialty swine or beef feedlot practice where clinical examination of individual animals is done only occasionally compared to dairy practice.

The clinical examination of the herd in which many animals may be affected with one or a number of clinical or subclinical diseases or in which the owner's complaint is that performance is suboptimal but the animals appear normal, has become a major and challenging task. This is particularly true in large swine herds, beef feedlots, lamb feedlots, and sheep flocks where the emphasis is on herd medicine. As mentioned earlier, modern intensified animal agriculture appears to have resulted in an increased frequency of herd problems including outbreaks of diseases such as pneumonic pasteurellosis or infectious bovine rhinotracheitis. Such well-known diseases are usually recognizable and a definitive etiological diagnosis can usually be made and in some cases the disease can be controlled by vaccination. However, in some cases of herd epidemics of respiratory disease or leptospirosis, for example, the veterinarian may have to make repeated visits to the herd and carry out an in-depth epidemiological investigation in order to develop effective treatment and control procedures.

There are alternatives to this strategy. In some countries, government supported field veterinarians will conduct extended on-farm investigations of complex disease problems encountered by private practitioners. In some situations, as in beef feedlot practice, it is a veterinary technician who identifies and treats cattle affected with acute undifferentiated respiratory disease and the veterinarian will only analyze the therapeutic responses, conduct necropsies and interpret the data which have been stored in a computer. However, in both of these systems only a veterinarian can make the important decisions.

For example, as animal agriculture continues to intensify, an increasing number of herd problems are evolving which have a multifactorial etiology and we are entering the era of the epidemiological diagnosis in which the definitive etiology may not be determined but in which manipulation of the epidemiological determinants may successfully and economically control the disease. For example, recent epidemiological observations revealed that certain congenital skeletal abnormalities of beef calves were associated with the use of grass or clover silage as the sole diet of pregnant beef cows during the winter months in Canada. The etiology was undetermined but in a controlled clinical trial supplementation of the silage with grain virtually eliminated the abnormality. This is an example of a modern-day epidemiological diagnosis comparable to the observation by John Snow that cholera in humans was associated with the use of the community water pump long before the causative bacterium was identified. It is clear that the next wave of development in food-producing animal practice will be associated with the increased use of applied and analytical epidemiology. This will allow the veterinarian to identify and quantify the risk factors associated with the disease, to provide a more accurate prognosis, to accurately assess treatment responses and not depend on clinical impressions, to scientifically evaluate control procedures and to conduct response trials. There is a large and challenging opportunity for veterinarians to become involved in clinical research in the field where the problems are occurring. It will necessitate that they become knowledgeable about the use of computerized data bases. These now provide an unlimited opportunity to capture and analyze data and generate useful information which heretofore was not considered possible. The technique of decision analysis is also a powerful tool for the veterinarian who is faced with making major decisions about treatment and control procedures.

It is clear from the foregoing that the collection, analysis and interpretation of animal health and production data will be a major activity of the successful food-producing animal practitioner. Livestock producers must keep and use good records if the veterinarian is to make informed decisions about animal health and production. The once tedious and unpopular work of recording and analyzing animal health and production data can now be done by the computer. Veterinarians will have to move in the direction of developing a computer-based animal health and production profile of each herd for which they are providing a service.

The veterinarian also has a major responsibility to ensure that the meat and milk produced by the animals under his care are free from pathogens, chemicals, antimicrobials and other drugs which may be harmful to man. In the past, veterinary public health was not an attractive career for veterinarians because it was perceived as an unimportant activity. However, because of the recent concern about the contamination of meat supplies and the potentially serious economic effects of such contamination on the export markets of a country, it is now clear that veterinarians, using a variety of testing techniques, will become involved in monitoring the use of veterinary drugs so that treated animals are not placed in the food-chain until the drugs have been excreted. The same principles apply to the contamination of milk supplies with antimicrobials, a major responsibility of the veterinarian.

The successful delivery of food-producing animal practice will depend on the ability of the veterinarian to provide those services which the producer wants at a price which is profitable to both the producer and the veterinarian. Several constraints interfere with this successful delivery. For example, maximizing net profit is not a high priority of many farmers. Being independent and making a living on the farm are commonly ranked higher than is maximizing net profit. Consequently when a veterinarian makes a recommendation to control a disease which optimizes production, his subsequent enthusiasm for giving advice may be dampened if the farmer does not adopt the control procedures because he is not profit-oriented, even though the advice is based on good information about expected economic returns. The frustrations which many veterinarians have experienced in attempting to get dairy producers to adopt the principles of an effective and economical mastitis control program are well known. Some producers do not use modern methods of production and disease control and do not use animal health and production records for their decision making because they are unaware of their importance. The variable financial return which farmers receive for their commodities, particularly the low prices received during times of oversupply of meat and milk, may also influence whether they purchase professional veterinary service or attempt to do the work themselves.

The inability or lack of the desire of the veterinarian to provide the high-level professional service which the producer needs will also limit the widespread use of the service by the livestock industry.

We have set out above our views on the state of food-producing animal medicine and what it requires of veterinarians who practice it. In summary, the veterinarian must become knowledgeable about all aspects of farm management, especially those which cause or contribute to clinical or subclinical disease and impaired animal production. Such veterinarians will become species–industry specialists who can provide totally integrated animal health and production management advice either to the dairy herd, the beef cow–calf herd, the beef feedlot, the swine herd or the sheep flock. To be able to do this the veterinarian will need to undertake a post-graduate clinical residency program or develop the expertise on his own by diligent self-education in a veterinary practice which is committed to the concept of a total animal health management and allows the veterinarian the time and the resources to develop the specialty. A prerequisite is that the livestock industry in the geographical area of the practice must be concentrated enough so that it will provide sufficient work at a specialty level.

All that we have said in this introduction is related to enhancing and improving the performance of the professional food-producing animal veterinarian. In developed countries this could mean greater utilization of each veterinarian by farmers and improved financial viability of their farming enterprises. In developing countries it could mean a greater volume of production at a time when malnutrition appears to be the fate of so many groups of the world community. These could be the outcomes if the world's agricultural situation was a stable one. As it is, there is currently a great upheaval in agriculture; developed countries are heavily overproduced and there is a sharp decline in farming as an industry and way of life. In developing countries, the decisions governing the health and welfare of animals and the people that depend on them often seem to depend more on political expediency than on the basic needs of humans and their animals. In these circumstances we do not feel sufficiently courageous and far-sighted to predict our individual futures but with the hindsight of how far the human population and their attendant agricultural and veterinary professions have come in the past 50 years we are confident that you will have an opportunity to properly pursue the objectives and principles that we have described.

How to Use this Book

We would like you to get the most out of this book.
To do that you should follow the directions below.
And if you keep doing this
every time you come to the book
you will develop a proper diagnostic routine
of going from:

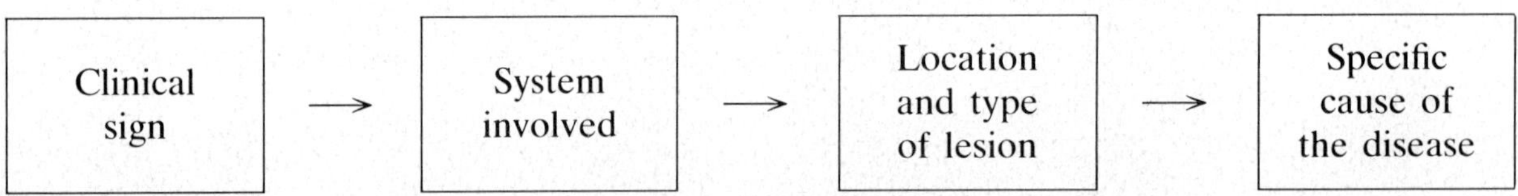

and become what we wish for every one of you:
a thinking clinician

FOR EXAMPLE

A yearling bull has a sudden onset of dyspnea, fever, anorexia, abnormal lung sounds and nasal discharge.

Step 1 The bull's problem is dyspnea. Go to the index and find the principal entry for dyspnea—p. 354.

Step 2 Go to p. 354. The discussion on dyspnea will lead you to respiratory tract dyspnea and cardiac dyspnea.

Step 3 Via the index consult these and decide that the system involved is the respiratory system and that the lungs are the location of the lesion in the system.

Step 4 Proceed to diseases of the lungs (p. 363) and decide on the basis of the clinical and other findings that the nature of the lesion is inflammatory and is pneumonia.

Step 5 Proceed to pneumonia, and on p. 367 consult the list of pneumonias which occur in cattle. Consult each of them via the index and decide that pneumonic pasteurellosis is the probable specific cause.

Step 6 Proceed to p. 663 and in the section on pneumonic pasteurellosis determine the appropriate treatment for the bull and the chances of saving it.

Step 7 Don't forget to turn to the end of the section on pneumonic pasteurellosis on p. 670 and remind yourself of what to do to protect the rest of the herd from sharing the illness.

PART ONE

GENERAL MEDICINE

1

Clinical Examination and Making a Diagnosis

THE focal point of any investigation of animal disease is the making of a diagnosis; and the critical part in making that decision is the clinical examination of the individual animal or group of animals. Therefore, it is appropriate that the first chapter of this book deals with this important subject.

However, before we begin that exercise, it is important that we be quite clear and agree upon what we mean by 'disease'. Let us assume that disease can be defined as 'inability to perform physiological functions at normal levels even though nutrition and other environmental requirements are provided at adequate levels'. Then not only does a clinically ill animal come into the area of examination, but also those animals or herds which are not clinically ill but which do not perform as expected. As veterinarians working with food-producing animals and horses, we are required to recognize individual animals which are affected with a particular, recognizable, pathological lesion, or biochemical or metabolic deficit, or nutritional deficiency which results in recognizable clinical signs like fever, dyspnea, convulsions or lameness. This is traditional veterinary medicine based on a transposition of attitudes and behavior from human medicine. However, it is also necessary for us to investigate disease which the owner recognizes simply as failure to perform or to reach predetermined objectives. This is not necessarily subclinical disease: it is recognizable clinically but perhaps only as poor performance such as unthriftiness without any specific system-oriented clinical signs. In other situations, the owner may not recognize any abnormality unless productivity is measured, e.g. milk production or growth rate per day.

There has been considerable emphasis on the clinical and laboratory examination of individual animals affected with clinical disease or which have not performed normally and the large body of information which is now available in laboratory medicine testifies to this preoccupation. Its greatest importance is in animals, such as companion and racing animals which are kept as singles, and unless the diagnosis is simple and readily obvious, if a laboratory is available there may be a tendency to make one or more laboratory examinations. The more valuable the animal, the greater the tendency towards some laboratory work. Many biochemical, hematological and biophysical examinations of each body system can yield valuable clues about system or organ function which usually lead to more accurate and detailed examination of that system or organ. In animals kept in herds or flocks these laboratory tests are also important but are equalled in importance overall by epidemiological investigations. There is little to be gained by this form of examination in animals kept as singles.

With a herd of animals affected with clinical disease, or which is failing to achieve expected objectives, an epidemiological investigation, in addition to the clinical examination of individual animals, may make a valuable contribution to the making of a diagnosis. This is not to suggest that clinical and laboratory examinations are de-emphasized in the examination of herd problems. In some instances, the clinical and laboratory examinations assume major importance to ensure that animals, in a herd which is not performing normally, are in fact not clinically ill. But when the presenting complaint is poor performance, it is necessary to collect all the pertinent epidemiological data, including accurate production measurements, and to decide whether or not an abnormality is present and if so its magnitude. It is at this point where veterinarians become the arbiters of what is health and what is illness (13). In herd health programs this is a continuing and positive service provided by veterinarians to farmer clients.

In this chapter on clinical examination and making a diagnosis, we have described the standard procedure for the clinical examination of an individual animal followed by some guidelines for the examination of the herd. The level of the examination set out is sufficient to enable the clinician to determine the nature of the abnormality and the system involved. For more detailed examination it is recommended that subsequent chapters which deal with individual systems be consulted. Each of them sets out a method for a special examination of the particular system.

CLINICAL EXAMINATION OF THE INDIVIDUAL ANIMAL

The expression 'clinical examination' should not be misunderstood. It has three aspects: the animal, the history and the environment. Inadequate examination of any of these may lead to error. The examination of the affected animal represents only a part of the complete investigation. Careful questioning of the owner or attendant can yield information about the diet or the prior diet, about recent vaccinations or surgery or about the introduction of animals into the group, that will provide the clues to a successful diagnosis. However, in certain instances, for example in arsenic poisoning, the most detailed examination of the animal and the most careful questioning of the owner may fail to elicit the evidence necessary for a correct diagnosis. Only a careful physical search of the environment for a source of arsenic can provide this information. Thus neglect of one aspect of the clinical examination can render valueless a great deal of work on the other aspects and lead to an error in diagnosis.

History-taking

In veterinary medicine history-taking is the most important of the three aspects of a clinical examination. The significance of the results obtained by examination of the patient and the environment are liable to be modified by a number of factors. Animals are unable to describe their clinical signs; they vary widely in their reaction to handling and examination, and a wide range of normality must be permitted in the criteria used in a physical examination. These variations are much greater in some species than in others. Dogs, horses and cattle, because of their size and because they are accustomed to human company, are relatively good subjects but sheep, goats and pigs are much more difficult. A satisfactory examination of the environment may prove difficult because of lack of knowledge of the factors concerned or because of the examiner's inability to assess their significance. Problems such as the measurement of the relative humidity of a barn and its importance as a predisposing factor in an outbreak of pneumonia or the determination of pH of the soil with reference to the spread of leptospirosis can present virtually insuperable difficulties to the veterinarian in the field. On the other hand a search for a specific factor such as a known poison may be relatively simple.

Nevertheless history-taking is the key to accurate diagnosis in veterinary medicine, and to be worth while it must be accurate and complete. Admittedly, human fallibility must be taken into consideration; there may be insufficient time, the importance of particular factors may not be appreciated, there may be misunderstanding. Although these are excusable to a point, failure to recognize the importance of the history can lead only to error. It is essential for the examiner to support and assess the accuracy of the history by careful examinations if he is not to be misled, but it is the inaccurate or incomplete history that can lead him furthest astray. For example, if the veterinarian rejects the possibility of erysipelatous endocarditis in a sow because there have never been cases of erysipelas on that particular farm, when in fact the patient has been purchased only 3 weeks previously, he is guilty of a cardinal error of omission.

The history should suggest not only the diagnostic possibilities but also the probabilities. A 1-year-old heifer is unlikely to have clinical Johne's disease; an adult cow is more likely to have parturient paresis than a first-calf heifer, which in turn is more likely to have maternal obstetric paralysis than is the adult cow. The history may often indicate that special attention should be paid to the examination of a particular system in the animal, or a particular factor in the environment. For example, in epilepsy the animal may be seen when it is clinically normal and the only means of reaching a diagnosis may be a consideration of the history.

History-taking method

Successful history-taking involves certain intangibles which cannot be discussed here. However, a number of suggestions follow, which may prove helpful to the clinician. The owner or attendant must be handled with diplomacy and tact. The use of non-technical terms is essential since stockowners are likely to be confused by technical expressions or be reluctant to express themselves when confronted with terms they do not understand. Statements, particularly those concerned with time, should be tested for accuracy. Owners, and more especially herdsmen and agents, often attempt to disguise their neglect by condensing time or varying the chronology of events. It is amazing how many cattle can lose 100 kg of body weight in a few hours! If a detailed cross-examination of the custodian seems likely to arouse his antagonism it is advisable for the veterinarian to forgo further questioning and be content with his own estimate of the dependability of the history. The clinician must try to separate the owner's observations from his interpretations. A statement that the horse had a bout of bladder trouble may, on closer examination, mean that the horse had an attack of abdominal pain in which it assumed a posture usually associated with urination. It is impossible to avoid the use of leading questions—'did the pigs scour?', 'was there any vomiting?'—but it is necessary to weigh the answers in accordance with the general veracity of the owner. Absence of a sign can only be determined by enquiring whether or not it occurred. Simply to ask for a complete history of what has happened almost invariably results in an incomplete history. The clinician must of course know the right questions to ask; this knowledge comes with experience and familiarity with disease. Laymen seldom describe clinical signs in their correct time sequence; part of the clinician's task is to establish the chronology of events.

For completeness and accuracy in history-taking the clinician should conform to a set routine. The system outlined below includes patient data, disease history and management history. The order in which these parts of the history are taken will vary. In general it is best to take the disease history first. The psychological effect is good: the owner appreciates the desire to get down to the facts about his animal's illness.

Patient data

If records are to be kept at all, even if only for financial purposes, accurate identification of the patient is essential. An animal's previous history can be referred to, the disease status of a herd can be examined, specimens for laboratory examination can be dispatched with the knowledge that the results can be related to the correct patient. And last but not least, financial statements will be sent, and to the correct owners, and will be correct in themselves. These points may have no importance in establishing the diagnosis but they are of first importance in the maintenance of a successful practice. The relevant data include: the owner's name and initials, postal address and telephone number; the species, type, breed (or estimate of parentage in a crossbred), sex, age, name or number, body weight and, if necessary, a description including color markings, polledness and other identifying marks of the patient. Such a list may appear formidable but many of the points, such as age, sex, breed, type (use made of animal, e.g. beef, dairy, mutton, wool), are often of importance in the diagnosis. A case history of a particular animal may suggest that further treatment is likely to be uneconomic because of age, or that a particular disease is assuming sufficient importance in a herd for different control measures to be warranted.

Disease history

History-taking will vary considerably depending on whether one animal or a group of animals is involved in the disease problem under examination. As a general rule in large animal work all disease states should be considered as herd problems until proved to be otherwise. It is often rewarding to examine the remainder of a group and find animals which are in the early stages of the disease.

Present disease

Attempts should be made to elicit the details of the clinical abnormalities observed by the owner in the sequence in which they occurred. If more than one animal is affected, a typical case should be chosen and the variations in history in other cases should then be noted. Variations from the normal in the physiological functions such as intake of food or drink, milk production, growth, respiration, defecation, urination, sweating, activity, gait, posture, voice and odor should be noted in all cases. There are many specific questions which need to be asked in each case but they are too numerous to list here and for the most part they are variations on the questions already suggested.

If a number of animals are affected information may be available from clinical pathological examinations carried out on living animals or necropsy examinations on fatal cases. The behavior of animals before death and the period of time elapsing between the first observable signs and death or recovery are important items of information. Prior surgical or medical procedures such as castration, docking, shearing, or vaccination may be important factors in the production of disease.

Morbidity and mortality rates

The morbidity rate is usually expressed as the percentage of animals which are clinically affected compared with the total number of animals exposed to the same risks. The case fatality rate is the percentage of affected animals which die. The population mortality rate is the percentage of all exposed animals which die. The estimates may be important in diagnosis because of the wide variations in morbidity, case fatality and population mortality rates which occur in different diseases. An equally important figure is the proportion of animals at risk which are clinically normal but which show abnormality on the basis of laboratory or other tests.

Prior treatment

The owner may have treated animals before calling for assistance. Exact details of the preparations used and doses given may be of value in eliminating some diagnostic possibilities. They will certainly be of importance when assessing the probable efficiency of the treatment, the significance of clinical pathological tests and in prescribing additional treatment. Drug withdrawal regulations now require that treated animals, or their products such as milk, be withheld from slaughter or market for varying lengths of time to allow drug residues to reach tolerable limits. This necessitates that owners reveal information about the drugs which they have used.

Prophylactic and control measures

It should be ascertained if preventive or control procedures have already been attempted. There may have been clinical pathological tests, the introduction of artificial insemination to control venereal disease, vaccination, or changes in nutrition, management or hygiene. For example, in an outbreak of bovine mastitis careful questioning should be pursued regarding the method of disinfecting the cows' teats after each milking with particular reference to the type and concentration of the disinfectant used, and whether or not back-flushing of teat cups is practiced. Spread of the disease may result from failure of the hygiene barrier at any one of a number of such points. When written reports are available they are more reliable than the memory of the owner.

Previous exposure

The history of the group relative to additions is of particular importance. Is the affected animal one of the group, or has it been introduced, and how long ago? If the affected animal has been in the group for some time, have there been recent additions? Is the herd a 'closed herd' or are animals introduced at frequent intervals? Not all herd additions are potential carriers of disease. They may have come from herds where control measures are adequate, they may have been tested before or after sale or kept in quarantine for an adequate period after arrival; or they may have received suitable biological or antibiotic prophylaxis. They may have come from areas where a particular disease does not occur, although a negative history of this type is less reliable than a positive history of derivation from an area where a particular disease is enzootic.

A reverse situation may occur where imported stock has no resistance to enzootic infection in the home herd, or has not become adapted to environmental stresses such as high altitudes, high environmental temperatures and particular feeding methods or is not used to poisonous plants occurring in the environment.

Transit
The possibility of infection during transit is a very real danger and pre-sale certificates of health may be of little value if an animal has passed through a sale barn, a show or communal trucking yards while in transit. Highly infectious diseases may be transmitted via trucks, railroad cars or other accommodation contaminated by previous inhabitants. Transient introductions, including animals brought in for work purposes, for mating or on temporary grazing, are often overlooked as possible vectors of disease. Other sources of infection are wild fauna which graze over the same area as domestic livestock, and inanimate objects such as human footwear, car tires and feeding utensils.

Culling rate
There may be considerable significance in the reasons for culling, and the number of animals disposed of for health reasons. Failure to grow well, poor productivity and short productive life will suggest the possible occurrence of a number of chronic diseases, including some caused by infectious agents, by nutritional deficiencies or by poisons.

Previous disease
Information elicited by questioning on previous history of illness may be illuminating. If there is a history of previous illness, enquiries should be made on the usual lines, including clinical observations, necropsy findings, morbidity, case fatality rates, the treatments and control measures used and the results obtained. If necessary, enquiries should be made about herds from which introduced animals have originated and also about herds to which other animals from the same source have been sent.

Management history
The management history includes nutrition, breeding policy and practice, housing, transport and general handling. It is most important to learn whether or not there has been any change in the prevailing practice prior to the appearance of disease. The fact that a disease has occurred when the affected animals have been receiving the same ration, deriving from the same source over a long period, suggests that the diet is not at fault, although errors in preparation of concentrate mixtures, particularly with the present-day practice of introducing additives to feeds, can cause variations which are not immediately apparent.

Nutrition
The major objective in the examination of the nutritional history is to determine how the *quantity* and *quality* of the diet, which the animals have been receiving, compares with the nutrient requirements which have been recommended for a similar class of animal. In some situations it may be necessary to submit feed and water samples for analyses to assess quality.

Livestock at pasture present a rather different problem from those being hand-fed in that they receive a diet which is less controlled and thus more difficult to assess. The risk of parasitic infestation and, in some cases, infectious disease is much greater in grazing animals. Enquiries should be made about the composition of the pasture, its probable nutritive value with particular reference to recent changes brought about by rain or drought, whether rotational grazing is practiced, the fertilizer program and whether or not minerals and trace elements are provided by top-dressing or mineral mixtures. The origin of mineral supplements, particularly phosphates which may contain excess fluorine, and home-made mixtures which may contain excessive quantities of other ingredients, should receive attention. Actual examination of the pasture area is usually more rewarding than a description of it.

Hand-fed animals are subjected to a more or less controlled food supply, but because of human error they are frequently exposed to dietary mistakes. Types and amounts of foods fed should be determined. Young pigs may be stunted because they have not been kept on a starting ration for a sufficiently long period and the growing ration has not been introduced sufficiently gradually. Further examples of disease produced by inadequate hand-fed diets include: osteodystrophia fibrosa in horses on diets containing excess grain; azoturia in the same species when heavy carbohydrate diets are fed during periods of rest; and lactic acid indigestion in cattle introduced to heavy grain diets too rapidly. The sources of the dietary ingredients may also be of importance. Grains from some areas are often much heavier and contain a much greater proportion of starch to husk than grains from other areas so that when feed is measured, rather than weighed, overfeeding or underfeeding may occur. Because the digestive enzyme capacity of newborn farm animals is most efficient in the digestion of whole milk, the use of non-milk sources of carbohydrates and proteins in the formulation of milk replacers may result in indigestion and nutritional diarrhea. Exotic diseases may be imported in feed materials; anthrax, foot-and-mouth disease and hog cholera are well-known examples. Variations in the preparation of ingredients of rations may produce variable diets. Overheating as in pelleting or the cooking of feeds can reduce their vitamin content; contamination with lubricating oil can result in poisoning by chlorinated naphthalene compounds; pressure extraction of linseed can leave considerable residues of hydrocyanic acid in the residual oil cake. Feeding practices may in themselves contribute to the production of disease. Pigs fed in large numbers with inadequate trough space or calves fed from communal troughs are likely to be affected by overeating or inanition depending on their size and vigor. High-level feeding and consequent rapid growth may create deficiency states by increasing the requirement for specific nutrients.

In both hand-fed and grazing animals *changes in diet* should be carefully noted. Removal of animals from one field to another, from pasture to cereal grazing, from unimproved to improved pasture may all precipitate the appearance of disease. Periods of sudden dietary deficiency can occur as a result of bad weather, transportation or during change to unfamiliar feeds. Rapid changes are more important than gradual alterations, particularly in pregnant and lactating ruminants when metabolic diseases, including those caused by hypocalcemia, hypoglycemia and hypomagnesemia, are likely to occur. The *availability of drinking water* must be determined; salt poisoning of swine occurs only when the supply of drinking water is inadequate.

Reproductive management and performance
In the examination of a single animal the breeding and parturition history may suggest or eliminate some diagnostic possibilities. For example, pregnancy toxemia occurs in sheep in late pregnancy while acetonemia in dairy cows occurs primarily between 2 and 6 weeks after parturition. Acute metritis is a possibility within a few days after parturition in any species but unlikely several weeks later.

The *breeding history* may be of importance with regard to inherited disease. The existence of a relationship between sires and dams should be noted. Hybrid vigor in crossbred animals should be considered when there is apparent variation in resistance to disease between groups maintained under similar environmental conditions. A general relationship between selection for high productivity and susceptibility to certain diseases is apparent in many breeds of animals and even in certain families. The possibility of genetotrophic disease, i.e. the inheritance of a greater requirement than normal of a specific nutrient, should be considered.

The examination of the herd *reproductive history* involves comparing past and present reproductive performance with certain optimum objectives. The mean length of the interval between parturition and conception, the mean number of services per conception and the percentage of young animals weaned relative to the number of females which were originally exposed for breeding (calf or lamb crop, pigs weaned) are general measures of reproductive performance and efficiency. Using cattle as an example, certain other observations may assist in determining the cause of failure to reach reproductive performance objectives. These are the percentage of abortions, length of breeding season, the percentage of females pregnant at specified times after the onset of breeding period, bull/cow ratio, size and topography of breeding pastures and the fertility status of the females and males at breeding time. The percentage of females which need assistance at parturition and the percentage of calves which die at birth are also indices of reproductive performance which are indicative of the level of reproductive management provided.

Climate
Many diseases are influenced by climate. Footrot in cattle and sheep reach their peak incidence in warm, wet summers and are relatively rare in dry seasons. Diseases spread by insects are encouraged when climatic conditions favor the propagation of the vector. Internal parasites are similarly influenced by climate. Cool, wet seasons favor the development of hypomagnesemia in pastured cattle. Anhidrosis in horses is specifically a disease of hot, humid countries. The direction of prevailing winds is of importance in many disease outbreaks, particularly in relation to the contamination of pasture and drinking water by fumes from factories and mines and the spread of diseases carried by insects.

General management
There are so many items in the proper management of livestock which if neglected can lead to the occurrence of disease that they cannot be related here; animal management in the prevention of disease is a subject in its own right and is dealt with in all parts of this book. Some of the more important factors include: hygiene, particularly in milking parlors and in parturition and rearing stalls; adequacy of housing in terms of space, ventilation, draining, situation and suitability of troughs; opportunity for exercise and the proper management of milking machines to avoid udder injury. The class of livestock under consideration is also of importance; for example, enterotoxemia is most common in fattening lambs and pigs, parturient paresis in milking cows, obstructive urolithiasis in lambs and steers in feedlots and pregnancy toxemia in ewes used for fat lamb production.

Examination of the environment

An examination of the environment is a necessary part of any clinical investigation because of the possible relationship between environmental factors and the incidence of disease. A satisfactory examination of the environment necessitates an adequate knowledge of animal husbandry and with the development of species specialization, it will be desirable for the veterinarian to understand the environmental needs of a particular species or class of farm animal.

Depending on the region of the world, some animals are kept outside year round, some are housed for part of the year during the winter months, and some are kept under total confinement. For animals raised on pasture, the effects of topography, plants, soil type, ground surface and protection from extremes of weather assume major importance. For animals housed indoors, hygiene, ventilation, and avoiding overcrowding are of major concern. Some of these items will be briefly presented here as guidelines.

Each observation should be recorded in detail for preparation of reports for submission to the owners. Detailed records and even photographs of environmental characteristics assume major importance when poisonings are suspected and where litigation proceedings appear possible.

Outdoor environment

Topography and soil type
The topography of grasslands, pastures and wooded areas can contribute to disease or inefficient production and reproduction. Flat, treeless plains offering no protection from wind predispose cattle to lactation tetany in inclement weather. Low marshy areas facilitate the spread of insect-borne diseases and soil-borne infections requiring damp conditions such as leptospirosis; Johne's disease and diseases associated with liver fluke infestation and lungworm pneumonia are more prevalent in such areas. Rough grasslands with extensive wooded areas can have an adverse effect on reproductive performance in beef herds because of the difficulty the bulls have in getting around to the females during peak periods of estrus activity.

The soil type of a district may provide important clues to the detection of nutritional deficiencies; copper and cobalt deficiencies are most common on littoral sands and the copper deficiency/molybdenum excess complex usually occurs on peat soils. The surface of the ground and its drainage characteristics are important in highly intensive beef feedlots and in large dairy herds where fattening cattle and dairy cows are kept and fed under total confinement.

Ground surfaces which are relatively impermeable and/or not adequately sloped for drainage can become a sea of mud following a heavy rainfall or snowstorm. Constant wetting of the feet and udders commonly result in outbreaks of footrot and mastitis. Dirty udders increase the time required for udder washing prior to milking and can seriously affect a mastitis control program. In some regions of the world, beef cows are calved in outdoor paddocks in the spring when it is wet and cool with an excess of surface water which increases the spread of infectious disease and results in a marked increase in neonatal mortality. A lack of sufficient protection from the prevailing winds, the heat of the sun, rain or snow can seriously affect production and exacerbate an existing disease condition or precipitate an outbreak. Dusty feedlots during the hot summer months may contribute to an increase in the incidence of respiratory disease or delay the response to treatment of diseases such as pneumonia.

Stocking rate (population density)

Overcrowding is a common predisposing cause of disease. There may be an excessive build-up of feces and urine which increases the level of infection. The relative humidity is usually increased and more difficult to control. Fighting and cannibalism are also more common in overcrowded pens than when there is adequate space for animals to move around comfortably. The detection and identification of animals for whatever reason (illness, estrus) can be difficult and inaccurate under crowded conditions.

Feed and water supplies

On *pastures*, the predominant plant types, both natural and introduced, should be observed as they are often associated with certain soil types and may be the cause of actual disease; the high estrogen content of some clovers, the occurrence of functional nervous diseases on pastures dominated by *Phalaris aquatica* (syn. *P. tuberosa*) and perennial rye grass, the presence of selective absorbing 'converter' plants on copper-rich and selenium-rich soils are all examples of the importance of the dominant vegetation. The presence of specific poisonous plants, evidence of overgrazing, the existence of a bone-chewing or bark-chewing habit can be determined by an examination of the environment. Vital clues in the investigation of possible poisoning in a herd may be the existence of a garbage dump or ergotized grass or rye in the pasture, or the chewing of lead-based painted walls in the barn, or careless handling of poisons in the feed area. The possibility that the forage may have been contaminated by environmental pollution from nearby factories or highways should be examined. In some cases the physical nature of the pasture plants may be important; mature, bleached grass pasture can be seriously deficient in carotene, whereas lush young pasture can have rachitogenic potency because of its high carotene content or it may be capable of causing hypomagnesemia if it is dominated by grasses. Lush legume pasture or heavy concentrate feeding with insufficient roughage can cause a serious bloat problem.

The feed supplies for animals raised in confinement outdoors must be examined for evidence of moldy feed, contamination with feces and urine and excessive moisture due to lack of protection from rain and snow. Empty feed troughs may confirm a suspicion that the feeding system is faulty.

The *drinking water supply* and its origin may be important in the production of disease. Water in ponds may be covered with algae containing neurotoxins or hepatotoxic agents and flowing streams may carry effluent from nearby industrial plants. In a feedlot, water may suddenly be unavailable because of frozen water lines or faulty water tank valves but should not go unnoticed if one recognizes the anxiety of a group of cattle trying to obtain water from a dry tank.

Waste disposal

The disposal of feces and urine has become a major problem for large intensified livestock operations. Slurry is now spread on pastures and may be important in the spread of infectious disease. Lagoons can provide ideal conditions for the breeding of flies which can be troublesome to a nearby livestock operation. The inadequate disposal of dead animals may be an important factor in the spread of certain diseases.

Indoor environment

There are few aspects of livestock production which have aroused more interest, development and controversy in the last few years than the housing and environmental needs of farm animals. Several textbooks on the subject have been written and only some of the important items will be mentioned here with the aid of some examples. The effects of housing on animal health have not received the consideration they deserve, due partly to insufficient knowledge of the animal's environmental needs and partly because there has been a failure to apply what is already known.

As a general statement it can be said that inadequate housing and ventilation, overcrowding and uncomfortable conditions are considered to have detrimental effects on housed animals which makes them not only more susceptible to infectious disease but also less productive. Moreover, this reduction in productive efficiency may be a greater cause of economic loss than losses caused by infectious disease. For this reason, the veterinarian must learn to examine and assess all aspects of an indoor environment which may be the primary cause of or a predisposing factor to disease.

By way of illustration, the major causes of preweaning mortality of piglets are chilling and crushing of piglets in the first few days of life and not infectious disease. These physical causes are commonly related to a combination of poorly designed farrowing crates, slippery floors, inadequate heating and perhaps overcrowding of the farrowing facilities.

One of the first things to observe is the level of *sanitation and hygiene*, which is usually a reliable indicator of the level of management; poor hygiene is often associated with a high level of infectious disease. For example, the incidence of diarrhea in piglets may be high because the farrowing crates are not suitably cleaned and disinfected before the pregnant sow is placed in the crate. A similar situation applies for lambing sheds, calving pens and foaling boxes. An excessive build-up of feces and urine with insufficient clean bedding will result in a high level of neonatal mortality. The methods used for cleaning and disinfection should be examined carefully. The removal of dried feces from animal pens which have been occupied for several months is a difficult and laborious task and often not done well. Undue reliance may be placed on the use of chemical disinfectants.

The total length of time which animals have occupied a pen without a cleaning and disinfection (*occupation time*) should be noted. As the occupation time increases, there is a marked increase in the infection rate and the morbidity and mortality from infectious disease often increase.

Inadequate ventilation is considered to be a major predisposing factor contributing to the severity of swine enzootic pneumonia in fattening pigs. The primary infection has a minimal effect on the pig, but inadequate ventilation results in overheating of the barn in the summer months, and chilling and dampness during the winter months, commonly results in subclinical and clinical pneumonia which severely affects productive efficiency. Similarly with young calves which are raised indoors in most of the temperate zones of the world, protection from the cold during the winter is necessary. The effects of enzootic pneumonia of housed calves are much more severe when ventilation is inadequate than when the calves are comfortable and have clean fresh air.

The evaluation of the adequacy of ventilation of a farm animal barn which is filled to economic capacity with animals is a difficult task and a major subject. Ventilation is assessed by a determination of the number of air changes per unit of time, the relative humidity during the day and night, the presence or absence of condensation on the hair coats of the animals or on the walls and ceilings, the presence of drafts, the building and insulation materials used, the positions and capacities of the fans and the size and location of the air inlets. The measurement of the concentration of noxious gases in animal barns, such as ammonia and hydrogen sulfide, may be a valuable aid in assessing the effectiveness of a ventilation system.

Animals raised indoors are frequently overcrowded which may predispose to disease, and measurements of *population density* and observations of animal behavior in such conditions assume major importance. When pigs are raised indoors in crowded conditions with inadequate ventilation their social habits may change drastically and they begin to defecate and urinate on the clean floor and on their pen mates rather than over the slatted floor over the gutter. This can result in outbreaks of diseases which are transmitted by the fecal–oral route.

The *quality of the floor* is often responsible for diseases of the musculoskeletal system and skin. Poorly finished concrete floors with an exposed aggregate can cause severe foot lesions and lameness in adult swine. Recently calved dairy cows are very susceptible to slipping on slippery floors in dairy barns, a common cause of the downer cow syndrome. Loose-housing systems, particularly those with slatted floors, have resulted in a new spectrum of diseases of the feet of cattle because of the sharp edges of some of the slats. The quality and quantity of bedding used should be noted. Bedding is now rarely used in intensified swine operations. The use of sawdust or shavings in loose-housing systems for dairy cattle may be associated with outbreaks of coliform mastitis. Wet bedding, particularly during the winter months, is commonly associated with endemic pneumonia in calves.

The *floor plan* and general layout of an animal house must be examined for evidence that the routine movements of animal attendants, the movements of animals and feeding facilities may actually be spreading disease. Communal gutters running through adjacent pens may promote the spread of disease through fecal or urinary contamination. The nature of the partitions between pens, whether solid or open grid type, may assist the control or spread of infectious disease. The building materials used will influence the ease with which pens, such as farrowing crates and calf pens, can be cleaned and disinfected for a new batch of piglets or calves.

The amount of light available in a barn should be noted. With insufficient light it may be difficult to maintain a sufficient level of sanitation and hygiene, sick animals may not be recognized early enough, and in general errors in management are likely to occur.

In the investigation of a herd problem of mastitis in dairy cattle the veterinarian should visit the farm at milking time and observe how the cows are prepared for milking, use of the milking machine, and the level of sanitation and hygiene practiced. Several successive visits may be necessary to reveal possible weaknesses in a mastitis control program.

Examination of the patient

A complete clinical examination of an animal patient includes, in addition to history-taking and an examination of the environment, physical and laboratory examinations. A complete clinical examination of every patient is unnecessary because of the simplicity of some diseases. However, a general clinical examination of every patient is necessary and the inexperienced clinician should spend as much time and effort as is practicable and economical in carrying it out. This will help to avoid the sort of embarrassing error in which a calf is operated on for umbilical hernia when it also has a congenital cardiac defect. As *learned* experience develops, the clinician will know the extent to which a clinical examination is necessary. All of the laboratory tests which are likely to be informative and which are practical and economical should be used. Because of the cost of laboratory tests, the clinician must be selective in the tests which are used. The most economical method is to examine the patient and then select those laboratory tests which will support or refute the tentative clinical diagnosis.

In this section a system for the examination of a patient is outlined in a general way. There is a great deal of difference between species in the ease with which this examination is carried out and the amount of information that can be collected. Special descriptions are available for cattle (10) and for sheep and goats (15). Also more detailed examination techniques are dealt with under the individual body systems. The examination of a patient consists of a general inspection carried out from a distance, followed by a physical examination in which the animal is examined at close quarters.

General inspection

The importance of a general inspection of the animal cannot be overemphasized, and yet it is often overlooked. Apart from the general impression gained from observation at a distance, there are some signs that can best be assessed before the animal is disturbed. The proximity of the examiner is particularly disturbing to animals that are unaccustomed to frequent handling.

Behavior and general appearance

The general impression of the health of an animal obtained by an examination from a distance is difficult to analyze but the following points are important.

Behavior Separation of an animal from its group is often an indication of illness. The behavior is also a reflection of the animal's health. If it responds normally to external stimuli such as sound and movement it is classified as bright. If the reactions are sluggish and the animal exhibits relative indifference to normal stimuli it is said to be dull or apathetic. A pronounced state of indifference in which the animal remains standing and is able to move but does not respond at all to external stimuli is usually referred to as the 'dummy' syndrome. This occurs in subacute lead poisoning, listeriosis and some cases of acetonemia in cattle and encephalomyelitis and hepatic cirrhosis in the horse. The terminal stage of apathy or depression is coma in which the animal is unconscious and cannot be roused.

Excitation states vary in severity. A state of anxiety or apprehension is the mildest form: here the animal is alert and looks about constantly but is normal in its movements. Such behavior is usually expressive of moderate constant pain or other abnormal sensation as in early parturient paresis or in recent blindness. A more severe manifestation is that of restlessness in which the animal moves about a good deal, lies down and gets up and may go through other abnormal movements such as looking at its flanks, kicking at its belly and rolling and bellowing. Again this demeanor is usually indicative of pain. More extreme degrees of excited demeanor include mania and frenzy. In mania the animal performs abnormal movements with vigor. Violent licking at its own body, licking or chewing inanimate objects, pressing forward with the head are typical examples. In frenzy, the actions are so wild and uncontrolled that the animals are a danger to anyone approaching them. In both mania and frenzy there is usually excitation of the brain as in rabies, acute lead poisoning and some cases of nervous acetonemia.

Voice Abnormality of the voice should be noted. It may be hoarse in rabies or weak in gut edema; there may be continuous lowing in nervous acetonemia or persistent bellowing indicative of acute pain. Soundless bellowing and yawning are commonly seen in rabid cattle and yawning is a common sign in animals affected with hepatic insufficiency.

Eating In a patient which has retained its appetite there may be abnormality of prehension, mastication or swallowing and, in ruminants, of belching and regurgitation. Prehension may be marred by inability to approach feed, as in cerebellar ataxia, osteomyelitis of cervical vertebrae and other painful conditions of the neck. When there is pain in the mouth prehension may be abnormal and affected animals may be able to take only certain types of feed. Mastication may be slow, one-sided or incomplete when mouth structures, particularly teeth, are affected. Periodic cessation of chewing when food is still in the mouth occurs commonly in the 'dummy' syndrome, when there are space-occupying lesions of the cranium or an encephalomyelitis exists. Swallowing may be painful because of inflammation of the pharynx or esophagus, as is found in strangles in the horse, in calf diphtheria, and where improper use of balling and drenching guns or bottles has caused laceration of the mucosa. Attempts at swallowing followed by coughing up of feed or regurgitation through the nostrils can also be the result of painful conditions but are most likely to be due to physical obstructions such as esophageal diverticula or stenosis, a foreign body in the pharynx, or to paralysis of the pharynx. It is important to differentiate between material that has reached the stomach and ingesta regurgitated from an esophageal site. Partial esophageal obstruction resulting in difficult swallowing is usually manifested by repeated swallowing movements often with associated flexion of the neck and grunting.

In ruminants there may be abnormalities of rumination and belching. Absence of cudding occurs in many diseases of cattle and sheep; violent efforts at regurgitation with grunting suggests esophageal or cardiac obstruction. There may be inability to control the cud—'cud-dropping'—due to pharyngeal paralysis or painful conditions of the mouth. Failure to belch is usually manifested by the appearance of bloat.

Defecation In constipation and rectal paralysis or stenosis the act of defecation may be difficult and be accompanied by much straining. When there is abdominal pain or laceration of the mucocutaneous junction at the anus defecation may cause obvious pain. Involuntary defecation occurs in severe diarrhea and when there is paralysis of the anal sphincter. Consideration of frequency, volume and character of feces is given later under the section on special examination of the digestive tract.

Urination Micturition may be difficult when there is partial obstruction of the urinary tract, painful when there is inflammation of the bladder or urethra. In cystitis and urethritis there is increased frequency with the passage of small amounts of fluid and the animal remains in the urination posture for some time after the flow ceases. Incontinence, with constant dribbling of urine, is usually due to partial obstruction of the urethra or paralysis of its sphincter.

Posture Abnormal posture is not necessarily indicative of disease, but when associated with other signs it may indicate the site and severity of a disease process. One of the simplest examples is resting of a limb in painful nditions of the extremities; if a horse continually shifts weight from limb to limb it may indicate the presence laminitis or early osteodystrophia fibrosa. Arching of e back with the limbs under the body usually indicates ild abdominal pain; downward arching of the back d 'saw horse' straddling of the legs is characteristic of vere abdominal pain, usually spasmodic in occurrence; 'dog-sitting' posture in the horse associated with rolling d kicking at the belly is usually associated with ab- ominal pain and pressure on the diaphragm such as curs in acute gastric dilatation after engorgement on rain. This posture is commonly adopted by normal ttle (1). Abduction of the elbows is usually synonymous ith chest pain or difficulty in breathing. Elevation and gidity of the tail, and rigidity of the ears and limbs, are ood indications of tetanus in animals. The carriage of e tail in pigs is a useful barometer of their state of ealth. Sheep that are blind, as in early pregnancy xemia, are immobile but stand with the head up and ear an expression of extreme alertness.

When the animal is recumbent there may also be bnormalities of posture. In cattle affected by dislocation f the hip or by sciatic nerve paralysis, the affected limb s not held flexed under the body but sticks straight out n an awkward position; unilateral pain in the chest may ause an animal to lie habitually on the other side, a veak hindleg may be kept under the animal. The head nay be carried around towards the flank in parturient aresis in cows and in colic in horses. Sheep affected vith hypocalcemia, and cattle with bilateral hip dis- ocation, often lie in sternal recumbency with the hind- egs extended behind in a frog-like attitude. Inability or ack of desire to rise are usually indicative of muscle weakness or of pain in the extremities as in enzootic muscular dystrophy or laminitis.

Gait Movements of the limbs can be expressed in terms of rate, range, force and direction of movement. Abnormalities may occur in one or more of these categories. For example, in true cerebellar ataxia all qualities of limb movement are affected. In louping-ill in sheep it is the range and force which are excessive giving a high-stepping gait and a bounding form of progression: in arthritis because of pain in the joints, or in laminitis because of pain in the feet, the range is diminished and the patient has a shuffling, stumbling walk. The direction of progress may be affected. Walking in circles is a common abnormality and is usually associated with rotation or deviation of the head; it may be a permanent state as in listeriosis or occur spasmodically as in acetonemia and pregnancy toxemia. Compulsive walking or walking directly ahead regardless of obstructions is part of the 'dummy' syndrome mentioned earlier and is characteristic of encephalomyelitis and hepatic insufficiency in the horse.

Condition The animal may be in normal bodily condition, or obese, thin or emaciated. The difference between thinness and emaciation is one of degree; the latter is more severe but there are additional signs that are usually taken into consideration. In an emaciated (cachectic) animal the coat is poor, the skin is dry and leathery and work performance is reduced. Thin animals on the other hand are physiologically normal. The difference between fatness and obesity is of the same order. Most beef cattle prepared for the show-ring are obese. In order to inject some degree of numerical assessment it is now customary in all farm animal species and in horses to use body condition on a scale of 1 to 5 or preferably 1 to 8 (16, 17).

Conformation The assessment of conformation or shape is based on the symmetry and the shape and size of the different body regions relative to other regions. An abdomen which is very large relative to the chest and hindquarters can be classified as an abnormality of conformation. To avoid repetition points of conformation are included in the description of body regions.

Skin Skin abnormalities can usually be seen at a distance. They include changes in the hair or wool, abnormal sweating, the presence of discrete or diffuse lesions, evidence of soiling by discharges and of itching. The normal luster of the coat may be absent: it may be dry as in most chronic debilitating diseases or excessively greasy as in seborrheic dermatitis. In debilitated animals the long winter coat may be retained past the normal time. Alopecia may be evident: in hyperkeratosis it is diffuse; in ringworm it may be diffuse but more commonly occurs in discrete areas. Sweating may be diminished, as in anhidrosis of horses; patchy as in peripheral nerve lesions; or excessive as in acute abdominal pain. Hypertrophy and folding of the skin may be evident, hyperkeratosis being the typical example. Discrete skin lesions range in type from urticarial plaques to the circumscribed scabs of ringworm, pox and impetigo. Diffuse lesions include the obvious enlargements due to subcutaneous edema, hemorrhage and emphysema. Enlargements of lymph nodes and lymphatics are also evident when examining an animal from a distance.

Inspection of body regions

As a general rule as much of a clinical examination as possible should be carried out before the animal is handled. This is partly to avoid unnecessary excitement of the patient but also because some abnormalities are better seen at a distance and in some cases cannot be discerned at close range. The general appearance of the animal should be noted and its behavior assessed. Some time should also be devoted to an inspection of the various body regions.

Head

The facial expression may be abnormal. The rigidity of tetanus, the cunning leer or maniacal expression of rabies and acute lead poisoning are cases in point. The symmetry and configuration of the bony structure should be examined. Doming of the forehead occurs in some cases of congenital hydrocephalus and in chondrodysplastic dwarfs, and in the latter there may be bilateral enlargement of the maxillae. Swelling of the maxillae and mandibles occurs in osteodystrophia fibrosa; in horses swelling of the facial bones is usually due to frontal sinusitis: in cattle enlargement of the maxilla or mandible is common in actinomycosis. Asymmetry of the soft structures may be evident and is most obvious in the carriage of the ears, degree of closure of the eyelids and situation of the muzzle and lower lip. Slackness of one side and drawing to the other are constant features in facial paralysis. Tetanus is accompanied by rigidity of the ears, prolapse of the third eyelid and dilatation of the nostrils. The carriage of the head is most important; rotation is usually associated with defects of the vestibular apparatus on one side: deviation with unilateral involvement of the medulla and cervical cord; opisthotonus is an excitation phenomenon associated with tetanus, strychnine poisoning, acute lead poisoning, hypomagnesemic tetany, polioencephalomalacia and encephalitis. The eyes merit attention: visible discharge should be noted; protrusion of the eyeball, as occurs in orbital lymphomatosis, and retraction of the bulb as occurs commonly in dehydration are important findings; spasm of the eyelids and excessive blinking usually indicate pain or peripheral nerve involvement; prolapse of the nictitating membrane usually characterizes central nervous system derangement, generally tetanus. Dilatation of the nostrils and nasal discharge suggest the advisability of closer examination of the nasal cavities at a later stage. Excessive salivation or frothing at the mouth denotes painful conditions of the mouth or pharynx or is associated with tremor of the jaw muscles due to nervous involvement. Swellings below the jaw may be inflammatory as in actinobacillosis and strangles, or edematous as in acute anemia, protein starvation or congestive heart failure. Unilateral or bilateral swelling of the cheeks in calves usually indicates necrotic stomatitis.

Neck

If there is enlargement of the throat this region should be more closely examined later to determine whether the cause is inflammatory and whether lymph nodes, salivary glands (or guttural pouches in the horse) or other soft tissues are involved. Goiter leads to local enlargement located further down the neck. A jugular pulse, jugular vein engorgement and edema should be looked for and local enlargement due to esophageal distension noted.

Thorax

The respiration should be examined from a distance, preferably with the animal in a standing position as recumbency is likely to modify it considerably. Allowance should be made for the effects of exercise, excitement, high environmental temperatures and fatness of the subject: obese cattle may have respiratory rates two to three times that of normal animals. The rate, rhythm, depth and type of respiration should be noted.

Respiratory rate In normal animals under average conditions the rate should fall within the following limits: horses 8–10, cattle 10–30, sheep and pigs 10–20 and goats 25–35/min. Increased respiratory rate is designated as polypnea, decreased rate as oligopnea and complete cessation as apnea. The rate may be counted by observation of rib or nostril movements, by feeling the nasal air movements or by auscultation of the thorax or trachea. A significant rise in environmental temperature or humidity may double the normal respiratory rate (2). Animals which are acclimatized to cold outdoor temperatures are susceptible to heat stress when exposed suddenly to warmer temperatures. When brought indoors the respiratory rate may increase to six or eight times the normal, and panting open-mouth breathing may be evident within 2 hours.

Respiratory rhythm The normal respiratory cycle consists of three phases of equal length: inspiration, expiration and pause; variation in the length of one or all phases constitutes an abnormality of rhythm. Prolongation of inspiration is usually due to obstruction of the upper respiratory tract, prolongation of the expiratory phase to failure of normal lung collapse as in emphysema. In most diseases of the lungs there is no pause and the rhythm consists of two beats instead of three. There may be variation between cycles: Cheyne–Stokes respiration, characteristic of advanced renal and cardiac disease, is a gradual increase and then a gradual decrease in the depth of respiration; Biot's breathing which occurs in meningitis affecting the medullary region, is characterized by alternating periods of hyperpnea and apnea, the periods often being of unequal length. Periodic breathing also occurs commonly in animals with electrolyte and acid–base imbalances—there are periods of apnea followed by short bursts of hyperventilation.

Respiratory depth The amplitude or depth of respiratory movements may be reduced in painful conditions of the chest or diaphragm and increased in any form of anoxia. Moderate increase in depth is referred to as hyperpnea and labored breathing as dyspnea. In dyspnea the accessory respiratory movements are brought into play; there is extension of the head and neck, dilatation of the nostrils, abduction of the elbows and breathing through the mouth plus increased movement of the thoracic and abdominal walls. Marked respiratory sounds, especially grunting, may also be heard.

Type of respiration In normal respiration there is movement of the thorax and abdomen. In painful conditions of the chest, e.g. acute pleurisy, and in paralysis of the intercostal muscles there is fixation of the thorax and a marked increase in the movements of the abdominal wall; there is usually an associated pleuritic ridge caused by thoracic immobility with the chest expanded. This syndrome is usually referred to as an abdominal-type respiration. The reverse situation is thoracic-type respiration in which the movements are largely confined to the chest, as in peritonitis, particularly when there is diaphragmatic involvement.

Chest symmetry This can also be gauged by inspection. Collapse or consolidation of one lung may lead to restriction of movements of the chest on the affected side. The 'rachitic rosary' of enlarged costochondral junctions is typical of rickets.

Respiratory noises or stridores These include: coughing due to irritation of the pharynx, trachea and bronchi; sneezing due to nasal irritation; wheezing due to stenosis of the nasal passages; snoring when there is pharyngeal obstruction as in tuberculous adenitis of the pharyngeal lymph nodes; roaring in paralysis of the vocal cords; and grunting, a forced expiration against a closed glottis, which happens in many types of painful and labored breathing.

An important part of the clinical examination of a horse that produces an externally audible noise, usually a grunt, while working is to determine when the noise occurs in the respiratory cycle. This can be related to limb movements, expiration occurring as the leading foot hits the ground at the canter or gallop. Flexion of the head by the rider will exacerbate the noise (8).

Abdomen
Variations in abdominal size are usually appreciated during the general inspection of the animal. An increase in size may be due to the presence of excess food, fluid, feces, flatus or fat, the presence of a fetus or a neoplasm. Further differentiation is usually possible only on close examination, although fetal movements may be visible; in severe distension of the intestines with gas the loops of bowel may be visible in the flank. Gaseous distension is usually uniform whereas fluid tends to give an increased distension ventrally. The term 'gaunt' is often used to describe a decrease in abdominal size. It occurs most commonly in starvation, in severe diarrhea and in many chronic diseases where appetite is reduced. Umbilical hernia or infection and dribbling from a pervious urachus may be apparent. Ventral edema is commonly associated with approaching parturition, gangrenous mastitis, congestive heart failure, infectious equine anemia, and rupture of the urethra due to obstructive urolithiasis. Ruminal movements are quite readily observed from a distance but are better examined at a later stage.

External genitalia
Gross enlargements of the sheath or scrotum are usually inflammatory in origin but varicocele or tumors can also be responsible. Degenerative changes in the testicles may result in a small scrotum. Discharges of pus and blood from the vagina indicate infection of the genito-urinary tract.

Mammary glands
Disproportionate size of the quarters of the udder suggests acute inflammation, atrophy or hypertrophy of a gland. These conditions can be differentiated only by palpation.

Limbs
Posture and gait have been described. Symmetry is important and comparison of pairs should be used when there is doubt of the significance of an apparent abnormality. Enlargement or distortion of bones, joints, tendons, sheaths and bursae should be noted and so should any enlargement of peripheral lymph nodes and lymphatic vessels.

Physical examination

Some of the techniques used in making a physical examination are set out below.

Palpation
Direct palpation with the fingers or indirect palpation with a probe is aimed at determining the size, consistency, temperature and sensitivity of a lesion or organ. Terms used to describe palpation findings include the following: doughy, when the structure pits on pressure as in edema; firm, when the structure has the consistency of normal liver; hard, when the consistency is bone-like; fluctuating, when the structure is soft, elastic and undulates on pressure but does not retain the imprint of the fingers; emphysematous, when the structure is puffy and swollen, and moves and crackles under pressure because of the presence of gas in the tissue.

Percussion
In percussion the body surface is struck so as to set deep parts in vibration and cause them to emit audible sounds. The sounds vary with the density of the parts set in vibration and may be classified as follows: resonant, the sound emitted by organs containing air, e.g. normal lung; tympanitic, a drum-like note emitted by an organ containing gas under pressure such as a tympanitic rumen or cecum; dull, the sound emitted by solid organs such as heart and liver.

The quality of the sound elicited is governed by a number of factors. The strength of the percussion blow must be kept constant as the sound volume increases with stronger percussion. Allowances must be made for the thickness and consistency of overlying tissues, the thinner the chest wall, the more resonant the lung; percussion on a rib must not be compared with percussion on an intercostal space; percussion in a fat animal may yield little information. The value of percussion as a diagnostic aid in large animals is limited. Man is the optimum size. Pigs and sheep are of a suitable size but the fatness of the pig and the wool coat of the sheep plus the uncooperative nature of both species make percussion impracticable. In cattle and horses the organs are too large and overlying tissue too thick for satisfactory outlining of organs or abnormal areas, unless the observer is highly skilled.

Percussion can be carried out with the fingers using one hand as a plexor and one as a pleximeter. In large animals a pleximeter hammer may be used on a finger or a pleximeter disk. The use of the fingers is preferable as they produce little or no additional sound.

Tactile percussion (ballottement)
By combining palpation and percussion it is possible to obtain information on the consistency and boundaries of organs not accessible by percussion alone. The technique consists essentially of an interrupted, firm, push stroke to push the organ away and allow it to rebound on to the fingertips. Ballottement of a fetus is a typical example. A modification of the method is fluid percussion when a cavity containing fluid is percussed on one side and the fluid wave thus set up is palpated on the other. The sensation created by the fluid wave is called a fluid thrill. It is felt most acutely by the palm of the hand at the base of the fingers.

Auscultation
Direct listening to the sounds produced by organ movement is performed by placing the ear to the body surface over the organ. Indirect auscultation by a stethoscope is much to be preferred. A considerable amount of work has been done to determine the most effective stethoscopic equipment including such things as the shape and proportions of bell chest pieces, the thickness of rubber tubes and the diameter and depth of phonendoscope chest pieces. A comparatively expensive unit from a reputable instrument firm is a wise investment. For large

animal work a stethoscope with interchangeable 5 cm diameter phonendoscope and rubber (to reduce hair friction sounds) bell chest pieces is all that is required. The details of the sounds heard on auscultations of the various organs are described in their respective sections.

Combined percussion and auscultation
The fact that sounds are transmitted more efficiently through solid tissue than through tissue containing air can be utilized by combining percussion and auscultation. The stethoscope bell is placed over the area to be examined and a percussion sound produced by tapping on the trachea or on another part of the chest. Since the objective is to produce a sharp sound, the tap should be short and forcible and be applied to tracheal cartilage or a prominent rib. An alternative method is to place one coin on the percussion site and strike it forcibly with the edge of another coin. When the tissue under examination is solid the percussion sound comes through sharply and loudly; when the tissue is air-filled it has an insulating effect and the sound produced is muffled and dull. The area of consolidation can be defined by comparing the sound with that heard in surrounding normal areas.

The sounds emitted on percussion of the abdomen and thorax of large animals are more easily audible with the aid of a stethoscope during the percussion procedures. The stethoscope is placed over the area to be examined and the areas around the stethoscope and radiating out from it are percussed. This is a valuable diagnostic aid for the detection and localization of a gas-filled viscus in the abdomen such as left-side displacement of the abomasum, dilatation and torsion of the abomasum, cecal torsion, or pneumoperitoneum. In diaphragmatic hernia the presence of gas-filled intestines in the thorax may be determined by this method. The technique of percussion to best determine the presence of a gas-filled viscus in the abdomen of a cow is critical. To elicit the diagnostic 'ping', it is necessary to percuss and auscultate side by side and to percuss with a quick, sharp, light and localized force. The obvious method is a quick tap with a percussion hammer or similar object. Another favored method is a 'flick' with the back of a forefinger suddenly released from behind the thumb. A gas-filled viscus gives a characteristic clear, sharp, high-pitched 'ping' which is distinctly different from the full, low-pitched noted of solid or fluid-filled viscera. The difference between the two is so dramatic that it is comparatively easy to define the borders of the gas-filled viscus.

Succussion, or shaking of the body to detect the presence of fluid, is an adaptation of the above method. By careful auscultation while the body is shaken, free fluid in the chest or abdomen can be heard to rattle and an estimate of the fluid level can be made. One drawback of the technique is that fluid in the gut, especially when gas is present, will also rattle and may be confused with free fluid.

Miscellaneous special physical techniques including biopsy and paracentesis are described under special examination of the various systems to which they apply. With suitable equipment and technique one of the most valuable adjuncts to a physical examination is a radiographic examination. The size, location and shape of soft tissue organs are often demonstrable in animals of up to moderate size. Ultrasound imaging, other than for pregnancy diagnosis, has had only limited use in food animals.

Examination method
The physical examination should be carried out as quietly and gently as possible to avoid disturbing the patient and thus increasing the resting heart and respiratory rates. At a later stage it may be necessary to examine certain organs after exercise, but resting measurements should be carried out first. If possible the animal should be standing, as recumbency is likely to cause variation in pulse rate, respiration and other functions.

Temperature
Normally the temperature is taken per rectum. When this is impossible the thermometer should be inserted into the vagina. Ensure that the mercury column is shaken down, moisten the bulb to facilitate entry and if the anus is flaccid or the rectum full of hard feces insert a finger also to ensure that the thermometer bulb is held against the mucosa. When the temperature is read immediately after defecation, or if the thermometer is stuck into a ball of feces or is left in the rectum for insufficient time, a false, low reading will result. As a general rule the thermometer should be left in place for 2 minutes. If there is doubt as to the accuracy of the reading, the temperature should again be taken. The normal average temperature range for the various species at average environmental temperature is as follows:

	Normal	*Critical point*
Horse	38·0°C (100·5°F)	39·0°C (102·0°F)
Cattle	38·5°C (101·5°F)	39·5°C (103·0°F)
Pig	39·0°C (102·0°F)	40·0°C (103·5°F)
Sheep	39·0°C (102·0°F)	40·0°C (104·0°F)
Goat	39·5°C (103·0°F)	40·5°C (105·0°F)

Temperature conversions are approximate

These figures indicate the average resting temperature for the species and the critical temperature above which hyperthermia can be said to be present. Normal physiological variations occur in body temperature and are not an indication of disease: a diurnal variation of up to 1°C (2°F) may occur with the low point in the morning and the peak in the late afternoon. There may be a mild rise of about 0·6°C (1°F) in late pregnancy, but a precipitate but insignificant decline just before calving is not uncommon in cows and ewes (3, 12) and lower temperatures than normal occur just before estrus and at ovulation (4) but the degree of change (about 0·3°C; 0·6°F) is unlikely to attract clinical attention. In sows the body temperature is subnormal before farrowing and there is a significant rise in body temperature coinciding with parturition. This rise is commonly high enough to exceed the critical temperature of 40°C and may be considered erroneously as evidence of disease (5). The elevation of temperature which occurs in sows at the time of parturition, of the order of 1°C, is maintained through lactation and disappears at weaning (11). High environmental humidity and temperature and exercise will cause elevation of the temperature; the deviation may be as much as 1·6°C (3°F) in the case of high environmental temperatures and as much as 2·5°C (4·5°F) after severe xercise: in horses, after racing, 2 hours may be required efore the temperature returns to normal.

If animals which have been acclimatized to cold outide temperatures are brought indoors to a warmer temerature their body temperatures may exceed the critical emperature within 2–4 hours (6).

Marked temperature variations are an indication of a athological process. *Hyperthermia* is simple elevation of he temperature past the critical point as in heat stroke. *Fever or pyrexia* is the state where hyperthermia is comined with toxemia as in most infectious diseases. *Hypohermia*, subnormal body temperature, occurs in shock, circulatory collapse (as in parturient paresis and acute rumen impaction of cattle), hypothyroidism and just before death in most diseases.

Pulse

The pulse should be taken at the middle coccygeal or facial arteries in cattle, the facial artery in the horse and the femoral artery in sheep and goats. With careful palpation a number of characters may be determined, including rate, rhythm, amplitude, tone, maximum and minimum and pulse pressures and the form of the arterial pulse. Some of these characters are more properly included in special examination of the circulatory system and are dealt with under that heading.

Rate The pulse rate is dependent on the heart alone and is not directly affected by changes in the peripheral vascular system. The pulse rate may or may not represent the heart rate; in cases with a pulse deficit where some heartbeats do not produce a pulse wave the rates will differ. Normal resting rates (per minute) for the various species are:

Horses	30–40
Colts up to a year old	70–80
Cattle	60–80
Young calves	100–120
Sheep and goats	70–90

Although there are significant differences in rate between breeds of dairy cows, and between high and low producing cows (9) the differences would not be noticeable to a clinician performing a routine examination. In newborn thoroughbred foals the pulse rate is 30–90 in the first 5 minutes, then 60–200 up to the first hour, and then 70–130 up to the first 48 hours after birth (7). No pulse is palpable in the pig but the comparable heart rate is 60–100 per minute.

Bradycardia or marked slowing of the heartbeat is unusual unless there is partial or complete heart block, but it does occur in cases of space-occupying lesions of the cranium and in cases of diaphragmatic adhesions after traumatic reticulitis in cattle. *Tachycardia* or increased pulse rate is common, and occurs in most cases of septicemia, toxemia, circulatory failure and in animals affected by pain and excitement. Counting should be carried out over a period of at least 30 seconds.

Rhythm The rhythm may be regular or irregular. All irregularities must be considered as abnormal except sinus arrhythmia, the phasic irregularity coinciding with the respiratory cycle. There are two components of the rhythm, namely the time between peaks of pulse waves and the amplitude of the waves. These are usually both irregular at the one time, variations in diastolic filling of the heart causing variation in the subsequent stroke volume. Regular irregularities occur with constant periodicity and are usually associated with partial heart block. Irregular irregularities are due to ventricular extrasystoles or atrial fibrillation. Most of these irregularities, except that due to atrial fibrillation, disappear with exercise. Their significance lies chiefly in indicating the presence of myocardial disease.

Amplitude The amplitude of the pulse is determined by the amount of digital pressure required to obliterate the pulse wave. It is largely a measure of cardiac stroke volume and may be considerably increased, as in the 'water harmmer' pulse of aortic semilunar valve incompetence, or decreased as in most cases of myocardial weakness.

Examination of body regions

After the examination of the pulse, temperature and respiration the physical examination proceeds with an examination of the various body regions. This is best carried out in orderly fashion beginning at the head.

Head and neck

Eyes Any discharge from the eyes should be noted: it may be watery in obstruction of the lacrimal duct, serous in the early stages of inflammation and purulent in the later stages. Whether the discharge is unilateral or bilateral is of considerable importance; a unilateral discharge may be due to local inflammation, a bilateral discharge may denote a systemic disease. Abnormalities of the eyelids include abnormal movement, position and thickness. Movement may be excessive in painful eye conditions or in cases of nervous irritability including hypomagnesemia, lead poisoning and encephalitis. The lids may be kept permanently closed when there is pain in the eye, or when the eyelids are swollen, as for instance in local edema due to photosensitization or allergy. The membrana nictitans may be carried across the eye when there is pain in the orbit or in tetanus or encephalitis. There may be tumors on the eyelids.

Examination of the conjunctiva is important because it is a good indicator of the state of the peripheral vascular system. The pallor of anemia and the yellow coloration of jaundice may be visible, although they are more readily observed on the oral or vaginal mucosae. Engorgement of the scleral vessels, petechial hemorrhages, edema of the conjunctiva as in gut edema of pigs or congestive heart failure, dryness due to acute pain or high fever are all readily observable abnormalities.

Corneal abnormalities include opacity varying from the faint cloudiness of early keratitis, to the solid white of advanced keratitis, often with associated vascularization, ulceration and scarring. Increased convexity of the cornea is usually due to increased pressure within the eyeball and may be due to glaucoma or hypopyon.

The *size of the eyeball* does not usually vary but protrusion is relatively common and when unilateral is due in most cases to pressure from behind the orbit. Periorbital lymphoma in cattle, dislocation of the mandible and periorbital hemorrhage are common causes. Retraction of the eyeballs is a common manifestation of reduction in volume of periorbital tissues, for example in starvation when there is disappearance of fat and in dehydration when there is loss of fluids.

Abnormal eyeball movements occur in nystagmus due to anoxia or to lesions of the cerebellum or vestibular tracts. In nystagmus there is periodic, involuntary movement with a slow component in one direction and a quick return to the original position. The movement may be horizontal, vertical or rotatory. In paralysis of the motor nerves to the orbital muscles there is restriction of movement and abnormal position of the eyeball at rest.

Examination of the deep structures of the eye can be satisfactorily carried out only with an ophthalmoscope but gross abnormalities may be observed by direct vision. Pus in the anterior chamber, hypopyon, is usually manifested by yellow to white opacity often with a horizontal upper border obscuring the iris. The pupil may be of abnormal shape or abnormal in position due to adhesions to the cornea or other structures. An abnormal degree of dilatation is an important sign, unilateral abnormality usually suggesting a lesion of the orbit. Bilateral excessive dilatation (mydriasis) occurs in local lesions of the central nervous system affecting the oculomotor nucleus, or in diffuse lesions including encephalopathies, or in functional disorders such as botulism and anoxia. Peripheral blindness due to bilateral lesions of the orbits may have a similar effect. Excessive constriction of the pupils (miosis) is unusual unless there has been overdose with organic phosphatic insecticides or parasympathomimetic drugs. Opacity of the lens is readily visible, especially in advanced cases.

Several tests of vision and of ocular reflexes are easily carried out, and when warranted should be done at this stage of the examination. Tests for blindness include the menace reflex and an obstacle test. In the former a blow at the eye is simulated, care being taken not to cause air currents. The objective is to elicit the eye preservation reflex manifested by reflex closure of the eyelids. This does not occur in peripheral or central blindness and in facial nerve paralysis there may be withdrawal of the head but no eyelid closure. An obstacle test in unfamiliar surroundings should be arranged and the animal's ability to avoid obstacles assessed. The results are often difficult to interpret if the animal is nervous. A similar test for night-blindness (nyctalopia) should be arranged in subdued light, either at dusk or on a moonlit night. Nyctalopia is one of the earliest indications of avitaminosis A. Total blindness is called amaurosis, partial blindness is called amblyopia. The pupillary light reflex, closure and dilatation of the iris in response to lightness and darkness, is best tested with a strong flashlight.

Nostrils Particular attention should be paid to the odor of the nasal breath. There may be a sweet sickly smell of ketosis in cattle or a fetid odor which may originate from any of a number of sources including gangrenous pneumonia, necrosis in the nasal cavities or the accumulation of nasal exudate. Odors originating in the respiratory tract are usually constant with each breath and may be unilateral. The sour smell of alimentary tract disturbance is detectable only periodically coinciding with eructation. Odors originating in the mouth from bad teeth or from necrotic ulcers caused by *Fusobacterium necrophorum* in calves may be smelled on the nasal breath but are stronger on the oral breath.

In certain circumstances it may be important to note the volume of the breath expelled through the nostrils. It may be the only way of determining if the animal is breathing and in some cases of counting the respiratory rate. Variation in volume between nostrils, as felt on the hands, may indicate obstruction or stenosis of one nasal cavity. This can be examined further by closing off the nostrils one at a time; if obstruction is present in one nostril, closure of the other causes severe respiratory embarrassment.

Any nasal discharge that is present should receive special attention and its examination should be carried out at the same time as an inspection of the nasal mucosa. Discharges may be restricted to one nostril in a local infection, or be bilateral in systemic infection. The color and consistency of the exudate will indicate its source. In the early stages of inflammation the discharge will be a clear, colorless fluid which later turns to a white to yellow exudate as leukocytes accumulate in it. In Channel Island cattle the color may be a deep orange, especially in allergic rhinitis. A rust or prune juice color indicates blood originating from the lower respiratory tract, as in pneumonia and in equine infectious anemia in the horse. Blood clots derived from the upper respiratory tract or pharynx may be in large quantities, or appear as small flecks. In general, blood from the upper respiratory tract is unevenly mixed with any discharge, whereas that from the lower tract comes through as an even color. The consistency of the nasal discharge will vary from watery in the early stages of inflammation, through thick, to cheesy in longstanding cases. Bubbles or foam may be present. When the bubbles are coarse it signifies that the discharge originates in the pharynx or nasal cavities; fine bubbles originate in the lower respiratory tract. In all species vomiting or regurgitation caused by pharyngitis or esophageal obstruction may be accompanied by the discharge of food material from the nose or the presence of food particles in the nostrils. In some cases the volume of nasal discharge varies from time to time, often increasing when the animal is feeding from the ground, infection of cranial sinuses.

Inflammation of the nasal mucosa varies from simple hyperemia, as in allergic rhinitis, to diffuse necrosis, as in bovine malignant catarrh and mucosal disease, to deep ulceration as in glanders. In hemorrhagic diseases variations in mucosal color can be observed and petechial hemorrhages may be present.

Mouth Excessive salivation, with ropes of saliva hanging from the mouth and usually accompanied by chewing movements, occurs when a foreign body is present in the mouth and also in many forms of inflammation of the oral mucosa or of the tongue. Actinobacillosis of the tongue, foot-and-mouth disease and mucosal disease are typical examples. Identical signs appear in disease of the central nervous system when the salivary nucleus is involved, or where there is an encephalopathy as in acute lead poisoning in young cattle. Hypersalivation is a characteristic sign in epidermic hyperthermia caused by the mycotoxins of *Acremonium coenophialum* and *Claviceps purpurea* and by the examination of the fungus

Rhizoctonia leguminicola sometimes found on red clover. Dryness of the mouth occurs in dehydration and poisoning with belladonna alkaloids, or when high levels of urea are fed.

Abnormalities of the buccal mucosa include local lesions, hemorrhages in purpuric diseases, the discolorations of jaundice and cyanosis and the pallor of anemia. Care must be taken to define the exact nature of lesions in the mouth, especially in cattle, differentiation between vesicles, erosive and ulcerative lesions is of diagnostic significance in the mucosal diseases of this species.

Examination of the teeth for individual defects is a surgical subject but a general examination of the dentition can yield useful medical information. Delayed eruption and uneven wear may signify mineral deficiency, especially calcium deficiency in sheep; excessive wear with mottling and pitting of the enamel is suggestive of chronic fluorosis.

The tongue may be swollen by local edema or by inflammation as in actinobacillosis of cattle, or shrunken and atrophied in postinflammatory or nervous atrophy. Lesions of the lingual mucosa are part of the general buccal mucosal response to injury.

Examination of the pharyngeal region is difficult in large animals. In cattle it is usually performed with the hand using a mouth speculum. Foreign bodies, diffuse cellulitis and pharyngeal lymph node enlargement can be detected by this means. A metal or Plexiglass cylindrical speculum combined with a flashlight may be used for detailed visual inspection of the pharynx and larynx in cattle. In horses, manual exploration can only be carried out under anesthesia. Endoscopy is a useful method of examination in this species, and the modern fiberoptiscope has made it possible to visualize lesions in the posterior nares and pharynx–esophagus, larynx–trachea in the standing, conscious horse or ox.

Submaxillary region Abnormalities of the submaxillary region which should be noted include enlargement of lymph nodes due to local foci of infection, subcutaneous edema as part of a general edema, local cellulitis with swelling and pain, enlargement of salivary glands or guttural pouch distension in the horse. Thyroid gland enlargement is often missed or mistaken for other lesions, but its site, pulsation and surrounding edema are characteristic.

Neck Examination of the neck is confined mainly to the jugular furrow. Engorgement of the jugular vein may be due to obstruction of the veins by compression or constriction, or to failure of the right side of the heart. A jugular pulse of small magnitude is normal in most animals but it must be differentiated from a transmitted carotid pulse which is not obliterated by compression of the jugular vein at a lower level. Variations in size of the vein may occur synchronously with deep respiratory movements but bear no relation to the cardiac cycles. When the pulse is associated with each cardiac movement it should be determined whether it is physiological or pathological. The physiological pulse is presystolic and due to atrial systole and is normal. The pathological pulse is systolic and occurs simultaneously with the arterial pulse and the first heart sound; it is characteristic of an insufficient tricuspid value.

Local or general enlargement of the esophagus associated with vomiting or dysphagia occurs in esophageal diverticulum, stenosis and paralysis, and in cardial obstructions. Passage of a stomach tube or probang can assist in the examination of esophageal abnormalities.

Tracheal auscultation is a useful diagnostic aid. Normally, the sounds which are audible are soft and low but in upper respiratory tract disease they are purring or rattling when inflammatory exudate is present, and whistling in the presence of stenosis. The abnormal tracheal sounds are usually transmitted down the bronchial tree and are audible on auscultation over the thorax, primarily during inspiration. They are commonly confused with abnormal lung sounds due to pneumonia but in pneumonia the abnormal sounds are usually present on both inspiration and expiration.

Thorax

Examination of the thorax includes palpation, auscultation and percussion of the cardiac area (precordium) and the lung area. The greatest difficulty is usually encountered with the examination of the chest of the horse. The difficulty arises because of the thickness of the chest wall and the normally slow respiratory rate. Both factors contribute to an almost soundless respiration in the normal horse. There is, too, the need to detect minor pulmonary lesions which may reduce the work performance of the horse only slightly, but because of the importance of perfect fitness in a racing animal, have major significance. Another important factor which emphasizes the care that must be taken with the examination of the respiratory system of the horse is the ability of racing animals to compensate for even major pulmonary lesions from their immense functional reserve. Because of this, one is likely to encounter horses with massive pulmonary involvement with little obvious impairment of respiratory function.

Cardiac area Palpation of the heart action has real value; the size of the cardiac impulses can be assessed and palpable thrills may on occasion be of more value than auscultation of murmurs. It is best carried out with the palm of the hand and should be performed on both sides. An increased cardiac impulse, the movements of the heart against the chest wall during systole, may be easily seen on close inspection of the left precordium and can be felt on both sides. It may be due to cardiac hypertrophy or dilatation associated with cardiac insufficiency or anemia or to distension of the pericardial sac with edema or inflammatory fluid. Care should be taken not to confuse a readily palpable cardiac impulse due to cardiac enlargement with one due to contraction of lung tissue and increased exposure of the heart to the chest wall. Normally the heart movements can be felt as distinct systolic and diastolic thumps. These thumps are replaced by thrills when valvular insufficiencies or stenoses or congenital defects are present. When the defects are large the murmur heard on auscultation may not be very loud but the thrill is readily palpable. Early pericarditis may also produce a friction thrill. The cardiac impulse should be much stronger on the left than the right side and reversal of this situation indicates displacement of the heart to the right side. Caudal or anterior displacement can also occur.

Auscultation of the heart is aimed at determining the character of normal heart sounds and detecting the presence of abnormal sounds. Optimum auscultation sites are the fourth and fifth intercostal spaces, and, because of the heavy shoulder muscles which cover the anterior border of the heart, the use of a flat phonendoscope chest piece pushed under the triceps muscles is necessary. Extension of the forelimb may facilitate auscultation if the animal is quiet. Areas where the various sounds are heard with maximum intensity are not directly over the anatomical sites of the cardiac orifices because conduction of the sound through the fluid in the chamber gives optimum auscultation at the point where the fluid is closest to the chest wall. The first (systolic) sound is heard best over the cardiac apex, the tricuspid closure being most audible over the right apex, and mitral closure over the left apex. The second (diastolic) sound is heard best over the base of the heart, the aortic semilunar closure posteriorly and the pulmonary semilunar anteriorly, both on the left side.

In auscultation of the heart the points to be noted are the rate, rhythm, intensity and quality of sounds and whether abnormal sounds are present. Comparison of the heart and pulse rates will determine whether there is a pulse deficit due to weak heart contractions failing to cause palpable pulse waves: this is most likely to occur in irregular hearts. Normally the rhythm is in three time and be described as LUBB-DUPP-pause, the first sound being dull, deep, long and loud and the second sound sharper and shorter. As the heart rate increases the cycle becomes shortened mainly at the expense of diastole and the rhythm assumes a two-time quality. More than two sounds per cycle is classified as a 'gallop' rhythm and may be due to reduplication of either the first or second sounds. Reduplication of the first sound is common in normal cattle and its significance in other species is discussed under diseases of the circulatory system. The rhythm between successive cycles should be regular except in the normal sinus arrhythmia associated with respiration. With irregularity there is usually variation in the time intervals between cycles and in the intensity of the sounds, louder sounds coming directly after prolonged pauses and softer than normal sounds after shortened intervals as in extrasystolic contractions. The intensity of the heart sounds may vary in two ways, absolutely or relatively: absolutely when the two sounds are louder than normal and relatively when one sound is increased compared to the other in the cycle. For example, there is increased absolute intensity in anemia and in cardiac hypertrophy. The intensity of the first sound depends on the force of ventricular contraction and is thus increased in ventricular hypertrophy and decreased in myocardial asthenia. The intensity of the second sound depends upon the semilunar closure, that is on the arterial blood pressure and is, therefore, increased when the blood pressure is high and decreased when the pressure is low.

Abnormal sounds may replace one or both of the normal sounds or may accompany them. The heart sounds are muffled when the pericardial sac is distended with fluid. Sounds which are related to events in the cardiac cycle are murmurs or bruits and are caused mainly by endocardial lesions such as valvular vegetations or adhesions, insufficiency of closure of valves and by abnormal orifices such as a patent interventricular septum or ductus arteriosus. Interference with normal blood flow causes the development of turbulence with resultant eddying and the creation of murmurs. In attempting to determine the site and type of the lesion it is necessary to identify its time of occurrence in the cardiac cycle; it may be presystolic, systolic or diastolic and it is usually necessary to palpate the arterial pulse and auscultate the heart simultaneously to determine accurately the time of occurrence. The site of maximum audibility may indicate the probable site of the lesion, but other observations including abnormalities of the arterial pulse wave should be taken into account. In many cases of advanced debility, anemia and toxemia soft murmurs which wax and wane with respiration (hemic murmurs) can be heard and are probably due to myocardial asthenia. In cases of local pressure on the heart by other organs, for example in diaphragmatic hernia in cattle, loud systolic murmurs may be heard, probably due to distortion of the valvular orifices.

Abnormal sounds not related to the cardiac cycle include pericardial friction rubs which occur with each heart cycle but are not specifically related to either systolic or diastolic sounds. They are more superficial, more distinctly heard than murmurs and have a to-and-fro character. Local pleuritic friction rubs may be confused with pericardial sounds especially if respiratory and cardiac rates are equal.

Percussion to determine the boundaries of the heart is of little value in large animal work because of the relatively large size of the heart and lungs and the depth of tissue involved. The area of cardiac dullness is increased in cardiac hypertrophy and dilatation and decreased when the heart is covered by more than the usual amount of lung as in pulmonary emphysema. More detailed examination of the heart by electrocardiography, radiographic examination, test puncture and blood pressure are described under diseases of the heart (Chapter 8, p. 307).

Lung area Palpation, percussion and auscultation are again the methods available for examination of the lung area. Palpation may reveal the presence of a pleuritic thrill, bulging of the intercostal spaces when fluid is present in the thoracic cavity, or narrowed intercostal spaces and decreased rib movement over areas of collapsed lung.

Percussion may be by the usual direct means, or indirectly by tracheal percussion when the trachea is tapped gently and the sound listened for over the lung area. By direct percussion within the intercostal spaces the area of normal lung resonance can be defined and abnormal dullness or resonance detected. Increased dullness may indicate the presence of a space-occupying mass, consolidated lung, edematous lung or an accumulation of fluid. An overloud normal percussion note is obtained over tissue containing more air than usual, for example emphysematous lung. A definite tympanitic note can be elicited over pneumothorax or a gas-filled viscus penetrating through a diaphragmatic hernia. For percussion to be a satisfactory diagnostic aid affected areas need to be large with maximum abnormality, and the chest wall must be thin.

The lung area available for satisfactory auscultation is

slightly larger than that available for percussion. The normal breath sound is heard over the bulk of lung tissue, particularly in the middle third anteriorly over the base of the lung and is a soft, sipping VEE-EFF, the latter, softer sound occurring at expiration. The sounds are heard with variable ease depending on the thickness of the chest wall and the amplitude of the respiratory excursion. In well-fleshed horses and fat beef cattle the sounds may not be discernible at rest. Increased breath sounds are heard in dyspnea and in early pulmonary congestion and inflammation. The breath sounds may be diminished or absent when the alveoli and small bronchi are not filling with air, as in the later stages of pneumonia, pulmonary edema and collapse. Bronchial sounds in normal animals are audible only at the base of the lung. If the lung is collapsed but there is no exudate in the bronchi, such as occurs in interstitial pneumonia, the area over which bronchial sounds may be heard is much increased.

Alterations in the breath and bronchial sounds are the most common abnormalities which are audible on auscultation of the lung area in animals with disease of the lower respiratory tract. Other abnormal sounds over the lung area include crackles, wheezes and friction rubs. They are the result of interference with the free movement of air in and out of the lungs, and of the presence of lesions which interfere with the normal movement of the lung and thus create additional respiratory sounds which are an indication of disease.

There is considerable variation in the descriptions of the characteristics and the interpretations of the significance of abnormal lung sounds. Our descriptions and interpretations are set out in Table 33 in Chapter 10.

The intensity of abnormal lung sounds may be increased and their clarity improved by measuring the rate and depth of respirations with forced mild exercise such as walking for a few minutes followed by immediate auscultation. If exercise is undesirable the occlusion of both nostrils for 30–45 seconds will be followed by some deep inspirations and accentuation of abnormal lungs. An alternative maneuver which is effective in both horses and cattle is to pull a plastic bag over the muzzle and lower face. When respiratory movements become exaggerated the bag is removed and the lungs auscultated immediately.

Sounds of peristalsis are normally heard over the lung area on the left side in cattle and in horses. In cattle these sounds are due to reticular movement and in horses to movements of the colon. Their presence is not of much significance in these species unless there are other signs. In cattle, too, sounds of swallowing, belching and regurgitation may be confused with peristaltic sounds; ruminal movements and the esophagus should be observed for the passage of gas or a bolus to identify these sounds. Other techniques for examination of the thorax are described under diseases of the respiratory system (Chapter 10).

Abdomen

Palpation and percussion through the abdominal wall
Because of the thickness and weight of the abdominal wall in mature cattle and horses, deep palpation of viscera and organs through the abdominal wall has limited value in these species compared to its usefulness in small animals. No viscera or organ, with the exception of the fetus, can be palpated with certainty through the abdominal wall in the horse. In cattle, the rumen and its contents can usually be palpated in the left paralumbar fossa. Ruminal distension is usually obvious while an inability to palpate the rumen may be due to a small relatively empty rumen or to medial displacement as in left-side displacement of the abomasum. A markedly enlarged liver in a cow may be palpable by ballottement immediately behind the right costal arch. Using a combination of palpation, percussion and simultaneous auscultation over the right paralumbar fossa and caudal to the entire length of the right costal arch it may be possible to detect any of the following in cattle: dilatation and torsion of the abomasum, cecal dilatation and torsion, impaction of the abomasum and omasum and torsion of the coiled colon. Percussion and auscultation over viscera which are distended with fluid and gas may be undertaken and the size and location of the tympanitic area will provide some indication of the viscera likely to be involved.

Tactile percussion of the abdomen aids detection of an excessive quantity of fluid in the peritoneal cavity: ascites due to a ruptured bladder, transudate in congestive heart failure and exudate in diffuse peritonitis. A sharp blow is struck on one side of the abdomen and a fluid wave, a 'blip' or undulation of the abdominal wall, can be seen and felt on the opposite side of the abdomen. The peritoneal cavity must be about one-third full of fluid before a fluid wave can be elicited.

The focus of abdominal pain may be located by external palpation in cattle and horses. Deep palpation with a firm uniform lift of the closed hand or with the aid of a horizontal bar held by two people under the animal is necessary to detect deepseated pain. Superficial pain may be elicited by a firm poke of the hand or extended finger. In cattle, pain may be elicited over the right costal arch when there are liver lesions, and immediately behind the xiphoid sternum in reticuloperitonitis or generally over the abdomen in diffuse peritonitis.

The response to palpation of a focus of abdominal pain in cattle is a 'grunt' which may be clearly audible. If there is doubt as to whether pain is produced, the simultaneous auscultation of the trachea will detect a perceptible grunt when the affected area is reached. In calves with abomasal ulceration, a focus of abdominal pain may be present on deep palpation over the area of the abomasum. In left-side displacement of the abomasum, percussion and simultaneous auscultation over the upper-third of the costal arch between the ninth and twelfth ribs may reveal the presence of high-pitched musical quality sounds. These may be mistaken for similar sounds present in ruminal atony.

In cases of severe abdominal distension (ruminal tympany in cattle, torsion of the large intestine) it is usually impossible to determine, by palpation and percussion, the viscera which are distended. Pneumoperitoneum is rare and thus gross distension of the abdomen is usually due to distension of viscera with gas, fluid or ingesta. A combination of rectal examination, passage of a stomach tube, paracentesis and exploratory laparotomy may be necessary to determine the cause.

The abdomen of pigs is difficult to examine by palpation because they are seldom sufficiently quiet or relaxed and the thickness of the abdominal wall limits the extent of deep palpation. In late pregnancy in sows the gravid uterus may be ballotted but it is usually not possible to palpate fetal prominences.

In sheep, the rumen, impacted abomasum and the gravid uterus are usually palpable through the abdominal wall. Positioning the sheep on its hindquarters will shift the viscera to a more easily palpable position.

Rectal examination Special care is necessary to avoid injuring the patient and causing it to strain. Suitable lubrication and avoidance of force are the two most important factors. Rectal examination enables observations to be made on the alimentary, urinary and genital tracts and on the vessels, peritoneum and pelvic structures. Palpable abnormalities of the digestive tract include paralysis and ballooning of the rectum, distension of the loops of the intestine with fluid or gas, the presence of hard masses of ingesta as in cecal and colonic impactions in the horse, and intestinal obstruction due to volvulus, intussusception or strangulation. The detection of tight bands of mesentery leading to displacement segments may be a valuable guide. In cattle the caudal sacs of the rumen are readily palpable. When the rumen is distended as in bloat or vagus indigestion they may push well into the pelvis or be only just within reach when the rumen is empty. A distended abomasum may be felt in the right half of the abdomen in cases of abomasal torsion and occasionally in vagus indigestion. In normal animals there is little to feel because of the space occupied by normal intestines. Palpable objects should be carefully examined.

The left kidney in the cow can be felt in the midline and distinct lobulations are evident. In the horse the caudal pole of the left kidney can often be felt, but the right organ is out of reach. There may be abnormalities of size in pyelonephritis, hydronephrosis and amyloidosis, and pain on pressure in pyelonephritis. The ureters are not normally palpable nor is the empty bladder. A distended bladder or chronic cystitis with thickening of the wall can be felt in the midline at the anterior end of the pelvic cavity. Large calculi have a stone-like hardness and are occasionally observed in horses in the same position. Pain with spasmodic jerking of the penis on palpation of the urethra occurs in urinary obstruction due to small calculi, cystitis and urethritis. Enlarged, thickened ureters such as occur in pyelonephritis can be felt between the kidney and the bladder.

In the peritoneum and mesentery one may feel the small, grape-like lesions of tuberculosis, the large, irregular, hard masses of fat necrosis and the enlarged lymph nodes of lymphomatosis. The abdominal aorta is palpable, and in horses the anterior mesenteric artery and some of its branches can be felt. This may be an important examination if a verminous aneurysm is suspected, in which case the vessels are thickened but still pulsate, have an uneven rough surface and may be painful. In horses the caudal edge of the spleen is usually palpable in the left abdomen. During a rectal examination in a horse it is advantageous in some cases to palpate the inguinal ring from inside the abdomen and, by pushing the other hand between the horse's thighs to palpate the external ring simultaneously. It is then easier to decide whether any abnormal structures are passing through the ring.

Examination of the genital organs is usually carried out at this stage but is not discussed here because it is dealt with adequately in texts on diseases of the genital system.

Auscultation Auscultation of the abdomen is an essential part of the clinical examination of cattle, horses and sheep. It is of limited value in pigs. The intestinal or stomach sounds will indicate the nature of the intraluminal contents and the frequency and amplitude of gastrointestinal movements which are valuable aids in clinical diagnosis. The intensity, duration and frequency of the sounds should be noted. All of these characteristics will be increased in animals which have just eaten or immediately following excitement.

Auscultation of the rumen of cattle and sheep is frequently a rewarding examination. In normal animals there are one to two primary contractions, involving the reticulum and the dorsal and ventral sacs of the rumen, per minute, depending on the amount of time which has elapsed since feeding, and the type of food consumed. Secondary contractions of the dorsal and ventral sacs of the rumen occur about 1 per minute and are commonly associated with eructation. The examination is made in the left paralumbar fossa and a normal sequence of sounds consists of a lift of the flank with a fluid gurgling sound, followed by a second more pronounced lift accompanied by a booming, gassy sound. Auscultation over the lower left ribs will reveal the fainter fluid sounds of reticular contractions just prior to the contractions of the dorsal and ventral ruminal sacs described above. The reticular and ruminal sounds are the predominant abdominal sounds in the normal ruminant.

A grunt, detectable by auscultation over the trachea, may occur during the reticular contraction phase of a primary contraction, in cattle with traumatic reticuloperitonitis. The factors which result in a decrease in the intensity and frequency of ruminal sounds are discussed in detail under diseases of the ruminant stomach.

The intestinal sounds which are audible on auscultation of the right flank of cattle and sheep consist of frequent faint gurgling sounds which are usually difficult to interpret. The contraction of the abomasum and the intestines result in a mixture of sounds which are difficult to distinguish.

The intestinal sounds of the horse are clearly audible and their assessment is one of the most vital parts of the clinical examination and surveillance of the horse with suspected abdominal disease. Over the right and ventral abdomen there are the loud, booming sounds (borborygmi) of the colon and cecum which are at peak intensity about every 15–20 seconds. Over the left abdomen there are the much fainter rushing fluid sounds of the small intestines. An increase in the intensity and frequency of sounds with a distinct fluid quality are heard in enteritis and loud, almost crackling, sounds in spasmodic colic. In impaction of the large intestine there is a decrease in the intensity and frequency of the bororygmi, and in thromboembolic colic due to verminous aneurysm and infarction of the colon there may be complete absence of sounds. In intestinal obstruction the intestinal sounds due to peristalsis are markedly decreased and usually absent and fluid tinkling sounds occur infrequently. In intestinal stasis in the horse, auscultation in the right flank often detects the tinkling sound of fluid dropping from the ileocecal valve through gas into the dorsal sac of the cecum.

A combination of auscultation and percussion is used in cattle for the detection of left-side displacement of the abomasum which is described under that heading.

MAKING A DIAGNOSIS

The practice of clinical veterinary medicine consists of two major facets, the making of a diagnosis and the provision of treatment and control measures. For treatment and control to be of optimum value the diagnosis must be as accurate as possible, so that diagnosis is the crux of all medical problems.

A diagnosis is the identification of the disease affecting the patient, and to be complete should include three parts:

- The specific cause.
- The abnormality of structure or function produced by the causative agent, and which is inimical to normal body processes.
- The clinical manifestation of that abnormality produced by the causative agent.

For recording purposes the animal species should also be included. For example, 'equine *Rhodococcus equi* pneumonia and lung abscess'. Many diagnoses fall short of this objective (10) because of lack of confirmatory laboratory assistance. So clinical signs (such as bovine chronic diarrhea) or necropsy lesions (such as bovine polioencephalomalacia) are often used.

Diagnostic methods

There are at least five distinctly recognizable methods that are used (18) and they are presented here in order of increasing complexity. As a general rule the experienced clinicians use more of the simpler strategies, the novice clinician more of the complex ones. This is because the simple method omits several steps in the clinical reasoning process, the sort of appropriate and safe cutting of corners that is done with confidence only after gaining wide experience and the payment of a good deal of attention to assessing one's personal competence as a clinician and especially as a diagnostician.

Method 1: The syndrome or pattern recognition

In the first few moments of viewing the patient, e.g. the pain-generated behavior of a horse with abdominal pain, the skin lesions of ecthyma in a sheep, or papillomatosis in a cow, the diagnosis is made instantaneously and reflexly. The same experience may occur while taking the history; one may have to rely entirely on the history in the case of a cow having an epileptic seizure to be able to diagnose it. This recognition is based on the comparison of the subject case and previous cases in the clinician's memory and the one is recognized as a replica of the other. There is no need to seek further supporting advice and the definitive diagnosis is made then and there. In the hands of the wise and experienced clinician the method is quick and accurate.

Method 2: Hypothetico-deductive reasoning method

As soon as the client commences to relate the presenting signs, usually commencing with the key clinical sign, the clinician begins to draw up a short list of diagnostic possibilities, usually three or four. This is the process of generating multiple plausible *hypotheses* from initial cues. The clinician then begins to ask questions and conduct clinical examinations which test the hypotheses. The questions and examinations may be directed at supporting or discounting the tentative diagnoses (the confirm–exclude technique) but they may lead to the addition of more hypotheses and the deletion of some others. (The questions used here are search ones, aimed at supporting a hypothesis and are distinctly different from scanning questions which are 'fishing' expeditions looking for more key signs about which to ask search questions.) This process of hypothesis and deduction is continued until one diagnosis is preferred to the others. The original list of hypotheses may be expanded, but usually not more than seven, and in the final stages is usually reduced to two or three. These are then arranged in order of preference and become the list of *diagnostic possibilities*.

In farm animal medicine there is usually a general absence of both hard primary data and ancillary data such as clinical pathology so that the clinician may be in the position of having to provide treatment for two or three possible illnesses. An example is the parturition syndrome of recently calved dairy cows in which the treatment of subacute mastitis, metritis and acetonemia is standard procedure because the clinician is uncertain about which disease is most accountable for the illness. In the more resourceful arena of a veterinary teaching hospital it may still be necessary to proceed in this way in the first instance but then to narrow down the list of hypotheses when additional information is received from the laboratory. This polypharmacy approach has a number of disadvantages amongst which are included the additional expense and the increased possibility of contamination of food products of animal origin by medications, especially antibiotics and sulfonamides, and with resistant strains of bacteria.

One of the important characteristics of this strategy is the dependence on the selection of a critical or key clinical sign or cue on which to base the original hypotheses. The selection of the key sign and additional supporting clinical findings is done instinctively by experienced clinicians on the basis of prior experience in similar situations. For novice clinicians it may be necessary to examine two or more key signs.

Method 3: The arborization or algorithm method

This is really an extension of method 2 but the hypothetico-deductive reasoning method is formalized and carried

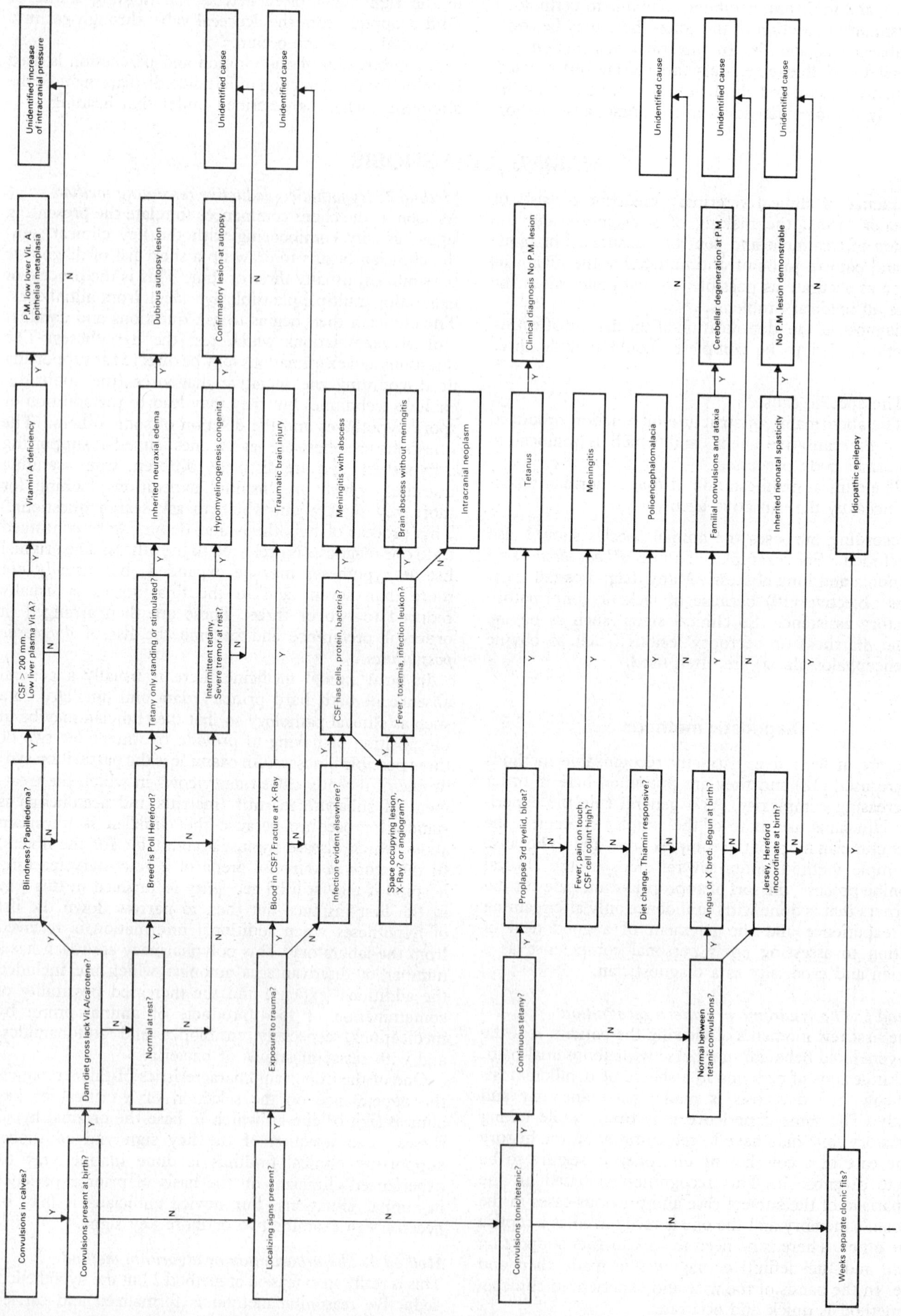
Convulsions in calves?
Convulsions present at birth?
Dam diet gross lack Vit A/carotene?
Blindness? Papilledema?
CSF > 200 mm. Low liver plasma Vit A?
Vitamin A deficiency
P.M. low lover Vit. A epithelial metaplasia
Unidentified increase of intracranial pressure
Normal at rest?
Breed is Poll Hereford?
Tetany only standing or stimulated?
Inherited neuraxial edema
Dubious autopsy lesion
Unidentified cause
Intermittent tetany. Severe tremor at rest?
Hypomyelinogenesis congenita
Confirmatory lesion at autopsy
Localizing signs present?
Exposure to trauma?
Blood in CSF? Fracture at X-Ray
Traumatic brain injury
Unidentified cause
Infection evident elsewhere?
CSF has cells, protein, bacteria?
Meningitis with abscess
Space occupying lesion, X-Ray? or angiogram?
Fever, toxemia, infection leukon?
Brain abscess without meningitis
Intracranial neoplasm
Convulsions tonic/tetanic?
Continuous tetany?
Proplapse 3rd eyelid, bloat?
Tetanus
Clinical diagnosis No P.M. lesion
Fever, pain on touch, CSF cell count high?
Meningitis
Diet change. Thiamin responsive?
Polioencephalomalacia
Normal between tetanic convulsions?
Angus or X bred. Begun at birth?
Familial convulsions and ataxia
Cerebellar degeneration at P.M.
Unidentified cause
Jersey, Hereford incoordinate at birth?
Inherited neonatal spasticity
No P.M. lesion demonstrable
Unidentified cause
Weeks separate clonic fits?
Idiopathic epilepsy
Unidentified cause

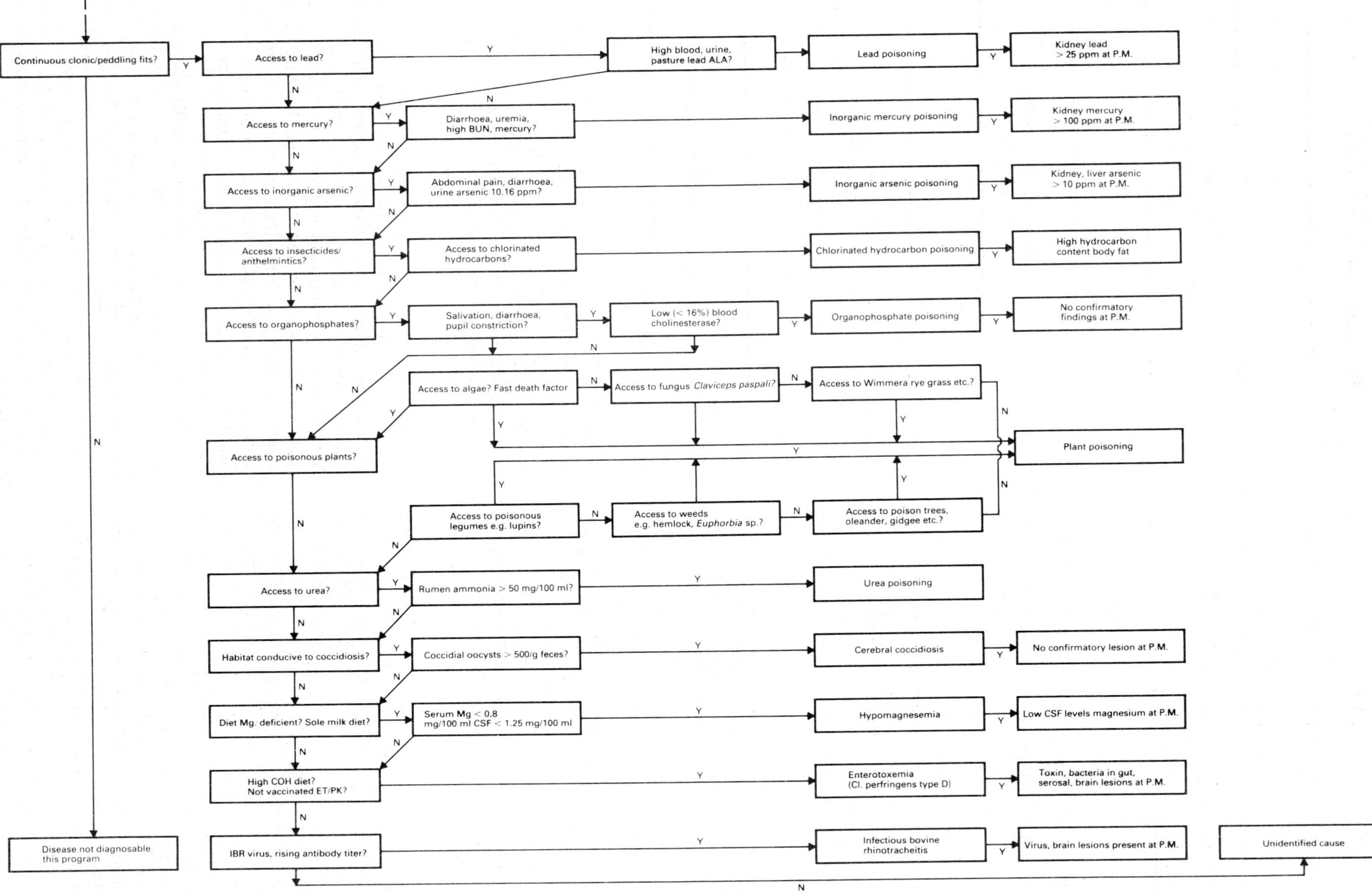

Fig. 1. Algorithm for the differential diagnosis of calves suffering from convulsive seizures

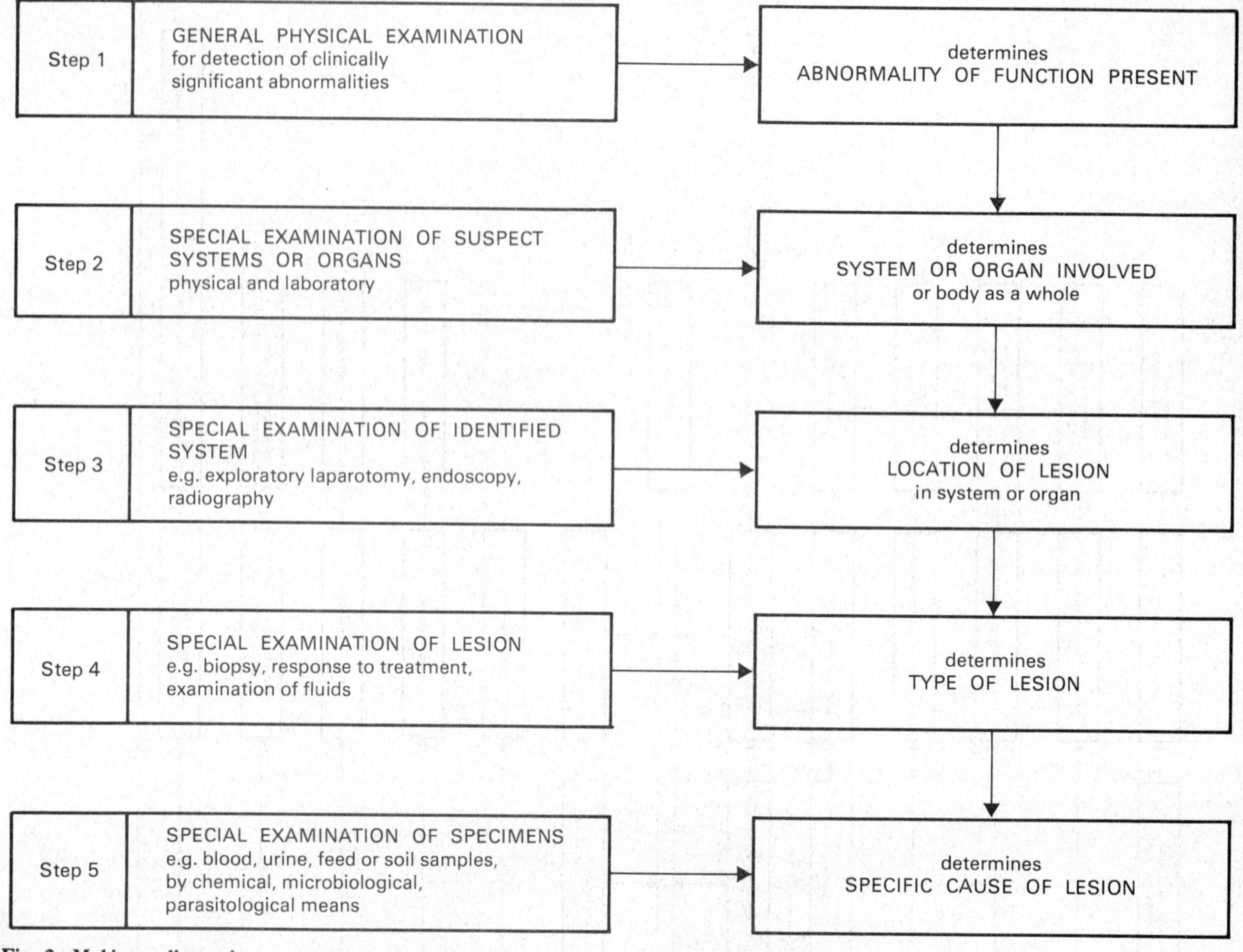

Fig. 2. Making a diagnosis

out according to a preplanned program. The hypothetico-deductive reasoning method depends on the clinician remembering and being aware of an all-inclusive list of diagnostic possibilities in the case under consideration. Because memory is unreliable and impressionistic the method is subject to error by omission. The arborization or algorithmic method similarly approaches a listed series of diagnoses and examines each one in turn with supporting or disproving questions; if they pass the proving test they stay in, if they fail it they are deleted. For example, a key sign of red urine in a cow promotes the question: has the cow had access to plant substances that color the urine red? If the answer is no, the next question is: is the red color caused by hemoglobinuria or hematuria? If the answer is hemoglobinuria, all of the diagnoses on the hematuria branch of the algorithm are deleted, and the questioner proceeds to the next question which will attempt to determine whether the cow has postparturient hemoglobinuria or any one of a number of diseases characterized by intravascular hemolysis.

Provided that the list of possible diagnoses is complete and is frequently updated as new diagnoses become available—and, just as importantly, as new ways of supporting or discounting each hypothesis are added as soon as they are published—the method works well. These algorithms (Fig. 1) are eminently suited to computerization and can be made available by the supply of floppy disks or by access to a central database via a modem, the online data base, or dialup information system.

The arborization method is well suited to the clinician who has not had the necessary experience for the memorization of long lists of potential diagnoses and the critical tests which confirm or exclude each of them. Because the algorithms are likely to include *all* the recorded diagnoses which have that particular key sign, error by omission is not a risk. Thus they are also valuable to the specialist who is less able to afford an omission than the general practitioner, and certainly cannot really afford to miss even the most obscure and unlikely diagnosis. Another major advantage is that they provide a system of tests which should be done and clinical findings which should be searched for which is really a form of a clinical protocol which acts as a reminder of the sequential diagnostic steps to be taken. The arrangement of the algorithm represents the clinical reasoning of the person who designed it and it should have considerable merit, assuming that the designer was an expert. This characteristic does arouse the comment that the method does away with the need for the clinicians to do their own clinical reasoning. That may be so but the interests of optimum clinical care of patients are probably better served by having first-year interns apply the clinical reasoning of a specialist and in fact achieve significantly better results (19).

Method 4: The key abnormality method

This is a more time-consuming method than the previous ones and requires that clinicians rely on their knowledge of normal structure and function to select the key abnormality or clinical cue. The method consists of five steps and is summarized in Fig. 2.

Determination of the abnormality of function present

Disease is abnormality of function which is harmful to the animal. The first step is to decide what abnormality of function is present. There may of course be more than one and some clinically insignificant abnormalities may be present, for example, a physiological cardiac murmur in a newborn foal. Definition of the abnormality is usually in general terms such as paralysis, state of the alimentary tract, hypoxia, respiratory insufficiency, nervous shock and so on. These terms are largely clinical, referring to abnormalities of normal physiological function, and their use requires a foreknowledge of normal physiology. It is at this point that the preclinical study of physiology merges into the clinical study of medicine.

The necessary familiarity with the normal, combined with observation of the case in hand, makes it possible to determine the physiological abnormality which may, for example, be hypoxia. The next step is to determine the body system or body as a whole or organ involved in the production of the hypoxia.

Determination of the system or body as a whole or organ involved

Having made a careful physical examination and noted any abnormalities it is then possible to consider which body system or organ is the cause of the abnormality. In some cases the body as a whole may be involved. This may not be difficult with some systems: for example, hypoxia may be due to failure of the respiratory or circulatory systems and examination of these is not difficult. However, special problems arise when attempting to examine the nervous system, the liver, kidney, endocrine glands, spleen and hemopoietic systems. Here, routine physical examination by palpation, auscultation and percussion is not very rewarding: special ancillary examination techniques with the aid of a laboratory are usually necessary. These are described under special examination methods for the various systems. As a guiding principle, all functions of the organ under examination should be observed and any abnormalities noted. For example, if the integrity of the central nervous system is to be examined, the clinician would look for abnormalities of mental state, gait, posture, muscle and sphincter tone and involuntary movements, abnormal posture and paralysis. Knowing the normal physiological functions of systems one looks for aberrations of them. When only simple physical examination is available it may be extremely difficult to choose between two or more systems as the possible location of the abnormality. For example, in an animal which is unable to rise from the recumbent position it may be difficult to decide if the nervous system or the musculoskeletal system or generalized weakness from a systemic illness is the origin of the clinical recumbency. If special diagnostic techniques and laboratory evaluations are inconclusive or not available it may be necessary to resort to probability as a guide. For example, paresis due to diseases of the muscles is most common in young calves, lambs and foals and uncommon in mature farm animals, with the exception of the myopathy associated with the downer cow syndrome in dairy cattle. However, paresis is common in mature cows affected with parturient hypocalcemia, peracute coliform mastitis and acute diffuse peritonitis.

Determination of the location of the lesion within the system or organ involved

The location of the lesion within the body system involved is not always obvious and may require special physical and laboratory examination techniques. For example, a detailed neurological examination may be necessary to localize the lesion in an animal with manifestation of disease of the nervous system. This may be combined with radiographic techniques such as myelography. An exploratory laparotomy with or without biopsy techniques may be necessary to determine the location of an intestinal lesion thought to be the cause of chronic diarrhea. Endoscopy is rapidly becoming standard practice for the localization of lesions of the respiratory tract of the horse. Radiography is often necessary to localize lesions of the musculoskeletal system and diseases of the feet of horses and cattle.

Determination of the type of lesion

The abnormality observed may be produced by lesions of different types. In general, lesions can be divided into anatomical or physical lesions and functional disturbances. The physical lesions can be further subdivided into inflammatory, degenerative or space-occupying. These classifications are not mutually exclusive, a lesion may be both inflammatory and space-occupying; abscesses in the spinal cord or lung are typical examples. In these circumstances it is necessary to modify the diagnosis and say that such and such a lesion is space-occupying and may or may not be inflammatory.

The differentiation between functional disturbances and physical lesions is often extremely difficult because the abnormalities produced may be identical. For example, in a case of hypomagnesemia in a cow there is no physical lesion but differentiation from the encephalitis of furious rabies may be impossible. As a rule, functional disturbances are transient, often recurrent or fluctuating and are readily reversible by treatment whereas structural lesions cause changes which are relatively static or at least change only gradually and are affected only gradually by treatment. This is by no means a regular rule; the acute abdominal pain of intestinal obstruction usually fluctuates but the lesion is a physical one whereas the paralysis of parturient paresis in cattle is static but the disturbance is functional only.

Differentiation between inflammatory, degenerative and space-occupying lesions is usually simpler. The latter produce signs characteristic of pressure on surrounding organs and can often be detected by physical means. Inflammatory lesions are characterized by heat, pain, swelling and a local or general leukocytosis and, in severe cases, a systemic toxemia. A total white blood cell count and differential is a *sensitive* but *non-specific* test for the presence of an infection. A leukopenia, neutropenia and a degenerative left shift suggests a severe infection. A neutrophilia and regenerative shift suggests an active chronic infection. The most common infections of cattle which are often not readily obvious are in the thoracic and abdominal cavities (pleuritis, pulmonary abscesses, pericarditis and peritonitis). Degenerative lesions produce the same loss or abnormality of function as lesions of the other types but are not usually accompanied by evidence of inflammation unless they are extensive. If the lesion is accessible biopsy should be considered as a means of determining its nature.

Determination of the specific cause of the lesion
If in the system involved, the nature of the abnormality and the type of lesion can be satisfactorily determined, it then remains to decide on the specific causative agent. If, for example, it could be said that a particular case of paralysis in a calf was caused by a degenerative lesion of the musculature only a few specific etiological agents would have to be considered to make a final diagnosis. In many, if not most, cases it is impossible to go beyond this stage without additional techniques of examination, particularly laboratory examinations, and it is a general practice to make a diagnosis without this confirmatory evidence because of limitations of time or facilities.

It is at this stage that a careful history-taking and examination of the environment show their real value. It is only by a detailed knowledge of specific disease entities, the conditions under which they occur, the epidemiology and the clinical characteristics of each disease that an informed judgment can be made with may degree of accuracy. If the diagnostic possibilities can be reduced to a small number, confirmation of the diagnosis by laboratory methods becomes so much easier because there are fewer examinations to be made and confirmation by response to treatment is easier to assess. If it is necessary to treat with a great many drugs serially, or in combination, to achieve a cure the expense is greater and the satisfaction of both the client and the veterinarian is diluted in proportion to the range of treatments. Accuracy in diagnosis means increased efficiency and this is the final criterion of veterinary practice.

Method 5: The database method
The basis of this method (also called also the *Weed or problem-oriented method*) is to conduct a complete clinical and clinicopathological examination of the patient in order to acquire a comprehensive patient *database*. The problems (key signs) in this database are then matched with the diagnostic database in which collections of signs or syndromes are labelled with diagnoses, to select the best fit with the patient's data.

This method also uses the *problem-oriented veterinary medical record system* which is an excellent system for the daily recording of clinical and laboratory data in an orderly, systematic and consistent manner which can be easily followed by the clinicians and their colleagues (43, 44). This system is now used widely by veterinary teaching hospitals. The system has four components based on the four phases of veterinary medical action: the *database*, the *problem list*, the *initial plans* and *progress notes*. The progress notes are created daily and divided into four parts known collectively by the acronym SOAP to designate *S*: subjective information, *O*: objective data, *A*: assessment of problem, and *P*: plans which may include diagnostic, therapeutic or client education (44). The method requires that clinicians be very painstaking in their examination and recording. It places great demands on the time spent by clinicians and clinical pathologists, on laboratory resources and on clinical record storage. Much of the data has no diagnostic significance because the diagnostic decisions are made largely on the presence or absence of relatively few key signs. It also has the disadvantage that there is a tendency to make the patient fit a category. It is the opposite of the *key abnormality* method in which only the signs and other indicants relevant to the proposed diagnosis are sought and recorded. Because of its requirement of time and data recording and storage this method is not suitable for use in food animal medicine where speed is a vital component of the diagnostic process. As mentioned earlier, however, it is an excellent system for the teaching of clinical veterinary medicine.

The method is really an expanded version of the *hypothetico-deductive* method, where the hypotheses are made sequentially as further information becomes available. In the *database* method all of the hypotheses are pursued in parallel because all the possible data has been collected into the patient's database. The source of error in the method is the possibility of undue importance being attached to a chance abnormality in, say, the clinical biochemistry. If the abnormality cannot be matched to a clinical sign it should be weighted downwards in value or marked for comment only. The same error may result from inclusion of an important sign, e.g. diarrhea, but which happens to be present at low intensity.

Computer-assisted diagnosis

In recent years there has been considerable interest in the concept of computer-assisted diagnosis (20–22). It was thought that the entry of the clinical and laboratory data from a patient into a computer program could result in the computer providing a differential diagnosis list of diseases in order of highest to lowest probability. However, despite over 20 years of interest in the use of computers for diagnosis, the impact of computer-assisted diagnosis in medical practice has been slight. Computerized programs have been useful in circumscribed areas such as the differential diagnosis of abdominal pain in man, and the diagnosis and treatment of meningitis (24). However, no program developed for use in a specific localized area of the body has been successfully adapted for generalized use. Theoretically, the computer could be expected to be useful to aid the clinician with the workup in order to make multiple and complex diagnoses.

Recent research on clinical decision-making has confirmed the importance of creating the list of differential diagnoses or diagnostic hypotheses. A clinician faced with a diagnostic problem must use clinical findings to develop a list of possible diagnoses. With a knowledge of the epidemiological and clinical characteristics of each disease the veterinarian can confirm or exclude certain diagnostic possibilities. Diagnostic acumen depends on the ability to recognize the most important clinical abnormalities and to generate a list of differential diagnoses, a task that becomes more efficient with experience.

Specialists can generate many differential diagnoses in

a narrow area of expertise, but the breadth of knowledge required in general practice makes it difficult for generalists to keep current on rare or unusual conditions (23). If a disease is not considered by the clinician faced with a presenting problem, it is frequently overlooked as a possibility and may not be 'stumbled-on' during the diagnostic process. This problem is complicated in veterinary education by the common practice of teaching according to disease entity. All of the nosology of a disease is presented in a standard format but the information must then be used in reverse order in clinical practice; the clinician generates a list of diseases based on the history and clinical findings. Textbooks that feature lists of differential diagnoses for animals with similar clinical findings assist in this task, but rapidly become outdated because of the many major and minor clinical findings which can be associated with a disease. The large storage capacity of computer databases and the ease of access to stored data makes the computer useful for handling this sort of information.

The success of a computer-assisted diagnosis will depend first on the clinician determining the important finding or *forceful feature* or *pivot* of the case which can be useful in separating possible look-alike diseases (1). The second most important requirement is to know the propensity for a certain clinical finding to occur in a disease syndrome. The algorithm is the center of a computer-aided diagnostic system (6). Statistical algorithms calculate the most likely diagnosis from explicit statistical analysis of disease probabilities and the frequency of clinical findings in a particular disease. A statistical algorithm is based on the Bayes theorem. The posterior probability that an animal has a given disease can be calculated if one has access to:

- The incidence (prior probability) of the disease
- The probability of a given clinical finding if the animal has the disease
- The probability of the same clinical finding occurring if the animal has the alternative disease.

After receiving the data, the computer uses this theory to calculate the likelihood of various diseases. However, a major problem of a Bayesian system is the availability of probabilities of the incidence of diseases and clinical findings associated with them. There is a need in veterinary medicine to generate comprehensive databases from which the probabilities of incidence and clinical finding for each disease can be determined from actual clinical practice.

In spite of these limitations, some progress is being made in the development of computer-assisted diagnosis in veterinary medicine.

Two independent computer-assisted diagnostic systems for veterinary medicine have been developed at Cornell University, Ithaca, New York. The CONSULTANT program is a system designed by M. E. White and J. Lewkowicz (20). The program contains a description of over 5600 diseases of dogs, cats, horses, cattle, sheep, pigs and goats. For each disease, there is a short description, including information on diagnostic testing, a list of current references, and a list of the clinical findings that might be present in the disease. The clinician enters one or more of the clinical findings present in a patient. The computer supplies a list of the diseases in which that clinical finding or combination of clinical findings are present. The complete description can be retrieved for any disease in the list of differential diagnoses. The program is available by long-distance telephone and a modem. A major limitation of the program to date is that the list of differential diagnoses is not in order of probability from highest to lowest. This is because the program does not include the probability of incidence and clinical findings for each disease, information which, as mentioned earlier, is not yet available.

Experience with the Cornell CONSULTANT program has shown that computer-assisted diagnosis is not used in day-to-day management of routine cases but is used primarily to provide assurance that a diagnosis was not overlooked when faced with an unusual problem (23). Computerized databases also offer a mechanism for the generalist to search through a complete list of differential diagnoses compiled from the recorded experience of many specialists and kept current as new information is published. Practitioners feel that having access to CONSULTANT is also a significant part of continuing education and a source of references. Experience with a computer-assisted diagnostic system has also confirmed the importance of an accurate history and an adequate clinical examination. If an important clinical finding is not detected, or not adequately recognized—for example, confusing weakness of a limb for lameness due to musculoskeletal pain—the computer program will be ineffective. Disagreement between observers about the meaning of a clinical finding will also continue to be a problem as computer-assisted diagnosis becomes more widely used.

The PROVIDES program is a computer-assisted diagnosis system for small animal medicine based on the principles of the *problem–knowledge coupler system* developed for human medicine by L. L. Weed (25). The system is constructed around clinical problems, for example, diarrhea, pruritus, coughing. The system is based on the algorithm and was called a problem–knowledge coupler because each bit of information on the patient is *coupled* to relevant information from the literature. It is based on a special matching algorithm known as pattern recognition (26). The PROVIDES system is designed to ask questions on signalment, history, clinical and laboratory findings. Positive responses are used to formulate a list of hypotheses or differential diagnoses. The findings of a specific patient are compared to a representative profile which has been stored in the computer. The computer generates a ranked list of disease hypotheses; the diseases whose discriminating signs most closely match those of the patient signs are listed first (26). For each disease in the differential diagnosis, the computer displays the propensities expected and whether they were observed or not observed in the patient. The relationship of each sign or demographic finding to a disease is supported by a full abstract and list of references. The database also suggests tests to aid the diagnosis of a disease, appropriate treatment and possible outcomes for each disease. The question-and-answer format of the PROVIDES program is designed to prevent errors of omission that may occur when clinicians obtain the history and perform a clinical examination.

The most important service the computer can provide in making a diagnosis is the generation of a hypotheses through the generation of a list of differential diagnoses and access to further information. Computers will probably not be able to make a definitive etiological diagnosis but they are able to remind the user of diagnoses which should be considered and to suggest the collection of additional data that might have diagnostic value.

Prognosis and therapeutic decision-making

The dilemma of whether or not to administer a certain drug or perform a certain operation in an animal patient with or without an established diagnosis, or when the outcome is uncertain, is familiar to veterinarians. Owners of animals with a disease, or merely a minor lesion, expect to receive a reasonably accurate prediction of the outcome and the cost of treatment but often considerable uncertainty exists about the presence or absence of a certain disease, or its severity, because confirmatory diagnostic information is not available.

The information which is required for a reasonably accurate prognosis includes: the expected morbidity and case fatality rates for that disease, the stage of the disease, whether or not a specific treatment or surgical operation is available or possible, and the cost of the treatment. If success is dependent on prolonged and intensive therapy, the high cost may be prohibitive to the owner who then may select euthanasia of the animal as the optimal choice. Veterinarians have an obligation to keep their clients informed about all the possible outcomes and the treatment which is deemed necessary, and should not hesitate to make strong recommendations regarding the treatment or disposal of a case. There are also different levels of outcome which may affect the prognosis and therapeutic decision-making. In the case of breeding animals, mere survival from a disease is insufficient and treatment is often not undertaken if it is unlikely that it will result in complete recovery and return to full breeding capacity. Slaughter for salvage may be the most economical choice. In other cases, like a pleasure horse, the return of sufficient health to permit light work may satisfy the owner.

Decision analysis

Veterinarians must routinely make decisions that have economic consequences for the client and the veterinarian. Questions such as whether to vaccinate or not, whether to treat an animal (29) or recommend slaughter for salvage value, whether or not to perform surgery, or even which surgical procedure to use to correct a case of left-side displacement of the abomasum, are common (30). Many of these questions are complex, requiring several successive decisions and each decision may have more than one outcome (27). Clinical decisions are not only unavoidable but also must be made under conditions of uncertainty. This uncertainty arises from several sources which include the following: errors in clinical and laboratory data; ambiguity of clinical data and variations in interpretations; uncertainty about the relationships between clinical information and presence of disease; uncertainty about the effects and costs of treatment; and uncertainty about the efficacy of control procedures such as vaccination or the medication of feed and water supplies in an attempt to control an infectious disease.

The process of selecting a management option from a range of options involves a mental assessment of the available options and their probable outcomes. Decision analysis provides a framework for handling complex decisions so that they can be more objectively evaluated. Decision analysis is a systematic approach to decision-making under conditions of uncertainty (33). Because the technique can be so useful in sorting out complex questions associated with the treatment and control of disease in individual animals, and in herds, it is almost certain to become more commonly used by large animal practitioners.

Decision analysis involves identifying all available choices and the potential outcomes of each, and structuring a model of the decision, usually in the form of a decision tree. Such a tree consists figuratively of nodes which describe choices and chances, and outcomes. The tree is used to represent the strategies available to the veterinarian and to calculate the likelihood that each outcome will occur if a particular strategy is employed. A probability value must be assigned to each possible outcome, and the sum of the probabilities assigned to the branches must equal 1·0. Objective estimates of these probabilities may be available from research studies or from a veterinarian's own personal records or it may be necessary to use subjective estimates. The monetary value associated with each possible outcome is then assigned followed by calculation of the expected value at each node in the tree. At each decision node the value of the branch with the best expected value is chosen and that becomes the expected value for that node. The expected value establishes a basis for the decision. An example of a decision tree without probability values assigned is shown in Fig. 3.

In the decision tree, choices such as the decision to use intervention no. 1 intervention or no. 2 are represented by squares, called *decision nodes*. Chance events such as favorable or unfavorable outcomes are represented by circles called *chance nodes*. When several decisions are made in sequence, the decision nodes must be placed from left to right in the same order in which the decisions would have to be made, based on information available at that time. The tree may become very complicated, but the basic units of choice and chance events represented by squares and circles remain the same. Lines, or *branches*, follow each node and lead to the next event. The branches following each decision node must be exhaustive; for example, they must include all possible outcomes, and the outcomes must be mutually exclusive (27). After each chance node there is a probability that an event occurs. The probabilities following a chance node must add up to 1·00. The probabilities are placed on the tree following the chance node. The expected outcomes (V_F and V_U in Fig. 3) are entered at the far right of the tree. The outcomes represent the value that would result of the events preceding them on the tree were to take place and must include the costs of the intervention. When a complete tree accurately representing the problem has been constructed, the next step is to solve it for the best decision to follow. This is done by starting at the right

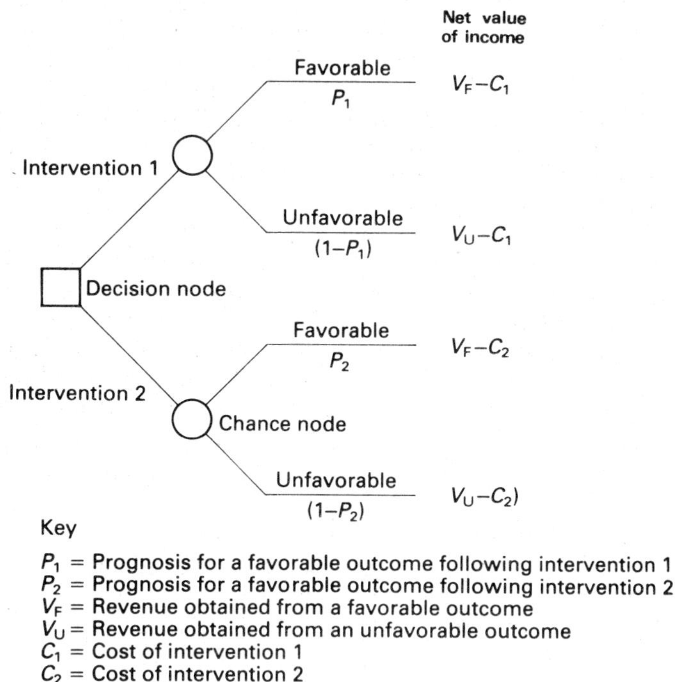

Fig. 3. A decision tree for choosing between two interventions. (Reprinted with permission from Fetrow, J. *et al.* (1985) *J. Am. vet. med. Assoc.*, *186*, 792–797)

of the tree, where outcome values are multiplied by the probabilities of outcome at the preceding chance node. The figures derived from this procedure are added together, to obtain the equivalent of a weighted average value at the chance node, known as the *expected value*, which by convention is circled with an oval. This procedure is repeated from right to left on the tree at each chance node. When a decision node is reached when moving from right to left, the most profitable path is chosen, and a double bar is drawn across the branches leading to the lesser cost-effective decisions. When the first decision node at the left of the tree is reached, a single path will be left which leads from left to right and has not been blocked by double bars. This path represents the best way to handle the problem according to the available information, including the outcome at the end of that path.

An example of the construction and use of a decision tree to assist in deciding at what day postpartum should an ovarian cyst be treated, as opposed to waiting for spontaneous recovery is illustrated in Fig. 4 (27). In structuring the problem, over time, the clinician knows that the cyst can be treated or left to be treated later. Retreatment is possible if the first treatment is ineffective. The structure must include all alternatives. The other information needed to solve the problem includes: the incidence or chances of spontaneous recovery; the response to treatment, both initially and following repeated treatments; when the response occurs; the cost of treatment and the cost of the disease (27).

The critical factor in each tree is the probability value for each possible outcome. The monetary value of each outcome can be estimated on a daily basis but unless the probability of the outcome can be assessed as accurately as possible, the decision analysis will be unreliable. Decision analysis has been used to determine the cost-effectiveness of heat mount detectors (36), the time at which to treat bovine ovarian cysts (28), the effectiveness of three alternative approaches to the control of hemophilus meningoencephalitis in feedlot cattle (31), the economically optimal control strategy among several alternatives for the control of infection with *Brucella ovis* in a sheep flock (37), and the relative merits of testing or not testing calves entering a feedlot with a metabolic and cellular profile test as predictors of performance in the feedlot (35). Decision analysis can now be done on microcomputers which makes the process highly suitable for assisting the veterinarian in daily decision-making (38).

The details of the steps used in decision analysis of several different problems in food-animal practice have been described and the reader is referred to the publications for further information (27–30, 34).

There are some limitations to using decision analysis in animal health programs (32). Decision analysis requires time and effort which practitioners are reluctant to provide unless the benefits are obvious. However, this problem can be overcome with the use of ready-made menu-driven programs like the ARBORIST which are now available (39). The estimates of the probabilities associated with the respective branches of the tree are seldom readily available. A number of techniques which can be used to derive these probabilities and incorporate them in decision-making have been recorded (14). The rapidly developing use of analytical veterinary clinical epidemiology can now provide the tools to generate the

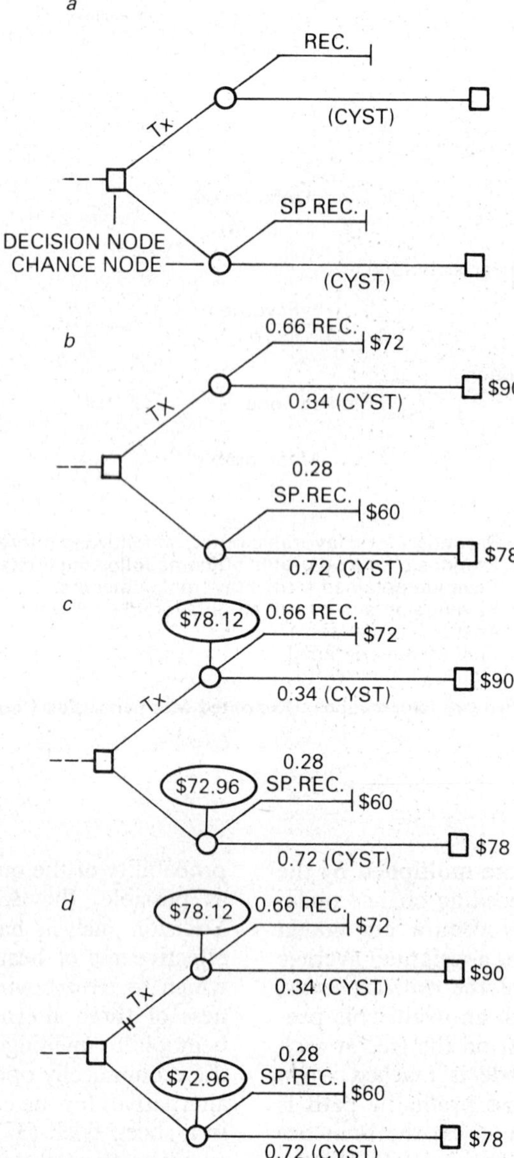

Fig. 4. Example of the construction and use of a decision tree. The sources of probabilities and dollar values are discussed in the text. (a) The skeleton of the decision tree with a decision (treat [T_x] versus do not treat) and chance outcomes (recovery [REC] or spontaneous recovery [SPREC] versus continued cyst [CYST]). (b) Probabilities and previously calculated outcome values are placed on the tree. (c) Expected costs of decision alternatives have been calculated and written in balloons above the chance nodes. (d) At this decision node, the correct choice is no treatment because it is cheaper ($72·96 versus $78·12). *Double bars* mark the pathway (treatment) that is not chosen. The value $72·96 is then the outcome cost for this decision node. This value is used in the calculation of the best alternative at the previous decision node, as the process is repeated from right to left (not shown). (Reprinted with permission from White, M. E. & Erb, H. N. (1982) *Comp. Cont. Educ.*, *4*, S426–S430)

numerical data necessary to make reliable decisions (40, 42). There is a need to apply epidemiological principles to prospective clinical studies to determine the most effective therapy or the efficacy of control procedures for the commonly occurring economically important diseases of food-producing animals. The inputs and outputs of a given strategy may not have a market value, or the market value may not be an appropriate measure, or they may not be tangible or measurable in the usual monetary units. For example, the market value of a dairy cow may not represent the true or real value of the cow to the farmer. The farmer may consider the value of the cow in relation to cattle replacement determinants such as herd size, the availability of replacements, and the genetic potential of the animal. The final selection of one option or the other is usually a complex process that will also vary from individual to individual depending on the decision criterion used.

In summary, decision analysis provides a systematic framework for making rational decisions about major questions in animal health and it is hoped that some veterinarians will adopt the technique for field use.

EXAMINATION OF THE HERD

Unless dealing with an outbreak of a specific disease, the making of a definitive etiological diagnosis may be more difficult, and elusive, in a herd than in an individual animal. The diseases which are encountered in herds may be clinically obscure and difficult to define because of the variation in response to disease by individual animals, more than one causative factor may be operating and the interactions which occur are not yet defined, records may be incomplete and there is a marked variation in the management from herd to herd. Thus in examination of the herd, all the factors which influence the behavior of a disease in that herd assume importance. It is the assessment of the relative importance of each of them which is the science of epidemiology.

Examination steps

The necessary steps for the examination of a herd are outlined in Fig. 5.

Step 1: defining the abnormality
It is necessary first to define the abnormality in either clinical or subclinical terms. In some cases the abnormalities will be obviously clinical, while in others the owner may complain about lowered production in the absence of clinical disease. The major problem will be in the collection of sufficient records on reproduction and production in order to define the complaint.

Step 2: defining the pattern of occurrence
After the identity of the abnormality has been established, all the available clinical, production and laboratory data are examined according to subgroups in the herd and according to time occurrence, genetic background, nutritional groups and relationship, if any, to other diseases and vaccination history. This attempts to determine if any associations exist between certain groups of animals and those factors which can influence the behavior of disease. In large dairy and swine herds, for example, the herd may be divided into different subunits and managed differently, and this can have a marked effect on production.

The pattern of occurrence of a disease in a population is therefore often of importance in suggesting which group of etiological agents is likely to be involved. For example, when all the animals in a population are exposed at the one time to a poison or a highly infectious agent, the pattern of occurrence will be that of a typical 'point outbreak', with many animals becoming affected at approximately the same time (14). When the infection has to be transferred from animal to animal after undergoing multiplication in each, delay results and the outbreak develops a bell-shaped occurrence graph. This information is also of value in indicating possible portals of entry of an infection or sources of a poison.

Step 3: defining the etiological group
Following characterization of the abnormality according to groups within the herd, and having made comparisons of the prevalence rates between groups, it may be possible to discern to which etiological category the abnormality most logically belongs. As mentioned previously the frequent occurrence of multiple causes of subclinical disease is a major consideration when examining a herd which is failing to achieve its production targets. For example, the failure to achieve expected levels of milk production in the absence of clinical disease could be due to the combined effects of subclinical mastitis, insufficient energy intake, use of a bull with a low production rating and long dry periods because of poor managerial expertise in the detection of estrus. Considerable difficulty may be encountered in deciding into which of the general areas of etiology the specific etiology is located. In so many cases herd problems are not the result of a single error but are multifactorial, with several causes contributing to a greater or lesser degree.

Step 4: defining specific etiology
The final step is to select the probable specific cause from within one or more of the general areas and prove the hypothesis by identifying the causative agent with the aid of the laboratory or a treatment response or control measure. It is becoming increasingly more difficult to obtain a clearly defined etiological diagnosis because of the complexity of disease. For example, certain *Leptospira* spp. many cause abortion in one herd and not in another and one is never certain of the significance of demonstrating the presence of the organism in the aborting herd. If nutritional inadequacy is suspected in a dairy herd, it may not be possible to determine if the cows are receiving an adequate intake if they are on pasture where an accurate measure of daily intake may not be possible. The frequency of occurrence of abnormalities in newborn animals may suggest inherited disease, but it is difficult to prove unless planned matings are conducted which is usually not practical or economical.

An assessment of the level of management expertise, or more importantly the intensity with which it is applied, is also impossible to do accurately in most circumstances. The ideal situation, if possible, is to use a statistical method, often an indirect one, to give an accurate expression of how well or poorly a certain technique is being applied. For example, the quarter infection rate with *Corynebacterium bovis* is a good indicator of the efficiency of teat dipping in a mastitis control program. In a dairy herd using artificial insemination, the percentage of cows presented for pregnancy diagnoses, but not pregnant, is a good indicator of the efficiency of estrus detection (except in rare circumstances where anestrus is a resident problem). The presence of diseases such as pregnancy toxemia in ewes and acute carbohydrate engorgement in cows is a rough measure of the degree of preventive medicine applied.

It will be apparent that the field veterinarian can be instrumental in examination and decisions in herd diseases which have significant clinical manifestations. The decisions made in diseases defined by clinicopathological measurements will need to be made by laboratory-based veterinarians but the field work could be done by non-veterinary persons collecting samples and applying tests. Diseases defined by the measurement of production are the province of persons who collect and analyze statistics

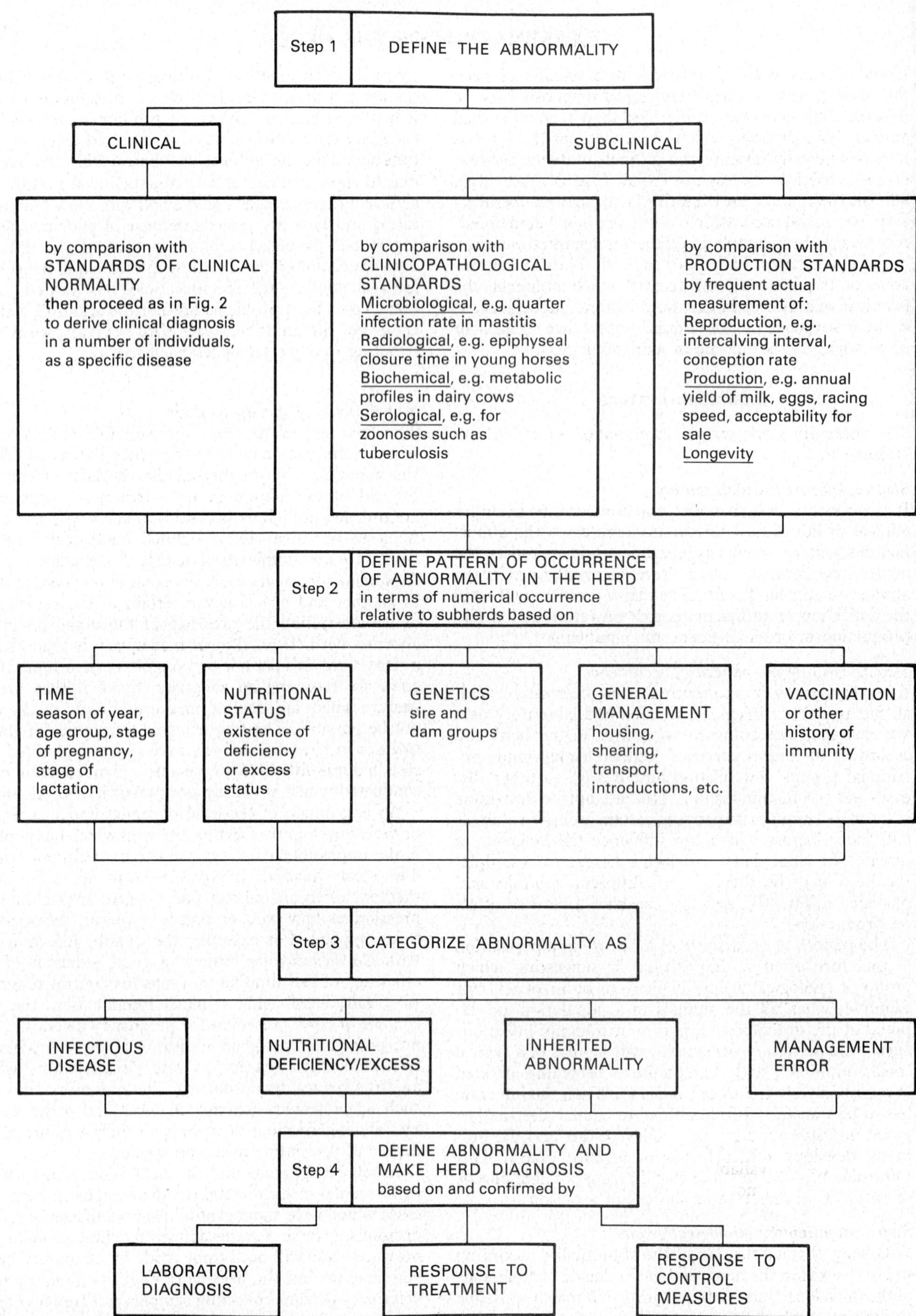

Fig. 5. Examination of the herd, with the objective of making a diagnosis

as far as field studies of them are concerned. But worthwhile decisions based on this data must come from someone knowledgeable in the relative importance of etiologically specific infectious diseases, as against nutrition, or genetics or managerial expertise. This level of authority can be achieved only by a veterinarian who is a species specialist, and knows the relevant industry, its practices and financial structure, and something about the cost–benefit relationship of individual diseases and their control.

Techniques in examination of the herd or flock

Set out below are some of the techniques used in examining a group or herd of animals. They are essentially the same as those used in the examination of an individual animal, but they are different because they are set in the context of a group. Any one or combination of the techniques can be used at the one time depending on the availability of such things as pathology laboratories and data analysis laboratories.

Clinical examination

A clinical examination is essential if clinical illness is a feature of the disease. Usually a representative sample of animals is examined and each submitted to a proper clinical examination. Recording the findings is a problem and is greatly assisted by a structured report form so that the same clinical features are recorded for each animal. For most species the recording of body weight would be an advantage, but is rarely possible. However, assessment of body condition score provides an almost equivalent criterion. The technique is based on visual recognition of body condition by contrast with a set of photographic standards.

Selection of the animals to be examined is vital. This should not be left to the farmer to do because his selection will be biased to include the sickest, the thinnest and the oldest, and not necessarily the animals which are representative of the disease under examination. This is particularly important if a group of animals is to be brought from the farm to a central site. Strict instructions should be given to a referring veterinarian to select ten to twelve animals as a minimum, and in larger groups about 10% of the total number. The groups should include eight sick animals, if possible four advanced and four early cases and four normal animals as controls. If the situation permits it the inclusion of animals that can be sacrificed for necropsy examination is an advantage.

It is customary to collect samples for clinicopathological examination at the time that the clinical examination is done. There will be occasions when this is the only profitable examination because there may be no animals clinically ill at the time of the visit. To defer a visit until clinical cases are available might be appropriate in some cases, but is usually not. The other most desirable activity which is carried out at the time of a visit is the examination of the environment which can provide so much more accurate a background of management than can a verbal account.

Clinical examinations on the farm are often difficult and sometimes misleading because of lack of proper facilities and management. Quiet cattle handled gently in a good crush or chute can present good clinical data, but wild cattle chased up in best rodeo style in an inaccessible chute are hardly worth examining clinically and their clinicopathological results need to be interpreted with caution.

Although a general clinical examination should be carried out on all animals the practical situation is usually satisfied by an examination of the cardinal signs of temperature, pulse, respiration, gut sounds, mucosae, mouth and skin plus more intensive examination of the system suspected of involvement on the basis of the information provided in the history. Thus, a history of a herd problem of red urine in cattle would lead to a special examination of the urine and a rectal examination of the bladder and left kidney and a search for ureters.

One other difficulty encountered in a herd examination is the availability of material for clinicopathological examination. For example, sheep and goats, and to a less extent cattle, which have just be brought into yards for examination commonly void their urine and evacuate their rectums. On the other hand, animals that have been standing around comfortably in yards for several hours usually have a full rectum—an embarrassment if one is to do pregnancy diagnosis of cattle by rectal examination, but a positive pleasure if the objective is to collect fecal samples for egg counts. Collection of urine samples presents a special problem in dairy herds because scared cows commonly urinate. If the cows can be kept away from the examination area until the veterinarian is quite ready to collect, the cow can be then brought in quietly, the perineum cleaned carefully and then stroked for a midstream sample or catheterized. At all times the sample vial is kept at the ready in case the cow urinates ahead of time.

Paraclinical examination

The expeditious, clean collection of blood, urine, and cerebrospinal fluid can be effected readily. What tests to ask for depends on the objective of the examination and recommendations are made for each disease in the ensuing chapters. There is no difficulty if the disease suspected is an obvious choice and the investigation is really one aimed at confirming the diagnosis. Even then, some thought should be given to alternative diagnoses, however remote, and samples collected or tests specified which will avoid the embarrassment of having to retest if the original decision was wrong.

A real difficulty exists if there is no obvious diagnosis or even that the list of diagnostic possibilities is bare. It is then necessary to collect blood samples in all types of storage media including clotted blood for serum (two specimens, one for serology, one for chemistry) and samples in EDTA, heparin and trichloroacetic acid. Duplicate samples of each are often desirable and storage of some is recommended so that second thoughts on tests to be accommodated can be carried out. This is particularly important in serological work where the hindsight may be at a long time interval and a serum bank is most profitable when one is attempting a retrospective examination of prevalence.

The principal consideration in a herd examination is the need to collect samples quickly, identify the animal and record the identity of the animal on the sample contained, and then record the clinical observations where they can be related to the clinicopathological findings. There are many suitable systems and it is not necessary to describe one, but the utmost care is required when planning or deciding the system because the ultimate embarrassment is to have the system fail and to have to go back and collect all the samples again.

The other consideration when planning a sampling system is how the results will be interpreted. If the laboratory has good data on normal standards for the area and the items being assayed that may be sufficient. However, it is usually safer to collect samples from normal animals, from animals which are not clinically abnormal but which have been exposed and are possibly in an incubation or subclinical stage, and from a third group of clinically affected animals. This system approximates the protocol for the Compton Metabolic Profile which is described in detail in Chapter 28. The only other matter for debate on this subject is the number of animals to be included in each group. The number required varies with the quality of the differences between the groups, but usually six to ten animals in each group will be adequate.

Numerical assessment of performance

Productivity indexes can be used as indicators of health; they can also be used to measure response to treatment or control measures. More and more they are being used as guides to husbandry and management questions to satisfy the present-day farmer's preoccupation with costs and returns.

In most instances this sort of data cannot be collected in a single visit. It is possible to eyeball a herd of cows and agree that they are in thin condition, or examine each cow individually and estimate her body condition, or use a weigh band or actually weigh each one. However, it is usually desirable to determine whether body weight or milk production, or wool yield, or racing performance is going up or down under a particular management or disease control program. So it is necessary to collect data over a period. The important decision is which criterion or production index should be monitored to give the best possible information on the criterion under examination. The answer will vary depending on the agricultural system which operates on the farm; for example, bulk milk cell count may be all that is possible unless the herd is production tested, in which case individual cow cell counts on milk will be possible on the samples collected for butter fat testing.

Having decided on the criterion to be used to measure the particular index you wish to examine it is necessary to compare the results with standards derived from comparable or peer farms either in an organized program or with standards created especially for the purpose.

This sort of numerical judgment provides not only a guide to diagnosis and an indicator of productivity trends, but also a mathematical expression of these results, and more and more we are coming around to giving our decisions on the basis of numerical and statistical-based information. This sort of work lends itself to use of a computer, and if there is any volume to it a computer is essential.

Response trial

Many herd situations are not correctable by making a diagnosis and then making adjustments to management, including health management, to avoid the predisposing causes. To a large extent this is due to the difficulty of making a diagnosis. This may result from a lack of laboratory and other resources or because the problem is a complex one, especially a disease or a shortfall in productivity with multiple causes. In that situation it is not unusual to conduct a response trial. The complexity of the trial will depend on the number of treatments that it is proposed to test. In a practical situation all that can be handled as a diagnostic trial is two treatments A and B, a combination AB and a control O.

There are two limitations. Where possible the animals must be housed or paddocked together to avoid biasing differences in nutritional and environmental stress. This requires that the treatment animals be treated individually, for example by a reticular residual pellet, or by a depot injection. The possibility that some of the treatment material will be excreted and contaminate the pasture exists, but is unlikely to be significant unless the trial is a long one. In those circumstances and with parasitic and infectious diseases it is necessary to run the controls and each of the three treatment groups separately from each other. This method creates the difficulty of introducing, between the groups, potential differences which are unrelated to the difference in effects of the treatments. The solution for that problem is to ensure that the differences are minimal and if possible replicate the groups and, better still, switch the groups between the paddocks halfway through the trial.

The second and big problem in response trials is to measure the response. The common need is to measure weight gain, although milk yield and other parameters are sometimes used. Weighing is an accurate enough measure under experimental conditions because the animals can be weighed frequently, and at the same time each day and in the same relationship to feeding and watering. In practical circumstances this is not so easy to arrange. Again, the solution is in terms of reducing error in assessment to a minimum, and by combining weighing with body condition score.

A diagnosis made in this way can only be presumptive and it has become customary to couch the diagnosis in terms of response to a treatment, for instance, 'a copper responsive diarrhea and poor weight gain of calves'. This is not a diagnosis in terms of satisfying Koch's postulates, but in today's complicated environment where the diseases are largely subclinical and difficult to identify exactly, and where they tend to be caused by a number of interacting factors of different genres including management, microbiology and minerals, the practical answer for the practical problem may be most economically derived by finding the cure rather than the cause. This is especially desirable if that course is cost-effective and finding the cause is more expensive than the wastage caused by the disease.

A complete examination of a herd

All of the above techniques are used when a complete and exhaustive initial examination of a herd or flock is conducted in order to arrive at a diagnosis. It consists of:

- A clinical examination
- A laboratory examination
- Examination of the statistically important numerical data—numerical data analysis
- Response trial.

It is outlined in graphical form in Fig. 5, p. 32.

There are, however, many circumstances in which some sort of herd surveillance is necessary, but short of a full examination. Some examples are:

1. When the diagnosis has been made and treatment or control measures instituted there is a need to monitor results by the simplest and most accurate means. This might entail measuring the percentage of animals that seroconvert after vaccination or conducting a necropsy examination on all pigs that die in a group.

2. When a diagnosis for the herd is made on the basis of the examination of one or two animals it is safest to determine the prevalence in the herd as a whole before recommending vaccination, or giving a prognosis on how many more animals will die. In this circumstance an examination of the herd as a whole, such as by a tuberculin test, is well advised, as with similar problems which are not disease problems, such as watery pork, steely wool, low-fat milk, sawdust livers.

3. When a diagnosis is made, for example that mannosidosis is present in a herd of cattle, a laboratory examination can be conducted which will decide the number of animals in the herd which are carrying the genes for the disease. This may be important in terms of clearing the disease from the herd. Carriers of *Salmonella* sp. bacteria or foot-and-mouth disease virus, or *Psorergates ovis* itch mite in sheep may be similarly important and require a sample survey of the herd to determine prevalence, and then a complete survey of the herd if the prevalence is low enough to warrant eradication by test and slaughter. The alternative would be slaughter or disposal of the herd as a whole.

4. In those circumstances where a diagnosis is not being attempted, but prevalence of a suspected disease is being monitored indirectly. An example is the estimation of the prevalence of subclinical mastitis in a dairy herd by periodic individual cow milk cell counting. Samples of milk from all cows in the milking herd are collected for another purpose and are also used for this one.

5. Examinations of herds not for the purpose of making a diagnosis, but with the objective of looking for prognostic indicators. For example, conducting Compton metabolic profiles on a herd in an attempt to predict an energy deficiency and a potential occurrence of reduced fertility and of acetonemia in recently calved cows.

6. Partial herd examinations are also conducted for the purpose of examining particular problems. Protocols for some of these are placed in several sections of this book, for example, protocols for examination of perinatal deaths in Chapter 3, and bovine mastitis in Chapter 15.

The place of the planned animal health and production program in the examination of a herd

Properly conducted herd health programs and planned animal health and production programs maintain accurate records on all matters of production and health. These are maintained against a background of epidemiological data including number of animals in the herd, numbers of animals in the reproductive cycle segment group, or age group which are therefore at risk. In many instances all the data that is required to effectively diagnose a disease or monitor its prevalence is already at hand in the records of these herds. It does put the veterinarian and the farmer in the position of almost being able to do a herd examination simply by consulting the records.

REVIEW LITERATURE

Blood, D. C. (1981) *The Clinical Examination of Cattle. Part 2: Examination of the Herd. Proc. 14th Ann. Conv. AABP*, pp. 14–21.

Kahrs, R. F. (1978) Techniques for investigating outbreaks of livestock disease. *J. Am. vet. med. Assoc.*, *73*, 101.

Weed, L. L. (1985) Knowledge coupling, medical education and patient care. *CRC Crit. Res. Med. Inform.*, *1*, 55–19.

REFERENCES

(1) Ewbank, R. (1964) *Vet. Rec.*, *76*, 388.
(2) Taneja, G. C. (1960) *Ind. J. vet. Sci.*, *30*, 107.
(3) Ewbank, R. (1969) *J. Reprod. Fertil.*, *19*, 569.
(4) Wrenn, T. R. (1958) *J. dairy Sci.*, *41*, 1071.
(5) King, G. J. et al. (1972) *Can. vet. J.*, *13*, 72.
(6) Webster, A. J. F. et al. (1970) *Can. J. anim. Sci.*, *50*, 89.
(7) Rossdale, P. D. (1967) *Br. vet. J.*, *123*, 521.
(8) Gerring, E. L. (1985) *In Pract.*, *7*, 109.
(9) King, J. O. L. (1983) *Br. vet. J.*, *139*, 15.
(10) Radostits, O. M. (1981) *Proc. 14th Ann. Conv. AABP*, pp. 2–12.
(11) Elmore, R. G. et al. (1979) *J. Am. vet med. Assoc.*, *174*, 620.
(12) Iketaki, T. et al. (1979) *Res. Bull. Okihiro Univ.*, *11*, 415.
(13) Rollin, B. E. (1983) *J. Am. vet. med. Assoc.*, *182*, 122.
(14) Kahrs, R. F. (1978) *J. Am. vet. med. Assoc.*, *173*, 101.
(15) Sherman, D. A. et al. (1983) *Vet. Clin. N. Am.*, *large Anim. Pract.*, *5*, 409.
(16) Radostits, O. M. and Blood, D. C. (1983) *Herd Health*, W.B. Saunders, Philadelphia.
(17) Henneke, D. R. (1983) *Equ. vet. J.*, *15*, 371.
(18) Sackett, D. L., Haynes, R. B. & Tugwell, P. (1985) *Clinical Epidemiology. A Basic Science for Clinical Medicine.* Little, Brown & Co., Toronto.
(19) de Dombal, F. T. (1976) In: *Decision Making and Medical Care*, eds F. T. deDombal and F. Gremy. Amer. Elsevier Co., New York, pp. 153–157.
(20) White, M. E. (1985) *J. Am. vet. med. Assoc.*, *187*, 475.
(21) Blois, M. S. (1984) *N. Engl. J. Med.*, *303*, 192.
(22) Blois, M. (1984) *Information and Medicine.* Berkley, Cal.; Univ. of Calif.
(23) White, M. E. et al. (1984) *Vet. Comput.*, *2*, 9.
(24) de Dombal, F. T. et al. (1974) *Br. vet. J.*, *1*, 376.
(25) Fessler, A. P. (1984) *Vet. Med.*, *79*, 409.
(26) Weed, L. L. (1985) *Mount Sinai J. Med.*, *52*, 94.
(27) White, M. E. & Erb, H. N. (1982) *Comp. cont. Educ. Pract. Vet.*, *4*, S426.
(28) White, M. E. & Erb, H. N. (1980) *Cornell Vet.*, *70*, 247.
(29) Madison, J. B. et al. (1984) *J. Am. vet. med. Assoc.*, *185*, 520.
(30) Fetrow, J. et al. (1985) *J. Am. vet. med. Assoc.*, *186*, 792.
(31) Davidson, J. N. et al. (1981) *Cornell Vet.*, *71*, 383.
(32) Ngategize, P. K. et al. (1986) *Prev. vet. Med.*, *4*, 187.
(33) Weinstein, M. C. & Fineberg, H. V. (1980) *Clinical Decision Analysis.* W. B. Saunders, Philadelphia.
(34) Dohoo, I. R. (1984) *Bov. Pract.*, *19*, 193.
(35) Carpenter, T. E. & Norman, B. B. (1983) *J. Amer. vet. med. Assoc.*, *183*, 72.
(36) Williamson, N. B. (1975) *Aust. vet. J.*, *51*, 114.
(37) Carpenter, T. E. et al. (1987) *J. Am. vet. med. Assoc.*, *190*, 983.
(38) Carpenter, T. E. (1986) *Am. J. Epidemiol.*, *124*, 843.
(39) Franke, D. W. & Carroll, R. H. (1984) ARBORIST Decision Tree Software. Texas Instruments, Inc. Technical Report. November, 1984; Austin, Texas.

(40) Davies, G. (1985) *Vet. Rec.*, *117*, 263.
(41) Martin, S. W. & Bonnett, B. (1987) *Can. vet. J.*, *28*, 318.
(42) Thrushfield, M. (1986) *Veterinary Epidemiology*. Butterworths, London.
(43) Weed, L. L. (1971) *Medical Records*, *Medical Education*, *and Patient Care*. Yearbook Publishers, Chicago.
(44) Saidla, J. E. (1978) *J. Am. Anim. Hosp. Assoc.*, *14*, 307.

2

General Systemic States

THERE are several general systemic states which contribute to the effects of many diseases. Because they are common to so many diseases they are considered here as a group to avoid unnecessary repetition. Toxemia, hyperthermia, fever and septicemia are closely related in their effects on the body, and an appreciation of them is necessary if they are not to be overlooked in the efforts to eliminate the causative agent.

TOXEMIA

Toxemia is caused by the presence of toxins deriving from bacteria or produced by body cells. It does not include the diseases caused by toxic substances produced by plants or insects or ingested organic or inorganic poisons. Theoretically a diagnosis of toxemia can be made only if toxins are demonstrable in the bloodstream. Practically, toxemia is often diagnosed when the syndrome described below is present. In most cases there is contributory evidence of a probable source of toxins which in many cases are virtually impossible to isolate or identify.

Etiology

Toxins can be classified as being metabolic or antigenic toxins.

Antigenic toxins

These are produced by bacteria and to a less extent by helminth parasites. Both groups of parasites act as antigens and stimulate the development of antibodies. Antigenic toxins are divided into exotoxins and endotoxins.

Exotoxins These are protein substances produced by bacteria which diffuse into the surrounding medium. They are very specific in their pharmacological effects and in the antibodies which they stimulate. The important bacterial exotoxins are those produced by *Clostridium* spp. and against which commercial antitoxins are available. They may be ingested preformed as in botulism, be produced in large quantities by heavy growth in the bowel, e.g., enterotoxemia, or from growth in tissue, e.g., in blackleg, black disease.

Enterotoxins These are exotoxins which exert their effect principally on the mucosa of the intestine causing disturbances of fluid and electrolyte balance. One of the potent members of this group is staphylococcal enterotoxin (3).

Endotoxins These have very similar pharmacological effects regardless of their specific bacteriological origin. They are lipopolysaccharides and are found within the cell, usually as part of the cell wall. They find their way into the medium, and into the systemic circulation only when the bacterial walls break down and liberate them. They are not ordinarily absorbed through the intestinal mucosa but if it is damaged, as in enteritis or more particularly in acute intestinal obstruction, the endotoxins are absorbed and may cause systemic intoxication. Ordinarily, small amounts of endotoxin which are absorbed into the circulation are detoxified in the liver, but if hepatic efficiency is reduced, or the amounts of toxin are large, a state of endotoxemia is produced. Endotoxins may also be absorbed in large amounts from sites other than intestine including mastitis, peritonitis, abscesses and other septic foci, or from large areas of burnt or otherwise traumatized tissue. The best known endotoxins are those of *Escherichia coli*, which have been used extensively as models for experimental endotoxemia, *Salmonella* spp. and *Corynebacterium* spp.

Metabolic toxins

These may accumulate as a result of incomplete elimination of toxic materials normally produced by body metabolism, or by abnormal metabolism. Normally, toxic products produced in the alimentary tract or tissues are excreted in the urine and feces or detoxified in the plasma and liver. When these normal mechanisms are disrupted, particularly in hepatic dysfunction, the toxins may accumulate beyond a critical point and the syndrome of toxemia appears (1, 2). In obstruction of the lower alimentary tract there may be increased absorption of toxic phenols, cresols and amines which are normally excreted with the feces, resulting in the development of the syndrome of autointoxication. In ordinary circumstances in monogastric animals these products of protein putrefaction are not absorbed by the mucosa of the large intestine but when regurgitation into the small intestine occurs there may be rapid absorption, apparently because of the absence of a protective barrier in the wall of the small intestine. In liver diseases many of the normal detoxification mechanisms, including oxidation, reduction, acetylation and conjugation with such substances as glycine, glucuronic acid, sulfuric acid and cysteine, are lost and substances are normally present in sufficient quantity to cause injury accumulate to the point where illness occurs. The production of toxins by abnormal metabolism is taken to include the production of histamine and histamine-like substances in damaged tissues. Ketonemia due to a disproportionate fat metabolism, and lacticacidemia caused by acute ruminal impaction are two common examples of toxemia caused by abnormal metabolism.

Pathogenesis

The specific effects of the particular bacterial exotoxins and metabolic toxins are dealt with in the relevant sections of the Special Medicine section of this book.

Of the endotoxins produced by bacteria most is known of those produced by *Escherichia coli* (4). These endotoxins are potent pyrogens and cause severe shock with resulting poor tissue perfusion, disseminated intravascular coagulation and a generalized Schwartzmann reaction. Hemoconcentration, neutropenia and subsequently neutrophilia, and thrombocytopenia are characteristic reactions. Hepatic dysfunction, hypoglycemia and abortion are also significant results of *E. coli* endotoxemia. Some information is also available about the toxins of *Salmonella* spp., these having been shown to cause fever and alimentary tract stasis (9).

In mycoplasmosis (*Mycoplasma mycoides* var. *mycoides*) at least part of the toxic effect is attributable to galactans contained in the toxins. These have a noticeably local effect in causing hemorrhages in alveolar ducts and pulmonary vessel walls so that pulmonary arterial blood pressure rises as systemic blood pressure falls (5). Later lesions are pulmonary edema and capillary thrombosis which are characteristic of the natural disease of pleuropneumonia. Disseminated intravascular coagulation is also a characteristic of the lesions caused by the toxin of *Pseudomonas* spp. (6).

The systemic effects of endotoxin toxemia, or endotoxicosis, can be demonstrated experimentally by the injection, or other administration, of purified toxin. In naturally occurring disease the total effect includes those of bacterial toxins plus those of other substances produced by tissues in response to the bacterial toxins. The following description relates to the clinically occurring toxemia.

The 'toxemia' produced by inflammatory stress affects carbohydrate, nitrogen, trace metal and hormone metabolism and distribution (11). At the peak of an illness these sequels may be to the advantage of the patient, but they usually create a deficit which subsequently needs to be repaired.

Carbohydrate metabolism

The effects on carbohydrate metabolism include a fall in blood sugar level, the rate and degree varying with the severity of the toxemia, a disappearance of liver glycogen and a decreased glucose tolerance of tissues so that administered glucose is not used rapidly (7). Blood pyruvate and lactate levels rise as a result of poor tissue perfusion and the anaerobic nature of the tissue metabolism which results. By extrapolation from the known pathogenesis of endotoxic shock in horses it is likely that the resulting accumulation of lactate has significant effects in causing mental depression and poor survival.

Protein metabolism

There is an increase in tissue breakdown and a rise in blood non-protein nitrogen levels. However, in spite of this tissue breakdown, there is likely to be an increase in total serum protein as a result of the stimulation of antibody production (10). There is also an alteration in the aminogram (the relative proportions of the amino acids present in blood) and the electrophoretic pattern of plasma proteins. The globulins are raised and albumin reduced.

Mineral metabolism

Negative mineral balances are caused. These include hypoferremia and hypozincemia, but blood copper levels are commonly raised concurrently with an increase in blood ceruloplasmin levels.

Effects on tissues

The means by which the changes are brought about have not been accurately defined, but a substance liberated by phagocytic cells when stimulated by infectious agents has been described. Such an agent could affect endocrine glands and enzyme systems especially those in the liver. Lesions are present in endocrine glands, particularly the anterior pituitary and adrenal glands, in most toxemias, and adrenocortical hormones do have protective and curative action in most toxemic states. Damage to the liver and kidney parenchyma is also apparent.

Effects on body systems

The combined effects of the hypoglycemia, high blood lactate (and low blood pH), interference with tissue enzyme systems and degenerative changes in the parenchyma reduce the functional activity of most tissues. Of these factors lactate is probably the most important except that in newborn animals glucose levels are probably as important as lactate. The myocardium is weakened, the stroke volume decreases and the response to cardiac stimulants is diminished. There is dilatation and in some cases damage to capillary walls so that the effective circulating blood volume is decreased; this decrease, in combination with diminished cardiac output, leads to a fall in blood pressure and the development of circulatory failure. The resulting decline in the perfusion of tissues and oxygen consumption contribute greatly to the animal's decline and to the clinical signs such as the dark red coloration of the oral mucosa. Respiration is little affected except in so far as it responds to the failing circulation.

There is decreased liver function, and the damage to renal tubules and glomeruli causes a rise in blood non-protein nitrogen and the appearance of albuminuria. The functional tone and motility of the alimentary tract is reduced and the appetite fails, digestion is impaired with constipation usually following. A similar loss of tone occurs in skeletal muscle and is manifested by weakness and terminally by prostration.

Apart from the effects of specific toxins on the nervous

system, such as those of *Cl. tetani* and *Cl. botulinum*, there is a general depression of function attended by dullness, depression and finally coma. Because of the suspected role of *E. coli* in the etiology of edema disease of swine it is noteworthy that some of the characteristic nervous system lesions of that disease are missing from experimentally induced porcine colitoxicosis (18). Changes in the hemopoietic system include depression of hemopoiesis and an increase in the number of leukocytes, the type of cells which increase often varying with the type and severity of the toxemia. Leukopenia may occur, but is usually associated with aplasia of the leukopoietic tissue caused by viruses or specific exogenous substances such as radioactive materials. Most of these pathophysiological effects of endotoxicosis have been produced experimentally, and it is apparent that very small amounts of endotoxin can contribute greatly to the serious effects of intestinal disease, especially in the horse.

Hypersensitivity

A secondary effect produced by some toxins is the creation of a state of hypersensitivity at the first infection so that a second infection, or administration of the same antigen causes anaphylaxis, or an allergic phenomenon such as purpura hemorrhagica. Also a generalized Schwartzmann reaction can be induced in pigs by an injection of *Escherichia coli* endotoxin, especially if there are two properly spaced (in time) injections. Pigs on a vitamin E-deficient diet are much more severely affected than pigs on a normal diet. Vitamin E is protective, selenium is not (12).

Antibiotic diffusion

A reduction in the volume of the extracellular fluid compartment reduces the amount of diffusion of antibiotics, e.g. gentamicin, into tissues (16).

Clinical findings

The clinical picture in most non-specific toxemias is approximately the same. It varies with the speed and severity of the toxic process but the variations in the syndrome are largely of degree. Depression, lethargy, separation from the group, anorexia, failure to grow or produce and emaciation are characteristic signs. Constipation is usual, the pulse is weak and rapid but regular and there may be albuminuria. The heart rate is increased, the sounds reduced and a 'hemic' murmur may appear. There may or may not be fever; in most toxemias due to bacterial infection or tissue destruction fever is present, but this is not so with metabolic toxins. Terminally there is muscular weakness to the point of collapse and death occurs in a coma or with convulsions.

Toxic shock

When toxin formation or liberation into the circulation is fast enough and the toxicity of the toxin high enough the onset of cardiovascular signs is rapid enough to cause a state of 'toxic' or 'septic' shock. Animals affected in this way have a severe peripheral vasodilatation with a consequent fall in blood pressure, pallor of mucosa, hypothermia, tachycardia, pulse of small amplitude, and muscle weakness. The syndrome is discussed also in the section on shock. It is most commonly associated with bacteremia or septicemia due to infection with Gram-negative organisms, especially *Escherichia coli*. Staphylococcal enterotoxin has the same effect in dwarf goats (3).

Localized infection

With localized infections there are, in addition to the general signs of toxemia, the clinical effects of the space occupation by the lesion. These are discussed on p. 50.

Clinical pathology

It may be possible to isolate and identify the specific exotoxin and its source. Non-specific endotoxins have been assayed in circulating blood by a biological technique based on horseshoe crab amebocytes, but the test has limited applicability in other than research investigation (13, 15). A low blood sugar, high blood NPN (non-protein nitrogen) and a high total serum protein, with globulins noticeably increased on electrophoretic examination, aplastic anemia, leukocytosis and albuminuria can be anticipated.

A glucose tolerance curve similar to that of diabetes mellitus in humans may be detectable in monogastric animals and there is little response to insulin in correcting this deficiency. The importance of this factor in ruminants is unknown.

Necropsy findings

Gross findings at necropsy are limited to those of the lesion which produces the toxin. Microscopically there is degeneration of the parenchyma of the liver, the glomeruli and tubules of the kidney and of the myocardium. There may also be degeneration or necrosis in the adrenal glands.

Diagnosis

A clinical diagnosis of toxemia is frequently made and often with little more basis than the rather ill-defined syndrome described above. This is largely unavoidable because of the difficulties encountered in isolating a toxin or in determining its origin. It is easily confused with subacute poisoning by arsenic and other metals which have a general depressing effect on most body enzyme systems. In this instance an examination of the environment for a source of poison, characteristic signs of each poison and assays of food, gut contents and tissues are necessary to make a definite diagnosis. Toxemia is a syndrome which forms part of many primary disease states, and it is largely in this secondary role that it requires recognition and adequate treatment. In all septicemias, extensive inflammations and tissue degenerations it is a contributory mechanism in the production of sickness and death.

Treatment

If possible, treatment should be directed at removal of the origin of the toxin, the provision of specific antitoxins and supportive treatment to counteract the effects of the toxemia. Intensive fluid and electrolyte therapy by continuous intravenous infusion is essential until the animal begins to eat and drink. The kinds and amounts of fluids used are described later in this chapter. If the appetite and digestion are impaired, parenteral nutrition may be indicated. Glucose, amino acids and emulsions of fat may be added to the fluid therapy. Insulin is unlikely to be of value, but concentrated vitamin preparations, particularly the B-complex group, may aid the utilization of glucose by supplementing impaired enzyme systems.

The use of glucocorticoids is now universally included in the treatment of toxemia, especially when shock is part of the pathogenesis. They are used most commonly in acute cases and in large doses (e.g. 1 mg/kg body weight of dexamethazone intravenously every 24 hours). Treatment after shock has been present for some time is likely to be ineffective. Non-steroidal anti-inflammatory drugs (NSAIDs) such as acetylsalicylic acid (8) and phenylbutazone which have adrenocorticoid-like activity are also used in this way. Phenylbutazone (15 mg/kg body weight initially and 10 mg/kg body weight at 6–12 hour intervals) is in routine use. Similar drugs of more recent introduction are indomethacin, sodium meclofenamate and flunixin meglumine (14). Naloxon, a specific opiate-antagonist has been used experimentally because of the probability that the endogenous opiate beta-endorphin is involved in the vascular lesion of toxemia. The effects are beneficial in dogs and pigs but not in ponies (17). Antibiotic therapy using an agent with a broad antibacterial spectrum is recommended if endotoxin formation by resident bacteria is a threat. Ampicillin and chloramphenicol are most widely used for this purpose, but sulfamethazine or a potentiated sulfonamide should be effective. If the endotoxin is likely to originate in the intestine the medication should be administered orally. Particular attention should be given to this possibility in the horse because of its tendency to develop endotoxemia and its susceptibility to it.

Preparations containing sodium thiosulfate and methylene blue are in general use in veterinary practice for the treatment of non-specific toxemias, but there seems to be little justification for their use except in specific poisonings caused by arsenic, hydrocyanic acid and nitrite.

REVIEW LITERATURE

Burrows, G. E. (1981) Endotoxaemia in the horse. *Equ. vet. J.*, *13*, 89.
Culbertson, R. & Osburn, B. I. (1980) The biological effects of bacterial endotoxin. A short review. *Vet. Sci. Commun.*, *4*, 3.
Mims, C. A. (1976) *The Pathogenesis of Infectious Disease*. London & New York: Academic Press.
Smith, H. (1976) *Modern Views on Microbiological Pathogenicity*. Shildon, UK: Meadowfield Press, Ltd.

REFERENCES

(1) Parke, D. V. & Williams, R. T. (1969) *Br. med. Bull.*, *25*, 256.
(2) Judah, J. D. (1969) *Br. med. Bull.*, *25*, 276.
(3) van Miert, A.S.J.P.A.M. et al. (1984) *Infect. Immun.*, *46*, 354.
(4) Hoffman, R. (1977) *J. comp. Pathol.*, *87*, 231.
(5) Buttery, S. H. et al. (1986) *J. med. Microbiol.*, *9* 379.
(6) Thomson, G. W. et al. (1974) *Can. J. comp. Med.*, *38*, 457.
(7) Holmes, E. (1939) *Physiol. Rev.*, *19*, 439.
(8) Schimmel, D. et al. (1976) *Arch. exp. Vet. Med.*, *30*, 951.
(9) Miert, A. et al. (1977) *Arch. int. Pharmaco-dyn. Therap.*, *225*, 39.
(10) Hibbitt, K. G. et al. (1977) *J. comp. Pathol.*, *87*, 195.
(11) Powanda, M. C. (1980) *Am. J. vet. Res.*, *41*, 1905.
(12) Teige, J. (1977) *Acta vet. Scand.*, *18*, 143.
(13) Duncan, S. G. et al. (1985) *Am. J. vet. Res.*, *46*, 1287.
(14) Moore, J. N. et al. (1986) *Am. J. vet. Res.*, *47*, 110.
(15) Mortensen, K. & Binder, M. (1985) *Acta. vet. Scand.*, *26*, 231 and 246.
(16) Wilson, R. C. et al. (1983) *Am. J. vet. Res.*, *44*, 1746.
(17) Moore, A. B. et al. (1983) *Am. J. vet. Res.*, *44*, 103.
(18) Kurtz, H. J. & Quast, J. (1982) *Am. J. vet. Res.*, *43*, 262.

Toxemia in the recently calved cow

A special occurrence of toxemia which is of great importance in food-animal medicine is that caused by a number of diseases in the period immediately after calving in the dairy cow. The syndrome is one of lack of appetite, seriously reduced milk yield, sluggish ruminal and intestinal activity, a dull expression, physical lethargy and a temperature in the high normal range. The syndrome is sometimes listed as the 'parturition syndrome', but the use of this term is not recommended because its general adoption could dissuade clinicians from seeking more accurate identification of the component disease.

The diseases which commonly fall into this broad category are the toxemias resulting from:

- Acetonemia
- The fat cow syndrome and pregnancy toxemia
- Mastitis
- Peritonitis
- Septic metritis,

and the non-toxic, physical diseases caused by:

- Left and right displacement of the abomasum.

All of these diseases, except septic metritis, are dealt with elsewhere in this book. Because of its importance to food-animal medicine, and without any desire to usurp a function traditionally performed by theriogenologists, a brief account of septic metritis in cattle is given here.

POSTPARTUM SEPTIC METRITIS IN CATTLE

Postpartum septic metritis occurs primarily in dairy cows within a few days after parturition and is characterized clinically by severe toxemia and a copious foul-smelling uterine discharge with or without retention of the fetal membranes.

Etiology

The etiology is multifactorial. It has been assumed that a combination of failure of normal postpartum uterine involution, often with retained fetal membranes and infection of the uterus precipitates the disease (1). A mixed bacterial flora is common which includes organisms such as *E. coli*, *Actinomyces (Corynebacterium) pyogenes*, *Staphylococcus* spp., *Streptococcus* spp., *Pseudomonas aeruginosa*, *Proteus* spp. and occasionally *Clostridium* spp.

Epidemiology
The disease occurs in cows of all ages, but is most common in mature dairy cows within 2–4 days after parturition. The disease is most common in cows when the placenta is retained for more than 24 hours following parturition. Retention of the placenta is associated most commonly with abortion, dystocia and multiple births.

In one study, the overall incidence of retained placenta was 11% with a range between herds of 3·5 to 27% (3). In single calvings the incidence was 9·5% and in twin calvings 46%. Metritis occurred in 55% of cows with retained placenta, and metritis is 25 times more likely to occur with retained placenta than without. Other less common associations include old age, increased gestation length, hormone-induced parturition, fetal anasarca, uterine prolapse and fetotomy. Thus, the factors which are associated with retention of the placenta are indirectly associated with the development of postpartum metritis. The forceful removal of retained placenta is also considered to be a major predisposing factor to septic metritis.

Uncomplicated cases of retained placenta in cattle have no significant effect on subsequent fertility and the calving-to-conception interval. However, the calving-to-conception interval is significantly increased in cows which develop clinical metritis as a sequel to retained placenta. Placentitis, vitamin E and selenium deficiency and vitamin A deficiency have also been suggested as factors (2).

Pathogenesis
Failure of normal uterine involution combined with retention of the fetal membranes and infection of the uterus with a mixed bacterial flora results in acute metritis and a severe toxemia. There is diffuse necrosis and edema of the mucosa and wall of the uterus. There is marked accumulation of foul-smelling fluid in the uterus and enlargement of the uterus. Absorption of toxins results in severe toxemia, particularly so in fat cows which may develop irreversible fatty degeneration of the liver.

Clinical findings
Affected cows become acutely anorexic and toxemic within 2–5 days after parturition. There is a marked drop in milk production. The temperature is usually elevated from 39·5 to 41°C, but may be normal in the presence of severe toxemia. The heart rate is usually elevated and may range from 96–120/min. The respiratory rate is commonly increased to 60–72/min and the vesicular sounds may be louder than normal. Rumen movements may be markedly depressed or absent. A foul-smelling fluid diarrhea may occur. Dehydration is common because affected cows do not drink normally.

Retention of the fetal membranes is common, and manual examination of the vagina reveals the presence of copious quantities of foul-smelling dark-brown to red fluid containing small pieces of placenta pooled in the vagina. When the fetal membranes are retained and protruding through the cervix, the hand can usually be inserted through the cervix and into the uterus. Manual exploration of the uterine cavity will usually reveal the state of adherence of the fetal membranes. Often the fetal cotyledons are firmly attached to the maternal caruncles, but occasionally, they have separated from the caruncles and the placenta can be removed by simple traction.

Rectal examination usually reveals that the uterus is large, flaccid and lacks the ridges which indicate involution. In large cows the enlarged flaccid uterus may be situated over the pelvic brim and extend into the ventral part of the abdomen and is then not easily palpable and examined. This is important because the fetal membranes may be fully retained in the uterus and no evidence of their presence may be detectable on examination of the cervix which may be almost closed, making examination of the uterus impossible. The presence of viscid non-odorous mucus in the cervix and anterior part of the vagina usually, but not always, indicates that the fetal membranes have been expelled. Tenesmus occurs most commonly when the fetal membranes are retained and this causes irritation in the vagina. Manual examination of the vagina may also stimulate tenesmus.

The course of the disease varies from 2 to 10 days. Those cases with retained fetal membranes may be toxemic and not return to normal appetite until the membranes are fully expelled which may take up to 10 days. Necrotic pieces of placenta may be passed for 10–14 days after treatment is begun.

Clinical pathology
A leukopenia, neutropenia and degenerative left shift occur in acute cases and the degree of change parallels the severity of the disease. Ketonuria may occur in animals which are overconditioned and mobilize excessive quantities of depot fat resulting in ketosis. Liver function tests reveal a decrease in liver function which may be irreversible in excessively fat cows. Samples of fluid from the vagina and uterus reveal a mixed bacterial flora including *E. coli*, *Proteus* sp., *Actinomyces (Corynebacterium) pyogenes*, *Staphylococcus* spp. and *Streptococcus* spp.

Necropsy findings
The uterus is enlarged, flaccid and may contain several liters of dark-brown colored foul-smelling fluid with decomposed fetal membranes. The uterine mucosa is necrotic and hemorrhagic and the wall of the uterus is thickened and edematous. In severe cases, fibrin may be present on the serosal surface of the uterus. The liver may be enlarged and fatty and there is mild degeneration of the myocardium and kidneys.

Diagnosis
The major characteristics of the disease are toxemia and the presence of large amounts of dark-brown foul-smelling fluid in an enlarged flaccid uterus within a few days after calving. However, the cervix is not open in all affected cows and the presence of septic metritis must not be excluded on the basis that a placenta is not protruding through the cervix.

The disease must be differentiated from other causes of toxemia, anorexia and loss of milk production in cows within a few days after parturition, and the major problem is to determine the significance of an abnormal uterine exudate, with or without retention of the fetal membranes. It is often impossible to decide if septic metritis is primary and is the real cause of the toxemia or if it is simply a partial failure of uterine involution in a cow affected with one of many other postpartum diseases. In such cases it is necessary to treat the animal for both diseases. The diseases likely to be confused with or associated with primary septic metritis are set out below.

The fat cow syndrome
This is characterized by excessive body condition, anorexia to inappetence, ketonuria, a marked loss in milk production, decreased rumen movements and delayed involution of the uterus. The temperature is usually normal, but the heart and respiratory rates may be increased. The prognosis is poor in cows which are totally anorexic; those which are inappetent will usually recover after 5–7 days of supportive therapy.

Left-sided displacement of the abomasum (LDA)
This is characterized by inappetence, rarely anorexia, ketosis, ketonuria and a ping on the left side from the 9th to the 12th rib. Retained fetal membranes and the presence of foul-smelling uterine fluid are not uncommon is recently calved cows with left-sided displacement of the abomasum. However, if there is septic metritis, varying degrees of toxemia are present.

Right-sided dilatation and displacement of the abomasum (RDA)
This results in inappetence to anorexia, drop in milk production, decreased ruminal activity and scant feces. A ping is usually audible on percussion of the area extending from the right paralumbar fossa to the normal anatomical position of the abomasum. On rectal examination the distended viscus may be palpable deep in the right lower quadrant of the abdomen.

A ping, unassociated with any major abnormality, may be audible on percussion of the right paralumbar fossa of dairy cows for 2–5 days following parturition. The pig may be due to gas trapped temporarily in the cecum, spiral colon or descending colon. The cause is unknown, but may be associated with indigestion at parturition. Its presence may suggest dilatation or torsion of the abomasum. However, there are usually no accompanying major abnormalities and conservative treatment with calcium borogluconate will result in recovery in a few days.

Acute diffuse peritonitis
This may occur in cows within a few days postpartum and is characterized by anorexia, toxemia, a spontaneous grunt or one which can be elicited by deep palpation, rumen stasis, fever and the presence of an inflammatory exudate in the peritoneal fluid.

Non-paretic parturient hypocalcemia
This may occur and not be easily recognizable clinically in cows within a few days postpartum. There is inappetence, normal temperature, a moderate drop in milk production, alimentary tract stasis and decreased rumination. The heart rate may be slightly elevated and the intensity of the heart sounds decreased. There is no toxemia and intravenous calcium borogluconate results in rapid recovery.

Simple indigestion
This is common in high-yielding dairy cows which are offered large amounts of a high-energy palatable diet shortly before and after parturition. Affected cows are inappetent, sometimes there is anorexia, the rumen is full and the contractions decreased. There are no systemic abnormalities and recovery usually occurs over a period of a few days.

Peracute and acute mastitis
This occurs in cows within a few days after parturition, is characterized by severe toxemia, swelling of the affected quarters and abnormal milk.

Treatment
Uncomplicated cases of retained placenta without any evidence of clinical toxemia usually require no parenteral and intrauterine treatment. The placenta will usually be expelled within 5–10 days. Cows with retained placenta which strain should be examined vaginally to ensure that there is no evidence of injury to the vagina or cervix. In the cows which strain, if the placenta is detached and loose it should be removed. *Forceful removal of the placenta should be avoided.*

Cows with retained placenta complicated by septic metritis develop clinical toxemia characterized by anorexia, depression, fever and agalactia. Antimicrobial agents such as penicillin, oxytetracycline or sulfamethazine must be given at therapeutic doses daily for several days or until recovery occurs. In severely affected cases, large amounts of fluids, electrolytes and glucose by continuous intravenous infusion may be necessary and often result in a marked beneficial response within 24–48 hours. The uterus should be examined vaginally if possible and by rectal palpation to determine the degree of involution. This can be done daily to assess progress. If parenteral antimicrobial and supportive therapy is provided the placenta will invariably be expelled within 10–12 days and usually within 5–7 days.

The necessity for intrauterine medication is controversial. There is limited evidence, if any, that the intrauterine infusion of antimicrobials with or without lytic enzyme and estrogens has any beneficial effect in the treatment of postpartum septic metritis. Nevertheless, a wide variety of antimicrobials are used for intrauterine medication for retained placenta and metritis in cows. Drugs used to improve uterine tone and involution and to assist in the expulsion of retained placentas include oxytocin, ergonovine maleate, estrogens and prostaglandins. However, there is only limited evidence that they have any beneficial effect compared to the conservative approach. The removal of large quantities of uterine exudate in cows with metritis, using a siphon tube, may promote uterine involution. However, this procedure is usually inefficient and rupture of the uterus with the siphon tube is a potential serious complication.

Affected cows should be identified and examined 30–40 days after parturition for evidence of further complications such as pyometra (4).

REFERENCES

(1) Arthur, G. H. (1979) *Vet. Ann.*, *19*, 26.
(2) Bierschwal, C. J. (1980) *Proc. Am. Assoc. bov. Pract.*, *12*, 102.
(3) Sandals, W. C. D. et al. (1980) *Bov. Pract.*, *15*, 8.
(4) Studer, E. & Morrow, D. A. (1978) *J. Am. vet. med. Assoc.*, *172*, 489.

HYPERTHERMIA, HYPOTHERMIA, FEVER

The symptom complexes characterized by significant changes in body temperature are dealt with together because they require some introduction in terms of the heat-regulating mechanisms of the body.

The body temperature is a reflection of the balance between heat gain (due to absorption from the environment and to metabolic activity) and heat loss. Absorption of heat from the environment occurs when the external temperature rises above that of the body. Most of the heat produced by the body derives from muscular movement and the maintenance of muscle tone. Heat losses occur by the standard physical phenomena of convection, conduction and radiation and the evaporation of moisture, including sweat, insensible perspiration and moisture vaporized by the respiratory tract. Losses by evaporation of moisture vary between species depending upon the development of the sweat gland system and are less important in animals than in man, beginning only at relatively high body temperatures. Horses sweat profusely, but in pigs, sheep and European cattle (1) sweating cannot be considered to be an effective mechanism of heat loss. In Zebu cattle the increased density of cutaneous sweat glands suggests that sweating may be more important (2). Profuse salivation and exaggerated respiration, including mouth breathing, are important mechanisms in the dissipation of excess body heat in animals. The tidal volume is decreased and the respiratory rate is increased so that heat is lost but alkalosis is avoided.

The balance between heat gain and heat loss is controlled by the heat-regulating functions of the hypothalamus. The afferent impulses derive from peripheral hot and cold receptors and the temperature of the blood flowing through the hypothalamus. The efferent impulses control respiratory centre activity, the caliber of skin blood vessels, sweat gland activity and muscle tone. Heat storage occurs and the body temperature rises when there is a decrease in rate and depth of respiration, constriction of skin blood vessels, cessation of perspiration and increased muscle tone. Heat loss occurs when these functions are reversed. These physiological changes occur in, and are the basis of, the increment and decrement stages of fever.

An important development in recent years has been the investigation of variability between and within races and breeds of farm livestock in their susceptibility to high environmental temperatures (3). Differences exist in coat and skin characters which affect heat absorption from solar radiation and heat loss by evaporative cooling, and also in metabolic rate which influences the basic heat load (4, 5). Interest in this subject has been aroused by the demands for classes of animals capable of high production in the developing countries of the tropical zone. As a result there has become available a sum of detailed information on the physiological effects of, and the mechanisms of adaptation to, high environmental temperatures (6–9).

As might have been expected, these findings have also aroused interest in more temperate climates where the demand for more economic animal husbandry methods has led to investigation of all avenues by which productivity might be increased. Such subjects as the provision of shelter in hot weather, the use of tranquilizers to reduce activity and therefore heat increment, and the optimum temperature in enclosed pig houses are subjects of vital importance to farming economy but are not dealt with in this book because they appear to have little relation to the production of clinical illness.

Extremes of environmental temperature are known to influence health in some instances. For example, low environmental temperature may predispose to hypothermia and hypoglycemia in neonates, and at high environmental temperatures pigs in pens lose their social-eliminative behavior which may predispose to enteric disease by facilitating the oral/fecal cycling of enteric pathogens. The influence of milder changes is recognized but poorly understood. Most clinicians would agree that fluctuations in temperature constitute a stress and may influence the incidence of such conditions as respiratory disease or esophagogastric ulceration in pigs, but the underlying mechanisms are not known.

The two clinical disorders of animals caused by exposure to high environmental temperatures are heat stroke, described below under hyperthermia, and anhidrosis described under diseases due to unknown causes. There appear to be no parallels to human prickly heat and heat syncope amongst animals. Heat exhaustion and anhidrotic asthenia, two well-recognized entities in human medicine, probably do occur in cattle and horses. The prominent features of these diseases in man are physical weakness, slight elevation of temperature, weight loss and dehydration, and these are seen often in large animals poorly adapted to tropical climates. Heat cramps have been described as a cause of equine colic after violent exercise and parenteral treatment with large volumes of normal saline solution has been recommended.

REFERENCES

(1) Brook, A. H. & Short, B. F. (1960) *Aust. J. agric. Res.*, *11*, 557.
(2) Taneja, G. C. (1960) *J. agric. Sci., Camb.*, *55*, 109.
(3) Robinson, D. W. (1969) *Br. vet. J.*, *125*, 112.
(4) Warwick, E. J. (1972) *Wld Rev. anim. Prod.*, *8*, 33.
(5) Rendel, J. (1972) *Wld Rev. anim. Prod.*, *8*, 16, 49.
(6) Bianca, W. (1965) *J. dairy Res.*, *32*, 291.
(7) Jones, E. W. et al. (1972) *Anaesthesiology*, *36*, 42.
(8) McFarlane, W. V. et al. (1958) *Aust. J. agric. Res.*, *9*, 217, 690.
(9) Singh, S. P. & Newton, W. M. (1978) *Am. J. vet. Res.*, *39*, 795, 799.

Hyperthermia (heat stroke)

Hyperthermia is the elevation of body temperature due to excessive heat production or absorption, or to deficient heat loss when the causes of these abnormalities are purely physical. Heat stroke is the most commonly encountered clinical entity.

Etiology

The major causes of hyperthermia are the physical ones of high environmental temperature and prolonged, severe muscular exertion especially when the humidity is high, the animals are fat, have a heavy hair coat, or are confined with inadequate ventilation, such as on board ship. Fat cattle, especially British beef breeds, can be overcome by the heat in feedlots. Brahman cattle in the same pen may be unaffected (8). Angora goats are much more sensitive to high environmental temperatures than sheep, especially when they are young (3).

High environmental temperature

The critical point in sheep with a light wool coat on board ship appears to be a temperature of 35°C (95°F) at a humidity of 33–39 mmHg (4·4–5·2 kPa) vapor pressure (1). Differences between breeds of animals in their tolerance to environmental high temperatures, exposure to sunlight and exercise are important in animal management and production. Water buffalo have been shown to be less heat-tolerant than Shorthorn steers, which were less tolerant than Javanese Banteng and Brahman crossbreds, which appear to be equally tolerant (2). The differences appear to be at least partly due to capacity to increase cutaneous evaporation under heat stress. There are similar differences in heat tolerance between lactating and non-lactating cows, the lactating animals showing significantly greater responses in rectal temperature and heart and respiratory rates when the environmental temperature is raised (4). Rested, hydrated horses are well able to maintain homeothermy in the hottest environmental conditions. Their most efficient mechanism in ensuring that body temperature is kept low is their capacity for heavy sweating (10). The original concept of sunstroke as being due to actinic irradiation of the medulla has now been discarded and all such cases are now classed as heat stroke.

Other causes of hyperthermia

- Neurogenic hyperthermia—damage to hypothalamus, e.g., spontaneous hemorrhage, may cause hyperthermia or poikilothermia
- Dehydration—due to insufficient tissue fluids to accommodate heat loss by evaporation
- Excessive muscular activity—e.g., strychnine poisoning
- Miscellaneous poisonings including levamisole and dinitrophenols
- Malignant hyperthermia in the porcine stress syndrome with rare occurrences in other species including horses (12)
- Cattle with hereditary bovine syndactyly (5)
- Administration of tranquilizing drugs to sheep in hot weather (6)
- Specific mycotoxins, e.g. *Claviceps purpurea*, *Acremonium coenophialum*, the causes of epidemic hyperthermia. These poisonings represent one of the most interesting new discoveries in food-animal medicine of recent times
- Iodism
- Sylade (possibly) poisoning.

Pathogenesis

The means by which hyperthermia is induced have already been described. The physiological effects of hyperthermia are important and are outlined briefly here. Unless the body temperature reaches a critical point a short period of hyperthermia is advantageous in an infectious disease because phagocytosis and immune body production are facilitated and the viability of most invading organisms is impaired. These changes provide justification for the use of artificial fever to control bacterial disease. However, the metabolic rate may be increased by as much as 40–50%, liver glycogen stores are rapidly depleted and extra energy is derived from increased endogenous metabolism of protein. If anorexia occurs because of respiratory embarrassment and dryness of the mouth, there will be considerable loss of body weight and lack of muscle strength accompanied by hypoglycemia and a rise in non-protein nitrogen.

There is increased thirst due in part to dryness of the mouth. An increase in heart rate occurs due directly to the rise in blood temperature and indirectly to the fall in blood pressure resulting from peripheral vasodilatation. Respiration increases in rate and depth due directly to the effect of the high temperature on the respiratory center. Urine secretion is decreased because of the reduced renal blood flow resulting from peripheral vasodilatation, and because of physicochemical changes in body cells which result in retention of water and chloride ions.

When the critical temperature is exceeded there is depression of nervous system activity, and depression of the respiratory center usually causes death by respiratory failure. Circulatory failure also occurs due to myocardial weakness, the heart rate becoming fast and irregular. If the period of hyperthermia is unduly prolonged, rather than excessive in degree, the deleterious effects are those of increased endogenous metabolism and deficient food intake. There is often an extensive degenerative change in most body tissues but this is more likely to be due to metabolic changes than to the direct effects of elevation of the body temperature.

Clinical findings

An elevation of body temperature is the primary requisite for a diagnosis of hyperthermia and in most species the first observable clinical reaction to hyperthermia occurs when the rectal temperature exceeds 39·5°C (103°F). In most instances the temperature exceeds 42°C (107°F) and may reach 43·5°C (110°F). An increase in heart and respiratory rates, with a weak pulse of large amplitude, sweating and salivation occur initially followed by a marked absence of sweating. The animal may be restless but soon becomes dull, stumbles while walking and tends to lie down. In the early stages there is increased thirst and the animal seeks cool places, often lying in water or attempting to splash itself. When the body temperature reaches 41°C (106°F) respiration is labored and general distress is evident. Beyond this point the respirations become shallow and irregular, the pulse becomes very rapid and weak and these signs are usually accompanied by collapse, convulsions and terminal coma. Death occurs in most species when a temperature of 41·5–42·5°C (106–108°F) is attained. Abortion may occur if the period of hyperthermia is prolonged and a high incidence of embryonic mortality has been recorded in sheep which were 3–6 weeks pregnant (7). In cattle breeding efficiency is adversely affected by prolonged heat stress and in intensively housed swine a syndrome known as summer infertility, manifested by a decrease in conception rate and litter size and an increase in anestrus, occurs during and following the hot summer months in most countries. Sudden exposure of cattle which are acclimatized to cold temperatures (−20°C; −4°F) to warmer temperature (20°C; 68°F) results in heat stress. The respiratory rate may increase from 20/min to 200/min within 1 hour, the heart rate will increase 10−20 beats/min, and the temperature will increase 0·5−1°C (33−34°F) (8).

Clinical pathology
No important clinicopathological change is observed in simple hyperthermia.

Necropsy findings
At necropsy there are only poorly defined gross changes. Peripheral vasodilatation may be evident, clotting of the blood is slow and incomplete, and rigor mortis and putrefaction occur early. There are no constant or specific histopathological changes.

Diagnosis
Simple hyperthermia must be differentiated from fever and septicemia. Clinically there may be little to distinguish between them. The toxemia which accompanies the latter conditions does not add much of significance to the clinical picture. In septicemia petechial hemorrhages in the mucosae and skin may be present and blood cultures may be positive in bacterial infections. In most cases of hyperthermia examination of the environment reveals the causative factor. In fever the temperature seldom exceeds 41°C (106°F), whereas in hyperthermia it frequently does.

Treatment
If treatment is necessary because of the severity or duration of the hyperthermia two methods are available. The intravenous administration of fluids, either normal saline or 5% dextrose, is indicated. Cold applications, including immersion, spraying, rectal enemas or cold packs, are also effective. Supportive treatment includes provision of adequate glucose and protein to compensate for increased utilization and in some cases deficient intake. The presence of adequate drinking water is essential and together with shade and air movement is of considerable assistance when animals are exposed to high air temperature. Shelter alone is a most important factor in maintaining the comfort of livestock (11). If animals have to be confined under conditions of high temperatures and humidity the use of tranquilizing drugs has been recommended to reduce unnecessary activity. However, care is needed because blood pressure falls and the animals may have difficulty losing heat if the environment is very hot and in some cases may gain it. Chlorpromazine, for example, has been shown to increase significantly the survival rate of pigs exposed to heat and humidity stress (9).

REFERENCES

(1) Hamilton, F. J. et al. (1961) *Aust. vet. J.*, *37*, 297.
(2) Moran, J. B. (1973) *Aust. J. agric. Res.*, *24*, 775.
(3) McGregor, B. (1985) *Aust. vet. J.*, *62*, 349.
(4) Huhnke, M. R. & Monty, D. E. (1976) *Am. J. vet. Res.*, *37*, 1301.
(5) Leipold, H. W. et al. (1974) *J. dairy Sci.*, *57*, 1401.
(6) Grosskopf, J. F. W. et al (1969) *J. S. Afr. vet. med. Assoc.*, *40*, 51.
(7) Smith, I. D. et al. (1966) *Aust. vet. J.*, *42*, 468.
(8) Edwards, W. C. & Kerr, L. A. (1982) *Vet. Med. SAC*, *77*, 805.
(9) Juszkiewicz, T. & Jones, L. M. (1961) *Am. J. vet. Res.*, *22*, 553.
(10) Honstein, R. N. & Monty, D. E. (1977) *Am. J. vet Res.*, *38*, 1041.
(11) Monty, D. E. & Garbareno, J. L. (1977) *Am. J. vet Res.*, *38*, 977.
(12) Waldron-Mease, E. (1981) *J. Am. vet. med. Assoc.*, *179*, 896.

Hypothermia

Hypothermia occurs when excess heat is lost or insufficient is produced so that the body temperature falls. It is of less importance than hyperthermia, but possibly is less recognized due to the limitations of clinical thermometry, and occurs for the opposite reasons. Exposure to excessively cold air temperatures will cause heat loss if increased metabolic activity, muscle tone and peripheral vasoconstriction are unable to compensate. Decrease of muscle tone as in parturient paresis and acute ruminal impaction and during anesthesia and sedation, associated with profuse diarrhea in the 'cold cow syndrome', peripheral vasodilatation in shock, and reduction of metabolic activity in the terminal stages of many diseases are common causes of hypothermia. In the latter case a sudden fall in temperature in a previously febrile animal, the so-called premortal fall, is a bad prognostic sign. Hypothermia may be a significant cause of postshearing mortality in sheep, especially where there has been a fall in body weight in the period immediately preceding shearing (1). Besides the absolute environmental temperature the factors which increase heat loss include wind speed, rainfall, sunshine versus cloud, and the depth of the wool cover. The speed of the wind at the location of the animals varies greatly depending on the presence of protective wind breaks such as timber.

Artificial hibernation or induced hypothermia has had experimental use as an anesthetic for extensive surgical operations in humans, but it is necessary initially to overcome the normal thermostatic mechanisms by the use of an anesthetic. In man, consciousness fails at rectal temperatures of 29·5−30·5°C (85−87°F), and fatal ventricular fibrillation is likely to occur at rectal temperatures of 25−26·6°C (77−80°F) (2). In dogs, the body temperature can be reduced to as low as 5°C (41°F) permitting complete exsanguination for 45 min and hypothermia is recommended as an anesthetic method in certain procedures in small-sized animals (3, 4).

Extensive reviews on acclimatization to cold environment are available (5, 6). During prolonged exposure of cattle and sheep to cold environments down to −10 to −20°C (−14 to −4°F) there is a reduction in the apparent digestibility of the diet (7). To offset the lowered digestibility, the animals would accordingly need to consume more feed to achieve a similar digestible energy intake when kept outdoors during winter than if they were kept in a heated barn. Hypothermia and environmental thermoregulatory interactions are of particular importance in the neonate (9, 10) especially piglets, but also in lambs and calves. Experimental chilling for long periods at only mildly cool levels (27·9°C (82·2°F) as against thermoneutrality of 34·6°C; 94·3°F) causes an increased death rate, at a younger age, and a poorer gain of body weight (8). Colder pigs have lower blood glucose levels and glycogen levels in liver and muscle than warm pigs. Cold pigs huddle more, neglect their food, are lethargic, disoriented and susceptible to environmental hazards. In calves experimental exposure to severe cold severely limits their intake of colostrum and may have importance in the field if the exposure is prolonged (11). The subject is further discussed in Chapter 3 on diseases of the newborn.

REVIEW LITERATURE

Webster, A. J. F. (1974) Heat loss from cattle with particular emphasis on the effects of cold. In: *Heat Loss from Animals and Man*, eds J. L. Monteith & L. E. Mount. London: Butterworths.

Ingram, D. L. (1974) Heat loss and its control in pigs. In: *Heat Loss from Animals and Man*, eds J. L. Monteith & L. E. Mount. London: Butterworths.

REFERENCES

(1) Hutchinson, K. J. & McRae, B. H. (1969) *Aust. J. agric. Res.*, *20*, 513.
(2) Pickering, G. (1958) *Lancet*, *1*, 59.
(3) Gilbert, G. H. (1972) *Bull. epizoot. Dis. Afr.*, *20*, 239.
(4) Northway, R. B. (1973) *Vet. Med.*, *68*, 1047.
(5) Ingram, D. L. (1974) In: *Heat Loss from Animals and Man*, ed. J. L. Monteith & L. E. Mount, pp. 233–54. London: Butterworths.
(6) Webster, A. J. F. (1974) In: *Heat Loss from Animals and Man*, ed. J. L. Monteith & L. E. Mount, pp. 205–31. London: Butterworths.
(7) Christopherson, R. J. (1976) *Can J. anim. Sci.*, *56*, 201.
(8) Stanton, H. C. & Mueller, A. L. (1977) *Am. J. vet. Res.*, *38*, 1003.
(9) Curtis, S. E. (1970) *J. anim. Sci.*, *31*, 576.
(10) Alexander, G. (1975) *Br. med. Bull.*, *31*, 62.
(11) Olson, D. P. et al. (1980) *Can. J. comp. Med.*, *44*, 11 & 19.

Fever

Fever is the syndrome in which hyperthermia and toxemia are produced by substances circulating in the bloodstream.

Etiology

Fevers may be septic, the more common type, or aseptic, depending on whether or not infection is present.

Septic

These include infection with bacteria, viruses, protozoa or fungi as:

- Localized infection such as abscess, cellulitis, empyema
- Intermittently systemic as in bacteremia
- Consistently systemic as in septicemia.

Aseptic

- Chemical fevers, caused by injection of foreign protein, intake of dinitrophenols
- Surgical fever due to breakdown of tissue and blood
- Fever from tissue necrosis, e.g.:
  - breakdown of muscle after injection of necrotizing material
  - severe intravascular hemolysis
  - extensive infarction
  - extensive necrosis in rapidly growing neoplasms
- Immune reactions—anaphylaxis, angioneurotic edema.

Pathogenesis

There is reasonable evidence that most fevers are mediated through the action of endogenous or leukocytic pyrogen produced by granulocytes, monocytes and macrophages. Interleukin-1, produced by monocytes and macrophages is the best known of these (4). The fall in temperature is accompanied by a decline in plasma zinc and plasma total iron concentrations (1). The production and release of endogenous pyrogen may be simulated directly by phagocytosis or by exposure of these cells to endogenous pyrogens such as endotoxin. In hypersensitivity states soluble antigen-antibody complexes may act as mediators. On the other hand the production of endogenous pyrogen by leukocytes may be activated by stimulation from lymphokinins released by activated lymphocytes exposed to antigen (5). The mediators between endogenous pyrogen and the hypothalamus appear to be prostaglandins and the level of calcium in the hypothalamus appears to regulate its activity (6).

It appears to be necessary for the physiological mechanisms involved in the production of fever after stimulation by pyrogens to be matured or sensitized by previous exposure to pyrogen (8). Injection of pyrogen into newborn lambs does not cause fever but subsequent injections do.

The effect of bacterial and tissue pyrogens is exerted on the thermoregulatory center of the hypothalamus so that the thermostatic level of the body is raised (9). The immediate response on the part of organs involved in heat regulation is the prevention of heat loss and the increased production of heat. This is the period of *increment* or chill which is manifested by cutaneous vasoconstriction, resulting coldness and dryness of the skin and an absence of sweating. Respiration is reduced and muscular shivering occurs while urine formation is minimal. Although the skin is cold the rectal temperature is elevated and the pulse rate increased. When the period of heat increment has raised the body temperature to a new thermostatic level the second period of fever, the *fastigium*, or period of constant temperature follows. In this stage the mechanisms of heat dissipation and production return to normal. Cutaneous vasodilatation causes flushing of the skin and mucosae, sweating occurs and may be severe and diuresis develops. During this period there is decreased ruminal motility (3), metabolism is increased considerably to maintain the body temperature, and tissue wasting may occur. There is also an inability to maintain a constant temperature when environmental temperatures vary.

When the effect of the pyrogenic substances is removed the stage of *decrement* or fever defervescence appears and the excess stored heat is dissipated. Vasodilatation, sweating and muscle flaccidity are marked and the body temperature falls. If the toxemia accompanying the hyperthermia is sufficiently severe the ability of tissues to respond to heat production or conservation needs may be lost and as death approaches there is a precipitate fall in body temperature.

The febrile reaction, and the altered behavior that accompanies it, are thought to be part of a total mechanism generated to conserve the resources of energy and tissue being wasted by the causative infection (2).

Clinical findings

The effects of fever are the combined effects of toxemia

nd hyperthermia. There is elevation of body temperaure, an increase in pulse rate with a diminution of amplitude and strength, hyperpnea, wasting, oliguria often with albuminuria, increased thirst, anorexia, constipation, depression and muscle weakness. The temperature elevation is always moderate and rarely goes above 42°C (107°F).

The form of the fever may vary. Thus the temperature rise may be *transient*, *continuous*, *remittent* when the diurnal variation is exaggerated, *intermittent* when fever peaks last for 2–3 days and are interspersed with normal periods, and *atypical* when temperature variations are irregular. A biphasic fever consisting of an initial rise, a fall to normal and a secondary rise, occurs in some diseases, e.g. in strangles in the horse and in erysipelas in swine. The outstanding example of intermittent fever in animal disease is equine infectious anemia.

Clinical pathology

There are no clinicopathological findings characteristic of fever.

Necropsy findings

The findings are a combination of those of hyperthermia, including vasodilatation, rapid onset of rigor mortis and putrefaction, and those of toxemia with microscopic evidence of degeneration in parenchymatous organs.

Diagnosis

Differentiation from hyperthermia, where there is no toxemia, and from septicemia, which is accompanied by infection of the bloodstream, is necessary. The characteristic findings of infectious fevers include:

- Sudden onset
- High fever (39·5–41°C; 103·1–105·8°F)
- Anorexia
- Dullness, depression, disinclination to move
- Vomiting or diarrhea
- Lymphadenopathy, possibly splenomegaly
- Marked changes in the total and differential leukocyte counts
- The isolation of a pathogen from blood or excreta

In the case of longstanding fevers the above signs are still characteristic but they may fluctuate in severity daily or over longer periods.

Treatment

The general principles of treatment of fever are to remove the source of the toxin and to treat the toxemia and the hyperthermia if the fever is excessive or prolonged. Stimulation of the circulation and respiration may be necessary if these are failing. Removal of the toxin necessitates control of infections by antibacterial drugs and removal of necrotic material in aseptic fevers and local infections. Specific antibodies and antitoxins find use in controlling infection and reducing the effects of bacterial toxins. Non-specific treatments include the use of adrenocortical hormones to facilitate repair processes and alleviate inflammation. These drugs must be used with great caution and be supported by large doses of broad-spectrum antibiotics. The need for caution arises because of the depression of resistance to infection which they induce. This disadvantage is not present with the use of the non-steroidal anti-inflammatory drugs, the antiprostaglandins, including salicylates and phenylbutazone (7). Inaccessible foci of infection may be benefitted by the systemic or local use of enzyme preparations but their use has been generally disappointing and they are no longer in general use. One aspect of the treatment of fever which has received little consideration has been the effect of fever, or hyperthermia, on the absorption and metabolism of drugs. It is apparent that the effect could be significant (10). Diuretics which have an important part to play in the removal of transudates are unlikely to have any effect on aggregations of inflammatory fluids.

REFERENCES

(1) Groothuis, D. G. et al. (1981) *Vet. Rec.*, *109*, 176.
(2) Hart, B. L. (1985) *J. Am. vet. med. Assoc.*, *187*, 998.
(3) van Miert, A. S. J. P. A. M. & van Duin, C. T. M. (1974) *Zentrabl. VetMed.*, *21A*, 692.
(4) Atkins, E. (1983) *New Engl. J. Med.*, *308*, 958.
(5) Atkins, E. et al. (1972) *J. exp. Med.*, *135*, 1113.
(6) Feldberg, W. (1975) *Proc. R. Soc. B*, *191*, 199.
(7) Jones, E. W. (1977) *J. Equ. med. Surg.*, *1*, 364.
(8) Pittman, Q. J. et al. (1974) *Clin. Sci. molec. Med.*, *46*, 591.
(9) Mitchell, D. et al. (1970) *Pflügers Arch. ges. Physiol.*, *321*, 293.
(10) van Miert, A. S. J. P. A. M. et al. (1976) *Vet. Rec.*, *99*, 480.

SEPTICEMIA/VIREMIA

Septicemia is the disease state compounded of toxemia, hyperthermia and the presence of large numbers of infectious microorganisms, including viruses, bacteria and protozoa in the bloodstream.

Etiology

Many infectious agents produce septicemias. The difference between septicemia and bacteremia is one of degree. In bacteremia bacteria are present in the bloodstream for only transitory periods and do not produce clinical signs; e.g. a clinically unimportant bacteremia probably occurs frequently after rectal examination or other manipulations in which mucosa is disturbed (4). In septicemia the causative agent is present throughout the course of the disease and is directly responsible for the signs which appear.

Some of the notable septicemias are as follows.

All species

- Anthrax, pasteurellosis, salmonellosis, *Pasteurella (Francisella) tularensis* (tularemia)
- *Pseudomonas pseudomallei*—melioidosis
- Rift Valley fever
- *Leptospira interrogans*
- Neonatal septicemias are listed separately in Chapter 3, p. 108.

Cattle, sheep and pigs

- *Pasteurella multocida*, *P. haemolytica*, *P.* (*Yersinia*) *pseudotuberculosis*.

Sheep (lambs)

- *Histophilus ovis*, *Haemophilus agni*

Pigs

- Hog cholera, African swine fever viruses
- *Streptococcus zooepidemicus*
- *Erysipelothrix insidiosa*

Horses, donkeys, mules

- *Pasteurella haemolytica*

Special septicemias

- The principal cause of death in subacute radiation injury is septicemia resulting from loss of leukocyte production because of injury to bone marrow
- Septicemia may result when there is a congenital defect in the immune system or when immunosuppression occurs in older animals as a result of corticosteroid therapy or toxin such as bracken, or infection, usually a virus such as bovine viral diarrhea virus.

Pathogenesis

Two mechanisms operate in septicemia. The exotoxins or endotoxins produced by the infectious agents produce a profound toxemia and high fever because of the rapidity with which they multiply and their rapid spread to all body tissues. Also localization occurs in many organs and may produce serious defects in animals which survive the toxemia. They also cause direct endothelial damage and hemorrhages into tissue commonly result. The same general principles apply to a viremia except that toxins are not produced by the virus. It is more likely that the general signs which occur are caused by the products of the tissue cells killed by the multiplying virus (1). Disseminated intravascular coagulation may occur in septicemic disease, especially that which terminates fatally. It is initiated by vascular injury with partial disruption of the intima caused by the circulation of foreign materials such as bacterial cell walls, antigen-antibody complexes and endotoxin, with subsequent platelet adherence and the formation of platelet thrombi. Once coagulation proceeds the initial hypercoagulable state changes to hypocoagulation, as clotting factors and platelets are consumed. The activation of the fibrinolysis system can be a major cause of the hemorrhagic diathesis present in this syndrome (2, 3).

Clinical findings

The clinical findings in septicemia are those of toxemia and hyperthermia and include fever and submucosal and subepidermal hemorrhages, usually petechial, or occasionally ecchymotic. The hemorrhages are best seen under the conjunctiva and in the mucosae of the mouth and vulva. Localizing signs may occur as the result of localization of the infection in joints, heart valves, meninges, eyes or other organs.

Clinical pathology

Isolation of the causative bacteria from the bloodstream should be attempted by culture or animal inoculation at the height of the fever. The presence of leukopenia or leukocytosis is an aid in diagnosis and the type and degree of leukocytic response may be of prognostic significance. Consumption coagulopathy is detected by falling platelet counts and prothrombin and fibrinogen values, and the presence of fibrin degradation products.

Necropsy findings

Apart from the changes caused by toxemia and hyperthermia there may be subserous and submucosal hemorrhages and embolic foci of infection in various organs but these are usually overshadowed by the lesions specific to the causative agent.

Diagnosis

Only by the isolation of the causative agent from the bloodstream can a positive diagnosis of septicemia be made. However, the presence of petechiae in mucosae and conjunctivae may suggest septicemia, and high environmental temperatures may suggest hyperthermia. Evidence of localization in individual organs is contributory evidence that septicemia is present or has occurred.

Treatment

The same general recommendations for treatment apply here as in fever, except that the need for treatment is more urgent and intravenous or parenteral treatment with antibacterial drugs or sera and antitoxins should be provided as soon as possible. Strict hygienic precautions to avoid spread of diseases may be necessary in many cases.

REVIEW LITERATURE

Schiefer, B. & Searcy, G. (1975) Disseminated intravascular coagulation and consumption coagulopathy. *Can. vet J.*, *16*, 151.

REFERENCES

(1) Downie, A. W. (1963) *Vet. Rec.*, *75*, 1125.
(2) Coe, N. P. & Salzman, E. W. (1976) *Surg. Clin. N. Am.*, *56*, 875.
(3) Sharp, A. A. (1977) *Br. med. Bull.*, *33*, 265.
(4) Stem, E. S. et al. (1984) *Vet. Rec.*, *114*, 638.

LOCALIZED INFECTIONS

A great number of animals presented to veterinarians have localized infections, many of them due to trauma. Because most of them have a surgical outcome, by incision and drainage, and by excision or amputation, they are not usually included in medical texbooks. They are dealt with briefly here because of their importance in the differential diagnosis of causes of toxemia and because of their space-occupying characteristic of compression of other structures. Also, the initial treatment is often medical, especially if the exact location of the lesion cannot be identified.

Etiology

Abscesses and similar aggregations of pyogenic material in special locations are dealt with in many other places in this book. The important ones include: pharyngeal, retroperitoneal, hepatic, splenic, pulmonary, brain, pituitary, spinal cord and subcutaneous abscesses. Other similar lesions include embolic nephritis, guttural pouch empyema, lymphadenitis, pharyngeal phlegmon, osteomyelitis and infections of the umbilicus and associated vessels.

More widespread accumulations of necrotic/toxic pyogenic debris occur and are dealt with under the headings of: pericarditis, pleurisy, peritonitis, metritis, mastitis, meningitis and pyelonephritis.

There still remain a few other pyogenic lesions which are worthy of note. These include:

- *Inguinal abscess in horses*. Some of these probably originate as postcastration infections, but some obviously have other origins, possibly as a lymphadenitis arising from drainage of a leg with a chronic skin infection
- *Traumatic cellulitis and phlegmon in soft tissue*, especially skeletal muscle. The neck is a common site of infection in the horse resulting from infected injection sites or the injection of escharotic materials, e.g., iron preparations intended only for intravenous injection. Penetrating traumatic wounds, often badly infected, are among the serious occurrences to the legs and hooves of horses and cattle. These commonly penetrate joint capsules, bursae and tendon sheaths, and underrun periosteum. In cattle the common causes are agricultural implements, in horses they are more commonly caused by galloping onto protruding objects including stakes
- *Abscessation and cellulitis of the tip or the proximal part of the tail*. Occurs in steers in feedlots and may extend to the hindquarters and the scrotum (1); the cause is unknown, the bacteria isolated being mixed infections
- *Perirectal abscess* occurs in horses caused usually by minor penetrations of the mucosa during rectal examination. Some of these rupture into the peritoneal cavity causing acute, fatal peritonitis. Others cause obstruction of the rectum and colic because of the pain and compression that they cause (2). They are readily palpable on rectal examination
- *Urachal abscess*. See omphalitis
- *Pituitary abscess* occurs in cattle as a single entity or in combination with other lesions (4). It causes a wide range of signs with emphasis on dysphagia due to jawdrop, blindness and absence of a pupillary light reflex, ataxia and terminal recumbency with nystagmus and opisthotonus (3). A high quality *Actinomyces (Cornyebacterium) pyogenes* vaccine against the disease is reported to have performed well (5).

Bacterial causes

These include those bacteria which are common skin contaminants in animals including *Actinomyces (Corynebacterium) pyogenes*, *Fusobacterium necrophorum*, streptococci and staphylococci. Clostridial infections are common but occur sporadically. They are dealt with under the heading of malignant edema. *Corynebacterium pseudotuberculosis* is quite common as a cause of local suppuration in horses and is the specific cause of caseous lymphadenitis of sheep. *Cor. (Rhodococcus) equi* also causes subcutaneous abscesses in horses and cervical lymphadenitis in pigs. Strangles, *Cor. equi* infection in foals, melioidosis and glanders are all characterized by extensive systemic abscess formation. *Histophilus ovis* causes systemic abscess formation in sheep. *Mycobacterium phlei* and other atypical mycobacteria are rare causes of local cellulitis and lymphadenitis/lymphangitis manifesting as 'skin tuberculosis' in cattle.

Streptococcal cervical abscesses in pigs is another specific abscess-forming disease.

Portal of entry

Most of the incidents being discussed arise because of penetrating wounds of the skin, caused accidentally, or neglectfully because of failure to disinfect adequately the skin before an injection or incision as in castration, tail docking.

Metastatic implantation from another infectious process, especially endocarditis, carried by blood or lymph, is the next most common cause. In this way a chain of lymph nodes can become infected. Cranial and caudal vena caval syndromes produce similar embolic showers in the lungs.

Pathogenesis

The local infection may take the form of a circumscribed aggregation of bacterial debris and necrotic tissue known as an *abscess*. This may be firmly walled off by a dense fibrotic wall, or be contiguous with normal tissue. When such an abscess occurs in a lymph node it is a *bubo*. When the infection material is purulent but diffusely spread through tissues, especially along fascial planes, it is known as a *phlegmon*, and when it is inflammatory but not purulent the same lesion is a *cellulitis*.

The species of bacteria in the abscess may dictate the type of pus present and the smell produced by it. Staphylococci produce much thick yellow pus, streptococci produce less pus and more serous-like exudates. Corynebacterial pus is deep-colored, yellow or green in color and very thick and tenacious. The pus of *Fusobacterium necrophorum* is very foul-smelling and usually accompanied by the presence of gas.

Deposition of bacteria in tissues is sufficient to establish infection there in most instances. Conditions which favor abscess development include ischemia, trauma, the presence of a cavity, a hematoma. A continuing process of pus formation results in enlargement to the stage of pointing and rupturing of an abscess, or spread along the path of least resistance into a nearby cavity or vessel or discharge to the exterior through a sinus. Continuing discharge through a sinus indicates the persistence of a septic focus usually as a foreign body such as a grass seed, or as a sequestrum of necrotic bone or an osteomyelitis lesion.

Clinical findings

The clinical signs of abscesses and other local aggregations of pyogenic lesions are described under each of the headings listed under etiology. General clinical signs which may suggest the presence of local infection without necessarily being present in any of them include the following:

- *Fever, depression, lack of appetite*—the signs of toxemia
- *Pain resulting in abnormal posture*, for example, arching of the back, or gait including severe lameness
- *Weight loss*, which can be dramatic in degree and rapidity
- *Obstruction of lymphatic and venous drainage*, which can cause local swelling and edema. Sequels to these developments include extensive cellulitis if there is a retrograde spread of infection along lymph drainage channels, and phlebitis and thrombophlebitis when there is stasis in the veins
- *Careful palpation under anesthesia or heavy sedation* may be necessary to overcome the muscle spasm caused by pain. Calves with extensive abscessation emanating from the navel, and horses with inguinal abscesses can only be satisfactorily examined by deep abdominal and rectal palpation
- *Radiological examination* may elicit evidence of osteomyelitis, and examination of a fistulous tract may be facilitated in this way especially if a radiopaque material is infused into the track.

Clinical pathology

A complete blood count is helpful in supporting a diagnosis of local abscess. Unless the infection is completely isolated by a fibrous tissue capsule there will be a leukocytosis with a left shift and an elevation of polymorphonuclear leukocytes in acute lesions or of lymphocytes and monocytes in more chronic ones. A moderate normochromic anemia is usual in chronic lesions, and mild proteinuria is common.

Attempts to identify the presence of an infectious agent and to establish its identity are usually undertaken but care is necessary to avoid spreading infection from a site in which it is presently contained. Techniques used include paracentesis, careful needle aspiration from an abscess, blood culture, with the chances of isolation of bacteria being very small unless there is phlebitis or endocarditis, and aspiration of CSF. The isolation of bacteria from a well-contained abscess may be difficult because of the paucity of organisms. Special techniques may be necessary and examination of a smear stained with Gram stain, perhaps also with Ziehl–Neelsen if the circumstances suggest it, is an essential part of the examination. Determination of sensitivity of the bacteria to antibiotics is usually undertaken.

Necropsy findings

In the event of the patient's demise the presence and location of the local infection can be demonstrated at necropsy. The location is not usually in doubt in a patient which is so severely affected.

Treatment

Medical treatment includes the systemic, and possibly local, administration of the appropriate antibiotic as indicated by a sensitivity test on a bacterial culture, or the use of a broad-spectrum antibacterial agent. The problems in therapy are related to poor diffusion of an antibacterial agent through a dense capsule and into a large accumulation of thick pus, and the relative resistance of organisms which are not actively dividing at the time. A common result with systemic antibacterial therapy in these circumstances is the conversion of what is a relatively active process into a very chronic one. There are three ways of avoiding this outcome:

1. Refrain from systemic treatment if suppuration is already taking place but the abscess is not yet ripe and has not pointed. Hot fomentations and hydrotherapy are difficult to apply in farm animals but will aid maturation of a superficial lesion. There may be need to use an analgesic during this stage.
2. Aspiration of the contents of the lesion and replacement with the antibacterial agent.
3. Surgical opening, flushing and drainage of the lesion with as much care as possible to avoid bacteremia and spread of infection to surrounding tissues.

When antibacterial agents are used systemically to treat a local suppurative lesion it is most important that the treatment regimen be vigorous. The dose rate of the agent needs to be high and treatment repeated often and over a long period, 1–2 weeks is usual, to ensure high blood levels continuously. The choice of an agent should take into account the likely sensitivity of the causative organism, and the ability of the agent to be effective in the presence of pus.

REFERENCES

(1) Buczek, J. et al. (1984) *Med. Wet.*, *40*, 643 and 707.
(2) Sanders-Sharis, M. (1985) *J. Am. vet. med. Assoc.*, *187*, 499.
(3) Perdrizet, J. A. (1986) *Comp. cont. Educ.*, *8*, S311.
(4) Taylor, P. A. & Meads, E. B. (1963) *Can. vet. J.*, *4*, 208.
(5) Cameron, C. M. et al. (1976) *Onderstepoort J. vet. Res.*, *43*, 97.

PAIN

Pain is a distressing sensation arising from stimulation of specific endorgans in particular parts of the body and perceived in the thalamus and cerebral cortex. It is basically a protective mechanism to ensure that the animal moves away from noxious (damaging) influences, but endogenous pain, arising from internal damaging influences, causes its own physiological and pathological problems that require the veterinarian's intervention. In man there is an additional psychological parameter to pain, and although it is customary to transpose attitudes rom pain in man to pain in animals it is a courtesy ather than an established scientific principle. To a large xtent this is due to the difficulty of measuring pain. It s a subjective sensation obviously known by experience nd describable by illustration, but measurement of it is ndirect and related to the effects of the pain and is herefore objective. In animals the measurement of pain s by observation of actions and by measurement of the physiological parameters of heart rate, blood pressure and so on, more accurately a measurement of nociception. Because of this lack of objectivity and accuracy the assessment of pain levels in animals is a problem area for veterinarians involved in animal experimentation but a program for measurement has been devised (1). It is based on the assumption that what is painful in humans causes pain in animals.

Pain in agricultural animals is a matter of increasing concern nowadays. Many agricultural practices which are thought to be necessary to avoid later painful disease or injury (e.g., the Mules operation in sheep, dehorning of cattle and sheep, tooth clipping in baby pigs), or to improve animal production (e.g., castration, spaying), are carried out by farmers without anesthetic. It is not our purpose to engage in a discussion on the subject of animal welfare or the prevention of cruelty to them. However, to be in pain is to suffer from a destructive body state and it is necessary to discuss it here in that clinical context.

Etiology

Pain sensations are aroused by different stimuli in different tissues and the agents that cause pain in one organ do not necessarily do so in another. In animals there are three types of pain, cutaneous, visceral and somatic (or musculoskeletal), and the causes of each are listed below.

Cutaneous or superficial pain

In general, the agents that cause pain are those which damage skin, such as burning, freezing, cutting and crushing. Thus, fire burns, frostbite, severe dermatitis, acute mastitis, laminitis, infected surgical wounds, foot-rot, crushing by trauma, conjunctivitis and foreign body in the conjunctival sac are familiar causes of pain.

Visceral pain

Causes are inflammation of serous surfaces including pleurisy, peritonitis and pericarditis, distention of viscera including stomach, intestines, ureters, bladder, swelling of organs as in hepatomegaly and splenomegaly. Inflammation as in nephritis, peripelvic cellulitis, and enteritis, stretching of mesentery and mediastinum are all causes of visceral pain. In the nervous system swelling of the brain caused by edema, or of the meninges caused by meningitis, are potent causes of pain. So is inflammation of (neuritis) or compression of (neuralgia) peripheral nerves or dorsal nerve roots.

Somatic or musculoskeletal pain

Muscular pain can be caused by tears and hematomas of muscle, myositis, and space-occupying lesions of muscle. Osteomyelitis, fractures, arthritis, joint dislocations, sprains of ligaments and tendons are also obvious causes of severe pain. Among the most painful of injuries are swollen, inflamed lesions of the limbs caused by deep penetrating injury or in cattle by extension from footrot. Amputation of a claw, laminitis and septic arthritis are in the same category. Ischemia of muscle and generalized muscle tetany, as occurs in electroimmobilization (6) also appear to cause pain.

The trauma of surgical wounds is a matter of debate in animal welfare considerations especially with reference to minor surgery such as tail-docking, dehorning and castration in food animals. From clinical observation supported by some laboratory examinations, e.g. salivary cortisol levels after castration in calves and lambs, it appears that the pain is very shortlived, up to about 3 hours (14).

Pathogenesis

Pain receptors are distributed as endorgans in all body systems and organs. They are connected to the central nervous system by their own sensory nerve fibers with their cell bodies in the dorsal root ganglion of each spinal nerve and via some of the cranial nerves. Intracord neurones connect the peripheral ones to the thalamus where pain is perceived and to the sensory cerebral cortex where the intensity and localization of the pain are appreciated, and the responses to pain are initiated and coordinated.

The stimuli which cause pain vary between organs. The important causes include:

- *Skin*—cutting, crushing, freezing, burning
- *Gastrointestinal tract*—distention, spasm, inflamed mucosa, stretching of mesentery
- *Skeletal muscle*—ischemia, traumatic swelling, tearing, rupture, hematoma
- *Joint cartilage*—by inflammation.

The physiological responses to pain are set out below. There are also normal responses including the morphine-like endorphin release from the brain (13), providing an endogenous analgesic system, and cortisol released by the adrenal cortex (15) in a reaction to any stress.

The clinical response to pain varies not only with the personality of the patient (some are more stoical than others), but also with other influences. For example, distraction, as in walking a horse with colic, application of an alternative pain in the forced elevation of the tail of a cow (tail jack), and application of local anesthetic agents all tend to relieve pain. In agricultural animals pain elicits behavioral and physiological responses. The behavioral responses can be interpreted as a form of distraction, a displacement activity, or as providing an alternative pain. The physiological responses appear to be part of the fight or flight phenomena and are accountable in terms of stimulation of the sympathetic system.

Clinical findings

Set out below are some of the general clinical signs of pain. Signs suggestive of pain in particular organs and systems are dealt with in each of them.

Physiological responses

Physiological responses to pain are manifested by the following signs, the severity of the pain determining the degree of response: tachycardia, polypnea, pupillary dilatation, hyperthermia and sweating. These cardiovascular responses may contribute to a fatal outcome, for example when dehydration, acid–base imbalance and endotoxic shock are also present.

Behavioral responses

These include abnormal posture and gait when the pain is musculoskeletal (i.e. somatic). The gait abnormalities include lameness, a shuffling gait, and rapid shifting of weight from one leg to another. These are subjects of importance in orthopedic surgery and are not dealt with further here.

The behavioral responses to pain may also include unrelated activities such as rolling, pawing, or crouching when the pain is visceral. However, the activities may be related to the site of the pain, e.g., flank watching in colic in horses, or to a particular function, e.g., pain on coughing, or walking, defecating, urinating. In general terms somatic pain is more localized and is therefore more easily identified than visceral pain. Injuries to limbs are usually identifiable by fractures or localized tendon strain or muscle injury. With severe pain as with a fracture, the limb is carried off the ground and no weight is taken on the limb. With lesser lesions more weight-bearing activity is undertaken.

One of the notable factors affecting pain in animals is the analgesic effect of laying the animal on its back or of its adopting a defeated, supine posture. This may be related to the release of endorphins (15).

More general behavioral responses to pain include failure to take adequate food and water, adoption of an anxious expression, disinclination to be examined and aversion to returning to a particular location where pain has been experienced previously. Moaning, grunting and grinding of the teeth (ondontophoresis or bruxism) are generally agreed to be indicative of pain. If the vocalization occurs with each respiration, or each rumination, the pain appears likely to arise from a lesion in the thoracic or abdominal cavities. When teeth-grinding is associated with head-pressing it is thought to indicate increased intracranial pressure such as occurs with brain edema, or lead poisoning. Grinding of the teeth as a sole sign of pain is usually associated with subacute distention of segments of the alimentary tract. More extreme kinds of vocalization caused by pain include moderate bellowing by cattle, bleating in sheep and squealing in pigs.

Elicitation of pain by the veterinarian

This is an essential part of a clinical examination. The techniques used are also generally surgical and are listed briefly here:

- Pressure by palpation, including firm ballottement with the fist, and use of a pole to depress the back in a horse, or to arch the back upwards by pressure from below in the cow, or by percussion, e.g., hoof hammer
- Movement by having the animal walk actively or by passively flexing or extending limbs or neck
- Stimulation of pain, which is related for example to coughing, by stimulating the animal to cough
- Relief of the pain by correction of the lesion

Periodicity and duration of pain

Limited duration of pain can be the result of natural recovery or of surgical or medical correction of the problem. Constant pain results from a static state whereas periodic or intermittent pain is often related to periodic peristaltic movement. In man and in companion animals some importance also attaches to observing the time of onset of pain, whether it is related to particular functions or happenings, and whether the patient gains relief by particular postures or activities. These factors are unlikely to be of importance as an aid to a diagnosis in agricultural animals.

Diagnosis

The objective in the clinical examination of an animal presented because its problem is thought to be one of pain is to:

- Ensure that pain is the cause of the signs observed
- Locate the site of the pain
- Determine the nature of the lesion and relieve it if possible
- Treat the pain symptomatically as a supportive treatment for the primary disease.

The differential diagnosis of pain should include restlessness due to paresthesia as in snakebite in horses, and to photosensitive dermatitis in ruminants, especially cattle.

Locating the site of the lesion and pain is more difficult than in man because the animal is unable to explain where it hurts. All of the techniques of observation and palpation and movement as set out in clinical findings are essential to locate the lesion properly.

Treatment

There are a number of aspects to the problems of relieving pain in agricultural animals. Not the least is the matter of cost. Relief of the causative lesion is number one priority and is dealt with under the various systems. Relief of pain as such should be one of the first tasks of the attending veterinarian, providing the following principles are followed:

- Relief of pain is a humane act
- Analgesia should not be used so as to obscure clinical signs which may be necessary to observe, to properly diagnose or maintain surveillance of a case
- It may be necessary to protect the animal from massive self-injury
- Analgesics for visceral pain are readily available and relatively effective
- A major problem in the clinical management of pain is for cases of severe, slowly healing, infected traumatic wounds of the musculoskeletal system in horses and cattle. Pain is likely to be very severe, continuous and to last for periods of up to several weeks. Affected animals cannot put the limb to the ground, have great difficulty getting around, lose much weight and lie down a lot. There is no suitable analgesic available and there is a major requirement for one which can be administered daily for 3 weeks without undesirable side-effects.

Analgesics

The analgesic agents and techniques available include the following items:

- *Neurectomy by surgical section* of peripheral nerves is practiced in horses. Local destruction of peripheral nerves by chemical means, e.g., the epidural injection of agents such as ethyl alcohol to prevent straining
- *Analgesia by non-opiate drugs* when sedation is not required.

The analgesics which are available for use in large animals have limitations to their use especially when the pain arises from severe inflammation of the limbs. For abdominal pain in horses the drugs available are adequate. Narcotics and anesthetics have limited use in large animals which are required to move around and eat and drink. The available analgesics are as follows.

Salicylates Aspirin or acetylsalicylic acid is the most extensively used analgesic in cattle, but there is limited clinical evidence of its efficacy. The recommended dose rate is 100 mg/kg body weight orally every 12 hours (2). Because there may be limited absorption from the small intestine the salicylates may be given intravenously (35 mg/kg every 6 hours in cattle, 25 mg/kg every 4 hours in horses). Salicylates are not very effective in alleviating severe pain. They act peripherally by blocking pain mediators which stimulate pain endorgans. They have no central depressant effect on the thalamus or cerebral cortex.

Phenylbutazone This agent is used extensively as an analgesic for horses, especially for musculoskeletal pain. It is most effective for the relief of mild to moderate pain caused by myositis, laminitis and so on. The half-life of the drug in plasma is about 3·5 hours so that repeated treatment is recommended. After oral use in horses the peak levels in plasma are reached at 2 hours, after intramuscular injection not until 6 hours so that oral or intravenous are the usual routes of administration. Unless care is taken to inject the drug slowly when using the intravenous route, severe phlebitis, sometimes causing complete obstruction of the jugular vein, may result. For horses the recommended dose rate is 4·4 mg/kg body weight daily for 5 days by oral or intravenous routes. Treatment on day 1 may be at 4·4 mg/kg twice, constituting a loading dose (10). Treatment beyond 5 days may be continued at minimal effective dose rates. However, prolonged use, especially in ponies, at a dose of 10–12 mg/kg body weight daily for 8–10 days, may be followed by ulceration of alimentary tract mucosa, including the oral mucosa, and fatal fluid retention due to hypoproteinemia (3). The pathogenesis of these lesions is thought to be due to a widespread phlebopathy (9). It should not be used if there is pre-existing gastrointestinal ulceration, clotting deficits or cardiac or renal dysfunction. Its use should be under close veterinary supervision so that the dose rate may be kept to a minimal effective level, and so that it is used only when there is a clear clinical indication to do so and that it can be withdrawn if there is no indication of a therapeutic response or if signs of toxicity appear. If there is doubt about toxicity or a prolonged course is advised periodic hematological examinations are recommended.

For cattle the recommended oral dosing regimen is 10–20 mg/kg body weight following by daily maintenance doses of 2·5–5·0 mg/kg (4). It is disappointing in cattle affected with painful conditions of the limbs. In most countries the drug is not approved for use in food-producing animals because of the risk of drug residues in the food chain, and the known toxicity of phenylbutazone in man.

Xylazine This has been shown to be the most effective analgesic for the relief of experimentally induced superficial, deep and visceral pain in ponies when compared to fentanyl, meperidine (pethidine) methadone, oxymorphone and pentazocine (5). Results in clinical cases are disappointing.

Flunixin meglumine This is a non-narcotic, non-steroidal anti-inflammatory antipyretic drug with analgesic properties. The dose rate is 1·1 mg/kg body weight with a peak response at 12 hours and a duration of effect of 30 hours (7). It is recommended as being effective for the relief of musculoskeletal pain. It can be administered orally or parenterally and has a wide margin of safety. Individual ponies may be poisoned but only with large doses (8). Toxic effects are similar to those with phenylbutazone and include ulceration of the colon, stomach and mouth.

Narcotic analgesics Meperidine (Demerol, pethidine) is extensively used as an analgesic for visceral pain in the horse. Methadone hydrochloride and pentazocine are also used to a limited extent and their use is detailed in the treatment of colic in the horse. Butorphanol, a synthetic narcotic used alone (11) or in combination with xylazine (12), provides highly effective analgesia in horses. They are used in somatic pain in man, and may have wider applicability in animals. A significant limitation to their use is that they are addictive drugs for man and must be kept under very strict control.

Chloral hydrate given intravenously to effect is used, but is a last resort because of its strong narcotic effect and the short duration of its effect.

Supportive therapy

The application of moist heat to a local lesion causing pain is effective and logical. Its value depends on how frequently and for how long it can be applied. Providing adequate bedding is important for an animal which is recumbent for long periods or which is likely to injure itself while rolling. A thick straw pack is most useful if it can be kept clean and densely packed. Sawdust is most practical, but has the problem that it gets into everything, especially dressings and wounds. Rubber floors and walls as in recovery wards, are effective but are usually available only for short periods.

Distracting a horse with colic by walking it continuously is a common device to avoid it injuring itself. It is valuable but has obvious limitations. The provision of adequate food and water is essential especially if the animal is immobilized and because appetite is often poor.

REFERENCES

(1) Morton, D. B. & Griffins, P.H.M. (1985) *Vet. Rec.*, *116*, 431.
(2) Davis, L. E. (1980) *J. Am. vet. med. Assoc.*, *176*, 65.
(3) Snow, D. H. et al. (1981) *Am. J. vet. Res.*, *42*, 1754.

(4) Backer, P. De et al. (1980) *J. vet. Pharm. Therap.*, *3*, 29.
(5) Pippi, N. L. & Lumb, W. V. (1979) *Am. J. vet. Res.*, *40*, 1082.
(6) Rushen, J. and Congdon, P. (1986) *Aust. vet. J.*, *63*, 373.
(7) Houdeshell, J. W. & Hennessey, P. W. (1977) *J. equ. Med. Surg.*, *1*, 57.
(8) Trillo, M. A. et al. (1984) *Equ. Pract.*, *6*(3), 21.
(9) Meschter, C. L. et al. (1984) *Cornell Vet.*, *74*, 282.
(10) Taylor, J. B. et al. (1983) *Vet. Rec.*, *113*, 183.
(11) Kalprvidh, M. et al. (1984) *Am. J. vet. Res.*, *45*, 211.
(12) Robertson, J. T. & Muir, W. W. (1983) *Am. J. vet. Res.*, *44*, 1667.
(13) van Ree, J. M. (1985) *Tijdschr. Diergeneeskd.*, *110*, 3.
(14) Fell, R. L. et al. (1986) *Aust. vet. J.*, *63*, 16.
(15) Schoental, R. (1986) *Vet. Rec.*, *119*, 223 (Corr).

STRESS

Stress is a systemic state which develops as a result of the longterm application of stressors. It includes pain which is discussed in detail in an earlier section.

Stressors are environmental factors which stimulate homeostatic, physiological and behavioral responses in excess of normal.

The only acceptable measurement of the presence or absence of stress is the blood level of adrenal corticosteroids. The importance of stress is that it may:

- Lead to the development of psychosomatic disease;
- Increase susceptibility to infection;
- Represent an unacceptable level of consideration for the welfare of animals;
- Reduce the efficiency of production.

The general adaptation syndrome described in man has no counterpart in our animals and it is lacking in accurate definitions, precise pathogenesis and general credibility.

Causes of stress

For animals a satisfactory environment is one that provides thermal comfort, physical comfort, control of disease and behavioral satisfaction. An environment which is short of these factors will lead to stress (21). The environmental influences which elicit physiological responses from animals are conveniently classified as set out below. The influences among them which put abnormally heavy strains on body systems, so much so that they can be classified as stressors, are presumably amongst them. The effects of most of these influences on production, reproductive activity and the like have been measured quantitatively (12) and many of them have been equated with blood levels of adrenal corticosteroids which quantitate them as stressors in the different species (13).

1. *Nutritional causes* including lack of energy, bulk and fluid.
2. *Climate*, especially temperature, either as excessive heat or cold, or more importantly comfort as expressed by the effects of wind and rain, and most importantly of all 'change'. A sudden change of climate in pastured animals can place great pressure on heat production and conservation mechanisms (8).
3. *Physical effort*, as in endurance rides for horses, staying upright in moving transports for long periods for cattle.
4. *Physical effort*, struggle, fear, excitement in capture, myopathy syndrome in wild life.
5. *Pain*, especially overriding pain as in severe colic in horses.
6. *Crowding* as distinct from temperature, humidity and the physical exhaustion associated with standing up for long periods, being walked on, difficulty getting to food and water. Two other factors could be important. One is the effect of crowding on behavior (10). For example, pigs in overcrowded pens appear to bite one another more than when they are thinned out, and are more restless than normal when temperatures in the pens are high. The biting is much more severe between males than between females (7). Also, it is known that pigs bite each other when establishing precedence in a group, for example after mixing of batches, and it is more severe when feed is short (3). The other possible factor which might affect the animal's response to crowding is psychological appreciation of the unattractiveness of crowding, or isolation. This seems an unlikely possibility in our animals.
7. *Presence or absence of bedding*. This is a comfort factor separate from temperature, wetness and so on, but whether comfort is a factor affecting physiological mechanisms is not identified.
8. *Housing* generally includes the matter of comfort as well as that of maintaining moderate temperatures, but whether there is a factor other than the physical ones is not known.
9. *Quietness versus excitement*. Harassment by man or other animals sufficient to cause fear does elicit stress responses in animals and this is thought to be one of the significant causes of stress-related diseases in animals. Thus, transportation, entry to saleyards, feedlots, fairs and shows, and simply the mixing of several groups so that competition for superiority in the social order of the group is stimulated, are causes of stress. Entry to an abattoir, which has the additional fear-inspiring factors of noise and smell, is likely to be very stressful for those reasons, but it is unlikely that fear of impending death is relevant. That it is stressful to the point of causing marked elevation of plasma adrenal levels has been established (11).
10. *Herding and flocking*. Animal species that are accustomed to be kept as herds or flocks may be distressed for a period if they are separated from the group (10).

Pathogenesis

Stress is thought to develop when the animal's mechanisms concerned with adapting its body to the environment are taxed beyond their normal capacities. The daily (circadian) rhythm of homeostatic and physiological changes in response to normal daily changes in environment require the least form of adaptation. Marked changes in environment, such as a dramatic change in weather, on the other hand, place a great strain on adaptation and are classified as stressors.

The body systems which are principally involved in the process of adaptation to the environment are the endocrine system for the long-term responses and the nervous system for the sensory inputs and the short-term responses. The endocrinal responses are principally the adrenal medullary response related to the 'flight or fight' situation which requires immediate response, and the adrenal cortical response which becomes operative if the stressful situation persists. In man, a large part of the 'stress' state is the result of stimuli arising in the cerebral cortex and is dependent on man's capacity to develop fear and anxiety about the effect of stressful situations, or even about the situations developing when they have not yet done so. Whether or not these psychological inputs play any part in animal disease is important but undecided. The evidence seems to suggest that psychic factors do play such a part, but that it is relatively minor.

The critical decision in relating 'stress' to disease is to decide when an environmental pressure exceeds that which the animal's adaptive mechanisms can reasonably accommodate. In other words, to define when each of the pressures outlined above does in fact become a stressor. There is a great dearth of definition in the subject. Probably the most serviceable is (1):

> Stress is any stimulus, internal or external, chemical or physical or emotional, that excites neurones of the hypothalamus to release corticotrophin-releasing hormone at rates greater than would occur at that time of the day in the absence of the stimulus.

The definition uses stress where stressor would have been more common usage. Other than that, it is acceptable. It lays the critical threshold of stress at the door of the adrenal cortex, and its physical determination is subject to a chemical assay of ACTH. This was the basis of the original 'Stress and the general adaptation syndrome' as set down by Selye (14). The original concept still has very great attraction because of its simplicity and logicality. However, finding hard evidence to support the theory has been a largely unfulfilled quest. The importance of the concept for our animals is unproven. The deficiency in evidence is that of obtaining a standard response to a standard application of a stimulus. There is a great deal of variation between animals, and stimuli which should be significant stressors appear to exert no effect at all on adrenocortical activity.

Clinical pathology

The direct criterion of stress is the assay of plasma ACTH, or indirectly of cortisol. Less direct assessment still is that of plasma fibrinogen. Salivary cortisol is also a good indicator in sheep (19). The sample is easy to collect and the laboratory assay easy to perform. It needs to be remembered that elevation of blood, and saliva cortisol levels is a normal physiological response and does not necessarily imply the existence of a damaging state of the environment (20).

Stress-related psychosomatic disease

In man there is a significant neuronal input from the cerebral cortex to the hypothalamus in response to the psychological pressure generated by stress. Inability to monitor anxiety and feelings of harassment in our animals makes it impossible to determine the presence or otherwise of psychological stress in them. However, psychosomatic diseases as they occur in man are almost unknown in farm animals. Two possible exceptions are esophagogastric ulcer in pigs and abomasal ulcer in adult cattle, especially bulls in insemination centers. However, in the former other factors are known to exert a very significant influence.

The pathogenesis of psychosomatic disease appears to be based on the ability of the cerebral cortex to effectively override the normal feedback mechanisms with which the pituitary gland regulates the secretion of corticosteroids from the adrenal cortex. In other words, the normal adaptive mechanisms do not operate and hyperadrenocorticism and adrenal exhaustion develop.

Stress and susceptibility to infection

Field observations very strongly support the view that stress reduces resistance to infection. This seems to be logical in the presence of higher than normal adrenocortical activity. The most intensively explored relationship of this kind has been that of exposure of calves to weaning and transportation, and their subsequent susceptibility to shipping fever. The prevalence appears to be increased and is still further enhanced by the introduction of other stress factors (2).

Stress and animal welfare

The harassment of domesticated animals by man has become a matter of great concern for the community at large. Intensive animal housing has become an accepted part of present-day agribusiness, but the consuming public is inclined to the view that these practices are cruel. The literature that has built up around the argument sets out to demonstrate that environmental stress in the shape of intensive housing, debeaking, detailing and so on is sufficient to cause a stress reaction as measured by increased corticosteroid secretion. Such has not been the case and this is understandable in the light of the known variation between animals in their response to environmental circumstances requiring their physiological adaptation. If it could be shown that this relationship did exist and that the increased adrenocortical activity caused reduction in resistance to infection the task of the responsible animal welfare person would be much easier. The absence of this experimental data makes the continuing argument less resolvable, but it is now generally accepted that the animal husbandman has a responsibility to his animals and to society generally to maintain an acceptable standard of humane care of animals (4). These arguments are usually expressed as *Codes of Animal Welfare* (9) to which most concerned people conform.

However, they are not statutory directives and are not capable of active enforcement. Some courts of law accept them as guidelines on what the human–animal relationship in agriculture should be. The codes themselves are quite arbitrary and are understandably heavily sprinkled with anthropomorphic sentiments (6). The study of ethology which has expanded greatly during the recent past may eventually provide some answers to this active, often bitterly fought-over field.

The status of animals used in experiments has always been a bone of contention between the experimenters and some sections of the general public. In general, these arguments revolve around anthropomorphic propositions that animals are subject to fear of pain, and illness and death in the same way as man is. There is no consistent evidence in physiological terms that supports these views. However, the public conscience has again achieved a good deal of acceptance to its view that animal experimentation should be controlled and restricted, and carefully policed to avoid unnecessary experiments and hardship in animals under our control.

Stress and metabolic disease

There is an inclination to label any disease caused by a strong pressure from an environmental factor as a 'stress' disease, for instance hypocalcemia of sheep and hypomagnesemia of cattle in cold weather, acetonemia and pregnancy toxemia of cattle and sheep on deficient diets, white muscle disease of calves and lambs on vigorous exercise. These diseases do have environmental origins, but their causes are much simpler than a complex interaction of the cerebral–cortical–hypothalamic–adrenocortical axis. They can be prevented and cured without any intervention in the 'stress' disease pathogenesis. This is not to say that there is no adrenocortical basis for the pathogenesis of the above-listed dieases, but attempts to establish the relationship have so far been unsuccessful (16). There is a good record of a number of dairy cows in one herd being affected by failure to let down their milk at milking time while being under the influence of a number of causes of stress; the cows had lower than normal serum cortisol levels (5).

Stress and its effect on economic performance

The constant struggle for domination of other animals in an animal population is most marked in chickens and pigs and the relationship between status in the hierarchy and productivity in these species has been established (13) with the low-status animals producing less well. It is also known (13) that birds which are highly sensitive and easily startled are poor producers and are easily identified and culled. The relationship between stress and production appears to be a real one. For example heat stress in the form of high environmental temperatures reduces roughage intake and hence milk production in dairy cows (18) and the relationships between stress and infertility (15) and stress and mastitis (17) in cattle are also well documented. The sensitivity of animals to environmental stress is greatest at times when they are already affected by metabolic stresses, e.g. late pregnancy and early lactation. At least the adoption of a policy of culling erratic, excitable animals appears to have an economic basis.

REVIEW LITERATURE

Dantzer, R. & Mormede, P. (1983) Stress in farm animals: a need for revaluation. *J. anim. Sci.*, *57*, 6.

Hails, M. R. (1978) Transport stress in animals. A review. *Anim. regulation Stud.*, *1*, 289.

Johnson, H. D. & Vanjonack, W. J. (1976) Symposium: stress and health of the dairy cow. *J. dairy Sci.*, *59*, 1603 & 1618.

Kilgour, J. (1978) The application of animal behaviour and the humane care of farm animals. *J. anim. Sci.*, *46*, 1478.

Ray, P. M. & Scott, W. N. (1973) Animal welfare legislation in the FFC. *Br. vet. J.*, *129*, 194.

Selye, H. (1973) The evaluation of the stress concept. *Am. Sci.*, *61*, 692.

Stephens, D. B. (1980) Stress and its measurement in domestic animals. *Adv. vet. Sci.*, *24*, 179.

REFERENCES

(1) Montcastle, V. B. (1974) *Medical Physiology*. St Louis: C. V. Mosby Co. *13*, 1697.
(2) Crookshank, H. R. et al. (1979) *J. anim. Sci.*, *48*, 4 & 439.
(3) Kelley, K. W. et al. (1980) *J. anim. Sci.*, *50*, 336.
(4) Kilgour, R. (1978) *J. anim. Sci.*, *46*, 1478.
(5) McCaughan, C. J. & Malecki, J. C. (1981) *Aust. vet. J.*, *57*, 203.
(6) Wood-Gush, D. G. M. (1973) *Br. vet. J.*, *129*, 167.
(7) Penny, R. H. C. et al. (1981) *Vet. Rec.*, 108, 35.
(8) Webster, A. J. F. (1981) *Vet. Rec.*, *108*, 183.
(9) Ministry for Agriculture, Food and Fisheries (1977) *Codes of Recommendations for the Welfare of Livestock*. Codes No. 1 to 5.
(10) Barnett, J. L. et al. (1984) *Appl. anim. Behav. Sci.*, *12*, 209.
(11) Pearson, A. J. et al. (1977) *Proc. NZ Soc. anim. Prod.*, *37*, 243.
(12) Johnson, H. D. & Vanjonack, W. J. (1976) *J. dairy Sci.*, *59*, 1603 & 1618.
(13) Stephens, D. B. (1980) *Adv. vet. Sci.*, *24*, 179.
(14) Selye, H. (1973) *Am. Sci.*, *61*, 692.
(15) Cowbrough, R. I. (1985) *Onderstepoort J. vet. Res.*, *52*, 153.
(16) Fraser, D. et al. (1975) *Br. vet. J.*, *131*, 653.
(17) Giesecke, W. H. (1985) *Onderstepoort J. vet. Res.*, *52*, 175.
(18) Collier, R. J. et al. (1982) *J. dairy Sci.*, *65*, 2213.
(19) Fell, L. R. et al. (1985) *Aust. vet. J.*, *62*, 403.
(20) Rushen, J. (1986) *Aust. vet. J.*, *63*, 359.
(21) Webster, A. J. F. (1986) *J. anim. Sci.*, *57*, 1584 et seq.

SUDDEN DEATH

When an animal is found dead without having been previously observed to be ill a diagnosis, even after necropsy examination, is often difficult because of the absence of clinical findings and epidemiology. Following is a checklist of diseases which could be considered when sudden death occurs. Details of each of the diseases listed are available in other sections of the book. The list applies particularly to cattle, but some occurrences in other species are noted. It is necessary to point out the difference between 'found dead' and 'sudden death'.

When animals are observed infrequently, for example at weekly intervals, it is possible for them to be ill with obvious clinical signs for some days without being observed. In these circumstances the list of possible diagnoses is very large. It is also correspondingly large when animals are run in large groups and are not observed as individuals. This is likely to happen in beef cattle, especially in feedlots or as calves with dams at pasture, when the animals are unaccustomed to human presence and move away when approached. The list below refers to animals that are closely observed as individuals at least once daily.

Sudden death in single animals

Spontaneous internal hemorrhage could be due to cardiac tamponade in cows, ruptured aorta or atrium or inherited aortic aneurysm or verminous mesenteric arterial aneurysm in horses, esophagogastric ulcer or intestinal hemorrhagic syndrome in pigs. In one survey of sudden deaths in horses while racing most (68%) were undiagnosed although it was assumed that they died of exercise-induced acute heart failure. Of those that were diagnosed most were due to spontaneous hemorrhage (1). Similar conclusions have resulted from other surveys (2).

Peracute endogenous toxemia, especially from rupture of stomach of horses, abomasum of cows, colon in mares at foaling, with large amounts of gastrointestinal contents deposited rapidly into the peritoneal cavity. In newborn animals, especially foals, fulminating infections are the commonest cause.

Peracute exogenous toxemia in a single animal could be snakebite, but the snake would have to be very large and potent to cause death without observable illness.

Trauma may cause death by either internal hemorrhage or damage to the central nervous system, especially brain or atlanto-occipital joint sufficient to damage medulla oblongata. In most cases the trauma is evident; there has been fighting, or a fall has occurred, or the animal has attempted to jump an obstacle. In horses a gallop while free may end in a crash when it is downhill, the ground is slippery and there is a wall at the end. Unapparent trauma usually occurs when animals are tied up by halter and rush backwards when frightened or are startled by an electric fence and the halter shank is long. Sometimes the animal will plunge forward and hit its forehead between the eyes on a protruding small object such as a bolt used in a fence. Sadism, especially by the insertion of whip handles or pitch fork handles into anus or vulva can also be unapparent.

Iatrogenic deaths may be due to overdose with intravenous solutions of calcium salts in an excited cow, too rapid fluid infusion in an animal with pulmonary edema, intravenous injection of procaine penicillin suspension, and intravenous injections of ivermectin in horses. These are not usually hard to diagnose. The farmer or the veterinarian are usually obviously embarrassed. One of the most sudden death occurrences is the anaphylactoid reaction in a horse to an intravenous injection of an allergen such as crystalline penicillin. Death occurs in about 60 seconds.

Sudden death in a group of animals

The diseases listed below could obviously affect single animals only if the animals were housed or run singly. It is also possible that only one animal would be affected if it were the only one exposed to the pathogenic agent, but group involvement is more likely.

Lightning strike or electrocution
This is usually accompanied by a number of animals all together in a pile or group. Rarely, electrical current only electrifies a contact object intermittently and deaths will be intermittent. In most cases the history and an examination of the environment reveals the cause.

Nutritional deficiency and poisoning
At pasture, sudden death may come from the sudden exposure of cattle to plants which cause bloat, hypomagnesemia, cyanide or nitrite poisoning, fluoroacetate poisoning (e.g., in the gidgee tree), fast death factor produced by algae in a lake or pond or acute interstitial pneumonia. Acute myocardiopathy in young animals on diets deficient in vitamin E or selenium are in this group, as is inherited myocardiopathy in Herefords. Gross nutritional deficiency of copper in cattle causes 'falling disease', a manifestation of acute myocardiopathy. Acute myocardiopathy and heart failure is caused by poisons in *Phalaris* sp. pasture, grass nematodes on *Lolium rigidum*, the hemlocks *Cicuta* and *Oenanthe* spp. and the weeds *Fadogia*, *Pachystigma*, *Pavette*, *Ascelapius* and *Aeriocarpa*, *Crytostegia* and *Albizia*, *Cassia* spp., also the trees oleander and yew (*Taxus* sp.) and those containing fluoroacetate such as the gidgee tree and the weeds *Gastrolobium*, *Oxylobium*, *Dichapetalum* and *Ixioloena* spp. There are a number of plants that cause cardiac irregularity and some sudden deaths, e.g. *Urginea*, *Kalanchoe* spp., but more commonly congestive heart failure. Monensin, lasolocid and salinomycin are increasingly common causes in horses, and to a less extent cows.

Access to potent poisons
Access to potent poisons is often found in prepared feeds in housed animals.

There are few poisons which cause sudden death without premonitory signs. Cyanide is one, but is an unlikely poison in these circumstances. Monensin, mixed in a feed for cattle which is then fed to horses, or fed in large excess to cattle, does cause death by heart failure. Organophosphates are more likely, but clinical signs are usually apparent. Lead is in a similar category, but very soluble lead salts can cause death quickly in young animals.

Diseases caused by infectious agents
These cause septicemia or toxemia, and include anthrax, blackleg, hemorrhagic septicemia, and peracute pasteurellosis especially in sheep, but occasionally in cattle. In pigs, mulberry heart disease and perhaps gut edema should be considered. In horses, colitis is about the only disease that will do this. In sheep and young cattle, enterotoxemia caused by *Clostridium perfringens* is on the list as it is, together with rumen overload in cattle in feedlots on heavy grain feed. Circumstances, feeding practices,

climate, season of the year usually give some clue as to cause.

Neonatal and young animals
In very young, including neonatal, animals congenital defects which are incompatible with life, prematurity, septicemia because of poor immune status or toxemia caused by particular pathogens, especially *Escherichia coli* and hypothyroidism, are important causes of sudden death.

Anaphylaxis
Anaphylaxis after injection of biological materials including vaccines and sera is usually an obvious diagnosis, but its occurrence in animals at pasture can cause obscure deaths. In these circumstances it is usually only one animal and clinical illness is usually observed. A similar occurrence is sudden death in a high proportion of a litter of newborn pigs injected with an iron preparation when their selenium–vitamin E status is low.

Procedure of examination of a sudden death incident

This is as follows:

1. Keep more than usually good records because of the probability of insurance enquiry or litigation.
2. Take a careful history which may indicate changes of feed or source of it, exposure to poisons, or administration of potentially toxic preparations.
3. Make a careful examination of the environment to look for potential sources of pathogens. Be especially careful of your personal welfare if electrocution is possible—wet concrete floors can be lethal when combined with electrical current unless you are wearing rubber boots.
4. Carefully examine the animals for signs of struggling, frothy nasal discharge, unclotted blood from natural orifices, bloat, pallor or otherwise of mucosae, burn marks on body especially on the feet or signs of trauma or of having been restrained. Pay particular attention to the forehead by palpating the frontal bones which may have been fractured with a heavy blunt object without much damage to the skin or hair.
5. Ensure that typical cadavers are examined at necropsy, preferably by specialist pathologists at independent laboratories, where opinions are more likely to be considered authoritative and unbiased.
6. Collect samples of suspect materials for analysis. Preferably, collect two samples, one to be made available to the opposition, e.g., a feed company, if this is appropriate.

REFERENCES

(1) Gelberg, H. B. et al. (1985) *J. Am. vet. med. Assoc.*, *187*, 1354.
(2) Platt, H. (1982) *Br. vet. J.*, *138*, 417.

DISTURBANCES OF BODY FLUIDS, ELECTROLYTES AND ACID–BASE BALANCE

There are many diseases of farm animals in which there are disturbances of body fluids, electrolytes and acid–base balance. A disturbance of body water balance in which more fluid is lost from the body than is absorbed results in reduction in circulating volume of the blood and in *dehydration* of tissues. *Electrolyte imbalances* occur commonly as a result of loss of electrolytes, shifts of certain electrolytes, or relative changes in concentrations due to loss of water. *Acid–base* imbalances, either *acidosis* or *alkalosis*, occur as a result of the addition of acid and depletion of alkali reserve or the loss of acid with a relative increase in bicarbonate. Under most conditions, all of the above disturbances of fluid and electrolyte balance will occur simultaneously, in varying degrees, depending on the initial cause. Each major abnormality will be described separately here with emphasis on etiology, pathogenesis, clinical pathology and treatment. However, it is important to remember that actual disease states in animals, in which treatments with fluids and electrolytes are contemplated, are rarely caused by single abnormalities. In most cases it is a combination of dehydration together with an electrolyte deficit, and often without a disturbance of the acid–base balance.

Dehydration

There are two major causes of dehydration. There is either failure of water intake or excessive loss. Deprivation of water, a lack of thirst due to toxemia and the inability to drink water as in esophageal obstruction are some common causes of dehydration. But the most common is when excessive fluid is lost. Diarrhea is the most common cause, although vomiting, polyuria and loss of fluid from extensive skin wounds or by copious sweating may be important in sporadic cases. Severe dehydration also occurs in acute carbohydrate engorgement in ruminants, acute intestinal obstruction and diffuse peritonitis in all species, and in dilatation and torsion of the abomasum. In most forms of dehydration, deprivation of drinking water being an exception, the serious loss, and the one that needs repair, is not the fluid but the electrolytes (Fig. 6).

The ability to survive for long periods without water in hot climates represents a form of animal adaptation which is of some importance. This adaptation has been examined in camels and in Merino sheep. In the latter, the ability to survive in dry, arid conditions depends on a number of factors, including insulation, the ability to carry water reserves in the rumen and extracellular fluid space, the ability to adjust electrolyte concentrations in the several fluid locations, the ability of the kidney to conserve water and the ability to maintain the circulation with a lower plasma volume.

Two factors are involved in the pathogenesis of dehydration: the depression of tissue fluid levels with resulting interference in tissue metabolism, and an-

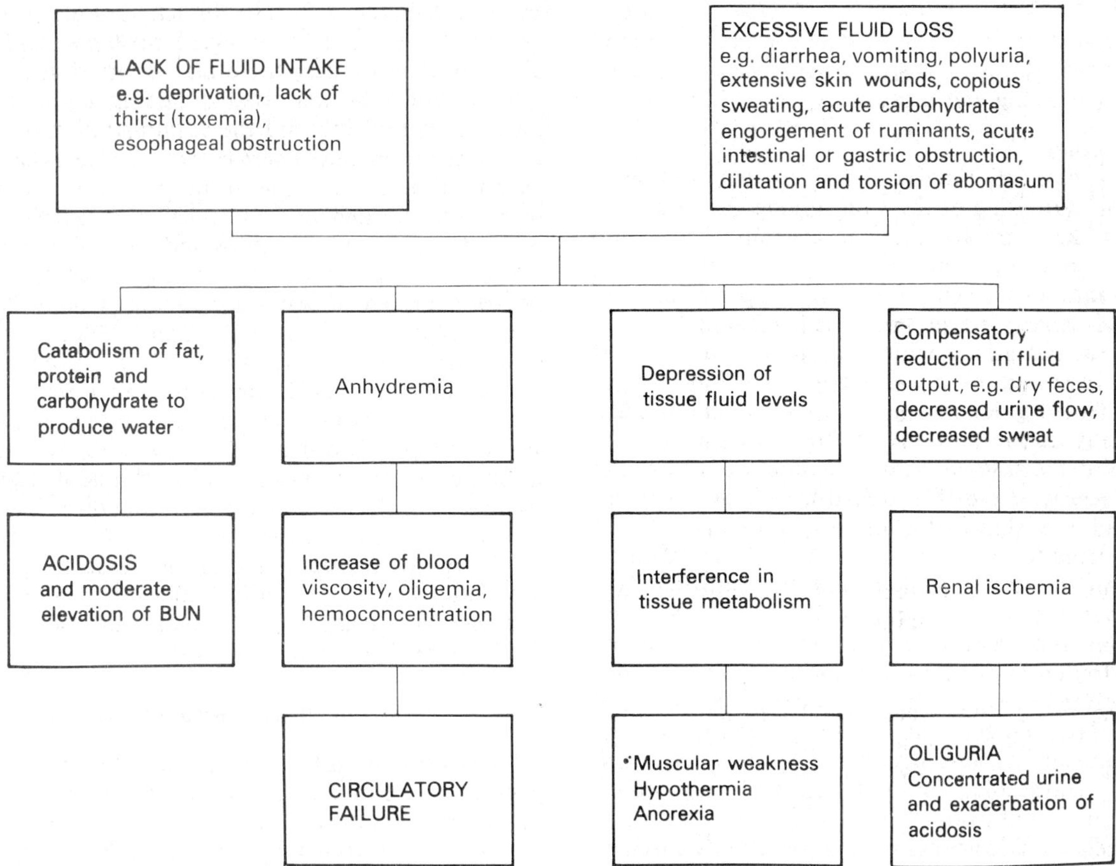

Fig. 6. Etiology and pathogenesis of dehydration

hydremia with reduction in the fluid content of the blood. The initial response to negative water balance is the withdrawal of fluid from the tissues and the maintenance of normal blood volume. The fluid is drained primarily from the intravascular compartment and the interstitial fluid space. Essential organs including the central nervous system, heart and skeleton contribute little and the major loss occurs from connective tissue, muscle and skin. In the goat, total body water may be reduced as much as 44% before death occurs (2).

The secondary response is a reduction in the fluid content of the blood causing a reduction in circulating blood volume (oligemia) and an increase in the concentration of the blood (hemoconcentration). Because of the hemoconcentration, there is an increase in the viscosity of the blood which impedes blood flow and further exacerbates the peripheral circulatory failure. In deprivation of water and electrolytes or in deprivation of water, or inability to consume water in an otherwise normal animal (esophageal obstruction), the dehydration is minimal because the kidney compensates effectively by decreasing output and increasing concentration. In addition, water is preserved by reduced fecal output and increased absorption, which results in dehydration of the contents of the rumen and large intestine which in turn results in dry scant feces.

In calves with acute diarrhea there is increased fecal output of water compared to normal calves but the total water losses are not significantly greater than in normal calves. In the diarrheic calf the kidney compensates very effectively (20) for fecal water loss, and the plasma volume can be maintained if there is an adequate oral fluid intake (4). This serves to illustrate the importance of oral fluid and electrolyte intake during diarrhea to compensate for continuous losses. The dehydration in horses used in endurance rides is hypotonic, which may account for the lack of thirst in some dehydrated horses with the exhaustion syndrome. Weight losses of 10–15 kg/hour may occur in horses exercising in high environmental temperatures exceeding 32°C (89°F). A horse weighing 450 kg can lose 45 liters of fluid in a 3-hour ride (39).

Dehydration exerts some important effects on tissue metabolism. There is an increase in breakdown of fat, then carbohydrate and finally protein, to produce water of metabolism. The increased endogenous metabolism under relatively anerobic conditions results in the formation of acid metabolites and the development of acidosis. Urine formation decreases because of the restriction of blood flow and this, together with the increased endogenous metabolism, causes a moderate increase in blood levels of non-protein nitrogen (5). The body temperature rises slightly—dehydration hyperthermia—because of insufficient fluid to maintain the loss of heat by evaporation. The onset of sweating in steers after exposure to high environmental temperatures has been shown to be delayed by dehydration (6).

Dehydration may cause death, especially in acute intestinal obstruction, vomiting and diarrhea, but it is chiefly a contributory cause of death when combined with other systemic states, such as acidosis, electrolyte imbalances, toxemia and septicemia.

Clinical findings

The first and most important sign in dehydration is dryness and wrinkling of the skin, giving the body and face a shrunken appearance. The eyeballs recede into the sockets and the skin subsides slowly after being picked up into a fold. The skin of the upper eyelid and of the neck gives one of the best indications of the degree of dehydration, which on a clinical basis is commonly assessed as a percentage of body weight (Table 1). Some guidelines are as follows. The mildest form of dehydration at 4–6% of body weight may be just barely detectable clinically but hemoconcentration may be present. At 6–8% dehydration, the eyes are sunken and the skin-fold ('tenting of the skin') will remain elevated for 2–4 seconds; at 8–10% dehydration the eyes are markedly sunken and the skin-fold will remain elevated for 6–10 seconds; at 10–12% dehydration the skin-fold may remain elevated for 20–45 seconds. The dehydration is usually much more marked if water and electrolyte losses have been occurring over a period of several days. Peracute and acute losses may not be obvious clinically because major loss will have occurred from the intravascular compartment and only minor shifts have occurred from the interstitial spaces. Sunken eyes and inelastic skin are not remarkable clinical findings of dehydration in the horse.

Loss of body weight occurs rapidly; there is muscular weakness and lack of appetite. The degree of thirst present will depend on the presence or absence of toxemia. In primary water deprivation, dehydrated animals are very thirsty when offered water. In cattle on pasture and deprived of water for up to 9 days and then given access to water there will be staggering, falling, convulsions and some death. This is similar to the syndrome of salt poisoning in pigs (40). Experimental restriction of the water intake in lactating dairy cattle for up to 4 days may reduce milk yield by 75% and decrease body weight by 14%. A 10% reduction in water intake causes a drop in milk production which may be difficult to detect. Behavioral changes are obvious; cows spend considerable time licking the water bowls (41, 42). In cold climates, cattle are often forced to eat snow as a source of water. The snow must be soft enough so that it can be scooped up by the cattle and 3–5 days are necessary for the animals to adjust to the absence of water and become dependent on snow. During this time there is some loss of body weight (43). Lactating ewes relying on snow as a source of free water reduce their total water turnover by approximately 35% (60). In dehydration secondary to enteritis associated with severe toxemia, acidosis and electrolyte imbalance, there may be no desire to drink. Horses which become dehydrated in endurance rides may refuse to drink and the administration of water by oral intubation and enemas may be necessary. Urine excretion decreases, the urine becomes progressively more concentrated and the renal insufficiency may accentuate pre-existing acidosis and electrolyte imbalance, hence the importance of restoring renal function. In horses deprived of water for 72 hours there is a mean body weight loss of about 15%, and 95% of the animals have a urine specific gravity of 1·042, a urine osmolality of 1310 mOsm/kg (1310 mmol/l) and a urine osmolality/serum osmolality ratio of 4:14 (59). Extrarenal azotemia also develops. The newborn calf is able to concentrate urine at almost the same level as the adult (20). Goats are more sensitive to water deprivation during pregnancy and lactation than during anestrus. Water deprivation for 30 hours causes a marked increase in the plasma osmolality and plasma sodium concentration in pregnant and lactating goats (3). Pregnant and lactating goats drink more than goats in anestrus.

Electrolyte imbalances

Most electrolyte imbalances are due to net loss of electrolytes due to disease of the alimentary tract. Sweating, exudation from burns, excessive salivation and vomiting are also accompanied by electrolyte losses, but are of minor importance in farm animals with the exception of losses which occur in sweating in the horse. The electrolytes of major concern are sodium, potassium, chloride and bicarbonate.

HYPONATREMIA

Sodium is the most abundant ion in the extracellular fluid and is chiefly responsible for maintenance of the osmotic pressure of the extracellular fluid. The most common cause of hyponatremia is increased loss of sodium through the intestinal tract in enteritis (Fig. 7). This is particularly marked in the horse with acute diarrhea (7). There is also loss of sodium in newborn calves with acute diarrhea (8, 9). The sodium is lost at the expense of the extracellular fluid. In calves with acute diarrhea due to enterotoxigenic *E. coli* the sodium concentration of the intestinal fluid produced in response to the enterotoxin is similar to that in plasma and hyponatremia usually occurs (hypotonic dehydration) (8). Animals affected with diarrhea of several days duration continue to lose large quantities of sodium and the hyponatremia may become severe. Hyponatremia can become severe

Table 1. Degrees of severity of dehydration and guidelines for assessment

Body weight loss (%)	*Sunken eyes, shrunken face*	*Skin fold test persists for* (*sec*)	*PCV* (%)	*Total serum solids* (*g/l*)	*Fluid required to replace volume deficit* (*ml/kg body weight*)
4–6	Barely detectable	—	40–45	70–80	20–25
6–8	++	2–4	50	80–90	30–50
8–10	+++	6–10	55	90–100	50–80
10–12	++++	20–45	60	120	80–120

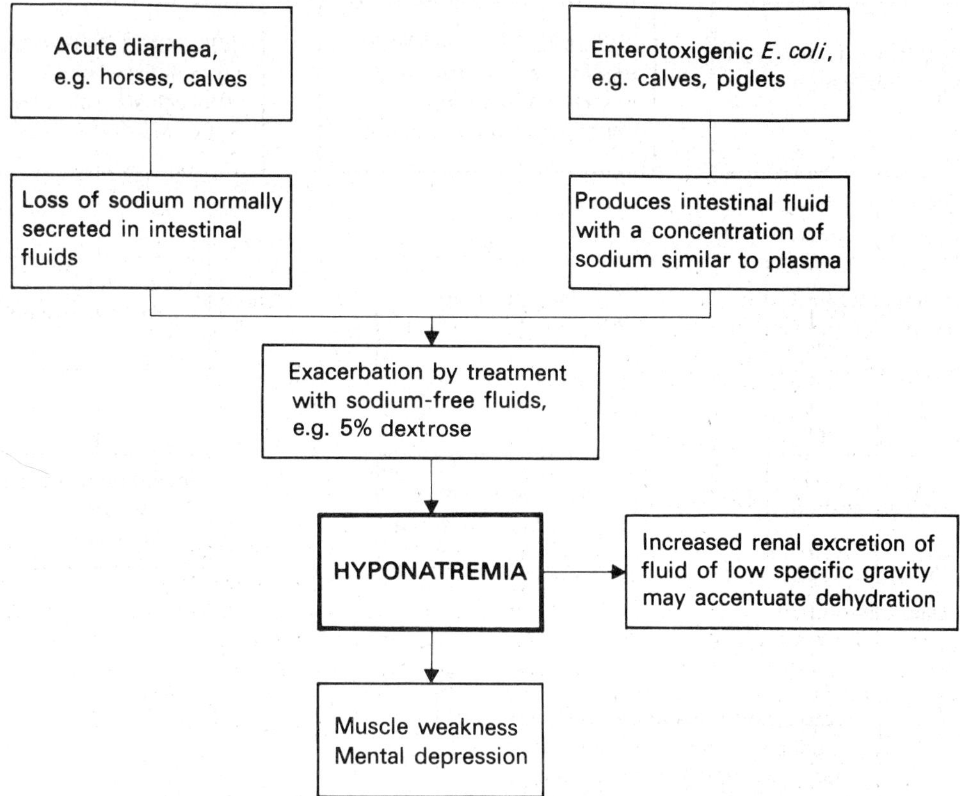

Fig. 7. Etiology and pathogenesis of hyponatremia

when sodium-free water or 5% dextrose are used as the only fluid therapy in animals already affected with hyponatremia.

Hyponatremia causes an increase in the renal excretion of water in an attempt to maintain normal osmotic pressure, which results in a decrease in the extracellular fluid space leading to a decreased circulating blood volume, hypotension, peripheral circulatory failure and ultimately renal failure. There is muscular weakness, hypothermia and marked dehydration.

Isotonic dehydration occurs when there is a parallel loss of water, and hypertonic dehydration, which is uncommon, when there is a loss or deprivation of water with minor losses or deprivation of sodium. The latter can occur in animals which are unable to consume water because of an esophageal obstruction. The dehydration in isotonic and hypertonic dehydration is mild compared to the marked clinical dehydration which can occur in hypotonic dehydration accompanied by marked loss of water and concentration of the extracellular space (Fig. 8).

There are no clinical signs which are characteristic of hyponatremia. There is usually dehydration, muscular weakness and mental depression, which occur with other disturbances of both water and electrolytes and with acid–base imbalance. Similarly there are no clinical signs characteristic of hypochloremia. However, hyponatremia affects the osmotic pressure of the extracellular fluid, and hypochloremia promotes the reabsorption of bicarbonate and further development of alkalosis. Polyuria and polydipsia occur in cattle with dietary sodium chloride deficiency (10).

HYPOCHLOREMIA

Hypochloremia occurs as a result of an increase in the net loss of the ion in the intestinal tract in acute intestinal obstruction, dilatation and impaction and torsion of the abomasum and in enteritis (Fig. 9). Normally a large amount of hydrochloric acid is secreted in the abomasum by the mucosal cells in exchange for sodium bicarbonate which moves into the plasma. The hydrogen, chloride and potassium ions of the gastric juice are normally absorbed by the small intestine (11). Failure of abomasal emptying and obstruction of the proximal part of the small intestine will result in the sequestration of large quantities of chloride, hydrogen and potassium ions which leads to a hypochloremic, hypokalemic alkalosis (12). A severe hypochloremia can be experimentally produced in calves by feeding them a low chloride diet and daily removal of abomasal contents. Clinical findings include anorexia, weight loss, lethargy, mild polydipsia and polyuria. A marked metabolic alkalosis occurs with hypokalemia, hyponatremia, azotemia and death (62).

HYPOKALEMIA AND HYPERKALEMIA

Hypokalemia may occur as a result of decreased dietary intake, increased renal excretion, abomasal stasis, intestinal obstruction and enteritis (Fig. 10). The prolonged administration of mineralocorticoids and the prolonged use of potassium-free solutions in fluid therapy for diarrheic animals may result in excessive renal excretion of potassium and hypokalemia. Alkalosis may result in an exchange of potassium ions for hydrogens ions in the

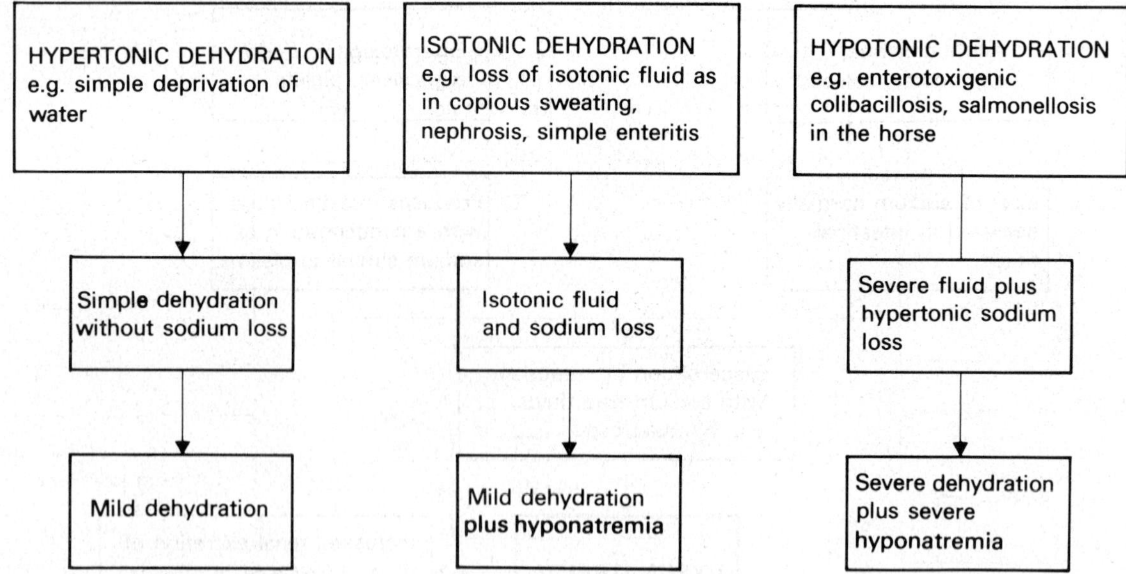

Fig. 8. Types of dehydration

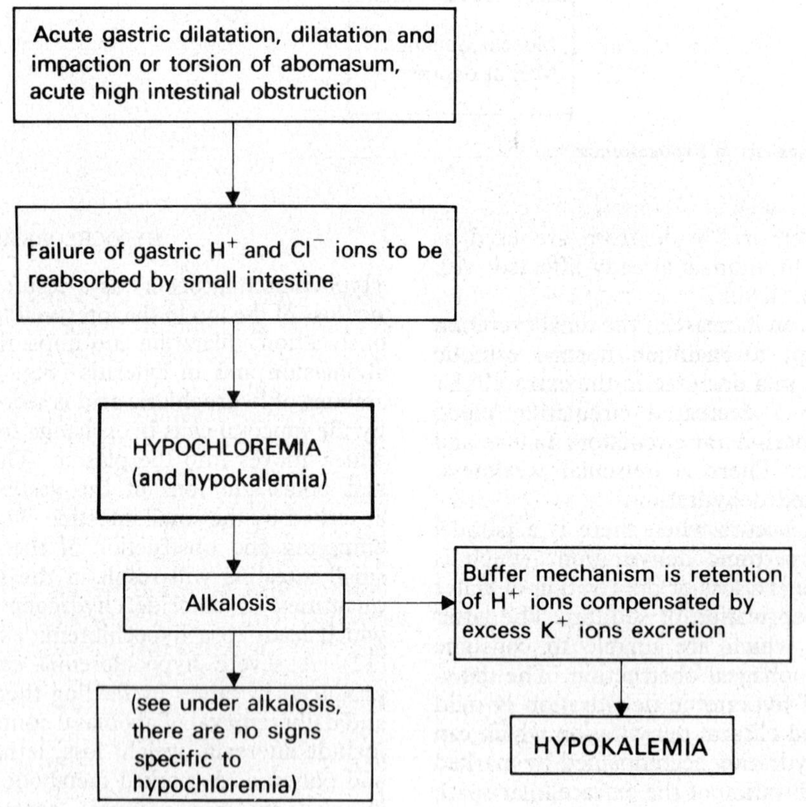

Fig. 9. Etiology and pathogenesis of hypochloremia

renal tubular fluid resulting in hypokalemia. The most common occurrence of hypokalemia is in diseases of the abomasum which cause stasis and the accumulation of fluid in the abomasum (11). Potassium becomes sequestered in the abomasum along with hydrogen and chloride, resulting in hypokalemia, hypochloremia and metabolic alkalosis.

The metabolic alkalosis and hypokalemia are often accompanied by muscular weakness and paradoxic aciduria (11). Hypokalemia causes muscle weakness by lowering the resting potential of membranes, resulting in decreased excitability of neuromuscular tissue. Thus, the differential diagnosis of the animal with muscle weakness should always include hypokalemia.

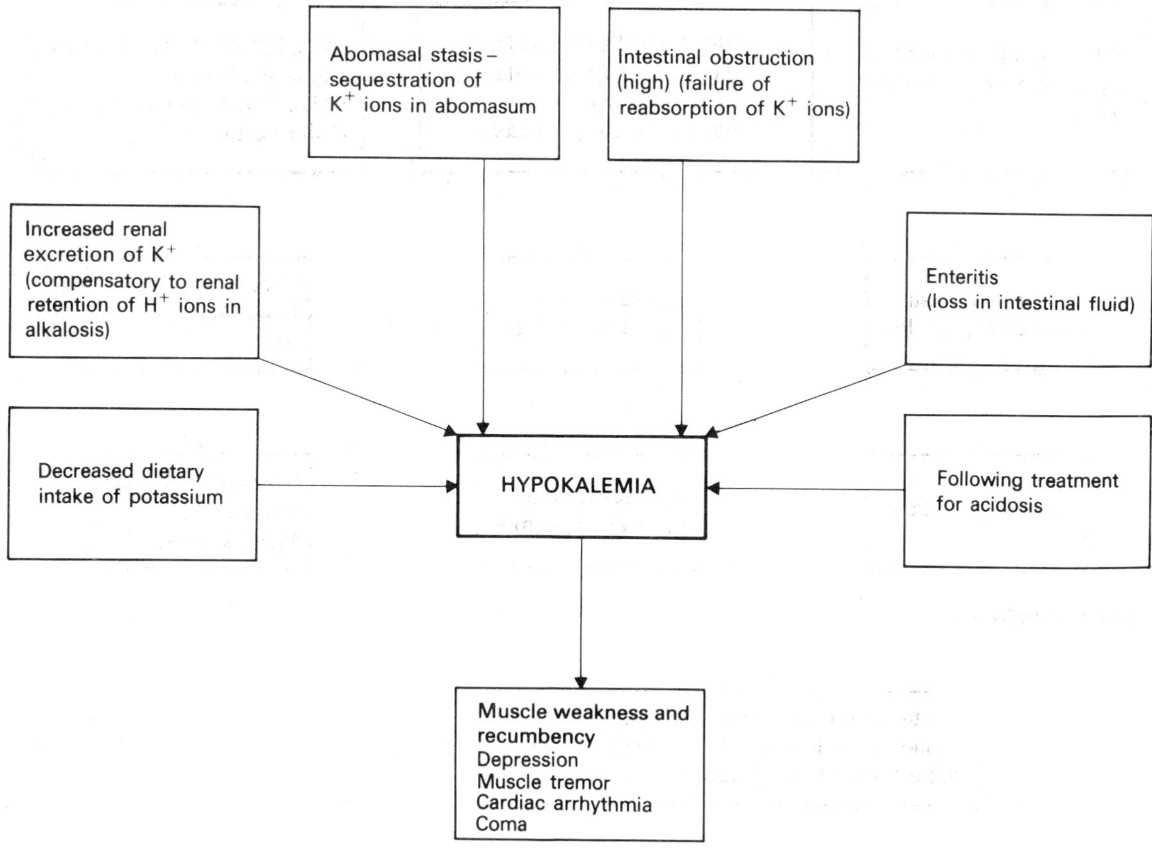

Fig. 10. Etiology and pathogenesis of hypokalemia

The hypokalemia and alkalosis are often directly related because of the renal response to either. Hypokalemia from true body deficits of potassium will cause decreased intracellular concentration of this ion. The intracellular deficit of potassium and excess of hydrogen will cause hydrogen secretion into the urine when distal sodium reabsorption is required. This situation exists in metabolic alkalosis where sodium bicarbonate reabsorption in the proximal nephron is decreased because of the excess of plasma bicarbonate. Distal nephron avidity for sodium is increased to protect extracellular fluid volume, and the increased distal sodium reabsorption is at the expense of hydrogen secretion, although it is contrary to the need of acid retention in the presence of alkalosis. The kidneys' function is to maintain electroneutrality of extracellular fluid by reabsorbing appropriate amounts of cations and anions. Since the major inorganic anions are chloride and bicarbonate, the reabsorption of these anions in the kidneys is inversely proportional to each other. Thus, with excess trapping of chloride in the abomasum, the kidneys will compensate for the resulting hypochloremia by increasing bicarbonate reabsorption which may proceed until metabolic alkalosis develops.

The treatment of hypochloremic, hypokalemic alkalosis requires only correction of extracellular fluid volume and sodium and chloride deficits with saline infusions (1). Providing adequate chloride ion allows sodium to be reabsorbed without bicarbonate. Increased proximal reabsorption of sodium will decrease distal acid secretion because less sodium is presented to the distal nephron. As less bicarbonate is reabsorbed and less acid secreted, plasma pH returns to normal. Concurrently, some intracellular potassium ions are replaced by hydrogen ions, and this pH-mediated cation shift also aids the return to normokalemia. Thus, saline infusions are usually sufficient to correct hypokalemic alkalosis. Only in cases of severe hypokalemia are the special formulated solutions containing potassium necessary. A similar situation occurs in obstruction of the upper intestinal tract (13). Hypokalemia also occurs following treatment of the horse affected with metabolic acidosis and hyponatremia. It has been suggested that correction of the acidosis results in an exchange of intracellular hydrogen and extracellular potassium (14). Horses used for endurance rides may be affected by hypokalemia, hypocalcemia and alkalosis due to loss of electrolytes during the competition (15). Synchronous diaphragmatic flutter also occurs, which may be the result of the electrolyte imbalance causing hyperirritability of the phrenic nerve (16) but the exact mechanism is not understood.

Since potassium is one of the major intracellular ions, the measurement of plasma or serum potassium is not a reliable indication of the potassium status of the body (17). Extremely low levels or high levels are usually indicative of a potassium imbalance, often associated with other electrolyte and acid–base imbalances. In severe alkalosis, for example, the potassium leaves the extracellular space and becomes concentrated in the cells. This may result in low serum potassium levels when, in fact, there might not be potassium depletion of the body. Conversely, in severe metabolic acidosis of calves with acute diarrhea, the potassium leaves the cells and moves into the extracellular fluid. This results in hyperkalemia in some cases where the body potassium is normal or even decreased. When changes occur in the concentration of intracellular and extracellular potassium, the ratio of intracellular to extracellular potassium may decrease by as much as 30–50%, which results in a decrease in the resting membrane potential (9). This is thought to be the explanation for the effects of hypokalemia and hyperkalemia on muscle function.

The potassium concentration of red blood cells may be a more accurate indicator of whole body potassium deficit in diarrheic horses and it provides a basis for a calculated oral dose of potassium chloride in horses with diarrhea which is a safe therapeutic procedure (66). Hypokalemia can cause muscle weakness, prolonged unexplained recumbency, inability to hold up the head, anorexia, muscular tremors and, if severe enough, coma.

Hyperkalemia is not as common in farm animals as is hypokalemia and occurs most commonly following severe metabolic acidosis. There is redistribution of potassium from the intracellular space to the extracellular space because a large proportion of the excess hydrogen ions are buffered intracellularly. Thus potassium and sodium leave to maintain neutrality (63). Hyperkalemia is potentially more dangerous than hypokalemia. Hyperkalemia (usually when over 7–8 mmol/l) has a marked effect on cardiac function. There is usually marked bradycardia and arrhythmia and sudden cardiac arrest may occur (18). The electrocardiographic changes in experimentally induced hyperkalemia in the horse have been described (64, 65). The ECG changes include four successive stages as hyperkalemia increased. There was a widening and lowering of amplitude followed by inversion and disappearance of the P wave, an increase in the amplitude of the T wave, an increase in the QRS interval, with some irregularity in the ventricular rate, and periods of cardiac arrest that became terminal or were followed by ventricular fibrillation (65). The minimum plasma potassium concentration required to induce ECG changes was 6–7 mmol/l and severe cardiotoxic effects occur at levels between 8 and 11 mmol/l (64, 65).

An episodic muscular weakness associated with serum hyperkalemia occurs in heavily muscled quarter horse-bred stock horses (74). Affected horses become weak, may stand base-wide and are reluctant to move. Sweating commonly occurs and generalized muscle fasciculations are apparent. Affected horses remain bright and alert but may yawn and do not eat or drink. Some horses become recumbent and may appear to be in a state of flaccidity. Attacks may occur in a rest period following exercise or at random. During the episode the serum potassium levels are elevated by two-fold and return to normal levels when the animal recovers. Treatment consists of sodium bicarbonate of 5% dextrose given intravenously.

The clinical findings associated with synchronous diaphragmatic flutter in the horse accompanied by an electrolyte imbalance consist of 'thumps' synchronous with each atrial contraction (16). There is usually some primary disorder which is causing the electrolyte imbalance.

HYPOCALCEMIA

Hypocalcemia may occur in recently calved mature dairy cows which have been inappetent or anorexic for a few days. The hypocalcemia can be due to a reduction in feed intake because of any illness which may have affected appetite, decreased absorption in diarrheic states or, it may be the earliest stages of hypocalcemic parturient paresis. The clinical findings include anorexia, tachycardia with a reduction in the intensity of the heart sounds and occasionally an arrhythmia, a decrease in the frequency and amplitude of rumen contractions or complete ruminal stasis, and a decrease or complete absence of feces which may last from 6 to 36 hours if untreated. These often mimic intestinal obstruction and create problems in the differential diagnosis. Affected cattle may not exhibit any evidence of muscular weakness and the detection of the hypocalcemic state can be elusive. The total serum calcium levels range from 1·5 to 2·0 mmol/l and the response to therapy with calcium borogluconate is usually good although recovery may require several hours before the appetite returns to normal and feces are passed.

HYPOPHOSPHATEMIA

Hypophosphatemia also occurs in cattle under conditions similar to those of hypocalcemia. A decrease in feed intake or alimentary tract states will result in a decrease in serum inorganic phosphate. There are no clinical signs attributed to the decreased levels which return to normal when feed intake and alimentary tract function are restored to normal.

Acid–base imbalance

The pH of the blood is maintained within the normal range of 7·35–7·45 by its buffer systems, of which the bicarbonate system is most important. The addition of relatively large amounts of acid or alkali to the blood is necessary before its buffering capacity is exhausted and its pH changed. The proportion of the dissolved carbon dioxide and the bicarbonate ion, which form the components of the buffer system, are maintained at a constant level either by increased pulmonary ventilation and discharge of carbon dioxide, or by increased urinary excretion of the bicarbonate radical.

Changes from normal acid–base balance towards either alkalosis or acidosis make significant contributions to ill-health and to clinical signs observed. Some information on acid–base balance is available for horses (19, 73) and for cattle (17, 73).

ACIDOSIS

The common causes of acidosis include: excessive loss of the bicarbonate ion in acute enteritis; the production and absorption of large quantities of fixed acid such as lactic acid in acute carbohydrate engorgement in ruminants; grain engorgement in horses and ketosis in ruminants (Fig. 11). Acidosis also occurs where there is retention of carbon dioxide in the blood due to interference with normal respiratory exchange. Thus pneumonia, severe pulmonary emphysema, depression of the

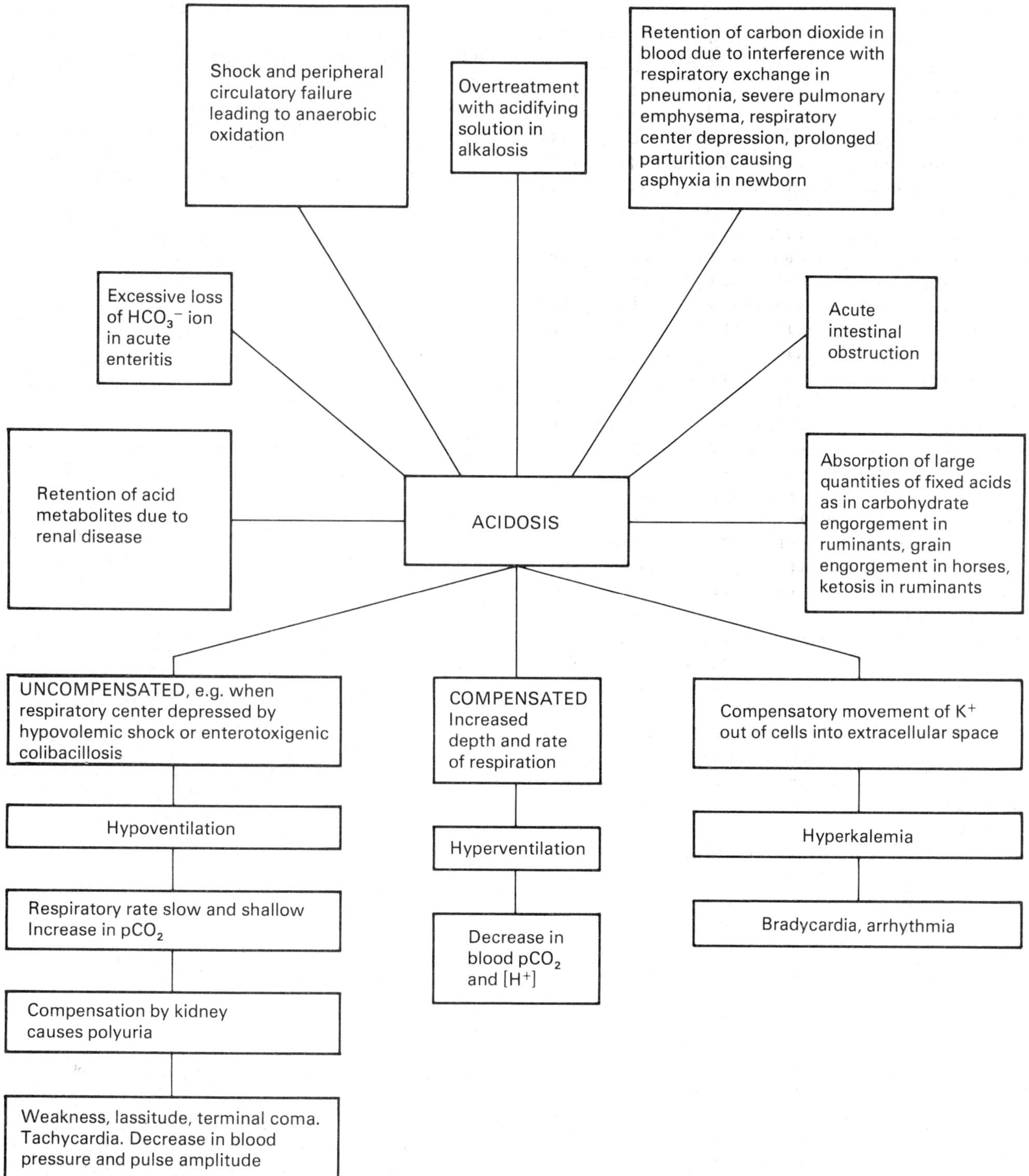

Fig. 11. Etiology and pathogenesis of acidosis

respiratory center and congestive heart failure may all be accompanied by acidosis. Acidosis also occurs in the newborn at the time of parturition if this is prolonged and difficult (21). It is also common in shock with peripheral circulatory failure and anerobic oxidation. A decrease in renal excretion of acid in renal insufficiency or renal failure also contributes to an acidotic state. The administration of excessive quantities of acidifying solutions for the treatment of alkalosis may cause acidosis. Acute intestinal obstruction in the horse is commonly accompanied by acidosis, whereas in other species alkalosis occurs at least initially.

In general, the body will tolerate a pH range of 7·0–7·8, although survival has been reported at pH values beyond these limits for short periods. Acidosis generally depresses cardiac contractility and cardiac output in the denervated heart. In the intact animal, however, activation of the sympathetic nervous system in response to acidosis causes increased cardiac contractility, increased heart rate, and increased cardiac output.

Acidosis increases catecholamine output in dogs and man. The myocardial response to catecholamines is not depressed until the blood pH is decreased to below 7·0–7·1 (44, 68).

Clinical findings

The clinically observable effects of acidosis are related chiefly to the respiratory system. The increased carbon dioxide tension of the blood and depletion of bicarbonate causes an increase in the depth and then the rate of respiration by stimulation of the respiratory centre (Kussmaul breathing). However, when hypovolemic shock is severe enough, there is often depressed respiratory function resulting in the additional accumulation of hydrogen ions and the acidosis is accentuated. Calves affected with severe acidosis and dehydration due to acute diarrhea may be unable to compensate because of depressed respiratory function. Their respiratory rate will be much slower and the depth of respiration much more shallow than normal. Respiratory compensation is normally evident when the bicarbonate level is diminished to 50% of normal. The increased urinary excretion of acids causes polyuria which may be sufficiently severe to cause dehydration or accentuate concomitant dehydration. There is usually tachycardia which becomes worse as the acidosis becomes more severe and the amplitude of the pulse and the blood pressure both decrease. Weakness, lassitude and terminal coma are other clinical findings. A concomitant hyperkalemia will cause bradycardia, heart block, sudden collapse and rapid death. This is particularly evident when animals with acidosis and hyperkalemia are transported and handled for treatment. The increased muscular activity appears to accentuate the abnormalities and sudden death is not uncommon.

A syndrome of metabolic acidosis with minimal signs of dehydration or diarrhea has been described in calves from 1 to 4 weeks of age (67, 71). Affected calves are depressed, weak, ataxic and the suck and menace reflexes may be weak or absent. Some calves appear comatose. On succussion of the abdomen fluid-splashing may be audible which suggests that the syndrome may be related to diarrhea which most of the calves have had but appeared to have recovered. The abnormal laboratory findings include a reduced venous blood pH, P_{CO_2} and bicarbonate ion concentration, elevated blood urea nitrogen, increased anion gap and a neutrophilic leukocytosis with a left shift. The intravenous administration of 2·5–4·5 litres of isotonic (1·3%) sodium bicarbonate solution intravenously, the amount depending on the severity of the condition (71), is necessary.

ALKALOSIS

Alkalosis can be caused by an increased absorption of alkali, excessive loss of acid or a deficit of carbon dioxide (Fig. 12). Abomasal atony due to dilatation, impaction or torsion of the abomasum is one of the commonest causes of alkalosis in cattle. There is continuous secretion of hydrochloric acid and potassium into the abomasum, with failure of evacuation of the abomasal contents into the duodenum for absorption. Sequestration of hydrochloric acid and potassium occurs in the abomasum along with reflux into the rumen, all of which results in a hypochloremic, hypokalemic alkalosis. In metabolic alkalosis, potassium will shift from the extracellular to the intracellular space, resulting in a hypokalemia when in fact there may not be depletion of body potassium (12, 22). In cattle with metabolic alkalosis there is a paradoxical aciduria, which is not well understood but may be due to severe electrolyte depletion placing limits on the kidney to regulate acid–base balance (23).

Clinical findings

As with acidosis, the clinical findings of alkalosis are not characteristic enough to be recognized clinically. Alkalosis results in slow, shallow respirations in an attempt to preserve carbon dioxide. Muscular tremors and tetany with tonic and clonic convulsions may occur because of depression of the ionized fraction of serum calcium. Hyperpnea and dyspnea may also occur in the terminal stages of alkalosis.

Naturally occurring combined abnormalities of fluid, electrolyte and acid–base balance

The disease states under discussion here are seldom primary. They are usually secondary to a serious disease state such as gastric torsion or rumen overload or acute intestinal obstruction, diseases which are in themselves life-threatening. The importance of fluid and electrolyte abnormalities is that they are also life-threatening and simple correction of the primary abnormality, for example removal of a large section of a horse's small intestine, is valueless unless the dehydration, hyponatremia and acidosis are also corrected. The variation which can occur in these naturally occurring errors of fluid, electrolyte and acid–base balance are what makes their diagnosis and treatment so difficult. If it were possible to have instant clinicopathological advice on what the abnormalities were, and how they were progressing as advised by constant monitoring, there would be little challenge in it. But the fact is that under normal clinical circumstances these services are not available and it is necessary to have enough understanding of the basic physiology and pathology of these diseases to be able to predict by clinical examination and examination of the history, the likely deficiencies, imbalances and the degree of their severity.

In the preceding paragraphs the individual errors of fluid and electrolyte homeostasis have been identified. It is now necessary to discuss the combined deficiencies which are the standard occurrence in naturally occurring disease. As an example, Fig. 13 sets out diagrammatically the probable developments in a case of acute diarrhea.

It is not possible to set down in such a diagram the constant variation in fluids and electrolytes which occurs as a result of compensatory changes by various organs including especially the respiratory and circulatory systems and the kidney. It is this volatility which makes chemical pathological monitoring so important. Some generalizations on this matter of the dynamics of fluid and electrolyte status are as follows.

The body water and electrolytes are maintained at a homeostatic level by the buffering system of the blood, the lungs and the kidney. In disturbances of body-water and electrolytes, the changes which occur are also dynamic and there is a constant reaction by the homeostatic mechanism to restore the water and electrolyte relationship to normal. With some exceptions, it is unusual to find an uncompensated acidosis or alkalosis. A partial compensation in the opposite direction of the primary acid–base imbalance is usually in progress and it is important to determine the nature of the primary disturbance for the selection of rational therapy. Often the nature of the primary disturbance can be determined from a consideration of the history and the clinical findings. The different compensations which can occur have been described (73).

The dehydration caused by deprivation of water and electrolytes (lack of water or inability to drink) is mild and animals may appear only mildly dehydrated even after several days of water deprivation. The feces are hard and dry, the rumen contents are firm and dry and urine volume is decreased considerably.

With the exception of clinical dehydration, the clinical findings of electrolyte and acid–base imbalances are not characteristic. Without laboratory evaluation, the nature and degree of electrolyte and acid–base imbalance must be assumed and estimated based on the history of the affected animal and the changes which are most likely to have occurred.

Clinical pathology

Some representative laboratory values in examples of body water and electrolyte disturbances are given in Table 2.

The packed cell volume (PCV) and the total serum proteins or total serum solids will indicate the severity of water loss. Anemic animals and those affected with diseases causing hypoproteinemia may provide misleading values.

The measurement of blood pH, P_{CO_2} (partial pressure of carbon dioxide) and hemoglobin will permit the determination of plasma bicarbonate (24). The plasma bicarbonate is a measure of alkali reserve, the quantity of which is usually referred to as base excess or base deficit. Blood for pH and P_{CO_2} must be taken anerobically, preferably in heparin, and should be submitted for analysis as soon as possible after collection.

In vitro dilution of the blood sample with anticoagulant should be avoided because it will alter the measured P_{CO_2} and base excess/deficit values. Arterial samples should be collected for meaningful pH and blood values. Central venous and free-flowing capillary blood can be used for screening procedures in normal animals, but are subject to considerable error (45).

In the horse, venous and central venous blood are equally suitable for establishing acid–base status (46). The acid–base status of bovine blood sampled and stored under different conditions is recorded (47). The magnitude of the changes present will depend on the compensation which has already occurred. The blood pH may be within the normal range, depending on the effectiveness of compensation. In metabolic acidosis there may be a compensatory decrease in P_{CO_2} due to hyperventilation. In metabolic alkalosis there may be an increase in P_{CO_2} due to hypoventilation (73).

The serum concentrations of sodium, potassium and chloride will depend on the initial cause and the severity of the disease. In most cases of acute diarrhea there is hyponatremia and metabolic acidosis. This is marked in the horse with acute diarrhea. The serum levels of chloride may be normal or subnormal in acute diarrhea. The serum levels of potassium will be below normal initially but as acidosis develops and becomes severe there may be hyperkalemia. In diseases causing abomasal atony there will be hypochloremic, hypokalemic, metabolic alkalosis. The blood urea nitrogen will be elevated, depending on the severity of the dehydration and decrease in circulating blood volume. The plasma osmolality may be decreased but the magnitude of the decrease will depend on the amount of water which was lost or which shifted into the intracellular space in response to the altered osmotic pressure. The specific gravity and total

Table 2. Representative laboratory values (mean ± SD) in body-water and electrolyte disturbances

Clinical pathology	*Acute diarrhea in horse*	*Acute diarrhea in calf*	*Metabolic alkalosis due to abomasal dilatation impaction/torsion in cattle*	*Acute intestinal obstruction*	*Acute carbohydrate engorgement in ruminants*
Packed cell volume (%)	60 ± 7	45·3 ± 7·0	42 ± 6	64 ± 5	45 ± 6
Total serum solids (g/dl)	10 ± 2	8·6 ± 1·5	8·2 ± 1·5	11·5 ± 1·5	8·5 ± 1·8
Blood pH (venous)	7·10 ± 0·15	7·08 ± 0·12	7·49 ± 0·04	7·15 ± 0·15	7·10 ± 0·05
Plasma bicarbonate (mmol/l)	12 ± 3	13·7 ± 4·2	35·4 ± 5·7	18 ± 6	12·5 ± 3·5
Partial pressure of carbon dioxide (mmHg)	45 ± 8	46·8 ± 6·4	46·4 ± 7·5	48 ± 6	40 ± 6
Serum sodium (mmol/l)	126 ± 3	138 ± 9·4	138·5 ± 5·4	135 ± 5	132 ± 4
Serum chloride (mmol/l)	99 ± 3	101·4 ± 7·5	88·6 ± 12·8	98 ± 4	93 ± 3
Serum potassium (mmol/l)	3·0 ± 1·2	7·4 ± 1·6	3·4 ± 0·6	3·8 ± 0·6	5·0 ± 2·5
Blood urea nitrogen (mg/dl)	60 ± 30	50·1 ± 30·5	40 ± 15	65 ± 35	55 ± 25

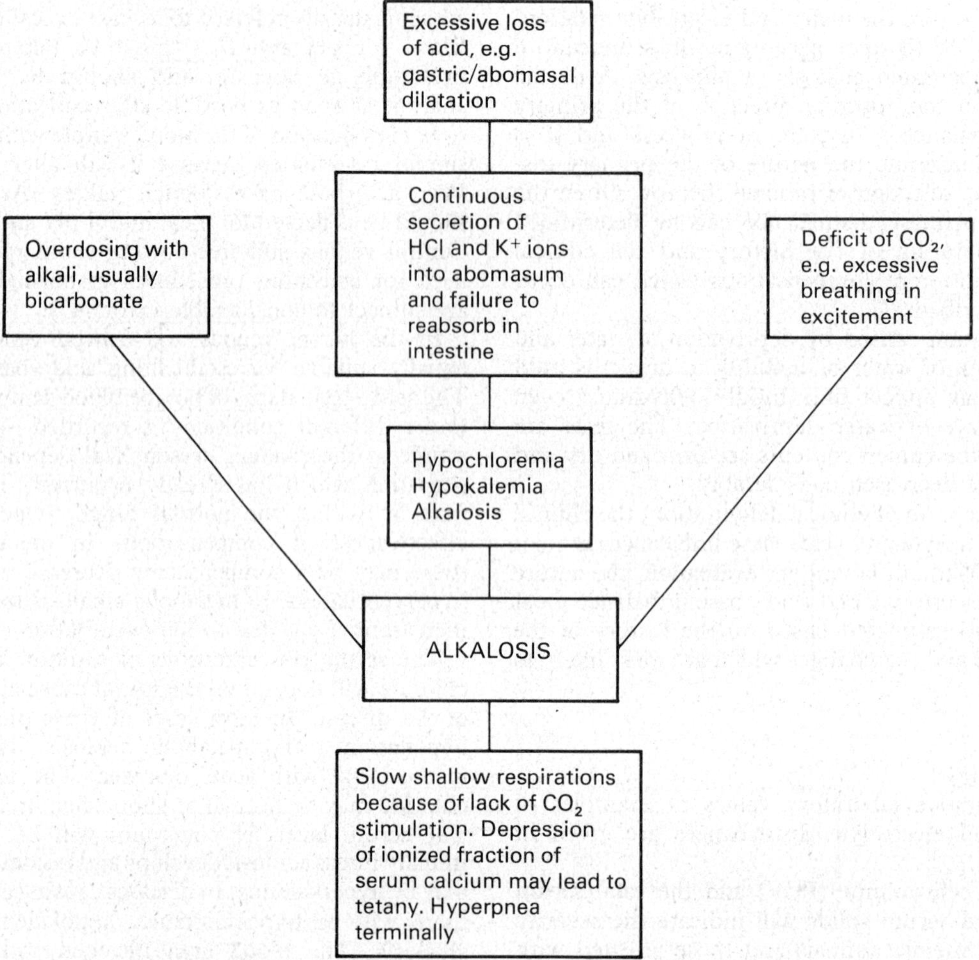

Fig. 12. Etiology and pathogenesis of alkalosis

osmolality of the urine of calves with diarrhea are both increased (25).

A complete laboratory evaluation would include the following: packed cell volume (PCV); total serum proteins; blood pH; P_{CO_2}; HCO_3; serum sodium, potassium and chloride; and blood urea nitrogen (73).

Necropsy findings

At necropsy there is a general appearance of dehydration but gross lesions are confined to those of the primary disease.

Diagnosis

There is usually little difficulty in determining the presence of dehydration. A reasonably accurate assessment of the degree of dehydration can also be made clinically and the determination of the PCV and total serum solids will improve the assessment. The extent of the electrolyte and acid–base imbalance cannot be easily evaluated clinically because the clinical findings are not characteristic. However, a consideration of the immediate history of the disease, the length of time the animal has been affected, and the tentative diagnosis will usually provide a clinical assessment of the possible nature and degree of electrolyte and acid–base imbalance. Animals affected with acute diarrhea due to infectious enteritis are likely to be in a state of metabolic acidosis and hyponatremia. In intestinal obstruction of the horse, there are varying degrees of dehydration and metabolic acidosis. In obstruction of the upper intestinal tract, or abomasal stasis, there are varying degrees of dehydration and metabolic alkalosis with hypochloremia and hypokalemia. A combination of the clinical assessment and the available laboratory evaluation will allow the clinician to make the most rational approach to treatment.

There is no single clinical or laboratory finding which will assess the severity or predict the outcome of an animal affected with water and electrolyte disturbances secondary to some other primary cause. In some cases the animal is in a stage of progressive shock, reversible or irreversible, the recognition of which would assist the clinician in deciding on a course of action. The assessment of severity and prognosis will depend on the integrated evaluation of the following.

- Nature of the disease causing the disturbances and knowledge of the history
- Clinical findings
- Packed cell volume or total serum proteins
- Total leukocyte and differential counts
- Blood pH, blood gases and serum electrolytes
- Anion and osmolal gaps

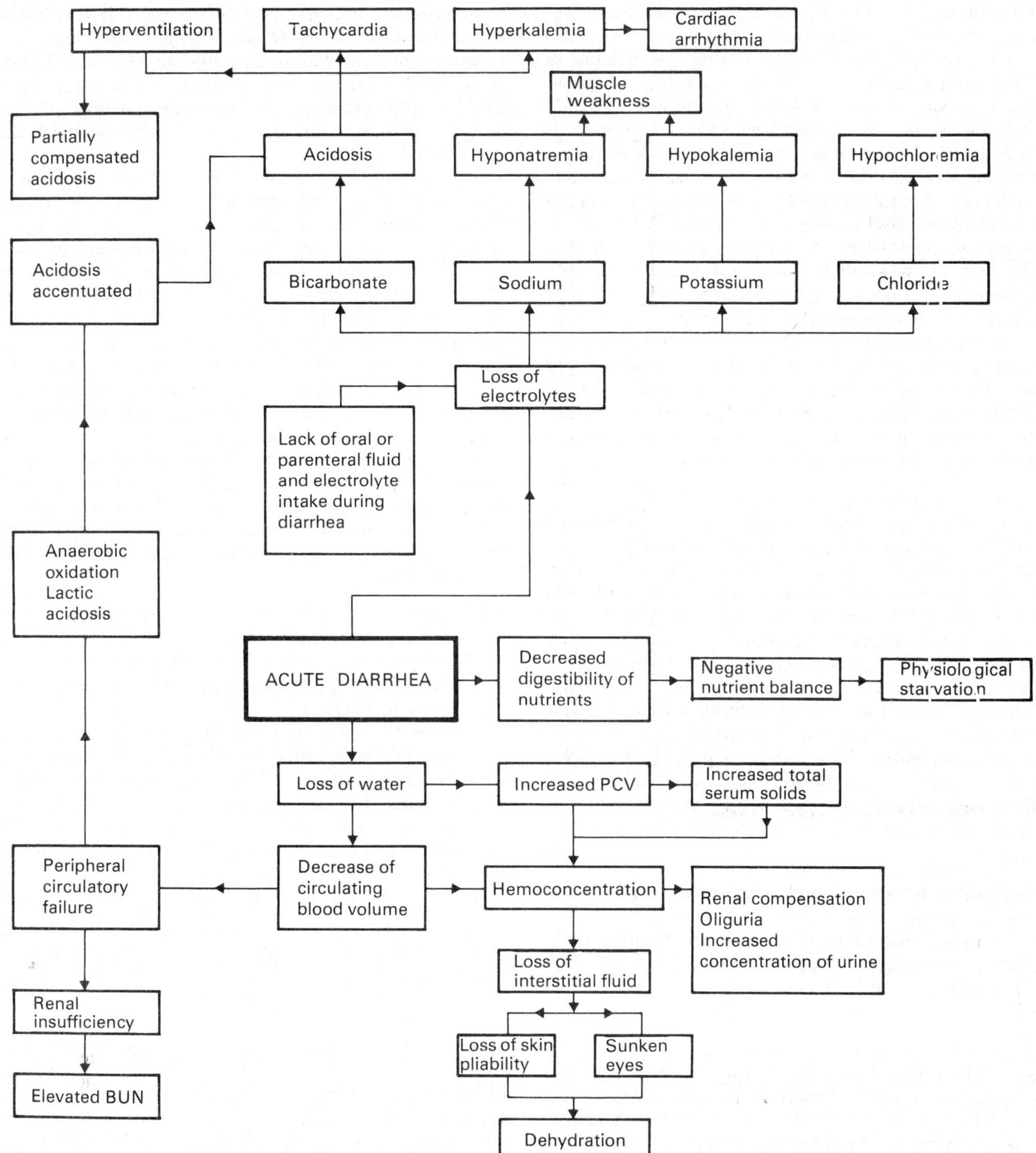

Fig. 13. The interrelationships of the changes in body-water, electrolytes and acid–base balance which can occur in diarrhea

- Arterial blood pressure
- Central venous pressure

Each of these is discussed below.

Nature of the disease and history
The information on the duration of illness must be accurate or it will be misleading. The sequence of clinical signs in the history may indicate the trend in severity. Animals which have had a profuse watery diarrhea for 18–24 hours may be severely acidotic. Acute intestinal obstruction in cattle is not as severe as in the horse. Acute gastric or intestinal rupture in the horse or in cattle is usually rapidly fatal. Acidosis in grain overload in cattle may be fatal in 24–48 hours; acidosis in the horse with grain overload may be much more rapidly fatal as electrolyte disturbances are more severe in the horse.

Clinical findings
A normal temperature is not a good prognostic guide

but a subnormal temperature suggests a worsening situation. A gradually progressive increase in heart rate also indicates that the patient is deteriorating. In general, in the horse, a heart rate up to 60/minute suggests a minor lesion (but not always), a heart rate between 60 and 80/minute is in the danger area, 80–100/minute is serious, and greater than 100/minute is commonly premortal (except in intestinal tympany which may be relieved). A cold clammy skin which remains tented for more than 30 seconds suggests severe dehydration. Cyanosis of the oral mucous membranes and a capillary refill time of more than 4 seconds suggests a poor prognosis, as does rapid respiration (three to four times normal) with intermittent hyperpnea and apnea. Muscular tremors and leg buckling are grave signs in the horse, and are commonly followed by collapse and death. The inability of any dehydrated animal to stand (other reasons being eliminated) is ominous. Severe depression and dullness are commonly observed in acute conditions, and coma is usually terminal.

Packed cell volume and total serum solids

The normal range depends on the age and species of animal, previous excitement, and the presence of anemia or hypoproteinemia. A packed cell volume between 30 and 40% is considered normal, between 40 and 50% fluids may or may not be necessary, between 50 and 60% fluids are necessary for recovery, and above 60% intensive fluid therapy is necessary and the prognosis is unfavorable. A total serum solids of 6–7·5 g/dl is usually considered normal; at 8–10 g/dl fluids are needed and the prognosis is favorable and above 12 g/dl the prognosis is unfavorable. In a review of published data on plasma protein concentration and packed cell volume during dehydration, the expected greater increase in plasma protein concentration was usually observed (77).

Total leukocyte and differential counts

A marked leukopenia and neutropenia with a degenerative left shift is an unfavorable prognosis. A regenerative left shift with a neutrophilia is a favorable prognosis. A marked lymphopenia indicates severe stress and the prognosis may be unfavorable.

Blood pH, blood gases and serum electrolytes

The normal blood pH varies from 7·35 to 7·45 (venous blood). The degree of *acidosis* encountered include moderate acidosis (7·30–7·25), severe acidosis (7·25–7·20), grave and commonly fatal (7·10–7·00). Horses with torsion or strangulation of the intestines generally have blood lactate levels over 75 mg/dl (8·2 mmol/l) whereas cases of impaction have levels of 5–9 mg/dl (0·55–1·0 mmol/l). The normal value is 6·0 mg/dl (0.78 mmol/l) with a range of 4–12 mg/dl (0·44–1·33 mmol/l). The survival rate in the series fell from 85% to zero as the lactate level increased from 75 to 155 mg/dl (8·3 to 17·2 mmol/l). The blood lactate levels increase following strenuous exercise which may make interpretation difficult in horses which develop colic immediately following exercise.

The normal range of *plasma bicarbonate* is 24–30 mmol/l. In mild acidosis the level is in the range of 20–24, moderate 14–18, and in severe cases below 10 mmol/l and a grave prognosis. The levels of P_{CO_2} and P_{O_2}, plasma bicarbonate and blood pH can be used to determine the degree of compensation, if any, which has taken place. In metabolic acidosis there may be a compensatory decrease in P_{CO_2} due to hyperventilation. In metabolic alkalosis there may be an increase in P_{CO_2} due to hypoventilation. In respiratory acidosis due to severe pneumonia the arterial P_{O_2} will be markedly decreased.

The severity and nature of the acidosis in diarrheic calves may vary depending on the age of the animal (78). Diarrheic calves under 8 days of age may have a lactic acidosis and those over 8 days of age may have a non-lactic acidosis. The base deficit was greater in diarrheic calves over 8 days of age than in those under 8 days, and the calculated amount of bicarbonate to correct the acidosis in the older calves was about twice the amount required in the calves under 8 days of age (78).

The *serum electrolyte* levels will usually indicate the severity of the electrolyte losses and the necessity for replacement with either balanced electrolyte solution or specific electrolyte solution. The total deficit for each electrolyte can be estimated using the standard formula presented under calculation of electrolyte requirements.

Water and electrolyte abnormalities are classified into three types based on the measurement of electrolytes and osmolality:

1. *hypertonic dehydration* (true dehydration desiccation), osmolality greater than 300 mOsm/kg (300 mmol/kg), associated with water deprivation, some acute gastrointestinal problems and some types of diarrhea;
2. *hypotonic dehydration* (acute desalting water loss), osmolalities less than 260 mOsm/kg (260 mmol/kg), associated with acute diarrhea, particularly secretory diarrheas such as salmonellosis;
3. *isotonic dehydration* (normal electrolyte and osmolality levels) as in horses losing electrolytes and water in almost equal porportions (61).

Evaluation of the *anion and osmolal gaps* has become routine in many medical institutions. Both calculations take little time, are essentially without cost, and have proven valuable in assessing a variety of clinical conditions in which electrolyte imbalances occur. The *anion gap* is defined as the difference between the sum of the serum concentration of sodium plus potassium and the sum of chloride plus bicarbonate, all concentrations expressed in milliequivalents per liter (mEq/l), but see p. 71. There are normal gaps for each species of animal. Significant changes in anion gaps are usually caused by a change in unmeasured anion concentration. Widening of the gap may be caused by lactic acid, inorganic phosphates and sulfates in uremia, toxins, nitrates, ethylene glycol and hyperproteinemia states. Laboratory error is also a cause of increased anion gap. The characterization of the causes of metabolic acidosis is a major clinical application of anion gap determination.

Evaluation of the osmolal gap is a means of detecting an increased amount of abnormal osmotically active solute in the blood. The *osmolal gap* is the difference between the measured plasma osmolality and the osmolality calculated from the plasma concentration of normally measured solutes. Sodium and potassium and their associated anions, along with glucose and urea constitute the majority of normal osmotically active solutes. The following formula is recommended:

$$1{\cdot}86\ (Na + K) + \frac{glucose}{18} + \frac{BUN}{2{\cdot}8} + 8{\cdot}6$$

Examination of the triad of calculated osmolality, measured osmolality and the osmolal gap is beneficial in the diagnosis and prognosis of a number of diseases (48, 49).

Arterial blood pressure

This provides a good guide for the presence and severity of shock but not for the severity or extent of the initiating lesion. Painful abdominal conditions may produce hypertension until shock intervenes. In the horse, a systolic pressure below 100 mmHg (13·3 kPa) suggests an unfavorable prognosis, 80–100 mmHg (10·6–13·3 kPa) a guarded prognosis, 50–80 mmHg (6·66–10·6 kPa) a grave prognosis and below 50 mmHg (6·66 kPa) is usually fatal. The normal systolic pressure in the horse is 125 mmHg (16·6 kPa).

Central venous pressure

This is more useful as a monitor during fluid replacement. Normal pressure is 6–10 cm of water (0·6–1·0 kPa). Below 6 cm (0·6 kPa) requires fluid; above 15 cm (1·5 kPa) indicates cardiac failure and volume overload.

Principles of fluid and electrolyte therapy

The most important principle is to prevent or minimize dehydration and electrolyte loss whenever possible. This means the provision of an adequate water supply, adequate drinking space and a continuous supply of salt and the necessary minerals. The next most important principle is to treat potential losses of fluid and electrolytes as quickly as possible to minimize the degree of dehydration and acid–base imbalance which may occur in animals with diseases in which losses are occurring.

The major objectives in fluid and electrolyte therapy are to correct the abnormalities which already exist and to monitor and provide maintenance therapy until the animal has recovered. Correction of the abnormalities may require 4–6 hours and maintenance therapy may require 2–4 days depending on the cause of the disease. There are at least four possible abnormalities which could exist at the same time which must be corrected. These include volume of fluid lost, plasma osmolar deficits, specific electrolyte imbalances and acid–base imbalance. The two major problems are to determine the nature and degree of the abnormalities present and to decide which fluid and electrolyte solution should be used (73). A practical approach to fluid therapy in the horse has been described (26). The fluid therapy of the horse with acute diarrhea has been reviewed (27).

The ideal situation would be to make both a clinical and laboratory evaluation of the animal. The history and the diagnosis will suggest the possibility of acidosis or alkalosis and the electrolyte imbalances which are likely to be present. The degree of dehydration can usually be recognized clinically. Severe dehydration and acidosis should be treated as quickly as possible. A summary of the disturbances of fluid and electrolyte balance which occur in some common diseases of cattle and horses, and the suggested fluid therapy, is presented in Table 3.

Calculation of electrolyte requirements

The electrolyte deficits can be estimated using the serum electrolyte values of the affected animal. The total deficit of the electrolyte in milliequivalents (mEq) is the product of the deficit of the electrolyte in mEq per liter (mEq/l) and the size of extracellular fluid space as a percentage of total body weight. Thus: deficit (mEq) = deficit of electrolyte mEq/l × 0·3 × body weight (kg). The size of the extracellular fluid (ECF) space is usually considered to be 30% of body weight (0·3 in the formula), but recent work suggests that the space is approximately 20%. Published values range from 17·7 to 22·1% (50, 51). The value of 0·3 has been used commonly for the size of the bicarbonate space and appears to be reliable and safe for sodium and chloride ions, but there is less certainty about the size of the potassium space because potassium is mainly an intracellular ion. Potassium solutions should not exceed 40 mEq/l (= 40 mmol/l; see below) and the heart should be closely monitored during administration; 1 or 2 days may be required for potassium to transfer from the extracellular to the intracellular space.

An example of the determination of the bicarbonate requirements in a 500 kg horse with acute diarrhea and acidosis is as follows:

- 500 kg body weight
- Blood pH 7·20
- Serum bicarbonate 12 mEq/l (12 mmol/l) (normal bicarbonate 26 mEq/l (26 mmol/l))
- Base deficit = 14 mEq/l (14 mmol/l)
- Total base deficit = 500 × 0·3 × 14 = 2100 mEq (2100 mmol/l)
- 1 g $NaHCO_3$ yields 12 mEq (12 mmol) HCO_3

Therefore, the horse needs 175 g $NaHCO_3$ which can be given intravenously as a 5% solution over a period of 30–45 minutes followed by the intravenous administration of isotonic electrolyte solutions as indicated.

For the preparation of electrolyte solutions certain formulae and the atomic and formula weights must be used and they are as follows.

Milligram–milliequivalent conversions The unit of measure of electrolytes is the milliequivalent (mEq) which expresses the chemical activity, or combining power, of a substance relative to the activity of 1 mg of hydrogen. Thus, 1 mEq is represented by 1 mg of hydrogen, 23 mg of sodium, 39 mg of potassium, 20 mg of calcium and 35 mg of chlorine. Conversion equations are as follows:

$$\text{mEq/l} = \frac{(\text{mg/l}) \times \text{valence}}{\text{formula weight}}$$

$$\text{mg/l} = \frac{(\text{mEq/l}) \times \text{formula weight}}{\text{valence}}$$

NOTE: Formula weight = atomic or molecular weight.

Using the International System of Units (SI) the milliequivalent (mEq) is equal to the millimole (mmol). Thus milliequivalents per liter (mEq/l) converts to millimoles per liter (mmol/l) without a numerical change if the valency of the ion is not greater than one. The atomic weights of the ions are as follows: hydrogen 1, carbon 12, nitrogen 14, oxygen 16, calcium 40, sodium 23,

Table 3. Summary of disturbances of body-water, electrolytes and acid–base balance in some common diseases of cattle and horses, and suggested fluid therapy

Disease	*Major abnormalities and deficits*	*Fluid and electrolyte requirements*
Neonatal calf diarrhea (including piglets and lambs)	*Metabolic acidosis*, low plasma bicarbonate, severe dehydration, loss of sodium, hyperkalemia when acidosis severe	Equal mixtures of isotonic saline and isotonic sodium bicarbonate with 5% dextrose. Balanced electrolytes too. Intravenously and orally. *See* Colibacillosis (p. 621) for details
D-Lactic acidosis (carbohydrate engorgement of ruminants)	*Metabolic acidosis*, low plasma bicarbonate, severe dehydration	Sodium bicarbonate initially followed by balanced electrolytes. Intravenously. *See* Rumen overload (p. 246) for details
Acute diffuse peritonitis	*Dehydration*. Slight metabolic alkalosis due to paralytic ileus	Balanced electrolyte solutions in large quantities intravenously for hydration and maintenance
Right-side dilatation/abomasal torsion of cattle, abomasal impaction (dietary or vagal nerve injury)	*Metabolic alkalosis*, marked *hypochloremia*, *hypokalemia*, severe *dehydration*	Balanced electrolyte solutions or high potassium and chloride acidifying solution intravenously. May give acidifying solutions orally. *See* Right-side displacement of abomasum for details; can also use mixture of 2 liters of isotonic saline (0·9%), 1 liter isotonic potassium chloride (1·1%) and 1 liter isotonic dextrose (5%)
Peracute coliform mastitis	Severe *dehydration*, mild electrolyte deficits including mild hypocalcemia. Acidosis if diarrhea present	Balanced electrolyte solutions intravenously in large quantities for hydration, and maintenance for 24–48 hours
Acute diarrhea in the horse (enteric salmonellosis, colitis-X)	Severe *dehydration*, marked *hyponatremia*, *metabolic acidosis*. Hypokalemia occurs following bicarbonate therapy	Hypertonic sodium bicarbonate (5%) 3–5 liters (500 kg body weight) followed by high sodium, high potassium alkalinizing solution to correct hypokalemia following bicarbonate therapy all by the intravenous route
Acute grain engorgement in the horse	*Metabolic acidosis*, *dehydration* and shock	Hypertonic sodium bicarbonate (5%) 3–5 liters (500 kg body weight) followed by balanced electrolytes intravenously
Water and electrolyte deprivation. Esophageal obstruction in horse	Moderate dehydration	Balanced electrolytes intravenously. When obstruction relieved provide electrolyte solution orally
Acute intestinal obstruction	Metabolic acidosis or alkalosis dependent on level of obstruction. Severe dehydration in horse, moderate in cow	Isotonic sodium bicarbonate initially, 3–5 liters (500 kg body weight) followed by balanced electrolytes intravenously. Horses may develop hypokalemia following bicarbonate therapy and must be given potassium chloride

magnesium 24, chloride 35, potassium 39. The formula weights and the mEq/l delivered by 1 g of substance are as follows:

NaCl	58.5–17
NaHCO	385–12
KCl	74–14

The isotonic concentrations of the commonly used solutions in percentages are as follows: NaCl 0·9, KCl 1·1, $NaHCO_3$ 1·3 and dextrose 5. Most laboratory values are expressed as amount per liter; e.g. mmol/l, mg/l. In the SI system, now in common use by diagnostic laboratories and scientific journals, if the molecular weight is known, it is preferable to express the amount of a substance as the amount in moles per liter (mol/l). Example: to convert 9·5 mg/100 ml Ca to mmol/l;

$$9{\cdot}5 \text{ mg/100 ml} = \frac{\text{mg/100 ml} \times 10}{\text{molecular weight}}$$

$$= \frac{9{\cdot}5 \times 10}{40} = 2{\cdot}375 \text{ mmol/l}$$

Composition of fluids

Under ideal conditions, with laboratory evaluation of the animal, the deficits can be more accurately assessed and fluids containing the deficient electrolytes could be used. However, this is not always possible and balanced electrolyte solutions are available and have been in general use. These usually contain sodium, potassium chloride and calcium at a concentration similar to the electrolyte composition of extracellular fluid and may contain lactate or acetate. The lactate and acetate are metabolized to bicarbonate and are indicated for the treatment of acidosis. Many also contain a source of dextrose. These balanced electrolyte solutions are considered to be safe and can usually be used in large quantities without creating electrolyte disturbances provided that circulating blood volume and renal function have been restored and are maintained. They can be used for most situations of dehydration and moderate acidosis or alkalosis and moderate electrolyte imbalances. They are usually not adequate for the treatment of severe acidosis or alkalosis, or severe hyponatremia, hypokalemia or hypochloremia. Sodium bicarbonate is superior to sodium L-lactate and sodium acetate for the treatment of metabolic acidosis in diarrheic calves (69, 70). Propionate, acetate and L-lactate are all good alkalinizing agents in healthy calves but may not be as effective in situations where tissue metabolism is impaired (72); D-gluconate, D-lactate and citrate are unsuitable for use as alkalinizing agents in intravenous fluids (72). In severe acidosis and dehydration the perfusion and metabolism of the liver may be inadequate and insufficient bicarbonate may be produced for the treatment of the acidosis. It is also possible that the lactate or acetate may accumulate in severe acidosis and accentuate the acidosis. However, this is not a common problem. Experimentally, in dogs, the use of lactate did not cause a prolonged or progressive elevation of arterial lactate in animals with severe hepatic dysfunction (28).

For the treatment of severe acidosis or alkalosis, and severe hyponatremia, hypokalemia and hypochloremia, several other specific electrolyte solutions may be necessary. These usually consist of a mixture of the common simple solutions with supplemented electrolytes to correct some major abnormality. These are considered necessary to correct abnormalities quickly which could not be corrected using balanced electrolyte solutions. These are summarized in Table 4.

The necessity for glucose in fluid therapy has been controversial. Hypoglycemia occurs in some cases of acute diarrhea in calves but it is uncommon in most other common diseases in which there is a fluid and electrolyte disturbance. Dextrose will promote the movement of extracellular potassium into the cell, it will provide metabolic water and is a source of carbohydrate. Large quantities of parenteral glucose are necessary to meet the maintenance energy requirements and every effort must be made to restore the animal's appetite and to provide the necessary requirements through dietary intake. The energy requirements for maintenance are calculated on the basis of metabolic body size, kg $W^{0 \cdot 73}$ which is a measure of fasting metabolism in an animal not eating and not doing any muscular work (29). If 1 g of dextrose given intravenously will provide 5 kcal (2·1 kJ) of energy, the following approximate amounts of 5% dextrose solution are needed to meet the energy needs for maintenance in cattle (Table 5). This is a rough estimate of the requirements and should be used as a guideline only. Every effort should be made to supply the energy needs through oral intake of energy-containing foods.

Hypertonic sodium bicarbonate (3–5 liters of 5%) may be necessary to correct severe hyponatremia and metabolic acidosis which occurs in the horse with acute diarrhea (30, 31). The rapid intravenous infusion of 5% sodium bicarbonate in 5% dextrose in the horse can cause metabolic alkalosis. Following this initial treatment, hypokalemia characterized by muscular weakness commonly occurs which can be treated using a high sodium, high potassium, alkalinizing solution (14). Hypertonic or isotonic solutions of sodium bicarbonate are also effective for the initial treatment of acidosis associated with D-lactic acidosis in cattle and acute diarrhea in calves. Solutions containing potassium have been recommended for the treatment of the potassium depletion which occurs in calves with acute diarrhea (32). However, in calves with severe acidosis and hyperkalemia, it is important to expand circulating blood volume, restore renal function and correct the acidosis before providing additional potassium which may be toxic. Solutions containing potassium may be indicated following correction of the acidosis and dehydration. However, if the animal's appetite is returned to normal, the potassium intake will usually correct any existing deficiencies. For the treatment of metabolic alkalosis, acidifying solutions can be used but should not be used unless constant laboratory evaluation of the animal is possible. The isotonic solution of potassium chloride

Table 4. Composition (mmol/liter) and indications for use of electrolyte solutions used in fluid therapy

Solutions	Na^+	K^+	Cl^-	Mg^{2+}	Ca^{2+}	HCO_3^-	*Lactate or acetate*	*Dextrose*	*Major indications*
0·9% Sodium chloride (isotonic saline)	155		155						Expand circulating blood volume
1·3% Sodium bicarbonate (isotonic)	155					156			Acidosis
1·3% Sodium bicarbonate in 5% dextrose	155					156		5%	Acidosis
5% Sodium bicarbonate (hypertonic)	600					600			Severe acidosis
Equal mixture or isotonic saline and isotonic sodium bicarbonate	155		78			78			Acidosis and dehydration
Balanced electrolyte solution (i.e. McSherry's solution)	138	12	100	5	3		50 (acetate)		Acidosis, alkalosis, electrolyte losses and dehydration
Lactated Ringer's solution	130	4	111		3		28 (lactate)		Acidosis
High sodium, alkalinizing solution. Lactated Ringer's solution plus sodium bicarbonate (5 g/l)	190	4	111			60	27 (lactate)		Acidosis and hyponatremia
High-sodium, high-potassium, alkalinizing solution. Lactated Ringer's solution plus 1 g/l potassium chloride and 5 g/l sodium bicarbonate	190	18	125			60	27 (lactate)		Acidosis, hyponatremia, hypokalemia
High-potassium acidifying solution. Isotonic saline plus 2·5 g potassium chloride/l	154	35	189						Alkalosis, hypochloremia, hypokalemia
Mixture of: 1 l isotonic potassium chloride (1·1%), 2 l isotonic saline (0·9%) and 1 l dextrose 5%									Metabolic alkalosis in cattle with abomasal disease

Table 5. Estimated daily energy requirements* of fasting cattle

Body weight (kg)	*Metabolic body size* (kg $W^{0.73}$)	*Metabolizable energy requirements* (kcal)	*Glucose 5%* (liters/day)
45 (1-month-old calf)	16	1760	7
90	27	2970	12
180	45	4950	20
360	74	8140	33
454	87	9510	38
544	100	12100	48

*Calculated on the basis of 110 kcal/kg $W^{0.73}$.

and ammonium chloride recommended for the treatment of the alkalosis associated with right-side displacement of the abomasum is relatively safe. Without laboratory evaluation, the use of balanced electrolyte solutions for alkalosis in cattle is recommended.

In general, there are three different kinds of solutions used in large animals. The balanced electrolyte solutions are indicated for dehydration and moderate degrees of acid–base and electrolyte imbalance. Hypertonic, high-sodium, alkalinizing solutions are used for severe acidosis and hyponatremia, and hypertonic high potassium acidifying solutions are used for alkalosis. Because economics is usually a major consideration in large animal fluid therapy, it is not usually possible to use sterile solutions. Most of the above solutions can be formulated using the necessary salt mixed with distilled water or a supply of boiled water or ordinary tap water.

Quantity of fluids required and routes of administration The amount of fluid required will depend on the degree of dehydration already present (an estimate of the volume losses which have already occurred), the amount of the continuous losses which are occurring during treatment and the maintenance requirements of the animal during treatment presuming its dietary intake of water, electrolytes and nutrients is minimal. The fluids are usually given in two stages. Hydration therapy in the first 4–6 hours and maintenance therapy (a combination of continuous losses and maintenance requirements) in the next 20–24 hours, depending on the severity and the course of the disease. Some examples of the large quantities of fluid which may be required in cases of acute diarrhea are outlined in Table 6. The maintenance requirements are calculated on the basis of 50–100 ml/kg body weight over a 24-hour period. In some cases of profuse diarrhea, the continuous losses and maintenance requirements will be about 150 ml/kg body weight over a 24-hour period.

Table 6. Examples of amounts of fluid required for hydration and maintenance therapy

Animal	*Degree of dehydration* (% of body weight)	*Fluid required for hydration* (liters)	*maintenance* (liters)
Mature horse (500 kg)	8	40	25–50
	12	60	25–50
Newborn calf (50 kg)	8	4	2·5–5
	12	6	2·5–5
Mature cow (700 kg)	8	56	35–70
	12	84	35–70

The total amount of the estimated necessary hydration therapy should be given intravenously using indwelling intravenous catheters in the first 4–6 hours in order to expand and maintain circulating blood volume. If acidosis or alkalosis is present, it also should be treated immediately. Thus the most important abnormalities—decreased circulating blood volume and acid–base imbalance—are treated first. Restoring circulating blood volume will restore renal function which will assist in acid–base and electrolyte balance. The immediate correction of acidosis will return the tissues to their normal physiological activity. The intravenous route is preferred for hydration therapy and for the correction of severe acid–base and electrolyte imbalances. All other routes (intraperitoneal, subcutaneous and oral) are unsatisfactory in the presence of decreased circulating blood volume. During the intravenous administration the animal must be monitored for clinical and laboratory evidence of improvement or deleterious effects. A favorable response is indicated by urination within 30–60 minutes, an improvement in mental attitude and some evidence of hydration. Unfavorable responses include dyspnea because of pre-existing pneumonia, pulmonary edema because of rapid administration, failure to urinate because of renal failure or paralysis of the bladder, and tetany because of the excessive administration of alkali. If a laboratory is available, the determination of PCV, bicarbonate and blood pH will provide an excellent monitoring system during the administration of the fluids.

The administration of large quantities of fluids intravenously to farm animals is best done with an indwelling, intravenous, flexible catheter which is appropriately secured to the animal's neck to prevent withdrawal from the vein. A plastic, spring-like, coiled tube and suitable rubber tubing are used to deliver the fluids from large 20–25 liter plastic containers (33). The use of a drip-chamber in the rubber tubing system will assist in determining the flow rate which can be adjusted with a clamp. The technique for long-term fluid administration in the calf has been described (34). Similarly, a technique for the long-term placement of an indwelling intravenous catheter in the horse is described. A long leader to the catheter is placed subcutaneously (54).

The rate of administration will depend on the size of the animal, the severity of the illness, the type of fluids being administered and the response of the animal to the fluids. In calves, isotonic saline and isotonic sodium bicarbonate can be given at the rate of 3–5 liters/hour; in a mature horse, fluids may be given at the rate of 10–12 liters/hour. Hypertonic solutions such as 5% sodium bicarbonate can be given to a mature horse at the rate of 3–5 liters/hour, followed by balanced electrolytes at 10–12 liters/hour. Solutions containing added potassium should be given cautiously at the rate of 3–5 liters/hour. In a cow with severe dehydration and acidosis due to carbohydrate engorgement, fluids may be given at the rate of 10–12 liters/hour. Adverse reactions in all species include: sudden muscle weakness (suggests hypokalemia) and sudden tachycardia and hyperventilation, which suggest overhydration. When these occur the fluids should be stopped and the clinical findings assessed. If laboratory assistance is available, the determination of blood pH and bicarbonate may provide an explanation for the reaction.

The maintenance requirement is also given by the intravenous route if extended intensive fluid therapy is necessary. Regular laboratory evaluations made every few hours will indicate the progress being made.

Whenever possible, the oral route can be used to deliver the maintenance requirements. Provided there are no abnormalities of the digestive tract which will interfere with the oral administration or the absorption of the fluids, the oral route is preferred for maintenance therapy. The total 24-hour maintenance requirement is calculated and given in divided doses every 2–4 hours. There is less danger from overhydration, electrolyte toxicity, and in acute diarrhea the maintenance of oral fluid and electrolyte intakes will replace continuous losses which are occurring during the diarrhea. In calves with diarrhea, the maintenance of plasma volume is directly related to continued oral intake of fluid (4). Oral electrolyte solutions and water should be made available at all times to animals affected with diarrhea and other diseases in which there are continuous losses of fluid and electrolytes. *Ad libitum* oral glucose–electrolyte therapy is successful for the treatment of acute diarrhea in children (35). The composition of oral fluids is similar to those used parenterally and has been given under the section on colibacillosis (p. 621). Calves affected with dehydration and diarrhea due to experimental colibacillosis absorb electrolyte solutions as effectively as healthy calves. The absorption of glucose and glycine is accompanied by the absorption of water and sodium and thus such a solution would have an advantage over an isotonic saline solution (55). Studies on the availability of oral carbohydrates to neonatal calves indicate that fruit pectin is equivalent to glucose, corn syrup is less effective than glucose, and sucrose is totally unavailable in their effect on plasma glucose concentration (56). The alkalinizing effects of several commercial and experimental oral electrolyte solutions have been compared in healthy calves (52). A bicarbonate-rich experimental solution induced the best alkalinization effect. Those oral electrolyte solutions which contain acid phosphate salts may cause net acidification of blood and may be undesirable for the treatment of acidosis in diarrheic calves (52). Bicarbonate-containing oral electrolyte solutions will restore acid–base imbalance in calves with viral-induced diarrhea much more effectively than solutions without bicarbonate (79). The use of oral electrolyte solutions without sodium bicarbonate for the treatment of acidosis in diarrheic calves may explain the syndrome of acidosis without dehydration. Others have also been described (36). The use of oral fluids in the horse with acute diarrhea, however, has not been successful (31). Apparently the diarrhea is exacerbated by the use of oral fluids. In experimentally induced dehydration in the horse without alimentary tract disease the oral administration of a glucose–glycine electrolyte solution at a rate of 10 liters every 30 minutes resulted in rapid correction of the dehydration and metabolic alkalosis (75). The intravenous administration of normal saline into horses dehydrated by fasting resulted in the urinary elimination of excessive quantities of sodium chloride because sodium and chloride were not the primary problems which thus required major renal adjustments and increased urinary water loss (76). This illustrates that the restoration of normal urine flow, which is generally taken as a guide to the adequacy of volume replacement, does not always indicate beneficial therapy. The close relationship between net fluid retention and urine output indicates that urinary excretion may eliminate most of the administration fluid and electrolytes in certain circumstances.

Parenteral nutrition (hyperalimentation)

In calves affected with persistent diarrhea due to chronic disease of the alimentary tract, or which cannot or will not eat, total intravenous feeding may be indicated. High concentrations of glucose, protein hydrolysates and electrolytes are given by continuous slow intravenous infusion over a period of several days. The total daily amounts given are calculated on the basis of daily caloric requirement (37). The intravenous catheter must be inserted down into the cranial vena cava where a large volume of blood will dilute the hypertonic concentration of the solution. The problems associated with parenteral nutrition include: the maintenance of a steady intravenous drip, hypertonicity of the solutions used, venous thrombosis, excessive diuresis, catheter sepsis and bacterial contamination of the solutions. The technique has been used successfully in dogs for periods up to 3 weeks without any oral feed or water intake (38). The details of parenteral nutrition in man are available in a comprehensive review (57).

Fluid and electrolyte therapy in newborn piglets and lambs

The most common cause of fluid and electrolyte imbalance in newborn piglets and lambs is acute neonatal diarrhea. There is severe dehydration, acidosis, hyponatremia and, in some cases, hyperkalemia due to the acidosis. Balanced electrolyte solutions or isotonic saline and sodium bicarbonate initially followed by balanced electrolytes are indicated and successful. These are given subcutaneously or intraperitoneally at the rate of 15 ml per piglet every 2 hours plus the same amount orally. The safe amount of sterilized porcine serum or saline and 5% dextrose which can be given to piglets is equivalent to about 8% of body weight intraperitoneally in two divided doses given 8 hours apart (58). Lambs are also treated subcutaneously (30–40 ml) and orally (50–100 ml) every 2 hours.

REVIEW LITERATURE

Brobst, D. (1986) Review of pathophysiology of alterations in potassium homeostasis. *J. Am. vet. med. Assoc.*, *188*, 1019–1025.

Hinton, M. (1978) On watering of horses: a review. *Equ. vet. J.*, *10*, 27–31.

Michell, A. R. (1985) Sodium in health and disease: A comparative review with emphasis on nerbivores. *Vet. Rec.*, *116*, 653–657.

Rose, R. J. (1981) A physiological approach to fluid and electrolyte therapy in the horse. *Equ. vet. J.*, *13*, 7–14.

Roussel, A. J. (1983) Principles and mechanics of fluid therapy in calves. *Compend. cont. Educ. pract. Vet.*, 5: S332–S339.

Tasker, J. B. (1971) Fluids, electrolytes and acid–base balance. In: *Clinical Biochemistry of Domestic Animals*, 2nd ed., vol. 2, ed. J. J. Kaneko & C. E. Cornelius. New York and London: Academic Press.

REFERENCES

(1) Easley, R. J. (1981) *J. Am. vet. med. Assoc.*, *178*, 4.
(2) Ohya, M. (1965) *Jap. J. vet. Sci.*, *27*, 41.
(3) Olsson, K. et al. (1982) *Acta Physiol. Scand.*, *115*, 361.
(4) Fisher, E. W. & Martinez, A. A. (1976) *Res. vet. Sci.*, *20*, 302.
(5) Thornton, J. R. et al. (1973) *Aust. vet. J.*, *49*, 20.
(6) Bianca, W. (1965) *Res. vet. Sci.*, *6*, 33, 38.
(7) Tasker, J. B. (1967) *Cornell Vet.*, *57*, 668.
(8) Tennant, B. et al. (1972) *J. Am. vet. med. Assoc.*, *161*, 993.
(9) Lewis, L. D. & Phillips, R. W. (1972) *Cornell Vet.*, *62*, 596.
(10) Whitlock, R. H. et al. (1975) *Cornell Vet.*, *65*, 512.
(11) McGuirk, S. M. & Butler, D. G. (1980) *J. Am. vet. med. Assoc.*, *177*, 151.
(12) Svendsen, E. (1969) *Nord. VetMed.*, *21*, 660.
(13) Hammond, P. B. (1964) *J. comp. Pathol.*, *74*, 210.
(14) Tasker, J. B. & Olson, N. E. (1964) *Proc. Am. Assoc. equ. Practnrs*, 63–70.
(15) Carlson, G. P. & Mansmann, R. A. (1974) *J. Am. vet. med. Assoc.*, *165*, 262.
(16) Mansmann, R. A. et al. (1974) *J. Am. vet. med. Assoc.*, *165*, 265.
(17) Schotman, A. J. H. (1970) *Tijdschr. Diergeneeskd.*, *95*, 331.
(18) Fisher, E. W. (1965) *Br. vet. J.*, *121*, 132.
(19) Rossdale, P. D. (1969) *Res. vet. Sci.*, *10*, 279.
(20) Dalton, R. G. (1967) *Br. vet. J.*, *123*, 237.
(21) Amman, H. et al. (1974) *Berl. Münch. Tierärztl. Wochenschr.*, *87*, 66.
(22) Tasker, J. B. (1969) *J. Am. vet. med. Assoc.*, *155*, 1906.
(23) Gingerich, D. A. & Murdick, P. W. (1975) *J. Am. vet. med. Assoc.*, *166*, 227.
(24) Brobst, D. (1975) *J. Am. vet. med. Assoc.*, *166*, 359.
(25) Thornton, J. R. & English, P. B. (1976) *Aust. vet. J.*, *52*, 335.
(26) Mason, T. A. (1972) *Aust. vet. J.*, *48*, 671.
(27) Whitlock, R.H. (1976) *Proc. 21st ann. Mtg Am. Assoc. equ. Practnrs*, 390.
(28) Goldstein, S. M. & MacLean, L. D. (1972) *Can. J. Surg.*, *15*, 318.
(29) Agricultural Research Council (1965) *The Nutrient Requirements of Farm Livestock*, No. 2. *Ruminants*. London.
(30) Donawick, W. J. & Alexander, J. T. (1970) *Proc. Am. Assoc. equ. Practnrs*, 343–53.
(31) Merritt, A. M. (1975) *J. S. Afr. vet. med. Assoc.*, *46*, 89.
(32) Lewis, L.D. & Phillips, R. W. (1971) *Proc. 4th ann. Mtg Am. Assoc. bovine Practnrs*, 109.
(33) Willoughby, R. A. & Butler, D. G. (1967) *Can. vet. J.*, *8*, 70.
(34) Sherman, D. M. et al. (1976) *J. Am. vet. med. Assoc.*, 169, 1310.
(35) Hirschhorn, N. et al. (1973) *J. Pediat.*, *83*, 562.
(36) Hamm, D. & Hicks, W. J. (1975) *Vet. Med. small Anim. Clin.*, *70*, 279.
(37) Hoffsis, G. F. et al. (1977) *J. Am. vet. med. Assoc.*, *171*, 67.
(38) Carter, J. M. & Freedman, a. B. (1977) *J. Am. vet. med. Assoc.*, *171*, 71.
(39) Fowler, M. E. (1980) *J. S. Afr. vet. med. Assoc.*, *51*, 87.
(40) Lindley, W. H. (1977) *J. Am. vet. med. Assoc.*, *171.*, 439.
(41) Little, W. et al. (1980) *Vet. Rec.*, *106*, 547.
(42) Litttle, W. et al. (1978) *Anim. Prod.*, 27, 79.
(43) Young, B. A. & Degen, A. A. (1980) *J. anim. Sci.*, *51*, 811.
(44) Haskins, S. C. (1977) *J. Am. vet. med. Assoc.*, *170*, 423.
(45) Haskins, S. C. (1977) *J. Am. vet. med. Assoc.*, *170*, 429.
(46) Speirs, V. C. (1980) *Am. J. vet. Res.*, *41*, 199.
(47) Poulsen, J. S. D. & Surynek, J. (1977) *Nord. VetMed.*, *29*, 271.
(48) Shull, R. M. (1978) *Vet. clin. Pathol.*, *8*, 12.
(49) Feldman, B. F. & Rosenberg, D. P. (1981) *J. Am. vet. med. Assoc.*, *178*, 396.
(50) Thornton, J. R. (1978) *Br. vet. J.*, *134*, 283.
(51) Carlson, G. P. *et al.* (1978) *Am. J. vet. Res.*, *40*, 587.
(52) Naylor, J. M. (1986) *Proc. 14th World Cong. Dis. of Cattle. Dublin, vol. 1*, pp. 362–367.
(53) Rumbaugh, G. E. et al. (1981) *J. Am. vet. med. Assoc.*, *178*, 267.
(54) Gulick, B. A. & Meagher, D. M. (1981) *J. Am. vet. med. Assoc.*, *178*, 272.
(55) Bywater, R. J. (1977) *Am. J. vet. Res.*, *38*, 1983.
(56) Cleek, J. L. et al. (1979) *J. Am. vet. med. Assoc.*, *174*, 373.
(57) Skenkin, A. & Wretline, A. (1978) Parenteral nutrition. In: Some aspects of human and veterinary nutrition. *World Rev. Nut. Diet*, *28*, 1.
(58) Staples, G. E. (1980) *Br. vet. J.*, *136*, 492.
(59) Brobst, D. F. & Bayly, W. M. (1982) *J. equ. vet. Sci.*, *2*, 51.
(60) Degen, A. A. & Young, B. A. (1981) *Can. J. anim. Sci.*, *61*, 73.
(61) Brownlow, M.A. & Hutchins, D. R. (1982) *Equ. vet. J.*, *14*, 106.
(62) Neathery, M. W. et al (1981) *J. dairy Sci.*, *64*, 2220.
(63) Brobst, D. (1986) *J. Am. vet med. Assoc.*, *188*, 1019.
(64) Epstein, V. (1984) *Equ. vet. J.*, *16*, 453.
(65) Glazier, D. B. et al. (1982) *Am. J. vet. Res.*, *43*, 1934.
(66) Muylle, E. et al. (1984) *Equ. vet. J.*, *16*, 447, 450.
(67) Kasari, T. R. & Naylor, J M. (1984) *Can. vet. J.*, *25*, 394.
(68) Brobst, D. (1983) *J. Am. vet. med. Assoc.*, *183*, 773.
(69) Hartsfield, S. M. et al. (1981) *J. Am. vet. med. Assoc.*, *179*, 914.
(70) Kasari, T. & Naylor, J. (1985) *J. Am. vet. med. Assoc.*, *187*, 392.
(71) Kasari, T. R. & Naylor, J. M. (1986) *Can. J. vet. Res.*, *50*, 502.
(72) Naylor, J. M. & Forsyth, G. W. (1986) *Can. J. vet. Res.*, *50*, 509.
(73) Tasker, J. B. (1971) In: *Clinical Biochemistry of Domestic Animals*, 2nd Ed. Vol. 2, eds, J. J. Kaneko & C. E. Cornelius. New York and London. Academic Press.
(74) Cox, J. H. (1985) *Proc. 21st Ann. Mtg Am. Assoc. Equ. Practrs*, (1986) pp. 383–391.
(75) Rose, R. J. et al. (1986) *Vet. Rec.*, *119*, 522.
(76) Carlson, G. P. & Rumbaugh, G. E. (1983) *Am. J. vet. Res.*, *44*, 964.
(77) Boyd, J. W. (1981) *Br. vet. J.*, *137*, 166.
(78) Naylor, J. M. (1987) *Can. vet. J.*, *28*, 168.
(79) Booth, A. J. & Naylor, J. M. (1987) *J. Am. vet. med. Assoc.*, *191*, 62.

DISTURBANCES OF APPETITE, FOOD INTAKE AND NUTRITIONAL STATUS

Hunger is a purely local subjective sensation arising from gastric hypermotility caused in most cases by lack of distension by food. *Appetite* is a conditioned reflex depending on past associations and experience of palatable foods, and is not dependent on hunger contractions of the stomach. The term appetite is used loosely with regard to animals and really expresses the degree of hunger as indicated by the food intake. When we speak of variations from normal appetite we mean variations from normal food intake, with the rare exception of the animal which demonstrates desire to eat but fails to do so because of a painful condition of the mouth or other disability. Variation in appetite includes increased, decreased or abnormal appetite.

Hyperorexia, or increased appetite, due to increased hunger contractions is manifested by *polyphagia* or increased food intake. Partial absence of appetite (*inappetence*) and complete absence of appetite (*anorexia*) are manifested by varying degrees of decreased food intake (*anophagia*). *Abnormal appetites* include cravings for substances, often normally offensive, other than usual foods. The abnormal appetite may be perverted, a temporary state, or depraved, the permanent or habit stage. Both are manifested by different forms of *pica* or *allotriophagia*.

Polyphagia

Starvation, functional diarrhea, chronic gastritis and abnormalities of digestion, particularly pancreatic deiciency, may result in polyphagia. Metabolic diseases, including diabetes mellitus and hyperthyroidism, are rare in large animals but are causes of polyphagia in other species. Internal parasitism is often associated with poor growth response to more than adequate food intakes.

Although appetite is difficult to assess in animals it seems to be the only explanation for the behavior of those which grossly overeat on concentrates or other palatable feed. The syndromes associated with overeating are dealt with under the diseases of the alimentary tract (Chapters 5 and 6).

Anophagia or aphagia

Decreased food intake may be due to physical factors such as painful conditions of the mouth and pharynx or to lack of desire to eat. Hyperthermia, toxemia and fever all decrease hunger contractions of the stomach. In species with a simple alimentary tract a deficiency of thiamin in the diet will cause atony of the gut and reduction in food intake. In ruminants a deficiency of cobalt and a heavy infestation with trichostrongylid helminths are common causes of anophagia, and low plasma levels of zinc have also been suggested as a cause. In fact alimentary tract stasis due to any cause results in anophagia. Some sensations, including severe pain, excitement and fear may override hunger sensations and animals used to open range conditions may temporarily refuse to eat when confined in feeding lots or experimental units. Some sheep which have been at pasture become completely anophagic if housed. The cause is unknown and treatment, other than turning out to pasture, ineffective (1).

A similar clinical sign is feed aversion, seen most commonly in pigs, which is rejection of particular batches of feed that are contaminated by fungal toxins e.g. *Fusarium* spp., or by the plant *Delphinium barbeyi*.

One of the important aims in veterinary medicine is to encourage an adequate food intake in sick and convalescent animals. Alimentary tract stimulants applied either locally or systemically are in common use but are of limited value unless the primary condition is corrected first. To administer strychnine orally or parasympathomimetic drugs parenterally when there is digestive tract atony due to peritonitis is unlikely to increase food intake. If the primary cause of the lack of appetite is corrected but the animal still refuses to take food these drugs and thiamin are more likely to achieve a response. In cattle, the intraruminal administration of 10–20 liters of rumen juice from a normal cow will often produce excellent results in adult cattle which have been anorexic for several days. The provision of the most palatable feed available is also of value. Parenteral or oral fluid and electrolyte therapy is indicated in animals which do not eat or drink after a few days. For animals which cannot or will not eat or with intractable intestinal disease the use of total intravenous feeding (parenteral nutrition) may be indicated. The subject of therapeutic nutrition for farm animals which cannot or will not eat appears to have been ignored. However, in most cases farm animals will begin to eat their normally preferred diets when the original cause of the anophagia or aphagia is removed or corrected. Intensive fluid therapy may be necessary during the convalescence stage of any disease which has affected feed intake. Reduced feed intake will result in a mild depression of serum electrolytes. A reduced feed intake in high-producing dairy cattle during the first few days or weeks of lactation and in fat beef cattle in late pregnancy may result in fatty infiltration and degeneration of the liver and high mortality. Cattle and sheep must be treated immediately with glucose parenterally and propylene glycol orally to minimize the mobilization of excessive amounts of body fat. In nervous anophagia the injection of insulin in amounts sufficient to cause hypoglycemia without causing convulsions is used in human practice, and in animals the use of tranquilizing drugs may achieve the same result. In ruminants the effects of blood glucose levels on food intake are debatable (2, 3), but it seems probable that neither blood glucose nor blood acetate levels are important factors in regulating the appetite (4, 5). The anorexia which is characteristic of acetonemia and pregnancy toxemia of ruminants appears to be the result of the metabolic toxemia in these diseases. Electrolytic lesions in the hypothalamic region can stimulate or depress food intake depending on the area affected (6, 7). This indicates the probable importance of the hypothalamus in the overall control of appetite.

REVIEW LITERATURE

Langhans, W. & Scharrer, E. (1986) Pathophysiology of inappetence. *J. vet. med. A.*, *33*, 401–413, 414–421.

REFERENCES

(1) Walker, K. H. et al. (1984) *Aust. vet. J.*, *61*, 193.
(2) Manning, R. et al. (1959) *Am. J. vet. Res.*, *20*, 242.
(3) Vallenas, G. A. (1956) *Am. J. vet. Res.*, *17*, 79.
(4) Bowen, J. M. (1962) *Am. J. vet. Res.*, *23*, 948; *24*, 73.
(5) Holder, J. M. (1963) *Nature, Lond.*, *200*, 1074.
(6) Baile, C. A. et al. (1968) *J. dairy Sci.*, *51*, 1474.
(7) Khalaf, F. & Robinson, D. W. (1972) *Res. vet. Sci.*, *31*, 1, 5.

Pica or allotriophagia

Pica refers to the ingestion of materials other than normal food and varies from licking to actual eating or drinking. It is due in most cases to dietary deficiency, either of bulk or in some cases more specifically fiber, or of individual nutrients, particularly salt, cobalt or phosphorus. It is considered as normal behavior in rabbits and foals (5) where it is thought to be a method of dietary supplementation or refection of the intestinal bacterial flora. Boredom, in the case of animals closely confined, often results in the development of pica. Chronic abdominal pain due to peritonitis or gastritis and central nervous system disturbances including rabies and nervous acetonemia are also causes of pica.

The type of pica may be defined as follows: *osteophagia* is the chewing of bones; *infantophagia* is the eating of young; *coprophagia* is the eating of feces. Other types include wood-eating in sheep, bark-eating, the eating of carrion and cannibalism and salt hunger resulting in coat-licking, leather-chewing and the eating of earth, and drinking of urine. Urine drinking may also occur if the urine is mixed with palatable material such as silage effluent. Bark-eating is a common vice in horses especially when their diet is lacking in fibre, e.g. when they are grazing irrigated pasture (18).

Cannibalism may become an important problem in housed animals, particularly swine, which bite one another's tails often resulting in severe local infections; and although some cases may be due to protein, iron or bulk deficiency in the diet many seem to be the result of boredom in animals given insufficient space for exercise. A high ambient temperature and generally limited availability of food also appear to contribute (1). Male castrates are much more often affected than females and the bites are also much more severe in males (13). Provision of larger pens or a hanging object to play with, removal of incisor teeth and the avoidance of mixing animals of different sizes in the same pen are common control measures in pigs. In many instances only one pig in the pen has the habit and his removal may prevent further cases. One common measure which is guaranteed to be successful in terms of tail-biting is surgical removal of all tails with scissors during the first few days of life, when the needle teeth are removed (2). Unfortunately the cannibalistic tendency may then be transferred to ears. As in all types of pica the habit may survive the correction of the causative factor.

Infantophagia can be important in pigs in two circumstances. In intensively housed sows, especially young gilts, hysterical savaging of each pig as it is born can cause heavy losses. When sows are grazed and housed at high density on pasture it is not uncommon to find 'cannibal' sows who protect their own litters but attack the young pigs of other sows. This diagnosis should be considered when there are unexplained disappearances of young pigs.

Pica may have serious consequences: cannibalism may be the cause of many deaths; poisonings, particularly lead poisoning and botulism are common sequels; foreign bodies lodging in the alimentary tract or accumulations of wool, fiber or sand may cause obstruction; perforation of the esophagus or stomach may result from the ingestion of sharp foreign bodies; grazing time is often reduced and livestock may wander away from normal grazing. In many cases the actual cause of the pica cannot be determined and corrective measures may have to be prescribed on a basis of trial and error.

Starvation

Complete deprivation of food causes rapid depletion of glycogen stores and a changeover in metabolism to fat and protein. In the early stages there is hunger, increase in muscle power and endurance, and a loss of body weight. In sheep there is often a depression of serum calcium levels sufficient to cause clinical hypocalcemia. The development of ketosis and acidosis follows quickly on the heels of increased fat utilization. A marked reduction in feed intake in pony mares in late pregnancy is often a precursor of hyperlipemia, a highly fatal disease discussed in Chapter 28 on metabolic diseases. The most pronounced biochemical change in ponies occurring as a result of experimental food deprivation is a lipemia which reaches a peak by the 8th day of fasting but quickly returns to normal when feeding is resumed (3). This degree of change in blood lipids appears to be a characteristic of ponies and horses (16); it is much higher than occurs in pigs. In lactating cows the effect of a short period of starvation is to significantly depress plasma glucose and raise plasma lipid concentrations. Milk yield falls by 70%. On refeeding most levels return to normal in 5 days but blood lipid and milk yield may take as long as 49 days to recover to normal levels (4, 14). In horses fecal output falls to zero at day 4 and water intake is virtually nil from that time on. However, urine volume is maintained (16). In spite of the apparent water imbalance there is no appreciable dehydration, plasma protein levels and PCV staying at normal levels. However, there may be a significant loss of skin turgor (increase in skin tenting) due to the disappearance of subcutaneous fat as cachexia develops (16). Muscular power and activity decrease and the loss of body weight may reach as high as 50–60%. The metabolic rate falls and is accompanied by a slowing of the heart and a reduction in stroke volume, amplitude of the pulse and blood pressure. The circulation is normal as indicated by mucosal color and capillary refill. In the final stages when fat stores are depleted massive protein mobilization occurs and a premortal rise in total urinary nitrogen is observed whereas blood and urine ketones are likely to diminish from their previous high level. Great weakness of skeletal and cardiac musculature is also present in the terminal stages and death is due to circulatory failure. During the period of fat utilization there is a considerable reduction in the ability of tissues to utilize glucose and its administration in large amounts is followed by glycosuria. In such circumstances readily assimilated carbohydrates and proteins should be given in small quantities at frequent intervals but fatty foods may exacerbate the existing ketosis. Diets for animals which have been through a period of great nutritional stress because of deprivation of food or because of illness are described below under *inanition*.

Inanition (malnutrition)

Incomplete starvation, inanition or malnutrition is a more common field condition than complete starvation. The diet is insufficient in quantity and all essential nutrients are present but in suboptimal amounts. The condition is compatible with life, and in general the same pattern of metabolic change occurs as in complete starvation but to a lesser degree. Thus ketosis, loss of body weight and muscular power and a fall in metabolic rate occur. As a result of the reduction in metabolic activity there is a fall in body temperature and respiratory and heart rates (15). In addition there is mental depression, anestrus in cows but not ewes, and increased susceptibility to infection. This increased susceptibility to infection which occurs in some cases of malnutrition cannot be accepted as a general rule. In the present state of knowledge it can only be said that 'some nutritional influences affect resistance to some forms of infection' (5, 6). A significantly reduced food intake also increases susceptibility to some poisons, and this has been related to the effects of starvation on hepatic function (7). In ruminants the effects of starvation on the activity of liver enzymes is delayed compared to that in monogastric animals, due apparently to the ability of the ruminal store of feed to cushion the effect of starvation for some days. The most striking effect of short-term malnutrition in sheep and cattle compared to rats was the very rapid and large accumulation of neutral fat in hepatocytes. If there is a relative lack of dietary protein over a long period of time, anasarca occurs, particularly in the intermandibular space. Malnutrition makes a significant contribution to a number of quasi-specific diseases, 'weaner ill-thrift' and 'thin sow syndrome' among them, and these are dealt with elsewhere. Controlled malnutrition in the form of providing submaintenance diets to animals during periods of severe feed shortage is now a nutritional exercise with an extensive supporting literature. For pastured animals it is a fact of economic life that significant loss of body weight is planned and tolerated for some parts of each year because the well-known phenomenon of compensatory growth (19) enables the animal to make up the lost weight, with no disadvantage during the times of plenty. Animals fed on submaintenance diets undergo metabolic changes reflected in blood and tissue values as well as the more significant changes in weight (8). Experimental restriction of feed intake to 65% of normal levels in non-lactating, non-pregnant heifers does not cause significant falls in serum calcium and phosphorus levels nor in plasma GOT (ASF), aspartate transferase; LDH, lactate dehydrogenase; CPK, creatine phosphokinase levels, nor in serum AP level (9). In sheep that are losing weight because of undernutrition there is a significant increase in plasma creatinine levels (17). Experimental feed restriction, followed by fasting, followed by *ad libitum* access to feed, such as might occur in nature, had no serious ill-effects on goats (10). The goats lost weight significantly but did not overeat on being allowed access to feed. A deficiency of one or more specific dietary essentials also causes a form of partial starvation and is dealt with in Chapter 29.

Outbreaks of incomplete starvation may occur in cattle, sheep and horses which are kept outdoors during the cold winter months in regions of the northern hemisphere. The feed usually consists of poor quality grass hay or cereal grain straw and no grain supplementation. During prolonged exposure to the cold environment the animals will increase their daily intake in an attempt to satisfy maintenance requirements and in cattle, abomasal impaction with a high case mortality may occur. Animals affected with severe inanition are usually weak and recumbent and may or may not eat when offered a palatable feed. Malnutrition and starvation may occur in calves under 1 month and fed poor quality milk replacers containing excessive quantities of non-milk carbohydrates and proteins. The diet is not well digested by young calves and chronic diarrhea and gradual malnutrition occur. Affected calves recover quickly when fed cow's whole milk for several days. At necropsy there is a marked reduction in muscle mass, lack of depot fat and serous atrophy of fat (11). Starvation may also occur in beef calves sucking poorly nourished heifer dams with an insufficient supply of milk. The mortality will be high during cold weather when the maintenance requirements are increased. Affected calves will initially suck vigorously and persistently, they will attempt to eat dry feed, drink surface water and urine and bawl for several hours. Eventually they lie in sternal recumbency with their head and neck turned into their flanks and die quietly. The response to therapy is usually unsatisfactory and the case fatality rate is high. The convalescence period in survivors is prolonged and treatment is usually uneconomical. Affected animals must be brought indoors and kept warm and well bedded during treatment and realimentation. Initially, fluid therapy using balanced electrolyte solutions containing glucose and amino acids may be necessary to restore the animal's strength and appetite. This is followed by the provision of controlled amounts of a highly palatable digestible diet. High-quality legume hay is excellent, small amounts of ground grain are of value and the daily administration of a multiple B vitamin and mineral mixture will replenish those lost during inanition. Skim-milk powder is an excellent source of carbohydrate and protein for young animals which have been partially starved. Adult animals cannot digest large quantities of milk powder because of the relative lack of the appropriate digestive enzymes.

Horses that have been ill and had poor appetite should be tempted with green grass first, and failing that tried with good quality hay—preferably alfalfa. It is best to dilute it with good grass hay to begin with, and increase the mix to 100% legume hay over a week. An average horse will require 1·5–2 kg/day. Grain can be added mixed with molasses or as a mash. Low-fiber diets are recommended to ensure maximum digestibility. A supplement of B vitamins may be advantageous until full appetite and intake are regained. Horses with broken jaws or which are unable to eat at all for some reason can be allowed to go without food for 3 days, but beyond that time they should be fed by stomach tube. A suitable ration (16) is:

- Electrolyte mixture (NaCl, 10 g; $NaHCO_3$, 15 g; KCl, 75 g; K_2HPO_4, 60 g; $CaCl_2$, 45 g; MgO, 24 g) — 210 g
- Water — 21 l
- Dextrose (increased from 300 g/day in 7 days to) — 900 g
- Dehydrated cottage cheese (increased from 300 g/day in 7 days to) — 900 g

The ration is divided into two or three equal amounts and fed during one day. Adult horses which are weak and recumbent may be supported in a sling to avoid decubitus ulceration and other secondary complications associated with prolonged recumbency. The rehabilitation of the recumbent malnourished (equine starvation syndrome) horse has been described (12).

REFERENCES

(1) Jericho, K. W. F. & Church, T. L. (1972) *Can. vet. J.*, *13*, 156.
(2) Penny, R. H. C. & Hill, F. W. G. (1974) *Vet. Rec.*, *94*, 174.
(3) Baetz, A. L. & Pearson, J. E. (1972) *Am. J. vet. Res.*, *33*, 1941.
(4) Reid, I. M. et al. (1977) *J. comp. Pathol.*, *87*, 241, 253.
(5) Crowell-Davis, S. L. & Houpt, K. A. (1985) *Equ. vet. J.*, *17*, 17.
(6) Hill, R. (1965) *Br. vet. J.*, *121*, 402.
(7) Manns, E. (1972) *Res. vet. Sci.*, *13*, 140.
(8) Payne, E. et al. (1970) *Aust. J. exp. Agric. Anim. Husb.*, *10*, 256.
(9) Reichmann, K. G. & May, R. I. (1976) *Aust. vet. J.*, *52*, 595.
(10) Fowle, K. E. & Church, D. V. (1973) *Am. J. et. Res*, 34, 849.
(11) Thomson, R. G. (1967) *Can. vet. J.*, *8*, 242.

(12) Finocchio, E. J. (1973) *Proc. 19th ann. Mtg Am. Assoc. equ. Practnrs*, 167.
(13) Penny, R. H. C. et al. (981) *Vet. Res.*, *108*, 35.
(14) Reid, I. M. et al. (1977) *J. comp. Pathol.*, *87*, 241.
(15) Ellis, R. N. W. & Lawrence, T. J. L. (1978) *Br. vet. J.*, *134*, 333.
(16) Naylor, J. M. (1967) *J. Equ. med. Surg.*, *1*, 64.
(17) Keenan, D. M. & Allardyce, C. J. (1986) *Aust. vet. J.*, *63*, 29.
(18) Keenan, D. M. (1986) *Aust. vet. J.*, *63*, 234.

Thirst

Thirst is an increased desire for water manifested by excessive water intake (polydipsia). There are two important causes of thirst: dryness of the pharyngeal and oral mucosae increases the desire for water, irrespective of the water status of body tissues; in addition cellular dehydration due to a rise in blood osmotic pressure causes increased thirst. Specific observations in ponies have shown that water intake is increased in response to either an increase in the osmotic pressure of tissue fluid or a decrease in the volume of their body fluids (8).

Cellular dehydration occurs commonly in many cases of dehydration due to vomiting, diarrhea, polyuria and excessive sweating. Increased thirst in early fever is due to changes in cell colloids leading to increased water retention. A marked polydipsia and polyuria occur in salt deficiency in lactating dairy cattle, in addition to weight loss, a fall in milk production and salt hunger. Salivary sodium levels are best used for diagnosis (1). A similar syndrome occurs in the 'thin sow syndrome'. In humans several other factors appear to exert some effect on water intake; a deficiency of potassium and an excess of calcium in tissue fluid both increase thirst; an increased thirst also occurs in uremia irrespective of the body's state of hydration. It has been suggested that these chemical factors may cause direct stimulation of the thirst center in the hypothalamus (2). Clinically diabetes insipidus produces by far the most exaggerated polydipsia.

The clinical syndrome produced by water deprivation is not well defined. Animals supplied with saline water will drink it with reluctance and, if the salinity is sufficiently great, die of salt poisoning.

Cattle at pasture which are totally deprived of water usually become quite excited and are likely to knock down fences and destroy watering points in their frenzy. On examination they exhibit a hollow abdomen, sunken eyes and the other signs of dehydration. There is excitability with trembling and slight frothing at the mouth. The gait is stiff and uncoordinated and recumbency follows. Abortion of decomposed calves, with dystocia due to failure of the cervix to dilate, may occur for some time after thirst have been relieved and cause death in survivors. At necropsy there is extensive liquefaction of fat deposits, dehydration and early fetal death in pregnant cows (3).

Experimental water deprivation has been recorded in camels (4) and lactating and non-lactating dairy cows (5). In camels death occurred on the seventh to ninth day of total deprivation; body weight loss was about 25%. Lactating cows allowed access to only 50% of their regular water supply become very aggressive about the water trough, spend more time near it and lie down less. After 4 days milk yield is depressed to 74% and body weight to 86% of original figures. There is a significant increase in serum osmolality with increased concentrations of urea, sodium, total protein and copper. The PCV is increased as are levels of creatinine kinase and SGOT (7). With complete deprivation for 72 hours the changes are similar but there are surprisingly few clinical signs at that time. The composition of the milk does not change markedly and blood levels return to normal in 48 hours. After deprivation of half of their water intake the cattle reduced their water loss by all routes, but plasma and total blood volumes were unchanged. Sheep, even pregnant ewes, are capable of surviving even though access to water is limited to only once each 72 hours, but there is a significant loss (26%) of body weight. Deprivation of water which allows access to water only once every 96 hours is not compatible with maintaining the pregnancy (6).

REFERENCES

(1) Ghosal, A. K. et al. (1973) *Ind. vet. J.*, 50, 518.
(2) Fourman, P. & Leeson, P. M. (1959) *Lancet*, *276*, 268.
(3) Knight, R. P. (1963–4) *Vict. vet. Proc.*, *22*, 45.
(4) Seif, S. M. et al. (1973) *J. dairy Sci.*, *56*, 581.
(5) Whitlock, R. H. et al. (1975) *Cornell Vet.*, *65*, 512.
(6) More, T. & Sahni, K. L. (1978) *J. agr. Sci. (UK)*, *90*, 435.
(7) Little, W. et al. (1984) *Res. vet. Sci.*, *37*, 283.
(8) Sufit, E. et al. (1985) *Equ. vet. J.*, *17*, 12.

WEIGHT LOSS OR FAILURE TO GAIN WEIGHT (ILL-THRIFT)

This section is concerned with the syndrome consisting of weight loss even though there is apparently adequate food supply and a normal appetite. In the absence of any primary disease an animal or group of animals presented with this as the problem requiring correction is a major diagnostic dilemma. Several semi-identified diseases in this category are 'weaner ill-thrift', 'thin sow syndrome', 'thin ewe syndrome', 'weak calf syndrome', all of which are dealt with in a later chapter. The problem is also encountered in horses, in stud animals of any species and in milking goats. It is most obvious when animals are kept as individuals, especially as companion animals.

A common source of error in clinical work in food and racing animals is with respect to estimating the animal's body weight. Scales are rarely available and estimations by weight-bands are subject to too much variability. A reasonably satisfactory alternative used in cattle and sheep (1) and described for horses (2) is a body condition score estimated on the basis of the amount of body covering of muscle, fat and connective tissue.

What follows is a checklist of causes which should be considered when an animal is presented with a weight loss problem and without signs indicative of a primary disease which is likely to be the cause of the problem.

Nutritional causes
These are as follows:

1. 'Hobby farm malnutrition', inanition or inadequate feed is a surprisingly common cause, especially in companion horses. Inexperienced owners who keep their animals where they are not able to graze pasture and are entirely dependent on stored feed often underfeed for economy's sake. The average 450 kg horse needs 20 kcal (84 kJ) a day for maintenance. A knowledge of the approximate energy and protein values of feeds is necessary to prepare an appropriate ration. In a hospital situation any horse presented with a weight loss problem and without a potential diagnosis on first examination should be weighed, fed an energy-rich diet *ad libitum* for 4 days, then weighed. A horse which has previously been underfed will gain 3–5 kg/day weight. The feed must be inspected. Mature meadow hay may be efficient only as a filler and poorly filled oat grain may be very poorly nutritive on a weight basis. Gentle horses that are fed in a group with others may be physically prevented from getting a fair share of available feed especially if trough space is inadequate.

   This problem is also common when urban people try to raise a few vealer calves or sheep to help defray the costs of their rural acreage. It is common in these circumstances to equate rough meadow grass with proper nutrition for young or pregnant ruminants.
2. Diets which are inadequate in total energy because they cannot replace the energy loss caused by the animal's level of production are now important causes of weight loss. This subject is discussed under the heading of production disease. An example is acetonemia of high-producing cows in which body stores of fat and protein are raided to repair the inadequacies of the diet.
3. Malnutrition as a result of a ration which is deficient in an essential trace element is unusual in the sort of situation being discussed. A nutritional deficiency of cobalt does cause weight loss in ruminants, but is likely to have an area effect and not cause weight loss in one animal. Copper salt, zinc, potassium, selenium, phosphorus, calcium and vitamin D deficiencies are in this category too. Experimental nutritional deficiencies of riboflavin, nicotinic acid, pyridoxine, pantothenic acid in calves and pigs are also characterized by ill-thrift.
4. Inadequate intake of an adequate supply of feed is dealt with under diseases of the mouth and pharynx and is not repeated here, but it is emphasized that the first place for a clinician to look in a thin animal is its mouth. So often the owner has forgotten just how old the animal is and one often finds a cow without any incisor teeth attempting to survive on pasture.
5. Other factors which reduce an animal's food intake when it is available in adequate amounts include anxiety, excitement of estrus, new surroundings, loss of newborn, bad weather, tick or other insect worry, and abomasal displacement.

Excessive loss of protein and carbohydrates
The following are causes:

1. Glucose loss in the urine in diabetes mellitus or chronic renal disease, the former indicated by hyperglycemia, and both by glycosuria, are obvious examples of weight loss as a result of excessive metabolic loss of energy.
2. Protein loss in the feces. Cases of protein-losing gastroenteropathy are unusual and are difficult to identify without access to a radioactive isotope laboratory. The loss may occur through an ulcerative lesion, via a generalized vascular discontinuity, or by exudation through intact mucosa as a result of hydrostatic pressure in blood vessels, e.g., in verminous aneurysm, or lymphatics in cases of lymphangiectasia of the intestine. The identification of a neoplasm (lymphosarcoma or intestinal or gastric adenocarcinoma are the usual ones), or of granulomatous enteritis, is not possible without laparotomy and biopsy of the alimentary segment. One is usually led to the possibility of this as a diagnosis by either a low serum total protein or low albumin level in a normal total protein level, and in the absence of other protein loss as set down in (3) below *et seq.*
3. Proteinuria for a lengthy period can cause depletion of body protein stores and resulting weight loss. Chronic renal disease with a significant tubular lesion is the usual cause. Glomerulonephritis is less common and more likely to be acute. Examination of the urine should be part of a clinical examination, but is not commonly so in horses because of the difficulty of obtaining a specimen without recourse to catheterization. Moving the horse into a box stall with fresh straw, or the intravenous injection of frusemide are used as alternative methods. The latter provides an abnormally dilute sample.
4. Internal and external parasitoses in which blood sucking is a significant pathogenetic mechanism can result in severe protein loss, as well as anemia *per se*.

Faulty absorption and digestion and metabolism
This is caused by the following:

1. Faulty digestion and absorption are commonly manifested by diarrhea, and diseases which have that effect are dealt with elsewhere under the heading of malabsorption syndromes—in the section on enteritis. In grazing ruminants the principal causes are the nematode worms *Ostertagia*, *Nematodirus*, *Trichostrongylus*, *Chabertia*, *Cooperia*, *Oesophagostomum* and the flukes *Fasciola* and *Paramphistomum*. In cattle there are, in addition, tuberculosis, coccidiosis, anaplasmosis, sarcosporidiosis and enzootic calcinosis. In sheep and goats there are Johne's disease, viral pneumonia without clinical pulmonary involvement, and hemonchosis. In horses there is strongylosis, diseases in foals, habronemiasis and heavy infestations with botfly larvae. In pigs there is stephanuriasis, hyostrongylosis (including the thin sow syndrome) infestation with

Macrocanthorhyncus hirudinaceus, ascariasis. Gastrointestinal neoplasia, as in (2) above, must be considered as a possible cause.
2. Chronic villous atrophy as occurs with intestinal parasitism or as a result of a viral infection is the most potent cause of long-term interference.
3. Other lesions caused by parasitic invasion and which affect digestion and absorption are gastric granuloma caused by *Habronema* spp. in horses, and verminous arteritis, also in horses. These are dealt with below.
4. Abnormal physical function of the alimentary tract, as typified in vagus indigestion of cattle and grass sickness in horses, can be a potent cause of failure to absorb nutrient, but the syndrome is usually manifested by poor food intake and grossly abnormal feces.
5. Inadequate utilization of absorbed nutriments is a characteristic of chronic liver disease. It is usually distinguishable by a low serum albumin level, by liver function tests and by serum enzyme estimations. A clinical syndrome including edema, jaundice, photosensitization and weight loss is a common accompaniment.
6. Neoplasia in any organ. The metabolism of the body as a whole is often unbalanced by the presence of a neoplasm so that the animal wastes even though its food intake seems adequate.
7. Chronic infection, including specific diseases such as tuberculosis, sarcocystosis, East Coast fever, trypanosomiasis (nagana), maedi-visna, caprine arthritis-encephalitis, enzootic pneumonia of swine and non-specific infections such as atrophic rhinitis of pigs, abscess, empyema and chronic peritonitis have the effect of reducing metabolic activity generally as well as reducing appetite. Both effects are the result of the toxemia caused by tissue breakdown and of toxins produced by the organisms present. Less well understood are the means by which systemic infections, e.g., equine infectious anemia, scrapie in sheep and other slow viruses, produce a state of weight loss progressing to emaciation.
8. Many diseases of other systems, e.g., congestive heart failure, are manifested by weight loss because of inadequate oxygenation of tissues. Determination of the specific cause of weight loss in an individual animal depends firstly on differentiation into one of the three major groups, nutritional causes by assessment of the food intake, protein or carbohydrate loss by clinicopathological laboratory tests, and faulty absorption by tests of digestion as set out in diseases of the alimentary tract.

REVIEW LITERATURE

Coffman, J. R. & Hammond, L. S. (1979) Weight loss and the digestive system in the horse: a problem specific data base. *Vet. Clin. N. Am.*, *1*(2), 237.

Scrutchfield, W. L. (1976) Protein losing gastroenteropathy. *Ann. Gen. Mtg Am. Assoc. Equ. Practnrs*, p. 203.

REFERENCES

(1) Radostits, O. M. & Blood, D. C. (1983) *Herd Health*. Philadelphia. W. B. Saunders.

(2) Henneke, D. R. (1983) *Equ. vet. J.*, *15*, 371.

POOR RACING PERFORMANCE IN HORSES (POOR PERFORMANCE SYNDROME)

This section deals with the problem of horses which have performed well and are now suffering from a series of poor performances without the intervention of a discernible disease or specific lamenesses including back injuries; it is the classical loss-of-form situation. Most clinical illnesses completely prevent any attempt to race because of the need to be as close as possible to 100% healthy to have any chance of winning. There are also many horses which, because of poor conformation and therefore poor running action, or poor chest capacity or small heart size, or even poor temperament, never do perform well. They present a different problem from the one under discussion. Some of the techniques described below will be applicable to that situation, but the whole scope of possible problems will not be covered.

One of the difficulties in conducting a performance test on a horse, other than a time trial, is the absence of a standard test with biochemical and physiological parameters by which to judge the results. Such a test has been described but the database on which criteria could be based still has not (3).

Some of the problems likely to be encountered when examining a horse for declining performance, and the techniques used to counter these problems are:

1. *Parasite infestation*—a fecal egg count will be the critical test if the prepatent period has been sufficiently long and if the horse has not been treated for worms in the preceding 5 weeks. There is no suitable test which will determine the presence or absence of migrating strongyle larvae.
2. *Anemia*—attempts to relate hemaglobin level to quality of racing performance have not been very successful. However, a detectable reduction in the erythron below the normal level for a horse's peers is likely to be the cause of at least some reduction in performance efficiency.
3. *Hepatic injury*—subacute, even subclinical, hepatitis due possibly to undetected fungal toxins in prepared feed may be a real cause of reduced performance level. There is a lack of appetite and a moderate increase in sorbitol dehydrogenase levels without an increase in bromsulfalein retention time. The diagnosis might be confirmed by liver biopsy, but the episode is often so transient that drastic measures are not undertaken.
4. *Myocarditis* caused by streptococci during a bacteremic phase of an upper respiratory tract infection, or by migrating strongyle larvae, is a common diagnosis for stopped horses. If an electrocardiographic examination identifies an abnormality

which is reconcilable with a recent myocarditis this is acceptable as confirming the diagnosis. An analysis of electrocardiography produced by racehorses and Olympic 3-day eventers showed that a high proportion of poorly performed horses had ECG abnormalities, especially of the T-wave and with intra-atrial block (2).

5. *A respiratory virus* may cause an 'outbreak' of poor performance in a stable, although there may be no outstanding clinical evidence of disease (1). The signs attributed to the infection are:

   - Poor performance in training gallops or races
   - 'Blowing' after cantering or faster work
   - Leaving some feed
   - Moderate transient fever
   - 'Starving', dandruffy coat
   - Serous to purulent nasal discharge and conjunctivitis
   - Enlarged submandibular lymph nodes
   - Intermittent cough
   - Small volume, foul-smelling feces
   - Stiffness of movement after exercise.

   Well-established cases with obvious signs as set out above will qualify as upper respiratory tract infections, either equine viral pneumonitis, equine influenza, or an infection with a rhinovirus or adenovirus, discussed in detail elsewhere. The subject is raised here because many cases are equivocal with respect to signs and this is to be expected in groups of horses that have some degree of immunity to the current infections.

6. *Endocarditis* in adult horses is usually readily identifiable by virtue of cardiac murmurs arising from stenotic or incompetent valves. However, such murmurs may be difficult to identify and the lesion may be missed especially if the heart is not carefully examined on both sides of the chest with a good-sized phonendoscope in a quiet box or stall where extraneous sounds do not interfere with auscultation.
7. *Chronic bronchitis and chronic obstructive respiratory disease* (COPD) are amongst the important causes of deteriorating exercise tolerance in horses especially when horses are stabled much of the time in poorly ventilated surroundings and with dusty feed. However, they are usually recognizable as overt disease. Early cases not showing clinical signs may present difficulties. Chronic lymphoid hyperplasia of the pharyngeal wall is in the same category and is a much more common problem than COPD in pastured horses.
8. *Subclinical osteodystrophia fibrosa*, an early stage of secondary nutritional hyperparathyroidism, is usually manifested by at least a shifting lameness, long before there are any detectable bony changes. As a result the 'poor performance' is accompanied by problems of gait, or not going freely, rather than just tiredness. The identity of the diagnosis is usually suspected when the history includes heavy grain, or grain byproduct, feeding without supplementation of the diet with calcium. 'Tying up' comes within the same category and is also discussed elsewhere.
9. *Hyponatremia, hypochloremia and hypokalemia* cause muscle tiredness and general fatigue, and horses in heavy work, losing a good deal of electrolytes in sweat, might conceivably develop these states, especially if they are overtrained. In veterinary work with racehorses a great deal of importance is attached to maintaining the serum electrolytes at exactly the correct levels. This is usually done by means of a 'saline drench' containing a mixture of various salts or by supplying a balanced electrolyte mixture in the feed or drinking water. Which salts to use and in what amounts depends to a very large extent on information gathered from biochemical analyses. An extension of this attitude towards tissue metabolism is the development of dependence on a full biochemical and hematological profile. There are no well-identified indices on which to base proper decisions and predictions although there is potentially a great deal of benefit to be derived from the system. Metabolic profiles as described for dairy cattle suggest themselves as a means of establishing normal parameters within a district or even within a stable provided the horse population is large enough.
10. *Inability to sweat*, as occurs in anhidrosis, so that incapacitating hyperthermia develops during exercise. In the developmental stages of the disease the cause may not be obvious.
11. *Inadequate feed supply*, especially in terms of carbohydrate content is a possible cause of poor performance and the diet of a horse does need to be evaluated, but the reverse is usually the case—most horses are overfed.
12. Other specific *nutritional deficiencies* are not much to the fore in horses, but selenium, folic acid and iron are often administered on the assumption that they will improve physical performance.
13. *Changes in temperament*, especially 'going sour', manifested by biting other horses while racing, and attendants in stables, are usually ascribed to overtraining, or training for too long periods. Mares with ovarian tumors probably behave worst of all.
14. *Thyroid carcinoma*—this is characterized by unilateral serious enlargement of one thyroid gland (14).

The hematological and biochemical abnormalities observed most commonly in two groups of Irish horses suffering from poor performance syndrome included leukopenia followed by leukocytosis, reversal of the ratios of neutrophils to lymphocytes and of albumin to globulin, elevation of the blood levels of amino aspartate transaminase and creatine kinase, and depression of serum levels of sodium and potassium (5).

REFERENCES

(1) Mumford, J. A. & Rossdale, P. D. (1980) *Equ. vet. J.*, *12*, 3.
(2) Rose, R. J. & Davis, P. E. (1978) *Aust. vet. J.*, *54*, 51.
(3) Isler, R. et al. (1982) *Schweiz. Arch. Tierheilkd.*, *124*, 603.
(4) Held, J. P. (1985) *J. Am. vet. med. Assoc.*, *187*, 104.
(5) Fogarty, U. & Leadon, D. (1987) *Irish vet. J.*, *41*, 203.

PHYSICAL EXERCISE AND EXHAUSTION

Most of the interest in this subject relates to horses. Of minor importance are the effects of violent and prolonged activity between fighting animals, especially boars and bulls. Part of the damage of these contests is due to lacerations caused by horns and tusks, but these are surprisingly superficial in most cases. Treatment consisting of topical application to lacerations, systemic antibiotic administration if these are severe, and treatment of shock with corticosteroids is appropriate.

In horses, there is obviously a great need for knowledge about the effects of arduous or violent exercise or of different training strategies on performance. There is some information available on racehorses, but most of the work relates to endurance rides (9, 10). There are two aspects to this rapidly developing area of veterinary sports medicine: one is the prevention of injury; the other is the desire to improve the quality of performance. In horses, it is necessary to give consideration to:

- Maintenance of muscle fiber integrity
- Restoration of electrolyte and fluid loss due to sweating
- Restoration of electrolyte imbalance between muscles and tissue fluids
- Replacement of utilized energy sources
- Replacement of hormones and enzymes depleted by prolonged and vigorous exercise
- Prophylactic administration of any of the above
- The effect of pre-exercise training in developing more rapid and better responses in metabolic systems related to the biophysical and biochemical effects of exercise
- Precompetition examinations, clinical and paraclinical, to estimate fitness for racing or performing.

Trotting and galloping races

Biochemical changes

After trotting races there are increases in blood levels of sodium, potassium, calcium and magnesium, but not chlorides. Plasma osmolarity increases due largely to rises in the levels of sodium and lactate (21). After galloping races there are rises, but these return to normal within an hour. At the same time there is a fall in plasma phosphate. Levels of creatinine, lactic acid and uric acid are elevated at the end of a race, and lactic acid and uric acid levels continue to be high at an hour afterwards (24). The high uric acid levels have not been explained (25), but could be a suitable benchmark for severity of physical activity. Cantering, as distinct from galloping, does not elevate blood lactate or uric acid levels. Because of the importance of selenium in the maintenance of muscle health, there has been a development of interest in its relationship to myositis, myoglobinuria and 'tying-up'. The effect of light exercise on relevant values in standardbred horses is to increase serum selenium, and hemoglobin and hematocrit levels immediately after a training job. Gluthathione peroxidase and reductase levels are not affected, but RBC-reduced glutathione is reduced (16). The increase in serum selenium may be related to the release of this selenium-containing enzyme from erythrocytes. Not all observers record these changes, especially the variations in selenium and peroxidase levels (17). The differences are between standardbreds and quarterhorses and may be due to breed differences or to different dietary practices.

In long-distance races, marathons as distinct from endurance rides, there are significant changes in biochemical parameters (17). There is an increase in blood lactate, up to 16-fold, a highly significant rise in blood glucose, free fatty acids and glycerol, a rise in plasma cortisol, a massive increase in glucagon and a variable effect on plasma insulin levels. Observations in an equine marathon indicate that of the electrolytes, potassium levels rise, sodium is unaffected and calcium is decreased. Bicarbonate is unaffected. Albumin and creatinine phosphokinase levels are increased, as are plasma urea, creatinine and uric acid.

Biophysical changes

The racehorse has a much greater capacity to consume oxygen during severe exercise than man or other domestic animals (11). This capacity is the result of greatly increased heart and respiratory rates and a large mobilization of erythrocytes from the spleen, where 30–50% of total erythrocytes are stored at rest. The horse's heart is, relatively speaking, much larger than man's so that the stroke volume is relatively greater. The respiratory system is similarly developed. All of these factors combined are capable of increasing oxygen consumption during strenuous exercise to 35 times the consumption at rest, i.e. about twice the increase which occurs in man.

Changes in biophysical parameters which occur in the horse with exercise include the following. Commencing at a resting heart rate of 30/min, heavy workloads result in peak heart rates in 45–120 secs; at the end of the exercise the rate falls rapidly and reaches prework rate at 2–20 minutes, depending on the severity of the workload. The peak rate may be 240/min. The duration of systole and diastole, and the cardiac output and stroke volume at rest and exercise show comparable responses to exercise. Arterial blood pressure also increases (10·7) markedly during exercise, prework pressures of 80 mmHg (16·0 kPa) (diastolic) to 120 (27·3 kPa) (systolic) rise with exercise, the systolic rising much higher, up to 205 mmHg (27·3 kPa) and diastolic to 116 mmHg (15·5 kPa). Very high systolic pressures, up to 240–260 mmHg (32·0–34·7 kPa) have been recorded. Respiratory rates rise from about 10/min to 80–100. The depth of respiration is also greatly increased.

The two factors in fatigue during exercise, which affect cardiovascular performance, are blood concentration of lactic acid and heart rate. Horses perform moderate exercise (300 m/min) completely aerobically. It is only during heavy exercise that blood lactic acid rises and the horse is performing anaerobically. At 600 m/min this rise in blood lactic acid is very steep. The heart rate is not easy to monitor in a galloping horse, but using telemetric techniques it is apparent that the heart rate can reach speeds at which the volume of ventricular ejection is compromised.

Trotters are given light exercise before a race to 'warm-up'; galloping horses are not. The warm-up has the functions of loosening up muscles and supporting structures, and of elevating body temperature which in turn enhances metabolic activity. Body temperature rises with exercise, the size of the rise being determined by the severity of the exercise. If heat generation exceeds capacity for heat loss, the body temperature rises, often as high as 41°C (105°F), and it can rise sufficiently high to stress the cardiovascular system. During extremes of environmental temperature and humidity, long-distance races and endurance rides may cause heat exhaustion because of the difficulty in losing the generated heat.

The effects of training include increased splenic storage of erythrocytes; this means that estimating work potential based on blood levels of hemoglobin is most accurate if carried out immediately after exercise (11), and increase in heart size and therefore stroke volume. Attempts to estimate heart size on the length of the QRS interval have not been universally acclaimed.

Recommendations about optimal training techniques are available, but careful comparisons of the effects of these are not available.

Endurance events

These events, ranging in length from 80 to 150 km to be completed in 1 or 2 days, have become very popular and because they are open to persons with little knowledge of physical exercise physiology and the need to prepare horses properly, the equine sports medicine groups, including veterinarians, have spent a lot of time and effort to ensure that the horses' welfare is protected. So there is a fairly extensive literature relating to the monitoring of biochemical and biophysical parameters of performance during rides. The relevant literature includes some of the following principles (30).

Clinical problems

Physical exhaustion

In endurance events the horses are under frequent surveillance for signs of injury or exhaustion. Clinical signs which suggest exhaustion (the exhausted horse syndrome) are depression, lethargy, dehydration, hyperthermia (40–41°C; 104–105°F), hyperpnea and tachycardia (both rates will be greater than 90/min), muscle tremor or spasms, and a degree of abdominal and respiratory distress which make the horse restless and anxious. Other bad signs are relaxed anal sphincter, unwillingness to stand but fidgeting when lying down, pale or cyanotic mucosae and a capillary refill time of more than 5 sec. One of the best indicators is the ratio of the respiratory to the cardiac rate. If it is of the order to 2 to 1, the horse is in a serious state, probably due to impending pulmonary edema. The severity of the exhaustion state in an individual horse can be judged fairly accurately on what happens when exercise is stopped. Significant remission of the signs and a return to almost normal should be achieved within 30–60 minutes after stopping work and some efforts being made to cool the horse down (2). As a further guide it is suggested that horses whose heart rates do not return to less than 60/min within 20 minutes of stopping work are unfit and should not be allowed to continue (9).

Heat exhaustion

A contributing or alternate disease problem to physical exhaustion is heat exhaustion which is likely to occur in physically stressed horses which are overfat and during hot weather. In these animals there is severe muscle weakness, recumbency, dyspnea, convulsions terminally and always a high temperature (42°C; 107·5°F) (14). A further problem at this time is the horse that develops exertional rhabdomyolysis manifested by muscle stiffness, tremor, weakness and possibly recumbency. There may be myoglobinuria if the disease is sufficiently severe and the serum enzymes (creatinine phosphokinase (CPK) and serum glutamic oxalate transaminase (SGOT)) levels are grossly increased. These horses are particularly vulnerable to further damage if they are immediately floated (boxed) long distances to home (29). Dehydration hyponatremia and hypokalemia are also occurrences at this time.

Horses which show signs of exhaustion usually recover within a few hours and the only treatment undertaken is the repair of fluid and electrolyte deficits as set down under biochemical changes. In physically fit horses completing an endurance or marathon ride of 80–100 km in a day at a rate of 10–12 km/hour, in ambient environmental temperatures of 10–20°C (50–68°F), the following biophysical parameters should be achieved:

- Rectal temperature—37·5°C (99°F) up to less than 40°C (104°F)
- Heart rate per minute—36 at rest to 80/min, but may reach 150 in circumstances of severe physical stress
- Respiratory rate per minute—12–20 at rest to 80–100 per minute after exercise
- Packed cell volume—35% at start, rising to 45% at finish. At 55% the horse is destined for exhaustion.

Synchronous diaphragmatic flutter occurs as part of the syndrome of physical exhaustion but in a number of diseases as well (p. 377).

Prediction of fitness for endurance rides is largely based on past performance, intensity of training and body condition. In a small group of horses the faster performers in an endurance ride had higher heart scores (longer QRS intervals) before the trial and had higher PCV values and heart rates during and at the end of it. These are logical findings and may provide some prognostic data (23). A lower than normal PCV at commencement of a trial may also be advantageous, and due to an increase in plasma volume as a result of training (26). In spite of their obvious fitness, horses performing well in 3-day events are observed to have more electrocardiographic abnormalities than other groups.

Biochemical changes

Horses participating in endurance rides, as distinct from long distance races, show a generally consistent pattern of hypoglycemia, and elevation of levels of free fatty acids and glycerol in plasma, hyperphosphatemia, and a reduction in plasma Na, K, Ca, Mg and Cl. Body fluid loss and clinical dehydration may or may not occur depending on the weather. Modest rises in levels of blood lactate, lactate dehydrogenase and creatinine phosphokinase are observed (1, 2, 13). Any tendency to acidosis, a feature of horses exercised at much greater speeds than in endurance rides, is compensated, restoring arterial pH and P_{CO_2}. The falls in serum calcium and magnesium levels occur earlier, about the middle of the ride, than those of sodium and potassium, which are not discernible until the end of the ride. Losses of sodium, potassium and chloride in sweat appear to be the cause of falls in blood levels of these electrolytes (18). Variations in the degree of alkalosis occur in direct proportion to increases in heart rate (19) and probably reflect the horse's fitness. Energy metabolism is reflected by falls in serum glucose and insulin levels while plasma corticosteroid levels rise (20). The level of lactate, which is usually moderately raised, is a good indicator of the horse's capacity to work without significant anaerobic glycolysis (17). A switch to fat metabolism is indicated by the rise in blood fatty acids and glycerol. Ketosis does not occur (17). Increased metabolic activity and decreased renal perfusion probably account for an observed increase in blood urea and other blood non-protein nitrogen levels (17). Any dehydration incurred during the ride is soon corrected by the voluntary intake of water, but the electrolyte deficit is unlikely to be corrected unless some positive supplementation of dietary intake is provided. Intravenous injection is a sure and rational means of doing this, but a saline drench is quite adequate and is the usual means. It should contain Na, K, Ca, and Mg ions (10). There is no objection to horses drinking during hard work of this sort, provided they are allowed to drink frequently, say every hour; with infrequent drinking the horse may drink too much at one time (29).

In addition to an increase in PCV and plasma protein indicative of hemoconcentration resulting from dehydration there is a stress leukon with a neutrophilic leukocytosis and a shift to the left. The degree of hemoconcentration is usually moderate but significant. Rises may be as great as 26% for PCV and 13% for plasma albumin, the former higher level resulting from splenic evacuation.

These changes in serum electrolytes, metabolites, enzymes and hormones reflect the muscle damage, tissue dehydration and increased anaerobic glycolysis and mobilization of lipids that the horses experience in this arduous form of competitive riding (33). The changes are greater in horses that complete a course at a faster speed, and in those that complete longer courses. All of the changes have disappeared within 24 hours (7).

Three-day events and other less demanding competitions

Competitions which contain a segment of cross-country riding on the flat and over jumps, and against a time limit, offer a degree of physical stress between those imposed by racing and by endurance rides. The standard format is: day 1—dressage; day 2—the speed and endurance tests, usually of road and track work, steeplechase, more road and track work and finally cross-country; day 3—show jumping. Thus, there are segments of endurance work, requiring aerobic energy metabolism, and segments of speed racing which depend heavily on anaerobic metabolism (28). The observed changes in horses competing in these 3-day events, are a combination of the effects of speed racing and endurance rides. The effects are of a lesser degree, and are most noticeable after the cross-country segment (22).

Effects of training

There is an expanding literature on the effects of exercise on clinical indexes, and the effects of training on these (3–6, 11). In general, training has the following physical effects on horses (11, 31):

- Enlargement of spleen and greater erythrocyte storage and mobilization
- Increase in cardiac output (stroke volume) and heart size
- Increased hemoglobin concentration in blood
- Slower utilization of muscle glycogen (up to 36% reduction in glycogen utilization in 7 weeks) (34)
- Partitioning of blood flow to provide a maximum flow rate to heart and muscles and a diminished flow rate to organs such as the kidney which are not immediately involved in the physical action (35).

All of these facilitate the perfusion of working muscles with oxygen, enhance aerobic metabolism and thus reduce the formation of lactic acid, the basic cause of muscle tiredness.

Attempts have been made in the past to relate height of training (and potential performance) to such things as blood hemoglobin levels, size of heart (heart score), bradycardia, lactic acid concentration in blood after exercise, heart rate (also after exercise), and blood pressure, but no worthwhile correlation has been demonstrated (11) and standardized exercise tolerance tests are the only suitable prospect.

As one might expect, gentle exercise produces little change in the efficiency of a horse's metabolic processes; to cope with the sudden demands on the animal which exercises violently (15), the training must be similarly vigorous. These comments apply only to the physical side of training. However, the psychological aspects of learning ability and emotional stability are also important.

Assessing performance potential (prediction of fitness)

In order to avoid overextending a horse physically and doing it some severe damage there is a growing interest in tests of performance potential. These tests are also of value in assessing an animal for sale. They include hematological (8), electrocardiographic (7) and biochemical (12) tests. The programs are available, but are as yet unproven. A complete profile including all of the above tests and a radiological examination of distal long bone epiphyses appears to be a highly desirable document to have as certification when buying a valuable horse.

Prediction of high performance potential is the dream of most horse owners and veterinarians. Prediction on the basis of progenitor performance is much used. More direct methods include measurement of heart score and the duration of QRS on an ECG (32). High enzyme levels in the blood (of gamma-glutamyl transferase (GGT), alkaline phosphatase (ACP), GOT, aspartate transferase (AST), creatinine phosphokinase (CPK) and lactate dehydrogenase (LD)) are reputed to foreshadow poor racing performance (27). However, none of these parameters predict racing performance of a horse with acceptable precision, although this is not to say that rough categorization is impossible.

The specific disease syndromes which arise as the result of physical exercise and which are dealt with elsewhere in this book (Chapter 35) are 'tying-up', exertional rhabdomyolysis, pulmonary hemorrhage and synchronous diaphragmatic flutter. Problems of an orthopedic nature are not our concern. Laryngeal hemiplegia and nasal bleeding are important to, but are not necessarily caused by, racing. Transit tetany and lactation tetany are metabolic diseases not usually related to exercise, but there is a relationship between the hypocalcemia which occurs in psychologically and physically stressed ponies and the synchronous diaphragmatic flutter already referred to. Besides the identifiable diseases dealt with in this book there is now a very large body of information under the heading 'equine exercise physiology' and no attempt is made to deal with it here. However, the biochemical biophysical and haematological reactions to physical exercise contained in it are of assistance in monitoring exhaustion levels, predicting fitness and perhaps indicating specific needs for prophylactic measures.

Treatment

The treatment of these diseases varies with the nature of the basic disturbance and has been dealt with elsewhere under such headings as dehydration, hyponatremia, etc. In most cases the problem is dehydration and the need is for the administration of large volumes (20–30 l) intravenously. A polyionic solution containing sodium, potassium, glucose and preferably calcium is usually used, especially if there is synchronous diaphragmatic flutter. The rate of flow needs to be slow, especially initially, to avoid overloading the heart, and the heart and respiratory rates and pulse amplitude need to be monitored carefully. There is usually no great disturbance of acid–base balance from neutrality. If the necessary services are available it is much the best if each patient receives the treatment most suited to its needs, as set out in the section of this chapter on disturbances of body fluids, electrolytes and acid–base balance (pp. 58–76). The greatest risk is that of precipitating pulmonary edema in a horse in which all cardiac reserve has already been utilized, and a further load, in the shape of a bolus of intravenous fluid, is added.

REVIEW LITERATURE

Carlson, G. (1985) Medical problems associated with protracted heat and work stress in horses. *Comp. cont. Educ.*, 7, S542.
Hinton, M. (1977) Long distance horse riding and the problem of dehydration and rhabdomyolysis. *Vet. Ann.*, *17*, 137.
Jeffcott, L. B. (1983) Equine exercise physiology, *Equ. vet. J.*, *15*, 87.
Rose, R. J. (1986) Endurance exercise in the horse. *Br. vet. J.*, *142*, 532, 542.

REFERENCES

(1) Lucke, J. N. & Hall, G. M. (1978) *Vet. Rec.*, *102*, 356.
(2) Snow, D. H. et al. (1982) *Vet. Rec.*, *110*, 377.
(3) Kohn, C. W. et al. (1978) *Am. J. vet. Res.*, *39*, 871.
(4) Thomas, D. P. et al. (1983) *Am. J. Physiol.*, *245*, R160.
(5) Mornicke, H. et al. (1977) *Pflügers Arch.*, *372*, 95.
(6) Milne, D. W. et al. (1976) *J. S. Afr. vet. Assoc.*, *45*, 345.
(7) Rose, R. J. et al. (1983) *Aust. vet. J.*, *60*, 101.
(8) Jeffcott, L. B. (1974) *J. S. Afr. vet. Assoc.*, *45*, 279.
(9) Kelly, C. M. (1977) *NZ vet. J.*, *25*, 393.
(10) Hinton, M. H. (1978) *Vet. Ann.*, *18*, 169.
(11) Rose, R. J. et al. (1983) *Vet. Rec.*, *113*, 612.
(12) McCashin, F. B. & von Solly, S. (1973) *Pract. Vet.*, *45*, 21.
(13) Carlson, G. P. & Mansmann, R. A. (1974) *J. Am. vet. med. Assoc.*, *165*, 262.
(14) Steere, J. H. (1975) *Mod. vet. Pract.*, *56*, 202.
(15) Snow, D. H. & MacKenzie, J. (1977) *Equ. vet. J.*, *9*, 226.
(16) Gallagher, K. & Stowe, H. D. (1980) *Am. J. vet. Res.*, *41*, 1333.
(17) Lucke, J. N. & Hall, G. M. (1980) *Vet. Rec.*, *106*, 405 & 523.
(18) Rose, R. J. et al. (1980) *Equ. vet. J.*, *12*, 19.
(19) Rose, R. J. et al. (1979) *Equ. vet. J.*, *11*, 56.
(20) Dybdal, N. O. et al. (1980) *Equ. vet. J.*, *12*, 137.
(21) Wittke, G. et al. (1974) *Berl. Munch. Tierärztl. Wochenschr.*, *87*, 425.
(22) Rose, R. J. et al. (1980) *Equ. vet J.*, *12*, 132.
(23) Rose, R. J. et al. (1979) *Equ. vet J.*, *55*, 247.
(24) Keenan, D. M. (1979) *Aust. vet. J.*, *55*, 54.
(25) Keenan, D. M. (1978) *Res. vet. Sci.*, *25*, 127.
(26) Rose, R. J. et al. (1980) *Aust. vet. J.*, *56*, 318.
(27) Sommer, H. et al. (1978) *Berl. Munch Tierärztl. Wochenschr.*, *91*, 433.
(28) Rose, R. J. et al. (1980) *Res. vet. Sci.*, *28*, 393.
(29) Hinton, M. (1977) *Vet. Ann.*, *17*, 136.
(30) Fowler, M. E. (1980) *J. S. Afr. vet. Assoc.*, *51*, 81, 85, 87.
(31) Engelhardt, W. V. (1979) *Dtsch Tierärztl. Wochenschr.*, *86*, 2.
(32) Steel, J. D. & Stewart, G. A. (1974) *J. S. Afr. vet. med. Assoc.*, *45*, 263.
(33) Deldar, A. et al. (1982) *Am. J. vet. Res.*, *43*, 2239.
(34) Hodgson, D. R. et al. (1985) *Am. J. vet. Res.*, *47*, 12.
(35) Parks, C. M. & Manohar, M. (1985) *Equ. vet. J.*, *17*, 311.

SHORTFALLS IN PERFORMANCE

The present-day emphasis on the need for economically efficient performance by farm animals introduces another set of criteria into consideration when deciding on an animal's future. The same comment applies, and much more importantly, when a herd's productivity is being assessed. This is usually done by comparing the subject herd's performances by peer herds, or animals, in similar environmental and managemental conditions.

It is usual to use the production indexes which are the essential outputs of the particular enterprise as the criteria of productivity. Thus, in dairy herds the criteria could be:

- Milk or butterfat production per cow per lactation (liters per cow or liters per hectare)
- Reproductive efficiency as mean intercalving interval
- Percent calf survival to 1 year of age
- Longevity as percent mortality per year or average age of cows in herd plus culling rate per year
- The culling rate needs to differentiate between sale

as reject because of disease or poor production and sale as a productive animal

- Acceptability of product at sale—as indicated by bulk milk cell count, rejection of milk because of poor quality, low fat content, low solids not fat content.

If it is decided that performance falls too far short of the target an investigation is warranted. Some targets for productivity in each of the animal industries are available, but they vary a great deal between countries depending on the levels of agriculture practiced and the standards of performance expected. So they are not set down here; nor is the degree of shortfall from the target which is acceptable. This depends heavily on the risk aversion or acceptability in the industry in that country. For example, if the enterprise is heavily capitalized by high-cost housing and land, the standard of performance would be expected to be higher than in a more exploitative situation where cattle are pastured all year. In the latter, a reasonable flexibility could be included in the assessment of productivity by permitting it to fall within the scope of two standard deviations of the mean productivity established by peer herds.

If it is decided that performance is below permissible standards an investigation should be conducted and should include the following groups of possible causes:

1. *Nutrition*—its adequacy in terms of energy, protein, minerals, vitamins and water.
2. *Inheritance*—the genetic background of the herd and the quality of its heritable performance.
3. *Accommodation*—to include protection from environmental stress by buildings for housed animals, terrain and tree cover for pastured animals, population density as affecting access to feed, water and bedding areas.
4. *General managerial expertise* and the degree of its application to the individual flock or herd. This is difficult to assess and then only indirectly, e.g., the efficiency of heat detection, achievement of planned calving pattern.
5. *Disease wastage*—as clinical disease or more particularly subclinical disease. The latter may include such things as quarter infection rate as an index of mastitis, fecal egg counts relative to parasite burden, metabolic profile relative to metabolic disease prevalence rate.

These investigations tend to require special techniques in addition to the clinical examination of individual animals. They are mostly self-evident, but attention is drawn to the section on examination of a herd or flock in Chapter 1 (p. 31). It will be apparent that there is a great deal of merit in having herds and flocks under constant surveillance for productivity and freedom from disease as is practiced in modern herd health programs. Monitoring performance and comparing it with targets is the basis of that system.

The specific syndromes that fall within this category of disease, and which are dealt with elsewhere in this book are ill-thrift of weaner sheep, thin sow syndrome, weak calf syndrome, poor performance syndrome of horses, low butterfat syndromes and summer slump of milk cows.

ALLERGY AND ANAPHYLAXIS

When exposure of an animal to an antigen produces a state of increased reactivity of the animals' tissues to that antigen a state of specific immune responsiveness is achieved. In most animals these responses are defensive and beneficial but, on occasion, they can be detrimental to the host. In these cases a state of hypersensitivity is said to exist which is clinically recognizable as allergy. When the reaction is sudden and clinically severe it is called anaphylaxis and if sufficiently severe it may result in anaphylactic shock.

There are a number of immune reactions which can be harmful to tissues but in large animals the immediate hypersensitivity reactions, especially those that result in severe anaphylaxis, pulmonary (especially chronic obstructive respiratory disease of horses), and dermatological (such as Queensland Itch) diseases, are most important. There are other immediate hypersensitivity reactions which should be noted. They include isoimmune erythrolysis of foals—a specific cytotoxic hypersensitivity, and the more generalized formation of circulating immune complexes which cause vasculitis, thrombosis, hemorrhage and consequent tissue damage. Purpura hemorrhagica is probably the best example.

In immediate hypersensitivity reactions the antigen, or allergen, reacts with antibody, which may be either circulating or cell-bound, to set in train a series of complex biochemical and pharmacological reactions which culminate in the release of pharmacologically active mediators. There are a number of recognized mediators and the importance of any one varies with the host species and possibly the nature of the hypersensitivity reaction. In general they act to contract smooth muscle and increase capillary permeability. These agents may act immediately at the site of antigen–antibody reaction or they may be carried in the blood to produce effects in susceptible tissues at sites remote from the primary focus. The difference in manifestation of acute, immediate-type hypersensitivity reactions between species appears to depend largely on differences in the tissue site of antibody binding and the distribution of susceptible smooth muscle as well as differences in the major pharmacological mediators of the reaction. The high incidence of atopic hypersensitivity with familial predisposition seen in man and dogs does not occur in large animals.

Immunological injury in the absence of significant release of pharmacological mediators also occurs but it is rarely approached from the clinical standpoint as a primary allergy and is generally considered in the disease complex in which it is occurring. The anemia and glomerulitis which accompany equine infectious anemia is an example. Serum sickness is rare in large animals.

Cell-mediated or delayed hypersensitivity is of importance in the tuberculin and other long-term skin sensitivity tests but similar delayed reactions to topically applied antigens are not common in farm animals. Queensland and Sweet itch are probably examples. Delayed hypersensitivity reactions may contribute to the pathology of many diseases such as mycoplasmal pneumonia in swine but those are considered clinically under their initiating etiology.

Autoimmune reactions appear to be rare in farm animals. They contribute to the formation of spermatic granulomas. Isoimmune hemolytic anemia and thrombocytopenic purpura could be considered as examples and are dealt with elsewhere under those headings.

The treatment of allergic states is by the use of functional antagonists which have opposing effects to those of the allergic mediators, and the specific pharmacological antagonists, especially antihistamines and corticosteroids. The functional antagonists include the sympathomimetic drugs, those related to epinephrine and, to a less extent, the anticholinergic drugs. Of the sympathomimetic drugs there is a choice between those with an alpha-response (vasoconstriction and maintaining vascular permeability) and those with a beta-response (bronchodilatory and cardiac-stimulatory). Of the pharmacological antagonists antihistamines have very limited usefulness being effective only when the allergic mediator is histamine, the corticosteroids have very wide applicability, and the non-steroid, anti-inflammatory drugs including acetylsalicylic acid, phenylbutazone and meclofenamic acid. All of these inhibit prostaglandin synthesis and thus reduce inflammation (12).

Anaphylaxis and anaphylactic shock

Anaphylaxis is an acute disease caused by antigen–antibody reaction. If severe it may result in anaphylactic shock.

Etiology

Most commonly, severe anaphylactic reactions are seen in farm animals following the parenteral administration of a drug or biological product. However, other routes of entry of the allergen such as via the respiratory or gastrointestinal tract may also result in anaphylactic reactions. The reaction may occur at the site of exposure or in other areas.

In general the reaction is due to sensitization to a protein substance entering the bloodstream and a second exposure to the same substance. In veterinary practice such incidents are not uncommon although the sensitizing substance cannot always be isolated.

Although severe anaphylactic reactions occur usually after a second exposure to a sensitizing agent, reactions of similar severity can occur with no known prior exposure. In large-animal work this is most likely to occur after the injection of sera and bacterins, particularly heterologous sera and bacterins in which heterologous serum has been used in the culture medium.

Hypersensitivity reactions are sometimes observed at a higher incidence than normal in certain families and herds of cattle.

Anaphylactic reactions can occur in the following circumstances:

1. Repeated intravenous injection of biological preparations such as glandular extracts.
2. Repeated blood transfusions from the same donor.
3. Repeated injections of vaccines, e.g., those against foot and mouth disease and rabies.
4. Rarely after a first injection of a conventional drug such as penicillin, usually procaine or benzathine penicillin, or test agent such as bromsulfalein. The reaction is reminiscent of 'serum sickness' in man because there has been no known previous exposure to the product, but occurs much earlier. It may be immediate and is usually within a few hours after injection.
5. Similar rare occurrences after the injection of lyophilized *Brucella abortus* strain 19 vaccine and salmonella vaccine (14). These, like the preceding group, are really anaphylactoid reactions because there has been no apparent previous exposure to the sensitizing antigen.
6. Assumed anaphylactic reaction to ingested protein occurs in animals at pasture or in the feedlot.
7. Cows, especially Channel Island cattle, may develop anaphylaxis when milking is stopped because the cows are being dried off, or being 'bagged-up' for a show—severe urticaria and respiratory distress occur 18–24 hours later (2).
8. A systemic reaction after *Hypoderma* sp. larvae are killed in their subcutaneous sites may be anaphylactic, but is more likely to be a toxic effect from breakdown products of the larvae.
9. Anaphylactic reactions can be produced experimentally in calves by injecting the endotoxin-like extract of ruminal contents. Acute toxemia develops about 30 minutes later, but an anaphylactic reaction occurs when the same extract is injected 15 days later (1).

Pathogenesis

Anaphylactic reactions occur as the result of antigen reacting with circulating or cell-bound antibody. In man and the dog a specific class of reaginic antibody, IgE, has been identified and has particular affinity for fixed tissue mast cells. The tissue distribution of mast cells in part accounts for the involvement of certain target organs in anaphylactic reactions in these species. Homocytotropic antibody has been detected in farm animals (3, 4) but the classes of antibodies involved in anaphylactic reactions have not been fully identified, and are likely to be diverse (5). Anaphylactic antibodies may be transferred via colostrum (6). Antigen–antibody reactions occurring in contact with, or in close proximity to, fixed tissue mast cells, basophils and neutrophil leukocytes result in the activation of these cells to release pharmacologically active substances that mediate the subsequent anaphylactic reaction. These include biogenic amines such as histamine, serotonin and catecholamines; vasoactive polypeptides such as kinins, cationic proteins and anaphylatoxins; vasoactive lipids such as prostaglandins and slow reacting substance of anaphylaxis (SRS-A); and others (7). Knowledge of the type and relative importance of pharmacological mediators of anaphylaxis in farm animals rests with studies of severe anaphylactic reactions which have been induced experimentally, but it is likely that these mediators are also of significance in less severe reactions. From these studies it appears that histamine is of less importance as a mediator in farm animals than in other species and that prostaglandins and SRS-A are of greater importance (9). Bradykinin and 5-hydroxytryptamine (5-HT) are also known to act as mediators in cattle (10) but the reactions in all species are complex and involve a sequence of mediator effects (11, 13).

It seems likely that the complexity of the pharmacodynamic picture will be resolved by the elucidation of the exact pattern of development of the reaction. In the horse, it is evident that there are four phases in the development of the anaphylactic response. The first is acute hypotension combined with pulmonary arterial hypertension 2–3 minutes after the injection of the triggering agent; it coincides with histamine release. In the second phase, blood plasma 5-HT levels rise, and central venous blood pressure rises sharply at about 3 minutes and onward. The third phase commences at about 8–12 minutes, and is largely reflex and manifested by a sharp rise in blood pressure, and alternating apnea and dyspnea. Subsequently there is a second and more protracted systemic hypotension due to prostaglandin and SRS-A influence which persists until the return to normality (9).

In cattle, there is a similar diphasic systemic hypotension with marked pulmonary venous constriction and pulmonary artery hypertension. An increase in mesenteric venous pressure and mesenteric vascular resistance causes considerable pooling of blood on the venous side of the mesenteric vessels (14, 15). In both species these reactions are accompanied by severe hemoconcentration, leukopenia, thrombocytopenia and hyperkalemia (9).

Sheep and pigs also show a largely pulmonary reaction. In horses and cattle the marked changes in vascular tone coupled with increased capillary permeability, increased secretion of mucous glands and bronchospasm are the primary reactions leading to the development of severe pulmonary congestion, edema and emphysema and edema of the gut wall. Death is due to anoxia.

Less severe reactions are also dependent upon the effect of mediators on capillary permeability, vascular tone and mucous gland secretion. The major manifestation depends on the distribution of antibody-sensitized cells and of susceptible smooth muscle in the various organs. In cattle reactions are generally referable to the respiratory tract but the alimentary tract and skin are also target organs. Sheep and pigs show largely a pulmonary reaction and horses manifest changes in the lungs, skin and feet.

Sensitization of a patient requires about 10 days after first exposure to the antigen, and persists for a very long time, months or years.

Clinical findings

In cattle the initial signs include a very sudden and severe dyspnea, muscle shivering, and anxiety. In some cases there is profuse salivation, in others moderate bloat and others diarrhea. After blood transfusions the first sign is often hiccough. Additional signs are urticaria, angioneurotic edema and rhinitis. Muscle tremor may be severe and a rise in temperature to 40·5°C (105°F) may be observed. On auscultation of the chest there may be increased vesicular murmur, crackling sounds if edema is present, and emphysema in the later stages if dyspnea has been severe. In most surviving cases the signs have usually subsided within 24 hours, although dyspnea may persist if emphysema has occurred.

In natural cases the time delay after injection of the reagin intravenously is about 15–20 minutes but in experimentally induced cases a severe reaction may be evident within 2 minutes, and death within 7–10 minutes after the injection. Clinical signs include collapse, dyspnea, wild paddling, nystagmus, cyanosis, cough, the discharge of a creamy, frothy fluid from the nostrils; recovery, if it occurs, is complete in about 2 hours (16).

Sheep and pigs show acute dyspnea and horses (17) may do the same, although laminitis and angioneurotic edema are also common signs in this species. Laminitis also occurs rarely in ruminants.

Naturally occurring anaphylactic shock in the horse is manifested by severe dyspnea, distress, recumbency and convulsions. Death may occur in as short a time as 5 minutes but it usually requires about an hour. Experimentally induced anaphylaxis may be fatal but not in such a short time (18, 19). Within 30 minutes of injecting the reagin the horse is showing anxiety, tachycardia, cyanosis and dyspnea. These signs are followed by congestion of conjunctival vessels, increased peristalsis, fluid diarrhea, generalized sweating and erection of the hair. If recovery occurs it is about 2 hours after the incident began. Death, if it occurs, takes place about 24 hours after the injection.

In pigs, experimentally produced anaphylactic shock can be fatal within a few minutes with systemic shock being severe within 2 minutes and death occurring in 5–10 minutes (20). The disease appears to occur in only one phase in contrast to the four fairly distinct states in horses. Labored respiration, severe cyanosis, vomiting and edema of the larynx, stomach and gallbladder are the usual outcome (8).

Clinical pathology

Blood histamine levels may or may not be increased and little data are available on blood eosinophil counts. Tests for sensitivity to determine the specific sensitizing substance are rarely carried out for diagnostic purposes but their use as an investigation tool is warranted. Serological tests to determine the presence of antibodies to plant proteins in the diet have been used in this way (21).

Some significant changes occur during immediate anaphylaxis in cattle and horses but whether they have diagnostic importance is uncertain. There is a marked increase in packed cell volume, a high plasma potassium concentration and a neutropenia (5).

Necropsy findings

In acute anaphylaxis in young cattle and sheep the necropsy findings are confined to the lungs and are in the form of severe pulmonary edema and vascular engorgement. In adult cattle there is edema and emphysema without engorgement. In protracted anaphylaxis produced experimentally in young calves the most prominent lesions are hyperemia and edema of the abomasum and small intestines. In pigs and sheep pulmonary emphysema is evident and vascular engorgement of the lungs is pronounced in the latter. Pulmonary emphysema and widespread petechiation in the horse may be accompanied by massive edema and extravasations of blood in the wall of the large bowel. There may also be subcutaneous edema and the lesions of laminitis.

Diagnosis

A diagnosis of anaphylaxis can be made with confidence if a foreign protein substance has been injected within the preceding hour, but should be made with reservation if the substance appears to have been ingested. Characteristic signs as described above should arouse suspicion and the response to treatment may be used as a test of the hypothesis. Acute pneumonia may be confused with anaphylaxis, but there is usually more toxemia and the lung changes are more marked in the ventral parts of the lung; in anaphylaxis there is general involvement of the entire lung.

Treatment

Treatment should be administered immediately; a few minutes' delay may result in the death of the patient. Adrenaline is still the most effective treatment for counteracting the effects of acute anaphylaxis and anaphylactic shock. Adrenaline administered intramuscularly (or one-fifth of the dose given intravenously) is often immediately effective, the signs abating while the injection is being made. Corticosteroids potentiate the effect of adrenaline and may be given immediately following the adrenaline. Antihistamines are in common use but provide variable results due to the presence of mediators other than histamine. Atropine is of little value.

The identification of mediators other than histamine in anaphylactic reactions in farm animals has led to studies of the effectiveness of drugs more active against these mediators than antihistamines. Acetylsalicylic acid, sodium meclofenamate and diethylcarbamazine have all shown ability to protect against experimentally induced anaphylaxis in cattle and horses (6, 9, 15) and warrant trial in anaphylactic reactions in these species.

One of the important clinical decisions, especially in horse work, is to decide whether an animal is sufficiently hypersensitive to be at risk when being treated. An acute anaphylactic reaction, and even death, can occur soon after intravenous injection of penicillin into a horse. In suspect cases it is customary to conduct an intradermal or a conjunctival test for hypersensitivity with a response time of about 20 minutes but these tests have their limitations. The types of sensitivities are not necessarily related and there is no sure relationship between anaphylactic sensitivity and either skin (or conjunctival) sensitivity or circulating antibody, and the test often gives false negatives (3). The reason why some animals develop systemic hypersensitivity and some develop cutaneous hypersensitivity does not appear to be related to the nature of the reagin, but it may be related to the size of the sensitizing dose (22).

REVIEW LITERATURE

Black, L. (1979) Hypersensitivity in cattle. Pt. 1. Mechanism of causation; Pt. 2. Clinical reactions; Pt. 3. Mediators of anaphylaxis. *Vet. Bull.*, *49*, 1, 77 & 303.

Eyre, P. (1980) Pharmacological aspects of hypersensitivity in domestic animals. A review. *Vet. Res. Commun.*, 4, 83.

REFERENCES

(1) Nagaraja, T. G. et al. (1979) *Norden News*, *54*, 22.
(2) Campbell, S. G. (1970) *Cornell Vet.*, *60*, 654.
(3) Aitken, M. M. et al. (1974) *Res. vet. Sci.*, *16*, 199.
(4) Burka, J. F. & Scarnell, J. (1976) *Vet. Rec.*, *102*, 483.
(5) Wells, P. W. et al. (1973) *Can. J. comp. Med.*, *37*, 119.
(6) Bentin, C. et al. (1976) *Zentralbl. vet. Med.*, *23B*, 200.
(7) Chand, N. & Eyre, P. (1977) *Can. J. comp. Med.*, *41*, 233.
(8) Teige, J. & Nordstoga, J. (1977) *Acta vet. Scand.*, *18*, 210.
(9) Eyre, P. (1976) *Can. J. comp. Med.*, *40*, 149.
(10) Aitken, M. M. & Sanford, J. (1972) *J. comp. Pathol.*, *82*, 247.
(11) Eyre, P. et al. (1973) *Br. J. Pharmacol.*, *47*, 504 & *48*, 426.
(12) Eyre, P. (1980) *Vet. Res. Commun.*, *4*, 83.
(13) Wray, C. & Tomlinson, J. R. (1974) *Br. vet. J.*, *130*, 466.
(14) Holroyde, M. C. & Eyre, P. (1975) *Eur. J. Pharmacol.*, *30*, 36, 43.
(15) Aitken, M. M. et al. (1975) *Res. vet. Sci.*, *18*, 41.
(16) Aitken, M. M. & Sanford, J. (1969) *J. comp. Pathol.*, *79*, 131.
(17) Hidalgo, R. J. & Linrode, P. A. (1969) *Proc. 15th ann. Conf. Am. Assoc. equ. Practnrs*, 293.
(18) McGavin, M. D. et al. (1972) *Am. J. vet. Res.*, *160*, 1632.
(19) Mansmann, R. A. (1972) *Fedn Proc. Fedn Am. Soc. exp. Biol.*, *31*, 661.
(20) Wells, P. W. et al. (1974) *Res. vet. Sci.*, *16*, 347.
(21) Brownlee, A. & Baigent, C. L. (1964) *Vet Rec.*, *76*, 1060.
(22) Aitken, M. M. et al. (1975) *J. comp. Pathol.*, *85*, 351.

Other hypersensitivity reactions

These reactions include anaphylaxis of a less severe degree than anaphylactic shock and cases of cell-mediated delayed hypersensitivity. The resulting clinical signs vary depending on the tissues involved, but are usually localized and mild.

Etiology

Exposure to any of the etiological agents described under anaphylaxis may result in this milder form of hypersensitivity. Exposure may occur by injection, by ingestion, by inhalation or by contact with the skin.

Pathogenesis

In anaphylactic reactions the clinical signs may depend on the portal of entry. Thus ingestion may lead to gastrointestinal signs of diarrhea, inhalation to conjunctivities, rhinitis, and laryngeal and bronchial edema. Cutaneous lesions can result from introduction of the reagin via any portal. They are usually manifested by angiedema, urticaria or a maculopapular reaction. All of the lesions result from the liberation of histamine, serotonin and plasma kinins as in anaphylactic shock.

Clinical findings

In ruminants inhalation of a sensitizing antigen may cause the development of allergic rhinitis. On ingestion of the sensitizing agent there may be a sharp attack of diarrhea and the appearance of urticaria or angioneurotic edema; in ruminants mild bloat may occur. Contact allergy is usually manifested by eczema. In farm animals the eczematous lesion is commonly restricted to the skin of the lower limbs, particularly behind the pastern, and at the bulbs of the heels, or to the midline of the back if the allergy is due to insect bites. In many cases of allergic disease the signs are very transient and often disappear spontaneously within a few hours. Cases vary in severity from mild signs in a single system to a systemic illness resembling anaphylactic shock. On the other hand cases of anaphylaxis may be accompanied by local allergic lesions.

Diagnosis

The transitory nature of allergic manifestations is often a good guide, as are the types of lesions and signs encountered. The response to antihistamine drugs is also a useful indicator. Skin test programmes as applied to man should be utilized when recurrent herd problems exist (1, 2). The differential diagnosis of allergy is discussed under the specific diseases listed above.

Treatment

A combination of adrenaline, antihistamines and corticosteroids is usually highly effective. Skin lesions other than edema may require frequent local applications of lotions containing antihistamine substances. Continued exposure to the allergen may result in recurrence or persistence of the signs. Keeping the animals indoors for a week often avoids this, probably because the allergen occurs only transiently in the environment. Hyposensitization therapy, as it is practiced in human allergy sufferers, may have a place in small animal practice but is unlikely to be practicable with farm animals.

REVIEW LITERATURE

Eyre, P. & Christopher, J. H. (1980) Equine allergies, *Equ. Pract.*, *2*, 40.

Eyre, P. (1980) Pharmacological aspects of hypersensitivity in domestic animals. A review. *Vet. Res. Commun.*, *4*, 83.

REFERENCES

(1) Scherr, M. S. (1964) *J. Am. vet. med. Assoc.*, *145*, 798.
(2) Campbell, S. G. (1970) *Cornell Vet.*, *60*, 240.

AMYLOIDOSIS

Amyloidosis usually occurs in association with a chronic suppurative process elsewhere in the body. Extensive infiltration of various body organs with amyloid causes depression of function of the organs involved.

Etiology

Amyloidosis occurs rarely and in animals exposed systemically and repeatedly to antigenic substances. Examples are: repeated injections of antigenic material for commercial production of hyperimmune serum; and long-standing suppurative diseases (1) or recurrent infection as in Chediak–Higashi syndrome (2). Most cases are without apparent cause (3).

Pathogenesis

How amyloid is formed is uncertain but a hyperglobulinemia is commonly present and this together with the circumstances under which it occurs suggest an abnormality of the antigen–antibody reaction. Extensive amyloid deposits may occur in the spleen, liver or kidneys and cause major enlargement of these organs and serious depression of their functions. The commonest form which is clinically recognizable in animals is renal amyloidosis (4). This presents as a nephrotic syndrome with massive proteinuria and a consequential hypoproteinemia and edema. In cattle the grossly enlarged left kidney should be palpable per rectum. Terminally the animal is uremic, becoming comatose and recumbent. Most cases appear soon after calving. The edema of the gut wall and its infiltration with amyloid create the conditions necessary for the development of diarrhea. In horses, cases of multiple cutaneous lesions are recorded. The amyloid is present in 5–25 mm diameter nodes in the skin of the head, neck and pectoral regions. Rare cases of involvement of the upper respiratory tract (nasal cavities, pharynx, larynx, guttural pouch and lymph nodes of the head and neck, and conjunctiva) are also recorded (5). The amyloid material deposited in the tissues is a glycoprotein and has specific staining reactions.

Clinical findings

Many cases of amyloidosis are detected incidentally at necropsy. The cutaneous form in horses is characterized by the presence of hard, non-painful, chronic plaques in the skin. Most lesions are on the sides of the neck, shoulders, and head. Respiratory tract involvement in the horse is usually limited to the nasal cavities, and this may cause dyspnea. Clinical cases in cattle are characterized by emaciation and enlargement of the spleen, liver or kidneys and involvement of the kidney causes proteinuria and is often accompanied by profuse, chronic diarrhea, polydipsia and anasarca (6, 7). Cases are recorded in cattle within 2 weeks of calving (8). They were characterized by anorexia, watery diarrhea, anasarca, rapid emaciation and death in 2–5 weeks.

Corpora amylacea are small, round concretions of amyloid material found in mammary tissue of cows. They are usually inert but may cause blockage of the teat canal.

Clinical pathology

An extreme, persistent proteinuria should suggest the presence of amyloidosis. Electrophoretic studies of serum may be of value in determining the presence of hyperglobulinemia. Alpha-globulin levels are usually elevated and albumin levels depressed. In cattle there is hypocalcemia, hyperfibrinogenemia, hypomagnesemia, high serum urea and creatinine concentration, low specific gravity urine and prolongation of the bromosulfalein clearance time (6). Biopsy of cutaneous plaques is an accurate diagnostic technique.

Necropsy findings

Affected organs are grossly enlarged and have a pale waxy appearance. In the spleen, the deposits are circumscribed, in the liver and kidneys they are diffuse. Deposits of amyloid in tissues may be made visible by staining with aqueous iodine. For histological reasons special stains such as Congo Red are used.

Diagnosis
Enlargement of parenchymatous organs associated with chronic suppurative processes should arouse suspicion of amyloidosis especially if there is emaciation and marked proteinuria. Pyelonephritis, non-specific nephritis and nephrosis bear a clinical similarity to amyloidosis.

Treatment
The course is often very long so that disposal is not an urgent matter.

REVIEW LITERATURE

Gruys, E. (1977) Amyloidosis in the bovine kidney. *Vet. Sci. Commun.*, *1*, 265.

REFERENCES

(1) Rooney, J. R. (1965) *Cornell Vet.*, *46*, 369.
(2) Burns, G. L. et al. (1984) *Can. comp. Med.*, *48*, 113.
(3) Radostits, O. M. & Palmer, N. (1965) *Can. vet. J.*, *6*, 208.
(4) Murray, M. et al. (1972) *Vet. Rec.*, *90*, 210.
(5) Jakob, W. (1971) *Vet. Pathol.*, *8*, 292.
(6) Johnson, R. & Jamison, K. (1984) *J. Am. vet. med. Assoc.*, *185*, 1538.
(7) Murray, M. et al. (1972) *Vet. Rec.*, *90*, 210.
(8) Konishi, T. et al. (1975) *Jap. J. vet. Sci.*, *37*, 227.

IMMUNE DEFICIENCY DISORDERS (LOWERED RESISTANCE TO INFECTION)

Increasingly, animals are encountered which are much more susceptible to infection than their cohorts. These animals may be suffering from a hypoimmune state and need to be identified as such. The history and signs which should suggest the possible presence of a hypoimmune state are:

- Infections developing in the first 6 weeks of life
- Repeated or continuous infections which respond poorly to treatment
- Increased susceptibility to low-grade pathogens and organisms not usually encountered in immunocompetent animals
- Administration of attenuated vaccines which leads to systemic illness
- Low leukocyte counts either generally or as lymphopenia, or neutropenia, perhaps within an associated low platelet count.

It is not proposed to detail the mechanisms of humoral and cellular immunity here; the subject is well reviewed (1). However, it is necessary to remember that the normal immune response is a very complicated process, including many sequential steps, and there are many sites at which defective development or function can occur.

The disorders of immunity may be *primary*, in which the animal is born with a congenital defect of one of the immune processes, or *secondary*, in which the animal has a normal complement of immunological processes at birth, but suffers a dysfunction of one of them, often temporarily, during later life. Toxicological and microbiological agents can have this effect.

Most of the diseases caused by immunological deficiency states are dealt with in systems or other categories of disease throughout this book and only a checklist of them is provided here.

Primary immune deficiency disorders

These are as follows:

1. Combined immunodeficiency (CID) of Arab horses due to an inherited failure to produce and differentiate lymphoid precursor cells into B and T lymphocytes.
2. Agammaglobulinemia of standardbred and thoroughbred horses, probably inherited, failure to produce B lymphocytes. These horses live much longer than those affected with CID.
3. Selective deficiencies of one or more globulins. A deficiency of IgM in Arab horses and quarterhorses is listed (3, 4). IgM and IgA-combined deficiencies with diminished but discernible levels of IgG is observed occasionally in horses (2). A transient hypogammaglobulinemia (absence of IgG) has been reported in one Arab foal which was immunodeficient until it was 3 months old and then became normal.
4. Lethal trait A46 (inherited parakeratosis) of cattle is a primary immunodeficiency influencing T lymphocytes with impairment of cellular immunity.
5. Selective IgG_2 deficiency of cattle causes increased susceptibility to gangrenous mastitis and other infections. It is a primary deficiency of IgG_2 synthesis, and is recorded in the Red Danish milk breed.
6. Chediak–Higashi syndrome, an inherited defect of many animal species, including cattle. This is a defect of phagocytic capacity via the neutrophils and monocytes, so that there is a weakened defense against infection rather than a deficient immunity *per se*.

Sheep and pigs: There do not appear to be any primary immunodeficiencies in these species.

Secondary immune deficiencies

These are as follows:

1. Failure of passive transfer (FPT), i.e., of antibodies from colostrum to the offspring, is well known as the commonest cause of deficient immunity in the newborn and is discussed in Chapter 3 on diseases of the newborn.
2. Atrophy of lymphoid tissue and resulting lymphopenia caused by:
   (a) Viral infections such as equine herpes virus in

newborn foals, rinderpest, bovine virus diarrhea, hog cholera, all cause lymphatic tissue suppression and a diminished immunoresponsiveness. The pathogenesis of the immunodeficiency caused by the BVD virus (7) may be due to impairment of the function of polymorphonuclear cells (8).

(b) Bacterial infections such as *Mycoplasma* spp., and *Mycobacterium paratuberculosis* have approximately the same effect.

(c) Physiological stress such as birth may cause immunosuppression in the fetus making it very susceptible to infection in the period right after birth (5). There is a similar depression of immunological efficiency in the dam immediately after parturition (11) which, for example, leads to periparturient rise of worm infestation in ewes. Psychological stress in experimental animals does increase susceptibility to infection, but the practical importance of this to animal production is not clear.

(d) Toxins such as bracken, tetrachlorethylene-extracted soybean meal, T_2 mycotoxin and atomic irradiation suppress leukopoiesis. Immunosuppression is also attributed to many environmental pollutants including polychlorinated biphenyls, 2,4,5-T contaminants, DDT, aflatoxin and the heavy metals (2).

3. General suppression of immune system responsiveness, e.g.:

(a) Glucocorticoids administered in large doses or over long periods reduce the activity of neutrophils, the numbers of circulating lymphocytes, although the reduction varies widely between species, and the production of antibodies (9).

(b) Nutritional deficiency (10) especially of zinc, pantothenic acid, calcium and vitamin E; a total caloric deficiency has a similar effect (12).

(c) Exposure to cold and heat stress for long periods of several weeks duration (6).

REVIEW LITERATURE

Porter, P. et al. (1979) Basic and clinical aspects of veterinary immunology. *Adv. vet. Sci.*, *23*, 1, 23, etc. (10 papers).

Hudson, R. J. et al. (1978) Physiological and environmental influences on immunity. *Vet. Bull.*, *44*, 119.

REFERENCES

(1) Perryman, L. E. (1979) *Adv. vet. Sci.*, *23*, 23.
(2) Koller, L. D. (1979) *Adv. vet. Sci.*, *23*, 267.
(3) Perryman, L. E. et al. (1977) *J. Am. vet med. Assoc.*, *170*, 212.
(4) Deem, D. A. et al. (1979) *J. Am. vet. med. Assoc.*, *175*, 469.
(5) O'Brien, B. et al. (1975) *Fed. Proc.*, *34*, 36.
(6) Kelley, K. W. et al. (1982) *Am. J. vet. Res.*, *43*, 775.
(7) Reggiardo, C. & Kaeberle, M. L. (1981) *Am. J. vet. Res.*, *42*, 218.
(8) Roth, J. A. et al. (1981) *Am. J. vet. Res.*, *42*, 244.
(9) Roth, J. A. et al. (1982) *J. Am. vet. med. Assoc.*, *180*, 894.
(10) Sheffey, B. E. & Williams, A. J. (1982) *J. Am. vet. med. Assoc.*, *180*, 1073.
(11) Lloyd, S. S. (1983) *Irish vet. J.*, *37*, 64.
(12) Naylor, J. M. et al. (1981) *Res. vet. Sci.*, *31*, 369.

3

Diseases of the Newborn

THIS chapter considers the principles of the diseases which occur during the first month of life in animals born alive at term. The diseases causing abortion and stillbirth are not included. The specific diseases referred to are presented separately under their own headings.

The inclusion of a chapter on diseases of the newborn and at this point in the book needs explanation. The need for the chapter arises out of the special sensitivities which the newborn have: their immunological incompetence; their dependence on adequate colostrum containing adequate antibodies at the right time; their dependence on frequent intake of readily available carbohydrate to maintain energy; and their relative inefficiency in maintaining normal body temperature, upwards or downwards; all of these points need emphasizing before proceeding to the study of each of the body systems.

There are no particular aspects of a clinical examination which pertain only to or mostly to neonates. It is the same clinical examination as is applied to adults with additional, careful examination for congenital defects and diseases which may involve the umbilicus, the liver, the heart valves, the joints and the tendon sheaths, eyes and meninges. Although it is necessary to avoid any suggestion that an examination of an adult could be cursory, it is necessary to ensure that an examination of a newborn animal is as complete as practically possible. This is partly for an emotional reason; the neonate always evokes a sentimental reaction. It is also important for the economic reason that in most species the offspring, when already on the ground, represents a very considerable part of the year's investment and productivity. There is also the much greater susceptibility to infectious disease, dehydration and death, and diagnosis and treatment must be reasonably accurate and rapid. Supportive therapy in the form of fluids, electrolytes and energy and nursing care are especially important in the newborn in order to maintain homeostasis.

PERINATAL DISEASES

One of the most unrewarding aspects of the study of these diseases is the almost unlimited number of classifications by which the diseases are categorized, so that it is very difficult to compare results and assessments. To ensure that our meanings are clear, we set out below what we think is the most satisfactory classification of all of the diseases of the fetus and the newborn—the perinatal diseases—adapted from a scheme proposed for lambs (1).

1. *Fetal diseases*. Diseases of the fetus during intrauterine life, e.g. prolonged gestation, congenital defects, abortion, fetal death with resorption or mummification, goiter.
2. *Parturient diseases*. Diseases associated with dystocia causing cerebral anoxia, injury to the skeleton or soft tissues, maladjustment syndrome of foals.
3. *Postnatal diseases*
   (a) *Early postnatal disease* (within 48 hours of birth), e.g. malnutrition due to poor mothering, hypothermia due to exposure to cold, low vigor in neonates due to malnutrition; special diseases, e.g. navel infection and colibacillosis.
   (b) *Delayed postnatal disease* (2–7 days of age). Desertion by mother, mammary incompetence resulting in starvation, and increased susceptibility to infection due to hypogammaglobulinemia, e.g. colibacillosis, lamb dysentery, foal septicemias.
   (c) *Late postnatal diseases* (1–4 weeks of age). White muscle disease, enterotoxemia.

General epidemiology

Diseases of the newborn and neonatal mortality are a major cause of economic loss in livestock production and every practical economical effort should be made to minimize disease and mortality.

Lambs

Perinatal lamb mortality is one of the major factors in impairment of productivity in sheep raising enterprises around the world (7–9). Total mortality varies from 9 to 25%; and from 30 to 50% of the losses are due to stillbirths and abortions of the lambs born alive. The weak lamb syndrome, accidents, hypothermia and starvation are the leading causes of mortality of lambs born alive. Approximately 75% of neonatal lamb mortality occurs in the first 3 days of life. During this period, nutritional, environmental and management factors resulting in weak lambs and starvation commonly account for approximately one-third of total mortality (6). Lambs found dead or missing may account for significant losses under some conditions such as mountain or hill pastures (8).

The mortality rate can differ between breeds and lambs from crossbred dams may have higher survival rates (2). Dystocia was the primary cause of death where it was recorded and usually in large single lambs (3). The weakly lamb syndrome is a major cause of lamb mortality and includes lambs which are light weight at birth, underdeveloped and die from a combination of starvation and exposure (4). The major infectious diseases of lambs which cause mortality are enteritis and pneumonia and there are differences in mortality rates between breeds (5).

A simple system for recording lamb mortality and relating the deaths to the weather and management system is available (10). It is effective in revealing the extent of lamb losses and the areas of management which require improvement.

Dairy calves

In dairy calves the mortality rate under 1 month of age averages about 10% and varies from 3 to 30% in individual herds. Losses up to 50% have occurred in large dairy herds. A calf mortality rate of 20% can reduce net profit by 38% (11). In well-managed dairy herds calf mortality usually does not exceed 5% from birth to 30 days of age. Dairy calf mortality increases significantly in larger herds. In an expansion program the numbers of cows and milking facilities are commonly enlarged without parallel changes in calf-rearing facilities or labor. Inadequate planning, overcrowding, the failure to feed colostrum early enough and labor shortages appear to be the most common problems associated with larger herds and high calf mortality (12). Mortality is also associated with the type of housing for calves, calving facilities, the person caring for the calves and attendance at calving (13). Certain meteorological influences may have an effect on dairy calf mortality rate (14). During the winter months, mortality may be associated with the effects of cold wet and windy weather, while during the summer months it may be the hot dry weather. The epidemiological observation that calf mortality is significantly lower when the owner manages the calves rather than when employees perform these duties suggests that owner-managers may be sufficiently motivated to provide the care necessary to ensure a high survival rate in calves (15).

Beef calves

In beef herds, mortality during the neonatal period averages about 5–6% but may exceed 50% during bad years when explosive outbreaks of neonatal diarrhea occur. The usual causes of mortality in beef calves include: hypoxia and traumatic injury at birth; exposure to extremely cold weather or being dropped at birth into deep snow or a gully; mismothering in calves born to heifers; and neonatal diarrhea. Accurate prospective studies have shown that 50–60% of the parturient deaths in beef calves are associated with slow or difficult birth and the mortality rate is much higher in calves born to heifers than from mature cows (16, 17). Thus dystocia is a major cause of mortality in beef calves at birth and neonatal diarrhea is the most important cause thereafter.

Piglets

Surveys of neonatal mortality in piglets have repeatedly indicated that the most important causes of death in piglets from birth to weaning are non-infectious in origin (18). Stillbirths account for 4–8% of all deaths of pigs born and, 70–90% are type II or intraparturient deaths in which the piglet was alive at the beginning of parturition. Preweaning mortality ranges from 5 to 48% with averages ranging from 12 to 19% of all pigs born alive (18). More than 50% of the preweaning losses occur before the end of the second day of life. The major causes of preweaning mortality are starvation and crushing (75–80%), congenital abnormalities (5%), and infectious disease (6%). The major congenital abnormalities are congenital splayleg, atresi ani and cardiac abnormalities. The large percentage of mortality caused by crushing and trampling probably includes piglets which were starved and weak and thus highly susceptible to being crushed. The estimated contribution of crushing and starvation to neonatal mortality varies from 50 to 80%. Thus it is clear that on an industry-wide basis, the major causes of neonatal mortality in piglets are related to environmental and nutritional factors. Minimizing the mortality rate of newborn piglets will depend on management techniques which include: proper selection of the breeding stock for teat numbers, milk production and mothering ability; surveillance at farrowing time to minimize the number of piglets suffering from hypoxia and dying at birth or a few days later (20); batch farrowing which allows for economical surveillance; fostering to equalize litter size; cross-fostering to equalize uniformity in birth weight within litters; and artificial rearing with milk substitutes containing purified porcine gammaglobulin to prevent enteric infection (21). Abattoir-derived porcine gammaglobulin administered at the rate of 10 g/kg body weight on the first day followed by 2 g/kg body weight on succeeding days, for a period of 10 days, is sufficient to confer passive immunity on the colostrum-deprived pig. The use of such a method to rear piglets artificially in a farm environment could have a major impact in reducing losses due to weakness, agalactia in the sow and supernumerary piglets which are not sufficiently competitive to secure a functional teat for themselves. The nursing behavior of the sow and her ability to expose the teats to all piglets, and the sucking behavior of piglets have a marked effect on survival (22).

The viability of newborn piglets can be accurately evaluated immediately after birth by scoring skin color, respiration, heart rate, muscle tone and ability to stand (21). Mortality increases as the mean litter size increases and as the mean birth weight of the pig decreases (19). The mean number of piglets weaned is related to the size of the litter up to an original size of 14 and increases with parity of sows up to their fifth farrowing (24).

A recent study of 32 randomly sampled farrow-finish swine herds over a 2-year period found the overall preweaning mortality rate (including stillbirths) to be 26% (27). Preweaning mortality was negatively correlated with herd size and farrowing crate utilization, and positively correlated with the number of farrowing crates per room. There was no relationship between preweaning mortality and housing and management characteristics such as the use of bedding or no bedding, batch farrowing versus continuous farrowing and single-use compared to multi-use farrowing rooms.

The provision of a warm and comfortable environment for the newborn piglet in the first few days of life is critical. The lower critical temperature of the single newborn piglet is 34°C (93°F) and when the ambient temperature falls below 34°C (93°F) the piglet is subjected to cold stress and must mobilize glycogen reserves from liver and muscle to maintain deep body temperature. The provision of heat lamps over the creep area and freedom from draughts are two major requirements.

Foals

Foals are usually well supervised and cared for as individual animals. In a large survey of thoroughbred mares in the UK only 2% of newborn foals died (25), only 41% of twins survived and 98% of singles survived.

The causes of mortality from birth to 2 months of age were: lack of maturity 36%, structural defect 23%, birth injury 5%, convulsive syndrome 5%, alimentary disorder 12%, generalized infection 11% and other (miscellaneous) 9%. There is a large growing literature on the neonatal aspects of foal physiology and medicine (26). Prematurity, immaturity, dysmaturity and neonatal maladjustment syndromes occur in newborn foals (28, 29). Diseases of the lungs of newborn foals appears to have assumed importance and has resulted in the development of critical care techniques to improve the survival rate in valuable foals (30–32). Gastrointestinal diseases (33) and immunologic abnormalities have also assumed some importance (34).

Bacterial septicemias are major causes of morbidity and mortality in newborn foals (35). The case fatality rate in foals with neonatal septicemia is more than 70% in spite of therapy.

Another statistic of importance in the analysis of neonatal mortality is the proportion which have lesions or clinical findings indicating that death is due either to a congenital defect, or to congenital or neonatal infection, or to external physical influences. It would seem reasonable to assume that this would vary greatly between species and between management systems. Thus in lambs 85% of parturient deaths appeared to be due to external physical influences such as dystocia and cold injury. Predators accounted for 5%, congenital deformities for 4%, infection 5% and miscellaneous causes 1%.

In summary, the cause of mortality in newborn lambs are largely physical and environmental and occur immediately at birth or shortly thereafter. In calves, the major causes of mortality are associated with dystocia and with neonatal diarrhea in postnatal life. Calves are not as susceptible to the physical and environmental influences as are lambs. The major causes of mortality of newborn pigs are weakness, starvation and crushing and tramping. Infectious diseases may be important on certain individual farms but do not account for a major cause of mortality. At the other end of the spectrum are foals in which neonatal deaths are infrequent, and inclement weather and infections are much less important than structural and functional abnormalities.

Special investigation of any neonatal deaths (illness)

The following protocol may be a useful guide when investigating deaths of newborn animals.

1. Determine the *duration of pregnancy* to ensure that the newborn animal was born at term. A *serum sample* should be collected from the dam for serological evidence of teratogenic pathogens. A precolostral serum sample from affected calves may assist in the diagnosis of intrauterine fetal infections.
2. Collect *epidemiological information* on prevalence in particular groups (maternal, paternal, nutritional, vaccinated etc.) At least get occurrence per 100 dams at risk! A complete epidemiological investigation will include the following:
   (a) What is the abnormality?
   (b) Who is affected?
   (c) When were the animals affected?
   (d) Where were the affected animals?
   (e) Why were the animals affected?
3. Conduct a *postmortem examination* of all available dead neonates. Note must be taken of whether the neonate breathed, walked or sucked. An estimate of body weight is vital.
4. *Specimens of fetal tissues and placenta* are to be sent for laboratory examination. Examinations requested are pathological and microbiological for known pathogens especially *Brucella abortus*, *Leptospira pomona* and *L. hardjo*, *Escherichia coli*, *Salmonella* sp. and rotavirus.
5. Investigate *management practices* operating at the time, with special attention to clemency of weather, feed supply, maternalism of dam, surveillance by owner—all factors which could influence the survival rate.
6. Ensure that the dam has a *milk supply*.

REVIEW LITERATURE

Edwards, B. L. (1972) Causes of death in new-born pigs. *Vet. Bull.*, *42*, 249.

English, P. R. & Morrison, V. (1984) Causes and prevention of piglet mortality. *Pig News Info.*, *4*, 369–376.

English, P. R. & Smith, W. J. (1975) Some causes of death in neonatal niglets. *Vet. Ann.*, *15*, 95.

Randall, G. C. B. (1978) Perinatal mortality. Some problems of adaptation at birth. *Adv. vet. Sci.*, *22*, 53.

Rossdale, P. D., Silver, M. and Rose, R. J. (1984). Equine perinatal physiology and medicine. *Equ. vet. J.*, *4*, 225–398.

REFERENCES

(1) Dennis, S. J. (1972) *Cornell Vet.*, *62*, 253.
(2) Wiener, G. et al. (1983) *J. agric. Sci.*, *100*, 539.
(3) Wooliams, C. et al. (1983) *J. agric. Sci.*, *100*, 553.
(4) Wooliams, C. et al. (1983) *J. agric. Sci.*, *100*, 563.
(5) Macleod, N. S. M. et al. (1983) *J. agric. Sci.*, *100*, 571.
(6) Ameghino, E. et al. (1984) *Prev. vet. Med.*, *2*, 833.
(7) Purvis, G. M. et al. (1985) *Vet. Rec.*, *116*, 293.
(8) Overas, J. et al. (1985) *Nord. VetMed.*, *97*, 469.
(9) Gumbrell, R. C. (1985) *Surveillance, NZ*, *12*, 5.
(10) Eales, F. A. et al. (1986) *Vet. Rec.*, *118*: 227.
(11) Martin, S. W. et al. (1973) *Am. J. vet. Res.*, *34*, 1027.
(12) Oxender, W. D. et al. (1973) *J. Am. vet. med. Assoc.*, *162*, 458.
(13) Speicher, J. A. & Hepp, R. E. (1975) *J. Am. vet. med. Assoc.*, *162*, 463.
(14) Martin, S. W. et al. (1975) *Am. J. vet. Res.*, *36*, 1105.
(15) Martin, S. W. et al. (1975) *Am. J. vet Res.*, *36*, 1111.
(16) Young, J. S. & Blair, J. M. (1974) *Aust. vet. J.*, *50*, 338.
(17) Patullo, D. A. (1973) *Aust. vet. J.*, *49*, 427.
(18) English, P. R. & Morrison, V. (1984) *Pig News Info.*, *4*, 369.
(19) Spicer, E. M. et al. (1986) *Aust. vet. J.*, *63*, 71.
(20) Randall, G. C. B. (1972) *Vet. Rec.*, *90*, 183.
(21) Whiting, R. et al. (1984) *Can. J. anim. Sci.*, *63*, 993.
(22) Fraser, D. (1973) *Br. vet. J.*, *129*, 324.
(23) DeRoth, L. & Downie, H. G. (1976) *Can. vet. J.*, *17*, 275.
(24) Glastonbury, J. R. W. (1976) *Aust. vet. J.*, *52*, 272.
(25) Platt, H. (1975) *Vet. Ann.*, *15*, 153.
(26) Rossdale, P. D., Silver, M. & Rose, R. J. (1984) Equine perinatal physiology and medicine. *Equ. vet. J.*, *4*, 225–398.
(27) Friendship, R. M. et al. (1986) *Can. vet. J.*, *27*, 307.
(28) Vaala, W. E. (1986) *Comp. cont. Educ. Pract. Vet.*, *8*, S211.
(29) Clabough, D. L. & Martens, R. J. (1985) *Comp. cont. Educ. Pract. Vet.*, *7*, S497.
(30) Beech, J. (1986) *Comp. cont. Educ. Pract. Vet.*, *8*, S284.
(31) Martens, R. J. (1982) *Comp. cont. Educ. Pract. Vet.*, *4*, S23.
(32) Sonea, I. (1985) *Comp. cont. Educ. Pract. Vet.*, *7*, S642.
(33) Becht, J. L. & Semrad, S. D. (1986) *Comp. cont. Educ. Pract. Vet.*, *8*, S367.
(34) Morris, D. D. (1986) *Comp. cont. Educ. Pract. Vet.*, *8*, S139.
(35) Carter, G. K. & Martens, R. J. (1986) *Comp. cont. Educ. Pract. Vet.*, *8*, S256.

CONGENITAL DEFECTS

Abnormalities of structure or function which are present at birth are obviously congenital defects. They may or may not be inherited, and inherited defects may or may not be present at birth.

Etiology

The effects of noxious insults applied to a pregnant female during the three major periods of gestation are summarized in Table 7. During the period of the ovum, an insult may cause death of the ovum and resorption. During the period of the embryo and organogenesis, the result may be death of the embryo with or without abortion, or congenital deformity or defective function of the embryo, depending upon the severity (dose size and duration of application) and the nature of the insult. Even within the period of organogenesis there is a gradation of response depending on the stage of development. When the insult is applied early the number and severity of the abnormalities will be greater than when one is applied later, in which case the response is likely to be focal. During the period of the fetus and fetal growth there may be death of the fetus followed by abortion or mummification or in the very late stages of gestation, just before normal term, stillbirths or weak neonates born alive may occur. The increased resistance of the fetus in its later stages of fetal growth is due to a gradually maturing immune system (1).

Although the type of noxious influence governs to a certain extent the type and severity of the defect which results, there is remarkable similarity between the defects observed after a wide range of insults. For example, the defects caused by vaccination of pregnant sows with attenuated hog cholera virus are similar to those caused by vitamin A deficiency in early pregnancy, and it seems therefore that the severity and time in gestation at which such influences are applied are of equal importance.

Table 7. Possible effects of noxious insults in the pregnant female during the three major periods of gestation

Period of gestation when noxious insult occurs	*Effects of insult on ovum, embryo, fetus and dam*	*Some examples*
Period of the ovum Cow 10–12 days following fertilization	Death of the ovum and resorption	Vibriosis
Period of the embryo and organogenesis Cow 15–45 days Ewe 11–34 days Mare 12–60 days	Depending on dosage or duration of insult: (1) Congential defects often carried to term as: structural abnormality functional deficit or (2) Death of the embryo and resorption or abortion	*Infectious.* Cerebellar hypoplasia in cattle affected with BVD virus *Nutritional deficiency.* Vitamin A *Toxic. Veratrum californicum* in pregnant ewes *Inherited defects.* Vibriosis
Period of the fetus and fetal growth Cow 45 days to term Cow 45–125 days Mare 55 days to term Ewe 34 days to term	Illness or death of the fetus resulting in: Abortion Mummification Stillbirths Weak neonates Persistent viremia and specific immunotolerance	 *Br. abortus*, IBR Bovine virus diarrhea (BVD) virus Inherited, infectious and unknown Dystocia hypoxia Infections in last week of gestation

Death of the dam may occur during any of the periods if the insult is severe enough. Death of the embryo with resorption or abortion does not always occur. In many cases abnormalities or disease of the fetus are carried to term which makes it difficult retrospectively to determine precisely when the insult occurred.

The time during gestation is important in determining the organ which is affected; those organs which are developing rapidly at the time are most likely to be affected. There is a tendency for the range of abnormalities, and correspondingly the organs affected, to be increased by an increase in the duration and severity of the insult. This suggests the possibility that there may be a final common pathway through which all noxious influences exert their deleterious influence on actively differentiating embryonic tissues. In man, most defects are attributed to defective blood supply to the fetus resulting from abnormal placentation, and in experimental animals, hypoxia produced by low atmospheric pressure causes a high incidence of embryonic defects (2). Hypoxia may be the cause in individual cases but is unlikely to be the cause in all. However, by an extension of the same principle, it is possible that a deficiency of an essential metabolite or the presence of a cytopathic agent (viral or chemical) in an unimpaired circulation could have the same effect as hypoxia by interfering with tissue metabolism at the same level. That is to say, the final common pathway may be the high rate of metabolism of rapidly dividing cells. On the other hand it is possible that increased activity of the adrenal cortex may be the final common path, the increased activity being due to deficiency of metabolites, hypoxia or other stress factors.

One of the remarkable features of non-inherited congenital defects in animals and man is their tendency to occur in 'outbreaks' (3). This is understandable if known viral infections (4) or nutritional deficiencies have a seasonal occurrence, but where the causative agent is not known the reason for the periodicity of the defect is obscure.

The noxious influences which are known to produce congenital defects are presented here.

Inheritance

There are many examples among domestic animals (see Chapter 34). It is possible that many inherited defects, which need not be congenital, are due to inheritance of a higher requirement of a specific metabolite than normal, the 'genetotrophic' diseases. Certainly some inherited defects including cleft palate can be reproduced by dietary deficiencies, the incidence of some inherited defects can be modified by dietary supplementation, and the effects of many noxious agents are modified by the genetic constitution of the animal.

Virus infection

Only seven viruses are known to cause congenital defects in man and animals under natural conditions, that is not only by experimental injection. They are the viruses of rubella and herpes simplex and the cytomegalovirus in man, and the viruses of swine fever, bluetongue, bovine virus diarrhea, and of Akabane disease in animals. Two other viruses, Rift Valley fever and Wesselsbron viruses, in their attenuated forms, can cause teratological changes in brain (37).

In animal diseases the details are:

Hog cholera virus
Vaccination of sows with modified vaccine virus between the 15th and 25th days of pregnancy produces piglets with edema, deformed noses and kidneys. Natural infection with field virus can cause cerebellar hypoplasia in piglets.

Bluetongue virus
Vaccination of ewes with attenuated vaccine virus between the 35th and 45th days of pregnancy causes high prevalence of porencephaly in lambs (4). Similar lesions occur after natural infection.

Bovine viral diarrhea (BVD) virus
Natural infection can cause cerebellar hypoplasia in calves. Experimental infection of susceptible pregnant heifers causes cerebellar hypoplasia, optic defects including cataracts, retinal degeneration, and hypoplasia and neuritis of the optic nerves (5). Other defects are brachygnathia, abortion, stillbirth and mummification. A closely related virus, *border disease virus*, causes 'hairy shaker' in lambs.

Infection of the bovine fetus between 45 and 125 days of gestation with the non-cytopathic biotype of the virus can result in the development of a persistently viremic and immunotolerant calf which is carried to term, born alive, remains persistently viremic and immunotolerant, will develop fatal mucosal disease at 6–8 months of age or later (up to 3 years of age) following superinfection with a cytopathic biotype of the virus (5).

Akabane virus
This infection of pregnant cows causes arthrogryposis and hydraencephaly. An impending epidemic of bovine congenital abnormalities due to the Akabane virus can be anticipated by serological surveys of young breeding cattle (4).

The means by which the viruses gain entrance to the fetus are not well defined (7). It seems likely that whether or not infection of the fetus occurs depends on the interaction of the nature of the virus, the timing of the infection relative to the age of the pregnancy, and the immunological status of the fetus.

Nutritional deficiency

There are many congenital defects in animals which are known to be caused by deficiencies of specific nutrients in the diet of the dam.

- Iodine—goiter in all species
- Copper—enzootic ataxia in lambs
- Manganese—limb deformities in calves
- Vitamin D—neonatal rickets
- Vitamin A—eye defects, harelip and other defects in piglets
- Experimental deficiencies in laboratory animals which have teratogenic effects are nutritional deficiencies of choline, riboflavin, pantothenic acid, cobalamin, folic acid (8), manganese and copper (9) and hypervitaminosis A
- Simple inanition or nutritional deficiency of protein do not cause congenital defects, but can increase prevalence of abortions and stillbirths

- Metabolic procedures have been used experimentally to produce congenital malformations (10).

Chemical poisons

Exposure to many toxic substances is capable of causing congenital defects.

Poisonous plants
Their teratogenic effects have been reviewed in detail (36).

- *Veratrum californicum* fed to ewes at about the 14th day of pregnancy can cause defects of the cranium and brain in lambs and prolonged gestation (13)
- *Astragalus* and *Oxytropis* spp.—locoweeds and lupins (*Lupinus sericeus*) causes limb contractures in calves and lambs (14)
- Tobacco plants—ingestion by sows can cause limb deformities in their piglets (15)
- *Conium maculatum*, poison hemlock fed to cows in the period from the 55th to 75th day of pregnancy, causes permanent flexure of carpal and elbow joints and scoliosis (16)
- *Leucaena leucocephala* (or mimosine, its toxic ingredient) cause forelimb polypodia (supernumerary feet) in piglets when fed experimentally to sows (36)
- Heliotrine, the pyrrolizidine alkaloid in *Heliotropium* sp. causes fetal anomalies in rats (12).

Farm chemicals
- Parbendazole and cambendazole are important teratogens for sheep (17, 18)
- Methallibure, a drug used to control estrus in sows causes deformities in the limbs and cranium of pigs (21, 22) when fed to sows in early pregnancy
- Apholate (24), an insect chemosterilant, is suspected of causing congenital defects in sheep
- Organophosphates have been extensively tested and found to be usually non-teratogenic (11). A supposed teratogenic effect is probably a reflection of the very common usage of these substances in agriculture (see under poisoning by organophosphates).

Miscellaneous chemicals and drugs
- Cortisone early in pregnancy to mice and humans causes increased incidence of cleft palate (19)
- Estrone and estradiol administered to mice (12th to 16th day of pregnancy) causes a high incidence of cleft palate (20)
- Bismuth (23), selenium, nitrogen mustards, tetanus toxin, sulfonamides, physostigmine, radium and x-ray irradiation all result in an increased incidence of congenital defects (2).

Physical insults

- *Severe exposure to beta or gamma irradiation*, for example, after an atomic explosion, can cause a high incidence of gross malformations in developing fetuses (25) including defective limb development (26)
- *Hyperthermia* applied to the dam experimentally causes congenital deformities (27), but this appears to have no practical application. The severest abnormalities occur after exposure during early pregnancy (18–25 days in ewes). Disturbances of CNS development are commonest. Defects of the spinal cord manifest themselves as arthrogryposis and exposure of ewes to high temperatures (42°C; 107·5°F) causes stunting of limbs; the lambs are not true miniatures, they have selective deformities with the metacarpals selectively shortened. The defect occurs whether nutrition is normal or not (28). Developmental abnormalities have been reproduced experimentally in explanted porcine embryos exposed to environmental temperatures similar to those which may be associated with high ambient temperatures and reproductive failure in swine herds (6).

Environmental influences

Currently, there is considerable interest in the possible teratogenic effects of manmade changes in the environment. The concern is understandable because the fetus is a sensitive biological indicator of the presence of some noxious influences in the environment. For example, during a recent accidental release of polybrominated biphenyls much of the angry commentary related to the probable occurrence of congenital defects. The noxious influences can be physical or chemical and the existing known pathogens are beta and gamma irradiation, and other than atomic pollution there are no identified teratogens. After one examination of the epidemiology of congenital defects in pigs it was apparent that any environmental causes were from the natural environment; manmade environmental changes, especially husbandry practices, had little effect (29).

Epidemiology
The determination of the cause of congenital defects in a particular case very often defies all methods of examination. Epidemiological considerations offer some of the best clues but are obviously of little advantage when the number of cases is limited. The possibility of inheritance playing a part is fairly easily examined if good breeding records are available. The chances of coming to a finite conclusion are much less probable. Some of the statistical techniques used are discussed in Chapter 34 on inherited diseases.

An expression of the prevalence of congenital defects is of very little value unless it is related to the size of the population at risk, and almost no records include this vital data. Furthermore, most of the records available are retrospective and based on the number of cases presented at a laboratory or hospital. In study, the registration, documentation and evaluation of abnormalities in calves and bovine fetuses has yielded some preliminary information (38). A carefully controlled prospective study of the congenital defects in a particular animal population would be more reliable and might make it possible to avoid the standard comment that, for example, 0·5–3·0% of all calves born have congenital defects. It should be possible to express a narrower range. That is not to say that a wider range cannot be observed. Some breeds and families have extraordinarily high prevalence rates because of intensive inbreeding. The prevalence rates of 0·5–3·0% for calves and 2% for lambs (30) are comparable with the human rate of 1–3%

(31). A much higher rate for animals of 5–6% is also quoted (32). A very extensive literature on congenital defects in animals exists and a bibliography is available (33, 39).

Checklists of recorded defects are included in the literature review.

Pathogenesis

Viruses which gain entry to the fetus are capable of destroying tissue. The viruses of bluetongue, bovine viral diarrhea and border disease have affinity for nervous tissue and cause extensive damage to the fetus. This can result in severe lesions not only in nervous tissue, but also in other tissues because of defects in their innervation. If the infection occurs early in gestation the virus may survive harmoniously with the tissue because no antibodies are produced. When organ and tissue differentiation begin, the virus is in a position to destroy the tissue. At a later stage, when the fetus acquires immunological maturity, the virus is disposed of and cannot subsequently be isolated from the fetus. The only technique which can then be used to make a presumptive diagnosis is the examination of precolostral serum from the newborn animal for virus neutralizing antibodies (35).

It has been suggested, with some good evidence, that the etiology and pathogenesis of congenital torticollis and head scoliosis in the equine fetus are related to an increased incidence of transverse presentation of the fetus (40, 41). This is an example of the necessity to consider mechanistic factors as well as others such as genetic when confronted with congenital defects of the newborn.

Clinical and necropsy findings

It is not intended to give details of the clinical signs of all the congenital defects here but some general comments are necessary. Approximately 50% of animals with congenital defects are stillborn. The defects are usually readily obvious clinically. Diseases of the nervous system and musculoskeletal system rate high in most published records and this may be related to the ease with which abnormalities of these systems can be observed. For example, in one survey of congenital defects in pigs (34) the percentage occurrence rates in the different body systems were as follows: bones and joints 23%, central nervous system 17%, special sense organs 12%, combined alimentary and respiratory tracts (mostly cleft palate and atresia ani) 27%, miscellaneous (mostly monsters) 9%, genitourinary and abdominal wall (hernias) each 5%, and cardiovascular system 3%. In a cattle survey the percentage occurrence rates were: musculoskeletal system 24%, respiratory and alimentary tracts 13%, central nervous system 22%, abdominal wall 9%, urogenital 4%, cardiovascular 3%, skin 2%, and others 4%. (Anomalous-joined twins and hydrops amnii accounted for 20%) (31).

Many animals with congenital defects have more than one anomaly; in pigs the average is two (34) and considerable care must be taken to avoid missing a second and third defect in the excitement of finding the first. In some instances, the combinations of defects are repeated often enough to become specific entities. Examples are microphthalmia and cleft palate which often occur together in piglets, and microphthalmia and patent interventricular septum in calves.

There are a number of defects which cannot be readily distinguished at birth and others which disappear subsequently. It is probably wise not to be too dogmatic in predicting the outcome in a patient with only a suspicion of a congenital defect or one in which the defect appears to be causing no apparent harm. A specific instance is the newborn foal with a cardiac murmur. Sporadic cases of congenital defects are usually impossible to define etiologically, but when the number of affected animals increases it becomes necessary and possible to attempt to determine the cause.

Clinical pathology

Blood samples should be collected from neonates before they suck and absorb gammaglobulins from colostrum. The gammaglobulin levels are assayed to determine if intrauterine infection has occurred. Specific antibodies against known antigens can be estimated. Serum should be stored for retrospective examination for other antibodies which subsequently appear important.

Diagnosis

The diagnostic challenge with congenital defects is to recognize and identify the defect and to determine the cause. Most congenital defects are recognized clinically immediately after birth or some time later. Their cause is almost never obvious. A detailed clinical and pathological examination can often determine that a defect such as a cardiac mural defect must have been congenital even though it may not have been recognized until some time after birth. On the other hand, the neurological signs may not appear until 2 months after birth in Arabian foals with inherited cerebellar hypoplasia. It is assumed that the lesion was present at birth (congenital) but the clinical signs did not become apparent until later.

The determination of the cause of a congenital defect is usually not undertaken unless more than a few newborn animals in a herd or area are affected in a short period of time with similar abnormalities. A detailed epidemiological investigation will be necessary which will include the following:

- Pedigree analysis. Does the frequency of occurrence of the defect suggest an inherited disease or is it characteristically non-hereditary?
- Nutritional history of dams of affected neonates and alterations in usual sources of feed
- Disease history of dams of affected neonates
- History of drugs used on dams
- Movement of dams during pregnancy to localities where contact with teratogens may have occurred
- Season of the year when insults may have occurred
- Introduction of animals to the herd.

The major difficulty in determining the cause of nonhereditary congenital defects is the long interval of time between when the causative agent was operative and when the animals are presented, often 6–8 months. The examination of precolostral sera from affected animals may assist in determining the presence of certain infectious agents; but the determination that specific nutritional deficiencies, toxins or environmental influences were causative is difficult. Detailed clinical and pathological examination of affected animals offers the best opportunity to determine the etiology based on the presence of lesions which are known to be caused by certain teratogens.

REVIEW LITERATURE

Dennis, S. M. & Leipold, H. W. (1979) Ovine congenital defects. *Vet. Bull.*, *49*, 233.
Done, J. T. (1978) Virus teratogens and domesticated animals. *Vet. Ann.*, *18*, 1.
Huston, R. et al. (1978) Congenital defects in pigs. *Vet. Bull.*, *48*, 645.
Huston, r. et al. (1977) Congenital defects in foals. *J. equ. med. Surg.*, *1*, 146.
Keeler, R. F. (1972) Known and suspected teratogenic hazards in range plants. *Clin. Toxicol.*, *5*, 529.
Leipold, H. W. (1978) Genetics and disease in cattle. *Proc. 11th Ann. Conv. Am. Assoc. Bov. Pract.*, p. 18.
Leipold, H. W., Huston, K. & Dennis, S. M. (1983) Bovine congenital defects. *Adv. vet. Sci. comp. Med.*, *27*, 197–271.
Parsonson, I.M., Della-Porta, A. J. & Snowdon, W. A. (1981) Developmental disorders of the fetus in some arthropod-bovine virus infection. *Am. J. trop. Med. Hyg.*, *30*, 600–673.
Pearson, H. (1979) Changing attitudes to congenital and inherited diseases. *Vet. Rec.*, *105*, 318.

REFERENCES

(1) Osburn, B. I. et al. (1970) *Fedn Proc. Fedn. Am. Socs exp. Biol.*, *29*, 286.
(2) Hogan, A. G. (1953) *Ann. Rev. Biochem.*, *22*, 299.
(3) Nicolson, T. B. et al. (1985) *Vet. Rec.*, *116*, 281.
(4) Kirkland, P. D. et al. (1983) *Aust. vet. J.*, *60*, 221.
(5) Duffell, S. J. & Harkness, J. W. (1985) *Vet. Rec.*, *117*, 240.
(6) Trujano, M. & Wrathall, A. E. *Br. vet. J.*, *141*, 603.
(7) Catalano, L. W. & Sever, J. L. (1971) *Ann. Rev. Microbiol.*, *25*, 255.
(8) Giroud, A. (1954) *Biol. Rev.*, *29*, 220.
(9) O'Dell, B. L. et al. (1961) *J. Nutr.*, *73*, 151.
(10) Kalter, J. & Warkany, J. (1959) *Physiol. Rev.*, *39*, 69.
(11) Bellows, R. A. et al. (1975) *Am. J. vet. Res.*, *36*, 1133.
(12) Queen, C. R. & Christie, C. S. (1961) *Br. J. exp. Pathol.*, *62*, 369.
(13) Binns, W. et al. (1965) *J. Am. vet. med. Assoc.*, *147*, 839.
(14) James, L. F. et al. (1967) *Am. J. vet. Res.*, *28*, 1379.
(15) Crowe, M. W. & Swerczek, T. W. (1974) *Am. J. vet. Res.*, *35*, 1071.
(16) Keeler, R. F. (1974) *Clin. Toxicol.*, *7*, 195.
(17) Szabo, K. T. et al. (1974) *Cornell Vet.*, *64*, Suppl. 4, 41.
(18) Saunders, L. Z. et al. (1974) *Cornell Vet.*, *64*, Suppl. 4, 7.
(19) Harris, J. W. S. & Ross, I. P. (1956) *Lancet.*, *270*, 1045.
(20) Nishihara, G. (1958) *Proc. Soc. exp. Biol. Med.*, *97*, 809.
(21) Schafer, J. H. et al. (1973) *J. anim. Sci.*, *36*, 722.
(22) Vente, J. P. et al. (1972) *Res. vet. Sci.*, *13*, 169.
(23) James, L. F. et al. (1966) *Am. J. vet. Res.*, *27*, 132.
(24) Younger, R. L. (1965) *Am. J. vet. Res.*, *26*, 991.
(25) Schjeide, O. A. (1957) *Nutr. Rev.*, *15*, 225.
(26) Erickson, B. H. & Murphree, R. L. (1964) *J. anim. Sci.*, *23*, 1066.
(27) Edwards, M. J. (1978) *Adv. vet. Sci.*, *22*, 29.
(28) Cartwright, G. A. & Thwaites, G. C. J. (1976) *J. agric. Sci., Camb.*, *86*, 573.
(29) Selby, L. A. et al. (1973) *Envir. Res.*, *6*, 77.
(30) Hughes, K. L. et al. (1972) *Teratology*, *5*, 5.
(31) Leipold, H. W. et al. (1972) *Adv. vet. Sci.*, *16*, 103.
(32) Preister, W. A. et al. (1970) *Am. J. vet. Res.*, *31*, 1871.
(33) WHO (1973) *Bibliography on Congenital Defects in Animals.* Veterinary Public Health Unit. Geneva: WHO.
(34) Selby, L. A. et al. (1971) *J. Am. vet. med. Assoc.*, *159*, 1485.
(35) Osburn, B. I. (1975) *Bov. Pract.*, No. 10, pp. 7–10.
(36) Keeler, R. F. (1972) *Clin. Toxicol.*, *5*, 529.
(37) Coetzer, J. A. W. (1980) *J. S. Afr. vet. Assoc.*, *51*, 153.
(38) Muller, W. et al. (1983) *Monat. vet. Med.*, *38*, 736.
(39) Crowe, M. W. & Swerczek, T. W. (1985) *Am. J. vet. Res.*, *46*, 353.
(40) Woolam, D. H. M. (1984) *Equ. vet. J.*, *16*, 399.
(41) Vadeplassche, M. et al. (1984) *Equ. vet. J.*, *16*, 419.

Intrauterine growth retardation

This is a special form of congenital defect. It is a failure to grow properly and is distinct from failure to gain body weight. It relates to stature, usually measured by the crown-to-rump length. Dwarfism in cattle and runting in pigs are the classical veterinary examples.

Runt piglets are defined as growth retardation without obvious cause such as fetal anomaly or maternal illness. Affected pigs are runts at birth so that the defect is more properly entitled fetal growth retardation. Runts are smaller, thinner and have disproportionately larger, domed heads than normal pigs. The stage or pregnancy at which runting occurs is debated, most views being that it occurs in the second half of pregnancy, but development at an earlier age has been demonstrated (1). Significant growth retardation *in utero* is recorded in the fetuses of cattle infected with bovine virus diarrhea. In the same group of animals there are likely to be abortions and mummifications (2).

Although body weight is not the best criterion, it is used because it is the most convenient measure. Because of the variety of species and breeds, the norm is established as the mean plus or minus two standard deviations from it (3). The same measure is used when determining the range of norm for length and weight of dorsal muscles and the weight of any individual organ.

REFERENCES

(1) Cooper, J. E. et al. (1978) *Vet. Rec.*, *102*, 529.
(2) Done, J. T. et al. (1980) *Vet. Rec.*, *106*, 473.
(3) Richardson, C. (1978) *Vet. Ann.*, *18*, 101.

Neonatal neoplasia

Neoplasms of the newborn are recorded rarely (1), but lymphosarcoma has been recorded in a foal which was weak at birth and died soon afterwards (2); both benign and malignant melanomas occur in foals and piglets (3), and myeloid leukosis is recorded in a 3-day-old piglet (4). Sporadic bovine leukosis of young calves may also be present at birth. It is described in the section on that disease (p. 816).

REFERENCES

(1) Misdorp, W. (1965) *Pathol. Vet.*, *2*, 328.
(2) Tomlinson, M. J. et al. (1979) *Vet. Pathol.*, *16*, 629.
(3) Hamilton, D. P. & Bryerley, C. S. (1973) *J. Am. vet. med. Assoc.*, *164*, 1040.
(4) Allsup, T. N. et al. (1981) *Vet Rec.*, *108*, 231.

DISEASES CAUSED BY PHYSICAL AND ENVIRONMENTAL INFLUENCES

Parturient injury and intrapartum death

As a result of dystocia, which may or may not be assisted by the farmer, there is the chance of physical trauma to limbs or the rib cage. More subtle is the possibility of damage to the brain by way of intracranial hemorrhages. A high proportion (70%) of non-surviving neonatal lambs at, or within 7 days of, birth have been shown to have single or multiple such hemorrhages, the highest incidence being in lambs of high birth weight (1). Similar lesions have been identified in foals (2) and calves (3). Experimentally controlled parturition in ewes showed that duration and vigor of the birth process affected the severity of intracranial hemorrhages. During a prolonged birth the head and neck are stretched resulting in trauma to meninges (5). Newborn foals which developed neurological signs within 5 days of birth had high protein and creatinine kinase activity, but few red blood cells in the cerebrospinal fluid. It is thought that these abnormalities may be due to changes occurring during foaling (11). Intracranial hemorrhage, especially subarachnoid hemorrhage, is a common occurrence in foals, born before full term (27). The highest incidence occurred in pony foals in which parturition was induced prior to 301 days of gestation. Similar hemorrhage occurred in pony foals born by cesarean section at 270 and 280 days of gestation.

In a prolonged birth, as distinct from dystocia, edema of parts of the body, such as the head and particularly the tongue, may also occur. However, the principal problem relative to neonatal disease is the effect of the often prolonged hypoxia to which the calf is subjected. There is interference with the placental circulation and failure of the calf to reach the external environment. The hypoxia may be sufficient to produce a stillborn calf, or the calf may be alive at birth but not survive because of irreparable brain damage (4). Intrapartum deaths due to prolonged parturition occur in piglets.

Fetal hypoxia

Most information about neonatal hypoxia relates to foals (26). Foals are born in a primary apneic state, but gasping respiration begins within 30–60 seconds. Failure to do so creates an urgent need for resuscitation measures. Placental dysfunction or occlusion of the umbilicus in the second stage of labor can result in a much more serious situation so that the foal is born in a state of terminal, as distinct from primary, apnea. It will be stillborn unless urgent and vigorous resuscitation is initiated immediately. Resuscitation includes:

- Extending the head and clearing the nostrils of mucus
- Sealing one nostril by hand and breathing forcibly into the other (or inflating with a rubber tube from an oxygen cylinder, delivering at a rate of 5 l/min), the chest wall to be moved only slightly with each positive breath. Continue at 25/min until respiration is spontaneous
- Administering 200 ml 5% sodium bicarbonate solution intravenously to counter the inevitable acidosis.

The syndromes in foals associated with neonatal hypoxia include 'barkers' and 'wanderers' (convulsive and dummy syndromes), which are dealt with elsewhere, and premature foals. These are foals less than 325 days of fetal age which are obviously of low birth weight, are weak and unable to stand and show respiratory distress and disinclination to suck, and a subnormal temperature. Treatment of these conditions is discussed elsewhere. Stomach tube feeding is often necessary and requires mare's milk (or reconstituted dried milk) at the rate of 80 ml/kg body weight/day in 10 divided feeds. This should provide 2250 calories (9414 J) per day to a 50 kg foal (26).

A simple device for resuscitation of newborn calves and lambs consists of a mouthpiece, a non-return valve, a flange which blocks the external nares and an oral tube (54).

Fetal anoxia may be an important cause of the *weak calf syndrome* described in Chapter 35 on specific diseases of unknown or uncertain etiology. Affected calves are fully developed at birth and may be born with or without assistance. They do not make the usual effort to sit up in sternal recumbency and usually cannot stand even when assisted. They are dull and inactive and the sucking reflex is poor or absent. They may die within 10–15 minutes after birth or live for several hours or a few days. There are usually no obvious clinical or pathological abnormalities detectable to account for the weakness. The cause is unknown, but intrapartum hypoxemia due to prolonged parturition, particularly in calves born to first-calf beef heifers, is considered as a possible cause. A similar syndrome has been produced experimentally by clamping the umbilical cord of the bovine fetus *in utero* for 6 or 8 minutes, followed by a cesarean section 30–40 minutes later. Calves born following this procedure may die in 10–15 minutes after birth or survive for only up to 2 days (4). During the experimental clamping of the umbilical cord, there is a decline in the blood pH, P_{O_2}, and standard bicarbonate levels and an increase in P_{CO_2} and lactate levels (4). During the clamping there is also increased fetal movement and a release of meconium which stains the calf and the amniotic fluid. Those which survive for a few hours or days are dull, depressed, cannot stand, have poor sucking and swallowing reflexes and their temperature is usually subnormal. They respond poorly to supportive therapy. A slight body tremor may be present and occasionally tetany and opisthotonus occur before death. Calves which are barely able to stand cannot find the teats of the dam because of uncontrolled head movements. At necropsy of these experimental cases, there are petechial and ecchymotic hemorrhages on the myocardium and endocardium, an excess of pericardial fluid, and the lungs are inflated. When the experimental clamping lasts only 4 minutes, the calves usually survive.

In lambs, severe hypoxia during birth results in metabolic acidosis and depressed heat production capacity which causes hyperthermia (9). Twins and triplets are more susceptible to hypothermia than are singles (13).

The prevention of intrapartum hypoxia depends on the provision of surveillance, and assistance if necessary, for first-calf heifers at the time of calving. Heifers which do not continue to show progress during the second stage of parturition should be examined for evidence of dystocia, and obstetrical assistance provided if necessary. There is no effective treatment for calves affected with intrapartum hypoxia. The provision of warmth, force feeding colostrum and fluid therapy are logical approaches.

The differential diagnosis includes:

1. *In utero* infections in late gestation, which can result in the birth of a toxemic calf which is weak and has a poor sucking reflex and death may occur in a few hours or a few days. The virus of infectious bovine rhinotracheitis usually causes a fatal viremia of the fetus followed by abortion. However, infection in the last 2 weeks of gestation can result in the birth of live weak calves.
2. Cold exposure may occur in lambs, calves and piglets that are born in cold environments. They may be born in inaccessible areas and be unable to reach the dam or the dam may be unable to reach its young.
3. Maternal deficiencies of the dam may result in weak neonates which may die within hours or a few days of birth. Examples include iodine deficiency and copper deficiency in lambs and kids. Congenital copper deficiency has not yet been documented as a cause of weak calves, but the possibility should be considered when several calves are born weak from cattle which are receiving a copper-deficient diet. A necropsy should be done on all weak calves which die for no obvious reason.

Environmental and nutritional factors

Two environmental factors which may predispose to infection, besides causing mortality themselves, are low environmental temperature and deprivation of carbohydrate leading to hypoglycemia (6).

Effects of temperature

Piglets are particularly susceptible to hypothermia and hypoglycemia. Their thermoregulation mechanism is highly inefficient during the first 9 days of life and is not fully functional until the 20th day (7). The preferred air temperature for neonatal pigs is 32°C (89·5°F) during the first day and 30°C (86°F) thereafter (8). Because of the importance of neonatal mortality in range lambs some observations have been made on their thermoregulation efficiency (10) and it is apparent that at high environmental temperatures it is not effective. Heat prostration and some deaths can occur when the environmental temperature is high especially if lambs have to perform prolonged physical exercise and if there is an absence of shade.

The major causes of *hypothermia* in newborn lambs are excessive heat loss, depressed heat production caused by intrapartum hypoxia and immaturity, and starvation (13). Excessive heat loss is the major cause when it occurs in lambs within a few hours after birth and some shelter is required. Wetness is considered to be an important factor determining whether or not lambs become hypothermic (28). Wet lambs suffer a reduction in coat insulation and an increase in evaporative heat loss which occurs as a result of wetting. Lightweight twin lambs also become hypothermic more quickly than heavier singles (28). Hypothermia occurring in lambs at 12 hours of age is usually due to starvation and the administration of glucose is necessary. Glucose is administered intraperitoneally at a dose of 2 g/kg body weight using a 20% solution. Following the administration of the glucose, the lambs are rewarmed in air at 40°C (104°F) and careful attention is given to the nutrition of the lambs after rewarming. A feeding of 100–200 ml of colostrum will also be beneficial. These factors are usually accompanied by a low plasma lactate, indicative of a low metabolic rate. Experimental hypothermia in lambs has shown little pathological effect, but there is a strong relationship between breed and the degree of hypothermia produced (16). Experimentally produced hypothermia in calves has also been shown to cause little overt injury except for peripheral damage to exterior tissues (21, 25). The physiological, hematological and serum biochemical responses to experimental hypothermia and rewarming in newborn calves has been examined (29). Loss of body heat occurred most rapidly from the peripheral tissue, but less rapidly from core body tissues during cooling.

There was no advantage of one method of rewarming over another, calves have a remarkable ability to resist and overcome the effects of severe cold temperatures. However, there is a relationship between the occurrence of cold weather and calf deaths, including those due to the 'weak calf syndrome'.

There is little information on thermoregulation in newborn *foals* but it is evident that healthy foals, within a normal environmental temperature range, are capable of homeothermic response (12). One of the effects produced by exposure to cold is a greatly increased metabolic rate and the subsequent development of acidosis. This has been demonstrated in *lambs* which maintained normal body temperature on exposure to extreme cold. The efficiency of the thermogenic response is considerably less in premature neonates than in full-term ones, whether the premature ones are delivered by cesarean section or by the administration of corticosteroids (14).

The effect of maternal nutrition on the newborn

Nutrition of the dam is important in relation to resistance of the offspring (15), but it is impossible to be specific in recommending the ration to be used.

Newborn lambs, calves and foals are much more capable of maintaining their blood glucose levels when starved than are piglets (17) although occasional cases of hypoglycemic coma may be seen in lambs. In the newborn piglet, liver glycogen is rapidly depleted postnatally (12–24 hours) for the maintenance of blood glucose. Because there is little lipid stored for utilization the piglets' capacity for gluconeogenesis is largely underdeveloped. Therefore, maintenance of the physiologically critical energy metabolite, glucose, depends largely on the neonate's ability to compete with littermates for regular nourishment from its dam. Piglets starved during the first week of life succumb quickly and manifest a specific syndrome known as neonatal hypoglycemia or baby pig disease. Calves are also highly resistant to insulin-produced hypoglycemia during the first 48 hours of life but are susceptible and respond convulsively to it at 7 days (18).

The effects of nutrition of the pregnant ewe on fetal growth rate, udder development, the availability of energy in the body reserves of fetuses at term, and the amount and energy content of colostrum has been examined (30–32). Fetal growth rate is much more sensitive to maternal underfeeding than previously thought. The weight of the placenta varies widely in uniformly treated ewes and much of this variation is unexplained. It appears that the survival of the fetus is jeopardized more by a small placenta than by maternal underfeeding. The underfeeding of hill sheep in late pregnancy markedly reduces the term weight of the udder and the prenatal accumulation and subsequent rates of secretion of colostrum (32). A low plane of nutrition in late pregnancy results in a marked decrease in fetal body lipid, and marked reductions in the total production of colostrum and in the concentration in colostrum during the first 18 hours after parturition (32).

Digestive enzyme capacities of newborn farm animals

All newborn farm animals are well endowed at birth with the digestive enzyme capacities to digest the nutrients of milk from their dams. In all species at birth, or within a few days, there are usually adequate quantities of lactase, pancreatic lipase and proteolytic enzymes with which to digest lactose, milk fat and milk proteins. Newborn calves digest the nutrients of cow's whole milk with a high degree of efficiency (19). The patterns of digestive enzyme capacity in newborn farm animals change with increasing age (20) as they become less dependent on milk and as other non-milk diets are introduced. Milk substitutes which contain excessive amounts of non-milk carbohydrates or non-milk proteins are not well digested by calves until they are about 3 weeks of age. In the calf, significant sucrase activity never develops with age; there are slight increases with age in amylase and maltase and the pepsin-HCl complex is not effective until about 2 weeks of age. Rennin activity in the abomasum is significant on the first day of life. The piglet develops significant sucrase activity by 2 weeks of age and thus sucrase may be added to preweaning rations. In the foal, lactase activity is maximal at birth and maintained until 4 months of age followed by a decline to nil levels at 4 years of age (23). Sucrase and maltase activities in the foal are barely detectable at birth but increase to adult levels at 7 months of age. All species have adequate levels of pancreatic lipase for the digestion of milk fat and added fats if they are properly homogenized, and the calf has salivary lipase too. All species have gastric proteolytic enzymes with which to digest milk proteins. Nutritional diarrhea and increased incidence of infectious diarrhea are common in calves fed poor quality milk replacers which contain relatively indigestible non-milk carbohydrates or non-milk proteins or heat-denatured skim-milk powder (19).

Poor mother–young relationship

Any examination of neonatal mortality suspected of being caused by hypothermia, starvation or infection due to hypogammaglobulinemia, and even trauma by crushing in piglets, must take into account the possibility that a poor mother–young bond may be the primary cause (12). The defect is most likely to be on the side of the dam, but may originate with the offspring. A poor relationship may be genetic or nutritional and, on the part of the offspring, be the result of birth trauma. For both the dam and the young there is a much greater chance of establishing a good bond if the animal has been reared in a group rather than as an individual. Because sight, smell, taste and sound are all important in the establishment of a seeking and posturing to suckle activity by the dam and a seeking, nuzzling and sucking activity by the offspring, any husbandry factor which interferes with the use of these senses predisposes to mortality. Weakness of the offspring due to poor nutrition of the dam, harassment at parturition by overzealous attendants, and high growth of pasture are obvious examples. This can be a problem in cattle, pigs and sheep, but rarely if ever in foals. In pigs it may be developed to an intense degree in the form of farrowing hysteria, and is dealt with under that heading. In sheep it can be a significant contributor to neonatal death from starvation especially in the highly strung breeds like the Merino.

The practical ways in which physical and environmental influences can result in illness and death in neonates are as follows. They apply principally to lambs but the same comments could apply generally to other species.

Malnutrition of lambs

This is caused by:

- Antepartum malnutrition of ewe reducing milk flow
- Inclement weather preventing lamb sucking or ewe mothering
- Inadequate maternal behaviour especially in some strains of Merino sheep and when there is too much human interference
- Ewes which are too old to have satisfactory milk flow
- Ewes too tired because of prolonged parturition

Inadequate mothering by ewe

This causes:

- Malnutrition of the lamb
- Lack of warmth and protection of lamb

Reduced vigor of the lamb

This is manifested by inadequate teat seeking and weak sucking, and caused by:

- Small lambs, especially during cold weather
- Malnutrition
- Intrauterine and postnatal infections
- Cold or hot weather
- Being one of multiple births; the lamb is small, and weak from prolonged parturition and fails to receive sufficient milk

Predation

Predation by foxes, eagles and crows is contributed to by weakness of the lamb resulting from above.

Treatment and control of neonatal hypothermia and malnutrition

Hypothermic neonates need careful warming by any

means available. They are very susceptible to overheating and severe tissue damage due to burning occurs easily because inert, comatose animals are unable to move off heated areas. Glucose (dextrose) intravenously is the quickest and surest way of raising the blood sugar. Solutions up to 20% concentration are satisfactory. For lambs, a dose rate of 2 g/kg body weight using a 20% solution of dextrose intraperitoneally is recommended. For oral medication through a stomach tube, glucose and either fruit pectin or corn syrup is satisfactory, but sucrose or starch should not be used (22). They are hypertonic until digested and this may be delayed; they are not digested at all by calves. Colostrum should also be given and the animal should be rewarmed in air at 40°C (104°F) at least.

Induction of premature parturition

Calves

The medical induction of parturition by the parenteral injection of corticosteroids into pregnant cows during the last 6 weeks of pregnancy has raised the question of the possible effects of prematurity on the disease resistance of the newborn calf.

The induction of premature parturition in cattle has found application in five main areas:

- Synchronization of the calving period with seasonal advantages
- Ensure that calving coincides with the availability of labor to facilitate observations and management of calving and to overcome the inconvenience caused by late-calving cows
- To minimize dystocias in small-sized heifers
- The therapeutic termination of pregnancy for various clinical reasons
- As an aid in the control of milk fever using vitamin D analogs (33).

A variety of short-acting and long-acting corticosteroids have been used. A single injection of a short-acting formulation is used when it is desirable to induce calving in the last 2–3 weeks of gestation. Earlier in pregnancy the long-acting formulations are more reliable. Parturition occurs 30–60 hours (mean 48 hours) after injection. Some reports indicated that the mortality rate of calves was higher than expected, and that the level of serum immunoglobulins was lower because of interference with absorption by the corticosteroids. Mortality in calves born as a result of induced parturition is primarily as a result of prematurity. The calves are usually lighter in weight. The health of calves which survive is generally good, provided they receive adequate quantities of colostrum. When short-acting corticosteroids are used to induce calving close to term, the ability of the calves to absorb immunoglobulins from colostrum is not impaired (24). However, calves born earlier in pregnancy after using long-acting corticosteroids are lethargic, slow to stand and to suck properly and their ability to absorb immunoglobulins is impaired (33). Up to 60% of calves born following induction with long-acting corticosteroids may be hypogammaglobulinemic. The colostrum available to such calves also has a reduced content of immunoglobulins, and there may also be a reduction in the total volume of colostrum available from the induced-calving cows. The incidence of retained placenta may be as high as 88% in some cases (24).

When parturition is induced in large herds of cattle, particularly with a high percentage of heifers, increased surveillance will be necessary after the calves are born to avoid mismothering. Every attempt must be made to establish the cow/calf pair (neonatal bond) and move them out of the main calving area. Heifers which disown their calves must be confined in a small pen and encouraged to accept the calf and let it suck—sometimes a very unrewarding chore for the cowman.

Foals

The induction of parturition in mares for reasons of economy, management convenience or research and teaching is now being practiced (35). However, it is not without risk and has been associated with the birth of foals which are weak, injured or susceptible to perinatal infections. In all spontaneous or induced parturitions in horses the adaptive ability of the newborn foal depends on an interaction between its maturity and the effects of the birth process and environment. Fetal maturity is the major prerequisite for successful induced parturition and the three essential criteria are a gestational length of more than 320 days, substantial mammary development, and the presence of colostrum in the mammary gland (35). Head lifting, sternal recumbency, and evidence of suck reflex occurs within 5 minutes of spontaneous full term deliveries. The foal can stand within 1 hour and suck the mare within 2 hours (36). The clinical and laboratory values which reflect normal adaptive responses of newborn foals have been determined (37–41).

The behavior and viability of the premature foal after induced parturition have been described (42). The overall survival rate of foals delivered from induced parturition before 320 days of gestation was 5% (42). Four patterns of neonatal adaptation were observed on the basis of righting, sucking and standing ability. If the suck reflex was weak or absent and the foals were unable to establish righting reflexes, the prognosis of survival was poor. Foals born before 300 days of gestation did not survive for more than 90 minutes; foals born closer to 320 days of gestation had a better chance of survival and exhibited behavioural patterns of adaptation.

The ionic concentrations of the mammary secretions of the mare may be useful in determining whether induction would be successful in terms of maturity of the newborn foal (43, 44). Calcium concentrations can be useful in predicting full term and also in the assessment of the chances of foal survival in prematurely induced parturition.

Piglets

The induction of parturition of gilts and sows on days 112, 113 or 114 of gestation is highly reliable and is an aid to management. Induction on day 110 may be associated with a slight increase in perinatal mortality.

Prematurity, immaturity and dysmaturity of foals

A large volume of literature has developed in the last 10 years on the subject of prematurity and dysmaturity in foals (52). Premature foals are those born before 320 days of gestation. They are characterized clinically by low birth weight, generalized muscle weakness, inability to stand, weak or no suck reflex, lack of righting ability, respiratory distress, short silky haircoat, pliant ears, soft lips, increased passive range of limb motion, and sloping pastern axis. Full term foals, born after 320 days of gestation, which exhibit signs of prematurity are described as immature. If there is evidence of placental dysfunction or intrauterine deprivation associated with signs of immaturity at full term, then the affected foal is described as dysmature.

An extensive collaborative investigation of equine prematurity is underway and includes topics such as the methodology (45), adrenocortical activity (46), insulin activity and carbohydrate metabolism (47), salt and water metabolism relative to the renin–angiotensin–aldosterone system (48), histology of the adrenal gland (49), and guidelines for clinical and laboratory assessment of foal maturity (50). Intracranial hemorrhage is a common occurrence in foals born before full term, not necessarily associated with the compression forces of parturition (51).

Details of the neurological examination of newborn foals have been described (53). In general, the behavior and response to neurological testing of apparently healthy newborn foals differ significantly from the adult horse. Foals respond to external stimulation with exaggerated movements although they sink into a relaxed state, a cataplectic response, when they are restrained. They assume a base wide stance and their head is more flexed than in the adult. The menace reflex is incomplete until 2 weeks of age even though within a few hours after birth they jerk their head away from movement.

In general, the foal's stride is short, rapid and dysmetric. In lateral recumbency, foals have increased extensor tone, hyperreflexive tendon reflexes, crossed extensor reflexes and recumbent extensor thrust reflexes in all four limbs.

These differences between the healthy newborn foal and the adult horse emphasize the importance of considering the neonate as a unique clinical entity rather than a small form of the adult (53).

REVIEW LITERATURE

Alexander, G., Barker, J. D. & Slee, J. (1986) Factors affecting the survival of newborn lambs. A seminar in the CEC programme of coordination of agricultural research held in Brussels, January 22–23, 1985. Commission of the European Communities, 1986.

MacDiarmid, S. C. (1983) Induction of parturition in cattle using corticosteroids: a review. Part 1. Reasons for induction, mechanisms of induction and preparations used. *Anim. Breed. Abst.*, *51*, 403–419.

MacDiarrmid, S. C. (1983) Induction of parturition in cattle using corticosteroids: a review. Part 2. Effects of induced calving on the calf and cow. *Anim. Breed. Abst.*, *51*, 499–508.

REFERENCES

(1) Haughey, K. G. (1973) *Aust. vet. J.*, *49*, 149
(2) Haughey, K. G. & Jones, R. T. (1976) *Vet. Rec.*, *98*, 518.
(3) Haughey, K. G. (1975) *Aust. vet. J.*, *51*, 22.
(4) Dufty, J. & Sloss, V. (1977) *Aust. vet J.*, *53*, 262.
(5) Haughey, K. G. (1980) *Aust. vet. J.*, *56*, 49.
(6) Shelley, H. J. & Neligan, G. A. (1966) *Br. med. Bull.*, *22*, 34.
(7) Holub, A. et al. (1957) *Nature, Lond.*, *180*, 858.
(8) Mount, L. E. (1963) *Nature, Lond.*, *199*, 1212.
(9) Eales, F. A. & Small, J. (1985) *Res. vet. Sci.*, *39*, 212.
(10) Alexander, G. (1962) *Aust. J. agric. Res.*, *13*, 82, 100, 122, 144.
(11) Rossdale, P. D. et al. (1979) *J. Reprod. Fertil.*, Suppl. 27, 593–599.
(12) Rossdale, P. D. (1968) *Br. vet. J.*, *124*, 18.
(13) Eales, F. A. et al. (1984) *Vet. Rec.*, *114*, 469.
(14) Alexander, G. et al. (1972) *Biol. Neonatol.*, *20*, 1 & 9.
(15) Wigglesworth, J. S. (1966) *Br. med. Bull.*, *22*, 13.
(16) Slee, J. et al. (1980) *Res. vet. Sci.*, *28*, 275.
(17) Dalton, R. G. (1967) *Br. vet. J.*, *123*, 237.
(18) Edwards, A. V. (1964) *J. Physiol., Lond*, *171*, 468.
(19) Roy, J. H. B. & Ternouth, J. H. (1972) *Proc. Nutr. Soc.*, *31*, 53.
(20) Toofanian, F. et al. (1974) *Res. vet. Sci.*, *16*, 382.
(21) Olson, D. et al. (1980) *Can. J. comp. Med.*, *44*, 11 & 19.
(22) Cleek, J. L. et al. (1979) *J. Am. vet. med. Assoc.*, *174*, 373.
(23) Roberts, M. C. et al. (1974) *Res. vet. Sci.*, *17*, 42.
(24) Hoerlein, A. B. & Jones, D. L. (1977) *J. Am. vet. med. Assoc.*, *170*, 325.
(25) Olson, D. P. et al. (1981) *Am. J. vet. Res.*, *42*, 758 & 876.
(26) Rossdale, P. D. (1979) *Vet Clin. N. Am., large Anim. Pract.*, *1*(1), 205.
(27) Palmer, A. C. et al. (1984) *Equ. vet. J.*, *16*, 383.
(28) McCutcheon, S. N. et al. (1983) *NZ J. agric. Res.*, *26*, 169, 175.
(29) Olson, D. P. et al. (1983) *Am. J. vet. Res.*, *44*, 564, 572, 577, 969.
(30) Mellar, D. J. (1983) *Br. vet. J.*, *139*, 307.
(31) Mellor, D. J. & Murray, L. (1982) *Res. vet. Sci.*, *32*, 177, 377.
(32) Mellor, D. J. & Murray L. (1985) *Res. vet. Sci.*, *39*, 230, 235.
(33) MacDiarmid, S. C. (1983) *Anim. Breed. Abst.*, *51*, 403, 499.
(34) Bailey, L. F. et al. (1973) *Aust. vet. J.*, *49*, 567.
(35) Jeffcott, L. B. & Rossdale, P. D. (1977) *Equ. vet. J.*, *9*, 208.
(36) Rossdale, P. D. (1967) *Br. vet. J.*, *123*, 470, 521.
(37) Rossdale, P. D. (1968) *Br. vet. J.*, *124*, 18.
(38) Rossdale, P. D. (1968) *Biol. Neonatol.*, *13*, 18.
(39) Rossdale, P. D. (1969) *Br. vet. J.*, *125*, 157.
(40) Rose, R. J. et al. (1982) *J. Reprod. Fertil.* (Suppl), *32*, 537.
(41) Jeffcott, L. B. et al. (1982) *J. Reprod. Fertil.* (Suppl).
(42) Leadon, D. P. et al. (1986) *Am. J. vet. Res.*, *47*, 1870.
(43) Ousey, J. C. et al. (1984) *Equ. vet. J.*, *16*, 259.
(44) Leadon, D. P. et al. (1984) *Equ. vet. J.*, *16*, 256.
(45) Rossdale, P. D. et al. (1984) *Equ. vet. J.*, *16*, 275.
(46) Silver, M. et al. (1984) *Equ. vet. J.*, *16*, 278.
(47) Fowden, A. L. et al. (1984) *Equ. vet. J.*, *16*, 286.
(48) Pipkin, F. B. et al. (1984) *Equ. vet. J.*, *16*, 292.
(49) Webb, P. D. et al. (1984) *Equ. vet. J.*, *16*, 297.
(50) Rossdale, P. D. (1984) *Equ. vet. J.*, *16*, 300.
(51) Palmer, A. C. et al. (1984) *Equ. vet. J.*, *16*, 383.
(52) Vaala, W. E. (1986) *Comp. cont. Educ. Pract. Vet.*, *8*, S211.
(53) Adams, R. & Mayhew, I. G. (1984) *Equ. vet. J.*, *16*, 306.
(54) Weaver, B. M. Q. & Angell-James, J. (1986) *Vet. Rec.*, *119*, 86.

NEONATAL INFECTION

Although there are specific infectious pathogens which commonly cause disease in the neonate it is evident that some infectious agents which are normally considered as non-pathogens can also cause disease if the immunological status of the animal is not at an optimum level, so that attention is currently being devoted to both the virulence of the pathogen and the resistance of the host.

Etiology

In domestic farm animals the common neonatal infections encountered are as follows.

Cattle

Bacteremia or septicemia which are caused by *Escherichia coli*, *Listeria monocytogenes*, *Pasteurella* spp., streptococci, or *Salmonella* spp.; enteritis caused by enterotoxigenic *E. coli*, *Salmonella* spp., rotavirus and coronavirus, *Cryptosporidia* spp. and *Clostridium perfringens* types A, B and C; respiratory tract disease caused by the virus of infectious bovine rhinotracheitis; persistent viremia with the bovine virus diarrhea virus, and leukosis caused by the virus of bovine viral leukosis.

Pigs
Septicemia with localization in joints, endocardium and meninges is caused by *Streptococcus suis* type 1, *Strep. equisimilis*, *Strep. zooepidemicus*; bacteremia, septicemia and enteritis is caused by *E. coli*; transmissible gastroenteritis, swine pox, and vomiting and wasting disease are caused by viruses; enteritis is caused by *Cl. perfringens* rotavirus and *Coccidia* spp.; arthritis and septicemia are caused by *E. insidiosa*; and septicemia by *L. monocytogenes*.

Horses
Septicemia with localization, particularly in joints, is caused by *E. coli*, *Actinobacillus equuli*, *S. abortivoequina*, *Strep. pyogenes equi* and *S. typhimurium*; septicemia with localization particularly in lungs is caused by *Corynebacterium equi*; enteritis by *Cl. perfringens* and rotavirus; and septicemia by *L. monocytogenes*.

Sheep
Bactermia with localization in joints is caused by streptococci, micrococci and *E. insidiosa*; gas gangrene of the navel is caused by *Cl. septicum* and *Cl. oedematiens*; lamb dysentery is caused by *Cl. perfringens* type B; and septicemia by *E. coli* and *L. monocytogenes*.

The following agents are recorded as causing neonatal infections, but are not considered to be of general importance:

Cattle *Pseudomonas aeruginosa*, *Strep. pyogenes*, *Strep. faecalis*, *Strep. zooepidemicus*, *Pneumococcus* sp.; enteritis due to *Providencia stuarte*, *Chlamydia* sp., *Actinobacillus equuli*.

Sheep *Staphylococcus aureus* (tick pyemia); enteritis due to *Escherichia coli*, rotavirus; pneumonia due to *Salmonella abortusovis*.

All species
Non-specific infections are caused by pyogenic organisms, including *Corynebacterium pyogenes* and *Sphaerophorus necrophorus*; *Streptococcus faecalis* and *Strep. zooepidemicus* and *Micrococcus* spp. and *Pasteurella* spp. occur in all species.

Epidemiology

Portal of infection
Considerable interest centers on the question of whether some infections of the newborn occur before or after birth and in many instances this has not been determined. The point is of particular importance in foals where infections due to *Actinobacillus equuli*, *Escherichia coli*, *Salmonella abortivoequina* and *Streptococcus pyogenes equi* cause heavy mortality. If the disease is intrauterine in origin it may influence the control measures to be used. If it is intrauterine the infection must gain entrance via the placenta, and probably by means of a placentitis due to a blood-borne infection or an existing endometritis. In the latter case disinfection of the uterus before mating becomes an important hygienic precaution and disinfection of the environment may have little effect on the incidence of the disease. If the disease is postnatal the portal of entry of the infection may be through the navel or by ingestion. Contamination of the environment can occur from soiling of the udder or bedding by uterine discharges from the dam, or from previous parturitions, or from discharges from other affected newborn animals. The rapidity with which signs appear and death occurs is not a satisfactory criterion on which to judge whether an infection has occurred before or after birth, as the incubation period in a virulent infection in a newborn animal may be less than 24 hours. If the causative agent can be detected in the uterine exudate of the dam and in the fetus at birth and if signs are observed at birth the infection can be classed as intrauterine. The presence of lesions in the fetus at birth, as in leptospiral abortion in pigs and *Act. equuli* infections in foals, is additional evidence that the infection gained entrance during intrauterine life. Septicemia in foals due to *Act. equuli* and *E. coli* can arise from infection *in utero* and sporadic cases of tuberculosis occur in newborn animals, but by far the greatest proportion of neonatal infections occur after birth. Intrauterine infections are more commonly associated with death of the dam or the fetus or with abortion. Infection of the bovine fetus between 45 and 125 days of gestation with the bovine virus diarrhea virus can result in persistent viremia, immunotolerance and birth of a clinically normal calf which may develop fetal mucosal disease at 6–8 months of age or older (118).

Bacteria and viruses are frequently found in the fetus in domestic animals and in man. Whether or not a placentitis must develop first is undecided and experimental work on the permeability of the placenta to virus particles is equivocal. It is possible that the restricted period during which the fetus is susceptible to infection is due to the need of the infection to gain entrance to the exposed trophoblast before closure of the amniotic folds, infection coming from the uterine contents via an existing metritis or blood-borne infection.

Resistance to infection
All newborn farm animals are more susceptible to infection than their adult counterparts, for some important reasons. The calf, lamb, piglet and foal are born without significant levels of gammaglobulin. They are born agammaglobulinemic and possess almost no resistance to infection until after they have ingested colostrum and absorbed sufficient quantities of lactoglobulins from the colostrum. The immune system of the newborn animal is also less mature than its adult counterpart and does not respond as effectively to antigen as does the older animal. In colostrum-fed animals, however, part of the inefficiency of the newborn to produce humoral antibody following injection of antigen is the interference by circulating colostral antibody. Colostrum-deprived calves respond actively to injected antigens (3) and are thus immunologically competent at birth. Immune competence

begins during fetal life and the age of gestation at which this occurs varies according to the nature of the antigen. The bovine fetus will produce antibody to some viruses beginning at 90–120 days (4) and by the third trimester of gestation it will respond to a variety of viruses and bacteria. The lamb will respond to some antigens beginning as early as 41 days and not until 120 days for others (5). The piglet at 55 days (6) and the fetal foal also responds to injected antigens (7). Normal foals are immunocompetent at birth and, before nursing, have detectable quantities of IgM, but little or no IgG. Functional T lymphocytes are present in the fetus by 100 days' gestational age and functional lymphocytes are present by 200 days. Immunoglobulins IgM and IgG are present in equine fetuses prior to 200 days' gestational age (7). The presence of high levels of antibody in the precolostral serum of newborn animals suggests that an *in utero* infection was present which is useful for diagnostic purposes. The detection of immunoglobulins and specific antibodies in aborted fetuses is a useful aid in the diagnosis of abortion in cattle (66–68).

Other factors may contribute to the lowered resistance to infection of the newborn. The fetal lamb produces large quantities of corticosteroid beginning 8–10 days before birth and there is evidence that a similar situation occurs in fetal calves (8). The high levels of corticosteroid result in a lymphopenia and a decrease in the phagocytic defences of the newborn which may affect the cellular immune mechanism and thereby decrease perinatal resistance (8). The concentration of cortisol and cortisone is high in calves at birth and declines until 15 days of age (8). There may also be a lowered level of neutrophil function in calves compared to adults (63). The relationship between the levels of serum colostral immunoglobulins achieved in newborn farm animals and the subsequent incidence of disease has been a major epidemiological activity for many years. The morbidity and mortality rates due to infectious diseases of the intestines and respiratory tract are significantly higher in calves with low levels of serum immunoglobulins than in calves with adequate levels (91–93).

There are now four recognizable immunological deficiency states in newborn foals. These include *combined immunodeficiency* (CID), which is inherited as an autosomal recessive trait in Arabian horses. There is marked lymphopenia, absence of lymphocytes in all lymphoid organs, hypogammaglobulinaemia or agammaglobulinemia and death at 2–20 weeks of age from a variety of infections, of which pneumonia is the most common. *Primary agammaglobulinemia* is described in a thoroughbred foal. In the horse this is characterized by animals which live much longer and are usually affected with a chronic infection intractable to treatment. Serum concentrations of IgG are low and IgM may not be detectable. There is failure of antibody production following injection of foreign antigens, but tests for cell-mediated immunity may be positive. Histologic examination of lymphoid tissues reveals absence of germinal centers and plasma cells (69). There is complete absence of B lymphocytes and immunoglobulins but normal T lymphocyte counts. *Hypogammaglobulinemia* following inadequate transfer of colostral immunoglobulin from dam to foal is the most common form of immunodeficiency and is associated with a high incidence of infection. *Selective immunoglobulin M (IgM) deficiency* associated with infections at 4–8 months of age is also recognized in foals (9).

Transfer of passive immunity

The transplacental transfer of immunoglobulins does not normally occur in calves, lambs, piglets or foals. There may be a rare possible exception in the mare which results in a foal with isoimmune hemolytic anemia. Any antibodies present in a newborn animal which has not ingested colostrum must have been produced by the immune system of the fetus.

After ingestion of colostrum by the newborn, colostral immunoglobulins are absorbed by the small intestine by a process of micropinocytosis, into the columnar cells of the epithelium. In the newborn calf this is a very rapid process and immunoglobulin can be detected in the thoracic duct lymph within 80–120 minutes of its being introduced into the duodenum. The period of absorption varies between species and the mechanism by which absorption ceases is not well understood. In the intestine of the fetal lamb exposed to large quantities of immunoglobulin, immediately after birth, the intestinal epithelium (fetal enterocytes) is gradually replaced by a digestive type of cell, and the layer of cells responsible for absorption of colostral antibodies progressively disappears from the villi, resulting in closure (95). The region of maximum absorption is in the lower small intestine (99). In calves, absorption continues for up to 24 hours but maximum absorption occurs within the first 6–8 hours after birth.

The details on colostral immunoglobulin transfer in calves are available (10). Termination or closure of intestinal permeability to colostral immunoglobulins in the calf occurs spontaneously with age at a progressively increased rate 12 hours after birth. The rate of absorption depends on the amount of colostrum fed and how soon after birth ingestion occurs. Increasing the amount fed up to 2 liters for the average-sized Holstein calf as early as possible after birth results in the highest levels of serum immunoglobulins in calves. Absorption is greater in calves which suck their dams than in calves which are bottle-fed.

The influence of prepartum stressors on the dam and on the calf, and the use of exogenous hormones to induce parturition on the absorption of colostral immunoglobulins has been examined. Shortacting corticosteroids used to induce parturition do not affect absorption but longacting corticosteroids do. This has been referred to earlier in the section on induced parturition (p. 106). The efficiency of absorption may be decreased in premature calves which are born following induced parturition (101). There are no significant effects of dystocia on the calf's ability to absorb colostral immunoglobulins. Calves affected with acidosis and hypoxemia from a different birth may fail to absorb adequate quantities of colostral immunoglobulins. However, high ambient temperature is a strong depressant of absorption and the provision of shade will obviate the problem (12).

In goats absorption continues for up to 4 days, and by way of comparison up to 12 days in dogs. In lambs it is considerably diminished by 15 hours but continues for up to 24–48 hours, in pigs absorption is markedly reduced between 12 and 27 hours and in foals (11) it terminates at about 24 hours. However, absorption of colostral immunoglobulins in newborn piglets may occur for up to 3 days (70). The period during which absorption of antibodies occurs through the intestinal epithelium is variable and the important factors governing it are the time at which colostrum is first taken and the amount of globulins taken. If colostrum is withheld, the capacity to absorb globulins is prolonged; the larger the amount taken, the shorter the absorptive period. This may have importance in closing the gut epithelium against pathogens too, so that early sustained ingestion of colostrum may be necessary for best results.

Absorption of colostral immunoglobulins is not specific; other proteins such as bovine serum globulins, serum albumin and even higher molecular weight polysaccharides are absorbed during the absorptive period. In the calf, there is evidence for differential absorption between individual classes of immunoglobulins and their duration of absorption. Approximately 90% of IgG is absorbed whereas only 59% of IgM and 48% of IgA are absorbed. IgG is absorbed for 27 hours after birth, IgA for 22 hours and IgM for 16 hours. But it must be re-emphasized that maximum absorption in the calf occurs during the first 6–8 hours after birth. In mare's colostrum IgG, IgM and IgA are all present and absorbed by the foal to produce similar concentrations in its serum to those in the mare (14) and the piglet/sow pair (15) within 24 hours of sucking. Maximum levels of serum immunoglobulins are usually achieved at 24 hours after birth in the calf.

The ultimate level of serum immunoglobulins achieved in the newborn will depend on the total mass of immunoglobulin absorbed, which is a function of the concentration of immunoglobulins in the colostrum and the total amount of colostrum ingested during the period of maximum absorption. There is a linear relationship between the concentration of immunoglobulin in the colostrum and the absorption in the immunoglobulins by the calf during the period of maximum absorption (100). If the concentration of immunoglobulins is low inadequate absorption occurs regardless of the volume fed. In cattle, the total amount of colostrum available and the concentration of colostral immunoglobulins increases with successive parturitions (16). Thus calves born to heifers may not obtain as much immunoglobulin as calves from mature cows. The concentration of immunoglobulins in colostrum is highest immediately at parturition in cattle and drops precipitously between 2 and 12 hours following parturition (17) which serves to emphasize the importance of early ingestion by the newborn.

There are seasonal and geographical variations in passive transfer of immunoglobulins in calves. In temperate climates the mean monthly serum IgG_1 concentrations are lowest in the winter, and increase during the spring and early summer to reach their peak in September after which they decrease (96, 97). In subtropical climates, peak levels occur in the winter months of February and March, while low levels are associated with elevated temperatures during the summer months of July and August (98).

Large single lambs may ingest much more colostrum than individual twins or triplets, but there is no significant difference in the serum immunoglobulins achieved. The amount of colostrum produced is also related to the demand by the lambs (72). Bovine colostrum can be used when necessary for the rearing of lambs (71). However, severe hemolytic anemia may occur because several bovine colostral proteins are present which after absorption by the lambs can produce immune complexes with the lambs' plasma proteins. These complexes attach to the surface of the red blood cells which are then sequestered by the reticuloendothelial system resulting in severe anemia (114). Treatment of the anemia consists of a blood transfusion. Bovine colostrum can be tested for 'antisheep' factors by a gel precipitation test on colostral whey (114).

In the sow, while the total concentration of colostral immunoglobulin falls in the first few days after parturition, mainly due to a decrease in the concentration of IgG, the concentration of IgA falls only slightly during the same period and it becomes a major immunoglobulin of sows' milk. IgA is synthesized by the mammary gland of the sow throughout lactation and serves as an important defense mechanism against enteric disease in the nursing piglet (15, 18). In the piglet, IgA is the most important mucosal defense mechanism whereas in the calf there is little IgA and its role is taken over by colostral and milk IgG, derived from serum and antigen stimulus probably from the intestines (18). Only low concentrations of IgA are secreted into the milk of the ruminant compared to monogastric species, and it is unlikely that milk immunoglobulins contribute much to alimentary tract defense after the initial phase of colostrum absorption (19). There are several factors which influence the availability of colostrum to piglets which may be unique because of modern pig production (115). Most of the colostrum received by newborn piglets is obtained in discrete injections rather than in a continuous manner. This suggests that piglets should lie close to the sow to take advantage of synchronized, episodic release of colostrum at irregular intervals. There is a large variation in colostrum supply from teat to teat which may explain variable health and performance. During farrowing, a strong coordinated sucking stimulus by the piglet is important for maximum release of colostrum and this requires that the ambient temperature and other environmental factors be conducive to optimum vigor of the piglets.

The practice of premilking cows beginning several days before calving in an attempt to reduce the effects of udder edema results in a marked drop in the concentration of immunoglobulin available in the colostrum immediately after parturition. Most of the immunoglobulins are concentrated in the colostrum about 3–9 days before parturition. Premilking can reduce the levels of immunoglobulins in the postpartum secretion from a normal of 68 g/l to 1·6 g/l. Therefore, the secretion produced after calving by cows that have been premilked is of less value to the calf than the same volume of normal colostrum (90). This can result in an increase in the morbidity and mortality in calves dependent on such colostrum.

The relative concentrations of the immunoglobulins

in serum, colostrum and milk of cattle and swine are summarized in Table 8. Most of the IgA (60%) is produced in the mammary gland, all of the IgG comes from the dam's serum and IgM originates from both sources but primarily from the dam's serum. By contrast the immunoglobulins in milk are produced primarily in the mammary gland (18).

Colostral immunoglobulins present in the intestine can prevent enteric disease. Circulating immunoglobulins are necessary for protection against septicemia; they do not prevent diarrhea, presumably because they are not able to reach the lumen of the intestine in protective amounts. Colostrum fed to the calf soon after birth provides protection from colisepticemia, but does not prevent the diarrhea of enteric colibacillosis. Colostrum provides serum immunoglobulins which prevent or minimize invasion of bacteria, but colostrum may also saturate the macromolecular transport system of the intestine and provide mechanical protection against invading organisms (73). However, high serum levels of IgG and IgA reduce the severity of diarrhea by preventing massive outpouring of fluids and electrolytes into the intestinal lumen (21). IgM may be the most important immunoglobulin for the prevention of diarrhea in calves (21). A serum IgM-rich fraction can be used experimentally, orally and intravenously as an excellent substitute for colostrum in calves (22).

Some absorbed colostral proteins are lost from the circulation through the kidney (23). In the calf and lamb there is a period of increased renal permeability to protein which is concurrent with the period of enhanced intestinal permeability. Only the low molecular weight proteins are excreted, the high molecular weight IgG and IgA globulins are not excreted by the kidney (25).

Agammaglobulinemia as described in man is not common in animals. However, hypogammaglobulinemia does occur commonly in newborn farm animals especially calves and lambs due to the reasons already discussed. Up to 25% of hand-fed dairy calves and single-suckled beef calves may be hypogammaglobulinemic (26). These animals are much more susceptible to infectious neonatal disease and the standard of hygiene and management must be correspondingly better to avoid losses. A similar situation exists in lambs raised naturally or artificially (28).

There is a marked variation in the serum levels of colostral immunoglobulins achieved in newborn farm animals. There are many important factors which influence the level of serum immunoglobulins achieved by the newborn and they are as follows:

1. Insufficient ingestion of immunoglobulins due to:
(a) Insufficient amount of colostrum produced by dam for many different reasons. Poor husbandry has a marked depressant effect on colostrum yield of beef cows with the result that calves born to such cows will receive insufficient colostrum. However, diets low in either protein or metabolizable energy during the second half of gestation appear to have no major effect on immunoglobulin (29). The yield of colostrum and colostral immunoglobulins in beef cows can vary widely (112). In one study, the volume of colostrum produced by beef cows at the first milking ranged from 700 ml to 7730 ml. Differences in yield may be due to breeds and nutritional status.
(b) Low concentration of immunoglobulin in the colostrum (100). Some foals are deficient in IgG because of low colostral IgG content (30). There can be a 10-fold difference in the concentration of IgG in colostrum from sows depending on the location of the farm, the parity of the sow, the nature of the diet, the number of sows raised on the farm and the type of farming (76). There may also be a wide variation in the concentration of colostral IgA, and the possible factors which influence concentration include breed of pig and parity of sow (77).
(c) Insufficient amount of colostrum ingested by the newborn due to:
(i) Poor mothering behavior which may prevent the newborn from sucking.
(ii) Poor udder and/or teat conformation so the newborn cannot suck normally.
(iii) The newborn may be weak, traumatized or unable to suck for other reasons.
(iv) Failure to allow newborn animals to ingest colostrum which may occur under some management systems.

2. Insufficient absorption of immunoglobulins from colostrum may be caused by:
(a) Delayed ingestion of colostrum. Calves must ingest sufficient colostrum before 6 hours after birth (88); every effort must be made to assist early sucking (94).
(b) Interference with the efficiency of absorption of immunoglobulins from colostrum may occur but this has not been well documented under practical conditions. Failure of transfer of colostral immunoglobulin IgG has occurred in up to 24% of

Table 8. Concentrations and relative percentage of immunoglobulins in serum and mammary secretions of cattle and swine (65)

		Concentration (mg/ml)			*Total immunoglobulins* (%)		
Animal	*Immunoglobulin*	*Serum*	*Colostrum*	*Milk*	*Serum*	*Colostrum*	*Milk*
Cow	IgG_1	11·0	47·6	0·59	50	81	73
	IgG_2	7·9	2·9	0·02	36	5	2·5
	IgM	2·6	4·2	0·05	12	7	6·5
	IgA	0·5	3·9	0·14	2	7	18
Sow	IgG	21·5	58·7	3·0	89	80	29
	IgM	1·1	3·2	0·3	4	6	1
	IgA	1·8	10·7	7·7	7	14	70

thoroughbred foals, in which subsequently there was a high prevalence of infection (30). The medical induction of parturition with short-acting corticosteroids in cattle does not interfere with the efficiency of absorption of immunoglobulins in calves (17). The influence of endogenous cortisol on the absorption of colostral immunoglobulins in newborn calves is uncertain. Calves which require assistance at parturition which lasts for more than 4 hours may have lower levels of serum glucucorticoids at birth than naturally born calves which may decrease the absorption of colostral immunoglobulins (78).

The presence of large numbers of intestinal bacteria may also interfere with the absorption of colostral immunoglobulins which emphasizes the need for the ingestion of colostrum as soon after birth as possible (79).

The movement of animals, either the dam just before parturition or the newborn animal during the first few days of life, is a special hazard. The dam may not have been exposed to, and thus have no circulating antibodies against, pathogens present in the new environment. The newborn animal may be in the same position with regard to both deficiency of antibodies and exposure to new infections.

Decline of passive immunity

Passive antibody levels fall quickly after birth and have usually disappeared by 6 months of age. In the foal, they have fallen to less than 50% of peak level by one month of age (11), and to a minimum level at 30–60 days. This is the point at which naturally immunodeficient foals are highly susceptible to fatal infection. In calves, the level of IgG declines slowly and reaches minimum values by 60 days (31), in contrast to IgM and IgA which decline more rapidly and reach minimum values by approximately 21 days of age (26, 32). The half-lives for IgG, IgM, and IgA are approximately 20, 4 and 2 days respectively (33). Immunological competence is present at birth but endogenous antibody production does not usually reach protective levels until 1 month, and maximum levels until 2–3 months of age (26). The endogenous production of intestinal IgA in the piglet begins at about 2 weeks of age, and does not reach significant levels until 5 weeks of age (15, 34).

Occasional foals experience a transitory hypogammaglobulinemia and do not develop autogenous antibodies until much later than normal. They are, as expected, more subject to infection than normal (35).

Other aspects of colostrum

The status of the newborn animal with regard to minerals and vitamins is dependent on the status of the dam. But in the case of vitamin A it is also dependent on placental permeability. Vitamin A in the alcohol form, as it occurs in the blood of the cow from the breakdown of carotene, does not pass the placental barrier. But in the form in which it occurs in cod liver oil it is transmissible. Thus a high intake of green feed does not increase the vitamin A content of the fetus, but markedly increases the content in colostrum.

Another function affected by colostrum intake is the degree of leukocytosis in the blood. Colostrum-deprived calves have a much lower total leukocyte count than those fed colostrum, and phagocytosis is much more active in colostrum-fed calves (36).

Isolation of the newborn animal from its dam may be necessary, for example, in foals produced by incompatible matings. In such cases it is necessary to provide an alternative source of antibodies and vitamin A, and prophylactic broad-spectrum antibodies.

Pathogenesis

The usual pattern of development in neonatal infections is a septicemia, with a severe systemic reaction, or a bacteremia with few or no systemic signs, followed by localization in various organs. If the portal of entry is the navel, local inflammation occurs—'navel ill'—which can be easily overlooked if clinical examination is not thorough. From the local infection at the navel, extension may occur to the liver or via the urachus to the bladder and result in chronic ill-health, or systemically to produce septicemia. In blood-borne infections, localization is most common in the joints producing a suppurative or non-suppurative arthritis. Less commonly there is localization in the eye to produce a panophthalmitis, in the heart valves to cause valvular endocarditis, or in the meninges to produce a meningitis. Most of these secondary lesions take some time to develop and signs usually appear at 1–2 weeks of age. Bacterial meningoventriculitis in newborn ungulates is preceded by a bacteremia followed by a fibrinopurulent inflammation of the leptomeninges, choroid plexuses and ventricle walls but does not affect the neuraxial parenchyma. It is proposed that the bacteria are transported monocytes which do not normally invade the neuraxial parenchyma (62).

Dehydration and electrolyte imbalance can occur very quickly in newborn animals whether diarrhea and vomiting are present or not. This is probably due to deprivation of fluid intake as much as to loss of fluid.

Clinical findings

The clinical findings depend on the rapidity of the spread of the infection. When it is slow spreading there is omphalophlebitis, fever, depression, anorexia, leukocytosis and signs referable to localization. These include endocarditis with a heart murmur; panophthalmitis with pus in the anterior chamber of the eye; meningitis with rigidity, pain and convulsion; and polyarthritis with lameness, and swollen joints which may rupture and discharge pus. When the spread is more rapid there are clinical signs of septicemia including fever, prostration, coma, petechiation of mucosae, dehydration, acidosis and rapid death.

The clinical and clinicopathological characteristics of the septicemic foal have been studied based on the clinical records of 38 septicemic foals admitted to a referral clinic (116). The survival rate of septicemic foals was only 26% which was much lower than the admissions. Blood cultures were valuable in diagnosis and treatment of septicemia which was due primarily to Gram-negative bacteria. There was evidence of failure of passive transfer of immunity in most septicemic foals—the range was 4·0–8·6 g/l, while the range in normal foals was 8·44–13·00 g/l. The major clinical findings included lethargy, unwillingness to suck, inability to stand without assistance but conscious, unawareness of environment and thrashing or convulsing, diarrhea, respiratory distress, joint distention, CNS abnormalities, uveitis and colic. Conditions in the mare prepartum which resulted in weak or diseased foals included bacterial placentitis, vaginal discharge, and premature lactation. Fever was not a consistent finding. Neutropenia and the presence of band neutrophils and toxic changes in the neutrophil population was a useful diagnostic aid. Hypoglycemia, metabolic acidosis and hypoxemia were also common findings.

Clinical pathology

The laboratory evaluation of the newborn animal is the same as for the adult but recently there has been considerable emphasis on the assessment of susceptibility of the host to infectious disease. The measurement of serum immunoglobulins in the newborn, in the intestinal fluids and mammary secretions and the further separation of these into immunoglobulin subclasses has expanded the understanding of susceptibility of the newborn to infectious disease. The quantitative determination of the levels of specific antibodies is now an important part of the investigation of neonatal disease, particularly when vaccines are being evaluated.

Serum

Precolostral blood should be collected from stillbirths and from neonates before they ingest colostrum if *in utero* infection is suspected.

Postcolostral blood is collected from neonates for an assessment of the level of serum immunoglobulins obtained from colostrum. The measurement of serum immunoglobulin is most reliable when done between 24–48 hours after birth, the time which will most accurately assess the amount of passive transfer which has occurred. Samples taken several days after birth may give spurious results because of the degradation of some of the immunoglobulins. This has been used most frequently in calves to determine whether or not the calf ingested sufficient colostrum early enough. This could be used as a monitoring technique where large numbers of calves are being purchased for rearing in one place or to investigate the causes of a high rate of morbidity and mortality in a newborn population. In individual calves the determination of the level of serum immunoglobulins may be useful in assessing the prognosis and/or in deciding whether gammaglobulin therapy is indicated. However, it must be emphasized that immunoglobulins are much more prophylactic than curative. Theoretically, it is attractive to determine the serum level of gammaglobulin in a 4-day-old calf and calculate the approximate deficit and attempt to replace the deficit using a concentrated source of gammaglobulin. However, very large quantities of gammaglobulin are necessary as is explained below.

The methods available for the evaluation of the level of serum immunoglobulins include the following:

1. *Indirect*
   (a) Refractometer which measures total serum proteins
   (b) Turbidity, precipitation and coagulation tests (zinc sulfate precipitation and the glutaraldehyde coagulation tests)
   (c) Latex agglutination tests in foals (107) and in calves (108).
2. *Direct*
   (a) Paper electrophoresis to determine serum protein profile
   (b) Radial diffusion test to quantitate immunoglobulin subclasses
   (c) Enzyme-linked immunosorbent assay (ELISA) for measurement of IgG concentration in porcine plasma and colostrum (111).

The refractometer is the most practical instrument for the field estimation of serum immunoglobulins in calves and lambs (37). There is a reliable correlation between the refractometer reading and the total immunoglobulin concentration (IgG and IgM), as measured by single radial diffusion test, and between the reading and the zinc sulfate test value which is a good estimation of serum immunoglobulins (38, 39). This relationship was examined and compared in home-raised dairy calves, market calves and single-suckled calves and is set out in Table 9.

The interpretation and implications of the results shown in Table 9 are as follows. The refractometer method is a useful and quick field method for estimating the level of immunoglobulins in calves before they become ill and dehydrated. Calves with levels of immunoglobulins similar to those of the home-reared dairy calves and purchased market calves have not ingested and absorbed sufficient immunoglobulins and are hypogammaglobulinemic. They are highly susceptible to infectious diarrhea and pneumonia and good management and hygiene are required to minimize morbidity and mortality. Sick calves from this group may require antibiotics and intensive supportive therapy. The immunoglobulin deficit in these two groups of calves cannot be corrected easily or economically. The deficit compared to the single-suckled calves is about 10 g/liter of serum and for a 45 kg calf

Table 9. Serum immunoglobulin levels (mean ± SE) in calves, assessed by three different methods (38)

	24 Dairy calves (home-reared)	*32 Market calves (purchased)*	*24 Single-suckled calves*
Refractometer (g/dl)	4·80 ± 0·16	5·08 ± 0·09	6·06 ± 0·23
Zinc sulfate turbidity test (units)	13·40 ± 2·20	21·47 ± 1·95	35·57 ± 3·17
Single radial diffusion test			
IgG (mg/ml)	6·25 ± 0·80	7·26 ± 0·65	14·20 ± 1·25
IgM (mg/ml)	0·97 ± 0·13	0·75 ± 0·08	1·98 ± 0·22
Total IgG and IgM (g/dl)	0·72	0·80	1·61

with a plasma volume of 78 ml/kg body weight (40) the total deficit is 35 g of gammaglobulin. This would be a minimum deficit because the gammaglobulin would be diffused more widely than merely in the circulating blood. To correct the above mathematical deficit would require approximately 2·5 litres of blood containing 1·5 g/dl of gammaglobulin. The administration of purified bovine gammaglobulin would be too expensive and no good evidence is available that the administration of even the necessary amounts would result in an increase in circulating gammaglobulins. A concentrated source of gammaglobulin from freeze-thawing of plasma and serum for the treatment of foals and calves deficient in gammaglobulin is described, but not yet adequately evaluated clinically (80).

The gammaglobulins achieved by the suckled calves are considered to be adequate and ideal for most management systems. These calves obviously received sufficient colostrum early enough.

The zinc sulfate turbidity test is also an excellent method for the rapid assessment of the immune globulin status of calves, lambs and foals before they become ill and dehydrated (41). The interpretation of the results are as follows:

ZST (units)	
0–5	Little or no absorption of immunoglobulins and no protection
6–15	Inadequate absorption and only minimal protection
16–20	Improved absorption and protection
above 20	Adequate absorption and good protection

The zinc sulfate turbidity test requires more time and facilities than the refractometer test, and hemolyzed blood samples will give artificially high readings (42). The major limitation of the above tests is that hemoconcentration in dehydrated animals will give artificially high readings.

The sodium sulfite precipitation test is also a rapid highly accurate field test to evaluate the immune status of neonatal calves (43). The glutaraldehyde coagulation test is also available for the detection of hypogammaglobulinemia in neonatal calves. It has practical application as a screening test in veal calf operations (83). Calves with low levels of gammaglobulin on entry to a vealer unit could be identified and managed separately or culled.

It must be emphasized that these tests are most valuable to assess the immunoglobulin status of animals before they become ill. It provides an excellent tool in epidemiological investigations to determine if newborn animals are receiving sufficient good-quality colostrum early enough.

For accurate measurements of the immunoglobulin status, the paper electrophoresis procedure or the single radial diffusion test are recommended.

The concentration of immunoglobulins in the colostrum of mares is highly correlated with the specific gravity of the colostrum which in turn is highly correlated with the serum immunoglobulin levels achieved in foals (81). The measurement of colostral immunoglobulin concentrations using a hydrometer is a rapid and easy method of identifying foals as a high risk for failure of passive transfer and to supplement these foals with colostrum of a higher Ig content. It is recommended that to prevent failure of passive transfer the colostral specific gravity be equal to or greater than 1·060 and the colostral IgG concentration be a minimum of 3000 mg/dl (81). The mean concentrations of IgG in colostrum of mares 3–28 days before foaling is greater than 1000 mg IgG/dl, while at parturition the mean concentrations may vary from 4000 to 9000 mg/dl. The concentrations will decrease markedly to 1000 mg/dl in 8–19 hours (106). In foals, the reliable tests for the determination of serum IgG include the zinc sulfate turbidity test, the single radial immunodiffusion test, and the latex agglutination test (82). If specific class or subclass immunoglobulin information is necessary, the single radial immunodiffusion test is the best available. The latex agglutination test is more accurate that the zinc sulfate turbidity test. Failure of passive transfer of immunoglobulin in foals can be detected by measuring serum IgG. Before foals suckle, they are hypogammaglobulinemic, with IgG usually low or absent or IgM present in low concentration. Levels of IgG below 200 mg/dl in postsuckle serum indicates failure of passive transfer; levels between 200 and 400 represent partial transfer failure, and levels over 400 represent transfer. Foals with adequate transfer commonly have IgG concentration of 800 mg/dl at 18–24 hours of age.

The incidence of failure of passive transfer in foals can be as high as 24%. The major mechanism by which failure of passive transfer occurs include failure of the foal to ingest an adequate volume of colostrum in the critical first 12 hours after parturition; loss of colostrum before parturition (premature lactation); inadequate Ig content of the colostrum; and insufficient Ig absorption by the intestinal epithelium (82). The induction of parturition in mares can affect passive transfer of immunity to foals (105).

The levels of immunoglobulins in colostrum can be estimated rapidly in the field using a hydrometer or a refractometer. Determination of the immunoglobulin concentration would permit selective feeding of colostrum containing an adequate amount of immunoglobulin. Also, colostrum from different cows could be pooled to obtain a mixture which would deliver the highest concentration of immunoglobulin per unit volume of colostrum fed. Excellent quality bovine colostrum would contain a whey immunoglobulin concentration of 80 mg/ml to ensure adequate passive transfer. Only colostrums that are within the excellent zone are recommended for precolostral neonates as soon after birth as possible to allow the successful transfer of immunity (84)

Certain enzymes are present in colostrum and are transferred to the newborn following ingestion of colostrum. Gamma glutamyl transferase occurs in both calves (109) and lambs (110).

Diagnosis

The principles of diagnosis of infectious disease in newborn animals are the same as for older animals. However, in outbreaks of suspected infectious disease in young animals there is usually a need for more diagnostic microbiology and pathology. Owners should be encouraged to submit all dead neonates as soon as possible for a meaningful necropsy examination. It is often difficult to identify the factors which may have contributed to an outbreak of disease in newborn calves, piglets or lambs.

and only detailed epidemiological investigation will reveal these.

Principles of treatment of infectious disease in newborn animals

The first principle is to obtain an etiological diagnosis if possible. Ideally a drug sensitivity of the causative bacteria should be obtained before treatment is given but this is not always possible. It may be necessary to choose an antibacterial based on the tentative diagnosis and previous experience with treatment of similar cases. Almost all of the antibacterials used in adult animals are used in neonates but the safe therapeutic doses for newborn farm animals are not known. The adult doses of antibacterials have been used with success in newborn animals but this practice should be evaluated. The drug metabolizing enzyme activities are generally lower in newborn mammals than in adults (44) because of the immaturity of the hepatic metabolism and renal excretion. Some characteristics of the neonatal period include greater absorption from the gastrointestinal tract, lower extent of plasma protein binding, increased apparent volume of distribution of drugs which distribute in extracellular fluid or body water, increased permeability of the blood–brain barrier and slower elimination of many drugs (44). The hepatic microsomal oxidative reactions and glucoronide conjugation are deficient metabolic pathways for a varying period of time, usually up to 6 weeks after birth or even longer in some species. Decreased metabolism can affect the duration of action of lipid-soluble drugs. Functional immaturity of the kidneys decreases the renal excretion of certain drugs and metabolites. Overall renal function appears to reach maturity within 2 weeks after birth in ruminants and pigs and up to 4 weeks in other species. Considerable physiological and biochemical development occurs during the first 5 days after birth and continues more slowly over the succeeding several weeks. The time it takes for any process to reach functional maturity depends on the particular process and varies with the species of animal (45). For example, in calves 3–7 days of age the half-life of chloramphenicol is 8·2 and 6·5 hours respectively which is substantially longer than the half-life of 4·2 hours in cows. In pigs, the half-life of chloramphenicol decreases from 6 hours in the newborn piglet to 2·3 hours 1 week after birth. At 5 weeks after birth, the half-life is similar to that in the adult pig, namely 1 hour.

Outbreaks of infectious disease are common in litters of piglets and groups of calves and lambs, and individual treatment is often necessary to maximize survival rate. There is usually no simple method of mass medicating the feed and water supply of sucking animals and each animal should be dosed individually as necessary. Supportive fluid therapy is usually necessary because of the delicate fluid and electrolyte balance of newborn animals and this has been described in detail under the discussion of body water and electrolyte disturbances and under the section on colibacillosis.

The provision of antibodies to sick and weak newborn animals through the use of blood transfusions or hyperimmune serum is often practiced, especially in newborn calves in which the immunoglobulin status is unknown. Whole blood given at the rate of 10–20 ml/kg body weight, preferably by the intravenous route, will often save a calf which appears to be in shock associated with neonatal diarrhea. The blood is usually followed by fluid therapy. Serum or plasma can also be given at half the dose rate. Blood should be taken from the oldest adult in the herd and from an animal not near parturition in which there is a drain of gammaglobulin into the mammary gland. Colostrum-deficient foals may be treated with equine plasma at doses of 20 ml/kg body weight given slowly intravenously (85). Blood may be collected, the RBC allowed to settle and the plasma removed and stored frozen. The donor blood should be prescreened serologically for lack of anti-RBC antibodies. Lyophilized hyperimmune equine serum as a source of antibodies may also be fed to foals within 4 hours after birth (86). In the special case of foals likely to develop isoimmunization hemolytic anemia, the dam's blood must not be used because of its high content of antibodies to which the foal is sensitized.

Good nursing care is often necessary and includes freedom from drafts, provision of heat lamps, and monitoring vital signs.

Principles of control and prevention of infectious diseases of newborn farm animals

The four principles are:

- Removal of the cause of the disease from the environment of the newborn
- Removal of the newborn from the infectious environment if necessary
- Increasing and maintaining the non-specific resistance of the newborn
- Increasing the specific resistance of the newborn through the use of vaccines

The application of each one of these principles will vary depending on the species, the spectrum of diseases which are common on that farm, the management system and success with any particular preventive method used previously.

Removal of the cause of the disease from the environment

The animal should be born in an environment which is clean, dry and conducive for the animal to get up after birth and suck the dam. Calving and lambing stalls or grounds, farrowing crates and foaling stalls should be prepared in advance for parturition. No conventional animal area can be sterilized but it can be made reasonably clean to minimize the infection rate before colostrum is ingested and during the first few weeks of life when the newborn animal is very susceptible to infectious disease.

The swabbing of the navel with tincture of iodine to prevent entry of infection is commonly practiced by some producers and seldom by others. In a heavily contaminated environment it is recommended, and ligation of umbilical vessels at the level of the abdomen using clean hands and clean cotton thread may be more effective. Plastic clamps are now available for this purpose. However, the efficiency of the disinfection of the umbilicus after birth is uncertain. It is often surprising how many cases of omphalophlebitis occur in calves in herds where swabbing with a solution of tincture of iodine is a routine practice. Severance of the umbilical cord too quickly during birth of thoroughbred foals has been suggested as a means by which foals are deprived of large quantities of blood, which may explain the pathogenesis of neonatal maladjustment syndrome. When attempting to remove the infection from the environment the problem of whether the infection derives from an intrauterine or extrauterine source must receive consideration. Intrauterine infection necessitates local uterine or systemic treatment of the dam to eliminate the infection from the uterus before conception occurs. Swabs of the uterine contents should be examined before and after treatment in suspected animals.

Removal of the newborn from the infectious environment
In some cases of high animal population density (e.g. a crowded dairy barn) and in the presence of known disease it may be necessary to transfer the newborn to a non-infectious environment temporarily or permanently. Thus dairy calves are often placed in individual pens inside or even outdoors after the colostral feeding period and reared in these pens separately from the main herd. This reduces the incidence of neonatal diarrhea and pneumonia.

The removal of the cow–calf pair from the main calving grounds to a 'nursery pasture' after the cow–calf relationship (neonatal bond) is well established at 2–3 days of age, has proved to be a successful management practice in beef herds (87). This system moves the newborn calf away from the main calving ground which may be heavily contaminated because of limited space. It necessitates that the producer plan the location of the calving grounds and nursery pastures well in advance of calving time. Calves which develop diarrhea in the calving grounds or nursery pasture are removed with their dams to a 'hospital pasture' during treatment and convalescence. The all-in all-out principle of successive population and depopulation of farrowing quarters and calf barns is an effective method of maintaining a low level of contamination pressure for the neonate (88).

Increasing and maintaining the non-specific resistance of the newborn
When deemed necessary, some surveillance should be provided for pregnant animals which are expected to give birth, and assistance provided if necessary. The major objective is to avoid or minimize the adverse effects of a difficult or slow parturition on the newborn. Physical injuries, hypoxia and edema of parts of the newborn will reduce the vigor and viability of the newborn and depending on the circumstances and the environment in which it is born it might die soon after birth. In other words the newborn must be given every chance possible to be born strong and vigorous.

When possible, every effort should be made to minimize exposure to extremes of temperature (heat, cold, snow). This again is achieved by surveillance at the time of parturition. In newborn calves exposed to a hot environment, the mortality was higher, the serum corticosteroid levels were higher and the immunoglobulins at 2 and 10 days of age were lower than calves which had some shade (12).

Following a successful birth the next important method of preventing neonatal disease is to ensure that the newborn ingests colostrum as soon after birth as possible. The minimum amount of colostrum which the newborn should ingest during the absorptive period in order to acquire adequate passive immunity varies somewhat with the species because of variation in the length of the absorptive period. The subject has been studied most intensively in the calf. The newborn calf should ingest colostrum at the rate of at least 5% of its body weight within the first 3–5 hours after birth. The amount which the calf ingests will depend on the amount available, the vigor of the calf, the acceptance of the calf by the dam and the management system used which may encourage or discourage the ingestion of liberal quantities of colostrum. The guideline recommended for calves is also recommended for the other species. The total amount of immunoglobulins absorbed from the colostrum is directly proportional to the total quantity ingested and inversely proportional to the time after birth the colostrum is ingested.

Leaving the newborn calf with the cow is no guarantee that the calf will obtain sufficient colostrum. Up to 42% of dairy calves left with their dams may fail to either suck or to absorb colostral immunoglobulins from ingested colostrum (89). This problem can be alleviated by the forced feeding of colostrum to every calf as soon after birth as possible. It is relatively easy to obtain 2 liters of colostrum from the cow and administer it to the calf by stomach tube preferably within minutes after birth or up to 6–12 hours after birth and leave the calf with the cow for 24 hours and allow it to suck voluntarily. At least 5 hours are required for the calf to reach half maximal saturation levels and under natural conditions there is a period of approximately 4 hours after birth during which a calf is agammaglobulinemic and presumably susceptible to systemic infection (58). A less satisfactory alternative is to administer the colostrum when the calf is removed from the cow at 24 hours. This practice will improve the immunoglobulin status of calves, but only 70% of calves will absorb significant quantities of colostral immunoglobulins when fed 1 liter of colostrum after being with their dams for 24 hours.

There are no significant differences in serum immunoglobulin levels achieved in calves which are force-fed colostrum by esophageal feeder or encouraged to suck from a nipple-bottle (102). Some workers contend that the force-feeding of beef calves is disruptive and of no practical benefit in terms of passive humoral antibody transfer (103, 109).

In suckled lambs there is a wide variation of serum immunoglobulin levels and despite the fact that lambs remain with their dams, a high proportion (20%) may have very low serum concentration of maternal immunoglobulin (113). Serum immunoglobulin levels in lambs are also influenced by size. The larger the number of lambs suckled, the lower the mean level and the greater the proportion of lambs which are markedly deficient in maternal immunoglobulin (55).

There is competition between siblings for colostrum and one large single lamb is capable of ingesting within a short period of birth all the available colostrum in the ewe's udder. An alternative source of immunoglobulin may be necessary to supplement the needs of multiple births. Lambs require a total of 180–210 ml colostrum/kg bodyweight during the first 18 hours after birth to provide sufficient energy for heat production (117). This amount will usually provide enough immunoglobulins for protection against infections. Ewes which are well fed during late pregnancy usually produce more colostrum than their lambs need. Lambs from underfed ewes can be supplemented on their first day after birth with surplus colostrum which can be obtained from suitable donor ewes (117). Oxytocin at a dose of 10–15 i.u. intramuscularly just prior to hand milking will assist in letdown of the colostrum.

Partial failure of passive transfer is defined as one SD below the normal mean, and failure of passive transfer as two SD below the normal mean at 24 hours after birth. Partial failure of transfer may occur in up to 14% of lambs which may remain normal. Failure of passive transfer is associated with increased mortality from 1 to 5 weeks of age and secondary starvation is a common cause of death (54).

Passive immunization and neonatal nutrition are closely related—immunoglobulin concentrations are a measure of both—and their relative importance depends on the environment at birth. Lambs born in a well-protected, clean and dry lambing barn have an advantage over lambs born on open range and exposed to cold windy weather (71).

Colostrum for frozen storage should be taken from the dam within 2 hours after birth to ensure a maximum concentration of immunoglobulins. Between the time of parturition and 8–12 hours later the concentration of immunoglobulins in cow colostrum may drop by as much as 100%. At 24 hours it may have decreased by a factor of 5 and at 36 hours by a factor of 10. Prepartum milking of cows to reduce the severity of udder edema should be avoided if possible because it results in a marked reduction in the concentration of immunoglobulins in the colostrum at parturition. Under some circumstances calves can be force fed colostrum with the use of a stomach tube or nipple bottle. The absorption of immunoglobulins from colostrum fed to calves using a stomach tube is very satisfactory. Calves fed approximately 80 ml/kg body weight of colostrum at 6 hours of age achieve total serum immunoglobulin levels of 3·17 g/dl at 24 hours of age (24, 27).

The placement of the stomach tube halfway down the esophagus will stimulate closure of the esophageal groove and delivery of the colostrum into the abomasum, thus bypassing the rumen (20). Dairy calves born under confinement, weak beef calves, calves with edematous tongues and calves which have been subjected to a difficult birth can be given colostrum within minutes after birth which will not interfere with subsequent desire to suck. The efficiency of absorption of immunoglobulins from colostrum is improved if the calf is left with its dam for 24–48 hours. For animals which have not ingested colostrum and none is available, blood transfusions are recommended. Freeze-dried colostrum (47) has been used experimentally and if made available commercially would be a major step forward. Surplus colostrum from dairy cattle is unmarketable and available in quantities sufficient to feed calves through 28 and 35 days of age. All of the available surplus colostrum can be stored at ambient temperatures in plastic containers, allowed to ferment which preserves its quality, and then fed to calves to replace an equal weight of whole milk in calf-feeding programs (46).

Colostrum often does not preserve properly, particularly in warm summer weather. Degradation of nutrients during summer storage as well as putrefaction of colostrum by acid-resistant molds and yeasts can be successfully lowered by application of 1000 ppm of sorbic acid during the first days of storage (47).

Fermented colostrum represents a rich source of nutrients which, if properly preserved, can serve as the only source of milk protein until weaning the dairy calf. Maintaining the quality, uniformity and palatability of colostrum often becomes difficult, particularly during hot weather. Efforts to control undesirable fermentation have included direct acidification with formic, acetic, propionic and lactic acids and use of preservatives such as formaldehyde. Propionic acid and formaldehyde are probably the most popular additives, but neither product controls mold and yeast growth in colostrum.

Waste milk from cows treated with antibiotics can be fed fresh or fermented to calves without detrimental effects. It can also be added to colostrum, allowed to ferment and fed to calves safely and effectively.

A major advantage of feeding fresh or stored colostrum to calves is the provision of specific antibodies to enteric pathogens such as enterotoxigenic *E. coli* and rotavirus and coronavirus. Colostrum from the first two milkings will be high in specific antibody to these pathogens if the dam was naturally exposed to them or if vaccinated in late pregnancy. The feeding of such colostrum will provide specific local immunity in the intestinal tract as long as the antibody containing colostrum is fed to the calves.

The ability of the newborn animal to get up, successfully find the teat, be accepted by its dam and successfully ingest sufficient colostrum early enough has been a very active area of investigation in the science of applied animal ethology (48). Some excellent work has shown the importance of establishing the neonatal bond which is vital particularly for those species such as the piglet and the beef calf which are not easily hand-reared. The reader is referred to many excellent references on this subject for the lamb (49, 50), the calf (51), the piglet (52, 53), and the foal (11).

Following the successful ingestion of colostrum and establishment of the neonatal bond, emphasis can then be given to provision, if necessary, of any special nutritional and housing requirements. Newborn piglets need supplemental heat, their eye teeth should be clipped and attention must be given to the special problems of intensive pig husbandry. Orphan and weak piglets can now be reared successfully under normal farm conditions with the use of milk replacers containing added porcine immunoglobulins. An immunoglobulin dose of 10 g/kg body weight on day 1 followed by 2 g/kg on succeeding days for 10 days is sufficient to confer passive immunity on the colostrum-deprived pig (56). Neonatal piglets can be successfully reared under practical, non-isolated conditions with limited suckling followed by a gammaglobulin supplemented milk replacer (56). Milk replacers for the newborn must contain high quality ingredients and a minimum amount of non-milk protein and carbohydrates (57). There may be a wide variation in the serum immunoglobulins achieved in newborn piglets. Early born and the heavier piglets of the litter may have higher levels than late born and smaller piglets (60). The mortality during the first 2 months of life is highest in piglets with low levels of serum immunoglobulin at 12–18 hours of age. Because small piglets are equal to their littermates in growing capacity it is necessary to protect small pigs from competition among littermates.

Newborn calves are commonly assembled and transported to calf-rearing units within a few days after birth. The effects of the transportation can have a deleterious effect on the defense mechanism of the animal and every effort should be made to reduce the stress of transportation by providing adequate bedding, avoiding long distances without a break and attempting to transport only calves which are healthy and have ingested sufficient colostrum. The incidence of hypogammaglobulinemia is high in calves which have been purchased at a few days of age for rearing in an intensive unit. Surveys have shown that 25–65% of such calves may be deficient in serum immunoglobulin (59). The incidence of infectious disease in these will be high unless hygiene, housing and ventilation, management and nutrition are excellent. The use of the field tests (refractometer or zinc sulfate turbidity tests) to identify immunoglobulin-deficient calves for immediate culling is suggested. If these deficient calves are kept they may require antibacterials prophylactically in their feed supply over a prolonged course.

Even after a large number of retrospective and prospective clinicopathological evaluations of the relationship between the levels of serum immunoglobulins in newborn farm animals at 24–48 hours of age and subsequent morbidity and mortality, there is still some controversy about the validity of the correlation. Some studies indicate that serum immune globulins in purchased calves at about 1 week of age are not a reliable indicator of viability and performance (1). Observations in some beef herds indicate that levels of serum immunoglobulins in calves at 48 hours of age are of no value in predicting the incidence of severity of acute undifferentiated diarrhea (2). However, the majority of surveys of neonatal calves have demonstrated a highly significant relationship between mortality usually from diarrhea, and low levels of serum immunoglobulins in calves measured at 24–48 hours of age. The factors which determine morbidity and mortality in neonatal farm animals are complex and interrelated. Some obvious ones include the vigor of the animal at birth, the amount of colostrum ingested, the amount of colostrum immunoglobulins absorbed, the spectrum of pathogens in the environment, the level of management, the ambient temperature especially for piglets and lambs, the feeds and feeding programs, the nature and severity of the stressors in the environment, the adequacy of housing, the maternal behavior of the dam, the size of the herd and the level of sanitation and hygiene provided for the newborn animals at birth.

An algorithm for minimizing financial losses due to immune deficiency in calves has been described (61).

Calves which are hypogammaglobulinemic are more susceptible to infectious disease and the effects of disease if they are subjected to physical and environmental factors which epidemiologically are known to predispose to disease. Thus, under good management conditions, hypogammaglobulinemic animals may perform normally.

In summary, the better the management and care provided for the newborn the lower the incidence of illness and mortality. The maintenance of a high level of non-specific resistance through regular feeding, proper feeding, and the provision of a comfortable environment will result in a high survival rate.

Increasing the specific resistance of the newborn

The specific resistance of the newborn to infectious disease may be enhanced by vaccination of the dam during pregnancy to stimulate the production of specific antibodies which are concentrated in the colostrum and transferred to the newborn after birth. The parenteral vaccination of the cow (5) or sow (64) before parturition with *E. coli* vaccines stimulates the production of specific colostral antibodies which provide specific protection against enteric pathogens. Vaccination of pregnant cattle with rotavirus and coronavirus vaccines can boost the level of antibody in the colostrum and provide passive lactogenic immunity within the lumen of the intestine for several days following cessation of absorption of colostral immunoglobulins (13). Combined vaccines containing *E. coli* and rotavirus given to pregnant cattle also provide protection against diarrhea in calves caused by these two enteropathogens (15).

Oral immunization of sows with *E. coli* antigen provides a primary stimulus which facilitates the rapid production of humoral IgM antibody following a single parenteral antigen dose. If the antigen is injected at a time close to parturition, antibody is transferred to the colostrum for subsequent absorption by the suckling newborn piglet (13). The vaccination of the late fetus *in utero* stimulates the production of antibody but its practical application has yet to be determined.

Vaccination of the newborn under 2 months of age has not been widely used because of the inefficient response due to the immature immune system.

REVIEW LITERATURE

Black, L., Francis, M. L. & Nicholls, M. J. (1985) Protecting young domestic animals from infectious disease. *Vet. Ann.*, *25*, 46–61.

Bourne, F. J. (1977) The mammary gland and neonatal immunity. *Vet. Sci. Commun.*, *1*, 141.

Butler, J. E. (1986) Biochemistry and biology of ruminant immunoglobulins. *Prog. vet. microbiol. Immunol.*, *2*, 1–53.

Foley, J. A. & Otterby, D. E. (1978) Availability, storage, treatment, composition, and feeding value of surplus colostrum. A review. *J. dairy Sci.*, *61*, 1033.

Gay, C. C. (1983) Failure of passive transfer of colostral immunoglobulins and neonatal disease in calves. A review. *Proc. 4th Int. Symp. Calf Diarrhea Vet. Inf. Dis. Org.*, pp. 346–364.

Halliday, R. (1978) Immunity and health in young lambs. *Vet. Rec.*, *103*, 489.

Jeffcott, L. B. (1974) Some practical aspects of the transfer of passive immunity to newborn foals. *Equ. vet. J.*, *5*, 109.

Morris, D. D. (1986) Immunologic disease of foals. *Comp. cont. Educ. Pract. Vet.*, *8*, S139–S150.

Norcross, N. L. (1982) Secretion and composition of colostrum and milk. *J. Am. vet. med. Assoc.*, *181*, 1057.

Osburn, B. I. (1973) Immune responsiveness of the fetus and neonate. *J. Am. vet. med. Assoc.*, *163*, 801.

Roberts, M. C. (1975) Equine immunoglobulins and the equine immune system. *Vet. Ann.*, *15*, 192.

Schultz, R. D. (1973) Developmental aspects of the fetal bovine immune response. *Cornell Vet.*, *63*, 507.

Sheldrake, R. F. & Husband, A. J. (1985) Immune defences at mucosal surfaces in ruminants. *J. dairy Res.*, *52*, 599–613.

Staley, T. E. & Bush, L. J. (1985) Receptor mechanism of the neonatal intestine and their relationship to immunoglobulin absorption and disease. *J. dairy Sci.*, *68*, 184–205.

REFERENCES

(1) Barber, D. M. L. (1978) *Vet. Rec.*, *102*, 418.
(2) Bradley, J. et al. (1979) *Can. vet. J.*, *20*, 227.
(3) Husband, A. J. & Lascelles, A. K. (1975) *Res. vet. Sci.*, *18*, 201.
(4) Schultz, R. D. (1973) *Cornell Vet.*, *63*, 507.
(5) Acres, S. D. (1985) *J. dairy sci.*, *68*, 229.
(6) Bourne, F. J. et al. (1974) *Res. vet. Sci.*, *16*, 223.
(7) Perryman, L. E. et al. (1980) *Am. J. vet. Res.*, *41*, 1197.
(8) Cabello, G. (1979) *Biol. Neonatol.*, *36*, 35.
(9) Perryman, L. E. et al. (1977) *J. Am. vet. med. Assoc.*, *170*, 212.
(10) Stott, G. H. et al. (1979) *J. dairy Sci.*, *62*, 1632, 1766, 1902 & 1908.
(11) Jeffcott, L. B. (1976) *J. Reprod. Fertil.*, Suppl. *23*, 727.
(12) Stott, J. H. (1980) *J. dairy Sci.*, *63*, 681.
(13) Saif, L. J. & Smith, K. L. (1985) *J. dairy Sci.*, *68*, 206.
(14) McGuire, T. C. & Crawford, T. B. (1973) *Am. J. vet. Res.*, *34*, 1299.
(15) Snodgrass, D. R. (1986) *Vet. Rec.*, *119*, 39.
(16) Kruse, V. (1970) *Anim. Prod.*, *12*, 619.
(17) Hoerlein, A. B. & Jones, D. L. (1977) *J. Am. vet. med. Assoc.*, *170*, 325.
(18) Bourne, F. J. (1977) *Vet. Sci. Commun.*, *1*, 141.
(19) Porter, P. (1973) *J. Am. vet. med. Assoc.*, *163*, 789.
(20) Wenham, G. & Robinson, J. J. (1977) *Vet. Rec.*, *104*, 199.
(21) Villouta, G. et al. (1980) *Br. vet. J.*, *136*, 394.
(22) Logan, E. F. et al. (1974) *Vet. Rec.*, *94*, 386.
(23) Gay, C. C. (1971) *Proc. 19th Wld Vet. Congr.*, *Mexico*, 1001.
(24) Logan, E. F. et al. (1981) *Vet. Rec.*, *108*, 283.
(25) Jeffcott, L. B. (1973) *Proc. 3rd Int. Conf. Equ. Infect. Dis.*, *Paris*, 419.
(26) Jensen, P. T. (1978) *Nord. VetMed.*, *30*, 145.
(27) Molla, A. (1978) *Vet. Rec.*, *103*, 377.
(28) Harkber, D. B. (1974) *Vet. Rec.*, *95*, 229.
(29) Logan, E. F. et al. (1978) *Anim. Prod.*, *26*, 93.
(30) McGuire, T. C. (1977) *J. Am. vet. med. Assoc.*, *170*, 1302.
(31) McGuire, T. C. et al. (1976) *J. Am. vet. med. Assoc.*, *169*, 713.
(32) Logan, E. F. et al. (1973) *Res. vet. Sci.*, *14*, 394.
(33) Porter, P. (1972) *Immunology*, *23*, 225.
(34) Allen, W. D. & Porter, P. (1973) *Immunology*, *24*, 365.
(35) McGuire, T. C. et al. (1975) *J. Am. vet. med. Assoc.*, *155*, 71.
(36) Lamotte, G. B. & Eberhart, R. J. (1976) *Am. J. vet. Res.*, *37*, 1189.
(37) Reid, J. F. S. & Martinez, A. A. (1975) *Vet. Rec.*, *96*, 177.
(38) McBeath, D. G. et al. (1970) *Vet. Rec.*, *88*, 266.
(39) Fisher, E. W. & Martinez, A. A. (1976) *Vet. Rec.*, *98*, 31.
(40) Haxton, J. A. et al. (1974) *Am. J. vet. Res.*, *35*, 835.
(41) Mullen, P. (1975) *Vet. Ann.*, *15*, 451.
(42) Fisher, E. W. & Martinez, A. A. (1975) *Vet. Rec.*, *96*, 113.
(43) Pfeiffer, N. E. & McGuire, T. C. (1977) *J. Am. vet. med. Assoc.*, *170*, 809.
(44) Baggott, J. D. & Short, C. R. (1984) *Equ. vet. J.*, *16*, 364.
(45) Short, C. R. (1980) *Proc. Symp. Vet. Pharmacol. Ther.*, *2*, 81.
(46) Foley, J. A. & Otterby, D. E. (1978) *J. dairy Sci.*, *61*, 1033.
(47) Larson, R. E. et al. (1974) *Am. J. vet. Res.*, *35*, 1061.
(48) Fraser, A. F. (1976) *Appl. anim. Ethol.*, *2*, 193.
(49) Arnold, G. W. & Morgan, P. D. (1975) *Appl. anim. Ethol.*, *2*, 25.
(50) Bareham, J. R. (1976) *Br. vet. J.*, *132*, 152.
(51) Edwards, S. A. & Broom, D. M. (1982) *Anim. Behav.*, *30*, 525.
(52) Harstock, T. G. & Graves, H. B. (1976) *J. anim. Sci.*, *42*, 235.
(53) Fraser, D. (1973) *Br. vet. J.*, *129*, 324.
(54) Sawyer, M. et al. (1977) *J. Am. vet. med. Assoc.*, *171*, 1255.
(55) Logan, E. F. & Irwin, D. (1977) *Res. vet. Sci.*, *23*, 389.
(56) Elliot, J. et al. (1978) *Can. J. anim. Sci.*, *58*, 799.
(57) Roy, J. H. B. & Ternouth, J. H. (1972) *Proc. Nutr. Soc.*, *31*, 53.
(58) Logan, E. F. et al. (1978) *Br. vet. J.*, *134*, 258.
(59) Logan, E. F. (1974) *Br. vet. J.*, *130*, 405.
(60) Yaguchi, H. et al. (1980) *Br. vet. J.*, *136*, 63.
(61) White, M. E. et al. (1983) *Cornell Vet.*, *73*, 76.
(62) Cordy, D. R. (1984) *Vet. Pathol.*, *21*, 587.
(63) Hauser, M. A. et al. (1986) *Am. J. vet. Res.*, *47*, 152.
(64) Nagy, L. K. et al. (1985) *Vet. Rec.*, *117*, 408.
(65) Butler, J. E. (1973) *J. Am. vet. med. Assoc.*, *163*, 795.
(66) Miller, R. B. & Wilkie, B. N. (1979) *Can. J. comp. Med.*, *43*, 255.
(67) Kirkbride, C. A. et al. (1977) *NZ vet. J.*, *25*, 180.
(68) Ohmann, H. B. (1981) *Acta vet. Scand.*, *22*, 428.
(69) Deem, C. A. et al. (1979) *J. Am. vet. med. Assoc.*, *175*, 469.
(70) Murata, H. & Namioka, S. (1977) *J. comp. Pathol.*, *87*, 431.
(71) Eales, F. A. et al. (1982) *Vet. Rec.*, *111*, 451.
(72) Shubber, A. H. et al. (1979) *Res. vet. Sci.*, *27*, 280, 283.
(73) Johnstone, N. E. et al. (1977) *Am. J. vet. Res.*, *38*, 1323.
(74) Olson, D. P. et al. (1981) *Res. vet. Sci.*, *30*, 49.
(75) Halliday, R. et al. (1977) *Res. vet. Sci.*, *24*, 26.
(76) Inoue, T. et al. (1980) *Am. J. vet. Res.*, *41*, 1134.
(77) Inoue, T. (1981) *Am. J. vet. Res.*, *42*, 533.
(78) Johnstone, T. E. & Oxender, W. D. (1979) *Am. J. vet. Res.*, *40*, 32.
(79) Staley, T. E. & Bush, L. J. (1985) *J. dairy Sci.*, *68*, 184.
(80) Thomas, K. W. & Pemberton, D. H. (1980) *Aust. J. exp. Biol. med. Sci.*, *58*, 133.
(81) LeBlanc, M. M. et al. (1986) *J. Am. vet. med. Assoc.*, *189*, 57.
(82) Morris, D. D. et al. (1985) *Am. J. vet. Res.*, *46*, S294.
(83) Tennant, B. et al. (1979) *J. Am. vet. med. Assoc.*, *174*, 848.
(84) Molla, W. A. & Stott, G. H. (1980) *J. dairy Sci.*, *63*, 973.
(85) Rumbaugh, G. E. et al. (1979) *J. Am. vet. med. Assoc.*, *174*, 273.
(86) Burton, S. C. (1981) *Am. J. vet. Res.*, *42*, 308.
(87) Radostits, O. M. & Acres, S. D. (1980) *Can. vet. J.*, *21*, 243.
(88) Edwards, S. A. et al. (1982) *Br. vet. J.*, *138*, 233.
(89) Brignole, R. J. & Stott, G. H. (1980) *J. dairy Sci.*, *63*, 451.
(90) Aschaffenberg, R. et al. (1951) *Br. J. Nutr.*, *5*, 343.
(91) Corbeil, L. B. et al. (1984) *Am. J. vet. Res.*, *45*, 773.
(92) Blom, J. Y. (1982) *Nord. VetMed.*, *34*, 276.
(93) Davidson, J. N. et al. (1981) *J. Am. vet. med. Assoc.*, *179*, 708.
(94) Petrie, L. (1984) *Vet. Rec.*, *114*, 157.
(95) Smeaton, T. C. & Simpson-Morgan, M. W. (1985) *Aust. J. exp. Biol. med. Sci.*, *63*, 41.
(96) Gay, C. C. et al. (1983) *J. Am. vet. med. Assoc.*, *183*, 566.
(97) Norheim, K. & Simensen, E. (1985) *Nord. VetMed.*, *37*, 121.
(98) Donovan, G. A. et al. (1986) *J. dairy Sci.*, *69*, 754.
(99) Fetcher, A. et al. (1983) *Am. J. vet. Res.*, *44*, 2149.
(100) Stott, G. H. & Fellah, A. (1983) *J. dairy Sci.*, 66, 1319.
(101) Johnston, N. E. & Stewart, J. A. (1986) *Aust. vet. J.*, *63*, 191.
(102) Adams, G. D. et al. (1985) *J. dairy Sci.*, *68*, 773.
(103) Bradley, J. A. & Niilo, L. (1984) *Can. vet. J.*, *25*, 121.
(104) Bradley, J. A. & Niilo, L. (1985) *Can. J. comp. Med.*, *49*, 152.
(105) Townsend, H. G. G. et al. (1983) *J. Am. vet. med. Assoc.*, *182*, 255.
(106) Pearson, R. C. et al. (1984) *Am. J. vet. Res.*, *45*, 186.
(107) Kent, J. E. & Blackmore, D. J. (1985) *Equ. vet. J.*, *17*, 125.
(108) White, D. G. (1986) *Vet. Rec.*, *118*, 68.
(109) Thompson, J. C. & Pauli, J. V. (1981) *NZ vet. J.*, *29*, 223.
(110) Pauli, J. V. (1983) *NZ vet. J.*, *31*, 150.
(111) Varley, M. A. et al. (1985) *Res. vet. Sci.*, *38*, 279.
(112) Petrie, L. et al. (1984) *Can. vet. J.*, *25*, 273.
(113) McGuire, T. C. et al. (1983) *Am. J. vet. Res.*, *44*, 1065.
(114) Bernadina, W. E. & Franken, P. (1985) *Vet. Immunol. Immunopathol.*, *10*, 297.
(115) Fraser, D. (1984) *Anim. Prod.*, *39*, 115.
(116) Koterba, A. M. et al. (1984) *Equ. vet. J.*, *16*, 376.
(117) Mellor, D. J. & Murray, L. (1986) *Vet. Rec.*, *118*, 351.
(118) Baker, J. C. (1987) *J. Am. vet. med. Assoc.*, *190*, 1449.

PRINCIPLES OF PROVIDING CRITICAL CARE TO THE NEWBORN

The provision of critical care to newborn farm animals, particularly foals affected with life-threatening abnormalities, has become a popular activity in veterinary teaching clinics and in specialty clinical practices. Potentially valuable foals affected with prematurity, dysmaturity, neonatal maladjustment syndrome, pneumonia and septicemia require intensive clinical care for survival. As a result of these conditions in the foal a large body of literature has been published which describes the extrapolation of intensive care methods used in neonatal infants to the newborn foal. The situation is not as critical in newborn calves, lambs and piglets. A follow-up evaluation of foals under 7 days of age admitted to a veterinary teaching clinic revealed that survival ranged from 0 to 67% dependent on disease. Neonatal maladjustment syndrome, neonatal isoerythrolysis, meconium impaction and ruptured bladder were associated with the most favorable survival rates (1). Foals affected with septicemia, pneumonia and failure of passive transfer were associated with much lower survival rates.

The information available on the foal can be used as a model for the development of the critical care for all newborn farm animals (3). The first step is the clinical and laboratory evaluation of the affected foal. The guidelines for assessment of maturity of the foal are summarized in Table 10.

Premature and mature foals may be distinguished by their behavioral and physical characteristics. Measurements of hematological parameters, pancreatic beta-cell activity (plasma glucose and insulin levels), adrenocorticoid–medullary activity and the renin–angiotensin system may be useful in evaluating the status of the newborn foal (2).

The evaluation of foals with respiratory distress consists of obtaining a detailed history such as gestational age of the foal at birth, a thorough clinical examination with emphasis on the respiratory and cardiomuscular systems, the determination of blood pH, arterial blood gas tensions, hematology and radiography (4). Respiratory measurements and blood–gas and acid–base values in term foals are available (7). The immunological status must also be determined and foals with failure of passive transfer treated accordingly (6).

The principles of critical care being used in newborn foals are outlined here and provide a basis for further development and refinement.

1. The abnormalities of function and the body system (5) involved must be determined; this requires appropriate clinical and laboratory evaluation and constant *monitoring* until full recovery occurs.
2. Every economical effort must be made to provide

Table 10. Criteria used to assess stage of maturity of the newborn foal

	Premature	*Full term*
Physical		
Gestational age	<320 days	Normally >320 days
Size	Small	Normal or large
Coat	Short and silky	Long
Fetlock	Overextended	Normal extension
Behavior		
First stand	>120 min	<120 min
First suck	>3 hours	<3 hours
Suck reflex	Poor	Good
Righting reflexes	Poor	Good
Adrenal activity		
Plasma cortisol values over first 2 hours postpartum	Low levels (<30 ng/ml)	Increasing levels (120–140 ng/ml) at 30–60 minutes postpartum
Plasma ACTH values over first 2 hours postpartum	Peak values (approx 650 pg/ml) at 30 minutes postpartum and declining subsequently	Declining values from peak (300 pg/ml at birth)
Response to synthetic ACTH (short-acting Synacthen), 1–24 dose 0·125 mg intramuscularly	Poor response shown by a 28% increase in plasma cortisol and no changes in neutrophil : lymphocyte ratio	Good response shown by a 208% increase in plasma cortisol and widening of neutrophil : lymphocyte ratio
Hematology		
Mean cell volume (fl)	>39	<39
White blood cell count ($\times 10^9$/litre)	6·0	8·0
Neutrophil : lymphocyte ratio	< 1·0	> 2·0
Carbohydrate metabolism		
Plasma glucose levels over first 2 hours postpartum	Low levels at birth (2·3 mmol/litre), subsequently declining	Higher levels at birth (4·1 mmol/litre) maintained
Plasma insulin levels over first 2 hours postpartum	Low levels at birth 8·6 μU/ml, declining	Higher levels at birth (16·1 μU/ml) maintained
Glucose tolerance test (0·5 mg/kg body weight intravenously)	Slight response demonstrated by a 100% increase in plasma insulin at 15 minutes postadministration	Clear response demonstrated by a 250% increase in plasma insulin at 5 minutes postadministration
Renin–angiotensin–aldosterone system		
Plasma renin substrate	Higher and/or increasing levels during 15–60 minutes postpartum	Low (<0·6 μg/ml) and declining levels during 15–30 minutes postpartum
Acid–base status (pH)	<7·25 and declining	>7·3 and maintaining or rising

comfortable surroundings which will prevent self-inflicted trauma from excessive activity such as paddling and convulsions. This may require 24-hour nursing care. Heat lamps and blankets should be provided as necessary.
3. An intravenous catheter should be inserted so that fluids and drugs can be administered easily and effectively.
4. Respiratory function should be evaluated and positive ventilation and oxygen provided as necessary.
5. Fluids and electrolytes should be given parenterally and orally as indicated.
6. Colostrum should be given by nipple-bottle or stomach tube to foals which did not suck the mare and are considered to be immune-deficient.
7. Mare's colostrum or milk, or cow's or goat's milk should be fed every few hours by nipple-bottle if the foal will suck or if necessary by stomach tube.
8. Foals which are convulsing or hyperesthetic should be sedated with phenobarbitol or diazepam.

REVIEW LITERATURE

Rossdale, P. D., Silver, M. & Rose, R. J. (1984) Equine perinatal physiology and medicine. *Equ. vet. J.*, *16*, 225–398.

REFERENCES

(1) Baker, S. M. et al. (1986) *J. Am. vet. med. Assoc.*, *189*, 1454.
(2) Rossdale, P. D. et al. (1984) *Equ. vet. J.*, *16*, 300.
(3) Rossdale, P. D. (1985) *Equ. vet. J.*, *17*, 343.
(4) Kosch, P. C. et al. (1984) *Equ. vet. J.*, *16*, 312.
(5) Webb, A. I. et al. (1984) *Equ. vet. J.*, *16*, 319.
(6) Morris, D. D. (1986) *Comp. cont. Educ. Pract. Vet.*, *8*, S139.
(7) Stewart, J. H. et al. (1984) *Equ. vet. J.*, *16*, 323.

OMPHALITIS, OMPHALOPHLEBITIS AND URACHITIS IN NEWBORN FARM ANIMALS (NAVEL-ILL)

Infection of the umbilicus and its associated structures occurs commonly in newborn farm animals and appears to be particularly common in calves. The umbilical cord consists of the amniotic membrane, the umbilical veins, the umbilical arteries and the urachus. The amniotic membrane of the umbilical cord is torn at birth and gradually the umbilical vein and the urachus close, but they remain temporarily outside the umbilicus. The umbilical arteries retract as far back as the top of the bladder. Normally, the umbilical cord dries up within 1 week after birth.

Infection of the umbilicus occurs soon after birth and may result in omphalitis, omphalophlebitis, omphaloarteritis or infection of the urachus with possible extension to the bladder, causing cystitis (1, 2). There is usually a mixed bacterial flora including *E. coli*, *Proteus* spp., *Staphylococcus* spp. and *Actinomyces (Corynebacterium) pyogenes*. Bacteremia and localization with infection may occur in joints, meninges, eyes, endocardium, and end arteries of the feet, ears and tail.

Omphalitis is inflammation of the external aspects of the umbilicus and occurs commonly in calves within 2–5 days after birth. The umbilicus is enlarged, painful on palpation and may be closed or draining purulent material through a small fistula. The affected umbilicus may become very large and cause subacute toxemia. The calf is moderately depressed, does not suck normally and is febrile. Treatment consists of surgical exploration and excision. A temporary drainage channel may be necessary.

Omphalophlebitis is inflammation of the umbilical veins which may involve only the distal parts or extend from the umbilicus to the liver. Large abscesses may develop along the course of the umbilical vein and spread to the liver with the development of a large hepatic abscess which may occupy up to one-half of the liver. Affected calves are usually 1–3 months of age and are unthrifty because of chronic toxemia. The umbilicus is usually enlarged with a purulent material. However, in some cases the external portion of the umbilicus is not enlarged. Placing the animal in dorsal recumbency and deep palpation of the abdomen dorsal to the umbilicus in the direction of the liver may reveal a space-occupying mass. The insertion of a probe and the use of contrast media and radiography may assist in the diagnosis. Affected calves are inactive, inappetent, unthrifty and may have a mild fever. Parenteral therapy with antibiotics is usually unsuccessful. Exploratory laparotomy and surgical removal of the abscess is necessary. Large hepatic abscesses are usually incurable, but the provision of a drain to the exterior and daily irrigation may be attempted.

In *omphaloarteritis*, which is less common, the abscesses occur along the course of the umbilical arteries from the umbilicus to the internal iliac arteries. The clinical findings are similar to those in omphalophlebitis: chronic toxemia, unthriftiness and failure to respond to antibiotic therapy. Treatment consists of surgical removal of the abscesses.

Infection of the urachus may occur anywhere along the urachus from the umbilicus to the bladder. The umbilicus is usually enlarged and draining purulent material, but may also appear normal. Deep palpation of the abdomen in a dorsocaudal direction from the umbilicus may reveal a space-occupying mass. Extension of the infection to the bladder can result in cystitis and pyuria. Contrast radiography of the fistulous tract and the bladder will reveal the presence of the lesion. The treatment of choice is also exploratory laparotomy and surgical removal of the abscesses. Recovery is usually uneventful.

The control of umbilical infection depends primarily on good sanitation and hygiene at the time of birth. The application of drying agents and residual disinfectants such as tincture of iodine is widely practiced. However, there is limited evidence that chemical disinfection is of significant value.

REFERENCES

(1) Bouckaert, J. H. & DeMoor, A. (1965) *Vet. Rec.*, *77*, 771.
(2) Cheli, R. (1968) *Clin. vet., Milano*, *91*, 141 & 173.

4

Practical Antimicrobial Therapeutics

THIS chapter is not intended as a treatise on pharmacology, pharmacodynamics and antibacterial activity of antimicrobial agents. There are textbooks to deal with those subjects. But the antibiotics and sulfonamides are the most commonly used group of drugs in large animal practice and their use is recommended on many occasions in the following chapters. To avoid repetition the principles of usage, the dose schedules and descriptions of the individual drugs are presented here. Particular attention is given to the selection of antibacterial agents for certain circumstances.

Some of the information or opinions presented are based on clinical use rather than experimental evidence. However, this is often unavoidable, because unfortunately many antimicrobial agents have been released for use in large animals with minimal pharmacological or clinical evaluation in large animals. As a result it has been assumed, often erroneously, that information obtained from studies in laboratory animals, dogs and man can be directly applied to the ruminant, horse and pig.

Only the more commonly used antimicrobial agents are presented in this chapter. Many have been excluded because, on the basis of cost, relative efficiency or limited application, they are of little current importance in large animal veterinary practice. Some of them, such as griseofulvin, are mentioned in their areas of specific application in the special medicine section.

PRINCIPLES OF ANTIMICROBIAL THERAPY

The success of antimicrobial therapy depends upon maintaining, at the site of infection, a drug concentration that will result, directly or indirectly, in the death or control of the infectious organism with minimal deleterious effect to the host. In order to achieve this aim the antimicrobial agent must have activity against the organism at its site of infection and it must be administered in such a way as to maintain an effective inhibitory or lethal concentration. These principles apply to therapy in all species and dictate the choice of antimicrobial agent to be used. However, in large animal veterinary practice cost is also critical. This consideration includes not only the primary cost of the drug but also related factors such as the ease and frequency of administration and the duration of treatment. Tissue residue problems and withdrawal periods must also be taken into consideration.

In the theoretically ideal situation the following steps would be taken before selecting an antimicrobial agent for therapy. Firstly, the site of infection would be located and the identity of the infecting organism established by culture. Secondly, the minimal inhibitory concentration (MIC) of each antimicrobial agent for the infecting organism would be identified. Then an initial selection would be made based on the sensitivity of the organism and the knowledge of the capacity of the individual antimicrobial agents to penetrate to the site of infection and to achieve and exceed these concentrations at non-toxic dose rates. The dose rates, route of administration and frequency of administration required to achieve these concentrations for each of the selected antibiotics would then be considered. The final selection would be based on a consideration of the potential toxicity to the host, the likely relative efficiency of each drug and on the cost and ease of administration.

It is obvious that for many clinical situations all of these steps cannot be followed before therapy is instituted. It may take several days to establish the identity of the infectious agent unless it can be established by clinical diagnosis. The identification of the organism helps in determining its potential sensitivity but even without identification the establishment of exact minimal inhibitory concentrations by tube dilution for each antimicrobial agent also takes several days and the results would frequently be historical by the time that they were received. Also a knowledge, for each antimicrobial agent, of the varying tissue and organ levels achieved following varying doses given by different routes of administration is not easily remembered and therefore not easily available in large animal field situations. Nor, unfortunately, is complete information of this type available for each antimicrobial agent in all large animal species. Because of this uncertainty some expedients are adopted in clinical antimicrobial therapy. One of them is the concept of the recommended dose and another is the use of disk sensitivity testing, both of which are discussed later in this section. Regardless of these expedients it should be recognized that rational antimicrobial therapy is based upon the principles outlined above. With some diseases the known clinical effectiveness of one antibiotic often dictates its use at a given dose for a given period, without the need for these considerations, although the treatment was based upon these principles in the first instance. In other situations a single treatment method may not be indicated from past clinical experience but it is frequently possible to quickly arrive at a choice of antibiotic based upon these principles. In others this cannot be done quickly and although initially empirical therapy is usually required, more rational therapy may be instituted subsequently as further information becomes available.

Because of the importance of these principles in antimicrobial therapy they are discussed in greater detail individually.

Identification of the infection by clinical examination

In infectious disease, clinical examination aims to identify the nature and site of the infection and its cause. The importance of making an accurate clinical diagnosis cannot be overemphasized as the first prerequisite for successful antimicrobial therapy. The establishment of a diagnosis in many instances immediately identifies the pathogen and makes possible a rational selection of an antimicrobial agent for therapy. Once the diagnosis is established, previous clinical experience may immediately suggest the exact antibiotic to be used and allow a confident prediction of success of the therapy. Equally it may indicate the likelihood of unsuccessful or prolonged therapy. For example, the diagnosis of erysipelas or Glasser's disease in pigs, or corynebacterial pneumonia in foals, or strangles in horses immediately identifies the etiological cause of the infection and the type of antimicrobial agent that will be required. It also gives some indication of the likely ease or difficulty of successful therapy and of the duration of therapy that might be required. The establishment of an accurate diagnosis is also important in animals where chemotherapeutic control of further disease may be required. Thus, in pigs, an accurate differentiation between the diarrhea of swine dysentery and that associated with coliform gastroenteritis is essential for effective prophylactic medication. The problems of the rational selection of an antimicrobial agent for therapy are minimal when a definitive diagnosis of the cause of the disease can be made. It is often not possible to do this at the first examination and yet in almost every instance it is essential that treatment be instituted at that time, not only for the wellbeing of the patient, but also for the maintenance of good client relationships. The lack of a definitive etiological diagnosis should never preclude the initiation of therapy during the period when further tests are being carried out to establish an exact diagnosis. Rational therapy in these circumstances depends very much on clinical acumen. A detailed examination leading to a determination of the site and nature of the infection can frequently allow an educated guess at the likely pathogen, and allow rational therapy during the period that this is being determined by culture. For example, a superficial examination may establish that a sick horse has respiratory disease and a detailed examination may establish that an effusive pleuritis is present. Clinical knowledge suggests that the most common pathogens causing this condition are streptococci, *Actinobacillus equuli* and *Pasteurella* spp. and that benzylpenicillin or ampicillin is indicated for treatment. Furthermore, the condition is more likely to respond to intrapleural as well as parenteral administration of antibiotic and both of these agents may be given intrapleurally with minimal irritation. Such therapy can be instituted while the exact cause of infection is being determined.

This approach is frequently used initially in field situations in large animal medicine but it requires good clinical knowledge. Clinicians should be familiar not only with the individual diseases of large animals but also with their differential diagnosis and with the relative prevalence of each condition in their area. They should also be familiar with the type of organisms which may produce infections in various body areas with similar clinical manifestations and the relative prevalence of each of these. Thus peracute mastitis in recently calved cows is most commonly associated with infection by staphylococci but can also be associated with coliform organisms or, more rarely, *Actinomyces (Corynebacterium) pyogenes* or *Pasteurella multocida*. Treatment must be initiated immediately if the gland or even the cow is to be saved. There are subtle clinical and epidemiological differences that may allow some clinical differentiation between these agents but frequently treatment must begin with no sure knowledge of which agent is involved. There are two approaches in this type of situation. Therapy may be directed at the most prevalent or likely agent and in situations where one particular infectious agent is the most prevalent cause of the condition, this is a rational approach. In other situations where the disease could be associated with any one of several different organisms, each with a different sensitivity, and where clinical experience suggests that no one organism is the predominant infectious agent, it is more common to initiate therapy with a broad-spectrum antimicrobial agent or a combination that will have activity against all of the possibilities. If indicated, the antibacterial agent being used for therapy may have to be changed to a more specific one if the actual pathogen and its sensitivity have been determined.

There are also clinical situations where therapy must begin when there is little knowledge of the site of infection and consequently no knowledge of the identity of the infecting agent. This occurs where infection, such as abscessation, occurs in deep-seated and clinically inaccessible organs such as the liver or spleen. Also in these situations it may not be possible to determine the nature and cause of the disease by laboratory examination although biochemical examinations may give some indication of the site. In these cases therapy is generally started with a broad-spectrum antimicrobial agent or a combination of lesser ones, and the accuracy of the selection determined by subsequent clinical response.

Taking samples for diagnosis

In cases where the etiological agent cannot be determined by clinical examination it is preferred that its identity and, if necessary, its antimicrobial sensitivity be determined from samples taken for laboratory examination. In teaching hospitals, there is ready access to bacteriology laboratories that frequently contain automated and rapid systems for sensitivity testing. However, in practice the taking of samples for this purpose is generally restricted and limited by such factors as the availability of a diagnostic laboratory and by cost. Furthermore in many cases the results of culture and sensitivity are frequently historical by the time that they are received in so far as any one case is concerned as the animal will have by this time responded to the therapy already given. Nevertheless, information of this type is of value for future, similar cases and it provides prevalence data and data of antimicrobial sensitivity that can be used for background clinical knowledge.

The recognition of when samples should be taken for microbiological examination and sensitivity testing comes with clinical experience. In general the approach is different when dealing with individual sick animals than when dealing with groups of animals and a contagious disease. In individual animals, cost and the time for processing usually limit the taking of samples to valuable stud animals and to horses. They should be taken from individual sick animals with life-threatening conditions so that if a response is not obtained to initial therapy the subsequent choice of antimicrobial agent can be based on laboratory data. They should also be taken from animals with disease syndromes that may be caused by one of several agents or by an organism that may show variable resistance patterns. Examples would be infective arthritis in foals or Gram-negative sepsis. The increasing emergence of variable resistance patterns in veterinary pathogens places an increasing importance on sampling and sensitivity testing and many practices have now established their own laboratories for this purpose.

Samples are also frequently taken from chronic, poorly responsive conditions to determine the best course of treatment. In groups of animals where there is contagious disease the taking of samples to establish or confirm the etiological diagnosis and to determine the best drug for chemotherapy is most important. Where there are a large number of animals at risk it is important to confirm the initial choice of therapy as soon as possible so that remedial steps can be taken if this was incorrect. With this approach the outbreak is more likely to be brought under control quickly and the losses minimized. It is also important in these situations to have a confirmed accurate etiological diagnosis so that control measures can be instigated to prevent future problems. Thus an outbreak of diarrhea in postweaned pigs may be due to coliform gastroenteritis, salmonellosis or swine dysentery. Clinical and pathological examination may eliminate swine dysentery but not allow complete differentiation between salmonellosis and coliform gastroenteritis. Neomycin sulfate could be used for the initial therapy of the outbreak but, at the same time, samples are taken for culture and sensitivity to determine the exact antimicrobial sensitivity of the infectious agent in case there is resistance to this antibiotic. Also by this procedure the exact etiological diagnosis will be determined which will then determine recommendations for future control of the disease.

Consideration should be given to the nature of the sample for examination. In outbreaks of diarrhea there is little point in taking fecal samples from chronically scouring and runted animals. Samples should be taken from animals at the onset of diarrhea. The site of sampling can also have an influence that may affect the relevance of the results. In animals with pneumonia, the nasal flora may not reflect that in the lung and lower airway isolates of *Pasteurella hemolytica* from pneumonic calves may have different sensitivity patterns to isolates from the nasal cavity (1).

Antimicrobial sensitivity tests

The need for sensitivity tests in large animal practice is limited. Many organisms are invariably sensitive to one or more antimicrobial agents and in most cases these can be used for therapy. The clinician should be familiar not only with the spectrum of each antimicrobial drug but also with the spectrum of sensitivity for the common organisms involved in diseases of large animals. Sensitivity testing is generally reserved for members of those groups of organisms that show considerable variation in sensitivity to individual antimicrobial agents and it is an invaluable test in these circumstances. Coliform organisms form one such group. There is considerable area-to-area variation in the sensitivity patterns of these groups and whereas, for example, the majority of *E. coli* isolates in one area or country may be susceptible to neomycin those from another area may show a greater proportion of resistant strains. Also isolates from different diseases within the same area may vary in sensitivity so that many *E. coli* isolated from coliform mastitis in cows may be sensitive to the tetracycline group of antibiotics whereas those associated with enteric disease in pigs are generally resistant. It is wise to establish the broad patterns of general sensitivity or resistance for these groups in any practice area and to monitor any change periodically so that initial therapy, when dealing with these groups, can be guided by this information.

The purpose of sensitivity testing is to attempt to determine if the organism under consideration is likely to be susceptible to the action of an antimicrobial agent at the drug levels that can be achieved using the usual therapeutic dose rates. In clinical terms organisms are considered either sensitive or resistant to the action of an antimicrobial. However, with many organism–antimicrobial associations, resistance or susceptibility is not an all-or-none phenomenon but is dependent upon drug concentration. Organisms which may be resistant to low levels of an antimicrobial agent are frequently susceptible to its action at higher concentrations. Thus an organism that is susceptible to the action of benzylpenicillin at a concentration of 0·1 μg/ml would be considered sensitive because equivalent levels of benzylpenicillin can be easily achieved in the blood and tissues. One that was susceptible only at a concentration above 50 μg/ml would be considered resistant because it is almost impossible to achieve and maintain the equivalent concentration of benzylpenicillin in the tissues.

Sensitivity tests may be quantitative or qualitative. Tube sensitivity tests using serial dilutions of the antimicrobial drug against a standard dose of the test organism provide quantitative information in terms of an exact minimal inhibitory concentration (MIC) of the drug being tested. With most antibiotics, a mean plasma level two to five times the MIC needs to be sustained through the dosing interval for effective therapy. These tests are laborious and time-consuming and are seldom used in practice situations for these reasons. Disk sensitivity tests provide more limited qualitative information. This is generally a very valuable adjunct in the choice of an antimicrobial agent for therapy. However, the limitations of the usual method of testing should be recognized by the clinician. The Kirby–Bauer technique is the most commonly used method of disk diffusion sensitivity testing (2). With this technique disks are impregnated with a standard amount of antibiotic that diffuses into the media to produce a zone of inhibition of growth. With a standard concentration of antibiotic in the disk and standard antibiotic sensitivity test media and test conditions, the concentration of the diffused antibiotic at any given distance from the disk is relatively predictable and constant. There is a linear relationship between the diameter of the zone of inhibition and the $\log_2$ of MIC. For each antibiotic MIC breakpoints have been established and corresponding zone size breakpoints established above or below which an organism is classified as resistant, susceptible, or of intermediate sensitivity (3).

Although the Kirby–Bauer disk sensitivity testing system has a quantitative genesis the results are qualitative—especially as used in most veterinary laboratories. The MIC breakpoints and thus the published reference zone sizes for resistance and susceptibility are based on the pharmacokinetic properties of each antimicrobial in man. These frequently have limited relationship to their pharmacokinetic properties in animals, particularly ruminants. Also, the use of specific zone diameters to establish resistance and susceptibility assumes a standard test with standard media and under standard conditions. These conditions are frequently not met in veterinary and practice laboratories (2–4). There are moves to establish parameters for disk sensitivity testing that will have their reference breakpoint based on antibiotic pharmacokinetics in animals, and there are indications of differences (5). Despite these limitations, disk sensitivity tests can be used as a guide to the selection of antimicrobials for therapy in large animal veterinary practice. They are of particular value in selecting a choice of antibiotic with organisms that exhibit variable patterns of resistance and where this pattern for any one antibiotic is essentially bimodal in distribution (7). They are also able to accurately predict unilateral sensitivity patterns (i.e., all sensitive or all resistant); however, sensitivity testing should not be necessary for this information. They may have limited value in the testing of organisms where the sensitivities are clustered around the MIC breakpoint. Also there should not be overreliance on the results of testing for sulfonamide sensitivity, as these are frequently misleading and a good clinical response can be achieved with therapy even though the sensitivity test suggests resistance.

Frequently with disk sensitivity tests, the organism proves sensitive to a number of different antimicrobial agents. The selection of one of these for therapy is based on such factors as ease of administration and cost. The relative efficacy of any one of the agents cannot be determined by comparison of the size of the zones of inhibition.

Disk sensitivity tests are usually conducted on subcultures from the initial isolation. However, when a rapid indication of sensitivity is required a direct sensitivity test can be conducted. This involves conducting a sensitivity test on the initial plating of the sample and frequently a result can be obtained within 8 hours. This can be of value in acute life-threatening diseases and those herd diseases where rapid treatment and control are required. Direct sensitivity tests are correctly criticized by bacteriologists because of the risk of misinterpretation when samples containing a mixed flora of varying sensitivities are examined. However, the method has considerable value where pure culture infections such as mastitis are being examined. It can also be very valuable in enteric diseases such as coliform gastroenteritis in pigs, provided care is taken in the sampling technique and in the interpretation of the test. The rapidity of the result outweighs potential disadvantages and the results can always be confirmed subsequently by the standard test method.

The limitations of the disk diffusion test suggest that direct determination of the MIC of isolates would be of greater value in predicting effective therapy. There have been limited studies on the correlation between the MIC suggested by disk diffusion tests and those determined by direct methods, but there is developing evidence that direct determination is more accurate (5, 6, 8, 9). This, and the development of semiautomated microtiter methodology for direct MIC determinations, suggests that many reference diagnostic laboratories and teaching hospitals will use directly determined MIC concentrations in bacterial sensitivity testing in the near future. The results from such laboratories will be more directly applicable to rational therapy and will have more relevance than disk diffusion tests for determining the sensitivity of organisms that cluster around the MIC breakpoint for a given antibiotic (5, 7).

A guide to the antimicrobial sensitivity of some microorganisms is shown in Table 11. It should be emphasized that this is only a guide. The antimicrobial sensitivity of an organism can vary considerably depending upon the species of animal from which it is isolated. *E. coli* isolates from pigs generally show a greater degree of antibiotic resistance than those isolated from horses. Similarly, *Campylobacter* spp. isolates from pigs show substantially different antibiotic sensitivity patterns than those from sheep. Isolates from the same species may also vary significantly in sensitivity so that *E. coli* isolated from mastitis in cattle generally have a broader sensitivity pattern than those isolated from enteric disease in calves. In addition there are area differences and changes with time. Low levels of antibiotic fed for growth promoting purposes may influence sensitivity patterns, and in herds where these are being used it is generally wise not to use

Table 11. Guide to antimicrobial sensitivity*

Organism	Benzylpenicillin	Methicillin	Cloxacillin	Ampicillin	Amoxycillin	Carbenicillin	Cephalosporins	Streptomycin	Neomycin	Paromomycin	Kanamycin	Gentamicin	Tetracyclines	Chloramphenicol	Erythromycin	Oleandomycin	Spiramycin	Tylosin	Lincomycin	Polymyxins	Colistin	Vancomycin	Bacitracin	Novobiocin	Sulfonamides	Sulfonamides + trimethoprim	Nitrofurans	Amikacin
Streptococci, β-hemolytic	S	MS	MS	MS	MS	MS	S	OR	OR	OR	OR	OR	OR	S	S	S	S	GS	GS			S	GS	GS	GS	GS	GS	
Strep. agalactiae	S	MS	MS	MS	MS	MS	S						S	S	S	S	S		S			S	GS	GS	GS	GS	S	
Streptococci non-agalactiae	GS	MS	OR	MS	MS	MS	S						GS	S	S	S	S		GS			S	GS	GS	GS	GS	OR	
Enterococci	OR	GR	GR	GS	GS	MS	MS		GR	GR	GR	MS	OR	MS	GS	GS	GS	GS	OR									
Diplococci	S	MS	MS	MS	MS	MS	S		GR	GR	GR	GR	GS	S	S	S	S					S	GS	GS				
Staphylococcus aureus	OR	GS	GS	OR	OR	MS	GS	OR	GS	GS	GS	GS	OR	GS	GS	GS	GS	MS	GS			GS	GS	GS	OR	GS	GS	GS
Staphylococci, penicillinase-positive		GS	GS					OR	GS	GS	GS	GS	OR	GS	GS	GS	GS	MS	GS			GS	GS	GS	OR	GS	GS	GS
Bacillus spp.	S	MS	MS	S	S	MS	S					GS	S	S	S	S	S	S	S			S	GS		GS	GS		
Clostridium spp.	S	MS	MS	S	S	MS	S						S	S	S	S	S	S	S			S	GS		GS	GS		
Corynebacterium spp.	S	MS	MS	S	S	MS	MS	MS	MS	MS	MS	MS	MS	MS	MS	MS	MS	MS	MS			S	GS					
Listeria spp.	S	MS	MS	S	S	MS	S						S	S	S	S	S	S	S					GS	GS	GS		
Erysipelothrix spp.	S	MS	MS	S	S	MS	S						MS	MS	MS	MS	MS	MS	MS				MS		GR	GS		
E. coli, gut				GS	GS	MS	OR	GR	GS	OR	OR	GS	GR	OR						GS	GS				OR	GS	GS	GS
E. coli, milk				GS	GS	MS	GS	OR	GS	GS	GS	GS	GS	GS						GS	GS				OR	GS	GS	GS
Salmonella spp.				GS	GS	MS	GR	OR	GS	GS	GS	GS	OR	GS						GS	GS				OR	GS	GS	GS
Klebsiella spp.				GR	GR	MS	GR	GR	GS	GS	GS	GS	OR	OR						GS	GS				OR	OR	GS	GS
Proteus spp.				GR	GR	MS		GR	OR	OR	OR	GS	GR	GR						OR	OR					GR	GR	GS
Pseudomonas spp.						MS			GR	GR	GR	GS	GR	GR						GS	GS					GR	GR	GS
Haemophilus spp.	GR	GR	GR	MS	MS	MS	MS	S	S	S	S	S	S	S	S	S	S	S	MS	GS	GS				GS	GS	S	S
Pasteurella spp.	OR	OR	OR	MS	MS	MS	MS	GR	GS	GS	GS	GS	OR	S	OR	MS	MS	MS	MS	GS	GS				OR	GS	GS	
Bordetella spp.						MS		OR	GS	GS	GS	GS	GS	MS	MS	MS	MS	GR	GR	GS	GS				GS	GS		
Actinobacillus spp.	S			MS	MS			GS	S	S	S	S	GS	GS	S	S	S		GR						GS			
Brucella spp.				GS	GS			MS					S	MS						GS	GS					GS	GS	
Bacteroides spp.				S	S	S								S	MS	MS	MS	MS	MS									
Fusobacterium spp.	S							GR	GS				S	S	MS			S								GS	GS	
Leptospira spp.	S						MS	S	S	S	S	S	MS	S	S													
Treponema spp.								GS	GS	GS	GS	GS		GS	MS	MS	MS	GS	MS				GS				GS	GS
Campylobacter spp.								GR	GS	GS	GS	GS	S	S	MS	MS	MS	MS	MS	CS	GS		GR			S		
Mycoplasma spp.								MS	MS	MS	MS	MS	MS	MS	GR	MS	MS	MS	MS									
Chlamydia	S												S	S	MS	MS	MS	MS										
Actinomyces spp.	S			S	S		S	S	S	S	S	S			S										GS	GS		
Dermatophilus	MS							MS	MS	MS	MS	MS	S		S	S	S	S	S									

*S = sensitive; GS = generally sensitive; MS = moderately sensitive (higher dose levels may be required); GR = generally resistant (many resistant strains in population); OR = often resistant. Blank spaces indicate that the organism is resistant or that information is not available.

the same drug or members of the same group for therapeutic purposes without prior testing.

Although in Table 11 some organisms are shown as sensitive to the activity of several antimicrobial agents in a given disease there is frequently a much superior clinical response to one particular drug, as is the case with benzylpenicillin and erysipelas in pigs, and the treatment sections for each disease should be consulted for these indications.

REVIEW LITERATURE

Baggot, J. D. & Prescott, J. F. (1987) Antimicrobial selection and dosage in the treatment of equine bacterial infections. *Eq. vet. J.*, *19*, 92–96.

Prescott, J. G. & Baggot, J. D. (1985) Antimicrobial susceptibility testing and antimicrobial drug dosage. *J. Am. vet. med. Assoc.*, *187*, 363–368.

Woolcock, J. B. & Mutimer, M. D. (1983) Antibiotic sensitivity testing: caeci caecos ducentes? *Vet. Res.*, *113*, 125–128.

REFERENCES

(1) Allan, M. E. et al. (1985) *Vet. Rec.*, *117*, 506.
(2) Linton, A. H. (1976) *Vet. Rec.*, *99*, 370.
(3) Woolcock, J. B. & Mutimer, M. D. (1983) *Vet. Rec.*, *113*, 125.
(4) McIntosh, M. E. (1981) *Vet. Rec.*, *108*, 52.
(5) Libal, M. C. (1985) *Am. J. vet. Res.*, *46*, 1200.
(6) Gilbride, K. A. & Rosendal, S. (1984) *Can. J. comp. Med.*, *48*, 47.
(7) Libal, M. C. et al. (1986) *Proc. Am. Assoc. vet. lab. Diag.*, *29*, 9.
(8) Fales, W. H. et al. (1986) *Proc. Am. Assoc. vet. lab. Diag.*, *29*, 1.
(9) Adamson, P. J. W. (1985) *Am. J. vet. Res.*, *46*, 447.

Antibiotic resistance

The introduction of antibiotics into clinical use has almost invariably been followed by the emergence of resistance to these drugs in bacterial populations. The resistance that can result from spontaneous mutation of chromosomal genes encoding a target site is probably of limited importance in clinical settings. It occurs more frequently with certain antibacterials, i.e. rifampicin, and may be combatted by the inclusion of a second antibacterial in the treatment regimen. Plasmid and transposon determined drug resistance is of much more importance in clinical situations and has led to widespread multi-resistance patterns in certain bacterial populations. Plasmids are extrachromosomal genetic elements that replicate independently of the chromosome. They can be transferred within, and in some cases between, bacterial species and may also act as vectors for transposons. They may encode for single or multiple patterns of antibiotic resistance and increasingly multiple patterns of resistance are emerging. With veterinary pathogens plasmid-determined resistance is particularly important in the Enterobacteriaceae, *Staphylococcus aureus* and to some extent with *Pasteurella* spp. (7–9). Virtually all antibiotics given in therapeutic doses cause marked changes in the microflora of sites in the host normally colonized by bacteria. There is suppression of the sensitive flora with subsequent colonization by resistant bacteria. Thus, the use of antibiotics for all purposes, but especially prolonging oral therapy, the feeding of antibiotics for growth promoting purposes and influences such as the feeding of antibiotic-treated milk to calves may select for resistance among organisms within the alimentary tract. These resistant organisms can persist in the animal and in the environment and subsequently form part of the normal colonizing flora of other animals so that it is not unusual to isolate organisms, *E. coli* for example, that are resistant to one or more antibiotics even though the animal from which they were isolated had never received antibiotic medication (2).

There is a higher prevalence of antibiotic resistant *E. coli* in the normal intestinal flora of young animal than adults. The prevalence is higher in young animals reared intensively such as veal calves and pigs and in environments where antibiotic usage has exerted selection pressure (1, 4, 5). The prevalence falls with increasing age and the intestinal flora of adults generally shows a broader sensitivity pattern (3). Although many of these resistant organisms are not pathogens, they contribute a pool of R plasmids that can be transmitted to pathogens. The importance of this pool in engendering multiple resistance in human pathogens from transmission via food products is the subject of considerable public health debate (6).

Escherichia coli that have multiple drug resistance patterns and that are part of the normal flora may invade to produce septicemia in calves and foals with failure of passive transfer. This creates problems in the selection of antibiotic therapy for Gram-negative sepsis in the neonate. Nosocomial infection with antibiotic-resistant organisms may be an emerging problem in veterinary hospitals (10). Plasmid-determined multiple antibiotic resistant strains of salmonella have emerged and have caused rapidly spreading epidemics of disease in young calves in England and Europe (11). However, these multiple resistance patterns have been associated with particular phage types and biotypes of *Salmonella typhimurium* and *Salmonella dublin* and other salmonella isolates continue to show relatively broad patterns of sensitivity (12, 13).

Plasmid-determined multiple patterns of resistance are likely to increase in organisms in environments where selection pressure is high due to frequent antibiotic usage. Procedures to limit its occurrence and to limit spread within animal industries and in human medicine are a subject of considerable debate (6, 12, 14). Recommendations to limit the spread of nosocomial infection with these strains in veterinary hospitals are available (10).

REVIEW LITERATURE

Hinton, M. (1986) The ecology of *Escherichia coli* in animals including man with particular reference to drug resistance. *Vet. Rec.*, *119*, 420–426.

Pohl, P. & Lintermann, P. (1986). R plasmid reservoirs and circulation. In: *Drug Residues in Animals. Vet. Sci. Comp. Med. A Series.* New York: Academic Press.

Saunders, J. R. (1984) Genetics and evaluation of antibiotic resistance. *Br. med. Bull.*, *40*, 54–60.

REFERENCES

(1) Hinton, M. et al. (1985) *J. appl. Bacteriol.*, *58*, 27.
(2) Hinton, M. et al. (1985) *J. appl. Bacteriol.*, *58*, 131.
(3) Linton, A. H. (1977) *Vet. Rec.*, *100*, 354.
(4) Jackson, G. (1981) *Vet. Rec.*, *108*, 325.

(5) Stabler, S. L. et al. (1982) *Am. J. vet. Res.*, *30*, 1763.
(6) Lacey, R. (1987) *Vet. Rec.*, *120*, 394.
(7) Hinckley, L. S. et al. (1985) *J. Am. vet. med. Assoc.*, *187*, 709.
(8) Boyce, J. R. & Morter, R. L. (1986) *Am. J. vet. Res.*, *47*, 1204.
(9) Libal, M. et al. (1982) *J. Am. vet. med. Assoc.*, *180*, 908.
(10) Koterba, A. et al. (1986) *J. Am. vet. Med. Assoc.*, *189*, 185.
(11) Threlfall, E. J. et al. (1985) *Vet. Rec.*, *117*, 355.
(12) Linton, A. H. (1984) *Br. med. Bull.*, *40*, 91.
(13) Mills, K.W. & Kelly, B.L. (1986) *Am. J. vet. Res.*, *47*, 2349.
(14) Raive, B. & Threlfall, E. J. (1984) *Br. med. Bull.*, *40*, 68.

Antibiotic dosage: the recommended dose

Theoretically there is no set dose for any antimicrobial agent. The concentration of an antimicrobial drug required for effective activity against different microorganisms varies and these requirements could be met by varying the dose rate of the drug. However, this is an impractical situation and in practice one works from the recommended dose. The recommended dose is one that will give blood and tissue levels which will be effective against very susceptible organisms, with minimal side-effects to the host. In this respect the recommended dose should be considered as a minimal dose. If one is dealing with organisms that require higher concentrations of the drug for therapeutic effectiveness the recommended dose can be exceeded. With low toxicity antibacterials this dose may be exceeded several-fold and with drugs such as benzylpenicillin this is a frequent therapeutic ploy. However, with antibacterials that have toxic potential the recommended dose should only be exceeded with caution and frequently it is wise to search for a different antimicrobial agent to which the organism is more sensitive.

Similarly, the recommended dose may be exceeded in an attempt to increase the concentration gradient in sensitive infections where necrotic tissue produces long diffusion paths. The recommended dose may also be exceeded for managemental reasons as in the case of the treatment of sheep with footrot or mycotic dermatitis where a single treatment is required for practical purposes.

The recommended doses for the common antibacterials and potential toxicities are given later for each of the antibacterial agents in common use.

The recommended doses are based on our expectations for therapeutic efficiency, and may exceed the label dose recommendations for the drugs. The problem of persisting tissue residues should be recognized when label recommendations are exceeded, especially when large doses of antibiotics are given for particular therapeutic reasons. Recommendations for withdrawal periods should be adjusted accordingly.

Suggested dose levels and dose intervals for many of the antimicrobial agents used in large animals are frequently lower and longer than those suggested and used in small animals and man, possibly for reasons of cost. In many cases there are no obvious pharmacological reasons for this and in fact, several antimicrobial agents have significantly shorter half-lives and faster excretion rates in ruminants and horses than in dogs and man, and probably should be used at higher dose rates or at shorter dose intervals. Some estimate of the dose required for an antimicrobial drug can be obtained by a comparison of the minimal inhibitory concentrations required for activity against various organisms with the blood and tissue levels of the drug obtained at various dose levels. Usually levels three to five times the minimal inhibitory concentration are considered necessary for effective therapy, and it is generally considered desirable to maintain these levels over the treatment period, especially with bacteriostatic antimicrobials, although this is probably not essential. Unfortunately pharmacokinetic studies of antimicrobial agents in large animal species have been limited and it would appear that in many instances antimicrobials have been released for use in large animals with insufficient evaluation. The ultimate proof for dose levels and dose intervals of an antimicrobial is by clinical trials of its efficacy in the treatment of infectious disease. It is apparent that antimicrobial drugs are effective in many diseases in large animals at the dose rates and intervals currently in use. Nevertheless, as the results of pharmacokinetic studies in farm animals become available it is quite probable that they will suggest changes in the dose levels and intervals for several of the antimicrobial drugs in use, which may result in more efficacious therapy and a broader spectrum of activity against disease.

Routes of administration

Intravenous injection

Intravenously administered antibiotics attain high and immediate blood and tissue levels and this route should be used in the treatment of septicemias and other life-threatening diseases. The levels obtained are much higher than those obtained with equivalent doses of the same drug given intramuscularly or orally, and consequently greater diffusion concentrations are achieved at sites of infection. For this reason this route of administration may also be used in an attempt to increase the drug concentration in areas where the antibiotic normally achieves only low concentrations and where areas of necrosis increase the length of the diffusion pathway. Intravenous administration may also be indicated in chronic infections such as corynebacterial pneumonia in foals where high diffusion concentrations are required in order to penetrate the abscess areas and the capsular material of the organism. An initial intravenous loading dose may combat the development of stepwise resistant mutants. Due to the initial higher blood and tissue levels the intravenous route may also be used for the treatment of infections that are only moderately sensitive to the antibacterial drug being used. This is because effective concentrations may be achieved by repeated intravenous dosing which would not be achieved by equivalent doses given intramuscularly or orally.

For practical reasons the intravenous route of administration is used for low-concentration high-volume antimicrobial agents such as sulfamethazine and oxytetracycline. It is also preferred to the intramuscular route in racehorses where there is a need to avoid muscular soreness or damage, and in beef cattle close to marketing.

Administration by this route is not without its dangers. Acute toxic reactions either to the drug or to its vehicle are more common when intravenous administration is used. Drugs specifically formulated for intravenous use should be used, or the manufacturer's recommendations on the advisability of the use of this route for any preparation followed. Severely toxemic terminal cases may die immediately following injection, and in the owner's mind death may be attributed to the therapy.

Injections should be given slowly and not as a bolus. Therapy by repeated intravenous administration is generally restricted to hospital situations and can be expensive due to the added cost of the intravenous preparations. In field situations an initial intravenous loading dose followed by sustaining intramuscularly administered doses is frequently indicated in the treatment of infectious diseases and is sound therapeutic policy. The jugular vein is used in all species except the pig where the inaccessibility of superficial veins other than the ear veins makes this route of administration generally impractical. Perivascular reactions and intravascular thrombosis are a hazard with this route especially following the administration of irritant drugs such as sulfonamides and tetracyclines.

Intramuscular injection

Intramuscular injection is the most commonly used method for antimicrobial administration in large animals. Where possible its use should be avoided in meat-producing animals for the 3 weeks prior to marketing, especially with irritant preparations. With certain antibiotics, drug residues may persist at these sites for long periods, and the label recommendation for withdrawal or withholding time should be followed. Irritant drugs should be used with care in horses or avoided as this species more commonly develops severe reactions at the site of injection. The development of such reactions is usually an indication to change to alternative therapy. Oil-based vehicles frequently produce severe reactions at the site of injection in horses and should not be used in this species. The muscles of the hindlimbs are the most commonly used site for intramuscular injections in all species except horses where the neck muscles are used for reasons of safety. The neck may also be used in pigs to avoid blemish to the hams. There is evidence, for some antibiotics at least, that the site of intramuscular administration can influence the rate of absorption, the bioavailability and the subsequent pharmacokinetics of the administered antibiotic. In both cattle and horses, injection in the neck gives more favorable pharmacokinetic parameters than does injection into the gluteal or shoulder muscles (1–3). Injection into the dewlap gives the poorest bioavailability. These differences presumably result from differences in the spread of the injected drug within and between the muscles and differences in blood supply. With intermuscular spread there is a greater absorption area and less compromise of capillary and lymphatic structures (3). Injection into the side of the neck of horses is considered malpractice in some countries. When irritant preparations must be given to horses it is wise to inject them into the muscle of the chest between the forelegs, as reactions in this area have less tendency to spread and are more accessible to drainage and treatment. At all sites care should be taken to ensure the injection is not inadvertently given intravascularly by applying negative pressure to the syringe prior to injection. In adult animals no more than 20 ml should be given at any injection site. With most antimicrobial drugs, excepting the repository forms and drugs of an irritant nature, peak blood concentrations are obtained within 30 minutes to 2 hours of injection. However, the bioavailability of drugs given by intramuscular injection is markedly influenced by their formulation and irritant nature. This is especially marked with oxytetracycline preparations. Peak blood and tissue levels are obtained within the first 2 hours following injection.

Intraperitoneal injection

Intraperitoneal injection is occasionally used for antimicrobial administration, especially in feedlot cattle close to market size, and where intravenous administration for various reasons may be impractical. It is also occasionally used in pigs with diarrhea where the antibacterial drug is combined with fluids for rehydration. In cattle the injection is given in the right flank midway between the last rib and the tuber coxae and at least 10 cm ventral to the lateral processes of the lumbar vertebrae so as to avoid retroperitoneal and perirenal deposition of the drug. An aseptic injection technique should be used. Animals with peritonitis are also occasionally additionally treated by this route of injection. In horses with peritonitis the peritoneal cavity can be drained through a cannula inserted in the ventral midline as used for abdominal paracentesis, and the antimicrobial agent is injected via this route. Intraperitoneal injection may also be used for the parenteral administration of the tetracycline group in acutely toxemic animals or in animals with severe respiratory distress where intravenous injection may result in collapse and even death.

Subcutaneous injection

Subcutaneous injection is seldom used in large animal practice. Providing the drug is not deposited in a fat depot it is probable that this route provides a reasonable alternative to intramuscular injection (16). With irritant preparations there is a danger of excessive reaction and the occurrence of sterile abscesses. Very small animals (piglets) are often treated by this route.

Oral administration

Oral administration of antimicrobial agents is generally restricted to pre-ruminant animals, young foals and pigs The blood and tissue levels achieved following oral administration are considerably less than those achieved by an equivalent dose of the same antimicrobial agent given parenterally, and for this reason the oral dose rate is generally two to five times greater than the parenteral dose. Also they are less reliable because absorption characteristics may vary with the volume of ingesta, the presence or absence of gastric and intestinal stasis or hypermotility and the nature of the ingesta which variably bind the orally administered drug. For example, oxytetracycline, chloramphenicol and trimethoprim have a much lower bioavailability to calves when administered in milk rather than in water due to the high degree of binding to milk (4, 17). There is some evidence that the oral administration of antibiotics to calves in glucose–glycine–electrolyte solutions is associated with more favorable absorption characteristics (4). The aminoglycoside and polymyxin groups of antimicrobial agents are not absorbed from the alimentary tract and benzylpenicillin is largely destroyed within the stomach.

The oral route is the easiest method for administration, and where the cost of revisits is a significant consideration this route is often chosen for continuing medication as it is within the capability of any owner. In general, however, systemic infections are better treated by parenteral injection and certainly treatment should be initiated by this route. The oral route is the one of choice for the treatment of enteric infections. Experimental studies have shown that the oral administration of antibiotics to healthy neonatal calves may induce villous atrophy within the intestine and a malabsorption diarrhea (13). This occurred particularly with chloramphenicol and neomycin and to a lesser extent with tetracycline and ampicillin. Although this does not negate the use of antibiotics for specific therapy of enteritis in young calves (when this is indicated), it does suggest that prophylactic use of oral antibiotics has a risk in young calves. Field studies have shown an increased risk for scours in calves given chloramphenicol prophylactically (14).

Antimicrobial drugs are seldom given orally to ruminant animals. Exceptions are the use of sulfonamides, especially as sustaining medication following initial parenteral treatment and low-level antibiotic therapy to feedlot animals to reduce the incidence of liver abscess and respiratory disease. Blood levels following oral administration in ruminants are variable and frequently not achieved until 12–18 hours after dosing. Also many antibacterials are destroyed or inactivated within the rumen. Orally administered antimicrobials cause a significant disruption to the ruminal flora and by itself this may result in a syndrome of ruminal stasis, anorexia and depression. If antibacterial agents are given orally to ruminants the course should be followed by re-establishment of the ruminal flora by cud transfer.

The inadvertent feeding of antibiotics to cattle and horses can result in clinical disease and the cause may not be immediately apparent to the investigating clinician. This can occur when cattle and horses are fed medicated pig feed, but can also occur when regular rations become contaminated with antibiotics. Antibiotic contamination of rations is a potential problem in feed mills that process medicated and non-medicated feeds consecutively. Residual carryover of medicated material into other feedstuffs can occur with feed-mixers of various types and also via residues in conveyors, hoppers and trucks (5). Within 24 hours of being fed medicated feed dairy cattle show anorexia, rumen stasis and subsequently pass custard-consistency feces containing undigested fiber. There is a precipitous fall in milk production. Dullness, muscle fasciculation, ketosis, hypocalcemia and recumbency have also been observed. Affected cattle usually recover when placed on non-medicated feed, but milk production may be adversely affected for the remainder of the lactation. Feeds contaminated with dimetridazole. lincomycin and tylosin have been incriminated (6, 7), although there is debate as to the role of tylosin in this syndrome (8). The carryover of medicated material into other feeds can also create violative tissue residues at slaughter. Sulfonamide contamination of swine rations is a particular problem (9).

The use of orally administered antimicrobial agents in horses over 3 months of age should be approached with great care. Their use is frequently followed by diarrhea which is often intractable and results in chronic debilitation or death. Tetracyclines and lincomycin are especially dangerous.

The oral route is the most common and convenient one for group medication of pigs (10). The antibacterial agent may be incorporated in the water or in the feed. For the treatment of disease in pigs, water medication is preferred as sick pigs may drink, whereas they frequently will not eat. Also water medication can usually be started immediately whereas the mixing of an antibacterial agent with the diet for piggeries purchasing prepared diets may take 1 or 2 days. Antibiotic bioavailability is also less in pelleted feeds (15). Dietary medication is generally used for longterm disease control. In outbreaks of contagious disease in pigs, the sick pigs within the group are usually initially treated individually by parenteral injection followed by mass medication of the water supply. With pigs using troughs, water medication is no problem. However, with automatic watering systems, medication must be through the header tank if this can be isolated, or more commonly the water is turned off and medicated water is provided for the pigs via portable 200 liter drums with a drinking bowl or nipple drinker inserted in the side. For determining the concentration of antibiotic required in the water the total daily dose of the drug is computed by multiplying the total weight of the group of pigs in kg by the daily dose of the drug in mg/kg. This dose must then be added to the amount of water which will be consumed on one day. It is obvious that this amount will vary according to climatic conditions and to the nature of the disease in the pigs. For example, diarrheic pigs may drink more than normal quantities. In practice a rule of thumb of 10% of body weight for water consumption of pigs between weaning and market age has been found satisfactory with estimates of 15% for situations in which high water consumption can be expected. The total daily dose is thus added to the number of liters of water equivalent to 10–15% of the estimated total body weight of the group. In pregnant sows, water consumption is usually 5–8 liters/day, but lactating sows may drink 15–20 liters/day. When there is doubt as to the exact water consumption the medication can be added to the lower estimate and, when consumed, fresh water provided for the remainder of the day. Water medication is generally continued for a period of at least 5 days. Antibiotics may deteriorate rapidly in water and a fresh mix should be prepared each day.

There are some major limitations in the mass medication of water supplies of cattle. The daily amount of water consumed is usually directly proportional to the amount of dry matter intake. Anorexia or inappetence will result in a marked decrease in water intake to mere maintenance requirements. Depending on the drug used, the palatability of the medicated water may affect intake. With large drinking water tanks which are replenished on a continuous basis, or even two or three times daily, it is difficult to determine how much drug should be added on a daily basis in order to maintain a reasonably steady concentration. On a theoretical basis, automatic inline water medicators should provide a uniform concentration of drug in the water supply. However, some medicators are extremely unreliable and regular surveillance and servicing may be necessary. In countries where below-freezing temperatures occur during the winter months, the medication of water supplies may be difficult and impractical under certain management conditions.

The concentration of antibiotic to be added to feed for feed medication is calculated in a similar fashion. The total daily dose of antibacterial drug required for the group is calculated, and this amount must then be added to the amount of food consumed daily by the group. Daily feed consumption varies with the level of restricted feeding practiced and can generally be determined from the owner. A rule of thumb for food consumption is 5% of body weight from weaning to 45 kg body weight with a fall to as low as 2·5% at 90 kg, depending on the level of feed restriction during the fattening period. The ratio of daily amount of drug required to daily feed consumption is generally then adjusted to give the drug concentration in mg/kg of feed or more commonly to grams per metric tonne of feed. An alternate method is to use the drug manufacturer's recommendations of 'therapeutic levels for inclusion in feed' which is usually stated in grams per metric tonne. However, this method does not allow an adjustment of dose to cover moderately resistant organisms, nor is it suitable or sufficient for oral medication of sows where feed intake may vary from approximately 2 kg in dry sows to 7 kg in the same sow during lactation.

Prolonged oral medication may result in superinfection in all animal species. Commonly a yeast, staphylococci or *Pseudomonas aeruginosa* is involved. It occurs most commonly in calves given courses of differing antimicrobial agents. It is more common following medication involving tetracyclines or chloramphenicol and usually a treatment period of at least 2 weeks is required for its development.

Other routes

Other routes of administration may be used to increase the level of antibacterial drug in areas where diffusion following parenteral administration of the drug may be limited and when high local levels are required. These include intra-articular, intrapleural and subconjunctival injection. Non-irritant preparations should be used with strict aseptic technique. In most cases these treatments should be supported by parenteral treatment. The indications are described in the special medicine section. Intramammary infusion of drugs is dealt with under mastitis.

Intratracheal administration of antibiotics has its advocates for the treatment of pneumonia in cattle. In theory, this could result in higher levels of antibiotics at the site of infection, although with many pneumonias diffusion through the affected lung must be minimal. The antibiotics are administered in sterile physiologic saline equivalent to 2·0 ml/kg body weight. An extensive study has shown variation in absorption and persistence between antibiotics administered by this route, when compared to parenteral administration, but has concluded that there is no potentially useful advantage to its use (11).

The local administration of antibiotics may not always be the preferred route despite historical precedence. For example, in the treatment of the genital tract, it has been shown that parenteral administration of antibiotics achieves tissue concentrations of drug in all areas of the genital tract, whereas intrauterine infusion results in comparable concentrations only in the endometrium and uterine secretions. Local and/or parenteral administration may be indicated in different cases of genital tract infection (12).

REFERENCES

(1) Hoffman, B. et al. (1986) *Dtsch Tierarztl. Wochenschr.*, *93*, 310
(2) Nouws, J. M. & Vree, T. B. (1983). *Vet. Q.*, *5*, 165.
(3) Firth, E. C. et al. (1986) *Am. J. vet. Res.*, *47*, 2380.
(4) Palmer, C. H. et al. (1983) *Am. J. vet. Res.*, *44*, 68.
(5) Anon (1979) *Feed Management*, *30*, 22.
(6) Crossman, P. J. & Payser, M. R. (1981) *Vet. Rec.*, *108*, 285.
(7) Anon (1984) *Vet. Res.*, *114*, 5 and 132.
(8) MacKinnon, J. D. et al. (1984) *Vet. Rec.*, *115*, 278.
(9) Rosenburg, M. C. (1985) *J. Am. vet. med. Assoc.*, *187*, 704.
(10) Walton, J. R. (1980) *In Pract.*, *2(6)*, 29.
(11) Hjerpe, C. A. (1979) *Bov. Pract.*, *14*, 18.
(12) Gustafsson, B. K. (1984) *J. Am. vet. med. Assoc.*, *185*, 1194.
(13) Mero, K. N. et al. (1985) *Vet. Clin. N. Am. food Anim. Pract.*, *1(3)*, 581.
(14) Waltner-Toews, D. et al. (1986) *Can. vet. J.*, *27*, 17.
(15) Mevius, D. J. et al. (1986) *Vet. Q.*, *8*, 274.
(16) Gilman, J. M. et al. (1987) *J. vet. Pharmacol. Therap.*, *10*, 101.
(17) Groothuis, D. G. & van Miert, A. S. J. P. A. M. (1987) *Vet. Q.*, *9*, 91.

Drug distribution

Antibiotics of the aminoglycoside group (streptomycin, neomycin etc.) and polymyxins are not absorbed from the alimentary tract and if circulating levels of these antibiotics are required they must be given by parenteral injection. Where both intestinal and systemic levels are required, as may be the case in neonatal colibacillosis, these drugs should be given both orally and parenterally. Benzylpenicillin and methicillin are destroyed by acid pH and significant blood levels are not achieved following oral administration. Certain sulfonamides (phthalylsulfathiazole, phthalylsulfacetamide, sulfaguanidine and succinyl sulfathiazole) are not absorbed from the alimentary tract. The remaining antibiotics and sulfonamides are absorbed following oral administration in pre-ruminant calves and lambs and in pigs and horses. However, in general, blood and tissue levels obtained are considerably lower than those achieved with equivalent doses given parenterally.

Factors governing the distribution of antimicrobial agents in the body fluids are complex, and distribution should be considered as involving a multicompartmental system with all body compartments being in contact directly or indirectly with the blood. The occurrence of exchange, and its rate, between the blood and the various tissue compartments is governed by the factors that influence the diffusion of solutes, such as the concentration of the drug and the volume of blood flow through the tissues and the volume of the tissue. It is also considerably influenced by the extent of protein binding of the drug in blood and in the tissues, the ionization constant of the drug, and pH differences in the compartments, and the lipid solubility of the drug. Drug distribution is also influenced by age and by the disease state of the animal. In most clinical therapeutic situations infection occurs in the extravascular tissue compartments and it is the concentration of the unbound drug at these sites that determines the efficacy of therapy. However, unfortunately, the experimental determination of drug concentration of these sites is extremely difficult and expensive and the majority of pharmacokinetic studies of antimicrobial agents in large animals have simply studied the kinetic behavior of the drug in blood. This gives only limited information. There may be significant differences in the tissue distribution of different antimicrobials within the same general group and also between different groups of antimicrobials. There may also be considerable interspecies differences in the distribution of the same antimicrobial agent and in its persistence in any one area. Unfortunately, for large animal species, information of this type is very sparse and where information is lacking one must assume, probably erroneously, that a given drug has the same pharmacokinetic properties in food-producing animals as those in small animals and man. The majority of antibiotics diffuse relatively freely in extracellular fluids but sulfonamides, tetracyclines and chloramphenicol have a distribution that more closely approximates total body water, and they can enter cells. There are several so-called barriers to antimicrobial diffusion and these include the brain and CSF, serous cavities, joints and synovial fluid, the eye and the placenta and fetus. In general sulfonamides, tetracyclines and chloramphenicol have some ability to penetrate these barriers in the normal state, whereas penicillin may not. Erythromycin has the ability to penetrate intracellularly and across most barriers but will not produce effective levels in the brain or CSF. Members of the aminoglycoside group of antibiotics generally achieve effective levels in synovial fluid and the pleural and peritoneal fluid but not in the brain or eye. The importance of these barriers, especially those of serous cavities and synovia, in the presence of inflammation is open to doubt and effective therapy can often be achieved by the use of antibiotics that do not in normal situations reach these areas unless they are inflamed. An exception to this rule is infections involving the eyes where, in order to achieve effective levels, high circulating levels of the antimicrobial agent are required and intravenous injection to achieve this is usually necessary. Lipophilic drugs diffuse into tears and parenterally administered chloramphenicol, erythromycin, oxytetracycline and gentamicin, for example, may achieve bacteriostatic concentrations in tears. In many areas, especially joints, and the peritoneal, pleural and pericardial cavities, high levels of the required antimicrobial agent can be achieved by local administration.

Almost all antimicrobial agents are excreted via the kidney, and the urine usually contains high levels of them. This feature is not of great significance in large animals where urinary tract infections are comparatively rare. Penicillins and tetracyclines have a significant enterohepatic cycle, and erythromycin also may obtain significant levels in bile. The duration of effective levels following a single dose is given for each antimicrobial agent later in this chapter.

REVIEW LITERATURE

Baggot, J. D. (1977) *Principles of Drug Distribution in Domestic Animals*. Philadelphia: W. B. Saunders.

Baggot, J. D. (1984) Factors involved in the choice of routes of administration of antimicrobial drugs. *J. Am. vet. med. Assoc.*, *185*, 1076–1082.

Koritz, G. D. (1984) Relevance of peak and trough concentrations to antimicrobial therapy. *J. Am. vet. med. Assoc.*, 185, 1072–1075.

Short, C. R. & Clark, C. R. (1984) Calculation of dosage regimens of antimicrobial drugs for the neonatal patient. *J. Am. vet. med. Assoc.*, *185*, 1088–1093.

Duration of treatment

For certain infectious diseases there is an established regimen of therapy which is known from clinical experience to be therapeutically effective, and where these are known they are stated in the treatment section for the individual diseases in the special medicine section As a rule of thumb in undifferentiated diseases therapy should be continued for a 3–5-day period, or longer if there is evidence of chronic infectious disease with localization. An alternative rule of thumb is that treatment should be continued for at least one day beyond the return of body temperature to normal, especially if bacteriostatic antibiotics are being used. Chronic pyogenic processes may require treatment for a 2–4-week period or even longer.

Drug combinations

Combinations of antimicrobial drugs are frequently used in veterinary practice and many mixtures are available commercially as fixed-dose combinations. In general, combinations of antimicrobial agents are used either to achieve a synergistic effect in the case of a single infection, or to achieve a broad spectrum of activity in the case of infections involving more than one agent. Combinations may also be of value in combatting the emergence of resistant mutants during therapy. The combination of two drugs may result in indifference, where the effect is either that of the single most effective drug or is equal to the sum of the effects of the two individual drugs, or it may result in synergism or antagonism (1). There are, however, no hard and fast rules for combinations that will result in any of these effects. Knowledge of these effects results largely from laboratory animal studies and from some human therapeutic trials. From these trials it is evident that the occurrence of synergism is very much dependent on the type of infectious organism, and to some extent the site of infection, and whereas two drugs may show a synergistic effect with one type of infection, the effect may be indifferent or even occasionally antagonistic with other infective agents (1). Antagonism is equally not easily predictable but the drugs which most commonly result in antagonistic effect when combined with others are the tetracycline group, chloramphenicol and the macrolide groups.

In general it can be stated that combinations of bactericidal drugs will generally result in an indifferent effect or in synergism; combinations of bacteriostatic drugs generally give an indifferent effect, whereas combinations of a bactericidal with a bacteriostatic drug may result in antagonism (Table 12). In farm animals, syn-

Table 12. Mode of action of antimicrobial drugs

Group 1: bactericidal	*Group 2: bacteriostatic*
Penicillins	All sulfonamides
Benzylpenicillin	Tetracyclines
Methicillin	Macrolides
Cloxacillin	Erythromycin
Ampicillin	Oleandomycin
Amoxycillin	Spiramycin
Carbenicillin	Tylosin
etc.	Carbomycin
Aminoglycosides	Chloramphenicol
Streptomycin	Lincomycin
Kanamycin	Trimethoprim
Neomycin	
Gentamicin	
Paromomycin	
Polymyxins	
Cephalosporins	
Vancomycin	
Bacitracin	
Novobiocin	
Nitrofurans	

ergistic activity between penicillin and streptomycin has been demonstrated in the therapy of mycotic dermatitis and footrot in sheep. Carbenicillin and gentamicin in combination can be of value in therapy against *Pseudomonas aeruginosa*, *Klebsiella* and *Proteus* spp., and tylosin and oxytetracycline can be of value in treating infection with *Pasteurella* spp. Trimethoprim and sulfonamide combinations are of special value in treating several infectious diseases in large animals. Rifampin and erythromycin show *in vitro* synergism against *Corynebacterium* (*Rhodococcus*) *equi* as does a combination of gentamicin and penicillin. Tiamutilin and tetracycline show *in vitro* synergism against several swine respiratory pathogens and herd studies show a measured response in the control of respiratory disease greater than that achieved by chlortetracycline alone (3).

Drug combinations are also used for broad-spectrum therapy. An accurate diagnosis with consequent recognition of the likely infectious organism allows specific antibacterial therapy, and obviates the need for broad-spectrum antibacterial therapy. However, there are clinical situations where broad-spectrum therapy including the possibility of combined drug therapy is indicated. These include such problems as the acute septicemias where a number of different organisms, with differing antibacterial sensitivities, can produce identical clinical disease, and those infections caused by organisms that have a varying sensitivity depending upon the isolate. The requirement for immediate treatment without knowledge of the bacterial sensitivity dictates the use of antimicrobial drugs designed to obtain a broad spectrum of activity. The availability of broad-spectrum drugs such as ampicillin or amoxycillin and trimethoprim-potentiated sulfonamides has lessened the need to use drug combinations but they may still be necessary in certain situations and are fully indicated. Although antagonism has not been demonstrated in clinical veterinary situations it is wise to avoid bacteriostatic and bactericidal drug combinations.

Other indications for the use of drug combinations include such factors as cost where a course of combined penicillin–streptomycin therapy, for example, is usually less costly than one with a broad-spectrum antibiotic such as oxytetracycline or ampicillin. Also, drug combinations may be less toxic at high doses than some broad-spectrum antibiotics such as tetracycline.

Where combinations of antibacterial drugs are used they should be given individually and at their respective recommended doses and repeats. Some antibiotics are physically incompatible when mixed together. The incompatibility may rest with the drugs or their vehicles and may be visible, as with crystalline benzylpenicillin and neomycin, or it may be inapparent as with gentamicin and carbenicillin. The two drugs should be given separately at separate sites. Incompatibilities can also occur with antibiotics and intravenous fluid solutions—especially those containing protein hydrolysates. Fixed-dose combinations have little to recommend them (2) as they suffer from the deficiency that the dose level of any one of the drugs in the combination is dictated by the level of the other. It is therefore not possible to increase the dose rate of one individual drug of the combination without increasing the other and this may have undesirable toxic effects and adds to the cost of treatment. Also the excretion rates of the two drugs may be markedly different. The most common of these, fixed dose procaine penicillin/streptomycin combinations, suffer from this deficiency where the effective therapeutic levels of the penicillin following a given dose may last for 24 hours whereas that of the streptomycin is generally only 8–12 hours.

Antibiotics may influence the activity of other drugs. In particular chloramphenicol and tetracyclines inhibit liver microsomal metabolism and may significantly increase the half-life of drugs metabolized by this mechanism, such as digitalis or barbiturates, with resultant potential toxicity.

REVIEW LITERATURE

Reilly, P. E. B. & Issacs, J. P. (1983) Adverse drug interactions of importance in veterinary practice. *Vet. Rec.*, *112*, 29–33.

REFERENCES

(1) Iowetz, E. (1975) *Vet. Clin. N. Am.*, *5*, 35.
(2) Parker, B. N. J. (1976) *Vet. Bull.*, *46*, 83.
(3) Burch, D. G. S. et al. (1986) *Vet. Rec.*, *119*, 108.

Additional factors determining the selection of an antimicrobial agent for therapy

In addition to the considerations of bacterial sensitivity to the antimicrobial agent there are other important factors that dictate the selection of the antimicrobial agent to be used in a particular case. In most clinical situations several agents would be effective and a choice needs to be made amongst them.

Cost

This is a major factor and includes not only the primary cost of the drug but also the ancillary costs that may be associated with its administration. This is a most important factor in agricultural animals but of less importance with pleasure horses. The importance of the primary cost of the drug is obvious. For example, in most countries a 5 day course of treatment with procaine benzylpenicillin will cost considerably less than one with, for example, oxytetracycline. If there is no specific indication for the use of the more expensive drug then the less expensive one should be used. The ancillary costs associated with administration of the drug may also be important. The decision to treat an animal with parenterally administered antibiotics for a 3 day period may in certain circumstances require revisits for the repeat treatments with mileage and other costs for each visit. Equivalent efficacy may well be obtained with sulfamethazine by an initial intravenous injection followed by subsequent oral treatments given by the owner. The practice of dispensing drugs for continuing intramuscular therapy varies between countries and veterinary practices and has an influence on this consideration.

Ease of administration
This is a further factor that influences the nature of the drug and treatment used. In general, one avoids starting a course of therapy with an antibacterial such as tetracycline which may require daily intravenous administration, in favor of one which can be administered more simply unless there are good therapeutic reasons for choosing the former. In situations where facilities are poor, where mustering or yarding is difficult, or where mass medication is required, long-acting repository preparations may be indicated. Irritant preparations are avoided where possible.

Toxicity
This is always a consideration when dealing with infections that may require high dose rates of antimicrobial drugs, or in chronic infections that require a prolonged course of therapy. Where a choice is available antimicrobial agents with a low incidence of toxic side-effects at high doses are chosen. There is comparatively little information of the toxicity of antimicrobial agents in large animal species. The potential toxicities which may be seen in practice are mentioned under each antimicrobial agent.

As in all clinical situations involving large animals it is essential to make an assessment of the case and to attempt a prognosis. The possible cost and duration of treatment should be estimated and the owner advised of this. When examined in this light the decision may be against treatment and for salvage slaughter.

Bactericidal or bacteriostatic antimicrobials
Antibiotics are either primarily bactericidal in their activity whereas others are bacteriostatic (see Table 12). Some of the bactericidal group are bacteriostatic at low concentration but bactericidal at higher concentrations. Both classes rely on intact and effective body defense mechanisms for full effect. Although in terms of clinical response little if any difference can be detected between the two groups in most diseases, in certain situations it is probably advisable to choose a bactericidal antibiotic for therapy. This is especially true when dealing with acute septicemic infection where there is frequently a significant leukopenia, and quick maximal bactericidal effect is required. There is also the need to prevent subsequent localization. Bactericidal antimicrobials are also indicated for antibacterial treatment of secondary infection in agranulocytopenic syndromes such as bracken fern poisoning or chronic furazolidone poisoning in calves. Bactericidal antibiotics are also preferable in the treatment of heavily capsulated organisms such as *Klebsiella* spp. and *Corynebacterium (Rhodococcus) equi* which show antiphagocytic activity. Infections in which significant intracellular parasitism occurs are a problem. The majority of antimicrobials that diffuse relatively freely into cells are bacteriostatic in activity and although the disease may be controlled by their use, infection may still persist in a latent carrier state.

Drug deterioration

Many antibacterials lose their activity rapidly when kept under adverse conditions. Quality control in terms of purity, efficacy and freedom from toxicity costs money but for these reasons it is preferable to purchase from known reputable companies and follow their recommendations with respect to storage and expiry periods. The use of cheap antibacterial preparations, often purchased in bulk and simply packaged, and distributed with little consideration for factors influencing drug stability, often results in poor therapeutic results. Crystalline or dry preparations which require reconstitution to a solution before parenteral administration are frequently presented this way because their activity degenerates rapidly once they are in solution. Therefore once they have been prepared they should be used immediately or the manufacturer's recommendations followed regarding storage and length of activity following reconstitution. Temperature and exposure to sunlight can be important factors in antibiotic stability and become important in farm ambulatory practice where car cold boxes should be used to store antibiotic preparations and other sensitive drugs.

Unfavorable response to therapy

In clinical cases that do not respond to antimicrobial therapy the initial consideration should be that the wrong antimicrobial agent has been chosen for therapy. This is especially true of infectious conditions of undertermined etiology where the drug has been chosen on the basis of an educated guess. In these circumstances adequate time should be given for an evaluation of the efficacy of the treatment before a change is made. In general a 3-day period of treatment is allowed for this evaluation provided there is no marked deterioration in the clinical state, or further elevation of temperature during this period. If there is no response to initial therapy then in the case of conditions of undetermined etiology it is generally best to change to an entirely different class of antimicrobial agent. However, the possibility of viral or non-infectious etiology should always be considered in these cases and the case and diagnosis should be reviewed before this change.

In any situation where there is a poor response to therapy the usual causes of this failure should be considered in any further adjustments to therapy or future therapy of similar cases. The first and most obvious of these is that the organism is either insensitive to the drug, or that it is not susceptible to the level of the drug that is being used for therapy. There are two possible approaches. The first is to increase the dose rate and dose frequency, and/or to change the route of administration so that higher and possibly effective levels will be achieved, bearing in mind the possible toxic consequences. The second and safer approach is to change the antimicrobial agent being used. This problem can be avoided if the organism and its potential sensitivity can be identified, either by clinical examination or by appropriate sampling with culture and sensitivity testing. The development of resistance during antimicrobial treatment of an individual animal is not a recognized problem in large animal medicine.

Another common cause of poor response is that the infection is situated in an area to which the drug is poorly accessible. If this is associated with an area behind a barrier to the entry of the antibiotic such as the joints or the eye it may be necessary to resort to higher dose rates and frequency, or intravenous administration of the drug, or to ancillary local treatment into this area. Alternatively another drug with superior penetrability may be used.

Organisms must be actively metabolizing in order for antimicrobial agents to exert their effect. This feature can result in poor response to therapy or relapse following discontinuation of therapy in chronic infections such as endocarditis or where there is excessive necrotic or fibrotic tissue associated with the infection. In these instances dormant organisms and the long diffusion tracks make effective cure difficult and high antimicrobial levels sustained over longer periods are required. In purulent conditions surgical drainage where possible is an essential adjunct to antimicrobial therapy.

The importance of ancillary and supportive therapy to counteract the effects of shock, toxemia and dehydration that may be associated with infection cannot be overemphasized and frequently such therapy may markedly influence the outcome of a case. It is obvious, for example, that 3 ml of antibiotic will do little to counter the effects of a 4 liter fluid deficit in a scouring calf.

Drug withdrawal requirements

In many countries there are requirements for the withdrawal of antimicrobial agents from the feed for specified periods prior to slaughter, and animals or their milk cannot be marketed for certain periods following antimicrobial therapy. Antibiotic contamination of food products can be a public health risk. An example would be allergic reactions to antibiotic residues—particularly penicillin. There are also commercial considerations where residues of antibiotics in milk can cause considerable problems in the manufacture of milk products. Effects on starter cultures for cheese and yoghurt can be particularly deleterious and can result in downgrading or total loss of large quantities of manufacturing milk. As important is the need to maintain the wholesomeness of meat and milk products, and to support the consumer demand for drug-free meat and milk. The purpose of withdrawal requirements is to ensure that meat and milk for human consumption are free of drug contamination.

A withdrawal period is the time when the animal must be held free of the drug before it can be marketed so as to allow the drug to be eliminated from the tissues. In the case of milk, the term withholding period is commonly used and states that period that milk cannot be sent for human consumption following the treatment of the animal with a drug so as to allow any residues in milk to be eliminated before it is placed on the market. It is obvious that the required withdrawal periods and withholding periods will vary between antimicrobial agents and also with the same antimicrobial agent depending upon the amount of drug given, and factors such as age and the disease state of the animal. Unfortunately, the required withdrawal and withholding periods to ensure freedom of food products from drug contamination are not known for the various antimicrobials at varying dose concentrations and dose intervals—nor are they likely to be known in the near future. In many countries this has lead to regulations that limit the quantity of antibiotics in drug products and that require label instructions explaining product usage and drug withdrawal times. These label instructions include what is generally called the label dose. The label dose (and dose interval) is a dose of an antimicrobial for which the specific withdrawal and withholding periods have been established and these are stated in conjunction with the label dose. The label dose is the officially approved or legal dose rate for that drug. *When an antimicrobial is used it is incumbent upon the practitioner to notify the owner than the animal cannot be marketed (or milk sent for human consumption) before the accompanying withdrawal (or withholding) period has expired. The practitioner may be legally liable if a violation occurs and this notification has not been given.* It is the intention that the label dose be one that is therapeutically effective for that drug. However, this is not always the case and the label dose should not be confused with the term 'recommended dose' as used elsewhere in this chapter.

There are also circumstances where, although the label dose may be therapeutically efficient in most cases, it is not for the particular case in hand. In these situations, antimicrobial drugs may need to be used at dose concentrations and dose intervals different from the label dose. This *extra-label* use of the drug may be therapeutically necessary for the successful treatment of the problem, but it is not officially approved and the establishment of the required withdrawal period is entirely incumbent upon the veterinarian. The withdrawal period in these circumstances cannot always be extrapolated from that for the label dose. Label dose withdrawal periods are determined from pharmacokinetic studies of excretion following administration of the label dose. However, the rate of drug elimination from the body can be influenced by drug dose and dose frequency. For example, the metabolism and excretion half-life of sulfonamides in cattle is dose-dependent. With repeated dosing of antibiotics such as tetracycline and the aminoglycosides there is deposition of the antibiotic in certain tissues and following cessation of drug administration there is a slow release from these tissues and a long washout period (1–4). During this washout period there are decreasing concentrations of the drug in tissues and in milk which, although not of therapeutic importance, are sufficiently high to be violative. This presents a dilemma to the veterinarian trying to establish withdrawal periods. The occurrence of significant washout periods following prolonged therapy with antibiotics has only recently been recognized and there is little data on their duration at different dose concentrations and dose frequencies. Computer-based data information banks with easy access are being established to resolve this dilemma (5). Currently the only way to ensure non-violation with extra-label use of antimicrobials is to test for residues. Tests such as the Delvotest-P and disk assay tests based on inhibition of growth of *Bacillus stearothermophilus* var. *calidolactes* or monoclonal antibody-base tests, are commercially available, rapidly performed and easily used in a practice laboratory (6, 7).

In most countries meat and milk is tested for antibiotic residues at frequent intervals by regulatory authorities and violations are likely to be detected. The concentrations for the various antibiotics that are violative are not stated in this chapter for two reasons. First, they vary from country to country (8). Second, the violative concentrations tend to be set by the sensitivity of the detection assay used by the regulatory authority and as assay technology improves legally acceptable minimal concentrations will be lowered. Local regulatory publications should be consulted for current requirements.

Antibiotic residues and violations may occur as the result of the selection of an inadequate withdrawal period following extra-label use of an antimicrobial. They may also occur with treatment modalities where they may not be considered as a risk. The local infusion of antibiotic solutions into the uterus of cows may result in circulating concentrations of antibiotic and residues in body tissues and in milk. This results from the absorption of the antibiotic through the endometrium and from the peritoneal cavity following passage through the fallopian tubes (9). Similarly, following infusion of antibiotic solutions into one-quarter of the udder, low concentrations of the antibiotic can occur in milk secreted from the remaining quarters.

In a retrospective study of reasons for the presence of violative antibiotic residues in milk (8) failure to withhold milk for the full withdrawal period and accidental inclusion of treated milk in the shipment were the most common. Accidental inclusion of treated milk can occur when there is inadequate identification of treated cows. The veterinarian should work with the producer to establish a system that easily identifies cows whose milk is subject to a withholding period. Colored leg markers are one system and are immediately seen by the milker.

Contamination of recorder jars and milking equipment with the high concentration of antibiotic secreted in milk in the first milking after treatment is a further reason for residue violations. Treated cows should be milked last and in large dairies are preferably kept separate as a hospital string. Other reasons for residue violations include: short dry periods where dry cow therapy has been used; the accidental milking of dry cows where the latter are not kept as a separate group; the withholding of milk from only treated quarters; and the use of dry cow infusion preparations for treatments during lactation (8).

In meat-producing animals tissue residues and violation can occur with individual animals that have been marketed after treatment with an inadequate withdrawal period. However, by far the more important problem is tissue residues resulting from antibiotic inclusions in feeds for growth promotion and disease control purposes. Non-observance of the required withdrawal period can result in the rejection of market batches of animals with a substantial financial loss to producers. If feed inclusions have been for the purposes of medication the prescribing veterinarian may be liable if adequate information on withdrawal periods has not been given. In the swine industry, there is also a potential problem with sulfonamide residues resulting from carryover of sulfonamides from medicated to non-medicated feeds at the feed mill. Carryover concentrations of sulfamethazine (sulfadimidine) of greater than 2 g/tonne in the finisher ration can result in violative residues in the liver at slaughter (10). The use of granular forms of sulfamethazine markedly reduces the potential for carryover (11).

Whenever possible, approved antimicrobials should be used at label dose for therapy in order to comply with regulatory requirements and to minimize the possibility of antibiotic residues in meat and milk. It may be necessary to use non-approved antimicrobial drugs in certain circumstances and in minor species. The use of an approved antibiotic in a minor species for which it is not approved constitutes an extra-label use of the drug. The legality of the use of unapproved drugs, or of approved drugs in minor species for which they are not approved, is questionable. If such use is contemplated it is probably wise to have culture and sensitivity data indicating that the use of the unapproved drug is therapeutically necessary. Certain non-approved antibiotics are totally banned for use in food-producing animals in some countries (such as chloramphenicol in the United States) and local regulations should be followed.

REVIEW LITERATURE

Bevill, R. F. (1984) Factors influencing the occurrence of drug residues in animal tissues after the use of antimicrobial agents. *J. Am. vet. med. Assoc.*, *185*, 1124.

Bishop, J. R. & White, C. H. (1984) Antibiotic residue detection in milk—a review. *J. Food Pract.*, *47*, 647.

Bishop, J. R. et al. (1984) Retention data for antibiotics commonly used for bovine infections. *J. dairy Sci.*, *67*, 437.

REFERENCES

(1) Nouws, J. F. M. et al. (1986) *Am. J. vet. Res.*, *47*, 642.
(2) Brown, S. A. et al. (1986) *Am. J. vet. Res.*, *47*, 789.
(3) Haddad, N. A. et al. (1987) *Am. J. vet. Res.*, *48*, 21.
(4) Toutain, P. L. & Raynaud, J. P. (1983) *Am. J. vet. Res.*, *44*, 1203.
(5) Sundlof, S. F. et al. (1986) *J. Vet. Pharmacol. Therap.*, *9*, 237.
(6) Bishop, J. R. et al. (1985) *J. dairy Sci.*, *68*, 3031.
(7) Ryan, J. J. et al. (1986) *J. dairy Sci.*, *69*, 1510.
(8) Booth, J. M. & Harding F. (1986) *Vet. Rec.*, *119*, 565.
(9) Ayliffe, T. R. & Noakes, D. E. (1986) *Vet. Rec.*, *118*, 243.
(10) Ashworth, R. B. et al. (1986) *Am. J. vet. Res.*, *47*, 2596.
(11) Rosenburg, M. C. (1985) *J. Am. vet. med. Assoc.*, *187*, 704.

ANTIMICROBIAL DRUGS

Although there is a large number of proprietary preparations available for therapy they represent a comparatively small number of groups of antimicrobial agents. For practical purposes it is easier to consider antimicrobial agents in these groups, because the broad pharmacokinetic properties and antimicrobial activities tend to be similar for member drugs within a group. Specific individual drug characteristics can be identified subsequently. Also if resistance to an organism is exhibited by a given antimicrobial agent it is, in most cases, sounder to attempt therapy with a drug from an unrelated group rather than to continue medication with other drugs within the same group. For general therapeutic purposes most practitioners attempt to achieve familiarity with one or two members in each group but for specific diseases they adhere to specific recommendations for individual drugs (Table 13).

Detailed pharmacokinetic studies for many of the antimicrobial agents are not available for large animals, and the large animal practitioner must assume that distribution and excretion characteristics are the same as in small animals and man. In many cases this is unlikely to be true. The recommended doses and dose intervals given below are based in part on pharmacokinetic studies in large animals where these are available. They are also heavily based on recommendations and results from clinical usage.

REVIEW LITERATURE

Brumbaugh, G. W. (1987) Rational selection of antimicrobial drugs for treatment of infection in horses. *Vet. Clin. N. Am., equ. Pract.*, *3(1)*, 191–220.

White, N. A. (1986) Symposium on antibiotics. *Proc. 32nd Ann. Conv. Am. Assoc., equ. Pract.*, 165–250.

Sulfonamides

The sulfonamides were the first group of antimicrobial agents available for chemotherapy of infectious disease. The progressive availability and promotion of an increasingly large number of antibiotics, many of which have more specific activity and greater ease of administration, has markedly reduced the use of sulfonamides in large animal practice and frequently they appear not even to be considered in the initial choice of an antimicrobial agent for therapy. The specificity of the activity of some antibiotics commends their use, but sulfonamides still have considerable value in the treatment of infectious disease in large animals, especially in food-producing animals. They are of proven efficacy in many diseases and members of the group can provide low-cost, effective therapy. Because of this they are still frequently the drugs of choice in the treatment of susceptible conditions in large animals, and the advent of the newer potentiated sulfonamides has further entrenched their position as effective antimicrobials. Sulfonamides are also more stable than antibiotics to the environmental fluctuations that occur in ambulatory dispensaries.

There are a large number of sulfonamides available for therapeutic use. The major differences between members of the group are in their absorption and excretion rates, their distribution and availability in active form within the body, and in their potential toxicity. Although there are some quantitative differences between members of the group in their activity against organisms there are only minor qualitative differences and the spectrum of activity of different sulfonamides can generally be considered to be the same. Some individual sulfonamides are promoted as having greater activity against certain sensitive organisms than other members of the group, i.e. sulfochloropyridazine and coliform organisms. Bacterial resistance to one sulfonamide implies resistance to the others and if this is encountered no sulfonamide should be used for therapy. Sulfonamides are bacteriostatic in activity and act by competitive inhibition. They are structurally related to *para*-aminobenzoic acid (PABA) which is required by most microorganisms for the production of folic acid for the subsequent synthesis of purines and nucleic acids. Sulfonamides compete with PABA and form non-functional analogs of folic acid. They are more effective at higher concentrations in achieving competitive inhibition and are less active or non-active in media that contain high concentrations of PABA, such as pus. The action of sulfonamides may be potentiated by benzylpyrimidines such as trimethoprim which inhibit the activity of bacterial dihydrofolic acid reductase and produce a sequential blocking of this metabolic pathway to effect a marked synergistic activity. Sulfonamides exhibit a broad spectrum of activity and are effective against most Gram-positive and many Gram-negative organisms. Coliform organisms with the exception of *Proteus* and *Pseudomonas* may be susceptible and there is also activity against chlamydia and some protozoa. Sulfonamides are of value in the control of coccidiosis. *In vitro* sensitivity is frequently a poor guide to therapeutic response.

Individual sulfonamides vary markedly in solubility, and absorption from the gut following oral administration varies. Some sulfonamides are not absorbed in any appreciable quantity and are given orally for local intestinal chemotherapy. Sulfonamides are usually given intravenously when administered parenterally because of their alkaline reaction and the large volume which is necessary to achieve adequate dose rates. Frequently these cannot be practically achieved by subcutaneous or intramuscular injection and schedules that recommend these routes of injection should be examined because they frequently recommend an inadequate dose. The sodium salt is usually used for parenteral administration of sulfonamides.

Sulfonamides are widely distributed throughout the body although the extent of penetration varies with individual sulfonamides. Activity is present in blood and extracellular fluid and also they penetrate intracellularly. Sulfonamides are able to cross physiological barriers and significant levels are present in synovial fluid, the serous cavities, the fetus, the CSF, and in milk, especially in mastitic glands. In cattle, tissue levels are generally lower than those of blood with most sulfonamides (1). The degree of activity depends upon the blood level, the extent of protein binding and the degree of acetylation.

Table 13. Recommended guidelines for the use of antimicrobial drugs in the treatment of etiologically undefined infections

Species	*Disease*	*Drug order of choice* First	*Drug order of choice* Second
All	Fever of unknown origin	Sulfadimidine or trimethoprim/sulfonamide	Benzylpenicillin and streptomycin or ampicillin or tetracycline (not horse)
	Prophylactic treatment of injured animals	Benzylpenicillin and streptomycin	
	Cystitis or urinary infections	Ampicillin or sulfonamide	Benzylpenicillin or gentamicin or erythromycin
Horse	Neonatal septicemia	Ampicillin or trimethoprim/sulfonamide	Benzylpenicillin + gentamicin or chloramphenicol or rolitetracycline
	Neonatal ophthalmitis	Chloramphenicol	Lincomycin or sulfacetamide
	Acute undifferentiated diarrhea	Ampicillin (parenteral)	Chloramphenicol (parenteral) or gentamicin or nitrofurans (orally)
	Chronic undifferentiated diarrhea	None recommended	Iodochlorhydroxyquin
	Acute hepatitis	Ampicillin	
	Pleurisy	Ampicillin	Trimethoprim/sulfonamide
	Acute undifferentiated upper respiratory tract infection	Benzylpenicillin	Trimethoprim/sulfonamide
	Pneumonia of foals	Benzylpenicillin or erythromycin + rifampin	Trimethoprim/sulfonamide or penicillin + gentamicin
Cattle	Neonatal septicemia	Ampicillin or trimethoprim/sulfonamide	Benzylpenicillin + neomycin or chloramphenicol
	Acute undifferentiated diarrhea of calves	Nifuraldezone or neomycin (parenteral and oral) or amoxycillin	Trimethoprim/sulfonamide or gentamicin
	Subacute calf diarrhea	Neomycin (oral) or amoxycillin	Nitrofurans or gentamicin
	Undifferentiated acute diarrhea of adult cattle	Sulfadimidine	Ampicillin or nitrofurans
	Peritonitis	Sulfadimidine	Trimethoprim/sulfonamide
	Acute undifferentiated pneumonia of calves	Trimethoprim/sulfonamide or tetracycline	Penethamate penicillin or chloramphenicol
	Acute undifferentiated pneumonia of adult cattle	Tetracycline	Sulfonamide
	Pinkeye	Chloramphenicol	Tetracycline
	Acute mastitis	Tetracyclines or chloramphenicol or gentamicin	Sulfonamide or trimethoprim/sulfonamide
Pig	Neonatal septicemia	Chloramphenicol	Trimethoprim/sulfonamide
	Acute undifferentiated diarrhea of		
	Piglets	Ampicillin or trimethoprim/sulfonamide	Neomycin or sulfonamide or chloramphenicol
	Weanlings	Nitrofurans	Sulfonamide or gentamicin
	Acute undifferentiated pneumonia	Tetracycline	Tylosin or spiramycin or trimethoprim/sulfonamide
Sheep	Acute mastitis with toxemia	Spiramycin or erythromycin	Sulfadimidine
	Drenching or dipping pneumonia	'Triple' penicillin	
	Pneumonia	Tetracycline	Tylosin or spiramycin

Recommendations for the antimicrobial therapy of etiologically undefined infections are always subject to considerable debate. The choice of drug will depend on (1) the history and epidemiological findings, (2) knowledge of bacterial statistics (their likely occurrence and drug sensitivity), and (3) the species of animal affected. Only some of the common diseases are listed, and the treatments of etiologically specific diseases are given under their relevant headings. Use of chloramphenicol in food animals is illegal in the USA.

The primary route of excretion is via the kidney where they are excreted unchanged or as acetylated or conjugated derivatives. Variations in the duration of activity are primarily influenced by the degree of protein binding, the extent of acetylation, lipid solubility and the extent of reabsorption of un-ionized drug by the renal tubules which can be markedly influenced by urine pH. These factors vary markedly between animal species for the same sulfonamide and the activity of a given sulfonamide in one animal species cannot be assumed for another.

There is a large and sometimes disconcerting number of sulfonamides available for use. Since the primary spectrum of activity of the group is essentially the same the differences within the group rest primarily with differences in absorption, distribution within the body, excretion and duration of activity (16). For farm animals the group can be conveniently considered in three main subgroups: enteric-acting sulfonamides, general sulfonamides, and potentiated sulfonamides. For practical therapeutic purposes in large animal practice it is only necessary to be familiar with the use of one or two members of each subgroup. The nomination of members within these subgroups below indicates our current preference but in no way excludes other sulfonamides for consideration in these areas.

Enteric-acting sulfonamides

Enteric-acting sulfonamides comprise those that are not absorbed from the alimentary tract following oral administration. They include sulfaguanidine, succinylsulfathiazole (sulfasuxidine), and phthalylsulfathiazole (sulfathalidine). They are used for the treatment of enteric infections, and proprietary preparations, containing one or more of these drugs, often in combination with an aminoglycoside antibiotic, are available for this purpose. Their use in large-animal practice is restricted because in most enteric diseases in neonatal animals or adults there is an intent to also achieve systemic levels of antibacterial activity and so other sulfonamides are used.

General sulfonamides

The general sulfonamide most in use in large animal practice is sulfadimidine (sulfamethazine). It has been used for many years and has proven efficacy in many diseases. It may be given orally and the sodium salt is given parenterally. It is recommended that all therapy should at least be initiated with parenteral administration. This is especially so in ruminant animals where rumen stasis may markedly influence the absorption (4) and peak blood levels may not occur for periods up to 15 hours following oral administration. Parenteral administration should be by intravenous injection. Subcutaneous or intraperitoneal injection is not recommended. Following intravenous injection, sulfadimidine rapidly equilibrates throughout the body and at a dose rate of 150 mg/kg effective levels are maintained for periods up to 24 hours. In cattle, dose rates of 200 mg/kg are usually recommended. This should be repeated at 150 mg/kg every 24 hours, or it can be maintained by the use of oral sulfadimidine 200 mg/kg given 12 hours later and repeated every 24 hours if circumstances do not allow repeat visits. The course of sulfonamide therapy is generally 3–5 days. In ruminants sulfadimidine is metabolized by hydroxylation and acetylation and the parent drug and its metabolites are excreted in the urine and saliva. Hydroxylation is capacity limited and at high dose rates the elimination half-life is extended and dose-dependent (18, 19). At dose rates of 100 mg/kg plasma and milk concentrations above 10 μg/ml are sustained for approximately 34 and 20 hours respectively. However, it can be argued that sustained higher plasma concentrations are important with sulfonamide therapy. It is a clinical impression that failure with sulfonamide therapy is more common at low dose rates, such as frequently occurs with owner-administered sulfadimidine given subcutaneously, and the higher dose rates above are still recommended.

Toxic reactions in cattle with sulfadimidine are rare provided the intravenous injection is given slowly. Sulfadimidine is frequently marketed as a 33·3% solution and the rapid intravenous administration of this concentration may produce respiratory distress and collapse in cattle. This is generally not fatal but may be alarming both to the clinician and owner. Sulfadimidine is preferably administered intravenously as a 15% solution and at this concentration toxic reactions are rare although many cattle show muscle trembling and urinate following dosing. At this concentration a 500 ml dose provides an effective therapetic dose to the majority of adult dairy cattle.

Sustained-release sulfonamide boluses are available for cattle which may provide effective therapeutic levels for periods up to 72 hours following a single dose (5). Sulfabromomethazine is also used for oral therapy in cattle at a dose of 200 mg/kg every 48 hours but should not be used intravenously.

Sulfadimidine is primarily used in swine for the control of atrophic rhinitis, but generally, proprietary compounds containing other sulfonamides are used for enteric infections such as colibacillosis in this species.

Other sulfonamides available for use in large animals include sulfamethylpyridazine, sulfamethylphenazole, sulfamethyldiazine, sulfadimethoxine, sulfaphenazole, sulfachloropyridazine, sulfathiazole and sulfamerazine. Very few of these differ favorably from sulfadimidine in terms of dose rate or dose interval when used in cattle.

Sulfamethylphenazole and sulfadimethoxine have a significantly longer excretion period than sulfadimidine in cattle (2, 6, 7) and at equivalent dose rates to those used with it, it is possible that the dose interval can be increased to 48 hours. Similarly at equivalent dose rates sulfamethoxypyridazine (8, 9) has a marginal advantage over sulfadimidine. However, in most countries the extra cost of these sulfonamides when compared to sulfadimidine outweighs these advantages. The use within this group is largely a matter of clinical preference with the consideration of primary cost of the drug being balanced against possible reduced costs with longer acting agents because of the need for fewer revisits.

Sulfonamides are used less frequently in horses. Sulfamethylphenazole or sulfamethoxypyridazine may be used at a dose rate of 100 mg/kg initially with subsequent daily doses of 50 mg/kg (6, 11).

In small animals and man some sulfonamides are called long-acting sulfonamides in that they are rapidly and efficiently absorbed following oral administration and are very slowly excreted. These features allow effective therapeutic levels to be achieved with low dose levels and long dose intervals in these species. Although information on these sulfonamides is limited there is little evidence that the excretion patterns seen in small animals and man occur in farm animals.

Pharmacokinetic studies in ruminants and horses (1–3, 20) suggest that the majority of these sulfonamides have little or no advantage over sulfadimidine at equivalent dose rates, in terms of longevity of action, and suggest that *many of the currently recommended doses for these drugs may be too low for effective therapy*. The faster elimination of long-acting sulfonamides in ruminants, when compared to man, may be due to the more alkaline urine in this species and this results in a smaller unionized fraction, and consequently less tubular resorption in the kidney. Although information is limited it is possible that these sulfonamides may show longer excretion patterns in suckling animals and they may therefore be effective at lower dose rates in this age group.

In swine the excretion rates of sulfonamides are generally slower than in ruminants and horses and dose rates may be somewhat lower (2). Sulfonamides are rarely administered parenterally to swine but may be incorporated in the feed or water or administered individually. They are primarily used for the treatment of enteric disease, especially that associated with *E. coli*. Sulfachloropyridazine is commonly used for this purpose. Dose rates of 50–100 mg/kg are generally used for sulfonamide therapy in swine.

Trimethoprim-potentiated sulfonamides

Trimethoprim-potentiated sulfonamides are also available

for therapy. Trimethoprim potentiates the antimicrobial activity of sulfonamides to produce a remarkable synergistic effect (10) so that antimicrobial efficiency can be obtained with very low levels of the drug combination. The optimal ratio for this synergistic effect varies considerably between pathogens. The combination appears bactericidal and is broad spectrum in activity. Trimethoprim is absorbed by the oral route and following both oral and parenteral administration, a high volume distribution and high levels in tissues are achieved which, with the exception of brain, generally exceed those in blood in ruminants (12). This penetration of tissues is much superior to that of the sulfonamides. It has an exceptionally short half-life and rapid excretion in adult cattle, goats and swine and only a moderate half-life in horses (13). Excretion rates are slower in neonates (14, 15) which suggests that greater therapeutic efficiency may be achieved in this age group with currently available preparations. Excretion is via the urine in swine and the urine and feces in horses and ruminants.

Trimethoprim-potentiated sulfonamides are currently available as fixed-dose preparations containing trimethoprim with either sulfadiazine, sulfadoxine, sulfamethoxazole or sulfafurazole, usually in a 1:5 ratio. The excretion rates of these sulfonamides in all farm animals varies markedly from that of trimethoprim and are much longer (13, 14). In view of the different pharmacokinetic properties of these drugs it is possible that different combinations would give better therapeutic efficiency. Even so the clinical response to these combinations demonstrate that they have considerable value in the therapy of infectious disease in large animals. Currently, the dose rates recommended by the manufacturers are used but much higher dose rates may be in order (12).

Toxicity following the use of sulfonamides is rare. As with sulfadimidine the rapid intravenous injection of any sulfonamide in concentrated solution can produce respiratory distress and collapse, and slow administration is advisable. Incorrect intravenous injection procedure can result in severe perivascular reactions and thrombophlebitis with all sulfonamides. Subcutaneous injection of concentrated solutions produces pain and subsequent swelling. Intramuscular injection of low dose volume sulfonamide preparations is followed by swelling and pain in a proportion of animals and this route should be avoided if possible in horses with these preparations although reactions with trimethoprim–sulfadiazine preparations are uncommon. Crystalluria is not a problem with sulfonamide therapy in large animals but all animals should have *ad libitum* access to water, and generally other drugs are used for therapy in severely dehydrated animals. Trimethoprim is reported as causing an acute anaphylactic reaction with death in an experimental horse that had possibly become sensitized to this drug by prior use (17). Diarrhea occasionally occurs in horses 3–5 days after initiation of therapy with trimethoprim-potentiated sulfonamides, but resolves following withdrawal.

REFERENCES

(1) Nielsen, P. & Rasmussen, F. (1977) *Res. vet. Sci.*, *22*, 205.
(2) Tschudi, P. (1973) *Zentralbl. VetMed.*, *20A*, 145 & 155.
(3) Nielsen, P. (1973) *Acta vet. Scand.*, *14*, 647.
(4) Bishop, C. R. et al. (1973) *Can. vet. J.*, *14*, 269.
(5) Miller, C. R. et al. (1972) *Vet. Med. small Anim. Clin.*, *67*, 513.
(6) Austin, F. H. & Kelly, W. R. (1966) *Vet. Rec.*, *78*, 122 & 192
(7) Rehm, W. F. & Rieder, J. (1965) *Arch. exp. Vet. Med.*, *19*, 807
(8) Stewart, G. A. & Parris, R. (1962) *Aust. vet. J.*, *38*, 535.
(9) Paul, B. S. et al. (1974) *Ind. J. anim. Sci.*, *43*, 618.
(10) Busby, S. R. M. (1980) *J. Am. vet. med. Assoc.*, *176*, 1049.
(11) Rasmussen, F. (1971) *Acta vet. Scand.*, *12*, 131.
(12) Nielsen, P. & Rasmussen, F. (1975) *Acta vet. Scand.*, *16*, 405.
(13) Rasmussen, F. et al. (1979) *J. vet. Pharmacol. Therap.*, 2, 245.
(14) Kovacs, J. et al. (1976) *Acta vet. Hung.*, *26*, 73.
(15) Nielsen, P. & Rasmussen, F. (1976) *Acta Pharmacol. Toxicol.*, *38*, 113.
(16) Van Gogh, H. (1980) *J. vet. Pharmacol. Therap.*, *3*, 69.
(17) Alexander, F. & Collett, R. A. (1975) *Equ. vet. J.*, 7, 203.
(18) Nouws, J. F. M. et al. (1985) *Vet. Q.*, 7, 177.
(19) Nouws, J. F. M. et al. (1986) *Am. J. vet. Res.*, *47*, 642.
(20) Odegaard, S. A. & Rostad, A. (1987) *J. vet. Pharmacol. Therap.*, *10*, 83.
(21) Shoaf, S. E. et al. (1986) *J. vet. Pharmacol. Therap.*, *9*, 446.

Penicillins

The penicillins have much to commend them as one of the most useful and effective groups of antimicrobial agents. They have low inherent toxicity because their bactericidal activity results from effects on the glycopeptide components of the bacterial cell wall. These are not present in mammalian cells and the drugs may be given in doses far exceeding the recommended dose when there are therapeutic indications for this. They should be considered as the drug of choice for the treatment of many infections in large animals.

Benzylpenicillin has had a long recognized value in large animal medicine but the development of the newer semisynthetic penicillins has greatly expanded the spectrum of activity of this group and the range of conditions for which they are of value. In many instances their use should be considered for the treatment of conditions traditionally treated with more toxic antimicrobial agents. From limited information there may be considerable differences between the pharmacokinetic properties of different penicillins (6, 10). The dose of benzylpenicillin is traditionally stated in units (1 unit ≡ 0.6 μg) whereas that of the newer penicillins is stated in more conventional metric units.

Benzylpenicillin

Benzylpenicillin (penicillin G) has essentially a Gram-positive spectrum of activity but is inactivated by penicillinase-producing staphylococci. At higher levels it has some activity against some Gram-negative organisms including *Pasteurella* spp. Benzylpenicillin is available in crystalline form as the sodium or potassium salt. It is unstable in solution and should not be kept for more than 24 hours following reconstitution. It is primarily used to achieve high and immediate blood and tissue levels of penicillin and for this purpose is given intravenously. This is recommended in acute septicemias or other acute infections, such as the clostridial toxemias, where the clinical course is short and immediate levels with high diffusion concentration to areas of infection are required. Intravenous administration to achieve high tissue levels is also indicated in chronic pyogenic infections such as *Corynebacterium* (*Rhodococcus*) *equi* pneumonia in foals and diseases such as tetanus where high levels may result in greater diffusion of effective concentrations of the antibiotic into the affected areas.

The sodium salt should be used for intravenous administration because the potassium content (1·6 mmol/million units) of the potassium salt may cause significant cardiac toxicity when the injection is given as a bolus. The dose given should be at least 8000 units/kg body weight and doses as high as 50 000 units/kg may be indicated. The drug is excreted rapidly and effective blood levels are only present for approximately 2–4 hours but tissue levels may persist slightly longer. In the horse the intravenous administration of 10 000 units/kg will give therapeutic blood values (above 0·5 μg/ml) for approximately $1\frac{1}{2}$ hours (1). The dose is repeated three times daily and although a continual antibacterial level is not achieved with this regimen clinical response suggests that it is sufficient. A single intramuscular dose of procaine penicillin is generally also given daily so as to achieve lower persistent levels. The use of this method of therapy is restricted to hospital situations or to extremely valuable stock, because of the need to repeat the treatments. A more common technique is to use crystalline benzylpenicillin to provide an initial intravenous loading dose at the beginning of more conventional penicillin therapy. A single intravenous loading dose of benzylpenicillin given at the same time as an intramuscular injection with procaine penicillin will provide high and immediate levels of penicillin, thus ensuring antibacterial activity during the period that absorption from the repository intramuscular proportion is occurring. Benzylpenicillin may also be given intramuscularly. The levels achieved are not as high as those which follow an equivalent dose intravenously, but are higher than those achieved by procaine penicillin. They persist for 4–6 hours. There are few indications for its use by this route.

Procaine benzylpenicillin is the most commonly used form of penicillin. It is a repository form of benzylpenicillin and a single intramuscular injection will provide maximal blood and tissue levels within 2–4 hours which persist at effective levels for up to 24 hours. Care should be taken to ensure that the drug is not inadvertently injected intravascularly as severe toxic reactions and death may result. The recommended dose is 8000 units/kg.

In the horse, blood levels may only marginally increase with higher dose rates but there may be greater persistence, whereas in cattle and sheep both level and persistence may be significantly increased with higher dose rates. In the horse there is variation in the peak serum concentration and bioavailability depending upon the muscle site of injection. They are highest with injection in the neck and biceps and lowest with injection in the gluteal muscles (12). Lower serum levels of penicillin are obtained in the horse than in other large animal species at equivalent dose rates (3), and the elimination half-life is shorter. Adequate serum concentration of penicillin in this species can be maintained by a dose rate of 15 000 i.u./kg every 12 hours or 30 000 i.u./kg every 24 hours (1). Procaine benzylpenicillin is used as standard therapy for penicillin-sensitive infections and is the least costly method of penicillin administration. In most clinical situations a daily intramuscular dose is sufficient for effective therapy but in acute infections an initial intravenous loading dose with sodium benzylpenicillin may be indicated.

Penethamate benzylpenicillin is a weak-base ester of benzylpenicillin which penetrates rapidly into milk to achieve high levels following parenteral administration (6).

Benethamine benzylpenicillin and *benzathene benzylpenicillin* are 'long-acting' repository forms of benzylpenicillin. They are given by intramuscular injection, and the slow absorption results in low but effective therapeutic levels for 4–6 days. Because of the low blood and tissue levels their use is restricted to infections that are highly susceptible to the action of penicillin. The recommended dose of each is 8000 units/kg body weight. Following administration of these forms of benzylpenicillin, effective levels may not be achieved for periods of 6–24 hours. Consequently they are frequently combined with procaine penicillin and occasionally crystalline benzylpenicillin. When used in these combinations the total dose given should equal the sum of the doses for each individual component. The long-acting repository forms of penicillin have especial merit in the therapy of individual or groups of animals where long-term therapy is required but where oral medication is contraindicated and where daily mustering for treatment may be inconvenient. For example, their use is valuable in an outbreak of post-dipping or post-drenching pneumonia in a group of sheep where mortality can be effectively reduced by a single injection given every 5 days for a period of 20 days. They are also of value in providing long-term treatment in individuals where the cost of daily revisits is not warranted. Pharmacokinetic studies suggest that there is little value to the use of these repository forms in horses as serum concentrations rapidly fall below that required for effective therapy even when high dose rates are used (1).

Benzylpenicillin is not given by the oral route. It is acid-susceptible and a significant proportion of the oral dose is destroyed in the stomach or abomasum so that exceptionally high doses are required for therapy. The acid-resistant phenoxymethyl and phenoxyethyl penicillins may be given orally to pre-ruminants and horses and pigs but are seldom used in practice. In calves there appear no indications for their use. Phenoxymethyl penicillin has a short half-life and 80% is bound to serum proteins requiring a minimal dose of 40 mg/kg to achieve short-time therapeutic serum concentrations (13). Phenoxymethyl penicillin does not achieve reasonable blood levels in the horse following oral administration of practical doses but 10 mg/kg given to pigs will achieve effective levels for periods of 4–6 hours.

Methicillin

Methicillin and the isoxazolyl penicillins *oxacillin*, *cloxacillin*, *dicloxacillin* and *floxacillin* are semisynthetic penicillins that have a similar spectrum of activity to benzylpenicillin but that are resistant to the action of bacterial penicillinase. Methicillin has lower intrinsic antibacterial activity than the isoxazolyl penicillins and benzylpenicillin. The isoxazolyl penicillins may be given orally to pre-ruminant calves and lambs and to pigs and horses but are seldom used by this route. Both may be given parenterally. The duration of activity following parenteral administration is 4–6 hours. The isoxazolyl penicillins have a similar distribution in the body to benzylpenicillin. Doses as high as 33–44 mg/kg given intravenously may be required to achieve effective therapeutic levels in areas such as synovial fluid (7). There are few indications for the use of these drugs in large animal medicine as the occurrence of staphylococcal infections is rare, and benzylpenicillin is more effective and less expensive for use against other penicillin-susceptible infections. The exception is their importance in the treatment and control of mastitis which is detailed under that heading. In the horse there may be indications for their use in the treatment of staphylococcal mastitis and staphylococcal dermatitis. Oxacillin is most frequently used for this purpose at a recommended dose of 25 mg/kg intravenously or intramuscularly repeated at 8–12 hour intervals. Other specific indications are detailed in the special medicine section of this text.

Ampicillin
This is a semisynthetic penicillin that has activity against both Gram-positive and Gram-negative organisms and can be considered as a broad-spectrum antibiotic. It achieves a significantly higher tissue penetration than benzylpenicillin in ruminants (6) and is excreted more slowly both in ruminants and the horse (4). However, its excretion rate is still very fast and this poses a limitation to practical therapy. Also it is less potent than benzylpenicillin and the latter should be used in preference in benzylpenicillin-sensitive infections. It is inactivated by penicillinase-producing staphylococci and has little activity against *Pseudomonas* spp. and *Klebsiella* spp. In large animal medicine it has been of especial value for the treatment of enteric infections associated with *Escherichia coli* and *Salmonella* spp. and pneumonic conditions. When given orally to pre-ruminant calves and lambs and to foals it achieves high levels within the intestinal tract and significant blood and tissue levels and high levels in the bile and urine. The oral route of administration is suitable for therapy of intestinal diseases of neonatal animals; however, the absorption of ampicillin from the intestine is inefficient, especially in the presence of milk, and if high blood and tissue levels are required it is advisable to use ampicillin by injection. *Pivampicillin* is absorbed with much greater efficiency from the alimentary tract, even in the presence of milk, and in calves 1 g given orally will give effective parenteral levels for 6 hours (8). Following parenteral administration there is a significant enterohepatic cycling and the drug has been found effective in eliminating *Salmonella* excretion in pigs. Ampicillin is also of exceptional value in the treatment of septicemic conditions associated with Gram-negative organisms, and is often the drug of choice in the initial treatment of acute infections of, as yet, undetermined etiology. It is often used in combination with gentamicin for the treatment of septic arthritis in foals, and a predictive formula for synovial fluid concentrations based on serum concentrations has been developed (15). Following oral or parenteral administration effective blood levels are obtained for periods of approximately 6 hours (4, 8). The recommended dose of ampicillin is 6–10 mg/kg by the oral or parenteral route and given twice or, if parenteral, preferably three times daily. Cost is a limiting factor in farm animals, but in horses dose rates of 22 mg/kg two or three times daily may be indicated. The sodium salt is used for intravenous injection. An injectable suspension in oil markedly prolongs the persistence of therapeutic levels following a single dose but adverse local reactions occur in a significant proportion of horses. Oral medication of pigs may be achieved by the addition of 100 mg ampicillin per liter of drinking water. For the treatment of enteric disease in young livestock the oral route is indicated; however, amoxycillin may have greater efficiency. For septicemic and internal infections ampicillin should be administered parenterally as this route will result in higher and more sustained tissue levels than orally administered equivalent doses.

Amoxycillin
This is a semisynthetic penicillin closely related to ampicillin and with a similar spectrum of activity. Following equivalent oral doses in most species it achieves higher serum concentrations than ampicillin and it possibly has higher intrinsic antibacterial activity than ampicillin (5). The recommended dose is 5–10 mg/kg repeated twice daily. Following oral administration in calves it achieves high levels in the intestinal wall and intestinal tract, and levels within the small intestine and colon are sufficient to be effective against the common enteric pathogens including *E. coli* and *Salmonella* spp. for 8 hours (5). Significant blood and tissue levels occur between 1 and 6 hours following oral administration. With both amoxycillin and ampicillin the bioavailability of an orally administered dose is improved by administration in glucose–glycine electrolyte solution rather than in water or milk (14).

The sodium salt can be used for intravenous and intramuscular injection and at a dose rate of 5–10 mg/kg three times daily effective concentrations are present in blood, liver, bile, urine and the intestinal wall and lumen of calves. The trihydrate salt can be used instead of the sodium salt for intramuscular administration and results in more prolonged levels; however, for satisfactory therapeutic levels, a dose of 20–25 mg/kg should be administered (9). Dose regimens for foals and horses are higher and it has been suggested that a dose of 22 mg/kg repeated every 8 hours should be used for sensitive organisms. Moderately sensitive organisms such as *Corynebacterium* (*Rhodococcus*) *equi* and non-beta-lactamase producing Gram-negative organisms should be treated with the same dose at 6 hour intervals (16). In large animals, the indications for the use of amoxycillin are similar to those for ampicillin.

Carbenicillin
This is a semisynthetic penicillin related to ampicillin and amoxycillin, with a similar spectrum of activity, but in addition it has activity against *Proteus* spp. and *Pseudomonas* spp. if used in high doses. Its activity against Gram-positive organisms is inferior to benzylpenicillin and it should not be used as a substitute for this purpose. Ticarcillin and piperacillin have even greater activity than carbenicillin against Gram-negative organisms. They have had little clinical application in large-animal medicine but may have an indication in conditions such

Pseudomonas-associated infertility in mares and septic thritis in foals (17). Pharmacokinetic studies are availle for ticarcillin in the horse and suggest that a dose 44 mg/kg repeated every 6 hours will achieve thera:utic concentrations against *Pseudomonas* spp. and other ram-negative infections (23). Therapy with ticarcillin markedly potentiated by combination with an aminoycoside such as gentamicin.

ephalosporins

ephalosporins are chemically similar to the penicillins id their antibacterial spectrum is similar to that of npicillin except that in addition they have some restance to the action of penicillinase which varies acording to the particular cephalosporin. To date, these itimicrobial agents have had limited use in large animal edicine.

Cephalothin, cephapirin and cefazolin are first generion cephalosporins for which there is some pharmaconetic data for the horse (10, 18, 19). Cephalothin and fazolin have a similar spectrum of activity and have a articular indication in the treatment of klebsiella and aphylococcal infections. They are not absorbed folwing oral administration but are rapidly absorbed and istributed following intramuscular injection. Both ephalothin and cefazolin show rapid elimination folwing intravenous administration (10, 18) and theraeutic concentrations are maintained for too short a me to make this route of administration of practical alue. The biological half-life following intramuscular ijection is considerably longer and at a dose of 11 mg/kg herapeutic concentrations are maintained in serum for hours with cephalothin and 3 hours with cefazolin. A roportion of the dose is excreted as the active form n the urine. Cephapirin is resistant to beta-lactamase roduced by Gram-positive organisms but is generally ensitive to those produced by Gram-negative bacteria. t shows similar pharmacokinetic characteristics and has ood penetrance into synovial, pleural and peritoneal luid and the endometrium (20). Based on minimal nhibitory concentrations of horse pathogens and pharnacokinetic studies the principal indication for the drug vould be staphylococcal infections (20). A dose of 0 mg/kg repeated every 8 hours for adult horses and hours for foals is suggested (19, 20). Considering the pectrum of activity, the extremely short biological life nd cost these cephalosporins have limited indications in eterinary practice. Cephalosporins are used in intranammary formulations for therapy in staphylococcal nastitis.

Third-generation cephalosporins show a broad spectrum of activity against Gram-positive organisms and a much wider spectrum of activity against Gram-negative bacteria than first-generation cephalosporins. They have good distribution within the body and achieve therapeutic concentrations in cerebrospinal fluid. They have particular value in the treatment of meningitis caused by resistant organisms and cefotaxime, at a dose rate of 40 mg/kg every 6 hours, has been used to treat meningitis in foals (21).

Toxicity in the penicillin group is low and adverse reactions are uncommon even at very high dose rates. Horses and cattle may show a hypersensitivity to procaine penicillin which may follow the initial injection or develop during a course of treatment. It is generally mild and manifested by the development of urticaria, moderate pruritus and a slight increase in respiratory rate. Providing the drug is immediately withdrawn no untoward effects result. Treatment with antihistamines and corticosteroids may be indicated. The reactivity of these individuals cannot be detected by conjunctival or intradermal challenge. More severe adverse reactions are seen in cattle and consist of the development of sweating with fever, staggering and severe respiratory distress 3–10 minutes after the intramuscular injection of procaine penicillin. Collapse with the passage of froth from the nostrils or mouth and cyanosis are rapidly followed by death in a significant proportion of cases despite treatment with adrenaline, antihistamines and corticosteroids. A similar effect has been seen in the horse. On postmortem examination there is severe pulmonary edema and emphysema. It is uncertain if this is an allergic manifestation or the result of inadvertent intravascular administration of the drug. A similar clinical syndrome with lassitude, vomiting, pyrexia, cyanosis of the extremities, but without death is occasionally seen in fattening pigs and adult sows following intramuscular injection with preparations containing benzathene and procaine penicillin and may result in embryonic death or abortion in pregnant sows (11). Sudden death immediately following the intravenous injection of sodium benzylpenicillin in horses has occurred although it is extremely uncommon. From limited experience it appears more common in horses with purpura hemorrhagica.

REFERENCES

(1) Love, D. D. et al. (1983) *Equ. vet. J.*, *15*, 43.
(2) Teske, R. H. (1972) *J. Am. vet. med. Assoc.*, *160*, 873.
(3) Rollins, L. D. et al. (1972) *J. Am. vet. med. Assoc.*, *161*, 490.
(4) Durr, A. (1976) *Res. vet. Sci.*, *20*, 24.
(5) Symposium on amoxicillin (1977) *Vet. Med. small Anim. Clin.*, *72*, 677–806.
(6) Ziv, G. et al. (1977) *Am. J. vet. Res.*, *38*, 1007.
(7) Martin, I. C. A. et al. (1980) *J. vet. Pharmacol. Therap.*, *3*, 21.
(8) Ziv, G. et al. (1977) *Am. J. vet. Res.*, *38*, 1007.
(9) Ziv, G. & Nouws, J. F. M. (1979) *Refuah Vet.*, *36*, 104.
(10) Ruoff, W. W. and Sams, R. A. (1985) *Am. J. vet. Res.*, *46*, 2085.
(11) Nurmio, P. & Schulman, A. (1980) *Vet. Rec.*, *106*, 97.
(12) Firth, E. C. et al. (1986) *Am. J. vet. Res.*, *47*, 2380.
(13) Soback, S. et al. (1987) *J. vet. Pharmacol. Therap.*, *10*, 17.
(14) Palmer, G. H. et al. (1983) *Am. J. vet. Res.*, *44*, 68.
(15) Bowman, K. F. (1986) *Am. J. vet. Res.*, *47*, 1590.
(16) Carter, G. K. (1986) *Am. J. vet. Res.*, *47*, 2126.
(17) Spensley, M. S. et al. (1986) *Am. J. vet. Res.*, *47*, 2587.
(18) Sams, R. A. & Rouff, W. W. (1985) *Am. J. vet. Res.*, *46*, 348.
(19) Brown, M. P. et al. (1987) *Am. J. vet. Res.*, *48*, 805.
(20) Brown, M. P. et al. (1986) *Am. J. vet. Res.*, *47*, 748.
(21) Morris, D. D. et al. (1982) *Equ. vet. J.*, *19*, 151.
(22) Embrechts, E. (1982) *Vet. Rec.*, *111*, 314.
(23) Sweeney, C. R. (1984) *Am. J. vet. Res.*, *45*, 1000.

Macrolide group

This group includes erythromycin, oleandomycin, spiramycin, tylosin and carbamycin. Of this group erythromycin, spiramycin and tylosin have common usage in large animal practice.

The spectrum of activity is almost identical to that of

penicillin. Its mode of action is by the inhibition of protein synthesis. The group is generally bacteriostatic in activity, and bactericidal at high concentration. Its members act predominantly against Gram-positive organisms including streptococci, staphylococci, corynebacteria and clostridia but *Haemophilus*, *Bordetella*, *Pasteurella* spp., chlamydiae, rickettsiae and *Mycoplasma* spp. may also be susceptible. These drugs are used primarily for the treatment of penicillin-resistant staphylococci and especially for the treatment of mycoplasmal diseases in swine and swine dysentery. They also have value in the treatment of respiratory disease. Erythromycin appears to have the greatest intrinsic antibacterial activity for most organisms, but other members of the group are superior in their activity against *Mycoplasma* spp. Cross-resistance within the group usually occurs. For this reason, when resistance is encountered, it is generally wise to choose an antibiotic from a different group for therapy. Resistance occurs by stepwise mutation, but plasmid R factor transfer occurs with staphylococci. The use of macrolides with aminoglycosides or chloramphenicol is inadvisable, but tylosin in combination with oxytetracycline may have synergistic activity against *Pasteurella* spp. (3).

Members of the group are absorbed following oral administration in pre-ruminants and swine, or may be administered parenterally, usually intramuscularly. Erythromycin is unpalatable to pigs, and growing pigs may refuse feed and water medication. Other macrolides should be used for administration by this route in swine. Due to their high lipid solubility, the macrolides are distributed widely throughout the body and they achieve good tissue and barrier penetration (1, 4). Following parenteral administration, serum levels may be deceptively low, but tissue concentrations several times larger than those in the blood are found in all areas with the possible exception of the eye, brain and skeletal muscle. Levels are dose-related, and there is some variation in distribution between members of the group (3). The majority of the administered dose is metabolized by the liver, but significant therapeutic levels of active drug are excreted in the bile, intestinal excretion and in urine (3, 8). The low pK of the macrolides results in ion-trapping in the milk, and therapeutic levels are achieved in milk following parenteral administration (2, 9). The group has value in the treatment of mastitis due to *Staphylococcus* spp., *Actinomyces (Corynebacterium) pyogenes* and *Mycoplasma* spp. The concentrations in milk following parenteral administration are high and persist for up to 24 hours; however, concentrations in mammary interstitial tissue fluids are transient and may not be sufficient for fully effective therapy of organisms invading udder tissue (9).

The recommended dose for the macrolide group is 10 mg/kg given by deep intramuscular injection preferably twice daily. This dose is usually sufficient for highly sensitive infections but 40 mg/kg may be required for moderately sensitive organisms such as pasteurellae. This is usually not practical. There do not appear to be major differences in the pharmacokinetics of the macrolide group in young ruminants, although information is limited (8), and the dose rates above should be followed. *Erythromycin* and *tylosin* may be injected as the base whereas *spiramycin* is injected as the adipate ester. Erythromycin may be administered as the ethyl succinate ester. Tylosin tartrate and tylosin phosphate are the usual macrolide antibiotics used for medication of the water or food respectively in swine. The inclusion rate in water is generally of the order of 250 mg/liter and in food 200–400 g/tonne.

Erythromycin and to some extent tylosin are extremely irritant and painful when given by intramuscular injection. This property distinctly limits their use, especially in the horse and in food-producing animals within 4 weeks of market. If used, no more than 10 ml should be injected in any one site and alternate sites should be used for subsequent injection. An outbreak of salt poisoning has followed attempts to medicate growing swine with erythromycin in the water. Tylosin has low toxicity but parenteral administration in swine has been followed by skin erythema, pruritus, rectal edema and transient diarrhea (5). Diarrhea may also occur during parenteral erythromycin therapy in horses and possibly with other macrolides. It is not fatal and stops after therapy is discontinued (6).

Lincomycin is structurally different to the macrolides but shows an almost identical spectrum of activity. *Clindamycin* is a newer derivative of lincomycin and has greater quantitative antimicrobial activity. From limited studies (3) in sheep these drugs have pharmacokinetic properties similar to the macrolide group following intramuscular injection. Peak blood levels are achieved within an hour of injection with both drugs. They have exceptional penetrability into areas such as the synovial fluid, aqueous and vitreous humors and milk. The levels achieved in milk are much higher than those achieved in blood.

The indications for lincomycin are essentially those for the use of the macrolide group of antibiotics. They are especially indicated for the treatment of mycoplasmal arthritis and mastitis in large animals. Lincomycin may show cross-resistance with erythromycin. The recommended dose is 10 mg/kg given twice daily but higher dose rates may be more effective. Currently cost limits its use. Lincomycin is commonly combined with *spectinomycin* for therapy against *Mycoplasma* spp. and *Pasteurella* spp. and *Treponema hyodysenteriae* in pigs. Lincomycin should not be administered orally to ruminants. Oral administration at high dose is rapidly followed by a syndrome of severe depression, diarrhea, collapse and there can be high mortality.

The contamination of cattle feed with lincomycin at levels as low as 6–10 ppm, or with macrolide antibiotics, can result in anorexia, diarrhea and a severe drop in milk production in lactating dairy cows (10). Tylosin contamination of feed has also been suspected of producing a similar syndrome but experimental challenge of lactating dairy cows with 60 and 240 mg/cow/day has shown no ill effect (11). Horses may develop intractable diarrhea during lincomycin therapy and it should not be used in this species. Diarrhea, manifest in some individuals as an acute and fatal hemorrhagic colitis resembling salmonellosis, and laminitis are recorded in horses fed grain inadvertently contaminated with lincomycin. An oral intake as low as 0·5 mg/kg for 2 days is sufficient to cause clinical illness (7).

REFERENCES

(1) Ziv, G. E. & Sulman, F. G. (1973) *Am. J. vet. Res.*, *34*, 329.
(2) Pignotteli, P. & Adreini, G. (1972) *Veterinaria, Milano*, *21*, 239.
(3) Burrows, G. E. (1980) *J. Am. vet. med. Assoc.*, *176*, 1072.
(4) Van Duyn, R. L. & Folkerts, T. M. (1979) *Vet. Med., small Anim. Clin.*, *74*, 375.
(5) Parker, B. N. J. (1976) *Vet. Bull.*, *46*, 83.
(6) Knight, H. D. (1975) *Proc. 21st Ann. Conv. Am. Assoc. Equ. Practnrs*, *131*.
(7) Raisbeck, M. F. et al. (1981) *J. Am. vet. med. Assoc.*, *179*, 362.
(8) Burrows, G. E. et al. (1983) *Am. J. vet. Res.*, *44*, 1053.
(9) Franklin, A. et al. (1986) *Am. J. vet. Res.*, *47*, 804.
10) Anon (1984) *Vet. Rec.*, *114*, 5 and 132.
11) Mackinnon, J. D. et al. (1984) *Vet. Rec.*, *115*, 278.

Aminoglycoside group

Members of the aminoglycoside group in common use in large animal practice include streptomycin, dihydrostreptomycin, neomycin, kanamycin, and gentamicin. Paromomycin, spectinomycin and the newer semisynthetic amikacin are also within the group. They are dealt with as one group as they have similar properties. The most commonly used member of the group has been streptomycin but with the emergence of resistance to this drug other members of the group are in use with increasing frequency. In some veterinary hospitals the prevalence of resistance to most aminoglycosides has made gentamicin and even amikacin the aminoglycoside of choice in treating Gram-negative sepsis, but this is unlikely to be the rule in rural veterinary practice.

The group is bactericidal in its activity and acts on the ribosome to inhibit protein synthesis. The spectrum of activity is essentially against Gram-negative organisms. The group also has some activity against staphylococci and streptococci but this is variable. Resistance to one member of the group does not necessarily imply resistance to other members. In general organisms that are resistant to either neomycin, kanamycin or paromomycin will be resistant to others of this triad and to streptomycin, but may be sensitive to gentamicin. Streptomycin-resistant organisms may still show sensitivity to other members of the groups. The incidence of resistance to streptomycin, especially amongst the coliform group of organisms, is quite high in some countries and the value of this drug for the treatment of these infections is now limited. *Streptomycin* has particular value in the treatment of leptospiral and *Haemophilus*-associated infections. *Amikacin* is the only member of the group that has significant activity against *Pseudomonas* (1) although gentamicin may show some activity. *Spectinomycin* has activity against *Mycoplasma*. The aminoglycoside group is primarily used in farm animals for the treatment of enteric diseases and colibacillosis, and in the treatment of septicemic disease in young animals, usually in conjunction with penicillin. Members of the group may show synergistic activity with benzylpenicillin and they are frequently used in combination with this drug to obtain low-cost, broad-spectrum antimicrobial activity.

The aminoglycosides show similar absorption, distribution and excretion characteristics although small differences do occur (2). Following oral administration members of this group are not absorbed in significant amounts from the intestinal tract, nor are they excreted into the intestinal tract following parenteral administration. If both systemic and enteric activity is required these drugs must be given by both oral and parenteral routes. The prime use of this group when administered orally is in the treatment of Gram-negative enteric infections in young animals and pigs and they have particular value for this purpose. In general, members other than streptomycin are used for this purpose due to the high incidence of coliform resistance to this drug. An oral dose of 5 mg/kg repeated twice or three times daily should be sufficient for enteric therapy.

Streptomycin, *dihydrostreptomycin*, *neomycin* and *kanamycin* are most commonly used for parenteral administration although with the increasing resistance of organisms to the traditionally used members of this group the use of *gentamicin* is becoming more common. They may be given intravenously or intramuscularly but are most commonly given intramuscularly. Following intramuscular injection, peak serum levels are achieved within about 1 hour and at effective dose rates they are maintained for an 8–12-hour period (1–3). There are only minor differences within the group for the time taken to reach maximal serum concentrations and in excretion rates. Distribution is largely restricted to the blood and extracellular fluid. Therapeutic drug levels occur in the pleural and peritoneal fluid and in pulmonary tissue and the endometrium, but the group does not reach intracellular sites and in the absence of inflammation has poor ability to penetrate CSF, the eye and the milk (11–13). Aminoglycosides achieve therapeutic concentrations in synovial fluid following parenteral administration (5, 13, 14). They are of little value for the parenteral treatment of mastitis although gentamicin has value in the treatment of coliform mastitis due to the extreme sensitivity of most coliforms to this antibiotic and the subsequent low levels of drug required in milk. Parenterally administered kanamycin is reported to achieve therapeutic levels in synovial fluid (5).

Excretion is via the urine and exceptionally high levels are present within the first 12 hours of therapy, and therapeutic levels may persist in urine for 24–36 hours (4). Aminoglycosides bind to renal tubular tissues with resultant persistent tissue residues which, in the case of neomycin, may last as long as 90 days.

Members of the group can also be given by intravenous injection. However, due to the high and rapid bioavailability from intramuscular sites, there are few indications for this that cannot be met by intramuscular administration. With most members of the group equilibration occurs within 30 minutes of injection, and elimination and excretion patterns are similar to those obtained following intramuscular injection.

The usual recommended dose for parenteral administration of this group is 10 mg/kg every 12 hours with the exception of gentamicin. However, pharmacokinetic studies suggest that more effective therapy would be achieved with an intramuscular dose of 25 mg/kg repeated at 6–10-hour intervals (1, 2). The use of this higher dose especially with neomycin should be approached with caution in view of potential toxicity. Kanamycin appears much less toxic than neomycin and is preferred for parenteral administration (5). The group is also commonly used in antibacterial preparations for topical use.

Main aminoglycosides in use

Gentamicin

Within the aminoglycoside group gentamicin is frequently selected for therapy because of its relatively wide spectrum of activity at relatively low concentrations. In addition to therapy for septicemic and enteric disease, gentamicin is commonly used to treat unresponsive conditions such as chronic endometritis and pneumonia. In ruminants, gentamicin is rapidly absorbed following intramuscular injection and is excreted via the kidneys with a half-life of between 1 and 3 hours depending on age (9–11). Pharmacokinetic studies suggest that a dose of 5 mg/kg administered intravenously or intramuscularly every 8 hours will achieve a mean circulating concentration of 5 μg/ml, which is required for activity against most sensitive organisms, and trough serum concentrations do not fall below 2 μg/ml (11). Gentamicin has poor penetration into areas such as the CSF, aqueous and vitreous humor and concentrations in milk at this dose rate are only marginally therapeutic (11, 12). Gentamicin is selectively bound in the renal cortex and achieves very high concentrations in this area.

With repeated dosing there is slow accumulation in other tissues and concentrations of gentamicin considerably in excess of those in serum are reached in the liver, lung, udder parenchyma and endometrium (9, 11). These concentrations have value for therapy of upper and lower respiratory tract infections and the concentrations in the endometrium are more sustained than those following intrauterine infusions (8). Following cessation of repeated dosing gentamicin is slowly released from tissue binding sites with an elimination or washout half-life of approximately 45 hours in adult cows (11). Serum, urine and milk concentrations during this washout period are subtherapeutic but may be violative. Gentamicin is not absorbed from the gastrointestinal tract but significant quantities can be absorbed following intrauterine infusions and subsequent serum, tissue and milk concentrations may also be violative (8). Similar tissue accumulation with a prolonged washout period is recorded in sheep (24). The washout period is dependent upon the dose interval and the dose frequency and presents a real problem for determining withdrawal periods when extra-label dose regimens are used. Gentamicin is not approved for use in food animals in many countries.

In the horse the indications for gentamicin are similar to those in ruminants. It is considered by some as the drug of choice for the treatment of Gram-negative bacterial sepsis and is also used widely for the treatment of arthritis. Gentamicin is rapidly absorbed following intramuscular injection with peak serum concentrations being reached within 1 hour. The biological half-life is approximately 2 hours and a dose of 5 mg/kg given every 8 hours will give mean serum concentration of approximately 6 μg/ml (14–16). Plasma concentrations and excretion following subcutaneous administration are similar to those following intramuscular injection at equivalent doses (16). The distribution of gentamicin in the horse appears similar to that in ruminants and significant concentrations are reached in endometrial tissues following parenteral injection (15). Gentamicin also penetrates into synovial fluid but therapy is commonly supplemented by intra-articular injection (13, 14). Synovial fluid concentrations relative to serum concentrations are available (23).

Gentamicin is nephrotoxic and there is concern that there is a narrow range between therapeutic and toxic doses. The dose rate of 5 mg/kg given every 8 hours for up to 7 days in healthy horses and 10 days in healthy cattle has not been associated with evidence of renal dysfunction (11, 15). However, electrolyte imbalance and volume depletion in sick animals can alter pharmacokinetic and toxic parameters (25, 26).

In view of the variability in gentamicin excretion in normal animals and its alteration in disease it has been suggested that dose rates of this drug should be individualized and based on gentamicin monitoring (26). The objective is to achieve peak serum concentrations of 10 μg/ml with trough concentrations of 1 μg/ml as prolonged trough concentrations greater than 2 μg/ml may be associated with greater risk of nephrotoxicity (26).

Obviously this is not a practical procedure for in practice situations but might be considered in valuable hospitalized horses. The potential for nephrotoxicity with gentamicin in large animals may be overstated; however until the risk is fully established the monitoring of renal function should be considered with prolonged administration of this drug. Urinary gamma glutamyl transpeptidase activity may be a sensitive early indicator of developing renal dysfunction (17).

Amikacin

Amikacin is a semisynthetic aminoglycoside derived from kanamycin. It has activity against *Pseudomonas aeruginosa* and its other main indication is in the treatment of infections with gentamicin-resistant organisms. Amikacin has similar pharmacokinetic properties to others within the aminoglycoside group and can be administered intravenously or intramuscularly. Absorption following intramuscular administration is rapid with peak serum concentrations within 1 hour (18–20). The biological half-life is 1·5–3·0 hours and is marginally longer in foals than in horses. There is good penetration into peritoneal and synovial fluid (19, 20). Based on the pharmacokinetic parameters and minimal inhibitory concentrations, dose rates of 7 mg/kg every 12 hours for foals and 5 mg/kg every 8 hours for adult horses have been proposed (18, 20).

Toxic effects of aminoglycosides

The aminoglycoside group is potentially one of the most toxic groups of antimicrobial agents. Their toxicity is well established in small animals, but is a less known quantity in large animals. Their toxic potential includes neuromuscular block and respiratory arrest, cardiovascular depression, nephrosis and vestibular and auditory toxicity.

Neuromuscular blockade is more likely following intravenous or intraperitoneal administration of members of this group. It occurs occasionally in calves following either intravenous or intramuscular administration of neomycin at routine recommended dose rates and is manifest by rapid collapse with paresis and apnea. It responds dramatically to intravenous calcium borogluconate given to effect. This syndrome is also reversible by neostigmine. In experimental animals the neuromuscular effects are potentiated by anesthetic agents and there are indications that this group should not be administered until after recovery from general anesthesia. Aminoglycosides also have a hypocalcemic action and may produce significant decreases in blood calcium levels. Caution should be used in the use of this group in periparturient dairy cattle—especially those with a history of milk fever (7).

The other toxic effects of the aminoglycosides are not commonly recognized as being a problem in large animal practice. Treatment periods with these drugs are probably too short to result in significant ototoxicity or vestibular damage, but treatment for periods longer than 7 days should be approached with caution. The possibility of cardiovascular depression and hypotension following the use of these drugs should be considered when treating severely toxemic animals or animals in shock. Renal toxicity is also possible and may occur in large animals treated with this group but remain unrecognized as renal function is rarely examined during the course of therapy. Nephrotoxicity and ototoxicity has been demonstrated in calves receiving parenteral neomycin at a dose rate of 2·5–4·5 mg/kg twice daily. Nephrotoxicity was detected after 5–7 days of treatment and there was marked azotemia and polyuria by 10 days. Deafness occurred after 2 weeks of treatment (6). Impaired excretion of this group, due to preexisting renal disease, is not generally a problem in large animals due to the relatively low prevalence of primary renal disease. However, in sick animals with electrolyte imbalance and circulatory volume depletion, there is always the potential for toxicity with the aminoglycoside group and the level and duration of therapy should be restricted to that which is compatible with effective therapy. Overenthusiastic and prolonged therapy should be avoided. An example of this is that despite the recognized clinical efficacy of the aminoglycoside group against enteric disease when used at recommended doses, the oral administration of neomycin at a high dose and prolonged dose regimen (25 mg/kg, four times a day for 5 days) has been shown to induce intestinal villous atrophy, an associated decreased absorption of glucose, and diarrhea in neonatal calves.

In addition to potential biological toxicities the aminoglycoside group has some chemical incompatibilities. One commonly encountered in practice involves gentamicin and neomycin which should not be mixed in solution with the penicillins or cephalosporins. In general, the chemical incompatabilities of the aminoglycoside group are such that they should not be mixed in solution with any other drug for administration.

REFERENCES

(1) Ziv, G. & Sulman, F. G. (1974) *Res. vet. Sci.*, *17*, 68.
(2) Conzelman, G. M. (1980) *J. Am. vet. med. Assoc.*, *176*, 1078.
(3) Ziv, G. (1976) *Am. J. vet. Res.*, *38*, 337.
(4) Stalheim, O. H. V. (1970) *Am. J. vet. Res.*, *31*, 497.
(5) Brown, M. P. et al. (1981) *Am. J. vet. Res.*, 42, 1823.
(6) Crowell, W. A. et al. (1981) *Am. J. vet. Res.*, *42*, 29.
(7) Crawford, L. M. et al. (1977) *Can. J. comp. Med.*, *41*, 251.
(8) Haddad, N.S. et al. (1986) *Am. J. vet. Res.*, *47*, 1597.
(9) Brown, S. A. et al. (1986) *Am. J. vet. Res.*, *47*, 2373.
(10) Clark, C. R. et al. (1985) *Am. J. vet. Res.*, *46*, 2461.
(11) Haddad, N. S. et al. (1987) *Am. J. vet Res.*, *48*, 21.
(12) Glaweschnig, E. et al. (1985) *Dtsch. Tierarztl. Wochenschr.*, *92*, 382.
(13) Stover, S.M. & Pool, R. P. (1985) *Am. J. vet. Res.*, *46*, 2485.
(14) Brown, M. P. et al. (1982) *J. vet. Pharmacol. Therap.*, *5*, 119.
(15) Haddad, N. S. et al. (1985) *Am. J. vet. Res.*, *46*, 1268.
(16) Gilman, J. M. et al. (1987) *J. vet. Pharmacol. Therap.*, *10*, 101.
(17) Adams, R. et al. (1987) *J. vet. Pharmacol. Therap.*, *8*, 194.
(18) Orsini, J. A. et al. (1985) *J. vet. Pharmacol. Therap.*, *8*, 194.
(19) Brown, M. P. et al. (1984) *Am. J. vet. Res.*, *45*, 1610.
(20) Brown, M. P. et al. (1986) *Am. J. vet. Res.*, *47*, 453.
(21) Mero, K. N. et al. (1985) *Vet. Clin. N. Am., food Anim. Pract.*, *1(3)*, 581.
(22) George, L. W. et al. (1986) *J. vet. Pharmacol. Therap.*, *9*, 183.
(23) Bowman, K. F. et al. (1986) *Am. J. vet. Res.*, *47*, 1590.
(24) Brown, S. A. et al. (1986) *Am. J. vet. Res.*, *47*, 789.
(25) Wilson, R. C. et al. (1983) *Am. J. vet. Res.*, *44*, 17.
(26) Sojka, J. E. and Brown, S. A. (1986) *J. Am. vet. med. Assoc.*, *189*, 784.

Tetracyclines

The four members of the tetracycline group commonly used in large animal practice are tetracycline, oxytetracycline, chlortetracycline and rolitetracycline (pyrrolidinomethyltetracycline). *Demethylchlortetracycline* (*demeclocycline*) *methacycline*, *doxycycline* and *minocycline* have usage in some areas. Individual members of this group have similar antibacterial properties but they differ pharmacokinetically (1). *Rolitetracycline* and demeclocycline, and probably doxycycline and minocycline, may give higher blood levels and greater persistence at equivalent doses than other members of the group (1, 2, 15). All tetracyclines have high affinity for tissues. *Tetracycline* and *chlortetracycline* are generally restricted to oral administration but parenteral preparations are available.

The tetracyclines are broad-spectrum antibiotics which are active against several different species of both Gram-positive and Gram-negative bacteria. They also show activity against some diseases associated with mycoplasma, rickettsia, chlamydia and diseases associated with babesia, anaplasma and eperythrozoa. Rolitetracycline may be combined with diminazene for the therapy of such diseases. Minocycline has special activity against *Nocardia* and *Staphylococcus aureus*, primarily bacteriostatic. In the case of protozoal infection and intracellular bacterial infections, treatment may result in control of the disease but not in total elimination of the infection. In general, resistance to one member of the group implies resistance to others and if this situation is encountered it is wise to consider the use of a completely different antimicrobial agent.

Tetracyclines have lipid solubility and with adequate doses therapeutic levels occur in pleural, peritoneal and synovial fluids and in the body organs and skeletal muscle. Moderate penetration of the eye, CSF and brain also occurs. There is variation within the group in this respect and the newer tetracyclines, minocycline and doxycycline achieve higher tissue levels at equivalent doses than other members of the group. Excretion occurs via the urine, bile and intestinal secretions.

Absorption following oral administration results in peak blood and tissue levels within 2–4 hours with excretion over a 12–24-hour period (3), largely in the urine. Absorption from the intestine is decreased by binding by calcium in milk, and other substances such as iron, bismuth and aluminium salts. It is generally recommended that in order to maintain high tissue levels the drug be administered three times daily, but twice daily appears satisfactory in most diseases. A significant proportion of the oral dose, which may reach 50% at high dose rates, is not absorbed from the intestine but is excreted via the feces. In pre-ruminant calves the administration of oxytetracycline in milk replacer is associated with a markedly reduced and delayed peak serum concentration and with significantly reduced bioavailability when compared with administration in water. This is due to binding to milk which is only partly reversible and so the bound oxytetracycline remaining in the intestine is unlikely to be biologically active at that site (14). Higher peak serum concentrations are achieved with administration in glucose–glycine–electrolyte solution than in water.

Significant blood levels are not easily achieved following oral dosing in ruminants, and because of this and its effect on the ruminal and intestinal flora in cattle and horses, oral administration of the tetracycline group is almost entirely restricted to pre-ruminants and foals, although oral low level (350–500 mg total dose) administration to feedlot cattle for disease control is used. The recommended oral therapeutic dose is 10 mg/kg given twice daily. The tetracyclines are commonly used in feed or water for medication in pig diseases at a level which will provide an intake of between 10–20 mg/kg body weight daily.

Oxytetracycline

Oxytetracycline is commonly administered parenterally. Two problems limit the use of this drug by intramuscular injection. First, injectable preparations are extremely irritant and the use of local anesthetics and special base carriers may minimize, but does not entirely eliminate, this problem. Second, the resultant local reaction and the persistence of the drug at the injection site strictly limits the use of this drug by this route during the 3-week period before marketing in meat-producing animals, and at all times in horses. Oxytetracycline is poorly soluble which necessitates low concentrations in injectable preparations and relatively large volumes must be injected which often requires several injection sites.

The bioavailability of oxytetracycline following intramuscular injection can vary with different commercial formulations. In a study of ten commercial products considerable differences were found between peak serum concentrations and time to peak concentration at the same dose. Differences in bioavailability could not be solely predicted on the solvent base as it was also influenced by factors such as the pH of the preparation and other manufacturing formulations (16). However, in general there was an inverse relationship between bioavailability and the degree of reaction at the injection site.

Peak blood concentrations and a modest plateau are achieved between 4 and 8 hours post-injection of oxytetracycline in polyvinyl pyrrolidone. The recommended dose is usually 10 mg/kg followed by a dose of 5–10 mg/kg at 12 hour intervals. However, pharmacokinetic studies suggest that 20 mg/kg would be more appropriate to achieve therapeutic concentrations against sensitive Gram-negative infections (5, 17, 18). Calves with pneumonia show a more rapid elimination half-life and if a dose of 10 mg/kg is used it must be repeated every 12 hours (20).

The higher dose rate is probably indicated in most instances but the irritant nature of the injection and the high volume of injection required at higher doses in conjunction with cost considerations, usually results in dose administration at the lower levels. In cattle, higher blood levels during the first 5 hours after therapy are achieved by the injection of the dose at multiple sites with no more than 10 ml being given at any one site. Intraperitoneal injection may obviate some of these problems. An intravenous loading dose can be used when high peak concentrations are required in the initial part of therapy.

A long-acting repository form of oxytetracycline containing 200 mg of oxytetracycline per ml in aqueous 2-pyrrolidone is available for use in ruminants and pigs. In cattle and sheep peak serum concentrations are achieved earlier with this preparation than with the conventional preparations and they persist for longer periods (5, 17, 18). This suggests that a portion of this preparation is available for immediate absorption while the remainder acts as a depot with absorption over a longer period (18). Following a dose of 20 mg/kg serum concentrations of 1 μg/ml or greater are maintained for $2\frac{1}{2}$–3 days (5, 18). This can be advantageous when treating sick animals where yarding and catching for the purposes of repeated therapy can itself be deleterious and it has been suggested that this long-acting form of tetracycline is the preparation of choice where intramuscular tetracycline is to be used. The dose rate of 20 mg/kg is considerably in excess of the manufacturer's recommended dose and the label dose.

Administration and complications of tetracyclines

The tetracyclines are most commonly given intravenously and they should be given slowly or diluted to a 1% solution to minimize acute toxic effects. Following parenteral injection there is a significant enterohepatic cycling and a proportion of the drug may be excreted in the feces and be active in the intestine. The recommended dose for intravenously administered oxytetracycline is 4–10 mg/kg. With highly sensitive organisms this can be repeated at 24 hour intervals but less sensitive infections require 12 hour dose intervals. There is pharmacokinetic evidence that higher dose rates and shorter dose intervals than these should be used in horses and cattle (7) for the treatment of many infections; however, the factors of cost and toxicity limit the recommendations to those above. Intravenous administration of oxytetracycline results in higher tissue concentrations of the drug than those achieved at equivalent dosage given intramuscularly (19). Concentrations are higher in kidney and liver than in serum and higher in pneumonic lung than normal lung (17, 18). Effective therapy against sensitive infections may be achieved with rolitetracycline given once daily at 3–5 mg/kg. The tetracyclines, especially oxytetracycline given parenterally, are indicated in the therapy of a variety of infectious diseases and because of their broad spectrum of activity they frequently result in a favorable response where other antimicrobials are less effective. Their special indications are given in the section on specific diseases. Because of its broad spectrum of activity, oxytetracycline is frequently the antibiotic of choice in the initial treatment of infectious disease of undetermined etiology or of those syndromes in which multiple infection occcurs. However, more recently, ampicillin or trimethoprim-potentiated sulfonamides have supplanted oxytetracycline from this role in many situations. The chief drawbacks to the use of tetracyclines are difficulty in administration and cost in cattle, and potential toxicity especially in horses. Tetracyclines are not used locally, such as in joint or pleural cavities, because of their irritant inflammatory nature.

Toxicity may occur following administration of tetracyclines. The problem of inflammation and necrosis following intramuscular injection has already been mentioned. An acute collapse syndrome is occasionally seen following intravenous administration. It occurs in horses and cattle, often following rapid injection, and in severely toxemic animals or in animals with dyspnea. It is manifested by rapid collapse within 1 minute of injection followed by a mild tonic–clonic convulsion, nystagmus, dyspnea, tachycardia and sweating. The majority of animals recover within a few minutes. Tetracyclines have the ability to induce neuromuscular block but it is unlikely that this is the mechanism of these toxic reactions in cattle and horses (8). The intravenous injection of tetracycline chloride has been shown to produce a similar syndrome in association with the occurrence of severe cardiac arrhythmias and conduction disturbances and a profound fall in systemic blood pressure (9). Most commonly there was marked bradycardia, associated with atrial tachycardia and pronounced heart block, followed by the occurrence of ventricular extrasystoles. The syndrome could be prevented by pretreatment with calcium and it appears that it is related to the ability of tetracycline to chelate the contractile calcium pool in heart muscle. However, it is possible that the cause of the collapse syndrome is multifactorial as the vehicles propylene glycol and polyvinyl pyrrolidone also have pronounced adverse cardiovascular effects when given intravenously (10). To avoid this syndrome slow administration is recommended. Antihistamines may be of value when propylene glycol is the cause.

Alimentary tract dysfunction may occur following either oral or parenteral administration. Doses greater than 350 mg daily when given orally to cattle may produce rumen dysfunction and atony. Prolonged oral treatment in calves may result in abomasal and intestinal superinfection. Hepatic and renal damage is recorded with high doses (33 mg/kg) of oxytetracycline sometimes used in the therapy of respiratory disease in feedlot cattle (13). Tetracyclines are deposited in bone and teeth with discoloration and fluorescence but this is not a problem in large animals. There are indications that the use of tetracyclines in horses should be approached with extreme caution. Its use in horses has always been limited because of the possibility of inducing diarrhea. However, high doses (15 g) given intravenously have been found to result in severe intractable diarrhea with death in 4–5 days (11). This syndrome also occurs in a significant proportion of horses given routine parenteral doses of tetracyclines following surgery (12) and can occur following tetracycline therapy in non-surgical situations. There appear to be no problems associated with the oral administration of tetracyclines to pigs but high parenteral doses may be associated with diarrhea. Superinfection in young animals following prolonged oral dosing can occur but is less common than following chloramphenicol. Nephrotoxicity has been associated with high and repeated doses of oxytetracycline in feedlot calves treated for pneumonia. Dose rates were 44 mg/kg intravenously followed by four daily doses of 22 mg/kg intramuscularly (21).

REFERENCES

(1) Aronson, A. L. (1980). *J. Am. vet. med. Assoc.*, *176*, 1061.
(2) Ziv, G. & Sulman, F. G. (1974) *Am. J. vet. Res.*, *35*, 1197.
(3) Owen, L. N. (1965) *Vet. Bull.*, *35*, 187 & 331.
(4) Clark, J. C. et al. (1974) *Vet. Med.*, *small Anim. Clin.*, *69*, 1542.
(5) Davey, L. A. et al. (1985) *Vet. Rec.*, *117*, 426.
(6) Eidt, E. et al. (1976) *Dtsch Tierärztl. Wochenschr.*, *83*, 489.
(7) Pilloud, M. (1973) *Res. vet. Sci.*, *15*, 224.
(8) Bowen, J. M. & McMullan, W. C. (1975) *Am. J. vet. Res.*, *36*, 1025.
(9) Gyrd-Hansen, R., et al. (1981) *J. vet. Pharmacol. Therap.*, *4*, 15.
(10) Gross, D. R. et al. (1981) *Am. J. vet. Res.*, *42*, 1371.
(11) Andersson, G. et al. (1971) *Nord VetMed.*, *23*, 9.
(12) Owen, R. ap R. (1975) *Vet. Rec.*, *96*, 267.
(13) Griffin, D. D. et al. (1979) *Bov. Pract.*, *14*, 29.
(14) Palmer, G. H. et al. (1983) *Am. J. vet. Res.*, *44*, 68.
(15) Shaw, D. H. & Rubin, S. I. (1986) *J. Am. vet. med. Assoc.*, *189*, 808.
(16) Nouws, J. F. M. et al. (1985) *Vet. Q.*, *7*, 306.
(17) Ames, T. R. & Patterson, E. B. (1985) *Am. J. vet. Res.*, *46*, 2471.
(18) Toutain, P. L. & Raynaud, J. P. (1985) *Am. J. vet. Res.*, *44*, 1203.
(19) Bengtsson, B. et al. (1986) *J. vet. Pharmacol. Therap.*, *9*, 71.
(20) Burrows, G. E. et al. (1986) *J. vet. Pharmacol. Therap.*, *9*, 213.
(21) Lairmore, M. D. et al. (1984) *J. Am. vet. med. Assoc.*, *185*, 793.

Chloramphenicol

Chloramphenicol has several theoretical advantages over other antimicrobial agents. It has a broad spectrum of activity in combination with excellent penetrability into body tissues, and its use in large animals has not been associated with any degree of toxic side activity. The drug is active against a number of Gram-positive and Gram-negative bacteria including staphylococci, pasteurellae, *Bordetella*, *Haemophilus* and coliform organisms which may be variably resistant to other antibacterial agents. It is frequently recommended for the treatment of salmonellosis. It also has activity against chlamydiae and rickettsiae. It has been used parenterally for the treatment of several infectious diseases and is also used topically especially in the treatment of infectious diseases of the eyes and skin and occasionally for footrot in sheep. In some countries, including the United States, there is an absolute ban on its use in food-producing animals.

Following intravenous injection chloramphenicol rapidly equilibrates throughout the body and is widely distributed. The serum levels following intravenous injection are dose-dependent. Studies in large animals (1–3) have shown that, as in other species, this drug has excellent tissue penetration including intracellular fluids, and that tissue levels equal or exceed those of serum. Chloramphenicol has the ability to cross physiological barriers; significant levels can be achieved in areas such as the brain, and it achieves high levels in liver and bile. It is one of the few antibiotics to penetrate into CSF and ocular fluids in significant amounts after parenteral administration and it also diffuses across the cornea following topical administration. Milk levels are approximately half blood levels in the normal udder, but may approach equivalence if the udder is inflamed. There is probably an enterohepatic circulation. Excretion is via the bile and urine. Significant blood levels can also be achieved with adequate dose rates administered orally in pre-ruminant animals and in foals but not in ruminants (4). Blood levels following oral administration are dose-dependent and can approach those obtained by equivalent doses given parenterally. Reports on blood levels following intramuscular injection are varied, depending upon the formulation of the preparation used. In the horse significant blood levels are not obtained following the intramuscular injection of chloramphenicol but significant levels can be obtained following the intramuscular injection of the succinate (1, 4). Similarly, in cattle the intramuscular administration of chloramphenicol succinate has therapeutic advantage over equivalent or greater doses of chloramphenicol base given by the same route (5).

The currently recommended dose rates for chloramphenicol in large animals range from 4 to 11 mg/kg intramuscularly and from 2 to 4 mg/kg of the succinate intravenously. There is considerable evidence that these dose rates will not achieve significant therapeutic levels in large animals and that much higher dose rates are required (1–3). Also currently used dose intervals appear too long. The pharmacokinetics of chloramphenicol in large animals differ considerably from those of other species. There is considerable species variation in the plasma half-life of chloramphenicol. It is extremely short in horses (1–2 hours) and is considerably less in cattle (2–3·5 hours), goats (1–2 hours) and pigs (1·3 hours) than in dogs, cats and man. Species variation results from variation in biotransformation of the drug (3, 6). From these findings it has been suggested that it is impossible to achieve a constant therapeutic level of chloramphenicol in the horse as the dose rate and dose frequency would be too high to be practical under field or even hospital situations. Plasma chloramphenicol concentrations of 5–8 μg/ml have been suggested as necessary for effective therapy (11). In ruminants a dose rate of 20–30 mg/kg given intramuscularly and repeated every 8 hours may be sufficient for therapy although higher doses may be required in goats (13), and a dose of 30–50 mg/kg every 8 hours is suggested for the horse (7, 10). In all cases the succinate ester should be used. Biotransformation of chloramphenicol in young neonatal animals may take significantly longer than in adults and it is probably more easy to maintain effective therapeutic blood levels in this age group in comparison to adults. For example, the half-life of chloramphenicol in day-old calves is 15 hours, and pharmacokinetic studies suggest an intramuscular dose of the succinate ester of 27·5 mg/kg daily at this age and 45 mg/kg twice daily for calves at 1 week of age (8). Chloramphenicol can be administered orally in monogastric animals and pre-ruminant calves and lambs. In the horse less than 50% of the orally administered dose is absorbed and even with dose rates of 50 mg/kg therapeutic serum, synovial and peritoneal fluid concentrations are barely achieved and persist for only short periods. There appears to be a decrease in the amount absorbed with repetitive oral dosing (10). Thus there appear to be limitations on the value of this route of administration.

The results of pharmacokinetic studies of chloramphenicol which indicate that high doses are necessary must be balanced against the apparent therapeutic value of chloramphenicol at lower dose rates. The ultimate test for any chemotherapeutic is the clinical outcome. However, with chloramphenicol, clinical experience also suggests that therapeutic failures appear to be much more frequent with this antibiotic than with others and this is probably related to inadequate dose rates which is largely a factor of cost. In horses, our current practice, when chloramphenicol is used, is to administer it as the succinate either intravenously or intramuscularly at a dose rate that approaches the high dose rate detailed above, if cost allows. The frequency of administration limits its use to hospital patients. We have experienced marked therapeutic inefficiency with chloramphenicol in organic solvents administered intramuscularly and prefer not to use chloramphenicol in cattle for systemic infections. In view of the limited information on variations in biotransformation within and between large animal species at young ages, it is difficult to recommend a dose for this age group. The dose rate in animals over 2 weeks of age should approximate that for adults, but lesser doses may suffice for those under 1 week of age. A reduced elimination rate, due to reduced hepatic biotransformation, has been shown in the newborn calf and pig. In calves the half-life at birth approximates 10 hours and decreases to reach adult values at about 6 weeks of age (12). However, there is considerable calf-to-calf variation.

Toxicity with chloramphenicol therapy in large animals is negligible with the possible exception of problems associated with oral administration in young animals. Depression, inappetence and diarrhea have been reported as occurring in initially healthy young calves following oral administration of chloramphenicol. The syndrome is possibly associated with the development of a malabsorption state associated with a local toxic effect of chloramphenicol on the intestinal epithelium in young calves (14). An equivalent syndrome could not be demonstrated in adult horses (10). Prolonged oral administration of chloramphenicol in young animals may also be followed by the development of superinfection within the intestine. In view of these associations the use of chloramphenicol by oral administration in young animals should be approached with caution.

The potential for chloramphenicol to prolong the action of general anesthetics that are inactivated by the liver should be considered and it is probably wise to avoid the use of this drug in these circumstances. Chloramphenicol, through its effect on protein synthesis, may be immunosuppressive and should not be used in temporal conjunction with vaccination procedures (4). There is some evidence that prolonged high doses (55 mg/kg b.i.d.) of chloramphenicol in very young calves may induce diarrhea and death (9). There are unpublished reports of toxicity in cattle following prolonged daily use of chloramphenicol containing propylene glycol as solvent and benzoic acid as a preservative.

There is considerable debate about the efficacy of chloramphenicol in large animals when used at current dose rates. The use of higher doses is expensive and it is held by some scientists that the use of this drug should be restricted in animals because of its potential for inducing multiple drug resistance in bacteria which may be transferred to man, and cause disease in man which may be difficult to treat effectively. It is recommended that other antimicrobials should be considered in preference to this drug for the treatment of disease in large animals except in circumstances where it has a specific indication. The use of chloramphenicol in food animals in the United States and Canada was banned primarily because of the potential for residues in food products coupled with the potential of chloramphenicol to induce non-dose related aplastic anemia in humans.

Thiamphenicol and florfenicol are structural analogs of chloramphenicol. It is possible that neither analog will induce aplastic anemia in man and that they could thus be used as substitutes for chloramphenicol in food animal practice (15). Florfenicol is of particular interest as it has only one site for bacterial acetylation as compared to two sites on both chloramphenicol and thiamphenicol. It shows equivalent antibacterial activity to chloramphenicol, but is also active against certain chloramphenicol-resistant organisms. Preliminary pharmacokinetic studies on florfenicol in cattle are available (15).

REFERENCES

(1) Sisodia, C. S. et al. (1975) *Can. J. comp. Med.*, *39*, 216.
(2) Sisodia, C. S. et al. (1973) *Am. J. vet. Res.*, *34*, 1147.
(3) Davis, L. E. et al. (1972) *Am. J. vet. Res.*, *33*, 2259.
(4) Sisodia, C. S. (1980) *J. Am. vet. med. Assoc.*, *176*, 1069.
(5) Ziv, G. (1980) *J. Am. vet. med. Assoc.*, *176*, 1122.
(6) Pilloud, M. (1973) *Res. vet. Sci.*, *15*, 231.
(7) Clark, C. H. (1978) *Mod. vet. Pract.*, *59*, 749.
(8) Reiche, R. et al. (1980) *J. vet. Pharmacol. Therap.*, *3*, 95.
(9) Huffman, E. M. (1981) *Proc. 42nd Ann. vet. Conf.*, *Fort Collins, Colorado*, 59.
(10) Gronwall, R. et al. (1986) *Am. J. vet. Res.*, *47*, 2591.
(11) Adamson, P. J. W. et al. (1985) *Am. J. vet. Res.*, *46*, 447.
(12) Burrows, G. E. et al. (1983) *Am. J. vet. Res.*, *44*, 1053.
(13) Kume, B. B. and Garg, R. C. (1986) *J. vet. Pharmacol. Therap.*, 9, 254.
(14) Rollin, R. E. et al. (1986) *Am. J. vet Res.*, *47*, 987.
(15) Varma, K. J. et al. (1986) *J. vet. Pharmacol. Therap.*, 9, 412.

Polymyxin B and colistin

Polymyxin B and colistin (polymyxin E) have essentially no activity against Gram-positive bacteria and are used primarily for their activity against coliform organisms, especially *Klebsiella* spp. and *Pseudomonas* spp., which may be resistant to other drugs. They are bactericidal in action. The therapeutic combination of polymyxins with tetracyclines, or chloramphenicol, or carbenicillin, has synergism against *P. aeruginosa*, and synergism with polymyxin and sulfonamides can occur against other Gram-negative organisms. Polymyxins are primarily used as topical preparations and are also given by oral administration. Significant blood levels are not achieved following oral administration and absorption from other mucous surfaces and the mammary gland is minimal (1).

These drugs are seldom used by parenteral administration in large animals. Limited information indicates that intramuscular administration of polymyxin B or colistin is followed by peak blood levels within 2 hours and that these levels are dose-dependent, with a half-life of 5–6 hours (2, 3). They are highly ionic weak bases with poor lipid solubility, and tissue penetration is poor. However, they have a high binding affinity for certain tissues and this is a dominant factor in their distribution in the body and elimination (1, 3). A high proportion of the drug in tissues is in a microbiologically inactive form. The strong affinity for muscle can result in drug residues persisting in edible tissue for several weeks. The methanesulfonate derivatives of these drugs give higher blood levels at equivalent dose rates and better tissue penetrability. They are also less toxic. Excretion with this group is via the urine. An intramuscular dose of 2·5 mg/kg will give active drug blood levels for 4–6 hours and with 5 mg/kg this period approaches 12 hours (2, 3). In view of their toxicity, tissue residue problems and poor penetrability there are probably few indications for the use of parenteral polymyxins in large animal practice that cannot be met by other antimicrobials. Tentative recommended dose rates for polymyxin and colistin are 2·5–5·0 mg/kg and for the methanesulfonate derivatives 5–7·5 mg/kg (1 mg = 10 000 units). This group has potential for serious neurotoxic and nephrotoxic side effects. Therapy at these doses for 3 days in calves has not been associated with detectable nephrotoxicity, but at the higher dose rate lethargy and mild ataxia may be present 2–4 hours after treatment (3). Toxicity and death associated with neuromuscular blocking activity has been observed with polymyxin B at 10 mg/kg (2). The usual dose for polymyxin B by oral administration is 5·0 mg/kg given twice daily.

The polymyxins have been shown to inactivate endotoxin and the pretreatment of the udder with 200 mg of polymyxin has been shown to reduce the febrile and inflammatory response to subsequent endotoxin infusion. Although this effect is not evident with treatment after endotoxin infusion the intramammary infusion of 100–200 mg of polymyxin may be of value in treating coliform mastitis if administered early in the course of the disease (1).

REFERENCES

(1) Ziv, G. (1981) *J. Am. vet. med. Assoc.*, *179*, 711.
(2) Ziv, G. & Sulman, F. G. (1973) *Am. J. vet. Res.*, *34*, 317.
(3) Ziv, G. et al. (1980) *J. vet. Pharmacol. Therap.*, *3*, 87.

Rifampin (rifamycin, rifampicin)

Rifampin is a complex macrocyclic semisynthetic antibiotic that is highly lipid soluble and able to penetrate many tissues including semisolid caseous material, neutrophils and macrophages. Historically rifampin has been used to treat tuberculosis in man; however, its penetrability and low minimal inhibitory concentrations for most Gram-positive organisms has excited interest for its value in veterinary medicine where it has been used for the treatment of *Corynebacterium* (*Rhodococcus*) *equi* pneumonia in foals (3). It is bactericidal in activity and inhibitis RNA synthesis by inhibition of bacterial DNA-dependent RNA polymerase. Rifampin can be given intravenously, intramuscularly or orally. The bioavailability following intramuscular injection is higher than that following oral administration but the rate of absorption is more rapid following oral administration and adequate circulating concentrations can be achieved following oral administration of moderate doses in the horse (1, 3). Rifampin is metabolized in the liver and has an enterohepatic circulation. The elimination half-life in adult horses is approximately 6 hours but considerably longer (approximately 17 hours) in foals. Minimal inhibitory concentrations for veterinary pathogens are poorly defined but pharmacokinetic studies suggest that an oral dose of 10 mg/kg for adults and 5 mg/kg for foals given once a day will achieve circulating concentrations active against most Gram-positive organisms. Therapy for Gram-negative organisms would require higher or more frequent dosing (1, 3). Resistance can develop in a stepwise fashion and it is suggested that rifampin should be used in combination with other antibacterials. Synergism with erythromycin, oleandomycin, vancomycin and nafcillin against Gram-positive organisms has been demonstrated (2). Toxicity of rifampin in large animals remains to be determined. Prolonged sweating and some intravascular hemolysis is recorded in horses following intravenous administration and the intramuscular injection is followed by tenderness at the injection site (1). Cost will likely preclude the use of this drug in large animals other than horses and its therapeutic value and spectrum in horses remains to be determined.

REFERENCES

(1) Burrows, G. E. et al. (1985) *Am. J. vet. Res.*, *46*, 442.
(2) Tuazon, C. V. et al. (1978) *Antimicrob. Agents Chemotherap.*, *13*, 759.
(3) Castro, L. A. et al. (1986) *Am. J. vet. Res.*, *47*, 2584.

Nitrofurans

The nitrofurans used as antimicrobial agents include furazolidone, nitrofurazone and furaltadone. Nitrofurantoin is used in small animals especially as a urinary antiseptic but is little used in large animals. The nitrofurans are bactericidal in activity and have a broad spectrum of activity against Gram-positive and Gram-negative bacteria and coccidia (1). Gram-negative activity extends to the coliform group but not to *Pseudomonas* or *Proteus* spp. In large animal practice, nitrofurans are used for their activity against staphylococci, especially for the treatment and prevention of colibacillosis in pigs and calves and the treatment of salmonellosis in growing pigs and adult cattle. They are also commonly used as bactericidal agents in topical preparations.

For the treatment of colibacillosis and salmonellosis the nitrofurans are given orally. Following oral administration of *furazolidone* in pigs there is good absorption but the drug is rapidly metabolized and excreted so that its persistence in tissues is low (2), and there is some doubt that significant systemic antibacterial activity is achieved with this group of drugs. Furazolidone is poorly water-soluble and is usually administered in the feed. *Furaltadone* and *nitrofurazone* may be administered in the water or the feed.

Dose rates recommended are usually in the order of 10–20 mg/kg body weight but dose rates as high as 100 mg/kg may be required for therapy in salmonellosis. Concentrations of furazolidone in the feed for growing pigs vary from 100 to 500 g/tonne with the higher level used for treatment. Medication of the water is usually in the order of 100 mg/liter.

Acute toxicity may be seen at high rates in pigs and calves and occasionally adult cattle. It usually develops on the second or third day of medication and is manifest by inappetence and hyperexcitability with incoordination, muscle twitching and severe tonic–clonic convulsions with excitement. The syndrome usually resolves if the animals are immediately removed from medication and kept quiet, but mortality may occur in pigs. Acute toxicity has been observed in calves with nitrofurazone intakes as low as 33 mg/kg fed twice daily (4).

Chronic toxicity has been observed in calves after several weeks of medication with furazolidone at dose levels as low as 4–10 mg/kg, usually in association with inclusion in milk replacers. It is manifest by an agranulocytopenia with the occurrence of extensive petechial hemorrhages and bleeding. The period of feeding required to induce the syndrome varies with the dose, varying from 8 weeks at intakes of 8 mg/kg to 15–22 weeks at intakes of 4 mg/kg (3). Despite the level of intake the onset is sudden and calves generally die within 3–7 days from overwhelming secondary infections.

REFERENCES

(1) Devriese, L. A. (1975) *Zentralbl. VetMed.*, *22B*, 220.
(2) Tennant, D. M. & Roy, W. H. (1971) *Proc. Soc. exp. Biol. Med.*, *138*, 808.
(3) Hofmann, W. et al. (1974) *Dtsch Tierärztl. Wochenschr.*, *81*, 53 & 59.
(4) Frankhauser, J. A. et al. (1981) *Vet. Med., small Anim. Clin.*, *76*, 861.

Metronidazole

Metronidazole is an antibacterial drug with activity against obligate anaerobic bacteria such as *Bacteroides* spp., fusobacteria, clostridia and anaerobic cocci and also against certain protozoa (1). Nitroimadiazoles such as metronidazole, dimetridazole and ronizadole have been used for several years in veterinary medicine for the treatment and control of swine dysentery; however there is now increasing interest in the use of metronidazole for the treatment of other anaerobic infections, especially in the horse. Anaerobic infections are common in conditions such as peritonitis, pleuritis, empyema, liver abscess, foot abscess and sinusitis. Obligate anaerobes frequently produce betalactamase active against penicillins and cephalosporins, and their presence in mixed aerobic and anaerobic pyogenic conditions may inhibit effective therapy against the aerobic organisms with the penicillin group. Metronidazole has no activity against the common aerobic infections associated with pyogenic infections and so is commonly used in conjunction with other drugs such as the penicillins. It can be administered either intravenously, orally or by infusion into body cavities. The drug has high lipid solubility and is widely distributed in tissues and body fluids including good penetration into abcesses and avascular areas. In the horse there is rapid absorption and high bioavailability following oral administration and a more prolonged therapeutic blood concentration than that following intravenous administration (2). Based on the available MIC for veterinary pathogens and pharmacokinetic data a dose of 15–25 mg/kg given orally four times a day has been recommended (1, 2). Metronidazole should not be administered in conjunction with anesthetic agents (3).

REFERENCES

(1) Hirsh, D. C. et al. (1985) *J. Am. vet. med. Assoc.*, *186*, 1086.
(2) Sweeney R. W. et al. (1986) *Am. J. vet. Res.*, *47*, 1726.
(3) Owen, R. R. et al. (1985) *Vet. Rec.*, *117*, 534.

Tiamutilin

Tiamutilin is a semisynthetic diterpine antibiotic with activity against *Mycoplasma* spp., *Ureaplasma* spp., *Treponema hyodysenteriae* and some Gram-positive organisms. It is available in injectable and oral preparations and is predominantly used in swine for the treatment and control of swine dysentery and mycoplasmal pneumonia. It has high activity against mycoplasma and is recorded as being capable of eliminating *Mycoplasma hyopneumoniae* from swine and *Ureaplasma* spp. from sheep (1, 2). In swine tiamutilin may be administered either orally in the feed (120 ppm) or by intramuscular injection (15 mg/kg). Tiamutilin may potentiate the toxicity of ionophores in swine and therapeutic doses of tiamutilin have precipitated ionophore toxicity in pigs being fed normally non-toxic concentrations of salinomycin for growth-promoting purposes (3).

REFERENCES

(1) Meszaros, J. et al. (1986) *Arch. exp. VetMed.*, *40*, 19.
(2) Ball, H. J. & McCaughey, W. S. (1985) *Vet. Rec.*, *117*, 640.
(3) Miller, D. J. S. et al. (1986) *Vet. Rec.*, *118*, 73.

5

Diseases of the Alimentary Tract—I

PRINCIPLES OF ALIMENTARY TRACT DYSFUNCTION

THE primary functions of the alimentary tract are the prehension, digestion and absorption of food and water and the maintenance of the internal environment by modification of the amount and nature of the materials absorbed.

The primary functions can be divided into four major modes and, correspondingly, there are four major modes of alimentary dysfunction. There may be abnormality of motility, of secretion, of digestion or of absorption. The procedure in diagnosis should be to determine which mode or modes of function is or are disturbed before proceeding to the determination of the site and nature of the lesion and ultimately of the specific cause.

Motor function

Hypermotility and hypomotility

The most important facets of alimentary tract motility are the peristaltic movements which move ingesta and feces from the esophagus to the rectum, the segmentation movements which churn and mix the ingesta, and the tone of the sphincters. In ruminants these movements are of major importance in the forestomachs. Prehension, mastication and swallowing are other facets of alimentary tract motility which are essential for normal functioning of the tract.

Abnormal motor function may take the form of increased or decreased motility. Peristalsis and segmenting movements are usually affected equally and in the same manner. Motility depends upon stimulation via the sympathetic and parasympathetic nervous systems and is thus dependent upon the activity of the central and peripheral parts of these systems, and upon the intestinal musculature and its intrinsic nervous plexuses. Autonomic imbalance, resulting in a relative dominance of one or other system, is manifested by hypermotility or hypomotility, and can arise as a result of stimulation or destruction of hypothalamic centers, the ganglia, or the efferent or afferent peripheral branches of the system. Debility, accompanied by weakness of the musculature, or severe inflammation, such as occurs in acute peritonitis or after trauma, results in atony of the gut wall. Less severe inflammation, such as occurs in mild gastritis and enteritis, causes an increase in muscular activity. Increased motility causes diarrhea, decreased motility causes constipation, and both have deleterious effects on digestion and absorption.

Increased irritability at a particular segment increases its activity and disturbs the normal downward gradient of activity which ensures that the ingesta is passed from the esophagus to the rectum. Not only is the gradient towards the rectum made steeper, thus increasing the rate of passage of ingesta in that direction, but the increased potential activity of an irritated segment may be sufficiently high to produce a reverse gradient to the oral segments so that the direction of the peristaltic waves is reversed, oral to the irritated segments. It is by this means that vomiting occurs and intestinal contents, even feces, are returned to the stomach and vomited.

Distension

One of the major results of abnormality of motility is distension of the tract which occurs in a number of disturbances including the rapid accumulation or inefficient expulsion of gas, complete occlusion of the lumen by intestinal accident or pyloric or ileocecal valve obstruction, and engorgement on solid or liquid foods. Fluids, and to a lesser extent gas, accumulate because of their failure to pass along the tract. Much of the accumulated fluid represents saliva and gastric and intestinal juices secreted during normal digestion. Distension causes pain and, reflexly, increased spasm and motility of adjoining gut segments. Distension also stimulates further secretion of fluid into the lumen of the gut and this exaggerates the distension. When the distension passes a critical point, the ability of the musculature of the wall to respond diminishes, the initial pain disappears, and a state of paralytic ileus develops in which all muscle tone is lost.

Abdominal pain

Visceral pain may arise in any organ but the mode of its development is always the same and it is discussed here because alimentary tract disease is the major cause of visceral and, more specifically, of abdominal pain. The most important mechanism is stretching of the wall of the organ which stimulates free pain endings of autonomic nerves in the wall. Contraction does not of itself cause pain but does so by causing direct and reflex distension of neighboring segments. Thus spasm, an exaggerated segmenting contraction of one section of bowel, will result in distension of the immediately oral segment of bowel when a peristaltic wave arrives. When there is increased motility for any reason, excessive segmentation and peristalsis cause abdominal pain, and the frequent occurrence of intermittent bouts of pain depends upon the periodic increases in muscle tone which are typical of alimentary tract wall. Other factors which have some stimulating effect on the pain end-organs are edema and failure of local blood supply such as occurs in local embolism or in intestinal accidents accompanied by twisting of the mesentery. A secondary mechanism in the production of abdominal pain is the stretching and inflammation of serous membranes.

Clinically, abdominal pain can be detected by palpation and the elicitation of pain responses. The question arises as to whether the response elicited is due to involvement of underlying organs or to referred pain. It is difficult to decide whether referred pain occurs in animals. In humans it is largely a subjective sensation although often accompanied by local hyperalgesia. At least there are no known examples of referred pain which are of diagnostic importance in animals and a local pain response on palpation of the abdomen is accepted as evidence of pain in the serous membranes or viscera which underlie the point of palpation.

Dehydration and shock

An immediate effect of distension of the stomach or small intestine by the accumulation of saliva and normal gastric and intestinal secretions is the stimulation of further secretion of fluid and electrolytes in the oral segments. The stimulation is self-perpetuating and creates a vicious cycle resulting in loss of fluid and electrolytes to the point where fatal dehydration can occur. The dehydration is accompanied by acidosis or alkalosis depending on whether the obstruction is in the intestine and accompanied by loss of alkali, or in the stomach and accompanied by heavy loss of acid radicals. The net effect is the same whether the fluid is lost by vomiting or is retained in the gut. The same cycle of events occurs in ruminants which gorge on grain but here the precipitating mechanism is not distension but a gross increase in osmotic pressure of the ingesta due to the accumulation of lactic acid. Dehydration is also of major importance in diarrhea irrespective of the cause. An important additional factor in the production of shock, when there is distension of alimentary segments, is a marked reflex depression of vasomotor, cardiovascular and respiratory functions. In diarrhea in calves in which there is no septicemia nor toxemia caused by bacteria, the end-point in the phase of dehydration can be cardiac failure due to severe metabolic acidosis. Renal ischemia leading to uremia may result from decreased circulating blood volume and also contribute to a fatal outcome. These matters are discussed in detail in the section on disturbances of body fluids, electrolytes and acid–base balance.

Secretory function

Diseases in which abnormalities of secretion occur are not generally recognized in farm animals. In humans, and to a less extent in small animals, defects of gastric and pancreatic secretion produce syndromes which are readily recognized but they depend upon clinical pathological examination for diagnosis. If they do occur in farm animals, they have so far only been recognized as aberrations of motility caused by the defects of secretion. However, it is reasonable to assume that some neonates may be deficient in lactase activity which results in dietetic diarrhea. Undigested lactose causes diarrhea by its hyperosmotic effect, and some of the lactose may be fermented in the large intestine, the products of which fermentation may exaggerate the diarrhea. A deficiency of lactase activity has been suspected in foals affected with diarrhea of undetermined origin but the definitive diagnosis has not been made. The intestinal lactase activity of foals is at its highest level at birth and gradually declines until the fourth month of age, and then disappears from adults before their fourth year (1).

Digestive function

The ability of the alimentary tract to digest food depends on its motor and secretory functions and, in herbivores, on the activity of the microflora which inhabit the forestomachs of ruminants, or cecum and colon of equidae. The flora of the forestomachs of ruminants are capable of digesting cellulose, of fermenting the end-products of other carbohydrates to volatile fatty acids, and converting nitrogenous substances to ammonia and protein. In a number of circumstances, the activity of the flora can be modified so that digestion is abnormal or ceases. Failure to provide the correct diet, prolonged starvation or inappetence, and hyperacidity as occurs in engorgement on grain all result in impairment of microbial digestion. The bacteria, yeasts and protozoa may also be adversely affected by the oral administration of antibiotic and sulfonamide drugs, or drugs which drastically alter the pH of the rumen contents.

Diseases of the stomach of ruminants are presented in Chapter 6. Information about the digestive and absorptive capacities of the equine gut is not exhaustive but some basic data are available (2, 3). The rate of passage of ingesta through the stomach and intestines is rapid but varies widely depending on the physical characteristics of the ingesta, dissolved passaging more rapidly than particulate material; 75% of a liquid marker can be emptied from the stomach in 30 minutes, and be in the cecum at 2 hours. Passage through the large bowel is much slower, especially in the latter part of the colon where much of the fluid is absorbed. There is an obvious relationship between the great activity of the small intestine and the effect of a complete obstruction of it; the pain is very severe and often uncontrollable with standard analgesics, fluid loss into the obstructed parts is rapid, and dehydration, loss of electrolytes and disturbances of acid–base balance are acute, severe and life-threatening.

Absorptive functions

Absorption of fluids and the dissolved end-products of digestion may be adversely affected by increased motility or by disease of the intestinal mucosa. In most instances, the two occur together but, occasionally, as with some helminth infestations, lesions occur in the intestinal wall without accompanying changes in motility.

Autointoxication

This mechanism is thought to operate when there is cessation of forward movement of ingesta. At one time it did enjoy a considerable vogue as a diagnosis in human medicine and was credited as the cause of many human ailments. It has largely been discarded as an important consequence of disease of the alimentary tract but, used in its widest sense, the term still retains an element of accuracy in that there are many clinical signs in these diseases which cannot be adequately explained or classified in any other way. The theory of autointoxication suggested that the toxic amines and phenols produced by putrefaction of protein in the large intestine but normally detoxified in the bowel wall could, if regurgitated into the small intestine, be absorbed and cause depression, anorexia and weakness.

MANIFESTATIONS OF ALIMENTARY TRACT DYSFUNCTION

Inanition is the major physiological effect of alimentary dysfunction when the disease is a chronic one, dehydration being the major effect in acute diseases, and shock is the important physiological disturbance in hyperacute diseases. Some degree of abdominal pain is usual in most diseases of the alimentary tract, the severity varying with the nature of the lesion. Other manifestations include abnormalities of prehension, mastication and swallowing, and vomiting, diarrhea, hemorrhage and constipation.

Abnormalities of prehension, mastication and swallowing

Prehension, including grazing and drinking, may be faulty. Causes are:

- Paralysis of muscles of jaw or tongue
- Malapposition of incisor teeth due to:
  - inherited skeletal defect (inherited displaced molar teeth, inherited mandibular prognathism, inherited congenital osteopetrosis)
  - rickets
- Absence of some incisor teeth
- Pain in mouth due to:
  - stomatitis, glossitis
  - foreign body in mouth
  - decayed teeth, e.g. fluorosis
- Congenital abnormalities of tongue and lips:
  - inherited harelip
  - inherited smooth tongue of cattle.

A simple examination of the mouth usually reveals the causative lesion. Paralysis is indicated by the behavior of the animal as it attempts to ingest feed without success. In all cases, unless there is anorexia due to systemic disease, the animal is hungry and attempts to feed but cannot do so.

Mastication may be painful and this is manifested by slow jaw movements interrupted by pauses and expressions of pain if the cause is a bad tooth, but in a painful stomatitis there is usually complete refusal to chew. Incomplete mastication is evidenced by the dropping of food from the mouth while eating and the passage of large quantities of undigested material in the feces.

Swallowing is a complex act governed by reflexes mediated through the glossopharyngeal, trigeminal, hypoglossal and vagal nerves. It has been described endoscopically and fluoroscopically in the horse (26). The mechanism of the act includes closure of all exits from the pharynx, the creation of pressure to force the bolus into the esophagus, and involuntary movements to the musculature of the esophageal wall to carry the bolus to the stomach. A defect in nervous control of the reflex or a narrowing of the lumen of the pharynx or esophagus may interfere with swallowing and it is difficult to differentiate clinically between physical and functional causes of dysphagia (difficulty in eating).

Dysphagia is manifested by forceful attempts to swallow accompanied by extension of the head at first, followed by forceful flexion and violent contractions of the muscles of the neck and abdomen.

Inability to swallow is usually caused by the same lesions as dysphagia, but in a greater degree. If the animal attempts to swallow, the results depend on the site of the obstruction. Lesions in the pharynx cause regurgitation through the nostrils or coughing up of the material. In the latter instance, there is danger that some of the material may be aspirated into the lungs and cause acute respiratory and cardiac failure or aspiration pneumonia. When the obstruction is at a low level in the esophagus, a large amount of material may be swallowed and then regurgitated. It is necessary to differentiate between material regurgitated from the esophagus and vomitus. The former is usually slightly alkaline, the latter acid.

Causes of dysphagia and inability to swallow

- Foreign body, tumor or inflammatory swelling in pharynx or esophagus
- Painful condition of pharynx or esophagus
- Esophageal dilatation due to paralysis
- Esophageal diverticulum
- Esophageal spasm at site of mucosal erosion (achalasia of cardia not encountered).

Excessive salivation

Drooling of excessive saliva from the mouth, distinct from frothing such as occurs during convulsions, may be caused by pain in the mouth, by inability to swallow, by stimulation of saliva production by systemic toxins, or by hyperthermia, especially that caused by fungal toxins. With systemic poisonings the increased salivation is often accompanied by lacrimation.

Local causes

- Foreign body in mouth or pharynx
- Ulceration, deep erosion or vesicular eruption of the oral mucosa
- Inability to swallow (*see above*).

Systemic causes

- Poisonous trees—*Oleander* sp., *Andromeda* sp. (rhododendron)
- Other poisonous plants—kikuyu grass (or an attendant fungus)
- Fungal toxins, e.g. slaframine and those causing hyperthermia e.g. *Claviceps purpurea*, *Acremonium coenophialum*
- Iodism
- Watery mouth of lambs
- Sweating sickness
- Methiocarb poisoning.

Diarrhea and constipation

Diarrhea and constipation are the most commonly observed abnormalities in fecal consistency, composition and frequency of passage. Cattle in which the sojourn of ingesta is prolonged in the forestomachs or abomasum pass characteristically pasty feces in small amounts. The details are available in Chapter 6. When there is complete intestinal stasis the rectum may be empty except for blood-tinged thick, pasty material.

Abnormalities of peristalsis and segmentation usually occur together and when there is a general increase in peristaltic activity, there is increased caudal flow resulting in a decrease in intestinal transit time and diarrhea. Because of a lack of absorption of fluid the feces are usually softer than normal, the dry matter content is below the normal range, and the total amount of feces passed per day is increased. The frequency of defecation is usually also increased. Common causes of diarrhea are:

- Enteritis, including secretory enteropathy
- Malabsorption, e.g., due to villous atrophy and in hypocuprosis (due to molybdenum excess)
- Functional diarrhea as in excitement
- Some cases of local structural lesions of the stomach or intestine, including:
  - ulcer, e.g. of abomasum, or stomach
  - tumor, e.g. intestinal adenocarcinoma
- Indigestible diet, e.g. lactose intolerance in foals, carbohydrate indigestion in cattle
- In some cases of ileal hypertrophy, ileitis, diverticulitis and adenomatosis
- Terminal stages of congestive heart failure
- Chronic and acute undifferentiated diarrhea in horses
- Vagus indigestion in cows causes pasty feces but bulk is reduced.

Malabsorption syndromes similar to those recognized in dogs are being recognized with increased frequency in monogastric farm animals. In many instances, especially in recently weaned pigs, there is a significant degree of villous atrophy with a resulting loss in secretory and absorptive function (4, 5). Inefficient digestion originating in this way may or may not be manifested by diarrhea, but in malabsorption there is usually diarrhea. There is always failure to grow or maintain body weight, in spite of an apparently normal appetite and an adequate diet. In horses, the lesions associated with malabsorption, which may be with or without diarrhea, include villous atrophy, edema and/or necrosis of the lamina propria of the gut wall, and nodular tracts and aggregations of eosinophils indicating damage by migrating strongyle larvae. It is possible also that some cases are caused by an atypical reaction of tissue to unknown allergens (possibly helminths) and are probably an abnormal immunological response (6). A common accompaniment in the horse is thin hair coat, patchy alopecia and focal areas of scaling and crusting. The pathogenesis is unknown. Special tests are now detailed for the examination of digestive efficiency in the horse. These are listed in the next section under special tests. Increased venous pressure in the portal circuit caused by congestive heart failure or hepatic fibrosis also causes diarrhea.

When the motility of the intestine is reduced, the alimentary transit time is prolonged and constipation occurs. Because of the increased time afforded for fluid absorption, the feces are dry, hard and of small bulk and are passed at infrequent intervals. Common causes of constipation are:

- Severe debility as in old age
- Deficient dietary bulk, usually fiber
- Chronic dehydration
- Partial obstruction of large intestine
- Painful conditions of the anus
- Paralytic ileus
- Grass sickness in horses
- Chronic zinc poisoning in cattle
- Terminal stages of pregnancy in cows.

The question of whether or not enteritis in animals causes intestinal hypermotility has been asked for many years and remains unresolved. It is an important question because the answer would help to determine whether or not anticholinergics should be used in acute infectious diarrheas. Current concepts on the pathophysiology of some of the common diarrheas caused by infectious agents (such as enterotoxigenic *E. coli*) indicate that there is a net increase in the flow of intestinal fluid into the lumen (and a decrease in outflow) which causes distension of the intestine with fluid. The mere hydraulic effect of the distension can cause diarrhea; hypermotility is probably not necessary. In addition, because of the temporary malabsorption which exists in infectious enteritides and the presence of infectious agents and enterotoxins in the lumen of the intestine the emphasis should be on evacuation of the intestinal contents and not on the use of anticholinergic drugs to inhibit evacuation. Furthermore, it is unlikely that the anticholinergics will have any significant effect on the secretory–absorptive mechanisms which have been altered by an enteropathogen.

Vomiting

Vomiting is the most complex of the motor disturbances of the alimentary tract. It is essentially a protective mechanism, in the nature of a reverse peristaltic movement, with the function of removing excessive quantities of ingesta or toxic materials from the stomach. It occurs in two forms. Projectile vomiting is based almost entirely on reverse peristalsis and is not accompanied by retching movements. Large amounts of fluid material are vomited with little effort. This is the common form of vomiting in horses and ruminants and occurs almost entirely as a result of overloading of the stomach or forestomachs with food or fluid. True vomiting is accompanied by retching movements including contraction of the abdominal wall and of the neck muscles and extension of the head. The movements are commonly prolonged and repeated and the vomitus is usually small in amount and of porridge-like or pasty consistency. It is most commonly a result of irritation of the gastric mucosa.

It is not proposed to deal extensively with vomiting here because it is not a common sign in farm animals. Examination of suspected vomitus to determine its site of origin should be undertaken. Vomiting is commonly designated as being either peripheral or central in origin depending on whether the stimulation arises centrally at the vomiting center or peripherally by overloading of the stomach or inflammation of the gastric mucosa, or by the presence of foreign bodies in the pharynx, esophagus or esophageal groove. Central stimulation of vomiting by apomorphine and in nephritis and hepatitis are typical examples but vomiting occurs rarely, if at all, in these diseases in farm animals. In young pigs, vomiting is a common accompaniment of many systemic diseases.

Vomiting may have serious effects in that fluid and electrolytes may be lost in large quantities. In horses and cattle it may be followed by aspiration pneumonia or acute laryngeal obstruction. In these animals true vomiting is usually accepted as an ominous sign of grave involvement of the alimentary tract. Causes of vomiting and regurgitation include:

- Vomiting in horses terminally in acute gastric dilatation
- 'Vomiting' in cattle is really regurgitation of large quantities of rumen contents out through the mouth. Causes include:
  - third-stage milk fever
  - arsenic poisoning
  - poisoning by plants including *Eupatorium rugosum*, *Geigeria* sp., *Hymenoxis* sp., *Andromeda* sp., *Oleander* sp., *Conium maculatum*
  - administration of large quantities of fluids into rumen
  - use of large-bore stomach tube
  - cud-dropping is a special case
- Vomiting in pigs in:
  - vomiting and wasting disease
  - acute chemical intoxications
  - poisoning by the fungus *Fusarium* sp., which also causes off-feed effects suspected analogous to nausea in man
- Regurgitation—in all diseases causing dysphagia or paralysis of swallowing.

Alimentary tract hemorrhage

Hemorrhage into the stomach or intestine is a common occurrence in farm animals. The main causes are:

- Gastric or abomasal (rarely duodenal) ulcers
- Severe enteritis
- Structural lesions of the intestinal wall, e.g., adenomatosis, neoplasia
- Infestation with blood-sucking nematodes, e.g. bunostomiasis
- Local vascular engorgement or obstruction as in intussusception, verminous thrombosis.

Hemorrhage into the stomach results in the formation of acid hematin which given vomitus a dark brown color like coffee grounds, and feces a black or very dark brown, tarry appearance (melena). The change in appearance of the feces caused by hemorrhage into the bowel varies with the level at which the hemorrhage occurs. If the blood originates in the small intestine, the feces may be brown-black, but if it originates in the colon or cecum, the blood is unchanged and gives the feces an even red color. Hemorrhage into the lower colon and rectum may cause the voiding of stools containing or consisting entirely of clots of whole blood.

Hemorrhage into the pharynx is unusual, but when it occurs the blood may be swallowed and appear in the feces or vomitus. If there is any doubt about the presence of blood in the feces or vomitus, biochemical tests should be performed. The hemorrhage may be sufficiently severe to cause anemia and, in more severe cases, acute peripheral circulatory failure. In cattle the most sensitive test is one using a dilute alcoholic solution of guiac as the test reagent. It is capable of detecting a daily blood loss into the abomasum of as small a volume as 70 ml. Transit time of blood from abomasum to rectum in normal cows varies from 7 to 19 hours (21).

Abdominal pain due to alimentary tract disease

The pain associated with diseases of the abdominal viscera causes similar signs irrespective of the organ involved and careful clinical examination is necessary to locate the site of the lesion. The manifestations of abdominal pain vary with the species, horses being particularly sensitive, but comprise largely abnormalities of behavior and posture. Pain as a systemic state is dealt with elsewhere in general terms including its effects on body systems and methods for its detection.

Readily identifiable syndromes of abdominal pain referable to the alimentary tract include the following.

Horse

Acute pain Pawing, flank-watching, rolling.

Subacute pain Lesser degree of flank-watching, often excessive pawing, lying down a lot without rolling, stretching out as if to urinate; males may extrude penis, walking backwards, dog-sitting posture, lying on back, impulsive walking.

Peritoneal pain Rigidity of abdominal wall, pain on palpation.

Cow

Acute pain Downward arching of back with paddling of hind feet, lying down, rolling is uncommon.

Subacute pain, including peritoneal pain Back arched upwards, grunt on walking or lying down, grunt on percussion of abdomen, immobility.

Differential diagnosis
The disease states likely to be mistaken for alimentary tract pain are:

Acute pain Paresthesia, e.g. in photosensitive dermatitis of cows, snakebite in horses, urticaria as in milk allergy in cows; renal and urethral colic; compulsive walking, e.g. in hepatic disease, lead poisoning; dysuria, obstruction of urinary tract generally; laminitis, lactation tetany in mares.

Subacute pain encephalopathy, possibly hepatic insufficiency.

Common causes of alimentary tract pain

Horses
Acute pain Colic including gastric dilatation, intestinal obstruction, enteritis generally, colitis X, rarely salmonellosis.

Subacute pain Thromboembolic colic, impaction of the large intestine, ileal hypertrophy.

Cattle
Acute pain Intestinal obstruction, especially phytobezoar; poisoning by kikuyu grass, *Andromeda* sp., *Oleander* sp., water hemlock (*Cicuta* sp.).

Subacute pain Traumatic reticuloperitonitis, peritonitis generally.

Tenesmus

Although tenesmus, or severe straining, is a common sign of many diseases of the organs of the pelvic cavity, it is not necessarily a diagnostic sign of disease in the lower alimentary tract; it is sometimes associated with frequent defecation caused by neurologic stimulation of peristalsis.

Cattle
- Lower alimentary tract disease, e.g., coccidiosis
- Genital tract disease, e.g., severe vaginitis, retained placenta
- Estrogen toxicity in steers, e.g., estrogen implantation, fusariotoxicosis
- 4-Aminopyridine poisoning, methiocarb poisoning
- Lower spinal cord lesions—spinal cord abscess, rabies.

In some cases the cause is unknown.

Horses
Does not usually occur except during parturition.

Pigs
Constipation in parturient sows; also dystocia.

Shock and dehydration

Acute rapid distension of the intestine or stomach causes reflex effects on heart, lungs and on blood vessels. The blood pressure falls abruptly, the temperature falls below normal and there is a marked increase in heart rate. In acute intestinal accidents in horses which terminate fatally in 6–12 hours, shock is probably the major cause of death. There appears to be some species difference in the susceptibility to shock because similar accidents in cattle rarely cause death in less than 3–4 days, although acute ruminal tympany may exert its effects in this way and cause death in a very short time. Less severe distension, and vomiting and diarrhea cause clinically recognizable dehydration and abnormalities of electrolyte concentration and acid–base balance. Determination of the relative importance in a particular case at a particular time of shock and dehydration is one of the challenges in gastroenterology. The subject is considered in detail under the heading of equine colic (p. 176) and under enteritis (p. 199).

Abdominal distension

Distension of the abdomen as a manifestation of disease of the alimentary tract is a common and important finding in ruminants and is dealt with in those species in Chapter 6. In horses and pigs it is not as common, but is of great intrinsic importance, bearing in mind that diseases of other systems may rarely cause similar distensions. The diseases in this category are ascites and chronic peritonitis. Pregnancy causes distension too, but is usually readily identified.

The alimentary tract diseases of simple-stomached animals in which abdominal distension may be a manifestation are:

Intestinal tympany due to excessive gas production caused by abnormal fermentation in the large bowel of horses and pigs.

Obstruction of the large intestine in horses and pigs as a result of their torsion or miscellaneous constrictions caused by adhesions, usually as a result of peritonitis.

Retention of the meconium in foals is often accompanied by severe distension of the colon and abdomen.

Obstruction of the small intestine causes its distension, but not to the degree that obvious abdominal enlargement occurs. Acute dilatation of the stomach is similarly undemonstrative.

In all the above diseases the principal sign is acute abdominal pain.

Abnormal nutrition

Failure of normal motor, secretory, digestive or absorptive functions causes impairment of nutrient supply to body tissues. Inanition or partial starvation results and the animal fails to grow, loses body weight or shows other signs of specific nutritional deficiencies. Ancillary effects include decreased appetite when motility is decreased; in many cases where motility is increased and there is no toxemia, the appetite is increased and may be voracious.

SPECIAL EXAMINATION

The greater part of the technique of the examination of the alimentary tract has been dealt with in Chapter 1 on clinical examination but there are some special aspects which require discussion here. Radiographic examination is difficult in horses and cattle and is little used in the examination of the alimentary tract of other species. It has been used extensively in the investigation of motor functions of the tract in sheep and can be used clinically in sheep, pigs, foals and calves if the expense is warranted. There is potential for further use of esophageal radiography in the diagnosis and research into disorders of swallowing in horses (34). Imaging by ultrasound is a less familiar technique but its use in pregnancy diagnosis should increase it usefulness, at least in the diagnosis of diseases of the reproductive system (7).

External palpation of the abdomen is of limited value in farm animals and is replaced by the passage of a stomach tube, by rectal examination and by auscultation of the abdomen. Attempts to pass a stomach tube will detect complete or partial obstruction of the esophagus. In gross distension of the stomach in the horse, there is an immediate rush of fluid contents as soon as the cardia is passed. Visual examination of the posterior fauces, pharynx and larynx of cattle is sometimes essential and general anesthesia to permit the examination is often unsatisfactory. With patience and proper restraint the examination is possible if a mouth speculum is illuminated with a flashlight. Fiberoptic gastroduodenoscopy is a practicable procedure in a sedated horse which has had no feed for 24–48 hours. A 275 cm × 13.5 cm fiberoptic instrument is passed via a nostril to the stomach which is then distended with air. The control of the objective of the endoscope is quite difficult and entry into the pylorus so much so that entry into the duodenum is not possible in all horses (31).

Examination of the feces may provide valuable information on the digestive and motor functions of the tract. They should be examined for volume, consistency, form, color, covering, odor and composition. Note should be made of the frequency and the time taken for material to pass through the tract. Laboratory examinations may be advisable to detect the presence of helminth eggs, occult blood, bile pigments, pathogenic bacteria or protozoa.

It is usually sufficient to say that the volume is scanty, normal or copious but, in special circumstances, it may be advisable to weigh or measure the daily output. Horses normally pass 15–20 kg/day, cattle 25–45 kg/day, pigs 1–2·5 kg/day and sheep and goats 0·5–1 kg/day. There is an increased bulk when much fiber is fed or during attacks of diarrhea. The consistency and form of the feces varies with each species and varies widely within a normal range, depending particularly on the nature of the food. Variations in consistency not explainable by changes in the character of the feed may indicate abnormalities of any of the functions of the tract. The consistency is more fluid in diarrhea and less fluid than normal in constipation. The consistency and form of the feces may provide some indication of the location of the dysfunction of the gastrointestinal tract. In general, large quantities of liquid feces suggest a dysfunction of the small intestine where normally most of the fluid is absorbed. If the feces contain large quantities of undigested feed this suggests overfeeding, incomplete mastication, a digestive enzyme deficiency or an acute disorder of the small intestine or stomachs. Large quantities of soft feces which contain well-digested ingesta suggest a dysfunction of the large intestine. However, these are only guidelines and are subject to error. Studies in man have shown a lack of correlation between the physical form of a stool and its water content. The water content in formed stools of man may range from 73·8 to 96% with a mean of 86·7%, and the water content of liquid stools may range from 80·3 to 99·8% with a mean of 94·3% (8). Thus the form of the stool as judged by gross examination is not a reliable measure of its water content.

The color of the feces also varies widely with the color of the food, but feces of a lighter color than normal may be caused by an insufficient secretion of bile or by simple dilution of the pigments as occurs in diarrhea. The effect of blood on the appearance of feces has already been described. Discoloration by drugs should be considered when the animal is undergoing treatment.

Fecal odor also depends largely on the nature of the food eaten but in severe enteritis the odor is characteristically one of putrefaction. The composition of the feces should be noted. In herbivorous animals, there is always a proportion of undigested fiber but excessive amounts suggest incomplete digestion due for example to bad teeth and faulty mastication. Excessively pasty feces are usually associated with a prolonged sojourn in the tract such as occurs in vagal indigestion or abomasal displacement in cattle. Foreign material of diagnostic significance includes sand or gravel, wool, and shreds of mucosa. Mucus is a normal constituent but, in excessive amounts, indicates either chronic inflammation when it is associated with fluid, copious feces, or constipation when the feces are small in volume and hard. Mucosal shreds or casts always indicate inflammation.

Frequency of defecation and the length of sojourn are usually closely allied, increased frequency and decreased sojourn occurring in diarrhea and the reverse in constipation. Most animals defecate eight to twelve times a day but the sojourn varies widely with the species. Omnivores and carnivores with simple stomachs have an alimentary sojourn of 12–35 hours. In ruminants it is 2–4 days and in horses 1–4 days depending on the type of feed.

Observation of other acts associated with the functions of the alimentary tract may provide information of diagnostic value. Prehension, mastication, swallowing, vomiting and defecation should be observed and an attempt made to analyse the behavior of the animal when there is evidence of abdominal pain.

Tests of digestion and absorption

Tests for digestive and absorptive efficiency are frequently used in small animal medicine. Recent interest in large animal medicine has been stimulated by the apparent increase in the frequency of chronic diarrhea in horses, related to diseases which appear to be characterized by malabsorption.

A suitable test for the evaluation of gastric and small intestinal and pancreatic function is the starch digestion test (9). The horse is fasted for 18 hours, and then given corn starch (1 kg in 4 liters of water or 2 g/kg body weight) by stomach tube. A pretreatment blood sample is matched with others taken at 15, 30, 60, 90 and 120 minutes and then hourly to 6 hours.

In the normal horse there is an increase in blood glucose levels of about 30 mg/dl (1·7 mmol/l) (from 90 up to 120 mg/dl (5·0 up to 6·7 mmol/l)) with the peak occurring at 1 hour and the curve returned to pretreatment level at 3 hours. This closely approximates the result obtained in a similar oral glucose absorption test (10). The glucose is administered by stomach tube at the rate of 1 g of anhydrous glucose (or comparable) per kg body weight. The blood sugar in the normal horse increases by 100% (up from 90–180 mg/dl (5·0–10·0 mmol/l)). The peak blood glucose level is about 2 hours and the pretreatment level is regained at 6 hours. The shape of the curve is affected by the horse's previous diet, the curve being much lower in horses fed on stored feeds such as hay and grain compared to horses eating pasture of clover and grass (30).

An oral lactose digestion test has been devised for foals (11). Lactose (1 g/kg body weight) is given by stomach tube in a 20% solution. In foals and young horses up to 3 years of age there is a rise in blood glucose levels from 86 ± 11 mg/dl (4·8 ± 0·1 mmol/l) up to 153 ± 24 mg/dl (8·5 ± 1·3 mmol/l), with a peak achieved in 90 minutes, and the level returns to pretreatment levels in 5 hours. In foals of 1–12 weeks of age the plasma glucose concentration should rise by at least 35 mg/dl (1·9 mmol/l) and peak within 40 minutes of the administration of the lactose (33). With this test no changes in blood sugar levels occur in horses over 4 years of age. Instead there is abdominal discomfort followed by diarrhea, with feces of the consistency of cow feces for the next 24 hours. Sucrose and maltose are readily digested by the intestine of the adult horse, but not by newborn foals. Maximum levels of the relevant intestinal disaccharidases (sucrase and maltase) are not achieved until 7 months of age. Details of the changes in intestinal enzymatic acitivity in the fetus and neonate are available for calves (12). The oral lactose digestion test is likely to be of value as a monitor of epithelial damage in young horses. In man the ability to hydrolyze lactose is one of the first functions of the intestinal mucosa to be lost where there is epithelial damage in the gut. It is also one of the last functions to return in the recovering patient. The loss of intestinal lactase may be the pathogenetic basis of the diarrhea which occurs in rotavirus infections in neonates.

An adaptation of the human xylose absorption test has been used in horses (13). D(+)-xylose, at a dose rate of 0·5 g/kg body weight as a 10% solution is administered by stomach tube after a starve of 18 hours. A maximum blood xylose level of 30 mg/dl (2·0 mmol/l) at 1·5 hours is a normal result in adult horses. In normal foals the peak blood concentration of xylose is reached in 30–60 minutes and the level attained varies with age being highest (47 mg/dl (3.14 mmol/l)) at 1 month of age and lowest (19 mg/dl (1·25 mmol/l)) at 3 months (36) (the pretreatment reading should be nil). In abnormal horses the xylose curve is flat (a peak of 7–13 mg/dl (0·5 mmol/l) at 60–210 minutes) contrasted with a peak of 20 mg/dl (1·3 mmol/l) at 60 minutes in normal horses (6). As an initial checking test, one postdosing sample at 2 hours is recommended. Theoretically, the test is preferred to the oral glucose absorption test because xylose is not a normal metabolite and blood levels are not affected by normal metabolic processes, although it is affected by prior diet, horses receiving a high energy diet having a lower absorption curve than horses on a low energy diet (29). But it is expensive, and the test is not without difficulties of manipulation and interpretation. For example, absorption can be recorded as being very low, and be caused by increased transit time through the gut, due perhaps to excitement.

A technique used for determining whether a protein-losing enteropathy is present is based on the examination of feces for radioactivity after the intravenous administration of radioactive material (22). The radioactive test agent $^{51}Cr^{13}C$-labeled plasma protein has been used for this purpose.

A D-xylose absorption curve has been determined for cattle (28). The xylose (0·5 g/kg body weight plus) is deposited in the abomasum by abomasocentesis, and a peak of blood glucose is attained in about 90 minutes.

Abdominal paracentesis

Collection of a sample of peritoneal fluid is a most useful aid in the diagnosis of diseases of the peritoneum and the abdominal segment of the alimentary tract (14–16, 25). It is of vital importance in horses in the differential diagnosis and prognosis of colic and in cattle in the diagnosis of peritonitis.

General comments applicable to peritoneal fluid of both horses and cattle

Normal peritoneal fluid is a transudate with values as set down in Tables 14 and 15 and has functions similar to those of other tissue fluids. It contains mesothelial cells, lymphocytes, neutrophils, a few erythrocytes and occasional monocytes and eosinophils. The following general comments apply:

1. It is capable of examination in terms of physical characteristics especially color, translucence, specific gravity and clotting time; biochemical composition; cellular volume, morphology and type.
2. Examination of the fluid may help in determining the presence in the peritoneal cavity of:
   - peritonitis (chemical or infectious)
   - infarction of a segment of gut wall
   - perforation of the alimentary tract wall
   - rupture of urinary bladder
   - leakage from biliary system
   - intraperitoneal hemorrhage
   - peritoneal neoplasia.
3. The reaction of the peritoneum varies with time and a single examination can be dangerously misleading. A series of examinations may be necessary, in acute cases at intervals as short as an hour.
4. A significant reaction in a peritoneal cavity may be quite localized and a sample of fluid collected

Table 14. Guidelines for the classification and interpretation of bovine peritoneal fluid

Classification of fluid	*Physical appearance*	*Total protein g/dl*	*Specific gravity*	*Total RBC × 10^6/μl*	*Total WBC × 10^3/μl*	*Differential WBC count*	*Bacteria*	*Particulate matter (plant fibers)*	*Interpretation*
Normal	Amber, crystal clear 1–5 ml per sample	0·1–3·1 (1·6) Does not clot	1·005–1·015	Few from puncture of capillaries during sampling	0·3–5·3	Polymorphonuclear and mononuclear cells, ratio 1:1	None	None	Increased amounts in late gestation, congestive heart failure
Moderate inflammation	Amber to pink, slightly turbid	2·8–7·3 (4·5) May clot	1·016–1·025	0·1–0·2	2·7–40·7 (8·7)	Non-toxic neutrophils, 50–90% macrophages may predominate in chronic peritonitis	None	None	Early stages of strangulation, destruction of intestine; traumatic reticuloperitonitis; ruptured bladder; chronic peritonitis
Severe inflammation	Serosanguineous, turbid, viscous 10–20 ml per sample	3·1–5·8 (4·2) Commonly clots	1·026–1·040	0·3–0·5	2·0–31·1 (8·0)	Segmented neutrophils, 70–90%. Presence of (toxic) degenerate neutrophils containing bacteria	Usually present	May be present	Advanced stages of strangulation obstruction; acute diffuse peritonitis; perforation of abomasal ulcer; rupture of uterus, stomachs or intestine

Table 15. Guidelines for the classification and interpretation of equine peritoneal fluid

Classification of fluid	*Physical appearance*	*Total protein g/dl*	*Specific gravity*	*Total RBC × $10^6/\mu l$*	*Total WBC × $10^3/\mu l$*	*Differential WBC count*	*Bacteria*	*Particulate matter (plant fibers)*	*Interpretation*
Normal	Pale yellow, crystal clear	0·5–1·5 Does not clot	1·000–1·015	None	0·5–5·0	Polymorphonuclear and mononuclear cells, ratio 1:1	None	None	Increased in late gestation, congestive heart failure
Suspected inflammation	Slightly cloudy, yellow	1·6–2·5 Usually does not clot	1·016–1·020	0·05–0·1	5·0–15·0	Segmented neutrophils, 50–60%; mesothelial cells	None	None	Modified transudate
Moderate inflammation	Yellow-pink turbid, viscous	2·6–4·0 May clot	1·021–1·025	1·0–0·2	15·0–60·0	Segmented neutrophils, 70–80%, few toxic neutrophils	May be present	None	Early stages of strangulation, obstruction uterine torsion, colonic torsion
Severe inflammation	Pink to serosanguineous, turbid, thick viscous	4·0–7·0 Commonly clots	Greater than 1·025	0·3–0·6	Greater than 60·0	Segmented neutrophils, 70–90%; toxic or degenerate neutrophils containing bacteria	Commonly present	May be present	Infarction of intestine; perforation or rupture of viscus

at one point in the cavity may not be representative of the entire cavity.

5. Changes in peritoneal fluid, especially its chemical composition, e.g., lactate level, may be a reflection of a systemic change. The examination of a concurrently collected peripheral blood sample will make it possible to determine whether the changes are in fact restricted to the peritoneal cavity.
6. As in any clinicopathological examination the results must be interpreted with caution and only in conjunction with the history and clinical findings.
7. Normal fluid is crystal clear; turbidity indicates the presence of increased leukocytes, and protein which may include fine strands of fibrin.
8. Normal fluid is straw-colored to yellow. A green color suggests food material, intense orange-green indicates rupture of the biliary system. Pink to red color indicates presence of hemoglobin, degenerated erythrocytes, entire erythrocytes and damage to vascular system by infarction, perforation or hydrostatic pressure. Red-brown color indicates the late stages of necrosis of the gut wall, and the presence of degenerated blood and hemoglobin and damage to gut wall containing blood.
9. Particulate matter in peritoneal fluid suggests either fibrin clots or strands or gut contents caused by leakage from a perforated or ruptured gut wall.
10. High specific gravity and high protein content are indicative of vascular damage and leakage of plasma protein as in peritonitis or mural infarction.
11. Volume of fluid varies. A normal flow is 1–5 ml per sample. A continuous flow with 10–20 ml per sample indicates excess fluid due to ruptured bladder or ascites (clear yellow), acute diffuse peritonitis (yellow, turbid), infarction or necrosis of gut wall (thin, red-tinged).
12. Whole blood, or clear fluid streaked with blood, or heavily bloodstained fluid indicate that the sample has been collected from the spleen or a blood vessel or that there is hemoperitoneum, or rupture of uterus, bladder or from dicoumarol poisoning.
13. Viscosity of fluid. The higher the protein content rises, as the peritoneal fluid shifts from being a transudate to being an inflammatory exudate, the fluid becomes increasingly viscous until it actually clots.
14. A rapid staining method, using a modified Wright's stain, gives a stained slide ready for examination within 5 minutes. The value of the technique is in indicating the number of leukocytes and other cells present, and in differentiating the type of cells (25).
15. An increase in total white cell count of the fluid including a disproportionate number of polymorphonuclear cells indicates acute inflammation which may have an infectious origin, or be sterile.
16. An increase in mononuclear phagocytes from the peritoneum is an indication of chronic peritonitis.
17. Degenerative changes in the neutrophils allow an informed estimate of the probability of infection being present, even though none are absorbed (27).
18. An increase in the number of mesothelial cells with the distinctive presence of actively dividing mitotic figures suggests neoplasia.
19. Bacteria found as phagocytosed inclusions in leukocytes or by culture of fluid indicate an infective peritonitis which may arise by hematogenous spread in which case the infection is likely to be a specific one. If there has been leakage from a peritoneal abscess the same comment applies, but if there is leakage through a segment of devitalized wall or a perforated wall there is likely to be a mixed infection.
20. Entire erythrocytes, often accompanied by some hemoglobin, indicate hemoperitoneum in which case there should be active phagocytosis of erythrocytes, or that the sample has been collected from the spleen. The blood is likely to be concentrated if there has been sufficient time for fluid resorption from the peritoneum. Splenic blood has a higher packed cell volume also, but there is no erythrophagocytosis.
21. A packed cell volume (PCV) of less than 5% in peritoneal fluid suggests extravasation of blood from an infarcted or inflamed gut wall; one of greater than 20% suggests a significant hemorrhage.
22. A dark green sample, containing motile protozoa, with very few leukocytes and no mesothelial cells indicates that the sample has been collected from the gut lumen. Enterocentesis has little apparent clinical effect in normal horses, although an occasional horse will show a transient fever. However, puncture of a devitalized loop of intestine may lead to extensive leakage of gut contents and a fatal peritonitis. The effect of enterocentesis of normal gut on peritoneal fluid is consistently to increase the neutrophilic count which persists for several days (32).

Technique for paracentesis in horses

In the horse the recommended site for paracentesis is on the ventral midline, 25 cm caudal to the xiphoid (midway between the xiphoid and the umbilicus). Following surgical preparation and subcutaneous infiltration of an anesthetic, a stab incision is made through the skin and subcutaneous tissues and into the linea alba. A 9 cm long blunt-pointed bovine teat cannula, with the tip wrapped in a sterile swab to avoid blood and skin contamination, is inserted into the wound and moved about until the cut into the linea alba can be felt. With a quick thrust the cannula is pushed through the linea alba into the peritoneal cavity. A 'pop' is often heard on entry into the peritoneal cavity. Failure to cut into the linea alba first will cause many of the cannulas to bend and break.

In most horses (about 75%) a sample of fluid is readily obtained. In others it takes a moment or two before the fluid runs out, usually spurting synchronously with the respiratory movements. Applying suction with a syringe may yield some fluid if there is no spontaneous flow. Normal fluid is clear, yellow and flows easily through an

18 gauge needle. Two samples are collected, one in a plain tube and one in a tube with an anticoagulant. In case the fluid clots readily a few drops should be placed and smeared out on a glass slide and allowed to dry for staining purposes. In peritonitis the total leukocyte count will increase markedly, but wide variation in the total count can occur between horses with similar conditions, and in the same horse within a period of hours. Variations are due to the nature and stage of the lesion and to the total amount of exudate in the peritoneal cavity which has a diluting effect on the total count. Total leukocyte counts ranging from 10 000 to 150 000/μl have been recorded in peritonitis and in infarction of the intestine in horses.

Paracentesis is not without some danger, especially by way of introducing fecal contents into the peritoneal cavity and causing peritonitis. This appears to be of major importance only if there are loops of distended atonic intestine situated on the ventral abdominal wall. This is a common occurrence in the later stages of intestinal obstruction which is still amenable to surgery. Puncture of a devitalized loop of intestine may cause a leakage of intestinal contents and acute diffuse peritonitis which is rapidly fatal. Penetration of a normal loop of intestine occurs often enough to know that it appears to have no ill-effects. If a sample of peritoneal fluid is an important diagnostic need in a particular case and the first attempt at paracentesis causes penetration of the gut, it is recommended that the attempt be repeated, if necessary two or three times, at more posterior sites. The technique most likely to cause bowel penetration is the use of a sharp needle instead of the blunt cannula recommended, and that of forcibly thrusting the cannula through the linea alba. Provided the suggested cut is made in the linea alba the cannula can be pushed gently through while rotating it.

Technique for paracentesis in cattle

There is less information about peritoneal fluid in cattle (23, 24). In this species the choice of sites for paracentesis is a problem because the rumen covers such a large portion of the ventral abdominal wall, and avoiding penetration of it is difficult. The most profitable sites are those in which, on an anatomical basis, there are recesses between the forestomachs, abomasum, diaphragm and liver. These are usually caudal to the xiphoid sternum and 4–10 cm lateral to the midline. Another recommended site is left of the midline and 3–4 cm medial and 5–7 cm cranial to the foramen for the left subcutaneous abdominal vein (10). A teat cannula similar to the one described for use in the horse is recommended, but with care and caution a 16 gauge 5 cm hypodermic needle may also be used. The needle or cannula is pushed carefully and slowly through the abdominal wall which will twitch when the peritoneum is punctured. When this happens the fluid will usually run out into a vial without the aid of a vacuum. However, if it does not, a syringe may be used and the needle moved backwards and forwards in a search for fluid, with the piston of the syringe withdrawn. Failure to obtain a sample does not preclude the possibility that peritonitis may be present, the exudate may be very thick and contain large masses of fibrin, or the peritonitis might be quite localized. Also, animals that are dehydrated may have less peritoneal fluid than normal. Most animals from which samples cannot be obtained are in fact normal. In animals in which peritonitis is strongly suspected for clinical reasons up to four attempts at paracentesis should be made before aborting the attempt. The fluid should be collected into an anticoagulant, preferably ethylenediaminetetra-acetate (EDTA), to avoid clotting.

Abnormal peritoneal fluid in the cow is a highly sensitive indicator of peritoneal disease, but it is not a particularly good indicator of the nature of the disease. The greatest abnormalities are found in acute diseases of the peritoneum, but chronic peritonitis may be accompanied by peritoneal fluid which is almost normal.

Examination of the fluid should take into account the following characteristics:

- Large amounts (10–20 ml) of serosanguineous fluid suggests infarction or necrosis of gut wall
- Heavily bloodstained fluid or whole blood, or fluid with streaks of blood through it are more likely to result from puncture of a blood vessel or from bleeding into the cavity as in dicoumarol poisoning or a neoplasm of the vascular system
- The same sort of bloodstained fluid may accompany a ruptured uterus or bladder, or severe congestive heart failure
- Large quantities of yellowish-colored turbid fluid suggests acute diffuse peritonitis. The degree of turbidity depends on the number of cells and the amount of fibrin present
- Particulate food material in the sample indicates perforation or rupture of the gut, except that penetration of the gut with the paracentesis instrument during collection may be misleading. Such samples are usually heavily fecal in appearance and contain no mesothelial cells
- Laboratory examination is necessary to derive full benefit from the paracentesis sample. This will include the number and kinds of leukocytes present—the number is increased in peritonitis, neutrophils predominating in acute peritonitis and monocytes in chronic forms; the number of erythrocytes present; whether bacteria are present inside or outside the neutrophils; total protein content.

The significant values for these items are included in Table 14.

Surgical visualization

Laparotomy for the purpose of palpating and inspecting the abdominal contents is a subject for surgery textbooks. How often it is used depends largely on the surgical proclivities of the individual veterinarian. An alternative is laparoscopy in which a small incision is made in the skin and an opening in the wall of the abdomen and a laparoscope passed into the peritoneal cavity. The instrument may be a rigid peritoneoscope requiring inflation of the cavity so that a view can be obtained (37), or a fiberoptiscope (35).

PRINCIPLES OF TREATMENT IN ALIMENTARY TRACT DISEASE

Removal of the primary cause of the disease is essential but the major part of the treatment of diseases of the alimentary tract is supportive and symptomatic, and aimed at relieving pain, correcting the abnormality and repairing the damage done. The specific treatments are discussed elsewhere and include antibacterial, coccidiostatic and antifungal agents, surgical correction of accidents and displacements, the provision of specific antidotes for poisons, and treatment of helminth infestations.

Correction of abnormal motility

Either excessive or depressed motility should be corrected. When motility is increased, the administration of atropine or other spasmolytics, such as Isaverin (dipyrone) or Myspamol (proquamezine) is usually followed by disappearance of the abdominal pain and a diminution of fluid loss. Benzetimide is a potent longacting anticholinergic agent which markedly depresses the secretion and motility of the entire gastrointestinal tract (17–20). Benzetimide has an effect for up to 48 hours in normal sheep (17) and is recommended as an adjunct to specific therapy for diarrhea in newborn calves and adult cattle (14, 16). The side-effects of mild bloat and dryness of the mucous membranes are not considered as significant. There is a need for some scientific clinical investigation into the desirability of treating intestinal hypermotility, if it does exist in enteritis for example, and the efficacy of anticholinergics. In human medicine, clinical trials have produced mixed results in evaluating the efficacy of anticholinergics in treating acute diarrhea. Studies of the use of intestinal paralytic agents (e.g. diphenoxylate–atropine) in children with non-specific diarrhea have shown no beneficial effect (8).

When motility is decreased the usual practice is to administer parasympathomimetic drugs or purgatives, usually combined with an analgesic. The use of atropine may relieve the pain transiently in these circumstances but has no effect in removing the distending material and is in fact likely to exacerbate the condition.

Replacement of fluids and electrolytes

In gastric or intestinal obstruction, or when diarrhea is severe, it may be necessary to replace lost fluids and electrolytes by the parenteral administration of large quantities of isotonic glucose–saline or other physiologically normal electrolyte solutions. The amount of fluid lost may be very large and fluids must be given in quantities of not less than 10 ml and preferably up to 20 ml/kg body weight daily, depending on severity. In acute, severe dehydration in horses, such as occurs in acute intestinal obstruction, the amount of fluid required before and during surgery is in the order of 50 ml/kg body weight. It is of great importance that the administration of fluid should be commenced at the earliest possible time because of the need to maintain homeostasis and thus avoid the almost impossible task of restoring animals to normal before surgery is to be attempted. The details of fluid therapy are given under the heading of disturbances of water, electrolytes and acid–base balance. In young animals the need is much greater still and amounts of 100 mg/kg body weight, given slowly intravenously, are probably not excessive. The treatment of shock is discussed elsewhere but should include the administration of fluids, plasma or blood and vasoconstrictor agents.

Relief of distension

This is one of the major principles of treatment in alimentary tract disease. It may be possible to relieve by medical means a distension caused by the accumulation of ingesta but surgical intervention is necessary in some cases. In purely functional distension, relief of the atony or spasm can be effected by the use of stimulants and spasmolytics respectively. Distension due to intestinal or gastric accidents usually requires surgical treatment.

Reconstitution of rumen flora and correction of acidity or alkalinity

When prolonged anorexia or acute indigestion occurs in ruminants, the rumen flora may be seriously reduced. In convalescence, the reconstitution of the flora can be hastened by the oral administration of a suspension of ruminal contents from a normal cow, or of dried ruminal contents which contain viable bacteria and yeasts and the substances necessary for growth of the organisms.

The pH of the rumen affects the growth of rumen organisms, and hyperacidity, such as occurs on overeating of grain, or hyperalkalinity, such as occurs on overeating of protein-rich feeds, should be corrected by the administration of alkalinizing or acidifying drugs as the case may be.

Relief of pain

The relief of pain is one of the major tasks in alimentary tract disease. No single drug is completely satisfactory and every effort should be made to correct the primary disease. Analgesics and narcotics are in general use and are discussed under the heading of pain, and the individual diseases.

Relief of tenesmus

This is a most difficult task. Commonly longacting epidural anesthesia and sedation are the aims and infusion of the rectum or vagina with a topical anesthetic may be added but in many cases are partly or completely ineffective. A suggested treatment in cattle is the production of artificial pneumoperitoneum by the insufflation of air into the peritoneal cavity via a cannula inserted at the paralumbar fossa. Insufflation is continued until both fossae are vaulted to the height of the costal arch.

REVIEW LITERATURE

Gerring, E. E. L. et al. (1986) Equine gastroenterology, *Equ. vet. J.*, *18*, 243, 249, 256, 261, 264, 271, 275.

Greatorex, J. C. (1968) Rectal exploration as an aid to the diagnosis of some medical conditions in the horse. *Equ. vet. J.*, *1*, 26–30.

Roberts, M. C. (1975) Carbohydrate digestion and absorption in the equine small intestine. *J. S. Afr. vet. med. Assoc.*, *46*, 19.

Weaver, A. D. (1985) Rectal examination in the diagnosis of gastro-intestinal disorders in the horse. *Vet. Ann. Educ.*, *25*, 211–216.

REFERENCES

(1) Roberts, M. C. et al. (1974) *Res. vet. Sci.*, *17*, 42.
(2) Argenzio, R. A. (1975) *Cornell Vet.*, *65*, 303.
(3) Alexander, F. (1972) *Equ. vet. J.*, *4*, 166.
(4) Arbuckle, J. B. R. (1977) *Vet. Ann.*, *17*, 123.
(5) Kenworthy, R. (1976) *Res. vet Sci.*, *21*, 69.
(6) Bolton, J. R. et al. (1976) *Cornell Vet.*, *66*, 183.
(7) White, R. A. S. & Allen, W. R. (1985) *Equ. vet. J.*, *17*, 401.
(8) Portnoy, B. L. et al. (1976) *J. Am. med. Assoc.*, *236*, 844.
(9) Loeb, W. F. et al. (1972) *Cornell Vet.*, *62*, 524.
(10) Roberts, M. C. & Hill, F. W. G. (1973) *Equ. vet. J.*, *5*, 171.
(11) Roberts, M. C. (1975) *Res. vet. Sci.*, *18*, 64.
(12) Toofanian, F. et al. (1974) *Res. vet. Sci.*, *16*, 375, 382.
(13) Roberts, M. C. (1979) *Equ. vet. J.*, *11*, 239.
(14) Coffman, J. R. (1973) *Mod. vet. Pract.*, *54*, 79.
(15) Swanwick, R. A. & Wilkinson, J. S. (1976) *Aust. vet. J.*, *52*, 109.
(16) Bach, L. G. & Ricketts, S. W. (1974) *Equ. vet. J.*, *6*, 116.
(17) Marsboom, R. & van Ravestyn, C. (1971) *Br. vet. J.*, *127*, 264.
(18) Symoens, J. H. et al. (1974) *Vet. Rec.*, *94*, 180.
(19) Fischer, W. (1975) *Tierärztl. Wochenschr.*, *82*, 102.
(20) Marsboom, R. et al. (1973) *Vet Rec.*, *93*, 382.
(21) Payton, A. J. & Glickman, L. T. (1980) *Am. J. vet. Res.*, *41*, 918.
(22) Snow, D. H. et al. (1980) *Vet Rec.*, *3*, 68.
(23) Oehme, F. W. (1969) *J. Am. vet. med. Assoc.*, *155*, 1923.
(24) Hirsch, V. M. & Townsend, H. G. G. (1982) *Can. vet. J.*, *23*, 348.
(25) Adams, S. B. et al. (1980) *Cornell Vet.*, *70*, 232.
(26) Heffron, C. J. & Baker, C. J. (1979) *Equ. vet. J.*, *11*, 137 & 148.
(27) Brownlow, M. A. (1983) *Equ. vet. J.*, *15*, 22.
(28) Pearson, E. G. & Baldwin, B. H. (1981) *Cornell Vet.*, *71*, 288.
(29) Jacobs, K. A. et al. (1982) *Am. J. vet. Res.*, *43*, 1856.
(30) Jacobs, K. A. et al. (1982) *J. Am. vet. Med. Assoc.*, *180*, 884.
(31) Brown, C. M. et al. (1985) *J. Am. vet. med. Assoc.*, *186*, 965.
(32) Schumacher, J. et al. (1985) *J. Am. vet. med. Assoc.*, *186*, 1301.
(33) Martens, R. J. et al. (1985) *Am. J. vet. Res.*, *46*, 2163.
(34) Greet, T. R. C. (1982) *Equ. vet. J.*, *14*, 73.
(35) Wilson, A. D. et al. (1984) *Can. vet. J.*, *25*, 229.
(36) Merritt, T. et al. (1986) *Equ. vet. J.*, *18*, 298.
(37) Fischer, A. T. et al. (1986) *J. Am. vet. med. Assoc.*, *189*, 289.

DISEASES OF THE BUCCAL CAVITY AND ASSOCIATED ORGANS

Diseases of the muzzle

The congenital defect of harelip may be contiguous with a cleft palate. Severe dermatitis with scab formation, development of fissures, and sloughing and gangrene of the skin are common lesions in cattle. The diseases in which these lesions occur are: photosensitive dermatitis; bovine malignant catarrh; bovine virus diarrhea; and rinderpest.

In sheep severe lesions of the muzzle are less common, but occur in: bluetongue; ecthyma.

In pigs only the vesicular diseases—vesicular exanthema of swine, swine vesicular disease, and foot and mouth disease—cause such lesions on the snout and on other sites. The lesions are vesicular initially and confusion has arisen in recent years because of the occurrence of isolated incidents in Australia and New Zealand in which such outbreaks occurred, but in which no pathogenic agent was identified.

Stomatitis

Stomatitis is inflammation of the oral mucosa and includes glossitis (inflammation of the lingual mucosa), palatitis (lampas) and gingivitis (inflammation of the mucosa of the gums). Clinically it is characterized by partial or complete loss of appetite, by smacking of the lips and profuse salivation. It is commonly an accompaniment of systemic disease.

Etiology

Stomatitis may be caused by physical, chemical or infectious agents, the latter being the largest group of causes. Under experimental conditions, stomatitis can be produced by some nutritional deficiencies but these are not known to cause clinical stomatitis under natural conditions.

Physical agents

- Trauma while dosing
- Foreign body injury
- Malocclusion of teeth
- Sharp awns or spines on plants. The commonest lesions are on the gums of cattle and sheep just below the corner incisors where tough grass is pulled around the corner of the incisor arcade. In spear grass country the alveoli are often stuffed full of grass seeds. Very young animals, e.g. 1–6 week old lambs, are particularly susceptible to traumatic injury from abrasive feed (3). Among the most dramatic lesions are the ones in the mouths of horses. They are large (2–3 cm long and 5 mm wide) and linear in shape. They may be caused by eating hairy caterpillars which infest pasture, or by the awns in hay or chaff made from triticale (a hybrid of wheat and rye) (4) and a yellow bristle grass (*Setaria lutescens*)
- Eating frozen feed and drinking hot water are recorded but seem highly improbable.

Chemical agents

- Irritant drugs administered in overstrong concentrations, e.g., chloral hydrate
- Counterirritants applied to skin, left unprotected and licked by the animal, including mercury and cantharides compounds
- Irritant substances administered by mistake including acids, alkalis, phenolic compounds
- Manifestation of systemic poisoning, e.g., chronic mercury. Poisoning with bracken, *Heraclum mantegazzianum*, furazolidone and some fungi (*Stachybotris*, *Fusarium* sp. and mushrooms) cause a combination of focal hemorrhages and necrotic

ulcers or erosions. They are a common cause of confusion with vesicular or erosive disease
- Included in syndrome of uremia in horses.

Infectious agents

Cattle They are as follows:

- Oral necrobacillosis caused by *Fusobacterium necrophorus*
- Actinobacillosis of the bovine tongue is not really a stomatitis, but there may be one or two ulcers on the dorsum and sides of the tongue and on the lips. The basic lesion is an acute diffuse myositis of the muscle of the tongue initially, followed by the development of multiple granulomas and subsequently fibrosis and shrinkage
- Ulcerative, granulomatous lesions may occur on the gums in cases of actinomycosis
- Vesicular stomatitis occurs in foot and mouth disease and vesicular stomatitis
- Erosive, with some secondary ulcerative, stomatitis occurs in bovine viral diarrhea (mucosal disease), bovine malignant catarrh, rinderpest and rarely in bluetongue. Cases of infectious bovine rhinotracheitis in young calves may have similar lesions
- Proliferative lesions occur in papular stomatitis, proliferative stomatitis and in rare cases of rhinosporidiosis and papillomatosis where the oral mucosa is invaded
- Oral mucosal necrosis in bovine sweating sickness
- Nondescript lesions varying from erosions to ulcers occur late in the stages of many of the above diseases when secondary bacteria have invaded the breaches in the mucosa. In some cases the involvement goes deeper still and a phlegmonous condition or a cellulitis may develop. Thus, lesions which were initially vesicular are converted to what look like bacterial ulcers. Secondary infection with fungi, especially *Monilia* sp., may also occur.

Sheep They are as follows:

- Erosive lesions in bluetongue, rinderpest and *peste de petits ruminantes*
- Vesicular lesions rarely in foot and mouth disease
- Granulomatous lesions due to ecthyma are not unusual in the mouth, especially in young lambs. Similarly, oral lesions occur in bad cases of sheep pox, ulcerative dermatosis, coital exanthema and mycotic dermatitis.

Horses They are as follows:

- Vesicular lesions in vesicular stomatitis
- Herpesvirus infections are commonly accompanied by small (1 mm diameter) vesicles surrounded by a zone of hyperemia. The lesions are in groups and at first glance appear to be hemorrhages
- Lingual abscess caused by *Actinobacillus* spp.

Pigs They are as follows:

- The vesicular diseases, foot and mouth disease, vesicular stomatitis, vesicular exanthema of swine and swine vesicular disease.

Many other causes of stomatitis have been suggested but the relationship of these conditions to the specific diseases listed above is unknown. It is common to find stomatitides that cannot be defined as belonging to any of these etiological groups. An example is necrotic glossitis reported in feeder steers in the United States (1, 2) in which the necrotic lesions are confined to the anterior part of the tongue.

Pathogenesis

The lesions of stomatitis are produced by the causative agents being applied directly to the mucosa, or gaining entrance to it by way of minor abrasions, or by localization in the mucosa from a viremia. In the first two instances, the stomatitis is designated as primary. In the third, it is usually described as secondary because of the common occurrence of similar lesions in other organs or on other parts of the body, and the presence of a systemic disease. The clinical signs of stomatitis are caused by the inflammation or erosion of the mucosa and the signs vary in severity with the degree of inflammation.

Clinical findings

There is partial or complete anorexia and slow, painful mastication. Chewing movements and smacking of the lips are accompanied by salivation, either frothy and in small amounts, or profuse and drooling if the animal does not swallow normally. The saliva may contain pus or shreds of epithelial tissue. A fetid odor is present on the breath only if bacterial invasion of the lesion has occurred. Enlargement of local lymph nodes may also occur if bacteria invade the lesions. Swelling of the face is observed only in cases where a cellulitis or phlegmon has extended to involve the soft tissues. An increased desire for water is apparent and the animal resents manipulation and examination of the mouth.

Toxemia may be present when the stomatitis is secondary to a systemic disease or where tissue necrosis occurs. This is a feature of oral necrobacillosis and many of the systemic viremias. In some of the specific diseases, lesions may be present on other parts of the body, especially at the coronets and mucocutaneous junctions.

The local lesions vary a great deal. Vesicular lesions are usually thin-walled vesicles 1–2 cm in diameter filled with clear serous fluid. The vesicles rupture readily to leave sharp-edged, shallow ulcers. Erosive lesions are shallow, usually discrete, areas of necrosis which are not readily seen in the early stages. They tend to occur most commonly on the lingual mucosa and at the commissures of the mouth. The necrotic tissue may remain *in situ* but is usually shed leaving a very shallow discontinuity of the mucosa with a dark-red base which is more readily seen. If recovery occurs, these lesions heal very quickly. Ulcerative lesions penetrate more deeply to the lamina propria. In lambs the tongue may be swollen and contain many microabscesses infected with *Actinomyces* (*Corynebacterium*) *pyogenes*. There is an accompanying abscessation of the pharyngeal lymph nodes (3).

Catarrhal stomatitis is manifested by a diffuse inflammation of the buccal mucosa and is commonly the result of direct injury by chemical or physical agents.

Mycotic stomatitis usually takes the form of a heavy, white, velvety deposit with little obvious inflammation or damage to the mucosa.

Deformity of or loss of tissue at the tip of the tongue may result in a chronic syndrome of chewing and swallowing food in such a way that food is always oozing from between the lips. In sheep this may cause permanent staining of the hair around the mouth, creating an appearance similar to that of a tobacco-chewer. Loss of the tip is usually the result of predator attack on a newborn or sick lamb.

Clinical pathology

Material collected from lesions of stomatitis should be examined for the presence of pathogenic bacteria and fungi. Transmission experiments may be undertaken with filtrates of swabs or scrapings if the disease is thought to be due to a viral agent.

Necropsy findings

The oral lesions are easily observed but complete necropsy examinations should be carried out on all fatally affected animals to determine whether the oral lesions are primary or are local manifestations of a systemic disease.

Diagnosis

Particularly in cattle, and to a less extent in sheep, the diagnosis of stomatitis is most important because of the occurrence of oral lesions in a number of highly infectious viral diseases. The diseases are listed under etiology and their differentiation is described under their specific headings. Careful clinical and necropsy examinations are necessary to define the type and extent of the lesions if any attempt at field diagnosis is to be made. In cattle, lymphoma of the ramus of the mandible may spread extensively through the submucosal tissues of the mouth causing marked swelling of the gums, spreading of the teeth, inability to close the mouth and profuse salivation. There is no discontinuity or inflammation of the buccal mucosa but gross enlargement of the cranial lymph nodes is usual.

The differentiation of causes of hypersalivation must depend on a careful examination of the mouth; the causative gingivitis is often surprisingly moderate in horses, and an awareness of the volume of increased saliva output caused by toxic hyperthermia, e.g. in fescue and ergot poisonings. Poisoning by the mycotoxin slaframine also causes hypersalivation.

Treatment

Affected animals should be isolated and fed and watered from separate utensils if an infectious agent is suspected. Specific treatments are dealt with under the headings of the specific diseases. Non-specific treatment includes frequent application of a mild antiseptic collutory such as a 2% solution of copper sulfate, a 2% suspension of borax or a 1% suspension of a sulfonamide in glycerin. Indolent ulcers require more vigorous treatment and respond well to curettage or cauterization with a silver nitrate stick or tincture of iodine.

In stomatitis due to trauma, the teeth may need attention. In all cases, soft, appetizing food should be offered and feeding by stomach tube or intravenous alimentation resorted to in severe, prolonged cases. If the disease is infectious, care should be exercised to ensure that it is not transmitted by the hands or dosing implements.

REFERENCES

(1) Wake, W. L. (1961) *J. Am. vet. med. Assoc.*, *138*, 7.
(2) Hill, J. K. & Herrick, J. B. (1961) *Vet. Med.*, *56*, 190.
(3) Rossiter, D. L. et al. (1984) *J. am. vet. med. Assoc.*, *185*, 1552.
(4) McCosker, J. E. & Keenan, D. M. (1983) *Aust. vet. J.*, *60*, 259.

Diseases of the teeth

Sporadic diseases of the teeth of animals are dealt with by surgeons and in textbooks of surgery. However, mention needs to be made here of those diseases which also have interest for students of medicine.

Etiology

The causes may be congenital or acquired.

Congenital defects

- Inherited
- Malocclusion of sufficient degree to interfere with prehension and mastication
- Red-brown staining of inherited porphyrinuria of cattle
- Defective enamel formation on all teeth combined with excessive mobility of joints in inherited defect of collagen metabolism in Holstein/Friesian cattle identified as bovine osteogenesis imperfecta. The teeth are pink and obviously deficient in substance. This defect is also recorded in a foal with severe epitheliogenesis imperfecta (13).

Dental fluorosis

The teeth are damaged before they erupt and show erosion of the enamel.

Premature wear and loss of teeth in sheep (periodontal disease)

Premature loss of teeth or 'broken mouth' causes concern because of the early age at which sheep have to be culled. The problem is particularly severe in New Zealand (1) and the hill country in Scotland (2) and is caused largely by periodontal disease and although the pathogenesis is not completely clear, some of the steps in its development have been identified. The primary lesion is an acute gingivitis around permanent incisors and premolars at the time of their eruption. This subsides leaving a chronic gingivitis and an accumulation of subgingival plaque. Molars and incisors are all affected. On some farms, for reasons not understood, this gingivitis penetrates down into the alveoli causing a severe periodontitis and eventual shedding of the teeth (4, 5). In some unusual circumstances the gingivitis appears to arise from heavy deposits of dental calculus (11). The occurrence of this periodontal disease is higher on some soil types than on others (6). The ingestion of irritating materials such as sand and spiny grass seeds (3) has been suggested as causes, but they are considered to be secondary complications in a pre-existing disease. On bacteriological examination spirochetes and *Fusobacterium* sp. are present and parenteral treatment in the early stages with penicillin leads to rapid recovery. Some affected sheep die. In the Scottish disease there is local alveolar bone loss but no accompanying general skeletal deficiency (2).

Another dental disease of sheep is also recorded on an extensive scale in New Zealand (7). There is excessive wear of deciduous incisors, but no change in the rate of wear of the molar teeth. The incisor wear is episodic and is not due to any change in the supportive tissues, nor is there any change in the intrinsic resistance to wear of the incisor teeth (10). The disease is not related to an inadequate dietary intake of copper or vitamin D and is thought to be caused by the ingestion of soil particles (12). There is a Russian report of a very similar disease in that country (8). The two New Zealand diseases do not occur together and have no apparent effect on body condition score (9).

Clinical findings

In food animals the syndrome is one of apparent starvation in the midst of plenty of feed. Inspection of the mouth may reveal the worn or damaged molar teeth but the molar teeth of sheep, the most commonly affected species, are not easily inspected in the living animal and tooth lesions are easily missed. It is common to find that incisors and molars are all affected and damage to incisors should indicate molar disease as well.

REVIEW LITERATURE

Spence, J. & Aitchison G. (1986) Clinical aspects of dental disease in sheep. *In Pract.*, *8*, 128.

REFERENCES

(1) McKinnon, M. M. (1959) *NZ vet. J.*, 7, 18.
(2) Aitchison, G. U. & Spence, J. A. (1984) *J. comp. Pathol.*, *94*, 285 and *95*, 505.
(3) Anderson, B. C. et al. (1984) *J. Am. vet. med. Assoc.*, *184*, 737.
(4) Morris, P. L. et al. (1985) *NZ vet. J.*, *33*, 87, 131.
(5) Spencer, J. A. et al. (1980) *J. comp. Pathol.*, *90*, 275.
(6) Steele, K. W. & Henderson, H. V. (1977) *NZ J. agric. Res.*, *20*, 301.
(7) Thurley, D. C. (1984) *NZ vet. J.*, *32*, 25; *33*, 25, 157.
(8) Isaev, V. V. & Lavrentev, I. I. (1980) *Veterinariya, Moscow*, *9*, 56.
(9) Orr, M. B. et al. (1986) *NZ vet. J.*, *34*, 111.
(10) Erasmuson, A. F. (1985) *NZ vet. J. agric. Res.*, *28*, 225.
(11) Baker, J. R. & Britt, D. P. (1984) *Vet. Rec.*, *115*, 411.
(12) Millar, K. R. et al. (1985) *NZ vet. J.*, *33*, 41.
(13) Dubielzig, R. R. et al. (1986) *Vet. Pathol.*, *23*, 325.

Parotitis

Parotitis is inflammation of any of the salivary glands.

Etiology

Parotitis may be parenchymatous when the glandular tissue is diffusely inflamed or it may be a local suppurative process. There are no specific causes in farm animals, cases occurring only sporadically and due usually to localization of a blood-borne infection, invasion up the salivary ducts associated with stomatitis, irritation by grass awns in the duct, or salivary calculi (1). Avitaminosis A often appears to be a predisposing cause.

Local suppurative lesions are caused usually by penetrating wounds or extension from a retropharyngeal cellulitis or lymph node abscess.

Pathogenesis

In most cases only one gland is involved. There is no loss of salivary function and the signs are restricted to those of inflammation of the gland.

Clinical findings

In the early stages, there is diffuse enlargement of the gland accompanied by warmth and pain on palpation. The pain may interfere with mastication and swallowing and induce abnormal carriage of the head and resentment when attempts are made to move the head. There may be marked local edema in severe cases. Diffuse parenchymatous parotitis usually subsides with systemic and local treatment within a few days but suppurative lesions may discharge externally and form permanent salivary fistulae.

Clinical pathology

Bacteriological examination of pus from discharging abscesses may aid the choice of a suitable antibacterial treatment.

Necropsy findings

Death occurs rarely and necropsy findings are restricted to local involvement of the gland or to primary lesions elsewhere in the case of secondary parotitis.

Diagnosis

Careful palpation is necessary to differentiate the condition from lymphadenitis, abscesses of the throat region, and metastases to the parotid lymph node in ocular carcinoma or mandibular lymphoma of cattle. Acute phlegmonous inflammation of the throat is relatively common in cattle and is accompanied by high fever, severe toxemia and rapid death. It may be mistaken for an acute parotitis but the swelling is more diffuse and causes pronounced obstruction to swallowing and respiration.

Treatment

Systemic treatment with sulfonamides or antibiotics is required in acute cases especially if there is a systemic reaction. Abscesses may require draining and, if discharge persists, the administration of enzymes either parenterally or locally. A salivary fistula is a common sequel.

REFERENCES

(1) Misk, N. A. & Nigam, J. M. (1984) *Equ. Pract.*, 6, 49.

DISEASES OF THE PHARYNX AND ESOPHAGUS

Pharyngitis

Pharyngitis is inflammation of the pharynx and is characterized clinically by coughing, painful swallowing and lack of appetite. Regurgitation through the nostrils and drooling of saliva may occur in severe cases.

Etiology

Pharyngitis in farm animals is usually traumatic or if it is infectious it is part of a syndrome with other more obvious signs.

Physical causes

- Injury while giving oral treatment with balling or drenching gun (3), or when performing endotracheal intubation (5)
- Accidental administration or ingestion of irritant or hot or cold substances
- Foreign bodies including grass and cereal awns, wire, bones, gelatin capsules lodged in the pharynx or suprapharyngeal diverticulum of pigs.

Infectious causes

Cattle These are:

- Oral necrobacillosis, actinobacillosis as a granuloma rather than the more usual lymphadenitis
- Infectious bovine rhinotracheitis (IBR)
- Pharyngeal phlegmon or intermandibular cellulitis is a severe, often fatal, necrosis of the wall of the pharynx and peripharyngeal tissues without actually causing pharyngitis. *Fusobacterium necrophorum* is a common isolate from the lesions.

Horse These are:

- As part of strangles, or anthrax
- The viral infections of the upper respiratory tract including equine herpesvirus 1, Hoppengarten cough, parainfluenza virus, adenovirus, rhinovirus, viral arteritis, influenza-1A/E1 and 1A/E2 cause pharyngitis
- Chronic follicular pharyngitis with hyperplasia of lymphoid tissue in pharyngeal mucosa giving it a granular, nodular appearance with whitish tips on the lymphoid follicles. An exaggerated form of the disease is a soft tissue mass hanging from the pharyngeal roof, and composed of lymphoid tissue (1).

Pigs These are:

- As part of anthrax in this species and some outbreaks of Aujeszky's disease.

Pathogenesis

Inflammation of the pharynx is attended by painful swallowing and disinclination to eat. If the swelling of the mucosa and wall is severe, there may be virtual obstruction of the pharynx. This is especially so if the retropharyngeal lymph node is enlarged, as it is likely to be in equine viral infections such as rhinovirus.

Clinical findings

The animal may refuse to eat or drink and, if it does so, swallows reluctantly and with evident pain. Opening of the jaws to examine the mouth is resented and manual compression of the throat from the exterior causes paroxysmal coughing. There may be a mucopurulent nasal discharge, sometimes containing blood, spontaneous cough and, in severe cases, regurgitation of fluid and food through the nostrils. Oral medication in such cases may be impossible. Affected animals often stand with the head extended, drool saliva and make frequent, tentative jaw movements. Severe toxemia may accompany the local lesions especially in oral necrobacillosis and, to a less extent, in strangles. Empyema of the guttural pouches may occur in horses. If the local swelling is severe, there may be obstruction to respiration and visible swelling of the throat. The retropharyngeal and parotid lymph nodes are commonly enlarged. In 'pharyngeal phlegmon' in cattle there is an acute onset with high fever (41–41·5°C, 106–107°F), rapid heart rate, profound depression and severe swelling of the soft tissues within and posterior to the mandible to the point where dyspnea is pronounced. Death usually occurs 36–48 hours after the first signs of illness.

Palpation of the pharynx may be undertaken in large animals with the use of a gag if a foreign body is suspected, and endoscopic examination through the nostril may be undertaken in the horse. Most acute cases subside in 3–4 days, but chronic cases may persist for many weeks especially if there is ulceration or a persistent foreign body. Pharyngitis has become one of the commonest respiratory system diseases of the horse (2) possibly because of its readier visualization with modern fiberoptiscopes.

In horses chronic pharyngitis after viral infections is relatively common. It causes a break in training which is very annoying and costly. On endoscopic examination there may be edema in early and relatively acute cases. In cases of longer standing there is lymphoid infiltration and follicular hyperplasia. This is more common and more severe in young horses who also suffer more attacks of upper respiratory tract disease. The condition does not appear to diminish racing performance (4) or respiratory efficiency (6). If secondary bacterial infection is present a purulent exudate is on the pharyngeal mucosa and in the nostrils. Affected horses cough persistently, especially during exercise, are dyspneic, and tire easily. Guttural pouch infections may occur secondarily. An occasional sequel is aspiration pneumonia when food is aspirated into the lungs.

Clinical pathology

Nasal discharge or swabs taken from accompanying oral lesions may assist in the identification of the causative agent.

Necropsy findings

Deaths are rare in primary pharyngitis and necropsy examinations are usually undertaken only in those animals dying of specific diseases. In 'pharyngeal phlegmon' there is edema, hemorrhage and abscessation of the affected area and on incision of the area a foul-smelling liquid and some gas usually escapes.

Diagnosis
The syndrome of pharyngitis is manifested by an acute onset and local pain. In pharyngeal paralysis and obstruction, the onset is usually slow except that obstruction by a foreign body may occur very acutely and cause severe distress and continuous, expulsive coughing but there are no systemic signs. Endoscopic examination of the pharyngeal mucous membranes is often of diagnostic value.

Treatment
The primary disease must be treated, usually parenterally, by the use of antibiotics or sulfonamides, although oral treatment with sulfonamides or iodides may be undertaken in chronic cases. In horses, drugs may be given mixed with syrup as an electuary or administered as a topical spray. 'Pharyngeal phlegmon' is highly fatal and early treatment, repeated at frequent intervals, with a broad-spectrum antibiotic is necessary if there is to be any chance of recovery.

Pharyngeal lymphoid hyperplasia is not susceptible to antibiotic or medical therapy generally. Surgical therapy including electrical and chemical cautery is indicated and has been successfully applied (2).

REFERENCES

(1) Meagher, D. M. & Brown, M. P. (1978) *Vet. Med. SAC*, *73*, 171.
(2) Raker, C. W. & Boles, C. L. (1978) *J. Equ. med. Surg.*, *2*, 202.
(3) Anderson, B. C. & Barrett, D. P. (1983) *Comp. cont. Educ.*, *5*, S431.
(4) Auer, D. E. et al. (1985) *Aust. vet. J.*, *62*, 124.
(5) Brock, K. A. (1985) *J. Am. vet. med. Assoc.*, *187*, 944.
(6) Bayly, W. M. et al. (1984) *Equ. vet. J.*, *16*, 435.

Pharyngeal obstruction

Obstruction of the pharynx is accompanied by stertorous respiration, coughing and difficult swallowing.

Etiology
Foreign bodies or tissue swellings are the usual causes.

Foreign bodies
Bones, corn cobs, pieces of wire.

Tissue swellings

Cattle These are:

- Retropharyngeal lymphadenopathy or abscess due to tuberculosis, actinobacillosis, bovine viral leukosis (5)
- Fibrous or mucoid polyps. These are usually pedunculated because of traction during swallowing and may cause intermittent obstruction of air and food intake.

Horse These are:

- Retropharyngeal lymph node hyperplasia and lymphoid granulomas as part of chronic follicular pharyngitis syndrome
- Retropharyngeal abscess and cellulitis (4)
- Retropharyngeal lymphadenitis caused by strangles
- Pharyngeal cysts in the subepiglottal area of the pharynx, probably of thyroglossal duct origin, and fibroma (1), and similar cysts on the soft palate and pharyngeal dorsum, the latter probably being remnants of the craniopharyngeal ducts (2)
- Dermoid cysts and goitrous thyroids (3).

Pigs These are:

- Diffuse lymphoid enlargement in the pharyngeal wall and soft palate
- Food and foreign body impaction in the suprapharyngeal diverticulum.

Pathogenesis
Reduction in caliber of the pharyngeal lumen interferes with swallowing and respiration.

Clinical signs
There is difficulty in swallowing and animals may be hungry enough to eat but, when they attempt to swallow, cannot do so and the food is coughed up through the mouth. Drinking is usually managed successfully. There is no dilatation of the esophagus and usually little or no regurgitation through the nostrils. An obvious sign is a snoring inspiration, often loud enough to be heard some yards away. The inspiration is prolonged and accompanied by marked abdominal effort. Auscultation over the pharynx reveals loud inspiratory stertor. Manual examination of the pharynx may reveal the nature of the lesion but an examination with a fiberoptic endoscope is likely to be much more informative. When the disease runs a long course, emaciation usually follows. Rupture of abscessed lymph nodes may occur when a nasal tube is passed and result in aspiration pneumonia.

Clinical pathology
A tuberculin test may be advisable in bovine cases. Nasal swabs may contain *Streptococcus equi* when there is streptococcal lymphadenitis in horses.

Necropsy findings
Death occurs rarely and in fatal cases the physical lesion is apparent.

Diagnosis
Signs of the primary disease may aid in the diagnosis in tuberculosis, actinobacillosis and strangles. Pharyngitis is accompanied by severe pain and commonly by systemic signs and there is usually stertor. It is of particular importance to differentiate between obstruction and pharyngeal paralysis when rabies occurs in the area. Esophageal obstruction is also accompanied by the rejection of ingested food but there is no respiratory distress. Laryngeal stenosis may cause a comparable stertor but swallowing is not impeded. Nasal obstruction is manifested by noisy breathing but the volume of breath from one or both nostrils is reduced and the respiratory noise is more wheezing than snoring.

Treatment
Removal of a foreign body may be accomplished through the mouth. Treatment of actinobacillary lymphadenitis with iodides is usually successful and some reduction in size often occurs in tuberculous enlargement of the glands but complete recovery is unlikely to occur. Parenteral treatment of strangles abscesses with penicillin may effect

a cure. Surgical treatment has been highly successful in cases caused by medial retropharyngeal abscess (6).

REFERENCES

(1) Speirs, V. C. et al. (1979) *J. equ. med. Surg.*, *3*, 473.
(2) Koch, D. B. & Tate, L. P. (1978) *J. Am. vet. med. Assoc.*, *173*, 860.
(3) Cermak, K. et al. (1979) *Tierärztl. Wochenschr.*, *86*, 485.
(4) Todhunter, R. J. et al. (1985) *J. Am. vet. med. Assoc.*, *187*, 600.
(5) Grymer, J. and Scott, E. A. (1982) *J. Am. vet med. Assoc.*, *180*, 942.
(6) Vestweber, G. & Roeder, B. (1986) *Comp. cont. Educ.*, *8*, F71.

Pharyngeal paralysis

Pharyngeal paralysis is manifested by inability to swallow and an absence of signs of pain and respiratory obstruction.

Etiology

Pharyngeal paralysis occurs sporadically in peripheral nerve injury and in some encephalitides with central lesions.

Peripheral nerve injury

- Guttural pouch infections in horses (1)
- Trauma to the throat region.

Secondary to specific diseases

- Rabies and other encephalitides
- Botulism
- African horse sickness
- A series of unexplained fatal cases in horses (2).

Pathogenesis

Inability to swallow and regurgitation are the major manifestations of the disease. There may be an associated laryngeal paralysis accompanied by 'roaring'. The condition known as 'cud-dropping' in cattle may be a partial pharyngeal paralysis as there is difficulty in controlling the regurgitated bolus which is often dropped from the mouth. In these circumstances, aspiration pneumonia is likely to develop.

Clinical findings

The animal is usually hungry but, on prehension of food or water, attempts at swallowing are followed by dropping of the food from the mouth, coughing and the expulsion of food or regurgitation through the nostrils. Salivation occurs constantly and swallowing cannot be stimulated by external compression of the pharynx. The swallowing reflex is a complex one controlled by a number of nerves and the signs can be expected to vary greatly depending on which nerves are involved and to what degree. There is rapid loss of condition and dehydration. Clinical signs of the primary disease may be evident but, in cases of primary pharyngeal paralysis, there is no systemic reaction. Pneumonia may follow aspiration of food material into the lungs and produces loud gurgling sounds on auscultation.

In 'cud-dropping' in cows, the animal is normal except that regurgitated boluses are dropped from the mouth, usually in the form of flattened disks of fibrous food material. Affected animals may lose weight but the condition is usually transient, lasting for only a few days. On the other hand, complete pharyngeal paralysis is usually permanent and fatal.

Clinical pathology

The use of clinicopathological examinations is restricted to the identification of the primary specific diseases.

Necropsy findings

If the primary lesion is physical, it may be detected on gross examination.

Diagnosis

In all species often the first impression gained is that there is a foreign body in the mouth or pharynx and this can only be determined by physical examination. Pharyngeal paralysis is a typical sign in rabies and botulism but there are other clinical findings which suggest the presence of these diseases. Absence of pain and respiratory obstruction are usually sufficient evidence to eliminate the possibility of pharyngitis or pharyngeal obstruction. Endoscopic examination of the guttural pouch is a useful diagnostic aid in the horse.

Treatment

Treatment is unlikely to have any effect. The local application of heat may be attempted. Feeding by nasal tube or intravenous alimentation may be tried if disappearance of the paralysis seems probable.

RFERENCES

(1) Cook, W. R. (1966) *Mod. vet. Pract.*, *47*, 41.
(2) Bjorck, G. et al. (1974) *Svenska Vet.*, *26*, 169.

Esophagitis

Inflammation of the esophagus is accompanied initially by signs of spasm and obstruction, pain on swallowing and palpation, and regurgitation of bloodstained, slimy material.

Etiology

Primary esophagitis caused by the ingestion of chemical or physical irritants is usually accompanied by stomatitis and pharyngitis. Laceration of the mucosa by a foreign body or too vigorous passing of a stomach tube or probang may cause esophagitis unaccompanied by lesions elsewhere. Death of *Hypoderma lineata* larvae in the submucosa of the esophagus of cattle may cause acute local inflammation and subsequent gangrene (1).

Inflammation of the esophagus occurs commonly in many specific diseases, particularly those which cause stomatitis, but the other clinical signs of these diseases overshadow those of esophagitis.

Pathogenesis

The first reaction of the esophagus to inflammation is an increase in muscle tone and involuntary movement and these, combined with local edema and swelling, create a functional obstruction.

Clinical signs

In the acute stages, there is salivation and attempts at swallowing which cause severe pain, particularly in horses. In some cases, swallowing is impossible and attempts to do so are followed by regurgitation and coughing, accompanied by pain, retching movements and vigorous contractions of the cervical and abdominal muscles. The regurgitus may contain much mucus and some fresh blood. If the esophagitis is in the cervical region, palpation in the jugular furrow causes pain and the swollen esophagus may be palpable. If perforation has occurred, there is local pain and swelling and often crepitus. Local cervical cellulitis may cause rupture to the exterior and development of an esophageal fistula, or infiltration along fascial planes with resulting compression obstruction of the esophagus, and toxemia. Perforation of the thoracic esophagus may lead to fatal pleurisy. Animals that recover from esophagitis are commonly affected by chronic esophageal stenosis with distension above the stenosis. Fistulae are usually persistent but spontaneous healing may occur (2). In the specific diseases such as mucosal disease and bovine malignant catarrh, there are no obvious clinical signs of esophagitis, the lesions being mainly erosive. Endoscopic examination of the esophagus with the fiberoptiscope will allow a full view of the esophageal mucosa.

Clinical pathology and necropsy findings

Antemortem laboratory examinations and necropsy findings are restricted to those pertaining to the various specific diseases in which esophagitis occurs. In traumatic lesions or those caused by irritant substances, there is gross edema, inflammation and, in some cases, perforation.

Diagnosis

Esophagitis may be mistaken for pharyngitis but, in the latter, the results of attempted swallowing are not so severe and coughing is more likely to occur. Local palpation may also help to localize the lesion. Pharyngitis and esophagitis commonly occur together. When the injury is caused by a foreign body, it may still be in the esophagus and, if suitable restraint and anesthesia can be arranged, the passage of a nasal tube may locate it. Complete esophageal obstruction is accompanied by bloat in ruminants, by palpable enlargement of the esophagus and by less pain on swallowing than in esophagitis although horses may show a great deal of discomfort.

In cattle perforation of the esophagus is not uncommon. There is a persistent, moderate toxemia, a moderate fever and a leukocytosis. Pus accumulates in surrounding fascial planes, but causes only slight physical enlargement which is easily missed on a physical examination.

Treatment

Food should be withheld for 2–3 days and the animal may need to be fed intravenously during this period. Parenteral antibacterial treatment should be administered, especially if laceration or perforation has occurred. Reintroduction to feed should be monitored carefully and all feed should be moistened to avoid the possible accumulation of dry feed in the esophagus which may not be fully functional.

REFERENCES

(1) Khan, M. A. (1971) *Can. J. anim. Sci.*, *51*, 411.
(2) Raker, C. W. & Sayers, A. (1958) *J. Am. vet. med. Assoc.*, *133*, 371.

Esophageal obstruction

Esophageal obstruction may be acute or chronic and the clinical signs of inability to swallow, regurgitation of food and water, and bloat in ruminants are accompanied in acute cases by severe distress.

Etiology

Obstruction may be internal by swallowed material or external by pressure on the esophagus by surrounding organs or tissues.

Ingested material

- Solid obstructions, especially in cattle, by turnips, potatoes, peaches, apples, oranges
- A particular occurrence of obstruction by 15 g gelatin capsules in Shetland ponies (1)
- Particulate material. This kind of obstruction is common in horses, e.g., when allowed to gulp dry hay or chop (chaff) immediately after a race. The horse eats ravenously, swallows large boluses without properly ensalivating it. The bolus lodges at the base of the neck or the cardia. Similar obstructions occur when horses are turned into stalls containing fresh bedding, including shavings
- A swallowed stomach tube (8).

Obstruction as a result of abnormality of local tissue

- Tuberculous or neoplastic lymph nodes in mediastinum or at base of lung
- Persistent right aortic arch
- Esophageal paralysis, diverticulum (5) or megaesophagus, which has been recorded in horses (10) and calves (14) and congenital hypertrophy of esophageal musculature (11) and esophagotracheal fistula (9) also in calves (18); congenital esophageal ectasia in foals (17) caused by degeneration of musculature and reduced ganglion cells in the myenteric plexus and congenital esophageal dysfunction in foals with no detectable histopathological lesion but with prolonged simultaneous contractions throughout the esophagus (6)
- Carcinoma of stomach causing obstruction of cardia (3)
- Esophageal hiatus hernia in cattle (4)
- Postesophagitis stenosis
- Esophageal mucosal granuloma (12)
- Thymoma
- Cervical or mediastinal abscess
- Traumatic rupture during treatment using a probang or nasogastric tube.

Pathogenesis

There is physical inability to swallow and, in cattle, inability to belch with resulting bloat. In acute obstruction, there is initial spasm at the site of obstruction and forceful, painful peristalsis and swallowing movements.

Clinical findings

Acute obstruction or choke

In cattle, the obstruction is usually in the cervical esophagus just above the larynx or at the thoracic inlet. The animal suddenly stops eating and shows anxiety and restlessness. There are forceful attempts to swallow and regurgitate, salivation, coughing and continuous chewing movements. If obstruction is complete, bloating occurs rapidly and adds to the animal's discomfort. Ruminal movements are continuous and forceful and there may be a systolic murmur audible on auscultation of the heart.

The acute signs, other than bloat, usually disappear within a few hours. This is due to relaxation of the initial esophageal spasm and may or may not be accompanied by onward passage of the obstruction. Many obstructions pass on spontaneously but others may persist for several days and up to a week. In these cases, there is inability to swallow, salivation and continued bloat. Passage of a nasal or stomach tube is impossible. Persistent obstruction causes pressure necrosis of the mucosa and may result in perforation or in subsequent stenosis due to fibrous tissue construction.

In horses, the obstruction is often in the terminal part of the thoracic esophagus and cannot be seen or palpated. The clinical signs are similar to those in the cow but are more severe and the horse's reaction may take the form of violent activity with very forceful attempts to swallow or retch. Persistent obstruction may also occur in the horse. Gelatin capsules are particularly liable to remain *in situ* for 3 or 4 days. Death may occur in either species from subsequent aspiration pneumonia or, when the obstruction persists, from dehydration.

Chronic obstruction

There is an absence of acute signs. In cattle, the earliest sign is chronic bloat which is usually of moderate severity and may persist for very long periods without the appearance of other signs. The rumen usually continues to move in an exaggerated manner for some weeks but, after prolonged distension, tone is usually depressed. In horses and in cattle in which the obstruction is sufficiently severe to interfere with swallowing, a characteristic syndrome develops. Swallowing movements are usually normal until the bolus reaches the obstruction when they are replaced by more forceful movements. Dilatation of the esophagus may cause a pronounced swelling at the base of the neck. The swallowed material either passes slowly through the stenotic area or accumulates and is then regurgitated. Projectile expulsion of ingested material occurs with esophageal diverticula, but water is retained and there is no impedance to the passage of the stomach tube. In the later stages, there may be no attempt made to eat solid food but fluids may be taken and swallowed satisfactorily.

When there is paralysis of the esophagus, regurgitation does not occur but the esophagus fills and overflows, and saliva drools from the mouth and nostrils. Aspiration into the lungs may follow. Passage of a stomach tube or probang is obstructed by stenosis but may be unimpeded by paralysis.

Clinical pathology

Laboratory tests are not used in diagnosis although radiographic examination is helpful to outline the site of stenosis, diverticulum or dilatation, even in animals as large as the horse. Radiological examination after a barium swallow is a practicable procedure if the obstruction is in the cervical esophagus. Viewing of the internal lumen of the esopnagus with a fiberoptiscope has completely revolutionized the diagnosis of esophageal malfunction.

Diagnosis

The clinical picture is typical but can be mistaken for that of esophagitis in which local pain is more apparent and there is often an accompanying stomatitis and pharyngitis. Differentiation of the causes of chronic obstruction may be difficult. A history of previous esophagitis or acute obstruction suggests cicatricial stenosis. Persistent right aortic arch is rare and confined to young animals. Mediastinal lymph node enlargement is usually accompanied by other signs of tuberculosis or lymphomatosis. Chronic ruminal tympany in cattle may be caused by ruminal atony in which case there is an absence of normal ruminal movements. Diaphragmatic hernia may also be a cause of chronic ruminal tympany in cattle and is sometimes accompanied by obstruction of the esophagus with incompletely regurgitated ingesta. This condition and vagus indigestion, another cause of chronic tympany, are usually accompanied by a systolic cardiac murmur but passage of a stomach tube is unimpeded. Dysphagia may also result from purely neurogenic defects. Thus, an early paralytic rabies 'choke' is often suspected with dire results for the examining veterinarian. Equine encephalomyelitis and botulism are other diseases in which difficulty is experienced with swallowing. Cleft palate is a common cause of nasal regurgitation in foals.

Treatment

In acute obstruction where there is marked distress, some attempt should be made to sedate the animal before proceeding with treatment. Administration of an ataractic drug or chloral hydrate may also help in relaxing the esophageal spasm. Other means of relaxing the spasm include the subcutaneous administration of atropine sulfate (16–32 mg) or the administration of fluid extract of belladonna (1–2 ml) by stomach tube. The passage of the stomach tube or probang is usually necessary to locate obstructions low down in the esophagus. Gentle attempts may be made to push the obstruction onward but care must be taken to avoid damage to the esophageal mucosa.

If the above simple procedures are unsuccessful it is then necessary to proceed to more vigorous methods. In cows, it is usual to attempt further measures immediately, partly because of the cow's distress and the risk of self-injury and partly because of the bloat. The important decision is whether to proceed and risk damaging the esophagus or to wait and allow the esophageal spasm to relax and the obstruction to pass spontaneously. This problem is most important in the horse. Attempts to push the obstruction may be so forceful as to damage the mucosa, a probably fatal lesion. Alternatively, leaving a large obstruction in place may restrict the circulation to the local area of mucosae and result in ischemic necrosis. In either case there will eventually be a constriction of the lumen requiring surgery which is not highly successful. As a guide in the horse it is suggested that conservative measures, principally sedation and waiting, be continued for 48 hours before attempting radical procedures such as general anesthesia and manipulation or esophagotomy.

Solid obstructions in the upper esophagus of cattle may be reached by passing the hand into the pharynx through a speculum and having an assistant press the foreign body up towards the mouth. It is often difficult to grasp the obstruction sufficiently strongly to be able to extricate it from the spastic esophagus. A long piece of strong wire bent into a loop may be passed over the object and an attempt made to pull it up into the pharynx. The use of Thygesen's probang with a cutting loop is a simple and effective method of relieving choke in cattle which have attempted to swallow beets and other similar-sized vegetables and fruits (7). If both methods fail, it is advisable to leave the object *in situ* and use treatments aimed at relaxing the esophagus. In such cases in cattle it is usually necessary to trocarize the rumen and leave the cannula in place until the obstruction is relieved. In horses, attempts to remove obstructions high up in the esophagus require a general anesthetic, a speculum in the mouth and a manipulator with a small hand. The fauces are much narrower in the horse than the cow and it is only with difficulty that the hand can be advanced through the pharynx to the beginning of the esophagus.

Accumulations of particulate material such as those which are commonly found in the lower esophagus of horses are more difficult to remove. Small quantities of warm saline should be introduced through a stomach tube passed to the point of obstruction and then pumped or siphoned out. This may be repeated a number of times until the fluid comes clear. If the obstruction is still present, fluid extract of belladonna should be administered before removal of the tube. Further attempts at irrigative removal should be attempted at short intervals. If the obstruction is palpable in the neck, vigorous squeezing from the exterior may break it up and aid its removal. Two tubes must be used, one in each nostril, to make faster irrigation possible, but care must be taken to avoid overflowing the esophagus and causing aspiration into the lungs. This is a constant hazard whenever irrigative removal is attempted and the animal's head must always be kept low to avoid aspiration. Surgical removal by esophagotomy may be necessary if other measures fail.

The animal must not be allowed access to water or food until the obstruction is removed. In chronic cases, especially those due to paralysis, repeated siphonage may be necessary to remove fluid accumulations. Successful results are reported in foals using resection and anastomosis of the esophagus (15) and in a horse using esophagomyotomy (16) but the treatment of chronic obstructions is usually unsuccessful. Tube feeding through a cervical esophagostomy has some disadvantages, but it is a reasonably satisfactory procedure in any situation where continued extraoral alimentation is required in the horse (2). However, the death rate is higher than with nasogastric tube feeding. When the obstruction is due to circumferential esophageal ulceration, the lumen is smallest at about 50 days and begins to dilate at that point so that it is normal again at about 60 days (13).

REFERENCES

(1) Lundvall, R. L. & Kingrey, B. W. (1985) *J. Am. vet. med. Assoc.*, *133*, 75.
(2) Todhunter, R. J. et al. (1986) *Cornell Vet.*, *76*, 16.
(3) Moore, J. N. & Kintner, L. D. (1976) *Cornell Vet.*, *66*, 590.
(4) Anderson, N. V. et al. (1984) *J. Am. vet. med. Assoc.*, *184*, 193.
(5) Frauenfelder, H. C. & Adams, S. B. (1982) *J. Am. vet. med. Assoc.*, *180*, 771.
(6) Clark, E. S. et al. (1987) *Cornell Vet.*, *77*, 151.
(7) Church, T. L. (1972) *Can. vet. J.*, *13*, 226.
(8) Travers, D. S. (1978) *Vet. med. SAC*, *73*, 783.
(9) Keane, D. P. et al. (1983) *Can vet. J.*, *24*, 57.
(10) Vrins, A. et al. (1983) *Can vet. J.*, *24*, 385.
(11) Wagner, P. C. et al. (1979) *Mod. vet. Pract.*, *60*, 1029.
(12) Meagher, D. M. & Mayhew, I. G. (1978) *Can. vet. J.*, *19*, 128.
(13) Todhunter, R. J. et al. (1984) *J. Am. vet. med. Assoc.*, *185*, 784.
(14) Vestweber, J. G. et al. (1985) *J. Am. vet. med. Assoc.*, *187*, 1369.
(15) Gideon, L. (1984) *J. Am. vet. med. Assoc.*, *184*, 1146.
(16) Nixon, A. J. et al. (1983) *J. Am. vet. med. Assoc.*, *183*, 794.
(17) Barber, S. M. et al. (1983) *Can. vet. J.*, *24*, 46.
(18) Kasari, T. R. (1984) *Can. vet. J.*, *25*, 177.

DISEASES OF THE STOMACH AND INTESTINES

Only those diseases which are accompanied by physical lesions or disturbances of motility are presented. Diseases caused by functional disturbances of secretion are not recognized in animals. In any case, disturbances of secretion are usually accompanied by disturbances of motility. Deficiencies of biliary secretion are dealt with in the chapter on diseases of the liver. Those diseases of the stomachs which are peculiar to ruminants are dealt with separately as they present rather special problems in diagnosis.

There are some other diseases of the alimentary tract which are not easily classified into the broad, pathologically based entities listed below, and which are dealt with as specific diseases in other sections of this book. They include gastric ulceration, rectal stricture, and acute intestinal hemorrhage, all of pigs.

Equine colic

Those diseases of the horse which cause abdominal pain, generally referred to as equine colic, are presented in the following sections.

Etiology

The known and suspected causes of colic are set out in summary form in Table 16.

Pathogenesis

Distension

The list of colics in Table 16 has been drawn up on the assumption that the primary disturbance in all colics is distension of the stomach or intestines. The distension may be static when there is an accumulation of ingesta, gas or fluid, or transient when local periodic distensions occur as the result of a spasm and increased peristalsis of intestinal segments. The static accumulations are classified as physical colics, requiring physical treatments, the transient distensions as functional colics for which the rational treatment is the relief of both spasm and increased peristalsis. A secondary cause of abdominal pain, of most importance in acute intestinal accidents, is stretching of the peritoneum, often for reasons other than simple distension of the viscus; for example, because of entrapment of a viscus and stretching of its mesentery.

Shock and dehydration

Although abdominal pain is a major problem in a case of colic, and although it can be exhausting and lead to the animal injuring itself, it is not what actually kills the animal. In acute fatal colics, such as an intestinal obstruction, it is dehydration and/or shock which kills; shock because of stretching and damage to tissues especially by infarction when the blood supply is occluded, and dehydration due to sequestration of fluid and electrolytes in the distended lumen of the intestine. Hyponatremia and acidosis are two other common life-threatening accompaniments. The secretion of fluid and electrolytes is a response to the prior presence of distension creating a self-perpetuating, fatal cycle. If the obstruction is at the pylorus, it is acidic fluid that is lost and alkalosis develops; more commonly the obstruction is in the lower intestine and the loss is of alkaline fluid

Table 16. Etiological classification of equine colic

Classification	*Primary etiological agent*	*Pathogenesis*	*Cause of distension*
PHYSICAL COLICS	Low-grade roughage Bad teeth Debility Exhaustion Excessive inspissation (e.g. retained meconium)	Distension	Accumulation of ingesta (*impaction of the large intestine*)
	Lush green feed *Clostridium perfringens* type A Secondary to acute intestinal obstruction	Distension of intestine	Accumulation of gas (*flatulent colic, intestinal tympany*)
	Gross feeding (engorgement on grain or other palatable food)	Distension of stomach	Accumulation of food (*gastric dilatation*)
	Engorgement on whey Pyloric obstruction Reflux from intestinal obstruction Spontaneous after racing	Distension of stomach	Accumulation of fluid (*acute gastric dilatation*)
	Impaction of ileocecal valve Fiber-balls, enteroliths, foreign bodies Volvulus, torsion, intussusception, strangulation in occlusive hernias, diaphragmatic hernia, pedunculated lipomas, congenital diverticula, Meckel's diverticulum, anomalous mesenteric bands, hematoma of gut wall*	Distension of intestine	Accumulation of fluid (*acute intestinal obstruction*)
	Verminous mesenteric arteritis (adhesions causing cicatricial constriction of lumen) Terminal ileal hypertrophy	Distension of intestine	Accumulation of fluid (*subacute intestinal obstruction*)
	Verminous mesenteric arteritis (infarction of gut wall) Peritonitis Grass sickness Sequel to acute intestinal obstruction	Distension of intestine due to paralytic ileus	Accumulation of fluid (*paralytic ileus*)
FUNCTIONAL COLICS	Parasitism (strongylosis) Bacterial (salmonellosis etc.) Rickettsial (equine intestinal ehrlichiosis) Idiopathic (hemorrhagic fibronecrotic duodenitis) Viral (equine viral arteritis) Physical (sand colic, enteroliths, phytobezoars) Chemical poison	Enteritis	Spasm and increased peristalsis
	Excitement Thunderstorms Cold drinks or chilling Reflex from other viscera Grass sickness *Verminous mesenteric arteritis*	Autonomic imbalance (*spasmodic colic*)	Spasm and increased peristalsis

*The variety of lesions causing intestinal distension is very great indeed (21, 22) and a complete listing is not possible. For example intussusception alone can come in four forms, small intestine into itself, or into cecum, cecum into itself or into colon.

resulting in acidosis. The horse is particularly susceptible to intestinal accidents and their fatal outcomes, and to colic generally, because of the great activity of the small intestine and the large amount of undigested material that it moves on to the large bowel. Ruminants are much better situated with the large fermentation compartments at the beginning of the alimentary tract, and with only the finer particulate material to convey through the long narrow reaches of the intestines.

Cause of death
Rupture of the stomach or intestine is also a characteristic termination of distension of the intestine in the horse. The resulting deposition of large quantities of highly toxic ingesta or fecal contents into the peritoneal cavity causes profound shock and death within a few hours. In the colics where impaction of ingesta occurs, the cause of death is assumed to be a combination of exhaustion due to pain, intoxication referred to earlier as autointoxication, deprivation of food due to failure to passage and digest it and the reflex effects of continuous distension of the intestines on the cardiovascular system. It is not usual for such colics to come to a fatal termination because of the satisfactory medical treatment available. Although the outcome in the more serious intestinal obstructions need not be fatal in most cases, provided the diagnosis is made and the surgery done early, and proper supportive therapy of fluid and electrolytes is supplied. It is well to remember that these facilities are not generally available to veterinarians in the field. The backup services required are sophisticated and therefore expensive, very expensive, and accordingly limited in their applicability.

Small intestine
When indigestible fiber cannot be digested in the intestine it is not difficult to imagine the pathogenesis of impaction of the large bowel. The pathogenesis is not so obvious when one is considering hypermotibility and spasmodic colic, and the almost certain participation of hypermotility in the development of volvulus, strangulation and intussusception. These account for almost half the colic cases encountered. Internal parasitism, specifically strongylosis, is credited with having this effect and any control program must take worms into account. *Strongylus vulgaris* larvae have this effect (36).

The frequency with which intestinal accidents affect the small intestine is often noted. So is the frequency with which they occur in the terminal part of the ileum. It is possible that with hypermotile movements the small intestine can move its loops through considerable distances but these movements are brought to a sudden halt when they approach the fixed point of the ileocecal valve; so that a whiplash effect is exerted, lending itself to displacements.

Large intestine
Colic emanating from disease of the large intestine is mostly due to impaction with undigested food fiber or infarction as a result of verminous arteritis. The colic is therefore inclined to be subacute and with a protracted course, and either amenable to medical treatment in the case of impactions, or incurable in the case of infarctions. But all of the acute intestinal accidents can occur, especially in small colon, and when they do the effects are as acute, and severe and lethal as they are when the small intestine is involved. The differences are that in the large bowel the distension is due to gas rather than fluid and is greater in degree. So that shock is likely to be more important than dehydration.

Epidemiology
The rate of occurrence of colic is not the same for all kinds of colic because the basic causes are different, but there are two principal etiological groups that do tend to have particular circumstances that affect their prevalence. Those colics which result from hypermotility, including spasmodic colics, and the displacements of volvulus and intussusception are much more common, in pastured horses, at times when strongyle larvae are active. Also, those farms which have an effective worm control program are much more free of the disease. On the other hand, impactions are much commoner in the drier times, rather than the spring season of succulent grass and its attendant hypermotility. The same comment applies to stabled horses which are fed too mature or coarse cereal, roughage. Horses, unlike cows, have an intestinal tract in which tough fiber has to pass through a simple stomach and small intestine, before reaching the fermentation chambers of the large bowel. An interesting analysis of types and causes of colics is available (30).

Clinical findings
The following description is generally applicable to colic of alimentary tract origin in the horse. Clinical findings characteristic of each etiological type of colic are dealt with under their individual headings.

Preliminary findings
Restlessness is evident and manifested by pawing or stamping or kicking at the belly or by getting up and lying down frequently. Pain is also manifested by looking at the flank, rolling, lying on the back, careful lying down and slowness in getting up, the horse often sitting like a dog for long periods. The posture is often abnormal, seen usually as a 'saw-horse' attitude. Geldings often protrude the penis without urinating. Frequent urination with small amounts being passed often results from irritation of the peritoneum such as occurs in the early stages of peritonitis after rupture of the gut. Another common sign in colic is continuous playing with the drinking water without actually drinking any—sham drinking. Water consumption may appear to be normal or increased if one measures it by how often the bucket is filled, but most of it ends up on the floor.

The pain is usually intermittent, especially in the early stages, often to the point where recovery is incorrectly diagnosed. Bouts of pain may last for over 10 minutes with like periods of relaxation. In general the level of pain, which may be subacute or acute, is of about the same severity for the duration of the illness; impaction of the ileocecal valve is an exception. In the most severe cases the pain is almost continuous and although it has the same general pattern as above there may be in addition obvious signs of shock, profuse sweating, sobbing respiration and uncontrolled movements of such violence that the horse quickly does itself serious injury. Although other diseases such as hepatitis are accompanied by pain because of stretching of the mesentery, the pain is very much less than in distension of the gut; rarely does it exceed pawing and flankwatching. A horse which goes down and rolls and which has elevations of respiratory and pulse rates due to pain almost certainly has alimentary tract colic.

Some indication of the site of the obstruction or impaction may be deduced from the behavior of the horse. For example, the adoption of a saw-horse posture with the legs stretched out behind usually accompanies impaction of the colon; lying down with legs in the air suggests a need to relieve tension on mesentery caused by the heavy gut contents of impaction or infarction of the gut wall (1).

Part of the pain syndrome is an increase in respiratory rate; it is common for it to increase from a normal of 18 per minute to as high as 40 per minute and in cases where the pain is intense it can reach 80 per minute. Sobbing dyspnea is a feature in the terminal stages when shock and dehydration are at their peak. An animal at this stage also shows marked muscle tremor, especially noticeable at the knees. Failure to respond to analgesia is a bad prognostic sign, and suggests a severe lesion in urgent need of correction.

Distension of the abdomen is not common in cases of colic in horses, and if it is obvious on cursory inspection it is probable that the cecum and colon are distended with gas. Maximum distension of stomach or small intestines is unlikely to cause obvious distension. Vomiting, or more usually regurgitation, of intestinal contents through the nose is a serious sign suggesting severe gastric distension and impending rupture.

Defecation should be observed but it is difficult to interpret (2). For example, it is often mistakenly assumed that there is no complete obstruction because feces are still being passed. But in the very early stages of acute intestinal obstruction there may be feces in the rectum and the animal may defecate several times before the more usual sign of an empty rectum with a sticky mucosa is achieved. It is our experience that as owners and veterinarians have come to appreciate the need for urgent and early action in severe cases of colic we get to examine them at an early stage when feces are still being passed, when gut sounds are still present and when there are no positive rectal findings. Because of the need to make an accurate diagnosis, and to avoid unnecessary expensive surgery we find that we need to adopt a pattern of case management where early cases are often admitted and then make their own history, as it were. They are monitored hourly for changes in heart rate and other cardiovascular signs, for clinicopathological parameters, especially hemoconcentration, and rectally for evidence of distending intestines, and by auscultation for the onset of atony and paralytic ileus. These findings, and the empty rectum with sticky mucosa are usually evident 12–18 hours after the intestinal accident appears. A protocol is set out below in this section.

Detailed clinical examination

Colic is one of the common disease complexes in the horse and its early recognition and accurate differentiation is very important (3). The clinical syndrome is described above. Having observed this, it is then necessary to carry out a more complete examination. The following is suggested as a minimum.

The pulse rate should be less than 80 per minute for a favorable prognosis; a rate of over 100 will probably indicate an early demise. A more accurate prediction scale is: pulse rates of less than 40 suggest the presence of other disease, 40–60 suggest a minor lesion such as impaction, 60–80 arouses suspicion of a major lesion such as an intestinal accident, and 80–100 is a positive indication of such a lesion, and over 100 suggests that irreversible damage has occurred. This scale should not be construed as an exact formula. All other clinical findings must also be taken into account; they may confirm or refute the pulse rate suggestions. Much can also be learned about the status of the circulatory system in a horse by examining the oral or other mucosa. A pale dry clammy mucosa suggests shock resulting from a compromised blood supply to a large section of intestine. A deeply congested dark red to purple mucosa with a long capillary-filling time of up to 8 seconds indicates very severe dehydration plus shock. The capillary filling time should be of the order of 1 second, certainly no more than 2. Palpation of the extremities to judge the efficiency of the peripheral circulation is also of value but only when the changes are great. A cold clammy feel suggests the existence of shock. The temperature is rarely above the normal range, in fact a subnormal temperature is more usual and when critically low, indicates the development of shock; fever suggests some other cause of the signs observed.

Auscultation of the abdomen is an essential part of the examination. The simplest statement is that continuous borborygmi suggest hypermotility, as occurs in spasmodic colic, or the early stages of both enteritis and peritonitis, and that absence of sounds indicates paralytic ileus or impaction. But there are many variations of this rule of thumb and the most important and overriding rule is that intestinal sounds can change precipitately, and continuous observation over a period, preferably in hospital, is the only way of making accurate observations and diagnoses. Probably the most critical area for auscultation is high up in the right flank, over the dorsal sac of the cecum, and aimed at listening to the ileocecal valve. If it is functioning there will be a periodic squirt of fluid contents into a gas-filled cavity with fluid at the bottom. The resulting sounds, a squelching, gassy rush, suggest this architecture.

The recognition and interpretation of a complete absence of sounds are also sometimes difficult. Even in the most serious of emergencies it is commonly possible to hear sounds caused by the movement of gas which is still being produced in the large intestine, and which moves through liquid ingesta as the respiratory movements of the abdominal wall and diaphragm cause movements of the loops of the bowel. These sounds are audible as isolated blips and tinkles, quite different from the long continuous rolls produced by normal peristaltic movements.

Palpation of the abdomen from the exterior has little application to the horse. Forceful upward ballottement with the heel of the hand to test the rigidity of the abdominal muscles and for a pain response is all that is attempted. It is a technique which is much too often neglected, and cases of peritonitis which could be simply identified by it escape the diagnostic net.

Rectal examination

A careful rectal examination is probably the most important part of the clinical examination in colic. The examiner must know the anatomy of the posterior abdomen in order to make reasonably accurate decisions about the location of various organs especially the large bowel. The abnormalities that need to be detected are three. One is firm enlargements of intestine in the form of long columns, caused by impaction of feces in the large colon, or ingesta in the terminal ileum at the ileocecal valve, or gross hypertrophy of the ileal wall at the same site. A second important finding is the distension of loops of intestine. The distension is usually fluid with some gas if the affected bowel is small intestine, or just gas if it is large bowel. The third finding which is noteworthy is very tight stretching of mesentery, indicating either a heavy bowel segment at the end of it, or a folding together of mesentery when intestine is twisted on itself or telescoped into itself. It is necessary to differentiate the mesentery of the cecum, which stretches from the right upper abdomen to the anterior left lower abdomen in normal horses.

Gas-filled loops of intestine indicate flatulent colic or, if they also contain much fluid, intestinal obstruction. Long columns of feces are a sure indication of impaction and are usually accompanied by a rectum full of dry, hard fecal balls. Predilection sites for impaction are the pelvic flexure, the right dorsal and the small colons. Differentiation between small and large intestines should be made if possible. The decision rests on whether taenia and sacculation are palpable. Isolated abnormal intestinal loops are often palpable in intussusception, strangulation, volvulus, and verminous mesenteric arteritis. In fact these diseases can only be positively diagnosed in this way. Although the affected segment may be out of reach from the rectum it is usually possible to pick up the tight-stretched band of mesentery, or adhesion, that leads to it. If the examiner is skilled and the horse is of the correct size and cooperative temperament, it is possible to palpate the caudal edge of the mesentery and the anterior mesenteric artery. An arteritis of significant size can be palpated as a lumpy enlargement on the artery and it can be felt to pulsate with the pulse wave, and sometimes to have fremitus. Similar lesions may be palpable elsewhere especially in the cecal artery on the dorsal surface of the cecum. In normal horses the edge of the fold is thin and distinct. When arteritis is present it is thick and lumpy and with a round, lumpy edge. It may be impossible to diagnose the nature of the lesion but it is often possible to predict its whereabouts, and this is most important in these highly fatal conditions because surgical intervention is the only means of salvage. A complete clinical examination must also include the passage of a nasal tube to determine whether the stomach is grossly distended with fluid, and paracentesis to determine whether there is inflammatory exudate in the peritoneal cavity, or whether there is any evidence of intestinal or gastric rupture (5). When rupture of the intestine does occur there is a sudden onset of shock and toxemia and the acute pain which preceded it disappears, and the horse becomes quiet and immobile. Even pain on palpation may no longer be evident. The terminal stages of colic due to rupture of the intestine or acute gastric dilatation or intestinal obstruction are very distressing. The horse may be recumbent but most continue to stand until the last few minutes when they literally drop dead. The respiration is sobbing and there is gross muscle tremor, sweating is profuse and sweat may actually drop from the horse, and there is often a delirious, staggering wandering.

Differentiation of types of colic

The differentiation of the specific lesions which cause colic is necessary because the prognosis varies so greatly with each and the choice of treatment used depends on the nature of the lesion. In general the prognosis is excellent for diseases caused by hypermotility, good for fecal impaction, and very bad in intestinal and vascular emergencies unless the diagnosis is accurate and surgery can be carried out immediately.

The most common colics are set out in Table 16 and details of the individual diseases are under their specific headings. Other less common causes, also listed elsewhere under their own headings, are neoplasms of the bowel, especially lymphosarcoma and gastric carcinoma, and terminal hypertrophy of the ileum. The possibility of psychogenic colic occurring in horses seems remote but at least one case has been reported (4).

In foals, intestinal colic, with or without intestinal tympany, is common immediately after birth and is discussed under the heading of retained meconium. Congenital atresia of the anus or a segment of gut is also relatively common in newborn thoroughbred horses and is dealt with elsewhere. The anal lesion is sometimes associated with absence of the tail (6). In older foals, acute intestinal obstructions are likely to be caused by torsion of the ileum close to the ileocecal valve, less commonly to intussusception at the same site. Pyloric stenosis, treated successfully surgically, has also been recorded but is very rare (6). Volvulus usually occurs in the 2–4-month age group and may be related to the commencement of roughage feeding in quantity and the resulting hypermotility. Cecal tympany is also recorded in foals of this age. The cause is not known.

Clinical pathology

Many tests are now used when making a diagnosis of colic and when attempting to assess the progress of a case (7, 24). Of particular value is the measurement of hemoconcentration so that the degree of dehydration can be estimated. Additional desirable assessments are of electrolytes and acid–base balance, and the tests used and their interpretation are discussed in the section under that heading to which the reader is referred. A total and differential leukocyte count may be valuable when peritonitis is suspected. A high count with a shift to the left is to be expected with acute local peritonitis, and a marked leukopenia when there is acute diffuse peritonitis.

The critical values of the laboratory measurements used most commonly in the horse are: total serum protein 7·5 g/dl or less, packed cell volume 45% or less, blood pH within the range of 7·25–7·3, plasma sodium not less than 132 mmol/l, and plasma bicarbonate not less than 24 mmol/l. These tests are aimed at determining the degree of dehydration and acidosis which exists. It is necessary to measure total protein and PCV together because the latter is likely to be influenced by sudden evacuation of the spleen leading to a PCV rise quite unrelated to a shock state. It is also important to conduct a series of tests over a period of time so that the development of a state of severe hemoconcentration can be recognized as it develops in spite of, for example, a preexisting anemia. The total serum protein level should also be watched carefully during the course of the disease because a great deal of protein may be lost into a damaged intestine, leaving the horse susceptible to the development of pulmonary edema if large volumes of fluid are administered parenterally.

A good correlation has also been established between the blood level of lactate and survival (8). Levels greater than 75 mg/dl (8·3 mmol/l) indicate a poor prognosis. Expressed differently, the blood lactate in normal horses is 6·13–7·30 mg/dl (0·68–0·81 mmol/l). The mean blood lactate levels in 12 horses which would have died without surgery was 43·6 mg/dl (4·84 mmol/l); six horses which recovered without surgery had a mean level of 10·1 mg/dl (1·21 mmol/l) at the time of acute colic. The blood lactate level is considered to have excellent prognostic value in terms of outcome and deciding when surgery is necessary (9). The levels are likely to be high only in those cases in which the small intestinal involvement is accompanied by severe abdominal pain. In large intestinal accidents, including torsions, blood lactate levels are only slightly elevated.

Other clinical chemical findings which may have diagnostic or prognostic relevance are:

- Low blood chloride levels with acute gastric dilatation
- Metabolic alkalosis in acute gastric dilatation and impactions of the large bowel
- Metabolic acidosis in most acute small intestinal obstructions
- Anion gap (total chloride and bicarbonate levels subtracted from total sodium and potassium levels) is an approximation of the lactate level, if that measurement is not available (24). Predicted survival rates are 81% survival at anion gap levels of $<$20 mEq/l (mmol/l), 47% at 20 to 24·9 mEq/l (mmol/l) and 0% at $\geq$25 mEq/l (mmol/l)
- The levels of the intestinal isoenzyme of alkaline phosphatase in plasma and peritoneal fluid (34).

Examination of stomach fluid is often helpful if regurgitation occurs. If there is duodenal regurgitation it will be alkaline (pH of about 7 usually), bile-stained and watery. The normal contents are thick with mucus, with a pH of about 2 and stained with bile.

Paracentesis abdominis is described in detail in an earlier section (p. 161). It is a most helpful test when trying to assess the degree of damage to the gut, but its indiscriminate use can be dangerous. Even if one uses the recommended technique in the most careful manner it is still possible to perforate an atonic loop of bowel filled with fluid and cause fatal peritonitis. On the other hand if there is no such distended loop and it is necessary to know whether there is peritonitis or that there is infarction of a loop of gut, or that there is neoplasia, paracentesis can be most helpful (10–12). In the horse, normal values are: nucleated cells 3000/μl (comprising 60% neutrophils and 10–20% lymphocytes) protein 1–1·5 g/dl and specific gravity 1·001. Devitalization of intestinal wall is manifested by elevations of the protein level, high cell count and blood staining, so that contamination of the sample by blood from the paracentesis incision must be avoided. The volume of fluid is characteristically increased in these circumstances but its volume is difficult to ascertain; a free flow of fluid under pressure suggests it. A stained smear is valuable in determining the presence of a preponderance of neutrophils suggesting peritonitis. Cell counts of over 5000/μl suggest inflammation and if this is present there is a tendency for a marked increase in the percentage of neutrophils to 75–95%. Such inflammation may of course be unassociated with intestine but it can also be the result of leakage from a section of intestine where verminous arteritis has caused venous infarction and necrosis of a section of the intestinal wall. If the fluid is bloodstained rather than contains blood it is reasonable to assume that a section of the intestine is necrotic. If it contains blood, it is more likely that there is hemorrhage into the peritoneal cavity or the paracentesis cannula has penetrated the spleen, or a blood vessel. On the other hand an absence of bloodstaining of the fluid does not mean that the intestinal wall is intact. It may be too early in the disease for leakage to occur, or the necrotic section may be outside the abdominal cavity, in the thorax through a diaphragmatic hernia, in the scrotum through the inguinal rings, into the omental bursa, or into the cecum in the case of intussusception of the terminal ileum through the ileocecal valve.

Central venous pressure is a valuable index of progress (5, 13) but the measurement is not likely to be applicable unless the animal is under general anesthesia. During surgery it is an excellent indicator of when to increase or decrease the flow of supplemental fluids. Normal levels are in the range of 6–10 mmH_2O (59–98·5 Pa), rising to about 15 mmH_2O (150 Pa) when sufficient fluids have been given.

Arterial blood pressure is a very good indicator of the degree of shock in colic, and the availability of a simple technique makes it a practical aid in assessing prognosis in a case of colic. If normal systolic pressure is about 100 mmHg (13·3 kPa), a pressure below 80 (11) indicates a critical situation (it can be as low as 50). In horses with very severe pain but not shock, the systolic pressure is likely to be very high, up to 250 mmHg (33·3 kPa) (25).

Protocol for evaluating a colic patient

For the horse with colic it has become vitally important to evaluate its physiologic–pathological state, as a separate exercise to making a diagnosis. There are at least three reasons why this is so important:

1. All cases of colic take time to resolve and it is most desirable to know whether the pain, which is so distressing esthetically to the client, and pathologically to the patient, is going to come to an end.
2. Now that so much abdominal surgery is done it is very important to the patient to perform it as early

as there are clear indications to do so. It is not infrequent that horses are operated on because there is intractable pain, and because the horse's physiological status in terms of standing up to surgical intervention is declining towards danger point.

3. If for some reason even exploratory surgery is not applicable to an individual case, the question of euthanasia arises. If a specific diagnosis, which identifies the critical lesion, is not available it is often necessary to make a decision on the basis of prognosis. This is always difficult for fear of putting a horse down which has a condition that is recoverable by medical means. It is necessary to have guidelines that take as much guessing as possible out of these decisions.

The suggested protocol for evaluating a horse with colic is set down below. How often it is conducted depends on a number of factors, including severity of the disease and the accessibility of the horse. For a horse with a possible intestinal obstruction this should be every hour; for a horse with probable colonic impaction examinations every 4 hours are adequate; for a chronic colic with ileal hypertrophy an examination every 1 or 2 days is usual. The following observations should be made.

Behavior
The following should be assessed: severity of pain, frequency and duration of attacks; whether food is taken; feces passed, piles should be removed from stall at every visit; urine passed, it is usually necessary to check under the straw.

Clinical and clinicopathological observations
The following should be noted:

1. Temperature, infrequently taken unless some positive indication, such as suspicion of peritonitis, to do so.
2. Respiratory rate, also of minor importance except as an indicator of severity of pain, or in terminal stages of endotoxic shock or dehydration, when it becomes gasping, because there are plenty of other indicators of these events.
3. Pulse rate, and fall in pulse amplitude, is one of the most reliable indicators of state of dehydration or shock, but it is still likely to be misleading in a horse which is excited because it is in strange surroundings, or separated from its dam, foal or close companion. It is also greatly influenced by pain so that a horse with a sharp pain of spasmodic colic, but without shock, may have a heart rate of 80, but not be in any serious danger. In a series of monitoring examinations it is the steady climb in heart rate of about 20 beats per minute at each hour which signals worsening of the situation. Skill at assessing pulse amplitude by touch is valuable in these circumstances. A small amplitude 'thready' pulse characterizes severe shock. Instrumental measurement of arterial blood pressure is more valuable still, but likely to be available only in a hospital.
4. Mucous membrane color and capillary refill time. Deep congestion (dark red) or cyanosis (purple) and capillary refill times much longer than 2 seconds are indicators of peripheral circulatory failure.
5. Auscultation of the abdomen. The disappearance of intestinal sounds indicates atony due to impaction or paralytic ileus, both serious lesions. Hypermotility is a less serious matter, usually susceptible to medical treatment.
6. Rectal examination. The development of gas and fluid-filled loops of small intestine, or large intestine, during a bout of colic, is one of the most ominous findings. It is so often the case that a decision on surgery is taken because of the appearance of this finding.
7. Amount and nature of feces is important. The empty rectum with the dry tacky feel, or with a smear of mucus and degenerated blood, some hours after the last defecation, presages a completely blocked intestine. The passage of oil but no feces suggest a partial blockage of large bowel which will permit the passage of oil, but not fecal balls. The use of plastic marker beads at the time of the first stomach tubing (as discussed under the heading of impaction of the large intestine) will help to establish whether or not the bowel is patent.
8. Passage of a stomach tube. Acute gastric dilatation or small intestinal regurgitation of fluid sufficient to cause reflux of fluid via the stomach tube is a grim development. This method of examination must be included in a monitoring examination if there is an indication of intestinal obstruction without a detectable finding on rectal examination.
9. Palpation of the abdomen from the exterior by firm upward thrusts of the heel of the hand, will elicit a pain response in early peritonitis caused by leakage from the bowel.
10. Abdominal paracentesis. Repeated examinations are without serious risk and can herald the development of infarction and necrosis of gut wall, leakage and the development of peritonitis, or rupture and death due to endotoxic shock.
11. Abdominal distension is a rare sign in equine colic. It may result from gaseous distension of the entire large bowel because of excessive fermentation and gas production. Entrapment of gas in the large bowel may also result from complete obstruction of the lumen. If this happens at the small colon the abdomen is distended symmetrically. If only the cecum is distended the abdomen will show an asymmetrical enlargement in the right sublumbar fossa.
12. Packed cell volume and plasma protein. Both estimations are desirable at least once, but provided total protein level has a normal ratio with PCV, repeat examinations may be restricted to PCV measurement. A rise in PCV of 5% (i.e., 55–60%) in an hour is a serious decline. Clinicopathological tests referable to damage to the cells of the intestinal wall are discussed under the clinical pathology of colic (p. 181).

13. Skin tenting on its own can be a very misleading indicator of the state of a horse's dehydration, but significant changes from one examination to another are likely to confirm deductions made on the basis of heart rate, mucosal color and so on.
14. Arterial blood pressure is one of the most reliable prognostic indicators in cases of colic. The use of promazine-type tranquilizers, which are of almost no value in colic, is contraindicated because of the misleading hypotension that they cause.
15. Response to analgesics. The best analgesics in horses are very valuable aids to treatment in colic, but they are almost entirely ineffective in relieving pain when intestinal distension goes beyond even a moderate degree. Decreasing relief of pain after administration of pethidine, pentazocine, or in desperation, chloral hydrate intravenously, can be interpreted as a serious decline in the status of the affected intestine.
16. During bouts of colic it is customary to have someone walk the horse. Having spent many hours doing this, it is possible to say that the gradual disappearance of pain, a willingness to walk, taking interest in surroundings and less inclination to roll or paw are welcome indications of relief and often foreshadow the physiological changes listed above. Alternatively, the sudden cessation of pain accompanied by a rapid deterioration in physiological parameters, the onset of polypnea leading to gasping, gross muscle tremor, profuse sweating and almost complete unwillingness to walk, all together these foreshadow rupture of the bowel and death from endotoxic shock within an hour. Many horses remain standing until the end, collapsing suddenly, making a few convulsive movements and dying quietly.

Necropsy findings

These vary widely depending on the nature and location of the lesion. There are two states which are common to many colics. Paralytic ileus is discussed under acute intestinal obstruction. A diffuse mucosal degeneration is also recorded in many colics, chiefly obstructive ones. The damage is general throughout the intestine and may be the cause of a poor response to treatment even after the primary lesion is removed surgically (38).

Diagnosis

The differential diagnosis of the different forms of colic is set out above and in summary form in Table 17. The specific details of each etiological entity are set out under the relevant headings.

Other diseases which have clinical signs reminiscent of colic are laminitis, hepatitis, lactation tetany, tetanus, urethral obstruction and peritonitis. In laminitis there is immobility rather than restlessness, the feet are held together and there is no evidence of abdominal pain, although the horse may be in great distress; the pain is obviously in the feet. In hepatitis, the horse may look at the flank and show abdominal pain but the pain is dull and continuous and the horse does not adopt an abnormal posture or roll or stamp its feet. There may be compulsive walking and evidence of delirium, and jaundice is common. Lactation tetany is not common but signs of tetany, incoordination and agitation in mares recently foaled or who have weaned their foals, or in horses of any type after great excitement or fatigue, should arouse suspicions of hypocalcemia. In tetanus, the extreme tetany, prolapse of the third eyelid and hypersensitivity are characteristic enough but if animals are down when they are first seen, the tetanic convulsions and gross sweating may suggest severe abdominal pain and lead to an incorrect diagnosis of colic. It is useful to remember that a horse with colic can always rise; a horse with tetanus that can rise has unmistakable clinical signs. Casual observation of a gelding with obstructive urolithiasis may lead to an incorrect diagnosis of colic. A simple clinical examination will reveal the frequent attempts to urinate and the passage of a few drops of bloody urine. In most cases the distended bladder is easily palpated on rectal examination. Horses affected with subacute or acute peritonitis may be flank-watchers, but pain is evident on percussion or deep palpation. Fever is characteristic and also immobility, instead of the restlessness of colic.

Abdominal pain is recorded in a 2-year-old filly due to distension of the uterus resulting from an imperforate hymen (33). The distension was palpable on rectal examination.

Pain in a testicle, e.g., in torsion of the spermatic cord (32) can cause abdominal pain, but the testicle is obviously swollen and painful and because the spermatic cord is stretched it can be palpated very easily as it enters the internal inguinal ring.

The severe distress of esophageal obstruction may suggest colic, especially gastric dilatation with overflow except that in that disease the fluid should be either acid or bile-stained. In choke, the fluid is alkaline and there are obvious attempts to vomit or swallow. Passage of a stomach tube will resolve the dilemma. Snakebite by tiger snake can be quite confusing because of the evident restlessness, but there is no pain generally although there is evident discomfort in the feet. The animal insists on getting up but the feet are so painful or paresthetic that the horse wanders about compulsively for a very short period and then slumps to the ground, assumes lateral recumbency, and is immediately relaxed and comfortable. The pupils are likely to be dilated and the serum creatinine phosphokinase level high. Recovery is prompt after treatment with antivenene.

In the early stages of enteritis caused by salmonellosis or colitis-X there are often obvious bouts of pain but these are transient and soon replaced by immobility and the weakness of severe dehydration. Diarrhea, fluid gut sounds, the presence of large amounts of fluid in the abdomen, and severe dehydration and hyponatremia are present in salmonellosis and acute obstruction of the small intestine. Sand colic presents a diagnostic problem unless the history or environment suggest it, because it is a combination of enteritis and impaction.

When there are mild signs of colic, especially flank-watching, but there are gut sounds, and feces are passed, other organs or systems must be examined. Acute enlargement of the spleen, liver or kidney could be the cause. If the pain is more than mild it is likely to be a partial obstruction due to compression from outside, such as that caused by hemorrhage into or edema of the gut wall. Purpura hemorrhagica and anthrax can cause severe colic in this way. Occasionally an intussusception can be intermittently obstructive and allow some feces to move past.

Treatment

The treatment of each case of colic depends upon the nature and situation of the lesion but the following principles apply. Analgesia is necessary to prevent self-inflicted injury without masking the signs necessary to determine the state of the disease, and also because the pain contributes to the degree of shock produced. For example, the experimental creation of volvulus in anesthetized horses results in less severe shock than in unanesthetized animals (28). It is assumed that elimination of the sympathoadrenal response to pain is the reason for this dampening effect. Pethidine (meperidine) or chloral hydrate, the latter given intravenously to effect, are satisfactory drugs for the purpose. Pethidine is subject to narcotics regulations and alternative analgesics would be advantageous. Pethidine has an estimated half-life of 66 minutes in normal horses (14). Pentazocine, a synthetic analgesic, is not a narcotic and has provided excellent pain relief in horses at a single dose rate of 0·3–0·6 mg/kg by any parenteral route (15). The drug is expensive so that the dose rates of 2 mg/kg body weight, which we have used, are not likely to become general. Pethidine at the recommended dose of 2 mg/kg body weight gives approximately the same effect. Dipyrone (Isaverin) has no significant analgesic function but does relieve gut spasm in some colics and is widely used, often without justification. Its most common use is in combination with the spasmolytic agent hyoscine butylbromide, which enjoys very wide popularity as Rx

Table 17. Differential diagnosis of equine colic

	Epidemiology and history	*Clinical findings*	*Clinical pathology*	*Response to treatment*
Acute gastric dilatation	Feeding on grain or whey. Eating immediately after race. Lipoma at pylorus	Acute severe pain, gut sounds negative, rectal negative. Stomach tube gives gush smelly, watery fluid and relief of pain. Regurgitation	Acid pH fluid from stomach. With intestinal reflux in intestinal accident pH is 7. Dehydration, alkalosis	Good to decompression. Permanent recovery depends on correcting lesion, e.g. removal of grain
Acute obstruction of small intestine	No history—just happens. Worm control usually poor	Acute, severe pain, no gut sounds, rectal reveals distended loops small intestine, tight bands mesentery at 12 hours. No feces after 12 hours. Pain intractable. Stomach fills and fluid gushes from stomach tube after 24 hours	Stomach tube fluid alkaline. Dehydration acidosis, hyponatremia, PCV 50% + after 12 hours. Paracentesis important to detect if blood supply damaged	Pain intractable. No response without surgery
Acute obstruction of large intestine	As above	As above except abdomen visibly distended. Rectal impeded by large loops distended bowel	As above	As above
Ileocecal valve impaction	Feed includes finely chopped oat straw, or sorghum, sudan grass	Subacute pain for 24 hours as small intestine distends. Then acute pain and as for small intestinal obstruction. Stomach fills with fluid. Solid impaction at ileocecal valve area palpable rectally	PCV normal first 24 hours—misleads. Must monitor it every 4 hours	Oil worth trying in first 24 hours. Usually surgical. Poor recovery rate
Spasmodic colic	Often spontaneous when worm control poor. Mostly excitement, unusual physical activity	Acute moderate pain but HR up to 80. Noisy gut sounds mostly loud and gassy. Rectal normal, feces normal, recovers spontaneously, quickly—last only 1–2 hours	Not usually carried out. Assume it would be normal	Excellent to atropine, proquamezine fumarate (Myspamol), dipyrone (Isaverin)
Impaction of large bowel	Old horse, debilitated, poor teeth, indigestible feed. Excessive consumption of low energy grass	Moderate pain, depressed or absent gut sounds, rectally long columns of dry hard fecal material, distinct from individual balls. Should not be able to feel shape of cecum or colons	Normal	Responds well to analgesic, and oil or dioctyl by stomach tube but takes 18 hours

Table 17. (cont.)

	Epidemiology and history	*Clinical findings*	*Clinical pathology*	*Response to treatment*
Verminous mesenteric arteritis				Thiabendazole 500 mg/kg body weight for all types
1. Neurogenic	Poor worm control. But 90% of horses have lesions and have to be very fortunate to escape infestation even when worm control appears to be adequate	Recurrent attacks often, are spasmodic colic as above, i.e. transient attacks of hypermotility	Nil	As for spasmodic colic—responds well. Recurs
2. Infarction of gut segments		Subacute pain continues for 3–4 days. No gut sounds. Rectally slightly distended loops; paralytic ileus	Slight leukocytosis and shift to left. Paracentesis, bloody fluid	Irreversible even if surgery performed
3. Infected verminous aneurysm		As for above but accompanied by fever and toxemia	As for above	Infection controllable by penicillin/streptomycin but colic may persist
4. Mesenteric hemorrhage		As for infarction of gut wall but massive hemorrhage subperitoneally	As for infarction of gut segments	Parenteral coagulant
Enteroliths	Endemic in some areas of United States (23)	Subacute or recurrent colic of moderate severity only. Masses about 8 cm diameter palpable in small colon	No changes	Surgery only
Subacute/chronic obstruction of small intestine*	History of recurrent moderate or persistent mild colic	No change in cardinal signs. Clinically limited to pawing, lying down frequently, flank watching. Rectally distinctive findings of thickened small intestinal wall and distended loops. Craniad point of obstruction may be palpable. Gut sounds normal to hypernormal	Normal	Excellent to surgery. Delay anesthesia for 24 hours after transport
Sand colic	Access to polluted feed. Grazing on sandy country when feed sparse. Salt deficiency or boredom leading to soil-eating or licking	May be severe pain with acute impaction as in the ileocecal valve impaction. Or chronic mild abdominal pain often with diarrhea for periods up to months when intake is low level and continuous. May palpate impacted loops containing sand	Normal. Mixture of feces and water allowed to stand shows heavy sand sediment	Analgesia and frequent oral oil gives good response
Flatulent colic	Mostly secondary to physical obstruction of large intestine	Severe acute pain. Visibly distended abdomen. Loud gut sounds usually present early. Rectal difficult because of size of loops	Not recorded	Usually an emergency. Trocarization through right flank or exploratory laparotomy

N.B.: The clinical picture varies with time: descriptions relate to clinical signs at 12–24 hours of illness.
*Chronic intussusception, terminal ileal hypertrophy, constrictive adhesions, Meckel's diverticulum, fibroma at the root of the mesentery (31).

Buscopan (16). Xviazine (Rx Rompun) at a dose rate of 1·0 mg/kg body weight is recommended, but appears to be inferior to pethidine in clinical trials. Alternative dose rates recommended to procure analgesia for 30–60 min are 0·2–0·4 mg/kg body weight intravenously or 0·4–0·8 mg/kg body weight subcutaneously (27). In spite of experimental evidence which rates the analgesic effects of the above drugs as being very low (26), clinical evidence for the efficacy of pethidine and pentazocine is moderately good. They have been generally superseded by flunixin meglumine (1·1 mg/kg body weight) which has a much longer period of analgesia, up to 8 hours. It has the added benefits of countering the effects of endotoxin and not reducing gastrointestinal motility. Another analgesic with good potential for the treatment of colic is the narcotic agonist-antagonist butorphanol tartrate. All drugs have an inability to control very severe pain when there is a rapidly increasing distension of the small intestine. The only recourse in such cases is laparotomy or euthanasia. Ataractic drugs are not generally sufficiently analgesic and are to be avoided. Phenylbutazone has relatively little analgesic effect on viscera and its use in colic cases is discouraged.

In impaction with fecal material there is a choice between lubricants, e.g. mineral oil, anthraquinone purgatives and dioctyl sodium sulfosuccinate. The anthraquinones are much smaller in bulk and easier to carry but they are variable in efficiency and inclined to overpurgate. Cholinergic drugs such as arecoline, physostigmine and a number of proprietary preparations have their place in the treatment of fecal impaction, but only as a follow-up or ancillary to a lubricant. A standard treatment is neostigmine 10–12 mg intramuscularly. The use of such drugs in horses whose colons are impacted by huge masses of very dry feces causes unnecessary pain. Antispasmodics, such as atropine, dipyrone or myspamol, have limited use because of the atony they produce in a normal gut. This often confuses the diagnosis and prognosis and may cause the development of colic (7). They should be avoided unless there is evidence of functional hypermotility when they are the drug of choice, and are rapidly and dramatically effective. Because of this efficiency they tend to be overused. Flunixin and dipyrone do not have this effect (17).

In many cases of colic, especially when there is fluid loss into the gut lumen, there is rapid and severe hemoconcentration and metabolic acidosis (1). In these cases the fluid and electrolyte status of the animals should be watched carefully, and the appropriate remedial measures, the parenteral administration of fluids and electrolytes, commenced early. The dose rates and composition of the solutions used are discussed elsewhere. Of particular importance in the horse is the need to avoid solutions containing lactate when the blood lactate is already perilously high, and the need to provide bicarbonate because most cases have such severe acidosis. When severe acidosis is suspected from the history and the clinical findings a handy guideline is to administer 50 g of sodium bicarbonate in 1 liter of water intravenously. This represents a 5% solution and 2–4 liters may be given in severe acidosis over a period of 1 hour. Very large doses of corticosteroids are currently fashionable in endotoxic shock and shock generally (5, 13, 27). A dose rate of 250 mg of dexamethasone intravenously is one which we have used but 1–2 g is recommended. The indication is where there is a large section of gut which has become necrotic because its blood supply has been occluded, and although the intestine has not ruptured there is obvious seepage of intestinal fluid into the peritoneal cavity. There is severe endotoxic shock and a fatal outcome seems likely. Administration of the corticosteroid before the shock develops would be a great deal more advantageous. In these and in all circumstances where peritoneal infection appears to have been possible, a broad-spectrum antibiotic directed against Gram-negative bacteria, for example neomycin, should be administered parenterally and orally (1).

Increasingly, surgery is being undertaken for the relief of physical colic with best results being obtained in the longer-standing lesions (18). The very acute, major lesions such as torsion of the cecum or colon present two problems: that of counteracting the severe shock and the difficulty of rearranging these voluminous viscera in their natural positions. These challenges are being taken up by our intrepid surgical colleagues who have made tremendous strides in the treatment of colic during the past decade. A number of surveys have been made of the recovery rate after surgical treatment and the recovery rate has been much lower than might have been anticipated (19); the percentage of cases returning to normal function may be as low as 35% (18) or as high as 88% (37). But if the results are looked at carefully it can be seen that many of the fatalities were unavoidable; neoplasms, rupture of the stomach or intestine with the peritoneal cavity full of feces and infarction of large segments of gut are all guaranteed to have fatal outcomes. As owners and veterinarians continue to appreciate the need for early action the recovery rate continues to improve. Those features of case management which have significantly improved the recovery rate include the following:

1. Early surgical treatment if this unavoidable and the case is acute.
2. If the case is chronic and surgery can wait, delay it for 24 hours after a long truck ride because precipitate anesthesia can lead to fatal cardiac arrest during induction.
3. Provide large volumes of fluids of appropriate composition intravenously to repair deficiencies in fluid, electrolyte and acid–base balance. If possible these are given before surgery commences, with a slower maintenance dosing being continued during surgery. In some horses it is not possible to continue the hydration procedure before surgery because of the horse's violent actions.
4. Constantly monitor biochemical and biophysical parameters before, during and after surgery to aid diagnosis, and to avoid durther deterioration in the horse's metabolic state and to indicate what supportive treatment is necessary.
5. Surgical intervention is used only when there is a positive indication for it. The positive indicators are acute gastric dilatation, indicated by regurgitation or a gush of fluid via stomach tube, acute or chronic obstruction of the small intestine indicated by distended loops of small intestine oral to the obstruction, or in rare cases the actual obstructed loop on rectal examination; acute obstruction of the large intestine defined in the same way but with the obstructed loop palpable, and intractable impactions of the large bowel which do not respond to medical treatment after 4 days.
6. For the best possible recovery rate do not operate on cases of intestinal infarction, ruptured rectum or other section of intestine or neoplasia. Recovery is not possible. However, in many cases the owner may insist on an attempt being made. The statistics should be kept separately under the heading of exploratory laparotomy. Recovery rates of 80–85%

are possible where the cases selected are those which are good surgical risks because they come early and the lesions can be diagnosed and repaired. In all cases, including those which are very exploratory and those known beforehand to be hopeless, a recovery rate of 40% is usual (29).

7. In the case of foals and young horses exception must be made to the above guidelines because a complete diagnosis is not possible in the absence of a rectal examination in a small animal.

Much of the hypermotility which leads to acute intestinal accidents is directly attributable to infestation with strongylid worms. It is generally conceded that the prevalence of surgical colics would be greatly reduced by control of these worms (20), and the incorporation of large doses of thiabendazole in the supportive treatment of clinically affected horses seems logical.

Prevention

Most cases of colic in the horse are caused either by impaction of indigestible feeds or by abnormalities of motility, including hypermotility or atony, as set out in Table 16. Prevention of the disease is largely possible in terms of good management, especially good care of the teeth, and feeding proper feeds that the horse's intestine can digest, and control of intestinal helminths, especially strongyles. The matter of teeth in colic is largely one of ensuring that the horse can chew properly. Annual examination of the molars with removal of their rough edges is desirable. Dietary care includes the avoidance of very mature coarse hay or straw, especially if it is finely chopped. Overeating on grain can cause either laminitis or gastric dilatation. But there is little that can be done to curb the gluttony of a gross feeder amongst horses fed as a group, except to take him out and feed him separately. The control of strongylosis is dealt with separately but attention is drawn to it here because of its significant involvement in causing colic (35).

REVIEW LITERATURE

Davis, L. E. & Knight, A. P. (1977) Review of the clinical pharmacology of the equine digestive system. *J. equ. Med. Surg.*, *1*, 27.
Parry, B. W. et al. (1983) Prognosis in equine colic. *Equ. vet. J.*, *15*, 337, 345.
Sellers, A. F. & Lowe, J. E. (1986) Review of large intestinal motility and mechanisms of impaction in the horse. *Equ. vet. J.*, *18*, 261–263.
Stashak, T. S. (1979) Clinical evaluation of the equine colic patient. *Vet. Clin. N. Am.*, *Gastroenterology*, *1*(2), 275.

REFERENCES

(1) Donawick, W. J. et al. (1975) *J. S. Afr. vet. med. Assoc.*, *46*, 101, 107, 111.
(2) Coffman, J. R. & Garner, H. E. (1972) *J. Am. vet. med. Assoc.*, *161*, 1195.
(3) Koal, F. et al. (1966) *Proc. 12th ann. Conv. Am. Assoc. equ. Practnrs*, 263.
(4) Murray, M. J. & Crowell-Davis, S. L. (1985) *J. Am. vet. med. Assoc.*, *186*, 381.
(5) Donawick, W. J. & Alexander, J. T. (1970) *Proc. 16th ann. Conv. Am. Assoc. equ. Practnrs*, 343.
(6) Crowhurst, R. C. et al. (1975) *J. S. Afr. vet. med. Assoc.*, *46*, 59.
(7) Ducharme, N. G. & Fabini, S. L. (1983) *J. Am. vet. med. Assoc.*, *182*, 229.
(8) Moore, J. N. et al. (1977) *Res. vet. Sci.*, *23*, 117.
(9) Donawick, W. J. et al. (1975) *J. S. Afr. vet. med. Assoc.*, *46*, 127.
(10) Swanick, R. A. & Wilkinson, J. S. (1976) *Aust. vet. J.*, *52*, 109.
(11) Nelson, A. W. (1979) *Vet. Clin. N. Am., large Anim. Pract., Gastroenterology*, *1*(2), 267.
(12) Bach, L. G. & Ricketts, S. W. (1974) *Equ. vet. J.*, *6*, 116.
(13) Gertsen, K. E. (1970) *Proc. 16th ann. Conv. Am. Assoc. equ. Practnrs*, 309.
(14) Alexander, F. & Collett, R. A. (1974) *Res. vet. Sci.*, *17*, 136.
(15) Drischer, L. K. et al. (1972) *Vet. Med. small Anim. Clin.*, *67*, 683.
(16) Keller, H. & Faulstich, A. (1985) *Tierärztl. Umschau*, *40*, 581.
(17) Adams, S. B. et al. (1984) *Am. J. vet. Res.*, *45*, 795.
(18) Ducharme, N. G. et al. (1983) *Vet. Surg.*, *12*, 206.
(19) Kersjes, A. W. & Bras, G. E. (1973) *Tijdschr. Diergeneeskd.*, *98*, 968.
(20) Bennett, D. G. (1972) *J. Am. vet. med. Assoc.*, *161*, 1198.
(21) Wheat, J. D. (1975) *J. S. Afr. vet. med. Assoc.*, *46*, 95.
(22) Pearson, H. et al. (1971) *J. Am. vet. med. Assoc.*, *159*, 1344.
(23) Ferraro, G. L. et al. (1973) *J. Am. vet. med. Assoc.*, *162*, 208.
(24) Bristol, D. G. (1982) *J. Am. vet. med. Assoc.*, *181*, 63.
(25) Gay, C. C. et al. (1977) *Equ. vet. J.*, *9*, 202.
(26) Lowe, J. E. (1978) *Equ. med. Surg.*, *2*, 286.
(27) Kohn, C. W. (1980) *Vet. Clin. N. Am., Gastroenterology*, *1*(2), 289.
(28) Hjortkjaier, R. R. & Svendsen, C. K. (1979) *Nord. VetMed.*, *31*, 466.
(29) Kopf, N. et al. (1979) *Wien. Tierärztl. Monatsschr.*, 66, 233.
(30) Tennant, B. (1976) *Proc. AGM Am. Assoc. Equ. Pract.*, p. 426.
(31) Wilson, T. D. & Sykes, G. P. (1981) *Vet. Rec.*, *108*, 334.
(32) Pascoe, J. R. et al. (1981) *J. Am. vet. med. Assoc.*, *178*, 242.
(33) Wright, I. M. (1982) *Vet. Rec.*, *111*, 283.
(34) Davies, J. V. et al. (1984) *Equ. vet. J.*, *16*, 215.
(35) Gerring, E. L. & Davies, J. V. (1984) *Equ. vet. J.*, *16*, 153.
(36) Berry, C. R. et al. (1986) *Am. J. vet. Res.*, *47*, 27.
(37) Huskamp, B. (1982) *Proc. equ. colic rese. symp. Athens, Georgia*, pp. 261–272.
(38) Meschta, C. L. et al. (1986) *Am. J. vet. Res.*, *47*, 598.

Gastric dilatation

Dilatation of the stomach is accompanied by signs of abdominal pain and occasionally by projectile vomiting.

Etiology

Acute gastric dilatation can be caused by:

- Obstruction of the pylorus
- Acutely by a foreign body or lipoma
- Subacutely by pressure of fat necrosis or lymphosarcoma from outside
- Chronically by cicatricial contraction or tumor mass resulting in stenosis (12)
- Gross overeating or drinking
- Torsion of the stomach
- By reflux of fluid from the small intestine in intestinal obstruction of postsurgical paralytic ileus
- By development of atony reflexly from intestinal disease
- Atony of the stomach wall in old age or horses that wind-suck
- In horses as a consequence of gastroduodenojejunitis (10, 13). This is a sporadic, often fatal transmural enteritis of the duodenum and proximal jejunitis of horses that presents as a mild to severe colic. The cause is unknown but the basic lesion appears to be vascular.

Gross overeating

This is particularly likely to occur in the horse, where the anatomy of the stomach lends itself to occlusion of the cardia. The ingestion of large amounts of grain is a common cause in horses but sporadic cases may also occur after drinking large quantities of whey or other palatable fluids. In the former circumstance, there may be the added effect of toxemia from the putrefactive breakdown of protein in the food. Acute spontaneous dilatation of the stomach also occurs in the horse. Sometimes it is related to feeding immediately after racing, at other times it occurs without apparent reason (1). In the horse gastric filling is more intense if roughage and grain are fed mixed together. The speed of emptying of the stomach depends on the particulate size of the feed, finer material passing on more rapidly, pellets are delayed longest (7); so gastric dilatation can occur if the rate of filling greatly exceeds the speed of emptying. That the stomach is distended may be suspected in these circumstances only when the stomach tube is passed and results in the evacuation of evil-smelling gas with or without fluid. In the pig, gastric distension is usually readily relieved by vomiting.

Obstruction of the pylorus
Obstruction by foreign bodies is not common in farm animals, but obstruction by fiber balls occurs commonly in cattle in some areas, and obstruction by ingested objects occurs occasionally in calves. External compression of the pylorus by lipoma in horses or abdominal fat necrosis or lymphoma may occur in cattle.

Acute torsion of the stomach
In sows this is much more severe (2). Death occurs 6–24 hours after the pig's last meal. Torsion is thought to occur because the sow eats a large sloppy meal very quickly. The occurrence is specifically related to intense excitement and activity occurring at feeding time.

Reflux from the intestine
Acute dilatation also occurs in all species secondarily to acute obstruction of the small intestine. The obstruction may be as far down as the ileocecal valve. The oral segment of intestine dilates and fills with fluid and refluxes into the stomach filling it. In the pig vomiting follows. The outcome depends on whether sufficient gastric motility returns to evacuate the stomach. Similar filling also occurs reflexly in combination with impaction of the small colon with a foreign body or enterolith. However, in this case the small intestine is empty; only the stomach is full.

Similar findings are also encountered in some horses in the early recovery stages after abdominal surgery involving the gut. The severe pain which occurs is relieved by the passage of the stomach tube and the evacuation of about 6 liters of normal gastric fluid. The accumulation appears to be the result of reflex dilatation after temporary ileus.

Subacute dilatation or gastric impaction
In these cases the stomach is enlarged with dry, fibrous feed material but is not grossly nor acutely distended.

Chronic dilatation
This may result from pyloric obstruction due to a tumor mass or cicatricial constriction (3), atony of the stomach wall in old or debilitated animals and those fed for long periods on coarse, indigestible roughage, and where ulceration causes pyloric spasm. The latter may occur in young calves about 3 months of age. Wind-sucking or crib-biting in horses may, in its advanced stages, cause chronic gastric dilatation.

Pathogenesis
Dilatation of the stomach stimulates vomition. In acute dilatation when vomition does not occur, the secretions accumulate and gastric motility is increased with powerful peristaltic waves passing towards the pylorus. The distension and hypermotility cause severe abdominal pain. Acute gastric dilatation is also accompanied by additional general effects. Reflex depression of the cardiac and peripheral vascular systems results in shock and there may be reflex depression of respiration. Excessive secretion and loss of fluid can result in fatal dehydration and alkalosis. Local damage to the gastric mucosa may cause additional shock and increase the permeability of the mucosa to toxic products produced by the abnormal digestion and putrefaction. Rupture of the stomach may occur, especially if the wall is weakened by existing ulcers. In chronic dilatation, the stomach is atonic, the reflex spasm and motility are reduced, the pain less severe, and onward passage of fluid is not completely prevented but the prolonged gastric sojourn causes indigestion and interference with nutrition. A secondary gastritis may develop in these circumstances. The appetite is reduced because of the chronic fullness of the stomach and the absence of hunger contractions.

Engorgement on wheat in the horse results in the production of large quantities of lactic acid in all parts of the intestine. The increase in osmotic pressure of the bowel contents causes passage of much fluid into the lumen and severe dehydration may result. Absorption of lactic acid is minor and only a mild acidosis develops. These changes occur at intakes of wheat of 10 g/kg body weight and they are not necessarily accompanied by laminitis but, at intakes of 7–9 g/kg body weight, severe laminitis occurs without the production of much lactic acid (4).

Clinical findings
In the horse acute gastric dilatation caused by grain engorgement may run a course of 2–3 days and the chronic condition may persist for a period of months. Vomiting is a cardinal sign in acute dilatation. It is usually projectile in nature and manifested by the vomiting of large quantities of fluid with little effort. In the horse, much of the material is passed through the nostrils and it is usually a terminal event, sometimes accompanied by gastric rupture. If the cause of dilatation is engorgement on grain, most of the fluid is absorbed by the mass of food and vomiting does not occur. Abdominal pain is usually severe and, in horses, is manifested by sweating, rolling, kicking at the belly, sitting on the haunches, and an increase in pulse and respiratory rates. Dehydration is severe and there is looseness of the skin and sinking of the eyes. If alkalosis is severe, the clinical signs may include tetany, tremor and rapid respiration. Passage of a stomach tube usually results in the evacuation of large quantities of foul-smelling fluid, except in cases of grain engorgement where it is absorbed by large

quantities of grain. Reflux is not an infallible indicator of primary gastric dilatation. It may be secondary to intestinal disease. Also some cases of dilatation do not produce reflux of contents and repeated attempts should be made if this diagnosis is strongly suspected (11). The distension is not visible or palpable. Laminitis may be a sequel of grain engorgement in horses.

Acute gastric dilatation in horses which occurs spontaneously or immediately after racing is accompanied by more serious and acute signs. There is abdominal distension, coughing and dyspnea. Tympany is also detectable on percussion of the anterior abdomen and large amounts of foul-smelling gas, and usually fluid, are passed via the stomach tube. This immediately relieves the animal's distress. Care is needed when the tube is being passed because fatal rupture of the stomach is a relatively common terminal event and it is best to avoid any suggestion that the passage of the tube had any causative relationship to the rupture. The syndrome is accompanied by severe pain, injected mucosae and markedly increased heart rate. There may also be signs indicative of esophageal choke, with violent retching and swallowing movements, and frothy saliva runs from the nostrils and mouth.

Acute gastric dilatation or torsion in sows is similar to the disease in dogs. The abdomen becomes greatly distended quickly. Pain is severe and the animal is soon in a state of shock with dyspnea. Death occurs within a very short time, an hour or two at most. Occasionally the stomach ruptures and the sow dies precipitately of shock. Gastric impaction is manifested by continuing subacute pain, an absence of shock and nasogastric reflux.

In chronic dilatation, there is anorexia, mild, continuous or recurrent pain, scanty feces and gradual loss of body weight. Vomiting and bouts of pain may occur after feeding but they are not usually severe. Dehydration may be present but is usually only of moderate degree. In affected horses, the distended stomach may be palpable on rectal examination and the feces are passed in small quantities and are usually of a soft, pasty consistency.

Clinical pathology

The vomitus should be checked for acidity to determine that it has originated in the stomach. Reflux of intestinal fluid may cause secondary gastric dilatation but the vomitus will be alkaline.

Necropsy findings

After grain engorgement in horses, the stomach is distended with a doughy, evil-smelling mass of food. In acute gastric dilatation due to other causes, the stomach is grossly distended with fluid and the wall shows patchy hemorrhages. Rupture may have occurred and the peritoneal cavity is then full of ingesta.

Torsion of the stomach in sows is marked by an enormous stomach (50–60 cm diameter), with engorgement of vessels and hemorrhagic effusion into the stomach which contains much gas and usually a lot of food. Rotation varies in degree from 90 to 360° and is usually to the right. The spleen is markedly displaced, the liver is bloodless and the diaphragm encroaches deeply into the chest (8).

Diagnosis

The vomiting in gastric dilatation is more profuse and projectile than that of gastritis or enteritis but may be simulated by that of obstruction of the upper part of the small intestine. Attention must be given to the possibility of an accumulation of fluid in the horse's stomach being related to the presence of an obstructing foreign body in the small colon. In both enteritis and intestinal obstruction, the vomitus may contain bile and is alkaline in reaction. A specific disease of horses, grass sickness, is characterized by an accumulation of fluid in the stomach and intestines.

When there is no history of overeating, and particularly in chronic cases, it is usually impossible to decide whether the pyloric obstruction is physical or functional but treatment with drugs likely to relax the pyloric sphincter may be of value in differentiating the two. The differential diagnosis is summarized in Table 17. Radiographic examination, with or without a barium meal, may be of diagnostic value in young animals.

Treatment

Treatment is palliative only, except in cases of overeating in horses in which case an attempt should be made to empty the stomach by the passage of a tube or by the administration of purgatives. Gastric lavage is often unsuccessful in cases of grain engorgement because of the pastiness of the ingesta. As large a tube as possible should be used and 5–10 liters of normal saline pumped in and then siphoned or pumped off. In many instances, the fluid cannot be recovered, or if it is recoverable, very little grain comes with it. The alternative is to administer mineral oil, preferably with a wetting agent, and follow this with a parasympathetic stimulant. There is danger that these latter drugs may cause rupture of an overdistended stomach. Surgery of the equine stomach is not easy because of difficult access to the organ but there are records of surgical relief of acute gastric dilatation in this species (5).

Periodic removal of fluid by stomach tube in cases of obstruction relieves the discomfort and prolongs the animal's life provided the fluid and electrolyte losses are replaced by the intravenous administration of electrolyte solutions. Final resolution of the problem depends on surgical correction of the small intestinal obstruction, and almost always of the impaction of the small colon. In the latter case the gastric dilatation does not occur until about 48 hours after the impaction becomes evident. Relaxation of the pylorus by the administration of 6–8 ml of 2% lignocaine orally (6), repeated if the regurgitation of fluid continues, should be attempted in case the obstruction is functional.

Physical obstructions due to tumors or foreign bodies are uncommon in farm animals but gastrotomy is sometimes advisable in pigs and young calves when the history suggests that a foreign body may have been ingested. Gastric impaction in horses is treated with an oral administration of normal saline but may require surgical intervention to confirm the diagnosis (9). Mineral oil is not usually satisfactory on its own because it does not moisten the impacted mass and is likely to bypass it. In cases caused by mild gastroduodenojejunitis repeated decompression is satisfactory but if the signs are still present after 24 hours a temporary duodenocecostomy is recommended (10). Chronic atony does not respond satisfactorily to treatment although stimulant strychnine preparations (14 ml tincture of nux vomica twice daily to horses) are usually advocated. The provision of soft, palatable, concentrated food may reduce the frequency and severity of attacks of abdominal pain in these cases.

REFERENCES

(1) Owen, R. R. (1975) *Vet. Rec.*, *96*, 437.
(2) Blackburn, P. W. et al. (1974) *Vet. Rec.*, *94*, 578.
(3) McGill, C. A. & Bolton, J. R. (1984) *J. Am. vet. med. Assoc.*, *61*, 190.
(4) Commonwealth Scientific and Industrial Research Organization (1954) *CSIRO, Aust., 6th ann. Rep.*
(5) Clayton-Jones, D. G. et al. (1972) *Equ. vet. J.*, *4*, 98.
(6) Coffman, J. R. (1975) *J. S. Afr. vet. med. Assoc.*, *46*, 111.
(7) Meyer, H. et al. (1980) *Tierärztl. Wochenschr.*, *87*, 43.
(8) Senk, L. (1977) *Vet. Glasnik*, *31*, 513.
(9) Barclay, W. P. et al. (1982) *J. Am. vet. med. Assoc.*, *181*, 682.
(10) Huskamp, B. (1985) *Equ. vet. J.*, *17*, 314.
(11) Todhunter, R. J. et al. (1986) *Equ. vet. J.*, *18*, 288.
(12) Munroe, G. A. (1984) *Equ. vet. J.*, *16*, 221.
(13) Tyler, D. E. et al. (1982) *Proc. equ. colic res. symp., Athens, Georgia*, 197–199.

Gastritis (inflammation of the monogastric stomach, abomasitis)

Inflammation of the stomach causes disorders of motility and is manifested clinically by vomiting. It is commonly associated with enteritis in the syndrome of gastroenteritis. Much of the discussion which follows, particularly on the subject of etiology, might be better dealt with under a separate heading of dyspepsia. The pathogenesis, clinical findings and necropsy lesions are poorly defined and could very well be functional rather than based on structural changes.

Etiology

Gastritis may be acute or chronic but both forms of the disease may be caused by the same etiological agents acting with varying degrees of severity and for varying periods. The inflammation may be caused by physical, chemical, bacterial, viral or metazoan agents.

Cattle and sheep

Diseases of the rumen and abomasum are dealt with in the next chapter. For comparative purposes the causes of abomasitis are listed here. For sheep there is no information other than about parasites. They are listed with cattle for convenience sake.

- *Physical agents* such as frosted feeds affect only the rumen. In calves gross overeating, and the ingestion of foreign materials may cause abomasitis. In adults, there is a very low incidence of foreign bodies in the abomasum (2), half the cases being associated with traumatic reticulitis
- *Chemical agents*. All of the irritant and caustic poisons including arsenic, mercury, copper, phosphorus and lead cause abomasitis. Fungal toxins cause abomasal irritation especially those of *Fusarium* sp. and *Stachybotris alternans*. Acute lactic acidosis due to engorgement on carbohydrate-rich food causes rumenitis with some runoff into the abomasum and the development of some abomasitis/enteritis
- *Infectious agents*. Only the viruses of rinderpest, bovine virus diarrhea (BVD) and bovine malignant catarrh cause abomasal erosions. Bacterial causes are very rare, sporadic cases of extension from oral necrobacillosis, hemorrhagic enterotoxemia due to *Clostridium perfringens* types A, B, C, rarely as an adjunct to colibacillosis and its enteric lesion in calves. Fungi, e.g., *Mucor* sp. and *Aspergillus* sp. complicate abomasal ulcer due to other causes
- *Metazoan agents*. Nematodes—*Trichostrongylus axei*, *Ostertagia* sp., *Haemonchus* sp. larval paramphistomes migrating to the rumen

Pigs

- *Physical agents*. Foreign bodies, bedding, frosted feeds, moldy and fermented feeds are all possible causes
- *Chemical agents*. As listed under cattle, these are also possible causes of gastritis in pigs
- *Infectious agents*. Venous hyperemia and infarction of the gastric mucosa occurs in erysipelas, salmonellosis, swine dysentery and acute colibacillosis in weaned pigs. Similar lesions occur in swine fever, African swine fever and swine influenza. Fungal gastritis also occurs secondarily
- *Metazoan agents*. The red stomach worm, *Hyostrongylus rubidus*, the thick stomach worms, *Ascarops strongylina* and *Physocephalus sexalatus*, are of low pathogenicity but cannot be disregarded as causes of gastritis in pigs.

Horses

Physical and chemical agents as listed under cattle may cause gastritis rarely. There are no infectious causes of gastritis in this species.

Metazoan agents causing gastritis in horses include massive infestation with botfly larvae (*Gasterophilus* sp.); *Habronema muscae* and *H. microstoma* infestation; *H. megastoma* causes granulomatous and ulcerative lesions and may lead to perforation and peritonitis.

Pathogenesis

Gastritis is an anatomical concept and does not often occur in animals without involvement of other parts of the alimentary tract. Even in parasitic infestations where the nematodes are relatively selective in their habitat, infestation with one nematode is usually accompanied by infestation with others so that gastroenteritis is produced. It is dealt with as a specific entity here because it may occur as such, and enteritis is common without gastric involvement. The net effects of gastroenteritis can be determined by a summation of the effects of gastritis and enteritis.

The reactions of the stomach to inflammation include increased motility and increased secretion. There is a particular increase in the secretion of mucus which does protect the mucosa to some extent but also delays digestion and permits putrefactive breakdown of the ingesta. This abnormal digestion may cause further inflammation and favors spread of the inflammation to the intestines. In acute gastritis, the major effect is on motility; in chronic gastritis, on secretion. In acute gastritis there is an increase in peristalsis causing abdominal pain and more rapid emptying of the stomach either by vomiting or via the pylorus in animals unable to vomit. In chronic gastritis, the emptying of the stomach is prolonged because of the delay in digestion caused by excessive secretion of mucus. This may reach the point where chronic gastric dilatation occurs. The motility is not necessarily diminished and there may be subacute abdominal pain or a depraved appetite due to increased stomach contractions equivalent to hunger pains.

Clinical findings

Acute gastritis

When the inflammation is severe, pigs and sometimes horses and ruminants vomit. The vomitus contains much mucus, sometimes blood, and is small in amount, and vomiting is repeated with forceful retching movements. The appetite is always reduced, often absent, but thirst is usually excessive and pigs affected with gastroenteritis may stand continually lapping water or even licking cool objects. The breath usually has a rank smell and there may be abdominal pain. Diarrhea is not marked unless there is an accompanying enteritis but the feces are usually pasty and soft. Additional signs are usually evident when gastritis is part of a primary disease syndrome. Dehydration and alkalosis with tetany and rapid breathing may develop if vomiting is excessive.

Chronic gastritis

Here the syndrome is much less severe. The appetite is depressed or depraved and vomiting occurs only sporadically, usually after feeding. The vomitus contains much viscid mucus. Abdominal pain is minor and dehydration is unlikely to occur but the animal becomes emaciated due to lack of food intake and incomplete digestion.

Anorexia, tympanites, gastritis, pyloric stenosis and gastric ulcers are the clinical manifestations of abomasal foreign body in cattle (2).

Clinical pathology

Specimens taken for laboratory examination are usually for the purpose of identifying the causative agent in specific diseases. Estimations of gastric acidity are not usually undertaken but samples of vomitus should be collected if a chemical poison is suspected.

Necropsy findings

The signs of inflammation vary in severity from a diffuse catarrhal gastritis to severe hemorrhagic and ulcerative erosion of the mucosa. In the mucosal diseases, there are discrete erosive lesions. In parasitic gastritis, there is usually marked thickening and edema of the wall if the process has been in existence for some time (1). Chemical inflammation is usually most marked on the tips of the rugae and in the pyloric region. In severe cases, the stomach contents may be hemorrhagic; in chronic cases the wall is thickened and the contents contain much mucus and have a rancid odor suggestive of a prolonged sojourn and putrefaction of the food.

It is important to differentiate between gastritis and the erythematous flush of normal gastric mucosa in animals which have died suddenly. Venous infarction in the stomach wall occurs in a number of bacterial and viral septicemias of pigs and causes extensive submucosal hemorrhages which may easily be mistaken for hemorrhagic gastritis.

Diagnosis

Gastritis and gastric dilatation have many similarities but, in the latter, the vomitus is more profuse and vomiting is of a more projectile nature although this difference is not so marked in the horse in which any form of vomiting is severe. Gastritis in the horse is not usually accompanied by vomiting but gastric dilatation may be. In esophageal obstruction the vomitus is neutral in reaction and does not have the rancid odor of stomach contents. Intestinal obstruction may be accompanied by vomiting and, although the vomitus is alkaline and may contain bile or even fecal material, this may also be the case in gastritis when intestinal contents are regurgitated into the stomach. Vomiting of central origin is extremely rare in farm animals.

Determination of the cause of gastritis may be difficult but the presence of signs of the specific diseases and history of access to poisons or physical agents listed under etiology above may provide the necessary clues. Analysis of vomitus or food materials may have diagnostic value if chemical poisoning is suspected.

Treatment

Treatment of the primary disease is the first principle and requires a specific diagnosis. Ancillary treatment includes the withholding of food, the use of gastric sedatives, the administration of electrolyte solutions to replace fluids and electrolytes lost by vomiting, and stimulation of normal stomach motility in the convalescent period.

In horses and pigs, gastric lavage may be attempted to remove irritant chemicals. Gastric sedatives usually contain insoluble magnesium hydroxide or carbonate, kaolin, pectin, or charcoal. Frequent dosing at intervals of 2–3 hours is advisable. If purgatives are used to empty the alimentary tract, they should be bland preparations such as mineral oil to avoid further irritation to the mucosa.

If vomiting is severe, large quantities of electrolyte solution should be administered parenterally. Details of the available solutions are given under the heading of disturbances of body water. If the liquids can be given orally without vomiting occurring, this route of administration is satisfactory.

During convalescence, the animal should be offered only soft, palatable, highly nutritious foods. Bran mashes for cattle and horses and gruels for calves and pigs are most adequate and are relished by the animal.

REFERENCES

(1) Martin, W. B. et al. (1957) *Vet. Rec.*, 69, 736.
(2) Haarenen, S. (1977) *Nord VetMed.*, 29, 482.

Gastric ulcer

Ulceration of the gastric mucosa causes a syndrome including anorexia, abdominal discomfort, abnormal intestinal motility leading to constipation or diarrhea, and in some cases gastric hemorrhage and melena.

Etiology

Gastric ulcers in farm animals are usually traumatic or associated with a primary erosive or ulcerative disease. The disease is much the most common in cattle and is described under the heading of abomasal ulcer in Chapter 6.

Horses

As a sequel to parasitic gastritis, ulcers may develop in horses infested with *Gasterophilus* spp., and *Habronema megastoma* larvae. Rupture of the ulcers may occur and cause local or diffuse peritonitis (2). Tumors of the mucosa may cause similar ulceration and perforation in this species. Ulcers are common in adult horses which have shown no clinical signs. They are more frequent and active in horses in training than those that are out of work (e.g. 80% as against 52%) (1).

Gastric ulcers occur in foals from 1 to 6 months of age (5). The etiology is not known. Some cases have been attributed to the ingestion of rough feed. The disease may appear to be primary in foals or associated with another disease of the gastrointestinal tract such as rotavirus enteritis (5). It is a known sequel to dosing with non-steroidal anti-inflammatory agents.

Pigs

In pigs, gastric ulceration with sudden death due to hemorrhage has become a disease of major proportions. It is dealt with separately under the heading of esophagogastric ulceration of swine. Ulcers have also been observed in association with hepatic dystrophy in vitamin E deficient pigs. In many cases the fungus *Rhizopus microspora* is present in the ulcer. They are probably contaminants rather than primary etiological agents and are important only in that they delay healing (3).

Pathogenesis

The effects of gastric ulcer are largely reflex, causing spasm of the pylorus and increased gastric motility. The resulting syndrome is similar to that caused by chronic gastritis except that rupture of blood vessels may lead to acute or chronic gastric hemorrhage or to perforation and fatal chronic peritonitis. Perforation is usually followed by the development of chronic peritonitis as the lesion is sealed off by the omentum. Healing ulcers may cause pyloric or duodenal obstruction. In horses secondary involvement of the spleen is common, the spleen being directly opposed to the stomach wall.

Clinical findings

Many gastric ulcers cause no apparent illness. In clinically affected animals the syndrome varies depending on whether ulceration is complicated by perforation, rupture of the stomach or hemorrhage. In uncomplicated ulcers there are mild and intermittent signs of abdominal pain and anorexia and either constipation or diarrhea. If hemorrhage results there may be sudden death or melena or a more chronic loss of blood in the feces with a severe hemorrhagic anemia developing in time. The feces are very black and tarry, and usually pasty and of small volume because of the accompanying pylorospasm. In the early stages there may be a short episode of profuse diarrhea. Perforation is usually followed by acute local peritonitis unless the stomach is overloaded and ruptures, when acute shock leads to death in a few hours (4). With acute local peritonitis, there is a chronic illness accompanied by a fluctuating fever, severe anorexia and intermittent diarrhea.

Involvement of the spleen in the horse results in the development of fever, anorexia, toxemia, a leukocytosis with a left shift and pain on deep palpation over the left flank. Squamous cell carcinomata of the gastric wall cause serious inappetence, and rapid weight loss, ventral edema and perhaps a mass which is palpable per rectum. Secondaries may be present in the lung and result in a massive pleural effusion which effectively masks the alimentary problem.

The common clinical findings of gastric ulcers in foals include: depression, abdominal pain, bruxism (grinding of the teeth), excessive salivation, gastric reflux, and a tendency to lie in dorsal recumbency for prolonged periods (5). The abdominal pain can also be localized by palpation either in the right (pyloric) or left (fundic) paracostal region.

Clinical pathology

Plasma pepsinogen levels are elevated in foals with gastric or duodenal ulcer but the test is not sufficiently accurate to be definitive (8). The dark brown to black color of the feces is usually sufficient proof of gastric hemorrhage but tests for blood may be necessary if pigmented pharmaceuticals are being used. In foals, blood may be detected in a sample of gastric fluid obtained by nasal tube. When perforation has occurred, there is a sharp rise in total leukocytes and neutrophils in the blood but these levels return to normal if the lesion is walled off. Abdominocentesis confirms the diagnosis. When splenitis develops in horses, they rise again to very high levels and are a diagnostic feature of the disease.

Necropsy findings

The ulcers are usually deep and well-defined but may be filled with blood clot or necrotic material and often contain fungal mycelia which may be of etiological significance. Lesions of the primary disease may be evident.

In horses, when there is an area of local peritonitis, the stomach wall is adherent to the tip of the spleen and an extensive suppurative splenitis may be present. In some cases, especially when the stomach is very full at the time of perforation, a long tear develops in the wall and large quantities of ingesta spill into the peritoneal cavity. Ulcers in young animals especially foals (6) and pigs (17) are commonly infected with *Candida* spp. or *Rhizopus* spp. fungi.

Diagnosis

Gastric ulceration is not usually diagnosed antemortem unless hemorrhage occurs, because of the clinical resemblance of the disease to chronic gastritis. When hemorrhage occurs, melena or hematemesis suggests the presence of ulcer but similar fecal discoloration may occur in acute intestinal obstruction. Gastroendoscopy with the fiberoptiscope is now possible and is useful for the diagnosis of gastric ulcers in the horse.

Treatment

Alkalinizing agents such as magnesium hydroxide, carbonate or trisilicate are indicated to neutralize the acidity and allow healing to occur. These must be given frequently over relatively long periods. The treatment of abomasal ulcers in cattle is covered under that heading. If hemorrhage is severe, blood transfusions or hematinic drugs are necessary and parenteral coagulants are usually administered. Food containing harsh material which is likely to be physically irritating should be avoided. Surgical repair has been undertaken satisfactorily in foals provided it is undertaken early in the development of the disease (9).

REVIEW LITERATURE

Becht, J. L. & Byars, T. D. (1986) Gastroduodenal ulceration in foals. *Equ. vet. J.*, *18*, 307–312.

REFERENCES

(1) Hammond, C. J. et al. (1986) *Equ. vet. J.*, *18*, 284.
(2) Rainey, J. W. (1948) *Aust. vet. J.*, *24*, 116.
(3) Gitter, M. & Austwick, P. K. C. (1957) *Vet. Rec.*, *69*, 924.
(4) Hemmingsen, I. (1967) *Nord. VetMed.*, *19*, 17.
(5) Rebhun, W. C. et al. (1982) *J. Am. vet. med. Assoc.*, *180*, 404.
(6) Gross, T. L. (1983) *J. Am. vet. med. Assoc.*, *182*, 1370.
(7) Mahanta, S. & Chaudhury, B. (1985) *Sabouradia*, *23*, 395.
(8) Wilson J. H. & Pearson, M. M. (1985) *Proc. 31 Ann. Conv. AAEP*, p. 149.
(9) Campbell-Thompson, M. L. et al. (1986) *J. Am. vet. med. Assoc.*, *188*, 840.

Acute intestinal obstruction

Intestinal obstruction includes volvulus, intussusception and strangulation. The clinical signs typical of these conditions include acute abdominal pain, severe shock, absence of defecation and often the passage of blood and mucus.

Etiology

The commonest causes are the intestinal accidents, volvulus, intussusception and strangulation, in which there is a physical occlusion of the intestinal lumen. Functional obstructive lesions, such as those which occur with local or general paralytic ileus, can be considered with physical occlusions, but are dealt with separately here. In many cases, the causes of the obstruction are bizarre and not readily diagnosed. There are three common groups of causes:

- Physical obstructions to the lumen of the intestine
- Physical luminal obstructions plus infarction of the affected section—intestinal accidents
- Functional obstructions with no passage of contents but with the lumen still patent—paralytic ileus.

Cattle

Intestinal accidents These are as follows:

- *Mesenteric torsion*. Commonest in calves and young cattle, e.g., coiled colon on its mesentery. As in cecal torsion, the colon may suffer from dilatation before torsion develops
- *Intussusception*. A common sporadic occurrence in adults. A series is recorded in cows with intestinal polyposis (24): polyps in the mucosa dragged a section of intestine into an invagination in the next section. There is also intussusception of colon into spiral colon (40)
- *Strangulation*—through a mesenteric tear (1) or behind a persistent vitelloumbilical band, the ventral ligament of the bladder, through the lateral ligament of a bull's bladder (55), an adhesion (7, 21) especially one between the omentum and an abscess of the umbilical artery in a young animal (9)
- *Compression stenosis* by, e.g., a blood clot from an expressed corpus luteum site on an ovary, or traumatic duodenitis caused by migration of a metallic foreign body (28)
- *Cecal dilatation* followed by *cecal torsion* (9). These two diseases are thought to be sequential stages in the one process created by heavy grain feeding. The two conditions have much in common clinically and are virtually indistinguishable without a laparotomy (11). Cattle fed heavily on grain have been shown to develop dilatation of the intestine (15).

Luminal blockages These are as follows:

- External pressure by fat necrosis of mesenteries and omenta, lipomas
- Fiber-balls or phytobezoars. May be very common in areas where fibrous feeds (e.g., *Romulea bulbocodium*) abound (18). The ability of the plant to survive dry autumns and dominate the pasture ensures that many fiber falls develop in the abomasum in autumn. Obstructions do not occur until the next spring when pasture is lush. Disease is common in late pregnancy or first 2 weeks of lactation or after a period of activity as at estrus (19). Bezoars pass at this time from abomasum into the first meter or two of intestine and then stick fast
- In cold climates a more common obstruction is by trichobezoars. Cattle confined outside have long shaggy haircoats and licking themselves and others probably leads to ingestion of the hair.

Summary—cattle There is a long list of causes in cattle and the common cause will vary from locality to locality depending on feeding and management programs. Cows on pasture have a low prevalence only unless phytobezoars are a local peculiarity. Cows on heavy grain feeding have a high prevalence of primary intestinal ileus resulting in intestinal dilatation and tympany leading to mesenteric or cecal torsion (17). Such cases are always in adult cows, usually during lactation.

Sheep

Intestinal obstructions are not commonly observed in sheep unless a series of them causes a noticeable mortality. The sheep's intestine does respond by dilating to heavy feeding with grain (15), as in cattle, but sheep are unlikely to be so heavily fed. Some notable occurrences have been:

- Heavy infestation with nodular worm (*Oesophagastomum columbianum*) leading to high prevalence of intussusception occlusion by adhesion
- High incidence of intussusception in traveling sheep for no apparent reason (22)
- Cecal torsion (red-gut) in sheep grazing pure (but not weedy) stands of alfalfa in New Zealand (23). Affected lambs survived only a few hours and up to 20% of a flock were affected
- Abomasal phytobezoars in South Africa (37) are

composed of plant hairs and have a striking velvety appearance.

Pigs
Heavy feeding on lactose (13) causes a dilatation and atony of the intestine in the same way as grain feeding does in ruminants. Some causes are:

- Torsion of the coiled colon about its mesentery occurs in adult pigs
- Obstruction of the terminal small colon in young piglets caused very hard fecal balls or barley chaff used as bedding (25).

Horses

Intestinal accidents These are as follows:

- *Mesenteric torsion*, of small intestine as a result of immobilization of a section of intestine by an adhesion or a Meckel's diverticulum adherent to the umbilicus (2), or a mesenteric defect produced by a congential mesodiverticular band. The band creates what is in effect a hernial sac, and entrapment of a loop of small intestine in it causes distension of the gut, rupture of the jejunal mesentery and incarceration of the gut loop (41). Torsion of the cecum or large colon may occur while rolling, especially when it is violent, for example during an attack of colic with another cause
- *Strangulation* of an inguinal hernia in stallions (45), of an umbilical hernia in a young horse (42) through an epiploic foramen (44), by bands of adhesions, by pedunculated lipomas, or via a diaphragmatic hernia. Hernias through the diaphragm are suspected much more commonly than they occur because of the frequent observation of loud gut sounds in the thorax of normal horses
- *Intussusception* is common including intussusception of the terminal ileum into the cecum, of colon into colon (5), and of cecum into cecum (53). Many intussceptions originate with local enlargements such as polyps, granulomatous cryptococcal lesions or leiomyomas (43) in the wall of the intestine, and a causal relationship to infestation with the tapeworm *Anoplocephala perfoliata* has been suggested (47). Most intussusceptions are of the small intestine and are acute obstructions. Those in the large intestine are less so. There are reports of chronic intussusception of the small intestine characterized by recurrent colic reminiscent of thromboembolic colic or obstruction by enterolith (51).

Luminal blockages These are as follows:

- Impaction of the ileocecal valve by fine dry indigestible fiber
- Linear foreign bodies, string, tail hair, ingested by foals with a licking–sucking–chewing habit. The string pulls the intestine into a concertina formation by acting as a drawstring (4)
- Enteroliths more likely to cause large bowel impaction and are dealt with there
- Phytobezoars occur and a high incidence of intestinal rupture caused by them is recorded (20).

Paralytic ileus
Excessive trauma, which may be unavoidable, to the intestines during surgical operations, distension for periods of up to several days and acute diffuse peritonitis cause a functional stasis of the intestine which is similar in many respects to that produced by a physical obstruction. This syndrome of paralytic ileus also occurs in grass sickness in horses, in peracute enteritis such as *colitis-X* and equine ehrlichial colitis, in watery mouth of lambs and it is also a prominent lesion in chlorpyrifos poisoning in adult cattle.

Although paralytic ileus occurs in all species it is most notable in horses in which it is the commonest cause of postoperative fatality in cases of surgical colic (52). The clinical picture is so similar to that of horses with physical obstruction of the gut that many horses are opened up again on the anticipation that a second intestinal accident has occurred. The basic lesion in paralytic ileus appears to be a loss of gastroduodenal coordination which may be mediated by dopamine (35).

Pathogenesis
The effects of intestinal obstruction differ considerably between species, and within species depending on the site and type of obstruction. In general, obstructions high in the small intestine cause a more acute and severe syndrome than those in the large intestine but the difference may not be great (26). For example, obstructions of the small intestine or colon in horses usually kill within 24 hours while similar obstructions in cattle are not usually fatal in less than a week. This generalization is not without exceptions, due possibly to the presence or absence of toxigenic bacteria in isolated loops of intestine. The type of lesion is important depending on whether the blood supply to a large section of intestine is occluded or whether circulatory effects are minimal. Obstructions caused by external pressure, such as occurs in fat necrosis, or caused by internal foreign bodies such as phytobezoars cause less acute signs than do torsion and intussusception.

There are several factors which are of importance in the production of clinical signs and in causing the death of the animals. Acute shock is the important factor in severe cases, particularly in the horse. Distension of the bowel causes reflex cardiovascular effects, and peripheral circulatory failure and collapse occur. In less severe cases, dehydration and loss of electrolytes are the important mechanisms as described under principles of alimentary tract dysfunction. The fluid and accompanying electrolytes are secreted into the lumen of the intestine in response to distension above the obstruction. It is this distension which is responsible for the abdominal pain observed. The greater severity of the disease in horses when obstruction occurs in the large intestine is probably due to the rapidity of the distension created by gas accumulation in this part of the alimentary tract. Distension is not a major factor in cattle or pigs unless there is occlusion of the lumen of the large intestine but, as compared to the horse, the syndrome produced is much less severe.

In the subacute cases which do not die from shock, there is the additional factor of interference with local blood supply when the vessels are occluded by twisting of the mesentery or by their passage into an intussusception. Because the veins are occluded most readily, there is usually considerable escape of fluid under pressure from the arteries into the intestinal wall and the peritoneal cavity. In the most severe lesion infarction devitalizes the gut completely, and the two factors of fluid loss and toxemia add further insults. In less severe lesions where the blood supply has been occluded for a relatively short period it has been shown experimentally that superficial necrosis affecting only the mucosa of a small segment of gut may result (10). This may explain why in some cases where displaced gut is replaced in a correct position and bowel wall is observed to return to apparent normality, fatal paralytic ileus develops.

Failure of ingesta to pass the obstruction and be absorbed is of little importance. Autointoxication may be a factor when feces accumulate in obstruction of the large intestine but the importance of this factor is debatable.

The pathogenesis of intestinal obstruction has been examined experimentally in horses (26, 29). Obstruction of the duodenum is most lethal; obstruction of the small colon has a much longer survival time, the signs are not nearly as severe and the blood chemistry is nearly normal. When the obstruction is in any part of the small intestine there is continuous pain, a fast, weak pulse, congestion of the conjunctiva and mucosa, acidosis, hyperkalemia, a decrease in plasma bicarbonate, sodium, chloride and blood ammonia, and an increase in hematocrit (PCV) and total protein.

Clinical signs

Horses

Acute obstruction of the small intestine There is usually an almost immediate onset of severe abdominal pain as the intestine begins to distend at the obstruction site, although the onset may be delayed for several hours, depending perhaps on the fullness of the gut at the time. What happens subsequently depends largely on whether the blood supply to the affected part of the intestine is compromised and whether or not infarction of the intestinal wall occurs. If there is no vascular involvement, the signs of pain begin to be accompanied by palpable intestinal distension and clinical and laboratory evidence of dehydration. If there is vascular involvement the signs are the same but in addition there is severe shock and toxemia, and on paracentesis there is evidence of bloodstained fluid leaking into the peritoneal cavity. The terminal stage is one of rupture of the gut with severe endotoxic shock and peracute diffuse peritonitis.

In the early stages there is severe pain, with an increase in pulse rate to 60–80/minute and the respiratory rate may be as high as 80/minute. Sweating may begin at this stage. It may be 8–12 hours in the case of obstruction of the small intestine, before distended loops of intestine are palpable on rectal examination and it is about the same time that clinical and laboratory evidence of dehydration begin to appear. At this time intestinal sounds are still present and feces are still passed. In the period 12–24 hours after obstruction commences, the pulse rate rises to 80–100, loops of distended intestine are easily palpable, defecation ceases and the rectum is empty and sticky to the touch. From 24 hours onwards, dehydration becomes marked and the pain may not worsen. However, the heart rate increases to 100–120, intestinal loops are easily palpable and reflux filling of the stomach occurs with much fluid being evacuated via the stomach tube and the horse may vomit. Rupture usually occurs at about 48 hours.

Acute obstruction of the large intestine There is also a sudden onset of severe pain as soon as the obstruction occurs. If the obstruction is incomplete, for example torsions of 180°, the signs are moderate only and remain so for up to 36 hours. If it is complete, e.g. complete torsions, and the blood supply to the obstructed loop is also blocked, shock with a high heart rate may be apparent within a few hours and soon there is panting respiration, profuse sweating and abdominal distension. Rectally the distended loops of large colon or cecum are large enough to completely block the pelvis and make further examination impossible. A distended small colon is difficult to differentiate from small intestine. All the clinicopathological indicators of shock and dehydration are now positive, pain is intense and the peritoneal fluid on paracentesis is bloodstained. The distension of the abdomen caused by the accumulation of gas is sufficiently severe to interfere with respiratory exchange and dyspnea follows. The course is acute and death follows within a few hours of the onset of signs. The mortality rate is high, reaching 60–80% even with surgical intervention. Without surgery death is inevitable (57).

Hernias and displacement of colons Some types of intestinal accident are recognized as specific entities (3, 5, 19). Strangulated scrotal hernia in the horse is such a one. They are often missed in the early stages because the distension is not gross, and the initially distended loops are out of reach. If distended loops of intestine are not palpable in a severe case of colic in a male, the inguinal canals should be searched for loops of intestine disappearing into one of them and every stallion with colic should be examined for inguinal hernia. Diaphragmatic hernia acquired after birth may have no distinguishing characteristics and may be identified only on exploratory laparotomy. Alternatively there may be a history of a fall in the not too distant past, maybe 3 or 4 months ago, distinct gut sounds are audible in a localized area of the chest, there is persistent walking backwards, lying on the left side for long periods and difficulty in lying down: the horse may attempt to lie down but aborts the attempt when the chest reaches a position which is lower than the abdomen (8). Diaphragmatic hernia acquired at birth, due to a traumatic or prolonged birth, may not cause clinical signs until several weeks later. At that time the syndrome resembles that of any other acute intestinal accident in the foal. Most diaphragmatic hernias have been identified during exploratory laparotomy.

In dorsal displacement of the left and right (12) colons the dorsal and ventral colons are displaced in the former to become enclosed in the space bounded by the base of the spleen, the dorsal aspect of the suspensory ligament of the spleen, the left kidney and the adjacent body wall. There is moderate to severe pain, individual signs of shock, medial displacement of the spleen and a consequential ease of penetrating the spleen when attempting paracentesis.

On rectal examination there may be a palpable tension of mesenteric bands in the dorsal anterior left abdomen, and the pelvic flexure is missing from its usual site in the lower left abdomen. In some cases there is an excessive accumulation of fluid in the stomach. Medical treatment is ineffective and surgical intervention to replace the organ is required. The displacement may recur.

In displacement of the right colon the large colon passes between the right body wall and the cecum in a cranial direction so that the pelvic flexure reaches the diaphragm. There are a number of variations in this general description. Clinically it is characterized by acute pain and severe distension of the right flank. The findings on rectal examination include a characteristic horizontal position of the gas-distended colon.

Obstruction of the small colon caused by hematoma in the gut wall This is also recorded (6). Clinically there was severe colic due to apparent intestinal obstruction, but the exact cause was identified only at laparotomy. *Strangulation* of small intestine through the epiploic foramen is characteristically a disease of older horses but is not identifiable without surgical intervention. The same comment applies to herniation through and strangulation by the nephrosplenic ligament. Tears in the mesentery are not uncommon and strangulation of a loop of bowel which passes through is a natural consequence. We have encountered similar hernias and strangulations behind the ventral ligament of the bladder and through a tear in the broad ligament of the uterus. *Intussusceptions* are amongst the most difficult to diagnose because they vary in the degree to which their blood supply is obstructed, and the degree to which the lumen is obliterated. In many, the obstruction is incomplete so that pain is constant and of moderate intensity and there is a disconcerting diarrhea. They are most common in young horses. *Strangulations by lipomas* only occur in old horses, usually aged ones.

Cattle

There is an initial attack of acute abdominal pain in which the animal kicks at its belly, treads uneasily with the hind feet, depresses the back and often groans or bellows with pain. The pain occurs spasmodically and at short, regular intervals and may occasionally be accompanied by rolling. This stage of acute pain usually passes off within a few (8–12) hours and during this time no food is taken and little or no feces are passed. The temperature and respiratory rates are relatively unaffected and the pulse rate may be normal or elevated depending on whether or not blood vessels are occluded. If there is infarction of a section of gut there will be signs of endotoxic shock including low blood pressure, very rapid heart rate, and muscle weakness and recumbency. These signs are absent in cases where the gut is not compromised. For example in cecal torsion the pulse rate may be normal (14). In all cases as the disease progresses and dehydration becomes serious the heart rate rises and may reach as high as 100 just before death.

The character of the feces is very variable. In the early stages they will be normal but passed frequently and in small amounts. It may be necessary to carry out a rectal examination because the feces may not be passed from the anus. In some cases they will be hard, turd-like lumps, usually covered with mucus. Blood is often present, not as melena, but as altered red blood, in the form of a thick red slurry leaving dried flakes of it around the anus, especially in intussusception. The last fecal material is more mucoid and may consist entirely of a plug of mucus. In some cases of obstruction caused by fiber balls the fecal material is pasty, evil-smelling and yellow-gray in color (30).

When the acute pain has subsided, the cow remains depressed, does not eat and passes no feces. The circulation, temperature and respiration circulation, are usually within normal limits and ruminal activity varies. In most cases there is complete stasis, but in exceptional cases, movements will continue though they are usually greatly reduced. Rumination ceases and there is usually complete anorexia. Rectal examination is important at this stage. The rectum remains empty except for the mucous or tarry exudate described above and insertion of the arm usually causes pain and vigorous straining and peristalsis. Distension of loops of intestine is not nearly as obvious as in horses and may not occur unless the colon or cecum is involved.

The abdomen is slightly distended in all cases. Where there is distension of bowel loops, as in ileus due to dietary error, this causes an obvious physical enlargement, especially of the right side of the abdomen. Splashing sounds can be elicited by ballottement in the left and right flanks over the rumen and abomasum when the obstruction is in the upper part of the small intestine. In obstruction of the pylorus the sounds can be produced only on the right side, just behind the costal arch and approximately half way down its length. Regurgitation of fluid ingesta through the nose is common (17). When there is intussusception or torsion of the small intestine, the affected loop is usually felt in the lower right abdomen but the site varies with the nature of the obstruction. A careful examination must be carried out. In intussusception the affected loop may be palpable, usually as an oblong, sausage-shaped mass of firm consistency, but if a long length of bowel is involved a spiral develops and is palpable as such. In torsion the loop may be small, soft and mobile. In many cases, it is possible to follow a tightly stretched mesenteric fold from the root of the mesentery to the loop. Palpation of the loop may cause distress especially in the early stages, and distension of a number of loops may increase intra-abdominal pressure to the point where entry of the hand beyond the pelvis is difficult.

Torsion of the coiled colon (mesenteric root torsion) can cause death in less than 24 hours. It is characterized by distension of the right abdomen and a number of distended loops can be palpated and these may be visible in the right flank (31). When there is torsion or dilatation of the cecum, there is usually one grossly distended loop running horizontally across the abdomen just anterior to the pelvis and posteriorly or medially to the rumen. It may be possible to palpate the blind end of the cecum, and in cases which have been affected for several days the organ may be so distended with fluid and gas that it can be seen through the right flank or fluid sounds produced by ballottement (14, 38) or simultaneous percussion and auscultation. One case is recorded in which the distended cecum was located in the left paralumbar fossa between the rumen and the abdominal wall, in a position reminiscent of a left displacement of the abomasum (39). The disease is likely to recur in the same cow in subsequent years, and a case of chronic dilatation which persisted for 10 months is recorded (32). Lipomas and fat necrosis are usually easily palpable as firm, lobulated masses which can be moved manually. They may encircle the rectum. An obstructing phytobezoar may be palpable on rectal examination in the right anterior abdomen. It is usually 5–15 cm in diameter and so mobile that when touched it may immediately pass out of reach. Affected cattle may remain in this state for 6–8 days but during this time there is a gradual development of a moderate, pendulous, abdominal enlargement, profound toxemia and an increase in heart rate. The animal becomes recumbent and dies at the end of 3–8 days.

Sheep

In sheep there is a special syndrome called 'red gut' (48, 49) which causes sudden death in sheep grazing on lush pasture, especially alfalfa or clover. The outstanding gross postmortem lesion is a distended, reddened cecum and/or colon which has undergone torsion. The rumen is smaller and the large intestine larger than normal because of the high digestibility of the diet. All ages, except sucking lambs, are affected and the mortality rate may be as high as 20%. Sheep that are seen alive have a distended abdomen, show abdominal pain and have tinkling sounds on auscultation of the right flank.

Pigs

In pigs, distension of the abdomen, absence of feces and complete anorexia are evident. The distension may be extreme in young pigs when the terminal colon is obstructed. Death usually occurs in 3–6 days.

Clinical pathology

While laboratory examinations of animals with intestinal obstruction may not be used in the diagnosis of the obstruction they are useful in assessing its severity. The details of the disturbances in body water, electrolytes and acid–base imbalance are given under that heading. In general, the laboratory findings in acute intestinal obstruction include the following:

- Hemoconcentration (the PCV seldom exceeds 50%)
- Acidosis
- Increase in blood urea nitrogen (BUN) depending on severity of the decrease in circulating blood volume
- Decreases in plasma bicarbonate, serum sodium and chloride. In cattle there may be a marked decrease in the concentration of serum chloride. The concentration of serum potassium usually declines initially but may increase if the acidosis becomes severe
- Leukopenia and neutropenia. This is due to devitalization of infarcted intestine, followed by necrosis and the development of peritonitis. This is a useful prognostic aid
- An increase in the total number of leukocytes and erythrocytes and the protein concentration (56), in the peritoneal fluid obtained by paracentesis. In acute intestinal obstruction with infarction, the peritoneal fluid will be bloodstained. As necrosis and gangrene develop there is an increase in the total number of leukocytes with an increase in the number of immature neutrophils. The total number will vary depending on the degree of dilution by the peritoneal fluid.

Necropsy findings

The physical lesions are readily observed and are accompanied by varying degrees of gaseous and fluid distension of the oral segments of the intestine compared to aboral segments, and varying degrees of congestion, edema, necrosis and gangrene of obstructed loops. In paralytic ileus, the same flaccidity of the gut and accumulation of fluid and gas occur but there is no physical obstruction.

Diagnosis

Acute intestinal obstruction must be differentiated from other causes of acute abdominal pain. These causes may be other diseases of the alimentary tract or diseases affecting other abdominal organs. Diseases affecting the alimentary tract include gastric dilatation caused by overeating or pyloric obstruction, particularly abomasal obstruction in calves. Vomiting or the passage of large quantities of gas or fluid through a nasal tube, followed by relief of pain, are more common in this condition but, in obstruction of the upper part of the intestine, fluid may also fill the stomach. Complete absence of feces and the passage of blood and mucus are more typical of intestinal obstruction and the obstructed segment of bowel can usually be felt on rectal examination in the cow and the horse. Abomasal torsion in cattle is a special case of gastric dilatation and may be accompanied by acute pain in the early stages.

In occasional cases of traumatic reticuloperitonitis in cattle there are early signs of acute abdominal pain but moderate fever, rumen stasis and abdominal tenderness are apparent and, although there may be constipation, some normal feces are passed. Acute enteritis and intestinal hypermotility are accompanied by severe pain but increased peristaltic sounds can be heard and, in the former condition, there is diarrhea. Intestinal hypermotility is transient and responds rapidly to treatment. Impaction of the ileocecal valve is a disease restricted to horses, and may be distinguishable on palpation per rectum. It is rapidly fatal but affected horses usually survive for 48 hours compared to the course of 12–24 hours in acute obstruction.

Two of the most difficult diseases to differentiate from intestinal obstruction in horses are mesenteric vessel thrombosis and intestinal tympany because distension of the intestines with gas is typical of all three. Intestinal tympany is not usually accompanied by such severe pain and the shock of obstruction is not present. No obstructed intestinal loop can be palpated and, in most cases, flatus is passed per rectum. The syndrome in mesenteric vessel thrombosis is less acute and there may be passage of feces containing blood rather than an absence of feces. Careful rectal palpation may reveal the thickened, obstructed mesenteric vessels (see Table 16 for a summary of causes of colic in horses).

Renal and ureteric colic may simulate intestinal obstruction. Passage of a calculus down the ureter is not known to occur but transient bouts of pain in cattle are often ascribed to this cause. Acute involvement of individual renal papillae in pyelonephritis in cattle is also thought to cause some of these attacks of colic. In steers and wethers, urethral obstruction causes abdominal pain but there are additional signs of grunting, straining, distension of the urinary bladder and tenderness of the urethra. Defecation is not impeded. Photosensitive dermatitis in cattle is also accompanied by kicking at the belly but the skin lesions are obvious and there are no other alimentary tract signs.

Treatment

Surgical removal of the obstruction is usually necessary. Resection of an intussusception may be followed by a period of intense and often painful peristalsis (33). Supportive treatment includes sedation in the early stages and the administration of antibiotics to control bacterial growth in the isolated section of gut, and of electrolyte solutions when dehydration has occurred. The administration of potassium by mouth is recommended to control the hypokalemia which occurs, and which may be responsible for the severe muscular weakness which characterizes this disease (34). Restoration of normal motility after surgery is often difficult, and cases which have been in existence for 4 or 5 days may show persistent paralytic ileus even though the displacement is corrected surgically. Based on experimental results the administration of metoclopramide should be effective, a combination of yohimbine and bethanechol less so, and propanolol not at all (35). Nasoduodenal intubation as practiced in human paralytic ileus is still in the experimental stage for horses (50) but some relief can be given to horses by draining the stomach when it has become filled with fluid regurgitated from the intestine. The long-term effect in horses of resection of a large proportion, over 50%, of the small intestine is a failure to maintain body weight (46). Resection of up to 75% of the colon is compatible with life and the maintenance of good body condition (54).

Conservative treatment has no logical place in acute intestinal obstruction. However, it is possible that ‘torsion’ of the cecum in cattle can be incomplete, and treatment by withholding food and administering saline purgatives can effect a cure (36). This adds weight to the suggestion that this disease is primarily an atony in which ingesta accumulates in the cecum to the point where it folds on itself. Spontaneous correction of a displacement may occur especially if the animal is exercised vigorously or driven in a truck over a rough road. Immediate passage of large quantities of feces heralds recovery. Spontaneous recovery has been recorded in intussusception when the gangrenous loop sloughs but subsequently fibrous constriction at the site may lead to a partial obstruction (33).

REVIEW LITERATURE

Edwards, G. B. (1981) Obstruction of the ileum in the horse. *Equ. vet. J.*, *13*, 158–166.

Moore, J. N., White, N. A. & Becht, J. L. (1986) *Equine Acute Abdomen Proc. Veterinary Seminar Univ. Georgia*, Vol. 1, Veterinary Learning Systems Co. Inc. Lawrenceville, New Jersey, 1–62.

Moore, J. N., White, N. A. & Becht, J. L. (1986) *Equine Colic Research Proc. Second Symposium Univ. Georgia*, Vol. 2, Veterinary Learning Systems Co. Inc. Lawrenceville, New Jersey, 1–349.

Pearson, H. & Pinsent, P. J. N. (1977) Intestinal obstruction in cattle. *Vet. Rec.*, *101*, 162.

Robertson, J. T. (1979) Differential diagnosis and surgical management of intestinal obstruction in cattle. *Vet. Clin. N.Am., large Anim. Pract.*, *1*(2), 377.

Smith, D. F. (1984) Bovine intestinal surgery. *Mod. vet. Pract.*, *65*, 705, 853, 909; *66*, 405, 443.

REFERENCES

(1) Velden, M. A. van der (1984) *Vet. Rec.*, *115*, 414.
(2) Grant, B. D. & Tennant, B. (1973) *J. Am. vet. med. Assoc.*, *162*, 550.
(3) Kopf, N. et al. (1980) *Wien. Tierärztl. Monatsschr.*, *66*, 233.
(4) Baker, G. J. (1974) *Vet. Rec.*, *95*, 293.
(5) Meagher, D. M. & Stirk, A. J. (1974) *Mod. vet. Pract.*, *55*, 951.
(6) Spiers, V. C. et al. (1981) *Aust. vet. J.*, *57*, 88.
(7) Richardson, D. W. (1984) *J. Am. vet. med. Assoc.*, *185*, 517.
(8) Hill, F. W. G. et al. (1987) *Vet. Rec.*, *120*, 127.
(9) Hylton, W. E. & Rousseaux, C. G. (1985) *J. Am. vet. med. Assoc.*, *186*, 1099.
(10) White, N. A. et al. (1980) *J. Am. vet. med. Assoc.*, *41*, 193.
(11) Pearson, H. (1963) *Vet. Rec.*, *75*, 961.
(12) Huskamp, B. & Kopf, N. (1980) *Tierärztl. Praxis*, *8*, 327.
(13) Shearer, I. J. & Dunkin, A. C. (1968) *NZ J. agric. Res.*, *11*, 923.
(14) Radostits, O. M. (1960) *Can. vet. J.*, *1*, 405.
(15) Svendsen, P. & Kristensen, B. (1970) *Nord. VetMed.*, *22*, 278.
(16) Huskamp, B. & Koff, N. (1983) *Equ. Pract.*, *5*(1), 20.
(17) Pearson, H. & Pinsent, P. J. N. (1977) *Vet. Rec.*, *101*, 162.
(18) Pitt, J. N. (1976) *Vict. vet. Proc.*, *34*, 27.
(19) Clem, R. R. & Johnston, P. H. (1977) *Aust. vet. Practnr*, *7*, 56.
(20) Maconochie, J. R. et al. (1968) *Aust. vet. J.*, *44*, 81.
(21) Koch, D. B. et al. (1978) *J. Am. vet. med. Assoc.*, *173*, 197.
(22) Osborne, H. G. (1958) *Aust. vet. J.*, *34*, 42.
(23) Gumbrell, R. C. (1973) *NZ vet J.*, *21*, 178.
(24) Crespeau, F. (1974) *Recl. Méd vét. Ec. Alfort*, *150*, 687.
(25) Roneus, O. (1957) *Nord. VetMed.*, *9*, 362.
(26) Datt, S. C. & Asenik, E. A. (1975) *Cornell Vet.*, *65*, 152.
(27) Weipers, W. L. (1963) *Bull. Off. int. Epizoot.*, *59*, 1419.
(28) Mullowney, P. C. & Whitlock, R. H. (1978) *Vet. Rec.*, *103*, 557.
(29) Moore, J. N. et al. (1981) *Can. J. comp. Med.*, *45*, 330.
(30) Christie, B. A. (1967–68) *Vict. vet. Proc.*, *26*, 61.
(31) Tulleners, E. P. (1981) *J. Am. vet. med. Assoc.*, *179*, 998.
(32) Duelke, E. & Whitlock, R. (1976) *Cornell Vet.*, *66*, 353.
(33) Pearson, H. (1971) *Vet. Rec.*, *89*, 426.
(34) Hammond, P. B. et al. (1964) *J. comp. Pathol.*, *74*, 210.
(35) Gerring, E. E. L. & Hunt, J. M. (1986) *Equ. vet. J.*, *18*, 249.
(36) Grunder, H. D. (1971) *Tierärztl. Wochenschr.*, *78*, 317.
(38) Pinsent, P. J. N. (1978) *Bov. Practnr*, *13*, 45.
(39) Toofanion, F. & Aliakbari, S. (1977) *Cornell Vet.*, *67*, 523.
(40) Hamilton, G. F. & Tulleners, E. P. (1980) *Can. vet. J.*, *21*, 32.
(41) Freeman, D. E. et al. (1979) *Am. vet. med. Assoc.*, *175*, 1089.
(42) Steckel, R. R. & Nugent, M. A. (1983) *J. Am. vet. med. Assoc.*, *182*, 818.
(43) Collier, M. A. & Trent, A. M. (1988) *J. Am. vet. med. Assoc.*, *182*, 819.
(44) Turner, J. A. et al. (1984) *J. Am. vet. med. Assoc.*, *184*, 731.
(45) Schneider, R. K. et al. (1982) *Am. J. vet. Res.*, *180*, 317.
(46) Tate, L. P. et al. (1983) *Am. J. vet. Res.*, *44*, 1187.
(47) Barclay, W. P. et al. (1982) *J. Am. vet. med. Assoc.*, *180*, 752.
(48) Barrell, G. K. et al. (1982) *J. Physiol.*, *330*, 92.
(49) Waldeland, H. (1982) *Vet. Rec.*, *111*, 455.
(50) Beroza, G. A. et al. (1985) *J. Am. vet. med. Assoc.*, *186*, 1304.
(51) Scott, E. A. & Todhunter, R. (1985) *J. Am. vet. med. Assoc.*, *186*, 383.
(52) Hunt, J. M. et al. (1986) *Equ. vet. J.*, *18*, 264.
(53) Semrad, S. D. & Moore, J. N. (1983) *Equ. vet. J.*, *15*, 62.
(54) Ducharm, N. G. et al. (1985) *Proc. 31 Ann. Conv. AAEP*, p. 505.
(55) Trent, A. M. & Bailey, J. V. (1985) *Can. vet. J.*, *26*, 16.

(56) Allen, D. et al. (1986) *J. Am. vet. med. Assoc.*, *189*, 777.
(57) Fischer, A. T. & Meagher, D. M. (1986) *Comp. cont. Educ.*, *8*, 525.

Rectal stricture

There are two notable occurrences, as part of an inherited rectovaginal constriction in Jersey cattle and a syndrome of acquired rectal stricture which occurs in feeder pigs at about 2–3 months of age. Although the latter is generally classed as a sequel to enteric salmonellosis caused by *Salmonella typhimurium* (1), it has been suggested that there is an inherited component in the etiology (3). The presumed pathogenesis is that a *prolonged enterocolitis with ulcerative proctitis* results in an annular cicatrization of the rectal wall 2–5 cm anterior to the anorectal junction. This results in colonic dilatation and compression atrophy of the abdominal and thoracic viscera. Clinically there is progressive abdominal distension, inappetence, emaciation, dehydration, and watery to pasty feces. The stricture of the rectum can be palpated on digital examination of the rectum. Most affected pigs die or are destroyed but a surgical technique for relief of the condition is described (2). Some pigs with incomplete strictures are unaffected clinically. The disease can be reproduced experimentally with *S. typhimurium* or the surgical manipulation of the rectal arterial blood supply resulting in ischemic ulcerative proctitis (1).

At necropsy there is a low-grade peritonitis, dilatation of the colon and sometimes the terminal ileum also. A stricture is present 2–5 cm from the anus, and may be so severe that it exists as a schirrous cord with or without a narrow luminal remnant in the centre. Histologically there is necrotic debris and granulation tissue at the site of the stricture.

REFERENCES

(1) Wilcock, B. P. & Olander, H. J. (1977) *Vet. Pathol.*, *14*, 36, 43.
(2) Boyd, J. S. & Taylor, D. J. (1984) *Vet. Rec.*, *114*, 386.
(3) Haskin, J. T. et al. (1982) *Aust. vet. J.*, *59*, 56.

Enteritis (including malabsorption, enteropathy and diarrhea)

The term enteritis has been used for many years to describe inflammation of the intestinal mucosa resulting in diarrhea and sometimes dysentery, abdominal pain occasionally, and varying degrees of dehydration and acid–base imbalance, depending on the cause of the lesion, its severity and location. In many cases, gastritis also occurs together with enteritis.

It is now evident that there are several diseases of the intestines of farm animals in which diarrhea and dehydration are major clinical findings, but classical inflammation of the mucosa may not be present. The best example of this is the diarrhea caused by enterotoxigenic *E. coli* which elaborate an enterotoxin which causes a large net increase of secretion of fluids into the lumen of the gut, with very minor, if any, structural change in the intestinal mucosa (1). This suggests that a word other than enteritis may be necessary to describe alterations in the intestinal secretory and absorptive mechanisms which result in diarrhea but in which pathologic lesions are not present. However, with the above qualifications, we have chosen, for convenience, to continue to use the term enteritis to describe those diseases in which diarrhea is a major clinical finding due to malabsorption in the intestinal tract.

Etiology

There are many causes of enteritis or malabsorption in farm animals and the disease varies considerably in its severity depending upon the causative agent. In addition to the primary etiological agent of enteritis, there are many influences exerted by the host and the environment which can play an important role in facilitating or suppressing the ability of the causative agent to cause enteritis. Thus newborn calves and piglets which are deficient in immunoglobulin are much more susceptible to diarrhea, and with a high mortality rate from diarrhea, than animals with adequate levels. Enteric salmonellosis is commonly precipitated by the stresses of transportation or deprivation of feed and water. The stress of weaning in pigs is considered an important contributory cause of weanling diarrhea. The prolonged use of antibacterial agents orally in all species may alter the intestinal microflora and permit the development of a superinfection by organisms which would not normally cause disease.

The salient features of the diseases in which diarrhea, due to enteritis or malabsorption, is a principal clinical finding are summarized by species in Tables 18 to 21. There are many other diseases in which diarrhea may be present but is only of minor importance.

Many additional different species of bacteria, other than those summarized in the tables, have been isolated from the intestinal tracts of horses and cattle, but it is not yet possible to conclude a cause and effect relationship (4).

Pathogenesis

Under normal conditions, a large quantity of fluid enters the small intestine from the saliva, stomach, pancreas, liver and intestinal mucosa. This fluid and its electrolytes and other nutrients must be absorbed chiefly by the small intestines, although large quantities move into the large intestine for digestion and absorption, especially in the horse. Any dysfunction of the intestines will result in failure of adequate absorption and diarrhea.

Depending on the causative agent, intestinal malabsorption may be the result of at least three different pathophysiological mechanisms. There may be an *osmotic effect* when substances within the lumen of the intestine increase the osmotic pressure over a greater than normal length of intestine, resulting in an osmotic movement of an excessive amount of fluid into the lumen of the intestine. The fluid is not reabsorbed and accumulates in the lumen. Examples include saline purgatives, overfeeding, indigestible feeds and disaccharidase deficiencies. A deficiency of a disaccharidase leads to incomplete digestion and the accumulation of large quantities of undigested material which acts as a hypertonic solution. Acute or chronic *inflammation* or *necrosis* of the intestinal mucosa will result in both a net increase in fluid production, inflammatory products, including loss of serum proteins and a reduction in absorption of fluids and electrolytes. Examples include many of the diseases caused by bacteria, viruses, fungi, protozoa, chemical agents and tumors which are summarized in Tables 18 to 21.

Malabsorption is caused by several epitheliotropic viruses which affect the villous absorptive cells. Examples include: the transmissible gastroenteritis (TGE) virus in newborn piglets, rotavirus and coronavirus infections in newborn calves and other species. The usual pathogenetic sequence of events is selective destruction of villous absorptive cells, villous atrophy, loss of digestive and absorptive capacities (malabsorption), diarrhea, crypt hyperplasia and recovery (36). Recovery depends on the severity of the lesion, the relative injury done to the villous cells and crypt epithelium, and the age of the animal. Newborn piglets affected with transmissible gastroenteritis commonly die of dehydration and starvation before there is sufficient time for regeneration of the villous cells from the crypt epithelium. In contrast, older pigs have greater capacity for regeneration of the villous cells and the diarrhea may be only transient.

A *secretory–absorptive* imbalance results in a large net increase in fluid secretion with little if any structural

Table 18. The epidemiological and clinical features of diseases of cattle in which diarrhea is a significant clinical finding

Etiological agent or disease	*Age and class of animal affected and important epidemiological factors*	*Major clinical findings and diagnostic criteria*
BACTERIA		
Enterotoxigenic *E. coli*	Newborn calves <3 to 5 days of age, colostral immune status determines survival. Outbreaks common	Acute profuse watery diarrhea, dehydration and acidosis. Culture feces for enteropathogenic type
Salmonella spp.	All ages. Outbreaks occur. Stress-induced	Acute diarrhea, dysentery, fever and high mortality possible. Culture feces
Clostridium perfringens types B and C	Young well nourished calves	Severe hemorrhagic enterotoxemia, rapid death. Fecal smear
Mycobacterium paratuberculosis	Mature cattle, sporadic, single animal	Chronic diarrhea with loss of weight, long course. No response to therapy. Special tests
Proteus spp. and *Pseudomonas* spp.	Calves treated for diarrhea with prolonged course of antibiotics	Chronic to subacute diarrhea, poor response to treatment, progressive loss of weight. Culture feces
FUNGI		
Candida spp.	Young calves following prolonged use of oral antibacterials	Chronic diarrhea, no response to treatment. Fecal smears
VIRUSES		
Rotavirus and coronavirus	Newborn calves, 5–21 days old, explosive outbreaks	Acute profuse watery diarrhea. Demonstrate virus in feces
Winter dysentery (*Coronavirus*)	Mature housed cows, explosive outbreaks	Acute epizootic of transient diarrhea and dysentery lasting 24 hours. Definitive diagnosis not possible currently
Bovine virus diarrhea (mucosal disease)	Young cattle 8 months to 2 years. Usually sporadic but epidemics occur	Erosive gastroenteritis and stomatitis. Usually fatal. Virus isolation
Rinderpest	Highly contagious, occurs in plague form	Erosive stomatitis and gastroenteritis. High morbidity and mortality
Bovine malignant catarrh	Usually mature cattle, sporadic but small outbreaks occur	Erosive stomatitis and gastroenteritis, enlarged lymph nodes, ocular lesions, hematuria and terminal encephalitis. Transmission with whole blood
HELMINTHS		
Ostertagiasis	Young cattle on pasture	Acute or chronic diarrhea, dehydration and hypoproteinemia. Fecal examination. Plasma pepsinogen
PROTOZOA		
Eimeria spp.	Calves over 3 weeks old and cattle up to 12 months of age. Outbreaks common	Dysentery, tenesmus, nervous signs. Fecal examination diagnostic
Cryptosporidium spp.	Calves 5–35 days of age	Diarrhea. Fecal smear and special stain
CHEMICAL AGENTS		
Arsenic, fluorine, copper, sodium chloride, mercury, molybdenum, nitrates, poisonous plants, mycotoxicoses	All ages, history of access to substance. Outbreaks occur	All severities of diarrhea, dysentery, abdominal pain, in some cases nervous signs, dehydration, toxemia. Fecal and tissue analyses

Table 18. (cont.)

Etiological agent or disease	*Age and class of animal affected and important epidemiological factors*	*Major clinical findings and diagnostic criteria*
PHYSICAL AGENTS		
Sand, soil, silage, feed containing lactic acid (sour brewers' grains)	Usually mature cattle, history of access. Outbreaks occur	Acute, subacute diarrhea and toxemia. See sand in feces. Rumen pH
NUTRITIONAL DEFICIENCY		
Copper deficiency, conditioned by excess molybdenum	Usually mature cattle on pasture with high levels of molybdenum	Subacute and chronic diarrhea, osteodystrophy, no systemic effects, hair color changes. Liver and blood analyses
DIETARY		
Overfeeding	Young calves overfed on milk	Mild diarrhea, feces voluminous and pale yellow. Clinical diagnosis
Simple indigestion	Change of ration of mature cows (hay to silage) or grain to feedlot cattle	Subacute diarrhea. Normal in 24 hours. Clinical diagnosis usually sufficient
Inferior milk replacers	Heat-denatured skim milk used in manufacturing of milk replacers for calves	Subacute to chronic diarrhea, progressive emaciation, no response to conventional treatment except cow's whole milk. Clotting tests on milk replacer
MISCELLANEOUS OR UNCERTAIN ETIOLOGY		
Intestinal disaccharidase deficiency	May occur in young calves. Sporadic	Subacute diarrhea unresponsive to usual therapy except withdrawal of milk. Lactose digestion tests
Congestive heart failure	Sporadic. Mature cattle	Profuse watery diarrhea associated with visceral edema
Toxemia (peracute coliform mastitis)	Sporadic	Acute diarrhea due to endotoxemia from peracute mastitis. Culture milk

change in the mucosal cells. The enterotoxin elaborated by enterotoxigenic *E. coli* is an example of such a mechanism (2).

Enteric enterotoxic colibacillosis is an example of a diarrheal disease resulting from intestinal hypersecretion. The villi, along with their digestive and absorptive capabilities, remain intact. The crypts also remain intact; however, their secretion is increased beyond the absorptive capacity of the intestines, resulting in diarrhea. The increased secretion is due to an increase in cyclic adenosine monophosphate which in turn may be stimulated by prostaglandins. The integrity of the mucosal structure is maintained and the secreted fluid is isotonic, electrolyte rich, alkaline and free of exudates. This is useful diagnostically in enterotoxic colibacillosis (36). A comprehensive review of the details of secretory diarrhea in man and experimental animals is available (40).

An important therapeutic principle can be applied in secretory diarrhea disease. Whenever possible, because of the cost of parenteral fluid therapy, fluids and electrolytes should be given orally. The mucosa remains relatively intact and retains normal absorptive capacity. Fluid replacement solutions containing water, glucose and amino acids can be given orally and are absorbed efficiently (37). Glucose and amino acids enhance the absorption of sodium and water, thus replacing or diminishing fluid and electrolyte losses.

Limited studies indicate that the presence of enteritis alters the pharmacodynamics of orally administered drugs. In acute diarrheal states there is delayed or impaired absorption resulting in subtherapeutic plasma concentration. In chronic malabsorption states, decreased, increased, or delayed absorption may occur, depending on the drug. Also, gastric antacids, anticholinergic drugs, and opiates, administered orally for the treatment of diarrhea may impair absorption of other drugs by altering solubility or delaying gastric emptying time (39).

The intestinal hypermotility and diarrhea associated with nervousness is an example of reduced intestinal absorption due to rapid passage of intestinal fluids in an otherwise normal intestine.

Most diarrheal diseases are primarily of small intestine origin although the colon may also participate in net fluid losses. This may not be just the consequence of overwhelming the functional capacity of the large intestine as has been commonly assumed. Instead, an important proportion of these losses may be due to a change in colonic function as a direct result of the composition of the fluid from the small intestine in the diarrheic animal (38). The colon is also capable of net electrolyte secretion similar to that which occurs in the small intestine.

There is also evidence that active electrolyte secretion occurs in enterocolitis due to salmonellosis in several species of animals (38). In diseases such as swine dysentery, the permeability of the colon may remain normal or even decrease, but the absorption of water and electrolytes is decreased. This suggests that the primary cause of fluid and electrolyte loss in some diseases of the colon may be due to failure of the affected epithelium to absorb fluids and electrolytes (38).

The net effect of an increase in the total amount of

Table 19. The epidemiological and clinical features of diseases of the horse in which diarrhea is a significant clinical finding

Etiological agent or disease	*Age and class of animal affected and important epidemiological factors*	*Major clinical findings and diagnostic criteria*
BACTERIA		
Salmonella spp.	Young foals. Mature horses, following stress	Acute profuse diarrhea, severe dehydration, foul smelling feces. Leukopenia and neutropenia. Culture feces. Hyponatremia
Actinobacillus equuli	Newborn foals. May be herd problem	Sudden onset of depression, diarrhea and death in 24 hours, renal microabscess
Corynebacterium equi	Young foals with history of respiratory disease	Diarrhea associated with *Cor. equi* pneumonia. Culture respiratory tract
Clostridiosis	Any age, similar to colitis-X. May be stress- and feed-induced	Acute profuse watery foul-smelling diarrhea, death in 24 hours. Large numbers of *Clostridim perfringens* type A in intestines and feces
VIRUSES AND *RICKETTSIA*		
Rotavirus (27), coronavirus and adenovirus	Newborn foals, herd outbreaks occur	Profuse watery diarrhea at few days of age. Recovery usually uneventful. Fecal isolation.
Rickettsia Potomac horse fever (*Ehrlichia risticii*)	Summer and fall in Potomac Valley. Any age. Sporadic or epidemic.	Depression, anorexia, fever, profuse watery diarrhea, leukopenia, case fatality rate 30%, serology
FUNGI		
Aspergillus fumigatus (28)	Foals and racehorses treated orally with antibiotics. Not common	Chronic diarrhea. Fecal smear
PARASITES		
Strongylus spp., *Trichonema* spp. and *Ascaris* spp.	Individual horses usually over 6 months of age. Must be massive infestation	Acute, subacute or chronic diarrhea; hypoproteinemia possible. Fecal examination
PHYSICAL		
Sand colic	Horses grazing on sandy pastures or consuming feed containing excessive quantity of sand or soil	Acute or chronic diarrhea, colic, impaction of large intestines. Feces contain sand
Stress-induced (29)	Usually follows prolonged surgical anesthesia	Acute profuse watery diarrhea, severe dehydration, death may occur in 24–48 hours. Leukopenia and neutropenia
Dioctyl poisoning (30)	Overdosage with dioctyl sodium sulfosuccinate used for treatment of impaction of large intestine	Acute onset of anorexia, paralytic ileus, *marked dehydration*, diarrhea 24 hours following overdose. Death may occur within 36 hours
TUMOR		
Lymphosarcoma (31)	Single horse affected	Chronic diarrhea, progressive loss of weight, no response to therapy. Intestinal biopsy necessary
MISCELLANEOUS OR UNKNOWN ETIOLOGY		
Colitis-X (32)	Single animal, usually mature horse but may affect yearlings too. May be stress-induced	Peracute profuse watery diarrhea, sudden onset, rapid collapse and death. Poor response to therapy
Granulomatous enteritis (33)	Single animal. Usually mature horse	Chronic weight loss. Diarrhea not a major clinical finding
Tetracycline-induced (34)	Horses treated with five to ten times usual dose of tetracycline	Acute profuse watery diarrhea, severe dehydration, death in 24–48 hours
Foal-heat diarrhea	Foals at 7–10 days of age coinciding with mare's first postpartum estrus	Mild diarrhea lasting 1–4 days. Minimal systemic effects. No specific treatment usually required
IDIOPATHIC OR UNKNOWN	Single horse, sporadic, no recognizable predisposing cause	Chronic intractable diarrhea, no response to standard treatments. Perhaps some slight villous atrophy at necropsy, nothing else diagnostic

Other sporadic causes of diarrhea in horses include those caused by: coronavirus, *Globidium leuckarti*, *Corynebacterium equi*, *Clostridium perfringens* types B and C.

Table 20. The epidemiological and clinical features of diseases of the pig in which diarrhea is a significant clinical finding

Etiological agent or disease	*Age and class of animal affected and important epidemiological factors*	*Major clinical findings and diagnostic criteria*
BACTERIA		
Enterotoxigenic *E. coli*	Common disease of newborn, 3-week-old and weaned piglets. Outbreaks. Colostral immune status important	Acute diarrhea, dehydration. Responds to early treatment. Fecal culture and serotype
Salmonella spp.	All ages. Most common in feeder pigs	Acute septicemia or chronic diarrhea. Responds to early treatment
Clostridium perfringens type C	Newborn piglets. High mortality	Acute and peracute hemorrhagic enterotoxemia
Treponema hyodysenteriae (swine dysentery)	Usually feeder pigs. Outbreaks common	Dysentery, acute to subacute, fever. Responds to treatment
VIRUSES		
Transmissible gastroenteritis (TGE)	Explosive outbreaks in newborn piglets. High morbidity and mortality	Acute diarrhea, vomition, dehydration and death. No response to treatment
Rotavirus and coronavirus	Outbreaks in newborn piglets and weaned piglets. May occur in well-managed herds	Acute diarrhea and dehydration. May continue to suck the sow. Death in 2–4 days. Virus isolation and pathology of gut
PROTOZOA		
Isospora spp.	Newborn piglets 5–14 days of age. High morbidity, low mortality	Acute diarrhea. Poor response to therapy with amprolium. Fecal examination for oocysts
PARASITES		
Ascaris lumbricoides	Young pigs	Mild diarrhea for few days
Trichuris suis	All ages usually older pigs	Diarrhea, dysentery and loss of weight. Fecal examination and gross pathology
NUTRITIONAL DEFICIENCY		
Iron deficiency	Young piglets 6–8 weeks. Not common in well-managed swine herds	Mild diarrhea and anemia
MISCELLANEOUS OR UNCERTAIN ETIOLOGY		
Proliferative hemorrhagic enteropathy (12)	Growing and mature pigs. Outbreaks common	Acute dysentery and death

fluid in the intestinal lumen and a reduction in intestinal absorption is a loss of fluids and electrolytes at the expense of body fluids and electrolytes and the normal intestinal juices (3). The fluid which is lost consists primarily of water, the electrolytes sodium, chloride, potassium and bicarbonate, and varying quantities of protein. Protein is lost (protein-losing enteropathy) in both acute and chronic inflammation leading to hypoproteinemia in some cases (5). The loss of bicarbonate results in metabolic acidosis which is of major importance in acute diarrhea. The loss of sodium, chloride and potassium results in serum electrolyte imbalances. In the horse with enteric salmonellosis, there is severe dehydration and marked hyponatremia (6). In the calf with neonatal diarrhea there are varying degrees of dehydration and a moderate loss of all electrolytes (7). With acute severe diarrhea, there is severe acidosis, reduced circulating blood volume resulting in reduced perfusion of the liver and kidney and of peripheral tissues. This results in uremia, anerobic oxidation and lactic acidosis, which accentuates the metabolic acidosis. Hyperventilation occurs in some animals in an attempt to compensate for the acidosis.

In acute diarrhea, large quantities of intestinal fluid are lost in the feces and large quantities are present in the intestinal lumen (intraluminal dehydration) which accounts for the remarkable clinical dehydration in some affected animals. The fluid moves out of the intravascular compartment first, then out of the extravascular compartment, followed lastly from the intracellular space. Thus in acute diarrhea of sudden onset the actual degree of dehydration present initially may be much more severe than is recognizable clinically; as the diarrhea continues, the degree of clinical dehydration becomes much more evident.

In chronic enteritis, as a sequel to acute enteritis or developing insidiously, the intestinal wall becomes thickened and mucus secretion is stimulated, the absorption of intestinal fluids is also decreased but not of the same magnitude as in acute enteritis. In chronic enteritis there is a negative nutrient balance because of decreased digestion of nutrients and decreased absorption,

Table 21. The epidemiological and clinical features of the diseases of sheep in which diarrhea is a significant clinical finding (35)

Etiological agent or disease	*Age and class of animal affected and important epidemiological factors*	*Major clinical findings and diagnostic criteria*
BACTERIA		
Enterotoxigenic *E. coli* (colibacillosis)	Newborn lambs in crowded lambing sheds. Cold chilling weather. Outbreaks. Inadequate colostrum. Mismothering problems. Poor udder development	Acute diarrhea (yellow feces), septicemia and rapid death. Culture feces for enterotoxigenic *E. coli*
Clostridium perfringens type B (lamb dysentery)	Newborn lambs up to 10 days of age. Overcrowded lambing sheds	Sudden death, diarrhea, dysentery, toxemia. Fecal smear
Salmonella spp.	Newborn lambs. Adult sheep in late pregnancy	Acute diarrhea and dysentery in lambs. Acute toxemia, diarrhea in ewes followed by abortion. Fecal culture and pathology
VIRUSES		
Rotavirus and coronavirus	Newborn lambs. Many lambs affected	Acute profuse watery diarrhea. No toxemia. Usually recover spontaneously if no secondary complications. Virus isolation
PARASITES		
Nematodirus spp.	Lambs 4–10 weeks of age on pasture. Sudden onset. Outbreaks. Ideal environmental conditions for parasite are necessary	Anorexia, diarrhea, thirsty, 10–20% of lambs may die if not treated. Fecal examination
Ostertagia spp.	Lambs 10 weeks of age and older lambs and young ewes on grass. Types I and II	Many lambs develop diarrhea, weight loss. Abomasitis
Trichostrongylus spp.	Older lambs 4–9 months of age	Dull, anorexic, loss of weight and chronic diarrhea. Fecal examination
PROTOZOA		
Eimeria spp.	Overstocking on pasture and overcrowding indoors, poor sanitation and hygiene. Commonly occurs following weaning and introduction into feedlot.	Acute and subacute diarrhea and dysentery. Loss of weight. Mortality may be high. Fecal examination
Cryptosporidium	Lambs 7–10 days of age	Dullness, anorexia, afebrile, diarrhea, may die in 2–3 days, survivors may be unthrifty. Examination of feces and intestinal mucosa. No specific treatment

resulting in body wasting. The animal may continue to drink and maintain almost normal hydration. In some cases of chronic enteritis, depending on the cause, there is continuous loss of protein leading to clinical hypoproteinemia. Intestinal helminthiasis (8) and other chronic diarrheas of the horse are examples (9). Lymphangiectasis of the intestine has been associated with hypoproteinemia in dogs (10). In other cases, lymphangiectasis may be the only lesion and probably contributes another cause of the so-called 'protein-losing' enteropathies (11).

Regional ileitis is a functional obstruction of the lower ileum associated with granulation tissue proliferation in the lamina propria and submucosa, with or without ulceration of the mucosa, and a massive muscular hypertrophy of the wall of affected areas of the intestine (12). It has been recognized with increased frequency in recent years in pigs, horses and lambs. The lesion undoubtedly interferes with normal digestion and absorption but diarrhea is not a common clinical finding.

The villous absorptive epithelial cells of the small intestine are involved in almost every type of enteritis or malabsorptive syndrome. These cells which line the villi and face the lumen of the intestine contain important digestive enzymes such as the disaccharidases (13). They are also involved in absorption of fluids, electrolytes, monosaccharides like glucose, and amino acids, and in the transport of fat micelles. Their replacement time is up to several days in the newborn calf and piglet, and only a few days when these animals are older (at 3 weeks) (1). This may explain the relatively greater susceptibility of the newborn to the viral enteritides, such as TGE in piglets and rotavirus infection in all newborn farm animal species. Almost any noxious influence can increase the rate of extrusion of these cells, which are then replaced by cells which are immature and not fully functional. The villi become shortened (villous atrophy) and chronic malabsorption similar to the 'sprue gut' of man may be the result (14). The destruction of villous epithelial cells explains the long recovery period of several days in some animals with acute enteritis and the chronic diarrhea in others with chronic villous atrophy (14).

The motility of the intestinal tract in animals with enteritis has not been sufficiently examined and little information is available. It was thought for many years that intestinal hypermotility was present in most enteritides as a response to the enteritis and that the hypermotility accounted for the reduced absorption. However, when the pathogenesis of the infectious enteritides is considered, for example, the unique secretory effect of enterotoxin, it seems more likely that if hypermotility is present, it is a response to the distension of the intestinal lumen with fluid rather than a response to irritation. With a fluid-filled intestinal lumen, very little intestinal peristalsis would be necessary to move large quantities of fluid down the intestinal tract. This may explain the fluid-rushing sounds which are audible on auscultation of the abdomen in animals with enteritis. It is possible that the intestines may be in a state of relative hypomotility rather than hypermotility, which makes the use of spasmolytics for the treatment of enteritis questionable.

The location of the lesion in the intestinal tract may also influence the severity of the enteritis or malabsorption. Lesions involving the small intestine are considered to be more acute and severe than those in the large intestine because approximately 75–80% of the intestinal fluids are absorbed by the small intestine and much lesser quantities by the large intestine. Thus, in general, when lesions of the large intestine predominate, the fluid and electrolyte losses are not as acute nor as severe as when the lesions of the small intestine predominate. However, the horse is an exception. The total amount of fluid entering the large intestine from the small intestine, plus the amount entering from the mucosa of the large intestine, is equal to the animal's total extracellular fluid volume, and 95% of this is reabsorbed by the large intestine (3). This illustrates the major importance of the large intestine of the horse in absorbing a large quantity of fluid originating from saliva, the stomach, liver, pancreas, small intestine and large intestine. Any significant dysfunction of the absorptive mechanism of the large intestine of the horse would result in large losses of fluids and electrolytes. This may explain the rapid dehydration and circulatory collapse which occurs in horses with colitis-X (3, 4).

Gastritis commonly accompanies enteritis but does not cause vomition except perhaps in the pig. Gastritis (or abomasitis) may also be the primary lesion resulting in a profuse diarrhea without lesions of the intestines. Examples are ostertagiasis and abomasal ulceration in cattle. Presumably the excessive amount of fluid secreted into the affected abomasum cannot be reabsorbed by the intestines. The comparative pathogenesis of some enteric diseases of animals has been reviewed (15).

Clinical findings

The major clinical finding in enteritis or malabsorption is diarrhea. Dehydration, abdominal pain, septicemia and toxemia with fever occur commonly and their degree of severity depends on the causative agent, the age and species of animal, and the stage of the disease.

In acute enteritis, the feces are soft or fluid in consistency and may have an unpleasant odor. They may contain blood, fibrinous casts and mucus or obvious foreign material such as sand. The color of the feces will vary considerably; they are usually pale yellow because of the dilution of the brown bile pigments but almost any color other than the normal is possible and, with the exception of the frank blood or melena, the color of the feces is usually not representative of a particular disease. When the feces are watery, they may escape notice on clinical examination. Some indication of the nature of the enteritis may be obtained from the distribution of the feces on the animal's perineum. Thus, in calves, the smudge pattern may suggest coccidiosis when both the staining that accompanies it and the feces are smeared horizontally across the ischial tuberosities and the adjoining tail, or helminth infestation when there is little smearing on the pinbones but the tail and insides of the hocks are liberally coated with feces. Straining may occur, especially in calves, and be followed by rectal prolapse, particularly when the lesions are present in the colon and rectum. Intussusception may occur when the enteritis involves the small intestine.

There are a number of diseases in which dysentery with or without toxemia occurs and death may occur rapidly. These include lamb dysentery, hemorrhagic enterotoxemia of calves, acute swine dysentery and hemorrhagic bowel syndrome of pigs.

The systemic effects in enteritis vary considerably. Septicemia, toxemia and fever are common in the infectious enteritides. An increased body temperature may return to normal following the onset of diarrhea or if circulatory collapse and shock are imminent. The clinical dehydration will vary from being just barely detectable at 4–6% of body weight up to 10–12% of body weight, when it is clinically very evident. The degree of dehydration can be best assessed by *tenting* the skin of the upper eyelid or neck and determining the time taken for the skin fold to return to normal. The degree of recession of the eyeball is also a useful aid. In the early stages of acute enteritis, the degree of clinical dehydration may be underestimated because of the time required for fluid to shift from the interstitial and intracellular spaces to the intravascular space to replace fluids already lost. Dehydration is usually evident by 10–12 hours following the onset of acute enteritis and clinically obvious by 18–24 hours. Peripheral circulatory collapse occurs commonly in acute and peracute cases. There may be tachycardia or bradycardia and arrhythmia depending on the degree of acidosis and electrolyte imbalance. In acute enteritis, there may be severe abdominal pain which is most severe in the horse and is often sufficient in this species to cause rolling and kicking at the abdomen. Abdominal pain in enteritis is unusual in the other species although it does occur in heavy inorganic metal poisonings, such as arsenic and lead, and in acute salmonellosis in cattle. Some severe cases of enteric colibacillosis in calves are characterized by abdominal pain evidenced by intermittent bouts of stretching and kicking at the abdomen. The passage of intestinal gas also occurs commonly in horses with acute and chronic diarrhea.

Auscultation of the abdomen usually reveals sounds of increased peristalsis and fluid-rushing sounds in the early stages of acute enteritis. Later there may be paralytic ileus and an absence of peristaltic sounds with only fluid and gas tinkling sounds. The abdomen may be distended in the early stages due to distension of intestines and gaunt in the later stages when the fluid has been passed out in the feces. Pain may be evidenced on palpation of the abdomen in young animals.

In chronic enteritis, the feces are usually soft, homogeneous in consistency, contain considerable mucus and usually do not have a grossly abnormal odor. Progressive weight loss and emaciation or 'runting' are common and there are usually no systemic abnormalities. Animals with chronic enteritis will often drink and absorb sufficient water to maintain clinical hydration but there may be laboratory evidence of dehydration and electrolyte loss. In parasitic enteritis and abomasitis there may be hypoproteinemia and subcutaneous edema. In terminal ileitis, there is usually chronic progressive weight loss and occasionally some mild diarrhea. The lesion is usually recognized only at necropsy. Intestinal adenomatosis of pigs, rectal strictures in pigs, granulomatous enteritis of horses and lymphosarcoma of the intestine of horses are examples of enteric disease causing chronic anorexia and progressive weight loss, usually without clinical evidence of diarrhea. These are commonly referred to as malabsorption syndromes.

Clinical pathology

Examination of the feces to determine the presence of causative bacteria, helminths, protozoa, viruses and chemical agents is described under the specific diseases. It is important that fecal specimens be taken as the differentiation of the etiological groups depends on laboratory examinations. In outbreaks of diarrhea, especially in neonates, it may be useful to do a necropsy on selected early untreated cases of acute diarrhea. The lesions associated with the enteropathogens are now well known and a provisional etiological diagnosis may be possible by gross and histopathological examination of the intestinal mucosa.

The examination of fecal leukocytes and epithelial cells can be helpful. Fecal leukocytes and epithelial cells occur in increased numbers in equine salmonellosis but also with other types of diarrhea (41).

With increasing sophistication in diagnostic laboratories and in large-animal practice, it is becoming common to do considerable laboratory evaluation to determine the actual changes which are present for purposes of a more rational approach to therapy. In most cases of acute enteritis there is hemoconcentration, metabolic acidosis, an increase in total serum solids concentration, a decrease in plasma bicarbonate, hyponatremia, hypochloremia and hypokalemia. Hyperkalemia is possible in severe acidosis. An increase in blood urea nitrogen is common due to inadequate renal perfusion associated with the dehydration and circulatory failure.

Digestion and absorption tests are available for the investigation of chronic malabsorptive conditions, particularly in the horse (17). Intestinal biopsy (18) may be necessary for a definitive diagnosis of chronic intestinal lesions which cannot be determined by the usual diagnostic tests. Examples include intestinal lymphosarcoma, granulomatous enteritis and perhaps Johne's disease. Serum electrophoresis and the administration of radioactive labeled albumin may be necessary to determine the presence of a protein-losing enteropathy (10).

Necropsy findings

The pathology of enteritis or malabsorption varies considerably dependent on the cause. There may be an absence of grossly visible changes of the mucosa, but the intestinal lumen will be fluid-filled or relatively empty, depending on the stage of examination in enterotoxigenic colibacillosis. When there is gross evidence of inflammation of the mucosa there will be varying degrees of edema, hyperemia, hemorrhage, foul-smelling intestinal contents, fibrinous inflammation, ulceration and necrosis of the mucosa. With acute necrosis there is evidence of frank blood, fibrinous casts and epithelial shreds. The mesenteric lymph nodes show varying degrees of enlargement, edema and congestion, and secondary involvement of spleen and liver is not unusual. In chronic enteritis, the epithelium may appear relatively normal but the wall is usually thickened and may be edematous. In some of the specific diseases, there are lesions typical of the particular disease (4).

Diagnosis

The approach to the diagnosis of diarrhea requires a consideration of the epidemiological history and the nature and severity of the clinical findings. With the exception of the acute enteritides in newborn farm animals, most of the other common enteritides have reasonably distinct epidemiological and clinical features. In some cases, a necropsy on an untreated case of diarrhea in the early stages of the disease can be very useful. If possible, a hemogram should be obtained to assist in determining the presence or absence of infection.

The gross appearance of the feces may provide some clues about the cause of the diarrhea (19). In general, the diarrheas caused by lesions of the *small* intestine are profuse and the feces are liquid and sometimes as clear as water. The diarrheas associated with lesions of the *large* intestine are characterized by small volumes of soft feces often containing excess quantities of mucus. The presence of toxemia and fever marked changes in the total and differential leukocyte count suggest bacterial enteritis, possibly with septicemia. This is of particular importance in horses and cattle with salmonellosis. The presence of frank blood and/or fibrinous casts in the feces usually indicates a severe inflammatory lesion of the intestines. In sand-induced diarrhea in horses the feces may contain sand (20). A chronic diarrhea with a history of chronic weight loss in a mature cow suggests Johne's disease. Chronic weight loss and chronic diarrhea, or even the absence of diarrhea, in the horse may indicate the presence of granulomatous enteritis, chronic eosinophilic gastroenteritis, alimentary lymphosarcoma, tuberculosis and histoplasmosis.

In dietary diarrhea the feces are usually voluminous, soft and odoriferous, the animal is usually bright and alert and there are minimal systemic effects. An examination of the diet will usually reveal if the composition of the diet or irregular feeding practices are responsible for the diarrhea. Analysis of samples of new feed may be necessary to determine the presence of toxic chemical agents. Arsenic poisoning is characterized by dysentery, toxemia, normal temperature and nervous signs. Copper deficiency conditioned by an excess of molybdenum causes a moderately profuse diarrhea with soft feces, moderate weight loss and there is usually normal hydration and possibly depigmentation of hair.

Intestinal helminthiasis such as ostertagiasis causes a profuse diarrhea and marked loss of weight and the temperature is normal and there is no toxemia.

In cattle it is important to examine the oral cavity for evidence of erosions which are characteristic of viral diseases such as mucosal disease.

Many diseases of the stomach, including ulceration, parasitism, gastritis, and tumors may result in diarrhea and must be considered in the differential diagnosis of chronic diarrhea. The soft scant feces associated with some cases of incomplete obstruction of the digestive tract of cattle affected with the complications of traumatic reticuloperitonitis must not be confused with diarrhea.

Treatment

The principles of treatment of enteritis are: removal of the causative agent, replacement of lost fluids and electrolytes, alteration of the diet if necessary and the possible use of drugs to inhibit secretion and control intestinal hypermotility if deemed necessary. Specific treatment is usually directed at intestinal helminthiasis with anthelmintics, antiprotozoan agents against diseases like coccidiosis and antibacterial agents against the bacterial enteritides. There are no specific treatments available for the viral enteritides in farm animals.

While considerable investigations have been done on the enteritides on farm animals, the emphasis has been on the immunology, pathology, microbiology, and body fluid dynamics, each with different emphasis in different species. For example, there is considerable information on the microbiology and immunology of the common enteritides in calves and piglets in addition to the extensive knowledge of the body fluid dynamics in calves. In the horse there is some information on body fluid dynamics but the microbiology of the diarrheas is not well understood. In none of the species is there sufficient information on the effects of antibiotics on the intestinal microflora.

Alteration of the diet

If the cause of the diarrhea is dietary in origin the feed should be removed until the animal has fully recovered and replaced by another source or reintroduced gradually. The question of whether or not a normally digestible diet should be removed temporarily or the total daily intake reduced in animals with acute enteritis is a difficult one. The rationale is that in acute enteritis the digestibility of nutrients is reduced considerably and undigested feed provides a substrate for fermentation and putrefaction to occur, the products of which may accentuate the malabsorptive state. However, temporary withdrawal of feed presents practical problems especially in the young. For example, the temporary removal from the sow of newborn piglets affected with acute enteritis presents practical problems and is of doubtful value, similarly with beef calves nursing cows on pasture. With foals it is relatively easy to muzzle them for 24 hours. With weaned piglets affected with weanling diarrhea and feeder pigs with swine dysentery, it is common practice to reduce the normal daily intake by half for a few days until recovery is apparent. Mature horses affected with diarrhea should not have access to any feed for at least 24 hours. During the period of temporary starvation, the oral intake of fluids containing glucose and electrolytes is desirable and necessary to assist in maintaining hydration. The exception is in diarrheic horses in which oral fluids may exacerbate the diarrhea, so parenteral fluid therapy is necessary. In newborn calves with diarrhea, providing oral fluid intake is maintained, the total loss of water from feces and through the kidney is not significantly greater than in normal calves because in diarrheic calves the kidney will effectively compensate for fecal losses (21). When recovery is apparent, the animal's usual diet may be reintroduced gradually over a period of a few days.

Antibacterials

The use of antibacterials either orally or parenterally, or by both routes simultaneously, for the treatment of bacterial enteritides is a controversial subject in both human and veterinary medicine (22). Those who support their use in acute bacterial enteritis claim that they are necessary to help reduce the overgrowth of pathogenic bacteria responsible for the enteritis and to prevent or treat bacteremia or septicemia which may occur secondary to an enteritis. Those who suggest that antibacterials are contraindicated or unnecessary in bacterial enteritis suggest that the drugs may eliminate a significant proportion of the intestinal flora in addition to the pathogenic flora. This may reduce the effect of competitive antagonism in the intestine which in turn may permit the development of a suprainfection (the appearance of bacteriological and clinical evidence of a new infection during the chemotherapy of a primary one). Also, the use of antibacterials in infectious enteric disease allows the development of multiple drug resistance which is of public health concern (23). The use of antibacterials may also increase the length of time over which affected animals excrete the organisms. This is a particular problem in enteric salmonellosis.

There is some experimental evidence that the oral administration of chloramphenicol, neomycin, ampicillin, or tetracycline for 3–5 days can cause diarrhea and malabsorption (16). The diarrhea is apparently mild and inconsequential and glucose absorption is decreased. The significance of these observations is unknown until additional studies are made available.

A large variety of antibacterial preparations for both oral and parenteral administration is available. The choice will depend on previous experience, the disease suspected and the results of a culture and drug sensitivity tests. Parenteral preparations are indicated in animals with acute diarrhea, toxemia and fever. Many antibacterials, when given parenterally, are excreted by the liver into the lumen of the intestine and oral preparations may not be necessary. In cases of subacute diarrhea with minimal systemic effects, the use of an oral preparation may be sufficient. However, oral preparations should not be used for more than 3 days to avoid suprainfection. The preparations and doses of the antibacterials commonly used in bacterial enteritides are described under each disease.

Mass medication of the drinking water supply with antibacterials for the treatment of outbreaks of specific infectious enteritides in animals is used commonly and with success. One of the best examples is the use of arsanilic acid or antibiotics in the drinking water of pigs affected with swine dysentery. Not all affected animals will drink sufficient quantity of the medicated water and daily intake must be monitored carefully. Severely affected animals in an outbreak need individual treatment.

Fluids and electrolytes

The initial goals of fluid and electrolyte therapy of the effects of enteritis are: the restoration of the body fluids to normal volume, effective osmolality, composition and acid–base balance. The quality and quantity of fluids required to achieve these goals depend on the characteristics of the dehydration and acid–base electrolyte imbalance. Under ideal conditions when a laboratory is available, the determination of packed cell volume, total serum proteins, plasma bicarbonate, blood pH, the serum electrolytes and a hemogram would provide the clinician with a laboratory evaluation initially and throughout the course of therapy, to assess the effectiveness of the treatment. However, such laboratory service is expensive and usually not readily available. The clinician must therefore assess the degree of clinical dehydration and, based on the history and clinical findings, estimate the degree of acidosis and electrolyte deficits which are likely to be present. A practical approach to fluid therapy in the horse has been described (24). Fluids should be given orally whenever possible to save time and expense and to avoid the complications which can arise from long-term parenteral fluid therapy. Also, fluids should be given as early as possible to minimize the degree of dehydration. With good kidney function there is a wider safe latitude in the solution used.

The three major abnormalities of dehydration, acidosis and electrolyte deficit are usually corrected simultaneously with fluid therapy. When severe acidosis is suspected, this should be corrected immediately with a hypertonic (5%) solution of bicarbonate given intravenously at the rate of 5–7 ml/kg body weight at a speed of about 100 ml/minute. This is followed by the administration of electrolyte solutions in quantities necessary to correct the dehydration. With severe dehydration, equivalent to 10% of body weight, large amounts of fluids are necessary. For example:

Animal	*Dehydration*	Fluid deficit
500 kg horse	10%	50 liters
75 kg foal	10%	7·5 liters
45 kg calf	10%	4·5 liters

The initial hydration therapy should be given over the first 4–6 hours by continuous intravenous infusion, followed by maintenance therapy for the next 20–24 hours, or for the duration of the diarrhea if severe, at a rate of 100–150 ml/kg body weight per 24 hours. Horses with acute enteritis have severe hyponatremia, and following fluid therapy may become severely hypokalemic, as evidenced by weakness and muscular tremors. The hypertonic solution of sodium bicarbonate will assist in correcting the hyponatremia but potassium chloride may need to be added to the large quantity of fluids given for dehydration; 1 g of potassium chloride added to each liter of fluid will provide an additional 14 mOsmol/l (14 mmol/l) of potassium. In preruminant calves with diarrhea, the fluids and electrolytes required for maintenance may be given orally in divided doses every few hours. In the early stage of acute diarrhea and for animals which are not severely dehydrated, the oral route can also be used successfully to correct dehydration and prevent it from becoming worse. The formulae of oral glucose–electrolyte solutions are given in the section under colibacillosis. Piglets and lambs affected with dehydration are most effectively treated using balanced electrolyte solutions given subcutaneously at the dose rates of 20 ml/kg every 4 hours and orally at 20 ml/kg every 2 hours. Those details of the treatment of fluid and electrolyte disturbances are given under that heading in Chapter 2.

Intestinal protectants and adsorbents

Kaolin and pectin mixtures are used widely to coat the intestinal mucosa, inhibit secretions and increase the bulk of the feces in animals with enteritis. In children with diarrhea, kaolin and pectin will result in formed rather than watery feces, but the water content of the feces is unchanged (25). It is not possible at this time to make a recommendation on their use in animals.

Antidiarrheal drugs

Anticholinergic drugs and opiates are available to decrease intestinal motility (25). The anticholinergic drugs block the action of acetylcholine on smooth muscle and glands. This results in decreased gastric secretion and emptying and a reduction on both segmental and propulsive movements of the intestines. Dosages of anticholinergics necessary to produce effectiveness may also cause side-effects such as xerostomia, photophobia, tachycardia, urinary retention and neuromuscular paralysis. The opiates function by producing an increase in segmentation while reducing propulsive movements in the intestine. The net effect is an increase in resistance to passage of intestinal contents and more complete absorption of both water and nutrients occurs with a subsequent decrease in the frequency of defecation. There are no published reports of clinical trials using anticholinergic drugs for the treatment of diarrhea in farm animals and, therefore, at the present time they cannot be recommended with any assurance of effectiveness.

Antisecretory drugs are also available for the treatment of diarrhea due to the hypersecretory activity of enterotoxin produced by bacteria such as enterotoxigenic *E. coli* (26). Antisecretory drugs include chlorpromazine, opiates, atropine and prostaglandin inhibitors. These also have not yet been adequately evaluated and the provision of balanced fluids and electrolytes, containing sodium chloride, sodium bicarbonate, potassium chloride and glucose, given both parenterally and orally are considered to be adequate and effective for treating the effects of the hypersecretion.

REVIEW LITERATURE

Arbuckle, J. B. R. (1977) Atrophy of small intestinal villi, with particular reference to the pig. *Vet. Ann.*, *17*, 123.

Argenzio, R. A. (1975) Function of the equine large intestine and their interrelationships in disease. *Cornell Vet.*, *65*, 303.

Argenzio, R. A. (1978) Physiology of diarrhea—large intestine. *J. Am. vet. med. Assoc.*, *173*, 667.

Bywater, R. J. (1975) Functional pathology of neonatal diarrhea in calves and piglets. *Vet. Ann.*, *15*, 425.
Michell, A. R. (1974) Body fluids and diarrhoea: dynamics of dysfunction. *Vet. Rec.*, *94*, 311.
Roberts, M. C. (1985) Malabsorption syndromes in the horse. *Comp. cont. Educ. Pract. Vet.*, 7, S637–S646.
Willard, M. D. (1985) Newer concepts in treatment of secretory diarrheas. *J. Am. Vet. Med. Assoc.*, *186*, 86–88.
Wilson, R. C. (1982) Antimotility drugs used in the treatment of diarrhea. *J. Am. vet. med. Assoc.*, *186*, 86–88.

REFERENCES

(1) Moon, H. W. & Joel, D. D. (1975) *Am. J. vet. Res.*, *36*, 187.
(2) Moon, H. W. (1974) *Adv. vet. Sci. comp. Med.*, *18*, 179.
(3) Argenzio, R. A. (1975) *Cornell Vet.*, *65*, 303.
(4) Al-Mashat, R. R. & Taylor, D. J. (1986) *Vet. Rec.*, *118*, 453.
(5) Targowski, S. P. (1975) *Infect. Immunol.*, *12*, 48.
(6) Whitlock, R. (1986) *Proc. 21st ann. Mtg Am. Assoc. equ. Practnrs*, 390.
(7) Fayet, J. C. (1971) *Br. vet. J.*, *127*, 37.
(8) Greatorex, J. C. (1975) *Vet. Rec.*, *97*, 221.
(9) Scrutchfield, W. (1976) *Proc. 21st ann. Mtg Am. Assoc. equ. Practnrs*, 203.
(10) Finco, D. R. et al. (1973) *J. Am. vet. med. Assoc.*, *163*, 262.
(11) Nansen, P. & Nielsen, K. (1967) *Nord. VetMed.*, *19*, 524.
(12) Rowland, A. C. & Lawson, G. H. K. (1975) *Vet. Rec.*, *97*, 178.
(13) Toofanian, F. et al. (1973) *Res. vet. Sci.*, *4*, 57.
(14) Arbuckle, J. B. R. (1977) *Vet. Ann.*, *17*, 123.
(15) Kent, T. H. & Moon, H. W. (1973) *Vet. Pathol.*, *10*, 414.
(16) Rollin, R. E. et al. (1986) *Am. J. vet. Res.*, *47*, 987.
(17) Roberts, M. C. (1975) *Res. vet. Sci.*, *18*, 64.
(18) Anderson, N. V. (1974) *Vet. Clin. N. Am.*, *4*, 317.
(19) Stober, M. & Serrano, H. S. (1974) *Vet. Med. Rev.*, *4*, 361.
(20) Ramey, D. W. & Reinerton, E. L. (1984) *J. Am. vet. med. Assoc.*, *185*, 537.
(21) Fisher, E. W. & Martinez, A. A. (1976) *Res. vet. Sci.*, *20*, 302.
(22) Radostits, O. M. et al. (1975) *Can. vet. J.*, *16*, 219.
(23) Williams-Smith, H. (1974) *Br. vet. J.*, *130*, 110.
(24) Mason, T. A. (1972) *Aust. vet. J.*, *48*, 671.
(25) Wilson, R. C. (1982) *J. Am. vet. med. Assoc.*, *180*, 776.
(26) Willard, M. D. (1985) *J. Am. vet. med. Assoc.*, *186*, 86.
(27) Conner, M. E. & Darlington, R. W. (1980) *Am. J. vet. Res.*, *41*, 1699.
(28) Lundvall, R. L. & Romberg, P. F. (1960) *J. Am. vet. med. Assoc.*, *137*, 481.
(29) Owen, P. ap R. (1975) *Vet. Rec.*, *96*, 267.
(30) Moffat, R. E. et al. (1975) *Can. J. comp. Med.*, *39*, 434.
(31) Wiseman, A. et al. (1974) *Vet. Rec.*, *95*, 454.
(32) Rooney, J. R. (1966) *Cornell Vet.*, *56*, 220.
(33) Cimprich, R. E. (1974) *Vet. Pathol.*, *11*, 535.
(34) Baker, J. R. (1975) *Vet. Ann.*, *15*, 178.
(35) Reid, J. F. S. (1976) *Vet. Rec.*, *98*, 496.
(36) Moon, H. W. (1978) *J. Am. vet. med. Assoc.*, *172*, 443.
(37) Whipp, S. C. (1978) *J. Am. vet. med. Assoc.*, *173*, 662.
(38) Argenzio, R. A. (1978) *J. Am. vet. med. Assoc.*, *173*, 667.
(39) Ahrens, F. A. (1978) *J. Am. vet. med. Assoc.*, *173*, 673.
(40) Field, M. et al. (1980) *Secretory Diarrhea*, Bethesda, Maryland: American Physiological Society, pp. 1–227.
(41) Morris, D. D. et al. (1983) *Cornell Vet.*, *73*, 265.

Intestinal hypermotility

A functional increase in intestinal motility seems to be the basis of a number of diseases of animals. Clinically there is some abdominal pain and, on auscultation, an increase in alimentary tract sounds and, in some cases, diarrhea. Affected animals do not usually die and necropsy lesions cannot be defined but it is probable that the classification as it is used here includes many of the diseases often referred to as catarrhal enteritis or indigestion.

The major occurrence of intestinal hypermotility is spasmodic colic of the horse.

Other circumstances in which hypermotility and diarrhea occur without evidence of enteritis include peat scours of cattle on pasture deficient in copper and containing an excess of molybdenum, allergic and anaphylactic states and a change of feed to very lush pasture.

Spasmodic colic

Etiology

Spasmodic colic occurs usually in horses which are predisposed to it by an excitable temperament. Precipitating causes include excitement, such as occurs during thunderstorms, preparations for showing or racing, and drinks of cold water when hot and sweating after work. Excitable cattle may suffer from transient attacks of diarrhea during periods of excitement. Mucosal penetration and submucosal migration of *Strongylus vulgaris* larvae are known to cause changes in ileal myoelectrical activity that could lead to the development of colic in horses (1).

Pathogenesis

The hypermotility of spasmodic colic in horses is thought to arise by an increase in parasympathetic tone under the influence of the causative factors mentioned above. This explanation is not particularly satisfying but the condition is comparable to the vague intestinal upsets which occur in children and excitable adults.

In calves, there may be a similar element of autonomic imbalance, particularly in cases of colic which occur transiently in calves in the 3–6 months age group and more rarely in adult cattle.

Clinical findings

Spasmodic colic of horses is characterized by short attacks of abdominal pain. The pain is intermittent, the horse rolling, pawing and kicking for a few minutes, then shaking itself and standing normally for a few minutes until the next bout of pain occurs. Intestinal sounds are often audible some distance from the horse and loud, rumbling borborygmi are heard on auscultation. The pulse is elevated moderately to about 60/minute and there may be some patchy sweating but rectal findings are negative and there is no scouring. The signs usually disappear spontaneously within a few hours. A similar syndrome occurs in cows and in calves although intestinal sounds are not usually increased.

Clinical pathology and necropsy findings

Laboratory examinations are not used in diagnosis and the disease is not fatal.

Diagnosis

Spasmodic colic may be confused with enteritis since both diseases are characterized by abdominal pain and increased intestinal sounds. Diarrhea is usually present in enteritis although an exception to this rule is acute parasitic enteritis in the horse. Confusion may also occur in cattle and in horses between spasmodic colic and acute intestinal obstruction especially in cattle where rectal examination may be negative in early cases of obstruction, but the failure to pass feces and the presence of blood and mucus in the rectum are typical of this condition. The disease has also been confused with obstructive urolithiasis because of the similar posture adopted by horses in both diseases. The causes of equine colic are summarized in Table 16.

Treatment

Acute hypermotility as manifested by spasmodic colic is best treated by a spasmolytic such as atropine. In horses, a standard treatment is 16–32 mg of atropine sulfate given subcutaneously followed by 2 liters of mineral oil by nasal tube. Pethidine (Demerol, isonipecaine hydrochloride or meperidine hydrochloride) injected parenterally at a dose rate of 2 mg/kg body weight is an effective analgesic and spasmolytic. Promazine derivatives have a tranquilizing and spasmolytic effect also and, followed by a mild purgative, appear to be the treatment of choice in this form of colic. Analgesics are not usually required but, if they are administered, they can be used as described under impaction of the large intestine.

REFERENCE

(1) Berry, C. R. et al. (1986) *Am. J. vet. Res.*, *47*, 27.

Dietary diarrhea

Dietary diarrhea occurs in all species and all ages but is most common in the newborn which ingests too much milk or a diet which is indigestible.

Etiology

The use of inferior quality milk replacers in young calves under 3 weeks of age is one of the commonest causes of dietary diarrhea. The quality of the milk replacer may be affected by the use of skim-milk powder which, during processing, was heat-denatured resulting in a decrease in the concentration of non-casein proteins (1). This results in ineffective clotting in the abomasum and reduced digestibility (2). The use of excessive quantities of non-milk carbohydrates and proteins in milk replacers for calves is also associated with a high incidence of diarrhea, loss of weight, emaciation and starvation (3). The use of large quantities of soybean protein and fish protein concentration in milk replacers for calves will result in chronic diarrhea and poor growth rates (5).

Most attempts to raise calves on diets based on large amounts of certain soybean products, such as heated soybean flour, have been unsuccessful because the animals developed diarrhea, loss of appetite and weight or inferior growth rate (4). Preruminant calves develop gastrointestinal hypersensitive responses to certain soybean products because major proteases of the digestive tract do not denature soluble antigenic constituents of the soybean protein.

Diarrhea of nutritional origin has become one of the most important problems where large numbers of calves are raised under intensive conditions. Because of the relatively high cost of good quality skim-milk powder, large quantities of both non-milk proteins and carbohydrates are used in formulating milk replacers. While some calves in these large units can satisfactorily digest the nutrients in these milk replacers, many cannot and this leads to a high incidence of diarrhea and secondary colibacillosis and enteric salmonellosis.

Milk replacers made from bovine milk and milk byproducts and used to feed orphan piglets, lambs and foals may cause nutritional diarrhea for the same reasons given above. In milk-replacer fed calves, increasing the total daily fluid intake as a percentage of body weight, causes a greater incidence of loose feces, dehydration and dullness than lower levels of fluid intake and higher dry matter concentration (7). This suggests that a greater amount of fluid intake increases the passage rate of dry matter and decreases absorption. The concentration of solids in the liquid diet should range between 10 and 13% and should be offered at 8% of body weight in calves fed milk replacer once daily and allowed free access to calf starter (6).

The feeding of excessive amounts of cows' whole milk to hand-fed calves will result in large amounts of abnormal feces but usually not a profuse watery diarrhea with dehydration and loss of weight (8). This suggests that simple overfeeding of milk may not be a cause of acute neonatal diarrhea of calves. However, it may predispose to secondary colibacillosis. There is some limited evidence that dietary diarrhea may occur in nursing beef calves ingesting milk which does not clot properly (17). Only the milk from cows with diarrheic calves showed evidence of impaired clotting in an *in vitro* test. The ingestion of excessive quantities of sows' milk by piglets at 3 weeks of age is thought to be a contributory cause of 3-week diarrhea of piglets. This may be due to the sow reaching peak production at 3 weeks. Beef calves sucking high-producing cows grazing on lush pasture are often affected with a mild diarrhea at about 3 weeks of age. The cause is thought to be simple overconsumption of milk. Similarly, vigorous lambs sucking high-producing ewes may develop diarrhea. Foals commonly have diarrhea at about 9 days of age which coincides with the foal heat of the mare. It has been thought for many years that the cause was a sudden change in the composition of the mares' milk but this has not been supported by analyses of mares' milk at that time (9). The fecal composition in foal heat diarrhea suggests that the diarrhea is a secretory-type hypersecretion of the small intestine mucosa which may not be controlled by an immature colon (19).

In recent years there has been considerable interest in determining the optimal conditions for feeding liquid diets to young calves. The temperature of the liquid when fed, feeding once or twice daily and the amount of dry matter intake can affect the performance of calves. However, there is a range of safety in which the performance of the calves will not be significantly affected if management is good (10). In one study, home-bred calves reared carefully in a good environment were relatively resistant to substantial changes in the composition and methods of feeding milk substitutes (11).

Dietary diarrhea also occurs in all species following a sudden change in diet but particularly in animals at weaning time. This is particularly important in the pig weaned at 3 weeks of age and not adjusted to the postweaning ration.

Pathogenesis

In calves, the ingestion of excessive quantities of cows' whole milk after several hours of no intake causes gross distension of the abomasum and possibly of the rumen. Under these conditions, the milk-clotting capacity of the abomasum may be limited, resulting in incomplete clotting. The flow of nutrients from the abomasum is more uniform in calves fed twice daily than once daily which suggests that twice daily feeding allows for more effective clotting and digestion (12).

Under normal conditions, the milk clot forms in the abomasum within minutes after feeding, and the whey moves to the duodenum within 5–10 minutes later. Overfeeding could result in whole milk or excessive quantities of whey entering the duodenum which cannot digest whole milk or satisfactorily digest and hydrolyze the substrates in whey. The presence of excessive quantities of such substrate, especially lactose, in the intestinal lumen would severe as a hydrogogue and result in a large increase in intestinal fluid, failure of complete absorption and abnormal feces. The speed of drinking is probably also important. Prolongation of drinking time results in dilution of the milk with saliva and the production of a more easily digested milk clot (13). Failure of the esophageal reflex in pail-fed calves may also be important. The milk enters the rumen where it undergoes putrefaction.

The pathogenesis of malabsorption and diarrhea in calves fed inferior quality milk replacers has been reasonably well examined (2). Heat-denatured skim-milk powder is incompletely clotted in the abomasum leading to reduced digestibility. Non-milk carbohydrates and non-milk proteins are not well digested by preruminant calves under 3 weeks of age because their amylase, maltase and sucrase activities are insignificant, and their pepsin-HCl activity is not well developed until at least 3 weeks of age. Following the ingestion of these nutrients, there is reduced digestibility, malabsorption and diarrhea. This results in a negative nutrient balance, loss of body weight and gradual starvation, all of which is reversible by the feeding of cows' whole milk. The digestion of fat is particularly affected resulting in varying degrees of steatorrhea.

The mechanism for the malabsorption and diarrhea which commonly occurs in all species following a sudden change in diet is not well understood. However, it is known that several days may be necessary for the necessary qualitative and quantitative changes to occur in the digestive enzyme capacity (14). Not much attention has been devoted to the study of development of intestinal enzymes in the fetus and newborn, but this is likely to be of importance in individual animals. Some work has been done in calves (15, 16) in which lactase activity is fully developed at birth. In the period between birth and weaning there are significant changes in enzyme activity, some of them influenced by the presence or absence of dietary substances.

Regardless of the cause of dietary diarrhea, the presence of undigested substrate in the intestine can lead to marked changes in the bacterial flora which may result in fermentation of carbohydrates and putrefaction of protein, the products of which accentuate the malabsorption (1). If enteropathogenic *E. coli* or *Salmonella* spp. are present they may colonize, proliferate in large numbers and cause enteric colibacillosis and salmonellosis.

Clinical findings

Dietary diarrhea of beef calves 3 weeks of age running at pasture is characterized by the passage of light-yellow feces which are foul-smelling and soft. The perineum and tail are usually smudged with feces. The calves are bright and alert and usually recover spontaneously without treatment in a few days.

Hand-fed calves overfed on cows' whole milk are usually dull, anorexic and their feces are voluminous, foul-smelling and contain considerable mucus. The abdomen may be distended due to distension of the abomasum and intestines. Secondary enteric colibacillosis and salmonellosis may occur resulting in severe dehydration. Most uncomplicated cases will respond with oral fluid therapy and withdrawal from or deprivation of milk.

In calves fed inferior quality milk replacers, there will be a chronic diarrhea with gradual weight loss. The calves are bright and alert, they usually drink normally, appear distended after drinking and spend considerable time in recumbency. Not uncommonly many treatments will have been tried unsuccessfully. The diarrhea and weight loss continues and in 2–4 weeks emaciation is evident and death from starvation may occur. Affected calves will often have a depraved appetite and eat bedding and other indigestible materials which further accentuates the condition. When large numbers of calves are involved, the incidence of enteric colibacillosis and salmonellosis may become high and the case mortality very high. This is a common situation in veal calf-rearing units.

Outbreaks of alopecia in calves fed a milk substitute have been observed but pathogenesis is not understood (18).

Clinical pathology

Laboratory evaluation of the animals is usually not necessary other than for elimination of other possible causes of the diarrhea. When milk-replacers are being used the determination of the rennet-clotting time of the milk replacer compared with whole milk is a useful aid in assessing the quality of the skim-milk powder for calves.

Necropsy findings

Emaciation, an absence of body fat, dehydration and serous atrophy are present in calves which have died from diarrhea and starvation while being fed inferior quality milk replacers (3).

Diagnosis

Dietary diarrhea occurs following a change in diet, the consumption of too much feed at once, or poor quality feed. There are usually no systemic signs and recovery occurs spontaneously when the dietary abnormality is corrected or the animal adapts to a new diet.

Treatment

In hand-fed calves affected with dietary diarrhea, milk feeding should be stopped and oral electrolyte solutions given for 24 hours. Milk is then gradually reintroduced. If milk replacers are being used their nutrient composition and quality should be examined for evidence of indigestible nutrients. Occasional cases of dietary diarrhea in calves will require intensive fluid therapy and antibacterials orally and parenterally. The feeding practices should be examined and the necessary adjustments made.

Beef calves affected with dietary diarrhea while sucking the cow and running on pasture do not usually require treatment unless complications develop. They must be observed daily for evidence of dullness, anorexia, inactivity and profuse watery diarrhea, at which point they need some medical care.

Foals with dietary diarrhea should be muzzled for 12 hours, which may require a hand-stripping of the mare to relieve tension in the udder and to prevent engorgement when the foal begins to suck again. Antidiarrheal compounds containing electrolytes, kaolin and pectin with or without antibiotics are used commonly but are probably not any more effective than oral electrolyte solutions for 24 hours.

The care and management of hand-fed calves to minimize the incidence of dietary diarrhea is an art. Much has been said about the use of slow-flowing nipple bottles and pails to reduce dietary diarrhea but they are not a replacement for good management. Calves which are raised for herd replacements should be fed on whole milk if possible for up to 3 weeks. When large numbers of calves are reared for veal or for feedlots the milk replacer used should be formulated using the highest quality milk and milk by-products which are economically possible. The more inferior the milk replacer the more impeccable must become the management, which is difficult given today's labor situation.

The problem of weanling diarrhea in pigs is discussed elsewhere.

REVIEW LITERATURE

Appleman, R. D. & Owen, F. G. (1975) Symposium: recent advances in calf rearing. Breeding, housing and feeding management. *J. dairy Sci.*, *58*, 447.

Radostits, O. M. & Bell, J. M. (1970) Nutrition of the preruminant dairy calf with special reference to the digestion and absorption of nutrients: A review. *Can. J. anim. Sci.*, *50*, 405.

Roy, J. H. B. (1969) Diarrhoea of nutritional origin. *Proc. Nutr. Soc.*, *28*, 160.

REFERENCES

(1) Roy, J. H. B. (1969) *Proc. Nutr. Soc.*, *28*, 160.
(2) Roy, J. H. B. & Ternouth, J. H. (1972) *Proc. Nutr. Soc.*, *31*, 53.
(3) Thomson, R. G. (1967) *Can. vet. J.*, *8*, 242.
(4) Sissons, J. W. & Thurston, S. M. (1984) *Res. vet. Sci.*, 37: 242.
(5) Huber, J. T. (1975) *J. dairy Sci.*, *58*, 441.
(6) Jenny, B. F. et al. (1982) *J. dairy Sci.*, 65: 2345.
(7) Stiles, R. P. et al. (1974) *Can. J. anim. Sci.*, *54*, 73.
(8) Mylrea, P. J. (1966) *Res. vet. Sci.*, *7*, 417.
(9) Johnston, R. H. et al. (1970) *J. anim. Sci.*, *31*, 549.
(10) Appleman, R. D. & Owen, F. G. (1975) *J. dairy Sci.*, *58*, 447.
(11) Burt, A. W. A. & Irvine, S. M. (1972) *Anim. Prod.*, *14*, 299.
(12) Leibolz, J. (1975) *Aust. J. agric. Res.*, *26*, 623.
(13) Wise, G. H. et al. (1947) *J. dairy Sci*, *30*, 499.
(14) Radostits, O. M. & Bell, J. M. (1968) *Can. J. anim. Sci.*, *48*, 293.
(15) Toofanian, F. et al. (1974) *Res. vet. Sci.*, *16*, 375.
(16) Toofanian, F. et al. (1974) *Res. vet. Sci.*, *16*, 382.
(17) Johnston, W. S. et al. (1980) *Vet. Rec.*, *106*, 174.
(18) Pritchard, G. C. et al. (1983) *Vet. Rec.*, *112*, 435.
(19) Masri, M. D. et al. (1986) *Equ. vet. J.*, *18*, 301.

Intestinal or duodenal ulceration

Intestinal ulceration occurs in animals only as a result of enteritis and clinically with manifestations of enteritis. As far as is known there is no counterpart of the psychosomatic disease which occurs in man. Ulceration does occur in many specific erosive diseases listed elsewhere, and in salmonellosis and swine fever, but the lesions are present in the terminal part of the ileum, and more commonly in the cecum and colon.

Duodenal ulcers in cattle and horses have a similar epidemiological distribution as gastric ulcers and also resemble them clinically. Occasionally they perforate, causing subacute peritonitis (3).

A perforated duodenal ulcer in a foal is recorded as causing acute, fatal peritonitis manifested by pain, dyspnea and vomiting (1). Moderate to severe ulceration of the mucosa of the cecum and colon is described in phenylbutazone toxicity in ponies. The dose rate of phenylbutazone was 12 mg/kg body weight/day for 8 days. There is significant hypoproteinemia due to protein loss from the gut (2). A similar hypoproteinemia has been produced in thoroughbred horses, but there was no clinical illness.

REFERENCES

(1) Orr, J. P. (1972) *Vet. Rec.*, *90*, 571.
(2) Snow, D. H. et al. (1980) *Vet. Rec.*, *106*, 68.
(3) Fatimah, I. et al. (1982) *Can. vet. J.*, *23*, 173.

Impaction of the ileocecal valve

Impaction of the ileocecal valve occurs commonly only in horses, causing a syndrome of subacute abdominal pain followed by one of acute pain. It is commonly fatal and is comparable in severity to acute intestinal obstruction.

Etiology

The common cause is feeding on low-grade, finely chopped roughage (1).

Pathogenesis

The finely chopped straw or poor hay passes through the stomach in an undigested form and collects in the terminal ileum at the ileocecal valve. The obstruction is complete and the further pathogenesis is identical with that of acute intestinal obstruction except that the local vascular occlusion which occurs in the latter disease is not present and shock does not occur. For this reason, the course of the disease is more prolonged.

Clinical findings

The syndrome develops in two stages (2). Initially there is a period of 8–12 hours in which subacute abdominal pain is evidenced, the horse doing some rolling and pawing and looking at the flank but there is no great increase in pulse rate or respiration. The intestinal sounds are increased in frequency and intensity. Rectal examination may reveal no abnormality although, with careful palpation, the enlarged, impacted ileum may be detectable in the upper right flank at the base of the cecum, although this is easily confused with an impaction of the small colon.

At the end of this phase, the pain increases in severity. There is severe depression, patchy sweating and coldness of the extremities and the animal stands with its head hung down, sits on its haunches and rolls and struggles violently. The abdominal pain becomes severe and continuous, the pulse rate rises to between 80 and 120/minute and the pulse is weak. Respirations are increased to 30–40/minute and the temperature up to 39·5°C (103°F). The abdominal sounds are almost entirely absent at this stage and passage of a nasal tube is followed by aspiration of sanguineous fluid, often in quantities up to several liters. On rectal examination, the large intestine is small and contracted but the small intestine is so tightly distended with gas and fluid that proper examination of the viscera is impossible although tightly stretched bands of mesentery may be palpable. Death usually occurs within 36–48 hours after the onset of illness.

Clinical pathology

Peritoneal fluid obtained by paracentesis is normal, serving to differentiate this disease from small intestinal obstruction in which the blood supply is compromised.

Necropsy findings

The distal 30–45 cm in the ileum are firmly packed with finely chopped fibrous material, and the small intestine and even the stomach are tightly distended with up to 90–135 liters of bloodstained fluid.

Diagnosis

In the early stages, the disease is easily mistaken for spasmodic colic or enteritis because of the moderate, acute pain and the increased intestinal sounds. The history of the diet and palpation of the impacted ileum are the principal differentiating features. In addition, the continuation of the illness suggests ileocecal valve impaction. In the second phase, the disease resembles acute tympany of the intestine except that the small rather than the large intestine is obstructed, or acute intestinal obstruction where shock is more severe and again it is the large intestine which is usually affected. Horses which develop an acute obstruction while rolling due to the pain of spasmodic colic or impaction of the large intestine present a clinical syndrome almost identical with that of ileocecal valve impaction. The characteristic features of ileocecal valve impaction are the gross accumulation of fluid and the relatively long course. See Table 16 for a summary of differentiation.

Treatment

Removal of fluid from the stomach prolongs the animal's life and eases the discomfort but intravenous alimentation is necessary to replace the lost fluids. Sedatives must be administered because of the severe bruising usually incurred during bouts of violent struggling. Removal of the obstruction is necessary if the patient is to survive but usually proves to be impossible without surgical interference. A large dose of mineral oil (2–4 liters), preferably containing a wetting agent, should be followed in 2–3 hours by a parasympathetic stimulant. The increased intestinal motility causes a reappearance of severe pain and rupture of the intestine may occur. Enterotomy carried out early in the development of the disease provides a satisfactory solution to the problem (1).

REFERENCES

(1) Embertson, R. M. et al. (1985) *J. Am. vet. med. Assoc.*, *186*, 570.
(2) Hutchins, D. R. (1952) *Aust. vet. J.*, *28*, 236.

Ileal hypertrophy

There are a number of weakly defined syndromes characterized by thickening of the wall of the terminal ileum.

Terminal ileal hypertrophy in horses

This is a long-term chronic or mild intermittent colic which persists over a period of weeks, sometimes months. The colicky pain is evidenced by crouching, flank-watching, and sometimes pawing, but nothing more serious than this. Pain is often worse after feeding. There are increased gut sounds especially over the ileocecal valve. On rectal examination the greatly thickened ileum can be palpated at the base of the cecum, and there are also distended loops of thick-walled ileum (1). On laparotomy the distended loops of intestine are found to have thick, hypertrophic walls. The cause is unknown.

Difficulty can be experienced in differentiating ileal hypertrophy from chronic intussusception, especially of the terminal ileum into the cecum. Fluid ingesta can pass the much constricted lumen so that mural hypertrophy occurs orally. A similar clinical picture results from stenosis of the small intestine by adhesions, usually resulting from verminous migration. In all three diseases there is increased mobility of the small intestine, and there is no interference with the blood supply.

Hypertrophy and diverticulosis in horses

There is hypertrophy of the wall of the terminal ileum apparently in response to increased resistance of the flow of ingesta. It seems probable that the resistance is at least partly provided by the diverticulosis, although that lesion is not always present (2). Colic is not recorded, the predominant clinical sign being chronic or intermittent diarrhea.

Diverticulitis and ileitis of pigs (proliferative ileitis)

In this disease there is thickening of the wall of the ileum, particularly in the terminal portion, so that the intestine becomes thick and rigid. There is a close clinical similarity to Crohn's disease in man and the etiology of both conditions is obscure. Familial predisposition is probable in man and has been suggested in pigs.

The signs are those of acute peritonitis due to ulceration and, sometimes, perforation of the affected ileum. Illness occurs suddenly with loss of appetite, excessive thirst, dullness and disinclination to rise. The temperature is subnormal, the respiration is distressed and there is a bluish discoloration of the skin. Death occurs in 24–36 hours.

Acute cases occur in young pigs up to 3 months of age, and chronic cases, due to ulceration and chronic peritonitis, in the 7–8 month age group.

At necropsy there may be diffuse peritonitis due to

leakage of alimentary tract contents through perforating ileal ulcers. Gross thickening of the ileal wall with nodular proliferation of the ileal mucosa (3) and enlargement of the mesenteric lymph nodes are common accompaniments. Although the macroscopic findings are similar to those of Crohn's disease in man, the histopathological findings differ markedly (4, 5). There is an obvious and significant protein loss through the intestinal lesion and a marked hypoproteinemia (6).

Terminal ileitis of lambs

This disease causes poor growth in lambs 4–6 months old (2, 7). The circumstances usually suggest parasitism or coccidiosis. The terminal 50–75 cm of the ileum is thickened and resembles the classical lesion of Johne's disease. Chronic inflammation is evident and there are some shallow ulcers in the epithelium. The terminal mesenteric lymph mode is enlarged. Histopathological examination of affected ileal wall shows mucosa thickened by epithelial hyperplasia, leukocytic infiltration and connective tissue infiltration. The cause is unknown, and the course of the disease has not been identified because most affected lambs are likely to be culled for ill-thrift.

REFERENCES

(1) Mason, T. A. et al. (1970) *Aust. vet. J.*, *46*, 349.
(2) Cordes, D. O. & Dewes, H. F. (1971) *NZ vet. J.*, *19*, 108.
(3) Dodd, D. C. (1968) *Pathol. Vet.*, *5*, 333.
(4) Field, H. I. et al. (1953) *J. comp. Pathol.*, *63*, 153.
(5) Rahkot, T. & Saloniemi, H. (1972) *Nord. VetMed.*, *24*, 132.
(6) Martinsson, K. et al. (1974) *Svensk VetTidn.*, *26*, 347.
(7) Cross, R. F. et al. (1973) *J. Am. vet. med. Assoc.*, *162*, 564.

Intestinal tympany

Intestinal tympany causes distension of the abdomen and severe abdominal pain and is sometimes accompanied by the passage of much flatus.

Etiology

Most cases of intestinal tympany occur in the horse and are secondary to obstruction of the intestinal lumen. All cases of tympany of the small intestine are caused by some form of intestinal obstruction. Tympany of the large intestine may be primary or secondary.

Primary large bowel tympany

- Ingestion of large quantities of highly fermentable green feed
- Ingestion of excess whey. Recorded in adult dry sows. Distension of proximal colon caused rupture with death from endotoxic shock (1).

Secondary large bowel tympany

- Horses—stenosis by constricting fibrous adhesions after castration, verminous aneurysm
- Pigs and ruminants—usually secondary to acute intestinal obstruction.

Pathogenesis

The excessive production of gas or its retention in a segment of bowel causes distension and acute abdominal pain. In primary tympany, the distension is periodically reduced by the evacuation of some gas and the course is relatively long. In secondary tympany, the pathogenesis depends largely on the primary cause, the distension adding a further burden. Some interference with circulation and respiration occurs and may contribute to death in cases which terminate fatally.

Clinical findings

Abdominal distension is evident in all species and the distended loops of intestine may be visible through the abdominal wall in thin animals. Pain is acute and affected horses may roll and paw violently. Peristaltic sounds are reduced but fluid may be heard moving in gas-filled, intestinal loops producing a tinkling, metallic sound. On rectal examination, gas-filled loops of intestine fill the abdominal cavity and make proper examination of its contents impossible. In primary tympany much flatus is passed and the anus may be in a state of continuous dilatation.

Clinical pathology

Laboratory examinations are of no value in diagnosis.

Necropsy findings

In cases of secondary tympany, the causative obstruction is evident. In primary cases, the intestines are filled with gas and the feces are usually pasty and loose.

Diagnosis

Primary tympany is always difficult to differentiate from secondary tympany and the presence of an intestinal obstruction may be difficult to determine as rectal examination is impeded. If flatus and feces are passed and if there is a history of engorgement on lush, legume pasture, primary tympany is probably the cause. Intestinal obstructions usually cause death in a much shorter time and the distension is often restricted to short lengths of intestine whereas primary tympany usually involves most if not all of the tract.

Treatment

In severe primary cases, trocarization with a long, small-caliber intestinal trocar and cannula may be necessary. This can be performed *per rectum* or through the upper right or left flank depending on the site of maximum distension. The distension is usually on the right-hand side, and the dorsal sac of the cecum suggests itself as a target of reasonable size. All cases should receive mineral oil (2–4 liters), containing an antiferment such as oil of turpentine (14–28 g), formalin (28 g) or chloroform (28 g). It may be necessary to administer a sedative if pain is acute.

In secondary tympany, permanent relief can be obtained only by correction of the obstruction.

REFERENCES

(1) McCausland, I. P. & Southgate, W. (1980) *Aust. vet. J.*, *56*, 190.

Verminous mesenteric arteritis (verminous aneurysm, thromboembolic colic)

Migration of the larvae of *Strongylus vulgaris* into the wall of the cranial mesenteric artery and its branches occurs commonly in horses and may cause restriction of the blood supply or damage to the nerve supply to the intestines, although experimentally induced vascular obstruction is not accompanied by colic (13). When horses are run at pasture for most of the year, none can be expected to escape strongylosis completely, even in those herds where moderately good worm control is practiced. In these circumstances about 90% of horses will show lesions of arteritis (1). The disease is basically an infarction of bowel wall without displacement of the bowel. The infarction is usually caused by thrombosis of mesenteric vessels due to invasion by *Strongylus vulgaris* larvae. It is difficult to diagnose without laparotomy and has a very high death rate (11). Resection of the affected bowel is usually not attempted because of the multiplicity of the lesions. Cases may occur in foals as young as 4–6 months. Complete vascular occlusion occurs in some cases and leads to infarction of sections of the large intestine. In these animals there is moderately severe abdominal pain for 3–4 days with almost complete cessation of defecation and absence of intestinal sounds due to stasis. However, in the early stages, there may be increased gut sounds, to the degree where spasmodic colic is suspected.

On rectal examination distended loops of intestines and tightly stretched mesentery may be felt, but the distension is neither severe nor general. If the horse is not too large, it is often possible to palpate the root of the cranial mesenteric artery as a fixed, firm swelling in the midline, level with the caudal pole of the left kidney. It will be much enlarged, have a rough, knobbly surface and it usually pulsates with each pulse wave. The colic and cecal arteries are usually thickened and enlarged to about 1 cm in diameter and have palpable lumps along them. These cases always terminate fatally, due either to peritonitis after rupture of the intestinal wall (4), or to toxemia caused by gangrene of the intestinal wall. Occasional cases with extensive occlusion die quickly, in 12–24 hours, due probably to shock from the massive infarction (5). Another (uncommon) syndrome is the development of a massive hemorrhage within the mesentery so that a large fold of it is virtually a sheet of blood. Clinically there is severe abdominal pain, and shock with pallor; paracentesis shows bloodstained fluid in the peritoneal cavity and the fluid will also have a high leukocyte count with a significant shift to the left. Because of obstruction of venous return there is also extensive hemorrhagic leakage into the lumen of the gut, so that feces may be passed, and they will be obviously bloodstained. Protein loss in the feces is considerable so that blood albumin levels are low. By contrast, the globulins are high, especially if the lesion is of long duration, so that the total serum protein level is often elevated (2). Radiological examination has been used to determine the presence of verminous aneurysms in Shetland ponies (10).

At necropsy, the arteries are partially or completely occluded along a large part of their course and larvae are usually found in the walls or free in the lumen. In severe cases, large patches of gangrene are present in the wall of atonic loops of bowel. Secondary bacterial invasion of the aneurysm may occur and cause gross enlargement and local peritonitis with the development of adhesions and eventual constriction of the intestine. In these cases there is usually a history of intermittent or continuous low-grade abdominal pain over a period as long as several months. The clinical signs are very similar to those of terminal ileal hypertrophy (8) but the two conditions may be distinguishable on the basis of rectal findings. In both diseases confirmation of the diagnosis and treatment can only be effected via a laparotomy incision.

Commonly the disease is not suspected until recurrent attacks of colic occur. Blood eosinophil counts and fecal examinations for worm eggs are of little value in diagnosis. Treatment with an anthelmintic such as thiabendazole (500 mg/kg), along with supportive treatment when indicated, is recommended (12). An unusually high recovery rate is recorded in affected horses treated with the plasma expander dextran 70. The treatment regimen is intravenous injection of 2·5 ml/kg body weight/day for 3 days followed by further injections at 4-day intervals for a total of nine injections (6). The preparation has marked anticoagulant properties. All forms of treatment, including parasympathetic stimulants, are ineffective. Surgical intervention is not usually recommended because a number of infarcted areas of intestine are usually present at the one time, and additional infarctions are likely to occur. Occasionally it is attempted (7).

Recurrent colic is commonly diagnosed as being due to strongylosis and chronic low-grade impairment of the vascular and nerve supply to the intestine (9). Such cases also occur when a secondary bacterial infection, usually *Streptococcus equi*, *Actinobacillus equuli* or *Salmonella typhimurium*, becomes established in the aneurysm. The signs produced by mesenteric abscess are similar to those of verminous aneurysm, but the temperature is usually elevated and rupture of the abscess may lead to the development of a diffuse peritonitis. This condition has been diagnosed by radiographic examination after the production of pneumoperitoneum, but it is more likely that these are cases of recurrent mesenteric embolism. Other causes of recurrent colic are continued overfeeding of horses that are prone to gorge, the gross eaters of the horse world, and adhesions due to previous peritonitis or embryonic retentions such as Meckel's diverticulum (3).

REVIEW LITERATURE

White, N. A. (1985) Thromboembolic colic in horses. *Comp. cont. Educ.*, 7, S156–S161.

REFERENCES

(1) Wright, A. I. (1971) *Equ. vet. J.*, *4*, 169.
(2) Ooms, L. et al. (1976) *Vlaams Diergeneeskd. Tijdschr.*, *45*, 290.
(3) Suann, C. J. & Livesey, M. A. (1986) *Vet. Rec.*, *118*, 230.
(4) Curtis, R. A. (1964) *Can. vet. J.*, *5*, 36.
(5) Nelson, A. W. et al. (1968) *Am. J. vet. Res.*, *29*, 315.
(6) Greatorex, J. C. (1977) *Vet. Rec.*, *101*, 184.
(7) Rau, D. (1973) *Prakt. Tierärztl.*, *54*, 435.
(8) Mason, T. A. et al. (1970) *Aust. vet. J.*, *46*, 349.
(9) Gay, C. C. & Spiers, V. C. (1978) *Aust. vet. J.*, *54*, 600.
(10) Slocombe, J. O. D. et al. (1977) *Proc. 23rd Ann. Conv. Am. Assoc. equ. Pract.*, p. 305.
(11) White, N. A. (1981) *J. Am. vet. med. Assoc.*, *178*, 259.

(12) Coffman, J. R. & Carlson, K. L. (1971) *J. Am. vet. med. Assoc.*, *158*, 1358.
(13) Sellers, A. F. et al. (1982) *Cornell Vet.*, *72*, 233.

Impaction of the large intestine

Impaction of the large intestine causes moderate abdominal pain, constipation and a syndrome of general depression and anorexia.

Etiology

In farm animals, the disease is common only in horses and pigs. Rare cases are recorded in cows and are discussed in Chapter 6. A number of causative factors are implicated in horses. For the most part, they are dietary causes and include feeding on low-grade, indigestible roughage, particularly old hay and sorghum, defective teeth causing improper mastication of the roughage, and feeding at overlong intervals.

Dietary causes

- Horses starved before surgery are likely to eat ravenously immediately after gaining their feet after surgery and should be restricted in their feed intake, especially by being deprived of the bedding. Impaction may occur as a result, manifesting itself next day, but esophageal obstruction, acute gastric dilatation and a colic manifested by hypermotility may occur within a few hours
- Horses which come into loose boxes and are offered hard feed after being on soft grass on pasture are also likely to develop impaction colic. Stored feeds and even bedding are likely to be palatable and they may eat excessively during the first few days. Impaction colic can also occur in horses accustomed to being housed indoors if the straw used as bedding is palatable, as it may be if the crop is harvested early leaving some grain in the straw which also has a green tint
- Overfed, fat horses and greedy feeders are particularly susceptible to recurrent attacks of the disease.

Other causes

- General debility is a predisposing cause in that the diminished intestinal muscle tone is incapable of moving the large bulk of ingesta
- Interference with the local blood supply to the intestine, short of complete occlusion of vessels such as occurs in verminous mesenteric arteritis, has the same effect
- Enteroliths and fiber balls may also cause obstruction of the large intestine and usually result in recurrent attacks of colic. They usually form in the small colon or are obstructed there or at the end of the right dorsal colon, when moving on from their development site in a lumen of larger diameter. Fiber balls (phytobezoars) occur rarely in horses, most physical obstructions of the lumen being enteroliths. Enteroliths are found only in horses which are more than 4 years old with the highest age incidence being 5–10 years (10). They are composed of ammonium magnesium phosphate. The mineral is deposited in concentric layers, alternating with food material, around some ingested foreign body (5). There may be several of them and some of them are passed in the feces. They are reported to be increasing in prevalence in some parts of the United States (15)
- Foreign bodies, especially pieces of rope, can also find their way to the small colon causing a severe impaction which requires enterotomy to correct. A large number of cases is now recorded of horses nibbling plastic or rubber covering from coated fence wire and developing colonic obstructions as a result (9, 13). The clinical syndrome includes moderate abdominal pain, distended loops of small colon on rectal examination and failure to pass feces. Reflux of fluid into the stomach is a common accompaniment. Medical treatment is ineffective and after a course of about 3 days the horses are usually operated on because of continuing pain
- Recurrent attacks may also be caused by persistence of any of the causative factors listed above
- An unusual, sometimes fetal impaction of the large intestine of horses is caused by the administration of Amitraz, a formamidine acaricide for cattle, but forbidden for use in horses (8)
- Retention of the meconium in foals is a common and special occurrence of impaction of the large intestine (2). Colt foals are more commonly affected than fillies, and foals carried over time and which have a narrow pelvis are most susceptible. Meconium retention is also part of the 'watery mouth' syndrome of lambs
- In cows and mares near parturition, an apparent rectal paralysis leading to constipation may occur. The cause is unknown but is considered to be the result of pressure by the fetus or fetuses on pelvic nerves
- In pigs impaction of the colon and rectum occurs sporadically, usually in adult sows which get little exercise and are fed wholly on grain. The disease also occurs in pigs which are overcrowded in sandy or gravelly outdoor yards
- A special occurrence in young weaned pigs causes obstruction of the coiled colon
- A presumed inherited megacolon of fattening pigs is reported as a cause of abdominal distension, constipation and wasting. There is no anal stricture (4)
- Rectal paralysis is also an occasional development in encephalitis of horses.

Pathogenesis

Continued overloading of the colon and cecum, either primarily, because of the nature of the food, or secondarily, because of poor intestinal motility, causes prolongation of the intestinal sojourn and excessive inspissation of fecal material so that movement of the mass by peristalsis is still further impaired. If the process is prolonged, the colon becomes insensitive to the stimuli caused by distension which normally provoke defecation. Chronic constipation results.

In horses, the effects of impaction of the large intestine are more serious than in other animals because of the tremendous capacity of the organ. Accumulation of fecal material occurs gradually until sufficient distension is present to cause pain. Autointoxication may also play a part in the production of clinical signs. Although impaction of the cecum and colon usually occur together, it is not uncommon to find maximum impaction in one particular region. Thus impaction may be restricted to the cecum, the small colon or the pelvic flexure of the large colon.

In pigs, the effects appear to be due largely to autointoxication although the commonly occurring posterior paresis seems more likely to be due to pressure from inspissated fecal material.

Clinical findings

Moderate abdominal pain is the typical sign in affected horses and pulse rate and respiration are relatively normal. This often continues for 3–4 days and sometimes for as long as 2 weeks. A very long course of more than 3–4 days is usually associated with enteroliths or cecal impaction. The horse is not violent, the principal manifestation of pain being stretching out and lying down and the bouts of pain are of moderate severity occurring at intervals of up to a half-hour. There is anorexia and constipation, and the feces are passed in small amounts and are hard and covered with thick, sticky mucus. Complete absence of defecation is common with enteroliths. Intestinal sounds are absent or much decreased in intensity. Rectal palpation usually enables one to detect the cause of the trouble.

Impaction of the pelvic flexure of the large colon is the commonest site and the distended, solid loop of the intestine often extends to the pelvic brim or even to the right of the midline. Lying on the floor of the abdomen, it is easily palpated, the fecal mass can be indented with the fingers and the curvature and groove between the dorsal and ventral loops of the left colon can be easily discerned.

Impaction of the cecum can be palpated in the right flank extending from high up and passing downwards and anteriorly. An impacted small colon may be felt dorsally to the right of the midline and almost at arm's length. Its diameter is much less than that of the other segments and it may be confused with an impacted terminal ileum. Cecal impactions have a bad prognosis (7). Some of them die of cecal rupture (14), most require surgical correction. It is possible that drugs used in anesthesia cause serious reduction in gut motility and thus predispose to these dilatations and ruptures (14).

Enteroliths and similar foreign bodies are usually located in the entrance to the small colon and may or may not be palpable per rectum. The cecum and colon are distended with gas and ingesta, and a reflux distension of the stomach with fluid is detectable in some cases by passing a nasal tube (13). The wall of the colon is usually tightly adhered to the foreign body and in the case of irregularly shaped or pitted ones pressure necrosis may develop so that the bowel ruptures.

The pulse rate may be moderately increased but does not usually rise above 50/minute and the temperature and respiratory rates are unaffected. Although the animal does not eat, it may drink small quantities of water at frequent intervals, often standing by the water trough and sipping or lapping the water continuously. Most cases respond satisfactorily to treatment although impaction of the cecum is difficult to relieve and may cause a fatal termination. Straining is an unusual sign except in foals with retention of meconium. It is usually an indication of an obstruction low down in the large intestine, often in the pelvis itself. Recurrence of impaction of the large intestine is common and is usually due to failure to correct the cause. When deaths occur, they are due to rupture of the intestine or from exhaustion after a long course.

Retention of the meconium in foals causes continuous straining with elevation of the tail, humping of the back with the feet under the body and even walking backwards. There is no toxemia and the colt continues to suck intermittently but is inclined to be restless and lie down for much of the time. Hard fecal balls can be palpated with the finger in the rectum.

In pigs, the syndrome has no specific signs. There is anorexia and dullness and the pig is recumbent much of the time. Feces passed are scanty, very hard and covered with mucus. Weakness to the point of inability to rise occurs in some cases. Hard balls of feces in the rectum are usually detected when a thermometer is inserted. In paralysis of the rectum, there is inability to defecate and usually some straining. The anus and rectum are ballooned and manual removal of the feces does not result in contraction of the rectum. Spontaneous recovery usually occurs 3–4 days after parturition.

Clinical pathology

Laboratory examinations are not usually undertaken except for fecal examinations for nematode eggs. Paracentesis and blood chemistry findings are normal and blood pressure is raised. A novel test which could qualify as clinical pathology consists of dosing the horse with 4 mm diameter plastic beads used as fecal markers, 50 of these being given in water by stomach tube. Failure of the markers to appear in the feces within 40 hours suggests that there is an unresolved impaction. The time of appearance of the markers may be as short as 24 hours. The size of the beads is critical, and those larger than 4 mm tend to stay caught up in the bowel. Oil and fluid may be passed around an enterolith or dense impaction, but the beads will not (6).

Necropsy findings

The large intestine is packed full of firm, dry fecal material and rupture may have occurred. Enteroliths are commonly located at the junction of the right dorsal colon and the small colon.

Diagnosis

Other causes of constipation such as peritonitis and dehydration must be considered when making a diagnosis of impaction of the large intestine.

Other forms of colic can be eliminated from consideration largely on the basis of rectal palpation, the absence of systemic signs and intestinal sounds (*see* Table 16 for a summary of causes). Acute gastric dilatation, acute intestinal obstruction and spasmodic colic are more severe and have a much shorter course. Palpation of the cranial mesenteric artery is necessary to make a diagnosis of verminous mesenteric arteritis. In foals, tympany of the large intestine occurs but is much more serious, with abdominal distension and acute abdominal pain the cardinal signs. Moderate straining, dullness and gradual distension of the abdomen are the main clinical features of rupture of the bladder in newborn foals and this can be mistaken for retention of the meconium.

Treatment

Many forms of treatment have been used in horses but one of the most satisfactory is the administration of 3–5 liters of mineral oil containing 15–30 g of chloral hydrate in 1 liter of water by nasal tube. A common alternative to the chloral is the parenteral administration of an ataractic drug. If the impaction is not relieved in 12 hours, the treatment is repeated, together with the subcutaneous injection of a parasympathetic stimulant. Parasympathetic stimulants, for example 10–12 mg neostigmine intramuscularly, should not be used without prior administration of oil to soften the fecal mass, or rupture of the overdistended intestine may result. Most cases respond to the first treatment but more severe cases may require a second treatment. Impactions of the cecum are the most intractable as soft feces may be passed through the dorsal sac without emptying the ventral sac. Surgical intervention is sometimes necessary (1). Linseed oil may be used instead of mineral oil but has no particular advantage and has the disadvantage that in some horses the usual dose of 600 ml causes superpurgation and the problem of correcting the fluid loss. Of the anthriquinone purgatives of 30 years ago only Istizin (Danthron Rx) is still in limited use, 10–30 g by bolus, avoiding overdosing because of the same awkward sequel of severe and continuing diarrhea. Saline purgatives are best avoided unless one is quite sure that there is no intestinal obstruction and therefore an already existing sequestration of fluid in the gut lumen. Detergents have been found to be of value when combined with mineral oil in severe constipation in humans (2) and are now used in the treatment of animals. Some interesting experimental observations have been made on the effects of large-volume enemas, up to 44 liters, on the small colon and its contents (11). However, the theoretical advantages of their use in cases of colic have not been demonstrated in clinical cases (12).

Dioctyl sodium sulfosuccinate (DOSS), an anionic surface-active substance and wetting agent, has been used extensively for the treatment of impaction of the large intestine in the horse. The dosage recommended ranges from 7·5 to 30 g per adult horse orally, with a maximum dose of 0·2 g/kg body weight. One-half of the original dose may be given on the second and third days. It is an effective fecal softening agent because of its wetting agent characteristics. Commonly it is given on the first day of treatment followed by the administration of mineral oil on the second day, or the drug may be mixed with the mineral oil. However, dioctyl sodium sulfosuccinate is toxic at levels from three to five times the recommended therapeutic doses. When given at the level of 1 g/kg body weight there is diarrhea, rapid dehydration, fluid distension of the intestinal tract and death in 14–72 hours following administration (3).

Some impactions do not respond to medical therapy alone and if the obstruction is not cleared by 72 hours, surgical correction should be considered.

Retention of the meconium in foals is treated by injecting mineral oil (60–80 g), glycerin (28 g) or dioctyl sodium sulfosuccinate (Coloxyl) into the rectum with a 30 cm rubber tube. The enemas are repeated until soft feces appear and the foal is comfortable. Oral doses of Coloxyl or 100–200 g of mineral oil are also advised. Affected foals should be treated regularly at 4-hour intervals until recovery. Some cases prove to be most obstinate and hard fecal masses continue to be passed for several days even though soft fecal material is being passed as well. Small doses of parasympathetic stimulants (one-eighth to one-sixteenth of the adult dose) may hasten recovery at this stage. In some cases, removal of the masses by traction with blunt forceps or by colostomy is necessary. Surgical removal is indicated when the foal has not sucked for more than 2 hours and its life is therefore endangered, or when the amount of meconium present is large, when the rectum has been damaged or is too small to permit manipulation.

REFERENCES

(1) Hekmati, P. & Shahrski, H. (1974) *Br. vet. J.*, *130*, 420.
(2) Annotation (1955) *Lancet*, *269*, 128.
(3) Moffatt, R. E. et al. (1975) *Can. J. comp. Med.*, *39*, 434.
(4) Ehrensberger, F. et al. (1978) *Schweiz Arch. Tierheelkd.*, *120*, 477.
(5) Tate, L. P. & Donawick, W. J. (1978) *J. Am. vet. med. Assoc.*, *172*, 830.
(6) Moore, J. N. et al. (1978) *J. equ. med. Surg.*, *2*, 541.
(7) Campbell, M. et al. (1984) *J. Am vet. med. Assoc.*, *184*, 950.
(8) Roberts, M. C. & Seawright, A. H. (1979) *Aust. vet. J.*, *55*, 553.
(9) Boles, C. L. & Kohn, C. W. (1977) *J. Am. vet. med. Assoc.*, *171*, 193.
(10) Blue, M. G. (1981) *J. Am. vet. med. Assoc.*, *179*, 79.
(11) Hjortkjaier, R. K. (1979) *Nord. VetMed.*, *31*, 508.
(12) Taylor, T. S. et al. (1979) *Equ. Pract.*, *1*, 22.
(13) Gay, C. C. et al. (1979) *Equ. vet. J.*, *11*, 60.
(14) Hilbert, B. J. et al. (1987) *Aust. vet. J.*, *64*, 85.
(15) Lloyd, K. et al. (1987) *Cornell Vet.*, *77*, 172.

Rectal prolapse

Prolapse of the rectum is commonplace in the pig, an occasional occurrence in cattle, and is rarely seen in the other species. In the pig the high prevalence is explained by the absence of appropriate supporting tissues for the rectum in the pelvis.

The common causes include enteritis with profuse diarrhea, violent straining such as occurs in coccidiosis in young cattle, in rabies sometimes, in spinal cord abscess and also when the pelvic organs are engorged. The use of estrogens as a growth stimulant and access to estrogenic fungal toxins predispose to rectal prolapse for this reason.

CONGENITAL DEFECTS OF THE ALIMENTARY TRACT

Congenital harelip and cleft palate

Harelip may be unilateral or bilateral and may involve only the lip or extend to the nostril (1). It may be associated with cleft palate and cause dysphagia and nasal regurgitation of milk and food, and a risk of inhalation pneumonia. It may be inherited or result from poisoning of lambs with *Veratrum californicum*. Cleft palate is difficult to correct surgically especially in foals in which it is a common congenital defect. Cleft palate (palatoschisis) is a common inherited defect in calves and is described under that heading.

REFERENCES

(1) Swartz, H. A. et al. (1982) *Am. J. vet. Res.*, *43*, 729.

Congenital artresia of the salivary ducts

Congenital atresia of salivary ducts usually results in distension of the gland followed by atrophy. Rarely the gland may continue secreting, resulting in a gross distension of the duct (1).

Agnathia and micrognathia

These are variations of a developmental deficiency of the mandible, relatively common in sheep. The mandible and its associated structures is partially or completely absent (2).

Persistence of the right aortic arch

Persistence of the right aortic arch as a fibrous band may occlude the esophagus and cause signs of obstruction, particularly chronic bloat in young calves.

Choanal atresia

Failure of the bucconasal membrane to rupture during fetal life prevents the animal breathing through the nostrils. The membrane separates the alimentary tract and the nasal cavities in the pharynx. It is incompatible with life in foals and lambs, the two species in which it is identified (16). The defect is usually bilateral, a unilateral lesion is tolerable. Surgical correction is likely to be only partially effective (18).

Congenital atresia of the intestine and anus

Atresia of the anus is recorded as a congenital defect in pigs, sheep (4) and calves (5, 6). Its occurrence is usually sporadic and no genetic or management factors can be indicated as causes. In other circumstances the occurrence can be suggestive of conditioning by inheritance, or be at such a rate as to suggest some environmental cause. Affected animals die at about 7–19 days of age unless the defect is corrected surgically. The intestine is grossly distended by then and the abdomen is obviously swollen as a result. There is marked absence of feces. When the defect is anal, and the rectal lumen in quite close to the perineum, surgical intervention is easy and the results, in terms of salvaging the animals for meat production, are good. These animals can usually be identified by the way in which the rectal distension bulges in the perineum where the anus should be; pressure on the abdomen provokes a tensing or further distension of this bulge (7). Other signs include tenesmus with anal pumping and inability to pass a proctoscope or other instrument.

Multiple atresia sites with segments of gut at various levels being atretic is rare in animals which usually have one defect, and the commonest zone affected is the colon. The atresia may be a membrane or cord (9). Atresia of the terminal colon occurs in foals (8), especially those of the Overoo breed, and the ileum and colon in calves (4, 6, 7, 12) and the small intestine in lambs (13, 14). The abdomen may be grossly distended before birth when the defect is in the small intestine and the distension may interfere with normal parturition. In defects of the large intestine distension usually occurs after birth. In these the anus is normal and the part of the intestine caudal to the obstructed section may be normal or absent. The passage of a rectal tube (10) or the infusion of barium and radiography will assist in the detection of atresia of the intestine. There are usually large quantities of thick tenacious mucus in the rectum with no evidence of meconium or feces. In the latter case only exploratory laparotomy can reveal the extent and nature of the defect. In many cases the animal has not sucked since the first day and 5–6-day-old animals are very weak and recumbent. The bowel may rupture and acute diffuse peritonitis develop (11). Intestinal segmental atresia has been produced experimentally by occluding the blood supply to the intestine in fetal lambs (3).

In many animals the congenital defects of the bowel are accompanied by defects in other organs (6, 7, 11) especially the lower urinary tract and reparative surgery is not possible. Atresia of the ileum and colon is probably conditioned by inheritance in Swedish highland cattle. Congenital construction of the anus and vagina is an inherited defect of Jersey cattle and is recorded under that heading. The defect may be combined with rectovaginal fistula manifested by the passage of feces via the vulva (15) or penile urethra (17). Congenital atresia of the intestine can be differentiated from retention of meconium in foals, and rarely calves, by the passage of some fecal color in the latter.

REVIEW LITERATURE

Gaag, I. van der & Tibboel, D. (1980) Intestinal atresia and stenosis in animals. *Vet. Pathol.*, *17*, 565.
Johnson, R. (1986) Intestinal atresia and stenosis: a review comparing its morphology. *Vet. res. Commun.*, *10*, 105–111.

REFERENCES

(1) Fowler, M. E. (1965) *J. Am. vet. med. Assoc.*, *146*, 1403.
(2) Smith, I. D. (1968) *Aust. vet. J.*, *44*, 510.
(3) Clark, W. T. et al. (1978) *NZ vet J.*, *44*, 510.
(4) Dennis, S. M. & Leipold, H. W. (1972) *Vet. Rec.*, *91*, 219.
(5) Cho, D. Y. & Taylor, H. W. (1986) *Cornell Vet.*, *76*, 11.
(6) Mobini, S. et al. (1983) *Comp. cont. Educ.*, *5*, S642.
(7) Steenhaut, M. et al. (1976) *Vet. Rec.*, *98*, 131.

(8) Vanderfecht, S. L. et al. (1983) *Vet. Pathol.*, *20*, 65.
(9) Gaag, I. van der & Tibboel, D. (1980) *Vet. Pathol.*, *17*, 565.
(10) Maclellan, M. & Martin, J. A. (1956) *Vet. Rec.*, *68*, 458.
(11) Johnson, R. et al. (1983) *J. Am. vet. med. Assoc.*, *182*, 1387.
(12) Hunter, A. G. (1974) *Vet. Rec.*, *94*, 170.
(13) Leipold, H. W. & Dennis, S. M. (1973) *Vet. Rec.*, *93*, 644.
(14) Littlejohn, A. (1974) *Vet. Rec.*, *93*, 363.
(15) Furie, W. S. (1983) *Equ. Pract.*, *5*(1), 30.
(16) Crouch, G. M. et al. (1983) *Comp. cont. Educ.*, *5*, S706.
(17) Kingston, R. S. & Park, R. D. (1982) *Equ. Pract.*, *4*, 32.
(18) Goring, R. L. et al. (1984) *Vet. Surg.*, *13*, 211.

NEOPLASMS OF THE ALIMENTARY TRACT

Mouth

Oral neoplasms in ruminants may be associated with heavy bracken intake. The tumors are usually squamous cell carcinomas arising from the gums and cause interference with mastication. They occur most commonly in aged animals and probably arise from alveolar epithelium after periodontitis has caused chronic hyperplasia. Sporadic occurrences of other tumors, e.g. adenocarcinoma, cause obvious local swelling and dysphagia.

Pharynx and esophagus

Papillomas sometimes involve the pharynx, esophagus, esophageal groove and reticulum and cause chronic ruminal tympany in cattle. A high incidence of malignant neoplasia affecting the pharynx, esophagus and rumen has been recorded in one area in South Africa (12). The tumors were multicentric in origin and showed evidence of malignancy on histological examination. The clinical disease was chronic and confined to adult animals with persistent, moderate tympany of the rumen and progressive emaciation as typical signs. A similar occurrence has been recorded in cattle in western Scotland (13) and related to the long-term consumption of bracken. The tumors were squamous-cell carcinoma in the pharynx and dorsal esophagus. The principal clinical abnormality was difficulty in eating and swallowing (13). Many of the carcinomas arise in pre-existing papillomas which are caused by a virus infection. The carcinomas occur only in cattle more than 6 years of age (18).

Stomach and rumen

Squamous-cell carcinomas occasionally develop in the mouth and stomach of horses and the rumen of cattle. In the stomach of the horse, they occur in the cardiac portion and may cause obscure indigestion syndromes, lack of appetite, weight loss, anemia, obstruction of the lower esophagus (2), dysphagia, colic and occasionally chronic diarrhea. Or it may ulcerate to terminate with perforation of the stomach wall and the development of peritonitis. Metastases may spread to abdominal and thoracic cavities with fluid accumulating there. Subcutaneous edema is a common accompanying sign (11). There may also be pleural effusion due to metastases in the pleura (10). Metastases in the female genital tract have also been noted (1). Most affected animals are euthanized because of anorexia and chronic weight loss (4). Large masses of metastatic tumor tissue may be palpable on rectal examination. In such cases an examination of paracentesis fluid sample cells should be valuable. Lymphosarcoma in horses is often manifested by chronic diarrhea due to massive infiltration of the intestinal wall (6). There is severe weight loss, even in the absence of diarrhea in some cases, usually a large appetite and often severe ascites, and anasarca and sometimes colic. The same signs are recorded in a case of mesothelioma in a horse (7). The oral glucose absorption test is abnormal with a poor absorption response (8). Rectal examination may reveal large masses of hard nodular tissue and hematological examination may be of assistance in diagnosis (9). Paracentesis and examination of cells in the fluid for the presence of mitotic figures is an essential part of an examination in suspected cases of neoplasia in the abdominal cavity. Nasal fibergastroscopy is an obvious technique for visualizing this tumour but suffers the limitation that standard instruments are not long enough (23). The course of this disease in horses is very variable with the period of illness lasting from 3 weeks to 3 months.

Ruminal tumors may obstruct the cardia and cause chronic tympany. In lymphomatosis of cattle, there is frequently gross involvement in the abomasal wall causing persistent diarrhea. Ulceration, hemorrhage and pyloric obstruction may also occur.

Intestines

A higher than normal rate of occurrence of carcinoma of the small intestine has been recorded in sheep in Iceland (14), Norway (21) and New Zealand (16) and in cows only in New Zealand (20). A series of intestinal carcinomas is also recorded in Europe (17), and another series in Australia (15). The Australian series were located at abattoirs and were causing intestinal stenosis. Metastasis to regional lymph nodes occurred readily. In New Zealand there appeared to be a much higher prevalence in British breed ewes (0·9–0·15%) compared to Merino and Corriedale ewes (0·2–0·4%), and significantly higher tumor rates were observed in sheep that had been pastured on feedstuffs sprayed recently with phenoxy or picolinic acid herbicides (24). The use of the herbicides 2, 4-D, 2, 4, 5-T, MCPA, piclorum and clopyralid has been associated with an increased incidence of these tumors. A higher prevalence in sheep kept at higher stocking rates was also suggested.

Occasional tumors of the intestine are recorded in abattoir findings but they can cause clinical signs such as chronic bloat and intermittent diarrhea (5) in cattle, persistent colic due to partial intestinal obstruction in horses (19), and anorexia and a distended abdomen in sheep (22). A series of cases of lymphoma in horses were characterized by malaborption without diarrhea but with anemia in some (25). Tumors of the anus are rare; a mucoepidermoid carcinoma is recorded in a goat (3) but most tumors of the perineal area are anogenital papillomata.

REFERENCES

(1) Pearson, G. R. & McCaughes, W. J. (1978) *NZ vet. J.*, *26*, 123.
(2) Tennant, B. et al. (1982) *Equ. vet. J.*, *14*, 238.
(3) Turk, J. R. et al. (1984) *Vet. Pathol.*, *21*, 364.
(4) Meagher, D. M. et al. (1974) *J. Am. vet. med. Assoc.*, *164*, 81.
(5) Cho, D. Y. & Archibald, L. F. (1985) *Vet. Pathol.*, *22*, 639.
(6) Gay, C. C. & Blood, D. C. (1976) *Proc. 53rd Ann. Conf. Aust. vet. Assoc.*, 130.
(7) Ricketts, S. W. & Peace, C. K. (1976) *Equ. vet. J.*, *8*, 78.
(8) Roberts, M. C. & Pinsent, P. J. N. (1975) *Equ. vet. J.*, *7*, 166.
(9) Neufeld, J. L. (1973) *Can. vet. J.*, *14*, 129.
(10) Wrigley, R. R. et al. (1981) *Equ. vet. J.*, *13*, 99.
(11) Meuten, D. J. et al. (1978) *Cornell Vet.*, *68*, 179.
(12) Plowright, W. et al. (1971) *Br. J. Cancer*, *25*, 72.
(13) Pirie, H. M. (1973) *Res. vet. Sci.*, *15*, 135.
(14) Georgsson, C. & Viglusson, H. (1973) *Acta vet. Scand.*, *14*, 392.
(15) Ross, A. D. (1980) *Aust. vet. J.*, *56*, 25.
(16) Simpson, B. H. (1974) *J. Pathol.*, *112*, 83.
(17) Vitovec, J. (1977) *Zentralbl. VetMed.*, *24A*, 413.
(18) Jarrett, W. F. H. (1978) *Bull. Cancer*, *65*, 191.
(19) Wright, J. A. & Edwards, G. B. (1984) *Equ. vet. J.*, *16*, 136.
(20) Johnstone, A. C. et al. (1983) *NZ vet. J.*, *31*, 147.
(21) Ulvund, M. (1983) *NZ vet. J.*, *31*, 177.
(22) Anderson, B. C. (1983) *J. Am. vet. Med. Assoc.*, *183*, 1467.
(23) Keirn, D. P. et al. (1982) *J. Am. vet. med. Assoc.*, *180*, 940.
(24) Newell, K. W. et al. (1984) *Lancet*, *2*, 1301.
(25) Platt, H. (1987) *J. comp. Pathol.*, *97*, 1.

DISEASES OF THE PERITONEUM

Peritonitis

Inflammation of the peritoneum is accompanied by abdominal pain which varies in degree with the severity and extent of the peritonitis. Tenderness on palpation and rigidity of the abdominal wall, fecal stasis and toxemia with fever are the typical manifestations.

Etiology

Peritonitis may occur as a primary disease or secondarily as part of an etiologically specific disease. As a primary disease it results most commonly by rupture of, or spread of infection from, an abdominal site or less commonly by perforation of the abdominal wall from the exterior. Some of the more common individual causes are as follows.

Cattle

- Traumatic reticuloperitonitis
- Perforation or leakage of abomasal ulcer
- Rupture of abomasum after torsion
- Rumenitis of cattle subsequent to acute carbohydrate indigestion
- Hepatic abscess of black disease in cattle and horses which survive the disease for more than 24 hours
- Rupture of vagina in young heifers during violent coitus with a young active bull
- Deposition of semen into the peritoneal cavity by any means
- Injection of sterile hypertonic solutions, e.g., calcium preparations for milk fever. The chemical peritonitis which results may lead to formation of constrictive adhesions between loops of the coiled colon
- Transection of small intestine which becomes pinched between the uterus and the pelvic cavity at parturition
- Intraperitoneal injection of non-sterile solutions
- Spontaneous uterine rupture during parturition, or during manual correction of dystocia
- Sadistic rupture of vagina
- Spontaneous rupture of rectum at calving (3)
- As part of specific diseases including tuberculosis, sporadic bovine encephalomyelitis.

Horses

- Rupture of dorsal sac of cecum or colon (1) at foaling, usually related to a large meal given just beforehand
- Administration of non-steroidal anti-inflammatory drugs (NSAIDs) causing cecal stasis and dilatation and eventually perforations (13)
- Rectal rupture or tear during rectal examination, predisposed to by inflammation of mucosa and overenthusiasm by the operator; this subject is dealt with separately under the heading of rectal tear
- Extension from a retroperitoneal infection, e.g., *Streptococcus equi* after an attack of strangles, *Corynebacterium* (*Rhodococcus*) *equi* in foals under 1 year of age, both probably assisted by migration of *Strongylus vulgaris* larvae
- Gastric erosion or rupture related to ulceration caused by larvae of *Gasterophilus* or *Habronema* spp.
- Leakage from a cecal perforation apparently caused by a heavy infestation of *Anoplocephala perfoliata* tapeworms (12)
- Spontaneous gastric rupture
- *Actinobacillus equuli* infection by unknown means (5).

Pigs

- Ileal perforation in regional ileitis
- Glasser's disease caused by *Haemophilus suis*.

Sheep

- Spread from intestinal wall abscess following infestation with *Oesophagostomum* sp. larvae
- Serositis-arthritis caused by *Mycoplasma* sp.

Goats

- Serositis-arthritis caused by *Mycoplasma* sp.

All species

- Traumatic perforation from the exterior of the abdominal wall by horn gore, stake wound

- Faulty asepsis at laparotomy, peritoneal injection, trocarization for tympany of rumen or cecum
- Leakage through wall of infarcted gut segment
- Spread from subperitoneal sites in spleen, liver, umbilical vessels.

Pathogenesis

At least six factors operate in the genesis of clinical signs in peritonitis. They are toxemia or septicemia, shock and hemorrhage, paralytic ileus, accumulation of fluid exudate, the development of adhesions and abdominal pain.

Toxemia

Toxins produced by bacteria and by the breakdown of tissue are absorbed readily through the peritoneum. The resulting toxemia is the most important factor in the production of clinical illness and its severity is usually governed by the size of the area of peritoneum involved. In acute diffuse peritonitis, the toxemia is profound; in local inflammation, it is negligible. The type of infection present is obviously important because of variations between bacteria in their virulence and toxin production.

With rupture of the alimentary tract wall and the spillage of a large quantity of gut contents into the peritoneal cavity, some acute peritonitis does develop, but death is usually too sudden, within 2 or 3 hours in horses, for more than an early lesion to develop. These animals really die of endotoxic shock due to absorption of toxins from the gut contents. In acute diffuse peritonitis due solely to bacterial contamination from the gut, the reaction depends on the bacteria which gain entry and the capacity of the omentum to deal with the peritonitis, and the amount of body movement that the animal has to perform. Cows which suffer penetration of the reticular wall at calving have lowered immunological competence, a greater than normal negative pressure in the peritoneal cavity, are invaded by *Fusobacterium necrophorum*, *Corynebacterium* sp. and *Escherichia coli*, and are required to walk to the milking parlor, to the feed supply and so on. They are likely to develop a massive diffuse purulent peritonitis and a profound toxemia and die within 24 hours. By contrast, horses which develop acute peritonitis due to streptococci or *Actinobacillus equuli* show little toxemia and manifest only abdominal pain due to the inflammatory reaction of the peritoneum.

Shock and hemorrhage

The shock caused by sudden deposition of gut contents, or infected uterine contents, into the peritoneal cavity, plus the hemorrhage resulting from the rupture, may be significant contributors to the common fatal outcome when an infected viscus ruptures. Following rupture of the uterus in cows the shock and hemorrhage may be minor and peritonitis may not develop if the uterine contents are not contaminated. Failure of the uterus to heal or be repaired may be followed by peritonitis several days later.

Paralytic ileus

Paralytic ileus arises as a result of reflex inhibition of alimentary tract tone and movement in acute peritonitis. It is also an important sequel to intestinal obstruction and to traumatic abdominal surgery in which much handling of viscera is unavoidable. Rarely it arises because of ganglionitis and a loss of neural control of peristalsis, similar to the idiopathic intestinal pseudo-obstruction of humans (11). The net effect is one of functional obstruction of the intestine and this may play a part in causing a fatal outcome of the case. Initially, there may be a temporary increase in motility, also mediated through extrinsic reflexes, but the resulting diarrhea is usually transient and of minor degree. The end result is a complete absence of defecation, often with no feces present in the rectum.

Adhesions

In chronic peritonitis, the formation of adhesions is more important than either of the two preceding factors. Adhesions are an essential part of the healing process and are important in that they localize infection to a particular segment of the peritoneum. If this healing process is developing satisfactorily and the signs of peritonitis are diminishing, it is a common experience to find that vigorous exercise may cause breakdown of the adhesions, spread of the peritonitis and return of the clinical signs. Thus, a cow treated conservatively for traumatic reticuloperitonitis by immobilization on an incline may show an excellent recovery by the third day, but if allowed to go out to pasture at this time, may suffer an acute relapse. The secondary role of adhesions is to cause partial or complete obstruction of the intestine or stomach, or by fixation to interfere with normal gut motility. Adhesions are of major importance in the production of vagus indigestion of cattle and may cause intestinal obstruction in horses as a sequel to mesenteric verminous arteritis or perforation of a gastric ulcer.

Accumulation of fluid exudate

Accumulation of large quantities of inflammatory exudate in the peritoneal cavity may cause visible abdominal distension and interfere with respiration by obstruction of diaphragmatic movement. It is a comparatively rare occurrence, but needs to be considered in the differential diagnosis of abdominal distension.

Abdominal pain

Abdominal pain is a variable sign in peritonitis. In acute, diffuse peritonitis, the toxemia may be sufficiently severe to depress the response of the animal to pain stimuli, but in less severe cases the animal usually adopts an arched-back posture and shows evidence of pain on palpation of the abdominal wall. Inflammation of the serous surfaces of the peritoneum causes pain, and a reflex effect is mediated through spinal cord reflex arcs to cause rigidity of the abdominal wall and the assumption of an abnormal posture.

Clinical findings

Peritonitis is common in cattle, less common in horses and rarely, if ever, identified clinically in sheep, pigs or goats. There are general signs applicable to all species and most forms of the disease in a general way. Then there are special findings peculiar to individual species of animals and to various forms of the disease.

Acute and subacute peritonitis

Inappetence and anorexia Inappetence occurs in less

severe, more chronic cases and complete anorexia in acute diffuse cases.

Toxemia and fever Toxemia usually with fever is always present, but its severity varies depending on the area of peritoneum involved, the identity of the pathogens and the amount of tissue destroyed. For example, in acute local peritonitis the temperature will be elevated (39·5°C; 103°F) for the first 24–36 hours, but then return to normal even though the animal may still be partly or completely anorectic. A high fever (up to 41·5°C; 106°F) suggests an acute diffuse peritonitis, but in the terminal stages the temperature usually falls to subnormal. It is most important to realize that a normal temperature does not preclude the presence of peritonitis. There is usually a moderate increase in pulse and respiratory rates, the latter contributed to by the relative fixation of the abdominal wall because of pain. In some cases there is spontaneous grunting at the end of each expiratory movement.

Feces The amount and composition of feces is always abnormal. The amount is reduced although in the early stages there may be increased frequency of passage of small volumes of diarrhea which may give the impression of increased fecal output; it is not sufficient to cause abnormality of fluid and electrolyte balance. Feces may be completely absent for periods up to 3 days, even in animals that recover, and the rectum may be so dry and tacky, due to the presence of small amounts of tenacious mucus, that it is difficult to conduct a rectal examination. This may suggest a complete intestinal obstruction.

The more common expression of longer alimentary sojourn in peritonitis in pastured cattle is the passage of scant, dark, hard turds accompanied by thick jelly-like mucus. The feces may alternatively have a thick sludge-like consistency, and be tenacious and difficult to remove from a rubber glove, and have a foul smell.

Alimentary tract stasis As well as absence of feces, there are other indicators of intestinal stasis. In cows with acute peritonitis ruminal contractions are reduced or absent; in chronic peritonitis the contractions may be present, but are weaker than normal. In the horse, gut stasis is evidenced by an absence or reduction of real gut sounds on auscultation, although the little tinkling sound of paralytic ileus may be audible. It is very important to differentiate the two.

Abdominal pain evidenced by posture and movement
In cattle with acute peritonitis there is a disinclination to move, disinclination to lie down, lying down with great care and grunting with pain. The posture includes a characteristically arched back, the gait is shambling and cautious, with the back held rigid and arched. Grunting at each step and when feces or urine are passed is a fairly standard sign, and when urine is eventually passed it is usually in a very large volume. Sudden movements are avoided and there is an absence of kicking or bellowing or licking the coat.

In horses, these overt signs of peritonitis which characterize the condition in cattle are uncommon which makes the diagnosis difficult. Also, the disease is often ushered in by a bout of abdominal pain including flank watching, kicking at the belly and going down and rolling which suggests colic caused by bowel obstruction (5, 8).

Abdominal pain as evidenced by palpation and percussion
In cattle, deep firm palpation of the abdominal wall elicits an easily recognized pain response. It may be possible to elicit pain over the entire abdominal wall if the peritonitis is widespread. If it is localized the response may be detectable over only a very small area. Increased tenseness of the abdominal wall is not usually detectable in the cow, although it is responsible for the characteristic arched back posture and apparent gauntness of the abdomen, because the wall is already tightly stretched anyway.

There are several methods of demonstrating abdominal pain in the cow by eliciting a grunt. In average-sized cows with acute local peritonitis, while listening over the trachea with a stethoscope, a controlled upward push with the closed fist of the ventral body wall caudal to the xiphoid sternum is most successful. In large bulls, especially if the peritonitis is subsiding, no pain response may be seen with this method. In these cases the best technique is a heavy pole held under the area of the xiphoid and a sharp lift given by assistants holding the pole on either side. Pinching of the withers or along the back and attempting to elicit a grunt has a mixed reputation; false positive reactions are easily aroused in very nervous, sensitive animals.

In horses, in acute or subacute peritonitis, it is usually easy to arouse a pain response manifested by the animal lifting its leg and turning its head with anger when its lower flank is firmly lifted, not punched. The abdominal wall also feels much stiffer if it is lifted firmly with the heel of the hand. In all cases of peritonitis in all species a pain response is always much more evident in the early stages of the disease and severe chronic peritonitis can be present without pain being detected on palpation.

Rectal examination The general absence of feces has already been noted. In cattle, it may be possible to palpate slightly distended, saggy, thick-walled loops of intestine in some cases. Also, it may be possible to feel fibrinous adhesions separating as the intestines are manipulated. This is not often palpable and its absence should not be interpreted as precluding the presence of peritonitis. Tough fibrous adhesions may be present in longstanding cases. In horses there are no rectal findings, other than a reduced fecal output, to indicate that peritonitis is likely to be present. However, there is a lack of clarity as to what can be felt in chronic cases due to fibrin deposits and thickening of the peritoneum. There may also be more than usual pain when an inflamed area is palpated or a mesenteric band or adhesion manipulated.

Peracute diffuse peritonitis
In those cases in which profound toxemia occurs, especially in cows immediately after calving or when rupture of the alimentary tract occurs, the syndrome is quite different. There is severe weakness, depression and circulatory failure. The animal is recumbent and often unable to rise, depressed almost to the point of coma, has a subnormal temperature of 37–37·5°C (99–100°F), a high heart rate (110–120/min), and a very weak pulse. No abdominal pain is evidenced spontane-

ously or on palplation. In mares that rupture the dorsal sac of the cecum during foaling, the owner observes that the mare has been straining and getting results when suddenly she stops making violent muscular constractions, and progress towards expelling the foal ceases (2). Moderate abdominal pain followed by shock are characteristic developments. Death follows 4–15 hours after the rupture.

The outcome in cases of acute, diffuse peritonitis varies with the severity. Peracute cases accompanied by severe toxemia usually die within 24–48 hours. The more common, less severe cases may be fatal in 4–7 days, but adequate treatment may result in recovery in about the same length of time.

Chronic peritonitis

Cattle The development of adhesions which interfere with normal alimentary tract movements, and gradual spread of infection as adhesions break down, combine to produce a chronic syndrome of indigestion and toxemia which is punctuated by short, recurrent attacks of more severe illness. The adhesions may be detectable on rectal examination, but they are usually situated in the anterior abdomen and are impalpable. If partial intestinal obstruction occurs, the bouts of pain are usually accompanied by a marked increase in alimentary tract sounds and palpable distension of intestinal loops with gas and fluid. The course in chronic peritonitis may be as long as some months and the prognosis is not favorable because of the presence of physical lesions caused by scar tissue and adhesions. In some cases there is marked abdominal distension with many liters of turbid-infected fluid present. This may be restricted in its location to the omental bursa (6). Detection of fluid in the peritoneal cavity of a cow is not easy because of the fluid nature of the ruminal contents. Results obtained by testing for a fluid wave should be interpreted cautiously. Collection of fluid by paracentesis abdominis is the critical test.

Horses Horses with chronic peritonitis usually have a history of ill-thrift for a period of several weeks. Weight loss is severe and there are usually intermittent episodes of abdominal pain suggesting intestinal colic. Gut sounds are greatly diminished or absent, and subcutaneous edema of the ventral abdominal wall occurs in some cases. There may also be a contiguous pleurisy. Identification of the cause of the colic depends on the examination of a sample of peritoneal fluid.

Clinical pathology

The total and differential leukocyte count is a useful aid in the diagnosis of peritonitis, and in assessing its severity. In acute diffuse peritonitis with toxemia there is usually a leukopenia, neutropenia and a marked increase in immature neutrophils (a degenerative left shift). There is 'toxic' granulation of neutrophils. In less severe forms of acute peritonitis of a few days' duration there may be a leukocytosis due to a neutrophilia with the appearance of immature neutrophils. In acute local peritonitis, commonly seen in acute traumatic reticuloperitonitis in cattle, there is commonly a normal total leukocyte count, or a slight increase, with regenerative left shift. In chronic peritonitis, depending on the extent of the lesion (diffuse or local), the total and differential leukocyte count may be normal, or there may be a leukocytosis with a marked neutrophilia and occasionally an increase in the total numbers of lymphocytes and monocytes. The plasma fibrinogen levels in cattle, in general, tend to increase as the severity of acute peritonitis increases and may be a useful adjunct to the cell counts for assessing severity (4).

Examination of peritoneal fluid obtained by paracentesis is a very valuable aid in the diagnosis of peritonitis and in assessing its severity. It may also provide an indication of the kind of antibacterial treatment required. It is dealt with in detail under the heading of special examination of the alimentary tract (p. 160). However, it is noted here that particular attention should be paid to:

- The ease of collection of the sample as a guide to the amount of fluid present
- Whether it is bloodstained, indicating damage to a wall of the viscus
- The presence of food or fecal material indicating bowel leaking or rupture
- Whether it clots and has a high protein content indicating inflammation rather than simple transudation
- The number and kinds of leukocytes present, also as an indication of the presence of inflammation, and also its duration
- Microbiological examination.

When these results are available they should be looked at not in isolation, but in conjunction with history, clinical signs, and with other paraclinical examinations including hematology, serum chemistry and possibly radiology. In particular, it must be noted that failure to obtain a sample does not preclude a possible diagnosis of peritonitis.

Necropsy findings

In acute diffuse peritonitis, the entire peritoneum is involved, but the most severe lesions are usually in the ventral abdomen. Gross hemorrhage into the subserosa, exudation and fibrin deposits in the peritoneal cavity and fresh adhesions which are easily broken down are present. In less acute cases, the exudate is purulent and may be less fluid, often forming a thick cheesy covering over most of the viscera. In cattle, ***Fusobacterium necrophorum*** and *Actinomyces* (*Corynebacterium*) *pyogenes* are often present in large numbers and produce a typical, nauseating odor. Acute local peritonitis and chronic peritonitis are not usually fatal and the lesions are discovered only if the animal dies of intercurrent disease such as traumatic pericarditis or intestinal obstruction.

Diagnosis

The diagnosis of peritonitis can be difficult because the predominant clinical findings are often common to other diseases. The clinical features which are the most reliable as indicators of peritonitis are:

- Abnormal feces—in amount and composition
- Alimentary tract stasis as judged by auscultation and passage of feces
- Abdominal pain evinced as a groan with each re-

spiration or on light or deep percussion of the abdomen
- Abnormality of intestines on rectal palpation
- Fibrinous or fibrous adhesions on rectal palpation
- Abnormal peritoneal fluid with an increased leukocyte count collected by paracentesis
- A normal or low blood leukocyte count with a degenerative left shift
- The peritonitis may be chemical so that although microbiological examination usually yields positive results these are not essential to a diagnosis of peritonitis.

Differential diagnosis

The diseases which could be considered in the differential diagnosis of peritonitis are as follows.

Cattle

Acute local peritonitis Traumatic reticuloperitonitis, acute intestinal obstruction, splenic or hepatic abscess, simple indigestion, abomasal displacement (right and left), postpartum metritis, ketosis.

Acute diffuse peritonitis Parturient paresis, coliform mastitis (peracute form), acute carbohydrate indigestion, perforation of or rupture at abomasal ulcer, acute intestinal obstruction, uterine rupture, postpartum metritis.

Chronic peritonitis Vagus indigestion, lipomatosis or extensive fat necrosis of the mesentery and omentum, persistent minor leakage from an intestinal lesion, large accumulations of fluid as in ascites, rupture of bladder, chronic pneumonia and chronic toxemias due to a great variety of causes.

Horses

Acute and subacute peritonitis Acute intestinal obstruction and thromboembolic colic.

Chronic peritonitis Repeated overeating causing colic, internal abdominal abscess (retroperitoneal or mesenteric abscess) may be classified as chronic peritonitis, but is dealt with separately under the heading of retroperitoneal abscess (9).

Pigs, sheep and goats

Peritonitis is not usually diagnosed antemortem in these species.

Treatment

The specific cause must be treated in each case and the treatments used are described under the specific diseases listed above. Horses with acute peritonitis caused by *Actinobacillus equuli* respond quickly to treatment with penicillin-streptomycin mixture or ampicillin administered systemically. The recovery rate in horses is very good, usually about 70%. Chronic cases are less responsive because of the serious involvement of gut with fibrous adhesions.

Non-specific treatment includes the administration of antibacterial drugs, including broad-spectrum antibiotics and sulfonamides to control the infection, and the treatment of the toxemia. Antibacterial drugs can be administered orally, parenterally or directly into the peritoneal cavity. Intraperitoneal injection may give maximum concentration of the drug at the site of inflammation, but there is no scientific evidence that it is superior to daily parenteral administration and there is some danger of causing adhesions and subsequent intestinal obstruction (10). The drug is usually administered in isotonic saline or electrolyte solutions and only non-irritating drugs should be used. Those which contain irritating bases such as propylene glycol must be avoided. If adhesions are likely to be present or the area of inflammation small, there is probably no advantage in the intraperitoneal route and, if the primary lesion is in the alimentary tract, there is probably an advantage in giving the drug by mouth, provided the alimentary tract flora is not unfavorably depressed. If large quantities of exudate are present in the peritoneal cavity, surgical drainage is advisable to remove the source of toxins. Peritoneal lavage with large volumes of fluid containing antibiotic is recommended when quantities of exudate are present (7), but it is not easy to maintain the patency of drains, especially in cattle. Some veterinarians use a more aggressive technique of perfusing the peritoneal cavity with dilute solutions of tamed iodine disinfectants. The peritoneum is a very sensitive tissue and chemical peritonitis is easy to produce. Great caution is required when foreign materials are introduced into the cavity in order to avoid causing more damage than already exists. The peritoneum is also a very vascular organ and absorption of toxic materials occurs rapidly from it.

No attempt should be made to prevent the development of adhesions although if they are extensive they may cause inconvenience later. The treatment of toxemia has been described elsewhere.

REVIEW LITERATURE

Dyson, S. (1983) Review of 30 cases of peritonitis in the horse. *Equ. vet. J.*, *15*, 25–30.

REFERENCES

(1) Platt, H. (1983) *J. comp. Pathol.*, *93*, 343.
(2) Littlejohn, A. & Ritchie, J. D. S. (1975) *J. S. Afr. vet. med. Assoc.*, *46*, 87.
(3) van Kruiningen, H. J. et al. (1961) *Cornell Vet.*, *51*, 557.
(4) Sutton, R. H. & Hobman, B. (1975) *Aust. vet. J.*, *23*, 21.
(5) Gay, C. C. & Lording, P. M. (1980) *Aust. vet. J.*, *56*, 296.
(6) van Beukelen, P. et al. (1979) *Tijdschr. Diergeenskd.*, *104*, 621.
(7) Kunesh, J. P. (1984) *J. Am. vet. med. Assoc.*, *185*, 1222.
(8) Traver, D. S. et al. (1977) *J. equ. med. Surg.*, *1*, 36.
(9) Rumbaugh, G. E. et al. (1978) *J. Am. vet med. Assoc.*, *172*, 304.
(10) Donawick, W. J. (1980) *J. Am. vet. med. Assoc.*, *177*, 458.
(11) Baker, J. S. et al. (1985) *Cornell Vet.*, *75*, 289.
(12) Beroza, G. A. (1983) *J. Am. vet. med. Assoc.*, *183*, 804.
(13) Ross, M. W. et al. (1985) *J. Am. vet. med. Assoc.*, *187*, 249.

Rectal tears

Tears in the wall of the rectum of horses are a very real hazard to both the practicing veterinarian and the experienced operator. The organ is sensitive and fragile, but powerful and peristaltically active, and the horse is often under only minimal restraint, so that it is no wonder that occasionally the rectal mucosa is damaged, and on some occasions the rectal wall is ruptured. By contrast, the bovine rectum is relatively durable and often traumatized, but rarely ruptured. There have been a number of reports on the problem in recent years (1, 2) reflecting the increased interest in the horse's abdomen, largely for reproductive reasons, but also because of more active diagnosis and treatment of cases of colic. Because of the difficulty encountered in creating tears experimentally it is suggested that there is as yet an undiscovered predisposing factor (6).

Most rectal tears are caused by veterinarians or owners while carrying out rectal examinations, rarely they are the result of dystocia or misdirection of the penis (1). Most tears are in a longitudinal direction in the dorsal aspect of the rectum and are located at about the level of the pelvic inlet. These are the least likely to lead to trouble. Lateral or ventral tears are more inclined to result in peritoneal contamination. Whether or not the rectum is full of feces at the time of the penetration is of obvious importance. The view has been expressed that plastic sleeves are more conducive to ruptures than are rubber ones. The inclusion of an anesthetic agent in the lubricant used on the sleeve has some advantages in preventing straining, thus reducing the chances of damage (3). The outcome of the damage is determined largely by the depth of the tear.

Mucosa-only tears
These are usually within the pelvic rectum and can be felt to occur when a peristaltic wave passes over one's knuckles. Infection of the deeper layers of the wall results, but provided a good antibiotic cover is supplied and the feces are kept soft and the diet is kept low on residue, a serious result will probably be avoided.

Tears of the wall into the pelvic fascia (retroperitoneal)
The pelvic fascia becomes infected, but the infection may remain contained within it for 7–10 days forming a local cellulitis or abscess. During this period, the horse is likely to be affected by milk chronic peritonitis, with mild abdominal pain, fever and mild toxemia. At the end of this time, the infection erodes through the peritoneum and an acute fatal diffuse peritonitis develops with death supervening in 24–36 hours.

Ruptures of the rectal wall into the peritoneal cavity (through the peritoneum)
Rupture is followed by deposition of fecal material directly into the peritoneal cavity, often in large quantities and causing acute endotoxic shock, and death within a few hours.

The prognosis in all rectal tears, with the possible exception of mucosa-only tears recognized immediately and treated vigorously, is unrelievedly bad. The few successful outcomes reported are in cases of minor tears in the pelvic area and where bypass colostomies have been maintained until the tear heals spontaneously. The following steps are recommended in treatment. If the person doing the rectal examination feels the mucosa tear, or if a horse which has had a rectal examination up to 2 hours previously starts to sweat and show abdominal pain, a rectal tear can be supposed. A thorough examination should be conducted immediately, but great care is necessary to avoid damaging the rectum further. Fecal balls need to be removed, if necessary with an epidural anesthetic to prevent straining. Suture of tears close to the anus is possible through the anus (2), but if the tear (4) is quite superficial a conservative approach is possible (1). Atropine is administered to stop peristalsis during examination and after treatment. Repair of the tear via a laparotomy, with or without a diverting colostomy, is the most comprehensive treatment. Drainage into the rectum or vagina is attempted (2). In cases where pelvic abscesses have formed, the owner should be advised immediately of what has happened and the subsequent treatment which is to be provided should be explained. A rectal tear is a very easy way to begin a malpractice suit and it is best avoided by giving the owner the opportunity of bringing in another opinion (5).

REFERENCES

(1) Speirs, V. C. et al. (1980) *Aust. vet. J.*, *56*, 313.
(2) Arnold, J. S. & Meagher, D. M. (1978) *J. equ. med. Surg.*, *2*, 55 & 64.
(3) Merkt, T. H. (1979) *Prakt. Tierärztl.*, *60*, 189.
(4) Stashak, T. S. & Knight, A. P. (1978) *J. equ. med. Surg.*, *2*, 196.
(5) Stauffer, V. D. (1981) *J. Am. vet. med. Assoc.*, *178*, 798.
(6) Jones, W. E. (1986) *J. equ. vet. Sci.*, *6*, 4.

Retroperitoneal abscess (internal abdominal abscess, chronic peritonitis, omental bursitis)

A recognized form of chronic or rarely intermittent colic is caused by an abscess in the abdominal cavity. The abscesses are usually retroperitoneal, sometimes involving the omental bursa (2), and chronic leakage from them into the peritoneal cavity causes chronic or recurrent peritonitis. Complete recovery is difficult to effect and there is a high failure rate in treatment. These abscesses result in any of the following:

- Infection of a verminous aneurysm, especially in young horses
- Post-strangles infection localizing anywhere, but particularly in pre-existing lesions such as verminous aneurysms
- Minor perforations of intestinal wall allowing minimal leakage of intestinal contents so that omental plugging is possible
- Erosion through a gastric granuloma caused by *Habronema* sp. or a squamous cell carcinoma of stomach wall
- In mares development of an abscess in the pelvic fascia commonly results after tearing of the rectal wall during pregnancy diagnosis.

Clinical signs suggestive of the disease include persistent or intermittent chronic colic and weight loss. There is fever and varying degrees of anorexia. Chronic anorexia due to bone marrow depression is always prominent and increased plasma fibrinogen and hypoalbuminemia occur. In cases with a concurrent chronic peritonitis or an omental bursitis the amount of inflammatory exudate is often so great that the abdomen is visibly distended (2). When the abscess is perirectal and in the pelvic fascia there may be straining and constipation due to voluntary retention of feces. These abscesses are easily palpated on rectal examination (3). Paracentesis abdominis produces turbid fluid with a protein content greater than 2·5 g/dl and an increase in leukocytes.

On rectal examination it may be possible to feel an abscess, or adhesions to one. They are often multiple and quite large and adherent to one another, so that tight bands of mesentery can be felt which will lead the hand to the site of the abscess. Pain is usually elicited by rectal palpation of the infected sites and by firm palpation of the external abdominal wall. Ultrasonography through the abdominal wall has been used to locate large retroperitoneal abscesses in a foal (4).

A hemogram, especially in acute cases, is characterized by a neutrophilia which may be as high as 30 000/dl with a significant left shift. If culture is possible the causative bacteria are usually determined to be *Streptococcus equi*, *Str. zooepidemicus*, *Corynebacterium* (*Rhodococcus*) *equi*, *Cor. pseudotuberculosis* or mixed infections if there has been intestinal leakage. It is common, even when there is an active infection in a retroperitoneal abscess, to fail to grow bacteria from a peritoneal effusion.

Leakages from stomach wall may result in adhesions to the spleen and development of splenic abscesses. In these animals a sharp pain response can be elicited on firm palpation of the abdomen in the left flank just behind the last rib. Abscesses in liver are not so easily located. Abscesses in pelvic fascia are usually not very discrete, but are instantly noticeable on inserting the hand into the rectum.

Response to treatment with a broad-spectrum antibiotic such as tetracycline or ampicillin or penicillin–streptomycin combination, or a potentiated sulfonamide is usually good, but often transitory if the usual course of treatment of 3–5 days' duration is administered. The prognosis must always be poor because of the difficulty of completely eliminating the infection. Treatment must be continued for at least 2 weeks and in some cases should be for a period of 2 to even 4 or 5 months (1). Surgical treatment may be possible, but is usually ineffectual because of the deformity of the area by adhesions and the usual outcome of gut tearing and spillage into the peritoneal cavity while attempting to exteriorize the lesion.

REFERENCES

(1) Rumbaugh, G. E. et al. (1978) *J. Am. vet. med. Assoc.*, *172*, 304.
(2) Baxter, G. M. (1986) *Mod. vet. Pract.*, *67*, 729.
(3) Saunders-Shamis, M. (1985) *J. Am. vet. med. Assoc.*, *187*, 499.
(4) Hanselaer, J. H. & Nyland, T. G. (1983) *J. Am. vet. med. Assoc.*, *183*, 1465.

Abdominal fat necrosis (lipomatosis)

The hard masses of necrotic fat which occur relatively commonly in the peritoneal cavity of adult cattle, especially the Channel Island breeds and possibly Aberdeen Angus, are commonly mistaken for a developing fetus and can cause intestinal obstruction. The latter usually develops slowly, resulting in the appearance of attacks of moderate abdominal pain and the passage of small amounts of feces (6). Many cases are detected during routine rectal examination of normal animals. The lipomatous masses are located in the small omentum, large omentum and mesentery in cattle and more diffusely to other parts of the body in sheep and goats (7). The composition of the fatty deposits is identical with the fat of normal cows (9) and there is no suggestion that the disease is neoplastic. One usually finds only sporadic cases but there are reports of a herd prevalence as high as 67% (2). The cause is unknown but there appears to be a relation between such high prevalence and the grazing of tall fescue grass (2), and an inherited predisposition is suggested (3). The rate of occurrence increases with age, the peak occurrence being at 7 years of age (8). An unusual form of the disease with many lesions in subcutaneous sites has been recorded in Holstein–Friesian cattle and is regarded as being inherited (4). There is no treatment and affected animals should be salvaged. A generalized steatitis has been reported in pony foals (5).

Pedunculated lipomas provide a special problem especially in older horses. Their pedicles may be 20–30 cm long, and during periods of active gut motility these pedicles can become tied around a loop of intestine anywhere from the pylorus to the rectum. At the pylorus they cause acute intestinal obstruction with gastric dilatation. At the rectum they cause subacute colic and a characteristic inability to enter the rectum with the hand. This is accompanied by a folded coning-down of the mucosa, not unlike that in a torsion of the uterus (1). Early diagnosis and surgical intervention can produce an early resolution, but delay is disastrous because the blood supply is always compromised; it is always a loop and its blood supply which are strangulated. The pedicle is always tied in a very tight knot.

REFERENCES

(1) Mason, T. A. (1978) *Equ. vet. J.*, *10*, 269.
(2) Stuedemann, J. A. et al. (1985) *Am. J. vet. Res.*, *46*, 1990.
(3) Bridge, P. S. & Spratling, F. R. (1962) *Vet. Rec.*, *74*, 1357.
(4) Albright, J. L. (1960) *J. Hered.*, *51*, 231.
(5) Platt, H. & Whitwell, K. E. (1971) *J. comp. Pathol.*, *81*, 499.
(6) Wallace, C. E. (1974) *Vet. Med. SAC*, *69*, 1113.
(7) Xu, L. R. (1986) *Acta. vet. Zootechnol. Sinica*, *17*, 113.
(8) Shimada, Y. & Morinaga, H. (1977) *J. Jap. vet. med. Assoc.*, *30*, 584.
(9) Rumsey, T. S. et al. (1979) *J. anim. Sci.*, *48*, 673.

6

Diseases of the Alimentary Tract—II

DISEASES OF THE FORESTOMACHS OF RUMINANTS

In the study of diseases of the ruminant stomachs the first consideration is the clinical and laboratory findings which attract special attention to the stomachs. The first step is the recognition that a basic syndrome of ruminant gastrointestinal dysfunction occurs without evidence of disease in another system which might suggest that the dysfunction is secondary.

The clinical findings which suggest primary ruminant gastrointestinal dysfunction include the following:

- Inappetence to anorexia, failure to regurgitate and chew the cud
- Ruminal atony or hypermotility observed visually, and detectable on auscultation
- Abnormal rumen contents palpable through the abdominal wall. The contents may feel dry or fluid splashing sounds may be detectable
- Visible abnormality of the abdomen, either distension or gauntness
- Abdominal pain, usually subacute, and characterized by humping of the back, or acute colicky signs of kicking at the belly and stretching. Pain may also be detectable on percussion or deep palpation of the abdomen if there is peritonitis either local or diffuse
- Abnormal feces. The feces are usually increased in amount and sweet-sour smelling in carbohydrate engorgement. In most other diseases of the ruminant stomach the amount of feces is reduced (scant) and the feces are pasty, foul-smelling and appear overdigested because of the long sojourn in the alimentary tract. A complete absence of feces for 24–48 hours is not uncommon with diseases of the ruminant stomach and may be confused with an intestinal obstruction or the earliest stages of hypocalcemia in a recently calved mature cow
- The temperature, heart rate and respirations are variable and often normal. If there is an associated acute peritonitis the temperature is usually elevated; in acute diffuse peritonitis with toxemia, it is commonly normal or subnormal; and in subacute and chronic peritonitis the temperature is usually normal. In most other diseases of the ruminant stomachs except carbohydrate engorgement and abomasal torsion where dehydration, acidosis, and gastric infarction occur, vital signs may be within the normal range.

Dropping regurgitated cuds occurs occasionally and is associated with straw impaction of the rumen, vagus indigestion, esophageal dilatation and rumenitis.

The stomachs of ruminants are closely associated anatomically and functionally, and disease of one usually affects the others (1). The rumen is easily examined clinically and experimentally and it is usually used as an indicator of the state of the other stomachs. Bacterial digestion and fermentation, and physical maceration by contraction of the stomach walls are the two main functions of the forestomachs and the two are interdependent. Thus abnormality of one leads to the abnormality of the other, and of the two the motility is most readily examinable. Ruminal motility is therefore used as an index of digestive function in the ruminant.

The plain muscle of the forestomachs has no intrinsic contractile power and the movement of the walls of these organs depends upon the integrity of both the afferent and efferent nerves and the reticuloruminal motor center of the medulla. Both afferent and efferent fibers are carried in the vagus nerves and damage to one or other branches of the nerve causes interference with normal movements and produces the syndrome of vagus indigestion.

When food enters the forestomachs it normally divides into layers, an upper layer of free gas and a lower layer of fluid containing gas bubbles and suspended food particles. A layer of undigested fiber floats on top and heavy material such as grain sinks to the bottom, often in the reticulum. Much mixing of the contents of the rumen and reticulum takes place during ruminal movements which occur at the rate of 1–3/minute, the more rapid rate occurring soon after feeding.

The movements occur in cycles commencing with a double reticular contraction, the second of which is accompanied by a strong contraction of the anterior dorsal sac of the rumen. These contractions pour the fluid reticular contents over the bulky food mass in the rumen. A contraction of the ventral sac follows and fluid is returned to the reticulum. The clinical evidence of this cycle of contractions has been dealt with in Chapter 1. During each reticular contraction fluid and food particles, particularly heavy grain, pass into the reticulo-omasal orifice and into the omasum and abomasum. It is this passage of heavy grain directly into the abomasum, without in many instances proper digestion in the rumen, which may lead to overloading of the abomasum and resultant displacement or torsion of this organ. It may also be important in the pathogenesis of enterotoxemia caused by *Clostridium perfringens* type D. If the floor of the reticulum is fixed to the ventral abdominal wall by adhesions it may be impossible for fluid to pass into the reticulo-omasal orifice. This may be a factor in the development of some forms of vagus indigestion.

Eructation contractions occur in the dorsal sacs, pass forward to the cardia of the esophagus and in conjunction with a reticular relaxation depress the level of the reticular fluid. The cardia relaxes and gas is expelled. If the ruminal contents are frothy it may be impossible for the cardia to be cleared and eructation to occur; ruminal tympany follows. Eructation contractions are independent of mixing contractions, their rate depending upon the pressure of the gas in the rumen. They occur for the most part immediately after the mixing contractions.

Rumination also depends upon additional ruminal contractions which are interposed before normal mixing movements of the rumen. These special contractions keep the area of the esophageal cardia flooded with reticular fluid. A voluntary movement by the animal follows; an inspiratory effort is made with the glottis closed: the negative pressure in the thorax is greatly increased and the reticular fluid, carrying some floating ingesta, is carried up to the pharynx. Defects of regurgitation are usually due to inability to create the necessary negative pressure in the thorax; this may occur in chronic pulmonary emphysema. In these circumstances there are usually visible efforts at regurgitation, often accompanied by grunting. Regurgitation ceases as soon as ruminal atony occurs because of absence of the ruminal contractions necessary to keep the cardiac region filled with fluid. However, regurgitation contractions play no part in the movement of the bolus up the esophagus. Regurgitation also diminishes when regurgitation contractions are not stimulated by coarse fiber in the rumen. Cattle on pelleted or finely ground diets ruminate little or not at all. Rumination is also depressed by excitement and fear.

The differential diagnosis of causes of gastrointestinal dysfunction in cattle is summarized in Table 22. The diseases of the ruminant stomachs and intestines with emphasis on differential diagnoses is reviewed (4).

In contrast with most other parts of the ruminant alimentary tract, and with the stomach of non-ruminants, specific lesions of the mucosa of the forestomachs are uncommon. Penetration of the wall by metallic foreign bodies is a common disease and dealt with below under the heading of traumatic reticuloperitonitis, but it is the peritonitis which causes interference with ruminal motility. Rarely there are actinomycotic or neoplastic lesions at the fundus of the reticulum which interfere with proper functioning of the esophageal groove and lead to a syndrome of vagus indigestion described later. Rumenitis does occur commonly but only as a secondary change in acute carbohydrate engorgement and it is this which has such damaging effects on gut motility and fluid and electrolyte status and eventually kills most cows. The rumenitis may have a long-term effect on ruminal motility but its main significance is as a portal for infection leading to the development of hepatic abscesses. Ingested animal hairs, and plant spicules and fibers are also credited with causing rumenitis but no clinical signs have been associated with the lesions (2). Because of the high prevalence of rumenitis lesions in cattle on heavy concentrated feed, especially when the feed is awned barley, the awns have been incriminated as traumatic agents (3). In acute arsenic poisoning there is an early postmortem dehiscence of the ruminal mucosa but no apparent lesions during life.

Other lesions of the forestomachs are parakeratosis, discussed below, and villous atrophy sometimes encountered in weanling ruminants on special diets low in fiber, even succulent young pasture, but these are not known to influence stomach function or motility. The factors which principally affect ruminal motility are those chemical and physical characteristics of its contents which are dealt with in simple indigestion and acute carbohydrate engorgement. Lesions in, and malfunctioning of, the abomasum are much more akin to abnormalities of the stomach in monogastric animals.

Some of the physiological factors which affect reticulorumen function and the clinical factors which cause reticulorumen dysfunction are summarized in Table 23. As mentioned earlier, when reticulorumen dysfunction is present, particularly hypomotility, the problem is to decide if the cause is directly associated with the stomachs and/or the other parts of the alimentary tract, or if the cause is due to an abnormality of another system. Differentiation requires a careful clinical examination including simple laboratory evaluation of the rumen contents.

The factors which affect the motility of the rumen are discussed in the section on simple indigestion, as are the principles of treatment in cases of ruminal atony.

REVIEW LITERATURE

Kay, R.N.B. (1983) Rumen function and physiology. *Vet. Rec.*, *113*, 6–9.

Leek, B.F. (1983) Clinical diseases of the rumen. A physiologist's view. *Vet. Rec.*, *113*, 10–14.

Radostits, O.M. (1981) Diseases of the ruminant stomachs and intestines of cattle. *Proc. 13th Annual Conv. Am. Assoc. Bov. Pract.*, 63–97.

REFERENCES

(1) Leek, B.F. (1969) *Vet. Rec.*, *84*, 238.
(2) Fell, R. et al. (1972) *Res. vet. Sci.*, *13*, 30.
(3) Kay, M. et al. (1969) *Res. vet. Sci.*, *10*, 181.
(4) Radostits, O. M. (1981) *Proc. 13th Ann. Conv. Am. Assoc. Bov. Pract.*, No. 13, 63–97.

Table 22. Differential diagnosis of causes of gastrointestinal dysfunction of cattle

Disease	*Epidemiology and history*	*Clinical findings*	*Clinical pathology*	*Response to treatment*
Simple indigestion	Dietary indiscretion, too much of a palatable, or indigestible or change of or damaged or frozen food. Can be outbreak. Consumption of excessive quantities of finely chopped straw	Simple gastrointestinal atony. Voluminous feces during recovery. Gross distension of the rumen and abdomen in straw impaction	All values normal. Slight changes in ruminal acidity, should be self-buffered	Excellent just with time. Usually a mild purgative. Rumenotomy necessary in case of straw impaction
Carbohydrate engorgement	Access to large amount readily fermentable carbohydrate when not accustomed. Enzootic in high grain rations in feedlots	Severe gastrointestinal atony with complete cessation of ruminal activity. Fluid splashing sounds in rumen. Severe dehydration, circulatory failure. Apparent blindness, then recumbency and too weak to rise. Soft odoriferous feces	Hemoconcentration with severe acidosis, pH of 4·5 in rumen, serum phosphorus levels up to 3·5 mmol/l. No living protozoa in rumen	Intensive fluid and electrolyte therapy necessary for survival. Rumenotomy or rumen lavage may be necessary. Alkalinizing agents
Ruminal tympany	Frothy bloat on lush legume pasture, or low roughage feedlot ration, especially lucerne hay. Free gas bloat secondary, occasionally primary on preserved feed	Gross distension of abdomen, especially high up on left. Sudden onset. Severe pain and respiratory distress. Rumen moves vigorously until end. Sloppy feces. Resonance on percussion over rumen	Nil	Excellent if in time, stomach tube for free gas. Froth-dispersing agent in frothy bloat. Severe cases may require trocarization or emergency rumenotomy
Acute traumatic reticuloperitonitis	Exposure to pieces of metal. Sporadic. Usually adult cattle	Sudden onset gastrointestinal atony with mild fever. Pain on movement and deep palpation on xiphoid, humped back. Constipation common. Lasts 3 days, then improvement begins	Neutrophilia and shift to left	Good to conservative medical treatment, or surgical treatment
Chronic traumatic reticuloperitonitis	Previous history of acute local peritonitis	Inappetence to anorexia; loss of weight; temperature, pulse and respirations normal; rumen small and atonic, chronic moderate bloat common, feces scant, grunt may be detectable on deep palpation over xiphoid, reticular adhesions on laparotomy	Hemogram depends on stage and extent of inflammation	Unfavorable
Vagus indigestion	May or may not have history of acute local peritonitis. Inappetence and progressive distension of abdomen during late pregnancy and no response to treatment with laxatives	Progressive distension of abdomen, scant soft feces, anorexia, rumen distended with well macerated and frothy contents, persistent moderate bloat, hypermotile initially and atonic later, temperature normal, heart rate variable, large L-shaped rumen rectally, abomasal impaction in some, large loss of weight, eventual recumbency, dehydration and weakness	Varying degree of dehydration, alkalosis, hypochloremia and hypokalemia	Inadequate response to treatment medically or surgically. Mild cases near term may respond spontaneously following parturition

Table 22 (cont.)

Disease	*Epidemiology and history*	*Clinical findings*	*Clinical pathology*	*Response to treatment*
Early hypocalcemia	Usually within 48 hours following parturition in a mature dairy cow susceptible to post parturient hypocalcemia	Anorexia, rumen hypotonic or static, scant or absence of feces for up to 24–36 hours, temperature normal, heart rate increased and possibly arrhythmia, still milking and may appear normal in all other aspects	Total serum calcium below 1·5 mmol/l	Good response to calcium administered intravenously or subcutaneously. May require several hours to return to normal
Abomasal impaction (dietary)	Excessive intake of poor quality roughage during cold weather. Outbreaks. Cattle eating crops contaminated with sand	Anorexia, moderate abdominal distension, weight loss, scant feces, weak, recumbent. Abomasum palpable through abdominal wall or rectally	Alkalosis, hypochloremia, hypokalemia and dehydration	High case fatality rate. Fluids, laxatives. Slaughter for salvage may be indicated
Left-side displacement of abomasum (LDA)	High-level grain diets, immediately postpartum, dairy cows, inactivity	Acetonemia in cow within days after parturition, inappetence, feces soft and amount variable (usually reduced). Ketonuria. Rumen sounds present but faint. Pinging sound on percussion and auscultation of left side	Ketonuria. Paracentesis into displaced abomasum yields pH of 2 and no protozoa	Good response following surgical correction
Right-side displacement of abomasum (RDA)	Usually 2–4 weeks postpartum	Anorexia, scant feces, poor milk production, moderate dehydration, rumen sluggish, fluid-filled viscus under right costal arch, ping commonly audible, may be palpable per rectum, progressive and commonly results in torsion	Alkalosis, hypochloremia, hypokalemia	Some recover spontaneously with medical therapy. Give calcium borogluconate and hay diet. Surgery may be required. Prognosis good if treated early. Fluid therapy
Torsion of abomasum	Sequel to right-side displacement of abomasum (RDA)	History of RDA followed by sudden onset of acute abdominal pain, distension of right abdomen, loud 'pinging' sound on percussion. Distended tense abomasum palpable per rectum, marked circulatory failure, weakness, bloodstained feces, death in 48–60 hours	Dehydrating alkalosis, hypochloremia	Laparotomy, abomasotomy and drainage. Survival rate about 75% if treated early. Fluid therapy required
Primary acetonemia (wasting form)	Overfat cows in late pregnancy or insufficient intake of energy in early lactation. May be high silage diet in heavy producing indoor cattle	Cow dull, off feed, small amounts firm balls of feces, not pasty, lose condition, milk yield down. Rumen activity depressed	Ketonuria and hypoglycemia	Dextrose intraveuously and propylene glycol orally, or corticosteroids intramuscularly. Usually excellent response
Acute intestinal obstruction	May be heightened activity, e.g. during sexual activity. Often no particular history	Sudden onset, short period acute pain. Kicking at belly, rolling. Complete anorexia, failure to drink and alimentary tract stasis. Dehydration commences. Distended loops of gut may be palpable. Gray to red foul-smelling rectal contents	Gradual development of dehydration and hemoconcentration over 3–4 days	Surgery is necessary
Idiopathic paralytic ileus	Few days postpartum, maybe change in diet	Anorexia, complete absence of feces for 24–48 hours	Nil	Usually recover spontanously

Table 22 (cont.)

Disease	*Epidemiology and history*	*Clinical findings*	*Clinical pathology*	*Response to treatment*
Obstruction of small intestine by phytobezoar	Single animal usually. Area prevalence may be high some years. Depends on frequency of fibrous plants, e.g. *Romulea* sp.	Sudden onset acute abdominal pain. Attack brief, often missed. Then anorexia, ruminal stasis, heart rate climbs to 120 over 3 or 4 days. Abdomen distends moderately, splashing sounds and tympany right flank. Rectal examination—distended loops if obstruction low down, mostly not, may feel 5–6 cm diameter, fiber ball, feces pasty, gray-yellow, smelly, small amount only. Untreated and fatal cases have course of 4–8 days	Hypochloremia, hypokalemia, severity depends on location	Depends on nature of phytobezoar, dense fiber balls require surgery, crumbly masses may pass after mineral oil for several days
Abomasal ulcer	Immediately after (2 weeks) parturition. High producers on heavy grain feed. In intensive feeding systems disease is becoming enzootic in some areas	Gastrointestinal atony with melena. May be sufficient blood loss to cause death. More likely prompt recovery after 4 days. Perforation and rupture of ulcer leads to death in a few hours	Melena or occult blood in feces. On perforation with local peritonitis may be leukocytosis and left shift. Anemia due to hemorrhage	Alkalinizing agents orally. Surgery if medical treatment unsuccessful
Pregnancy toxemia of beef cattle	Fat beef cattle, deprived of feed in last month of pregnancy. Commonly have twin pregnancy	Complete anorexia, rumen stasis, scant feces, ketonuria, weak and commonly recumbent	Ketonemia, increase in non-esterified fatty acids, ketonuria, increase in liver enzymes	Poor response to therapy. Fluids, anabolic steroids, insulin
Fatty liver (fat cow) syndrome	Fat dairy cow, few days following parturition or may have had LDA for several days	Complete anorexia, rumen stasis, almost no milk yield, ketonuria initially but may have more later	Ketonemia, increase in liver enzymes	Poor response to therapy. Glucose, insulin, anabolic steroids
Cecal dilatation and/or torsion	Single case. Dairy cow, early lactation, inappetence, feces may be scant. Severe cases have history of mild abdominal pain	Systemically normal. Rumen only slightly sluggish, tympanic sounds over right upper flank which may be distended. Rectally enlarged cylindrical movable cecum with blind end can be felt	Nothing diagnostic, but has hemoconcentration, compensated hypochloremia, hypokalemia and alkalosis	Good response to surgical correction. Unfavorable prognosis with severe torsion and gangrene
Acute diffuse peritonitis	Following acute traumatic reticuloperitonitis, uterine rupture at parturition, rupture of rectum, postsurgical	Acute toxemia, fever followed by hypothermia, weakness, tachycardia, recumbency, groaning, moderate distension, scant feces, palpate fibrinous adhesions rectally	Leukopenia, neutropenia, degenerative left shift. Hemoconcentration. Paracentesis positive	Usually die
Chronic ruminal tympany	Beef calves 6–8 months of age following weaning; feeder cattle after arrival in feedlot	Chronic free-gas bloat, relapses after treatment, no other clinical findings	Nil	Good response to surgical ruminal fistula or insertion of corkscrew-type trocar and cannula and leave in place for few weeks
Omasal impaction	Uncommon. Single cases in pregnant cows with vagus indigestion. Feedlot cattle with abomasal impaction dietary in orgin	Inappetence to anorexia. Scant feces, abdominal distension. Rectally large distended round hard viscus below kidney can be felt	Nil	Slaughter for salvage. Treat as for abomasal impaction

Table 23. The effects of some common clinical excitatory and inhibitory influences on primary cycle movements of the reticulorumen*

Clinical afferent input	*Clinical findings and responses to treatment*
EXCITATORY INPUTS	
Low threshold reticular tension receptors	
Increased reticular tension	
After feeding Mild ruminal tympany	Increases frequency, duration and amplitude of primary cycle contractions and mixing promotes fermentation
Decreased reticular tension	
Starvation Anorexia	Decreases frequency, duration and amplitude of primary cycle contractions and decreases fermentation
Lesions of medial wall of reticulum	
Chronic induration and fibrosis due to traumatic reticuloperitonitis	Causes hypomotility of rumen contractions and may be explanation for atony in some cases of vagus indigestion. Some cases are characterized by erratic hypermotility
Acid receptors in abomasum	
Increases in abomasal acidity following emptying of organ	Increase primary cycle movements which increases flow of ruminal contents into abomasum to maintain optimum volume and to decrease acidity
Buccal cavity receptors	
Following eating	Increased reticulorumen activity
INHIBITORY INPUTS	
High threshold reticular tension receptors	
Peak of reticular contraction Severe ruminal tympany Ruminal impaction with forage, hay, straw (not necessarily grain overload)	Depression of primary cycle movements, ruminal hypomotility, depression of fermentation because of failure of mixing
Abomasal tension receptors	
Impaction, distension or displacement of abomasum	Abomasal impaction, dilatation and torsion may result in complete ruminal stasis. Left-side displacement of abomasum (LDA) usually does not cause clinically significant hypomotility
Pain	
Visceral pain due to distension of abomasum or intestines. Severe pain from anywhere in body	Moderate to total inhibition of reticulorumen movements possible with visceral pain. The degree of inhibition from pain elsewhere will vary
Depressant drugs	
Anesthetics, central nervous system depressants Prostaglandin E	Inhibition of primary and secondary cycle movements, and eructation resulting in ruminal tympany
Changes in rumen contents	
Marked decrease (below 5) or increase (above 8) in pH of ruminal fluid. Engorgement with carbohydrates or protein-rich feeds. Absence of protozoa in ruminal acidosis and in lead and other chemical poisoning	Inhibition of primary and secondary cycle movement and lack of fermentation. Cud transfer promotes return to normal activity
Changes in body water, electrolytes and acid–base balance	
Hypocalcemia	Inhibition of primary and secondary cycle movements and of eructation resulting in ruminal tympany which responds to treatment with calcium
Dehydration and electrolyte losses, acidosis, alkalosis	Inhibition of reticulorumen movements which gradually return to normal with fluid and electrolyte therapy
Peritonitis	
Traumatic reticuloperitonitis	Inhibition of primary and secondary cycle movements and of eructation resulting in ruminal tympany. Return of primary movements is good prognostic sign. Lesions must heal without involvement of nerve receptors or adhesions which will interfere with normal motility
Toxemia/fever	
Peracute coliform mastitis Acute bacterial pneumonia	Inhibition of primary and secondary cycle movements which return to normal with treatment of toxemia
Ruminal distension	
Early ruminal tympany	Increased frequency of secondary cycle movements and of eructation
Covering of cardia (fluid or foam)	
Ruminal tympany Recumbent animal	Cardia does not open, failure of eructation resulting in ruminal tympany. Clearance of cardia results in eructation

*Most of the sensory inputs are transmitted to gastric centers in the dorsal vagal nerve nuclei from which the efferent outputs originate and pass down the vagal motor nerve fibers. Modified according to Leek (1).

SPECIAL EXAMINATION OF THE ALIMENTARY TRACT AND ABDOMEN OF CATTLE

When gastrointestinal dysfunction is suspected a complete special clinical examination is necessary to determine the location and nature of the lesion. A systematic method of examination is presented here.

History

Obtain a complete history with as much detail as is available. The stage of the pregnancy–lactation cycle, the days since parturition, the nature of the diet, the speed of onset and the duration of illness will often suggest diagnostic possibilities. An accurate description of the appetite will suggest whether the disease is acute or chronic. The previous treatments used and the response obtained should be determined. Any evidence of abdominal pain and its characteristics should be determined. The nature and the volume of the feces may suggest enteritis or alimentary tract stasis.

Systemic state, habitus and appetite

The vital signs will indicate the severity of the disease and suggest if it is acute, subacute or chronic. In acute intestinal obstruction, abomasal torsion, acute diffuse peritonitis and acute carbohydrate engorgement, the heart rate may be 100–120/minute and dehydration is usually obvious. Anemia is an important indicator of alimentary tract hemorrhage especially if there is concurrent melena. If cattle with any of the above diseases are recumbent and unable to rise the prognosis is usually unfavorable. A marked increase in the rate and depth of respirations associated with alimentary tract disease usually indicates the presence of fluid or electrolyte disturbances and possible subacute pain. Grunting or moaning suggests abdominal pain associated with distension of a viscus or acute diffuse peritonitis.

The degree of appetite and the presence or absence of rumination are very reliable indicators of the state of the alimentary tract including the liver. Complete anorexia persisting for more than 3–5 days is unfavorable. The return of appetite and chewing of the cud following alimentary tract disease or surgery is a favorable prognostic sign. Persistent inappetence suggests a chronic lesion usually with an unfavourable prognosis.

Visual inspection of the abdomen

The contour or silhouette of the abdomen should be examined from the rear, and each lateral region veiwed from an oblique angle. Examination of the contour will assist in determining the cause of abdominal distension. Abdominal distension may be unilateral, bilaterally symmetrical or asymmetrical or more prominent in the dorsal half or ventral half. Recognition of the area of maximum distension suggests diagnostic possibilities which are set out in Fig. 14. The differential diagnosis of abdominal distension of cattle is summarized in Table 24.

The cause of distension of the abdomen of cattle is determined by a combination of the following examinations:

- Visual inspection of the contour or silhouette of the abdomen to determine the site of maximum distension
- If necessary, relief of rumen contents with a stomach tube to determine if the distension is due to an enlarged rumen. The ruminal contents can also be examined grossly at the same time
- Auscultation and percussion of the abdomen to detect the presence and location of gas-filled viscuses
- Rectal examination to identify any obvious enlargements
- Paracentesis abdominis to examine the amount and nature of the peritoneal fluid which may indicate the presence of ischemic necrosis of intestines or peritonitis
- Trocarization of severe gas-filled swellings such as an abomasal torsion in a calf.

Oral cavity and esophagus

The oral cavity is easily inspected visually and by digital palpation with the aid of a suitable mouth speculum. The patency of the esophagus is determined by passage of a stomach tube into the rumen.

Left abdomen and rumen

Visual inspection and palpation

The primary and secondary cycle contractions of ruminal motility can be identified by simultaneous auscultation, palpation and observation of the left paralumbar fossa and the left lateral abdominal region. During contractions of the rumen there is an alternate rising and sinking of the left paralumbar fossa in conjunction with abdominal surface ripples. The ripples reflect ruminal motility and occur during both the primary (or mixing) cycle and the secondary (or eructation) cycle of ruminal motility (2). As the left paralumbar fossa rises during the first part of the primary cycle there are two horizontal ripples which move from the lower left abdominal region up to the paralumbar fossa. When the paralumbar fossa sinks, during the second part of the primary cycle, the ripple moves ventrally and fades out at the lower part of the left abdominal region. Similar ripples follow up and down after the rising and sinking of the paralumbar fossa associated with the secondary cycle movements. In vagus indigestion, there may be three to seven vigorous incomplete contractions of the rumen per minute. These contractions may not be audible because the rumen contents are porridge-like and do not cause the normal crackling sounds. However, the contractions are visible and palpable as waves of undulations of the left flank.

The nature of the contents of the rumen can be assessed by palpation of the rumen through the left paralumbar fossa. In the roughage-fed animal, the rumen contents are doughy and pit on pressure. In cattle which have consumed large quantities of long cereal grain straw the rumen is large and the contents palpated through the abdominal wall feel very firm. In the dehydrated animal the contents may feel almost firm. In the grain-fed animal the contents may be soft and porridge-like. When the rumen contains excessive quantities of fluid the left flank will fluctuate on deep palpation. In the atonic rumen filled with excess gas the left flank will be tense, resilient and tympanitic on percussion.

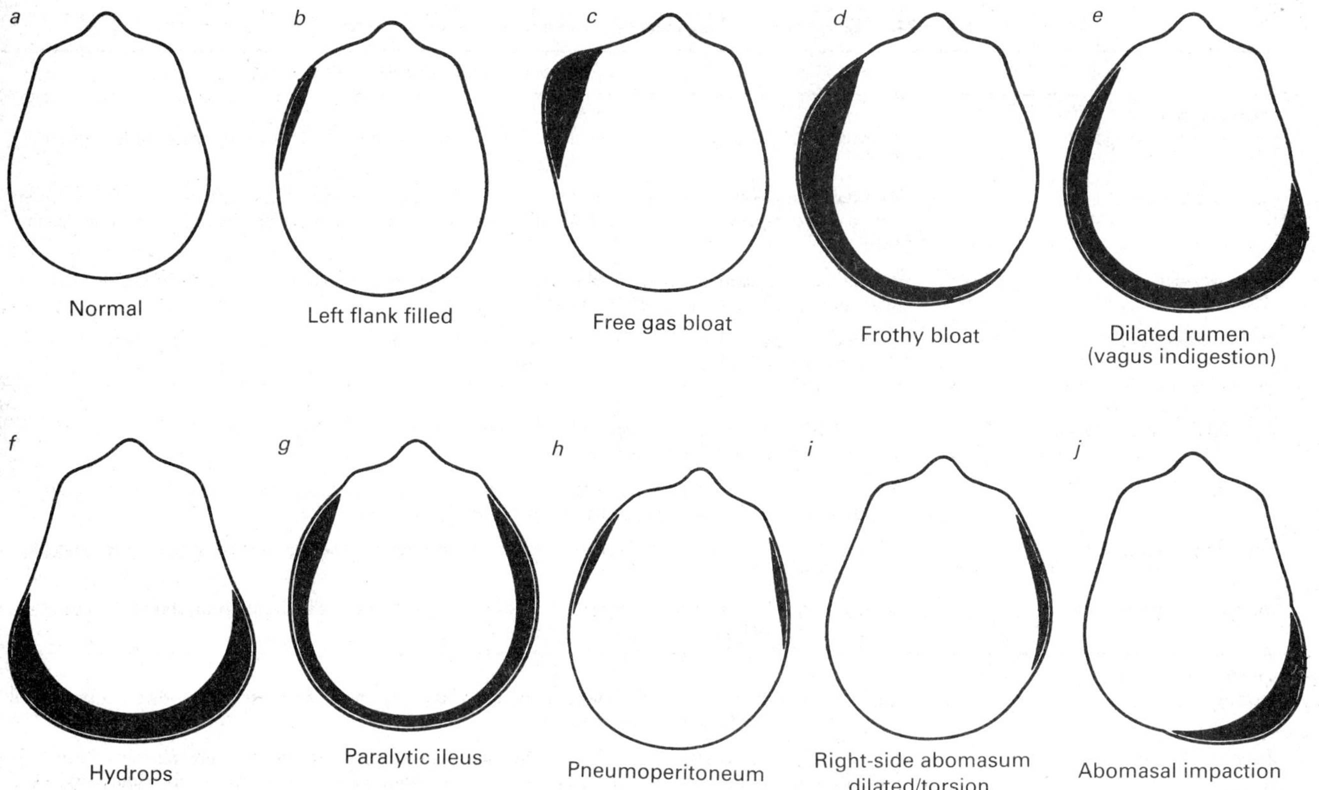

Fig. 14. Silhouettes of the contour of the abdomen of cattle, viewed from the rear, with different diseases of the abdominal viscera. (After Stober and Dirksen (1), courtesy of the authors and the editor of *Bovine Practitioner*.)

Auscultation of the rumen and left flank

In the normal animal on a roughage diet there are two independent contraction sequences of the reticulorumen. The *primary cycle*, which recurs approximately every minute, consists of a diphasic contraction of the reticulum followed by a monophasic contraction of the dorsal ruminal sac and then by a monophasic contraction of the ventral ruminal sac. These movements appear to be concerned primarily with 'mixing' the rumen contents and with assisting the passage of rumen contents into the omasum. The *secondary cycle* movements, which occur at intervals of about 2 minutes, are confined to the rumen and consist of a contraction of the dorsal sac followed by a contraction of the ventral sac. The former causes the fluid contents of the dorsal sac to be forced ventrally and the gas layer to be forced cranially to the region of the cardia where eructation takes place. Contractions of the dorsal and ventral sacs cause undulations of the left paralumbar fossa and lower flanks which are readily visible and palpable.

The clinical recognition of the presence or absence of either the primary cycle or secondary cycle contractions or both may aid in determining the cause and severity of the disease and the prognosis. These are outlined in Table 23.

In auscultation of the rumen, the stethoscope is placed in the middle of the left paralumbar fossa area. After sufficient contractions have occurred, the stethoscope should then be moved anteriorly to determine if rumen contractions can be heard in the region that becomes occupied with a left displacement of the abomasum. In the normal animal, rumen movement will be heard in this area which is in the second last intercostal space. The type, strength and frequency of rumen movements should be noted. The rumen sounds of the normal animal consuming roughage are booming-crackling sounds. When the rumen contains less coarse roughage or primarily grain, the sounds may be much less distinct but still possess a crackling characteristic.

The presence of fluid-tinkling or fluid-splashing sounds, usually along with a static rumen, suggests that the rumen contains an excessive quantity of fluid, and that the coarse ingesta is not floating on the fluid layer of the rumen contents as in the normal animal. Fluid-splashing sounds suggest diseases such as grain overload, or an atonic rumen associated with prolonged anorexia (chronic diffuse peritonitis, abomasal or omasal impaction). The sounds are similar to those present in left-side displacement of the abomasum. To assist in the differential diagnosis, the outline of the rumen can be percussed to observe a much wider area of metallic sound than normally expected in left-side displacement of the abomasum.

In *vagus indigestion* with an enlarged hypermotile rumen, the contractions of the rumen will usually be obvious and frequent (3–6/minute). The contractions are visible as prominent undulations of the wall of the left flank which are visible and palpable but may not be audible because the rumen contents are homogeneous and porridge-like due to prolonged maceration in the rumen. Complete atony of the rumen also occurs in vagus indigestion.

Table 24. The differential diagnosis of abdominal distension in cattle

Cause	*Major clinical findings and methods of diagnosis*
Distension of rumen	
Acute ruminal tympany	Marked distension of left abdomen, less of right. Pass stomach tube and attempt to relieve gas or froth
Vagus indigestion	Marked distension of left abdomen, less of right. Fluctuating rumen on palpation. Excessive rumen activity or complete atony. Large L-shaped rumen on rectal examination. Pass large-bore stomach tube
Grain overload	Moderate distension of left flank, less of right. Rumen contents are doughy or fluctuate. Rumen static and systemic acidosis. Rumen pH below 6–5
Simple indigestion	Marked distension of rumen. Contractions may be present or absent depending on severity. Systemically normal. May be dropping cuds
Distension of abomasum	
Right dilatation and torsion	Right flank and paralumbar fossa normal to severely distended. Ping on percussion. Rectal palpation of fluctating or tense viscus in right abdomen
Impaction	Right lower flank normal to moderately distended. Doughy viscus palpable caudal to costal arch. Rectal palpation feel doughy viscus in right lower flank
Left-side displacement	Abdomen usually gaunt. Occasionally left paralumbar fossa distended due to displaced abomasum. Ping on percussion
Abomasal trichobezoars	Older calves (2–4 months of age). Right lower flank distended. Fluid-splashing sounds. Painful grunt on deep palpation. Confirm by laparotomy
Distension of intestines	
Enteritis	Slight to moderate distension of right abdomen. Fluid-rushing and splashing sounds on auscultation and ballottement. Diarrhea and dehydration
Intestinal obstruction	Slight to moderate distension of right abdomen. Fluid tinkling, percolating and splashing sounds on auscultation and ballottement. May palpate rectally. Scant dark feces. Paracentesis abdominis
Paralytic ileus	Slight to moderate distension of right abdomen. Tinkling sounds on auscultation. Tympanitic ping on percussion. Loops of distended intestine palpable per rectum
Cecal dilatation and torsion	Right flank may be normal or moderately distended. Ping present. Palpate movable blind end cecum on rectal examination. Confirm by laparotomy
Englargement of uterus	
Physiological	Gross distension of both flanks, especially right. Normal pregnancy with more than one fetus. May palpate rectally
Pathological	
Hydrops amnion	Gradual enlargement of lower half of abdomen in late gestation. Flaccid uterus, fetus and placentomes are easily palpable per rectum
Hydrops allantosis	Gradual distension of lower half of abdomen in late gestation. Palpable uterus rectally, cannot palpate placentomes or fetus
Fetal emphysema	History of dystocia or recent birth of one calf, twin in uterus and emphysematous. Diagnosis obvious on vaginal and rectal examination
Fluid accumulation in peritoneal cavity	
Ascites Congestive heart failure, peritonitis, ruptured bladder	Bilateral distension of lower abdomen. Positive fluid waves. Paracentesis abdominis
Pneumoperitoneum Perforated abomasal ulcer, postsurgical laparotomy	Not common. Bilateral distension of dorsal half of abdomen. Ping both sides

Auscultation and percussion of the left paralumbar fossa over an area extending from the mid-point of the 9th rib to the 13th rib is used to detect the presence of a 'ping' associated with left-sided displacement of the abomasum. Percussion can be accomplished with a flick of the finger or most reliably with a percussion hammer. The causes of 'pings' on percussion of the left abdomen in mature cattle include: left-side displacement of the abomasum, atonic rumen and, rarely, pneumoperitoneum.

For special investigations of reticulorumen motility radio telemetry capsules can be placed in the rumen (3).

Auscultation, percussion and palpation of the right abdomen

The contour of the right flank should be examined by *visual adspection* for evidence of distension which may be due to a viscus filled with fluid, gas or ingesta, ascites or a gravid uterus. In severe distension of the rumen, the ventral sac may also distend the lower half of the right flank.

A combination of deep palpation, ballottement, and simultaneous percussion and auscultation, and succussion (shaking the animal) is used to detect the presence of viscera which are distended with gas and/or fluid, or ingesta.

The causes of '*pings*' on percussion of the right abdomen include:

- Right-sided dilatation and torsion of the abomasum
- Cecal dilatation and torsion
- Torsion of the coiled colon
- Descending colon and rectum filled with gas in a cow with tenesmus
- Intestinal tympany of uncertain etiology
- Torsion of the root of the mesentery in young calves
- Intussusception
- Pneumoperitoneum
- Intestinal tympany in the postparturient cow (for first few days following parturition).

The causes of fluid-splashing sounds on ballottement and auscultation of the right flank include: fluid-filled intestines in acute intestinal obstruction and enteritis, and a fluid-filled abomasum in right-side dilatation. Palpation of a firm viscus in the right flank caudal or ventral to the right costal arch may be due to: omasal impaction, abomasal impaction, an enlarged ventral sac of the rumen which extends over to the right abdominal wall and enlargement of the liver. The liver must be grossly enlarged before it is palpable caudal to the right costal arch. A rectal examination is necessary to identify the distended viscus and a laparotomy may be necessary to positively identify the lesion and correct it.

The area of liver dullness can be outlined by percussion over the abdominal part of the right rib cage. In abomasal torsion the area of liver dullness may be moved caudally and be smaller than normal because of medial and caudal displacement of the liver.

Examination of rumen contents

Examination of the rumen contents is often essential to establish an accurate diagnosis of diseases of the rumen. The color, depending on the feed to a limited extent, will be a green, olive green or brown green. At pasture, the color is very green, with root crops the color tends to be gray, and with silage or straw the color is mostly of a yellow-brown nature. The color of the rumen contents will be a milky-gray in grain overload, and greenish-black in cases where rumen stasis is of long duration and where putrefaction is occurring within the rumen. The consistency of the rumen contents is normally slightly viscid, and watery rumen contents is indicative of inactive bacteria and protozoa. Excess froth is associated with frothy bloat as in primary ruminal tympany or vagus indigestion. The odor of the rumen contents is normally aromatic and, although somewhat pungent, not objectionable to the nose. A moldy, rotting odor usually indicates protein putrefaction, and an intensely sour odor indicates an excess of lactic acid formation, due to grain or carbohydrate engorgement. The pH of the rumen varies according to the type of feed and the time interval between the last feeding and taking a sample for pH examination. The normal range, however, is between 6·2 and 7·2. The pH of rumen fluid should be examined immediately after the sample is obtained, using a wide range pH (1–11) paper. High pH values (8–10) will be observed when putrefaction of protein is occurring in the rumen or if the sample is mixed with saliva. Low pH values (4–5) are found after the feeding of carbohydrates. In general, a value below 5 indicates carbohydrate engorgement and this pH level will be maintained for between 6 and 24 hours after the animal has actually consumed the carbohydrate diet. Microscopic examination of a few drops of rumen fluid on a glass slide with a low-power field will reveal the level of protozoan activity. Normally five to seven protozoans are active per low power field. In lactic acidosis the protozoa are usually absent or a few dead ones are visible.

In adult cattle presented with severe abdominal distension due to gross distension of the rumen it is difficult, if not impossible, to assess the status of the abdomen. To determine if the rumen is distended and/or to relieve the pressure a large-bore stomach tube should be passed. In vagus indigestion, the rumen may be grossly distended with fluid contents which will gush out through a large-bore tube. In some cases 100–150 liters of rumen contents may be released. If no contents are released the contents may be frothy or mushy and the rumen end of the tube will plug almost instantly. Rumen lavage may then be attempted using a water hose to deliver from 20–40 liters of water at a time followed by back drainage by gravity flow. After the rumen is partially emptied it is usually possible to more accurately assess the rumen and the abdomen.

Rectal exploration of the abdomen

Some of the specific abnormalities of the digestive tract, which are commonly palpable on rectal examinations, include the following. (See Fig. 15*a* to *l* which illustrate the abnormalities through a transverse section of the abdomen.)

(*a*) Normal.
(*b*) L-shaped rumen (occurs commonly in vagus indigestion and other diseases of the rumen characterized by gradual distension of the rumen).
(*c*) Cecal torsion (commonly palpable as long distended organ usually movable, may feel blind end).
(*d*) Abomasal torsion (commonly palpable as tense viscus in lower right half of abdomen).
(*e*) Abomasal impaction (not palpable in late pregnancy).
(*f*) Left-side displacement of the abomasum (usually cannot palpate the displaced abomasum but can often feel rumen which is usually smaller than normal).
(*g*) Intussusception (not always palpable, dependent on location of intussusception and the size of the animal).
(*h*) Mesenteric torsion—usually palpable.
(*i*) Intestinal incarceration—commonly palpable.
(*j*) Peritonitis—only palpable if peritoneum of posterior aspect of abdomen affected.
(*k*) Lipomatosis—commonly palpable as 'lumps' in the abdomen and pelvic cavity.
(*l*) Omental bursitis—not common.

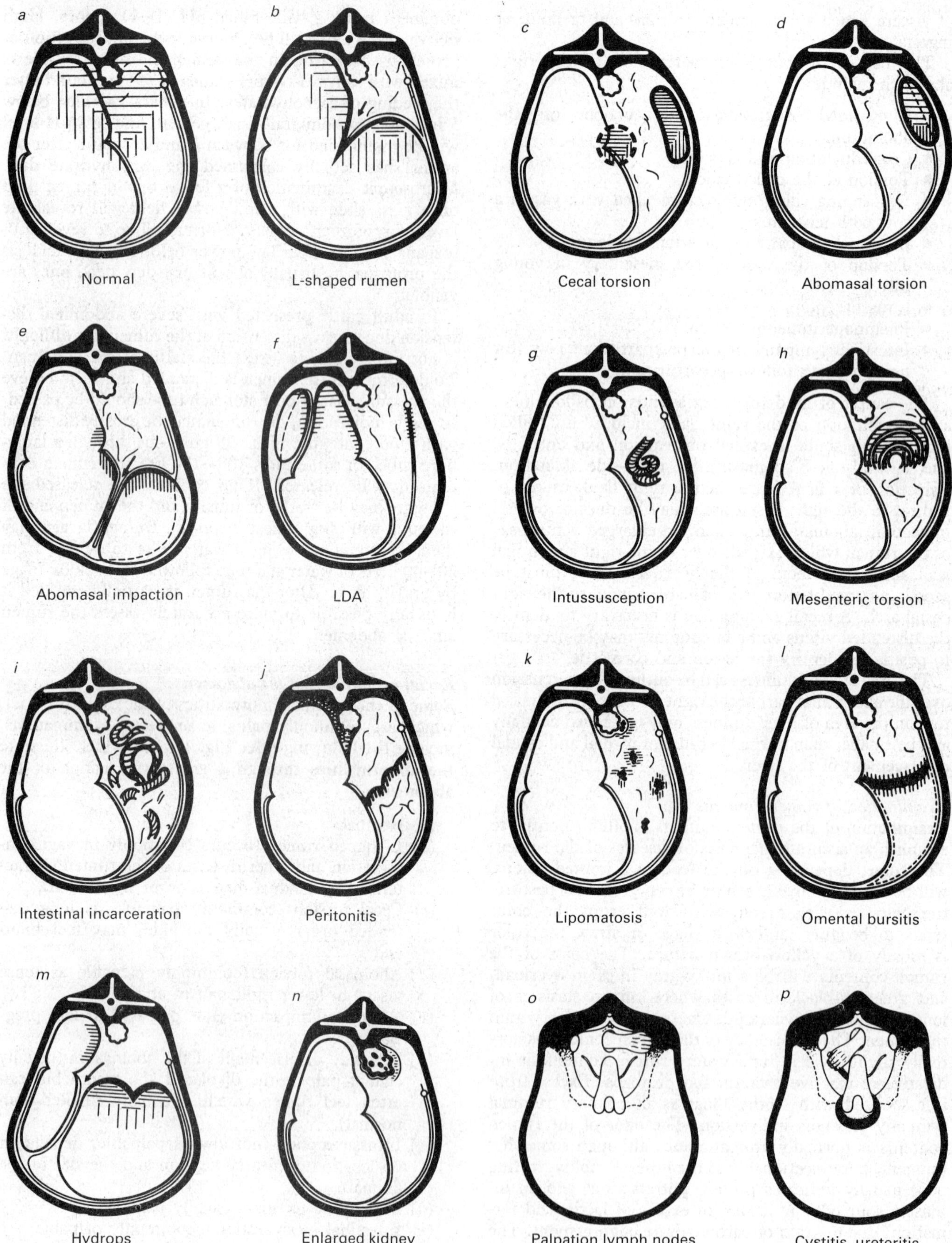

Fig. 15. Schematic illustrations of the rectal findings in cattle affected with different diseases of the abdominal viscera. (After Stober and Dirksen (1), courtesy of the authors and the editor of *Bovine Practitioner*.)

Figure 15 *m*, *n*, *o* and *p* are included for the differential diagnosis of the diseases each represents.

As part of the differential diagnosis of digestive tract disease in the postparturient cow, the uterus should be examined carefully for evidence of retained placenta and metritis. Both vaginal and rectal examinations should be done. The toxemia caused by retained fetal membranes and postpartum metritis may cause anorexia, rumen stasis, paralytic ileus, scant feces and sometimes a 'ping' in the right flank all of which may be interpreted as primary digestive tract diseases.

Gross examination of feces

The gross appearance of the feces of cattle is not only an indicator of disease of the digestive tract but can provide valuable clues for the differential diagnosis of disease elsewhere.

Amount of feces

In adult cattle, the passage of ingesta through the digestive tract takes $1\frac{1}{2}$–4 days. Mature cattle generally pass some feces every 1·5–2 hours, amounting to a total of 30–50 kg/day in ten to 24 portions.

A reduction in the bulk of feces can be due to: a decrease in feed or water intake or a retardation of the passage through the alimentary tract. In diarrhea, the feces are passed more frequently and in greater amounts than normal and contain a higher water content (over 90%) than normal.

Failure to pass any feces for 24 hours or more is abnormal and the continued absence of feces may be due to a physical intestinal obstruction. However, in many cases the intestine is not physically obstructed but rather there is a functional obstruction. Diseases causing disturbances of motility of the rumen and abomasum often result in a relative absence of feces. Paralytic ileus of the intestines due to peritonitis or idiopathic intestinal tympany also result in a marked reduction in feces, sometimes a complete absence, for up to 3 days. The marked reduction of feces which occurs in functional obstruction is a major source of diagnostic confusion because it resembles physical obstructions of the intestines. The causes of physical and functional obstruction of the alimentary tract of cattle are summarized in Fig. 16.

Color of the feces

The color of the feces is influenced by: the nature of the feed, the concentration of bile in the feces, and the passage rate through the digestive tract. Calves reared on cow's milk normally produce gold-yellow feces which become pale brown when hay or straw is eaten. The feeding of milk substitutes adds a gray component to a varying degree.

The feces of adult cattle on green forage are dark olive-green, on a hay ration, more brown-olive, while the ingestion of large amounts of grain produces gray-olive feces. A retardation of the ingesta causes the color to darken. The feces become ball-shaped and dark brown with a shining surface due to the coating with mucus. Diarrheic feces tend to be paler than normal because of their higher water content and lower concentration of bile.

The presence of large amounts of bile produces a dark olive-green to black-green color such as in cattle with hemolytic anemia. In cattle with obstruction of the common bile duct, the feces are pale olive-green because of the absence of bile pigments.

Hemorrhage into the digestive tract, depending on the amount, location and rate of passage, will result in feces which vary from chocolate-brown to blackish-tarry (melena). Hemorrhage in the abomasum and small intestine usually causes black, tarry feces. Hemorrhage in the rectum usually causes a red-brown discoloration distributed throughout the feces or red streaks of frank blood adhering to the fecal particles (dysentery).

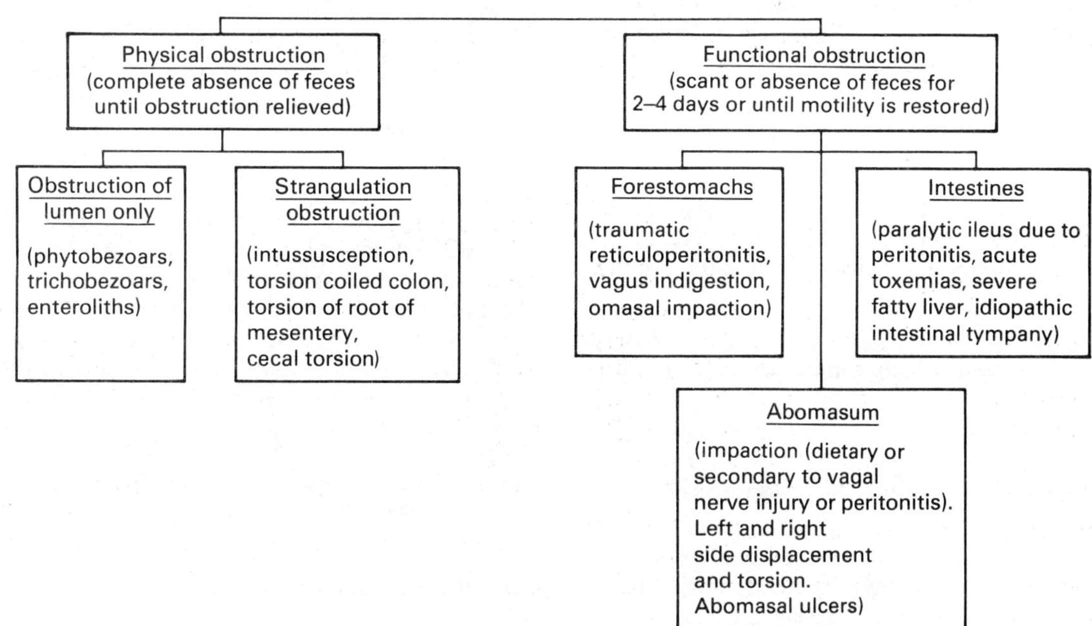

Fig. 16. Some common causes of physical and functional obstruction of the alimentary tract of cattle

Odor of the feces

Fresh bovine feces are not normally malodorous. Objectionable odors are usually due to putrefaction or fermentation of ingesta which are usually associated with inflammation. The feces in cattle with salmonellosis may be fetid while in advanced pericarditis with visceral edema due to passive congestion the feces are profuse but do not possess a grossly abnormal odor.

Consistency of feces

The consistency of the feces is dependent on the water content, the type of feed and the length of time the ingesta has remained in the digestive tract. Normally, milk-fed calves excrete feces of a medium to firm porridge-like consistency. After transition to a plant diet, the first solid particles begin to appear. Normal bovine feces are of a medium porridge-like consistency. A moderate thickening leads to the passage of fecal disks of a more solid consistency and severe dehydration causes the formation of firm balls of feces arranged in facets inside the rectum, the surfaces of which are dark and coated with mucus. The feces of cows with left-side displacement of the abomasum commonly are pasty in appearance. Sticky and tenacious feces are commonly seen in obstruction of the forestomachs (vagus indigestion, chronic peritonitis).

Degree of comminution of feces

The proportion of insufficiently comminuted (poorly digested) plant particles in the feces is dependent on the duration and thoroughness of rumination and the rate of passage of ingesta through the forestomachs. The length of time the ingesta is in the postruminal digestive tract seems to have no appreciable influence on its trituration. Poor comminution of feces indicates failure in rumination and/or accelerated passage of ingesta through the forestomachs. Thus in some cattle with acute traumatic reticuloperitonitis, the feces may contain small walnut-sized chunks of undigested plant fibers which presumably have escaped the cellulose digestive processes of the forestomachs. The presence of large numbers of kernels of grain in the feces is associated with the ingestion of large quantities of unprocessed grain like whole wheat or barley.

Other substances in the feces

Mucus The presence of mucus on the surface of fecal balls suggests a prolonged sojourn of the ingesta in the large intestine. The presence of a plug of mucus in the rectum is suggestive of a functional obstruction (paralytic ileus).

Fibrin In enteritis, large quantities of clear watery mucus may be passed which sometimes clot to form gelatinous masses.

In fibrinous enteritis, fibrin may be excreted in the form of long strands which may mold into a print of the intestinal lumen (intestinal fibrinous casts).

Blood Blood in the feces may originate from the following locations: (1) the swallowing of blood coughed up from pulmonary hemorrhage (not common, usually detected as *occult blood* with *Hemetest tablets*); (2) hemorrhage into the abomasum; acute hemorrhage usually appears as black-tarry feces (melena); chronic hemorrhage as occult blood; (3) hemorrhagic enteritis of small intestines; the feces are uniformly dark red; (4) hemorrhagic enteritis of the large intestines. Blood originating in the cecum or colon appears as frank blood evenly distributed throughout the feces. Blood originating in the rectum appears as streaks or chunks of frank blood unevenly distributed throughout the feces.

Detection of abdominal pain

Cattle with acute local or diffuse peritonitis may *grunt* with almost every expiration. The grunt is exaggerated in the recumbent position. However, grunting may also be caused by severe pneumonia, pleurisy and severe pulmonary emphysema. Careful auscultation and percussion of the lungs is therefore necessary to exclude the presence of pulmonary disease.

Not all *grunts* occur spontaneously. Deep palpation of the abdomen using the closed hand or knee is often necessary to elicit a grunt. Auscultation over the trachea is often necessary to hear the grunt. The grunt is best produced if pressure is applied to the abdomen at the end of inspiration and the beginning of expiration. The inspiratory and expiratory sounds are auscultated for six to eight respirations and then without any particular warning the pressure is applied to the abdomen. The presence of a grunt means the presence of a peritoneal lesion (stretching, inflammation, edema). The absence of a grunt does not exclude the presence of a peritoneal lesion. In acute traumatic reticuloperitonitis the grunt may be absent in 3–5 days after the initial penetration of the reticulum.

A rigid bar or wooden pole may be necessary to apply pressure in large cattle (large cows and bulls). The bar is held by two people in a horizontal position just behind the xiphoid sternum while a third person auscultates over the trachea when the bar is lifted quickly up into the abdomen. Several attempts should be made to elicit a grunt before concluding the absence of a grunt. The ventral and both sides of the abdomen should be examined beginning at the level of the xiphoid sternum and moving caudally to a point caudal to the umbilicus. In this way the anterior and caudal aspects of the abdomen will be examined for evidence of painful points.

Pinching of the withers is also used to elicit a grunt. In the average-sized cow, pinching of the withers causes the animal to depress its back. In an animal with an inflammatory lesion of the peritoneum, depression of its back will commonly result in a grunt which may be audible without auscultation over the trachea but auscultation will usually be necessary.

The term *anterior abdominal pain* is now being used to characterize the pain associated with several diseases of anterior abdomens of cattle which would include traumatic reticuloperitonitis, hepatic abscesses, abomasal ulcers, and intestinal obstruction. The differential diagnosis of the anterior abdominal pain would include diseases which cause thoracic pain such as pleuritis, pericarditis and severe pulmonary disease (5).

Clinical examination of the digestive tract and abdomen of the calf

The clinical examination of the digestive tract and abdomen of the calf may be more difficult than in the adult animal. The rumen in the preruminant calf is not yet functional, and thus cannot be used as an indicator of the state of the alimentary tract as is possible in the adult animal. Also, a rectal examination of the abdomen is not usually possible until the animal is about 10–12 months of age, depending on the breed. A digital examination of the rectum of young calves is useful to determine the nature and amount of feces. This may provide an indication of the presence of diarrhea which may not yet have begun. A complete absence of feces may suggest the presence of an acute intestinal obstruction, acute diffuse peritonitis or atresia coli.

The oral cavity of the calf is easily examined and should be part of the clinical examination of every sick calf.

A common problem in calves under 2 months of age is acute abdominal distension. The distension may appear to be symmetrical and it is difficult to determine if the distension is in the rumen, abomasum, intestines or peritoneal cavity. A rectal examination of abdomen is not possible. The differential diagnosis of the common causes of abdominal distension in the calf are set out in Table 25.

Examination of the abdomen of the young calf includes visual inspection of the contour of the abdomen to determine the maximum area of any distension, deep palpation and ballottement of each flank to determine the presence of fluid-splashing sounds which indicates a fluid-filled viscus, and percussion and auscultation to determine the presence of a gas-filled viscus. Placing the calf's hindquarters on the ground and allowing the viscera to move to the caudal part of the abdomen may allow visual adspection and palpation of a distended abomasum below the xiphoid sternum. With the calf in lateral recumbency, careful palpation and simultaneous auscultation may reveal the location of the distended viscus. However, it is often necessary to do an exploratory laparotomy to determine the cause. A stomach tube should always be passed into the rumen to relieve any pressure caused by the accumulation of gas or fluid. In the case of severe distension of the abdomen accompanied by severe abdominal pain (kicking, bellowing, rolling, getting up and lying down) it may be necessary to relieve pressure with a large gauge needle (12–14 gauge, 75–100 mm; 3–4 in.). The most common cause of severe abdominal distension in a young calf which can be relieved by trocarization is abomasal torsion.

Paracentesis abdominis is easily done in the calf and at least three taps should be done before concluding a negative tap. To avoid puncture of the abomasum, choose sites which are caudal to the umbilicus.

Paracentesis of the peritoneal cavity

This is presented in Chapter 5, page 161.

Table 25. Differential diagnosis of diseases of the digestive tract and abdomen of young calves presented with distension of the abdomen

Disease	*History, clinical and laboratory findings, treatment*
Abomasal torsion	Always acute to peracute, 1 week to 6 months of age, acute abdominal pain, bellowing, up and down, severe tight distension of abdomen, loud ping and fluid-splashing right side, emergency surgery necessary
Abomasal dilatation (fluid, milk, hair balls and often abomasal ulcers)	Chronic or acute onset, calves 1–6 months of age, history of abnormal feces, may be unthrifty, mild to moderate abdominal distension and pain, fluid-splashing sounds over right flank, dehydration, negative peritoneal fluid, surgery
Perforated abomasal ulcers	Acute onset, sudden collapse, calves 2 weeks to 3 months, hand-fed or nursing calves, weakness, recumbency, tachycardia, mild to moderate abdominal distension, mild or no abdominal pain, abdominal splinting occasionally, *positive paracentesis*, feces variable
Torsion of root of mesentery	Sudden onset, found in state of collapse, abdominal pain common, moderate abdominal distension, distended loops of intestine visible and palpable over right flank, bloodstained peritoneal tap, fluid-splashing sounds on palpation and auscultation, scant feces, emergency surgery
Acute diffuse peritonitis (not due to perforated abomasal ulcer)	Usually in calves under 3 weeks of age. Toxemia, temperature variable, weak, may be grunting, splinting of abdominal wall, mild abdominal distension, scant feces, fluid-splashing sounds over right flank (due to paralytic ileus), *positive paracentesis*, commonly associated with enteric colibacillosis, polyarthritis and umbilical and urachal abscess
Atresia coli	Calf usually under 10 days of age, progressive distension of abdomen, bright and alert for first few days then becomes depressed, no feces only thick mucus from rectum, insertion of tube into rectum may lead to blind end but often blind end is near spiral colon. Surgery indicated but often unrewarding
Intussusception	May have history of diarrhea, now scant bloodstained feces, depressed, will not suck or drink, dehydrated, contour of abdomen may appear normal or slightly distended, fluid-splashing sounds and small 'ping' may be audible, bloodstained peritoneal fluid, presurgical diagnosis often difficult, surgery necessary
Peracute to acute enteritis	Usually in calves under 3 weeks of age, acute onset of abdominal pain (kicking, stretching), will not suck or drink, may not yet appear dehydrated, temperature variable (if elevated is reliable), mild to moderate abdominal distension, fluid-splashing sounds, continuous loud peristaltic sounds on auscultation, digital examination of rectum may stimulate defecation of foul-smelling, soft, watery feces, peritoneal tap negative
Omphalitis, omphalophlebitis, umbilical abscess	Single calf, usually 2–6 weeks of age. May be unthrifty, chronic toxemia. Large painful swelling of umbilicus which may be obvious externally or deep palpation dorsal to umbilicus reveals firm swellings directed towards liver or bladder. Surgical excision required

Interpretation of clinical findings

The interpretation of the clinical findings associated with diseases of the digestive tract and abdomen of cattle are set out in Table 26. These must be considered in conjunction with the history and the laboratory findings before a list of tentative diagnoses is made.

Exploratory laparoscopy

A flexible fiberoptic colonoscope, 14 mm diameter and 1120 mm working length is very useful as an aid for the diagnosis of traumatic reticuloperitonitis (4). The instrument has been used through the right flank of cattle and was not useful for the detection of left-side displacement of the abomasum (LDA).

Exploratory laparotomy

An exploratory laparotomy may assist in the diagnosis of diseases of the digestive tract or abdomen. When a significant lesion is found at laparotomy the surgery is usually justifiable whether or not the outcome is favorable.

Table 26. The pathogenesis and interpretation of clinical findings associated with diseases of the digestive tract and abdomen of cattle

Clinical Findings	*Pathogenesis, interpretation*
Anorexia, inappetence	Toxemia, distension of intestines and stomachs, enteritis, peritonitis
Scant feces, includes small volume diarrhea	Reduced feed intake, functional obstruction of forestomachs and abomasum, paralytic ileus, strangulation obstruction or obstruction of lumen of intestine with phytobezoar or trichobezoar
Large volume diarrhea	Profuse watery diarrhea usually associated with enteritis, simple indigestion or carbohydrate engorgement
Dehydration	Failure to drink adequate amounts of water (due to toxemia or lesions of oral cavity), malabsorption due to enteritis, diseases of the forestomachs interfering with absorption of water, e.g. vagus indigestion
Tachycardia	Toxemia, acid–base imbalance, abdominal pain, distension of intestines
Polypnea	Acid–base imbalance (torsion of the abomasum, severe enteritis, vagus indigestion), distension of the abdomen due to gas or fluid-filled intestines
Weakness and recumbency	Toxemia, severe dehydration, severe distension of abdomen, peritonitis
Colic (abdominal pain)	Sudden onset of distension of forestomachs, abomasum or intestines. Stretching of mesenteric bands. Strangulation of intestine in mesenteric tear or scrotal hernia
Grunting with every respiration	Diffuse peritonitis (also pleuritis, pulmonary emphysema and advanced pneumonia), distension of stomachs or intestines
Presence of grunt on deep palpation of ventral abdominal wall	Presence of a peritoneal lesion (stretching of the peritoneum, inflammation, edema, recent adhesions)
Abdominal distension	Most commonly due to gas or fluid-filled intestines and/or forestomachs and abomasum. Rarely due to pneumoperitoneum. Also due to ascites and hydrops–allantois–amnion
Rumen distension	May be distended with gas, fluid or ingesta. Primary dietary ruminal tympany and grain overload. Secondary ruminal tympany due to peritonitis, vagus indigestion
Rumen stasis	Toxemia, metabolic (hypocalcemia), fever, ruminal acidosis, distension of omasum or abomasum, peritonitis, vagal nerve injury
Hyperactive rumen	Early stages of primary dietary ruminal tympany; vagal nerve injury
Acidic rumen pH	Ruminal acidosis associated with carbohydate engorgement; almost no other cause known
Alkaline rumen pH	Ruminal alkalosis associated with accidental consumption of high protein diet, urea poisoning
Reduced or absent rumen protozoan activity	Ruminal acidosis (lactic acid inactivates protozoa); primary starvation lasting more than 2–3 days; ingestion of lead, arsenic and other poisonous substances
Abnormal foul-smelling rumen contents	Putrefaction of rumen contents in static and defaunated rumen
Presence of 'ping' over left flank	Left-side displacement of abomasum, atonic rumen with a gas cap, pneumoperitoneum (rarely)
Presence of loud or clear 'ping' over right flank	Right-side dilatation displacement and torsion of the abomasum, cecal dilatation and torsion, torsion of the spiral colon, gas in distended colon and rectum
Presence of low pitched 'pings' not clearly distinct over right flank	Tympany of right paralumbar fossa in recently calved cows (2–3 days). Gas in distended colon and rectum. Fluid and gas-filled intestines with enteritis
Distended upper right flank	Dilatation and torsion of abomasum. Cecal dilatation and torsion. Torsion of spiral colon
Distended lower right flank	Impaction of the abomasum. Enlarged L-shaped rumen and distension of ventral sac to the right flank. Advanced pregnancy
Fluid splashing sounds on ballottement of abdomen or succussion	Fluid-filled intestines or forestomachs or abomasum. Usually associated with enteritis, paralytic ileus, or obstruction. Fluid-splashing sounds are *rarely* due to fluid in the peritoneal cavity. Percolating fluid sounds audible over right flank are common in cattle with acute intestinal obstruction
Dropping cuds	Cattle rarely regurgitate uncontrollably (dropping cuds). It is usually associated with chronic inflammatory lesions of the reticulum and cardia resulting in lack of control of regurgitation and a larger than normal bolus of rumen contents is regurgitated which cannot be controlled by the animal. Also occurs in certain heavy metal poisonings like arsenic poisoning. Cattle affected with straw impaction of the rumen will also drop large dry fibrous cuds

However, because a properly done laparotomy is time-consuming and expensive, the veterinarian would like to minimize the number of laparotomies in which no significant lesions are present. The challenge is, therefore, to improve the accuracy of diagnosis before doing a laparotomy unnecessarily.

There are some well-recognized diseases in which, if a clinical diagnosis can be made, a laparotomy is indicated (Table 27). (In some cases slaughter for salvage may be more economical.)

Other than the rumenotomy for the treatment of grain overload and the cesarean section, the most common indication for a laparotomy in cattle is for the surgical correction of displacement or obstructions of parts of the digestive tract (i.e., abomasal displacement, abomasal dilatation and torsion, intussusception and volvulus, torsion of the root of the mesentery, torsion of spiral colon, cecal dilatation and torsion). If any of these diagnoses can be made, a laparotomy or slaughter is indicated.

In other cases, the diagnosis may be suspected, but is not obvious and the indications for a *laparotomy*, *slaughter*, *euthanasia* or *conservative medical treatment* are not clear.

The major question is, 'under what conditions is a laparotomy indicated if the history and clinical and laboratory findings *suggest* an obstruction (strangulation obstruction or functional), but the obstruction cannot be located on clinical examination?'

Some diseases which may elude diagnosis before laparotomy, and which are or may be amenable to surgical correction include the following.

Intussusception and other strangulation obstruction of the small intestines

This is an indication if located in the anterior aspect of the abdomen (not palpable per rectum) and depending on a history of acute onset of colic, absence of feces and serosanguineous exudate in peritoneal tap. However, phytobezoars and trichobezoars can cause acute intestinal obstruction which may not be palpable rectally and which becomes progressively more severe with time, and only

Table 27. Diseases of the digestive tract and abdomen of cattle in which a laparotomy is indicated *if* the diagnosis can be made

Disease	*Major clinical findings*
Left-side displacement of the abomasum (LDA)	'Ping' over 9th to 12th ribs and other well recognized findings
Right-side displacement (RDA) and torsion of the abomasum	Distension of upper right flank, 'ping', palpable per rectum
Cecal dilatation and torsion	Distension of upper right flank, 'ping', long cylindrical mass palpable per rectum
Torsion of spiral colon	Distension of upper right flank, 'ping', distended loops of intestine easily palpable
Intussusception	Abdominal pain, absence of feces, distended loops of intestine, palpable intussusception
Phytobezoars or trichobezoars	Scant feces, subacute abdominal pain, distended loops of intestine and hard lumps palpable rectally
Severe life-threatening ruminal tympany	Severe distension of rumen, skin over rumen cannot be picked up, animal grunting, is lying down, mouth breathing, cannot relieve with stomach tube or trocar
Unidentifiable lumps palpable on rectal examination, i.e., fat necrosis	Chronic gastrointestinal atony, scant feces, large hard lumps palpable per rectum
Peracute grain overload	Weakness, recumbency, dehydration, tachycardia, rumen pH 5 (see Table 29 for guidelines in the treatment of grain overload)

Table 28. Clinical and laboratory indications for an exploratory laparotomy in cattle when the diagnosis is not obvious

Parameter/criterion	*Significance and interpretation of criteria*
History	Does the history suggest an acute surgically correctable condition?
Abdominal distension	Laparotomy indicated if distension of abdomen caused by distension of abomasum, cecum or intestines with fluid and gas
Volume and nature of feces	Scant or absence of feces for more than 36–48 hours indicates a *physical* or *functional* obstruction. In *functional obstruction* (i.e., peritonitis) some dark feces are usually present. In *physical obstruction* (intussusception) feces are very scant and dark red due to leakage of blood into intussusceptus. Laparotomy indicated unless can determine that cause of absence of feces is not surgically correctable (diffuse peritonitis or impaction of abomasum or omasum)
Rectal findings	Distended viscera other than rumen (abomasum, cecum, small and large intestines) warrant laparotomy. Palpable 'bread and butter' fibrinous inflammation in caudal part of abdomen suggests acute diffuse peritonitis and laparotomy would not be rewarding
Peritoneal fluid and hemogram	Bloodstained peritoneal exudate and a degenerative left shift in the leukocyte count suggest leakage of the intestinal wall and warrants laparotomy if history and clinical findings suggest a strangulation obstruction
Abdominal pain (colic) and grunting	Behavioral and postural signs of acute abdominal pain (colic) such as kicking at the belly, stretching the body, suggest acute distension of the stomachs or intestines with fluid and gas. Spontaneous grunting with each respiration, which usually becomes pronounced in sternal recumbency, or the presence of a grunt on deep palpation of the abdomen suggests inflammation or stretching of the peritoneum

minimal, if any, changes may occur in the peritoneal fluid. A progressively worsening systemic state warrants a laparotomy.

'Atypical' left-sided displacement of the abomasum
A small percentage of cases are difficult to detect on auscultation and percussion. When the typical LDA 'ping' cannot be detected after several examinations over a period of a few days, a presumptive diagnosis may be made on the basis of ketosis in a recently calved cow (within the last week), the presence of rumen contractions, but reduced intensity, normal vital signs (unless fatty liver is present) and fluid-gurgling sounds over the left flank.

Traumatic reticuloperitonitis
In traumatic reticuloperitonitis with a persistently penetrating foreign body conservative medical treatment of immobilization in a stanchion, antibiotics and a magnet has not resulted in a beneficial response. Diagnosis depends on continued anorexia, mild fever, grunt, rumen stasis, a hemogram indicating infection and peritoneal fluid containing exudate.

The guidelines for the indications of an exploratory laparotomy when a firm diagnosis is not available are set out in Table 28.

REFERENCES

(1) Stober, M. & Dirksen, G. (1977) *Bov. Practnr*, *12*, 35–38.
(2) McCarthy, P. H. (1981) *Am. vet. Res.*, *42*, 255.
(3) Kath, G. S. et al. (1985) *Am. J. vet. Res.*, *46*, 136.
(4) Wilson, A. D. & Ferguson, J. G. (1984) *Can. vet. J.*, *25*, 229.
(5) Henninger, R. W. & Mullowney, P. C. (1984) *Comp. cont. Educ.*, 6, S453.

DISEASES OF THE RUMEN, RETICULUM AND OMASUM

Simple indigestion

Simple indigestion occurs commonly in hand-fed ruminants and is characterized clinically by inappetence to anorexia, decreased ruminal movements and abnormal feces; the feces may be scant or voluminous and diarrheic. The disease is usually associated with some dietary abnormality.

Etiology
The disease is common in dairy cattle and stall-fed beef cattle because of the variability in quality and the large amounts of food consumed. It is not commonly observed in pastured beef cattle or sheep because they are less heavily fed. The common causes are dietary abnormalities of minor degree including indigestible roughage, particularly when the protein intake is low, moldy, overheated and frosted feeds, and moderate excesses of grain and concentrate intake (1). Cases occur under excellent feeding regimens and are usually ascribed to overfeeding with grain. Although the difference between simple indigestion and acute impaction of the rumen is largely one of degree, their separation can be justified by the marked clinical difference between the two syndromes. Gross overfeeding usually occurs when cattle or sheep gain accidental access to large quantities of grain or are suddenly introduced to high grain diets in feedlots. Indigestion is more common when heavily fed cows are fed a little more concentrate than they can digest properly. Sudden change to a new source of grain, especially from oats to wheat or barley, may have the same effect.

Indigestible roughage may include straw, bedding or scrub fed during drought periods. It is probable that limitation of the available drinking water may contribute to the occurrence of the disease during dry seasons. Depraved appetite may also contribute to the ingestion of coarse indigestible material. Although good quality ensilage cannot be considered an indigestible roughage, cases of indigestion can occur in cattle which are allowed unlimited access to it. This is most likely to happen in heavy-producing cows running outside in cold weather and whose hay and grain rations are limited. It is not uncommon for large Holstein cows to eat 45–50 kg of ensilage daily in such circumstances and the high intake of acetate and acetic acid (2) may be sufficient to depress their appetite. Prolonged or heavy oral dosing with sulfonamides or antibiotics may cause indigestion due to inhibition of the normal ruminal flora. An unusual circumstance is the feeding of a special diet to produce milk, and dairy products, with a high content of polyunsaturatd fats for special diets in humans. Fats in the diet are protected against hydrogenation in the rumen by a coating of formalin. The efficiency and safety of the diet depends on a thorough mixing of the formalin with the concentrates. If this is not done the free formalin causes severe rumenitis.

Pathogenesis
Primary atony caused by dietary abnormality is difficult to explain. Changes in the pH of its contents markedly affect the motility of the rumen and in cases caused by overeating on grain an increase in acidity is probably of importance. High-protein diets including the feeding of excessively large quantities of legumes or urea, also depress motility because of the sharp increase in alkalinity which results (3). Atony which occurs after feeding on damaged feeds may have the same basis or be due to other unidentified agents in the food. The simple accumulation of indigestible food may physically impede ruminal activity. Putrefaction of protein may also play a part in the production of atony. The toxic amides and amines produced may include histamine which is known to cause ruminal atony when given intravenously and to be reversed by the administration of antihistamine drugs (4, 5). Histamine may contribute to the ruminal atony which occurs in allergy, or after heavy grain feeding, but the absorption of histamine from the forestomachs in any circumstances is probably very limited (6).

Affected cattle usually show a pronounced fall in milk yield caused probably by the sharp fall in volatile fatty acid production in that atonic rumen (7). Rumen contractions appear to play the same role as hunger contractions in simple stomachs and the decreased food intake is probably due to the ruminal atony.

Clinical findings
A reduction in appetite is the first sign and is followed closely in milking cows by a slight drop in milk production. Both occur suddenly, the anorexia may be partial or complete but the fall in milk yield is relatively slight. The animal's posture is unaffected but there is mild depression and dullness. Rumination ceases and the ruminal movements are depressed in frequency and amplitude and sometimes are absent. The rumen may be larger than normal if the cause is sudden access to an unlimited supply of palatable feed. There may be moderate tympany, especially with frozen or damaged feeds or in allergy, but the usual finding is a firm, doughy rumen without obvious distension. The feces are usually reduced in quantity and are drier than normal on the first day. However, 24–48 hours later the animal is commonly diarrheic; the feces are softer than normal, voluminous and commonly malodorous.

There is no systemic reaction and the pulse, temperature and respiration rates are unaffected. Pain cannot be elicited by percussion of the abdominal wall; although cows which have consumed an excessive quantity of a highly palatable feed like silage, after not having had any for a long period of time, will have a grossly distended rumen, and mild abdominal pain may be present for several hours. The pain usually disappears when the rumen movements return to normal and the rumen returns to its normal size. Most cases recover spontaneously or with simple treatments in about 48 hours.

Clinical pathology
Examination of the urine for ketone bodies is usually necessary to differentiate indigestion from acetonemia.

Two simple laboratory tests have been introduced to assess the activity of the ruminal microflora (8). The sediment activity test is carried out on aspirated ruminal fluid strained to remove coarse particles. The strained fluid is allowed to stand in a glass vessel at body temperature and the time required for flotation of the particulate material recorded. The time in normal animals varies between 3 minutes, if the animal has just been fed and 9 minutes if the last feeding has occurred some time previously. Settling of the particulate material indicates gross inactivity, less severe degrees being manifested by prolongation of the time required for flotation. The cellulose digestion test is also performed on aspirated rumen fluid and depends upon the time required to digest a thread of cotton. A bead is tied to the end of the thread to indicate when separation occurs. Digestion times in excess of 30 hours indicate abnormality. The rumen juice can be examined for pH using wide range indicator paper. Values between 6.5 and 7 are considered normal. In cattle on grain diets, the pH may range from 5.5 to 6 normally but in cattle which have been on roughage diets such low values should arouse suspicion of lactic acidosis and careful monitoring is necessary.

Necropsy findings
The disease is not a fatal one.

Diagnosis
Simple indigestion must be differentiated from all of the diseases of the forestomachs and abomasum in which ruminal atony is a common clinical finding, and from diseases of other body systems which cause secondary ruminal atony. In acetonemia, the appetite and milk production decrease over a few days, there is ketonuria and the rumen contractions are present but weaker than normal. In traumatic reticuloperitonitis there is a sudden onset of anorexia and agalactia, a mild fever, a painful grunt on deep palpation of the xiphoid sternum, and the rumen is static with an increase in the size of the gas cap. Carbohydrate engorgement is characterized by depression, dehydration, tachycardia, staggering, recumbency, diarrhea, ruminal stasis with the presence of fluid-splashing sounds, and the pH of the ruminal fluid is usually below 6 and commonly down to 5. Left-side displacement of the abomasum (LDA) usually occurs within a few days after parturition and the rumen is usually smaller than normal, the contractions are usually reduced in amplitude, there is a ping on percussion over the lower left flank, and ketonuria. In dilatation and torsion of abomasum the rumen becomes progressively more hypotonic as the abomasum distends and is displaced and twisted. Vagus indigestion is characterized by gradual distention of the rumen over a a period of several days and there is hypomotility or hypermotility of the rumen, dehydration and scant feces. Phytobezoars cause inappetence to anorexia, scant feces, and on rectal examination distended loops of intestine and the firm masses may be palpable.

Secondary ruminal atony occurs in many diseases especially when septicemia or toxemia are present, but there are usually additional clinical findings to indicate their presence. Ruminal stasis is common in the early stages of hypocalcemia which is usually accompanied by anorexia and a decreased amount of feces, and the motility and appetite return to normal following treatment with calcium borogluconate. The rumen is also static in allergic and anaphylactic states and returns to normal following treatment.

Treatment
Rational treatment is often difficult because of lack of knowledge of the etiology, and for the most part treatment is symptomatic, consisting primarily of the use of rumenatoric drugs. Many drugs are used for this purpose. A number of these have little justification for their use (4, 5, 9) and their reputation depends to a large extent on the tendency of affected animals to recover spontaneously. Tartar emetic (10–12 g) may be effective when given orally but causes chemical reticulitis if given in concentrated form in a static rumen (10).

Parasympathetic stimulants are widely used as rumenatorics but have the disadvantage of creating undesirable side-effects and being very transitory in their action. Large doses depress rumen activity but small doses repeated at short intervals increase ruminal activity and promote violent emptying of the colon. The normal flow of rumen contents from the reticulorumen to the abomasum is the result of a complex of synchronized contractions and relaxations of various parts of the forestomachs, orifices and abomasum occurring simultaneously. One of the major limitations of injectable parasympathomimetics used as rumenatorics is that they do not provide these synchronized movements and therefore little movement of ingesta can occur. Carbamylcholine chloride, physostigmine and neostigmine are most commonly used. The last is the most effective and should be given at a dose rate of 2·5 mg/45 kg body weight (9). Carbamylcholine acts on the musculature only and causes uncoordinated and functionless movements (11). These drugs are not without danger, especially in very sick animals or those with peritonitis, and are *specifically contraindicated* during late pregnancy.

Epsom salts (0·5–1·0 kg per adult cow) and other magnesium salts are reasonably effective and have the merit of simplicity and cheapness (12).

More rational therapy should include the use of alkalizers, such as magnesium hydroxide, at the rate of 400 g per adult cow (450 kg body weight) when the rumen contents are excessively acid, or of an acid, such as acetic acid or vinegar 5–10 liters, when the reaction is alkaline. Magnesium oxide or hydroxide should be used only if ruminal acidosis is present (14). The administration of 400 g of magnesium oxide to normal, mature, non-fasted cattle weighing 450 kg can cause metabolic alkalosis and electrolyte disturbances for up to 24 hours following treatment. A sample of rumen fluid can be readily obtained and the pH determined approximately by the use of reagent paper. If there is inspissation of ruminal contents 15–20 liters of normal saline should be administered by stomach tube.

Cases of indigestion which have run a course of more than a few days, and animals suffering from prolonged anorexia due to any cause suffer an appreciable loss of ruminal microflora, especially if there have been marked changes in pH. Reconstitution of the flora by the use of cud transfers is highly effective. An abattoir is the best source of material but it can be obtained from living animals by reaching into the mouth or kneeing the animal in the ribs as a bolus is regurgitated. Fluid may also be removed by siphoning or sucking with a special pump. Best results are obtained if 10–15 liters of normal saline are pumped into the rumen and then withdrawn. The material to be transferred should be mixed with water, strained and administered as a drench or by stomach tube. Repeated dosing is advisable. The infusion will keep for several days at room temperature. Commercial products comprising dried rumen solids are available and provide some bacteria and substrate for their activity. They are of most value as adjuncts to cud transfer and have not been found to be highly effective in restoring gastric motility in lambs whose appetite has been reduced by oral administration of chloromycetin (13).

When affected animals resume eating they are best tempted by good, stalky meadow or cereal hay. Good quality alfalfa or clover hay, green feed and concentrate may be added to the diet as the appetite improves.

REFERENCES

(1) Hoflund, S. (1967) *Vet. Bull.*, *37*, 701.
(2) Dowden, D. R. & Jacobson, D. R. (1960) *Nature (Lond.)*, *188*, 148.
(3) Miklovich, N. (1972) *Tierärztl. Umschau*, *27*, 329.
(4) Dougherty, R. W. (1942) *Cornell Vet.*, *32*, 269.
(5) Clark, R. (1950) *J. S. Afr. vet. med. Assoc.*, *21*, 13, 49.
(6) Dickinson, J. E. & Hubra, W. G. (1972) *Am. J. vet. Res.*, *33*, 1789.
(7) Stone, E. C. (1949) *Am. J. vet. Res.*, *10*, 26.
(8) Nichols, R. E. & Penn, K. E. (1958) *J. Am. vet. med. Assoc.*, *133*, 275.
(9) Clark, R. & Weiss, K. E. (1954) *Onderstepoort J. vet. Res.*, *26*, 285.
(10) Stevens, C. E. et al. (1959) *J. Am. vet. med. Assoc.*, *27*, 79.
(11) Clark, R. (1956) *J. S. Afr. vet. med. Assoc.*, *27*, 79.
(12) Lamberth, J. L. (1969) *Aust. vet. J.*, *45*, 223.
(13) Tucker, J. O. et al. (1956) *Am. J. vet. Res.*, *17*, 498.
(14) Ogilvie, T. H. et al. (1983) *Can. J. comp. Med.*, *47*, 108.

Acute carbohydrate engorgement of ruminants (rumen overload)

The ingestion of large amounts of highly fermentable carbohydrate rich feeds causes an acute disease due to the excessive production of lactic acid in the rumen. Clinically the disease is characterized by severe toxemia, dehydration, ruminal stasis, weakness and recumbency, and a high mortality rate. The terms carbohydrate engorgement, grain overload, rumen overload, founder and acidosis are all commonly used and for practical purposes are synonymous.

Etiology

The sudden ingestion of toxic doses of carbohydrate-rich feed, such as grain, is the most common cause of the disease. Less common causes include engorgement of apples, grapes, bread, baker's dough, sugar beet, mangels, sour wet brewers' grain which was incompletely fermented in the brewery, and concentrated sucrose solutions used in apiculture (2). The different kinds of feeds which have caused the disease in ruminants have been reviewed (1).

Epidemiology

Species

All types of ruminant cattle and sheep are susceptible, but the disease occurs most commonly in feedlot cattle fed on high-level grain diets. The disease has been recorded in goats and in wild deer (3).

Types and toxic doses of feeds

Wheat, barley and corn grains are considered to be the most toxic when ingested in large quantities. Oats and grain sorghum are least toxic. All of the grains are considered much more toxic when ground finely or even crushed or just cracked, processes which expose the starch component of the grain to the ruminal microflora. The experimental feeding of unprocessed barley to cattle did not result in rumenitis, whereas feeding rolled barley was associated with ruminal lesions (4). An unrestricted supply of stale bread can cause outbreaks (23).

The amount of a feed which is required to produce acute illness depends on the kind of grain, previous experience of the animal with that grain, the nutritional status of the animal and its bodily condition, and the nature of the microflora. Dairy cattle accustomed to heavy grain diets may consume 15–20 kg of grain and develop only moderate illness, while beef cows or feedlot cattle may become acutely ill and die after eating 10 kg of grain. Doses of feed reported to be lethal in experimental engorgement, range from 50–60 g of crushed wheat per kg body weight in undernourished sheep to 75–80 g/kg in well nourished sheep, and in cattle doses ranging from 25 to 62 g/kg of ground cereal grain or corn produced severe acidosis (1).

Susceptibility
Because the type and level of ration consumed by a ruminant affects the numbers and species of bacteria and protozoa in the rumen, when a change from one ration to another occurs, a period of microbial adaptation occurs which is a variable interval of time before stabilization occurs (5). Animals which are on a low carbohydrate level ration are thus considered to be most susceptible to a rapid change because satisfactory adaptation cannot occur quickly enough, but instead there is the rapid onset of abnormal fermentation.

Occurrence
The disease occurs commonly following accidental consumption of toxic levels of grain by cattle which gain sudden access to large quantities of stored grain. A single animal or a group of hungry cows may break into a grain storage bin or simply come across a large supply of unprotected grain, as not uncommonly happens on a mixed cattle-grain farm. Another common occurrence is when cattle are left under the care of an assistant, who because he is unaware of the feeding habits of the animals, gives the cattle an unaccustomed quantity of grain.

The disease has also occurred when cattle have been turned into unripe, green corn standing in the field, when cattle or sheep have been placed on stubble fields in which considerable grain lost by the harvester was available on the ground, and following the irregular feeding of large quantities of other less common animal feeds and byproducts, such as bread, baker's dough and wet brewers' grain. Problems usually arise with these feeds when a larger than usual amount is fed to cattle either for the first time or because the usual supplementary feed was in short supply.

The occurrence of grain overload in feedlot cattle, however, has gained the most attention, presumably because of its economic impact. The economics of feedlot beef production dictate that cattle should gain weight at their maximum potential rate and this usually involves getting them onto a full feed of a high concentration of grain quickly. Economics also favor the processing of grain by one of several methods available which will increase the availability of starch and thereby increase the rate of degradation in the rumen. All of these factors set the stage for a high incidence of grain overload in feedlot cattle (6).

There are some critical periods during which grain overload occurs in feedlot cattle. When starting cattle on feed, those with some previous experience with grain will commonly consume a toxic dose if offered a high level grain ration. The disease occurs commonly in feedlot cattle in which their total daily feed intake has been brought up to what is considered the same feed on an *ad libitum* basis, they engorge themselves. When increasing the concentration of grain in the ration from one level to another, if the increment is too high the total amount of grain consumed by some cattle will be excessive. Rapid changes in barometric pressures may affect the voluntary intake of cattle. A rapid change to cold weather may result in a moderate increase in feed intake in animals which are fed *ad libitum* and outbreaks of grain overload may occur. When rain is involved and feed becomes wet and possibly even moldy, feed intake will drop, but when fresh dry feed is offered again there may be a marked increase in feed intake which results in grain overload.

The diseases also occurs when cattle which have been on a high-level grain ration (full feed) have become hungry because they have been out of feed for 12–24 hours due to a breakdown in the feed mill or handling facilities. Offering an unlimited supply of feed to these cattle will often result in severe cases of grain overload. In large feedlots, where communications can be a problem, the accidental feeding of a high-level grain ration to cattle which are on a high-level roughage ration is a common cause of the disease.

Outbreaks of the disease occur in lamb feedlots in which lambs are started on a high-level grain ration without a period of adjustment. The disease is not as common in lambs as in cattle, perhaps because lambs are usually fed on oats.

The ruminal lesions of rumenitis and ruminal hyperkeratosis, which are commonly present in feedlot cattle at slaughter, are thought to be associated with the continuous feeding of grain (7). These lesions are often remarkable at slaughter in well-nourished cattle and their effect on live weight gain and feed conversion is not known.

Morbidity and mortality
Outbreaks of the disease occur in cattle herds kept on grain farms and in feedlots. Depending on the species of grain, the total amount eaten and the previous experience of the animals, the morbidity will vary from 10 to 50%. The case mortality rate may be up to 90% in untreated cases, while in treated cases it may still be up to 30–40%.

Pathogenesis
The details of the pathogenesis of ruminant lactic acidosis have been reviewed (1, 8, 9). A summary of the events which occur in the rumen and the systemic effects on the animal will follow. The disease is a good example of metabolic acidosis.

The ingestion of excessive quantities of highly fermentable feeds by the ruminant is followed within 2–6 hours by a marked change in the microbial population in the rumen. There is marked increase in the number of *Streptococcus bovis* which utilizes the carbohydrate to produce large quantities of lactic acid. In the presence of a sufficient amount of carbohydrate (a toxic or a lethal dose) the *Strep. bovis* will continue to produce lactic acid which decreases the rumen pH down to 5 or less, at which point the cellulolytic bacteria and protozoa are destroyed. When large amounts of starch are added to the diet, growth of *Strep. bovis* is no longer restricted by energy source and grows faster than any other species of bacteria (10). The concentration of volatile fatty acids (VFA) is also increased initially and contributes to the fall in ruminal pH. The low pH allows the lactobacilli to use the large quantities of carbohydrate in the rumen to produce excessive quantities of lactic acid. Both D and L forms of the acid are produced which markedly increase ruminal osmolality and water is drawn in from the systemic circulation causing hemoconcentration and dehydration.

Some of the lactic acid is buffered by ruminal buffers but considerable amounts are absorbed through the wall of the rumen and some undoubtedly moves into and is absorbed by the intestinal tract. Lactate is a ten times stronger acid than the volatile fatty acids, and accumulation of lactate eventually exceeds the buffering capacity of rumen fluid (10). As the ruminal pH is lowered, the amplitude and frequency of the rumen movements are decreased and at about a pH of 5 there is complete ruminal stasis. Recent evidence suggests that the increased molar concentration of butyrate causes the ruminal stasis and not the lactic acid. Inhibition of ruminal activity may also be due to lactic acid entering the duodenum and exerting a reflex inhibitory action on the rumen (30). Experimentally, ruminal stasis occurs in sheep within 8–12 hours after grain engorgement (49). The non-dissociated volatile fatty acid concentrations may have been responsible for the reduced reticulorumen motility. The diarrhea is considered to be due to the reduction in net absorption of water from the colon (32).

The absorbed lactic acid is buffered by the plasma bicarbonate buffering system. With non-toxic amounts of lactic acid, the acid–base balance is maintained by utilization of bicarbonate and elimination of carbon dioxide by increased respirations. In those which survive an acute form of the disease, this compensatory mechanism may overcompensate, resulting in alkalosis. In severe cases of lactic acidosis the reserves of plasma bicarbonate are reduced, the blood pH declines steadily, the blood pressure declines, causing a decrease in perfusion pressure and oxygen supply to peripheral tissues resulting in a further increase in lactic acid from cellular respiration. Lactic acid given intravenously to cattle causes hypertension, increased responses to norepinephrine, slight bradycardia and slight hyperventilation (38).

Both D- and L-lactic acids are produced. The L-lactic acid is utilized much more rapidly than the D-isomer which accumulates and causes a severe D-lactic acidosis (11). If the rate of entry of lactic acid into body fluids is not too rapid, compensatory mechanisms are able to maintain the blood pH at a compatible level until the crisis is over and recovery is usually rapid. This may explain the common observation that feedlot cattle may be ill for a few days after being introduced to a grain ration but quickly recover, while in other cases when the rate of entry is rapid the compensatory mechanisms are overcome and urgent treatment is necessary (12). In experimental lactic acidosis using sucrose in sheep, feed intake does not resume until rumen pH has returned to 6·0 or higher and when lactic acid is no longer detectable in the rumen (33). Renal blood flow and glomerular filtration rate are also decreased, resulting in anuria. Eventually there is shock and death. All of these events can occur within 24 hours after engorgement of a lethal dose of carbohydrate; with toxic doses the course of events may be from 24 to 48 hours.

The high concentration of lactic acid in the rumen is considered to be the cause of the chemical rumenitis which sets the stage for the development of mycotic rumenitis in those which survive, about 4–6 days later. The low pH of the rumen favors the growth of *Mucor*, *Rhizopus* and *Absidia* spp. which multiply and invade the ruminal vessels, causing thrombosis and infarction. Spread also occurs directly to the liver. Severe bacterial rumenitis also occurs. Widespread necrosis and gangrene may affect the entire ventral half of the ruminal walls and lead to the development of an acute peritonitis. The damage to the viscus causes complete atony and this, together with the toxemia resulting from the gangrene, is usually sufficient to kill the animal.

In uncomplicated chemical rumenitis the ruminal mucosae will slough and heal with scar tissue and some mucosal regeneration. In this connection, the pathogenesis of hepatic abscesses, so common in feedlot cattle, is considered to be the result of a combination of rumenitis caused by lactic acidosis, and allowing *Fusobacterium necrophorum* and *Actinobacillus* (*Corynebacterium*) *pyogenes* to enter directly into ruminal vessels and spread to the liver, which may have also undergone injury from the lactic acidosis (13). Severe diffuse coagulation necrosis and hyperplasia of the bile duct epithelium and degeneration of renal tubules may also be present histologically (31).

Chronic rumenitis and ruminal hyperkeratosis are common in cattle fed for long periods on grain rations, and the lesions are attributed to the chronic acidosis but it is possible that barley awns and ingested hair may contribute to the severity of the lesions (14).

In cattle being placed on a grain ration, it has been shown that even with control of the daily intake, hepatic cell damage and liver dysfunction occurred (15, 16) even though dietary adaptation may have occurred in 2–3 weeks. The biochemical profile indicated that complete metabolic adaptation required at least 40 days following the start of grain feeding (17).

Several toxic substances other than lactic acid have been proposed as contributory to the disease. Increased concentrations of histamine have been found in the rumen of experimentally engorged cattle, but its possible role in the disease remains unknown. Histamine is not absorbed from the rumen except at abnormally high pH values, but is absorbed from intestinal loops. Laminitis occurs in some cases of rumen overload but the cause is unknown. Other substances which have been recovered from the rumen in grain overload include a suspected endotoxin (18, 35, 36), ethanol and methanol (8). However, the role of the endotoxin is still uncertain; endotoxin administered into the intestine of lactic acidotic sheep is not absorbed (37). *Clostridium perfringens* and coliform bacteria have also been found in increased numbers but their significance is uncertain (19). The electrolyte changes which occur include a mild hypocalcemia due to temporary malabsorption, loss of serum chloride due to sequestration in the rumen, and an increase in serum phosphate due to renal failure.

The experimental disease has been produced in cattle and sheep with a variety of grains, fruits, sugars and pure solutions of lactic acid (1, 8). The severity of the experimental disease and the magnitude of the pathophysiological changes vary depending on the substance used, but changes similar to the natural disease occur (20). Lesions in the brain have been recorded in the experimental disease in sheep (21) and naturally occurring cases in cattle (22), but their pathogenesis and significance are uncertain. There are detectable changes in the cellular and biochemical composition of the cerebrospinal fluid which suggests the blood–brain barrier may be affected (34). Experimentally, sublethal doses of volatile fatty acids, lactate, and succinate have an effect on liver function (47). Toxic and lethal doses of butyrate can cause sudden flaccid paralysis and death from asphyxia (48).

Clinical findings

The speed of onset of the illness varies with the nature of the feed, being faster with ground feed than whole grain. The severity increases with the amount of feed eaten. If cattle are examined clinically within a few hours after engorgement, the only abnormality which may be detectable is a full rumen and occasionally some abdominal pain, evidenced by kicking at the belly. In the mild form, affected cattle are anorexic, but still fairly bright and alert and a soft feces diarrhea is common. The rumen movements are reduced but not entirely absent. They do not ruminate for a few days but usually begin to eat on the third or fourth day without any specific treatment.

When a large number of cattle are affected with the severe form, within 24–48 hours animals will be found down, some staggering and others standing quietly by themselves. All affected cattle are completely off feed. Once they are ill they usually do not drink water, but cattle may engorge themselves on water if it is readily available immediately after consuming large quantities of dry grain. In an outbreak, a visual examination of the feces on the ground will usually reveal many spots of soft to watery feces.

On clinical examination the temperature is usually below normal, 36·5–38·5°C (98–101°F), but animals exposed to hot sun may have temperatures up to 41°C (106°F). The heart rate is usually increased and continues to increase with the severity of the acidosis and circulatory failure. In general, those with heart rates below 100/minute are considered much better treatment risks than those with rates up to 120–140/minute. This is a useful prognostic aid. The respirations are usually shallow and increased up to 69–90/minute. Diarrhea is almost always present and is usually profuse; the feces are light-colored with an obvious sweet-sour odor. The feces commonly contain an excessive quantity of kernels of grain in grain overload, and pips and skins when grapes or apples have been eaten (23). An absence of feces is considered by some veterinarians as a grave prognostic sign but diarrhea is much more common. The dehydration is severe and progressive. In mild cases the dehydration will be equal to 4–6% of body weight, and with severe involvement up to 10–12% of body weight. The rumen contents palpated through the left paralumbar fossa may feel firm and doughy in cattle which were previously on a roughage diet and have consumed a large amount of grain. In cattle which have become ill on smaller amounts of grain, the rumen will not necessarily feel full with rumen contents, but rather it feels resilient because the excessive fluid contents are being palpated. Thus the findings on palpation may be deceptive and a source of error. The primary contractions of the rumen are completely absent although the gurgling sounds of gas rising through the large quantity of fluid which accumulates in the rumen are usually audible on auscultation. Severely affected animals have a staggery, drunken gait and their eyesight is impaired. They bump into objects and their palpebral eye preservation reflex is sluggish or absent. The pupillary light reflex is usually present but slower than normal. Acute laminitis may be present and is most common in cases which are not severely affected and appear to be good treatment risks. Chronic laminitis may occur several weeks or months later. Anuria is a common finding in acute cases and diuresis following fluid therapy is a good prognostic sign.

Recumbency usually follows after about 48 hours but it may be present as an early sign. Affected animals lie quietly, often with the head turned into the flank and their response to any stimulus is much decreased so that they resemble parturient paresis. Rapid development of acute signs, particularly recumbency, suggests an unfavorable prognosis and the necessity for urgent, radical treatment. Death may occur in 24–72 hours and improvement during this time is best measured in terms of a fall in heart rate, rise in temperature, return of ruminal movement and passage of large amounts of soft feces. Some animals appear to make a temporary improvement but become severely ill again on the third or fourth day. These are probably animals in which severe fungal rumenitis has occurred and death usually follows in 2–3 days due to acute diffuse peritonitis.

The syndrome described above is the commonest and most dramatic but when a number of animals have been exposed to overfeeding there are all degrees of severity from this to simple indigestion which responds readily to treatment. The prognosis varies with the severity, and those clinical parameters which are useful in deciding on a course of treatment are summarized in Table 29. In pregnant cattle which survive the severe form of the disease, abortion may occur from 10 days to 2 weeks later.

Clinical pathology

The severity of the disease can usually be determined by physical examination but field and laboratory tests are of some additional value.

The pH of the ruminal fluid obtained by stomach tube or by paracentesis through the left paralumbar fossa can be measured in the field using wide-range pH indicator paper. The ruminal fluid must be examined immediately because the pH will increase upon exposure to air. Cattle which have been fed a roughage diet will have a ruminal pH between 6 and 7; those on a grain diet between 5·5 and 6. A ruminal pH of between 5 and 6 in roughage-fed cattle suggests a moderate degree of abnormality, but a pH of less than 5 suggests severe involvement and the need for energetic treatment. Feedlot cattle which have been on grain for several days

Table 29. Guidelines for the use of clinical findings in assessing the severity of grain overload in cattle for the selection of the treatment of choice

Degree of illness	*Clinical parameters* Mental state and muscular strength	Degree of dehydration (% of body weight)	Abdominal distension	Heart rate (min.)	Body temp. (°C)	State of rumen; fullness, consistency of contents, movements and pH	Treatment
Peracute	Severely depressed, weak, in lateral recumbency, unable to stand, apparent blindness, pupils dilated and slow response	8–12	Prominent	110–130	35·5–38	Distended with fluid, complete stasis, sweet-sour smelling fluid contents. Rumen juice pH below 5 and usually about 4. No protozoa	Rumenotomy. Sodium bicarbonate 5 liters (5%) intravenously in 30 min (for 450 kg body weight) followed by isotonic (1·3%) at 150 ml/kg body weight for 6–12 hours
Acute	Depressed, still able to walk but ataxic, complete anorexia, may want to drink water, pupils slightly dilated and slow response	8–10	Moderate	90–100	38·5–39·5	Distended with fluid, complete stasis, sweet-sour smelling fluid contents. Rumen pH between 5 and 6. No protozoa	Consider immediate slaughter. Rumen lavage or rumenotomy. Sodium bicarbonate intravenously as in peracute case. Feed hay
Subacute	Fairly bright and alert. Able to walk. No ataxia. May eat, usually wants to drink. Pupils normal	4–6 Just barely detectable clinically	Mild or none	72–84	38·5–39	Moderate distension with fluid, some doughy ruminal ingesta palpable, some weak ruminal contractions, rumen pH between 5·5 and 6·5. Some protozoa alive	Magnesium hydroxide 500 g/450 kg body weight into rumen. Fluids if indicated. Feed hay. Should begin eating 24–36 hours
Mild	Bright and alert. Able to walk, no ataxia, eats and drinks normally	Not detectable clinically	Not significant	Normal	Normal 38·5–39	No detectable distension, ruminal contents palpable, ruminal contractions still present but not as strong as normal, rumen pH 6·5–7. Almost normal protozoan activity	Feed hay and observe for 48 hours. Watch for anorexia

or weeks and are affected with grain overload usually have a pH below 5.

The microscopic examination of a few drops of ruminal fluid on a glass slide (with a coverslip) at low power will reveal the absence of ruminal protozoa, which is a reliable indication of an abnormal state of the rumen, usually acidosis. The predominantly Gram-negative bacterial flora of the rumen is replaced by a Gram-positive one.

The degree of hemoconcentration, as indicated by hematocrit, increases with the amount of fluid withdrawn from the extracellular fluid space into the rumen. The hematocrit rises from a normal of 30–32% to 50–60% in the terminal stages and is accompanied by a fall in blood pressure. The urine pH falls to about 5 and becomes progressively more concentrated, and terminally there is anuria. Blood lactate and inorganic phosphate levels rise and blood pH and bicarbonate fall markedly. In almost all cases there is a mild hypocalcemia which is presumably due to a temporary malabsorption. Serum levels may drop to between 6 and 8 mg/dl (1·5 and 2 mmol/l).

The serum enzyme activities of cattle fed on barley for several months has been measured and suggest that hepatocellular damage occurs during the early stages of feeding grain but that recovery occurs after about 1 month (13).

Necropsy findings

In acute cases which die in 24–48 hours the contents of the rumen and reticulum are thin and porridge-like and have a typical odor suggestive of fermentation. The cornified epithelium may be mushy and easily wiped off leaving a dark, hemorrhagic surface beneath. This change may be patchy, caused probably by the production of excess lactic acid in pockets where the grain collects, but is generaly restricted to the ventral half of the sacs. Abomasitis and enteritis are also evident in many cases. The abomasum may contain large quantities of grain. There is a pronounced thickening and darkening of the blood and the visceral veins stand out prominently.

In cases which have persisted for 3–4 days the wall of the reticulum and rumen may be gangrenous. This change is again patchy but may be widespread. In affected areas the wall may be three or four times the normal thickness, show a soft black mucosal surface raised above surrounding normal areas and a dark red appearance visible through the serous surface. The thickened area is very friable and on cutting has a gelatinous appearance. Histological preparations show infiltration of the area by fungal mycelia and a severe hemorrhagic necrosis. A fungal hepatitis is common in those with fungal rumenitis. In the nervous system, in cases of 72 hours or more duration, demyelination has been reported (22). A terminal ischemic nephrosis is present in varying degrees in most fatal cases of more than several days' duration (31).

If the examination is less than an hour after death, estimation of ruminal pH may be of value in confirming the diagnosis but after 1 hour the pH of the rumen contents begins to increase and its measurement may not be reliable. A secondary enteritis is common in animals which have been ill for several days.

Diagnosis

When outbreaks of the disease with an appropriate history are encountered, the diagnosis is usually readily obvious and confirmed by the clinical findings and examination of the ruminal fluid for pH and rumen protozoa. When the disease occurs in a single animal without a history of engorgement, the diagnosis may not be so readily obvious. The anorexia, depression, ruminal stasis with gurgling fluid sounds from the rumen, diarrhea and a staggery gait with a normal temperature are characteristics of rumen overload.

Severe cases which are recumbent may resemble parturient paresis, but in the latter the feces are usually firm and dry, marked dehydration does not occur, the absolute intensity of the heart sounds is reduced, and the response to calcium injection is favorable. Other common toxemias of cattle which may resemble ruminal overload include peracute coliform mastitis and acute diffuse peritonitis, but a careful clinical examination will usually reveal the cause of the toxemia.

The consumption of large quantities of palatable feed, such as ensiled green feed offered to cattle for the first time, may cause simple indigestion which may resemble grain overload. The rumen is full, the movements are reduced in frequency and amplitude, there may be mild abdominal pain due to the distension, but the ruminal pH and protozoan numbers and activity are normal.

Treatment

The principles of treatment of carbohydrate engorgement in ruminants are:

- Correct the ruminal and systemic acidosis and prevent further production of lactic acid
- Restore fluid and electrolyte losses and maintain circulating blood volumes
- Restore forestomach and intestinal motility to normal

There are at least two common clinical situations encountered. One is when cattle have been found accidentally eating large quantities of grain and the animals are not yet ill and they all appear the same clinically, except perhaps for varying degrees of distension depending on the amount each animal has consumed. In the other situation, the engorgement occurred some 24–48 hours previously and the animals are presented with the clinical signs of lactic acidosis.

When cattle are found engorging themselves, the following procedures are recommended. Prevent further access to feed, provide no water for 12–24 hours but offer a supply of good quality palatable hay equal to one-half of the daily allowance per head. All animals should be exercised every hour for 12–24 hours to encourage movement of the ingesta through the digestive tract. Those cattle which have consumed a toxic dose of grain will show signs of anorexia, inactivity and depression in approximately 6–8 hours and they should be identified and removed from the group for individual treatment. Those cattle which did not consume a toxic dose of grain will usually remain bright and alert and will usually eat hay if offered a supply. Not all cattle found engorging themselves with grain will have consumed a toxic dose and careful monitoring over a 24–48-hour period will usually distinguish between those which need treatment and those which do not.

After 18–24 hours those cattle which have continued to eat hay may be allowed free access to water. Those with clinical evidence of grain overload must be separated out and treated accordingly. They will engorge themselves if allowed free access to water. The rumen becomes grossly distended with fluid and affected cattle may die 18–24 hours later from electrolyte disturbances and acid–base imbalance.

In certain situations, if feasible and warranted by economics, such as when fattened cattle have accidentally engorged on grain, emergency slaughter may be the most economical course of action (46).

The recommendations for treatment which are given here are guidelines (Table 29). In an outbreak, some animals will not require any treatment while severely affected cases will obviously need a rumenotomy. For those which are not severely affected, it is often difficult to decide whether to treat them only medically with antacids orally and systemically or to do a rumenotomy. Each case must be examined clinically and the most appropriate treatment selected. The degree of mental depression, muscular strength, degree of dehydration, heart rate, body temperature, and rumen pH are clinical parameters which can be used to assess severity and to determine the treatment likely to be most successful.

In severe cases, in which there is recumbency, severe depression, hypothermia, prominent ruminal distension with fluid, a heart rate from 110–130/minute and a rumen pH of 5 or below, a rumenotomy is the best course of action. The rumen is emptied, washed out with a siphon, examined for evidence of and the extent of chemical rumenitis and a cud transfer (10–20 liters of rumen juice) is placed in the rumen along with a few handfuls of hay. The rumenotomy will usually correct the ruminal acidosis and an alkalinizing agent is not necessary. A large quantity of the lactic acid and its substrate can be removed. The oral or intraruminal administration of compounds such as magnesium oxide or magnesium hydroxide to cattle following complete evacuation of the rumen may cause metabolic alkalosis for up to 24–36 hours (39). Not all of the feed consumed will be removed because considerable quantities may have passed into the omasum and abomasum, where fermentation may also occur. The major disadvantages of a rumenotomy are time and cost, particularly when many animals are involved. The systemic acidosis is treated with intravenous solutions of 5% sodium bicarbonate at the rate of 5 liters for a 450 kg animal given initially over a period of about 30 minutes. This will usually correct the systemic acidosis. This is followed by isotonic sodium bicarbonate (1·3%) at 150 ml/kg body weight given over the next 6–12 hours. Cattle which respond favorably to the rumenotomy and fluid therapy will show improved muscular strength, begin to urinate within 1 hour and attempt to stand with 6–12 hours.

In less severe cases, in which affected cattle are still standing but are depressed, their heart rate is 90–100/minute, there is moderate ruminal distension and the rumen pH is between 5 and 6, an alternative to a rumenotomy is rumen lavage if the necessary facilities are available (24). A large 25–28 mm inside diameter rubber tube is passed into the rumen and warm water is pumped in until there is an obvious distension of the left paralumbar fossa, and then the rumen is allowed to empty by gravity flow. The rumen may be almost completely emptied by 10–15 irrigations, which may require about the same length of time as taken for a rumenotomy. With successful gastric lavage, alkalinizing agents are not placed in the rumen but the systemic acidosis is treated as described above.

In moderately affected cases, the use of 500 g of magnesium hydroxide per 450 kg body weight, or magnesium oxide in 10 liters of warm water pumped into the rumen and followed by kneading of the rumen to promote mixing, will usually suffice. Dehydration and acidosis in these can be treated with isotonic sodium bicarbonate or balanced electrolyte solution.

Ancillary treatment has included antihistamines for laminitis, corticosteroids for shock therapy, thiamin or brewer's yeast to promote the metabolism of lactic acid, and parasympathomimetics to stimulate gut motility. Their efficacy has been difficult to evaluate and it is unlikely any of them would be of much value. Calcium borogluconate is used widely because there is a mild hypocalcemia and a beneficial but temporary response does occur.

Regardless of the treatment used, all cases must be monitored several times daily until recovery is obvious for evidence of unexpected deterioration. Following treatment, cattle should begin eating hay by the third day, some ruminal movements should be present, large quantities of soft feces should be passed and they should maintain hydration. In those which become worse, the heart rate increases, depression is marked, the rumen fills with fluid and weakness and recumbency occur. During treatment, the water supply should be restricted because some cattle, either immediately after they have engorged themselves or once they become ill, appear to have an intense thirst and will drink excessive quantities of water and die precipitously within a few hours.

Orally administered antibiotics including penicillin, the tetracyclines and chloramphenicol have been used to control growth of the bacteria which produce lactic acid but appear to be of limited value.

The fungal rumenitis which may occur about 3–5 days after engorgement is best prevented by early effective treatment of the ruminal acidosis.

Prevention

Cattle can be started, grown and fattened on high-level grain rations successfully, providing they are allowed a gradual period of adaptation during the critical period of introduction. The important principle of prevention is that the ruminant can adapt to an all-concentrate ration. For animals which have just arrived in the feedlot, the length of the adaptation period required will depend on the immediate nutritional history of the animals, their appetite and the composition of the ration to be used.

One of the safest procedures is to feed a milled mixed ration, consisting of 50–60% roughage and 40–50% grain, as the starting ration for 7–10 days and monitor the response. If results are satisfactory, begin decreasing the level of roughage by 10% every 2–4 days down to a level of 10–15% roughage, with the remainder grain and vitamins–mineral–salt supplement. The use of roughage–grain mixtures ensures that cattle do not engorge themselves on grain and adaptation can occur in about 21 days. A system of adding 25% grain to a mixed ration every 5 days was a safe method of introducing cattle to a ration containing 85% wheat (25).

Another method is to begin with small amounts of grain, 8–10 g/kg body weight, which is increased every 2–4 days by increments of 10–12%. A source of roughage is supplied separately. The disadvantages of this system are that hungry or dominant cattle may eat much more than their calculated share and there is no assurance that sufficient roughage will be consumed. In this system, on a practical basis, the cattle are usually fed twice daily and brought up to a daily intake of grain which satisfies their appetite and then the grain ration is offered free choice from self-feeders. Unless there is sufficient feeding space in the self-feeders, competitive and dominant animals will often overeat and careful monitoring is necessary.

Feedlot starter rations consisting of a mixture of roughage and grain and offered free choice along with hay and gradually replaced by a finishing ration have successful adapted cattle in 10 days (26). The starter ration contained about 2500 kcal (10 460 kJ) DE (digestible energy) per kg of feed. The finishing ration about 3100 kcal (12 970 kJ) and controlling the rate of increase of DE concentration of the ration was a major factor in getting cattle on feed.

The incorporation of buffers, such as sodium bicarbonate, into the ration of feedlot cattle has been studied extensively but to date the results are inconclusive and reliable recommendations cannot be made (27, 28, 40). A level of 2% dietary sodium bicarbonate, sodium bentonite, or limestone provided some protection from acidosis during the early adaptation phase of high-concentrate feeding; but they were no more effective than 10% alfalfa hay (27). Buffers have been most effective in reducing acidosis early in the feeding period and have little or no effect later (40). They may be associated with an increased incidence of urinary calculi, bloat and vitamin deficiencies. The experimental results to date are conflicting. Some trials indicate that buffers maintain a Gram-negative rumen flora in sheep fed grain compared to a shift to Gram-positive rumen flora in animals not fed buffers (42). Liveweight performance is also improved in some trials (42) but not in others (41) fed 0·75, 1·0 or 2·25% of diet as sodium bicarbonate.

The inclusion of thiopeptin, a sulfur-containing peptide antibiotic, at the rate of 11 ppm in a lactic acidosis-inducing diet (wheat) of sheep will prevent the disease (43). Ruminal lactate is reduced by 68% and volatile fatty acids are increased by 33%. Feed efficiency and growth rate are also increased in sheep (43) and cattle. Thiopeptin and sodium bicarbonate may also be used in combination (45). The ionophore antibiotics salinomycin, monensin and lasalocid have been compared for their protective effects, and salinomycin is more effective than the other two (44); monensin also shows some promise (50).

An interesting new approach for the prevention of acidosis is to inoculate unadapted cattle with ruminal fluid from adapted animals which contains a large population of lactic acid utilizing bacteria (29). The rate of gain and feed efficiency over a 21-day trial were improved when cattle were inoculated with ruminal bacteria from adapted cattle before they were changed to a high-level grain ration (8).

REVIEW LITERATURE

Dunlop, R. H. (1972) Pathogenesis of ruminant lactic acidosis. *Adv. vet. Sci. comp. Med.*, *16*, 259.
Loew, F. M. & Chaplin, R. k. (1976) Abnormal acid production in the rumen: newer findings from around the world. *Proc. Am. ann. Mtg Am. Assoc. bov. Practnrs*, 161.
Scanlan, C. M. & Hathcock, T. L. (1983) Bovine rumenitis—liver abscess complex: a bacteriological review. *Cornell Vet.*, *73*, 288–297.
Symposium on acidosis in feedlot cattle (1976) *J. anim. Sci.*, *43*, 898.
Weinberg, M. S. & Sheffner, A. L. (1976) *Buffers in Ruminant Physiology and Metabolism.* New York: Church & Dwight.
Wheeler, W. E. (1980) Gastrointestinal tract pH environment and the influence of buffering materials on the performance of ruminants *J. anim. Sci.*, *51*, 224.

REFERENCES

(1) Dunlop, R. H. (1972) *Adv. vet. Sci. comp. Med.*, *16*, 259.
(2) Stowe, C. M. et al. (1983) *J. Am. vet. med. Assoc.*, *182*, 415.
(3) Wobeser, G. & Runge, W. (1975) *J. Wildl. Mgmt*, *29*, 596.
(4) Orskov, E. R. (1973) *Res. vet. Sci.*, *14*, 110.
(5) Grubb, J. A. & Dehority, B. A. (1975) *Appl. Microbiol. 30*, 404.
(6) Elam, C. J. (1976) *J. anim. Sci.*, *43*, 898.
(7) Mullen, P. A. (1972) *Vet. Bull.*, *42*, 119.
(8) Slyter, L. L. (1976) *J. anim. Sci.*, *43*, 910.
(9) Huber, J. L. (1976) *J. anim. Sci.*, *43*, 902.
(10) Russell, J. B. & Hino, J. (1985) *J. dairy Sci.*, *68*, 1712.
(11) Dunlop, R. H. & Hammond, P. B. (1965) *Ann. NY Acad Sci.*, *119*, 1109.
(12) Huber, J. L. (1976) In: *Buffers in Ruminant Physiology and Metabolism*, eds M. S. Weinberg & A. S. Sheffner. New York: Church & Dwight.
(13) Scanlan, C. M. & Hathcock, J. L. (1983) *Cornell Vet.*, *73*, 288.
(14) Fell, B. F. et al. (1972) *Res. vet. Sci.*, *13*, 30.
(15) Mullen, P. A. (1976) *Vet. Rec.*, *98*, 439.
(16) Bide, R. W. & Dorwood, W. J. (1975) *Can. J. anim. Sci.*, *55*, 23.
(17) Bide, R W. et al. (1973) *Can. J. anim. Sci.*, *53*, 697.
(18) Nagaraja, J. G. et al. (1978) *Can. J. Microbiol.*, *24*, 1253.
(19) Allison, M. J. et al. (1974) *Am. J. vet. Res.*, *35*, 1587.
(20) Morrow, L. L. et al. (1973) *Am. J. vet. Res.*, *34*, 1305.
(21) Vestweber, J. G. E. & Leipold, H. W. (1974) *Am. J. vet. Res.*, *35*, 1537.
(22) Strafuss, A. C. & Monlux, W. S. (1966) *Cornell Vet.*, *56*, 128.
(23) Schukken, A. et al. (1985) *Tijdschr. Diergeneeskd.*, *110*, 69.
(24) Radostits, O. M. & Magnusson, R. A. (1971) *Can vet J.*, *12*, 150.
(25) Pryor, W. J. & Laws, L. (1972) *Aust. vet. T.*, *48*, 500.
(26) Hironaka, R. (1968) *Can. J. anim. Sci.*, *49*, 181.
(27) Ha, J. K. et al. (1983) *J. dairy Sci.*, *56*, 698.
(28) Emerick, R. J. (1976) In: *Buffers in Ruminant Physiology and Metabolism*, eds M. S. Weinberg & A. S. Sheffner. New York: Church & Dwight.
(29) Huber, J. L. et al. (1976) *Am. J. vet. Res.*, *37*, 611.
(30) Smith, C. M. et al. (1979) *Can. J. anim. Sci.*, *59*, 255.
(31) Nauriyal, D. C. et al. (1978) *Zentralbl. vet. Med.*, *25A*, 383.
(32) Lee, G. J. (1977) *Aust. J. agric. Res.*, *28*, 1075
(33) Kezar, W. W. & Church, D. C. (1979) *J. anim. Sci.*, *49*, 567.
(34) Randhawa, S. S. et al. (1980) *Res. vet. Sci.*, *29*, 118.
(35) Nagaraja, J. G. et al. (1979) *J. anim. Sci.*, *49*, 567.
(36) McManus, W. R. et al. (1978) *Res. vet. Sci.*, *24*, 388.
(37) Huber, J. L. et al. (1979) *Am. J. vet. Res.*, *40*, 792.
(38) Svendsen, C. K. (1979) *Nord. VetMed.*, *31*, 497.
(39) Ogilvie, J. H. et al. (1983) *Can. J. comp. Med.*, *47*, 108.
(40) Wheeler, W. E. (1980) *J. anim. Sci.*, *51*, 224.
(41) McKnight, D. R. et al. (1979) *Can. J. anim. Sci.*, *59*, 805.
(42) McManus, W. R. & Bigham, M. L. (1978) *Res. vet. Sci.*, *24*, 129.
(43) Muir, L. A. et al. (1981) *J. anim. Sci.*, *52*, 635.
(44) Nagaraja, T. G. et al. (1985) *Am. J. vet. Res.*, *46*, 2444.
(45) Kezar, W. W. & Church, D. C. (1979) *J. anim. Sci.*, *49*, 1396.
(46) Bauck, S. W. (1981) *Can. vet. J.*, *22*, 243.
(47) Bide, R. W. (1983) *Can. J. comp. Med.*, *47*, 222.
(48) Bide, R. W. & Dorward, W. J. (1983) *Can. J. comp. Med.*, *47*, 230.
(49) Crichlow, E. C. & Chaplin, R. K. (1985) *Am. J. vet. Res.*, *46*, 1908.
(50) Burrin, D. G. & Brittton, R. A. (1986) *J. anim. Sci.*, *63*, 888.

Ruminal parakeratosis

Parakeratosis of the ruminal epithelium does not, as far as is known, cause clinical illness but opinions on its effects on weight gains and productivity vary. There is evidence that the development of parakeratosis increases and then reduces the absorption of volatile fatty acids from the rumen (1) and that the addition of volatile fatty acids to a calf starter increases the incidence of the condition (2). The abnormality has been observed most commonly in cattle and sheep fed high-concentrate rations of alfalfa pellets which have been subjected to heat treatment, and does not occur in cattle fed on rations containing normal quantities of unpelleted roughage (3). The incidence of the disease does not appear to be related to the feeding of antibiotics or protein concentrates.

In affected rumens the papillae are enlarged, leathery, dark in color and often adhered to form clumps. Histologically there is an increase in thickness of the cornified portion of the ruminal epithelium and a persistence of nuclei in the cornified cells (4). Some of the affected cells contain vacuoles. The greatest severity of lesions are present on the dorsal surface of the rumen about the level of the fluid ruminal contents. It is thought that they are caused by the lowered pH and the increased volatile fatty acid content in the rumen liquor (5). The fact that unprocessed, whole grain, on which animals gain weight as readily, does not lead to the development of the disease is probably related to the higher pH and higher concentration of acetic, as against longer chain VFAs, in the ruminal liquor (6). The incidence of affected animals in a group may be as high as 40% (4, 7).

REFERENCES

(1) Hinders, R. F. & Owen, F G. (1965) *J. dairy Sci.*, *48*, 1069.
(2) Gilliland, R. L. et al. (1962) *J. dairy Sci.*, *45*, 1211.
(3) Harvey, R. W. et al. (1968) *J. anim. Sci.*, *27*, 1438.
(4) Jensen, R. et al. (1958) *Am. vet. Res.*, *19*, 277.
(5) Fell, B. F. et al. (1968) *Res. vet. Sci.*, *9*, 458.
(6) Orskov, E. R. (1973) *Res. vet. Sci.*, *14*, 110.
(7) Hopkins, H. A. et al. (1960) *J. anim. Sci.*, *19*, 652.

Traumatic reticuloperitonitis and allied syndromes

Perforation of the wall of the reticulum by a sharp foreign body produces initially an acute local peritonitis which may spread to cause acute diffuse peritonitis or remain localized to cause subsequent damage including vagal indigestion and diaphragmatic hernia. The penetration of the foreign body may proceed beyond the peritoneum and cause involvement of other organs resulting in pericarditis, cardiac tamponade, pneumonia, pleurisy and mediastinitis, and hepatic, splenic or diaphragmatic abscess (1).

These sequelae of traumatic perforation of the reticular wall are set out diagrammatically in Fig. 17.

This complexity of development makes diagnosis and prognosis difficult, and the possibility that a number of syndromes may occur together further complicates the picture. All of these entities except endocarditis are dealt with together here, even though many of them are diseases of other systems.

Traumatic reticuloperitonitis

Here the acute local peritonitis is characterized clinically by sudden anorexia and fall in milk yield, mild fever, ruminal stasis and local pain in the abdomen. Rapid recovery may occur, or the disease may persist in a chronic form or spread widely to produce an acute, diffuse peritonitis.

Etiology

Most cases are caused by the ingestion of foreign bodies in prepared feed. Baling or fencing wire which has passed through a chaff-cutter, feed chopper or forage harvester is the commonest cause of injury. In one series of 1400 necropsies, 58% of lesions were caused by wire, 36% by nails and 6% by miscellaneous objects (2). The foreign bodies may be in the roughage or concentrate or may originate on the farm when repairs are made to fences, yards and in the vicinity of feed troughs. Adult dairy cattle are most commonly affected because of their more frequent exposure but cases occur infrequently in yearlings, beef cattle, dairy bulls, sheep and goats. In the series of 1400 necropsies referred to, 93% were in cattle over 2 years old and 87% were in dairy cattle. The disease is much more common in cattle fed on stored feeds, especially those penned up inside for part of the year. It is almost unknown in cattle fed entirely on pasture. Accordingly, it is much more common in the winter months in the northern hemisphere (9).

The disease is of great economic importance because of the severe loss of production it causes and the high mortality rate. Many cases go unrecognized and many more make spontaneous recoveries. In industrialized countries, metallic foreign bodies may be present in the reticulum in up to 90% of normal cattle (3) and residual traumatic lesions may be present in as many as 70% of dairy cows (4). Amongst those animals seen clinically as being sick, about 25% develop serious complications that make their prognoses poor. The other 75% can be expected to recover completely with conservative treat-

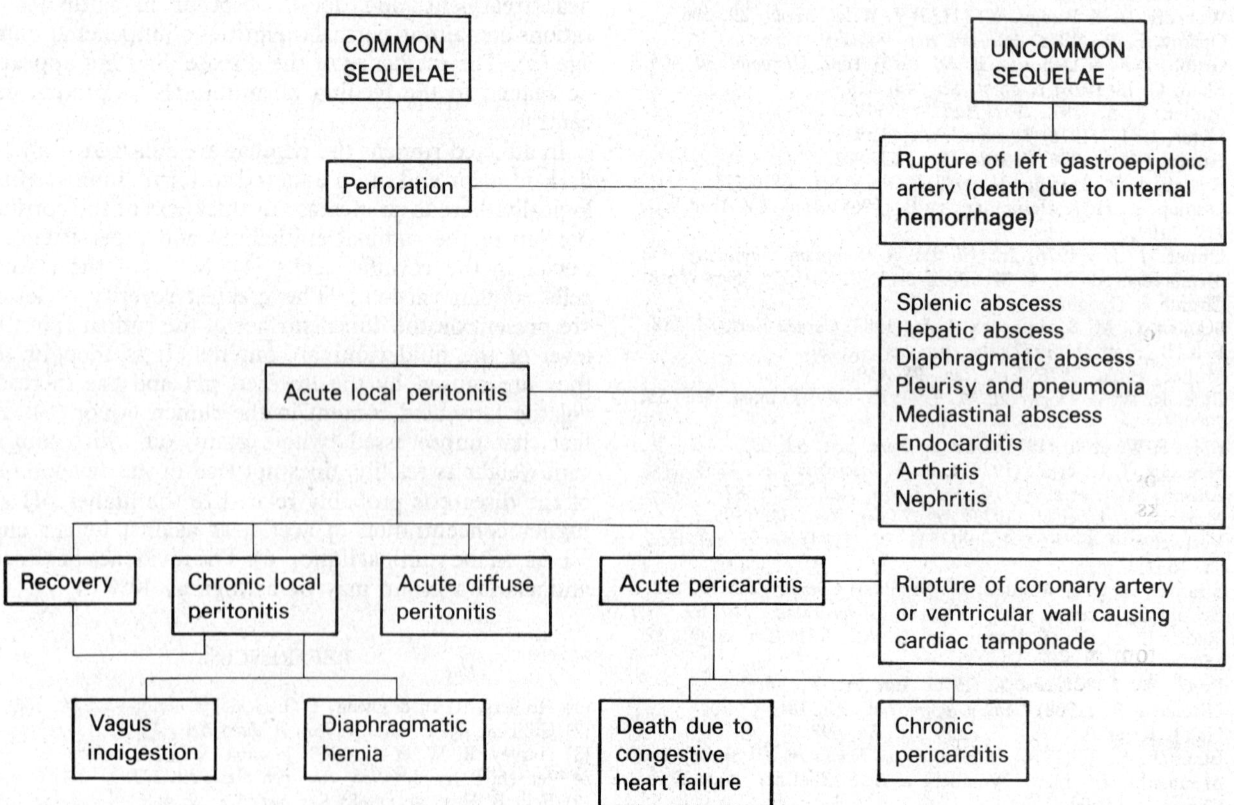

Fig. 17. Sequelae of traumatic perforation of the reticular wall

ment or routine surgical intervention. In a survey in sheep and goats there was one case in 17 goats examined and an incidence of 2% in adult sheep and 0·1% in lambs (5). The disease also occurs in camels, but only rarely, and presents a syndrome identical with that seen in cattle (6). The natural and experimental disease in goats is also identical with that seen in cattle (7). The disease is also recorded in the buffalo (17).

Pathogenesis

Lack of oral discrimination in cattle leads to the ingestion of foreign bodies which would be rejected by other species. Swallowed foreign bodies may lodge in the upper esophagus and cause obstruction, or in the esophageal groove and cause vomiting but in most instances they pass to the reticulum. Radiological examination of goats which have been fed foreign bodies experimentally indicate that they may first enter various sacs of the forestomachs before reaching the reticulum (13). Many lie there without causing harm but the cell-like structure of the lining provides many spots for fixation of the foreign body and the vigorous contractions of the reticulum are sufficient to push a sharp-pointed object through the wall. Most perforations occur in the lower part of the anterior wall but some occur laterally in the direction of the spleen and medially towards the liver.

If the wall is injured without penetration to the serous surface no detectable illness occurs, and the foreign body may remain fixed in the site for long periods and gradually be corroded away. This applies particularly to wire which can disappear in a period as short as 6 weeks, but nails last much longer and are unlikely to disappear in less than 1 year. The ease with which perforation occurs has been illustrated by the artificial production of the disease (3). Sharpened foreign bodies were given to ten cows in gelatin capsules. Of 20 pieces of wire and ten nails, 25 were found in the reticulum. Of the 20 pieces of wire 18 had perforated or were embedded in the wall or plicae. Only one of the nails was embedded. Complete perforations were caused by 13 foreign bodies and incomplete by six. All cows suffered at least one perforation, showed clinical signs of acute local peritonitis, and recovered after surgical removal of the foreign bodies.

Many foreign bodies do not remain embedded and are found lying free in the reticulum if surgery is delayed until about 72 hours after illness commences. This is probably due to necrosis around the penetrating object and the returning reticular movements manipulating it from its position (8). Objects which are deeply embedded, have kinks or barbs, or have large diameters tend to remain *in situ* and cause persistent chronic peritonitis.

The initial reaction to perforation is one of acute local peritonitis, and in experimentally induced cases, clinical signs commence about 24 hours after penetration (3). The peritonitis causes ruminal atony and abdominal pain. If the foreign body falls back into the reticulum spontaneous recovery may occur, although spread of the inflammation to affect most of the peritoneal cavity is likely to occur in cows which calve at the time of perforation, and in cattle which are forced to exercise. Immobility is a prominent sign of the disease and it serves as a protective mechanism in that adhesions are able to form and localize the peritonitis. Animals made to walk or transported long distances frequently suffer relapses when these adhesions are broken down during body movements.

During the initial penetration the foreign body may penetrate beyond the peritoneal cavity and into the pleural or pericardial sacs to set up inflammation there. It is often stated that foreign bodies which remain embedded in the reticular wall may be pushed further by the pressure of the calf during late pregnancy or the efforts of parturition. This may occur in some cases but the more common train of events is that in cows in advanced pregnancy the initial perforation is likely to extend further than in non-pregnant cows. At least it can be said that serious complications including pericarditis are more likely to occur in cows after the sixth month of pregnancy (8).

The pathogenesis of the more common complications are discussed under traumatic pericarditis, vagus indigestion, diaphragmatic hernia and traumatic abscess of the spleen and liver (pp. 265, 263, 259, and 265). Less common sequelae include rupture of the left gastroepiploic artery causing sudden death due to internal hemorrhage and the development of a diaphragmatic abscess which infiltrates tissues to the ventral abdominal wall at the xiphoid process, rupturing to the exterior and sometimes discharging the foreign body. Hematogenous spread of infection from a diaphragmatic abscess or chronic local peritonitis is one of the commonest causes of endocarditis and its attendant lesions of arthritis, nephritis and pulmonary abscess. Penetration into the pleural cavity causes development of an acute suppurative pleurisy and pneumonia. In rare cases the infection is localized chiefly to the mediastinum with the development of an extensive abscess which causes pressure on the pericardial sac and resulting cardiac embarrassment and congestive heart failure. Rarely the foreign body penetrates to the abomasum (16) causing gastritis, abomasitis, pyloric stenosis and abomasal ulcer, manifested clinically by anorexia and gaseous distension.

Clinical findings

Acute local peritonitis

The onset is sudden with complete anorexia and a sharp fall in milk yield usually to about a third or less of the previous yield. These changes occur within a 12-hour period and their abrupt appearance is typical of this disease. There is subacute abdominal pain in all cases. The animal is reluctant to move and does so slowly. Walking, particularly downhill, is often accompanied by grunting. Most animals prefer to remain standing for long periods and lie down with great care; habitual recumbency is characteristic in others. Arching of the back is marked in about half the cases but there is always rigidity of the back and of the abdominal muscles so that the animal appears gaunt or 'tucked-up'. Defecation and urination cause pain and the acts are performed infrequently and usually with grunting. In rare cases an attack of acute abdominal pain with kicking at the belly, stretching and rolling is the earliest sign. In others there is recumbency and inability to rise.

A moderate systemic reaction occurs, the temperature rising usually to 39·5–40°C (103–104°F), rarely higher, the pulse rate to about 80/minute and the respiratory rate to about 30/minute. Temperatures above 40°C (104°F) accompanied by heart rates greater than 90/minute should arouse suspicion of serious complications. The respirations are usually shallow and, if the pleural cavity has been penetrated, are painful and accompanied by an audible expiratory grunt. Rumination is suspended and ruminal movements are absent, or at least severely depressed to a rate of about one per 2 minutes with the sounds much reduced in intensity. The rumen may appear to be full because of the presence of mild tympany and in some cases there is moderate distension of the left flank. On palpation a typical cap of gas can be felt before the firm doughy ruminal contents are reached. The presence of this cap is caused by the separation of the gas from the solid and fluid contents and may occur in other forms of acute ruminal atony. Constipation or scant feces is common.

Pain can be elicited by deep palpation of the abdominal wall just behind the xiphoid process of the sternum. Pressure can be exerted by a short, sharp jab with the closed fist or knee. Pinching the withers to cause depression of the back is not reliable in large adult cows and bulls, and for these the sharp elevation of a rail held under the abdomen is a useful method for detecting pain. A positive response to any of these tests is a grunt of pain which may be audible some distance away but is best detected by auscultation of the trachea. Pain may also be manifested when the infrequent reticular contractions occur. Observation of pain or uneasiness coinciding with the primary ruminal movement or just prior to it is suggested as an aid to making a diagnosis (11). The palpation of significant enlargement of the lymph nodes in the medial, ruminal, longitudinal furrow, during a rectal examination or on exploratory laparotomy, is thought to be of help in diagnosing the condition (10).

The stage of acute local peritonitis is quite short and the signs described above are at their maximum on the first day and in most cases subside quickly thereafter so that they may be difficult to detect by the third day. The most constant sign is the abdominal pain which may require deep palpation for its demonstration. In cases which recover spontaneously or respond satisfactorily to conservative treatment there may be no detectable signs of illness by the fourth day.

Chronic local peritonitis

When chronic peritonitis persists the appetite and milk yield do not return completely to normal. Pain is not evident although the gait may be slow and careful, and grunting may occur during rumination, defecation and urination. Rumination is depressed and chronic moderate bloat may be present although ruminal movements are usually normal.

Rectal examination is not revealing although the feces are usually firm and dry and indicative of a prolonged sojourn in the gut. The amount of peritoneal fluid is usually increased and paracentesis abdominis is easily carried out. Fluid spurts out and on examination suggests chronic inflammation, as set out above. In rare cases the amount of fluid which accumulates is very great and causes obvious distension of the abdomen. In some animals the abdomen is gaunt and little or no fluid is present. The peritoneal cavity in these animals is a mass of tight fibrous adhesions. A more common syndrome is chronic intoxication, alimentary tract stasis and subacute abdominal pain in which a greater part of the serous surface is covered with a coagulated mixture of protein and pus. In some cases there are extensive lesions well walled off from the remainder of the peritoneal cavity by adhesions. These can be misleading because paracentesis abdominis can produce a negative result.

In none of these animals is treatment likely to be effective or the prognosis favorable.

Acute diffuse peritonitis

The development of acute, diffuse peritonitis is manifested by the appearance of a profound toxemia within a day or two of the onset of local peritonitis. Alimentary tract movements cease entirely, there is severe depression and the temperature may be higher than normal, or subnormal in fulminating cases, especially those which occur immediately after calving. The pulse rate rises to 100–120/minute and pain can be elicited by palpation anywhere over the ventral abdominal wall. Usually this stage is followed by one of acute collapse and peripheral circulatory failure with all pain responses having disappeared. A terminal stage of recumbency and coma produces a clinical picture not unlike that of parturient paresis.

Metal detectors have come to be widely used in the diagnosis of traumatic reticuloperitonitis. The presence of ferrous, metallic foreign bodies and their whereabouts can be accurately determined through the body wall but the instruments are of limited usefulness because most normal dairy cows (about 80%) give positive results. Being able to locate the foreign body well above the floor of the reticulum and in association with a pain response on percussion may have diagnostic significance, but locating the foreign body on the floor of the viscus is of little importance because most cows will have them in that location (15). However, it is agreed that these detectors do lend themselves to the accumulation of a great deal of data (12).

Clinical pathology

The total and differential leukocyte counts provide good diagnostic and prognostic data. The differential leukocyte count is usually considerably more indicative of the acute peritonitis than the total count. In acute local peritonitis there is commonly a neutrophilia (mature neutrophils above 400/μl) and a left shift (immature neutrophils above 200/μl). This is a regenerative left shift. Both the neutrophilia and the left shift will be increased on the first day and will last for up to 3 days, when in uncomplicated cases the count begins to return to normal (3). In chronic cases the levels do not return completely to normal for several days or longer periods and there is usually a moderate leukocytosis, neutrophilia and a monocytosis.

The determination of total plasma protein has been used as an aid to the diagnosis of traumatic reticuloperitonitis (28). There is a significant difference in total plasma protein levels between cattle with traumatic reticuloperitonits and those with other diseases of the gastrointestinal tract which might be confused with the former. The mean plasma protein concentrations, measured before surgery, were 88 ± 13 g/l for traumatic reticuloperitonitis and 77 ± 12 g/l for controls.

In acute diffuse peritonitis there is often a leukopenia (total count below 4000/μl) with a greater absolute number of immature neutrophils than mature neutrophils (degenerative left shift) which suggests an unfavorable prognosis if severe. The degree of lymphopenia (lymphocyte count below 2500–3000/μl) is an indication of the stress reaction to the infection. In cases of severe diffuse peritonitis the fibrinogen levels may be increased up to 10–20 g/l.

Abdominocentesis is a valuable aid for the diagnosis and should be done whenever possible. A reliable site for obtaining peritoneal fluid from mature cattle is 10 cm cranial and 10 cm to the right-hand side of the umbilicus (33). A regular blunt-ended teat cannula is commonly used with satisfactory results. If no fluid can be obtained, a trocar and cannula 80 mm long and with a 4 mm internal diameter can be used with success. The trocar and cannula are inserted into the abdomen, the trocar removed and an 80 cm long 10 French gauge infant feeding tube is inserted into the abdomen through the cannula leaving about 10–20 cm outside. The tube acts as a wick and within several minutes fluid can be collected into vials (33). Laboratory evaluation of peritoneal fluid consists of determinations of total white blood (WBC) cell count, differential cell count, total protein and culture for pathogens. The interpretations of the analysis of the peritoneal fluid can be unreliable because to date only a few correlations have been made between the laboratory findings and the presence or absence of peritoneal lesions. In one retrospective study a nucleated cell count of greater than 6000 cells/μl and total protein content of greater than 3 g/dl is consistent with the diagnosis of peritonitis in 80% of cases (34). However, one study indicated that a relative neutrophil count greater than 40% and a relative eosinophil count of less than 10% was frequently associated with the diagnosis of peritonitis (34).

Right flank laparoscopy using a flexible fiberoptic laparoscope, 14 mm diameter and 1120 mm working length, is a reliable diagnostic aid for the presence of traumatic reticuloperitonitis (29).

Radiological examination of the reticulum with the animal in dorsal recumbency (dorsal reticulography) is considered to be an accurate diagnostic method for the evaluation of cattle with suspected traumatic reticuloperitonitis (30).

Necropsy findings

Neither acute local nor chronic local peritonitis is fatal. In acute diffuse peritonitis a fibrinous or suppurative inflammation affects the whole of the peritoneal surface. There is a characteristic smell and large quantities of fluid are usually present. The foreign body can usually be found perforating the anterior lower wall of the reticulum, although it may have fallen back into the reticulum leaving only the perforation site and its surrounding inflammation as evidence of the site of penetration.

Diagnosis

In traumatic reticuloperitonitis, the classical syndrome is one of sudden onset of grunting pain, ruminal stasis, complete anorexia, severe fall in milk yield, pain on percussion of the abdomen, slight but significant fever, an elevated leukocyte count with a left shift in the hemogram and a peritoneal fluid sample which has the same characteristics. No other disease, with the exception of ephemeral fever causes a syndrome which is similar, and ephemeral fever always occurs in outbreak form. However, the times at which cases of traumatic reticuloperitonitis are seen for the first varies from day 1 when the syndrome is classical to day 3 or 4 by which time it has subsided so much clinically that confusion with other diseases is a significant possibility.

A sudden onset of ruminal stasis, lack of appetite and fall in milk yield is also characteristic of acute intestinal obstruction, simple indigestion, abomasal displacement or torsion, acute carbohydrate indigestion and postpartum metritis. Grunting pain is an important sign in cattle and occurs in many diseases other than traumatic reticuloperitonitis. Some of them, like bloat and pyelonephritis have obvious localizing signs, and some, such as chronic peritonitis, do not. The differential diagnosis of grunting is set out in Fig. 18. There are other diseases which can resemble traumatic reticuloperitonitis when its original sharp image has faded by the third day. These are diseases in which toxemia and moderate, less well-defined pain are significant parts of the disease. Included are pyelonephritis, hepatic abscess or distension due to other causes including fascioliasis, pneumonia and pleurisy and less obviously, primary ketosis and fat cow syndrome.

Acute local peritonitis due to penetration of the uterine wall by a catheter or of the rectal wall by a foreign body thrust sadistically into the rectum may be difficult to differentiate unless the painful area of the peritoneum can be determined. Acute local peritonitis can be differentiated from indigestion, acute ruminal impaction and acetonemia by the presence of fever, local abdominal pain and the abrupt fall in milk yield and appetite. Pyelonephritis can be distinguished by the presence of pus and blood in the urine and abomasal displacement by the presence of abomasal sounds in the left flank. Hepatic lesions may be distinguishable by the elicitation of pain over the posterior ribs on the right side and are not necessarily accompanied by ruminal stasis. Acute ruminal impaction is a much more serious disease and is usually accompanied by a marked increase in heart rate, staggering, recumbency, blindness and hypothermia. Acute diffuse peritonitis may present a similar clinical picture but there is no history of engorgement and no sign of hemoconcentration.

Traumatic reticuloperitonitis usually causes a secondary acetonemia when it occurs during early lactation and the presence of ketonuria should not be used as the sole basis for differentiation of the diseases. Differentiation may be extremely difficult if the peritonitis is of 3–4 days' duration and leukocyte counts and blood sugar estimations may be necessary in many cases. Response to treatment may also serve as a guide. The history is often helpful; the appetite and milk yield fall abruptly in traumatic reticuloperitonitis, but slowly over a period

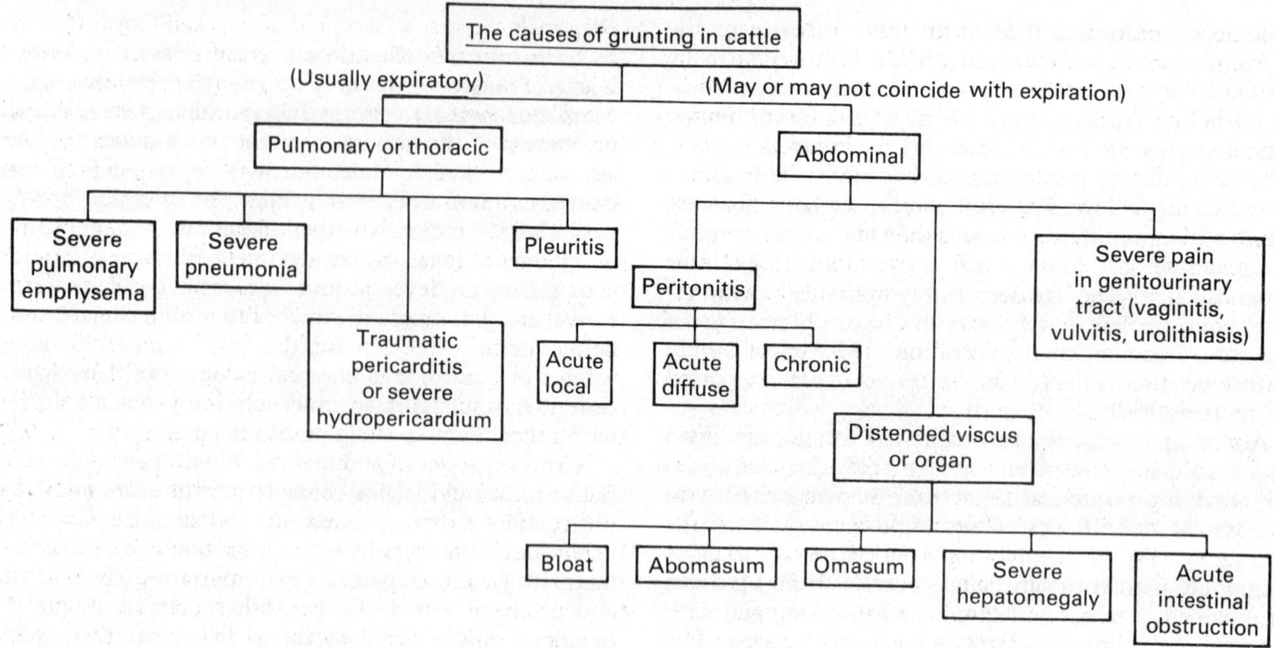

Fig. 18. The causes of grunting in cattle

of several days, and not to the same degree in acetonemia.

Continued high fever, high pulse rate and toxemia suggest involvement of the pericardial sac, liver or spleen as traumatic pericarditis or traumatic splenitis and hepatitis. All are marked by high total leukocyte and neutrophil counts. Typical sounds are heard on auscultation of the heart in the former and signs of congestive heart failure are present. Pain responses can be elicited by deep palpation over the respective organs when hepatic or splenic involvement occur.

Traumatic reticuloperitonitis is clinically indistinguishable from ephemeral fever although there is a more marked tendency to recumbency in the latter. Peritonitis due to perforation of an abomasal ulcer is characterized by evidence of pain on palpation over a much larger area of the abdominal wall and in the early stages this is most marked on the right-hand side. If, as is usual, the peritonitis becomes diffuse the syndrome cannot be distinguished clinically from that caused by traumatic reticuloperitonitis. Extension from a metritis to involve the peritoneum is suggested by other signs of the primary disease.

Treatment

Two methods of treatment are in general use, conservative treatment with or without the use of a magnet, and rumenotomy. Both have advantages and each case must be considered when deciding on the form of treatment to be used.

Conservative treatment

Conservative treatment comprises immobilization of the animal, administration of antibacterial drugs to control the infection and possibly the oral administration of a magnet to immobilize the foreign body. The cow is tied or stanchioned and not moved for 10–14 days. Milking, feeding and watering are carried out on the spot. The immobilization facilitates the formation of adhesions and this, and removal of the foreign body, may be further aided by standing the animal on an inclined plane (14) made of a door or planks or by packing earth under the front feet of the cow. The front feet should be elevated about 25 cm above the floor. Feed, particularly the roughage, should be reduced to about half. The response is often so good that the farmer is tempted to turn the cow loose before the allotted time and relapses frequently occur.

Sulfamethazine at the rate of 150 mg/kg body weight daily for 3–5 days provides good results in uncomplicated cases and is recommended as a first preference. The first dose should be given intravenously followed by oral daily doses for 3–4 days. Oral sulfonamides depress the activity of rumen bacteria (15) but give a high concentration of drug in the vicinity of the lesion. The general effect appears to be good and a high rate of recovery is recorded with this treatment combined with immobilization (3) provided treatment is begun in the early stages of the disease. Cows past their 6th month of pregnancy are likely to show incomplete recovery or relapse. Penicillin or broad-spectrum antimicrobials given parenterally daily for 3–5 days are also widely used with empirical success. Because of the high probability that mixed gastrointestinal flora will be present in the lesion it seems more rational to use a broad-spectrum antimicrobial rather than penicillin which is commonly used now because of cost and a short withdrawal period in the event that the animal does not respond favorably in a few days. However, there are no published clinical trials to indicate the preferential value of any particular antimicrobial. The objective of the treatment is to control the peritoneal contamination by the mixed bacterial flora from the reticulum, so a strong recommendation has been made for the intraperitoneal administration of broad-spectrum antibiotics (3). This technique is not much favored because of the risks of causing intestinal obstruction by fibrous adhesions resulting from the injections.

Small cylindrical or bar magnets, 7·5 cm long by 1–2·5 cm diameter with rounded ends, have been developed as a prophylactic measure against traumatic reticuloperitonitis (18) but they have also come into fairly general use as an aid to treatment. It is unlikely that they will extract a firmly embedded foreign body from the wall of the reticulum but loosely embedded ones with long free ends may be returned to the reticulum and loose foreign bodies will be immobilized. Used prophylactically they reduce the incidence of the disease a great deal provided they lodge in the reticulum. However, many pass straight through into the rumen unless the amount of roughage fed is reduced for 24 hours beforehand (19). The majority of these do relocate in the reticulum within the subsequent 48 hours (15). Premedication with atropine at a dose of 0·1 mg/kg body weight subcutaneously will ensure that the magnet moves into the reticulum soon after its administration (31). There have been only a few reports of physical harm to the wall of the reticulum being caused by the magnets and the incidence of traumatic reticuloperitonitis is very greatly reduced (20, 21). To completely avoid any chance of damage to the reticular wall by the magnet and its attached foreign body, the magnets are now available in plastic cages. A compass can be used to check that the magnet is correctly sited in the reticulum (23). A magnetic probe for placement in the reticulum by a wire passing through the nasal cavity and esophagus is available (32). In the reticulum the instrument attracts foreign bodies and is then retracted with the foreign bodies attached. The extensive prophylactic use of these magnets has been shown to reduce the prevalence of traumatic indigestion by 90–98% (22). It is common practice to administer the magnet to herd replacement heifers at 18 months to 2 years of age as part of a herd health program.

Rumenotomy

Surgical removal of the foreign body through a rumenotomy incision is widely used as a primary treatment. It has the advantage of being both a satisfactory treatment and diagnostic procedure. The recovery rate varies, depending largely upon the time at which surgery is undertaken, but is approximately the same as that obtained with the conservative treatment described above. In both instances 80–90% of animals recover compared with about 60% in untreated animals (2, 3, 24–26). Failure to improve is usually due to involvement of other organs or to the development of diffuse peritonitis or to persistent penetration by the foreign body, necessitating removal via a rumenotomy.

The recovery rate after surgery is likely to be much lower if only complicated cases are operated on and conservative treatment is given to the early mild cases. In one series (27) the recovery rate in the cases treated conservatively was 84% and in those difficult cases treated surgically it was 47%.

The choice of treatment is largely governed by economics and the facilities and time available for surgery. A rumenotomy, satisfactorily performed, is the best treatment but is unnecessary in many cases because of the tendency of the foreign body to fall back into the reticulum. The best general policy is to treat the animal conservatively for 3 days and if marked improvement has not occurred by that time to perform a rumenotomy. Cows in the last 3 months of pregnancy probably need a rumenotomy if serious sequels are to be avoided. Movement of the cow during the early stages of the disease is most undesirable because of the risk of breaking down the adhesions which localize the infection.

As a preventive measure all chopped feed should be passed over magnets to remove metallic material before being fed to cattle. The practice of tying bales of hay with string instead of wire has led to a major decrease in the incidence of the disease.

Cases of chronic traumatic reticuloperitonitis are best treated by rumenotomy because of the probability that the foreign body is still embedded in the wall. Acute diffuse peritonitis is highly fatal but if detected early vigorous treatment with broad-spectrum antibiotics results in recovery in a good proportion of cases. The best route of administation is in normal saline by intraperitoneal injection. About 2–3 g of oxytetracycline or tetracycline in 4 liters of saline or electrolyte solution provide needed fluids and good distribution of the antibiotic through the cavity. The treatment is repeated daily for 3 days.

REFERENCES

(1) Pinsent, P. J. N. (1962) *Vet. Rec.*, *74*, 1282.
(2) Editorial (1954) *J. Am. vet. med. Assoc.*, *125*, 331.
(3) Kingrey, B. W. (1955) *J. Am. vet. med. Assoc.*, *127*, 477.
(4) Maddy, K. T. (1954) *J. Am. vet. med. Assoc.*, *124*, 113.
(5) Maddy, K. T. (1954) *J. Am. vet. med. Assoc.*, *124*, 124.
(6) Dunn, H. O. et al. (1965) *Cornell Vet.*, *55*, 204.
(7) Stober, M. (1976) *Vet. med. Rev.*, *276*, 166.
(8) Blood, D. C. & Hutchins, D. R. (1955) *Aust. vet. J.*, *31*, 113.
(9) Leunenberger, W. et al. (1978) *Schweiz. Arch. Tierheilkd.*, *120*, 213 & 281.
(10) Stober, M. et al. (1978) *Tierärztl. Umschau*, *33*, 315.
(11) Williams, E. I. (1955) *Vet. Rec.*, *67*, 907, 922; *68*, 835.
(12) Roztocil, V. et al. (1968) *Vet. Rec.*, *83*, 667.
(13) Hague, M. A. et al. (1976) *Acta vet. Brno*, *45*, 141.
(14) Jensen, H. E. (1945) *N. Am. Vet.*, *26*, 213.
(15) Oyaert, W. et al. (1951) *Onderstepoort J. vet. Sci.*, *25*, 59.
(16) Haaranen, S. (1977) *Nord. VetMed.*, *29*, 482.
(17) Lethuraman, V. & Rathor, S. S. (1979) *Ind. J. vet. Sci.*, *49*, 703.
(18) Carroll, R. E. (1956) *J. Am. vet. med. Assoc.*, *129*, 376.
(19) Lundvall, R. L. (1957) *J. Am. vet. med. Assoc.*, *131*, 471.
(20) Said, A. H. (1963) *Vet. Rec.*, *75*, 966.
(21) Fuhrimann, H. (1966) *Schweiz. Arch. Tierheilkd.*, *108*, 190.
(22) Anderson, G. & Gillund, P. (1980) *Norsk. Veterinaertidsschr.*, *92*, 93.
(23) Poulsen, J. S. D. (1976) *Vet. Rec.*, *98*, 149.
(24) Blaser, E. (1980) *Schweiz. Arch. Tierheilkd.*, *122*, 169.
(25) Fraser, C. M. (1961) *Can. vet. J.*, *2*, 65.
(26) Albright, J. L. et al. (1962) *J. dairy Sci.*, *45*, 547.
(27) Fabian, M. & Palfi, J. (1971) *Magy. Allatorv. Lap.*, *26*, 104.
(28) Dubensky, R. A. & White, M. E. (1983) *Can. J. comp. Med.*, *47*, 241.
(29) Wilson, A. D. & Ferguson, J. G. (1984) *Can. vet. J.*, *25*, 229.
(30) Ducharme, N. G. et al. (1983) *J. Am. vet. med. Assoc.*, *182*, 585.
(31) Schneider, E. (1982) *Schweiz. Arch. Tierheilkd.*, *124*, 97.
(32) Hekmati, P. et al. (1985) *Nord. VetMed.*, *37*, 338.
(33) Wilson, A. D. et al. (1985) *Can. vet. J.*, *26*, 74.
(34) Hirsch, V. M. & Townsend, H. G. G. (1982) *Can. vet. J.*, *23*, 348.

Vagus indigestion

Lesions which involve the vagus nerve supply to the forestomachs and abomasum cause varying degrees of paralysis of the stomachs resulting in syndromes characterized by delayed passage of ingesta, distension, anorexia and the passage of soft pasty feces in small quantities. It is a common disease in cattle and has been recorded in sheep.

Etiology

In cattle, traumatic reticuloperitonitis is the commonest cause, the inflammatory and scar tissue lesions affecting the ventral branch of the vagus nerve as it ramifies over the anterior wall of the reticulum (1). Some cases have adhesions, for example between the rumen and abomasum, which do not appear to involve the vagus nerve (2). Induration of the medial reticular wall where vagal stretch receptors are located is sufficient to interfere with normal esophageal groove reflexes (3). In most cases the lesions are situated on the right hand wall of the reticulum (4). Actinobacillosis of the rumen and reticulum is a less common cause (5). In sheep peritonitis caused by *Sarcosporidia* and *Cysticercus tenuicollis* has been found to be an apparent cause (6). Abomasal impaction in sheep has been recorded (18). The etiology and pathogenesis were not determined. Disturbances similar to those which occur under natural conditions have been produced by sectioning the vagus nerve (17). The possibility that naturally occurring lesions may exert their effects by physical impairment of stomach movement and interference with the functioning of the esophageal groove rather than by actual involvement of the vagus nerve has also been suggested (7) but not received with enthusiasm (4). Some cases have been associated with liver abscesses (15).

Involvement of the vagus nerve in the thorax may occur as a result of enlargement of lymph nodes affected by tuberculosis or lymphomatosis. Similar disturbances may occur as a result of diaphragmatic hernia.

Pathogenesis

A number of syndromes develop depending upon the branches of the nerve which are involved and possibly upon the degree of immobilization caused by adhesion of the reticulum to the diaphragm. The major abnormality appears to be in the development of achalasia of the reticulo-omasal and the pyloric sphincters, although paralysis of the forestomach and abomasal walls also plays a part.

When there is achalasia of the reticulo-omasal sphincter, ingesta accumulates in the rumen. If the ruminal wall is atonic the ingesta accumulates without bloat occurring; if it has normal motility the ruminal wall responds to the distension by increased motility and the production of frothy bloat. When there is achalasia of the pylorus there is blockage of ingesta at this point and a syndrome of pyloric obstruction develops, often accompanied by pyloric ulceration. Associated with pyloric achalasia there is in some cases an apparent failure of the esophageal groove to permit the passage of ingesta into the rumen, this organ containing only fluid. It is possible that the different syndromes represent stages in the development of the one disease but for satisfactory definition they are dealt with separately here. It is often difficult to reconcile the apparent defects in motility of the stomachs, as evidenced by clinical and necropsy findings with the effects of experimental vagotomy (8, 10). The probable sequence of events is that hypermotility is the initial reaction and that atony occurs in the later stages. The syndrome observed depends on the stage of the disease at which the veterinarian is called to examine the cow.

Depending on the location and severity of the functional obstruction, distension or impaction there will be varying degrees of dehydration and a tendency towards a hypochloremic, hypokalemic alkalosis. In pyloric achalasia there is sequestration of abomasal juice in the abomasum and a reflux of abomasal contents into the forestomachs resulting in metabolic alkalosis, dehydration and an increase in the chloride concentration in the reticulorumen (11). In reticulomasal achalasia, also refferred to as *'failure of omasal transport'*, the abomasal juice can pass onto the duodenum and neither metabolic alkalosis or dehydration can be expected (11). In a series of 43 cases of vagus indigestion in cattle, only nine had pathological evidence of vagal nerve injury while in 30 there were adhesions or abscesses involving the medial wall of the reticulum (4). It is possible that chronic inflammation of this area may affect the reticular tension receptors which are responsible for sensory stimulation of the gastric centers via the vagal nerves (3). This could account for the ruminal dysfunction in cases not accompanied by significant injury to the vagal nerves.

Pyloric achalasia can also occur as part of a secondary indigestion due to septicemia and toxemia (16). There is also ruminal distension with fluid material, abomasal reflux into the reticulorumen, dehydration, hypochloremia, hypokalemic metabolic alkalosis and uremia.

Clinical findings

A number of syndromes have been described (4, 12) but the following arbitrary division into three is considered to be sufficiently descriptive.

The general clinical picture characteristic of all three includes:

- Inappetence for several days
- Scant feces
- An enlarging *'papple'*-shaped abdomen (pear-shaped on the right and apple-shaped on the left) with or without bloat
- Enlarged impacted abomasum palpable through right flank or on rectal examination
- Enlarged rumen palpable on rectal examination
- Vital signs and responses to stimuli within the normal range
- No response to treatment.

Ruminal distension with hypermotility

The occurrence of this type is not particularly related to pregnancy or parturition. The first obvious sign is moderate to severe ruminal tympany although the animal is usually thin and has not been eating well for some time. The abdomen is distended but the rumen is moving forcefully and almost continuously with the sounds much reduced in volume. The rumen contents are usually well macerated and frothy, which accounts for the relative absence of normal rumen sounds in spite of the hyperactivity of the rumen. The feces are normal or pasty but scanty. There is no fever and the heart rate is usually slower than normal and the sounds are often accompanied by a systolic murmur which waxes and wanes with respiration, being loudest at the peak of inspiration. The murmur disappears when the tympany is relieved. Ruminal distension is apparent on rectal examination. The dorsal sac of the rumen is grossly distended and is pushed back against the brim of the pelvis and the ventral sac is also enlarged and occupies much of the right lower quadrant of the abdomen. Viewed from the rear the enlarged rumen is L-shaped giving an external silhouette with the left flank distended from top to bottom, and the right flank distended only in the lower half—the 'papple'-shaped abdomen. Standard treatments for ruminal tympany and impaction have no effect on the course of the disease.

Ruminal distension with atony

This type occurs most commonly in late pregnancy and may persist after calving. The cow is clinically normal in all respects of soft pasty feces, has a distended abdomen and will not respond to treatment with purgatives, lubricants or parasympathetic stimulants. Ruminal movements are seriously reduced or absent and there may be persistent mild bloat. There is no fever or increase in heart rate and no pain on percussion of the abdomen. On rectal examination the only abnormality is gross distension of the rumen which may almost block the pelvic inlet. The animal loses weight rapidly, becomes very weak and eventually recumbent. At this stage the heart rate increases markedly. The animal dies slowly of inanition.

Pyloric obstruction and abomasal impaction

Most cases of this type also occur late in pregnancy and are manifested by anorexia and a reduced volume of pasty feces. There may be no abdominal distension and no systemic reaction until the late stages when the pulse rate rises rapidly. The distended abomasum may be palpable on the abdominal floor on rectal examination but this is impossible if the cow is pregnant. The abomasum is firm and not distended with gas or fluid. Rumen movements are usually completely absent. As in the first type death occurs slowly due to inanition, although the impacted abomasum may rupture and cause death in a few hours.

Combinations of these types may occur; in particular, distension of the rumen with atony combined with abomasal obstruction is the most commonly observed syndrome (13).

Clinical pathology

In most cases there are no abnormalities on hematological examination although a moderate neutrophilia, a shift to the left and a relative monocytosis may suggest the presence of chronic traumatic reticuloperitonitis. With abomasal distension and/or impaction there are varying degrees of hypochloremic, hypokalemic alkalosis. Hemoconcentration is also common in those cases in which there is fluid accumulation in the rumen. There may be high levels of chloride in the ruminal fluid because of reflux of abomasal contents (11).

Necropsy findings

Cases of the disease in which there is ruminal hypermotility do not usually come to necropsy. In both of the other types there is impaction of the abomasum. The pyloric region contains a solid mass of sand or impacted, fine, partly digested fiber. The remainder of the organ is filled with coarse undigested material similar to that usually found in the rumen. Ulcers of the pyloric mucosa are a common accompaniment. When there is ruminal distension the contents are usually in an advanced state of digestion and may have undergone some putrefaction. Cases in which ruminal distension was absent before death have a contracted rumen containing thin clear fluid and a few particles of feed. In both types the intestines are relatively empty and the feces have a thick, pasty consistency and are dark green in color (14).

Lesions are usually present on the anterior wall of the reticulum which suggests that traumatic reticuloperitonitis occurred some time previously. The lesions comprise extensive adhesions, fibrous fistulae, sometimes containing a foreign body, or abscesses. The situation of these lesions is often such that physical involvement of the vagus nerve does not appear likely.

Diagnosis

The salient clinical features of vagus indigestion in cattle are inappetence for several days leading to anorexia, a gradually enlarging abdomen especially on the left side, scant feces, failure to respond to common medical therapy, loss of body condition, and varying degrees of dehydration. Obtaining an accurate history is of paramount importance. Most cases of vagus indigestion have been affected for at least several days or a few weeks. The diagnosis can be perplexing in those cases which occur in late pregnancy because the animal has usually been housed and fed with other dry cows, and daily observation of feed intake and fecal output have not been made, so it is difficult to obtain an accurate and helpful history. The clinical examination should focus on the state of the rumen and the abomasum. In valuable animals a left-side exploratory laparotomy and rumenotomy will often be necessary in order to make a diagnosis. This will allow the determination of the presence of reticular adhesions, obstructions of the reticulo-omasal orifice and the state of the abomasum.

There are no other diseases of cattle which resemble ruminal distention with hyperactivity of the rumen.

Ruminal distention with atony may resemble several diseases of the forestomachs and abomasum which include chronic traumatic reticuloperitonitis, abomasal impaction due to ingestion of straw or sand, omasal impaction phytobezoars blocking the abomasal pylorus and abomasal ulceration without melena. Obstruction of the reticulo-omasal orifice by baling twine, plastic sleeves and bags may cause distension of the rumen indistinguishable from vagus indigestion.

Treatment

The prognosis in most cases in unfavorable but also unpredictable. The problem is to determine the location and extent of the lesion which may be difficult or impossible even on exploratory laparotomy or rumenotomy. If the rumen is grossly distended with fluid or mushy rumen contents, it may be emptied using a large-bore (25 mm inside diameter) stomach tube and gravity flow. The contents are usually well macerated and foul-smelling. Emptying the rumen in this way not only relieves the pressure but allows for easier examination of the abdomen. Some cases respond beneficially following fluid and balanced electrolyte therapy for 3 days combined with the oral administration of mineral oil (5–10 liters) daily for 3 days or dioctyl sodium sulfosuccinate as described under the treatment of abomasal impaction of dietary origin. Others do not respond but there is no reliable method of knowing which ones will respond other than by treatment for a few days. Valuable pregnant cows near parturition may be maintained on fluid and electrolyte therapy for several days or until near enough to term to induce parturition with dexamethazone (20 mg intramuscularly) and hopefully obtain a live calf. Some cows will recover following parturition but the condition may recur in the next pregnancy.

Rumenotomy and emptying of the rumen is usually followed by slow recovery over a period of 7–10 days when there is ruminal hypermotility. The creation of a permanent ruminal fistula to permit the escape of gas in cases where gas retention is a problem may cause dramatic improvement (9). In our hands they have been unsuccessful because a fistula plug cannot be kept in place, and leaving the fistula open results in the loss of much ruminal content to the exterior. Surgical interference, including abomasotomy, in the other types is usually unsatisfactory because the motility of the abomasum does not return (4, 13). The most satisfactory procedure is to slaughter affected animals for meat.

REFERENCES

(1) Hoflund, S. (1940) *Svensk. vet. Tidskr.*, Supp. zum. 45 Band.
(2) Jones, R. S. & Pirie, H. M. (1962) *Vet. Rec.*, *74*, 582.
(3) Leek, B. F. (1968) *Vet. Rec.*, *82*, 498.
(4) Neal, P. A. & Edwards. G. B. (1968) *Vet. Rec.*, *82*, 396.
(5) Begg, H. (1950) *Vet. Rec.*, *62*, 797.
(6) Naerland, D. G. & Helle, O. (1962) *Vet. Rec.*, *74*, 85.
(7) Hutchins, D. R. et al. (1957) *Aust. vet. J.*, *33*, 77.
(8) Habel, R. E. (1956) *Cornell Vet.*, *46*, 555.
(9) Rebhun, W. C. (1980) *J. Am. vet. med. Assoc.*, *176*, 506.
(10) Stevens, C. E. & Sellers, A. F. (1956) *Am. J. vet. Res.*, *17*, 588.
(11) Kuiper, R. & Breukink, J. J. (1986) *Vet. Rec.*, *119*, 169
(12) Kubin, G. (1955) *Wien. Tierärztl. Monatsschr.*, *42*, 170.
(13) Pope, D. C. (1961) *Vet. Rec.*, *73*, 1174.
(14) Clark, C. H. (1953) *Vet. Med.*, *48*, 389.
(15) Fubini, S. L. et al. (1985) *J. Am. vet. med. Assoc.*, *186*, 1297.
(16) Kuiper, R. & Breukink, H. J. (1986) *Vet. Rec.*, *119*, 404.
(17) Gregory, P. C. (1982) *J. Physiol.*, *328*, 431.
(18) Kline, E. E. et al. (1983) *Vet. Rec.*, *113*, 177.

Diaphragmatic hernia

Herniation of a portion of the reticulum through a diaphragmatic rupture causes chronic ruminal tympany, anorexia and displacement of the heart.

Etiology

Most cases occur because of weakening of the diaphragm by lesions of traumatic reticuloperitonitis (3), but diaphragmatic rupture can occur independently of a foreign body (5) and congenital defects of the diaphragm may be a cause in some animals (6). An unusually high incidence of herniation of the reticulum through the diaphragm, sometimes accompanied by the abomasum, has been recorded in buffalo in India (2).

Pathogenesis

The usual syndrome produced is identical with that caused by vagus indigestion in which ruminal hypermotility is present. It seems probable that there is either achalasia of the reticulo-omasal sphincter due to involvement of the vagus nerve or impairment of function of the esophageal groove caused by the fixation of the reticulum to the ventral diaphragm. The disturbance of function in the forestomachs suggests that food can get ito the rumen but cannot pass from there to the abomasum. The hypermotility is thought to be due to overdistension of the rumen and be the cause of the frothy bloat.

There is usually no interference with respiration without major herniation but displacement and compression of the heart occur commonly.

Clinical findings

There is a capricious appetite and loss of condition for several weeks before abdominal distension due to accumulation of fluid and froth in the rumen, and persistent moderate tympany of the rumen occur. Grinding of the teeth may be conspicuous and the feces are usually pasty and reduced in volume. Rumination does not occur but occasional animals vomit especially when a stomach tube is passed.

There is no fever and the pulse rate is usually slower than normal (40–60/minute). Respiration is unaffected in most cases. A systolic murmur is usually audible on auscultation, and the intensity of the heart sounds may suggest displacement of the heart, usually anteriorly or to the left. Reticular sounds are audible just posterior to the cardiac area in many normal cows and they are not significantly increased in diaphragmatic hernia.

A more severe syndrome is recorded in cases where viscera other than a portion of the reticulum is herniated. Peristaltic sounds may be audible in the thorax and there may be interference with respiration and signs of pain with each reticular contraction (5). Affected animals usually die from inanition in 3–4 weeks after the onset of bloat.

Clinical pathology

Laboratory examinations are of no value in diagnosis. Radiological examination after a barium meal has facilitated diagnosis (1).

Necropsy findings

The majority of cases are sequels to traumatic reticuloperitonitis and a fistulous tract is often found in the vicinity of the diaphragmatic rupture which is usually 15–20 cm in diameter. A portion of the reticulum protrudes into the right pleural cavity to form a spherical distension usually 20–30 cm in diameter, but more extensive in some cases. The reticulum is very tightly adherent to the hernial ring which is thickened by fibrous tissue. The omasum and abomasum are relatively empty but the rumen is overfilled with frothy, porridge-like material which contains very little fiber. Less common cases are those in which part of the reticulum, the omasum and part of the abomasum are herniated.

Diagnosis

Other causes of chronic bloat must be considered in the

differential diagnosis, especially vagus indigestion with hypermotility which is also often accompanied by a systolic murmur. The two can only be differentiated by rumenotomy but there is the hazard that cases of diaphragmatic hernia are not relieved by the operation and tympany returns rapidly, sometimes necessitating a permanent ruminal fistula.

Passage of a stomach tube is usually necessary to determine whether or not a physical obstruction is present in the esophagus. Regurgitation is likely to occur in cases of diaphragmatic hernia and this occasionally causes blockage of the esophagus with ingesta, simulating choke.

Causes of diaphragmatic hernia other than traumatic reticuloperitonitis include violent trauma to the abdomen and straining at parturition. In both instances there is probably a primary weakness of the diaphragm. In buffalo this is thought to be an anatomical characteristic of the species, the weakness being located in the right half of the diaphragm (4).

Treatment

Most recorded attempts at surgical repair in cattle have been unsuccessful (6) and treatment has not usually been recommended. The animals could not be left as they were, so salvage by slaughter has been the usual outcome. There is a report of a high recovery rate after surgery in buffalo (7).

The ruminal contents are frothy, and trocarization or passing a stomach tube has virtually no effect in reducing the tympany, nor have standard antifrothing agents. The tympany is usually not sufficiently severe to require emergency rumenotomy. The signs may be partly relieved by keeping the animal confined with the forequarters elevated.

REFERENCES

(1) Divers, J. J. & Smith, B. P. (1979) *J. Am. vet. med. Assoc.*, *175*, 1099.
(2) Prasad, B. et al. (1979) *Can. vet. J.*, *20*, 26.
(3) Hutchins, D. R. et al. (1959) *Aust. vet. J.*, *33*, 77.
(4) Singh, J. et al. (1980) *Jap. J. vet. Sci.*, *42*, 89.
(5) Robison, R. W. (1956) *N. Am. Vet.*, *37*, 375.
(6) Done, S. H. & Drew, R. A. (1972) *Br. vet. J.*, *128*, 553.
(7) Singh, J. et al. (1977) *Aust. vet. J.*, *53*, 473.

Traumatic pericarditis

Perforation of the pericardial sac by a sharp foreign body originating in the reticulum causes pericarditis with the development of toxemia and congestive heart failure. Tachycardia, fever, engorgement of the jugular veins, anasarca, hydrothorax and ascites, and abnormalities of the heart sounds are the diagnostic features of the disease.

Etiology

The etiology has already been described. There is a greater tendency for perforation of the pericardial sac to occur during the last 3 months of pregnancy and at parturition than at other times. Approximately 8% of all cases of traumatic reticuloperitonitis will develop pericarditis (1). Most affected animals die or suffer from chronic pericarditis and do not return to completely normal health. The disease has been produced experimentally in cattle (2) and buffalo (8) by penetration from the reticulum.

Pathogenesis

The penetration of the pericardial sac may occur with the initial perforation of the reticular wall. On the other hand the animal may have a history of traumatic reticuloperitonitis some time previously, followed by a subsequent attack of pericarditis, usually during late pregnancy or at parturition. In this case it is probable that the foreign body remains in a sinus in the reticular wall after the initial perforation and penetrates the pericardial sac at a later date. Physical penetration of the sac is not essential to the development of pericarditis, infection sometimes penetrating through the pericardium from a traumatic mediastinitis. The introduction of a mixed bacterial infection from the reticulum causes a severe local inflammation, and persistence of the foreign body in the tissues is not essential for the further progress of the disease. The first effect of the inflammation is hyperemia of the pericardial surfaces and the production of friction sounds synchronous with the heart beats. Two mechanisms then operate to produce signs: the toxemia due to the infection and the pressure on the heart of the fluid which accumulates in the sac and produces congestive heart failure. In individual cases one or other of these two factors may be more important. Profound depression is characteristic of the first and edema of the second. Thus an affected animal may be severely ill for several weeks with edema developing only gradually, or extreme edema may develop within 2–3 days. The rapid development of edema usually indicates early death.

If chronic pericarditis persists there is restriction of the heart action due to adhesion of the pericardium to the heart. Chronic congestive heart failure results in most cases but some animals show a relatively good recovery. An uncommon sequel after perforation of the pericardial sac by a foreign body is rupture of a coronary artery or the ventricular wall. Death usually occurs suddenly due to acute, congestive heart failure from compression of the heart by the hemopericardium, and often without premonitory illness (3).

Clinical findings

Profound depression, complete anorexia, habitual recumbency and rapid weight loss are common. Diarrhea or scant feces may be present and grinding of the teeth, salivation and nasal discharge are occasionally observed. The cow stands with the back arched and the elbows abducted. Respiratory movements are more obvious, being mainly abdominal, shallow, increased in rate to 40–50/minute and often accompanied by grunting. Engorgement of the jugular vein, and edema of the brisket and ventral abdominal wall occur and in severe cases there may even be edema of the conjuctiva with grape-like masses of edematous conjunctiva hanging over the eyelids. A prominent jugular pulse is usually visible and extends well up into the neck. Pyrexia (40–41°C, 104–106°F) is always present in the early stages and an increase in the pulse rate to the vicinity of 100/minute and a diminution in the pulse amplitude are constant. Rumen movements are usually present but depressed.

Pinching of the back and abdominal palpation produce a marked pain response. An even more pronounced grunt and an increased area of cardiac dullness can be detected by percussion over the precordial area, preferably with a pleximeter and hammer.

Auscultation of the chest reveals the diagnostic signs. In the early stages before effusion commences the heart sounds are normal but are accompanied by a pericardial friction rub which may wax and wane with respiratory movements. Care must be taken to differentiate this from a pleural friction rub due to inflammation of the mediastinum. In this case the rub is much louder and the heart rate will not be so high. Several days later when there is marked effusion the heart sounds are muffled and there may be gurgling, splashing or tinkling sounds. The cardiac impulse is increased in amplitude and is palpable over a larger area than usual. In all cases of suspected pericarditis careful auscultation of the entire precordium on both sides of the chest is essential as abnormal sounds may be audible only over restricted areas. This is especially so in chronic cases.

Most affected animals die within a period of 1–2 weeks although a small proportion persist with chronic pericarditis. The obvious clinical signs in the terminal stages are gross edema, dyspnea, severe watery diarrhea, depression, recumbency and complete anorexia. Death is usually due to asphyxia and toxemia.

Animals which have recovered from an initial pericarditis are usually affected by the chronic form of the disease. The animal is in poor condition and has a variable appetite although there is no systemic reaction and the demeanor is bright. Edema of the brisket is usually not present but there is jugular engorgement. Auscultation reveals variable findings. The heart sounds are muffled and fluid splashing sounds may be heard over small discrete areas corresponding to the loculi of fluid in the sac, or there may be irregularity of the heart beat. The pulse rate is rapid (90–100/minute) and the pulse is small in amplitude. These animals never do well and are unlikely to withstand the strain of another pregnancy or lactation.

Clinical pathology

A pronounced leukocytosis with a total count of 16 000–30 000/μl accompanied by a neutrophilia and eosinopenia is usual although less dramatic changes are recorded in one series of cases (4). When gross effusion is present the pericardial fluid may be sampled by paracentesis with a 10 cm 18 gauge needle over the site of maximum audibility of the heart sound, usually in the fourth or fifth intercostal space on the left side. In mid-stage pericarditis the fluid is usually easily obtained, and is foul-smelling and turbid. In chronic pericarditis only small amounts may be present and a sample may not be obtainable.

Necropsy findings

In acute cases there is gross distension of the pericardial sac with foul-smelling, grayish fluid containing flakes of fibrin, and the serous surface of the sac carries very heavy deposits of newly formed fibrin. A cord-like, fibrous sinus tract usually connects the reticulum with the pericardium. Additional lesions of pleurisy and pneumonia are commonly present. In chronic cases the pericardial sac is grossly thickened and fused to the pericardium by strong fibrous adhesions surrounding loculi of varying size which contain pus or thin straw-colored fluid.

Diagnosis

Endocarditis, lymphomatosis with cardiac involvement and congenital cardiac defects are all likely to be confused with traumatic pericarditis because of the similarity of the abnormal heart sounds. Endocarditis is usually associated with a suppurative process in another organ, particularly the uterus or udder, and although the abnormal heart sounds are typical bruits rather than pericardial friction sounds, this may be difficult to determine when extensive pericardial effusion has occurred (5). The diagnosis of lymphomatosis depends upon the detection of lymphomatous lesions in other organs or the presence of a marked leukocytosis and lymphocytosis. Congenital cardiac defects may not cause clinical abnormality until the first pregnancy but can be diagnosed by the presence of loud murmurs, a pronounced cardiac thrill and an absence of toxemia. Sporadic bovine encephalomyelitis is accompanied by a severe fibrinous pericarditis and a pericardial friction rub but usually no signs of heart failure.

Less common causes of abnormal heart sounds include thoracic tumors and abscesses, diaphragmatic hernia and chronic bloat which cause distortion of the atria and atrioventricular orifices. They are associated with other diagnostic signs, particularly displacement of the heart. In severely debilitated animals or those suffering from severe anemia a hemic murmur which fluctuates with respiration may be audible. Occasional cases of hematogenous pericarditis are encountered, and in some cases of pasteurellosis a fibrinous pericarditis may be present, but there is usually serious involvement of other organs and the pericarditis is only secondary.

Treatment

The results of treatment are usually unsatisfactory but salvage of up to 50% of cases can be achieved by longterm treatment with sulfonamides or antibiotics (1). The prognosis is much better in cases where toxemia is the major factor, rapidly developing edema presaging death in a short time. In these cases drainage of the pericardial sac may temporarily relieve the edema and respiratory embarrassment but relapse is usually complete in about 24 hours. Selected cases of traumatic pericarditis have been treated satisfactorily by pericardiotomy (7, 8).

REFERENCES

(1) Blood, D. C. & Hutchins, D. R. (1955) *Aust. vet. J.*, *31*, 229.
(2) Simeonov, S. P. (1978) *Vet. Nauki*, *15*, 114.
(3) Awadhiya, R. et al. (1974) *Vet. Rec.*, *95*, 260.
(4) Holme, J. R. (1960) *Vet. Rec.*, *72*, 355.
(5) Johns, F. V. (1974) *Vet. Rec.*, *59*, 214.
(6) Ramakrishna, O. et al. (1978) *Haryana Vet.*, *17*, 29.
(7) Mason, T. A. (1979) *Vet. Rec.*, *105*, 350.
(8) Krishnamurthy, D. et al. (1979) *J. Am. vet. med. Assoc.*, *175*, 714.

Traumatic splenitis and hepatitis

These conditions occur relatively uncommonly as sequels to traumatic reticuloperitonitis and are manifested either by continuation of the illness caused by the initial perforation or by apparent recovery followed by relapse several weeks later (1). The prominent clinical signs include fever (39·5–40·5°C, 103–105°F), an increase in heart rate and a gradual fall in food intake and milk yield but ruminal movements are present and may be normal. Percussion of the abdomen over the site, usually used to detect the pain of traumatic reticuloperitonitis, gives a negative response although deep, forceful palpation may elicit a mild grunt. The diagnostic sign is pain on palpation with the thumb in the last two intercostal spaces halfway down the abdomen, on the right side when there is hepatic involvement, and on the left side when the spleen is affected.

Hematological examination is important, the total leukocyte count being greatly increased (above 12 000/μl) and the differential count showing a marked neutrophilia and a shift to the left. Rumenotomy is not usually undertaken except for diagnostic purposes. Treatment with antibacterial drugs is effective if commenced sufficiently early. Oral treatment with sulfadimidine has been effective in some cases.

REFERENCE

(1) Blood, D. C. & Hutchins, D. R. (1955) *Aust. vet. J.*, *31*, 233.

Ruminal tympany (bloat)

Ruminal tympany is overdistension of the rumen and reticulum with the gases of fermentation, either in the form of a persistent foam mixed with the rumen contents or in the form of free gas separated from the ingesta. Primary ruminal tympany (frothy bloat) is dietary in origin and occurs in cattle on legume pasture and in feedlot cattle on high level grain diets. Secondary ruminal tympany (free gas bloat) is usually due to failure of eructation of free gas because of a physical interference with eructation.

Etiology

Primary ruminal tympany (frothy bloat)
The cause of primary ruminal tympany or frothy bloat is the production of a stable foam which traps the normal gases of fermentation in the rumen. The essential feature is that coalescence of the small gas bubbles is inhibited and intraruminal pressure increases because eructation cannot occur. Leguminous bloat is due to the foaming qualities of the soluble leaf proteins in legumes and other bloating forages.

The cause of feedlot or grain bloat is uncertain. Associative evidence suggests that the feeding of finely ground grain promotes frothiness of rumen contents (1). The feeding of large quantities of grain to cattle results in marked changes in the total numbers and proportions of certain ruminal protozoa and bacteria. Some species of encapsulated bacteria increase in numbers and produce a slime which may result in a stable foam but there is no firm evidence that this is the cause of feedlot bloat (2).

There is some evidence that some cases of feedlot bloat may be of the free-gas type based on the observations that gas may be released with a stomach tube. Feedlot cattle are susceptible to esophagitis, ruminal acidosis and rumenitis, overfill and ruminal atony. Each of these may interfere with eructation and cause secondary ruminal tympany and free-gas bloat which is discussed later.

Foaming or frothiness Foaming or frothiness of the ruminal contents is the vital factor in causing primary pasture bloat. This may be caused by any one of a number of factors and probably in many instances by a combination of them. The cause of the frothing is the formation of a stable persistent foam in the rumen. In pasture bloat, many factors in the fluid contents, including saponins, pectins and hemicelluloses have in the past been advanced as contributory causes. The soluble leaf cytoplasmic proteins were once considered to be the principal foaming agents but their role is now questionable (3). Recent observations indicate that bloat-causing legumes are more rapidly digested by rumen microorganisms than non-bloat-causing forages and that rupture of leaf mesophyll cells leads to the release of chloroplast particles. These particles are readily colonized by rumen microorganisms and gas bubbles are trapped among the particles which prevent coalescence of bubbles by preventing drainage of rumen fluid from the liquid lamellae between the bubbles. The condition of the rumen prior to feeding is an important factor in the immediate susceptibility of an animal to pasture bloat. A predisposed rumen is characterized by an excess of dispersed particulate matter with adherent microorganisms, which provides an active inoculum for the fermentation of incoming feedstuffs (4). The soluble leaf protein may contribute to the frothiness but is not the primary foaming agent. The chloroplast particles in the rumen have a slower rate of clearance in bloating animals than in non-bloating ones (29, 31, 32).

The cause of the foam in feedlot bloat is uncertain and not all cases of feedlot bloat are of the frothy type; some are free-gas bloat. In frothy feedlot bloat the viscosity of the ruminal fluid is markedly increased and may be due to the production of insoluble slime by certain species of bacteria which proliferate to large numbers in cattle on a high carbohydrate diet (2). The slime may entrap the gases of fermentation. The delay in occurrence of feedlot bloat suggests that a gradual change in the microbial population of the rumen may be an important factor in explaining the cause. The physical form of a grain ration appears to be related to grain bloat. As in frothy legume bloat, where too rapid release of leaf nutrients appears to be instrumental in producing bloat, it seems likely that the small particle size of ground feed could have the same effect (30). It is known that fine particulate matter can markedly increase foam stability (1). The feeding of ground grain of fine particle size (geometric mean particle size, 388 μm) was associated with more rumen froth than the use of a coarse particle size (715 μm). The pH of the rumen contents also plays an important part in the stability of the foam (maximum stability occurs at a pH of about 6) and the composition of the diet and the activity and composition of the rumen microflora are known to influence this factor.

The rate of flow and composition of the saliva has an effect on the tendency for tympany to occur. This effect may be exerted by means of the buffering effect of the saliva on the pH of the rumen contents or because of variation in its content of mucoproteins. The physical effects of dilution of ruminal ingesta by saliva may also be important; there is a negative correlation between the proportion of liquid present and the incidence of tympany, and feed of a low fiber and high water content depresses the volume of saliva secreted. Also susceptible cows secrete significantly less saliva than non-susceptible cows and there are differences in the composition of saliva which are genetically determined (7).

In summary, it is suggested that primary frothy pasture bloat occurs when there is rapid digestion of leaf material by rumen microorganisms leading to the release of chloroplast particles into the liquid phase of the rumen contents which prevents the coalescence of the gas bubbles. In primary frothy feedlot bloat, the fine particle size of the feed and the presence of rumen microorganisms which produce slime may be important factors.

Secondary ruminal tympany (free-gas bloat)

Physical obstruction to eructation occurs in esophageal obstruction caused by a foreign body, by stenosis or by pressure from enlargements outside the esophagus, such as tuberculous lymphadenitis or bovine viral leukosis involvement of bronchial lymph nodes, or by obstruction of the cardia from the interior. Interference with esophageal groove function in vagus indigestion and diaphragmatic hernia may cause chronic ruminal tympany and the condition also occurs in tetanus particularly in young animals and in poisoning with the fungus *Rhizoctonia leguminicola* due probably to spasm of esophageal musculature. Carcinoma, granulomatous lesions caused by *Actinomyces bovis* near the esophageal groove and in the reticular wall and papillomata of the esophageal groove and reticulum are less common causes of obstructive bloat.

There may also be interference with the nerve pathways responsible for maintenance of the eructation reflex. The receptor organs in this reflex are situated in the dorsal pouch of the reticulum and are capable of discriminating between gas, foam and liquid. The afferent and efferent nerve fibers are contained in the vagus nerve but the location of the central coordinating mechanism has not been defined. Depression of this center or lesions of the vagus nerve can interrupt the reflex which is essential for removal of gas from the rumen.

Normal tone and motility of the musculature of the rumen and reticulum are also necessary for eructation. In anaphylaxis, bloat occurs commonly because of muscle atony and is relieved by the administration of adrenaline or antihistamine drugs. A sudden marked change in pH of the rumen contents due to either acidity or alkalinity causes ruminal atony but the tympany which results is usually of a minor degree only, probably because the gas-producing activity of the microflora is greatly reduced.

While most cases of feedlot bloat associated with outbreaks are of the frothy type (primary) and cannot be easily relieved with a stomach tube, it is apparent that sporadic cases are of the free-gas type which suggests that they are secondary. Possible causes of the ruminal atony and failure of eructation include: esophagitis, acidosis, rumenitis and failure of rumination because of an all-grain diet. It is known that feedlot cattle on high-level grain diets for long periods will not ruminate normally and their rumen movements are significantly reduced.

Chronic ruminal tympany occurs relatively frequently in calves up to 6 months of age without apparent cause. Persistence of an enlarge thymus, chronic ruminal atony caused by a continued feeding on coarse indigestible roughage, and the passage of unpalatable milk replacer into the rumen, where it undergoes fermentation and gas production, instead of into the abomasum (21), have all been suggested as causes but the condition usually disappears spontaneously in time and the cause in most cases is undetermined. Necropsy examination of a number of fatal cases has failed to detect any physical abnormality although a developmental defect appears to be likely because of the age at which it occurs. One case of chronic tympany in a calf has been recorded as caused by a partial rotation of the rumen about its long axis (8). Unusual postures, particularly lateral recumbency, are commonly characterized by secondary tympany. Cattle may die from secondary tympany if they become accidentally cast in dorsal recumbency in handling facilities, crowded transportation vehicles, irrigation ditches and other restrictive positions.

In some cases of vagus indigestion characterized by ruminal hyperactivity the secondary bloat may be of the frothy type because of ruminal hyperactivity.

Epidemiology

Incidence, occurrence and economic importance

Primary ruminal tympany causes heavy losses through death, severe loss of production, and the strict limitations placed on the use of some high-producing pastures for grazing. The incidence of the disease has increased markedly with the improvement of pastures by heavy applications of fertilizers and the use of high-producing leguminous pasture plants, and losses in cattle at times have reached enormous proportions (9).

Pasture bloat Pasture bloat has a seasonal occurrence when the pasture is lushest. Dry hot conditions and matured plants, and thus midsummer, are the forerunners of a decline in prevalence. Spring and autumn are the most dangerous seasons when the pastures are lush, young and the leaves of the plants contain a high concentration of soluble proteins.

The most obvious form of loss is sudden death. And although this is the dramatic loss, especially when a large number of cattle are unexpectedly found dead, an equivalent loss occurs as the result of reduced food intake. For example, on clover dominant pasture (60–80% white clover) where bloat was common the weight gains of cattle grazing it were 20–30% less than normal (10). It has been argued that the returns achieved by good bloat prevention in pastured cattle would not compensate for the costs incurred (22), but the opposite view is strongly held. Sheep can also be affected but appear to be much less susceptible than cattle.

Feedlot bloat or grain bloat occurs in feedlot cattle during the 50–100 days when cattle are fed large quantities of grain and small quantities of roughage. In some cases the use of pelleted, finely ground feed has been associated with outbreaks of feedlot bloat. High-producing dairy cows which are fed 12–22 kg of grain daily may also develop grain bloat. In a survey of Kansas feedlots (60 lots totalling 450 000 head of cattle) the incidence of deaths due to bloat was 0·1%, 0·2% of cattle had severe bloat and 0·6% moderate bloat (2). In a Colorado feedlot, during one full year, bloat was the cause of 3% of all mortalities (11). In the same study, bloat was among the four most common causes of sudden death or of cattle found dead without having been seen ill (12). Outbreaks of feedlot bloat are usually of the frothy type (primary) while the sporadic cases are of the free-gas type and secondary to lesions which cause dysfunction of eructation.

Factors which influence the occurrence of primary ruminal tympany

Many factors are known to have an influence on the occurrence of primary bloat and possibly to contribute to its causation. The dietary and animal factors have received most attention.

Dietary factors Of dietary factors, grazing on very succulent pasture, immature rapidly growing legumes in the pre-bloom stage, is the biggest single cause of bloat in cattle. The disease also occurs occasionally when cattle are grazed on cereal crops, rape, cabbages, leguminous vegetable crops including peas and beans, and young grass pasture with a high protein content. An increasing occurrence of bloat is noted when cattle are grazed on young green cereal crops such as wheat, especially if it is heavily fertilized and irrigated (14). Of the commonly grown legumes, alfalfa and ladino clover are classified as highly dangerous, white and red clovers are in the intermediate position of moderately dangerous, and crimson and subterranean clovers as only mildly dangerous. Ingestion of the more succulent parts of plants and avoidance of the more mature portions can be a precipitating factor and tympany is less likely to occur if the crop is harvested and fed than if it is grazed. Restriction of the grazing area, by forcing the cattle to eat the entire plants, has a similar effect. A high incidence is recorded when pasture is wet but this is probably due to the rapid growth of the plants during heavy rainfall periods rather than to physical wetness of the crop. Under experimental conditions the production of tympany is not influenced by the water content of clover or by wilting. Other plant factors which are known to be associated with an increased tendency to bloat are liberal administration of urea to the pasture, a high intake of glucose, calcium and magnesium and a high nitrogen intake.

Those legumes which do not cause bloat, commonly contain tannins which inhibit microbial digestion rather than by precipitation of soluble proteins in the rumen as was previously accepted (3). Sainfoin and *Lotus* spp. contain tannins and may be used in mixtures with bloating legumes. White and red clovers and alfalfa contain very little tannin and the challenge for agronomists and plant biochemists is to genetically increase the concentration of tannins in these plants while preserving their other beneficial characteristics (15).

Feedlot or grain bloat occurs most commonly in hand-fed animals confined in feedlots and barns and when insufficient roughage is fed or the feed is too finely ground. Two separate sets of circumstances conducive to feedlot bloat have been identified. In one the cattle are being fed a high-level grain finishing ration in which grain comprises more than 80% of the weight of the ration. The effect of these rations on the rumen is a tendency to acidity and a shortage of rumen-stimulating roughage which may interfere with motility and eructation. The other circumstance is where grain comprises 30–70% of the ration with the same but less marked effect, as above, but in which the roughage component is alfalfa hay with its own bloat-inducing capacity (3).

Animal factors Cattle vary in their susceptibility to primary ruminal tympany, especially that caused by legumes, and this individual idiosyncrasy may be inherited. Recent work has shown that some cows can be classified according to their susceptibility to pasture bloat into high or low susceptibility and the offspring show influences of their parentage (7). A number of inherited characteristics are related to bloat (9). They include ruminal structure and motility, composition of salivary proteins, rate of salivation, and the greater capacity of the rumen contents of high-susceptibility animals to degrade mucoproteins which would either reduce antifoaming activity or increase foam-stabilizing activity (18). There may also be differences between animals in the rate and extent of physical breakdown of feed in the rumen, and the rate of passage of solids out of the rumen (33).

Under experimental conditions the production of tympany is not influenced by the rate of intake, or the total intake of dry matter. Susceptibility increases with time when a tympany producing diet is fed for a relatively short period (16). However, animals accustomed over very long periods to grazing bloating pastures may be less susceptible than other animals. Accordingly the mortality rate in young cattle is much higher than in mature animals (15).

Pathogenesis

Normally, gas bubbles produced in the rumen fluid coalesce, separate from the rumen contents to form pockets of free gas above the level of the contents, and are finally eliminated by eructation.

In frothy bloat, the gas bubbles remain dispersed throughout the rumen contents, producing an abnormal increase in the volume of the ruminoreticular contents and, consequently, inhibiting eructation. The characteristic frothiness of ruminal contents is caused by inadequate coalescence of gas bubbles.

In free-gas bloat the gas bubbles coalesce and separate from the rumen fluid, but the animals cannot eructate the pockets of free gas because of abnormalities of the reticulorumen or esophagus.

Most interest centers on the pathogenesis of primary bloat on legume pasture. Two major groups of factors have received most attention—those factors which cause foaming of the ruminal contents and those which cause ruminal atony. Most cases of naturally occurring pasture or feedlot bloat are not accompanied by ruminal atony; in fact in the early stages there is unusually pronounced hypermotility. If atony were an important cause one would expect to find large quantities of gas free in the rumen but this does not occur. Almost without exception the great bulk of the gas is intimately mixed with the solid and fluid ruminal contents to form a dense froth. Some free gas is present but the amount which can be removed by a stomach tube or trocar and cannula does little to relieve the distension of the rumen. As a general rule it can be accepted that ruminal tympany characterized by the accumulation of free gas is due to esophageal obstruction or ruminal atony.

If the eructation reflex can operate, the experimental introduction of very large amounts of gas does not cause tympany since eructation removes the excess. Tympanogenetic feeds do not produce noticeably more gas than safe feeds and the simple production of excessive gas is known not to be a precipitating factor.

Frothiness of the ruminal contents causes physical obstruction of the cardia and inhibits the eructation reflex, and vomiting or eructation of the froth rarely occurs because the caudal sphincter of the esophagus fails to open. Rumen movements are intitially stimulated by the distension and the resulting hypermotility exacerbates the frothiness of the ruminal contents. Terminally there is a loss of muscle tone and ruminal motility.

The cause of death in bloat is obscure. The absorption of toxic gases, particularly hydrogen sulfide, or toxic amines, particularly histamine, has been suggested but is likely to be only a contributory factor. Distension probably plays an important part by reflexly depressing the cardiovascular and respiratory systems but experimental works shows a great deal of variation in the susceptibility of animals to ruminal distension.

Clinical findings

Bloat is a common cause of sudden death (or found dead) in cattle. Pastured beef cattle which die of bloat are usually found dead because they are not observed as regularly as dairy cattle. Feedlot cattle which die of bloat are commonly found dead in the morning, which may be due to the relative inactivity during the night or the lack of observation, detection and treatment. Dairy cattle which are being milked and observed regularly will commonly begin to bloat within 1 hour after being turned into a bloat-producing pasture. There is commonly a lag period of 24–48 hours before bloating occurs in cattle which have been placed on a bloat-producing pasture for the first time. They may bloat on the first day but more commonly they bloat on the second and third days. A similar situation has been observed in pastured beef cattle which have been on a particular pasture for several days or weeks before bloat occurs. This is always a surprise to the owner and the veterinarian who find it difficult to explain why bloat suddenly becomes a problem on a pasture which cattle have grazed with impunity for some time.

In primary pasture bloat, obvious distension of the rumen occurs suddenly, sometimes as soon as 15 minutes after going on to bloat-producing pasture. The distension is usually more obvious in the upper left flank but the whole of the abdomen is enlarged. There is discomfort and the animal may get up and lie down frequently, kick at the belly and even roll. Dyspnea is marked and is accompanied by mouth breathing, protrusion of the tongue, salivation and extension of the head. The respiratory rate is increased up to 60/minute. Occasionally projectile vomiting occurs and soft feces may be expelled in a stream. Ruminal movements are usually much increased in the early stages and may be almost continuous but the sounds are reduced in volume because of the frothy nature of the ingesta. Later, when the distension is extreme, the movements are decreased and may be completely absent. The tympanic note produced by percussion is characteristic. Before clinical tympany occurs there is a temporary increase in eructation and rumination but both disappear in the acute stages. The course in ruminal tympany is short but death does not usually occur within 3–4 hours of the onset of clinical signs. Collapse and death almost without struggle occur quickly.

If animals are treated by trocarization or the passage of a stomach tube, only small amounts of gas are obtained before frothy material blocks the tube.

In a group of affected cattle there is usually a number of animals with clinical tympany and the remainder have mild to moderate distension of the abdomen. These animals are uncomfortable, graze for only short periods and suffer considerably in their milk production. This drop in production may be caused by depression of food intake or by failure of milk letdown.

In secondary bloat, the excess gas is usually present as a free gas cap on top of the solid and fluid ruminal contents although frothy bloat may occur in vagus indigestion when there is increased ruminal motility. As in pasture bloat there is usually an increase in rate and force of ruminal movements in the early stages followed by atony. Passage of a stomach tube or trocarization results in the expulsion of large quantities of gas and subsidence of the ruminal distension. If an esophageal obstruction is present it will be detected when the stomach tube is passed.

In both forms of bloat there is dyspnea and a marked elevation of the heart rate up to 100–120/minute in the acute stages. A systolic murmur is often audible, caused probably by distortion of the base of the heart by the forward displacement of the diaphragm. This murmur has been observed in ruminal tympany caused by tetanus, diaphragmatic hernia, vagus indigestion and esophageal obstruction and disappears immediately if the tympany is relieved.

Clinical pathology

Laboratory tests are not necessary in the diagnosis of ruminal tympany but a great deal of useful information about the pathogenesis of the disease can be obtained if estimations of ruminal pressure and examinations of ruminal microflora and the physical and chemical properties of rumen fluids are carried out.

Necropsy findings

Animals that have died about an hour previously show

protrusion and congestion of the tongue, marked congestion and hemorrhage of lymph nodes to the head and neck, epicardium and upper respiratory tract, friable kidneys and mucosal hyperemia in the small intestine. The lungs are compressed, the cervical esophagus shows congestion and hemorrhage, but the thoracic portion of the esophagus is pale and blanched (17). In general, congestion is marked in the front quarters and less marked or absent in the hindquarters. The rumen is distended but the contents are much less frothy than before death. A marked erythema is evident beneath the ruminal mucosa especially in the ventral sacs. The liver is pale due to expulsion of blood from the organ. Occasionally the rumen or diaphragm have ruptured. Animals that have been dead for some hours show subcutaneous emphysema, almost complete absence of froth in the rumen, and exfoliation of the cornified epithelium of the rumen with marked congestion of submucosal tissues.

Diagnosis

A diagnosis of ruminal tympany can be arrived at fairly easily and determination of the cause in primary bloat is in most cases a simple matter but in secondary bloat, particular when it is chronic, this decision is often difficult to make. If the case is severe enough it is usually necessary to carry out emergency treatment without complete examination of the animal. Passage of a stomach tube will detect esophageal obstruction or stenosis, both of which are accompanied by difficult swallowing, and in acute cases by violent attempts at vomiting. Vagus indigestion and diaphragmatic hernia have a prior history of traumatic reticuloperitonitis and partial anorexia. Tetanus is manifested by limb rigidity, prolapse of the third eyelid and hyperesthesia. Carcinoma and papillomata of the esophageal groove and reticulum and actinobacillosis of the reticulum cannot usually be diagnosed antemortem without exploratory rumenotomy.

One of the difficult situations encountered in veterinary practice is the postmortem diagnosis of bloat, especially in animals found dead at pasture in warm weather. Blackleg, lightning stroke, anthrax and snakebite are common alternatives. A diagnosis of bloat must depend on an absence of local lesions characteristic of these diseases, the presence of marked ruminal tympany in the absence of other signs of postmortem decomposition, the relative pallor of the liver and the other lesions described above.

Treatment

The approach to treatment depends very much on the circumstances in which bloat occurs, whether the bloat is frothy or due to free gas, and whether or not the bloat is life-threatening. It is often necessary to advise an owner on some first-aid measures before professional attention can be provided. All animals should be removed immediately from the source of the bloating pasture or feed if possible. In severe cases in which there is gross distension, mouth-breathing with protrusion of the tongue and staggering, an emergency rumenotomy is necessary to save the life of the animal. Once the animals falls down it will die in a few minutes and many animals have died unnecessarily because owners are unable or reluctant to do an emergency rumenotomy. Using a sharp knife a quick incision 10–20 cm in length is made over the midpoint of the left paralumbar fossa. This will be followed by an explosive release of ruminal contents and marked relief for the cow. There is remarkably little contamination of the peritioneal cavity and irrigation and cleansing of the wound followed by standard surgical closure usually results in uneventful recovery with only occasional minor complications. The trocar and cannula has been used for many years for the emergency release of rumen contents and gas in bloat. However, the standard sized trocar and cannula does not have a large enough diameter to allow the very viscous stable foam in peracute frothy bloat to escape quickly enough to save an animal's life. A larger bore instrument (2·5 cm in diameter) is necessary and an incision with a scalpel or knife must be made through the skin before it can be inserted into the rumen. If any sized trocar and cannula fails to reduce the intraruminal pressure and the animal's life is being compromised by the pressure, an emergency rumenotomy should be performed. If the trocar is successful in reducing the pressure, the antifoaming agent of choice can be administered through the cannula which can be left in place, until the animal has returned to normal in a few hours. Owners should be advised on the proper use of the trocar and cannula; the method of insertion and the need for a small incision in the skin and the care of cannulas left in place for several hours or days. A corkscrew type trocar and cannula has been recommended for long-term insertion in cases of chronic bloat which occur in feedlot cattle and in beef calves following weaning (19). The etiology of these is often not understood but leaving a cannula in place for several days or the surgical preparation of a rumen fistula will often yield good results.

For less severe cases, owners may be advised to tie a stick in the mouth like a bit on a horse bridle to promote the production of excessive saliva which is alkaline and may assist in denaturation of the stable foam. Careful drenching with sodium bicarbonate (150–200 g in 1 liter of water) or any non-toxic oil as described below is also satisfactory.

The passage of a stomach tube of the largest bore possible is recommended for cases in which the animal's life is not being threatened. The use of a Frick oral speculum and passage of the tube through the oral cavity permits the passage of tubes measuring up to 2 cm in diameter whereas this may not be possible if passed through the nasal cavity. In free gas bloat, there will be a sudden release of gas and the intraruminal pressure may return to normal. While the tube is in place, the antifoaming agent can be administered. In frothy bloat, the tube may become plugged up immediately on entering the rumen. A few attempts should be made to clear the tube by blowing and moving it back and forth in an attempt to find large pocketes of rumen gas which can be released. However, in frothy bloat it may be impossible to reduce the pressure with the tube and the antifoaming agent should be administered while the tube is in place.

In every case in which the bloat has not been relieved but an antifoaming agent has been administered, the animal must be observed carefully for the next hour to determine if the treatment has been successful or if the bloat is becoming worse and something else must be done.

In an outbreak of feedlot bloat, the acute and peracute cases should be treated individually as necessary. There will be many 'swellers' which are affected with moderate bloat which will usually relieve itself if the cattle are forcefully walked. After a few minutes of walking they usually begin to eructate. Shaking of experimentally reproduced foam results in loss of stability of foam and coalescence into large bubbles and it is thought that forced moving of moderately bloated cattle has the same effect. If walking is effective in reducing the foam, the animals should be kept under close surveillance for several hours in case the frothing returns.

Details of the oils and synthetic surfactants used as antifoaming agents in treatment are given in the section on control because the same compounds are used in prevention. Any non-toxic oil, especially a mineral one which persists in the rumen, not being biodegradable, is effective and there are no other significant differences between them. The dose rate needed is not great (250 ml for cattle and 50 ml for sheep) but one usually errs on the side of generosity with these safe compounds in this dangerous situation, and 500 ml would be a more conventional dose. An emulsified oil or one containing a detergent such as dioctyl sodium sulfosuccinate is preferred because it mixes better with ruminal contents. Of the synthetic surfactants, poloxalene is the one in most general use for leguminous bloat and a dose of 25–50 g is recommended for treatment (20). It is not as effective for feedlot or grain bloat. Alcohol ethoxylates are a promising new group of compounds as bloat remedies and both poloxalene and the ethoxylates are more effective and faster than oil, which is relatively slow and better suited to prevention than treatment. All three are recommended as being satisfactory for legume hay bloat, but poloxalene is not recommended for feedlot bloat. All of them can be given by drench, stomach tube or through a ruminal cannula. The effect of all is enhanced if they are thoroughly mixed with the ruminal contents, and if rumen movements are still present mixing will occur. If the rumen is static it should be kneaded through the left flank.

Following the treatment of the individual cases of bloat the major problem remaining is the decision about whether or not, or when, or under what conditions, to return the cattle to the bloat-producing pasture or to the concentrate ration in the case of feedlot cattle. The possible preventive measures are presented under control but unless one of the reliable ones can be instituted, the cattle should not be returned until the hazardous period has passed. This is difficult on some farms because the bloat-producing pasture may be the sole source of feed.

Control

Pasture bloat

On pasture, prevention of frothy bloat is a difficult problem. In the past many husbandry practices have been recommended including the prior feeding of dry, scabrous hay, particularly sudan grass, cereal hay and straw, restricting the grazing to 20 minutes at a time or until the first cow stops eating, cutting the crop and feeding it in troughs, and strip grazing to ensure that all available pasture is utilized each day. These methods have value when the pasture is only moderately dangerous but may be ineffective when the tympany-producing potential is high. In these circumstances the use of simple management procedures can be highly unreliable because the occurrence of bloat can be so unpredictable. Generally, the farmer does not know for certain that his pastures are dangerous until bloat actually occurs and once he starts using effective prophylactic methods, he cannot be certain when he can safely stop (15). The bloat-producing potential of a pasture can change dramatically almost overnight and the management strategy can be quickly overpowered. The only satisfactory method available for the prevention of bloat in cattle on a bloating pasture is the administration of antifoaming agents as described below. The questions at issue are not related to the strategies but rather which of the compounds to use in a given situation in terms of cost of the product, the method and ease of administration and the absence of side-effects.

Oils and fats

These have achieved great success in New Zealand and Australia. Individual drenching is sometimes practiced but because of the time and labor involved it is most suited to short-term prophylaxis. It is popular as an effective standard practice in New Zealand (15) in pastured cattle. The common practice is to administer the antifoaming agent at the time of milking using an automatic dose syringe which is moved up and down to reach each cow in the milking parlor. Cows will become conditioned quickly and turn their heads to the operator to receive their twice daily dose of 60–120 ml of the oil. The duration of the foam-preventing effect is short, lasting only a few hours and increasing the dose does not significantly lengthen the period of protection. If the oil or fat is emulsified with water it can then be sprayed on to a limited pasture area which provides part or all of the anticipated food requirements for the day. Backgrazing must be prevented and care is required during rainy periods when the oil is likely to be washed from the pasture. The method is ideal where strip-grazing is practiced on irrigated pasture but is ineffective when grazing is uncontrolled. Under these conditions the oil can be administered at the rate of 120 g per head in concentrates fed before the cattle go on to the pasture or by addition to the drinking water to make a 2% emulsion. The latter practice can be satisfactorily carried out by mixing a mineral oil with the water in all available troughs, turning off the water supply and refilling the troughs when they are emptied. The serious disadvantage of this method is that the actual intake of the oil cannot be guaranteed and cattle which fail to drink after becoming accustomed to drinking the oil appear to be more susceptible than those which are not so accustomed. Climatic conditions also cause variations in the amount of water which is taken with consequent variation in the oil intake. It is probably safest to make provision for the daily intake of 240–300 g of oil per head during those periods when the pasture is at its most dangerous stage. The recommended procedure (15) is to provide an automatic watering pump which injects antifrothing agents into all the drinking water supplies to which the cattle have access, and in such amounts as to maintain a concentration of 1% of the antifrothing agent. Hand replenishment means that the preparation must be added twice daily. Surfactants are preferred to oils because of their faster action and the smaller dose rates (5–8 ml in 10–20 ml of water) and their longer period of effectiveness (10–18 hours). A recently introduced method of administering antifoaming agents is their application to the flanks of cows with a large paint brush as they go out of the milking shed. A preparation which is palatable to cattle and which encourages them to lick their flanks is preferred. Although this is the most popular method of controlling bloat in dairy cows in Australia, failures are not infrequent, especially in individual cows.

Many oils have been used and all vegetable oils, mineral oil and emulsified tallow are effective. The choice of oil to be used depends on local availability and cost. If the oils are to be used over an extended period some consideration must be given to the effects of the oil on the animal. Continued administration of mineral oil causes restriction of carotene absorption and reduces the carotene and tocopherol content of the butter produced. Linseed oil, soya oil and whale oil have undesirable effects on the quality and flavor of the milk and butter. Peanut oil and tallow are the most satisfactory. In most areas the tympany-producing effect of pasture is short-lived and may last for only 2–3 weeks. During this time the pasture can be grazed under the sheltering umbrella of oil administration until the bloat-producing period is passed.

Synthetic non-ionic surfactants

These, especially poloxalene (polyoxythylene polyoxypropylene block polymer), are highly effective, more so in cattle than sheep and their use in cattle grazing lush legume pasture or young cereal crops is recommended. In cattle daily intakes of poloxalene of 10–20 g are recommended and daily dose rates of up to 40 g are without deleterious effect. In very high risk situations it may be advisable to administer the drug at least twice daily. Poloxalene is rather unpalatable and its use in drinking water was not possible until the introduction of the pluronic L64 which is suitable for mixing with drinking water and is effective. It needs to be introduced to the cattle several weeks before the bloat season commences (24). It is in most general use as an additive to grain mixtures but it is also used in feed pellets and in mineral blocks (25). The use of pluronics administered by mixing with molasses and allowing them to be licked from a roller drum had a brief popularity for control of bloat in beef cattle but the erratic rate of consumption has brought the method into disfavor (26). The alternative of mixing pluronics with the drinking water is also undependable.

Alcohol ethoxylate detergents are known to have equal foam-reducing qualities to poloxalene, and have the advantage of better palatability so that they can be administered by a voluntary intake method such as medicated blocks. Small-scale field trials (6) show that these blocks are palatable and attractive and should be satisfactory in reducing the severity and prevalence of bloat. Not all cattle visit them voluntarily so that some cases are likely to occur. The blocks contain 10% of the alcohol ethoxylate, known as Teric, and a daily consumption of 17–19 g of it is usual. Application of Teric to the flanks of cows has not been as successful as a bloat prevention as have oils (13).

Sustained release techniques

Sustained release capsules have been under investigation for some time (27). A large capsule is administered into the rumen via a flexible large-bore tube. In the rumen the capsule opens exposing an antifoaming agent, which diffuses slowly from a matrix of ethylcellulose gel. The duration of effect is about 2 weeks.

Feedlot bloat

This is more resistant to the above-mentioned preventive measures than is pasture bloat and continues to be a problem. Feedlot high-level grain rations should contain at least 10–15% roughage which is cut or chopped and mixed into a complete feed. This ensures that cattle will consume a minimum amount of roughage. The roughage should be a cereal grain straw or grass hay. The use of leafy alfalfa hay may be hazardous. The roughage may be fed separately in the long form as a supplement to the grain ration but this practice is dangerous because the voluntary intake of roughage will vary considerably. The more palatable the grain ration, the less total amount of roughage will be eaten and outbreaks of feedlot bloat may occur. Grains for feedlot rations should be only rolled or cracked, not finely ground. If the grain is very dry, the addition of water during processing will prevent pulverization to fine particles. The use of pelleted rations for feedlot cattle cannot be recommended because a fine grind of the grain is normally necessary to process a solid pellet. When the pellet dissolves in the rumen, a fine pasty rumen content forms which may be associated with the development of a stable foam. In addition, it is difficult to incorporate sufficient quantity of roughage into a pellet.

The use of dietary antifoaming agents for the prevention of feedlot bloat has had variable success. The addition of tallow at the level of 3–5% of the total ration has been used with success judged empirically, but controlled trials did not reduce bloat scores (3). If animal fats were effective in preventing feedlot bloat they would be attractive for other reasons. They are a source of concentrated energy and they control dust in dusty feeds. The possibility that the long-term use of animal fats or oils could interfere with the absorption of vitamin A has not been examined. Poloxalene has had an unsatisfactory reputation in the prevention of feedlot bloat. A non-toxic dimethyl dialkyl quaternary ammonium compound is effective (28) but requires additional field testing. The addition of a 4% salt to feedlot rations has been recommended when other methods are not readily available, but it will, of course, also reduce feed intake and rate of gain of body weight. The effect of the high salt diet, as distinct from a low salt content in a largely concentrate ration, is to oppose the development of conditions in the rumen which are conducive to bloat (23). The effects of the high salt diet include an increase in water intake, an alteration in the proportion of disrupted cells in the forage due to changes in fermentation, and an increase in the rate of flow of material out of the rumen. Other management factors considered to be important in the prevention of feedlot bloat generally include the following: avoid overfeeding after a period of temporary starvation, for example after bad weather, or machinery failure or transportation and feed handling failure; and ensure that the water supply is available at all times.

General comments

Apart from the impressive reduction in clinical and fatal cases of ruminal tympany resulting from the prophylactic use of oils, there are the added advantages of being able to utilize dangerous pasture with impunity, and the reduction of subclinical bloat and its attendant lowering of food intake. Production may rise by as much as 25% in 24 hours after the use of oil. Nevertheless, these preventive methods should be considered as temporary measures only. The ultimate aim should be the development of a pasture of high net productivity where the maximum productivity is consistent with a low incidence of bloat and diarrhea. At present, a pasture comprising equal quantities of clovers and grasses comes closest to achieving this ideal but with available pasture plants and current methods of pasture management this clover/grass ratio is not easy to maintain. Research work in this area is directed towards selecting cattle which are less susceptible to bloat. More practical are the moves being made to breed varieties of legumes which are low on bloat-producing potential.

Two pasture management techniques are worthy of note. The usual 5–10-year period of clover dominance after a mixed pasture is established and the period of bloat susceptibility can be reduced to about 2 years by the administration of high levels of superphosphate (250–350 kg/ha per year). Also the use of high levels of nitrogen administration to pasture may reduce the risk of bloat during the development period of a pasture. One procedure which does have value is to concentrate on making dangerous pasture into hay and utilizing safer fields for grazing during dangerous periods.

Recommendations

The only reliable methods for the prevention of bloat in dairy cows are either strip grazing of pasture sprayed daily with oil or pluronics, or twice daily drenching with the same preparations. For beef cattle at pasture the only safe precaution is the daily feeding of hay, which is supplemented with a surfactant during dangerous periods. Best results in feedlot bloat are obtained by the incorporation of non-bloating roughages in the grain ration at a level of at least 10% and avoiding fine grinding of the grain.

REVIEW LITERATURE

Bartley, E. E., Meyer, R. M. & Fina, L. R. (1975) Feedlot or grain bloat. In: *Digestion and Metabolism in the Ruminant*, eds I. W. McDonald & A. C. I. Warner, pp. 551–562. University of New England Publishing Unit.

Clark, R. T. J. & Reid, C. S. W. (1974) Foamy bloat of cattle: a review. *J. dairy Sci.*, 57, 753.

Howarth, R. E., Cheng, K. J., Majak, W. & Costerton, J. W. (1986). Ruminant bloat. In *Control of Digestion and Metabolism in Ruminants. Proc. 6th Int. Symp. Ruminant Physiol.* Banff, Canada, Sept. 10–14, 1984, eds L. P. Milligan, W. L. Grovum & A. Dobson, pp. 516–527.

Leng, R. A. & McWilliam, J. R. (1973) Bloat. Proceedings of a symposium held at the University of New England, Armidale, NSW, Australia. *Rev. rural Sci.*, *1*, 103.

Reid, C. S. W., Clarke, R. T. J., Cockrem, F. R. M., Jones, W. T., McIntosh, J. T. & Wright, D. E. (1975) Physiological and genetical aspects of pasture (legume) bloat. In: *Digestion and Metabolism in the Ruminant*, eds I. W. McDonald & A. C. I. Warner, pp. 525–536. University of New England Publishing Unit.

REFERENCES

(1) Hironaka, R. J. E. et al. (1973) *Can. J. anim. Sci.*, *53* 75.
(2) Bartley, E. E et al. (1975) In: *Digestion and Metabolism in the Ruminant*, eds I. W. McDonald & A. C. I. Warner, pp. 551–562. University of New England Pulishing Unit.
(3) Howarth, R. E., Cheng, K. J., Majak, W. & Costerton, J. W. (1986). In: *Control of Digestion and Metabolism in Ruminants. Proc. 6th Int. Symp. Ruminant Physiol.* Banff, Canada, Sept. 10–14, 1984, eds L. P. Milligan, W. L. Grovum & A. Dobson, pp. 516–527.
(4) Majak, W. et al. (1983). *J. dairy Sci.*, 66, 1683.
(5) Jones, W. T. & Lyttelton, J. W. (1973) *NZ J. agric. Res.*, *16*, 161.
(6) Barr, D. A. & Graham, C. A. (1978) *NZ vet. J.*, 26, 117.
(7) Reid, C. S. W. et al. (1975) In: *Digestion and Metabolism in the Ruminant*, eds I. W. McDonald & A. C. I. Warner, pp. 525–536. University of New England Publishing Unit.
(8) Neal, P. A. & Edwards, G. B. (1963) *Vet. Rec.*, 75, 672.
(9) Reid, C. S. W. et al. (1975) *Proc. NZ Soc. Anim. Prod.*, *35*, 13.
(10) Wolfe, E. C. & Lazenby, A. (1972) *Aust. J. exp. Agric. anim. Husb.*, *12*, 119.
(11) Jensen, R. et al. (1976) *J. Am. vet. med. Assoc.*, *169*, 497.
(12) Pierson, R. E. et al. (1976) *J. Am. vet. med. Assoc.*, *169*, 527.
(13) Flynn, K. L. et al. (1976) *Proc. Aust. Soc. Anim. Prod.*, *11*, 31P.
(14) Bartley, E. E. et al. (1975) *J. anim. Sci.*, *41*, 752.
(15) Reid, C. S. W. (1976) *Bov. Practnr*, *11*, 24.
(16) Clarke, R. T. J. & Reid, C. S. W. (1974) *J. dairy Sci.*, *57*, 753.
(17) Mills, J. H. L. & Christian, R. G. (1970) *J. Am. vet. med. Assoc.*, *157*, 947.
(18) Jones, W. T. & Lyttleton, J. W. (1978) *NZ J. agric. Res.*, *21*, 401.
(19) Breukink, H. J. et al. (1974) *Tijdschr. Diergeneeskd.*, *99*, 913.
(20) Bartley, E. E. et al. (1967) *J. Am. vet. med. Assoc.*, *151*, 339.
(21) Jayne-Williams, D. J. (1979) *J. appl. Bacteriol.*, *47*, 271.
(22) Stockdale, C. R. et al. (1980) *Aust. J. exp. Agric. anim. Husb.*, *20*, 265.
(23) Cheng, K. J. et al. (1979) *Can. J. anim. Sci.*, *59*, 737.
(24) Phillips, D. S. M. (1968) *N. Am. J. agric. Res.*, *11*, 85.
(25) Foote, L. E. et al. (1968) *J. dairy Sci.*, *51*, 584.
(26) Langlands, J. P. & Holmes, C. R. (1975) *Aust. J. exp. Agric. anim. Husb.*, *15*, 5.
(27) Gyles, A. (1970) *J. Agric. Vict., Dept. Agric.*, *68*, 156, 158.
(28) Meyer, R. M. & Bartley, E. E. (1972) *J. anim. Sci.*, *34*, 234.
(29) Majak, W. et al. (1985). *Can. J. anim. Sci.*, *65*, 147.
(30) Cheng, K. J. et al. (1976) *Can. J. Microbiol.*, *22*, 450.
(31) Majak, W. et al. (1986). *Can. J. anim. Sci.*, *66*, 97.
(32) Majak, W. et al. (1986). *J. dairy Sci.*, *69*, 1560.
(33) Carruthers, V. R. (1984). *Proc. NZ Soc. Anim. Prod.*, *44*, 79.

Impaction of the omasum

Chronic omasal impaction as a clinical entity is difficult to define and is usually diagnosed at necropsy when the omasum is enlarged and excessively hard (1). It seems unlikely that it could cause death and is frequently observed in animals dying of other disease. It is reputed to occur when feed is tough and fibrous, particularly alfalfa stalks and loppings from fodder trees, or under drought feeding conditions in sheep which are fed on the ground. In the latter, the impaction is due to the accumulation of soil in the omasum. Chronic recurrent bouts of indigestion occur and are manifested by decreased rumen motility, infrequent and scanty feces, refusal to eat grain and a negative ketone test (2). Pain may be elicited and the hard distended viscus palpated on deep pressure under the right costal arch or in the seventh to ninth intercostal spaces on the right side. It may also be palpable per rectum as a large, round, firm mass with a checkered surface to distinguish it from the smooth surface of the abomasum. Repeated dosing with mineral oil is recommended as treatment.

The omasum is grossly distended, the leaves and in some cases the wall of the organ show patches of necrosis and an associated peritonitis. Necrosis of the ruminal lining may also be present. Clinically the disease is manifested by complete anorexia, cessation of defecation, an empty rectum and subacute abdominal pain with disinclination to move or lie down.

REFERENCES

(1) Hughes, W. A. & Cartwright, J. R. (1962) *Vet. Rec.*, *74*, 676.
(2) McDonald, J. S. & Witzel, D. A. (1968) *J. Am. vet. med. Assoc.*, *152*, 638.

DISEASES OF THE ABOMASUM OF CATTLE

Diseases of the abomasum of cattle associated with metabolic disturbances, stress and nutritional disorders are being recognized more frequently now than ever before. These diseases include left-side displacement of the abomasum (LDA), right-side displacement of the abomasum (RDA), abomasal torsion, abomasal ulcers and dietary abomasal impaction. Their recognition is due in part to improved diagnostic techniques and increased awareness of their occurrence, but perhaps there is a real increase in their frequency because of economic pressures. Dairy cattle are being selected for high milk production and being fed large quantities of grain, kept more commonly in total confinement where exercise is limited, all of which may contribute to abomasal atony which is considered to be the precursor of abomasal displacements.

Abomasal ulcers occur in high-producing dairy cows, usually following parturition, which suggests that stress may be an important factor. Abomasal ulcers also occur in young milk-fed calves following the introduction of a dry ration, and in well-nourished thrifty sucking beef calves from 2 to 4 months of age running on pasture. Abomasal impaction, dietary in origin, is caused by the feeding of poor quality roughage, usually chopped, to pregnant beef cattle during the cold winter months. Abomasal phytobezoars occur in sheep and goats causing chronic alimentary tract stasis and abdominal distension (4). Early diagnosis and slaughter for salvage is considered as the best method of management. Metal foreign bodies occur occasionally in the abomasum of cattle (5). Clinical findings are similar to those of traumatic reticuloperitonitis. The metal may be detectable by exploring the abomasal area with a metal detector. The foreign body will move with movements of the abomasum and the metal detector will detect a moving metal signal in contrast to the fixed signal from a fixed foreign body.

The normal abomasum cannot usually be examined by the standard techniques of clinical examination, with perhaps the exception of auscultation and paracentesis. In left-side displacement of the abomasum, the tympanitic sounds on auscultation and percussion between the ninth and twelfth rib are characterisitc. In right-side dilatation and displacement the tympanitic and fluid-splashing sounds on percussion, auscultation and succussion are characteristic. The distended organ may be palpable on rectal examination. In abomasal torsion, the clinical findings are similar but much more severe. In abomasal impaction, the enlarged firm doughy viscus can usually be palpated behind the lower aspect of the right costal arch but the gravid uterus of later pregnancy commonly makes this difficult. Following parturition it is more readily detectable by palpation through the abdominal wall or rectally.

Diseases of the abomasum which cause stasis and accumulation of ingesta, fluid and gas in the organ, result in varying degrees of *dehydration*, *metabolic alkalosis*, *hypochloremia* and *hypokalemia*. The metabolic alkalosis and hypokalemia are often accompanied by muscular weakness and paradoxic aciduria (3). When these changes are severe as in right-side dilatation, abomasal torsion and abomasal impaction intensive fluid therapy is necessary for a favorable response. However, in spite of exhaustive efforts, because of irreversible abomasal atony, the recovery rate is low. The abomasum of young calves can be intubated (6).

Abomasal reflux

Reflux of abomasal fluid into the omasum and reticulorumen occurs when the abomasal fluid fails to move normally through the pylorus into the small intestine (1). This occurs most commonly in diseases of the abomasum, left-side displacement, right-side dilatation and vagus indigestion. Reflux may also occur in peritonitis, compression of the abomasum in advanced pregnancy, intussusception and toxemias. The rumen chloride levels increase from a normal of 10–25 mmol/l to 80–100 mmol/l and the buffering capacity of the rumen is decreased from 80–110 mmol/l to less than 50. Hypochloremic, hypokalemic metabolic alkalosis occurs. Treatment consists of removing excessive quantities of fluid from the rumen and the administration of large quantities of balanced electrolytes or simply saline intravenously.

A series of abomasal emptying defects in sheep were characterized by weight loss, anorexia, variable degrees of abdominal distension, increased concentrations of rumen chloride and grossly enlarged abomasa (7). No explanation for the emptying defect was found at necropsy.

The administration of apomorphine to sheep causes expulsion of acidic abomasal contents back into the pre-abomasal compartments without expulsion of gastric contents through the mouth—'internal vomiting' (2). In sheep, it is estimated that approximately 280 g of sodium bicarbonate given orally would be necessary to return the ruminal pH to the neutral range.

REFERENCES

(1) Breukink, H. J. & Kuiper, R. (1980) *Bov. Pract.*, *15*, 139.
(2) Eiler, H. et al. (1981) *Am. J. vet. Res.*, *42*, 202.
(3) McGuirk, S. M. & Butler, D. G. (1980) *J. Am. vet. med. Assoc.*, *177*, 551.
(4) Bath, G. F. (1978) *J. S. Afr. vet. Assoc.*, *49*, 133.
(5) Haaranen, S. (1977) *Nord. VetMed.*, *29*, 482.
(6) Chapman, H. W. (1986) *Can. J. vet. Res.*, *50*, 291.
(7) Rings, D. M. et al. (1985) *J. Am. vet. med. Assoc.*, *185*, 1520.

Left-side displacement of the abomasum (LDA)

In this disease the abomasum is displaced from its normal position on the abdominal floor (extending from the midline and to the right) to the left side of the abdomen between the rumen and the left abdominal wall.

Etiology and epidemiology

Left-side displacement of the abomasum (LDA) occurs most commonly in large-sized, high-producing adult dairy cows immediately after parturition. In a case study of 315 cases, 91% occurred within 6 weeks following parturition (1). Occasional cases occur a few to several weeks before parturition and the clinical findings are similar to those occurring after parturition. High-producing dairy cattle are usually fed large quantities of grain and there is general agreement that heavy grain feeding including corn and corn silage is an important etiological factor (2–4). A crude fiber concentration of less than 16–17% in the diet of dairy cows is a significant risk factor for left-side displacement of the abomasum (5). Epidemiological studies have shown that cows affected with LDA were higher producers than their herdmates, and they were from higher producing herds than herds without LDAs (2). The affected cows were also older and heavier than the average of cows examined in the survey (2, 6, 7). The disease has been called a disorder of *throughput* because of its relationship to diseases associated with high milk production and concentrate feeding. The association between milk production and occurrence of left-side displacement of the abomasum is a two-way interaction; high-yielding cows are at greater risk of the disease, which in turn leads to decreased milk production during the lactation in which the disease occurs (9).

Heavy grain feeding is thought to increase the flow of ruminal ingesta to the abomasum which causes an increase in the concentration of volatile fatty acids which can inhibit the motility of the abomasum (4, 9, 10). This inhibits the flow of digesta from the abomasum to the duodenum so that ingesta accumulates in the abomasum. The large volume of gas (methane) produced in the abomasum following grain feeding may become trapped there, causing its distension and displacement (11). However, other experimental work does not support the explanation that an increase in abomasal volatile fatty acid concentration is the cause of the abomasal atony (31). High protein feeding may also be a contributing factor (32). The prevalence of the disease did not change over a period of 13 years in an area where radical changes in feeding and housing of dairy cattle occurred (29).

Because parturition appears to be the most common precipitating factor, it has been postulated that during late pregnancy the rumen is lifted from the abdominal floor by the expanding uterus and the abomasum is pushed forward and to the left under the rumen. Following parturition, the rumen subsides, trapping the abomasum, especially if it is atonic or distended with feed as it is likely to be if the cow is fed heavily on grain (6, 12). Hypocalcemia which occurs commonly in mature dairy cows at the time of parturition has been suggested as an important contributing factor in LDA (13). However, it is not known whether the hypocalcemia is primary, or secondary to the inappetence. Unusual activity, including jumping on other cows during estrus, is a common history in cases not associated with parturition. Occasional cases occur in calves and bulls but the disease occurs only rarely in beef cattle. Retained fetal membranes, metritis and mastitis occur commonly with LDA (1, 6, 14) but a cause-and-effect relationship has been difficult to establish. In one retrospective study the disease was associated in terms of increased relative risk with periparturient factors such as stillbirth, twins, retained placenta, metritis, aciduria, ketonuria and low milk yield in the previous lactation (28).

The disease has been recorded in calves between 8 and 14 weeks of age (26).

The disease is common in the United Kingdom and North America where dairy cattle are fed grain for milk production and the animals are usually housed for part of the year or kept under confinement (zero grazing, loose housing). The disease is uncommon in Australia and New Zealand where grain is not normally fed to dairy cattle and the animals are usually out on pasture for most of the year. The importance of exercise in the etiology of LDA has not been explored. The incidence of LDA is higher during the winter months which may be a reflection of either a higher frequency of calving or relative inactivity (1, 6, 7).

In one survey of the prevalence of disease in dairy herds, during a 3-year period, 24% of herds reported at least one case of LDA and there was a prevalence of 1·16% among the affected herds and 0·35% when all herds surveyed were considered (2). The mean rate of occurrence in a cow population over a period of years in Denmark was 0·62% with a range of 0·2–1·6% (33). In Norway 88% of the abomasal displacements are left side and 12% are right side (34). The economic losses from the disease include lost milk production during the illness and postoperatively, and the cost of the surgery. The mean total cost per case has been estimated at US $150 (2). The interrelationships between displacement and milk production and survivorship have been examined (30). An average 80% of cows with left-side displacement of the abomasum produced 250–500 kg less milk during the lactation when the displacement occurred, whereas 9–18% produced at least 2000 kg less milk than expected. There was no effect on survivorship.

An inherited and breed predisposition to LDA has been suggested and examined but the results are inconclusive. No differences have been found between the pedigrees of affected and non-affected cows (15).

Another interesting recent observation is the shift in acid–base balance which occurs in cattle during the year. In high-producing dairy cows, the acid–base balance changed in the alkaline direction from summer to spring and was most alkaline during the winter months (16, 17) when the cattle were housed and fed concentrates. After the cattle were put out to grass in the spring the acid–base balance changed in the acid direction. Experimentally, metabolic alkalosis causes abomasal atony and decreased emptying rate (18).

Pathogenesis

Abomasal atony is considered to be the primary dysfunction in LDA. The atonic, perhaps partially gas-filled abomasum, becomes displaced upward along the left abdominal wall, usually lateral to the spleen and the dorsal sac of the rumen. It is primarily the fundus and greater curvature of the abomasum which becomes displaced, which in turn causes displacement of the pylorus and duodenum. The omasum, reticulum and liver are also rotated to varying degrees (19). The displacement invariably results in rupture of the attachment of the greater omentum to the abomasum. Compression by the rumen of the impounded part of the abomasum causes a great decrease in the volume of the organ and interference with normal movements. There is probably some interference with the function of the esophageal groove due to slight rotation of all the stomachs in a clockwise direction and this impedes forward passage of digesta. The obstruction of the displaced segment is incomplete and although it contains some gas and fluid a certain amount is still able to escape and the distension rarely becomes severe. In occasional cases the abomasum becomes trapped anteriorly between the reticulum and diaphragm—anterior displacement of the abomasum. There is no interference with blood supply to the trapped portion so that effects of the displacement are entirely those of interference with digestion and movement of the ingesta, leading to a state of chronic inanition. A mild metabolic alkalosis with hypochloremia and hypokalemia are common due probably to the abomasal atony, continued secretion of hydrochloric acid into the abomasum, and impairment of flow into the duodenum (4). Affected cattle usually develop secondary ketosis which in fat cows may be complicated by the development of the fatty liver syndrome. Abomasal ulceration and adhesions also occur in cases of long standing. The ulcers may perforate and cause sudden death (20). Polymorphonuclear leukocyle function may be depressed in cattle with LDA (36).

Clinical findings

Usually within a few days or a week following parturition there will be inappetence, sometimes almost complete anorexia, a marked drop in milk production and varying degrees of ketosis. It is not uncommon to stumble onto the disease in a cow which was treated for ketosis, improved for a few days and then relapsed. On visual inspection the left lateral abdomen is usually 'slab-sided' because the rumen is smaller than normal and displaced medially. The temperature, heart rate and respirations are usually within normal ranges. The feces are usually reduced in volume and softer than normal but periods of profuse diarrhea may occur.

In one study, the mortality rate was much higher (21%) in cows with LDA and diarrhea than in cows with LDA and normal feces (8%) (21). The diarrhea was not necessarily associated with the LDA but in some cases was due to concurrent disease.

Ruminal movements are present but may be decreased in frequency and are always decreased in intensity, often to the point where no sounds are heard. Auscultation of an area below a line from the center of the left paralumbar fossa to just behind the left elbow reveals the presence of abnormal sounds of a much higher pitch and of a tinkling or splashing and more fluid nature than ruminal sounds. They often have a progressive peristaltic character. These are abomasal sounds and may occur frequently or as long as 15 minutes apart. They are not related in occurrence to ruminal movements and this can be ascertained by simultaneous auscultation of the left lower abdomen and palpation of the dorsal sac of the rumen. Auscultation in the tenth left intercostal space may reveal splashing sounds.

Simultaneous percussion, using a flick of the finger or a plexor, and auscultation over an area between the 9th and 12th ribs of the upper third of the abdominal wall commonly reveal the high-pitched tympanitic sounds which are characteristic of LDA. Not uncommonly these characteristic sounds will disappear if the cow is transported to a clinic for surgery and reappear in 24–48 hours. Occasionally, a careful time-consuming examination using percussion and auscultation is necessary to detect the sounds.

In rare cases there is initially a sudden onset of anorexia accompanied in occasional cases by signs of moderate abdominal pain and abdominal distension. These are the acute cases which are uncommon. An obvious bulge caused by the distended abomasum may develop in the anterior part of the upper left paralumbar fossa and this may extend up behind the costal arch almost to the top of the fossa. The swelling is tympanitic and gives a resonant note on percussion. In acute cases the temperature may rise to 39·5°C (103°F) and the heart rate to 100/minute but in the more common subacute cases the temperature and pulse rate are normal. The appetite returns but is intermittent and selective, the animal eating only certain feeds, particularly hay.

Care must be taken not to mistake an atonic distended rumen for a displaced abomasum. This can best be done be carefully delimiting the area over which the characteristic resonant note can be heard on percussion. There may be transitory periods of improvement in appetite and disappearance of these sounds especially after transport or vigorous exercise.

On rectal examination a sense of emptiness in the upper right abdomen may be appreciated. The rumen is small when the case is of several weeks' duration and the distended abomasum is only rarely palpable to its left. In occasional cases there is chronic ruminal tympany and the rumen is distended. Untreated animals usually reach a certain level of inanition and then remain static for long periods.

Cows which were fat at the time of parturition may develop severe ketosis and the fatty liver syndrome. The disease is not usually fatal but affected animals are usually less than satisfactory production units (22).

Occasional cases occur in cows which are clinically normal in all other respects. In one case, a cow had an LDA, which was confirmed at necropsy, for 1·5 years, during which time she calved twice and ate and produced milk normally (22).

In anterior displacement the clinical findings are very similar to those described above except that normal ruminal sounds can be heard in the usual position and gurgling sounds characteristic of a distended abomasum are heard just behind and above the heart and on both sides of the chest. If a rumenotomy is performed the distended abomasum can be felt between the reticulum and diaphragm (23).

The course of the disease is extremely variable. Untreated animals usually reach a certain level of inanition and then remain static for several weeks or even a few months. Milk production decreases to a small volume and the animals becomes thin with the abdomen greatly reduced in size.

A paroxysmal atrial fibrillation is present in some cases which is considered to be caused by a concurrent metabolic alkalosis. Following surgical correction the arrhythmia usually disappears.

In calves, the clinical findings include inappetence, reduced weight gain, recurrent distension of the left paralumbar fossa and a metabolic 'ping' and fluid-splashing sounds on auscultation and percussion of the left flank (26).

Clinical pathology

There are no marked changes in the blood picture unless there is intercurrent disease, particularly traumatic reticuloperitonitis or abomasal ulcer. A moderate to severe ketonuria is always present but the blood glucose level is within the normal range.

Paracentesis of the displaced abomasum through the tenth or eleventh intercostal space in the middle third of the abdominal wall will reveal the presence of fluid with no protozoa and a pH of 2. Ruminal fluid will have protozoa and a pH of between 6 and 7. There is usually a mild hemoconcentration evidenced by elevations of the PCV, hemoglobin and total serum protein. A mild metabolic alkalosis with slight hypochloremia and hypokalemia may also be present (24). A mild hypocalcemia is usually present but parturient hypocalcemia is uncommon. Fluid is not always present in appreciable quantity in the abomasum and a negative result on puncture cannot be interpreted as eliminating the possibility of abomasal displacement.

Necropsy findings

The disease is not usually fatal but carcasses of affected animals are sometimes observed at abattoirs. The displaced abomasum is trapped between the rumen and the ventral abdominal floor and contains variable amounts of fluid and gas. In occasional cases it is fixed in position by adhesions which usually arise from an abomasal ulcer.

Diagnosis

Left-side displacement of the abomasum occurs most commonly in cows within a few days after parturition and is characterized by gauntness, a relatively slab-sided left abdomen and secondary ketosis. The characteristic tympanitic sounds are usually audible with percussion and auscultation. The presence of secondary ketosis in a cow immediately after parturition should arouse suspicion of the disease. Primary ketosis usually occurs in cows 2–6 weeks after calving with a history that they have produced well since calving. The response to treatment of primary ketosis is usually permanent when treated early, while the response to treatment of the ketosis due to LDA is temporary and a relapse in a few days is common.

Traumatic reticuloperitonitis is accompanied by ruminal stasis, mild fever, a grunt on deep palpation over the xiphoid sternum and possibly a slight neutrophilia with a regenerative left shift. However, in subacute and chronic traumatic reticuloperitonitis a painful grunt may be absent, the temperature and hemogram may be normal and on auscultation and percussion the atonic rumen may be mistaken for an LDA. The tympanitic sounds from an atonic rumen, however, are usually not as high-pitched and occur over a larger area than with an LDA. In some cases an exploratory laparotomy is necessary to distinguish between the two, although peritoneoscopy and abdominocentesis may be alternatives. Vagus indigestion is usually manifested by abdominal distension due to a grossly distended rumen with or without an enlarged abomasum and is more common before parturition. Diaphragmatic hernia is characterized by chronic ruminal tympany and abdominal enlargement.

Treatment

Surgical replacement is now commonly practiced and many techniques have been devised with emphasis on avoidance of recurrence of the displacement (1, 25). A right flank laparotomy and omentopexy are now in common use and excellent results are claimed (27). A right paramedian abomasopexy is also used. A few closed suturing abomasopexy techniques have been advocated (37), but the complications which can occur indicate that laparotomy and omentopexy are desirable (38, 39). Complications include peritonitis, cellulitis, abomasal displacement or evisceration, complete forestomach obstruction, and thrombophlebitis of the subscutaneous abdominal vein (39). In the blind suture technique, the precise location of insertion of the sutures is unknown. The surgical repair of the common diseases of the abomasum of cattle has been reviewed (14). The surgical correction of left-side displacement of the abomasum is reviewed (35).

Rolling and manipulation have produced moderately good results for some workers but relapses occur. The cow is cast and laid on her back, then rolled vigorously to the right and the roll stopped abruptly in the hope that the abomasum will free itself. Chances of success are greatest in the advanced stages when the rumen is small. Starvation and restriction of fluid for 2 days before may be advisable. Violent exercise and transport over bumpy roads has on occasion caused spontaneous recovery. The use of parenteral glucose and oral propylene glycol is necessary for the treatment of the ketosis and to avoid fatty liver as a complication. All cases of LDA should be corrected as soon as possible to minimize the incidence of peritoneal adhesions and abomasal ulcers which may perforate and cause sudden death (20).

Control

Because the etiology and pathogenesis of LDA are uncertain it is not possible to make definitive recommendations for the control or prevention of the disease. However, if abomasal atony due to grain feeding in late pregnancy combined with the relative inactivity of late pregnancy, especially in housed cows, are important predisposing causes, it would seem logical to approach prevention by feeding large quantities of forage during late pregnancy and ensuring that housed cows are exercised daily. Every effort should be used to minimize dietary alterations near parturition which could result in indigestion. The amount of grain and corn silage fed prepartum should be at minimum, while other forages are fed *ad libitum* (2). Several experiments have shown no response in production to lead feeding, started before parturition, when cows were in good condition at drying-off and were fed well following parturition (2). Consequently, there seems little reason to continue the practice of steaming-up cows before parturition.

REFERENCES

(1) Wallace, C. E. (1975) *Bov. Practnr*, *10*, 50, 56.
(2) Coppock, C. E. (1974) *J. dairy Sci.*, *57*, 926.
(3) Svendsen, P. (1970) *Nord. VetMed.*, *22*, 571.
(4) Svendsen, P. (1969) *Nord. VetMed.*, *21*, Suppl. 1, viii.
(5) Grymer, J. et al. (1981). *Nord. VetMed.*, *33*, 306.
(6) Robertson, J. McD. (1968) *Am. J. vet. Res.*, *29*, 421.
(7) Martin, W (1972) *Can. vet. J.*, *13*, 61.
(8) Willeberg, P. et al (1982). *Nord. VetMed.*, *34*, 404.
(9) Grymer, J. et al. (1982). *Nord. VetMed.*, *34*, 412.
(10) Sack, W. O. (1968) *Am. J. vet. Res.*, *31*, 1539.
(11) Svendsen, P. E. (1975) In: *Proc. 4th int. Symp. Ruminant Physiol.*, 563.
(12) Pinsent, P. J. N. et al. (1961) *Vet. Rec.*, *73*, 729
(13) Hull, B. L. & Wass, W. M. (1973) *Vet. Med. small Anim. Clin.*, *412*, 414.
(14) Pearson, H. (1973) *Vet. Rec.*, *92*, 245.
(15) Martin, S. W. et al. (1978) *Can. J. comp. Med.*, *42*, 511.
(16) Poulsen, J. S. D. (1976) *Nord. VetMed.*, *28*, 299.
(17) Poulsen, J. S. D. (1974) *Nord. VetMed.*, *26*, 1.
(18) Poulsen, J. S. D. & Jones, B. E. V. (1974) *Nord. VetMed.*, *26*, 22.
(19) Sack, W. O. (1968) *Am. J. vet. Res.*, *29*, 567.
(20) Stewart, D. H. (1973) *Vet. Rec.*, *92*, 462.
(21) Wallace, C. E. (1976) *Bov. Practnr*, *11*, 62.
(22) Ingling, A. L. et al. (1975) *J. Am. vet. med. Assoc.*, *166*, 601.
(23) Watering, C. C. v. d. et al. (1975) *Tijdschr. Diergeneeskd.*, *90*, 1478.
(24) Poulsen, J. S. D. (1974) *Nord. VetMed.*, *26*, 91.
(25) Gabel, A. A. & Heath, R. B. (1969) *J. Am. vet. med. Assoc.*, *155*, 632.
(26) Dirksen, G. (1982) *Bov. Pract.*, *17*, 75.
(27) Lagerweij, E. & Numans, S. R. (1968) *Tijdschr. Diergeneeskd.*, *93*, 366.
(28) Markusfield, O. (1986). *Prev. vet. Med. 4*, 173.
(29) Sutherland, F. R. (1984). *Vet. Rec.*, *115*, 33.
(30) Martin, S. W. et al. (1978) *Can. vet. J.*, *19*, 250.
(31) Breukink, H. J. & de Ruyter, T. (1976) *Am. J. vet. Res. 37*, 1181.
(32) Markusfield, O. (1977) *Refuah Vet.*, *34*, 11.
(33) Hesselholt, M. & Grymer, J. (1978) *Dansk Vet.*, *61*, 853.
(34) Varden, S. A. (1979) *Nord. VetMed.*, *31*, 106.
(35) Edwards, G. B. (1979) *Vet. Ann.*, *19*, 61.
(36) Gyang, E. O. et al., (1986). *Am. J. vet. Res.*, *47*, 429.
(37) Grymer, J. & Sterner, K. E. (1982). *J. Am. vet. med. Assoc.*, *180*, 1458.
(38) Rutgers, L. J. E. & Van DerVelden, M. A. (1983). *Vet. Rec.*, *113*, 225.
(39) Tithoff, P. K. & Rebbun, W. C. (1986). *J. Am. vet. med. Assoc.*, *189*, 1489.

Dilatation and right-side displacement and torsion of the abomasum

Abomasal dilatation, or right-side displacement as it is sometimes called, is a subacute disease which occurs in mature cows within a few weeks after calving and is characterized by inappetence, depression, dehydration and gradual distension of the right side of the abdomen, due to accumulation of fluid and gas in the abomasum. It is probably a common, but not a necessary, precursor to abomasal torsion, which is an acute obstruction of the alimentary tract and is manifested by severe abdominal pain, a short course and a high mortality rate.

Etiology and epidemiology

Dilatation and torsion of the abomasum occur in adult dairy cows usually within the period 3–6 weeks after calving (1–4). The disease is being recognized with increased frequency because of improvements in diagnostic techniques, and perhaps because more cows are being fed intensively for milk production. The cause of the dilatation is thought to be that a primary distension of the abomasum occurs because of either obstruction of the pylorus or primary atony of the abomasal musculature. Most cases have no apparent obstruction at the pylorus and atony of the abomasum seems to be the more likely cause. It seems likely that the atony is caused by an interplay of grain feeding, relative inactivity during winter housing and the stress of parturition. The frequency of the disease appears to be higher in Scandinavia than elsewhere. The epidemiological factors have not been identified but it is thought that indoor winter feeding and the shift of the acid–base balance to an alkalotic state during the winter months may be important factors (5). In Denmark, the ingestion of large quantities of soil particles on unwashed root crops used as feed is thought to be significant. This may be the reason for the higher incidence of the disease in the later part of the winter (4). However, attempts to reproduce the condition by feeding large quantities of sand have been unsuccessful (6). Because atony is often associated with vagus indigestion, a relationship between the two has been suspected but there are usually no lesions affecting the reticulum or vagus nerves. The disease occurs in young calves from a few weeks of age up to 6 months and there may not be a history of previous illness, which suggests that the cause may be accidental (7, 8).

Pathogenesis

In right-side displacement of the abomasum it would appear that abomasal atony occurs initially, resulting in the accumulation of fluid and gas in the viscus leading to gradual distension and displacement in a caudal direction on the right side (dilatation phase). During the dilatation phase which commonly extends over several days, there is continuous secretion of hydrochloric acid, sodium chloride, and potassium into the abomasum, which becomes gradually distended and does not evacuate its contents into the duodenum (4, 9). This leads to dehydration and metabolic alkalosis with hypochloremia and hypokalemia (10). These changes are representative of a functional obstruction (paralytic ileus) of the upper part of the intestinal tract and occur in experimental right-side displacement of the abomasum (11) and experimental obstruction of the duodenum in calves (12). Up to 35 liters of fluid may accumulate in the dilated abomasum of a mature 450 kg cow and the dehydration will vary from 5 to 12% of body weight. In uncomplicated cases, there is only slight hemoconcentration and a mild electrolyte and acid–base imbalance, with moderate distension of the abomasum. These cases are reversible with fluid therapy. In complicated cases there is severe hemoconcentration and marked metabolic alkalosis with a severely distended abomasum. In cattle with severe and prolonged abomasal torsion, a metabolic acidosis may develop and be superimposed on the metabolic alkalosis leading to a low base excess concentration of extracellular fluid (26). These require surgery and intensive fluid therapy. A paradoxic aciduria may occur in cattle affected with metabolic alkalosis associated with abomasal disease (13). This may be due to the excretion of acid by the kidney in response to severe potassium depletion or the excretion of acid metabolites as a result of starvation, dehydration and impaired renal function.

Following the dilatation phase, the distended abomasum may twist in a clockwise or anticlockwise (viewed from the right side) direction in a vertical plane around a horizontal axis passing transversely across the body in the vicinity of the omasoabomasal orifice. The torsion will usually be of the order of 180–270° and causes a syndrome of acute obstruction with local circulatory impairment and ischemic necrosis of the abomasum. Detailed examinations of necropsy specimens of torsion of the abomasum indicate that the displacements can occur in a dual axial system (22). One system relates to displacements of the abomasum on a pendulum model, the point of suspension being situated on the visceral surface of the liver and the arms consisting of parts of the digestive tract adjacent to the abomasum. The other system comprises axes centered on the abomasum, about which this organ is able to rotate without changing its position in the abdomen. A theoretical analysis of the types of displacement of the abomasum which can occur is described (22).

In some cases the abomasum and omasum are greatly distended and form a loop with the cranial part of the duodenum (24). This loop may twist up to 360° in a counterclockwise direction as viewed from the rear or from the right side of the cow. The reticulum is drawn caudally on the right side of the rumen by its attachment to the fundus of the abomasum. The probable mode of rotation is in a sagittal plane. Pressure and tension damage to the ventral vagal nerve trunk and to the blood vessels are in part responsible for the poor prognosis in severe cases even after successful surgical correction.

There are varying degrees of dehydration, hypochloremia, alkalosis and circulatory failure (14).

There is speculation that violent exercise and transportation may be contributory factors in the pathogenesis of acute abomasal torsion which occurs occasionally in mature cows and young calves without a history of immediate previous illness associated with the dilatation phase. The metabolic changes which occur are similar to those described above.

Clinical findings

In right-side dilatation and displacement of the abomasum (4, 9) there is usually a history of calving within the last few weeks and inappetence, poor milk production and abnormal feces. The cow may have been treated for an uncertain disorder of the digestive tract. Anorexia is usually complete when the abomasum is distended. There is usually depression, dehydration, no interest in feed, perhaps increased thirst and sometimes muscular weakness. Many affected cows will sip water continuously from a water bowl. The temperature is usually normal, the heart rate will vary from normal to 100/minute, and the respirations are usually within the normal range. The mucous membrances are usually a pale, muddy color. The rumen is usually static. The distended abomasum may be detectable on palpation immediately behind and below the right costal arch. Deep palpation and percussion will reveal what feels and sounds like a fluid-filled viscus because of the fluid-splashing sounds. In many cases the distension continues and after 3–4 days the abdomen becomes obviously distended on the right side and the abomasum can be palpated on rectal examination. It may completely fill the right lower half of the abdomen. The wall of the distended abomasum is fairly tense and is filled with fluid and gas. Auscultation and simultaneous percussion will commonly elicit high-pitched tympanitic sounds in those which contain considerable quantities of gas. This dilatation phase may last as long as 10–14 days before torsion of the abomasum occurs. In severely distended cases, affected cattle become recumbent with a grossly distended abdomen and grunt with each respiration. A rectal examination is very important at this stage. In the dilatation stage the partially distended abomasum may be palpable with the tips of the fingers in the right lower quadrant of the abdomen. It may not be palpable in large-sized cows. In the torsion phase, the distended tense resilient viscus is usually palpable in the right abdomen anywhere from the upper to the lower quadrant.

The feces are usually scant, soft and dark in color. The soft feces must not be mistaken for a diarrhea, as is commonly done by the owner of the animal. Cattle with abomasal torsion usually become recumbent within 24 hours after the onset of the torsion. Death usually occurs in 48–96 hours from shock and dehydration. Rupture of the abomasum may occur and cause sudden death.

In calves with acute abomasal torsion, there is a sudden onset of anorexia, acute abdominal pain with kicking at the belly, depression of the back, bellowing and straining. The heart rate is usually 120–160/minute, the abdomen is distended and tense, and auscultation and percussion over the right flank reveal distinct highpitched tympanitic sounds. Palpation behind the right costal arch reveals a tense viscus and the animal resents the palpation.

In acute abomasal torsion in adult cattle there is a

sudden onset of abdominal pain with kicking at the abdomen, depression of the back and crouching. The heart rate is usually increased to 100–120/minute, the temperature is subnormal, and there is peripheral circulatory failure. The animal feels cold, the mucous membrances are pale, dry and cold. The abdomen is grossly distended on the right side and auscultation and percussion reveal the tympanitic sounds of a gas-filled viscus. Fluid-splashing sounds are audible on percussion. Paracentesis of the distended abomasum will usually reveal large quantities of blood-tinged fluid with a pH from 2 to 4. The distended abomasum can usually be palpated on rectal examination but the torsion may have moved it in a cranial direction and not uncommonly these are not as readily palpable as when only dilated. The feces are scant, soft and dark in color and become bloodstained or melenic in the ensuing 48 hours if the cow lives long enough. In some cases there is profuse watery diarrhea.

The severity of torsion of the abomasum can be classified, and the prognosis evaluated, according to the amount of fluid in the abomasum and the concentration of serum chloride and the heart rate (18). Group 1—abomasum distended principally with gas; group 2—abomasum distended with gas and fluid, and surgical reduction possible without removal of fluid; group 3—abomasum distended with gas and fluid, 1–29 liters of fluid removed before reduction of abomasum; group 4—abomasum distended with gas and fluid, more than 30 liters of fluid removed before reduction of torsion. The serum chloride levels and heart rates before surgery are also valuable prognostic aids. Cows classified as groups 3 or 4 or those having presurgical chloride levels equal to or below 79 mEq/l (79 mmol/l) or pulse rates equal to or greater than 100/minute have a poor prognosis. The base excess concentration of the extracellular fluid can be a useful prognostic and diagnostic indicator in cows with abomasal torsion or right displacement of the abomasum (26). In one retrospective study cows with a base excess of ≤ −5·0 mEq/l (−5·0 mmol/l) had abomasal torsion rather than displacement. The survival rate of cows with abomasal torsion was 50% with a base excess ≤ −0·1 mEq/l (−0·1 mmol/l) whereas it was 84% if the base excess was ≤ 10·0 mEq/l (10·0 mmol/l) (26).

The evaluation of the degree of circulatory insufficiency, dehydration and the levels of base excess and blood lactates are also used (19) but less reliable. Postoperatively decreased gastrointestinal motility is an unfavorable prognostic sign.

Clinical pathology

There are varying degrees of hemoconcentration (increased PCV and total serum proteins), metabolic alkalosis, hypochloremia and hypokalemia (5). Paradoxic aciduria may also be present. The total and differential leukocyte count may indicate a stress reaction in the early stages, and in the later stages of torsion there may be leukopenia with a neutropenia and degenerative left shift due to ischemic necrosis of the abomasum and early peritonitis. Paracentesis of the distended abomasum will yield large quantities of fluid without protozoa and a pH of from 2 to 4. The fluid may be serosanguineous when torsion is present.

Necropsy findings

In abomasal dilatation the abomasum is grossly distended with fluid and some gas. The rumen may contain an excessive amount of fluid. In some cases there may be impaction of the pylorus with particles of soil or sand and there may be an accompanying pyloric ulcer. In acute torsion the abomasum is grossly distended with brownish, sanguineous fluid and is twisted usually in a clockwise direction (viewed from the right side), often with displacement of the omasum, reticulum and abomasum. In complete torsion the wall of the abomasum is grossly hemorrhagic and gangrenous and may have ruptured.

Diagnosis

Conditions responsible for right-side tympanitic resonance (ping) include dilatation and distension of the abomasum, cecum, cranial duodenum, parts of the small intestine, descending colon and rectum and pneumoperitoneum (25).

The evaluation of pings audible over the right abdomen is dependent upon the size and location of the sound elicited by percussion and simultaneous auscultation (25). In dilatation and right-side displacement of the abomasum the ping is usually audible between the 9th and 12th ribs extending from the costochondral junction of the ribs to their proximal third aspects. Rarely will the ping extend into the paralumbar fossa in right-side dilatation and displacement. In torsion of the abomasum, the area of the ping is typically larger than that of the right-side displacement and extends more cranially and caudally, often extending into the right paralumbar fossa but not completely filling the fossa. Also, the ventral border of the ping area in a torsion is variable, often horizontal because of the level of fluid within the abomasum. In a cecal dilatation, the ping is usually confined to the dorsal paralumbar fossa and caudal one or two intercostal spaces. In dilatation and torsion of the cecum the ping usually fills the paralumbar fossa and extends cranially and caudally the equivalent of two rib spaces. The ascending colon is often involved in a torsion of the cecum which will result in an enlarged ping area extending from the paralumbar fossa. Dilatation of the ascending colon may yield a ping centered over the proximal aspects of the 12th and 13th ribs. The presence of multiple, small areas of ping which varies in pitch and intensity is characteristic of dilatation of the jejunoileum caused by intussusception or intestinal volvulus. A ping in the right caudal abdomen just ventral to the transverse processes of the vertebrae indicates dilatation of the descending colon and rectum which is commonly heard following rectal examination. In pneumoperitoneum, pings may be audible over a wide area of the dorsal third of the abdomen bilaterally. In one study, the sensitivity and predictive values of abomasum as the source of the ping were 98% and 96% respectively; for cecum and/or ascending colon, the sensitivity and predictive values were both 87%.

The important clinical features of dilatation and right-side displacement of the abomasum are: recent calving, an uncertain indigestion since calving, soft scant feces, and the presence of the distended organ in the right lower flank. Impaction of the abomasum with vagus indigestion presents a similar clinical picture but the rumen is usually distended with fluid and the impacted abomasum may be palpable as a firm, doughy mass behind the lower aspect of the costal arch, situated on the floor of the abdomen, whereas most cases of dilatation are situated more dorsally adjacent to the right paralumbar fossa. Tympanitic sounds are audible on percussion and auscultation of dilatation and torsion of the abomasum and not in abomasal impaction. At laparotomy the difference is obvious. Subacute abomasal ulceration with moderate dilatation of the abomasum in a recently calved cow may not be distinguishable clinically from right-side displacement of the abomasum. The presence of melena suggests abomasal ulcers but these may be present as secondary complications in dilatation and right-side displacement. In cecal torsion there may be distension of the right flank, tympanitic sounds on auscultation and percussion, and the cecum can usually be palpated and identified tentatively, on rectal examination, as a long (60–80 cm), usually easily movable, cylindrical, tense tube (10–20 cm in diameter), with a blind sac. In fetal hydrops, the distended gravid uterus can be palpated on rectal examination. Some cases of abomasal dilatation will resemble chronic or subacute traumatic reticuloperitonitis, but in the latter there may be a grunt on deep palpation, the feces are usually firm and dry, the abdomen is gaunt and a mild fever may be present. However, a laparotomy may be necessary to make the diagnosis. A paracentesis may be useful.

In abomasal torsion there is abdominal distension of the right side, tympanitic sounds on percussion, muscular weakness and circulatory failure with heart rate up to 120/minute. In intestinal obstruction, there is usually a history of sudden onset, the feces are scant and may be blood-tinged and the affected portion of the intestines or loops of distended intestines may be palpable rectally. Acute diffuse peritonitis as a sequel to local peritonitis in a cow soon after calving may be indistinguishable from acute torsion of the abomasum. There is severe toxemia, dehydration, abdominal distension, grunting, weakness, recumbency and rapid death. Paracentesis of the peritoneal cavity will assist in the diagnosis.

Treatment

The prognosis in right-side dilatation, displacement and torsion is favorable if the diagnosis is made within a few days after the onset of clinical signs before large quantities of fluid accumulate in the abomasum. Slaughter and salvage may be the best course of action for cattle of commercial value. Cows with considerable economic worth can be treated as outlined here. Not all cases require surgical correction; medical treatment is possible in mild cases.

In mild cases with minimal systemic disturbance, treatment with 500–1000 ml of 25% calcium borogluconate intravenously will yield good results. Affected cows are offered good quality hay but no grain for 3–5 days and monitored daily. Surgical correction may not be necessary if the appetite and movements of the alimentary tract return to normal in a few days. The ping in the right flank may gradually become smaller in 2–3 days and eventually disappear. In mild cases of dilatation with only slight hemoconcentration and metabolic alkalosis, early treatment with fluids and electrolytes intravenously and orally will often yield good results. The fluid therapy is essential to restore motility of the gastrointestinal tract, particularly the abomasum which is distended with fluid and must begin evacuating its contents into the duodenum for absorption of the electrolytes to occur. The cow will usually not regain her appetite until the abomasal atony has been corrected. Mineral oil (5–10 litres/day orally) and magnesium hydroxide (500 g per adult cow orally every 2 days) are used commonly in an attempt to evacuate the contents of the abomasum. However, it is probably more important to restore the fluid and electrolyte imbalances.

In the more advanced cases of dilatation, displacement and torsion, a right flank laparotomy for drainage of the distended abomasum and correction of the torsion if present is necessary (15). The surgical techniques in common use have been described (16). Intensive fluid therapy is usually necessary preoperatively and for several days postoperatively to correct the dehydration, metabolic alkalosis and to restore normal abomasal motility. Electromyographic studies of the postoperative abomasal and duodenal motility reveal loss of motility, some retrograde motility and loss of spike activity (23). Cholinergics have been used to help restore motility (17) but are not reliable. Rumen transplants to restore rumen function and appetite will provide a more effective stimulus to restore gastrointestinal tract motility.

The composition of the fluids and electrolyte solutions which are indicated in right-side displacement and abomasal torsion has been a subject of much investigation. There are varying degrees of dehydration, metabolic alkalosis, hypochloremia and hypokalemia. With the aid of a laboratory it is possible to monitor the serum biochemistry during the administration of the fluids and electrolytes and to correct certain electrolyte deficits by adding ('spiking') the appropriate electrolytes to the fluids. Without a laboratory, the veterinarian has no choice but to use the solutions which are considered safe and judicious. Balanced electrolyte solutions containing sodium, chloride, potassium, calcium and a source of glucose will commonly suffice. Isotonic solutions of potassium chloride and ammonium chloride (KCl 108 g, NH_4Cl 80 g, H_2O 20 liters) will provide a source of potassium and chloride and will correct the alkalosis. This solution can be given intravenously at the rate of 20 liters over 4 hours to a 450 kg cow. This may be followed by the use of balanced electrolyte solutions at the rate of 100–150 ml/kg body weight over a 24-hour period. However, acidifying solutions such as potassium and ammonium chloride must be used carefully and ideally the serum biochemistry should be monitored every hour to ensure that acidosis does not occur. The above solutions are considered safe when given as described. A mixture of 2 liters of isotonic saline (0·85%), 1 liter of isotonic potassium chloride (1·1%) and 1 liter isotonic dextrose (5%) given at the rate of 4–6 l/hour intravenously is also recommended and reliable (20). Normal saline is also effective and potassium solutions may not be necessary unless there is severe hypokalemia (21). Oral electrolyte therapy has been recommended, particularly in the postoperative period following surgical drainage of the distended abomasum.

A mixture of sodium chloride (50–100 g), potassium chloride (50 g) and ammonium chloride (50–100 g) is given daily for a few days postoperatively along with the parenteral fluids as necessary (4). Treatment with potassium chloride (50 g/day) orally can be continued daily until the cow resumes her normal appetite.

REFERENCES

(1) Ide, P. R. & Henry, J. H. (1964) *Can. vet. J.*, *5*, 46.q
(2) Espersen, G. (1964) *Vet. Res.*, *76*, 1423.
(3) Neal, P. A. & Pinsent, P. J. N. (1960) *Vet. Rec.*, *72*, 175.
(4) Poulsen, J. S. D. (1974) *Nord. VetMed.*, *26*, 65.
(5) Poulsen, J. S. D. (1976) *Nord. VetMed.*, *28*, 299.
(6) Svendsen, P. (1965) *Nord. VetMed.*, *17*, 500.
(7) Macleod, N. S. M. (1964) *Vet. Rec.*, *76*, 223.
(8) Martin, J. A. (1964) *Vet. Rec.*, *76*, 297.
(9) Espersen, G. & Simesen, M. G. (1961) *Nord. VetMed.*, *13*, 147.
(10) Whitlock, R. H. et al. (1975) *Am. J. digest. Dis.*, *20*, 595.
(11) Svenden, P. (1969) *Nord. VetMed.*, *21*, Suppl. I, 1–60.
(12) Hammond, P. B. et al. (1964) *J. comp. Pathol. Therap.*, *74*, 210.
(13) Gingerich, D. A. & Murdick, P. W. (1975) *J. Am. vet. med. Assoc.*, *166*, 227.
(14) Pearson, H. (1973) *Vet. Rec.*, *92*, 245.
(15) Baker, J. S. (1976) *Bov. Practnr*, *11*, 58.
(16) Hofmeyer, C. F. B. (1974) In: *Textbook of Large Animal Surgery*, eds F. W. Oehme & J. S. Prier. Baltimore: Williams and Wilkins.
(17) Olson, V. E. & Krumm, D. (1876) *Mod. vet. Pract.*, *57*, 195.
(18) Smith, S. D. (1978) *J. Am. vet. med. Assoc.*, *173*, 108.
(19) Hjortkjaer, R. K. & Svendsen, C. K. (1979) *Nord. VetMed.*, *31*, Suppl. II, 1.
(20) McGuirk, S. M. & Butler, D. G. (1980) *J. Am. vet. med. Assoc.*, *177*, 551.
(21) Easley, R. (1981) *J. Am. vet. med. Assoc.*, *178*, 4.
(22) Wensvoort, P. & van der Veldrn, M. A. (1980) *Vet. Q.* *2*, 125.
(23) Ooms, L. et al. (1978) *Vlaams Diergeneeskd. Tijdschr.*, *47*, 113.
(24) Habel, R. E. & Smith, D. F. (1981) *J. Am. vet. med. Assoc.*, *179*, 447.
(25) Smith, D. F. et al. (1982) *Cornell Vet.*, *72*, 180.
(26) Simpson, D. F. et al. (1985). *Am. J. vet. Res.*, *46*, 796.
(27) Frazee, L. S. (1984). *Can. vet. J.*, *25*, 293.

Dietary abomasal impaction in cattle

Dietary abomasal impaction occurs in cattle in the prairie provinces of western Canada during the cold winter months and elsewhere when the animals are fed poor quality roughage. The disease is most common in pregnant beef cattle which increase their feed intake during extremely cold weather in an attempt to meet the increased needs of a higher metabolic rate (1). The disease has also occurred in feedlot cattle fed a variety of mixed rations containing chopped or ground roughage (straw, hay) and cereal grains and in late pregnant dairy cows on similar feeds.

Etiology and epidemiology

The cause of the disease is considered to be the consumption of excessive quantities of poor quality roughages which are low in both digestible protein and energy (7). Cattle can also become affected with impaction of the abomasum with sand if they are fed hay on sandy soils or root crops which are sandy or dirty (2). Outbreaks of impaction with sand have occurred in which up to 10% of cattle at risk were affected.

The disease occurs most commonly in young pregnant beef cows which are kept outdoors year round, including during the cold winter months, when they are fed roughages consisting of either grass or legume hay or cereal straw, which may or may not be supplemented with some grain. In these circumstances cows commonly lose 10–15% of their total body weight from October to May and even more during very cold winters. In one retrospective study of the necropsy reports of cattle which died with abomasal impaction, 20% of the animals had lesions of traumatic reticuloperitonitis, 60% were thought to be due to the ingestion of too much poor quality roughage without a supplement of concentrate, and 20% did not fit into either category (8).

When large quantities of long roughage without sufficient grain are fed during very cold weather, the cattle cannot eat sufficient feed to satisfy energy needs so that the roughage is then provided in a chopped form. The chopped roughage is commonly mixed with some grain in a mix mill but usually at an insufficient level to meet the energy requirements. Cattle can and do eat more of these chopped roughage–grain mixtures than of long roughage because the smaller particles pass through the forestomachs at a more rapid rate. But impaction of the abomasum, omasum and rumen may occur because of the relative indigestibility of the roughage. Outbreaks may occur affecting up to 15% of all pregnant cattle on individual farms when the ambient temperature drops down to −10 to −30°C (14 to −22°F) for several days.

The disease has also occurred in feedlot cattle fed similar rations (e.g. 80% roughage, 20% grain) in an attempt to reduce the high cost of grain feeding and to satisfy beef grading standards which put the emphasis on producing a smaller amount of fat cover. With these constraints and the increased emphasis on roughage feeding, it is possible that the incidence of abomasal impaction may increase in feedlot cattle.

Pathogenesis

Chopped roughage and finely ground feeds pass through the forestomachs of ruminants more quickly than long roughage and perhaps in this situation the combination of low digestibility and excessive intake leads to excessive accumulation in the forestomachs and abomasum.

When large quantities of sand are ingested, the omasum, abomasum, large intestine and cecum can become impacted. The sand which accumulates in the abomasum causes abomasal atony and chronic dilatation.

Once impaction of the abomasum occurs a state of subacute obstruction of the upper alimentary tract develops. The hydrogen and chloride ions are continually secreted into the abomasum in spite of the impaction and atony and an alkalosis with hypochloremia results. Varying degrees of dehydration occur because fluids are not moving beyond the abomasum into the duodenum for absorption. The potassium ions are also sequestered in the abomasum resulting in a hypokalemia. Almost no ingesta or fluids move beyond the pylorus, and dehydration, alkalosis, electrolyte imbalance and progressive starvation occur. The impaction of the abomasum is usually severe enough to cause permanent abomasal atony.

Clinical findings

Complete anorexia, scant feces and moderate distension of the abdomen are the usual presenting complaints given by the owner. Cattle which have been affected for several days have lost considerable weight and are too weak to rise. The body temperature is usually normal but may be subnormal during cold weather which suggests that the specific dynamic action of the rumen is not sufficient to meet energy needs of basal metabolism. The heart rate varies from normal to 90–100/minute and may increase to 120/minute in advanced cases where alkalosis, hypochloremia and dehydration are marked. The respiratory rate is commonly increased and an expiratory grunt due to the abdominal distension may be audible especially in recumbent cattle. A mucoid nasal discharge usually collects on the external nares and muzzle which is usually dry and cracking due to the failure of the animal to lick its nostrils, and to the effects of the dehydration.

The rumen is usually static and full of dry rumen contents, or it may contain an excessive quantity of fluid in those cattle which have been fed finely ground feed. The pH of the ruminal fluid is usually within the normal range (6·5–7·0). The rumen protozoan activity ranges from normal to a marked reduction in numbers and activity as assessed on a low power field. The impacted abomasum is usually situated in the right lower quadrant of the abdomen on the floor of the abdominal wall. It usually extends caudally beyond the right costal arch but may or may not be easily palpable because of the gravid uterus, but an impacted omasum may also be palpable. It may be impossible, however, to distinguish between an impacted abomasum and an impacted omasum. In feedlot steers and non-pregnant heifers the impacted abomasum and omasum may be easily palpable on rectal examination. Deep palpation and strong percussion of the right flank may elicit a 'grunt' as is common in acute traumatic reticuloperitonitis and this is probably due to overdistension of the abomasum and stretching of serosa of the abomasum.

The course of the disease depends on the extent of the impaction when the animal is first examined and the severity of the acid–base and electrolyte imbalance. Severely affected cattle will die in 3–6 days after the onset of signs. Rupture of the abomasum has occurred in some cases and death from acute diffuse peritonitis and shock occurs precipitously in a few hours. In sand impaction, there is considerable weight loss, chronic diarrhea with sand in the feces, weakness, recumbency and death within a few weeks.

Severe impaction and distension of the rumen and the abomasum can occur in cattle given access to large quantities of finely chopped straw during the cold winter months. There is gross distension of the abdomen, anorexia, scant dry feces, and affected animals will drop large dry fibrous cuds. The rumen is grossly distended and usually static.

Clinical pathology

A metabolic alkalosis, hypochloremia, hypokalemia, hemoconcentration and a total and differential leukocyte count within the normal range are common.

Necropsy findings

At necropsy the abomasum is commonly grossly enlarged to up to twice normal size and impacted with dry rumen-like contents. The omasum may be similarly enlarged and impacted with the same contents as in the abomasum. The rumen is usually grossly enlarged and filled with dry ruminal contents or ruminal fluid. The intestinal tract beyond the pylorus is characteristically empty and has a dry appearance. Varying degrees of dehydration and emaciation are also present. If rupture of the abomasum occurs, lesions of acute diffuse peritonitis are present. Abomasal tears, ulcers, and necrosis of the walls of the rumen, omasum or abomasum may occur (8).

Diagnosis

The clinical diagnosis of impacted abomasum depends on the nutritional history, the clinical evidence of impaction of the abomasum and the laboratory results. The disease must be differentiated from abomasal impaction as a complication of vagus indigestion, omasal impaction (3), diffuse peritonitis and acute intestinal obstruction due to intestinal accidents or enteroliths and lipomas.

Impaction of the abomasum as a complication of traumatic reticuloperitonitis usually occurs in late pregnancy, commonly only in one animal, a mild fever may or may not be present and there may be a grunt on deep palpation of the xiphoid. The rumen is usually enlarged and may be atonic or hypermotile. Depending on the lesion present a neutrophilia may be present, suggestive of a chronic infection. A hypochloremia is common as in dietary impaction. In many cases it is impossible to distinguish between the two causes of impacted abomasum and a laparotomy may be necessary to explore the abdomen for evidence of peritoneal lesions. Cattle with abomasal impaction as a complication of traumatic reticuloperitonitis are usually a single incident, and have usually been ill for several days, whereas those with dietary impaction have usually been ill for only a few days and more than one may be affected (8). Impaction of the omasum (3) occurs in advanced pregnancy and is characterized by anorexia, scant feces, normal rumen movements, moderate dehydration, and an enlarged omasum which may be palpable per rectum or behind the right costal arch. The serum electrolytes may be within normal limits if the abomasum is normal.

Diffuse peritonitis is characterized by anorexia, toxemia, dehydration, scant feces and a grunt on deep palpation and percussion. However, in peracute cases the abdominal pain may be absent. Fibrinous adhesions may be palpable on rectal examination, and paracentesis may yield some diagnostic peritoneal exudate, but a negative result cannot rule out peritonitis. The presence of a marked leukopenia and neutropenia or a neutrophilia may assist in the diagnosis, but it is often necessary to perform an exploratory laparotomy to confirm the diagnosis. Intestinal obstructions due to intestinal accidents or enteroliths result in anorexia, scant feces, dehydration and abdominal pain, and the abnormality may be palpable on rectal examination. The rumen is usually static and filled with doughy contents. Fluid and gas accumulations in the intestines anterior to the obstruction may be detectable as fluid-splashing sounds by using simultaneous auscultation and succussion of the abdomen.

Treatment

The challenge in treatment is to be able to recognize the cases which will respond to treatment and those which will not and which should, therefore, be slaughtered immediately for salvage. Those which have a severely impacted abomasum and are weak with a marked tachycardia (100–120/minute) are poor treatment risks and should be slaughtered. Rational treatment would appear to consist of correcting the metabolic alkalosis, hypochloremia, hypokalemia and the dehydration, and attempting to move the impacted material with lubricants and cathartics or surgically emptying the abomasum. Balanced electrolyte solutions are infused intravenously on a continuous basis for up to 72 hours at a rate of 100–150 ml/kg body weight over a 24-hour period. Some cases will respond remarkably well to this fluid therapy and begin ruminating and passing feces in 48 hours. The use of acidifying isotonic solutions of mixtures of ammonium chloride and potassium chloride at a rate of 20 liters per 24-hour period for a 450 kg animal as described under the treatment for right-side displacement is also recommended.

Dioctyl sodium sulfosuccinate is administered into the rumen by stomach tube at a dose rate of 120–180 ml of a 25% solution for a 450 kg animal repeated daily for 3–5 days. It is mixed with 10 liters of warm water and 10 liters of mineral oil. The amount of mineral oil can be increased to 15 liters/day after the third day and for a few days until recovery is apparent. A beneficial response cannot be expected in less than 24 hours and most cattle which do respond will show improvement by the end of the third day after treatment begins. Cholinergics such as neostigmine, physostigmine, and carbamylcholine have been used but appear not to alter the outcome.

Surgical correction consists of an abomasotomy through a right paramedian approach and removal of the contents of the abomasum. The results are often unsuccessful probably because of abomasal atony which exists and which appears to worsen following surgery. An alternative approach may be to do a rumenotomy, empty the rumen and infuse dioctyl sodium sulfosuccinate directly into the abomasum through the reticulo-omasal orifice in an attempt to soften and promote the evacuation of the contents of the abomasum. The placement of a nasogastric tube into the omasal groove and into the abomasum through a rumenotomy procedure is described (6). Mineral oil can then be pumped into the abomasum at the rate of 2 liters/day for several days. Recovery should occur within 5 to 7 days. A rumenotomy and emptying of the rumen is necessary in the case of severe straw impaction of the rumen.

The induction of parturition using 20 mg of dexamethasone intramuscularly may be indicated in affected cattle which are within 2 weeks of term and in which the response to treatment for a few days has been unsuccessful. Parturition may assist recovery because of a reduction in intra-abdominal volume. In sand impaction, affected cattle should be moved off the sandy soil and fed good hay and a grass mixture containing molasses and minerals. Severely affected cattle should be treated with large daily doses of mineral oil, at least 15 liters/day.

Control

Prevention of the disease is possible by providing the necessary nutrient requirements for wintering pregnant beef cattle with added allowances for cold windy weather when energy needs for maintenance are increased. When low quality roughage is to be used for wintering pregnant beef cattle, it should be analyzed for crude protein and digestible energy. Based on the analysis, grain is usually added to the ration to meet the energy and protein requirements (7). Pregnant beef cows fed a diet of 94% barley straw for 83 days during the cold winter months may consume only 70% of their energy requirements (7). Such straw-based diets must be supplemented with protein and energy (7). During prolonged periods of cold weather, wintering pregnant beef cattle should be given additional amounts of feed to meet the increased feed requirements for maintenance which has been estimated to be 30–40% greater during the colder months than during the warmer months. These increased requirements are due almost equally to both the effects of reduced feed digestibility and the increased maintenance requirements (4).

The published nutrient requirements of beef cattle are guidelines for the nutrition of cattle under average conditions and higher nutrient levels than those indicated may be necessary to provide for maintenance requirements particularly during periods of cold stress (5). Adequate amounts of fresh drinking water should be supplied at all times and the practice of forcing wintering cows to obtain their water requirements from eating snow while on low quality roughage is extremely hazardous. The question of whether or not low-quality roughages should be chopped or ground for wintering pregnant beef cattle is controversial. The daily voluntary intake of low-quality roughage can be increased by chopping or grinding but neither processing method increases quality or digestibility; in fact digestibility is usually decreased. If increased consumption during cold weather exceeds physical capacity and the nutrient requirements are still not satisfied, impaction of the abomasum may occur. Thus during the coldest period of the winter low-quality roughages must be supplemented with concentrated sources of energy such as cereal grains.

REFERENCES

(1) Young, B. A. (1975) *Proc. 3rd Wld Conf. Anim. Prod.*, ed. R. L. Reid. Sydney: Sydney University Press.
(2) Hunter, R. (1975) *J. am. vet. med. Assoc.*, *166*, 1179,
(3) McDonald, J. S. & Witzel, D. A. (1968) *J. Am. vet. med. Assoc.*, *152*, 638.
(4) Christopherson, R. J. (1976) *Can. J. anim. Sci.*, *56*, 201.
(5) National Research Council (1976) *Nutrient Requirements of Beef Cattle*, No. 4, 5th ed. Washington, DC: National Academy of Sciences.
(6) Baker, J. S. (1979) *J. Am. vet. med. Assoc.*, *175*, 1250.
(7) Mathison, G. W. et al. (1981) *Can. J. anim. Sci.*, *61*, 375.
(8) Ashcroft, R. A. (1983) *Can. vet. J.*, *24*, 375.

Abomasal ulcers of cattle

Abomasal ulceration occurs in mature cattle and calves and may cause an acute gastric hemorrhage with indigestion, melena and sometimes perforation resulting in a painful acute local peritonitis or acute diffuse peritonitis and rapid death or a chronic indigestion with only minimal gastric hemorrhage. Some calves have abomasal ulceration at necropsy or slaughter which were subclinical.

Etiology and epidemiology

Many different causes of abomasal ulceration in cattle have been suggested. With the exception of lymphoma of the abomasum and the erosions of the abomasal mucosa which occur in the viral diseases such as bovine virus diarrhea, rinderpest and bovine malignant catarrh, the causes of abomsal ulceration are not well understood. Some studies have shown that acute hemorrhagic abomasal ulcers occur in high-producing mature dairy cows within the first few weeks following parturition (1), while others have found that most acute bleeding ulcers occurred in cows 3–6 months after parturition (2). The close relationship of the disease to parturition has led to the speculation that a combination of the stress of parturition, the onset of lactation and heavy grain feeding is the cause of acute ulceration in dairy cows.

In a recent epidemiological study of acute hemorrhagic abomasal ulceration in cattle there was no association with the stress of calving (2, 3). The incidence was highest in dairy cows during the summer months when the animals were grazing on pasture. There was also a direct association between amount of rainfall, amount of fertilizer used, and stocking rate and the amount of milk produced by affected cows. This suggests that some factor in grass may play an important role in the acute disease in mature dairy cattle.

The prevalence of abomasal ulcers in mature cattle varies depending on the population of animals surveyed. Of cattle admitted to a veterinary teaching hospital over a 4-year period, 2·17% had confirmed abomasal ulcers (14). In surveys at abattoirs the prevalence may reach 6% (1). The case fatality rate for mature cattle with confirmed abomasal ulcers is about 50%, for those with severe blood loss or diffuse peritonitis the case fatality rate is usually 100% (14). Concurrent disease conditions are common in cattle with abomasal ulcers unassociated with lymphosarcoma of the abomasum (16).

The acute disease occurs occasionally in mature dairy and beef bulls particularly following long transportation, prolonged surgical procedures and in painful conditions such as a fractured limb or rupture of the cruciate ligaments of the stifle joint. It is not uncommon for mature high-producing dairy cows in early lactation to develop acute hemorrhagic ulceration of the abomasum following a prolonged illness such as pneumonia or after having been to a cattle show and sale. This suggests that stress may be an important contributing cause. Abomasal ulcers have also been the cause of sudden death in yearling feedlot cattle (4).

Ulcers of the abomasum are common in hand-fed calves when they are weaned from milk or milk replacer and begin to eat roughage (5). Most of these are subclinical and non-hemorrhagic. Non-hemorrhagic abomasal ulcers are also found commonly in veal calves at the time of slaughter. The incidence of abomasal ulcers in milk-fed calves veal calves is higher when the animals have access to roughage than when roughage is not provided (18, 19). The type of roughage may also be a factor; pellets produced from corn silage caused more lesions than pellets produced from barley straw or alfalfa hay (18). Occasionally milk-fed calves under 2 weeks of age are affected by acute hemorrhagic abomasal ulcers which may perforate and cause rapid death. Well-nourished sucking beef calves, 2–4 months of age, may be affected by acute hemorrhagic and perforating abomasal ulcers while they are on summer pasture. Abomasal trichobezoars are commonly present in these calves (12), but whether the hair balls initiated the ulcers or developed after the ulcers is uncertain. The causes of the acute disease in young calves are unknown but by association it appears that some calves are susceptible when they are changing from a diet of low dry matter content (milk or milk replacer) to one of a higher dry matter content (grass, hay, grain). Abomasal ulcers may arise in association with abomasal displacements, impaction or torsion, lymphomatosis, vagus indigestion, or apparently unrelated to other disease. They are a common finding in calves with abomasal hair balls and in calves which have pica as a sequal to chronic enteritis.

Pathogenesis

In man it is thought that any injury to the gastric mucosa allows diffusion of hydrogen ions from the lumen into the tissues of the mucosa and also permits diffusion of pepsin into the different layers of the mucosa resulting in further damage (6, 7). It is probable that the pathogenesis is similar in cattle. There may be only one large ulcer but more commonly there is evidence of many acute and chronic ulcers.

A classification of abomasal ulcers in cattle has been proposed (14) and is presented modified as follows.

Type 1: non-perforating ulcer

There is incomplete penetration of the abomasal wall resulting in a minimal degree of intraluminal hemorrhage, focal abomasal thickening, or local serositis. Non-bleeding chronic ulcers commonly cause a chronic gastritis.

Type 2: ulcer causing severe blood loss

There is penetration of the wall of a major abomasal vessel usually in the submucosa, resulting in severe intraluminal hemorrhage and anemia. In acute ulceration with erosion of a blood vessel there is acute gastric hemorrhage with reflex spasm of the pylorus and accumulation of fluid in the abomasum resulting in distension, metabolic alkalosis and hypochloremia and hypokalemia and hemorrhagic anemia. Usually within 24 hours there is release of some of the abomasal contents into the intestine resulting in melena.

Type 3: perforating ulcer with acute, local peritonitis

There is penetration of the full thickness of the abomasal wall resulting in leakage of abomasal contents. Resulting peritonitis is localized to the region of the perforation by adhesion of the involved portion of abomasum to adjacent viscera, omentum, or the peritoneal surface. Omental bursitis and empyema may develop with the accumulation of a large quantity of exudate and necrotic debris in the omental cavity.

Type 4: perforating ulcer with diffuse peritonitis

There is penetration of the full thickness of the abomasal wall resulting in leakage of abomasal contents. Resulting peritonitis is not localized to the region of the perforation, thus digesta is spread throughout the peritoneal cavity.

In some calves the ulcers are subclinical and the factors which determine how large or how deep an ulcer will become are unknown. Based on abattoir studies it is evident that abomasal ulcers will heal by scar formation.

Clinical findings

The clinical syndrome varies depending on whether ulceration is complicated by hemorrhage or perforation. The pertinent clinical findings of abomasal ulcers in cattle are abdominal pain, melena and pale mucous membranes (14). At least one of these clinical findings will be present in about 70% of cattle with abomasal ulcers. The case fatality rates for cattle with types 1, 2, 3, or 4 are 25, 100, 50 and 100% respectively (14). In the common clinical form of bleeding abomasal ulcers there is a sudden onset of anorexia, mild abdominal pain, tachycardia (90–100/minute), severely depressed milk production and melena. Acute hemorrhage may be severe enough to cause death in less than 24 hours. More commonly there is subacute blood loss over a period of a few days with the development of hemorrhagic anemia. The feces are usually scant, black and tarry. There are occasional bouts of diarrhea. Melena may be present from 4 to 6 days, after which time the cow usually begins to recover or lapses into a stage of chronic ulceration without evidence of hemorrhage.

Perforation is usually followed by acute local peritonitis unless the stomach is overloaded and ruptures, when acute diffuse peritonitis and shock results in death in a few hours (9). With the development of local peritonitis, with or without omental adhesions, there is a chronic illness accompanied by a fluctuating fever, anorexia and intermittent diarrhea. This is common in dairy cows in the immediate postpartum period (17). Pain may be detectable on deep palpation of the abdomen and the distended, fluid-filled abomasum may be palpable behind the right costal arch. In some cases the abomasum is grossly distended and fluid-splashing sounds are audible on succussion similar to those in right-side displacement of the abomasum. Moderate dehydration is common and affected cows commonly sip water continuously and grind their teeth frequently (8). The prognosis in chronic ulceration is poor because of the presence of several ulcers and the development of chronic abomasal atony. Some cows improve temporarily but relapse several days later and fail to recover permanently.

Calves with abomasal ulceration secondary to hair balls may have a distended gas-filled and fluid-filled abomasum which is palpable behind the right costal arch. Deep palpation may reveal abdominal pain associated with local peritonitis due to a perforated ulcer. Unless an abomasal ulcer has extended to the serosa it is unlikely that it can be detected by deep palpation. Many cases of abomasal ulcers particularly in calves cause no apparent illness. Melena is almost a pathognomonic sign of an acute bleeding ulcer of the abomasum; however, the presence of normal colored feces does not preclude the presence of chronic non-bleeding ulcers which may be the cause of an intractable indigestion. The use of an occult blood test on the feces will aid in differentiating those which are equivocal. Abomasal ulceration secondary to lymphoma of the abomasum is characterized by chronic diarrhea and melena. The ulcer does not heal.

Clinical pathology

The dark brown to black color of the feces is usually sufficient indication of gastric hemorrhage but tests for occult blood may be necessary. Results from experiments simulating abomasal hemorrhage indicate that the transit time for blood to move from the abomasum to the rectum ranges from 7 to 19 hours (13). The available fecal occult blood tests may not detect slow abomasal hemorrhage at any one sampling. This can be overcome by testing several fecal samples over a 2–4 day period and reading multiple smears per specimen. The sensitivity of the occult blood tests increases after the fecal samples have been stored at room temperature for 2 days. The predictive value of the occult blood test may be a more reliable diagnostic indicator of abomasal disease than abdominal pain or the presence of anemia (15). When perforation has occurred, with acute local peritonitis, there is neutrophilia with a regenerative left shift for a few days after which time the total leukocyte and differential count may be normal. In acute gastric hemorrhage there is acute hemorrhagic anemia.

Necropsy findings

Ulceration is most common along the greater curvature of the abomasum. There is a distinct preference for most of the ulcers to occur on the most ventral part of the fundic region with a few on the border between the fundic and pyloric regions. The ulcers are usually deep and well-defined but may be filled with blood clot or necrotic material and often contain fungal mycelia which may be of etiological significance in calves. The ulcers will measure from a few millimeters to 5 cm in diameter and are either round or oval with the longest dimension usually parallel to the long axis of the abomasum. In bleeding ulcers the affected artery is usually visible after the ulcer is cleaned out. Most cases of perforation in cattle are walled off by omentum with the formation of a large cavity 12–15 cm in diameter in the peritoneal cavity which contains degenerated blood and necrotic debris. Material from this cavity may infiltrate widely through the omental fat. Adhesions may form between the ulcer and surrounding organs or the abdominal wall (8, 9) (omental bursitis and omental empysema). Multiple phytobezoars are commonly present in the abomasum of beef calves with abomasal ulcers.

Diagnosis

A sudden onset of anorexia, ruminal stasis, depressed milk production and melena are characteristic of acute hemorrhagic abomasal ulceration. In some cases the melena may not be evident for 18–24 hours after the onset of hemorrhage because of the pylorospasm. An examination of the right flank may reveal a distended abomasum and a grunt on deep palpation over the abomasum, caudal to the xiphoid sternum on the right side. The presence of tachycardia may also be useful. Duodenal ulceration may cause melena and a syndrome indistinguishable from hemorrhagic abomasal ulceration.

The diagnosis of chronic abomasal ulceration without sufficient hemorrhage to result in melena is difficult and commonly not possible without surgical exploration or necropsy examination. The clinical findings of chronic ulceration can resemble many other diseases of the alimentary tract but the presence of occult blood in the feces and hematological evidence of hemorrhagic anemia are suggestive. The hemorrhage may be intermittent and repeated tests may be necessary. A positive result for occult blood may also be due to hematemesis, abomasal torsion, intestinal obstruction or blood-sucking parasites. Abomasal ulceration with perforation and local peritonitis may be indistinguishable from chronic traumatic reticuloperitonitis unless hemorrhage and melena occur. Chronic abomasal ulceration in calves associated with hair balls and chronic abomasitis from eating sand and dirt cannot usually be diagnosed as a separate entity.

Treatment

Blood transfusions and fluid therapy may be necessary for acute hemorrhagic ulceration. Parenteral coagulants are commonly used but are of doubtful value. Large doses of liquid mixtures of kaolin and pectin (2–3 liters twice daily for a mature cow) have been used with limited success. The use of antacids appears to be the most rational approach. The elevation of the pH of the abomasal contents would abolish the proteolytic activity of pepsin and reduce the damaging effect of the acidity on the mucosa. Magnesium oxide (500–800 g/450 kg body weight daily for 2–4 days) has been successful in some cases. The use of 100 g/day magnesium silicate has been recommended (10). The injection or infusion of the antacid directly into the abomasum would probably be much more effective but injections of the abomasum through the abdominal wall are not complete reliable. An abomasal cannula placed through the abdominal wall may provide a means of ensuring the infusion of antacids directly into the abomasum (11).

Surgical correction of abomasal ulcers has been attempted with some limited success (1, 8). The presence of multiple ulcers may require the radical excision of a large portion of the abomasal mucosa and hemorrhage is usually considerable. The conservative medical approach is usually used for the treatment of abomasal ulcers in cattle. The surgical approach requires a laparotomy and exploratory abomastomy to determine the presence and location of the ulcer. Thus one of the major problems is to decide when to elect surgical correction. Valuable animals with clinical evidence of chronic ulceration or those which relapse should be considered for surgical correction. Surgical correction of perforated abomasal ulcers in calves is described with some success (12). Recommendations for the prevention of abomasal ulceration in cattle cannot be given because the etiology is so poorly understood.

REFERENCES

(1) Tasker, J. B. et al. (1958) *J. Am. vet. med. Assoc.*, *133*, 365.
(2) Aukema, J. J. & Breukink, H. J. (1974) *Cornell Vet.*, *64*, 303.
(3) Breukink, H. J. (1976) *9th Cong. int. Maladies Betail*, Paris, pp. 447–452.
(4) Jensen, R. et al. (1976) *J. Am. vet. med. Assoc.*, *169*, 524.
(5) Groth, W. & Berner, H. (1971) *Zentralbl. VetMed.*, *18A*, 481.
(6) Davenport, H. W. (1972) *Digestion*, *5*, 162.
(7) Davenport, H. W. (1966) *Gastroenterology*, *50*, 487.
(8) Pinsent, P. J. N. (1968) *Vet. Rev.*, *19*, 17.
(9) Hemmingsen, J. (1967) *Nord. VetMed.*, *19*, 17.
(10) Espersen, G. (1977) *Vet. Ann.*, *17*, 44.
(11) Alonso, F. R. et al. (1973) *Am. J. vet. Res.*, *34*, 447.
(12) Tulleners, E. P. & Hamilton, G. F. (1980) *Can. vet. J.*, *21*, 262.
(13) Payton, A. J. & Glickman, L. T. (1980) *Am. J. vet. Res.*, *41*, 918.
(14) Smith, D. F. et al. (1983). *Cornell Vet.*, *73*, 213.
(15) Smith, D. F. et al. (1986). *Prev. vet. Med.*, *3*, 573.
(16) Palmer, J. E. & Whitlock, R. h. (1983). *J. Am. vet. med. Assoc.*, *183*, 448.
(17) Palmer, J. E. & Whitlock, R. H. (1984). *J. Am. vet. med. Assoc.*, *184*, 171.
(18) Wensing, T. et al. (1986) *Vet. Res. Commun.*, *10*, 1985.
(19) Welchman, D. de B. & Baust, G. N. (1986) *Proc. nutr. Soc.*, *45*, 32A.

Omental bursitis

Inflammation of the omental bursa occurs rarely, usually in dairy cattle. The causes include perforated abomasal ulcers of the medial wall of the abomasum, penetration of the ventral wall of the blind sac of the rumen, penetration of the reticulum by a foreign body, spread of an umbilical infection to the greater omentum, extension of an abdominal abscess, and localized peritonitis, with subsequent spread to omental bursa secondary to postpartum parametritis (1, 2). Inflammation of the bursa results in the accumulation of inflammatory exudate in the bursal cavity which enlarges beyond its normal capacity. There may also be rupture of the leaves of the greater omentum, resulting in diffuse peritonitis, ileus or functional obstruction of the intestines. Clinical findings include anorexia of several days duration, chronic toxemia, dehydration, and abdominal distension particularly of the right lower flank. Fluid-splashing sounds may be audible on auscultation and percussion of the right flank. On rectal examintion a large amorphous spongy mass may be palpable anterior to the pelvic brim in the right upper quadrant of the abdomen. The peritoneal fluid may reveal evidence of a chronic suppurative inflammation. A neutrophilia and an increase in the serum fibrinogen are common. There may also be a metabolic alkalosis with hypochloremia and hypokalemia. Treatment consists of surgical drainage and long-term therapy with antibiotics. At necropsy there is diffuse fibrinous and necrotizing peritonitis and a large accumulation of purulent exudate in the omental bursa.

REFERENCES

(1) Grymer, J. & Johnson, R. (1982). *J. Am. vet. med. Assoc.*, *181*, 174.
(2) Baxter, G. M. (1986). *Mod. vet. Pract.*, *67*, 729.

Abomasal bloat in lambs and calves

Abomasal bloat occurs in lambs and calves fed milk replacer diets. Feeding systems which allow lambs to drink large quantities of milk replacer at infrequent intervals predispose them to abomasal bloat (1). This situation can occur under *ad libitum* feeding when the supply of milk replacer is kept at about 15°C (59°F) or higher, and particularly if it is not available for several hours. Lambs fed warm milk replacer to appetite twice daily appear to be very susceptible to abomasal bloat.

Ad libitum feeding of cold milk replacers containing few or no insoluble ingredients, and adequately refrigerated, results in little or no bloating. The pathogenesis of the abomasal tympany is thought to be associated with a sudden overfilling of the abomasum followed by the proliferation of gas-forming organisms which release an excessive quantity of gas which cannot escape from the abomasum (3). The severe distension causes compression of the thoracic and abdominal viscera and blood vessels leading to them. This results in asphyxia and acute heart failure. Affected lambs and calves will become grossly distended within 1 hour after feeding and die in a few minutes after the distension of the abdomen is clinically obvious. At necropsy, the abomasum is grossly distended with gas, fluid and milk replacer which is usually not clotted. The abomasal mucosa is hyperemic.

Abomasal bloat also occurs in lambs 15–30 days of age just prior to being turned onto pasture in Norway (4). Housing these lambs on floors with built-up litter when silage is used as a roughage is a predisposing epidemiological factor. It is postulated that affected lambs eat fecal contaminated bedding which may result in the growth of an abnormal gas-producing microflora in the abomasum.

The addition of formalin (37% formaldehyde) at the rate of 0·1%, to a 20% solids milk replacer will minimize the incidence of abomasal bloat without adversely affecting the performance of artificially reared lambs (2).

REFERENCES

(1) Gorrill, A. D. L. et al. (1975) *Can. J. anim. Sci.*, *55*, 731.
(2) Gorrill, A. D. L. et al. (1975) *Can. J. anim. Sci.*, *55*, 557.
(3) Arsenault, G. et al. (1980) *Can. J. anim. Sci.*, *60*, 303.
(4) Lutanaes, B. & Simensen, E. (1982–83) *Prev. vet. Med.*, *1*, 335.

Cecal dilatation and torsion in cattle

Dilatation and torsion of the cecum occurs sporadically in cattle usually within a few weeks after calving in well-fed dairy cows. The etiology is not clear but experimentally a rise in the concentration of undissociated volatile fatty acids in the ingesta of the cecum will result in cecal atony (1). Dietary carbohydrates which have not been completely fermented in the rumen will be fermented in the cecum resulting in an increase in the concentration of volatile fatty acids, a drop in pH and cecal atony.

Butyric acid has the greatest depressant effect on cecal motility while acetic has the least. Inhibition of cecal motility may lead to accumulation of ingesta and gas in the organ and consequently dilatation, displacement and possible torsion.

Clinically there are varying degrees of anorexia, mild abdominal discomfort, a decline of milk production over a period of few days and a decreased amount of feces. The temperature, pulse and respirations are usually normal. A gas-filled viscus may be detectable on percussion and simultaneous auscultation in the upper right flank. There may be slight distension of the upper right flank but in some cases the flank is normal. On rectal examination the distended cecum can usually be palpated as a long cylindrical movable organ measuring up to 20 cm in diameter and 90 cm in length. Palpation and identification of the blind end of the cecum is diagnostic. Varying degrees of distension of the colon and ileum may occur dependent on the degree of displacement or torsion present. Rupture of the distended cecum may occur following rectal palpation or transportation of the animal. This is followed by shock and death within a few hours.

A mild degree of dehydration may be present and a compensated hypochloremia and hypokalemia occur (2). The treatment of choice is surgical correction and the prognosis is usually good. A recurrence rate of 10% is recorded (2). Mild cases may be treated conservatively by withholding feed for a few days and administering saline purgatives (3). Severe cases require surgical correction through a right flank laparotomy and in some cases amputation is necessary if ischemic necrosis and gangrene are present.

REFERENCES

(1) Svendsen. P. (1974) *Gastrointestinal Atony in Ruminants*. Copenhagen: Royal Veterinary and Agricultural University.
(2) Whitlock, R. H. (1976) *Proc. 9th int. Mtg Dis. Cattle*, Paris, 1, pp. 69–74.
(3) Grunder, H. D. (1972) *Tierärztl. Wochenschr.*, *78*, 317.

7

Diseases of the Liver and Pancreas

Diseases of the Liver

INTRODUCTION

Primary diseases of the liver, with the exception of the fat cow syndrome of cows in early lactation, seldom occurs in farm animals except as a result of poisonings. Liver metabolism in late pregnancy and early lactation in dairy cows is under a great deal of stress. The metabolic demands at these times are very much increased and require that the liver synthesize more glucose from non-carbohydrate precursors, harvest and metabolize butyrate and, because the cow is so often in negative energy balance, to mobilize body fat resulting in an increase in deposition of fat in the liver; a fatty liver and the fat cow syndrome may result (1, 18).

Secondary disease of the liver, arising as part of a generalized disease process or by spread from another organ, occurs more commonly. In primary hepatic disease the clinical manifestations are caused solely by the lesions in the liver while in secondary involvement the syndrome may include clinical signs unrelated to the hepatic lesions. This chapter is devoted to a consideration of primary diseases of the liver and to those aspects of other diseases in which manifestations of hepatic involvement occur.

Diseases of the liver are in general neglected by agricultural animal clinicians and clinical descriptions of them are meager.

PRINCIPLES OF HEPATIC DYSFUNCTION

Diffuse and focal hepatic disease

The liver has a very large reserve of function and approximately three-quarters of its parenchyma must be rendered inactive before clinical signs of hepatic dysfunction appear. Diffuse diseases of the liver are more commonly accompanied by signs of insufficiency than are focal diseases, which produce their effects either by the toxins formed in the lesions or by pressure on other organs, including the biliary system. The origin of a toxemia is often difficult to localize to the liver because of the physical difficulty of examining the organ.

Diffuse diseases of the liver can be classified as hepatitis and hepatosis according to the pathological change which occurs, and the classification also corresponds roughly with the type of causative agent. Clinically the differences between these two diseases is not marked, although some assistance can be obtained from clinicopathological examination.

Hepatic dysfunction

There are no specific modes of hepatic dysfunction. The liver has a great many functions and any diffuse disease of the organ interferes with most or all of the functions to the same degree. Variations occur in the acuteness and severity of the damage but the effects are the same and the clinical manifestations vary in degree only. The major hepatic functions which, when disordered, are responsible for clinical signs include the maintenance of normal blood sugar levels by providing the source as glycogen, the formation of some of the plasma proteins, the formation and excretion of bile salts and the excretion of bile pigments, the formation of prothrombin, and the detoxification and excretion of many toxic substances including photodynamic agents. The clinical signs produced by interference with each of these functions are dealt with under manifestations of hepatic dysfunction. A rather special aspect is the role of the liver in the genesis of primary ketosis of cattle.

The portal circulation

The portal circulation and the liver are mutually interdependent, the liver depending upon the portal vein for its supply of nutrients and the portal flow depending upon the patency of the hepatic sinusoids. The portal flow is unusual in that blood from the gastrosplenic area and the lower part of the large intestine passes to the left half of the liver and the blood from the two intestines to the right half, without mixing of the two streams in the portal vein. The restriction of toxipathic hepatitis to one half of the liver and the localization of metastatic abscesses and neoplasms in specific lobes results from the failure of portal vein blood from different gut segments to mix. The localization of toxipathic hepatitis may be because of selective distribution of the toxin or of protective metabolites. The passage of blood from the portal circuit through the liver to the caudal vena cava is dependent upon the patency of the hepatic vascular bed, and obstruction results in damming back of blood in the portal system, portal hypertension, interference with digestion and absorption, and in the final stages the development of ascites.

MANIFESTATIONS OF LIVER AND BILIARY DISEASE

Jaundice

Jaundice is a clinical sign which often arises in diseases of the liver and biliary system but also in diseases in which there are no lesions of these organs. It does not always occur and may be conspicuously absent in acute hepatitis. Although jaundice is a result of the accumulation of bilirubin, the staining is much more pronounced with direct than with indirect bilirubin. Thus the jaundice is more intense in cases of obstructive and hepatocellular jaundice than in hemolytic jaundice. The levels of bilirubin in blood also affect the intensity of the jaundice, the obstructive form often being associated with levels of bilirubin which are ten times higher than those commonly seen in hemolytic anemia. The staining of jaundice is due to staining of tissues, especially elastic tissue, and not to accumulation in tissue fluids, so that it is best detected clinically in the sclera, and jaundice which may be detectable easily at necropsy may not be visible on clinical examination. Many classifications have been suggested but the simplest is that proposed by Popper and Schaffner (2) and illustrated in Fig. 19.

The primary differentiation has to be made between jaundice with and without impairment of bile flow. Some indication of the type of jaundice can be derived from clinical examination. Thus jaundice is usually much more severe when impairment of flow occurs and when bile pigments are absent from the feces. However, obstructive jaundice can occur with only partial occlusion of hepatic flow provided at least half of the bile flow is obstructed. In such cases jaundice may occur even though bile pigments are still present in the feces. With lesser obstruction the portion of the liver and biliary tract which is functioning normally excretes the extra load of bile pigments. The only accurate basis for the differentiation between jaundice with impaired bile flow, and jaundice without impaired flow is the examination of the urine for the presence of bilirubin and urobilinogen and

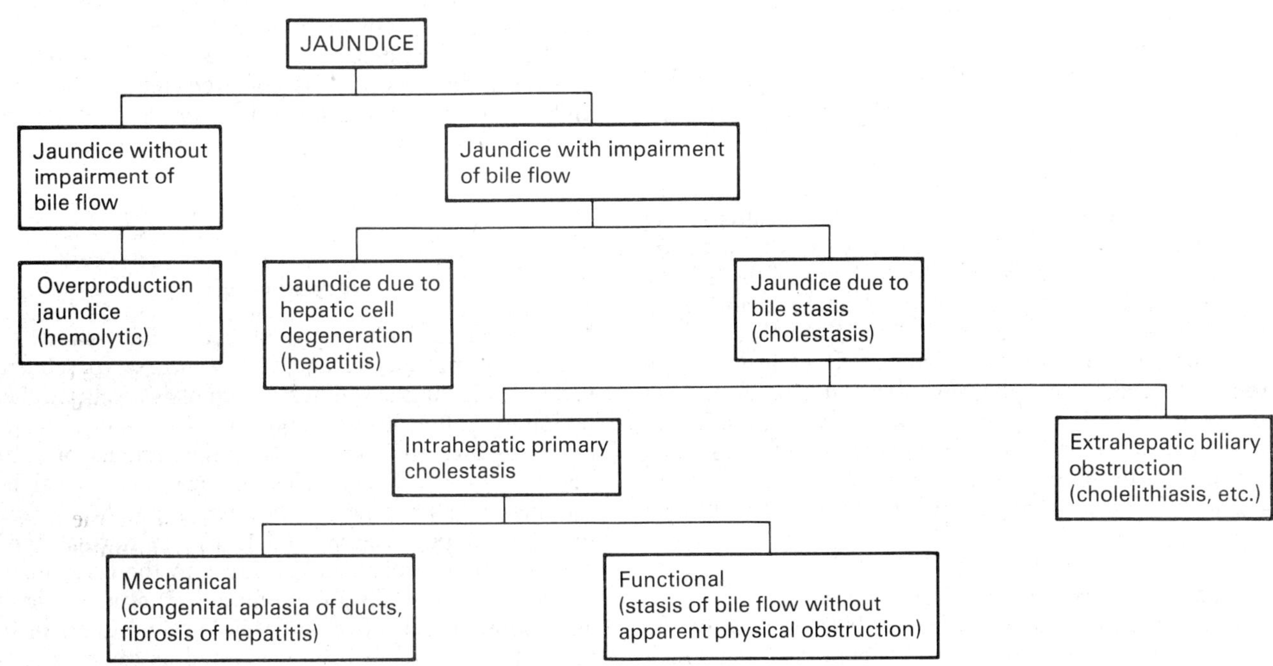

Fig. 19. Classification of jaundice

the determination of the relative amounts of direct and indirect bilirubin present in the serum. Indirect bilirubin which has not passed through hepatic cells is not excreted by the kidney, so that in hemolytic jaundice the indirect bilirubin content of serum is increased markedly and although the urine contains an increased amount of urobilinogen, no bilirubin is present. In those cases in which jaundice is caused by impairment of bile flow there is a marked increase in the serum level of direct bilirubin, and the bilirubin content of the urine is greatly increased. The amount of urobilinogen varies depending on whether any bilirubin reaches the intestine to be metabolized to urobilinogen and reabsorbed. In complete extrahepatic biliary obstruction urobilinogen is not present in the urine.

Overproduction or hemolytic jaundice

Hemolytic jaundice is common in animals and may be caused by bacterial toxins, invasion of erythrocytes by protozoa or viruses, inorganic and organic poisons and immunological reactions. Diseases in which bacterial toxins cause intravascular hemolysis are bacillary hemoglobinuria of cattle and leptospirosis although the mechanism by which hemolysis is produced in the latter disease does not seem to have been accurately determined. The common protozoan and viral diseases in which hemolysis occurs include babesiosis, anaplasmosis, eperythrozoonosis and equine infectious anemia. Chronic copper poisoning, selenium poisoning in sheep (3), phenothiazine poisoning in horses, pasturing on rape and other cruciferous plants and bites by some snakes are other common causes. Postparturient hemoglobinuria has an uncertain etiology but is usually attributed to a deficiency of phosphorus in the diet and the feeding of cruciferous plants. Isoimmunization hemolytic anemia of the newborn is caused by an immunological reaction between the sensitized cells of the newborn and antibodies in the colostrum of the dam. The occurrence of acute hemolytic anemia and jaundice in calves which drink large quantities of cold water may also be of the nature of an immunological response.

Neonatal jaundice is relatively common in babies and is regarded as a benign condition. It is rarely, if ever, observed clinically in newborn animals but may be noticeable at necropsy. Although it is generally stated that the jaundice is hemolytic and results from the destruction of excess erythrocytes when postnatal life begins, it appears more probable that it is due to retention of bile pigments because of the immaturity of the hepatic excretion mechanism. It does occur in foals and is an important differential diagnosis from isoerythrolysis.

Hemolytic jaundice is characterized clinically by a moderate degree of yellowing of the mucosae, and by the presence of hemoglobinuria in severe cases. Clinicopathological findings indicate the presence of anemia, an increase in urobilinogen and an absence of bilirubin in the urine, and a preponderance of indirect bilirubin in the serum.

Jaundice due to hepatic cell degeneration

The cause may be any of those diffuse diseases of the liver which cause degeneration of hepatic cells and which are listed under hepatitis. Because there is only partial obstruction of biliary excretion, the change in serum and urine lie between those of hemolytic jaundice and extrahepatic biliary obstruction. Serum levels of total bilirubin are increased because of retention of direct bilirubin which also passes out in the urine, causing an elevation of urine levels. The urobilinogen levels in the urine also rise.

Extrahepatic biliary obstruction

Obstruction of the bile ducts or common bile duct by biliary calculi or compression by tumor masses is a rare occurrence in farm animals. Commonly listed causes are obstruction of the common duct by nematodes and inflammation of the bile ducts by extension from an enteritis or by infestation with trematodes.

A significant number of pigs die with biliary obstruction and purulent cholangitis secondary to invasion of the ducts by *Ascaris lumbricoides*. Parasitic cholangitis and cholecystitis also occur due to fascioliasis and infestation with *Dicrocoelium dendriticum*. In horses an ascending cholangitis may develop from a parasitic duodenal catarrh and cause signs of biliary obstruction.

Obstruction is usually complete and results in the disappearance of bile pigments from the feces. Serum levels of direct bilirubin rise causing a marked elevation of total bilirubin in the serum. Excretion of the direct bilirubin in urine occurs on a large scale but there is no urobilinogen because of the failure of excretion into the alimentary tract. Partial obstruction of the common bile duct or occlusion of a number of major bile ducts may cause variations in serum and urine similar to those observed in complete obstruction except that the feces do contain bile pigments and urobilinogen appears in the urine. In this circumstance it is difficult to differentiate between partial extrahepatic biliary obstruction and jaundice caused by hepatic cell degeneration (see above).

Jaundice due to intrahepatic primary cholestasis

The mechanical stasis of biliary flow caused by fibrous tissue constriction and obliteration of the small biliary canaliculi may occur after hepatitis and in many forms of fibrosis. Functional stasis is a major problem in hepatic disease in humans but has not been defined in animals. In both instances the defect is the same as in extrahepatic biliary obstruction and the two diseases cannot be differentiated by laboratory tests.

Nervous signs

Nervous signs, including hyperexcitability, convulsions and coma, muscle tremor and weakness, psychic disturbances including dullness, compulsive walking, head-pressing, failure to respond to signals and, in some cases, mania, are common accompaniments of diffuse hepatic disease. The biochemical and anatomical basis for these signs has not been determined. Many factors including hypoglycemia, and failure of normal hepatic detoxification mechanisms, leading to the accumulation of excess amino acids and ammonia, or of acetylcholine, and the liberation of toxic breakdown products of liver parenchyma have all been suggested as causes and it is probable that more than one factor is involved.

One of the primary effects of severe, acute liver damage is a precipitate fall in blood sugar accompanied by nervous signs including hyperexcitability, convulsions and terminal coma. If the hepatic damage occurs more slowly the hypoglycemia is less marked and less precipitous and is accompanied by inability to perform work, drowsiness, yawning and lethargy. With persistent hypoglycemia, structural changes may occur in the brain (hypoglycemic encephalopathy) and these may be the basis for the chronically drowsy animals or dummies. However, hypoglycemia does not always occur in acute hepatitis and cannot be considered to be the only or even the most important factor in producing the cerebral signs. Because of this there is great interest in the observation that high blood levels of ammonia occur in pyrrolizidine poisoning in sheep, and are reflected in the development of spongy degeneration in the brain, and the clinical signs of hepatic encephalopathy (4, 5). The same status spongiosa has also been reproduced experimentally in sheep (6) and calves (11) by the intravenous infusion of ammonia (6). This role of ammonia as a cerebrotoxicant can be important in hepatopathies in which the detoxicating function of the liver is lost, and also in congenital defects of hepatic vasculature in which blood is bypassed around the liver. In the latter case ammonia and similar toxic byproducts of protein degradation in the large bowel avoid the detoxication filter of the liver. Blood ammonia levels are increased and bromosulfalein dye clearance is delayed. The clinical signs in an affected horse included aimless wandering and chewing and somnolence (13).

Edema and emaciation

Failure of the liver to anabolize amino acids and protein during hepatic insufficiency is manifested by tissue wasting and a fall in plasma protein. This may be sufficiently severe to cause edema because of the lowered osmotic pressure of the plasma. Hepatic edema is not usually very marked and is manifested most commonly in the intermandibular space (bottle jaw). If there is obstruction to the portal circulation, as may occur in hepatic fibrosis, the edema is much more severe but is largely limited to the abdominal cavity.

Diarrhea and constipation

In hepatitis, hepatic fibrosis, and in obstruction or stasis of the biliary system the partial or complete absence of bile salts from the alimentary tract deprives it of the laxative and mildly disinfectant qualities of these salts. This, together with the reflex effects from the distended liver in acute hepatitis, produces an alimentary tract syndrome comprising anorexia, vomition in some species, and constipation punctuated by attacks of diarrhea. The feces are pale in color and, if there is an appreciable amount of fat in the diet, there is steatorrhea.

Photosensitization

Most photosensitizing substances including phylloerythrin, the normal breakdown product of chlorophyll in the alimentary tract, are excreted in the bile. In hepatic or biliary insufficiency excretion of these substances is retarded and photosensitization occurs.

Hemorrhagic diathesis

In severe diffuse diseases of the liver there is a deficiency in prothrombin formation and a consequent prolongation of the clotting time of the blood. Abnormality of the prothrombin complex is not the only defect, deficiencies of fibrinogen and thromboplastin also occurring. Prothrombin and other factors in the prothrombin complex depend upon the presence of vitamin K for their formation and an absence of bile salts from the intestine retards the absorption of this fat-soluble vitamin. Parenteral administration of vitamin K is advisable before surgery is undertaken in patients with severe hepatic dysfunction.

Abdominal pain

Two mechanisms cause the pain in diseases of the liver: distension of the organ with increased tension of the capsule, and lesions of the capsule. Acute swelling of the liver occurs as a result of engorgement with blood in congestive heart failure and in acute inflammation. Inflammatory and neoplastic lesions of the capsule, or of the liver parenchyma just beneath the capsule, cause local irritation to its pain endorgans. The pain is usually subacute, causing abnormal posture, particularly arching the back and disinclination to move. Tenseness of the abdominal wall and pain on deep palpation over the liver area may also be detected in the majority of cases.

Alteration in size of the liver

Great variation in the size of the liver is often seen at necropsy but clinical detection is not easy unless the liver is grossly enlarged. This is most likely to occur in advanced congestion of the liver due to congestive heart failure, in some plant poisonings in horses and when multiple abscesses or neoplastic metastases occur. In acute hepatitis the swelling is not sufficiently large to be detected clinically and in terminal fibrosis the liver is much smaller than normal.

Displacement of the liver

The liver may be displaced from its normal position and protrude into the thoracic cavity through a diaphragmatic hernia causing respiratory distress and abnormal findings on percussion of the chest. Torsion of a lobe of the liver has been recorded in aged sows in the early part of lactation (7). Inappetence, uneasiness and unwillingness to suckle the young were followed by severe, prolonged vomiting, acute abdominal pain and dyspnea. The twisted lobe was greatly increased in size and in one case the capsule was ruptured leading to severe internal hemorrhage.

Rupture of the liver

Rupture of the liver is an occasional accident in animals occurring usually as a result of trauma. In most instances rupture results in death from hemorrhage although small breaks in the capsule may heal. Horses used for the production of serum frequently develop hepatic amyloidosis, presumably as a reaction to repeated injection of foreign protein, and the death rate from rupture of the liver is relatively high in this group (8). A specially high prevalence is recorded in newborn lambs of the North Country Cheviot breed. The lambs are stillborn or are born alive but become anemic and weak and die within 12 hours of birth from internal hemorrhage. It is thought that the cause of the fatal anemia is an inherited short length of the sternum which exposes the liver to compresion and rupture of its capsule (32).

Black livers of sheep

Dark brown to black pigmentation of the liver and kidneys occurs commonly in sheep in certain parts of Australia. No illness is associated with the condition but the livers are not used for human consumption for esthetic reasons and extensive financial loss may result. Commonly referred to as 'melanosis' the pigmentation has been determined to be the result of deposition of the pigment lipofuscin at various stages of oxidation (9). Areas in which the disease occurs carry many mulga trees (*Acacia aneura*) the leaves of which are fed to sheep in drought times.

The above condition should not be confused with the black livers found in a mutant strain of Corriedales in California (10). In these mutant sheep there is photosensitization following retention of phylloerythrin. The darkening of the liver is due to melanin.

SPECIAL EXAMINATION OF THE LIVER

When disease of the liver is suspected after a general clinical examination, special techniques of palpation, biopsy and biochemical tests of function can be used to determine further the status of the liver.

Palpation and percussion

In farm animals the liver is well concealed by the rib cage on the right-hand side and its edge cannot be palpated. A general impression of the size of the liver can be obtained by percussion of the area of liver dullness but accurate definition is not usually attempted. Deep percussion or palpation to detect the presence of hepatic pain can be carried out over the area of liver dullness in the posterior thoracic region on the right-hand side. Percussion over the entire area is necessary as the pain of a discrete lesion may be quite localized.

If the liver is grossly enlarged its edge can be felt on deep palpation behind the costal arch and the edge is usually rounded and thickened in contradistinction to the sharp edge of the normal liver. This type of palpation is relatively easy in ruminants but is unrewarding in horses and pigs because of the thickness of the abdominal wall and the shortness of the flank.

Biopsy

Biopsy of the liver has been used extensively as a diagnostic procedure in infectious equine anemia, and poisoning by *Crotalaria* spp. and other species of plants, and in experimental work on copper and vitamin A deficiency. The technique requires some skill and anatomical knowledge. The most satisfactory instrument is a long, small-caliber trocar and cannula to which is screwed a syringe capable of producing good negative pressure. The sharp point of the instrument is introduced in an intercostal space on the right-hand side, the number depending on the species, and advanced across the pleural cavity so that it will reach the diaphragm and diaphragmatic surface of the liver at an approximately vertical position. The point of insertion is made high up in the intercostal space so that the liver is punctured at the thickest part of its edge. The instrument is rotated until the edge of the cannula approximates the liver capsule; the trocar is then withdrawn, the syringe is attached and strong suction applied; the cannula is twisted vigorously and advanced until it reaches the visceral surface of the liver. If its edge is sufficiently sharp the cannula will now contain a core of liver parenchyma and if the instrument is withdrawn with the suction still applied a sample sufficient for histological examination and microassay of vitamin A, glycogen or other nutrient is obtained. Details of the technique for cattle (12, 33), sheep (14) and horses (16) are available. A disposable biopsy needle suitable for use in animals is available and a needle has also been designed which includes a device that ensures that the core of tissue in the cannula is in fact detached from the parenchyma of the organ (16).

The major deficiency of the method lies in the small sample which is obtained, and unless the liver change is diffuse the sample may not be representative. The procedure has been repeated many times on one animal without injury. The principal danger is that if the direction of the instrument is at fault it may approach the hilus and damage the large blood vessels or bile ducts. If the liver is shrunken or the approach too caudal no sample is obtained. Fatal hemoperitoneum may result if a hemorrhagic tendency is present and peritonitis may occur if the liver lesion is an abscess containing viable bacteria. Biliary peritonitis results if a large bile duct is perforated. It seems possible that the technique would precipitate a fatal attack of 'black disease', but many thousands of biopsies are performed without such incident. Compared to the human patient who can voluntarily restrain respiratory movements, the animal patient will traumatize its diaphragm and liver if the needle is not withdrawn quickly.

An alternative technique involving peritoneoscopy and visualization of the liver's edge is recommended for pigs (15).

Radiographic examination

The application of radiography to examination of the liver and biliary system in large animals is limited to experimental work. Cholecystography after the oral administration of a halogenated phenolphthalein permits visualization of the gall bladder but cholangiography can only be satisfactorily performed by direct injection of radiopaque materials into the ducts after laparotomy.

Biochemical tests of hepatic function

Laboratory tests of hepatic function are exacting and time-consuming and are seldom undertaken at present in routine diagnostic work in farm animals. They find a place in the investigation of disease problems but in general insufficient work has been done with them to determine standards for normality and the relative usefulness of the different tests (17). The tests in use in human medicine can be classified in three groups, those that measure the excretory rate of parenterally administered substances such as bromosulfalein; those that measure the metabolic activity of the organ by its capacity to metabolize such substances as galactose; and those which test detoxification functions including the hippuric acid synthesis test and the glucuronic acid test. Apart from tests designed specifically for these particular functions, there is also a great deal of information to be gained from examination of body constituents which may however vary from causes which are not hepatic. These include serum bilirubin (direct and indirect), plasma protein, the albumin/globulin ratio and the non-specific serum protein reactions on which the flocculation or turbidity tests are based. Electrophoresis has largely displaced other means of estimating proteins and segregating them, but as a diagnostic technique it may be too expensive for general laboratory use. For full details of these tests and their comparative values up-to-date reviews should be consulted (31).

In animals the bromosulfalein clearance test has been used in cattle (19), sheep (20), and horses (21) and although little information is available the test appears to have diagnostic value (22). It is time-consuming and care is needed with prepared solutions in open containers; anaphylactoid reactions have occurred after injection of solutions which are 10 days old (23). The time required by normal livers to reduce the plasma concentration of BSP to half the initial concentration is taken as the standard (the $t_{\frac{1}{2}}$) in cattle and is 2·5–5·5 minutes. The results are modified by the ability of the liver to excrete BSP via the biliary system and to store it in hepatocytes. Factors other than liver disease which increase the $t_{\frac{1}{2}}$ significantly are starvation in horses (24), competition with bilirubin for excretory capacity, and youth, foals less than 6 months of age having a significantly slower clearance time. Precise timing of samples is needed because of the rapid excretion rate.

Of the tests based on carbohydrate metabolism the galactose tolerance and adrenaline response tests appear to show some promise. However, the galactose tolerance test in undependable in goats, being much too dependent on renal efficiency and fluid homeostasis (25). Variations in urine bilirubin levels are not sufficiently great to indicate the presence or absence of hepatic disease in cattle unless the insufficiency is of extreme degree. An increase in the concentration of porphyrins (mainly coproporphyrin) in the urine also occurs and should not be mistaken for the porphyrins of inherited porphyria.

In sheep, where severe hepatic dysfunction is accompanied by a steep rise in blood ammonia levels, and where this is reflected in the development of spongy degeneration in the brain, the level of glutamine in the cerebrospinal fluid is also elevated (4). Glutamine is a byproduct of the metabolism of ammonia in brain cells. Acute ammonia toxicity is manifested by tetany, ataxia and pulmonary edema, and affected animals are likely to die before the effects of subacute poisoning, hepatic encephalopathy, are seen.

Determination of serum levels of liver enzymes is now much used in the detection of hepatic injury. Sorbitol dehydrogenase (SDH) is almost completely selective as an indicator of liver damage and is the preferred test for it. Serum alkaline phosphate levels increase markedly when there is damage to biliary tissue but there is a similar response to damage in other tissues (26).

The levels of aspartate aminotransferase (AST, previously known as SGOT) or L-alanine aminotransferase (ALT, previously known as SGPT) in serum have some value as indicators of liver damage because of their high content in liver, but they are generally considered to be too non-specific to be of great diagnostic value. Gamma-glutamyl transferase is a better indicator especially of acute liver damage and biliary tract lesions.

In ruminants glutamate dehydrogenase (GLDH) occurs in high concentration in the liver and rises appreciably in serum when liver damage occurs. Serum levels of ornithine and carbamyl transferase (OCT) are also elevated even in chronic diseases (27), but only when there is active liver necrosis, and not when the lesions are healing. Sorbitol dehydrogenase has been shown specifically to be a good indicator of hepatic damage in sheep and cattle (28). Significant variations occur in serum levels of alkaline phosphatase but the variations in normal cattle have such a wide range that results are difficult to interpret. Serum alkaline phosphatase levels in plasma are used as a test of hepatic excretory function in the horse and are of value in that species. Of the tests available for testing of biliary obstruction the serum alkaline phosphatase test is preferred.

Measurement of the icteric index of plasma, by comparing its color with a standard solution of potassium dichromate, cannot be considered to be a liver function test but it is used commonly as a measure of the degree of jaundice present. The color of normal plasma varies widely between species depending upon the concentration of carotene. Horse, and to a less extent cattle, plasma is quite deeply colored, but sheep plasma is normally very pale. The color index needs to be corrected for this factor before the icteric index is computed.

In the early stages of hepatic dysfunction in cattle the serum enzyme tests, particularly sorbitol dehydrogenase, are efficient and sensitive tests. In the later stages when tests of biliary excretion are more applicable, estimations of serum bilirubin and phylloerythrin and the bromosulfalein test are indicated (29). In horses the estimation of sorbitol dehydrogenase is preferred (26). In goats the BSP test is recommended (30). A satisfactory combination of tests for liver function is bromosulfalein clearance, OCT test and prothrombin time.

PRINCIPLES OF TREATMENT IN DISEASES OF THE LIVER

In diffuse diseases of the liver no general treatment is satisfactory and the main aim should be to remove the source of the damaging agent. The most that can be attempted in acute hepatitis is to tide the animal over the danger period of acute hepatic insufficiency until the subsidence of the acute change and the normal regeneration of the liver restores its function. Death may occur during this stage because of hypoglycemia, and the blood glucose level must be maintained by oral or intravenous injections of glucose. Because of the danger of guanidine intoxication an adequate calcium intake should be ensured by oral or parenteral administration of calcium salts.

There is some doubt as to whether protein intake should be maintained at a high level, as incomplete metabolism of the protein may result in toxic effects particularly in the kidney. However, amino acid mixtures, especially those containing methionine, are used with apparently good results. The same general recommendations apply in prevention as in the treatment of acute diffuse liver disease. Diets high in carbohydrate, calcium and protein of high biological value and a number of specific substances are known to have a protective effect against hepatotoxic agents.

In chronic, diffuse hepatic disease fibrous tissue replacement causes compression of the sinusoids and is irreversible except in the very early stages, when removal of fat from the liver by the administration of lipotrophic factors including choline, and maintenance on a diet low in fat and protein, may reduce the compressive effects of fibrous tissue contraction. A high protein diet at this stage causes stimulation of the metabolic activity of the liver and an increased deposit of fat, further retarding hepatic function.

Local diseases of the liver require surgical or medical treatment depending upon the cause, and specific treatments are discussed under the respective diseases.

REVIEW LITERATURE

Person, E. G. & Craig, A. M. (1980) The diagnosis of liver disease in equine and food animals. *Mod. vet. Pract.*, *61*, 233 & 315.

Pinsent, P. J. N. (1982) Diagnosis of the diseases of the bovine liver. *Bov. Pract.*, *17*, 165.

REFERENCES

(1) Baird, G. D. (1982) *Bov. Pract.*, *17*, 147.
(2) Popper, H. & Schaffner, F. (1957) *Liver: Structure and Function.* New York: McGraw-Hill.
(3) De Boom, H. P. A. & Brown. J. M. M. (1968) *J. S. Afr. vet. Med. Assoc.*, *39*, 21.
(4) Hooper, P. T. et al. (1974) *Res. vet Sci.*, *16*, 216.
(5) Finn, J. P. & Tennant, B. (1974) *Cornell Vet.*, *64*, 136.
(6) Hooper, P. T. (1972) *Vet. Rec.*, *90*, 37.
(7) Hamir, A. N. (1980) *Vet. Rec.*, *106*, 362.
(8) Schützler, H. & Beyer, J. (1964) *Arch. exp. vet. Med.*, *18*, 1119.
(9) Winter, H. (1966) *Aust. vet. J.*, *42*, 40.
(10) Arias, I. et al. (1964) *J. clin. Invest.*, *43*, 1249.
(11) Cho, D. Y. & Leipold. H. W. (1977) *Acta Neuropathol.*, *39*, 115.
(12) Smart, M. E. (1985) *Comp. Cont. Educ.*, *7*, 5327.
(13) Beech, J. et al. (1977) *J. Am. vet. med. Assoc.*, *170*, 164.
(14) Harvey, R. B. et al. (1984) *Cornell Vet.*, *74*, 322.
(15) Shiels, I. A. (1983) *Aust. vet. J.*, *60*, 317.
(16) Simpson, J. W. (1985) *Vet. Rec.*, *117*, 639.
(17) Harvey, D. G. (1958) *Vet. Rec.*, *70*, 616.
(18) Reid, I. M. (1982) *Bov. Pract.*, *17*, 149.
(19) Cornelius, C. E. et al. (1958) *Am. J. vet. Res.*, *19*, 560.
(20) Forbes, T. J. & Singleton, A. G. (1966) *Br. vet. J.*, *122*, 55.
(21) Cornelius, C. E. & Wheat, J. D. (1957) *Am. J. vet. Res.*, *18*, 369.
(22) Caple, I. W. et al. (1976) *Aust. vet. J.*, *52*, 192.
(23) Morgan, H. C. et al. (1960) *Vet. Med.*, *55*, No. 8, 28.
(24) Gronwall, R. (1975) *Am. J. vet. Res.*, *36*, 145.
(25) Treacher, R. J. (1972) *Res. vet. Sci.*, *13*, 427.
(26) Pinsent, P. J. N. (1982) *Bov. Pract.*, *17*, 165.
(27) Holtenius, P. & Jacobsson, S.-O. (1964) *Rep. 3rd int. Mtg Dis. Cattle, Copenhagen.*
(28) Shaw, F. D. (1974) *Aust. vet. J.*, *50*, 277.
(29) Ford, E. J. H. & Boyd, J. W. (1962) *J. Pathol. Bacteriol.*, *83*, 39.
(30) Sen, M. M. et al. (1976) *Ind. vet. J.*, *53*, 504.
(31) Pearson, E. G. & Craig, A. M. (1980) *Mod. vet. Pract.*, *61*, 233 & 315.
(32) Johnston, W. S. & Maclachlan, G. K. (1986) *Vet. Rec.*, *118*, 610.
(33) Buckley, W. T. et al. (1986) *Can. J. Anim. Sci.*, *66*, 1137.

DIFFUSE DISEASES OF THE LIVER

Hepatitis

The differentiation of hepatic diseases into two groups of hepatitis and hepatosis has not achieved general acceptance and non-specific terms such as hepatic injury have been suggested to avoid the connotation of inflammation associated with the word hepatitis. To facilitate ease of reading, the word hepatitis is used throughout this chapter to include all diffuse, degenerative and inflammatory diseases which affect the liver. It is used here also to include the common pathological classification of cirrhosis. Clinically the syndrome caused by fibrosis of the liver is the same as that caused by hepatitis and the etiology is the same, the only difference being that the onset of the disease is slower and less acute than in hepatitis.

Etiology

Although there is an extensive list of causes of hepatitis there is still a number of unknown factors. At least there are many sporadic cases of hepatic insufficiency, especially in horses, in which the cause is not determined. An approximately similar situation exists in dogs. In most cases the clinical disease has an acute onset and a fatal outcome, the lesion is of a much longer duration.

Toxic hepatitis

The usual lesion is centrilobular and may be mild in degree and manifested by cloudy swelling, or severe and accompanied by extensive necrosis. If the necrosis is severe enough or repeated a sufficient number of times fibrosis develops. The common causes of toxic hepatitis in farm animals are *inorganic poisons*—copper, phosphorus, arsenic, possibly selenium; or *organic poisons*—carbon tetrachloride, hexachloroethane, Gossypol, creosols and coal tar pitch, chloroform, and copper diethylamine quinoline sulfonate. Ferrous fumarate administered in a digestive inoculate to newborn foals is also recorded as a cause (1–3).

Poisonous plants These include the following:

- Weeds including *Senecio*, *Crotalaria*, *Heliotropum*, *Amsinckia*, *Tribulus* spp., *Encephalartos lanatus*, *Trachyandra* spp., *Tribulus terrestris*
- Pasture and cultivated plants, *Panicum effusum*, lupins, Alsike clover, water-damaged alfalfa hay (14)
- Trees and shrubs—*Lantana camara*, Yellow wood—*Terminalia oblongata*, Ngaio tree—*Myoporum* sp., Australian boobialla—*M. tetrandrun*, seeds of *Zamia* sp.
- Fungi—*Pithomyces chartarum*, *Aspergillus flavus*, *Penicillium rubrum*, *Phomopsis leptostromiformis*, *Fusarium* sp., *Myrothecium* sp., *Periconia* sp.
- Algae—the slow death factor
- Insects—ingestion of sawfly larvae (*Lophyrotoma interrupta*).

Miscellaneous farm chemicals These include dried poultry waste, cottonseed cake, herring meal (3).

Drugs The hepatotoxicity of veterinary drugs has been reviewed (5).

Toxemia/perfusion hepatitis
Moderate degrees of hepatitis occur in many bacterial infections irrespective of their location in the body and the hepatitis is usually classified as toxic, but whether the lesions are caused by bacterial toxins or by shock, anoxia or vascular insufficiency is unknown. The same position applies in hepatitis caused by extensive tissue damage occurring after burns, injury and infarction.

Infectious hepatitis
Diffuse hepatic lesions in animals are rarely caused by infectious agents. The significant ones are:

- The virus of Rift Valley fever
- *Bacillus piliformis* as the cause of Tyzzer's disease in foals
- The equid herpesvirus 1 of viral rhinopneumonitis as a cause of abortion in foals
- *Chlamydia* sp. as a cause of epizootic abortion of cattle in California
- Postvaccinal hepatitis, probably caused by a virus, but this has not been identified
- Severe cases of equine viral arteritis manifest signs of hepatitis
- Systemic mycoses, e.g., histoplasmosis, may be accompanied by multiple granulomatous lesions of the liver
- Other diseases in which hepatic lesions may be common at necropsy, but in which there are no overt signs of clinical disease during life. Some of these are infectious equine anemia, salmonellosis, septicemic listeriosis, leptospirosis.

Parasitic hepatitis

- Acute and chronic liver fluke infestation
- Migrating larvae of *Ascaris* sp.

Nutritional hepatitis (trophopathic hepatitis)
The cirrhosis of the liver caused by methionine deficiency, and acute hepatic necrosis caused by cystine deficiency in the diet of rats (7) are not known to have any importance in farm animals. The knowledge that vitamin E prevents acute hepatic necrosis in rats on cystine-deficient diets has led to the suggestion that the vitamin may be important in the prevention of dietary hepatic necrosis in pigs. There is an interesting relationship between the so-called factor 3, which contains selenium and protects against trophopathic hepatitis (8), and vitamin E, both agents protecting also against enzootic muscular dystrophy. Selenium and alpha-tocopherol have been shown capable of preventing dietary hepatic necrosis in pigs. A multiple dietary deficiency has also been suggested as the cause of a massive hepatic necrosis observed in lambs and adult sheep on trefoil pasture in California (9).

'White liver disease' is a well-identified clinical entity occurring in young sheep in the warmer parts of New Zealand (4). The cause is unknown, but the disease affects only cobalt-deficient sheep. The disease occurs on leafy pastures with lots of leaf litter, and in spring and early summer. Affected sheep show photosensitivity, anorexia, weight loss, sometimes jaundice and blindness. At necropsy there is a very much enlarged, light-colored, fatty liver. Most deaths occur in a chronic phase after the acute signs have passed. A similar disease, suspected to be caused by a mycotoxin, has been observed in Norway (6).

Congestive hepatitis
Increased pressure in the sinusoids of the liver causes anoxia and compression of surrounding hepatic parenchyma. Congestive heart failure is the common cause and leads to centrilobular degeneration.

Inherited hepatic insufficiency in Southdown and Corriedale sheep is described later (p. 1401). It is a functional disease and not hepatitis.

Pathogenesis
Hepatitis may be caused by a number of agents but the clinical effects are approximately the same in all instances as set out under manifestations of liver disease above. The usual lesion in toxipathic hepatitis is centrilobular and varies from cloudy swelling to acute necrosis with a terminal veno-occlusive lesion in some plant poisonings. In infectious hepatitis the lesions vary from necrosis of isolated cells to diffuse necrosis affecting all or most of the hepatic parenchyma. In parasitic hepatitis the changes depend upon the number and type of migrating parasites. In massive fluke infestations sufficient damage may occur to cause acute hepatic insufficiency, manifested particularly by submandibular edema. In more chronic cases extension from a cholangitis may also cause chronic insufficiency. Trophopathic hepatitis in experimental animals is characterized by massive or submassive necrosis, and congestive hepatitis by dilatation of central veins and sinusoids with compression of the parenchymal cells. Hepatic fibrosis develops particularly if there is

massive hepatic necrosis which destroys entire lobules. Degeneration is not possible as it is when the necrosis is zonal, and fibrous tissue replacement occurs. Thus fibrosis is a terminal stage of hepatitis which may have developed acutely or chronically and is manifested by the same clinical syndrome as that of hepatitis except that the signs develop more slowly. Fibrosis may also develop from a cholangitis. The term cirrhosis has been avoided because it carries connotations from human medicine which may be misleading when applied to animals.

The pathogenesis of lesions to clinical signs is dealt with earlier in this chapter under the heading of manifestations of hepatic disease.

Clinical findings

The cardinal signs of hepatitis are anorexia, mental depression, with excitement in some cases, muscular weakness, jaundice and in the terminal stages somnolence, recumbency and coma with intermittent convulsion. Hemoglobinuria is also a variable sign in horses (10). The hemolytic crisis with which it is associated is always a precursor to a fatal outcome. The pathogenesis is unexplained. Animals which survive the early acute stages may evidence photosensitization, a break in the wool or hair leading to shedding of the coat and susceptibility to metabolic strain for up to a year.

The initial anorexia is often accompanied by constipation and punctuated by attacks of diarrhea. The feces are lighter in color than normal and if the diet contains much fat there may be steatorrhea. Vomiting may occur in pigs. The nervous signs are often pronounced and vary from ataxia and lethargy with yawning, or coma, to hyperexcitability with muscle tremor, mania, including aggressive behavior, and convulsions. A characteristic syndrome is the dummy syndrome in which affected animals push with the head, do not respond to normal stimuli and may be blind (11). There may be subacute abdominal pain, usually manifested by arching of the back, and pain on palpation of the liver. The enlargement of the liver is usually not palpable.

Jaundice and edema may or may not be present and are more commonly associated with the less acute stages of the disease. Photosensitization may also occur but only when the animals are on a diet containing green feed and are exposed to sunlight. A tendency to bleed more freely than usual may be observed. In chronic hepatic fibrosis the signs are similar to those of hepatitis but develop more slowly, and persist for longer periods, often months. Ascites and the dummy syndrome are more common than in hepatitis.

Clinical pathology

Urine and blood samples and liver biopsy specimens may be submitted for laboratory examination as outlined under the discussion of jaundice and tests of hepatic dysfunction.

Necropsy findings

The liver in hepatitis is usually enlarged and the edges swollen but the appearance of the hepatic surface and cross-section varies with the cause. In acute toxic and trophopathic hepatitis the lobulation is more pronounced and the liver is paler and redder in color. The accentuation of the lobular appearance is caused by engorgement of the centrilobular vessels or centrilobular necrosis. There may be accompanying lesions of jaundice, edema and photosensitization. In infectious hepatitis the lesions are inclined to be patchy and even focal in their distribution. Parasitic hepatitis is obviously traumatic with focal hemorrhages under the capsule and the necrosis and traumatic injury definable as tracks. Congestive hepatitis is marked by severe enlargement of the liver, a greatly increased content of blood, and marked accentuation of the lobular pattern caused by vascular engorgement and fatty infiltration of the parenchyma. In hepatic fibrosis the necropsy findings vary widely depending on the causative agent, the duration of its action and on its severity. The liver may be grossly enlarged or be much reduced in size with marked lobulation of the surface.

Diagnosis

Hepatitis is easily misdiagnosed as an encephalopathy unless jaundice or photosensitization is present. The nervous signs are suggestive of encephalomyelitis, encephalomalacia and cerebral edema. Congestive hepatitis is usually not manifested by nervous signs and, being a secondary lesion in congestive heart failure, is usually accompanied by ascites and edema in other regions and by signs of cardiac involvement. Hepatic fibrosis may produce ascites without evidence of cardiac disease.

Acute diseases affecting the alimentary tract, particularly engorgement on grain in cattle and horses, may be manifested by signs of nervous derangement resembling those of acute hepatic dysfunction but the history and clinical examination usually suggests a primary involvement with the alimentary tract. Anorexic hepatic insufficiency may be mirrored by an adenocarcinoma of the pancreas which is unlikely to be diagnosed during life (13).

Treatment

The principles of treatment of hepatitis have already been outlined. Results are seldom good (11). Protein and protein hydrolysates are probably best avoided because of the danger of ammonia intoxication. The diet should be high in carbohydrate and calcium, and low in protein and fat but affected animals are usually completely anorectic. Because of the failure of detoxification of ammonia and other nitrogenous substances by the damaged liver and their importance in the production of nervous signs, the oral administration of broad-spectrum antibiotics has been introduced in man to control protein digestion and putrefaction. The results have been excellent with neomycin and chlortetracycline (12, 13), the disappearance of hepatic coma coinciding with depression of blood ammonia levels. Purgation and enemas have also been used in combination with oral administration of antibiotics but mild purgation is recommended to avoid unnecessary fluid loss. Supplementation of the feed or periodic injections of the water-soluble vitamins are desirable. Hepatic fibrosis is considered to be a final stage in hepatitis and treatment is not usually undertaken.

REVIEW LITERATURE

Ross, M. A. (1982) The relationship of hepatic drug metabolism to hepatotoxicity with some examples in sheep. *Vet. Ann.*, *22*, 129–134.

REFERENCES

(1) Divers, T. T. et al. (1983) *J. Am. vet. med. Assoc.*, *183*, 1407.
(2) Mullaney, T. P. et al. (1984) *Vet. Rec.*, *114*, 115.
(3) Acland, H. M. et al. (1984) *Vet. Pathol.*, *21*, 3.
(4) Sutherland, R. J. et al. (1979) *NZ vet. J..* *29*, 227.
(5) Adam, S. E. I. (1972) *Vet. Bull.*, *42*, 683.
(6) Ulvund, M. J. & Overas, J. (1980) *NZ vet. J.*, *28*, 19.
(7) Schwarz, L. (1954) *Ann. NY Acad. Sci.*, *57*, 617.
(8) Bunyan, J. et al. (1958) *Nature (Lond.)*, *181*, 1801.
(9) Cordy, D. r. & McGowan, B. (1956) *Cornell Vet.*, *46*, 422.
(10) Tennant, B. et al. (1972) *Mod. vet. Pract.*, *53*, 40.
(11) Fowler, M. E. (1965) *J. Am. vet. med. Assoc.*, *147*, 55.
(12) Annotation (1957) *Lancet*, *273*, 280, 1263.
(13) Kerr, O. M. et al. (1982) *Equ. vet. J.*, *14*, 338.
(14) Putnam, M. R. et al. (1986) *J. Am. vet. med. Assoc.*, *189*, 77.

FOCAL DISEASES OF THE LIVER

Hepatic abscess

Local suppurative infections of the liver do not cause clinical signs of hepatic dysfunction unless they are particularly massive or extensively metastatic. They do cause significant losses in feedlot and grain-fed cattle because of the frequency of rumenitis in those cattle leading to hepatic abscess formation and the rejection of the affected livers at the abattoir. Some abscesses may, however, cause signs of toxemia because of the destruction of hepatic tissue or the liberation of potent toxins. The toxemia of traumatic hepatitis is usually due to toxins from *Actinomyces (Corynebacterium) pyogenes*, *Streptococcus* and *Staphylococcus* spp. and *Fusobacterium necrophorum* which are implanted in the lesions by the perforating foreign body; of the *F. necrophorum* isolates most will be of the A biotype, although the B biotype does occur usually in combination with other bacteria (1).

Omphalophlebitis, ruminal parakeratosis, or rumenitis may also lead to hepatic invasions by *F. necrophorum* or other organisms and abscessed livers are common in cattle fed heavily on concentrates. Black disease is a profound toxemia caused by the liberation of potent exotoxin from *Clostridium novyi*. *Cl. sordelli* causes hepatic abscesses in neonatal lambs and bacillary hemoglobinuria by a toxin from *Cl. haemolyticum* in focal hepatic necroses. A focal bacterial hepatitis, identified as 'Tyzzer's disease', and caused by *Bacillus piliformis*, and yersiniosis caused by *Yersinia pseudotuberculosis* are listed elsewhere. Occasional cases of strangles which develop bacteremic spread may also develop hepatic abscesses, as may septicemia in lambs caused by *Haemophilus agni*.

The clinical signs of these specific diseases are included under the discussion of each disease and the only finding common to all is local pain on palpation or percussion over the liver.

A most important relationship is that between liver abscess and caudal vena caval syndrome. Sudden death, or any death, of cattle due to pulmonary hemorrhage should be examined with this possibility in mind. Liver abscesses have been produced experimentally in cattle by injecting *Fusobacterium necrophorum* into the hepatic portal vein (4). They are characterized by an elevation of blood levels of sialic acid and mucoprotein (5).

Tumors of the liver

Metastatic lesions of lymphomatosis in calves are the commonest neoplasms encountered in the liver of animals although primary adenoma, adenocarcinoma and metastases of other neoplasms in the area drained by the portal tract are not uncommon especially in ruminants. For the most part, they produce no signs of hepatic dysfunction but they may cause sufficient swelling to be palpable, and some abdominal pain by stretching of the liver capsule. Primary tumors of the gallbladder and bile ducts also occur rarely and do not as a rule cause clinical signs. A primary hepatic fibrosarcoma in a goat has caused loss of body weight, although appetite was maintained, anemia and jaundice. There is a record of 40 neoplasms in 358 846 livers examined in abattoirs (3). At a prevalence of 0·011% they are unlikely to excite much interest.

REFERENCES

(1) Scanlan, C. M. & Hathcock, C. L. (1983) *Cornell Vet.*, *73*, 288.
(2) Higgins, R. J. et al. (1985) *Vet. Rec.*, *116*, 444.
(3) Johnstone, A. C. (1972) *Vet. Pathol.*, *9*, 159.
(4) Scanlan, C. M. & Berg, J. N. (1983) *Cornell Vet.*, *73*, 117.
(5) Motoi, Y. et al. (1985) *Jap. J. vet. Sci.*, *47*, 341.

Diseases of the biliary system

Cases of biliary tract disease with clinical manifestations are very rare in food animals and horses but deserve a brief mention. Occasional cases of cholangitis occur in cattle and horses. Associated clinical signs include fever, pain over the liver, jaundice and photosensitization. There is usually an accompanying leukocytosis and a left shift. In horses a sequel to cholangitis may be a diffuse bacterial hepatitis with signs of hepatic insufficiency (8).

Concretions in the biliary system of cattle are usually a sequel to fascioliasis. Mild cases show anorexia and pain over the liver. Severe cases show recurrent attacks of severe abdominal pain, alimentary tract stasis and pain on percussion over the liver. Jaundice occurs only in the terminal stages of fatal cases and is accompanied by recumbency, depression and coma (1). Other causes of biliary tract disease include gallbladder empyema (7) and a bile duct carcinoma. In the latter case there was severe loss of body weight and signs referable to metastases in other organs but there were no clinical or postmortem signs of biliary malfunction (6). Biliary atresia in young foals (9, 10) is manifested by an early period of normality for 2–3 weeks after birth followed by the development of listlessness, anorexia, the passage of grey, pasty feces, and jaundice. Death occurs about a week later.

Obstructive cholelithiasis in horses may cause intermittent colic (2, 3) or continuous pain and sometimes jaundice (4, 5). A delay in bromosulfalein clearance is also recorded (8). Clinical signs suggestive of biliary disease in adult horses may be due to neoplasia of the pancreas (see below).

REFERENCES

(1) Stober, M. (1963) *Dtsch Tierärztl. Wochenschr.*, *68*, 608, 647.
(2) van der Luer, R. J. T. & Kroneman, J. (1982) *Equ. vet. J.*, *14*, 251.
(3) Traub, T. L. et al. (1983) *J. Am. vet. med. Assoc.*, *182*, 714.
(4) Roussel, A. J. et al. (1984) *Cornell Vet.*. *74*, 166.
(5) Scarratt, W. K. et al. (1985) *Comp. cont. Educ.*, *7*, S428.
(6) Warner, A. E. (1985) *J. Am. vet. med. Assoc.*, *187*, 177.
(7) Tulleners, E. P. (1983) *J. Am. vet. med. Assoc.*, *182*, 410.
(8) McDole, M. G. (1980) *Equ. Pract.*, *2*, 37.
(9) Bastienello, S. S. & Nesbit, J. W. (1986) *J. S. Afr. vet. Assoc.*, *57*, 117.
(10) van der Luer, R. T. J. & Kroneman, J. (1982) *Equ. vet. J.*, *14*, 91.

Diseases of the Pancreas

Pancreatic disease in food animals and horses are not sufficiently common to warrant a full-scale exposition.

Diabetes mellitus

Lesions of the pancreas causing diabetes mellitus are recorded in cows (4, 6) and horses and donkeys (7, 8). The clinical syndrome in horses includes weight loss, polydipsia, polyuria, intense hyperlipemia and high blood levels of cholesterol, triglycerides and glucose. Clinical observations suggest that the disease is most likely to occur in old horses and may be due to pancreatic injury related to migration of strongyle larvae (5). In cows there is afebrile emaciation, polydipsia, ketonuria, glucosuria and hyperglycemia.

Pancreatic adenocarcinoma

The pancreatic duct of the horse is anatomically close to the common bile duct and it is not unexpected that a tumor mass should cause a syndrome of biliary duct pathology (1, 2) although there is a surprising absence of jaundice at some stages of the disease. There is emaciation, concomitant moderate abdominal pain and variable fecal texture up to diarrhea. Gamma-glutamyl transferase and blood ammonia levels are greatly increased.

Pancreatic adenoma

Convulsions due to hypoglycemia are recorded in a pony with a pancreatic adenoma (3). It is assumed that the hypoglycemia resulted from hyperinsulinism generated by the beta-cell adenoma.

REFERENCES

(1) Kerr, O. M. et al. (1982) *Equ. vet. J.*, *14*, 338.
(2) Church, S. et al. (1987) *Equ. vet. J.*, *19*, 77.
(3) Ross, M. W. et al. (1983) *Cornell Vet.*, *73*, 151.
(4) Mostaghni, K. & Ivoghli, B. (1977) *Cornell Vet.*, *67*, 24.
(5) Bulgin, M. S. & Anderson, B. C. (1983) *Comp. cont. Educ.*, *5*, S482.
(6) Kaneko, J. J. & Rhode, E. A. (1964) *J. Am. vet. med. Assoc.*, *144*, 367.
(7) Jeffrey, J. R. (1968) *J. Am. vet. med. Assoc.*, *153*, 1168.
(8) Moore, J. N. et al. (1979) *Endocrinology*, *104*, 576.

8

Diseases of the Cardiovascular System

PRINCIPLES OF CIRCULATORY FAILURE

THE primary function of the cardiovascular system is to maintain the circulation of the blood so that normal exchanges of fluid, electrolytes, oxygen, and other nutrient and excretory substances can be made between the vascular system and tissues. Failure of the circulation in any degree interferes with these exchanges and is the basis for circulatory failure, the primary concept in diseases of the cardiovascular system. The two functional units of the system are the heart and the blood vessels and either may fail independently of the other, giving rise to two forms of circulatory failure—heart failure and peripheral failure. In heart failure the inadequacy is due to involvement of the heart itself; in peripheral circulatory failure the deficiency is in the vascular system which fails to return the blood to the heart.

Heart failure

The failure of the heart as a pump can result from a defect in filling of the heart, an abnormality in the myocardium or conducting system, an excessive workload, or a combination of any of the three. The two criteria used in assessing cardiac efficiency are the maintenance of circulatory equilibrium and the maintenance of the nutritional requirements of tissues. The maintenance of oxygen requirements is the most important, the nervous system in particular being very susceptible to deprivation of oxygen. Although both factors usually operate together, one of them is dominant in a particular case. It is therefore usual to subdivide heart failure into two types, acute heart failure and chronic or congestive heart failure, depending on which of the two factors is more important. However, a complete range of syndromes occurs and some of them do not fit neatly into one or other of the categories. Circulatory equilibrium is not maintained when cardiac output is deficient. If this develops sufficiently slowly, compensatory mechanisms, plus the failure of the heart itself as a pump, result in an increase in venous pressure and congestive heart failure. If on the other hand there is an acute reduction of cardiac output, as is caused by sudden cessation of the heart beat, the effect is to deprive tissues of their oxygen supplies and the syndrome of acute heart failure develops.

Peripheral circulatory failure

In peripheral circulatory failure the effective blood volume is decreased because of loss of fluid from the vascular system or by pooling of blood in peripheral vessels. The failure of venous return results in incomplete filling of the heart and a reduction in its minute volume, although there is no primary defect in cardiac ejection. The effects are the same as those of congestive heart failure in that the supply of nutrients and oxygen to tissues is reduced but there is no cardiac failure and backward congestion of the venous system does not occur. Peripheral circulatory failure is unaccompanied by engorgement of any sort except where there is splanchnic vasodilatation and pooling of the blood in the visceral vessels.

Cardiac reserve and compensatory mechanisms in heart failure

The normal heart has the capacity to increase its output several-fold in response to normal physiological demands created by exercise and to a less extent by pregnancy, by lactation and by digestion. Collectively, these responses comprise the cardiac reserve. Similar responses are utilized by the failing heart in an attempt to maintain cardiac output. Cardiac reserve and its response in heart failure have not been studied extensively in large domestic animals and consequently its description must rely heavily on studies on cardiac failure in small domestic animals and studies of the effect of exercise on cardiovascular performance in the horse (1, 7). Clinical observations on cardiac insufficiency and cardiac failure in large animals suggest that the processes are very similar to those in small animals and man.

The major mechanisms whereby cardiac output can be increased and circulatory efficiency improved are an increase in heart rate, an increase in stroke volume, increased extraction of oxygen from the blood and redistribution of blood to vital organs, or organs with particularly high requirements at the time. All of these mechanisms act synergistically and are interrelated. Heart rate and stroke volume are the determinants of cardiac output.

There is a great deal of cardiac reserve in the heart rate, and an elevation of heart rate alone is a significant factor in increasing cardiac output in the exercising horse. There is a limitation to heart rate reserve, because with increasing heart rates there is a decrease in diastolic filling time, and stroke volume falls at excessive heart rates. Effective heart rate reserve can be increased with exercise training, and maximal heart rate in trained exercising horses is six to seven times resting values (1). An increase in heart rate is also used to maintain cardiac output by the failing heart. In congestive syndromes associated with disorders of filling, such as constrictive pericarditis, this may be the principal reserve mechanism. With cardiac insufficiency in the horse and the cow it is rare for the heart rate to exceed 120/min, and rates higher than this are frequently due to tachyarrhythmias. Stroke volume is variable and depends upon the amount of shortening that the myocardial fibers can attain when working against arterial pressure. It is determined by an interplay of three factors: the ventricular distending or filling pressure (preload), the contractility of the myocardium (inotropic state), and the tension that the ventricular myocardium must develop during contraction (afterload).

An increase in ventricular distending pressure (end-diastolic pressure or volume) will increase ventricular end-diastolic fiber length which, by the Frank–Starling mechanism, will result in increased stroke work and a larger stroke volume. Ventricular distending pressure is influenced by atrial contraction and is greatly augmented by increased venous return associated with exercise and increased sympathetic activity. Contractility is most influenced by adrenergic activity and circulating catecholamines. An increase in stroke volume is achieved primarily by an increase in the ejection fraction and a reduction in the end-systolic volume, but can also be achieved by a decrease in afterload, which is primarily a function of aortic, or pulmonary, impedance and peripheral vascular resistance.

In cardiac insufficiency the principal defect is in the contractile state of the myocardium, and ventricular performance at any given end-diastolic volume or pressure is diminished. The heart still maintains to some degree its intrinsic propensity to alter its contractile properties in response to changes in filling pressure and its ability to increase its contractility under sympathetic nerve activity.

In early failure, cardiac output may still be maintained in the normal range by an increase in filling pressure and, through utilization of the Frank–Starling principle, the ventricles can eject a normal stroke volume despite the depression in contractility. Thus, early in the course of cardiac failure, the end-diastolic pressure may be elevated only during periods with heavy demands on the heart, such as during exercise.

However, as myocardial function becomes increasingly impaired, this mechanism is increasingly utilized for lesser work demands until end-diastolic pressure is elevated even at rest or with normal activity. Ventricular filling pressure is augmented by increased venous return associated with contraction of the venous capacitance vessels under increased sympathetic tone, and by an increase in blood volume as the result of salt and water retention by the kidney. Although the increase in ventricular end-diastolic pressure acts to maintain cardiac output, it is also reflected in a marked increase in systemic or pulmonary venous pressure, producing secondary effects that result in many of the clinical abnormalities associated with congestive heart failure. Where the contractile state of the heart is markedly reduced, the increased end-diastolic pressure is unable to maintain normal stroke volume, even at normal activity, and cardiac output is reduced even at rest—the state of uncompensated heart failure.

In normal animals, at rest, the oxygen tension of mixed venous blood is above 40 mmHg (5·3 kPa) which represents a considerable reserve. Increased extraction of oxygen from the blood by various tissues, with a subsequent increase in arterial venous oxygen difference, occurs during exercise and also in states of cardiac insufficiency. In uncompensated heart failure where stroke volume is reduced the arterial venous oxygen difference is large. There is also a redistribution of blood flow to vital organs. In the horse the splenic storage capacity for erythrocytes is large and the spleen may contain one-third of the total red cell volume. Maximal emptying of the spleen under adrenergic activity can significantly influence the oxygen-transporting capacity of the blood and, in the horse, the splenic reservoir contributes significantly to cardiovascular reserve.

It is evident that increased sympathetic nerve activity also plays a significant role in compensating for the failing ventricle, but one that is not readily determined clinically. An increase in sympathetic activity acts to augment cardiac output by increasing the heart rate, by improving the contractility of the myocardium, and by augmenting venous return to the heart. Autonomic nerve activity also regulates blood flow to more essential organs even when faced with insufficient cardiac output. Cardiac reserve is reduced by many pathological processes, and in many cases by the use of pharmacological agents. A stage of diminished cardiac reserve is the first step in heart disease and is manifested by inability of the animal to respond normally when called upon for extra effort. The compensatory mechanisms operate but not to the normal extent. The second stage in heart disease is one of decompensation when the heart is unable to maintain circulatory equilibrium at rest and all cardiac reserve is lost.

From a clinical standpoint it would be desirable to be able to detect incipient cardiac insufficiency at a very early stage. Unfortunately, the present state of the art is such that this is impracticable in usual clinical situations. Measurements to detect cardiac insufficiency center on attempts to determine the presence of a reduction in cardiac reserve. Since the fundamental problem in heart failure is a reduction in the contractile state of the heart, these measurements must reflect myocardial force–velocity relationships and length–active tension curves. Force, length, time and the derived variable velocity are the four factors that determine contractility. However, they are complexly interrelated and no one single clinical measurement can adequately define them. Measurements used to assess cardiac contractility are available. Values for large domestic animals are available (2–5), but their determination requires sophisticated instrumentation and is restricted to research laboratories. Other measurement assessments of cardiac performance such as cardiac output and ventricular end-diastolic pressure are, in general, too insensitive and too influenced by other variables to be of value in the assessment of cardiac insufficiency, especially at its early stages (6). Consequently, the current level of activity in veterinary medicine is such that the detection of heart failure must rely on the assessment of the effects of cardiac insufficiency rather than on a direct determination of impaired myocardial performance. The measurement of the ratio of cardiopulmonary blood volume to stroke volume, determined from a radiocardiogram following the injection of technetium 99^m pertechnetate, shows promise as a measure of cardiac function and for the detection of heart disease in horses (9).

The estimation of cardiac reserve is important when a prognosis is to be made on an animal with heart disease. Some of the important criteria used in making this assessment include the heart rate, the intensity of its sounds, the size of the heart, the characters of the pulse, and the tolerance to exercise. A resting heart rate above normal indicates loss of cardiac reserve because the ability to raise the minute volume of the heart is thereby reduced. Heart rates above a certain limit (e.g. 100–120/min in adult horses and cattle) result in lesser diastolic filling and decreased minute volume. The absolute intensity of the heart sounds suggests the strength of the ventricular contraction, soft sounds suggesting weak contractions, and sounds which are louder than normal suggesting cardiac dilatation and possibly hypertrophy. The interpretation of variation in intensity must be modified by recognition of other factors, such as pericardial effusion, which interfere with audibility of the heart sounds. An increase in heart size may occur in dilatation or hypertrophy of the ventricles. Both of these are compensatory mechanisms and the presence of either suggests that the cardiac reserve is waning, but hypertrophy, when it is accompanied by a heart rate which is slower than normal, is an indication that reserve has been reinstated. Dilatation up to a critical point is a compensatory mechanism, but beyond this the contractile power of the myocardium is reduced and decompensation and congestive heart failure result.

Pulse characters are of value in determining the cardiac reserve but they are greatly affected by factors other than cardiac activity. An increased amplitude of the pulse occurs when the cardiac stroke volume is increased, but a decreased amplitude may result from reduced venous return as well as from reduced contractile power of cardiac muscle.

Exercise tolerance is a good guide to cardiac reserve. It is best measured by estimation of the maximum heart rate attained after a standard exercise test, and the speed with which the heart rate returns to normal (7). An increase in respiratory rate and depth is also a good guide but is modified by changes in the respiratory system as well as by changes in the cardiovascular system. Signs of congestive heart failure occur only when all cardiac reserve is lost. Other indications of cardiac disease, including cardiac irregularity, heart murmurs and the presence of pericarditis, are not signs of reduced cardiac reserve but it can usually be accepted that some loss of reserve must be present. A knowledge of the etiology of the cardiac disease may be of value in prognosis in that a disease such as cardiac lymphomatosis, which is known to be progressive, must lead to further loss of reserve and eventually to congestive heart failure.

Cardiac enlargement

The ratio of heart weight to body weight is greater in athletic animals than in non-athletic animals, and the heart–weight ratio in horses can be modestly increased during training as a result of physiologic hypertrophy. Cardiac enlargement is also a compensatory response to persistent increased workloads that are associated with cardiovascular disease. The heart may respond by dilatation, hypertrophy or a combination of both. Cardiac hypertrophy is the usual response to an increased pressure load, and there is hypertrophy of individual fibers with an increase in the number of contractile units and an increase in total muscle mass. In states of cardiac insufficiency coronary blood flow reserve places limitations on this compensatory mechanism. Cardiac dilatation is the usual response to an increased volume load and probably results from fiber rearrangement. Contractions occurring in a dilated chamber can eject a larger volume of blood per unit of myocardial shortening. However, the limitation to this compensatory mechanism is evident in the law of Laplace which shows that in the dilated chamber greater myocardial wall tension is required to produce an equivalent elevation of intrachamber pressure during ejection.

The significance of finding cardiac enlargement on clinical examination is that it indicates the presence of a significant volume or flow load on the heart, or the presence of myocardial disease and a reduction of cardiac reserve.

The degree of enlargement is a good indication of the degree of cardiac embarrassment but accurate measurement is not usually undertaken in farm animals. Detection of cardiac enlargement is aided by careful auscultation of the heart and palpation of the apex beat. A palpable and audible increase in the apex beat and area of audibility, backward displacement of the apex beat, and increased visibility of the cardiac impulse at the base of the neck and behind the elbow are all indications of cardiac enlargement. Care must be taken that the abnormalities observed are not due to displacement of the heart by a space-occupying lesion of the thorax, or to collapse of the ventral part of the lung and withdrawal of lung tissue from the costal aspects of the heart. Careful percussion may also be of value but enlargement is only detectable by this method when it is extreme because of the situation of the heart behind the heavy shoulder muscles. Radiographic examination is a satisfactory method of measurement if the animal's size permits it. Echocardiographic examination can also be used to measure cardiac enlargement, and antemortem measurements correlate well with postmortem measurements (8). Treatment of cardiac enlargement depends upon the treatment of the primary condition.

REFERENCES

(1) Engelhardt, W. W. (1977) *Adv. vet., Sci.*, *21*, 173.

(2) Buss, D. D. & Bisgard, G. E. (1976) *Am. J. vet. Res.*, *38*, 365.
(3) Buss, D. D. & Bisgard, G. E. (1976) *Basic Res. Cardiol.*, *71*, 456.
(4) Hillidge, C. J. & Lees, P. (1976) *Res. vet. Sci.*, *21*, 176.
(5) Brown, C. M. & Holmes, J. R. (1979) *Equ. vet. J.*, *11*, 244 & 248.
(6) Hamlin, R. L. (1977) *Adv. vet. Sci.*, *21*, 19.
(7) Physick-Sheard, P. W. (1985) *Vet. Clin. Am. equ. Pract.*, *1(2)*, 383.
(8) O'Callaghan, M. W. (1985) *Equ. vet. J.*, *17*, 361.
(9) Van Aarde, M. N. (1984) *Vet. Res. Commun.*, *9*, 293.

MANIFESTATIONS OF CIRCULATORY FAILURE

The manifestations of circulatory failure depend on the manner and rapidity of its onset, and on its duration. They are best illustrated by a description of the three basic syndromes—congestive heart failure, acute heart failure or cardiac syncope, and peripheral circulatory failure.

Congestive heart failure

In congestive heart failure, the heart, due to some intrinsic defect, is unable to maintain circulatory equilibrium at rest and congestion of the venous circuit occurs, accompanied by dilatation of vessels, edema of the lungs or periphery, enlargement of the heart and an increase in heart rate.

Etiology

Diseases of the endocardium, myocardium and pericardium, diseases which primarily interfere with the flow of blood into or away from the heart and diseases which impede heart action may all result in congestive heart failure. The broad categories of causes of congestive heart failure are as follows:

Valvular disease

- Endocarditis resulting in either valvular stenosis or valvular insufficiency
- Congenital valvular defects—most commonly valvular stenosis
- Rupture of valve or valve chordae.

Myocardial disease

- Myocarditis—bacterial, viral, or parasitic
- Myocardial degeneration—toxic or nutritional
- Congenital and hereditary cardiomyopathy
- Chemicals affecting cardiac conduction.

Pericardial disease

- Pericarditis
- Pericardial tamponade.

Hypertension

- Pulmonary hypertension—high altitude disease, cor pulmonale
- Systemic hypertension—rare cause of heart failure in large animals.

Congenital defects producing shunts

- Defects of myocardium, such as septal defects
- Vascular abnormalities.

Diseases that produce cardiac insufficiency commonly do so by increasing the workload on the heart, and its increase can be due to either a pressure load or a flow load. Pressure loads occur with lesions that produce an obstruction to outflow such as aortic or pulmonary valve stenosis where the heart is required to perform more work to eject an equivalent amount of blood. Pressure loads are not necessarily associated with lesions in the heart. For example, systemic hypertension or pulmonary hypertension, such as occurs in high altitude disease of cattle due to an increase in pulmonary vascular resistance, may result in significant cardiac insufficiency. In general, the left ventricle can tolerate a pressure load to a much greater extent without overt signs of cardiac insufficiency than the right ventricle.

Volume loads or flow loads occur commonly with both acquired and congenital heart defects. In both aortic valve insufficiency and mitral valve insufficiency the volume of blood delivered to the body tissues does not differ significantly from normal. However, in order to achieve this, the stroke volume of the ventricle is markedly increased and the heart is much more inefficient for the same amount of effective work. In a similar manner a patent ductus arteriosus or an interventricular septal defect with a large shunt of blood can place a considerable flow load on the left ventricle. In general, the right ventricle is more capable of sustaining a flow load than the left ventricle.

Cardiac insufficiency may occur without any increase in workload if there is a primary weakness in the myocardium or defect in its rhythmic and coordinated contraction. Myocarditis, myocardial dystrophy and neoplasms of the heart, especially bovine viral leukosis lesions of the right atrium, are the common causes of myocardial asthenia and irregularity. Anoxia and toxemia cause myocardial asthenia and these syndromes are accompanied by signs of reduced cardiac reserve but the reduction is not sufficiently severe to result in congestive heart failure.

Pericardial diseases comprise pericarditis, cardiac tamponade and hydropericardium. They may result in cardiac insufficiency through interference with filling of the heart during diastole.

Pathogenesis

When an increased load is placed upon ejection of the blood from the heart, or the contractile power of the myocardium is reduced, compensatory mechanisms including increased heart rate, increased ventricular filling, redistribution of blood flow, dilatation and hypertrophy come into play to maintain circulatory equilibrium. However, cardiac reserve is reduced and the animal is not able to cope with circulatory emergencies as well as a normal animal. This is the stage of waning cardiac reserve in which the animal is comparatively normal at rest but is incapable of performing exercise, the phase of poor exercise tolerance. When these compensatory mechanisms reach their physiologic limit and the heart is unable to cope with the circulatory requirement at rest, congestive heart failure develops.

Early compensatory mechanisms in cardiac insufficiency include an increase in ventricular filling pressure, resulting in an increased ventricular end-diastolic volume, and improved cardiac performance by the Frank–Starling principle. Increased filling pressure is achieved by an increase in venous return and a shift in blood volume distribution under sympathetic nerve activity, but in the longer term is also facilitated by an increase in total blood volume, resulting from sodium and water retention by the kidneys. Sodium retention appears to be a consequence of decreased renal blood flow which can result either from increased renal vascular resistance due to sympathetic vasoconstriction of the efferent arterioles of the glomerulus or from decreased cardiac output in later stages of failure. There is a resultant increase in the filtration fraction and in sodium resorption from the proximal tubules. Sodium retention may also be favored by activation of the renin–angiotensin system and increased aldosterone activity. The increase in ventricular end-diastolic pressure is reflected in the atrial and input venous systems.

Many of the signs which appear during the stage of developing cardiac insufficiency, as well as those associated with decompensated heart failure, can be explained by the increase in venous pressure that arises either via these mechanisms or, more acutely, by the failure of the heart to pump blood. These signs are the consequence of congestion or edema due to increased venous hydrostatic pressure. A decreased forward output of blood from the heart also contributes to the clinical signs by the production of tissue hypoxia.

In animals, congestive heart failure may occur in either the right or left ventricles or in both together. With failure of the right side venous congestion is manifested only in the greater circulation, and with failure of the left side the resulting engorgement and edema are restricted to the lesser pulmonary circulation. Right-sided failure causes involvement of the liver and kidneys and reduces their normal function. In the kidneys the increase in hydrostatic pressure is offset by the reduced flow of blood through the kidney and urine output is reduced. Anoxic damage to the glomeruli causes increased permeability and escape of plasma protein into the urine. Venous congestion in the portal system is an inevitable sequel of hepatic congestion and is accompanied by impaired digestion and absorption and eventually by transudation into the intestinal lumen and diarrhea.

The net force for filtration of fluid across the capillary bed is greatly increased resulting in a potential for the production of edema in dependent subcutaneous body areas and in body cavities. Increased pulmonary venous pressure results in venous congestion, which decreases the compliance of the lung and leads to an increase in respiratory rate, an increase in the work of breathing, and to exercise intolerance. Similarly, bronchial capillary congestion and edema result in encroachment on airways and a decrease in ventilatory efficiency. Where venous hydrostatic pressure is exceptionally high, the increased transudation may lead to pulmonary edema, with the presence of fluid around the septal vessels and in the alveolar spaces, with marked impairment of gas exchange. The development of clinical pulmonary edema depends to some extent on the rapidity of the onset of cardiac failure. In chronic failure syndromes, the development of a capacious lymphatic drainage system may limit the occurrence of clinical edema, and in large animals, pulmonary edema is usually limited to cardiac failure where there is a relatively sudden onset of a volume load on the left ventricle.

Clinical findings

In the very early stages when cardiac reserve is reduced but decompensation has not yet occurred there is respiratory distress on light exertion. The time required for return to the normal respiratory and pulse rates is prolonged. In affected animals there may be evidence of cardiac enlargement and the resting heart rate is moderately increased.

Congestive heart failure referable to failure of the left side is manifested by an increase in the rate and depth of respiration at rest, cough, the presence of moist crackles at the base of the lungs and increased dullness on percussion of the ventral borders of the lungs. Terminally there is severe dyspnea and cyanosis. The heart rate is increased and there may be a murmur referable to the left atrioventricular or aortic semilunar valves.

In congestive heart failure of the right side the heart rate is increased and there is edema, usually anasarca, ascites, hydrothorax and hydropericardium. The anasarca is characteristically limited to the ventral surface of the body, the neck and the jaw. If the congestion is sufficiently severe the liver is palpably enlarged, protruding beyond the right costal arch and the edge is thickened and rounded. The respiration is deeper than normal and the rate may be slightly increased. Urine flow is usually reduced and the urine is concentrated and contains a small amount of albumen. The feces are usually normal at first but in the late stages diarrhea may be profuse. Body weight may increase because of edema but the appetite is poor and condition is lost rapidly. The superficial veins are dilated, particularly the jugular vein. The normal right atrial and right ventricular diastolic pressures will support a column of blood 5–8 cm high. The level of the jugular vein that this will distend will depend upon head position. Since the jugular vein communicates directly with the right ventricle, an increase in right ventricular end-diastolic pressure will be reflected in the height of the jugular vein distension and can be crudely estimated in this manner. The normal jugular pulse will transmit through this heightened column of blood and will appear more visible. Accentuation of the atrial component of the jugular pulse may occur in situations where there is decreased ventricular distensibility or atrial hypertrophy, and a jugular pulse associated with ventricular contraction occurs with tricuspid insufficiency. Epistaxis may occur in the horse but is rare in other species. The attitude and behavior of the animal is one of listlessness and depression, exercise is undertaken reluctantly, and the gait is shuffling and staggery due to weakness.

The prognosis in congestive heart failure varies to a certain extent with the cause but in most cases in large animals it is unfavorable. With a defect of the neuromyocardium the possibility of recovery exists but when the myocardium or endocardium are involved complete recovery rarely if ever occurs, although the animal may survive with a permanently reduced cardiac reserve. Uncomplicated defects of rhythm occur commonly only in the horse and these defects are more compatible with life than are extensive anatomical lesions.

Clinical pathology

Clinicopathological examinations are usually of value only in differentiating the causes of congestive heart failure. Venous pressure is increased and on venepuncture the pressure of blood from the needle is much greater than normal although it is not usually measured. Aspiration of fluid from accumulations in any of the cavities may be thought necessary if the origin of the fluid is in doubt. Classically the fluid is described as an edematous transudate. In most cases protein is present in large amounts due to leakage of plasma from damaged capillary walls. Proteinuria is often present for the same reason.

Necropsy findings

Lesions characteristic of the specific cause are present and may comprise abnormalities of the endocardium, myocardium, lungs or large vessels. Space-occupying lesions of the thorax may also exert pressure on the heart and interfere with its function. The lesions which occur in all cases of congestive heart failure, irrespective of cause, are pulmonary congestion and edema if the failure is left-sided, and anasarca, ascites, hydrothorax and hydropericardium, and enlargement and engorgement of the liver if the failure is right-sided.

Diagnosis

Accumulations of free fluid in the abdomen may also occur in peritonitis, rupture of the bladder and hepatic fibrosis. In chronic peritonitis, fluid removed by paracentesis contains bacteria and many leukocytes and there is an absence of signs of cardiac involvement. A normal heart is characteristic of the other two conditions also and when the bladder is ruptured, minimal urine is passed, the blood urea nitrogen and peritoneal fluid urea nitrogen are grossly elevated and there is usually a history of abdominal pain and straining to urinate. Fibrosis of the liver is usually accompanied by other signs of hepatic insufficiency including jaundice and photosensitization.

Edema may occur without cardiac insufficiency in mares and cows near the end of pregnancy but it characteristically commences at the udder and reaches its maximum degree in this region. It may be sufficiently severe to extend to the brisket but there is no engorgement of the jugular veins and no evidence of cardiac involvement. Other causes of generalized edema include particularly hypoproteinemia, as it occurs in parasitism, but the edema is not usually severe, is most apparent in the intermandibular space, and is usually accompanied by anemia. Bottle-jaw, as it is called, is most noticeable in grazing animals and it may disappear when the animal is fed from the trough, the dependence of the part being reduced.

Dyspnea has many causes but when it is accompanied by pulmonary edema it is usually due either to left-sided congestive heart failure or to acute pulmonary edema as it occurs in fog fever of cattle or other allergic and anaphylactic states. Poisoning with organic phosphates may have the same effect. It may be difficult to differentiate acute pulmonary emphysema from pulmonary edema, especially since emphysema often occurs as a complication of edema.

Treatment

The primary cause may be amenable to specific treatment. Non-specific treatment of congestive heart failure is applicable in most cases irrespective of the cause. It consists of attempts to reduce demands on cardiac output by restriction of activity, the reduction of the effects of altered preload by diuretic agents, and improvement of contractility by the administration of positive inotropic agents such as digitalis glycosides and theophylline derivatives. The use of agents to specifically reduce afterload has not received attention in large animal practice. Rest, or at least avoidance of violent exercise, is the primary consideration. If edema is present the salt intake should be reduced to as low as possible. Diuretics, mercurials, acetazolamide, chlorothiazide or frusemide, may reduce the embarrassment caused by large accumulations of fluid in body cavities.

Venesection can be used as an emergency treatment in acute pulmonary edema and 4–8 ml of blood per kg body weight may be withdrawn at a time. The immediate embarrassment to respiration is removed but the hydrostatic pressure usually returns to pretreatment levels within 24 hours. The same applies to drainage of the serous cavities by paracentesis, and the fluid loss should not be permitted to reach the point where dehydration occurs. If venesection is required at intervals of less than 7 days it is probably inadvisable to persist.

The use of drugs which increase the contractile power of the myocardium, e.g. digitalis and ouabain, has not received much attention in large animals. Oral administration in ruminants is probably of little value because of digestion of the glucosides. Intramuscular administration of purified extracts gives erratic results and intravenous injections must be given cautiously because of the danger of acute toxicity. The use of these drugs is also dangerous when there is severe infection, toxic myocarditis, or vegetative lesions of the valves and since these constitute the majority of conditions in which congestive heart failure occurs in farm animals the drugs do not find wide application. If they are used it is essential that the dosage be arranged in accordance with the principle of digitalization in which large, loading doses are given initially to obtain maximum improvement in cardiac output in a short time, followed by small maintenance doses to avoid intoxication. Unless myocardial damage is transient administration of the drug will probably have to be continued for life and this is unlikely to be a practicable procedure. No dosing regime is absolute and the dose may need adjustment based on clinical response, evidence of toxicity, or from the results of plasma digoxin assay. The half-life of digoxin in the horse has been determined at 17–23 hours (1, 2) and a plasma therapeutic range for digoxin of 0·5–2·0 ng/ml has been suggested (2).

Pharmacokinetic studies suggest that therapeutic but non-toxic plasma concentrations of digoxin in the horse will be achieved by an initial intravenous loading dose of 10–15 μg/kg followed by a maintenance dose of 5–7·5 μg/kg every 24 hours (1). An alternate schedule suggests 3·6–5·6 μg/kg as the loading dose followed by 1·4–2·2 μg/kg every 12 hours (3). The half-life of digoxin in cattle is reported as being 7·2 hours and an initial loading dose of 22 μg/kg followed by 3·4 μg/kg every 4 hours has been suggested (4).

In the horse the bioavailability of powdered digoxin given *per os* is low, being less than 20% of the administered dose. An oral loading dose of 7 mg/100 kg, followed by a daily oral maintenance dose of 3·5 mg/100 kg is suggested by pharmacokinetic studies (2).

REVIEW LITERATURE

Muir, M. W. & McQuirk, S. M. (1985) Pharmacology and pharmacokinetics of drugs to treat cardiac disease in horses. *Vet. Clin. N. Am. equ. Pract*, *1*, 353.

REFERENCES

(1) Francfort, P. & Schotzmann, H. J. (1976) *Res. vet. Sci.*, *20*, 84.
(2) Button, C. et al. (1980) *Am. J. vet. Res.*, *41*, 1388.
(3) Brumbaugh, G. W. et al. (1983) *J. vet. Pharmacol. Therap.*, 6, 163.
(4) Koritz, G. D. et al. (1983) *J. vet. Pharmacol. Therap.*, 6, 141.

Acute heart failure

In acute heart failure there is sudden loss of consciousness, falling with or without convulsions, severe pallor of the mucosae and either death or complete recovery from the episode. Acute heart failure should be a major consideration as a cause of sudden death in large animals, especially when death is associated with exertion or excitement.

Etiology

Acute heart failure can occur when there is a severe defect in filling, when there is failure of the heart as a pump, either due to severe tachycardia or bradycardia, and where there is a sudden increase in workload. The nature of the syndrome suggests a sudden catastrophic event from causes such as cardiac rupture or rupture of the aortic valve. However, these occurrences are usually predisposed by preexisting pathology of the affected area (2). Acute heart failure can also result from the sudden development of tachyarrhythmias secondary to myocardial disease resulting from infection or certain nutritional deficiencies. Commonly acute heart failure and death associated with these syndromes immediately follows periods of excitement or activity. The sudden occurrence of tachyarrhythmias in association with excitement and severe enough to cause acute heart failure presumably results from the exacerbating influence of catecholamines (3, 4). These are released in association with episodes of excitement and act to heighten the discharge potential of ectopic excitatory foci associated with myocardial disease.

Acute heart failure can also occur in the absence of primary cardiac disease under the influence of pharmacologic agents that affect cardiac conduction. These are associated with the ingestion of certain poisonous plants.

The many causes of acute heart failure are listed in greater detail under myocardial diseases. Some examples are as follows:

Disorders of filling
- Pericardial tamponade—atrial and ventricular rupture
- Aortic and pulmonary artery rupture.

Tachyarrhythmia
- Myocarditis, e.g., encephalomyocarditis virus, foot and mouth disease
- Nutritional deficiency myopathy, e.g., copper or selenium deficiency
- Plant poisoning, e.g., *Phalaris* spp.
- Electrocution and lightning strike.

Bradycardia
- Iatrogenic, e.g., intravenous calcium preparations, xylazine, concentrated solutions of potassium chloride
- Plant poisoning, e.g., *Taxus* spp.

Increase in workload
- Rupture of aortic valve
- Acute anaphylaxis.

Bradycardia caused by hypersensitivity of the carotid sinus is a specific syndrome in man but there appears to be no parallel in animals. Occlusion of a coronary vessel is another common cause of acute heart failure in man which is recorded rarely in animals. In the horse, arrhythmias and cardiac arrest may occur during the induction of anesthesia with barbiturates and may occur without premonitory signs in horses under halothane anesthesia (11).

Pathogenesis

With excessive tachycardia the diastolic period is so short that filling of the ventricles is impossible and cardiac output is grossly reduced. In ventricular fibrillation no coordinated contractions occur and no blood is ejected from the heart. The cardiac output is also seriously reduced when the heart rate slows to beyond a critical point. In all of these circumstances there is a precipitate fall in minute volume of the heart and a severe degree of tissue anoxia. In peracute cases the most sensitive organ, the brain, is affected first and the clinical signs are principally nervous in type. Pallor is also a prominent sign in these cases because of the reduction in arterial blood flow.

In less acute cases respiratory distress is more obvious because of pulmonary edema and although these can be classified as acute heart failure they are more accurately described as acute congestive heart failure.

Clinical findings

The acute syndrome may occur while the animal is at rest, but commonly occurs during periods of excitement or activity. The animal usually shows dyspnea, staggering and falling, and death often follows within seconds or minutes of the first appearance of signs. There is marked pallor of the mucosae. Although clonic convulsions may occur they are never severe and consist mainly of sporadic incoordinated movements of the limbs. Death usually is accompanied by deep, asphyxial gasps. If there is time for physical examination, absence of a palpable pulse and bradycardia, tachycardia or absence of heart sounds are observed.

In less acute cases, such as those which occur in enzootic muscular dystrophy in calves the course may be as long as 12–24 hours, and the clinical syndrome is one of acute left-sided heart failure. There is a marked elevation in heart rate usually associated with a severe tachyarrhythmia such as multiple ventricular extrasystoles. The specific findings in the heart and vascular system depend upon the arrhythmia and are detailed in the section on arrhythmias in this chapter (p. 312). There is an increase in respiratory rate and depth and evidence of pulmonary edema on auscultation of the lungs. Hydrothorax and mild ascites may develop if the animal lives long enough. The major presenting sign in acute heart failure is respiratory distress.

Acute heart failure was considered to be the cause of death in a significant proportion of horses that died suddenly during training or racing (5). The diagnosis was based primarily on the findings of significant pulmonary hemorrhage and edema although myocardial pathology was absent in most. Severe arrhythmic disturbances secondary to myocardial fibrosis and catecholamine influence were considered a possible cause.

Clinical pathology

In general, there is insufficient time available in which to conduct laboratory tests before the animal dies. The demonstration of elevated serum concentrations of tissue enzymes released in association with myocardial damage confirms the presence of myocardial disease. Laboratory tests may also be used to elucidate the specific etiology.

Necropsy findings

In typical acute cases engorgement of visceral veins may be present if the attack has lasted for a few minutes but there may be no gross lesions characteristic of congestive heart failure. Microscopic examination may show evidence of pulmonary congestion and early pulmonary edema. In more prolonged cases, venous engorgement with pulmonary congestion and edema are evident along with hydrothorax but these are more accurately described as acute congestive heart failure. The primary cause may be evidenced by macroscopic or microscopic lesions of the myocardium.

Diagnosis

Acute heart failure may be mistaken for primary disease of the nervous system but is characterized by excessive bradycardia or tachycardia, pallor of mucosae, absence of the pulse, and the mildness of the convulsions. Epilepsy is usually transient and repetitive and has a characteristic pattern of development. Similarly, horses with rupture of the aortic valve, rupture of mitral valve chordae, sudden onset of atrial fibrillation or multiple ventricular extrasystoles show a syndrome where sudden onset of respiratory distress is the prominent manifestation. However, examination of the heart will allow a diagnosis of the underlying cause.

Treatment

Treatment of acute heart failure is not usually practicable in large animals because of the short course of the disease. Deaths due to sudden cardiac arrest or ventricular fibrillation while under anesthesia can be avoided to a limited extent in animals by direct cardiac massage or electrical stimulation but these techniques are generally restricted to the more sophisticated institutional surgical units. Also, the electrical energy required for defibrillation of large animals is beyond the capabilities of conventional defibrillators (1). Intracardiac injections of very small doses of adrenalin are used but are likely to do as much harm as good, especially if ventricular fibrillation is present.

Peripheral circulatory failure

Peripheral circulatory failure occurs when the cardiac output is reduced because of the failure of venous return to the heart. The decreased blood flow to tissues and the resulting hypoxia causes depression of tissue function. Clinical manifestations include muscle weakness, subnormal temperature, decreased arterial blood pressure, increased respiratory and heart rates, and depression, coma, and in some cases mild clonic convulsions.

Etiology

Failure of venous return occurs when there is peripheral vasodilatation and pooling of blood in the vessels, and when there is a reduction in circulating blood volume. When the defect is vascular the failure is termed vasogenic and when due to reduced blood volume it is termed hematogenic or hypovolemic.

In vasogenic failure, blood collects in dilated splanchnic vessels. In the initial stages the total blood volume is normal but the circulating blood volume is greatly reduced. In later stages there is reduction of total blood volume and irreversible shock develops as the peripheral circulatory failure progresses to the hematogenic type. Alternate classifications of peripheral circulatory failure based on mechanistic circumstances include: hypovolemic, cardiogenic, defects in distribution of blood flow, vascular obstruction to blood flow.

Common causes of peripheral circulatory failure in large animals are as follows.

Vasogenic failure

- Parturient paresis in dairy cattle
- Septic shock—acute diffuse peritonitis, acute gangrenous mastitis, acute metritis
- Endotoxic shock—peracute coliform mastitis; this is contributory to shock associated with acute intestinal accidents
- Acute intestinal accidents; in the horse severe pain associated with acute intestinal accidents may contribute to the development of peripheral circulatory failure.

Hematogenic failure

- Hemorrhage

- Dehydration, such as in colitis-X, neonatal calf diarrhea, or stress-induced dehydration.

Pathogenesis

When cardiac output falls due to a decrease in circulating blood volume in hypovolemic states, the carotid and aortic baroreceptors stimulate the sympathetic nerves and adrenal medulla to release catecholamines resulting in vasoconstriction in vessels with alpha-adrenergic receptors. There is contraction of the spleen and venous capacitance vessels, tachycardia, and increased peripheral vascular resistance, all in an attempt to maintain cardiac output and blood perfusion through the coronary and cerebral blood vessels. Perfusion through these vessels is largely autoregulatory and relies principally on pressure. Peripheral vasoconstriction in the face of falling cardiac output results in a fall in blood pressure and in decreased perfusion of many organ systems, with resultant damage from hypoxia and tissue acidosis. Lowered renal perfusion results in oliguria and there may be a fall in blood pH from metabolic and lactic acidosis. If the circulating blood volume can be restored to normal by treatment before permanent damage occurs recovery may be complete. Endorphins that are released in response to the stress of shock may mediate the decrease in systemic blood pressure. The opiate antagonist naloxone shows promise in the prevention of experimental shock induced by endotoxin or hemorrhage in horses (6). However, with a continued fall in cardiac output, coronary and cerebral artery perfusion may be reduced sufficiently to cause damage to the myocardium and central nervous system. At this stage there may also be severe damage to other organ systems and further complications from the occurrence of disseminated intravascular coagulation (DIC). In these circumstances the restoration of circulating blood volume by treatment is ineffectual and death may intervene.

In vasogenic shock there is a fall in effective circulating blood volume with decreased tissue perfusion due to changes in peripheral arterial resistance and venous capacitance, and also due to peripheral arteriovenous shunting.

The speed with which fluid loss or splanchnic vasodilatation occurs has some bearing on the severity of the illness, as the compensatory mechanisms are capable of a continued response and are more readily overcome by acute than chronic stress. It is in circumstances where the failure is acute that damage to the central nervous system is most likely to occur. The major response to decreased venous return is observable clinically in the circulatory system where there is a fall in blood pressure and an increase in heart rate. Failure of the circulation also stimulates respiratory activity.

Clinical findings

A general depression, weakness and listlessness are accompanied by a fall in temperature to below normal, an increase in heart rate with abnormalities of the pulse including small amplitude, weak pressures and an increased vessel tone, although this latter is decreased in the terminal stages. Arterial blood pressure, measured either directly by arterial puncture or by indirect methods, will be low, and provides a valuable monitor of the severity and progression of circulatory inefficiency. The absolute intensity of the heart sounds may also be reduced because of the fall in blood pressure. The skin is cold and the mucosae pale with a prolonged capillary refill time. The respiratory rate is increased and respirations are usually shallow. Anorexia is usual but thirst may be evident. Nervous signs include depression and listlessness, and coma in the terminal stages. Clonic convulsions may occur but they are not a prominent part of the syndrome. Acute vasogenic failure, as it occurs in vasovagal syncope in man, is manifested by fainting and falling but this syndrome does not appear to occur in animals except possibly as a cause of death when vomitus is aspirated during anesthesia.

Clinical pathology

Clinicopathological examinations to determine the severity of a hemorrhagic anemia, or the degree of hemoconcentration in cases of shock or dehydration, give an excellent estimate of the severity of the primary condition. Blood examination usually shows an eosinopenia, lymphocytopenia, thrombocytopenia and hyperkalemia. Commonly, there are alterations in the acid–base status with both a metabolic and lactic acidosis.

Necropsy findings

The findings at necropsy examinations vary with the cause and there are no lesions which are characteristic of peripheral circulatory failure.

Diagnosis

Peripheral circulatory failure can be diagnosed when there is evidence of circulatory failure but no detectable cardiac abnormality, and when a primary cause, such as hemorrhage, shock or dehydration, is known to be present. It is only by inclusion of the latter proviso that peripheral failure can be differentiated from severe toxemia. Differentiation of the causes of peripheral failure depends upon ability to recognize the existence of shock, dehydration and hemorrhage and these subjects are discussed elsewhere.

Treatment

Regardless of cause, the main principle of treatment in peripheral circulatory failure is to restore the circulating blood volume to normal and maintain it so that tissue anoxia is avoided. The method of doing this varies with the cause. In hematogenic failure lost fluids should be replaced, the type of replacement depending on how the loss has occurred; in shock, plasma is required; in dehydration, isotonic fluids; and in hemorrhage, whole blood. The preparations used and the methods of administration are discussed in more detail under the headings of specific forms of fluid loss. In general, acute hemorrhage which reduces the packed cell volume to less than 20% makes blood replacement essential, and blood or fluid loss that results in total protein concentrations below 3·5 g/dl requires plasma.

Large quantities of fluid may be required to restore circulating blood volume. Because of the volume required, overhydration and pulmonary edema are not usually problems; in fact, the more common problem exists in being able to administer adequate amounts.

Measurement of central venous pressure can be used to monitor the adequacy of fluid replacement. The normal central venous pressure of the standing horse is recorded as 11·5 ± 5·6 cm H_2O (1130 ± 550 Pa), but is markedly influenced by factors such as head position and excitement (12). A rule of thumb is to administer fluids as long as the CVP remains below 5 cm H_2O. Indirect arterial blood pressure measurement can also be used as a monitor. In the absence of these monitors, the clinical observations of jugular venous pressure, quality of the palpable arterial pulse, and the restoration of urine flow, give some guide that peripheral perfusion is being reestablished. Disturbances in acid-base status are usually corrected by the reestablishment of adequate tissue perfusion; however, where there is marked lactic acidosis, or a blood pH of less than 7·1, specific bicarbonate therapy should also be included.

There appears to be little indication for the use of cardiac stimulants and inotropic drugs in peripheral circulatory failure in large animals as there is no primary cardiac deficiency. Cardiogenic shock in large animals is not documented. In general, vasoconstricting agents should be avoided, as they further restrict blood flow and decrease tissue perfusion. A large dose of corticosteroids (dexamethasone, 5–10 mgkg or methylprednisolone, 30 mg/kg) may be beneficial. The side-effects of a single massive dose of intravenous corticosteroids appear to be minimal, even in septic shock. The cyclo-oxygenase inhibitors flunixin, meglumine and phenylbutazone and the administration of corticosteroids may be of value in endotoxic shock (7–10) but need to be given early in the course for maximum benefit.

REVIEW LITERATURE

Muir, W. W. (1987) Equine shock: the need for prospective clinical studies. *Equ. vet. J.*, *19*, 1–7.

REFERENCES

(1) Geddes, L. A. et al. (1974) *J. clin. Invest.*, *53*, 310
(2) Van Vleet, J. F. & Ferrans, V. J. (1986) *Am. J. Pathol.*, *124*, 98.
(3) Van Vleet, J. F. et al. (1977) *Am. J. vet. Res.*, *38*, 991.
(4) Rona, G. (1985) *J. Mol. Cell Cardiol.*, *17*, 291.
(5) Gelberg, H. B. et al. (1985), *J. Am. vet. med. Assoc.*, *187*, 1354
(6) Weld, J. M. (1984) *Res. Commun. Chem. Pharmocol.*, *44*, 227.
(7) Olson, N. C. & Brown, T. T. (1986) *Am. J. vet. Res.*, *47*, 2187.
(8) Fessler, J. F. et al. (1982) *Am. J. vet. Res.*, *43*, 140.
(9) Olson, N. C. et al. (1985) *J. appl. Physiol.*, *59*, 1464.
(10) Turek, J. J. (1985) *Am. J. vet. Res.*, *46*, 591.
(11) Kellagher, R. E. B. & Watney, G. C. G. (1980) *Vet. Rec.*, *119*, 347.
(12) Schatzmann, U. & Battier, B. (1987). *Dtsch Tierärztl. Wochenschr.*, *4*, 137.

SPECIAL EXAMINATION OF THE CARDIOVASCULAR SYSTEM

The more commonly used techniques of examination of the heart and pulse are described in Chapter 1 but special techniques are available which may be of value in some cases. With the possible exception of electrocardiography and methods for indirect determination of blood pressure, these techniques currently have limited application in practice situations. Sophisticated and expensive equipment is required for many of these examinations. The prevalence and economic importance of cardiovascular disease in large animals that requires examination by these methods is generally not significant enough to warrant their use. Furthermore, spurious and misleading readings can be obtained with such equipment if the principles underlying its use are not appreciated. Examination of the cardiovascular system of large animals using these techniques has been limited and generally confined to teaching hospitals and investigative units. For this reason these techniques of examination and their interpretation are not dealt with in detail in this section.

Electrocardiography

The electrocardiogram (ECG) provides a record and measure of the varying potential difference that occurs over the surface of the body as the result of electrical activity within the heart. This is associated with depolarization and repolarization of the myocardium. At any one instant during depolarization and repolarization there are generally several fronts of electrical activity within the heart. However, at the body surface the potential difference is generally the sum of this activity and at any one instant the electrical activity in the heart registers as a single dipole vector that has polarity, magnitude and direction.

The polarity is determined by the charge on the surface of the cells while the magnitude and direction is determined by the mass of muscle being depolarized or repolarized and the sum of the instantaneous vectors. Thus a wave of depolarization or repolarization over a muscle mass such as the atria or the ventricles is presented at the body surface as a sequence of instantaneous vectors with changing magnitude and direction.

The electrocardiograph is used to detect these characters. In simple terms it can be considered as a voltmeter consisting of two input terminals, an amplifier to allow the recording of low input signals and a galvanometer with an attached recording device such as a heated stylus on heat sensitive paper or an ink pen or ink squirter. When a potential difference exists across the input terminals (electrodes), current flows through the coils of the electromagnet suspended between the poles of the permanent magnet to cause a deflection of the recording pen. The electrocardiograph can therefore detect the polarity of the cardiac electrical vectors and by calibration of the machine and appropriate placement of electrodes on the body surface it can detect their magnitude and direction.

The calibration of most electrocardiographs is such that an input of 1 mV produces a 1 cm deflection of the recording pen. Recording speeds are generally 25 or 50 mm/second. In recording an ECG, certain standard electrode positions are used for recording. A lead is the recording or circuit between two recording points. Depending upon the wiring within the electrocardiograph the same potential difference across a lead could result in an upward or downward deflection of the recording pen. In order to allow standard recording and comparison between recordings the polarity of the electrodes for standard leads has been established by convention and the leads are always recorded at these polarities. The electrodes of a lead are commonly called positive or negative. A positive electrode in a lead is one which when electrically positive relative to the other, due to a potential difference between them, yields an upward or positive deflection of the recording pen.

In the normal heart, depolarization and repolarization of the myocardium occurs in a definite pattern and sequence and the electrocardiograph can be used to measure and time these events. Thus discharge of the sinoatrial node results in a wave of depolarization over the atria to produce a P wave in the ECG. The delay in conduction at the AV node is registered by no electrical activity at the body surface and an isoelectric P–R interval on the ECG. Depolarization of the ventricles occurs with several sequential fronts to produce the QRS complex which is followed by another isoelectric period before repolarization represented by the T wave.

In view of these characteristics the electrocardiogram is primarily used for two purposes. The prime use is in the detection and diagnosis of conduction abnormalities and arrhythmic heart disease. This is detected by measurement of the various waveforms and intervals in the ECG that represent conduction and depolarization in the heart, and by observation of their absence or abnormality. The ECG can also be used to detect changes in the state of the myocardium. In so far as the magnitude and direction of the electrical vectors can be influenced by factors such as cardiac hypertrophy and by the health of the myocardium, measurements of vector changes from normal may detect these abnormalities. The electrocardiogram cannot be used for the primary detection of valvular disease or congenital cardiac defects but may detect the secondary myocardial hypertrophic changes that result from such diseases.

Lead systems used in electrocardiography in large animals have generally been based on Einthoven's triangle as used in man. The standard bipolar limb leads (I, II and III) and the augmented unipolar limb leads (aVR, aVL, aVF) are commonly used in conjunction with an exploring unipolar chest lead (2, 3). Variations in the position of the feet may produce changes in ECG waveforms with this lead system and recordings should be taken with the animal standing square or with the left front foot set slightly in advance of the right front foot. The requirements for recording satisfactory electrocardiograms using this lead system have been described (4). This lead system is quite satisfactory for the detection of conduction disturbances and arrhythmic heart disease. Other simpler lead systems, less subject to movement artefact, have also been used for this purpose (5). There are, however, deficiencies associated with its use for the detection of change in the magnitude and direction of electrical vectors that may result from hypertrophy or myocardial disease (6). Nevertheless it has been used extensively for this purpose and there is now a considerable body of information on the normal and abnormal electrocardiogram in horses (2, 4, 7–9) and ruminants (1, 9, 11, 12). These are set out in summary form in Table 30.

Table 30. Electrocardiographic parameters in cattle and horses

	Holstein (52)*	*Jersey* (39)	*Thoroughbred* (2, 3)
Duration (secs)			
Lead II			
P	0·1 ± 0·011	0·08 ± 0·022	0·132 ± 0·012
P–R	0·208 ± 0·022	0·16 ± 0·006	0·325 ± 0·065
QRS	0·088 ± 0·008	0·070 ± 0·003	0·110 ± 0·009
Q–T	0·398 ± 0·034	0·38 ± 0·010	0·524 ± 0·034
T	0·114 ± 0·081	0·10 ± 0·011	—
Mean electrical axis–frontal plane			
P	+23·5 ± 12	—	Majority +50–+90
QRS	+196 ± 70	—	Majority +30–+90
T	+129 ± 76	—	Majority +60–+160

*Numbers in parentheses are references.

Lead systems based on the standard limb leads are not particularly suited for detection of vector changes associated with myocardial change. These systems are primarily influenced by vectors in the frontal plane (longitudinal and transverse) whereas early and late forces in the myocardium are significantly directed in the vertical direction. Furthermore the heart is not electrically equidistant from the electrodes of each lead and distortion of recorded vector loops can result (3, 6). A partial correction of these deficiencies can result from the recording of a lead using an exploring electrode at the V10 position over the dorsal spinous processes in addition to the standard limb leads. However, for proper representation of the vector changes associated with electrical activity within the heart completely different electrode placement is required. A number of systems have been proposed. The electrode placement varies and is quite complicated but electrocardiographic studies using these methods are available for the horse (3, 15, 16), ruminants (17, 18) and swine (19).

The order of ventricular activation in horses, cattle, sheep and swine differs from that of man and dogs in that ventricular depolarization is represented by only two fronts of activity (21). Depolarization of a large proportion of the myocardial mass in large animals is not recognized by the surface electrocardiogram due to the fact that the Purkinje fibers penetrate much more deeply in these species and depolarization occurs over multiple minor fronts that tend to cancel out, rather than a large single front as in dogs. For this reason, the detection of cardiac hypertrophy and myocardial abnormality by vector analysis of the electrocardiogram is less reliable in large animals than in other species.

Electrocardiograms are of limited practical value for the assessment of electrolyte imbalances in large animal species. Nevertheless, changes do occur. For example, there is a linear correlation between Q–T interval and plasma calcium in cattle, with elongation of the interval in hypocalcemic and shortening in hypercalcemic states.

Increased amplitude and prolongation of the P wave and QRS complex may occur with hypokalaemia and metabolic alkalosis.

The fetal ECG may be recorded, and can be of value in determining if the fetus is alive, the presence of a singleton or twins, and as a monitor for fetal distress during difficult or prolonged parturition. A modified lead system is required with the RA and LA electrodes being placed over the ventral abdomen below the flank on the right and left sides respectively, and LL being placed just behind the sternum in the midline. RL can be situated anywhere. All bipolar and augmented leads should be recorded using increased sensitivity. Fetal heart rate decreases logarithmically from approximately 110 beats/minute at 150 days before term to 75 beats/minute near to term (77). Continued monitoring traces may be needed to assess fetal distress. Following birth and during early growth of the foal there are age-dependent increases in the electrocardiographic intervals and changes in the orientation of the mean electrical axis (63, 64). In the horse, estimates of heart size have been made from measurements of the electrocardiogram and may be of value in assessing the potential performance (4, 6). Postexercise electrocardiograms frequently deliver information additional to that of the resting ECG, and methods for radiotelemetry have been described (23).

Phonocardiography

Phonocardiography allows the recording and measurement of heart sounds. A special microphone is placed over the various auscultatory areas of the heart and the heart sounds are recorded graphically on moving paper or on an oscilloscope. Prior to recording they are usually passed through high pass, low pass or band pass filters to allow better discrimination of the individual sounds and to allow a crude frequency examination. Phonocardiograms are usually recorded in conjunction with an electrocardiogram which allows timing of their occurrence in relationship to the electrical activity within the heart.

Phonocardiograms can provide considerable information on heart sounds additional to that acquired by stethoscopic examination. In the horse, up to eleven sound events can be detected in each cardiac cycle and figures of the occurrence and duration of normal heart sounds in large animals are available (10, 25, 26, 28).

In cardiovascular disease, phonocardiograms are primarily used for the characterization and timing of murmurs (32) especially at fast heart rates where simple stethoscopic examination may not allow this.

In conjunction with an electrocardiogram the phonocardiogram can be used to measure systolic time intervals which may be altered in congenital and acquired cardiovascular abnormalities (33, 34).

Exercise tolerance

Dyspnea, fatigue and a prolonged elevation in heart rate following exercise are signs suggestive of cardiac insufficiency. Frequently animals with suspect cardiac disease are exercised in an attempt to elicit these signs and to get an estimate of exercise tolerance. In most practice situations the assessment of exercise tolerance is subjective. There is obviously a considerable difference in the amount of exercise that a beef bull or trained racehorse can tolerate under normal conditions, and the amount of exercise given to any one animal is determined by the clinician's judgment. In the horse, there have been attempts to develop a standard exercise test and to study the relationship between fitness and cardiovascular function. In terms of the heart, these have largely been concerned with the relationship between the heart rate and the velocity of movement of the horse and have been determined on horses on a treadmill or by means of telemetry from horses timed over a measured distance on race tracks (36, 37). Working capacity is generally expressed as the velocity in metres/second related to heart rate, and there is a linear relationship between the speed of work and heart rate at all gaits (35–37). The slope of the regression line between heart rate and velocity, and the heart rate at a given velocity, i.e., HR 400, can be used to estimate fitness in the horse and also can be used as a measure for determining the significance of cardiopulmonary disease (13, 14). Significant differences are observed in the heart rate/velocity relationships between normal horses and horses with chronic respiratory disease (14, 36) or conduction abnormalities on resting electrocardiograms (37), but the method is not capable of detecting the presence of heart disease in every instance (14). The rate of fall in heart rate following exercise and the time required to reach resting levels depends upon the severity of the exercise even in fit horses (37). Heart rate falls rapidly over the first minute and then more slowly over the ensuing 10–15 minute period.

Criteria for cardiovascular performance in endurance rides are described and the rapidity of heart rate decline following completion of each section of the ride can be used for field assessment of this function (20).

Cardiac output

There are several techniques available for the measurement of cardiac output but the one almost universally applied in large animals is the dye dilution technique using such dyes as Evans' blue or indocyanine green. It involves the injection of an exact amount of dye into the jugular vein or pulmonary artery via a catheter and the serial collection of blood samples from a suitable proximally located artery (40–42). Cardiac output can be calculated manually from a dye dilution curve by determining the mean concentration of the dye and the time taken for one circulation through the heart (40). Automated cardiodensitometers are also available for this estimation. Cardiac output is expressed as liters per minute (l/min) but obviously varies according to size and is usually corrected to the cardiac index on the basis of weight or body surface area. The cardiac index for horses (43), sheep (44) and cattle (40) at rest has been determined as 86 ± 13, 131 ± 39 and 113 ± 11 ml/min/kg, respectively, but other determinations are available (41, 42, 45). Stroke volume estimates can also be derived by a correction for heart rate.

In general the normal variation between animals in indexes of cardiac output is too great to allow it to be used as a diagnostic measure in individual animals with suspected cardiac disease. It can be of considerable value in experimental studies where the effects of certain procedures can be followed within the same animal. The monitoring of cardiac output would be of value during anesthetic procedures; however, indicator dilution techniques are too cumbersome for use in routine clinical practice. There is a significant correlation between mixed venous O_2 tension, measured in blood collected via a pulmonary artery catheter, and cardiac output in anesthetized horses, and it has been suggested that this measure may provide a facile method for the monitoring of cardiac output during clinical anesthesia (78).

The estimation of cardiac output has been of value in determining the myocardial depressant activity of such drugs as anesthetics (46) and has also been used in the study of the effects of primary cardiac and other disease (48). Indicator dilution curves using dyes or thermodilution methodology can be used to detect the presence of intracardiac defects such as septal defects and to quantify their significance (47).

Cardiac catheterization

The measurement of pressure within the various chambers of the heart and in the inflow and outflow vessels can provide diagnostic information in both acquired and congenital heart disease in large animals. Generally pressure is determined by means of fluid-filled catheters introduced into these areas and connected to an external pressure transducer. These systems are generally satisfactory for the measurement of pressure and the detection of changes with abnormality. However, because of their transmission characteristics they are less suitable for the precise timing of pressure events, and catheter tip manometers should be used for this purpose.

Catheterization of the right side of the heart is a comparatively simple procedure in large animals but is not without risk to the animal. It can be done in the standing position. Flow-directed catheters are used and can be introduced through a needle inserted into the jugular vein. Balloon-tipped catheters aid the flow of the catheter into the pulmonary artery (49). Catheterization of the left side of the heart is more complicated and less commonly performed. It generally requires the use of a stiff catheter that is introduced into the carotid or femoral artery by surgical methods and subsequently manipulated to the left ventricle. The techniques of catheterization for large animals have been described (50).

The systematic determination of the pressure within each area of the heart and in the inflow and outflow vessels can allow a determination of the type of abnormality that is present. Valvular stenosis or incompetence is associated with abnormal pressure differences across the affected valve during systole or diastole (51). Cardiac hypertrophy is generally accompanied by an increase in pressure during systole of the affected chamber. With high fidelity equipment, pressure waveforms can also have diagnostic values (34).

During catheterization blood may be withdrawn through the catheter and subjected to blood gas analysis. In right-sided catheterization an increase in oxygen saturation in the right ventricle or pulmonary artery can be diagnostic for the presence of a left-to-right shunt with interventricular septal defects or a patent ductus arteriosus (51, 52). Shunts can also be demonstrated by dye or thermodilution techniques (65).

Myocardial force-velocity relationships can also be examined by this procedure with suitable instrumentation (53–55).

Radiographic examination

Because of the size of horses and cattle this method of examination is more common in neonates of these species. Angiocardiography can be a diagnostic method of examination in congenital cardiac defects where the passage of contrast media through abnormal routes can be detected (56, 57).

Although standard data are not available for heart size as estimated on radiographic examination, significant enlargement of the heart as a whole or of one or other of the ventricles or displacement can be detected by this means, as can a dilated posterior vena cava.

Echocardiography

In echocardiography, high frequency sound waves are pulsed through tissues at known velocities. When the sound waves encounter an acoustic tissue interface echoes are reflected back to the transducer. In M (motion) mode echocardiography these reflections are displayed on an oscilloscope in conjunction with an ECG, and determinations of ventricular wall thickness, luminal dimensions and value motion can be made. Alternatively, two-dimensional (real time) echocardiograms can be achieved that have depth and width. The echocardiogram is capable of determining spatial orientation and distance of the returning echo. It provides a non-invasive method of cardiac examination that has considerable potential for use in veterinary medicine. Measurements of cardiac and individual chamber dimensions (24, 27, 68, 69) can be of value in assessing effects of cardiac lesions on cardiac response and function and can also be used to predict the type of lesion likely to result in these changes. Valvular defects and endocarditis may be diagnosed by imaging abnormal valve motion, incompetent valve orifices or vegetative masses associated with the valves (70–72). Similarly echocardiography can be of value in the diagnosis of congenital cardiovascular defects (75) and the injection of echogenic materials such as microbubble-laden saline may aid in the detection of shunts (76). Echocardiography can also be used to determine indexes of contractility; it has detected the presence of tumor mass within the heart (73) and can be used to determine the presence and extent of pleural and precardial effusion. In the examination of the vascular system ultrasound shows significant promise in the early detection of iliac thrombosis in horses and is more sensitive than manual palpation per rectum (74). The use of echocardiography in the horse (22), cow (24) and pig (27) is recorded and reference values for echocardiography in normal horses are available (67).

Special examination of the pulse

The more commonly used criteria for examination of the pulse have been described in Chapter 1. Additional information on blood pressure may be obtained by careful palpation. An estimate of the systolic pressure can be made by determining the amount of pressure that has to be exerted with a proximal finger to obliterate the pulse felt by a distal finger. Care must be taken that sufficient pressure is exerted with the distal finger to obtain maximum amplitude.

An estimate of the diastolic pressure can be obtained by gradually increasing pressure with one finger and determining the amount of pressure required to obtain the maximum amplitude of the pulse wave. An artery with a low diastolic pressure is flattened by light pressure between pulse waves and the maximum amplitude is felt with little digital pressure. Conversely a high diastolic pressure in an artery requires much pressure to flatten it and the maximum amplitude is only obtained by the exertion of considerable digital pressure.

The form of the pulse wave may have significance. A rapid rise and fall in the wave and a large amplitude are usually associated with aortic semilunar insufficiency and patent ductus arteriosus. In such cases there may be visible pulsation of small arteries. Low blood pressure, arteriovenous fistulae and anemia are also accompanied by a rapid rise and fall of the pulse wave and an increased amplitude of the pulse. A slow-rising pulse is characteristic of stenosis of the aortic semilunar valves.

Special examinations of the arterial pulse include palpation of the external iliac and volar digital arteries in iliac thrombosis of horses, of the middle uterine arteries in pregnancy diagnosis of cattle, and the cranial mesenteric arteries of horses affected by verminous arteritis.

Examination of the arteriolar–capillary circulation

The warmth and color of the skin, mucosae and conjunctivae give some information on the state of the circulation in the smaller vessels. The color of these surfaces depends upon the amount of blood present in the capillaries, pallor indicating emptiness of the capillaries, reddening indicating engorgement. Temperature of the skin depends largely upon the degree of arteriolar flow, warmth indicating good arteriolar flow, coldness suggesting poor flow.

In man, fragility of capillary walls can be measured by the amount of negative pressure, applied through a suction cup, required to cause petechiation in the underlying skin. Standard data are not available for such tests in animals. The spontaneous occurrence of petechiae usually indicates increased capillary fragility but defects in the clotting mechanisms may also cause apparently spontaneous hemorrhages of varying sizes.

Ophthalmoscopic examination may reveal the presence of hemorrhages in the retina and, provided trauma to the orbit has not occurred, these may suggest increased vascular fragility. The hemorrhages may appear as red patches of various size which become brown to orange with increasing age. Discontinuities of vessels or lack of definition of their walls may also suggest vascular disease. Gross hemorrhage into the anterior chamber may also occur and is usually visible on direct examination of the eye.

Measurement of arterial blood pressure

Blood pressure may be determined directly by arterial puncture and pressure measurement but this is impractical in clinical cases. The development of simple methods for the indirect determination of arterial blood pressure has proved difficult in large animals due to the paucity of suitably located arteries where a pressure cuff can be applied and to problems in detecting pulse return by simple auscultatory or palpatory methods. Most methods have concentrated on the tail as the site for measurement but pulse return has been detected by a variety of cumbersome or expensive equipment methods (58). Frequently only systolic pressure can be determined by these methods.

In the horse a simple and relatively inexpensive method for indirect determination of systolic and diastolic blood pressure is described using the Doppler ultrasound principle to detect pulse return characters (60, 61). For adult horses, the method uses a rectangular self-adhesive sphygmomanometer cuff 37 x 12.5 cm containing an inflatable rubber bag of 19 x 11 cm as the occlusive cuff in conjunction with a standard rubber pump and aneroid manometer. The cuff is applied snugly to the base of the tail and pulse sounds are detected in the ventral coccygeal artery. On deflation of the cuff the pressure at emergence of the first sound is read as the systolic pressure. Diastolic pressure can be identified by a number of criteria (60) but the occurrence of a distinct second sound can be used as a satisfactory detection point (61). Systolic and diastolic blood pressure of a large series of trained thoroughbred horses were 112 ± 16 mmHg (14·9 ± 2·1 kPa) and 77 ± 14 mmHg (10·2 ± 1·9 kPa) respectively (59). Equivalent values have been recorded in other breeds (62). These values are coccygeal uncorrected values and can be corrected to heart level by adding 0·7 mmHg (0·93 kPa) for every centimeter in height between the base of the heart and the tail. Posture of the horse is important as lowering of the head significantly lowers systolic, diastolic and pulse pressure (38).

The clinical diagnostic value of indirect blood pressure determination has yet to be determined. Hypertension has been found in association with epistaxis, laminitis in horses, and with painful fractures of the distal bones of the limb. It is also of value in the assessment of the degree of shock and possibly may prove of value in the differential diagnosis of conditions such as colitis-X and acute salmonellosis and in assessing the prognosis of colics. Blood pressure readings can be obtained by equivalent techniques from the tails of cattle. However, due to anatomical differences these do not always correlate well with true blood pressure. Pressures have been observed to be 100–140 mmHg (13·3–18·7 kPa) systolic and 50–85 mmHg (6·7–11·3 kPa) diastolic (31).

Measurement of blood volume

The rate of disappearance from the circulation of intravenously injected Evans blue is an accurate enough method for clinical purposes. However, errors are likely unless age and recent physical activity are taken into account (29).

REVIEW LITERATURE

Bonagura, J. D., Herring, D. S. & Welker, F. (1985) Echocardiography. *Vet. Clin. N. Am. equ. Pract.*, *1(2)*, 311–333.

REFERENCES

(1) Buss, D. D. et al. (1980) *J. Am. vet. med. Assoc.*, *177*, 174.
(2) Steel, J. D. (1963) *Studies on the Electrocardiogram of the Racehorse*. Sydney: Australasian Medical Publishing Co.
(3) Miller, P. J. & Holmes, J. R. (1984) *Res. vet. Sci.*, *36*, 370.
(4) Steel, J. D. & Stewart, G. A. (1974) *J. S. Afr. vet. Assoc.*, *45*, 263.
(5) Helwig, R. W. (1977) *J. Am. vet. med. Assoc.*, *170*, 153.
(6) Nielsen, K. & Vibe Petersen, G. (1980) *Equ. vet. J.*, *12*, 81.
(7) Kurger, J. M. & Jenkins, W. L. (1974) *J. S. Afr. vet. Assoc.*, *45*, 139.
(8) Gross, D. R. (1971) *J. Am. vet. med. Assoc.*, *159*, 1335.
(9) Fregin, G. F. (1985) *Vet. Clin. N. Am. equ. Pract.*, *1(2)*, 419.
(10) Vanselow, B. et al. (1978) *Aust. vet. J.*, *54*, 161.
(11) Littledike, E. T. et al. (1976) *Am. J. vet. Res.*, *37*, 383.
(12) Unshelm, J. et al. (1974). *Zentralbl. VetMed.*, *21A*, 479.
(13) Engelhardt, W. (1977) *Adv. vet. Sci.*, *21*, 173.
(14) Maier-Bock, H. & Erhlein, H–J. (1978) *Equ. vet. J.*, *10*, 235.
(15) Miller, P. J. & Holmes, J. R. (1984) *Res. vet. Sci.*, *37*, 334.
(16) Deegen, E. & Reinhard, H. J. (1974) *Dtsch Tierärztl. Wochenschr.*, *81*, 257.
(17) Schultz, R. A. & Pretorius, P. J. (1972) *Onderstepoort J. vet. Res.*, *39*, 209.
(18) Thielscher, H. H. & Flock, D. (1968) *Zentralbl. VetMed.*, *15A*, 401.
(19) Thielscher, H. H. (1969) *Zentralbl. VetMed.*, *16A*, 370.
(20) Rose, R. J. et al. (1979) *Equ. vet. J.*, *11*, 56.
(21) Muylle, E. & Oyaert, W. (1975) *Zentralbl. VetMed.*, *22A*, 463, 474.
(22) Wingfield, S. et al. (1980) *Equ. vet. J.*, *12*, 181.
(23) Hall, M. C. et al. (1976) *Aust. vet. J.*, *52*, 1, 6.
(24) Pipers, S. F. et al. (1978) *J. Am. vet. med. Assoc.*, *172*, 1313.
(25) Bornert, G. & Bornert, D. (1971) *Arch. exp. VetMed.*, *25*, 549, 565, 619, 635.
(26) Leurada, A. A. et al. (1970) *Am. J. vet. Res.*, *31*, 1695.
(27) Pipers, S. F. et al. (1978) *Am. J. vet. Res.*, *39*, 707.
(28) Paterson, D. F. et al. (1965) *Ann. NY Acad. Sci.*, *127*, 242.
(29) Persson, S. G. B. & Ulberg, L. E. (1979) *Acta vet. Scand.*, *20*, 10.
(30) Parry, B. W. (1984) *J. equ. vet. Sci.*, *4*, 49.
(31) Olsen, J. D. & Booth, G. D. (1972) *Cornell Vet.*, *62*, 85.
(32) Glazier, D. B. et al. (1975) *J. Am. vet. med. Assoc.*, *167*, 49.
(33) Amend, J. F. et al. (1975) *Can. J. comp. Med.*, *39*, 62.
(34) Miller, P. J. & Holmes, J. R. (1985). *Equ. vet. J.*, 17, 181.
(35) Persson, S. G. B. (1967) *Acta vet. Scand.*, Suppl. *19*, 127.
(36) Littlejohn, A. et al. (1977) *Equ. vet. J.*, *9*, 75.
(37) Hall, M. C. et al. (1976) *Aust. vet. J.*, *52*, 1, 6.
(38) Parry, B. W. et al. (1980) *Am. J. vet. Res.*, *41*, 1626.
(39) Uphadyay, R. C. et al. (1976) *Ind. vet. J.*, *53*, 953.
(40) Fisher, E. W. & Dalton, R. G. (1961) *Br. vet. J.*, *117*, 143.
(41) Orr, J. A. et al. (1975) *Am. J. vet. Res.*, *36*, 1667.
(42) Bergsten, G. (1974) *Acta vet. Scand.*, Suppl. 48.
(43) Eberly, V. E. (1966) *J. appl. Physiol.*, *21*, 883.
(44) Hamlin, R. L. & Smith, R. C. (1962) *Am. J. vet. Res.*, *23*, 711.
(45) Garner, H. E. et al. (1971) *Cardiac Res. Centre Bull.*, *9*, 91.
(46) Hilledge, C. J. & Lees, P. (1975) *Equ. vet. J.*, 7, 16.
(47) McGuirk, S. M. et al. (1984) *J. Am. vet. med. Assoc.*, *184*, 1141.
(48) Garner, R. et al. (1977) *Am. J. vet. Res.*, *38*, 725.
(49) Milne, D. W. et al. (1975) *Am. J. vet. Res.*, *36*, 1431.
(50) Will, J. A. & Bisgard, G. E. (1972) *J. appl. Physiol.*, *33*, 400.
(51) Lombard, C. W. et al. (1983). *J. Am. vet. med. Assoc.*, *183*, 562.
(52) DeRoth, R. (1980) *Can. vet. J.*, *21*, 271.
(53) Miller, P. J. & Holmes, J. R. (1984) *Res. vet. Sci.*, *37*, 18.
(54) Miller, P. J. & Holmes, J. R. (1984). *Equ. vet. J.*, *16*, 210.
(55) Brown, C. M. & Holmes, J. R. (1978) *Equ. vet. J.*, *10*, 188, 207 & 216.
(56) Scott, E. A. et al. (1975) *Am. J. vet. Res.*, *36*, 1021.
(57) Farrow, C. S. (1981) *J. Am. vet. med. Assoc.*, *179*, 776.
(58) Geddes, L. A. (1970) *The Direct and Indirect Measurement of Blood Pressure*. Chicago: Year Book Medical Publishers.
(59) Parry, B. W. et al. (1984) *Equ. vet. J.*, *16*, 53.
(60) Johnson, J. H. et al. (1976) *Equ. vet. J.*, 7, 55.
(61) Gay, C. C. et al. (1977) *Aust. vet. J.*, *53*, 163.
(62) Ostlund, C. et al. (1983) *Comp. Biochem. Physiol.*, *74*, 11.
(63) Lombard, C. W. et al. (1984) *Equ. vet. J.*, *16*, 342.
(64) Stewart, J. H. et al. (1984) *Equ. vet. J.*, *16*, 332.
(65) McQuirk, S. M. et al. (1984) *J. Am. vet. med. Assoc.*, *184*, 1141.
(66) Koblik, P. D. & Hornoff, W. J. (1985). *Vet. Clin. N. Am. equ. Pract.*, *1(2)*, 289.
(67) Lescure, F. & Tamzali, J. (1984) *Rev. med. Vet.*, *135*, 405.
(68) Lombard, C. W. et al. (1984) *Equ. vet. J.*, *16*, 342.
(69) Yamaga, Y. and Too, K. (1984) *Jap. J. vet. Sci.*, *6*, 493.
(70) Ware, W. A. et al. (1986) *J. Am. vet. med. Assoc.*, *188*, 185.
(71) Bonagura, J. D. et al. (1983) *J. Am. vet. med. Assoc.*, *182*, 595.
(72) Yamaga, Y. & Too, K. (1987) *Jap. J. vet. Res.*, *35*, 49.
(73) Dill, S. G. (1986) *Equ. vet. J.*, *19*, 414.
(74) Reef, V. B. (1987) *J. Am. vet med. Assoc.*, *190*, 286.
(75) Pipers, S. F. et al. (1985) *J. Am. vet. med. Assoc.*, *187*, 810.
(76) Kvart, C. et al. (1985) *Equ. vet. J.*, *17*, 361.
(77) Matsui, K. et al. (1985) *Jap. J. vet. Sci.*, *47*, 597.
(78) Wetmore, L. A. et al. (1987) *Am. J. vet. Res.*, *48*, 971.

ARRHYTHMIAS

Variations in cardiac rate and rhythm include tachycardia (increased rate), bradycardia (decreased rate), arrhythmia (irregularity in rate and rhythm) and gallop rhythms. The rate and rhythm of the heart is influenced primarily by the integrity of the pacemaker, the conducting system and the myocardium and also by the influence of the autonomic nervous system. Variation in the rate and rhythm can occur in normal animals due to strong or varying autonomic influence but can also be a reflection of primary myocardial disease. Other factors such as electrolyte imbalance can influence rate and rhythm. These factors must be taken into consideration in the assessment of apparent abnormalities detected on clinical examination of the cardiovascular system.

The majority of arrhythmias and conduction disturbances can be detected on clinical examination. However, some may be unsuspected on clinical examination and be found only on electrocardiographic examination. The occurrence of conduction and myocardial disturbances is probably more common than generally recognized, because an electrocardiogram is usually only taken from animals in which there have been prior clinical indications of conduction abnormalities.

A definitive categorization of an arrhythmia is difficult purely on clinical examination and in general an electrocardiogram is required for this purpose, especially if specific antiarrhythmic therapy is to be instituted. However, a tentative diagnosis of the nature of the arrhythmia can frequently be reached by clinical examination and this can be important in field situations where an electrocardiograph is not readily available. It is also important to be able to recognize those forms of arrhythmia which are not indicative of pathological heart disease but which are normal physiological variations. These occur especially in the horse.

In the examination of the heart with arrhythmic heart disease especial attention should be given to the rate, rhythm and intensity of the individual heart sounds and the rate, rhythm and amplitude of the arterial pulse, and venous pulsations at the jugular inlet.

Examination of the heart sounds

In the horse it is not uncommon to hear four heart sounds on auscultation. The first heart sound is associated with mitral and tricuspid valve closure and is most audible at the fourth intercostal space on the left side approximately 10 cm above the sternum, and on the right side at the third intercostal space at the level of the costochondral junction. The second sound is associated with aortic and pulmonic valve closure. The aortic component is most audible in the left third intercostal space at the level of the scapular/humeral joint while the pulmonic component is most audible ventrally and anteriorly at the left second or third intercostal space at the level of the costochondral junction. These two components of the second sound have the same temporal occurrence on auscultation but frequently tonal differences can be detected at the two areas of maximal audibility. In addition to the first and the second heart sound two further sounds are frequently heard. The third heart sound is associated with rapid filling of the ventricle in early diastole and is heard as a dull thudding sound occurring immediately after the second sound. It is usually most audible in the left fifth intercostal space posterior to the area of maximal audibility of the first heart sound. However it is frequently heard over the base and also over the area of cardiac auscultation on the right side. Phonocardiographically there are two components to this sound but these are not usually detectable on clinical auscultation.

The third heart sound is very common in horses and can be detected in the majority of fit racing animals. It is more audible at heart rates slightly elevated above resting normal.

The fourth heart sound is associated with atrial contraction. It occurs immediately before the first heart sound and is a soft sound most audible over the base of the heart on the left and right hand side. It is also common in horses but its clear separation from the first heart sound is dependent upon the length of the P–R interval which varies between horses. At resting heart rates it is detectable on clinical examination in at least 60% of horses.

The sequence of occurrence of these sounds is thus 4–1–2–3. The intensity of the third and fourth sounds is less than that of the first and second and the complex can be described as du LUBB DUP boo. In some horses, the third and/or fourth sound may be inaudible so that 1–2, 4–1–2 and 1–2–3 variations occur. The name *gallop rhythm* is frequently applied when these extra sounds occur.

Gallop rhythms also occur in cattle and may be due to the occurrence of a fourth or third sound or to true splitting of the components of the first heart sound. In sheep, goats and pigs only two heart sounds are normally heard. The occurrence of a third or fourth heart sound in horses and cattle is not an indication of cardiovascular abnormality as it is in other species.

The relative temporal occurrence and the intensity of the third and fourth heart sounds changes with heart rate. At moderately elevated heart rates the third heart sound becomes more audible. At faster heart rates the third sound may merge and sum with the fourth sound or the fourth sound may merge with the first sound if the P–R interval decreases. During periods of a rapid change in heart rate, such as during the increase in rate that occurs following sudden noise or similar stimuli in excitable horses or the subsequent decrease in rate, the variation in the occurrence and the intensity of the third and fourth sound coupled with the variation in intensity of the first and second sound during this change can give the impression of a gross arrhythmia. Such impressions should be ignored if they occur only at times of rapid *change* of rate which is obviously induced by external influences and if there is no arrhythmia at the resting rate or the intervening stable elevated rate. Examination of the pulse during these periods of rapid change is also of value.

Variations in the intensity of the individual heart sounds or complete absence of some of them can occur in conduction disturbances and arrhythmic heart disease and can provide valuable clinical information. In several of these disturbances there is variation in the intensity of the first and third heart sounds associated with variation in the time of the preceding diastolic period and variations in diastolic filling. The intensity of the first heart sound may also vary with variations in the P-R interval or where there is complete atrioventricular dissociation. In several of the arrhythmias there is absence of one or more of the heart sounds. These findings are detailed below under the specific abnormalities.

Examination of the arterial pulse

In arrhythmic heart disease the arterial pulse should be examined in more detail than that applied during routine clinical examination. The pulse rate should be examined over a period to determine if there is any sudden change in rate such as can occur with a shift in pacemaker to an irritable myocardial focus. At some stage during the examination of animals with tachyarrhythmias the heart rate and pulse rate should be taken synchronously to determine the presence of a pulse deficit. A convenient artery for this purpose is located on the posterior medial aspect of the carpus in the horse and cow.

When a 'dropped pulse' or arrhythmia is detectable in the pulse the basic underlying rhythm should be established in order to determine if the heart is under regular sinus pacemaker influence. This is best done by mentally or physically tapping out the basic rhythm of the heart and to continue this rhythm when irregularity occurs. With conditions such as second-degree heart block where there is a basic underlying sinus rhythm it is possible to tap through the irregularity and reestablish synchrony with the pulse when it is over. However, in conditions such as atrial fibrillation where there is no regular pacemaker it is not possible to establish any basic rhythm. This examination of rhythm can alternatively be conducted by auscultation and allows an immediate categorization of the arrhythmia into one of two groups, those superimposed on a regular pacemaker influence and those in which there is no regular pacemaker.

The amplitude of the pulse should also be carefully examined. Variations in pulse amplitude are associated with those arrhythmias that produce a variation in diastolic filling period within the heart. The extreme of this is a pulse deficit.

Examination of the jugular inlet

This is primarily examined for the pulsations in the jugular vein that result from atrial contraction and thus gives some idea of atrial activity. Jugular atrial contraction waves may be seen in second-degree heart block in the absence of heart sounds. Cannon atrial waves occur periodically in complete heart block when atrial contraction occurs against a closed atrioventricular valve. This examination is done in conjunction with auscultation of the heart. Depending upon the P–R interval the pulsation associated with atrial contraction occurs immediately preceding or essentially synchronous with the first heart sound due to the delay in transmission. A second pulsation associated with valve and heart movement during contraction is usually also visible occurring at about the time of the second heart sound.

The diagnosis of cardiac arrhythmias

The specific findings associated with conduction disturbances and arrhythmias (Table 31) are given below. At slow heart rates many of these conditions can be detected by clinical examination. However, at fast heart rates this can be extremely difficult due to the speed of mental and physical correlation that is required. In these instances an electrocardiogram is the only method of diagnosis. Because of the importance of electrocardiography in the diagnosis of arrhythmias the salient electrocardiographic findings are also given. For more detail the reader is referred to the references.

There are several arrhythmias that can occur in the absence of heart disease and which appear to result from excess vagal tone. These occur especially in the horse and include sinus arrhythmia, wandering pacemaker, sinoatrial block, first-degree and also second-degree atrioventricular block. They occur in animals that are at rest and can frequently be induced by the application of a nose twitch in horses or by forceful elevation of the tail in young ruminants. There is some debate as to the significance of these disturbances in animals but it is generally believed that if they are abolished by exercise and if there is no evidence of cardiac insufficiency they are not of pathological significance. Perinodal myocardial fibrosis and microvascular abnormality have been observed in horses with sinoatrial and atrioventricular block and considered as the excitatory cause (37). However, myocardial fibrosis is common in horses and in one study was detected in 79% of horse hearts examined at random (38). All animals with evidence of arrhythmic heart disease should be examined following exercise as should any animal in which cardiac disease is suspected. The occurrence of cardiac irregularities following exercise is highly indicative of serious cardiac disease (1, 2).

The treatment of arrhythmic heart disease generally relies on the treatment of the underlying clinical condition inducing the problem. This may vary from electrolyte and acid–base disturbance and toxicities to primary myocardial disease resulting from infective myocarditis, myocardial anoxia and changes resulting from heart failure or myopathies resulting from nutritional deficiency (3). These are detailed in later sections in this text. Racing and work horses should be rested for periods up to 3 months following evidence of myocardial disease. Frequently a course of corticosteroids is given to attempt to reduce the severity of myocardial damage if this is not contraindicated by the initiating cause. Specific antiarrhythmic therapy may be applied in certain conditions and is detailed below.

Table 31. Common conduction disturbances and arrhythmias in the horse and cow

Horses	*Cattle*
First degree heart block	Ventricular extrasystoles
Second degree heart block	Atrial fibrillation
Sinoatrial block	Atrial extrasystoles
Ventricular extrasystoles	
Atrial extrasystoles	
Atrial fibrillation	

Sinus tachycardia and sinus bradycardia

The heart rate results from the discharge of impulses from the sinoatrial node which has its own intrinsic rate of discharge but which is also modified by external influences, particularly the vagus nerve.

The term sinus tachycardia or simple tachycardia is used to describe an increase in heart rate caused by detectable influences such as pain, excitement, exercise, hyperthermia, a fall in arterial blood pressure or the administration of adrenergic drugs. The heart rate returns to normal when the influence is removed or relieved.

Sinus bradycardia or simple bradycardia is a normal heart action at a decreased rate due to a decreased rate of discharge from the sinoatrial node. It is most commonly associated with highly trained, fit animals and can be differentiated from the pathological bradycardias by its abolition by exercise or the administration of atropine. Simple bradycardia may also occur in association with an increase in arterial blood pressure, space-occupying lesions of the cranium and increased intracranial pressure, hypothermia and hypoglycemia. Bradycardia is sometimes associated with vagus indigestion and diaphragmatic hernia in cattle. Sinus arrhythmia may be present in some animals with sinus bradycardia.

The resting heart rate seldom falls below 26 beats/min in adult horses and 48 beats/min in adult cattle. Rates below this are suggestive of pathological bradycardias, and an intrinsic cardiac problem should be suspected. In resting horses and cattle which are used to being handled heart rates are not usually elevated above 48 and 80 beats/min respectively and rates above this are usually classified as tachycardia. In the cow and horse it is rare for the causes of sinus tachycardia to elevate the heart rate above 120 beats/min in the resting animal, and at heart rates above this an intrinsic pathological tachycardia should be sought.

Arrhythmias with normal heart rates or bradycardia

Sinus arrhythmia

Sinus arrhythmia is a normal physiological arrhythmia which occurs at slow resting heart rates and is associated with variation in the rate of discharge from the sinoatrial node associated with variation in the intensity of vagal stimulation. It is commonly correlated with respiration so that the discharge rate and heart rate increases during inspiration and decreases during expiration. In the horse, sinus arrhythmia unassociated with respiration also occurs. In the majority of large animals, sinus arrhythmia is much less overt than in the dog and generally it is not detected except on very careful clinical examination or examination of the electrocardiogram. It is more clinically obvious in tame sheep and goats and in the young of all species and is correlated with respiration. It is abolished by exercise or by the administration of atropine.

In the electrocardiogram it is detected by variations in the P–P intervals with or without variation in the P–R interval and is frequently associated with a *wandering pacemaker*. This is associated with differences in the site of discharge from the sinoatrial node with subsequent minor variations in the vector of atrial depolarization with subsequent minor variations in the configuration of the P wave (4). In the horse there may be an abrupt change in the contour of the P wave so that the normal biphasic positive P wave in lead II, for example, changes to one with an initial negative deflection. There may or may not be a change in P–R interval. This is not pathological and is present in as many as 30% of normal horses at rest (5–7). If sinus arrhythmia is not abolished by exercise it is considered pathological (8). Sinus arrhythmia may be induced in the early stages of hypercalcemia during treatment for milk fever in cattle.

Sinoatrial block

In sinoatrial block the sinus node fails to discharge or its impulse is not transmitted over the atrial myocardium (9). It is associated with the complete absence of heart sounds, of jugular atrial wave and of an arterial pulse for one beat period. The underlying rhythm is regular unless sinus arrhythmia is present. In the electrocardiogram there is complete absence of the P, QRS and T complex for one beat. The distance between the preblock and postblock P waves is twice the normal P–P interval or sometimes slightly shorter. This arrhythmia is not uncommon in fit racing horses at rest and can be induced in horses and cattle by procedures that increase vagal tone. Provided it does not persist during and following exercise it is considered as a physiological variant of normal rhythm.

Atrioventricular block

Atrioventricular block is divided into three categories depending upon the degree of interference with conduction at the atrioventricular node.

First-degree atrioventricular block This is an electrocardiographic diagnosis and cannot be detected clinically. It occurs when conduction is delayed at the atrioventricular node. The P–R interval is prolonged beyond normal limits and the condition may be transient due to waxing and waning vagal tone. It is generally considered to have little significance.

Second-degree atrioventricular block Also called partial heart block this occurs when there is periodic interference with conduction at the atrioventricular node so that some atrial contractions are not followed by ventricular contraction. This may occur apparently at random or occur in a regular pattern, for example at every third or fourth beat. At the blocked beat there is complete absence of the first and second heart sounds and no palpable pulse. The underlying rhythm is still sinus in origin and is thus regular. In horses the presence of a fourth heart sound can be a valuable aid to diagnosis as with careful auscultation it can be heard during the block period in the manner of du LUBB DUPP, du , du LUBB DUPP. This is diagnostic for this condition. An atrial jugular impulse can also be detected during the block period. The intensity of the first sound in the immediate postblock beat is usually intensified.

The electrocardiogram shows the presence of a P wave but complete absence of the subsequent QRS and T waves at the blocked beat. There may be variations in the P–R intervals preceding and following the block and first-degree heart block may also be present in the horse. Depending upon the pattern of these variations it is possible to subcategorize second-degree atrioventricular block on electrocardiographic examination (8, 10–12) but the clinical significance of these variations has not been established.

Second-degree atrioventricular block is extremely common in horses. The application of a twitch to the upper lip of a horse will frequently slow the heart rate and allow the expression of second-degree heart block. It is more common in thoroughbreds and standardbreds than in heavy horses and may be detected in as high as 20% of such animals when they are examined in quiet surroundings at rest. In this species it can occur as a normal physiological variation due to variations in vagal tone (9, 10) and in this instance will be abolished by exercise or the administration of atropine. Second-degree atrioventricular block can be associated with myocarditis in the horse (13, 14) and its presence has been associated with decreased racing performance (14).

Methods for the clinical differentiation of physiologic versus pathologic second-degree heart block in the horse have not been established. However, the persistence of the arrhythmia at heart rates above resting normal should be considered to be abnormal. In all other species the presence of this arrhythmia should probably be considered as an indication of myocardial disease. Atrioventricular conduction disturbances can also be associated with electrolyte imbalance in all species (15, 16), overdosing with calcium salts, digitalis poisoning, cardiomyopathy and myocarditis associated with nutritional and infectious disease. There is usually no necessity to treat this arrhythmia specifically and treatment is generally directed at the underlying cause. In cases where the block is frequent and syncopal episodes are likely, atropine may give some alleviation of the frequency of the block; however, this is only short-term therapy. Second-degree heart block may progress to complete heart block.

Third-degree or complete heart block This occurs rarely in large animals, or perhaps is seen only infrequently because it is almost invariably fatal. In complete heart block there is no conduction at the atrioventricular node. The ventricle establishes a pacemaker in the nodal or conducting system and the atria and ventricles beat independently. The ventricular rate is regular but very slow. Bradycardia is the prominent feature and it is unresponsive to exercise or atropine. Atrial contractions are much faster than the ventricle. Atrial contraction sounds are rarely heard on auscultation but evidence of the rate may be detected by examination of the jugular inlet. Periodically, as the atrium contracts during the period that the atrioventricular valves are closed, atrial cannon waves may occur up the jugular vein. There is usually variation in the intensity of the first heart sound due to variation in ventricular filling. Affected animals show extremely poor exercise tolerance and usually have evidence of generalized heart failure. There is frequently a history of syncopal attacks. The electrocardiogram shows a slow and independent ventricular rate characterized by QRS complexes which are completely dissociated from the faster P waves (6).

The prognosis in complete heart block is extremely grave unless it is associated with a correctable electrolyte imbalance. The animal should be kept at rest in quiet surroundings while every effort is made to correct the underlying cause. Corticosteroids and dextrose are usually given intravenously in an attempt to reduce the severity of the initiating myocardial lesion. Isoprenaline may stimulate higher nodal tissue and may increase the heart rate. It is usually infused intravenously at a concentration of 1 mg/liter of infusion fluid and the rate of infusion is adjusted to effect. It is not a practical treatment in most situations. The use of an internal pacemaker has been reported in the horse (17).

Atrioventricular block may develop during anesthesia and can be associated with arrhythmogenic anesthetic drugs, hypercarbia, hypoxia, and electrolyte and acid–base imbalances. In these circumstances, the administration of regular doses of atropine (0·02 mg/kg) may not alleviate the arrhythmia. Dopamine HCl infusions (3–5 μg/kg/min) have been effective (40).

Premature beats

Premature beats or extrasystoles arise by the discharge of impulses from irritable foci within the myocardium. They are classified according to the site of their origin (3) as atrial, junctional and ventricular premature beats. Frequently it is not possible to clinically distinguish between these.

Atrial premature beats These arise from the discharge of an ectopic atrial pacemaker outside of the sinus node. The occurrence of an atrial premature beat cannot itself be clinically detected unless it has an effect on the ventricular rhythm and the effect can vary (3). If the stimulus from the premature atrial contraction falls outside of the refractory period of the ventricle it will initiate a ventricular contraction which occurs earlier than expected. The heart sounds and pulse will therefore occur earlier than that expected from the normal rhythm. In some instances the sinus node becomes reset from the atrial premature beat so that a regular rhythm is established from this contraction. In this case atrial premature beats are characterized by the occurrence of periods of regular rhythm interrupted by beats with exceptionally short interbeat periods. In other instances the sinus node is not reset following the atrial premature contraction and if its discharge occurs during the refractory period of the atrium then no atrial or subsequent ventricular contraction will occur. This will be detected clinically as an early ventricular contraction followed by a compensatory pause following which normal rhythm is continued. This character is identical to that produced by many ventricular premature beats. If the stimulus from the atrial premature contraction falls within the refractory period of the ventricle it will have no effect on ventricular rhythm and may go undetected.

Junctional premature beats These arise from the region of the atrioventricular node or conducting tissue. They produce a premature ventricular contraction which is usually followed by a compensatory pause due to the fact that the following normal discharge from the sinus node usually falls upon the ventricle during its refractory period.

Ventricular premature beats These usually result in a similar pattern. They may arise from an irritable process anywhere within the ventricular myocardium. In both cases the normal rhythm is interrupted by a beat that occurs earlier than expected but the initial rhythm is established following a compensatory pause. This can be established by tapping through the arrhythmia as described earlier. The heart sounds associated with the premature beat are usually markedly decreased in amplitude while the first sound following the compensatory pause is usually accentuated. Occasionally, ventricular premature beats may be interpolated in the normal rhythm and not followed by a compensatory pause.

If the diastolic filling period preceding the premature beat is short the pulse associated with it will be markedly decreased in amplitude or even absent.

With atrial premature beats the P wave of the premature beat occurs earlier than expected from the basic rhythm and is abnormal in configuration. QRS complexes associated with atrial premature beats are normal in configuration. Junctional premature beats produce

QRS configurations that are similar to those of normal beats but they may produce a P wave that has a vector opposite to normal. Ventricular premature beats are characterized on the electrocardiogram by QRS complexes which are bizarre. Conduction over nonspecialized pathways results in a complex of greater duration and amplitude to normal and the complex slurs into a T wave that is also of increased duration and magnitude. The vector orientation depends on the site of the ectopic foci initiating the contraction but it is invariably different from that of normal contractions (6, 18). Electrocardiographic examination allows a differentiation of the site of origin of premature beats and further subclassification within the categories (6).

Failure in clinical differentiation between the sites of origin of premature beats is of little concern as in all cases their occurrence is indicative of cardiac abnormality (2, 19, 20). At slow heart rates their presence is suggested by periodic interruption of an underlying sinus rhythm and by the occurrence of a 'dropped pulse' or a pulse which is markedly decreased in amplitude. The prime differentiation is from sinoatrial block and second-degree atrioventricular block, which have distinguishing characteristics. Animals in which premature beats are detected or suspected should be examined after careful exercise which will usually increase the occurrence and severity of the arrhythmia. They are most easily detected during the period of slowing of heart rate after exercise (9).

Arrhythmias with tachycardia

An excitable focus within the myocardium may spontaneously discharge and cause depolarization of the remaining myocardium. If the discharge rate approaches that of the sinus node or exceeds it the focus may transiently take over as the pacemaker of the heart. If the onset of tachycardia is rapid and stops abruptly this condition may be called paroxysmal tachycardia.

Paroxysmal tachycardia may arise from an irritant focus within the atria or the ventricles (14, 22, 23). These cannot be differentiated on clinical grounds. In large animals ventricular paroxysmal tachycardia is seen more commonly (14, 22, 24). Atrial paroxysmal tachycardia and atrial flutter are very rare and are transients leading to atrial fibrillation.

Paroxysmal tachycardia

Paroxysmal tachycardia may occur spontaneously or may follow an increase in sympathetic tone caused by factors such as excitement. In paroxysmal tachycardia the increase in heart rate is abrupt and the fall to normal is equally sudden. This characteristic usually serves to distinguish this arrhythmia from the transient increases in heart rate that may normally follow such factors as excitement. Also the heart rate is elevated to a rate far in excess of that which would be normally expected from such stimuli.

More commonly the excitable focus discharges repetitively over a long period of time to produce more continual ventricular tachycardia associated with ventricular extrasystoles.

Ventricular tachycardia

Ventricular tachycardias may produce either a regular heart rate or an irregular heart rate and rhythm. When the discharge rate or the irritant focus far exceeds that of the sinoatrial pacemaker the ectopic focus will take over completely as the pacemaker of the heart. On examination of the cardiovascular system a rapid but regular heart rate and pulse is detected and there is no irregularity of rhythm or of pulse amplitude or intensity of heart sounds and this abnormality is easily overlooked clinically. It should be suspected in any adult horse or cow where the heart rate exceeds 100 beats/min and is frequently the cause of heart rates in excess of 120 beats/min. It should also be suspected where the heart rate is elevated to a level that is higher than that expected from the animal's clinical condition. The diagnosis can be made from an electrocardiogram based on the occurrence of multiple regular extrasystoles with abnormal amplitude and duration of the QRS and T complexes. P waves may be detected on the electrocardiogram but they have no relationship to the QRS–T complex and are frequently lost within them. This is known as ventricular tachycardia with atrioventricular dissociation.

When the discharge rate of the irritant focus within the myocardium is similar to that of the sinoatrial node the ventricular tachycardia can be manifested by a gross irregularity in rhythm. This is a common manifestation in large animals. In this situation many of the discharges which originate in the sinus fall on the ventricle during a refractory period from a previous extrasystole, but some reach the ventricle when it is not in a refractory state and are conducted normally. At some periods ventricular contractions may be initiated by the discharges from both sites. The varying influence of each pacemaker on ventricular contraction produces a marked irregularity in cardiac rhythm and it is frequently not possible to establish clinically a regular pattern to the heart rhythm. Variations between beats in the degree of atrial filling and in the diastolic filling period will result in a marked variation in the intensity of the heart sounds and in the amplitude of the pulse. Frequently at fast heart rates there is a pulse deficit. Cannon atrial waves can be observed in the jugular vein when atrial contraction occurs at the same time as a ventricular extrasystole. The electrocardiogram shows runs of extrasystoles interspersed with normally conducted complexes and usually the presence of fusion beats (6, 23).

Ventricular tachycardias are evidence of severe cardiac disease. They are usually accompanied by signs of acute heart failure. They may result from primary myocarditis or nutritional cardiomyopathy, or be secondary to valvular disease and myocardial anoxia and are common in certain plant poisonings and other toxicities, in colitis-X and in severe electrolyte and acid–base disturbance. They also commonly occur in the final stages of heart failure. If uncorrected they may lead to ventricular fibrillation and death and frequently specific antiarrhythmic therapy is indicated during the period that the prime cause is being corrected.

Quinidine sulfate is the drug of choice for use in horses. An initial dose of 20 mg/kg is given orally followed by a dose of 10 mg/kg given every 8 hours. The drug is not effective until 1–2 hours following administration. Intravenous lignocaine (without epinephrine) infused as a 2% solution at a dose of 4 mg/kg gives an immediate but shortlived control of ventricular tachyarrhythmias in small animals which may cover this period and has been effective for this purpose in young calves and goats. In horses it can be administered as an intravenous bolus at a dose of 0·5 mg/kg, which is repeated every 5 minutes to achieve the required effect (39). Muscular weakness and temporary recumbency may occur during administration. Also in horses high doses are reported to produce central nervous system irritation with excitement, sweating, and convulsions (39). We have not found lidocaine particularly efficacious in relieving ventricular tachycardia and its duration of action is short. Intravenous quinidine may be of greater value in those rare instances when oral quinidine is not indicated. The severity of ventricular tachycardias is augmented by factors which increase sympathetic tone, and affected animals should be kept in quiet surroundings.

Ventricular fibrillation

Ventricular fibrillation is not usually observed clinically because the incoordinated twitching of the myocardium does not result in ventricular ejection and the animal dies very quickly. Ventricular fibrillation occurs in the terminal stages of most suddenly fatal diseases including lightning stroke, plant poisonings such as acute *Phalaris* toxicity, overdose with anesthetics, severe toxemia and in the terminal phases of most acquired cardiac diseases. There is complete absence of the pulse and heart sounds, the blood pressure falls precipitously and the animal rapidly becomes unconscious and dies within a minute or two of onset. Treatment is usually impractical although deaths during anesthesia may be prevented by cardiac massage. Electrical defibrillation is not feasible in large animals due to the bulk of the animal and the current required. Intracardiac injections of adrenalin are often used in acute cardiac arrest but do not correct fibrillation and are of little value.

Atrial fibrillation

In atrial fibrillation atrial depolarization is characterized by numerous independent fronts of excitation that course continuously and haphazardly through the atria (25). There is no synchronous atrial contraction (21) and atrioventricular nodal stimulation occurs in an irregular and random fashion. The effects within the atria cannot be appreciated clinically and the clinical detection of this arrhythmia occurs through its effects on ventricular function. The random stimulation of the ventricles produces a heart rate and pulse that is grossly irregular. It is not possible to establish any basic rhythm by tapping out this arrhythmia and the rate varies from period to period. Because there is no atrial contraction, filling of the ventricles is entirely passive and very much dependent on diastolic filling time. Some contractions occur very quickly following the preceding contraction with little time for diastolic filling and this produces a marked variation in the intensity of the heart sounds and in the amplitude of the pulse. At fast heart rates there will be a pulse deficit. There is no atrial fourth sound or atrial wave at the jugular inlet, but the third heart sound is usually grossly accentuated. The degree of cardiac insufficiency that results from this arrhythmia varies and depends upon the general rate at which the ventricles beat at rest. This is determined primarily by vagal activity. In the horse, vagal tone may be high and conduction through the atrioventricular node is suppressed to result in heart rates in the region of approximately 26–48 beats/min. At this rate there is no cardiac insufficiency at rest and hemodynamic parameters are normal (32). The horse can elevate its heart rate with exercise to allow moderate performance, although it will never perform satisfactorily as a racehorse. This is the most common manifestation in this species and it is typified by a gross irregularity in rate, rhythm and intensity of the heart sounds and by the occurrence, at rest, of occasional periods lasting for 3–6 seconds where there is no ventricular activity. At very slow rates periodic syncopy may occur.

Occasionally in the horse, and more commonly in other species, the ventricular rate at rest is much higher and the arrhythmia presents as a tachycardia. In the horse ventricular filling is impaired at heart valve rates above 70 (39) and at resting heart rates above 80–100 min there is gross cardiac inefficiency and the animal rapidly develops signs of cardiac insufficiency and cardiac failure. At fast heart rates the syndrome is clinically similar to ventricular tachycardia associated with multiple ventricular extrasystoles and electrocardiographic differentiation is required.

In atrial fibrillation there are no P waves discernible on the electrocardiogram but the base line shows multiple waveforms (f waves) that occur with a frequency of between 300 and 600 beats/min. QRS–T complexes are normal in configuration but there is wide variation and no pattern in the Q–Q intervals.

Atrial fibrillation is common in large animal species. In the *horse* it occurs not infrequently in draft horses and is also seen in racehorses. Commonly these have a history of normality at rest but poor exercise tolerance following a race in which the horse ran well for the first 200–300 m but subsequently faded badly and finished a long way behind the field. Paroxysmal atrial fibrillation has also been observed in the horse under these circumstances. Horses with paroxysmal atrial fibrillation show atrial fibrillation when examined immediately following the race, but convert to normal sinus rhythm shortly after and have normal cardiovascular function if the examination as to cause of poor racing performance is delayed (26, 27).

In the horse, there is some debate as to the cause of atrial fibrillation. Myocardial and vascular lesions have been found in the atria of a significant proportion of animals with this arrhythmia (28, 29). However, the frequency with which this arrhythmia can be converted to be followed by successful racing performance suggests that this arrhythmia may occur spontaneously in the horse or in the absence of significant atrial pathology. A recent survey of 106 cases of atrial fibrillation in horses revealed the following (36): the disease was diagnosed most commonly in standardbred and thoroughbred horses under 7 years of age which may have been a reflection of the admissions to the clinic rather than real breed incidence. Exercise intolerance was the most common clinical history. All horses had an irregular heart rate and rhythm and the pulse and intensity of the heart sounds were variable. Horses with evidence of congestive heart failure, edema and cardiac murmurs had advanced myocardial disease. Approximately 80% of horses with atrial fibrillation converted and returned to previous performance levels following treatment with quinidine sulfate.

In the *cow* atrial fibrillation may occur secondary to myocardial disease or endocarditis resulting in atrial hypertrophy, but more commonly is functional in occurrence and not associated with cardiac lesions (25, 30). It is frequently paroxysmal and most commonly occurs in association with gastrointestinal disease, abnormalities causing abdominal pain, and metabolic disease. Abnormalities as diverse as acute enteritis, left displacement of the abomasum and torsion of the uterus may be accompanied by this arrhythmia. Heightened excitation of the atria, in association with electrolyte and acid–base disturbances or due to change in vagal tone, has been postulated as a cause, but none has been proved. The arrhythmia regresses spontaneously with correction of the abdominal disorder.

In the *goat* atrial fibrillation is a sequel to interstitial pneumonia along with cor pulmonale. The presenting signs are those of respiratory distress and heart failure. Ascites is prominent and there is marked jugular distension with an irregular jugular pulse. Response to treatment is poor (30). In all species, atrial fibrillation can occur where there is atrial hypertrophy secondary to other cardiac lesions. In general, ruminants with atrial fibrillation are not treated with specific antiarrhythmic drugs. The treatment of horses with atrial fibrillation at high heart rates is generally unsuccessful as serious cardiac pathology is usually present. Digitalis and quinidine sulfate are used. The decision to treat a horse with atrial fibrillation at low heart rates depends upon the requirement for the horse to perform work because horses with this arrhythmia can be retired and will live for several years. They may be used successfully as brood mares.

There are several reports of the successful conversion of racehorses with atrial fibrillation with subsequent return to successful racing performance (27, 31, 33). Oral quinidine sulfate is usually used. Several dose regimens have been used, but the administration of an oral dose of 20 mg/kg every 2 hours until conversion is achieved or toxicity is manifest has proved effective (31, 36). In the majority of cases, conversion will occur before the total dose exceeds 40 g. Toxicity is likely when the total dose exceed 60 g and the decision to continue with therapy once this dose has been reached should be considered carefully. Toxicity is not uncommon with quinidine therapy and in one study 48% of horses showed some form of adverse reaction (36). Depression, lassitude, anorexia, urticaria, congestion of the mucous membranes, colic, and death are recorded. Prolongation of the QRS interval to 25% greater than pretreatment values has been considered a monitor for cardiovascular toxicity. Some prefer to digitalize the horse intravenously prior to medication with quinidine in an attempt to reduce tachyarrhythmias at the point of conversion and those associated with quinidine toxicity. Nephrotoxicity with uremia and diarrhea can occur at lower doses. It is transient and repairs rapidly following withdrawal of the drug but the blood urea nitrogen (BUN) and urine should be monitored during therapy in addition to cardiovascular function. There is a much greater success rate with conversion in young horses and when it is attempted shortly following the onset of the arrhythmia. In horses older than 5 years, or where the arrhythmia has been present for more than 3 months, successful conversion is much less common. Following cardioversion the horse should be rested for 3 months. In some horses the conditions recurs after a period of racing and repeated conversions with quinidine are possible. Conversion by the use of intravenous quinidine preparations has been reported in the cow (25) and horse (34, 35).

REVIEW LITERATURE

McQuirk, S. M. & Muir, W. W. (1985). Diagnosis and treatment of cardiac arrhythmias. Symposium on Cardiology. *Vet. Clin. N. Am. equ. Pract.*, *1(2)*, 353–370

REFERENCES

(1) Fisher, E. W. et al. (1970) *Vet. Rec.*, *86*, 499.
(2) Deegen, E. (1974) *Dtsch Tierärztl. Wochenschr.*, *81*, 532.
(3) Deengen, E. (1976) *Dtsch Tierärztl. Wochenschr.*, *83*, 361, 483.
(4) Hamlin, R. L. et al. (1970) *Am. J. vet. Res.*, *31*, 1027.
(5) Hamlin, R. L. et al. (1970) *Am. J. Physiol.*, *219*, 306.
(6) Hilwig, R. W. (1977) *J. Am. vet. med. Assoc.*, *70*, 153.
(7) Muylle, E. & Oyaert, W. (1975) *Zentralbl. VetMed.*, *22A*, 474.
(8) Kruger, J. M. & Jenkins, W. L. (1974) *J. S. Afr. vet. med. Assoc.*, *45*, 139.
(9) Holmes, J. R. (1980) *In Practice*, *2*, 15.
(10) Smetzer, D. L. et al. (1969) *Am. J. vet. Res.*, *30*, 933.
(11) Sporri, H. (1952) *Schweiz. Arch. Tierheilkd.*, *94*, 337.
(12) Holmes, J. R. & Alps, B. J. (1966) *Can. vet. J.*, *7*, 280.
(13) Smetzer, D. L. et al. (1969) *Am. J. vet. Res.*, *30*, 337.
(14) Steel, J. D. (1963) *Studies on the Electrocardiogram of the Racehorse.* Sydney: Australasian Medical Publishing.
(15) Littledike, E. T. et al. (1976) *Am. J. vet. Res.*, *37*, 383.
(16) White, N. A. & White, S. L. (1975) *Vet Med. small Anim. Clin.*, *70*, 967.
(17) Taylor, D. H. & Mero, M. A. (1967) *J. Am. vet. med. Assoc.*, *151*, 1172.
(18) Holmes, J. R. & Alps, B. J. (1967) *Can. J. comp. Med.*, *31*, 219.
(19) Holmes, J. R. & Alps, B. J. (1966) *Vet. Rec.*, *78*, 672.
(20) Noor, J. (1924) *Mschr. Tierheilkd*, *34*, 177.
(21) Wingfield, S. et al. (1980) *Equ. vet. J.*, *12*, 181.
(22) Buchanan, J. W. (1965) *Ann. NY Acad. Sci*, *127*, 224.
(23) Clarke, D. R. et al. (1966) *Vet. Med. small Anim. Clin.*, *60*, 861.
(24) Senta, T. et al. (1971) *Exp. Rep. equ. Hlth Lab.*, Tokyo, *8*, 61.
(25) Brightling, P. & Townsend, H. G. G. (1983) *Can. vet. J.*, *24*, 331.
(26) Holmes, J. R. et al. (1986) *Equ. vet. J.*, *19*, 37.
(27) Amada, A. & Kurita, A. (1975) *Exp. Rep. equ. Hlth Lab., Tokyo*, *12*, 89.
(28) Kiryu, K. et al. (1974) *Exp. Rep. equ. Hlth Lab., Tokyo*, *11*, 70.
(29) Else, R. W. & Holmes, J. R. (1971) *Equ. vet. J.*, *3*, 56.
(30) Gay, C. C. and Richards, W. P. C. (1983) *Aust. vet. J*, *60*, 274.
(31) Rose, R. J. & Davis, P. E. (1977) *Equ. vet. J.*, *9*, 68.
(32) Muir, W. W. & McQuirk, S. M. (1986) *J. Am. vet. med Assoc.*, *184*, 965.
(33) Deegen, E. & Buntenkotter, S. (1976) *Equ. vet. J.*, *8*, 26.
(34) Deegen, E. & Buntenkotter, S. (1974) *Dtsch Tierärztl. Wochenschr*, *81*, 161.
(35) Gerber, H. et al. (1971) *Equ. vet. J.*, *3*, 10.

(36) Deem, D. A. & Fregin, G. F. (1982) *J. Am. vet. med. Assoc.*, *180*, 261.
(37) Kiri, K. et al. (1985) *Jap. J. vet. Sci.*, *47*, 45.
(38) Dudan, F. et al. (1985) *Schweiz. Arch. Tierhlkd.*, *127*, 319.
(39) Muir, W. W. & McQuirk, S. M. (1985) *Vet. Clin. N. Am. equ. Pract.*, *1(2)*: 335.
(40) Whitton, D. L. & Trim, C. M. (1985) *J. Am. vet. med. Assoc.*, *187*, 1357.

DISEASES OF THE HEART

Myocardial disease, myocardial asthenia, cardiomyopathy

Myocardial disease, cardiomyopathy and myocardial asthenia or weakness are manifest by decreased power of contraction resulting in reduction of cardiac reserve and, in severe cases, in congestive heart failure or acute heart failure.

Etiology

A number of diseases are accompanied by inflammation, necrosis or degeneration of the myocardium. These include several bacterial, viral, or parasitic infections and some nutritional deficiencies. In most cases, the involvement of the myocardium is only part of the total spectrum of these diseases although the cardiac manifestations may be clinically preeminent. The term cardiomyopathy is generally restricted to those diseases where myocardial damage is the sole manifestation. Most commonly, myocardial disease results in conduction disturbances or arrhythmias. These may be minor and contribute minimally to the clinical disease or they may be major and result in death from severe arrhythmic disturbances and acute heart failure. Myocardial asthenia occurs with many diseases. The reduction in cardiac efficiency due to physical or functional disturbances of the myocardium, and the resulting circulatory insufficiency, contribute to the illness or to death, but in most cases do not produce a syndrome characteristic of acute or congestive heart failure. An example is the myocardial asthenia that occurs in milk fever in cows, which is entirely reversible by the administration of calcium salts parenterally, and the myocardial asthenia that occurs with toxemias.

Toxicities can also produce cardiac disease in farm animals. Some of these, such as fluoroacetate, are cardiotoxic because they result in myocardial damage, but others act through pharmacologic effects on the conduction system without direct myocardial damage. Causes of myocardial dysfunction include the following.

Bacterial myocarditis

- Following bacteremia, as in strangles or from navel ill
- Tuberculosis—especially horses
- Tick pyemia in lambs
- *Clostridum chauvoei*
- Extension from pericarditis or endocarditis.

Viral myocarditis

- Foot and mouth disease—especially young animals
- African horse sicknesss
- Equine viral arteritis
- Equine infectious anemia
- Swine vesicular disease (SVD)
- Encephalomyocarditis virus infection in pigs
- Bluetongue in sheep.

Parasitic myocarditis

This is primarily caused by *Strongylus* spp. (migrating larvae) Cysticercosis, Sarcosporidiosis. In a recent post-mortem study of over 2000 equine hearts, 15% showed myocardial fibrosis in association with occlusive angiopathic change (3). No age association was found, but recent infarcts were more common in yearlings. It was postulated that these lesions result from thromboemboli from verminous plaques in the proximal thoracic aorta.

Nutritional deficiency

- Vitamin E/selenium deficiency in all large animal species
- Some forms of chronic copper deficiency in cattle (falling disease)—experimental copper deficiency in swine
- Iron deficiency in piglets and veal calves
- Copper/cobalt deficiency in lambs.

Poisoning

- Inorganic poisons—selenium, arsenic, mercury, phosphorus, thallium
- Gossypol from cotton seed cake
- Fluoroacetate (1080) and poisoning by *Acacia georgina*, *Gastrolobium, and Oxylobium* spp., *Dichapetalum cymosum*
- Plants and weeds including members of *Ixiolena*, *Pachystigma*, *Pavette*, *Ascelapias*, *Geriocarpa*, *Cryptostigia*, *Albizia*, *Cassia*, *Digitalis*, *Pimelea*, *Astragalus*, *Fadogia*, *Cicuta*, *Karwinskia*, *Vicia*, *Trigonella*, *Palicourea*, *Lupinus*, *Lantana*, *Kalanchoe*, *Homeria* spp.
- Trees including gidgee, yew, oleander
- Grasses including *Phalaris tuberosa* and grass nematodes infesting *Lolium rigidum*, hay infested with blister beetles (horses)
- Drugs including succinylcholine, catecholamines, xylazine (ruminants) monensin—especially in horses, but also cattle, sheep, and pigs, lasalocid in horses and cattle, and Adriamycin (used experimentally to produce cardiomyopathy)
- Vitamin D and myocardial and endocardial calcification following ingestion of *Cestrum diurnum*, *Solanum malacoxylon*, *Trisetum flavescens* (see enzootic calcinosis); calcification also occurs with hypomagnesemia in milkfed calves.

Embolic infarction

- Emboli from vegetative endocarditis or other embolic disease such as brackenfern poisoning in cattle.

Tumor

- Viral leukosis of cattle.

Inherited

- Malignant hyperthermia of swine

- Congenital cardiomyopathy of Polled Herefords with dense curly coats and Japanese Black calves
- Suspected inherited cardiomyopathy (2) in Holstein-Friesian, Red Holstein and Simmental cattle (see inherited cardiomyopathy)
- Glycogen storage disease—α-1,4-glucosidase deficiency in Shorthorn and Brahman cattle and Corriedale sheep.

Unknown or uncertain etiology

- Myocardial necrosis and hemorrhage secondary to acute lesions in the central nervous system (4)
- Exertional rhabdomyolysis of horses, capture myopathy of wild ruminants, restraint stress in swine (5)
- Sudden death in young calves associated with acute heart failure and myocardial necrosis and precipitated by periods of intense excitement such as that at feeding time (6)
- Myocardial lipofuscinosis (brown atrophy) occurs in aged or cachectic cattle, especially Ayrshires, but often is found in healthy animals at slaughter (7)
- Myocardial disease following mild upper respiratory disease in horses, especially when training or exercise is continued through the respiratory disease episode.

Pathogenesis

The primary effect of any myocardial lesion is to reduce cardiac reserve and restrict compensation in circulatory emergencies. Minor lesions may only reduce performance efficiency (1) while more severe lesions may produce greater clinical effect. Most commonly, myocardial disease results in conduction disturbances and/or arrhythmias. These can result from primary involvement of the conduction system or from the establishment of excitatory foci within the myocardium. While the animal is at rest, there may be minimal disturbances to the function of the heart and the presence of myocardial disease may be manifest clinically only by the occurrence of occasional extrasystoles, other arrhythmic disturbances or be detected only by techniques of special examination. However, these effects are markedly exacerbated by adrenergic influences such as exercise or excitement and under these influences catastrophic disturbances in cardiac conduction may occur. Consequently, extensive myocardial disease may be clinically silent in animals at rest but can result in sudden death from acute heart failure when exercise or excitement occurs.

Endogenous or synthetic catecholamines, in their own right, can produce multifocal myocardial necrosis, especially in the left ventricle (8). Sympathetic overactivity and local catecholamine release in the myocardium has been postulated as the cause of myocardial disease accompanying acute brain lesions in domestic animals and myocardial disease associated with some forms of stress and overexertion (4, 9). Catecholamine release may exacerbate preexisting myocardial disease, and the effects of pharmacologic cardiotoxic agents in poisonous plants are frequently also initially manifest when the animals are moved or otherwise excited. Myocardial disease may also result in congestive heart failure through its primary effect on the myocardium and the function of the heart as a pump. The clinical abnormalities associated with myocardial disease consequently include many of the manifestations of heart disease described earlier, including cardiac enlargement, arrhythmia, or abnormalities of rate, and in the terminal stages a syndrome of congestive heart failure or acute heart failure develops, depending upon the rate at which failure occurs.

Clinical findings

In early cases, or cases with mild or moderate myocardial damage, a decreased exercise tolerance is the usual initial presenting sign. This is usually accompanied by an increase in heart rate and heart size although the latter may not be detectable. There may be clinically recognizable abnormalities of rate or rhythm, particularly tachyarrhythmias associated with multiple ventricular extrasystoles. The characters of the pulse and heart sounds are also changed but these changes can also occur due to extracardiac influences.

Animals with suspect myocardial disease but with no or minimal arrhythmic disturbances at rest can be judiciously exercised, which will frequently result in the expression of conduction or arrhythmic abnormality. Exercise or excitement should be avoided in animals with overt arrhythmias at rest.

In the late stages, or in cases with more severe myocardial damage, there may be sudden death or attacks of cardiac syncope due to acute heart failure, or severe dyspnea or general edema due to congestive heart failure. Details of the clinical findings associated with conduction disturbances, arrhythmias and heart failure have been given earlier. Myocardial weakness is frequently accompanied by a hemic murmur which occurs with the first heart sound and reaches maximum intensity at the peak of inspiration and diminishes or disappears with expiration.

Clinical pathology

Electrocardiography should be carried out when possible as it gives a good indication of the status of the myocardium even though the type of lesion cannot be diagnosed. Other tests as outlined in special examination of the cardiovascular system are not generally practicable. Myocardial infarction and necrosis may be associated with the release of cell enzymes into the bloodstream during the acute phase. Elevated transaminase (SGOT, SGPT) and lactic dehydrogenase levels may be of diagnostic significance. These enzymes are not specific for heart muscle but greater specificity and a measure of the degree of damage to the myocardium can be achieved by the measurement of creatine kinase and lactic dehydrogenase isoenzymes (11). Toxicologic examination and tests for nutritional trace element deficiencies may be indicated.

Necropsy findings

Bacterial infections may cause discrete abscesses or areas of inflammation in the myocardium but viral infections and degenerations due to nutritional deficiencies and poisonings usually produce a visible pallor of the muscle which may be uniform or present as streaks between apparently normal bundles of muscle. In acute cases, there may be petechial or linear hemorrhages in the myocardium. Calcification may occur in areas of myocardial damage and with enzootic calcinosis and vitamin D toxicity. The nature and distribution of myocardial damage within the heart can vary according to the inciting agent and this can be an aid to diagnosis. The degenerated muscle may also be present in only the inner layers of the wall, leaving the external layers with a normal appearance. In coronary thrombosis infarction of a large area of the wall may have occurred but this is not visible unless the animal survives for at least 24 hours afterwards. Careful examination of the coronary arteries is usually necessary to detect the causative embolus. In horses infarction occurs most commonly in the right atrium.

The terminal stage of myocardial degeneration or myocarditis is often fibrous tissue replacement of the damaged tissue. The heart is flabby and thin-walled and shows patches of shrunken, tough fibrous tissue. Rupture of the atrial walls may result, with sudden death occurring due to the pressure of blood in the pericardial sac. The lesions of lymphomatosis are characteristic of this disease: large, uneven masses of pale, firm, undifferentiated tissue with the consistency of lymphoid tissue.

Focal myocardial fibrosis, possibly resulting from microembolism from strongyle-induced endarteritis, is common in healthy horses but has also been ascribed as the predisposing factor to conduction disturbances such as atrial fibrillation and heart block (10).

Diagnosis

Myocardial disease should always be part of the differential diagnosis of any animal showing decreased exercise tolerance or signs of heart failure. Myocardial disease is a major consideration in the differential diagnosis of sudden death in livestock. Most cases of myocardial disease will present with clinical or electrocardiographic evidence of conduction disturbances or arrhythmias, either at rest or following exercise, and with biochemical evidence of myocardial damage. The primary differential diagnosis is from other cardiac defects that may produce heart failure. Endocardial lesions and congenital defects of the heart or large vessels are usually accompanied by an audible murmur, and in some cases a palpable cardiac thrill, and abnormalities of the pulse. Pericarditis causes muffling of the heart sounds and is accompanied in the early stages by a pericardial friction rub and in the later stages by fluid sounds on auscultation. Hydropericardium is also accompanied by muffling of the heart beat. Cardiac rupture and tamponade may cause acute heart failure but affected animals die so quickly that clinical examination is usually not possible.

The cardiac dilatation of myocardial asthenia needs to be differentiated from increased audibility of heart sounds caused by retraction of the lung, and decreased audibility of the sounds from muffling by expanded lungs in pulmonary emphysema. Space-occupying lesions of the chest, including diaphragmatic hernia, mediastinal abscess and tumor, may also cause a degree of congestive heart failure and displacement of the heart, and are probably the commonest cause of error in the diagnosis of myocardial disease. They can be diagnosed only by careful auscultation and percussion. Myocardial asthenia associated with conditions such as hypocalcemia and toxemia is a clinical finding secondary to the primary cause.

The diagnosis of the specific etiology of myocardial disease rests with the epidemiologic and other considerations of the individual causes and may require specific bacteriological and virological examinations, toxicologic and nutritional analyses or an examination of the environment.

Treatment

The primary cause must be treated and details are given under the specific diseases listed above. When possible, the primary cause of the myocardial damage must be corrected or treated, and details are given elsewhere for the various etiologies listed above. The treatment of conduction disturbances, arrhythmias and heart failure is given elsewhere in this chapter.

REVIEW LITERATURE

Van Vleet, J. F. & Ferrans, V. J. (1986) Myocardial diseases of animals. *Am. J. Pathol.*, *124*, 98–178.

REFERENCES

(1) Hall, M. C. et al. (1976) *Aust. vet. J.*, *52*, 1, 6.
(2) Baird, J. D. et al. (1986) *Proc. 14th, Wld Cong. Dis. Cattle*, *1*, 89.
(3) Baker, J. R. & Ellis, C. E. (1981) *Equ. vet. J.*, *123*, 43 & 47.
(4) King, J. M. et al. (1982) *J. Am. vet. med. Assoc.*, *180*, 144.
(5) Johannson, G. et al. (1982) *Can. J. comp. Med.*, *6*, 176.
(6) Rogers, P. A. M. & Poole, D. B. R. (1978) *Vet. Rec.*, *103*, 366.
(7) Bradley, R. & Duffell, S. J. (1982) *J. comp. Pathol.*, *92*, 85.
(8) Van Vleet, J. F. et al. (1977) *Am. J. vet. Res.*, *38*, 991.
(9) Van Vleet, J. F. & Ferrans, V. J. (1986) *Am. J. Pathol.*, *124*, 98.
(10) Cranley, J. J. & McCullagh, K. C. (1981) *Equ. vet. J.*, *13*, 35.
(11) Fujii, Y. et al. (1983) *Bull. equ. Res. Inst.*, *20*, 87.

Rupture of the heart

Rupture of the heart occurs rarely in animals. It is recorded in cattle where a foreign body penetrating from the reticulum perforates the ventricular wall and in the left atrium of horses as a consequence of chronic fibrotic myocarditis (6). Rupture of the base of the aorta is not uncommon in horses and has the same effect as cardiac rupture. The pericardial sac immediately fills with blood and the animal dies of acute heart failure. A similar cardiac tamponade occurs when reticular foreign bodies lacerate a coronary artery or when foals suffer severe laceration of the epicardium during a difficult parturition (1).

When the aorta ruptures it may do so through its wall just above the aortic valves. The wall may have been weakened previously by verminous arteritis associated with migrating strongyles in horses (5) or onchocerciasis in cattle (2) or by the development of medionecrosis. Another form of rupture occurs through the aortic ring (3). Death occurs very suddenly; all cases reported by one author affected stallions and coincided with the time of breeding. Cardiac tamponade may occur but the common finding is a dissecting aneurysm into the ventricular myocardium. Rupture of the aortic arch and the pulmonary artery near the ligamentum arteriosum occurs occasionally in horses. The resultant fistula between the aorta and the pulmonary artery produces severe cardiac embarrassment with sudden onset of cardiac failure and respiratory distress. Affected horses usually die shortly after the onset of clinical signs but can survive up to 8 days. The rupture is predisposed by abnormalities in the vasa vasorum of the vessels and may have a familial occurrence (4). Rupture of the aorta above the cardiac arch is a more common cause of sudden death in horses.

REFERENCES

(1) Awadhiya, R. P. et al. (1974) *Vet. Rec.*, *95*, 260.
(2) Kolte, G. N. et al. (1976) *Vet. Rec.*, *98*, 460.
(3) Rooney, J. R. et al. (1967) *Pathol. vet.*, *4*, 268.
(4) Van der Linde-Sipman, J. S. (1985) *Vet. Pathol*, *22*, 51.
(5) Deegen, E. et al. (1980) *Tierärztl. Praxis*, *8*, 211.
(6) Haaland, M. A. & Davidson, J. P. (1983) *Vet. Clin. N. Am.*, *78*, 1284.

Cor pulmonale

Cor pulmonale is the syndrome of right heart failure resulting from an increase in right heart workload secondary to increased pulmonary vascular resistance and pulmonary hypertension.

The most documented cause of pulmonary hypertension in livestock is alveolar hypoxia (1). Acute alveolar hypoxia (lowered alveolar Po_2) is a potent cause of pulmonary hypertension in several species, but cattle are especially reactive and there is a genetic predisposition that determines the magnitude of the response. Pulmonary hypertension results from contraction of the precapillary pulmonary vessels; however, the mechanism whereby alveolar hypoxia induces this response is uncertain. Prolonged hypoxia and persistent pulmonary vasoconstriction can lead to medial muscular hypertrophy of the small pulmonary arteries and arterioles with a further increase in pulmonary vascular resistance. This mechanism by itself may produce insufficiency and right heart failure in cattle living at high altitudes.

Cattle residing above 1500 m are predisposed to cor pulmonale and at altitudes above 2200 m an annual incidence of 0.5–2% is recorded (2). The incidence is highest in calves and in cattle newly introduced to these altitudes. Recovery occurs if cattle are moved to lower altitudes. Cattle grazing locoweed (*Oxytropis sericea*) at high altitude are particularly predisposed to cor pulmonale and the annual incidence may approach 100% with high case fatality (4). It has been shown experimentally that the ingestion of locoweed intensifies the effect of high altitude on the development of congestive heart failure but the mechanism is unknown (5). The syndrome of cor pulmonale in cattle at high altitudes, bovine brisket disease, is described in more detail elsewhere in this text (p. 1230).

Pulmonary hypertension can also result from partial destruction of the pulmonary vascular bed and a reduction in its total cross-sectional area. Pulmonary thromboembolic disease can produce right heart failure by this mechanism. Chronic interstitial pneumonia and emphysema may also induce cor pulmonale by the same mechanism.

Chronic obstructive pneumonias, where there is airway constriction and accumulation of fluid in distal airways, may induce pulmonary hypertension by a combination of chronic hypoxia and reduction of the pulmonary vascular bed (3). However, although pulmonary hypertension and right heart hypertrophy may be present in livestock with primary pulmonary disease, clinical cardiac insufficiency is minor, and right heart failure rare. Heart failure may occur when additional cardiac stress in superimposed, such as by pregnancy or moderate altitude anoxia in cattle, or the development of atrial fibrillation in goats.

In highly conditioned feedlot cattle, increased intra-abdominal pressure resulting from excessive abdominal fat, forestomach engorgement and recumbency can lead to pulmonary hypoventilation, with decreased alveolar Po_2 and subsequent right heart failure, a syndrome analogous to the Pickwickian syndrome in man (2).

Chronic severe elevations in pulmonary venous pressure can lead to constriction and hypertrophy of the vascular smooth muscle of precapillary vessels with resultant pulmonary hypertension. An elevated left ventricular filling pressure is perhaps the more common cause and can set the stage for right heart failure in the left heart failure situations. The toxic principle in poisoning by *Pimelea* spp. appears to act in part by constricting the pulmonary venules producing pulmonary hypertension which contributes to the clinical syndrome.

REFERENCES

(1) Bisgard, G. E. (1977) *Adv. vet. Sci.*, *21*, 151.
(2) Alexander, A. F. (1978) In: *Effects of Poisonous Plants on Livestock*, p. 285. New York: Academic Press.
(3) Nuytten, J. et al. (1985) *Zentralbl. Vet. Med. A*, *32*, 81.
(4) James, L. F., et al. (1983) *Am. J. vet. Rec.* *44*, 254.
(5) James, L. F., et al. (1986) *J. Am. vet. med. Assoc.*, *189*, 1549.

Valvular disease

Disease of the heart valves interferes with the normal flow of blood through the cardiac orifices, causing murmurs and, in severe cases, congestive heart failure.

Etiology

Valvular disease may be either acquired or congenital. Congenital valvular disease is rare in large domestic animals.

Endocarditis, in its acute or chronic form, is the commonest cause of valvular disease in animals and is described in detail below. Laceration or detachment of valves during severe exercise may occur but probably only when there is prior disease of the endocardium. Fenestration of the aortic and pulmonary semilunar valves has been observed commonly in horses. The cause of the lesions is unknown although their presence in very young animals, including newborn foals, suggests that some may be congenital defects. The importance of these lesions as causes of valvular insufficiency is doubtful although they may cause valvular murmurs if they are present close to the attachments of the cusps. Congenital hematocysts in the atrioventricular valves are also common (2) but are considered of no functional significance. A systolic murmur most audible on the left side behind the shoulder joint is common in normal newborn foals and is caused by patency of the ductus arteriosus. The persistence of this murmur to the fifth day suggests the presence of a congenital defect (3). Excessive cardiac dilatation in any form of myocardial asthenia or when there is excessive overloading of the arterial flow may result in dilatation of the orifices and functional insufficiency of the valves. Careful examination of the heart sounds is most commonly performed in the horse but the incidence of significant valvular lesions is remarkably low. Verrucose endocarditis of the atrioventricular valves occurs occasionally (4) and degenerative lesions of the aortic valves resulting in insufficiency have been observed in this species (5). An extensive abattoir survey (6) suggests that valvular lesions may be more common in the horse than is clinically appreciated. Approximately 25% of horses had lesions, the majority being nodular or distorting lesions on the valves or chordae tendinae of the left side, and in a significant proportion murmurs were detected prior to slaughter. Chronic trauma of the valve leaflets was considered an important initiating factor.

Cardiac murmurs are common in old horses, as they are in newborn foals, and it is often difficult to know how much importance one should attach to them. The commonest murmur is a diastolic murmur loudest over the aortic valve area and in most cases there is some evidence of aortic valvular insufficiency (3).

Pathogenesis

The presence of valvular lesions and murmurs may mean little except that some degree of cardiac reserve is lost. This may be small in degree, and moderate stenosis or incompetence can be compensated and supported for long periods provided myocardial asthenia does not develop. The importance of valvular lesions lies in their possible contribution to disease in other organs by the liberation of emboli, and the necessity for close examination of the heart when they are present. The purpose for which the animal is maintained also has some bearing on the significance of a murmur. Valvular lesions are of much greater importance in racing animals than in those kept for breeding purposes.

The important clinical indications of valvular disease are audible murmurs and palpable thrills. Both are caused by turbulence and eddying in blood flow and possibly also by the vibrations produced by abnormally directed flow impinging on the heart and vessel walls. Turbulence in flow may be produced by a sudden change in the diameter of the vessel through which the blood is flowing. Its occurrence is directly related to the velocity of flow and inversely related to blood viscosity. With murmurs associated with valvular lesions the valve lesion produces a sufficient change in stream bed diameter to result in turbulent flow. However, the severity of the turbulence and hence the murmur can be increased with higher flow velocities such as occur with exercise and by factors that decrease blood viscosity such as anemia or hypoproteinemia. In general, the loudest murmurs are produced by leaks of only moderate size but a cardiac thrill always indicates the presence of a large leak. The turbulence may occur when the valves do not close properly (insufficiency) and blood is forced through atrioventricular orifices during ventricular systole, or through semilunar orifices during ventricular diastole. Turbulence may also occur when the valves do not open completely (stenosis) and blood enters the ventricle through a narrow atrioventricular orifice during its diastolic phase or is forced through a stenotic semilunar orifice during ventricular systole. In general acquired lesions produce an insufficiency of the affected valve whereas stenosis is more commonly associated with congenital valvular disease. Simple stenosis or insufficiency may occur independently but in many cases in animals, especially those in which there are vegetative lesions, insufficiency and stenosis of the one group of valves occur at the same time.

Murmurs may occur in the absence of valvular disease. A change in vessel diameter such as occurs with dilatation of the aorta or pulmonary artery can produce turbulence and a murmur. Turbulent flow may also occur in the absence of a change in stream bed diameter if a certain critical velocity of flow is exceeded. This is believed to be the cause of functional or ejection murmurs that occur commonly in horses during the rapid ejection phase even at rest and especially following exercise (1). A reduction in blood viscosity contributes to the frequency of murmurs occurring in anemic and hypoproteinemic states.

The presence of a significant valvular lesion will induce compensatory responses by the myocardium. Stenosis of the outflow valves results in an increased pressure load on the heart and compensatory hypertrophy. Insufficiency of the semilunar valves or of the aortic or pulmonic valve produces a volume load on the heart and is followed by compensatory dilatation and hypertrophy. If the valves on the left side of the heart are affected, especially the aortic valve, the changes in ejection of the blood from the ventricle produce changes in the character of the peripheral pulse. Involvement of the tricuspid valve will produce changes in the jugular pulse.

Clinical findings

Only the clinical findings referable to valvular disease are discussed here. The clinical findings in congestive heart failure, which may coexist, are discussed elsewhere. There is an obvious need for very careful auscultation if accurate observations are to be made. The need is perhaps greatest in the horse in which minimal lesions may be of great importance. Good equipment and a knowledge of the optimum areas of auscultation and the significance of the murmurs encountered are essential (7–9). When a murmur is detected it should be categorized according to its timing and duration, intensity, location and frequency pattern.

Timing allows a subdivision into systolic, diastolic and continuous murmurs and immediately shortens the list of possible defects present. It is done with reference to the arterial pulse which occurs in early to mid-systole if a proximal artery is examined. A convenient artery is on the posterior-medial aspect of the carpus in cattle and horses. A less satisfactory alternative is timing with the occurrence of the apex beat. Timing by relation to the heart sounds is unreliable as these are frequently altered in character and at fast heart rates a diastolic murmur may be mistaken for a systolic one. Systolic murmurs are associated with stenosis of the outflow valves or insufficiency of the atrioventricular valves. Diastolic murmurs are associated with insufficiency of the outflow valves or stenosis of the atrioventricular valves. A continuous murmur or one that occurs during both systole and diastole may be associated with both stenosis and insufficiency of the same valve or with multiple valvular lesions but more commonly results from the turbulent flow of blood from a high pressure to a low pressure system with no intervening valve such as occurs with a patent ductus arteriosus.

Duration during systole or diastole is determined by a careful examination of the murmur with relationship to the period between the heart sounds. Pansystolic and pandiastolic murmurs, occurring throughout the systole or diastole, have greater significance than murmurs that occur for example only in early systole and early diastole. The intensity or loudness of the murmur provides a guide to its significance. A system of grading the intensity of murmurs that has been found to be of clinical value is as follows (9).

Grade I The faintest audible murmur. Generally only detected after careful auscultation

Grade II A faint murmur that is clearly heard after only a few seconds auscultation

Grade III A murmur which is immediately audible as soon as auscultation begins and is heard over a reasonably large area

Grade IV An extremely loud murmur accompanied by a thrill. The murmur becomes inaudible if the stethoscope is held with only light pressure on the chest

Grade V An extremely loud murmur accompanied by a thrill. The murmur can still be heard when the stethoscope is held with only light pressure against the chest

Grade I murmurs are not clinically significant whereas grade IV and V invariably are. The significance of grade II and III murmurs varies according to their cause.

The location of murmurs is related to their areas of generation and transmission. Low intensity murmurs are generally restricted to the auscultatory area overlying their area of generation. The auscultatory areas of the heart and of the individual heart sounds have been described earlier in the section on arrhythmias. The vibrations associated with very loud murmurs may be transmitted to other auscultatory areas but generally they are most intense near the area of generation as is any associated thrill. Murmurs and thrills can be restricted to local areas and it is essential to examine several auscultatory areas over both sides of the heart.

The frequency pattern of murmurs is crudely described by the characters of pitch and quality. Murmurs may be described as high or low pitched and by terms such as harsh, blowing, musical, sighing. This is the least useful clinical characteristic in large animals. Murmurs may also vary in intensity and frequency and have crescendo or decrescendo characteristics.

Following this examination the functional defect producing the murmur and the valve involved is determined from the characteristics of timing and duration, location, and also any secondary effects that may be present in arterial or venous pulse characteristics. The severity of the lesion is judged in part on the intensity of the murmur but also on the degree of cardiac insufficiency that is present. The cause of the lesion cannot be determined from auscultation but may be determined from the results of general clinical and special pathological examinations and by a consideration of the common causes of valvular disease that involve the particular valve affected in the animal species being examined.

The salient features of functional lesions on the various heart valves are as follows.

Stenosis of the aortic valve

There is a harsh systolic murmur, most audible high up over the base of the heart on the left side and posteriorly. The murmur replaces or modifies the first heart sound. A systolic thrill may be palpable over the base of the heart and the cardiac impulse is increased due to ventricular hypertrophy. The stenosis has no functional significance unless the pulse is abnormal, with a small amplitude rising slowly to a delayed peak. There may be signs of left-sided heart failure (10).

Insufficiency of the aortic valve

This is the most common acquired valvular defect in horses (5, 8, 11, 12). There is a loud holodiastolic murmur, frequently accompanied by a thrill caused by the reflux of blood from the aorta into the left ventricle during diastole. The murmur is generally audible over the left cardiac area and is most intense at the aortic valve area and radiates to the apex. It may modify the second heart sound or start immediately following. The murmur may be noisy or musical and the relative intensity varies from horse to horse. Frequently it is decrescendo in character but other variations in its intensity occur. Valvular insufficiency of a sufficient degree to have functional significance is accompanied by an arterial pulse of very large amplitude and high systolic and low diastolic blood pressures. The pulse wave may be great enough to cause a visible pulse in small vessels and even in capillaries. Rarely this lesion is accompanied by a diastolic jugular pulse due to transmission of the impact of the reflex wave across the ventricular septum to the right side of the heart.

Stenosis and insufficiency of the pulmonary valve

Acquired lesions of this valve are rare in large animals (6, 8, 9). The signs are similar to those produced by aortic valve lesions except that there are no abnormalities of the pulse. Differentiation may be difficult when aortic valve lesions are small and produce no pulse changes. Pulmonary valve lesions are more audible anterior to the aortic valve area and heart failure, if it occurs, is right-sided.

Insufficiency of the left atrioventricular valve

This is the second most common acquired valvular disease in horses, cattle and pigs (15). The insufficiency may result from endocarditis or rupture of the mitral valve chordae (14). There is a loud harsh pansystolic murmur that is most intense in the mitral area. The murmur transmits dorsally and in severe cases may also be heard on the right side. There is frequently modification of the first and second heart sounds with marked accentuation or the occurrence of a third heart sound which may be mistaken for the second. The pulse characters are unchanged until the stage of cardiac failure. Cases of mitral insufficiency may compensate at rest and may be only evidenced by decreased work tolerance. Failure, if it occurs, will be initially associated with left ventricular volume overload; however, in some cases the retrograde flow of blood through the mitral valve may lead to pulmonary hypertension and the additional occurrence of right-sided heart failure. Acute onset heart failure is usually associated with rupture of the valve chordae (16). In the horse mitral insufficiency may predispose to atrial fibrillation.

Insufficiency of the right atrioventricular valve
This is the most common acquired valvular lesion in cattle, pigs and sheep. Insufficiency may also result from dilatation of the valve annulus in myocardial asthenia associated with chronic anemia and from cor pulmonale in conditions such as high altitude disease in cattle. There is a harsh pansystolic murmur which usually modifies the first heart sound as it is most audible over the tricuspid valve area. Loud murmurs project dorsally and to the cranial part of the thoracic cavity on both right and left sides. It is usually accompanied by an exaggeration of the systolic component of the jugular pulse. Congestive heart failure, if it occurs, will be manifest in the greater circulation.

Stenosis of the right or left atrioventricular valves
Stenosis of either atrioventricular valve is uncommon. There is a diastolic murmur caused by passage of blood through a stenosed valve during diastolic filling and audible over the base of the heart on the relevant side. The severity of the lesion will govern the duration of the murmur but there is likely to be a presystolic accentuation due to atrial contraction. Right atrioventricular valve stenosis may be accompanied by accentuation of the atrial component of the jugular pulse. It is possible that some degree of mitral stenosis may occur in acquired lesions that manifest primarily as an insufficiency (8).

Clinical pathology
Clinicopathological findings will reflect the changes caused by the primary disease and are significant only when there is endocarditis.

Necropsy findings
Care is needed when the heart is opened to ensure that the valves can be viewed properly from both upper and lower aspects. Lesions of endocarditis may be visible or there may be perforations, distortion or thickening of the valves or breakage of the chordae tendinae. The lesions of congestive heart failure may also be present.

Diagnosis
Diagnosis of valvular disease depends largely on recognition of an endocardial murmur. Murmurs must be differentiated from pericardial and pleural friction sounds and from murmurs due to congenital defects. Valvular murmurs always accompany or replace the normal heart sounds and although a systolic and a diastolic murmur may be present in the one animal there is a strict relation to the cardiac cycle. Pleural friction rubs may be localized to the cardiac area but can be distinguished by their occurrence with each respiratory cycle. Pericardial friction sounds are more clearly audible and are present throughout the cardiac cycle, waxing and waning in intensity during diastole and systole. Murmurs caused by congenital valvular defects may be impossible to differentiate clinically from acquired lesions and especial reference is made to history and age of the animal. Those associated with shunts are usually very loud, do not displace the normal heart sounds and can be heard in specific sites. A thrill is more commonly felt in congenital defects but may occur in valvular disease.

Special attention should be given to the differentiation of functional hemic murmurs and those due to structural lesions of the valves. Hemic murmurs can be expected in animals suffering from anemia and in emaciated and debilitated animals. The murmur is soft and usually only discernible by careful auscultation and characteristically waxes and wanes with each respiratory cycle, reaching maximum intensity at the height of inspiration.

Murmurs are commonly encountered in normal animals (9). In the horse, an early systolic decrescendo or crescendo–decrescendo murmur is commonly heard over the aortic valve area. It is of grade I or II in intensity and is considered a functional or ejection murmur. Ejection murmurs can be associated with the rapid ejection phase at both the pulmonary and the aortic valve in horses (1). Also a grade I or II early diastolic decrescendo murmur localized to the aortic valve region is frequently present in the horse, possibly associated with the rapid filling phase of the heart in early diastole. Systolic ejection clicks may occur in the horse but have not been associated with lesions on postmortem (8). Systolic murmurs are heard in many animals during recumbency which disappear on standing. In newborn calves and foals a systolic murmur is frequently audible over the base of the heart and it is believed to be due to a partial temporary patency of the closing ductus arteriosus. In newborn pigs a continuous murmur may be heard and this is often replaced by an early systolic murmur audible for the first week of life. The murmur is thought to be caused by patency of the ductus arteriosus which subsequently disappears (13).

Treatment
There is no specific treatment for valvular disease. Methods for the treatment of congestive heart failure and endocarditis are discussed under those headings.

REVIEW LITERATURE

Brown, C. M. (1985) Acquired cardiovascular disease. Symposium on cardiology. *Vet. Clin. N. Am. equ. Pract.*, *1 (2)*, 371–382.

REFERENCES

(1) Brown, C. M. & Holmes, J. R. (1979) *Equ. vet.J.*, *11*, 11.
(2) Kemler, A. G. & Martin, J. E. (1972) *Am. J. vet. Res.*, *32*, 249.
(3) Rossdale, P. D. (1967) *Br. vet. J.*, *123*, 521.

(4) Miller, W. C. (1962) *Vet. Rec.*, *74*, 825.
(5) Bishop, S. P. et al. (1966) *Pathol. vet.*, *3*, 137.
(6) Else, R. W. & Holmes, J. R. (1972) *Equ. vet. J.*, *4*, 1, 57.
(7) Littlewort, M. C. G. (1962) *Vet. Rec.*, *74*, 1247.
(8) Holmes, J. R. & Else, R. W. (1972) *Equ. vet. J.*, *4*, 195.
(9) Glendinning, E. S. A. (1972) *Equ. vet. J.*, *4*, 21.
(10) Fisher, E. W. (1968) *Vet. Rec.*, *82*, 618.
(11) Smetzer, D. L. et al. (1966) *Am. Heart J.*, *72*, 489.
(12) Sporri, H. & Leemann, W. (1972) *Berl. Tierärztl. Wochenschr.*, *23*, 441.
(13) Evans, J. R. et al. (1963) *Circ. Res.*, *12*, 85
(14) Holmes, J. R. & Miller, P. J. (1984) *Equ. vet. J.*, *16*, 125.
(15) Miller, P. J. & Holmes, J. R. (1985) *Equ. vet. J.*, *17*, 181.
(16) Brown , C. M. et al. (1983). *J Am. vet. med. Assoc.*, *182*, 281.

Endocarditis

Inflammation of the endocardium may interfere with the ejection of blood from the heart by causing insufficiency or stenosis of the valves. Murmurs associated with the heart sounds are the major clinical manifestation and, if interference with blood flow is sufficiently severe, congestive heart failure develops.

Etiology

Most cases of endocarditis in farm animals are caused by bacterial infection but whether the infection gains entrance by direct adhesion to undamaged endothelium, or through minor discontinuities of the valvular surfaces, or by hematogenous spread through the capillaries at the base of the valve is uncertain. The common infectious causes of endocarditis in animals are listed below (1–4, 6).

Cattle

- Alpha-hemolytic streptococci
- *Corynebacterium (Actinomyces) pyogenes*
- *Clostridium chauvoei* (blackleg)
- *Myoplasma mycoides*
- *Erysipelothrix rhusiopathia (insidiosa)* (rare).

Horses

- *Actinobacillus equuli*
- *Streptococcus* spp., including *Strep. equi*
- Migrating *Strongylus* spp. larvae

Pigs and sheep

- *Erysipelothrix rhusiopathia (insidiosa)*
- *Streptococcus* spp.
- *Escherichia coli*.

Pathogenesis

Endocarditis may arise from implantation of bacteria onto the valves from the bloodstream or by bacterial embolism of the valve capillaries. It is most commonly a sequel of chronic infection at some distant site and a persistent bacteremia. Myocardial disease may lead to edema of the valves and predispose to endothelial damage. Endocarditis is also a common sequel on valves that are subject to flow-associated stress as the result of congenital cardiac defects.

Vegetative or ulcerative lesions may develop and interfere with the normal passage of blood through the cardiac orifices, resulting in congestive heart failure. Fragments of vegetative lesions may become detached and cause embolic endarteritis, with the production of miliary pulmonary abscesses, or abscesses in other organs including myocardium, kidneys and joints.

Chronic lesions are less crumbly and less likely to release emboli but adhesions between cusps develop and retraction of scar tissue causes shrinking, distortion, and thickening of the valve cusps. At this stage interference with blood flow is severe and congestive heart failure almost always follows.

In cattle, valvular lesions occur most commonly on the right atrioventricular valve and venous congestion is most marked in the general systemic vessels but bilateral or left-sided involvement of the atrioventricular valves is not uncommon (7). In horses, aortic semilunar valves are most commonly affected although the left atrioventricular valves may also be involved (8).

Clinical findings

In cattle there is frequently a history of ill thrift with periodic, dramatic, but temporary fall in milk production.

The important finding is a murmur on auscultation or a thrill on palpation of the cardiac area. The area of maximum intensity of the murmur varies with the situation of the affected valves (7) and this also governs whether or not there are abnormalities of the amplitude and pressure of the arterial pulse and abnormality of the jugular pulse. Details of the specific findings for individual valve abnormalities can be found in the preceding section on valvular disease. Phonocardiography can be of value as an aid to diagnosis, and echocardiography may show reflected echoes from vegetative lesions and detect abnormal valve movement (5).

In compensated cases there may be poor exercise tolerance. In advanced cases, particularly where a concurrent myocardial asthenia reduces cardiac compensation, congestive failure develops. At all stages a moderate, fluctuating fever is common and secondary involvement of other organs may cause the appearance of signs of peripheral lymphadenitis, embolic pneumonia, nephritis, arthritis, tenosynovitis or myocarditis. There is usually much loss of condition, pallor of mucosae and an increase in heart rate. In cattle, additional signs observed include a grunting respiration as though the animal was in pain, moderate ruminal tympany, scouring or constipation, blindness, facial paralysis, muscle weakness to the point of tremor or recumbency, jaundice and sudden death (2). Distension of the jugular vein, general edema and a systolic or diastolic murmur are also present in many cases. In horses, edema occurs rarely and jugular engorgement is not a marked sign until the terminal stages.

The course in endocarditis may be as long as several weeks or months, or animals may drop dead without premonitory signs. In sows it is common for agalactia to develop in the first 2–3 weeks after farrowing, followed by a loss of weight, intolerance to exercise and dyspnea at rest.

Clinical pathology

A marked leukocytosis and a shift to the left occurs in acute cases (9). A significant increase in monocytes and macrophages and a severe anemia have been observed in cattle at this time (1). In chronic cases where the lesions are due largely to scarring of the valves hematological findings are usually normal. Hypergammaglobulinemia is common and an indication of chronic bacterial infection. Blood cultures should be attempted at the peaks of the fever but may have to be repeated on a number of occasions. Determination of the sensitivity of the organism to antibacterial drugs may aid in treatment. Repeated examination of the urine may reveal transient episodes of proteinuria and the shedding of bacteria.

Necropsy findings

The lesions are termed vegetative when they are large and cauliflower-like and verrucose when they are small and wart-like. The former are present on the valves in most fatal cases. In the later stages the valves are shrunken, distorted and often thickened along the edges. This stage of recovery is rare in farm animals but may be observed in the semilunar valves in horses. Spontaneous healing is rare and in most cases treatment is commenced at too late a stage.

Embolic lesions may be present in any other organ. Culture of the valvular lesions should be undertaken but in many cases no growth is obtained. The causative bacteria may be dead or not cultivable and the examination of direct smears should always be undertaken.

Diagnosis

The differentiation of valvular disease from other conditions in which heart murmurs occur has already been discussed. Failure to observe a valvular murmur may result in confusion between endocarditis and pericarditis or other causes of congestive heart failure. The commonest error in cattle is in differentiation of the disease from lymphomatosis.

Treatment

Treatment is not highly successful because of the difficulty encountered in completely controlling the infection. The thickness of the lesions prevents adequate penetration of the drugs and unless the sensitivity of the causative organism is known a range of antibacterial drugs may have to be tried. The streptococci which cause endocarditis in cattle are often resistant to most antibiotics but the parenteral administration of procaine benzylpenicillin is occasionally effective. Large doses (20 000 units/kg daily) should be given for at least 7–10 days and preferably longer. This is frequently combined with treatment with an aminoglycoside antibiotic for the initial 5 days of treatment. If treatment is attempted a fall in temperature can be taken as an indication that infection is being brought under control but treatment should be continued for at least another 7 days. Ampicillin or a macrolide antibiotic such as erythromycin is more effective but the cost of prolonged treatment restricts their use for all but valuable animals. Relapse is common and treatment of endocarditis should be approached with reservation. If signs of congestive heart failure are present the prognosis is poor.

The sequelae of embolic lesions in other organs and permanent distortion of valves resulting in valvular insufficiency also militate against a satisfactory outcome. The use of parenteral anticoagulants, as used in man to prevent further deposition of material on vegetative lesions, has not been found to be practicable in animals.

REFERENCES

(1) Power, H. T. & Rebhun, W. C. (1983) *J. Am. vet. med. Assoc.*, *182*, 806.
(2) John, F. V. (1947) *Vet. Rec.*, *59*, 214.
(3) Larsen, H. E. et al. (1963) *Nord. VetMed.*, *15*, 645, 668, 691.
(4) Innes, J. R. M. et al. (1950) *Br. vet. J.*, *106*, 245.
(5) Lacuata, A. Q. et al. (1980) *J. Am. vet. med. Assoc.*, *176*, 1355.
(6) Narucka, U. & Westendorp, J. F. (1973) *Tijdschr. Diergeneeskd.*, *98*, 655.
(7) Wagenaar, G. (1963) *Tijdschr. Diergeneeskd.*, *88*, 1760.
(8) Detweiler, D. K. (1958) *Univ. Pennsylvania Bull.*, *Vet. Ext. Q.*, *59*, 4.
(9) Kroneman, J. (1970) *Tijdschr. Diergeneeskd.*, *95*, 862.

Pericarditis

Inflammation of the pericardial sac causes an audible friction rub initially, followed by muffling of the heart sounds and congestive heart failure as fluid accumulates in the sac, or the exudate organizes to form obliterating and restrictive adhesions.

Etiology

Perforation of the pericardial sac by an infected foreign body occurs commonly only in cattle. The resulting syndrome of traumatic pericarditis has already been discussed. Localization of a blood-borne infection occurs sporadically in many diseases. Direct extension of infection from pleurisy or myocarditis may also occur in all animals but the clinical signs of pericarditis in such cases are usually dominated by those of the primary disease.

Cattle

- Pasteurellosis
- Black disease—if patients survive more than 24 hours
- Sporadic bovine encephalomyelitis
- *Haemophilus* spp., including *Haem. somnus*
- Tuberculosis
- *Pseudomonas aeruginosa*
- *Mycoplasma* spp.

Horses

- *Streptococcus* spp., including *Strep. equi*, *Strep. zooepidemicus* and *Strep. fecalis*
- Tuberculosis
- Idiopathic fibrinous pericarditis (4).

Sheep

- Pasteurellosis
- *Staphylococcus aureus*
- *Mycoplasma* spp.

Pigs

- Pasteurellosis
- *Mycoplasma* spp., especially *M. hyorhinis*
- *Haemophilus* spp.—Glasser's disease and pleuropneumonia
- *Streptococcus* spp.
- Salmonellosis.

Pathogenesis

In the early stages inflammation of the pericardium is accompanied by hyperemia and the deposition of fibrinous exudate which produces a friction rub when the pericardium and epicardium rub together during cardiac movement. As effusion develops the inflamed surfaces are separated, the friction rub is replaced by muffling of the heart sounds, and the accumulated fluid compresses the atria and right ventricle, preventing their complete filling. Congestive heart failure follows. A severe toxemia is usually present in suppurative pericarditis because of the toxins produced by the bacteria in the pericardial sac.

In the recovery stage of non-suppurative pericarditis the fluid is resorbed, and adhesions form between the pericardium and epicardium to cause an adhesive pericarditis but the adhesions are usually not sufficiently strong to impair cardiac movement. In suppurative pericarditis the adhesions which form become organized and may cause complete attachment of the pericardium to the epicardium, or this may occur only patchily to leave some loculi which are filled with serous fluid. In either case restriction of cardiac movement will probably be followed by the appearance of congestive heart failure.

Clinical findings

In the early stages there is pain, avoidance of movement, abduction of the elbows, arching of the back and shallow, abdominal respiration. Pain is evidenced on percussion or firm palpation over the cardiac area of the chest wall, and the animal lies down carefully. A pericardial friction sound is detectable on auscultation of the cardiac area. The temperature is elevated to 39·5–41°C (103–106°F) and the pulse rate is increased. Associated signs of pleurisy, pneumonia and peritonitis may be present.

In most cases of pericarditis caused by traumatic reticuloperitonitis, hematogenous infection, or spread from pleurisy, the second stage of effusion is manifested by muffling of the heart sounds, decreased palpability of the apex beat and an increase in the area of cardiac dullness with decreased amplitude of the peripheral pulse. If gas is present in the pericardial sac each cardiac cycle may be accompanied by splashing sounds. Signs of congestive heart failure become evident. Fever is present, the heart rate is markedly increased and toxemia is severe, although this varies with the types of bacteria present. This is the most dangerous period and affected animals usually die of congestive heart failure, or of toxemia, in 1–3 weeks. Those that survive pass through a long period of chronic ill health during which the toxemia subsides relatively quickly but congestive heart failure diminishes slowly. In this stage of chronic pericarditis additional signs of myocarditis, particularly irregularity, may appear. The heart sounds become less muffled and fluid sounds disappear altogether or persist in restricted areas. Complete recovery is not common but with suitable antibacterial treatment relative normality may be regained.

In fibrinous pericarditis in the horse, there is marked muffling of the heart sounds, tachycardia, distension of the jugular veins and subcutaneous edema of the ventral body wall (4).

Clinical pathology

A marked leukocytosis and shift to the left is detectable on hematological examination in traumatic pericarditis. In the other forms of pericarditis changes in the blood depend upon the other lesions present and on the causative agent. In the stage in which effusion occurs a sample of fluid may be aspirated from the pericardial sac and submitted for bacteriological examination. The technique is not without danger as infection may be spread to the pleural cavity.

Necropsy findings

In the early stages there is hyperemia of the pericardial lining and a deposit of fibrin. When effusion occurs there is an accumulation of turbid fluid and tags of fibrin are present on the greatly thickened epicardium and pericardium. Gas may also be present and the fluid may have a putrid odor if *Fusobacterium necrophorus* or *Actinomyces (Corynebacterium) pyogenes* are present. When the pericarditis has reached a chronic stage the pericardium is adherent to the epicardium over a greater or lesser part of the cardiac surface. Loculi containing serous fluid often remain. Embolic abscesses may be present in other organs. Lesions typical of the specific causative diseases listed above are described under their specific headings.

Diagnosis

Pericardial friction sounds may be mistaken for the friction sounds of early pleurisy. Synchronization of friction sounds with respiratory cycles indicates that the sounds are pleural in origin. Cardiac movement may produce friction sounds when pleurisy is localized to the pleural surface of the pericardial sac but there is an absence of other signs of pericardial involvement. Pericardial sounds may also be confused with valvular murmurs, or murmurs caused by congenital defects, but pericardial sounds are usually present throughout the cardiac cycle rather than accompanying or displacing one or other of the heart sounds.

Muffling of the heart sounds may also occur in pleurisy with effusion and in pulmonary emphysema but there are prominent signs of respiratory involvement. Hydropericardium is usually found in association with edema and an increase in the cardiac impulse. It occurs commonly in congestive heart failure, in mulberry heart disease of pigs, in *Herztod* of pigs, gossypol poisoning, clostridial intoxications of sheep and in lymphomatosis. Mediastinal abscess may also cause signs of congestive heart failure and local pleurisy.

Treatment

Antibacterial treatment of the specific infection should be undertaken if possible. Non-specific treatment should include broad-spectrum antibiotics or sulfonamides. Intravenous alimentation is usually not indicated because of the long course. Repeated paracentesis to relieve the fluid pressure in the pericardial sac affords only temporary relief of the cardiac embarrassment, the fluid returning quickly. If the infection can be brought under control paracentesis of the pericardial sac followed by the administration of diuretics is recommended, but digitalization is usually not very effective and is dangerous if infection is still present. Surgical treatment, to provide continuous drainage of the sac, has been used, but is not usually successful (3).

REFERENCES

(1) Rainey, J. W. (1944) *Aus. vet. J.*, *20*, 204.
(2) Ryan, A. F. & Rainey, J. W. (1945) *Aust. vet. J.*, *21*, 146.
(3) Horney, F. D. (1960) *Can. vet. J.*, *1*, 363.
(4) Dill, S. G. et al. (1982) *J. Am. vet. med. Assoc.*, *180*, 266.

Congenital cardiac defects

Some of the defects described in this section are actually defects of the peripheral vascular system but are described here for convenience. The defects often produce clinical signs at birth and cause severe illness or death in the first few weeks of life but in a number of cases adequate compensation occurs and the defect may not be observed until a comparatively late age. It is probably wise to avoid giving a too unfavorable prognosis in newborn animals which have a cardiac murmur, especially in foals and baby pigs and when the murmur is minimal. It is possible that in many such cases there is no structural defect and the murmur is innocent and functional and will disappear early in life.

The important factor in the pathogenesis of most congenital cardiac defects is the mixing of oxygenated and reduced blood through an anastomosis between the pulmonary and systemic circuits. The blood leaving the left ventricle or aorta therefore includes some oxygenated and some reduced blood. The resulting anoxic anoxia causes severe dyspnea, and cyanosis may be marked if the proportion of unsaturated blood is high. This is most likely to occur when there is obstruction of the pulmonary artery. There is a notable absence of fever and toxemia if intercurrent disease does not develop. Cardiac enlargement is usually detectable.

In animals which survive to maturity, sudden death due to acute heart failure or congestive heart failure is likely to occur when the animals are subjected to a physical stress such as the first pregnancy. The primary appearance of signs of cardiac disease when an animal is 2 or 3 years of age should not eliminate congenital defects from consideration. One of the major difficulties in clinical cardiology is to distinguish between the congenital anomalies themselves. An accurate diagnosis can be made only by the utilization of the special techniques for examination of the cardiovascular system which have been outlined earlier.

Congenital cardiac anomalies occur in all species but are not common in any one of them. The prevalence is probably highest in cattle and lowest in horses (3). The relative frequency of individual cardiac defects in 36 calves at postmortem in one study (1) was: interventricular septal defect—14%; ectopia cordis—13%; right ventricular hypoplasia—13%; left ventricular hypoplasia—13%; dextraposed aorta—10%; valvular hematomas—9%; patent ductus arteriosus—6%; patent foramen ovale—6%; endocardial fibroelastosis—4%; common aortic trunk—4%; and other cardiac defects—10%. The animals were neonatal calves and the relative frequencies are biased towards defects that are incompatible with longer life. In a large series of necropsy examinations on lambs (4), 1·3% had cardiac anomalies of which approximately 90% were interventricular septal defects. The relative frequency of congenital cardiac malformations in pigs (2) has been reported as: dysplasia of the tricuspid valve— 34%; atrial septal defect—25%; subaortic stenosis—18%; ventricular septal defect—9%; persistent common atrioventricular canal—9%; and other defects—10%. The cause of congenital cardiac defects is unknown, but it is assumed they result from prenatal insults during development or from single recessive genes or polygenic sets that have lesion-specific effects on cardiac development.

An increasing number of clinical reports on congenital cardiovascular defects are appearing in the veterinary literature. However, their general importance is low. A general description of the more common defects is given below; there are many variations in the exact nature of these defects.

Ectopia cordis

An abnormal position of the heart outside the thoracic cavity is most common in cattle, the displacement usually being to the lower cervical region (5). The heart is easily seen and palpated and there is an accompanying divergence of the first ribs and a ventrodorsal compression of the sternum giving the appearance of absence of the brisket. Affected animals may survive for periods of years, as they also may with an abdominal displacement, but those with a displacement through a defective sternum or ribs rarely survive for more than a few days.

Patent foramen ovale

This defect of the atrial septum is reasonably common in cattle but usually causes no clinical signs when it is present as an isolated defect and is detected incidentally at necropsy. Normally a flap-like opening allows only a shunt from right to left but large defects may allow a shunt in both directions. Relative resistance to outflow from the atria is greater in the left than the right and the shunt, if it occurs, is from left to right. This induces a moderate flow load on the right side of the heart which is well tolerated. Large flows will generally increase pulmonary vascular resistance and result in moderate right ventricular hypertrophy. The increase in outflow resistance from the right atrium results in a decreased flow across the shunt and control of the effects of the defect. Atrial septal defects are of more significance when they are present with other cardiac defects. If these result in a severe right ventricular hypertrophy the shunt may reverse from right to left and cyanosis will occur.

Ventricular septal defects

These are probably the most common congenital cardiac defects in sheep, cattle and horses (1, 3, 4, 6). They are almost invariably subaortal defects occurring high in the septum at the pars membranaceae. In the absence of other defects their presence results in the shunting of blood from the left to the right ventricle. The magnitude of the shunt and the fate of the animal is determined by the size of the defect and the degree of resistance to flow from the right ventricle as determined by pulmonary vascular resistance. With large defects the shunt of blood can be considerable and the animal may die at birth or show clinical signs at a few weeks to a few months of age (6, 7). The major presenting signs during this period are lassitude, failure to grow well and dyspnea with moderate exercise. The shunt may be less severe and allow an apparently normal existence until maturity (6, 9–11) or cause no apparent problem during life and be detected incidentally on necropsy or abattoir examination. On auscultation there is a loud blowing pansystolic murmur audible over both sides of the chest (6, 11, 12). It is usually audible over a large area on both sides but most intense at the left fourth intercostal and the right third intercostal space and more intense on the right than left side. The murmur in this defect is one of the loudest and most obvious murmurs encountered. It does not modify the heart sounds which are usually increased in intensity. A pronounced cardiac thrill is frequently palpable on both the left and the right-hand side. Echocardiography is of limited value in detecting ventricular septal defects (11), but the diagnosis can be confirmed by right-sided catheterization with the finding of an elevation of right ventricular and pulmonary artery pressure in conjunction with an increase in the percentage oxygen saturation of blood between the right atrium and the right ventricle or pulmonary artery (10, 11). Indicator dilution techniques including dye dilution and thermodilution curves are also of value in diagnosis (37). The signs of heart failure, if present, vary. The defect produces a flow load on the left and the right ventricle and, depending on the degree of increase in pulmonary vascular resistance, a pressure load on the right ventricle. Signs of acute left-sided failure are usually evident in animals dying with this defect at or shortly following birth, whereas in cattle right-sided congestive heart failure is more common in later life.

An increase in pulmonary vascular resistance occurs as the result of increased pulmonary blood flow. In cattle, this increase may be sufficient to cause reversal of the shunt, and cyanosis develops. This syndrome, sometimes referred to as an Eisenmenger complex (13, 14), develops most commonly between 1 and 3 years of age and should always be suspected where there is a sudden onset of cyanosis and exercise intolerance in an animal of this age.

The turbulence associated with flow across the defect may produce secondary changes in the valves closely located to the defect, which may complicate the clinical picture. Cattle are prone to develop endocarditis in the region of the septal cusp of the right atrioventricular valve.

In horses, the medial cusp of the aortic valve is more commonly involved. Other complications are prolapse of the cusps into the septal defect due to lack of aortic root support with the development of signs of aortic insufficiency (39). Rupture of the valve may occur to produce a severe additional flow load on the left ventricle with rapid onset of acute left heart failure and death.

Ventricular septal defects may occur in association with other congenital cardiac or vascular defects and the clinical findings are varied (6, 38). Special examination of the heart by techniques outlined earlier in this section is generally required for the antemortem diagnosis of these complex defects.

There is no practical correction for ventricular septal defects in large animals, and meat animals in which it is detected should be sent for early slaughter. It should be emphasized that small defects can produce dramatic auscultatory findings, and unless signs of cardiac insufficiency are present care should be taken in giving an unfavorable prognosis in pleasure or breeding animals. Pleasure animals with this defect should never be ridden but it is possible for them to live a reasonable life span and to breed. There is insufficient information on the advisability of breeding animals which have this defect. An inheritable predisposition has been suspected in Hereford cattle (7), and chromosomal abnormalities have been demonstrated in association with this defect in cattle (15). Ventricular septal defects have high prevalence in calves and lambs with microphthalmia.

Tetralogy of Fallot

This is almost always a lethal defect in farm animals. The tetralogy consists of a ventricular septal defect, pulmonary stenosis, dextral position of the aorta so that it overrides both ventricles, and secondary right ventricular hypertrophy. The marked increase in resistance to outflow into the pulmonary artery results in a shunt of blood from the right to left with the major outflow of blood through the aorta. The condition presents with clinical signs very early in life, frequently results in death at or shortly following birth (6, 16–19) and has been reported predominantly in foals and calves. Affected animals show lassitude and dyspnea after minor exertion such as suckling. Cyanosis may or may not be present depending upon the degree of pulmonary stenosis, but is usually prominent, especially following exercise. On auscultation a murmur and sometimes a thrill is present and most intense in the left third or fourth intercostal space. Diagnosis can be confirmed by the detection of a pressure differential across the pulmonary valve, if the pulmonary artery can be entered, and the detection of a shunt by the dye dilution curve, blood gas analysis and angiocardiography (20).

Patent ductus arteriosus

This defect results from a failure of closure of the ductus arteriosus following birth and is probably the second most common defect in horses after ventricular septal defect. There is some controversy over the period of time involved in normal closure in large animals (21–23). Clinically, murmurs associated with a patent ductus arteriosus are frequently heard during the first day after birth in normal animals and may persist for periods up to 5 days. Physiological studies in foals (23) suggest that closure occurs before 24 hours after birth. Patent ductus arteriosus is not a common clinical cardiac defect in older animals. Clinically it produces a loud continuous murmur associated with the shunting of blood from the aorta to the pulmonary artery (24, 25). The intensity of the murmur waxes and wanes with each cycle due to the effects of normal pressure changes on blood flow, giving rise to the name of 'machinery murmur'. The systolic component of the murmur is very loud and usually audible over most of the cardiac auscultatory area, but the diastolic component is much softer and confined to the base of the heart. The pulse is large in amplitude but has a low diastolic pressure. Diagnosis is by the demonstration of an increase in the percentage oxygen saturation of the blood distal to the shunt, and by angiocardiography. Surgical correction is possible.

Coarctation of the aorta

Constriction of the aorta at the site of entrance of the ductus arteriosus causes a syndrome similar to that of stenosis of the aortic semilunar valves; there is a systolic murmur and a slow-rising pulse of small amplitude.

Persistence of the right aortic arch

Persistence of the right fourth aortic arch causes constriction of the esophagus with dysphagia and regurgitation. The aorta is situated to the right of the esophagus and trachea and the ligamentum arteriosum in its connection to the pulmonary artery encloses the esophagus in a vascular ring and compresses it against the trachea. Clinical signs are usually evident soon after birth and consist primarily of regurgitation of milk from the mouth and nostrils after suckling (26) but survival until 5 years of age has been recorded in a bull which showed chronic bloat and visible esophageal dilatation (27). Resistance to the passage of a stomach tube is encountered just behind the first rib and the diagnosis can be confirmed by radiological examination following a barium swallow. Medical treatment is concerned with the control of aspiration pneumonia but the correction of the defect is surgical.

Persistent truncus arteriosus

This defect (8, 28, 29) and other defects of the outflow vessels including pulmonary and aortic hypoplasia (29, 30) have been recorded in animals but their prevalence is low. Congenital absence of the aortic arch is recorded in two foals (34).

Fibroelastosis

Congenital fibroelastosis has been observed in calves and pigs. The endocardium is converted into a thick fibroelastic coat, and although the wall of the left ventricle is hypertrophied the capacity of the ventricle is reduced. The aortic valves may be thickened and irregular and obviously stenosed. A similar condition occurs in humans but the cause in all species is unknown. The syndrome is one of congestive heart failure but there are no signs which indicate the presence of specific lesions of the myocardium, endocardium or pericardium. The defect may cause no clinical abnormalily until the animal is mature.

Subvalvular aortic stenosis

Stenosis of the aorta at or just below the point of attachment of the aortic semilunar valves has been recorded as a common defect in pigs (31, 32) but its differentiation from other causes of heart failure is difficult. A heritable predisposition has been suggested (33). Clinically affected animals may die suddenly with asphyxia, dyspnea and foaming at the mouth and nostrils, or after a long period of ill-health with recurrent attacks of dyspnea. In the acute form death may occur after exercise or be unassociated with exertion.

Anomalous origin of coronary arteries

Either or both coronary arteries may originate from the pulmonary artery instead of the aorta. The resulting anoxia causes myocardial weakness in the ventricle of the affected side. Congestive heart failure usually follows. Congenital deformities of the coronary arteries have been recorded in cattle and pigs (33, 35).

REFERENCES

(1) Gopal, T. et al. (1986) *Am. J. vet. Res.*, *47* 1120.
(2) Hsu, F. S. & Du, S. J. (1982) *Vet. Pathol.*, *19*, 676.
(3) Rooney, J. R. & Franks, W. C. (1964) *Pathol. vet.*, *1*, 454.
(4) Dennis, S. M. &. Leipold, H. W. (1968) *Am. J. vet. Res.*, *29*, 2337.
(5) Bowen, J. M. & Adrian, R. W. (1962) *J. Am. vet. med. Assoc.*, *141*, 1162.
(6) Fisher, E. W. & Pirie, H. M. (1964) *Br. vet. J.*, *120*, 253.
(7) Lombard, C. W. et al. (1983) *J. Am. vet. med. Assoc.*, *183*, 562.
(8) Sandusky, G. E. & Smith, C. W. (1981) *Vet. Rec.*, *108*, 163.
(9) Blood, D. C. (1960) *Can. vet. J.*, *1*, 104.
(10) Muylle, E. et al. (1974) *Equ. vet. J.*, 6, 174.
(11) Lombard, C. W. et al. (1983) *J. Am. vet. med. Assoc.*, *183*, 562
(12) Blood, D. C. & Steel, J. D. (1946) *Aust. vet. J.*, *22*, 22.
(13) Fisher, E. W. et al. (1962) *Vet. Rec.*, *74*, 447.
(14) Machida, N. (1986) *Jap. J. vet. Sci.*, *48*, 1031.
(15) Tschudi, P. (1975) *Schweiz. Arch. Tierheilkd.*, *117*, 335.
(16) Dear, M. G. & Price, E. K. (1970) *Vet. Rec.*, *86*, 219.
(17) Kieth, J. C. (1981) *Vet. Med. small. Anim. Clin.*, *76*, 889.
(18) Oshima, K. & Muira, S. (1972) *Jap. J. vet. Sci.*, *34*, 333.
(19) Greene, H. J. et al. (1975) *Irish vet. J.*, *29*, 115.
(20) Prickette, M. E. et al. (1973) *J. Am. vet. med. Assoc.*, *162*, 552.
(21) Amoroso, E. C. et al. (1958) *Br. Heart J.*, *20*, 92.
(22) Rossdale, P. D. (1967) *Br. vet. J.*, *123*, 521.
(23) Scott, E. A. et al. (1975) *Am. J. vet. Res.*, *36*, 1021.
(24) Buergelt, C. D. et al. (1970) *J. Am. vet. med. Assoc.*, *157*, 313.
(25) Carmicheal, J. A. et al. (1971) *J. Am. vet. med. Assoc.*, *158*, 767.
(26) Bartels, J. E. & Vaughan, J. T. (1969) *J. Am. vet. med. Assoc.*, *154*, 406.
(27) Roberts, S. J. et al. (1953) *Cornell Vet.*, *43*, 537.
(28) Rang, H. & Hurtienne, H. (1976) *Tierärztl. Praxis*, *4*, 55.
(29) Linde-Sipman, J. S. & Wensing, C. J. G. (1972) *Vet. Med.*, *19A*, 15.
(30) Vitums, A. et al. (1973) *Cornell Vet.*, *63*, 41.
(31) Van Nie, C. J. & Vincent, J. (1980) *Vet. Q.*, 2, 160.
(32) Hofmann, W. (1974) *Zentralbl. VetMed.*, *21A*, 417.
(33) Baker, J. R. (1976) *Vet. Rec.*, *98*, 485.
(34) Scott, E. A. et al. (1978) *J. Am. vet. med. Assoc.*, *172*, 347.
(35) Dennis, S. M. & Gardiner, M. R. (1972) *Vet. Rec.*, *90*, 10.
(36) Bayly, W. M. et al. (1982) *J. Am. vet. med. Assoc.*, *181*, 684.
(37) McQuirk, S. M. et al. (1984) *J. Am. vet. med. Assoc.*, *184*, 1141.
(38) Wilson, R. B. & Hoffner, J. C. (1987) *Cornell Vet.*, *77*, 187.
(39) Reef, V. B. & Spencer, P. (1987) *Am. J. vet. Res.*, *48*, 904.

Cardiac neoplasia

Primary neoplasia of the heart is exceedingly rare and cardiac disease secondary to metastatic neoplasms occurs infrequently. Aortic body adenoma and pericardial mesothelioma are reported (1, 2). Lymphosarcoma is probably the most common metastatic tumor in both cattle and horses but cardiac involvement by melanoma, hemangiosarcoma, testicular embryonal carcinoma, squamous cell carcinoma and other tumors is also recorded (3).

REFERENCES

(1) Carnine, B. L. et al. (1977) *Vet. Pathol.*, *14*, 513.
(2) Barros, C. S. L. & Santos, M. N. D. (1983) *Aust. vet. J.*, *60*, 61.
(3) Dill, S. G. et al. (1986) *Equ. vet. J.*, *18*, 414.

DISEASES OF THE BLOOD VESSELS

Arterial thrombosis and embolism

Arteritis leading to thrombus formation causes ischemia of the tissues supplied by the affected artery. Clinical signs of reduced function or ischemic necrosis vary with the site of the obstruction.

Etiology

Parasitic arteritis

- *Strongylus vulgaris*—horses. Migrating larvae cause arteritis of the anterior mesenteric artery, iliac arteries, base of aorta, and occasionally cerebral, renal, or coronary arteries. This is a major cause of arteritis and associated clinical disease in horses
- Onchocerciasis and eleophoriasis in cattle, sheep, goats, and horses.

Viral arteritis

- Important in pathogenesis of several viral diseases, including malignant catarrhal fever, equine viral arteritis, African swine fever, hog cholera, African horse sickness.

Bacterial arteritis

- Septicemic salmonellosis, erysipelas.

Embolic arteritis and thromboembolism

- From vegetative endocarditis or emboli from arterial thrombus in various sites
- Hyperlipemia and hyperlipidemia in horses
- Fat emboli following surgery
- Associated with subclinical *Salmonella dublin* infection in calves
- Rupture of abscesses into blood vessels—pulmonary embolism resulting from caudal vena caval thrombosis or jugular thrombosis.

Microangiopathy

- Vitamin E/selenium deficiency
- Cerebrospinal angiopathy
- Terminal in most septicemic disease (1).

Calcification

- Enzootic calcinosis
- Vitamin D toxicity.

Vasoconstrictive agents

- Ergot poisoning
- Fescue poisoning.

Pathogenesis

In parasitic arteritis, inflammation and thickening of the arterial wall result in the formation of thrombi which may partially or completely occlude the artery. The common site is in the anterior mesenteric artery, obstruction of the vessel causing recurrent colic or fatal ischemic necrosis of a segment of the intestine. Less common sites include the origin of the iliac artery at the abdominal aorta causing iliac thrombosis, the base of the aorta leading to rupture and hemopericardium, and the coronary arteries causing myocardial infarction. With other causes of arteritis, the clinical syndrome is dependent upon the site of arteritis or embolism. Arteritis associated with bacterial and viral infections is usually widespread and several organ systems are involved. Cerebrospinal angiopathy following subclinical edema disease produces a variety of neurological signs. Bacterial emboli have a predilection to lodge in vascular plexuses in the kidney to produce renal disease, the synovial membranes to produce arthritis and tenosynovitis, and in the endocardium to produce endocarditis. Less commonly, they may lodge in other vascular plexuses such as the rete cerebri. Vasoconstrictive alkaloids produced by *Claviceps purpurea* infestation of grass seed heads cause arteriolar constriction and result in ischemic necrosis and gangrene of distal extremities in cattle. The hindlimbs below the fetlocks and the tip of the tail are most commonly involved with the forelimbs and the tips of the ear being involved in some cases. A similar syndrome occurs associated with grazing of *Festuca arundinacea* and may be associated with a vasoconstrictive alkaloid in tall fescue (21) or ergopeptide alkaloids produced by infestations of fescue by the claviceptaceous fungus *Sphacelia typhena* (22). Frostbite produces a similar syndrome.

Sporadic cases of dry gangrene of the extremities are seen in calves which resemble the lesions seen in ergotism but in situations where contact with the fungus is not possible. The calves are usually chronically affected with diarrhea and infection with *Salmonella* sp. has been suggested as a cause of the gangrene (4). Periarteritis nodosa and embolic endarteritis cause a variety of syndromes depending on the localization of the lesions. Large emboli which lodge in the pulmonary arteries cause anoxic anoxia, and emboli arising from the pulmonary veins may lodge in any organ, particularly the brain and kidneys. Embolism in the renal artery causes acute cortical necrosis and gross hematuria. An aneurysm of the abdominal aorta which involved a ureter in a horse caused recurrent hemorrhage into the urinary tract (5).

Clinical findings

The clinical findings in mesenteric verminous arteritis of horses and renal and myocardial infarction, gangrene associated with *Claviceps purpurea* or tall fescue grass and other diseases listed above are described elsewhere under those headings. Arteritis may lead to arterial rupture and thromboembolism contributes to the clinical syndrome in a large number of diseases. Two of particular significance are described here.

Iliac thrombosis in the horse

Iliac thrombosis (6, 7) is reported most commonly in racehorses, but occurs in other breeds. It is primarily a disease of horses of over 3 years of age. Either one or both hindlegs may be involved. The clinical manifestations vary according to the stage of progression of the disease and are associated with ischemia of the hindlimbs. Early mild cases are usually detected in racehorses or horses subjected to maximal exertion where the disease may be a cause of poor performance. In early cases there is lameness only on exercise, the animal returning to normal after a short rest. If the horse is forced to work when lameness develops the signs may increase to resemble those of the acute form. The lameness takes the form of weakness, usually of one hindlimb which tends to give way especially when the animal turns on it. Frequent lifting of the foot or cow-kicking may also be shown. In more severe cases, lameness or refusal to work may be evident after minimal exercise. The disease is chronic and progressive, but occasionally the onset may be acute.

In the acute form there is great pain and anxiety and the pulse and respiration rates are markedly increased. Profuse sweating may be evident, but the affected limb is usually dry and may be cooler than the rest of the body. The pain is often sufficiently severe to cause the animal to go down and refuse to get up. Suspect animals should be examined following exercise. The affected limb is cool from the mid-gaskin distally and there is usually diminished or variable sweating over this area. The amplitude of the pulse in the common digital artery is less in the affected limb than in the normal limb or the front limbs and slow filling of the saphenous vein of the affected limb can usually be detected. Palpable abnormalities on rectal examination include enlargement and firmness of the aortic quadrifucation, irregularity and asymmetry of the internal and external iliac arteries and decreased amplitude or absence of an arterial pulse. Recovery by the development of collateral circulation or shrinkage of the thrombus is unlikely to occur and the disease is usually chronically progressive with a poor prognosis.

There is some controversy over the etiology of this disease. Current thought suggests that it results from strongyle-related thromboembolism with organization of thrombi and their incorporation into the arterial wall with centripetal development of progressive thrombosis. Alternatively spontaneous degenerative vascular disease of unknown etiology, but particularly at the aortic quadrifucation may result in thrombosis in the area and subsequently thromboembolism of more distal vessels (6). Until recently the detection and diagnosis of the occurrence of this abnormality has been limited to horses showing clinical signs and horses where abnormality could be palpated on rectal examination. Ultrasonography shows promise as a method for detection of iliac thrombosis and is more sensitive than rectal palpation (23). Its use as a diagnostic technique may lead to a better definition of the occurrence of this disease and ultimately its pathogenesis.

Iliac thrombosis may also be associated with impotence in stallions (7).

Pulmonary embolism

Severe dyspnea develops suddenly and is accompanied by profuse sweating and anxiety. The temperature and pulse rate are elevated but the lungs are normal on auscultation. In horses the signs usually pass off gradually in 12–24 hours but in cattle the anoxia may be more severe and cause persistent blindness and imbecility. Infected emboli may lead to more severe pulmonary embolic disease with arteritis and pulmonary abscessation. There is pulmonary hypertension, and cor pulmonale is a possible sequel. Pulmonary arteritis and aneurysm may be followed by rupture and pulmonary hemorrhage. The emboli usually arise from tricuspid valve endocarditis, caudal vena caval thrombosis or jugular vein phlebitis and thrombosis (3, 8). The general syndrome is described in greater detail under caudal vena caval thrombosis. That associated with endocarditis or jugular vein thrombosis has, in addition, specific clinical findings associated with these abnormalities.

Clinical pathology

Extensive thrombus formation is usually associated with a leukocytosis and a shift to the left and there is an increase in serum fibrinogen concentration. In the majority of cases of iliac thrombosis serum muscle enzyme concentrations are within the normal range both preexercise and postexercise (6), but in severe cases there may be enzymic evidence of myonecrosis with secondary hyperkalemia and uremia (9).

Necropsy findings

Obstruction of the affected artery is easily seen when it is opened. The thrombus or embolus is adherent to the intima and is usually laminated. Local or diffuse ischemia or infarction may be evident if the embolus has been present for some time and may have progressed to the point of abscess formation.

Diagnosis

Iliac thrombosis in its acute form may be confused with azoturia but the muscles of the thigh and rump are not hard, there is no myoglobinuria and usually no history of working after a period of rest on full rations. In the less acute form it resembles a number of non-specific lamenesses and enzootic incoordination of horses. The fact that it commonly affects only one limb may be of assistance in identifying the vascular lesion. In early mild cases, the primary differential is from other causes of poor performance and tying up. Pulmonary embolism may be confused with pneumonia but the onset is more sudden, and with acute emphysema, although this disease is accompanied by characteristic pulmonary signs.

Causes of arterial rupture other than verminous arteritis include a possibly inherited tendency to aneurysm of the abdominal aorta in cattle (10), and copper deficiency in pigs causing rupture of major blood vessels and the heart wall (11). Aneurysm of the aortic arch and bicarotid trunk is reported in the horse. The clinical manifestations were aortic valve insufficiency and severe heart failure (20).

Although clinical atherosclerosis occurs rarely in farm animals, it has been recorded in a horse in which sufficient vascular obstruction occurred to cause severe central nervous signs and a fatal outcome (12). Spontaneous atherosclerosis is a common necropsy finding in swine, cattle, goats, horses and wild animals but its relationship to disease has not been established (13–17). Arteriosclerosis and calcification are major findings in enzootic calcinosis and occur following overdosing with vitamin D or its analogs in the prevention of milk fever in cattle.

Treatment

Treatment with parenteral anticoagulants or enzymes is carried out only rarely. There are several records of good results in iliac thrombosis in horses after the intravenous injection of sodium gluconate or fibrinolytic enzymes (18, 19), and retrograde catheterization of the ventral coccygeal artery can allow the deposition of these materials at high local concentration. The use of antibiotics has merit if a bacterial arteritis or endocarditis is suspected.

REFERENCES

(1) Schulz, L. C. et al. (1971) *Dtsch Tierärztl. Wochenschr.*, *78*, 563.
(2) Baker, J. R. & Ellis, C. E. (1981) *Equ. vet. J.*, *13*, 43 & 47.
(3) Rebhun, W. C. (1980) *J. Am. vet. med. Assoc.*, *176*, 1366.
(4) Mouwen, J. M. V. M. (1967) *Tijdschr. Diergeneeskd.*, *92*, 1282.
(5) Nolan, V. J. & Henigan, M. J. (1964) *Vet. Rec.*, *76*, 298.
(6) Maxie, M. G. & Physick-Sheard, P. W. (1985) *Vet. Pathol.*, *2*, 238.
(7) Azzie, M. A. J. (1972) *Proc. 18th ann. Conv. Am. Assoc. equ. Practnrs*, 43.
(8) Breeze, R. G. et al. (1976) *Vet. Ann.*, *16*, 52.
(9) Mayhew, I. G. & Kryger, M. D. (1975) *Vet. Med.*, *70*, 1281.
(10) Schuiringa-Sybesma, A. M. (1961) *Tijdschr. Diergeneeskd.*, *86*, 1192.
(11) Anonymous (1962) *NZ J. Agric.*, *105*, 261.
(12) Rothenbacher, H. J. & Tufts, S. (1964) *J. Am. vet. med. Assoc.*, *145*, 132.
(13) Skold, B. et al. (1966) *Am. J. vet. Res.*, *27*, 257.
(14) French, J. E. et al. (1965) *Ann. NY Acad. Sci.*, *127*, 780.
(15) McKinney, B. (1962) *Lancet*, *2*, 281.
(16) Prasad, M. C. et al. (1973) *Exp. mol. Pathol.*, *19*, 328.
(17) Pauli, B. (1973) *Schweiz. Arch. Tierheilkd.*, *115*, 517.
(18) Moffett, F. S. & Vaden, P. (1978) *Vet. Med.*, *73*, 184.
(19) Branscomb, B. L. (1968) *J. Am. vet. med. Assoc.*, *152*, 1643.
(20) Derksen, F. J. et al. (1981) *J. Am. vet. med. Assoc.*, *179*, 692.
(21) Davis, C. B. (1983) *Vet. hum. Toxicol.*, *25*, 408.
(22) Lyons, P. C. et al. (1986) *Science*, *232*, 487.
(23) Reef, V. B. et al. (1987) *J. Am. vet. med. Assoc.*, *190*, 286.

Venous thrombosis

The development of thrombi in veins may result in local obstruction to venous drainage or in liberation of emboli which lodge in the lungs, liver or other organs.

Phlebitis is the common origin of thrombi and may be caused by localization of a blood-borne infection, by extension of infection from surrounding diseased tissues, by infection of the umbilical veins in the newborn, and by irritant injections into the major veins. Especially troublesome in equine medicine is the obstruction of the jugular vein which results from prolonged (3–4 days) venous catheterization in some animals. The cause is not explained, but irritation to the vascular endothelium by the catheter seems likely. Intravenous injections of irritating materials, such as tetracycline, phenylbutazone or solutions of calcium chloride, may also cause endothelial damage followed by cicatricial contraction, with or without thrombus formation. Jugular phlebitis with thrombosis is not uncommon in feedlot cattle that have received repeated intravenous antibiotic medication and may lead to thromboembolic respiratory disease.

Phenylbutazone is commonly used as a non-steroidal anti-inflammatory drug (NSAID). Its use in horses may be associated with toxicity, which is manifest with oral and gastrointestinal ulceration and renal medullary crest necrosis (4–6). Affected horses show depression, anorexia, and neutropenia with ulcers in the mouth, especially on the ventral aspect of the tongue. Ulcers in the fundic and pyloric portion of the stomach also develop, but are usually subclinical although they may be evident on gastroscopic examination or at postmortem. More severe cases show signs of colic and diarrhea in association with intestinal ulceration and duodenitis and show evidence of renal disease. Toxicity may develop following either intravenous or oral administration of the drug. Intravenous administration is frequently associated with the development of phlebitis and jugular thrombosis at the site of injection. Phlebitis may also develop at sites of venepuncture performed for purposes other than phenylbutazone administration. Experimental studies (5) suggest that a phlebopathy induced by phenylbutazone is central to the development of all of these lesions including the oral and gastrointestinal ulceration and the renal crest necrosis. The exact pathogenesis of the vein damage in phenylbutazone toxicity has not been elucidated, but experimentally toxicity can be prevented by the concurrent administration of prostagladin E_2 (6). Clinical pathological examination for leukopenia and a fall in serum aspartate aminotransferase may be of value as a monitoring technique for the development of toxicity during phenylbutazone therapy of disease.

Accidental injection of irritating materials around the vein usually cause a marked local swelling, sometimes with necrosis and local sloughing of tissue which may be followed by cicatricial contraction of local tissues. Venous thrombi are relatively common in strangles in the horse, and may affect the jugular veins or the caudal vena cava. Thrombosis of the caudal vena cava due to hepatic abscessation and resulting in embolic pneumonia and pulmonary arterial lesions occurs in cows and is described together with cranial vena caval thrombosis in Chapter 10 on diseases of the respiratory tract.

Less common examples of venous thrombosis are those occurring in the cerebral sinuses either by drainage of an infection from the face or those caused by the migration of parasite larvae. Purpling and later sloughing of the ears which occur in many septicemias in pigs are also caused by phlebitis and venous thrombosis.

Engorgement of the vein, pain on palpation and local edema are the important signs. In unsupported tissues rupture may occur and lead to fatal internal or external hemorrhage. There are no typical findings on clinicopathological examination and at necropsy the obstructed vessel and thrombus are usually easily located by the situation of the edema and local hemorrhage.

The diagnosis depends on the presence of signs of local venous obstruction in the absence of obvious external pressure by tumor, enlarged lymph nodes, hematomas or fibrous tissue constriction. Angiography can assist in diagnosis (2). Pressure of a fetus may cause edema of the perineum, udder and ventral abdominal wall during late pregnancy. Local edema due to infective processes such as blackleg, malignant edema and peracute staphylococcal mastitis are accompanied by fever, severe toxemia, acute local inflammation and necrosis.

Parenteral treatment with antibacterial drugs and surgical measures, such as hot fomentations to external veins, are usually instituted to remove the obstruction or allay the swelling. Persistent bleeding from the vulva in association with ulcerated varicose veins on the dorsal wall of the vagina is also recorded in horses (3). Resection or ligation of the affected veins was curative.

Congenital venous aneurysm is rare but has been recorded in the horse (1).

REFERENCES

(1) Hilbert, B. J. & Rendano, V . T. (1975) *J. Am. vet. med. Assoc.*, *167*, 394.
(2) Scott, E. A. et al. (1978) *J. equ. Surg.*, *2*, 270.
(3) White, R. A. S. et al. (1984) *Vet. Rec.*, *115*, 263.
(4) Tobin, T. et al. (1986) *J. vet. Pharmacol. Therap.*, 9, 1.
(5) Meschter, C. L. et al. (1984) *Cornell Vet.*, *74*, 282.
(6) Collins, L. G & Tyler, D. E. (1985) *Am. J. vet. Res.*, *46*, 1605.

Hemorrhagic disease

Petechial and ecchymotic hemorrhage, spontaneous hemorrhage or excessive bleeding after minor injury may result from increased capillary fragility or from defects in the coagulation mechanism of the blood. The latter would be more properly considered in the next chapter but for convenience it is dealt with here.

Examples of diseases with hemorrhagic tendencies include the following.

Vasculitis

- *Septicemic and viremic diseases*. The vasculitis is associated with endothelial damage from the direct inflammatory or degenerative effects of the infection. It may be complicated by defects in blood coagulation and platelet disorders depending upon the infection (1, 16). In many instances coagulation defects are a manifestation of early disseminated intravascular coagulation. Clinically, petechial and ecchymotic hemorrhages associated with septicemia are most obvious in the mucous membrane of the mouth, vulva and conjunctiva or in the sclera but they are widely distributed throughout the body on postmortem examination
- *Purpura hemorrhagica* is a hemorrhagic disease of horses associated with a leukocyclastic vasculitis. The majority of cases occur as a sequel to strangles. Cases also occur following immunization against *Streptococcus equi* and as a sequel to infection with other streptococci. The disease appears to be an immune complex-mediated disease with deposition of IgA containing immune complexes on vessel walls (17, 18). Hemorrhagic tendencies in the disease include petechial and ecchymotic hemorrhages but also may result in large extravasations of blood and serum into tissues. The hemorrhage and exudation of serum may result in anemia and a depression in the circulating blood volume. Hemorrhage associated with purpura is usually treated with blood transfusions and corticosteroids. A fuller description of the syndrome is given elsewhere
- *Necrotizing vasculitis* of unknown etiology, but possibly immune mediated, occurs in all species (19, 20). The syndrome is similar to purpura and may be local or generalized with petechial hemorrhage and serosanguineous exudation subcutaneously and into tissue spaces. Hemorrhagic tendencies associated with vasculitis may be confused with those associated with a defect in the clotting mechanism as the primary cause. Differentiation depends on accurate laboratory examination. Treatment other than that of the primary condition is largely empirical. Antihistamines are used when allergy appears to be an important mechanism but response is poor when the extravasations have already occurred. Corticosteroids are also of value in immunologically mediated hemorrhagic disease. Adrenalin applied locally on a pad may be of assistance when bleeding occurs from the nostrils. Agents which enhance coagulability of the blood are extensively used when the clotting mechanism is at fault but effect little response when endothelial damage has occurred.

Coagulation defects

- Prothrombin deficiency resulting from coumarol poisoning following ingestion of coumarol-containing plants such as *Melilotus alba*, *Anthoxanthum odoratum*, *Apium nodiflorum*, *Ferula communis* (7, 21) or warfarin and related compounds
- *Factor VIII deficiency*. Factor VIII is a glycoprotein complex composed of two distinct polypeptide components VIII:C and VIII:vWF. Factor VIII participates in coagulation and is involved in adhesion of platelets to damaged surfaces. Lack of synthesis of the whole or part of the complex results in a bleeding diathesis. In hemophilia the activities of both the VIII:C and VIII:vWF components are reduced, whereas in von Willebrand's disease VIII:vWF is reduced. Hemophilia is recorded in thoroughbreds (2, 3), standardbreds (4), and Arab (5) colt foals associated with a deficiency in factor VIII (2, 4) and factors VIII, IX and XI (5). Clinically affected foals show signs of a hemorrhagic tendency within a few weeks of birth with the development of hematomas, persistent nasal bleeding, bleeding from injection sites, and sudden death from massive internal hemorrhage. Affected foals are anemic. Two variations of von Willebrand's disease are recorded in pigs (11, 24)—both inherited as simple autosomal recessive traits. Suspect factor VIII deficiency has also been reported in Hereford calves (25). The prime manifestation was mortality shortly following castration with bleeding from the surgical site, intra-abdominal hemorrhage and severe anemia
- *Other factor deficiencies*. Factor XI deficiency is recorded in Holstein-Friesian cattle and is transmitted as an autosomal recessive gene. Affected cattle show prolonged or repeated bleeding episodes after trauma such as dehorning and hemorrhage and thrombosis following venepuncture. There are occasional deaths associated with multiple hemorrhages. Heterozygote carriers have decreased factor XI coagulant activity (26). Prekallikrein deficiency is recorded in a family of miniature horses (27). The condition is not associated with clinical disease but blood samples fail to clot
- *Snake venoms* may have procoagulant or anticoagulant action (22). In both cases coagulation

defects may occur as procoagulant toxins and result in the activation, consumption and depletion of prothrombin and fibrinogen leading to a coagulopathy and prolonged clotting times

- Carcass hemorrhage or blood splash in slaughter lambs has been associated with extended prothrombin times caused by prior grazing of coumarin producing plants (7). The method of electrical stunning at slaughter can also result in carcass hemorrhage (23)
- *Parafilaria bovicola* produces large extravasations of blood under the skin of cattle and to some extent in tissue spaces (28). Bleeding from the skin may be the presenting sign of infestation
- A hemorrhagic syndrome in postweaned early grower pigs is recorded from the United States, New Zealand, France, Japan and South Africa (29, 30). The syndrome occurs as an outbreak with anemia, hemarthrosis, spontaneous hemorrhage under the skin of the legs and body and hemorrhage following management procedures such as castration. There is a high case fatality. There is prolongation of the prothrombin time and activated partial thromboplastin time. The outbreaks resolve promptly following the injection of vitamin K or its inclusion in the diet. The disease is believed to be due to vitamin K deficiency possibly resulting from decreased synthesis in the gut as a result of antibiotics in the feed or due to some unidentified antagonist
- A number of *fungal toxins* can cause hemorrhagic disease when ingested (12). Aflatoxins produced by *Aspergillus* spp. do so in association with increased prothrombin time in cattle, swine and horses. Trichothecene toxins produced by fungal infestations of feed by *Fusarium* spp., *Myrothecium* spp., *Cephalosporium* spp., and *Trichothecium* spp. also produce hemorrhagic disease as do toxins associated with *Penicillium rubrum* and the grass nematodes that infest *Lolium rigidum*.

Platelet disorders

- Thrombocytopenia may result from decreased production of platelets in the bone marrow or by increased consumption or destruction. These can be differentiated by examination of bone marrow
- *Thrombocytopenic purpura* is rarely diagnosed in farm animals but has been observed in newborn pigs due to maternal isoimmunization (6–8), and has been reproduced experimentally (9). Piglets are normal at birth but become thrombocytopenic after suckling colostrum containing antiplatelet antibody. Clinical signs do not develop until after the fourth day of life. There is a heavy mortality rate, death being preceded by a generalized development of submucosal and subcutaneous hemorrhages, drowsiness, weakness and pallor. There is no treatment. The sow should be culled
- *Idiopathic thrombocytopenia* is recorded in horses (13). Petechiation and hemorrhage may be confined to single systems, such as the respiratory system with epistaxis and hematomas in the nasal sinuses, or the genital tract producing a bloody vulval discharge, with no detectable abnormality at other mucous membranes. More generalized involvement with widespread petechiation of mucous membranes, epistaxis and melena has occurred within 2–3 weeks of routine deworming and vaccination (40). Dexamethasone is effective in controlling the syndrome
- *Megakaryocyte infection* such as occurs in hog cholera and African swine fever may result in thrombocytopenia and contributes to the hemorrhagic tendency seen in these diseases (31)
- *Granulocytopenia* with associated thrombocytopenia occurs with poisonings by *Pteridium* spp., *Cheilanthes seiberi* or the fungus *Stachybotrys* spp. in cattle, chronic furazolidone poisoning in calves, poisoning caused by trichloroethylene extracted soybean meal and radiation injury. The syndrome is predominantly one of spontaneous hemorrhage but is complicated by bacteremia and fulminant infections facilitated by the severe leukopenia. A granulocytopenic syndrome of unknown origin, occurring in all ages of cattle and manifest with a severe hemorrhagic diathesis, high morbidity and high case fatality, has been reported on various occasions in Australia (32)
- *Drug-induced platelet disorders* occur, such as the prolonged bleeding time produced by the antiplatelet activity of acetylsalicylic acid in horses (33)
- *Thrombocytopenia* of autoimmune origin has been observed with lymphosarcoma (39)
- *Navel bleeding or umbilical hemorrhage* is a syndrome of unknown etiology in newborn piglets. Following birth and for periods up to 2 days afterwards blood drips or oozes from the umbilicus of affected pigs to produce severe anemia with death frequently occurring from crushing. A variable number of piglets within the litter may be affected and the syndrome may have high incidence on certain problem farms. The addition of vitamin K and folic acid to the sows' ration may be followed by a drop in incidence but controlled trials with menadione have shown no effect (10). Dosing pregnant sows with vitamin C has been found to be effective (14). The defect appears to be one of immaturity of collagen so that a proper platelet clot does not form. The navel cords are abnormally large and fleshy and fail to shrink after birth. Ear-notching for identification is also followed by excessive bleeding. To be completely effective vitamin C must be given for at least 6 days before farrowing. Shorter periods of supplementation reduce the severity of bleeding, but do not completely prevent it. Ascorbic acid is given at the rate of 1 g daily. Pigs from treated sows are significantly heavier at 3 weeks of age than control pigs
- *Non-thrombocytopenic purpuras* which are not due to vascular lesions may theoretically be due to faulty platelet function (thrombopathia and thrombasthenia) or other faults in the coagulation mechanism. An example is the bleeding tendency present in the Chediak–Higashi syndrome in cattle. A prolonged bleeding time is demonstrable despite the presence of normal soluble coagulation factors and platelet

numbers, and is due to a defect in platelet aggregation associated with a platelet storage abnormality.

The treatment of coagulation defects can only be effected rationally if the missing factor can be defined.

Disseminated intravascular coagulopathy (DIC)

A hemorrhagic diathesis may develop in a number of diseases which, in themselves, are not diseases that primarily affect hemostatic mechanisms. This syndrome is called disseminated intravascular coagulopathy (DIC) or consumption coagulopathy, and it complicates a variety of primary disorders. It is characterized by an augmentation of normal clotting mechanisms which result in depletion of coagulation factors, deposition of fibrin clots in the microvasculature, and the secondary activation of fibrinolytic mechanisms. The augmentation of clotting mechanisms can result in a depletion of platelets and factors V, VIII and XIII, and the depletion of fibrinogen in association with the formation of fibrin clots in the microvasculature. These fibrin clots decrease tissue perfusion which may lead to further activation and depletion of clotting factors by the release of tissue thromboplastin as a result of tissue hypoxia. The bleeding tendency occasioned by the depletion of these clotting factors is further accentuated by the secondary activation of the thrombolytic system with the production of fibrin degradatory products which have anticoagulant properties.

Disseminated intravascular coagulation can be initiated by a variety of different mechanisms. Extensive tissue necrosis such as occurs in trauma, rapidly growing neoplasms, acute intravascular hemolysis and infective diseases such as blackleg, can cause extensive release of tissue thromboplastin and initiate exuberant coagulation via the extrinsic coagulation pathway. Exuberant activation of the intrinsic pathway can occur when there is activation of the Hageman factor by extensive contact with vascular collagen, as occurs in disease with vasculitis, or those associated with poor tissue perfusion and tissue hypoxia with resultant endothelial damage. Factors that initiate platelet aggregation such as endotoxin, that cause reticuloendothelial blockage such as excessive iron administration to piglets, or that cause hepatic damage to interfere with clearance of activated clotting factors, can contribute to the occurrence of disseminated intravascular coagulation. Clinically the syndrome has been recorded as occurring in diseases as diverse as those associated with acute sepsis, neoplasia, endotoxemia, enteropathies and parasitism (34–36). Hemorrhage, thrombosis and multiorgan failure are consequences of clotting factor depletion and microcirculation occlusion.

Clinically overt disseminated intravascular coagulation is manifested by local or generalized bleeding tendencies varying from the occurrence of petechial hemorrhages in mucous membranes to life-threatening hemorrhage. Subclinical disseminated intravascular coagulation may only be detected by the presence of altered hematological indices. There is little doubt that disseminated intravascular coagulation contributes to the clinical manifestations, especially the terminal clinical manifestations, of many diseases of large animal species. It is also possible that it mediates some local diseases such as laminitis in horses. The importance of DIC in veterinary medicine is the subject of current clinical investigation. Certainly this syndrome should be suspected when there is an untoward bleeding tendency in any clinical situation.

The detection of the presence of a consumptive coagulopathy depends heavily on laboratory examination of blood. Early detection in the hypercoagulable state can allow early corrective therapy. Unfortunately, DIC is usually diagnosed when the syndrome has progressed to the hemorrhagic state at which stage the prognosis is generally poor. Early detection requires monitoring for its development in cases of high risk. In view of the fact that there are a number of mechanisms whereby the coagulation system can be activated, one must expect differences in hemostatic profiles with different initiating mechanisms and no single laboratory test is definitive. The occurrence of disseminated intravascular coagulation can be suspected where there is a combination of the following: red blood cell distortion and fragmentation (produced by damage of red blood cells during passage through microvascular thrombi), a decrease in fibrinogen concentration relative to initial values during the disease process—hypofibrinogenemia may not be a good indicator of impending or current DIC in horses (38), abnormality in the prothrombin time (extrinsic system) or the activated partial thromboplastin time, the presence of fibrin degradation products and the demonstration of thrombocytopenia. The findings in these tests will also vary according to the severity and fulminant nature of the process and the time of sampling. Preferably repeated monitoring and assessment should be used. A reduction in antithrombin III concentration has been shown to be one of the more reliable indicators of DIC in the horse (38).

Disseminated intravascular coagulation is invariably secondary to an initiating primary disease. The most vigorous therapy should consequently be directed towards correction of the primary initiating disease. In human medicine, heparin therapy is used to reduce blood coagulation, and streptokinase and urokinase are used to help resolve clots, but their use in large animal medicine has been too limited to allow recommendations. Massive doses of corticosteroids may aid in reestablishing tissue perfusion, and where the primary aggregation of platelets is involved in the initiation of disseminated intravascular coagulation, such as occurs with endotoxin-induced endothelial damage or immune complex disease, corticosteroids or the antiplatelet agents such as aspirin (15) may be of value. Fresh plasma transfusion replacement of coagulant factors is also used in therapy and the decision for replacement may be aided by specific laboratory monitoring (37, 38). Component therapy to combat depletion of specific coagulation factors is also used in man, but currently in large animal medicine is not possible other than by whole blood transfusion.

REVIEW LITERATURE

Mason, R. G. (1978) Normal and abnormal hemostasis—an integrated view. *Am. J. Pathol.*, 92, 775–811.

McFarlane, R. G. et al. (1977) Haemostasis. *Br. med. Bull.*, *33*, 183 (16 papers).

Moore, D. J. (1979) Disseminated intravascular coagulation: a review of its pathogenesis, manifestations and treatment. *J.S. Afr. vet. Assoc.*, *50*, 259–264.

REFERENCES

(1) Tsai, K. & Karstad, L. (1973) *Am. J. Pathol.*, *70*, 379.
(2) Archer, R. K. & Allen, B. V. (1972) *Vet. Rec.*, *91*, 655.
(3) Sanger, V. L. et al. (1964) *J. Am. vet. med. Assoc.*, *144*, 259.
(4) Hutchins, D. R. et al. (1967) *Aust. vet. J.*, *43*, 83.
(5) Hinton, M. et al. (1977) *Equ. vet. J.*, *9*, 1.
(6) Hani, H. (1976) *Schweiz. Arch. Tierheilkd.*, *118*, 347.
(7) Restall, D. J. (1980) *Meat Sci.*, *5*, 125.
(8) Andersen, S. & Nielsen, R. (1973) *Nord. VetMed.*, *25*, 211.
(9) Linklater, K. A. (1975) *Res. vet. Sci.*, *18*, 127.
(10) Simensen, M. G. et al. (1973) *Medlemsbl. danske Dyrlaegeforen.*, *56*, 1049.
(11) Bowie, E. J. W. (1973) *Am. J. vet. Res.*, *34*, 1045.
(12) Schimoda, W. (1980) *Conference on Mycotoxins in Animal Feeds and Grains Related to Animal Health.* FDA, Nat. Tech. Info. Serv., USA.
(13) Valdez, H. & Peyton, L. C. (1978) *J. equ. med. Surg.*, *2*, 379.
(14) Sandholm, M. et al. (1979) *Vet. Rec.*, *104*, 337.
(15) Judson, D. G. & Barton, M. (1981) *Res. vet. Sci.*, *30*, 241.
(16) Edwards, J. F., et al. (1985) *Vet. Pathol.*, *22*, 171.
(17) Roberts, M. C. & Kelley, W. R. (1982) *Vet. Rec.*, *110*, 144.
(18) Galan, J. E. & Timoney, J. F. (1985) *J. Immunol.*, *13*, 3134.
(19) Easley, J. R. (1979) *J. Am. anim. Hosp. Assoc.*, *15*, 207.
(20) Werner, L. L. et al. (1984) *J. Am. vet. med. Assoc.*, *185*, 87.
(21) Schlosberg, A. & Egyed, M. N. (1986) *Res. vet. Sci.*, *40*, 141.
(22) Crawford, A. M. & Mills, J. N. (1985) *Aust. vet. J.* , *62*, 185.
(23) Devine, C. E. et al. (1983) *Meat Sci.*, *9*, 247.
(24) Thiele, G. L. et al. (1986) *J. Hered.*, *77*, 179.
(25) Healy, P. J. et al. (1984) *Aust. vet. J.*, *61*, 132.
(26) Gentry, P. A. (1984) *Can. J. comp. Med.*, *48*, 58.
(27) Turrentine, M. A. et al. (1986) *Am. J. vet. Res.*, *47*, 2464.
(28) Lundquist, H. (1983) *Nord. VetMed.*, *35*, 57.
(29) Sasaki, Y., et al. (1985) *Jap. J. vet. Sci.*, *47*, 435.
(30) Nuwsholme, S. J. et al. (1985) *J. S. Afr. vet. Assoc.*, *56*, 101.
(31) Edwards, J. F. et al. (1985) *Vet. Pathol.*, *22*, 171.
(32) Nicholls, T. J. et al. (1985) *Aust. vet. J.*, *62*, 67.
(33) Kopp, K. J. et al. (1985) *Equ. vet. J.*, *17*, 322.
(34) Morris, D. D. & Beech, J. (1983) *J. Am. vet. med. Assoc.*, *183*, 1067.
(35) Duncan, S. G., et al. (1985) *Am. J. vet. Res.*, *46*, 1287.
(36) Johnstone, I. B. & Crane, S. (1986) *Am. J. vet. Res. 47*, 356.
(37) Bernard, W. et al. (1987) *Am. J. vet. Res.*, *48*, 866.
(38) Johnstone, I. B. et al. (1986) *Equ. vet. J.*, *18*, 337.
(39) Reef, V. B. et al. (1984) *J. Am. vet. med. Assoc.*, *184*, 313.
(40) Larson, V. L. et al. (1983) *J. Am. vet. med. Assoc.*, *183* 328.

Hemangiosarcoma

Vascular neoplasms

Hemangioma and hemangiosarcoma are of rare occurrence in large animals, but are described and may be associated with hemorrhage related to the site of the tumor (2, 3). Hemangiomas in the skin occur most commonly in young animals and may be congenital (3, 4). The tumors grow with age; those on the skin may ulcerate and bleed and may necessitate euthanasia due to their eventual size. Similar tumors may occur in the mouth as pedunculated pink granular masses that ulcerate and bleed. Local hemangiomas on the skin and in the mouth may respond to surgical excision, thermocautery, or radiation therapy. Widespread disseminated hemangioma is also recorded with multiorgan involvement (6). Hemangioma has also been reported with moderate prevalence affecting the ovaries of sows (5). Hemangiosarcoma is more prevalent in middle-aged and older animals.

Disseminated hemangiosarcomas in horses cause anemia due to hemorrhage into the tumor or into body cavities. In the pleural cavity they may produce sufficient hemorrhage to cause respiratory embarrassment and a clinical picture which in general resembles pleurisy without the toxemia. In addition to the severe hemorrhagic anemia there is weight loss, but good appetite, and weakness. Metastasis is extensive to lung, myocardium, brain, retroperitoneum and skeletal muscle (1). The primary site is usually the spleen. Lesions in skeletal muscle cause difficulties in movement. Hemoperitoneum, detectable by paracentesis, is present with peritoneal tumors. All of the tumors are cavitatious and bleed profusely if incised.

REFERENCES

(1) Waugh, S. L. et al. (1977) *J. equ. med. Surg.*, *1*, 311.
(2) Green, H. J. & O'Connor, J. P. (1986) *Vet. Rec.*, *118*, 445.
(3) Hargis, A. M. & McElwain, T. F. (1984) *J. Am. vet. med. Assoc.*, *184*, 1121.
(4) Sartin, E. A. & Hodge, T. G. (1982) *Vet. Pathol.*, *19*, 569.
(5) Sheik-Omar, A. R. & Jaffar, M. (1985) *Vet. Rec.*, *117*, 110.
(6) Baker, J. C. et al. (1982) *J. Am. vet. med. Assoc.*, *181*, 172.

9

Diseases of the Blood and Blood-forming Organs

INTERFERENCE with the normal functions of the blood can occur in a number of ways. There may be a decrease in the circulating blood volume, abnormalities of the cellular constituents, and abnormalities of the non-cellular constituents including protein, electrolytes and the buffering systems. In all of these dysfunctions there is a failure of one or more of the transportation mechanisms of the blood and the tissues are deprived of their essential nutrients or are not relieved of their excretory products. Because of the multiplicity of the modes of dysfunction which can occur it is not possible to summarize the physiological basis and major manifestations of diseases of the blood and these aspects are dealt with in the discussion of the individual diseases. The common diseases of the system are dealt with individually below. Rarer diseases are polycythemia vera, which is an inherited disease of Jersey cattle, inappropriate secondary polycythemia (1) and inherited congenital methemoglobinemia in horses. Dyspnea is the prominent sign in both.

Diseases characterized by abnormalities of body fluids, electrolytes and acid–base balance are presented in Chapter 2.

REFERENCE

(1) Beech, J. et al. (1984) *J. Am. vet. med. Assoc.*, *184*, 986.

HEMORRHAGE

The rapid loss of whole blood from the vascular system causes peripheral circulatory failure and anemia.

Etiology

Spontaneous rupture or traumatic injury to large blood vessels are the common reasons for acute severe hemorrhage. Primary hemorrhagic disease occurs less commonly. Important causes include the following.

All species

- Thrombocytopenia, e.g. induced by drugs that cause bone-marrow suppression (13) or premature destruction of circulating platelets; a similar thrombocytopenia is caused by toxins, probably mycotoxins, in pasture plants (14).

Cattle

- Spontaneous pulmonary hemorrhage associated with the caudal vena caval syndrome
- Abomasal ulcer, sometimes originating from a bovine viral leukosis lesion
- Enzootic hematuria with bleeding from a bladder lesion
- Pyelonephritis with bleeding from a renal lesion
- Ruptured middle uterine artery during prolapse of uterus
- Any sort of minor surgical wound, e.g., castration, dehorning, when cattle are being fed moldy sweet clover hay
- Cardiac tamponade due to rupture of coronary artery or ventricular chamber, sometimes due to traumatic pericarditis
- Hemorrhagic diseases, the only significant one being moldy sweet clover poisoning; warfarin and bracken fern poisoning are rare causes
- Massive hookworm or *Haemonchus* sp. infestations, also *Fasciola hepatica*
- Heavy infestations with ticks and sucking lice are quoted as causes, but would have to be extremely heavy
- Coccidiosis in calves and yearlings.

Horses

- Nasal bleeding at rest usually as a result of a guttural pouch lesion; can also result from pulmonary abscess, but usually during vigorous exercise
- Pulmonary hemorrhage associated with pre-existing lesions of the lung
- Massive infestation with strongyles

- Traumatic injury by collision while running
- Hemophilia (5) or other clotting defect, e.g. idiopathic thrombocytopenia (11), disseminated intravascular coagulopathy (12).

Pigs

- Esophagogastric ulceration
- Congenital neonatal bleeding, e.g. umbilical hemorrhage.

Pathogenesis

The major effects of hemorrhage are loss of blood volume, loss of plasma protein and loss of erythrocytes. If the rate of blood loss is rapid the loss of circulating blood volume results in peripheral circulatory failure, and anemic anoxia results from the loss of erythrocytes. The combination of these two factors is often fatal. If the rate of blood loss is less rapid the normal compensatory mechanisms, including evacuation of blood stored in the spleen and liver and the withdrawal of fluid from the tissue spaces may maintain a sufficient circulating blood volume but the anemia is not relieved and the osmotic pressure of the blood is reduced by dilution of residual plasma protein. The resulting anemia and edema are repaired with time provided the blood loss is halted.

Clinical findings

Pallor of the mucosae is the outstanding sign but there is in addition, weakness, staggering and recumbency, a rapid heart rate and a subnormal temperature. The respirations are deep but not dyspneic. There is listlessness and dullness and in fatal cases the animal dies in a coma in lateral recumbency.

Clinical pathology

Examination of the blood for hemoglobin and hematocrit levels, and the erythrocyte count are of value in indicating the severity of the blood loss and provide an index to the progress of the disease. Estimation of clotting and prothrombin times should be undertaken in cases in which unexplained spontaneous hemorrhages occur.

Necropsy findings

Extreme pallor of all tissues and a thin watery appearance of the blood may be accompanied by large extravasations of blood if the hemorrhage has been internal. Where the hemorrhage has been chronic, anemia and edema are characteristic findings.

Diagnosis

Other forms of peripheral circulatory failure include shock and dehydration but they can usually be differentiated on history alone. Anemia due to other causes is not accompanied by signs of peripheral circulatory failure.

Treatment

All elements of the blood should be replaced and in severe cases blood transfusion is the most satisfactory treatment. In large animal practice donors are usually readily available and the need for storing blood does not arise.

Blood can be collected into an anticoagulant solution in an open-mouthed vessel. Venepuncture into the jugular vein is the method of choice, using a 12- or 14-gauge needle or a small diameter trocar and cannula. A choke-rope to increase the venous blood pressure facilitates collection in cattle. Bottles from which air has been evacuated reduce the collection time and avoid clotting in the needle, which usually occurs after about a liter has been collected by the open method. An excellent method is to use a milking machine to create a negative pressure in the flask which is fitted up so that the blood passes through the anticoagulant solution as it flows into the flask. In dairy cattle 4 liters of blood can be collected in 10–15 minutes by this method. Sodium citrate (10 ml of a 3.85% solution to each 100 ml of blood collected) is the standard anticoagulant used in cattle work. More sophisticated mixtures are used in horses (2). There is usually little risk to the donor if it is in good health, and 10–15 ml of blood per kg body weight can be drawn off at one time without danger. Special anticoagulants are available for special purposes.

Blood is usually administered intravenously but there are occasions when this is very difficult to do, especially in shocked or uncooperative animals, and intraperitoneal injections are then used. The only criticism of this method is that absorption is delayed. However, in dogs 48% of the cells are absorbed in 24 hours, 65% in 48 hours and 82% in 1 to 2 weeks (1), but the erythrocytes are taken up by the bloodstream in an unaltered state. From our own observations the absorption of erythrocytes from the bovine peritoneal cavity appears to be rapid and complete. The method has particular advantages for newborn calves and baby pigs with isoimmune hemolytic anemia. It is used extensively in human infants and is considered to be safe and effective. Its use is contraindicated when the animal is in a state of oligemic shock, when intravenous transfusion is obligatory. It is not recommended in cases with ascites, peritonitis, abdominal distension, peritoneal adhesions, recent abdominal surgery or abdominal distension due to any cause.

If the blood is properly mixed with anticoagulant during collection there is little need to filter it and the urgency in most cases precludes this. Clotted blood inevitably blocks the needle and the blood has to be discarded. Crossmatching of bloods to determine compatibility is not often practiced in animals other than the horse, although repeated transfusions from one donor may provoke anaphylactic shock. Even in horses an initial transfusion from any donor can be made without much risk except in the special case of isoimmunization hemolytic anemia. To avoid any possibility of producing an agglutination–hemolysis reaction a matching test should be carried out by mixing the serum of the recipient with the cells of the donor. Two drops of donor blood are mixed in 2 ml of a 3·85% citrate solution and 2 drops of the mixture are added to 2 drops of the recipient's serum on a glass slide, which is then gently rocked. Agglutination between incompatible samples is readily seen. A reasonably satisfactory alternative is to inject a small amount of blood (200 ml in an adult cow) and wait for 10 minutes. If no transfusion reaction occurs, the remainder of the blood can then be injected without risk. In an emergency, interspecies transfusion may be used but is limited in value because of the poor longevity of the transfused erythrocytes particularly when the horse is used as a donor. Transfusion reactions are unlikely except with horse blood transfused into other species (3). In cattle the incidence of transfusion reactions is greatest in young animals (14% incidence but sufficiently severe to require treatment in only 6%) and in pregnant cattle (41% incidence with a high proportion of cows aborting within 8 days). There is no individual blood group factor in cattle which is more important than others in transfusion reaction (4).

Anaphylactic reactions occur more commonly and are more severe when repeated transfusions from one donor are given more than a week after the initial transfusion (6). Sensitization to the blood of a particular donor may persist for more than a year. At the third transfusion almost 50% of cattle will show a moderate to severe reaction. Signs may appear while the transfusion is in progress or within a few minutes afterwards. Hiccough usually occurs first, followed by dyspnea, muscle tremor, salivation, frequent coughing, lacrimation, fever (40–40·5°C, 104–105°F) and in some cases ruminal tympany. Hemoglobinuria and abortion may also occur. The illness in cattle is often mild and responds within a few minutes to the administration of adrenaline hydrochloride (4–5 ml of 1:1000 solution injected intramuscularly or 0·2–0·5 ml intravenously in large animals). Intramuscular injection is safest and produces an effect within 3–4 minutes. Necropsy findings in animals dying of transfusion reaction are similar to those seen in acute anaphylaxis and include pulmonary edema and subserosal petechiation. Horses which develop a sensitivity at a first transfusion are likely to have a serious anaphylactic reaction to the second transfusion from the same donor (10). An increase in respiratory rate, anxious demeanor and restless treading commence soon after the start of administration, and by as little as 200 ml. Large doses of adrenalin, antihistamine or corticosteroid should be administered, preferably intravenously, but even then the horse may not survive.

A third reaction to transfusion, the pyrogenic reaction, occurs in man and in small animals but has not been recorded in farm animals. Administration of the blood at too rapid a rate may cause overloading of the circulation and acute heart failure. This is most likely to occur if blood is administered when there is myocardial asthenia due to toxemia. The heart rate increases rapidly and weakness and dyspnea precede collapse. A gallon (4·5 liters) of blood usually requires an hour to administer to a cow and comparable rates in the smaller species are advisable; 10–15 ml of blood per kg body weight is an average figure worth remembering but in severe cases it is probably better to continue transfusion until improvement is apparent. In the event of cardiac failure during transfusion the blood flow should be stopped immediately.

The most common causes of failure in treatment by blood transfusion are failure to administer sufficient blood, and the irreversible changes which may have occurred in the patient before treatment commences. The survival of red blood cells transfused from a donor cow into a recipient cow is limited (7). Following a first transfusion the red blood cells remained in the recipient's circulation for only up to 72 hours. The main sites of red blood cell destruction are the lung and spleen. Following a second transfusion at a later date the donor's cells circulate for less than an hour and sometimes for only a few minutes. Such rapid destruction of red blood cells might lead to the conclusion that blood transfusions in cattle may be of doubtful value unless given to correct an acute, anemic hypoxia. However, clinical experience suggests that blood transfusions are useful and perhaps the major beneficial effect is derived from the transfused plasma. In horses, survival of erythrocytes varies from 60 to 100% at 4 days to other horses in which the erythrocytes have all disappeared by 48 hours. At a second transfusion the survival time of erythrocytes is much shorter still. Erythrocyte compatibility tests are not good indicators of survival time of the cells (10).

Alternatives to blood transfusion include the infusion of blood plasma, or plasma extenders such as acacia (6% solution in 0·9% saline), gelatin (6% solution of special gelatin of known molecular size and capable of being retained in the circulation, in a solution of 0·85% saline) or dextran, a neutral polysaccharide. These preparations find little place in large animal work because of the ready availability of whole blood and the possible toxicity of dextran in the horse (8). Intravenous injections of those fluids used in the treatment of dehydration have some value in that they help to restore the circulating blood volume but the important deficit of hemoglobin is not made good. There are some advantages to the use of stored plasma because it can be frozen and stored for a long period (9).

Cardiac stimulants are of no value because the efficiency of the heart is unimpaired. Vasoconstrictor drugs should not be used as they tend to further aggravate the existing anoxia. Parenterally administered coagulants have found favor in recent years and many proprietary preparations are available. Their value is open to doubt but they are in general use because in most cases the situation is sufficiently serious to encourage the use of all available forms of treatment.

REFERENCES

(1) Clark, C. H. & Woodley, C. H. (1959) *Am. J. vet. Res.*, *20*, 1062.
(2) Schmotzer, W. B. et al. (1985) *Vet. Med.*, *80*, 89.
(3) Clark, C. H. & Kiesel, G. K. (1963) *J. Am. vet. med. Assoc.*, *143*, 400.
(4) Walt, K. V. D. & Osterhoff, D. R. (1969) *J. S. Afr. vet. med. Assoc.*, *40*, 107.
(5) Feldman, B. F. & Giacopuzzi, R. L. (1982) *Vet. Med.*, *4(10)*, 24.
(6) Lachmann, G. et al. (1973) *Arch. exp. VetMed.*, *27*, 871.
(7) McSherry, B. J. et al. (1966) *Can. vet. J.*, *7*, 271.
(8) Archer, R. K. & Franks, D. (1961) *Vet. Rec.*, *73*, 657.
(9) Eicker, S. W. & Ainsworth, D. M. (1984) *J. Am. vet. med. Assoc.*, *185*, 772.
(10) Kallfelz, F. A. et al. (1978) *Am. J. vet. Res.*, *39*, 617.
(11) Hammill, D. & Helton, M. (1981) *Mod. vet. Pract.*, *62*, 392.
(12) Morris, D. D. & Beech, J. (1983) *J. Am. vet. med. Assoc.*, *183*, 1067.
(13) Handagama, P. J. & Feldman, B. F. (1986) *Vet. Res. Commun.*, *10*, 1.
(14) Jeffers, M. & Lenghaus, C. (1986) *Aust. vet. J.*, *63*, 262.

SHOCK

Shock is defined as the state in which there is a generalized, acute, and serious reduction in the perfusion of tissues, and is characterized principally by a severe reduction in the effective circulating blood volume and a severe reduction in arterial blood pressure. The failure of the circulation to maintain the perfusion of tissues quickly leads to irreversible loss of tissue viability.

Etiology

Acute failure of tissue perfusion can occur because of a severe reduction in blood volume such as occurs in hypovolemic shock. It can also occur when the blood volume is normal or even high but where the effective circulating volume is markedly reduced. It is more effective to classify shock into pathogenic forms rather than etiological ones, as the basis of treatment then becomes more apparent.

Hypovolemic shock

The volume of circulating fluid is significantly reduced as in:

- Severe hemorrhage with loss of 35% or more of total blood volume
- Dehydration from severe diarrhea, intestinal obstruction, especially if fluid loss is severe and over a short period.

Distributive shock

This form includes the vascular abnormalities that were at one time referred to as vasogenic shock, although that term usually referred to peripheral dilatation in which a large bulk of the circulating fluid was pooled in one part of the vasculature, usually the splanchnic vessels. The term distribution includes not only low peripheral resistance forms but also high resistance vascular abnormalities, e.g. those caused by endotoxemia, in which circulating blood is directed away from particular tissues or organs. The extreme form of distributive shock is the obstructive distributive form — such as a massive pulmonary embolism.

Examples of causes of distributive shock are:

- After severe trauma or burn injury
- Following extensive surgery
- After prolapse of uterus
- Acute diffuse peritonitis after intestinal rupture
- Too sudden reduction of pressure in a body cavity, e.g. by rapid withdrawal of ascitic fluid. In acute gastric dilatation and high obstruction of the small intestine, fluid loss into the intestine may not appear to be very great. In these cases vasogenic and toxic shock also contribute heavily
- Severe pain as in colic in horses.

Toxic shock

The special class of this group is toxic or septic shock where large numbers of bacteria exert their effect via toxins, either endotoxins or exotoxins. Some examples are:

- Septicemia in which the vascular response depends on the nature of the toxin produced and the organism involved
- Absorption of toxin from the intestine, e.g. in enterotoxic colibacillosis of calves, grain engorgement in horses and cattle, infarction of a large segment of intestinal wall in horses
- Absorption of toxins of gram-negative bacteria, e.g. *Escherichia coli*, from the mammary gland in coliform mastitis, from abscesses, e.g. *Shigella*, *Pseudomonas* spp. In this case the form of distributive shock is likely to be high or normal peripheral resistance.

Cardiogenic shock

This occurs as a result of an acute reduction of cardiac output due either to myocardial asthenia with loss of muscular power, or cardiac arrhythmia with loss of coordinated contraction. Either of these abnormalities causes failure of perfusion to tissues generally. They represent a significant segment of occurrences of shock.

Pathogenesis

The salient feature with all forms of shock is a marked reduction in effective circulating blood volume with consequent lowered cardiac output, hypotension and impaired tissue perfusion. Compensatory mechanisms include the release of catecholamines which act to maintain perfusion through vital areas such as the heart and brain (1, 2) by reducing flow in other tissues through their action on terminal arterioles, precapillary sphincters and venules. This accentuates further the degree of tissue anoxia. Oxidative phosphorylation is blocked and anerobic glycolysis results in lactic acid production, acidemia and intracellular acidosis (3). Sustained arteriolar constriction leads eventually to the local accumulation of vasoactive substances and the precapillary sphincters relax in defiance of neural tone to result in capillary pooling of blood and further exacerbation of the circulating blood volume deficit. Hypoxia causes changes in the capillary endothelium to alter its permeability and eventually its viability (4).

In its early stages, shock can be reversed by transfusion of fluids and the restoration of an effective circulating blood volume. However, later in its course it may become irreversible. The irreversible lesion is the loss of cellular integrity in all tissues. The functions of cell membranes are lost and intracellular constituents, especially enzymes and potassium ions are released into the tissue fluids and the circulation. Because of the loss of tissue function and the loss of local defense mechanisms the barrier between intestinal contents and tissues is disrupted and toxins, and even bacteria, may gain entrance to the systemic circulation.

Clinical findings

Coldness of the skin, a subnormal temperature, rapid, shallow breathing, and a rapid heart rate accompanied by a weak pulse of small amplitude and low pressures are characteristic of shock. Venous blood pressure is greatly reduced and the veins are difficult to raise. The mucosae are pale but not to the severe degree of blanching observed in hemorrhage. Capillary refill time is extended beyond 3–4 seconds. The animal is dull, weak, often recumbent, and if the condition is fatal dies in a coma.

Clinical pathology

Measurement of the circulating blood volume is possible by the use of dyes or radioactive substances but the techniques are unlikely to be used in clinical practice. Hemoconcentration may or may not occur, depending on whether the fluid loss is in the form of plasma or whole blood, but measurement of the hematocrit may be of value in individual cases to determine the progress of the disease. Similar limitations apply with plasma protein analysis. Blood lactate concentrations are elevated and blood gas analysis shows a lowered pH in conjunction with a low $P\text{CO}_2$ (5). A high eosinophil count may suggest that adrenal cortical dysfunction has occurred and that treatment with adrenocorticotropic hormones or adrenal corticosteroids may be necessary.

Estimation of the arterial blood pressure is one of the best methods of measuring the severity of shock. In severe shock the systolic blood pressure will fall from a normal of approximately 120 mmHg (15·6 kPa) to below 60 mmHg (8·0 kPa) and this usually indicates a fatal outcome. A more accurate method of assessment is the insertion of a catheter into the right atrium and monitoring the central venous pressure (6). A marked decline from the normal of 12 ± 6 cmH_2O (120 ± 60 Pa) (measured at the sternal manubrium) is usually an indication of severe shock.

Necropsy findings

There may be evidence of trauma and the capillaries and small vessels of the splanchnic area may be congested.

Diagnosis

Shock is usually anticipated when severe trauma occurs, and is diagnosed when peripheral circulatory failure is present without evidence of hemorrhage or dehydration.

Treatment

There is some merit in trying to match treatment to the form of the shock to be treated, but there are still basic generalities that refer to all kinds of shock. The most important principle is to anticipate its occurrence and treat the animal prophylactically before a serious stage of shock is reached. The administration of intravenous fluids or a blood transfusion is now standard prophylaxis in potentially dangerous situations. Besides attempting to improve the mechanisms for carrying oxygen and metabolites to and from tissues it is also imperative to ensure an adequate supply of oxygen by maintaining a good supply of fresh air, or oxygen, in the immediate environment, and by ensuring that the animal's airway is unobstructed. Avoiding chilling the animal is critical but overheating, because it causes peripheral vasodilatation and a further decrease in circulating blood pressure, needs to be avoided.

Circulating fluid volume enhancement

The primary objective is to restore the circulating blood volume either by a blood transfusion or plasma or plasma expander; because of the difficulty of supplying either in sufficient quantities and in a brief time it is customary in food animals to resort to the use of isotonic fluids, in ruminants often by stomach tube. The techniques for the administration of fluids or blood are dealt with in the sections on dehydration and hemorrhage.

Antiprostaglandins and corticosteroids

These two groups of drugs are now in common use in shock and their use is based on good pharmacological principles relating to the maintenance of cell membranes and the protection of tissues against damage by metabolites. There is a notable deficit of controlled trials relating to the use of these compounds, but the very wide experience of a large number of veterinarians indicates that drugs in both groups can play a large part in prolonging survival of shocked patients and, provided tissues are not irreversibly damaged by a delay in commencing treatment, the recovery rate is improved. Flunixin meglumine and phenylbutazone are in common use, and corticosteroids given in large doses (5–10 mg/kg body weight of dexamethazone intravenously) are especially useful in cases of septic shock.

Vasoactive drugs

The intelligent use of vasoconstrictors and vasodilators in cases of shock presents a major problem unless the patient's cardiovascular status is known and can be continuously monitored. The administration of a vasoconstrictor substance in a case of low pressure distributive shock would be rational because blood pressure would be elevated but it could reduce tissue perfusion still further. Conversely beta-adrenergic stimulators such as isoproterenol are valuable once the circulating blood volume has been restored but if hypotension is already present it will be further exacerbated. In experimentally induced shock in horses the opioid antagonist naloxone has been effective in reducing some of the damaging cardiovascular responses in shock and should be of value in clinical cases (7). The combination of fluids, antiprostaglandins, corticosteroids and antibiotics, which are always included in shock therapy for fear that bacteria may escape from damaged visci and invade healthy tissue, is widely accepted and used by field veterinarians.

REVIEW LITERATURE

Muir, W. W. (1987) Equine shock; the need for prospective clinical studies. *Equ. vet. J.*, *19*, 1–5.

Symposium on Shock (1976) *Vet. Clin. N. Am.*, 6, 171.

REFERENCES

(1) Kovack, A. G. et al. (1976) *Ann. Rev. Physiol.*, *38*, 571.
(2) Brasmer, T. H. (1972) *Vet. Clin. N. Am.*, 2, 219.
(3) Schumer, W. & Erve, P. R. (1975) *Circ. Shock*, *2*, 109.
(4) Michell, A. R. (1974) *J. small Anim. Pract.*, *15*, 279.
(5) Stevens, J. B. (1976) *Vet. Clin. N. Am.*, *6*, 203.
(6) Hall, L. W. & Nigam, J. M. (1975) *Vet. Rec.*, 97, 66.
(7) Weld, J. M. et al. (1984) *Res. Commun. Chem. Pathol. Pharmacol.*, *44*, 227.

WATER INTOXICATION

The ingestion of excessive quantities of water when animals are very thirsty may result in water intoxication, especially if there has been much loss of salt due to severe exercise or high environmental temperatures (1). Experimentally the condition is difficult to reproduce unless the antidiuretic principle of the pituitary gland is administered, since the normal excretory mechanisms remove the bulk of the administered fluid. Under field conditions calves are most commonly affected (2, 3).

Cellular hydration occurs and in organized tissues the cells increase in turgor. This is particularly noticeable in the brain where a condition analogous to cerebral edema occurs and causes nervous signs including muscle weakness and tremor, restlessness, ataxia, tonic and clonic convulsions and terminal coma. In unorganized tissues, particularly the erythrocytes, lysis occurs and the resulting hemolysis may cause severe hemolytic anemia and hemoglobinuria. Additional signs include hypothermia and salivation.

Water intoxication does not occur commonly and can be avoided by allowing thirsty animals to have only limited access to water. Treatment of affected animals should include sedation, the administration of diuretics and in severe cases the intravenous injection of hypertonic solutions.

REFERENCES

(1) Lawrence, J. A. (1965) *J. S. Afr. vet. med. Assoc.*, *36*, 277.
(2) Hannan, J. (1965) *Irish vet. J.*, *19*, 211.
(3) Kirkbride, C. A. & Frey, R. A. (1967) *J. Am. vet. med. Assoc.*, *151*, 742.

EDEMA

Edema is the excessive accumulation of fluid in tissue spaces caused by a disturbance in the mechanism of fluid interchange between capillaries, the tissue spaces and the lymphatic vessels.

Etiology

Edema results mainly from an increase in hydrostatic pressure in the capillaries, from a fall in osmotic pressure of the blood, from obstruction to lymphatic drainage or from damage to capillary walls.

Increased hydrostatic pressure

- Generally in congestive heart failure
- Locally in portal hypertension due to hepatic fibrosis causing ascites
- Locally by compression of mammary veins by a large fetus causing mammary or ventral edema in mares and cows in late pregnancy. Similar edema in hyperlipemia of ponies is unexplained.

Decreased plasma osmotic pressure—hypoproteinemia

- Continued blood loss especially in heavy infestations with blood-sucking parasites such as *Strongylus* sp. in the horse, *Fasciola* sp. in ruminants, *Bunostomum* sp. in calves, *Haemonchus* sp. in ruminants of all ages, especially goats; loss of osmolality is due to protein loss
- Renal disease causing continued loss of protein, but nephritic edema occurs rarely in our animals. Examples are poisoning by shin oak (*Quercus* sp.) and yellow-wood (*Terminalia oblongata*)
- Protein-losing enteropathy as in enterocolitis (1); heavy infestation with nematode parasites in ruminants, particularly *Ostertagia* sp. in young cattle, causes such anasarca, but with minimal damage to enteric epithelium
- Liver damage causing failure of synthesis of plasma proteins; congestive heart failure contributes to this
- Malnutrition with diets low in protein, e.g., ruminants at range in drought time, or in feedlots with poor nutritional management
- Edema of newborn piglets caused by inadequate protein nutrition of sows (2).

Obstruction of lymphatic flow

- Part of the edema caused by tumors or inflammatory swellings is lymphatic obstruction. Extensive fluid loss also originates from granulomatous lesions on serous surfaces. Ascites or hydrothorax may result. Lymphosarcoma in buffalo has a marked tendency to do this
- Congenital in inherited lymphatic obstruction edema of Ayrshire calves. Occurs also in pigs
- Sporadic lymphangitis of horses
- Edema in enzootic calcinosis of cattle
- Edema of the lower limbs of horses immobilized because of injury or illness is usually ascribed to poor lymphatic and/or venous return. It may also be related to variations in hematocrit, plasma protein, and erythrocyte sedimentation rate (ESR) which alter significantly after activity (3).

Vascular damage to small vessels

- Allergic edema—urticaria, angioneurotic edema, purpura hemorrhagica—caused by local liberation of vasodilators
- Toxic damage—in anthrax, gas gangrene, malignant edema, gut edema, mulberry heart disease, viral arteritis, equine infectious anemia, heartwater, intravenous ivermectin to horses, and the poisonous plants *Verbesina encelioides*, *Galega officinalis* and *Wedelia asperimma*.

Pathogenesis

At the arterial end of the capillaries the hydrostatic pressure of the blood is sufficient to overcome its osmotic pressure and fluid tends to pass into the tissue spaces. At the venous end of the capillaries the position is reversed and fluid tends to return to the vascular system. The pressure differences are not great and a small increase in hydrostatic pressure or decrease in osmotic pressure leads to failure of the fluid to return to the capillaries. The resulting accumulation of fluid in the tissue spaces, or by escape into serous cavities, constitutes edema.

Clinical findings

Accumulations of edematous transudate in subcutaneous tissues are referred to as anasarca, in the peritoneal cavity as ascites, in the pleural cavities as hydrothorax and in the pericardial sac as hydropericardium. Anasarca in large animals is usually confined to the ventral wall of the abdomen and thorax, the brisket and, if the animal is grazing, the intermandibular space. Intermandibular edema may be less evident in animals which do not have to lower their heads to graze. Edema of the limbs is uncommon in cattle, sheep and pigs but occurs in horses quite commonly when the venous rerurn is obstructed or there is a lack of muscular movement. Local edema of the head in the horse is a common lesion in African horse sickness and purpura hemorrhagica.

Edematous swellings are soft, painless and pit on pressure. In ascites there is distension of the abdomen and the fluid can be detected by a fluid thrill on tactile percussion, fluid sounds on succussion and by paracentesis. A level top line of fluid may be detectable by any of these means. In the pleural cavities and pericardial sac the clinical signs produced by the fluid accumulation include restriction of cardiac movements, embarrassment of respiration and collapse of the ventral parts of the lungs. The heart sounds and respiratory sounds are muffled and the presence of fluid may be ascertained by percussion, succussion and paracentesis.

More localized edemas cause more localized signs; pulmonary edema is accompanied by respiratory distress, loud, harsh breath sounds with crackles and in some cases by an outpouring of froth from the nose; cerebral edema is manifested by severe nervous signs. A not uncommon entity is a large edematous plaque around the umbilicus in yearling horses. The plaque develops rapidly, causes no apparent illness and subsides spontaneously after about 7 days.

Clinical pathology

Examination of a sample of fluid reveals an absence of signs of inflammation. In some instances the transudate is free of protein but in advanced cases much protein may be present because of the capillary damage which has occurred. The fluid may clot, have a high specific gravity and even contain free blood, particularly if the edema is caused by increased hydrostatic pressure.

Necropsy findings

The cause of the accumulation of fluid is obvious in many cases but estimations of the concentration of protein in the plasma may be necessary if hypoproteinemia is thought to be the cause. If the primary cause is endothelial damage this will probably be detectable only on histological examination.

Diagnosis

Differentiation of the specific causes of edema listed in etiology above depends upon identification of the primary disease. Subcutaneous and peritoneal accumulations of urine occur when the urethra or bladder ruptures after urethral obstruction by calculi. Peritonitis, pleurisy and pericarditis are also characterized by local accumulations of fluid but toxemia and other signs of inflammation are usually present. When there is doubt, paracentesis is an obvious way of determining the composition of the fluid. The number and type of inflammatory cells present, and whether or not bacteria can be isolated, are the best indicators of the origin of the fluid. In diseases causing hypoproteinemia the total serum protein concentration will be decreased and there may be a severe hypoalbuminemia. In renal amyloidosis there is a marked proteinuria. Liver function tests may be indicated when liver disease is the suspected cause of the edema.

Treatment

The treatment of edema should be aimed at correcting the primary disease. Myocardial asthenia should be relieved by the use of digitalis, pericarditis by drainage of the sac, and hypoproteinemia by the administration of plasma or plasma substitutes and the feeding of high quality protein. Ancillary measures include restriction of water intake and the amount of salt in the diet, the use of diuretics and aspiration of fluid. Diuretics may relieve the effects of pressure temporarily but are of little value if the transudate has a high content of protein. Aspiration of fluid must be carried out slowly to avoid acute dilatation of splanchnic vessels and subsequent peripheral circulatory failure. The technique usually gives only temporary relief because the fluid rapidly accumulates again causing further withdrawal of fluids from tissues.

REFERENCES

(1) Nansen, P. & Nielsen, K. (1967) *Nord. VetMed.*, *19*, 524.
(2) Edwards, B. L. (1961) *Vet. Rec.*, *73*, 540.
(3) Dalton, R. G. (1973) *Equ. vet. J.*, *5*, 81.

DISEASES CHARACTERIZED BY ABNORMALITIES OF THE CELLULAR ELEMENTS OF THE BLOOD

Anemia

Anemia is defined as a deficiency of erythrocytes, or hemorrhage, or by increased destruction or the inefficient production of erythrocytes. Anemias are therefore usually classified as hemorrhagic or hemolytic anemia, or anemia due to decreased production of erythrocytes.

Etiology

Anemia may be caused by excessive loss of blood by hemorrhage, or by increased destruction or the in-

efficient production of erythrocytes. Anemias are therefore usually classified as hemorrhagic or hemolytic anemia, or anemia due to decreased production of erythrocytes.

Hemorrhagic anemia

The causes are the same as those listed under the heading 'hemorrhage' on page 341.

Hemolytic anemia

Cattle

- **Babesiosis, anaplasmosis, eperythrozoonosis trypanosomiasis (*Trypanosoma theileri*), Nagana, theileriosis**
- **Bacillary hemoglobinuria**
- **Leptospirosis (*L. interrogans* serovar *pomona*)**
- **Postparturient hemoglobinuria**
- **Poisoning by rape (canola), kale, chou moellier**
- **Poisoning by weeds—*Mercurialis* and *Allium* spp.**
- **Poisoning by miscellaneous agents including cannery offal, especially tomatoes and onions (4), onions as a steady diet, phenothiazine**
- **Poisoning—chronic copper poisoning can occur, but cattle are much less susceptible than sheep**
- **Treatment with longacting oxytetracycline (7)**
- **Calves which drink a large volume of cold water**
- **Part of a transfusion reaction**
- **Rare cases of isoerythrolysis in calves**
- **Rarer cases (2, 21) of autoimmune hemolytic anemia**
- **Inherited intracorpuscular defects leading to hemolytic anemia, as in dogs and cats, do occur.**

Sheep

- **Chronic copper poisoning (as in toxemic jaundice) is the most important cause**
- **Eperythrozoonosis and babesiosis**
- **Poisoning by cruciferous plants including rape, etc.**

Pigs

- **Eperythrozoonosis is recorded, but hemolytic anemia is rare**
- **Isoerythrolysis, with concurrent neutropenia and thrombocytopenia occurs, but is uncommon (6)**
- **Willebrand's and other similar hemorrhagic diseases (6).**

Horses

- **Equine infectious anemia**
- **Babesiosis**
- **Phenothiazine poisoning. This anthelmintic is rarely used in horses now**
- **Isoerythrolysis in foals**
- **Autoimmune hemolytic anemias. Several series have been recorded (1, 8, 9, 22). The direct antiequine globulin test is often positive and some of the horses develop purpura hemorrhagica or neoplasms of the lymphoreticular series (10). Others resemble the cold agglutinin disease of man with cold-induced hemoglobinuria (4, 11)**
- **Some snake envenomations cause intravascular hemolysis in dogs and cats. Some clinical accounts** record hemoglobinuria in snakebite in horses and calves.

Anemia due to decreased production of erythrocytes or hemoglobin

The diseases in this group tend to affect all species equally so that they are divided up according to cause rather than according to animal species.

Nutritional deficiency

- Cobalt and copper. These elements are necessary for all animals, but clinically occurring anemia is observed only in ruminants
- Iron, but as a clinical occurrence this is limited to baby pigs and possibly to young calves designated for the white veal market. In more general terms perhaps, iron deficiency should be considered as a possible cause of failure to perform well in housed calves. Male calves up to 8 weeks of age and on a generally suitable diet can show less than optimum performance in erythron levels, and the calves with subclinical anemia have deficits in growth rate and resistance to diarrhea and pneumonia (18). A great deal of attention is paid to providing adequate iron to racehorses, often by periodic injection of iron compounds regularly during the racing season
- Potassium deficiency is implicated in causing anemia in calves
- Pyridoxine deficiency, produced experimentally, can contribute to the development of anemia in calves
- Folic acid deficiency. Anemia in racing horses attracts a good deal of attention, and much nonsense is talked and practiced. However, stabled horses, especially pregnant mares who have no access to pasture, respond well to folic acid (12).

Chronic disease

- Chronic suppurative processes can cause severe anemia by depression of erythropoiesis
- Radiation injury
- Poisoning by bracken, trichlorethylene-extracted soybean meal, arsenic, phenylbutazone (19) cause depression of bone marrow activity
- A sequel to inclusion body rhinitis infection in pigs
- Intestinal parasitism, e.g., ostertagiasis, trichostrongylosis in calves and sheep, have this effect (4)
- An idiopatic hypoplastic anemia in a foal (14)
- Temporarily for several weeks after sudden movement to high altitude (13).

Myelophthisic anemias, in which the bone marrow cavities are occupied by other, usually neoplastic, tissues, are rare in farm animals. Plasma cell myelomatosis has been observed as a cause of such anemia in pigs, calves and a horse (15). Clinical signs, other than of the anemia, which is macrocytic and normochromic, includes skeletal pain, pathological fractures and paresis due to the osteolytic lesions produced by the invading neoplasm. Cavitation of the bone may be detected on radiographic examination.

Pathogenesis

Irrespective of the cause of anemia the primary abnormality of function is the anemic anoxia which follows. In acute hemorrhagic anemia there is in addition a loss of circulating blood volume and plasma proteins. The fluid loss is quickly repaired by equilibration with tissue fluids and by absorption and, provided hemorrhage does not continue, the plasma proteins are quickly restored to normal by synthesis in the liver. However, erythropoiesis requires a longer time interval to alleviate the anemia. Hemolytic anemia is often sufficiently severe to cause hemoglobinuria and may result in hemoglobinuric nephrosis and depression of renal function. Aplastic anemia caused by toxins from a suppurative process is a secondary manifestation and is relieved by removal of the cause, and anemia due to nutritional deficiency is similarly reversible. In the situation where erythrolysis occurs immediately after drinking a large volume of cold water, the hemolysis occurs in the capillaries in the intestinal wall. The plasma osmotic pressure decreases as a result of the fluid intake, and hemolysis occurs because this is below the minimum osmotic tolerance of the erythrocytes (3).

The primary responses to tissue anoxia caused by anemia are an increase in cardiac output due to increases in stroke volume and heart rate, and a decrease in circulation time. A diversion of blood from the peripheral to the splanchnic circulation also occurs. In the terminal stages when the tissue anoxia is sufficiently severe there may be a moderate increase in respiratory activity. Provided the activity of the bone marrow is not reduced, erythropoiesis is stimulated by lowering of the tissue oxygen tension.

Clinical findings

Pallor of the mucosae is the outstanding clinical sign but appreciable degrees of anemia can occur without clinically visible change in mucosal or skin color. These degrees of anemia are usually not sufficient to cause signs of illness but they may interfere with performance, particularly in racehorses, and this aspect of equine medicine has come into prominence in recent years (16). Many horses suffer from moderate anemia, due probably in most cases to strongylosis, and respond spectacularly to treatment with hematinic drugs.

In clinical cases of anemia there are signs of pallor, muscular weakness, depression and anorexia. The heart rate is increased, the pulse has a large amplitude and the absolute intensity of the heart sounds is markedly increased. Terminally the moderate tachycardia of the compensatory phase is replaced by a severe tachycardia, a decrease in the intensity of the heart sounds and a weak pulse. The initial increase in intensity of heart sounds is caused by cardiac dilatation and an increase in blood pressure. If the dilatation is sufficiently severe the atrioventricular orifices become dilated causing relative insufficiency of the valves and a hemic systolic murmur which waxes and wanes with each respiratory cycle, reaching its maximum at the peak of inspiration. This type of murmur is not pathognomonic of anemia and may be present in any form of myocardial asthenia or when the viscosity of the blood is reduced for any other reason.

Dyspnea is not pronounced in anemia, the most severe degree of respiratory distress appearing as an increase in depth of respiration without much increase in rate. Labored breathing occurs only in the terminal stages. Additional signs which often accompany anemia but are not essential parts of the syndrome are edema, jaundice and hemoglobinuria. Cyanosis does not occur because of the relative deficiency of hemoglobin.

Clinical pathology

Clinical signs do not appear until the hemoglobin level of the blood falls below about 50% of normal, and a hemoglobin level as low as 20% of normal is compatible with life, as long as its development is prolonged. The erythrocyte count and the hematocrit are usually depressed. In hemorrhagic and hemolytic anemias there is an increase in the number of immature red cells in the blood. This is not apparent in the horse and there is great difficulty in that species in determining whether there is an erythropoietic response or not. In hemorrhagic anemia there is a fall in total serum protein, an unlikely event in hemolytic anemia. In the latter the serum or plasma is usually discolored due to the presence of hemoglobin, but the serum is clear in hemorrhagic anemias. A biopsy of bone marrow is the only satisfactory method available but the estimation of the adenosine-5-triphosphate content of erythrocytes is suggested as an additional technique (11). The characteristic finding in anemia caused by a deficiency of iron is hypochromasia caused by a reduction in mean corpuscular hemoglobin concentration; the hemoglobin level is low but the erythrocyte count may be normal.

Necropsy findings

Necropsy findings include those specific to the primary cause. Findings indicative of anemia include pallor of tissues, thin, watery blood and contraction of the spleen. Centrilobular hepatic necrosis is commonly present in cattle, and probably in other animals, if the anemia has existed for some time (17).

Diagnosis

A diagnosis of anemia is usually suggested by the obvious clinical signs. Differentiation between hemorrhagic and hemolytic anemias and those caused by deficient production of erythrocytes or hemoglobin depends upon the history of hemorrhage, hemoglobinuria, jaundice, or diet, and upon clinical evidence of these signs. The clinicopathological findings may also suggest the origin of the anemia. Hemorrhagic and hemolytic anemias are manifested by the presence of immature erythrocytes in the blood; deficiency anemias by hypochromasia; and aplastic anemia caused by toxins is manifested by low erythrocyte counts without evidence of regeneration. These generalizations are often not of much assistance in urgent situations where an animal is seriously ill, as so often happens with anemia, or a number are affected. More accurate methods of determining the classification of the anemia would be an advantage.

Treatment

Treatment of the primary cause of the anemia is essential. Non-specific treatment includes blood transfusion in acute hemorrhage and even in chronic anemia of severe degree. The subject is dealt with in detail under the heading of hemorrhage. Hematinic preparations are used in less severe cases and as supportive treatment after transfusion. Iron administered by mouth or parenterally is in common use and in horses is much superior to other more expensive substances (20). Preparations injected intravenously give a rapid response and intramuscular injections of organic-iron preparations give less rapid but more prolonged results. Vitamin B_{12} is widely used as a non-specific hematinic, particularly in horses, but there is no evidence that it is a rational procedure if traces of cobalt are available in the diet. In extreme cases of anemia irreversible changes caused by anoxia of kidneys and heart muscle may prevent complete recovery in spite of adequate treatment.

REFERENCES

(1) Sutton, R. H. et al. (1978) *NZ vet. J.*, *26*, 311.
(2) Valli, V. E. O. & Erb, H. N. (1977) *Can. vet. J.*, *18*, 222.
(3) Shimizu, Y. et al. (1979) *Jap. J. vet. Sci.*, *41*, 583.
(4) Schalm, O. W. (1972) *J. Am. vet. med. Assoc.*, *161*, 1269.
(5) Lachmann, G. et al. (1973) *Arch. exp. VetMed.*, *27*, 871.
(6) Thiele, G.L. et al. (1986) *J. Hered.*, *77*, 179.
(7) Anderson, W. I. et al. (1983) *Mod. vet. Pract.*, *12*, 997.
(8) Lobhorst, H. M. & Breukink, H. J. (1975) *Tijdschr. Diergeneeskd.*, *100*, 752.
(9) Moriarty, K. M. et al. (1976) *NZ vet. J.*, *24*, 85.
(10) Dixon, J. B. & Archer, R. K. (1975) *Vet. Ann.*, *15*, 185.
(11) Smith, J. E. & Agar, N. S. (1976) *Equ. vet. J.*, *8*, 34.
(12) Seekington, I. M. et al. (1967) *Vet. Rec.*, *81*, 158.
(13) Collins, J. D. et al. (1969) *Irish vet. J.*, *23*, 42.
(14) Archer, R. K. & Miller, W. C. (1965) *Vet. Rec.*, *77*, 538.
(15) Cornelius, C. E. et al. (1959) *Cornell Vet.*, *49*, 478.
(16) Lumsden, J. H. et al. (1975) *Can J. comp. Med.*, *39*, 324, 332.
(17) Urbaneck, D. & Rossow, N. (1962) *Mh. VetMed.*, *17*, 941.
(18) Bunger, U. et al. (1979) *Arch. Tierenahrung*, *29*, 703.
(19) Dunavant, M. L. & Murry, E. S. (1977) *Proc. 1st Inter. Symp. Equ. Haematol., 28–30th May, USA*, p. 383.
(20) Kirkham, W. W. et al. (1971) *J. Am. vet. med. Assoc.*, *159*, 1136.
(21) Dixon, P. M. et al. (1978) *Vet. Rec.*, *103*, 155.
(22) Sockett, D. et al. (1987) *J. Am. vet. med. Assoc.*, *190*, 308.

Leukemia

Leukemia is manifested by abnormal proliferation of myelogenous or lymphatic tissues causing a marked increase in the number of circulating leukocytes. The disease is probably neoplastic in origin and is usually accompanied by enlargement of the spleen, lymph nodes and bone marrow, singly or in combination. The persistent lymphocytosis which is a characteristic response by some cattle to infection with the bovine viral leukosis virus is the only leukemia known to be caused by an infectious agent.

In leukemic leukemia, immature leukocytes appear in the blood, in aleukemic leukemia the total leukocyte count may or may not be increased. In leukemia the differential leukocyte count may be distorted, a preponderance of immature granulocytes occurring in myelogenous leukemia and a relative increase in lymphocytes occurring in lymphatic leukemia. There may be an accompanying aplastic anemia if erythropoiesis is depressed by expansion of myeloid tissue in the bone marrow—a myelophthisic anemia. Examination of smears of bone marrow has become commonplace in cases of leukemia in large animals. Samples of bone marrow contents are easily obtained from the sternum of animals in the standing position. In the horse specimens can be readily obtained from the ilium, entrance being made through the tuber coxae (1). Bone marrow biopsy techniques have also been described for cows (2) and goats (4).

In farm animals the only common form of leukemia is lymphomatosis. Myelogenous leukemia is rare but has been recorded in all species. Erythroblastic and plasma cell tumors and monocytic leukemia are still less frequent. Information on hemopoietic tissue tumors has been reviewed recently (5) and is not recapitulated here. When the leukemia is leukemic there is usually no difficulty in making a diagnosis because of the very high total white cell count, the distortion of the differential count, and the presence of immature cells. Most cases of lymphomatosis in farm animals are subleukemic, at least when the disease is clinically recognizable, and the differentiation from lymphadenitis may be difficult. In lymphadenitis enlargement of the nodes usually occurs rapidly and asymmetrically and the enlargement may fluctuate or completely regress. A case of primary lymphoid leukemia in a horse showed poor performance, unthriftiness, ventral edema and dullness. There were high levels of immature lymphocytes in peripheral blood and bone marrow, but no tumor masses anywhere, and no lymph node enlargement (6). Several cases of equine monomyelocytic leukemia have presented with ventral edema, weight loss, splenomegaly and some lymph node enlargement (7, 9). Eosinophilic myeloproliferative disease is also recorded in a horse (8). Clinical signs included a systolic murmur, pallor, mucosal petechiation and ventral edema. There was also a severe thrombocytopenia.

The leukocytosis associated with local or generalized infections is usually less severe in degree than that of leukemic leukemia and the distortion of the differential count is not so marked, following a standard pattern. There is a neutrophilia with a relative increase in band forms in acute generalized or local inflammatory processes, and a lymphocytosis or monocytosis in chronic suppurative infections.

A number of leukopenia-producing drugs, including nitrogen and sulfur mustards, urethane and antifolic acid compounds have been used in the treatment of leukemia in human and small animal practice but the poor results obtained do not justify their use in farm animals.

REFERENCES

(1) Archer, R. K. (1964) *Vet. Rec.*, *76*, 465.
(2) Lawrence, W. C. et al. (1962) *Cornell Vet.*, *52*, 297.
(3) Brumbaugh, G. W. et al. (1982) *J. Am. vet. med. Assoc.*, *180*, 313.
(4) Wilkins, J. H. (1961) *Vet. Rec.*, *74*, 244.
(5) Squire, R. A. (1964) *Cornell Vet.*, *54*, 97.
(6) Roberts, M. C. (1977) *Equ. vet. J.*, *9*, 216.
(7) Burkhardt, E. et al. (1984) *Vet. Pathol.*, *21*, 394.
(8) Morris, D. D. et al. (1984) *J. Am. vet. med. Assoc.*, *185*, 993.
(9) Spier, S. J. et al. (1986) *J. Am. vet. med. Assoc.*, *188*, 861.

Leukopenia

Leukopenia does not occur as a specific disease entity but is a common manifestation of a number of diseases. Virus diseases, particularly hog cholera, are frequently accompanied by a panleukopenia in the early acute stages. Leukopenia has also been observed in leptospirosis in cattle although bacterial infections are usually accompanied by a leukocytosis. Acute local inflammations may cause a transient fall in the leukocyte count because of withdrawal of the circulating cells to the septic focus.

Leukopenia may also occur as part of a pancytopenia in which all cellular elements of the blood are depressed. Agents which depress the activity of the bone marrow, spleen and lymph nodes and result in pancytopenia occur in poisonings caused by trichloroethylene-extracted soybean meal, toluene, fungal toxins e.g. fusaritoxicosis, notably that of *Stachybotrys alternans*, and bracken fern. Pancytopenia occurs also in radiation disease and in an increasingly common disease of calves ascribed to furazolidone poisoning. The disease is discussed under the title of granulocytopenic calf disease. Chronic arsenical poisoning, and poisoning by sulfonamides, chlorpromazine and chloramphenicol cause similar blood dyscrasias in man but do not appear to have this effect in animals. Depression of the blood level of granulocytes also occurs occasionally but the cases are mostly idiopathic unless they are part of a wider specific disease, such as Chediak–Higashi syndrome (1, 2).

The importance of leukopenia is that it reduces the resistance of the animal to bacterial infection and may be followed by a highly fatal, fulminating septicemia. Treament of the condition should include the administration of broad-spectrum antibiotics to prevent bacterial invasion. Drugs, including pentnucleotide, which have been used to stimulate leukopoietic activity, have not been shown materially to affect most leukopenias.

REFERENCES

(1) Hagemoser, W. A. et al. (1983) *J. Am. vet. med. Assoc.*, *183*, 1093.
(2) Searcy, G. P. & Orr, J. P (1981) *Can. vet. J.*, *22*, 148.

DISEASES OF THE SPLEEN AND LYMPH NODES

Splenomegaly

Diffuse diseases of the spleen which result in enlargement are usually secondary to diseases in other organs. Splenomegaly with complete destruction of splenic function is virtually symptomless, especially if the involvement occurs gradually, and in most cases clinical signs are restricted to those caused by involvement of other organs. An enlarged spleen may be palpable on rectal examination in the horse and careful percussion may detect enlargement of the spleen in cattle but in most instances involvement of the organ is not diagnosed at antemortem examination unless laparotomy is performed. Left dorsal displacement of the colon in the horse is a colic in which the spleen is displaced caudally and this may give the impression that the organ is enlarged. Rupture of a grossly enlarged spleen may cause sudden death due to internal hemorrhage. This is sometimes the cause of death in bovine viral leukosis.

Moderate degrees of splenomegaly occur in many infectious diseases, especially salmonellosis, anthrax, babesiosis, and equine infectious anemia. Animals which die suddenly because of lightning stroke, electrocution and euthanasia may also show a moderate degree of splenomegaly but the enlargement is minor compared to that observed in congestive heart failure, portal obstruction or neoplastic change. Neoplasms of the spleen are not common in large animals but may include lymphosarcoma (1) myelocytic leukemia (2) or malignant melanoma in horses. They may be discovered incidentally during rectal examination or because of colic resulting from displacement of the bowel by the enlarged spleen.

REFERENCES

(1) Browning, A. P. (1986) *Vet. Rec.*, *119*, 178.
(2) Brumbaugh, G. W. et al. (1982) *J. Am. vet. med. Assoc.*, *180*, 313.

Splenic abscess

Splenic abscess may result when a septic embolus lodges in the spleen, but is more commonly caused by extension of infection from a neighboring organ. Perforation by a foreign body in the reticulum of cattle is the commonest cause of the disease in large animals and penetrations by sharp metal have caused splenitis in the horse (1). Perforation of a gastric ulcer or an erosion of the gastric wall caused by *Gasterophilus intestinalis* (3) or extension of a granuloma caused by larvae of *Habronema* sp. in horses may lead, by extension, to development of a suppurative lesion in the spleen. In those occasional cases of strangles in horses in which systemic spread occurs, splenic abscess is a common localization.

If the abscess is extensive and acute there are systemic signs of fever, anorexia and increased heart rate. Pain is evidenced on palpation over the area of the spleen and hematological examination reveals a marked increase in the total white cell count and a distinct shift to the left in the differential count. Paracentesis usually provides evidence of chronic peritonitis by the presence of a large amount of inflammatory exudate. Peritonitis is often coexistent and produces signs of mild abdominal pain with arching of the back and disinclination to move. Mild recurrent colic may also occur. Anemia, with marked pallor of mucosae, and terminal ventral edema are also recorded (1). The spleen may be sufficiently enlarged to be palpable per rectum (2).

Treatment of splenic abscess is often unrewarding because of the extensive nature of the lesion before clinical signs appear. The systemic signs can usually be brought under control by treatment with sulfonamides or antibiotics over a period of about 7 days but relapses are common and death is the almost certain outcome. Splenectomy is recommended if adhesions and associated peritonitis are absent.

REFERENCES

(1) Swan, R. A. (1968) *Aust. vet. J.*, *44*, 459.
(2) Spier, S. et al. (1986) *J. Am. vet. med. Assoc.*, *189*, 557.
(3) Dart, A. J. et al. (1987) *Aust. vet. J.*, *64*, 155.

Enlargement of the lymph nodes

Enlargement of peripheral nodes causes visible and palpable swellings and in some cases obstruction to lymphatic drainage and subsequent local edema as in sporadic lymphangitis of horses. Enlargement of internal nodes may cause obstruction of the esophagus or pharynx, trachea, or bronchi.

Enlargement of the lymph nodes may occur as a result of infection or of neoplastic invasion.

Neoplasia
Metastases may develop as a result of spread from neoplasms in surrounding tissues. Primary neoplasms involving lymph nodes include lymphomatosis (bovine viral leukosis is a particular example), lymphosarcoma and myeloid leukemia.

In lymphomatosis and myeloid leukemia, and in bacterial endocarditis simultaneous enlargement of a number of lymph nodes is characteristic. Generalized lymphadenopathy is not a characteristic of lymphosarcoma in horses although it may occur and is recorded in an aborted foal. In adults there may be multiple cutaneous nodules (6) or a major involvement of the organs of the thoracic cavity, of the abdomen or in other individual locations, e.g. the palate, in which it is characterized by dysphagia (8).

The commonest syndrome in horses is that of weight loss, ventral edema of the neck and thorax, sometimes accompanied by pleural or peritoneal effusion, anemia, dyspnea, cough and abdominal masses palpable per rectum (2–4). In cases where the lesions are predominantly in the thorax the syndrome is that produced by a space-occupying lesion (9) manifested by pectoral edema, jugular vein engorgement but an absence of the jugular pulse and dyspnea. The heart may be displaced and there may be cardiac murmurs. If there is compression of the esophagus dysphagia is present. Weight loss, anorexia and pleural effusion are other incidental clinical signs. Involvement of the intestinal wall is usually accompanied by colic or diarrhea (7) and the disease is listed as a common cause of chronic undifferentiated diarrhea of horses; involvement of the spinal cord causes spinal cord compression.

Only a small proportion of horses with lymphadenopathy due to lymphosarcoma have concurrent leukemic blood changes (10). Those cases which do have changes show a marked lymphocytosis and possibly thrombocytopenia and anemia.

Infection
Lymphadenitis accompanies other signs in many specific diseases including strangles, bovine malignant catarrh, sporadic bovine encephalomyelitis, East Coast fever, Ondiri disease, glanders, melioidosis, enzootic lymphangitis and ephemeral fever, but as a sole presenting sign it occurs commonly in tuberculosis, caseous lymphadenitis of sheep, Morel's disease of sheep caused by an unidentified micrococcus, cervical adenitis of pigs caused principally by *Streptococcus* sp., and an uncommon lymphadenitis in lambs caused by *Pasteurella multocida*, and in some cases of actinobacillosis. In acute lymphadenitis there may be pain and heat on palpation but the nodes are for the most part painless. Cervical adenitis is a common finding in slaughtered pigs, but the lesions rarely cause clinical illness. As well as the streptococcal lesions mentioned above, there is a variety of bacterial causes including *Corynebacterium (Rhodococcus) equi, Mycobacterium tuberculosis, M.avium, M. bovis*, and other atypical mycobacteria.

Lymphadenopathy which causes enlargement of abdominal lymph nodes is a characteristic of infection with *Streptococcus equi* in the burro. Differentiation between lymphadenitis and neoplastic enlargement may require examination of a biopsy specimen. Retropharyngeal lymph node enlargement up to three or four times normal, and colored bright green, have been identified in cattle as resulting from infection with the algae *Prototheca* spp. (1).

REFERENCES

(1) Rogers, R. J. et al. (1980) *J. comp. Pathol.*, *90*, 1.
(2) Schalm, O. W. (1981) *Equ. Pract.*, *3*, 23.
(3) Hoven, R. van der & Franken, P. (1983) *Equ. vet. J.*, *15*, 49.
(4) Rebhun, W. C. & Bertone, A. (1984) *J. Am. vet. med. Assoc*, *184*, 720.
(5) Haley, P. J. & Spraker, T. (1983) *Vet. Pathol.*, *20*, 647.
(6) Humphrey, M. et al. (1984) *Equ. vet. J.*, *16*, 547.
(7) Wilson, R. G. et al. (1985) *Equ. vet. J.*, *17*, 148.
(8) Lane, J. G. (1985) *Equ. vet. J.*, *17*, 465.
(9) Mair, T. S. et al. (1985) *Equ. vet. J.*, *17*, 428.
(10) Allen, B. V. et al. (1984) *Vet. Rec.*, *115*, 130.

10

Diseases of the Respiratory System

PRINCIPLES OF RESPIRATORY INSUFFICIENCY

THE functional efficiency of the respiratory system depends on its ability to oxygenate and to remove carbon dioxide from the blood as it passes through in the respiratory circulation. Interference with these functions can occur in a number of ways but the underlying defect in all instances is lack of adequate oxygen supply to tissues. The anoxia (or more correctly hypoxia) of respiratory insufficiency is responsible for most of the clinical signs of respiratory disease and for respiratory failure, the terminal event of fatal cases. An understanding of anoxia and respiratory failure is essential to the study of clinical respiratory disease.

Anoxia

Failure of the tissues to receive an adequate supply of oxygen occurs in a number of ways. *Anoxic anoxia* occurs when there is defective oxygenation of blood in the pulmonary circuit and is usually caused by primary disease of the respiratory tract. *Anemic anoxia* occurs when there is a deficiency of hemoglobin per unit volume of blood. The percentage saturation of the available hemoglobin and the oxygen tension are normal but the oxygen-carrying capacity of the blood is reduced. Anemia due to any cause has these characteristics. Alteration of hemoglobin to pigments which are not capable of carrying oxygen has the same effect. Thus in poisoning caused by nitrite, in which hemoglobin is converted to methemoglobin, and that due to carbon monoxide, when the hemoglobin is converted to carboxyhemoglobin, there is an anemic anoxia. *Stagnant anoxia* is the state in which the rate of blood flow through the capillaries is reduced. The oxygen saturation of arterial blood, the total oxygen load and the oxygen tension of arterial blood are normal, but because of the prolonged sojourn in the tissues the oxygen tension there falls to a very low level, reducing the rate of oxygen exchange. A relative anoxia of tissues results. Stagnant anoxia is the basic defect in congestive heart failure, peripheral circulatory failure and local venous obstruction. *Histotoxic anoxia* occurs when the blood is fully oxygenated but because of failure of tissue oxidation systems the tissues cannot take up oxygen. Cyanide poisoning is the only common cause of this form of anoxia.

Anoxic anoxia may occur when the oxygen tension in the inspired air is too low to oxygenate the pulmonary blood efficiently, but the common causes in animal disease are lesions or dysfunctions of the respiratory tract which reduce the supply of alveolar air. Abnormalities of the alveolar epithelium such as occur in pneumonia, decreased vital capacity as it occurs in pulmonary atelectasis, pneumonia, pneumothorax, pulmonary edema and congestion, and decreased amplitude of chest movement due to pain of the chest wall all reduce the oxygen tension of the blood leaving the lungs. Obstruction of the air passages by the accumulation of exudate and depression of the respiratory center by drugs or toxins have the same effect. Anoxic anoxia is also the basic defect in congenital defects of the heart and large blood vessels when mixing of arterial and venous blood occurs through shunts between the two circulations. Anoxic anoxia also occurs when there is paralysis of the respiratory muscles in tick paralysis, botulism, tetanus and strychnine poisoning.

If the development of anoxia is sufficiently slow several compensatory mechanisms operate. An increase in depth of the respiratory movements (hyperpnea) occurs as a result of the anoxia and is mediated by the chemoreceptors of the carotid and aortic bodies. Stimulation of splenic contraction and erythropoiesis in the bone marrow are produced by the anoxia and may result in polycythemia. An increase in heart rate and stroke volume results in an increased minute volume of the heart. If these compensatory mechanisms are insufficient to maintain an adequate supply of oxygen to tissues, signs of dysfunction appear in the various organs. The central nervous system is most susceptible to anoxia and signs referable to cerebral anoxia are usually the first to appear. Myocardial asthenia, renal and hepatic dysfunction and reduction of motility and secretory activity of the alimentary tract also occur.

Carbon dioxide retention (hypercapnia)

Respiratory insufficiency results in faulty elimination of carbon dioxide and its accumulation in blood and tissues. This appears to have little effect other than to stimulate an increase in respiratory effort by its action on the respiratory center.

Respiratory failure

Respiratory movements are involuntary and are stimulated and modified by the respiratory centers in the medulla. The centers appear, at least in some species, to have spontaneous activity which is modified by afferent impulses from higher centers including cerebral cortex and the heat-regulating center in the hypothalamus, from the stretch receptors in the lungs via the pulmonary vagus nerves, and from the chemoreceptors in the carotid bodies. The activity of the center is also regulated directly by the pH and oxygen and carbon dioxide tensions of the cranial arterial blood supply. Stimulation of almost all afferent nerves may also cause reflex change in respiration, stimulation of pain fibers being particularly effective.

Respiratory failure is the terminal stage of respiratory insufficiency in which the activity of the respiratory centers diminishes to the point where movements of respiratory muscles cease. Respiratory failure can be paralytic, dyspneic or asphyxial, or tachypneic, depending on the primary disease. In asphyxial failure, which occurs in pneumonia, pulmonary edema, and upper respiratory tract obstruction there is hypercapnia and anoxia. The hypercapnia stimulates the respiratory center, and the anoxia the chemoreceptors of the carotid body so that respiratory movements are dyspneic, followed by alternating periods of gasping and apnea just before death. Paralytic respiratory failure is caused by poisoning with respiratory center depressants or by nervous shock. Acute heart failure or hemorrhage may cause paralytic respiratory failure but there is usually a variable degree of dyspnea and gasping, although not usually as severe as in typical asphyxial failure. In typical paralytic failure the respiratory centers are paralyzed so that the respirations rapidly become more shallow and less frequent and then cease altogether without the appearance of dyspnea or gasping.

Tachypneic respiratory failure is the least common form and arises when pulmonary ventilation is increased as in hyperthermia so that there is hypoxia but no carbon dioxide retention (acapnia). Because of the lack of carbon dioxide to stimulate the respiratory movements they are rapid and shallow—tachypnea. The differentiation of these types of failure is of some importance in determining the type of treatment which is necessary. In the paralytic form a respiratory center stimulant is required, in the asphyxial form oxygen is the rational treatment, and in the tachypneic form oxygen and carbon dioxide should be provided.

PRINCIPAL MANIFESTATIONS OF RESPIRATORY INSUFFICIENCY

The principal manifestations of respiratory dysfunction are those which derive from anoxia but in infectious diseases or where tissue destruction is extensive there is the added effect of toxemia, the manifestations of which have been discussed elsewhere. The toxemia may be so intense, for example in calf diphtheria, aspiration pneumonia and equine pleurisy, as to kill the patient although its oxygen and carbon dioxide exchange are not greatly impaired.

Hyperpnea, dyspnea and poor exercise tolerance

Hyperpnea is defined as increased pulmonary ventilation. Dyspnea has a subjective element in that it is defined as the consciousness of the necessity for increased respiratory effort, and is loosely applied to animals to include increased respiratory movement which appears to cause distress to the animal. Hyperpnea becomes dyspnea at an arbitrary dyspneic point and the two are discussed together.

Dyspnea is a physiologic occurrence after strenuous exercise and is abnormal only when it occurs at rest or with little exercise. It is usually caused by anoxia and hypercapnia arising most commonly from diseases of the respiratory tract. In pulmonary dyspnea one other factor may be of contributory importance; there may be an abnormally sensitive Hering–Breuer reflex. This is most likely to occur when there is inflammation or congestion of the lungs or pleura. Rapid, shallow breathing results. The dyspnea of pulmonary emphysema is characteristically expiratory in form and is caused by anoxic anoxia and the need for forced expiration to achieve successful expulsion of the tidal air. The abnormalities of the respiratory cycle such as prolongation of expiration or inspiration and disproportionate movements of the thoracic walls are presented under clinical examination of the thorax in Chapter 1.

Cardiac dyspnea results from backward failure of the left ventricle with congestion and edema of the lungs. Stagnant anoxia plays some part in the production of this form of dyspnea but diminished ability of the lungs to distend, with increased sensitivity of the Hering–Breuer reflex, and the effect of increased venous pressure on the respiratory center are probably more important.

Dyspnea is never marked in anemic anoxia when the patient is at rest because of the absence of hypercapnia. In acidosis the liberation of carbon dioxide stimulates the respiratory center and dyspnea may occur, and in some cases of encephalitis or space-occupying lesions of the cranial cavity stimulation of the center may cause neurogenic dyspnea.

Dyspnea, and hyperpnea, is the clinical sign most likely to attract attention to the possible presence of disease in the respiratory system. A brief summary of the causes of dyspnea are set down below and in Fig. 20. It is most important when attempting to differentiate diseases that cause it to include diseases of systems other than the respiratory system. The differentiation is between those diseases which cause dyspnea at rest or lack of exercise tolerance, the latter being a mild form of the former.

Diseases causing dyspnea at rest or lack of exercise tolerance

Respiratory tract disease
This causes interference with oxygen supply to and carbon dioxide discharge from the alveolar epithelium:

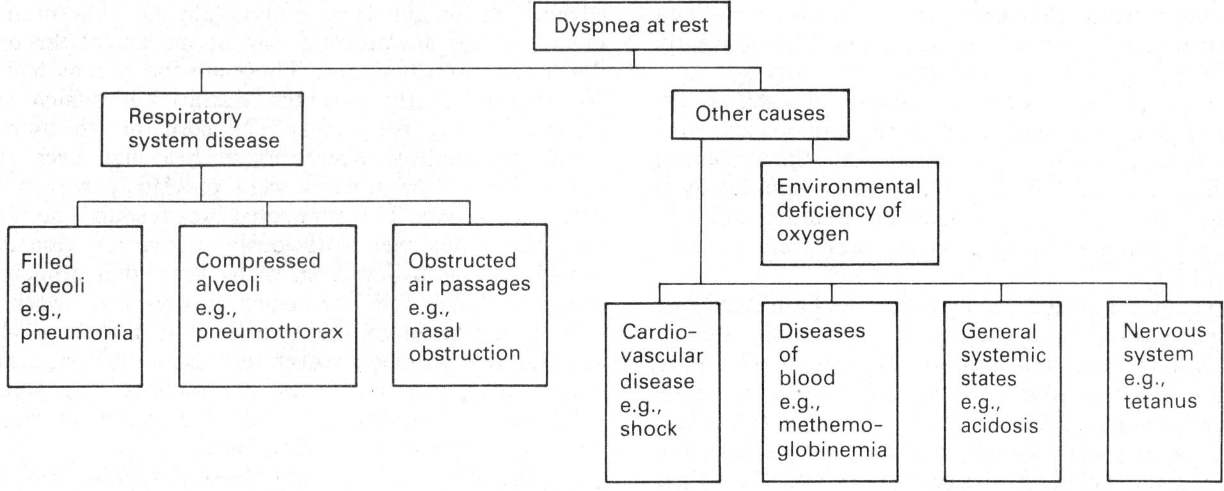

Fig. 20. The causes of dyspnea

- *Characterized by filled alveoli*—pneumonia and pulmonary edema
- *Compressed alveoli*—pleural effusion, hemothorax, hydrothorax, pneumothorax, emphysema and diaphragmatic hernia
- *Blocked air passages*—nasal obstruction, pharyngeal/laryngeal obstruction, tracheal/bronchial obstruction and bronchiolar obstruction.

Cardiovascular disease
This causes inadequate perfusion of lung:

- *Cardiac disease*—including congestive heart failure and acute heart failure
- *Peripheral circulatory failure*—shock and dehydration
- *Increased blood viscosity*—hemoconcentration including polycythemia vera (e.g. the inherited disease in cattle), and disseminated intravascular coagulopathy (DIC).

Diseases of the blood
These cause inadequate supply of oxygen to tissues and carbon dioxide discharge from tissues as a result of inadequate supply of hemoglobin:

- *Anemia*—an insufficient supply of hemoglobin
- *Altered hemoglobin*—methemoglobinemia (e.g. in nitrite poisoning, inherited methemoglobinemia of horses), carboxyhemoglobinemia.

Nervous system diseases
These affect movement of respiratory muscles by impairment of their nerve supply. In most cases the effect is one of paralysis so that hyperpnea does not occur. However, the patient is aware of the respiratory embarrassment and, technically speaking, is dyspneic. However, respiratory movements may just gradually fade away or take the form of infrequent convulsive gasps.

- *Paralysis of respiratory muscles*—in tetanus, tick paralysis, botulism
- *Paralysis of the respiratory center*—as in poisoning by nicotine sulfate
- *Stimulation of the respiratory center—neurogenic dyspnea*—stimulation of the center by a small irritative lesion, e.g. in encephalitis, in its vicinity.

General systemic states
- Pain
- Hyperthermia
- Acidosis.

Environmental causes
- Oxygen lack in altitude diseases
- Oxygen lack in fires or exposure to toxic gases.

Miscellaneous poisons
A number of poisons cause dyspnea as a prominent sign, but in most cases the pathogenesis has not been identified. *Farm chemicals* including methaldehyde and dinitrophenols (probable mechanism is stimulation of respiratory center). Organophosphates and carbamates (probable mechanism is alteration of pulmonary epithelium), urea (probably effective as ammonia poisoning). Nicotine depresses the respiratory center. *Poisonous plants*, including *fast-death* factor of algae, the weeds *Albizia, Helenium, Eupatorium, Ipomoea, Taxus* spp., and *Laburnum* and ironwood (*Erythrophloeum* sp.), also appear to act by central stimulation.

Abnormal respiratory sounds

Auscultation of the lungs and air passages is the most critical of the physical examinations made of the respiratory system. It is preferable to begin the examination by auscultating the larynx, trachea and the area of the tracheal bifurcation in order to assess the rate of air flow, and the volume of air sound to be heard over the lungs. To be effective and reliable diagnostically, auscultation must be systematic. Both the upper and lower parts of the respiratory tract must be examined in each case. Because air movement through the airways is necessary for proper auscultation it may be necessary to make the animal hyperventilate which can be done by 'bagging off' its breathing. Holding a plastic bag over the head of the animal for 1–2 minutes will usually cause hyperventilation and accentuate both normal and abnormal respiratory sounds which may not be clearly audible if the animal is breathing with less depth.

The terminology used to describe normal and abnormal lung sounds has now become much more clear than formerly and should hence be more reliable and useful as a diagnostic aid (24–27). The revised terminology is summarized in Table 32, and the identification and clinical significance of respiratory sounds are summarized in Table 33.

The clinician must carefully auscultate both the upper respiratory tract (larynx, trachea) and the entire aspects of both lung fields and interpret the sounds which are audible or not audible. The variables which must be interpreted include the nature of the sounds (increased or decreased breath sounds, crackles or wheezes), the timing of the sounds in the respiratory cycle and their anatomical location. Interpretation of these variables should indicate the nature of the lesion. Examples are summarized in Table 33.

Lung sounds can be divided into breath sounds and adventitious or abnormal sounds (25, 26). The normal breath sounds are produced by air movement through the tracheobronchial tree. These are the sounds which are audible clearly over the trachea and which are attenuated over the lungs. The clear breath sounds which are audible over the trachea and over the bifurcation of the trachea were previously known as bronchial sounds. The attenuated breath sounds audible over the lungs were previously known as vesicular sounds. It was believed for many years that bronchial sounds originated in the major airways and vesicular sounds originated in the alveoli. It is now generally accepted that air movement in terminal airways does not appear to contribute to breath sounds. The terms bronchial and vesicular sounds are gradually being replaced by the term *breath sounds*.

Abnormally loud or soft breath sounds can be attributed to either changes in sound production in the airways by changes in flow rate or altered transmission of sound through various normal or abnormal tissues or fluids in the thorax.

Table 32. Terminology for normal and abnormal lung and chest sounds (adapted from Curtis *et al.*, 1986)

Sounds	*Terms which have been replaced*	*Significance*
Normal lung sounds		
Normal breath sounds	Alveolar sounds Vesicular sounds Bronchovesicular sounds Bronchial sounds/tones	
Increased breath sounds	Increased bronchial sounds	Occurs in fever, after exercise, high environmental temperature, early pneumonia
Decreased or absent breath sounds		Shallow breathing, extreme fatness, space-occupying lesions of the thorax
Abnormal lung and chest sounds		
Increased breath sounds	Hard bronchial tones	Severe pneumonia in cattle, sheep and goats with consolidation; chronic obstructive pulmonary disease in horses (expiration)
Crackles	Moist râles Coarse crackles Fine crackles Crepitation	Acute atypical interstitial pneumonia in cattle; pulmonary adenomatosis in sheep
Wheezes	Dry râles Rhonchi	Chronic obstructive pulmonary disease in horses; chronic atypical interstitial pneumonia in cattle
Pleural friction rub		Pneumonic pasteurellosis in cattle (advanced case); pleurisy in horses (rarely); acute atypical interstitial pneumonia in cattle
Absence of breath sounds (silent lung)		Pneumothorax; pleural effusion; space-occupying mass in thorax
Stridors (due to laryngeal lesion)		Bovine diphtheria; infectious bovine rhinotracheitis (IBR) (respiratory form)
Miscellaneous sounds from thoracic area		
Crepitation in subcutaneous emphysema Expiratory grunt Heart sounds Rumen sounds Skin sounds Peristaltic sounds		

Table 33. Identification and clinical significance of respiratory sounds

Sounds	*Identifying characteristics*	*Significance*
Increased breath sounds	Increased breath sounds audible on inspiration and expiration	Occurs in fevers, after exercise, high environmental temperatures, early pneumonia
Decreased breath sounds	Decreased amplitude of breath sounds	Obese animal, cold ambient temperature
Loud breath sounds	Increased amplitude of breath sounds, begin and end abruptly, on inspiration and expiration	Any disease resulting in collapse or filling of alveoli and leaving bronchial lumen open; consolidation and atelectasis; heard commonly in cattle with severe pneumonia and calves with enzootic pneumonia where there is consolidation of the cranial lobes of the lungs
Crackles	Discontinuous, bubbling, sizzling, moist sounds primarily on inspiration; may be characterized as coarse or fine crackles	Suggests the presence of secretions and exudate in airways and edematous bronchial mucosa as in exudative bronchopneumonia, exudative tracheobronchitis, aspiration pneumonia
Loud crackling sounds	Harsh crackling sounds on inspiration and expiration	Interstitial pulmonary emphysema in cattle
Wheezes (replaces rhonchus and dry râles)	Continuous musical-type squeaking and whistling, occur primarily on expiration although they are frequently heard during both inspiration and expiration	Indicates narrowing of airways; expiratory polyphonic wheezing common in animals with chronic obstructive pulmonary disease, chronic bronchopneumonia, any species; inspiratory monophonic wheezing occurs when upper extrathoracic airways are constricted, such as in laryngeal disease
Pleuritic friction rubs	'Sandpapery' sound; dry, grating, sounds close to the surface, on inspiration and expiration, tend to be jerky and not influenced by dry coughing	Pleuritis, diffuse pulmonary emphysema in cattle with dry pleural surfaces; diminish or disappear with pleural effusion
Absence of lung sounds (silent lung)	Lung sounds not audible	Bronchial lumen filled with exudate, space-occupying mass, pleural effusion, diaphragmatic hernia
Peristaltic sounds	Intermittent intestinal sounds	Normal in cattle thoraces after eating. Does not indicate diaphragmatic hernia unless other signs present
Expiratory grunting	Loud grunting on expiration which is usually forced against a closed glottis with sudden release, audible on auscultation of the thorax, over the trachea and often audible without the aid of a stethoscope	Severe diffuse pulmonary emphysema, extensive consolidation; in acute pleurisy and peritonitis a groan is more characteristic
Laryngeal stertor (stridor)	Loud stenotic sounds on inspiration audible with or without stethoscope over the trachea	Obstruction of larynx (due to edema, laryngitis, paralysis of vocal cord); prime example is calf diphtheria

Normal breath sounds

Normal breath sounds vary in quality depending on where the stethoscope is placed over the respiratory tract. They are loudest over the trachea and base of the lung and quietest over the diaphragmatic lobes of the lung. Normal breath sounds are louder on inspiration than expiration because inspiration is active and expiration is passive in normal animals. Breath sounds may be barely audible in obese animals or in noisy surroundings which are common in field conditions. Increased breath sounds are heard in normal animals with increased respiratory rate and depth of respiration. This can occur for physiological reasons such as exercise, excitement, or a high environmental temperature. They can also occur in abnormal states such as fever, acidosis or pulmonary congestion in early pneumonia or myocardial disease.

The normal breath sounds heard over the trachea may sound abnormally loud (or soft) over the lungs due to changes in the transmission properties of the respiratory system (26). This is because when sound waves pass through structures of different physical properties, the amount of sound transmitted depends on the matching of acoustic properties of the different structure. Consolidation results in less reflection of sound at the thoracic wall and consequently more transmission to the stethoscope. Thus in consolidation the breath sounds are much louder than normal (loud bronchial sounds). Hyperinflation of the lungs can result in quiet breath sounds because of the same mechanism. In pleural effusion or pneumothorax there is almost a complete absence of breath sounds because of almost complete reflection of the breath sounds at the pleural surface due to the mismatching of the acoustic properties of the pleural tissues and fluids. Space-occupying masses between the lung and the thoracic wall also cause a relative absence of breath sounds over the site.

Abnormal (adventitious) lung and thoracic sounds

Abnormal lung sounds include increased breath sounds (increased bronchial sounds), crackles and wheezes. Crackles are discontinuous sounds and wheezes are continuous sounds (24).

Increased breath or bronchial sounds These are harsh breath sounds which approximate those heard over the trachea. They are audible on inspiration and expiration but become louder on expiration in abnormal states such as consolidation or atelectasis. Any disease in which the bronchial lumen remains open and the surrounding lung tissue has been replaced by cells, exudate or tissues (consolidation) which transmits sound without reflection will result in increased bronchial sounds.

Crackles Crackles are abnormal lung sounds described as clicking, popping or bubbling sounds. They were formerly known as moist râles and it was thought that they were due to air being forced through exudate. It is now suggested that they are caused by airways which remain closed for a portion of inspiration, and then suddenly open. The crackling is caused by the sudden equalization of pressure between the proximal and distal part of the airway (24). Crackles may thus be caused by the presence of exudate and secretions in the airways edematous bronchial mucosa. Crackling lung sounds are also audible in cattle with interstitial pulmonary emphysema. Crackling sounds may move their point of maximum intensity following coughing presumably due to movement of exudate.

Wheezes Wheezes are continuous whistling, squeaking sounds caused by vibrations of airways or air passing through a narrowed airway. They were formerly known as dry râles or rhonchi. They can be characterized as monophonic (single tone) or polyphonic (multiple tones) and by the timing of their occurrence in the respiratory cycle. Inspiratory wheezing suggests obstruction of the upper airways, usually extrathoracic. Expiratory wheezing usually indicates intrathoracic airway obstruction such as chronic obstructive pulmonary disease and distal airways which are narrowed because of tenacious exudate.

A pleuritic friction rub is a combination of continuous and discontinuous sounds produced by the rubbing together of inflammed parietal and visceral pleura. The sound is loud, coarse and usually not influenced by coughing. Pleuritic friction rubs are not common and their absence does not preclude the presence of pleuritis, particularly in the horse. Pleuritic friction rubs may also occur in cattle with severe diffuse pulmonary emphysema and the relatively dry parietal and visceral surfaces rub together during the respiratory cycle.

Absence of lung sounds A complete absence of lung sounds occurs when the breath sounds are reflected at the interface between the lung and thoracic wall by the presence of a medium such as a space-occupying mass, fluid or air. The common causes of the 'silent lung' include pleural effusion, space-occupying masses of the thorax, large pulmonary abscess, complete destruction of a lobe of lung including the terminal airways and diaphragmatic hernia (24).

Miscellaneous sounds Miscellaneous unexpected sounds which are occasionally audible over the thorax include peristaltic sounds, skin and hair sounds caused by the stethoscope, crepitating sounds due to subcutaneous emphysema and muscular contractions.

Thoracic pain

Spontaneous pain, evidenced by grunting with each respiratory cycle, usually means pleural pain, from a fractured rib, torn intercostal muscle or traumatic injury including hematoma, of the pleura, or pleurisy. A similar grunt may be obtained by thumping the animal on the chest, over the affected area, with a closed fist or a percussion hammer. Pain due to a chronic deepseated lesion cannot be detected in this way. The use of a pole under the sternum, as described under traumatic reticuloperitonitis, provides a useful alternative.

Respiratory noises

These noises—cough, sneeze, snort, snore, wheeze and roar—are also discussed in Chapter 1. Coughing and sneezing are highly coordinated reflex acts. Coughing is initiated by irritation of the respiratory mucosa of the pharynx, larynx, trachea, bronchi and bronchioles; sneezing is initiated by stimulation of the nasal mucosa. Both have the primary function of expelling material by explosive force. However, material of low viscosity may be spread further back into smaller bronchial passages, thus spreading the infection further. Coughing and sneezing are usually recorded as spontaneous acts. However, a cough test is valuable. It consists of squeezing the first few rings of the trachea—instant coughing indicates inflammation of the larynx–trachea. Sneezing is not a common occurrence in animals, but a forceful expulsion of air through the nostrils as a snort is very common.

A wheeze is a high-pitched sound made by air coming through a narrow passage, such as a stenotic nasal passage. A snore is a deeper, more guttural sound originating from the pharynx and larynx. Snoring is often intermittent, depending on the animal's posture. For example, a fat young bull will often snore when he is dozing half asleep, with his head hung down, but the snore will disappear when he is alert and his head is held up in a more normal position. A grunt, so often synonymous with pain, comes from expiring against a partly closed larynx. Common causes of respiratory noises are

- Wheezing—rhinitis, obstruction of nasal cavities
- Sneezing and snorting—rhinitis, obstruction of nasal cavities
- Cough—pharyngitis, laryngitis, tracheitis, bronchitis, pneumonia, lung abscess, pulmonary edema. The differential diagnosis of coughing in horses is of particular importance and is dealt with in some detail in the section on equine viral influenza
- Snoring—usually a chronic, obstructive lesion of the pharynx
- Stridor—laryngeal edema, laryngeal abscess
- Roar—during exercise is caused by air passing through a larynx with a small lumen, e.g. laryngeal hemiplegia in horses
- Grunt—when spontaneous occurs in pain of any sort, but usually visceral and often thoracic. When stimulated by menace it is the result of forced expulsion of air against a partly closed larynx.

Cyanosis

Cyanosis is a bluish discoloration of the skin, conjunctivae and visible mucosae caused by an increase in the absolute amount of reduced hemoglobin in the blood. It can occur only when the hemoglobin concentration of the blood is normal or nearly so, and when there is incomplete oxygenation of the hemoglobin. It can occur in all types of anoxic anoxia and in stagnant anoxia but not in anemic patients because there is insufficient hemoglobin present. On the other hand polycythemia predisposes to cyanosis. To satisfy all criteria of cyanosis the bluish discoloration should disappear when pressure is exerted on the skin or mucosa and blood flow is stopped temporarily. Methemoglobinemia is accompanied by discoloration of the skin and mucosae but the color is more brown than blue and cannot be accurately described as cyanosis. The most marked cyanosis occurs in congenital cardiac defects and is never marked in acquired heart disease. It is not usually marked in pulmonary disease unless the degree of pulmonary collapse is severe without the circulation being impeded so that blood flows through large sections of lungs without being oxygenated—a right-to-left shunt. It is also a common and life-threatening sign in severe cases of laryngeal obstruction as occurs in severe laryngitis in calves with necrotic laryngitis.

Nasal discharge

Excessive or abnormal nasal discharge is usually an indication of respiratory tract disease. Nasal discharges are common in all of the farm animal species. Cattle may remove some or all of the nasal discharge by licking with their tongue while horses do not remove any.

The nasal discharge is usually obvious but the determination of its origin and significance can be difficult and elusive. The history should determine the duration of the nasal discharge and if it has been unilateral or bilateral. The characteristics of the discharge are then noted carefully by visual inspection. The discharge may be copious, serous, mucoid, purulent, caseous, streaked with blood, foul-smelling (ozena), contain feed particles.

Nasal discharges may originate from lesions in the nasal cavities, congenital defects of the hard palate such as cleft palate in the newborn, paranasal sinuses, guttural pouch in the horse, pharynx, larynx, trachea and lungs. Diseases of the esophagus and stomach which cause dysphagia and regurgitation or vomition can also cause a nasal discharge.

A copious bilateral serous nasal discharge is characteristic of early inflammation of the nasal cavities such as in viral rhinitis. A bilateral mucoid discharge suggests inflammation of a few days duration. A bilateral purulent discharge can indicate inflammation in the upper or lower respiratory tract. A copious bilateral caseous discharge suggests an allergic or bacterial rhinitis. Foul-smelling nasal discharges (ozena) are usually associated with necrosis of tissues anywhere in the nasal cavities, the guttural pouch in the horse, or severe necrotic and gangrenous pneumonia. A bilateral foul-smelling discharge containing feed particles suggests dysphagia, regurgitation or vomition. In most cases, a chronic unilateral nasal discharge suggests a lesion of one nasal cavity. A bilateral nasal discharge suggests a lesion posterior to the nasal system.

There is not necessarily a correlation between the characteristics of a nasal discharge and the nature of any pulmonary lesions. In exudative pneumonias in cattle, mucopus is produced and is moved up the trachea and into the pharynx by the mucociliary mechanism or by coughing. Some of it is then swallowed and some may be deposited in the nasal cavities and moved forward to the external nares by ciliary action. In the horse with its long soft palate most purulent material from the lungs will be deposited in the nasal cavities and appear as a nasal discharge.

In animals with evidence of an infectious disease of the respiratory tract accompanied by a bilateral serous to mucopurulent nasal discharge it is usually assumed that the discharge is primary or secondary.

When infectious disease is suspected nasal swabs can be collected and submitted for microbiological examination. However, the mixed flora obtained may be difficult to interpret and pharyngeal swabs or transtracheal aspirates may be more reliable and representative of the lesion. Cytological examination of the discharge may reveal exfoliated cells in the case of nasal tumors or eosinophils when allergic rhinitis is present.

The determination of the anatomical origin of a nasal discharge is done by detailed visual inspection of the external nares and anterior parts of the nasal cavities using a pointed source of light. However, only a small percentage of cases will be solved by this simple method.

Physical examination of the paranasal sinuses for evidence of pain and facial deformity will assist in the diagnosis of sinusitis. Examination of the pharynx and larynx of cattle can be done simply through the oral cavity. The use of a flexible fiberoptic endoscope is necessary for detailed examination of the upper and lower respiratory tract of the horse with an undetermined nasal discharge. Radiographic examination of the strictures of the head may also be necessary.

Epistaxis and hemoptysis

Epistaxis or nosebleed is in most instances a result of disease of the mucosae of the upper respiratory tract.

However, pulmonary hemorrhage, particularly in the horse, may be manifested as epistaxis. This is discussed later under the heading of epistaxis and hemoptysis.

A small amount of serosanguineous fluid in the nostrils, as occurs in equine infectious anemia and infectious equine pneumonia, does not represent epistaxis, which must also be differentiated from the passage of blood-stained froth caused by acute pulmonary edema. In this instance the bubbles in the froth are very small in size and passage of the froth is accompanied by severe dyspnea, coughing and auscultatory evidence of pulmonary edema.

SPECIAL EXAMINATION OF THE RESPIRATORY SYSTEM

Opportunities for examination of the respiratory system by special techniques do not often arise and are not often used because of the need for expensive facilities. Nevertheless, special examinations are carried out on valuable young farm animals, horses and smaller species. For example, methods are available for measuring tidal and minute respiratory volumes in foals as an aid to the assessment of pulmonary efficiency (1).

Radiographic examination of the thorax is valuable for the differential diagnosis of diseases of the lungs of young farm animals (20). As cattle and horses become mature the increased thickness of the thoracic wall and size of the thorax results in considerable magnification of normal and abnormal tissues which makes interpretation difficult and unreliable. Radiography can assist in the recognition and differentiation of atelectasis and consolidation, intersitial and exudative pneumonias, the alveolar pattern of pulmonary disease (18), neoplasms, pleural effusions, hydropericardium and space-occupying lesions of the thorax. The radiological features of bovine respiratory disease are described (15). Bronchography, utilizing contrast agents, is of value in determining the patency of the trachea and bronchi, but general anesthesia is required to overcome the coughing stimulated by the passage of the tracheal catheter (16). Using a fluoroscope to determine the location of the catheter tip, the contrast agent can be deposited in each dependent lobe in turn. Angiocardiographic techniques are also available for the detailed investigation of diseases of the lung. Such studies may supplement pathologic studies of chronic bronchopneumonia and help to explain why treatment is ineffective (16).

When an infectious process is suspected in the respiratory system it is customary to collect samples for examination. A direct swab from the nasal passages is the simplest but least satisfactory test. The resulting bacteriological examination usually reveals a large population of normal flora. Nevertheless, the method is not without value. For example, using a special nasal swab frequent isolations of *Pasteurella haemolytica* in young bulls were associated with frequent cases of bacterial pneumonia, but the isolation was not related to the development of pneumonia in the individual calf (2). For virological purposes nasal washings are usually collected, the simplest technique being irrigation of the nasal cavities and collection into an open dish. For more reliable results swabs of the laryngeal–pharyngeal area are collected. A swab in a long covering sheath, of the type used for collecting cervical swabs from mares, is easily passed up the nostril and provides a suitable sampling method.

Nasal swabs frequently provide an unsatisfactory specimen which bears insufficient cells and secretion, and they rapidly deteriorate in transit. The development of immunofluorescent and enzyme-linked antibody methods has provided reliable systems for the diagnosis of a variety of virus diseases in the early stages of infection. A technique and apparatus is available which obtains much better samples than the conventional cotton-wool swab provides. A vacuum pump aspirates epithelial cells and secretion from the nasal passages and pharynx. Cell smears are then prepared for microscopic examination and the mucus and cells are used for conventional microbiological isolation (17).

A sputum cup is sometimes of value in obtaining a sample of tracheal mucus for bacteriological examination. The technique is practicable in cattle but good restraint and a heavy dose of an ataractic drug are necessary so that the tongue can be fully drawn and the laryngeal orifice brought into view.

Transtracheal aspiration is a highly successful method of examining the air passages for infectious agents and of aspirates for cytological examination (3–5). It is reported in horses and we find the technique adaptable to cattle, sheep and goats. A long (60 cm in horses) No. 280 polyethylene tube is passed through a 9 gauge bleeding cannula inserted into the trachea between two rings, and as low on the neck as the trachea can be palpated and where it is not obviously covered by other tissue. The skin site is prepared aseptically and an incision made after the area has been anesthetized. The cannula is removed to avoid cutting the tube and the tube pushed in as far as possible. When it passes into a bronchus it usually induces paroxysmal coughing. Then 30 ml of sterile saline are introduced from a syringe, and aspiration is attempted while withdrawing the catheter slightly. Several volumes of air may have to be discarded from the syringe in the process. Complications such as subcutaneous emphysema, pneumomediastinum (20) and cellulitis can occur which necessitates care and asepsis. Sudden movement of the cannula during the insertion of the tubing may cause part of the tube to be cut off and to fall into the bronchi but without exception this is immediately coughed up through the nose or mouth. A flexible fiberoptic endoscope may be used to visualize directly the amount of fluid which is present in the trachea and at the same time to obtain a sample (33).

The aspirates from normal horses contain ciliated columnar epithelial cells, mononuclear cell and a few neutrophils with some mucus. In suppurative pneumonia and bronchiolitis the cells are more numerous and are predominantly neutrophils, and there is much mucus. Eosinophils are rare even when allergy is suspected. Horses with hemoptysis have aspirates containing macrophages with intracytoplasmic green globules of hemosiderin. Sometimes the aspirates indicate the presence of subclinical disease of the lung.

While evaluation of tracheobronchial aspirates is now widely used in an attempt to make an etiological diagnosis of pulmonary disease for purposes of specific therapy, there are no reports which support the validity of the procedure. In one study there was little, if any, correlation between the cytological features of the individual lavage sample and the pathologic status of the lung as determined by histopathologic examination. The presence of pathogens along with evidence of cytologic changes may give useful information (4, 5). The relationships between the cytology of bronchoalveolar lavage fluid and clinical disease are variable. For example, in ponies with heaves, acute disease exacerbation is associated with increased neutrophil numbers in the bronchoalveolar fluid and a decrease during periods of disease remission (35). More clinicopathologic studies are needed in order to improve the interpretation of the laboratory analysis of tracheal aspirates (34). Inclusions and cellular changes in bronchial aspirates in horses with respiratory tract disease similar to equine herpes virus type I (EHV−1) infection have been described (36). The aspirates contained detached ciliated tufts and cytoplasmic inclusions characteristic of the specific degenerative process called ciliocytophthoria.

Paracentesis of the pleural cavity is of value when the presence of fluid in the sac is suspected. The needle should be introduced in the sixth or seventh intercostal space, below the anticipated level of fluid, and aspiration effected with a syringe. Care must be taken to avoid the pericardial sac unless a sample of pericardial fluid is specifically required. Collected fluid may be obviously purulent or bloody. Microscopic examination may be necessary to demonstrate a cellular reaction to chronic infection, or neoplastic cells, such as in diffuse mesothelioma in the horse (6).

Needle puncture of a suspected lung abscess to determine the species of bacteria present is sometimes practiced but there is the risk that infection will be spread to the pleura by this technique.

A beginning has been made in the formidable task of devising tests which will allow a calibration to be made of an animal's respiratory efficiency (7, 21). This is most important in the horse and the greyhound dog where it is necessary to know that efficiency is impaired before it becomes clinically evident. Determination of arterial levels of oxygen before, immediately after, and well after hard exercise is a highly profitable test. Biophysical tests using a spirogram and a treadmill for stationary exercise are also effective aids but their use is likely to be restricted to large research centers.

A portable system for monitoring cardiovascular and respiratory function in large animals is available (28). Pulmonary function testing of cattle is also being examined and may provide some understanding of the pathophysiology of respiratory tract disease (29).

A rigid metal or flexible fiberoptic endoscope is now standard equipment for the examination of the respiratory tract of the horse. Diseases of the guttural pouch, nasal cavity, nasopharynx, larynx and major bronchi can be identified (8).

The techniques of auscultation and percussion used in examination of the thorax are discussed in Chapter 1.

PRINCIPLES OF TREATMENT AND CONTROL OF RESPIRATORY TRACT DISEASE

Treatment of respiratory disease

Antimicrobial therapy

Bacterial infections of the respiratory tract of all species are treated with antimicrobial agents. Individual treatment is usually necessary and the duration of treatment will depend on the causative agent and the severity when treatment was begun. In outbreaks of infectious respiratory disease the use of mass medication of the feed and water supplies may be advisable for the treatment of subacute cases and for convalescent therapy. The response to mass medication will depend on the total amount of the drug ingested by the animal which is a reflection of the appetite or thirst of the animal, and the palatability of the drug and its concentration in the feed or water. The choice of drug used will depend on its cost, previous experience on similar cases and the results of drug sensitivity tests if available.

Environmental alterations

One of the most seriously neglected aspects of the treatment of respiratory tract disease in farm animals, is the failure to provide a comfortable well-ventilated environment during and after the disease episode. Affected animals should be placed in a draft-free area, which is adequately ventilated and with an abundance of bedding for comfort and warmth, particularly during their convalescence. Feed and water should be readily available and dusty feeds avoided.

Oxygen therapy

The principal ancillary treatment in diseases of the lungs should be the administration of oxygen. Oxygen therapy is not often used in large animal work but the use of a portable oxygen cylinder may find a place in tiding animals over a period of critical hypoxia until inflammatory lesions of the lungs subside. It has been used most often in valuable calves and foals. The disadvantages of oxygen therapy are that it must be given continuously, requiring constant attendance on the animal, and suitable apparatus is required or much oxygen is wasted. The use of an oxygen tent is impractical and a mask must be used, or a tube introduced into the pharynx via the nostril. An oxygen therapy mask for cattle has been adapted from a human one and is successful (9) if used with a minimum flow rate of 12 liters/min.

In cattle the nasal tube must be inserted to the correct point because passage short of this causes excessive waste of oxygen and beyond this much is swallowed (10). The length of tube inserted should equal the distance from the nostril to a point one-third of the way from the lateral canthus of the eye to the base of the ear. Insertion of a nebulizer in the system permits the simultaneous administration of antibiotics and moisture to prevent drying of the pharyngeal mucosa. The volume of oxygen used should be about 4−8 liters/min for an animal of 90 kg (200 lb) weight. In foals a flow rate of 4 liters/min appears adequate (22). In newborn foals there is no difference in $Pa\text{O}_2$ when oxygen is administered via a face mask, compared to administration at 10 litres/min via an intranasal tube (30). The ability to elevate arterial oxygen increases with age from birth to 7 days of age because of the existence of right-to-left shunts in the newborn foal (30).

Oxygen therapy is of value only when anoxic anoxia is present and oxygen saturation of the available hemoglobin is incomplete. Cases of pneumonia, pleurisy, and edema and congestion of the lungs are the ones most likely to benefit. Relief may also be obtained in emphysema but the disease is incurable and no real advantage is gained. Anemic and histotoxic anoxia are unlikely to respond and the response in stagnant anoxia is small because, although the degree of saturation of hemoglobin may be increased, the rate of blood flow through capillaries is slow and the rate of oxygen transfer to tissues is not greatly increased.

Respiratory stimulants

When depression of the respiratory center occurs the use of respiratory stimulants is advisable, but these drugs are unlikely to effect any improvement in animals in which the respiration is already deep. The most effective respiratory stimulant is carbon dioxide and this can be administered most efficiently as a mixture with oxygen containing 5–10% of carbon dioxide. Increase in the depth of respiration results and improves the intake of oxygen. Improvement in the pulmonary circulation also occurs and the chances of pulmonary congestion in recumbent animals are correspondingly reduced. The impracticability of carrying gas cylinders and supervising continuous administration of the gas reduces the suitability of the technique in large animal work and parenterally administered stimulants are generally used. Picrotoxin, leptazol (Metrazol), nikethamide (Coramine), caffeine and amphetamine sulfate are widely used for this purpose. Artificial respiration should not be neglected in acute cases and should be performed until respiration recommences or until failure to respond to the administration of a parenteral stimulant is apparent.

There is a simple device for respiratory resuscitation of newborn calves and lambs consisting of a mouthpiece, a non-return valve, a flange and an oral tube (31).

Expectorants

These are commonly used in farm animals, especially horses, and the choice of the most suitable drug for each case may improve the response obtained. Knowledge of the nature of the lesion, the character of the bronchial exudate and the type of cough are necessary before the choice can be made. When the cough is painful and exhausting and the secretion tenacious, sedative expectorants, such as ammonium or potassium salts, stimulate secretion of protective mucus and lessen the coughing. In chronic bronchitis when the cough is soft and the bronchial exudate voluminous a stimulant expectorant is more valuable. These drugs cause slight irritation and hyperemia of the respiratory mucosa and tend to stimulate healing and diminish bronchial secretions. Chronic bronchitis or bronchopneumonia is a continuous problem in horses as a forerunner to chronic obstructive respiratory disease. A proprietary product Bisolven® is much favored by horse people as a mucolytic and is well reported (23). When the cough is exhausting and interferes with activity but there is little exudation an anodyne expectorant such as morphine, codeine or heroin, or belladonna is indicated. This situation is most commonly encountered in infectious equine bronchitis.

Bronchodilators

Bronchodilatation improves ventilation and tends to correct perfusion imbalances with a resulting net improvement in oxygen exchange. The most commonly used agents are aminophylline and theophylline. However their efficacy has not been documented with clinical trials. Sympathomimetic drugs such as epinephrine and isoprotenerol are effective but little used because of their short-term action. The beta-2-adrenergic receptor selective bronchodilators, such as Clenbuterol, a new long-acting beta-2-receptor stimulant, are now being used in chronic obstructive pulmonary disease, and exert a very strong beneficial effect, temporarily at least (32). They have minimal if any cardiovascular stimulating effect.

Relief of obstructions to respiration

Obstruction of the upper respiratory tract by inflammatory or non-inflammatory lesions may necessitate a tracheotomy to permit respiratory exchange until such time as the lesions are effectively treated. The tracheotomy cannula used should fit just slightly loose to avoid the necrosis which can occur when it fits too tightly against the tracheal mucosa. The cannula must be removed and cleaned out frequently because of the formation and accumulation of dried mucus plugs. Large accumulations of fluid in the pleural cavity which may interfere with the expansion of the lungs should be removed when practicable.

Control of respiratory disease

Infectious diseases of the respiratory tract of farm animals are caused by a combination of infectious agents and predisposing causes such as inclement weather, the stress of weaning or transportation and poorly ventilated housing, each of which can weaken the defense mechanisms of the animal.

A rational approach to the control of respiratory disease would include: (*a*) obtaining an accurate clinical and laboratory diagnosis of clinically affected animals; (*b*) attempting to predict the possible occurrence of specific disease based on previous experience and introducing management techniques which minimize the effects of stressors; and (*c*) introducing immunization programs for specific diseases if deemed necessary.

It is becoming increasingly more difficult to obtain a definitive etiological diagnosis because some of the common diseases appear to be caused by multiple infections rather than a single one. Most of the infective agents which cause respiratory disease are ubiquitous in the environment and are present as normal residents in the nasal cavities of normal animals. This often creates difficulty with the interpretation of the microbiological findings in outbreaks of respiratory disease because the infectious agents can commonly be isolated from both sick and well animals (11). Thus there may be no well defined cause-and-effect relationship and the predisposing causes begin to assume major importance in any control program.

Most of the common respiratory diseases occur at certain times under certain conditions and successful control will depend on the use of management techniques before the disease is likely to occur. For example, in beef cattle, pneumonic pasteurellosis can be kept to a minimum with the use of certain management procedures which minimize stress at weaning. The incidence of pneumonia can be minimized in young bulls destined for performance testing station if they are weaned well in advance of movement to the test center (12). In

North America, bovine respiratory disease is most common in feedlots where young cattle from several different backgrounds have been mingled after having been transported long distances. Outbreaks of equine respiratory disease occur in young horses which are assembled at the racetrack for training or at horse shows.

Cattle and swine barns which are overcrowded, damp and cold during the cold winter months, and hot and stuffy during the summer months can predispose to a high incidence of pneumonia. The morbidity and mortality from pneumonia may be much higher when the ammonia concentration of the air is high or if it is dusty. The incidence of pulmonary emphysema and coughing in horses is much higher in those which are housed in barns which are dusty and not ventilated compared to horses kept outdoors (13). Bad stabling management as a major cause of coughing in horses was described almost 200 years ago but there is still a major emphasis on the clinical management of chronic coughing in housed horses using a wide spectrum of antibiotics, expectorants and other drugs (14). More consideration of good housing and ventilation is necessary. In swine, enzootic pneumonia is widespread but the effects of the pneumonia can be maintained at an insignificant level with adequate housing, ventilation and nutrition. Too much emphasis has been placed on the attempted eradication of *Mycoplasma* sp., which is extremely difficult, and insufficient on building design and ventilation methods.

Vaccines are available for the immunization of farm animals against some of the common infectious diseases of the respiratory tract. Their advantages and disadvantages are discussed under each specific disease.

In effect, the principles of control and prevention of airborne respiratory disease are based largely on keeping the levels of pathogens in the air at a low level. This can be accomplished by a combination of the following practices (19):

- The use of filtered-air positive pressure ventilation systems
- The removal of affected animals from the group
- Increasing the ventilation rate of the building unit
- Subdivision of the unit into small units each with its own ventilation system
- Continual disinfection system where appropriate and practicable
- The provision of supplemental heat so that during cold weather the ventilation can be maintained and animals will not huddle together to keep warm and thereby increase the exposure rate of infection
- The use of vaccines for specific diseases of the respiratory tract
- Effective dust control.

REVIEW LITERATURE

Adams, R. H. (1984) New perspectives in cardiopulmonary therapeutics: receptor selective adrenergic drugs. *J. Am. vet. med. Assoc.*, *185*, 966.

Beech, J. (1979) Evaluation of the horse with pulmonary disease. *Vet. Clin. N. Am.*, *1(1)*, 43.

Donaldson, A. I. (1978) Factors influencing the dispersal, survival and deposition of airborne pathogens of farm animals. *Vet. Bull.*, *48*, 83–94.

Kotlikoff, M. I. & Gillespie, J. R. (1983) Lung sounds in veterinary medicine. Part 1: Terminology and mechanisms of sound production. *Comp. cont. Educ. pract. Vet.*, 5, 634–1, 639.

Kotlikoff, M. I. & Gillespie, J. R. (1983) Lung sounds in veterinary medicine. Part 2: Deriving clinical information from lung sounds. *Comp. cont. Educ. pract. Vet.*, 6, 462–467.

Roudebush, P. (1982) Lung sounds. *J. Am. vet. Med. Assoc.*, *181*, 122–126.

REFERENCES

(1) Rossdale, P. D. (1969) *Br. vet. J.*, *125*, 157.
(2) Magwood, S. F. et al. (1969) *Can. J. comp. Med.*, *33*, 237.
(3) Larson, V. L. & Busch, R. H. (1985) *Am. J. vet. Res.*, *46*, 144.
(4) Sweeney, C. R. et al. (1985) *Am. J. vet. Res.*, *46*, 2562.
(5) Morris, D. D. (1984) *J. Am. vet. med. Assoc.*, *184*, 340.
(6) Kramer, J. W. et al. (1976) *Equ. vet. J.*, *8*, 81.
(7) Sasse, H. H. L. (1972) *Tijdschr. Diergeneeskd.*, *97*, 593.
(8) Cook, W. R. (1974) *Vet. Rec.*, *94*, 533.
(9) Weaver, B. M. Q. (1973) *Vet. Rec.*, *92*, 133.
(10) Kowalczyk, T. (1957) *J. Am. vet. med. Assoc.*, *131*, 333.
(11) Little, T. W. A. (1967) *Vet. Rec.*, *96*, 540.
(12) Andrews, A. H. (1976) *Vet. Rec.*, *98*, 146.
(13) Cook, W. R. (1976) *Vet. Rec.*, *99*, 448.
(14) Hall, S. A. (1977) *Equ. vet. J.*, *9*, 37.
(15) Lee, R. (1975) *J. Am. vet. Radiol. Soc.*, *15*, 41.
(16) Vestweber, G. E. (1977) *Bov. Pract.*, No. *12*, 55.
(17) Baskerville, A. & Lloyd, G. (1977) *Vet. Rec.*, *101*, 168.
(18) Myer, W. J. (1979) *J. Am. vet. Radiol. Soc.*, *20*, 10.
(19) Donaldson, A. I. (1978) *Vet. Bull.*, *48*, 83.
(20) Farrow, C. S. (1976) *J. Am. vet. Radiol. Soc.*, *17*, 192.
(21) Willoughby, R. A. & McDonell, W. N. (1979) *Vet. Clin. N. Am., large Anim. Pract.*, *1*(1), 171.
(22) Rose, R. J. et al. (1979) *Vet. Rec.*, *104*, 437.
(23) Pearce, H. G. et al. (1978) *NZ vet. J.*, *26*, 28.
(24) Roudebush, P. (1982) *J. Am. vet. met. Assoc.*, *181*, 122.
(25) Kotlikoff, M. I. & Gillespie, J. R. (1983) *Comp. cont. Educ. pract. Vet.*, *5*, 634.
(26) Kotlikoff, M. I. & Gillespie, J. R. (1984) *J. Am. vet. med. Assoc.*, 6, 426.
(27) Curtis, R. A. et al. (1986) *Can. vet. J.*, *27*, 170.
(28) Kvart, C. et al. (1982) *J. Am. vet. med. Assoc.*, *180*, 1227.
(29) LeKeux, P. et al. (1984) *Am. J. vet. Res.*, *45*, 342, 2003.
(30) Stewart, J. H. et al. (1984) *Equ. vet. J.*, *16*, 329.
(31) Weaver, B. M. Q. & Angell-James, J. (1986) *Vet. Rec.*, *119*, 86.
(32) Adams, R. H. (1984) *J. Am. vet. med. Assoc.*, *185*, 966.
(33) Whitwell, K. E. & Greet, T. C. (1984) *Equ. vet. J.*, *16*, 499.
(34) Lane, J. G. (1984) *Equ. vet. J.*, *16*, 483.
(35) Derksen, F. J. et al. (1985) *Am. Rev. resp. Dis.*, *132*, 1066.
(36) Freeman, K. P. et al. (1985) *J. Am. vet. med. Assoc.*, *186*, 359.

DISEASES OF THE LUNGS

Pulmonary congestion and edema

Pulmonary congestion is caused by an increase in the amount of blood in the lungs due to engorgement of the pulmonary vascular bed. It is sometimes followed by pulmonary edema when intravascular fluid escapes into the parenchyma and alveoli. The various stages of the vascular disturbance are characterized by respiratory embarrassment, the degree depending upon the amount of alveolar air space which is lost.

Etiology

Pulmonary congestion and edema is a common terminal event in many diseases but is frequently overshadowed by other disturbances. Congestion which is clinically apparent may be primary when the basic lesion is in the lungs or secondary when it is in some other organ, most commonly the heart.

Primary congestion

- Early stages of most cases of pneumonia
- Inhalation of smoke and fumes
- Anaphylactic reactions
- Hypostasis in recumbent animals.

Secondary congestion

- Congestive heart failure
- Severe overexertion in horses.

In man 'heart-strain' due to overexertion is considered to be an unlikely development, muscular activity failing when the circulation is overtaxed, but horses which are forcibly driven appear to develop this syndrome.

Pulmonary edema

This occurs chiefly as a sequel to congestion in cases of:

- Acute anaphylaxis
- Acute interstitial pneumonia
- Congestive heart failure and acute heart failure, e.g. the myocardial form of enzootic muscular dystrophy in inherited myocardiopathy of Hereford calves
- Inhalation of smoke or manure gas (6)
- Specific diseases including mulberry heart disease of swine, the pulmonary form of African horse sickness, poisoning with organophosphates, ANTU (alphanaphthyl thiourea), plant poisonings with the weeds *Hymenoxis* sp. and *Phenosciadium* sp.
- Barker and wanderer syndrome in foals, the barker syndrome in young pigs.

Pathogenesis

In pulmonary congestion much of the effective alveolar air space is lost because of engorgement of the pulmonary capillaries. The vital capacity is reduced and oxygenation of the blood is impaired. Oxygenation is further reduced by the decreased rate of blood flow through the pulmonary vascular bed. Anoxic anoxia develops and is the cause of most of the clinical signs that appear.

The vital capacity is still further reduced when edema, the second stage, occurs. The edema is caused by damage to the capillary walls by toxins or anoxia or by transudation of fluid due to increased hydrostatic pressure in the capillaries. Filling of the alveoli, and in severe cases the bronchi, effectively prevents gaseous exchange.

Clinical findings

All degrees of severity occur and only the most severe form is described here. The depth of respiration is increased to the point of extreme dyspnea with the head extended, the nostrils flared and mouth-breathing. The respiratory movements are greatly exaggerated and can be best described as heaving; there is marked abdominal and thoracic movement during inspiration and expiration. A typical stance is usually adopted, with the front legs spread wide apart, the elbows abducted and the head hung low. The respiratory rate is usually increased especially if there is hyperthermia which occurs in acute anaphylaxis and after violent exercise as well as in the early stages of pneumonia. The pulse rate is usually elevated (up to 100/min) and the nasal mucosa is bright red or cyanotic in terminal cases. In acute congestion there are hard breath sounds but no crackles are present on auscultation. When edema develops there may be little air entry so that increased breath sounds and crackles are the only audible sounds, particularly in the ventral parts of the lungs. In cases of long standing there may be emphysema with crackles and wheezes of the dorsal parts of the lungs, especially if the lesion is caused by allergy. Percussion sounds vary from normal in early congestion to dullness when there is edema.

Coughing is usually present but it is soft and moist and appears to cause little discomfort. A slight to moderate serous nasal discharge occurs in the early stage of congestion but in severe pulmonary edema this increases to a voluminous, frothy nasal discharge which is often blood-tinged.

The main importance of pulmonary congestion is as an indicator of early pathological changes in the lung or heart. Spontaneous recovery occurs quickly unless there is damage to alveolar epithelium, or myocardial asthenia develops. Severe pulmonary edema has much greater significance and usually indicates a stage of irreversibility. Death in cases of pulmonary edema is accompanied by asphyxial respiratory failure.

Clinical pathology

Laboratory examinations are of value only in differentiating the causes of the congestion or edema. Bacteriological examination of nasal swabs and a complete hematological examination, looking particularly for the presence of eosinophilia are the standard examinations which are carried out.

Necropsy findings

In acute pulmonary congestion the lungs are dark red in color. Excessive quantities of venous blood exude from the cut surface. Similar but less marked changes occur in milder forms of congestion but are only seen in those animals which die from intercurrent disease. Histologically the pulmonary capillaries are markedly engorged and some transudation and hemorrhage into alveoli is evident.

Macroscopic findings in pulmonary edema include swelling and loss of elasticity of the lungs which pit on pressure. They are usually paler than normal. Excessive quantities of serous fluid exude from the cut surface of the lung. Histologically there are accumulations of fluid in the alveoli and parenchyma.

Diagnosis

The diagnosis of pulmonary congestion and edema is always difficult unless there is a history of a precipitating cause such as overexertion or inhalation of smoke or fumes. Pneumonia usually presents itself as an alternative diagnosis and a decision cannot be based entirely on the presence or absence of hyperthermia. The best indication is usually the presence of toxemia but this again is not entirely dependable. Bacterial pneumonia is usually accompanied by some toxemia but cases of viral pneumonia are often free of it. Response to antibacterial treatment is one of the best indications, the only variable being the tendency for congestion and edema of allergic origin to recover spontaneously. In many instances there will be doubt and it is then advisable to treat the animal for both conditions.

Treatment

The treatment of pulmonary congestion and edema must first be directed at correction of the primary cause as listed under etiology. Affected animals should be confined at rest in a clean, dry environment and exercise avoided. Adrenalin is recommended in pulmonary edema due to anaphylaxis. It will have an immediate pharmacological effect which may be followed by the use of a corticosteroid to maintain vascular integrity and to decrease permeability of pulmonary vessels. Antihistamines are commonly used in conjunction with adrenaline for the treatment of acute pulmonary edema due to anaphylaxis. However, recent studies of experimental anaphylaxis in cattle and horses have shown that the antihistamines may be of limited value because histamine and serotonin are of relatively low significance as mediating substances (1). On the other hand, the kinins, prostaglandins and slow release substances may be more important (2). Studies in cattle have shown that antihistamines and 5-hydroxytryptamine (5-HT) antagonists failed to protect cattle in experimental hypersensitivity (3). Sodium meclofenamate has been more successful in antagonizing experimental anaphylaxis in cattle and horses (2, 3). Acetylsalicylic acid was more effective than antihistamines or antiserotonin agents in providing symptomatic relief in experimental acute interstitial pneumonia of calves (4). It is difficult, however, to extrapolate the results of these studies in which the drugs were usually given before or at the same time as the experimental disease was produced. There is a need for the development of the most effective antianaphylactic drugs for the treatment of acute anaphylaxis in farm animals which invariably results in pulmonary edema and emphysema. Thus adrenalin and antihistamines, which are readily available, are still the drugs of choice for the emergency treatment of pulmonary edema due to anaphylaxis.

Oxygen therapy may effectively reduce the anoxia but administration of carbon dioxide or parenteral respiratory stimulants is unlikely to have any beneficial effect. In large animals, oxygen therapy is limited to the use of a nasal catheter as described in principles of treatment in respiratory system disease. The slow intravenous administration of aminophylline will help by dilating bronchioles. Removal of fluid from the lungs may be assisted by intravenous treatment with furosemide or other quick-acting diuretic. Morphine is recommended (5), but is not a common drug in large animal dispensaries. Large doses of corticosteroids intravenously may help reduce capillary wall permeability. Reduction of foaming in the airways may be achieved with nebulized 20% ethanol.

When edema is due to organophosphate poisoning prompt administration of atropine may reduce fluid transudation. In these cases the animal is in considerable danger and repeated injections may be necessary. Details of the recommended treatment regimen are given in the section on treatment of poisoning by organophosphorus compounds.

REFERENCES

(1) Eyre, P. (1972) *Vet. Rev.*, *23*, 3.
(2) Eyre, P. (1976) *Can. J. comp. Med.*, *40*, 149.
(3) Eyre, P. et al. (1973) *Br. J. Pharmacol.*, *47*, 504.
(4) Eyre, P. et al. (1976) *Vet. Rec.*, *98*, 64.
(5) Davis, L. E. (1979) *J. Am. vet. med. Assoc.*, *175*, 97.
(6) Schoon, M. A. et al. (1985) *Dtsch Tierärztl. Wochenschr.*, *92*, 372.

Pulmonary hemorrhage

Pulmonary hemorrhage is uncommon in farm animals but does occur occasionally in cattle, and exercise-induced pulmonary hemorrhage (EIPH) occurs in 45–75% of exercised horses (1–3).

In cattle the most common cause is erosion of pulmonary vessels adjacent to lesions of embolic pneumonia. The onset of hemorrhage is usually sudden and affected animals hemorrhage profusely and die after a short course of less than 1 hour. Marked epistaxis and hemoptysis, severe dyspnea, muscular weakness, and pallor of the mucous membranes are characteristic.

Exercise-induced pulmonary hemorrhage following exercise occurs in racing Thoroughbreds, Standardbreds, Quarter Horses, Appaloosas and Polo ponies (1). It is usually first noted in 2-year-olds when they begin training. The lung is the source of the hemorrhage but the mechanism of hemorrhage is uncertain. The presence of preexisting lung disease such as chronic obstructive lung disease is thought to be a predisposing factor. It is proposed that in horses with small airway disease the vessels adjacent to the diseased areas of the lung are subjected to tremendous increase in local perivascular pressures to produce vessel rupture or tissue tearing and subsequent hemorrhage.

While up to 75% of horses may be affected by EIPH following exercise only 0·5–2·5% exhibit epistaxis. Most horses show no apparent discomfort during bleeding episodes. Swallowing is often the first indication of pulmonary hemorrhage seen by experienced trainers. If the horse lowers its head to the ground within 90 min after a race, epistaxis may be visible. The examination of the trachea with a flexible fiberoptic endoscope is necessary to detect pulmonary hemorrhage. Rarely, a horse will develop fatal pulmonary hemorrhage during a race. Because of this possibility horses with a history of epistaxis are disqualified from racing. A variety of drugs has been used for the treatment of EIPH but none has had any significant beneficial effect. The use of furosemide has been evaluated, and it may be effective in reducing the severity of the hemorrhage but does not stop it.

REVIEW LITERATURE

Clarke, A. F. (1985) Review of exercise-induced pulmonary hemorrhage and its possible relationship with mechanical stress. *Equ. vet. J.*, *17*, 166–172.

Pascoe, J. R. (1986) Pulmonary hemorrhage in exercising horses: a review. In: *Lung Function and Respiratory Diseases in the Horse. Int. Symp. Hanover, June 27–29, 1985*. Eds E. Deegen & R.E. Beadle, pp. 81–83.

REFERENCES

(1) Clarke, A. F. (1985) *Equ. vet. J.*, *17*, 166.
(2) Cook, W. R. (1974) *Equ. vet. J.*, 6, 45.
(3) Pascoe, J. R. & Rapel, C. F. (1982) *Comp. cont. Educ. pract. Vet.*, *4*, 411.

Pulmonary emphysema

Pulmonary emphysema is distension of the lung caused by overdistension of alveoli with rupture of alveolar walls with or without escape of air into the interstitial spaces. Pulmonary emphysema is always secondary to some primary lesion which effectively traps an excessive amount of air in the alveoli. It is a common clinicopathological finding in many diseases of the lungs of all species and is characterized clinically by dyspnea, hyperpnea, poor exercise tolerance and forced expiration.

Etiology

One of the most common forms of pulmonary emphysema in farm animals is chronic obstructive pulmonary disease (COPD) formerly known as 'heaves' in horses (7). COPD of horses is presented in Chapter 35 dealing with disease of unknown or uncertain etiology. The cause of the disease in horses is uncertain, but the highest incidence is in horses over 5 years of age and is usually associated with prolonged feeding of moldy or dusty feed. It is most common where horses are housed in barns for long periods and is virtually unknown where horses are kept on pasture or outdoors all year round.

In the other species pulmonary emphysema is an important lesion only in cattle although occasional cases occur in pigs. The bovine lung is highly susceptible to the development of emphysema from many different causes, not all of them respiratory in origin. In those of respiratory origin it is common to find pulmonary emphysema when the primary lesion in the lung causes trapping of air in alveoli or terminal bronchioles. A toxemia, for example, may weaken the supporting structures of the alveolar wall. Some causes of emphysema are as follows:

Cattle

- Acute interstitial pneumonia
- Parasitic pneumonia with pulmonary edema in acute anaphylaxis
- Perforation of the lung by foreign body as in traumatic reticuloperitonitis
- Poisoning by the plants *Senecio quadridentatus*, rape, *Zeieria arborescens*, *Perilla frutescens* and the fungus *Periconia* sp. are recorded as causing pulmonary emphysema in cattle
- Pulmonary abscess.

All species

- Secondary to bronchopneumonia
- Acute chemical injury—as in inhalation of welding fumes (3)
- Chlorine gas poisoning (4)
- Local or perifocal emphysema is also a common necropsy finding around local pulmonary lesions, especially atelectasis, often with no respiratory dysfunction. In calves and pigs the emphysema is sometimes sufficiently extensive to kill the animal.

Emphysema may also occur secondary to foreign body pneumonia in pigs which may inhale actual starch granules when the environment is very poorly ventilated (1). Sporadic cases of pulmonary cystic emphysema of unknown etiology occur in newborn piglets (8).

Pathogenesis

Excessive dilatation of alveoli can only occur by overstretching of the supporting and elastic tissue of the pulmonary parenchyma. There are in the main two schools of thought on the pathogenesis of pulmonary emphysema. One proposes that there is a primary deficiency in the strength of the supporting tissues which are thus unable to support the alveolar walls during coughing or exertion. The other hypothesis is that chronic bronchitis and bronchiolitis or bronchial spasm due to allergy cause obstruction of the air passages but air still enters the alveoli through the communications between them. This air accumulates, causes overdistension and finally rupture of the alveoli (5). In either case an initial lesion probably leads to an area of weakness from which emphysema spreads during coughing or exertion. In interstitial emphysema there is the additional factor of distension of the connective tissue with air and compression collapse of the alveoli. The development of interstitial emphysema depends largely upon the amount of interstitial tissue which is present and is most common in cattle and pigs. In horses the emphysema is usually purely alveolar. Whether there is simple overdistension of alveoli, or whether their walls are also ruptured, is very important in prognosis and treatment. Excellent response is often obtained in cases of apparent emphysema, especially those occurring acutely at pasture. In this circumstance one can only conclude that the lesion is functional and that the alveoli are not substantially damaged.

Emphysema which develops in association with another lesion such as atelectasis or edema is often spoken of as compensatory, as though overdistension of residual lung causes alveolar dilatation. This may be the case but it seems probable that an agent which causes the primary lesion may also reduce the strength of the surrounding, supporting tissue and cause obstruction of neighboring bronchioles with emphysema developing in the usual way as set out above.

The pathophysiology of emphysema depends upon the inefficiency of evacuation of pulmonary airspace and failure of normal gaseous exchange in the lungs. The elastic recoil of the tissue is diminished, and when the chest subsides during expiration incomplete evacuation occurs. Because of the increase in residual volume the tidal volume must be increased to maintain normal gaseous exchange. Retention of carbon dioxide stimulates an increase in the depth of respiration but maximum respiratory effort necessitated by exercise cannot be achieved. Anoxia develops and metabolism of all body tissues is reduced (6). The characteristic effect of emphysema is to produce an increase in expiratory effort necessitated by the failure of normal elastic recoil.

Interference with the pulmonary circulation results from collapse of much of the alveolar wall area and a consequent diminution of the capillary bed. The decreased negative pressure in the chest and the abnormally wide respiratory excursion also cause a general restriction of the rate of blood flow into the thorax. The combined effect of these factors may be sufficient to cause failure of the right ventricle especially if there is a primary defect of the myocardium. Acidosis may also result because of the retention of carbon dioxide.

Clinical findings

The clinical finding of chronic obstructive pulmonary disease in horses is presented in Chapter 35 on diseases of unknown or uncertain etiology.

In cattle and pigs the presence of pulmonary emphysema in pulmonary disease is not always detectable clinically. Characteristically, diffuse pulmonary emphysema causes severe expiratory dyspnea with a grunt on expiration and loud crackling lung sounds on auscultation over the emphysematous lungs. In severe cases in cattle, the emphysema is commonly interstitial and dissection of the mediastinum and fascial planes results in subcutaneous emphysema over the withers.

Clinical pathology

The retention of carbon dioxide may cause an increase in alkali reserve, and a compensatory polycythemia may develop. There are no characteristic hematological findings, but if there is a significant secondary bronchopneumonia a leukocytosis and left shift may be evident. In the appropriate location, an examination of feces for lungworm larvae may be desirable. In cases suspected of an allergic origin, swabs of nasal secretion may reveal a high proportion of eosinophils and a hematological examination may show eosinophilia. Precipitins against the fungus *Micropolyspora faeni* have also been identified in the serum of affected horses (2) and allergic stain tests have also been used (1).

Necropsy findings

The lungs are distended and pale in color and may bear imprints of the ribs. In interstitial emphysema the interalveolar septae are distended with air which may spread to beneath the pleura, to the mediastinum and under the parietal pleura. There may be evidence of congestive heart failure. On histopathological examination a bronchiolitis is present in most cases. This may be diffuse and apparently primary or orginate by spread from a nearby pneumonia.

Diagnosis

Acute emphysema in cattle and horses is often accompanied by pulmonary edema with the presence of consolidation and crackles in the ventral parts of the lungs. It may be confused with acute pulmonary congestion and edema caused by anaphylaxis but forced expiration is not a characteristic of these latter conditions.

Those cases of severe dyspnea which occur acutely and spontaneously in horses at pasture, and in which there is a marked double expiratory effort, and no febrile or toxemic response, present a problem in diagnosis. They are usually classified as acute emphysema, but they can also be considered as bronchial spasm due to acute bronchiolitis due either to infection or to allergy. Treatment with an antihistamine, or antibiotic followed by corticosteroid, can produce a dramatic improvement. Pneumonia is characterized by fever and localization of abnormal respiratory sounds which are not as marked nor as widely distributed as those of emphysema. Crackles and wheezes may occur in chronic pneumonia and are loudest at the periphery of areas of consolidation. Pneumothorax is accompanied by forced inspiration and an absence of normal breath sounds.

In young animals the diagnostic dilemma is always to decide whether or not the disease is a lungworm infestation. Mingling with donkeys is a good way of fostering the spread of lungworms in horses, and a fecal examination for larvae and response to treatment with an anthelmintic are necessary steps to a diagnosis.

Treatment

The treatment of pulmonary emphysema will depend on the species affected, the cause of the emphysema and the stage of the disease.

There is no known specific treatment for the pulmonary emphysema associated with acute interstitial pneumonia in cattle. This is discussed under that heading. The emphysema secondary to the infectious pneumonias will usually resolve spontaneously if the primary lesion of the lung is treated effectively. In valuable animals, the administration of oxygen may be warranted if the hypoxia is severe and life-threatening (6). Antihistamines, atropine and corticosteroids have been used for the treatment of pulmonary emphysema in cattle but their efficacy has been difficult to evaluate.

REVIEW LITERATURE

Cook, W. R. (1976) Chronic bronchitis and alveolar emphysema in the horse. *Vet. Rec.*, *99*, 448.

Littlejohn, A. (1979) Chronic obstructive pulmonary disease in horses. *Vet. Bull.*, *49*, 907–917.

REFERENCES

(1) Eyre, P. (1972) *Vet. Rec.*, *91*, 134
(2) Schatzmann, U. et al. (1973) *Proc. 3rd int. Conf. equ. infect. Dis., Paris*, 448.
(3) Hilderman, E. & Taylor, P. A. (1974) *Can. vet. J.*,*15*, 173.
(4) MacDonald, E. W. et al. (1971) *Can. vet. J.*, *12*, 33.
(5) Lister, W. A. (1958) *Lancet*, *276*, 66.
(6) Simpson, T. (1955) *Lancet*, *273*, 105.
(7) Littlejohn, A. (1979) *Vet. Bull.*, *49*, 907.
(8) Cooper, J. E. (1978) *Vet. Rec.*, *103*, 195.

Pneumonia

Pneumonia is inflammation of the pulmonary parenchyma usually accompanied by inflammation of the bronchioles and often by pleurisy. It is manifested clinically by an increase in respiratory rate, cough, abnormal breath sounds on auscultation and, in most bacterial pneumonias, by evidence of toxemia.

Etiology

In addition to the infectious agents which cause the pneumonia, there are predisposing factors which contribute to the susceptibility of the animal. These are of paramount importance in any consideration of pneumonia and are discussed under the headings of control of diseases of the respiratory tract and the pathogenesis of pneumonia.

Pneumonia may be caused by viruses, bacteria, or a combination of both, fungi, metazoan parasites and physical and chemical agents. Most of the pneumonias in animals are bronchogenic in origin but some originate by the hematogenous route. The pneumonias which occur in farm animals are grouped here according to species.

Cattle

- Pneumonic pasteurellosis (shipping fever)—*Pasteurella haemolytica*, *P. multocida* with or without parainfluenza-3 virus
- Enzootic pneumonia of calves—parainfluenza-3, adenovirus 1, 2 and 3, rhinovirus, bovine respiratory syncytial virus, reovirus, bovine herpesvirus 1 (the IBR virus), plus *Chlamydia* sp., *Mycoplasma* sp., *Pasteurella* sp., *Actinomyces (Corynebacterium) pyogenes*, *Streptococcus* sp. and *Bedsonia* sp., *Actinobacillus actinoides*
- Viral interstitial pneumonia in recently weaned beef calves caused by bovine respiratory syncytial virus; it may also occur in yearling and adult cattle
- Contagious bovine pleuropneumonia—*Mycoplasma mycoides*
- Acute and chronic interstitial pneumonia
- Massive infestation with pig ascarid larvae
- Lungworm pneumonia—*Dictyocaulus viviparus*
- *Klebsiella pneumoniae* infection in calves and nursing cows with mastitis caused by this organism
- Sporadically in tuberculosis caused by *Mycobacterium bovis*
- Sporadically in calf diphtheria—*Fusobacterium necrophorus*
- *Haemophilus somnus*, possibly in young cattle affected with the more common septicemic form of the disease. Its role as a primary cause is uncertain.

Pigs

- Enzootic pneumonia—*Mycoplasma* sp. with *Pasteurella* sp. secondarily
- Pneumonic pasteurellosis—*Past. multocida*
- Pleuropneumonia—*Actinobacillus (Haemophilus) pleuropneumoniae*
- Interstitial pneumonia—septicemic salmonellosis
- *Bordetella bronchiseptica, Salmonella cholerae-suis*
- Uncommonly, lungworm pneumonia
- Anthrax by inhalation causing pulmonary anthrax.

Horses

- Pleuropneumonia in mature horses due to anaerobic bacteria (7, 8)
- Newborn foals—any of the septicemias which occur at this time: *Streptococcus* sp., *Escherichia coli*, *Actinobacillus equuli*
- In immunodeficient foals, pneumonia caused by adenovirus or *Pneumocystis carinii*
- Older foals—*Corynebacterium (Rhodococcus) equi*, equine herpesvirus-1 (the EVR virus), 1A/E2 equine influenza virus
- *Dictyocaulus arnfeldi* and *Parascaris equorum* rarely cause a significant pneumonia
- As a sequel to strangles
- Rarely, as a sequel to equine viral arteritis or equine viral rhinopneumonitis in adult animals
- Glanders and epizootic lymphangitis (*Histomonas farcinicus*) usually include pneumonic lesions.

Sheep

- Pneumonic pasteurellosis (*Pasteurella* sp.) as acute primary pneumonia in feedlot lambs, or secondary to parainfluenza-3 or *Chlamydia* sp. infection
- Newborn lambs—uncommonly *Streptococcus zooepidemicus*, *Salmonella abortus-ovis*
- Severe pneumonia due to *Mycoplasma* sp. in lambs—Kageda in Iceland and Switzerland
- Symptomless pneumonias without secondary infection—adenovirus, respiratory syncytial virus, reovirus, *Mycoplasma* sp. (including *M. ovipneumoniae, M. dispar)*
- *Corynebacterium pseudotuberculosis*—sporadic cases only
- Melioidosis (*Pseudomonas pseudomallei*)
- Lungworm (*Dictyocaulus filaria*)
- Progressive interstitial pneumonia (maedi) and pulmonary adenomatosis (jaagsiekte)
- Carbolic dip toxicity.

Goats

- Pleuropneumonia caused by *Mycoplasma* strain F 38 or *M. capri* is a devastating disease
- Chronic interstitial pneumonia with cor pulmonale as a common sequel may be caused by a number of *Mycoplasma* sp., but *M. mycoides* var. *mycoides* appears to be the most commonly recorded
- Retrovirus infection.

All species

- Toxoplasmosis—rare, sporadic cases
- Systemic mycoses—lesions are focal only
- Aspiration pneumonia is dealt with as a separate entity
- Sporadic secondary pneumonia caused by *Streptococcus* sp., *Corynebacterium* sp., *Dermatophilus* sp.
- Interstitial pneumonia, pulmonary consolidation and fibrosis by toxins in plants—*Eupatorium glandulosum* in horses, *Zieria arborescens* (stinkwood) in cattle, *Astragalus* sp. in all species.

Pathogenesis

Pulmonary defense mechanisms

Under normal conditions the major airways and the lung parenchyma prevent the entry of and neutralize or remove injurious agents, so that the lung contains very few, if any, organisms beyond the terminal lung units. Many infections of the respiratory tract originate from aerosolized particles carrying infectious agents which arise external to or within the respiratory tract. In order to induce an infection by the aerosol route, an etiological agent must be aerosolized, survive in the aerosol, be deposited at a vulnerable site in the respiratory tract of a susceptible host, and then multiply. Thus the pathogenesis of these respiratory infections is related to the deposition of particles and infectious agents within the respiratory tract.

Under normal conditions a complex of biochemical, physiological and immunological defense mechanisms protects the respiratory tract from inhaled particles which could be injurious or infectious. The major defense mechanisms of the respiratory tract include aerodynamic filtration by the nasal cavities, sneezing, local nasal antibody, the laryngeal reflex, the cough reflex, the mucociliary transport mechanisms, the alveolar macrophages and the systemic and local antibody systems. Most of the research on defense mechanisms has been done in man and in laboratory animals.

Large aerosolized particles which are inhaled are removed by the nasal cavities and only small ones are able to get into the lung. In the upper respiratory tract, essentially 100% of particles more than 10 μm in diameter and 80% of particles of the 5 μm size, are removed by gravitational settling on mucosal surfaces. Particles deposited between the posterior two-thirds of the nasal cavity and the nasopharynx and from the larynx to the terminal bronchioles, land on airways lined by mucus-covered, ciliated epithelium and are removed by means of mucociliary transport mechanism. The nasopharyngeal and tracheobronchial portions of the ciliated airways transport mucus toward the pharynx where it can be eliminated by swallowing. The cilia beat most effectively in mucus at a certain elasticity, viscosity and chemical composition. Anything which interferes with the secretion and maintenance of normal mucus will interfere with the clearance of particles from the upper respiratory tract. The damaging effect of viruses on mucociliary clearance has been demonstrated in laboratory animals and in man.

Mycoplasma pneumoniae infection slows tracheobronchial clearance for as long as 1 year, suggesting a possible explanation for the predisposition to bacterial pneumonia commonly observed after these infections. Viral diseases of the upper respiratory tract of farm animals are common and a similar interference in the mucociliary transport mechanism may explain the occurrence of secondary bacterial pneumonia.

The cough reflex provides an important mechanism by which excess secretions and inflammatory exudates from the lungs and major airways can be removed from the airways and disposed of by expectoration or swallowing. In animals with relatively normal lungs, coughing represents a very effective means of expelling material. In the presence of severe tracheitis and pneumonia, coughing may result in retrograde movement of infected material to the terminal respiratory bronchioles and actually promote spread of the infection to distal parts of the lung.

Particles of the 1–2 μm size settle in the lungs through the action of gravity in the alveolar spaces, and particles below 0–2 μm settle through diffusion of air. The alveolar macrophage plays a major role in clearing inhaled particles from the lung. Under normal conditions bacteria which gain entry into the alveoli are cleared quickly and effectively in a matter of hours. Debilitating factors which interfere with the normal bacterial clearance mechanism of the lung have received considerable attention in laboratory animals and man. Very little attention has been directed to the factors which may impair bacterial clearance in domestic animals. Recent studies in calves have shown that an experimental parainfluenza-3 infection has the greatest adverse effect on the pulmonary clearance of *Past. haemolytica* which was administered by intranasal aerosol on the 7th day following the viral infection. The effect on pulmonary clearance was much less when the bacteria were given on the 3rd or 11th day following the initial viral infection.

The presence of preexisting antibody to *Past. haemolytica* eliminated the effect of the viral infection on pulmonary clearance. This represents the first scientific evidence in domestic animals that the lung clearance mechanism may be affected by a concurrent viral infection. This may have major implications in the control of some of the common infectious respiratory diseases of farm animals.

Several stressors have been associated as predisposing factors to pneumonia in farm animals. It is postulated that these stressors deleteriously affect the pulmonary defense mechanism and allow the pneumonia to develop. The commonly recognized stressors include: the weaning of beef calves in northern climates; the long transportation of beef cattle to feedlots; the collection and mixing of animals at auction marts where they may be deprived of feed and water for prolonged periods; the transportation of horses to races and shows; the housing of dairy calves in poorly ventilated overcrowded barns; and marked changes in weather.

Species susceptibility

The anatomical and physiological features of the respiratory system of cattle may predispose them to the development of pulmonary lesions much more than the other farm animal species (2). Cattle have a small physiological gaseous exchange capacity and greater resultant basal ventilatory activity. The small gaseous exchange capacity may predispose cattle to low bronchiolar or alveolar oxygen levels during exposure to high altitudes and during periods of active physical or metabolic activity. During these times, low oxygen tension or hypoxia may slow mucociliary and alveolar macrophage activity and decrease pulmonary clearance rates. The basal ventilatory activity is comparatively greater than other mammals which results in the inspired air becoming progressively more contaminated with infectious, allergenic, or noxious substances.

The bovine lung also has a higher degree of compartmentalization than other species. This may predispose to airway hypoxia peripheral to airways which become occluded. This results in reduced phagocytic activity and the retention or multiplication of infectious agents. In addition, because of the low numbers of alveolar macrophages in the bovine lung the pulmonary clearance mechanism may not be as effective as in other species. There is also a low level or atypical bioactivity of lysozyme in bovine respiratory mucus which may make cattle more susceptible to infection of the respiratory tract than other species.

Development of the disease

The process by which pneumonia develops varies with the causative agent and its virulence and with the portal by which it is introduced into the lung. Bacteria are introduced largely by way of the respiratory passages and cause a primary bronchiolitis which spreads to involve surrounding pulmonary parenchyma. The reaction of the lung tissue may be in the form of an acute fibrinous process as in pasteurellosis and contagious bovine pleuropneumonia, a necrotizing lesion as in infection with *Fusobacterium necrophorus*, or as a more chronic caseous or granulomatous lesion in mycobacterial or mycotic infections. Spread of the lesion through the lung occurs by extension but also by passage of infective material along bronchioles and lymphatics. Spread along the air passages is facilitated by the normal movements of the bronchiolar epithelium and by coughing. Hematogenous infection by bacteria results in a varying number of septic foci which may enlarge to form lung abscesses. Pneumonia occurs when these abscesses rupture into air passages and spread as a secondary bronchopneumonia.

Viral infections are also introduced chiefly by inhalation and cause a primary bronchiolitis but there is an absence of the acute inflammatory reaction which occurs in bacterial pneumonia. Spread to the alveoli causes enlargement and proliferation of the alveolar epithelial cells and the development of alveolar edema. Consolidation of the affected tissue results but again there is an absence of acute inflammation and tissue necrosis so that toxemia is not a characteristic development. Histologically the reaction is manifested by enlargement and proliferation of the alveolar epithelium, alveolar edema, thickening of the interstitial tissue and lymphocytic aggregations around the alveoli, blood vessels and bronchioles. This interstitial type of reaction is characteristic of pneumonias.

Irrespective of the way in which lesions develop, the pathological physiology of all pneumonias is based upon interference with gaseous exchange between the alveolar air and the blood. Anoxia and hypercapnia develop. In bacterial pneumonias there is the added effect of toxins produced by the bacteria and necrotic tissue, and the accumulation of inflammatory exudate in the bronchi is manifested by moist râles on auscultation. Interstitial pneumonia results in consolidation of pulmonary parenchyma without involvement of the bronchi and on auscultation loud bronchial tones are heard. These are caused by the passage of air through unobstructed bronchioles and are made more audible by the consolidation of the surrounding tissue. The presence of pleurisy is not necessarily indicative of either form of pneumonia. It occurs in both and its development depends more on the etiological agent than on the mode of development of the lesion.

Restriction of gaseous exchange occurs because of the obliteration of alveolar spaces and obstruction of air passages. In the stage before blood flow through the affected part ceases, the reduction in oxygenation of the blood is made more severe by failure of part of the circulating blood to come into contact with oxygen. Cyanosis is most likely to develop at this stage and be less pronounced when hepatization is complete and blood flow through the part ceases. An additional factor in the production of anoxia is the shallow breathing which occurs. Pleuritic pain causes reduction in the respiratory excursion of the chest wall but when no pleurisy is present the explanation of the shallow breathing probably lies in the increased sensitivity of the Hering–Breuer reflex. Retention of carbon dioxide with resulting acidosis is most likely to occur in the early stages of pneumonia because of this shallow breathing.

Clinical findings

Rapid, shallow respiration is the cardinal sign of early pneumonia, dyspnea occurring in the later stages when much of the lung tissue is non-functional. Polypnea may be quite marked with only minor pneumonic lesions and the rapidity of the respiration is an inaccurate guide to the degree of pulmonary involvement. Cough is another important sign, the type of cough varying with the nature of the lesion. Bronchopneumonia is usually accompanied by a moist, painful cough, interstitial pneumonia by frequent, dry, hacking coughs, often in paroxysms. Auscultation of the thorax before and after coughing may detect exudate in the air passages. Cyanosis is not a common sign and occurs only when large areas of the lung are affected. A nasal discharge may or may not be present, depending upon the amount of exudate present in the bronchioles and whether or not there is accompanying inflammation of the upper respiratory tract. The odor of the breath may be informative: it may have an odor of decay when there is a large accumulation of inspissated pus present in the air passages; or it may be putrid, especially in horses, when pulmonary gangrene is present.

Auscultation of the lungs is a valuable aid to diagnosis. The stage of development and the nature of the lesion can be determined and the area of lung tissue affected can be outlined. In the early congestive stages of bronchopneumonia and interstitial pneumonia the breath sounds are increased especially over the cranioventral aspects of the lungs. Crackles (moist râles) develop in bronchopneumonia as bronchiolar exudation increases, but in uncomplicated interstitial pneumonia, clear, harsh breath sounds (bronchial sounds) are audible. In viral interstitial pneumonia, wheezes may be audible due to the presence of bronchiolitis. When complete consolidation occurs in either form, loud breath sounds are the most obvious sound audible over the affected lung but crackles may be heard at the periphery of the affected area in bronchopneumonia. Consolidation also causes increased audibility of the heart sounds. When pleurisy is also present a pleuritic friction rub may be audible in the early stages, and muffling of the breath sounds in the late exudative stages. Consolidation can be detected also by percussion of the thorax or trachea.

In acute bacterial bronchopneumonia, toxemia, anorexia, depression, tachycardia and a reluctance to lie down are common. In the terminal stages, mania and a tendency to attack are not uncommon, especially in cattle.

In chronic bronchopneumonia in cattle there is chronic toxemia, rough hair coat and a gaunt appearance. The respiratory and heart rates are above normal and there is usually a moderate persistent fever. However, the temperature may have returned to within a normal range even though the animal continues to have chronic incurable pneumonia. The depth of respiration is increased and both inspiration and expiration are prolonged. A grunt on expiration and open-mouth breathing indicate advanced pulmonary disease. A copious bilateral mucopurulent nasal discharge and a chronic moist productive cough are common. On auscultation of the lungs, loud breath sounds are usually audible over the ventral half of the lungs, and crackles and wheezes are commonly audible over the entire lung fields but are most pronounced over the ventral half.

With adequate treatment in the early stages, bacterial pneumonia usually responds quickly and completely but viral pneumonia may not respond at all or may relapse after an initial response. The transient response is probably due to control of secondary bacterial invaders. In some bacterial pneumonias the same course is apparent due either to reinfection or to persistence of the infection in necrotic foci out of reach of usual therapeutic measures. The final outcome depends on the susceptibility of the causative agent to the treatments available and the severity of the lesions when treatment is undertaken. Although pleurisy is a common accompaniment of pneumonia and rarely occurs independently of it, it has been dealt with separately to facilitate the description of the two conditions. Pleuropneumonia in mature horses is now being recognized with increasing frequency.

Congestive heart failure or cor pulmonale may occur in some animals which survive a chronic pneumonia for several weeks or months (10).

Clinical pathology

Antemortem laboratory examinations consist largely of cultural examinations of nasal swabs or tracheal sputum and determination of the sensitivity of isolated bacteria to antibacterial agents. In suspected cases of pleuropneumonia the collection and culture of pleural fluid is a valuable aid to diagnosis (8). In equine pleuropneumonia both anaerobic and aerobic bacteria must be considered (7, 8). Transtracheal aspiration has been described earlier and is a valuable tool for an intensive investigation of a respiratory tract infection. It needs to be remembered that the tract is normally highly contaminated, and the quality and quantity of the contaminants varies with the environment (1). Radiographic examination is undertaken only in animals of suitable size. Hematological observations usually reveal a leukocytosis and a shift to the left in bacterial pneumonias. A leukopenia and lymphopenia occurs in some cases of acute viral pneumonia. In viral pneumonia, the serological testing of acute and convalescent sera, in addition to isolation of the virus, is useful supporting evidence of the presence of an active infection.

Necropsy findings

Gross lesions are usually observed in the anterior and dependent parts of the lobes, and even in fatal cases where much of the lung is destroyed, the dorsal parts of the lobes may be unaffected. The gross lesions vary a great deal depending upon the type of pneumonia present. Bronchopneumonia is characterized by the presence of serofibrinous or purulent exudate in the bronchioles, and lobular congestion or hepatization. In the more severe, fibrinous forms of pneumonia there is gelatinous exudation in the interlobular septae and an acute pleurisy, with shreds of fibrin present between the lobes. In interstitial pneumonia the bronchioles are clean and the affected lung is sunken, dark red in color and has a granular appearance under the pleura and on the cut surface. There is often an apparent, firm thickening of the interlobular septae. These differences are readily detected on histological examination. In chronic bronchopneumonia of cattle there is consolidation, fibrosis, fibrinous pleuritis, interstitial and bullous emphysema, bronchi filled with exudate, bronchiectasis and pulmonary abscessation (3). Lesions typical of the specific infections listed under etiology are described under the headings of the specific diseases.

Diagnosis

There are two major difficulties in the clinical diagnosis of pneumonia. The first is to decide that the animal has pneumonia, the second problem is to determine the nature of the pneumonia and its cause. The suspected cause will dictate the clinical management and more particularly in infectious pneumonias the kind of antimicrobial therapy used.

There are two kinds of errors made in the clinical diagnosis of pneumonia. One is that the pneumonia is not detected clinically because the abnormal lung sounds are apparently not obvious. The other is to make a diagnosis of pneumonia, because of the presence of dyspnea which was due to disease in some other body system.

The major clinical findings of pneumonia are polypnea in the early stages and dyspnea later, abnormal lung sounds, and fever and toxemia in bacterial pneumonia. Polypnea and dyspnea may result from involvement of other body systems. Congestive heart failure, the terminal stages of anemia, poisoning by histotoxic agents such as hydrocyanic acid, hyperthermia and acidosis are accompanied by respiratory embarrassment, but not by the abnormal sounds typical of pulmonary involvement. Pulmonary edema and congestion, embolism of the pulmonary artery and emphysema are often mistaken for pneumonia, but can usually be differentiated by the absence of fever and toxemia, on the basis of the history and on auscultation findings.

Once the clinician has decided that pneumonia is present the next step is to determine the nature and cause of the pneumonia. All of the practical laboratory aids described earlier should be used when necessary. This is of particular importance when outbreaks of pneumonia are encountered in which case necropsy examination of selected cases is indicated. In single routine cases of pneumonia the cause is usually not determined. However, the age and class of the animal, the history and epidemiological findings and the clinical findings can usually be correlated and a presumptive etiological diagnosis made.

Pleuritis is characterized by shallow, abdominal-type respiration, by pleuritic friction sounds when effusion is minimal, and a muffling of lung sounds and a fluid line detectable by auscultation and percussion when fluid is plentiful. Thoracocentesis reveals the presence of fluid.

Pulmonary consolidation, which may include fibrosis, also occurs in some plant poisonings, e.g. *Eupatorium glandulosum* in horses, *Zieria arborescens* (stinkwood) in cattle and *Astragalus* sp. in all species.

In pneumothorax there is inspiratory dyspnea and on the affected side the abnormalities include: an absence of breath sounds over the lobes but still audible over the base of the lung; an increase in the absolute intensity of the heart sounds; and increased resonance on percussion.

Diseases of the upper respiratory tract such as laryngitis

and tracheitis are accompanied by varying degrees of inspiratory dyspnea which is often loud enough to be audible without a stethoscope. In less severe cases, auscultation of the mid-cervical trachea will reveal moist wheezing sounds on inspiration. These sounds are transmitted down into the lungs and are audible on auscultation of the thorax. These transmitted sounds must not be interpreted as due to pneumonia. In some cases of severe laryngitis and tracheitis the inspiratory sounds audible over the trachea and lungs are markedly reduced because of almost total obliteration of these organs. In laryngitis and tracheitis there is usually a more frequent cough than in pneumonia and the cough can be readily stimulated by squeezing the larynx or trachea. In pneumonia the abnormal lung sounds are audible on both inspiration and expiration. Examination of the larynx through the oral cavity in cattle and with the aid of a rhinolaryngoscope in the horse will usually reveal the lesions.

Treatment

In specific infections as listed above, isolation of affected animals and careful surveillance of the remainder of the group to detect cases in the early stages should accompany the administration of specific antibacterial drugs or biological preparations to affected animals. The choice of antibacterial agent will depend on the tentative diagnosis, the experience with the drug in previous cases and the results of drug sensitivity tests. The common bacterial pneumonias of all species will usually recover quickly (24 hours) if treated with an adequate dose of the drug of choice early in the course of the disease. Animals with severe pneumonia will require daily treatment for several days until recovery occurs. Those with bacterial pneumonia and toxemia must be treated early on an individual basis. Each case should be identified and carefully monitored for failure to recover, and an assessment made.

Antimicrobial agents in a longacting base may be used to provide therapy over a 4–6 day period instead of the daily administration of the shorter-acting preparations. However, the blood levels from the longacting preparations are not as high as the shorter-acting preparations and may not be as effective in severely affected animals. The common causes for failure to respond favorably to treatment for bacterial pneumonia include: advanced disease when treatment was undertaken; the development of pleurisy and pulmonary abscesses; drug-resistant bacteria; inadequate dosage of drug, and the presence of other lesions or diseases which do not respond to antibacterial drugs.

There is no specific treatment for the viral pneumonias and while many of the *Mycoplasma* spp. are sensitive to antibiotics *in vitro*, the pneumonias caused by them do not respond favorably to treatment. This may be due to the intracellular location of the *Mycoplasma* making them inaccessible to the drugs. Because viral and mycoplasmal pneumonias are commonly complicated by secondary bacterial infections, it is common practice to treat acute viral and mycoplasmal pneumonias with antibacterials until recovery is apparent.

In outbreaks of pneumonia where many animals are affected and new cases occur each day for several days, the use of mass medication of the feed and/or water supplies should be considered. Outbreaks of pneumonia in swine herds, lamb feedlots, veal calf enterprises and beef feedlots are usually ideal situations for mass medication through the feed or water. Mass medication may assist in the early treatment of subclinical pneumonia and is a labor-saving method of providing convalescent therapy to animals which have been treated individually. The major limitation of mass medication is the uncertainty that those animals which need the drug will actually get the drug in the amounts necessary to be effective. Total daily water intake by animals is a function of total dry matter intake and wellbeing, and the water consumption is therefore markedly reduced in toxemic animals. The provision of a reliable concentration of the drug in the water supply on a 24 hour basis is also a problem. However, with careful calculation and monitoring, mass medication can be a valuable and economical method of treating large numbers of animals. The method of calculating the amount of antimicrobials to be added to the feed or water supplies is presented in Chapter 4 on antimicrobial therapy.

When outbreaks of pneumonia occur and new cases are being recognized at the rate of 5–10% per day of the total in the group, all the remaining in-contact animals may be injected with an antimicrobial in a longacting base. This may help to treat subclinical cases before they become clinical and thus 'abort' the outbreak. A brief review of the principles of antibacterial therapy for pulmonary infection is available (5).

Corticosteroids have been used for their anti-inflammatory effect in the treatment of acute pneumonia. However, there is no clinical evidence that they are beneficial. When used as supportive therapy in bronchopneumonia in feedlot cattle there was no beneficial effect and the treatment response was not as good as when antibiotics alone were used (4).

Bronchodilators such as Clenbuterol (11) and non-steroidal anti-inflammatory drugs (NSAIDs) (12) are being evaluated as adjunctive therapy in the treatment of pneumonia in cattle and horses. In some cases there may appear to be a temporary beneficial effect but additional clinical trials are necessary to determine the cost effectiveness. In calves with bronchopneumonia the main effect of Clenbuterol is to increase dynamic compliance (13). Beta-adrenergic receptors are present in bovine lung airways and Clenbuterol may be effective in alleviating some of the respiratory distress associated with bronchopneumonia (14).

Affected animals should be housed in warm, well-ventilated, draft-free accommodation, provided with ample fresh water, and light nourishing food. During convalescence premature return to work or exposure to inclement weather should be avoided. If the animal does not eat, oral or parenteral force-feeding should be instituted. If fluids are given intravenously care should be exercised in the speed with which they are administered. Injection at too rapid a rate may cause overloading of the right ventricle and death due to acute heart failure.

Supportive treatment may include the provision of oxygen, if it is available, especially in the critical stages when hypoxia is severe. In foals the oxygen can be administered through an intranasal tube passed back to the nasopharynx and delivered at the rate of about 8 liters/min for several hours (6). Respiratory stimulants serve no useful purpose in pneumonia but expectorants may have value in chronic cases and during convalescence.

REVIEW LITERATURE

Cohen, A. V. & Gold, W. M. (1975) Defense mechanisms of the lungs. *Am. Rev. Physiol.*, *37*, 325.

Newhouse, M. et al. (1976) Lung defense mechanisms. *N. Engl. J. Med.*, *295*, 990, 1045.

Thomson, R. G. & Gilka, F. (1974) A brief review of pulmonary clearance of bacterial aerosols emphasizing aspects of particular relevance to veterinary medicine. *Can. vet. J.*, *15*, 99.

REFERENCES

(1) Mansmann, R. A. & Strouss, A. A. (1976) *J. Am. vet. med. Assoc.*, *169*, 631.
(2) Veit, H. P. & Farrell, R. L. (1978) *Cornell Vet.*, *68*, 555.
(3) Vestweber, G. E. (1977) *Bov. Pract.*, No. *12*, 55.
(4) Christie, B. M. et al. (1977) *Bov. Pract.*, No. *12*, 115.
(5) Larson, V. L. (1980) *J. Am. vet. med. Assoc.*, *176*, 1091.
(6) Rose, R. J. et al. (1979) *Vet. Rec.*, *104*, 437.
(7) Sweeney, C. R. et al. (1985) *J. Am. vet. med. Assoc.*, *187*, 721.
(8) Bernard-Strother, S. & Mansmann, R. A. (1985) *Comp. cont. Educ. pract. Vet.*, *7*, S341.
(9) Linklater, K. A. et al. (1982) *Vet. Rec.* *110*, 33.
(10) Gay, C. C. & Richards, W. P. C. (1983) *Aust. vet. J.*, *60*, 274.
(11) Behrens, H. J. (1983) *Tierarztl. Umschau*, *38*, 628.
(12) Selman, I. E. et al. (1984) *Vet. Rec.*, *115*, 101.
(13) Nuytten, J. et al. (1986) *Vet. res. Commun.*, *10*, 463.
(14) Nuytten, J. et al. (1986) *Vet. res. Commun.*, *10*, 453.

Aspiration pneumonia

Aspiration or inhalation pneumonia is a common and serious disease of farm animals. Most cases occur after careless drenching or passage of a stomach tube during treatment for other illness. Even when care is taken these procedures are not without risk. Other causes include the feeding of calves and pigs on fluid feeds in inadequate troughing, inhalation occurring in the struggle for food. Dipping of sheep and cattle when they are weak, or by keeping their heads under for too long, also results in inhalation of fluid. Vomiting in ruminants and horses may be followed by aspiration, especially in cattle with parturient paresis or during the passage of a stomach tube if the head is held high. Rupture of a pharyngeal abscess during palpation of the pharynx or passage of a nasal tube may cause sudden aspiration of infective material. Animals suffering from paralysis or obstruction of the larynx, pharynx or esophagus may aspirate food or water when attemping to swallow. Aspiration pneumonia is the constant lesion of crude oil poisoning in cattle and probably results from vomiting or regurgitation.

Although farm animals fed on dusty feeds inhale many dust particles and bacteria which can be readily isolated from the lung, this form of infection rarely results in the development of pneumonia. Much of the dust is filtered out in the bronchial tree and does not reach the alveoli. However, this may be of importance in the production of the primary bronchiolitis which so often precedes alveolar emphysema in horses. The inhalation of feed particles in pigs in a very poorly ventilated environment has been demonstrated to cause foreign body pneumonia (1). Also a dry, dusty atmosphere can be created in a piggery by overfrequent changing of wood shavings used as bedding, and this can lead to the production of foreign body pneumonia (2). Liquids and droplets penetrate to the depths of the alveoli and run freely into the dependent portions, and aspiration pneumonia often results. An uncommon but important effect of aspiration with lodgement of food at the glottis is the production of asphyxia or sudden death due to vagal inhibition and cessation of respiration and circulation.

If large quantities of fluid are aspirated after passage of a stomach tube into the trachea death may be almost instantaneous, but with smaller quantities the outcome may depend on the composition of the aspirated material. Absorption from the lungs is very rapid and soluble substances such as chloral hydrate and magnesium sulfate exert their systemic pharmacologic effects very rapidly. With insoluble substances and vomitus the more common occurrence is the development of a pneumonia with profound toxemia which is usually fatal in 48–72 hours. Signs of pneumonia, including polypnea, cough and the presence of râles, consolidation and an associated pleuritic friction rub, are present but the latter may be localized. The severity of aspiration pneumonia depends largely upon the bacteria which are introduced although in animals the infection is usually mixed, causing in many cases an acute gangrenous pneumonia which may be manifested by a putrid odor on the breath, or extensive pulmonary suppuration. Occasionally animals survive the acute stages but persist in a state of chronic ill-health due to the presence of pulmonary abscess.

If the lesion is well advanced treatment is not often effective but treatment with a broad-spectrum antibiotic or sulfonamide may prevent development of the disease if administered soon after aspiration occurs.

REFERENCES

(1) Jericho, K. W. F. & Harries, N. (1975) *Can. vet. J.*, *16*, 360.
(2) Jericho, K. W. F. (1975) *Vet. Pathol.*, *12*, 415.

Caudal vena caval thrombosis and embolic pneumonia in cattle (posterior vena caval thrombosis, PVCT)

Embolic pneumonia as a sequel to thrombosis of the posterior vena cava is a relatively common disease of cattle in Europe and the United Kingdom (1–4). The disease is rare in cattle less than 1 year old although it can occur at any age. A preponderance of affected animals are in feedlots on heavy grain diets and there are peaks of incidence at those times of the year when most cattle are on such diets (8). There is an obvious relationship between the occurrence of this disease and that of hepatic abscessation arising from lactic acid-induced rumenitis on heavy grain diets.

The etiology and pathogenesis of the disease are based on the development of a thrombus in the posterior vena cava, and the subsequent shedding of emboli which lodge in the pulmonary artery causing embolism, endarteritis, multiple pulmonary abscesses and chronic suppurative pneumonia (5). Pulmonary hypertension develops in the pulmonary artery, leading to the development of aneurysms, which may rupture causing massive intrapulmonary or intrabronchi hemorrhage. In most cases the thrombi in the vena cava originate from hepatic abscesses, or postdiaphragmatic abscesses. Usually there is an initial phlebitis and the subsequent thrombus extends into the thoracic part of the vessel. When the thrombus occludes the openings of the hepatic veins into the vena cava, there is congestion of the liver and hepatomegaly, and ascites and abdominal distension in some of these cases.

The most common form of the disease is characterized by manifestations of respiratory tract disease (10). Commonly there is a history of respiratory tract disease for a few weeks or longer but some animals are 'found dead' without prior recorded illness. There is usually an increase in the rate and depth of respiration, coughing, epistaxis and hemoptysis, anemia with pallor, a hemic murmur and a low PCV. Respirations are painful and a mild expiratory grunt or groan may be audible with each respiration. Subcutaneous emphysema and frothing at the mouth are evident in some. Deep palpation in the intercostal spaces and over the xiphoid sternum may elicit a painful grunt. The lung sounds may be normal in the early stages but with the development of pulmonary arterial lesions, embolic pneumonia and collapse of affected lung there are widespread rhonchi audible on auscultation. In one series of cases the presence of anemia, hemoptysis and widespread rhonchi were considered to be characteristic features of the disease (7). There are accompanying non-specific signs of inappetence, ruminal stasis and scant feces.

About one-third of affected cattle become progressively worse over a period of 2–18 days with moderate to severe dyspnea, and die of acute or chronic anemia, or are euthanized on humane grounds. Almost half of the cases die suddenly due to voluminous intrabronchial hemorrhage. It is probably the only common cause in cattle of acute hemorrhage from the respiratory tract which causes the animal to literally drop dead. The remainder have a brief, acute illness of about 24 hours.

Some evidence of hepatic involvement is often present, including enlargement of the liver, ascites, and melena. Chronic cor pulmonale develops in some with attendant signs of congestive heart failure.

Radiographic examination of the thorax of some affected animals (3) have revealed an increase in lung density and markings. These are irregular, focal or diffuse, and non-specific. More distinct opacities are present in some and are referable to embolic infarcts and larger pulmonary hemorrhages.

A neutrophilia with a regenerative left shift and a hypergammaglobulinemia due to chronic infection are common.

The necropsy findings include a large pale thrombus in the posterior vena cava between the liver and the right atrium. Occlusion of the posterior vena cava results in hepatomegaly and ascites. Hepatic abscesses of varying size and number are common and often near the wall of the thrombosed posterior vena cava. Pulmonary thromboembolism with multiple pulmonary abscesses, suppurative pneumonia and erosion of pulmonary arterial walls with intrapulmonary hemorrhage are also common. The lungs reveal emphysema, edema and hemorrhage. A variety of bacteria including streptococci, *Escherichia coli,* staphylococci and *Fusobacterium necrophorum* are found in the abscesses in the liver (9).

Animals which die suddenly are found lying in a pool of blood and necropsy reveals large amounts of clotted blood in the bronchi and trachea.

The disease must be differentiated from verminous pneumonia, chronic aspiration pneumonia, pulmonary endarteritis due to endocarditis, chronic atypical interstitial pneumonia. There is no treatment which is likely to have any effect on the disease and the principal task is to recognize the disease early and slaughter the animal for salvage if possible.

REVIEW LITERATURE

Gudmundson, J., Radostits, O. M. & Doige, C. E. (1980) Pulmonary thromboembolism in cattle due to thrombosis of the posterior vena cava associated with hepatic abscessation. *Can. vet. J.*, *19*, 304.

REFERENCES

(1) Wagenaar, G. (1965) *Tijdschr. Diergeneeskd.*, *90*, 873.
(2) Stober, V. M. (1966) *Schweiz. Arch. Tierheilkd.* *108*, 631.
(3) Breeze, R. G. et al. (1976) *Bov. Practnr*, *11*, 64.
(4) Breeze, R. G. et al. (1976) *Vet. Ann.*, *16*, 52.
(5) Breeze, R. G. et al. (1976) *J. Pathol.*, *119*, 229.
(6) Rebhun, W. et al. (1980) *J. Am. vet. med. Assoc.*, *176*, 1366.
(7) Selman, I. E. et al. (1974) *Vet. Rec.*, *94*, 459.
(8) Gudmundson, J. et al. (1980) *Can. vet. J.*, *19*,304.
(9) Fautsch, R. P. D. (1978) *Vet. Mexico*, *9*, 77.

Cranial vena caval thrombosis

Several cases of thrombosis have been recorded in the cranial vena cava in cows. As in caudal vena caval thrombosis a number of pulmonary abscesses develop causing respiratory signs including cough, hyperpnea and poor exercise tolerance. Pulmonary hypertension is not a feature as it is in the caudal lesion. However, increased jugular vein pressure, dilatation of the jugular vein and local edema may all occur (1). Cases in young animals are also recorded and it is suggested that they arise from navel infection.

REFERENCE

(1) Breeze, R. G. & Petrie, L. (1977) *Vet. Rec.*, *101*, 130.

Pulmonary abscess

The development of single or multiple abscesses in the lung causes a syndrome of chronic toxemia, cough and emaciation. Suppurative bronchopneumonia may follow.

Etiology

Pulmonary abscesses may be part of a primary disease or arise secondarily to diseases in other parts of the body.

Primary diseases

- Tuberculosis
- Actinomycosis rarely occurs as granulomatous pulmonary lesions
- Aerogenous infections with 'systemic' mycoses, e.g.

coccidioidomycosis, aspergillosis, histoplasmosis, cryptococcosis and moniliasis
- Sequestration of an infected focus, e.g. strangles in horses, caseous lymphadenitis in sheep
- *Corynebacterium (Rhodococcus) equi* pulmonary abcesses of foals (13).

Secondary diseases
- Sequestration of an infected focus of pneumonia, e.g. bovine pleuropneumonia, often after prolonged antibiotic therapy
- Emboli from endocarditis, caudal or cranial vena caval thrombosis, metritis, mastitis, omphalophlebitis
- Aspiration pneumonia from milk fever in cows, drenching accident in sheep—residual abscess
- Penetration by foreign body in traumatic reticuloperitonitis.

Pathogenesis

Pulmonary abscesses may be present in many cases of pneumonia and are not recognizable clinically. In the absence of pneumonia, pulmonary abscess is usually a chronic disease, clinical signs being produced by toxemia rather than by interference with respiration. However, when the spread is hematogenous and large numbers of small abscesses develop simultaneously, polypnea and hyperpnea appear, caused probably by stimulation of stretch receptors in the alveolar walls or by the sudden development of extensive embolic endarteritis. In these animals the respiratory embarrassment cannot be explained by the reduction in vital capacity of the lung. However, in more chronic cases the abscesses may reach a tremendous size and cause respiratory difficulty by obliteration of large areas of lung tissue. In rare cases, erosion of a pulmonary vessel may occur resulting in pulmonary hemorrhage and hemoptysis.

In many cases there is a period of chronic illness of varying degree when the necrotic focus is walled off by connective tissue. Exposure to environmental stress or other infection may result in a sudden extension from the abscess to produce a fatal, suppurative bronchopneumonia, pleurisy or empyema.

Clinical findings

In typical cases there is dullness, anorexia, emaciation and a fall in milk yield in cattle. The temperature is usually moderately elevated and fluctuating. Coughing is marked. The cough is short and harsh and usually not accompanied by signs of pain. Intermittent episodes of bilateral epistaxis and hemoptysis may occur which may terminate in fatal pulmonary hemorrhage following erosion of an adjacent large pulmonary vessel. Respiratory signs are variable depending on the size of the lesions, and although there is usually some increase in the rate and depth this may be so slight as to escape notice. When the abscesses are large (2–4 cm in diameter) careful auscultation and percussion will reveal the presence of a circumscribed area of dullness over which no breath sounds are audible. Crackles are often audible at the periphery of the lesion.

Multiple small abscesses may not be detectable on physical examination but the dyspnea is usually more pronounced. There may be a purulent nasal discharge and fetid breath but these are unusual unless bronchopneumonia has developed from extension of the abscess.

Most cases progress slowly and many affected animals have to be discarded because of chronic ill health; others terminate as a bronchopneumonia or emphysema. A rare sequel is the development of hypertrophic pulmonary osteoarthropathy.

The clinical findings of *Corynebacterium (Rhodococcus) equi* pulmonary abscessation in young foals is presented under that disease.

Clinical pathology

Examination of nasal or tracheal mucus may determine the causative bacteria, but the infection is usually mixed and interpretation of the bacteriological findings is difficult. Radiographic examination in young animals can be used to detect the presence of the abscess and give some information on its size and location. Hematological examination may give an indication of the severity of the inflammatory process but the usual leukocytosis and shift to the left may not be present when the lesion is well encapsulated.

Necropsy findings

An accumulation of necrotic material in a thick walled fibrous capsule is usually present in the ventral border of a lung, surrounded by a zone of bronchopneumonia or pressure atelectasis. In sheep there is often an associated emphysema. In rare cases the abscess may be sufficiently large to virtually obliterate the lung. A well-encapsulated lesion may show evidence of recent rupture of the capsule and extension as an acute bronchopneumonia. Multiple small abscesses may be present when hematogenous spread has occurred.

Diagnosis

The diagnosis may not be obvious when respiratory distress is minimal and especially when multiple, small abscesses are present. These cases present a syndrome of chronic toxemia which may be mistaken for splenic or hepatic abscess. Differentiation between tuberculous lesions and non-specific infections may require the use of the tuberculin test. Focal parasitic lesions, such as hydatid cysts, may cause a similar syndrome, but are not usually accompanied by toxemia or hematological changes. Pulmonary neoplasms usually cause chronic respiratory disease, a progressive loss of weight and lack of toxemia.

Treatment

Treatment is not usually successful. The daily administration of large doses of antibiotics for several days may be attempted but is usually not effective and slaughter for salvage or euthanasia is necessary. The recommended treatment for pulmonary abscessation due to *Corynebacterium (Rhodococcus) equi* infection in foals is a combination of erythromycin 25 mg/kg three times daily and rifampicin 5 mg/kg twice daily for 4–9 weeks (13).

Pulmonary neoplasms

Primary neoplasms of the lungs, including carcinomas and adenocarcinomas, are rare in animals (1–3) and metastatic tumors also are relatively uncommon in large animals. Pulmonary adenocarcinoma is the most commonly reported primary lung tumor in cattle (10). The ultrastructure and origin of some of these have been characterized (12). An asymptomatic, squamous-cell type tumor, thought to be a benign papilloma, has been observed in 10 of a series of 1600 adult angora goats (4). The lesions were mostly in the diaphragmatic lobes, were multiple in 50% of the cases and showed no evidence of malignancy although some had necrotic centers. Six cases of 'granular-cell myoblastoma' have been reported in horses, none of whom showed any clinical signs of illness (5). Malignant melanomas in adult gray horses and lymphomatosis in young cattle may be accompanied by pulmonary localization. Clinical findings are those usually associated with the decrease in vital capacity of the lungs, and include dyspnea which develops gradually, cough and evidence of local consolidation on percussion and auscultation. There is no fever or toxemia and a neoplasm may be mistaken for a chronic, encapsulated, pulmonary abscess. In the latter there may be no evidence of inflammation, and the total and differential white cell counts may be normal.

A pleural mesothelioma in a 13-year-old Thoroughbred stallion caused a similar syndrome plus accumulation of a large volume of clear serous fluid in the thorax (6). A myoblastoma in the lung of a 13-year-old mare also caused coughing, anorexia, weight loss, muffled lung sounds and edema of the legs (8). A mesothelioma causing dyspnea and cyanosis is described in an aged goat. Respiratory and cardiac sounds were absent from one side of the chest (9).

Thymoma, or lymphosarcoma as a part of the disease bovine viral leukosis, is not uncommon in cattle and may resemble pulmonary neoplasm but there is usually displacement and compression of the heart resulting in displacement of the apex beat and congestive heart failure. The presence of jugular engorgement, ventral edema, tachycardia, chronic tympany and hydropericardium may cause a mistaken diagnosis of traumatic pericarditis. Mediastinal tumor or abscess may have a similar effect. Metastasis to the bronchial lymph nodes may cause obstruction of the esophagus with dysphagia, and in cattle chronic ruminal tympany. This tumor is also common in goats, many of which show no clinical illness (1).

Occasional intrathoracic space-occupying masses occur in the thorax, and radiographic techniques and nuclear scientigraphy can be used to characterize their nature (11).

REFERENCES

(1) Monlux, A. W. et al. (1956) *Am. J. vet. Res.*, *17*, 646.
(2) Cotchin, E. (1956) *Neoplasms of the Domesticated Animals*. Farnham Royal, Bucks: Commonwealth Agricultural Bureau.
(3) Swoboda, R. (1964) *Pathol. vet.*, *1*, 409.
(4) Pearson, E. G. (1961) *Cornell Vet.*, *51*, 13.
(5) Misdorp, W. & Gelder, H. L. N. (1968) *Pathol. vet.*, *5*, 385.
(6) Kolbl, S. (1979) *Wien Tierarztl. Monatsschr.* *66*, 22.
(7) Hadlow, W. J. (1978) *Vet. Pathol.*, *15*, 153.
(8) Parker, G. A. et al. (1979) *J. comp. Pathol.*, *89*, 421.
(9) McCullogh, K. G. et al. (1979) *Vet. Pathol.*, *16*, 119.
(10) Scarratt, K. W. et al. (1984) *J. Am. vet. med. Assoc.*, *185*, 1549.
(11) Hornof, W. J. et al. (1982) *J. Am. vet. med. Assoc.*, *180*, 1319.
(12) Kadota, K. et al. (1986) *J. comp. Pathol.*, *96*, 407.
(13) Hillidge, C. J. (1986) *Vet. Rec.*, *119*, 261.

DISEASES OF THE PLEURA AND DIAPHRAGM

Hydrothorax and hemothorax

The accumulation of edematous transudate or whole blood in the pleural sacs is manifested by respiratory embarrassment caused by collapse of the ventral parts of the lungs.

Etiology

Hydrothorax and hemothorax are lesions occurring as part of a number of diseases.

Hydrothorax

- As part of a general edema due to congestive heart failure or hypoproteinemia
- As part of African horse sickness or bovine viral leukosis
- Chylous hydrothorax, very rarely due to ruptured thoracic duct.

Hemothorax

- Traumatic injury to chest wall
- Hemangiosarcoma of pleura.

Pathogenesis

Accumulation of fluid in the pleural sac causes compression atelectasis of the ventral portions of the lungs and the degree of atelectasis governs the severity of the resulting dyspnea. Compression of the atria by fluid may cause an increase in venous pressure in the great veins.

Clinical findings

In both diseases there is an absence of systemic signs although acute hemorrhagic anemia may be present when extensive bleeding occurs in the pleural cavity. There is dyspnea, which usually develops gradually, and an absence of breath sounds accompanied by dullness on percussion over the lower parts of the chest. These conditions are always bilateral in the horse but may be unilateral in other species, causing an absence of movement of the ribs on the affected side. In thin animals the intercostal spaces may be observed to bulge. If sufficient fluid is present it may cause compression of the atria, engorgement of the jugular veins, and a jugular pulse of increased amplitude may be present. The cardiac embarrassment is not usually sufficiently severe to cause congestive heart failure although this disease may already be present.

Clinical pathology

Thoracic puncture will be followed by a flow of clear serous fluid in hydrothorax, or blood in recent cases of hemothorax. The fluid is bacteriologically negative but may contain protein.

Necropsy findings
In animals which die of acute hemorrhagic anemia resulting from hemothorax, the pleural cavity is filled with blood which usually has not clotted, the clot having been broken down by the constant respiratory movement. Hydrothorax is not usually fatal but is a common accompaniment of other diseases which are evidenced by their specific necropsy findings.

Diagnosis
Hydrothorax and hemothorax can be differentiated from pleurisy by the absence of pain, toxemia and fever and by the sterility of an aspirated fluid sample. Other space-occupying lesions of the thorax, including tumors, are not characterized by an accumulation of fluid unless the tumors have implanted on the pleura.

Treatment
Treatment of the primary condition is necessary. If the dyspnea is severe, aspiration of fluid from the pleural sac causes a temporary improvement but the fluid usually reaccumulates rapidly. Parenteral coagulants and blood transfusion are rational treatments in severe hemothorax.

Pneumothorax

Entry of air into the pleural cavity in sufficient quantity causes collapse of the lung and respiratory embarrassment.

Etiology
Rupture of the lung is the most common cause. Rarely there is puncture of the chest wall from the exterior.

Rupture of lung
- Traumatic rib fracture perforates lung
- Spontaneous rupture precipitated by coughing or exercise from primary parenchymal weakness, usually emphysematous bullae
- Thoracotomy usually for drainage of pericardial sac, or pleural drainage.

Pathogenesis
Pneumothorax is unilateral except in the horse. Collapse of the lung on the affected side occurs because of the absence of negative pressure in the pleural sac. The degree of collapse varies with the amount of air which enters the cavity, small amounts being absorbed very quickly but large amounts may cause fatal anoxia. Hemothorax may occur simultaneously and pleurisy is a common sequel.

Clinical findings
There is an acute onset of inspiratory dyspnea which may terminate fatally within a few minutes in the horse. If the collapse occurs in only one pleural sac, the rib cage on the affected side collapses and shows decreased movement. There is a compensatory increase in movement and bulging of the chest wall on the unaffected side. On auscultation there is complete absence of the normal vesicular murmur but bronchial tones are still audible over the base of the lung. The mediastinum bulges toward the unaffected side and may cause moderate displacement of the heart and the apex beat. The heart sounds on the affected side have a metallic note and the apex beat may be absent. On percussion of the thorax on the affected side the sound is metallic rather than tympanitic. The same sound can be heard with auscultatory percussion.

The entry of air into the sac usually ceases within a short time and the air is absorbed, the lung returning to its normal functional state. The introduction of infection at the time of injury usually causes a serious pleurisy.

Clinical pathology
Laboratory examinations are of no assistance in diagnosis but radiographic examination of animals of suitable size shows displacement of the mediastinum and heart, and collapse of the lung.

Necropsy findings
The lung in the affected sac is collapsed. In cases where spontaneous rupture occurs there is discontinuity of the pleura usually over an emphysematous bulla. Hemothorax may also be evident.

Diagnosis
The clinical findings are usually diagnostic. Diaphragmatic hernia may cause similar clinical signs in small animals but is relatively rare in farm animals. In cattle, herniation is usually associated with traumatic reticulitis and is not usually manifested by respiratory distress. Large herniae with entry of liver, stomach and intestines cause respiratory embarrassment, a tympanitic note on percussion and audible peristaltic sounds on auscultation. Radiographic examination is of value in differentiation if the animal is sufficiently small.

Treatment
Every effort should be made to determine the cause of the pneumothorax. An open pneumothorax, due to a thoracic wound should be surgically closed and sealed. Emergency decompression of the pleural cavity using a needle into the pleural cavity, connected to a tubing and submerged into a flask of saline or water, creates a water-seal drainage. A simple one-way flutter valve has been used successfully in small animals (1) and the Heimlich chest drainage valve is also useful. The animal should be kept as quiet as possible and permitted no exercise. Prophylactic treatment to avoid the development of pleurisy is advisable.

REFERENCE

(1) Butler, W. B. (1975) *J. Am. vet. med. Assoc.*, *166*, 473.

Diaphragmatic hernia

Diaphragmatic hernia is uncommon in farm animals. It occurs in cattle, especially in association with traumatic reticuloperitonitis. Here the hernia is small and causes no respiratory distress, and there may be no abnormal sounds in the chest. Occasional cases of acquired hernia not caused by foreign body perforation also occur in cattle and horses (1). Some of the acquired diaphragmatic hernias in the horse are of long duration with an additional factor, such as the passage of a stomach tube or transportation, precipitating acute abdominal pain. One case of traumatic hernia in a foal is described in which lack of exercise tolerance was the only clinical sign (9).

Colic and dyspnea are recorded as prominent clinical findings and these are usually as acute attacks (2, 10). In some there is a history of recent thoracic trauma (3). Affected horses may have one or all of the following: tachypnea, painful or forced respirations (2), but often there is no interference with it (4). The colic is a severe one, with the herniated bowel likely to become necrotic. All of the indications for exploratory laparotomy may be present except that the rectal findings are negative. However, fluid gushes from the stomach when the nasal tube is passed, and vomiting may occur terminally. Although the intestine may be incarcerated, paracentesis of the abdomen is likely to be negative but bloodstained fluid is present in the thoracic cavity. Clinical signs suggesting that the blood supply to the herniated intestine is compromised, but which are not accompanied by positive paracentesis findings, suggest that the lesion is in the chest, the scrotum or the omental bursa (5). The presence of intestinal sounds in the thorax can be misleading; they are often present in the normal animal, but their presence, accompanied by dyspnea and resonance on percussion, should arouse suspicion. Radiography and exploratory laparotomy are the most useful diagnostic procedures.

Congenital herniae occur in all species and the defects are usually large, in the dorsal tendinous part of the diaphragm, and have thin edges. Because of the large size of the defect much of the abdominal viscera including liver, stomach and intestines, enter the thorax and dyspnea is evident at birth. In some cases the pericardial sac is incomplete and the diaphragm is rudimentary and in the form of a small fold projecting from the chest wall (6, 11). Affected animals usually survive for a few hours to several weeks. In pigs a number of animals in each litter may be affected (7). Surgical repair has been performed in neonates, and successful surgical intervention is recorded in one horse (8) but the prognosis is usually poor (2).

REFERENCES

(1) Sasse, H. H. L. & Kalsbeek, H. C. (1965) *Tijdschr. Diergeneeskd.*, *90*, 1327.
(2) Wimberly, H. C. et al. (1977) *J. Am. vet. med. Assoc.*, *170*, 1404.
(3) Pearson, H. et al. (1977) *Equ. vet. J.*, *9*, 32.
(4) Coffman, J. R. & Kinther, L. D. (1972) *Vet. Med. small Anim. Clin.* *67*, 423.
(5) Firth, E. (1976) *Cornell Vet.*, *66*, 353.
(6) Horney, F. D. & Cote, J. (1961) *Can. vet. J.*, *2*, 422.
(7) Griffin, R. M. (1965) *Vet. Rec.*, *77*, 492.
(8) Scott, E. A. & Fishbank, W. A. (1976) *J. Am. vet. med. Assoc.*, *168*, 45.
(9) Speirs, V. C. & Reynolds, W. T. (1976) *Equ. vet. J.*, *8*, 170.
(10) Wyn-Jones, G. & Baker, J. R. (1979) *Vet. Rec.*, *105*, 251.
(11) Mitchell, G. & McFadden, G. (1980) *Aust. vet. J.*, *56*, 610.

Synchronous diaphragmatic flutter in horses (thumps)

This disease occurs sporadically, and for no apparent reason in many horses, usually adult ponies used for pleasure riding. Recently a tendency for the disease to occur more frequently than normal has been recorded in horses subjected to stress of long duration, and possibly to accompanying electrolyte imbalance of the blood, by reason of participation in endurance rides (1–3).

The syndrome is characteristic with a violent hiccough occurring synchronously with every heart beat. It is often unilateral, the contraction being felt very much more strongly on one side than the other. The horse is distressed because the hiccough interferes with eating, and to an extent with respiration. In all cases in our experience the disease has resolved spontaneously in 24 hours. However, based on laboratory findings of hypocalcemia, hemoconcentration, alkalosis and hypokalemia, hypochloremia, and elevation of creatinine phosphokinase levels, treatment with calcium borogluconate slowly and intravenously has been followed by rapid recovery (4). In some cases there are additional signs suggestive of hypocalcemia. These include muscular rigidity and fasciculation, and a high-stepping gait. These are cases of lactation tetany in which hiccough is a prominent sign.

The pathogenesis is thought to be related to hyperirritability of the phrenic nerve caused by metabolic disturbances including hypocalcemia, and the phrenic nerve being stimulated by each atrial depolarization to fire with each heart beat. The stimulation occurs because of the close physical promixity of the heart to the nerve in the horse. Dietary supplementation with calcium and other electrolytes during a ride is recommended but excessive calcium feeding beforehand may reduce the activity of calcium homeostatic mechanisms, and is to be avoided.

Regular veterinary inspection of all horses at the mandatory stops of endurance rides will reveal those animals with 'thumps' which should not be allowed to proceed in the event (5).

REFERENCES

(1) Mansmann, R. A. et al. (1974) *J. Am. med. Assoc.*, *165*, 265.
(2) White, N. A. & White, S. L. (1975) *Vet. Med. small Anim. Clin.*, *70*, 967.
(3) Ellis, P. M. (1976) *Vet. Rec.*, *99*, 403.
(4) Hinton, M. et al. (1976) *Vet. Rec.*, *99*, 402.
(5) Hall-Patch, P. K. et al. (1977) *Vet. Rec.*, *100*, 192.

Pleurisy

Acute inflammation of the pleura causes pain during respiratory movements, manifested clinically by shallow, rapid respiration. Subacute inflammation is accompanied by empyema causing collapse of the lung and respiratory embarrassment. Chronic pleurisy is usually manifested by the development of fibrous adhesions and minor interference with respiratory movement.

Etiology

Pleurisy is almost always part of a primary disease of the lungs.

Primary

- Penetration, usually traumatic, of the chest wall.

Secondary

- As part of specific infectious diseases including:
  all species—Pasteurella multocida and *Past. haemolytica*;
  in swine—Glasser's disease, pleuropneumonia

caused by *Actinobacillus (Haemophilus) pleuropneumoniae*;
in cattle—tuberculosis, sporadic bovine encephalomyelitis, contagious bovine pleuropneumonia, *Haemophilus somnus* infection;
in sheep and goats—pleuropneumonia caused by *Mycoplasma* sp. and *Haemophilus* sp.

- As part of a sporadic, non-specific disease, e.g.: septicemias, e.g., *Pseudomonas aeruginosa*; bacteremia with localization causing a primary septic pleural effusion (1); by extension, bacterial pneumonias or lung abscesses with spread occurring from the pulmonary parenchyma. In horses, the infection is usually *Streptococcus equi* and the original disease is strangles. In goats, it is usually spread from a mycoplasmal pneumonia
- By perforation of the diaphragm in traumatic reticuloperitonitis in cattle and goats. Spread into the pleural cavity can occur without actual penetration of the diaphragm, as it occurs via the lymphatics. Septic pleuritis has occurred in a pony which inhaled a plant stem that became lodged in the bronchi causing suppurative pneumonia which spread to the pleura (3)
- *In horses* the disease may be caused by rupture or extension to the plasma of a preexisting pulmonary abscess, granuloma or chronic pneumonic lesion. In one study of 122 horses with pleural effusions, 74% had pleuritis secondary to pneumonia or lung abscessation (13). Pleuropneumonia in mature horses was due to anaerobic bacteria (*Bacteroides* spp.) (7, 8) and *Klebsiella pneumoniae* and *Streptococcus zooepidemicus* (11). *Mycoplasma felis* has been identified as a causative agent from a naturally occurring case and was reproduced experimentally using the organism (9). A second list of rare causes of pleurisy and pleural effusion in animals includes lymphosarcoma and equine infectious anemia. However, culture results have been negative for bacteria, mycoplasms and viruses in a significant number of cases. Mesothelioma of the pleura causing persistent dyspnea, pleural effusion and death is also recorded in the horse (2).

Pathogenesis

In the early, acute, dry stage of pleurisy, contact and movement between the parietal and visceral pleurae causes pain due to stimulation of pain endorgans in the pleura. Respiratory movements are restricted and the respiration is rapid and shallow. The second stage of pleurisy is characterized by the production of serofibrinous inflammatory exudate which collects in the pleural sacs and causes collapse of the ventral parts of the lungs, thus reducing vital capacity and interfering with gaseous exchange. If the accumulation is sufficiently severe there may be pressure on the atria and a damming back of blood in the great veins. Clinical signs may be restricted to one side of the chest in all species with an imperforate mediastinum. In the third stage, the fluid is resorbed and adhesions develop, restricting movement of the lungs and chest wall but interference with respiratory exchange is usually minor and disappears gradually as the adhesions stretch with continuous movement.

In all bacterial pleuritides there is an element of toxemia caused by toxins produced by the bacteria and by tissue breakdown. The toxemia may be severe when large amounts of pus accumulate.

Clinical findings

In the early stages the respirations are rapid and shallow and the animal shows evidence of pain and anxiety. Respiratory movements are markedly abdominal and movement of the thoracic wall is restricted. The animal stands with its elbows abducted and is disinclined to move. On auscultation pleuritic friction sounds may be audible. These have a continuous to and fro character, are dry and abrasive, and do not abate with coughing. They may be difficult to identify if there is a coincident pneumonia accompanied by râles and increased vesicular murmur. When the pleurisy involves the pleural surface of the pericardial sac a friction rub may be heard with each cardiac cycle and be confused with the friction rub of pericarditis. However, there is usually in addition a rub synchronous with respiratory movements and the pericardial rub waxes and wanes with expiration and inspiration. Pressure on the thoracic wall and deep digital palpitation of the intercostal spaces usually causes pain. The temperature and pulse rate are usually elevated, the degree varying with the virulence of the causative agent. Toxemia, with anorexia and depression, is also present in most cases. Acute pleuritis in the horse may be manifested by colicky signs. Affected horses are often reluctant to move or lie down and stand quietly with an anxious expression (1). Subcutaneous edema of the ventral body wall extending from the pectorals to the prepubic area is common in the horse with advanced pleurisy. Presumably this is due to blockage of lymphatics normally drained through the sternal lymph nodes. Horses may be affected with pleuropneumonia for several weeks and lose considerable weight in spite of therapy (7, 11).

As exudation causes separation of the inflamed pleural surfaces, the pain and friction rub diminish but do not completely disappear. The respiratory rate decreases but is still above normal. On auscultation there may still be friction sounds but they are less evident and usually localized to small areas. Both normal and abnormal lung sounds are diminished in intensity according to the amount of pleural effusion present. There is dullness on percussion over the fluid-filled area of the thorax and the dull area has a level topline—a fluid line. Dyspnea is evident, particularly during inspiration, and a pleuritic ridge develops at the costal arch due to elevation of the ribs and the abdominal-type respiration. If the pleurisy is unilateral, movement of the affected side of the chest is restricted as compared to the normal side. Pain is still evident on percussion on deep palpation of the intercostal spaces and the animal still stands with its elbows abducted, is disinclined to lie down or move but is not as apprehensive as in the early stages. Toxemia is often more severe during this stage, the temperature and the pulse rate are usually above normal and the animal eats poorly. Cough is usually present because of the concurrent pneumonia and is painful, short and shallow. Extension of the inflammation to the pericardium may occur. Death may occur at any time and is due to a combination of toxemia and anoxia caused by pressure atelectasis.

Animals that recover do so slowly. The toxemia usually disappears first but residual respiratory embarrassment of moderate degree remains for some time because of the presence of adhesions. Rupture of the adhesions during severe exertion may cause fatal hemothorax. Some impairment of respiratory function can be expected to persist and racing animals do not usually regain complete efficiency. Chronic pleurisy, such as that which occurs in tuberculosis in cattle, is usually symptomless, no acute inflammation or fluid exudation occurring. Weight loss is one of the most common presenting complaints of chronic pleuritis in the horse and the disease may not be noticed on initial clinical examination because dyspnea may not be a prominent clinical finding.

Clinical pathology

Thoracentesis to obtain a sample of the fluid for laboratory examination is necessary. The fluid should be examined for its odor, color and viscosity, protein concentration, presence of blood or tumor cells and cultured for bacteria. It is important to determine whether the fluid is an exudate or a transudate. Pleural fluid from horses affected with anaerobic bacterial pleuropneumonia may be foul-smelling (8). Laboratory analysis of pleural fluid invariably reveals a remarkable increase in leukocytes up to 40 000–100 000 μl and protein concentrations of up to 50 g/l (6, 13). The fluid should be cultured for both aerobic and anaerobic bacteria (7, 8) and *Mycoplasma* sp. (9). Radiographic examination may reveal the presence of a fluid line and fluid displacement of the mediastinum and heart to the unaffected side and collapse of the lung. Pleuroscopy using a rigid or flexible fiberoptic endoscope is now available for direct visual inspection of the pleural cavity (5, 12).

Necropsy findings

In early acute pleurisy there is marked edema, thickening and hyperemia of the pleura, with engorgement of small vessels and the presence of tags and shreds of fibrin. These can be most readily seen between the lobes of the lung. In the exudative stage the pleural cavity contains an excessive quantity of turbid fluid containing flakes and clots of fibrin. The pleura is thickened and the central parts of the lung collapsed and dark red in color. A concurrent pneumonia is usually present and there may be an associated pericarditis. In the later healing stages adhesions connect the parietal and visceral pleurae. The pathology and pathogenesis of pleural adhesions in sheep has been examined (4). Type I fibrinous adhesions appear to be associated with pneumonia while type II fibrinous proliferative adhesions are idiopathic (4).

Diagnosis

Identification of pleurisy depends upon the presence of a friction rub or inflammatory exudate in the pleural sac. Pleurisy usually occurs in conjunction with pneumonia and differentiation is difficult and often unnecessary. The crackles and wheezes of pneumonia are less distinct and abrasive, and fluctuate with coughing. Emphysema, especially when bullae are present under the pleura, may be manifested by a friction rub but loud crackles are present and the dyspnea has a characteristic prolongation of expiration. In pleurisy the dyspnea is largely inspiratory. A tympanitic note on percussion is typical of emphysema, dullness on percussion is typical of pleurisy, and fever and toxemia usually accompany the latter.

Hydrothorax and hemothorax are not usually accompanied by fever or toxemia and pain and pleuritic friction sounds are not present. Aspiration of fluid by needle puncture can be attempted if doubt exists. Pulmonary congestion and edema are manifested by increased vesicular murmur and ventral consolidation without hydrothorax or pleural inflammation.

Treatment

The prognosis in horses and cattle is unfavorable. The presence of more than about 6 h of pleural fluid suggests an unfavorable prognosis (16). The disease is commonly in an advanced stage when first recognized and the extensive fibrinous inflammation is unresponsive to treatment. Also, the common failure to culture the primary causative agent, particularly in horses, makes specific therapy difficult.

The primary aim of treatment is to control the infection in the pleural sac. This is best achieved by the parenteral or oral administration of antibiotics or sulfonamides, the choice of drug preferably being dictated by bacteriological examination of the pleuritic exudate. The treatment of anaerobic bacterial pleuropneumonia in horses may require the use of antimicrobials such as chloramphenicol or metronidazole if *Bacteroides fragilis* is present which is a penicillinase producer (14). Long-term therapy daily for several weeks may be necessary.

Treatment of pleuritis and pleural effusion should include drainage of pleural fluid and the use of appropriate antimicrobial therapy parenterally and directly into the pleural cavity. Clinical experience suggests that drainage improves. When the amount of fluid present is excessive, aspiration may cause temporary improvement and the antibacterial agent can be injected directly into the pleural sac. Aspiration is not easy as the drainage needle or cannula tends to become blocked with fibrin, and respiratory movements may result in laceration of the lung. Drainage may be difficult or almost impossible in cases in which adhesion of visceral and parietal pleura are extensive and fluid is loculated. Diuretics are unlikely to aid in the removal of this or any other inflammatory exudate. Large quantities of pleural fluid may be removed initially followed by the use of drainage tubes with one-way valves which are sutured into place in the dorsal and ventral aspects of the pleural cavity on both sides. Following drainage each day, antibiotics may be placed directly into the pleural cavities. Claims are made for the use of dexamethazone at 0·1 mg/kg body weight to reduce the degree of pleural effusion (1). In acute cases of pleurisy in the horse analgesics such as phenylbutazone are valuable to relieve pain and anxiety, allowing the horse to eat and drink more normally.

Pleural adhesions are usually unavoidable and may become quite thick and extensive with the formation of loculation which traps pleural fluid, all of which prevents full recovery. However, some animals will stabilize at a certain level of chronicity, survive for long periods and may be useful for light work or as breeding animals.

REFERENCES

(1) Smith, B. P. (1977) *J. Am. vet. med. Assoc.*, *170*, 208.
(2) Kolbl, S. (1979) *Wien Tierärztl. Monatsschr.*, *66*, 22.
(3) O'Brien, J. K. (1986) *Vet. Rec.*, *119*, 274.
(4) Pfeffer, A. (1986) *NZ vet. J.*, *34*, 85.
(5) Mansmann, R. A. & Bernard-Strother, S. (1985) *Mod. vet. Pract.*, *99*, 9.
(6) Wagner, A. E. & Bennett, D. G. (1982) *Vet. clin. Pathol.*, *11*, 13.
(7) Sweeney, C. R. et al. (1985) *J. Am. vet. med. Assoc.*, *187*, 721.
(8) Bernard-Strother, S. & Mansmann, R. A. (1985) *Comp. cont. Educ. pract. Vet.*, *7*, S341.
(9) Ogilvie, T. H. et al. (1983) *J. Am. vet. med. Assoc.*, *182*, 1374.
(10) Sweeney, R. W. et al. (1986) *Am. J. vet. Res.*, *47*, 1726.
(11) Purdy, C. M. (1985) *Com. cont. Educ. pract. Vet.*, *7*, S361.
(12) MacKey, V. S. & Wheat, J. D. (1985) *Equ. vet. J.*, *17*, 140.
(13) Raphel, C. F. & Beech, J. (1982) *J. Am. vet. med. Assoc.*, *181*, 808.
(14) Sweeney, R. W. et al. (1986). *Am. J. vet. Res.*, *47*, 1726.
(15) Hultgren, B. D. et al. (1986). *J. Am. vet. med. Assoc.*, *189*, 797.
(16) Bennet, D. G. (1986) *J. Am. Vet. med. Assoc.*, *188*, 814.

DISEASES OF THE UPPER RESPIRATORY TRACT

Rhinitis

Rhinitis is characterized clinically by varying degrees of sneezing, wheezing and stertor during inspiration and a nasal discharge which may be serous, mucoid or purulent in consistency depending on the cause.

Etiology

Rhinitis usually occurs in conjunction with inflammation of other parts of the respiratory tract. It is present as a minor lesion in most bacterial and viral pneumonias but the diseases listed are those in which it occurs as an obvious and important part of the syndrome.

Cattle

Ulcerative/erosive rhinitis in bovine malignant catarrh, mucosal disease, rinderpest. Catarrhal rhinitis in infectious bovine rhinotracheitis, adenoviruses 1, 2 and 3 and respiratory syncytial virus infections. Rhinosporidiosis caused by fungi, the blood fluke *Schistosoma nasalis*, and the supposedly allergic 'summer snuffles' also known as atopic rhinitis (15).

Horses

Glanders, strangles and epizootic lymphangitis. Infections with the viruses of equine viral rhinopneumonitis (herpesvirus 1), equine viral arteritis, influenza viruses 1A/E1 and 1A/E2, equine rhinovirus, parainfluenza virus, reovirus, adenovirus, virus of Hoppengarten cough.

Chronic rhinitis is claimed to be caused by dust in dusty stables, and acute rhinitis occurs after inhalation of smoke and fumes. Nasal granuloma due to chronic infection with *Pseudoallescheria boydii* is reported in the horse (14).

Sheep

Melioidosis, bluetongue, rarely contagious ecthyma and sheep pox; also *Oestrus ovis* and *Elaeophora schneideri* infestations; and allergic rhinitis.

Pigs

Atrophic rhinitis, inclusion body rhinitis, swine influenza, some outbreaks of Aujeszky's disease.

Pathogenesis

Rhinitis is of minor importance as a disease process except in severe cases when it causes obstruction of the passage of air through the nasal cavities. Its major importance is as an indication of the presence of some specific diseases. The type of lesion produced is important. The erosive and ulcerative lesions of rinderpest, bovine malignant catarrh and mucosal disease, the ulcerative lesions of glanders, melioidosis and epizootic lymphangitis and the granular rhinitis of the anterior nares in allergic rhinitis all have diagnostic significance.

In atrophic rhinitis of pigs the destruction of the turbinate bones and distortion of the face appear to be a form of devitalization and atrophy of bone caused by a primary, inflammatory rhinitis. Secondary bacterial invasion of facial tissues of swine appears to be the basis of necrotic rhinitis.

Clinical findings

The cardinal sign in rhinitis is a nasal discharge which is usually serous initially but soon becomes mucoid and, in bacterial infections, purulent. Erythema, erosion or ulceration may be visible on inspection. The inflammation may be unilateral or bilateral. Sneezing is characteristic in the early acute stages and this is followed in the later stages by snorting and the expulsion of large amounts of mucopurulent discharge. A chronic unilateral purulent nasal discharge lasting several weeks or months may suggest nasal mycosis (14).

'Summer snuffles' of cattle presents a characteristic syndrome. Cases occur in the spring and autumn when the pasture is in flower and are most common in Channel Island breeds. There is a sudden onset of dyspnea with a profuse nasal discharge of thick, orange to yellow material which varies from a mucopurulent to caseous consistency. Sneezing, irritation and obstruction are severe. The irritation may cause the animal to shake its head, rub its nose along the ground or poke its muzzle repeatedly into hedges and bushes. Sticks and twigs may be pushed up into the nostrils as a result and cause laceration and bleeding. Stertorous, difficult respiration, accompanied by mouth breathing may be evident when both nostrils are obstructed. In the most severe cases a distinct pseudomembrane is formed which is later snorted out as a complete nasal cast. In the chronic stages multiple nodules about 1 cm in diameter are present in the anterior nares.

Clinical pathology

Examination of nasal swabs of scrapings for bacteria, inclusion bodies or fungi may aid in diagnosis. Discharges in allergic rhinitis usually contain many more eosinophils than normal.

Endoscopic examination using a flexible fiberoptic endoscope or a rigid endoscope is very useful for the visual inspection of lesions affecting the nasal mucosae which are not visible externally.

Necropsy findings
Rhinitis is not a fatal condition although animals may die of specific diseases in which rhinitis is a prominent lesion.

Diagnosis
Rhinitis is readily recognizable on clinical grounds. Differentiation of the specific diseases listed under etiology above is discussed under their respective headings. Rhinitis may be confused with inflammation of the facial sinuses or guttural pouches in the horse in which the nasal discharge is usually purulent and persistent and often unilateral, and there is an absence of signs of nasal irritation.

Treatment
Specific treatment aimed at control of individual causative agents is described under the specific diseases. Thick tenacious exudate which is causing nasal obstruction may be removed gently and the nasal cavities irrigated with saline. A nasal decongestant sprayed up into the nostrils may provide some relief. Newborn piglets with inclusion body rhinitis may be affected with severe inspiratory dyspnea and mouth breathing which interferes with sucking. The removal of the exudate from each nostril followed by irrigations with a mixture of saline and antibiotics will provide symptomatic relief and minimize the development of a secondary bacterial rhinitis. Animals affected with allergic rhinitis should be taken off the pasture for about a week and treated with antihistamine preparations.

Obstruction of the nasal cavities

Nasal obstruction occurs commonly in cattle and sheep. Cystic enlargement of the ventral nasal conchae in cattle can cause bilateral nasal obstruction (9). Chronic obstruction in cattle is most often due to enzootic nasal granuloma, acute obstruction to the allergic condition 'summer snuffles'. The disease is usually chronic in sheep and due to infestation with *Oestrus ovis*. Minor occurrences include the following: large mucus-filled polyps may develop in the posterior nares of cattle and sheep and cause unilateral or bilateral obstruction. Granulomatous lesions caused by a fungus, *Rhinosporidium* spp. and by the blood fluke, *Schistosoma nasalis* may cause chronic obstruction. A chronic pyogranuloma due to *Coccidioides immitis* infection has occurred in the horse (11). Foreign bodies may enter the cavities when cattle rub their muzzles in bushes in an attempt to relieve the irritation of acute allergic rhinitis. Neoplasms of the olfactory mucosa are not common but do occur, particularly in sheep and cattle where the incidence in individual flocks and herds may be sufficiently high to suggest an infectious cause (1, 2, 4, 6). The lesions are usually situated just in front of the ethmoid bone, are usually unilateral but may be bilateral and have the appearance of adenocarcinomas of moderate malignancy. An angiosarcoma of the nasal cavity of a mature horse (10) and congenital ethmoid carcinoma in a foal (13) have been recorded.

In cattle, the disease is commonest in 6–9 year olds and may be sufficiently extensive to cause bulging of the facial bones. The tumors are adenocarcinomas arising from the ethmoidal mucosa, and they metastasize in lungs and lymph nodes. Clinical signs include nasal discharge, often bloody, mouth breathing, assumption of a stretched-neck posture. There is evidence to suggest that a virus may be associated (3, 6, 7). A similar syndrome is observed in cattle with other nasal tumors such as osteoma (5).

Enzootic nasal adenocarcinoma occurs in sheep in Canada (8) and elsewhere (12). The disease is sporadic but has occurred in related flocks which suggests that it may be an enzootic problem. The clinical findings include a persistent serous, mucous or mucopurulent nasal discharge and stridor. Affected sheep progressively develop anorexia, dyspnea and mouth breathing and most die within 90 days after the onset of signs. The tumors originate unilaterally or occasionally bilaterally in the olfactory mucosa of the ethmoid turbinates. They are locally invasive but not metastatic. Histologically the tumors are classified as adenomas or more frequently, adenocarcinomas. The etiology is unknown, but a retrovirus may be involved.

In cattle, sheep and pigs there is severe inspiratory dyspnea when both cavities are blocked. The animals may show great distress and anxiety and breathe in gasps through the mouth. Obstruction is usually not complete and a loud, wheezing sound occurs with each inspiration. A nasal discharge is usually present but varies from a small amount of bloodstained serous discharge when there is a foreign body present, to large quantities of purulent exudate in allergic rhinitis. Shaking of the head and snorting are also common signs. If the obstruction is unilateral the distress is not so marked and the difference in breath streams between the two nostrils can be detected by holding the hands in front of the nose. The magnitude of the air currents from each nostril on expiration can be assessed with the aid of a piece of cotton thread (watching the degree of deflection). The passage of a stomach tube through each nasal cavity may reveal evidence of a space-occupying lesion. The diameter of the tube to be used should be one size smaller than would normally be used on that animal to ensure that the tube passes easily. The signs may be intermittent when the obstruction is caused by a pedunculated polyp in the posterior nares.

Treatment must be directed at the primary cause of the obstruction. Removal of foreign bodies can usually be effected with the aid of long forceps although strong traction is often necessary when the obstructions have been in position for a few days. As an empirical treatment in cattle oral or parenteral administration of iodine preparations is in general use in chronic nasal obstruction.

REFERENCES

(1) Young, S. et al. (1961) *Cornell Vet.*, *51*, 96.
(2) Dunan, J. R. et al. (1967) *J. Am. vet. med. Assoc.*, *151*, 732.
(3) Nairn, M. K. et al. (1980) *Aust. Adv. vet. Sci.*, p. 15.
(4) Njoku, C. O. et al. (1978) *Am. J. vet. Res.*, *39* 1850.
(5) Rumbaugh, G. E. et al. (1978) *Cornell Vet.*, *68*, 544.
(6) Yonemichi, H. et al. (1978) *Am. J. vet. Res.*, *39*, 1599.
(7) Popischil, A. et al. (1979) *Vet. Pathol.*, *16*, 180.
(8) McKinnon, A. O. et al. (1982) *Can vet. J.*, *23*, 88.
(9) Ross , M. W. et al. (1986) *J. Am. vet. med. Assoc.*, *188*, 857.

(10) Chan, C. W. & Collins, E. A. (1985) *Equ. vet. J.*, *17*, 214.
(11) Hodgin, E. C. et al. (1984) *J. Am. vet. med. Assoc.*, *184*, 339.
(12) Rings, D. M. & Roijko, J. (1985) *Cornell Vet.*, *75*, 269.
(13) Acland, H. M. et al. (1984) *J. Am. vet. med. Assoc.*, *184*, 979.
(14) Brearley, J. C. et al. (1986) *Equ. vet. J. 18*, 151.
(15) Wiseman, A. et al. (1982) *Vet. Rec.*, *110*, 420

Epistaxis and hemoptysis

Epistaxis as used here means bleeding from the nostrils regardless of the origin of the hemorrhage, and hemoptysis means the coughing-up of blood with the hemorrhage usually originating in the lungs. Both epistaxis and hemoptysis are important clinical signs in cattle and horses. The bleeding may be in the form of a small volume of bloodstained serous discharge coming from the nose only, or it can be a large volume of whole blood coming precipitously from both nostrils and sometimes the mouth. The first and most important decision is to determine the exact location of the bleeding point.

Epistaxis occurs commonly in the horse and may be due to lesions in the nasal cavity, nasopharynx, auditory tube diverticulum (guttural pouch) or lungs. Hemorrhagic lesions of the nasal cavity, nasopharynx and guttural pouch in the horse usually cause unilateral epistaxis of varying degree depending on the severity of the lesions. Pulmonary lesions in the horse resulting in hemorrhage into the lumen of the bronchi also result in epistaxis. Blood originating from the lungs of the horse is discharged most commonly from the nostrils and not the mouth because of the horse's long soft palate. Also, blood from the lungs of the horse is not foamy when seen at the nose because the horizontal position of the major bronchi allows blood to flow out freely without being coughed-up and made foamy. It was previously thought that upper respiratory tract hemorrhage could be distinguished from lower respiratory tract hemorrhage by the blood in the latter case being foamy. This does not apply in the horse. Froth is usually the result of pulmonary edema in which case it is a very fine pink stable froth.

Exercise-induced pulmonary hemorrhage with or without epistaxis is a problem in Thoroughbred race horses (17). It also occurs in polo horses (18) and mixed breed horses exercised competitively at speeds of 520 m/min which contrasts greatly with the average speed of a thoroughbred racing horse at 1050 m/min (19). The incidence of bleeding based on the presence of blood at the nostrils is less than 10%, but depending on the age of the horse, the distance exercised and the speed 40–75% of horses will have evidence of exercise-induced pulmonary hemorrhage as determined by endoscopic examination of the tracheal lumen within 2 hours after racing (20). The cause is bleeding from the lungs due to the mechanical stress of exercise (17). The presence of preexisting lung disease such as the lesions of chronic obstructive pulmonary disease (1) has also been considered to be a precursor but there is declining support for this explanation. An increase in pulmonary vascular pressure may also be a factor (13). The hemorrhage occurs primarily in the dorsocaudal area of the diaphragmatic lobes of the lung invariably with the start of fast work in 2-year-olds (17). It always occurs at the same position in the lung, it has a worldwide distribution regardless of such factors as climate, housing or management procedures and follows a certain type and level of exertion.

The upper respiratory tract of the horse from the nares to the tracheal bifurcation can be examined with a flexible fiberoptic endoscope and the degree of hemorrhage graded based on the following numerical grading system: grade O, no blood observed; grade I, traces of blood including spots and discontinuous streaking of blood in tracheal mucus; grade II, a streak of blood < 5 mm wide; grade III, a streak of blood > 5 mm wide (21). An endoscope 140 cm in length is required.

Epistaxis is a problem in racehorses which bleed from the nostrils during a race. Horses which do so are usually disqualified from further racing so that owners often require an accurate diagnosis, prognosis, and preferably treatment. Affected horses bleed during the last part of a race and may bleed to death very quickly, literally dropping dead during a race. However, most of them just slow down, but precipitably, thus causing later horses to collide with them. Because of the dangers in the situation disqualification is essential. Horses that bleed from the nostrils have historically been considered the most severe bleeders. However, the presence of blood at the nostrils is not a reflection of the severity of pulmonary hemorrhage, since more than half of the horses with blood at the nostrils did not receive the maximum grading based on the degree of blood within the trachea (20).

The therapeutic agents which have been recommended for the treatment of exercise-induced pulmonary hemorrhage in the horse includes coagulants, estrogens, furosemide, Clenbuterol, atropine and others (17). However, all of these drugs have been used without a full understanding of the pathophysiology of the disease and without knowledge of the pharmacological effects on the horse and without adequate clinical trials (17). The efficacy of furosemide has been evaluated extensively (13, 15, 16). When given prior to racing it had no beneficial effect (22, 23). In one study, furosemide did not stop the hemorrhage but it did reduce the intensity of hemorrhage (21). The effect of furosemide on the racing times of horses with exercise-induced pulmonary hemorrhage has been examined (23). The effect of furosemide administration on systemic circulation of ponies during severe exercise indicates it does not significantly modify the fundamental circulatory adaptation to severe exercise (24). Furosemide is a potent diuretic which causes marked circulatory volume contraction in horses. Right atrial pressure and mean pulmonary arterial pressure increase to a lower level when exercise is performed after furosemide administration (25). Mean aortic pressure during exercise after furosemide administration remains less than during exercise before furosemide is administrated (24). Hesperidin-citrus bioflavinoids administered orally to horses did not alter the prevalence of the hemorrhage (26). In any case, the rules of racing would prevent its use in most countries. Treatment for chronic obstructure pulmonary disease, based on dust-free stable management, appears to be beneficial and prevents epistaxis and reduces its frequency (1).

Epistaxis caused by lesions of the upper respiratory tract usually occur spontaneously while the horse is at rest. One of the commonest causes of unilateral epistaxis in the horse is mycotic ulceration of the blood vessels in the wall of the guttural pouch (3–5). If it occurs during exercise it is slow exercise (1).

Other less common causes of nasal bleeding include hemorrhagic polyps of the mucosa of the nasal cavity or paranasal sinuses (6), and encapsulated hematomas which look like hemorrhagic polyps commencing near the ethmoidal labyrinth, and expanding into the nasal cavity and the pharynx (2, 7). There is respiratory obstruction, coughing, choking and persistent unilateral epistaxis. The capsule of the hematoma is respiratory epithelium. Surgical correction has been achieved. Another cause, most uncommonly, is a parasitic arteritis of the internal carotid artery as it courses around the guttural pouch (8). A generalized bleeding tendency originating from a thrombocytopenia is also recorded (9). Erosions of the nasal mucosa in glanders, granulomatous and neoplastic diseases and trauma due to passage of a nasal tube or endoscope, or from physical trauma externally, are other obvious causes. A case of fibrous dysplasia in the ventral meatus of a horse with epistaxis is recorded (14). Similarly, in congestive heart failure and purpura hemorrhagica there may be a mild epistaxis.

Bracken fern or moldy sweet clover poisoning are two common causes of spontaneous epistaxis in cattle. The epistaxis may be bilateral, and hemorrhages of other visible and subcutaneous mucous membranes are common. An enzootic ethmoidal tumor has been described in cattle in Brazil, and was at one time a disease of some importance in Sweden (10). The lesion occupies the nasal cavities, causes epistaxis and may invade paranasal sinuses.

In hemoptysis in horses the blood flows along the horizontal trachea and pools in the larynx until the swallowing reflex is stimulated and swallowing occurs, or coughing is stimulated and blood is expelled through the mouth and nostrils. In some horses repeated swallowing, without eating or drinking can be a good indicator that bleeding is occurring (16). Some of the blood is usually swallowed, resulting in melena or occult blood in the feces. The origin of the hemorrhage is usually in the lungs and in cattle the usual cause is a pulmonary arterial aneurysm and thromboembolism from a posterior vena caval thrombosis usually originating from an hepatic abscess. Recurrent attacks of hemoptysis with anemia and abnormal lung sounds usually culminate in an acute intrapulmonary hemorrhage and rapid death.

The origin of the hemorrhage in epistaxis and hemoptysis may be obvious, as in traumatic injury to the turbinates during passage of a stomach tube intranasally, or if a systemic disease with bleeding defects is present. In many other cases, however, the origin of the hemorrhage is not obvious and special examination procedures may be required. Careful auscultation of the lungs for evidence of abnormal lung sounds associated with pulmonary diseases is necessary. In racechorses with the 'bleeder syndrome' due to pulmonary disease, the lungs are usually normal on auscultation and the diagnosis is made on the basis of history and endoscopic examination to eliminate non-pulmonary causes.

In epistaxis the nasal cavities should be examined visually with the aid of a strong pointed source of light through the external nares. Only the first part of the nasal cavities can be examined directly but an assessment of the integrity of the nasal mucosa can usually be made. In epistaxis due to systemic disease or clotting defects the blood on the nasal mucosa will usually not be clotted. When there has been recent traumatic injury to the nasal mucosa or erosion of a blood vessel by a space-occupying lesion such as tumor or nasal polyp, the blood will usually be found in clots in the external nares.

The nasal cavities should then be examined for any evidence of obstruction as set out in the previous section. When the blood originates from a pharyngeal lesion there are frequent swallowing movements and a short explosive cough which may be accompanied by the expulsion of blood from the mouth. Hematological examinations are indicated to assist in the diagnosis of systemic disease or clotting defects. Radiological examinations of the head are indicated when space-occupying lesions are suspected.

In the horse, the use of the flexible fiberoptic endoscope will permit a thorough examination of the nasal cavities, nasopharynx, guttural pouch, and larynx, trachea and major bronchi (11). Such an endoscope is considered essential in equine practice to identify several diseases of the respiratory tract which cannot be detected with conventional diagnostic techniques (12).

The treatment of epistaxis and hemoptysis depends on the cause. Hemorrhage from traumatic injuries to the nasal mucosa does not usually require any treatment. Space-occupying lesions of the nasal mucosa may warrant surgical therapy and epistaxis associated with guttural pouch mycosis may require ligation of the affected artery. The ineffectiveness of therapy for exercise-induced pulmonary hemorrhage has been presented above. There is no successful treatment for the hemoptysis due to pulmonary aneurysm and posterior vena caval thrombosis in cattle. General supportive therapy is as for any spontaneous hemorrhage and includes rest, blood transfusions and hematinics.

REVIEW LITERATURE

Clarke, A. F. (1985) Review of exercise-induced pulmonary haemorrhage and its possible relationship with mechanical stress. *Equ. vet. J.*, *17* 166–172.

Robinson, N. E. (1979) Functional abnormalities caused by upper airway obstruction and heaves: their relationship to the etiology of epistaxis. *Vet. Clin. N. Am. large Anim. Pract.*, *1(1)*, 17.

REFERENCES

(1) Cook, W. R. (1974) *Equ. vet. J.*, 6, 45.
(2) Etherington, W. B. et al. (1982) *Can. vet. J.*, 23, 231.
(3) McIlwraith, C. W. (1978) *Vet. med. SAC*, 73, 67.
(4) Nation, P. N. (1978) *Can. vet. J.*, *19*, 194.
(5) Lingard, D. R. et al. (1974) *J. Am. vet. med. Assoc.*, *164*, 1038.
(6) Platt, H. (1975) *J. Pathol.*, *115*, 51.
(7) Cook, W. R. & Littlewort, M. C. G. (1974) *Equ. vet. J.*, 6, 101.
(8) Owen, R. R. (1974) *Equ. vet. J.*, 6, 143.
(9) Franco, D. A. (1969) *Vet. Med. small Anim. Clin.*, *64*, 1071.
(10) Tokarnia, C. H. et al. (1972) *Pesquisa agro. Brasileira, Ser. vet.*, 7, 41.
(11) Cook, W. R. (1970) *Equ. vet. J.*, 2, 137.
(12) Cook, W. R. (1974) *Vet. Rec.*, *94*, 533.

(13) Robinson, N. E. (1979) *Vet. Clin. N. Am. large Anim. Pract.*, *1*, 17.
(14) Livesey, M. A. et al. (1984) *Equ. vet. J.*, *16*, 144.
(15) Dixon, P. M. (1980) *Equ. vet. J.*, *12*, 28.
(16) Pascoe, J. R. et al. (1981) *Am. J. vet. Res.*, *42*, 203.
(17) Clarke, A. F. (1985) *Equ. vet. J.*, *17*, 166.
(18) Voynick, B. T. & Sweeney, C. R. (1986) *J. Am. vet. med. Assoc.*, *188*, 301.
(19) Sweeney, C. R. & Soma, L. (1982) *Proc. ann. Mtg Am. Assoc. equ. Pract.*, 51
(20) Raphel, C. F. & Soma, L. R. (1982) *Am. J. vet. Res.*, *43*, 1123.
(21) Pascoe, J. R. et al. (1985) *Am. J. vet. Res.*, *46*, 2000.
(22) Sweeney, C. R. et al. (1984) *Cornell Vet.*, *74*, 263.
(23) Soma, L. R. et al. (1985) *Am. J. vet. Res.*, *46*, 263.
(24) Manohar, M. (1986) *Am. J. vet. Res.*, *47*, 1387.
(25) Goetz, T. & Manohar, M. (1986) *Am. J. vet. Res.*, *47*, 270.
(26) Sweeney, C. R. & Soma, L. R. (1984) *J. Am. vet. med. Assoc.*, *185*, 195.

Laryngitis, tracheitis, bronchitis

Inflammation of the air passages usually involves all levels and no attempt is made here to differentiate between inflammations of various parts of the tract. They are all characterized by cough, noisy inspiration and some degree of inspiratory embarrassment.

Etiology

All infections of the upper respiratory tract cause inflammation, either acutely or as chronic diseases. In most diseases the laryngitis, tracheitis and bronchitis form only a part of the syndrome and the causes listed below are those diseases in which upper respiratory infection is a prominent feature.

Cattle
Infectious bovine rhinotracheitis (bovine herpesvirus 1), calf diphtheria, *Haemophilus somnus*. Congenital cavitation of the arytenoid may contribute to laryngeal abscess development (1).

Sheep
Chronic infection with *Actinomyces (Corynebacterium) pyogenes* (2).

Horses
Equine herpesvirus (EVR), equine viral arteritis (EVA), equine viral influenza (EVI), strangles (*Streptococcus equi*).

Pigs
Swine influenza.

Pathogenesis

Irritation of the mucosa causes frequent coughing, and swelling causes partial obstruction of the air passages with resulting inspiratory dyspnea.

Clinical findings

Coughing and inspiratory dyspnea are the common clinical signs.

In the early stages of acute infections the cough is usually dry and non-productive and is easily induced by grasping the trachea or larynx, or by exposure to cold air or dusty atmospheres. In acute laryngitis, the soft tissues around the larynx are usually enlarged and painful on palpation. In chronic affections, the cough may be less frequent and distressing and is usually dry and harsh. If the lesions cause much exudation or ulceration of the mucosa, as in bacterial tracheobronchitis secondary to infectious bovine rhinotracheitis in cattle, the cough is moist, and thick mucus, flecks of blood and fibrin may be coughed up. The cough is very painful and the animal makes attempts to suppress it. Fever and toxemia are common and affected animals cannot eat or drink normally.

Inspiratory dyspnea varies with the degree of obstruction and is usually accompanied by a loud stridor and harsh breath sounds on each inspiration. These are best heard over the trachea although they are quite audible over the base of the lung, being most distinct on inspiration. The respiratory movements are usually deeper than normal and the inspiratory phase more prolonged and forceful. Additional signs, indicative of the presence of a primary specific disease, may also be present.

Examination of the larynx is usually possible through the oral cavity using a cylindrical speculum of appropriate size and a bright pointed source of light. This is done relatively easily in cattle, sheep and pigs but is difficult in the horse. Lesions of the mucosae of the arytenoid cartilages and the vault of the larynx are usually visible if care and time are taken. In laryngitis, there is usually an excessive quantity of mucus, which may contain flecks of blood or pus in the pharynx. Palpation of the pharyngeal and laryngeal areas may reveal lesions not readily visible through a speculum. During opening of the larynx, lesions in the upper part of the trachea are sometimes visible. The use of a fiberoptic endoscope in the horse allows a detailed examination of the upper respiratory tract.

Inflammation or lesions of the larynx may be severe enough to cause marked inspiratory dyspnea and death from asphyxia. In calves and young cattle with diphtheria the lesion may be large enough, or have a pedicle and act like a valve, to cause severe inspiratory dyspnea, cyanosis, anxiety and rapid death. The excitement associated with loading for transportation to a clinic or of a clinical examination, particularly the oral examination of the larynx, can exaggerate the dyspnea and necessitate an emergency tracheotomy.

Most cases of bacterial laryngitis will heal without obvious residual sign after several days of antibiotic treatment. Some cases in cattle become chronic in spite of therapy due to the inflammation extending down into the arytenoid cartilages resulting in a chronic chondritis due to a sequestrum similar to osteomyelitis. Abscess formation is another common cause of chronicity. Secondary bacterial infection of primary viral diseases, or extension of bacterial infections to the lungs commonly results in pneumonia.

Clinical pathology

Laboratory examinations may be of value in determining the presence of specific diseases.

Necropsy findings

Upper respiratory infections are not usually fatal but lesions vary from acute catarrhal inflammation to chronic granulomatous lesions depending upon the duration and severity of the infection. When secondary bacterial invasion occurs a diphtheritic pseudomembrane may be present and be accompanied by an accumulation of exudate and necrotic material at the tracheal bifurcation and in the dependent bronchi.

Diagnosis

Infections of the larynx usually result in coughing, and inspiratory dyspnea with a stertor and loud abnormal laryngeal sounds on auscultation over the trachea and over the base of the lungs on inspiration. Lesions of the larynx are usually visible by laryngoscopic examination, those of the trachea and major bronchi are not so obvious unless special endoscopic procedures are used. Every reasonable effort should be used to visually examine the larynx and trachea. Differentiation from pneumonia, especially viral pneumonia, may be difficult if râles are absent and abnormal pulmonary sounds consist solely of bronchial tones. Differentiation is usually necessary in terms of the specific diseases. Obstruction of the upper respiratory tract due to other causes may also be difficult to distinguish unless other signs are present.

Treatment

Most of the common viral infections of larynx, trachea and major bronchi will resolve spontaneously if the affected animals are rested, not worked and not exposed to inclement weather and dusty feeds. Secondary bacterial complications must be recognized and treated with the appropriate antibacterial agent.

The bacterial infections can result in severe inflammation with necrosis and granulomatous lesions and must be treated with antibiotics or sulfonamides. Calves with calf diphtheria are treated with sulfamethazine intravenously initially followed by oral therapy daily for 3–5 days. Several days are usually required for the animal to return to normal. A broad-spectrum antimicrobial daily or more often for up to 3 weeks or more may be necessary for treatment of the chondritis. Animals with severe lesions and marked inspiratory dyspnea may require a tracheotomy and insertion of a tracheotomy tube for several days until the lesion heals. The tube must be removed, cleaned out and replaced at least once daily because of the accumulation of dried mucus plugs which interfere with respiration.

A corticosteroid (dexamethasone) may be used in an attempt to reduce the laryngeal edema associated with some severe cases of bacterial laryngitis in cattle. If successful, a tracheotomy may be unnecessary. Surgical excision of chronic granulomatous lesions and abscesses of the larynx may be indicated following failure of long-term antibiotic therapy but postoperative complications of laryngeal and pharyngeal paralysis are common. A combination of dexamethasone and antibiotic therapy is reported to be of value in chronic cases in horses (3).

REFERENCES

(1) Lawrence, J. A. (1967) *Vet. Rec.*, *81*, 540.
(2) Salisbury, R. M. (1956) *NZ vet. J.*, *4*, 144.
(3) Gerber, H. (1968) *Schweiz. Arch. Tierheilkd.*, *110*, 139.

Traumatic laryngotracheitis, tracheal compression and tracheal collapse

Traumatic laryngotracheal injury can occur following endotracheal intubation used for general anaesthesia (1, 2). Nasotracheal intubation can result in mucosal injury to the nasal meatus, the arytenoid cartilages, the trachea, the dorsal pharyngeal recess, the vocal cords and the entrance to the guttural pouches (1). The laryngeal injury is attributed to the tube pressure on the arytenoid cartilages and vocal folds and the tracheal damage is due to the pressure exerted by the inflated cuff on the tracheal mucosa.

Tracheal collapse is reported in the goat (3), and cow (5) and results in stridor, exercise intolerance and coughing. Tracheal rupture due to blunt trauma in the horse may result in severe subcutaneous emphysema and pneumomediastinum (5). Conservative therapy is usually successful. Tracheal compression secondary to enlargement of the cranial mediastinal lymph nodes can also cause inspiratory dyspnea (6) and conservative treatment with antimicrobials is successful.

REFERENCES

(1) Holland, M. et al. (1986) *J. Am. vet. med. Assoc.*, *189*, 1447.
(2) Trim, C. N. (1984) *J. Am. vet. med. Assoc.*, *185*, 541.
(3) Jackson, P. G. G. et al. (1986) *Vet. Rec.*, *119*, 160.
(4) Watt, B. R. (1983) *Aust. vet. J.*, *60*, 309.
(5) Fubini, S. L. et al. (1985) *J. Am. vet. med. Assoc.*, *187*, 69.
(6) Rigg, D. L. et al. (1985) *J. Am. vet. med. Assoc.*, *186*, 283.

Obstruction of the larynx

Structural obstruction with impairment of air flow at rest

Acute obstruction Edema of the larynx may occur as part of an allergic syndrome or because of the inhalation of smoke or fumes and cause upper respiratory tract obstruction. The edema which occurs in gut edema of swine is usually not sufficiently severe to do this. Acute cellulitis of the throat (pharyngeal phlegmon) and anthrax in horses and pigs commonly cause acute peripharyngeal cellulitis and edema. Swelling is readily visible from the exterior and is accompanied by a high fever and profound toxemia. Obstruction may occur accidentally when cattle or horses vomit and solid food material lodges in the larynx or when sharp pointed foreign bodies lodge in the region of the pharynx or larynx. A specific form of obstruction in sheep is caused by chronic laryngitis associated with *Actinomyces (Corynebacterium) pyogenes* infection. One of the most important causes of nasal obstruction in farm animals is enzootic nasal granuloma which is discussed under that heading. Acute bilateral paralysis of the vocal cords has occurred in a group of foals apparently as a result of poisoning with an organophosphate anthelmintic (1). A similar ocurrence in a group of 2-year-old thoroughbred horses given minerals thought to be contaminated with trichlorphon has been described (6). Clinical signs were severe dyspnea, especially when stressed, prolonged inspiration with inspiratory stridor, and collapse of the thorax. Tracheotomy provided temporary relief, but complete recovery did not occur.

Clinically there is marked inspiratory dyspnea with forceful prolonged elevation of the ribs and sinking of the flanks. Distress is often evident and cyanosis may be marked. Mouth breathing, respiratory stridor, salivation and extension of the head are prominent signs and manipulation of the head or exercise may cause fatal asphyxia.

Chronic obstruction The common causes of obstruction are: *cattle*—retropharyngeal lymphadenitis caused by tuberculosis, actinobacillosis, non-specific infection, usually *Actinomyces (Corynebacterium) pyogenes* (3); *horse*—pharyngeal lymphoid hyperplasia. Rare causes include neoplasm, e.g. chondroma of larynx in a horse (2), and laryngeal papillomatosis due to *Besnoitia bennetti* (4). A tracheobronchial foreign body in a horse caused chronic coughing (5).

Auscultation of the larynx reveals loud, stenotic sounds and fremitus may be detectable on palpation. Tracheotomy or laryngotomy may be necessary to prevent fatal asphyxia until the obstruction subsides or is relieved.

REFERENCES

(1) Rose, R. J. (1978) *Aust. vet. J.*, *54*, 154.
(2) Trotter, G. W. et al. (1981) *J. Am. vet. med. Assoc.*, *178*, 829.
(3) Vestweber, J. G. & Roeder, B. (1986) *Comp. cont. Educ. pract. Vet.*, *8*, F71.
(4) Lane, J. G. et al. (1986) *Vet. Rec.*, *119*, 591.
(5) Brown, C. M. & Collier, M. A. (1983) *J. Am. vet. med. Assoc.*, *182*, 280.
(6) Duncan, I. D. & Brook, D. (1985) *Equ. vet. J.*, *17*, 228.

Impairment of air flow through upper respiratory tract evident only during exercise

These disease problems are restricted almost entirely to the horse. They represent a very special group which affect racing performance rather than health, and have surgical outcomes rather than medical ones. Accordingly, they are not dealt with in this book. The list of diseases with indications of source material is as follows.

Pharyngeal lymphoid hyperplasia This provides a structural rather than a functional obstruction. It can be found in up to 65% of 2-year-old horses (10). It is dealt with under the heading of pharyngitis.

Left laryngeal hemiplegia This is a disease of unknown cause in which degeneration of nerve fibers in the left recurrent laryngeal nerve (4) is followed by atrophy of one or more of the intrinsic muscles of the left half of the larynx (1). The severity of the clinical signs is related to the number of muscles affected. In some cases the nerve is affected by guttural pouch mycosis; in others there is no such lesion. Partial respiratory obstruction during exercise renders the horse unfit for fast work; when work is attempted the respiratory distress is accompanied by a loud roaring sound from the larynx. The interpretation of laryngeal function tests in the horse have been described (11).

Soft palate paresis This provides an anatomical basis for a nondescript clinical entity of functional pharyngeal obstruction in which the horse chokes up during exercise. No organic lesion is detectable, but there is a general consensus that failure to control the soft palate during exercise causes obstruction of the airway. It often occurs together with laryngeal hemiplegia.

Dorsal displacement of the soft palate may be associated with palatal myositis (8). The lesions may result in muscular weakness which contributes to dorsal displacement of the soft palate. These horses also have a high frequency of pharyngeal lymphoid hyperplasia. However, the lesions may be secondary to trauma associated with mechanical displacement of the soft palate. In some cases the dorsal displacement may be due to a shortened epiglottis incapable of maintaining the soft palate in abnormal subepiglottic position (9).

Entrapment of the epiglottis This is caused by the development of large, abnormally mobile aryepiglottic folds which enfold the epiglottis and prevent its normal movement (3, 5). Affected horses commonly have a good racing career behind them and develop respiratory obstruction at a mature age.

Subepiglottic cysts In adult horses (6). These cause respiratory stridor, choking and decreased exercise tolerance. A few have nasal discharge. Foals (7) present a different syndrome including the abnormal respiratory sounds of adult horses, but also dysphagia, chronic cough, bilateral nasal discharge and aspiration pneumonia.

There are still more ill-defined functional obstructions of the horse's upper respiratory tract (2).

REVIEW LITERATURE

Boles, C. (1979) Abnormalities of the upper respiratory tract. *Vet. Clin. N. Am. large Anim. Pract.* *1(1)*, 89 & 127.

REFERENCES

(1) Anderson, L. J. (1977) *NZ vet J.*, *25*, 387.
(2) Goulden, B. E. (1977) *NZ vet. J.*, *25*, 389.
(3) Speirs, V. C. (1977) *J. Equ. med. Surg.*, *1*, 267.
(4) Duncan, I. D. et al. (1978) *Neuropathol. appl. Neurobiol.*, *4*, 483.
(5) Boles, C. L. et al. (1978) *J. Am. vet. med. Assoc.*, *172*, 338.
(6) Boles, C. L. (1979) *Vet. Clin. N. Am.*, *1(1)*, 89 & 127.
(7) Stick, J. A. & Boles, C. L. (1980) *J. Am. vet. med. Assoc.*, *177*, 62.
(8) Blythe, L. L. et al. (1983) *J. Am. vet. med. Assoc.*, *183*, 781.
(9) Haynes, P. F. (1981) *J. Am. vet. med. Assoc.*, *179*, 677.
(10) Raphel, C. F. (1982) *J. Am. vet. med. Assoc.*, *181*, 470.
(11) Hillidge, C. J. (1986) *Vet. Rec.*, *118*, 535.

Diseases of the guttural pouch

The guttural pouch of the horse is the province of the surgeon and it is not intended to deal with its diseases in detail. However, they do produce clinical signs which also occur in diseases which are usually dealt with medically. To assist in the differential diagnosis of them some brief notes are provided.

Guttural pouch mycosis

Mycotic lesions arise in the guttural pouch of the horse as a result of an infection entering the eustachian tube via its pharyngeal orifice. At least three different sequels may result:

- Erosion of internal carotid artery with the sudden development of profuse epistaxis usually in a horse at rest. The maxillary artery may also be involved (8)
- Thrombus development in the internal carotid

artery with emboli being shed to locate unilaterally in the brain resulting in blindness and ataxia (1)

- Mycotic encephalitis may be a sequelae of guttural pouch mycosis (6). The development of a fistula between the dorsal pharyngeal recess and the guttural pouches has also been described (7)
- Inflammation of the cranial neveres anatomically close to the wall of the guttural pouch (2). The common effects of damage to these nerves are:
  - dysphagia due to involvement of pharyngeal branches of the hypoglossal and vagal nerves;
  - laryngeal hemiplegia due to involvement of laryngeal branches of the vagus;
  - facial paresis due to involvement of facial nerve;
  - Horner's syndrome (ipsilateral facial sweating and hyperthermia, smaller palpebral fissure, mild miosis) due to involvement of sympathetic neurons.

Carotid and cerebral angiography are available for diagnosis (11). Treatment of the disease is surgical (3). Palliative treatment by the systemic administration of iodides to control the mycosis may effect a cure (4). Indwelling catheters and povidone-iodine flushes of the guttural pouches have been evaluated (12).

Guttural pouch empyema
The accumulation of pus in a pouch causes chronic toxemia, distension of one or both pouches, pain on swallowing and palpation, coughing and in some cases a purulent nasal discharge, especially if the horse is eating off the ground.

Guttural pouch tympany
The disease is limited in occurrence to foals a few days old. A congenital defect of closure of the eustachian tube allows the pouch or pouches to fill with air and distend obviously, and to an enormous size (5). The condition is not an acute one nor life-threatening, and foals survive well for several weeks before swallowing and respiration become impaired.

Miscellaneous diseases of the guttural pouch include hemangiomas (9) and foreign body penetration causing epistaxis (10).

REFERENCES

(1) Wagner, P. C. et al. (1978) *J. equ. Med. Surg.*, *2*, 355.
(2) Delahunta, A. (1978) *Cornell Vet.*, *68*, 122.
(3) Owen, R. R. & McKelvey, W. A. C. (1979) *Vet. Rec.*, *104*, 100.
(4) Rawlinson, R. J. & Jones, R. T. (1978) *Aust. vet. J.*, *54*, 135.
(5) Boles, C. L. (1979) *Vet. Clin. N. Am. large Anim. Pract.* *1(1)*, 89 & 127.
(6) McLaughlin, B. G. & O'Brien, J. L. (1986) *Can. vet. J.*, *27*, 109.
(7) Jacobs, K. A. & Fretz, P. B. (1982) *Can. vet. J*, *23*, 117.
(8) Smith, K. M. & Barber, S. M. (1984) *Can. vet. J.*, *25*, 239.
(9) Greene, H. J. & O'Connor, J. P. (1986) *Vet. Rec.*, *118*, 445.
(10) Bayly, W. M. (1982) *J. Am. vet. med. Assoc.*, *180*, 1232.
(11) Colles, C. M. & Cook, W. R. (1983) *Vet. Rec.*, *113*, 483.
(12) Wilson, J. (1985) *Equ. vet. J.*, *17*, 242.

Congenital defects

Primary congenital defects are rare in the respiratory tracts of animals. Secondary defects, which are associated with major defects in other systems, are more common. Most of the defects in lambs are associated with defects of the oral cavity, face and cranial vault (1). Accessory lungs are recorded occasionally (2, 3) and if their bronchi are vestigial the lungs can present themselves as tumor-like masses occupying most of the chest.

REFERENCES

(1) Dennis, S. M. (1975) *Aust. vet. J.*, *51*, 347.
(2) Smith, R. E. & McEntee, C. (1974) *Cornell Vet.*, *64*, 335.
(3) Osborne, J. C. & Troutt, H. F. (1977) *Cornell Vet.*, *67*, 222.

11

Diseases of the Urinary System

INTRODUCTION

DISEASES of the bladder and urethra are more common and more important in farm animals than diseases of the kidneys but some discussion of renal insufficiency is necessary because of the sporadic cases of pyelonephritis, embolic nephritis, amyloidoisis and nephrosis that occur in these species. A knowledge of the physiology of urinary secretion and excretion is also required for a proper understanding of diseases of the bladder and urethra. The principles of renal insufficiency as set out below are derived largely from human medicine and, although they probably apply in general terms to farm animals, the details of renal function and failure in these animals have not been extensively examined. In the section on manifestations of renal insufficiency only those abnormalities which are known to occur in farm animals are discussed.

Diseases of the reproductive tract are not presented in this book and details of them should be sought in the textbooks on the subject. Inevitably, some of the diseases are mentioned in the differential diagnosis of the medical diseases included here and in circumstances in which the reproductive tract is affected coincidentally. Reference to these entries in the text can be made through the index.

PRINCIPLES OF RENAL INSUFFICIENCY

The two functions of the kidneys are to excrete the end-products of tissue metabolism (except for carbon dioxide), and to maintain homeostasis with respect to fluids and solutes by selective excretion of these substances. This latter function is controlled by the capacity of the kidney to vary the volume of fluid excreted and the concentration of solutes. This capacity is dependent upon the functional activity of the tubules while control of excretion of metabolic end products is vested in the glomeruli. Glomerular filtrate is derived from plasma by a process of simple filtration and is identical with it except that it contains little protein or lipids. The absolute volume of filtrate, and therefore its content of metabolic end-products, depends upon the hydrostatic pressure and the plasma osmotic pressure in the glomerular capillaries and the proportion of glomeruli which are functional. These factors are not under the control of renal mechanisms and in the absence of disease the rate of filtration through the glomeruli varies little.

It is the function of the tubules actively to reabsorb from the glomerular filtrate those substances which need to be retained for utilization and participation in metabolic processes, while permitting the excretion of waste products. The retention of water by reabsorption in the proximal tubules is the main means whereby control of water homeostasis is achieved. As a result the concentration of solutes in the urine varies widely when the kidneys are functioning normally. The principal mechanism which governs reabsorption of water is the antidiuretic hormone (ADH) of the posterior pituitary gland, the secretion of which is stimulated by tissue dehydration and an increase in effective osmotic pressure of the tissue fluid. This control is not limitless, functioning only within a restricted range, and can be overcome by the use of diuretics whereby the flow of urine is so increased that maximum tubular reabsorption cannot sufficiently reduce the volume. Thus, an animal in a state of dehydration can be still further dehydrated by the use of diuretics. The tubular epithelium also selectively reabsorbs the solutes in the glomerular filtrate. Glucose is reabsorbed entirely, within the normal range of blood levels; phosphate is reabsorbed in varying amounts depending upon the needs of the body to conserve it; other substances such as inorganic sulfates and creatinine are not reabsorbed at all.

Diseases of the kidneys, and in some instances of the ureters, bladder and urethra, reduce the efficiency of these two functions and causes disturbances in protein, solute and water homeostasis and the excretion of metabolic end-products. A relative loss of function is described as renal insufficiency, complete or fatal loss as renal failure.

Renal insufficiency and renal failure

Renal efficiency depends upon the functional integrity of the individual nephrons, and insufficiency can occur because of abnormality in the rate of renal blood flow, the glomerular filtration rate, and the efficiency of tubular reabsorption. Of these, the latter two are those which are intrinsic functions of the kidney, the first depending largely upon vasomotor control and in animals is affected only by emergencies in circulatory dynamics such as shock, dehydration and hemorrhage. Although in these diseases there may be a serious reduction in glomerular filtration the cause is extrarenal and cannot be considered as a true cause of renal insufficiency. However, tubular necrosis may follow prolonged renal ischemia and cause renal insufficiency.

Glomerular filtration and tubular reabsorption may be affected independently of each other in disease states such as hemoglobinuric nephrosis, where glomerular filtration is unaffected but tubular reabsorption is seriously depressed. However, because of the common blood supply of the glomerulus and tubule, damage to any part of the nephron is followed by damage to the remaining parts and it is probably more accurate to think in terms of loss of entire nephrons rather than loss of tubular or glomerular function. At least this is true when the prognosis in a particular case is under discussion. Even when there is loss of entire nephrons rather than selective depression of tubular function, the end result may be the same because of disproportionate compensatory response on the part of the residual nephrons, resulting in an imbalance of glomerular and tubular functions. The progress and the end result of renal disease of any kind thus tend to be very similar. In glomerulonephritis the primary reaction is glomerular but a secondary involvement of the tubules occurs. In nephrosis the primary lesion is in the tubules and in the interstitial nephritis tubular degeneration is probably the primary and major lesion but glomerular dysfunction commonly follows.

The development of renal dysfunction is dependent upon the loss of functional renal tissue. If the degree of loss, and therefore the degree of dysfunction, is such that the animal's continued existence is not possible it is said to be in a state of renal failure and the clinical syndrome of uremia is manifest.

In contrast to the degree of renal dysfunction there is the concept of the form of the insufficiency. The form, including the clinical and clinicopathological manifestations of the dysfunction, depends upon the anatomical location of the lesion and thus upon the imbalance of residual function between glomeruli and tubules. Renal dysfunction tends to be a dynamic process and the degree and form of the dysfunction are likely to vary from time to time.

Pathological physiology of renal insufficiency

Damage to the glomerular epithelium permits the passage of plasma proteins into the capsular fluid. The protein is principally albumin, probably because it has a smaller molecule than globulin. Complete cessation of glomerular filtration may occur when there is extensive damage to glomeruli, particularly if there is acute swelling of the kidney, but it is believed that in many instances the anuria of the terminal stages of acute renal disease is caused by back diffusion of all glomerular filtrate through the damaged tubular epithelium. When the kidney damage is of a less severe degree, the compensatory response on the part of residual nephrons is to maintain total glomerular filtration by an increase in filtration per nephron. This may be in excess of the capacity of the tubular epithelium to reabsorb fluid and solutes and achieve normal urine concentration, and therefore urine of a constant specific gravity and daily volume passes into renal pelvis. This defect may be further exaggerated if there is tubular damage. It is this lack of ability to concentrate urine (isothenuria), in spite of variations in fluid and electrolyte intake, which is characteristic of developing renal insufficiency.

Loss of glomerular filtration is also reflected by a retention in the blood of urea and other nitrogenous end-products of metabolism. Although blood levels of urea are probably not significant in the production of clinical signs they are used as a measure of glomerular filtration rate. This is becoming a disease of some importance in horses usually as a result of renal tubular dysfunction in which there is bicarbonate loss via the tubular epithelium without a corresponding loss of chloride leading to hyperchloremia (29). Phosphate and sulfate retention also occurs when total glomerular filtration is reduced and may precipitate renal acidosis. Phosphate retention also causes a secondary hypocalcemia, due in part to an increase in calcium excretion in the urine. Variations in serum potassium levels also occur and appear to depend on potassium intake. Hyperpotassemia is a serious complication in renal insufficiency in man and is one of the principal causes of the myocardial asthenia and fatal heart failure which occurs in uremia in this species.

Loss of tubular reabsorptive function is evidenced by a continued loss of sodium and a resultant hyponatremia which eventually occurs in all cases of nephritis. The continued loss of large quantities of fluid in the poorly concentrated urine may cause clinical dehydration but more commonly puts the patient in a position of being particularly susceptible to further fluid loss or to shock or other circulatory emergency.

Pathogenesis of renal failure

The terminal stage of renal insufficiency—renal failure—is the result of the accumulated effects of disturbed renal excretory and homeostatic functions. Continued excretion of large volumes of urine of low concentration causes a degree of dehydration, and if other circulatory emergencies arise acute renal ischemia results, and is followed by acute renal failure. Hypoproteinemia may be prolonged and results in rapid loss of body condition and muscle weakness. Acidosis is also a contributing factor. Hyponatremia and hyperpotassemia cause skeletal muscle weakness and myocardial asthenia. The hypocalcemia may be of sufficient degree to increase circulatory failure further and contribute to nervous signs. All of these factors play some part in the production of clinical signs. In some cases one or other of them may be of major importance and the clinical syndrome is therefore subject to a great deal of variation.

Renal failure is manifested by the clinical state of uremia which can also occur in urinary tract obstruction. It is characterized biochemically by an increase in blood levels of total and urea nitrogen (azotemia) and by retention of other solutes as described above.

Causes of renal insufficiency and uremia

The causes of renal insufficiency, and therefore of renal failure and uremia, can be divided into prerenal and renal groups. Prerenal causes include congestive heart failure and acute circulatory failure, either cardiac or peripheral, in which acute renal ischemia occurs. Hemoglobinuric and myoglobinuric nephrosis are also included in this category. Renal causes include glomerulonephritis, interstitial nephritis, pyelonephritis, embolic nephritis and amyloidosis.

Acute renal failure due to nephrosis has been produced experimentally in ponies by the administration of mercuric chloride and potassium dichromate (31). Experimental uremia has also been induced by surgical removal of both kidneys but the results, especially in ruminants, are quite different to those in naturally occurring renal failure. The clinical pathology is similar but there is a prolonged period of normality after the surgery (30).

Uremia may also occur due to postrenal causes, specifically complete obstruction of the urinary tract by vesical or urethral calculus or more rarely by bilateral ureteral obstruction. Internal rupture of any part of the urinary tract will have the same effect.

PRINCIPAL MANIFESTATIONS OF URINARY TRACT DISEASE

The principal manifestations of disease of the urinary tract include abnormal constituents of the urine, abnormalities of volume, pain and dysuria, rupture of the renal pelvis, bladder and urethra, and defects of nervous control of the bladder.

There are also general signs of toxemia which vary with the rate of development of the disease. In acute renal failure the characteristic syndrome is that of uremia as set out below. In chronic renal disease there is a severe loss of body weight, polyuria, polydipsia and pitting edema (19–21). Lethargy, anorexia and emaciation are terminal signs.

Abnormal constituents of the urine

Proteinuria

Normal urine contains very small amounts of protein derived from desquamating epithelial cells but the amount is insufficient to produce a positive reaction to standard tests for proteinuria. One exception to this rule is the proteinuria observed in normal calves up to 40 hours old if they have received colostrum and in newborn kids and lambs (1). Protein may be present in appreciable amount in hemoglobinuria, myoglobinuria, and hematuria and when the sample contains necrotic material from the urinary tract. These possibilities should be eliminated as causes before a diagnosis of renal disease is made.

Proteinuria, often designated as albuminuria because of the high proportion of albumin present, occurs in congestive heart failure, glomerulonephritis, renal infarction, nephrosis and amyloidosis. It is also a common finding in cows affected by the 'downer cow' syndrome. The degree of proteinuria varies, the greatest concentration occurring in amyloidosis. Small amounts may be present when mild glomerular damage occurs in fever and toxemia. In renal disease the concentration may vary during different phases of the disease. Not all of the protein derives from the passage of plasma albumin through damaged glomerular capillaries; appreciable amounts may be contributed by the degeneration of the cells of the tubules in acute cortical necrosis. The significance of proteinuria as an indication of renal disease is much greater when formed elements, including casts, are present in the urine.

If the proteinuria persists there may be sufficient loss to cause hypoproteinemia but edema of renal origin as it occurs in man is uncommon in animals. If the protein originates from the lesions of pyelonephritis or cystitis clinical evidence of these diseases can usually be detected.

Casts and cells

Casts appear as organized, tubular structures which vary in appearance according to their composition. They occur only in nephritis and their presence is an indication of inflammatory or degenerative changes in the kidney, the casts having been formed by the agglomeration of desquamated cells and protein. Erythrocytes, leukocytes and epithelial cells may originate in any part of the urinary tract.

Hematuria

Prerenal causes of hematuria include trauma to the kidney, septicemias and purpura hemorrhagica accompanied by vascular damage. Renal causes include acute glomerulonephritis, renal infarction, embolism of the renal artery, tubular damage as caused by sulfonamide intoxication, and pyelonephritis. Postrenal hematuria occurs particularly in urolithiasis and cystitis. A special instance is enzootic hematuria of cattle.

In severe cases the blood may be voided in the form of clots but more commonly causes a deep red to brown coloration of the urine. Less severe cases may show only cloudiness which settles to form a red deposit on standing, or the hematuria may be so slight as to be detectable only on microscopic examination of a centrifuged sediment. The origin of the blood may be ascertained by collection of the urine in stages. Blood which originates from the kidneys is usually intimately mixed with the urine and is present in equal concentration in all samples. When the blood originates from a vesical lesion it is usually most concentrated in the final sample and blood from a urethral lesion is most evident in the first part of the flow. It may be necessary to collect a sample by catheterization in females to avoid the chance of contamination of the urine occurring in the vagina.

Urine containing blood gives positive results in biochemical tests for hemoglobin and myoglobin, and as the erythrocytes are often lysed, it is necessary to examine all red-colored urine for the presence of erythrocytes. The presence of a heavy brown deposit is not sufficient basis for a diagnosis of hematuria as this may also occur in hemoglobinuria. Involvement of the bladder or urethra may be detectable on physical examination of the patient. Gross hematuria persisting for long periods may result in severe hemorrhagic anemia.

Hemoglobinuria

False hemoglobinuria occurs in hematuria when the erythrocytes are broken down and liberate their hemoglobin. Its presence can be determined only by microscopic examination of the urinary sediment for the presence of cellular debris.

True hemoglobinuria is manifested by a deep red coloration of the urine, a positive reaction to chemical tests for hemoglobin and protein, and the absence of cellular debris. A positive hemeglobin test, using test-dip papers will not give a positive protein test unless the concentration of the hemoglobin is very high (27). There are many causes of intravascular hemolysis, the source of hemoglobinuria. The specific causes are listed under hemolytic anemia.

Normally, hemoglobin liberated from effete erythrocytes is converted to bile pigments in the cells of the reticuloendothelial system. When hemolysis occurs in excess of the capacity of this system to remove the hemoglobin, it increases in concentration in the blood until it exceeds a certain renal threshold and then escapes with the urine. There is no evidence as to why the large hemoglobin molecule passes the glomerular filter when smaller molecules are retained. Some hemoglobin is reabsorbed from the glomerular filtrate by the tubular epithelium but probably not in sufficient amounts to appreciably affect the hemoglobin content of the urine. Precipitation of hemoglobin to form casts occurs in the tubules, especially if the urine is acid and some plugging of tubules results, but the chief cause for the development of uremia in hemolytic anemia is the tubular nephrosis which occurs.

Myoglobinuria

The presence of myoglobin (myohemoglobin) in the urine is evidence of severe muscle dystrophy. The only notable occurrence in animals is azoturia of horses. In enzootic muscular dystrophy, myoglobinuria may occur but there is usually insufficient myoglobin in the muscles of young animals to cause an appreciable degree of abnormality. The myoglobin molecule is much smaller than that of hemoglobin and passes the glomerular filter much more readily so that a detectable dark brown staining of the urine occurs without very high levels of myoglobin being attained in the serum. Thus a detectable discoloration of the serum does not occur as it does in hemoglobinemia. In inherited congenital porphyria, the other disease in which the urine is discolored a reddish brown, the plasma is also normal in color. Differentiation from myoglobinuria is made on the negative reaction to the guaiac test and the characteristic spectrograph. The porphyrins in this disease are the only pigments which fluoresce when illuminated by ultraviolet light.

The presence of the pigment in the urine can be determined accurately by spectrographic examination. The abnormality of the urine is usually accompanied by clinical signs of acute myopathy. Precipitation of myoglobin in the tubules occurs as with hemoglobin and may contribute towards a terminal uremia.

Pyuria

Pus in the urine indicates inflammatory exudation at some point in the urinary tract, usually the renal pelvis or bladder. It may occur as macroscopically visible clots or shreds, or be detectable only by microscopic examination as leukocytic casts, or as individual cells which are most readily observed in a centrifuged deposit. Pyuria is usually accompanied by the presence of bacteria in the urine.

Crystalluria

The presence of crystals in the urine of herbivorous animals has no special significance unless they occur in very large numbers and are associated with clinical signs of irritation of the urinary tract. Crystals of calcium carbonate and triple phosphate are commonly present in normal urine. Their presence in large numbers may suggest that the concentration of the urine is above normal and the possible future development of urolithiasis.

Glycosuria and ketonuria

Glycosuria together with ketonuria occurs only in diabetes mellitus, a rare disease in large animals. Glycosuria is not common but is associated with enterotoxemia due to *Clostridium perfringens* type D and occurs after parenteral treatment with dextrose solutions, adrenocorticotrophic hormones or cortisone analogs. It occurs also in nephrosis due to failure of tubular resorption. Ketonuria is a more common finding and occurs in starvation, acetonemia of cattle and pregnancy toxemia of ewes and cows.

Indicanuria

The presence of indican (potassium indoxyl sulfonate) in excessive amounts indicates increased absorption of this detoxification product of indole from the large intestine. Indicanuria occurs when the alimentary sojourn is prolonged for any reason.

Creatinuria

Excessive endogenous breakdown of muscle causes an increased concentration of creatinine in the urine and some use has been made of this in the detection of muscular dystrophy. However, a degree of creatinuria may be found in normal sheep, cattle and pigs suggesting caution in the use of the creatinine-to-creatinine ratio as a diagnostic aid in these species (2, 3).

Variations in daily urine flow

An increase or decrease in urine flow is often described in animals but accuracy demands physical measurement of the amount of urine voided over a 24-hour period. This is not often practicable in clinical work and it is often necessary to guess whether the flow is increased or decreased. Care should be taken to differentiate between increased daily flow increased frequency without increased flow. The latter is much more common. Decreased urine output rarely if ever presents as a clinical problem in agricultural animals although the volume may be reduced by 50% in horses denied all access to water (23).

Polyuria
A transient increase in urine volume may be apparent with excessive water intake or a diet deficient in sodium chloride. It also occurs in normal animals, especially horses which for reasons of boredom or other psychological aberration eat more than the usual amount of salt or drink excessive amounts of water (18). The time taken to excrete an oral water load varies widely between individual animals and between species, being longer in cattle than in the dog (4). Continued polyuria is in most instances the result of decreased tubular reabsorption. This may occur because of absence of the antidiuretic hormone (diabetes insipidus), because of an increase in solutes in the glomerular filtrate beyond the resorptive capacity of the tubular epithelium, or because of damage to the tubules. A transient increase in urine volume may occur due to fear or emotional stress. Diabetes insipidus is rare in farm animals, being reported most commonly in horses in which it is usually caused by a tumor of the pituitary gland. Cases are recorded in a young ram (28) and in a cow (14) in which all the criteria for the diagnosis of diabetes insipidus were present but the cow recovered gradually over a period of a year. It is characterized by excessive thirst, the passage of a very large volume of urine of low specific gravity (1·002–1·006), and a temporary response to the parenteral administration of pitressin. Osmotic diuresis, caused by an increase in solutes in the glomerular filtrate, may result from administration of diuretics comprising substances not reabsorbed by the tubules, or by the excretion of naturally occurring substances such as urea and glucose in amounts larger than the tubular epithelium can reabsorb. Fluid is lost in both instances because of the osmotic relationship between solutes and water in the urine. Polyuria has been demonstrated to occur in vitamin A deficiency in sheep but the mechanism is uncertain (5).

Damage to the tubular epithelium and failure of tubular resorption occur in nephrosis and nephritis. This form of polyuria is characterized by inability of the kidney to vary the concentration of the urine with varying intakes of fluid (isosthenuria or hyposthenuria), so that dehydration occurs if fluid intake is reduced. The specific gravity also varies only within narrow limits (1·006–1·016) and is usually about 1·010. Specific gravity is a relatively crude method of measuring renal concentrating function and a more accurate, and nowadays more commonly used, technique is the measurement of renal osmolality. Renal osmolalities of 300 mOsm/kg of urine are in the normal range.

Oliguria and anuria
Reduction in the daily output (oliguria) and complete absence of urine (anuria) occur under the same conditions and vary only in degree. Complete anuria occurs most commonly in urethral obstruction, although it may result from acute tubular necrosis such as is caused by mercury poisoning. The anuria of acute glomerulonephritis which is a familiar syndrome in man rarely if ever occurs in animals. Oliguria occurs in the terminal stages of all forms of nephritis. The retention of solutes and disturbances of acid–base balance that follow anuria or severe oliguria contribute to the development of uremia. In dehydration urine flow decreases due to increased osmotic pressure of the plasma, and congestive heart failure and peripheral circulatory failure may cause such a reduction in renal blood flow that oliguria follows.

Pain and dysuria

Abdominal pain and dysuria are both expressions of discomfort caused by disease of the urinary tract. Acute abdominal pain due to disease of the urinary tract occurs rarely and is usually associated with sudden distension of the renal pelvis or ureter, or infarction of the kidney. None of these conditions is common in animals, but occasionally in cattle affected with pyelonephritis attacks of acute abdominal pain occur which are thought to be due to either renal infarction or obstruction of the pelvis by necrotic debris. The attacks of pain are acute with downward arching of the back, paddling with the hind feet, rolling and bellowing. Subacute abdominal pain occurs with urethral obstruction and distension of the bladder and is manifested by tail-switching, kicking at the belly, and efforts at urination accompanied by grunting.

Painful or difficult urination occurs in cystitis, vesical calculus and urethritis and is manifested by the frequent passage of small amounts of urine. Grunting may occur with urination and the animal remains in the typical posture after the act is completed. Differentiation of pain caused by urinary disease from that due to other causes depends largely upon detection of other signs indicative of involvement of the urinary tract.

Uremia

The term uremia is poorly defined but is used here to describe the clinical syndrome which occurs in the terminal stages of renal insufficiency. The physiological basis of the various signs observed is uncertain, and in dogs and humans varies from case to case and from time to time in the one patient. This subject has been discussed in general terms under principles of renal failure.

Clinical signs include anuria or oliguria, the latter being more common unless there is complete obstruction of the urinary tract. Chronic renal disease may be manifested by polyuria but this is essentially a compensatory phenomenon and oliguria always appears in the terminal stages when clinical uremia develops. The animal is depressed, shows muscular weakness and muscle tremor and the respiration is usually deep and labored. If the disease has been in progress for some time body condition is poor, due probably to continued loss of protein in the urine, to dehydration and to the anorexia which is characteristic of the disease. The respiration is usually increased in rate and depth but is not dyspneic; in the terminal stages it may become periodic in character. The heart rate is markedly increased because of the terminal dehydration and myocardial asthenia but the temperature remains normal unless an infectious process is present. An ammoniacal or uriniferous smell on the breath is often described but is usually undetectable.

In the terminal stages the animal becomes recumbent and comatose, the temperature falls to below normal and death occurs quietly, the whole course of the disease having been one of gradual but inexorable intoxication. Necropsy findings apart from those of the primary disease are non-specific and include degeneration of parenchymatous organs, sometimes accompanied by emaciation and moderate gastroenteritis. There are rare reports of encephalopathy caused by renal insufficiency (12).

Uremia has been produced experimentally in cattle by bilateral nephrectomy (15) and urethral ligation (16). There is a progressive metabolic alkalosis, hypercapnia and an elevation of blood urea nitrogen (up to 250 mg/100 ml) and creatinine. However, similar findings are reported in prerenal uremia in cattle (11).

SPECIAL EXAMINATION OF THE URINARY SYSTEM

Rectal examination in horses and cattle is essential for examination of the urinary tract and is described in Chapter 1. Radiographic examination is not usually undertaken but special examination techniques including catheterization, and biochemical and microscopic examination of urine are in routine use. Tests of renal function are available but have not been generally adopted in large animal practice because of the infrequent occurrence of renal disease. Percutaneous biopsy of the kidney has been successfully carried out in cows and a horse. The left kidney is fixed in position by rectal manipulation and a biopsy needle introduced through the upper flank (6). Special attention has been given in recent years to the study of the functional performance of the equine kidney. The estimation of glomerular filtration rate, the effective renal plasma flow and plasma renin activity are feasible techniques and scintigraphic imaging using ^{99m}Tc-glucoheptonate[h] has been carried out (22).

Collection of urine samples can cause difficulties. Catheterized samples are preferred especially for microbiological examination but failing this, other techniques are worth trying. For horses, walking them indoors into a box stall freshly floored with clean straw works in most cases. Cows oblige if they are relaxed and have their perineum and vulval tip massaged upwards very gently, without moving the tail. Steers and bulls may urinate if the preputial orifice is massaged and splashed with water. Ewes urinate if their nostrils are occluded and asphyxia threatened. They often urinate just as they are released and allowed to breathe again. An intravenous injection of furosemide (0·5–0·8 mg/kg body weight) produces a urination in most animals in about 20 min in all species. The sample is useful for microbiological examination, but its composition has been drastically altered by the diuretic. In experimental situations special apparatuses are used on animals that are accustomed to them.

Catheterization

Rams and boars cannot be catheterized because of inaccessibility of the penis and the small diameter of the urethra. A lead wire is used in steers and bulls but is not sufficiently flexible to make the passage easy. Ewes and sows have vulvas which are too small to allow easy access to the urethra. Passage of a catheter in a cow is relatively simple provided a fairly rigid catheter of small diameter (0–5 cm) is used and a finger can be inserted into the suburethral diverticulum to direct the tip of the catheter into the external urethral orifice. Mares are catheterized with ease, the external urethral orifice being large and readily accessible. There is difficulty in bringing the penis of the male horse into view, although the penis is usually relaxed when urethral obstruction occurs. Administration of an ataractic drug makes manipulation of the penis easier and often results in its complete relaxation. A proper male horse catheter, well lubricated, should be used as sufficient rigidity is necessary to pass through the long urethra and around the ischial arch.

Urinalysis

The reader is referred to a textbook of veterinary clinical pathology for details of the biochemical and microscopic examination of the urine. The occurrence and significance of the more common abnormalities of the urine are described under manifestations of diseases of the urinary system.

Renal function tests

The simplest and most important test of urinary function is that aimed at determining whether or not urine is being voided. This is generally accomplished in large animals by restraining them on a clean, dry floor which is examined periodically.

The term renal function tests includes those tests in which various functions of the kidney are measured by biochemical means. They can be considered in groups depending on whether they are based on the examination of blood, urine or both.

Tests conducted on urine

The simplest test is that which measures the capacity of the kidneys to vary the specific gravity of the urine. The normal specific gravity is of the order of 1·028–1·032. In chronic nephritis this falls to about 1·010 and is not appreciably altered by either deprivation of water for 24 hours or the administration of large quantities of water by stomach tube. Other more complicated tests require the administration of urea or the intravenous injection of a dye such as phenolsulfonphthalein which is excreted in urine. Periodic catheter samples are taken and the time required for excretion of the administered compound determined. Excretion is delayed in renal disease but standards for normality in large animals are not generally available, and results obtained after surgical extirpation of all or part of the kidneys do not necessarily reflect the situation provided by diseased tubules (26). The measurement of the concentration of enzymes in urine is presently proving to be an advantageous method of assessing renal tubular function, as described in the section on nephrosis. The concentration of these substances in urine is unrelated to their concentration in urine (24).

Tests conducted on blood
These tests depend on the accumulation, in cases of renal insufficiency, of metabolites normally excreted by the kidney. The estimation of the level of urea in the blood is most commonly used but tests for non-protein nitrogen or creatinine are also available. All suffer from the disadvantage that blood levels of these substances vary with the rate of protein catabolism and are not dependent entirely on renal function (7). For example in cattle, blood urea nitrogen levels caused by prerenal lesions may be higher than the levels resulting from renal disease (11). In renal disease the levels do not rise appreciably above the normal range until 60–75% of nephrons are destroyed. The fractional clearance of phenolsulfonphthalein has been suggested as a suitable test for the measurement of renal function in animals and some data are available for cattle (8, 9). The renal clearance of sodium sulfanilate (10 mg/kg body weight as a 20% solution in water injected intravenously) measured at 10, 15, 30, 60 and 90 min after injection shows a $t_{\frac{1}{2}}$ value of 39·5 ± 4·4 min (13).

Tests conducted on urine and blood
The capacity of the kidneys to transfer administered urea from the bloodstream to the urine is measured against time and is probably the most efficient clearance test available. It suffers from the deficiency that urine samples are often not readily obtainable, especially in male ruminants. This test, together with a test of the ability to increase and decrease the specific gravity of the urine, provides most information on renal efficiency. A good deal of information is available on renal function in the calf (10).

The urine urea nitrogen/plasma urea nitrogen ratio (Uun/Pun), urine creatinine/plasma creatinine ratio (Ucr/Pcr), urine osmolality/plasma osmolality ratio (Uosm/Posm), and fractional excretion of filtered sodium (FE_{Na}) is being used to differentiate between prerenal and renal azotemia in the horse (17).

PRINCIPLES OF TREATMENT OF DISEASES OF THE URINARY SYSTEM

Little can be done other than to treat the primary disease. If an inflammatory or infectious process can be halted the animal may be able to survive on its residual, functional, renal tissue; reversible renal failure is not a common occurrence in animals but the rational treatment of dehydration, hemorrhagic anemia and shock may prevent renal ischemia and resulting renal insufficiency.

Supportive treatment, including the parenteral administration of fluid and sodium and possibly calcium salts, may enable an animal to survive an acute renal insufficiency until an infectious process is brought under control. Continuous peritoneal or vascular dialyzation as is practiced in human medicine has not yet achieved any significant place in veterinary medicine except in small animal work. Once the destruction of nephrons has passed the critical point there is little that can be done other than temporarily to prolong the animal's life. Emergency slaughter is not recommended as the carcass is usually graded as unsuitable for human consumption.

The use of diuretics has no place in renal disease. In chronic uremia solute diuresis is already in operation and the stimulation of further water flow can only exacerbate the dehydration. In acute uremia the defect is one of glomerular filtration which is not improved by diuretics, and in the terminal stages of chronic uremia too many nephrons have been destroyed to enable any functional improvement in nephron efficiency to exert an appreciable effect on the course of the disease.

REVIEW LITERATURE

Fletcher, A. (1985) Renal disease in cattle. *Comp. cont. Educ.*, Part 1, 7, S701–S707; Part 2 (1986), *8*, S338–S345.

Koterba, A. M. & Coffman, J. R. (1981) Renal disease in the horse. *Proc. 27th Ann. Conf. Am. Assoc. Equ. Practnrs*, 313–321.

REFERENCES

(1) Pierce, A. B. (1961) *Proc. R. Soc. Med.*, *54*, 996.
(2) Blanch, E. & Setchell, B. P. (1960) *Aust. J. biol. Sci.*, *13*, 356.
(3) Aafjes, J. H. & de Groot, T. (1961) *Br. vet. J.*, *117*, 201.
(4) Dalton, R. G. (1964) *Br. vet. J.*, *120*, 69.
(5) Webb, K. E., Jr et al. (1968) *J. anim. Sci.*, *27*, 1657.
(6) Osborne, C. A. et al. (1968) *J. Am. vet. med. Assoc.*, *153*, 563.
(7) Campbell, J. R. & Watts, C. (1970) *Vet. Rec.*, *87*, 127.
(8) Mixner, J. P. & Anderson, R. R. (1958) *J. dairy Sci.*, *41*, 306.
(9) Osbaldiston, G. W. & Moore, W. E. (1971) *J. Am. vet. med. Assoc.*, *159*, 292.
(10) Dalton, R. G. (1968) *Br. vet. J.*, *124*, 371, 451, 498, *125*, 367.
(11) Brobst, D. F. et al. (1978) *J. Am. vet. med. Assoc.* *173*, 481.
(12) Summers, B. A. et al. (1985) *Cornell Vet.*, *75*, 524.
(13) Brobst, D. L. et al. (1978) *J. equ. med. Surg.*, *2*, 500.
(14) Wallace, C. E. & Kociba, G. J. (1979) *J. Am. vet. med. Assoc.*, *175*, 809.
(15) Watts, C. & Campbell, J. R. (1970) *Res. vet. Sci.*, *11*, 508 & *12*, 234.
(16) Sharma, S. N. et al. (1981) *Am. J. vet. Res.*, *42*, 333.
(17) Grossman, B. S. et al. (1982) *J. Am. vet. med. Assoc.*, *180*, 284.
(18) Buntain, B. J. & Coffman, J. R. (1981) *Equ. vet. J.*, *13*, 26.
(19) Divers, T. J. (1983) *Comp. cont. Educ.*, *5*, S310.
(20) Snyder, J. R. (1983) *Comp. cont. Educ.*, *5*, S134.
(21) Koterba, A. M. et al. (1981) *Proc. 27th Ann. Conv. Am. Assoc. Equ. Practnrs*, p. 313.
(22) Hood, D. M. et al. (1982) *Southwestern Vet.*, *35*, 19.
(23) Rumbaugh, G. E. et al. (1982) *Am. J. vet. Res.*, *43*, 735.
(24) Brobst, D. F. et al. (1986) *Cornell Vet.*, *76*, 299.
(25) Paulson, G. D. et al. (1984) *Am. J. vet. Res.*, *45*, 2150.
(26) Filippich, L. J. et al. (1985) *Am. J. vet. Res.*, *46*, 733.
(27) Jansen, B. S. & Lumsden, J. H. (1985) *Can. vet. J.*, *26*, 221.
(28) Thomson, J. R. (1986) *J. comp. Pathol.*, *96*, 119.
(29) Ziemer, E. L. et al. (1987) *J. Am. vet. med. Assoc.*, *190*, 294.
(30) Singh, J. et al. (1983) *Can. J. comp. med.*, *47*, 217.
(31) Bayly, W. M. et al. (1986) *Cornell Vet.*, *76*, 287.

DISEASES OF THE KIDNEY

Renal ischemia

Reduction in the flow of blood through the kidneys is usually the result of a general circulatory failure. There is transitory oliguria followed by anuria and uremia if the circulatory failure is not corrected.

Etiology
Ischemia may be acute or chronic.

Acute renal ischemia

- General circulatory emergencies such as shock, dehydration, acute hemorrhagic anemia, acute heart failure
- Embolism of renal artery, recorded in horses.

Chronic renal ischemia

- Chronic circulatory insufficiency such as congestive heart failure.

Pathogenesis
Acute ischemia of the kidneys occurs when compensatory vasoconstriction affects the renal blood vessels in response to a sudden reduction in circulating blood volume. There is an immediate reduction in glomerular filtration and an elevation of levels of normally excreted metabolites in the bloodstream. For example, an elevation of blood urea nitrogen occurs and gives rise to the name prerenal uremia. There is a concomitant reduction in urine flow. If the ischemia is severe enough and persists for long enough the reduction in glomerular filtration, which has been reversible by a return of normal blood flow, becomes irreversible because of anoxic degenerative lesions in the renal parenchyma. This is most likely to occur in acute circulatory disturbances and is an unlikely event in chronic congestive heart failure.

The parenchymatous lesions vary from tubular necrosis to cortical necrosis in which both tubules and glomeruli are affected. The nephrosis of hemoglobinuria is caused by the vasoconstriction of renal vessels. The uremia which contributes to a fatal termination in acute hemolytic anemia and in acute muscular dystrophy with myoglobinuria may be exacerbated by plugging of the tubules with casts of coagulated protein, but the nephrosis is the more important factor.

Clinical findings
Renal ischemia does not usually appear as a disease entity, largely because it is masked by the clinical signs of a primary disease. However, bilateral cortical necrosis, with anuria and renal colic, has been reported in a mare (1). The oliguria and azotemia which occur will in most cases go unnoticed if the circulatory defect is corrected in the early stages. However, failure to respond completely to treatment with transfusion or the infusion of other fluids in hemorrhagic or hemolytic anemia, or in shock or dehydration, may be caused by renal insufficiency. The general clinical picture has been described under uremia.

Clinical pathology
Laboratory examinations are of value particularly in determining the degree of residual renal damage after the circulatory defect has been corrected. Estimation of urea nitrogen levels in the blood are most commonly used as an index. Hematological examinations may be undertaken to determine the degree and type of circulatory insufficiency. In the irreversible stage when damage to the parenchyma has occurred there will be proteinuria if the lesion is primarily glomerular. The passage of large volumes of urine of low specific gravity after a period of oliguria is usually a good indication of a return of normal glomerular and tubular function.

Necropsy findings
Renal ischemia is manifested chiefly in the cortex which is pale and swollen and there may be a distinct line of necrosis visible macroscopically at the corticomedullary junction. Histologically there is necrosis of tubular epithelium and, in severe cases, of the glomeruli. In hemoglobinuria and myoglobinuria hyaline casts are present in the tubules.

Diagnosis
Evidence of oliguria and azotemia in the presence of circulatory failure suggests renal ischemia with the possibility of permanent renal damage. It is important to differentiate the early reversible stage from primary renal disease. In the latter instance there are abnormalities of the urine as described above. When irreversible ischemic changes have occurred it is impossible to differentiate the disease from glomerulonephritis and nephrosis.

Treatment
Treatment must be directed at correction of the circulatory disturbance at the earliest opportunity. If renal damage has occurred, supportive treatment as suggested for the treatment of renal failure should be instituted.

REFERENCE

(1) Nordstoga, K. (1967) *Pathol. vet.*, *4*, 233.

Glomerulonephritis

Glomerulonephritis occurs in association with many primary diseases of animals such as equine infectious anemia and chronic swine fever. As a primary disease, involving only the kidney, and affecting principally the glomeruli and extending secondarily into the surrounding interstitial tissue and blood vessels, it is a rare disease in animals. A relatively high incidence of proliferative glomerulonephritis has been recorded in normal sheep and also in cattle and goats (1, 2) and pigs (4). Chronic renal failure, most commonly due to proliferative glomerulonephritis, is becoming a common diagnosis in horses (5, 8–12). Other less common causes in this species are pyelonephritis and chronic interstitial nephritis (13) usually subsequent to acute nephrosis. The earliest and most consistent sign of chronic renal failure in horses is weight loss; additional signs are anorexia, polyuria, polydipsia and ventral edema. The consistent clinical pathological finding is a high blood urea nitrogen (BUN) or serum urea nitrogen and a serum:creatinine ratio of > 10:1. Urinalysis findings vary with the nature and stage of the disease. In horses the glomerular lesion is thought to be caused by the deposition of circulating antigen–antibody complexes. The origin of these complexes is uncertain, the only known causes being prior infection with streptococci or equine infectious anemia virus, neither of which are likely to be involved in the majority of cases.

In animals the disease is most common in dogs, but it is principally a disease of humans.

The suspected cause in humans, in which species the disease occurs commonly, is the development of hypersensitivity to streptococcal protein, and the relative infrequency of systemic streptococcal infections in animals other than the horse and pig may be responsible for the rarity of the disease.

An apparently inherited disease in Finnish Landrace lambs less than 4 months of age is remarkably similar to forms of human glomerulonephritis (3). In it lambs which suckle their dams appear to absorb an agent from the colostrum which causes an immunologic response in the lamb and the deposition of immune complexes within the glomerular capillary walls; this initiates a fatal mesangiocapillary glomerulitis. Many affected lambs are asymptomatic and are found dead. Some have been observed with tachycardia, edema of the conjunctiva, and nystagmus, walking in circles and convulsions. Enlarged tender kidneys are palpable and there is severe proteinuria, low plasma albumin, and high blood levels of blood urea nitrogen (greater than 100 mg/100 ml). There is also hyperphosphatemia and hypocalcemia. At postmortem the kidneys are large and pale and have a fleabitten appearance. On histopathological examination there are severe vascular lesions in the choroid plexuses and the lateral ventricles of the brain.

The disease is thought to be conditioned in its occurrence by inheritance (1) and to be limited to the Finnish Landrace breed. However, cases have also occurred in crossbred lambs (6).

A necrotizing glomerulonephritis is listed as occurring in pigs fed a waste product from an industrial plant producing a proteolytic enzyme (7). Glomerulonephritis has also been recorded in pigs without clinical illness being evident although an association with the 'thin-sow' syndrome is suggested (4).

REVIEW LITERATURE

Osborne, C. A. et al. (1977) The glomerulus in health and disease. A comparative review of domestic animals and man. *Adv. vet. Sci.*, *21*, 207.

Slauson, D. O. & Lewis, R. M. (1979) Comparative pathology of glomerulonephritis in animals. *Vet. Pathol.*, *16*, 135.

REFERENCES

(1) Young, G. B. et al. (1981) *Br. vet. J.*, *137*, 368.
(2) Lerner, R. A. (1968) *Fedn Proc. Fedn. Am. Soc. exp. Biol.*, *27*, 363.
(3) Angus, K. W. et al. (1974) *J. comp. Pathol.*, *84*, 309.
(4) Leigh, L. C. (1978) *Res. vet. Sci.*, *24*, 205.
(5) Tennant, B. et al. (1982) *J. Am. vet. med. Assoc.*, *180*, 630.
(6) Frelier, P. F. et al. (1984) *Can. J. comp. Med.*, *48*, 215.
(7) Elling, G. (1979) *Acta vet. Microbiol. Scand.*, *87A*, 387.
(8) Buntain, B. et al. (1979) *Vet. Rec.*, *104*, 307.
(9) Wimberly, H. C. (1981) *Vet. Pathol.*, *18*, 692.
(10) Waldvogel, A. et al. (1983) *Vet. Pathol.*, *20*, 500.
(11) Divers, T. J. (1983) *Comp. cont. Educ.*, *5*, S310.
(12) Snyder, J. R. & Cruzda, J. B. (1984) *Comp. cont. Educ.*, *6*, S134.
(13) Alders, R. G. & Hutchins, D. R. (1987) *Aust. vet. J.*, *64*, 151.

Nephrosis

Nephrosis includes degenerative and inflammatory lesions of the renal tubules. Uremia may develop acutely or as the terminal stage after a chronic illness manifested by polyuria, dehydration and loss of weight.

Etiology

Most cases of nephrosis are caused by toxins with some influence being exerted by hemodynamic changes.

Toxins

- Mercury, arsenic, cadmium, selenium, organic copper compounds; nephrosis can be reproduced experimentally in horses by the oral administration of potassium dichromate and mercuric chloride (3)
- Horses treated with vitamin K_3 (menadione sodium bisulfite) administered by intramuscular or intravenous injection (1)
- Oxalate as oxalate in plants—listed under the heading of oxalate poisoning
- Oxalate in fungi, e.g., *Penicillium* sp. and mushrooms
- Oxalate in ethylene glycol
- Benzimidazole compounds used as anthelmintics; only some of them but including thiabendazole (4)
- Unidentified toxin in *Amaranthus retroflexus* in pigs (5) and cattle (6) in *Narthecium asiaticum* fed to cattle (16) and in the foliage of oak trees and acorns (1); also the plant *Isotropis forrestii*
- Ingestion of *Lophyrotoma interrupta* (sawfly) larvae by cattle
- Overdosing with neomycin (7) and gentamicin (14) and treatment of calves with tetracycline preparations accidentally contaminated by tetracycline degradation compounds (2)
- Low level aldrin poisoning in goats
- Treatment of horses with non-steroidal anti-inflammatory drugs including phenylbutazone and flunixin meglumine (10). Dose rates of more than 8·8 mg/kg body weight of phenylbutazone per day for 4 days are likely to cause nephrosis (10). Doses of 4·4 mg/kg body weight are considered to be safe but the toxicity is enhanced by water deprivation (18) and horses which have been poisoned may have been taking the drug for periods varying between 6 days and 2 years (17)
- Highly chlorinated naphthalenes
- Overdosing with sulfonamides or solutions of calcium salts intravenously; these are unlikely to be significant causes of illness
- Most non-specific endogenous or exogenous toxemias cause some degree of temporary nephrosis.

Hemodynamic factors

- Dehydration leading to concentration of toxic substances in the tubules
- Renal ischemia, only when it is severe
- Hemoglobinuria causing hemoglobinuric nephrosis.

Pathogenesis

In acute nephrosis there is obstruction to the flow of glomerular filtrate through the tubules and an obstructive oliguria and uremia develop. In subacute cases there may be impairment of tubular resorption of solutes and fluids with an attendant polyuria. The total daily excretions of calcium and phosphorus are increased in horses and there may be an accompanying hypophosphatemia and a consequential hypercalcemia (15).

Clinical findings

Clinical signs are often masked by other signs of the primary disease. In peracute cases, such as those caused by vitamin K_3 administered by injection there may be colic and strangury. In acute nephrosis there is oliguria and proteinuria and the clinical signs of uremia in the terminal stages. These signs include anorexia, hypothermia, depression, slow heart rate, small weak pulse and inappetence and diarrhea. The diarrhea may be sufficiently intense to cause severe clinical dehydration. In cows there is a continuous mild hypocalcemia with signs reminiscent of that disease and which respond, in a limited way, to treatment with calcium. Polyuria is characteristic of chronic cases but oliguria usually follows when secondary glomerular damage prevents glomerular filtration.

In many illnesses there is sufficient toxemia to cause temporary tubular nephrosis. The degree of renal epithelial loss is not sufficient to cause complete renal failure and, provided the degree of renal damage is small, complete function can be restored. Two possible mechanisms for this are adaptation by residual nephrons, and repair of damaged tubular epithelium as part of the normal replacement of exfoliated epithelium.

Clinical pathology

The presence of protein in a urine of high specific gravity is accompanied by high levels of urea nitrogen and leucine aminopeptidase in the blood in acute nephrosis. Hypoproteinemia is a common accompaniment (19). Acute cases may show hematuria. Work on ponies with experimentally induced nephrosis has shown that the earliest clinicopathological indication of the development of proximal renal tubular disease is provided by the measurement of the urine concentration of gamma-glutamyl transferase (8). In the chronic stages the urine is of low specific gravity and may or may not contain protein, but no azotemia occurs until the terminal stages when uremia is present.

Necropsy findings

In acute cases the kidney is swollen and wet on the cut surface and edema, especially of perirenal tissues, may be apparent. Histologically there is necrosis and desquamation of tubular epithelium, and hyaline casts are present in the dilated tubules. In phenylbutazone poisoning the renal lesion is specifically a renal medullary necrosis (17). There may also be ulcers in all or any part of the alimentary tract from the mouth to the colon (18). Double contrast radiography has been used successfully to diagnose the gastric ulcers (9).

Diagnosis

Clinical differentiation from glomerulonephritis is difficult except in terms of the specific causes listed above. A combination of polyuria and glycosuria is an uncommon finding in large animals and is usually caused by nephrosis, but occasional cases of diabetes mellitus have been recorded in horses (12) and cattle (11). Rare cases of Cushing's syndrome (chronic hyperadrenocorticism) are recorded in horses (13). Besides debilitation, polyuria and glycosuria the clinical syndrome includes hirsutism, polyphagia and hyperglycemia. A terminal case of uremia in a horse may have diarrhea so badly that it can be confused with colitis-X or the other acute diarrheas. It requires a blood urea nitrogen estimation to identify its presence.

Treatment

Only those treatments directed at correction of the primary disease and those indicated as supportive treatment during acute uremia can be recommended.

REFERENCES

(1) Rebhun, W. C. et al. (1984) *J. Am. vet. med. Assoc.*, *184*, 1237.
(2) Teuscher, E. et al. (1982) *Can. vet. J.*, *23*, 327.
(3) Bayly, W. M. et al. (1986) *Cornell Vet.*, *76*, 287.
(4) Benson, J. A. & Williams, B. M. (1974) *Br. vet. J.*, *130*, 475.
(5) Buck, W. B. et al. (1966) *J. Am. vet. med. Assoc.*, *148*, 1525.
(6) Jeppesen. O. E. (1966) *J. Am. vet. med. Assoc.*, *149*, 22.
(7) Divers, T. J. et al. (1982) *J. Am. vet. med. Assoc.*, *181*, 694.
(8) Bayly, W. M. et al. (1986) *Cornell Vet.*, *76*, 306.
(9) Traub, J. L. et al. (1983) *Am. J. vet. Res.*, *44*, 1410.
(10) Faulkner, J. W. et al. (1984) *Bull. env. Contamination Toxicol.*, *33*, 379.
(11) Kaneko, J. J. & Rhode, E. A. (1964) *J. Am. vet. med. Assoc.*, *144*, 367.
(12) Moore, J. N. et al. (1979) *Endocrinology*, *104*, 576.
(13) Baker, J. R. & Ritchie, H. E. (1974) *Equ. vet. J.*, *1*, 7.
(14) Riviere, J. E. et al. (1982) *J. Am. vet. med. Assoc.*, *180*, 648.
(15) Elfers, R. S. et al. (1986) *Cornell Vet.*, *76*, 317.
(16) Suzuki, K. et al. (1985) *Cornell Vet.*, *75*, 348.
(17) Read, W. K. (1983) *Vet. Pathol.*, *20*, 662.
(18) Gunson, D. E. & Soma, L. R. (1983) *Vet. Pathol.*, *20*, 603.
(19) Collins, L. G. & Tyler, D. E. (1984) *J. Am. vet. med. Assoc.*, *184*, 699.

Interstitial nephritis

Interstitial nephritis is a common disease of the dog but less so in other animals. It may be diffuse or focal but is always non-suppurative. Focal interstitial nephritis (white-spotted kidney) is a common incidental finding at necropsy but has no known clinical significance (2). Diffuse interstitial nephritis is usually associated with infection by *Leptospira* spp. and is important clinically because of the resultant destruction of nephrons which occurs. Chronic poisoning resulting from feeding cows on caustic-treated roughage causes interstitial nephritis. In the acute stages affected nephrons show chiefly tubular degeneration, and fatal uremia is uncommon. In the chronic stages much of the renal parenchyma is gradually replaced by scar tissue, and although many glomeruli are unaffected the destruction of tubules is eventually almost complete and results in death due to uremia. Clinically the disease is characterized by a gradual onset of polyuria, urine of low specific gravity, isosthenuria and terminal uremia. The renal lesion is also important in relation to the renal excretion of the organism and the effect of this on the epidemiology of the disease, rather than to the pathogenesis of renal insufficiency in the affected animals (1).

REFERENCES

(1) Armatredjo, A. et al. (1976) *Aust. vet. J.*, *52*, 398.
(2) Monaghan, M. (1985) *Irish. vet. J.*, *39*, 15.

Embolic nephritis

Embolic lesions in the kidney cause no clinical signs unless they are very extensive, when toxemia may be followed by terminal uremia. Transitory periods during which proteinuria and pyuria occur may be observed if urine samples are examined at frequent intervals.

Etiology

Embolic suppurative nephritis or renal abscess may occur after any septicemia or bacteremia when bacteria lodge in renal tissue.

The origin of the emboli may be in *sporadic cases* such as:

- Valvular endocarditis, in all species
- Suppurative lesions in uterus, udder, navel, peritoneal cavity in cattle;

or associated with systemic infections such as:

- Shigellosis in foals
- Erysipelas in pigs
- Septicemic or bacteremic strangles in horses.

Pathogenesis

Localization of single bacterial cells or bacteria in small clumps in renal tissue causes the development of embolic suppurative lesions. Emboli which block vessels larger than capillaries cause infarction in which portions of kidney, the size varying with the caliber of the vessel which is occluded, are rendered acutely ischemic. These infarcts are not usually so large that the residual renal tissue cannot compensate fully and they usually cause no clinical signs. If the urine is checked repeatedly for the presence of protein and erythrocytes, the sudden appearance of proteinuria, casts, and microscopic hematuria, without other signs of renal disease, suggests the occurrence of a renal infarct. The gradual enlargement of focal embolic lesions leads to the development of toxemia and gradual loss of renal function. Clinical signs usually develop only when the embolic are multiple and destroy much of the renal parenchyma, although the same result can be produced by one or more large infected infarcts.

Clinical findings

Usually there is insufficient renal damage to cause signs of renal dysfunction but signs of toxemia and the primary disease are usually present. Enlargement of the kidney may be palpable on rectal examination. Repeated showers of emboli or gradual spread from several large, suppurative infarcts may cause fatal uremia. Spread to the renal pelvis may cause a syndrome very similar to that of pyelonephritis. The development of large infarcts may cause bouts of transient abdominal pain.

Clinical pathology

The urine may contain pus and blood which are visible macroscopically although microscopic examination may be necessary to detect the presence of these abnormalities when the lesions are minor. Culture of urine at the time when proteinuria occurs may reveal the identity of the bacteria infecting the embolus.

Necropsy findings

In animals which die of intercurrent disease the early lesions are seen as small grayish spots in the cortex. In the later stages these lesions may have developed into large abscesses, which may be confluent and in some cases extend into the pelvis. Much fibrous tissue may surround lesions of long standing and healed lesions consist of areas of scar tissues in the cortex. These areas have depressed surfaces and indicate that destruction of cortical tissue has occurred. When many such lesions are present the shrinking of the cortex may cause an obvious reduction in the size of the kidney.

Diagnosis

Differentiation from pyelonephritis is difficult unless the latter is accompanied by detectable cystitis or urethritis. Enlargement of the kidney occurs in both conditions and the findings on urinalysis are the same when embolic nephritis invades the renal pelvis. Many cases of embolic nephritis go unrecognized clinically because of the absence of overt signs of renal involvement.

The sudden occurrence of bouts of acute abdominal pain in some cases of renal infarction may suggest acute intestinal obstruction but defecation is usually unaffected and rectal examination of the intestines is negative.

Treatment

If the causative bacteria can be isolated and their sensitivity to standard antibiotics and sulfonamides determined, control of early cases of embolic nephritis can usually be effected. However, unless the primary disease is controlled renal lesions may recur. Antibiotic treatment is usually required over a fairly lengthy period (7–10 days) and can be supplemented by the administration of parenteral enzymes during this time. Bacteriological examination of the urine is advisable at intervals after treatment is completed to ensure that the infection has been completely controlled.

Pyelonephritis

Pyelonephritis develops by ascending infection from the lower urinary tract. Clinically it is characterized by pyuria, suppurative nephritis, cystitis and ureteritis.

Etiology

Pyelonephritis may develop in a number of ways:

- Secondary to bacterial infections of the lower urinary tract
- Spread from embolic nephritis of hematological origin such as septicemia in cattle caused by *Pseudomonas aeruginosa*
- Specific pyelonephritides caused by
  Corynebacterium renale in cattle
  Cor. (Eubacterium) suis in pigs.

Pathogenesis

The development of pyelonephritis depends upon the common presence of infection in the urinary tract and the stagnation of urine, permitting the multiplication and progression of the infection up the tract (1) and possibly enhanced by reflux up the ureters from the bladder (2). Urinary stasis may occur as a result of bacterial infection and the blocking of ureters by inflammatory swelling or debris, by pressure from the uterus in pregnant females, and by obstructive urolithiasis. The infection ascends the ureters, not always bilaterally, and invades the renal pelvis. Involvement of the papillae occurs and lesions develop in the renal medulla although the lesions may extend to the cortex. Toxemia and fever result and if renal involvement is bilateral and sufficiently extensive uremia develops. Pyelonephritis is always accompanied by pyuria and hematuria because of the inflammatory lesions of the ureters and bladder.

Clinical findings

The clinical findings in pyelonephritis vary between species. In sows there may be an initial period during which a vaginal discharge is noted but most affected animals die without premonitory illness. The disease in cattle is described in detail in the section on bovine pyelonephritis.

Clinical pathology

Erythrocytes, leukocytes and cell debris are found in the urine on microscopic examination and there may be gross evidence of their presence in severe cases. Culture of the urine is necessary to determine the causative bacteria.

Necropsy findings

The kidney is usually enlarged and lesions in the parenchyma are in varying stages of development. The characteristic lesions are necrosis and ulceration of the pelvis and papillae and the pelvis is usually dilated and contains clots of pus and turbid urine. Streaks of gray, necrotic material radiate out through the medulla and may extend to the cortex. The affected parenchyma is necrotic but suppuration is unusual and healed lesions appear as contracted scar tissue. Infarction of lobules may also be present, especially in cattle. Histologically the lesions are similar to those of embolic nephritis except that there is extensive necrosis of the apices of the papillae. Necrotic, suppurative lesions are usually present in the bladder and ureters.

Diagnosis

The presence of pus and blood in the urine may suggest cystitis or embolic nephritis, as well as pyelonephritis, and it may be difficult to distinguish between these diseases. Renal enlargement or pain on rectal palpation of the kidney will indicate the presence of renal involvement and if the urine is abnormal at all times pyelonephritis is the more likely cause. Diagnosis at necropsy will depend on the principal location of the lesions; they are most common in the medulla in pyelonephritis, and in the cortex in embolic nephritis.

Treatment

The treatment prescribed for cases of suppurative embolic nephritis applies equally well in this disease and is discussed in more detail under bovine pyelonephritis.

REFERENCES

(1) Brumfitt, H. W. & Heptinstall, R. H. (1958) *Br. J. exp. Pathol.*, *39*, 610.
(2) Heptinstall, R. H. (1964) *Br. J. exp. Pathol.*, *45*, 436.

Hydronephrosis

Cystic enlargement of the kidney due to obstruction of the ureter is a relatively common finding at necropsy but is seldom detected clinically in farm animals, because it is usually unilateral and the unaffected kidney compensates fully for the loss of function. Obstructive urolithiasis is the most common cause although congenital obstructive anomalies of the ureter may have the same effect. Partial obstruction of the ureters by papillomas of the urinary bladder has been recorded in a series of cows (1). The bladder lesions were proliferative rather than neoplastic. Compression by neoplastic tissue in cases of bovine viral leukosis may cause hydronephrosis. Complete obstruction of the urethra causes dilatation and rupture of the bladder. Back pressure in the ureters causes distension of the pelvis and pressure atrophy of the renal parenchyma but this effect is greatest when the obstruction is only partial and develops slowly. Bilateral hydronephrosis results in terminal uremia; unilateral obstruction may be detectable on palpation per rectum of a grossly distended kidney.

REFERENCE

(1) Skye, D. V. (1975) *J. Am. vet. med. Assoc.*, *166*, 596.

Renal neoplasms

Primary neoplasms of the kidney are uncommon. Adenomas occur in cattle and horses and nephroblastomas in pigs but they may cause little clinical disturbance. Enlargement of the kidney is the characteristic sign and in cattle and horses neoplasms must be considered in the differential diagnosis of renal enlargement. Nephroblastomas in particular may reach a tremendous size and cause visible abdominal enlargement in the pig. Renal adenocarcinomas are very slowgrowing but cause weight loss, intermittent bouts of abdominal pain and are readily palpable in the horse on rectal examination (1). They may be accompanied by massive ascites, hemoperitoneum, or hematuria (2, 3, 5) and may cause a number of syndromes if they metastasize widely (4).

Metastatic neoplasms occur fairly commonly in the kidney, especially in lymphomatosis but again cause little clinical disturbance. They may be palpable as discrete enlargements in the kidneys of cattle but the lesion may be diffuse and cause a general enlargement of the organ.

REFERENCES

(1) Mol, K. A. C. von & Fransen, J. A. (1986) *Vet. Rec.*, *119*, 238.
(2) Hascheek, W. M. et al. (1981) *J. Am. vet. med. Assoc.* *179*, 992.
(3) Pomroy, W. (1981) *Equ. vet. J.*, *13*, 198.
(4) Van Amstel, S. R. et al. (1984) *J. S. Afr. vet. Assoc.*, *55*, 35.
(5) Brown, P. S. & Holt, P. E. (1985) *Equ. vet. J.*, *17*, 473.

DISEASES OF THE BLADDER, URETERS AND URETHRA

Cystitis

Inflammation of the bladder is usually caused by bacterial infection and is characterized clinically by frequent, painful urination and the presence of blood, inflammatory cells, and bacteria in the urine.

Etiology

Cystitis occurs sporadically due to the introduction of infection into the bladder when trauma to the bladder has occurred or when there is stagnation of the urine. In agricultural animals the common associations are:

- Vesical calculus
- Difficult parturition
- Contaminated catheterization
- Late pregnancy
- As a sequel to paralysis of the bladder (rarely).

The bacterial population in the above cases is usually mixed but predominantly *Escherichia coli*.

- Accompaniment of specific pyelonephritides in cattle and pig, caused by *Corynebacterium renale* and *Corynebacterium (Eubacterium) suis*, respectively; many sporadic cases also occur in pigs, especially after farrowing. Common isolates from these are *Escherichia coli*, *Streptococcus* and *Pseudomonas* spp. (4)
- A special case in horses grazing sudax or sudan grass (1, 2) is recorded. The disease occurs as outbreaks, manifested by incontinence and hematuria, in some cases by incoordination in the hindlimbs, in Australian horses (3). It is caused possibly by a fungal toxin
- Enzootic hematuria of cattle resembles but is not a cystitis.

Pathogenesis

Bacteria frequently gain entrance to the bladder but are removed before they invade the mucosa by the physical emptying of the urine. Injury to the mucosa facilitates invasion but stagnation of urine is the most important predisposing cause. Introduction of bacteria occurs chiefly via the urethra but descending infection from an embolic suppurative nephritis may also occur.

Clinical findings

The urethritis which usually accompanies a cystitis causes painful sensations and the desire to urinate. Urination occurs frequently and is accompanied by pain and sometimes grunting; the animal remains in the posture adopted for urination for some minutes after the flow has ceased, often manifesting additional expulsive efforts. The volume of urine passed on each occasion is usually small. In very acute cases there may be moderate abdominal pain as evidenced by treading with the hind-feet, kicking at the belly and swishing with the tail, and a moderate febrile reaction. Acute retention may develop if the urethra becomes blocked with pus or blood but this is unusual.

Chronic cases show the same syndrome but the abnormalities are less marked. Frequent urination and small volume are the characteristic signs. The small volume is in part due to the inflammatory thickening of the bladder wall which is palpable on rectal examination. In acute cases no palpable abnormality may be detected but pain may be evidenced.

Clinical pathology

The presence of blood and pus in the urine is typical of acute cases and the urine may have a strong odor. In less severe cases the urine may be only turbid and in chronic cases there may be no abnormality on gross inspection. Microscopic examination for erythrocytes, leukocytes and desquamated epithelial cells, carried out on sedimented or centrifuged deposits, and bacteriological examination, may be necessary to confirm the diagnosis.

Necropsy findings

Acute cystitis is manifested by hyperemia, hemorrhage, swelling and edema of the mucosa. The urine is cloudy and contains mucus. In subacute and chronic cases the wall is grossly thickened and the mucosal surface is rough and coarsely granular. Highly vascular papillary projections may have eroded causing the urine to be bloodstained or contain large clots of blood. In the cystitis associated with sudan grass, soft masses of calcium carbonate may be found in the bladder and the vaginal wall may be inflamed and coated with the same material.

Diagnosis

The syndrome caused by cystitis resembles that of pyelonephritis and vesical urolithiasis. Pyelonephritis is commonly accompanied by vesical involvement and differentiation depends on whether there are lesions in the kidney. This may be determined by rectal examination but in many cases it is not possible to make a firm decision. Provided the causative bacteria can be identified this is probably not of major importance as the treatment will be the same in either case. However, the prognosis in pyelonephritis is less favorable than in cystitis. Thickening of the bladder wall, which may suggest a diagnosis of cystitis, occurs also in enzootic hematuria and in poisoning by the yellow-wood tree (*Terminalia oblongata*) in cattle and by sorghum in horses.

The presence of calculi in the bladder can usually be detected by rectal examination or by radiographic examination in smaller animals. Urethral obstruction may also cause frequent attempts at urination but the urine flow is greatly restricted, usually only drops are voided, and the distended bladder can be felt on rectal examination.

Treatment

Irrigation of the bladder has been largely discarded as a method of treatment and the usual technique is to depend entirely on parenteral treatment. Antibiotics offer the best chance of controlling the infection and determination of the drug sensitivity of the causative bacteria is virtually essential if recovery is to be anticipated. Sulfonamides, and drugs such as hexamine and mandelic acid which alter the pH of the urine, are at best bacteriostatic and their use is often followed by relapse. Even with antibiotics relapses are common unless the treatment is continued for a minimum of 7 and preferably for 14 days. Persistence of the infection is usually due to failure to destroy small foci of infection in the accessory glands and in the bladder wall.

The prognosis in chronic cases is poor because of the difficulty of completely eradicating the infection and the common secondary involvement of the kidney. Free access to water should be permitted at all times to ensure a free flow of urine.

REFERENCES

(1) Adams, L. G. et al. (1969) *J. Am. vet. med. Assoc.*, *155*, 518.
(2) Knight, P. R. (1968) *Aust. vet. J.*, *44*, 257.
(3) Hooper, P. T. (1968) *Aust. vet. J.*, *44*, 11.
(4) Stirnimann, J. (1984) *Schweiz. Arch. Tierheilkd.*, *126*, 597.

Paralysis of the bladder

Vesical paralysis is uncommon in large animals, the main cause being lesions in the lumbosacral part of the spinal cord. Lack of tone of the bladder wall may persist for some days after correction of obstructive distension.

In the early stages of paralysis of neurogenic origin the bladder remains full, and dribbling occurs especially during movement although a good flow of urine can be obtained by manual compression of the bladder per rectum or through the abdominal wall. At a later stage the bladder will begin to empty involuntarily although the evacuation is usually incomplete and some urine is retained. The stagnation causes ideal conditions for the multiplication of bacteria, and cystitis is a common sequel. The prognosis in paralysis of the bladder is therefore poor. Regular catheterization is essential and adequate care must be taken to avoid the introduction of infection. The administration of antibiotics as a prophylaxis against the development of cystitis is advisable.

Rupture of the bladder

This occurs most commonly in castrated male ruminants because of urethral obstruction by calculi. Rare cases are recorded in cows as sequels to difficult parturition (1) and in mares after normal parturition (5), possibly because of compression of a full bladder during foaling. Congenital rupture is dealt with elsewhere. The resulting syndrome includes a gradual development of ascites, ruminal stasis, constipation, depression of consciousness, the syndrome of uremia but which may take 1–2 weeks to develop to the point where euthanasia is obligatory. Not all animals become uremic and the survival rate in one study was 49·2%. The best indicator of viability among clinical pathology tests was the serum phosphate level; all animals with levels greater than 9·0 mg/dl (2·9 mmol/l) died (2).

It is often critical to decide whether or not the bladder has ruptured. Paracentesis gives preliminary information, the ratio of urea in peritoneal fluid to that in serum is also a good guide in the early stages but after 40 hours the ratio of the peritoneal to serum creatinine is more certain (3). Experimentally induced bladder rupture in steers has been monitored in terms of biochemical responses (4). Treatment is surgical and most satisfactorily consists of a bladder repair. To avoid the costs involved the preferred procedure in feedlot animals is to create a urethrostomy or install an indwelling catheter and allow the rupture to repair itself.

REFERENCES

(1) Smith, J. A. et al. (1983) *Cornell Vet.*, *73*, 3.
(2) Donecker, J. M. & Bellamy, J.E.C. (1982) *Can. vet. J.*, *23*, 355.
(3) Genetzky, R. M. & Hagemoser, W. A. (1985) *Can. vet. J.*, *26*, 391.
(4) Sockett, D. C. et al. (1986) *Cornell Vet.*, *76*, 198.
(5) Nyrop, K. A. et al. (1984) *Comp. cont. Educ.*, *6*, S510.

Urolithiasis

Urolithiasis is an important disease of castrated male ruminants, because of the common occurrence of urethral obstruction. Obstruction of the urethra is characterized clinically by complete retention of urine, unsuccessful efforts to urinate, distension of the bladder and the sequelae of urethral perforation and rupture of the bladder.

Etiology

The formation of urinary calculi, or uroliths, results when urinary solutes, mostly inorganic but sometimes organic, are precipitated out of solution. The precipitates can occur as crystals, or in the case of organic substances as amorphous 'deposits'. However, because the precipitation occurs slowly and over a long period, there is a common physical tendency for precipitation to occur around a nidus, resulting in the formation of a calculus. Factors which affect the urinary concentration of specific solutes, the ease with which the solutes are precipitated out of solution, the provision of a nidus, the tendency to concretion, all affect the rate of occurrence of urolithiasis, and are dealt with under the heading of epidemiology. The epidemiology of obstructive urolithiasis, the obvious disease manifestion of urolithiasis, is dealt with separately.

Factors known to be important in the etiology of urolithiasis and obstructive urolithiasis are presented here. A diagrammatic summary is included in Fig. 21.

Epidemiology

Urolithiasis occurs in all species but is of greatest economic importance in feeder steers and lambs being fed heavy concentrate rations, and stock running at range in particular problem areas. The latter areas may be associated with the presence of pasture plants containing large quantities of oxalate, estrogens or silica. At pasture the incidence of obstructive urolithiasis often varies with the seasons; this variation is probably related to variation in one or a number of etiological factors described below. In cattle on pasture containing high levels of silica, which may be as high as 6% (35), uroliths occur in animals of all ages and sexes. The incidence of uroliths is about the same in cows, heifers, bulls and steers grazing on the same pasture. They are even present in newborn calves. However, females and bulls usually pass the calculi and obstructive urolithiasis is primarily a problem in castrated male animals.

There are three main groups of causes of urolithiasis; those which favor the development of a nidus about which concretion can occur, those which facilitate precipitation of solutes on to the nidus, and those which favor concretion by cementing the precipitated salts to the developing calculus.

Nidus formation
A nidus, usually in the form of a group of desquamated epithelial cells or necrotic tissue, favors the deposition of crystals about itself. The nidus may result from local infection in the urinary tract in occasional cases but when large numbers of animals are affected it is probable that some other factor such as a deficiency of vitamin A or the administration of estrogens is the cause of excessive epithelial desquamation. A mortality rate of 20% due to obstructive urolithiasis has been recorded in wethers implanted with 30 mg of stilbestrol compared with no mortalities in a control group (1). Diets low in vitamin A have been implicated as a cause of urolithiasis but vitamin A deficiency does not appear to be a major causative factor (2).

Precipitation of solutes
Urine is a highly saturated solution containing a large number of solutes, many of them in higher concentrations than their individual solubilities permit in a simple solution. The reasons why the solutes remain in solution are improperly understood but several factors are known to be important. Probably the most important factor in preventing precipitation is the presence of protective colloids which convert urine into a gel. These colloids are efficient up to a point but their capacity to maintain the solution may be overcome by abnormalities in one or more of a number of other factors. Even in normal animals crystals of a number of solutes may be present in the urine from time to time and urine must be considered to be an unstable solution.

The pH of urine affects the solubility of some solutes, mixed phosphate and carbonate calculi being more readily formed in an alkaline than an acid medium. Addition of ammonium chloride or phosphoric acid to the rations of steers increases the acidity of the urine and reduces the incidence of calculi (3). The mechanism is uncertain but is probably related to the effect of pH on the stability of the urinary colloids. The most important factor in the development of siliceous calculi is the precipitation of silicic acid in the urine of cattle consuming grass or roughage containing a high level of silica (4). The ingestion of certain quantities of sodium chloride prevents the formation of silica calculi by reducing the concentration of silicic acid in the urine and maintaining it below the saturation concentration (5). The fate of silica in prairie hay and alfalfa hay consumed by cattle has been examined (6). Citrate acts as a buffer in urine, maintaining calcium in solution by the formation of soluble citrate complexes which are not dissociated. Depression of the citrate content of the urine thus favors the precipitation of calcium salts.

Concentration of the urine may occur in several ways and also favors precipitation of salts. Continued deprivation of water is often exacerbated by heavy fluid loss by sweating in hot, arid climates. An excessive intake of minerals may occur on highly mineralized artesian water, or on diets containing high concentrations, particularly of phosphates on heavy concentrate diets

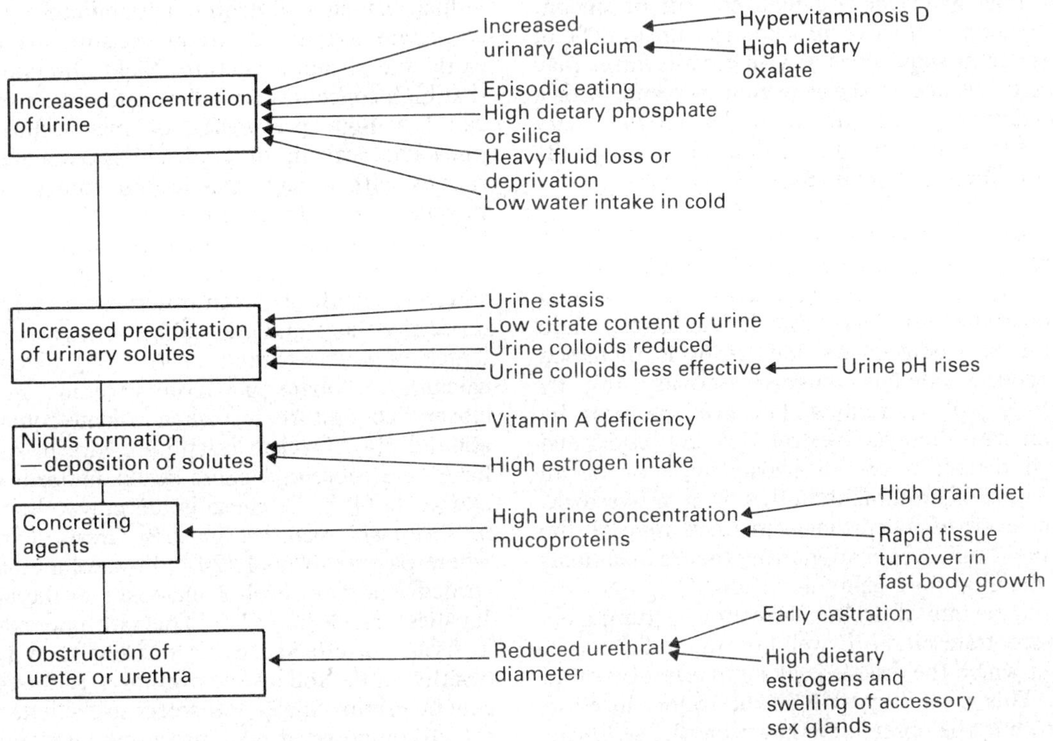

Fig. 21. Factors affecting occurrence of obstructive urolithiasis in ruminants

(7). It has been shown in sheep that a high dietary intake of phosphorus causes an increase in concentration of phosphorus in the urine and an increased development of calculi. Diets high in magnesium have the same effect of increasing the incidence of obstructive urolithiasis. Additional calcium in the diet is protective (43) against the high magnesium intake and also in a general context (8).

One of the important factors in the development of uroliths in ruminants is the episodic nature of their feeding—short periods of eating followed by long periods of rumination. Urinary function, with respect to concentration and pH, changes markedly depending on whether or not the animal is eating. This is thought to have a considerable influence on the precipitation and concretion of minerals in the urine of sheep (9).

Metabolic defects may also cause increased concentration of the urine. Hypervitaminosis D has been suggested as a cause of excessive urine concentration of calcium especially in hot climates where dehydration may also be a contributing factor. The ingestion of large quantities of oxalic acid, and possibly other organic acids, results in an increased concentration of calcium in the urine, and the oxalates formed in the tubules are relatively insoluble and readily precipitate out of solution. The oxalates are usually ingested in certain herbaceous plants which have an unusually high concentration and these plants may dominate a pasture at certain times of the year. Although pasture of this type appears to be capable of causing a high incidence of urolithiasis without the apparent intervention of other factors (10), the simple feeding of oxalate does not have this effect. A similar comment applies to the occurrences of siliceous calculi which occur much more commonly in wethers and steers when they are pastured on wheat and oat stubble which have a high content of silicon. The high incidence of siliceous calculi in up to 80% of calves on range in some areas and on certain farms may or may not be related to the ingestion of plants with a high silica content (11, 12). It appears that a high urinary level of silicon is not the only factor involved in the formation of siliceous calculi (2).

Factors favoring concretion

It has been suggested that mucoprotein, particularly its mucopolysaccharide fraction, may act as a cementing agent and favor the formation of calculi. The mucoprotein in the urine of feeder steers and lambs is increased by heavy concentrate-low roughage rations (13), by the feeding of pelleted rations (14), even more so by implantation with diethylstilbestrol (15) and, combined with a high dietary intake of phosphate, may be an important cause of urolithiasis in this class of livestock. These high levels of mucoprotein in urine may be the result of a rapid turnover of supporting tissues in animals which are making rapid gains in weight.

The increased rate of urolith formation in ruminants on high concentrate rations is well known, and the level of feeding at which the disease is likely to occur becomes important. This must vary with all the factors listed in this section, but one observation has been that sediment begins to appear in steer's urine when concentrates reach 1·5% of the body weight, and urolithiasis formation begins when concentrates have been fed for 2 months at the rate of 2·5% of the animal's body weight (16).

Miscellaneous factors in the development of urolithiasis

Stasis of urine favors precipitation of the solutes, probably by virtue of the infection which commonly follows and provides cellular material for a nidus. Certain feeds, including cottonseed meal and milo sorghum, are credited with causing more urolithiasis than other feeds. Alfalfa is in an indeterminate position: by some observers it is thought to cause the formation of calculi, by others to be a valuable aid in preventing their formation. Pelleting appears to increase calculi formation if the ration already has this tendency.

Attempts to produce urolithiasis experimentally by varying any one of the above factors are usually unsuccessful and natural cases most probably occur as a result of the interaction of several factors. In feedlots a combination of high mineral feeding and a high level of mucoprotein in the urine associated with rapid growth are probably the important factors in most instances, but a dietary deficiency of vitamin A or the use of estrogens as implants may be contributing factors in some. In range animals a high intake of mineralized water, or oxalates or silica in plants, are most commonly associated with a high incidence of urinary calculi, but again other predisposing factors, including deprivation or excessive loss of water, or vitamin A deficiency may contribute to the development of the disease. Restriction of water intake in very cold weather may also be a contributory factor.

Composition of calculi

The chemical composition of urethral calculi varies and appears to depend largely on the dietary intake of individual elements. Calcium, ammonium and magnesium carbonate are the common constituents of calculi in cattle and sheep at pasture. Field observations indicate that high concentrations of magnesium in feedlot rations cause a high prevalence of magnesium ammonium phosphate calculi in lambs. Experimental feeding of rations with a high magnesium content increases the prevalence of calcium apatite urolithiasis in calves. The occurrence is prevented by supplementary feeding with calcium (17). In particular areas a high incidence of siliceous calculi has been observed in steers and sheep, especially those grazing stubble and pastures consisting largely of grasses without clovers (35). Calculi containing calcium carbonate are more common in animals on clover-rich pasture, or when oxalate-containing plants abound (19). Oxalate calculi are rare in ruminants but have been observed sporadically in feedlot cattle (18) and goats (45); the cause is unknown. Xanthine calculi in sheep are recorded in some areas in New Zealand where pasture is poor (20) and xanthine calculi are recorded at a high level of incidence in the offspring of a Japanese Black bull (10). The xanthine oxidase activity in tissues of affected cattle was less than 1% of that of healthy cattle and the xanthinuria is thought to be of genetic origin. Sheep and steers in feedlots usually have calculi composed of calcium, ammonium and magnesium phosphate, the latter being especially prevalent when sorghum products form a major part of the ration. The calculi are usually present as individual stones of varying size. Less commonly there is a sludge-like sediment but no formed calculi. An amorphous sediment is less likely to cause obstruction than a stone but may do so when the animal is shaken up by driving or transport. Although the greatest field problem is that of obstructive urolithiasis caused by mineralized calculi or sediment, obstruction can also be caused by materials containing very little mineral. Soft, moist, yellow calculi containing 2 benzocoumarins (21), and isoflavones and indigotin-indirubin have been observed in sheep grazing pasture dominated by subterranean clover, which has a high content of an estrogenic substance. Estrogenic subterranean clover can cause urinary tract obstruction in wethers in a number of ways. Calculi or unformed sediments of benzocoumarins (urolithins) and 4^1-*O*-methylequol, either singly or in various combinations with equol, formonentin, biochanin A, indigotin and indirubin occur. So does obstruction promoted by estrogenic stimulation of glandular enlargement and mucus secretion. Pastures containing these plants are also reputed to cause urinary obstruction by calculi consisting of calcium carbonate (44). A 10% incidence of obstructive urolithiasis has also been recorded in feedlot lambs receiving a supplement of stilbestrol (1 mg/kg of feed or 2 mg per lamb daily), the obstruction being caused by plugs of mucoprotein (22). The accessory sex glands were enlarged.

Epidemiology of obstructive urolithiasis

The size of individual calculi, and the total bulk of calculous material are both important in the final development of urethral obstruction. But usually the obstruction is caused by one stone, rather than by a sabulous deposit such as occurs in cats. The most important factor contributing to obstruction is the bore size of the urethra, and as set out later, deferment of castration is a recognized preventive measure. A statistical assessment has been made of the effects of castration on the bore size of the urethra in steers (23). For example, it was estimated that bulls could expel calculi which were twice the size of those which could be passed by a steer. However the urethral bore of castrates increased by only 14% in late castrates (6 months old) and early castrates (2 months). In spite of these statistics, the greater susceptibility of early castrates is still apparent. In North America, obstructive urolithiasis due to siliceous calculi is most common in beef feeder cattle during the fall and winter months. The calves are weaned at 6–8 months and moved from pasture to a dry lot situation where they are fed roughage and grain. The incidence of obstructive urolithiasis appears to be highest during the early part of the feeding period and during cold weather when the consumption of water may be decreased.

The common occurrence of urethral obstruction in wethers and steers is due to the relatively small diameter of the urethra in these animals. The obstruction may occur at any site but is most common at the sigmoid flexure in steers (68% of one series of 193 cases (42)), and in the vermiform appendage or at the sigmoid flexure in wethers, all sites at which the urethra narrows. The mortality rate in these animals may reach as high as 10% and in special circumstances may be as high as 20% (1). Bulls are not infrequently affected and a high incidence has been observed in rams. An emerging problem is urolithiasis in Angora goat bucks because of their current popularity as fiber producers. The management of these animals is often one of gross overcrowding on pastures so that the males tend to be kept indoors and fed commercial feed pellets for sheep. On this diet goats can develop a significant incidence of fatal obstructive urolithiasis (41) and a diet containing less concentrate is recommended. Urethral obstruction occurs rarely in horses, most cases being seen in geldings with the calculus lodged in the scrotal region. Urolithiasis is as common in females as in males but obstruction rarely if ever occurs because of the shortness and large diameter of the urethra. Repeated attacks of obstructive urolithiasis are not uncommon in wethers and steers and at necropsy up to 200 calculi may be found in various parts of the tract of one animal.

Although the occurrence of obstructive urolithiasis is usually sporadic, cases occurring at irregular intervals in a group of animals, outbreaks have been recorded in which a large number of animals are affected in a short time (1). In these outbreaks it is probable that some factor operates which favors the development of calculi, as well as the development of obstruction. For example, large numbers of animals grazing on pasture dominated by clover, especially subterranean clover, can become affected during a short period. It is known that such diets produce 'deposits' which originate in the kidney and can block ureters and urethras. These are probably the principal causes of the obstructive urolithiasis. Swelling of the accessory sex glands may also contribute by means of constricting the urethral bore, but it is unlikely to be a significant factor (24). Obstructive urolithiasis increases in occurrence with age but it is recorded in lambs as young as 1 month of age (25). There are also records of fatal uremia in newborn pigs which exhibited nervous signs at 3–4 days of age. Depression, paralysis and convulsions comprised the syndrome (43, 45). Heavy sabulous deposits were present in kidneys, bladder and ureters.

Pathogenesis

Urinary calculi are commonly observed at necropsy in normal animals, and in many appear to cause little or no harm. In a few animals pyelonephritis, cystitis, and ureteral obstruction may occur. Obstruction of one ureter causes death from uremia. The important effect of urolithiasis is in the production of urethral obstruction, particularly in wethers and steers. This difference between urolithiasis and obstructive urolithiasis is an important one. Simple urolithiasis has relatively little importance but obstructive urolithiasis is a fatal disease unless the obstruction is relieved. Rupture of the urethra or bladder occurs and the animal dies of uremia or secondary bacterial infection. Rupture of the bladder is more likely to occur with a spherical smooth calculus which causes complete obstruction of the urethra. Rupture of the urethra is more common with irregularly shaped stones which cause partial obstruction and pressure necrosis of the urethral wall.

Clinical findings

Calculi in the renal pelvis or ureters are not usually diagnosed antemortem although obstruction of a ureter may be detectable on rectal examination, especially if it is accompanied by hydronephrosis. Occasionally the exit from the renal pelvis is blocked and the acute distension which results may cause acute pain, accompanied by stiffness of the gait and pain on pressure over the loins. Calculi in the bladder commonly cause cystitis and are manifested by signs of that disease (26). Rectal palpation usually reveals the presence of the calculi and in male horses these may reach a diameter of 15–22 cm.

Obstruction of the urethra by a calculus is a common occurrence in steers and wethers and causes a characteristic syndrome of abdominal pain with kicking at the belly, treading with the hindfeet and swishing of the tail. Repeated twitching of the penis, sufficient to shake the prepuce, is often observed and the animal may make strenuous efforts to urinate, accompanied by straining, grunting and grating of the teeth, but these result in the passage of only a few drops of bloodstained urine. On rectal examination the urethra and bladder are palpably distended and the urethra is painful and pulsates on manipulation. A heavy precipitate of saline crystals is often visible on the preputial hairs or on the inside of the thighs. The passage of a lead wire up the urethra, after relaxing the penis by epidural anesthesia or by administering an ataractic drug, may make it possible to locate the site of obstruction. Cattle with incomplete obstruction—'dribblers'—will pass small amounts of bloodstained urine frequently. Occasionally a small stream of urine will be voided followed by a complete blockage. This confuses the diagnosis. In these the calculus is triangular in shape and allows small amounts of urine to move past the obstruction at irregular intervals. However, these are rare.

In horses the syndrome is similar but in addition the penis is relaxed during efforts at urination. Passage of a catheter enables the site of obstruction to be determined, the end of the catheter grating on the rough surface of the calculus. Horses may also develop a sabulous deposit in the bladder especially when it is atonic. The clinical signs which result include fullness of the bladder, hematuria, and frequent urination (28). Prospects for recovery in these cases is poor.

If the obstruction is not relieved perforation of the urethra or rupture of the bladder occurs in about 48 hours. In the first instance the urine leaks into the connective tissue of the ventral abdominal wall and prepuce and causes an obvious fluid swelling which may spread as far as the thorax. The urine is often infected and severe cellulitis may occur with an attendant toxemia. In occasional animals an area of skin over the swelling sloughs permitting drainage, and the course is rather more protracted in these cases. When the bladder ruptures there is an immediate disappearance of discomfort but anorexia and depression develop as uremia appears. Distension of the abdomen soon becomes apparent and a fluid thrill is detectable on tactile percussion. The animal may continue in this state for as long as 2–3 days before it dies in a coma. In occasional cases death occurs soon after rupture of the bladder due to severe internal hemorrhage.

Rupture of the bladder is a common sequel in horses. There is usually complete emptying of the bladder into the peritoneal cavity but if the rupture occurs at the neck of the bladder the urine accumulates retroperitoneally with the production of a large diffuse, fluid swelling which is palpable per rectum. When rupture occurs the acute signs disappear and are replaced by immobility and pain on palpation of the abdominal wall. The pulse rate rises rapidly and the temperature falls to below normal.

In occasional cases calculi may form in the prepuce of steers. The calculi are top-shaped and, by acting as floating valves, cause obstruction of the preputial orifice, distension of the prepuce and infiltration of the abdominal wall with urine (1). These cases may be mistaken for cases of urethral perforation.

Clinical pathology

Laboratory examinations may be utilized in the diagnosis of the disease in its early stages when the calculi are present in the kidney or bladder. The urine usually contains erythrocytes and epithelial cells and a higher than normal number of crystals, sometimes accompanied by larger aggregations described as sand or sabulous deposit. The examination of the urinary sediment (27) and the chemical analysis of the calculi is considered necessary because control procedures will vary dependent on the chemical composition of the calculus. Bacteria may also be present if secondary invasion of the traumatic cystitis and pyelonephritis has occurred. The blood urea nitrogen will be increased before either urethral or bladder rupture occurs and will increase even further afterwards.

Aspiration of fluid from the abdominal cavity after rupture of the bladder or from a subcutaneous aggregation is often practiced as an aid to diagnosis but there is some difficulty in identifying the fluid as urine other than by appearance and smell, or by exhaustive biochemical examination.

Necropsy findings

Calculi may be found in the renal pelvis or bladder of normal animals, or of those dying of other diseases. In the renal pelvis they may cause no abnormality although in occasional cases there is an accompanying pyelonephritis. Unilateral ureteral obstruction is usually accompanied by dilatation of the ureter and hydronephrosis. Bilateral obstruction causes fatal uremia. Calculi in the bladder are usually accompanied by varying degrees of chronic cystitis. The urethra may be obstructed by one or more stones, or may be impacted for up to 35 cm with fine sabulous deposit.

When rupture of the urethra has occurred the urethra is eroded at the site of obstruction and extensive cellulitis and accumulation of urine are present in the ventral abdominal wall. When the bladder has ruptured the peritoneal cavity is distended with urine and there is a mild to moderate chemical peritonitis which is more marked in horses than in cattle or sheep. In areas where urolithiasis is a problem it is an advantage to determine the chemical composition of the calculi.

Diagnosis

Obstruction of the urethra in agricultural animals and horses is rare unless the obstructing agent is a calculus but a fibroepithelial polyp has caused obstruction in the urethra of a horse (46). Non-obstructive urolithiasis may be confused with pyelonephritis or cystitis, and differentiation may be possible only by rectal examination in the case of vesical calculi or by radiographical examination in small animals. The same comments apply to the diagnosis of obstructive urolithiasis in the ureter which on physical examination is indistinguishable from other causes of abdominal pain. Subsequent development of hydronephrosis may enable a diagnosis to be made in cattle.

The syndrome caused by obstruction of the urethra in cattle and sheep is characteristic but if there is doubt a rectal examination should be carried out or the animal kept under observation to see if urine is passed. The syndrome in horses is also typical but the condition is uncommon and the attempted passage of a catheter is necessary for diagnosis.

In adults rupture of the bladder is usually the result of obstructive urolithiasis although other occasional causes of urethral obstruction are observed. In the newborn the most common cause is defective closure of the dorsal bladder wall.

Treatment

The treatment of obstructive urolithiasis is primarily surgical. Fat cattle or lambs affected with obstructive urolithiasis should be slaughtered for salvage if the result of an antemortem inspection is satisfactory. It is not practicable to expect that calculi can be dissolved by medical means although further increase in size of existing stones and the development of new ones may be prevented. The use of agents to relax the urethral muscle and permit the onward passage of an obstructing calculus has not received much attention. In cattle the injection of a protein-free extract of mammalian pancreas (5–10 ml repeated once or twice on successive days) has been reported to produce this effect provided some urine is still dribbling from the urethra (29). Similar doses have been used in sheep with good results (30). Other specific relaxants of plain muscle, e.g. aminopromazine, have given excellent results in feedlot cattle (31). Animals treated medically should be in the early stages of the disease and kept under close observation to ensure that urination continues.

Surgical treatment includes urethrostomy to relieve bladder pressure and for the removal of calculi, and pelvic or prepubic cystotomy with a long catheter (38).

Prevention

A number of agents and management procedures have been recommended in the prevention of urolithiasis in feeder lambs and steers. First, and probably most important, the diet should contain an adequate balance of calcium and phosphorus to avoid precipitation of excess phosphorus in the urine. The ration should have a Ca:P ratio of 1·2:1, but higher calcium inputs (1·5–2·0:1) have been recommended (32, 33). The control of siliceous calculi in cattle which are fed native range grass hay, which may contain a high level of silica, is dependent primarily on manipulation of the water intake. Every practical effort must be used to increase and maintain water intake in feeder steers which have just been moved into a feedlot situation. The feeding of alfalfa hay is considered to increase urine flow and lower the incidence of urolithiasis but the important reason may be that it contains considerably less silica. The addition of salt at the level of 4% of the total ration of feeder calves has been shown experimentally to have this effect on both steers (11) and lambs (34).Under practical conditions salt is usually fed at a concentration of 3–5%, higher concentrations causing lack of appetite. For yearling (300 kg) steers the daily consumption of 50 g of salt is without effect on the formation of siliceous calculi; at 200 g daily intake the occurrence of calculi is significantly reduced, and at 300 g daily calculus formation is almost eliminated (5). For calves on native range the provision of supplements containing up to 12% salt is effective in eliminating siliceous calculi (35). This effect is caused solely by the physical diluting effect on the urine, which is the result of the salt-induced diuresis (40). If the calves consume sufficient quantities of salt to increase the water intake above 200 g/kg body weight$^{0·82}$ day the formation of siliceous calculi will be completely suppressed. Since siliceous calculi form primarily in the last 60 days before weaning, it is recommended that calves on range during this time be started on salt-free supplements and gradually increase the concentration of salt up to 12% which would encourage consumption of sufficient salt to control the disease. It is usually necessary to increase the salt gradually to this level over a period of several weeks and incorporate it in pellets to facilitate mixing. It is thought that supplementary feeding with sodium chloride helps to prevent urolithiasis by decreasing the rate of deposition of magnesium and phosphate around the nidus of a calculus (36). The feeding of ammonium chloride (45 g/day to steers and 10 g daily to sheep) has also been found to be satisfactory in the prevention of urolithiasis due to phosphate calculi (37). For range animals the drug can be incorporated in a protein supplement and fed at about two-thirds of the above dosage.

The observation that the addition of chlortetracyline to the ration (20 mg/kg) significantly reduced deaths from obstructive urolithiasis may be due to alteration in the pH of the urine subsequent to changes in ruminal digestion or the control of urinary tract infection. The latter is not known to be a factor of importance in the etiology of urolithiasis in animals, except in sporadic cases.

Dangerous pastures can usually be grazed with impunity by females. In areas where the oxalate content of the pasture is high wethers and steers should be permitted only limited access to pasture dominated by herbaceous plants. Adequate water supplies should be available and highly saline waters should be regarded with suspicion. Sheep on lush pasture commonly drink little if any water, apparently because they obtain sufficient in the feed. Although the importance of vitamin A in the production of the disease has been decried in recent years an adequate intake should be ensured, especially during drought periods and when animals are fed grain rations in feedlots. Deferment of castration, by permitting greater urethral dilatation, may reduce the incidence of obstrutive urolithiasis (2) but the improvement is unlikely to be significant (23). Ammonium chloride has no effect on the formation of siliceous urinary calculi in calves (39).

REVIEW LITERATURE

Bailey, C. B. (1981) Silica metabolism and silica urolithiasis in ruminants: a review. *Can. J. anim. Sci.*, *61*, 219–235.

REFERENCES

(1) Udall, R. H. & Jensen, R. (1958) *J. Am. vet. med. Assoc.*, *133*, 514.
(2) Hawkins, W. W. et al. (1965) *J. Am. vet. med. Assoc.*, *147*, 132.
(3) Crookshank, H. R. et al. (1960) *J. anim. Sci.*, *19*, 595.
(4) Bailey, C. B. (1967) *Science, NY*,*155*, 696.
(5) Bailey, C. B. (1973) *Can. J. anim. Sci.*, *53*, 55.
(6) Bailey, C. B. (1976) *Can. J. anim. Sci.*, *56*, 213.
(7) Robbins, J. D. et al. (1965) *J. anim. Sci.*, *24*, 76.
(8) Godwin, I. R. & Williams, V. J. (1982) *Aust. J. agric. Res.*, *33*, 843.
(9) Stacy, B. D. (1969) *Aust. vet. J.*, *45*, 395.
(10) Sutherland, A. K. (1958) *Aust. vet. J.*, *34*, 44.
(11) Whiting, F. et al. (1958) *Can. J. comp. Med.*, *22*, 332.
(12) Mathams, R. H. & Sutherland, A. R. (1951) *Aust. vet. J.*, *27*, 68.
(13) Udall, R. H. et al. (1958) *Am. J. vet. Res.*, *19*, 825.
(14) Crookshank, R. H. et al. (1965) *J. anim. Sci.*, *24*, 638.
(15) Cornelius, C. E. (1963) *Ann. NY Acad. Sci.*, *104*, 638.
(16) Munakata, K. et al. (1974) *Natl Inst. anim. Hlth Q., Tokyo*, *14*, 31.
(17) Kallfelz, F. A. et al. (1985) *Dtsch Tierarztl. Wochenschr*, *92*, 407.
(18) Huntington, G. B. & Emerick, R. J. (1984) *Am. J. vet. Res.*, *45*, 180.
(19) Bennetts, H. W. (1956) *J. Dep. Agric. W. Aust.*, *5*, 421, 425, 429, 433.
(20) Askew, H. O. (1957) *Rep. Cawthron Inst. sci. Res.*, 28
(21) Pope, G. A. (1964) *Biochem. J.*, *93*, 474.
(22) Marsh, H. (1961) *J. Am. vet. med. Assoc.*, *139*, 1019.
(23) Bailey, C. B. (1975) *Can. J. anim. Sci.*, *55*, 187.
(24) White, R. R. et al. (1972) *Aust. J. agric. Res.*, *23*, 693.
(25) Jones, J. O. (1976) *Vet. Rec.*, *99*, 337.
(26) Mair, T. S. & McCaig, J. (1983) *Equ. vet. J.*, *15*, 173.
(27) Munakata, K. et al. (1974) *Natl Inst. anim. Hlth Q., Tokyo*, *14*, 33 and 89.
(28) Holt, P. C. & Pearson, H. (1984) *Equ. vet. J.*, *16*, 31.
(29) Tonkin, B. W. (1958) *Can. J. comp. Med.*, *22*, 347.
(30) Prier, J. E. et al. (1952) *Vet. Med.*, *47*, 459.
(31) Scheel, E. H. & Paton, I. M. (1960) *J. Am. vet. med. Assoc.*, *137*, 665.
(32) Hoar, D. W. et al. (1970) *J. anim. Sci.*, *30*, 597; *31*, 118.
(33) Vipperman, P. E. et al. (1969) *J. Nutr.*, *97*, 449.
(34) Udall, R. H. (1962) *Am. J. vet. Res.*, *23*, 1241.
(35) Bailey, C. B. (1981) *Can. J. anim. Sci.*, *61*, 219.
(36) Udall, R. H. et al. (1965) *Cornell Vet.*, *55*, 198, 538.
(37) Crookshank, R. H. (1970) *J. anim. Sci.*, *30*, 1002.
(38) Bhaskar Singh, K. (1984) *Ind. vet. J.*, *61*, 336.
(39) Bailey, C. B. (1976) *Can. J. anim. Sci.*, *56*, 359.
(40) Bailey, C. B. (1978) *Can. J. anim. Sci.*, *58*, 513 & 651.
(41) Bellenger, C. D. et al. (1981) *Aust. vet. J.*, *57*, 56.
(42) Gera, K. L. & Nigam, J. M. (1979) *Ind. vet. J.*, *56*, 417.
(43) Kallfelz, F. A. et al. (1987) *Cornell Vet.*, *77*, 33
(44) Nortle, M. C. (1976) *Aust. J. agric. Res.*, *27*, 867.
(45) Fliess, D. G. (1981) *Vet. Rec.*, *108*, 568.
(46) Ricketts, S. W. et al. (1983) *Equ. vet. J.*, *15*, 170.

Urinary bladder neoplasms

Tumors of the urinary bladder are common only in cattle where they are associated with bracken poisoning, but they do occur in other circumstances. For example, 18 cows are recorded in one series with angioma, transitional epithelial carcinoma, and vascular endothelioma being the most common tumors (2). Six cases of vesical neoplasia are also recorded in horses (1). Clinical signs included hematuria, weight loss, strangury and the secondary development of cystitis.

REFERENCES

(1) Fischer, A. T. et al. (1985) *J. Am. vet. med. Assoc.*, *186*, 1294.
(2) Maeda, T. (1978) *J. Jap. vet. med. Assoc.*, *31*, 78.

CONGENITAL DEFECTS OF THE URINARY TRACT

A small number of urinary tract defects is recorded in farm animals (1). The uncommon ones include congenital urethral obstruction in female calves (10) causing anuria, rupture of the bladder and uroperitoneum.

Pervious urachus

Failure of the urachus to obliterate at birth occurs most commonly in foals. Urine is discharged through the umbilicus as a continuous dribble and cystitis is a common sequel. The umbilicus fails to heal and urachal abscess, omphalophlebitis and polyarthritis may also develop (4).

Urachal abscess is a subgroup of umbilical abscess discussed in Chapter 3. When the infection is localized in the urachus there are all of the signs of cystitis, especially that of frequency of urination (19).

Rupture of the bladder

This condition has been described as rupture of the bladder (2–4) and in some cases this etiology is supported by the presence of several tears with obviously recently traumatized edges. In others the general appearance of the lesion suggests that there is a congenital, defective closure of the bladder wall. In rare cases the defect is in the urachus (16). It is observed only in newborn colt foals, clinical signs appearing 24–36 hours after birth. There is subacute colic which bears some resemblance to that which occurs in retention of the meconium. The foal sucks in a half-hearted manner and makes frequent, moderate straining movements during which the penis may be protruded but no urine is passed, there is upward humping of the back and the legs are bunched under the body. Catheterization is not obstructed but urine does not flow. The temperature and pulse rate are normal in the early stages. The course of the disease is not acute and during the subsequent 48 hours the foal becomes progressively more dull, the temperature falls as uremia develops, and the abdomen becomes distended. Fluid can be heard in the abdomen if the foal is shaken and paracentesis through the posteroventral abdominal wall, lateral to the umbilicus, reveals free urine in the peritoneal cavity. Surgical repair of the discontinuity has been successfully carried out (5).

Some foals present problems in diagnosis because

they look so bright and clinically normal, and if the rupture is small they may pass apparently normal volumes of urine from the urethra. In these cases diagnosis can be based on the injection of radiopaque or dye into the bladder. In the latter a positive test is collection of dye-stained urine from the peritoneal cavity. In the early stages the blood, urea and nitrogen (BUN) levels are normal but there is a marked hyponatremia, hypochloremia and hyperkalemia (13). A similar clinicopathological picture is presented by a congenital defect of a ureter (14) and the true nature of the problem may only become apparent when the abdomen is opened surgically.

Urethral atresia

This is recorded rarely in calves (20) and is manifested by failure to pass urine and distension of the patent portion of the urethra.

Polycystic kidneys

In most species this is the most common congenital defect. If it is extensive and bilateral the affected animal is usually stillborn or dies soon after birth. If it is unilateral no clinical signs appear because of compensatory activity in the other kidney, but in cattle and horses the enormously enlarged kidney may be encountered during rectal examination. A high incidence of renal defects has been recorded in sucking pigs from sows vaccinated during early pregnancy with attenuated hog cholera virus, and a bilateral renal hypoplasia has been observed as a probably inherited defect in Large White pigs (12). Most polycystic kidneys in pigs are inherited and have no effect on the pig's health or renal function (8). However, there is a record of the defect in newborn pigs in one herd in which it caused gross abdominal distension due to moderate ascites and gross cystic distension of the kidneys and tract. There was no evidence that the disease was inherited and a toxic origin was surmised (6). It is possible that a congenital renal defect is compatible with life and may not present clinical signs until the residual nephron mass is exhausted and the animal is adult (18).

Hypospadias

Imperfect closure of the external male urethra in a series of newborn lambs is recorded with other neonatal defects including atresia ani and diaphragmatic hernia. No genetic influence was suspected and the cause was unidentified (7).

Renal hypoplasia and dysplasia

Bilateral renal hypoplasia with or without agenesis is recorded in Large White piglets, the piglets being dead at birth (21). Cortical dysplasia has been recorded in a yearling pony (9). There was a gradual onset of anorexia, weight loss and lethargy. Blood urea nitrogen and creatinine levels were raised and at necropsy the kidneys were shrunken and nodular.

Ectopic ureter

Clinical signs suggestive of ectopic ureter are constant dribbling of urine and pyuria. The ectopic ureter opens into the urogenital tract at a place other than the bladder, e.g. the cervix (11), so that retrograde infection occurs readily (17). Definite diagnosis is difficult without radiology (15).

REFERENCES

(1) Pearson, H. & Gibbs, C. (1973) *Vet. Rec.*, *92*, 463.
(2) Cosgrove, J. S. M. (1955) *Vet. Rec.*, *67*, 961.
(3) du Plessis, J. L. (1958) *J. S. Afr. vet. med. Assoc.*, *29*, 261.
(4) Turner, T. A. et al. (1982) *Equ. Pract.*, *4*, (1) 24.
(5) Darbishire, H. B. (1961) *Vet. Rec.*, *73*, 693.
(6) Webster, W. R. & Summers, P. M. (1978) *Aust. vet. J.*, *54*, 451.
(7) Dennis, S. M. (1979) *Vet. Rec.*, *105*, 94.
(8) Wijeratne, W. V. S. & Wells, G. A. H. (1980) *Vet. Rec.*, *107*, 484.
(9) Roberts, M. C. & Kelly, W. R. (1980) *Aust. vet. J.*, *56*, 599.
(10) Hylton, W. E. & Trent, A. M. (1987) *J. Am. vet. med. Assoc.*, *190*, 433.
(11) Barclay, W. P. (1978) *J. Am. vet. med. Assoc.*, *173*, 485.
(12) Cordes, D. O. & Dodd, D. C. (1965) *Pathol. vet.*, 2, 37.
(13) Behr, M. J. et al. (1981) *J. Am. vet. med. Assoc.*, *178*, 263.
(14) Robertson, J. T. (1983) *Am. J. vet. Res.*, *183*, 799.
(15) Christie, B. et al. (1981) *Aust. vet. J.*, *57*, 336.
(16) Ford, J. et al. (1982) *Vet. Med.*, *77*, 94.
(17) Mondransky, P. D. et al. (1983) *Vet. Surg*, *12*, 141.
(18) Scott, P. C. & Vasey, J. (1986) *Aust. vet. J.*, *63*, 92.
(19) Trent, A. M. & Smith, D. F. (1984) *J. Am. vet. med. Assoc.*, *184*, 984.
(20) Rifat, J. F. (1985) *Agri-Practice*, 6 (3), 28.
(21) Mason, R. W. et al. (1985) *Aust. vet. J.*, *62*, 413.

12

DISEASES OF THE NERVOUS SYSTEM

INTRODUCTION

This chapter contains the principles of clinical neurology and their application to large animal practice. In general, this activity has not kept pace with the study of neurology in humans and small animals, although some advances are being made in horses. To a large extent this shortfall is due to the failure of large animal clinicians to relate observed clinical signs to the subsequently determined location of the lesion. In many cases this failure has been because of the environmental circumstances, or the size or nature of the beast, all of which can react adversely on the quality of the neurological examination which is conducted. It may be impossible to conduct a neurological examination on an ataxic belligerent beef cow which is still able to walk and attack the examiner. An angry, paretic bull in broad sunlight can be a daunting subject if one wants to examine a pupillary light reflex; ophthalmoscopic examination of the fundus of the eye in a convulsing steer in a feedlot pen can be an exasperating assignment. Therefore, the conduct of a careful clinical examination of the nervous system of an animal is often impossible. Even if it is made the information available to make a satisfactory interpretation of the findings is usually not adequate to the task.

Fortunately, discrete lesions of the central nervous system resulting in well-defined neurological signs are not common in agricultural animals. Most of the diseases encountered are characterized by diffuse lesions caused by viruses, bacteria, toxins, nutritional disorders and embryological defects, and the clinical signs presented by each disease are very similar to the others. Rather than attempting to localize lesions in the nervous system, large animal practitioners more commonly devote much of their time attempting to identify whether an animal has meningoencephalitis, or cerebral edema, or increased intracranial fluid, as occurs in hypovitaminosis A, or whether the dysfunction is at the neuromuscular level, as occurs in hypomagnesemic tetany. Radiographical examination, including myelography, is not routinely used or available as a diagnostic aid in large animal neurology. If it is available, economics severely limits its use. The collection of cerebrospinal fluid from the different species and ages of large animals, without causing damage to the animal or contaminating the sample with blood, is a technique which few large animal veterinarians have mastered. However, provided that adult cattle are well restrained, cisternal taps can be done, and the information that can be obtained is so valuable that greater use of the technique could be very profitable. Following successful collection, the CSF should be examined as soon as possible, which creates difficulties for the veterinarian in the field.

Nevertheless, the large animal practitioner has an obligation to attempt to make the best diagnosis possible with all the available aids at his disposal. The principles of large animal neurology are presented in this chapter and the major objective is to recognize the common diseases of the nervous system. Some of these, such as rabies, have public health importance. It is also important to be able to recognize the treatable diseases such as polioencephalomalacia, hypovitaminosis A, *Haemophilus* meningoencephalitis, and hypomagnesemic tetany, and to institute treatment immediately. The non-treatable diseases must also be recognized as such, and slaughter for salvage or euthanasia recommended if necessary. There must be a major emphasis on prognosis because it is inhumane and uneconomic to hospitalize an adult cow or horse with neurological disease for an indefinite period. They are usually recumbent and develop decubitus ulcers, and often should have been destroyed in the first place. Very few diseases of the nervous system of farm animals are treatable successfully over an extended period of time. This has become particularly important in recent years with the introduction of legislation which prohibits the slaughter of animals which have been treated with antibiotics until after a certain withdrawal period which may vary from 5 to 30 days. This creates even greater pressure on the clinician to make a fast, reliable field diagnosis.

Because of limitations in the neurological examination of large animals, there must be much more emphasis on the history and epidemiological findings. Many of the diseases have epidemiological characteristics which give the clinician a clue to the possible causes thus helping to narrow the number of possibilities. For example, viral encephalomyelitis of horses occurs with a peak incidence during the insect season, lead poisoning is most common in calves after they have been turned out onto pasture and polioencephalomalacia occurs in grain-fed feedlot cattle.

The functions of the nervous system are directed at the maintenance of the body's spatial relation with its environment. These functions are performed by the several divisions of the nervous system including: the sensorimotor system responsible for the maintenance of normal posture and gait; the autonomic nervous system controlling the activity of smooth muscle and endocrine glands, and thereby the internal environment of the body; the largely sensory system of special senses; and the psychic system which controls the animal's mental state. The system is essentially a reactive one geared to the reception of internal and external stimuli and their translation into activity and consciousness, and is dependent upon the integrity of both the afferent and efferent pathways.

It is because of this integrative function that it is often difficult to determine in a sick animal whether it is the nervous system, or the musculoskeletal or even endocrinal system which is abnormal. Accordingly, the first step in considering the diagnosis in a case in which the nervous system is thought to be involved is to determine whether other relevant systems are functioning normally. In this way a decision to implicate the nervous system is often made on the exclusion of other systems.

The nervous system itself is not independent of other organs and its functional capacity is regulated to a large extent by the function of other systems, particularly the cardiovascular system. Hypoxia (anoxia), due to cardiovascular disease, quite commonly leads to altered cerebral function because of the dependence of the brain on an adequate oxygen supply. It is important to distinguish between primary and secondary disease of the nervous system since both the prognosis and the treatment will differ with the cause. In primary disease of the nervous system the lesion is usually an anatomical one with serious, long-range consequences; in secondary disease the lesion, at least in its early stages, is more likely to be functional and therefore more responsive to treatment, provided the defect in the primary organ can be corrected.

The clinical signs which should arouse suspicion of neurological disturbance include abnormalities in the three main functions of the system.

Posture and gait

An animal's ability to maintain a normal posture and to proceed with a normal gait are dependent largely upon the tone of skeletal muscle but also upon the efficiency of its postural reflexes. Abnormalities of posture and gait are among the best indications of nervous system disease because these functions are governed largely by the coordination of nervous activity. Besides contributing to posture and gait, skeletal muscle tone is characteristic in its own right. However, its assessment in animals is subject to great inaccuracy because of our inability to request complete voluntary relaxation by the patient. In man it is a very valuable index of nervous system efficiency, but in animals it has serious limitations. The most difficult step when there is a defect of gait or posture is to decide whether it originates in the skeleton, or the muscles or the nerve supply.

Sensory perceptivity

Tests of sensory perception in animals can only be objective, and never subjective as they can be in man, and any test used in animals presupposes integrity of the motor system.

Mental state

Depression or enhancement of the psychic state is not difficult to judge, particularly if the animal's owner is observant and accurate. The difficulty usually lies in deciding whether the abnormality is due to primary or secondary changes in the brain.

Disease of the nervous system should be suspected when there are abnormalities of posture or gait, involuntary muscle movements, aberration of muscle tone including that of viscera and sphincters, abnormality of sensory perceptivity including that of skin and special senses, and mental disturbances.

Although one or more of these abnormalities is suggestive of neurological disease the interpretation of them is subject to the principles given below.

PRINCIPLES OF NERVOUS DYSFUNCTION

Nervous tissue is limited in the ways in which it can respond to noxious influences because of its essentially coordinating function. The transmission of impulses along nerve fibers can be enhanced or depressed in varying degrees, the extreme degree being complete failure of transmission. Because of the structure of the system, in which nerve impulses are passed from neuron to neuron by relays at the nerve cells, there may also be excessive or decreased intrinsic activity of individual cells giving rise to an increase or decrease in nerve impulses discharged by the cells. The end result is the same whether the disturbance be one of conduction or discharge and these are the only two ways in which disease of the nervous system is manifested. Nervous dysfunction can thus be broadly divided into two forms, depressed activity and exaggerated activity. These can be further subdivided into the four common modes of nervous dysfunction given below.

Modes of nervous dysfunction

Excitation or irritation signs

Increased activity of the reactor organ occurs because of an increase in the number of nerve impulses received either because of excitation of neurons or by facilitation of passage of stimuli. The excitability of nerve cells can be increased by many factors including stimulant drugs, inflammation, and mild degrees of those influences which in a more severe form may cause depression of excitability. Thus early or mild anoxia may result in increased excitability while continued or severe anoxia will cause depression of function or even death of the nerve cell.

Hypoglycemia also may cause increased excitability, as manifested by hypoglycemic convulsion in insulin therapy, but if sufficiently severe or prolonged causes a fatal hypoglycemic encephalopathy. Irritation phenomena may result from many causes including inflammation of nervous tissue caused by bacteria or viruses, certain nerve poisons and anoxia. In those diseases which cause an increase in pressure within the cranial cavity, irritation phenomena result from interference with circulation and the development of local anemic anoxia. The major manifestations of irritation of nervous tissue are convulsions and muscle tremor in the motor system and hyperesthesia and paresthesia in the sensory system. For the most part the signs produced fluctuate in intensity and may occur periodically as nervous energy is discharged and reaccumulated in the nerve cells.

The area of increased excitability may be local or sufficiently generalized to affect the entire body. Thus a local lesion in the brain may cause signs of excitatory nervous dysfunction in one limb and a more extensive lesion may cause a complete convulsion.

Release signs

Exaggeration of normal nervous system activity occurs when lower nervous centers are released from the inhibitory effects of higher centers. Cerebellar ataxia is a classical example. In the absence of cerebellar control combined limb movements are exaggerated in all modes of action including rate, range, force and direction. In general, release phenomena are present constantly while the causative lesion operates, whereas excitatory phenomena fluctuate with the building up and exhaustion of energy in the nerve cells.

Paralysis due to tissue destruction

Degrees of depression of activity can occur with depression of metabolic activity of nerve cells, the terminal stage being complete paralysis when nervous tissue is destroyed. Such depression of activity may result from failure of supply of oxygen and other essential nutrients either directly from their general absence or indirectly because of failure of the local circulation. Infection of the nerve cell itself may cause initial excitation, then depression of function, and finally complete paralysis when the nerve cell dies.

Signs of paralysis are constant and are manifested by muscular paresis or paralysis when the motor system is affected and by hypoesthesia or anesthesia when the sensory system is involved. Deprivation of metabolites and impairment of function by actual invasion of nerve cells or by toxic depression of their activity produce temporary, partial depression of function which is completely lost when the neurons are destroyed.

Nervous shock

An acute lesion of the nervous system causes damage to nerve cells in the immediate vicinity of the lesion but there may be, in addition, a temporary cessation of function in parts of the nervous system not directly affected. The loss of function in these areas is temporary and usually persists for only a few hours. Stunning is the obvious example. Recovery from the flaccid unconsciousness of nervous shock may reveal the presence of permanent residual signs caused by the destruction of nervous tissue.

It is because of this limited range of modes of reaction to injury in the nervous system that determination of the type of lesion is so difficult. Irritation signs may be caused by bacterial or virus infection, by pressure, vascular disturbance or general anoxia, by poisons and by hypoglycemia. It is often impossible to determine whether the disturbance is structural or functional. Degenerative lesions produce mainly signs of paralysis but unless there are signs of local nervous tissue injury, such as facial nerve paralysis, paraplegia or local tremor, the disturbance may only be definable as a general disturbance of a part of the nervous system. Encephalopathy is an all-embracing diagnosis, but it is often impossible to go beyond it unless other clinical data, including epizootiology and systemic signs, are assessed or special tests including radiographical examination and examination of the cerebrospinal fluid are undertaken.

Some information can be derived from a study of the time relationships in the development of nervous disease. A lesion which develops suddenly tends to produce maximum disturbance of function, sometimes accompanied by nervous shock. Slowly developing lesions permit a form of compensation in that undamaged pathways and centers may assume some of the functions of the damaged areas. Even in rapidly developing lesions partial recovery may occur in time but the emphasis is on maximum depression of function at the beginning of the disease. Thus a slowly developing tumor of the spinal cord will have a different pattern of clinical development to that resulting from an acute traumatic lesion. Another aspect of the rapidity of onset of the lesion is that irritation phenomena are more likely to occur when the onset is rapid and less common when the onset is slow.

MANIFESTATIONS OF DISEASE OF THE NERVOUS SYSTEM

The major manifestations of nervous dysfunction include aberrations of mental state, posture, movement, perception and sphincter activity.

Mental state

Excitation states include mania and frenzy. Both are probably manifestations of general excitation of the cerebral cortex. The areas of the cortex which govern behavior, intellect and personality traits in humans are the frontal lobes and temporal cortex. The importance of these areas, which are poorly developed in animals, is not likely to be great. They, and the limbic system associated with them, are highly susceptible to influences such as anoxia and increased intracranial pressure which affect the brain generally.

Mania

In mania the animal acts in a bizarre way and appears to be unaware of its surroundings. Maniacal actions include licking, chewing of foreign material, sometimes themselves, abnormal voice, constant bellowing, apparent blindness, walking into strange surroundings, drunken gait and aggressiveness in normally docile animals. A state of delirium cannot be diagnosed in animals, but mental disorientation is an obvious component of mania as we see it. Diseases characterized by mania include:

- Encephalitis, e.g. the furious form of rabies, Aujeszky's disease in cattle (mad itch)
- Degenerative diseases of brain, e.g. mannosidosis, early polioencephalomalacia, poisoning by *Astragalus* sp.
- Toxic and metabolic diseases of brain, e.g. nervous acetonemia, pregnancy toxemia, acute lead poisoning, poisoning with carbon tetrachloride, severe hepatic insufficiency, especially in horses.

Frenzy

Frenzy is characterized by violent activity and with little regard for surroundings. The animal's movements are uncontrolled and dangerous to other animals in the group and to human attendants, and are often accompanied by aggressive physical attacks.

Nervous system diseases These can occur in frenzy:

- Encephalomyelitides, e.g. Aujeszky's disease
- Toxic and metabolic brain disease, e.g. hypomagnesemic tetany of cattle and sheep, poisoning with ammoniated roughage in cattle.

Diseases of other systems The following can occur:

- Acute pain of colic in horses
- Extreme cutaneous irritation, e.g. photosensitization in cattle.

Apparently reasonless panic, especially in individual horses or groups of cattle, is difficult to differentiate from real mania. A horse taking fright at a botfly or a swarm of bees, a herd of cattle stampeding at night are examples.

Aggression and other personality changes

Aggression and a willingness to attack other animals, humans and inert objects is characteristic in the early stages of rabies and Aujeszky's disease in cattle, in sows during postparturient hysteria, in the later stages of chronic anoxia in any species, and in some mares and cows with granulosa-cell tumors of the ovary. The latter are accompanied by signs of masculinization and erratic or continuous estrus (27). It is often difficult to differentiate between an animal with a genuine change in personality and one which is in pain or is physically handicapped, for example, pigs and cattle with atlanto-axial arthroses (31).

Depressive mental states

Depressive mental states include somnolence, lassitude, narcolepsy/catalepsy, syncope and coma. They are all manifestations of depression of cerebral cortical function in various degrees and occur as a result of those influences which depress nervous system function generally, as well as those which specifically affect behavior, probably via the limbic system. It is not possible to classify accurately the types of depressive abnormality and relate them to specific causes, but the common occurrences in farm animals are listed below.

Depression leading to coma In all species this may result from:

- Encephalomyelitis and encephalomalacia
- Toxic and metabolic diseases of brain such as uremia, hypoglycemia, hepatic insufficiency, toxemia, septicemia and most toxins which damage tissues generally
- Hypoxia of brain as in peripheral circulatory failure of milk fever
- Heat stroke
- Specific poisons which cause somnolence include bromides, Amitraz in horses, methyl alcohol, *Filix mas* (male fern), kikuyu grass.

Syncope The sudden onset of fainting (syncope) may occur as a result of:

- Acute heart failure leading to acute cerebral anoxia
- Spontaneous cerebral hemorrhage, a most unlikely event in our animals
- Traumatic concussion and contusion
- Lightning stroke, electrocution.

Narcolepsy (catalepsy) Affected animals experience episodes of uncontrollable sleep and literally 'fall' asleep. The disease is recorded in Shetland ponies and is thought to be inherited in them, in other horses, and in cattle (28).

Compulsive walking or head-pressing

Head-pressing is a syndrome characterized by the animal pushing its head against fixed objects, leaning into a stanchion or between fence posts. A variation of the syndrome is probably compulsive walking. Affected animals put their heads down and walk. Often they appear blind. If they walk into an object they lean forward and indulge in head pressing; if confined to a stall they will often walk around the pen continuously or head-press into a corner. The syndrome represents a change in behavior pattern due to an unsatisfied compulsive drive characteristic of a disorder of the limbic system. Causes include:

- Toxic and metabolic brain disease, especially hepatic encephalopathy
- Diseases manifested by increased intracranial pressure
- Encephalomyelitides.

Aimless wandering

A similar but less severe syndrome to compulsive walking is aimless walking, severe mental depression, apparent blindness, with tongue protrusion, continuous chewing movements, but the animal is unable to ingest feed or drink water. Causes include:

- Toxic and metabolic diseases of brain including poisoning by *Helichrysum* sp. and tansy mustard

- Degenerative brain diseases, e.g. nigropallidal encephalomalacia in horses, ceroid lipofuscinosis in sheep, hydrocephalus in the newborn.

Involuntary movements

Involuntary movements include convulsions and tremor.

Tremor
This is a continuous, repetitive twitching of skeletal muscles which is usually visible and palpable. The muscle units involved may be small and cause only local skin movement in which case the tremor is described as fibrillary, or the muscle units may be extensive, the movement much coarser and sufficient to move the extremities, eyes or parts of the trunk. The tremor may become intensified when the animal undertakes some positive action, this usually being indicative of cerebellar involvement and is the counterpart of intention tremor in humans. True tremor is often sufficiently severe to cause incoordination and severe disability in gait. Causes of tremor include:

- Degenerative nervous system disease, e.g. hypomyelinogenesis of the newborn as in congenital tremor of pigs and calves, poisoning by *Swainsona* sp.
- Toxic and metabolic nervous disease caused by a large number of poisons, especially poisonous plants and fungi, and probably bacterial toxins as in shaker foal syndrome, and an occasional metabolic defect such as hyperkalaemic periodic paralysis in a horse (48).

Tics
Tics are spasmodic twitching movements made at much longer intervals than in tremor, the intervals being usually at least several seconds duration and often much longer. The movements are sufficiently widespread to be easily visible and are caused by muscles which are ordinarily under voluntary control. They are rare in large animals but may occur after traumatic injury to a spinal nerve (37).

Convulsions
Convulsions are violent muscular contractions affecting part or all of the body and occurring for relatively short periods as a rule, although in the late stages of encephalitis they may recur with such rapidity as to give the impression of being continuous. They may be clonic, the typical 'paddling' convulsions in which repeated muscle spasms alternate with periods of relaxation. Tetanic or tonic convulsions are less common and are manifested by prolonged muscular spasm without intervening periods of relaxation. True tetanic convulsions occur only rarely, chiefly in strychnine poisoning and in tetanus, and in most cases they are a brief introduction to a clonic convulsion. Convulsions can originate from disturbances anywhere in the prosencephalon, including cerebrum, thalamus or even hypothalamus. However, the initiating cause may be in the nervous system outside the cranium or in some other system altogether, so that convulsions are therefore often subdivided into intracranial and extracranial types. Causes are many and include the following.

Intracranial convulsions These are caused by:

- Encephalomyelitis, meningitis
- Encephalomalacia
- Acute brain edema
- Brain ischemia, including increased intracranial pressure
- Local lesions caused by trauma (concussion, contusion), abscess, tumor, parasitic injury, hemorrhage
- Inherited idiopathic epilepsy.

Extracranial convulsions These are caused by:

- Brain hypoxia as in acute cardiac failure
- Toxic and metabolic diseases of the nervous system including:
  - hepatic encephalopathy
  - hypoglycemia (as in newborn piglets and in hyperinsulinism due to islet cell adenoma of the pancreas as described in a pony (46))
  - hypomagnesemia (as in lactation tetany in cows and mares)
  - inorganic poisons, poisonous plants and fungi. There are too many to give a complete list but well-known examples are the chlorinated hydrocarbons, pluronics used in bloat control, *Clostridium* spp. intoxications, e.g. *C. perfringens* type D and *C. sordelli*, and subacute fluoracetate poisoning
- Congenital and inherited defects without lesions, e.g. familial convulsions and ataxia in Angus cattle.

Involuntary spastic pareses
Involuntary, intermittent contractions of large muscle masses may result in spasmodic movements of individual limbs or parts of the body. In most, contractions occur when voluntary movement is attempted. Diseases in this category are:

- Stringhalt and Australian stringhalt of horses
- Inherited spastic paresis (Elso-heel) of cattle
- Inherited periodic spasticity (stall-cramp) of cattle
- Inherited neuraxial edema of cattle
- Inherited myotonia of goats.

Posture and gait

Abnormal postures may be adopted intermittently by animals in pain but in diseases of the nervous system the abnormality is usually continuous. Deviation or rotation of the head and drooping of the lips, eyelids, cheeks and ears, and opisthotonus and orthotonus are examples, although the latter two are often intermittent in that they occur as part of a convulsive seizure. Head-pressing and assumption of a dog-sitting posture are further examples.

Disturbances of posture, other than those more accurately defined as disturbances of balance caused by lesions of the cerebellum and vestibular tract, are rarely diagnosed in farm animals and are not discussed here. The importance of vision and thalamic and cortical control in the maintenance of posture by statotonic and statokinetic reflexes have not been extensively studied in animals other than the dog and cat. Blindfolding an animal during an examination may be profitable because it removes the compensating effect of visual adaptation, and may thus accentuate an abnormality of gait. However, the effect of blindfolding on the gait of a normal horse must also be considered.

Miscellaneous causes of abnormal posture include some poisonings by plants including *Swainsona* sp. and *Astragalus* sp.

One of the major clinical syndromes encountered by food animal veterinarians is ataxia or incoordination of gait. Some cases are due to specific pathoanatomic lesions, but in animals at pasture most of them are transient abnormalities caused by fungal and plant toxins as set out below. A bizarre disease in this category is 'kangaroo gait' in lactating ewes (41, 42). In the latter the ewes are unable to move their forefeet except by a synchronized bounding action of them. The hindlimbs are rarely affected also. There is slow recovery at the end of lactation. At necropsy there is a generalized polyneuropathy affecting principally the radial nerves. A secondary nutritional deficiency of thiamin and nicotinic acid has been suggested as a cause.

An unusual ataxia syndrome in horses is dysmetria of the hindlimbs due to neuraxonal dystrophy originating in the accessory cuneate nuclei and possibly of genetic origin (19). Badly affected horses lift their feet excessively high and stamp them to the ground.

Vestibular disease

The vestibular influence on balance can be affected at the inner ear, along the vestibular nerve or at the vestibular nucleus in the medulla. Unilateral excitation or loss of function can be caused by lesions at any of these points. Rotation of the head occurs and the animal falls to one side. When the lesion affects the inner ear, as it may do in otitis media, the affected side is turned down, the animal falls to that side and there is usually facial paralysis on the same side. When the vestibular nucleus is affected, which may occur in listeriosis, the animal falls to the opposite or normal side. Nystagmus and forced circling are common when there is irritation of the vestibular nucleus or the medial longitudinal fasciculus.

Causes of vestibular disease include:

- Otitis media with involvement of the inner ear
- Focal lesion at the vestibular nucleus, e.g. listeriosis
- Traumatic injury to the vestibular apparatus in the horse caused by fracture of the basisphenoid bone in a fall. The clinical signs include lack of control of balance, rotation of the head, nystagmus and facial paralysis.

Cerebellar disease

When cerebellar function is abnormal there is ataxia which is an incoordination of muscular action or gait. In general terms there are defects in the rate, range, force and direction of movement. In true cerebellar ataxia (e.g. cerebellar hypoplasia) the affected animal stands with the legs wide apart, sways and falls in any direction. The head oscillates and cannot be maintained in the normal spatial relationship with the rest of the body. The limbs do not move in unison, the movements are grossly exaggerated, muscular strength is usually preserved, and there is a lack of proper placement of the feet (hypermetria and hypometria) so that falling is common. The fault in placement is the result of poor motor coordination and not related in any way to muscle weakness or proprioceptive deficit. Attempts to proceed to a particular point are usually unsuccessful and the animal cannot accurately reach its feed or drinking bowl. Nystagmus may also be present. Head tremor (nodding) may be the most obvious sign in mild cases of cerebellar hypoplasia in young foals.

Causes of cerebellar disease include:

- Encephalomyelitis in which other localizing signs also occur
- Inherited defects of cerebellar structure or abiotrophy (1) in most breeds of cattle, and in Arab horses
- Congenital cerebellar defects resulting from maternal viral infections such as bovine virus diarrhea infection in cattle
- Traumatic injury, e.g. by parasite larvae such as *Hypoderma bovis* which have caused unilateral cerebellar ataxia in adult cattle
- Poisoning by *Claviceps paspali*.

Spinal cord disease

Ataxia due to cerebellar dysfunction can be difficult to differentiate from the proprioceptive defects and partial motor paralysis (weakness) which occur in animals with spinal cord lesions and it is most important that this differentiation be made. The weakness is caused by damage to the upper motor neurons and the proprioceptive deficit to the ascending sensory neurons. Signs of weakness and/or ataxia may be elicited by gently pushing the hindquarters to one side or pulling it by the tail to one side, as the animal is walked (the sway response). The normal animal resists these movements or steps briskly to the side as it is pushed or pulled. The weak animal can be easily pulled to one side and may stumble or fall. The weak animal may also tend to buckle or collapse when strong pressure is applied with the hand over the withers and loin regions. The ataxic animal may sway to one side, be slow to protract a limb, cross its hindlegs or step on its opposite limb. It is often difficult to distinguish paresis from ataxia but in most instances it is unimportant because of the close anatomical relationship of the ascending general proprioceptive and descending upper motor neuron tracts in the white matter of the spinal cord. These same abnormal sway responses can be elicited in the standing animal. The ataxic animal may abduct too far the outside pelvic limb as it is pushed to one side or moved in a small circle. This may appear as a hypermetric movement similar to a stringhalt action and is assumed to be a sign of a general proprioceptive tract lesion. The pushed or circled animal may keep a clinically affected pelvic limb planted in one position on the ground and pivot around it without moving it. The same failure to protract the limb may be seen on backing. It may even force the animal into a 'dog-sitting' posture.

Causes of ataxia due to spinal cord disease include:

- Limited trauma to the spinal cord
- In the early stages of a developing compression lesion in the vertebral canal
- Degenerative and inflammatory diseases of the nervous system, especially those causing enzootic incoordination in horses and staggers in sheep (both of them dealt with under their respective headings)
- Functional diseases in toxic and metabolic diseases of the nervous system in which lesions have not yet been identified and caused mainly by poisons, especially plant materials. Typical examples are poisoning by the fungi *Claviceps paspali*, *Diplodia* spp., *Acremonium lolii*, the grass *Phalaris aquatica*, the ferns *Zamia* and *Xanthorrhea* spp. and herbaceous plants such as *Kallstroemia*, *Vicia*, *Baccharis*, *Solanum*, *Aesculus* and *Ficus* spp.
- Nutritional deficiency especially of thiamin, occurring naturally in horses poisoned by bracken and horsetail, and experimentally in pigs
- Developmental defects including congenital abnormalities and abiotrophic abnormalities that develop some time after birth. Examples are Brown Swiss weavers and Pietrain pig creepers.

In many of these diseases incoordination and paresis are a stage in the development of paresis and paraplegia.

Paralysis

The motor system comprises the pyramidal tracts, originating in the motor cortex, the extrapyramidal system originating in the corpus striatum, red nucleus, the vestibular nucleus and the roof of the midbrain, and the peripheral nerves originating in the ventral horn cells. In hoofed animals (ungulates) the pyramidal tracts are of minor importance, reaching only to the fourth cervical segment. Accordingly, lesions of the motor cortex in farm animals do not produce any deficit of gait. Neither is there any paresis, although in an acute lesion weakness may be evident for the first day or two. If the lesion is unilateral the paresis will be on the contralateral side. This is in marked contradistinction to the severe abnormalities of gait and posture which occur with lesions of the pons, medulla and spinal cord. The main motor nuclei in these animals are subcortical and comprise the extrapyramidal system and most combined movements are controlled by nerve stimuli originating in the corpus striatum. The pyramidal and extrapyramidal tracts comprise the upper motor neurons which reach to the ventral horn cells of the spinal cord, which cells together with their peripheral axons form the lower motor neurons. Paralysis is a physiological end result in all cases of motor nerve injury, which if severe enough is expressed clinically. The type of paralysis is often indicative of the site of the lesion. A lesion of the upper motor neuron causes a spastic paralysis with loss of voluntary movement, increased tone of limb muscles and increased tendon jerks or clonus. These are all release phenomena resulting from liberation of spinal reflex arcs from higher control. A lesion of the lower motor neuron causes a flaccid paralysis, with loss of voluntary movement, decreased tone of the limb muscles, absence of the tendon jerks and wasting of the affected muscle (*neurogenic atrophy*). As injuries to specific peripheral nerves are treated surgically, these are dealt with in surgical textbooks and not repeated here (2).

A special form of paralysis is the *Schiff–Sherrington syndrome* which is common in dogs but recorded rarely in large animals (38). It is caused by acute, severe, compressive injury of the thoracolumbar spinal cord and manifested by extensor rigidity or hypertonia of the forelimbs and hypotonic paralysis of the hindlimbs.

The spasticity of an upper motor neuron lesion usually occurs with the affected limb in extension.

The degree of paralysis needs to be defined. Paralysis is identified as an inability to make purposeful movements. Thus convulsive, uncontrolled movements as they occur in polioencephalomalacia may still fit a description of paralysis. Paresis, or weakness short of paralysis, can be classified into four categories, one in which the animal can support itself if helped but cannot rise, and another group in which the animal cannot rise nor support itself if helped up, but can make purposeful movements in attempting to rise. Animals that can rise but are paretic can be subdivided into those which can move the limbs well and stumble only slightly on walking, and those which move with difficulty and have severe incoordination and stumbling.

Probably the most difficult decision in farm animal neurology is whether a patient's inability to move is because of a nervous or muscular deficit. For example, the horse recumbent because of exertional rhabdomyolysis often resembles a horse with an injured spinal cord. Causes of paralysis are:

- Final stages of encephalomyelitis, encephalomalacia and similar spinal lesions, meningitis
- Toxic and metabolic diseases of the nervous system in their most severe form, e.g. flaccid paralysis is caused by tick (*Ixodes holocyclus*, *Ornithodorus* sp.), poisoning, botulism, snakebite. Comparable tetanic paralyses include tetanus, lactation tetany of mares, hypomagnesemic tetany of cows and calves
- Focal inflammatory, neoplastic, traumatic lesions in the motor pathway.

Neurogenic muscular atrophy

Destruction of the lower motor neurons either within the vertebral canal or peripheral to it causes neurogenic atrophy. Whether or not the lesion is visible depends on how many neurons and therefore how many muscle fibers are affected.

Disturbances in sensation

Lesions of the sensory system are rarely diagnosed in animals, except for those affecting sight and the vestibular apparatus, because of the impossibility of measuring subjective responses.

Thus, although animals must experience paresthesia, as in rabies in sheep, in pseudorabies and acetonemia in cattle, the response by the animal of licking or scratching does not make it possible to decide whether the diagnosis should be paresthesia or pruritus. Lesions of the peripheral sensory neurons cause hypersensitivity or decreased sensitivity of the area supplied by the nerve. Lesions of the spinal cord may affect only motor or only sensory fiber tracts or both, or may be unilateral.

Although it is often difficult to decide whether failure to respond to a normally painful stimulus is due to failure to perceive or inability to respond, certain tests may give valuable information. The test commonly used is pricking with a pin or needle and observing the reaction. In exceptional circumstances light stroking may elicit an exaggerated response. The reaction in sheep affected with scrapie is a striking example of hypersensitivity.

In every test of sensitivity it must be remembered that there is considerable variation between animals and in an individual animal from time to time, and much discretion must be exercised when assessing the response. In any animal there are also cutaneous areas which are more sensitive than others. The face and the cranial cervical region are highly sensitive, the caudal cervical and shoulder regions less so, with sensitivity increasing over the caudal thorax and lumbar region to a high degree on the perineum. The proximal parts of the limbs are much less sensitive than the distal parts and sensitivity is highest over the digits, particularly on the medial aspect.

Absence of a response to the application of a painful stimulus to the limbs (absence of the withdrawal reflex) indicates interruption of the reflex arc; absence of the reflex with persistence of central perception, as demonstrated by groaning or body movement, indicates interruption of motor pathways and that central perception of pain persists. In the horse the response can be much more subtle than in other species, with movements of the ears and eyelids being the best indicators of pain perception. Increased sensitivity is described as hyperesthesia, decreased as hypoesthesia and complete absence as anesthesia. Special cutaneous reflexes include the anal reflex, in which spasmodic contraction of the anus occurs when it is touched, and the corneal reflex, in which there is closure of the eyelids on touching it. The panniculus reflex is valuable in that the sensory pathways, detected by the prick of a pin, enter the cord at T1–L3, but the motor pathways leave the cord only at C8, T1 and T2. The quick twitch of the superficial cutaneous muscle along the whole back, which is the positive response, is quite unmistakable. Examination of the eye reflexes and hearing are discussed under examination of the cranial nerves (see below).

Manifestations of disease of the autonomic nervous system

Lesions affecting the cranial parasympathetic outflow do so by involvement of the oculomotor, facial, vagus and glossopharyngeal nerves or their nuclei and the effects produced are discussed under examination of the individual nerves. In general the lesions cause abnormality of pupillary constriction, salivation and involuntary muscular activity in the upper part of the alimentary and respiratory tracts. Lesions affecting the craniocervical branch of the sympathetic system also cause abnormalities of salivation and pupillary constriction. Lesions of the spinal sympathetic system interfere with normal motility of all viscera including heart and alimentary tract. For the most part, affections of the autonomic nervous system are of minor importance in farm animals. Central lesions of the hypothalamus can cause abnormalities of heat exchange, manifested as neurogenic hyperthermia or hypothermia and obesity, but they are also of minor importance.

Some manifestations of autonomic disease are important. Autonomic imbalance is usually described as the physiological basis for spasmodic colic of horses; grass sickness of horses is characterized by degenerative lesions in the sympathetic ganglia; involvement of the vagus nerve in traumatic reticulitis of cattle causes impairment of motility of the stomachs and the development of vagus indigestion.

Defects of sphincter control and motility of the bladder and rectum may also be of importance in the diagnosis of defects of lumbosacral parasympathetic outflow and the spinal sympathetic system. The sacral segments of the cord are the critical ones, and loss of their function will cause incontinence of urine and filling of the rectum. The parasympathetic nerve supply to the bladder stimulates the detrusor muscle and relaxes the sphincter; the sympathetic nerve supply has the reverse function. A spinal cord lesion may cause loss of the parasympathetic control and result in urinary retention. Incontinence, if it occurs, does so from overflow. When the sympathetic control is removed incontinence occurs but the bladder should empty. Similar disturbances of defecation occur. Both micturition and defecation are controlled by medullary and spinal centers but some measure of control is regained even when the extrinsic nerve supply to the bladder and rectum is completely removed. Incontinence of feces and urine is almost impossible to determine, except in housetrained cats and dogs.

Blindness

Blindness is manifested as a clinical abnormality by the patient walking into objects which it should avoid. The critical test is that of the menace reflex in which the animal should blink when a menacing gesture is made at the eye with the hand without touching the tactile hairs of the eyelids or creating a wind which can be felt by the patient. It may be necessary to alert the patient to the risk of injury by touching the cornea first. In very alert and young animals a good test is to drop a light object (a feather is best, or a cotton ball) in such a way as to attract the patient's gaze. The patient should watch the object fall to the ground and continue to watch it afterwards.

A further test is to make the patient run an obstacle course. A similar procedure is the only way to test for night blindness. The area should be dimly lit, but the observer should be able to see the obstructions clearly. A decision that the animal is blind creates a need for the examination of the visual pathways. Causes of blindness include:

- Diseases of the orbit including keratoconjunctivitis, hypopyon, cataract, panophthalmia, mixed ocular defects inherited in white Shorthorn and Jersey cattle, night blindness in Appaloosa horses (14), sporadic cases of blindness due to idiopathic retinal degenerative disease in cattle (21)

- Congenital retinal dysplasia of goats (9). Lenticular cataracts caused by poisoning with hygromycin in pigs (13); congenital ocular malformations in calves after intrauterine infection with bovine virus diarrhea virus, usually accompanying cerebellar defects (44)
- Diseases of optic nerve and chiasma, e.g. abscess of pituitary rete mirabile, constriction of optic nerve by diet deficient in vitamin A. Tumor of pituitary gland, injury to the optic nerve especially in horses after rearing and falling backwards. There is a sudden onset of unilateral or bilateral blindness with no ophthalmologic change until 3–4 weeks after the injury, when the optic disc becomes paler and less vascular (43)
- Traumatic or ischemic lesions of optic cortex as in polioencephalomalacia, cerebral edema, hydrocephalus
- Localized infectious or parasitic lesions caused by abscesses, migrating larvae
- Functional blindness in which there is complete, often temporary, blindness in the absence of any physical lesions. Causes are acetonemia, pregnancy toxemia and acute carbohydrate indigestion of ruminants
- Specific poisonings causing blindness include *Filix mas* (male fern), *Cheilanthes* sp. (rockfern) and rape. *Stypandra* sp. causes a specific degeneration of the optic nerves. Lead poisoning in cattle.

SPECIAL EXAMINATION OF THE NERVOUS SYSTEM

Many of the techniques used in the special examination of the nervous system in humans and in dogs or cats are not applicable to farm animals because of their size and because they are unaccustomed to being handled. Young calves, lambs and pigs may be satisfactory subjects because of their size but the result of many tests, particularly those involving tonic and kinetic postural reflexes, cannot be interpreted and are not dealt with here. The neurological examination of the newborn foal is fraught with hazards because of the different responses elicited from those in adults. The differences relate mostly to the temporary dysmetria of gait and exaggerated responses of reflexes (25).

History

Special attention should be given to the recording of an accurate history. The duration of signs, the mode of onset—particularly whether acute with later subsidence, or chronic with gradual onset—the progression of involvement and the description of signs which occur only intermittently should be ascertained. When the disease is a herd problem the morbidity and mortality rates and the method of spread may indicate an intoxication when all affected animals show signs within a very short period. Changes in behavior and mental state can often be assessed only on the history. Traumatic injury is often a cause of nervous disease and may not be detectable other than from the history.

When obtaining a history of convulsive episodes an estimate should be made of their duration and frequency. The pattern is also of importance, and may be diagnostic, for example in salt poisoning in swine. The occurrence of pallor or cyanosis during the convulsion is of particular importance in the differentiation of cardiac syncope and a convulsion originating in the nervous system.

General examination

Many of the general techniques of examination of the central nervous system have already been dealt with in Chapter 1 and in the section on manifestations of nervous system disease in this chapter. They include assessment of the mental state, gait, posture, balance and sensory perception and the presence of involuntary and compulsive movements. Special aspects of examination of the nervous system include examination of gait, muscle tone, muscle wasting, reflex arcs, cranial and spinal nerves and the bony encasement of the central nervous system (CNS). Examination of the cerebrospinal fluid and radiographical examination are also included.

Gait

The more sophisticated tests are suitable for use only in the horse. The best observations are made when the animal is running free, preferably at a fast gait, to avoid abnormalities conferred by being led. Also slight abnormalities such as a high-stepping gait, slight incoordination of movement, errors of placement of feet, stumbling, failure to flex joints properly, are all better observed in a free animal. The primary decision is to decide whether there is a proprioceptive deficit as indicated by the animal not knowing where its feet are, or a cerebellar, coordinative deficit when the legs do not end up where the animal obviously intended them to go. It is often not possible to be sure and the decision is often subjective.

With the animal on a lead it is possible to get it to perform special movements. These include backing, quick pivoting to observe placement and movement at the right time, pushing laterally on the hindquarters when walking (a version of the placing reflexes used in dogs), and moving when blindfolded to determine the importance of sight in compensating for a vestibular deficit.

Spontaneous walking in circles is an important sign. It can be the result of a head rotation (or tilt), or deviation of the head. When the head is held in a rotated position and there is a loss of balance while walking the lesion is vestibular. If there is no loss of balance the lesion is more likely to be in the frontal lobe of the cortex. If the head is rigidly deviated and cannot be voluntarily held straight out in front the lesion is medullary or in the upper cervical cord; if it can be held straight the lesion is probably in the frontal lobe of the cerebral cortex.

Balance
Balance control is not usually measurable in a large animal other than by simple observation of it carrying out its normal physical functions. Of particular importance are the animal's actions when it is lying down or getting up. Particular note should be made of any tendency to fall to a particular side, or to be unable to get up or have difficulty getting up when lying on a particular side, and whether there is a tendency to walk in circles to a particular side.

Muscle tone
The tone of skeletal muscle may be examined by passively flexing and extending the limbs and moving the neck from side to side and up and down. Increased muscle tone, spasticity or tetany may be so great that the limb cannot be flexed without considerable effort. If the spastic-extended limb does begin to flex but the resistance remains this is known as 'lead-pipe' rigidity which is seen in tetanus. If after beginning to flex an extended spastic limb, the resistance suddenly disappears ('clasp-knife release') this suggests an upper motor neuron lesion spastic paralysis as occurs in polioencephalomalacia.

Flaccidity, or decreased muscle tone, indicates the presence of a lower motor neuron lesion with interruption of the spinal reflex arc.

Muscle wasting
Localized atrophy of muscles may be myogenic or neurogenic and the difference can be determined only by electromyography, a technique not well suited to large animal practice. If the atrophic muscle corresponds to the distribution of a peripheral nerve it is usually assumed that the atrophy is neurogenic. In addition, neurogenic atrophy is usually rapid (will be clinically obvious in a few days) and much more marked than either disuse or myogenic atrophy.

Reflex arcs
Much of the examination already described depends upon the integrity of reflex arcs. Additional tests include the pupillary light reflex (see below), postural reflexes which are not described here because of their limited use in farm animals, and the tendon reflexes. Of the tendon reflexes, the patella reflex is the only one which can be consistently applied and then only to the smaller species and when they are recumbent. A light tap on the patella tendon elicits reflex extension of the limb. Absence of the response is caused by interruption of the reflex arc by damage to the peripheral nerve or to the relevant spinal cord segment. An enhanced response, characterized by an exaggeration of the limb extension, or by clonus, a rapid series of muscle twitches, is caused by an upper motor neuron lesion in which the relevant spinal cord segment is not directly involved but is released from the inhibitory effects of higher centers.

The laryngeal adductory reflex is of special interest in the examination of ataxic horses. In normal horses a slap on the saddle region just caudal to the withers causes a flickering adductory movement of the contralateral arytenoid cartilage which is visible by an endoscope. The reflex is absent when there is damage to afferent tracts up the spinal cord, when there is damage to the recurrent laryngeal nerves, and in tense or frightened horses (34). Elicitation of the reflex is called the slap test.

Special regional examination

One of the very important parts of a clinical examination of the nervous system is the examination of regions in an attempt to localize the site of the lesion. To an extent this is more important to an academic study than to a practical clinical one. However, there are many occasions in which a knowledge of the localization of the lesion can materially help in making the diagnosis. Because of pressures of space this section is dealt with principally in tabular form (Tables 34–39). More detailed examination is given here to the cranial nerve, spinal cord and peripheral nerves.

Examination of the cranial nerves

Olfactory nerve
Tests of smell are unsatisfactory in animals because of their response to food by sight and sound.

Optic nerve
The only tests of visual acuity applicable in animals are testing the eye preservation (menace) reflex, consisting of provoking closure of the eyelids and withdrawal of the head by stabbing the finger at the eye, and by making the animal run a contrived obstacle course. Both tests are often difficult to interpret and must be carried out in such a way that other senses are not used to determine the presence of the obstacles or threatened injury. In more intelligent species, a good test is to drop some light object such as a handkerchief or feather in front of the animal. It should gaze at the object while it is falling and continue to watch it on the ground. The same comment applies to young ruminants which demonstrate normal vision by following the examiner's moving hand at an age so early that they have not yet developed a menace reflex. Ophthalmoscopic examination is an integral part of an examination of the optic nerve.

Oculomotor nerve
This nerve supplies the pupilloconstrictor muscles of the iris and all of the extrinsic muscles of the eyeball except the dorsal oblique, the lateral rectus and the retractor muscles. Loss of function of the nerve results in pupillary dilatation and defective pupillary constriction when the light intensity is increased, abnormal position (ventrolateral deviation) or defective movement of the eyeballs and palpebral ptosis.

The pupillary light reflex is best tested by shining a bright point source of light into the eye which causes constriction of the iris of that eye (direct pupillary reflex). Constriction of the opposite eye (consensual pupillary light reflex) will also occur but is not as marked in farm animals as in the dog and man. The consensual

Table 34. Correlation between clinical findings and location of the lesions in the nervous system of farm animals: abnormalities of mental state (behavior)

Principal sign	*Secondary sign*	*Location of lesion*	*Example*
Mania/hysteria/ hyperexcitability	Continuous, leading to paralysis; aggressive, convulsions	Cerebrum-limbic system	Peracute lead poisoning, rabies, acute dilatation of lateral ventricles in cholesteatoma, encephalitis
	Intermittent, acetonuria, signs of hepatic insufficiency	Cerebrum-limbic system	Hypoglycemia, hypoxia
Coma (recumbency with no response to stimuli; dilated pupils)	Gradual development. Hypothermia, peripheral vascular collapse. Clinicopathological tests	Cerebral-brainstem reticular formation (ascending reticular activating system)	Hepatic insufficiency, uremia, toxemia, septicemia
	Sudden onset. Normal temperature, pulse/heart rate slow to normal, nose bleed, skin laceration, bruising middle of forehead or poll	Cerebral-brainstem reticular formation (ascending reticular activating system)	Accidental, severe blunt trauma with edema, concussion, contusion of brain
Narcolepsy ± catalepsy. Uncontrollable sleep	With or without sudden, intermittent falling due to loss of voluntary motor function	Brainstem control of cerebral cortex	Inherited in Shetland ponies (16) and Suffolk horses (20)
Compulsive walking and head-pressing, aggressive behavior, grinding of teeth.	Apparent blindness, nystagmus	Cerebral-visual cortex and limbic system	Increased intracranial pressure in polioencephalomalacia
No ataxia	Apparent blindness, no nystagmus, hepatic insufficiency shown on clinical pathology tests	Cerebral-visual cortex and limbic system	Hepatic insufficiency (i.e. ammonia intoxication) in pyrrolizidine poisoning
Imbecility in neonate; lack of response to normal stimuli; can walk, stand	Blindness	Cerebral cortex absent; hydranencephaly	Intrauterine infection with Akabane or bovine virus diarrhea (BVD) virus (39) in calves

light reflex may be used to localize lesions of the optic pathways.

Examination of the menace reflex (eye preservation reflex to a menace) and the results of the pupillary light reflex can be used to distinguish between blindness due to a cortical lesion (central blindness) and that due to lesions in the optic nerve or other peripheral parts of the optic pathways (peripheral blindness). As an example, in polioencephalomalacia (central blindness) the menace reflex is absent but the pupillary light reflex is usually present. In the ocular form of hypovitaminosis A (peripheral blindness) in cattle the menace reflex is also absent, the pupils are widely dilated and the pupillary light reflex is absent. In polioencephalomalacia, the optic nerve, oculomotor nucleus and oculomotor nerve are usually intact but the visual cortex is not; in hypovitaminosis A the optic nerve is usually degenerate which interferes with both the menace and pupillary light reflexes. Testing of ocular movements can be carried out by moving the hand about in front of the face. In paralysis of the oculomotor nerve there may also be deviation from the normal ocular axes and rotation of the eyeball. There will also be an absence of the normal horizontal nystagmus reaction with a medial jerk of the eyeball in response to quick passive movement of the head. Failure to jerk laterally indicates a defect of the abducens nerve. An inherited exophthalmos and strabismus occurs in Jersey cattle.

Trochlear nerve

This nerve supplies only the dorsal oblique muscle of the eye so that external movements and position of the eyeball are abnormal (dorsolateral fixation) when the nerve is injured. This is common in polioencephalomalacia in cattle resulting in a dorsomedial fixation of the eyeball. The medial angle of the pupil is displaced dorsally when the head is held in normal extension.

Trigeminal nerve

The sensory part of the trigeminal nerve supplies sensory fibers to the face and can be examined by testing the palpebral reflex and the sensitivity of the face. The motor part of the nerve supplies the muscles of mastication and observation of the act of chewing may reveal abnormal jaw movements and asymmetry of muscle contractions. There may also be atrophy of the muscles, which is best observed when the lesion is unilateral.

Abducent nerve

Because the abducent nerve supplies motor fibers to the retractor and lateral rectus muscles of the eyeball, injury to the nerve may result in protrusion and medial deviation of the globe. This is not readily observable clinically.

Facial nerve

The 7th cranial nerve supplies motor fibers to the muscles of the face and ears. The symmetry and posture of the ears, eyelids and lips are the best criteria for assessing

Table 35. Correlation between clinical findings and location of the lesion in the nervous system of farm animals: involuntary movements

Principal sign	*Secondary sign*	*Location of lesion*	*Example*
Tremor	Moderate rigidity, combined movement	No specific focal lesion. Generalized disease, e.g. hypomyelinogenesis	Congenital tremor of Herefords. Hypomyelinogenesis, shaker pigs, lambs with border disease
	Paralysis with spasticity		
	Intention tremor, sensory ataxia	Cerebellum	Cerebellar hypoplasia
Nystagmus	With head rotation	Vestibular apparatus	Otitis media and interna. Fracture of petrous temporal bone
	Usually with tetraparesis, impaired consciousness, abnormal pupils, opisthotonus, facial palsy, dysphagia	Cerebellopontine and midbrain areas	Injury, increased intracranial pressure, polioencephalomalacia, listeriosis
	Pendular nystagmus	No lesion	Benign sporadic occurrence in cattle (22), inherited in Finnish Ayrshire bulls (30)
Convulsions	Independent episodes	Focus of irritation in cerebral cortex or thalamus, with spread of excitation	Idiopathic or traumatic epilepsy
	Continuous, leading to paralysis	Cerebral cortex	Increased intracranial pressure, encephalitis
	Intermittent, related to periods of metabolic stress	Cerebral cortex	Hypomagnesemia (lactation tetany) hypoglycemia (e.g. of baby pigs)
Tenesmus (straining)	Later paralysis of anus, sometimes tail head. Sexual precocity in male	Caudal cord segments and cauda equina, stimulation of nerve cells, later paralysis	Rabies, subacute local meningitis
Compulsive rolling	Disturbance of balance, cannot stand, must lie on one side. Nystagmus	Vestibular apparatus	Brain abscess, otitis media
Compulsive walking and head-pressing	See Table 34		

the function of the nerve. Ability to move the muscles in question can be determined by creating a noise or stabbing a finger at the eye. Absence of the eye preservation reflex may be due to facial nerve paralysis or blindness. Facial paralysis includes dropped ear and eyelid, lack of lip tone and perhaps drooling of saliva. The common causes of damage to the nerve are fracture of the petrous temporal bone, guttural pouch mycosis and damage to the peripheral nerve at the mandible. A common accompaniment is injury to the vestibular nerve or centre.

Vestibulocochlear nerve
The cochlear part of the vestibulocochlear nerve is not easily tested by simple clinical examination, but failure to respond to sudden sharp sounds, created out of sight and without creating air currents, suggests deafness. It can be tested electronically (the brainstem auditory evoked response, or BAER, test) to diagnose a lesion of the auditory nerve, eliminating the possibility of a central brain lesion (24). Abnormalities of balance and carriage of the head (rotation around the long axis and not deviation laterally) usually accompany lesions of the vestibular part of the vestibulocochlear nerve and nystagmus is usually present. In severe cases, rotation of the head is extreme, the animal is unable to stand and lies in dorsal recumbency with its legs pointed upwards; rolling to achieve this posture is compulsive and forceful. There is no loss of strength (17). In most species there is a relatively common occurrence of paralysis of the facial and the vestibular nerves as a result of otitis interna or otitis media. This does occur in the horse but less commonly than traumatic injury to the skull as a result of falling (23). There is also what appears to be a chronic inflammatory, infectious disease of calves manifested by space-occupying granulomatous lesions on the roots of the facial and vestibulocochlear nerves and an attending syndrome of facial paralysis and disturbance of balance (36). Benign, pendular nystagmus should not be mistaken as a sign of serious neurological disease. It is characterized by oscillations of the eyeball which are always the same speed and amplitude and which appear in response to a visual stimulus, e.g. a flashing light. It is common in cattle and is not accompanied by other signs and there is no lesion (22).

Glossopharyngeal nerve
Because of its motor function for the muscles of the pharynx and larynx, defects in this nerve are usually accompanied by paralysis of these organs with signs of dysphagia or inability to swallow, regurgitation through

Table 36. Correlation between clinical findings and location of the lesion in the nervous system of farm animals: abnormalities of posture

Principal sign	*Secondary sign*	*Location lesion*	*Example*
Paresis (difficulty in rising, staggering gait, easily falling)	Persistent recumbency, muscle tone and reflexes variable depending on site of lesion	Loss of function in nervous tissue, e.g. spinal cord, may be upper or motor neuron lesion	Bovine viral leukosis affecting spinal cord
	General loss of muscle tone including vascular, alimentary systems	Depression of synaptic or neuromuscular transmission for metabolic reasons or toxic reasons	Milk fever, botulism, peracute coliform mastitis, tick paralysis
Flaccid paralysis (1) Hindlimbs only	Forelimbs normal. Hindlimbs flaccid, no tone, or reflexes, no anal reflex, urinary incontinence, straining initially	Tissue destruction, myelomalacia at lumbosacral cord segments L4 to end	Paralytic rabies. Spinal cord local meningitis, vertebral body osteomyelitis, fracture
	Fore limbs normal. Hindlimbs normal tone and reflexes, anal reflex normal. No withdrawal reflex caudally	Cord damage at thoracolumbar segments T3–L3	Spinal cord local meningitis as above, damage by vertebral fracture, lymphosarcoma
(2)Fore and hindlimbs	Flaccid paralysis, normal tone and reflexes hindlimbs. Absent tone and reflexes in front limbs. Atrophy only in front. Anal reflex all right. No withdrawal reflex caudally	Cord damage at cervicothoracic segments C6–T2	Fracture of vertebra, lymphosarcoma, abscess
	Flaccid paralysis all four legs and neck. Unable to lift head off ground. Normal tone and reflexes all legs. Pain perception persists. No withdrawal reflex caudally	Cord damage at upper cervical segments C1–C5	Injury while running or falling, abscess or lymphosarcoma
Spastic paralysis (permanent, no variation, all four limbs in extension, increased tone, exaggerated reflexes, opisthotonus)	Cranial nerve deficits trigeminal to hypoglossal. Loss of central perception of pain. Depression	Medulla, pons and midbrain	Abscess, listeriosis
Tremor	Tremor (fine or coarse) no convulsions	Red nucleus and reticular apparatus and midbrain/basal ganglia area tracts	Congenital diseases of calves, e.g. hypomyelinogenesis, neuraxial edema
Tetany (all four limbs extended, opisthotonus). Variable intensity modifiable by treatment	Intense hyperesthesia, prolapse 3rd eyelid	Decreased synaptic resistance generally	Tetanus
	Exaggerated response to all external stimuli, i.e. hyperesthesia	Increased neuromuscular transmission	Hypomagnesemia
Paralysis of anus	No anal or perineal reflex. May be straining	Damage to spinal cord at segments S1–S3	Injury or local meningitis, early rabies
Paralysis of tail	Flaccid tail with anesthesia	Injury to caudal segments	Injury or local meningitis, early rabies
Opisthotonus	With spastic paralysis, tremor, nystagmus, blindness	Cerebrum, cerebellum and midbrain	Polioencephalomalacia, trauma
	Part of generalized tetanic state or convulsion	Neuromuscular transmission defect, tetanus, hypomagnesemia	Tetanus
Falling to one side	Mostly with circling (see below). Also with deviation of tail	No detectable lesion in spinal cord	*Xanthorrhea hastile* poisoning

the nostrils, abnormality of the voice and interference with respiration.

Vagus nerve

The motor nerve supply to the pharynx and larynx also contains fibers from the vagus nerve and abnormalities of swallowing, voice and respiration may also occur when the vagus nerve is injured. Because of the additional role of this nerve in supplying nerve fibers to the upper alimentary tract, loss of its function will lead to paralysis of the pharynx and esophagus. Parasympathetic nerve fibers to the stomach are also carried in the vagus and

Table 37. Correlation between clinical findings and location of the lesion in the nervous system of farm animals: abnormalities of gait

Principal sign	*Secondary sign*	*Location of lesion*	*Example*
Circling			
(1) Rotation of the head	Nystagmus, circles, muscle weakness, falls easily, may roll, other cranial nerves affected	Vestibular nucleus	Brain abscess, listeriosis
	Nystagmus, walks in circles, falls occasionally, animal strong. Falls easily if blindfolded, sometimes facial paralysis	Inner ear (vestibular canals), VIIIth cranial nerve, facial nerve	Otitis media, otitis interna, fracture petrous temporal bone (horse)
(2) Deviation of the head	Deviation of head and gaze, compulsive walking, depression. Can walk straight. Balance may be normal	Cerebrum	Brain abscess in calf (infection from dehorning or umbilicus)
	Unable to walk straight. Facial paralysis, other cranial nerve deficits, head may be rotated	Medulla	Listeriosis
Cerebellar ataxia	Exaggerated strength and distance of movement, direction wrong. Hypermetria. Incoordination because of exaggerated movement. No paresis	Cerebellum	Inherited cerebellar hypoplasia in all species especially Arab horses; *Claviceps paspali* poisoning; Gomen disease (32, 33) a probable plant poisoning; destruction by a virus especially bovine virus diarrhea in cattle; hematoma in the fourth ventricle causing cerebellar displacement (18). Idiopathic cerebellar degeneration in adult cattle (26)
Sensory ataxia	No loss of movement or strength but timing movement wrong, legs get crossed, feet badly placed when pivoting	Damage to sensory tracts in spinal cord	Cervical cord lesion, thoracolumbar if just pelvic limb
Sensorimotor ataxia	Weakness of movement, e.g. scuffing toes, knuckling, incomplete flexion, extension causes wobbly, wandering gait, falls down easily, difficulty in rising	Moderate lesion to spinal cord tracts	Plant poisonings, e.g. sorghum. Cervical vertebral compression of spinal cord. Degenerative myelopathy

damage to them could cause hypomotility of that organ. The principal clinical finding in vagus nerve injury is laryngeal and pharyngeal paralysis.

Spinal accessory nerve

Damage to this nerve is infrequent and the effects are not documented. Based on its anatomical distribution loss of function of this nerve could be expected to lead to paralysis of the trapezius, brachiocephalic and sternocephalic muscles and lack of resistance to lifting the head.

Hypoglossal nerve

As the motor supply to the tongue the function of this nerve can be best examined by observing the motor activity of the tongue. There may be protrusion, deviation or fibrillation of the organ, all resulting in difficulty in prehending food and drinking water. The most obvious abnormality is the ease with which the tongue can be pulled out. The animal also has difficulty in getting it back into its normal position in the mouth. In lesions of some duration there may be obvious unilateral atrophy.

Examination of the spinal cord

The testing of individual cord segments and their peripheral nerves depends upon a knowledge of the anatomical distribution of each nerve. The tests usually used are the skin reflexes tested with a pin, and tendon reflexes where they are applicable.

The tendon reflexes have been described above. The response to pricking with a pin is manifested by a quick movement of the cutaneous muscle—the panniculus reflex. The motor arm of this reflex emanates from spinal cord segments C8–T1. Deeper pressure causes obvious central recognition of pain, and this may include local muscular movement. Tests applicable to specific zones of the cord are set out below. The usual procedure is to prick with a pin beside the backbone, and on both sides of the vertebral column, looking for differences between sides and between different levels of the one side in terms of sensitivity and degree of response. There are zones where natural sensitivity is less or greater than other zones, so that only dramatic differences should be classified as abnormal.

Specific tests applicable to examining spinal cord

Table 38. Correlation between clinical findings and location of the lesion in the nervous system of farm animals: abnormalities of the visual system

Principal sign	*Secondary sign*	*Location of lesion*	*Example*
Blindness (bumps into objects)	Pupillary dilatation. No pupillary light reflex. No menace reflex	Optic nerve (examine fundus of eye)	Toxoplasmosis (retina). Vitamin A deficiency. Pituitary rete mirabile abscess. Congenital retinal dysplasia of goats
	Pupil normal size. Pupillary light reflexes normal	Cerebral cortex	Polioencephalomalacia, lead poisoning
Night blindness	—	Retina	Nutritional deficiency of vitamin A. Inherited defect Appaloosa foals
Abnormal dilatation of pupil (mydriasis)	Absence of pupillary light reflex. Can see—does not bump into objects	Motor path of oculomotor nerve	Snakebite, atropine poisoning, milk fever
	Absent pupillary light reflex. No vision. Retinal damage on ophthalmoscopic examination	Retinal lesion	Toxoplasmosis, trauma, ophthalmitis
	Absent pupillary light reflex. No vision. Retina normal	Optic nerve atrophy and fibrosis	Avitaminosis A in cattle
Abnormal constriction of pupil (miosis)	Diarrhea, dyspnea	Failure to inactivate acetylcholine	Specific for organophosphate poisoning
	Blindness, coma, semicoma, spastic paralysis	Diffuse lesion	Polioencephalomalacia, acute lead poisoning
Horner's syndrome. Drooping upper eyelid, miosis, enophthalmos (15)	Hemilateral sweating and temperature rise side of face and upper neck. Unilateral exophthalmus; nasal obstruction	Damage to cranial thoracic and cervical sympathetic trunks	Mediastinal tumor (12), Guttural pouch mycosis. Neoplastic space-occupying lesions of the cranium involving the periorbit (35); perivascular injection around jugular vein or normal intravenous injection of xylazine hydrochloride in normal horses (40), melanoma at the thoracic inlet in a horse (45)
Nystagmus	See Table 35		
Abnormal position of eyeball and eyelids	Dorsomedial deviation of eyeball	Trochlear (IVth)	Polioencephalomalacia
Eyelid	Facial nerve	Listeriosis	
Ventrolateral fixation	Oculomotor (IIIrd)	Abscess/tumor, e.g. bovine viral leukosis	
Protrusion and medial deviation	Abducent (VIth)		
No palpebral reflex	—	Deficit sensory branch of Vth nerve	Trauma
Absence of menace response	—	Facial nerve (provided vision is all right)	Listeriosis
Absence of pupillary light reflex	—	Oculomotor (provided vision is present)	

segments of horses have been described (3). Segmental motor relationships are C1–C6, movements of head and neck; C5–T2, movements of forelimbs; C7–T2, withdrawal reflex front limb; L4–L6, hindlimb withdrawal reflex; L5–L6, patellar reflex; and the sacrocaudal segments, the anal reflex including contraction of the external sphincter and clamping of the tail. All of these reflexes depend on the presence of a motor path, and absence of a response means only that one or other of the sensory or motor paths is not functioning. It is possible, by watching the patient's head while testing, to determine whether there is any central perception of pain, e.g. laying back of the ears, and thus determining whether there is conscious perception.

The spinal cord of the calf has less control of basic physical functions than in humans, dogs and horses. For example, calves are able to retain control of the pelvic limb in spite of experimentally induced lesions which cause hemiplegia in dogs and humans. Also transection of the spinothalamic tract in the calf cord does not produce an area of hypalgesia or analgesia on the controlateral side as such a lesion would do in a human (47).

Observation of defecation and urination movements

Table 39. Correlation between clinical findings and location of the lesion in the nervous system of farm animals: disturbances of prehension, chewing or swallowing

Principal sign	*Secondary sign*	*Location of lesion*	*Example*
Inability to prehend or inability to chew	Sensory/proprioceptive, deficiency approaching feed	Sensory branch of trigeminal (Vth) dysfunction	Poisoning by *Phalaris aquatica* in cattle. Local medullary lesion
	Inappropriate movements of tongue	Hypoglossal nerve (XIIth) dysfunction	Poisoning by *Phalaris aquatica* in cattle. Listeriosis, local medullary lesion
	Inappropriate movements of lips	Facial nerve (VIIth) dysfunction	Traumatic injury to petrous temporal bone, otitis media and interna, listeriosis, guttural pouch mycosis
	Inadequate chewing movements of jaw	Motor branch of the (Vth) trigeminal dysfunction	Poisoning by *Phalaris aquatica* in cattle, listeriosis
Inability to swallow (in absence of physical foreign body) is pharyngeal paresis or paralysis	Regurgitation through nose, inhalation into lungs causing aspiration pneumonia	Glossopharyngeal (IXth) nerve dysfunction. Nuclei in medulla	Abscess or tumor adjacent to nerve. Listeriosis, abscess in medulla
	Inappropriate all swallowing movements	Globus pallidus and substantia nigra	Poisoning *Centaurea* sp.

and postures contributes to knowledge of the state of the cauda equina. Thus neuritis of the cauda equina is characterized by flaccid paralysis and analgesia of the tail, anus and perineum, and the rectum and bladder. There is no paresis or paralysis of the hindlimbs unless lumbosacral segments of the cord are damaged.

Examination of peripheral nerves

Peripheral nerves, other than the cranial nerves already dealt with, are examined by observing the relevant parts of the body for muscle tone, strength and atrophy, and by warmth and posture. Specific tests are used relating to sensitivity to external stimuli and the movements they produce, e.g. the patellar reflex. If the expected reaction is absent or greatly reduced the peripheral nerve or the relevant spinal cord segment is hypofunctional. If it is the cord which is affected, there should be a related deficit of cord function below and sometimes above the lesion.

The bulk of the work done and expertise available on diseases affecting the peripheral nerves is regarded as being within the discipline of surgery and is not presented here.

Palpation of the bony encasement of the central nervous system

Palpable or visible abnormalities of the cranium or spinal column are not commonly encountered in diseases of the nervous system but this examination should not be neglected. There may be displacement, abnormal configuration or pain on deep palpation. These abnormalities are much more readily palpable in the vertebral column and if vertebrae are fractured. Abnormal rigidity or flexibility of the vertebral column, such as occurs in atlanto-occipital malformations in cattle and Arabian horses, may also be detectable by manipulation.

Examination of cerebrospinal fluid (CSF)

CSF can be collected from the cerebellomedullary cistern or the lumbosacral space. Provided the animal is well restrained and care is exercised in introducing the needle, little difficulty should be encountered. The site should be carefully prepared and the procedure carried out in an aseptic manner. A special spinal needle containing a stillete should be used as ordinary hypodermic needles readily block with tissue. For collection from the lumbosacral space the needle must be introduced in a perfectly vertical position relative to the plane of the animal's vertebral column because of the danger of entering one of the lateral blood vessels in the vertebral canal. A mature cow in sternal recumbency can be restrained with a pair of nosetongs and tethering the head to the upper pelvic limb. For a lumbar puncture, local anesthesia is adequate (4). Collection from the cysterna magna is much easier and is the preferred site if the lesion is considered to be in the cranial vault because the CSF is produced in the subarchnoid space and flows caudally down the spinal cord. Ventriflexion of the head and neck of cattle enlarges the space of the cysterna magna and allows easy entry using an 8 cm spinal needle inserted at a point created by the transection of the transverse line of the base of the ears and the dorsal midline, and directed at angle towards the symphysis of the lower jaw. Xylazine is effective in providing sedation and analgesia for this procedure in cattle; in the horse, a general anesthetic is recommended. The laboratory values for the CSF of normal horses are recorded (5).

CSF can be collected and examined for the presence of protein, cells and bacteria. The number of cells present in normal animals is usually less than 5/μl but they may be present in large numbers in cases of meningitis. Samples which show visible turbidity usually contain large numbers of cells and much protein. Blood contamination appears to have little effect on the leukocyte numbers (7). Variations in CSF pressure are not of much use in clinical investigations except in the diagnosis of hypovitaminosis A. Care is needed in interpreting results because the pressure is greatly affected by voluntary movement such as straining. The CSF pressure can be determined by the use of a manometer attached to the spinal needle. When the fluid system is properly connected occlusion of both jugular veins causes a marked rise in a water manometer. CSF pressure is increased in a number of diseases including polioencephalomalacia, bacterial meningitis and hypovitaminosis A. As a rule pressures are higher during the early stages of the disease (6). Normal pressures are of the order of 120 mm of Ringer's solution.

Brain biopsy

A technique for obtaining small samples of brain from cattle has been described (8) and may have value in clinical work when animals have to be salvaged for meat.

Radiographic examination

Examination of the bony skeleton of the head and vertebral column to detect abnormalities which are affecting the nervous system is used only to a limited extent in large animals such as the mature horse or cow. In smaller animals such as sheep, pigs and young horses and cattle the detection of fractures radiographically is a useful aid to diagnosis. The injection of contrast media into the cerebrospinal fluid system is useful for the detection of hydrocephalus and spinal cord compression. In cases of peripheral nerve injury the radiograph of the appropriate limb may reveal the presence of a fracture or space-occupying lesion which has caused dysfunction of the peripheral nerve.

Electroencephalography (EEG) and electromyography (EMG)

These biophysical techniques have not been utilized to any significant degree in large animals. The EEG is impractical although recommendations have been made in order to standardize EEG techniques for animals (9–11). Electromyography seems likely to have more potential and practicality, especially for peripheral nerve injury in horses.

PRINCIPLES OF TREATMENT IN DISEASES OF THE NERVOUS SYSTEM

Treatment of disease of the nervous system presents some particular problems because of the failure of nervous tissue in the brain and spinal cord to regenerate and because of the impermeability of the blood–brain barrier to many antibiotics.

When peripheral nerves are severed, regeneration occurs if the damage is not extensive but no specific treatment, other than surgical intervention, can be provided to facilitate repair. When neurons are destroyed in the brain and spinal cord no regeneration occurs and the provision of nervous system stimulants can have no effect on the loss of function that occurs. The emphasis in treatment of diseases of the nervous system must be on prevention of further damage. On occasion this can be done by providing specific or ancillary treatments.

Elimination and control of infection

Most of the viral infections of the nervous system are not susceptible to antibiotics or chemotherapeutics. Some of the larger organisms like *Chlamydia* spp. are susceptible to the broad-spectrum antibiotics like the tetracyclines and chloramphenicol. Bacterial infections of the central nervous system are usually manifestations of a general systemic infection as either bacteremia or septicemia. Treatment of such infections is limited by the existence of the blood–brain and blood–CSF barriers which prevent penetration of some substances into nervous tissue and into the cerebrospinal fluid. Very little, if any, useful data exist on the penetration of parenterally administered antibiotics into the central nervous system of either normal farm animals or in those in which there is inflammation of the nervous system. In humans it is considered that most antibiotics do not enter the subarachnoid space in therapeutic concentrations unless inflammation is present, and the degree of penetration varies between drugs. Chloramphenicol is an exception; levels of one-third to one-half of the blood level are commonly achieved in normal individuals (11). The most promising antimicrobial agents for the treatment of bacterial meningitis in farm animals are the third-generation cephalosporins, trimethoprim–sulfonamide combinations and gentamicin (49).

The relative diffusion of Gram-negative antimicrobial agents from blood into cerebrospinal fluid in humans (11) is shown in Table 40.

In most instances of bacterial encephalitis or meningitis in farm animals it is likely that the blood–brain barrier is not intact and that parenterally administered drugs will diffuse into the nervous tissue and cerebrospinal fluid. Certainly, the dramatic beneficial response achieved by the early parenteral treatment of *Haemophilus* meningoencephalitis in cattle using a penicillin–streptomycin mixture or the broad-spectrum antibiotics suggests that the blood–brain barrier may not be a major limiting factor when inflammation is present. Another example of an antibiotic which does not pass the blood–brain barrier normally, but which is able to do so when the barrier is damaged is penicillin in the treatment of listeriosis. However, the levels of chloramphenicol required in the CSF for bactericidal activity of most Gram-negative enteric bacteria which cause meningitis in farm animals are not attainable and therefore it is not considered to be the drug of choice (49). When cases of bacterial meningoencephalitis fail to respond to antibacterial agents, to which the organisms are sensitive, other reasons should also be considered. Often the lesion is irreversibly

Table 40. Relative diffusion of Gram-negative antimicrobial agents

Excellent with or without inflammation	*Good only with inflammation*
Chloramphenicol Sulfonamides Third generation cephalosporins (Cefoperazone, Cefotaxime, Moxalactam)	Ampicillin Carbenicillin Cephalothin Cephaloridine
Minimal or not good with inflammation	***No passage with inflammation***
Tetracycline Streptomycin Kanamycin Gentamicin	Polymyxin B Colistin

advanced or there is a chronic suppurative process which is unlikely to respond.

Injection of antibacterial agents directly into the CSF is used when parenteral therapy appears to be unsuccessful. For cerebral meningoencephalitis the injections should be made into the cerebellomedullary cistern rather than the lumbosacral space. The normal flow of CSF is mostly unidirectional out of the ventricle and into the CSF spaces of the spinal cord. Some flow occurs from the caudal part of the cord to the cerebellomedullary cistern, but the flow is much slower. Thus, although the lumbar puncture is an ideal sampling route for CSF, antibiotics administered via the lumbar intrathecal space may not enter the cerebral ventricular system in therapeutic concentration. For intrathecal injection, only those antibiotic preparations which are safe for use by direct injection into the subarachnoid space should be used. Antibiotic preparations incorporated in an irritating base (i.e. propylene glycol) may cause rapid death when injected into the cerebellomedullary cistern. It may be necessary to repeat intrathecal injections daily for several days—a technique which can be very difficult to repeat successfully. This is a major disadvantage of the procedure which may restrict its use to valuable animals.

Decompression

Increased intracranial pressure probably occurs in most cases of inflammation of the brain but it is only likely to be severe enough to cause physical damage in acute cerebral edema, space-occupying lesions such as abscesses, and hypovitaminosis A. In these circumstances some treatment should be given to withdraw fluid from the brain tissue and reduce the pressure.

One treatment which may be attempted is the combination of mannitol and corticosteroids used in man and in small animals (4). Mannitol given as a 20% solution intravenously over a 30–60-minute period is a successful intracranial decompressant with an effect lasting about 4 hours which can be prolonged by the intravenous administration of dexamethazone 3 hours after the mannitol. The treatment has been used in calves with polioencephalomalacia, combined with thiamin, with excellent results to relieve the effects of acute cerebral edema. The dose rates have been those recommended for dogs and are very expensive: mannitol 2 g/kg body weight, dexamethazone 1 mg/kg body weight, both intravenously. There are dangers with mannitol: it should not be repeated often; it must not be given to an animal in shock; it should be given intravenously slowly. Dexamethazone on its own is safe and has a good effect but does not decompress sufficiently. Hypertonic glucose given intravenously is dangerous because an initial temporary decompression is followed after a 4–6-hour interval by an elevation of CSF pressure.

Central nervous system stimulants

These substances are used to excess in many instances. They exert only a transitory improvement in nervous function and are indicated only in nervous shock and after anesthesia or other short-term reversible anoxias such as cyanide or nitrate poisoning. It is unlikely that terminal respiratory failure caused by anoxia over a long period, and in which anoxia is likely to continue, will respond permanently to their use.

Central nervous system depressants

Animals with convulsions should be sedated to avoid inflicting traumatic injuries on themselves. Most of the general anesthetic agents in common use will satisfactorily control convulsions, and allow some time to properly examine the animal, and thus assess the diagnosis and institute specific therapy if possible.

REVIEW LITERATURE

Brewer, B. (1984) Therapeutic strategies involving antimicrobial treatment of the central nervous system in large animals. *J. Am. vet. med. Assoc.*, *185*, 1217.

de Lahunta, A. (1979) *Veterinary Neuroanatomy and Clinical Neurology*. Philadelphia: Saunders.

Rooney, J. R. (1971) *Clinical Neurology of the Horse*. Philadelphia: KNA Press.

REFERENCES

(1) Dungworth, D. L. & Fowler, M. E. (1966) *Cornell Vet.*, *61*, 17.
(2) Vaughn, L. C. (1964) *Vet. Rec.*, 76, 1293.
(3) Rooney, J. R. (1973) *J. Am. vet. med. Assoc.*, *162*, 117.
(4) Beech, J. (1983) *Vet. Pathol.*, *20*, 553.
(5) Mayhew, I. G. et al. (1977) *Am. J. vet. Res.*, *38*, 1271.
(6) Howard, J. R. (1969) *J. Am. vet. med. Assoc.*, *154*, 1174.
(7) Wilson, J. W. & Stevens, J. B. (1977) *J. Am. vet. med. Assoc.*, *171*, 256.
(8) Johnston, L. A. & Callow, L. L. (1963) *Aust. vet. J.*, *39*, 22.
(9) Klemm, W. R. & Hall, C. L. (1974) *J. Am. vet. med. Assoc.*, *164*, 529.
(10) Klemm, W. R. (1968) *Am. J. vet. Res.*, *29*, 1895.
(11) Rahal, J. J. (1972) *Ann. intern. Med.*, *77*, 295.
(12) Firth, E. C. (1978) *Equ. vet. J.*, *10*, 9.
(13) Sanford, S. E. & Dukes, T. W. (1978) *J. Am. vet. med. Assoc.*, *173*, 852.
(14) Witzel, D. A. et al. (1977) *J. equ. med. Surg.*, *1*, 226 & 383.
(15) Smith, J. S. & Mayhew, I. G. (1977) *Cornell Vet.*, *67*, 529.
(16) de Lahunta, A. (1978) *Cornell Vet.*, *68*, 122.
(17) Firth, E. C. (1977) *Aust. vet. J.*, *53*, 560.
(18) Miller, L. M. et al. (1985) *J. Am. vet. med. Assoc.*, *186*, 601.
(19) Beech, J. (1987) *Am. J. vet. Res.*, *48*, 109.
(20) Sheather, A. L. (1924) *J. comp. Pathol.*, *37*, 106.
(21) Clegg, F. G. et al. (1981) *Vet. Rec.*, *109*, 101.
(22) McConnon, J. M. et al. (1983) *J. Am. vet. med. Assoc.*, *182*, 812.
(23) Power, H. T. et al. (1983) *J. Am. vet. med. Assoc.*, *183*, 1076.
(24) Marshall, A. E. et al. (1981) *J. Am. vet. med. Assoc.*, *178*, 282.
(25) Adams, R. & Mayhew, I. G. (1984) *Equ. vet. J.*, *16*, 306.
(26) Oz, H. H. et al. (1986) *Can. vet. J.*, *27*, 13.
(27) Perino, L. J. et al. (1985) *Equ. Pract.*, *7(4)*, 14.
(28) Strain, G. M. et al. (1984) *J. Am. vet. med. Assoc.*, *185*, 538.
(29) Sweeney, C. R. et al. (1983) *J. Am. vet. med. Assoc.*, *183*, 126.
(30) Nurmio, P. et al. (1982) *Nord. VetMed.*, *34*, 130.
(31) Stedding-Jessen, H. (1982) *Dansk Veterinaertidsskr.*, *65*, 201.
(32) LeGonidek, G. et al. (1981) *Aust. vet. J.*, *57*, 194.
(33) Hartley, W. J. et al. (1982) *Vet. Pathol.*, *19*, 399.
(34) Greet, T. R. C. et al. (1980) *Equ. vet. J.*, *12*, 127.
(35) Guard, C. L. et al. (1984) *Cornell Vet.*, *74*, 361.
(36) Maenhout, D. et al. (1984) *Vet. Rec.*, *115*, 407.
(37) Beech, J. (1982) *J. Am. vet. med. Assoc.*, *180*, 258.
(38) Chiapetta, J. R. et al. (1985) *J. Am. vet. med. Assoc.*, *186*, 387.
(39) Badman, R. T. et al. (1981) *Aust. vet. J.*, *57*, 307.

(40) Sweeney, R. W. & Sweeney, C. R. (1984) *J. Am. vet. med. Assoc.*, *185*, 802.
(41) Duffel, S. J. et al. (1986) *Vet. Rec.*, *118*, 296.
(42) Barlow, R. M. & Greig, A. (1986) *Vet. Rec.*, *119*, 174.
(43) Martin, L. et al. (1986) *Equ. vet. J.*, *18*, 133.
(44) Ohmann, H. B. (1984) *Acta vet. Scand.*, *25*, 36.
(45) Milne, J. C. (1986) *Equ. vet. J.*, *18*, 74.
(46) Ross, M. W. et al. (1983) *Cornell Vet.*, *73*, 151.
(47) Cash, W. C. et al. (1986) *J. vet. Med.*, *A*, *33*, 491.
(48) Steiss, J. E. et al. (1986) *Can. vet. J.*, *27*, 332.
(49) Jamison, J. M. & Prescott, J. F. (1988) *Comp. Cont. Educ.*, *10*, 225.

DIFFUSE DISEASES OF THE BRAIN*

Cerebral anoxia

Cerebral anoxia occurs when the supply of oxygen to the brain is reduced for any reason. An acute or chronic syndrome develops depending on the acuteness of the deprivation. Initially there are irritation signs followed terminally by signs of loss of function.

Etiology

All forms of anoxia, including anemic, anoxic, histotoxic and stagnant forms cause some degree of cerebral anoxia but signs referable to cerebral dysfunction occur only when the anoxia is severe. The anoxia of the brain may be secondary to a general systemic anoxia or be caused by lesions restricted to the cranial cavity.

Cerebral anoxia secondary to general anoxia

- Poisoning by hydrocyanic acid or nitrite
- Acute heart failure in severe copper deficiency in cattle
- Terminally in pneumonia, congestive heart failure
- During or at birth in foals, respiratory maladjustment syndrome, or calves due to prolonged parturition (2).

Cerebral anoxia secondary to intracranial lesion

- In increased intracranial pressure
- In brain edema.

Pathogenesis

The central nervous system is extremely sensitive to anoxia, and degeneration occurs if the deprivation is extreme and prolonged for more than a few minutes. The effects of the anoxia vary with the speed of onset and with the severity (1). When the onset is sudden there is usually a transitory period during which excitation phenomena occur and this is followed by a period of loss of function. If recovery occurs a second period of excitation usually develops as function returns. In more chronic cases the excitation phase is not observed, the signs being mainly those of loss of function. These signs include dullness and lethargy when deprivation is moderate, and unconsciousness when it is severe. All forms of nervous activity are depressed but the higher centers are more susceptible than medullary centers and the pattern of development of signs may suggest this.

Clinical findings

Acute and chronic syndromes occur depending on the severity of the anoxia. Acute cerebral anoxia is manifested by a sudden onset of signs referable to paralysis of all brain functions, including flaccid paralysis and unconsciousness. Muscle tremor, beginning about the head and spreading to the trunk and limbs, followed by recumbency, clonic convulsions and death or recovery after further clonic convulsions is the most common pattern although affected animals may fall to the ground without premonitory signs. In chronic anoxia there is lethargy, dullness, ataxia, weakness, blindness and in some cases muscle tremor or convulsions. In both acute and chronic anoxia the signs of the primary disease will also be evident. Cerebral anoxia of fetal calves is thought to be a cause of weakness and failure to suck after birth, leading to the eventual death of the calf from starvation (2). Such hypoxia can occur during the birth process, especially if it is difficult or delayed, or during late pregnancy.

Clinical pathology and necropsy findings

There is no distinctive clinical pathology or characteristic necropsy lesions other than those of the primary disease. Lesions of cerebrocortical necrosis very similar to those of polioencephalomalacia develop if the hypoxia persists for a sufficient period.

Diagnosis

Clinically there is little to differentiate cerebral anoxia from hypoglycemia or polioencephalomalacia in which similar signs occur. Irritation and paralytic signs follow one another in many poisonings including lead and arsenic and in most diffuse diseases of the brain including encephalitis and encephalomalacia. The differential diagnosis of cerebral anoxia depends upon the detection of the cause of the anoxia.

Treatment

The provision of oxygen is essential and can usually only be provided by removing the causative agent. A respiratory stimulant may be advantageous in acute cases and artificial respiration may keep the animal alive for a few minutes.

REFERENCES

(1) Terlecki, S. et al. (1967) *Acta Neuropathol.*, 7, 185.
(2) Dufty, J. H. & Sloss, V. (1977) *Aust. vet. J.*, *53*, 262.

Hydrocephalus

Obstructive hydrocephalus may be congenital or acquired and is manifested in both cases by a syndrome referable to a general increase in intracranial pressure. Irritation signs of mania, head-pressing, muscle tremor and convulsions occur when the onset is rapid, and signs of paralysis including dullness, blindness and muscular weakness are present when the increased pressure develops slowly.

*In the following discussion of diseases of the brain, the terms 'irritation', 'release', 'paralysis' and 'nervous shock' are used to describe groups of signs. These terms are used in accordance with their definitions under the principles of nervous dysfunction (p. 412).

Etiology

Obstructive hydrocephalus may be congenital or acquired but in both instances it is due to defective drainage or absorption of cerebrospinal fluid. In the congenital disease there is an embryological defect in the drainage canals and foraminae between the individual ventricles or between the ventricles and the subarachnoid space, or in the absorptive mechanism, the arachnoid villi.

Congenital hydrocephalus

Causes are:

- Alone, with lateral narrowing of the mesencephalon (1)
- Inherited defects of Hereford, Holstein, Ayrshire and Jersey cattle (2)
- Inherited combined defects with chondrodysplasia, or in white Shorthorn cattle combined with hydrocephalus, microphthalmia and retinal dysplasia
- Virus infections of the fetus suggest themselves as possible causes of embryological defects in the drainage system, but there are no verified examples of this. The cavitation of brain tissue and subsequent accumulation of fluid, hydranencephaly, which occurs after infection with bluetongue virus in lambs and Akabane virus in calves, is compensatory, not obstructive
- Vitamin A deficiency may contribute
- Other occurrences, sometimes at high levels of prevalence, but without known cause (1).

Acquired hydrocephalus

Causes include:

- Hypovitaminosis A in young growing calves causing impaired absorption of fluid by the arachnoid villi (3)
- Cholesteatoma in choroid plexuses of the lateral ventricles in the horse. These may produce an acute, transient hydrocephalus on a number of occasions before the tumor reaches sufficient size to cause permanent obstruction
- Other tumor or chronic inflammatory lesion obstructing drainage from the lateral ventricles.

Pathogenesis

Increased intracranial pressure in the fetus and before the syndemoses of the skull have fused causes hydrocephalus with enlargement of the cranium. After fusion of the suture lines the skull acts as a rigid container and an increase in the volume of its contents increases intracranial pressure. Although the increase in volume of the contents may be caused by the development of a local lesion such as an abscess, tumor, hematoma, or cestode cyst, which interferes with drainage of the CSF, the more common lesion is a congenital defect of CSF drainage. Clinical and pathological hydrocephalus has been produced experimentally in animals by creating granulomatous meningitis (4). The clinical signs included depression, stiffness of gait, recumbency and opisthotonus with paddling convulsions. The general effects in all cases are the same, the only difference being that local lesions may produce localizing signs as well as signs of increased intracranial pressure. These latter signs are caused by compression atrophy of nervous tissue and ischemic anoxia due to compression of blood vessels and impairment of blood supply to the brain. In congenital hydrocephalus the signs observed are usually those of paralysis of function, while acquired hydrocephalus, being more acute, is usually manifested first by irritation phenomena followed by signs of paralysis. Edema of the optic papilla is a sign of increased intracranial pressure and may be detected ophthalmoscopically. Bradycardia occurs inconstantly and cannot be considered to be diagnostic.

Clinical findings

In acquired hydrocephalus there is, in most cases, a gradual onset of general paralysis. Initially there is depression, disinclination to move, central blindness, an expressionless stare and a lack of precision in acquired movements. A stage of somnolence follows and is most marked in horses. The animal stands with half-closed eyes, lowered head and a vacant expression and often leans against or supports itself upon some solid object. Chewing is slow, intermittent and incomplete and animals are often observed standing with food hanging from their mouths. The reaction to cutaneous stimulation is reduced, and abnormal postures are frequently adopted. Frequent stumbling, faulty placement of the feet and incoordination are evidenced when the animal moves, and circling may occur in some cases. Bradycardia and cardiac arrhythmia have been observed.

Although the emphasis is on depression and paralysis, signs of brain irritation may occur particularly in the early stages. These signs often occur in isolated episodes during which a wild expression, charging, head-pressing, circling, tremor and convulsions appear. These episodes may be separated by quite long intervals, sometimes of several weeks duration. In vitamin A deficiency in calves blindness and papilledema are the early signs and an acute convulsive stage occurs terminally.

Congenitally affected animals are usually alive at birth but are unable to stand and most die within 48 hours. The cranium is sometimes domed, the eyes protrude and nystagmus is often evident. Meningocele is an infrequent accompaniment.

Clinical pathology

Examination of the composition and pressure of the CSF will be of value. The fluid is usually normal biochemically and cytologically but the pressure is increased. A marked increase in serum muscle enzyme levels has been observed in calves with congenital hydrocephalus, due probably to an accompanying muscular dystrophy (5). Convulsions, if they occur, may contribute to this increase.

Necropsy findings

The cranium may be enlarged and soft in congenital hydrocephalus. The ventricles are distended with CSF under pressure and the overlying cerebral tissue is thinned if the pressure has been present for some time.

Diagnosis

Congenital hydrocephalus may be mistaken for vitamin A deficiency in newborn pigs, toxoplasmosis and hydranencephaly if there is no distortion of the cranium.

Acquired hydrocephalus needs to be differentiated

from other diffuse diseases of the brain, including encephalitis and encephalomalacia, and from hepatic dystrophies which resemble it very closely. In these latter diseases there may be other signs of diagnostic value, including fever in encephalitis, and jaundice in hepatic dystrophy. In most cases it is necessary to depend largely on the history and recognition of individual disease entities.

REFERENCES

(1) Barlow, R. M. & Donald, L. G. (1963) *J. comp. Pathol.*, *73*, 410.
(2) Greene, H. J. et al. (1974) *Cornell Vet.*, *64*, 596.
(3) Okamoto, M. et al. (1962) *J. dairy Sci.*, *45*, 882.
(4) Greene, H. J. et al. (1974) *Am. J. vet. Res.*, *35*, 945.
(5) Rhodes, M. B. et al. (1962) *Proc. Soc. exp. Biol., NY*, *111*, 735.

Diffuse edema of the brain

Diffuse edema of the brain always occurs acutely and causes a general increase in intracranial pressure. It is rarely a primary disease, but commonly an accompaniment of other diseases. It is commonly a transient phenomenon and may be fatal but complete recovery or recovery with residual nervous signs also occurs. It is manifested clinically by blindness, opisthotonus, muscle tremor, paralysis and clonic convulsions.

Etiology

Edema of the brain may be vasogenic, when there is increased permeability of capillary endothelium, cytotoxic when all the elements of brain tissue, glia, neurons and endothelial cells undergo swelling, or interstitial. Causes include the following.

Vasogenic edema of brain

- Brain abscess, hemorrhage, lead encephalopathy, purulent meningitis
- Minor edema occurs after most traumatic injuries, in many encephalitides and many poisonings, including propylene glycol in the horse, and probably contributes to the pathogenesis
- Accidental intracarotid injection of promazine in horses.

Cytotoxic edema of brain

- Hypoxia
- Polioencephalomalacia of ruminants
- Salt poisoning of swine.

Interstitial edema of brain

- Hydrocephalus (1).

Pathogenesis

The extracellular fluid volume in vasogenic edema is increased by the edema fluid which is a plasma filtrate containing plasma protein. In cytotoxic edema it is the cellular elements which increase in size. In hypoxia this is because of failure of the ATP-dependent sodium pump within the cells. As a result sodium accumulates within the cells and water follows to maintain osmotic equilibrium. In polioencephalomalacia and salt poisoning the edema of the brain is primary. In salt poisoning in pigs there is an increase in concentration of cations in brain tissue with a sudden passage of water into the brain to maintain osmotic equilibrium. The cause of the edema in polioencephalomalacia of ruminants, associated with a thiamin inadequacy, is unknown. When promazine is injected accidentally into the carotid artery of the horse it produces a vasogenic edema and infarction generally, but especially in the thalamus and corpora quadrigemina on the injected side (2). The vasogenic edema surrounding an abscess is localized and is not evident in the white matter.

An increase in intracranial pressure occurs suddenly and, as in hydrocephalus, there is a resulting ischemic anoxia of the brain due to compression of blood vessels and impairment of blood supply. This may not be the only factor which interferes with cerebral activity in polioencephalomalacia and salt poisoning. The clinical syndrome produced by the rapid rise in intracranial pressure is manifested by irritation phenomena followed by signs of paralysis. If the compression of the brain is severe enough and of sufficient duration ischemic necrosis of the superficial layers of the cortical gray matter may occur, resulting in permanent nervous defects in those animals which recover. Opisthotonus and nystagmus are commonly observed and are probably due to the partial herniation of the cerebellum into the foramen magnum.

Clinical findings

Although the rise of intracranial pressure in diffuse edema of the brain is usually more acute than in hydrocephalus, the development of clinical signs takes place over a period of 12–24 hours and cerebral shock does not occur. There is central blindness, and periodic attacks of abnormality occur in which opisthotonus, nystagmus, muscle tremor and convulsions are prominent. In the intervening periods the animal is dull, depressed, and blind and papilledema can be observed on ophthalmoscopic examination. The irritation signs of tremor, convulsions and opisthotonus are usually not extreme but this varies with the rapidity of onset of the edema. Because of the involvement of the brainstem in severe cases muscle weakness appears, the animal becomes ataxic, goes down and is unable to rise and the early signs persist. Clonic convulsions occur terminally and animals that survive may have residual defects of mentality and vision.

Clinical pathology

Clinicopathological observations will depend on the specific disease causing the edema.

Necropsy findings

Macroscopically the gyrae are flattened and the cerebellum is partially herniated into the foramen magnum with consequent distortion of its caudal aspect. The brain has a soft, swollen appearance and tends to sag over the edges of the cranium when the top has been removed. Posterior portions of the occipital lobes herniate ventral to the tentorium cerebelli.

Diagnosis

Diffuse brain edema causes a syndrome not unlike that of encephalitis although there are fewer irritation phenomena. Differentiation from encephalomalacia and vitamin A deficiency may be difficult if the history does not give a clue to the cause of the disease. Metabolic diseases, particularly pregnancy toxemia, hypomagnesemic tetany of calves and lactation tetany resemble it closely, as do some cases of acute ruminal impaction. In the history of each of these diseases there are distinguishing features which aid in making a tentative diagnosis. Some of the poisonings, particularly lead, organic mercurials and arsenicals and enterotoxemia caused by *Clostridium perfringens* type D produce similar nervous signs and gut edema of swine may be mistaken for diffuse cerebral edema.

Treatment

Decompression of the brain is desirable in acute edema. The treatment will depend in part on the cause; the edema associated with polioencephalomalacia will respond to early treatment with thiamin. In general terms, edema of the brain responds to parenteral treatment with hypertonic solutions and corticosteroids. Hypertonic solutions are most applicable to cytotoxic edema and corticosteroids to vasogenic edema. This is in addition to treatment for the primary cause of the disease. Mannitol at 2 g/kg body weight and dexamethazone at 1 mg/kg body weight, both intravenously, are recommended. The mannitol is given as a 20% solution intravenously and followed 3 hours later by the dexamethazone also intravenously. Diuretics usually produce tissue dehydration too slowly to be of much value in acute cases, but they may be of value as an adjunct to hypertonic solutions or in early or chronic cases. The removal of cerebrospinal fluid from the cerebellomedullary cistern (cysterna magna) in an attempt to provide relief is hazardous. In some cases the removal of 25–75 ml of CSF provides some temporary relief but the condition becomes worse later because portions of the swollen brain herniate into the foramen magnum. There is no published information available on how much fluid can be safely removed and recommendations cannot be made.

REFERENCES

(1) Fishman, R. A. (1975) *New Engl. J. Med.*, *293*, 706.
(2) Christian, R. G. et al. (1974) *Can. vet. J.*, *15*, 29.

Encephalitis

Encephalitis is, by definition, inflammation of the brain but in general usage it is taken to include those diseases in which inflammatory lesions occur in the brain, whether there is inflammation of the nervous tissue or primarily of the vessel walls. Clinically encephalitis is characterized by initial irritation signs followed by signs caused by loss of nervous function. Encephalomyelitis is included in the following description of encephalitis.

Etiology

Most animal encephalitides are caused by viruses. Causes are as follows.

All species

- Toxoplasmosis is not a common cause in any species
- Sarcocystosis
- Viral infections—rabies, pseudorabies, Japanese B encephalitis.

Cattle

- Bacterial infections including *Listeria monocytogenes*, *Haemophilus somnus*, heartwater
- Viral infections—bovine malignant catarrh, sporadic bovine encephalomyelitis, infectious bovine rhinotracheitis virus in young calves.

Sheep

- Viral infections—louping ill, scrapie, visna, an idiopathic meningoencephalitis of sheep in the United Kingdom (1).

Goats

- The viral caprine arthritis-encephalitis

Pigs

- Bacterial infections—as part of systemic infections with *Salmonella* and *Erysipelas* spp., rarely *Listeria monocytogenes*
- Viral infections—hog cholera, African swine fever, encephalomyocarditis, swine vesicular disease, vomiting and wasting disease.

Horses

- Viral infections—infectious equine encephalomyelitis, Borna disease, equine herpes virus, near eastern and west Nile equine encephalomyelitides, rarely louping ill virus
- Protozoal encephalomyelitis.

Parasitic invasion of the central nervous system is presented under the heading of traumatic injury to the brain.

Pathogenesis

With the exception of the viruses of bovine malignant catarrh and equine herpesvirus 1, which exert their effects principally on the vasculature, those viruses which cause encephalitis do so by invasion of cellular elements, usually the neurons, and cause initial stimulation and then death of the cells. Those bacteria which cause diffuse encephalitis also exert their effects primarily on vascular endothelium. *Listeria monocytogenes* does so by the formation of microabscesses.

Entrance of the viruses into the nervous tissue occurs in several ways. Normally the blood–brain barrier is an effective filtering agent but when there is damage to the endothelium infection readily occurs. The synergistic relationship between the rickettsiae of tickborne fever and the virus of louping ill probably has this basis. Entry may also occur by progression of the agent up a peripheral nerve trunk as occurs with the viruses of rabies and pseudorabies and with *L. monocytogenes*. Entry via the olfactory nerves is also possible.

The clinical signs of encephalitis are usually referable to a general stimulatory or lethal effect on neurons in the brain. This may be in part due to the general effect of inflammatory edema and partly due to the direct effects of the agent on nerve cells. In any particular case one or other of these factors may predominate but the tissue damage and therefore the signs are generalized. This is not the case in listeriosis in which damage is usually localized in the pons-medulla. Localizing signs may appear in the early stages of generalized encephalitis and remain as residual defects during the stage of convalescence. Visna is a demyelinating encephalitis, and caprine leukoencephalomyelitis is both demyelinating and inflammatory and also invades other tissues including joints and lung.

Clinical findings

Because the encephalitides are caused by infectious agents they are sometimes accompanied by fever and its attendant signs of anorexia, depression and increased heart rate. This is not the case in the very chronic diseases such as scrapie. In those diseases caused by agents which are not truly neurotropic there are characteristic signs which are not described here.

There may be an initial period of excitement or mania. The animal is easily startled and responds excessively to normal stimuli. It may exhibit viciousness and uncontrolled activity including blind charging, bellowing and pawing. Mental depression, including head-pressing, may occur between episodes. Irritations are very variable in their occurrence and may not appear at all. When they do occur they include convulsions, usually clonic and accompanied by nystagmus, champing of the jaws and excessive frothy salivation, and muscle tremor especially of the face and limbs. Unusual irritation phenomena are the paresthesia and hyperesthesia of pseudorabies and scrapie. Signs caused by loss of nervous function follow and may be the only signs in some instances. The loss of function varies in degree from paresis with knuckling at the lower limb joints, to spasticity of the limbs with resultant ataxia, to complete paralysis. More restricted pareses do occur and may be manifested by deviation of the head, walking in circles, abnormalities of posture, ataxia and incoordination but these are more commonly residual signs after recovery from the acute stages. Residual lesions affecting the cranial nerves do not commonly occur, except in listeriosis and protozoal encephalitis of horses, both infections predominating in the caudal brainstem.

Clinical pathology

Clinical pathology may be of considerable assistance in the diagnosis of encephalitis but the techniques used are for the most part specific to the individual diseases.

Necropsy findings

There are no gross lesions in most encephalitides apart from those which occur in organs other than the brain and which are typical of the specific disease. On transverse section extensive areas of necrosis may be visible. Histological lesions vary with the type and mode of action of the causative agent. Material for laboratory diagnosis should include the fixed brain and portions of fresh brain material for culture and for transmission experiments.

Diagnosis

The diagnosis of encephalitis cannot depend entirely on the recognition of the typical syndrome because similar syndromes may be caused by many other brain diseases. Acute cerebral edema and focal space-occupying lesions of the cranial cavity, a number of poisonings, including salt, lead, arsenic, mercury, rotenone and chlorinated hydrocarbons all cause similar syndromes as do hypovitaminosis A, hypoglycemia, encephalomalacia and meningitis. Fever is common in encephalitis but does not occur for example in rabies and scrapie, but it may occur in the non-inflammatory diseases if convulsions are severe. To a great extent, the clinical diagnosis rests upon the recognition of the specific encephalitides and the elimination of the other possible causes on the basis of the history and clinical pathology, especially in poisonings, and on clinical findings characteristic of the particular disease. In many cases a definite diagnosis can only be made on necropsy. For differentiation of the specific encephalitides reference should be made to the diseases listed under etiology above.

Treatment

Specific treatments are dealt with under each disease. Generally the aim should be to provide supportive treatment by intravenous or stomach tube feeding during the acute phase. Sedation during the excitement stage may prevent the animal from injuring itself, and nervous system stimulants during the period of depression may maintain life through the critical phase. Although there is an increase in intracranial pressure no attempt is usually made to relieve this because of the deleterious effects of the procedure on other affected tissues.

REFERENCE

(1) Duffel, S. J. (1984) *Vet. Rec.*, *115*, 547.

Encephalomalacia

The degenerative diseases of the brain are grouped together under the name encephalomalacia. By definition encephalomalacia means softening. Here it is used to include all degenerative changes. Leukoencephalomalacia and polioencephalomalacia refer to softening of the white and gray matter respectively. The syndrome produced is essentially one of loss of function.

Etiology

Some indication of the diversity of causes of encephalomalacia can be obtained from the examples which follow but many sporadic cases occur in which the cause cannot be defined.

All species

- Hepatic encephalopathy thought to be due to high blood levels of ammonia consequent upon severe liver damage. This is recorded in experimental pyrrolizidine alkaloid poisoning in sheep (2), in hepatic arteriovenous anomaly and thrombosis of the portal vein in the horse (1)
- Poisoning by organic mercurials and, in some instances, lead; possibly also selenium poisoning; a bilateral multifocal cerebrospinal poliomalacia of sheep in Ghana (4)
- Cerebrovascular disorders corresponding to the main categories in man are observed in animals, but their occurrence is chiefly in pigs and their clinical importance is minor
- Congenital hypomyelinogenesis and dysmyelinogenesis are recorded in lambs (hairy shakers), piglets

(myoclonia congenita) and calves (hypomyelinogenesis congenita). All are caused by viral infections *in utero*. Equine herpes virus 1 infections in horses cause ischemic infarcts
- The inherited defect of Brown Swiss cattle known as 'weavers', and discussed elsewhere, is a degenerative myeloencephalopathy (5).

Ruminants
- Plant poisons, e.g., *Astragalus* sp., *Oxytropis* sp., *Swainsona* spp., *Vicia* sp., *Kochia scoparia*
- Focal symmetrical encephalomalacia of sheep, thought to be a residual lesion after intoxication with *Clostridium perfringens* type D toxin
- Polioencephalomalacia caused by thiamin inadequacy in cattle and sheep; poliomalacia of sheep caused possibly by an antimetabolite of nicotinic acid (4)
- The abiotrophic lysosomal storage diseases—progressive ataxia of Charolais cattle, mannosidosis, gangliosidosis, globoid cell leukodystrophy of sheep
- Swayback and enzootic ataxia due to nutritional deficiency of copper in lambs
- Prolonged parturition of calves.

Horses
- Leukoencephalomalacia caused by feeding moldy corn infested with *Fusarium moniliforme*
- Nigropallidal encephalomalacia caused by feeding on yellow star thistle (*Centaurea solstitialis*)
- Poisoning by bracken and horsetail causing a conditioned deficiency of thiamin
- Ischemic encephalopathy of neonatal maladjustment syndrome of foals.

Pigs
- Leukoencephalomalacia in mulberry heart disease
- Subclinical attacks of enterotoxemia similar to edema disease (3)
- Poisoning by organic arsenicals, and salt.

Pathogenesis

The pathogenesis of leukoencephalomalacia is obscure although there is some indication that it may occur as a result of endothelial injury. Polioencephalomalacia appears to be, in some cases at least, a consequence of acute edematous swelling of the brain and cortical ischemia. The principal defect in swayback appears to be one of defective myelination probably caused by interference with phospholipid formation. However, some lesions in the newborn are more extensive, and show cavitation with loss of axons and neurons rather than simply demyelination.

Whether the lesion is in the gray matter (polioencephalomalacia) or in the white matter (leukoencephalomalacia) the syndrome is largely one of loss of function although as might be expected irritation signs are more likely to occur when the gray matter is damaged.

Clinical findings

Paralysis of varying degree is accompanied by dullness or somnolence, blindness, ataxia, head-pressing, circling and terminal coma. In the early stages, particularly in polioencephalomalacia, there are irritation signs including muscle tremor, opisthotonus, nystagmus and convulsions. The course may be one of gradual progression of signs, or more commonly a level of abnormality is reached and maintained for a long period, often necessitating sacrifice of the animal.

Clinical pathology

There are no clinicopathological tests specific for encephalomalacia but various tests may aid in the diagnosis of some of the specific diseases mentioned above under etiology.

Necropsy findings

Gross lesions including areas of softening, cavitation and laminar necrosis of the cortex may be visible. The important lesions are described under each of the specific diseases.

Diagnosis

The syndromes produced by encephalomalacia resemble very closely those caused by most lesions which elevate intracranial pressure. The onset is quite sudden and there is depression of consciousness and loss of motor function. One major difference is that the lesions tend to be non-progressive and affected animals may continue to survive in an impaired state for long periods.

Treatment

Encephalomalacia is irreversible and the best that can be hoped for is that the patient can be maintained by supportive treatment through the initial stages so that it can be fattened for slaughter.

REFERENCES

(1) Beech, J. et al. (1977) *J. Am. vet. med. Assoc.*, *170*, 164.
(2) Hooper, P. T. et al. (1974) *Res. vet. Sci.*, *16*, 216.
(3) Harding, J. D. J. (1966) *Pathol. vet.*, *3*, 83.
(4) Bonniwell, M. A. & Barlow, R. M. (1985) *Vet. Rec.*, *116*, 94.
(5) Stuart, L. D. & Leipold, H. W. (1985) *Vet. Pathol.*, *22*, 13.

Traumatic injury to the brain

The effects of trauma to the brain vary with the site and extent of the injury but initially nervous shock is likely to occur followed by death, recovery, or the persistence of residual nervous signs.

Etiology

Traumatic injury to the brain may result from direct trauma applied externally, by violent stretching or flexing of the head and neck or by migration of parasitic larvae internally. Recorded causes include the following.

- Direct trauma is an uncommon cause because of the force required to damage the cranium. Accidental collisions, rearing forwards, falling over backwards after rearing are the usual reasons
- Injury by heat in goat kids achieved with a hot iron used for debudding (2)
- Pulling back violently when tethered may cause problems at the atlanto-occipital junction
- Animals trapped in bogs, sumps, cellars, waterholes and dragged out by the head, or recumbent animals pulled onto trailers may suffer dire consequences

to the medulla and cervical cord, but the great majority of them come to surprisingly little harm

- The violent reaction of animals to lightning stroke and electrocution may cause damage to central nervous tissue, and the traumatic effect of the electrical current itself may also cause neuronal destruction
- Migration of larvae of parasitic species that normally have a somatic migration route, e.g. *Micronema deletrix* (11), *Setaria* spp. (1), *Paraelaphostrongylus tenuis* (3) in all species and *Draschia megastoma* (7) and *Strongylus vulgaris* (4) in horses
- Migration of parasitic insect larvae, *Hypoderma bovis* and *Oestrus ovis* occasionally migrate to brain and spinal cord
- Spontaneous hemorrhage into the brain is rare but can occur in cows at parturition, multiple small hemorrhages occurring in the medulla and brainstem
- Brain injury at parturition is recorded in lambs and calves (5) and foals (6, 8) and may be a significant cause of mortality in the former.

Pathogenesis

The initial reaction in severe trauma or hemorrhage is nervous shock. Slowly developing subdural hematoma, a common development in man, is accompanied by the gradual onset of signs of a space-occupying lesion of the cranial cavity but this seems to be a rare occurrence in animals (7).

If structural injury to nervous tissue does not occur there are no residual effects, but in most cases damage has been done and the residual signs vary with the site and extent of the lesion. There may be hemorrhage or a depressed fracture, both of which cause local pressure effects; there may be bruising (contusion) or damage to nerve cells without macroscopic change (concussion). In nematodiasis, traumatic destruction of nervous tissue may occur in many parts of the brain and in general the severity of the signs depends upon the size and mobility of the parasites and the route of entry. One exception to this generalization is the experimental 'visceral larva migrans' produced by *Toxocara canis* in pigs when the nervous signs occur at a time when lesions in most other organs are healing. The signs are apparently provoked by a reaction of the host to static larvae rather than trauma due to migration (9). Nematodes not resident in nervous tissues may cause nervous signs due possibly to allergy or the formation of toxins. In birth injury the lesion is principally one of hemorrhage subdurally and under the arachnoid.

Clinical findings

The syndrome usually follows the pattern of greatest severity initially with recovery occurring quickly but incompletely to a point where a residual defect is evident, this defect persisting unchanged for a long period and often permanently. This failure to improve or worsen after the initial phase is a characteristic of traumatic injury.

With severe injury there is cerebral shock in which the animal falls unconscious with or without a transient clonic convulsion. Consciousness may never be regained but in animals that recover it returns in from a few minutes up to several hours. During the period of unconsciousness, clinical examination reveals dilatation of the pupils, absence of the eye preservation and pupillary light reflexes, and a slow, irregular respiration, the irregularity being phasic in many cases. There may be evidence of bleeding from the nose and ears and palpation of the cranium may reveal a site of injury. Residual signs vary a great deal, blindness is present if the optic cortex is damaged; hemiplegia may be associated with lesions in the midbrain; traumatic epilepsy may occur with lesions in the motor cortex.

Fracture of the petrous temporal bone is a classical injury in horses caused by rearing and falling over backwards. Both the facial and the vestibular nerves are likely to be damaged so that at first the animal may be unable to stand and there may be blood from the ear and nostril of the affected side. When the animal does stand the head is rotated with damaged side down. There may be nystagmus, especially early in the course of the disease. The ear, eyelid and lip on the affected side are also paralyzed and sag. Ataxia with a tendency to fall is common. Some improvement occurs in the subsequent 2 or 3 weeks as the horse compensates for the deficit, but there is rarely permanent recovery. An identical syndrome is recorded in horses in which there has been a stress fracture of the petrous temporal bone resulting from a preexisting inflammation of the bone (12). The onset of signs is acute but unassociated with trauma.

The other common fracture is that of the *basisphenoid* and or *basioccipital bones* (10). These fractures can seriously damage the jugular vein, carotid artery and the glossopharyngeal, hypoglossal and vagus nerves. The cavernous sinus and the basilar artery may also be damaged and lead to massive hemorrhage within the cranium. Large vessels in the area are easily damaged by fragments of the fractured bones causing fatal hemorrhage. A midline fracture of the frontal bones can also have this effect.

Other signs of severe trauma to the brain include opisthotonus with blindness and nystagmus, and if the brainstem has been damaged, quadriplegia. There may also be localizing signs including head rotation, circling and falling backwards. Less common manifestations of resulting hemorrhage include bleeding into the retropharyngeal area which may cause pressure on guttural pouches and the airways and cause asphyxia. Bleeding may take place into the guttural pouches themselves.

Newborn lambs affected by birth injury to the brain are mostly dead at birth, or die soon afterwards. Surviving lambs drink poorly and are very susceptible to cold stress. In some flocks it may be the principal mechanism causing perinatal mortality.

In the horse with cerebral nematodiasis due to *Strongylus vulgaris* the clinical signs are referable to migration of the parasite in the thalamus, brainstem and cerebellum. There is incoordination, leaning and head-pressing, dysmetria, intermittent clonic convulsions, unilateral or bilateral blindness and paralyses of some cranial nerves. The onset may be gradual or sudden. The clinical diagnosis is extremely difficult because examination of cerebrospinal fluid and hematology are of limited value. A pathological diagnosis is necessary.

Clinical pathology
Cerebrospinal fluid should be sampled from the cerebellomedullary cistern and examined for evidence of red blood cells. Extreme care must be taken to ensure that blood vessels are not punctured during the sampling procedure as this would confound the interpretation of the presence of red blood cells. The presence of heme pigments in the cerebrospinal fluid suggests the presence of preexisting hemorrhage, the presence of eosinophils suggests parasitic invasion.

Necropsy findings
In most cases a gross hemorrhagic lesion will be evident but in concussion and nematodiasis the lesions may be detectable only on histological examination.

Diagnosis
Unless a history of trauma is available diagnosis may be difficult. Infestation with nematode larvae causes a great variety of signs depending on the number of invading larvae and the amount and location of the damage.

Treatment
In those animals which recover consciousness within a few hours or earlier, the prognosis is favorable and little or no specific treatment may be necessary other than nursing care. When coma lasts for more than 3–6 hours the prognosis is unfavorable and slaughter for salvage or euthanasia is recommended. Treatment for edema of the brain as previously outlined may be indicated when treatment for valuable animals is requested by the owner. Animals which are still in a coma 6–12 hours following treatment are unlikely to improve and continued treatment is not warranted.

REVIEW LITERATURE

Palmer, A. C. (1982) Concussion; the result of impact injury to the brain. *Vet. Rec.*, *111*, 575.

REFERENCES

(1) Innes, J. R. M. (1951) *Br. vet. J.*, *107*, 187.
(2) Dickson, J. (1984) *Vet. Rec.*, *114*, 387.
(3) Whitlock, J. (1959) *Cornell Vet.*, *49*, 3.
(4) Little, P. B. et al. (1974) *Am. J. vet. Res.*, *35*, 1501.
(5) Haughey, K. G. (1975) *Aust. vet. J.*, *51*, 22.
(6) Mayhew, I. G. (1982) *J. Reprod. Fertil.*, no 32, Suppl, 569–575.
(7) Mayhew, I. G. et al (1982) *J. Am. vet. med. Assoc.*, *180*, 1306.
(8) Palmer, A. C. et al. (1984) *Equ. vet. J.*, *16*, 383.
(9) Done, J. T. et al. (1960) *Res. vet. Sci.*, *1*, 133.
(10) Stick, J. A. et al. (1980) *J. Am. vet. med. Assoc.*, *176*, 228.
(11) Powers, R. D. & Benz, G. W. (1977) *J. Am. vet. med. Assoc.*, *170*, 175.
(12) Blythe, L. L. et al. (1984) *J. Am. vet. med. Assoc.*, *185*, 775.

FOCAL DISEASES OF THE BRAIN

Brain abscess

Abscesses of the brain occur most commonly in young farm animals under one year of age and only occasionally in older animals. Brain abscesses produce a variety of clinical signs depending on their location and size. Basically the syndrome produced is one of a space-occupying lesion of the cranial cavity with some motor irritation signs.

Etiology
Abscesses in the brain originate in a number of ways. Hematogenous infections are common, but direct spread from injury to the cranium or via the nasopharynx may also occur.

Hematogenous spread
The lesions may be single, but are often multiple, and are usually accompanied by meningitis. The infection usually originates elsewhere.

- *Actinobacillus mallei* from glanders lesions in lung
- *Streptococcus equi* as a complication of strangles in horses
- *Actinomyces bovis* and *Mycobacterium bovis* from visceral lesions in cattle
- *Fusobacterium necrophorum* from lesions in the oropharynx of calves
- *Pseudomonas pseudomallei* in melioidosis in sheep
- *Staphylococcus aureus* in tick pyemia of lambs
- Systemic fungal infections such as cryptococcosis may include granulomatous lesions in brain (3).

Local spread
- Via peripheral nerves from oropharynx, the one specific disease is listeriosis in all species
- Abscesses of rete mirabile of pituitary gland secondary to nasal septal infection after nose-ringing (2). Similar abscesses, usually containing *Actinomyces (Corynebacterium) pyogenes*, occur in the pituitary gland itself (4)
- Extensions from local suppurative processes in cranial signs after dehorning, from otitis media. The lesions are single, most commonly contain *A. (Corynebacterium) pyogenes* and are accompanied by meningitis.

Pathogenesis
Single abscesses cause local pressure effects on nervous tissue and may produce some signs of irritation including head-pressing and mania but the predominant effect is one of loss of function due to destruction of nerve cells. Multiple abscesses have much the same effect but whereas in single abscesses the signs usually make it possible to define the location of the lesion, multiple lesions present a confusing multiplicity of signs and variation in their severity from day to day suggesting that damage has occurred at a number of widely distributed points and at different times.

Clinical findings
General signs include mental depression, clumsiness, head-pressing and blindness, often preceded or interrupted by transient attacks of motor irritation including

excitement, uncontrolled activity and convulsions. A mild fever is usually present but the temperature may be normal. The degree of blindness varies depending on the location of the abscess and the extent of adjacent edema and meningoencephalitis. The animal may be blind in one eye and have normal eyesight in the other eye or have normal eyesight in both eyes. Unequal pupils and abnormalities in the pupillary light reflex, both direct and consensual, are common. Nystagmus is common when the lesion is near the vestibular nucleus. Localizing signs depend on the location of lesions and may include cerebellar ataxia, deviation of the head with circling and falling, hemiplegia or paralysis of individual or groups of cranial nerves often in a unilateral pattern. In the later stages there is usually papilledema.

These localizing signs may be intermittent especially in the early stages and may develop slowly or acutely (1). Alternatively there may be an acute necrotizing hemorrhagic encephalitis of the cerebral cortex appearing 4 days after the dehorning with death commonly 48 hours after clinical signs appeared. This syndrome is probably caused by *Clostridium* spp. infection of the dehorning wound (7).

In abscesses of the pituitary rete mirabile, there is depression, dysphagia and difficulty in chewing and swallowing, with resulting drooling of saliva. Characteristically the animal stands with his mouth not quite closed. There may also be ptosis and prolapse of the tongue. Blindness and absence of the pupillary light reflex are also to be expected because of pressure on the optic chiasma. Terminally there is opisthotonus, nystagmus and loss of balance, followed by recumbency (6).

Clinical pathology

Radiographic examination will not detect brain abscesses unless they are calcified or cause erosion of bone. Leukocytes, protein and bacteria may be present in the CSF and it may be possible to determine the drug sensitivity of the causative organisms.

Necropsy findings

The abscess or abscesses may be visible on gross examination and if superficial are usually accompanied by local meningitis. Large abscesses may penetrate to the ventricles and result in a diffuse ependymitis. Microabscesses may be visible only on histological examination. A general necropsy examination may reveal the primary lesion.

Diagnosis

Brain abscess is manifested by signs of irritation and loss of function which can occur in many other diseases of the brain especially when local lesions develop slowly. This occurs more frequently with tumors and parasitic cysts but it may occur in encephalitis. There may be evidence of the existence of a suppurative lesion in another organ, and a high cell count and detectable infection in the cerebrospinal fluid to support the diagnosis of abscess. Fever may or may not be present. The only specific disease in which abscess occurs is listeriosis in which the lesions are largely confined to the medulla and the characteristic signs include circling and unilateral facial paralysis. Occasional cases may be caused by fungal infections including cryptococcosis. Toxoplasmosis is an uncommon cause of granulomatous lesions in the brain of most species.

Many cases have a superficial resemblance to otitis media but there is, in the latter, rotation of the head, a commonly associated facial paralysis and an absence of signs of cerebral depression (5).

Treatment

Parenteral treatment with antibacterial drugs offers the best chance of curing the animal but the results are generally unsatisfactory because of the inaccessibility of the lesion.

REFERENCES

(1) Raphel, C. F. (1982) *J. Am. vet. med. Assoc.*, *180*, 874.
(2) Moriwaki, M. et al. (1973) *Natl Inst. anim. Hlth Q.*, *Tokyo*, *13*, 14.
(3) Teuscher, E. et al. (1984) *Zentralbl. VetMed*, *A*, *31*, 132.
(4) Moller, T. & Espersen, G. (1975) *Nord. VetMed.*, *27*, 465, 552, 627.
(5) Blood, D. C. (1960) *Can. vet. J.*, *1*, 437, 476.
(6) Perl, S. et al. (1978) *Refuah Vet.*, *35*, 175.
(7) Nation, P. B. & Calder, W. A. (1985) *Can. vet. J.*, *26*, 378.

Neoplasms of the brain

Neoplasms in the brain or meninges produce a syndrome indicative of a general increase in intracranial pressure and local destruction of nervous tissue.

Etiology

The reader is referred to references (1) and (2) for a summary of available reports on the neoplasms of the brain in animals. Subsequent reports include:

- Bovine viral leukosis with brain lesions
- Cholesteomata of horses (a chronic granulomatous lesion containing massive deposits of cholesterol and growing sufficiently slowly to cause a syndrome similar to that produced by a brain tumor (10, 11))
- Pituitary carcinomata as a series of cases (13, 14); malignant neuroblastoma of the bovine pituitary gland (19)
- A long list of individual neoplasms as single occurrences (3–9, 12, 15, 17, 18, 20, 22)
- Most nervous tissue neoplasms in animals are on peripheral nerves, and have a very low overall prevalence (16).

Pathogenesis

The development of the disease parallels that of any space-occupying lesion with the concurrent appearance of signs of increased intracranial pressure and local tissue destruction. Many lesions found incidentally at autopsy have had no clinical manifestation.

Clinical findings

The clinical picture is very similar to that produced by a slowly developing abscess and localizing signs depend on the location, size and speed of development of the tumor. Clinical signs are usually representative of increased intracranial pressure, including opisthotonus, convulsions, nystagmus, dullness, head-pressing, and hyperexcitability. Common localizing signs include circling, deviation of the head, disturbance of balance. Lesions close to the pituitary gland may cause diabetes insipidus and Cushing's syndrome (21). Cholesteomata are manifested by a standardized syndrome similar to that of a brain tumor (10). There is incoordination, intermittent convulsions, followed by paralysis and recumbency. There are often serious changes in temperament with previously placid animals becoming violent and aggressive. In others there are outbursts of frenzied activity followed by coma. The horse may be normal between attacks and these may be precipitated by moving the head rapidly.

Clinical pathology
There are no positive findings in clinicopathological examination which aid in diagnosis.

Necropsy findings
The brain should be carefully sectioned after fixation if the tumor is deep-seated.

Diagnosis
Differentiation is required from the other diseases in which space-occupying lesions of the cranial cavity occur. The rate of development is usually much slower in tumor than with the other lesions.

Treatment
Surgical removal of a tumor is unlikely to be attempted in a farm animal.

REFERENCES

(1) Innes, J. R. M. & Saunders, L. Z. (1957) *Adv. vet. Sci.*, *3*.
(2) Luginbuhl, H. (1963) *Ann. NY Acad. Sci.*, *108*, 702.
(3) Rees Evans, E. T. & Palmer, A. C. (1960) *J. comp. Pathol.*, *70*, 305.
(4) Luginbuhl, H. (1956) *Vet. Rec.*, *68*, 1032.
(5) Peterson, J. E. (1963) *J. comp. Pathol.*, *73*, 163.
(6) Palmer, A. C. & Spratling, F. R (1964) *Br. vet. J.*, *120*, 105.
(7) McGavin, M. D. (1961) *Aust. vet. J.*, *37*, 390.
(8) Kelly, D. F. & Watson, W. J. B. (1976) *Equ. vet. J.*, *8*, 110.
(9) Sullivan D. J. & Anderson, W. A. (1958) *Am. J. vet. Res.*, *19*, 848.
(10) Ooms, L. et al. (1976) *Vlaams Diergeneeskd, Tijdschr.*, *45*, 87.
(11) Ivoghli, B. et al. (1977) *Vet.Med. SAC*, *72*, 602.
(12) Summers. B. A. (1979) *Vet. Pathol.*, *16*, 132.
(13) Powers, R. D. et al. (1977) *Vet. Pathol.*, *14*, 524.
(14) Holscher, M. A. et al. (1978) *Vet. Med. SAC*, *73*, 1197.
(15) Reynolds, B. L. et al. (1979) *J. Am. vet. med. Assoc.*, *174*, 734.
(16) Hayes, H. M. et al. (1975) *Int. J. Cancer*, *15*, 39.
(17) Zeman, D. H. & Cho, D. Y. (1986) *Cornell Vet.*, *76*, 236.
(18) Saunders, G. K. (1984) *Vet. Pathol.*, *21*, 528.
(19) Haynes, J. S. & Leininger, J. R. (1984) *Vet. Pathol.*, *21*, 610.
(20) Hodgin, E. C. (1985) *Vet. Pathol.*, *22*, 420.
(21) Green, E. M. & Hunt, E. L. (1985) *Comp. cont. Educ.*, *7*, S249.
(22) Sweeney, R. W. et al. (1986) *J. Am. vet. med. Assoc.*, *189*, 555.

Coenurosis (gid, sturdy)

Coenurosis is the disease caused by invasion of the brain and spinal cord by the intermediate stage of *Taenia multiceps*. The syndrome produced is one of localized, space-occupying lesions of the central nervous system. In most countries the disease is much less common than it used to be and relatively few losses occur.

Etiology
The disease is caused by *Coenurus cerebralis* which is the intermediate stage of the tapeworm *Taenia multiceps* which inhabits the intestine of dogs and wild Canidae. The embryos, which hatch from eggs ingested in feed contaminated by the feces of infested dogs, hatch in the intestine and pass into the bloodstream. Only those embryos which lodge in the brain or spinal cord survive and continue to grow to the coenurid stage. *Coenurus cerebralis* can mature in the brain and spinal cords of sheep, goats, cattle, horses and wild ruminants and occasionally man but clinical coenurosis is primarily a disease of sheep and occasionally cattle (2). Infection in newborn calves, acquired prenatally, has been observed occasionally (3).

Pathogenesis
The early stages of migration through nervous tissue usually passes unnoticed, but in heavy infections an encephalitis may be produced (1). Most signs are caused by the mature *Coenurus* which may take 6–8 months to develop to its full size of about 5 cm. The cyst-like *Coenurus* develops gradually and causes pressure on nervous tissue resulting in its irritation and eventual destruction. It may cause sufficient pressure to rarefy and soften cranial bones.

Clinical findings
In acute outbreaks due to migration of larval stages, sheep show varying degrees of blindness, ataxia, muscle tremors, nystagmus, excitability and collapse (1). Sheep affected with the mature *Coenurus* show an acute onset of irritation phenomena including a wild expression, salivation, frenzied running and convulsions. Deviation of the eyes and head may also occur. Some animals may die in this stage but the greater proportion go on to the second stage of loss of function phenomena, the only stage in most affected animals. The most obvious sign is slowly developing partial or complete blindness in one eye. Dullness, clumsiness, head-pressing, ataxia, incomplete mastication and periodic epileptiform convulsions are the usual signs. Papilledema may be present. Localizing signs comprise chiefly deviation of the head and circling; there is rotation of the head with the blind eye down, and deviation of the head with circling in the direction of the eye blind (5). In young animals local softening of the cranium may occur over a superficial cyst and rupture of the cyst to the exterior may follow with final recovery. When the spinal cord is involved there is a gradual development of paresis and eventually inability to rise. Death usually occurs after a long course of several months.

Clinical pathology
Clinicopathological examinations are not generally used in diagnosis in animals and serologic tests are not sufficiently specific to be of value (1). Radiological examinations are helpful in defining the location of the cyst especially if there is a prospect of surgical intervention (5).

Necropsy findings
Thin-walled cysts may be present anywhere in the brain but are most commonly found on the external surface of the cerebral hemispheres. In the spinal cord the lesions are most common in the lumbar region but can be

present in the cervical area. Local pressure atrophy of nervous tissue is apparent and softening of the overlying bone may occur.

Diagnosis

The condition needs to be differentiated from other local space-occupying lesions of the cranial cavity and spinal cord including abscess, tumor and hemorrhage. In the early stages the disease may be confused with encephalitis because of the signs of brain irritation. Clinically there is little difference between them and while clinical signs and local knowledge may lead to a presumptive diagnosis, demonstration of the metacestode is essential.

Treatment and control

Surgical drainage of the cyst may make it possible to fatten the animal for slaughter (4), and surgical removal with complete recovery is possible in a majority of cases. The life cycle can be broken most satisfactorily by control of mature tapeworm infestation in dogs. Periodic treatment with a tenicide of all farm dogs is essential for control of this and other more pathogenic tapeworms. Carcasses of livestock infested with the intermediate stages should not be available to dogs.

REVIEW LITERATURE

Skerritt, G. C. & Stallbaumer, M. F. (1984) Diagnosis and treatment of coenuriasis (gid) in sheep. *Vet. Rec.*, *115*, 399.

REFERENCES

(1) Dyson, D. A. & Linklater, K. A. (1979) *Vet. Rec.*, *104*, 528.
(2) Greig, A. & Holmes, E. (1977) *Vet. Rec.*, *100*, 266.
(3) McManus, D. (1963) *Vet. Rec.*, *75*, 697.
(4) Skerritt, G. C. & Stallbaumer, M. F. (1984) *Vet. Rec.*, *115*, 399.
(5) Tirgari, M. et al. (1987) *Vet. Rec.*, *120*, 173.

Otitis media/interna

Infection of the middle ear occurs in young animals of all species, but especially pigs, and to a lesser extent calves and lambs, and rarely foals. The infection may gain entrance from the external ear, for example caused by ear mite infestation (2), but the spread is chiefly hematogenous in a young animal from an infected navel. Newborn animals are not affected and the peak of occurrence in calves and lambs is 1–4 weeks (1). The highest prevalence is in calves (3) and lambs (4) in feedlots and the disease is probably secondary to pasteurellosis.

Clinically there is rotation of the head, with the affected side down, facial paralysis may occur on the same side, and walking in circles with a tendency to fall to the affected sides. In most cases the animals are normal in other respects. At necropsy the tympanic bulla contains pus, and a variety of organisms such as staphylococci, streptococci, *Pasteurella haemolytica* and *Neisseria catarrhalis* may be isolated. Medical treatment is likely to be unsuccessful. The disease needs to be differentiated from otitis externa in which the head may be carried in a rotated position, but usually intermittently, and this is accompanied by head shaking and the presence of exudate and an offensive smell in the ear canal, and from cerebral injury or abscess, and similar lesions of the upper cervical cord. All of these are characterized by deviation of the head, not rotation.

REFERENCES

(1) McLeod, N. S. et al. (1972) *Vet. Rec.*, *91*, 360.
(2) Wilson, J. (1984) *Comp. cont. Educ.*, *6*, S179.
(3) Jensen, R. et al. (1983) *J. Am. vet. med. Assoc.*, *182*, 967.
(4) Jensen, R. et al. (1982) *J. Am. vet. med. Assoc.*, *181*, 805.

DISEASES OF THE MENINGES

Meningitis

Inflammation of the meninges occurs most commonly as a complication of a preexisting disease. It is usually caused by a bacterial infection and clinically is manifested by fever, cutaneous hyperesthesia and rigidity of muscles. Although it may affect the spinal cord or brain specifically it commonly affects both and is dealt with here as a single entity.

Etiology

Most significant meningitides are bacterial, although most viral encephalitides have some meningitic component.

Cattle

- Viral diseases—bovine malignant catarrh, sporadic bovine encephalomyelitis
- Bacterial diseases—listeriosis, *Haemophilus somnus*, rarely tuberculosis and leptospirosis.

Horses

- Strangles, *Pasteurella haemolytica* (also donkeys and mules).

Sheep

- Melioidosis, *Staphylococcus aureus* (tick pyemia) in newborn lambs
- *Pasteurella multocida* in lambs
- *Past. haemolytica* in lambs.

Pigs

- Glasser's disease, erysipelas, salmonellosis; *Streptococcus suis* type 2 in weaned and feeder pigs.

Young animals generally

Streptococcal and coliform septicemias. Probably the commonest cause of meningitis in animals is hematogenous infection deriving from omphalophlebitis of the newborn. It occurs in all species, especially calves, and may be accompanied by joint-ill, endocarditis and hypopyon. The causative bacteria are usually a mixed flora (1). Hematogenous infection occurs from other sites also (2). In neonates some of the common infections are:

- Piglet—*Str. zooepidemicus, Str. suis* type 1
- Lamb—*Str. zooepidemicus.*

Pathogenesis

Inflammation of the meninges causes local swelling, interference with blood supply to the brain and spinal cord, but as a rule penetration of the inflammation along blood vessels and into nervous tissue is of minor importance and causes only superficial encephalitis. Failure to treat meningitis caused by pyogenic bacteria often permits the development of a fatal choroiditis, with exudation into CSF, and ependymitis. There is also inflammation around the nerve trunks as they pass across the subarachnoid space. The signs produced by meningitis are thus a combination of those resulting from irritation of both central and peripheral nervous systems. In spinal meningitis there is muscular spasm with rigidity of the limbs and neck, arching of the back and hyperesthesia with pain on light touching of the skin. When the cerebral meninges are affected, irritation signs, including muscle tremor and convulsions are the common manifestations. Since meningitis is usually bacterial in origin, fever and toxemia can be expected if the lesion is sufficiently extensive.

Defects of drainage of CSF occur in both acute and chronic inflammation of the meninges and produce signs of increased intracranial pressure. The signs are general although the accumulation of fluid may be localized to particular sites such as the lateral ventriles.

Clinical findings

Acute meningitis usually develops suddenly and is accompanied by fever and toxemia in addition to nervous signs. Vomiting is common in the early stages in pigs. There is trismus, opisthotonus and rigidity of the neck and back. Motor irritation signs include tonic spasms of the muscles of the neck causing retraction of the head, muscle tremor and paddling movements. Cutaneous hyperesthesia is present in varying degrees, even light touching of the skin causing severe pain in some cases. There may be disturbance of consciousness manifested by excitement or mania in the early stages, followed by drowsiness and eventual coma. Blindness is common in cerebral meningitis but not a constant clinical finding. In young animals, ophthalmitis with hypopyon may occur, which supports the diagnosis of meningitis. The pupillary light reflex is usually much slower than normal. Examination of the fundus of the eyes may reveal evidence of optic disk edema, congestion of the retinal vessels and exudation. In uncomplicated meningitis the respiration is usually slow and deep, and often phasic in the form of Cheyne-Stokes's or Biot's breathing. Terminally there is quadriplegia and clonic convulsions.

Although meningitis in farm animals is usually diffuse, affecting particularly the brainstem and upper cervical cord, it may be quite localized and produce localizing signs including involvement of the cranial or spinal nerves. Localized muscle tremor, hyperesthesia and rigidity may result. Muscles in the affected area are firm and board-like on palpation. Anesthesia and paralysis usually develop caudal to the meningitic area. Spread of the inflammation along the cord is usual.

Reference should be made to the specific diseases cited under etiology for a more complete description of their clinical manifestations.

Clinical pathology

Cerebrospinal fluid collected aseptically under anesthesia contains elevated protein levels, has a high cell count and usually contains bacteria (1). Culture and determination of drug sensitivity of the bacteria is advisable because of the low concentrations of antibacterial drugs achieved in CSF.

Necropsy findings

Hyperemia, the presence of hemorrhages, thickening and opacity of the meninges, especially over the base of the brain, are the usual macroscopic findings. The CSF is often turbid and may contain fibrin. A local, superficial encephalitis is a common accompaniment. Additional morbid changes are described under the specific diseases and are often of importance in differential diagnosis.

Diagnosis

Hyperesthesia, severe depression, muscle rigidity and blindness are the common clinical findings in cerebral meningitis but it is often difficult to differentiate it from encephalitis and acute cerebral edema. Examination of the CSF is the only means of confirming the diagnosis before death. The total white cell count and differential may provide an indication of an infection. Subacute or chronic meningitis is difficult to recognize clinically. The clinical findings may be restricted to recumbency, apathy, anorexia, slight incoordination if forced to walk and some impairment of the eyesight. Spinal cord compression is usually more insidious in onset and is seldom accompanied by fever; hyperesthesia is less marked or absent and there is flaccidity rather than spasticity.

Treatment

The infection is usually bacterial, and parenteral treatment with antibiotics is necessary. Large doses daily for several days are required. The levels of antibiotics which are achieved in the meninges and cerebrospinal fluid following parenteral administration to farm animals are not known. Presumably, the blood–brain and blood–cerebrospinal fluid barriers are not intact in meningitis and minimum inhibitory concentrations of some drugs may be achieved. The injection of antibiotics into the cerebromedullary cistern or into the lumbosacral space has been recommended but the technique is difficult to repeat on a daily basis. Also, some antibiotics may be irritating when injected directly into the cerebromedullary cistern and may cause rapid death. If parenteral treatment with the antibiotic of choice, determined by a drug sensitivity test, does not result in a beneficial response in 3–5 days the prognosis is unfavorable.

The choice of antimicrobial agent will depend on the suspected cause of the meningitis. The common antibiotics such as penicillin and oxytetracycline are effective for the treatment of meningoencephalitis in cattle due to *Haemophilus somnus* when treatment is begun early.

Neonatal streptococcal infections also respond beneficially to penicillin when treated early before irreparable injury has occurred.

The response to therapy will depend on the causative pathogen and the severity of the inflammation present. Some cases of meningitis such as that in swine caused by *Streptococcus suis* type 2 commonly do not respond to treatment when clinical signs are obvious. Conversely, the meningoencephalitis in cattle caused by *Haemophilus somnus* will respond dramatically if treatment is begun as soon as clinical signs are apparent.

Chloramphenicol has been considered the antimicrobial drug of choice for the treatment of meningitis because it readily crosses the blood–CSF–barrier whether or not inflammation is present (1). However, the CSF concentrations necessary for bactericidal activity against most of the Gram-negative enteric bacteria which cause meningitits, particularly in neonatal animals, are not attainable (1). Therefore, because of its bacteriostatic effects it is not the drug of choice for the treatment of meningitis commonly encountered in neonatal farm animals. Furthermore, the use of chloramphenicol in food-producing animals is prohibited in some countries. Based on recent experiences in human medicine, the most promising antimicrobials for the treatment of meningitis in farm animals, particularly the neonates, may be the new third-generation cephalosporins which resist hydrolysis by beta-lactamases, have enhanced penetration into the CSF and are bactericidal at very low concentrations (1). Moxalactam and cefotaxime are used widely for the treatment of Gram-negative bacillary meningitis in man and ceftazidime is equally effective (1). Trimethoprim-sulfonamide combinations, with or without gentamicin which is synergistic with the former, are also recommended. The principles of the pharmacotherapeutics of bacterial meningitis in farm animals has been reviewed (1).

REFERENCES

(1) Jamison, J. M. & Prescott, J. F. (1988) *Comp. Cont. Educ.*, *10*, 225.
(2) Rumbaugh, G. E. (1977) *J. Am. vet. med. Assoc.*, *171*, 452.

TOXIC AND METABOLIC DISEASES OF THE NERVOUS SYSTEM

There are a very large number of poisons, especially poisonous plants and farm chemicals, and some metabolic defects which cause abnormalities of function of the nervous system. Those plants which cause degenerative nervous system disease are listed under encephalomalacia; those which cause no detectable degenerative change in tissue are listed here. So too are those which are the subject of debate. Inevitably there will be some in the wrong group, but the principal point is that there are some poisons which cause a functional encephalopathy.

A partial list of toxins and metabolic errors which cause nervous system dysfunction are as follows.

Abnormalities of consciousness and behavior

- Hypoglycemia and ketonemia of pregnancy toxemia (with degenerative lesions in some) and acetonemia
- Hypomagnesemia of lactation tetany
- High blood levels of ammonia in hepatic insufficiency
- Unspecified toxic substances in uremic animals
- Exogenous toxins including carbon tetrachloride, hexachloroethane and trichlorethylene
- Plants causing anemic and histotoxic hypoxia especially plants causing cyanide or nitrite poisoning
- Poison plants including *Helichrysum* sp., tansy mustard, male fern, kikuyu grass (or a fungus, *Myrothecium* sp. on the grass).

Abnormality characterized by tremor and ataxia

- Weeds including *Conium* sp. (hemlock), *Eupatorium* sp. (snakeroot), *Sarcostemma* sp., *Euphorbia* sp. and *Karwinskia* sp.
- Bacterial toxins in shaker foal syndrome (probably)
- Fungal toxins, e.g. *Penicillium cyclopium.*

Convulsions

- Metabolic deficits including hypoglycemia (piglets, ewes with pregnancy toxemia), hypomagnesemia (of whole milk tetany of calves, lactation tetany, cows and mares)
- Nutritional deficiencies of vitamin A (brain compression in calves and pigs), pyridoxine (experimentally in calves)
- Inorganic poisons including lead (calves), mercury (calves), farm chemicals such as organic arsenicals (pigs), organophosphates, chlorinated hydrocarbons, strychnine, urea, metaldehyde
- Bacterial toxins including *Clostridium tetani*, *Cl. perfringens* type D
- Fungal toxins, e.g. *Claviceps purpurea*, *Penicillium cyclopium* (the fungus of ryegrass staggers)
- Grasses including Wimmera ryegrass (*Lolium rigidum*) or the nematode on it; *Echinopogon ovatus*
- Pasture legumes—lupins
- Weeds—*Oenanthe* sp. (hemlock water dropwort), *Indigophera* sp. (in horses), *Cicuta* sp. (water hemlock), *Albizia tanganyinicus*, *Sarcostemma* sp. and *Euphorbia* sp.
- Trees—laburnum, oleander, supplejack (*Ventilago* sp.).

Ataxia apparently due to proprioceptive defect

- Grasses—*Phalaris tuberosa (aquatica)* (and other *Phalaris* sp.), *Lolium rigidum*, *Echinopogon ovatus*
- Weeds—*Romulea bulbocidum*, sneezeweed (*Helenium* sp.), *Indigophera* sp., Iceland poppy (*Papaver nudicaule*), *Gomphrena* sp., *Malva* sp., *Stachys* sp., *Ipomoea* sp., *Solanum esuriale*
- Trees—*Kalmia* sp., *Erythrophloeum* sp., *Eupatorium rugosum*
- Ferns—*Xanthorrhea* sp., *Zamia* sp. Induced thiamin deficiency caused by bracken and horsetail poisoning.

Involuntary spastic contraction of large muscle masses
This includes, for example, Australian stringhalt caused by *Arctotheca calendula* (flatweed).

Tremor, incoordination and convulsions
There is an additional long list of plants which cause diarrhea and nervous signs, especially ataxia, together, but whether the latter are due to the former or caused by neurotoxins is not identified.

The nervous signs include tremor, incoordination and convulsions.

Paralysis
Many of the toxic substances and metabolic defects listed above cause ataxia when their influence is mild and paralysis when it is severe. Some of the items appear in both lists. Because an agent appears in one list and not the other is not meant to suggest that it does not cause the other. It is more likely that it occurs in circumstances which are almost always conducive to the development of a mild syndrome (or a severe one as the case may be).

- Disturbance of function at neuromuscular junctions, e.g., hypocalcemia, hypomagnesemia, tetanus, botulism, possibly hypophosphatemia and hypokalemia (as in downer cows), hypoglycemia of pregnancy toxemia in cows and ewes, and tick paralysis
- Nutritional deficiency, but including only experimentally induced deficiency of nicotinic and pantothenic acids, biotin and choline, cause posterior paresis and paralysis in pigs and calves
- Toxic diseases of the nervous system including disease caused by many chemicals used in agriculture, e.g., piperazine, rotenone, 2,4-D and 2,4,5-T, organophosphates, carbamates, chlorinated hydrocarbons, propylene glycol, metaldehyde, levamisole, toluene, carbon tetrachloride, strychnine, and nicotine sulfate.

Psychoses or neuroses

Psychoses or neuroses are extremely rare in farm animals although the vices of crib-biting and weaving in horses could be included in this category.

Crib-biting and windsucking
Crib-biting is an acquired habit in which the horse grasps an object, usually the feed box or any solid projection, with the incisor teeth, then arches the neck and, by depressing the tongue and elevating the larynx, pulls upwards and backwards and swallows air emitting a loud grunt at the same time. This results in erosion of the incisor teeth, intermittent bouts of colic and flatulence. It must be distinguished from chewing wood due to boredom and from pica due to a mineral deficiency. Some horses perform similarly but do not actually seize the object with their teeth; they must just rest their teeth or their chin on it (9). *Windsucking* is the vice in which the horse flexes and arches the neck and swallows air and grunts but there is no grasping of objects. *Grasping* is the seizing of an object with the teeth but without swallowing of air.

Kicking, pawing, circling, weaving
Persistent kicking of the stall, in the absence of pruritic lesions of the lower limbs, continuous circling of a stall, pawing of the floor with a forefoot and weaving, standing at the window looking out while rocking from one forefoot to the other and swinging the head and neck to the same side, are all neurotic vices caused by boredom in active horses. The extreme case is the animal that bites itself and causes cutaneous and subcutaneous mutilation.

Farrowing hysteria
Hysteria in sows at farrowing is a common occurrence. This syndrome occurs most commonly in gilts. Affected animals are hyperactive and restless and they attack and savage their piglets as they approach the head during the initial teat sucking activity after birth. Serious and often fatal injuries result. Cannibalism is not a feature. When the syndrome occurs, the remaining piglets and freshly born piglets should be removed from the sow and placed in a warm environment until parturition is finished. The sow should then be tested to see if she will accept the piglets. If not, ataractic or neuroleptic drugs should be administered to allow initial sucking after which the sow will usually continue to accept the piglets. Azaperone (2 mg/kg) is usually satisfactory (1) and pentobarbitone sodium administered intravenously until the pedal reflex is lost has been recommended (2). Promazine derivatives are effective but subsequent incoordination may result in a higher crushing loss of piglets. The piglets' teeth should be clipped. It is generally recommended that affected gilts be culled subsequently as the syndrome may recur at subsequent farrowing. Where possible, gilts should be placed in their farrowing accommodation 4–6 days before parturition and the farrowing environment should be kept quiet at the time of parturition.

Tail-biting, ear-chewing, snout-rubbing
The incidence of cannibalism has increased with intensification of pig rearing and it is now a significant problem in many pig-rearing enterprises (3, 4). Tail-biting is the most common and occurs in groups of pigs, especially males, from weaning to market age. Ear-chewing is less common and is generally restricted to pigs in the immediate postweaning and early growing period although both syndromes may occur concurrently. The incidence of ear-chewing has increased with the practice of docking piglet tails at birth (3). Tail-biting usually begins with one or two pigs sucking or chewing the tails of pen-mates. Initially the practice causes no resentment but as the tail becomes raw and eroded, pain is shown. Rarely, if the offending agonists are removed at this stage, the problem will not progress. Generally the raw eroded tail becomes attractive to other individuals within the group and the vice spreads within the group to involve the majority of pigs. Most of the tail may eventually be removed, leaving a raw bleeding stump. Productivity is affected by severe lesions and sequelae such as spinal abscessation with paralysis and abscessation or pyemia with partial or total carcass condemnation are not uncommon (4).

Ear-biting occurs in similar fashion. The lesions are

usually bilateral and most commonly involve the ventral part of the ear. Lesions from bite wounds may also occur on the flanks of pigs. There is frequently an association with mange infestation with both of these vices.

A syndrome of snout-rubbing to produce eroded necrotic areas on the flanks of pigs has been described (5). Affected pigs were invariably colored although both white and colored pigs acted as agonists.

The causes of these forms of cannibalism in pigs are poorly understood but they are undoubtedly related to an inadequate total environment. Affected groups are usually more restless and have a heightened activity. Factors such as a high population density, both in terms of high pen density and large group size, limited food and competition for food, low protein and inadequate nutrition, boredom, and inadequate environment in terms of temperature, draft and ventilation have been incriminated in precipitating the onset of these vices (3, 4, 6–8).

When a problem is encountered each of these factors should be examined and corrected or changed if necessary. Prevention is through the same measures. Chains or tires are frequently hung for displacement activity but are not particularly effective.

The problem may recur despite all attempts at prevention. Also for economic reasons it is not always possible to implement the radical changes in housing and management that may be necessary to avoid the occurrence of these vices. Because of this, the practice of tipping or docking the piglets' tails at birth has become common as a method of circumventing the major manifestation of cannibalism.

Idiopathic epilepsy

This appears to be very rare in farm animals. It is recorded as an inherited condition in Brown Swiss cattle. Residual lesions after encephalitis may cause symptomatic epileptiform seizures but there are usually other localizing signs. A generalized seizure is manifested by an initial period of alertness, the counterpart of the aura in human seizures, followed by falling in a state of tetany which gives way after a few seconds to a clonic convulsion with paddling, opisthotonus and champing of the jaws. The clonic convulsions may last for some minutes and are followed by a period of relaxation. The animal is unconscious throughout the seizure, but appears normal shortly afterwards. Some seizures may be preceded by a local motor phenomenon such as tetany or tremor of one limb or of the face. The convulsion may spread from this initial area to the rest of the body. This form is referred to as Jacksonian epilepsy and the local sign may indicate the whereabouts of the local lesion or point of excitation. Such signs are recorded very rarely in dogs and not at all in agricultural animals. The seizures are recurrent and the animal is normal in the intervening periods.

REVIEW LITERATURE

Henry, J. P. (1976) Mechanisms of psychosomatic disease in animals. *Adv. vet. Sci.*, *20*, 115.

REFERENCES

(1) Symoens, J. & Gestel, J. V. (1972) *Tierarztl. Umschau*, *27*, 170.
(2) Lewis, C. J. & Oakley, G. A. (1970) *Vet. Rec.*, *87*, 616.
(3) Penny, R. H. C. & Mullen, P. A. (1976) *Vet. Ann.*, *16*, 103.
(4) Penny, R. H. C. & Hill, F. W. G. (1974) *Vet. Rec.*, *94*, 174.
(5) Allison, C. J. (1976) *Vet. Rec.*, *98*, 254.
(6) Jericho, K. W. F. & Church, T. L. (1972) *Can. vet. J.*, *13*, 156.
(7) Anon. (1974) *Vet. Rec.*, *95*, 123.
(8) Putten, G. (1969) *Br. vet. J.*, *125*, 511.
(9) Owen, R. R. (1982) *Vet. Ann.*, *22*, 159.

DISEASES OF THE SPINAL CORD

Traumatic injury

Sudden severe trauma to the spinal cord causes a syndrome of immediate, complete, flaccid paralysis caudal to the injury because of spinal shock. This is so brief in animals as to be hardly recognizable clinically. It is soon followed by flaccid paralysis in the area supplied by the injured segment and spastic paralysis caudal to it.

Etiology

Most cases of traumatic injury to the cord arise because of external injury. Some are caused by invasion by parasitic elements. Concussion and contusion can occur without structural damage to bones.

External trauma

- Falling off vehicles, through barn floors
- Osteoporotic or osteodystrophic animals, especially aged brood mares and sows, spontaneously while jumping or leaning on fences
- Spondylosis and fracture in old bulls in insemination centers
- Trauma due to excessive mobility of upper cervical vertebrae may contribute to the spinal cord lesion in wobbles in horses
- Dislocations of the atlanto-occipital joint are being reported increasingly (6, 7)
- Stenosis of the cervical vertebral canal at C2–C4 in young rams probably as a result of head-butting (2)
- Fracture of T1 vertebra in calves turning violently in an alleyway wide enough to admit cows (9)
- Lightning strike may cause tissue destruction within the vertebral canal.

Parasitic invasion

- Cerebrospinal nematodiasis, e.g., *Paraelaphostrongylus tenuis*, *Setaria* sp. in goats and sheep, *Stephanurus dentatus* in pigs. *P. tenuis* in moose causing moose sickness
- *Toxocara canis* experimentally in pigs (4)
- *Strongylus vulgaris* in horses and donkeys
- *Hypoderma bovis* larvae in cattle.

Local ischaemia of the spinal cord

Obstruction to blood flow to the cord by embolism, or of drainage by compression of the caudal vena cava, for example, in horses during prolonged dorsal recumbency under general anesthesia (11, 13), in pigs due to fibrocartilaginous emboli, probably originating in injury to the nucleus pulposus of an intervertebral disk (12).

Pathogenesis
The lesion may consist of disruption of nervous tissue or its compression by displaced bone or hematoma. Minor degrees of damage may result in local edema or hyperemia, or in the absence of macroscopic lesions, transitory injury to nerve cells classified as concussion. The initial response is that of spinal shock which affects a variable number of segments on both sides of the injured segment, and is manifested by complete flaccid paralysis. The lesion must affect at least the ventral third of the cord before spinal shock occurs. When the shock wears off the effects of the residual lesion remain. These may be temporary in themselves and completely normal function may return as the edema or the hemorrhage is resorbed. In man, if structural damage persists, there is usually hyperesthesia in the area of the lesion, flaccid paralysis in the same general area and spastic paralysis caudally. Whether the same pattern holds for animals, especially ruminants, is open to doubt. In sheep extensive experimental damage to the cord may be followed by recovery to the point of being able to walk (5), but not sufficiently to be of any practical significance.

Traumatic lesions usually affect the whole cross-section of the cord and produce a syndrome typical of complete transection. Partial transection signs are more common in slowly developing lesions.

Clinical findings
Spinal shock develops immediately after severe injury and is manifested by flaccid paralysis to a variable degree up and down the cord. There is a concurrent fall in local blood pressure due to vasodilatation and there may be local sweating. Stretch and flexor reflexes and cutaneous sensitivity disappear but reappear within a half to several hours, although hypotonia may remain. The extremities are affected in most cases and the animal is unable to rise and may be in sternal or lateral recumbency. The muscles of respiration may also be affected resulting in interference with respiration. The body area supplied by the affected segments will eventually show flaccid paralysis, disappearance of reflexes and muscle wasting—a lower motor neurone lesion.

When the condition is caused by invasion by parasitic larvae there is no stage of spinal shock but the onset is acute although there may be subsequent increments of paralysis as the larvae moves to a new site (10).

Fracture of the cervical vertebra—horse
In horses fracture/dislocation of anterior cervical vertebrae occurs fairly commonly (6, 7). Affected animals are recumbent and unable to lift the head from the ground. However, they may be fully conscious and be able to eat and drink. It may be possible to palpate the lesion, but a radiograph is usually necessary. Lesions of the lower cervical vertebrae may permit lifting of the head, but the legs are not moved voluntarily. In all cases the tendon and withdrawal reflexes in the limbs are normal to supernormal.

Spondylosis in bulls
Old bulls in artificial insemination centers develop calcification of the ventral vertebral ligaments and subsequent spondylosis or rigidity of the lumbar area of the backbone. When the bull ejaculates vigorously the calcified ligaments may fracture and this discontinuity may extend upward through the vertebral body. The ossification is extensive, usually from about T2 to L3, but the fractures are restricted to the midlumbar region. There is partial displacement of the vertebral canal and compression of the cord. The bull is usually recumbent immediately after the fracture occurs but may rise and walk stiffly several days later. Arching of the back, slow movement, trunk rigidity and sometimes unilateral lameness are characteristic signs. Less severe degrees of spondylosis have been recorded in a high proportion of much younger (2–3 years) bulls, but the lesions do not appear to cause clinical signs (1).

Sensation may be reduced at and caudal to the lesion and hyperesthesia may be observed in a girdle-like zone at the cranial edge of the lesion due to irritation of sensory fibers by local inflammation and edema. Because of interference with the sacral autonomic nerve outflow there may be paralysis of the bladder and rectum although this is not usually apparent in large animals. The vertebral column should be examined carefully for signs of injury. Excessive mobility, pain on pressure, and malalignment of spinous processes may indicate bone displacements or fractures. Rectal examination may also reveal damage or displacement particularly in fractures of vertebral bodies and in old bulls with spondylosis. Residual signs may remain when the shock passes off. This usually consists of paralysis which varies in extent and severity with the lesion. The paralysis is apparent caudal to and at the site of the lesion. The reflexes return except at the site of the lesion. There is usually no systemic disturbance but pain may be sufficiently severe to cause an increase in heart rate and prevent eating.

Recovery may occur in 1–3 weeks if nervous tissue is not destroyed but when extensive damage has been done to a significantly large section of the cord there is no recovery and disposal is advisable. In rare cases animals which suffer a severe injury continue to be ambulatory for up to 12 hours before paralysis occurs. In such instances it may be that a fracture occurs but displacement follows at a later stage during more active movement. Recovered animals may be left with residual nervous deficits or with structural changes such as torticollis (8).

Clinical pathology
Radiological examination may reveal the site and extent of the injury. Cerebrospinal fluid obtained from the lumbosacral space may reveal the presence of red blood cells suggesting pre-existing hemorrhage.

Necropsy findings
The abnormality is always visible on macroscopic examination.

Diagnosis
Differentiation from other spinal cord diseases is not usually difficult because of the speed of onset and the history of trauma, although spinal myelitis and meningitis

may also develop rapidly. Other causes of recumbency may be confused with trauma especially if the animal is not observed in the immediate preclinical period. In most diseases characterized by recumbency, such as azoturia, acute rumen impaction and acute coliform mastitis there are other signs to indicate the existence of a lesion other than spinal cord trauma. White muscle disease in foals is a confusing syndrome and unless tests for muscle enzymes are carried out on serum the diagnosis may be missed.

Treatment

Treatment is expectant only, surgical treatment rarely being attempted. Careful nursing on deep bedding with turning at 3-hourly intervals, massage of bony prominences and periodic slinging may help to carry an animal with concussion or other minor lesion through a long period of recumbency. In cattle especially, recumbency beyond a period of about 48 hours is likely to result in widespread necrosis of the posterior muscles of the thigh and recovery in such cases is improbable.

REFERENCES

(1) Bane, A. & Hansen H. I. (1962) *Cornell Vet.*, *52*, 362.
(2) Jackson, P. G. G. & Palmer, A. C. (1983) *Vet. Rec.*, *112*, 65.
(3) Zink, M. C. (1985) *Can. vet. J.*, *26*, 275.
(4) Done. J. T. et al. (1960) *Res. vet. Sci.*, *1*, 133.
(5) Tietz, W. J. (1964) *Am. J. vet. Res.*, *25*, 1500.
(6) Owen, R. R. & Maxie, L. L. S. (1978) *J. Am. vet. med. Assoc.*, *173*, 854.
(7) White, M. E. et al. (1978) *Can. vet. J.*, *19*, 79.
(8) McKelvey, W. A. C. & Owen, R. R. (1979) *J. Am. vet. med. Assoc.*, *175*, 295.
(9) Anderson, B. C. (1982) *Vet. Med. SAC*, *77*, 1254.
(10) Mayhew, I. G. et al. (1984) *Cornell Vet.*, *74*, 30.
(11) Blakemore, W. F. et al. (1984) *Vet. Rec.*, *114*, 569.
(12) Tessaro, S. V. et al. (1983) *Can. J. comp. Med.*, *47*, 124.

Spinal cord compression

The gradual development of a space-occupying lesion in the vertebral canal produces a syndrome of progressive paralysis.

Etiology

Compression of the spinal cord occurs from space-occupying lesions in the vertebral canal, the common ones being as follows.

Tumors

- Bovine viral leukosis is the only one which occurs more than very rarely
- Rare tumors include fibrosarcomas, metastases (1), plasma cell myeloma (2), angioma (3), melanoma (10), neurofibroma (19) and lymphosarcoma, e.g. in horses (22).

Abscess

- Hematogenous spread from actinomycosis in cattle, *Corynebacterium pseudotuberculosis* in sheep, and *Actinomyces (Corynebacterium) pyogenes* generally
- Young animals from infected navels in calves, docking wounds in lambs, bite wounds in pigs (4), pneumonia in calves (5); compression is caused by a vertebral body abscess and there may or may not be deviation of the vertebral canal and its contents (5, 15). The original site of infection may have long since disappeared when the clinical signs referable to the spinal cord abscess appear (5)
- Spinal cord abscesses usually originate from vertebral osteomyelitis, e.g. in severe brucellosis, and are associated with local meningitis
- Spinal cord abscesses not associated with vertebral bodies also occur in lambs (6).

Bony lesions

- Exostoses over fractures with no displacement of vertebral bodies
- Similar exostoses on vertebral bodies of lambs grazing around old lead mines
- Hypovitaminosis A in young growing pigs causing crowding of vertebral canal
- Congenital deformity or fusion of the atlanto-occipital-axial joints in calves, foals and goats (see congenital defects, p. 447)
- Rarely there is protrusion of an intervertebral disc, identifiable by myelogram (21, 26), and progressive paresis and ataxia also occur rarely in diskospondylitis in horses (24). Cervical pain is a more common sign in the latter. The degenerative lesions in disks in the neck of the horse resemble the Hansen type 2 disk prolapses in dogs (25)
- Adult sows and boars may have degeneration of intervertebral disks and surrounding vertebral osteophytes. Less commonly ankylosing spondylosis, arthrosis of articular facets, defects in annulus fibrosus and vertebral end plates, and vertebral osteomyelitis or fracture (12). These lesions of diskospondylitis cause lameness in boars and sows rather than compression of cord and paresis/paralysis (16). These are not to be confused with the many extravertebral causes of posterior lameness or paralysis in adult pigs, which are discussed in Chapter 13 on the musculoskeletal system.

Ataxia in horses

This is a major problem and is dealt with more extensively under the heading of enzootic incoordination of horses. For purposes of comparison the diseases involved (11) are listed here.

- Non-fatal fractures of the skull (basisphenoid, basioccipital, and petrous temporal bones)
- Non-fatal cervical fractures
- Atlanto-occipital instability
- Stenosis of cranial vertebral orifice of C3–C7; this may be effective as a compression mechanism only if the vertebrae adopt exaggerated positions
- Abnormal growth of interarticular surfaces
- Dorsal enlargement of caudal vertebral epiphyses and bulging of intervertebral disks
- Formation and protrusion of false joint capsules and extrasynovial bursae
- Spinal myelitis due to parasitic invasion or equine herpes virus 1 virus, even louping-ill virus and probably others
- Spinal abscess usually in a vertebral body
- Cerebellar hypoplasia—most commonly the inherited version in Arabian foals

- Degenerative myelomalacia/myelopathy—cause unknown
- Fusion of occipital bone with the atlas, which is fused with the axis
- Thromboembolic ischemic myeloencephalopathy (as in iliac thrombosis) which appears during exercise
- Tumors of the meninges.

Pathogenesis

The development of any of the lesions listed above results in the gradual appearance of motor paralysis or hypoesthesia depending on whether the lesion is ventrally or dorsally situated. In most cases there is involvement of all tracts but care is necessary in examination if the more bizarre lesions are to be accurately diagnosed. There may be hemiparesis or hemiplegia if the lesion is laterally situated. Paraparesis or paraplegia is caused by a bilateral lesion in the thoracic or lumbar cord and monoplegia by a unilateral lesion in the same area. Bilateral lesions in the cervical region cause tetraparesis to tetraplegia (quadriplegia).

Clinical findings

Pain and hyperesthesia may be evident before motor paralysis appears. The pain may be constant or occur only with movement. In most cases the motor paralysis gets gradually worse as the tumor enlarges. However, a sudden onset of signs often occurs even though growth of the lesion is slow. Difficulty in rising is the first sign, then unsteadiness during walking due to weakness which may be more marked in one of a pair of limbs. The toes are dragged along the ground while walking and the animal knuckles over on the fetlocks when standing. Finally the animal can rise only with assistance and then becomes permanently recumbent. These stages may be passed through in a period of 4–5 days. The paralysis will be flaccid or spastic depending on the site of the lesion and reflexes will be absent or exaggerated in the respective states.

Considerable variation in signs occurs depending on the site of the lesion. There may be local hyperesthesia around the site of the lesion and straining to defecate may be pronounced. Retention of the urine and feces may occur. There is usually no detectable abnormality of the vertebrae on physical examination.

Clinical pathology

Radiographic examination of the vertebral column should be carried out if the animal is of a suitable size. The cerebrospinal fluid may show a cellular reaction if there is some invasion of the spinal canal.

Necropsy findings

The abnormality is usually visible.

Diagnosis

Differentiation between abscess, tumor and exostosis in the vertebral canal is usually not practicable without radiographic examination. In lymphomatosis of cattle there may be signs caused by lesions in other organs. A history of previous trauma may suggest exostosis. The history usually serves to differentiate the lesion from acute trauma. Spinal myelitis, myelomalacia and meningitis may resemble cord compression but are much less common. They are usually associated with encephalitis, encephalomalacia and cerebral meningitis respectively. Meningitis is characterized by much more severe hyperesthesia and muscle rigidity. Rabies in the dumb form may be characterized by a similar syndrome but ascends the cord and is fatal within a 6-day period. In the newborn there are many congenital defects in which there is defective development of the spinal cord. Most of them are not characterized by compression of the cord, the diminished function being caused in most cases by an absence of tissue. Spina bifida, syringomyelia and dysraphism are characterized by hindquarter paralysis or, if the animal is able to stand, by a wide-based stance and overextension of the legs when walking. Some animals are clinically normal (13, 14).

A generalized degeneration of peripheral nerves such as that described in pigs (7) and cattle (9) causes a similar clinical syndrome; so does polyradiculoneuritis (8). A non-suppurative ependymitis, meningitis and encephalomyelitis, such as occurs in equine infectious anemia (20), may also cause an ataxia syndrome in horses.

The subject of back pain, and its relationship to lameness, is a very important one in horses. There is often a lesion in the vertebral canal and by pressing on the cord or peripheral nerves it causes gait abnormalities which suggest the presence of pain, or they actually cause pain. Spondylosis, injury to dorsal spinous processes, and sprain of back muscles are common causes of the same pattern of signs. Because these problems are largely orthopedic ones, and therefore surgical, their exposition is left to other authorities (9, 17, 18). Also it is necessary in horses to differentiate spinal cord lesions from acute nutritional myodystrophy, and subacute tying-up syndrome. Those diseases are characterized by high serum CPK and SGOT levels.

Treatment

Successful treatment of partially collapsed lumbar vertebra by dorsal laminectomy has been performed in a calf (23) and in horses (27), but in farm animals treatment is usually not possible and in most cases it is advisable to sacrifice the animal for meat.

REVIEW LITERATURE

Jeffcott, L. B. & Dalin, G. (1983) Bibliography of thoracolumbar conditions in the horse. *Equ. vet. J.*, *15*, 155–157.

REFERENCES

(1) Reinertson, E. L. (1974) *Cornell Vet.*, *64*, 617.
(2) Drew, R. A. & Greatorex, J. C. (1974) *Equ. vet. J.*, *6*, 131.
(3) Palmer, A. C. & Hickman, J. (1960) *Vet. Rec.*, *72*, 611.
(4) Finley, G. C. (1975) *Can. vet. J.*, *16*, 114.
(5) Sherman, D. M. & Amos, T. R. (1986) *J. Am. vet. med. Assoc.*, *188*, 608.
(6) Dodd, D. C. & Cordes, D. O. (1964) *NZ vet. J.*, *12*,1.
(7) Higgins, R. J. et al. (1983) *Acta Neuropathol.*, *54*, 288.
(8) MacLachlan, N. J. et al. (1982) *J. Am. vet. med. Assoc.*, *180*, 166.
(9) Rousseaux, C. G. et al. (1983) *Can. vet. J.*, *24*, 296.
(10) Traver, D. S. et al. (1970) *Am. vet. med. Assoc.*, *170*, 1400.
(11) Whitwell, K. E. (1980) *Vet Rec. In Practice*, *2(4)*, 17.

(12) Doige, C. E. (1979) *Can. J. comp. Med.*, *43*, 142.
(13) Cho, D. Y. & Leipold, H. W. (1977) *Zentralbl. VetMed.*, *24A*, 680.
(14) Cho, D. Y. & Leipold, H. W. (1977) *Equ. vet. J.*, *9*, 195.
(15) Markel, M. D. et al. (1986) *J. Am. vet. med. Assoc.*, *188*, 632.
(16) Doige, C. E. (1980) *Can. J. comp. Med.*, *44*, 121 & 382.
(17) Jeffcott, L. B. & Dalin, G. (1980) *Equ. vet. J.*, *12*, 101.
(18) Koch, D. B. (1980) *Calif. vet.*, *34*, 28.
(19) Helfer, D. H. & Stevens, D. R. (1978) *Vet. Pathol.*, *15*, 784.
(20) McClure, J. J. et al. (1982) *J. Am. vet. med. Assoc.*, *180*, 279.
(21) Nixon, A. J. et al. (1984) *Vet. Surg.*, *13*, 154.
(22) Shamish, L. D. (1984) *J. Am. vet. med. Assoc.*, *184*, 1517.
(23) Smith, K. D. & Miller, C. (1984) *J. Am. vet. med. Assoc.*, *184*, 1508.
(24) Adams, B. A. et al. (1985) *J. Am. vet. med. Assoc.*, *186*, 270.
(25) Yovich, J. V. et al. (1985) *Am. J. vet. Res.*, *46*, 2372.
(26) Foss, R. R. et al. (1983) *Can. vet. J.*, *24*,188.
(27) Grant, B. D. et al. (1985) *Equ. Pract.*, *7*, 19.

Myelitis

Inflammation of the spinal cord is usually associated with viral encephalitis. The signs are referable to the loss of function although there may be signs of irritation. For example hyperesthesia or paresthesia may result if the dorsal nerve nuclei are involved. This is particularly noticeable in pseudorabies and to a lesser extent in rabies. Paralysis is the more usual result. There are no specific myelitides in animals. Listeriosis is sometimes confined in its lesion distribution to the spinal cord in sheep. Viral myelitis caused by equine herpes virus 1 (the equine rhinopneumonitis virus) is now commonplace and equine infectious anemia and dourine include incoordination and paresis in their syndromes. In goats, caprine arthritis encephalitis is principally a myelitis, involving mostly the white matter. Protozoal encephalomyelitis of horses causes serious lesions in the spinal cord and is included in the group of diseases causing 'wobbles'. Myelitis resembles myelomalacia and space-occupying lesions of the vertebral canal. A rather more topographically specific entity than most is neuritis of the cauda equina discussed elsewhere.

Myelomalacia

Myelomalacia occurs rarely as an entity separate from encephalomalacia. One recorded occurrence is focal spinal poliomalacia of sheep and in enzootic ataxia the lesions of degeneration are often restricted to the spinal cord. In both instances there is a gradual development of paralysis without signs of irritation and with no indication of brain involvement. Progressive paresis in young goats may be caused by the virus of caprine arthritis encephalitis, and other unidentified, possibly inherited causes of myelomalacia (2). Degeneration of spinal cord tracts has also been recorded in poisoning by *Phalaris aquatica* in cattle and sheep, and sorghum in horses, by 3-nitro-4-hydroxyphenylarsonic acid in pigs (9), and by selenium in ruminants; the lesion is a symmetrical spinal poliomalacia. Poisoning of cattle by plants of *Zamia* spp. produces a syndrome suggestive of injury to the spinal cord but no lesions have been reported. Pantothenic acid or pyridoxine deficiencies also cause degeneration of spinal cord tract in swine. A disease of obscure etiology in sheep with spinal cord degeneration is Murrurrundi disease. A spinal myelinopathy, possibly of genetic origin is recorded in Murray Grey calves (8). Affected animals develop ataxia of the hindlegs, swaying of the hindquarters and collapse of one hindleg with falling to one side. Clinical signs become worse over an extended period.

Sporadic cases of degeneration of spinal tracts have been observed in pigs. One outbreak is recorded in the litters of sows on lush clover pasture (1). The piglets were unable to stand, struggled violently on their sides with rigid extension of the limbs and although able to drink usually died of starvation. Several other outbreaks in pigs have been attributed to selenium poisoning (7).

A degenerative myeloencephalopathy of unknown etiology of young horses is recorded also in the United States (3). The major clinical signs are referable to bilateral leukomyelopathy involving the cervical spinal cord. There is abnormal positioning and decreased strength and spasticity of the limbs as a result of upper motor neuron and general proprioceptive tract lesions. Hypalgesia, hypotonia, hyporeflexia, muscle atrophy or vestibular signs are not present and there is no evidence of cranial nerve, cerebral or cerebellar involvement clinically. Abnormal gait and posture are evident usually initially in the pelvic but eventually also in the thoracic limbs. There are no gross lesions but histologically there is degeneration of neuronal processes in the white matter of all spinal cord funiculi, especially the dorsal spinocerebellar and sulcomarginal tracts. The lesion is most severe in the thoracic segments. The disease is progressive and there is no known treatment.

Sporadic cases of spinal cord damage in horses include spontaneous hemorrhage during surgery (4), a hemorrhagic infarct assumed due to cartilage emboli (5), and a venous malformation causing tissue destruction (6). The disease requires to be differentiated from myelitis and spinal cord compression caused by space-occupying lesions of the vertebral canal, and cervical, vertebral malformation/malarticulation.

REFERENCES

(1) McClymont, G. L. (1954) *Aust. vet. J.*, *30* , 345.
(2) Lancaster, M. J. et al. (1987) *Aust. vet. J.*, *64*, 123.
(3) Mayhew, I. G. et al. (1977) *J. Am. vet. med. Assoc.*, *170*, 195.
(4) Schatzmann, U. et al. (1979) *Schweiz. Arch. Tierheilkd.*, *121*, 149.
(5) Taylor, W. H. et al. (1977) *Vet. Pathol.*, *14*, 479.
(6) Gilmour, J. S. & Fraser, J. A. (1977) *Equ. vet. J.*, *9*, 40.
(7) Harrison, L. H. et al. (1983) *Vet. Pathol.*, *20*, 265.
(8) Richards, R. B. & Edwards, J. R. (1986) *Vet. Pathol.*, *23*, 35.
(9) Kennedy, S. et al. (1986) *Vet. Pathol.*, *23*, 454.

Spinal meningitis

Spinal meningitis is usually an accompaniment of cerebral meningitis and when it does occur locally in association with spinal cord abscess it produces paraplegia, or severe incoordination, local hyperesthesia and rigidity characteristic of meningitis. The commonest occurrence is in lambs after infection of docking wounds. The treatment is as for cerebral meningitis.

CONGENITAL DEFECTS OF THE CENTRAL NERVOUS SYSTEM

Developmental defects of the central nervous system

The pathogenesis of congenital defects, including those of the central nervous system, has been dealt with in general terms in Chapter 3 on diseases of the newborn. Inheritance, nutrition, virus infection in early pregnancy and some toxins can all play a part in the genesis of these defects and the purpose of this section is to guide the diagnostician through the recognition of the defect to the possible causes. However, there are many such cases which occur sporadically but for which no specific cause can be identified.

Although most developmental defects are present at birth there are a few which appear later in life, especially the abiotrophic diseases in which an essential metabolic process, essential that is for cellular structure and function, is missing and the tissue undergoes degeneration.

The diseases to be identified are listed under the headings of the principal clinical signs and syndromes which they produce. Many affected neonates are weak and either die during birth or soon afterwards so that they tend to be diagnoses for pathologists rather than clinicians. There may be an unintentional bias towards more clinically conspicuous diseases in the following material. Checklists of familial and inherited diseases of the CNS of pigs (9), lambs (13) and all species (10) are available.

Defects with obvious structural errors

- Hydrocephalus, sporadic or inherited, with obvious enlargement of the cranium
- Meningocele with protrusion of a fluid-filled sac through the open fontanelle in the cranial vault. The defect is inherited in some pigs
- Hydrocephalus with spina bifida combination—the Arnold–Chiari syndrome—in cattle (17)
- Hydrocephalus with congenital achondroplasia (bulldog calf syndrome)
- Cranium bifidum (may include meningocele) of pigs
- Microphthalmia. In microcephaly the cranium is usually of normal size
- Some cases of failure of closure of neural tube, e.g. spina bifida. There is a defect in the skin and dorsal arch of the vertebra in the lumbosacral area in some cases
- Exophthalmos with or without strabismus, an inherited form in Jersey and Shorthorn cattle does not appear until the animal is more than 6 months of age
- Neurofibromas occur as enlargements on peripheral nerves and are seen as subcutaneous swellings. They are passed from cow to calf (7)
- Hydranencephaly, porencephaly and other structural defects due to intrauterine infection with Akabane, bluetongue and Wesselsbron viruses.

Diseases characterized by congenital paresis/paralysis

- Enzootic ataxia due to nutritional deficiency of copper. It may also develop later, within the first month of postnatal life
- Inherited congenital posterior paralysis of calves, and of pigs
- Spina bifida (18) may be accompanied by flexion and contracture and atrophy of hindlegs and most are stillborn. In rare cases the affected calf is ambulatory (27)
- Spinal dysraphism in Charolais and Angus calves (22), syringomyelia and hydromyelia in calves
- Tetraparesis, tetraplegia, progressive ataxia with head deviation in foals with congenital occipito-atlanto-axial malformations. A familial tendency to the defects occurs in Arab (20) and non-Arabian (26) horses. Additional signs include stiffness of the neck, palpable abnormalities at the site, a clicking sound on passive movement. Foals may be affected at birth or develop signs later. The defect is identifiable radiographically. A congenital dysplasia of the atlanto-occipital joint with excessive mobility is recorded in Angora goats and causes a compressive myelopathy (21). Devon calves may be affected by the same deformity (2) and similar ones have been recorded in calves which were recumbent at birth (6, 25) and others in which ataxia developed subsequently (6). More widespread malacic changes have been recorded in the spinal vertebrae of calves (28) but without the specific etiology being determined.

Diseases characterized by cerebellar ataxia

- Inherited cerebellar hypoplasia of calves, Arab foals, lambs
- Cerebellar hypoplasia and hypomyelinogenesis in calves from cows infected with bovine viral diarrhea virus (24) and possibly Akabane virus (32) during pregnancy
- Cerebellar hypoplasia in piglets after hog cholera vaccination of dams
- Inherited cerebellar ataxia in pigs and foals (19)
- Familial convulsions and ataxia of Angus cattle
- Mannosidosis of cattle
- Intracranial hemorrhage in newborn foals, discussed in more detail under neonatal maladjustment syndrome
- Spinal cord hypoplasia in Akabane virus infection in ruminants.

Diseases characterized by tremor

- Congenital paresis and tremor of piglets
- Inherited congenital spasms of cattle
- Inherited neonatal spasticity (Jersey and Hereford cattle) develops at 2–5 days old
- Border disease (hairy shakers) in lambs due to bovine virus diarrhea virus
- Inherited neuraxial edema (now inherited congenital myoclonus) of polled Hereford cattle and congenital brain edema of Herefords (14)
- Myoclonia congenita as a result of infection with hog cholera or Aujeszky's disease viruses
- Tremor with rigidity (23) due to hydranencephaly and porencephaly in calves infected *in utero* with bovine viral diarrhea (BVD) virus
- 'Shaker calves' in Herefords.

Neurogenic arthrogryposis and muscle atrophy

- Akabane virus infection of calves, kids, possibly lambs, *in utero*
- There are many other causes of arthrogryposis listed under congenital abnormalities of joints, but they are not known to be neurogenic.

Spasms of muscle masses

- Inherited spastic paresis (Elso-heel) of calves
- Inherited periodic spasticity (stall-cramp).

Convulsions

- Brain injury during birth in calves and lambs
- Brain compression due to hypovitaminosis A in calves and pigs
- Neonatal maladjustment syndrome (barkers and wanderers) in thoroughbred foals
- Congenital toxoplasmosis in calves, bluetongue virus infection in lambs
- Tetanic convulsion in inherited neuraxial edema (now inherited congenital myoclonus) of Hereford calves, but only when lifted to standing position
- Inherited idiopathic epilepsy of Brown Swiss cattle
- Familial convulsions and ataxia of Angus cattle
- Inherited narcolepsy/catalepsy in Shetland ponies and Suffolk horses (not really a convulsion)
- Doddler calves.

Imbecility

- Microcephaly (3) in calves, probably inherited, with no abnormality of the cranium, but the cerebral hemispheres, cerebellum and brainstem are reduced in size and the corpus callosum and fornix are absent
- Microcephaly is recorded in sheep (4, 5); many dead at birth, viable ones unable to stand, blind, incoordinate and have a constant tremor
- Anencephaly in calves with absence of cerebral hemispheres, rostral midbrain, occurs sporadically in calves (16)
- Hydranencephaly caused by Akabane virus infection of calf, kid and possibly lamb *in utero*
- Congenital porencephaly in lambs after intrauterine infection with bluetongue virus.

Eyes

- Spontaneous microphthalmia and anophthalmia in calves, usually due to unknown cause
- Congenital lenticular cataracts in cattle (15) and lambs (29)
- Blindness developing after birth in gangliosidosis of cattle and ceroid lipofuscinosis of sheep
- Constriction of optic nerve by vitamin A deficiency causing blindness in calves and pigs
- Constriction of optic nerve and blindness with bovine viral diarrhea virus infection in calves *in utero*
- Inherited exophthalmos with strabismus of cattle
- Familial undulatory nystagmus.

Lists of congenital ocular defects of cattle (12), and of congenital eye defects in all species (11) are available.

Defects conditioned by inheritance but not present at birth

- Cerebellar atrophy (abiotrophy) in calves and foals (8) and a probably inherited cerebellar abiotrophy in sheep aged 3·5–6 years (30)
- Inherited idiopathic epilepsy of Jerseys and Shorthorns
- Mannosidosis of cattle
- Gangliosidosis of cattle
- Bovine generalized glycogenosis
- Globoid cell leukodystrophy of sheep
- Ceroid lipofuscinosis of sheep
- Inherited myotonia of goats
- Progressive ataxia of Charolais cattle
- Inherited citrullinemia of calves
- Inherited maple syrup urine disease.

REVIEW LITERATURE

Cho, D. Y. & Leipold, H. W. (1977) Congenital defects of the bovine central nervous system. *Vet. Bull.*, *47*, 489.

Done, J. T. (1976) Developmental disorders of the nervous system in animals. *Adv. vet. Sci.*, *20*, 69.

REFERENCES

(1) Umemura, T. et al. (1987) *Jap. J. vet. Sci.*, *49*, 95.
(2) McCoy, D. J. et al. (1986) *Cornell Vet.*, *76*, 277.
(3) Fielden, E. D. (1959) *NZ vet. J.*, 7,80
(4) Hartley, W. J. & Kater, J. C. (1965) *Aust. vet. J.*, *41*, 107.
(5) Hartley, W. J. & Haughey, K. G. (1974) *Aust. vet. J.*, *50*, 55, 323.
(6) Boyd, J. S. & McNeil, P. E. (1987) *Vet. Rec.*, *120*, 34.
(7) Simon, J. & Brewer, R. L. (1963) *J. Am. vet. med. Assoc.*, *142* 1102.
(8) Dungworth, D. L. & Fowler, M.E. (1966) *Cornell Vet.*, *61*, 17.
(9) Done, J. T. (1968) *Lab. Anim.*, *2*, 207.
(10) Saunders, L. Z. (1952) *Cornell Vet.*, *42*, 592.
(11) Priester, W. A. (1972) *J. Am. vet. med. Assoc.*, *160*, 1504.
(12) Gelatt, K. N. (1976) *Mod. vet. Pract.*, *57*, 105.
(13) Dennis, S. M. (1975) *Aust. vet. J.*, *51*, 385.
(14) Cho, D. Y. & Leipold, H. W. (1977) *Vet. Bull.*, *47*, 489.
(15) Ashton, N. et al. (1977) *Vet. Rec.*, *100*, 505.
(16) Cho, D. Y. & Leipold, H. W. (1978) *Cornell Vet.*, *68*, 60 & 99.
(17) Cho, D. Y. & Leipold, H. W. (1977) *Acta Neuropathol.*, *39*, 129.
(18) Cho, D. Y. & Leipold, H. W. (1977) *Zentralbl. VetMed.*, *24A*, 680.
(19) Beech, J. (1976) *Proc. 22nd Ann. Conv. Am. Assoc. equ. Practrs*, p. 77.
(20) Mayhew, I. G. et al. (1978) *Equ. vet. J.*, *10*, 103 and 125.
(21) Robinson, W. F. et al. (1982) *Aust. vet. J.*, *58*, 105.
(22) Johnson, M. I. et al. (1978) *Bov. Pract.*, *13*, 109.
(23) Axthelm, M. K. et al. (1981) *Cornell Vet.*, *71*, 164.
(24) Wilson, T. M. et al. (1983) *J. Am. vet. med. Assoc.*, *183*, 544.
(25) Watson, A. G. et al. (1985) *J. Am. vet. med. Assoc.*, *187*, 740.
(26) Wilson, W. D. et al. (1985) *J. Am. vet. med. Assoc.*, *187*, 36.
(27) Boyd, J. S. (1985) *Vet. Rec.*, *116*, 203.
(28) Orr, J. P. & McKenzie, G. C. (1981) *Can. vet. J.*, *22*, 121.
(29) Brooks, H. V. et al. (1982) *NZ vet. J.*, *30*, 113.
(30) Harper, P. A. W. et al. (1986) *Aust. vet. J.*, *63*, 18.

13

Diseases of the Musculoskeletal System

DISEASES of the organs of support, including muscles, bones and joints, have much in common in that the major clinical manifestations of diseases which affect them are lameness, failure of support, insufficiency of movement and deformity. Insufficiency of movement affects all voluntary muscles, including those responsible for respiratory movement and mastication, but lameness and failure of support are manifestations of involvement of the limbs.

Various classifications of the diseases of the musculoskeletal system, based on clinical, pathological and etiological differences are in use, but the simplest is that which divides the diseases into degenerative and inflammatory types. The degenerative diseases of muscles, bones and joints are distinguished as myopathy, osteodystrophy and arthropathy, respectively, and the inflammatory diseases as myositis, osteomyelitis and arthritis.

PRINCIPAL MANIFESTATIONS OF MUSCULOSKELETAL DISEASE

Lameness

Because of the difficulty inherent in the differentiation of diseases causing lameness, and other abnormalities of gait and posture, a summary is presented in Table 41. It does not include lameness in racing horses which is described voluminously elsewhere, or diseases of the nervous system which interfere with normal movement and posture. These are dealt with in the previous chapter.

Abnormal posture and movement

As a group the diseases are characterized by reduced activity in rising and moving, and the adoption of unusual postures. Abnormal movements include limpness, sagging or stiffness and lack of flexion. Abnormal postures include persistent recumbency, including lateral recumbency. There may be signs of pain on standing, moving or palpation. There is an absence of signs specifically referable to the nervous system. For example, there are no signs of brain damage, the spinal cord reflexes are present, but may be only partly elicitable (the sensory pathway is intact, but the motor response may be diminished). Differentiation from diseases of the nervous system and from each other may be aided by specific biochemical, radiological or hematological findings which indicate the system involved. Specific epidemiological findings may indicate the location of the lesion (which may be secondary) in muscle, bones or joints, as set out in Table 41.

Deformity

Atypical disposition, shape or size of a part of the musculoskeletal system constitutes a deformity. This may occur in a number of ways, and be caused by the following.

Muscle and tendon defects
These include:

- Congenital hypermobility of joints, inherited and sporadic
- Congenital flexed or stretched tendons of limbs causing contracture of joints or hyperextension
- Inherited congenital splayleg of pigs
- Muscle hypertrophy (Doppelender, Culard) of cattle
- Acquired asymmetric hindquarters of pigs.

Joint defects

- Inherited congenital ankylosis of cattle causing fixation in flexion
- Joint enlargement of rickets and chronic arthritis.

Defects of the skeleton

- Dwarfism—inherited miniature calves, achondroplastic dwarfs; short legs of inherited congenital osteopetrosis; nutritional deficiency of manganese; acorn calves
- Giant stature—inherited prolonged gestation, not really giantism, only large at birth

Table 41. Differential diagnosis of diseases of the musculoskeletal system

Clinical findings	*Epidemiological findings*	*Clinical pathology*	*Necropsy findings*	*Examples*
MYASTHENIA				
Paresis, paralysis and incoordination	Ischemia or reduced supply of energy or electrolytes	Hypoglycemia, hypocalcemia, hypokalemia, hypomagnesemia	Reversible malfunction	Iliac thrombosis, toxemia generally, poisonous plants, milk fever, lactic acidosis
MYOPATHY				
Either stiff gait, disinclination to move, boardlike muscles *or* weakness, pseudoparesis or paralysis, difficult rising, staggery gait, flabby muscles. Always bilateral, mostly hindlimbs	Often precipitated by sudden increase in muscular work. Usually diet-dependent on: (1) High carbohydrate intake (2) Deficiency in selenium/vitamin E intake (3) Ingestion myopathic agents, e.g. in poison plants, cod liver oil	Marked elevations in serum levels of CPK and SGOT Myoglobinemia and possibly myoglobinuria	White, waxy, swollen, 'fish flesh' muscle	*Horses*: Azoturia ('equine paralytic myoglobinuria', 'tying-up', 'equine rhabdomyolysis') Postanesthetic myositis *Pigs*: Porcine stress syndrome, selenium deficiency, inherited splaylegs *Cattle*: Selenium/vitamin E deficiency (enzootic muscular dystrophy), poisoning by *Cassia occidentalis*, *Karwinskia humboldtiana*, ischemic necrosis of recumbency *Sheep*: Approximately the same. Exertional rhabdomyolysis in sheep
MYOSITIS				
Acute inflammation, swelling, pain, may be associated systemic signs if infectious. Chronic manifested by atrophy, contracture of joint, incomplete extension	Related to trauma or specific infectious disease	As for myopathy plus hematological response when infection present	Bruising, edema and hemorrhage in acute. Atrophy, pallor in chronic	Blackleg, false blackleg (malignant edema). Eosinophilic myositis in beef cattle. Traumatic injury by strain of muscle or forceful impact
OSTEODYSTROPHY				
Stiff gait, moderate lameness often shifting from leg to leg, arched back, crackling sounds in joints while walking. Disinclination to move; horses affected early race very poorly. Severely affected animals disinclined to stand, recumbent much of time. Fractures common. Bones soft, e.g. frontal bones to digital pressure. Deformities of bones, e.g. bowing, pelvic collapse. Ready detachment of tendons and ligaments	Absolute deficiency and/or relative imbalance of dietary calcium, phosphorus and vitamin D. Most apparent in rapidly growing or in working animals and in heavy milk-producing animals	Radiographic evidence of osteoporosis, deformed epiphyseal lines, broadness of epiphyses. Subperiosteal unossified osteoid	Osteoporosis, subepiphyseal collapse of bone at pressure points. Fracture of soft bones. Bone ash determinations of Ca, P and Mg content of bones	*Cattle*: Phosphorus deficiency, Marie's disease. Hypovitaminosis D. Calcium deficiency. Poisoning by *Trachymene glaucifolia* (bowie or bentleg) *Horses*: Osteodystrophia fibrosa due to low calcium diet, or to poison plants containing large amounts of oxalate (see under oxalate poisoning) *Pigs*: Osteodystrophia fibrosa due to low Ca high P in diet
OSTEOMYELITIS				
Pain, swelling (little), toxemia, fever, may be discharge through sinus	Only of specific disease	Radiographic evidence of rarefaction, new bone growth	Osteomyelitis	Actinomycosis, brucellosis in pigs and cattle. Necrotic and atrophic rhinitis diseases in pigs
ARTHROPATHY (OSTEOARTHRITIS)				
Lameness with pain on walking, standing, palpation. Some enlargement but not gross. Slackness in joints, may be ligament rupture, crepitus	(1) Inherited predisposition in cattle (2) Dietary excess of phosphorus, relative deficiency of calcium (3) Very rapid increase in body weight in young (4) Heavy milk production during many lactations	Excessive sterile brownish fluid with floccules. Radiological evidence of joint erosion, epiphyseal deformity, new bone growth peripherally	Erosion of cartilage and bone, ligament rupture, new bone growth (epiphytes) around edge of joint. Excess brownish sterile clear fluid containing floccules	*Cattle*: Degenerative joint disease (of young beef bulls), inherited osteoarthritis *Horses*: As early part of osteodystrophy syndrome *Pigs*: Epiphyseolysis of femurs of young breeding boars. Osteochondrosis

Table 41—cont.

Clinical findings	*Epidemiological findings*	*Clinical pathology*	*Necropsy findings*	*Examples*
ARTHRITIS *Acute*. Sudden onset, severe pain, very lame, sore to touch, swelling, heat in joint *Chronic*. Continuous pain, recumbency, may be toxemia if infectious. Joint may be visibly swollen but may be normal appearance. Pain may be evident only when animal stands on joint	Most commonly in young via navel infection and bacteremia, or residual from septicemia of neonate	Aspiration of fluid under very sterile conditions shows leukocytes and somatic cells in large numbers. Culture may be positive but often negative. Joint fluid may appear normal in chronic case	*Acute*. Inflammation or suppuration increased fluid content *Chronic*. Thickened synovial membrane. Increased amount clear fluid. Erosion of articular cartilage	*Cattle*: *Mycoplasma* sp., *Erysipelothrix insidiosa*, *Streptococcus* and *Staphylococcus* spp., *Escherichia coli*, *Salmonella* sp. in newborn. *Brucella abortus*, *Mycoplasma* sp. and *Chlamydia* sp. *Swine*: *Erysipelothrix insidiosa*, *Mycoplasma* sp. *Sheep*: *Corynebacterium pseudotuberculosis*, *E. insidiosa*, *Haemophilus agni*, *Pasteurella haemolytica*, *Actinobacillus seminis*, *Chlamydia* sp., *Mycoplasma* sp. *Horses*: Foal septicemias
TENOSYNOVITIS, CELLULITIS, LYMPHANGITIS, BURSITIS Inflammation of other supporting tissues. Visible, painful enlargements	Sporadic due to trauma or localization of systemic infection	Culture of aspirate from local lesion	Inflammation of affected part. Acute hemorrhagic or chronic, suppurative	*Horse and cattle:* Bursitis—*Brucella abortus*. Taeniosynovitis—*Haemophilus somnus* cattle, *Strep. equi*—horse; *Histophilus ovis*—sheep
FOOTROT Severe foot lameness. Visible local lesion at skin horn junction, necrotic smell, horn underrun. Allied similar conditions have less severe lesions	Severe epidemics in wet, warm weather in sheep. Infection soil-borne. Some farms have disease persistently	Culture of infectious agent, swab from depth of lesion	Necrosis of soft tissue	*Sheep*: Footrot—*Bacteroides nodosus*; footscald—avirulent B. *nodosus*; foot abscess—*F. necrophorus*; *Cor. pyogenes*; interdigital dermatitis—*F. necrophorus* *Cattle*: Footrot—*F. necrophorus*, *B. nodosus*
LAMINITIS Severe foot pain, separation of horn from sensitive laminae, rotation pedal bone. Metabolic, traumatic or infectious types	Sporadic except infectious type in sheep related to dipping. Possibly inherited susceptibility to metabolic laminitis in cattle	Very high blood pressure. Radiological demonstration of P_3 rotation	Infection or hemorrhage/edema, sensitive laminae	*Sheep*: *Erysipelothrix insidiosa*—postdipping laminitis. *Horses*—traumatic due to continuous pawing *All species*: Metabolic associated with heavy grain feeding—in mares with retained placenta and metritis
DAMAGE TO HORN OF HOOF Severe foot pain if sensitive laminae affected. Horn damage obvious	Related to hard abrasive surfaces—pigs and dairy cattle; soft underfoot—cows indoors on wet bedding	Nil	Foothorn lesion only	*Cattle*: Stable footrot on soft footing; sole wear on rough concrete *Pigs*: Sole wear on rough concrete, predisposed by biotin deficiency in diet *Horses*: Thrush and canker on soft wet underfoot

Table 41—cont.

Clinical findings	*Epidemiological findings*	*Clinical pathology*	*Necropsy findings*	*Examples*
TRAUMATIC INJURIES OF FEET OF NEWBORN PIGLETS				
Severe lameness in piglets from 1 to 8 days of age. Bruising of sole congestion and swelling followed by peeling, erosion and cracking of horn of sole; both claws and accessory digits injured more often on medial aspect and incidence in hindfeet twice that of forefeet; abrasions of skin of carpal joints common; accessory digits involved too. Ascending secondary bacterial infection resulting in tenosynovitis and septic arthritis. Most piglets recover following antibacterial therapy	Newborn piglets raised on concrete or slatted floors. Distribution of lesions related to sucking behavior of piglets, the backwards, outwards and downwards thrusting movements of the hindlegs while sucking	Nil	Erosion, necrosis, congestion, fissures and hemorrhage of horn of sole and sensitive laminae of digit. Secondary tenosynovitis and arthritis	*Piglets*: Newborn piglets raised on concrete expanded metal or plastic slatted floors
CORONITIS DERMATITIS AT CORONET				
Lesions vary from granuloma through vesicles, erosions. Lameness in all, but severity varies with type of lesion. Essential to examine oral mucosa	Acute outbreaks of lameness due to coronitis in any species raises specter of foot-and-mouth disease	Microbiology of material from local lesion	Local lesions only	*Sheep*: Bluetongue, foot-and-mouth disease, vesicular stomatitis, ecthyma, strawberry footrot, ulcerative dermatosis, heel dermatitis (*B. nodosus*), strongyloidosis. *Cattle*: Foot-and-mouth disease, vesicular stomatitis, bovine virus diarrhea, bovine malignant catarrh, epitheliogenesis imperfecta *Pigs*: Foot-and-mouth disease, vesicular exanthema of swine, swine vesicular disease, vesicular stomatitis *Horses*: Vesicular stomatitis, greasy heel, chorioptic mange

- Asymmetry—high withers, low pelvis of hyena disease of cattle
- Limbs—complete or partial absence, inherited or sporadic amputates; curvature of limbs in rickets; bowie or bentleg of sheep poisoned by *Trachymene* sp.
- Head—inherited and sporadic cyclopean deformity; inherited probatocephaly (sheeps head) of calves; inherited moles, bulldog calves; acquired atrophic rhinitis of pigs.

Ease of fracture

An uncommon field finding in farm animals is ease of fracture of bones. Disease states which could contribute are:

- Nutritional excess of phosphorus causing osteodystrophia in horses
- Nutritional deficiency of calcium causing osteodystrophia in pigs
- Nutritional deficiency of phosphorus or vitamin D in ruminants causing rickets and/or osteomalacia; hypervitaminosis A may contribute to this
- Nutritional deficiency of copper
- Chronic fluorine intoxication.

Economics of lameness

Diseases of the musculoskeletal system and feet which cause lameness cause major economic losses. Loss of production occurs because animals which are in pain have difficulty moving around and do not eat and milk normally. Reproductive performance may be reduced because of failure to come into heat normally. The culling rate may be higher than desirable because so many of the lesions of the feet and legs are incurable. The direct monetary costs for the treatment of lame animals are not high, but the actual treatment of either individual animals or groups of animals is time-consuming and laborious. The condemnation of animals at slaughter because of lesions of the musculoskeletal system also contributes to the total economic losses (3). When lameness is a herd problem not only are the economic losses increased, but clinical management becomes very difficult.

The epidemiological factors which contribute to lameness include: injuries due to floor surfaces (1, 5), persistently wet, unhygienic ground conditions, overcrowding and trampling during transportation and handling (4), nutritional inadequacies, undesirable skeletal conformation and failure to provide regular foot-trimming. Certain breeds may be more susceptible to diseases of the feet and legs than others. Osteoarthritis occurs most commonly in old animals. Diseases of the legs of dairy cattle occur most commonly at the time of parturition and during the first 50 days of lactation. Diseases of the feet of dairy cattle occur most commonly from 50 to 150 days of the lactation period (2). Often the etiology is complex and a definitive etiological diagnosis cannot be made. This makes clinical management difficult and often unrewarding.

REFERENCES

(1) Animal Housing Injuries Due to Floor Surfaces. *Proc. Symp. Cement and Concrete Assoc., Fulmer Grange, Slough, Berks, England, November 1978*, pp. 1–177.
(2) Baggott, D. G. & Russell, A. M. (1981) *Br. vet. J.*, *137*, 113.
(3) Weaver, A. D. (1977) *Vet. Rec.*, *100*, 172.
(4) Jensen, R. et al. (1980) *Cornell Vet.*, *70*, 329.
(5) Dewes, H. F. (1978) *NZ vet. J.*, *26*, 147 & 157.

Special examinations of the musculoskeletal system

The clinical and laboratory examination of the musculoskeletal system and the feet of farm animals would include the following special examinations.

Analysis of gait and conformation

Inspection of the gait of the animal is necessary to localize the site of lameness. Evaluation of its conformation may provide clues about factors which may contribute to lameness.

Close examination

A detailed physical examination of the affected area is necessary to localize the lesion. This includes passive movements of limbs to identify fractures, dislocations and pain on movement. Muscles can be palpated for evidence of enlargement, pain or atrophy.

Radiography

Radiography is useful for the diagnosis of diseases of bones, joints and soft tissue swelling of limbs, which cannot be easily defined. Detailed radiographic information about the joint capsule, joint cavity or articular cartilage can be obtained using negative (air), positive, or double contrast arthrography (2).

Muscle biopsy

A muscle biopsy may be useful for microscopic and histochemical evaluations.

Arthrocentesis and arthroscopy

Joint fluid is collected by needle puncture of the joint cavity (arthrocentesis) and examined for the presence of cells, biochemical changes in the joint fluid and the presence of infectious agents. The techniques and application of arthrocentesis for some of the joints commonly sampled in the horse have been reviewed (3). Special endoscopes are available for visceral inspection of the joint cavity and articular surfaces (arthroscopy). Diagnostic and surgical arthroscopy is now commonplace in specialized equine practice (4). Surgical arthroscopy is rapidly replacing conventional arthrotomy for the correction of several common surgical conditions of the musculoskeletal system of the horse. Accurate quantitation of equine carpal lesions is possible when the procedure is performed by an experienced arthroscopist (6). Convalescent time following surgery is decreased and the cosmetic appearance improved compared to arthrotomy. The arthroscopic anatomy of the intercarpal and radiocarpal joints of the horse have been described (5). A synovial membrane biopsy can be examined histologically and for infectious agents and may yield useful diagnostic information.

Serum biochemistry and enzymology

When disease of bone or muscle is suspected, the serum levels of calcium, phosphorus, alkaline phosphatase, and the muscle enzymes, creatinine phosphokinase (CPK) and serum glutamic oxaloacetic transaminase (SGOT) may be useful. The muscle enzymes are sensitive indicators of muscle cell damage; the serum levels of calcium, phosphorus and alkaline phosphatase are much less sensitive indicators of osteodystrophy.

Nutritional history

Because the most important osteodystrophies and myopathies are nutritional in origin a complete nutritional history must be obtained. This should include an analysis of the feed and determination of the total amount of intake of each nutrient, including the ratio of one nutrient to another in the diet.

Environment and housing

When outbreaks of lameness occur in housed cattle and swine the quality of the floor must be examined to evaluate the possibility of floor injuries.

REFERENCES

(1) McIlwraith, C. & Fessler, J. F. (1978) *J. Am. vet. med. Assoc.*, *172*, 263.
(2) Dik, K. J. (1984) *Vet. Radiol.*, *25*, 93.
(3) Rose, R. J. & Frauenfelder, H. C. (1982) *Equ. vet. J.*, *14*, 173.
(4) McIlwraith, C. W. (1984) *Equ. vet. J.*, *16*, 11.
(5) Martin, G. S. & McIlwraith, C. W. (1985) *Equ. vet. J.*, *17*, 373.
(6) Hurtig, M. B. et al. (1985) *Vet. Surg.*, *14*, 93.

DISEASES OF MUSCLES

Myasthenia (skeletal muscle asthenia)

The differential diagnosis of paresis, paralysis and incoordination should include a consideration of skeletal muscle weakness unrelated to primary neurogenic hypotonia or to permanent muscle injury including myopathy and myositis. Most of the syndromes which fall into this group of myasthenia have been described in detail elsewhere in this book and they are referred to briefly here only to complete the list of abnormalities of skeletal muscle which affect gait and posture. Distinct from myopathy and myositis they are reversible states.

The common causes of myasthenia in farm animals are:

- *Ischemia* in iliac thrombosis in the horse and after recumbency in cows with parturient paresis. The end stage is myonecrosis and is not reversible
- *Metabolic effect on muscle fibers*—causes include hypokalemia, hypocalcemia and possibly hypophosphatemia (in parturient paresis of dairy cows), hypomagnesemia (in lactation tetany), hypoglycemia of newborn pigs and lactic acidemia after engorgement on grain
- *Poisons*—general toxemia is a cause. Also, many plant poisons exert an effect on skeletal muscle activity. Although in most cases the mode of action of the poison is unknown, the poisons have been listed as neurotoxins.

Myopathy

The term myopathy describes the non-inflammatory degeneration of skeletal muscle which is characterized clinically by muscle weakness and pathologically by hyaline degeneration of the muscle fibers. The serum levels of some muscle enzymes are elevated and myoglobinuria is a common accompaniment.

Etiology and epidemiology

The most important myopathies in farm animals are due to nutritional deficiencies of vitamin E and selenium and the effects of unaccustomed exercise (1). In man, in contrast, the muscular dystrophies occur as inherited defects of muscle or degenerative lesions caused by interruption of their nerve supply. The skeletal myopathies can be classified into primary and secondary myopathies (27).

The major causes of myopathy in farm animals and their epidemiological determinants are as follows.

Enzootic nutritional muscular dystrophy
A nutritional deficiency of vitamin E and/or selenium is a common cause in young calves, lambs, foals and piglets. Factors enhancing or precipitating onset include: rapid growth, highly unsaturated fatty acids in diet and unaccustomed exercise. The disease also occurs in adult horses (2).

Exertional or postexercise rhabdomyolyses
This is not known to be conditioned by vitamin E (selenium deficiency) and occurs as equine paralytic myoglobinuria (tying-up syndrome, azoturia) in horses after unaccustomed exercise or insufficient training (3), in sheep chased by dogs (26), and in cattle after running wildly for several minutes, and as capture myopathy during capture of wildlife (4, 5).

Congenital myopathies
These are inherited diseases and include 'double-muscling' in cattle (7) and possibly congenital splaylegs of newborn pigs.

Degenerative myopathy
This occurs in newborn calves, sheep and goats affected by Akabane virus infected *in utero*.

Other inherited diseases
The porcine stress syndrome (*Herztod*, pale, soft exudative pork, malignant hyperthermia following halothane anesthesia) is predisposed to by an inherited factor and precipitated by transportation, overcrowding and handling at slaughter. Dystrophy of the diaphragmatic muscles in adult Meuse–Rhine–Yessel cattle is thought to be inherited (28).

Chemical agents and drugs
This is caused by poisonous plants including *Cassia occidentalis*, *Karwinskia humboldtiana* (6), *Ixioloena* sp., *Geigeria* sp. and lupins. A special case is enzootic calcinosis of all tissues especially muscle and the principal signs are muscular. It is caused by poisoning by *Solanum malacoxylon*, *Tricetum* sp. and *Cestrum* sp.

Ischemia
Ischemic myonecrosis occurs in the thigh muscles of cattle recumbent for about 48 hours or more and is discussed in detail under the heading 'downer-cow syndrome'.

Neurogenic
Neurogenic muscular atrophy occurs sporadically due to traumatic injury and subsequent degeneration or complete severance of the nerve supply to skeletal muscle. The myopathy in arthrogryposis caused by the Akabane virus is thought to be due to lesions of the lower motor neurons supplying the affected muscles. It has been suggested that cattle with muscular hypertrophy may be more susceptible to the effects of exercise and the occurrence of acute muscular dystrophy (7).

Other causes
The porcine stress syndrome, which is discussed under that heading, now includes *Herztod*, pale soft exudative pork encountered at slaughter and malignant hyperthermia following halothane anesthesia. Certain blood types in pigs have been used as predictors of stress susceptibility (8) and malignant hyperthermia in Pietrain pigs is genetically predetermined (9). Most of these myopathies of swine thus have an inherited basis and the stress of transportation, overcrowding and handling at slaughter precipitates the lesion and rapid death (10, 11). Xanthosis occurs in the skeletal and cardiac muscles of cattle and is characterized grossly by a green iridescence (29).

Neoplasms
Neoplasms of striated muscle are uncommon in animals. Rhabdomyosarcomas are reported in the horses affecting the diaphragm and causing loss of body weight, anorexia and respiratory distress (30).

Pathogenesis
In most animals skeletal muscle is composed of a mixture of fibers with different contractile and metabolic characteristics. Fibers with slow contraction times have been called slow twitch or type I fibers, and those with fast contraction time are fast twitch or type II. Histochemically, types I and II fibers can be differentiated by staining for myofibrillar ATPase. Type II fibers can be subgrouped into type IIA and IIB on the basis of acid preincubations (31). Several different characteristics of these muscle fibers have been studied in the horse. There are variations in the percentage of each type of fiber present and in composition of muscle fibers dependent on genetic background, age and stage of training (31). There are variations in the muscle fibers within one muscle (33) and between different muscles (34). The histochemical characteristics of equine muscle fibers have been examined (35, 36). Type I fibers are characterized by strong aerobic capacity, compared with type IIA fibers which are more glycolytic and have strong aerobic and moderate-to-strong anaerobic capacities. Type IIB fibers are characterized by a relatively low aerobic and a relatively high anaerobic capacity and are glycolytic (35). The histochemical staining characteristics of normal equine skeletal muscle have been examined and serve as a standard for comparison with data obtained from skeletal muscles with lesions (36).

In primary nutritional muscular dystrophy associated with a deficiency of vitamin E and/or selenium there is lipoperoxidation of the cellular membranes of muscle fibers resulting in degeneration and necrosis (12). The lesion is present only in muscle fibers and the histological and biochemical changes which occur in the muscle are remarkably similar irrespective of the cause. Variations in the histological lesion occur but indicate variation in the severity and rapidity of onset of the change rather than different causes.

In exertional rhabdomyolysis in horses there is enhanced glycolysis with depletion of muscle glycogen, the accumulation of large amounts of lactate in muscle and blood and the development of hyaline degeneration of myofibers (3). Affected muscle fibers are richer in glycogen in the acute stage of 'tying-up' than in the late stages, suggesting an increased glycogen storage in the early phase of the disease compared with normal healthy horses. During enforced exercise there is local muscle hypoxia and anerobic oxidation resulting in the accumulation of lactate and myofibrillar degeneration. The pathogenesis of postanesthetic myositis in horses is uncertain (24). However, prolonged lack of adequate tissue perfusion, the partitioning of the calcium ion, leading to tetany and death of muscle cells are plausible hypotheses (24).

The characteristic change in most cases of primary myopathy varies from hyaline degeneration to coagulative necrosis, affecting particularly the heavy thigh muscles and the muscles of the diaphragm. Myocardial lesions are also commonly associated with the degeneration of skeletal muscle and when severe will cause rapid death within a few hours or days. The visible effects of the lesions are varying degrees of muscle weakness, muscle pain, recumbency, stiff gait, inability to move the limbs and the development of respiratory and circulatory insufficiency.

Because of the necrosis of muscle, myoglobin is excreted in the urine and myoglobinuric nephrosis is an important complication, particularly of acute primary myopathy. The degree of myoglobinuria depends on the severity of the lesion, acute cases resulting in marked myoglobinuria, and on the age and species of animal affected. Adult horses with myopathy may liberate large quantities of myoglobin resulting in dark brown urine. Yearling cattle with myopathy release moderate amounts and the urine may or may not be colored and calves with severe enzootic nutritional muscular dystrophy may have grossly normal urine. In all species the renal threshold of myoglobin is so low that discoloration of the serum does not occur.

An important biochemical manifestation of myopathy is the increased release of muscle cell enzymes which occurs during muscle cell destruction. Creatinine phosphokinase (CPK) and serum glutamic oxaloacetate transaminase are both elevated in myopathy and CPK, particularly, is a more specific and reliable indication of acute muscle damage. Increased amounts of creatinine are also released into the urine following myopathy.

In secondary myopathy due to ischemia there may be multiple focal areas of necrosis which causes muscle weakness and results in an increase of muscle enzymes in the serum. The degree of regeneration with myofibers depends on the severity of the lesion. Some regeneration occurs but there is considerable tissue replacement.

In neurogenic atrophy there is flaccid paralysis, a marked decrease in total muscle mass and degeneration of myofibers with failure to regenerate unless the nerve supply is at least partially restored.

Clinical findings
The nutritional myopathies associated with a deficiency of vitamin E and/or selenium occur most commonly in young growing animals and may occur in outbreak form particularly in calves and lambs. The details are presented under the heading of vitamin E and selenium deficiency.

In general terms in acute primary myopathy there is a sudden onset of weakness and pseudoparalysis of the affected muscles causing paresis and recumbency and, in many cases, accompanying respiratory and circulatory insufficiency. The affected animals will usually remain bright and alert but may appear to be in pain. The temperature is usually normal but may be slightly elevated in severe cases of primary myopathy. Cardiac irregularity and tachycardia may be evident, and myoglobinuria occurs in adult horses and yearling cattle. The affected skeletal muscles in acute cases may feel swollen, hard and rubbery but in most cases it is difficult to detect significant abnormality by palpation. Acute cases of primary myopathy may die within 24 hours after the onset of signs.

Acute nutritional myopathy
While acute nutritional myopathy in horses occurs most commonly in foals from birth to 7 months of age, acute dystrophic myodegeneration also occurs in adult horses (2). There is muscle stiffness and pain, myoglobinuria, edema of the head and neck, recumbency and death in a few days. A special occurrence of myopathy has been recorded in sucking thoroughbred foals up to 5 months of age (13). The disease occurs in the spring and summer in foals running at pasture with their dams and is unassociated with excessive exercise. In peracute cases there is a sudden onset of dejection, stiffness, disinclination to move, prostration and death 3–7 days later. Lethargy and stiffness of gait are characteristic of less acute cases. There is also a pronounced swelling and firmness of the subcutaneous tissue at the base of the mane and over the gluteal muscles. There may be excessive salivation, desquamation of lingual epithelium and board-like firmness of the masseter muscles. The foals are unable to suck because of inability to bend their necks. Spontaneous recovery occurs in mild cases but most severely affected foals die.

Tying-up
In tying-up in horses there is a very sudden onset of muscle soreness 10–20 minutes following exercise. There is profuse sweating and the degree of soreness varies from mild, in which the horse moves with a short, shuffling gait, to acute, in which there is a great disinclination to move at all. In severe cases, horses are unable to move their hindlegs, and swelling and rigidity of the croup muscles develops. Myoglobinuria is common.

Postanesthetic myositis
In postanesthetic myositis affected horses experience considerable difficulty during recovery from anesthesia (23, 24). Recovery is prolonged and when initial attempts are made to stand there is lumbar rigidity, pain and reluctance to bear weight. The limbs may be rigid and the muscles firm on palpation. In severe cases the temperature begins to rise reminiscent of malignant hyperthermia (23). Other clinical findings include anxiety, tachycardia, profuse sweating, myoglobinuria and tachypnea. Death may occur in 6–12 hours. Euthanasia is the only course for some horses. In the milder form of the syndrome, affected horses are able to stand, but are stiff and in severe pain for a few days.

Exertional rhabdomyolysis
In exertional rhabdomyolysis in sheep chased by dogs, affected animals are recumbent, cannot stand, appear exhausted, and myoglobinuria is common (26). Death usually follows. A similar clinical picture occurs in cattle which have run wildly for several minutes.

Secondary myopathy due to ischemia
In secondary myopathy due to ischemia, e.g. the downer-cow syndrome, the affected animal is unable to rise and the affected hindlegs are commonly directed behind the cow in the frogleg attitude. The appetite and mental attitude are usually normal. No abnormality of the muscles can be palpated. With supportive therapy, good bedding and the prevention of further ischemia by frequent rolling of the animal, most cows will recover in a few days.

Neurological atrophy
With neurological atrophy there is marked loss of total mass of muscle, flaccid paralysis, loss of tendon reflexes and failure of regeneration. When large muscle masses are affected, e.g. quadriceps femoris in femoral nerve paralysis in calves at birth, the animal is unable to bear normal weight on the affected leg.

Dystrophy of the diaphragmatic muscles
In dystrophy of the diaphragmatic muscles in adult Meuse–Rhine–Yessel cattle there is loss of appetite, decreased rumination, decreased eructation and recurrent bloat. The respiratory rate is increased and there are forced abdominal respirations, forced movement of the nostrils and death from asphyxia in a few weeks (28).

Clinical pathology
The serum levels of the muscle enzymes are characteristically elevated following myopathy due to release of the enzymes from altered muscle cell membranes. Creatinine phosphokinase (CPK) is a highly specific indication of both myocardial and skeletal muscle degeneration. CPK has a half-life of about 4–6 hours and following an initial episode of acute myopathy, serum levels of the enzyme may return to normal within 3–4 days if no further muscle degeneration is occurring. The levels of serum glutamic oxaloacetic transaminase (SGOT) are also increased following myopathy but because the enzyme is present in other tissues such as liver, it is not a reliable indicator of primary muscle tissue degeneration.

Because SGOT has a longer half-life than CPK, the levels of SGOT may remain elevated for several days following acute myopathy. The daily monitoring of both the CPK and SGOT levels should provide an indication if active muscle degeneration is occurring. A marked drop in CPK levels and a slow decline in SGOT levels suggests that no further degeneration is occurring whereas a constant elevation of CPK suggests active degeneration.

In acute nutritional muscular dystrophy in calves, lambs and foals the CPK levels will increase from normal values of below 100 IU/liter to levels ranging from 1000 to 5000 IU/liter and even higher.

In calves the levels of CPK will increase from a normal of 50 IU/liter to 4700 IU/liter within a few days after being placed outdoors followed by unconditioned exercise (14).

The measurement of serum levels of glutathione peroxidase is a useful aid in the diagnosis of myopathy due to selenium deficiency.

In downer cows and ischemic necrosis of the thigh muscles the CPK and SGOT levels will be markedly elevated and will remain elevated if muscle necrosis is progressive in cows which were not well bedded and rolled from side to side several times daily to minimize the degree and extent of ischemic necrosis.

High levels of serum muscle enzymes (1000 IU/liter and greater) usually indicate acute primary myopathy. Levels from 500 to 1000 IU/liter may be difficult to interpret in animals recumbent for reasons other than primary myopathy. This will necessitate a careful reassessment of the clinical findings, history and epidemiology.

In horses with acute exertional rhabdomyolysis (paralytic myoglobinuria) the CPK levels will range from 5000 to 10 000 IU/liter. Following vigorous exercise in unconditioned horses, the CPK and SGOT levels will rise due to increased cell membrane permeability associated with the hypoxia of muscles subjected to excessive exercise (15–17). Lactate dehydrogenase (LDH) has also been used as a biochemical measurement of the degree of physical work done by horses in training. With progressive training in previously unconditioned horses there is no significant change between rest and exercise in the levels of serum CPK, SGOT and LDH (15). In horses with postanesthetic myositis the creatinine phosphokinase (CPK) levels may exceed 100 000 IU/liter, the serum calcium is decreased and the serum inorganic phosphorus is increased. In naturally occurring cases of exertional rhabdomyolysis in horses the most consistent acid–base abnormality may be a hypochloremia rather than metabolic acidosis as has been assumed (38).

Investigation of the structural and biochemical alterations of muscle tissue in myopathy include biopsy techniques which have been described (14, 18, 19).

Myoglobinuria is a common finding in adult horses with acute paralytic myoglobinuria but is not a common finding in acute nutritional muscular dystrophy in young farm animals, except perhaps in yearling cattle with acute muscular dystrophy. The myoglobinuria may be clinically detectable as a red or chocolate brown discoloration of the urine. This discoloration can be differentiated from that caused by hemoglobin by spectrographic examination or with the use of orthotolidine paper strips (20). Urine becomes dark when myoglobin levels exceed 40 mg/dl of urine (21). Discoloration of the plasma suggests hemoglobinuria. Both myoglobin and hemoglobin give positive results for the presence of protein in urine. Porphyria causes a similar discoloration although this may not be evident until the urine has been exposed to light for some minutes. The coloration is lighter, pink to red rather than brown, and the urine is negative to the guaiac test and fluoresces with ultraviolet light. Creatinuria accompanies acute myopathy but has not been used routinely as a diagnostic aid.

Electromyography is a special technique for the evaluation of the degree of neurogenic atrophy.

Necropsy findings

Affected areas of skeletal muscle have a white, waxy, swollen appearance like fish flesh. Commonly only linear strips of large muscle masses are affected and the distribution of lesions is characteristically bilaterally symmetrical. Histologically the lesion varies from a hyaline degeneration to a severe myonecrosis, with subsequently the disappearance of large groups of muscle fibers and replacement by connective tissue. Calcification of the affected tissue may be present to a mild degree in these cases.

The lesions in exertional rhabdomyolysis in the horse are of a focal distribution and consist of hyaline degeneration with insignificant inflammatory reaction and slight calcification. The degenerative changes affect primarily the fast twitch fibers which have a low oxidative capacity and are used when the horse trots at very close to its maximal speed (3).

Diagnosis

Most myopathies in farm animals occur in rapidly growing young animals and are characterized clinically by a sudden onset of acute muscular weakness, and pain often precipitated by unaccustomed exercise. There may be evidence of a dietary deficiency of vitamin and selenium in the case of nutritional muscular dystrophy. A sudden onset of recumbency or stiffness in young farm animals which are bright and alert should arouse suspicion of acute muscular dystrophy. Primary myopathies are not common in adult cattle, sheep or swine but myopathy secondary to recumbency for other reasons does occur. The exertional myopathies in the horse in training are usually readily obvious. The determinations of CPK and SGOT levels are valuable aids to diagnosis. In special circumstances, such as neurogenic myopathy, muscle biopsy and electromyography may be useful additional diagnostic aids. The histological and histochemical staining characteristics of equine muscle have been described and serve as a standard for comparison with abnormal muscle (36).

Myositis may present a similar syndrome but is usually present as a secondary lesion in a clinically distinguishable primary disease or is accompanied by obvious trauma or toxemia.

Treatment

Vitamin E and selenium are indicated for the treatment of nutritional muscular dystrophy and the details are provided under that heading. The treatment of exertional rhabdomyolysis in horses has not been well defined because of the uncertain etiology, but enforced rest and the relief of pain, if necessary, seems logical. Supportive therapy for any case of myopathy, particularly severe cases in which there is persistent recumbency, consists of liberal quantities of thick bedding, removal from solid floors to softer ground, frequent turning from side to side to minimize secondary myopathy, the provision of fluid therapy to prevent myoglobinuric nephrosis and a palatable, nutritious diet. With the exception of the sporadically occurring congenital and inherited myopathies of farm animals, all of the nutritional and exertional myopathies are amenable to treatment if it is begun early and if adequate supportive therapy is provided.

In myopathies associated with systemic acidosis the use of solution of sodium bicarbonate may be indicated (22). Dietary sodium bicarbonate at the rate of 2% of total dry matter intake has been used for the treatment of exertional rhabdomyolysis in a horse (37). Horses with postanesthetic myositis must be considered as critical care patients for 18–24 hours. Maintenance of adequate renal perfusion is vital. Large quantities of intravenous polyionic balanced electrolyte fluids (50–100 liters) must be given over a 24-hour period. Dantrolene sodium at 4 mg/kg body weight given orally immediately upon recognition of clinical signs is efficacious (25).

Control

The nutritional myopathies in farm animals can be satisfactorily prevented by the provision of adequate quantities of dietary vitamin E and selenium. The prevention of exertional myopathy in the horse depends on a progressive training program and avoidance of sudden unaccustomed exercise in animals which are in good body condition and have been inactive. Similarly, in general terms, the prevention of the porcine stress syndrome will depend on careful handling and transportation techniques combined with genetic selection of resistant pigs.

REVIEW LITERATURE

Bartsch, R. C., McConnell, E. E., Imes, G. D. & Schmidt, J. M. (1977) A review of exertional rhabdomyolysis in wild and domestic animals. *Vet. Pathol.*, *14*, 314.

Blaxter, K. L. (1974) Myopathies in animals. In: *Disorders of Voluntary Muscles*, ed. J. N. Walton, 3rd edn, pp. 907–940. Edinburgh: Churchill Livingstone.

Breazile, J. E. (1976) Electrolyte and energy metabolism of muscle: basic concepts. *Proc. 22nd ann. Conv. Am. Assoc. equ. Practnrs*, p. 187.

Carlson, G. P. & Nelson, T. (1976) Exercise-related muscle problems in endurance horses. *Proc. 22nd ann. Conv. Am. Assoc. equ. Practnrs*, p. 223.

Coffman, J. D. et al. (1978) Pathophysiologic evaluation of neuromuscular disorders in horses. *J. equ. med. Surg.*, *2*, 85.

McLean, J. G. (1973) Equine paralytic myoglobinuria ('azoturia'): a review. *Aust. vet. J.*, *49*, 341.

Milne, D. W., Gabel, A. A., Muir, W. W. & Skarda, R. T. (1976) Effects of exercise and training on cardiovascular and biochemical values in the horse. *Proc. 22nd ann. Conv. Am. Assoc. equ. Practnrs*, p. 211.

Snow, D. H. & Guy, P. S. (1976) The structure and biochemistry of equine muscle. *Proc. 22nd ann. Conv. Am. Assoc. Equ. Practnrs*, p. 199.

REFERENCES

(1) Blaxter, K. L. (1974) In: *Disorders of Voluntary Muscle*, ed. J. N. Walton, 3rd edn, pp. 907–946. Edinburgh: Churchill Livingstone.
(2) ap Owen, R. R. et al. (1977) *J. Am.vet. med. Assoc.*, *171*, 343.
(3) Lindholm, A. et al. (1974) *Acta vet. Scand.*, *15*, 325.
(4) Wobeser, G . et al. (1976) *J. Am. vet. med. Assoc.*, *169*, 1971.
(5) Bartsch, R. C. et al. (1977) *Vet. Pathol.*, *14*, 314.
(6) Dollahite, J. W. & Henson, J. B. (1965) *Am. J.vet. Res.*, *26*, 749.
(7) Holmes, J. H. G. et al. (1972) *Vet. Rec.*, *90*, 625.
(8) Rasmusen, B. A. & Christian, L. L. (1976) *Science, NY*, *191*, 947.
(9) Ollivier, L. et al. (1975) *Ann. Génét.*, *7*, 159.
(10) Steinhardt, M. et al. (1976) *Mh. VetMed.*, *31*, 449, 606, 655.
(11) Lannek, N. (1976) *Svensk VetTidskr.*, *28*, 3.
(12) Hoekstra, W. G. (1975) *Fedn Proc. Fedn Am. Soc. exp. Biol.*, *34*, 2090.
(13) Hartley, W. J. & Dodd, D. C. (1957) *NZ vet. J.*, *5*, 61.
(14) Anderson, P. H. et al. (1977) *Br. vet. J.*, *133*, 160.
(15) Milne, D. W. et al. (1976) *Am. J vet. Res.*, *37*, 285.
(16) Anderson, M. G. (1975) *Equ. vet. J.*, *7*, 160.
(17) Milne, D. W. (1975) *J. S. Afr. vet. med. Assoc.*, *45*, 345.
(18) Snow, D. H. & Guy, P. S. (1976) *Equ. vet. J.*, *8*, 150.
(19) Climie, A. R. W. (1973) *Am. J. clin. Pathol*, *60*, 753.
(20) Carlson, G. P. & Nelson, T. (1976) *Proc. 22nd ann. Conv. Am. Assoc. equ. Practnrs*, p. 223.
(21) McLean, J. G. (1973) *Aust. vet. J.*, *49*, 341.
(22) Harthorn, A. M. & Young, E. (1974) *Vet. Rec.*, *95*, 337.
(23) Waldron-Mease, E. & Rosenberg, H. (1979) *Vet. Sci. Commun.*, *3*, 45.
(24) Johnson, B. D. et al. (1978) *J. equ. med. Surg.*, *2*, 109.
(25) Klein, L. (1978) *Proc. 24th Conv. Am. Assoc. equ. Pract.*, p. 89.
(26) Peet, R. L. et al. (1980) *Aust. vet. J.*, *56*, 155.
(27) Bradley, R. (1981) *In Practice*, *3(2)*, 5.
(28) Goedegebuure, S. A. et al. (1983) *Vet. Pathol.*, *20*, 32.
(29) Bradley, R. and Duffell, S. J. (1982) *J. comp. Pathol.*, *92*, 85.
(30) Hamir, A. N. (1982) *Vet. Rec.*, *111*, 367.
(31) Essen-Gustavsson, B. & Lindholm, A. (1985) *Equ. vet. J.*, *17*, 434.
(32) Valberg, S. et al. (1985) *Equ. vet. J.*, *17*, 439.
(33) Bruce, V. & Turek, R. J. (1985) *Equ. vet. J.*, *17.*, 317.
(34) van den Hoven, R. et al. (1985) *Am. J. vet. Res.*, *46*, 939.
(35) van den Hoven, R. et al. (1985) *Am. J. vet. Res.*, *46*, 1755.
(36) Andrews, F. M. & Spurgeon, T. L. (1986) *Am. J. vet. Res.*, *47*, 1843.
(37) Robb, E. J. & Kronfeld, D. S. (1986) *J. Am. vet. med. Assoc.*, *188*, 602.
(38) Koterba, A. & Carlson, G. P. (1982) *J. Am. vet. med. Assoc.*, *180*, 303.

Myositis

Myositis may arise from direct or indirect trauma to muscle and occurs as part of a syndrome in a number of specific diseases including blackleg, foot-and-mouth disease, bluetongue, ephemeral fever, swine influenza, sarcosporidiosis and trichinosis, although clinical signs of myositis are not usually evident in the latter. An asymptomatic eosinophilic myositis is not uncommon in beef cattle and may cause economic loss through carcass condemnation (1). The cause has not been determined.

Acute myositis of limb muscles is accompanied by severe lameness, swelling, heat and pain on palpation. There may be accompanying toxemia and fever. In chronic myositis there is much wasting of the affected muscles and this is difficult to differentiate clinically from atrophy due to other causes. Biopsy of the muscle may be necessary to confirm the diagnosis. In horses traumatic myositis of the posterior thigh muscles may be followed by the formation of fibrous adhesions between the muscles (fibrotic myopathy) and by subsequent calcification of the adhesions (ossifying myopathy). External trauma can result in fibrotic myopathy, but it may also be associated with excessive exercise or secondary to intramuscular injections (4). Occasionally similar lesions may be seen in the foreleg. The lesions cause a characteristic abnormality of the gait in that the stride is short in extension and the foot is suddenly withdrawn as it is about to reach the ground. The affected area is abnormal on palpation (2). An inherited disease of pigs, generalized myositis ossificans, is also characterized by deposition of bone in soft tissues (3). In traumatic injuries caused by penetration of foreign bodies into muscle masses, ultrasonography may be used to detect fistulous tracts and the foreign bodies (5).

Extensive damage to or loss of muscle occurs in screwworm and sometimes blowfly infestation, although the latter is more of a cutaneous lesion, and by the injection of necrotizing agents. For example, massive cavities can be induced in the cervical muscles of horses by the intramuscular injection of escharotic iron preparations intended only for slow intravenous injection. Similarly, necrotic lesions can result from the intramuscular injection of infected or irritant substances. Horses are particularly sensitive to tissue injury, or are at least most commonly affected. Some common causes are chloral hydrate, antibiotics suspended in propylene glycol, and even antibiotics by themselves in some horses.

REFERENCES

(1) Reitten, A. C. et al. (1966) *Am. J. vet. Res.*, *27*, 903.
(2) Adams, O. R. (1961) *J. Am. vet. med. Assoc.*, *139*, 1089.
(3) Seibold, H. R. & Davis, C. L. (1967) *Pathol. vet.*, *4*, 79.
(4) Turner, A. S. & Trotter, G. W. (1984) *J. Am. vet. med. Assoc.*, *184*, 335.
(5) Cartee, R. E. & Rumph, P. F. (1984) *J. Am. vet. med. Assoc.*, *184*, 1127.

DISEASES OF BONES

Osteodystrophy

Osteodystrophy is a general term used to describe those diseases of bones in which there is a failure of normal bone development, or abnormal metabolism of bone which is already mature. The major clinical manifestations include distortion and enlargement of the bones, susceptibility to fractures and interference with gait and posture.

Etiology

The common causes of osteodystrophy in farm animals include the following.

Nutritional causes

- Calcium, phosphorus and vitamin D. Absolute deficiencies or imbalances in calcium-phosphorus ratios in diets cause
  - rickets in young animals (1), for example, growing lambs fed a diet rich in wheat bran (24)
  - osteomalacia in adult ruminants (4)
  - osteodystrophia in adult pigs and horses
- Copper deficiency in diet can cause
  - osteoporosis in lambs (3)
  - epiphysitis in young cattle (4)
- Inadequate dietary protein (5) and general undernutrition of cattle (6) and sheep can result in severe osteoporosis and a great increase in ease of fracture
- Chronic parasitism can cause osteodystrophy in young growing ruminants (25)
- Hypovitaminosis A (8) and hypervitaminosis A (7) can cause osteodystrophic changes in cattle and swine
- Prolonged feeding of a diet high in calcium to bulls can cause nutritional hypercalcitoninism combined with replacement of trabecular bone in the vertebrae and long bones with compact bone, and neoplasms of the ultimobranchial gland (9). Similar lesions occur in the dog (10)
- Multiple vitamin and mineral deficiencies are recorded as causing osteodystrophy in cattle (11). The mineral demands of lactation in cattle can result in a decrease in bone mineral content during lactation with a subsequent increase during the dry period (32).

Chemical agents

- Chronic lead poisoning is reputed to cause osteoporosis in lambs and foals
- Chronic fluorine poisoning causes the characteristic lesions of osteofluorosis including osteoporosis and exostoses
- Grazing the poisonous plant *Setaria sphaceleta*, *Cenchrus ciliaris*, *Panicum maximum* var. *trichoglume* (21, 22) causes osteodystrophia in horses
- Enzootic calcinosis of muscles and other tissues is caused by the ingestion of *Solanum malacoxylon* (23), *S. torvum* (34), *Trisetum flavescens* (yellow outgrass) and *Cestrum diurnum* which exert a vitamin D-like activity. The subject has been reviewed (26)
- Bowie or bentleg, a disease caused by poisoning with *Trachymene glaucifolia* is characterized by extreme outward bowing of the bones of the front limbs.

Inherited and congenital causes

There are many inherited and congenital defects of bones of newborn farm animals which are described on pp. 1388–1394, and presented in detail in Chapter 34 on inherited diseases. A summary of them includes:

- Achondroplasia and chondrodystrophy in dwarf calves and some cases of prolonged gestation
- Osteogenesis imperfecta in lambs (31) and Charolais cattle (27). There is marked bone fragility and characteristic changes on radiological examination
- Osteopetrosis in Hereford and Angus calves (28, 29)
- Chondrodystrophy in 'acorn' calves
- Inherited exostoses in horses, inherited thicklegs and inherited rickets of pigs are well-established entities
- Angular deformities of joints of long bones due to asymmetric growth plate activity (30) are common in foals and are commonly repaired surgically. The distal radius and distal metacarpus are most often affected, distal tibia and metatarsal less commonly (20). Physiologically immature foals subjected to exercise may develop compression-type fractures of the central or third tarsal bones (35). Some of these foals are born prematurely or are of twin pregnancies. Retained cartilage in the distal radial physis of foals from 3 to 70 days of age presents without apparent clinical signs (37).

Physical

In recent years there has been an obvious increase in cases of moderate osteodystrophy and arthropathy in rapidly growing pigs and cattle fed diets which contain adequate amounts of calcium, phosphorus and vitamin D. Cattle and pigs raised indoors on slatted floors or concrete floors are most commonly affected and it is thought that traumatic injury of the epiphyses and condyles of long bones may be the mitigating factor resulting in osteochondrosis and arthrosis in the pig (leg weakness) (12, 13) and epiphysitis in cattle (15). Experimentally, raising young calves on metal slatted floors may result in more severe and more numerous lesions of the epiphysis than occurs in calves raised on clay floors (14). Total confinement rearing of lambs can result in the development of epiphysiolysis and limb deformities (38). However, the importance of weight-bearing injury as a cause of osteodystrophy in farm animals is still obscure. In most reports of such osteodystrophy, all other known causes have not been eliminated. Abnormal bone growth can be induced experimentally by unilateral hip excision arthroplasty in skeletally immature lambs (39) which indicates that altered weight-bearing can affect endochondral bone growth (39). This may partially explain the deformities which are associated with abnormal conformation. Chronic osteodystrophy and arthropathy have been associated with undesirable conformation in the horse (16). Vertebral exostoses are not uncommon in old bulls and usually affect the thoracic vertebrae (T2 and T12) and the lumbar vertebrae (L2–L3) which are subjected to increased pressure during the bending of the vertebral columns during breeding. The exostoses occur mainly on the ventral aspects of the vertebrae, fusing them to cause immobility of the region. Fracture of the ossification may occur resulting in partial displacement of the vertebral column and spinal cord compression (17). The disease is commonly referred to as spondylitis or vertebral osteochondrosis and also occurs less commonly in adult cows and in pigs. The pathogenesis suggested for the disease is that the annulus fibrosus degenerates and the resulting malfunctioning of the disk allows excessive mobility of the vertebral bodies leading to the stimulation of new bone formation (17). A similar lesion occurs commonly in horses and may affect performance, particularly in hurdle races and crosscountry events (18). The initial lesion may be a degeneration of the intervertebral disk (19). Some types of growth plate defects occur in young growing foals and these are considered to be traumatic in origin (20). Failure of chondrogenesis of the growth plate may be the result of crush injuries in heavy rapidly growing foals with interruption of the vascular supply to the germinal cells of the growth plate. Asymmetrical pressures due to abnormal muscle pull or joint laxity may slow growth on the affected side and result in limb angulation (20).

Pathogenesis

There are some species differences in the abnormalities which occur with dietary deficiencies of calcium, phosphorus and vitamin D. Rickets and osteomalacia occur primarily in ruminants and osteodystrophia fibrosa in horses, and all three may occur in pigs.

Osteodystrophia fibrosa occurs most commonly in the horse receiving a diet low in calcium and high in phosphorus. Osteodystrophia fibrosa occurs commonly in swine as a sequel to rickets and osteomalacia which may occur together in young growing swine which are placed on rations deficient in calcium, phosphorus and vitamin D following weaning.

In rickets, which occurs in the young growing animal, there is a failure of provisional calcification of the osteoid plus a failure of mineralization of the cartilaginous matrix of developing bone. There is also failure of degeneration of growing cartilage, formation of osteoid on persistent cartilage with irregularity of osteochondral junctions and overgrowth of fibrous tissue in the osteochondral zone. Failure of provisional calcification of cartilage results in an increased depth and width of the epiphyseal plates of particularly the long bones (humerus, radius and ulna and tibia) and the costal cartilages of the ribs. The uncalcified, and therefore soft, tissues of the metaphyses and epiphyses become distorted under the pressure of weight-bearing which also causes medial or lateral deviation of the shafts of long bones. There is a decreased rate of longitudinal growth of long bones and enlargement of the ends of long bones due to the effects of weight causing flaring of the diaphysis adjacent to the epiphyseal plate. Within the thickened and widened epiphyseal plate there may be hemorrhages, minute fractures of adjacent trabecular bone of the metaphyses and in chronic cases the hemorrhagic zone may be largely replaced by fibrous tissue. These changes can be seen radiographically as '*epiphysitis*' and clinically as enlargements of the ends of long bones and costochondral junctions the ribs. These changes at the epiphyses may result in separation of the epiphysis which commonly affects the femoral head. The articular cartilages may remain normal or there may be subarticular collapse resulting in grooving and folding of the articular cartilage and ultimately degenerative arthropathy and osteochondrosis. Eruption of the teeth in rickets is irregular and dental attrition is rapid. Growth of the mandibles is retarded and combined with abnormal dentition. There may be marked malocclusion of the teeth.

In osteomalacia there is softening of mature bone due to extensive resorption of mineral deposits in bone and failure of mineralization of newly formed matrix. There are no enlargement of the ends of long bones or distortions of long bones but spontaneous fractures of any bone subjected to weight-bearing are common.

Osteodystrophia fibrosa may be superimposed on rickets or osteomalacia and occurs in secondary hyperparathyroidism. Diets low in calcium or which contain a relative excess of phosphorus cause secondary hyperparathyroidism. There is extensive resorption of bone and replacement by connective tissue. The disease is best known in the horse and results in swelling of the mandibles, the maxillae and frontal bones (the 'bighead' syndrome). Spontaneous fracture of long bones and ribs occurs commonly. Radiographically there is extreme porosity of the entire skeleton.

Osteoporosis is due to failure or inadequacy of the formation of the organic matrix of bone and the bone becomes porous, light, fragile and fractures easily. Osteoporosis is not common in farm animals and is usually associated with general undernutrition rather than specifically a deficiency of calcium, phosphorus or vitamin D. Copper deficiency in lambs may result in osteoporosis due to impaired osteoblastic activity (3).

Chronic lead poisoning in lambs also results in osteoporosis due to deficient production of osteoid. In a series of 19 lactating or recently weaned sows with a history of lameness, weakness or paralysis, ten had osteoporosis and pathological fractures while six had lumbar vertebral osteomyelitis (42). Bone ash, specific gravity of bone and the cortical-to-total ratio were significantly reduced in sows with osteoporosis and pathological fractures.

The osteodystrophy of chronic fluorosis is characterized by the development of exostoses on the shafts of long bones due to periosteal hyperostosis. The articular surfaces remain essentially normal but there is severe lameness due to the involvement of the periosteum and encroachment of the osteophytes on the tendons and ligaments.

Congenital defects of bone include complete (achondroplasia) and partial (chondrodystrophy) failure of normal development of cartilage. Growth of the cartilage is restricted and disorganized and mineralization is reduced. The affected bones fail to grow, leading to gross deformity, particularly of the bones of the head.

Clinical findings

In general terms there is weakening of the bones due to defective mineralization and osteoporosis, which results in the bending of bones which probably causes pain and shifting lameness which is one of the earliest clinical signs of acquired osteodystrophy. The normal weight and tension stresses cause distortion of the normal axial relationships of the bones which results in the bowing of long bones. The distortions occur most commonly in young growing animals. The distal ends of the long bones are commonly enlarged at the level of the epiphyseal plate and circumscribed swellings of the soft tissue around the epiphyses may be prominent and painful on palpation.

The effects of osteodystrophy on appetite and body weight will depend on the severity of the lesions and their distribution. In the early stages of rickets in calves and pigs the appetite and growth rate may not be grossly affected until the disease is advanced and causes considerable pain. Persistent recumbency due to pain will indirectly affect feed intake unless animals are hand-fed.

Unexpected fractures occur commonly and usually in mature animals. Common sites for fractures include the long bones of the limbs, pelvic girdle femoral head, vertebrae, ribs and transverse processes of the vertebrae. Ordinary hand pressure or moderate restraint of animals with osteomalacia and osteodystrophia fibrosa is often sufficient to cause a fracture. The rib cage tends to become flattened and in the late stages affected animals have a slab-sided appearance of the thorax and abdomen. Separations of tendons from their bony insertions also occur more frequently and cause severe lameness. The osteoporotic state of the bone makes such separations easy. Any muscle group may be affected but in young cattle in feedlots, separation of the gastrocnemius is the most common. Thickening of the bones may be detectable clinically if the deposition of osteoid or fibrous tissue is excessive, or if exostoses develop as in fluorosis. Compression of the spinal cord or spinal nerves may lead to paresthesia, paresis or paralysis which may be localized in distribution. Details of the clinical findings in the osteodystrophies caused by nutritional deficiencies are provided in Chapter 29.

Calcinosis of cattle is characterized clinically by chronic wasting, lameness, ectopic calcifications of the cardiovascular system, lungs and kidneys, ulceration of joint cartilage and extensive calcification of bones.

Clinical pathology

The laboratory analyses which may be indicated include the following: serum calcium and phosphorus, serum alkaline phosphatase, feed analysis for calcium, phosphorus, vitamin D and other minerals when indicated (such as copper, molybdenum and fluorine), bone ash chemical analysis, histopathology of bone biopsy and radiographic examination of the skeleton. Single photon absorptiometry, a safe and non-invasive method for the measurement of bone mineral content is now available (32, 40).

The serum calcium and phosphorus concentrations in nutritional osteodystrophies may remain within the normal range for long periods and not until the lesions are well advanced will abnormal levels be found. Several successive samplings may be necessary to identify an abnormal trend. The serum alkaline phosphatase levels may be increased in the presence of increased bone resorption but is not a reliable indicator of osteodystrophy. Increased serum levels of alkaline phosphatase may originate from osseous tissues, intestine or liver (41) but osseous tissue appears to be the major source of activity. The nutritional history and results of analyses of feed will often provide the best circumstantial evidence of osteodystrophy. The definitive diagnosis is best made by a combination of chemical analysis of bone, histopathological examination of bone and radiography. The details for each of the common osteodystrophies are discussed under the appropriate headings.

Necropsy findings

The pathological findings vary with the cause, and the details are described under each of the osteodystrophies elsewhere in the book. In general terms, the nutritional osteodystrophies are characterized by bone deformities, bones which may cut easily with a knife and bend or break easily with hand pressure and the presence in prolonged cases of degenerative joint disease. In young growing animals the ends of long bones may be enlarged and the epiphyses may be prominent and circumscribed by periosteal and fibrous tissue thickening. On longitudinal cut sections the cortices may appear thinner than normal and the trabecular bone may have been resorbed leaving an enlarged marrow cavity. The epiphyseal plate may be increased in depth and width and appear grossly irregular, and small fractures involving the epiphyseal plate and adjacent metaphysis may be present. Separation of epiphyses are common, particularly of the femoral head. The calluses of healed fractures of long bones, ribs, vertebrae and pelvic girdle are common in pigs with osteodystrophy. On histological examination there are varying degrees of severity of rickets in young growing animals, osteomalacia in adult animals and osteodystrophia fibrosa is possible in both young and adult animals.

Diagnosis

In both congenital and acquired osteodystrophy the clinical findings are usually suggestive. There are varying degrees of lameness, stiff gait, long periods of recumbency, failure to perform physical work normally, progressive loss of body weight in some cases and there may be obvious contortions of long bones, ribs, head and vertebral column. The most common cause of osteodystrophy in young growing animals is a dietary deficiency or imbalance of calcium, phosphorus and vitamin D. If the details of the nutritional history are available and if a representative sample of the feed which was fed is analyzed, a clinical diagnosis can be made on the basis of clinical findings, nutritional history and response to treatment. In some cases, it may be due to overfeeding such as might occur in rapidly growing large foals.

However, often the nutritional history may indicate that the animals have been receiving adequate quantities of calcium, phosphorus and vitamin D which necessitates that other less common cause of osteodystrophy be considered. Often the first clue is an unfavorable response to treatment with calcium, phosphorus and vitamin D. Examples include copper deficiency in cattle, leg-weakness in swine of uncertain etiology but perhaps due to weight-bearing trauma and a relative lack of exercise due to confinement, chemical poisoning such as enzootic calcinosis or fluorosis. These will require laboratory evaluation of serum biochemistry, radiography of affected bones and pathological examination. The presence of bony deformities at birth suggests congenital chondrodystrophy, some cases of which appear to be inherited and some due to environmental influences.

Treatment

The common nutritional osteodystrophies due to a dietary deficiency or imbalance of calcium, phosphorus and vitamin D will usually respond favorably following the oral adminstration of a suitable source of calcium and phosphorus combined with parenteral injections of vitamin D. The oral administration of dicalcium phosphate at the rate of three to four times the daily requirement, daily for 6 days followed by a reduction to the daily requirement by the tenth day, combined with one injection of vitamin D at the rate of 10 000 IU/kg body weight is recommended. Affected animals are placed on a diet which contains the required levels and ratios of calcium, phosphorus and vitamin D. The oral administration of the calcium and phosphorus will result in increased absorption of the minerals which will restore depleted skeletal reserves. Calcium absorption is increased in adult animals following a period of calcium deficiency and young animals with high growth requirements absorb and retain calcium in direct relation to intake (33). General supportive measures include adequate bedding for animals which are recumbent.

The treatment of the osteodystrophies due to causes other than calcium and phosphorus deficiencies will depend on the cause. Copper deficiency will respond gradually to copper supplementation. There is no specific treatment for the osteodystrophy associated with leg-weakness in pigs and slaughter for salvage is often necessary. Overnutrition in young rapidly growing foals may require a marked reduction in the total amount of feed made available daily.

REFERENCES

(1) Nisbet, D. I. et al. (1966) *J. comp. Pathol.*, *76*, 159.
(2) Nisbet, D. I. et al. (1970) *J. comp. Pathol.*, *80*, 535.
(3) Suttle, N. F. et al. (1972) *J. comp. Pathol.*, *82*, 93.
(4) Smith, B. P. et al. (1975) *J. Am. vet. med. Assoc.*, *166*, 682.
(5) Siebert, B. D. et al. (1975) *Aust. J. exp. Agric. Anim. Husb.*, *15*, 321.
(6) Herrmann, H. J. (1965) *Pathol. vet.*, *2*, 468.
(7) Davis, T. E. et al. (1970) *Cornell Vet.*, *60*, 90.
(8) Dobson, K. J. (1969) *Aust. vet. J.*, *45*, 570.
(9) Krook, L. et al. (1971) *Cornell Vet.*, *61*, 625.
(10) Hedhammer, A. et al. (1974) *Cornell Vet.*, *64*, suppl. 5.
(11) Massip, A. & Pondant, A. (1975) *Zentralbl. VetMed.*, *22A*, 265.
(12) Grondalen, T. (1974) *Nord. VetMed.*, *26*, 534.
(13) Reiland, S. (1974) *Svensk VetTidn.*, 2628.
(14) White, S. et al. (1984) *Am. J. vet. Res.*, *45*, 633.
(15) Murphy, P. A. et al. (1975) *Vet. Rec.*, *97*, 445.
(16) Haakenstad, L. H. (1969) *Equ. vet. J.*, *1*, 248.
(17) Thomson, R. G. (1969) *Pathol. vet.*, *6*, Suppl. 46.
(18) Smythe, R. (1962) *Mod. vet. Pract.*, *43*, 50.
(19) Hansen, H. J. (1959) *Lab Invest.*, *8*, 1242.
(20) Vaughan, L. C. (1976) *Vet. Rec.*, *98*, 165.
(21) Groenendyk, S. & Seawright, A. A. (1974) *Aust. vet. J.*, *50*, 131.
(22) Walthall, J. C. & McKenzie, R. A. (1976) *Aust. vet. J.*, *52*, 11.
(23) Dobereiner, J. et al. (1975) *Br. vet. J.*, *131*, 175.
(24) Mahin, L. (1984) *Vet. Rec.*, *115*, 355.
(25) Frandsen, J. C. (1982) *Am J. vet. Rec.*, *43*, 1951.
(26) Simesen, M. G. (1977) *Nord. VetMed.*, *29*, 76.
(27) Jensen, P. T. et al. (1976) *Nord. VetMed.*, *28*, 304.
(28) Ojo, S. A. et al. (1975) *J. Am. vet. med. Assoc.*, *166*, 781.
(29) Greene, H. J. et al. (1974) *J. Am. vet. med. Assoc.*, *164*, 389.
(30) Brown, M. P. & MacCallum, F. J. (1976) *Vet. Rec.*, *98*, 443.
(31) Kater, J. C . et al. (1963) *NZ vet. J.*, *11*, 41.
(32) Holmberg, T. et al. (1985) *Acta vet. Scand.*, *26*, 49.
(33) Braithwaite, G. D. (1976) *J. dairy Res.*, *43*, 501.
(34) Morris, K. M. L. et al. (1979) *Res. vet. Sci.*, *27*, 264.
(35) Dewes, H. F. (1982) *NZ vet. J.*, *30*, 129.
(36) Wasserman, R. H. (1977) *Cornell Vet.*, *67*, 333.
(37) Firth, E. C. & Poulos, P. W. (1984). *Vet. Pathol.*, *21*, 10.
(38) Uhthoff, H. K. et al. (1982) *Ann. réch. vét.*, *13*, 237.
(39) Duff, S. R. I. (1986) *J. comp. Pathol.*, *96*, 3, 15 & 25.
(40) Jeffcott, L. B. et al. (1986) *Vet. Rec.*, *118*, 499.
(41) Trueman, K. F. et al. (1983) *Can. vet. J.*, *24*, 108.
(42) Doige, C. E. (1982) *Can. J. comp. Med.*, *46*, 1.

Hypertrophic pulmonary osteoarthropathy (Marie's disease, achropachia ossea)

Although hypertrophic pulmonary osteoarthropathy is more common in dogs than in the other domestic animals it has been observed in horses (1–3), cattle (4, 5) and sheep (6). The disease is characterized by proliferation of the periosteum leading to the formation of periosteal bone, and bilateral symmetrical enlargement of bones, usually the long bones of limbs. The enlargement is quite obvious, and in the early stages is usually painful and often accompanied by local edema. On radiographical examination there is a shaggy periostitis and evidence of periosteal exostosis. The pathogenesis is obscure but the lesion appears to be neurogenic in origin, unilateral vagotomy causing regression of the bony changes (7). Stiffness of gait and reluctance to move are usually present, and there may be clinical evidence of the pulmonary lesion with which the disease is almost always associated. Such lesions are usually chronic, neoplastic or suppurative processes such as tuberculosis (8). The disease is considered to be incurable, unless the thoracic lesion can be removed, and affected animals are usually euthanized. At necropsy the periostitis, exostosis and pulmonary disease are evident. There is no involvement of the joints.

REFERENCES

(1) Alexander, J. E. et al. (1965) *J. Am. vet. med. Assoc.*, *146*, 703.
(2) Goodbarry, R. F. & Hage, T. J. (1960) *J. Am. vet. med. Assoc.*, *137*. 602.
(3) Holmes, J. R. (1961) *Vet. Rec.*, *73*, 333.
(4) Hofmeyr, C. F. B. (1964) *Berl. Munch. Tierarztl. Wochenschr.*, *77*, 319.
(5) Merritt, A. M. et al. (1971) *J. Am. vet. med. Assoc.*, *159*, 443.
(6) Carre, H. et al. (1936) *C.R. Séances Soc. Biol.*, *123*, 557.
(7) Holling, H. E. et al. (1961) *Lancet*, *7215*, 1269.
(8) Kersjes, A. W. et al. (1968) *Neth. J. vet. Sci.*, *1*, 55.

Osteomyelitis

Inflammation of bone is uncommon in farm animals except when infection is introduced by traumatic injury or by the hematogenous route. Focal metaphyseal osteomyelitis can occur following open fractures in the horse (9). Specific diseases which may be accompanied by osteomyelitis include actinomycosis of cattle and brucellosis, atrophic rhinitis, and necrotic rhinitis of pigs. Non-specific, hematogenous infection with other bacteria occurs sporadically and is often associated with omphalitis, abscesses from tail-biting in pigs or infection of castration or docking wounds in lambs.

Osteomyelitis is characteristically accompanied by severe, persistent pain. Erosion of bone occurs and pus discharges into surrounding tissues causing a cellulitis or phlegmon, and to the exterior through sinuses which persist for long periods. The affected bone is often swollen and fractures easily because of weakening of its structure. When the bones of the jaw are involved, the teeth are often shed and this, together with pain and the distortion of the jaw, interferes with prehension and mastication. Involvement of vertebral bodies may lead to the secondary involvement of the meninges and the development of paralysis. Lameness and local swelling are the major manifestations of involvement of the limb bones.

Foals and calves under one month of age (6) and growing cattle from 6 to 12 months of age may be affected by osteomyelitis in one or more bones (2, 4, 5). The majority of foals with suppurative polyarthritis have a polyosteomyelitis of the bones adjacent to the affected joints. In a series of cases of tarsal osteomyelitis in foals there was usually evidence of infectious arthritis (7). The infections occur commonly in the metaphysis, physis and epiphysis which are sites of bony growth and thus susceptible to blood-borne infections. The metaphyseal blood vessels loop towards the physis and ramify into sinusoids which spread throughout the metaphyseal region. Blood flow through the sinusoids is sluggish and presents an ideal environment for propagation of bacteria (6). Lesions occur on both sides of the physis—in both the metaphysis and the epiphysis. Multiple lesions are common and support the explanation that septic emboli are released from a central focus.

Hematogenous osteomyelitis in cattle can be of the physeal type in which an infection generally of metaphyseal bone originates at or near the growth plate usually affecting the distal metacarpus, metatarsus, radius or tibia (10); or the epiphyseal type in which an infection originates near the junction of the subchondral bone and the immature epiphyseal joint cartilage most often affecting the distal femoral condyle epiphysis, the patellar and the distal radius. The epiphyseal osteomyelitides are usually due to infection with *Salmonella* spp. and are most common in calves under 12 weeks of age. The physeal infections are usually due to *Actinomyces (Corynebacterium) pyogenes* and occur most commonly in cattle over 6 months of age.

The lesions are typically destructive of bone and cause severe pain and lameness. Those caused by *Salmonella* spp. are characteristic radiographically in foals and calves (6). *A. pyogenes*, *Corynebacterium* spp. and *Escherichia coli* may also be causative agents. Affected animals are very lame and the origin of the lameness may not be obvious. A painful discrete soft tissue swelling over the ends of the long bones is often the first indication. The lameness characteristically persists in spite of medical therapy and the animal may become lame in two or more limbs and spend long periods recumbent. Radiographic changes include: a necrotic sequestrum initially, new bone formation and loss of bone density. The lesions are characteristically centered at the growth and extend into both metaphysis and epiphysis. At necropsy the osteomyelitis may not be obvious unless the bones are opened longitudinally and the cut surfaces of the metaphysis and epiphysis examined.

A differential diagnosis for a destructive lesion in the end of a long bone of a foal or calf would include: a healing fracture, traumatic periostitis or osteitis, bone tumor, nutritional osteodystrophy and infection of the bone due to external trauma, fracture, extension from adjacent infection, or hematogenous spread. The absence of equal pathologic involvement in the comparable parts of long bones and the young age of the animal will usually suggest infection on bone. The pathologic features of multiple bone infection in foals is described (4).

Medical therapy is rarely completely successful because of the poor vascularity of the affected solid bone and the inaccessibility of the infection. A long course of antibiotics administered parenterally may control the infection, but local surgical treatment and drainage is much more effective (1–3). Good results are obtained when the affected bone is removed and the affected area irrigated daily through a temporary drainage tube (3). The exudate should be cultured and antibiotic sensitivity tests done to determine the drug of choice. Parenteral antibiotic therapy should be continued for 4–6 weeks following surgical curettage.

Anaerobic bacteria are frequently associated with osteomyelitis and should be considered when submitting samples for culture (8). Specimens should consist of sequestra and soft tissues immediately adjacent to bone thought to be infected. Special transport media are desirable for optimum culture results. Most anaerobic bacteria are sensitive to penicillin and the cephalosporins, but some species of *Bacteroides fragilis* and *B. asaccharolyticus* and other species of *Bacteroides* are known to produce beta-lactamases which can inactivate penicillin and cephalosporin. Metronidazole, chloramphenicol and clindamycin will penetrate bone and can be considered.

A special osteomyelitis is that which affects the cervical vertebrae, usually the 4th to the 6th vertebra, and causes a reasonably standard syndrome of abnormal posture and difficulty with ambulation. Initially there is a stumbling gait, which then becomes stiff and restricted and with a reluctance to bend the neck. Soon the animal has difficulty eating off the ground and must kneel to graze pasture. At this stage there is obvious atrophy of the cervical muscles and pain can be elicited by deep, forceful compression of the vertebrae with the fists. There is no response to treatment and at necropsy there is irreparable osteomyelitis of the vertebral body and compression of the cervical spinal cord. Radiological examination is usually confirmatory.

REFERENCES

(1) Weaver, A. D. (1972) *Br. vet. J.*, *128*, 470.
(2) Funk, K. A. (1978) *Berl. Munch. Tierarztl. Wochenschr.*, *91*, 276.
(3) Rose, R. J. (1978) *Vet. Rec.*, *102*, 498.
(4) Bennett, D. (1978) *Vet. Rec.*, *103*, 482.
(5) Moss, E. et al. (1971) *J. Am. vet. med. Assoc.*, *158*, 1369.
(6) Morgan, J. P. et al. (1974) *J. Am. vet. radiol. Soc.*, *15*, 66.
(7) Firth, E. C. et al. (1985) *Vet. Rec.*, *116*, 261.
(8) Walker, R. D. et al. (1983) *J. Am. vet. med. Assoc.*, *182*, 814.
(9) Stickle, R. L. et al. (1983) *J. Am. vet. med. Assoc.*, *183*, 797.
(10) Firth, E. C. et al. (1987) *Vet. Rec.*, *120*, 148.

DISEASES OF JOINTS

Arthropathy (osteoarthropathy, degenerative joint disease)

The terms osteoarthropathy and degenerative joint disease are used here to describe non-inflammatory lesions of the articular surfaces of joints characterized by degeneration and erosion of articular cartilage, eburnation of subchondral bones, and hypertrophy of bone surrounding the articular cartilage resulting in lipping and spur formation at the joint margins. Osteochondrosis is a degeneration of both the deep layers of the articular cartilage and the epiphyseal plate—a defect in endochondral ossification—which is now being recognized in pigs (1) and horses (2, 3) and is similar to the well-recognized disease in dogs. The current concepts of equine degenerative joint disease including pathogenesis, diagnosis, and treatment have been reviewed (3).

Etiology and epidemiology

The etiology is not clear but in most of the commonly occurring cases the lesions are considered to be secondary to conformational defects resulting in excessive joint laxity, acute traumatic injury of a joint, the normal aging process and nutritional deficiencies. The etiological information is primarily circumstantial and some of the epidemiological observations which have been associated with osteoarthritis of farm animals will be presented here.

Nutritional causes

- Secondary to, or associated with, rickets, osteomalacia, bowie and osteodystrophia fibrosa (14)
- Coxofemoral arthropathy in dairy cattle associated with aphosphorosis (4)
- Copper deficiency thought to be related to enlargement of limb joints in foals on pasture and pigs fed experimental copper-deficient diets
- Experimental diets deficient in manganese or magnesium can cause arthropathy and joint deformity in calves
- Experimental riboflavin deficiency in pigs.

Poisonings

- Chronic zinc poisoning in pigs and foals (2)
- Fluorosis in cattle (15)
- As part of the enzootic calcinosis syndrome caused by poisoning with *Solanum malacoxylon* and others.

Corticosteroid-induced

The intra-articular injection (17) or prolonged parenteral administration of corticosteroids (19) in horses can result in degenerative joint disease.

Trauma

- Acute traumatic injury, e.g. injury to joint surfaces, menisci and ligaments, especially the cruciate ligaments of the stifle joints of breeding bulls, may lead to chronic progressive osteoarthritis (5)
- Repeated subacute trauma to joint surfaces can lead to degenerative arthropathy. This is common in young racehorses in training which may have their joint surfaces and surrounding tissues made susceptible to injury because of conformational defects and subtle deficiencies of calcium and phosphorus. Degenerative joint disease of the proximal interphalangeal joints of young horses (20) and bilateral degenerative coxofemoral joint disease in a foal are recorded (21). Hard running surfaces may also contribute
- Trauma caused by movement is suspected of contributing to the erosive lesions on the articular surfaces of some horses affected by enzootic incoordination, the intervertebral joints of caudal thoracic and cranial lumbar vertebrae of old bulls with spondylitis, and in bulls with inherited spasticity.

Inheritance

- Degenerative arthropathy in aged dairy cows and bulls (16) which may be a manifestation of the normal aging process. Osteochondrosis, degenerative joint disease and vertebral osteophysis occurs in middle-aged bulls (40)
- Degenerative coxofemoral arthropathy in young beef bulls as early as 9 months of age. A congenital shallow acetabulum may predispose (11). It may be secondary to hip dysplasia (18), but in some cases is no evidence of this. The large, weight-bearing joints subjected to the greatest movement and concussion appear to be most susceptible. Rapidly growing bull calves appear to be most susceptible and some of them have an inherited susceptibility

(13). Osteoarthritis of the tarsal joint (spavin) of cattle may have an inherited basis but other factors such as housing and feeding intensity may be predisposing factors (38).

Conformation
Osteochondrosis is now described in growing pigs (34), horses (30–32) and young growing bulls (33). Osteochondrosis dissecans has become regarded as an important cause of lameness in horses. It is usually seen in young rapidly growing animals, and affects males more commonly than females (45). The stifle, hock and shoulder joints are more commonly affected, but many other joints may also be affected including the metatarsal and metacarpal bones (43) and rarely the acetabula of a 3-week old foal (44). The most common sites of equine osteochondrosis, the tali and proximal humeri, are also the sites of thickest cartilage in these bones.

There is an increasing recognition of osteoarthropathy in rapidly growing cattle and pigs raised in confinement on hard, usually concrete, floors and with minimal exercise. Osteochondrosis in feedlot cattle may be associated with a high-caloric diet and rapid growth rate (39). It is thought that weight-bearing trauma in these rapidly growing animals is sufficient to cause degenerative lesions of certain joints, especially in animals with a skeletal conformation which results in abnormal stress on certain weight-bearing condyles of long bones (1). In pigs, osteochondrosis and arthrosis are considered to be major causes of 'leg weakness' in rapidly growing animals (6–9). Recent work has shown a significant relationship between body conformation and the presence of joint lesions. Pigs with a narrow lumbar region, broad hams and a large relative width between the stifle joints were highly susceptible to poor locomotor ability due to lesion in the elbow and stifle joints, the lumbar intervertebral joints and the hip joint (7). This excellent work represents real progress in understanding the relationship between skeletal conformation and bone and joint lesions. It is postulated that inherited weakness of muscle, ligaments, cartilage, and exterior joint conformation results in local overloading in the joint and the development of osteochondrosis and arthrosis (10).

The influence of breed and level of feeding on the normal skeletal growth and the development of lesions of the bones of dairy cattle over a lifetime has been examined (54). In general, breed had the greatest influence on the traits studied which included age of closure of growth plates and lesions of growth plates. During the rearing period numerous lesions of the growth plate were detectable radiographically but these were not visible following closure of the growth plates (54).

Pathogenesis
The details of the pathogenesis of degenerative joint disease have been reviewed (3, 41). A brief review of the structure and biochemistry of the normal articular joint will serve as background for understanding the pathogenesis of osteoarthropathy (41). Articular cartilage is a tissue consisting of chondrocytes scattered in a matrix of collagen fibers and an amorphous intercellular substance containing proteoglycans. Articular cartilage contains no nerves, is avascular and has a high matrix-to-cell ratio. The chondrocytes are the only living matter in cartilage and produce the fine strands of collagen and are engaged in protein and proteoglycan synthesis. The matrix of the cartilage consists of water-soluble proteoglycans interspersed with collagen fibers which are arranged in parallel rows superficially and crisscross rows closer to the calcified layer. This enables the cartilage to withstand shearing stresses superficially and compression more deeply. The proteoglycans are glycosaminoglycan–protein complexes, bound by a link glycoprotein to a linear hyaluronic acid molecule. The glycosaminoglycans in articular cartilage are chondroitin 4-sulfate and chondroitin 6-sulfate and keratan sulfate. About 75% of the proteoglycans exist on aggregates which protect them from degradation and, because of their high content of water, form large polyanionic complexes which have considerable elastic resistance to compression. Nutrition of the articular cartilage is provided via the synovial fluid and is dependent on the capillary flow to the synovial membrane. Nutrients flow through the synovial fluid and diffuse through the cartilage to the chondrocytes. Proteoglycans are synthesized by the chondrocytes and secreted to the cell exterior. Proteoglycans are also degraded intracellularly by lysosomes. The normal equilibrium between anabolism and catabolism is maintained by several different low molecular proteins. When the equilibrium is disturbed and shifts towards catabolism, degeneration occurs.

Primary osteoarthropathy
This is due to normal aging processes and ordinary joint usage (21). The initial lesions occur in the superficial layers of the articular cartilages where, with increasing age, there is loss in the normal resilience of the cartilage, a lowering of the content of chondroitin sulfate and reduction in the permeability of the cartilaginous matrix which results in progressive degeneration of the articular cartilage. There is grooving of the articular cartilage and eburnation of subchondral bone and secondary hypertrophy of marginal cartilage and bone with the formation of pearl-like osteophytes (22). In experimentally induced arthritis in the horse the major changes include synovitis, increased synovial effusion (36) and superficial fibrillation with chondrocyte necrosis in the articular cartilage. These are comparable to the early changes in naturally occurring degenerative joint disease (37).

Secondary osteoarthropathy
This appears to be initiated by injuries or congenital conformational defects which create greater shearing stresses, on particular points, in contrast to the intermittent compressive stresses typical of ordinary weight-bearing. These irregular stresses result in cartilaginous erosion, increased density of subchondral bone at points of physical stress and proliferation of bone and cartilage at the articular margins.

Following acute trauma, the initial changes are often characterized by acute synovitis and capsulitis. As a result of the inflammatory response, leukocytes, prostaglandins, lysosomal enzymes and hyaluronidase enter the synovial fluid which becomes less viscous and affects the nutrition of the cartilage. The cartilage matrix undergoes a variety of changes, possibly because of chondrocyte damage with lysosomal enzyme release, or to collagen fiber injury. There is an increase in water content and loss of orientation of the collagen fibers. Proteoglycans are lost and while increased chondrocyte activity synthesizes proteoglycans they are of lower molecular weight and altered glycosaminoglycan composition. This leads to loss of elasticity and surface integrity of the cartilage, resulting in increased friction and blistering and ulceration. There is additional lysosomal enzyme release from the chondrocytes, resulting in matrix destruction and further proteoglycan destruction. The degrading enzymes enter the altered matrix and cause further degradation. The first stage of matrix degradation involves discoloration, softening and blistering of the tangential layer of the cartilage surface, a process known as early fibrillation. As the fissuring extends to the radial layer, microfractures occur with loss of cartilage fragment (detritus) into the synovial fluid. As the cartilage is destroyed the underlying bone is exposed and becomes sclerotic. Bony proliferation occurs in the floor of the cartilage lesions, while at the joint margins osteophyte formation occurs. The pathogenesis of degenerative joint disease indicates that the ideal treatment would be the use of a substance which would promote synthesis of matrix components and retard catabolic processes (41).

In femoral–tibial osteoarthrosis of bulls, the secondary degenerative joint lesions are due to rupture of the attachments of the lateral meniscus resulting in mechanical instability in the joint with unusual mechanical stresses on the articular cartilage leading to degeneration (5). The cranial cruciate ligament becomes progressively worn and eventually ruptures, resulting in loss of all joint stability and the development of gross arthrosis. In cattle with severe degenerative joint disease of the coxofemoral joints, an acetabular osseous bulla may develop at the cranial margin of the obturator foramen (42).

Osteochondrosis

Osteochondrosis (dyschondroplasia) is characterized by disturbance of the normal differentiation of the cells in the growing cartilage (35). Both the metaphyseal growth plate (the growth zone of the diaphysis) and immature joint cartilage (the growth zone of the epiphysis) are affected. The loss of normal differentiation of the cartilage cells results in failure of provisional calcification of the matrix and endochondral ossification ceases. An osteochondrotic lesion in the metaphyseal growth plate may disturb growth to such a degree that the whole shape of the bone is altered. Epiphysiolysis may also occur. Osteochondrosis of joint cartilage may lead to osteochondritis dessicans and secondary osteoarthrosis. The lesion may heal and only the sequels are present once the period of growth is over.

In osteochondrosis and arthrosis in rapidly growing swine raised in confinement with minimal exercise there is degeneration of the deep layer of the articular cartilage and adjacent subchondral bone with degenerative lesions of the epiphyseal plate (10, 23). Lesions in the epiphyseal plate may result in epiphysiolysis which occurs most commonly in the femoral head. The typical lesions are usually symmetrical and commonly involve the elbow, stifle and hip joints and the distal epiphyseal plate of the ulna. Lesions also occur in the intervertebral articulations. The lesions are common in pigs when they are examined at slaughter (90–100 kg body weight) and there may have been no evidence of clinical abnormality or a proportion of the pigs with severe lesions may have been affected with the leg-weakness syndrome. Osteochondrosis and *Erysipelothrix rhusiopathiae* are the most common causes of non-suppurative joint disease of pigs examined at the abattoir (52). Thus not all lesions are clinical.

Clinical findings

The major clinical characteristic is a chronic lameness which becomes progressively worse over a long period of time and usually does not respond to treatment. The disease is insidious and generally not clinically apparent in the early stages. A common clinical history is that the affected animal becomes progressively more lame over a period of weeks and months and prefers long periods of recumbency. The lesion may develop slowly over a period of weeks and months during the convalescent stages of an acute traumatic injury to the joint when recovery is expected but the animal continues to be lame. Young breeding bulls in the early stages of coxofemoral arthropathy may be reluctant to perform the breeding act and yet appear to have sufficient libido. One of the first clinical abnormalities of osteochondrosis and epiphyseolysis in young breeding boars may be inability to mount the sow—'*impotentia coeundi*' (10).

There is usually difficulty in flexing affected joints normally which results in a stiff and stilted gait. In cattle confined to stanchions one of the earliest and persistent signs is shifting weight from limb to limb. In dairy cattle, as the lesions become more painful, there is a decline in appetite and milk production, prolonged recumbency and considerable difficulty in rising from the recumbent state. In the early stages there may be an apparent remission of the lameness but relapses are common. The bony prominences of the joint eventually appear more prominent than normal which is due to the disuse muscle atrophy of the affected limbs. Distension of the joint capsule is not a characteristic as it is in an infectious or suppurative arthritis. The joint capsule of palpable joints is usually not painful on palpation. Passive flexion of affected joints may be painful and it may be possible to elicit crepitus due to detached pieces of cartilage and bone and osteophytes surrounding the articular cartilage. However, crepitus is most common in the large movable joints, such as the stifle, and commonly in the osteoarthropathy secondary to acute traumatic injury of the meniscus and cranial cruciate ligament of the joint.

Epiphysiolysis of the head of the femur occurs in young pigs from 5 months to 1 year of age. There is usually a history of slight to moderate lameness sudden in onset, affecting one or both hindlimbs (25). The onset of lameness may coincide with some physical activity such as breeding, farrowing or transportation. The lameness is progressive and in about 7–10 days the animal is unable to use its hindlegs. Crepitus may be audible on circumduction of the affected limb and radiography may reveal the separation.

In leg weakness associated with osteochondrosis and

arthrosis of pigs the common clinical findings are hyperflexion of the carpus, limb bowing, adduction of both forelegs at the level of the carpus, hyperextension of the fore and hind phalanges, and anterior curvature of the tarsus. Locomotory dysfunction involves primarily the hindlegs. There is pronounced swaying of the hindquarters, and crossing the hindlegs with each step which makes the pig appear incoordinated.

In osteochondrosis in young growing bulls there is reluctance to move, stiffness, enlargement of the ends of long bones and straightened joint (33).

In the horse with osteochondrosis of the shoulder joint there is intermittent lameness characterized by a swinging leg, shoulder lameness with pain elicited by extension, flexion or abduction of the limb. Secondary joint disease is also a common finding (29). In a retrospective study of osteochondrosis dissecans in 21 horses, affected animals were 8 months to 5 years of age (45). The usual age of onset of clinical abnormalities was 18–24 months. The common presenting complaints included joint effusion and lameness of either gradual or suddent onset. The prevalence was higher in males than in females.

Clinical pathology

The changes in the synovial fluid of joints affected with degenerative arthropathy are usually unremarkable and can be distinguished from the changes in infectious arthritis. A summary of the laboratory evaluation of synovial fluid in diseases of the joints is set out in Table 42. This should be combined with appropriate hematology and serum biochemistry where indicated. The concentration of hyaluronic acid in synovial fluid can be determined using an assay technigue (49). The determination of serum calcium and phosphorus may reveal the existence of a dietary deficiency or imbalance of minerals. The isolation of an infectious agent from the synovial fluid of a diseased joint suggests the presence of an infectious arthritis but failure to isolate an organism must not be interpreted as the presence of a non-infectious arthritis. In well-advanced cases of infectious arthritis the number of organisms may be small or they have been phagocytosed by neutrophils in the joint fluid.

Necropsy findings

In degenerative joint disease the joint cartilage is thin or patchily absent and polished subchondral bone is evident. The articular surfaces are irregular and sometimes folded. Exposed bone may be extensively eroded and osteophytes (small bony excrescences, like pearls) may be present on the non-articular parts of the joint on the circumference of the articular cartilage. The synovial fluid is usually only slightly increased in volume and appears amber-colored. Menisci, intra-articular cartilages and ligaments may be entirely absent and there may be areas of calcification in the joint capsule and cartilages free in the synovium. When the stifle is affected, fractures of the head of the tibia occur commonly, usually a chip of the lateral condyle having become separated. In such cases, fractures of the lateral condyle of the distal end of the femur may follow. With either of these fractures, lameness is extreme and the animal may often refuse to rise. The radiographic and pathological findings of femoral–tibial osteoarthrosis in bulls is described (5). When the hip joint of bulls is affected, the head of the femur becomes smaller and more flattened than normal, the acetabulum is shallower and the round ligament is usually ruptured. The pathology of coxofemoral arthropathy in young bulls is described (17). The pathologic changes in experimentally induced osteoarthritis in the horse are similar to the early changes of naturally occurring degenerative joint disease (31).

In osteochondrosis there is splitting and invagination of articular cartilage, loss of articular cartilage, chip fractures of condyles, exposed and collapsed subchondral bone, osteophyte formation around the circumference of the articular cartilage and loose pieces of cartilage in the joint. In the epiphyseal plates (for example, the distal ulna in pigs with leg-weakness) the cartilage is uneven and thickened with hemorrhage, fibrous tissue,

Table 42. Laboratory evaluation of synovial fluid in diseases of the joints* (see references 22, 26–28)

Synovial fluid analysis	*Normal joint*	*Degenerative arthropathy*	*Infectious arthritis*
Gross appearance	Colorless, clear	Pale yellow, may contain flocculent debris	Turbid, yellow
Total volume	—	Normal or slight increase	Usually marked increase
Clot formation	No clot	No clot	May clot within minutes after collection
Erythrocytes (/μl)	<4000	6000–12 000	4000–8000
Leukocytes(/μl)	<250	250–1000	50 000–150 000
Neutrophils (%)	7	10–15	80–90
Lymphocytes (%)	35–40	45–50	4–8
Monocytes (%)	45–50	35–40	1–3
Microbiology	—	—	May be able to culture bacteria, mycoplasma or virus, but not always
Total protein (g/dl)	1·2–1·8	1·6–1·8	3·20–4·5
Relative viscosity	—	Slightly reduced	Decreased

*Other laboratory analyses of synovial fluid include: sugar content, alkaline phosphatase activity, lactic dehydrogenase activity, aldolase activity, glutamic oxaloacetic transaminase activity, glutamic pyruvic transaminase activity, mucinous precipitate quality.

collapse of bone tissue in the metaphysis and epiphyseal separation. Complete separation of the epiphysis occurs most commonly at the head of the femur (24). The ultrastructural appearance of normal epiphyseal cartilage of the articular–epiphyseal cartilage complex in growing swine has been examined and serves as a standard for comparison with the lesions in affected pigs (46). The lesions may be present in pigs at an early age as part of the usual growth pattern of cartilages (47).

Diagnosis

Osteoarthropathy is characterized clinically by a chronic lameness which becomes progressively worse and usually does not respond to treatment. The gait is stiff, there is disuse muscle atrophy, the bony prominences of the joint are more apparent but usually there is no marked distension and pain of the joint capsule as in infectious arthritis. Examination of synovial fluid may aid in differentiation from infectious arthritis. Radiographically there is erosion of articular cartilage, sclerosis of subchondral bone and periarticular accumulations of osteophytes. In the early stages of the disease, in large animals, radiographic changes may not be visible and repeated examinations may be necessary. Radiographic changes of osteochondrosis in the shoulder joint of the horse consist of: alteration in the contour of the humeral head and glenoid cavity, periarticular osteophyte formation, sclerosis of the subchondral bone, and bone cyst formation (29). The radiological findings of osteochondrosis of the hock joints in horses has been described (48).

Treatment

The treatment of arthropathy depends largely upon correction of the cause, but in most cases the lesions are progressive and irreparable and food-producing animals should be slaughtered for salvage. Tarsal degenerative joint disease in cattle has been treated with intra-articular injections of corticosteroids (27) and has provided temporary relief from pain and discomfort. However, the corticosteroids do not promote healing of the joint and their use in arthropathy may actually accelerate erosion of articular cartilage, loss of joint sensation and the development of 'steroid arthropathy'. Large doses of acetylsalicylic acid may be given to reduce the pain in animals which are kept for breeding purposes.

Several modalities of the treatment of degenerative joint disease in the horse have been examined (3). Treatment is symptomatic and non-specific. Primary causes such as infectious arthritis should be treated specifically. The prevention of further trauma should be assured and possible nutritional causes corrected. The treatment of active disease, particularly in soft tissues which is contributing to articular degeneration, includes rest, immobilization, physical therapy, intra-articular injections of corticosteroids, non-steroidal anti-inflammatory agents (NSAIDs), joint lavage, and intra-articular injection of sodium hyaluronate which have all been used with variable success (3). The changes in the synovia following the intra-articular injection of sodium hyaluronate into normal equine joints and after arthrotomy and experimental cartilage damage have been examined, but in general the results are inconclusive (50). Surgical therapy includes curettage of articular cartilage, removal of osteophytes, and surgical arthrodesis (3). In a retrospective study of stifle lameness in 42 cattle admitted to two veterinary teaching hospitals over a period of 6 years, 18 had radiographic evidence of subchondral bone cyst (51) without radiographic evidence of degenerative joint disease. The prognosis in those with a subchondral bone cyst was favorable, 75% returning to their intended function, while in septic arthritis only 22% returned to normal (51).

The prevention of osteoarthropathy will depend upon recognition and elimination of the predisposing causes. These include the provision of an adequate diet and the avoidance of overnutrition, regular exercise for confined animals, the provision of suitable flooring to minimize persistent concussion and the use of breeding stock which have suitable body conformation that does not predispose to joint lesions.

REVIEW LITERATURE

Clyne, M. J. (1987) Pathogenesis of degenerative joint disease. *Equ. vet. J.*, *19*, 15–18.
McIlwraith, C. W. (1982) Current concepts in equine degenerative joint disease. *J. Am. vet. med. Assoc.*, *180*, 239–250.
Nizolek, D. J. H. & White, K. K. (1981) Corticosteroid and hyaluronic acid treatments in equine degenerative joint disease: a review. *Cornell Vet.*, *71*, 355–375.
Olsson, S. E. (1978) Osteochondrosis in domestic animals, I. *Acta Radiol.* Suppl. 358, pp. 1–306, Stockholm.
Stromberg, B. (1979) A review of the salient features of osteochondrosis in the horse. *Equ. vet. J.*, *11*, 211–214.

REFERENCES

(1) Grondalen, T. (1974) *Nord VetMed.*, *26*, 534.
(2) Moore, J. N. & McIlwraith, C. W. (1977) *Vet. Rec.*, *100*, 133.
(3) McIlwraith, C. W. (1982) *J. Am. vet. med. Assoc.*, *180*, 239.
(4) McTaggart, H. S. (1959) *Vet. Rec.*, *71*, 709.
(5) Bartels, J. E. (1975) *J. Am. vet. Radiol. Soc.*, *16*, 151, 159.
(6) Reiland, S. (1974) *Svensk. VetTidskr.*, *26*, 28.
(7) Grondalen, T. (1974) *Acta vet. Scand.*, *15*, 555, 574.
(8) Nielsen, N. C. (1973) *Nord. VetMed.*, *25*, 17.
(9) Schaffer, E. & Bombard, D. (1973) *Berl. Muñch. Tierärztl. Wochenschr.*, *86*, 64.
(10) Grondalen, T. (1974) *Acta vet. Scand.*, Suppl. 46, 1.
(11) Howlett. C. R. (1973) *Pathology*, *2*, 135.
(12) Radostits, O. M. et al. (1976) *Can. vet. J.*, *17*, 48.
(13) Howlett, C. R. (1972) *Aust. vet. J.*, *48*, 562.
(14) Hedhammer, A. et al. (1974) *Cornell Vet.*, *65*, suppl. 5.
(15) Jones, W. G. (1972) *Vet. Rec.*, *90*, 503.
(16) Shupe, J. L. (1961) *Can. vet. J.*, *2*, 369.
(17) Owens, Rh. ap Rh. et al. (1984) *J. Am. vet. med. Assoc.*, *184*, 302.
(18) Wood. A. K. W. et al. (1974) *Aust. vet. J.*, *50*, 275.
(19) Glade, M. J. et al. (1983) *Cornell Vet.*, *73*, 170.
(20) Ellis, D. R. & Greenwood, R. E. S. (1985) *Equ. vet. J.*, *17*, 66.
(21) Hoffman, K. D. et al. (1984) *Equ. vet. J.*, *16*, 135.
(22) Van Pelt, R. W. (1975) *Am. J. vet. Res.*, *36*, 1009.
(23) Grondalen, T. (1974) *Acta vet. Scand.*, *15*, 1, 26, 43, 53, 61.
(24) Trent, A. M. & Krook, L. (1985), *J. Am. vet. med. Assoc.*, *186*, 284.
(25) Vaughan, L. C. (1969) *Br. vet. J.*, *125*, 354.
(26) Van Pelt, R. W. (1975) *J. Am. vet. med. Assoc.*, *166*, 239.
(27) Van Pelt, R. W. (1974) *J. Am. vet. med. Assoc.*, *165*, 91.
(28) Van Pelt, R. W. (1968) *Am. J. vet. Res.*, *29*, 507.
(29) Nyack, B. et al. (1981) *Cornell Vet.*, *71*, 149.
(30) Stromberg, B. & Rejno, S. (1978) *Acta Radiol.*, Suppl. 358, 139.
(31) Rejno, S. & Stromberg, B. (1978) *Acta Radiol.*, Suppl. 358, 153.
(32) Stromberg, B. (1979) *Equ. vet. J.*, *11*, 211.
(33) Reiland, S. et al. (1978) *Acta Radiol.*, Suppl. 358, 179.

(34) Reiland, S. (1978) *Acta Radiol.*, Suppl. 358, 45.
(35) Olsson, S. E. & Reiland, S. (1978) *Acta Radiol.*, Suppl. 358, 299.
(36) McIlwraith, C. W. et al. (1979) *Am. J. vet. Res.*, *40*, 11.
(37) McIlwraith, C. W. & VanSickle, D. C. (1981) *Am. J. vet. Res.*, *42*, 209.
(38) Holmberg, T. & Reiland, S. (1984) *Acta. vet. Scand.*, *25*, 113.
(39) Jensen, R. et al. (1981) *Vet. Pathol.*, *18*, 529.
(40) Weisbrode. S. E. et al. (1982) *J. Am. vet. med. Assoc.*, *181*, 700.
(41) Clyne, M. J. (1987) *Equ. vet. J.*, *19*, 15.
(42) Weaver, A. D. (1982) *Br. vet. J.*, *138*, 123.
(43) Yovich. J. V. et al. (1985) *J. Am. vet. med. Assoc.*, *186*, 1186.
(44) Miller, C. L. & Todhunter, R. (1987) *Cornell Vet.*, *77*, 75.
(45) Lindsell, C. E. et al. (1983) *Aust. vet. J.*, *60*, 291.
(46) Carlson, C. S. et al. (1985) *Am. J. vet. Res.*, *46*, 306.
(47) Hill, M. A. et al. (1985) *Vet. Rec.*, *116*, 46.
(48) Hoppe, F. (1984) *Equ. vet. J.*, *16*, 425.
(49) Rowley, G. et al. (1982) *Am. J. vet. Res.*, *43*, 1096.
(50) Hilbert, B. J. et al. (1985) *Aust. vet. J.*, *62*, 182.
(51) Ducharme. N. G. et al. (1985) *Can. vet. J.*, *26*, 212.
(52) Johnston, K. M. et al. (1987) *Can. vet. J.*, *28*, 174.
(53) Firth, E. C. & Greydanus, Y. (1987) *Res. vet. Sci.*, *42*, 35.
(54) Holmberg, T. et al. (1984) *Zentralbl. VetMed.*, *A 31*, 193.

Arthritis

Inflammation of the synovial membrane and articular surfaces occurs commonly in animals as a result of infection. It is characterized by lameness and local pain, heat and swelling of the joint.

Etiology and epidemiology
Specific infections in farm animals in which localization occurs in joints from bacteremia or septicemia include particularly the infections of newborn animals which arise from navel or intrauterine infection. Surveys of thoroughbred studs have shown that the incidence of infectious arthritis is higher in foals with other perinatal abnormalities and in which the ingestion of colostrum was delayed for more than 4 hours after birth (1). Calves with hypogammaglobulinemia are particularly susceptible to bacteremia and meningitis, ophthalmitis and arthritis. Some of the important infectious causes of arthritis are as follows.

Calves
- Non-specific joint ill from omphalophlebitis caused by *Actinomyces (Corynebacterium) pyogenes*, *Fusobacterium necrophorum*, *Staphylococcus* sp.
- *Erysipelothrix insidiosa* sporadically in older calves
- *Salmonella dublin*, *Salmonella typhimurium* and *Mycoplasma bovis* (9).

Lambs
- *Erysipelothrix insidiosa* in newborn and recently docked lambs (2)
- Sporadic cases caused by *Fusobacterium necrophorum*, *Staphylococcus* sp., *Cor. pseudotuberculosis*, *Haemophilus agni*, *Pasteurella hemolytica*
- *Chlamydia* sp. causes polyarthritis extensively in feedlot lambs (5, 6)
- In tick pyemia caused by *Staphylococcus aureus*.

Foals
- *Actinobacillus equuli*, *Cor. equi*, *Salmonella abortivoequina* in the newborn
- *Chlamydia* sp. has caused polyarthritis in foals.

Young pigs
- *Erysipelothrix insidiosa* in pigs of any age. Up to 65% of joints of pigs at slaughter are affected (3) and up to 80% of the farms from which the pigs come do not vaccinate for erysipelas. Mortality in preweaning groups of pigs may affect 18% of litters, 3·3% of the piglets and a herd mortality of 1·5% (4).

Cattle
- *Haemophilus somnus* is a cause of synovitis
- *Mycoplasma agalactia* var. *bovis* is a common cause of synovitis, arthritis and pneumonia in young feedlot cattle (8)
- *Mycoplasma bovigenitalium* may cause mastitis in cows with some animals developing arthritis
- *M. mycoides* may cause arthritis in calves vaccinated with the organism against contagious bovine pleuropneumonia. Calves already sensitive to the organism develop an immediate-type allergic reaction of the synovial membrane (10)
- *Brucella abortus*: occasional cows with brucellosis develop an arthrodial synovitis
- Some cases of ephemeral fever have a sterile arthritis
- Bovine virus diarrhea virus in young bulls, rarely (7).

Sheep
- As part of melioidosis
- *Mycoplasma* sp. of serositis-arthritis

Pigs
- Glasser's disease
- *Mycoplasma* sp. in synovitis and arthritis of growing pigs (10) especially in housed pigs
- *Brucella suis* commonly infects bones, especially vertebrae, and joints.

Horses
- Rare cases of generalized strangles
- Rare case of non-erosive polysynovitis in a horse, possibly immunological (31).

All species
Sporadic cases are due to:

- Traumatic perforation of the joint capsule
- Spread from surrounding tissues, e.g. footrot to interphalangeal joints in cattle and pigs (11), interdigital abscess in sheep
- Hematogenous spread from suppurative lesions commonly in udder, uterus, diaphragmatic abscess, infected navel or tail, castration wound
- Idiopathic septic arthritis in cows within weeks of calving—cause unknown (12).

Pathogenesis
In infectious arthritis which is hematogenous in origin there is usually a synovitis initially, followed by changes in the articular cartilages and sometimes bone. With almost any systemic infection there may be localization of the infectious agent in the synovial membrane and joint cavity. The synovial membrane is inflamed, edematous and there are varying degrees of villous hypertrophy and deposition of fibrin. Bacteria colonize in

synovial membranes which makes treatment difficult. The synovitis causes distension of the joint capsule with fluid and the joint is painful and warm. Successful treatment in the early stages of synovitis will minimize or avoid changes in articular cartilage and bone and healing will result. A progressive infectious synovitis commonly results in pannus formation between articular surfaces with erosion of articular cartilage, infection of subchondral bone and osteomyelitis. In the chronic stage there is extensive granulation tissue formation, chronic synovitis and degenerative joint disease with osteophyte formation and ankylosis is possible. Depending on the organism, the arthritis may be suppurative or sero-fibrinous. Suppurative arthritis is particularly destructive of cartilage and bone and commonly there is rupture of the joint capsule. In foals with septic arthritis there may be a concurrent polyosteomyelitis usually in either the epiphysis and or the metaphysis of the long bones (31).

Septicemic foals may develop infectious arthritis and a concurrent polyosteomyelitis because of the patency of transphyseal vessels in the newborn foal which allows spread of infection across the physes with the development of lesions in the metaphysis, epiphysis and adjacent to the articular cartilage (32, 33). The syndrome is classified according to the location of the lesions. A foal with S-type septic arthritis–osteomyelitis has synovitis, without macroscopic evidence of osteomyelitis. Foals with E-type have osteomyelitis of the epiphysis at the subchondral bone–cartilage junction. Those with P-type have osteomyelitis directly adjacent to the physis. The same joint may have a single type or any combination of types but most foals with the S-type have concurrent bone lesions (33).

Infectious arthritis may occur following traumatic injury to a joint but the pathogenesis is obscure. Traumatic injury of the joint capsule resulting in edema and inflammation may allow latent organisms to localize, proliferate and initiate an arthritis.

There is considerable interest in the possibility that rheumatoid-like arthritis may occur in farm animals. The disease is now described in dogs (13, 14) and chronic arthritis due to infection with *Erysipelothrix insidiosa* in pigs appears to be a suitable experimental animal model of the disease (15, 16). A rheumatoid-like arthritis is described in calves (17) and a bovine rheumatoid factor occurs in experimental infection of deer with *Erysipelothrix insidiosa* (18). It is postulated that following infection of the joint, there is formation of IgG and IgM antibodies (rheumatoid factor) which have reacted with altered IgG antigen. These complexes activate the complement sequence which generates the leukotactic factor and leukocytes enter the joint in large numbers. The neutrophils phagocytose the immune complexes and in the process release lysozymal enzymes which cause destructive changes in the joint. This sequence of events could explain why the disease persists long after the organism cannot be recovered. In experimentally induced arthritis in pigs, using *Erysipelothrix insidiosa*, the joints become sterile 6 months after the experimental infection but the antigen of the organism can be demonstrated in the synovial fluid with the fluorescent antibody technique (15). There are increased concentrations of lysozymal activity in the joints of swine affected with arthritis due to *Erysipelothrix insidiosa* (19) but their exact origin is uncertain. Acute synovitis may be induced with killed *Erysipelothrix insidiosa* injected parenterally into lambs possessing colostral antibody to the same organism (20). There are marked proliferative changes in the synovial membrane leading to pannus formation, destruction of cartilage and ankylosis. This suggests that prior sensitization to an organism may make newborn animals more susceptible to severe and chronic arthritis if they are exposed to the homologous strains of bacteria to which their dams were immune and transferred to the colostrum.

Clinical findings

Inflammation of the synovial membrane causes pain and lameness in the affected limb, sometimes to the point that the animal will not put it to the ground. Pain and heat are usually detectable on palpation and passive movement of the joint is resented. The joint may be swollen but the degree will depend on the type of infection. Pyogenic bacteria cause the greatest degree of swelling and may result in rupture of the joint capsule. Some enlargement of the epiphysis is usual and this may be the only enlargement in non-pyogenic infections, particularly that caused by *Erysipelothrix insidiosa*.

In many of the neonatal infections there will also be an accompanying omphalophlebitis and evidence of lesions in other organs, particularly the liver, endocardium and meninges. Arthritis in older animals may also be accompanied by signs of inflammation of the serous membranes and endocardium when the infection is the result of hematogenous localization.

The joints most commonly involved are the hock, stifle and knee but infection of the fetlock, interphalangeal and intervertebral joints is not uncommon. In chronic cases there may be physical impairment of joint movement because of fibrous thickening of the joint capsule, periarticular ossification, and rarely ankylosis of the joints. Crepitus may be detectable in joints where much erosion has occurred. In newborn and young animals, involvement of several joints is common. The joints may become inflamed simultaneously or serially. Lameness is often so severe that affected foals lie down in lateral recumbency most of the time and may have to be assisted to rise. The gait may be so impaired as to suggest ataxia of central origin.

The prognosis in cases of acute suppurative arthritis is never good. Neglected animals may die or have to be destroyed because of open joints or pressure sores. The subsequent development of chronic arthritis and ankylosis may greatly impede locomotion and interfere with the usefulness of the animal.

Clinical pathology

Aspiration of joint fluid from the joint may be attempted if the swelling is marked and free fluid is present. Careful disinfection of the skin and the use of sterile equipment is essential to avoid the introduction of further infection. The laboratory examinations of joint fluid which are commonly done include: culturing for the presence of bacteria and viruses and total and differential leukocyte counts and erythrocyte counts. Synovial fluid must be cultured for aerobic and anaerobic bacteria and on specific media when *Mycoplasma* sp. are suspected. In infectious arthritis the volume of joint fluid is increased, the total leukocyte count is increased with a high percentage (80–90) of neutrophils. The severity of infectious arthritis may be manifested systemically by a leukocytosis with a marked regenerative left shift. In degenerative joint disease, the volume may be normal or only slightly increased and the total and differential leukocyte count may be within the normal range. In traumatic arthritis there may be a marked increase in the number of erythrocytes. The laboratory findings in examination of the joint fluid are summarized in Table 42.

Serological tests may be of value in determining the presence of specific infections with *Mycobacterium mycoides*, *Salmonella* spp., *Brucella* spp. and *Erysipelothrix insidiosa*. Special biochemical examinations of joint fluid are available which measure for viscosity, strength of the mucin clot and concentrations of certain enzymes (21). Radiographic examination may aid in the detection of joint lesions and can be used to differentiate between inflammatory and degenerative changes. In foals with arthritis and suspected osteomyelitis there may be radiographic evidence of osteolysis of the metaphysis or epiphysis (32). A series of radiographs taken several days apart may be necessary to detect lesions of the bone (33). Contrast arthroscopy is sometimes used to define joint abnormalities more clearly (22). Although its application may be limited to experimental studies, the measurement of joint movements by electronic means—electrogoniometry—offers an opportunity for advancement in the study of diseases of joints (23).

Necropsy findings

The nature of the lesions varies with the causative organism. The synovial membrane is thickened and roughened and there is inflammation and erosion of the articular cartilage. There is usually an increase in the amount of synovial fluid present, varying from a thin, clear, serous, brownish fluid through a thicker, serofibrinous fluid to pus. There may be some inflammation of the periarticular tissues in acute cases and proliferation of the synovial membrane in chronic cases. In the latter, plaques of inspissated necrotic material and fibrin may be floating free in the synovial fluid. Infectious arthritis due to *A. pyogenes* is characterized by extensive erosion and destruction of articular cartilage and extensive suppuration (24). There may be a primary omphalophlebitis in newborn animals and metastatic abscesses may be present in other organs.

Diagnosis

Infectious arthritis is characterized clinically by swollen joints which are painful and warm to touch, and lameness of varying degrees of severity. The volume of joint fluid is usually markedly increased and the leukocyte count is increased with a high percentage of neutrophils. In the early stages of synovitis and in chronic nonsuppurative arthritis, the joint may not be visibly enlarged and careful examination by palpation may be necessary to reveal abnormalities of the joint capsule. Lameness is common, however, even though only slight in some cases, and should arouse suspicion of the possibility of arthritis. The diseases of the musculoskeletal system which cause lameness and stiffness of gait include: degenerative joint disease, osteodystrophy and epiphysitis, osteomyelitis, degenerative myopathy, myositis and traumatic injuries of tendons and ligaments. Also, diseases of the nervous system, especially the peripheral nerves and spinal cord, may be confused with arthritis unless the joints are examined carefully. Some severe cases of polyarthritis may cause recumbency which may be erroneously attributed to the nervous system.

Degenerative joint disease is characterized by an insidious onset of moderate lameness and stiffness of gait which becomes progressively worse over several weeks. The joint capsule is usually not grossly enlarged, not painful and there is usually no systemic reaction. The total leukocyte count in the joint fluid is only slightly increased and the differential count may be normal. Chronic arthritis is often difficult to differentiate clinically from degenerative joint disease. Chronic arthritis is more common in young animals than in adults like rapidly growing yearling bulls, adult bulls, aged dairy cows and horses in which degenerative arthropathy is most common. A sudden onset of acute lameness and marked swelling of a joint with severe pain suggests an infectious arthritis or traumatic injury to the joint. Marked swelling of several joints suggests infectious polyarthritis. Osteodystrophy is characterized by lameness and stiffness of gait, usually an absence of joint capsule abnormalities, enlargements and deformities of the long bones in growing animals, and a number of animals may be affected at about the same time. Radiography may reveal the abnormal bones and the nutritional history may explain the cause.

Degenerative myopathy causes acute lameness, a stiff and trembling gait, often leading to recumbency and absence of joint or bone involvement.

Traumatic sprains of tendons or ligaments, and fractures of the epiphyses may cause lameness and local pain, and when they involve periarticular tissues may be difficult to differentiate from arthritis.

Arthritis is never present at birth and apparent fixation of the joints should arouse suspicion of a congenital anomaly.

The differentiation between arthritis and diseases of the peripheral nerves or spinal cord, both of which can cause lameness and/or recumbency may be difficult if the arthritis is not clinically obvious. Diseases of the peripheral nerves cause lameness due to flaccid paralysis and neurogenic atrophy. Lesions of the spinal cord usually result in weakness of the hindlimbs, weak or absent withdrawal reflexes and loss of skin sensation.

Treatment

Acute infectious arthritis should be treated as quickly as possible to avoid irreversible changes in the joint. The conservative approach is the use of antimicrobial agents given parenterally daily for several days. The selection of the drug of choice will depend on the suspected cause of the arthritis. The antibiotics which are known to perfuse into the joint in therapeutic concentrations include the natural and synthetic penicillins, tetracycline, streptomycin, neomycin, gentamicin and kanamycin (28).

Cloxacillin, methicillin or penicillin have been used successfully for the treatment of staphylococcal septic arthritis in the horse (30). In piglets at 2 weeks of age, streptococcal arthritis is most likely and it will respond quickly to penicillin, given parenterally. Likewise acute arthritis associated with erysipelas in pigs will respond beneficially if treated early before there is pannus formation. The synovitis due to *Haemophilus somnus* infection responds quickly to systemic treatment. However, in other specific types of infectious arthritis the response is poor and recovery, if it does occur, requires several days or a week. Mycoplasmal arthritis in cattle is relatively non-responsive to treatment and affected cattle may be lame for up to several weeks before inprovement occurs and complete recovery may not occur. Chronic arthritis due to infection of pigs with *Erysipelothrix insidiosa* will commonly develop into a rheumatoid-like arthritis and be refractory to treatment.

The local application of heat, by hot fomentations or other physical means, is laborious, but if practiced frequently and vigorously will reduce the pain and local swelling. The local application of liniments may also be advantageous in chronic cases. Analgesics are often advisable if the animal is recumbent much of the time. Sodium salicylate (25–50 g twice daily in large animals) can be left for administration by the owner. Persistent recumbency is one of the problems in the treatment of arthritis, particularly in foals. The animal spends little time feeding or sucking and loses much condition. Compression necrosis over bony prominences is a common complication and requires vigorous preventive measures.

Failure to respond to conservative therapy has been attributed to the inadequate concentrations of antibiotic achieved in the joint cavity, the presence of excessive amounts of exudate and fibrin in the joint which makes the infectious agent inaccessible to the antibiotic, drug-resistant infections or the development of rheumatoid-like arthritis which is chronic and progressive. It is often not possible to determine which situation is responsible.

If conservative treatment is not providing sufficient improvement and the value of the animal warrants extended therapy, a joint sample should be obtained for culture and drug sensitivity. The most suitable antibiotic may then be given parenterally and/or by intra-articular injection. Injection directly into the joint is presumed to overcome the inadequate levels of antibiotic in the joint following parenteral administration. Strict asepsis is necessary to avoid further introduction of infection.

The parenteral or intra-articular administration of corticosteroids and the oral or parenteral administration of phenylbutazone are used in an attempt to reduce pain and facilitate healing by permitting movement of the affected joint. However, corticosteroids are contra-indicated in infectious arthritis particularly if the infection is not under control when the corticosteroids are administered. Aspiration and distension—irrigation using polyionic electrolyte solutions buffered to 7.4 may be beneficial (28). The rationale is that irrigation removes exudates which may contain lysozymes which destroy articular cartilage. A through and through lavage system may also be used with drainage tubes.

Failure to respond to parenteral and intra-articular medication may require surgical opening of the joint capsule, careful debridement, excision of synovium and infected cartilage and bone (25, 28, 29). This may be followed by daily irrigation of the joint cavity with antibiotics and saline and joint immobilization for several weeks to promote ankylosis. The major difficulty is to obtain a bacteriological cure. Infected sequestrae and osteomyelitis of subchondral bone will prevent proper healing. Septic pedal arthritis in cattle may be treated successfully by the creation of a drainage track (26).

A combination of antimicrobials given by the parenteral and intra-articular routes along with radiation and surgical drainage had been evaluated with moderate success (34).

Control

The control of infectious arthritis is of major importance in newborn farm animals. The early ingestion of colostrum and a clean environment for the neonate are necessary. The prophylactic use of antibiotics in newborn piglets (27) and foals (1) significantly reduced the incidence of infectious arthritis. Some of the infectious arthritides associated with specific diseases can be controlled through immunization programs. For example, vaccination of piglets at 6–8 weeks of age will provide protection against both the systemic and arthritic forms of erysipelas.

REVIEW LITERATURE

Firth, E. C. (1983) Current concepts of infectious polyarthritis in foals. *Equ. vet. J.*, *15*, 5–9.

Martens, R. J., Aver, J. A. & Carter, K. (1986) Equine pediatrics: septic arthritis and osteomyelitis. *J. Am. vet. med. Assoc.*, *188*, 582–585.

REFERENCES

(1) Platt, H. (1977) *Equ. vet. J.*, *9*, 141.
(2) Tontis, A. et al. (1977) *Tierärztl. Wochenschr.*, *84*, 113.
(3) Bond, M. P. (1966) *Aust. vet. J.*, *52*, 462.
(4) Nielsen, N. C. et al. (1975) *Nord. VetMed.*, 27, 529.
(5) McChesney, A. E. et al. (1974) *J. Am. vet. med. Assoc.*, *165*, 259.
(6) Hopkins, J. B. et al. (1973) *J. Am. vet. med. Assoc.*, *163*, 1157.
(7) Hanly, G. J. & Mossman, D. H. (1977) *NZ vet. J.*, *25*, 38.
(8) Langford, E. V. (1977) *Can. J. comp. Med.*, *41*, 89.
(9) Piercy, D. W. T. (1972) *J. comp. Pathol.*, *82*, 279, 291.
(10) Ross, R. F. et al. (1971) *Am. J. vet. Res.*, *32*, 1743.
(11) Penny, R. H. C. et al. (1963) *Vet. Rec.*, *75*, 1225.
(12) Van Pelt, R. W. (1973) *J. Am. vet. med. Assoc.*, *162*, 284.
(13) Newton, C. D. et al. (1976) *J. Am. vet. med. Assoc.*, *168*, 113.
(14) Pedersen, N. C. et al. (1976) *J. Am. vet. med. Assoc.*, *169*, 295.
(15) Seidler, D. et al. (1976) In: *Infection and Immunology in the Rheumatic Diseases*, ed. D. C. Dumonde, pp. 201–204. Oxford: Blackwell Scientific.
(16) O'Brien, J. J. et al. (1973) *Irish vet. J.*, 27,21.
(17) Wright-George, J. et al. (1976) *Cornell Vet.*, 66, 110.
(18) Sikes, D. et al. (1972) *Am. J. vet. Res.*, *33*, 2545.
(19) Timoney, J. F., Jr (1976) *Am. J. vet. Res.*, *37*, 295.
(20) Piercy, D. W. T. (1971) *J. comp. Pathol.*, *81*, 557.
(21) Van Pelt, R. W. (1975) *J. Am. vet. med. Assoc.*, *166*, 239.
(22) Knezevic, V. P. & Wruhs, O. (1975) *Wien. Tierärztl. Monatsschr.*, 62, 300.
(23) Taylor, B. M. et al. (1974) *Am. J. vet. Res.*, 27, 85.
(24) Van Pelt, R. W. (1966) *J. Am. vet. med. Assoc.*, *149*, 303.

(25) Verschooten, F. et al. (1974) *J. Am. vet. med. Assoc.*, *165*, 271.
(26) Merkens, H. W. (1977) *Tijdschr. Diergeneeskd.*, *102*, 326.
(27) Horugel, K. (1975) *Mh. VetMed.*, *30*, 688.
(28) Leitch, M. (1979) *J. Am. vet. med. Assoc.*, *175*, 701.
(29) Edwards, G. B. & Vaughan, L. C. (1978) *Vet. Rec.*, *103*, 227.
(30) Rose, R. J. & Love, D. N. (1979) *Equ. vet. J.*, *11*, 85.
(31) Byars, T. D. et al. (1984) *Equ. vet. J.*, *16*, 141.
(32) Martens, R. J. et al. (1986) *J. Am. vet. med. Assoc.*, *188*, 582.
(33) Firth, E. C. (1983) *Equ. vet. J.*, *15*, 5.
(34) Merkens, H. W. et al. (1984) *Vet. Rec.*, *114*, 212.

CONGENITAL DEFECTS OF MUSCLES, BONES AND JOINTS

Defects of the musculoskeletal system are amongst the most common congenital abnormalities in farm animals. In cattle 476 such defects are listed (1). Many of them are lethal, and most of the remainder are life-threatening because of interference with grazing, or the prehension of food. Many of them occur in combinations so that single defects are uncommon. For example, most axial skeletal defects and cleft palates occur in calves which already have arthrogryposis. Two reviews of congenital defects of the skeleton of animals are available (2, 3).

Because of the very large volume of literature involved it is not possible to deal with all the recorded defects here, and the text is limited to those defects which are thought to be of general importance. Whether or not they are inherited or have an environmental cause is often not known so that an etiological classification is not very effective. Nor is an anatomical or pathological classification, so we are reduced to a classification based on abnormal function.

Congenital defects characterized by fixation of joints

Because arthrogryposis, which has been used to convey the description of joint fixation, strictly means fixation in flexion the term congenital articular rigidity has been introduced (4). The immobilization of the joint may be due to lack of extensibility of muscles, tendons, ligaments or other tissues around the joint, or to deformity of articular surfaces, or theoretically to fusion between the bones at the articular surface. Muscle contracture, which is the principal cause of joint fixation, has been produced experimentally, and occurs naturally, as a result of primary muscle atrophy or of atrophy resulting from denervation. Articular surface deformity is usually associated with gross deformity of the limb bones and is usually identifiable but the principal problem in the diagnosis of congenital articular rigidity is to determine what the pathogenesis might have been, and beyond that, what was the specific cause.

Congenital fixation of joints can be caused by some well-known entities, as follows.

Cattle

- Hereditary congenital articular rigidity (HCAR) with cleft palate in Charolais
- HCAR with normal palates in Friesian, Danish Red, Swedish, Shorthorns
- Inherited arthrogryposis
- Inherited multiple tendon contracture
- Inherited multiple ankylosis of Holstein/Friesian cattle
- Environmentally induced CAR caused by:
  - intrauterine infection with Akabane virus
  - ingestion of lupins (6, 7)
  - ingestion of *Astragalus* and *Oxytropis* spp. (locoweeds)
  - sorghum, Johnson grass, sudan grass
  - dietary deficiency of manganese.

Sheep and goats

- Inherited congenital articular rigidity in Merino sheep (5)
- Infection with Akabane virus
- Poison plants as for cattle
- Poisoning with parbendazole and cambendazole.

Piglets

- Inherited congenital articular rigidity
- Nutritional deficiency of vitamin A
- Poisonous plants, hemlock (*Conium maculatum*), *Prunus serotina*, Jimson weed (*Daturia stramonium*), tobacco wastes.

Foals

- 'Contracted' foals—congenital axial and appendicular contractures of joints in the United States, cause unknown (8), not thought to be inherited. Deformities include torticollis, scoliosis, thinning of ventral abdominal wall, sometimes accompanied by eventration, asymmetry of the skull, flexion contracture distal limb joints
- CAR also occurs in foals from mares fed on hybrid sudan grass pastures (9).

Sporadic cases of congenital joint deformity occur in foals and calves. They are manifested usually by excessive flexion of the metacarpophalangeal joints causing affected animals to 'knuckle' at the fetlocks and sometimes walk on the anterior aspect of the pastern. A similar defect occurs in the hindlegs. Many mild cases recover spontaneously but surgical treatment may be required in badly affected animals. The cause in these sporadic cases is unknown and necropsy examination fails to reveal lesions other than excessive flexion of the joints caused by shortening of the flexor tendons. Rarely such fixations are associated with spina bifida or absence of ventral horn cells of the spinal cord.

Congenital defects characterized by hypermobility of joints

It is also recorded as an inherited defect in Jersey cattle. Affected animals are unable to rise or stand because of the lack of fixation of limb joints. The joints and limbs are usually all affected simultaneously and are so flexible that the limbs can be tied in knots. Causes include:

- Inherited joint hypermobility in Jersey cattle
- Inherited in Holstein/Friesian cattle which also have pink teeth due to absence of enamel
- In inherited congenital defects of collagen formation

including dermatosparaxia, hyperelastosis cutis and Ehlers-Danlos syndrome in cattle
- Sporadically in newborn animals (4).

Congenital defects characterized by weakness of skeletal muscles

A number of sporadic myopathies are recorded in cattle and sheep (4). Causes have not been determined in most of them. Splayleg in pigs has been well described and occurs in most countries.

Congenital hyperplasia of myofiber

There is only one identified state; it is the inherited form of Doppelender, double muscling or culard of cattle described in Chapter 34 on inherited diseases. The principal cause of the bulging muscles is an increase in the number of myofibers in the muscle.

Congenital defects characterized by obvious absence or deformity of specific parts of the musculoskeletal system

A number of these defects are known to be inherited and are dealt with in Chapter 34. They include:

- Achondroplastic dwarfism, inherited miniature calves, bulldog calves
- Umbilical, scrotal hernia, cryptorchidism
- Tail deformity (kinking) taillessness
- Reduced phalanges including hemimelia (individual bones missing), amputates (entire limbs missing), vestigial limbs (all parts present, but limbs miniaturized). Amputates in outbreak form recorded in cattle (10) and produced experimentally by irradiation injury of sows, cows and ewes during early pregnancy (11). Inherited arachnomyelia (spidery limbs) of calves
- Congenital thickleg of pigs, (13) osteopetrosis calves, muscular hypertrophy of calves
- Cyclopian deformity. Inherited form associated with prolonged gestation. Toxic form caused by ingestion of *Veratrum californicum*
- Displaced molar teeth, mandibular prognathism. Agnathia in lambs takes a variety of forms including complete absence of lower jaw and tongue (11, 12).

REVIEW LITERATURE

Done, J. T. (1976) Developmental nervous disorders of animals. *Adv. vet. Sci.*, *20*, 104.

Swatland, H. J. (1974) Developmental disorders of skeletal muscle in cattle, pigs and sheep. *Vet. Bull.*, *44*, 179.

REFERENCES

(1) Greene, H. J. et al. (1974) *Zentralbl. VetMed.*, *21A*, 789.
(2) Greeneberg, H. (1963) *The Pathology of Development. A Study of Inherited Skeletal Disorders in Animals*. Oxford: Blackwell Scientific.
(3) Hutt, F. B. (1968) *Cornell Vet.*, *58*, Suppl. 104.
(4) Swatland, H. J. (1974) *Vet. Bull.*, *44*, 179.
(5) Morley, F. H. W. (1954) *Aust. vet. J.*, *30*, 237.
(6) King, J. A. (1965) *J. Am. vet. med. Assoc.*, *147*, 239.
(7) Shupe, J. L. et al. (1967) *J. Am. vet. med. Assoc.*, *151*, 191, 198.
(8) Rooney, J. R. (1966) *Cornell Vet.*, *56*, 172.
(9) Pritchard, J. T. & Voss, J. L. (1967) *J. Am. vet. med. Assoc.*, *150*, 871.
(10) Harbutt, P. R. et al. (1965) *Aust. vet. J.*, *41*, 173.
(11) McFee, A. F. et al. (1965) *J. anim. Sci.*, *24*, 1130.
(12) Dennis, S. M. & Leipold, H. W. (1972) *Am. J. vet. Res.*, *33*, 339.
(13) Doige, B. & Martineau, G. P. (1984) *Can. J. comp. Med.*, *48*, 414.

14

Diseases of the Skin and Conjunctiva

INTRODUCTION

DISEASES of the skin may be primary or secondary in origin. In primary skin disease the lesions are restricted initially to the skin although they may spread from the skin to involve other organs. On the other hand cutaneous lesions may be secondary to disease originating in other organs. Differentiation between primary and secondary skin diseases can be accomplished by making a complete clinical examination of the patient. If there is no evidence that organs other than the skin are affected it can be assumed that the disease is primary. When involvement of other organs is suspected, it is necessary to determine whether the involvement constitutes the primary state or whether it has developed secondarily to the skin disease. The chronology of the signs, elicited by careful history-taking, is the most efficient guide in making a correct decision, although a detailed knowledge of the individual diseases likely to be encountered is of the utmost importance. When a careful clinical examination has been made and an accurate history taken it is then necessary to make a careful examination of the skin itself. Using the proper technique of examination and making accurate observations, then applying one's knowledge of pathology of the skin make it possible to determine the basic defect, whether it be inflammatory or due to malfunction, and thus to define the type of lesion present.

The purpose of this chapter is to describe the basic skin lesions so that the differential diagnosis up to the point of defining the type of lesion can be accomplished. Final determination of the exact cause requires further examination and is included in the discussion of the specific disease. The present section describes in sequence the various steps in clinical examination of the skin, beginning with the exact definition of the lesions, then the interpretation of the findings, and finally the physiological effects of the disease and the consequential principles of treatment.

CLINICAL SIGNS AND SPECIAL EXAMINATION

A general clinical examination should be carried out first. This is followed by the special examination of the skin and must include inspection, and in many cases, palpation. Additional information can be provided by the taking of swabs for bacteriological examinations, by taking scrapings for examination for dermatophytes and metazoan parasites and by biopsy for histological examination. The biopsy material should include abnormal, marginal, and normal skin. Special staining techniques are of considerable assistance in the histological examination of skin. There are a good many sources of potential error in biopsy specimens, especially the taking of a non-representative sample, crushing the specimen by forceps or hemostat and inadequate fixation (4). The use of Wood's lamp in the examination of the skin for dermatophytes is discussed under ringworm.

The description of lesions should include their size, the depth to which they penetrate, their distribution over the body surface, and the area covered. Abnormalities of sebaceous and sweat secretion, or changes in the hair or wool coat, and alterations in color of the skin should be noted. The presence or absence of pain or pruritus should be observed. The manifestations of skin disease are set out below and the common lesions are defined.

Lesions

An accurate definition of the lesions is an essential part of a clinical record of a patient with a skin disease. A summary of the common terms used is in Table 43. Although it makes a primary differentiation into discrete and diffuse lesions, these categories frequently overlap. The differentiation then requires one to categorize the diseases as having limited diffuse lesions or extensive localized ones.

Table 43. Terms used to identify skin lesions

Name of lesion	*Nature of lesion*	*Relation to skin surface*	*Skin surface*
		Diffuse Lesions	
Scales	Dry, flaky exfoliations	On surface, no penetration of skin	Unbroken
Excoriations	Traumatic abrasions and scratches	Penetration below surface	Variable skin surface damage—depends on severity
Fissures	Deep cracks	Penetrate into subcutis	Disrupted
Dry gangrene	Dry, horny, black avascular, shield-like	Above skin, usually all layers affected	Removed
Early moist gangrene	Blue, black, cold, oozing serum	In plane of skin or below	Complete depth of subcutis
Keratosis	Overgrowth of dry horny keratinized epithelium	Above skin	Undamaged; stratum corneum is retained
Acanthosis	Like keratosis but moist soft	Above skin	Prickle cell layer swollen; is really part of skin
Hyperkeratosis	Excessive overgrowth of keratinized epithelium-like scab	Above skin	Skin surface unbroken
Parakeratosis	Adherent to skin	Above skin	Cells of stratum corneum nucleated and retained; really part of skin
Eczema	Erythematous, itching dermatitis	Superficial layer of epidermis affected	Weeping, scabby disruption of surface
		Discrete Lesions	
Vesicle, bleb, bullae, blister	Fluid (serum or lymph)-filled blister 1–2 cm diameter	Above surface, superficial	Unbroken, but will slough
Pustule	Pus-filled blister, 1–5 mm	Above, superficial	Will rupture
Wheals	Edematous, erythematous swellings, transitory	Above; all layers affected	Undamaged
Papules (pimples)	Elevated, inflamed, necrotic center; up to 1 cm	Above surface, all layers affected	Points and ruptures
Nodules nodes	Elevated, solid, up to 1 cm acute or chronic inflammation. No necrotic center	Above surface; all layers affected	Surface unbroken
Plaque	A larger nodule, up to 3–4 cm diameter	All layers affected; raised above surface	Unbroken surface
Acne	Used synonymously with pimple, but strictly means infection of sebaceous gland	Above surface of skin; all layers affected	May point and rupture
Impetigo	Flaccid vesicle, then pustule then scab, up to 1 cm diameter	Raised above skin. Very superficial	Upper layers destroyed
Scab	Crust of coagulated serum, blood, pus and skin debris	Raised above skin	Disrupted, depth varying with original lesion

Pyoderma: any pyogenic infection of skin, includes impetigo, acne, pimple, pustule

Abnormal coloration

Abnormal colorations including jaundice, pallor and erythema may be visible. These signs are best seen in the oral or vaginal mucosae or in the conjunctiva. In animals with light-colored skins they may be visible at first glance. The red to purple discoloration of the skin of white pigs affected by various septicemias may be extreme and no diagnostic significance can be attached to its degree because the same color can be observed in cases of salmonellosis, pasteurellosis, erysipelas and hog cholera. Early erythema is a common finding where more definite skin lesions are to develop, as in early photosensitization. The blue coloration of early gangrene is characterized by coldness and loss of elasticity. This is particularly evident on the udder and teat skin of cows in the early stages of acute mastitis caused by *Staphylococcus aureus*.

Pruritus

Pruritus or itching is the sensation which gives rise to the desire to scratch. It must be differentiated from hyperesthesia, which is increased sensitivity to normal stimuli. Paresthesia or perverted sensation is subjective in nature and can hardly be defined in animals. All sensations which give rise to rubbing or scratching are therefore included with pruritus. The abnormality is more properly defined as scratching.

Itching can arise from peripheral or central stimulation. Itching of peripheral origin is a primary cutaneous sensation along with heat, cold, pain and touch (1). It has similarities to pain but differs from it, especially in that it is purely epidermal, whereas pain can still be felt in areas of skin denuded of epidermis. Thus itching does not occur in the center of deep ulcerations nor in very superficial lesions, such as those of ringworm, where only the hair fibers and keratinized epithelium are involved. Although itching can be elicited over the entire skin surface, it is most severe at the mucocutaneous junctions. Common causes include the following.

Cattle

- Sarcoptic and chorioptic manges
- Aujeszky's disease
- Nervous acetonemia
- Lice infestation.

Sheep

- Lice, ked and itch-mite infestations
- Scrapie.

Pigs

- Sarcoptic and chorioptic mange
- Lice infestation.

Horses

- Chorioptic mange on the legs
- Queensland (Sweet) itch along the dorsum of the body
- Lice infestation
- Perianal pruritus due to *Oxyuris equi* infestation.

All species

- The early stages of photosensitive dermatitis
- Urticarial wheals in an allergic reaction
- 'Licking syndromes' such as occur in cattle on copper-deficient diets are accompanied by pica and the licking of others as well as themselves. They are classified as depraved appetites as a response to nutritional deficiency and are not a response to pruritus.

Itching of central origin derives in the main from the scratch center below the acoustic nucleus in the medulla. It may have a structural basis as in scrapie and pseudorabies, or it may be functional in origin as in the nervous form of acetonemia. The only lesions observed are those of a traumatic dermatitis with removal of the superficial layers to a variable depth, breakage or removal of the hairs, and a distribution of lesions in places where the animal can bite or rub easily.

One other cause for scratching is mnemodermia or 'skin memory'. This is a special form of hyperesthesia in which hypersensitivity to innocuous stimuli persists after the initial lesions have subsided. There are numerous examples of this in humans as a result of plant and insect stings. It would be difficult to make a diagnosis of mnemodermia in animals.

Effective treatment of pruritus depends upon the reduction of central perception of itch sensations, or on successful restraint of the mediator between the lesion and the sensory endorgan (1). Reduction of central perception of pruritus is usually achieved by the use of ataractic, sedative or narcotic drugs administered systemically. However, boredom contributes significantly to an animal's response to itch stimuli, and close confinement of affected animals is best avoided. Little is known of the mediating substances which stimulate itch endorgans but proteolytic enzymes are thought to be instrumental. In the absence of accurate knowledge of the pathogenesis it is usual to resort to local anesthetic agents which are short-lived in their activity, and corticosteroids which are longer acting, and effective provided that vascular engorgement is part of the pruritus-stimulating mechanism.

Abnormalities of sweat secretion

The activity of the sweat glands is controlled by the sympathetic nervous system and is for the most part a reflection of body temperature. Excitement and pain may cause sweating before the body temperature rises; here the sweating is due to cerebral cortical activity. A form of hyperhydrosis, apparently inherited, has been recorded in Shorthorn calves (2). Local areas of abnormal sweating may arise from peripheral nerve lesions or obstruction of sweat gland ducts. A generalized anhidrosis is recorded in horses and occasionally in cattle.

Abnormalities of sebaceous gland secretion

Excess sebum secretion causes oiliness of the skin. It occurs in several diseases of animals including greasy heel of horses and exudative epidermitis of pigs but the pathogenesis of seborrhea is poorly understood.

Abnormalities of wool and hair fibers

Deficiency of hair or wool in comparison to the normal pilosity of the skin area is referred to as alopecia. There are two kinds of alopecia. One is caused by follicle dysfunction and the other by injury to the fiber, as in ringworm and trauma. The capacity of the follicular epithelium to produce a fiber may be congenitally defective or may be temporarily reduced because of nutritional deficiency or severe systemic disease. Bands of weak fiber through a hair coat or fleece may result in 'breaks' and loss of the major part of the coat. Special note should be taken of whether the fibre is completely absent or has been broken off along the shaft.

The character of the fiber may also vary with variations in the internal environment. In copper deficiency the crimp of fine wool fibers is lost and the wool becomes straight and 'steely'. Alteration in coat color, often segmentally or in patches, is an important diagnostic sign in agricultural animals. It is discussed under the heading of achromotrichia (p. 488).

SPECIAL PATHOLOGY

The reaction of the skin to noxious stimuli varies with the severity and depth of the injury (3). In the corium or dermis the reaction is the same as that in other tissues because of the presence of blood and lymphatic vessels, nerve fibers, and connective tissue. The epidermis, because of its purely cellular composition, reacts differently. If the reaction is acute, the development of lesions begins with swelling and edema of the cells of the prickle cell layer—the so-called 'spongiosis'. If the edema is severe enough, cells rupture and fluid collects to form foci which gradually emerge through the stratum corneum and appear on the surface as vesicles. Should the foci rupture before reaching the surface the result is weeping of the affected area. In less acute inflammations, the intracellular edema in the prickle cell layer interferes with the normal functioning of the granular layer and gives rise to abnormal formation of cornified epithelium. As a result the epidermis becomes thickened. All layers are affected, particularly the stratum corneum, because of improper keratinization and failure of exfoliation. The lesion is described histologically as parakeratosis. It may be accompanied by acanthosis which consists of pronounced thickening of the prickle cell layer and prolongation of the interpapillary processes. The disease state is usually described as pachydermia. Acanthosis in conjunction with the deposition of melanin is known as acanthosis nigricans, a disease in dogs and man commonly associated with thyroid dysfunction.

It should be possible to distinguish clinically between acute inflammatory changes and those caused by chronic inflammation or malfunction of skin tissue due to other causes by observing the type of reaction in the skin. Both acute and chronic inflammation may be caused by bacterial, viral, metazoan and protozoan agents, and also by chemical and physical agents including light-sensitization and allergy. Chronic inflammation may also arise from any of these causes and the inflammation interferes with normal skin metabolism. Similar lesions can be produced by nutritional deficiency; thus parakeratosis may arise from chronic inflammation or from a dietary deficiency of zinc. Further identification of the type of lesion necessitates classification and the various categories are set out in the subsequent parts of this chapter.

Skin diseases of allergic origin are not well understood, but two manifestations require mention here. When an allergen is applied to skin sensitized to it, it causes a local increase in tissue histamine levels and an accumulation of eosinophils. If the quantity of histamine liberated is in excess of the detoxifying capacity of the eosinophil aggregation, histamine escapes into the vascular system, and the blood histamine levels rise. This elevation of total blood histamine levels and the accompanying eosinophilia are quite transitory. The levels return to normal in 1–8 hours after removal of the allergen, the time varying with the severity and duration of the allergic reaction. Examination of histamine levels or eosinophil counts in the blood may be of diagnostic value although negative results do not preclude the possibility of an allergic etiology. The local skin reaction to the allergen is due to the vasodilatory effects of histamine. If the reaction is severe enough, other organs may show the effects of histamine toxicity. An ingested allergen may produce reactions in other organs in addition to those in the skin.

PHYSIOLOGICAL EFFECTS OF DISEASES OF THE SKIN

The major functions of the skin are to maintain a normal body temperature and a normal fluid and electrolyte balance within the animal. In general these functions are not greatly impeded by most diseases of the skin although failure of the sweating mechanism does seriously interfere with body temperature regulation, and severe burns or other skin trauma may cause fatal fluid and electrolyte loss.

The major effects of skin diseases in animals are esthetic and economic. The unsightly appearance of the animal distresses the owner. Discomfort and scratching interfere with normal rest and feeding and when the lips are affected there may be interference with prehension. There is loss of the economic coat and the protective function of the skin is reduced.

Another cause of loss may be the serious depletion of protein stores when extensive loss of epithelium occurs. The epithelial cells and appendages have a high content of sulfur-containing amino acids and if these are not available in the diet they will be withdrawn from protein molecules in other tissues and serious tissue wasting may result. The intervention of secondary infection may, of course, lead to grave consequences.

PRINCIPLES OF TREATMENT OF DISEASES OF THE SKIN

Removal of hair coat and debris to enable topical applications to come into contact with the causative agent is desirable. Accurate diagnosis of the cause must precede the selection of any topical or systemic treatment. In bacterial diseases sensitivity tests on cultures of the organism are advisable. Specific skin diseases due to bacteria, fungi and metazoan parasites are reasonably amenable to treatment. Removal of the causative agent in allergic diseases and photosensitization may be impossible and symptomatic treatment may be the only practicable solution. In many cases, too, the primary disease may be confounded by the presence of a secondary agent, which can lead to confusion in diagnosis. Treatment may be unsuccessful if both agents are not treated. In addition to specific treatments the following measures should be considered:

- Prevent secondary infection by the use of bacteriostatic ointments or dressings
- Prevent further damage from scratching by the application of local anesthetic ointments or the administration of centrally acting sedatives
- When large areas of skin are involved prevent the absorption of toxic products by continuous irrigation or the application of absorptive dressings. Losses of fluid and electrolytes should be made good by the parenteral administration of isotonic fluids containing the necessary electrolytes
- Ensure an adequate dietary intake of protein, particularly sulfur-containing amino acids to facilitate the repair of skin tissues.

Many preparations are used empirically in the treatment of skin diseases. Preparations containing arsenic, antimony, gold, and manganese given orally or, more commonly, parenterally, are also in common use in human medicine. Arsenic, sulfur and antimony are deposited preferentially in the skin and hair in high concentrations, and in addition arsenic has activity against spirochetes and protozoa.

REVIEW LITERATURE

Montes, L. F. & Vaughan, J. T. (1983) *Atlas of Skin Diseases of the Horse*. Philadelphia: W. B. Saunders.

Mullowney, P. C. (1984) Symposium on large animal dermatology. *Vet. Clin. N. Am. large Anim. Pract.*, 6(1) 1–226.

Mullowney, P. C. & Fadok, V. A. (1984) Dermatologic diseases of the horse. *Comp. cont. Educ.*, 6, S16–S20, S22–S26.

Pascoe, R. R. (1974) Equine dermatoses. *Univ. of Sydney Postgrad. Found. Vet. Sci.*. Review no. 22.

REFERENCES

(1) Halliwell, R. E. W. (1974) *J. Am. vet. med. Assoc.*, *164*, 793.

(2) Larson, P. W. & Prior, R. W. (1971) *Vet. Med. small Anim. Clin.*, 66, 667.

(3) Head, K. W. (1970) *Vet. Rec.*, *87*, 460.

(4) McGavin, M. D. et al. (1984) *Vet. Clin. N. Am. large Anim. Pract.*, *6(1)*, 203.

DISEASES OF THE EPIDERMIS AND DERMIS

Pityriasis

Pityriasis or dandruff is a condition characterized by the presence of bran-like scales on the skin surface.

Etiology

Pityriasis may be of dietary, parasitic, fungal or chemical origin. Causes in all species are follows.

Dietary causes

- Hypovitaminosis A
- Nutritional deficiency of B vitamins, especially riboflavin and nicotinic acid, and especially in pigs
- Nutritional deficiency of linolenic acid, and probably other essential unsaturated fatty acids
- Poisoning by iodine (probably be causing a secondary fatty acid deficiency).

Parasitic pityriasis

- Flea, louse and mange infestations.

Infectious causes

- Especially keratolytic agents as in ringworm.

Pathogenesis

The scales of pityriasis are keratinized epithelial cells. These are sometimes softened and made greasy by the exudation of serum or sebum. Overproduction of keratinized epithelial cells, as in vitamin A deficiency, or excessive desquamation, caused for example by scratching in parasitic infestations, lead to the accumulation of scales on the skin surface. When hyperkeratinization occurs it begins around the orifices of the hair follicles and spreads to the surrounding stratum corneum.

Clinical findings

Primary pityriasis comprises the accumulation of scales without itching or other skin lesions. The scales are superficial in origin. They accumulate most readily where the coat is long and their presence is usually associated with a dry lusterless coat. Secondary pityriasis is usually accompanied by the lesions of the primary disease.

Clinical pathology

The definition of primary pityriasis depends upon the examination of skin scrapings to eliminate other primary agents, particularly parasites and fungi.

Diagnosis

Pityriasis is one of the commonest accompaniments of skin disease. Further differentiation of primary causes will not be discussed here although it is necessary to distinguish pityriasis from hyperkeratosis and parakeratosis.

Treatment

Correction of the primary cause is the first necessity. Non-specific treament should commence with a thorough washing. This is followed by alternating applications of a bland, emollient ointment and an alcoholic lotion. Salicylic acid is frequently incorporated into a lotion or ointment with a lanolin base.

Parakeratosis

Parakeratosis is a condition of the skin in which keratinization of the epithelial cells is incomplete.

Etiology
Causes in animals include:

- Non-specific chronic inflammation of cellular epidermis, causing faulty keratinization of the horny cells
- Dietary deficiency of zinc
- Inherited as Adema disease in cattle
- Inherited as dermatosis vegetans in pigs.

Pathogenesis
The initial lesion comprises edema of the prickle cell layer, dilatation of the intercellular lymphatics, and leukocyte infiltration. Imperfect keratinization of epithelial cells at the granular layer of the epidermis follows. When keratinization is thus interfered with the horn cells produced are sticky and soft and retain their nuclei. They tend to stick together to form large masses. These either stay fixed to the underlying tissues or fall off as large scales.

Clinical findings
The lesions may be extensive and diffuse but are often confined to the flexor aspects of joints. Initially there is reddening followed by thickening of the skin and the development of a gray coloration. The scales are often held in place by hairs. The lesions usually crack and fissure, and removal of the scales leaves a raw, red surface. Psoriasis, mallenders and sallenders are clinical terms describing various forms of parakeratosis.

Clinical pathology
For a definite diagnosis of parakeratosis a biopsy or a skin section at necropsy is necessary.

Diagnosis
Histologically, the imperfect keratinization is evident and differentiates the condition from hyperkeratosis. In contrast to hyperkeratosis the crusts are soft and have a raw skin surface beneath them.

Treatment
In nutritional parakeratosis the deficiency must be corrected. The abnormal tissue is first removed by the use of a keratolytic ointment (e.g. salicylic acid ointment) or by vigorous washing with soapy water. This is followed by the application of an astringent preparation (e.g. white lotion paste). The astringent preparation must be applied frequently and for some time after the lesions have disappeared.

Hyperkeratosis

Hyperkeratosis is a condition in which excessively keratinized epithelial cells accumulate on the surface of the skin.

Etiology
Hyperkeratosis may be local at pressure points, for example elbows, when animals lie habitually on hard surfaces. Generalized hyperkeratosis may be caused by:

- Poisoning with highly chlorinated naphthalene compounds used in industry
- Chronic arsenic poisoning
- Inherited congenital ichthyosis (fish-scale disease) of cattle.

Pathogenesis
The continued adhesion of epithelial scales, which is characteristic of hyperkeratosis, is caused by excessive keratinization of epithelial cells and intercellular bridges and by hypertrophy of the stratum corneum. The excessive keratinization encountered in cases of poisoning with highly chlorinated naphthalenes is due to a deficiency of vitamin A and interference with normal cell division in the granular layer of the epidermis. Local compression also leads to the accumulation of keratinized epithelial cells.

Clinical findings
The skin becomes thicker than normal and is usually corrugated and hairless. Dryness and scaliness of the external surface are characteristic. Fissures develop in a grid-like fashion giving a scaly appearance. Secondary infection of the fissures may occur if the area is continually wet. However, the lesion is usually dry and the plugs of hyperkeratotic material can be removed leaving the underlying skin intact.

Clinical pathology
Histological examination of a biopsy section shows the characteristically thickened stratum corneum.

Diagnosis
The differentiation of hyperkeratosis from parakeratosis has already been described.

Treatment
Treatment of the primary condition is essential. The use of keratolytic agents (e.g. salicylic acid ointment) may effect some improvement.

Pachydermia

Pachydermia is a thickening of the skin affecting all layers. Frequently the subcutaneous tissue is also involved. Scleroderma is also included in this classification.

Etiology
Non-specific chronic or recurrent inflammation of the skin is the cause of most cases of pachydermia. The lesion is usually local in origin although the affected area may be of considerable size as in lymphangitis and greasy heel in the horse and in baldy calves. There are no specific causes of pachydermia.

Pathogenesis
The cells in all layers are usually normal but the individual layers are increased in thickness. There is hypertrophy of the prickle cell layer of the epidermis and enlargement of the interpapillary processes.

Clinical findings
The hair coat is thin or absent and the affected skin is thicker and tougher than usual. The skin appears tight and, because of its thickness and the diminution of subcutaneous tissue, cannot be picked into folds or moved over underlying tissue as readily as in normal areas. There are no discontinuities in the skin surface.

Diagnosis
In pachydermia the thickening of the skin is usually confined to localized areas. There are no superficial skin lesions and no accumulation of cell debris. These findings serve to differentiate the condition from the other chronic skin thickenings, parakeratosis and hyperkeratosis.

Treatment
In chronic cases little improvement can be anticipated. The administration of cortisone preparations locally or parenterally in the early stages of the disease may cause recovery. When small areas are involved surgical removal may be attempted.

Impetigo

Impetigo is a superficial eruption of thin-walled, usually small, vesicles surrounded by a zone of erythema. The vesicles develop into pustules and rupture to form scabs.

Etiology
In humans, impetigo is specifically a streptococcal infection but lesions are often invaded secondarily by staphylococci. In animals the main organism found is usually a staphylococcus. The only specific causes of impetigo in animals are:

- Udder impetigo of cows
- Infectious dermatitis or 'contagious pyoderma' of baby pigs, caused by unspecified streptococci and staphylococci.

Pathogenesis
The causative organism appears to gain entry through minor abrasions. Rupture of lesions causes contamination of the surrounding skin and the appearance of more lesions. Spread from animal to animal occurs readily. Udder impetigo in cows is particularly infectious.

Clinical findings
Vesicles appear chiefly on the relatively hairless parts of the body. They remain as small (3–6 mm) discrete lesions and do not become confluent. In the early stages a zone of erythema is evident around the vesicle. There is no irritation. Rupture of the vesicles occurs readily although they may persist and become pustules which form yellow scabs. Involvement of hair follicles is common and leads to the development of acne and much deeper, more extensive lesions. Individual lesions heal rapidly in about a week but successive crops of vesicles may occur and prolong the duration of the disease.

Clinical pathology
Culture of vesicular fluid should be carried out to determine the causative bacterium and its sensitivity.

Diagnosis
Impetigo must be differentiated from pox lesions particularly in cattle. Cowpox lesions occur mainly on the teats and pass through the characteristic stages of pox. Pseudocowpox is unlikely to develop as a true pox lesion and its distribution on the udder is its major diagnostic feature. The early, vesicular stages of eczema may be confused with impetigo but in eczema irritation is intense and the lesions show a marked tendency to coalesce. The vesicles are also much smaller in size.

Treatment
Local treatment is usually all that is required. Individual lesions heal so rapidly that the main aim of treatment is to prevent the occurrence of new lesions and spread of the disease to other animals. Twice daily bathing with an efficient germicidal skin wash is usually adequate.

Urticaria

Urticaria is an allergic condition characterized by the appearance of wheals on the skin surface.

Etiology
Urticaria may be primary resulting directly from the effect of the pathogen, or secondary as part of a syndrome.

Primary urticaria

- Insect stings, contact with stinging plants
- Ingestion of unusual food, with the allergen usually a protein; a recent change of diet is a common precursor
- Administration of a particular drug, e.g., penicillin
- Death of warble fly larvae in tissue
- Milk allergy when Jersey cows dried off.

Secondary urticaria

- Respiratory tract infections in horses, including strangles and the viral infections
- During erysipelas in pigs.

Pathogenesis
The lesions of urticaria are characteristic of an allergic reaction. A primary dilatation of capillaries causes erythema of the skin. Exudation from the damaged capillary walls results in local edema of the dermis, with swelling and pallor due to compression of the capillaries. The lesion usually remains red at the edges. Only the dermis, and sometimes the epidermis, is involved.

Clinical findings
Urticarial lesions appear very rapidly and often in large numbers, particularly on the body. They vary from 0·5 to 5 cm in diameter, are elevated with a flat top and are tense to the touch. There is usually no itching, except with plant or insect stings, nor discontinuity of the epithelial surface. Color changes in the wheals can be observed only in unpigmented skin. No exudation or weeping occurs. Other allergic phenomena, including diarrhea and slight fever, may accompany the eruption. Subsidence of the lesions within a few hours is common but the disease may persist for 3–4 days. Such persistence is usually due to the appearance of fresh lesions.

Clinical pathology
Tissue histamine levels are increased and there is a local accumulation of eosinophils. Blood histamine levels and eosinophil counts may show transient elevation.

Diagnosis
Urticaria can be differentiated from angioneurotic edema because in urticaria the lesions can be palpated

in the skin itself. Angioneurotic edema involves the subcutaneous tissue rather than the skin and the lesions are much larger and more diffuse.

Treatment

Spontaneous recovery is common. Antihistamines provide the best and most rational treatment. Parenteral injections of adrenaline may also be used. One treatment is usually sufficient. Lesions may recur if the diet is not changed or exposure to the causal insects or plants not prevented. A mild purgative is recommended, and the local application of cooling astringent lotions such as calamine or white lotion or a dilute solution of sodium bicarbonate is favored. In large animal practice parenteral injections of calcium salts are used with apparently good results.

Eczema

Eczema is an inflammatory reaction of the epidermal cells to substances to which the cells are sensitized. These substances may be present in the external or internal environment.

Etiology

Eczema occurs when the skin cells are brought into contact with allergens (1). These allergens are described as exogenous when they are applied to the skin surface or as endogenous when they are carried in the bloodstream.

Endogenous allergens

These are absorbed via the gut but not identifiable in most animals, and probably occur in the following categories:

- Ingested as proteins
- Formed in the gut, mostly amines as in autointoxication due to overeating or bowel stasis and reflux, digestion of internal parasites.

Exogenous allergens

- External parasites
- Antiseptic and disinfectant washes.

Predisposing causes

Some animals are much more susceptible than the rest of group. Possible causes include:

- Inherited susceptibility
- Repeated wetting or dampness as in continued sweating
- Constant scratching due to external parasite infestation
- Long-term soiling and accumulation of skin debris.

Pathogenesis

The primary lesion is erythema, followed by intercellular and intracellular edema, the characteristic 'spongiosis' lesion of eczema. The accumulation of edematous fluid causes the formation of small vesicles which are characteristic of the early stages of eczema. Rupture of the vesicles and exfoliation of epidermal cells result in weeping and the subsequent development of scabs. In some cases a general outpouring of fluid without the appearance of vesicles occurs. This acute stage may disappear quickly or a chronic inflammation may persist with either parakeratosis or, in the very chronic form, pachydermia.

Clinical findings

True eczema is rare in large animals. In the acute form the earliest observable change is a patch of erythema, followed by the appearance of small vesicles which rupture and cause weeping of the surface. Scab formation follows. The lesions may occur in isolated patches or be diffuse over large areas and in some cases are symmetrical. In sheep, outbreaks are recorded of periorbital eczema in which 50% of a flock may be affected (2). Itching and irritation are usually intense and scratching and rubbing exacerbate the condition. Chronic eczema may follow an acute attack or, because of a persistent low-grade irritation, be chronic from the beginning. Because of the scratching and rubbing there is alopecia, some scaling and hypertrophy of all skin layers with resultant pachydermia, but there is no discontinuity of the skin.

Clinical pathology

Because of the expense involved, skin tests to determine the sensitizing agent are not used. The clinical pathology of the condition consists of the elimination of other causes of superficial dermatitis, particularly ectoparasites.

Diagnosis

A definite diagnosis of eczema is difficult to make because differentiation between it and dermatitis poses a problem, especially in an individual case. In eczema the lesions are superficial, follow a fairly regular pattern of development and recur when the skin is exposed to the same or other sensitizing substances which are not recognized irritants and are innocuous to normal animals.

Treatment

The basis of treatment is to prevent exposure to the sensitizing substance. Because detection of the allergen is often impossible, changes in environment, including a change in diet, changes of bedding and in the surroundings, the removal of internal and external parasites, the avoidance of wetting and unnecessary irritation, and the protection of the skin are often instituted. A light, high-protein, laxative diet is generally recommended. In the early acute stages sedation is an advantage because it avoids further damage by scratching. Antihistamine preparations are used extensively in the treatment of eczema and give good results in acute cases. Non-specific protein injections, including autogenous whole blood or boiled skim milk, and cortisone preparations are also used to stimulate healing.

Local treatment varies with the stage of development of the disease. In the early, weeping stage astringent antiseptic lotions are required. In the later, scabby stage, protective ointments or pastes, particularly those containing local anesthetic agents, should be applied at frequent intervals.

REFERENCES

(1) Walton, G. S. (1968) *Vet. Rec.*, *82*, 204.
(2) O Brien, J. J. & McCracken, R. M. (1971) *Irish vet. J.*, *25*, 69.

Dermatitis

The term dermatitis includes those conditions characterized by inflammation of the dermis and epidermis.

Etiology

Some of the identifiable occurrences of food animals and horses are as follows.

All species

- Mycotic dermatitis due to *Dermatophilus congolensis*, horses, cattle, sheep
- Ringworm
- Burns and frostbite
- Photosensitive dermatitis
- Beta-irradiation
- Chemical irritation topically
- Arsenic—systemic poisoning
- Mange mite infestation—sarcoptic, psoroptic, chorioptic, demodectic mange
- Trombidiform mite infestation (tyroglyphosis) e.g. *Pyemotes tritici* (4) and *Acarus (Tyroglyphus) farinae* (5) in horses
- *Stephanofilaria* sp. dermatitis
- *Strongyloides* sp. dermatitis
- Screw-worm infestation
- Infection with the protozoan (*Besnoitia* sp.).

Cattle

- Udder impetigo—*Staphylococcus aureus*
- Cutaneous botryomycosis of the udder caused by a combination of trauma and infection by *Pseudomonas aeruginosa* (6)
- Cowpox
- Ulcerative mammillitis—udder and teats only
- Lumpy skin disease—Allerton and Neethling 'strains'
- Foot-and-mouth disease—vesicles around maternal orifices and vesicular stomatitis, teats and coronet
- Rinderpest, bovine diarrhea, bovine malignant catarrh, bluetongue—erosive lesions around natural orifices, eyes, coronets
- Sweating sickness
- Dermatitis (vesicular, necrotic) around anus—mushroom poisoning
- Dermatitis on legs—potato poisoning, topical application irritants or defatting agents, e.g. diesoline
- Dermatitis due to the ingestion of *Vicia villosa* and *V. dasycarpa*
- Experimental nutritional deficiency of B vitamins—calves (as listed under pigs)
- Flexural seborrhea—cause unknown.

Sheep

- Strawberry footrot—*Dermatophilus pedis*
- Facial or limb pyoderma (syn. staphylococcal dermatitis)—*Staphylococcus aureus*
- Sheep pox
- Contagious ecthyma
- Ulcerative dermatosis
- Rinderpest PPR, bluetongue—as for cattle
- Foot-and-mouth disease and vesicular stomatitis
- Fleece rot—constant wetting
- Lumpy wool—*Dermatophilus congolensis*
- Itch-mite (*Psorergates ovis*) infestation
- Blowfly infestation (cutaneous myiasis)
- 'Cockle' (probably parasitic)
- Elaeophoriasis (*Elaeophora* sp. infestation).

Pigs

- Infectious pyoderma—*Streptococcus* sp. and *Staphylococcus aureus*
- Ulcerative granuloma—*Borrelia suilla*
- Exudative epidermitis—*Staphylococcus hyicus* (greasy pig disease)
- Pig pox
- Swine vesicular disease, vesicular exanthema of swine, foot-and-mouth disease—vesicles around natural orifices
- Sunburn
- Trauma or contact dermatitis—carpal necrosis and other sites
- Porcine necrotic ear syndrome; there is extensive necrosis of the edges of the ears. The cause is unknown but the possibility of a combination of *Staphylococcus hyicus* infection and trauma by biting being the cause seems high (7)
- Non-specific nutritional dermatitis—experimental nutritional deficiency of nicotinic acid, riboflavin, pantothenic acid, biotin
- Pityriasis rosea—cause unknown.

Horses

- Staphylococcal dermatitis—*Staphylococcus aureus* and *S. intermedius*, rarely *S. hyicus* (3) in a syndrome reminiscent of greasy heel
- Horsepox
- Canadian horsepox
- Viral papular dermatitis
- Vesicular stomatitis—vesicles around natural orifices
- Sporotrichosis
- Dermatophytes—follicular dermatitis (as well as standard ringworm); also tinea versicolor dermatitis
- Scald—constant wetting
- Queensland (Sweet) itch—sensitivity to *Culicoides* sp., sandflies
- Chronic eosinophilic dermatitis, cause unknown. There is marked acanthosis and hyperkeratosis and eosinophilic granulomas in pancreas, salivary glands and other epithelial organs. The systemic involvement is accompanied by severe weight loss. The disease is chronic (2)
- Pemphigus
- Nodular necrobiosis (8). Firm, small (up to 1 cm diameter) nodules, usually a number of them, occurring on the sides of the trunk and neck. The cause is unknown. The lesions consist largely of an accumulation of eosinophils (9)
- Ear plaque (8). Multiple white plaques, about 1 cm in diameter on the inner surface of the ear pinna of horses and resembling papilloma
- Uasin gishu disease
- Molluscum contagiosum of horses characterized by multiple cutaneous nodules with distinctive histopathology (10)

- Hyperplastic dermatitis (1)—cause unknown
- Cutaneous habronemiasis.

Special local dermatidites
These include dermatitis of the teats and udder, the bovine muzzle, and the coronet, and flexural seborrhea and are dealt with under their respective headings.

Pathogenesis
Dermatitis is basically an inflammation of the deeper layers of the skin involving the blood vessels and lymphatics. The purely cellular layers of the epidermis are involved only secondarily. The noxious agent causes cellular damage, often to the point of necrosis and, depending on the type of agent responsible, the resulting dermatitis varies in its manifestations. It may be acute or chronic, suppurative, weeping, seborrheic, ulcerative or gangrenous. In all cases there is increased thickness and increased temperature of the part. Pain or itching is present and erythema is evident in unpigmented skin. Histologically there is vasodilatation and infiltration with leukocytes and cellular necrosis. These changes are much less marked in chronic dermatitis.

Clinical findings
Affected skin areas first show erythema and increased warmth. The subsequent stages vary according to the type and severity of the causative agent. There may be development of discrete vesicular lesions or diffuse weeping. Edema of the skin and subcutaneous tissues may occur in severe cases. The next stage may be the healing stage of scab formation or, if the injury is more severe, there may be necrosis or even gangrene of the affected skin area. Spread of infection to subcutaneous tissues may result in a diffuse cellulitis or phlegmonous lesion. A distinctive suppurative lesion is usually classified as pyoderma.

Staphylococcal dermatitis is a serious disease of horses because the lesions are intractable to treatment and are so painful to touch that the horse is hard to handle, and the presence of the lesions under harness, where they commonly are, prevents the horse from working kindly. Harness horses are at a particular disadvantage. Individual lesions are 3–5 mm in diameter, are raised nodules with a small, easily removed scab on top. When these lift they take a tuft of hair with them and a small crater is left. Only a little pus exudes and only a red serous fluid can be expressed. Individual lesions last a long time, at least several weeks, and fresh crops occur causing the disease to spread slowly on the animal.

A systemic reaction is likely to occur when the affected skin area is extensive. Shock, with peripheral circulatory failure, may be present in the early stages. Toxemia, due to absorption of tissue breakdown products, or septicemia, due to invasion via unprotected tissues, may occur in the later stages.

Clinical pathology
Examination of skin scrapings or swabs for parasitic, bacterial or other agents is essential. Culture and sensitivity tests for bacteria are advisable to enable the best treatment to be selected. Skin biopsy may be of value in determining the causal agent. In allergic or parasitic states there is usually an accumulation of eosinophils in the inflamed area. In mycotic dermatitis organisms are usually detectable in the deep skin layers although they may not be cultivable from superficial specimens.

Diagnosis
The clinical features of dermatitis are apparent. Differentiation from eczema may be difficult unless there is a history of exposure to a probable allergen. The characteristic features of the etiological types of dermatitis are described under each specific disease.

Treatment
The primary aim of treatment must be to remove the noxious stimulus. Removal of the physical or chemical agent from the environment or supplementation of the diet to repair a nutritional deficiency are an essential basis for treatment. The choice of a suitable treatment for infectious skin disease will depend upon the accurate identification of the etiological agent. For example, in bacterial infections the sensitivity of the organism will influence the choice of antibacterial drugs.

Supportive treatment includes both local and systemic therapy. Local applications may need to be astringent either as powders or lotions in the weeping stage or as greasy salves in the scabby stage. The inclusion of antihistamine preparation is recommended in allergic states and it is desirable to prescribe anesthetic agents when pain or itching is severe.

If shock is present, parenteral fluids should be administered. When tissue destruction is extensive or the dermatitis is allergic in origin, antihistamines are of value. If the lesions are extensive or secondary bacterial invasion is likely to occur, parenterally administered antibiotics or antifungal agents may be preferred to topical applications. To facilitate skin repair, a high protein diet or the administration of protein hydrolysates or amino acid combinations may find a place in the treatment of valuable animals.

The use of vaccines as prophylaxis in viral and bacterial dermatitides must not be neglected. Autogenous vaccines may be most satisfactory in bacterial infections. A particular recommended use of an autogenous vaccine is in the treatment of staphylococcal dermatitis in horses. Long and repeated courses of treatment with penicillin produce only temporary remission. An autogenous vaccine produces a cure in many cases. Bovine udder impetigo responds similarly.

REFERENCES

(1) Binninger, C. E. & Piper, R. C. (1968) *J. Am. vet. med. Assoc.*, *153*, 69.
(2) Wilkie, J. S. N. et al. (1985) *Vet. Pathol.*, *22*, 297.
(3) Devriese, L. A. et al. (1983) *Equ. vet. J.*, *15*, 263.
(4) Kunkle, G. A. & Greiner, E. G. (1982) *J. Am. vet. med. Assoc.*, *181*, 467.
(5) Norval, J. & McPherson, E. A. (1983) *Vet. Rec.* *112*, 385.
(6) Donovan, G. A. & Gross, T. L. (1984) *J. Am. vet. med. Assoc.*, *184*, 197.
(7) Richardson, J. A. et al (1984) *Vet. Pathol.*, *21*, 152.
(8) Thomsett, L. R. (1984) *Vet. Clin. N. Am. large Anim. Pract.*, *6(1)*, 59.
(9) Nicolls, T. J. et al. (1983) *Aust. vet. J.*, *60*, 148.
(10) Cooley, A. J. et al. (1987) *J. comp. Pathol.*, *97*, 29.

Pemphigus

This is an autoimmune disease of the skin, sometimes affecting mucosae, and characterized by the presence of vesicles or bullae, which are usually very difficult to find, and subsequent erosions and ulcerations. There are a number of manifestations including pemphigus vulgaris and pemphigus foliaceous. It is a chronic autoimmune disease often accompanied by severe weight loss (6).

Pemphigus foliaceous is recorded in goats (1, 7) as a widespread disease characterized by the presence of scales, sometimes in heavy crusts, and involvement of the coronets. It occurs also in horses (2) as a generalized disease (3, 4) but it may be localized as circumscribed, circular lesions in the mouth and vulva and on the skin at mucocutaneous junctions (5). The lesions are sore to the touch, are subepidermal bullae from which the top layer can be pulled away. In some cases the lesions are around the coronary bands on all limbs.

REFERENCES

(1) Jackson, P. G. G. et al. (1984) *Vet. Rec.*, *114*, 479.
(2) George, L. W. & White, S. L. (1984) *Vet. Clin. N. Am.*, *6(1)*, 79.
(3) Power, H. T. et al. (1982) *J. Am. vet. med. Assoc.*, *180*, 400.
(4) Messer, N. T. & Knight, A. P. (1982) *J. Am. vet. med. Assoc.*, *180*, 939.
(5) Manning, T. O. et al. (1981) *Equ. Pract.*, *3*, 38.
(6) Peter, J. E. et al. (1981) *Vet. Med. SAC*, 76, 1203.
(7) Scott, D. W. et al. (1984) *Agri-Practice*, 5, 38 & 44.

Photosensitization

Photosensitization is the disease caused by the sensitization of the superficial layers of lightly pigmented skin to light of certain wavelengths. Dermatitis develops when the sensitized skin is exposed to strong light.

Etiology

If photosensitizing substances (photodynamic agents) are present in sufficient concentration in the skin, dermatitis occurs when the skin is exposed to light (1). Photodynamic agents are substances which are activated by light and may be ingested preformed (and cause primary photosensitization), be products of abnormal metabolism (and cause photosentization due to aberrant synthesis of pigment) or be normal metabolic products which accumulate in tissues, because of faulty excretion through the liver (and cause hepatogenous photosensitization). Faulty excretion through the liver is usually due to hepatitis, caused in most instances by poisonous plants, but in rare cases is due to biliary obstruction by cholangiohepatitis or biliary calculus.

Primary photosensitization

Photosensitization due to the ingestion of exogenous photodynamic agents usually occurs when the plant is in the lush green stage and is growing rapidly. Livestock are affected within 4–5 days of going onto pasture and new cases cease to appear soon after the animals are removed. In most cases the plant responsible must be eaten in large amounts and will therefore usually be found to be a dominant inhabitant of the pasture. All species of animals are affected by photodynamic agents although susceptibility may vary between species and between animals of the same species. Photosensitizing substances which occur naturally in plants include:

- Hypericin in *Hypericum perforatum* (St John's wort), and other *Hypericum* sp.
- Fagopyrin in seeds and dried plants of *Polygonum fagopyrum* (buckwheat), and *F. esculentum* (7)
- Unidentified photodynamic substances in *Cynopterus* sp. (wild carrot) and the tree *Agave lecheguilla*
- The weeds *Ammi majus* and *Thamnosma texana* are thought to cause photosensitization even by physical contact (8)
- Perloline from perennial ryegrass (*Lolium perenne*) and an unidentified photodynamic agent in the aphids that infest *Medicago denticulata* (burr trefoil). The plant itself may also be photosensitizing
- Miscellaneous chemicals including phenothiazine (its metabolic end-product phenothiazine sulfoxide is photosensitizing to calves), rose bengal and acridine dyes
- Cows treated with corticosteroids to induce calving may develop a photosensitive dermatitis of the teats, escutcheon and udder (9). Its occurrence is sporadic and does not appear to be related to a particular drug (2).

Photosensitization due to aberrant pigment synthesis

The only known example in domestic animals is inherited congenital porphyria in which there is an excessive production in the body of porphyrins which are photodynamic.

Hepatogenous photosensitization

The photosensitizing substance is in all instances phylloerythrin—a normal end-product of chlorophyll metabolism excreted in the bile. When biliary secretion is obstructed by hepatitis or biliary duct obstruction phylloerythrin accumulates in the body and may reach levels in the skin which make it sensitive to light. Although hepatogenous photosensitization is more common in animals grazing green pasture it can occur in animals fed entirely on hay or other stored feeds. There appears to be sufficient chlorophyll, or breakdown products of it, in such feed to produce critical tissue levels of phylloerythrin in affected animals (1). The following list includes those substances or plants which are common causes of hepatogenous photosensitization. The individual plants are discussed in more detail in the section on poisonous plants.

Plants

- *Pithomyces chartarum* fungus on perennial ryegrass—causing facial eczema
- *Periconia* sp. fungus on Bermuda grass (3)
- Algae (water bloom) on drinking water in ponds, dams and dugouts—*Microcystis flosaquae*
- Pasture and crop plants
  - panic and millet grasses—*Panicum* sp.
  - lupins—*Lupinus angustifolium* (or accompanying fungi)
  - weeds including lantana (*Lantana camara*), *Lippia rehmannii*, caltrops (*Tribulus terrestris*), sacahuiste (*Nolina texana*), coal oil bush (*Tetradymia* sp.),

alecrim (*Holocalyx glaziovii*), ngaio (*Myoporum laetum*), *Crotolaria retusa*, ragwort (*Senecio jacobaeum*), *Phenosciadium* sp.

Chemicals

- Carbon tetrachloride poisoning
- Corticosteroids used systemically to terminate parturition in cows
- Phenanthridium used in the treatment of trypanosomiases

Congenitally defective hepatic function

- Inherited congenital photosensitivity in Corriedale and Southdown lambs—an inherited defect in the excretion of bile pigment.

Infections

- Leptospirosis is suspected of being a preliminary to photosensitization (7).

Photosensitization of uncertain etiology

In the following diseases it has not been possible to ascertain whether the photosensitization is primary or due to hepatic insufficiency.

- Feeding on rape or canola (*Brassica rapa*), kale, lucerne or alfalfa (*Medicago sativa*), burr medic or burr trefoil (*Medicago denticulata*), *Medicago minima*, *Trifolium hybridum* (Alsike or Swedish clover), *Erodium cicutarium* and *E. moschatum* (lamb's tongue, plantain)
- Extensive outbreaks in cattle fed on water-damaged alfalfa hay (4) which may have been heavily contaminated by fungi
- Many clinical cases occur sporadically in cattle grazing lush pasture, in sheep (5) and in horses in the disease known as bluenose (6).

Pathogenesis

Sensitization of skin tissues to light of particular wavelengths can only result in dermatitis if the skin is exposed to sunlight and if the light rays can penetrate the superficial layers of skin. Thus lesions occur only on the unpigmented skin areas and on these only when they are not covered with a heavy coat of hair or wool. Lesions are thus more severe on the dorsal parts of the body and on those underparts exposed to sunlight when the animal lies down. The penetration of light rays to sensitized tissues causes the liberation of histamine, local cell death and tissue edema. Irritation is intense because of the edema of the lower skin level and loss of skin is common in the terminal stages. Nervous signs may occur and are caused either by the photodynamic agent as in buckwheat poisoning or by liver dysfunction.

Clinical findings

The clinical findings in liver insufficiency are described elsewhere and may accompany photosensitive dermatitis when it is secondary to liver damage. The skin lesions show a characteristic distribution. They are restricted to the unpigmented areas of the skin and to those parts which are exposed to solar rays. They are most pronounced on the dorsum of the body, diminishing in degree down the sides and are absent from the ventral surface. The demarcation between lesions and normal skin is often very clearcut, particularly in animals with broken-colored coats. Predilection sites for lesions are the ears, eyelids, muzzle, face, the lateral aspects of the teats and, to a lesser extent, the vulva and perineum. The first sign is erythema followed by edema. Irritation is intense and the animal rubs the affected parts, often lacerating the face by rubbing it in bushes. When the teats are affected the cow will often kick at her belly and will walk into ponds to immerse the teats in water, sometimes rocking backwards and forwards to cool the affected parts. In nursing ewes there may be resentment to the lambs sucking and heavy mortalities due to starvation can occur. The edema is often severe and may cause drooping of the ears, dyspnea due to nasal obstruction and dysphagia due to swelling of the lips. Exudation commonly occurs and results in matting of the hair and, in severe cases, closure of the eyelids and nostrils. In extreme cases, necrosis and gangrene, sometimes with sloughing of affected parts, is the terminal stage.

The skin lesions may be severe enough to cause shock in the early stages. There is an increase in the pulse rate with ataxia and weakness. Subsequently a considerable elevation of temperature (41–42°C, 106–107°F) may occur. Dyspnea is often marked, and nervous signs including ataxia, posterior paralysis, blindness and depression or excitement are often observed. A peculiar sensitivity to water is sometimes seen in sheep with facial eczema.

Clinical pathology

There are no suitable field tests to determine whether or not photosensitivity is present. In experimental work the application of filter-containing screens to the skin is used to determine which light wavelengths activate the sensitized cells. An important step in diagnosis is the differentiation of primary from hepatogenous photosensitization. The use of serum enzyme tests, as described under the heading of diseases of the liver, is recommended as the most valuable procedure.

Necropsy findings

Liver lesions may be present if the photodynamic agent is phylloerythrin. In congenital bovine porphyria there is a characteristic pink-brown pigmentation of the teeth and bones. In other forms of the disease the lesions are confined to the skin and are manifested by dermatitis of varying degree.

Diagnosis

The determination of photosensitivity depends almost entirely on the distribution of the lesions. It can be readily confused with other dermatitides if this restriction to unpigmented and hairless parts is not kept in mind. Mycotic dermatitis is often mistaken for photosensitization because of its tendency to commence along the backline and over the rump. Bighead of rams caused by *Clostridium novyi* infection may also be confused with this disease but the local swelling is an acute inflammatory edema and many clostridia are present in the lesion.

To differentiate between the etiological types of photosensitization one must first determine whether the photodynamic agent is exogenous or endogenous and, if it is exogenous, whether or not its accumulation is due to liver damage.

Treatment

In cases of photosensitization, general treatment includes immediate removal from direct sunlight, prevention of ingestion of further toxic material and the administration of laxatives to eliminate toxic materials already eaten. In areas where the disease is enzootic the use of dark-skinned breeds may make it possible to utilize pastures which would otherwise be too dangerous.

Local treatment will be governed by the stage of the lesions. Antihistamines should be administered immediately and adequate doses maintained. To avoid septicemia the prophylactic administration of antibiotics may be worth while in some instances.

REFERENCES

(1) Clare, N. T. (1955) *Adv. vet. Sci.*, *2*, 182.
(2) Tyndel, J. (1984) *NZ vet. J.*, *32*, 119.
(3) Kidder, R. W. et al. (1961) *Bull. Fla. agric. Exp. Stn*, *630*, 21.
(4) Monlux, A. W. et al. (1963) *J. Am. vet. med. Assoc.*, *142*, 989.
(5) Ford, E. J. H. (1964) *J. comp. Pathol.*, *74*, 37.
(6) Greatorex, J. C. (1969) *Equ. vet. J.*, *1*, 157.
(7) Smith, B. L. & O'Hara, P. J. (1978) *NZ vet. J.*, *26*, 2.
(8) Egyed, M. N. et al. (1974) *Refuah vet.*, *31*, 128.
(9) Malmo, J. & Brightling, P. (1982) *Aust. Adv. vet. Sci.*, p. 152.

DISEASES OF THE HAIR, WOOL, FOLLICLES, SKIN GLANDS, HORNS AND HOOVES

Alopecia

Alopecia or baldness is deficiency of the hair or wool coat.

Etiology

Alopecia may be due to lack of hair production or to damage to hairs already produced.

Failure of follicles to develop

The number of secondary wool follicles that develop in ovine fetuses is significantly decreased by underfeeding during the period of 110–130 days of gestation. This has been an observation limited to a research project and is not recorded as having reduced wool yield (3).

Failure of the follicle to produce a fiber

- Inherited hypotrichoses, symmetrical alopecia
- In baldy calves and adenohypophyseal hypoplasia
- Hypothyroidism (goiter) congenitally due to iodine deficiency in the dam
- After viral infection of the dam, alopecia congenitally in the newborn, e.g. after bovine virus diarrhea in cattle and sheep (border disease)
- Neurogenic alopecia due to peripheral nerve damage
- Infection in the follicle
- Cicatricial alopecia due to scarring after deep skin wounds which destroy follicles.

Loss of preformed fibers

- Dermatomycoses—ringworm
- Mycotic dermatitis in all species due to *Dermatophilus congolensis*
- Metabolic alopecia subsequent to a period of malnutrition or severe illness—'a break in the wool', e.g. excessive whale, palm, or soya oil in milk replacers to calves (1)—the fibers grown during the period of nutritional or metabolic stress have a zone of weakness and are easily broken. A nutritional deficiency of vitamin E has been suspected in herds where enzootic muscular dystrophy also occurs (4)
- Traumatic alopecia occurs when there is excessive scratching or rubbing, e.g. in Queensland (Sweet) itch
- Poisoning by thallium or the tree *Leucaena leucocephala*
- Loss of hair from the tail-switch of well-fed beef bulls in the United States-cause unknown
- As part of the syndrome of sterile eosinophilic folliculitis of cattle (5); asymptomatic papules, nodules and annular areas of alopecia and crusting develop on the face, neck and trunk
- Wool slip of housed sheep.

Pathogenesis

Normal shedding of hair fibers is a constant process. It occurs most rapidly when there are changes in environmental temperature. The long winter coat is shed in response to warmer spring temperatures and increased hours of sunlight. The hair coat rapidly grows again as environmental temperatures fall in the autumn. Whether these variations in growth rate are due to the effects of temperature variations, of longer sunlight hours or of specific light wavelengths is unknown. Nor is it certain in what manner the response is mediated. Possibilities that suggest themselves are variations in capillary blood supply to the skin, or variations in the nutritive quality of the blood of the hairs. The fact that alopecia areata of humans occurs without diminution in capillary blood supply and is often associated with psychic disturbances suggests that there is at least some element of nervous control. In most cases of congenital alopecia there is reduction of all cellular elements of the epidermis. In some congenital conditions there is an absence of hair follicles. Chemical depilation produced by cytotoxic agents, such as cyclophosphamide, occurs as a result of induced cytoplasmic degeneration in some of the germinative cells of the bulb of the wool follicle. The alteration in cell function is temporary so that regrowth of the fiber should follow (2).

Clinical findings

When alopecia is due to breakage of the fiber, the stumps of old fibers or developing new ones may be seen. When fibers fail to grow the skin is shiny and in most cases is thinner than normal. In cases of congenital follicular aplasia, the ordinary covering hairs are absent but the coarser tactile hairs about the eyes, lips and extremities are often present. Absence of the hair coat makes the animal more susceptible to sudden changes of environmental temperature. There may be manifestations of a primary disease and evidence of scratching or rubbing.

Clinical pathology

Unless the cause of the alopecia is apparent after the examination of skin scrapings or swabs, a skin biopsy should be taken to determine the status of the follicular epithelium.

Diagnosis

Alopecia is readily recognizable, the main diagnostic problem being to determine the primary cause of the hair or fiber loss.

Treatment

The primary condition should be treated but in most animal cases little is done to stimulate hair growth. The most logical treatment is to improve the blood supply to the skin by the use of an ultraviolet lamp or mild rubefacients (e.g. 1 in 20 parts biniodide of mercury or cantharides).

REFERENCES

(1) Grunder, H. D. & Musche, R. (1962) *Dtsch Tierärztl. Wochenschr.*, *69*, 437.
(2) Brinsfield, T. H. et al. (1972) *J. anim. Sci.*, *34*, 273.
(3) Hutchison, G. & Mellor, D. J. (1983) *J. comp. Pathol.*, *93*, 577.
(4) Pritchard, G. C. (1983) *Vet. Rec.*, *112*, 435.
(5) Scott, D. W. et al. (1986) *Agri-Practice*, *7(3)*, 8.

Achromotrichia

Bands of depigmentation in an otherwise black wool fleece are the result of a transitory deficiency of copper in the diet. Cattle on diets containing excess molybdenum and deficient copper show a peculiar speckling of the coat caused by an absence of pigment in a proportion of hair fibers. The speckling is often most marked around the eyes giving the animal the appearance of wearing spectacles. There is also a general loss of density of pigmentation in all coat colors. Hereford cattle, for example, shade off from their normal deep red to a washed-out orange. Vitiligo, premature graying of the hair, is not uncommon in cattle and horses (1). The usual manifestation is the appearance of patches of gray or white hair—'snowflakes'—in an otherwise pigmented coat. The defect is esthetic only. The cause is unknown but the condition may be inherited. Depigmentation can only be brought about by the application of 'supercooled' instruments which selectively destroy melanocytes (2). Pressure and x-irradiation may have a similar effect. In horses, patchy depigmentation of skin on the prepuce, perineum, underneath the tail, and on the face occurs quite commonly. It usually accompanies a debilitating disease. There is no discontinuity of the skin and the horse suffers no harm but owners are often disturbed. No treatment can be recommended.

REFERENCES

(1) Meijer, W. C. P. (1965) *Vet. Rec.*, *77*, 1046.
(2) Farrell, R. K. et al. (1966) *J. Am. vet. med. Assoc.*, *149*, 745.

Seborrhea

Seborrhea is an excessive secretion of sebum on to the skin surface.

Etiology

Primary or true seborrhea as it occurs in humans is rarely recorded in animals. Secondary seborrhea associated with dermatitis and skin irritation, e.g. in some types of eczema, appears to be more common. The common forms of seborrhea encountered in animals are:

- Exudative epidermitis of pigs (*Staphylococcus hyicus*)
- Greasy heel of horses. *Staphylococcus hyicus* is capable of causing a similar lesion (2)
- Flexural seborrhea of cattle.

All of these conditions probably originate as a dermatitis or eczema, the increased sebaceous exudate being secondary rather than primary.

Pathogenesis

Increased blood supply to the skin and increased hair growth appear to stimulate the production of sebum. The reason why skin irritation should provoke seborrhea in some individuals and not in others is unknown.

Clinical findings

In primary seborrhea there are no lesions, the only manifestation being excessive greasiness of the skin. The sebum may be spread over the body surface like a film of oil or be dried into crusts which can be removed easily. Hypertrophy of the sebaceous glands may be visible. Secondary infection can lead to the development of acne.

Flexural seborrhea

Flexural seborrhea of cattle occurs most commonly in young dairy cows which have calved recently. Lesions are present in the groin between the udder and the medial surface of the thigh, or in the median fissure between the two halves of the udder. There is severe inflammation and a profuse outpouring of sebum. Extensive skin necrosis may develop and it is the pronounced odor of decay which may first attract the owner's attention. Irritation may cause lameness and the cow may attempt to lick the part. Shedding of the oily, malodorous skin leaves a raw surface beneath; healing follows in 3–4 weeks.

Greasy heel

Greasy heel occurs most commonly in the hindlegs of horses which are allowed to stand for long periods in wet unsanitary stables, athough cases do occur under good management conditions. Cattle, especially those animals kept on muddy pasture or in dirty barns, may develop lesions similar to those in horses. The first signs seen are lameness and soreness due to excoriations called 'scratches' which appear on the back of the pastern and extend down to the coronary band. There is thickening and pronounced greasiness of the skin of the part which is painful to the touch and causes lameness. If the disease is neglected, it usually spreads around to the front and up the back of the leg. When the thickening of the skin and subcutaneous tissue is very marked it can interfere with normal movements of the limbs.

Clinical pathology
The primary cause of the seborrhea may be parasitic or bacterial and suitable diagnostic procedures should be employed.

Diagnosis
The principal difficulty is to determine whether the seborrhea is primary or secondary. The safest procedure is to treat all cases as being secondary and to search carefully for the primary cause. Flexural seborrhea of cattle may be mistaken for injury, and greasy heel of horses for chorioptic mange.

Treatment
The skin must be kept clean and dry. Affected areas should be defatted with hot soap and water washes, then properly dried, and an astringent lotion, e.g. white lotion, applied daily. In acute cases of greasy heel the application of an ointment made up of 5 parts salicylic acid, 3 parts boric acid, 2 parts phenol, 2 parts mineral oil and 2 parts petroleum jelly at 5-day intervals is recommended.

REFERENCES

(1) Sigmund, H. M. et al. (1982) *Tierärztl. Umschau.*, *37*, 618.
(2) Devriese, L. A. et al. (1983) *Equ. vet. J.*, *15*, 263.

Acne

When correctly used the term acne refers specifically to an infection of hair follicles by the acne bacillus—a diphtheroid organism. In the present context 'acne' is used to include all infections of hair follicles caused by suppurative organisms, including staphylococci (more properly termed sycosis). Boils or furuncles are acneiform lesions which progress to penetrate the deeper skin layers and subcutaneous tissue.

Etiology
Acnes identifiable as individual diseases include:

- Staphylococcal dermatitis of horses
- Canadian 'horse-pox' caused by *Corynebacterium pseudotuberculosis*
- Demodectic mange.

Pathogenesis
When sebaceous gland ducts are blocked by inspissated secretion and epithelial debris they are predisposed to infection. Pressure is likely to cause such obstruction. Seborrhea with hypertrophy of the glands and dilatation of the ducts also predisposes to acne.

Clinical findings
Lesions begin as nodules around the base of the hair and then develop into pustules. The lesions are painful and rupture under pressure. This leads to contamination of the surrounding skin and the lesions spread as further follicles become infected. The hair in the affected follicle is usually shed.

Clinical pathology
Swabs should be taken for bacteriological and parasitological examination.

Diagnosis
Acne is an infection of the hair follicles and should not be confused with impetigo in which the lesions arise on the surface of the skin.

Treatment
Clean the skin by washing and follow this with a disinfectant rinse. Affected areas should be treated with antibacterial ointments or lotions. If the lesions are extensive the parenteral administration of antibiotics is recommended. In stubborn cases an autogenous vaccine may be helpful. Infected animals should be isolated and grooming tools and blankets disinfected.

Diseases of hooves and horns

Most of the diseases of the horny appendages are, by common usage, dealt with by surgeons and textbooks on surgery. However, some of them have medical importance, largely from the point of differential diagnosis. Thus, horn cancer has been dealt with under the heading of squamous cell carcinoma of the skin, and diseases of the foot causing lameness are listed in Table 41 in diseases of the musculoskeletal system.

Sloughing of the hooves and dewclaws (chestnuts)
Separation of the hooves from the sensitive laminae and, in severe cases, sloughing of the horn occur in:

- Severe edema of the legs causing capillary dilatation and fluid effusion into the laminar tissues. The edema may result from lymphangitis in the leg or to severe external trauma, commonly after a horse is caught up in a wire fence
- Burns in grass fires where only the undersurface of the body is burned. Separation may appear to be very severe at the coronet, but the recovery rate is high
- Coronitis occurring as part of a pemphigus-like lesion in horses. The initial lesion is a weeping, granulomatous lesion at the coronet, and later around the dewclaws. Separation around the coronets is soon evident and in very bad cases the horn sloughs. Accompanying lesions are a severe dermatitis around all the body orifices including the eyes. A severe, scabby and weeping dermatitis becomes generalized. The horse is apathetic, eats little and loses weight rapidly. There may be a temporary response to corticosteroids, but the progress is inexorable and the horse usually has to be destroyed for humane reasons
- Horses poisoned by eating mushrooms
- Terminally in laminitis.

There is no treatment once the hooves have sloughed and all attempts should be made to avoid it if separation is evident at the coronet. Reduction of the swelling in the limb requires that lymphatic and vascular drainage from the area be encouraged.

DISEASES OF THE SUBCUTIS

Subcutaneous edema (anasarca)

The accumulation of edema fluid in the subcutaneous tissue is called anasarca when the accumulation is extensive.

Etiology

The causes of subcutaneous edema include those of edema generally plus some additional ones. A summary of the common causes is set out below.

Increased vascular resistance

- Congestive heart failure
- Vascular compression by tumor, e.g. anterior mediastinal lymphosarcoma, udder engorgement in heifer about to calve
- Inherited absence of lymph nodes and some lymph channels in Ayrshire calves causing edema to be present at birth.

Hypoproteinemia

- In liver damage with reduced albumin production due to liver insufficiency, especially fascioliasis
- Renal damage with protein loss into urine occurs rarely in animals; renal amyloidosis may also have this effect
- Protein-losing enteropathy but rarely, for example, in intestinal lymphosarcoma
- Intestinal nematodiasis
- Protein starvation.

Vascular damage

- In purpura hemorrhagica there are extensive subcutaneous aggregations of protein-rich fluid due to vascular damage
- Anasarca observed in conjunction with hypovitaminosis A is unexplained
- Angioneurotic edema has an allergic origin and is due to vascular damage
- The edematous plaques of equine infectious anemia result from an immune reaction lesion in the vessel walls
- Subcutaneous plaques in dourine
- Horses standing in black walnut shavings as bedding.

Inflammatory edema

Many bacteria cause local edema due to infection. *Clostridium* sp. are the most noted of them; *Anthrax* in swine and horses often takes the form of local inflammatory edema of the neck and brisket; insect bites, especially bee stings are also a cause.

Myxedema

Some pigs with congenital goiter also have myxedema, especially of the neck.

Pathogenesis

The accumulation of fluids symptomatic of edema may be due either to increased venous pressure, to decreased osmotic pressure of the blood or to damage to capillary walls. Reduced osmotic pressure is often associated with hypoproteinemia. When capillary walls are damaged, as in malignant edema and angioneurotic edema, there is leakage of fluid or plasma into local tissue spaces.

Clinical findings

There is visible swelling, either local or diffuse. The skin is puffy and pits on pressure; there is no pain unless inflammation is also present. In large animals the edema is usually confined to the ventral aspects of the trunk and is seldom seen on the limbs.

Clinical pathology

The differentiation between obstructive and inflammatory edema can be made on the basis of the location of the edematous area, and the presence or absence of fever, anorexia or local pain, and by bacteriological examination of the fluid.

Diagnosis

Subcutaneous edema may be confused with infiltration of the belly wall with urine as a result of urethral obstruction and with subcutaneous hemorrhage.

Treatment

Unless the primary condition is repaired, removal of the fluid by drainage methods such as intubation or multiple incision, or by the use of a diuretic, will be of little value.

Angioneurotic edema

The sudden appearance of transient subcutaneous edema due to allergic cause is known as angioneurotic edema.

Etiology

Endogenous and exogenous allergens provoke either local or diffuse lesions. Angioneurotic edema occurs most frequently in cattle and horses on pasture, especially during the period when the pasture is in flower. This suggests that the allergen is a plant protein. Fish meals may also provoke an attack. Recurrence in individual animals is common.

Pathogenesis

Local vascular dilatation with damage to capillary walls is apparently caused by the liberation of histamine. Leakage of plasma through damaged vessels produces edema after an initial erythema.

Clinical findings

There are usually no general signs except in rare cases where bloat, diarrhea and dyspnea are manifest. In angioneurotic edema local lesions most commonly affect the head although the perineum and udder are also involved in some cases. There is diffuse edema of the muzzle, eyelids and sometimes the conjunctiva and cheeks. Occasionally the conjunctiva is the only part affected, and in this case the eyelids are puffy, the nictitating membrane is swollen and protrudes, and lacrimation is profuse. There is no pain on touching affected parts but there is some irritation, evidenced by shaking the head and rubbing against objects. There may be salivation and nasal discharge.

When the perineum is involved, the vulva is swollen, often asymmetrically, and the perianal skin, and sometimes the skin of the udder, is swollen and edematous. When the udder alone is affected, the teats and base of the udder are edematous. There is some irritation and the cow may paddle with the hindlegs. Sometimes there is edema of the lower limbs, usually from the knees or hocks down to the coronets.

Clinical pathology

The blood eosinophil count is often within the normal range, but may be elevated from a normal level of 4–5% up to 12–15%.

Diagnosis

The sudden onset and equally sudden disappearance of edema at the predilection sites typifies this condition. Subcutaneous edema due to vascular pressure occurs mostly in dependent parts and is not irritating. In horses, and rarely in cattle, angioneurotic edema may be simulated by purpura hemorrhagica but in the latter disease hemorrhages are usually visible in the mucosae.

Treatment

Local applications are seldom necessary. Spontaneous recovery is the rule, but treatment is often administered. Antihistamine drugs are favored, and usually one injection of 0·5–1·0 g intramuscularly is adequate for an adult cow or horse. For more rapid response intravenous injection is advisable. Adrenalin or epinephrine (3–5 ml of a 1:1000 solution intramuscularly) is also satisfactory. A purgative may be administered to hasten the elimination of exogenous allergens.

Affected animals should be removed from the source of allergens. Cattle running at pasture should be confined and fed on dry feed for at least a week to prevent a recurrence.

Emphysema

The term emphysema denotes the presence of free gas in the subcutaneous tissue.

Etiology

Emphysema occurs when air or gas accumulates in the subcutaneous tissue. This may be the result of:

- Air entering through a cutaneous wound made surgically or accidentally
- Lung puncture by the end of a fractured rib
- Internal penetrating wounds, e.g. traumatic reticulitis; penetration of tracheal mucosa (1)
- Rumen gases migrating from a rumenotomy or ruminal trocharization
- Extension from a pulmonary emphysema
- Gas gangrene infections, but severe systemic signs are also present.

Pathogenesis

When a lung is punctured air escapes under the visceral pleura and passes to the hilus of the lung, hence to beneath the parietal pleura, between the muscles and into the subcutis. The extension of an interstitial pulmonary emphysema occurs in the same way.

Clinical findings

Visible swellings occur over the body. They are soft, fluctuating and obviously crepitant to the touch. There is no pain and no external skin lesion except in gas gangrene, when discoloration, coldness and oozing of serum may be evident. The emphysema may be sufficiently widespread to cause stiffness of the gait and interference with feeding and respiration.

Clinical pathology

If a severe systemic reaction is evident a bacteriological examination of fluid from the swelling should be carried out to determine the organism present.

Diagnosis

The crepitus and the extreme mobility of the swelling distinguish emphysema from other superficial swellings.

Treatment

Sterile emphysema requires no treatment, unless it is extensive and incapacitating when multiple skin incisions may be necessary. The primary cause of the condition should be ascertained and treated. Gas gangrene requires immediate and drastic treatment with antibiotics.

REFERENCE

(1) Caron, J. P. & Townsend, H. G. G. (1984) *Can. vet. J.*, *25*, 339.

Lymphangitis

The term lymphangitis denotes inflammation and enlargement of the lymph vessels and is usually associated with lymphadenitis.

Etiology

Lymphangitis is due in most cases to local skin infection with subsequent spread to the lymphatic system. The common causes in the various species are as follows.

Horse

- Glanders, epizootic lymphangitis, sporadic lymphangitis, ulcerative lymphangitis due to *Corynebacterium pseudotuberculosis*
- Strangles in cases where bizarre location sites occur
- In foals *Streptococcus zooepidemicus* has been observed as a cause of ulcerative lymphangitis.

Cattle

- Skin farcy caused by *Nocardia farcinica*, rarely *Corynebacterium (Rhodococcus) equi*
- Cutaneous tuberculosis and other allied infections.

Pathogenesis

Spread of infection along the lymphatic vessels causes chronic inflammation of the vessel walls. Abscesses often develop and discharge to the skin surface through sinuses.

Clinical findings

An indolent ulcer usually exists at the original site of infection. The lymph vessels leaving this ulcer are enlarged, thickened and tortuous and often have secondary ulcers or sinuses along their course. Local edema may result from lymphatic obstruction. In chronic cases considerable fibrous tissue may be laid down in the subcutis and chronic thickening of the skin may follow. The medial surface of the hindleg is the most frequent site, particularly in horses.

Clinical pathology
In lymphangitis laboratory examination is largely a matter of the bacteriological examination of discharges for the presence of the specific bacteria or fungi which commonly cause the disease.

Treatment
The focus of infection must be removed by surgical excision or specific medical treatment. Early treatment is essential to prevent the widespread involvement of lymphatic vessels and nodes.

Hemorrhage

Subcutaneous hemorrhage occurs as a result of extravasations of whole blood into the subcutaneous tissues.

Etiology
Accumulation of blood in the subcutaneous tissues beyond the limit of that normally caused by trauma may be due to defects in the coagulation mechanism or to increased permeability of the vessel wall. Included in the common causes of subcutaneous hemorrhage in farm animals are:

- Dicoumarol poisoning from moldy sweet clover hay
- Purpura hemorrhagica in horses
- Bracken poisoning in cattle, and other granulocytopenic diseases. These diseases are manifested principally by petechiation and the lesions are observed only in mucosae
- Hemangiosarcoma are often in subcutaneous sites.

Pathogenesis
Defects in the clotting system are seldom encountered except in dicoumarol poisoning. The damage to capillary walls which occurs in allergic states such as purpura hemorrhagica is probably due to liberation of histamine.

Clinical findings
Subcutaneous swellings resulting from hemorrhage are diffuse and soft with no visible effect on the skin surface. There may be no evidence of trauma and the diagnosis can only be confirmed by opening the swelling.

Clinical pathology
In cases where hemorrhage is excessive the determination of the primary cause may be helped by ascertaining platelet counts, the levels of histamine in the blood, and prothrombin, clotting and bleeding times.

Diagnosis
Subcutaneous hemorrhages are usually associated with hemorrhages into other tissues, both manifestations being due to defects in clotting or capillary wall continuity as listed above.

Treatment
Removal of the cause is of first importance. The hemorrhages should not be opened until clotting is completed. If blood loss is severe, blood transfusions may be required. Parenteral injection of coagulants is advisable if the hemorrhages are recent.

Gangrene

Gangrene is the result of death of tissues with subsequent sloughing of the affected part and when it occurs in the skin it usually involves the dermis, epidermis and the subcutaneous tissue.

Etiology
Severe damage to the skin in the following categories causes gangrene:

- Severe or continued trauma, e.g pressure sores, saddle and harness galls
- Strong caustic chemicals, e.g. creosote
- Severe cold or heat, bushfires and stable fires being the worst offenders
- Bacterial infections, especially:
  - erysipelas and salmonellosis in pigs
  - clostridial infections in cattle affecting subcutis and muscle
  - staphylococcal mastitis in cattle, pasteurella mastitis in sheep
  - bovine ulcerative mammillitis of the udder and teats
- Local vascular obstruction by thrombi or arterial spasm causing skin gangrene, but includes deeper structures also:
  - poisoning by *Claviceps purpurea*
  - *Festuca arundinacea* (or an accompanying fungus)
  - *Aspergillus terreus*
  - mushrooms
- Similar cutaneous and deeper structure involvement occurs in systemic infections in which bacterial emboli block local vessels, e.g. in salmonellosis in calves, and after tail vaccination of calves with *Mycoplasma mycoides*
- Final stages of photosensitive dermatitis and flexural seborrhea.

Pathogenesis
The basic cause of gangrene is interference with local blood supply. This is often brought about by external pressure or by severe swelling of the skin, as in photosensitization. Arteriolar spasm or damage to vessels by bacterial toxins has the same effect.

Clinical findings
If the arterial supply and drainage systems are involved the initial lesion will be moist. The area is swollen, raised, discolored and cold. Separation occurs at the margin and sloughing may occur before drying of the affected skin is apparent. The underlying surface is raw and weeping. If, on the other hand, the veins and lymphatics remain patent, the lesion is dry from the beginning and the area is cold, discolored and sunken. Sloughing may take a considerable time and the underlying surface usually consists of granulation tissue. Secondary bacterial invasion may occur in either type of gangrene.

Treatment

Local treatment comprises the application of astringent and antibacterial ointments to facilitate separation of the gangrenous tissue and to prevent bacterial infection. The primary condition must also be treated.

Subcutaneous abscess

Boils or furuncles, as they occur in man, do not occur in animals. Most subcutaneous abscesses are the result of traumatic skin penetration with infection resulting. On rare occasions, the infection may reach the site by hematogenous means or from an internal organ, e.g. from traumatic reticuloperitonitis.

What appears to be a specific disease characterized by multiple subcutaneous abscesses occurs in horses and is recorded only in the United States. The lesions are in the pectoral area for the most part and the constant infection is *Corynebacterium pseudotuberculosis*. Many of the abscesses originate in deeper sites and in some cases there is systemic spread.

Subcutaneous abscesses, as part of a general suppurative process, occur in foals infected with *Corynebacterium (Rhodococcus) equi*, and in all species in infections with *Pasteurella pseudotuberculosis*, and in lambs with *Histophilus ovis* infection. Multiple subcutaneous abscesses may also be a feature of melioidosis in this species. In cases of acne, pyoderma and impetigo, the infection in some lesions spreads to subcutaneous sites (subcutaneous abscess). Facial subcutaneous abscesses are common in cattle eating roughage containing squirreltail grass, or foxtail grass (*Hordeum jubatum*). Several animals in a herd may be affected at one time. The awns of these plants migrate into the cheek mucosa, followed by the development of multiple subcutaneous abscesses containing *Corynebacterium (Actinomyces) pyogenes* and *Actinobacillus* sp. The abscesses contain purulent material, are well encapsulated and must be surgically drained and treated as an open wound. Medical therapy with parenteral antimicrobials and iodine are ineffective.

GRANULOMATOUS LESIONS OF THE SKIN

Granulomatous lesions of the skin are manifested by chronic inflammatory nodules, plaques and ulcers. The lesions are cold, hard and progress slowly and are often accompanied by lymphangitis and lymphadenitis. In many cases there is no discontinuity of the skin, nor loss of hair. Some of the common causes in animals are as follows.

Cattle

- *Mycobacterium* sp. especially *M. farcinogenes*
- *Nocardia farcinica*
- *Actinobacillus lignieresi* (rarely)
- Infestation with *Onchocerca* sp.
- *Hypoderma* sp. larvae and their connective tissue reaction.

Sheep

- Strawberry footrot—*Dermatophilus congolensis*
- Ecthyma
- Ulcerative lesions of lower jaw and dewlap caused by *Actinobacillus lignieresi*

Pigs

- Actinomyces sp. and *Borrelia suilla* cause lesions which are often very extensive on the skin of the udder.

Horses

- *Actinobacillus mallei*—cutaneous farcy or glanders
- *Actinomadura* sp. and *Nocardia brasiliensis*—painless mycetomas
- *Histomonas farcinicus*—epizootic lymphangitis
- *Corynebacterium pseudotuberculosis*—ulcerative lymphangitis
- *Habronema megastoma, Hyphomyces destruens* as causes of swamp cancer, bursattee, Florida horse leech and blackgrain mycetoma
- Infestation with *Onchocerca* sp.

CUTANEOUS NEOPLASMS

Neoplasms arising from the epidermis, dermis and subcutaneous tissue are not rare in animals (1). In this species the bulk of neoplasms are found in the skin, and most of them are fibroblastic. In horses the common ones are equine sarcoid, squamous cell carcinoma of the eye region, the prepuce and the glans penis, and melanoma (28). A brief description of the more common types is given here.

Papilloma and sarcoid

Sarcoid of horses and cutaneous papillomatosis of horses, goats and cattle have been described in other sections as specific diseases. The lesions are characteristically nodular growths of viable tissue with no discontinuity of the covering epidermis.

Squamous cell carcinoma

This neoplasm is common on the eyelids and the eyeball in horses and cattle. The specific disease of cattle known colloquially as 'cancer-eye' is dealt with separately elsewhere. In cattle the initial lesion may be on the third eyelid, the cornea or the eyelid. The tumors grow rapidly and show considerable invasiveness, often metastasizing to the local lymph nodes. In horses, the nictitating membrane is the most common site with some lesions occurring on the orbit and the lids. Metastases to local lymph nodes occur in a few horses; the susceptible age group is over 10 years (4).

Squamous cell carcinomas are also common on the penis and prepuce of horses, and can occur anywhere on the skin (26) including the genitalia and also in the mouth and maxillary sinus and on the third eyelid and the cornea (36).

The common 'cancer of the horn core' in cattle is a squamous cell carcinoma arising from the mucosa of the frontal sinus and invading the horn core (5, 6). The horn becomes loosened and falls off leaving the tumor exposed. Cancer of the ear in sheep is in most cases a squamous cell carcinoma. The lesion commences around the free edge of the ear and then invades the entire ear which becomes a large cauliflower-shaped mass. A high incidence may occur in some flocks (20) but the cause is not known. Less commonly the perineum and muzzle are involved. A high incidence of epitheliomas has been recorded in some families of merino sheep in Australia. The lesions occurred on the woolled skin and were accompanied by many cutaneous cysts. It has been suggested that predisposition to the neoplasm is inherited (7). Metastasis is common with both epitheliomas and squamous cell carcinomata. The latter also occur on the vulva of cattle and a greater incidence has been observed on unpigmented than on pigmented vulvas (8).

In Merino ewes a high prevalence of vulvar squamous cell carcinoma has been attributed to increased exposure of vulvar skin to sunlight, after radical surgery to the perineal area has been carried out to help control blowfly strike (3, 9). During the radical Mules operation for blowfly strike prevention there is also a good deal of skin removed from the tail and the tail is shortened. The occurrence of granulomatous, necrotic lesions on the tails treated in this way led to the suspicion that more squamous cell carcinomas were being encouraged and these lesions are now confirmed as precursors of squamous cell carcinomas (23). Papilloma virus has been isolated from them and it is thought may have some etiological significance (2). The so-called 'brand cancer', which occurs as a granulomatous mass at the site of a skin fire brand, is of chronic inflammatory rather than neoplastic origin. In goats, the perineum is a common site for squamous cell carcinoma. The udder, ears, and base of the horns may also be affected. Ulceration, fly strike, matting of hair are unattractive sequels. A bilaterally symmetrical vulvar swelling due to ectopic mammary tissue which enlarges at parturition is likely to be confused with squamous cell carcinoma. Milk can be aspirated from the swellings (32).

The tumor tissue of squamous cell carcinoma on injection can cause immunosuppression (21) and it is thought that this prevents rejection of the neoplasm by tissues (30). By way of contrast, a phenol extract of horn core tissue is immunogenic, and immunotherapy may be a successful treatment technique (22, 24). Other forms of therapy are also recommended, including surgical excision, preferably by cryotherapy (34) and radiofrequency hyperthermia (25).

Melanoma

Superficially situated melanomata are most often seen in aged, gray horses and also occur rarely in darkskinned cattle. Those of horses are usually malignant and metastasize widely, in the first instance to the local lymph nodes. In horses the common site is at the root of the tail. The skin is usually intact but ulceration may occur if the tumor is growing rapidly. Melanomata in cattle are usually benign and are only removed if they spoil the animal's appearance. Malignant melanomata have been observed rarely in sheep (10) and goats (11, 39). In pigs the incidence is low, but a very high rate of occurrence has been observed in young pigs of the Duroc-Jersey breed (12). In some cases the tumors are congenital and malignant (13, 33). Melanomas and kindred neoplasms occur commonly in Sinclair miniature swine but they frequently regress spontaneously (14).

Cutaneous angiomatosis

This condition is recorded only in dairy cattle in the United Kingdom (15) and France (16). It is manifested clinically by recurrent profuse hemorrhage from small single cutaneous lesions usually situated along the dorsum of the back. The lesions are relatively inconspicuous and consist of what appears to be protruding granulation tissue about 1–1·5 cm in diameter. In most instances the life of the cow does not appear to be endangered. Surgical excision is an effective treatment.

Lymphomatosis

In this disease of cattle and horses the skin lesions commonly occur as nodules under the skin. They are situated in the subcutaneous tissue and are most common in the paralumbar fossae and the perineum. In the cow the lesions are a secondary manifestation of the disease and are associated with lesions in other organs. Biopsy of a node may reveal a considerable increase in immature lymphocytes. A diffuse thickening of the skin itself is a rare form of this neoplasm. All forms are malignant. In cattle the neoplasm is caused by the virus of bovine viral leukosis and the disease is irreversible. In horses there are no leukemic lesions in lymph nodes or visceral organs (31).

Mast cell tumors

Cutaneous mastocytoma is recorded rarely in cattle (17, 42). It appears as a rapidly growing intradermal nodule, which may become widely disseminated if excised or there may be multiple tumors in the first instance. They show no tendency to metastasize internally and are compatible with life provided they do not ulcerate and become repulsive.

Cutaneous mastocytomas (mastocytosis) is a cutaneous neoplasm recorded in horses of all ages (18). The neonatal form is manifested by multiple cutaneous nodules up to 3 cm in diameter. The skin surface is intact except for larger lesions which are sometimes ulcerated. Lesions occur all over the body, but especially on the flanks. Each nodule appears, enlarges, and then regresses during a period of about 30 days. Fresh lesions may appear for up to about a year. Histologically the lesions contain aggregations of mast cells.

Congenital neurofibromatosis

A particularly high prevalence of this disease is recorded in European pied cattle. Tumor-like lumps develop between the eyes and on the cheeks. They are flat, round tumors up to 8 cm in diameter and of a lumpy elastic consistency. Virological tests are negative and the condition is not fatal (27).

Histiocytoma

This is a rare neoplasm in farm animals but is recorded as a discoid plaque on the scrotum of a goat (40). The lesions regress spontaneously.

Hemangioma and hemangiosarcoma

Benign hemangiomas are most common in horses less than 1 year old and some are present at birth. They are also recorded on the scrotum of mature pigs (29). The lesions are small (1–3 cm in diameter) round, black lumps that bleed easily and are morphologically the same as bovine cutaneous angiomatosis lesions (43).

Hemangiosarcomas occur in senior horses (38). They are large, subcutaneous masses, usually associated with one or more internal lesions. A similar lesion in a newborn foal has been diagnosed as a vascular nevus (19). The lesion is also referred to as an hemangioepithelioma (41).

Reticulum cell sarcoma

Like lipomas these are not neoplasms of skin but when they are in subcutaneous sites they cause multiple lumps on the skin surface in horses (35) and cattle.

Lipoma

External lipomas are not cutaneous neoplasms but they do occur as large subcutaneous masses and invade fascia and muscle. They are generally susceptible to surgical removal (37).

REVIEW LITERATURE

Daniels, P. W. & Johnson, R. H. (1987) Ovine squamous cell carcinoma. *Vet. Bull.* 57, 153.

REFERENCES

(1) Cotchin, E. (1956) *Neoplasms of the Domesticated Mammals*, Review Series No. 4. Farnham Royal, Bucks: Commonwealth Bureau of Animal Health.
(2) Vanselow, B. A. & Spradbrow, P. B. (1983) *Aust. vet. J.*, *60*, 194.
(3) Tustin, R. C. et al. (1982) *J. S. Afr. vet. Assoc.*, *53*, 141.
(4) Gelatt, K. N. et al. (1974) *J. Am. vet. med. Assoc.*, *165*, 617.
(5) Pachauri, S. P. & Pathak, R. C. (1969) *Am. J. vet. Res.*, *30*, 475.
(6) Dhingra, V. K. et al. (1982) *Ind. J. anim. Sci.*, *52*, 1177.
(7) Carne, H. R. et al. (1963) *J. Pathol. Bacteriol.*, *86*, 305.
(8) Burdin, M. L. (1964) *Res. vet, Sci.*, *5*, 497.
(9) Vandegraaff, R. (1976) *Aust. vet. J.*, *52*, 21.
(10) Baxter, J. T. (1960) *Br. vet. J.*, *116*, 67.
(11) Omar, A. R. & Collins, G. W. (1961) *J. comp. Pathol.*, *71*, 183.
(12) Hjerpe, C. A. & Theilen, G. H. (1964) *J. Am. vet. med. Assoc.*, *144*, 1129.
(13) Jáyasekara, U. & Leipold, H. W. (1981) *Bov. Pract.*, *2(4)*, 25.
(14) Manning, P. J. et al. (1974) *J. Natl Cancer Inst.*, *52*, 1559.
(15) Cotchin, E. & Swarbrick, O. (1963) *Vet. Rec.*, *75*, 437.
(16) Lombard, C. & Levesque, L. (1964) *C. R. hebd. Séances. Acad. Sci., Paris*, *258*, 3137.
(17) Stephens, K. A. & Mullowney, P. C. (1986) *Comp. cont. Educ.*, *8*, S309.
(18) Prasse, K. W. et al. (1975) *J. Am. vet. med. Assoc.*, *166*, 68.
(19) Jabara, A. G. et al. (1984) *Aust. vet. J.*, *61*, 286.
(20) Nobel, T. A. et al. (1982) *Refuah Vet.*, *39*, 166.
(21) Johnson, R. H. et al. (1980) *Aust. Adv. vet. Sci.*, p. 12.
(22) Batra, U. K. et al. (1986) *Aust. vet. J.*, *63*, 251.
(23) Swan, R. A. et al. (1980) *Aust. vet. J.*, *61*, 146.
(24) Chauhan, H. V. S. et al. (1980) *Aust. vet. J.*, *56*, 509.
(25) Grier, R. L. et al. (1980) *J. Am. vet. med. Assoc.*, *177*, 55.
(26) Akerejola, O. O. et al. (1978) *Vet. Rec.*, *103*, 336.
(27) Slanina, L. et al. (1978) *Dtsch Tierärztl. Wochenschr.*, *85*, 41.
(28) Cotchin, E. (1977) *Equ. vet. J.*, *9*, 16.
(29) Munro, R. et al. (1982) *J. comp. Pathol.*, *92*, 109.
(30) Jun, M. H. et al. (1979) *Res. vet. Sci.*, *27*, 144, 149, 155 & 161.
(31) Rutgers, H. C. et al. (1979) *Neth. J. vet. Sci.*, *104*, 511.
(32) Smith, M. C. (1981) *J. Am. vet. med. Assoc.*, *178*, 728.
(33) Case, M. T. (1964) *J. Am. vet. med. Assoc.*, *144*, 254.
(34) Omara-Opyene, S. et al. (1985) *Vet. Rec.*, *117*, 518.
(35) Gay, C. C. & Richards, W. P. C. (1983) *Aust. vet. J.*, *60*, 189.
(36) Junge, R. E. et al. (1984) *J. Am. vet. med. Assoc.*, *185*, 656.
(37) Bristol, D. G. & Fubini, S. (1984) *J. Am. vet. med. Assoc.*, *185*, 791.
(38) Hargis, A. M. & McElwain, T. F. (1984) *J. Am. vet. med. Assoc.*, *84*, 1121.
(39) Sockett, D. C. et al. (1984) *J. Am. vet. med. Assoc.*, *185*, 907.
(40) Roth, L. &, Perdrizet, J. (1985) *Cornell Vet.*, *75*, 303.
(41) Scott, D. W. & Hackett, R. P. (1983) *Equ. Pract.*, *5*, 8.
(42) Ames, T. R. & O'Leary, T. P. (1984) *Can. J. comp. Med.*, *48*, 115.
(43) Vos, J. H. et al. (1986) *J. comp. Pathol.*, *96*, 637.

CONGENITAL DEFECTS OF THE SKIN

The common diseases are inherited. Examples are:

- Inherited parakeratosis (Adema disease) of cattle
- Dermatosis vegetans of pigs
- Inherited congenital ichthyosis (fish-scale disease) of calves
- Inherited hypotrichoses and alopecias in cattle
- Inherited congenital absence of skin (epitheliogenesis imperfecta) in all species. The lesions commonly involve the coronet. There are also records of congenital, possibly inherited, absence of the hooves of all four limbs in calves (3)

- Epitheliogenesis imperfecta in piglets due to ingestion of *Fusarium* spp. toxin
- Familial acantholysis and dermatosparaxias. In familial bovine acantholysis the skin is normal at birth, but is shed later at the carpus and the coronet
- There are two similar diseases of sheep, inherited epidermolysis bullosa where mucosa, skin and horn are shed from bullous lesions at these sites, and inherited redfoot with similar shedding of skin at 2–3 days of age
- In dermatosparaxia, hyperelastosis cutis and the Ehlers–Danlos syndrome, all in cattle, there is a defect in collagen synthesis due to a deficiency of procollagen peptidase. The skin is therefore very loosely connected to underlying tissues and may be friable and fragile. There may be also a concurrent hypermobility of joints. A mild form of dermatosparaxia is recorded in sheep (1, 2) and rare cases in horses (4).

REFERENCES

(1) Ramshaw, J. A. M. et al. (1983) *Aust. vet. J.*, *60*, 149.
(2) Bavinton, J. H. et al. (1985) *J. invest. Dermatol.*, *84*, 391.
(3) Dass, L. L. et al. (1984) *Vet. Rec.*, *114*, 404.
(4) Solomons, B. (1984) *Equ. vet. J.*, *16*, 541.

DISEASES OF THE CONJUNCTIVA

Some of the common diseases of the conjunctiva are listed here because they are often treated medically, and because they are often secondary to the presence of some other diseases. Also, an examination of the conjunctiva often provides additional information on which to base a diagnosis. General practitioners need to know something of the common diseases of the eye for these reasons.

The following notes are intended only to provide guidelines to the relevant sections of Part 2 (Special Medicine), where specific conjunctivitides have been set out in detail.

Conjunctivitis and keratoconjunctivitis

This is inflammation of the covering mucosa of the eye, including the orbit and the inner surface of the eyelids. The inflammation commonly extends to layers below the conjunctiva, hence keratoconjunctivitis.

Etiology

Specific conjunctivitis

Cattle Infectious bovine keratoconjunctivitis is caused by:

- *Moraxella bovis* is the only significant cause
- *Moraxella bovis* with infectious bovine rhinotracheitis virus
- *Neisseria catarrhalis*
- *Mycoplasma* sp.
- *Chlamydia* sp.

Sheep

- *Rickettsia conjunctivae* is the important infection
- *Neisseria catarrhalis*
- *Mycoplasma conjunctivae*
- *Acholeplasma oculi* are also listed
- *Chlamydia* sp.

Goats *Rickettsia conjunctiva*

Pigs *Rickettsia* sp.

Horses There is no well-identified specific conjunctivitis in this species but *Moraxella equi* has been recorded as a cause on several occasions (1). There is also infestation with *Thelazia* sp. and *Habronema* sp.

Specific keratitis lesions

- *Thelazia* spp. in cattle and horses
- *Onchocerca* spp. in cattle
- *Elaeophora schneideri* in sheep and goats
- *Habronema* spp. in horses.

Diseases in which conjunctivitis is a significant but secondary part of the syndrome

Cattle

- Bovine viral diarrhea
- Bovine malignant catarrh
- Rinderpest
- Infectious bovine rhinotracheitis
- Viral pneumonia due to various viruses.

Sheep Bluetongue.

Pigs

- Swine influenza
- Inclusion body rhinitis.

Horses

- Equine viral arteritis
- Equine viral rhinopneumonitis.

Non-specific conjunctivitis
Inflammation caused by foreign bodies or chemicals, or secondarily as exposure keratitis and conjunctivitis/keratitis in paralysis of eyelids as in listeriosis. Ant-bite conjunctivitis occurs in similar circumstances.

Clinical findings

Initially there is blepharospasm and weeping from the affected eye. The watery tears are followed by the appearance of mucopurulent, then purulent ocular discharge if the lesion extends below the conjunctiva. There will be varying degrees of opacity of the conjunctiva depending on the severity of the infection. In the severest lesions there is underrunning of the conjunctiva with pus. At this stage there is considerable vascularization of the cornea. During the recovery stage there is often longlasting, diffuse opacity of the eye and terminally a chronic white scar in some.

Clinical pathology

In herd or flock outbreaks conjunctival swabs and/or scrapings should be taken for culture and examination of cells using special stains and histological techniques.

Treatment and control

These are set out under the headings of the individual diseases.

REFERENCE

(1) Huntington, P. J. et al. (1987) *Aust. vet. J.*, *64*, 110.

PART TWO

SPECIAL MEDICINE

15

Mastitis

THE term mastitis refers to inflammation of the mammary gland regardless of the cause. It is characterized by physical, chemical and usually bacteriological changes in the milk and by pathological changes in the glandular tissue. The most important changes in the milk include discoloration, the presence of clots and the presence of large numbers of leukocytes. Although there is swelling, heat, pain and induration in the mammary gland in many cases, a large proportion of mastitic glands are not readily detectable by manual palpation nor by visual examination of the milk using a strip cup. Because of the very large numbers of such subclinical cases the diagnosis of mastitis has come to depend largely on indirect tests which depend, in turn, on the leukocyte content of the milk. In the present state of knowledge it seems practicable and reasonable to define mastitis as a disease characterized by the presence of a significantly increased leukocyte content in milk from affected glands. Because the increased leukocyte count is a reaction of tissue to trauma, and because it is preceded by changes in the milk which are the direct result of damage to tissue, the possibility exists that the definition of mastitis might in fact change. But until such time as it becomes common usage to define the disease in terms of the sodium or chloride content of the milk, or the electrical conductivity, or the bovine serum albumin content, we see no need to change. More exact definition of the type of mastitis depends on the identification of the causative agent whether it be physical or infectious.

GENERAL FEATURES OF MASTITIS

Etiology

Many infective agents have been implicated as causes of mastitis and these are dealt with separately as specific entities. The common causes in cattle are *Streptococcus agalactiae* and *Staphylococcus aureus* with *Escherichia coli* becoming a significant cause in housed or confined cattle, principally in the northern hemisphere. The following are recorded but less frequent causes.

Cattle

Streptococcus uberis, *Str. dysgalactiae*, *Str. zooepidemicus*, *Str. faecalis*, *Str. pyogenes*, *Campylobacter jejuni*, *Haemophilus somnus*, *Str. pneumoniae*, *Corynebacterium (Actinomyces) pyogenes*, *Cor. ulcerans*, *Klebsiella* sp., *Enterobacter aerogenes*, *Mycobacterium bovis*, *M. lacticola*, *M. fortuitum*, *Bacillus cereus*, *Pasteurella multocida*, *P. haemolytica*, *Pseudomonas pyocyaneus*, *Bacteroides funduliformis*, *Serratia marcescens*, *Mycoplasma bovis*, *M. canadensis*, *M. bovigenitalium*, *M. alkalescens*, *Acholeplasma laidlawii*, *Nocardia asteroides*, *Nocardia brasiliensis*, *N. farcinica* have all been found.

There are not many recorded isolations of anaerobic bacteria. Exhaustive laboratory investigations for them have resulted in some isolations, usually in association with other facultative bacteria (110). Some of the more common organisms are *Peptococcus indolicus*, *Bacteroides melaniogenicus*, *Eubacterium combesii*, *Clostridium sporogenes* and *Fusobacterium necrophorum* (111).

Fungal infections include *Trichosporon* sp., *Aspergillus fumigatus*, *A. nidulans*, and *Pichia* sp.; and yeast infections include *Candida* sp., *Cryptococcus neoformans*, *Saccharomyces* sp. and *Torulopsis* sp. Algal infections include *Protetheca trispora* and *P. zopfii*.

Leptospirae, including *Leptospira interrogans* serovar. *pomona* and especially *L. interrogans hardjo* cause damage to blood vessels in the mammary gland and gross abnormality of the milk. They are more correctly classified as systemic diseases with mammary gland manifestations, and are dealt with elsewhere under the headings of the causative organisms. Two bacteria, *Corynebacterium bovis* and *Staphylococcus epidermidis* are commonly found as constant inhabitants of mammary glands, but they are not regarded as significant pathogens because of their low pathogenicity. Experimentally induced infection of quarters with *C. bovis* causes a mild but significant rise in the milk cell count and a persistent infection of the teat duct epithelium but there is no clinical abnormality nor change in milk composition (8). Naturally occurring infections have similar effects (88, 95). The disease in buffalo in India (1) and in Iraq (104) is caused by the same bacteria as in cattle. Some viruses may also cause mastitis in cattle and buffalo, but present knowledge suggests that this has very little significance.

Sheep
Pasteurella haemolytica, *Staph. aureus*, *Actinobacillus lignieresi*, *E. coli*, *Str. uberis* and *Str. agalactiae* are recorded. Sheep used for milk production show subclinical mastitis in about 7% of ewes. *Staph. aureus* is the commonest infection with *Str. agalactiae*, *Str. dysgalactiae*, *Str. uberis* (2), and *Staph. epidermidis* and *Actinomyces (Corynebacterium) pyogenes* also occurring (83). *Histophilus ovis* is a rare cause of acute mastitis (93). Suppurative lesions caused by *Cor. pseudotuberculosis* are found commonly in ovine mammary glands, but they usually involve only the supramammary lymph nodes and are not true mastitis, although the function of the mammary gland may be lost. In some rare cases the infection has spread from the lymph node to mammary tissue. Clinically normal quarters show a high rate of infection with coagulase-negative staphylococcus (80).

Goats
Goats are much less affected by mastitis than cattle and details of the infections encountered are inconsistent; coliform organisms, for example, are listed as not occurring (59) or being most common (112). *Staph. aureus* is usually considered to be the most important pathogen (81). Other infections are *Mycoplasma agalactia*, *M. mycoides* var. *mycoides*, *Str. agalactiae*, *Str. dysgalactiae*, *Str. pyogenes*, and *Yersinia pseudotuberculosis* (66).

Pigs
Aerobacter aerogenes, *E. coli*, *Klebsiella* sp., *Pseudomonas aeruginosa*, coagulase-positive staphylococci, *Str. agalactiae*, *Str. dysgalactiae*, *Str. uberis* have been found. Mammary actinomycosis is not a true mastitis and is dealt with under the heading of actinomycosis. Clinically inapparent mammary abscess is a much more common disease in sows than clinical mastitis.

Horses
Mastitis in mares is rare (78). *Corynebacterium pseudotuberculosis* (3), *Pseudomonas aeruginosa* (109), *Str. zooepidemicus* (4) and *Str. equi* (5) are recorded. Severe swelling and soreness of the udder, but without abnormal milk, is a common enough finding when a sick foal, which does not suck for 24 hours, goes unobserved. Gangrenous mastitis similar to that in cows has been observed.

Other species
A surprisingly high occurrence of mastitis is recorded in deer in Russia (6); draught yaks have a high prevalence of mastitis caused by streptococci (97).

Epidemiology

Spread of infection
Infection of each mammary gland occurs via the teat canal, the infection originating from two main sources, the infected udder and the environment. In dairy cattle and milking goats, the important infections are those which persist readily in the udder, especially *Str. agalactiae* and *Staph. aureus*. Bacteria which are normal inhabitants of the environment, such as *E. coli* and *Ps. pyocyaneus*, cause mastitis much less frequently but, when they do, the disease is much more resistant to hygienic control measures. The contamination of milkers' hands, wash cloths and milking machine cups by milk from infected quarters may quickly lead to the spread of infection to the teats of other animals.

In sheep, the only other species in which outbreaks occur, spread appears to be due to contamination of sheep bedding grounds by discharges from affected glands. The number of new cases which occur during lactation increases with age, and number and weight of lambs (67). This suggests that trauma due to very vigorous sucking by big lambs may be an important cause of mammary inflammation.

The frequency of occurrence of each of the etiological types of mastitis set out above depends on the ability of the bacteria or fungus to set up infection in the mammary tissue. The differences between bacteria in their ability to set up a mastitic state is dependent on at least two important groups of factors: bacterial characteristics and transmission mechanisms.

Bacterial characteristics These are as follows:

- The ability of the organism to survive in the cow's immediate environment—that is, its resistance to environmental influences including cleaning and disinfection procedures
- Its ability to colonize the teat duct (61)
- Its ability to adhere to mammary epithelium and set up a mastitis reaction (58)
- Its resistance to antibiotic therapy.

Transmission mechanisms These depend on the following:

- Bulk of the infection in the environment including infected quarters
- Efficiency of milking personnel, milking machines, including high milking speed (60), and especially hygiene in the milking parlor
- Susceptibility of the cow which is related to:
  - stage of lactation, early (first 2 months) being most susceptible
  - age of cow, older (more than four lactations) being more susceptible
  - level of inherited resistance, possibly related to teat shape and anatomy of the teat canal
  - lesions on teat skin, especially the orifice
  - immunological, including leukocytic, status of each mammary gland, including prior infections, especially with *Staph. aureus*. Infections with other bacteria of low pathogenicity, e.g. *Cor. bovis* and *Staph. epidermidis* (62) increase resistance to mastitis-producing pathogens by provoking an increase in the polymorphonuclear cell content of the milk.

These matters are dealt with later under the heading of control of mastitis (p. 537).

Prevalence
In most countries, surveys of the incidence of mastitis, irrespective of cause, show comparable figures of about

40% morbidity amongst dairy cows and a quarter infection rate of about 25%. A major survey of dairy herds in the United Kingdom revealed a quarter infection rate, in terms of a positive cell count, of 27%, but the actual quarter infection rate, as indicated by infection with a significant pathogen, of only 9·6% (32). A Canadian study in one herd over a long period has shown an incidence rate of episodes of clinical mastitis of about 10% (4), the highest incidence rate of any clinical disease in the herd. The incidence is similar in goat and buffalo kept in dairies (1). Surveys of beef cattle show prevalence figures as low as 1·8% of infected quarters (7) and as high as 18% (8), so that the possibility of a severe mastitis problem occurring in a beef herd should not be discounted.

Surveys of the prevalence of the various infections in cattle show remarkable similarity in different countries. The predominant position of *Str. agalactiae* as a cause of bovine mastitis has been usurped by *Staph. aureus* (32, 45), especially in areas where the treatment of mastitis with penicillin has been practiced intensively and where machine milking has replaced hand milking. In such areas a relative incidence of *Str. agalactiae*, other streptococci and *Staph. aureus* of 1: 1: 2 is a common finding. Although *Staph. aureus* is still preeminent as a cause of subclinical mastitis its prevalence has been significantly curbed by modern control programs based on teat dipping and dry period treatment. These programs have also led to a higher proportion of bacteriologically sterilized quarters and a corresponding, and perhaps consequent, increase in infections by *Escherichia coli*, *Pseudomonas*, *Aerobacter aerogenes*, and *Klebsiella* spp. The change in the balance away from Gram-positive cocci to Gram-negative bacteria has been significant, and in the United Kingdom it was the commonest single infection encountered in a survey of clinical cases (18). There may be an effect on relative prevalence by size of herd and quality of management. Large, zero-grazed herds in feedlots are likely to encounter more hygiene problems than conventionally housed herds. The problems relate mainly to fouling of the udder caused by inadequate or improper bedding in the larger units. In some large units there is a much higher prevalence than usual of mastitis caused by *Escherichia coli* and *Streptococcus uberis* (74).

Although *Corynebacterium bovis* is rarely a cause of udder disease it is frequently found in random milk samples. Because it is highly infectious and is susceptible to teat disinfection it has been suggested that its prevalence could be used as an indicator of teat-dipping efficiency in a herd, either of the intensity of the dipping or of the efficacy of the dip. Examination of milk from a sample or cows, looking expressly for *Cor. bovis*, could also be used as a secondary screening test, after a bulk milk cell count has shown to be positive, to determine its possible origin (17). The fact that *Cor. bovis* is limited in its colonization to the streak canal makes it valuable as a monitor.

Surveys of the incidence of the disease in sheep show varying results. In the United Kingdom one survey showed that 8·4% of ewe deaths and up to 34% of lamb deaths were due to mastitis (84). One Norwegian survey (19) records a total incidence of mastitis in 6000 sheep at 2% per year, 86% of these being caused by *Staph. aureus*, 10% by *E. coli*, 3% by *Str. agalactiae*, and 1% by *Past. haemolytica*. In a New Zealand survey the incidence of mastitis was 1·65%. In recently lambed ewes streptococci were most common (20). In sheep, the prevalence of mastitis may also affect the lamb survival rate. The same effect is produced by a diffuse homogeneous induration of the udder in ewes which is unrelated to the age of the ewe and which is not characterized by the presence of bacteria in the milk (2). This indurative form of mastitis is associated with the occurrence of maedi in ewes and caprine arthritis-encephalitis in goat does.

Economic losses

Although mastitis occurs sporadically in all species, it assumes major economic importance only in dairy cattle. In milking buffalo the epidemiological pattern is similar (1), and similar patterns of loss could be expected. In terms of economic loss it is undoubtedly the most important disease with which the dairy industry has to contend. This loss is occasioned much less by fatalities, although fatal cases do occur, than from the reduction in milk production from affected quarters.

The clinical syndrome may vary from a peracute inflammation with toxemia to a fibrosis which develops so gradually that it may escape observation until most of the secretory tissue has been destroyed. There is the additional danger that the bacterial contamination of milk from affected cows may render it unsuitable for human consumption, or interfere with manufacturing process or, in rare cases, provide a mechanism of spread of disease to humans. Tuberculosis, streptococcal sore throat and brucellosis may be spread in this way.

Most estimates show that on the average an affected quarter suffers a 30% reduction in productivity and an affected cow is estimated to lose 15% of its production (22). Experimental infection of quarters during the dry period causes 35% reduction in yield in these quarters during the next lactation. Quarters found to be infected in late lactation had a 48% reduction in yield, but if the infection occurred in the dry period the depression of yield after calving was only 11% (9). It is evident that the loss in production by an infected quarter may be largely compensated by increased production in the other quarters so that the net loss to the cow may be less than that set out above. These losses are supplemented by a loss of about 1% of total solids by changes in composition (fat, casein and lactose are reduced and glycogen, whey proteins, pH and chlorides are increased) which interfere with manufacturing processes (10), loss due to increased culling rates and costs of treatment.

It is suggested that the total economic losses caused by mastitis are composed of the following items:

	Percent of total
Value of milk production host	70
Value of cows lost by premature culling	14
Value of milk discarded or downgraded	7
Treatment and veterinary expenses	8

A comparison between low and high prevalence herds in

the United Kingdom has shown an advantage to the low prevalence herds of £29 per cow per year, a gain of 22% over the high prevalence herds (11). An American figure (76) suggests that mastitis costs $90 to $250 per cow per year in that country.

A good deal more has been written on the biological effects of mastitis on total milk production and the chemical composition of milk from mastitic quarters (12). This information is of very great importance when attempting to plan a control program, but its compilation and analysis awaits a chapter on quantitative pathology in a textbook of preventive veterinary medicine. If, as has been suggested, it is necessary to control mastitis to maintain or increase the solids not fat content of milk to comply with minimum legal standards for milk as a food, the control programs may well be in operation before too long.

Modes of wastage caused by mastitis have been outlined above. These vary in occurrence with the species of bacteria and are described in the following sections which describe etiologically specific mastitides. In general terms it is *Staph. aureus*, *E. coli* and lesser coliforms which cause loss of life; *Corynebacterium* (*Actinomyces*) *pyogenes* causes complete loss of quarters, staphylococci and streptococci cause acute clinical mastitis, particularly the latter, but their principal role is in causing subclinical mastitis resulting in a reduction of milk produced and a downgrading of its quality. Of these *Str. agalactiae* causes the greatest production loss, for example a decrease in quarter infection rate from 28% down to 7% was followed by an increase in average annual production of 477 kg/cow (21), whereas *Staph. aureus* causes the higher infection rate, greater resistance to treatment and longer duration of infection. At one time it represented the impassable barrier to mastitis control programs.

Pathogenesis

The mechanisms by which mastitis pathogens produce the lesions of the disease are dealt with under the headings of the individual mastitides. The general principles of pathogenesis have been well described (77) and are not repeated here, but a description of the mode of infection is included below because of its relevance to the control of the disease.

Except in the case of tuberculosis, where the method of spread may be hematogenous, infection of the mammary gland always occurs via the teat canal and on first impression the development of inflammation after infection seems a natural sequence. However, the development of mastitis is more complex than this and can be most satisfactorily explained in terms of the three stages—invasion, infection, inflammation. Invasion is the stage at which organisms pass from the exterior of the teat to the milk inside the teat canal. Infection is the stage in which the organisms multiply rapidly and invade the mammary tissue. After invasion a bacterial population may be established in the teat canal and, using this as a base, a series of multiplications and extensions into mammary tissue may occur, with infection of mammary tissue occurring frequently or occasionally depending on its susceptibility. This in turn causes inflammation, the stage at which clinical mastitis appears or a greatly increased leukocyte count is apparent in the milk.

In the context of the above general description of the development of mastitis the following factors suggest themselves as being involved in the development of the disease in individual cows and in the herd.

Invasion phase

1. The presence and population density of the causative bacteria in the milking shed environment. The quarter infection rate and the degree of contamination of the teat skin are commonly used as indices of this factor.
2. The frequency with which the cow's teats, particularly the apices, are contaminated with these bacteria. This depends largely on the efficiency of milking hygiene (63).
3. The degree of damage to the teat sphincters facilitating entry of bacteria into the teat canal. Milking machine design, adjustment, maintenance and proper use, and teat care are the important contributors to this factor and to the possible reflux of milk back into the udder from the liner of the milking cup during milking.
4. Tone of the teat sphincter, particularly in the period directly after milking when the sphincter is most relaxed. Slackness of the sphincter facilitates invasion by permitting both suction and growth of bacteria into the teat.
5. The presence of antibacterial substances in the teat duct.

Infection phase

6. The type of bacteria which determines its capacity to multiply in the milk and to adhere to the mammary epithelium. The virulence of individual bacterial species appears to depend, at least in part, on this capacity of adherence (91).
7. The susceptibility of the bacteria to the commonly used antibiotics. This may depend on natural or acquired resistance resulting from the improper use of antibiotics.
8. The presence of protective substances in the milk. Immune substances may be natural or be present as a result of previous infection or vaccination.
9. A pre-existing high leukocyte count due to intercurrent mastitis or physical trauma.
10. The stage of lactation, infection occurring more readily in the dry period because of the absence of physical flushing. There has been general acceptance that this is so but a careful analysis suggests that susceptibility is high at drying off, but is much less in the quarter which has been dried off for some time (3).

Inflammation phase

11. The pathogenicity and tissue-invasive powers of the causative bacteria. These differ widely between bacteria. For example, streptococci cause little pathological change in secretory cells, while staphylococci cause gross degenerative changes.
12. The susceptibility of the mammary tissue to the bacteria. This may vary from resistance, due to

the presence of fixed tissue antibody, to hypersensitivity as a result of previous infection.

Of the three phases, prevention of the invasion phase offers the greatest potential for reducing the incidence of mastitis by good management, notably in the use of good hygienic procedures.

Because of the difficulties encountered in the control of the disease any factor capable of reducing the severity of the response to infection is worthy of examination. Immunity to infection, because of the promise it holds as a control measure, has attracted much attention but in spite of the resistance to mammary infection which is known to occur naturally in a small proportion of cows little is known of its mechanism. The artificial production of immunity is at present of no practical value.

Clinical findings

Bovine mastitis

Dependent upon the resistance of the mammary tissue and the virulence of the invading bacteria, there may be all degrees of variation in signs from the gradual onset of fibrosis, through acute inflammation without systemic signs, to severe toxemia with systemic signs.

Details of the clinical findings are provided under each bacteriological type of mastitis. These may be taken as a guide but because many species of bacteria can cause chronic, acute and peracute forms of the disease, clinical differentiation of bacteriological types of mastitis is generally impossible. In one analysis of clinical accuracy in predicting microbiological findings the positive predictive value for coliform mastitis was 42% and the negative value 79%. These results were significantly better than would be expected by chance (47).

The clinical findings in mastitis include abnormalities of secretion, abnormalities of the size, consistency and temperature of the mammary glands and frequently a systemic reaction. The clinical forms of mastitis are usually classified according to their severity; severe inflammation of the quarter with a marked systemic reaction is classified as peracute; severe inflammation without a marked systemic reaction as acute; mild inflammation with persistent abnormality of the milk as subacute; and recurrent attacks of inflammation with little change in the milk as chronic.

Mastitis is said to be subclinical when there is evidence of inflammation, e.g. a high somatic cell count in the milk without any visible abnormality of the milk or udder.

Abnormalities of milk

Proper examination of the milk requires the use of a strip cup, preferably one which has a shiny, black plate permitting the detection of discoloration as well as clots, flakes and pus. Milk is drawn on to the plate in pools and comparisons made between the milk of different quarters. Discoloration may be in the form of bloodstaining or wateriness, the latter usually indicating chronic mastitis when the quarter is lactating. Little significance is attached to barely discernible wateriness in the first few streams but if this persists for ten streams or more, it can be considered to be an abnormality. Clots or flakes are usually accompanied by discoloration and they are always significant, usually indicating a severe degree of inflammation, even when small and present only in the first few streams. Blood clots are of little significance, neither are the small plugs of wax which are often present in the milk during the first few days after calving, especially in heifers. Flakes at the end of milking may be indicative of mammary tuberculosis in cattle. During the dry period in normal cows, the secretion changes from normal milk to a clear watery fluid, then to a secretion the color and consistency of honey and finally to colostrum in the last few days before parturition. Some variation may occur between individual quarters in the one cow and if this is marked, it should arouse suspicion of infection.

The strip cup has been a valuable adjunct to the detection of mastitis and still has its place in the cursory examination of suspicious quarters. However, it has been almost completely superseded by the more accurate indirect tests listed below. Because the herdsman frequently has little time to examine milk for evidence of mastitis it is customary to milk the first few streams onto the floor, in some parlors onto black plates in the floor. The practice does not appear to be harmful, especially where the floor is kept washed down. To avoid the difficulties arising from foremilk stripping inline filters are sometimes used to detect the presence of clots in the milk.

Abnormalities of udder

Abnormalities of size and consistency of the quarters may be seen and felt. Palpation is of greatest value when the udder has been recently milked, whereas visual examination of both the full and empty udder may be useful. The udder should be viewed from behind and the two back quarters examined for symmetry. By lifting up the back quarters, the front quarters can be viewed. A decision on which quarter of a pair is abnormal may depend on palpation, which should be carried out on adjacent quarters simultaneously. Although in most forms of mastitis the observed abnormalities are mainly in the region of the milk cistern, the whole of the quarter must be palpated, particularly if tuberculosis is suspected. Moreover, the teats and supramammary lymph nodes should be palpated and the teats examined for sores especially about the sphincter.

Palpation and inspection of the udder are directed at the detection of fibrosis, inflammatory swelling and the atrophy of mammary tissue. Fibrosis occurs in various forms. There may be a diffuse increase in connective tissue, giving the quarter a firmer feel than its opposite number and usually a more nodular surface on light palpation. Local areas of fibrosis may also occur in a quarter, and vary in size from peak-like lesions to masses as large as a fist. Acute inflammatory swelling is always diffuse and is accompanied by heat and pain and marked abnormality of the secretion. In severe cases there may be areas of gangrene, or abscesses may develop in the glandular tissue. The terminal stage of chronic mastitis is atrophy of the gland. On casual examination an atrophied quarter may be classed as normal because of its small size, while the normal quarter is judged to be hypertrophic. Careful palpation may reveal that, in the atrophic quarter, little functioning mammary tissue remains (24).

Systemic reaction

A systemic reaction comprising toxemia, fever, general depression and anorexia may or may not be present, depending on the type and severity of the infection. The details of the different types of mastitis in cattle are given in the subsequent sections.

Mastitis in other species

The disease in sheep and goats is similar to that in cattle. Particular care is needed in the clinical examination of goat's milk because of its apparent normality when there are severe inflammatory changes in the udder. In pigs it is almost always a disease of recently farrowed sows, usually within 48 hours of farrowing. It is most often a part of the mastitis–metritis–agalactia syndrome, described elsewhere. There is systemic involvement with fever, anorexia, recumbency and agalactia. One or more mammary glands are swollen, hot, painful and red. The appearance of the milk is hard to establish because of the small volume of the secretion. It often seems surprisingly normal, but it may contain clots. Many piglets die; some sows may too.

In mares there is swelling, pain and heat in the affected half, the milk is clotted, and lameness in the leg on the affected side is common. Gangrene and sloughing of the ventral floor of a gland may occur.

Clinical pathology

In the diagnosis and control of mastitis, laboratory procedures are of value in the examination of milk samples for cells, bacteria and chemical changes, and for testing for sensitivity of bacteria to specific drugs. Because of the expense of laboratory examination of large numbers of milk samples, much attention has been given to the development of field tests based on physical and chemical changes in the milk. These tests are indirect and detect only the presence of inflammatory changes, they are of value only as screening tests and may need to be supplemented by bacteriological examination for determination of the causative organism and, if necessary, its sensitivity to antibiotics and chemotherapeutic agents. The physical tests carried out on milk in a mastitis examination are limited to the cell count and its immediate development, the bulk milk cell count. Indirect tests are also limited almost entirely to tests such as the California mastitis test (CMT) and the Whiteside test which are dependent on the cell count. Other indirect tests are the chloride content and electrical conductivity, and the test for bovine serum albumin. The latter tests are more accurately diagnostic of damage to mammary epithelium.

The present day emphasis in mastitis control is to maintain a particular program of hygiene and to monitor it continuously. Because the surveillance is on the prevalence of subclinical mastitis, clinicopathological tests must be used. The logistics of providing surveillance is defeated by the very large number of cows that must be checked routinely. The situation is worsened because farmers in many areas milk their cows for only a limited period of the year. Currently the tendency is to dispense with any bacteriological examination and limit the program to identifying cows with 'cell-countosis' rather than mastitis. Because more traditional strategies are still in operation in many parts of the world they are dealt with extensively below, as in the past.

Bacteriological culturing of milk

Culturing of milk samples is a standard method of examination for mastitis. It may be carried out on individual quarter samples or on composite samples including milk from all four quarters. Individual quarter samples are preferred because the costs of treatment require that the least possible number of quarters be treated. With the former technique only affected quarters are treated and if the quarter infection rate is low the saving could be great. In mastitis control programs the costs of bacteriological culture in the laboratory can be greatly reduced by screening the cows with an indirect test first and then culturing the positive reactors. Unless bacteriological identification is necessary, it may be the first examination of the herd, or the prevalence or clinical picture may have changed, further economy can be achieved by spot checks on small samples of cows.

The culture of milk samples from bulk milk supplies has also been examined as a means of monitoring the mastitis status of herds. Mastitis caused by *Streptococcus agalactiae* lends itself to this kind of surveillance, but mastitis due to *Staphylococcus aureus* does not, because of the ubiquitous nature of the organism.

The culturing of milk samples from quarters that have been recently treated carries the hazard that the important bacteria may have been eliminated. However, provided that the sampling is delayed until at least 12 hours after treatment, such samples are mostly culturally positive (53).

Milk sampling for cultural examination

This must be carried out with due attention to cleanliness since samples contaminated during collection are worthless. The technique of cleaning the teat is of considerable importance. If the teats are dirty, ensure that they are properly dried after washing or water will run down the teat and infect the milk sample. Cleanse the end of the teat with a swab dipped in 70% alcohol, extruding the external sphincter by pressure to ensure that dirt and wax are removed from the orifice. Brisk rubbing is advisable, especially of teats with inverted ends. The first streams used to be collected as the bacterial population is usually higher in these than in later samples. The question is still hotly debated, but the tide of opinion has now turned, to recommend that the first few streams be rejected because their cell count and bacterial count are likely to be a reflection of the disease situation within the teat, rather than the udder as a whole. If tuberculosis is suspected, the last few streams should be collected. By contrast, the indirect tests and chemical tests for mastitis (concentration of immunoglobulins, serum albumin, total protein, pH, fat percentage, Wisconsin mastitis test) can be carried out as accurately on foremilk as on later milk (29). In sows where the amount of secretion may be small, a few drops of milk may be collected on to a sterile swab.

If individual quarter samples are collected, screw-cap vials with rubber wads are most satisfactory. During collection the vial is canted to avoid as far as possible the entrance of dust, skin scales and hair. If there is delay between the collection of samples and laboratory examinations, the specimens should be kept cool. The laboratory techniques used vary widely and depend to a large extent on the facilities available. Incubation on blood agar is most satisfactory, selective media for *Str. agalactiae* having the disadvantage that other pathogens may go undetected. Smears of incubated milk are generally unsatisfactory as not all bacteria grow equally well in milk.

Cell counts in milk

Cell counts in milk are coming to be the most favored method of determining the freedom or otherwise of a quarter, or a cow or a herd from mastitis. The counts used include the direct microscopic somatic cell count (DMSCC), the electronic somatic cell count (ESCC), the bulk milk cell count (BMCC) and the individual cow cell count (ICCC). There is a good deal of variation in the number and type of cells at different times during the lactation and especially at the beginning and end of lactation (33). There are also consistent and significant differences in actual cell counts between cows and individual cows tend to maintain the same class of count throughout their lives. Cows that have consistently low counts do not seem to be more susceptible to mastitis than others (23). Cell counts are usually performed on the same sample as that used for cultural examination and serious errors are avoided if the samples are always taken at the same stage of milking. There is a great deal of variation in the cell counts at various times during milking and the most significant sample is the one taken just before the evening milking (25). In chronic mastitis the highest counts are in the strippings. When foremilk counts are highest the lesion is probably in the teat. These variations need to be taken into account when assessing the mastitis status of a quarter or a cow. To overcome the difficulty in decision-making created by this variability it is customary to set arbitrary threshold levels beyond which a positive diagnosis of mastitis is made.

Leukocytes break down readily in stored milk, and for preference smears should be made, fixed and stained within an hour or two of collection of the sample. Formalin added to the milk (0–1 ml to 5–10 ml of 40% formaldehyde solution) within 24 hours of collection will prevent lysis of cells. Multiple cell counts, now a practical reality because of the development of electronic cell-counting machines (26), are of considerable value in determining the presence of inflammation. Counts of less than 250 000/ml are considered to be below the limit indicative of inflammation although most normal quarters show less than 100 000/ml. Cows in early and late lactation may show high counts but all four quarters are equally affected, an unusual state in mastitis. The degree of elevation also varies with the type of mastitis, *Str. agalactiae* infections being associated with higher counts than other types of infection.

Differential counts have not received much attention because of the difficulty of identifying the cell types. The total count reflects the amount of gland involved in the inflammatory process, whereas the neutrophil count reflects the stage of the inflammation. A high total count (e.g. 10^6/ml) and a high proportion of neutrophils (e.g. 90%) indicate acute inflammation affecting much of the quarter. A low total count (e.g. 500 000/ml) and a low proportion of neutrophils (e.g. less than 40%) indicate a small, chronic lesion. Attempts to carry out differential leukocyte counts on the automatic cell counting machines, using cell size as the differentiating criterion, have not provided greater accuracy in selecting infected quarters than the regular somatic cell count (16).

There is not much call for milk cell counts in species other than cattle. In goats the counts are higher, but vary more widely than in cows (52) although they have a similar relationship to the CMT as does cows' milk. A count of greater than 1 million cells/ml can be regarded as positive for mastitis (86). There may be some value in doing a differential count, which differentiates as the count of nucleated and non-nucleated cells, because of the variability in normal ewes in the number of cells other than leukocytes (56). In milking ewes the threshold for a diagnosis of mastitis is 300 000 somatic cells and 100 000 neutrophils/ml (79). Using a Coulter counter for the cell count means using a threshold level of 1 million cells/ml (92).

Bulk milk cell counts

Cell counts on bulked milk from a herd, collected at the farm or at the milk depot, have become universally adopted as a screening test for herds. It is most useful in creating awareness in the mind of the farmer of the existence of a mastitis problem in his herd. So that when the bulk milk cell count exceeds permissible limits a further investigation using other techniques is indicated. Its most frequent use is in herds that have no present problem with mastitis but which wish to monitor their status on a continuing basis (57). Most developed countries now provide such a service to all herds and usually on a monthly basis.

It is not possible to determine the number of cows in a herd affected by mastitis with a bulk milk cell count but it is possible to estimate fairly accurately the number of infected quarters (27). And now that electronic laboratory cell counters are generally available the procedure has attractions logistically. A number of constraints apply to the use of the test. Only somatic cells must be counted; if bacteria are included the relationship of the test and mastitis occurrence is distorted. Also the relationship between cell count and bacterial status is not very high. If, however, mastitis is defined as cell count plus bacterial infection the relationship between it and bulk milk cell count is high. The relationship is more accurate still if the standards of CMT reaction 2 plus isolation of 26 colonies of pathogenic bacteria per 0–05 ml of inoculum are accepted as positive reactions for mastitis. These criteria depend on the prerequisite that the foremilk is discarded before the testing sample is taken.

None of the above matters are relevant to the technique of bulk milk cell counting, but only to the justification for using it. The test itself is simple enough, requiring only that the sample for examination be taken randomly, that it be prepared with the correct reagent, the laboratory counter be set at the right calibration, the sample be examined quickly or preserved with formalin because of changes in cell count which occur in storage (28), and that the count be interpreted in relation to a scale of predetermined levels. In some countries a bulk milk cell count of more than 300 000/ml is considered to indicate a level of mastitis in the herd that warrants examination of individual cows. For standard use a count of 500 000/ml is probably sufficiently stringent. The levels in European countries are lower than elsewhere. In goats the range of normal levels of cell counts in milk seems to be higher than the level in cows in spite of the lower prevalence of infection (87).

The bulk milk itself will vary in composition, irrespective of sampling errors, and this must be taken into account when attempting to interpret cell counts. For example, the number of clinical cases which are occurring, the kind of infection, because *Str. agalactiae* is a more potent stimulator of cellular reaction than *Staph. aureus*, the strictness with which clinically affected milk is kept out of the bulk supply, and the stage of lactation should all be considered. With respect to the latter it is obvious that in a seasonal herd in which all cows are at the same stage of lactation the bulk milk cell count will normally be high in early lactation and just before drying off. To overcome these, and other factors which are likely to transiently influence bulk milk cell counts, it has become standard practice to use a standard rolling cell count in which monthly data are averaged for the preceding 3 months. Consideration of this figure will avoid too hasty conclusion on a temporarily high count caused by an extraneous factor.

A sampling and counting program is of little value on its own, and a system of reporting results back to farmers is an essential part of the program, and if this can be supplemented by an educational program the results in reducing mastitis prevalence can be dramatic (11).

Cell counts in milk of individual cows or quarters
There is a strong relationship between the somatic cell count of quarter samples of milk and the milk yield of the quarter. The relationship extends to include a high prevalence of clinical cases and a high mean CMT result in quarters with high cell counts (72, 75). Nowadays, because of the time and labor saved, there is great interest in selecting individual affected cows by a total somatic cell count of a composite milk sample, which has already been collected for testing for butterfat. It is more economical still to use an automatic electronic cell counter, either a Coulter Counter or a Fossomatic. The diagnosis that the cow is affected by mastitis could then, theoretically, be used as a base on which to make a decision to cull or to treat during lactation, or as a basis on which to administer selective dry period treatment. The problems are these:

- Results are for a cow so that a positive test requires that all four quarters be treated unless a further examination of quarter samples is carried out to determine which of the quarters is/are affected
- Cell counts are high for quarters infected with *Strep. agalactiae* and an individual cow cell count picks out the affected cows, but the important and common infection of *Staph. aureus* is often accompanied by low cell counts. Thus, the threshold for a positive diagnosis has to be set so low that many unaffected cows are diagnosed as positive
- High lactation age and hand milking increase the cell count in milk without the intervention of mastitis. Cows near the end of lactation also have higher cell counts due to shedding of mammary epithelium
- The CMT, or other suitable indirect test, is more accurate as a method of diagnosis, but requires a special collection of milk, whereas the cell count technique uses milk already collected for other purposes, usually butterfat testing
- The automatic cell counters are very accurate in measuring total cell counts in milk, but the importance of the cell count depends on the proportion of them which are inflammatory cells (leukocytes) and those which are exfoliated epithelial cells from the mammary tissue. An attachment to some type of cell counter which differentiates cells into these two categories is under test and may make these cell counts more useful as indicators of infection (5, 13–15, 56, 71). The procedure shows promise for monitoring the level of infection in either dairy herds or individual cows, but requires further refinement before it can be recommended for general use.

At the present time it is possible only to recommend that individual cow cell counts which do not differentiate between leukocytes and epithelial cells should be used as follows (55):

- A threshold of 400 000 cells/ml be used to identify affected quarters
- Positive results will indicate the cow's mastitis status over a period
- Treatment during lactation should not be based solely on the results from automatic cell counts. Positive cows should have individual quarters examined by the CMT, preferably at a laboratory to avoid inconsistency in results. Quarters positive to CMT should be treated and quarters not responding to treatment should be cultured. The alternative is to culture all CMT-positive quarters immediately. A strip cup or similar technique should be used at all times to detect clinical cases
- Cows in early lactation which have cell counts exceeding 400 000/ml should be treated during lactation. Cows in mid to late lactation should not be treated until drying off
- A record of chronic mastitis and severe fibrosis detected on deep udder palpation should be the basis of a recommendation to cull
- Selection of cows for dry period treatment solely by the use of individual cow cell counts is widely used. The recommended procedure is the examination of each quarter by the CMT and the treatment of those giving a positive reaction. Prior culture is recommended of the CMT-positive quarters. Such selective dry cow therapy is recommended only when the quarter infection rate is at a suitably low level, say 15%.

Indirect tests for the detection of mastitis, and designed principally for use in the field, are now restricted almost entirely to those which determine the quantity of DNA, and therefore approximately the number of leukocytes, in the sample. The California (rapid) mastitis test is most commonly used and has proved to be highly efficient, especially in the hands of a skilled operator. It reflects accurately the total leukocyte and the polymorph count of the milk (50). After mixing milk and the prepared reagent in a white container, the result is read as a negative, trace, 1, 2 or 3 reaction depending on the amount of gel formation in the sample. Cows in the first week after calving or in the last stages of lactation always give a strong positive reaction. The alternative technique to the CMT is the rolling-ball viscometer which is based on the same principles as the CMT and gives a numerical answer but is slow to operate (101).

The relationship between the CMT reaction and the leukocyte count of milk and the reduced productivity of affected cows is set out in the table below (30) as an example, and is recorded by many large-scale investigations (96). The test has also been shown to be a reliable indicator of the cell count of ewe's milk (31).

CMT reaction	*Leukocyte count* (/ml)	*Loss of milk yield for lactation* (%)
Trace	500 000	6·0
1	1 000 000	10·0
2	2 000 000	16·0
3	4 000 000	24·5

Other field tests are available and comparisons of their relative efficiencies have been made.

The CMT has been used extensively in the laboratory as well as in the field. Other laboratory tests depending on the development of gels and the measurement of their viscosity have been used. They include the Brabant, Wisconsin (87) and the NAGase mastitis tests. The latter test is suited to the rapid handling of large numbers of samples because of the ease of its automation. It is based on the measurement of a cell-associated enzyme (N-acetyl-B-D-glucosaminidase) in the milk, a high level of the enzyme indicating a high cell count. It is reputed to have the same accuracy as milk cell counts and requires a less sophisticated reading instrument than the average automatic cell counter (82).

The CMT has the advantage that it can be used on the bulk milk from the cow, from individual cans and from a herd bulk tank as well as on individual quarters (34). Of course the results become less accurate as greater dilution occurs and permissible counts should be less for herds producing larger volumes of milk (51). Bulk samples from the herd will tolerate on the average about 18% of positive cows before showing a grade 1 reaction. A grade 1 reaction on herd milk suggests that mastitis is present, a grade 2 or 3 that a serious situation exists. CMT scores of N, T, 1, 2 and 3 have been found to equate to mean cow cell counts of 100 000, 300 000, 900 000, 2 700 000 and 8 100 000 respectively. When a positive test is obtained on a herd or individual sample a bacteriological examination of those quarters showing a positive CMT is indicated.

The CMT has been done in lactating ewes and found to be highly accurate in diagnosing infections with the major pathogens (103).

Indirect chemical tests

The chemical test which has received most attention is the one based on the increase in sodium and chloride ions, and the consequent increase in electrical conductivity which occurs in mastitic milk (35). The chemical changes in milk are the first to occur in mastitis and the test has attractions for this reason. But a number of factors affect these characteristics, and to derive much benefit from the test it is necessary to examine all quarters and use differences between quarters to indicate affected quarters. For greater accuracy all quarters need to be monitored each day. Because the test measures actual damage to the udder, rather than the cow's response to the damage as the cell count does, it has attractions. However, its limitations probably restrict its use to very high-producing cows kept in small herds, or to laboratories which have autoanalyzers (36). The most commonly promoted device based on measuring the electrical conductivity of milk is a hand-held device with a built-in cup into which milk is squirted (98). It has been suggested that the incorporation of Na^+ and electrical conductivity sensors into milking machines would permit daily monitoring of cows and the detection of deviations from normal in individual quarters, permitting the early identification of quarters with mastitis (37). However, compared to other indirect tests the electronic sensor in the milk line detecting electrical conductivity of milk is much too inaccurate (54).

Other indirect tests set out to assess the integrity of the mammary mucosa. One is the estimation of serum albumin concentration in milk, a high concentration indicating epithelial damage. The commercially available test is a radial immunodiffusion test, called the 'monomastest' (38). A second is the antitrypsin test which measures the trypsin-inhibitor capacity of milk. This is high at the beginning of lactation due to the antitrypsin activity of colostrum, but after the first month of lactation this activity is due solely to serum antitrypsin activity which has leaked through damaged epithelium. The technique has the virtue that it can be automated easily (85, 102). A comparison of all the indirect tests available suggests that the cell count tests are the best indicators of udder health, especially when bulk milk is used (39).

Summary reports on milk samples should include identification of the organisms and some estimate of their numbers. Additional valuable information includes an estimate of the pathogenicity and drug sensitivity of the bacteria. Some information on the presence of inflammation is required either in the form of a cell count or the result of one of the indirect tests mentioned above. In about 10% of clinical cases a negative bacterial result will be obtained because the infection is at the time under control by natural defense mechanisms. Resampling in such cases is recommended. A suggested addition is a microbiological assessment of the prevalence of *Corynebacterium bovis*, a high count suggesting inadequate teat dipping (17).

Necropsy findings

Necropsy findings are not of major interest in the diagnosis of mastitis and are omitted here, but included in the description of specific infections.

Diagnosis

The diagnosis of mastitis presents little difficulty if a careful clinical examination is carried out. Examination of the udder is often omitted unless called for, particularly when the animals are recumbent. The diagnosis of mastitis depends largely upon the detection of clinical abnormality of the milk. Other mammary abnormalities, including edema, passive congestion, rupture of the suspensory ligament and hematomata, are not accompanied by abnormality of the milk unless there is hemorrhage into the udder. The presence of 'free' electricity in the milking plant should not be overlooked in herds where the sudden lowering of production arouses an unfounded suspicion of mastitis. Clinical differentiation of the various bacteriological types of mastitis is not easy but may have to be attempted, especially in peracute cases, as specific treatment has to be given before results of laboratory examinations are available.

Treatment

Special bacterial types of mastitis require specific treatments and these are discussed under the etiological entities, but there are some general principles that apply to all forms.

Degree of response

The treatment of mastitis can be highly effective in removing infection from the quarter and returning the milk to normal composition. However, the yield of milk, although it can be improved by the removal of congestion in the gland and inflammatory debris from the duct system, is unlikely to be returned to normal, at least until the next lactation. The degree of response obtained depends particularly on the type of causative agent, the speed with which treatment is commenced and other factors as set out below.

The first decision is whether to treat a particular case systemically by parenteral injection or locally by intramammary infusion. Having decided that, there is still the serious problem of selecting the best antibacterial agent for the particular pathogen involved. In the past the bulk of these decisions have been based on *in vitro* tests and although some *in vivo* data is now available the choice of drugs is still largely dependent on findings about the actual effectiveness of each drug in particular circumstances (26).

Parenteral treatment This is advisable in all cases of mastitis in which there is a marked systemic reaction, to control or prevent the development of a septicemia or bacteremia and to assist in the treatment of the infection in the gland. The systemic reaction can usually be brought under control by standard doses of antibiotics or sulfonamides but complete sterilization of the affected quarters is seldom achieved because of the relatively poor diffusion of the antibiotic from the bloodstream into the milk. The rate of diffusion is greater in damaged than in normal quarters. Parenteral treatment is also advisable when the gland is badly swollen and intramammary antibiotic is unlikely to diffuse properly. Those most likely to diffuse well are erythromycin, tylosin, penethemate, chloramphenicol and trimethoprim. Poor diffusers include neomycin and streptomycin. The penicillins, tetracycline and novobiocin are medium performers.

To produce therapeutic levels of antibiotic in the mammary gland by parenteral treatment it is necessary, for the above reasons, to use higher-than-normal dose rates (69). Recommended levels per kg body weight are penicillin 16 500 units, oxytetracycline 10 mg, tylosin or erythromycin 12·5 mg, sulfadimidine 200 g. Of these, the tetracyclines and tylosin are preferred because of their broad antibacterial spectrum and ability to reach high levels in milk after parenteral injection; drugs of the penicillin family are not highly regarded for this purpose (73). Streptomycin, neomycin, chloramphenicol and the sulfadoxine–trimethoprim combination are not recommended either.

Udder infusions

Because of convenience and efficiency, udder infusions are the preferred method of treatment. Disposable tubes containing suitable drugs in a water-soluble ointment base are best suited for dispensing and the treatment of individual cows but aqueous infusions are adequate, are much cheaper and are indicated when large numbers of quarters are to be treated. The degree of diffusion into glandular tissue is the same when either water or ointment is used as a vehicle for infusion.

Strict hygiene is necessary during treatment to avoid the introduction of bacteria, yeasts and fungi into the treated quarters. Care must be taken to ensure that bulk containers of mastitis infusions are not contaminated by frequent withdrawals and that individual, sterilized teat cannulae are used for each quarter. Because of the bad record of spread of pathogens by bulk treatments they are best avoided if possible.

Diffusion of infused drugs is often impeded by the blockage of lactiferous ducts and alveoli with inflammatory debris. Complete emptying of the quarter before infusion by the parenteral injection of oxytocin is advisable in cases of acute mastitis. This can be further aided by hourly stripping of the quarter, the intramammary infusion being left until right after the last stripping has been carried out.

After an intramammary infusion avoid emptying the gland, and thus losing the antibiotic or other drug, for as long as possible by treating immediately after milking, preferably in the evening. The choice of drugs to be used for intramammary infusion in the lactating cow is set down in Table 44. The drugs which have the best record of diffusion through the udder after intramammary infusion are penethemate, ampicillin, amoxycillin, chloramphenicol, novobiocin, erythromycin and tylosin. Those of medium performance are penicillin G, cloxacillin and tetracyclines. Poor diffusers include streptomycin and neomycin (26). Less well known drug combinations which appear to have good performance (94) have a mixture of kanamycin (250 mg) and procaine penicillin G (300 000 units), and a mixture of ampicillin sodium (100 mg) and cephalothin sodium (200 mg).

Treatment of dry cows

Chronic cases, particularly those caused by *Staph. aureus*, are often cleared up most satisfactorily by treatment when the cow is not lactating. Treatment at this time is

Table 44. Comparative efficiencies of intramammary treatment of mastitis in lactating quarters (48)

Preparation	*Dose*	*Cure rate (%)*			*Recommended use*
		Staphylococcus	*Streptococcus*	*Coliform*	
Penicillin G	100 000 units	40–70	100	Nil	In slow-release base; 2 infusions at 48-hour intervals Many are resistant
Cloxacillin	500 mg	30–60	Up to 100	—	In long-acting base, 1 infusion
Cloxacillin + ampicillin	200 mg 75 mg	64	94	97	3 infusions, once daily for 3 days (49)
Spiramycin	250 mg	45–82	56	—	3 infusions at 24-hour intervals
Rifamycin	100 mg	59–73	74	—	2 infusions at 24-hour intervals
Streptomycin + penicillin	1 mg 100 000 units	40–70	100	80	3 infusions at 24-hour intervals
Tetracyclines	200–400 mg	50	Up to 100	Poor	Daily for 2–3 days
Chloramphenicol	200 mg	28	24	50	Daily for 4 days
Neomycin	500 mg	36	30–67	25	Daily (or 48-hour intervals) for 2 infusions

Additives in intramammary infusions. Materials other than antibacterial agents included in mastitis infusions have been many and varied. Hyaluronidase has been included to promote diffusion through the udder, enzymes such as streptodornase have been used to encourage the discharge of pus, corticosteroids to reduce inflammation, immunoglobulins to control bacterial growth, cobalt to enhance antibiotic activity and many others. Few investigations have been made of their worth and what has been done has been largely to discredit the claims made for them. They have no place in treatment and are no longer actively promoted (43)

also a good prophylaxis. Because of interference with diffusion of an infused drug by the viscid secretion of much of the dry period, infusion at the time of the last milking or at the beginning or end of the dry period is recommended. The material is introduced and allowed to remain permanently. Dry period treatment is a part of the control program for bovine mastitis and is discussed under that heading and in Table 44.

Intraparenchymal injections

Intraparenchymal injection of drugs into mammary tissue by passing a needle through the skin into the mass of the gland is not widely used. It is sometimes recommended when the gland is so swollen that no diffusion is likely to occur from the milk cistern, but in this case diffusion from a parenchymal injection may also be greatly impeded.

Choice of drug

In vitro laboratory testing of bacterial sensitivity is not necessarily a justifiable basis for selecting the antibacterial agent to be used in individual cows, and the response to treatment in clinical cases is often unrelated to the results of *in vitro* sensitivity tests (60). However, a treatment program for a herd which is under continuous surveillance as part of the herd health program must take a good deal of notice of the antibiotic susceptibility of the current infections (99). Much of the earlier difficulty with drug evaluation has been overcome by the development of an induced infection model as a means of *in vivo* testing (49). Present-day knowledge of the pharmacokinetics of parenterally administered drugs, and their diffusion into mammary tissue, and on drugs administered by intramammary infusion includes knowledge of the importance of other factors: the degree of binding of a drug to mammary tissues and secretions, its ability to pass through the lipid phase of milk, and the degree of ionization have a great deal of influence on the duration of the minimum inhibitory concentration, the critical level of the antibiotic in the mammary gland. It is apparent that the most successful drugs for dry period treatment are those which persist in the udder longest, and for lactating quarters it is the drugs with the short milk-out time, to avoid contamination of milk, that are required (41).

Until recently the emphasis was on the elimination of Gram-positive cocci from the udder, but in recent years Gram-negative infections, especially *E. coli*, have increased in prevalence to the point where a broad spectrum preparation is almost essential. For lactating quarters penicillin alone (100 000 units) or in combination with streptomycin (1 g) or neomycin (500 mg) is standard treatment, but a preparation containing ampicillin 75 mg and sodium cloxacillin 200 mg is also effective (42).

The treatment of lactating quarters still presents a problem. Clinical cases have to be treated and the recovery rate with streptococci is good. For staphylococci a cure rate of 65% is about the best that can be expected and unless there are good reasons for doing otherwise it is recommended that treatment be postponed until the cow is dry. The recommended treatment is sodium cloxacillin in a slow-release base with an expected cure rate of 80% against streptococci and 60% against *Staph. aureus* (44). Although there are contrary views it is generally held to be necessary to maintain an effective concentration of antibiotic in the quarter for at least 3 and preferably 6 days to obtain good results in terms of bacteriological cure. This can be done either by multiple infusions in a quick-release base or one or two infusions in a slow release base. Either recommendation is opposed by farmers because of the long milk-out time and the amount of milk that has to be discarded, and by dairying administrators because of the inevitable increase in the number of infringements of health regulations relating to antibody residues in milk. A summary of the most common treatment for lactating quarters is shown in Table 44.

All of the above recommendations are subject to the general comment that very little good research and development work has been done on the subject and most of the products available have been developed with very little scientific support. They also tend to place attractiveness to the consumer above efficiency resulting in intramammary preparations containing a battery of antibacterial agents, one or more of a long list of generally unhelpful adjuvants, and inappropriate recommendations about their use, especially with regard to frequency of administration and length of time after treatment for which milk has to be withheld from sale. The indiscriminate and improper use of antibiotics for the treatment of clinical mastitis in lactating cows which has resulted from inaccurate promotion and uninformed use by farmers has meant that the control of mastitis has really received little assistance. Drug-resistant organisms, especially *Staph. aureus*, have been encouraged, the bacterial population in the environment has not been significantly reduced, and the chances of human consumers of dairy products being exposed to antibiotic residues has been increased.

Because of the widespread and often indiscriminate use of penicillin a large part of the mastitis which occurs is caused by penicillin-resistant bacteria, especially *Staph. aureus*. For this reason other antibiotic preparations such as the penicillin/cephoxazole combination (64), nafcillin (65), cefuroxime, cefoperazone (105) and cephacetrile (68) are now being tried. Cefoperazone at a dose rate of 250 mg per infusion is effective against a wide range of bacteria with single treatments (106).

Treatment to reduce high milk cell counts

It is apparent that farmers are using antibiotic udder infusions to reduce milk cell counts and thus satisfy quality requirements of a health authority or milk shipper, rather than to control mastitis. The effect is likely to be an increase in the indiscriminate use of antibiotics and failure to attend to the managemental and environmental factors which are likely to be as important as bacterial infection. Some drugs likely to be used, e.g. tetracyclines, chloramphenicol, gentamicin, rifampicin and nitrofurantoin are also detrimental to leukocyte function and may increase a quarter's susceptibility (100).

Sheep Although ewes probably require smaller doses of intramammary infusions than cows it is customary to use ordinary cow-type treatments (70). The treatment of ewes with peracute gangrenous mastitis is as unsatisfactory in terms of results as in cows. Systemic treatment is necessary and requires larger doses than normal to achieve significant levels in the mammary secretion.

Antibiotic residues in milk

Of great consequence is the effect of antibiotics in milk on the manufacture of dairy products and the development of sensitivity syndromes in human beings. In most countries the maximum intramammary dose of antibiotics is limited by legislation and the presence of detectable quantities of antibiotics in milk constitutes adulteration. Attention has also been directed to the excretion of antibiotics in milk from untreated quarters, after treatment of infected quarters and after their administration by parenteral injection or by insertion into the uterus. The degree to which this excretion occurs varies widely between animals and in the same animal at different points in the lactation period, and differs from one antibiotic to another. Milk from cows subjected to dry period treatment is usually required to be withheld for 4 days after calving. The use of any dry-period treatments in lactating cows is a most serious error.

Veterinarians have the responsibility of warning farmers of the need to withhold milk and they should be aware of the withholding times of each product, details of which are usually required to be included on its label. Marking the cow in some way to remind the farmer is advisable. The alternative is to include a dye marker in the intramammary infusion, preferably one that persists in the udder at least as long as the antibiotic (107, 108).

Acid-resistant penicillins, e.g. phenoxymethylpenicillin, are probably best not used as mammary infusions because of their ability to pass through the human stomach, thus presenting a more serious potential threat to humans drinking contaminated milk. Recommended periods for which milk should be withheld from sale after different methods of antibiotic administration are:

- Udder infusion in a lactating cow—72 hours
- Parenteral injection, one only—36 hours
- Parenteral injections, series of—72 hours
- Antiobiotics parenterally in longacting bases—10 days
- Intrauterine tablet—72 hours
- Dry cow intramammary infusion—to be administered at least 4 weeks before calving and the milk withheld for at least 96 hours afterwards.

Drying-off chronically affected quarters

If a quarter does not respond to treatment and is classified as incurable, the affected animal should be isolated from the milking herd or the affected quarter may be permanently dried-off by producing a chemical mastitis. Methods of doing this, arranged in decreasing order of severity, are infusions of 30–60 ml of 3% silver nitrate solution, 20 ml of 5% copper sulfate solution, 100–300 ml of 1 in 500, or 300–500 ml of a 1: 2000 acriflavine solution. If a severe local reaction occurs, the quarter should be milked out and stripped frequently until the reaction subsides. If no reaction occurs, the quarter is stripped out 10–14 days later. Two infusions may be necessary.

Supportive therapy

Supportive treatment, including the parenteral injection of large quantities of isotonic fluids, particularly those containing glucose, and of antihistamine drugs, is indicated in cases where extensive tissue damage and severe toxemia are present. The application of cold, usually in the form of crushed ice in a canvas bag suspended around the udder, may reduce absorption of toxins in such cases.

Alternative therapy

Treatment of mastitis by conventional methods is highly

satisfactory with only a few of the most badly damaged quarters failing to respond. Good results are also claimed for the intramammary infusion of oxygen (89), and for acupoint laser irradiation (90), but these techniques are not in general use.

Control

A discussion of the methods used in the control of all types of bovine mastitis is included at the end of this chapter.

REVIEW LITERATURE

Allison, J. R. D. (1985) Antibiotic residues in milk, *Br. vet. J.*, *141*, 9.
Booth, J. (1982) Antibiotic residues in milk. *In Practice*, *4*, 100.
Brolund, L. (1985) Cell counts in bovine milk. *Acta. vet. Scand.*, Suppl. 80, pp 1–123.
East, N. E. & Birnie. E. F. (1983) Diseases of the udder of sheep and goats. *Vet. Clin. N. Am. large Anim. Pract.*, *5(3)*, 591–600.
Kitchen, B. J. (1981) Bovine mastitis. Milk compositional changes and diagnostic tests. *J. dairy Res.*, *48*, 167.
McDonald, J. S. et al. (1979) Symposium. Bovine mastitis. *J. dairy Sci.*, *62*, 117 (7 papers).
Moore, G. A. & Heider, L. E. (1984) Treatment of mastitis. *Vet. Clin. N. Am. large Anim. Pract.*, *6 (2)*, 323.
Shotto, E. B. & Leard, A. T. (1984) Microbiologic aspects of mastitis diagnosis. *Vet. Clin. N. Am. large Anim. Pract.*, *6 (2)*, 247–255.
Watson, D. J. & Buswell, J. F. (1984) Modern aspects of sheep mastitis. *Br. vet. J.*, *140*, 529.
Ziv, G. (1980) Practical pharmacokinetic aspects of mastitis therapy. Pts 1, 2 & 3. *Vet. Med. SAC*, *75*, 277, 469, 657.
Ziv, G. (1980) Drug selection and use in mastitis. Systemic versus local therapy. *J. Am. vet. med. Assoc.*, *176*, 1109.

REFERENCES

(1) Paranjape, V. L. & Das, A. M. (1986) *Ind. vet. J.*, *63*, 438.
(2) Kirk, J. H. et al. (1980) *J. anim. Sci.*, *50*, 610.
(3) Addo, P. B. et al. (1974) *Vet. Rec.*, *95*, 193.
(4) Al-Graibawi, M. A. A. et al. (1984) *Vet. Rec.*, *115*, 383.
(5) Hoare, R. J. T. et al. (1980) *J. dairy Res.*, *47*, 167.
(6) Torasenko, T. A. (1973) *Veterinariya, Moscow*, *4*, 81.
(7) Sobari, S. et al. (1976) *Aust. vet. J.*, *52*, 458.
(8) Hunter, A. C. & Jeffrey, D. C. (1975) *Vet. Rec.*, *96*, 442.
(9) Smith, A. et al. (1968) *J. dairy Res.*, *35*, 287.
(10) Redaelli, G. & Ruffo, O. (1976) *Arch. Lebensmittelhyg.*, *27*, 19.
(11) Pearson, J. K. L. (1977) *Vet. Rec.*, *101*, 3.
(12) Janzen, J. J. (1970) *J. dairy Sci.*, *53*, 1151.
(13) Ron, I. & Syrstad, O. (1980) *Norsk VetTidsskr*, *92*, 11.
(14) Syrstad, O. & Ron, I. (1979) *Acta vet. Scand.*, *20*, 555.
(15) Titterton, M. & Oliver, J. (1979) *Rhodesian J. agric. Res.*, *17*, 89.
(16) Dohoo, I. R. et al. (1981) *Can. J. comp. Med.*, *45*, 8.
(17) Bramley, A. J. et al. (1976) *Vet. Rec.*, *99*, 275.
(18) Wilesmith, J. W. et al. (1986) *Vet. Rec.*, *118*, 199.
(19) Saeter, E. A. & Eieland, E. (1961) *Nord. VetMed.*, *13*, 32.
(20) Quinlivan, T. D. (1968) *NZ vet. J.*, *16*, 149, 153.
(21) Natzke, R. P. et al. (1972) *J. dairy Sci.*, *55*, 1256.
(22) Morris, R. S. (1973) *Aust. vet. J.*, *49*, 153.
(23) Coffey, E. M. et al. (1986) *J. dairy Sci.*, *69*, 552.
(24) Grootenhurs, G. (1980) *Tijdschr. Diergeneeskd.*, *105*, 121.
(25) Schalm, O. W. & Lasmanis, J. (1968) *J. Am. vet. med. Assoc.*, *153*, 1688.
(26) Ziv, G. (1980) *J. Am. vet. med. Assoc.*, *176*, 1109.
(27) Pearson, J. K. L. & Greer, D. O. (1974) *Vet. Rec.*, *95*, 252.
(28) Sweetscer, A. W. M. & Phillips, J. D. (1976) *J. dairy Res.*, *43*, 53.
(29) Guidry, A. J. et al. (1980) *J. dairy Sci.*, *63*, 611.
(30) Schneider, R. & Jasper, D. E. (1964) *Am. J. vet. Res.*, *25*, 1635.
(31) Ziv, G. et al. (1968) *Refuah vet.*, *25*, 133, 179.
(32) Wilson, C. D. & Richards, M. S. (1980) *Vet. Rec.*, *106*, 431.
(33) McDonald, J. S. & Anderson, A. J. (1981) *Am. J. vet. Res.*, *42*, 1360 & 1366.
(34) Pearson, J. K. L. et al. (1971) *Vet. Rec.*, *88*, 488.
(35) Chamings, R. J. et al. (1984) *Vet. Rec.*, *114*, 243.
(36) Fleet, I. R. et al. (1972) *Br. vet. J.*, *128*, 297.
(37) Linzell, J. L. & Peaker, M. (1972) *Br. vet. J.*, *128*, 284.
(38) Bakken, G. & Thorburn, M. (1985) *Acta vet. Scand.*, *26*, 273.
(39) Sheldrake, R. F. et al. (1983) *J. dairy Sci.*, *66*, 548.
(41) Ziv, G. (1975) *Int. Dairy Fedn, Proc. Seminar Mastitis Control, Bull. Document* No. 85, 314.
(42) Watkins, J. H. et al. (1975) *Vet. Rec.*, *96*, 289.
(43) Black, W. D. (1977) *J. Am. vet. med. Assoc.*, *170*, 1187.
(44) Wilson, C. D. (1972) *Br. vet. J.*, *128*, 71.
(45) Brooks, B. W. et al. (1982) *Can. vet. J.*, *23*, 156.
(47) White, M. E. et al. (1986) *Can. vet. J.*, *27*, 218.
(48) LeLoudec, C. (1978) *Ann. réch. vét.*, *9*, 63.
(49) Newbould, F. H. S. (1977) *J. Am. vet. med. Assoc.*, *170*, 1208.
(50) Milne, J. R. & de Langen, H. (1977) *NZ J. dairy Sci. Technol.*, *12*, 44.
(51) Devos, O. J. et al. (1977) *Tijdschr. Diergeneeskd.*, *102*, 795.
(52) Nesbakken, T. (1978) *Nord. VetMed.*, *30*, 21.
(53) Stem, E. S. et al. (1984) *J. Am. vet. med. Assoc.*, *184*, 161.
(54) Gebre-Egziabher, A. et al. (1979) *J. dairy Sci.*, *62*, 1108.
(55) Jones, G. M. et al. (1977) *J. Food Protection*, *40*, 490.
(56) Hinckley, L. S. (1982) *Vet. Med. SAC*, *78*, 1267.
(57) Guterbock, W. M. (1984) *Comp. cont. Educ.*, *6*, S601.
(58) Brooks, B. W. & Barnum, D. A. (1984) *Can. J. comp. Med.*, *48*, 141.
(59) Hunter, A. C. (1984) *Vet. Rec.*, *114*, 318.
(60) Pearson, J. K. L. & Mackie, D. P. (1979) *Vet. Rec.*, *105*, 456.
(61) Bramley, A. J. et al. (1979) *Br. vet. J.*, *135*, 149.
(62) Bramley, A. J. (1978) *Br. vet. J.*, *134*, 146.
(63) Zarkower, A. & Scheuchenberger, W. J. (1978) *Cornell Vet.*, *68*, 40.
(64) Harris, A. M. et al. (1977) *Vet. Rec.*, *101*, 4.
(65) Phillips, J. M. (1979) *Vet. Rec.*, *104*, 371.
(66) Cappucci, D. T. et al. (1978) *J. Am. vet. med. Assoc.*, *173*, 1589.
(67) Gross, S. J. et al. (1978) *J. anim. Sci.*, *46*, 1.
(68) Schluep, J. et al. (1979) *Zentralbl. VetMed.*, *26B*, 304.
(69) McDiarmid, S. C. (1978) *NZ vet. J.*, *26*, 290.
(70) Landau, M. & Tamarin, R. (1974) *Refuah vet.*, *31*, 134.
(71) Meek, A. H. et al. (1980) *J. Food Protection*, *43*, 10.
(72) Meijering, A. et al. (1978) *J. dairy Res.*, *45*, 5.
(73) Gingerich, D. A. (1977) *Proc. 10th ann. Conv. Am. Assoc. Bov. Practnrs*, p. 64.
(74) Faull, W. B. et al. (1983) *Vet. Rec.*, *113*, 415.
(75) Gill, M. S. & Holmes, C. W. (1978) *NZ J. dairy Sci. Technol.*, *13*, 157.
(76) Dobbins, C. N. (1977) *J. Am. vet. med. Assoc.*, *170*, 1129.
(77) Schalm, O. W. (1977) *J. Am. vet. med. Assoc.*, *170*, 1137.
(78) Jackson, P. G. G. (1986) *Equ. vet. J.*, *18*, 88.
(79) Fruganti, G. et al. (1985) *Clin. Vet.*, *108*, 286.
(80) Hueston, W. D. et al. (1986) *J. Am. vet. med. Assoc.*, *188*, 170.
(81) Manser, P. A. (1986) *Vet. Rec.*, *118*, 552.
(82) Kitchen, B. J. et al. (1984) *J. dairy Res.*, *51*, 11.
(83) Al-Samarrae, S. A. G. et al. (1985) *Vet. Rec.*, *116*, 323.
(84) Watson, D. J. (1982) *Ann. Proc. vet. Sheep Soc.*, *6*, 88.
(85) Sandholm, M. et al. (1984) *J. dairy Res.*, *51*, 1.
(86) Poutrel, B. & Lerondelle, C. (1983) *J. dairy Sci.*, *66*, 2575.
(87) Heider, L. E. (1984) *Bov. Pract.*, *18*, 7.
(88) Brooks, B. W. et al. (1983) *Can. J. comp. Med.*, *47*, 73.
(89) Khilkevich, N. M. & Khilkevich, S. N. (1986) *Veterinariya, Moscow*, *8*, 60.
(90) Wei, Z. L. et al. (1983) *Chin. J. vet. Med.*, *9*, 39.
(91) Wanasinghe, D. D. (1981) *Acta vet. Scand.*, *22*, 109.
(92) Green, T. J. (1984) *Vet. Rec.*, *114*, 43.
(93) Beauregard, M. & Higgins, R. (1983) *Can. vet. J.*, *24*, 284.
(94) Storper, M. et al. (1981) *Refuah Vet.*, *38*, 154.
(95) LeVan, P. L. et al. (1985) *J. dairy Sci.*, *68*, 3329.
(96) Jones, G. M. et al. (1984) *J. dairy Sci.*, *67*, 1523.
(97) Shen, W. Q. (1983) *Chin. J. vet. Med.*, *9*, 12.
(98) Green, T. J. & Middleton, L. (1984) *Vet. Rec.*, *114*, 616.
(99) Hinckley, L. S. et al. (1985) *J. Am. vet. med. Assoc.*, *187*, 709.
(100) Nickerson, S. C. et al. (1986) *J. dairy Sci.*, *69*, 1733.
(101) Whittlestone, W. G. (1984) *Agri-Practice*, *5(9)*, p. 6.
(102) Mattila, T. et al. (1985) *J. dairy Sci.*, *68*, 114.

(103) Hueston, W. D. et al. (1986) *J. Am. vet. med. Assoc.*, *188*, 522.
(104) Khalaf, A. M. (1983) *Proc. 3rd int. Symp. World Assoc. Vet. Lab Diagnostns, Ames, Iowa, Vol. 2*, 198.
(105) Wilson, C. D. & Gilbert, G. A. (1986) *Vet. Rec.*, *118*, 607.
(106) Wilson, C. D. et al. (1986) *Vet. Rec.*, *118*, 17.
(107) Novak, N. F. et al. (1984) *J. dairy Sci.*, 67, 1841.
(108) Gilmore, T. M. et al. (1986) *J. dairy Sci.*, *69*, 1128.
(109) Roberts, M. C. (1986) *Equ. vet. J.*, *18*, 146.
(110) Preez, J. H. du and Greeff, F. S. (1984) *Proc. 13th World Congress, Dis. Cattle, Durban, Vol. 2*, pp. 226— 231.
(111) McGillivery, D. J. et al. (1984) *Aust. vet. J.*, *61*, 325.
(112) Lewter, M. M. (1984) *Comp. cont. Educ.*, 6, S417.

MAJOR MASTITIDES

Mastitis caused by *Streptococcus agalactiae*

Infection of the mammary gland with *Streptococcus agalactiae* produces a specific mastitis in cattle, sheep and goats.

Etiology

The disease can be reproduced by the introduction of *Str. agalactiae* into the mammary glands of cattle, goats and sheep.

Epidemiology

The disease occurs in cattle wherever dairying is practiced and usually at about the same level of incidence. In any large cattle population where the disease is not controlled in any way, most herds will be found to be infected and the average morbidity rate among the cows will be about 25%. Where good hygienic measures and efficient treatments are in general use, the morbidity rate in the cattle population will be considerably below this. In fact, since the advent of antibiotic treatment, *Str. agalactiae* has been supplanted by *Staphylococcus aureus* as the major cause of bovine mastitis. This is not to say the infection is uncommon. Where mastitis control and the treatment of clinically affected and lactating quarters are actively prosecuted the morbidity will be low. But in other circumstances, and particularly in herds with a high bulk milk cell count, the probability is that *Str. agalactiae* infection will be common (3, 4).

This disease is of major importance as a brake on the economic production of milk. In individual cows, the loss of production caused by *Str. agalactiae* mastitis is about 25% during the infected lactation, and in affected herds the loss may be of the order of 10–15% of the potential production. Reduction of the productive life probably represents approximately an average loss of one lactation per cow in an affected herd. Deaths rarely if ever occur due to *Str. agalactiae* infection and complete loss of productivity of a quarter is uncommon, the losses being incurred in the less dramatic but no less important fashion of decreased production per cow.

Goats are uniformly susceptible but only about 50% of cows can be infected experimentally. Although the disease is most common under natural conditions in cattle, it occurs to a lesser extent in goats and has been recorded in pigs, and in sheep used as milking animals (5). The mortality in the latter species may be severe, approaching 10% in some herds. In cattle there is no particular breed susceptibility but infection does become established more readily in older cows (6) and in the early part of each lactation.

The main source of the infection is the udder of infected cows although, when hygiene is poor, contamination of the environment may provide a ready source of infection. The teats and skin of cattle, milkers' hands, floors, utensils and clothes are often heavily contaminated. Sores on teats are the commonest sites outside the udder for persistence of the organism. The infection may persist for up to 3 weeks on hair and skin and on inanimate materials such as dung and bricks. The importance of environmental contamination as a source of infection is given due recognition in the general disinfection technique of eradication. Transmission of infection from animal to animal occurs most commonly by the medium of milking machine liners, hands, udder cloths and possibly bedding.

Only the teat canal is important as a portal of entry, although there is doubt as to how the invasion occurs through the sphincter. Suction into the teat during milking or immediately afterwards does occur, but growth of the bacteria into the canal between milkings also appears to be an important method of entry (5). It is difficult to explain why heifers which have never been milked may be found to be infected with *Str. agalactiae* although sucking between calves after ingestion of infected milk or contact with infected inanimate materials are the probable sources of infection.

Pathogenesis

When the primary barrier of the teat sphincter is passed, either naturally or experimentally, many of the introduced bacteria are washed out by the physical act of milking. In many animals the bacteria proliferate, and in some invasion of the udder tissue follows. There is considerable variation between cows in the developments which occur at each of these three stages. The reasons for this variation are not clear but resistance appears to depend largely on the continuity of the lining of the teat cistern (6). After the introduction of infection into the teat, the invasion, if it occurs, takes 1–4 days and the appearance of inflammation 3–5 days. Again there is much variation between cows in the response to tissue invasion, and a balance may be set up between the virulence of the organism and the undefined defense mechanisms of the host so that very little clinically detectable inflammation may develop, despite the persistence of a permanent bacterial flora.

The development of mastitis caused by *Str. agalactiae* is essentially a process of invasion and inflammation of lobules of mammary tissue in a series of crises, particularly during the first month after infection, each crisis developing in the same general pattern (7). Initially there is a rapid multiplication of the organism in the lactiferous ducts, followed by passage of the bacteria through the duct walls into lymphatic vessels and to the supramammary lymph nodes, and an outpouring of neutrophils into the milk ducts. At this stage of tissue invasion, a shortlived systemic reaction occurs and the milk yield falls sharply due to inhibition and stasis of secretion caused by damage to acinar and ductal epithelium. Fibrosis of the interalveolar tissue and involution of acini result even though the tissue invasion is quickly cleared. Subsequently, similar crises develop and more lobules are affected in the same way resulting in a stepwise loss of secretory function with increasing fibrosis of the quarter and eventual atrophy.

The clinicopathological findings vary with the stage of development of the disease. Bacterial counts in the milk are high in the early stages but fall when the cell count rises at the same time as swelling of the quarter becomes apparent. In some cases bacteria are not detectable culturally at this acute stage. The cell count rises by 10–100 times normal during the first 2 days after infection and returns to normal over the next 10 days (1). The febrile reaction is often sufficiently mild and shortlived enough to escape notice. When the inflammatory changes in the epithelial lining of the acini and ducts begin to subside, the shedding of the lining results in the clinical appearance of clots in the milk. Thus the major damage has already been done when clots are first observed. At the stage of acute swelling, it is the combination of inflamed interalveolar tissue and retained secretion in distended alveoli which causes the swelling. Removal of the retained secretion at this stage may considerably reduce the swelling and permit better diffusion of drugs infused into the quarter. Inflammmatory reactions also occur in the teat wall of affected quarters.

The variation in resistance between cows and the increased susceptibility with advancing age are unexplained. Hormonal changes and hypersensitivity of mammary tissue to streptococcal protein have both been advanced as possible causes of the latter. Local immunity of mammary tissue after an attack probably does not occur but there is some evidence to suggest that a low degree of general immunity may develop. At least in goats, vaccination causes a rise in serum antibodies which may provide a degree of immunity. The rapid disappearance of the infection in a small proportion of cows in contrast to the recurrent crises which are the normal pattern of development suggests that immunity does develop in some animals (8). The antibodies are hyaluronidase inhibitors and are markedly specific for specific strains of the organism. A non-specific rise in other antibodies may occur simultaneously and this is thought to account for the field observations that coincident streptococcal and staphylococcal infections are unusual and that the elimination of one infection may lead to an increased incidence of the other.

Difficulty is likely to be encountered in the application of the known facts about immunity to the artificial production of immunity in the field because of the multiplicity of strains involved and the known variability between animals in their reaction to mammary infection.

Clinical findings

In the experimentally produced disease, there is initially a sudden attack of acute mastitis, accompanied by a transient fever, followed at intervals by similar attacks, usually of less severity. In natural cases, fever, lasting for a day or two, is occasionally observed with the initial attack, but the inflammation of the gland persists and the subsequent crises are usually of a relatively mild nature. These degrees of severity may be classified as peracute when the animal is febrile and off its feed, acute when the inflammation of the gland is severe but there is no marked systemic reaction, and chronic when the inflammation is mild. In the latter instance, the gland is not greatly swollen, pain and heat are absent, and the presence of clots in watery foremilk may be the only apparent abnormality. The induration is most readily palpable at the cistern and in the lower part of the udder and varies in degree with the stage of development of the disease.

The milk yield of affected glands is markedly reduced during each crisis but with proper treatment administered early, the yield may return to almost normal. Even without treatment the appearance of the milk soon becomes normal but the yield is significantly reduced and subsequent crises are likely to reduce it further.

Clinical pathology

Most of the information on the clinical pathology of mastitis in general applies in this form of the disease. The number of bacteria present in the milk sample is of importance, infected glands usually yielding more than 200 colonies/ml of milk, with smaller counts suggesting the invasion phase before the infection becomes established, or contamination of the sample from the skin of the teat (9). It is characteristic of mastitis caused by *Str. agalactiae* that bacteria may virtually disappear from the milk during the acute phase when they invade mammary tissue, the count subsequently rising and then falling as involution and fibrosis develop. Conversely the cell counts of milk from infected quarters are highest at the acute inflammatory stage.

Large scale mastitis programs are faced with the problem of deciding which of the available methods to use in order to determine the type of streptococci present. Agglutination tests are most accurate but are laborious. Selective media, such as the sodium hippurate–arginine–aesculin (HAA) medium, are simple to use but the results may require confirmation. An ELISA test is also available (25), and a commercial latex agglutination test (12) suitable for laboratory use is reported favorably in preliminary trials. The CAMP test, which utilizes the lytic phenomenon shown by Lancefield's group B streptococci in the presence of staphylococcal beta-toxin, is sufficiently accurate for the routine presumptive identification of *Str. agalactiae* in large-scale eradication schemes.

The critical judgment is that of deciding the point at which the quarter infection rate is so high that control or eradication measures are necessary. A decision can be made on the basis of the bulk milk cell count as an indicator of prevalence of mastitis, and on culture of the bulk milk sample to indicate that *Strep. agalactiae* is the important pathogen, but the technique is too inaccurate to be effective (24). There seems to be no alternative to carrying out cell counts and cultural examinations on milk samples from individual cows or quarters.

Necropsy findings

The gross and microscopic pathology of mastitis caused by *Str. agalactiae* is not of importance in the diagnosis of the disease and is not reported here, although detailed information is available (9).

Diagnosis

The diagnosis of mastitis has already been described and the identification of this particular form of the disease depends entirely on the isolation of *Str. agalactiae* from the milk. Differentiation from other types of acute and chronic mastitis is not possible clinically.

Treatment

Procaine penicillin G is universally used as a mammary infusion at a dose rate of 100 000 units. There seems to be advantage in using higher dose rates especially as they have the disadvantage of increasing penicillin residues in the milk (10). A moderate increase in efficiency is obtained by using procaine penicillin rather than crystalline penicillin and a significant increase can be obtained by the use of a slow-release base, particularly mineral oil and aluminum monostearate. Using 100 000 units of penicillin in a long-acting base the cure rate (95·5%) was significantly better than with quickacting preparations (83%). There is a place for both preparations (11), the short-acting being best in a contaminated environment when reinfection is likely, and the long-acting when a control program is in operation. To provide a broader spectrum of antibiotic efficiency penicillin is often combined with other drugs which are more effective against Gram-negative organisms. A mixture of penicillin (100 000 units) and neomycin sulfate (0·5g) is recommended.

The duration and frequency of treatment are subject to variation. On the understanding that it is necessary to maintain adequate milk levels for 72 hours, three infusions at intervals of 24 hours are recommended but dosing with two infusions 72 hours apart, or one infusion of 100 000 units in a base containing mineral oil and aluminum monostearate (13) give similar results. As a general rule clinical cases should be treated with three infusions and subclinical cases, particularly those detected by routine examination in a control program, with one infusion. If a combined infection with streptococci and staphylococci is encountered, four infusions of 100 000 units each, at 48-hour intervals, may be administered. Infusions of procaine penicillin give more prolonged levels in the milk than the crystalline salts but the proportion of cures effected is approximately the same for each.

Recovery, both clinically and bacteriologically, should be achieved in at least 90% of quarters if treatment has been efficient. In dry cows, one infusion is sufficient, milk levels of penicillin remaining high for 72 hours. Failure of penicillin to cure *Str. agalactiae* infections is encountered occasionally. On rare occasions a penicillin-resistant strain of streptococci is encountered, a mixed infection with bacteria which produce penicillinase, e.g. *E. coli*, *B. subtilis*, may inactivate the penicillin, and treatments administered after the morning milking in highly productive cows may not maintain an adequate milk level of penicillin for long enough if the morning and evening milkings are close together. Failure to respond to treatment may be countered as follows. Quarters treated previously with one infusion of penicillin G should be retreated with a two or three-infusion course of penicillin. In the absence of a laboratory diagnosis of drug sensitivity, quarters which do not respond to a three-infusion course of treatment with penicillin G should be treated with one of the tetracylines (0·6 g) or with spiramycin (0·25 g).

Penicillin can be administered parenterally and is effective against this form of mastitis but it is expensive as compared to intramammary infusions. An initial dose of 6 million units of procaine penicillin G injected intramuscularly, followed by 12 injections of three million units at 12-hour intervals, is an efficient treatment regimen (14) but lighter doses of three daily injections of 10 000 units/kg body weight are also claimed to be satisfactory (15). Benzathine penicillin administered parenterally has been only moderately effective when given at an initial dose level of 6 million units followed by two injections of 3 million units each at 24-hour intervals (16).

Other drugs used in the treatment of *Str. agalactiae* infections include the tetracyclines, which are as effective as penicillin and have the added advantage of a wider antibacterial spectrum, an obvious advantage when the type of infection is unknown. Neomycin (15) and chlorhexidine (Hibitane) are reported to be inferior to penicillin in the treatment of *Str. agalactiae* mastitis, while tylosin (17) and erythromycin (18) appear to have equal efficiency. A single treatment with 300 mg of erythromycin (as intramammary erythromycin cerate) is recommended as curing 100% of quarters infected with *Str. agalactiae* (19) but this result would need to be confirmed. Lincomycin (200 mg) combined with neomycin (286 mg) and administered twice at 12-hour intervals also has a good record (2).

Treatment of mastitis in other animal species can utilize the same drugs. Ewes and does can be treated locally with infusion tubes prepared for bovine use but sows are best treated parenterally.

Control

Eradication on a herd basis of mastitis caused by *Str. agalactiae* is an accepted procedure and has been undertaken on a large scale in some countries. The control measures as outlined elsewhere in this chapter are applicable to this disease and should be adopted in detail. If suitable hygienic barriers against infection can be introduced and if the infection can be eliminated from individual quarters by treatment, the disease is eradicable fairly simply and economically (10, 13).

In general it can be anticipated that about 80% of herds can be rid of infection within a year of commencing the program. In herds where the initial incidence of infection is very high, the reinfection rate may be too rapid to permit elimination of the infection by this means, and in these circumstances a general disinfection technique (20) has given good results.

As with any eradication program a high degree of vigilance is required to maintain a 'clean' status . This is particularly so with mastitis due to *Str. agalactiae*. Breakdowns are usually due to the introduction of infected animals, even heifers which have not yet calved (21), or the employment of milkers who carry infection with them.

There are many reports of breakdowns in herds in which the disease has been eradicated. The cause is always the introduction of an infected animal and the relaxation of hygienic precautions (22). With increasing awareness of the need for continuous prophylaxis such breakdowns should diminish greatly.

Vaccination against *Str. agalactiae* has been attempted and elicits a systemic hyperimmunity but no apparent intramammary resistance (23).

REFERENCES

(1) Commandeur, M. A. M. (1985) *Kiel. Milchwirtsch. Forschungsber*, *37*, 629.
(2) Milojevic, Z. et al. (1985) *Veterinarski, Glasnik*, *39*, 523.
(3) Greer, D. O. & Pearson, J. K. L. (1973) *Br. vet. J.*, *129*, 543.
(4) Pearson, J. K. et al. (1976) *Br. vet. J.*, *132*, 588.
(5) Murphy, J. M. & Stuart, O. M. (1955) *Cornell Vet.*, *45*, 262.
(6) Murphy, J. M. (1959) *Cornell Vet.*, *49*, 411.
(7) Pattison, I. H. (1958) *Vet. Rec.* *70*, 114.
(8) Howell, D. G. et al. (1954), *J. comp. Pathol.*, *64*, 335.
(9) Neave, F. K. et al. (1952) *J. dairy Res.*, *19*, 14.
(10) Roberts, S. J. et al. (1963) *J. Am. vet. med. Assoc.*, *143*, 1193.
(11) Sanderson, C. J. (1966) *Vet. Rec.*, *79*, 328.
(12) Daniel, R. C. W. & Barnum, D. H. (1986) *Am. J. vet. Res.*, *50*, 133.
(13) Frost, A. J. & Sanderson, C. J. (1965) *Aust. vet. J.*, *41*, 97.
(14) Murphy, J. M. & Stuart, O. M. (1954) *Cornell Vet.*, *44*, 139.
(15) Simon, J. et al. (1954) *J. Am. vet. med. Assoc.*, *124*, 89.
(16) Quadri, C. A. D. et al. (1959) *J. Am. vet. med. Assoc.*, *135*, 224.
(17) Barnes, L. E. & Hennessey, J. A. (1961) *J. Am. vet. med. Assoc.*, *139*, 548.
(18) Schultz, E. J. (1968) *J. Am. vet. med. Assoc.*, *152*, 376.
(19) Johnston, W. S. (1975) *Vet. Rec.*, *96*, 430.
(20) Stableforth, A. W. (1950) *Vet. Rec.*, *62*, 219.
(21) Hale, H. H. et al. (1961) *Cornell Vet.*, *51*, 200.
(22) Hassman, S. & Thieme, D. (1974) *Mh. VetMed.*, *29*, 94.
(23) Mackie, D. P. et al. (1983) *Vet. Rec.*, *112*, 472.
(24) Pearson, J. K. L. et al. (1979) *Br. vet. J.*, *135*, 119.
(25) Logan, E. F. et al. (1982) *Vet. Rec.*, *110*, 247.

Mastitis caused by miscellaneous streptococci

Mastitis caused by these streptococci assumes increased importance in dairy herds where infection with *Str. agalactiae* has been greatly reduced or eliminated.

Etiology

Cattle

Streptococcus dysgalactiae and *Str. uberis* are the common infections. Uncommon ones include streptococci of Lancefield's group O, *Str. zooepidemicus, Str. viridans* (10), *Streptococcus* sp., group G (3), *Str. pyogenes* and *Str. pneumoniae*. None of these bacteria is a common inhabitant of the bovine udder and infections in other species, including humans, e.g. group B-streptococci (15) may provide a reservoir.

Other species

These infections are recorded most commonly in cattle, but sporadic cases occur in sows, and female goats can be infected experimentally with *Str. agalactiae. Str. zooepidemicus* is recorded as a cause of chronic suppurative mastitis in female goats (2). *Str. pyogenes* is recorded as a cause of mastitis in mares (7).

Epidemiology

Streptococcus dysgalactiae and *Str. uberis* are the only specific bovine parasites in this group and there appears to be a definite causal relationship between infection and teat injuries and bad milking technique and housing (1). *Str. uberis* is a common inhabitant of the skin, lips and tonsils of cows in infected herds, the skin of the belly often carrying the largest population (8). Some cows become permanently colonized with *Str. uberis* and may pass very large numbers of the organism in the feces. This observation is also linked with the finding of large numbers of the organism in straw bedding on farms where this form of mastitis persists (9). Infection of the mammary gland appears to be secondary to infection of the skin and both appear to be more prevalent during the cool months of the year (4).

None of the other bacteria are common residents of the bovine udder and some are suspected of originating in the respiratory tracts of human attendants. *Str. pneumoniae* and *Str. pyogenes* infections are known to originate in this way, and in spite of this apparently chance transmission serious outbreaks are recorded, with 50% of a herd becoming affected. The disease resembles mastitis caused by *Str. agalactiae*, and losses from it are due to loss of production, not to fatalities. *Streptococcus uberis* is the most common cause of clinical mastitis occurring during the dry period (12), and the chances of this happening during the dry period is greater during the month before parturition (13), but most clinical cases occur during the first part of lactation.

Pathogenesis

Infections with *Str. dysgalactiae*, artificially induced in goats, are indistinguishable from mastitis caused by *Str. agalactiae* and the pathogenesis is probably similar in all streptococcal mastitides.

Clinical findings

In bovine mastitis caused by *Str. dysgalactiae*, *Str. uberis*, *Str. viridans*, and streptococci of Lancefield's group O the syndrome is usually acute, with severe swelling of the quarter and abnormality of the milk, and occasional cases show a moderate systemic reaction. Mastitis caused by *Str. zooepidemicus* is usually subacute or chronic, and that caused by *Str. pneumoniae* is peracute with a high fever in most cases but can result in chronic disease (5). In the mare there may be severe local pain and moderate systemic signs.

Diagnosis

There are no significant differences between the clinicopathological and necropsy findings in mastitis caused by these streptococci and those in mastitis caused by *Str. agalactiae. Streptococcus uberis* mastitis in dry cows may be mistaken for mastitis caused by *Actinomyces (Corynebacterium) pyogenes*. Diagnosis depends on cultural examination of the milk.

Treatment

Mastitis caused by *Str. dysgalactiae* and *Str. uberis* responds well to penicillin, erythromycin or tetracyclines but reinfection may occur quickly if the contributory causes are not corrected. Infections with *Str. zooepidemicus* do not respond well to treatment with penicillin. Mastitis caused by *Str. pneumoniae* responds well to local treatment with penicillin in large doses (300 000 units per infusion) but complete loss of function results in quarters allowed to go without treatment for any length of time. All cases of mastitis caused by this organism should receive parenteral treatment with penicillin (6).

Control

Although general control measures as set out later in this chapter are recommended for all forms of mastitis the results in the control of *Str. uberis* are poor (11) probably because infection occurs at times other than during milking. A selective-therapy dry cow program may result in an increase in the infection rate and treatment of all dry cows seems to be necessary (14). Once the infection has become established in a herd, sporadic cases are likely to occur in spite of good hygienic precautions. Because of the failure of the general control program to restrain the spread of the infection it is more than usually necessary to treat infected quarters vigorously. In herds where the disease is a problem in dry cows a second dry period treatment is recommended 3–4 weeks after drying off. Experimental vaccination techniques have been unsuccessful.

REVIEW LITERATURE

Bramley, A. J. (1984) *Streptococcus uberis* udder infection; a major barrier to reducing mastitis incidence. *Br. vet. J.*, *140*, 328.

REFERENCES

(1) Cullen. G. A. (1969) *Vet. Bull.*, *39*, 155.
(2) Nesbakken, T. (1975) *Norsk VetTidsskr.*, *87*, 188.
(3) Watts, J. L. et al. (1984) *Vet. Microbiol.*, *9*, 571.
(4) Cullen, G. A. & Little, T. W. A. (1969) *Vet. Rec.*, *85*, 115.
(5) Romer, O. (1962) *Pneumococcus Infections of Animals.* Copenhagen: Mortensen.
(6) Smith, H. W. & Stables, J. W. (1958) *Vet. Rec.*, *70*, 986.
(7) Reese, G. L. & Lock, T. F. (1978) *J. Am. vet. med. Assoc.*, *173*, 83.
(8) Bramley, A. J. et al. (1979) *Br. vet. J.*, *135*, 262.
(9) Bramley, A. J. (1982) *J. dairy Res.* *49*, 369, 375.
(10) Groothuis, D. G. (1981) *Tidschr. Diergeeneeskd.*, *106*, 367.
(11) King. J. S. (1981) *Br. vet. J.*, *137*, 160.
(12) Francis, P. G. et al. (1986) *Vet. Rec.*, *118*, 549.
(13) Smith, K. L. et al. (1985) *J. dairy Sci.*, *68*, 1531.
(14) Robinson, T. C. et al. (1985) *Br. vet. J.*, *141*, 635.
(15) Nielsen, L. (1987) *Dansk Vet. Tidskr.*, *70*, 154.

Mastitis caused by *Staphylococcus aureus*

Mastitis caused by *Staph. aureus* occurs in cattle, sheep, goats and pigs. In the former it may be a peracute or an acute or a chronic disease.

Etiology

Hemolytic, coagulase-positive *Staph. aureus* is the usual cause, although it may be difficult to demonstrate the presence of the organism in peracute cases especially when necrotic tissue is invaded by *E. coli* and *Clostridium* spp. The beta-toxin, or a combination of alpha-toxins and beta-toxins, is produced by most pathogenic strains isolated from cattle but its pathogenic significance is doubtful. The mechanisms of virulence in staphylococcal infections generally appear to be related to their capacity to invade tissues rather than to excrete substances. Coagulase is an exception but it appears to assist the invasion of tissues (1).

Epidemiology

Staphylococcal mastitis in cattle assumes equal importance with mastitis caused by *Str. agalactiae* or other miscellaneous streptococci in most surveys of the disease. As in other forms of mastitis, loss of production is the major cause of economic loss, but in some herds there may be fairly heavy death losses. Response to treatment is comparatively poor and satisfactory methods for the eradication of staphylococcal mastitis from infected herds have yet to be devised. The pressure of *Staph. aureus* in market milk may be considered to present a degree of risk to the consumer.

In sheep the disease can be a serious problem because the morbidity rate may be as high as 20%; the mortality rate varies between 25 and 50% and affected quarters in surviving ewes are usually destroyed. The disease can be a very important one in those countries in which ewes' milk is a staple article of diet. Sporadic cases occur in sows.

Staphylococcal antibodies are found in the blood of infected cows but they appear to afford little protection against mastitis due to these bacteria. This may be due to the low titer of the antibodies in the milk. Antibody titers in the serum rise with age and after an attack of mastitis. Experimental mastitis caused by *Staph. aureus* causes a significant reduction in milk yield and rate of milking (3).

Non-hemolytic, coagulase-negative staphylococci, especially *Staph. epidermidis* and micrococci, have in general been disregarded as mammary pathogens, but because of the intense investigation of staphylococcal mastitis they have come under closer scrutiny (5). It does appear that although these bacteria are capable of causing microscopic lesions, and in some cases increased leukocyte counts in the milk, they are not nearly as pathogenic as hemolytic staphylococci (6). The tissue reaction is usually so mild that the CMT is negative. If the infection is capable of causing loss of productivity, current standards for the diagnosis of mastitis will need to be reassessed. They appear to have the advantage that they resist colonization of the teat duct and teat skin by coagulase-positive staphylococci (6).

All the evidence suggests that in cattle this form of mastitis is infectious, the main source of the infection being the quarter infected with the organism, and the method of spread being by infected hands and teat cups. Although staphylococci can multiply on the surface of the skin and provide a source of infection for the udder, the cutaneous lesions are usually infected originally from the udder (7). There is some doubt about the age susceptibility to this type of mastitis in cattle but there does not seem to be an increase in susceptibility with advancing age as there is in *Str. agalactiae* mastitis, the disease tending to reach a peak in the younger age groups (8). In sows the infection appears to gain entrance most commonly through cutaneous wounds.

Pathogenesis

Although the disease can be reproduced experimentally by the injection of *Staph. aureus* organisms into the udder of cattle and sheep, there is considerable variation in the type of mastitis produced. This does not seem to be due to differences in virulence of the strains used, although strain variations do occur (9), but it may be related to the size of the inoculum used or more probably the lactational status of the udder at the time of infection. Infection during early lactation often results in the appearance of the peracute form, with gangrene of the udder due to the acute necrotizing action of the alpha-toxin. During the later stages of lactation or during the dry period new infections are not usually accompanied by a systemic reaction but result in the chronic or acute forms. Chronic staphylococcal mastitis in cows has been converted to the peracute, gangrenous form by the experimental production of systemic neutropenia (11).

The pathogenesis of acute and chronic staphylococcal mastitis in the cow is the same, the variation occurring only in degree of involvement of mammary tissue. In the chronic form there are less foci of inflammation and the reaction is milder. In both forms each focus commences with an acute stage characterized by proliferation of the bacteria in the collecting ducts and, to a lesser extent, in the alveoli. In acute mastitis the small ducts are quickly blocked by fibrin clots leading to more severe involvement of the obstructed area. In chronic mastitis the inflammation is restricted to the epithelium of the ducts. The inflammation subsides within a few days and is replaced by connective tissue proliferations around the ducts, leading to their blockage and atrophy of the drained area (10).

In the experimentally produced disease in goats the pathogenesis is very similar except that there is a marked tendency for the staphylococci to invade and persist in foci in the interacinar tissue (12). In some cases abscesses develop and botryomycosis of the udder, in which granulomata develop containing Gram-positive cocci in an amorphous eosinophilic mass, is also seen. In the gangrenous form the death of tissue is precipitated by thrombosis of veins causing local edema and congestion of the udder. Staphylococci are the only bacteria which commonly cause this reaction in the udder of the cow, and the resulting toxemia is due to bacterial toxins and tissue destruction. Staphylococcal gangrenous mastitis in ewes is identical to that in cattle.

Clinical findings

In cows the peracute form is more dramatic, but the most important losses are caused by the *chronic form*. Although 50% of cattle in a herd may be affected by the latter, only a few may show sufficient signs to be recognized by the average dairyman. Many cases are characterized by a slowly developing induration and atrophy with the occasional appearance of clots in the milk or wateriness of the first streams. The cell count of the milk is increased but, unless strip cup or indirect tests and palpation of the udder are carried out regularly, the disease may go unnoticed until much of the functional capacity of the gland is lost. The infection can persist and the disease progress slowly over a period of many months.

Acute staphylococcal mastitis occurs most commonly in early lactation. There is severe swelling of the gland and the milk is purulent or contains many thick clots. Extensive fibrosis and severe loss of function always result.

The peracute form occurs usually in the first few days after calving and is highly fatal. There is a severe systemic reaction with elevation of the temperature to 41–42°C (106–107°F), rapid heart rate (100–120/min), complete anorexia, profound depression, absence of ruminal movements, and muscular weakness, often to the point of recumbency. The onset of the systemic and local reactions is sudden. The cow may be normal at one milking and recumbent and comatose at the next. The affected quarter is grossly swollen, hard and sore to touch, and causes severe lameness on the affected side. Gangrene is a constant development and may be evident very early. A bluish discoloration may develop and this may eventually spread to involve the floor of the udder and the whole or part of the teat, but may be restricted to patches on the sides and floor of the udder. Within 24 hours the gangrenous areas become black and ooze serum and may be accompanied by subcutaneous emphysema and the formation of blisters. The secretion is reduced to a small amount of bloodstained serous fluid without odor, clots or flakes. Unaffected quarters in the same cow are often swollen, and there may be extensive subcutaneous edema in front of the udder caused by thrombosis of the mammary veins. Toxemia is profound and death usually occurs if early, appropriate treatment is not provided. Even with early treatment the quarter is invariably lost and the gangrenous areas slough. Separation begins after 6–7 days, but without interference the gangrenous part may remain attached for weeks. After separation, pus drains from the site for many more weeks before healing finally occurs.

Ewes

Staphylococcal mastitis in ewes is clinically identical with the peracute form in cattle and the edema and gangrene often spread along the belly as far as the front legs.

Goat does

The disease is clinically identical with peracute staphylococcal mastitis of cows (22).

Pigs

The disease in sows is always chronic and is characterized by the presence of large, fibrous nodules in the gland and the discharge through sinuses of thin pus, containing granules.

Clinical pathology

The laboratory diagnosis of staphylococcal mastitis has been made much easier by the observation that pathogenic staphylococci grown on sheep or cow blood-agar plates produce alpha-hemolysis, beta-hemolysis or alpha–beta-hemolysis. Such bacteria are always coagulase-positive and produce alpha-toxins and beta-toxins of high potency. Bacterial counts of more than 200/ml are commonly used as a criterion for a positive diagnosis of infection and leukocyte counts of more than 500 000/ml of milk are usually considered to indicate the presence of inflammation. The CMT, although not specific to any causative agent, is of great value in attracting attention to a chronically infected quarter which may show no clinical abnormality.

Necropsy findings

Necropsy examinations are not often carried out on mastitis cases except where an animal dies of acute toxemia. In acute mastitis there is necrosis of parenchymal epithelium and many foci of epithelial erosions and ulcerations in the ductal system. Neutrophils accumulate in large numbers on and below the epithelium and in the secretion (10). In peracute staphylococcal mastitis, the affected quarter is grossly swollen, may contain bloodstained milk in the upper part of the udder but only serosanguineous fluid in the ventral part. There is extreme vascular engorgement and swelling, and hemorrhage of the mammary lymph nodes. Bacteria are not isolated from the bloodstream or tissues other than the mammary tissue or regional lymph nodes. Histologically there is severe coagulation necrosis and thrombosis of veins.

Diagnosis

Because of the occurrence of the peracute form in the first few days after parturition, the intense depression and inability to rise, the owner may conclude that the cow or ewe has parturient paresis. The heart rate is much faster than in parturient paresis and a cursory examination of the udder will indicate the true source of the trouble. Other bacterial types of mastitis, particularly *E. coli* and *Actinomyces (Corynebacterium) pyogenes*, may cause severe systemic reactions but gangrene of the quarter does not occur. Coliform mastitis is a much commoner cause of death than staphylococcal mastitis (14). The chronic and acute forms are indistinguishable clinically from many other bacterial types of mastitis and bacteriological examination is necessary for identification.

In sheep there is a strong similarity between this form of mastitis and that caused by *Pasteurella haemolytica*. They are both peracute, gangrenous infections. In sows the disease is chronic and has to be differentiated from the granulomatous lesions of the ventral abdominal wall caused by *Actinomyces* spp.

Treatment

Although most staphylococci isolated from quarters affected with mastitis are sensitive to penicillin and tetracyclines *in vitro*, the results of treatment with these drugs in infected quarters are often disappointing. The poor results are probably due to the inaccessibility of the bacteria in the interacinar tissue (26) or obstructed ducts and alveoli. Resistant strains of staphylococci appear to be increasing but their incidence varies from 70 to 100% (13).

Because of the increasing incidence of staphylococcal mastitis, and the high proportion of bacteria which are resistant to penicillin and streptomycin, considerable work has been directed to finding a satisfactory program of treatment for chronic and acute cases in lactating cows. Novobiocin (250 mg per infusion for three infusions) or sodium cloxacillin (0·2–0·6 g in a slow-release base per infusion for three infusions at 12-hour or 48-hour intervals) appear to be most effective and in early cases can be expected to achieve cure rates of 50–80% (17, 18). A single treatment with 250 000 units of benzathine penicillin plus 125 mg of streptomycin in a longacting base gives a 55% cure rate (19).

The following treatment programs, all of three infusions at 24-hour intervals, appear to be about 60–80% effective in lactating cows:

Tetracyclines (400 mg), penicillin–streptomycin combination (100 000 units—250 mg), penicillin–nitrofurazone combination (100 000 units—150 mg), penicillin–tylosin combination (100 000 units—240 mg), furaltadone (500 mg), erythromycin (300–600 mg), spiramycin (250 mg).

Because of the increasing availability of laboratory services the final choice of the antibiotic to be used can often be decided on a drug sensitivity test. One of the major problems in mastitis control is the variation in response to treatment or control between herds. Examination of this problem with respect to *Staph. aureus* shows that this infection is less likely to respond when it occurs in an older cow, when the cow has several infected quarters and in cows treated in early lactation and so on. A high success rate can be achieved by using higher than normal doses of antibiotic by intramammary infusion, e.g. 1·22 g of spiramycin adipate (17), but the withholding time is significantly prolonged.

It has become a common practice to leave chronic cases until they are dried off before attempting to eliminate the infection. Milk need not be discarded and results are always better in non-lactating quarters. All of the above preparations can be used provided they are combined with slow-release bases and can be expected to achieve about 80% of cures. The material is infused either early or late in the dry period and left *in situ*. The treatment of chronic cases by parenteral injection is unlikely to achieve popularity but has been used in valuable animals that do not respond to intramammary infusion.

Early parenteral treatment of peracute cases with adequate doses of sulfonamides or penicillin or a tetracycline will save the lives of most animals. When penicillin is used the initial intramuscular injection should be supported by an intravenous injection of crystalline penicillin, and subsequent intramuscular injections should aim at maintaining the highest possible blood level of the drug over a 4–6 day period. To achieve this tamethicillin or penthemate hydriodide are preferred (20). Intramammary infusions or intraparenchymal injections appear to be of little value in such cases because of failure of the drugs to diffuse into the gland. Transient improvement may follow the injection of large doses of antihistamine drugs, and their administration may help to combat the effects of toxemia. The administration of large quantities of electrolyte solutions is also recommended. Frequent massage and stripping exert a beneficial effect by aiding drainage of the quarter; the administration of pitressin gives little effect. Total amputation of the quarter or ligation of the mammary vessels is often indicated, but the animal may be a poor surgical risk because of toxemia. Amputation of the teat is frequently practiced to encourage drainage but multiple incision of the gland has little beneficial effect.

Control

Because of the relatively poor results obtained in the treatment of staphylococcal mastitis, any attempt at control must depend heavily on effective methods of preventing the transmission of infection from cow to cow. Hygiene in the milking shed attains great importance, especially as the organism is capable of such persistence in the environment, and considerable attention is being devoted to possible production of a suitable method of vaccination. Eradication is not possible and only control programs aimed at restraining the infection rate should be instituted.

Until recent years satisfactory control of staphylococcal mastitis was impossible. At the present time the quarter infection rate can be rapidly and profitably reduced from the average level of 30% to 10% or less. The measures set down for control of bovine mastitis (p. 537) must be intensively applied (4) and the disinfection of hands or use of rubber gloves provides additional advantages. The program helps to eliminate infected quarters and reduces the new infection rate by 50–65% compared to controls.

The inconclusive nature of the results of experimental work on vaccines against staphylococcal mastitis (15) is not reflected by the claims of the manufacturers of commercial vaccines nor by the very large quantities of their products used in dairy cows. Antibodies and antitoxins present in the serum of vaccinated cows do not appear in the milk, other than in the colostrum or during drying off, unless the mammary epithelium is damaged. Thus any parenteral vaccine is unlikely to be completely effective, although it could reduce the severity of an attack—a common finding in field practice (21). A combination of vaccination and an intramammary polyethylene retention device is also ineffective as a prophylactic procedure (23, 24). Injections of levamisole, used to enhance immunity at drying-off, have not had any preventive action in cows (2).

The disease in ewes is probably spread from infected bedding grounds, the infection gaining entry through teat injuries caused by sucking lambs. It is possible that vaccination could be an effective method of control. A bacterin-toxoid has proved moderately effective in reducing the incidence of the disease. Two injections of the vaccine were necessary (16). Prophylactic infusion of each half of the udder within a few days of weaning, using half of a tube of dry cow treatment of penicillin and streptomycin, has also given good results (25). The frequent changing of pasture areas and culling of affected ewes should also help to control the spread of infection.

REVIEW LITERATURE

Buddle, B. M., Cooper, M. G. (1978) Aspects of the epidemiology of bovine staphylococcal mastitis. *NZ vet. J.*, *26*, 296.

REFERENCES

(1) Anderson, J. C. (1976) *Br. vet. J.*, *132*, 229.
(2) Buddle, B. M. & Pulford, H. D. (1985) *NZ vet. J.*, *33*, 177.
(3) Prasad, L. B. M. & Newbould, F. H. S. (1968) *Can. vet. J.*, *9*, 170.
(4) Ziv, G. & Sompolinsky, D. (1976) *Res. vet. Sci.*, *20*, 281, 288.
(5) Brown, R. W. (1973) *Cornell Vet.*, *63*, 630.
(6) Linde, C. et al. (1975) *Acta vet. Scand.*, *16*, 146.
(7) Stableforth, A. W. (1953) *Vet. Rec.*, *65*, 709.
(8) Edwards, S. J. (1958) *Vet. Rec.*, *70*, 139.
(9) Schalm, O. W. (1944) *Vet. Med.*, *39*, 279.
(10) Gudding, R. et al. (1984) *Am. J. vet. Res.*, *45*, 2525.
(11) Schalm, O. W. et al. (1976) *Am. J. vet. Res.*, *37*, 885.
(12) Derbyshire, J. B. (1958) *J. com. Pathol.*, *68*, 449.
(13) Sanderson, C. J. (1965) *Aust. vet. J.*, *42*, 47.
(14) Hazlett, M. J. et al. (1984) *Can. J. comp. Med.*, *48*, 125.
(15) Watson, D. L. (1984) *J. dairy Sci.*, *67*, 2608.
(16) Plommet, M. & Bezard, G. (1974) *Ann. rech. vét.*, *5*, 29.
(17) Ziv, G. & Storper, M. (1984) *Schweiz. Arch. Tierheilkd.*, *126*, 479.
(18) Davis, W. T. et al. (1975) *J. dairy Sci.*, *58*, 1822.
(19) Newbould, F. H. S. (1974) *Can. J. comp. Med.*, *38*, 411.
(20) Ziv, G. & Storper, M. (1985) *J. vet. Pharmocol. Therap.*, *8*, 276.
(21) Yoshida, K. et al. (1984) *J. dairy Sci.*, *67*, 620.
(22) Sasshofer, K. & Schlerka, G. (1984) *Prakt. Tierärztl.*, *65*, 157.
(23) Poutrel, B. et al. (1983) *Ann. réch vét.*, *14*, 13.
(24) Schultze, W. D. & Paape, M. J. (1984) *Am. J. vet. Res.*, *45*, 420.
(25) Hendy, P. G. et al. (1981) *Vet. Res.*, *109*, 56.
(26) Craven, N. & Anderson, J. C. (1984) *J. dairy Res.*, *51*, 513.

Mastitis caused by *Corynebacterium* spp.

Sporadic cases of mastitis caused by *Actinomyces (Corynebacterium) pyogenes* occur but its major importance is in relation to endemic 'summer mastitis' of cattle.

Etiology

Actinomyces (Corynebacterium) pyogenes can cause sporadic cases of suppurative mastitis and successful transmissions have been effected (6), but the specific cause of 'summer mastitis' is not this bacterium alone. *Peptococcus indolicus*, *Streptococcus dysgalactiae*, *Bacillus melaninogenicus*, and other Bacterioidaceae and *Micrococcus* spp. are also found and *Actinomyces (Corynebacterium) pyogenes* is seldom found in pure culture (1). All of these bacteria are capable of causing suppurative mastitis when infused into the udder (19). *Cor. bovis* is a common inhabitant of the bovine udder and is usually considered to be nonpathogenic. It selectively colonizes the epithelium of the teat canal and causes a small rise in the milk cell count. It is commonly held that its presence in a quarter reduces the chances of infection by pathogens, but the evidence for this view is inconclusive (3, 20) and the effect may be different for different pathogens (10). The level of infection is low in herds where teat dipping and dry period treatment are practiced. *Cor. ulcerans* is an uncommon cause of a subacute mastitis (4).

Epidemiology

Bovine mastitis caused by *Actinomyces (Corynebacterium) pyogenes* occurs only sporadically and is most common in dry cows or pregnant heifers, although lactating cows may also be affected. A high prevalence is also recorded in heifer calves as young as 5 months (7). In the United Kingdom, Japan (5), the United States and Europe there is a much higher incidence of suppurative 'summer mastitis' during the summer months when non-lactating females are left at pasture and not kept under close observation. The incidence is much higher in wet summers and on heavily wooded and low lying farms when the fly population is high (5). The infection rate of *Actinomyces (Corynebacterium) pyogenes* in udders is much less in housed cattle than in the same cattle at pasture. In Australia the disease occurs mostly in lactating cows and usually after injury or the development of black spot on the teat (17). The disease is a serious one in that the mortality rate without adequate treatment is probably about 50% and the affected quarters of surviving cows are always totally destroyed.

The method of spread is uncertain in sporadic cases but insects, especially biting ones such as *Hydrotoea irritans*, appear to play an important role in outbreaks of 'summer mastitis' (13, 16). The prevalence of the disease is related to the peaks of the fly populations and the prevailing climate, especially the wind force and direction (14).

Pathogenesis

It is suggested that the infection is carried from udder to udder by flies and that massive invasion of the mammary tissue occurs via the teat canal. The greater part of the gland is affected at the first attack causing a severe systemic reaction and loss of function of the entire quarter. The disease has been produced experimentally in goats with udder lesions being typical of acute suppurative mastitis (8). Non-lactating goats developed a severe mastitis, lactating animals only a moderate one. A diffuse suppurative mastitis has also been produced experimentally in sheep (9).

Clinical findings

Corynebacterial mastitis is always peracute with a severe systemic reaction, including fever (40–41°C, 105–106°F), rapid heart rate, complete anorexia, severe depression and weakness. Abortion may occur during this stage. The quarter is very hard, swollen and sore and the secretion is watery and later purulent, with a typical, putrid odor. If the cow survives the severe toxemia, the quarter becomes extremely indurated and abscesses develop, later rupturing through the floor of the udder, commonly at the base of the teat. These may be presented as being chronic ones but they are usually residual after an acute episode. True gangrene, such as occurs in staphylococcal mastitis, rarely if ever occurs in uncomplicated infections with *Actinomyces (Corynebacterium) pyogenes* but quarters may be so severely affected that sloughing occurs. The function of the quarter is permanently lost and cows which have calved recently may go completely dry. Severe thelitis with obstruction of the teat is a common sequel. Partial or complete obstruction of the teat and damage to the teat cistern can also occur independently of an acute attack of mastitis. Fetal growth retardation is thought to be a feature of calves born to cows affected by summer mastitis during pregnancy (2).

Clinical pathology

Isolation of the organism and determination of its sensitivity to antibacterial drugs is the only special examination required.

Necropsy findings

Details of the pathology of the disease are not available.

Diagnosis

The seasonal incidence of the disease in some areas, the acute inflammation of the quarter, the suppurative nature and putrid odor of the milk, the development of abscesses and the severe systemic reaction makes this form of mastitis one of the easiest to diagnose clinically in cattle.

Treatment

Although the organism is usually susceptible to penicillin *in vitro*, response to treatment with this drug is poor. In peracute cases parenteral treatment with sodium sulfadimidine or one of the tetracyclines is preferable and should be accompanied by repeated stripping of the quarter. Broad-spectrum antibiotics are usually given by intramammary infusion but the quarter is almost always rendered functionless. Clearing of proteinaceous debris from the affected quarter may be aided by the intramammary application of proteolytic enzymes but the outcome as far as the quarter is concerned is unlikely to be much altered. Treatment with *Actinomyces (Corynebacterium) pyogenes* antiserum in the acute stages and toxoid in the later, chronic, suppurative stage has been used but with little effect. Even with intensive therapy at least 50% of quarters are rendered useless and many of those which respond are greatly reduced in productivity.

Control

The question of control of this form of mastitis centers largely on 'summer mastitis'. Many prophylactic measures, including infusion of the quarter when the cow is dried off, sealing the teat ends with collodion and vaccination with toxoid, have been tried but with inconclusive results. The most favored technique is intramammary infusion with a dry cow preparation (e.g. cloxacillin 500 mg and ampicillin 250 mg in a long-acting base) at 3-week intervals. Less frequent administration offers less protection (12). Repeated spraying of the udder, for example, automatically at watering points, with a contact insecticide (15) is also most helpful. An alternative intramammary infusion procedure is to use cefalonium at 4-weekly intervals (11). An alternative to spraying is the use of insecticide-impregnated eartags (18). Careful, daily examination of dry cows during the summer may enable affected quarters to be identified and treated at an early stage and thus limit the spread of infection.

REVIEW LITERATURE

Sol, J. (1984) Control methods in summer mastitis: the importance of fly control. *Proc. 13th World Cong. Dis. Cattle, Durban, South Africa, Vol. 1*, pp. 236–242.

Yeoman, G. H. & Warren, B. C. (1984) Summer mastitis. *Br. vet. J.*, *140*, 232–243.

REFERENCES

(1) Tolle, A. et al. (1983) *Tierarztl. Wochenschr.*, *90*, 256.
(2) Richardson, C. et al. (1982) *Proc. 12th World Cong. Dis. Cattle, Vol. 11*, p. 1063.
(3) Brooks, B. W. et al. (1983) *Can. J. comp. Med.*, *47*, 73.
(4) Higgs, T. M. et al. (1967) *Vet. Rec.*, *81*, 34.
(5) Hamana, K. et al. (1978) *Bull. Faculty Agric., Miyazaki Univ.*, *25*, 307, 315, 329.
(6) Tarry, D. W. et al. (1978) *Vet. Rec.*, *102*, 91.
(7) Bramley. A. J. et al. (1977) *Vet. Rec.*, *100*, 464.
(8) Jain, N. C. & Sharma, G. L. (1964) *Ind. vet. J.*, *41*, 379, 516 and *42*, 231.

(9) El Etreby, M. F. & Abdel-Hamid, Y. M. (1970) *Pathol. vet.*, 7, 246.
(10) Pankey, J. W. et al. (1985) *J. dairy Sci.* 68, 2684.
(11) Sol, J. & Vardy, A. (1982) *Tijdschr. Diergeneeskd.*, *107*, 466.
(12) Egan, J. (1986) *Irish J. agric. Res.*, *25*, 173.
(13) Brummerstedt, E. & Nielsen, S. A. (1986) *Acta vet. Scand.*, *27*, 138.
(14) Olesen, J. E. et al. (1985) *Acta vet. Scand.*, *26*, 466.
(15) Bertels, G. & Robijns, J. M. (1983) *Vlaams Diergeneeskd. Tijdschr.*, *52*, 77.
(16) Bramley, A. J. et al. (1985) *Br. vet. J.*, *141*, 618.
(17) Slee, K. J. & McOrist, S. (1985) *Aust. vet. J.*, *62*, 63.
(18) Ron, I. & Bakken, G. (1986) *Norsk VetTiddskr.*, *98*, 445.
(19) Preez, J. H. du et al. (1982) *J. S. Afr. vet. Assoc.*, *53*, 157.
(20) Honkanen-Buzalski, T. et al. (1984) *J. dairy Res.*, *51*, 371 & 379.

Mastitis caused by *Escherichia coli, Klebsiella* spp. and *Enterobacter aerogenes* (Environmental mastitis)

The term coliform mastitis is used here to include the mastitides in cattle caused by *E. coli*, *Klebsiella* spp. and *Enterobacter aerogenes*. Each of these can cause a peracute mastitis, sometimes in outbreak form, resulting in large economic losses. The term environmental mastitis is used to mean mastitis caused by bacteria which are transferred from the environment to the cow rather than from other infected quarters.

The prevalence of coliform mastitis has increased considerably in recent years and is a cause for concern in the dairy industry and among dairy practitioners.

Etiology

Many different serotypes of *E. coli* (1), numerous capsular types of *Klebsiella pneumoniae* (2) and *Enterobacter aerogenes* are responsible for coliform mastitis in cattle (3). *E. coli* isolated from the milk of cows with acute mastitis cannot be distinguished as a specific pathogenic group on the basis of biochemical and serological test reactions (1). In one study, out of 290 *E. coli* isolates, there were 63 O-serogroups which indicates that coliform mastitis is not caused by a limited number of specific pathogenic strains (3). The incidence of antibiotic resistance was also low presumably because the organisms are opportunists originating from the alimentary tract from which antibiotic-resistant *E. coli* are rarely found in adults.

Coliform mastitis has been reported worldwide and is most common in dairy cattle which are housed during the winter months or kept in total confinement in a dry lot (5). The disease is uncommon in dairy cattle which are continuously in pasture but it has been reported on pastured dairy cattle in New Zealand (9).

Epidemiology

The incidence of both intramammary infection and clinical mastitis due to coliform bacteria has increased, particularly in dairy herds in which there has been a marked reduction in the incidence of mastitis due to streptococci and staphylococci as a result of an effective mastitis control program. Compared to other forms of mastitis, coliform infections are relatively uncommon and in data based on herd surveys, the percentage of quarters infected with these organisms is low.

In the United Kingdom, about 0·2% of quarters of cows may be infected at any one time (4) and surveillance of a dairy herd in total confinement in the United States indicated that infection with coliform bacteria by either day of lactation or day of the year never exceeded 3·5 % of quarters, and this maximum was reached on the day of calving (5). Percent quarters infected by day of the year varied from less than 1 to a maximum of 3 (5). However, in herds with a problem, up to 8% of cows have been infected with coliform bacteria and 80% of the cases of clinical mastitis were due to coliform. The number of clinical cases of coliform mastitis varies from 3 to 32 per 100 cows per year but the average incidence in dairy herds can be as low as 6–8 per 100 cows per year (4). It has been suggested that the incidence of coliform mastitis is higher in high-yielding cows but the effect may be due to increasing age rather than milk yield alone (7). Coliform mastitis is the most common cause of fatal mastitis (6). The case fatality rate from peracute coliform mastitis is commonly high and may reach 80% in spite of intensive therapy.

The disease occurs most commonly within a few days of calving and in herds which concentrate calvings over a short period. Outbreaks of the disease can occur in which up to 25% of recently calved cows become affected within a few weeks. Cows affected with the downer cow syndrome following parturient paresis, or recently calved cows which are clinically recumbent for any reason, are susceptible to coliform mastitis because of the gross contamination of the udder and teats with feces and bedding.

All of the environmental components which come in contact with the udder of the cow are considered potential sources of the organisms. The coliform bacteria are considered as opportunists, and contamination of the skin of the udder and teats probably occurs primarily between milkings when the cow is in contact with contaminated bedding rather than at the time of the milking (43). Feces, which commonly provide the source of *E. coli*, can contaminate the perineum and the udder directly or indirectly through bedding, calving stalls, dry lot grounds, udder wash water, udder wash sponges and cloth rags, teat cups and milkers' hands (43). Cows with chronic coliform mastitis also provide an important source of the organism and direct transmission probably occurs through the milking machine (43). Inadequate drying of the base of the udder and the teats after washing them prior to milking can lead to a drainage of coliform-contaminated water down into the teat cups and subsequent infection.

Sawdust and shavings used as bedding, which are contaminated and harboring *E. coli*, and particularly *Klebsiella pneumoniae*, are considered to play a major role in the epidemiology of coliform mastitis (10). Cows bedded on sawdust had the largest teat end population of total coliforms and klebsiellae; those bedded on shavings had an intermediate number and those on straw had the least (11). Experimentally, the incubation of bedding samples at 30–44°C (86–111°F) resulted in an increase in the coliform count; at 22°C (71° F) the count was maintained, and at 50°C (122° F) the organisms were killed (12). Wet bedding, particularly sawdust and shavings, promote the growth of coliform bacteria, especially *Klebsiella* spp. (27).

The relationship between the bedding populations of Enterobacteriaceae was studied over a 12-month period in a dairy herd (40). The analyses revealed that rainfall bedding populations of *E. coli* and coliform mastitis incidence were statistically independent, while there was a strong association between rainfall and *Klebsiella pneumoniae* bedding populations and the incidence of *K. pneumoniae* mastitis (40). The lack of an association between bedding population of *E. coli* and coliform mastitis along with the observation that cows are most susceptible immediately after parturition suggest that the ability of the bacteria to penetrate the streak canal may be a factor of resistance in the cow and not a characteristic of the organism. Also, it appears that the cow in early lactation is not as susceptible to *K. pneumoniae* as to *E. coli*.

The ability of several different bedding materials to support the growth of environmental pathogens has been outlined under controlled conditions (41). Bedding materials vary in their ability to support growth of different pathogens, and under barn conditions it appears that high bacterial counts are influenced by factors more complex than type of bedding alone. Even clean damp bedding may support bacterial growth (41).

High populations of coliform bacteria on the teat end, unless accompanied by actual chronic quarter infection, are probably transitory and represent recent environmental contamination which would usually be eliminated by an effective sanitation program at milking time. However, any teat skin population, whether associated with infection in another quarter, from contaminated teat cup liners or from other environmental sources, must be considered as a potential source of new infections.

Several teat factors are important in the epidemiology of *E. coli* mastitis (42). It is generally accepted that *E. coli* is common in the environment of housed dairy cows and that mastitis can be produced experimentally by the introduction of as few as 20 organisms into the teat cistern via the teat duct. However, the processes by which this occurs under natural conditions are unknown. *E. coli* does not colonize the healthy skin of the udder on the teat duct.

The teat duct normally provides an effective barrier to invasion of the mammary gland by bacteria. As a result of machine milking there is some relaxation of the papillary duct followed by gradual reduction in the duct lumen diameter in the next 2 hours following milking (52). This period of relaxation after milking may be a risk factor predisposing to new intramammary infection.

However, experimentally repeated wet contact of the teat ends with a high concentration of coliform bacteria does not necessarily result in an increase in new intramammary infection (13). The experimental application of high levels of teat end contamination with *E. coli* after milking repeatedly led to high rates of intramammary infection which suggests that penetration of the teat duct by *E. coli* occurs in the period between contamination and milking (44). Milking machines which produce cyclic and irregular vacuum fluctuations during milking can result in impacts of milk against the teat ends which may propel bacteria through the streak canal and increase the rate of new infections due to *E. coli* and outbreaks of peracute coliform mastitis (45).

In summary, there appears to be a relationship between the population of coliform bacteria in the environment and coliform new infection rate (14).

Not all coliform bacteria will cause mastitis. Coliform bacteria isolated from the milk of cows or from their environment were found to have different degrees of susceptibility to the bactericidal action of bovine sera, with almost all of the isolates which cause severe mastitis being serum-resistant (15). Serum-sensitive organisms are unable to multiply in normal glands due to the activity of bactericidins reaching milk from the blood (15, 46). There are also somatic and capsular factors of coliforms which affect resistance to bovine bactericidal activity (15). Strains of *Klebsiella* which cause mastitis are also resistant to bovine serum (47).

The factors which influence the susceptibility of cows to coliform mastitis include the level of leukocytes in the milk and the stage of lactation. Experimentally, somatic cell counts of 250 000/ml in the milk of a quarter may limit significant growth of bacteria and development of mastitis when small inocula of coliform organisms are experimentally introduced into it (16). Counts of 500 000/ml provided complete protection. Thus cows in herds with a low incidence of streptococcal and staphylococcal mastitis would have a low level of pre-existing leukocytosis and be more susceptible to coliform mastitis.

Coliform mastitis occurs almost entirely in the lactating cow and rarely in the dry cow, and experimentally the disease can be produced in lactating quarters much more readily than in dry quarters (17). The difference in the susceptibility may be due to the much higher somatic cell counts in the secretion of dry quarters than in the milk of lactating quarters. It has been a common observation that cows with known uninfected quarters at drying-off developed peracute coliform mastitis at calving, which suggests that infection occurred during the dry period. New intramammary infections can occur during the non-lactating period, especially during the last 30 days, remain latent until parturition and cause peracute mastitis after parturition (26).

In a study of a dairy herd in total confinement, the intramammary infection rate was higher during the dry period than during lactation, increased progressively as parity increased and was maximal during the summer which coincided with maximum exposure to coliforms in the bedding (5). The rate of coliform intramammary infection is highest during the 2 weeks following drying-off and in the 2 weeks prior to calving. The fully involuted mammary gland appears to be highly resistant to experimental challenge by *E. coli* (7) but it becomes susceptible during the immediate prepartum period. There are several environmental and physiological factors which might influence the level of resistance of the non-lactating gland to coliform infection. The rate of new intramammary infection is highest during transitions of the mammary gland from lactation to involution and during the period of colostrum production to lactation. The differences in susceptibility or resistance to new intramammary infection may be due, in part, to changes in concentration of lactoferrin, IgG, bovine serum albumin and citrate which are correlated with *in vitro* growth inhibition of *Klebsiella pneumoniae*, *E. coli* and *Streptococcus uberis* (49). Surveys now reveal that environmental mastitis pathogens can account for more than 50% of bacteria isolated during lactation in *Str. agalactiae*-negative herds in which postmilking teat disinfection and dry cow therapy are practiced (50). During the dry period, the rate of intramammary infection by coliform bacteria and species of streptococci other than *Str. agalactiae* is high and many of these infections persist and may cause mastitis in early lactation.

The failure of lactoferrin within mammary secretions to prevent new infections and mastitis near and after parturition might be due to a decrease in lactoferrin before parturition. Lactoferrin normally binds iron needed by iron-dependent organisms which multiply excessively in the absence of lactoferrin. Also, citrate concentration increases in mammary secretions at parturition and may interfere with iron-binding by lactoferrin. There is also a slower increase in polymorphonuclear neutrophils in milk after new intramammary infection in early lactation than in mid- and late lactation (26). These conditions may explain the peracute coliform mastitis which occurs in early lactation. This suggests latent infection or, more likely, that infection occurred at a critical time just a few days before and after calving, when the streak canal became patent and the population of coliform bacteria on the teat end was persistently high because the cow was not being milked routinely and thus would not be subjected to udder washing and teat dipping. Coliform bacteria do have the ability to pass through the streak canal unaided by machine milking (12). The higher relative susceptibility of older cows may be related to the increased patency of the streak canal which occurs with age. The presence of a fatty liver in a recently calved cow does not appear to increase the susceptibility of the animal to coliform mastitis (51).

The sporadic occurrence of the disease may be associated with the use of contaminated teat siphons and mastitis tubes and infection following traumatic injury to teats or following teat surgery.

Pathogenesis

After invasion and infection of the mammary gland, *E. coli* proliferates in large numbers and elaborates a potent endotoxin which causes a change in vascular permeability, resulting in edema and acute swelling of the gland and a marked increase in the number of neutrophils in the milk (18). The polymorphonuclear leukocytes may increase 40 to 250 times and strongly inhibit the survival of the *E. coli* (18). This marked diapedesis of neutrophils accounts for the remarkable leukopenia and neutropenia which occurs in peracute coliform mastitis. The severity of the disease is influenced by the degree of the pre-existing leukocytosis in the milk and the number of neutrophils which invade the affected gland to control growth of the organism and the susceptibility of the organism to serum bactericidins which are secreted into the gland and the amount of endotoxin produced (15). The neutrophil kinetics in naturally occurring cases have been reproduced experimentally (28, 29).

The severity of the disease may also be dependent on the stage of lactation. Experimental infection of the mammary gland of recently calved cows with *E. coli* produces a more severe mastitis when compared with animals in mid-lactation. This may be due to a delay of 10–12 hours in diapedesis of neutrophils into the mammary gland of recently calved cows (30). Furthermore, because of this delay there may be no visible changes in the milk for up to 15 hours after infection but the systemic effects of the endotoxin released by the bacteria are evident in the cow (anorexia, fever and severe diarrhea). The net result is endotoxemia which presumably persists as long as organisms are multiplying and releasing endotoxin. This persistent endotoxemia is probably a major cause of failure to respond to therapy compared to the transient endotoxemia in the experimental inoculation of one dose of endotoxin.

Newly calved cows tend to be refractory to the presence of irritants, such as endotoxin, and are thus slow to mobilize defense mechanisms following infection (30). Also, those glands which are sensitive to small amounts of irritant and produce milk which is opsonic for *E. coli* can promote the rapid elimination of the organism before clinical signs develop (30). The ability of polymorphonuclear leukocytes to kill *E. coli* varies among cows (53). Experimental infection of the mammary gland of cows with *E. coli* results in the stimulation of a longlasting opsonic activity for the phagocytosis and killing of the homologous strain of the organism by polymorphonuclear (PMN) leukocytes (48). Thus opsonic deficiency is not a problem in early lactation but rather a failure of rapid migration of polymorphonuclear leukocytes into the gland cistern (54).

The organisms are not always readily eliminated from the infected gland by the neutrophils. Serum-resistant *E. coli* may be eliminated from experimentally infected single mammary glands of healthy cows before the appearance of clinical signs (32). Following infection of two quarters, the organism may persist for several days (31). It is thought the organism may remain latent in neutrophils and reappear as long as 40 days later and cause a recurrence of mastitis. In naturally occurring cases, it is not uncommon to be able to culture the organism from the mammary gland during and after both parenteral and intramammary antibacterial therapy.

The experimental introduction of *E. coli* into the mammary glands of lactating goats and cows results in necrosis and sloughing of the epithelial cells of the teat and lactiferous sinuses. Tissue damage is confined to the basement membrane which may explain the rapid resolution of most natural infection (38).

The final outcome is probably dependent on the degree of neutrophil response. If the neutrophil response is delayed and growth of the organisms is unrestricted, the high levels of toxin produced could cause severe destruction of udder tissue and general toxemia. If the animal responds quickly there is often little effect on milk yield because the injury is confined to the sinuses without involvement of secretory tissues (18). In an attempt to further understand the pathogenesis of coliform mastitis the effect of experimentally introducing *E. coli* endotoxin into the mammary gland has been examined. The involuted dry mammary gland is refractory to the presence of *E. coli* endotoxin due to changes which occur in the ductular epithelium during involution (55). An absence of complement activity in milk has been identified in some cows in which mastitis was induced with *E. coli* or endotoxin (56). The intramammary infusion of *E. coli* endotoxin in cows and goats may result in the release of inflammatory endogenous mediators in the udder and their subsequent absorption into the circulation rather than the absorption of endotoxin (57); an observation which challenges the assumption that the systemic clinical signs in peracute coliform mastitis are due to absorbed endotoxin. The zinc concentration in milk and plasma decrease in spontaneous and induced *E. coli* endotoxin mastitis (62) but the significance is unknown.

The intramammary infusion of either *E. coli* endotoxin or the sterile culture of the medium in which the organism had been grown results in a rapid intense inflammatory response in 4 hours. The culture filtrate, in addition to inflammation, causes degeneration and necrosis of ductular walls which suggests that two toxins may be involved (29).

The intramammary infusion of endotoxin results in sequential increase of immunoglobulin in milk whey and of phagocytosis of staphylococci by milk polymorphonuclear cells which is consistent with spontaneous recovery of cows with acute coliform mastitis which can occur (58). Endotoxin infusion can also result in increases in arachidonic acid metabolites such as thromboxanes which may be involved in mediation of local quarter inflammation and systemic signs observed in acute coliform mastitis (59, 60). There is also a marked increase in prostaglandin concentrations which indicates that they may play a role in the pathogenesis of endotoxin-induced mastitis and that the use of non-steroidal anti-inflammatory drugs may be of value therapeutically. Flunixin meglumine at a dose of 1·1 mg 1 kg body weight, the first given intravenously 2 hours after endotoxin infusion and six additional doses at 8-hour intervals intramuscularly had some beneficial effect (61).

The experimental intravenous infusion of an *E. coli* ectotoxin into non-lactating or low-producing cows resulted in a marked decrease in serum calcium and phosphorus which was associated with recumbency (63) suggesting that toxemia can cause hypocalcemic paresis.

In the peracute form, severe toxemia with fever, shivering, weakness leading to recumbency in a few hours, and diarrhea are all common and thought to be due to the absorption of large quantities of endotoxin. In experimental endotoxemia in cattle there was leukopenia, a mild hypocalcemia and elevation in plasma corticosteroids (19). The endotoxin appears to exert its effect beginning at about 6 hours after infusing into the mammary gland (33). Experimentally infused endotoxin is detoxified very rapidly after absorption into the circulation. The hypocalcemia also occurs in naturally occurring cases and is thought to be due to decreased intestinal absorption associated with the endotoxemia. In the acute form the systemic changes are usually less severe. In both forms, there is marked agalactia and the secretions in the affected quarter become serous and contain small flakes. Coliform organisms are not active tissue invaders, and in affected cattle which survive the systemic effects of the endotoxin the affected quarter(s) will usually return to partial production in the same lactation and even full production in the next. However, in some cows which survive the peracute form, subsequent milk production in the current lactation is very poor and cows are commonly culled.

The prognosis for coliform mastitis in cows is largely dependent on the speed and extent of the host response rather than the pathogenicity and dose of the organism. Initially, the bacteria multiply within the teat sinus and produce toxins which cause severe but local epithelial damage. Within a few hours, the bacteria move into the lactiferous sinuses and the larger ducts. If the infection persists, the secretory glands gradually reduce their output, and histologically show changes of involution. Even if only one quarter is affected the other quarters may also dry off. The final outcome depends on the speed and ability of the neutrophils to decrease the bacterial population before long-term secretion is affected. The numbers of bacteria in the milk also influence the outcome. If bacterial numbers exceed 10^6/ml, the ability of the neutrophil to phagocytose is impaired. If the bacterial count is less than 10^3/ml at 12 hours post-infection, the organisms will be rapidly eliminated and the prognosis will be favorable. This response is seen as a subacute form of the disease. With spontaneous self-cure of the neutrophil response is slow or delayed. The cow will exhibit more severe signs of coliform mastitis due to toxemia. These are most common in recently calved cows and are characterized clinically by a serous secretion in the affected quarter (5) which later becomes watery, fever, depression, ruminal hypomotility and diarrhea. The prognosis for these is unfavorable. These more severe forms of coliform mastitis usually occur between calving and the first 6 weeks of lactation. Cows with coliform mastitis in mid- to late lactation generally generate a rapid neutrophil response rate and their prognosis is likely to be favorable.

A retrospective analysis of cows with clinical and laboratory features of coliform mastitis revealed that 60% returned to produce a milk-like secretion in the affected quarters (5) in the current lactation and 40% did not (67). However, only 63% of the former group and 14% of the latter group remained in the herd and produced milk in the next lactation (67). Some cows were culled during the current lactation for low milk production and other reasons, some died and others were culled for mastitis. Of the original 88 cows with coliform mastitis, only 38 (43%) remained in the herd and produced milk in the next lactation.

Clinical findings

Peracute coliform mastitis in the cow is a severe disease characterized by a sudden onset of agalactia and toxemia. The cow may be normal at one milking and be acutely ill at the next. Complete anorexia, severe depression, shivering and trembling and a fever of 40–42°C (104–108°F) are common. Within 6–8 hours after the onset of signs the cow may be recumbent and unable to get up. The temperature may be normal or even subnormal, all of which may superficially resemble parturient paresis. The heart rate is usually increased up to 100–120/min, the rumen static, there may be a profuse watery diarrhea, and dehydration is common. The respiratory rate is commonly increased and in severe cases an expiratory grunt may be audible due to pulmonary congestion and edema.

The affected quarter(s) is usually swollen and warm but not remarkably, and for this reason coliform mastitis is not uncommonly missed on initial clinical examination. The cow may be severely toxemic, febrile and have diarrhea before there are visible changes in the mammary gland or the milk. The secretion is considered characteristic, and changes from the consistency of watery milk initially to a thin, yellow serous fluid, containing small meal-like flakes which are barely visible to the naked eye and are best seen on a black strip plate. Additional quarters may become affected within a day or two of the initial infection.

The course of peracute coliform mastitis is rapid; some affected cows will die in 6–8 hours after the onset of signs, others will live for 24–48 hours. Those which survive the peracute crisis will either return to normal in a few days or remain weak and recumbent for several days and eventually develop the complications associated with prolonged recumbency and may need to be destroyed. Intensive fluid therapy may prolong the life of the cow for up to several days but significant improvement may not occur and eventually euthanasia appears to be the best course of action.

In the acute form, the systemic signs are mild, the affected quarter is slightly swollen and the secretions are watery to serous in consistency and contain flakes. Recovery with treatment usually occurs in a few days.

Because of the severity of peracute coliform mastitis and the necessity for expensive and narrow-spectrum antimicrobials it is desirable to be able to make a clinical diagnosis of the disease in the field with a high degree of accuracy if possible. A discriminant analysis of clinical indicants revealed that only a history of previous mastitis in the affected quarter, muscle weakness, clear or white color of milk, swelling of the udder, watery consistency of the milk, lack of previous mastitis in other quarters, lack of palpable udder abscesses and fever were significantly associated with coliform mastitis (69). Using these variables 78% of cases were correctly classified. A prospective discriminant analysis of these variables, in cows with mastitis, to determine if they would show coliform organisms cultured from affected quarters, resulted in an accuracy of 71% (sensitivity = 0·42, specificity = 0·61) compared to an accuracy of 62% (sensitivity = 0·64, specificity = 0·61) for cowside prediction by the attending clinician (68). Analysis of the clinical findings used to diagnose coliform mastitis indicates that clinicians rely on watery consistency of milk, shivering, firmness of udder, heart rate, fever, and respiratory rate to make a diagnosis of coliform mastitis. Inclusion of weakness of the cow, swelling of the udder, decreased temperature of the cow, and duration of mastitis less than 24 hours increased accuracy over clinical prediction alone (70).

Chronic coliform mastitis is characterized by repeated episodes of subacute mastitis which cannot be readily clinically distinguished from other common causes of mastitis.

Subclinical coliform mastitis is characterized by the presence of coliform organisms in the milk samples of cows without clinical evidence of mastitis. There is a background level of coliform infection which varies from 0·9 to 1·2% in quarters (14).

The disease produced experimentally with the organism or the endotoxin has been well documented (18) and is usually not as severe as the peracute form which occurs naturally.

Clinical pathology

Milk samples should be submitted for culture and drug sensitivity. The milk samples will usually yield a positive culture. However, in some cases the organism cannot be cultured when clinical signs are evident. Presumably the neutrophils have cleared the organisms. It may also be possible to culture the organism during the period of intensive therapy and for several days after recovery in spite of using antimicrobials to which the organism is sensitive (31). The CMT on secretions from affected quarters is usually 3+.

In the peracute form of the disease the total and differential leukocyte count are characteristic and a useful diagnostic aid. There is a marked leukopenia, neutropenia and a degenerative left shift due to the migration of large numbers of neutrophils into the affected quarter. If the degenerative left shift, leukopenia and neutropenia become worse on the second day after the onset of clinical signs the prognosis is unfavorable. An improvement in the differential white count on the second day is a good prognosis. In the experimental disease the cell count of the milk ranges from 14 to 25 million cells per ml of milk at 5 hours after inoculation.

Necropsy findings

There is edema and hyperemia of the mammary tissue. In severe cases hemorrhages are present and are accompanied by thrombus formation in the blood and lymphatic vessels and there is necrosis of the parenchyma (21).

A study of the progressive pathological changes in experimental and natural cases of *E. coli* mastitis in cows reveals that pathological changes are most marked in the epithelium of the teat and lactiferous sinuses and diminish rapidly towards the ducts (65). Tissue invasion by the bacteria is not a feature despite the presence of large numbers of organisms. There is minimal involvement of secretory tissue. There is intense neutrophil infiltration, subepithelial edema and epithelial hyperplasia of the sinuses and large ducts. There is no evidence that bacteremia occurs in coliform mastitis; the culturing of blood of cows with the disease revealed no evidence of bacteria (66).

Diagnosis

Peracute coliform mastitis in cattle is characterized clinically by a sudden onset of toxemia, weakness, shivering, often recumbency, fever in the early stages followed by a normal temperature or hypothermia in several hours and characteristic gross changes in the milk which usually is watery and contains some particles barely visible to the unaided eye. The peracute form of the disease is most common in recently calved cows.

In recently calved cows the weakness and recumbency resembles parturient hypocalcemia paresis but the tachycardia, and dehydration and diarrhea if present, are not characteristic of parturient paresis and should prompt further clinical examination particularly of the udder. In the early stages of coliform mastitis the changes in the milk may be just barely visible. Those clinical findings which are most useful to predict peracute coliform mastitis include watery consistency of milk, shivering, firmness of udder, tachycardia, polypnea, fever, weakness, and mastitis of less than 24 hours duration (70). A marked leukopenia and neutropenia are characteristic of coliform mastitis, whereas in parturient paresis there is usually a neutrophilia and stress reaction. The *Limulus* amebocyte lysate test for the detection of endotoxins in milk and serum may be a useful test for experimentally induced coliform mastitis (33).

The differential diagnosis of recumbency in the immediate postpartum period is discussed under parturient paresis (p. 1104).

Treatment

The prognosis in the peracute form of the disease is unfavorable if severe clinical toxemia is present. Severe depression, weakness, recumbency, a heart rate over 120/min are indicators of an unfavorable prognosis.

The successful treatment of peracute coliform mastitis requires the earliest possible action, and clinical surveillance until recovery is apparent.

Broad-spectrum *antibiotics* are indicated parenterally, preferably by the intravenous route initially, followed by intramuscular injections to maintain blood levels. The antimicrobial sensitivities of aerobic Gram-negative bacteria isolated from udder infections in one survey indicate that 90% are sensitive to chloramphenicol, gentamicin and polymyxin B (35).

However, chloramphenicol has now been banned for use in food-producing animals in some countries, and there has been moderate increases in the level of resistance of *E. coli* from acute mastitis to chloramphenicol (71). Some surveys also reveal a high degree of resistance of *E. coli* from cases of mastitis to tetracycline and spectinomycin which are considered as alternatives to chloramphenicol. The newer antimicrobials such as beta-lactams, amoxicillin–clavulanic acid combination, and the new quinolone norfloxacin have excellent activity and are worthy of clinical trials (71). Polymyxin B, gentamicin, nalidixic acid and the second generation cephalosporin, cefoxitin, were also highly effective *in vitro* (71). There was evidence of resistance to ampicillin and amoxicillin, trimethoprim, trimethoprim–sulfamethoxanine and the first generation cephalosporin, cephalothin. In nine surveys in Denmark the most active antimicrobials against *E. coli* from acute and chronic cases of mastitis in cattle included colistin, gentamicin, and polymyxin B (72).

It is clear that the antimicrobial sensitivities of *E. coli* isolates from coliform mastitis will vary considerably which suggest that drug sensitivity determination and surveillance are necessary in order to select the drug of choice.

Where allowed by drug use legislation, and when drug sensitivities indicate their use, the following antimicrobials and their dosages are recommended for parenteral administration to cattle with peracute coliform mastitis.

Chloramphenicol	20–30 mg/kg body weight every 12 hours intravenously
Oxytetracycline	10 mg/kg body weight every 24 hours intravenously
Trimethoprim–sulfadoxine (24% solution trimethoprim 4 g/100 ml, sulfadoxine 20 g/100 ml)	1 ml/10 kg body weight every 24 hours intravenously
Gentamicin	2–5 mg/kg body weight every 12 hours intravenously

Oxytocin at the rate 30 IU per adult cow given intravenously, followed by vigorous hand massage and stripping of the affected quarter, may assist in removing inflammatory debris. The affected gland should be stripped out hourly.

Intramammary antibiotic preparations of choice should be infused after the affected quarter has been stripped out completely for the last time at the end of the day. The choice of antibiotic will depend on previous experience initially, until the results of the culture and drug sensitivity are available.

Polymyxin B has the potential to inactivate bacterial endotoxins, and evaluation of the intramammary infusion of the drug for the treatment of coliform mastitis has been attempted (20). The results indicate that the drug will not alter the clinicopathological course of endotoxin-induced mastitis. Thus at the present time there is little evidence available to recommend its use in clinical cases (20, 34).

Antimicrobials such as the cephalosporins, gentamicin, colistin, and polymyxin B should be evaluated for their effectiveness as intramammary infusions for the treatment of coliform mastitis.

Fluid and electrolyte therapy are essential. Balanced electrolyte solutions containing 5% glucose are given at the rate of 100–150 ml/kg body weight per 24 hours by continuous intravenous infusion. For a mature cow (400 kg) a total of 40–60 liters are indicated over a 24-hour period with 20–30 liters given during the first 4–6 hours and the remainder over the next 20 hours. A favorable response is usually clinically evident in 6–8 hours.

Anti-inflammatory agents are used widely but their efficacy has been difficult to evaluate. The use of massive doses of 9 alpha-fluoro-prednisolone acetate infused into the mammary gland or given intramuscularly was ineffective in inhibiting or delaying the inflammatory response associated with experimental coliform mastitis (22).

Experimentally, corticosteroids provide optimum protection against a measured dose of endotoxin when animals are pretreated or treated simultaneously with the steroids relative to the administration of the endotoxin (23). The apparent failure of corticosteroids to provide a consistent beneficial effect in peracute coliform mastitis may be due to the small doses which are commonly used compared to those used for septic shock in man and dog. The use of such large doses in cattle may be economically prohibitive. A dose of at least 1 mg/kg body weight given intravenously twice daily is recommended in peracute cases. Presumably, the continued absorption of large quantities of endotoxin from the mammary gland is difficult to counteract with even large doses of corticosteroids. There is a need for an experimental model which evaluates the effectiveness of corticosteroids in animals which are absorbing endotoxin into their systemic circulation over a period of 24–48 hours.

The therapeutic effect of flunixin meglumine for the treatment of endotoxin-induced mastitis has been evaluated (59). The multiple use of flunixin meglumine may result in a reduction of the febrile response, the clinical signs of quarter inflammation and depression scores, but there is no improvement in milk production or the laboratory indicators of inflammation in milk (59).

The use of dimethylsulfoxide (DMSO) as a carrier vehicle for antibiotics and corticosteroids has no beneficial effect (23).

Control

The control of coliform mastitis can be difficult, unreliable and frustrating. Several cases of fatal peracute coliform mastitis may occur in a herd of 100 cows during a period of 1 year in spite of the existence of apparently excellent management. No control methods have effectively reduced the incidence of coliform injections in carefully controlled trials under field conditions. The principles of mastitis control which have been effective for the control of streptococcal and staphylococcal mastitis have been unsuccessful for the control of coliform mastitis. This is because the epidemiology of coliform mastitis is different from that caused by the coccal bacteria. In the control of coliform mastitis, the emphasis is on the prevention of new infection.

When an outbreak of peracute coliform mastitis is encountered the following procedures are recommended in an attempt to prevent new cases:

- Culture milk samples and obtain a definitive etiological diagnosis
- Examine the bedding for evidence of heavy contamination with coliform bacteria. If sawdust or shavings are being used replace them with straw, if possible
- Conduct a general clean-up of the stall and lounging areas
- Improve premilking hygiene (37)
- Examine milking machine function
- Culture milk samples of cows immediately before parturition and treat infected quarters. Place prepartum cows in clean, dry boxstalls (36).

The normal presence of coliform bacteria in every aspect of the cow's environment must be recognized but every effort must be made to avoid situations which will allow a build-up of organisms. This is especially important in dairy herds which have been on a mastitis control program resulting in a high percentage of cows with a low level of preexisting leukocytosis in their milk which makes them susceptible to coliform mastitis. The overall level of sanitation and hygiene must be improved and maintained in these herds.

While no reliable recommendations are available, cows which are housed during part or all of the day or night should be bedded on dry bedding and not overcrowded to prevent heavy fecal contamination. There is an urgent need for the determination of optimum space and bedding requirements for the lounging areas of dairy cows kept under loose housing. Bedding should be kept as dry as possible by adding fresh bedding as necessary (27). Excessively wet bedding should be removed. Sawdust and shavings harbor more coliform bacteria than straw, and require special attention. The build-up of high numbers of coliform bacteria in the bedding of cow cubicles can be controlled by the daily removal of the sawdust from the rear of the cubicle and rebedding with clean sawdust which is usually of low coliform count. The use of a paraformaldehyde spray on sawdust bedding reduced the coliform count for 2–3 days but it returned to its predisinfection level in 7 days (12). When outbreaks of coliform mastitis are encountered which are possibly associated with heavily contaminated sawdust or shavings, they should be removed immediately and replaced with clean, fresh, dry straw (25). The use of sawdust or shavings as bedding should be avoided if possible. Sand may be a suitable alternative (12) and has been successful. The use of dried manure or composted dried manure makes excellent safe bedding for cows. Mixing dirt with dried manure solids may improve characteristics of the bedding and help maintain low bacterial counts (27).

Regular daily cleaning of barns is necessary to minimize contamination of teats. In free-stall and loose-housing dairy barns, every management technique available must be used to ensure that cows do not defecate in their stalls which will increase the level of contamination. This requires daily raking of the bedding in free-stall barns and adjusting head rails to ensure that cows do not lie too far forward in the stall and to ensure that they defecate in the alleyway.

In dairy herds which are confined for all or part of the year, as herd size increases the level of contamination usually increases and commonly the ventilation is inadequate. This leads to excessive humid conditions which promote the development of coliform bacteria in wet bedding. This will require increased attention to sanitation and hygiene.

It must be emphasized that postmilking teat dipping with a disinfectant will have little effect on reducing the incidence of coliform mastitis because contamination of the teats occurs between milking rather than at milking. Thus one logical approach to the control of coliform mastitis is to reduce environmental contamination (25). In the event of gross fecal contamination of the udder and teats, additional time and care will be required at milking time. Udders and teats must be washed thoroughly, perhaps with soap, and dried completely with individual paper towels. Because irregular vacuum fluctuations in the milking machine may induce coliform mastitis in quarters exposed to a high level of contamination, the operation and sanitation of the milking machine, especially those parts in direct contact with the teats, must be examined. Because considerable movement of coliform bacteria can occur from the teat apex into the teat sinus in cows which are not being milked, cows which are due to calve should be kept on grass or moved into a clean area at least 2 weeks before calving and their udders and teats washed daily if necessary, and a teat dipping with a teat disinfectant begun 10 days before calving. This is particularly necessary for older cows and those which are known to be easy milkers. The teats of those cows which are 'leakers' just before calving may have to be sealed with adhesive tape or collodion to minimize the chance of infection.

Cows which are recumbent and unable to get up (e.g. the downer cow) should be well bedded on clean dry straw and their udders washed twice daily and teats dipped with a teat disinfectant. Strict hygiene must be practiced when using teat siphons, teat creams, and strict asepsis when doing teat surgery.

The use of autogenous vaccines in problem herds has been considered but no results are yet available.

REVIEW LITERATURE

Eberhart, R. J., Natzke, R. P., Newbould, F. H. S., Nonnecker, B. & Thompson, P. (1979). Coliform mastitis: a review. *J. dairy Sci.*, *62*, 1–22.

Golodetz, C. L. (1985). Prognosis of cows with coliform mastitis. *Vet. Ann.*, *25*, 78–83.

Jackson, E. & Bramley, J. (1983) Coliform mastitis. *Vet. Rec. Suppl., No. 4, In Practice*, *5*, 135–146.

Jones, T. O. (1986) A review of teat factors in bovine *E. coli* mastitis. *Vet. Rec.*, *118*, 507–509.

Oz, H. H., Farnsworth, R. J. & Larson, V. L. (1985) Environmental mastitis. *Vet. Bull.*, *55*, 829–840.

Smith, K. L., Todhunter, D. A. & Schoenberger, D. S. (1985) Environmental mastitis: cause, prevalence, prevention. *J. dairy Sci.*, *68*, 1531–1553.

REFERENCES

(1) Sanchez-Carlo, V. et al. (1984). *Am. J. vet. Res.*, *45*, 1771.
(2) Bramman, S. K. et al. (1973) *J. Am. vet. med. Assoc.*, *162*, 109.
(3) Linton, A. H. and Robinson, T. C. (1984) *Br. vet. J.*, *140*, 368.
(4) Jackson, E. & Bramley, J. (1983). *Vet. Rec. Suppl. In Practice*, *5*, 135.
(5) Smith, K. L. et al. (1985) *J. dairy Sci.*, *68*, 1531.
(6) Hazlett, M. J. et al. (1984) *Can. J. comp. Med.*, *48*, 125.
(7) Smith, K. L. et al. (1985) *J. dairy Sci.*, *68*, 402.
(8) Jasper, D. E. et al. (1975) *J. Am. vet. med. Assoc.*, *166*, 175.
(9) Jasper, D. E. (1976). *Theriogenology*, *6*, 175.
(10) Newman, L. E. & Kowalski, J. J. (1973) *Am. J. vet Res.*, *34*, 979.
(11) Rendos, J. J. et al. (1975) *J. dairy Sci.*, *58*, 1492.
(12) Bramley, A. J. & Neave, F. K. (1975) *Br. vet. J.*, *131*, 160.
(13) Thiel, C. C. et al. (1973) *J. dairy Res.*, *40*, 117.
(14) Eberhart, R. J. et al. (1979) *J. dairy Sci.*, *62*.
(15) Ward, G. E. & Sebunya, T. K. (1981) *Am. J. vet. Res.*, *42*, 1937, 1947.
(16) Schalm, O. W. et al. (1964) *Am. J. vet. Res.*, *25*, 83.
(17) Bramley, A. J. (1976) *J. dairy Res.*, *43*, 205.
(18) Frost, A. J. et al. (1982) *Res. vet. Sci.*, *33*, 105.
(19) Griel, L. C. et al. (1975) *Can. J. comp. Med.*, *39*, 1.
(20) Ziv, G. & Schultze, W. D. (1983) *Am. J. vet. Res.*, *44*, 1446.
(21) Renk, W. (1962) *Zentralbl. VetMed.*, *9*, 264.
(22) Carroll, E. J. et al. (1965) *Am. J. vet. Res.*, *26*, 858.
(23) Carroll, E. J. et al. (1974) *Am. J. vet. Res.*, *35*, 781.
(24) Jones, T. O. & Jones, P. C. (1986) *Vet. Rec.*, *119*, 319.
(25) Eberhart, R. J. (1975) *Proc. int. dairy Fedn Seminar Mastitis Control*, pp. 371–376.
(26) McDonald, J. S. & Anderson, A. J. (1981) *Am. J. vet. Res.*, *42*, 229.
(27) Jasper, D. E. (1980) *Bov. Pract.*, No. 15, 39.
(28) Jain, N. C. & Lasmanis, J. (1978) *Res. vet. Sci.*, *24*, 386.
(29) Frost, A. J. et al. (1984) *Aust. vet. J.*, *61*, 77.
(30) Frost, A. J. & Brooker, B. E. (1986) *Aust. vet. J.*, *63*, 327.
(31) Hill, A. W. et al. (1979) *Res. vet. Sci.*, *26*, 32.
(32) Hill, A. W. et al. (1978) *Res. vet. Sci.*, *25*, 89.
(33) Liu, G. et al. (1976) *Theriogenology*, *6*, 343.
(34) Liu, G. et al. (1978) *J. vet. Pharmacol. Therap.*, *1*, 213.
(35) McDonald, J. S. et al. (1977) *Am. J. vet. Res.*, *38*, 1503.
(36) Armstrong, K. R. (1977) *Bov. Pract.*, *12*, 85.
(37) Bushnell, R. B. (1980) *J. Am. vet. med. Assoc.*, *176*, 746.
(38) Schultze, W. D. & Thompson, P. D. (1980) *Am. J. vet. Res.*, *41*, 1396.
(39) Frost, A. J. et al. (1980) *Proc. Royal Soc., London, B (Biol. Sci.)*, *209*, 431.
(40) Thomas, C. B. et al. (1982–83). *Prev. vet. Med.*, *1*, 227.
(41) Zehner, M. M. et al. (1986) *J. dairy Sci.*, *69*, 1932.
(42) Jones, T. O. (1986) *Vet. Rec.*, *118*, 507.
(43) Jasper, D. E. & Dellinger, J. D. (1973) *Cornell Vet.*, *65*, 380.
(44) Bramley, A. J. et al. (1980) *J. dairy Res.*, *48*, 379.
(45) Huffman, E. M. & Lucas, M. (1983) *J. Am. vet. med. Assoc.*, *183*, 570.
(46) Sanchez-Carlo, V. et al. (1984) *Am. J. vet. Res.*, *45*, 1775.
(47) Nonnecke, B. J. & Newbould, F. H. S. (1984) *Am. J. vet. Res.*, *45*, 12451.
(48) Hill, A. W. et al. (1983) *Vet. Microbiol.*, *8*, 293.
(49) Breau, W. C. & Oliver, S. P. (1986) *Am. J. vet. Res.*, *47*, 218.
(50) Oliver, S. P. & Mitchell, B. A. (1984) *J. dairy Sci.*, *67*, 2436.
(51) Hill, A. W. et al. (1985) *Vet. Rec.*, *117*, 549.
(52) Schultze, W. D. & Bright, S. (1983) *Am. J. vet. Res.*, *44*, 2373.
(53) Williams, M. R. & Bunch, K. J. (1981) *Res. vet. Sci.*, *30*, 298.
(54) Hill, A. W. et al. (1983) *Res. vet. Sci.*, *35*, 222.
(55) Frost, A. J. & Brooker, B. E. (1983) *J. comp. Pathol.*, *93*, 211.
(56) Mueller, R. et al. (1983) *Am. J. vet. Res.*, *44*, 1442.
(57) Verheijden, J. H. M. et al. (1983) *Vet. res. Commun.*, *7*, 229.
(58) Anderson, K. L. et al. (1986) *Am. J. vet. Res.*, *47*, 2405.
(59) Anderson, K. L. et al. (1986) *Am. J. vet. Res.*, *47*, 1373.
(60) Giri, S. N. et al. (1984) *Am. J. vet. Res.*, *45*, 586.
(61) Anderson, K. L. et al. (1986) *Am. J. vet. Res.*, *47*, 1366.
(62) Verheijden, J. H. M. et al. (1983) *Am. J. vet. Res.*, *44*, 1637.
(63) Sandstedt, H. (1984) *Nord. VetMed.*, *36*, 406.
(64) Burvenich, C. et al. (1983) *Vet. res. Commun.*, *7*, 237.
(65) Hill, A. W. et al. (1984) *Res. vet. Sci.*, *37*, 179.
(66) Powers, M. S. et al. (1984) *J. Am. vet. med. Assoc.*, *189*, 440.
(67) Golodetz, C. L. & White, M. E. (1983) *Vet. Rec.*, *112*, 402.
(68) White, M. E. et al. (1986) *Cornell Vet.*, *76*, 342.
(69) White, M. E. et al. (1986) *Cornell Vet.*, *76*, 335.
(70) White, M. E. et al. (1987) *Cornell Vet.*, *77*, 13.
(71) Muckle, C. A. et al. (1986) *Cornell Vet.*, *76*, 13.
(72) Sogaard, H. (1982) *Nord. VetMed.*, *34*, 248.
(73) Dodd, F. H. et al. (1984) *Vet. Res.*, *114*, 522.

Mastitis caused by *Pasteurella* spp.

Mastitis caused by *Pasteurella* spp. is common in ewes, occurring in a peracute gangrenous form, but it is comparatively rare in cattle and goats.

Etiology

Past. hemolytica, the causative organism in ewes, can be isolated from affected quarters and the disease can be reproduced by the intramammary infusion of cultures of the organism (1). *Staph. aureus*, *Cor. (Actinomyces) pyogenes* and streptococci are often present as secondary invaders (2). In cattle *Past. multocida* is the causative organism; in goats it is tentatively identified as *Past. hemolytica* (3).

Epidemiology

In sheep the disease occurs in the western United States, Australia and in Europe in ewes kept under systems of husbandry varying from open mountain pasture to enclosed barns. It is most common in ewes suckling big lambs 2–3 months old. In cattle the disease is encountered rarely but may be a problem in individual herds, particularly where calves are reared by nurse cows (4).

Infection is thought to occur through injuries to teats perhaps caused by overvigorous sucking by big lambs or calves. The occurrence of this form of mastitis is not related to hygiene, many outbreaks occurring in sheep at range, but because of the sheep's habit of sleeping at night on bedding grounds, it is possible that transmission occurs by contact with infected soil or bedding. The disease in both sheep and cattle is sporadic in occurrence.

Clinical findings

In ewes an acute systemic disturbance, with a high fever (40–42°C, 105–107°F), anorexia and dyspnea, accompanies acute swelling of the gland and severe lameness on the affected side. This lameness is an important early sign and is useful in picking affected animals from a group. The udder is at first hot, swollen and painful and the milk watery, but within 24 hours the quarter becomes blue and cold, the milk shows clots and a profound toxemia is evident. The temperature subsides in 2–4 days, the secretion dries up entirely and the animal either dies of toxemia in 3–7 days or survives with sloughing of a gangrenous portion of the udder, followed by the development of abscesses and the continual draining of pus. Usually only one side is affected. During outbreaks of this type of mastitis, cases of pneumonia due to the same organism may occur in lambs.

In cattle the mastitis is severe with fever, marked swelling, abnormal secretion, complete cessation of milk flow in affected and unaffected quarters and subsequent fibrosis and atrophy. Calves allowed to suck affected cows may die of pasteurellosis (5).

Clinical pathology

Culture of the organism in the milk is necessary to confirm the diagnosis.

Necropsy findings

The disease is not fatal in cows but in ewes there is marked edema of the ventral abdominal wall and severe engorgement and edema of the mammary tissue.

Diagnosis

In sheep the peracute nature of the disease makes it similar to mastitis caused by *Staph. aureus* although gangrene of the udder is more typical in the latter disease. A similar disease in ewes has been ascribed to *Actinobacillus lignieresi* but the causative organism closely resembles the *Pasteurella* spp. described here (6). Suppurative mastitis caused by *Cor. pseudotuberculosis* is chronic in type and no systemic signs occur. Mastitis caused by *Str. agalactiae* in ewes resembles the same disease in cattle. Bovine mastitis caused by *Past. multocida* must be differentiated from the many other forms of acute mastitis in this species and this can be done only by bacteriological examination of the milk.

Treatment

Sulfadimidine administered intravenously and orally is effective in ewes if given in the early stages of the disease (1). Streptomycin and the broad-spectrum antibiotics should be equally effective. In cattle, streptomycin administered by intramammary infusion is effective but a tetracycline is preferred. Recurrence in quarters which appear to have recovered is not infrequent (7) and poor response to treatment has been observed (8).

Control

Removal of sources of infection in sheep flocks necessitates culling some ewes with affected udders but even rigid culling usually fails to completely eradicate the disease. Polyvalent hyperimmune serum and a formolized vaccine have been shown to be of value in prophylaxis (9) and an autogenous vaccine may be effective in a flock where the disease is occurring.

REFERENCES

(1) Tunnicliff, E. A. (1949) *Vet. Med.*, *44*, 498.
(2) Simmons, G. C. & Ryley, J. W. (1954) *Q. J. agric. Sci.*, *11*, 29.
(3) Bagadi, H. O. & Razig, S. E. (1976) *Vet. Rec.*, *99*, 13.
(4) Barnum, D. A. (1954) *Can. J. comp. Med.*, *18*, 113.
(5) Packer, R. A. & Merchant, I. A. (1946) *N. Am. Vet.*, 27, 496.
(6) Laws, L. & Elder, J. K. (1969) *Aust. vet. J.*, *45*, 401.
(7) Pascoe, R. R. (1960) *Aust. vet. J.*, *36*, 408.
(8) Pepper, T. A. et al. (1968) *Vet. Rec.*. 83, 211.
(9) Mura, D. & Manca, A. (1955) *Vet. ital.*, 6, 1003.

Mastitis caused by *Nocardia* spp.

Nocardial mastitis is an uncommon occurrence in cattle and is manifested as an acute or subacute mastitis accompanied by extensive granulomatous lesions in the udder.

Etiology

Nocardia asteroides can be cultured from the milk of affected quarters and the disease can be produced experimentally by this organism. One case of chronic mastitis caused by *N. brasiliensis* (1) and two caused by *N. farcinicus* (2) have also been recorded.

Epidemiology

Nocardial mastitis is a sporadic disease affecting only one or two cows in a herd, unless there is accidental introduction of the causative bacteria into udders when infusions are being administered when it may appear as a herd problem (4). It is recorded as being a relatively common chronic mastitis in Cuba (5).

With rare exceptions, nocardial mastitis in cattle had been recorded only as a sporadic infection. The disease is a serious one in that there is extensive destruction of tissue, loss of production and occasionally death of a cow. Also, there is a possibility that human infection may occur as the organism may not be destroyed by usual pasteurization procedures.

The organism is a common soil contaminant and probably gains entrance to the udder when udder washing is ineffective or udder infusion is not carried out aseptically. The disease is most common in freshly calved adult cows particularly if infusion of the udder with contaminated materials is carried out in the dry period (6). *N. asteroides* is capable of surviving in mixtures used for intramammary infusion for up to 7 weeks. There is one record of a massive outbreak with many deaths probably due to the use of a contaminated homemade udder infusion (11).

Pathogenesis

The inflammation of the teat sinus and lower parts of the gland suggest invasion via the teat canal. Infection of mammary tissue results in the formation of discrete granulomatous lesions and the development of extensive fibrosis, the spread of inflammation occurring from lobule to lobule. Infected animals are not sensitive to tuberculin.

When infection occurs early in lactation (the first 15 days) the reaction is a systemic one with fever and anorexia. At other times the lesions take the form of circumscribed abscesses and fibrosis. There may also be infected foci in supramammary and mesenteric lymph nodes (8).

Clinical findings

Affected animals may show a systemic reaction with high fever, depression and anorexia but an acute or subacute inflammation is more usual. Fibrosis of the gland and the appearance of clots in grayish, viscid secretion, which also contains small, white particles, is the usual clinical picture. The fibrosis may be diffuse but is usually in the form of discrete masses 2–5 cm in diameter. Badly affected glands may rupture or develop sinus tracts to the exterior.

Laboratory examinations of herds in which cases occur may also reveal subclinical cases which have intermittent flareups (3).

Clinical pathology

The organism can be detected on culture of the milk. Small (1 mm diameter) specks are visible in the milk and, on microscopical examination, these prove to be felted masses of mycelia. Intradermal injection of antigens prepared from the organism has shown some promise as a diagnostic test (9).

Necropsy findings

Grossly diffuse fibrosis and granulomatous lesions containing pus are present in mammary tissue. The lining of milk ducts and the teat sinus are thick and roughened. On histological examination the granulomatous nature of the lesions is evident. Metastatic pulmonary lesions have been found in occasional longstanding cases (10).

Diagnosis

The appearance of the milk is distinctive but cultural examination is necessary for positive identification.

Treatment

The disease does not respond well to treatment. Erythromycin and miconizol are most effective but need to be used for 1–2 weeks (3). Neomycin and chloramphenicol (7) have moderate efficiency.

Control

Because of the probable invasion via the teat canal from a soil-borne infection, proper hygiene at milking and strict cleanliness during intramammary infusion are necessary on farms where the disease is enzootic. The organism appears to be sensitive to sodium hypochlorite (200 ppm of free chlorine). Treatment in late cases is unlikely to be of value because of the nature of the lesions, and in affected herds particular attention should be given to the early diagnosis of the disease. Dry period treatment with cloxacillin or novobiocin is ineffective.

REFERENCES

(1) Ditchfield, J. et al. (1959) *Can. J. comp. Med.*, *23*, 93.
(2) Awad, F. I. (1960) *Vet. Rec.*, *72*, 341.
(3) Sears, P. M. (1983) *Bov. Pract.*, *18*, 4.
(4) Argente, G. et. al. (1983) *Pointe vet.*, *14*, 7.
(5) Merino, N. et al. (1973) *Revta cub. Cienc. vet.*, *4* 19.
(6) Pier, A. C. et al. (1961) *Am. J. vet. Res.*, *22*, 698.
(7) Schulz, W. & Wester, G. (1968) *Mh. VetMed.*, *23*, 601.
(8) Nicolet, J. et al. (1968) *Schweiz. Arch. Tierheilkd.*, *110*, 289.
(9) Salman, M. D. et al. (1982) *Am. J. vet. Res.*, *43*, 332.
(10) Pier, A. C. (1961) *Am. J. vet. Res.*, *22*, 502.
(11) Hibbs, C. M. et al. (1980) *Proc. ann. Mtg. Am. Assoc. vet. Lab. Diag.*, *23*, 73.

Bovine mastitis caused by *Mycoplasma* spp.

Bovine mastitis caused by *Mycoplasma* spp. is characterized by sudden onset, involvement of all four quarters usually, a precipitous drop in milk production, severe swelling of the udder and gross abnormality of the milk without obvious signs of systemic illness.

Etiology

At least seven species of *Mycoplasma*, especially *M. bovis*, unnamed species ST–6, and group 7 (2). Occasionally *M. canadense*, *M. bovigenitalium*, *M. alkalescens* (13), *M. capricolum* (9), *M. californicum* (4, 17) and *M. dispar* (21) have been isolated from clinical cases. Other mycoplasmas, not usually associated with the development of mastitis, also cause the disease when injected into the udder (6). There is also evidence of mastitis caused by *Ureaplasma* spp. (1). A striking characteristic of the mycoplasmas is that they seem to be able to survive, or even prosper, in the presence of large numbers of leukocytes in the milk. Antibodies to the bacteria have not been detectable in sera or whey from animals infected with some strains, but complement-fixing antibodies are present in the sera of animals recovered from infection with other strains.

Acholeplasma laidlawii is not a mastitis pathogen, but it has been observed that a high proportion of bulk tanks will give positive cultural tests for it, especially during wet, rainy weather (15). This increase is accompanied by an increase of clinical mycoplasmal mastitis due to pathogenic mycoplasms. *A. laidlawii* is considered to be a milk contaminant in these circumstances.

The group of diseases, including mastitis, which are caused by *Mycoplasma* spp. in sheep and goats are dealt with separately.

Epidemiology

The disease has been recorded in the United Kingdom, the United States, Canada and Israel and has been observed in Australia. The first recordings of the disease were in the mid-1960s. The disease is a disastrous one because of the high incidence in affected herds and the almost complete cessation of production for the lactation and failure in many cows to ever return to milking. The quarter infection rate in infected herds varies widely (5) and as many as 75% of affected cows may have to be culled.

Cows of all ages and at any stage of lactation are affected, cows which have recently calved showing the most severe signs, and dry cows the least. There are several recorded outbreaks in dairy herds in dry cows (18), one of them immediately after mammary infusions of dry period treatment which affected all quarters of all cows (20).

Little is known of the epidemiology of the disease. It occurs most commonly in large herds (22) and in herds where milking hygiene is poor and when cows are brought in from other farms or from public saleyards. *Mycoplasma* mastitis usually breaks out subsequently after a delay of weeks or even months. The delay in development of an outbreak may be related to the long-term persistence of the organism (up to 13 months) in some quarters, and some cows become shedders of the organism without ever evidencing severe clinical mastitis. There is also evidence that the causative organism is capable of colonizing, and surviving in, the upper respiratory tract and the vagina (7). If this is a common habitat for the organism it would explain many of its epidemiological paradoxes. Another interesting epidemiological observation is the detection of mycoplasmas and the virus of infectious bovine rhinotracheitis in affected udders at the same time. Because the virus is difficult to isolate and is not commonly looked for it could be the much sought-after unknown factor in the etiology of the disease (8). Outbreaks of mastitis are recorded with outbreaks of vaginitis and vestibulitis (19).

The use of bulk mastitis treatments using a common syringe and cannula may be included in the immediate past history. The disease is readily transmitted by inoculation of the bacteria into a quarter or by external application of infected secretion to the teat skin. Although the disease occurs first in the inoculated quarter there is usually rapid spread to all other quarters. It seems likely that the infection is spread between cows in the same manner as are other mastitis organisms, by contamination of the teats during milking, but other means, particularly inhalation, have been suggested.

Mycoplasma spp. group 7 has also been isolated from cases of pneumonia and polyarthritis in calves fed milk from cows with mycoplasmal mastitis (2).

Pathogenesis

This is a purulent interstitial mastitis and although infection probably occurs via the teat canal, the rapid spread of the disease to other quarters of the udder and occasionally to joints suggests that systemic invasion may occur. The presence of the infection in heifers milked for the first time also suggests that systemic invasion may be followed by localization in the udder (9).

Experimental production of the disease (10) with *M. bovis* causes severe loss of milk production and a positive California mastitis test reaction and clots in the milk (11). It produces little tissue necrosis but *Mycoplasma* are detectable in many tissues including blood, vagina and fetus, suggesting again that systemic invasion occurs. It is also apparent that spread of infection between quarters in one cow can be hematogenous (3). There are no significant pathological differences between the mastitides produced by *M. bovigenitalium* and *M. bovis* (12).

Clinical findings

In lactating cows there is a sudden onset of swelling of the udder, a sharp drop in milk production and grossly abnormal secretion in one or more quarters. In most cases all four quarters are affected and a high-producing cow may fall in yield to almost nil between one milking and the next. Dry cows show little swelling of the udder. Although there is no overt evidence of systemic illness, and febrile reactions are not observed in most field cases in lactating cows, those which have recently calved show most obvious swelling of the udder and may be off their feed and have a mild fever. However, cows infected experimentally show fever up to 41°C (105·5°F) on the third or fourth day after inoculation, at the same time as the udder changes appear. The temperature returns to normal in 24–96 hours. In some cases the supramammary lymph nodes are greatly enlarged. A few cows, with or without mastitis, develop arthritis in the knees and fetlocks. The affected joints are swollen, with the swelling extending up and down the leg. Lameness may be so severe that the foot is not put to the ground. *Mycoplasma* may be present in the joint.

The secretion from affected quarters is deceptive in the early stages in that it appears fairly normal at collection, but on standing a deposit which may be in the form of fine, sandy material, flakes or floccules settles out leaving a turbid whey-like supernatant. Subsequently the secretion becomes scanty and resembles colostrum or soft cheese curd in thin serum. It may be tinged pink with blood or show a gray or brown discoloration. Within a few days the secretion is frankly purulent or curdy but there is an absence of large, firm clots. This abnormal secretion persists for weeks or even months.

Affected quarters are grossly swollen but the swelling is smooth, hard and almost painless and quite unlike the uneven fibrosis which occurs in most other types of mastitis, except that caused by *Mycobacterium lacticola*. Response to treatment is very poor and the swollen udders become grossly atrophied. In infection with one strain of the *Mycoplasma*, many cows do not subsequently come back into production although some may produce moderately well at the next lactation. With other strains there is clinical recovery in 1–4 weeks without apparent residual damage to the quarter.

Clinical pathology

The causative organism can be cultured without great difficulty and concurrent infection with other bacteria is common. A marked leukopenia, with counts as low as 1800–2500/μl, is present when clinical signs appear and persists for up to 2 weeks. Leukocyte counts in the milk are very high, usually over 20 million/ml. In the acute stages the organisms can usually be demonstrated by the examination of a milk film stained with Giemsa or Wright-Leishman stain. The fluorescent antibody technique may also be of value.

Necropsy findings

The disease is a purulent interstitial mastitis with granuloma formation as a common feature. There is cortical hyperplasia in the local lymph nodes and organisms are plentiful in the mammary tissue, subcutaneous edema fluid and in the lymph nodes.

Diagnosis

A presumptive diagnosis can be made on clinical grounds because of the unusual clinical findings but laboratory confirmation by culture of the organism is desirable.

The fact that the organism does not grow on standard media and other pathogenic bacteria are commonly present may lead to errors in the laboratory unless attention is drawn to the characteristic field findings.

Mycoplasma mastitis resembles that caused by *Mycobacterium lacticola*. They both occur commonly after intramammary infusion with oily materials and both show marked, smooth, painless hypertrophy of the udder. The secretions differ, however, and cultural examination serves to differentiate them accurately.

Treatment

None of the commonly used antibiotics are effective and oil–water emulsions used as infusions appear to increase the severity of the disease. Parenteral treatment with oxytetracycline (5 g daily for 3 days intravenously) has been shown to cause only temporary improvement. Because of the general sensitivity of *Mycoplasma* spp. to tylosin and erythromycin these two antibiotics should be tried, but unless treatment is administered very early the damage will already have been done.

Control

Prevention of introduction of the disease into a herd appears to depend upon avoidance of introductions, or of isolating introduced cows until they can be checked for mastitis. The disease spreads rapidly in a herd and affected animals should be culled immediately or placed in strict isolation until sale. Eradication of the disease from a large dairy herd has been achieved by culling infected cows identified by culture of milk and nasal swabs, especially at drying-off and calving (22). When eradication is completed the bulk milk cell count is the best single monitoring device to guard against reinfection. Intramammary infusions must be carried out with great attention to hygiene and preferably with individual tubes rather than multidose syringes. Most commercial teat dips are effective in control (14). Vaccination is a possible development (10) but is unlikely to be a satisfactory control measure because the observed resistance of a quarter to infection after a natural clinical episode is less than 1 year. There appears to be merit in the frequent culturing of bulk milk samples as a surveillance strategy for problem herds and areas (22).

REVIEW LITERATURE

Boughton, E. (1979) Mycoplasma bovis mastitis. *Vet. Bull.*, *49*, 377.
Bushnell, R. B. (1984) Mycoplasma mastitis. *Vet. Clin. N. Am. large Anim. Pract.*, *6(2)*, 301–312.
Jasper, D. E. (1981) Bovine mycoplasmal mastitis. *Adv. vet. Sci.*, *25*, 122–159.
Pfutzner, H. et al. (1983) Investigations on *Mycoplasma* mastitis in cattle. *Arch. exp. vet. Med.*, *37*, 361, 375, 383, 415.

REFERENCES

(1) Jurmanova, K. et al. (1986) *Arch. exp. vet. Med.*, *40*, 67.
(2) Alexander, P. G. et al. (1985) *Aust. vet. J.*, *62*, 135.
(3) Bennett, R. H. & Jasper, D. E. (1977) *Vet. Microbiol.*, *2*, 341.
(4) Pfutzner, H. et al. (1986) *Arch. exp. vet. Med.*, *40*, 56.
(5) Ruhnke, H. L. et al. (1976) *Can. J. comp. Med.*, *40*, 142.
(6) Vandeplassche, M. et al. (1979) *Vlaams Diergeneeskd. Tijdschr.*, *48*, 467.
(7) Jasper, D. E. et al. (1974) *Cornell Vet.*, *64*, 407.
(8) Gourlay, R. N. et al. (1974) *Vet. Rec.*, *95*, 534.
(9) Taoudi, A. & Kirchhoff, H. (1986) *Vet. Rec.*, *119*, 247.
(10) Boothby, J. T. et al. (1986) *Cornell Vet.*, *76*, 188.
(11) Boothby, J. T. et al. (1986) *Can. J. vet. Res.*, *50*, 200.
(12) Gourlay, R. N. (1973) *J. Am. vet. med. Assoc.*, *163*, 905.
(13) Jackson, G. et al. (1981) *Vet. Rec.*, *108*, 31.
(14) Jasper, D. E. et al. (1976) *Cornell Vet.*, *66*, 164.
(15) Jasper, D. E. et al. *(1979) Am. J. vet. Res.*, *40*, 1043.
(16) Ball, H. J. & Mackie, D. P. (1986) *Vet. Rec.*, *118*, 72.
(17) Mackie, D. P. et al. (1982) *Vet. Rec.*, *110*, 578.
(18) Mackie, D. P. et al. (1986) *Vet. Rec.*, *119*, 350.
(19) Pfutzner, H. et al. (1986) *Monatsh. VetMed.*, *41*, 382.
(20) Poumarat, F. et al. (1985) *Rec. Med. vet.*, *161*, 649.
(21) Hodges, R. T. et al. (1983) *NZ Vet. J.*, *31*, 60.
(22) Bicknell, S. R. et al. (1983) *Vet. Rec.*, *112*, 294.

MISCELLANEOUS MASTITIDES

Mastitis caused by *Fusobacterium necrophorum*

A high incidence of mastitis in one dairy herd has been attributed to infection with *Fusobacterium necrophorum*. Affected quarters showed viscid, clotty, stringy secretion but little fibrosis. No systemic reaction was apparent but treatment with a variety of antibiotics was unsuccessful (1).

Mastitis caused by *Pseudomonas aeruginosa*

Mastitis in cattle and sheep caused by *Pseudomonas aeruginosa* is rare and occurs usually as sporadic cases after intramammary infusion with contaminated material, *Pseudomonas* spp. being common in the environment of cattle. Occasionally it may be encountered as a herd problem with a number of animals affected and in this instance the infection may originate in contaminated water used for washing udders (4). An outbreak in ewes followed a milking machine breakdown (44). Serious outbreaks in cows have also occurred in association with the use of a suspected contaminated mastitis infusion (13, 26). The mastitis was clinically severe and the mortality rate was as high as 17% of affected cows. The contaminated material had been used as a dry-period treatment and the cows became affected soon after calving. Clinically there is a severe systemic reaction, acute swelling of the gland, and the appearance of clotted, discolored milk; function of the gland is usually completely lost at the first attack but recurrent crises may occur. Rarely, strains of this organism are highly virulent and cause fatal mastitis with generalized lesions. Less commonly still there is a high level of infection in a herd due to a contaminated water supply but with no clinical cases. Reinfection is common unless the source of infection is removed, even though there is apparent cure by treatment with spectinomycin (45). Experimentally the disease in goats is acute with extensive necrosis and fatal septicemia in some (6), and the natural disease in ewes is likely to be gangrenous and lethal (38) and accompanied by severe lameness in the hindlimb on the affected side (22). Treatment with antibiotics is generally unsuccessful. Daily infusions of streptomycin (1 g) or neomycin (0·5 g), or both combined with polymixin B, for 4 days are most commonly employed. Carbenicillin (Pyopen) should be effective but has given variable results (4). It is the best drug available for intramammary use. Gentamicin has some activity (8). The oral administration of an organic iodine compound and vaccination with a killed autogenous vaccine are credited with bringing the disease under control in one herd (9).

Mastitis caused by *Mycobacterium* spp.

Tuberculous mastitis has been dealt with under tuberculosis. Other mycobacteria, especially *Mycobacterium lacticola*, have been isolated from cases of mastitis in cattle which occur after the intramammary infusion of therapeutic agents in oils (11). The disease can be reproduced by the intramammary injection of the organism in oil but not in watery suspension. Subsequent oily infusions exacerbate the condition. Clinically there is tremendous hypertrophy of the quarter with the appearance of clots in discolored milk but there is no systemic reaction. Affected animals do not show sensitivity to avian or mammalian tuberculin. No effective treatment is recorded. It is suggested that the treatment of injured teats and quarters with oil-based intramammary preparations is inadvisable because of the risk of them already being infected with *Mycobacteria*.

A mild, acute mastitis, self-terminating and unresponsive to treatment has occurred in outbreak form (48). It may be unassociated with intramammary infusion but apparently predisposed to by stress and caused by an unidentified mycobacterium.

Mycobacterium fortuitum has been encountered as a cause of a severe outbreak of bovine mastitis (12). Infected quarters were seriously damaged, did not respond to treatment and affected cows died or were salvaged. The disease was reproduced experimentally and affected animals showed positive reactions to mammalian and avian tuberculosis and some sensitivity to johnin. Similar experiences are recorded with *M. smegmatis* (34) and *M. chelonei* (39). The mammary secretion of affected quarters varied from pus to a watery fluid containing flakes and there was a high milk loss and irreparable damage to quarters.

Mastitis caused by *Bacillus* spp.

Bacillus cereus and *B. subtilis* are saprophytic organisms and only chance pathogens. They have caused an acute hemorrhagic mastitis in cattle. *B. cereus* cases are often associated with contamination associated with teat injuries or surgery. Recent reports have described the occurrence of the mastitis in cows at the time of calving and associated with the feeding of brewers' grains in which the spores of *B. cereus* were present. In the former, the infection is thought to have occurred during the dry period following the use of dry cow therapy preparations which may have been contaminated with the organism (14, 16). Infection probably occurs at the time of infusion but the acute mastitis does not occur until after parturition. *Bacillus cereus* is a spore-former and may remain dormant in the mammary gland for long periods, unaffected by the presence of the antibiotic. In one outbreak, 62 of 67 cows infused with a dry cow infusion product contaminated with the organism developed acute hemorrhagic mastitis. Six cows died and the remainder survived but were subsequently culled and slaughtered due to recurrent mastitis, inadequate milk production and loss of weight.

Clinically there is peracute to acute mastitis affecting one or more quarters. There is severe swelling and pain and the secretions are red-tinged and serous in consistency. Initially there is a high fever (40–41°C, 104–106°F) and severe toxemia. Affected cows are weak and quickly become recumbent and death may occur in 24–36 hours. Gangrene may occur and in cows which survive, portions of affected gland will slough out and a chronic relapsing mastitis will persist. Experimentally produced mastitis due to *B. cereus* causes toxemia, acute swelling of the quarter and clots in the milk. The mastitis persists in a chronic form and the quarter eventually dries up (51).

The organism can usually be cultured from milk samples from affected quarters. At necropsy there is focal hemorrhagic necrosis of the mammary tissue, acute lymphadenitis and disseminated intravascular coagulation (17).

Treatment consists of intensive fluid therapy, chloramphenicol intravenously, and vigorous massage and stripping of the affected gland. Intramammary infusion of the most suitable antibiotic determined by culture and sensitivity is indicated but the results are often not good because of the presence of severe hemorrhage and necrosis and plugging of the lactiferous ducts. Prevention depends on the use of sterile techniques during teat surgery and the use of sterile intramammary infusions and instruments. In problem herds, autogenous bacterins have been prepared but not extensively evaluated (15). If *B. cereus* infection is identified in the mammary glands of dry cows the recommended prevention program is infusion of each quarter with 750 mg neomycin and 375 mg framycetin (27).

Bacillus subtilis is recorded less frequently as a cause of acute mastitis. It is also characterized by yellow or bloody milk, sometimes with clots, and the cow is febrile (50).

Mastitis caused by *Serratia* spp.

Serratia marcescens causes mild chronic mastitis in which clinical signs of swelling of the quarters with the presence of the clots in the milk appears periodically. It has been observed to occur naturally and has been produced experimentally (18, 41). Neomycin (2 g initially followed by three daily doses of 1 g by intramammary infusion) was successful as a treatment. *Serratia liquefaciens* has caused a similar mastitis (40). Most cases are sporadic but a herd outbreak is recorded (49) caused probably by the use of contaminated sawdust as bedding and inadequate cleaning of the teats before milking.

Mastitis caused by *Clostridium perfringens* type A

This is a rare form of mastitis (37) characterized by high fever, swelling and superficial hyperemia of the affected quarter, later followed by gangrene, enlargement of the supramammary lymph nodes, a thin brown secretion containing gas and subcutaneous emphysema.

Mastitis caused by *Campylobacter jejuni*

Only one case has been recorded (35) but the incident is of some importance because of its zoonotic impact. Infection of the udder by the organism is easy to establish and the infection is persistent but subclinical for the most part. Other experimental cases have been recorded (15) and campylobacters which have not been further identified (7) have also been observed in naturally occurring cases. These were characterized by fine granular clots in the milk, very high cell counts and a very transient episode of fever and swelling of the quarter.

Miscellaneous bacterial mastitides

Yersinia pseudotuberculosis has caused mastitis in an aborting goat doe which probably experienced a bout of systemic yersiniosis. The infection would have had zoonotic implications (42).

Haemophilus somnus has caused mild, chronic mastitis, an acute form with high fever and bloodstained milk, and a gangrenous form (43, 52).

Mastitis caused by fungi, yeasts and algae

Trichosporon spp. can cause mastitis in cattle and is manifested clinically by swelling of the gland and clots in the milk. The infection rate is low and the fungi disappear spontaneously. Experimental transmission of the disease has been effected (19).

Cryptococcus neoformans, the yeast which causes human cryptococcosis, has caused acute mastitis in cattle (21) and buffaloes (25). Contaminated infusion material and spread from other infected quarters are the probable source of infection. Infection in humans drinking the milk is unlikely to occur because the yeast does not withstand pasteurization but there may be some hazard to farm families. While there is no systemic reaction, the mastitis may be acute with marked swelling of the affected quarter and the supramammary lymph node, a severe fall in milk yield and the appearance of viscid, mucoid, gray-white secretion. Clinical mastitis persists for some weeks and, in many cases, subsides spontaneously, but in others the udder is so severely damaged that the cow has to be slaughtered. Systemic involvement occurs rarely. At necropsy, there is dissolution of the acinar epithelium and in chronic cases a diffuse or granulomatous reaction in the mammary tissue and lymph node. Similar lesions have been found in the lungs. Similar lesions in the mammary glands and in internal organs have also been observed in goats infected with *Cryptococcus neoformans* experimentally via the teat canal (31).

Many other yeasts including *Candida* sp., *Saccharomyces* sp., *Pichia* sp. and *Torulopsis* sp. (23), and *Aspergillus fumigatus* (20, 30) have also caused mastitis in cattle. A US survey of 91 bovine cases of fungal mastitis showed that 78% belonged to *Candida* sp. (10). The infection is probably introduced with contaminated intramammary infusions or teat cup liners (26). Establishment of the infection is encouraged by damage to the mammary epithelium and stimulated by antibiotic therapy; for example *Candida* spp. utilize penicillin and tetracylines as sources of nitrogen. A fever (41°C, 106°F) is accompanied by a severe inflammation of the quarter, enlargement of the supramammary lymph nodes, and a marked fall in milk yield. The secretion consists of large yellow clots in a watery, supernatant fluid. Lesions are limited to the walls of the milk cistern and there is no invasion of the mammary gland itself (46). Usually the disease is benign and spontaneous recovery following in about a week is the rule. With infection by *Aspergillus fumigatus* or *A. nidulans* there are multiple abscesses in the quarter. These are surrounded by granulation tissue, but the milk ducts are generally unaffected (20).

None of these infections respond well to antibiotic therapy but treatment with iodides, either sodium iodide intravenously, organic iodides by mouth, or iodine in oil as an intramammary infusion, might be of value. A number of drugs, including cycloheximide (Actidione), nystatin, polymixin B, neomycin and isoniazid, have been tested for efficiency against mastitis in cattle produced experimentally by the infusion of *Cryptococcus neoformans* but did not alter the clinical course of the disease (28). Merthiolate (20 ml of a 0·1% solution) as an infusion daily for 2–3 days is reported to have a beneficial effect if administered early in the course of the disease (29). Actinomycotic agents tested *in vitro* against fungi, mostly *Candida* sp. from cases of mastitis, showed sensitivity to clomitrazole, nystatin, polymyxin, miconazole, amphotericin B, and least sensitivity to 5 fluorocytosine (5). Miconazole (100 mg/l as an intramammary infusion, possibly supplemented by 400 mg doses given intravenously) is reported to produce good results (36). Sulfamethoxypyridazine given parenterally (22 mg/kg body weight for 2 or 3 days) has resulted in better than 50% clinical cures in quarters infected with *Candida krusei* (2).

Prototheca trispora and *P. zopfii* are algae which have been identified as causes of chronic bovine mastitis (24, 33). Reduced milk yield, large clots in watery milk and induration of the affected quarter may be the only clinical signs. Cases of this disease are usually sporadic but one severe outbreak is recorded (3). The organisms are common isolates from animal environments (47). Treatment is usually unsuccessful and affected cows should be culled. Because of a high prevalence rate in many affected herds the loss to the farmer can be considerable (3). Experimental transmission of the disease causes a progressive pyogranulomatous lesion in the gland and the organism can be isolated from draining lymph nodes (32).

Traumatic mastitis

Injuries to the teats or udder which penetrate to the teat cistern or milk ducts, or involve the external sphincter are commonly followed by mastitis. Any of the organisms which cause mastitis may invade the udder after such injury and in such cases mixed infections are usual. All injuries to the teat or udder, including surgical interference, should be treated prophylactically with wide-spectrum antibiotics.

REVIEW LITERATURE

Kirk, J. H. & Bartlett, P. C. (1968) Bovine mycotic mastitis. *Comp. cont. Educ.*, *8*, F106.

REFERENCES

(1) Simon, J. & McCoy, E. (1958) *J. Am. vet. med. Assoc.*, *133*, 165.
(2) Mackie, D. P. et al. (1987) *Vet. Rec.*, *120*, 48.
(3) Spalton, D. E. (1985) *Vet. Rec.*, *116*, 347.
(4) Malmo, J. et al. (1972) *Aust. vet. J.*, *48*, 137.
(5) McDonald, J. S. (1980) *Am. J. vet. Res.*, *41*, 1987
(6) Lepper, A. W. D. & Matthews, P. R. J. (1966) *Res. vet. Sci.*, *7*, 151.
(7) Logan, E. F. et al. (1982) *Vet. Rec.*, *110*, 229.
(8) Ziv, G. & Risenberg-Tirer, R. (1970) *Zentralbl. VetMed.*, *17B*, 963.
(9) van Kruiningen, H. J. (1963) *Cornell Vet.*, *53*, 240.
(10) Richards, J. L. et al. (1980) *Am. J. vet. Res.*, *41*, 1991.
(11) Richardson, A. (1971) *Cornell Vet.*, *61*, 640.
(12) Peterson, K. J. (1965) *J. Am. vet. med. Assoc.*, *147*, 1600.
(13) Osborne, A. D. et al. (1981) *Can. vet. J.*, *22*, 215.
(14) Gedek, W. (1986) *Tierärztl. Umschau*, *41*, 526.
(15) Lander, K. P. & Gill, K. P. W. (1980) *J. Hyg.*, *84*, 421.
(16) Perrin, D. et al. (1976) *Can. vet. J.*, *17*, 244.
(17) Schiefer, B. et al. (1976) *Can. vet. J.*, *17*, 239.
(18) Bowman, G. L. et al. (1986) *J. Am. vet. med. Assoc.*, *189*, 913.
(19) Murphy, J. M. & Drake, C. H. (1947) *Am. J. vet. Res.*, *8*, 43.
(20) Thompson, K. G. et al. (1978) *NZ vet. J.*, *26*, 176.
(21) Pal, M. & Mehrotra, B. S. (1983) *Mykosen*, *26*, 615.
(22) Honhold, N. & Carter, M. E. (1987) *Vet. Rec.*, *120*, 16.
(23) Bolck, G. et al. (1967) *Mh. VetMed.*, *22*, 289.
(24) Dion, W. M. (1982) *Can. vet. J.*, *23*, 272.
(25) Rahman, H. et al. (1983) *Vet. Rec.*, *112*, 16.
(26) Nicholls, T. J. et al. (1981) *Vet. Rec.*, *108*, 93.
(27) Heer, A. et al. (1987) *Prakt. Tierärztl.*, *68*, 40.
(28) Redaelli, G. & Rosaschino, F. (1957) *Arch. vet. ital.*, *8*, 311.
(29) Immer, J. (1965) *Schweiz. Arch. Tierheilkd.*, *107*, 206.
(30) Walser, K. & Kleinschroth, E. (1979) *Berl. Münch. Tierärztl. Wochenschr.*, *92*, 129.
(31) Lohan, C. B. et al. (1977) *Haryana agric. Univ. J. Res.*, *7*, 67.
(32) McDonald, J. S. et al. (1984) *Am. J. vet. Res.*, *45*, 592.
(33) Schick, W. & Kutzer, H. (1982) *Monatsh. VetMed.*, *37*, 295.
(34) Heide, L. et al. (1978) *Monatsh. VetMed.*, *33*, 164.
(35) Morgan, G. et al. (1985) *Vet. Rec.*, *116*, 111.
(36) VanDamme, D. M. (1983) *Vet. Med. SAC*, *78*, 1425.
(37) Johnston, A. M. (1986) *Vet. Rec.*, *118*, 728.
(38) Bachh, A. S. & Pathak, R. C. (1986) *Ind. J. anim Sci.*, *56*, 391.
(39) Menard, L. et al. (1983) *Can. vet. J.*, *24*, 305.
(40) Nicholls, T. J. & Barton, M. G. (1981) *Vet. Rec.*, *109*, 288.
(41) Isaksson, A. & Holmberg, O. (1984) *Nord. vet. Med.*, *36*, 354.
(42) Jones, T. O. (1982) *Vet. Rec.*, *110*, 231.
(43) Hazlett, M. J. et al. (1983) *Can. vet. J.*, *24*, 135.
(44) Rapoport, E. & Bar-Moshe, B. (1986) *Israel J. vet. Med.*, *42*, 203.
(45) Kirk, J. H. & Bartlett, P. C. (1984) *J. Am. vet. med. Assoc.*, *184*, 671.
(46) Dion, W. M. & Dukes, T. W. (1982) *Sabouraudia*, *20*, 95.
(47) Schuster, H. & Blaschke-Hellmessen, R. (1983) *Monatsh. VetMed.*, *38*, 24.
(48) Schultze, W. D. et al. (1985) *Am. J. vet. Res.*, *46*, 42.
(49) Holmgren, O. (1984) *Nord. vet. Med.*, *36*, 354.
(50) Fossum, K. (1986) *Nord. vet. Med.*, *38*, 233.
(51) Horvath, G. et al. (1986) *Acta vet. Hung.*, *34*, 29.
(52) Armstrong, K. R. et al. (1986) *Can. vet. J.*, *27*, 211.

THE CONTROL OF BOVINE MASTITIS

During the 1970s there were good developments in the techniques for controlling bovine mastitis. These developments were teamed with existing techniques for the maintenance of reproductive efficiency and promoted as the basis for total herd health programs which would provide a schedule of regular visits to dairy herds to conduct disease prevention work. What has happened in intensive dairy areas has been an almost complete elimination of food animal veterinarians from the mastitis control part of the program during the past few years, and they now find themselves relegated again to the familiar role of problem-solvers when mastitis outbreaks occur in individual herds.

Two major influences have guided the development of mastitis control and brought about this change. The NIRD program, the basis of all current mastitis control, was designed to function without participation by veterinarians but it could be supplemented by having a veterinarian in attendance to monitor progress and predict danger. The monitoring procedure was based on the collection of milk samples and the laboratory assessment of the status of all quarters of all cows. The advent, first of bulk milk cell counts, followed by individual cow cell counts, has made the process of monitoring much less expensive and laborious and has eliminated any need for participation in the program by veterinarians unless a problem arises. It is still feasible for veterinarians to include a monitoring and advisory system in a computerized herd health program (106) and the rewards to the farmer are high. However, veterinarians are not involved in actual mastitis work with the cows, and practitioners generally find difficulty in charging without physically performing a service for which a fee can be charged.

In the following section of the text the control program which utilizes veterinarians is included because the more advanced system based on individual cow cell counts and the NIRD program is not available everywhere. The text also provides a program suitable for use in problem herds.

Limitation of infection versus eradication

Although mastitis due to *Str. agalactiae* has been eradicated from individual herds, bovine mastitis is not, in terms of practicality, an eradicable disease at the herd or area level. For this reason it does not lend itself to legislative control but rather to voluntary involvement by dairymen in programs aimed at reducing its incidence and maintaining the infection rate at a low level. Because the justification for control of the disease is purely economic, any control program must be based on its applicability on each individual farm. Generally area controls is not a feasible objective and a national program can only be in the form of providing incentives and assistance to individual dairymen who wish to participate.

A difference of opinion exists about the desirability of complete eradication versus limitation of infection rate in relation to the occurrence of coliform mastitis, and the matter is dealt with in some detail under that heading. In general the argument revolves around the concept that subclinical mastitis causes a continuous low level leukocytosis in the milk which acts as a protective mechanism against other infections. Present-day knowledge about immunity in the mammary gland suggests that control programs that reduce milk cell counts to unrealistically low levels may reduce the glands' resistance (60). Correspondingly the complete elimination of common udder pathogens such as *Str. agalactiae* and *Staph. aureus* is thought to increase the susceptibility of the udder to the normally chance pathogens, especially the coliforms. Another point of view is that the commonly encountered intramammary resident, but lowly pathogenic *Corynebacterium bovis* may be the significant microbial agent in maintaining the resistance of udders. The mastitic effect of this organism is too low to warrant action against it but the infection rate with pathogenic bacteria is significantly lower in quarters that harbor it than in those that do not (1). An intensive program to disinfect udders could well eliminate *Cor. bovis* and increase susceptibility to other pathogens. There is good field evidence to suggest that this is in fact happening in North America and the United Kingdom. It is likely to be more important where cows are housed, and therefore more exposed to teat contamination with coliforms. All of the criticism about the increasing numbers of clinical cases which occur in herds on the control program and which have achieved very low levels of udder infection, as indicated by very low bulk milk cell counts, comes from the United Kingdom where the most durable program, the NIRD program, originated. The matter is still unresolved (61, 62).

One of the characteristics of the NIRD program is that it is effective especially in herds where infections with *Str. agalactiae* and *Staph. aureus* predominate. *Str. uberis* and *Str. dysgalactiae* infections are not significantly affected (67).

Modern mastitis control programs—general principles

Current mastitis control programs have as their objective the limitation of prevalence of mastitis to a level which in the particular circumstances is economically achievable. Nowhere has complete eradication been shown to be the appropriate target.

Modern day policy with respect to mastitis control is to approach it in two stages:

- A *mastitis awareness scheme* (57) that sets out to alert dairy farmers generally to the losses caused by mastitis and to identify those herds which have a problem. Almost universally this is done by conducting somatic cell counts on bulk milk from the herd
- Having alerted individual farmers to the fact that they have a mastitis problem it is necessary to be prepared with a mastitis control program known to be effective in limiting the occurrence of the disease
- Although mastitis is identified as a cause of massive wastage in dairying, and in spite of the existence of these highly effective control programs, the awareness by farmers of the importance of mastitis, especially subclinical mastitis, is poor (11, 66). The adoption of basis procedures such as teat dipping and dry period treatment is usually only about 25%. Partly as a means of overcoming this reluctance, mastitis control has been incorporated into planned health and production programs which promote control of reproduction, mastitis and other diseases, and maintenance of milk production at financially optimal levels.

To be effective a mastitis control program must

- Provide an economic advantage
- Be within the scope of the dairyman's technical skill and understanding
- Be capable of introduction into the management system employed
- Encourage farmers by rapidly reducing the occurrence of clinical mastitis.

Most of the control programs of the past have not satisfied these criteria, and on most dairy farms in developed areas, even today, mastitis control depends on the treatment of clinical cases and the use of relatively ineffective hygiene techniques in the milking parlor. As a result, subclinical cases go undetected and the continuous spread to further quarters goes on relatively unchecked. In most dairy populations the percentage of quarters infected is in the range of 25–50% and the resulting financial losses are very heavy. What is required is a control program which satisfies the above criteria and is capable of being applied at various levels of intensity to accommodate various levels of profitability, with the object of limiting the quarter infection rate to a predetermined level. The two criteria necessary to limit the quarter infection rate are (*a*) reduction of the new infection rate and (*b*) reduction of the infected status of infected quarters.

All of these criteria are satisfied in the NIRD mastitis control program which has the capacity of quickly reducing the quarter infection rate (from 30 to 10%) and the number of clinical cases by half (67). As a generalization it would be fair to say that the program is capable of reducing the quarter infection rate (QIR) by 50% in one year and by 75% by the end of the second or third years, depending on the energy with which the program is applied. This is subject, of course, to the preexistence of a standard QIR of 25–30%. The net value of the program will depend on the value of the increased production and the cost of implementation of the program. Where whole milk for human consumption is the end-product these values are likely to be of the order of $40–80 and $10–15 respectively, giving a return to investment of 250–500% (4, 67).

The NIRD program

The basic control program is the one developed at the National Institute for Research in Dairying at Reading, England (6). It has the virtues of simplicity, profitability and widespread applicability because it does not depend on laboratory diagnosis. It is set out in detail below but it is also suggested that the program is susceptible to desirable modification for individual farms by the inclusion of veterinary surveillance and laboratory diagnosis (8). Most countries with a significant dairy industry have devised their own variant of the NIRD program to suit their own local needs.

There is no doubt from the many reports available and from our personal experience of the NIRD program that its application for a very large population of dairy cattle could be very rapid indeed and could reduce the wastage due to mastitis by 65% within the space of a year and at very low cost. Without doubt the program is one of the most profitable ever offered to farmers. It is our experience that the average return to investment can be 300–500%. However, three problems can arise and, in the provision of an individually tailored service to a farmer, some attempt should be made to overcome them, provided this can be done in a financially rewarding manner. The most important problem is that the NIRD program is unsupervised and the average farmer, having witnessed the dramatic reduction in clinical cases which usually occurs, is likely to relax the intensity of the several techniques and allow a recrudescence of the disease. A monitoring system is desirable, if not essential. Bulk milk cell counts do provide such a system but they are seriously inaccurate, and a bad mastitis situation could develop in a herd before a warning was given. Periodic sampling of a portion of the herd is a suitable alternative.

The second problem with the NIRD program is that it is designed for the control of the common mastitis pathogens and at the average level of incidence. Absence of a diagnostic examination could result in the application of a control program to a herd with a 'free electricity' problem rather than mastitis, or to infection with *Nocardia* spp. or with a quarter infection of less than 10%, in none of which is measurable improvement likely to occur. The frequency of such occurrences will be so small that they will be nationally insignificant but they could be very significant to individual farmers. Whether the problem herds are revealed by the failure of the program or by a preliminary diagnostic examination may be immaterial, but in terms of providing the best available veterinary service to a client the latter course is recommended.

A third problem arises when the program is not supervised, or at least serviced, by a veterinarian. It is the same problem that occurs in any disease control program unless there is someone in a supervisory capacity to cajole, chide and encourage the farmer and the milker into maintaining the very few labor inputs that the system needs. Without this supervision progress can be achieved, however, but in a limited rather than a dramatic manner (10).

The control program was devised to attack the occurrence of mastitis at those points at which the quarter infection rate (QIR) was multiplied (the QIR having been established as the index of severity of the disease in the herd). The points of attack were to reduce the new infection rate by hygienic measures, and to reduce the duration of infections by therapeutic means.

The basic program is:

1. Reduction of duration of infection.
   (*a*) Treat all quarters of all cows at drying off.
   (*b*) Treat clinical cases as they occur; detect clinical cases by inline filter.
   (*c*) Cull chronic clinical cases.
2. Reduction of new infection rate.
   (*d*) Dip all teats after each milking.
   (*e*) Adequately service and maintain milking machine.
   (*f*) Backflush cups after each milking and rinse off udder before milking, both with running water.

There are many additional options and these are set down in the following paragraphs.

Reducing the duration of the infection

To properly reduce the source of infection for the herd includes treatment and culling of infected cows. This can be done effectively by treating all quarters of all cows. The alternative is to identify the affected quarters. Attitudes to how this should be done have altered dramatically during the past few years, especially with respect to subclinically infected quarters.

Detection of infected quarters

Clinical cases

When cows are tied in and milked *in situ* the use of a strip cup is mandatory. In a milking parlor, especially when there is plenty of running water, squirting of the first streams of milk onto a black tile on the floor is adequate. Before recommending this as an additional measure, it should be remembered that in herds where the quarter infection rate is already high this may, in fact, cause an exacerbation of the number of clinical cases in the herd unless special instruction is given on how to squirt milk without causing reflux of milk up into the milk cistern. The matter is further discussed below. An alternative is the installation of in-milk-line stainless steel filters (25). These pick out clots in the milk so that they are readily seen. They have the disadvantages that the clots block the milk-line and the cups fall off, which keeps mastitic milk out of the milk vat, but upsets work flow in a busy shed, and they do not pick up the cows with watery milk but very few clots.

Subclinical infected quarters

Whether or not to embark on a strategy of attempting to detect these subclinical quarters has become a very important option in mastitis control. When the NIRD program was developed it was designed on the presumption that laboratory services were not available, perhaps not even necessary, and that veterinarians were not available to participate in at least the decision-making of the program. It is now evident that dry-period treatment of all quarters is under critical review and that selective treatment is likely to be universally adopted. Also, the balance of occurrence rate of individual pathogens is swinging gradually away from *Streptococcus agalactiae* and *Staphylococcus aureus* and towards the Gram-negative and exotic pathogens. Both changes make a bacteriological diagnosis much more desirable. It is still the case that a laboratory examination is expensive and if they are adopted generally the logistic strain on laboratories will be heavy.

Two strategies are in use; both include the use of a preliminary screening test using minimal laboratory facilities and minimal labor. *Strategy No. 1* is to make use of milk samples collected for herd (butterfat and yield) testing. These are suitable for submission to the individual cow milk cell count (ICMCC) which can be carried out on an automatic cell counter at low cost. Details are provided under the heading of clinical pathology, but specifically those quarters with cell counts of over 800 000 cells/ml are considered to be positive. Positive quarters may be classified as affected and no further investigation undertaken, lending itself to the criticism that the diagnosis is one of 'cell countosis' rather than mastitis. To proceed beyond this point follow steps 2–4 in *strategy No. 2*. A decision on whether to attempt microbiological identification of the pathogen can be made on the following grounds. If a herd owner has a problem and calls for assistance it is obligatory to carry out a full laboratory examination of at least a representative sample of the herd. However, where it is intended to encourage a widespread use of a control program, it is reasonable practice to omit any examination at all in the first instance. At the end of the first year of the program it will be apparent on the basis of bulk milk cell count and prevalence of clinical cases which farmers have a successful operation and which do not. *Strategy 2* can then be applied to these problem herds. It gives satisfactory results at reasonable cost, and includes:

- Screening all quarter samples by submitting them to the California mastitis test (CMT)
- Identifying infected quarters by microbiological examination of quarters giving a CMT reading of 1 or higher
- Identifying bacteria generally on simple culture, but *Streptococcus agalactiae* identified as cAMP–positive and the pathogenicity of *Staphylococcus aureus* identified by determining whether it is coagulase-positive
- Determining the microbiological sensitivity of the pathogens.

Choosing between the CMT and ICMCC presents problems at the present time (1983) because the CM test is well understood, but is labor-intensive and very subject to variation in interpretation; ICMCC avoids both of these disadvantages, but is still not completely documented.

Reducing the new infection rate

Treatment

Treatment of infected quarters in lactating cows

These cows and quarters may be identified because they are presented as clinical cases in which situation treatment is obligatory. The preferred treatments for each bacterial type of mastitis are set down under the respective headings. On the other hand, if the quarters are identified as being infected during an across-the-herd survey, or a representative sampling either during a routine check or because there is a mastitis problem, a number of options are available. In general terms, infected quarters are best left untreated until the dry period. This policy is derived from the need to avoid loss of milk withheld from sale because of antibiotic content. However, withholding milk from a high-producing cow for 72 hours during treatment and for 72 hours afterwards represents a significant loss, especially if there is no alternative use for the milk. Two unhappy outcomes may result; the farmer may give an incomplete course of treatment or he may return the milk to the human food chain before time. The penalty for the latter can be very severe.

If the cow is a heavy producer and is in early lactation, and if the infection is *Str. agalactiae* in which the recovery rate is high, treatment during lactation needs to be considered. The decision will be based on whether the gain of additional milk production for the lactation will compensate for the cost of treatment and the need to withhold milk. Most observers agree that the milk gained by treating subclinical but infected quarters during lactation does little more than pay for the costs of treatment, but that in some instances where further spread is likely treatment of these cases may be desirable (89). Another reason for departing from the policy of delaying treatment until the dry period could be a very high prevalence of infection, in which case it is necessary to reduce the degree of environmental contamination quickly or even face the extreme situation of a threat to discontinue acceptance of the milk at the receiving depot because of its poor quality.

If the infection in the herd is predominantly *Staphylococcus aureus*, the recovery rate for treatment during lactation is so small that only pressing arguments should lead to introducing it. The Scandinavian countries have always persisted with treatment during lactation, but there is no cost-benefit analysis of the system available (5).

Dry-period treatment

This is carried out at the end of the last milking before the cow is turned out. In seasonal dairying areas farmers would prefer to dry off their cows over a 2 or 3-week period, bring them all in when the last one is dry and treat them all. This method permits a large number of infections to develop in the period right after drying-off, the most dangerous period. It also provides an opportunity for a flare-up of chemical mastitis when the treatment is infused into a quarter which has no secretion in it. Although chlortetracycline is extensively used in the treatment of lactating cows it should not be used in dry cows because of its tendency to cause chemical mastitis especially when the udder is competely dry.

The target of dry-period treatments is the group of significant pathogens that reside in the udder, for example, *Staphylococcus aureus*, *Streptococcus agalactiae*, *Str. dysgalactiae*, *Str. uberis* and *Corynebacterium (Actinomyces) pyogenes*. Incidentally, there is a significant cure rate in infections of *Corynebacterium bovis* and coagulase-negative *Staphylococcus* spp. (76) but whether this is desirable or not is open to debate.

Standard dry-period treatment is not an adequate protection against new infections that occur in the few days before calving. Only a second treatment during the last 1 or 2 weeks of pregnancy is effective against that occurrence, but great care is required with the administration of the treatment because of the high susceptibility to infection of the mammary gland at this time. The second intramammary infusion should be a low persistency product in contrast to the high persistency product used at the beginning of the drying-off period (100) otherwise there is a strong possibility that there will be antibiotic contamination of the first milk of the lactation (78).

Choice of intramammary infusion

Because of the preponderance of *Staphylococcus aureus* infection the recommended antibiotics are benzathine cloxacillin, neomycin and novobiocin, but more important is the need for the antibiotic to be in a longacting base because most dry-period new infections arise in the first 3 weeks of the drying-off period, and a good slow-release base with a suitable antibiotic will maintain a minimum effective concentration (MEC) for 25 days. Besides the base in which the drug is suspended it is desirable to use an antibiotic which has an affinity for binding to mammary tissue and secretions, and is therefore likely to remain in the udder rather than be absorbed into the bloodstream. The antibiotics most likely to be satisfactory in this respect are neomycin, dihydrostreptomycin, spiramycin, polymyxin B, cloxacillin, novobiocin and phenoxymethyl penicillin (12).

A present preoccupation in dry-period treatment is the inclusion of a dye in the infusion with the objective of marking the first milking of the ensuing lactation as being contaminated with antibiotics. This has not been finally achieved because of the difficulty of matching the milk-out times of the dye and the antibiotic and infusion vehicle (15). The possibility of antibiotic being carried over into the first milk for the lactation is high if the infusion has been administered during the last 6 weeks of pregnancy (59).

The range of suitable products for use as dry-cow therapy is not wide. They are set down in Table 45. Benzathine cloxacillin (0·5–1·0 g) in a longacting base gives excellent results. A mixture of sodium novobiocin (500 mg) and penicillin (500 000 units) is equally effective (80). Procaine penicillin G alone has a mixed reputation. In a longacting base it does prevent new infections with *Cor. (Actinomyces) pyogenes* during the dry period (18), but it is of mediocre efficiency in eliminating staphylococci and streptococci (19). These results are achieved with standard dose rates of 100 000 units procaine penicillin plus 0·5 or 1·0 g of streptomycin; increasing the amount of penicillin to 1 million units (MU) greatly enhances the activity of the product against staphylococci (21). These products are now in general use for dry-period treatment largely because of their cheapness. Errors can creep in if a smaller dose rate of penicillin is used in an attempt to reduce costs even further. Spiramycin (500 mg) is less effective (15). Neomycin (500 mg) or furaltadone (500 mg) in procaine penicillin (500 mg) are also extensively used, especially because of their activity against Gram-negative bacteria, but their efficiency against the totality of bacteria likely to be encountered is relatively low (22). Cephalonium (250 mg) has also shown excellent results against a wide range of bacteria especially staphylococci (101).

Technique of mammary infusion

One of the serious problems associated with dry-period treatment is the high prevalence of new infections, some of them disastrous to the cow or to the quarter, after the infusion. It is essential that maximum asepsis be observed for the operation, especially to avoid introduction of skin-based infections. It is also recommended that the infusion be introduced only into the teat canal and not into the teat sinus, the common practice in treatment during lactation (14). The infusion of amounts of penicillin–streptomycin longacting preparation as small as 0·25 and 0·1 ml into the teat canal at drying-off significantly reduces the new infection rate during the

Table 45. Comparative efficiencies of intramammary treatments of mastitis in dry cows

		Cure rate (%)			
Preparation	*Dose*	*Staphylococcus*	*Streptococcus*	*Coliform*	*Recommended use*
Benzathine cloxacillin	500 mg	84	94	Not effective	Effective, expensive, use for infected quarters, cheaper preparation for non-infected
Procaine penicillin + novobiocin	1 million units (MU) 500 mg	84	94	Not effective	Identical results to benzathine cloxacillin; identical recommendation
Procaine penicillin + dihydrostreptomycin	1 million units (MU) 1 g	87	96	Effective	Should be of advantage against coliforms
Procaine penicillin + dihydrostreptomycin	100 000 units (U) 100 mg	54	90	Unknown	Dose of dihydrostreptomycin is small; cheap; use for non-infected quarters
Neomycin (Neodry)	500 mg	62	65	89	Use for quarters infected with coliforms
Procaine penicillin + furaltadone	100 000 units (U) 500 mg	67	94	100	Good broad-spectrum result

dry period (79), but the technique has not been tested in a large-scale field trial.

Selective versus all-quarter dry-period treatment
One of the undecided questions about dry-period treatment is whether or not all quarters should be treated. The general recommendation is that all quarters be treated and this is fine when the infection rate is 40–50% of quarters. But the resulting complete sterilization of quarters and a fall in leukocyte count possibly leading to infection just before or at calving with a potent pathogen such as *Escherichia coli* is what the herd owner fears most. There is no proof that this is a significant occurrence (5) but there is evidence of an increase in coliform infections compared to other pathogens after dry-period treatment (13). The subject of the role of *Corynebacterium bovis* in the prevention of infection by other bacteria is discussed under the heading of mastitis caused by *Corynebacterium* spp. Also the treatments are not inexpensive and if the infected quarters are 10% or less the reduction of the treatment cost by 75% would be a useful saving. In herds with *Streptococcus uberis* infection as a problem selective therapy appears to enhance the prospects of new infections with this bacteria (99). In herds with a low prevalence of infection and low average cell count no significant gain in production or profitability is achieved (105). The alternative method is to sample the cows before drying-off and treat only the infected quarters. A middle-of-the-road strategy is to treat all infected quarters with a high efficiency product such as benzathine cloxacillin (500 mg), and the uninfected with a less effective but much cheaper product such as procaine penicillin 100 000 units with streptomycin (500 mg).

Selective dry-period therapy
The advantages of treating only infected quarters at drying-off are the saving in cost, especially when only 8–10% of quarters are infected, and the avoidance of total sterilization of all quarters, with a resulting possible increase in susceptibility to infection. This appears to have been realized in New Zealand where cows with low cell counts, and which have been treated during the dry period, have had a higher level of clinical mastitis than untreated controls (94). The disadvantages are that selecting the quarters to treat at drying-off will mean that new infections which develop between then and calving will be missed, and the accuracy of the methods used to select infected quarters varies widely. In spite of the conclusion from an intensive examination of selective treatment programs that none of them has been shown to be superior to the treatment of all quarters at drying-off (58), there are many programs which do precisely that and which are in use. Some samples are quoted.

One method used satisfactorily in herd health programs where herds are visited regularly each month, is the testing of quarter milk samples with a CMT and microbiological examination of those quarters which return a positive CMT at a score of 1 or greater. Only quarters infected with coagulase-positive *Staph. aureus* and *Str. agalactiae*, *Str. dysgalactiae* and *Str. uberis* are treated. A similar program in which the California mastitis test is administered 8 weeks before drying off is found to be very discriminating, simple and economic. It avoids the false positives (about 23%) which develop in the last 8 weeks of lactation as a result of normal desquamation of mammary epithelium. To avoid too much laboratory work the results of the CMT are taken as diagnostic without the need for bacteriological culture (7). A further variant of treating all quarters in all cows treated is that it doubles the number of quarters treated. There are two options using the CMT: to carry out the test at the cow, or back at a laboratory where the results are likely to be more consistent and reproducible.

Another method of detecting infected cows, as set out in detail in clinical pathology, is by the use of individual cow somatic milk cell counts (81). This has the great advantage of economy because the test is carried out on a composite milk sample which has already been collected for milk fat testing. It has the disadvantage of inaccuracy unless several tests are run and the results averaged, two tests 1 month apart being suggested as minimum. The method identifies infected cows and if selective therapy is to be applied only to infected quarters it is necessary to re-examine the nominated cows using a CMT to identify the quarters. This is usually done at drying-off (56). Another disadvantage is that cell counts differ widely in affected quarters depending largely on the type of infection present. Thus, *Streptococcus agalactiae* infections are associated with high cell counts and *Staphylococcus aureus* with low ones so that quarters and cows with this infection are more likely to be missed by this technique unless the threshold is set so low that many unaffected cows are classified as positive. The method is not as accurate as the CMT and cannot be used for individual quarter sampling as can this test, but it does not require a special visit to the farm. Much remains to be done with this technique before an exact protocol can be spelled out, but all the indications are that it will become a permanent part of mastitis control programs. It has the advantage that it may pinpoint badly affected cows during lactation and be a guide to lactation-period treatment.

As a general recommendation for the present, the following guidelines should be used when only one test is applied: normal counts are less than 400 000 cells/ml; suspicious counts are 400 000–800 000 cells/ml; positive counts are more than 800 000 cells/ml. The recommended target for a herd is 90% of the herd with counts less than 400 000/ml. Cows with counts greater than 400 000/ml should be treated during the dry period. Treatment of such quarters during lactation should only be done if the positive cell count is supported by a positive CMT and a positive cultural result obtained from CMT-positive quarters (55).

Many variants of the protocol, particularly relating to the number of tests carried out, the timing of the last one, and the cell counts which are regarded as being critical, have been and are still being tried with the objective of finding the most accurate and least expensive program. Provided sampling is done for another purpose and is not chargeable to the program, frequent testing is acceptable. One program with 86% accuracy in detecting infected quarters is based on two ICMCCs, with a critical count of 500 000 cells/ml or greater, and a CMT result at drying-off of two or greater (56). A New Zealand system (9) based on five tests during lactation and the treatment with a dry-cow preparation of those cows with mean cell counts of over 300 000 cells/ml was gainful in terms of subsequent production. A subsequent trial in the United States fixes the threshold at 400 000 cells/ml. Below this the program could be financially disadvantageous (90).

Cell counts in the milk of individual cows or quarters
Cell counts in the milk of individual cows are easily performed with automatic equipment. They are subject to a great deal of variation over quite short periods so that they lack dependability as a diagnostic tool. Nevertheless, they are being used in this way and also included in a computerized herd health program as an indicator of udder health (75). To overcome the variability of the count requires frequent sampling and averaging the samples. There is a strong positive correlation between cell counts estimated in this way and the number of clinical cases which will occur, with milk yield of individual quarters (72) and between cell count and California mastitis test reaction. The value of the ICMCC in mastitis control is set out under that heading.

Monitoring quarter infection rate
Once a program is under way it becomes a matter of importance to monitor the results. This is for two purposes. One is to check that the program is working against the causative agents in the particular herd; the other is to check that the program is being properly applied. There are three ways of applying such surveillance. The cheapest and least satisfactory is to keep check on the number of clinical cases treated, often by monitoring consumption of treatment tubes. A more effective method is to have cell counts or California mastitis tests carried out on bulk milk samples at regular, say weekly, intervals. This probably should be done at the milk depot anyway as a check point in quality milk control. The technique is not inexpensive and although it is generally favored (6) as a monitoring system it lacks accuracy (24) for individual herds. For a control program which is under veterinary supervision the method is not good enough. Suitable alternatives are the sampling of cows being dried off and individual cow milk cell counts as set out under selective dry-period treatment.

Teat dipping or spraying
Excellent results in preventing new infections are obtained by the use of suitable teat dips (26, 70). This effectiveness includes herds infected with *Staph. aureus* and the technique is the basis of modern control programs. Teat dips are in general only effective against streptococci and staphylococci and the increasing importance of coliforms is creating a need for new agents. Caution is needed when recommending a teat dip because some commercially available products may be ineffective, due either to overdilution of the disinfectant agent (68), to a formulation that renders it ineffective, or because of skin irritation. All teats of all cows are dipped or sprayed after each milking. The most satisfactory method of application is complete immersion of the teat and the base of the udder in the solution. But dipping is just too time-consuming in fast herringbone sheds and diluted dipping solutions are sprayed on (69). Spraying does not really reduce disinfection time, coverage of the teat is incomplete and much of the costly solution is wasted; up to five times as much spray may be used compared to teat dipping (28). What comparisons have been done (27) suggest that there is not a great deal of difference between spraying and dipping, because the sphincter is covered whichever method is used (71). There is a great need for an efficient automatic method.

The teat dipping solution must be as cheap as possible, be effective at killing bacteria on the teat skin and remain effective until the next milking (35) even if cows are walking through long, wet grass, but be non-irritant to the skin of teats and hands. Iodophor solutions containing 1% of available iodine, hypochlorite solutions containing 4% of free chlorine and with negligible free alkali, and chlorhexidine (Hibitane) 0·5 or 1% in polyvinylpyrrolidone solution or as 0·3% aqueous solution have been shown to be effective. Iodophor dips are expensive but efficient. A commercial bleach (Chlorox) in the United States meets the requirements of a 4% available chlorine dip (of 0·08% sodium hydroxide, 0·3% sodium carbonate, 0·17% sodium chlorate and 4·5% sodium chloride), but other commercially available products generally contain too much alkali and cause severe skin irritation. The choice between iodophors and chlorine teat dips, used at recommended concentrations of 4% and 1%, depends on price and susceptibility of the herd to teat chapping; there is no difference in efficiency (29). Chlorhexidine (0·2%) has similar efficiency (30), and 1·94% linear dodecylbenzene sulfonic acid (48) and 1·5% dodecylaminoalkyl glycine (38) have performed well experimentally.

Chapping of teats is a common sequel to constant use of teat dips. The usual remedy is to add a skin emollient to the dip; mineral (paraffin) oil or lanolin are the usual products and when these are added by the farmer they can seriously reduce the bactericidal effectiveness of the dip. Glycerin is a common additive in commercial dips, but at the usual levels of admixing, 15–33 %, it also reduces the dip's bactericidal effect (39). Soluble lanolin appears not to have this effect and is recommended (26). What appears to be an even greater improvement is a mixture of methylglucoside and urea instead of lanolin.

Teat dipping in iodophors does increase the iodine content of the milk (38). The permissible level varies with countries: in Europe the limit is 1000 μg/liter; in Australia it is 500 μg/liter (31). Concern about this pollution of milk has generated investigation of the minimum effective concentration which appears to be 0·1% iodine (3·5 ppm of free iodine) rather than the 1·0% usually recommended (16). The use of the 0·1% dip significantly reduces the milk iodine content compared to the 1·0% preparation (39). This has attracted the attention of organizations concerned with maintaining the purity of foods to the extent that iodophor teat dips are now prohibited in some areas. For this and financial reasons the choice of teat dip is an important one. There is no rule of thumb available as a guide to efficiency except that oily teat dips are the least successful (2). Teat sealants of several types and used at drying-off are discussed under that heading.

Udder washing and teat stripping

It has been adequately shown that the new infection rate is reduced significantly if the teats are stripped (a few squirts milked out) before premilking washing rather than after (28), and if the stripping is done in such a way that there is no chance of refluxing milk from the teat cup into the udder (29). It is generally accepted that before-milking and after-milking strippings do tend to reduce the new infection rate, but the effect is not likely to be significant unless the rate is already high (65).

Udder washing and teat sanitization (or disinfection)

At the present time the commonest procedure to prepare the cow for milking and to improve the milk quality is to wash the teats and lower udder with running water, preferably warmed. The dilution of contamination on the skin appears to be sufficient to reduce intramammary infection to a suitable level (102). Physical manipulation during washing and drying of the teats on a single-use paper towel reduce bacterial contamination of the teats, but the addition of standard teat sanitizers to the wash-water does not. In fully automated milking sheds the wash-water is sprayed from fixed nozzles in the floor. The procedure is also calculated to promote milk letdown, although this probably needs the application of squeezing pressure to the teat rather than just wetting. Manual stimulation of the udder encourages speedy letdown, but not necessarily complete letdown. In areas where water supplies are limited chemical sanitization is necessary. Individual paper towels are used, or cloth towels boiled after each use on one cow. The same procedure may also be adopted in addition to udder washing when a 'partial hygiene' program is attempted. In these circumstances it is usual to wear disinfected rubber gloves during milking.

The chemical to be used is important but more harm is usually done by the inappropriate use of an effective agent than by the use of poor preparations. Some recommendations are generally applicable. The cost of some highly efficient disinfectants for application to the udder is prohibitive in some circumstances. Chlorhexidine (Hibitane), a diguanide compound, in a solution containing a detergent (alkylaryl polyether alcohol) is highly efficient when used in the proportion of 4–8 g/liter of water, i.e. 1:5000. Quaternary ammonium compounds as 0·2% solutions, compounds containing iodine and phosphorus (iodophors) used in solutions containing at least 100 ppm of available iodine, and sodium hypochlorite solutions containing 800–1200 ppm of free chlorine are efficient against *Str. agalactiae*. Since all of these compounds are likely to lose much of their efficiency when contaminated with organic matter, udders should be cleaned carefully before disinfection and the wash-water changed frequently.

Teat cup disinfection/back-flushing

Three methods are available. The conventional method is to rinse the cups and dip them in disinfectant wash-water between cows, ensuring that the disinfectant gets well up into the cups by dipping a pair of each cluster in turn. Short-term immersion in hot water (76·5–82°C (170–180°F) for 10 seconds) is effective, but has physical disadvantages in a fast-moving line. Back-flushing with water at 85°C (185°F) for 5 seconds greatly reduces bacterial contamination of cups; a mechanism for doing this without significantly increasing milking time has been designed for use in herringbone milking parlors (64). Chemical sanitization has the same disadvantages as those for udder washing and the same alternative procedure is now extensively used—the back-flushing of the milking tube and cups with cold water for 15 seconds after each cow. In herringbone sheds automatic equipment is available and very little time is wasted. The general tendency is to omit this procedure from central programs because of the time and cost required to carry it out. It is safe to eliminate it if the prevalence is low, and especially if teat dipping and dry-period treatment are carried out meticulously. If the prevalence in the herd is high, and heifers are milked in the same group as the cows, their quarter infection rate may be as high as 50%, and be reducible to 10% if the cups are disinfected and the heifers are milked separately from the cows (32).

Milking machine design and management

The milking machine is an essential part of the dairying industry but it is assumed that its use, proper or improper, has been the principal factor in the increase of subclinical (largely staphylococcal) mastitis in recent years. The following features of machine milking are generally accepted as those which need to be examined in a control program. An annual examination by a qualified technician is the minimum. It is worth noting that some specialist dairy cattle veterinarians now include milking machine surveillance in the herd health service they provide. Some knowledge of the milking machine is essential for all veterinarians working with cattle and details of the examinations carried out and a list of the common errors found is available (75).

With respect to failure of the control program described here it will be found that most failures are due to machine faults. The desirable standards for machines are: reserve vacuum pump capacity 28 liters/min (1 cfm, cubic feet per minute) free air per unit; vacuum level 50 kPa (38 cmHg); pulsation rate 40–60/min; ratio vacuum/rest 50:67; clawpiece air-bleed 7 liters/min ($\frac{1}{4}$ cfm) free air per unit; vacuum level high-line 48–50 kPa (35·5–38 cmHg), low-line 43–5 kPa (32–34·5 cmHg); milking vacuum at teat cup under full load 40–42 kPa (28–30·5 cmHg) minimum vacuum residual for massage 20 kPa (15 cmHg); milk-to-rest ratio 35:65 to 65:35 (33).

Developments in milking machine design could influence the level of mastitis in a herd. Automatic teat cup removers are helpful in that they avoid overmilking. Teat cup deflector shields (32) which divert milk that refluxes into all cups in a cluster from the common milk-line prevents the milk from impacting on the open teat orifice, and thus reduces the spread of infection between the quarters of the one cow. Prolonging the length of the milking tube from each teat cup before combining all four into a common milking tube also reduces cross-infection between quarters. So does the proper design of the metal handpiece of the cluster which can prevent transfer of infection altogether (81). A one-way valve for the milk-line is also now available.

It prevents milk from one quarter refluxing back into other teat cups during milking. For it to operate efficiently the air inlet valve at the end of the milking machine handpiece must be open at all times and the teat cups must not be pulled off before the vacuum is released.

Vacuum pressure in milking machines
Although excessive vacuum level is generally considered to be the most obvious cause of injury by milking machines, there is much conflicting evidence about it and no general agreement that vacuum pressure *per se* is associated with the incidence of infection. However, there are many clinical reports which indicate that an unsuspected high vacuum has resulted in outbreaks of severe clinical mastitis and that a reduction in vacuum level was followed by an improvement in the disease situation. These conflicting views probably depend on differences in the rate of infection in the respective herds initially.

Vacuum pressure in a machine should not exceed that recommended by the manufacturer. With most machines a pressure of 50 kPa (37·5 cmHg) is sufficient and pressures in excess of this are likely to cause injury, as are large fluctuations of pressure caused by inadequate vacuum reserve. In any eradication or control program the milking technique should be observed and the pressure checked, as obstructions may be present in the airline permitting the pressure between the obstruction and the pump to be greatly in excess of normal. The gauge on the machine should also be checked. The small air vent at the end of the claw which permits onward movement of the milk may be blocked, causing milk to accumulate in the liner and exert excessive pressure on the teat. When this occurs the teat ends show redness and prominence of the external meatus, and in severe cases, sores or chapped, rosette formations at the tip. This may progress to eversion of the teat lining with fissuring of the teat sphincter and warty or hair-like growths around it. Such teats are extremely sore at milking and predispose to permanent obstruction or mastitis caused by mixed bacterial infections. Small, firm teats are most susceptible to this form of trauma (95). The maintenance of teat health is a profitable objective because of the frequency with which teat sores are infected with mastitis pathogens and act as sources of infection for their respective quarters. There is a positive correlation between infection rate and teat end sores provided the sores are acute or if the teat leaks, but chronic teat end lesions do not appear to have this effect (92).

Vacuum stability and reserve
Excessive variation in vacuum level is of great importance (34). Fluctuation of more than 0·7 kPa (5 cmHg) in bucket systems and more than 1 kPa (7·5 cmHg) in pipeline systems is considered to be undesirable. Vacuum stability can be checked by inserting a vacuum gauge in one cup of a cluster on a cow while the rest of the units are in use. Excessive fluctuations in vacuum pressure which last for 5 seconds should indicate the need for a close check on the equipment by a serviceman.

Reverse flow of milk in high-line milkers, when the milk-line is too small in caliber to take peak milk flows, can result in the transfer of contaminated milk from one set of cups to another during the milk process. In the same way reflux back into the udder may also be encouraged. Such errors can occur suddenly when a dairyman changes to Friesians from Jerseys or increases the size of his shed without increasing milking machine capacity. A similar error can occur with infection being transferred between quarters of the same udder. This is most likely to occur when the milk flow rate is low near the end of milking. This may play a part in the observed lower prevalence of mastitis in quarters milked by machines equipped with automatic take-off devices, which remove milking machines as soon as the milk flow rate falls below a critical level (37). Reverse flow of milk within the milking machine is a characteristic of high-line milkers; it does not occur in low-line milkers where the milk collecting line is below floor level (36).

Design and management of teat cup liners/inflations
Abnormalities in the size and shape of teat cup liners are likely to cause damage. Small diameter (2 cm) tension liners are preferable to wide (2·5–3 cm) moulded slack liners as they cause less injury (96). In the same way, liners which are allowed to lose their resilience and shape are also dangerous.

Proper care of liners includes rinsing after milking, weekly boiling in caustic soda or lye solution (7 g/liter) for 15 minutes, followed by rinsing in boiling water. Teat cup liners are usually made of synthetic rubber which has a porous surface. Not only is such a surface hard to disinfect, but it is susceptible to filling with milk fat and other solids so that cleaning, which is essential to a prolonged life of the article, cannot be complete. For these reasons the inflations should be discarded after the number of uses recommended by the maker. Liners should also be discarded when they lose shape or become rough or cracked. When one liner is discarded, the others in the set should also be changed because a new liner will milk more efficiently and may work on a dry teat for some time while the inefficient liners are still milking. Alternative materials such as silicon rubber, which is not porous, are likely to be longer-lasting (40).

Milking technique
Machine stripping has the virtue that it significantly increases milk yield and may reduce the incidence of mastitis (41), but excessive machine stripping and removal of the teat cups too violently or before the vacuum is released are two common causes of teat injury. Such errors can only be detected if the milking shed is visited at milking time.

Removal of the cups at the appropriate time is important since if the cups are left on too long the teat is sucked into the cup and the lining of the teat canal may be injured. This can be adequately controlled by having a sight-glass between each cup and the claw, and removing the cups individually from each quarter as milk ceases to flow. Cups are apt to be left on too long when too many cows are being milked by one person. One of the best measures of milking machine efficiency is the average milking time per cow; 4 minutes is considered to be optimum and 6 minutes can be considered as evidence of defective procedure or inefficient equipment or both. Provided adequate hygienic precautions are taken, careful hand-milking is probably the technique least likely to cause damage to the udder and predisposition to mastitis.

The number of sets of teat cups that one person can handle is critical. Labor costs demand that it be high. Mastitis control requires it to be sufficiently low that significant overmilking does not occur. What determines how many sets can be handled by one person is the time required for the necessary chores for each cow, bringing in, preparation and so on. Under existing conditions one person can look after two sets in a long static milk line, up to four sets in a doubled-up walk-through, and six sets in a herringbone. To increase this number automation of the chores, e.g. automatic cluster removers, are necessary.

Although there are conflicting reports on the relationship between overmilking and mastitis it is generally assumed that if a milking machine is adjusted so that it is likely to cause damage, then the effect will be aggravated by any delay in removing the cups after milk flow has ceased. Overmilking, particularly for long periods, causes severe damage to the lining of the teat cistern and streak canal and could contribute to the development of mastitis. Also, overmilking which accompanies pulsation failure, as exemplified by the use of too short inflations, does result in a significant increase in the new infection rate (17). Overmilking also prolongs exposure time to infection and has the effect of increasing the number of quarters of one cow that are infected rather than any effect on increasing the number of cows with new infections (91).

Another potentially important factor in the milking process is the development of a higher negative pressure in the udder than at the apex of the teat. This can occur during overmilking, with vacuum fluctuation and because of failure of letdown. In this event there is a possibility of a reflux of contaminated milk back into the udder. One of the important recent advances in milking machine technology is the automatic teat cup remover which operates on the rate of milk flow and completely avoids overmilking.

Pulsation rate

The pulsation rate is of doubtful importance in so far as mastitis is concerned. Too rapid pulsation (the optimum is about 40/min but varies with different machines) results in incomplete filling of the teat and a tendency for the teats to be crammed into the cup with resulting injury to the soft tissues.

In recent years more and more attention has been given to the construction, installation and handling of the milking machine in such a way as to avoid mastitis.

Milking order

Known infected cows should be milked last and in general young cows should be milked before older ones. Newly introduced animals should be milked separately until their status is determined. The CMT offers a quick and efficient method of screening cows before admitting them to the milking herd. The procedure is practicable only in small herds which are managed intensively or in herds which have large cheap labor resources.

Drying-off

Cows are commonly dried off at the end of a lactation by abrupt cessation of milking or by milking them at gradually increasing intervals. Many new infections occur during this period due to flare-ups of infections not apparent during lactation or to the fall in bactericidal and bacteriostatic qualities of the milk which are at their lowest ebb during the dry period. The method of drying-off has no effect on subsequent milk yields but in herds where mastitis is common the incidence of infection during the dry period is higher when milking is terminated abruptly, particularly if the cow is milking well when she is dried-off (63). Under normal conditions there appears to be little difference between the stop system and intermittent milking (42) but care is advised when cows giving 10 kg or more of milk are dried-off; the stop method may cause severe swelling and encourage the development of mastitis. This difficulty is minimized by confinement and complete restriction of food and water for 24–36 hours. Withdrawal of milk during the dry period does not appear to increase the chance of infection. These factors are of considerable importance as many of the infections, particularly those caused by *Str.agalactiae*, which commence during the dry period, persist and cause clinical mastitis when the next lactation begins. These is good evidence that unmilked quarters are much more susceptible to infection than quarters that are being milked, due probably to the flushing out of pathogens from the teat canal during milking of the latter (3). Dipping of the teats for 20 seconds in 5% tincture of iodine, after preliminary washing with sodium hypochlorite, on several occasions at drying-off effectively reduces the subsequent rate of new infections with *Staph. aureus*. A potentially important contribution to drying-off maneuvers is the infusion of a teat-sealer, with or without antibiotic, at drying-off to avoid further invasion of quarters. Although sealers appear to persist for only 3 weeks in dry quarters there is a significant reduction in the number of new infections (43). One of the disadvantages of these sealers, some of which have bismuth as a base, is that they may fragment and be discharged in the milk for some days after calving. Dipping of the teats in a latex teat sealer has also been advocated, but the protection provided appears to be minimal for Gram-positive infections (74) though significant against coliforms (85).

The entire policy related to hygiene and treatment at drying-off needs to be reviewed in the light of the identifiable variations in new infections as the dry period progresses. The most recent information is that the period immediately after cessation of milking is the most susceptible time. This decline in susceptibility and infection rate depends on the gradual decrease in the ease with which infection penetrates the teat (82) and colonizes mammary tissue (44, 48). In the latter part of the dry period the susceptibility increases again. Several factors affect this ease of infection; one is the presence of milk in the gland, the greater the dilatation of the teat duct and cistern the greater the susceptibility, and the cell count, which is at its maximum when secretion is least

(48). The degree to which the teat skin is infected will also have a big influence on the number of quarters that become infected.

This information is relevant to the procedures adopted at drying-off. Disinfection of teat skin at drying-off is obviously important. Intramammary infusion should be done immediately each cow is dried-off. If a second infusion is used it could reasonably be administered about 3 weeks before calving, but the milk must be withheld for 4 weeks afterward.

Nutrition and inheritance

It is commonly believed that the incidence of mastitis increases when cattle go on to lush pasture or are fed diets high in protein. There is no proof of either contention but reduction of diet is commonly practiced when clinical mastitis occurs. The commonly reported increased incidence of mastitis when cows are turned out to pasture has led to the suggestion that a high intake of estrogenic compounds may precipitate mastitis but investigations into the role of these substances have been inconclusive. Vitamin E, often supplemented with selenium, is administered 21 days before the expected calving date as a prophylaxis against mastitis (87).

Genetic variations in resistance to mastitis have been proven with regard to *Str. agalactiae* mastitis and high milk cell counts in cows (36). It may well hold for other forms of the disease (45) but it is unlikely that selection for resistance to mastitis will ever be of very great importance. This is not to say that it should not be included in a genetic profile used as a basis for selection. There do seem to be differences in susceptibility between Dutch and Swedish breeds of cattle (53). Only slight differences were observed between Holstein and Friesian breeds in Canada (54). American (83) and English (82) work is similarly equivocal. Attempts to find an indicator test which would serve to indentify cows of high or low inherent resistance have been unsuccessful (51) and there seems little hope of progress without such an aid.

One of the inherited characteristics which may affect susceptibility to mastitis is teat shape; the characteristic is inherited and cows with cylindrical teats become affected more commonly than cows with funnel-shaped teats (46). The latter would be less susceptible to teat cup crawl. The shape of the teat end may also be important. Those with inverted, funnel-shaped ends, or with a recessed plate-like end appear to be more susceptible (49). Cows which are habitually fast milkers and therefore presumably have more dilated orifices (50) are also reported to be more susceptible, but on the information available it would seem to be imprudent to select against fast milkers. Other characters which should be selected against are deep udders, excessively low hindquarters, widely placed teats, rear teats too far back and short wide teats (23).

The somatic cell count during the first lactation has also been examined as a basis for selection against mastitis (97). The rate of infection in subsequent lactations favours low initial cell counts.

Vaccination

Vaccination has so far proved to be of no significant value in the control of mastitis (55). Its efficiency will depend largely upon the antigenicity of the causative organisms. While the vaccination story is by no means complete and further research is indicated, it seems safe to say that vaccination against *Str. agalactiae* mastitis is unlikely to be effective since most recovered animals have little if any immunity. The use of an autogenous bacterin against *Staph. aureus* may be of some value in herds where the infecting organism is highly antigenic. In these herds it is unlikely to be sufficiently effective to completely prevent infection but it may reduce the incidence and severity of clinical mastitis. Recent developments in vaccines against staphylococcal mastitis are discussed under that heading and the possible use of vaccination in the control of mastitis in sows caused by the coliform organisms, and in ewes caused by staphylococci and pasteurellae is discussed under those headings.

Bedding

As set out under coliform mastitis, the nature and condition of bedding can significantly affect mastitis prevalence, wet sawdust being worst, shavings in an intermediate position and straw the least predisposing to coliform mastitis. The opposite findings with these materials in laboratory trials suggest that factors other than the bedding materials alone determine how much growth occurs in them (26). Danish experience (2) is that there is less clinical mastitis in bedding cubicles than in tiestalls, which in turn had less than loose housing on a strawpack. Cubicles need to be long enough, with a higher prevalence occurring when cubicles are too short. Cubicles with no bedding, that is to say wet concrete, predispose to mastitis.

Miscellaneous husbandry and milking procedures

Some of the most dramatic wastage due to mastitis is caused by deaths of cows due to gangrenous or coliform endotoxic mastitis. The greatest care is needed to ensure that new infections do not occur during the first few days of lactation when the udder is most susceptible to peracute mastitis. Even heifers which have never been inside a milking parlor come into lactation for the first time with a high prevalence of infection (88). The only recommended prophylaxis is to ensure that calves do not suck each other in early life. Mastitic milk fed to calves from a bucket causes no disease in the calves provided the milk contains antibiotics or formalin (104).

The maintenance of a *high culling rate* of senior cows with lumpy udders or a history of repeated attacks of mastitis is probably the most important tactic in herds where the prevalence of mastitis is high.

Insertion of a smooth, coiled, plastic *intramammary device* has been widely tested in commercial herds as a prevention against infection of the mammary gland. The objective is to create sufficient injury to the teat duct and cistern lining to create a high leukocyte count in the milk and thus enhance its protective properties. There is an increase in the cell count of the udder but the level of protection against infection remains unchanged (93, 98). The use of an abraded or roughened coil (52), or one with copper impregnated in it (20) produces a greater, but still acceptable, cell count in the milk but still only a modest increase in resistance to infection. The device is still undergoing extensive field testing.

Parenteral levamisole administered during the dry period has been promoted as a preventive measure because of its known role as an immunomodulator. It does not appear to affect existing infections, nor prevent new ones, but it may reduce the severity of staphylococcal mastitis (84). The ability of certain bacteria to colonize the teat skin, and thus be in advantageous position to invade the mammary gland, is well recognized. *Teat sores* are common sites for such colonization but few dairymen appreciate their importance in mastitis control. Vigorous treatment with a suitable antiseptic cream after each milking is recommended. The preferred antiseptics are chlorhexidine and iodophors. Iodophor teat dip containing glycerin often clears up sore and chapped teats. *Disinfection of the hands* is necessary only where hand stripping or hand milking is practiced. In these circumstances the hands should be dipped in a disinfectant wash-water between cows and rubbed with a disinfectant cream at the end of the milking period. The latter procedure is most important because of the persistence of the causative organism on the skin.

Hand stripping should be avoided when possible and only machine stripping by bearing down on the milking cups permitted. Sucking by calves may spread infection from quarter to quarter or cow to cow and may also be a factor in the spread of the disease to other calves if they are allowed to suck each other. Infected milk must be disposed of hygienically. The addition of 5% phenol or an equivalent disinfectant is a satisfactory method of destroying the infectivity of small quantities of milk.

Quarters which do not respond to treatment should be permanently dried up as described above or the affected cows culled. Valuable breeding cows may be retained if they are isolated and milked with strict hygienic precautions.

Amputation of the tail has been used in an attempt to reduce the prevalence of mastitis but without apparent effect (47).

Mastitis control programs for unusual pathogens

Mastitis problems created by the occurrence of unusual pathogens including *Escherichia coli*, *Mycoplasma* sp., *Nocardia* sp., yeasts and fungi have not been matched by the development of effective, specific control programs. The most serious group is that which has come to be called environmental mastitis because the causal bacteria are not common inhabitants of the mammary gland but colonize it infrequently from sites in the environment where they normally persist. The subject is discussed in detail under the heading of mastitis caused by *Escherichia coli* but the following recommendations (11, 103) apply:

- Microbiological identification of the causative agent
- Intensive examination of the environment in search of unusual methods of spread, e.g. bedding, homemade or proprietary intramammary infusions which are likely to be contaminated or administered in an unusual way, or wash-water
- Applying intensive hygiene including maximum concentration of teat dip, proper application of it, disinfection of teats before milking, disinfection or back-flush of teat cups between cows
- Segregating and culling or milking last the infected cows. If the cows are kept they should be milked separately and under strict conditions of hygiene.

Causes of error in mastitis control programs

As in most biological systems there are circumstances in which the outcome is not as planned. In the mastitis control program outlined above the errors encountered may be manifested in one of the six following modes.

1. Antibiotic residue in bulk tank milk.
2. High bacteria count.
3. High bulk milk cell count at factory or depot.
4. Increase in quarter infection rate at sampling of cows at drying-off (based on presence of pathogenic bacteria in quarter samples positive to the CMT).
5. An increased number of clinical cases of mastitis.
6. An increased number of infected quarters during the succeeding lactation because the program does not control new infections in late pregnancy and early lactation.

Antibiotic residues in milk are actually less likely in this control program than in ordinary circumstances because the emphasis in it is on avoiding treating lactating cows.

High bacteria counts

Milk for human consumption is required to contain no more than a specified number, usually 100 000 of bacteria/ml on arrival at the processing depot. Counts in excess of this are almost always due to improper cleaning of milking machines or transport containers, but mastitis, especially *Str. agalactiae* infections, can cause them. It would of course be a dreadful indictment of the control program if it allowed such a thing to happen, because it occurs only when the prevalence is high and the farmer is incautious in keeping mastitic milk out of the bulk tank. Visual examination supplemented by bacteriological examination of equipment is usually sufficient to identify the source of trouble.

High bulk milk cell count: increase in QIR: increase in clinical cases

As a criterion in quality control, the bulk milk cell count should not exceed 500 000/ml of milk. Counts above this level may result from a large number of fresh cows, or a large number of cows in late lactation so that no action is usually taken by the milk depot at one infringement. However, such an infringement on one occasion would warrant an investigation in a herd which was on a control program. A QIR of less than 10% is the usual target in a mastitis control program, and an increase to above 12% in a 3-monthly rolling average will indicate a problem in the control program. The prevalence of clinical cases is directly proportional to the QIR and it is unlikely that attention will be drawn to a fault by an increase in them. A trouble-shooting examination of an erring dairy should include an examination of the environment to detect possible precipitating causes such as deep mud in gateways and too narrow stall beds, examination of a sample of cows by the CMT, or other similar test, and bacteriological culture of positive samples, if this is not part of standard procedure. An ad hoc check of the milking machine is recommended because mechanical faults can occur accidentally. A veterinarian offering herd health services to dairy herds should be aware of the ways in which milking machine function can be at fault, and how the faults can be detected (77, 78).

The usual faults encountered in an existing control program are included in the following list:

- Use of an inefficient or too dilute teat dip. These can be easily checked but it is more difficult to detect the hired milker who is just not dipping teats for the sake of speed. An occasional cultural check for *Corynebacterium bovis* in the foremilk will indicate the efficiency of teat dipping. If an iodophor is used the degree of coloration of teats, or the reaction produced in a starch-impregnated swab rubbed on the teat, can be used as a determinant. The use of sprays instead of dips is suspect unless sufficient spray is used to run down the teat and surround the orifice
- The use of infected water for udder washing, or infected bedding, should be suspected if cultural examination turns up an unusual infection such as *Pseudomonas* or *Klebsiella* spp.
- Contaminated infusion materials are likely to be unsuspected if commercial preparations are used but if homemade preparations are used they and the equipment used to make, store and infuse them need to be carefully examined. They are suspect if yeasts or fungi are present in milk samples
- Naturally occurring or induced resistant strains of bacteria are common but they present a problem only if the antibiotic therapy regimens are inadequate: low doses or insufficient duration of treatment will encourage the development of resistance but they will also allow an increase in QIR and that is more likely to create a problem
- Inadequate treatment of lactating cows. This is usually the result of too low doses, or insufficient duration of minimum inhibitory concentration of the antibiotic in the quarter. The latter usually results from the use of quick release antibiotic preparation at one milking only
- Failure to properly disinfect the teats when the drying-off treatment is given may result in an outbreak of mastitis due to an exotic bacterium (73)
- Inadequate treatment of dry cows, again because of too small a dose or an insufficiently slow-release base, is probably the commonest cause of error. It is simply misplaced economy
- Insufficient culling pressure, especially in the early stages of a control program in a badly infected herd, may cause a significant delay in apparent progress. As a result too many old cows with severe lesions are left to contaminate the environment to a point where the sanitation procedures in use are swamped
- The control program outlined above is aimed at *Staphylococcus aureus* and *Streptococcus agalactiae*. As already indicated it may not be effective against other exotic bacteria. This is causing great concern in some countries where the virtual eradication of the normal mastitis-producing Gram-positive bacteria is being followed by an increase in infections by Gram-negative coliforms. This development will mean some modification of recommendations about teat dips and dry period treatments.

Control of ovine and caprine mastitis

It is assumed that the principles of a bovine mastitis control program could be adapted for use in milking goat does and ewes. A common recommendation for suckling ewes in flocks with a bad history of mastitis is the infusion of each half with sodium cloxacillin at weaning (86).

REVIEW LITERATURE

American Veterinary Medical Association Colloquium (1977) Bovine mastitis. *J. Am. vet. med. Assoc.*, *170*, 1119.

Boyer, F. E. (1983) Milking equipment components, function and evaluation. *Bov. Pract.*, *18*, 25–29.

Dodd, F. H. (1981) Advances in understanding mastitis; progress on control. *J. dairy Sci.*, *66*, 1773, 1781, 1790–1794.

Guterbock, W. M. (1984) Mastitis control in large dairy herds. *Comp. cont. Educ.*, 6, S601–605, S651–658, 692–696 & 7, S601.

Hoare, R. J. J. et al. (1979) Mastitis control. A survey of farm practices and their relationship to bulk milk cell count. *Aust. J. dairy Tech.*, *34*, 91.

Jackson, E. R. (1980) The control of bovine mastitis. *Vet. Rec.*, *107*, 37.

Jarrett, J. A. (1984) Bovine mastitis. *Vet. Clin. N. Am. large Anim. Pract.*, *6 (2)*, 233–241.

Seykora, A. J. & McDaniel, B. T. (1985) Udder and teat morphology related to mastitis resistance. *J. dairy Sci.*, *68*, 2807–2093.

Thiel, C. C. & Dodd, F.H. (1977) Machine milking. *Natl Inst. Res. Dairying*, Reading, U.K.

REFERENCES

(1) Black, R. T. et al. (1972) *J. dairy Sci.*, *55*, 1016.
(2) Klastrup, O. (1981) *Proc. 20th Ann. Mtg US Natl Mastitis Ccl Inc.*, p. 38.
(3) Muller, R. H. & Schultze, W. D. (1981) *Proc. 20th Ann. Mtg US Natl Mastitis Ccl Inc.*, p. 51.
(4) Asby, C. B. et al. (1975) *Benefits and Costs of Mastitis Control in Individual Herds*. Reading: Department of Agriculture and Horticulture, University of Reading, England.
(5) Klastrup, O. (1981) *Proc. 20th Ann. Mtg US Natl Mastitis Ccl Inc.*, p. 116.
(6) Dodd, F. H. & Jackson, E. R. (1971) *Mastitis Control*. Reading: British Veterinary Cattle Association.
(7) Poutrel, B. & Rainard, P. (1981) *J. dairy Sci.*, *64*, 241.
(8) Blood, D. C. (1974) *Bov. Pract.*, 9, 2.
(9) McMillan, K. L. et al. (1980) *Proc. NZ Soc. anim. Prod.*, *40*, 180.
(10) Thornton, D. A. K. (1973) *Vet. Rec.*, *93*, 284.
(11) Bushnell, R. B. (1980) *J. Am. vet. med. Assoc.*, *176*, 746.
(12) Ziv, G. et al. (1976) *Br. vet. J.*, *132*, 318.
(13) Oliver, S. P. & Mitchell, B. A. (1983) *J. dairy Sci.*, *66*, 1162.
(14) Boddie, R. L. & Nickerson, S. C. (1986) *J. dairy Sci.*, *69*, 253.
(15) Gilmore, T. M. et al. (1986) *J. dairy Sci.*, *69*, 1128.
(17) Mein, G. A. et al. (1986) *J. dairy Res.*, *53*, 17.
(18) Edwards, S. J. & Smith, G. S. (1967) *Vet. Rec.*, *80*, 486.
(19) Daniel, R. C. W. & Seffert, I. J. (1969) *Aust. vet. J.*, *45*, 530.
(20) Paape, M. J. & Corlett, N. J. (1984) *Am. J. vet. Res.*, *45*, 1572.
(21) Evans, J. M. et al. (1972) *Vet. Rec.*, *90*, 542.
(22) Ward, G. E. & Schultz, L. H. (1974) *J. dairy Sci.*, *57*, 1341.
(23) Thomas, C. L. et al. (1984) *J. dairy Sci.*, *67*, 1281.
(24) Pearson, J. K. L. et al. (1971) *Vet. Rec.*, *88*, 488.
(25) Hoyle, J. B. & Dodd, F. H. (1970) *J. dairy Res.*, *37*, 133.
(26) Zehner, M. M. et al. (1986) *J. dairy Sci.*, *69*, 1932.

(27) Meek, A. H. et al. (1981) *Can. vet. J.*, *22*, 46.
(28) Sheldrake, R. F. & Hoare, R. J. T. (1982) *Aust. J. dairy Technol.*, *37*, 95.
(29) Natzke, R. P. & Bray, D. R. (1973) *J. dairy Sci.*, *56*, 148.
(30) Schultze, W. D. & Smith, J. W. (1972) *J. dairy Sci.*, *55*, 426.
(31) Ryssen, van J. B. J. et al. (1985) *J. S. Afr. vet. Assoc.*, *56*, 181.
(32) Griffin, T. K. et al. (1983) *J. dairy Res.*, *50*, 397.
(33) Schroder, R. J. et al. (1968) *J. Am. vet. med. Assoc.*, *153*, 1676.
(34) Thiel, C. L. et al. (1973) *J. dairy Res.*, *40*, 117.
(35) Godinho, K. S. & Bramley, A. J. (1980) *Br. vet. J.*, *136*, 574.
(36) Grootenhuis, G. (1981) *Vet. Rec.*, *108*, 258.
(37) Philpott, W. N. (1972) *J. Milk Fd Technol.*, *35*, 544.
(38) Boddie, R. L. & Nickerson, S. C. (1986) *J. dairy Sci.*, *69*, 258.
(39) Galton, D. M. et al. (1986) *J. dairy Sci.*, *69*, 267.
(40) Heckman, R. et al. (1985) *Mod. vet. Pract.*, *66*, 437.
(41) Ebendorff, W. et al. (1987) *Milchwissenschaft*, *42*, 23.
(42) Natzke, R. P. et al. (1975) *J. dairy Sci.*, *58*, 1828.
(43) Meaney, W. J. (1977) *Irish J. agric. Res.*, *16*, 293.
(44) Macdonald, J. & Anderson, A. J. (1981) *Am. J. vet. Res.*, *42*, 462.
(45) Grootenhuis, G. (1976) *Tijdschr. Diergeneeskd.*, *101*, 779.
(46) Rathore, A. K. (1976) *Br. vet. J.*, *132*, 389.
(47) Elliott, R. E. W. (1969) *NZ vet. J.*, *17*, 89.
(48) Pankey, J. W. et al. (1985) *J. dairy Sci.*, *68*, 1523.
(49) Lojda, L. et al. (1976) *Acta vet. Brno*, *45*, 181.
(50) Pearson, J. K. L. & Mackie, D. P. (1979) *Vet. Rec.*, *105*, 456.
(51) Hibbit, K. G. (1983) *Vet. Ann.*, *23*, 65.
(52) Ziv, G. et al. (1985) *Bov. Pract.*, *20*, 102.
(53) Schwan, O. & Holmberg, O. (1979) *Vet. Microbiol.*, *3*, 213.
(54) Batra, T. R. (1979) *Can. J. anim. Sci.*, *59*, 597.
(55) Adlam, C. et al. (1981) *J. comp. Pathol.*, *91*, 105.
(56) Rindsig, R. B. et al. (1979) *J. dairy Sci.*, *62*, 1335.
(57) Francis, P. G. (1984) *Proc. 13th World Cong. Dis. Cattle, Durban, Vol. 1.* pp. 193–198.
(58) Philpot, W. N. (1977) *Proc. 10th Ann. Conv. Amer. Assoc. Bov. Practrs*, p. 55.
(59) Hill, B. M. & Small, J. M. (1985) *NZ vet. J.*, *33*, 105.
(60) Colditz, I. G. & Watson, D. L. (1985) *Aust. vet. J.*, *62*, 145.
(61) Pearson, J. K. L. et al. (1978) *Vet. Rec.*, *102*, 447.
(62) Wilson, C. D. et al. (1978) *Vet. Rec.*, *102*, 468.
(63) Hirsch, H. P. (1984) *Monatsh. VetMed.*, *39*, 579.
(64) Box, P. G. & Ellis, K. R. (1979) *Vet. Rec.*, *102*, 35.
(65) Roguinsky, M. (1978) *Ann. rech. vét.*, *9*, 465.
(66) Mein, G. A. et al. (1977) *Aust. J. dairy Techol.*, *32*, 81.
(67) Hoare, R. J. T. et al. (1977) *Aust. vet. J.*, *53*, 529, 534 & 538.
(68) King, J. S. et al. (1977) *Vet. Rec.*, *101*, 421.
(69) Hayward, P. J. & Webster, A. N. (1977) *NZ J. dairy Sci. Technol.*, *12*, 78.
(70) Philpot, W. N. & Pankey, J. W. (1978) *J. dairy Sci.*, *61*, 950, 956 & 964.
(71) Pankey, J. W. & Watts, J. L. (1983) *J. dairy Sci.*, *66*, 355.
(72) Curtis, R. et al. (1977) *Vet. Rec.*, *100*, 557.
(73) Wilson, C. D. & Fitton, J. (1979) *Vet. Rec.*, *104*, 375.
(74) McArthur, B. J. et al. (1984) *J. dairy Sci.* 67, 1331.
(75) Noordhuizen, J. P. T. M. et al. (1987) *Vet. Q.*, *9*, 60.
(76) Harmon, R. J. et al. (1986) *J. dairy Sci*, *69*, 843.
(77) Heider, L. E. & Barr, H. L. (1977) *J. Am. vet. med. Assoc.*, *170*, 1236.
(78) Hill, B. M. & Small, J. M. (1985) *NZ vet. J.*, *33*, 105.
(79) duPreez, J. H. & Greeff, A. S. (1985) *J. S. Afr. vet. Assoc.* 56, 191.
(80) Heald, C. W. et al. (1977) *Can. vet. J.*, *18*, 171.
(81) Hamann, J. et al. (1980) *Milchwissenschaft*, *35*, 411.
(82) Cousins, C. L. et al. (1980) *J. dairy Res.*, *47*, 11.
(83) Alrawi, A. A. et al. (1979) *J. dairy Sci.*, *62*, 1115.
(84) Buddle, B. M. & Pulford, H. D. (1985) *NZ vet. J.*, *33*, 177.
(85) Farnsworth, R. J. et al. (1980) *J. Am. vet. med. Assoc.*, *177*, 441.
(86) Watson, D. J. (1982) *Ann. Proc. Sheep vet. Soc.*, 6, 88.
(87) Ivandija, L. (1985) *Praxis Vet.*, *33*, 263.
(88) Oliver, S. P. & Mitchell, B. A. (1983) *J. dairy Sci.*, *66*, 1180.
(89) Mwakipesile, S. M. et al. (1983) *NZ vet. J.*, *31*, 192.
(90) McDermott, M. P. et al. (1983) *J. dairy Sci.*, 66, 1198.
(91) Natzke, R. P. et al. (1982) *J. dairy Sci.*, *65*, 117.
(92) Sieber, R. L. & Farnsworth, R. J. (1981) *J. Am. vet. med. Assoc.*, *178*, 1263.
(93) Baran, V. et al. (1986) *Vet. Med.*, *31*, 393.
(94) Macmillan, K. L. et al. (1983) *J. dairy Sci.*, *66*, 259.
(95) Binde, M. & Bakke, H. (1984) *Nord. VetMed.*, *36*, 111.
(96) Bakke, H. & Binde, M. (1984) *Nord. VetMed.*, *36*, 117.
(97) Coffey, E. M. et al. (1986) *J. dairy Sci.*, *69*, 2163.
(98) Corlett, N. J. et al. (1984) *J. dairy Sci.*, *67*, 2571.
(99) Robinson, T. C. et al. (1985) *Br. vet. J.*, *141*, 635.
(100) Pankey, J. W. et al. (1982) *NZ vet. J.*, *30*, 13.
(101) Ziv, G. et al. (1981) *Vet Q.*, *3*, 75; in *Tijdschr. Diergeneeskd.*, *106(8)*.
(102) Galton, D. M. et al. (1984) *J. dairy Sci.*, 67, 260, 2580.
(103) Oz, H. H. et al. (1985) *Vet. Bull.*, *55*, 829.
(104) Kesler, E. M. (1981) *J. dairy Sci.*, *64*, 719.
(105) McMillan, K. L. et al. (1983) *J. dairy Sci.*, 66, 259.
(106) Williamson, N. B. (1987) *Proc. 26th ann. Mtg Natl Mastitis Ccl Inc.*, p. 51.

MISCELLANEOUS ABNORMALITIES OF THE UDDER AND TEATS

Lesions of the teat and udder skin

Specific diseases of teat skin are dealt with individually under the headings of papillomatosis, cowpox, pseudo-cowpox, bovine ulcerative mammillitis, blackpox and udder impetigo. Cows burned in grass fires where most of the damage is done to the ventral part of the body may suffer very severe burns to the teats which may slough altogether or be blocked subsequently by scar tissue. As a part of other diseases there may be vesicles on the teats in foot-and-mouth disease, vesicular exanthema of swine, and swine vesicular disease. Sloughing of the epidermis occurs in peracute bovine malignant catarrh, dermatitis of the lateral aspects of the teats occurs in photosensitive dermatitis. Ringworm and mycotic dermatitis are other diseases of teat skin encountered in cows. Flexural seborrhea in cows is often manifested by lesions extending from the groin on to udder skin and is described under the heading of seborrhea. In ewes ecthyma may be manifested by lesions on the teats accompanying facial lesions in lambs.

Thelitis (Mammillitis)

Inflammation of the wall of the teat is a non-specific lesion usually associated with traumatic injury to the lining of the teat cistern. The wall of the cistern is thickened, hardened, painful and, in chronic lesions, irregular in its internal lining. It can be felt as a dense, vertical cord in the cord of the teat tip. The lesions are intractable to treatment which usually consists of intra-mammary antibiotics and refraining from milking.

In photosensitive dermatitis in cows with white teats there is a characteristic erythema and hardness of the white parts of the lateral aspects of each teat. The medial aspect is soft and cool. The teats are also painful and in the early stages apparently irritable, because affected cows will also stand in ponds or waterholes in such a way that the teats are immersed and then rock backwards and forwards. They will also brush the sides of the udder with the hindfeet in a way that could suggest the stamping movements of abdominal pain. In cases where the photosensitization is related to the induction of parturition by the administration of corticosteroids, the skin lesions are usually restricted to the teats. In cases due to other causes there are usually obvious lesions of photosensitive dermatitis on the dorsal aspects of the body but confined to the white parts.

An enzootic mammillitis of alpine cows in Switzerland (25) is characterized by nodular lesions in the teat wall. The lesions are multicentric nodules containing atypical mycobacteria.

Teat necrosis

Abrasion of nipples of baby pigs on rough non-slip concrete may be observed as acute lesions or be apparent only when the piglets mature and are found to have deficient teat numbers as set out below.

Blood in the milk

Blood in the milk is usually an indication of a rupture of a blood vessel in the gland by direct trauma, or of capillary bleeding in a congested udder soon after calving. Although in the latter circumstance the bleeding usually ceases in 2–3 days it may persist beyond this period and render the milk unfit for human consumption. The discoloration varies from a pale pink to a dark chocolate brown and may still be present 7–8 days after parturition. Rarely the blood loss may be sufficiently severe to require treatment for anemia (19). Treatment is often requested although the cow is clinically normal in all other respects. Calcium borogluconate injected intravenously is a standard treatment but better results are likely to be obtained by the injection of parenteral coagulants. Difficulty may be experienced in milking the clots out of the teats but if they are broken up by compressing them inside the teat, they will usually pass easily. The presence of bloodstained milk in all four quarters at times other than immediately postpartum should arouse suspicion of leptospirosis, and possibly other diseases in which intravascular hemolysis or capillary damage occurs.

Edema and congestion of the udder

Congestion of the udder at parturition is physiological but it may be sufficiently severe to cause edema of the belly, udder and teats in cows and mares. In most cases the edema disappears within a day or two of calving, but if it is extensive and persistent, it may interfere with sucking and milking (1). It is a prominent sign in inherited rectovaginal constriction of Jersey cows described under that heading.

If the edema is severe one or more of the following treatments is recommended. Milking may be started some days before parturition. After parturition, frequent milking, massage and the use of diuretics are recommended. Corticosteroids appear to exert no beneficial effect (2). Acetazolamide (1–2 g twice daily orally or parenterally for 1–6 days) gives excellent results in a high proportion of cases, the edema often disappearing within 24 hours. Chlorothiazide (2 g twice daily by mouth or 0·5 g twice daily by intravenous or intramuscular injection, each for 3–4 days) is also effective (4). The use of diuretics before calving may be dangerous if considerable fluid is lost. Interference with venous drainage resulting from pressure of the fetus in the pelvic cavity is thought to be the primary cause in individual cows which recover spontaneously at calving. When there is a herd problem detection of the cause is often difficult, hypoproteinemia has been proposed as a predisposing cause but biochemical examinations do not support this view (28). It is a common recommendation that the amount of grain fed in the last few weeks of pregnancy be limited and there is evidence that heavy grain feeding predisposes to the condition, at least in heifers (1). High sodium (26) or potassium (14) intakes have been shown to cause the defect, especially in housed cattle; the disease often disappears when the cows are turned out to pasture. The tendency to udder edema may be heritable in some herds and selection against bulls that sire edematous daughters is thought to be worthwhile (16). Such a tendency could be mediated through a complex interaction between sex steroids which are thought to play a role in the etiology (17). There is also a reduction in blood flow through, and an increase in blood pressure in, the superficial epigastric or milk veins of cows with chronic edema (27). There is no explanation of this apparent venous impedance.

Simple congestion causing a hard, localized plaque along the floor of a quarter is most common after parturition in heifers and is relatively innocuous but may interfere with milking. If repeated for a number of lactations it may cause permanent thickening of the skin (scleroderma) of the lateral aspect of the udder (6). Hot fomentations, massage and the application of liniments are of value in reducing the hardness and swelling. A chronic form of the disease is recorded from New Zealand, but no credible etiological agent has been proposed (4).

Hard udder or indurative mastitis is described in goats under the heading of caprine arthritis–encephalitis and in ewes in maedi.

Rupture of the suspensory ligaments of the udder

Rupture of the suspensory ligaments occurs most commonly in adult cows and develops gradually over a number of years. When it occurs acutely, just before or after parturition, the udder drops markedly, is swollen and hard, and serum oozes through the skin. Severe edema occurs at the base of the udder. It may be confused with gangrenous mastitis on cursory examination. Partial relief may be obtained with a suspensory apparatus but complete recovery does not occur.

Agalactia

The most important cause of agalactia in farm animals is mastitis–metritis–agalactia (MMA) in sows. The general principles that apply there apply also to the less common cases of agalactia that occur in all species. In them there is partial or complete absence of milk flow which may affect one or more mammary glands and is of major importance in sows although it occurs occasionally in cattle. The importance of the disease in sows derives from the fact that piglets are very susceptible to hypoglycemia. The condition may be due to failure of letdown or absence of milk secretion (8).

The causes of failure of letdown include painful conditions of the teat, sharp teeth in the piglets, inverted nipples which interfere with sucking, primary failure of milk ejection especially in gilts and excessive engorgement and edema of the udder. In many sows the major disturbance seems to be hysteria which is readily cured by the use of ataractic drugs. Treatment of the primary condition and the parenteral administration of oxytocin, repeated if necessary, is usually adequate.

Ergotism may be a specific cause of agalactia in sows and has been recorded in animals fed on bullrush millet infested with ergot (9).

Apparent hormonal defects do occur, particularly in cattle. Sporadic cases occur in which cows calve normally and have a normal udder full of milk but fail to let it down when stimulated in the normal way. A single injection of oxytocin is often sufficient to start the lactation. In rare cases repeated injections at successive milkings are required. There is one report of a number of cows in a herd being affected (15). The cows were under severe stress for a number of reasons and had depressed serum cortisol levels. In heifers and gilts there may be complete absence of mammary development and, in such cases, no treatment is likely to be of value. In animals which have lactated normally after previous parturitions, the parenteral administration of chorionic gonadotrophin has been recommended but often produces no apparent improvement.

Antibiotics in milk

This problem arises principally as a result of treatment for mastitis and is dealt with under that heading.

Milk drop

This is a herd syndrome in which the milk yield falls precipitately without there being any clinical evidence of disease, especially mastitis, or obvious deprivation of food or water. Leptospirosis due to *Leptospira hardjo* and summer fescue toxicosis are among the more common causes.

Milk fat depression

The butter fat percentage overall in a herd may drop precipitately from the normal of 3·6% to below 3% and in bad cases to below 1%. The cows appear healthy, eat well and total milk yield is undisturbed. In almost all cases there is a dietary error of insufficient fiber, to below 17% crude fiber on a dry matter basis (22).

'Free' or 'stray' electricity as a cause of failure of letdown

Free electrical current is common in dairies, especially recently built ones. The problem is most common when a herd moves into a new shed, but it also occurs with alterations to electrical equipment and wiring or to ordinary wear and tear to it. The stray current is present in the metallic part of the building construction, much of which is interconnected. Cows are very sensitive to even small amperages and are highly susceptible because they make good, often wet contact with the metal and with wet concrete on the floor. People working in the dairy are not likely to notice the electrical contact because they are usually wearing rubber boots. The voltage present would be too low to be of much interest to the local power authority and an independent technician may be necessary to carry out the work. The examination should be carried out while the milking machine is working and more than one visit may need to be made. The effects of free electricity in the milking shed may be:

- Fatal electrocution, stunning causing unconsciousness, frantic kicking and bellowing, all manifested when the animal contacts the electrified metal, all as set down under the heading of electrocution
- Restlessness, frequent urination, defecation, failure to let milk down, in tie stalls frequent lapping at water bowl but refusing to drink. This abnormality may be apparent only when cow is in a particular position or posture
- Startled, alert appearance with anxiety, balking, refusal to enter milking parlor
- Failure of letdown leads to lower milk production, recrudescence of existing subclinical mastitis leading to appearance of clinical signs.

In spite of the many field observations of these abnormalities experimental application of AC current up to 8 MÅ causes changes in behaviour but not in milk yield or letdown (32).

Recommended guidelines for diagnosis of free electricity problems are set out below (13). For simplicity it can be assumed that cows will behave abnormally if the free voltage exceeds 1 volt AC (20). A safer threshold is 0.35 volts AC as a maximum (10). A proper voltmeter is necessary to make a diagnosis and in most circumstances a qualified electrician is necessary for the exercise.

	Volts
Normal	0–0·50
Suspicious	0·50–0·75
Milk reactions	0·75–1·50
Strong reactions	1·50–3·50
Critical reactions	3·50–5·0
Life at risk	>5·0

The development of voltages in the metalwork of the milking shed can arise from many factors. Obvious short circuits from faulty wiring are the least common cause. Most cases are due to accumulation of relatively low voltages because of increased resistance in the earth or ground system—thus neutral to earth voltages. Reasons for the accumulation include poor earthing or grounding system, grounding rods too short to reach the water table, insufficient grounding rods, dry seasons lowering the water table. The problem may be intermittent and even seasonal depending on climatic conditions which facilitate the passage of current through the cow as an alternative grounding system.

'Black pox' (black spot)

This is an abnormality of the teat tip caused in most cases by excessive vacuum pressure or overmilking in teats that are naturally firm and have pointed ends. There is no specific bacteriology although *Fusobacterium necrophorum* is commonly present and *Staphylococcus aureus* is frequently isolated from the lesions. The latter occur only on the teats and take the form of deep, crater-shaped ulcers with raised edges and a black spot in the center. The lesions are confined almost entirely to the tip of the teat, usually invade the sphincter and are responsible for a great deal of mastitis. Lesser lesions of teat sphincters are listed under vacuum pressure in bovine mastitis control.

The lesions are painful leading to kicking by the cows, sometimes repeated kicking off of the teat cups, and to blockage of the sphincter. Coliform mastitis is a common sequel (24). The lesions are poorly responsive to treatment even if the machine error is corrected.

Treatment of black spot is usually by topical application of ointments. Whitfield's, 10% salicylic, 5% sulfathiazole and 5% salicylic, 5% copper sulfate are all recommended. An iodophor ointment, or iodophor teat dip with 35% added glycerol, are also effective but treatment needs to be thorough and repeated and milking machine errors need to be corrected.

Udder impetigo

This disease is of importance because of the discomfort it causes, its common association with staphylococcal mastitis, its not uncommon spread to milkers' hands (11) and the frequency with which it is mistaken for cowpox. The lesions are usually small pustules (2–4 mm diameter) but in occasional animals they extend to the subcutaneous tissue and appear as furuncles or boils. The commonest site is the hairless skin at the base of the teats but the lesions may spread from here on to the teats and over the udder generally. Spread in the herd appears to occur during milking and a large proportion of a herd may become affected over a relatively long period. The institution of suitable sanitation procedures, such as dipping teats after milking, washing of udders before milking and treatment of individual lesions with a suitable antiseptic ointment as described under the control of mastitis usually stops further spread. An ancillary measure is to vaccinate all cows in the herd with an autogenous bacterin produced from the *Staph. aureus* which is always present. Good immunity is produced for about 6 months but the disease recurs unless satisfactory sanitation measures are introduced.

What appears to have been an exaggerated form of this disease has been reported in a recently gathered herd of cows. It is assumed that the cows were very susceptible and the *Staphylococcus aureus* present was very virulent. In addition to the signs described above, there was a high prevalence of clinical mastitis and a generalized exudative epidermitis reaching from the escutcheon to the thighs (6).

Sores of bovine teat skin in Norway, characterized by the presence of *Staph. aureus*, and referred to as 'bovine teat skin summer sore' are thought to be caused by cutaneous invasion by *Stephanofilaria* sp. nematodes (3). The differential diagnosis of discrete lesions on bovine teat skin is dealt with in the subject of cowpox.

Neoplasms of the udder

Neoplasms of the bovine udder are particularly rare and have moderate malignancy (12). A fibrosarcoma originating within or close to a mammary gland has been observed to have high malignancy (30). Mammary carcinoma occurs occasionally in mares and is characterized by great malignancy. Neoplasms of the skin of the udder may spread to involve mammary tissue. The commonest neoplasm of cows' teats is viral papillomatosis. It is esthetically unattractive and may play a part in harboring mastitis organisms on the teat skin. It is dealt with in detail under the heading of papillomatosis. Similar papillomata occur on the teat and udder skin of lactating Saanen goats. Rarely these lesions may develop a squamous cell carcinoma lesion of low malignancy (18).

Corpora amylacea

These inert concretions of amyloid may become calcified and detached from the mammary tissue so that they cause blockage of the teat canal and cessation of milk flow. They are formed as the result of stasis due to blocked mammary tissue ducts and resorption of the milk fluids (7).

Teat and udder congenital defects

The common sporadic defects in cows are supernumerary teats, fused teats with two teat canals opening into one teat sinus, hypomastia, absence of a teat canal and sinus (29), and absence of a connection between the teat sinus and the udder sinus; in sows insufficient and inverted teats are the common errors. A high prevalence of defects is recorded in Murrah buffaloes (23) and inheritance of hypomastia, rudimentary teats and angulation of teats are suspected in cows (31).

Traditionally sows are required to have at least 12 functional teats (5) and sows deficient in this regard are likely to be culled. Reasons for the deficit include inherited shortage (teat number is highly heritable), misplaced teats, usually too far posteriorly to be accessible to the piglets, or unevenly placed, inverted teats either congenital or acquired as a result of injury, vestigial nipples which do not acquire a lumen, cistern or gland, and normal-sized teats which are occluded. Inverted teats in sows may be so because they lack a teat upturn, the teat duct opening directly into the mammary gland cistern (21).

REVIEW LITERATURE

Al-Ani, F. K. & Vestweber, J. G. E. (1986) Udder edema; an updated review. *Vet. Bull.*, *56*, 763–769.

Francis, P. G. (1984) Teat skin lesions and mastitis. *Br. vet. J.*, *140*, 430.

Sieber, R. L. & Farnsworth, R. J. (1984) Differential diagnosis of bovine teat lesions. *Vet. Clin. N. Am. large Anim. Pract.*, *6(2)*, 313–321.

REFERENCES

(1) Emery, R. S. et al. (1969) *J. dairy Sci.*, *52*, 345.
(2) Mitchell, R. G. et al. (1976) *J. dairy Sci.*, *59*, 109.
(3) Bakker, G. (1980) *Vet. Rec.*, *106*, 178.
(4) Hicks. J. D. & Pauli, J. V. (1976) *NZ vet. J.*, *24*, 225.
(5) Done, J. T. (1980) *Vet. Ann.*, *20*, 246.
(6) Nicholls, T. J. & Rubira, R. J. (1981) *Aust. vet. J.*, *57*, 54.
(7) Lokvancic, H. et al. (1979) *Vet. Glasnik*, *33*, 443.
(8) Loveday, R. K. (1964) *J. S. Afr. vet. med. Assoc.*, *35*, 229.
(9) Shone, D. K. et al. (1959) *Vet. Rec.*, *71*, 129.
(10) Appleman, R. D. & Gustafson, R. J. (1985) *J. dairy Sci.*, *68*, 1554.
(11) Zinn, R. D. (1961) *J. Am. vet. med. Assoc.*, *138*, 382.
(12) Beamer, P. D. & Simon, J. (1983) *Vet. Pathol.*, *20*, 509.
(13) Williams, G. F. H. et al. (1981) *Proc. 20th Ann. Mtg U.S. Natl Mastitis Ccl Inc.*, pp. 13, 18, 25, 31, 36.
(14) Sanders, D. E. & Sanders, J. A. (1981) *J. Am. vet. med. Assoc.*, *178*, 1274.
(15) McCaughan, C. J. & Malecki, J. C. (1981) *Aust. vet. J.*, 57, 203.
(16) Dentine, M. R. et al. (1983) *J. dairy Sci.*, *66*, 2391.
(17) Malvern, P. V. et al. (1983) *J. dairy Sci.*, *66*, 246.
(18) Ficken, M. D. & Andrews, J. J. (1983) *J. Am. vet. med. Assoc.*, *183*, 467.
(19) Eddy, R. G. & Clark, P. J. (1982) *Vet. Rec.*, *110*, 482.
(20) Kirk, J. H. et al. (1984) *J. Am. vet. med. Assoc.*, *185*, 426.
(21) Gunther, C. et al. (1985) *Zuchtungskunde*, 57, 256.
(22) Olson, W. G. (1984) *Bov. Pract.*, *19*, 125.
(23) Rao, A. V. N. & Murthy, T. S. (1983) *Ind. vet. Med. J.*, 7, 217.
(24) Ogden, N. H. (1986) *Vet. Rec.*, *118*, 674.
(25) Rusch, P. et al. (1984) *Schweiz. Arch. Tierheilkd.*, *126*, 467.
(26) Jones, T. O. et al. (1984) *Vet. Rec.*, 115, 218.
(27) Al-Ani, F. K. et al. (1985) *Vet. Rec.*, *116*, 156.
(28) Vestweber, J. G. E. & Al-Ani, F. K. (1984) *Cornell Vet.*, *74*, 366.
(29) Duraes, M. C. et al. (1982) *J. dairy Sci.*, *65*, 1804.
(30) Orr, J. P. (1984) *Can. J. comp. Med.*, 48, 219.
(31) Crinion, R. A. P. (1984) *Irish vet. J.*, *38*, 116.
(32) Drenkard, D. V. H. et al. (1985) *J. dairy Sci.*, *68*, 2694.

MASTITIS–METRITIS–AGALACTIA (MMA) SYNDROME IN SOWS (TOXEMIC AGALACTIA, FARROWING FEVER, LACTATION FAILURE)

The MMA syndrome occurs in sows between 12 and 48 hours after farrowing and is characterized clinically by anorexia, lethargy, disinterest in the piglets, fever, swelling of the mammary glands and agalactia. Most affected animals respond to therapy within 12–24 hours. Pathologically there are varying degrees of mastitis. The disease is of major economic importance when outbreaks occur because of the high piglet mortality from starvation and secondary infectious diseases. Ringarp (1) studied 1180 cases of postparturient illness in sows in which agalactia was present, and recognized at least five causes of agalactia or hypogalactia which are as follows (the incidence of each group as a percentage of the total cases is given in brackets):

1. *Eclampsia* (0·6%) usually of older sows, responding to calcium and magnesium therapy.
2. *Failure of milk ejection reflex* (3·3%) affecting primarily first litter gilts and usually treated satisfactorily with oxytocin.
3. *Mammary hypoplasia* (1·5%) in gilts and resulting in deficient milk secretion.
4. *Primary agalactia* (6%) in which reduced milk supply is the only abnormality.
5. *Toxic agalactia* (88·6%) was the most important numerically and economically. It is characterized by anorexia, depression, fever, swelling of the mammary glands and a course of 2–4 days. Mastitis was commonly present while metritis was not.

The term mastitis–metritis–agalactia (MMA) was originally developed to describe sows with agalactia which had swollen udders, assumed to be due to mastitis, and the appearance of a vulvar discharge, assumed to be due to metritis. Necropsy of spontaneously occurring cases has frequently confirmed the presence of mastitis but the incidence of metritis has been insignificant.

Etiology

The etiology has not yet been adequately determined. Several different cause-and-effect relationships have been proposed based on clinical and epidemiological observations but only infectious mastitis has been adequately substantiated. The list of proposed causes includes infectious mastitis, metritis, overfeeding during pregnancy, nutritional deficiencies, constipation and endocrine dysfunction (1, 2).

A major problem in the determination of the etiology is the difficulty of being precise in the description of the clinical findings of the abnormal mammary glands of affected sows. The common clinical findings are swelling of the glands, agalactia, toxemia, and a fever. There is considerable overlap in the clinical findings from one affected sow to another but the lesion present in the mammary glands may vary from uncomplicated physiological congestion and edema to severe necrotizing mastitis.

Infectious mastitis is suggested as a major cause in many clinicopathological investigations and there is a greater incidence of infection of the mammary glands of affected sows compared to normal sows. A cumulative tabulation of several necropsy examinations of affected sows reveals that 82% had gross lesions of mastitis (2). Mastitis may also be present in normal lactating sows, but at a much lower level. Peracute mastitis in sows is readily recognized as a clinical entity but less severe infections may result in small foci of inflammation within the gland which cannot be detected on clinical examination. *E. coli* and *Klebsiella pneumoniae* have been recovered from the mammary glands of naturally affected cases and both bacterial species are associated with histopathologic changes of mastitis (2, 9–11). Experimental intramammary inoculation of sows with field isolates of *E. coli* (12) and *K. pneumoniae* has resulted in cases of lactation failure and mastitis which closely resembles naturally occurring cases (11). *Streptococcus* sp. and *Staphylococcus* sp. have also been isolated, but these are frequently isolated from healthy glands unassociated with pathologic changes. Based on bacteriological studies of field cases of sow agalactia it is unlikely that *Mycoplasma* spp. are the significant causative agents they were once considered to be (2).

Coliforms are probably the most significant bacteria isolated from sows with mastitis (2). Pathological examination of affected sows which were euthanized within

3 days after parturition revealed the presence of varying degrees of mastitis (13) and *E. coli* and *Klebsiella* spp. were the most common organisms recovered (10). Toxic agalactia can be produced experimentally by the introduction of *E. coli* endotoxin into the mammary gland of sows at parturition and the clinical, hematological and serum biochemical changes are similar to those which occur in naturally occurring cases of toxic agalactia (6, 14, 15). *E. coli* endotoxin acting at the level of hypothalamus can suppress prolactin release which results in a pronounced decline in milk production (31). Experimental *Klebsiella* mastitis in sows is an excellent model for the study of toxic agalactia due to infectious mastitis (11).

Thus there is sufficient scientific evidence to support the conclusion that infectious mastitis is a major cause of toxic agalactia in sows. Each mammary gland of the sow is divided into a separate anterior and posterior section, each with its own teat cistern and teat canal. In a sow with 14 teats there are 28 potential portals of entry for environmental infectious agents and perhaps it is little wonder that mastitis should occur commonly immediately after parturition when the teat canals have become patent.

Some clinicopathological examinations of affected sows have revealed the presence of a slightly enlarged flaccid uterus from which coliform and streptococcal organisms can be recovered. However, pathological evidence of metritis in affected sows is uncommon and the organisms which can be recovered are commonly present in the reproductive tract of normal sows after parturition, and their recovery from vaginal mucus is difficult to interpret. In other studies, there are no differences between the state of the uterus in affected sows and normal sows (13).

Some excellent studies on the nursing behavior of the sow and the sucking behavior of the piglets are recorded (16–18) and may provide an explanation for the pathogenesis and clinical findings of some cases of agalactia in sows. These studies emphasize that successful ejection of milk by the sow is dependent on proper stimulation of the sow's udder by the piglets followed by a complex response by the sow. A period of time ranging from 15 to 45 minutes must elapse from the last successful milk ejection to the next. Failure of milk ejection may occur in up to 27 % of sows which attempt to suckle their piglets within 40 minutes after the previous milk ejection (19). The failure of milk ejection in sows within the first few crucial adjustment days after farrowing might possibly contribute to the cause of mastitis and engorgement of the mammary glands. The possible causes of failure of milk ejection, even when a suitable interval has elapsed since the previous milk ejection, include: environmental or other animal noises and disturbances; uncomfortable farrowing crates; high environmental temperatures; and insufficient time to adjust to the farrowing crate.

Digestive disturbances and certain feeding practices have been associated with the disease. Sows that have been on high-level feeding during pregnancy appear to be susceptible to the disease, especially if they are subjected to a change of feed immediately prior to parturition. Also any management practice which results in a marked change in feed intake at or near farrowing may appear to precipitate the disease. A sudden change of feed severe enough to result in gastrointestinal stasis has been used to reproduce the condition experimentally (1). Constipation of sows at farrowing time has been suggested as a cause but has not been substantiated. However, clinical and pathological examinations of both spontaneously occurring cases of agalactia and experimental agalactia induced by the introduction of *E. coli* endotoxin into the mammary gland have been unable to support the observation of constipation (15). Both sick and normal sows defecate less frequently from 1 day before farrowing until 2 days later. There is no difference in the weight of feces in the terminal colon and rectum between sick and normal sows. Mycotoxins in feed (21) and deficiencies of vitamin E and selenium (22) have also been incriminated but the evidence is not sufficiently supportive.

It is thought that certain sows are more susceptible than others and an abnormality in thyroid function during gestation of sows which subsequently developed the syndrome has been reported (15). Agalactia may also be the result of a deficiency of prolactin. Any factor which interferes with the release of prostaglandin from the uterus may affect the increase in prolactin which must occur to stimulate lactogenesis immediately prior to parturition (5).

An unusual cause of agalactia and secondary mastitis in sows is that due to the migration of *Sarcopsylla penetrans* into the streak canal (25).

In summary, the etiology is not clear. Field observations have suggested many different causes and predisposing factors including infectious mastitis, nutritional disturbances, metabolic disorders and the stress of farrowing in total confinement in a crate. Based on the examination of spontaneously occurring cases infectious mastitis appears to be a major cause. Most of the other suggested causes have not been substantiated.

Epidemiology

The disease occurs most commonly in sows which are farrowed in crates indoors and only occasionally in sows farrowed outdoors, which may be a reflection of the greater number of pigs raised in confinement. Morbidity and mortality data are not readily available nor precise because of the difficulty of making a reliable clinical diagnosis. The population incidence of toxic agalactia ranges from 4 to 10% of all farrowings while the herd incidence may vary from 0 to 100%. Some surveys report an overall incidence of 6·9% of all farrowings with a range from 1·1 to 37·2% (32). In one single, large, closed herd, over a period of 24 months, 31% of 1360 farrowings were associated with postparturient disease, 25% due to mastitis and 75% due to farrowing fever (33). Sporadic outbreaks of the disease may occur in which almost all sows farrowing over a period of several weeks or a few months may be affected and then suddenly no further cases develop for no apparent reason. The mortality of sows affected with toxic agalactia is usually less than 2%, but piglet losses due to starvation and crushing may be as high as 80%. Epidemiological observations indicate that the risk of sows developing toxic mastitis increases with increasing age up to the third or fourth litter (33). In one study the incidence of the disease was 4·2% in gilts and 13·0% in pluriparous sows (32). A peak incidence during the summer months has also be observed (32). However, none of these has been substantiated. The disease does not usually recur in the same animal which may suggest that immunity develops, and possibly that affected sows should not necessarily be culled because of the disease.

The predisposing factors which have been proposed based on field observations include overfeeding during pregnancy, a drastic change of feed at farrowing, insufficient time for the sow to adjust to the farrowing crate after being transferred from the gestation unit and constipation of the sow at farrowing. The incidence of the disease may also be higher in sows with larger litters than sows in the same herd which remain healthy, and in those with a higher number of stillbirths and pigs found dead after birth (32). The disease has been observed under management, environmental and sanitation conditions ranging from very poor to excellent. However, the possible relationship between the level of bacterial contamination in the farrowing barn and on the skin of the sow and the incidence of the disease has apparently not been examined. If infectious mastitis is the most common cause of the disease then it would appear logical to study the ecology of the organisms in the sow's environment. This requires an interdisciplinary investigation of the microbiological, immunological and pathological aspects of the disease under naturally occurring circumstances.

Pathogenesis

The pathogenesis of infectious mastitis due to *E. coli* or *Klebsiella* spp. is probably similar to that of bovine mastitis in which the infection gains entry through the teat canal and invades the mammary tissue causing mastitis. Susceptibility of some sows to *E. coli* induced mastitis may be associated with a depressed function of polymorphonuclear cell function of uncertain cause (20). In one study susceptible sows were from a conventional herd and the resistant sows from a specific-pathogen-free (SPF) herd (12). Endotoxemia occurs accounting for the fever initially, and the depression, anorexia and agalactia, even in glands which are unaffected (6). The lipopolysaccharide endotoxins acting at the level of the hypothalamus and hypophysis suppress the release of prolactin which results in a marked decline in milk production (34, 35). The endotoxin may also have a direct inhibitory effect on the mammary gland. There is a higher prevalence of bacterial endotoxin in the blood of affected sows compared to control animals (24). Experimentally, mastitis can be produced in sows by contamination of the skin of the teats with *Klebsiella pneumoniae* either shortly before or after parturition (11). The clinical signs are similar to those described for MMA; mastitis is present in more than 50% of the mammary gland subsections and a marked leukopenia and degenerative left shift occurs. A total of 120 organisms is sufficient to produce the mastitis when the organisms are inoculated into the teats.

If non-infectious acute painful swelling of the mammary glands accompanied by agalactia occurs in the sow due to the possible non-infectious factors which are described earlier, the pathogenesis is unclear. It is difficult to synthesize a pathophysiological mechanism which would explain how stress, overfeeding, changes in diet or constipation could result in acute swelling of the mammary gland in sows.

Clinical findings

The sow is usually normal with a normal milk flow for the first 12–18 hours after farrowing. One of the first indications of the disease is the failure of the sow to suckle her piglets. She is disinterested in the piglets, generally lies in sternal recumbency and is unresponsive to their squealing and sucking demands. Litters of affected sows are more noisy and are generally scattered around the pen searching for an alternative food supply. Such piglets may drink surface water or urine in the pen and infectious diarrhea may occur. If sucking is permitted, it does not progress from the vigorous nosing phase to the quiet letdown stage, and it is accompanied by much teat-to-teat movement by the piglets. Many piglets may die from starvation and hypoglycemia. Some sows are initially restless and stand up and lie down frequently which contributes to a high mortality from crushing and trampling.

Affected sows do not eat, drink very little and are generally lethargic. The body temperature is usually elevated and ranges from 39·5 to 41°C (103·1 to 105·8°F). Mild elevations in body temperatures of sows in the first 2 days after parturition are difficult to interpret because a slight elevation occurs in normal healthy sows (26). This is known as uncomplicated farrowing fever. However, temperatures above 40°C (104°F) are usually associated with acute mastitis which requires treatment. The heart and respiratory rates are usually increased.

Initial temperatures greater than 40·5°C (104·9°F) are usually followed by severe illness and toxemia.

The characteristic findings are present in the mammary glands and consist of varying degrees of swelling and inflammation (3). In most cases, several sections are affected which results in the appearance of diffuse involvement of the entire udder. Individual sections are enlarged, warm and painful, and may feel 'meaty' and lack the resilience of normal mammary tissue. There may be extensive subcutaneous edema around and between each section which results in a ridge of edema on the lateral aspects of the udder extending for its entire length. The skin overlying the sections is usually reddened and is easily blanched by finger pressure. The teats are usually empty and may be slightly edematous. A few drops of milk may be expressed out of some teats after gentle massage of the section or the administration of oxytocin but rarely can a normal stream of milk be obtained. In severe cases of mastitis the milk contains flakes and pus or is watery.

The feces are usually scant and drier than normal but whether or not constipation is present in most cases is uncertain. The inappetence and anorexia and failure to drink normally could account for the reduced volume of feces. Constipation with impaction of the rectum with large quantities of feces is uncommon in sows and when it does occur as the only abnormality it has little effect on appetite and milk production.

A vaginal discharge is normal following parturition, and normal sows frequently expel up to 50 ml of a viscid non-odorous clear mucus which contains variable amounts of white material within the first 3 days following farrowing. Tenacious strands of this discharge may also be observed within the vagina. The presence of this discharge has been misleading and interpreted as evidence of the presence of metritis. Necropsy examination after euthanasia of affected sows has failed to reveal evidence of significant metritis (27). The clinical diagnosis of metritis in sows is difficult but generally large quantities of dark-brown foul-smelling fluid are expelled several times daily accompanied by severe toxemia. This is uncommon in sows.

Clinical pathology

Some hematological and biochemical changes are present in affected sows but may not be marked enough to be a routine reliable diagnostic aid. In severe cases of infectious mastitis, a marked leukopenia with a degenerative left shift is common (4). In moderate cases there is a leukocytosis and a regenerative left shift. The serum biochemical changes which occur in naturally occurring cases and in the experimental disease, are recorded (14, 15). The plasma cortisol levels are commonly elevated which may be due to a combination of the stress of parturition and infectious mastitis (4, 15). The plasma protein-to-fibrinogen ratio is lower than normal and the plasma fibrinogen levels are commonly increased in severe cases which occur 8–16 hours after parturition.

The pH of the milk from affected sows with mastitis ranges from 7 to 7·8, whereas in normal sows the pH ranges from 6·4 to 6·5. The number of somatic cells in the milk from sows with mastitis will range from 2 to 20 million/ml compared to the normal of less than 2 million/ml (28). Milk obtained for laboratory examination and culture should be taken after thorough cleaning and disinfection of the teats to minimize contamination by skin flora. However, because mastitis may be present in only one or a few of the mammary gland subsections in the sow and because it is often impossible to clinically identify affected subsections and distinguish them from unaffected adjacent glands which may be swollen and agalactic because of continuous swelling, a valid assessment of intramammary infection is not possible unless milk samples are obtained from each subsection.

Necropsy findings

The most important lesions are present in the mammary gland (2). There may be extensive edema and some slight hemorrhage of the subcutaneous tissue. Grossly on cross-section of the mammary tissue there is focal to diffuse reddening and often only one subsection of a mammary gland may be affected. Histologically, the mastitis may be focal or diffuse in distribution and the intensity of the lesion varies from a mild catarrhal inflammation to a severe purulent and necrotizing mastitis involving usually more than 50% of all the mammary glands. There are no significant lesions of the uterus when compared with the state of the uterus in normal healthy sows immediately after parturition (13). The adrenal gland is enlarged and heavier than normal presumably due to adrenocortical hyperactivity. In a series of spontaneous cases, *E. coli* and *Klebsiella* spp. were most commonly isolated from the mammary tissues (10). The disease can be reproduced experimentally by contamination of the skin of the teats of sows with *Klebsiella* spp. immediately before and after parturition (11). The abscesses of the mammary glands of sows examined at slaughter are not sequelae to coliform mastitis but rather probably due to injuries and secondary infection (23).

Diagnosis

The characteristic clinical findings in toxic agalactia are a sudden onset of anorexia and disinterest in the piglets, acute swelling of the mammary gland, hypogalactia or agalactia, a moderate fever and a course of about 2 days. In severe cases of infectious mastitis there may be a leukopenia and a degenerative left shift. The mammary secretion from mastitic glands may be watery or thickened and contain pus, and the cell count will be increased up to 20 million ml.

The major problem in the clinical diagnosis is to differentiate the acute swelling and agalactia of infectious mastitis from other non-infectious causes of acute swelling or 'caking' of the mammary glands which also results in agalactia. Agalactia due to a failure in milk letdown is most common in first litter gilts and is characterized by a fullness of the mammary glands but an inability of the gilt to suckle her piglets in spite of her grunting at them. The gilt is usually bright and alert and systemically normal. The response to oxytocin is dramatic and repeat treatment is rarely necessary. Farrowing fever is characterized clinically by loss of appetite, inactivity, a body temperature from 39·3 to 39·9°C (102·7 to 103·8°F) with minimal detectable changes of the mammary gland (32).

Parturient psychosis of sows is characterized by an aggressive and nervous behavior of the sow after the piglets are born. The sow does not call the piglets and does not allow them to suck. When the piglets approach the sow's head, she will back away, snap and make noisy staccato nasal expirations. Some sows will bite and kill their piglets. The mammary gland is usually full of milk but the sow will not let it down (29). Ataractic drugs and/or short-term general anesthesia are indicated and the response is usually excellent. Some sows need repeated tranquillization or sedation for the first few days until the maternal–neonatal bond is established. Other causes of agalactia accompanied by enlargement of the mammary gland include inherited inverted teats, and blind teats due to necrosis of the teats occurring when the gilt was a piglet. These are readily obvious on clinical examination. The sharp needle teeth of piglets may cause the sow to refuse to suckle her piglets. The sow attempts to suckle but leaps up suddenly, grunting and snapping at the piglets. The piglets squeal and fight to retain a teat, thus causing more damage to the teats which is obvious on clinical examination. Other causes of agalactia accompanied by systemic illness include retained piglets and infectious disease such as outbreaks of transmissible gastroenteritis and erysipelas. The common causes of agalactia in swine where there is lack of mammary development include ergotism, immature gilts and inherited lack of mammary development. These are set out in Fig. 22.

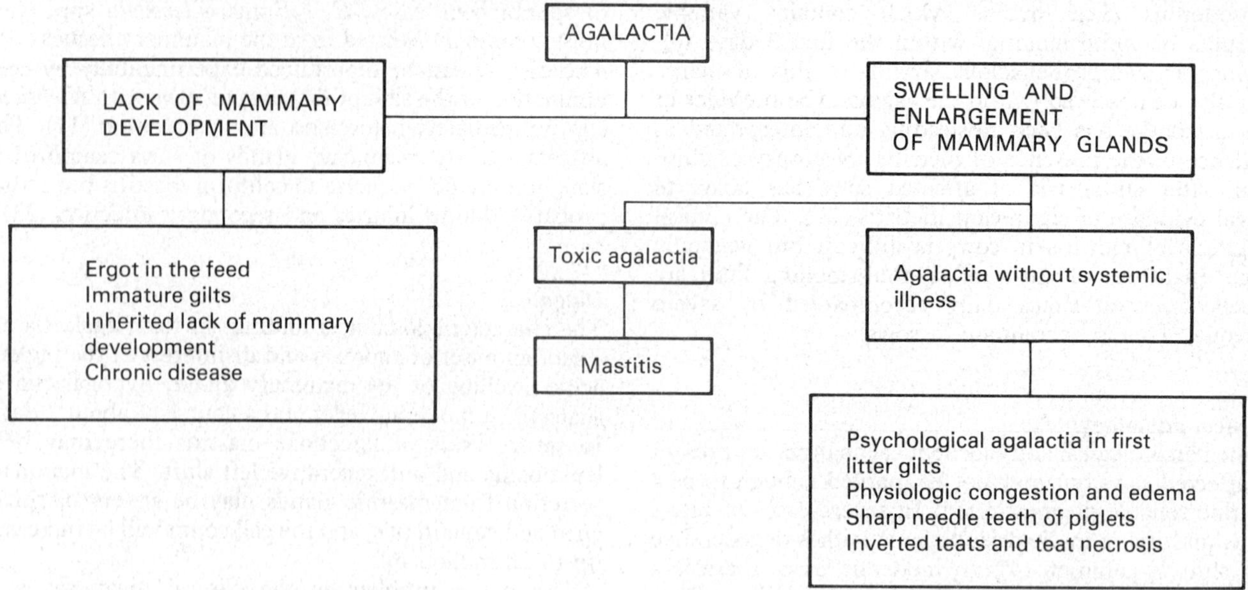

Fig. 22. The causes of porcine agalactia

Treatment

Most affected sows will recover within 24–48 hours if treated with a combination of antibiotics, oxytocin and corticosteroids (1).

Antibiotics are indicated in most cases because infectious mastitis is one of the most common causes of the disease. The choice of antibiotic is generally determined by previous experience in the herd or region but broad-spectrum antibiotics are indicated because *E. coli* and *Klebsiella* spp. are the most common pathogens involved. They should be given daily for at least 3 days.

As soon as possible after the disease is recognized every effort must be made to restore normal mammary function through the use of oxytocin and warm water massaging of the affected mammary glands. Oxytocin, 30–40 units intramuscularly or 20–30 units intravenously, is given to promote the letdown of milk. If there is a beneficial response the piglets should be placed on the sow if she is willing to allow them to suck. This will assist in promoting milk flow. Massage of the mammary glands with warm water soaked towels and hand milking for 10–15 minutes every few hours may assist in reducing the swelling and inflammation and promote the flow of milk. It will also relieve the pain and encourage the sow to suckle her piglets. Intramuscular injections of oxytocin may be repeated every hour along with massaging of the glands with warm water. Failure of milk letdown or a low response following the use of oxytocin may be due to a reduced sensitivity of the sow to oxytocin during the first week of lactation (7). In the normal healthy sow the peak response to oxytocin occurs in the second week of lactation and gradually decreases to a low response at the eighth week.

The use of a longacting synthetic analog of oxytocin d (COMOT) is being explored as a possible substitute for oxytocin (34). Oxytocin has an effect for about 14 minutes, while the analog has an effect for about 6 hours. Preliminary results of its use in agalactic sows indicate superior results compared to oxytocin (36).

Corticosteroids are used regularly, presumably for their anti-inflammatory effect. Plasma cortisol levels are increased in the experimental disease (6) and for this reason may be contraindicated. But field reports suggest that their use along with antibiotics and oxytocin provides a better response than when they are not used. Corticosteroids used alone do not appear to prevent the disease or enhance recovery (30). To be effective they must be used in combination with antibiotics and oxytocin. Dexamethazone at the rate of 20 mg intramuscularly daily for 3 days for sows weighing 150–200 kg is recommended.

The piglets must be given a supply of milk and or balanced electrolytes and dextrose until the milk flow of the sow is resumed, which may take 2–4 days. Piglets should receive from 300 to 500 ml of milk per day divided into hourly doses of 40–50 ml given through a 12–14 F gauge plastic tube passed orally into the stomach. A solution of balanced electrolytes containing 5% glucose can also be given for 1 or 2 days if a supply of cows' milk is not available. Condensed canned milk diluted with water 1:1 is a satisfactory and readily available supply of milk. In severe cases where the return to milk production and flow are unlikely, the piglets should be fostered onto other sows. If these are unavailable, the use of porcine gammaglobulin fortified milk substitute is recommended to prevent the common enteric diseases. This is discussed under colibacillosis.

The indication for the use of laxatives and cathartics in this disease is questionable. Their use is recommended if constipation is present but constipation is uncommon in this disease and, indeed, is uncommon in sows at any time. For this reason they are not recommended for routine use.

Control

It has been difficult to develop a rational approach to control because the disease has been considered as a complex syndrome caused by several different factors. However, the control of infectious mastitis would seem to be of major importance. Farrowing crates should be vacated, cleaned, disinfected and left vacant for a few days before pregnant sows are transferred from the dry sow barn and placed in the crates. Pregnant sows should be washed with soap and water before being placed in the crate. Farrowing crates must be kept clean and hosed down if necessary, particularly a few days before and after farrowing to minimize the level of intramammary infection. In problem herds, it may be necessary to wash and disinfect the skin over the mammary glands immediately after farrowing.

To minimize the stress on the sow of adjusting to the farrowing crate and the farrowing facilities, the sow should be placed in the crates at least 1 week before the expected date of farrowing. The nature and composition of the diet fed to the sow while in the farrowing crate should not be changed. The only change which is necessary is to increase the daily intake (compared to the intake during the dry period) beginning on the day after the sow has farrowed and in increments thereafter as the stage of lactation proceeds. The inclusion of bran at the rate of one-third to one-half of the total diet for 2 days before and after farrowing has been recommended to prevent constipation. In some herds the use of lucerne meal at the rate of 15% of the diet at all times appears to be necessary to control the disease. However, under intensified conditions it may be impractical to prepare and provide these special diets on a regular basis. While field observations suggest that a bulky diet at the time of farrowing will minimize the incidence of toxic agalactia, there is little scientific evidence to support the practice.

Antimicrobial agents used prophylactically have apparently been successful in controlling some outbreaks. A sulfadimidine–trimethoprim and sulfathiazole combination fed for 3–5 days before the expected farrowing date may reduce the incidence of the disease in problem herds (8).

The use of prostaglandins for the induction of parturition in sows has not been associated with a marked consistent change in the incidence of the disease. Some field trials have shown a reduction (9) while others have had no effect (22).

REVIEW LITERATURE

Smith, B. P. (1985) Pathogenesis and therapeutic management of lactation failure in periparturient sows. *Comp. cont. E duc. Pract. Vet.*, 9, S523–S532.

REFERENCES

(1) Ringarp, N. (1960) *Acta agric. Scand.*, Suppl. 7.
(2) Ross, R. F. et al. (1981) *Am. J. vet. Res.*, *42*, 949.
(3) Hermansson, I. et al. (1978) *Nord. VetMed.*, *30*, 465.
(4) Hermansson, I. et al. (1978) *Nord. VetMed.*, *30*, 474.
(5) Peter, A. T. et al. (1985) *Res. vet. Sci.*, *39*, 222.
(6) Elmore, R. G. et al. (1978) *Theriogenology*, *10*, 439.
(7) Sims, M. H. & Eilen, H. (1979) *Am. J. vet. Res.*, *40*, 1104.
(8) Sorensen C. P. & Wittenburg, J. (1978) *Dansk Vet.*, *61*, 287.
(9) Ehrvall, R. et al. (1977) *Nord. VetMed.*, 29.
(10) Bertschinger, H. U. et al. (1977) *Schweiz. Arch. Tierheilkd.*, *119*, 223.
(11) Bertschinger, H. U. et al. (1977) *Schweiz. Arch. Tierheilkd.*, *119*, 265.
(12) Ross, R. F. et al. (1983) *Am. J. vet. Res.*, *44*, 949.
(13) Von Middleton-Williams, D. M. et al. (1977) *Schweiz. Arch. Tierheilkd.*, *119*, 213.
(14) Nachreiner, R. F & Ginther, O. J. (1974) *Am. J.vet. Res.*, *35*, 619.
(15) Nachreiner, R. F & Ginther, O. J. (1972) *Am. J. vet. Res.*, *33*, 799, 2233, 2489.
(16) Fraser, D. (1973) *Br. vet. J.*, *129*, 324.
(17) Whittemore, C. T. & Fraser, D. (1974) *Br. vet. J.*, *130*, 346.
(18) Fraser, D. (1975) *Br. vet. J.*, *131*, 416.
(19) Fraser, D. (1977) *Br. vet. J.*, *133*, 126.
(20) Lofstedt, J. et al. (1983) *Am. J. vet. Res.*, *44*, 1224.
(21) Anderson, J. F. & Werdin, R. E. (1977) *J. Am. vet. med. Assoc.*, *170*, 1089.
(22) Hansen, L. H. (1979) *Nord VetMed.*, *31*, 122.
(23) Delgado, J. A. & Jones, J. E. T. (1981) *Br. vet. J.*, *137*, 639.
(24) Morkoc, A. et al. (1983) *J. Am. vet. med. Assoc.*, *183*, 786.
(25) Verhulst, A. (1976) *Vet. Rec.*, *98*, 384.
(26) King, G. J. et al. (1972) *Can. vet. J.*, *13*, 72.
(27) Jones, J. E. T. (1971) *Vet. Rec.*, *89*, 72.
(28) Jones, J. E. T. (1976) *Proc. 4th int. Congr. Pig vet. Soc.*, E6.
(29) Henry, D. P. (1969) *Aust. vet. J.*, *45*, 344.
(30) Martin, C. E. & Threlfall, W. R. (1970) *Vet. Rec.*, *87*, 768.
(31) Smith, B. B. & Wagner, W. C. (1984) *Science*, *224*, 605.
(32) Backstrom, L. et al. (1984) *J. Am. vet. med. Assoc.*, *183*, 70.
(33) Halgaard, C. (1983) *Nord. VetMed.*, *35*, 161.
(34) Smith, B. B. (1985) *Comp. cont. Educ. Pract. Vet.*, 9, S523.
(35) Smith, B. B. & Wagner, W. C. (1985) *Am. J. vet. Res.*, *46*, 175.
(36) Cort, N. et al. (1982) *Am. J. vet. Res.*, *43*, 1283.

16

Diseases Caused by Bacteria—I

INTRODUCTION TO INFECTIOUS DISEASES

THE infectious diseases are of major importance in agricultural animals. The bacterial, viral, fungal, protozoal and parasitic diseases account for a major portion of this book. The infectious diseases are capable of affecting many animals in a short period of time and the case fatality rate in some diseases can be very high and the economic losses may be very large. Certain infectious diseases, especially the viral diseases, are endemic in some countries and pose a threat to other countries considered free of the disease. The veterinary profession has made a major contribution in developing reliable diagnostic techniques and effective control procedures for many of these diseases. Some of the infectious diseases assume major importance because they are directly transmissible to man.

The clinical and laboratory diagnosis of the infectious diseases can be difficult. However, with the appropriate laboratory support and suitable samples, most of them can be diagnosed definitively. For each disease certain samples must be submitted to the laboratory for isolation or demonstration of the specific pathogen.

When herd or area population epidemics occur, a detailed examination of the epidemiological characteristics of the disease is often useful in helping to make a diagnosis and in treatment and control. Particular attention should be given to the epidemiological aspects of the history, for example: the descriptive epidemiology including the distribution in age or other groups; the morbidity and case fatality and population mortality rates; the seasonal incidence; relationship to other species; recent changes in management; vaccination history; nutritional history; disease in previous years; source of imported animals; and the treatments used and the success rate. The epidemiological behavior of the epidemic includes an examination of the manner of spread of disease between individual and groups of animals, the age of animals affected, the length of the course of the disease and the estimated incubation period. It may be necessary to establish a prospective survey or surveillance studies on sentinel herds to monitor the spread of the disease. Field investigation may include the examination of nearby herds or other species such as wildlife or man, which may be sources of the infection.

When an infectious disease is suspected it is customary to undertake certain kinds of laboratory investigations in addition to the general clinical examinations. The recommended techniques of investigation are given for each disease. A general protocol for the detailed examination of a suspected infectious disease would include the following:

- Clinical, hematological, and immunological examinations should be done on as many clinically affected animals as possible. Similar examinations should be conducted on normal animals which have been in close contact with the affected animals. The detection of latent carriers among clinically normal animals may require special laboratory tests. Repeated visits and examinations may be necessary to determine the presence and rate of seroconversion in an affected herd as an indication of the rate and direction of spread
- Tissue samples from necropsies and from live animals (biopsies) and discharges, feces and urine should be submitted for isolation or demonstration of the suspected pathogen.

The responsibility of the veterinarian in the case of infectious diseases is to advise the owner of the risks of spread to other animals or population and the need for treatment and/or control. In the case of notifiable diseases, the government regulatory authorities must be notified immediately. Every precaution must be taken to prevent the spread of the disease to nearby herds or other geographical areas. Veterinarians also have a responsibility to alert their clients of the possibility that an infectious disease may be approaching geographically and to take the necessary precautions.

The control of infectious diseases is dependent on a knowledge of the etiology and epidemiological characteristics of the disease. Any one or a combination of the following principles may be effective for the control of a specific infectious disease.

- Ensure adequate colostral immunity in the newborn
- Identify affected animals, isolated from normal

animals, treat or dispose of as indicated and return to the herd if considered safe

- Prevent the introduction of infected animals into herds previously considered free of the disease. Quarantine all animals imported into a herd for a period of 30–60 days. Serological testing may be done on imported animals
- Determine the source of the infection and remove if possible. Sources include infected animals, feed and water supplies, wildlife and contaminated environments
- Control use of mass medication of feed and water supplies, which may be effective in swine dysentery and coccidiosis
- Clean and disinfect animal houses and grounds regularly—this is essential. When animals occupy a barn for prolonged periods (weeks or months) without a clean-out and disinfection, the build-up of infectious agents increases almost geometrically and the incidence of disease will increase
- Provide an optimal environment for housed animals. This includes adequate ventilation, the prevention of overcrowding and effective removal of manure
- Establish primary breeding stock through the use of specific-pathogen-free animals obtained by hysterectomy or cesarean section and rearing under controlled conditions; may be indicated for the control of diseases such as enzootic pneumonia of swine
- Vaccinate susceptible animals against endemic diseases; this should be part of a regularly scheduled herd health program which includes vaccination of the pregnant dam for the enhancement of colostral immunity in the newborn
- Avoid stress associated with long transportation, inclement weather and undernutrition
- Base effective control of intestinal parasites on measures designed to prevent or limit contact between parasite and host. The strategies are to: (*a*) prevent the build-up of dangerous numbers of larvae on pastures; (*b*) anticipate the periods during which large numbers of larvae are likely to occur and remove susceptible animals from heavily contaminated pastures before these periods. These aims can be achieved using three interrelated approaches: by grazing management, by the use of anthelmintics, and by dependence on the acquisition of immunity.

DISEASES CAUSED BY *STREPTOCOCCUS* spp.

Mastitis caused by *Streptococcus agalactiae*, *Str. dysgalactiae*, *Str. uberis* and *Str. zooepidemicus* is dealt with in Chapter 15. Strangles in horses, neonatal streptococcal infections and streptococcal cervical abscesses of pigs are dealt with in this section.

Other miscellaneous diseases in which streptococci appear to have etiological significance include septicemic infections of swine, sheep and calves, pneumonia in calves, meningoencephalitis and otitis media in feeder pigs, lymphangitis in foals, and infectious dermatitis of piglets.

Septicemia

- Acute streptococcal septicemia of adult sows and their litters occurs sporadically (1). The onset is sudden and death occurs in 12–48 hours. Clinically there is weakness, prostration, fever, dyspnea, dysentery and hematuria. At necropsy, petechial and ecchymotic hemorrhages are present throughout all organs. Animals which survive for several days show extensive edema and consolidation of the lungs. The infection spreads rapidly and the mortality rate may be very high unless the drug sensitivity of the organism, usually *Str. zooepidemicus*, is determined and appropriate treatment instituted
- Septicemia with sudden death in calves has also been recorded in which *Strep. pneumoniae* was the apparent cause (2)
- In sheep flocks septicemia due to *Strep. zooepidemicus* has caused up to 90% mortality in lambs (3).

Enteritis

Streptococcus durans has been isolated from a foal with enteritis and has caused mild enteritis and diarrhea in foals infected orally. A similar disease was produced in gnotobiotic piglets (7).

Pneumonia

- A syndrome of pneumonia and fibrinous pleuritis and pericarditis is recorded in lambs as being caused by *Str. zooepidemicus* (4)
- Pneumonia in calves may be caused commonly by *Str. pneumoniae* in some areas (5) and unidentified streptococci are common invaders in viral pneumonia of calves. Infections in calves with *Str. pneumoniae* may have public health significance; the isolation of identical strains of the organism from the lungs of calves dying of the disease and from the throats of their human attendants suggests that interspecies transmission may occur (6). Calves may be immunized either by the use of antiserum or through vaccination of their dams with a polyvalent aluminum hydroxide-adsorbed vaccine (8). *Streptococcus pneumoniae* is also associated with inflammatory disease of the lower respiratory tract of horses, sometimes in association with *Str. zooepidemicus* (13).

Meningoencephalitis

Meningoencephalitis is a common complication of streptococcal septicemia of the newborn but it has also occurred in weaned pigs 10–14 weeks of age and in feeder pigs of 5–6 months of age (9). In the former the causative organism is identified as *Str. suis* type 2 as distinct from type 1 which affects only newborn piglets (10). These *Str. suis* type 2 bacteria are probably identical with the Lancefield group R streptococci isolated from some cases of porcine pneumonia in the United Kingdom (12).

Lymphangitis

An ulcerative lymphangitis caused in many instances by *Str. zooepidemicus*, has been observed in foals from 6 months to 2 years of age and may be confused with ulcerative lymphangitis caused by *Corynebacterium pseudotuberculosis*.

Dermatitis

Infectious dermatitis (contagious pyoderma) of pigs is characterized by the formation of pustules about the face and neck, and to a lesser extent the trunk. Streptococci and staphylococci are present in the lesions and spread appears to occur through abrasions, especially in young pigs which fight and have not had their needle teeth removed. The disease may be confused with exudative epidermitis.

Genital tract infections

Streptococcal infections of the genital tract occur commonly, especially in mares, in which the disease is thought to be spread by coitus, and is accompanied by a high incidence of abortion, sterility and neonatal infection in foals. Foals from infected mares may be affected each year. Although streptococcal metritis occurs in sows, there appears to be no relationship between uterine infection and neonatal septicemia. Abortions in sows may be due in some instances to infection with beta-hemolytic streptococci (11).

One of the important features of streptococcal diseases is their lack of susceptibility to control by vaccination. Vaccines against strangles of horses and cervical adenitis of pigs are available, but results with them are equivocal. When the vaccines are properly prepared and carefully and intelligently applied the results are very good. However, it is apparent that the streptococci are not good antigens and the vaccines made with them lack the ease of application and safety that one expects with, say, the clostridial vaccines.

REVIEW LITERATURE

Wood, R. D. & Ross, R. F. (1976) Streptococcosis of swine. *Vet. Bull.*, *46*, 397.

REFERENCES

(1) Baker, W. L. (1960) *Vet. Med.*, *55*, 32.
(2) Donald, I. G. & Mann, S. O. (1950) *Vet. Rec.*, *62*, 257.
(3) Rafyi, A. & Mir Chamsey, H. (1953) *Bull. Acad. vét. Fr.*, *26*, 145.
(4) Stevenson, R. G. (1974) *Can J. comp. Med.*, *38*, 243.
(5) Hammer, D. (1956) *Zentralbl. Bakteriol.*, *161*, 269.
(6) Romer, O. (1960) *Nord. VetMed.*, *12*, 73.
(7) Tzipori. S. (1984) *J. Infect. Dis.*, *150*, 589.
(8) Fey, H. & Richle, J. (1961) *Schweiz. Arch. Tierheilkd.*, *103*, 349.
(9) Jansen, J. A. C. & van Dorssen, C. A. (1951) *Tijdschr. Diergeneeskd.*, *76*, 815.
(10) Windsor, R. S. (1977) *Vet. Rec.*, *101*, 378.
(11) Saunders, C. N. (1958) *Vet. Rec.*, *70*, 965.
(12) Koehne, G. et al. (1978) *Am. J. vet. Res.*, *40*, 1640.
(13) Burrell, M. H. et al. (1986) *Equ. vet. J.*, *18*, 183.

Strangles (distemper)

Strangles is an acute disease of horses caused by infection with *Streptococcus equi*. It is characterized by inflammation of the upper respiratory tract and abscessation in the adjacent lymph nodes.

Etiology

Streptococcus equi is present in the nasal discharge and abscesses and young, pure cultures of the organism are capable of producing the disease in susceptible horses (1). An atypical milder form of the disease is caused by a capsule-deficient variant of *Str. equi* (11).

Epidemiology

Horses are the only species affected, the disease occurring in animals of any age but particularly in the 1–5-year age group. Outbreaks can occur at any time of the year but are most likely to happen in cold, wet weather. However, the movement of horses has more influence on the occurrence of outbreaks than the climate. Although strong immunity occurs immediately after an attack, a horse may suffer repeated attacks at intervals of about 6 months if the infection is a virulent one and persists in the group.

The source of infection in strangles is the nasal discharge from infected animals which contaminates pasture and feed and water troughs. Such animals can spread infection for at least 4 weeks after a clinical attack. The organism is relatively resistant to environmental influences and mediate contagion can occur in infected premises for about a month after affected animals have been removed. Infection occurs by ingestion or by inhalation of droplets.

The infection is capable of persisting in the pharynx of clinically normal horses for up to 10 months and this provides a means of carrying the infection through periods when the disease is dormant (2). There is evidence that infection with *Str. equi* causes strong immunity in horses and the immunity can be detected by a hypersensitivity skin test (1). However, serum bactericidal activity is not considered to be a good indicator of resistance to the infection (11).

Antibodies are passed to foals via the colostrum and are secreted into the foal's nasopharyngeal mucosa and also physically coat the oral and upper respiratory mucosae during the first few months of life (15).

The distribution of strangles is worldwide although, with the decline in horse numbers and improvement in therapy, it has become of minor importance in most countries. The major epidemics which used to occur in mounted units of the armed forces, in remount depots and draft horse stables are now reduced for the most part to minor outbreaks in polo and racing stables and to individual horses taken to fairs and riding schools.

When an outbreak does occur in a large group of horses, it is usually restricted to the younger age groups and the morbidity rate may be as low as 10%. Under adverse climatic conditions, and when shelter is inadequate, or when the group is made up of predominantly young horses, up to 100% may be affected. Such a high incidence is often encountered soon after large numbers of susceptible horses, which may have come from many localities, are stabled together.

The mortality rate with adequate early treatment is very low but may reach 1–2% due to occasional extension of infection to other organs. Purpura hemorrhagica may also be an important sequel.

Pathogenesis

Infection of the pharyngeal and nasal mucosae causes an acute pharyngitis and rhinitis. Empyema of the guttural pouches is an uncommon sequel of strangles, and most cases involving them have no etiological relationship to strangles. However, experimental intranasal inoculation of horses with *Str. equi* has led to a high rate of occurrence of guttural pouch empyema (3). Drainage to local lymph nodes results in abscessation and the infection may spread to other organs causing the development of suppurative processes in the kidney, brain, liver, spleen, tendon sheaths and joints (8). After an attack of strangles has subsided purpura hemorrhagica may occur, due to the development of sensitivity to streptococcal protein.

Clinical findings

After an incubation period of 4–8 days, the disease develops suddenly with complete anorexia, fever (39·5–40·5°C, 103–105°F), a serous nasal discharge, which rapidly becomes copious and purulent, and a severe pharyngitis and laryngitis. Rarely there is a mild conjunctivitis. The pharyngitis may be so severe that the animal is unable to swallow, and attempts to swallow food or water are often followed by regurgitation through the nostrils. A soft, moist cough which causes apparent pain and is easily stimulated by compression of the pharynx is constant. The head may be extended to ease the pain in throat.

The febrile reaction commonly subsides in 2–3 days but soon returns as the characteristic abscesses develop in the lymph nodes of the throat region. The affected nodes become hot, swollen and painful. The purulent nasal discharge increases and there may be obstruction to swallowing and respiration. Obvious swelling of the nodes may take 3–4 days to develop and, in many cases, if treatment is not effective, the glands begin to exude serum at about 10 days and rupture to discharge thick, cream-yellow pus soon afterwards.

If the infection is particularly severe, many other lymph nodes, including the pharyngeal, submaxillary and parotid nodes, may abscess at the same time. Local abscesses may also occur at any point on the body surface, particularly on the face and limbs, and the infection may spread to local lymphatic vessels causing obstructive edema. This occurs most frequently in the lower limbs where extreme edema may cause the part to swell to three or four times the normal size. It is probable that abscess formation in other organs also occurs at this time.

Complications of the disease occur as a result of metastasis and abscess formation in other organs; metastatic spread to the lungs may cause the development of acute pneumonia; cerebral involvement usually takes the form of purulent meningitis with signs of excitation, hyperesthesia, rigidity of the neck and terminal paralysis; infected thrombi in veins occur rarely and cause local signs of vascular obstruction; abscesses may develop in the liver, spleen or visceral lymph nodes and may cause death if rupture occurs weeks or months after apparent recovery from the acute form of the disease. A specific syndrome has been described in which pericarditis and arthritis occur and from which *Str. faecalis* has been isolated. Clinically there are severe lameness, dyspnea and an increased cardiac impulse.

An atypical form of the disease may occur and is characterized by widespread subclinical infection and a mild disease. Affected horses have a transient fever for 24–48 hours, a profuse nasal discharge and are anorexic. A moderate enlargement of the mandibular lymph nodes occurs in only about one-half of the affected horses (10).

Strangles in burros is a slowly developing debilitating disease. At postmortem examination the characteristic lesions consist of caseation and calcification of abdominal lymph nodes (4).

Clinical pathology

Nasal swabs and discharges from abscesses can be examined for the presence of *Str. equi* and sensitivity tests carried out on the cultures. The serological response to the natural infection or vaccination can be measured using the passive hemagglutination and long chain and bactericidal tests (9). There is leukocytosis with a neutrophilia reaching a peak as the lymph nodes abscess. There may or may not be an anemia due to the hemolytic effect of the streptococci or to toxic depression of hemopoiesis.

Necropsy findings

In the rare fatalities that occur, necropsy examination usually reveals extensive suppuration in internal organs, especially the liver, spleen, lungs, pleura, large vessels and the peritoneum. When the latter is involved, it is usually due to extension from abscesses in the mesenteric lymph nodes.

Diagnosis

An upper respiratory tract infection with purulent nasal discharge and enlargement of the lymph nodes of the throat region are diagnostic of strangles. In the early stages of the disease it may be confused with equine viral rhinopneumonitis, equine viral arteritis and equine influenza but in these diseases there is usually no marked enlargement of the lymph nodes. Occasionally non-specific syndromes with purulent nasal discharges but no enlargement of the lymph nodes are found to be associated with infection by *Str. zooepidemicus* (see also Table 46). Experimental infection of horses by the intravenous injection of this organism causes fever, anorexia, pain in joints, lameness and emaciation (14).

Treatment

Infected horses should be isolated and treatment commenced as soon as possible. Specific treatment comprises

Table 46. Differential diagnosis of diseases of the upper respiratory tract of horses

Disease	Epidemiology	Clinical signs: Respiratory tract	Clinical signs: Other	Clinical pathology	Treatment and/or control
Strangles	Incubation period 4–8 days. Course 10–21 days. Spreads rapidly by contact (inhalation) or mediate (ingestion). Mostly young horses, especially in large comingled groups	Nasal discharge—serous then copious purulent. Cranial lymphadenitis and rupture. Moist severe cough. Rarely conjunctivitis. Obstruction of pharynx can cause dyspnea	Severe illness with emphasis on suppuration. Fever 39·5–40·5°C (103–104·5°F). Atypical cases show involvement of other organs. No abortion or diarrhea. Serious sequelae, e.g. purpura hemorrhagica	*Str. equi* in oropharyngeal pus or lymph node abscess pus. Leukocytosis	Penicillin, ampicillin early and in sufficient dosage. Good vaccine available.
Equine viral arteritis	Incubation period 1–6 days. Course 3–8 days. Some deaths	Serous nasal discharge, may become purulent. Slight cranial lymphadenitis, moderate cough. Severe conjunctivitis, purulent with edema or petechiae. Severe respiratory distress	Severe disease, emphasis on anasarca. Temperature 39–41°C (102–105°F). Severe edema of ventral abdomen, prepuce, legs, scrotum. May be severe diarrhea and jaundice. Up to 50% of mares abort	Virus in blood at fever peak. Serology and tissue culture techniques available. Leukopenia	Nil treatment. Tissue culture vaccine possible but infrequent need means unlikely to be available
Equine viral rhinopneumonitis (equid herpesvirus 1)	Incubation period 2–10 days. Course 2–5 days. Cough may last as long as 3 weeks	Serous nasal discharge, may become purulent. Slight degree of cranial lymphadenitis, coughing and conjunctivitis	Mild disease; emphasis on respiratory tract infection in young, abortion in mares. Up to 90% abort from 5 months up	Virus in nasal discharge. Tissue culture and serological tests well documented. Leukopenia. Hepatic lesions in aborted foals contain the virus. Intranuclear inclusions in fetal liver	Nil treatment. Vaccination where indicated
Equine influenza (influenza A equi 1 and influenza A equi 2)	Incubation period 2–3 days. Course 7 days. Cough may persist 3–4 weeks. Enzootic, world-wide. Explosive outbreaks. 80–100% morbidity in young	Nasal discharge slight, serous only. Slight cranial lymphadenitis. Severe barking dry cough. No conjunctivitis and no respiratory distress	Mild disease; emphasis on coughing. Temperature 39–41°C (102–105°F)	Virus in nasal discharge. Good serological tests available	Nil. Successful bivalent vaccines
Equine rhinovirus	Incubation period 3–8 days. Rapid spread, high morbidity (70%). Solid immunity after natural infection	Pharyngitis, pharyngeal lymphadenitis, nasal discharge serous to mucopurulent. Cough persists 2–3 weeks	Mild disease. Emphasis on coughing. Fever to 39·5°C (103°F)	Equine rhinovirus on tissue culture. Serological tests available	Planned exposure of young horses recommended. No vaccine
Equine adenovirus	Many inapparent infections. High proportion of population serologically positive	Mild respiratory signs in adults. In foals can cause severe non-fatal pneumonia. In Arab foals with combined immunodeficiency may cause fatal pneumonia	Transient softness of feces. In mares can cause abortion without clinical illness	Adenovirus in oropharyngeal swabs. Serological tests available	Nil
Guttural pouch disease	Single horse. Etiology unknown	Intermittent or fatal epistaxis, nasal catarrh, abnormal respiratory noises	Dysphagia, parotid pain, abnormal head posture, sweating and shivering, Horner's syndrome, colic and facial paralysis	Nil	Ligate internal carotid artery. Irrigation of pouches with antimicrobial agent practiced but of doubtful value

the parenteral administration of suitable antibiotics. The sulfonamides are quite effective but have been largely replaced by penicillin. The first injection should combine crystalline and procaine penicillin (2000 and 5000 units/kg body weight respectively is not excessive) and be followed by procaine penicillin alone for two further injections at 24-hour intervals. Provided treatment is commenced early, penicillin is quite adequate but at a later stage intravenous injections of one of the tetracyclines (10 mg/kg body weight/daily) will be more effective but must be continued over a longer time, say 4–5 days. The systemic involvement at least can be controlled but if abscessation in lymph nodes is advanced, the nodes may continue to enlarge and eventually rupture. There is a tendency to restrict the use of tetracylines because of the risk of causing severe diarrhea.

There is controversy about treatment, one school of thought maintaining that horses should not be treated. This view is based on the undesirable outcomes which are likely to occur if cases are well advanced when first seen. Treatment of these horses when lymph nodes are severely abscessed and the infection has spread to a number of sites in the body is likely to result in a temporary improvement and then a recrudescence of the disease. These cases should not be treated other than in a supportive way. On the other hand, failure to treat any cases in an outbreak will return us to the preantibiotic era when massive outbreaks spread through the horse population in a community, increasing in virulence as they went. Morbidity rates would be 90% or more and disability and mortality rates would be 5–10%. A very important matter which has a bearing on a policy of treatment versus non-treatment is that *Str. equi* is not a good antigen and the protection achieved by even the best vaccination regimen is not strong. To subject it to the assault of a massive, high virulence outbreak originating with a program of withholding treatment would be disastrous.

General treatment consists in providing good warm shelter, blanketing if necessary, a soft, palatable diet, keeping the nostrils and muzzle clean and, if time is available, giving steam inhalation. Surgical treatment of abscessed nodes is usually not necessary unless pressure causes dyspnea.

Control

Infected animals should be isolated immediately. If the animal has been housed the stall should be thoroughly cleaned and disinfected and the bedding burned. Pails, brooms, grooming brushes and blankets should also be disinfected.

Vaccination should be considered if a number of horses are exposed but infected horses should not be vaccinated as they are likely to suffer hypersensitivity reactions. Although these reactions are usually restricted to a local one at the injection site they can be very severe and require drainage. For this reason vaccination in the brisket is safest. Occasional cases of a general hypersensitivity reaction including anaphylaxis and purpura hemorrhagica are also reported. The efficiency of strangles vaccination has always been in doubt and there are many records of breakdowns in vaccination programs. This has led to a search for vaccines of greater antigenicity which are less damaging to tissues (13).

A commercial vaccine prepared by carefully killing young cultures of *Str. equi* (5–7), is administered in gradually increasing doses on two or three occasions at 10–14 day intervals. Three injections are recommended for satisfactory protection. Following a series of three vaccinations satisfactory immunity lasts for 12 months and an annual booster dose is recommended (7). Vaccination of foals from 2 to 12 months of age with a commercial bacterin or an autogenous vaccine consisting of whole cells and an acid extract of *Str. equi*, three times at 10-day intervals, results in good protection from natural or experimental challenge (9). Reactions at the site of vaccination are common and cause discomfort to the horse which may alarm the owner, but an explanation that other complications will not occur will usually suffice. Careful skin preparation and massage after injection are strongly recommended. Vaccination should not be commenced until foals are 12 weeks of age. The most that can be expected from such a vaccination program is a reduction in the number of cases and in the severity of the illness in the cases that do occur. On the other hand the immunity produced may be sufficient to slow down or stop an outbreak. Satisfactory protection against strangles is also provided by an M-like protein extracted from *Str. equi* by enzyme treatment and which is injected intramuscularly (12, 13).

REVIEW LITERATURE

Yelle, M. (1987) Clinical aspects of *Streptococcus equi* infection. *Equ. vet. J.*, *19*, 158–162.

REFERENCES

(1) Nara, P. L. et al. (1983) *Am. J. vet. Res.*, *44*, 529.
(2) George, J. L. et al. (1983) *J. Am. vet. med. Assoc.*, *183*, 80.
(3) Knight, A. P. et al. (1973) *Vet Med.*, *70*, 1194, 1198.
(4) Wisecup, W. G. et al. (1967) *J. Am. vet. med. Assoc.*, *150*, 303.
(5) Bazeley, P. L. (1942) *Aust. vet. J.*, *18*, 141, 189; (1943) *19*, 62.
(6) Engelbrecht, H. (1969). *J. Am. vet. med. Assoc.*, *155*, 425.
(7) Woolcock, J. B. (1975) *Aust. vet. J.*, *51*, 554.
(8) Neibauer, G. W. et al. (1979) *Wien. Tierarztl. Monatsschr.*, *66*, 321.
(9) Srivastava, S. K. & Barnum, D. A. (1981) *Can J. comp. Med.*, *45*, 20.
(10) Pres, J. F. et al. (1982) *J. Am. vet. med. Assoc.*, *180*, 293.
(11) Timoney, J. F. & Eggers, D. (1985) *Equ. vet. J.*, *17*, 306.
(12) Bryant, S. et al. (1985) *Vet. Med.*, *80*, 58.
(13) Srivastava, S. K. & Barnum, D. A. (1985) *Can. J. comp. Med.*, *49*, 351.
(14) Varma, K. J. et al. (1984) *J. vet. Pharmacol. Therap.*, *7*, 183.
(15) Galan, J. E. et al. (1986) *Infect. Immun.*, *54*, 202.

Neonatal streptococcal infection

Streptococcal infection of the newborn is characterized by bacteremia and septicemia resulting in localization of the infection in other organs, particularly joints, meninges and endocardium.

Etiology

Str. genitalium (*Str. pyogenes equi*) is usually recovered from the joints of infected foals and may also be present in the uterus of the mare and in aborted fetuses. The streptococci isolated from pigs are in Lancefield's groups C, E and L and are responsible for sporadic disease in young piglets (1, 11). *Streptococcus suis* type 1 and *Streptococcus suis* type 2 are subgroups of Lancefield's group D (11) and cause epidemic disease, principally meningitis. *Streptococcus suis* type 2 is a common cause of meningitis, arthritis and septicema in growing pigs (13). *Str. equisimilis* is also capable of causing disease in piglets (2). Group C streptoccoci and *Str. faecalis* have been isolated from cases of polyarthritis and endocarditis in lambs (3) and *Str. pyogenes* from swollen joints in calves (1).

Epidemiology

The source of the infection is usually the environment which may be contaminated by uterine discharges from infected dams or by discharges from lesions in other animals. The organism can be isolated from the nasopharynx of the sow, and direct infection from the sow to the piglet is suggested by some epidemiological data. The portal of infection in most instances appears to be the umbilicus, and continued patency of the urachus is thought to be a contributing factor in that it delays healing of the navel. Contamination of the umbilicus may result from infected soil or bedding, although in the special occurrence of the disease in calves in the southern United States, the screwworm fly (*Cochlyomyia americana*) is known to act as a passive carrier. The palatine tonsil has been shown to be a portal of entry for the infection in piglets (5) and infection may also occur through skin abrasions such as carpal necrosis or facial lesions following fighting.

Streptococci are the commonest cause of postnatal infections of foals, representing 50% of such cases in some surveys (6). Up to 20% of abortions in mares are found in similar surveys to be due to streptococci. Affected foals may die or be worthless because of permanent injury to joints. Streptococcal septicemia due to beta-hemolytic streptococci may occur in foals under 5 days of age which have been stressed and did not receive colostrum early enough (10).

In pigs, lambs (7) and calves the disease is sporadic but a high incidence may occur on individual farms. In an extensive Danish survey streptococcal arthritis was recorded in 18% of litters and the average morbidity was 3·3% and the mortality 1·5% (8). Sporadic disease in piglets, caused by Lancefield's groups C, E and L occur soon after birth and cause septicemia, arthritis, endocarditis, meningitis, abscesses and lymphadenitis (11). In a survey of bacterial endocarditis in pigs, 77% were due to Lancefield's groups C and L (15). The sporadic occurrence of the disease in some litters of pigs suggests that an increased susceptibility of the piglet could affect the epidemiological pattern of the disease (4). The common occurrence after tail-docking and teethclipping suggests that they may precipitate attacks. The sow is considered to be the main source of infection.

Epidemic disease caused by *Strep. suis* type 2 causes outbreaks of meningitis in young pigs 10–14 days after weaning. The disease occurs most commonly in weaned pigs raised in intensive systems of high population density, such as flat-deck rooms and fattening pens (29). The incidence of clinical disease can range from 0 to 15%. In a 2-year survey of a breeding herd, the morbidity and mortality rates due to meningitis from *Str. suis* type 2 was 3, 8 and 9·1% respectively (26). The incidence of the disease has increased markedly in recent years in the United Kingdom (14). In Canada, pigs may be affected from 3 to 24 weeks of age with most cases occurring between 6 and 12 weeks of age (18). *Strep. suis* type 2 can infect man and cause disease and the potential exists for man to be the source of infection in herds with no previous history of the disease or no introduction of replacement stock (14). Mixing and moving pigs are common predisposing factors (12). The infection is transmitted directly from the carrier sow to the young piglet which transmits it to susceptible piglets following weaning (13).

The organism is carried in the tonsils and occasionally in the nose of healthy pigs and transmission to uninfected pigs can occur within 5 days after mixing (13). The introduction of breeding gilts from infected herds results in disease appearing subsequently in weanlings and growing pigs in the recipient herds (13). The detectable carrier rates in different groups of pigs can vary from 0 to 80% and are highest in weaned pigs aged 4–10 weeks (30). There may be no correlation between the prevalence of infection in herds and the incidence of clinical disease (31). Weaned detectable tonsil carriers transmit the infection to previously uninfected pigs after mixing following weaning. The organism can persist in the tonsils of carrier pigs for more than 1 year, and in the presence of circulating opsonic and binding antibodies, and in pigs receiving penicillin-medicated feed (15, 33). Thus the organism can be endemic in some herds without causing recognizable clinical disease. *Streptococcus suis* type 2 can be isolated from pigs from infected herds when they are sampled at slaughter at the abattoir (32). The carrier rate in some surveys of slaughtered pigs ranged from 32 to 50% of pigs 4–6 months of age (21). This may explain the high incidence of *Str. suis* type 2 meningitis in humans in the Netherlands (22). The organism is a potential hazard for abattoir workers, particularly eviscerators who remove the larynx and lungs from carcasses. They have a significantly higher risk of exposure to *Str. suis* than other abattoir workers (35). *Str. suis* type 2 can survive in feces for 104 days at 0°C (32°F), up to 10 days at 9°C (48°F) and up to 8 days at 22–25°C (71–77°F) (19). It can survive in dust for up to 25 days at 9°C (48°F) but could not be isolated from dust stored at room temperature for 24 hours (19). The organism is rapidly inactivated by disinfections commonly used on farms. Liquid soap inactivates *Str. suis* type 2 in less than 1 min at a dilution in water of 1 in 500 (19). The organism can survive in pig carcasses at 40°C (39°F) for 6 weeks which may be an important source of the organisms for infection in man (13, 20).

Streptococcus suis type 2 has also been isolated from pigs affected with bronchopneumonia, usually secondary to enzootic pneumonia, from cases of pleuropneumonia, arthritis, vaginitis, aborted fetuses and in neonatal piglets 1–2 days of age affected with fatal septicemia (23). It appears that the organism is found in the lungs of pigs affected with pneumonia more frequently in North America than in other countries (23, 24). Several capsular serotypes of *Streptococcus suis* have been identified (34). Valvular endocarditis due to *Str. suis* type 2 has also been reported in a 13-week-old fattening pig in a breeding herd which had a long history of streptococcal meningitis (25).

Pathogenesis

The infection spreads from the portal of entry to produce a bacteremia which is not detectable clinically. The period of bacteremia is variable but it may last several days in piglets. A terminal acute fatal septicemia is the common outcome in animals under 1 week of age but in older animals suppurative localization in various organs is more common. Arthritis is the most common manifestation but other complications may be encountered. These include ophthalmitis in foals, meningitis and endocarditis in piglets, meningitis in calves and endocarditis in lambs. Streptococcal endocarditis can be produced by the intravenous inoculation of group L *Streptococcus* (16). Lesions are well established within 5 days, the left heart is most commonly affected and myocardial and renal infarction occur.

Clinical findings

Horses

Foals do not usually show signs until 2–3 weeks of age. The initial sign is usually a painful swelling of the navel and surrounding abdominal wall, often in the form of a flat plaque which may be 15–20 cm in diameter. A discharge of pus may or may not be present and a patent urachus is a frequent accompaniment. A systemic reaction occurs but this is often mild with the temperature remaining at about 39·5 °C (103°F). Lameness becomes apparent and is accompanied by obvious swelling and tenderness in one or more of the joints. The hock, stifle and knee joints are most commonly affected but in severe cases the distal joints are involved and there is occasionally extension to tendon sheaths. Lameness may be so severe that the foal lies down most of the time, sucks rarely and becomes extremely emaciated. There may be hypopyon in one or both eyes.

If treatment is begun in the early stages, recovery occurs but when joint involvement is severe, particularly if the abscesses have ruptured, the animal may have to be destroyed because of the resulting ankylosis. Death from septicemia may occur in the early stages of the disease.

Pigs

Arthritis and meningitis may occur alone or together and are most common in the 2–6-week age group. More commonly several piglets within a litter are affected. The arthritis is identical with that described in foals above. With meningitis there is a systemic reaction comprising fever, anorexia and depression. The gait is stiff, the piglets standing on their toes and there is swaying of the hindquarters. The ears are often retracted against the head. Blindness and gross muscular tremor develop followed by inability to maintain balance, lateral recumbency, violent paddling and death. In many cases there is little clinical evidence of omphalophlebitis. With endocarditis the young pigs are usually found comatose or dead without premonitory signs having been observed.

In epidemics of meningitis due to *Str. suis* type 2, sudden death in one or more pigs may be the first sign. Affected pigs found alive are incoordinated and rapidly become recumbent. There is opisthotonus, paddling and convulsions and death in less than 4 hours. A fever of up to 41°C (105°F) is common. In the United Kingdom meningitis of recently weaned pigs is the most striking feature of *Str. suis* type 2 infection. Arthritis is common in younger pigs.

Sheep

The incubation period is short, usually 2–3 days, and outbreaks occur soon after birth or docking. There is intense lameness with swelling of one or more joints appearing in a day or two. Pus accumulates and the joint capsule often ruptures. Recovery usually occurs with little residual enlargement of the joints, although there may be occasional deaths due to toxemia.

Calves

These show polyarthritis, meningitis, ophthalmitis and omphalophlebitis. The ophthalmitis may appear very soon after birth. The arthritis is often chronic and causes little systemic illness. Calves with meningitis show hyperesthesia, rigidity and fever.

Clinical pathology

Pus from any source may be cultured to determine the organism present and its sensitivity to the drugs available. Bacteriological examination of the uterine discharges of the dam may be of value in determining the source of infection. The success rate with blood cultures is not very high but an attempt is worthwhile. The identification of the causative bacteria is important but the sensitivity of the organism may mean the difference between success and failure in treatment. The specific identity of the streptococcus should be determined; serological methods are necessary to identify the presence of *Str. suis*. The organism can be cultured from the cerebrospinal fluid, brain and lungs of affected pigs (18).

Examination of synovial fluid may be of value in estimating the extent of joint damage.

Necropsy findings

In affected foals, calves and lambs, suppuration at the navel and severe suppurative arthritis affecting one or more joints are usual, and multiple abscesses may also be present in the liver, kidneys, spleen and lungs. Valvular endocarditis may be present in the lambs. Acute cases may die without suppurative lesions having had time to develop. Pigs show the same range of necropsy findings but in addition there will be large vegetative lesions on the heart valves in those dying of endocarditis. Necropsy findings in the meningitic form in pigs include turbidity of the cerebrospinal fluid, congestion and inflammation of the meninges and an accumulation of whitish, purulent material in the subarachnoid space. In most cases the choroid plexuses are severely affected and the ventricles, aqueduct and central canal of the medulla and the cord may be blocked by exudate, in some cases sufficient to cause internal hydrocephalus. The nervous tissue of the spinal cord, cerebellum and brain stem may show liquefaction necrosis. In pigs dying from *Str. suis* type 2 infection, the gross and microscopic findings include one or more of fibrinous polyserositis, fibrinous or hemorrhagic bronchopneumonia, purulent meningitis, myocardial necrosis, focal myocarditis and valvular endocarditis (18).

Diagnosis

Omphalophlebitis and suppurative arthritis in foals may be due to infection with *Escherichia coli, Actinobacillus equuli* or *Salmonella abortivoequina*, but these infections tend to take the form of a fatal septicemia within a few days of birth whereas streptococcal infections are delayed in their onset and usually produce a polyarthritis. In pigs there may be sporadic cases of arthritis due to staphylococci but the streptococcal infection is the common one. Arthritis due to *Mycoplasma hyorhinis* is less suppurative but may require cultural differentiation. Glasser's disease occurs usually in older pigs and is accompanied by pleurisy, pericarditis and peritonitis. Erysipelas in very young pigs is usually manifested by septicemia. Nervous disease of piglets may resemble arthritis on cursory examination but there is an absence of joint enlargement and lameness. However, the meningitic form of the streptococcal infection can easily be confused with viral encephalitides. Meningitis in young calves may also be caused by *Pasteurella multocida*. Polyarthritis in calves, lambs and piglets may also be caused by infection with *Actinomyces* (*Corynebacterium*) *pyogenes* and *Fusobacterium necrophorum*. *Streptococcus suis* type 2 can also be the cause of meningitis in older pigs of 10–14 weeks of age (9).

The response of streptococcal infections to treatment with penicillin may be of value in the differentiation of the arthritides, and the microscopic and histological findings at necropsy enable exact differentiation to be made. In lambs suppurative arthritis occurs soon after birth and after docking. The other common arthritis in the newborn lamb is that caused by *Erysipelothrix insidiosa* but this usually occurs later and is manifested by lameness without pronounced joint enlargement. Calves may also develop erysipelatous arthritis.

Treatment

Penicillin is successful as treatment in all forms of the disease provided irreparable structural damage has not occurred. In newborn animals the dosage rate should be high (20 000 units kg body weight) and should be repeated at least once daily for 3 days. If suppuration is already present, a longer course of antibiotics will be necessary, preferably 7–10 days. Piglets treated early in the course of the disease will survive but may runt. Because of the common litter incidence in piglets and the occurrence of subclinical bacteremia it is wise to also treat all littermates of affected piglets. Benzathine or benethamine penicillins can be used in conjunction with shorter-acting penicillins. Treatment of pigs affected with meningitis due to *Str. suis* type 2 with either trimethoprim-sulfadiazine or penicillin reduced the case fatality rate from 55 to 21% (28). General aspects of treatment of the newborn are dealt within Chapter 3 on diseases of the newborn.

Control

The principles of control of diseases of the newborn are dealt with elsewhere. Because the most frequent source of infection in foals is the genital tract of the dam, some attempt should be made to treat the mare and limit the contamination of the environment. Mixed bacterins have been widely used to establish immunity in mares and foals against this infection but no proof has been presented that they are effective. On heavily infected premises the administration of long-acting penicillin at birth may be advisable. A major factor in the control of navel and joint-ill in lambs is the use of clean fields or pens for lambing, as umbilical infection originating from the environment seems to be more important than infection from the dam in this species. Docking should also be done in clean surroundings and, if necessary, temporary yards should be erected. Instruments should be chemically sterilized between lambs. Regardless of species and where practicable, all parturition stalls and pens should be kept clean and disinfected and the navels of all newborn animals disinfected at birth. Where screwworms are prevalent, the unhealed navels should be treated with a reliable repellent.

Eradiction of *Str. suis* type 2 infection can be attempted by depopulation of suspected carrier sows and replacement with non-infected breeding stock (12). However, there are no reliable tests for the detection of carrier animals. Often the infection is self-limiting and special control procedures are unnecessary. Studies are being conducted on the use of vaccines containing the immunogenic polysaccharide from *Str. suis* type 2 (17).

Outbreaks in sucking piglets have been controlled by a single injection of benethamine penicillin to all piglets given 5 days before the average age of onset of clinical signs. The feeding of oxytetracycline (400 g/tonne) for 14 days immediately prior to the usual onset prevented the occurrence of the disease in weaned pigs (9). The use of a medicated feed containing trimethoprim-sulfadiazine (1:5) at a rate of 500 g/tonne for the first 6 weeks after weaning did not significantly reduce the incidence of disease (27).

At the present time there are no known specific methods for the prevention of meningitis due to infection of weaning pigs with *Str. suis* type 2. Good management and hygiene techniques should be emphasized. Medicated early weaning and classical SPF techniques applied to infected herds appears to be most effective in producing pigs free of infection (33).

REVIEW LITERATURE

Clifton-Hadley, F. A. (1983) *Streptococcus suis* type 2 infections. *Br. vet. J.*, 139, 1–5.

Windsor, R. S. (1978) Streptococcal infections in young pigs. *Vet. Ann.*, *18*, 134.

REFERENCES

(1) Elliott, S. D. (1966) *J. Hyg., Camb.*, *64*, 205, 213.

(2) Woods, R. D. & Ross, R. F. (1976) *Vet. Bull..*, *46*, 397.

(3) Jamieson, S. & Stuart, J. (1950) *J. Pathol. Bacteriol.*, *62*, 235.
(4) Riising, H. J. et al. (1976) *Nord. VetMed.*, *28*, 65, 87.
(5) Williams, D. M. et al. (1973) *Res. vet. Sci.*, *15*, 352.
(6) Platt, H. (1973) *Br. vet J.*, *129*, 221.
(7) Dennis, S. M. (1968) *Vet. Rec.*, *82*, 403.
(8) Nielsen, N. C. et al. (1975) *Nord. VetMed.*, *27*, 529.
(9) Windsor, R. S. & Elliott, S. D. (1975) *J. Hyg.*, *Camb.*, *75*, 69.
(10) Dubielzig, R. R. (1978) *J. equ. med. Surg.*, *2*, 28.
(11) Windsor, R. (1978) *Vet. Ann*, *10*, 134.
(12) Windsor, R. S. (1977) *Vet. Rec.*, *101*, 378.
(13) Clifton-Hadley, F. A. (1983) *Br. vet. J.*, *139*, 1.
(14) Lamont, M. H. et al. (1980) *Vet. Rec.*, *107*, 467.
(15) Jones, J. E. T. (1980) *J. comp. Pathol.*, *90*, 11.
(16) Jones, J. E. T. (1981) *J. comp. Pathol.*, *91*, 51.
(17) Elliott, S. D. et al. (1980) *J. Hyg.*, *Camb.*, *85*, 275.
(18) St John, V. S. et al. (1982) *Can. vet. J.*, *23*, 95.
(19) Clifton-Hadley, F. A. & Enright, M. R. (1984) *Vet. Rec.*, *114*, 584.
(20) Clifton-Hadley, F. A. et al. (1986) *Vet. Rec.*, *118*, 275.
(21) Arends, J. P. et al. (1984) *J. clin. Microbiol.*, *20*, 945.
(22) Zanen, H. C. & Engel, H. W. B. (1975) *Lancet*, i, 1286.
(23) Sanford, S. E. & Tilker, M. E. (1982) *J. Am. vet. med. Assoc.*, *181*, 673.
(24) Erickson, E. D. et al. (1984) *J. Am. vet. med. Assoc.*, *185*, 666.
(25) Lamont, M. H. et al. (1984) *Vet. Rec.*, *115*, 22.
(26) Guise, H. J. et al. (1985) *Vet. Rec.*, *117*, 43.
(27) Guise, H. J. et al. (1986) *Vet. Rec.*, *119*, 395.
(28) Guise, H. J. et al. (1985) *Vet. Rec.*, *117*, 65.
(29) Clifton-Hadley, F. A. & Alexander, T. J. L. (1981) *Pig vet. Soc. Proc.*, *8*, 8.
(30) Clifton-Hadley, F. A. et al. (1984) *Vet. Rec.*, *114*, 513.
(31) Clifton-Hadley, F. A. et al. (1984) *Vet. Rec.*, *115*, 562.
(32) Clifton-Hadley, F. A. & Alexander, T. J. L. (1986) *Vet. Rec.*, *118*, 274.
(33) Clifton-Hadley, F. A. (1984) *Vet. Res. Commun.*, *8*, 217.
(34) Perch, B. et al. (1983) *J. clin. Microbiol.*, *17*, 993.
(35) Breton, L. et al. (1986) *Can. J. vet. Res.*, *50*, 338.

Streptococcal lymphadenitis of swine (jowl abscesses, cervical abscesses)

Cervical or 'jowl' abscess of pigs is observed mainly at slaughter. Clinically there is obvious enlargement of the lymph nodes of the throat region, particularly the mandibular nodes. It is of considerable importance because of the losses due to rejection of infected carcasses at meat inspection.

The condemnation rate of heads at slaughter pigs may be as high as 78–94% in some herds. However, based on annual reports from the Federal Meat and Poultry Inspection Service in the United States, the incidence of jowl abscesses in pigs has declined steadily to a level in 1981 less than one-third of the peak incidence 20 years earlier (13). This may be due to changes in management of swine herds and the use of antibiotic feeding.

Most jowl abscesses in swine are caused by beta-hemolytic streptococci of Lancefield's group E type IV (1, 13) although *Pasteurella multocida*, *Escherichia coli* and *Actinomyces* (*Corynebacterium*) *pyogenes* may also be present. Some additional serotypes have been isolated (14). The disease occurs primarily in postweaning and fattening swine. Piglets under 28 days of age are relatively resistant and even colostrum-deprived piglets are resistant to clinical disease following experimental infection (15).

The disease has been produced by feeding or the intranasal or intrapharyngeal instillation of streptococci (2) and they are thought to be the cause, infection occurring through the pharyngeal mucosa from contaminated food and water (3). In herds where cervical abscess is a problem, streptococci can commonly be isolated from the vaginas of pregnant sows and the pharynges of normal young pigs (4). The persistence of the infection in herds is thought to depend on the presence of carrier animals (5). Transmission occurs via feed and drinking water. After infection has occurred a bacteremia develops and abscesses are initiated in the cervical lymph nodes in a high proportion of pigs (6). Infrequently, abscesses occur in atypical sites other than the head and neck. Pigs which have recovered from the natural disease are immune to experimental challenge (12). A microtitration agglutination test is available to detect infections caused by type IV streptococci (17). Vaccination of pregnant sows with an autogenous or commercial bacterin containing streptococci and staphylococci is thought to be of value in protecting the litters of the vaccinated sows (7). Vaccination of young pigs with a whole-culture bacterin has provided some protection, but the use of an oral vaccine prepared from an avirulent strain of group E streptococci, and sprayed into the oropharynx, is highly effective as a preventive measure (9). A number of prophylactic regimens based on the feeding of antibiotics have been proposed and generally give good results. Chlortetracycline fed to young pigs at the rate of 220 g/tonne for 1 month is an example (10). Treatment of breeding pigs at the same time is likely to have a beneficial effect in reducing the severity of exposure of the young pigs to infection. A similar advantage can be gained by keeping the treated groups isolated from untreated groups of older pigs. Because piglets under 28 days of age are relatively resistant to clinical disease, the weaning and isolation from older pigs is a successful control program.

REFERENCES

(1) Collier, J. R. & Noel, J. (1971) *Am. J. vet. Res.*, *32*, 1501.
(2) Armstrong, C. H. (1971) *J. Am. vet. med. Assoc.*, *160*, 655.
(3) Collier, J. R. & Noel, J. (1974) *Am. J. vet. Res.*, *35*, 799.
(4) Jones, J. E. T. (1976) *Br. vet. J.*, *132*, 276.
(5) Schmitz, J. A. & Olson, L. D. (1973) *Am. J. vet. Res.*, *34*, 189.
(6) Schmitz, J. A. et al. (1972) *Am. J. vet. Res.*, *33*, 449.
(7) Conner, G. H. et al. (1965) *J. Am. vet. med. Assoc.*, *147*, 479.
(8) Wood, R. L. & Wessman, G. E. (1984) *Am. J. vet. Res.*, *45*, 1933.
(9) Collier, J. R. et al. (1976) *J. Am. vet. med. Assoc.*, *169*, 697.
(10) Schmitz, J. A. & Olson, L. D. (1973) *J. Am. vet. med. Assoc.*, *162*, 55, 58.
(11) Miller, R. B. & Olson, L. D. (1983) *Am. J. vet. Res.*, *44*, 945.
(12) Jenkins, E. M. & Collier, J. R. (1978) *Am. J. vet. Res.*, *39*, 325.
(13) Wood, R. L. (1982) *Proc. US Anim. Hlth Assoc.*, *86*, 503.
(14) Wessman, G. E. et al. (1983) *Cornell Vet.*, *73*, 307.
(15) Wood, R. L. et al. (1986) *Am. J. vet. Res.*, *47*, 1722.
(16) Miller, R. G. & Olson, L. D. (1983) *Am. J. vet. Res.*, *44*, 937.
(17) Armstrong, C. H. et al. (1982) *Can. J. comp. Med.*, *46*, 201.

DISEASES CAUSED BY *STAPHYLOCOCCUS* spp.

Mastitis caused by *Staphylococcus aureus* is dealt with in Chapter 15, udder impetigo of cattle in the section on miscellaneous abnormalities of the udder, and staphylococcal pyoderma of horses under the heading of dermatitis. Other miscellaneous infections include:

- Tick pyemia of lambs (see below)
- Exudative epidermitis of pigs (see below)
- Staphylococcal septicemia of the newborn, especially lambs. This is a relatively common disease and may have a significant mortality rate, due partly to a high incidence of myocardial lesions. In most cases the navel appears to be the portal of infection (1), but infection may also occur through marking wounds
- A severe ulcerative dermatitis affecting particularly the face is recorded in adult sheep (2, 3). The disease is caused by *Staph. aureus*
- A benign folliculitis of the face of sucking lambs (4, 5)
- Dermatitis of the legs of sheep with most lesions close to the coronet (6)
- *Staphylococcus hyicus*, the causative organism of exudative epidermitis of pigs, is also an occasional cause of a scabby dermatitis, accompanied by itching and alopecia, on the skin of the neck and back of donkeys and horses (7).

REFERENCES

(1) Dennis, S. J. (1966) *Vet. Rec.*, *79*, 38.
(2) Scott, F. M. M. et al. (1980) *Vet. Rec.*, *107*, 572.
(3) Savey, M. et al. (1983) *Rec. med. Vet.*, *159*, 701.
(4) Scott, F. M. M. & Scott, G. R. (1984) *Vet. Rec.*, *114*, 23.
(5) Parker, B. N. J. et al. (1983) *Vet. Rec.*, *113*, 570.
(6) Synge, B. A. et al. (1985) *Vet. Rec.*, *116*, 459.
(7) Devriese, L. A. & Thelissen, M. (1986) *Vet. Rec.*, *118*, 76.

Tick pyemia of lambs (enzootic staphylococcosis of lambs)

Tick pyemia is a staphylococcal infection of lambs spread by the bites of ticks and is manifested by septicemia, or by bacteremia with subsequent localization occurring in many organs. The disease has been recorded only in the United Kingdom (1). It occurs in the early summer and causes serious losses in areas where tick infestations are heavy. Lambs are affected soon after birth and die quickly of septicemia or show signs of arthritis or meningitis in the period between the second and fourth weeks of life. In cases where localization has occurred, suppurative lesions may be found in the skin, muscles, tendon sheaths, joints, viscera and meninges.

Tick pyemia may occur in association with a number of other diseases including enterotoxemia, louping-ill, lamb dysentery and tick-borne fever, and a concurrent infection with the last is thought to predispose to its development (2). The disease has been produced experimentally using *Ixodes ricinus* ticks as vectors (4).

Tick pyemia resembles other suppurative infections of the newborn, including those infections caused by *Streptococcus* spp., but the lesions are much more extensive, and infection enters through bites of the ticks rather than navel or docking wounds. The ticks are not thought to provide portals of entry for, nor to act as carriers of, the infection but to act as a precipitating cause possibly by causing intercurrent disease. *Staph. aureus* can be isolated from the lesions, and in affected flocks there is a high incidence of lambs carrying the same infection on their nasal mucosa (5). Cutaneous infection shows no such relationship. Although spread of the infection from the ewes to the lambs is not proven, the lambs acquire the infection during the first few days of life and the incidence of infection is highest in flocks kept in confined quarters. Control of the tick population is the obvious method of controlling the disease, and dipping the lambs every 3 weeks in an organophosphatic insecticide is capable of greatly reducing the incidence of the clinical disease and increasing the weight gains of clinically normal lambs (6). Failing this, vaccination of the ewes with an autogenous bacterin during late pregnancy may be practiced but is of doubtful value (3). Treatment with penicillin should be effective, provided lesions are not too advanced. Effective prophylaxis is obtained by the injection of 1 million units of benzathine penicillin but administration has to be timed at just before the period of greatest risk (7).

REFERENCES

(1) Watson, W. A. (1964) *Vet. Rec.*, *76*, 743, 793.
(2) Foster, W. M. N. & Cameron, A. E. (1968) *J. comp. Pathol.*, *78*, 243.
(3) Foggie, A. (1948) *J. comp. Pathol.*, *58*, 24.
(4) Webster, K. A. & Mitchell, G. B. B. (1986) *Vet. Rec.*, *119*, 186.
(5) Watson, W. A. (1965) *Vet. Rec.*, *77*, 477.
(6) Watson, W. A. (1966) *Vet. Rec.*, *79*, 101.
(7) Watt, J. A. (1968) *Vet. Rec.*, *83*, 507.

Exudative epidermitis (greasy pig disease)

Exudative epidermitis of sucking pigs is a poorly defined disease thought to be caused by a bacterium provisionally identified as *Staphylococcus hyicus (hyos)*. Clinically it is distinguished by the appearance of an acute, generalized, seborrheic dermatitis.

Etiology

The disease can be reproduced by the inoculation of a Gram-positive organism designated as *Staphylococcus hyos* or *Staph. hyicus* (1, 2). It resembles closely a nonpathogenic staphylococcus but can be differentiated serologically (3).

Epidemiology

Field evidence suggests that environmental stress of various kinds, including agalactia in the sow and intercurrent infection, predisposes to the disease.

In many cases lesions develop first about the head, apparently in association with bite wounds which occur when the needle teeth have not been cut. Within litters the incidence is high, often all piglets being affected. The morbidity will vary from 20 to 100% and the case

Table 47. Differential diagnosis of diseases of swine with skin lesions

Disease	*Epidemiology*	*Clinical and laboratory findings*	*Response to treatment*
Swine pox	Mainly suckling piglets. High morbidity but low mortality except in very young piglets. Usually associated with swine louse infestation	Papules, vesicles and circular redbrown scabs on ventral belly wall and over the sides and back. Pox characteristics	None required except for insect and louse control. Spontaneous recovery in 3 weeks
Skin necrosis	Suckling piglets. High morbidity with abrasive flooring	Abrasion and necrosis starting shortly after birth and reaching maximum severity at about 1 week. Anterior aspect of carpus more common site but also fetlock, hock, elbow and coronet. Bilateral. Necrosis and erosion of anterior two or three pairs of teats	Usually none required. Recovery 3–5 weeks. Protect area with tape if severe, plus topical antiseptics. Teat necrosis will render animal unsuitable for selection and breeding. Correction of flooring
Exudative epidermitis (greasy pig disease)	Entire litters of suckling pigs, most severe under 1 week of age, occurs up to 10 weeks, high case fatality in younger pigs	Marked cutaneous erythema with seborrhea, severe dehydration, weakness and death in piglets under 10 days. Older piglets covered with greasy exudate and recover. *Staph. hyos* on culture	Piglets under 10 days of age die in spite of therapy. Older pigs may survive with penicillin treatment topically and parenterally
Dermatosis vegetans	Inherited and congenital, high morbidity. High case fatality by 8 weeks	Erythema and edema of coronets, uneven brittle hooves, dry brown crusts on belly wall, giant cell pneumonia. Club foot	None indicated. Genetic control
Pityriasis rosea	One or more piglets in litter after weaning. High morbidity, nil mortality	Lesions begin as small red flat plaques which enlarge from 1 to 2 cm diameter with a prominent ring of erythematous skin covered in center by thin, dry, brown, loose scales. Lesions usually coalesce forming a mosaic pattern, especially on belly. Scraping negative. No growth depression	None required. Emollient to soothe the lesion. Recovery occurs in 4–8 weeks
Parakeratosis (zinc deficiency)	Weaners and feeder pigs on diet low in zinc and high in calcium. Herd problem, high morbidity, no mortality	Erythematous areas on ventral abdomen and symmetrically over back and legs. Develop into thick crusts and fissures. No pruritus. Skin scrapings negative. Growth rate depression	Add zinc to diet 100 ppm. Adjust calcium. Recovery in 2–6 weeks
Ringworm	Feeder and mature pigs. Usually several pigs within pen or shed. High morbidity with *M. nanum* in sows	Centrifugally progressing ring of inflammation surrounding an area with scabs, crusts and brown or black exudate. May reach large size. Bristles usually intact. No pruritus. Positive skin scrapings and hair. No growth depression	Fungicides. In growers spontaneous recovery in 8–10 weeks if well nourished. *M. nanum* in sows is persistent and responds poorly
Facial dermatitis	Suckling piglets. High incidence in litters associated with fighting. Low mortality	Lesions on cheeks—usually bilateral abrasions which become infected. Scabs hard and brown and difficult to remove. Overlie a raw shallow bleeding ulcer. Occasional extension to other areas	Usually none indicated. Topical antibacterials. Clip teeth at birth
Ulcerative granuloma	Young pigs but all ages. Sporadic. Infection following abrasion. Poor hygiene	Large swollen tumorous mass with several discharging sinuses. Central slough and ulcer	Fair, depending on site. Surgical removal and/or sulfadimidine and streptomycin
Sarcoptic mange	All ages of pigs. Herd problem. Reservoir of infection in sows. High morbidity. Nil mortality	Intense pruritus. Mites on scraping. Erythematous spots with scale and minor brown exudation. Especially evident in thin skin areas. Secondary trauma to skin and bristles from rubbing. If severe, intense erythema. Chronic infections, thickening and wrinkling of skin. Depression of weight gain	Good response to vigorous therapy with acaricides. Treat on a herd basis

Table 47. (cont.)

Disease	*Epidemiology*	*Clinical and laboratory findings*	*Response to treatment*
Allergic dermatoses due to *Tyroglyphus* spp. (harvest mites)	Weaner and feeder pigs few weeks after eating dry ground feed from autonomic feeders	Pinpoint erythematous spots and fragile scales. Intense pruritus. Skin scraping positive for mites	Spontaneous recovery common. Insecticide effective
Erysipelas	Feeder and adult pigs, occasionally weaners. Variable morbidity. Low mortality if treated early	Small red spots developing to characteristic rhomboidal lesion raised and red in color. Lesions may become joined and lose their characteristic shape. Progress to necrosis and desquamation. Fever and other signs of septicemia	Penicillin

Acute septicemias in pigs may be manifest with skin discoloration that varies from mild hyperemia to an intense purple discoloration especially of the ears, jaws, underside of neck, belly, inside of limbs and tail. Lesions on the snout, skin horn junction of the claws and accessory digits and the interdigital skin occur in viral vesicular diseases in swine. Skin lesions also occur with deficiencies of niacin, biotin, riboflavin and pantothenic acid, with sunburn and photosensitivity, and following vices of tail-biting and ear-chewing.

fatality rate from 50 to 75%. Most cases occur in animals under 6 weeks of age, with a peak incidence in piglets under 1 week. Occasionally groups of pigs up to 3 months of age suffer from the disease. The presence of the disease in a swine herd can account for a 35% reduction in the margin of output over feed and veterinary costs over a 2-month period (7).

The source of the organism is unknown but the gilt or sow are probably inapparent carriers. It can be isolated from the skin of healthy in-contact piglets and healthy sows (11). The organism has also been isolated from the atmosphere of buildings housing affected pigs (11). Bacteriophage typing of *Staph. hyicus* subsp. *hyicus* isolated from pigs with or without exudative epidermitis revealed two or more phage patterns in the isolates from each pig with the disease and a single-phage pattern in isolates from healthy pigs (12). The organism has been found as a frequent inhabitant of the skin of cattle (9). Naturally occurring lesions of dermatitis of the lower limbs of horses (15) and similar lesions over the neck and back of donkeys (14) have been recorded. Experimentally, the organism can cause lesions in horses similar to those of exudative epidermitis. A concurrent infection with *Dermatophilus congolensis* has also been reported (13).

The disease appears under various names. It is referred to as non-specific 'eczema' in the United Kingdom, as exudative dermatitis and seborrhea oleosa in the United States. It has also been recorded in Australia and Europe. The incidence is not high but many of the affected pigs die.

Pathogenesis

Although the principal lesion is an inflammatory-exudative reaction in the corium and upper layers of the epidermis (4), the disease is probably a systemic rather than local one. Experimental infection of gnotobiotic pigs leads to dermatitis of the snout and ears, then the medial aspect of the thighs, the abdominal wall and the coronets. At autopsy there are lesions in most organs, especially the kidneys, ureters and brain (4, 5). The organism has been isolated from a pig with septic polyarthritis (8).

Clinical findings

In the peracute form which occurs most commonly in piglets only a few days of age, there is a sudden onset of marked cutaneous erythema, with severe pain on palpation evidenced by squealing. Anorexia, severe dehydration and weakness are present and death occurs in 24–48 hours. The entire skin coat appears wrinkled and reddened and is covered with a greasy, gray-brown exudate which accumulates in thick clumps around the eyes, behind the ears, and over the abdominal wall. In the less acute form, seen in older pigs from 3 to 10 weeks of age, the greasy exudate becomes thickened and brown and peels off in scabs leaving a deep pink-colored to normal skin surface. There is no irritation or pruritus. In the subacute form, the exudate dries into brown scales which are most prominent on the face, around the eyes, and behind the ears. In a small percentage of pigs the chronic form occurs and the course is much longer and there is thickening with wrinkling of the skin and thick scabs which crack along flexion lines, forming deep fissures. Most peracute cases die, while piglets with the less severe forms will survive if treated. Some pigs are affected with ulcerative glossitis and stomatitis (10).

Clinical pathology

Bacterial examination of skin swabs may reveal the presence of staphylococci.

Necropsy findings

At necropsy there are macroscopic lesions in the skin and kidneys. A white precipitate is found in the papillary ducts and the renal pelvis and kidneys are pale and wet. There are degenerative changes in the renal tubular epithelium, retention of urine within the kidneys and blockage of the ureters. Lesions in the central nervous system have also been described (5).

Diagnosis

Exudative epidermitis may resemble several skin diseases of pigs of all age groups (Table 47). Careful gross examination of the lesions, particularly their distribution, the state of the hair shaft, the character of the exudate, and the presence or absence of pruritus must be considered along with skin scrapings and biopsies.

Treatment

Experimentally infected piglets respond favorably to a topical application of cloxacillin 10 000 units/g of lanolin base and 1% hydrocortisone combined with parenteral cloxacillin (6). Treatment must be administered as soon as the lesions are visible. Procaine benzylpenicillin at a dose of 20 000 units/kg body weight intramuscularly daily for 3 days is also recommended. The antimicrobial sensitivities determined in one field investigation revealed that all isolates were sensitive to novobiocin, neomycin, and cloxacillin (11). Novobiocin may be the antimicrobial of choice since staphylococci are universally sensitive to this antibiotic. However, there is no available information on the efficacy of antimicrobials for naturally occurring cases of exudative epidermitis. Naturally occurring cases in piglets under 10 days of age respond poorly while older pigs recover with a skin wash using a suitable disinfectant soap.

Control

The infected accommodation should be cleaned, disinfected and left vacant before another farrowing sow is placed in the pen. Strict isolation of the affected piglets and their dam is necessary to prevent spread throughout the herd. Dead piglets should be promptly removed from the premises and in-contact sows should be washed with a suitable disinfectant soap.

REFERENCES

(1) Van Os, J. L. (1967) *Tijdschr. Diergeneeskd.*, *92*, 662.
(2) Schulz, W. (1969) *Arch. exp. VetMed.*, *23*, 415.
(3) Hunter, D. et al. (1970) *Br. vet. J.*, *126*, 225.
(4) Schmidt, U. et al. (1972) *Berl. Munch. Tierärztl. Wochenschr.*, *85*, 181.
(5) Amtsberg, G. et al. (1973) *Dtsch Tierärztl. Wochenschr.*, *80*, 496, 421.
(6) L'Ecuyer, C. & Alexander, D. C. (1969) *Can. vet. J.*, *10*, 227.
(7) Pepper, T. A. & Taylor, D. J. (1977) *Vet. Rec.*, *101*, 204.
(8) Phillips, W. E. et al. (1980) *Am J. vet. Res.*, *41*, 274.
(9) Devriese, L. A. & Derycke, J. (1979) *Res. vet. Sci.*, *26*, 356.
(10) Andrews, J. J. (1979) *Vet. Pathol.*, *16, 432.*
(11) Holland, J. T. S. & Hodges, R. T. (1981) *NZ vet J.*, *29*, 57.
(12) Kawano, J. et al. (1983) *Am. J. vet. Res.*, *44*, 1476.
(13) Loman, L. G. & Cole, J. R. (1983) *J. Am. vet. med. Assoc.*, *183*, 1091.
(14) Devriese, L. A. & Thelis en, M. (1986] *Vet. Rec.*, *118*, 1091.
(15) Devriese, L. A. et al. (1983) *Equ. vet. J.*, *15*, 263.

DISEASES CAUSED BY *CORYNEBACTERIUM* spp.

Actinomyces (*Corynebacterium*) *pyogenes* is an ubiquitous organism and occurs in many animal diseases either as a primary cause or as a secondary invader. Its role in the production of mastitis in cattle is described in the section on mastitis, and as a secondary invader in calf and sheep pneumonia in the descriptions of the viral pneumonias of calves and sheep and in foot abscess of sheep under that heading. The important specific diseases caused by *Corynebacterium* spp. are described later in this section. There are also a number of minor diseases caused by corynebacteria. They include the following.

Metritis

Infection of the uterus of mares and cows is commonly associated with sterility and abortion or with the birth of infected young. Although many uterine infections with *Actinomyces* (*Corynebacterium*) *pyogenes* are secondary, primary ones resulting in abortion do occur. It is thought that the uterus becomes infected via the bloodstream (1). The disease must be differentiated from those caused by *Salmonella abortivoequina* and *Str. genitalium*, and equine viral rhinopneumonitis and equine viral arteritis. The bacteriology, occurrence, method of transmission and susceptibility of the organism to various drugs have been reviewed (2).

Perinatal disease

Most corynebacteria have been recorded as causes of perinatal deaths in lambs (3).

Arthritis and bursitis

Corynebacterium pseudotuberculosis has been determined to cause a non-suppurative arthritis and bursitis in lambs. The joints are only slightly enlarged and many animals show only mild clinical signs. Recovery occurs if the lambs are fed and confined.

Infections in wildlife

Corynebacterium pseudotuberculosis has been isolated from deer and from engorged female ticks (*Dermacentor albipictus*) feeding on the deer. Transmissibility between sheep and deer, possibly by means of the bites of ticks, is suggested (5). The occurrence of ulcerative lymphangitis in an isolated group of horses has also suggested that wild animals may act as vectors of the organism (6).

Orchitis

Suppurative orchitis in rams caused by *Cor. pseudotuberculosis* may be confused with epididymitis caused by *Brucella ovis*. The corynebacterial infection is considered to be a specific transmissible disease of sheep.

Chronic pectoral abscess

In horses in California (7, 8), *Cor. pseudotuberculosis* infections have also been associated with a high incidence of chronic abscesses, chiefly in the pectoral region but in some animals extending as far back as the mammary gland. The abscesses appear to develop in a deep site and may reach a diameter of 10–20 cm, with a surrounding area of edema, before they rupture 1–4 weeks later. Clinical signs include local swelling, lameness, pain on palpation, ventral edema, reluctance to move, midline dermatitis, fever and depression in the early stage, eventually rupture of the abscesses (4). Occasional generalized cases occur, the internal lesions being located chiefly in the abdominal cavity and being palpable rectally particularly in and around the kidney (9). The disease occurs in an area where caseous lymphadenitis is common in sheep but the portal of entry of infection is unknown. Because of the seasonal occurrence of the disease its transmission by insect vectors has been suggested but not confirmed (4). A serological test of some value in diagnosing the infection has been developed, but gives many false-positive reactions (7).

REFERENCES

(1) Hinton, M. (1972) *Vet. Bull.*, *42*, 1753.
(2) Purdom, M. R. et al. (1958) *Vet. Rev. A.*, *4*, 55.
(3) Dennis, S. M. & Bamford, V. W. (1966) *Vet. Rec.*, *79*, 105.
(4) Miers, K. C. & Ley, W. B. (1980) *J. Am. vet. med. Assoc.*, *155*, 446.
(5) Humphreys, F. A. & Gibbons, R. J. (1942) *Can J. comp. Med.*, *6*, 35.
(6) Mitchell, C. A. & Walker, R. V. L. (1944) *Can. J. comp. Med.*, *8*, 3.
(7) Knight, H. D. (1978) *Cornell Vet.*, *68*, 220.
(8) Knight, H. D. (1969) *J. Am. vet. med. Assoc.*, *155*, 446.
(9) Cameron, C. M. (1976) *Onderstepoort J. vet. Res.*, *43*, 97.
(10) Brumbaugh, G. W. & Ekman, T. L. (1981) *J. Am. vet. med. Assoc.*, *178*, 300.

Contagious bovine pyelonephritis

Contagious bovine pyelonephritis is a specific infection of the urinary tract of cattle caused by *Cor. renale* and characterized by chronic purulent inflammation in the bladder, ureters and kidneys.

Etiology

Corynebacterium renale, the specific etiological agent, has three, possibly four, serotypes (1). Type 1 appears to be most pathogenic, and all four types are capable of stimulating production of complement-fixing antibodies which give cross-reactions with *Mycobacterium johnei*. *Corynebacterium renale* has little apparent resistance to physical or chemical agents and is readily isolated from the urine of affected or carrier animals. *Cor. pseudotuberculosis*, *Actinomyces* (*Corynebacterium*) *pyogenes*, *Act. equuli*, *E. coli* and *Staph. aureus* are sometimes found in the urinary tract of cattle and pigs affected with pyelonephritis, either alone or associated with *Cor. renale*. Because of the ease with which pyelonephritis can be produced by causing stagnation of urine, it is likely that the primary cause of the disease is temporary or permanent obstruction of part of the urinary tract. *Cor. renale*, because of its particular ability to grow in urine, is the most common pathogen present in these circumstances.

Epidemiology

The disease is widespread in Europe and North America although it seldom constitutes an important problem in any herd or area. As a rule, clinical cases appear sporadically, even in herds found to harbor a significant number of carriers. Unless appropriate treatment is instituted early, the disease is highly fatal and economic loss is due mainly to deaths of the affected animals.

Although pyelonephritis is considered to be essentially a bovine disease, sheep are occasionally affected (2). Cattle are seldom affected before maturity and cows appear to be much more susceptible than bulls. An increase in clinical cases is usually found in the colder seasons of the year and heavily fed, high-producing dairy herds appear to show an increased susceptibility.

Although the intravenous injection of *Cor. renale* has been shown to produce renal lesions in mice (3), the vulva is thought to be the portal of entry in the cow. This view is supported by the very firm adhesion of *Cor. renale* to the epithelial cells of the bovine vulva (9). Typical lesions can be established in some animals by the introduction of the organism into the bladder (4). Clinically affected or clinically normal 'carrier' cows are probably the principal source of infection, the disease being transmitted by direct contact, brushing the vulva of clean cows with contaminated bulls or by the careless use of catheters. The incidence of cows excreting *Cor. renale* in their urine is higher in herds where the disease occurs than in herds where the disease is unknown (5). There is a strong inference that in some circumstances the disease, or the infection, can be spread venereally. This is suggested by the occasional occurrence of a series of cases in a herd, usually related to the use of a particular bull, and the cessation of cases when artificial insemination is used. The organism can often be isolated from the prepuce and urethra of bulls, but not from other organs, nor are there detectable lesions in the prepuce (6), that is in the absence of balanoposthitis, of which *Cor. renale* is thought to be the cause.

Pathogenesis

Pyelonephritis usually appears to develop as an ascending infection involving successively the bladder, ureters and kidneys. The destruction of renal tissue and obstruction of urinary outflow ultimately result in uremia and the death of the animal.

Clinical findings

Early signs vary considerably from case to case. The first sign observed may be the passage of bloodstained urine in an otherwise normal cow. In other cases, the first sign may be an attack of acute colic, passing off in a few hours. Such attacks are caused by obstruction of a ureter or renal calyx by pus or tissue debris and may be confused with acute intestinal obstruction. More often the onset is gradual with a fluctuating temperature (about 39·5°C, 103°F), capricious appetite, loss of condition and fall in milk yield over a period of weeks. Other than this, there is little systemic reaction and the diagnostic signs are associated with the urinary tract. The most obvious sign is the presence of blood, pus, mucus and tissue debris in the urine, particularly in the last portion voided. Urination is frequent and may be painful. Periods during which the urine is abnormal may be followed by apparent recovery with later remissions. In the early stages, rectal examinaton may be negative but later there is usually detectable thickening and contraction of the bladder wall and enlargement of one or both ureters. The terminal portion of the latter may be palpated through the floor of the vagina over the neck of the bladder. One or both of the kidneys may show enlargement, absence of lobulation and pain on palpation. The course is usually several weeks or even months and the terminal signs are those of uremia.

Clinical pathology

The presence of *Cor. renale* in suspected urine can be confirmed by culture, specific immunofluorescence (7) or by direct microscopic examination. Blood constituents remain normal until the later stages when the waste products ordinarily eliminated by the kidneys will be increased. The urine will contain blood cells and protein. A diagnostic serological test has been reported (4).

Necropsy findings
Characteristic necropsy findings are limited to the kidneys, ureters and bladder. The kidneys are usually enlarged and the lobulation less evident than normal. Light-colored necrotic areas may be observed on the surface, and the pelvis and grossly enlarged ureters will contain blood, pus and mucus. Abscesses and necrotic areas may be observed in the cut lobules. The bladder and urethra are thick-walled and their mucous membranes are hemorrhagic, edematous and eroded.

Diagnosis
The gross changes in urine, together with palpable abnormalities in the urinary tract and the presence of bacteria including *Cor. renale* in the urine, are sufficient basis for a diagnosis of contagious bovine pyelonephritis. Cases characterized by acute colic can be differentiated from acute intestinal obstruction by the absence of a palpable obstruction and the disappearance of abdominal pain within a few hours. Chronic cases may be confused with traumatic reticulitis but may be differentiated by the urine changes present in pyelonephritis. Sporadic cases of non-specific cystitis can only be differentiated by culture of the urine. Other causes of hematuria must be considered but, for the most part, they are not associated with pyuria. Enzootic hematuria resembles contagious bovine pyelonephritis clinically but it occurs only in certain areas, the lesions are confined to the bladder, and the urine is sterile. Death in this disease usually results from hemorrhagic anemia.

Treatment
Prior to the introduction of penicillin, treatment of pyelonephritis was seldom undertaken successfully. Acidification of the urine by the administration of monobasic sodium phosphate (100 g daily for several days) was frequently followed by clinical improvement but seldom by permanent recovery.

Although several antibiotics appear to inhibit *Cor. renale*, penicillin remains the antibiotic of choice for treatment of pyelonephritis. Large doses (15 000 IU/kg body weight of procaine penicillin G) are recommended daily for 10 days. In early cases where little structural damage has occurred, permanent recovery can be expected following such a course of treatment. In general, a good prognosis is suggested by an improvement in condition, appetite and milk yield and clearing of the urine. However, in well-established cases, relapse is not uncommon and, where tissue destruction has been extensive, relief through antibiotic therapy is only temporary. In valuable animals, unilateral nephrectomy may be an alternative and the surgical technique has been described (8).

Control
No specific control measures are usually practiced but isolation of affected animals and destruction of infected litter and bedding should reduce the population of the organism in the local environment and minimize the opportunity for transmission. Where natural breeding is practiced, some reduction in occurrence may be achieved by the introduction of artificial insemination.

REFERENCES

(1) Goudswaard, J. & Budhai, S. (1975) *Zentralbl. VetMed.*, *22B*, 473.
(2) Higgins, R. J. & Weaver, C. R. (1981) *Vet. Rec.*, *109*, 256.
(3) Lovell, R. & Cotchin, E. (1952) *J. comp. Pathol.*, *62*, 245.
(4) Hitamune, T. et al. (1972) *Res. vet. Sci.*, *13*, 82.
(5) Morse, E. V. (1950) *Cornell Vet.*, *40*, 178.
(6) Hitamune, T. et al. (1975) *Natl Inst., Anim. Hlth Q., Tokyo*, *15*, 116.
(7) Addo, P. B. & Cook, J. E. (1979) *Br. vet. J.*, *135*, 50.
(8) Tulleners, E. P. et al. (1981) *J. Am. vet. med. Assoc.*, *179*, 696.
(9) Hayashi, A. et al. (1985) *Am. J. vet. Res.*, *46*, 409.

Cystitis and pyelonephritis of pigs

This disease is caused by *Corynebacterium suis*, an anaerobic diphtheroid recently renamed *Eubacterium suis* (7). The organism can be isolated from the preputial diverticulum of boars of various ages (9, 10). The prevalence of infection in adult males can be as high as 90% (10). Infection and colonization of the preputial diverticulum may occur in pigs as early as 5 weeks of age if they are housed with older pigs.

The disease tends to occur in small outbreaks, with a small number of sows, which have been mated to a single boar, becoming affected. More serious outbreaks can occur in large intensive piggeries in which stress enhances susceptibility (1). In many cases adult sows become ill quite suddenly, show profound depression and circulatory collapse and die within 12 hours. In the early stages of the disease, the frequent passage of bloodstained, turbid urine accompanied by vaginal discharge, occurs in sows usually 3–4 weeks after service (2). However, clinical signs may not be apparent until the end of pregnancy (3). Infection may be introduced at mating or be residual from the previous farrowing. The relationship to mating has been well-established and it has been suggested that sows which bleed or show pain after service should be treated prophylactically with a broad-spectrum antibiotic (4). Affected sows often go unobserved until they are found dead. Where surveillance is good the sows are observed to be depressed, anorectic, mildly febrile (normal to 39·5°C, 103°F), and sometimes show arching of the back and painful urination. Because of the occurrence of the disease after mating and the presence of the organism in the urine, semen and sheath of normal boars but only in association with pathological condition in sows (5), and the apparent ascending nature of the disease, venereal transmission seems likely (6). The diagnostic sign is the passage of turbid, bloodstained urine. Boars are usually unaffected clinically, but intermittent, hematuric episodes lasting several days are recorded. At necropsy, cystitis is the main lesion with ureteritis and pyelonephritis occurring in some pigs.

The organism can usually be cultured from the lesions at necropsy. However, isolation of the organism from the prepuce requires special cultural media because of the anaerobic requirements and the mixed bacterial flora present in the prepuce (8). Early treatment with penicillin is recommended but, if lesions are well advanced, the case fatality rate is high and relapse commonly occurs.

REFERENCES

(1) Larsen, J. L. (1973) *Medlemsbl. danske Dyrlaegeforen.*, *56*, 509.
(2) Soltys, M. A. & Spratling, F. R. (1957) *Vet. Rec.*, *69*, 500.
(3) Glazebrook, J. S. et al. (1973) *Aust. vet. J.*, *49*, 546.
(4) Biering-Sorenson, U. (1967) *Medlemsbl. danske Dyrlaegeforen.*, *24*, 1103.
(5) Soltys, M. A. (1961) *J. Pathol. Bacteriol.*, *81*, 441.
(6) Narucka, U. & Westerndorp, J. F. (1972) *Tijdschr. Diergeneeskd.*, *97*, 647.
(7) Wegienek, J. & Reddy, C. A. (1982) *Int. J. system. Bacteriol.*, *32*, 218.
(8) Dagnall, G. J. R. & Jones, J. E. T. (1982) *Res. vet. Sci.*, *32*, 389.
(9) Pijoan, C. et al. (1983) *J. Am. vet. med. Assoc.*, *183*, 428.
(10) Jones, J. E. T. & Dagnall, G. J. R. (1984) *J. Hyg.*, *Camb.*, *93*, 381.

Enzootic posthitis (pizzle rot, sheath rot, balanoposthitis)

This enzootic inflammation of the prepuce and penis of principally castrated male sheep is caused by a diphtheroid organism which produces lesions which themselves become severe only in certain circumstances of management and urinary composition.

Etiology

Although the disease fluctuates in its incidence, depending upon climate and feed conditions, it was considered for many years to be non-infectious. The two factors considered to be most important were a high alkalinity of the urine causing irritation of the preputial and surrounding skin and a high intake of estrogens in pasture causing swelling and congestion of the prepuce. Factors of lesser, and largely unknown, importance were considered to be continued wetness of the area around the prepuce due to removal of preputial hairs at shearing, a high-calcium, low-phosphorus diet and the ingestion of large quantities of alkaline water. In spite of the finding that the disease is caused by a diphtheroid organism, now identified as *Cor. renale* (1), the above factors appear to be of major importance as predisposing causes because their removal has such a beneficial effect on the occurrence of posthitis (2).

The causative organism can be recovered from lesions and from clinically normal prepuces and has also been found in the lesions of vulvitis in ewes and posthitis in bulls (3, 4) and Angora goat wethers (5). Implantation of the organism on a scarified prepuce in the presence of urine is capable of causing the external ulceration which is characteristic of the disease. Its growth on the prepuce is prevented by the prior systemic implantation of testosterone but the mechanism of interaction is unclear; at least it is known that the testosterone does not alter the biochemical composition of the urine (6). The organism is capable of hydrolyzing urea and proliferates more rapidly in high concentrations of urea which probably accounts for its pathogenicity in this situation. It has been suggested that the exact cytotoxic agent may be the ammonia produced by the bacteria rather than any destructive capacity of the bacterium itself (7). Factors likely to increase the urinary concentration of urea include the provision of a high-protein diet such as would be available on lush, improved pasture, the circumstance in which the disease occurs most commonly.

Epidemiology

Enzootic posthitis occurs in epizootic proportions in wethers in conditions of excellent pasture growth especially when legumes are plentiful. The incidence in affected flocks may be as high as 40% and in some areas the disease is so common that it is not possible to maintain bands of wethers. Many deaths occur because of uremia and secondary bacterial infections and all affected sheep show a severe setback in growth rate and wool production. Young rams are sometimes affected and are subsequently incapable of mating.

In Australia, enzootic posthitis occurs most commonly in Merino sheep, particularly wethers over 3 years of age and young rams, but in a severe outbreak young wethers and old rams may also be affected. The high incidence in castrates and young rams is probably related to the close adherence of the preputial and penile skins which separate in mature entire animals.

An ulcerative vulvitis occurs in ewes in the same flocks in which posthitis occurs in wethers and is thought to be a venereal extension of that disease. The causative bacterium is transmissible to the prepuce of male cattle and an ulcerative posthitis occurs naturally in bulls and is thought to be caused by the agent of ovine posthitis (8, 9). There appears to be no counterpart to ovine vulvitis in cows. In Uruguay the rate of ocurrence of the disease in bulls appears to have reached a very high level (14) and the economic effects are considerable.

The causative bacterium persists for 3–6 months in the laboratory at room temperature but details of its persistence in the normal ovine environment are not available.

Enzootic posthitis occurs most extensively on lush, improved pasture with a high legume content and reaches its highest incidence in autumn in summer rainfall areas and in spring where the major rainfall is in winter. In the early stages the progress of the disease can be halted or reversed by starvation for several days.

Transmission of the causative organism could occur in a number of ways. Infection at dipping or shearing seems not to be important but flies are considered to be probable mechanical vectors and contact with infected soil and herbage is a likely method of spread. Transmission to ewes appears to occur venereally from infected rams (9). Although the natural disease in cattle is usually benign they may act as vectors of infection for sheep on the same farm.

Pathogenesis

It is generally believed that the initial lesion in the wether (the external lesion) is caused by ammonia produced from urea in the urine by the causative bacteria (10). This lesion may be maintained in a static condition for a long period but, if satisfactory conditions of high urea content of the urine and continued wetting of the wool around the prepuce are maintained, the lesion proceeds to invade the interior of the prepuce, producing the 'internal lesion'. A similar pathogenesis is postulated for vulvar lesions.

Clinical findings

The primary lesion is a small scab on the skin dorsal to the preputial orifice (the external lesion) and this may persist for long periods without the appearance of any clinical signs. The scab is thick, adherent and tenacious. If extension to the interior of the prepuce occurs (the internal lesion) ulceration and scabbing of the preputial opening appear and the sheep may show restlessness, kicking at the belly and dribbling of the urine as in urethral obstruction. Swelling of the prepuce occurs commonly and the area is often infested by blowfly maggots. The development of pus and fibrous tissue adhesions may interfere with urination and protrusion of the penis, and cause permanent impairment of function in rams.

Some deaths occur due to obstructive uremia, toxemia and septicemia. During an outbreak many sheep may be affected without showing clinical signs and are detected only when they are subjected to a physical examination. Others recover spontaneously when feed conditions deteriorate. In ewes the lesions are confined to the lips of the vulva and consist of ulcers and scabs. They may cause an increased susceptibility to blowfly-strike.

The lesions in bulls are similar to the external lesions which occur in wethers but rarely there may be invasion of the interior of the prepuce. The external lesions occur at any point around the urethral orifice and may encircle it (9). Their severity varies from local excoriation to marked ulceration with exudation and edema. There is a tendency for the lesions to persist for several months without treatment and with highly alkaline urine (4, 11).

Clinical pathology

Isolation of the causative diphtheroid bacterium may be necessary if there is doubt as to the identity of the disease (3).

Diagnosis

The occurrence of other forms of enzootic posthitis in cattle and sheep seems likely but ulcerative dermatosis of sheep and infectious pustular vulvovaginitis of cattle, caused by viruses, are the only common ones. Obstructive urolithiasis in wethers may superficially resemble posthitis but there is no preputial lesion.

Treatment

In bad outbreaks the sheep can be removed on to dry pasture and their feed intake restricted to that required for subsistence only. They should be inspected at regular intervals, the wool shorn from around the prepuce and affected animals treated individually. Weekly application of a 10% copper sulfate ointment is recommended for external lesions and when the interior of the prepuce is involved, it should be irrigated twice weekly with a 5% solution of copper sulfate. Cetrimide (20% in alcohol or water with or without 0·25% acid fuchsin) or alcohol alone (90%) are about as effective as copper sulfate preparations. Penicillin topically or parenterally may effect a temporary response. Thiabendazole by mouth appears to have a beneficial effect on the lesions but does not eliminate them (12). In severe cases the only satisfactory treatment is surgical, antibiotics effecting no response and testosterone implants producing a good weight gain without affecting the lesions (13). Surgical treatment may be necessary if the prepuce is obstructed. The recommended procedure is to open the sheath by inserting one blade of a pair of scissors into the external preputial orifice and cutting the prepuce back as far as the end of the urethral process; extension beyond this leads to trauma of the penis. Badly affected rams should be disposed of as they are unlikely to be of value for breeding.

Control

The principal control measures are restriction of the diet to reduce the urea content of the urine, removal of the wool around the prepuce or vulva to avoid a local accumulation of urine, segregation of affected sheep and disinfection of the preputial area. The latter measure may be necessary only if the causative bacterium is present in the environment but it is likely to be a ubiquitous organism. As a preventive measure it is carried out on three occasions over a period of a year commencing at 6 months of age. In wethers the antiseptic is infused into the prepuce and smeared over the skin around the prepuce. In ewes it is swabbed on to the vulva and surrounding skin (9).

Subcutaneous implantation with testosterone propionate is highly effective as a preventive and a treatment especially against the internal lesion, but response in affected animals is improved by the simultaneous application of one of the local treatments listed above. At the dose rate used there is no appreciable deterioration in the quality of the carcass and there is a marked increase in the rate of gain. A slight disadvantage is that there is an increase in the growth of horn. A single implantation of 60–90 mg is effective for 3 months and although the treatments can be repeated four times a year, it is more economical to time them to coincide with periods of maximum incidence which will vary from district to district. Three implantations in autumn, winter and spring provide an effective control program in most areas (12). The tablets are implanted subcutaneously, preferably at the base of the ear, using preloaded tubes to avoid undue contact to the operator.

REVIEW LITERATURE

Dent, C. H. R. (1971) Ulcerative vulvitis and posthitis in Australian sheep and cattle. *Vet. Bull.*, *41*, 719.

REFERENCES

(1) Rojas, J. A. & Biberstein, E. L. (1974) *J. comp. Pathol.*, *84*, 301.
(2) Johnstone, I. L. (1963) *Aust. vet. J.*, *39*, 371.
(3) Southcott, W. H. (1965) *Aust. vet. J.*, *41*, 193.
(4) Nielsen, I. (1972) *Aust. vet. J.*, *48*, 39.
(5) Shelton, M. & Livingston, C. W. (1975) *J. Am. vet. med. Assoc.*, *167*, 154.
(6) McMillan, K. R. et al. (1974) *Aust. vet. J.*, *50*, 298.
(7) Brook, A. H. et al. (1965) *Aust. vet. J.*, *42*, 9.
(8) Bassett, C. R. (1963–64) *Vict. vet. Proc.*, 38.
(9) Southcott, W. H. (1965) *Aust. vet. J.*, *41*, 225.
(10) McMillan, K. R. & Southcott, W. H. (1973) *Aust. vet. J.*, *49*, 405.
(11) Parsonson, I. M. & Clark, B. L. (1972) *Aust. vet. J.*, *48*, 125.

(12) Southcott, W. H. (1968) *Aust. vet. J.*, *44*, 526.
(13) Swan, R. A. (1971) *Vet. Rec.*, *88*, 304.
(14) Correa, F. R. et al. (1979) *Cornell Vet.*, *69*, 33.

Caseous lymphadenitis of sheep

Caseous lymphadenitis is a chronic disease of sheep characterized by the formation of abscesses in lymph nodes and exerting little effect on the general health of the sheep unless the disease becomes generalized.

Etiology

Corynebacterium pseudotuberculosis is the specific cause of the disease which can be produced experimentally by injection into tissues, lymphatics or intravenously (12). It is also the cause of ulcerative lymphangitis of cattle and horses, contagious and suppurative arthritis of lambs, suppurative orchitis of rams and contagious acne of horses, but these have been dealt with as separate diseases because they do not occur in association with caseous lymphadenitis.

Epidemiology

Caseous lymphadenitis in sheep reaches a peak of incidence in adults because of repeated exposure to infection at each shearing. In one Australian population the frequency of infected sheep at abattoir inspection was 3·4% for lambs and 54% for adult ewes (10) and similar levels of prevalence are recorded in North (3) and South America (19). The disease is recorded also in domesticated goats at a prevalence rate of 8% in a large population (5). In some goat flocks it has become established as a very significant cause of wastage. A similar prevalence is recorded in feral goats (21).

The source of infection is the discharges from ruptured lymph nodes. Contamination of the soil on bedding grounds or in shelters may result in persistence of the organism in the environment for very long periods. It has been commonly assumed that infection occurs via wounds created by shearing, docking and castration, the infection deriving from contaminated soil, or being transported by surgical equipment which has been contaminated by pus from freshly ruptured abscesses. However, it has now been shown that there is at least one other important source of infection, the sheep dip. The bacterium can survive in commercial sheep dips for at least 24 hours, and infection can occur through the intact skin. Sheep dipped in infected dipping fluid within 2 weeks of having been shorn are especially susceptible to infection because of ease of contact between the bacteria and the skin (2). This places a different perspective on the control program.

The disease appears to be of importance wherever sheep are raised in large numbers. In most cases the disease has little effect on the health or body weight gains (7) of affected sheep but in rare instances generalization may occur and cause death. The important losses are caused by restriction on the use of affected carcasses.

Pathogenesis

Spread of infection from infected skin sites leads to involvement of local lymph nodes and the development of abscesses. Less commonly, blood-borne infection may result in the development of septicemia in lambs and in adults in abscess formation in many organs including lung, liver, kidney, brain and spinal cord. This may be in the absence of peripheral lesions. Up to 25% of affected sheep at abattoirs are recorded as having lesions only in thoracic viscera (2). This tendency for a high incidence of lesions in the lung appears to be general but varies significantly between geographic areas (3). The abdominal visceral and somatic tissues are also commonly affected. In goats there is a much greater proportion of affected goats having lesions in the head, related possibly to a high rate of superficial injury during browsing (21).

Experimental induction of caseous lymphadenitis in goats (10) has shown that the incubation period for the development of abscesses after injection averaged 95 days, and the shedding of *Cor. pseudotuberculosis* from open abscesses averaged 20 days. The abscesses were in regional peripheral lymph nodes; there were none in mesenteric lymph nodes and no bacteria were found in nasal secretions or feces.

Clinical findings

There is palpable enlargement of one or more of the superficial lymph nodes. Those most commonly affected are the submaxillary, prescapular, prefemoral, supramammary and popliteal nodes. The abscesses commonly rupture and thick, green pus is discharged. In cases in which systemic involvement occurs, chronic pneumonia, pyelonephritis, ataxia and paraplegia may be present. The debilitating disease of adult ewes commonly referred to as 'thin ewe syndrome' is often associated with the occurrence of internal abscesses (81% of ewes), many of which contain *Cor. pseudotuberculosis* (86%). Other bacteria, especially *Moraxella* sp., are also commonly present. The abscesses may be a factor in producing the disease or be a secondary consequence of it. In ewes, local spread from the supramammary lymph node to the mammary tissue is common. The resulting fall in milk yields leads to poor growth and even death of lambs and this may be a serious economic feature in badly affected flocks. Intrascrotal lesions are common in rams, but do not involve the testicles or semen (8).

In goats the disease is common and identical with the disease in sheep including the high prevalence of thoracic disease which may take the form of a highly fatal, acute bronchopneumonia (4).

Clinical pathology

Examination of pus for the presence of *Cor. pseudotuberculosis* is the usual laboratory aid available. Allergic tests have been used but are unreliable as diagnostic tools (13) but may be useful in following the course of the disease (16). Serological tests including tube agglutination, complement fixation, gel diffusion, antihemolysin inhibition, and indirect agglutination tests were not completely accurate in diagnosing the disease (6). Of the tests the indirect hemagglutination test is the most satisfactory in sheep (2, 11), and in goats the bacterial agglutination and haemolysis inhibition tests are satisfactory (18). An ELISA test has also been developed (14).

Necropsy findings

Caseous abscesses filled with greenish-yellow pus occur chiefly in lymph nodes and to a lesser extent in internal organs. In the early stages the pus is soft and pasty but in the later stages it is firm and dry and has a characteristic laminated appearance. Diffuse bronchopneumonia, with more fluid pus of a similar color, may also be present.

Diagnosis

Palpable enlargements of peripheral lymph nodes as a flock problem in sheep are usually due to this disease. The caseous greenish pus is diagnostic. Caseous lymphadenitis runs a much more chronic course than that of melioidosis although the lesions in the two diseases have a superficial similarity. Suppurative lymphadenitis in lambs has also been found to be caused by infection with *Past. multocida* and a disease characterized by the presence of yellow-green pus in abscesses situated in close proximity to the lymph nodes of sheep is caused by a Gram-positive micrococcus. The latter disease occurs in France and Kenya and is referred to as Morel's disease.

Treatment

Treatment is not usually attempted although the organism is susceptible to penicillin. The local formation of abscesses is unlikely to respond to other than surgical treatment and the usual non-progressive nature of this disease makes treatment unnecessary in most cases.

Control

Attempts at producing an effective vaccine against caseous lymphadenitis in sheep have been largely unsuccessful. What is achieved by vaccination is protection against the lethal effects of the bacterial toxin (9), but without much restriction of systemic spread and abscess development. Inclusion of adjuvants in killed vaccines, and the use of live vaccines, seem unlikely to improve the efficiency of a vaccination program (9). Vaccination of goats is recorded as providing good but not complete protection against experimentally induced systemic development of abscesses (16). Cutaneous infection is unimpeded (1). Based on findings in goat kids it is recommended that immunoprophylaxis commences at 2–3 months of age when passive immunity from the dam disappears (17).

Immunization by vaccination with BCG vaccine against tuberculosis has been reported on favorably in sheep, especially if they were vaccinated as lambs about 1 month old (15). A disadvantage is that the vaccinated sheep react positively to a tuberculin test for very long periods.

Control must depend upon elimination of the source of infection by culling all sheep with enlarged lymph nodes, preferably at shearing time when palpation is easier. Although this is a logical procedure it is worth noting that it is not capable of detecting early lesions, especially in the prescapular lymph node (2). Lambing and docking should be carried out in clean surroundings or in fresh fields. All docking implements and shears used for the Mules operation should be dipped in strong disinfectant before each use. Similar attention should be given to shears at shearing time and pus spilled on the shearing floor should be cleaned up and all shearing cuts disinfected. *Cor. tuberculosis* has been known to survive for up to 7 weeks in soil but for only a few days on surfaces (20). The younger age groups should be shorn first as the chance of infection is less among the lambs. All efforts must also be directed to avoid contaminating dipping fluid; one discharging abscess is capable of contaminating an entire tank of fluid. Dipping after shearing may be undesirable in badly affected flocks. The addition of an efficient bactericidal agent to the dipping fluid is worthy of consideration.

REVIEW LITERATURE

Batey, R. G. (1896) Pathogenesis of caseous lymphadenitis in sheep and goats. *Aust. vet. J.*, *63*, 269.

Brown, C. C. & Olander, H. J. (1987) Caseous lymphadenitis of goats and sheep: a review. *Vet. Bull.*, *57*, 1.

REFERENCES

(1) Nairn, M. E. et al. (1977) *Aust. Adv. Vet. Sci.*, *Aust. vet. Assoc. Ann. Conf. Prog. Pathol.*, p. 159.
(2) Nairn, M. E. & Robertson, J. P. (1974) *Aust. vet. J.*, *50*, 537.
(3) Stoops, S. G. et al. (1984) *Am. J. vet. Res.*, *45*, 557.
(4) Williams, C. S. F. (1980) *Vet. Med. SAC*, *75*, 1165.
(5) Ashfaq, M. K. & Campbell, S. G. (1979) *Vet. Med. SAC*, *74*, 1161.
(6) Brown, C. C. et al. (1986) *Am. J. vet. Res.*, *47*, 1461, 2322.
(7) Batey, R. G. (1986) *Aust. vet. J.*, *63*, 268.
(8) Williamson, P. E. & Nairn, M. E. (1980) *Aust. vet. J.*, *56*, 496.
(9) Cameron, C. M. & Bester, F. J. (1984) *Onderstepoort J. vet. Res.*, *51*, 263.
(10) Batey, R. G. (1986) *Am. J. vet. Res.*, *47*, 482.
(11) Shigidi, M. T. A. (1979) *Br. vet. J.*, *135*, 172.
(12) Brogden, K. A. (1984) *Am. J. vet. Res.*, *45*, 1532.
(13) Renshaw, H. W. et al. (1979) *Am. J. vet. Res.*, *40*, 1110.
(14) Brown, C. C. & Olander, H. J. (1987) *Vet. Bull.*, *57*, 1.
(15) Barakat, A. A. (1979) *Bull. Off. int. Epizootol.*, *91*, 679.
(16) Brown, C. C. et al. (1986) *Am. J. vet. Res.*, *47*, 1116.
(17) Lund, A. et al. (1982) *Acta vet. Scand.*, *23*, 483.
(18) Lund, A. et al. (1982) *Acta vet. Scand.*, *23*, 473.
(19) Unanian, M. M. et al. (1985) *Trop. Anim. Hlth Prod.*, *17*, 57.
(20) Augustine, J. L. (1986) *Am. J. vet. Res.*, *47*, 713.
(21) Batey, R. G. et al. (1986) *Aust. vet. J.*, *63*, 33.

Ulcerative lymphangitis of horses and cattle

Ulcerative lymphangitis is a mildly contagious disease of horses and cattle characterized by lymphangitis of the lower limbs.

Etiology

Corynebacterium pseudotuberculosis causes the classical disease and the disease has been produced experimentally in buffalo (1). Similar lesions may be due to infection with other pyogenic organisms including streptococci, staphylococci, *Cor.* (*Rhodococcus*) *equi* (2), and *Pseudomonas aeruginosa* (3).

Epidemiology

Infection occurs through abrasions on the lower limbs and is more likely when horses are crowded together in dirty, unhygienic quarters. Contact is the obvious means of spread but passive transmission by flies is probable (5). As a rule only sporadic cases occur in a stable.

The disease was of considerable importance and widely distributed during the horse era. The mortality rate was negligible but among the affected horses there was interference with their ability to perform. Ulcerative lymphangitis has also been recorded in cattle (4).

Pathogenesis

Infection of skin wounds is followed by invasion of lymphatic vessels and the development of abscesses along their course. Lymph node involvement is unusual.

Clinical findings

In horses the initial wound infection is followed by swelling and pain of the pastern, often sufficient to cause severe lameness. Nodules develop in the subcutaneous tissue particularly around the fetlock, but can spread to subcutaneous sites on all parts of the body (7). These may enlarge to 5–7 cm in diameter and rupture to discharge a creamy green pus. The resulting ulcer has ragged edges and a necrotic base. Lymphatics draining the area become enlarged and hard and secondary ulcers may develop along them. Lesions heal in 1–2 weeks but fresh crops may occur and cause persistence of the disease for up to 12 months. The lesions in cattle are similar to those in horses except that there may be lymph node enlargement and the ulcers discharge a gelatinous clear exudate (4).

Clinical pathology

The isolation of *Cor. pseudotuberculosis* from discharging lesions is necessary to confirm the diagnosis.

Diagnosis

Differentiation of ulcerative lymphangitis from the other diseases causing similar lesions is important because of the serious nature of such diseases as glanders and epizootic lymphangitis in horses. Restriction of the lesion to the lower limbs and absence of lymph node involvement are important features although these are shared by sporotrichosis.

Treatment

Local treatment of ulcers is the usual procedure but parenteral injections of penicillin or tetracycline may be necessary in severe cases (6). In the early stages an autogenous bacterin may have value as treatment.

Control

Good hygiene in stables and careful disinfection of injuries to the lower limbs usually afford adequate protection against the disease.

REFERENCES

(1) Khater, A. R. et al. (1983) *Assiut. vet. Med. J.*, *10*, 47.
(2) Bain, A. M. (1963) *Aust. vet. J.*, *39*, 116.
(3) Azizuddin, I. M. & Chandrasekharan, N. K. P. (1954) *Madras vet. Coll. Ann.*, *12*, 17.
(4) Purchase, H. S. (1944) *J. comp. Pathol.*, *54*, 238.
(5) Addo, P. B. (1983) *Vet. Rec.*, *113*, 496.
(6) Adeyefa, C. A. O. (1983) *Trop. Vet.*, *1*, 56.
(7) Abu-Samra, M. T. et al. (1980) *Equ. vet. J.*, *12*, 149.

Contagious acne of horses (Canadian horse pox, contagious pustular dermatitis)

Contagious acne of horses is characterized by the development of pustules particularly where the skin comes in contact with harness.

Etiology

Corynebacterium pseudotuberculosis is the specific cause of this disease.

Epidemiology

The disease is spread from animal to animal by means of contaminated grooming utensils or harness. An existing seborrhea or folliculitis due to blockage of sebaceous gland ducts by pressure from harness probably predisposes to infection. Inefficient grooming may also be a contributing cause.

Contagious acne is of limited occurrence and causes temporary inconvenience when affected horses are unable to work.

Pathogenesis

Infection of the hair follicle leads to local suppuration and the formation of pustules which rupture and contaminate surrounding skin areas. Occasional lesions penetrate deeply and develop into indolent ulcers.

Clinical findings

The skin lesions usually develop in groups in areas which come into contact with harness. The lesions take the form of papules which develop into pustules varying in diameter from 1 to 2·5 cm. There is no pruritus but the lesions may be painful to touch. Rupture of the pustules leads to crust formation over an accumulation of greenish-tinged pus. Healing of lesions occurs in about 1 week but the disease may persist for 4 or more weeks if successive crops of lesions develop.

Clinical pathology

Swabs of the lesions can be taken to determine the presence of *Cor. pseudotuberculosis*.

Diagnosis

Contagious acne bears some similarity to other skin diseases, particularly some forms of ringworm, bursatti and non-specific pyogenic infections including those caused by staphylococci. Bursatti, or swamp cancer, is caused by the larvae of the nematode worm, *Habronema megastoma*. Nodules which develop into ulcers occur below the eyes, and on the legs and belly. Isolation of *Cor. pseudotuberculosis* from lesions is necessary to confirm the diagnosis of contagious acne.

Treatment

Affected animals should be rested until all lesions are healed. Frequent washing with a mild skin disinfectant solution followed by the application of antibacterial ointments to the lesions should facilitate healing and prevent the development of further lesions. Parenteral administration of antibiotics may be advisable in severe cases.

Control

Infected horses should be rigidly isolated and all grooming equipment, harness and blankets disinfected. Grooming tools must be disinfected before each use. Vaccination is not likely to be effective because of the poor antigenicity of the organism.

Corynebacterial pneumonia of foals

This is a well-recognized infectious disease of young foals with localization in many organs but particularly in the lungs with clinical manifestations of pneumonia.

Etiology

Corynebacterium (*Rhodococcus*) *equi* is the cause of this disease. The organism has been found to have at least seven serotypes (25). It affects horses principally but may also be found in lymph node abscesses in the pig and in ulcerative lymphangitis in cattle. *Cor. pseudotuberculosis* and *Actinomyces* (*Corynebacterium*) *pyogenes* can also cause the disease.

Epidemiology

This disease usually causes sporadic foal deaths on farms where it recurs. The morbidity is usually low but it can reach epidemic proportions with most of a year's foal crop being lost (3). The organism is not highly resistant but it has been found to survive in moist soil for periods of longer than 12 months. The infection is considered to be soil associated and to be maintained through a soil–horse cycle (16). The bacterium appears to be so widespread that it must be considered to be a part of the normal flora of the gut of pastured horses, as distinct from those kept in stables (9, 21) and occurs also in the gut of other species and in lymph nodes of pigs (5).

The modes of transmission of the infection include ingestion and inhalation. Intrauterine infection is considered to be of no importance. Because of the ubiquitous nature of *Cor. (Rhodococcus) equi* most foals on infected farms become infected but only a few develop the disease. This view of the pathogenesis includes the concept of reduced immunological resistance in individual foals to explain the sporadic occurrence of clinical cases (8). However, it seems unlikely that intestinal lesions are commonly precursors of pulmonary disease (13) and inhalation is considered to be the principal portal of entry; the disease has been initiated by inhalation of aerosols containing *Cor. (Rhodococcus) equi* (20).

The disease appears to occur in most countries, comprising about 5% of infectious disease in foals in the United Kingdom and probably a similar proportion in other countries. A mortality of about 80% is usual, although the number of deaths decreases markedly in foals more than 3 months of age. The disease is most common in foals 1–2 months of age but can occur in older foals up to 6 months old (3). Foals which survive the acute stages of the disease seldom develop normally. Rare cases occur in adults (2).

Pathogenesis

Although the method of development of this disease is not completely clear it is evident that there are at least two important pathways by which infection occurs. Most cases result from inhalation of *Cor.* (*Rhodococcus*) *equi* in dusty surroundings in heavily contaminated environments around stables. The resulting disease is manifested by pneumonia and pulmonary abscesses. Foals running at pasture are more likely to be infected orally and to develop the ulcerative lesions of the mucosa of the large intestine. In rare cases there is an initial bacteremia and subsequently suppurative foci may develop in many organs, particularly the lungs and to a lesser extent in the joints and subcutaneous tissues. When the pulmonary involvement reaches a sufficiently advanced stage, the standard clinical picture becomes apparent. Intestinal lesions result from massive exposure to infection over a sustained period (24). In cases with severe intestinal lesions diarrhea may be the main presenting sign.

The disease has a chronic course and is resistant to treatment, largely because of the ability of *Cor.* (*Rhodococcus*) *equi* to survive within macrophages and escape the usual defense mechanism of the pulmonary tissue. In immunocompromised animals the disease may be acutely fatal.

Clinical findings

The clinical picture in foals varies with the age at which foals become affected. Those affected at a month of age have a more acute form of the disease than those affected subsequently. Thus young foals may suddenly become acutely ill with the appearance of signs of pneumonia, fever, anorexia and in some cases acute arthritis affecting one or more joints. Subcutaneous abscesses may develop. In older foals the disease assumes a characteristic clinical syndrome marked by a serious development of lesions without apparent abnormality in the foal. Then a subacute pneumonia develops slowly with coughing, an increase in the depth of respiration with obvious dyspnea developing in the late stages and characteristic loud, moist crackles, or 'rattles', on auscultation. The foal continues to suck and the temperature is normal but the foal becomes emaciated. Severe diarrhea may follow or accompany the respiratory signs. Nasal discharge and lymph node enlargement in the throat regions are absent. In most cases there is continued emaciation even with treatment and severely affected animals die in 1–2 weeks.

Radiographic examination is a valuable aid in diagnosis and in monitoring progress in hospitalized foals (18). Affected animals show evidence of consolidation of lung tissue, lymphadenopathy and cavitation of the lungs.

When lesions are confined to the intestinal wall the predominant clinical sign will be diarrhea which may be acute or chronic (10).

Clinical pathology

Cervical swabs for cultural purposes could be taken from the cervix of repeat-breeding mares and those that abort or produce infected foals. Nasal swabs or tracheal washings from infected foals in the later stages of the disease may reveal the presence of respiratory tract infection with *Cor.* (*Rhodococcus*) *equi*. A drug sensitivity should be obtained. The use of a filtrate from a culture of the organism has been used as an allergic skin test, a positive result being an edematous plaque at the injection site 18 hours later (2). A lymphocyte immunostimulation test can be used to distinguish infected foals from normal foals at 2 months of age (12); an ELISA test has proven useful for the early diagnosis of the disease (15) and an anti-*equi* factor test is also recommended (17). Weekly qualitative culture of feces may have merit in the early diagnosis of the disease; affected animals show a large increase in bacterial numbers (23).

Necropsy findings

The predominant lesion is suppurative pyogranulomatous pneumonia with multiple abscesses along the ventral borders of the lungs and in the bronchial lymph nodes (6). Many cases also have ulcerative enterocolitis and some have abscesses in mesenteric lymph nodes, and subcutaneous tissue, and there is sometimes suppurative arthritis. In spite of the severity of the lesions many cases are subclinical.

Diagnosis

The age group affected, the suppurative bronchopneumonia, the long subacute course and the association with infected mares all help in field diagnosis of the disease. Other respiratory tract infections including equine viral rhinopneumonitis, equine viral arteritis and strangles have a short course and affect upper respiratory tract rather than lungs. The other foal septicemias and bacteremias including infections with *Act. equuli*, *E. coli*, *Str. pyogenes equi*, *S. abortivoequina* and *S. typhimurium* may show joint lesions but there is rarely serious involvement of the lungs.

The differentiation from other similar diseases is outlined in Table 48. Other diseases of foals of this age (1–3 months) which are clinically dissimilar are joint ill, chronic diarrhea and shaker foals.

Treatment

Because of the chronic suppurative nature of the lesion, treatment is often not successful. To have any chances of success the program must begin early in the disease and be aggressive and based on bacterial sensitivity tests (14). Even that is not too satisfactory because clinical results with patients often do not reflect the laboratory findings. For example *Cor.* (*Rhodococcus*) *equi* is not very susceptible to penicillin but an intensive program of treatment with penicillin is reported to have had some success (1) but is not recommended.

There is a wide variation in the susceptibility of isolates of *C. equi* to antimicrobial agents. Some studies indicate that the most effective antibiotics are benzylpenicillin, erythromycin, lincomycin and the aminoglycosides (11) while other reports indicate that isolates of *Cor.* (*Rhodococcus*) *equi* are resistant to penicillin, ampicillin, streptomycin, tetracyclines and sulfonamides, but sensitive to erythromycin and neomycin (4). Some antibiotic mixtures have synergic effects (for example, penicillin with erythromycin). Others have additive effects (for instance, penicillin–rifampicin–erythromycin) and some have antagonistic effects (for example, gentamicin and erythromycin). The position is too confusing to make a general recommendation but excellent results are reported with a combination of erythromycin (25 mg/kg body weight, three times a day and rifampicin (5 mg/kg twice a day) (19). Neomycin is also an effective treatment but is disliked because of possible toxic effects which may be overestimated (22).

Control

Provision of colostrum in appropriate amounts at the earliest possible time after birth must be the first part of the program. If the infection can be shown to be present in the mares, control of the disease should aim at removal of the infection from the group, by either treating or culling affected animals. On present epidemiological evidence the most important recommendation is to reduce dust in the yards and around the stables. In badly affected studs, hygiene at foaling, particularly muzzling the foal and allowing it to suckle only when the mare has been washed down, is recommended. When an outbreak is in progress on a farm prophylactic injections of longacting penicillin for the first week of each foal's life appear to prevent further cases. A program to reduce infestation with helminth parasites is recommended as a control measure (3). Vaccination has been attempted but seems an unlikely prospect (7).

REVIEW LITERATURE

Barton, M. D. & Hughes, K. L. (1980) *Corynebacterium equi*. A review. *Vet. Bull.*, *50*, 65.

Hillidge, C. J. (1986) Review of *Corynebacterium* (*Rhodococcus*) *equi* lung abscesses in foals: pathogenesis, diagnosis, treatment. *Vet. Rec.*, *119*, 26.

REFERENCES

(1) Gay, C. C. et al. (1981) *Aust. vet. J.*, *57*, 150.
(2) Roberts, M. C. et al. (1980) *Aust. vet. J.*, *56*, 96.
(3) Campero, C. M. et al. (1981) *Gaceta Vet.*, *43*, 775.
(4) Barton, M. D. & Fulton, L. C. (1980) *Aust. vet. J.*, *56*, 339.
(5) Takai, S. & Tsubaki, S. (1985) *Jap. J. vet. Sci.*, *47*, 493.
(6) Zinc, M. C. et al. (1986) *Can. vet. J.*, *27*, 213.
(7) Prescott, J. F. et al. (1979) *Can. J. comp. Med.*, *43*, 356.
(8) Wilks, C. R. et al. (1982) *J. Reprod. Fertil.*, 32, Suppl. 497.
(9) Barton, M. D. & Hughes, K. L. (1984) *Vet. Microbiol.*, *9*, 65.
(10) Smith, K. D. & Butler, D. G. (1984) *Can. vet. J.*, *25*, 180.
(11) Woolcock, J. B. & Mutimer, M. D. (1980) *Antimicrob. Agents Chemotherap.*, *18*, 976.
(12) Prescott, J. F. et al. (1980) *Am. J. vet Res.*, *41*, 2073.
(13) Johnson, J. A. et al. (1983) *Vet. Pathol.*, *20*, 440, 450.
(14) Prescott, J. F. et al. (1984) *J. vet. Pharmacol. Therap.*, 7, 61.
(15) Takai, S. et al. (1985) *Am. J. vet. Res.*, *46*, 2166.
(16) Takai, S. et al. (1986) *Vet. Microbiol.*, *12*, 169.
(17) Prescott, J. F. et al. (1984) *Can. J. comp. Med.*, *48*, 370.
(18) Falcon, J. et al. (1985) *J. Am. vet. med. Assoc.*, *186*, 593.
(19) Hillidge, C. J. (1986) *Vet. Rec.*, *119*, 26.
(20) Martins, R. J. et al. (1982) *Equ. vet. J.*, *14*, 111.
(21) Prescott, J. F. et al. (1984) *Equ. vet. J.*, *48*, 10.
(22) Barton, M. D. (1986) *Aust. vet. J.*, *63*, 163.
(23) Takai, S. et al. (1986) *Can. J. vet. Res.*, *50*, 479.
(24) Prescott, J. F. et al. (1980) *Can. J. comp. Med.*, *44*, 280.
(25) Prescott, J. F. (1981) *Can. J. comp. Med.*, *45*, 130.

DISEASES CAUSED BY *LISTERIA* spp.

Listeriosis

Listeriosis is an infectious disease caused by *Listeria monocytogenes* and characterized by meningoencephalitis, abortion or septicemia.

Etiology

Listeria monocytogenes is the causative organism and can be isolated in pure culture from affected animals. Five serotypes labeled 1 to 5, and a number of subtypes, have been identified. The commonest serotype in natur-

Table 48. Differential diagnosis of diseases of older (not newborn) foals

Disease	*Epidemiology*	*Clinical findings*	*Clinical pathology*	*Necropsy findings*	*Treatment and response*
Corynebacterium (*Rhodococcus*)	Enzootic to a farm. Foals up to 3 months. Infection by inhalation of dust or ingestion of infected pasture plants. Case mortality high	Septicemia in 1-month-old foals. Pneumonia in 3-month-olds. May be diarrhea too	ELISA or anti-*equi* factor tests	Suppurative bronchopneumonia. May be mesenteric and other lymph node abscess. Rarely septicemia	Erythromycin plus rifampicin. Treatment must begin early in disease
Shigellosis (*Actinobacillus equuli*)	Enzootic to particular farms. Foals up to 3 months old. Recurs in foals from same mare	Sudden onset, recumbency, anorexia, fever, diarrhea, comatose, peripheral circulatory collapse. Death in 24 hours	Blood culture. Cervical swab of mare	Pinpoint abscesses in kidney, septicemia, enteritis. Longstanding cases have joint lesions	Chloramphenicol plus fluids. Excellent results if early. Maybe blood transfusion
Tyzzer's disease (*Bacillus piliformis*)	Foals 3–5 weeks old	Sudden onset, high fever, death in a few hours	Nil	Miliary necrotic foci in enlarged liver	Not known
Combined immunodeficiency of Arabian foals	Enzootic to Arab pony studs. Ponies sick at 4 weeks. Dead at 7 weeks	Poor condition, tire easily, cough, ocular and nasal discharge, diarrhea in some	Severe lymphopenia. Failure to synthesize immunoglobulin	Lymphocytes absent from lymphoid tissue. Adenoviral pneumonia	Nil
Abscess of urachus	Sporadic. Related to occurrence of navel ill	Foals 2 months, chronic ill health, frequent urination, patent urachus	Nil	Abscesses in old umbilicus and urachus	Surgical excision gives good recovery
Muscular dystrophy	Enzootic to a farm or area. May occur in twos of threes. Few days to yearlings	Sudden onset. Stiff, difficulty in moving. Many die at 7 days. Terminal recumbency	Serum level glutathione peroxidase and creatinine phosphokinase	Muscular dystrophy	Selenium. Poor response but good preventive
Upper respiratory tract infection with *Str. zooepidemicus*	Outbreaks in foals up to weaning	Identical to strangles in adults. Nasal discharge, enlarged lymph nodes, fever	*Str. zooepidemicus* in nasal swabs	Nil	Penicillin. Good recovery rate

ally occurring cases in farm animals is 4B. Serotype 5 has been identified as a cause of abortion in sheep (1) but is apparently of low pathogenicity. The infectivity and pathogenicity of all serotypes is sufficiently low to require a reduction in the host's resistance before disease is produced.

Epidemiology

Many animals carry *L. monocytogenes* in their feces as a normal bowel inhabitant (8) and many develop a systemic infection but only a small proportion of these develop clinical disease. A number of predisposing agents has been proposed as causing a lowering of the host animal's resistance, and thus initiating the disease. Heavy silage feeding is the commonest precursor of outbreaks. Other circumstances thought to contribute to a high incidence are sudden changes of weather to very cold and wet, and long periods of flooding with resulting poor access to pasture. Overcrowding and unsanitary conditions in housed sheep also cause poor access to feed supplies (28). Silage may exert its effect by increasing the susceptibility of the host or by providing a suitable medium for the growth and maintenance of the bacteria. *L. monocytogenes* is a common inhabitant of silage (8), but it does not multiply in good ensilage (pH 4·0–4·5) and it may not be killed. In spoiled silage with incomplete fermentation and a pH above 5·5 the bacteria survive and may multiply (2). Outbreaks which occur in sheep after introduction to silage usually commence about 3 weeks later. Experimental work with mice suggests that a diet containing *Pinus ponderosa* pine needles may also enhance infection with *L. monocytogenes* (5).

Sheep, cattle, buffalo, goats, horses, pigs, dogs, cats, rabbits and some wild animals and man are susceptible to infection. There is one report of the isolation of *L. monocytogenes* from the brain of a moose and it is suggested that the disease may be prevalent in this species and cause many losses. The presence of listeria in mice and deer in association with its presence in sheep and ensilage (6) and its frequent occurrence in birds suggest possible feral reservoirs of infection.

Experimentally meningoencephalitis can be produced

by intranasal instillation, inoculation of the conjunctival sac, or intraneural, intracerebral or intracarotid injections of the organism. Intravenous and subcutaneous injections have caused septicemia, oral dosing has produced visceral infection and intravenous injection in pregnant heifers has caused abortion. Experimental inoculation into rams has resulted in localization in testis and epididymis and suggests the possibility of venereal transmission (11).

The portal of infection in natural cases is uncertain but the prevalence of the particular forms of the disease under different environmental conditions suggests that infection may gain entrance by several portals. It seems probable that meningoencephalitis results from inhalation or conjunctival contamination, and the visceral infection with abortion from ingestion of infected material. Venereal transmission may also lead to abortion.

Infective material derives from infected animals in the feces, urine, aborted fetuses and uterine discharge and in the milk. Although immediate spread among animals in a group has been demonstrated, field observations suggest that mediate contagion by means of inanimate objects also occurs and this has been substantiated under experimental conditions (12). The organism persists for as long as 3 months in sheep feces and has been shown to survive for up to 11½ months in damp soil, up to 16½ months in cattle feces, up to 207 days on dry straw and for more than 2 years in dry soil and feces. The bacterium is also resistant to temperatures of −20°C (−6°F) for 2 years and is still viable after repeated freezing and thawing. It appears from the epizootiological pattern of the disease that carrier animals play a part in its transmission and normal animals from infected herds appear to bring the disease into herds to which they are introduced (7).

The disease has been of most importance in New Zealand, North America, Europe, the United Kingdom and Australia. It is much less common in tropical and subtropical than in temperate climates. Losses due to this disease, from both abortion and fatal meningoencephalitis, have been reported more frequently in recent years. The disease is of greatest economic importance in sheep and cattle but its host range includes 37 mammals in addition to man, 17 fowls, a fly, fish and crustaceans. The disease in goats, especially angoras, has leaped into prominence in recent years. Serious epidemics occur in young weaner and yearling goats (4), especially when there is a period of cold stress. Introduction to the flock appears to be via a carrier animal, although birds, such as seagulls, may carry a heavy population of the bacteria (27). In man the disease is serious, often fatal, and the fact that the organism occurs commonly in the milk of infected animals and may withstand pasteurization adds a further reason for the prompt recognition and control of this disease (7). Extreme care should be exercised by veterinarians when infected material, particularly from abortions, is handled. However, in spite of the importance of listeriosis as a zoonosis, an observed relationship between infected animals and humans is rare. It occurs most commonly after drinking infected milk that may have been pasteurized (13). Animals of any age, including the newborn, may be affected and in a herd the infection rate may reach 10%. The mortality rate without treatment in listerial septicemia and listerial meningoencephalitis approaches 100%.

Pathogenesis

There are a number of manifestations of the disease and these have an irregular distribution among the animal species. In naturally occurring cases, visceral (septicemic) listeriosis, with or without meningitis occurs most commonly in monogastric animals and young ruminants, especially the fetus and the neonate. The meningoencephalitic form of the disease is more common in adult ruminants (7). Infection of the uterus causing abortion and intrauterine infection occurs in all mammals. Visceral listeriosis affects organs other than the brain and the principal clinical manifestations are those of abortion or septicemia. In listerial meningoencephalitis the lesions are confined to the brain and the clinical picture is referable only to these lesions. *L. monocytogenes* is found rarely as a cause of chronic mastitis in cattle (9). It can be found as a probable cause of catarrhal conjunctivitis of cattle (10).

When the disease is produced experimentally by injection, both visceral and meningoencephalitic forms may occur in the one animal and organisms can be isolated from brain, spinal cord and viscera. Pregnant ewes abort in 7–11 days, the fetuses are often decomposed and *L. monocytogenes* is present in the fetal tissues and placenta.

In naturally occurring cases usually only the one clinical form, either the meningoencephalitic or the visceral, occurs in a particular group of animals. In the nervous form the organism is present in the brain only, in most cases, but a localized myelitis, manifested clinically by posterior paralysis of one limb, has been recorded in lambs (14). In the visceral form the viscera and sometimes the spinal cord, but never the brain, are infected. These observations lend weight to the hypothesis that different portals of entry may result in involvement of different organs. The pathway by which *L. monocytogenes* enters the brain is still under debate. It has been shown experimentally that the bacteria can ascend the trigeminal nerve to produce meningoencephalitis, in which the lesions are confined to the brain-stem in the region of the trigeminal nerve nucleus, and lesions occur along the nerve trunk and its branches (11). It is presumed that the organism reaches peripheral branches of the nerve by way of wounds in the oral mucosa or more probably by exposed terminals of the trigeminal nerve which became accessible when teeth are being shed or are penetrating the mucosa (25). A study of natural cases suggests that the pathogenesis of the disease can be viewed in two ways. The lesions are consistent with centripetal migration of the bacteria along peripheral nerves (15). It is also possible to interpret the location of the lesions as indicating that spread of the infection occurs along blood vessels, the bacteria lodging in and about the reticular formation of the brain-stem with lesions developing in the midbrain, pons and medulla with subsequent extension to the meninges, ependyma and occasionally the eye.

Ingestion of the organism, with penetration of the

mucosa of the intestine, is thought to lead either to an inapparent infection with prolonged fecal excretion of the organism (16) which occurs in a large proportion of infected animals; or to a bacteremia with localization in various organs; or to development to a fatal septicemia. The pregnant uterus appears to be particularly susceptible to infection. Infection early in pregnancy causes abortion, but infection late in pregnancy results in stillbirths or the delivery of young which rapidly develop a fatal septicemia. Maternal metritis is constant and if the fetus is retained a fatal listerial septicemia may follow. The fetus is infected via the maternal circulation and the amniotic fluid (17).

The peculiar localization of the infection to the brainstem in cases of meningoencephalitis is often unilateral and accounts for the localizing signs of facial paralysis and circling. The lesions may be bilateral causing bilateral facial and jaw paralysis. The additional signs of dullness, head-pressing and delirium are referable to the more general effects of inflammation of the brain. Spread of the infection along the optic nerve may result in endophthalmitis in sheep and cattle.

Clinical findings

One can expect to find the meningoencephalitic form and the visceral form (chiefly as abortion or neonatal septicemia) in different outbreaks of the disease, and rarely the two forms together in the one outbreak although the dual occurrence is recorded (26). The encephalitic form is the commonest one.

Listerial meningoencephalitis

This form has been observed in all species and presents a standard syndrome except that in pigs there are more involuntary muscle movements of the jaws and salivation than in the other species. In adult cattle the course of the disease is usually 1–2 weeks but in sheep and calves the disease is more acute, death occurring in 3–4 days. In goats also the disease is similar to that in the other species, but in the young goat the onset is very sudden and the course short with death occurring in 2–3 days.

Basically the clinical picture combines the signs of the 'dummy' syndrome, with pressing against fixed objects, and unilateral facial paralysis (24). Affected animals are dull, often to the point of somnolence, and isolate themselves from the rest of the group. There may be dropped jaw, in which case prehension and mastication are slow and the animal may stand for long periods drooling saliva and with food hanging from its mouth. Such cases probably have bilateral lesions in the medulla (12). Facial hypalgesia accompanies this paralysis and there may be lingual hypotonia and protrusion. Animals affected in this way are unable to eat and drink. The position of the head and neck varies. In most cases there is deviation of the head to one side with the poll–nose relationship undisturbed (i.e. there is no rotation of the head as in a middle ear infection). However, the head may be retroflexed or ventroflexed depending on the localization of the lesions in the brain-stem and in some cases may be in a normal position. The deviation of the head cannot be corrected actively by the animal and if it is corrected passively the head returns to its previous position as soon as it is released. Progression is usually in a circle in the direction of the deviation and the circle is of small diameter. There is ataxia, often with consistent falling to one or the other side.

Unilateral facial paralysis is also a common localizing sign, the ear, eyelids and lips on the affected side showing a flaccid paralysis. This may be accompanied by exposure keratitis, often severe enough to cause corneal ulceration. Strabismus and nystagmus occur in some. Panophthalmitis, with pus evident in the anterior chamber of one or both eyes, is not uncommon in cattle which have been affected for a number of days. The affected animal becomes recumbent and is unable to rise although often still able to move its legs. Death is due to respiratory failure. Fever (usually 40°C, 104°F, but occasionally as high as 42°C, 107°F) is usual in the early stages of the disease but the temperature is usually normal when frank clinical signs are present.

Listerial abortion

In cattle many sporadic abortions due to *L. monocytogenes* are recorded and outbreaks of abortion due to this organism are recorded in cattle, sheep and in goats. It is recorded rarely in pigs. In cattle there may be stillbirths or abortions at about the month of pregnancy or later, retention of the afterbirth occurs commonly, there is no evidence of clinical meningoencephalitis but there is commonly clinical illness and fever of up to 40·5°C (105°F) and *L. monocytogenes* is present in the fetal stomach. The disease has been observed soon after the commencement of silage feeding. In sheep and goats abortions occur from the 12th week of pregnancy onwards and the afterbirth is retained; meningoencephalitis does not occur although there may be some deaths of ewes due to septicemia if the fetus is retained. In both species the incidence of abortion in a group is low but may reach as high as 15% and on some farms recurs each year, sometimes more than once in the one animal. In infections with serotype 5 in sheep flocks there are no illnesses and when abortions occur the lambs are still alive and the ewes show no systemic reaction (1).

Septicemic listeriosis

Acute septicemia due to *L. monocytogenes* is not common in adult ruminants but does occur in monogastric animals including newborn lambs and calves. There are no signs suggestive of nervous system involvement, the syndrome being a general one comprising depression, weakness, emaciation, pyrexia and diarrhea in some cases, with hepatic necrosis and gastroenteritis at necropsy. The same syndrome is also seen in ewes and goats after abortion if the fetus is retained. A rather better defined but less common syndrome has been described in calves 3–7 days old. Corneal opacity is accompanied by dyspnea, nystagmus and mild opisthotonus. Death follows in about 12 hours. At necropsy there is ophthalmitis and serofibrinous meningitis.

Clinical pathology

Attempts may be made to isolate the organism from the feces, urine and milk of infected animals and from aborted fetuses. All organs of the fetus, including the stomach, should be examined as well as the placenta and uterine discharges, if they are available, because the organisms tend to be very patchy in their distribution. The organism can be cultivated from vaginal secretions for up to 2 weeks after abortion and a proportion of aborting cows also have *L. monocytogenes* in the milk and feces (20). Reculture of tissues is recommended if listeriosis is suspected.

Hematological examination is not of much value as the monocytosis of laboratory animals does not occur in the domestic animals. A non-diagnostic neutrophilia does occur in sheep. Examination of the cerebrospinal fluid for inflammatory cells and the presence of bacteria is an essential part of the examination of a suspected case. The cerebrospinal fluid usually contains an increased number of leukocytes most of which are mononuclear cells or lymphocytes (24). Serological tests (agglutination and complement fixation tests) are used but are unreliable because of a high proportion of false negatives (20). The interpretation of serological tests for antibodies against *L. monocytogenes* is made difficult by the presence of positive reactions of up to 1:200 in clinically normal animals. Titers higher than this are usually associated with listerial infection but are commonly encountered in normal cattle in herds where clinical cases have been seen. In sheep the antibody titer may persist for several years but after abortion in cattle it may return to normal in as short a time as 1 month.

Necropsy findings

The cerebrospinal fluid may be cloudy, there may be some congestion of meningeal vessels and in some bovine cases there is panophthalmitis but in general the macroscopic findings are not marked. Histological examination of brain tissue is necessary to demonstrate the microabscesses which are characteristic of the disease. Heavy inoculation of media with material which has been macerated and refrigerated for long periods is advisable when attempting to isolate the organisms which are often present in small numbers (12). Visceral lesions occur as multiple foci of necrosis in the liver, spleen, endocardium and myocardium especially in the septicemic form and in aborted fetuses. Gross lesions suggested as being almost pathognomonic for listeriosis in aborted lambs are small yellow foci of necrosis in the liver, small abomasal erosions and yellow-orange meconium (21). Macroscopically, aborted fetuses are usually edematous, rarely mummified, and autolyzed. In animals which abort there is placentitis and endometritis in addition to the lesions in the fetus (22).

A characteristic of the pathology of the disease is the formation of granulomas as well as foci of necrosis, and these appear at the beginning of the disease, rather than as sequels to necrosis.

Diagnosis

Listerial meningoencephalitis may be confused with the nervous form of acetonemia in cattle and with early cases of pregnancy toxemia in sheep. In these diseases dullness, isolation, apparent blindness and circling are also characteristic but there is no facial nerve paralysis and no endophthalmitis. However, acetonemia occurs in cattle soon after parturition and in ewes pregnancy toxemia is observed only during late pregnancy and usually in association with multiple pregnancy and a declining nutritional status. Also circling in these diseases is accompanied by muscle twitching, particularly of the face, champing of the jaw and blinking of the eyelids and these signs appear only intermittently. As soon as the convulsive episode has passed a normal posture is adopted and the animal can walk in a straight line. Pregnancy toxemia may be accompanied by a rise in body temperature if muscular activity is much increased. Both these metabolic diseases are accompanied by marked ketonuria. Brain abscess, while rare, may be clinically indistinguishable from listeriosis. Cerebrospinal fluid and blood leukocyte examinations may yield little or no basis for differentiation. The course is usually much longer, the animal often surviving for some weeks. Rabies should be considered in the differential diagnosis but there are no localizing signs as there are in listeriosis.

Listerial abortion must be differentiated from the other causes of abortion in cattle and sheep and in goats from *Br. melitensis* infection. Acute septicemias of newborn animals are due to many causes but association with abortion and stillbirths may suggest the possible presence of listeriosis. The necropsy lesions are distinctive and positive cultural findings confirm the diagnosis.

Treatment

Listeria monocytogenes is resistant to many drugs but is sensitive to chlortetracycline. The intravenous injection of chlortetracycline (10 mg/kg body weight/day for 5 days) is reasonably effective in meningoencephalitis of cattle but less so in sheep. Penicillin at a dosage of 44 000 units/kg body weight given intramuscularly daily for 7 days, and in many cases for 10–14 days, is reported to give good results (24). The recovery rate depends largely on the speed with which treatment is commenced. If severe clinical signs are already evident death usually follows in spite of treatment. Usually the course of events in an outbreak is that the first case dies but subsequent cases are picked out sufficiently early for treatment to arrest further development of the disease. Chloramphenicol and a combination of streptomycin and penicillin (0·25 g and 0·3 million units) have also been used successfully in the septicemic form in lambs. Dehydration, acid–base imbalances and electrolyte disturbances must also be corrected.

Control

Most attempts to produce a satisfactory killed vaccine have been unsuccessful although field trials with a killed bacterin are reported to reduce the incidence in sheep flocks. Living attenuated bacteria are also under investigation as immunizing agents and appear to exert significant protection (18, 23). A common recommendation is to reduce the amount of ensilage fed and in animals in the feedlot the constant feeding of low levels of tetracyclines is recommended for the duration of the fattening period. There may be some merit in the recommendation that a change of diet to include heavy feeding of ensilage should be made slowly, particularly if the ensilage is spoiled or if listeriosis has occurred on the premises previously. Other recommendations on the feeding of silage include: avoidance of silage contaminated by earth; silage that is obviously decayed; silage with a pH of greater than 5 or an ash content of more than 70 mg/kg of dry matter; or obviously moldy silage.

REVIEW LITERATURE

Gray, M. L. & Killinger, A. H. (1966) *Listeria monocytogenes* and listeric infections. *Bact. Rev.*, *30*, 309.

Ladds, P. W., Dennis, S. M. & Njoku, C. O. (1974) Pathology of listeric infections in animals. *Vet. Bull.*, *44*, 67.

REFERENCES

(1) Macleod, N. S. M. et al. (1974) *Vet. Rec.*, *95*, 365.
(2) Irvin, A. D. (1968) *Vet. Rec.*, *82*, 115
(3) Wilesmith, J. W. & Gitter, M. (1986) *Vet. Rec.*, *119*, 467.
(4) du Toit, I. F. (1977) *J. S. Afr. vet. Assoc.*, *48*, 39.
(5) Adams, C. J. et al. (1979) *Inf. Immun.*, *25*, 117.
(6) Killinger, A. H. & Mansfield, M. E. (1970) *J. Am. vet. med. Assoc.*, *157*, 1318.
(7) Garayzabal, J. F. F. et al. (1987) *Vet. Rec.*, *120*, 258.
(8) Gronstol, H. (1970) *Acta vet. Scand.*, *20*, 168, 417, 492 & *21*, 1.
(9) Gitter, M. et al. (1980) *Vet. Rec.*, *107*, 890.
(10) Morgan, J. H. (1977) *Vet. Rec.*, *100*, 113.
(11) Smith R. E. et al. (1968) *Cornell Vet.*, *58*, 389.
(12) West, H. J. & Obwolo, M. (1987) *Vet. Rec.*, *120*, 258.
(13) Fleming, D. W. et al. (1985) *New Engl. J. Med.*, *312*, 404.
(14) Gates, G. A. et al. (1967) *J. Am. vet. med. Assoc.*, *150*, 200.
(15) Charlton, K. M. & Garcia, M. M. (1977) *Vet. Pathol.*, *14*, 297.
(16) Gitter, M. (1986) *Vet. Rec.*, *118*, 575.
(17) Njoku, C. O. & Dennis, S. M. (1973) *Cornell Vet.*, *63*, 171, 213.
(18) Kloster, D. & Gudding, R. (1987) *Vet. Rec.*, *120*, 563.
(19) Long, J. R. & Dukes, T. W. (1972) *Can vet. J.*, *13*, 49.
(20) Dijksra, R. G. (1967) *Proc. 3rd int. Symp. Listeriosis, Bilthoven*, *215*, 275.
(21) Dennis, S. M. (1975) *Aust. vet. J.*, *51*, 75.
(22) Ladds, P. W. et al. (1974) *Am. J. vet. Res.*, *35*, 155, 161.
(23) Gudding, R. et al. (1985) *Vet. Rec.*, *117*, 89.
(24) Rebhun, W. C. & deLahunta, A. J. (1982) *J. Am. vet. med. Assoc.*, *180*, 395.
(25) Barlow, R. M. & McGrorum, B. (1985) *Vet. Rec.*, *116*, 233.
(26) Low, J. C. & Renton, C. P. (1985) *Vet. Rec.*, *116*, 147.
(27) Fenton, D. R. (1985) *J. appl. Bacteriol.*, *59*, 537.
(28) Meredith, C. D. et al. (1984) *J. S. Afr. vet. Assoc.*, *55*, 55.

DISEASES CAUSED BY *ERYSIPELOTHRIX RHUSIOPATHIAE* (*INSIDIOSA*)

Erysipelas of pigs is the major disease of animals caused by this bacterium but there are several other minor conditions which require mention.

Erysipelas in cattle

Erysipelas occurs rarely in cattle. It is recorded in isolated incidents, such as an outbreak of septicemia with postmortem lesions of abscesses in liver and lungs (11). Infection with *Erysipelothrix rhusiopathiae* has also been associated with arthritis in calves (1). There is a non-suppurative arthritis with ulceration of articular cartilages. Polyarthritis is manifested by lameness, recumbency, fluctuating joint capsules and severe loss of condition. Clinical erysipelas in adult cattle has not been recorded but the organism has been isolated from the tonsils of healthy cattle and from endocardial lesions at postmortem examination (2).

Erysipelas in sheep

Erysipelas in sheep is manifested as arthritis or laminitis, and rarely as endocarditis (3). However, sheep other than colostrum-deprived lambs are strongly resistant to *Ery. rhusiopathiae* (*insidiosa*) (4) and generalized infections are unlikely. If the infection rate in sheep were sufficiently high vaccination against it seems likely to be a fruitful procedure and would be worth investigating (10).

Arthritis in lambs

Two forms of arthritis are recorded in lambs, one acute and one chronic, and both non-suppurative. The chronic form is now much the commoner of the two (12).

Acute, non-suppurative arthritis of lambs caused by *Ery. rhusiopathiae* (*insidiosa*) occurs commonly after docking, less commonly after birth as an umbilical infection and has occurred accidentally by the use of contaminating serum (5). Phenol in the concentration ordinarily used in serum will not kill the organism. It persists for long periods in soil and if lambing or docking are carried out in an infected environment the organism gains entry through wounds or the umbilicus and causes polyarthritis. Up to 50% of a flock may become affected and although the mortality rate is low, about 5% of the affected lambs lose much weight and may have permanently swollen joints. This is of importance in the level of rejection of meat at abattoirs. More importantly there is a high level of infection in other tissues, often without gross indications of pathological change (6).

Signs appear about 14 days after birth or docking. Lameness develops suddenly with minor swelling of affected joints, usually the carpal, hock and stifle joints. Recovery is slow and there is a high incidence of swollen joints and chronic lameness. At necropsy the synovium is turbid and present in excessive amounts but there is no suppuration as in arthritis of lambs due to streptococcal infection. There is thickening of the joint capsule and erosion of articular cartilages. Penicillin is effective in treatment if given early. Hygiene in lambing and docking areas and the use of clean instruments will reduce the incidence of the disease considerably. Vaccination could be considered on farms where the disease is a problem but this has been shown experimentally to prolong the arthritic reaction. Lambs from vaccinated ewes develop a proliferative synovitis rather than the acute fibrinous synovitis produced in non-immunized lambs (7).

Chronic polyarthritis also occurs in lambs between 2 and 6 months of age (12). Usually several joints are affected and not uncommonly the lamb is lame on all four legs. The morbidity rate is usually 10%, up to 30%, and where infected pig slurry has been used on the pastures, up to 50% of lambs are affected. The mortality rate, including animals sent for slaughter, is almost 100%. Spread is probably by means of infection from contaminated soil through fresh umbilical and docking wounds. Introduction to a farm can be easily effected by carrier animals, usually pigs. The response to treatment with antiserum, antibiotics and corticosteroids is poor. Protection by vaccination, especially of the ewes during pregnancy, is at the experimental stage.

Laminitis after dipping

The use of plunge baths as dips for sheep may be followed by a high incidence of laminitis if the insecticide solution used does not contain a suitable disinfectant. Dips that become grossly contaminated with organic matter are most likely to cause the disease. Infection occurs through skin abrasions and causes a cellulitis with extension to the laminae of the feet but without involving the joints. Up to 90% of a flock may be affected although the incidence is usually about 25%. Similar outbreaks of laminitis caused by *Ery. rhusiopathiae* (*insidiosa*) have occurred unassociated with dipping and usually in circumstances where sheep have to walk through muddy areas likely to be contaminated with the organism (8).

Severe lameness begins 2–4 days after exposure, usually in one leg, sometimes in all four. The affected legs are hot and slightly swollen from the coronet to halfway up the metatarsus or metacarpus and the hair over the affected area usually falls out. Much bodily condition is lost but deaths are rare, except in recently weaned lambs where a septicemia may develop. The lambs show fever, malaise and anorexia.

At necropsy there is subcutaneous edema of the area, sometimes accompanied by hemorrhage. The inflammation usually extends into the laminae of the feet. Most cases recover spontaneously in 10–14 days but penicillin should facilitate recovery. Inclusion of a bacteriostatic agent such as copper sulfate (0·04%) in the dipping fluid is usually sufficient to prevent spread of the disease (9). There is no underrunning of the hoof as in foot rot, no abscessation as in foot abscess and no proliferative dermatitis as in strawberry foot rot.

REVIEW LITERATURE

Jones, T. D. (1978) Aspects of epidemiology and control of *Erysipelothrix insidiosa* polyarthritis in lambs. *Vet. Ann.*, *18*, 88.

Lamont, M. H. (1979) *Erysipelothrix insidiosa:* epidemiology and infection in sheep. *Vet Bull.*, *49*, 479 & 735.

REFERENCES

(1) Moulton, J. E. et al. (1953) *J. Am. vet. med. Assoc.*, *123*, 335.
(2) Roemmele, O. (1952) *Lebensmittelierärztl*, *3*, 43.
(3) Chimene, C. N. et al. (1973) *J. Am. vet. med. Assoc.*, *162*, 278.
(4) Piercy, D. W. T. (1974) *Res. vet. Sci.*, *17*, 210.
(5) Rowlands, W. T. & Edwards, C. M. (1950) *Vet. Rec.*, *62*, 213.
(6) Kaferstein, K. F. et al. (1972) *NZ vet. J.*, *20*, 49.
(7) Piercy, D. W. T. (1971) *J. comp. Pathol.*, *81*, 557.
(8) Whitten, L. K. et al. (1952) *Aust. vet. J.*, *28*, 6.
(9) Thompson, G. E. et al. (1968) *J. S. Afr. vet. med. Assoc.*, *38*, 420.
(10) Lamont, M. H. (1979) *Vet. Bull.*, *49*, 735.
(11) Rebhun, W. E. (1976) *Vet. Med. SAC*, *71*, 684, 686.
(12) Jones, T. D. (1978) *Vet. Ann.*, *18*, 88.

Erysipelas in swine

Erysipelas is an infectious disease of pigs and appears in an acute, septicemic form often accompanied by diamond-shaped skin lesions, and a chronic form manifested by a non-suppurative arthritis and a vegetative endocarditis.

Etiology

Erysipelothrix rhusiopathiae (*insidiosa*) is the causative bacterium and the disease can be produced in either chronic or acute, septicemic forms by the injection of cultures of the organism. A number of different serotypes have been identified (1).

Epidemiology

At least 22 serotypes are known to exist; however, serotypes 1 and 2 are the most common types isolated from swine affected with clinical erysipelas and are generally believed to the only serotypes that cause the acute disease (1, 2). The other serotypes are relatively uncommon and none of them has yet been a cause of acute epidemics, but some has been isolated from lesions of chronic erysipelas (4). Serotypes 1a, 3, 5, 6, 8, 11, 21 and type N have been isolated from pigs with chronic erysipelas, mainly arthritis and lymphadenitis (33). In the United States 19 of the 22 serotypes have been found and the most frequent are serotypes 1, 2, 5, 6 and 21 (35). Serotypes 1 (subtypes 1a and 1b), 2, 5, 6, and 4 have been found in Puerto Rico (35).

The serotype antigens of *Ery. rhusiopathiae* (*insidiosa*) are immunologically distinct and commercial bacterins prepared from the common serotypes will not provide protection against other pathogenic serotypes. This may be an explanation for the epidemics that may occur in vaccinated swine (3). Also, a variety of serotypes may be recovered from pigs affected with the septicemic and arthritic forms of the disease (6).

There is considerable variation in the ease with which the disease can be reproduced, and in its severity. Many factors such as age, health and intercurrent disease, exposure to erysipelas, and heredity govern the ease of both natural and artificial transmission. Virulence of the strain is probably the most important factor. Smooth strains can be used successfully to produce the disease experimentally but rough strains appear to be non-pathogenic. This variation in virulence between strains of the organism has been utilized in the production of living, avirulent vaccines.

Pigs of all ages are susceptible although adult pigs are most likely to be affected if the local strain is of relatively low virulence. Recently farrowed sows seem to be particularly susceptible. When the strain is virulent, pigs of all ages, even sucklings a few weeks old, develop the disease. Almost entire litters under 2 weeks of age may be affected (34). Piglets from an immune sow may get sufficient antibodies in the colostrum to give them immunity for some weeks.

Soil contamination occurs through the feces of affected or carrier pigs. Other sources of infection include infected animals of other species, and birds. The clinically normal carrier group represents the most important source of infection, the tonsils being the predilection site for the organism in such cases (5). Young pigs in contact with carrier sows rapidly acquire the status of carriers and shedders (9). Since the organism can pass through the stomach without loss of viability, carrier animals may reinfect the soil continuously (10) and this, rather than survival of the organism, appears to be the main cause of environmental contamination (11). The organism can survive in feces for several months (9). However its persistence in soil is variable and may be governed by many factors including temperature, pH and the presence of other bacteria (10, 11). *Ery. rhusiopathiae* (*insidiosa*) can be isolated from the effluent of commercial piggeries and from the soil and pasture of effluent disposal sites for up to 2 weeks after application of the effluent containing the organism (7). Although the environment is considered secondary to animals as a reservoir of infection, the survival of the organism in the environment could create an infection hazard.

The organism is resistant to most environmental influences and is not readily destroyed by chemical disinfection.

Experimentally the disease can be produced by oral dosing, by intradermal, intravenous and intra-articular injection and by application to scarified skin, conjunctiva and nasal mucosa. Under natural conditions, skin abrasions and the alimentary tract mucosa are considered to be the probable portals of entry and transmission is by ingestion of contaminated food. Flies are known to transmit the disease (12) and a lowered prevalence has been attributed to the use of insecticides (13). Occasional outbreaks occur after the use of virulent and incomplete avirulent culture as vaccines. Abortion storms in late pregnant sows with septicemic death in sucklers may herald its introduction into SPF herds.

Erysipelas in pigs occurs generally throughout the world and in most countries reached a level of incidence sufficient to cause serious economic loss due to deaths of pigs and devaluation of pig carcasses due to arthritis. The importance of the disease is increased by the difficulties encountered in controlling and eradicating it. Because of man's susceptibility, swine erysipelas has some public health significance. Veterinarians particularly are exposed to infection when vaccinating with virulent culture.

Spread of the infection to most other species can also occur. Morbidity and mortality rate in swine vary considerably from place to place largely due to variations in virulence of the particular strain of the organism involved. On individual farms or in areas the disease may occur as a chronic arthritis in fattening pigs, or as extensive outbreaks of the acute septicemia, or both forms may occur together. The organism has been recovered from sylvatic mammals in north-western Canada (14). The organism has been isolated from a horse affected with vegetative endocarditis (36).

Pathogenesis

Invasion of the bloodstream occurs in all infected animals in the first instance. The subsequent development of either an acute septicemia, or a bacteremia with localization in organs and joints, is dependent on undetermined factors. Virulence of the particular strain may be important and this may depend upon the number of recent pig passages experienced (15). Concurrent viral infection, especially hog cholera, may increase susceptibility of the host.

Localization in the chronic form is commonly in the skin, joints and on other heart valves with probable subsequent bacteremic episodes. Selective adherence of some strains of *Ery. rhusiopathiae* (*insidiosa*) to heart valves may be a factor in the pathogenesis of endocarditis (37). In joints, the initial lesion is an increase in synovial fluid and hyperemia of the synovial membrane followed in several weeks by the proliferation of synovial villi, thickening of the joint capsule and enlargement of the local lymph nodes (16). Diskospondylitis also occurs in association with chronic polyarthritis due to erysipelas (8). Amyloidosis may occur in pigs with chronic erysipelas polyarthritis (21).

There has been some controversy over whether the arthrodial lesions result from primary infection or whether they result from hypersensitivity to the *Erysipelothrix* or other antigen (18–20). Current opinion suggests that the former is the case but that the lesions are enhanced by immunological mechanisms to persistent antigen at the site. There are increased levels of immunoglobulins IgG and IgM in the synovial fluids of pigs with polyarthritis due to *Ery. rhusiopathiae* (*insidiosa*) (17) and the levels are considered only partly due to serum and increased permeability.

Clinical findings

Acute form

After an incubation period of 1–7 days there is a sudden onset of high fever (up to 42°C, 108°F) which is followed some time later by severe prostration, complete anorexia, thirst and occasional vomiting. Initially, affected pigs may be quite active and continue to eat even though the temperature is high. However, generally in an outbreak one is initially presented with one or two dead or severely affected pigs showing marked red to purple discoloration of the skin of the jowl and ventral surface with others in the group showing high fever, reluctance to rise and some incoordination while walking. A conjunctivitis with ocular discharge may be present. Skin lesions are almost pathognomonic but may not always be apparent. These may take the form of the classical diamond-shaped, red, urticarial plaques of about 2·5–5 cm square or a more diffuse edematous eruption with the same appearance. In the early stages the lesions are often palpable before they are visible. The lesions are most common on the belly, inside the thighs, on the throat, neck and the ears and appear usually about 24 hours after the initial signs of illness. After a course of 2–4 days the pig recovers or dies with diarrhea, dyspnea and cyanosis evident terminally. The mortality rate may reach 75% but wide variation occurs.

The so-called 'skin' form is usually the acute form with more prominent skin localization but less severe signs of septicemia and with a low mortality. The skin lesions disappear in about 10 days without residual effects. In the more serious cases the plaques spread and coalesce, often over the back, to form a continuous, deep purple area extending over a greater part of the skin surface. The affected skin becomes black and hard, the edges curl up and separate from an underlying, raw surface. The dry skin may hang on for a considerable time and rattle while the pig walks.

Chronic form

Signs are vague and indistinct except for the joint lesions characteristic of this form of the disease. There may be alopecia, sloughing of the tail and tips of the ears, and a dermatitis in the form of hyperkeratosis of the skin of the back, shoulders and legs, and growth may be retarded. Joint lesions are commonest in the elbow, hip, hock, stifle and knee joints and cause lameness and stiffness. The joints are obviously enlarged and are usually hot and painful at first but in 2–3 weeks are quite firm and without heat. This is especially the case when the arthritis has been present for some time, allowing healing and ankylosis to develop. Paraplegia may occur when intervertebral joints are involved or when there is gross distortion of limb joints.

Endocarditis also occurs as a chronic form of the disease with or without arthritis. Suggestive clinical signs are often absent, the animals dying suddenly without previous illness, especially at times of exertion such as mating, or movement between pens. In others there is progressive emaciation and inability to perform exercise. With forced exercise dyspnea and cyanosis occur. The cardiac impulse is usually markedly increased, the heart rate is faster and a loud murmur is audible on auscultation.

Clinical pathology

In the acute form, examination of blood smears may reveal the presence of the bacteria, particularly in the leukocytes, but blood culture is likely to be more successful as a method of diagnosis. Repeated examinations in the chronic forms of the disease may by chance give a positive result during a bacteremic phase. Final identification of the organism necessitates mouse or pigeon inoculation tests, and protection tests in these animals using antierysipelas serum.

In the early stages of acute form there is first a leukoyctosis followed by a leukopenia and a monocytosis (22). The leukopenia is of moderate degree (40% reduction in total leukocyte count at most) compared with that occurring in hog cholera. The monocytosis is quite marked, varying from a 5–10-fold increase (2·5–4·5% normal levels rise to 25%). The efficiency of agglutination tests for *Ery. rhusiopathiae* (*insidiosa*) is not clear. They appear to be satisfactory for herd diagnosis but not sufficiently accurate for identification of individual affected pigs, particularly clinically normal carrier animals. A more accurate complement fixation test is available but an enzyme immunoassay test is much quicker, easier and more economical to perform (23).

Necropsy findings

Acute form

Skin lesions may be absent although the 'diamond skin' lesions are pathognomonic when they occur. The more diffuse, purplish edema of the belly is common to other septicemic diseases of pigs. Large ecchymotic hemorrhages throughout the body are reported by some observers but others find only minor degrees of petechiation. They are best observed under the kidney capsule, pleura and peritoneum. Venous infarction of the stomach is accompanied by swollen, hemorrhagic mesenteric lymph nodes and there is congestion of the lungs and liver. Infarcts may be present in the spleen and kidney. The organism can be isolated from blood and tissues.

Chronic form

A non-suppurative proliferative arthritis involving limb and intervertebral joints is characteristic. A synovitis, with a serous or serofibrinous, amber-colored, intra-articular effusion occurs first and degenerative changes in the subendochondral bone, cartilages and ligaments follow. When the synovial changes predominate, the joint capsule and villi are thickened. They are enlarged, dark red pedunculations or patches of vascular granulation tissue which spread as a pannus onto the articular surface. When bony changes predominate, the articular cartilages are detached from the underlying bone causing abnormal mobility of the joint. Ulceration of the articular cartilages may also be present. Local lymph node enlargement is usual. The joint lesions in time often repair by fibrosis, adhesions and ankylosis sufficiently to permit use of the limb. Such joints are often sterile on bacteriological examinations. Joints in which changes are still progressing may also be sterile.

Endocardial lesions, when present, are large, crumbly vegetations on the valves, often sufficiently large to apparently block the valvular orifice. *Ery. rhusiopathiae* (*insidiosa*) was the most frequent isolate from cases of endocarditis seen in slaughtered pigs (38). Infarcts occur in the kidney.

Isolation of *Ery. rhusiopathiae* (*insidiosa*) from the joints should be attempted. Many affected joints may be sterile and secondary bacterial invaders may cause an atypical necrosis and an excess of turbid joint fluid. The probability of positive isolation increases with the number of joints sampled, and isolations are more frequent from the smaller, distal joints (24). The frequency of isolation may be increased by storage of joint fluid and synovial membranes in media for 4 weeks at 4°C (39°F) (32). Endocardial vegetations and kidney infarcts yield pure cultures of the organism as a rule.

Diagnosis

Erysipelas in pigs is not ordinarily difficult to diagnose because of the characteristic clinical and necropsy findings. The acute disease may be confused with the other septicemias affecting pigs, but pigs with erysipelas usually show the characteristic skin lesions and are less depressed than pigs with hog cholera or salmonellosis. In salmonellosis there is usually gross skin discoloration, some evidence of enteritis, and respiratory difficulty. In both hog cholera and salmonellosis signs of cerebral involvement including muscle tremor and convulsions are also common.

The chronic disease occurs in pigs of all ages but less commonly in adults. Streptococcal septicemia and arthritis is almost entirely confined to sucking pigs in the first few weeks of life. Streptococcal endocarditis has a similar age distribution to erysipelas endocarditis and bacteriological examination is necessary to differentiate them. Glasser's disease in pigs is accompanied by a severe painful dyspnea and at necropsy there is serositis and meningitis. *Mycoplasma hyorhinis* generally affects pigs less than 10 weeks of age and produces a polyserositis as well as polyarthritis. However, *Myocoplasma hyosynoviae* can produce simple polyarthritis in growing pigs. In general the periarticular, synovial and cartilaginous changes are less severe in these infections when compared to erysipelas; however, cultural differentiation is frequently necessary (18). Rickets and chronic zinc poisoning produce lameness in pigs but they occur under special circumstances, are not associated with fever, and rickets is accompanied by abnormalities of posture and gait which are not seen in erysipelas. Foot rot of pigs is easily differentiated by the swelling of the hoof and the development of discharging sinuses at the coronet.

In recent years there has been a marked increase in chronic osteoarthritis and various forms of 'leg weakness' in growing swine, probably related to the increased growth rate resulting from modern feeding and management practices. In many instances differentiation from erysipelas can be accomplished only by bacteriological methods (18).

Treatment

Penicillin and antierysipelas serum comprise the standard treatment, often administered together by dissolving the penicillin in the serum. Penicillin alone is usually adequate when the strain has only mild virulence. Standard dose rates give a good response in the field but experimental studies suggest that 50 000 units/kg body weight of procaine penicillin for 3 days are required for complete chemotherapeutic effect (25). Chronic cases do not respond well to either treatment because of the structural damage which occurs to the joints and the inaccessibility of the organism in the endocardial lesions. Cortisone (75 mg daily) administered subcutaneously produces marked clinical improvement of the arthritis without complete recovery but adrenocorticotrophic hormones appear to be of no therapeutic value (26).

Control

Eradication is virtually impossible because of the ubiquitous nature of the organism and its resistance to adverse environmental conditions. Complete removal of all pigs and leaving the pens unstocked is seldom satisfactory and eradication by slaughter of reactors to the agglutination test is not recommended because of the uncertain status of the test.

General hygienic precautions should be adopted. Clinically affected animals should be disposed of quickly and all introductions isolated and examined for signs of arthritis and endocarditis. This procedure will not prevent the introduction of clinically normal carrier animals. All animals dying of the disease should be properly incinerated to avoid contamination of the environment. Although thorough cleaning of the premises and the use of very strong disinfectant solutions are advisable, these measures are unlikely to be completely effective. Whenever practicable contaminated feedlots or paddocks should be cultivated.

Specific-pathogen-free (SPF) piggeries established on virgin soil may remain clinically free of erysipelas for several years. However, because of the high risk of introduction of the organism it is advisable to vaccinate routinely.

Immunization

Because of the difficulty of eradication biological prophylactic methods are in common use. Immunizing agents available include hyperimmune serum and vaccines.

Antierysipelas serum

The parenteral administration of 5–20 ml of serum, the amount depending on age, will protect in-contact pigs for 1–2 weeks during on outbreak. Sucking pigs in herds where the disease is endemic should receive 10 ml during the first week of life and at monthly intervals until they are actively vaccinated which can be done as early as 6 weeks provided the sows have not been vaccinated. Repeated administration of the serum may cause anaphylaxis because of its equine origin.

Vaccination

There is no fully satisfactory vaccine available for erysipelas. Serum-simultaneous vaccination (27) has been largely replaced by the use of bacterins, for which lysate and absorbate preparations are available, or by the use of attenuated or avirulent live-culture vaccines which are administered orally or by injection. The use of live-culture vaccines is prohibited in many countries due to the risk of variation in virulence of the strains used and the possibility of spreading infection.

None of these vaccines gives lifelong protection from a single vaccination and the actual duration of protection achieved following vaccination varies considerably. There is considerable difficulty in the experimental evaluation of the efficacy of erysipelas vaccines. Strain differences in immunogenicity, and variation in host response to vaccination due to innate and acquired factors influence this evaluation, as does variation in virulence of the challenge strain and the method of challenge (3, 4). Similar factors are involved in the variations seen in field response to the use of these vaccines. Cross-protection of mice and pigs given a live-organism vaccine against 10 serovars of *E. rhusiopathiae (insidiosa)* has been demonstrated (39). Vaccination will reduce the incidence of polyarthritis due to erysipelas, but not mild cases of arthritis (31). Passively acquired maternal immunity may significantly affect the immune response to vaccination in the young piglet (30). Also the immunity engendered by standard vaccines is not uniformly effective against all strains. Under certain conditions, some unusual serotypes have the potential for causing disease in animals vaccinated with vaccines containing the common serotypes (4). This possibility cannot be ignored and must be considered when vaccination failures occur. Nevertheless, these vaccines are valuable immunizing agents in field situations (3, 4).

Following a single vaccination at 6–10 weeks of age significant protection is provided to market age. However, a second 'booster' vaccination given 2–4 weeks later is advisable (30). In herds where sows are routinely vaccinated prior to farrowing, a persisting maternal passive immunity may require that piglet vaccination be delayed until 10–12 weeks of age for an effective active immunity.

It is also advisable to vaccinate replacement gilts and adults in the herd. Bacterins are effective, and field evidence suggests that vaccination provides immunity for approximately 6 months. Sows should be vaccinated twice yearly, preferably 3–6 weeks before farrowing, as this will also provide significant protection against the septicemic form in young sucklers. If possible a closed herd should be maintained. Abortion may occur sporadically following the use of live vaccines (29).

Vaccination is subcutaneous in the skin behind the ear, or the axilla and the flank. Reactions at the site of injection are not uncommon. Swelling with subsequent nodule formation and occasional abscessation may occur following the injection of bacterins, and modified live vaccines may produce hemorrhage in the skin at the injection site. Granulomatous lesions may occur following the use of oil-based vaccines (28). There is little evidence that vaccination increases the incidence of arthritis.

REVIEW LITERATURE

Wood, R. L. (1984). Swine erysipelas—a review of prevalence and research. *J. Am. vet. med. Assoc.*, *184*, 944–949.

REFERENCES

(1) Nørrung, V. (1979) *Nord. VetMed.*, *31*, 462.
(2) Wood, R. L. et al. (1978) *Am. J. vet. Res.*, *39*, 1833.
(3) Wood, R. L. (1979) *Am. J. vet. Res.*, *40*, 795.
(4) Wood, R. L. et al. (1981) *Am. J. vet. Res.*, *42*, 608.
(5) Stephenson, E. H. & Berman, D. T. (1978) *Am. J. vet. Res.*, *39*, 187.
(6) Cross, G. M. J. & Claxton, P. D. (1979) *Aust. vet. J.*, *55*, 77.
(7) Chandler, D. S. & Craven, J. A. (1980) *J. appl. Bacteriol.*, *48*, 367.
(8) Doige, C. E. (1980) *Can. J. comp. Med.*, *44*, 121.
(9) Wood, R. L. (1974) *Am. J. vet. Res.*, *35*, 41.
(10) Rowsell, H. C. (1958) *J. Am. vet. med. Assoc.*, *13*, 357.
(11) Wood, R. L. (1973) *Cornell Vet.*, *63*, 370.
(12) Wellman, G. (1966) *Zentralbl. Bakteriol.*, *162*, 261, 265.
(13) Meyer, P. (1975) *Tijdschr. Diergeneeskd.*, *100*, 1109.
(14) Langford, E. V. & Dorward, W. J. (1977) *Can. vet. J.*, *18*, 101.
(15) Rowsell, H. C. (1955) *Proc. 92nd ann. Mtg. Am. vet. med. Assoc.*, 143.
(16) Cohrs, P. & Schulz, L. C. (1960) *Mh. VetMed.*, *15*, 608.
(17) Timoney, J. F. & Yarkoni, U. (1976) *Vet. Microbiol.*, *1*, 467.
(18) Cross, G. M. & Edwards, M. J. (1976) *Vet. Ann.*, *16*, 117.
(19) Ajmal, M. (1970) *Vet. Bull.*, *40*, 1.
(20) Timoney, J. & Berman, D. T. (1970) *Am. J. vet. Res.*, *31*, 1411.
(21) Winkelman, J. et al. (1979) *Dtsch Tierärztl. Wochenschr.*, *86*, 131.
(22) Dougherty, R. W. et al. (1965) *Cornell Vet.*, *55*, 87.
(23) Kirchoff, H. et al. (1985) *Vet. Microbiol.*, *10*, 549.
(24) Bond, M. P. (1976) *Aust. vet J.*, *52*, 462.
(25) Azechi, H. et al. (1972) *Am J. vet. Res.*, *33*, 1963.
(26) Sikes, D. et al. (1955) *Am J. vet. Res.*, *16*, 367.
(27) Shuman, R. D. (1953) *J. Am. vet. Med. Assoc.*, *123*, 304, 307.
(28) Summers, P. M. & Webster, W. R. (1977) *Aust. vet. J.*, *53*, 593.
(29) Henry, S. (1979) *J. Am. vet. med. Assoc.*, *45*, 453.
(30) Ose, E. E. (1972) *J. Am. vet. med. Assoc.*, *160*, 603.
(31) Mercy, A. R. & Bord, M. P. (1978) *Aust. vet. J.*, *53*, 600.
(32) Blackall, P. J. & Summers, P. M. (1978) *Queensland J. Agric. anim. Sci.*, *35*, 1.
(33) Takahashi, T. et al. (1985) *Jap. J. vet. Sci.*, *47*, 1.
(34) Bastianello, S. S. & Spencer, B. T. (1984) *J. S. Afr. vet. Assoc.*, *55*, 195.
(35) Wood, R. L. et al. (1981) *Am. J. vet. Res.*, *42*, 1248.
(36) McCormick, B. S. et al. (1985) *Aust. vet. J.*, *62*, 392.
(37) Bratberg, A. M. (1981) *Acta vet. Scand.*, *22*, 39.
(38) Pedersen, K. B. et al. (1984) *Acta Pathol. Microbiol. Immunol. Scand.*, *3*, 92, 237.
(39) Sawada, T. & Takahashi, T. (1987) *Am. J. vet. Res.*, *48*, 81.

DISEASES CAUSED BY *BACILLUS* spp.

Anthrax

Anthrax is a peracute disease characterized by septicemia and sudden death with the exudation of tarry blood from the body orifices of the cadaver. Failure of the blood to clot, absence of rigor mortis and the presence of splenomegaly are the most important necropsy findings.

Etiology

Bacillus anthracis is the specific cause of the disease. When material containing anthrax bacilli is exposed to the air, spores are formed which protract the infectivity of the environment for very long periods. The spores are resistant to most external influences including the salting of hides, normal environmental temperatures and standard disinfectants. Anthrax bacilli have remained viable in soil stored for 60 years in a rubberstoppered bottle (1), and field observations indicate a similar duration of viability in exposed soil, particularly in the presence of organic matter, in an undrained alkaline soil and in a warm climate. However, acid soils reduce the survival of *B. anthracis*.

Epidemiology

Outbreaks originating from a soil-borne infection always occur after a major climate change, for example heavy rain after a prolonged drought and always in warm weather when the environmental temperature is over 15°C (60°F) (2). The occurrence of outbreaks at isolated points when environmental conditions are warm and humid has made it possible to predict 'anthrax years' (3) and has led to the suggestion that vegetative proliferation may occur in the soil. The characteristic epidemiology of anthrax in developed countries currently is the sudden occurrence of multicentric foci of infection with many sudden deaths without observed illness, in an area which has recently had appropriate climatic conditions, and in which the disease has occurred previously, although it may be as long ago as 30 years (4). Putrefaction in the carcass destroys the bacteria and provided the carcass is unopened and no discharges appear, contamination of the soil will not occur.

Predisposing causes include close grazing of tough scratchy feed in dry times, which results in abrasions of the oral mucosa, and confined grazing on heavily contaminated areas around water holes. The disease occurs in all vertebrates but is most common in cattle and sheep and occurs less frequently in goats and horses. There are several records which indicate a higher infection rate in horses than in cattle, in the same outbreak (4, 5). Man occupies an intermediate position between this group and the relatively resistant swine, dogs and cats. Algerian sheep are said to be resistant and, within all species, certain individuals seem to possess sufficient immunity to resist natural exposure. Whether or not this immunity has a genetic basis has not been determined. The most interesting example of natural resistance is the dwarf pig in which it is impossible to establish the disease (6). Spores remain in tissues ungerminated and there is complete clearance from all organs by 48 hours. This ability to prevent spore germination appears to be inherited in this species.

An atypical form of anthrax has been observed in pigs in Papua-New Guinea (7). Severe outbreaks with heavy mortalities occur in pigs but, except for guinea-pigs, the disease is not transmissible to other species in spite of the apparent classical identity of the bacteria.

In most developed countries anthrax is no longer a significant cause of livestock wastage because of appropriate control measures. However, it still holds an important political position and, largely because of its potential as a zoonosis, the cry 'anthrax' is almost as evocative as 'mad dog'.

Infection gains entrance to the body by ingestion, inhalation or through the skin. While the exact mode of infection is often in doubt, it is generally considered that animals are infected by the ingestion of contaminated food or water. It is true that experimental transmission by the ingestion of virulent anthrax spores has not always been successful. Injury to the mucous membrane of the digestive tract will facilitate infection but there is little doubt that infection can take place without such injury. The increased incidence of the disease on sparse pasture is probably due both to the ingestion of contaminated soil and to injury to the oral mucosa facilitating invasion by the organism. Spores can be picked up directly from the soil or from fodder grown on infected soil, from contaminated bone meal or protein concentrates or from infected excreta, blood or other material. Outbreaks in swine can usually be traced to the ingestion of infected bone meal or carcasses. Water can be contaminated by the effluent from tanneries, infected carcasses and by flooding anthrax-infected soil.

Inhalation infection is thought to be of minor importance in animals although the possibility of infection through contaminated dust must always be considered. 'Woolsorter's disease' in man is due to the inhalation of anthrax spores by workers in the wool and hair industries, but even in these industries cutaneous anthrax is much more common.

Biting flies and other insects have often been found to harbor anthrax organisms and their ability to transmit the infection has been demonstrated experimentally. The transmission is mechanical only and a local inflammatory reaction is evident at the site of the bite. The tendency in infected districts for the heaviest incidence to occur in the late summer and autumn may be due to the increase in the fly population at that time but an effect of higher temperature on vegetative proliferation of *B. anthracis* in the soil is more likely. An outbreak of anthrax has been recorded following the injection of infected blood for the purpose of immunization against anaplasmosis. There have been a number of reports of the occurrence of anthrax after vaccination, due probably to inadequately attenuated spores. Wound infection occurs occasionally.

Spread of the organism within an area may be accomplished by streams, insects, dogs and other carnivores, and wild birds and by fecal contamination from infected animals. Introduction of infection into a new area is usually through contaminated animal products such as bone meal, fertilizers, hides, hair and wool or by contaminated concentrates or forage.

In an outbreak where control is not practiced there are two series of cases. The first cases, which may be only one animal, are those which have been exposed to the primary source of infection, such as soil turned up from an old anthrax grave. The secondary cases are those which become infected by the discharge of other animals; these may be spread extensively if the affected animal is still mobile just before death (10).

The disease is worldwide in distribution although the incidence varies with the soil, climate and the efforts put forward to suppress it. It is often restricted to particular areas, the so-called 'anthrax belts', where it is enzootic. In most countries vaccination of susceptible animals in affected areas has reduced the prevalence of the disease to negligible proportions on a national basis but heavy losses may still occur in individual herds. The morbidity rate may be high among all farm animals although susceptibility is highest among ruminants followed by horses and swine in that order. The disease is almost invariably fatal except in swine and even in this species the death rate is high. Anthrax in man takes the form of a localized cutaneous infection although a fatal septicemic form does occur. Serious outbreaks of anthrax and persistence of the infection in the soil are most commonly encountered in tropical and subtropical countries. In temperature cool climates sporadic outbreaks due to accidental ingestion of contaminated bone meal or tannery effluent are more common although permanently infected areas do exist. In this circumstance outbreaks are few and the number of animals affected is small (12). As many as 50% of consignments of bone meal imported into the United Kingdom have been shown to be contaminated with the anthrax bacillus (13). This is obviously related to the common observation in the United Kingdom that most outbreaks of the disease are caused by feeding infected feedstuffs, usually bone meal (14).

Pathogenesis

Upon ingestion of the spores, infection may occur through the intact mucous membrane, through defects in the epithelium around erupting teeth or through scratches from tough, fibrous food materials. After entry the bacteria are moved to the local lymph nodes by motile phagocytes. After proliferation in this site the bacilli pass via the lymphatic vessels into the blood stream and septicemia, with massive invasion of all body tissues, follows (15). *B. anthracis* produces a lethal toxin which causes edema and tissue damage, death resulting from shock and acute renal failure (16), and terminal anoxia mediated by the central nervous system (17). The pathology of anthrax and the mode of action of the toxin have always been matters of great scientific interest, largely because of the great speed with which the infection kills animals. For further information on these subjects two reviews should be consulted (15, 18).

In pigs, localization occurs in the lymph nodes of the throat after invasion through the upper part of the digestive tract. Local lesions often lead to a fatal septicemia.

Clinical findings

The incubation period after field infection is not easy to determine but is probably 1–2 weeks.

Cattle and sheep

Only two forms of the disease occur in these species, the peracute and the acute. The peracute form of the disease is most common at the beginning of an outbreak. The animals are usually found dead without premonitory signs, the course being probably only 1–2 hours, but fever, muscle tremor, dyspnea and congestion of the mucosae may be observed. The animal soon collapses, and dies after terminal convulsions. After death, discharges of blood from the nostrils, mouth, anus and vulva are common. The acute form runs a course of about 48 hours. Severe depression and listlessness are usually observed first although they are sometimes preceded by a short period of excitement. The body temperature is high, up to 42°C (107°F), the respiration rapid and deep, the mucosae congested and hemorrhagic and the heart rate much increased. No food is taken and ruminal stasis is evident. Pregnant cows may abort. In milking cows the yield is very much reduced and the milk may be bloodstained or deep yellow in color. Alimentary tract involvement is usual and is characterized by diarrhea and dysentery. Local edema of the tongue and edematous lesions in the region of the throat, sternum, perineum and flanks may occur.

Pigs

In pigs anthrax may be acute or subacute. There is fever, with dullness and anorexia and a characteristic inflammatory edema of the throat and face. The swellings are hot but not painful and may cause obstruction to swallowing and respiration. Bloodstained froth may be present at the mouth when pharyngeal involvement occurs. Petechial hemorrhages are present in the skin and when localization occurs in the intestinal wall there is dysentery, often without edema of the throat. An outbreak of a pulmonary form of the disease has been observed in baby pigs which inhaled infected dust. Lobar pneumonia and exudative pleurisy were characteristic (19). Death usually occurs after a course of 12–36 hours although individual cases may linger for several days.

Horses

Anthrax in the horse is always acute but varies in its manifestations with the mode of infection (20). When infection is by ingestion there is septicemia with enteritis and colic. When infection is by insect transmission, hot, painful, edematous, subcutaneous swellings appear about the throat, lower neck, floor of the thorax and abdomen, prepuce and mammary gland. There is high fever and severe depression and there may be dyspnea due to swelling of the throat or colic due to intestinal irritation. The course is usually 48–96 hours.

Clinical pathology

In the living animal the organism may be detected in a stained smear of peripheral blood. The blood should be carefully collected in a syringe to avoid contamination of the environment. When local edema is evident smears may be made from the edema fluid. For a more certain diagnosis, especially in the early stages when bacilli may not be present in the bloodstream in great numbers, blood culture or the injection of syringe-collected blood into guinea-pigs is satisfactory. Fluorescent antibody techniques are available for use on blood smears and tissue sections. In cases where antibiotic therapy has been used the identification from blood smears or culture may be difficult and animal passage may be necessary. Isolation of anthrax bacilli from infected soil may be difficult unless the proper technique is used (21).

Necropsy findings

At necropsy there is a striking absence of rigor mortis and the carcass undergoes gaseous decomposition and quickly assumes the characteristic 'sawhorse' attitude. All natural orifices usually exude dark, tarry blood which does not clot and putrefaction and bloating are rapid. If there is a good reason to suspect the existence of anthrax the carcass should not be opened. However, if a necropsy is carried out, the failure of the blood to clot, the presence of ecchymotic hemorrhages throughout the body tissues, the presence of bloodstained serous fluid in the body cavities, severe enteritis and gross enlargement of the spleen with softening and liquefaction of its structure are almost certain indications of the presence of anthrax. Subcutaneous swellings containing gelatinous material and enlargement of the local lymph nodes are features of the disease as it occurs in horses and pigs.

To confirm the diagnosis on an unopened carcass smears of peripheral blood or local edema fluid should be collected by needle puncture (9). If possible, blood or edema fluid should also be collected for guinea-pig or mouse inoculation. If decomposition of a carcass is advanced an ear or a portion of spleen should be sent to the laboratory for the preparation of an Ascoli precipitin test and for culture. If experimental animal inoculation is not possible, microscopic examination of smears should be supported by blood culture (22). Care must be taken when suspected material is sent through the mail to ensure that no hazard is created for persons handling the package.

Diagnosis

There are many causes of sudden death in farm animals and differentiation is often difficult. Lightning strike is usually evidenced by singeing of the hair and by a history of electrical storms. Peracute blackleg may resemble anthrax but it is largely restricted to young animals and the crepitating swellings which are characteristic of blackleg do not occur in anthrax. Other clostridial infections may simulate anthrax, especially in pigs.

Acute leptospirosis usually occurs only sporadically and is characterized by hemoglobinuria. Bacillary hemoglobinuria is featured by hemoglobinuria and the presence of characteristic infarcts in the liver. Blood culture and smear will serve to differentiate the conditions. Peracute lead poisoning and hypomagnesemic tetany are usually accompanied by obvious nervous signs and a completely different necropsy picture.

Animals dying of acute bloat show gaseous distension and exudation of blood from orifices as in anthrax. The probability of either disease occurring can usually be assessed and laboratory examination must be used if there is any doubt.

Treatment

Antibiotics and antianthrax serum are most commonly used in treatment. Severely ill animals are unlikely to recover but in the early stages, particularly when fever is detected before other signs are evident, recovery can be anticipated. Penicillin (10 000 units/kg body weight twice daily) has had considerable vogue (9, 23) but streptomycin (8–10 g/day in two doses intramuscularly for cattle) is much more effective (24). Oxytetracycline (5 mg/kg body weight/day) parenterally has also proved superior to penicillin in the treatment of clinical cases after vaccination in cattle (3, 25) and sheep (26). In spite of the observations made on clinically affected animals, a strong case has been made for the use of procaine penicillin and streptomycin in large doses at 12-hour intervals plus antiserum for at least 5 days (15). The need to prolong treatment to at least 5 days to avoid a recrudescence of the disease is stressed (27). While antianthrax serum intravenously in doses of 100–250 ml daily is effective and may be given in conjunction with an antibiotic, it is too expensive for routine use.

Control

The control of meat and milk-producing animals in infected herds in such a way as to avoid any risk to the human population is a special aspect of the control of anthrax. It is necessary at the time to avoid unnecessary waste and the imposition of unnecessarily harsh prohibitions on the farmer. These matters are the province of public health veterinarians and are documented (8), but they are not dealt with here. When an outbreak occurs, the placing of the farm in quarantine, the destruction of discharges and cadavers, and the vaccination of survivors, are part of the animal disease control program and indirectly reduce human exposure. Prohibition of movement of milk and meat from the farm during the quarantine period should prevent entry of the infection into the human food chain. Vaccination of animals, although the vaccine is a live one, does not present a hazard to man.

Hygiene is the biggest single factor in the prevention of spread of the disease. Careful disposal of infected material is most important. Infected carcasses should not be opened but immediately burned or buried, together with bedding and soil contaminated by discharges. Burial should be at least 2 m deep with an ample supply of quicklime added. All suspected cases and in-contact animals must be segregated until cases cease and for 2 weeks thereafter the affected farm placed in quarantine to prevent the movement of livestock. The administration of hyperimmune serum to in-contact animals may prevent further losses during the quarantine period. The disinfection of premises, hides, bone meal, fertilizer, wool and hair requires special care. When disinfection can be carried out immediately, before spore formation can occur, ordinary disinfectants or heat (60°C, 140°F for a few minutes) are sufficient to kill vegetative forms. This is satisfactory when necropsy room or abattoir floors are contaminated. When spore formation occurs (i.e. within a few hours of exposure to the air), disinfection is almost impossible by ordinary means. Strong disinfectants such as 5% lysol require to be in contact with spores for at least 2 days. Strong solutions of formalin or sodium hydroxide (5–10%) are probably most effective. Peracetic acid (3% solution) is an effective sporicide, and if applied to the soil in appropriate amounts (8 liters/m^2) is an effective sterilant (28). Infected clothing should be sterilized by soaking in 10% formaldehyde. Shoes may present difficulty and sterilization is most efficiently achieved by placing them in a plastic bag and introducing ethylene oxide. Contaminated materials should be damp and left in contact with the gas for 18 hours (15). Hides, wool and mohair are sterilized commercially by gamma-irradiation, usually from a radioactive cobalt source. Special care must be taken to avoid human contact with infected material and if such contact does occur the contaminated skin must be thoroughly disinfected. The source of the infection must be traced and steps taken to prevent further spread of the disease. Control of the disease in a feral animal population presents major problems. Attempts to control anthrax in wild bison have been recorded (29).

Immunization

Immunization of animals as a control measure is extensively used and many types of vaccine are available. Those vaccines which consist of living attenuated strains of the organism with low virulence but capable of forming spores, have been most successful. The sporulation character has the advantage of keeping the living vaccine viable over long periods. These vaccines have the disadvantage that the various animal species show varying susceptibility to the vaccine and anthrax may result in some cases from vaccination. This has been largely overcome by preparing vaccines of differing degrees of virulence for use in different species and in varying circumstances. Another method of overcoming the virulence is the use of saponin or saturated saline solution in the vehicle to delay absorption (30). This is the basis of the Carbozo vaccine. The avirulent spore vaccine described by Stern has overcome the risk of causing anthrax by vaccination and produces a strong immunity which lasts for at least 26 months in sheep (31). It appears probable that this vaccine will supersede others in current use. Although two doses are recommended, only one appears to be necessary, and cases cease about 8 days after vaccination (32). A febrile reaction does occur after vaccination and the milk yield of dairy cows will be depressed and pregnant sows will probably abort. The injection of penicillin, and probably other antibiotics, at this time should be avoided as it may interfere with the development of immunity (34).

An additional vaccination method utilizes a cell-free filtrate of a culture of a non-encapsulated, spore-forming strain of *B. anthracis*, either injected as an aqueous solution intradermally, or injected subcutaneously as an antigen adsorbed on to colloidal aluminum hydroxide. The vaccine is incapable of causing anthrax but the duration of the immunity produced in cattle (3–6 months) leaves something to be desired (35). Two injections of the vaccine produce a longer period of immunity but the procedure is rather costly.

In enzootic areas annual revaccination of all stock is necessary. When the disease occurs for the first time in a previously clean area, all in-contact animals should either be treated with hyperimmune serum or be vaccinated. Vaccination before this is not usually recommended because of the possibility of introducing infection on to the farm. This is unlikely to happen with the newer, avirulent vaccines. The measures used to control outbreaks and the choice of a vaccine depend largely on local legislation and experience. If a large feed supply becomes suspect of being contaminated by anthrax spores, a reasonable procedure is to vaccinate the livestock and resume feeding the material 2–3 weeks later. There is some risk of contamination of the environment if this is done.

Milk from vaccinated cows is usually discarded for 72 hours after the injection in case the organisms in the vaccine should be excreted in the milk. Organisms of the Stern vaccine do not appear in the milk nor can they be isolated from the blood for 10 and 7 days respectively after vaccination (11).

Prophylactic treatment

A single injection of an appropriate longacting antibiotic is credited with reducing the mortality rate in a herd in which cases are still occurring during the few days after vaccination before the vaccine has time to exert any significant protection (33).

REFERENCES

(1) Wilson, J. B. & Russell, K. E. (1964) *J. Bacteriol.*, *87*, 237.
(2) van Ness, G. B. (1961) *Southwestern Vet.*, *14*, 290.
(3) Flynn, D. M. (1968/69) *Vict. vet. Proc.*, *27*, 32.
(4) Fox, M. D. et al. (1977) *J. Am. vet. med. Assoc.*, *170*, 327.
(5) Young, J. B. (1975) *J. Am. vet. med. Assoc.*, *167*, 842.
(6) Walker, J. S. et al. (1967) *J. Bacteriol.*, *93*, 2031.
(7) Egerton, J. R. (1966) *Papua-New Guinea agric. J.*, *17*, 136, 141.
(8) Baxter, R. G. (1977) *J. S. Afr. vet. Assoc.*, *48*, 293.
(9) Whitford, H. W. (1978) *J. Am. vet. med. Assoc.*, *173*, 1467.
(10) Hugh-Jones, M. E. (1974) *Vet. Rec.*, *94*, 228.
(11) Tanner, W. B. et al. (1978) *J. Am. vet. med. Assoc.*, *173*, 1465.
(12) Campbell, A. D. (1969) *Vet. Rec.*, *85*, 89.
(13) Davies, D. G. & Harvey, R. W. S. (1972) *J. Hyg., Camb.*, *70*, 455.
(14) Hugh-Jones, M. E. & Hussaini, S. N. (1975) *Vet. Rec.*, *97*, 256.
(15) Lincoln, R. E. et al. (1964) *Adv. vet. Sci.*, *9*.
(16) Harris-Smith, P. W. et al. (1958) *J. gen. Microbiol.*, *19*, 91.
(17) Remmele, N. S. et al. (1968) *J. infect. Dis.*, *118*, 104.
(18) Nungester, W. J. (1967) *Fedn Proc. Fedn Am. Socs exp. Biol.*, *26*, 1483.
(19) Ratalics, L. & Toth, L. (1964) *Magy. Allatorv. Lap*, *19*, 203.
(20) McNellis, R. (1943) *Bull. US Army med. Dept*, *71*, 84–86.
(21) Manchee, R. J. et al. (1981) *Nature (Lond.)*, *294*, (5835) 254.
(22) Thompson, P. D. (1955) *J. comp. Pathol.*, *65*, 1.
(23) Riggs, C. W. & Tew, A. C. (1947) *J. Am vet. med. Assoc.*, *111*, 44.
(24) Miller, E. S. et al. (1946) *J. Immunol.*, *53*, 371.
(25) Bailey, W. W. (1954) *J. Am. vet. med. Assoc.*, *124*, 296.
(26) Johnson, W. P. & Percival, R. C. (1955) *J. Am. vet. med. Assoc.*, *127*, 142.
(27) Greenough, P. R. (1965) *Vet. Rec.*, *77*, 784.
(28) Hussaini, S. N. & Ruby, K. R. (1976) *Vet. Rec.*, *98*, 257.
(29) Cousineau, J. G. & McClenaghan, R. J. (1965) *Can. vet. J.*, *6*, 22.
(30) Bone, J. R. (1957) *N. Am. Vet.*, *38*, 10, 12a.
(31) Israil, M. & Quader, M. A. (1955) *Pakist. J. sci. Res.*, *7*, 38.
(32) Kaufman, A. F. et al. (1973) *J. Am. vet. med. Assoc.*, *163*, 442.
(33) Gill, I. J. (1982) *Aust. vet. J.*, *58*, 214.
(34) Webster, A. (1973) *Aust. vet. J.*, *49*, 545.
(35) Jackson, F. C. et al. (1957) *Am. J. vet. Res.*, *18*, 771.

Tyzzer's disease

This is a fatal necrotizing hepatitis caused by *Bacillus piliformis* and recorded in several rodents, the rhesus monkey, cats and foals (1–3). It is a disease of foals 1–5 weeks of age and marked by a sudden onset, high fever (to 40·5°C, 113°F), shock, terminal coma and a short course of a few hours to 2 days. Foals running with mares are difficult to assess in terms of health and it is probable that foals with Tyzzer's disease have clinical signs of fever, tachycardia and tachypnea for up to 48 hours before the observable depression appears (6). Jaundice and severe diarrhea occur in some. Clinicopathological examination shows severe leukopenia with leukocyte counts in the range of 2000–4000/μl. Serum enzymes, SGOT, SGPT and LDH are highly elevated. At necropsy examination the liver is grossly enlarged and has miliary necrotic foci, and jaundice is present. There is also a necrotizing colitis (4). Culture of the causative organism is sufficiently difficult to encourage diagnosis by staining a smear to demonstrate the characteristic bacteria (1). The disease is likely to be confused with shigellosis, septicemia caused by *Corynebacterium (Rhodococcus) equi*, pneumonia of immunodeficient Arab foals caused by adenovirus, chronic abscess in the urachus and idiopathic myopathy. It has been recorded concurrently with combined immune deficiency in Arab foals (5). Tetracycline is thought to be the most successful therapy.

The disease appears to be increasing in prevalence in the United States although the prevalence is still very low (2) and the occurrence is sporadic. Originally the disease probably came from muskrats but adult horses become inapparent carriers and infect newborn foals, which are normally coprophagous. Only newborn foals are susceptible to the infection.

REFERENCES

(1) Brown, C. M. (1983) *Equ. vet. J.*, *15*, 375.
(2) Swerczek, T. W. (1977) *Vet. Ann.*, *17*, 130.
(3) Thomson, G. W. et al. (1977) *Can. vet. J.*, *18*, 41.
(4) Yates, W. D. G. & Hayes, M. A. (1980) *Can. vet. J.*, *21*, 63.
(5) Turk, M. A. M. et al. (1981) *J. Am. vet. med. Assoc.*, *178*, 279.
(6) Trent, A. & Walsh, K. M. (1983) *Equ. Pract.*, 5.8.

17

Diseases Caused by Bacteria—II

DISEASES CAUSED BY *CLOSTRIDIUM* spp.

THE clostridia are of major importance in farm animals as primary causes of disease. They rarely act as secondary invaders except where gangrene is already present. They are all potent producers of exotoxins upon which their pathogenicity depends. The toxins of the different organisms vary in their effects and in the manner in which they gain entry to the circulation; they may be ingested preformed in the feed as in botulism; be absorbed from the gut after abnormal proliferation of the causative organism in the alimentary tract as in enterotoxemia; or be elaborated in a more proper infection of the tissues such as blackleg. Other clostridial infections develop as local infections with elaboration of toxins in minor lesions such as in tetanus, black disease, braxy and bacillary hemoglobinuria.

As well as the specific disease entities set out below there are some less well-known occurrences of pathogenic clostridia. For example, *Cl. sordelli* can cause a fatal myositis and be identified as blackleg or malignant edema. It has also been found to be a cause of a fatal hepatitis in newborn lambs (1), of enteritis with hemorrhagic diarrhea in calves (2), and of the syndrome of opisthotonus and convulsions usually associated with *Cl. perfringens* type D (4).

Pathogenic clostridia are commonly present in soils rich in humus. They are also found in the intestinal contents of normal animals and cause disease only in special circumstances. The ubiquitous character of these organisms makes eradication of the clostridial diseases virtually impossible and necessitates control by prophylactic measures. Fortunately, diseases of this group are unique among bacterial diseases in that they can be effectively prevented in almost all instances by vaccination with killed culture vaccines. Because of the common occurrence of a number of clostridial infections in an area, it has become a common practice in recent years to use multiple vaccines capable of immunizing against as many as five separate diseases. The vaccines, if carefully prepared, appear to be highly effective and, in situations where the extra expense can be justified, worthy of recommendation. In high-risk situations such as feedlots they appear to be very cost-effective (3). There appears to be a difference between sheep and goats with respect to their response to clostridial infections. Goats in general suffer more severe forms of these diseases than do sheep and the protection afforded to goats by multivalent vaccines is less than that to sheep (5).

REFERENCES

(1) Richards, S. M. & Hunt, B. W. (1982) *Vet. Rec.*, *111*, 22.
(2) Al-mashat, R. R. et al. (1983) *Vet. Rec.*, *112*, 141.
(3) Knott, G. K. L. et al. (1985) *Vet. Med.*, *80*, 95.
(4) Popoff, M. R. (1984) *Vet. Rec.*, *114*, 324.
(5) Green, D. S. et al. (1987) *Vet. Rec.*, *120*, 435.

Tetanus

Tetanus is a highly fatal, infectious disease of all species of domestic animals caused by the toxin of *Clostridium tetani*. It is characterized clinically by hyperesthesia, tetany and convulsions.

Etiology

Clostridium tetani forms spores which are capable of persisting in soil for many years. The spores are resistant to many standard disinfection procedures including steam heat at 100°C (212°F) for 30–60 minutes but can be destroyed by heating at 115°C (239°F) for 20 minutes.

Epidemiology

The neurotoxin of *Cl. tetani* is exceedingly potent but there is considerable variation in susceptibility between the animal species, the horse being the most susceptible and cattle the least. The variation in incidence of the disease in the different species is partly due to this variation in susceptibility but also because exposure is more likely to occur in some species than in others.

Cl. tetani organisms are commonly present in the feces of animals, especially horses, and in the soil contaminated by these feces. What determines the survival period of the organism in soil, and this varies very widely from soil to soil, is unknown but the climate and the soil type appear not to be important. The portal of entry is usually through deep puncture wounds but the spores may lie dormant in the tissues for some time and produce clinical illness only when tissue conditions favor their proliferation. For this reason the portal of entry is often difficult to determine. Puncture wounds of the hooves are common sites of entry in horses. Introduction to the genital tract at the time of parturition is the usual portal of entry in cattle. A high incidence of tetanus may occur in young pigs following castration, and in lambs following castration, shearing, docking and vaccination for other diseases (9). Docking by the use of elastic band ligatures is reputed to be especially hazardous.

Tetanus occurs in all parts of the world and is most common in closely settled areas under intensive cultivation. It occurs in all farm animals mainly as individual, sporadic cases, although outbreaks are occasionally observed in cattle (2), young pigs and lambs. The mortality in young ruminants is over 80%, but the recovery rate is high in adult cattle. In horses it varies widely between areas. In some areas almost all animals die acutely. In others the mortality rate is consistently about 50% (3).

When outbreaks of tetanus occur in cattle it is possible that toxin is produced in the gut, or is ingested preformed in the feed. The grazing of rough, fibrous feeds before these outbreaks is a common finding and suggests that entry of infection may occur via wounds in the mouth.

Pathogenesis

The tetanus bacilli remain localized at their site of introduction and do not invade surrounding tissues. They start to proliferate and produce neurotoxin only if certain environmental conditions are attained, particularly a lowering of the local tissue oxygen tension. This may occur immediately after introduction if the accompanying trauma has been sufficiently severe, or may be delayed for several months until subsequent trauma to the site causes tissue damage. The original injury may have completely healed by this time.

The toxin reaches the central nervous system by passing up peripheral nerve trunks and not by passage from the bloodstream through the blood–brain barrier. The exact means by which the toxin exerts its effects on nervous tissue is not known. No structural lesions are produced but there is central potentiation of normal sensory stimuli so that a state of constant muscular spasticity is produced and normally innocuous stimuli cause exaggerated responses. Death occurs by asphyxiation due to fixation of the muscles of respiration.

Clinical findings

The incubation period varies between 1 and 3 weeks with occasional cases occurring as long as several months after the infection is introduced. In sheep and lambs cases appear 3–10 days after shearing or docking. The clinical picture is similar in all animal species. A general increase in muscle stiffness is observed first and is accompanied by muscle tremor. There is trismus with restriction of jaw movements, prolapse of the third eyelid, stiffness of the hindlegs causing an unsteady, straddling gait and the tail is held out stiffly especially when backing or turning. The prolapse of the third eyelid is one of the earliest signs and can be exaggerated by sharp lifting of the muzzle or tapping the face below the eye. Additional signs include an anxious and alert expression contributed to by an erect carriage of the ears, retraction of the eyelids and dilatation of the nostrils, and exaggerated responses to normal stimuli. The animal may continue to eat and drink in the early stages but mastication is soon prevented by tetany of the masseter muscles and saliva may drool from the mouth. If food or water are taken, attempts at swallowing are followed by regurgitation from the nose. Constipation is usual and the urine is retained, due in part to inability to assume the normal position for urination. The temperature and pulse rate are within the normal range in the early stages but may rise later when muscular tone and activity are further increased. In cattle, particularly young animals, bloat is an early sign, but is not usually severe and is accompanied by strong, frequent rumen contractions.

As the disease progresses, muscular tetany increases and the animal adopts a 'sawhorse' posture. Uneven muscular contractions may cause the development of a curve in the spine and deviation of the tail to one side. There is great difficulty in walking and the animal is inclined to fall, expecially when startled. Falling occurs with the limbs still in a state of tetany and the animal can cause itself severe injury. Once down it is almost impossible to get a large animal to its feet again. Tetanic convulsions begin in which the tetany is still further exaggerated. Opisthotonus is marked, the hindlimbs are stuck out stiffly behind and the forelegs forward. Sweating may be profuse and the temperature rises, often to 42°C (107°F). The convulsions are at first only stimulated by sound or touch but soon occur spontaneously.

The course of the disease varies both between and within species. The duration of a fatal illness in horses and cattle is usually 5–10 days but sheep usually die about the third or fourth day. Although tetanus is almost always fatal a long incubation period is usually associated with a mild syndrome, a long course and a favorable prognosis. In fatal cases there is often a transient period of improvement for several hours before a final, severe tetanic spasm during which respiration is arrested. Mild cases which recover usually do so slowly, the stiffness disappearing gradually over a period of weeks or even months.

Clinical pathology

There is no satisfactory antemortem test which is of any value in confirming or refuting the diagnosis. It can only be made on clinical grounds. Blood levels of tetanus antitoxin can be measured but the significance of any results is open to question (14).

Necropsy findings

There are no gross or histological findings by which a diagnosis can be confirmed although a search should be made for the site of infection, and culture of the organism attempted.

Diagnosis

Fully developed tetanus is so distinctive clinically that it is seldom confused with other diseases. The muscular spasms, the prolapse of the third eyelid and a recent history of accidental injury or surgery are characteristic findings. However, in its early stages, tetanus may be confused with other diseases. Strychnine poisoning is uncommon in farm animals, usually affects a number at one time or results from overdosing, and the tetany between convulsive episodes is not so marked. Hypocalcemic tetany (eclampsia) of mares also resembles tetanus but is confined to lactating mares and responds to treatment with calcium salts. Acute laminitis also resembles tetanus, but there is no tetany or prolapse of the third eyelid. Cerebrospinal meningitis causes rigidity, particularly of the neck, and hyperesthesia to touch but the general effect is one of depression and immobility rather than excitement and hypersensitivity to sound and movement. Lactation tetany of cattle and whole milk tetany of calves are accompanied by tetany and convulsions but these are more severe than those seen in tetanus, and prolapse of the third eyelid and bloat are absent. Enzootic muscular dystrophy may be mistaken for tetanus because of the marked stiffness but there is an absence of tetany. Enterotoxemia of lambs is accompanied by other more marked nervous signs. Polioencephalomalacia may also resemble tetanus in cattle, especially when the animals are recumbent, but there is no prolapse of the third eyelid, and the increased tone in leg muscles is not nearly as rigid.

Treatment

The response to treatment in horses and sheep is poor but cattle frequently recover. The demand for treatment by horse owners is high and they should be aware of the high mortality rate and the long and intensive course of treatment required; the average course is 27 days, the prospects are not good and the costs are high (4).

The main principles in the treatment of tetanus are to eliminate the causative bacteria, neutralize residual toxin, relax the muscle tetany to avoid asphyxia, and maintain the relaxation until the toxin is eliminated or destroyed. There are no structural changes in the nervous system, and the management of cases of tetanus depends largely on keeping the animal alive through the critical stages.

Elimination of the organism is usually attempted by the parenteral administration of penicillin in large doses. If the infection site is found it should be treated locally but preferably only after antitoxin has been administered, because debridement, irrigation with hydrogen peroxide and the local application of penicillin may facilitate the absorption of the toxin.

Tetanus antitoxin is usually administered but is of little value once signs have appeared. For example, after the experimental administration of toxin, antitoxin is of limited value at 10 hours and ineffective by 48 hours (5). For optimum results horses should receive 300 000 units 12-hourly for three injections (6). Local injection of some of the antitoxin around the wound is advised. There have been a number of attempts to justify the treatment of early cases of equine tetanus by the injection of antitoxin into the subarachnoid space. The latest recommendation is supported by convincing results after the injection of 50 000 units of antitoxin into the cerebrospinal fluid at the foramen magnum (7).

Relaxation of the muscle tetany can be attempted with various drugs. Chloral hydrate and magnesium sulfate injections have been in use for many years but suffer from the deficiency of short-term action and depression of the respiratory center. Ataractic drugs have given excellent results in horses and cattle. Chlorpromazine (0·4 mg/kg body weight intravenously, 1·0 mg/kg body weight intramuscularly) and acetyl promazine (0·05 mg/kg body weight) twice daily for 8–10 days until severe signs subside are widely used.

Additional supportive treatment includes slinging of horses during the recovery period when hyperesthesia is diminishing, and intravenous or stomach-tube feeding during the critical stages when the animal cannot eat or drink. Because of the disturbance caused each time the stomach tube is passed, the use of an indwelling tube should be considered. Positive respiratory control by tracheal intubation is an important feature of treatment in humans but is unlikely to be attempted in animals. Affected animals should be kept as quiet as possible and provided with dark, well-bedded quarters with plenty of room to avoid injury if convulsions occur. Administration of enemas and catheterization may relieve the animal's discomfort.

Control

Many cases of tetanus could be avoided by proper skin and instrument disinfection at castrating, docking and shearing time. These operations should be carried out in clean surroundings and in the case of lambs docked in the field, temporary pens are to be preferred to permanent yards for catching and penning.

For short-term prophylaxis, passive immunity can be achieved by the injection of antitoxin. Doses of 1500–3000 IU of antitoxin are injected subcutaneously in horses, the dose varying with the extent and duration of the injury. On farms where the incidence of tetanus in lambs is high, antitoxin is usually given at docking and a dose rate of 200 IU has been shown to be effective (8). The immunity is transient, persisting for only 10–14 days. The antitoxin can be administered at the same time as the toxoid, provided they are injected at different sites and using different syringes. And the toxoid can also be combined with pulpy kidney vaccine without reduction of the antibody response to either vaccine.

In enzootic areas all susceptible animals should be actively immunized with 'toxoid', an alum-precipitated, formalin-treated toxin. One injection gives immunity in 10–14 days lasting for a year and revaccination in 12 months gives solid immunity for life. A more vigorous program of two vaccinations 6–8 weeks apart followed by annual booster vaccinations is preferred (10). A transient phase of reduction of antibody titer occurs after this booster injection in horses and the animal may be more susceptible at this time (12). However, the fall in level of antibodies is unlikely to leave the horse unprotected. An alternative to alum-precipitated toxoid is one precipitated on aluminum phosphate (11).

In spite of the known efficiency of vaccination, animals which suffer injury subsequently are usually given an injection of antitoxin to ensure complete protection. Antitoxin does not interfere with the production of antibodies by toxoid so that both can be administered at the one time, the antitoxin providing short-term passive immunity until an active immune status is attained. The procedure is also strongly recommended after all surgery in horses. It avoids those cases of tetanus which develop after the prophylactic effect of antitoxin disappears. Care is needed with the technique—the two materials must not be mixed in the one syringe, but must be administered from separate syringes on opposite sides of the neck.

All horses which suffer wounds which could possibly be contaminated with the spores of *Cl. tetani* should receive a combined injection of toxoid and antitoxin as above. An injection of longacting penicillin is commonly given at the same time. In some areas the incidence of tetanus in young foals is high and repeated doses of antitoxin at weekly intervals is not always completely effective. Provided foals get an adequate supply of colostrum they can be passively immunized during the first 10 weeks of life by active vaccination of the mare during the last weeks of pregnancy. The foal should be vaccinated with toxoid at 10 weeks of age and revaccinated 12 weeks later (1). The poor response of foals to toxoid creates some difficulties in ensuring their protection. The toxoid is usually injected subcutanously but intramuscular injection produces less local inflammation and an increased immune response (13). Reactions to absorbed toxoid in horses, which take the form of severe local swelling, can be avoided by using a product containing minimal amounts of aluminum hydroxide (9).

Prevention of tetanus in newborn lambs is also best effected by vaccination of the ewe in late pregnancy. Because the duration and degree of immunity are dependent on the titer of antibodies in the ewe's serum, optimum protection is obtained by vaccinating the ewes in the last 2 or 3 weeks of pregnancy. The greatest response is obtained in ewes which have received a prior vaccination, for example as a lamb or in a preceding pregnancy (13), and annual revaccination of late-pregnant ewes is highly recommended (8). Vaccination of cattle is usually not considered unless an outbreak of the disease has occurred in the immediate past and further cases may be anticipated.

REFERENCES

(1) Jansen, B. C. & Knoetz, P. C. (1979) *Onderstepoort J. vet. Res.*, *46*, 211.
(2) Ramsay, W. R. (1973) *Aust. vet. J.*, *49*, 188.
(3) Neilsen, K. (1976) *Dansk VetTijdschr.*, *59*, 469.
(4) Komarek, J. (1986) *Veterinarstvi*, *36*, 543.
(5) Habermann, E. & Wellhoner, H. H. (1972) Studies on pathogenesis of tetanus with radioactive toxin. In: *Radioactive Tracers in Microbial Immunology*. Vienna: International Atomic Energy Agency.
(6) Radvilla, P. & Lohrer, J. (1965) *Schweiz. Arch. Tierheilkd.*, *107*, 123, 319.
(7) Muylle, E. et al. (1975) *J. Am. vet. med. Assoc.*, *167*, 47.
(8) Cooper, B. S. (1966) *NZ vet. J.*, *14*, 186.
(9) Rao, M. et al. (1978) *Ind. vet. J.*, *55*, 363.
(10) Lohrer, L. & Radvila, P. (1970) *Schweiz. Arch. Tierheilkd.*, *112*, 307.
(11) Cameron, C. M. et al. (1983) *Onderstepoort J. vet. Res.*, *50*, 229.
(12) Liefman, C. E. (1981) *Aust. vet. J.* 57, 57.
(13) Wallace, G. V. (1964) *NZ vet. J.*, *12*, 61.
(14) Power, E. P. & O'Callaghan, M. (1986) *Irish vet. J.*, *40*, 132.

Botulism

Botulism is a rapidly fatal, motor paralysis caused by the ingestion of the toxin of *Clostridium botulinum*, which organism proliferates in decomposing animal matter and sometimes in plant material.

Etiology

The causative organism is *Cl. botulinum*, a spore-forming anaerobe which proliferates only in decaying animal or plant material. There are a number of antigenically distinct types of *Cl. botulinum* classified as A, B, C, D and E. The geographical distribution of these types varies considerably. Under favorable conditions of warmth and moisture the spores multiply rapidly elaborating a stable and highly lethal toxin which, when ingested, causes the disease.

Epidemiology

The spores of *Cl. botulinum* are extremely resistant and survive for long periods in most environmental circumstances. The toxin is also capable of surviving for long periods particularly in bones or if protected from leaching.

In its vegetative form the organism is a common inhabitant of the alimentary tract of herbivores and may be introduced into new areas in this way. It occurs commonly in soils in affected areas, and soil and water contamination occurs from feces and decomposing carcases. A careful study of soils to determine the conditions which favor the presence of *Cl. botulinum* showed a regional distribution for the various types in the United States (4). Type A was found in neutral or alkaline soils in the west, types B and E were in damp or wet soil all over except that B was not found in the south. Type C was found in acid soils in the Gulf Coast, and type D in alkaline soils in the west. Microorganisms capable of inhibiting *Cl. botulinum* were present, with or without the clostridia, in many soils.

The source of infection for animals is almost always carrion, which includes domestic and wild animals and birds. Where cattle subsist on a phosphorus-deficient diet, and manifest osteophagia and the ingestion of carrion, the disease is likely to occur in outbreak form. In sheep, pica is more usually associated with a dietary deficiency of protein or net energy. Occasional outbreaks occur due to drinking of water contaminated by carcasses of dead animals. A not uncommon occurrence is in livestock drinking lake water contaminated by the carcasses of ducks and other waterfowl which have died of botulism. The disease has also occurred in horses fed on spoiled vegetables and potatoes contaminated by *Cl. botulinum*. Dead rodents in haystacks or ensilage pits may provide a source of toxin. Chicken manure used as cattle feed (7) or pastoral fertilizer (8) and chicken house litter used as bedding in cattle loose housing (5) have also caused mortality when the organism was present in the intestinal tract of the birds. Dried poultry waste is a very important source of protein supplement in some countries, but poisoning due to botulism has caused very heavy losses after its use. Factors which affect the toxicity of the product are the efficiency of the heat sterilization used in making it, and the amount fed (7).

Although decomposing animal carcasses are by far the commonest source of toxin, proliferation of the organism can occur in decaying vegetable material. Decaying grass at the base of old tussocks and in trampled stubble are reputed to be suitable sites for growth of *Cl. botuli-*

num. Silage and hay may spoil to a stage suitable for the growth of *Cl. botulinum*. This is most likely if the forage is very succulent or is wet by rain when it is made (25). Grass clippings allowed to accumulate and decay in a pile have poisoned horses (6). Grass ensilage, provided the pH is not too low, can be a suitable substrate for the growth of the organism and so provide a large amount of toxin in the diet (1). The use of wilted grass to make the ensilage may be a critical factor in the epidemiology of the disease in all species and outbreaks in horses have been related to the feeding of big bale silage (26) and of hay polluted by rodent carcasses (27). This ability to grow in such material may be limited to the proteolytic strains of *Cl. botulinum* types A and B (2). The commonest source in Australia is hay made at the time of a mouse plague. At such times even good fresh hay can contain a great deal of carrion. Brewer's grains can also be contaminated and cause serious outbreaks (6, 24). Toxin has also been demonstrated in oat grain which caused toxic effects when fed to horses. High moisture grain has a high potential toxicity.

Botulism has no geographical limitations, sporadic outbreaks occurring in most countries. In farm animals it assumes major economic importance, however, only in areas where sheep and cattle suffer from a phosphorus or protein deficiency on range. Most such outbreaks have been reported from South Africa, Australia and the Gulf Coast area of the United States. The disease usually occurs in a number of animals at one time and is almost invariably fatal.

Botulism is most common in birds, particularly the domestic chicken and wild waterfowl. Cattle, sheep and horses are susceptible, but pigs (8), dogs and cats appear to be resistant. Cattle are usually affected by types C and D. The variation which occurs in the geographical distribution of the various types is an important factor when considering prophylactic vaccination programs. Botulism in range animals has a seasonal distribution. Outbreaks are most likely to occur during drought periods when feed is sparse, phosphorus intake is low and carrion is plentiful.

Spread of the infection from place to place is possible in most of the simple ways, including carriage by birds and blowflies (22).

Pathogenesis

The toxins of *Cl. botulinum* are neurotoxins and produce functional paralysis without the development of histological lesions. When toxin is injected parenterally much smaller doses are required to cause death than when it is ingested. This is probably due to digestion of some of the toxin by proteolytic enzymes in the alimentary tract. The site at which neuromuscular transmission is impeded is probably at the synapses of efferent parasympathetic and somatic motor nerves where there is interference with the secretion of acetylcholine, the chemical mediator of nerve impulse transmission (9). A true flaccid paralysis develops and the animal dies of respiratory paralysis.

After the experimental administration of botulinus toxin to goats clinical signs appear on the second or third day. Small doses of toxin administered over a number of days can produce a cumulative effect (10).

Toxicoinfectious botulism is described as the disease in which *Cl. botulinum* is present in tissues and produces toxins there (23). The toxins are liberated from the lesions and cause typical botulism. This has been suggested as a means of producing the 'shaker foal syndrome' discussed in Chapter 35. Toxicoinfectious botulism has been produced experimentally (3).

Clinical findings

Cattle and horses

Signs usually appear 3–17 days after the animals gain access to the toxic material, the incubation period being shorter as the amount of toxin available is increased. Peracute cases die without prior signs of illness although a few fail to take water or food for a day beforehand. The disease is not accompanied by fever and the characteristic clinical picture is one of progressive muscular paralysis affecting particularly the limb muscles and the muscles of the jaw and throat. Muscle weakness and paralysis commence in the hindquarters and progress to the forequarters, the head and the neck.

The onset is marked by very obvious muscle tremor and fasciculation, often sufficient to make the whole limb tremble.

In most cases the disease is subacute. Restlessness, incoordination, stumbling, knuckling, and ataxia are followed by inability to rise or to lift the head. Skin sensation is retained. Affected animals lie in sternal recumbency with the head on the ground or turned into the flank, not unlike the posture of a cow with parturient paresis. In some cases the tongue becomes paralyzed and hangs from the mouth, the animal is unable to chew or swallow and drools saliva. In others there is no impairment of swallowing or mastication and the animal continues to eat until the end. This variation in signs is often a characteristic of an outbreak, all of the cases having tongue paralysis or all of them not having it. Ruminal movements are depressed. Defecation and urination are usually unaffected although cattle may be constipated. Paralysis of the chest muscles results in a terminal abdominal-type respiration. Sensation and consciousness are retained until the end which usually occurs quietly, and with the animal in lateral recumbency, 1–4 days after the commencement of illness.

Occasional field cases and some experimental cases in cattle show mild signs and recover after an illness of 3–4 weeks (12). These chronic cases show restlessness and respiratory distress followed by knuckling, stumbling and disinclination to rise. Anorexia and adipsia are important early signs but are often not observed in pastured animals. In some there is a pronounced roaring sound with each respiration. The roaring persists for up to 3 months. During the major part of the illness the animals spend most of their time in sternal recumbency. In some animals there is difficulty in prehending hay but concentrate and ensilage may be taken. This disability may persist for 3 weeks.

Sheep

Sheep do not show the typical flaccid paralysis of other species until the final stages of the disease. There is stiffness while walking, incoordination and some excitability in the early stages. The head may be held on one side or bobbed up and down while walking. Lateral switching of the tail, salivation, and serous, nasal discharge are also common. In the terminal stages there is abdominal respiration, limb paralysis and rapid death.

Pigs
Authentic reports in this species are rare (8, 13). Clinical signs include staggering followed by recumbency, vomiting, and pupillary dilatation. The muscular paralysis is flaccid and affected animals do not eat or drink.

Clinical pathology

Little if any antemortem data can be assembled to aid in diagnosis, although mild to marked indicanuria, albuminuria and glycosuria have been observed in cattle (14) and albuminuria and glycosuria in pigs (15). Animals that have been recumbent for a period will have a non-specific creatine phosphokinasemia. In cattle, these biochemical changes occur intermittently and only in some animals and they do not provide satisfactory clinicopathological tests. However, their presence can be used to support a tentative diagnosis in disputed cases (17). In peracute cases, toxin can be detected in the blood by mouse inoculation tests (11, 21) but is often not detectable in the average field case in farm animals (18).

A time-consuming and sometimes necessary exercise is to examine the feed culturally and for the presence of the toxin. The simplest method of detecting toxin is to feed the feed to experimental animals, of the same species preferably. Alternatively one can make an infusion of the feed sample and use this as the sole drinking water supply for experimental animals. Failure to produce the disease in animals vaccinated against botulism, when deaths are occurring in the unvaccinated controls is also a standard diagnostic procedure. The problem with all feeding experiments is that the botulinus toxin is likely to be very patchy in its distribution in the feed. Therefore, particular attention should be given to parts of the feed near carrion, or which have obviously been soiled by animals.

Necropsy findings

There are no specific changes detectable at necropsy although the presence of suspicious, foreign material in the forestomachs or stomach may be suggestive. There may be non-specific subendocardial and subepicardial hemorrhages and congestion of the intestinal mucosa and serosa. Perivascular hemorrhages have been recorded in the brain, especially in the corpus striatum, cerebellum and cerebrum and there may be destruction of Purkinje cells in the cerebellum. The presence of *Cl. botulinum* in the alimentary tract is of little significance and examination of gut contents for the presence of toxin is often misleading because the toxin may have already been absorbed. The presence of the toxin in the liver at postmortem examination is taken as evidence that the disease has occurred (16).

Diagnosis

Although sporadic cases of botulism are often suspected it is seldom possible to establish the diagnosis by demonstrating the presence of toxin in the suspected food (7). Filtrates of the stomach and intestinal contents should be tested for toxicity to experimental animals but a negative answer may not be proof that the disease has not occurred. The main contributory evidence is provided by the feeding of suspect material to susceptible animals. When the disease occurs in ruminants at pasture the occurrence of pica is of diagnostic significance. Clinically and at necropsy the disease resembles parturient paresis in cattle, and hypocalcemia in sheep but the conditions under which the diseases occur are quite different. Many other diseases of the nervous system may present a clinical picture similar to that of botulism. Paralytic rabies and poisoning by *Phalaris aquatica* grass in cattle and equine encephalomyelitis, encephalomyelitis caused by herpes virus 1, and ragwort poisoning in horses may present similar clinical pictures. In sheep, louping-ill, some cases of scrapie, and miscellaneous plant poisonings may also be confused with botulism.

Treatment

Specific or polyvalent antitoxic serum may be used in very early cases but their efficacy is questionable. Purgatives to remove the toxin from the alimentary tract, and central nervous system stimulants are sometimes administered. These treatments are usually confined to horses which may also be supported in slings and fed by stomach tube. In general, treatment should only be undertaken in subacute cases in which signs develop slowly and which have some chance of recovery. The remainder of the animals in the group should be vaccinated immediately.

Control

In range animals, correction of dietary deficiencies by supplementation with phosphorus or protein should be implemented if conditions permit. Hygienic disposal of carcasses is advisable to prevent further pasture contamination but may not be practicable under range conditions. Vaccination with type-specific or combined (bivalent C and D) toxoid is practiced in enzootic areas. A single dose, precipitated toxoid is available which gives good immunity after 2 weeks and the immunity is solid for about 24 months (19). A common problem which arises when the disease appears to have resulted from feeding contaminated silage, hay or other feed is what to do with the residue of the feed; there may be a large quantity of it. What had been done in these circumstances has been to vigorously vaccinate the stock with a toxoid on three occasions at 2-week intervals and then recommence feeding the same material (28). The disease in horses is usually due to accidental contamination of feed or water, and the incidence is low; vaccination is seldom practiced in this species. Some local reactions are encountered after vaccination in horses but they are seldom serious (20).

REVIEW LITERATURE

Hariharan, H. & Mitchell, W. R. (1977) Type C botulism: the agent, host spectrum and environment. *Vet. Bull.*, *47*, 95.
Smith, L. D. S. (1979) *Botulism, the Organisms, its Toxins, the Disease.* Springfield, Illinois: Charles C. Thomas.

REFERENCES

(1) Notermans, S. et al. (1985) *Tijdschr. Diergeneeskd.*, *110*, 175.
(2) Notermans, S. et al. (1979) *Appl. envir. Microbiol.*, *38*, 767.
(3) MacKay, R. J. et al. (1982) *J. Am. vet. med. Assoc.*, *180*, 163.
(4) Smith, L. D. (1978) *Hlth Lab. Sci.*, *15*, 74.
(5) Haagsma, J. et al. (1977). *Tijdschr. Diergeneeskd.*, *102*, 330 & *103*, 1317 & 1327.
(6) Switzer, J. W. et al. (1984) *Calif. Vet.*, *38*, 14.
(7) Egyed, M. N. et al. (1978) *Refuah Vet.*, *35*, 91, 93 *et seq.*
(8) Smart, J. L. et al. (1987) *Epidemiol. Infect.*, *98*, 73.
(9) Wright, G. P. (1955) *Mechanisms of Microbial Pathogenicity*, pp. 78–102. London: Cambridge University Press.
(10) Fjolstad, M. (1973) *Acta vet. Scand.*, *14*, 69.
(11) Smith, G. R. & Murray, L. G. (1984) *Vet. Rec.*, *114*, 75.
(12) Davies, A. B. et al. (1974) *Vet. Rec.*, *94*, 412.
(13) Beiers, P. R. & Simmons, G. C. (1967) *Aust. vet. J.*, *43*, 270.
(14) Noyan, A. (1958) *Am. J. vet. Res.*, *19*, 840.
(15) Simintzis, G. & Durin, L. (1950) *Bull. Soc. Sci. vet. Med. comp. Lyon*, *52*, 71.
(16) Muller, J. (1981) *Nord. VetMed.*, *33*, 33.
(17) Egyed, M. N. (1973) *Vet. Med. small Anim. Clin.*, *68*, 854.
(18) Ektvedt, R. & Hanssen, I. (1974) *Norsk. VetTidsskr.*, *86*, 286.
(19) Tammemagi, L. & Grant, K. McD. (1967) *Aust. vet. J.*, *43*, 368.
(20) White, P. G. & Appleton, G. S. (1960) *J. Am. vet. med. Assoc.*, *137*, 652.
(21) Gruys, E. et al. (1977) *Tijdschr. Diergeneeskd.*, *102*, 983.
(22) Graham, J. M. (1978) *Vet. Rec.*, *102*, 242.
(23) Swerczek, T. W. (1980) *J. Am. vet. med. Assoc.*, *176*, 217.
(24) Breukink, H. J. et al. (1978) *Tijdschr. Diergeneeskd.*, *103*, 303 & 1327.
(25) Whitlock, R. H. et al. (1985) *Proc. 18th Ann. Conv. Am. Assoc. Bov. Pract.*, p. 164.
(26) Ricketts, S. W. et al. (1984) *Equ. vet. J.*, *16*, 515.
(27) Kelly, A. P. et al. (1984) *Equ. vet. J.*, *16*, 519.
(28) Divers, T. J. (1986) *J. Am. vet. med. Assoc.*, *188*, 382.

Blackleg

Blackleg is an acute, infectious disease caused by *Clostridium chauvoei* and characterized by inflammation of muscles, severe toxemia and a high mortality. True blackleg is common only in cattle but infection initiated by trauma occurs occasionally in other animals.

Etiology

True blackleg is caused by *Cl.* (*feseri*) *chauvoei*, a Gram-positive spore-forming, rod-shaped bacterium. The spores are highly resistant to environmental changes and disinfectants and persist in soil for many years. 'False blackleg' may be caused by *Cl. septicum* and *Cl. novyi* but this disease is more accurately classified as malignant edema. Mixed infections with *Cl. chauvoei* and *Cl. septicum* are not uncommon but the significance of *Cl. septicum* as a cause of the disease is debated (3). However, in a study of 176 cases of clostridial myositis in cattle, *Cl. chauvoei* either alone or with *Cl. septicum* was demonstrated in 56%. In 36%, *Cl. novyi* was found alone or with *Cl. septicum* (4). This indicates that maximum protection to cattle can be provided only by a multivalent vaccine which contains the antigens of *Cl. chauvoei*, *Cl. novyi* and *Cl. septicum*.

Epidemiology

Blackleg is a soil-borne infection but the portal by which the organism enters the body is still in dispute. However, it is presumed that the portal of entry is through the alimentary mucosa after ingestion of contaminated feed. The bacteria may be found in the spleen, liver and alimentary tract of normal animals, and contamination of the soil and pasture may occur from infected feces or decomposition of carcasses of animals dying of the disease. True blackleg develops when spores which are not lodged in normal tissues are caused to proliferate by mechanisms which have not been identified.

True blackleg is usually thought of as a disease of cattle and occasionally sheep but outbreaks of the disease have been recorded in deer (6) and in one case in a horse (2). In cattle the disease is largely confined to young stock between the ages of 6 months and 2 years. In the field the disease appears to occur most frequently in rapidly growing cattle on a high plane of nutrition. Elevation of the nutritional status of sheep by increased protein feeding increases their susceptibility to blackleg. In sheep there is no restriction to age group.

In pigs, blackleg does not occur commonly, although a gas gangrene type of lesion may be caused by *Cl. chauvoei* (8, 9) or *Cl. septicum* (10) infection. Typical blackleg of cattle has a seasonal incidence with most cases occurring in the warm months of the year. The highest incidence may vary from spring to autumn, depending probably on when calves reach the susceptible age group. Some outbreaks of blackleg in cattle have occurred following excavation of soil which suggests that disturbances in soil may expose and activate latent spores (11).

In sheep the disease is almost always a wound infection. Infection of skin wounds at shearing and docking and of the navel at birth may cause the development of local lesions. Infections of the vulva and vagina of the ewe at lambing may cause serious outbreaks and the disease has occurred in groups of young ewes and rams up to a year old, usually as a result of infection of skin wounds caused by fighting. Occasional outbreaks have occurred in sheep after vaccination against enterotoxemia (12). Presumably the formalinized vaccine causes sufficient tissue damage to permit latent spores of the organism to proliferate. A special occurrence has been recorded in fetal lambs (13). Ewes exposed to infection at shearing developed typical lesions but ewes treated with penicillin were unaffected except that the pregnant ewes in the latter group showed distended abdomens, weakness and recumbency due to edema and gas formation in the fetus from which *Cl. chauvoei* was isolated.

Blackleg is a cause of severe financial loss to cattle raisers in many parts of the world. For the most part major outbreaks are prevented by vaccination although outbreaks still occur, occasionally in vaccinated herds but more frequently in herds where vaccination has been neglected. When the disease occurs it is usual for a number of animals to be affected within the space of a few days. The disease is enzootic in particular areas, especially when they are subject to flooding; such an area may vary in size from a group of farms to an individual field. The case fatality rate in blackleg approaches 100%.

Pathogenesis

In true blackleg the stimulus which results in growth of the latent bacterial spores is unknown. Toxin formed by the organism produces a severe necrotizing myositis locally, and a systemic toxemia which is usually fatal.

Clinical findings

Cattle

If the animal is observed before death there is marked lameness, usually with pronounced swelling of the upper part of the affected leg. On closer examination the animal will be found to be very depressed, have complete anorexia and ruminal stasis and a high temperature (41°C, 106°F) and pulse rate (100–120/min). In the early stages the swelling is hot and painful to the touch but soon becomes cold and painless, and edema and emphysema can be felt. The skin is discolored and soon becomes dry and cracked. Although the lesions are usually confined to the upper part of one limb, occasional cases are seen where the lesions are present in other locations such as the base of the tongue, the heart muscle, the diaphragm and psoas muscles, the brisket and udder. Lesions are sometimes present in more than one of these locations in the one animal. The condition develops rapidly and the animal dies quietly 12–36 hours after the appearance of signs. Many animals die without signs having been observed.

Sheep

When blackleg lesions occur in the limb musculature in sheep, there is a stiff gait and the sheep is disinclined to move due to severe lameness in one or, more commonly, in several limbs. The lameness may be severe enough to prevent walking in some animals but be only moderate in others. Subcutaneous edema is not common and gaseous crepitation cannot be felt before death. Discoloration of the skin may be evident but skin necrosis and gangrene do not occur.

In those cases where infection occurs through wounds of the skin, vulva or vagina there is an extensive local lesion. Lesions of the head may be accompanied by severe local swelling due to edema and there may be bleeding from the nose. In all instances there is high fever, anorexia, depression and death occurs very quickly (14).

The clinical syndrome in horses is not well defined. Pectoral edema, stiff gait and incoordination are recorded (2).

Clinical pathology

The disease is usually so acute that necropsy material is readily available but, failing this, it may be possible to obtain material suitable for cultural examination by needle puncture or swabs from wounds. As might be expected serum levels of lactic dehydrogenase, SGPT and SGOT are significantly increased during the course of the disease, and hypovolemia occurs in the later stages (15).

Necropsy findings

Cattle found dead of blackleg are often in a characteristic position, lying on the side with the affected hindlimb stuck out stiffly. Bloating and putrefaction occur quickly and bloodstained froth exudes from the nostrils and anus. Clotting of the blood occurs rapidly. Incision of the affected muscle mass reveals the presence of dark, discolored, swollen tissue with a rancid odor, a metallic sheen on the cut surface and an excess of thin, sanguineous fluid containing bubbles of gas. In some cases the myocardial muscle and diaphragm may be the only tissues affected. All skeletal muscles of the body including those of the lumbar region must be examined for evidence of the lesion, which may be small and escape cursory examination. All body cavities contain excess fluid which contains variable amounts of fibrin and is usually bloodstained. The solid organs show some degree of degeneration, and postmortem decomposition with the production of gas in the liver occurs rapidly.

Sheep show a similar picture at necropsy but the muscle lesions are more localized and deeper and the subcutaneous edema is not so marked except around the head. Gas is present in the affected muscles but not in such large amounts as in cattle. When the disease has resulted from infection of skin wounds the lesions are more obvious superficially, with subcutaneous edema and swelling, and involvement of the underlying musculature. When invasion of the genital tract occurs, typical lesions are found in the perineal tissues and in the walls of the vagina and occasionally the uterus. In the special case of pregnant ewes which develop infection of the fetus, typical lesions involve the entire fetus and cause marked abdominal distension in the ewe.

In all cases of suspected blackleg smears of affected tissue should be made and material collected for bacteriological examination. Pasteur pipettes from muscle tissue and heart blood, and sections of muscle removed aseptically are suitable specimens for laboratory examination. The isolation and identification of the causal organisms from muscle lesions is difficult because of the rapidity with which clostridia invade the tissues from the gastrointestinal tract after death and the fastidiousness in culture of certain clostridial species such as *Cl. chauvoei* and *Cl. novyi*. Thus it is essential that tissues be examined as soon after death as possible and that special precautions be taken to ensure the isolation of *Cl. chauvoei* and *Cl. novyi* (4).

Diagnosis

In typical cases of blackleg in cattle a definite diagnosis can be made on the clinical signs and the necropsy findings. However, positive identification on gross postmortem findings of which one of the clostridial myositides is present is hazardous except by an experienced pathologist. This is an important matter if all the common infections are likely to occur in the area. For example, one survey (7) has shown the following isolations from cases of bovine myositis:

Cl. chauvoei (+ *Cl. septicum*) 56%
Cl. novyi (+ *Cl. septicum*) 36%
Cl. septicum only 6%
Cl. sordellii only 1·7%

In many cases the diagnosis may be in doubt because of failure to find extensive, typical lesions. Such cases may be confused with other acute clostridial infections, with lightning strike and with anthrax although in the latter the characteristic splenic lesion is usually present. Bacillary hemoglobinuria produces a rather similar necropsy picture with rapidly developing postmortem changes in muscle but the liver infarcts and hemoglobinuria should identify the disease. Lactation tetany and acute lead poisoning may also cause sudden deaths in a number of cattle but the typical lesions of blackleg are not present.

In establishing a diagnosis when a number of animals are found dead in a group not kept under close observation one must depend on one's knowledge of local disease incidence, season of the year, age group affected and pasture conditions, and on a close inspection of the environment in which the animals have been maintained. Necropsy findings are most valuable if the cadavers are still fresh but, on many occasions, postmortem decomposition is so advanced that little information can be obtained.

Treatment

Treatment of affected animals with penicillin is logical if the animal is not moribund but results are generally only fair because of the extensive nature of the lesions. Large doses (10 000 units/kg body weight) should be administered, commencing with crystalline penicillin intravenously and followed by longer-acting preparations some of which should be given into the affected tissue if it is accessible. Blackleg antiserum is unlikely to be of much value in treatment unless very large doses are given.

Control

On farms where the disease is enzootic annual vaccination of all cattle between 6 months and 2 years of age should be carried out just prior to the anticipated danger period, usually spring and summer. Vaccination of calves at 3 weeks of age has been recommended when the incidence of the disease is very high. Subsequent revaccination will be advisable (16). Of the available preparations the formalin-killed, alum-precipitated bacterin is most satisfactory. Immunity does not develop for 14 days and deaths may continue for some days if vaccination is carried out during an outbreak. When the disease is present in a group other measures are necessary to protect the remainder of the group until immunity has developed. Movement of the cattle from the affected pasture is advisable. In an outbreak all cattle in the remainder of the herd should be vaccinated immediately and injected with penicillin at a dose of 6000 units/kg body weight intramuscularly or a combination of penicillin and benzathine penicillin. If the antibiotics are not given, new cases of blackleg may occur for up to 14 days until immunity develops. Constant surveillance and the early treatment of cases is about all that can be done.

In sheep, the use of alum-precipitated bacterin is also highly recommended but a good immunity does not develop in sheep vaccinated when less than a year old (17). In areas where the disease is enzootic the following vaccination program is recommended. To prevent infection of the ewes at lambing they are vaccinated 3 weeks before lambing on one occasion only. This vaccination will give permanent protection. In subsequent years the young ewes are vaccinated. This vaccination will also protect lambs against umbilical infection at birth (18) and infection of the tail wound at docking, provided the tail is docked before the lamb is 3 weeks old. Vaccination can also be carried out 2–3 weeks before shearing or crutching if infection is anticipated. Because of the common occurrences of the disease in young sheep, vaccination before they go on to pasture and are exposed to infection of skin wounds from fighting is recommended in danger areas. The duration of the immunity in these animals, vaccinated at about 7 months of age, is relatively short and ewes in particular must be revaccinated before they lamb for the first time. If an outbreak commences in a flock of ewes at lambing time prophylactic injections of penicillin and antiserum to ewes requiring assistance has been recommended (14, 19).

The constitution of the vaccine is important. A bacterin prepared from a local strain of *Cl. chauvoei* is preferred. If deaths continue after an approved vaccination program has been used an investigation should be made of the antigenic composition of the vaccine relative to the isolates found in dead vaccinated animals. If necessary, the spectrum of the antigens in the vaccine should be expanded (1). The improvement to be expected would be greater still if the toxin composition of each isolate were known rather than its identifying antigenicity. It is advisable to use a combined bacterin containing *Cl. chauvoei*, *Cl. septicum* and *Cl. novyi*, if these organisms occur in the area and cause clostridial myositis (4). Attenuated organisms are also used in the preparation of vaccines for use in cattle and the same attenuated strain of bovine origin or a recently isolated, virulent, ovine strain may be used to prepare vaccines for use in sheep. Multiple clostridial vaccines are now the vogue, in preference to separate vaccines for each disease. It is also possible to administer a polyvalent vaccine—anthelmintic combination (5). The polyvalent vaccine is highly recommended for the extra protection acquired at very little extra cost.

It is important that carcasses of animals dying of blackleg be destroyed by burning or deep burial to limit soil contamination.

REFERENCES

(1) Reed, G. A. & Reynolds, I. (1977) *Aust. vet. J.*, *53*, 393.
(2) Hagemoser, W. A. et al. (1980) *J. Am. vet. med. Assoc.*, *176*, 631.
(3) Barnes, D. M. et al. (1975) *Can. vet. J.*, *16*, 357.
(4) Williams, B. M. (1977) *Vet. Rec.*, *100*, 90.
(5) Hogarth-Scott, R. S. et al. (1980) *Aust. vet. J.*, *56*, 285 & 292.
(6) Armstrong, H. L. & MacNamee, J. K. (1950) *J. Am. vet. med. Assoc.*, *117*, 212.
(7) Williams, A. M. (1977) *Vet. Rec.*, *100*, 90.
(8) Sterne, M. & Edwards, J. B. (1955) *Vet. Rec.*, *67*, 314.
(9) Gualandi, G. L. (1955) *Arch. vet. ital.*, *6*, 57.
(10) Clay, H. A. (1960) *Vet. Rec.*, *72*, 265.
(11) Barnes, D. M. et al. (1975) *Can. vet. J.*, *16*, 257.
(12) Seddon, H. R. et al. (1931) *Aust. vet. J.*, *7*, 2.
(13) Butler, H. C. & Marsh, H. (1956) *J. Am. vet. med. Assoc.*, *128*, 401.
(14) Watt, J. A. A. (1960) *Vet. Rec.*, *72*, 998.
(15) Pemberton, J. R. et al. (1974) *Am. J. vet. Res.*, *35*, 1037, 1041.
(16) Wayt, L. K. (1953) *N. Am. Vet.*, *34*, 506.
(17) Buddle, M. B. (1954) *NZ J. Sci. Technol.*, *35*, 395.
(18) Oxer, D. T. et al. (1967) *Aust. vet. J.*, *43*, 25.
(19) Buddle, M. B. (1952) *NZ vet. J.*, *1*, 13.

Malignant edema (gas gangrene)

Malignant edema is an acute wound infection caused by organisms of the genus *Clostridium*. There is acute inflammation at the site of infection and a profound systemic toxemia.

Etiology

Clostridium septicum, Cl. chauvoei, Cl. perfringens, Cl. sordellii and *Cl. novyi* have all been isolated from lesions typical of malignant edema of animals. *Cl. sordellii* has been associated chiefly with malignant edema of cattle but it has been found to be a cause of malignant edema and swelled head in sheep (1). *Cl. fallax* has caused gas gangrene in a horse (4). Swelled head of rams, in which the lesions of malignant edema are restricted to the head, is almost always caused by *Cl. novyi* infection.

Epidemiology

All ages and species of animals are affected. In most cases a wound is the portal of entry and a dirty environment which permits contamination of wounds with soil is the common predisposing cause. The occurrence of malignant edema due to *Cl. chauvoei* has been discussed in the section on blackleg.

The infection is usually soil-borne and the resistance of spores of the causative clostridia to environmental influence leads to persistence of the infection for long periods in a local area. Deep puncture wounds accompanied by severe trauma provide the most favorable conditions for growth of anaerobes, and malignant edema occurs most frequently under such conditions. Infection may occur through surgical or accidental wounds, following vaccination or venepuncture, or through the umbilical cord in the newborn. The current popularity of intramuscular injection as a means of administering medicaments including anthelmintics and nutritional supplements, some of which can cause significant tissue damage at the site, can be expected to result in a higher incidence of this disease unless proper asepsis is practiced (2, 5, 7). Outbreaks have been observed in both cattle and sheep following parturition, sometimes, though not always, associated with lacerations of the vulva. An unusual method of infection occurs when crows which have eaten infected carrion carry the infection to live, weak sheep and to lambs when they attack their eyes. The practice of dipping sheep immediately they are shorn may cause a high incidence of malignant edema if the dip is heavily contaminated.

The clostridia which cause malignant edema are common inhabitants of the animal environment and intestinal tract and although some of the causative species have a restricted distribution, the disease is general in most parts of the world. The disease occurs sporadically, affecting individual animals except in special circumstances when outbreaks may occur. The disease 'swelled head', a form of malignant edema, occurs in young rams 6 months to 2 years old when they are run in bands and fight among themselves. After shearing, docking or lambing a high incidence may occur in sheep especially if they are dipped soon afterwards. Castration wounds in pigs and cattle may also become infected. Unless treatment is instituted in the early stages the death rate is extremely high.

Pathogenesis

Potent toxins are produced in the local lesion and cause death when absorbed into the bloodstream. Locally the exotoxins cause extensive edema and necrosis followed by gangrene.

Clinical findings

Clinical signs appear within 12–48 hours of infection. There is always a local lesion at the site of infection consisting of a soft, doughy swelling with marked local erythema accompanied by severe pain on palpation. At a later stage the swelling becomes tense and the skin dark and taut. Emphysema may or may not be present depending on the type of infection and may be so marked as to cause extensive frothy exudation from the wound. With *Cl. novyi* infections there is no emphysema. A high fever (41–42°C, 106–107°F) is always present and affected animals are depressed, weak, show muscle tremor and usually stiffness or lameness. In horses the mucosae are dry and congested and have very poor capillary refill. The illness is of short duration and affected animals die within 24–48 hours of the first appearance of signs. New cases continue to appear for 3–4 days after shearing or other precipitating cause.

When infection occurs at parturition swelling of the vulva accompanied by the discharge of a reddish-brown fluid occurs within 2–3 days. The swelling extends to involve the pelvic tissues and perineal region. The local lesions are accompanied by a profound toxemia and death occurs within 1–2 days.

In 'swelled head' of rams the edema is restricted initially to the head. It occurs first under the eyes, spreads to the subcutaneous tissues of the head and down the neck. In pigs the lesions are usually restricted to the axilla, limbs and throat and are edematous with very little evidence of emphysema. Local skin lesions consisting of raised, dull red plaques distended with clear serous fluid containing *Cl. septicum*, and causing no systemic illness have also been observed in pigs at abattoirs (3).

Clinical pathology

Antemortem examination of affected animals is not usually undertaken in the laboratory although aspirated fluid from edematous swellings or swabs from wounds may give an early diagnosis of the type of infection involved.

Necropsy findings

Tissue changes occur rapidly after death, particularly in warm weather, and this must be kept in mind when evaluating postmortem findings. There is usually gangrene of the skin with edema of the subcutaneous and intermuscular connective tissue around the site of infection. There may be some involvement of underlying muscle but this is not marked. The edema fluid varies from thin serum to a gelatinous deposit. It is usually bloodstained and contains bubbles of gas except in *Cl. novyi* infections when the deposit is gelatinous, clear and contains no gas. A foul, putrid odor is often present in infections with *Cl. perfringens* and *Cl. sordellii*.

Subserous hemorrhages and accumulations of serosanguineous fluid in body cavities are usual. In 'swelled head' of rams the edema of the head and neck may extend into the pleural cavity and also involve the lungs. Material from local lesions should be examined bacteriologically to determine the specific bacteria present.

Diagnosis

The association of profound toxemia with local inflammation and emphysema is characteristic. The disease is differentiated from blackleg by the absence of typical muscle involvement and the presence of wounds. A history of prior vaccination against blackleg and the age of the animal may be of assistance in diagnosis. Anthrax in pigs is often accompanied by subcutaneous gelatinous edema of the throat region. The problem in malignant edema is to determine the identity of the organism or organisms and this can only be done by laboratory procedures. Clostridia are present in the alimentary tract of normal animals, and under favorable conditions postmortem invasion of the tissues may occur rapidly.

Treatment

Affected animals should be treated as emergency cases because of the acute nature of the disease. Specific treatment requires the administration of penicillin or a broad-spectrum antibiotic. Antitoxin is effective in controlling the toxemia, but is usually too expensive for practical use and must be given very early in the course of the disease. Injection of penicillin directly into and around the periphery of the lesions may be of value in some cases. Local treatment consists of surgical incision to provide drainage, and irrigation with hydrogen peroxide.

Control

Hygiene at lambing, shearing, castration and docking is essential to the control of the infection in sheep. Vaccination with the specific or combined, formalinized bacterin is satisfactory in preventing the occurrence of the disease in enzootic areas. Vaccines against all the common pathogens are generally available, and an effective vaccine against *Cl. sordellii* has been produced (6). If the probability of infection appears great the administration of adequate doses of penicillin will prevent its occurrence.

REFERENCES

(1) Smith, L. D. et al. (1962) *Cornell Vet.*, *52*, 63.
(2) Harwood, D. G. (1984) *Vet. Rec.*, *115*, 412.
(3) McDonald, I. W. & Collins, F. V. (1947) *Aust. vet. J.*, *23*, 50.
(4) Coloe, P. J. et al. (1983) *J. comp. Pathol.*, *93*, 597.
(5) Rebhun, W. C. et al. (1985) *J. Am. vet. med. Assoc.*, *187*, 732.
(6) Coleman, J. D. et al. (1975) *Vet. Med. small Anim. Clin.*, *70*, 191.
(7) Breuhas, B. A. et al. (1983) *J. Equ. vet. Sci.*, *3*, 42.

Braxy (bradsot)

Braxy is an acute infectious disease of sheep characterized by inflammation of the abomasal wall, toxemia and a high mortality rate.

Etiology

Clostridium septicum, the common cause of malignant edema in animals, is generally regarded as the causative bacterium.

Epidemiology

The disease occurs only in midwinter when there are heavy frosts and snow and usually only in weaner and yearling sheep. It has occurred in experimental sheep receiving infusion of acetic acid into the abomasum. These were thought to cause abomasitis (4). Adult animals in an enzootic area appear to have acquired immunity.

Cl. septicum is a soil-borne organism and in many areas can be considered as a normal inhabitant of the ovine intestinal tract.

The disease occurs in the United Kingdom, various parts of Europe and has been reported in the southern part of Australia (1) but appears to be rare in North America. It is not of major importance because of its low incidence, although at one time it was sufficiently common to be an important cause of loss in some countries. In affected sheep the mortality rate is usually about 50% and in enzootic areas an annual loss of 8% has been reported (2).

Pathogenesis

Presumably a primary abomasitis, caused by the ingestion of frozen grass or other feed, permits invasion by *Cl. septicum* resulting in a fatal toxemia.

Clinical findings

There is a sudden onset of illness with segregation from the group, complete anorexia, depression and high fever (42°C, 107°F or more). The abdomen may be distended with gas and there may be signs of abdominal pain. The sheep becomes recumbent, comatose and dies within a few hours of first becoming ill.

Clinical pathology

Antemortem laboratory examinations are of little value in establishing a diagnosis.

Necropsy findings

There are localized areas of edema, congestion, necrosis and ulceration of the abomasal wall. Congestion of the mucosa of the small intestine may also be present and there may be a few subepicardial petechiae. *Cl. septicum* can be isolated by smear from the cut surface of the abomasal wall or by culture from the heart blood and other organs of fresh carcasses. Bacteriological examinations of tissues must be carried out within an hour of death if the diagnosis is to be confirmed.

Diagnosis

Clinically the diagnosis of braxy is most difficult. At necropsy the lesions of abomasitis are characteristic especially if the disease occurs under conditions of severe cold. Overeating on grain may cause local patches of rumenitis and reticulitis but there are no lesions in the abomasum. Braxy may resemble infectious necrotic hepatitis but there are no liver lesions in braxy. The final diagnosis depends on isolation of *Cl. septicum* from typical alimentary tract lesions.

Treatment

No treatment has been found to be of value.

Control

Management of the flock is important. The sheep should be yarded at night, and fed hay before being let out to the frosted pasture each morning. Vaccination with a formalin-killed whole culture of *Cl. septicum* (3), preferably two injections 2 weeks apart, is also an effective preventive.

REFERENCES

(1) Dumaresq, J. A. (1939) *Aust. vet. J.*, *15*, 252.
(2) Gaiger, S. H. (1922) *J. comp. Pathol.*, *35*, 191, 235.
(3) Gordon, W. S. (1934) *Vet. Rec.*, *14*, 1.
(4) Ellis, T. M. et al. (1983) *Aust. vet. J.*, *60*, 308.

Infectious necrotic hepatitis (black disease)

Infectious necrotic hepatitis is an acute toxemia of sheep, cattle and sometimes of pigs caused by the toxin of *Clostridium novyi* elaborated in damaged liver tissue. Under field conditions it is usually associated with fascioliasis.

Etiology

The disease occurs in sheep and cattle and rarely in pigs and in horses (3, 13). *Cl. novyi*, especially type B, is the cause of the disease but the intervention of a necrotic process in the liver, which causes the organism to proliferate and produce lethal amounts of toxin, is commonly stated to be the precipitating cause. The disease has been produced experimentally in sheep by the administration of spores of *Cl. novyi* after prior infection with fluke metacercariae (1). Although field outbreaks of the disease are usually precipitated by invasion of the liver by immature liver fluke (2) it is possible that other causes of local hepatic injury, e.g. invasion by cysts of *Cysticercus tenuicollis*, and liver biopsy (16), may precipitate the disease.

There is an increasing number of cases being reported in which no specific precipitating lesions are detected (4, 5). These are being advanced as an explanation of sudden deaths in cattle and pigs heavily fed on grain. Although *Cl. novyi* should be considered in the differential diagnosis of animals dying in these circumstances there is no definitive evidence that this disease is a cause of sudden death in feedlot cattle unless there are lesions in the liver which allow the organism to proliferate (6, 7).

Epidemiology

Well-nourished adult sheep in the 2–4-year age group are particularly susceptible, lambs and yearlings rarely being affected. A seasonal occurrence is marked because of fluctuation in the liver fluke and host snail population. Outbreaks are most common in the summer or autumn months and cease soon after frosts occur because of destruction of encysted metacercariae. Exposure to fluke infestation, as occurs when sheep graze on marshy ground during drought, is commonly associated with outbreaks of black disease, although they can occur in winter (8). Fatal infection with *Cl. novyi* can also occur through the navel in lambs and the uterus in ewes (9). The epidemiological association between liver fluke and *Cl. novyi* has been supported by the observation that both are more prevalent in the soil in areas where black disease occurs than in other areas (10). Moreover the survival of both the bacteria and the fluke is favored by the same type of soil environment (11).

Fecal contamination of the pasture by carrier animals is the most important source of infection although the cadavers of sheep dead of the disease may cause heavy contamination. Many normal animals in flocks in which the disease occurs carry *Cl. novyi* in their livers, not all strains being pathogenic (12). The spread of the infection from farm to farm occurs via these sheep and probably also by infected wild animals and birds and by the carriage of contaminated soil during flooding. Spores of the causative clostridia are ingested and are carried to the liver in the lymphatic system (14). Sheep removed from a black disease farm may die of the disease up to 6 weeks later because of the timelag required for migration of the flukes. Heavy irrigation of pastures, by creating favorable conditions for the development of flukes, lends itself to a high incidence of the disease and the occurrence of the disease in cattle is limited largely to irrigated farms (15).

The disease is worldwide in distribution but is of particular importance in Australia and New Zealand, and to a lesser extent in the United Kingdom, the United States and in Europe. In sheep, the morbidity rate is usually about 5% in affected flocks but may be as high as 10–30% and in rare cases up to 50%. The disease is always fatal in both sheep and cattle. Details of the incidence in cattle (15, 16) and pigs (4, 17) are scanty but the disease is becoming more common in some areas.

Pathogenesis

Under local anaerobic conditions, such as occur in the liver when migrating fluke cause severe tissue destruction, the organisms already present in the liver proliferate, liberating toxins which cause local liver necrosis and more diffuse damage to the vascular system. The nervous signs observed may be due to this general vascular disturbance or to a specific neurotoxin.

Clinical findings

Affected sheep commonly die during the night and are found dead without having exhibited any previous signs of illness. When observation is possible, clinically affected sheep are seen to segregate from the rest of the flock, lag behind and fall down if driven. There is fever (40–42°C, 105–107°F) which subsides to a premortal (subnormal) level, some hyperesthesia, respiration is rapid and shallow, the sheep remains in sternal recumbency and often dies within a few minutes while still in this position. The course from first illness to death is never more than a few hours and death usually occurs quietly, without evidence of struggling.

Clinical findings are the same in cattle as in sheep but the course is longer, the illness lasting for 1–2 days (15). Outstanding clinical findings in cattle include a sudden severe depression, reluctance to move, coldness of the skin, absence of rumen sounds, a low or normal temperature, and weakness and muffling of the heart sounds. There is abdominal pain, especially on deep palpation of the liver, and the feces are semifluid. Periorbital edema may also develop.

Cl. novyi is becoming more frequently recognized as a cause of sudden death in pigs. Descriptions of the clinical disease in horses are scant. They include reluctance to walk, pain on palpation of the abdomen, frequent straining and recumbency. The syndrome presents as a peritonitis accompanied by severe toxemia (13).

Clinical pathology

Antemortem laboratory examinations are not usually possible because of the peracute nature of the disease.

Necropsy findings

Bloodstained froth may exude from the nostrils. The carcass undergoes rapid putrefaction. There is pronounced engorgement of the subcutaneous vessels and a variable degree of subcutaneous edema. The dark appearance of the inside of the skin, particularly noticeable on drying, has given rise to the name black disease. Gelatinous exudate may be present in moderate quantities in the fascial planes of the abdominal musculature. There is a general engorgement of the liver which has a dark, gray-brown appearance and exhibits characteristic areas of necrosis. These are yellow areas, 1–2 cm in diameter, and surrounded by a zone of bright red hyperemia. They occur mostly under the capsule of the diaphragmatic surface of the organ but may be more deeply seated and can easily be missed unless the liver is sliced carefully. In cattle they are linear in shape and may be difficult to find (15). There is usually evidence of recent invasion with liver fluke with channels of damaged liver tissue evident on the cut surface of the liver. These may be mistaken for subcapsular hemorrhages when viewed from the surface. Mature flukes are not ordinarily observed. Bloodstained serous fluid is always present in abnormally large amounts in the pericardial, pleural and peritoneal cavities. Subendocardial and subepicardial hemorrhages are frequent. Unusual lesions such as a large area of inflammation in the wall of the abomasum (18) and congestion of the subcutaneous tissue and muscle in the shoulder and withers (4) have been observed in some cattle dying of the disease.

Material for laboratory examination should include a piece of necrotic liver removed aseptically and packed in a sterile jar, impression smears made from the periphery of the lesion, and a piece of liver packed in formalin for histological examination. The critical observation in the diagnosis of black disease is the finding of *Cl. novyi* in the typical liver lesion and the demonstration of preformed toxin in peritoneal fluid and the liver lesion (19). However, the use of fluorescent antibody techniques is almost as accurate and much less time-consuming (4).

The most difficult diagnostic situation is the cadaver of the animal which has been dead for sufficient time to permit autolysis to cloud the postmortem findings. Errors are likely if the simple presence of *Cl. novyi* or its toxin in the liver or spleen are considered as positive evidence. If the carcass is more than 24 hours old the bacteria may have multiplied after death from an innocuous premortal level (14). Another problem is the relatively common occurrences in livers of strains of *Cl. novyi* B which are of insignificant pathogenicity (10). These strains are detected by the fluorescent antibody technique and this may lead to a false positive identification of black disease.

Diagnosis

In sheep, acute fascioliasis can cause heavy mortalities due to massive liver destruction at the same time and under the same conditions as does black disease. The course in fascioliasis is longer, affected sheep showing depression and anorexia for 2–3 days before death. At necropsy excess serous fluid is present only in the peritoneal cavity, the necrotic areas characteristic of black disease are absent and the liver is enlarged, friable and mottled, and penetrated by many small blood-filled channels of liver destruction and these may perforate through the liver capsule producing small, subcapsular hemorrhages. Young flukes may be visible through the capsule. Other acute clostridial infections such as enterotoxemia, blackleg and malignant edema, and also anthrax cause similar heavy mortalities in sheep with a brief period of illness and specific lesions may be sufficient to make a diagnosis possible at necropsy. However, laboratory examination is necessary for a definite diagnosis.

Treatment

No effective treatment is available. In cattle the longer course of the disease suggests the possibility of controlling the clostridial infection by the parenteral use of penicillin or wide-spectrum antibiotics.

Control

Control of the disease can be effected by control of the liver fluke. The host snail must be destroyed in streams and marshes by the use of a molluscicide and the flukes eliminated from the sheep by treatment with carbon tetrachloride or other drug. Pasture contamination from cadavers should be minimized by burning the carcasses.

Vaccination with an alum-precipitated toxoid is highly effective and can be carried out during the course of an outbreak. The mortality begins to subside within 2 weeks. On an affected farm the initial vaccination is followed by a second vaccination 1 month later and subsequently by annual vaccinations. To provide maximum immunity at the time when the disease is most likely to occur, vaccination as a prophylactic measure should be carried out in early summer. A single vaccination of toxoid has also been reported to give lifelong immunity (20).

REVIEW LITERATURE

Bagadi, H. O. (1974) Infectious necrotic hepatitis (black disease) of sheep. *Vet. Bull.*, *44*, 385.

REFERENCES

(1) Bagadi, H. O. & Sewell, M. M. H. (1974) *Res. vet. Sci.*, *17*, 179.
(2) Turner, A. W. (1931) *Counc. sci. industr. Res. Aust.*, Pamphlet No. 19.
(3) Hollingsworth, T. C. & Green, V. J. D. (1978) *Aust. vet. J.*, *54*, 48.
(4) Batty, I. et al. (1964) *Vet. Rec.*, 76, 115.
(5) Williams, B. M. (1964) *Vet. Rec.*, 76, 591.
(6) Niilo, L. et al. (1969) *Can. vet. J.*, *10*, 159.
(7) Thomson, R. G. et al. (1968) *Can. vet. J.*, 9, 263.
(8) Osborne, H. G. (1958) *Aust. vet. J.*, *34*, 301.
(9) Wallace, G. V. (1966) *NZ vet. J.*, *14*, 24.
(10) Williams, B. M. (1976) *Br. vet. J.*, *132*, 221.
(11) Bagadi, H. O. & Sewell, M. M. H. (1973) *Res. vet. Sci.*, *15*, 49.

(12) Roberts, R. S. et al. (1970) *Vet. Rec.*, *86*, 628.
(13) Gay, C. C. et al. (1980) *Equ. vet. J.*, *12*, 26.
(14) Bagadi, H. O. & Sewell, M. M. H. (1974) *Res. vet. Sci.*, *17*, 320.
(15) Gee, R. W. (1958) *Aust. vet. J.*, *34*, 352.
(16) Duncan, I. F. (1984) *Aust. vet. J.*, *61*, 272.
(17) Bourne, F. J. & Kerry (1965) *Vet. Rec.*, *77*, 1463.
(18) Ditchfield, J. & Julian, R. J. (1960) *Can. vet. J.*, *1*, 542.
(19) Williams, B. M. (1962) *Vet. Rec.*, *74*, 1536.
(20) Tunnicliff, E. A. (1943) *J. Am. vet. med. Assoc.*, *103*, 368.

Bacillary hemoglobinuria

This acute, highly fatal toxemia of cattle and sheep is characterized clinically by a high fever, hemoglobinuria and jaundice, and by the presence of necrotic infarcts in the liver.

Etiology

Cl. hemolyticum (*Cl. novyi* type D), a soil-borne anaerobe, is present in the lesions. Cultures of the organism produce severe muscle necrosis and hemoglobinuria when injected intramuscularly into cattle and experimental animals. In infected areas the organism is often found in the livers of healthy cattle. The high incidence on irrigated pasture suggests an environmental precipitating cause. Telangiectasis, necrobacillosis caused by *Fusobacterium necrophorum* and fascioliasis have been suggested as precipitating causes but evidence on this point is incomplete (1, 2). The disease has been produced experimentally by infecting calves orally and precipitating a clostridial toxemia by carrying out liver biopsy (3), or by implanting the organism in the liver (4, 8).

Cl. hemolyticum is serologically identifiable by an agglutination reaction between specific antiserum and young cultures of the organism. However, antigenically similar but less virulent organisms may produce a positive agglutination test and a positive reaction is not proof of the presence of the disease. Immunity appears to develop as a result of subclinical infection or continued exposure under field conditions.

Epidemiology

As is the case in many clostridial diseases, animals in good condition are more susceptible. The longevity of the spores in soil is unknown but the isolation of the organism from bones at least a year after the death of an animal from bacillary hemoglobinuria has been reported (5).

The disease is spread from infected to non-infected areas by flooding, natural drainage, by contaminated hay from infected areas or by carrier animals. The carriage of bones or meat by dogs or other carnivores could also effect spread of the infection. Contamination of pasture may occur from feces or from decomposing cadavers. Although attempts to produce the disease by feeding the organism have been unsuccessful it is probable that under natural conditions invasion occurs from the alimentary tract after ingestion of contaminated material. In field outbreaks cattle are the usual species involved although occasional cases occur in sheep and rare cases in pigs. It is a disease of the summer and autumn months.

Bacillary hemoglobinuria has been reported principally from the western part of the United States (6), although the disease has also been observed in the southern states, Mexico, Venezuela, Chile, Turkey (9), Australia (10), New Zealand (11) and Great Britain (12). The disease is not a common one but on infected farms death losses, which are usually less than 5%, may reach as high as 25%. Recovery without treatment is rare. The highest incidence of bacillary hemoglobinuria is on irrigated or poorly drained pasture, especially if the soil is alkaline in reaction (13). Some outbreaks have occurred in feedlots where hay cut from infected fields was fed. The disease is rare on dry, open range country. Heavy mortalities may occur when cattle from an uninfected area are brought on to an infected farm, cases beginning to occur 7–10 days later.

Pathogenesis

As in black disease of sheep the bacteria are carried to the liver and lodge there until damage to the parenchyma of the liver and the resulting hypoxia create conditions suitable for their proliferation. The development of an organized thrombus in a subterminal branch of the portal vein produces the large anemic infarct which is characteristic of the disease. Most of the bacteria are to be found in this infarct and it is presumed that under the anaerobic conditions prevailing there, toxin is elaborated in large amounts and causes the severe toxemia which is the basis of the signs produced. Two toxins, a hemolysin and a necrotizing agent, are formed by the bacterium, the hemolytic agent being responsible for the acute hemolytic anemia which develops (1). In the later stages bacteremia also develops and, combined with the anoxia resulting from the severe hemolysis, results in endothelial damage, and extravasations of blood into the tissues, and plasma into serous cavities (14).

Clinical findings

The experimental disease occurs as early as 15 hours following the intramuscular injection of cultures. When animals are brought into contact with the infection in the field, losses seldom start until 7–10 days later. The illness is of short duration and cattle at pasture may be found dead without signs having been observed. More often there is a sudden onset, with complete cessation of rumination, feeding, lactation and defecation. Abdominal pain is evidenced by disinclination to move and an arched-back posture. Grunting may be evident on walking. Respiration is shallow and labored and the pulse is weak and rapid. Fever (39·5–41°C, 103–106°F) is evident in the early stages but the temperature subsides to subnormal before death. Edema of the brisket is a common finding. The feces are dark brown; there may be diarrhea with much mucus and some blood. The urine is dark red. Jaundice is present but is never very obvious. The duration of the illness varies from 12 hours in dairy cows in advanced pregnancy, to 4 days in dry stock. Pregnant cows often abort. Severe dyspnea is evident just before death.

Clinical pathology

The red color of the urine is due to the presence of hemoglobin: there are no free red cells. In the later stages the blood is thin, the erythrocyte count being depressed to between 1 and 4 million/mm^3 and the hemoglobin to 3–8 g/dl. Leukocyte counts vary considerably from 6700 to 34 800/mm^3. Differential counts vary similarly with a tendency to neutrophilia in severe cases. Serum calcium and phosphorus levels are normal but blood glucose levels may be elevated (100–120 mg/dl) in some cases.

Blood cultures during the acute stages of the disease may be positive. Serum agglutinins against *Cl. hemolyticum* may be detectable at low levels (1:25 or 1:50) during the clinical illness and if the animal recovers rise to appreciable levels (1:50 to 1:800) a week later. Titers greater than 1:400 are usual at this time. As pointed out previously a positive agglutination test is not conclusive evidence of the presence of the disease.

Necropsy findings

Rigor mortis develops quickly. The perineum is soiled with bloodstained urine and feces. Subcutaneous, gelatinous edema which tends to become crepitant in a few hours, and extensive petechial or diffuse hemorrhages in subcutaneous tissue are characteristic. There is a variable degree of jaundice. Excessive amounts of fluid, varying from clear to bloodstained and turbid, are present in the pleural, pericardial and peritoneal cavities. Generalized subserous hemorrhages are also present. Similar hemorrhages appear under the endocardium. Hemorrhagic abomasitis and enteritis are accompanied by the presence of bloodstained ingesta or free blood. The characteristic lesion of bacillary hemoglobinuria is an anemic infarct in the liver. One or more may be present in any part of the organ and vary from 5 to 20 cm in diameter. The infarct is pale, surrounded by a zone of hyperemia and has the general appearance of local necrosis. Red urine is present in the kidneys and bladder and petechiation is evident throughout the kidney.

Cl. hemolyticum can be isolated from heart blood, the liver infarct and many other organs from a fresh carcass although postmortem invaders quickly obscure its presence.

Diagnosis

The diagnosis of bacillary hemoglobinuria is largely a question of differentiation from other diseases in which hemoglobinuria, myoglobinuria and hematuria are cardinal signs. Acute leptospirosis is likely to occur under the same environmental conditions and present a similar clinical picture. Necropsy findings will differentiate the two and clinical pathology may help but in acute outbreaks it may be impossible to make a positive clinical diagnosis in time to save individual animals. Postparturient hemoglobinuria, hemolytic anemia caused by cruciferous plants including rape, kale and *chou moellier* are not accompanied by a severe febrile reaction. Babesiosis and anaplasmosis are geographically limited and the causative protozoa are detectable in blood smears. The course of all the above diseases may be as short as that of bacillary hemoglobinuria.

Enzootic hematuria, pyelonephritis and cystitis are recognizable by the presence of red cells in the urine. In sheep chronic copper poisoning presents a clinical picture similar to that of bacillary hemoglobinuria but there are no infarcts in the liver. Other causes of sudden death in cattle and sheep including anthrax, blackleg and infectious necrotic hepatitis may confuse the diagnosis especially if terminal hematuria occurs.

Treatment

Specific treatment includes the immediate use of penicillin or tetracyclines in full doses and antitoxic serum (500–1000 ml). Prompt treatment is essential and provided the serum is administered in the early stages of the disease, hemoglobinuria may disappear within 12 hours. Supportive treatment, including blood transfusion, parenteral fluid and electrolyte solutions, is of considerable importance. Care is required during treatment and examination as undue excitement or exercise may cause sudden death. Bulls should not be used for service until at least 3 weeks after recovery because of the danger of liver rupture. Convalescence is often prolonged and animals should be protected from nutritional and climatic stress until they are fully recovered. Hemopoiesis should be facilitated by the provision of mineral supplements containing iron, copper and cobalt.

Control

It has been the practice to use a formalin-killed whole culture adsorbed on aluminum hydroxide which gives good protection for a year in cattle. Vaccination is carried out 4–6 weeks before the expected occurrence of the disease. Annual revaccination of all animals over 6 months of age is necessary in enzootic areas. In some locations of extreme risk a second vaccination during the grazing season is recommended. To obviate the local reaction which occurs at the site of injection the inoculum may be administered at several sites and distributed under the skin by massage. The injection must be subcutaneous, as intradermal and intramuscular injections are likely to produce severe reactions. Modern vaccines prepared so as to avoid these local reactions, lack immunogenicity and require to be administered twice a year (7). In the absence of a type-specific vaccine the use of black disease vaccine appears to be a satisfactory alternative. The carcasses of animals dying of the disease should be disposed of by burning or deep burial.

REFERENCES

(1) Orr, J. P. et al. (1982) *Can. vet. J.*, *23*, 177.
(2) Smith, L. D. S. (1957) *Adv. vet. Sci.*, *3*, 465.
(3) Olander, H. J. et al. (1966) *Pathol. vet.*, *3*, 421.
(4) Joa, R. & Cabrera, J. (1981) *Rev. Salud Anim.*, *3*, 55.
(5) Jasmin, A. M. (1947) *Am. J. vet. Res.*, *8*, 341.
(6) Records, E. & Vawter, L. R. (1945) *Bull. Nev. agric. Exp. Stn*, *173*, 9.
(7) Lozano, E. A. (1981) *Am. J. vet. Res.*, *42*, 1641.
(8) Erwin, B. G. (1977) *Am J. vet. Res.*, *38*, 1625.
(9) Gurturk, S. (1952) *Z. ImmunForsch. exp. Therap.*, *109*, 462.
(10) Wellington, N. A. M. & Perceval, A. (1966) *Aust. vet. J.*, *42*, 128.
(11) Quinlivan, T. D. & Wedderburn, J. F. (1959) *NZ vet. J.*, *7*, 113, 115.
(12) Soltys, M. A. & Jennings, A. R. (1950) *Vet. Rec.*, *62*, 5.
(13) van Ness, G. B. & Erickson, K. (1964) *J. Am. vet. med. Assoc.*, *144*, 492.
(14) Williams, B. M. (1964) *Vet. Rec.*, *76*, 591.

Enterotoxemia caused by *Clostridium perfringens* type A

The role of *Cl. perfringens* type A in the pathogenesis of diseases of animals is uncertain because the organism forms part of the bacterial flora of the alimentary tract in many normal animals. However, there are isolated reports of mortalities caused by the organism. There are reports of a highly fatal hemolytic disease in sheep and cattle in Australia (1) and in lambs in California (2). An acute hemorrhagic enteritis in calves and adult cattle (4) has been recorded in the United Kingdom. There is also an equine intestinal clostridiosis which is characterized by an acute profuse watery diarrhea and high mortality in adult horses. There is hemorrhagic cecitis and colitis similar to colitis-X (5).

In the hemolytic disease there is an acute onset of severe depression, collapse, mucosal pallor, jaundice, hemoglobinuria and dyspnea. Temperatures range from normal to 41°C (106°F). The disease is highly fatal, most affected animals dying within 12 hours of the onset of illness although occasional animals survive for several days. Large numbers of colonies of *Cl. perfringens* in fecal cultures are thought to provide a positive diagnosis of the disease in horses (3, 5), and the presence of the specific toxin in feces is also used to make presumptive diagnoses (1). At necropsy the cardinal features are pallor, jaundice and hemoglobinuria. The kidneys are swollen, dark brown in color and may contain infarcts; the liver is pale and swollen and there may be hydropericardium and pulmonary edema. Clostridia dominate the bacterial population of the small intestine as indicated by smears made from the contents and alpha toxin is present in large quantities. The toxin is a lecithinase and is actively hemolytic, and its presence in large quantities in the intestine is indicative of the existence of the disease. The syndrome is very similar to that caused by chronic copper poisoning and leptospirosis in calves.

In the hemorrhagic enteritis of calves and adult cattle the syndrome observed is indistinguishable from that caused by *Cl. perfringens* types B and C. The disease in adult cattle occurs most commonly in the period shortly after calving. The experimental disease in lambs (6) and calves (7) produced by the intravenous injection of toxin, is characterized by transitory diarrhea and hyperemia of the intestinal mucosa. Type A antiserum has been effective in prevention of the disease in calves and a formalinized vaccine has shown some immunizing capacity in sheep (8).

REFERENCES

(1) Senf, W. (1983) *Mh. Vet. Med.*, *38*, 528.
(2) McGowan, B. et al. (1958) *J. Am. vet. med. Assoc.*, *133*, 219.
(3) Wierup, M. & DiPietro, J. A. (1981) *Am. J. vet. Res.*, *42*, 2167.
(4) Shirley, G. N. (1958) *Vet. Rec.*, *70*, 478.
(5) Wierup, M. (1977) *Acta vet. Scand.*, Suppl. *62*, 1.
(6) Niilo, L. (1971) *Infect. Immun.* *3*, 100.
(7) Niilo, L. (1973) *J. comp. Pathol.*, *83*, 265.
(8) Niilo, L. et al. (1971) *Can. J. Microbiol.*, *17*, 391.

Enterotoxemia caused by *Clostridium perfringens* types B, C and E

Infection with *Cl. perfringens* types B and C results in severe enteritis with diarrhea and dysentery in young lambs, calves, pigs and foals. A number of diseases caused by these clostridia occur in different parts of the world and are given specific names but are dealt with here as a group. They include lamb dysentery (*Cl. perfringens* type B), struck (*Cl. perfringens* type C), and hemorrhagic enterotoxemia (*Cl. perfringens* type C). Necrotic hemorrhagic enteritis due to *Cl. perfringens* type E has been recorded in calves (1).

Etiology

The causative clostridia occur commonly in soil and the alimentary tract of normal animals, and, as in enterotoxemia caused by *Cl. perfringens* type D, the disease appears to be precipitated by factors still incompletely understood. The bacteria are capable of forming spores which survive for long periods in soil. In general rapidly growing, well-nourished animals are most susceptible.

The diseases as they occur in the different animal species are as follows:

- *Lamb dysentery* caused by *Cl. perfringens* type B occurs in young lambs up to 3 weeks of age. An enterotoxemia of young lambs may also be caused by *Cl. perfringens* type C (2)
- *Struck* (3) caused by *Cl. perfringens* type C affects adult sheep, particularly when feed is abundant
- *Goat enterotoxemia* has been caused by *Cl. perfringens* type C (4)
- *Calf enterotoxemia* caused by *Cl. perfringens* types B and C (6) occurs in young calves up to 10 days of age
- *Pig enterotoxemia* caused by *Cl. perfringens* type C is recorded in sucking pigs during the first week of life (10, 11) and has been produced experimentally by feeding whole cultures of *Cl. perfringens* type C (7, 12)
- *Foal enterotoxemia* caused by *Cl. perfringens* (type C) (8, 12) and type B has occurred in foals within the first few days of life (5).

Epidemiology

Enterotoxemia caused by *Cl. perfringens* type B is encountered only sporadically except for lamb dysentery which occurs fairly extensively in Britain, Europe and South Africa. In affected groups of lambs, the morbidity may reach as high as 20–30%. A characteristic of the disease is the tendency for the morbidity rate on infected farms to increase year by year and to affect older lambs up to 2–3 weeks of age. The mortality rate approaches 100%. Lamb dysentery is most prevalent in cold weather and on farms where ewes are kept closely confined in small yards or fields for lambing. Gross contamination of the surroundings with the causative bacteria is likely to occur in these circumstances. Hemorrhagic enterotoxemia caused by *Cl. perfringens* type C has been reported most commonly from certain areas in the United States and Britain. Struck is limited in its occurrence to certain localities in Britain. In all species, these diseases are likely to occur in outbreaks affecting a number of animals and death losses are high. Outbreaks in pigs usually affect most susceptible litters on the farm and the majority of pigs in each litter are affected.

The organisms occur in the feces of infected animals and contamination of the soil and pasture is followed by ingestion of the bacteria. The toxins produced are *alpha*, *beta* and *epsilon* in type B, and *alpha* and *beta* in type C. In pigs the organisms are recoverable from the skin of sows and the feces of affected piglets and infection probably occurs during suckling (10). The predominance of these diseases in very young animals may be due to the immaturity of their alimentary tracts, the beta-toxin being readily inactivated by trypsin. It is probable that many animals become infected but do not show clinical illness as antitoxin has been detected in clinically normal animals (9).

Pathogenesis

The characteristic effect of the beta-toxin, the important toxin produced by *Cl. perfringens* types B and C, is the production of hemorrhagic enteritis and ulceration of the intestinal mucosa (14). Even in non-immune animals protection is provided by the presence of pancreatic proteases in the intestine which digest the toxin. These are decreased or absent in affected swine (15). Experimentally administered soybean flour used as a protease inhibitor converts experimentally induced clostridial enteritis from a non-fatal to a fatal disease.

Clinical findings

Lamb dysentery usually occurs in lambs less than 2 weeks old and is manifested by sudden death without premonitory signs in peracute cases. In the more common acute form, there is severe abdominal pain, recumbency, failure to suck and the passing of brown, fluid feces sometimes containing blood. Death usually occurs after a period of coma and within 24 hours of the onset of illness. On farms where the disease has become established, cases may occur in older lambs up to 3 weeks of age and occasional cases may survive for several days.

Struck in adult sheep is manifested only by sudden death, clinical signs not being observed beforehand. Occasionally death is preceded by abdominal pain and convulsions.

In calves, the disease usually occurs as outbreaks of severe dysentery with some deaths in calves 7–10 days old although calves up to 10 weeks of age may be affected. The signs include diarrhea, dysentery and acute abdominal pain accompanied by violent bellowing and aimless running. There may be additional nervous signs including tetany and opisthotonus. In very acute cases, death occurs in a few hours, sometimes without diarrhea being evident. In less severe cases, the illness lasts for about 4 days and recovery is slow, usually requiring 10–14 days.

Affected pigs are normal at birth but become dull and depressed and exhibit diarrhea, dysentery and gross reddening of the anus. Most affected pigs die within 24 hours. Frequently the majority of litters born during an outbreak will be affected although affected litters may include some normal pigs. The disease tends to recur on the same premises in succeeding years (16). Occasionally weaned pigs are affected. Foals usually show severe depression, abdominal pain, diarrhea and dysentery, and die within a few hours. In both piglets and foals, the disease occurs in the first few days of life. Affected foals are a few days old and have an acute attack of collapse with bloody feces, subnormal temperature, fast pulse and respiratory rate and death within a few hours (12). Colic may be evident (18).

The disease is a toxemia and there is usually no fever in any of the species.

Clinical pathology

The disease in all species is so acute and highly fatal that the diagnosis is usually made on necropsy material. Antemortem laboratory examinations are not widely used in diagnosis but the predominance of clostridia in a fecal smear may suggest a diagnosis of hemorrhagic enterotoxemia. Specific antitoxins are detectable in the sera of recovered animals, an ELISA test being most favored. A severe hypoglycemia has been observed in baby pigs dying of the disease but this is not specific in this infection.

Necropsy findings

A hemorrhagic enteritis, with ulceration of the mucosa in some cases, is the major lesion in all species (18). The intestinal mucosa is congested and dark red, and the ulcers are large (2·5 cm in diameter) and penetrate almost to the serosa. The lesions are usually most severe in the ileum. Bloodstained contents are present in the intestine and there is an excess of serous fluid in the peritoneal cavity. Subendocardial and subepicardial hemorrhages are often present. In sheep affected with struck, in addition to the above lesions there is often peritonitis and the skeletal muscles have the appearance of malignant edema if necropsy is delayed for several hours. In pigs in the 7–10 days age group, in which the disease is less acute than in newborn pigs, the hemorrhagic enteritis is not so evident, the major lesion being a yellow, fibrinous deposit on the intestinal mucosa accompanied by large quantities of watery, lightly bloodstained ingesta in the lumen.

A portion of small intestine with its contents is suitable for laboratory diagnosis. Smears of intestinal contents can be stained and examined for large numbers of clostridia, and filtrates of the contents tested for toxin content. Cultural examination of the ingesta may also be attempted.

Diagnosis

The early age at which this disease occurs, the rapid course and typical necropsy findings suggest the diagnosis, which can be readily confirmed by laboratory examination. Other acute diseases of newborn animals which may be confused with lamb dysentery and hemorrhagic enterotoxemia include particularly enteritis and septicemia caused by *Escherichia coli* and *Salmonella* spp., *Actinobacillus equuli* and porcine transmissible gastroenteritis. In most instances, it is necessary to confirm the diagnosis of these diseases by laboratory examination of fecal material or intestinal contents collected at necropsy. Struck is strictly regional in distribution and in affected areas can usually be diagnosed on the basis of necropsy lesions.

Treatment

Hyperimmune antiserum is the only treatment likely to be of value. Doses of 25 ml of type C antiserum have been used successfully in calves (9) but in other species death usually occurs too quickly for treatment to be effective. Oral administration of penicillin may prevent further proliferation of organisms and production of toxins. Chelating agents as described in the section on enterotoxemia may offer some promise in treatment.

Control

Vaccination, preferably with type-specific toxoid or bacterin, is the only preventive measure available. Because of the need for rapid action, it is usually necessary to proceed with vaccination before typing of the organism can be carried out. Cross-protection occurs between *Cl. perfringens* types B and C because of the importance of beta-toxin in both strains, and the efficiency of lamb dysentery antiserum in protection against type C infections has been recorded. Type C toxoid and antiserum are also available (13).

When an outbreak occurs, active vaccination may be impracticable because of the acute nature of the disease and the immaturity of the exposed animals. Antiserum will protect susceptible animals and should be administered immediately after birth. When the disease is enzootic in a herd, vaccination of the dams should be carried out. To initiate the program two injections of vaccine are necessary 1 month apart, the second injection being given 2 weeks before parturition. For the prevention of lamb dysentery the two vaccinations of ewes may be spaced from 2 to 5 weeks apart and the second injection can be given as early as 2 months before lambing, thus avoiding handling of heavily pregnant ewes (19). In subsequent years, cows and ewes require only one booster injection immediately prior to parturition. For the protection of piglets two sow vaccinations 5 and 3 weeks before farrowing are used (7), but vaccination at mating and repeated 2–3 weeks before farrowing is adequate (9). With the use of clostridial toxoids and antisera, attention should be given to the unitage of the antigen or antitoxin present in the preparation used. These vary widely and the manufacturer's instructions should be followed closely. Anaphylaxis may occur because of the equine origin of the antisera and treated animals should be kept under close observation for 24 hours and treated quickly if signs of dyspnea and muscle shivering occur.

REFERENCES

(1) Hart, B. & Hooper, P. T. (1967) *Aust. vet. J.*, *43*, 360.
(2) Griner, L. A. & Johnson, H. W. (1954) *J. Am. vet. med. Assoc.*, *125*, 125.
(3) Jayaraman, M. S. et al. (1972) *Ind. vet. J.*, *49*, 357, 1075.
(4) Barron, N. S. (1942) *Vet. Rec.*, *54*, 82.
(5) Dickie, C. W. et al. (1978) *J. Am. vet. med. Assoc.*, *173*, 306.
(6) Niilo, L. et al. (1974) *Can. vet. J.*, *15*, 224.
(7) Kohler, B. et al. (1978) *Arch. exp. Vet. Med.*, *32*, 69 & 841, and *33*, 313, 595 & 621.
(8) Sims, L. D. et al. (1985) *Aust. vet. J.*, *62*, 194.
(9) Ripley, P. H. & Gush, A. F. (1983) *Vet. Rec.*, *112*, 201.
(10) Azuma, R. et al. (1983) *Jap. J. vet. Sci.*, *45*, 135.
(11) Högh, P. (1969) *Acta vet. Scand.*, *10*, 57, 84.
(12) Pearson, E. G. et al. (1986) *J. Am. vet. med. Assoc.*, *188*, 1309.
(13) Kennedy, K. K. et al. (1977) *Vet. Med. SAC*, *72*, 1213.
(14) Niilo, L. (1986) *Can. J. vet. Res.*, *50*, 32.
(15) Bergeland, M. E. (1972) *J. Am. vet. med. Assoc.*, *160*, 568.
(16) Boon, H. W. & Bergeland, M. E. (1965) *Can. vet. J.*, *6*, 159.
(17) Niilo, L. & Cho, H. J. (1984) *Can. J. comp. Med.*, *48*, 111.
(18) Howard-Martin, M. et al. (1986) *J. Am. vet. med. Assoc.*, *189*, 564.
(19) Jansen, B. C. (1961) *Onderstepoort J. vet. Res.*, *28*, 495.

Enterotoxemia caused by *Clostridium perfringens* type D (pulpy kidney)

This is an acute toxemia of ruminants caused by the proliferation of *Cl. perfringens* type D in the intestines and the liberation of toxins. Clinically the disease is characterized by diarrhea, convulsions, paralysis and sudden death.

Etiology

Enterotoxemia is not a contagious disease in that the presence of the causative bacteria, *Cl. perfringens* type D, in the intestine does not in itself produce the disease. Under natural conditions the ingestion of feed contaminated by infected feces introduces the organism into the alimentary tract but the disease does not occur unless other factors intercede.

Epidemiology

Clostridium perfringens type D normally inhabits the alimentary tract of sheep (1) and probably other ruminants but only in small numbers. The extent to which it occurs in the alimentary tract varies widely between flocks, although this accounts only in part for the variable incidence. The organism does not persist for very long in the soil. Under certain conditions, the organisms proliferate rapidly in the intestines and produce lethal quantities of toxin (1). The husbandry conditions in which the disease occurs include grazing on lush, rapidly growing pasture or young cereal crops, and heavy grain feeding in feedlots. Lambs on well-fed heavy-milking ewes are particularly susceptible. The high incidence under these conditions has given rise to the name of 'overeating' disease. An increased incidence of the disease has been reported after dosing with phenothiazine and experimental evidence suggests that such dosing may precipitate outbreaks in lambs (2). The disease can be produced experimentally in susceptible sheep and cattle by the injection into the duodenum of whole culture of *Cl. perfringens* type D and dextrin (3, 4).

While enterotoxemia is most common in lambs it also occurs in adult sheep, in goats (5, 6), in calves (7–9) and rarely in adult cattle (10, 11) and domesticated camels. In most, if not all circumstances, the affected animals are on highly nutritious diets and are in very good condition. The highest incidence of the disease is in sucking lambs between 3 and 10 weeks of age and single lambs are more susceptible than twins. Feeder lambs are most commonly affected soon after they are introduced into feedlots. Immunity is readily produced by suitable vaccination and a degree of natural immunity may be attained by non-lethal exposure to the toxin (12). A blood level of 0·15 Wellcome unit of epsilon antitoxin per ml of serum is sufficient to protect sheep against further doses of toxin (3).

Enterotoxemia caused by *Cl. perfringens* type D is worldwide in its distribution principally as a disease of lambs. It causes heavy losses particularly in flocks managed for lamb and mutton production. In North America it ranks as one of the main causes of loss among feedlot lambs. Morbidity rates vary a great deal but seldom exceed 10%. The mortality rate approximates

100%. A proportion of lambs and calves appear to be exposed to subclinical but antigenic levels of *Cl. perfringens* toxin so that they become immune without having shown signs of illness or without having been vaccinated (13). It is a common belief among cattlemen and veterinarians that many unexplained sudden deaths in feedlot cattle are due to this type of enterotoxemia. However, there is no laboratory evidence to support such field observations.

Pathogenesis

In the normal course of events, ingested *Cl. perfringens* type D are destroyed in large numbers in the rumen and abomasum although some survive to reach the duodenum where multiplication occurs and toxin is produced. Toxemia does not occur because the movement of ingesta keeps the bacterial population and toxin content down to a low level. In certain circumstances, this does not hold and multiplication of the organisms and the production of toxin proceeds to the point where toxemia occurs. One of the circumstances has been shown to be the passage of large quantities of starch granules into the duodenum when sheep overeat on grain diets or are changed suddenly from a ration consisting largely of roughage to one consisting mainly of grain (14). Other factors such as heavy milk feeding may have the same effect. A slowing of alimentary tract movement has also been thought to permit excess toxin accumulation (15) and it may be that any factor which causes intestinal stasis will predispose to the disease. The importance of diet in the production of ruminal stasis has been discussed in diseases of the forestomachs of ruminants. In a number of instances outbreaks have followed the administration of phenothiazine. A high incidence has been observed in association with heavy tapeworm infestation (16).

The epsilon-toxin of *Cl. perfringens* type D increases the permeability of the intestinal mucosa to this and other toxins, thereby facilitating its own absorption (17). The first effect of the toxin is to cause a profuse, mucoid diarrhea, and secondarily, to produce a stimulation and then depression of the central nervous system. In sheep, acute cases are characterized by the development in the brain of degeneration of vascular endothelium, perivascular and intercellular edema and microscopic foci of necrosis in the basal ganglia, thalamus, internal capsule, substantia nigra, subcortical white matter and cerebellum (18). The situation of the lesions is similar to those which can be seen macroscopically in the brains of sheep affected by focal symmetrical encephalomalacia, a disease thought to be a sequel to enterotoxemia. Most of the clinical and pathological findings in enterotoxemia due to *Cl. perfringens* type D endotoxin are explainable in terms of the observed widespread vascular damage (19). There is a severe hyperglycemia due to depletion of hepatic stores, severe hemoconcentration, and elevation of blood concentrations of pyruvate, lactate and alpha-ketoglutarate. The damage to the vascular endothelium leads to the accumulation of protein-rich fluid effusions observable in heart, brain and lung. The post-mortem autolysis of kidney tissue which occurs so rapidly, and is the characteristic of 'pulpy kidney', has the same basis.

Clinical findings

In lambs, the course of the illness is very short, often less than 2 hours and never more than 12 hours, and many are found dead without previously manifesting signs. In closely observed flocks the first signs may be dullness, depression, yawning, facial movements and loss of interest in feed. Acute cases may show little more than severe clonic convulsions with frothing at the mouth and sudden death. Cases which survive for a few hours show a green, pasty diarrhea, staggering, recumbency, opisthotonus and severe clonic convulsions. The temperature is usually normal but may be elevated if convulsions are severe. Death occurs during a convulsion or after a short period of coma.

Adult sheep usually survive for longer periods, up to 24 hours. They lag behind the flock, show staggering and knuckling, champing of the jaws, salivation and rapid, shallow, irregular respiration. There may be bloat in the terminal stages. Irritation signs, including convulsions, muscle tremor, grinding of the teeth and salivation, may occur but are less common than in lambs.

In calves the syndrome is similar to that seen in adult sheep, with nervous signs predominating. Peracute cases are found dead without having shown premonitory signs of illness and with no evidence of struggling. The more common, acute cases show a sudden onset of bellowing, mania and convulsions, the convulsions persisting until death occurs 1–2 hours later. Subacute cases, many of which recover, do not drink, are quiet and docile and appear to be blind, although the eyes preservation reflex persists. They may continue in this state for 2–3 days and then recover quickly and completely. In an outbreak of the disease in calves all three forms of the disease may be seen. Diarrhea is a prominent sign in affected goats especially in those which survive for more than a few days (20). In acute cases, there are convulsions after an initial attack of fever (40·5°C, 105°F) with severe abdominal pain and dysentery, and death occurs in 4–36 hours. In subacute cases, the goats may be ill for several weeks and show anorexia, intermittent severe diarrhea and, in some cases, dysentery and the presence of epithelial shreds in the feces. Chronic cases manifested by emaciation, anemia and chronic diarrhea are also recorded in goats.

Clinical pathology

A high blood sugar level of 150–200 mg/dl and marked glycosuria are characteristic of the terminal stages of enterotoxemia in sheep (21). However, similar observations can be made in sheep dying of a number of diseases, especially when there is hepatic injury. The detection of large numbers of clostridia or specific toxins in the feces of suspected cases is also used to make presumptive diagnoses (22).

Necropsy findings

The carcass is usually in good condition. In peracute cases there may be no gross lesions. More frequently there is an excess of clear, straw-colored pericardial fluid and many petechiae are present in the epicardium and endocardium. Patchy congestion of the abomasal and intestinal mucosae is characteristic and the intestine usually contains a moderate amount of thin, custardy ingesta. If the examination is delayed for a few hours, there is rapid decomposition, purple discoloration of the woolless skin, and the wool is easily plucked. A characteristic change is the presence of soft, pulpy kidneys a few hours after death. The liver is dark and congested and the pericardial fluid may be gelatinous and blood-stained. The rumen and abomasum of feedlot lambs may be overloaded with concentrates. In goats there is acute hemorrhagic inflammation of the mucosae of the omasum and small intestine (23). In sheep that have not died acutely there may be brain lesions. These are characteristically symmetrical areas of hemorrhage, edema and liquefaction, especially in the area of the basal ganglia. Inclusion of the brain in the specimens submitted can be very helpful.

Smears of ingesta should be taken from several levels in the small intestine and stained to determine the presence of Gram-positive rods. In affected animals the short, fat, Gram-positive rods dominate the slide to the almost complete exclusion of other bacteria. Attempts should be made to isolate the clostridia by cultural means and bowel filtrates should be tested for toxicity by injection into mice. If the filtrate is toxic, the type of toxin can be determined by protection of the mice with specific antisera but this does not determine the type of clostridia. The presence of beta-toxin indicates the presence of types B and C and epsilon-toxin the presence of B or D. Final identification depends upon agglutination tests with specific antisera (24). Intestinal contents to be examined for the presence of toxin should be milked out into a glass container, not left in a loop of intestine. At average temperatures one can expect to be able to isolate the toxin from the intestine of a sheep dead for up to 12 hours. The addition of one drop of chloroform to each 10 ml of ingesta will stabilize the toxin for periods of up to a month (22). Hyperglycemia and glycosuria may also be detected in necropsy material.

Diagnosis

In lambs, the circumstances and the clinical and necropsy findings are diagnostic. Other causes of sudden death in lambs include acute pasteurellosis, hypocalcemia with hypomagnesemia, and septicemia caused by *Hemophilus agni*. Focal symmetrical encephalomalacia, which may be a chronic form of enterotoxemia, is accompanied by blindness, incoordination and paralysis. In live animals, enterotoxemia may be confused with polioencephalomalacia in which the syndrome is similar but less acute and the course longer. There is no hyperglycemia or glycosuria. Acute rumen impaction due to overeating may occur in the same circumstances but there are no convulsions or glycosuria although the animals may be recumbent. The course in acute ruminal impaction is much longer (1–3 days) than in enterotoxemia (about 1 hour). In adult sheep and calves, the syndrome is readily confused with rabies, acute lead poisoning, hypomagnesemic tetany, pregnancy toxemia or louping-ill. Clinically there may be little difference between these diseases although generally they are less acute and are not restricted to lambs. The history should be examined carefully. In rabies, there is usually a history of exposure; in acute lead poisoning access to toxic material should be evident; pregnancy toxemia occurs only in late pregnancy in ewes on a falling plane of nutrition, and louping-ill has a seasonal occurrence related to the activities of the vector ticks. Biochemical tests are of value in determining the presence of ketonuria in pregnancy toxemia and the hypomagnesemia of hypomagnesemic tetany. Chemical tests of feces, urine and blood aid in the diagnosis of lead poisoning.

The disease is rare in adult cattle.

Treatment

Hyperimmune serum is an efficient short-term prophylactic but is unlikely to be of much value in sick animals because of the acute nature of the disease, although serum (50 ml twice daily) combined with orally administered sulfadimidine is reported to be effective in goats (20). Chelating agents are highly effective in neutralizing the toxins of *Cl. perfringens* in experimental animals. The mode of action is the temporary removal of metallic ions necessary for toxin activity. The toxins are capable of causing irreversible effects and the chelating compounds must be given soon after the administration of the toxin (25).

Control

There are two major control measures available, reduction of the food intake and vaccination. Vaccination is highly effective but not completely so and it is often necessary to reduce the food intake if best results are to be obtained (26). This will cause a setback in the growth of the lambs and for this reason farmers tend to rely more on vaccination as a control measure. The best advice is to both adjust the food intake and vaccinate, but to avoid interference with growth as much as possible.

Vaccination

Alum-precipitated, formalin-killed, whole culture (anaculture) is in general use but a similar vaccine activated by trypsin (activated alum-precipitated toxoid) is thought to give better results (27). All vaccines in current use are alum-precipitated but the advantage gained by alum precipitation has been questioned (29). Many multiple vaccines are in use and the latest variation in the battle of vaccination against clostridia is the use of combined vaccines suspended in oil-water emulsions (30) and injected intraperitoneally. The vehicle ensures a continuing high level of antibodies, the route avoids local lesions in muscle. Single injections of individual toxins in Freund adjuvant give protection for as long as 2 years (31). The simultaneous administration of enterotoxemia vaccine by injection and vitamin E by mouth or injection greatly increases the immune response to the vaccination (28).

Activated alum-precipitated toxoid is used in the same manner but smaller doses are required (2 ml as against 5 ml) and the response to vaccination in young lambs immunized passively via the ewe is better (32). The standard anaculture produces no immunity in very young lambs but the activated toxoid administered when the lambs are 3 days old produces good immunity, although a second injection at 1 month of age is recommended (27). The simultaneous administration of hyperimmune serum with this vaccine does not interfere with the stimulation of antibody production. Revaccination at 6-monthly intervals provides permanent protection. Sheep vaccinated for three consecutive years can be considered to be permanently immune and to require no further vaccination (33).

The recommended vaccination program for fat lamb flocks which are exposed to maximum risk is as follows (34). If an outbreak occurs administer antiserum and toxoid (preferably the activated alum-precipitated product) immediately and repeat the toxoid in a month's time. Revaccinate breeding ewes with toxoid at 6-month intervals thereafter attempting to time one of the two annual injections to fall during the penultimate month of pregnancy. The lambs will derive passive immunity from the colostrum but should be vaccinated with toxoid when 4–10 weeks of age and again a month later. If a vaccination program is initiated at a time other than when an outbreak is in progress the initial injection of antitoxin can be omitted. Most vaccination programs fall far short of this ideal and recommendations need to be adapted to suit local conditions of economy and degree of risk; for example, in New Zealand vaccination of the ewes before lambing is often sufficient to protect fat lambs through to sale time (35). In areas where the disease occurs only sporadically it is customary to administer serum to all sheep as soon as an outbreak commences. Although the immunity lasts for only 2 weeks further immediate losses are prevented, and in most instances the disease does not recur. Toxoid is cheaper, but to administer it alone at such times may result in further serious losses before active immunity develops.

Any vaccination of sheep is not without danger of precipitating blackleg or other clostridial disease and if these are a severe problem in an area it may be wise to vaccinate a portion of the flock as a pilot test and proceed with vaccination of the remainder only when no complications arise. A multiple vaccine (including toxoids of enterotoxemia, tetanus, blackleg and braxy) is recommended for use in sheep in those circumstances where all of these diseases are likely to occur (36). Effective responses are obtained and the only difficulty is the additional cost (37).

Vaccination with toxoid has been effective in calves (7) but is not highly effective in goats (5, 20) and should be repeated in this species at 6-monthly intervals. The antibody titer is variable and reactions at vaccination sites are often large and longlasting (20). The use of serum must be carried out with caution in goats, particularly Saanens, which are very prone to anaphylactic reactions. Kids should be vaccinated twice, a month apart, commencing at 4 weeks of age. Subsequent vaccinations are at 6-month intervals (38).

REVIEW LITERATURE

Niilo, L. (1980) *Clostridium perfringens* in animal disease. *Can. vet. J.*, *21*, 141.

REFERENCES

(1) Bullen, J. J. (1952) *J. Pathol. Bacteriol.*, *64*, 201.
(2) Jansen, B. C. (1960) *J. S. Afr. vet. med. Assoc.*, *31*, 209.
(3) Jansen, B. C. (1960) *J. S. Afr. vet. med. Assoc.*, *31*, 205.
(4) Niilo, L. et al. (1963) *Can. vet. J.*, *4*, 31, 288.
(5) Oxer, D. T. (1956) *Aust. vet. J.*, *32*, 62.
(6) Wanasingle, D. D. (1973) *Ceylon vet. J.*, *21*, 62.
(7) Blood, D. C. & Helwig, D. M. (1957) *Aust. vet. J.*, *33*, 144.
(8) Griner, L. A. et al. (1956) *J. Am. vet. med. Assoc.*, *129*, 375.
(9) Munday, B. (1973) *Aust. vet. J.*, *49*, 451.
(10) Keast, J. C. & McBarron, E. J. (1954) *Aust. vet. J.*, *30*, 305.
(11) Mumford, D. H. (1961) *Aust. vet. J.*, *37*, 122.
(12) Griner, L. A. (1961) *Am. J. vet. Res.*, *22*, 447.
(13) Griner, L. A. (1963) *Bull. Off. int. Epizoot.*, *59*, 1443.
(14) Bullen, J. J. & Batty, I. (1957) *Vet. Rec.*, *69*, 1268.
(15) Bennetts, H. W. (1932) *Bull. Coun. sci. indust. Res. Melb.*, *57*, 72.
(16) Thomas, P. L. et al. (1956) *NZ vet. J.*, *4*, 161.
(17) Bullen, J. J. & Batty, I. (1957) *J. Pathol. Bacteriol.*, *73*, 511.
(18) Griner, L. A. (1961) *Am. J. vet. Res.*, *22*, 429, 443.
(19) Gardiner, D. E. (1973) *J. comp. Pathol.*, *83*, 499, 509, 525.
(20) Blackwell, T. E. et al. (1988) *Can. J. comp. Med.*, *47*, 127.
(21) Gordon, W. S. et al. (1940) *J. Pathol. Bacteriol.*, *50*, 251.
(22) Senf, W. (1983) *Mh. VetMed.*, *38*, 528.
(23) Winter, J. et al. (1974) *Mh. VetMed.*, *29*, 223.
(24) Frank, F. W. (1956) *Am. J. vet. Res.*, *17*, 492.
(25) Moskowitz, M. (1958) *Nature, Lond.*, *181*, 550.
(26) Whitlock, J. H. & Fabricant, J. (1947) *Cornell Vet.*, *37*, 211.
(27) Cameron, C. M. (1980) *Onderstepoort J. vet. Res.*, *47*, 287.
(28) Tengerdy, R. P. (1983) *Br. vet. J.*, *139*, 147.
(29) Smith, L. D. S. (1957) *Adv. vet. Sci.*, *3*, 465.
(30) Thomson, R. O. et al. (1969) *Vet. Rec.*, *85*, 81, 84.
(31) Jansen, B. C. (1967) *Bull. Off. int. Epizoot.*, *67*, 1539.
(32) Batty, I. et al. (1954) *Vet. Rec.*, *66*, 249.
(33) Jansen, B. C. (1967) *Onderstepoort J. vet. Res.*, *34*, 333.
(34) Montgomerie, R. F. (1960) *Vet. Rec.*, *72*, 995.
(35) Wallace, G. V. (1963) *NZ vet. J.*, *11*, 39.
(36) Hepple, J. R. et al. (1960) *Vet. Rec.*, *72*, 766.
(37) Oxer, D. T. et al. (1971) *Aust. vet. J.*, *47*, 134.
(38) Smith, H. V. & Klose, J. B. (1980) *Vict. vet. Proc.*, *38*, 46.

Focal symmetrical encephalomalacia

Focal symmetrical encephalomalacia is a sporadic disease of sheep in which aimless wandering, an inability to eat and a dummy syndrome are predominant findings. The disease is almost certainly a chronic neurological manifestation of enterotoxemia. However, it is included under separate title as the clinical course and necropsy findings are not those typically associated with enterotoxemia.

Etiology

Lesions of focal symmetrical encephalomalacia have been produced in experimental enterotoxemia and by infusion with epsilon-toxin of *Cl. perfringens* type D (1, 2).

Epidemiology

The disease occurs in lambs, weaners and mature sheep (3–5), and suspected cases have also been reported in calves (1). In grazing sheep it has the same seasonal occurrence as enterotoxemia but may occur in sheep of poor body condition. In weaners and mature sheep there is often a history of a move to fresh pasture or of anthelmintic administration 5–14 days preceding the occurrence of initial cases. Several outbreaks have been associated with the grazing of young green cereal crops (4, 5). The morbidity is usually low but may approach 15%. The case fatality rate is high.

Clinical findings

Most commonly the finding of dead sheep is the first indication of the disease. Clinically affected sheep are separate from the group or can be detected by slow movement of the flock. They show no fear of man or dogs and can be examined without restraint. Blindness, aimless wandering, head-pressing and incoordination are the predominant findings. More severely affected sheep lie quietly in lateral recumbency with moderate dorsiflexion of the head and show infrequent nystagmus with paddling convulsions. The sheep are unable to eat and most cannot drink although some affected lambs may still retain a suck reflex. The feces of affected sheep are unformed, as are those of a significant number of other apparently normal sheep within the group. The clinical course varies from 1 to 14 days with the majority of affected sheep surviving for 5–7 days.

Necropsy findings

Lesions are confined to the brain. In the majority of cases these can be detected on macroscopic examination and consist of areas of hemorrhage and softening in the internal capsule, lateral thalamus and cerebellar peduncles. Glycosuria is not a feature and toxin cannot be demonstrated in gut contents.

Treatment and control

There is no treatment. Less severely affected cases may recover if they are maintained with fluids and nutrients given by stomach tube. Outbreaks cease if the sheep are vaccinated with pulpy kidney vaccine (4, 5).

REFERENCES

(1) Buxton, D. et al. (1981) *Vet. Rec.*, *108*, 459.
(2) Gardner, D. E. (1973) *J. comp. Pathol.*, *83*, 509.
(3) Hartley, W. J. (1956) *NZ vet. J.*, *4*, 129.
(4) Pienaar, J. G. & Thornton, D. J. (1964) *J. S. Afr. vet. med. Assoc.*, *35*, 351.
(5) Gay, C. C. et al. (1975) *Aust. vet. J.*, *51*, 266.

18

Diseases Caused by Bacteria—III

DISEASES CAUSED BY *ESCHERICHIA COLI*

COLIBACILLOSIS occurs in all species of newborn farm animals and is a major cause of losses in this age group. Gut edema, enteric colibacillosis of feeder pigs and mastitis caused by *Escherichia coli* are also important diseases commonly caused by this organism.

Acute undifferentiated diarrhea of newborn farm animals (particularly calves)

Diarrhea in newborn farm animals under 15 days of age is one of the most common diseases which the large animal clinician is faced with in practice. It is a significant cause of economic loss in cattle and swine herds and may assume even greater importance in the future as livestock production becomes more intensified. The effective treatment and control of diarrhea in calves and piglets has been frustrating and usually empirical because the precise etiology cannot usually be determined quickly enough. Field and laboratory investigations have indicated that there is not a single etiology of calf and piglet diarrhea but rather the cause is complex and usually involves an interplay between enteropathogenic bacteria and viruses, the immunity of the animal and the effects of the environment. Thus we use the term *acute undifferentiated diarrhea of newborn calves* to describe the acute diarrhea which occurs in newborn calves usually under 15 days of age, and sometimes older up to 35 days, which is characterized clinically by acute profuse watery diarrhea, progressive dehydration and acidosis and death in a few days or earlier after the onset. On a clinical basis it is not usually possible to differentiate between the common known causes of diarrhea in newborn calves which includes enterotoxigenic *Escherichia coli* (ENTEC), rotavirus, coronavirus, *Cryptosporidia* spp. and *Salmonella* spp. (2). The common pathological lesions are dehydration, emaciation and a fluid-filled intestinal tract with no other obvious gross lesions.

For many years following the early work of Smith and Little in which they indicated that *E. coli* was the causative agent of calf diarrhea, it has been accepted that this was the primary pathogen in diarrheic calves and the term *colibacillosis* has been in common use. We still recognize the existence of colibacillosis in calves, piglets and lambs as a disease, but wish to emphasize that diarrhea in newborn calves, for example, can be caused by many different enteropathogens influenced by several epidemiological factors (Table 49). Thus colibacillosis is presented in its usual section and the viral diarrheas of newborn farm animals has been expanded in the light of new information. The other causes of diarrhea such as *Cryptosporidia* are found in their respective sections. This section outlines the general picture of acute undifferentiated diarrhea of newborn farm animals with emphasis on the disease in calves.

The distribution and occurrence of enteropathogens in the feces of diarrheic and normal healthy calves varies depending on the geographical location, the farm, the age and type of calves being examined and the extent to which the diagnostic laboratory is capable of isolating or demonstrating the pathogens. The relative importance of enteric pathogens affecting neonates of domestic animals has been reviewed (8). The rotavirus, *Cryptosporidium* sp., coronavirus and enterotoxigenic *E. coli* are responsible for 75–95% of infections in neonatal calves worldwide (6, 8). The relative frequency of each of the four differ between locations and between seasons and years (1). Any one of the common pathogens may predominate or be absent in a certain group of animals. The rotavirus will be most common in some groups (8–10, 16), the coronavirus may predominate in beef calves in some countries (13) and not in others (12), and *Cryptosporidium* may occur in 30–50% of diarrheic calves on a worldwide basis (8). In some countries, enterotoxigenic K99^{+} *E. coli* may occur in 30–40% of diarrheic calves (8) while in the United Kingdom the incidence may be as low as 3–6% (9, 16). The combination of *Cryptosporidium* sp. and rotavirus may predominate in some situations (12). *Cryptosporidium* were the second most commonly detected pathogens next to rotavirus, and case-control studies indicated a highly significant association with diarrhea (9). Enteropathogens may not be detectable in up to 30% of diarrheic calves (9).

The age occurrence of the common enteropathogens associated with diarrhea in calves is shown in Table 50. Case-control studies of diarrheic and healthy calves from the same groups indicate that the enteropathogens commonly found in diarrheic calves can also be found in

Table 49. Summary of the relationship between the primary etiological agents and the epidemiology of acute undifferentiated diarrhea of newborn calves

Primary etiological agents	*Epidemiological factors*	*Possible role of epidemiological factor*
COMMON Enterotoxigenic *E. coli*	Colostral immunity of calf	Low levels of serum immunoglobulins render calves highly susceptible to death from diarrhea
Rotavirus and coronavirus *Cryptosporidium*	Overcrowding	Increased population density increases infection rate and high morbidity and mortality
Dietary abnormalities	Parity of dam	Calves born from heifers may not acquire sufficient level of colostral immunoglobulins
LESS COMMON *Salmonella* spp. *Chlamydia* sp.	Meteorological	Changes in weather; wet, windy and cold weather commonly precedes outbreaks of diarrhea in beef calves (3). Higher mortality in dairy calves exposed to hot environmental temperatures (4). High environmental temperatures precipitate outbreaks
Adenovirus Infectious bovine rhinotracheitis (IBR)	Quality of diet	Heat denatured skim-milk used in milk replacers is less digestible than whole milk and precipitates diarrhea
Bovine virus diarrhea (BVD) *Clostridium perfringens* types B and C *Providentia stuarti*	Calf rearer	The concern and care provided by the calf rearer will have a direct effect on morbidity and mortality associated with diarrhea

healthy calves but at a lower frequency with the exception of rotavirus which may be excreted by up to 50% of healthy calves (7, 10). The prevalence of enteropathogens in healthy calves on farms where there is no recent history of diarrhea indicates an absence of *Salmonella* spp., enterotoxigenic *E. coli*, *Cryptosporidium* and coronavirus, but the presence of rotavirus in some calves (11). It appears that healthy calves may be infected more often with enterotoxigenic *E. coli*, *Cryptosporidium*, coronavirus and rotavirus in herds in which some calves have or recently have had enteric disease than in herds free from major enteric disease (11).

The rotavirus and coronavirus occur with almost equal frequency in the intestinal tracts of normal and diarrheic calves of some studies (7). Intestinal lesions compatible with the viral infections are found in about 70% of diarrheic calves. Thus, these viruses are widespread in the bovine population and only under some circumstances will the infection be severe enough to cause lesions and diarrhea. Other viruses such as parvovirus, astrovirus, Breda virus, and calici-like virus have been isolated from the feces of diarrheic calves, but their role in the etiology is yet to be defined.

Table 50. Age occurrence of the common enteropathogens

Enteropathogen	*Age (days)*
Enterotoxigenic *E. coli* (ENTEC)	<3
Rotavirus	5–15
Coronavirus	5–21
Cryptosporidium	5–35
Salmonella spp.	5–42
Clostridium perfringens types B and C	5–15

Certain management procedures may be associated with differences in the prevalence of enteropathogens. In dairy calves fed on nipple feeders there was an increased probability of the calves shedding detectable fecal levels of *Salmonella*, *E. coli* or rotavirus or coronavirus (14). The use of group pens was associated with an increased odds of finding *Campylobacter jejuni*. Calves with diarrhea on these farms tended to have increased odds of shedding rotavirus and K99$^+$ *E. coli* (14).

Campylobacter jejuni is well adapted to the bovine host and can be found in the feces of diarrheic and healthy calves at a similar prevalence (11). Its significance as a pathogen in newborn calves is questionable (8). They are probably part of the normal enteric flora of ruminants.

To confound the issue, intensive studies have been done on the effects of colostral immunity on acute diarrhea in calves. Earlier work centered on the protective effect of colostrum against colibacillosis and recently on protection against rotavirus infection. The importance of colostral immunity is well established, and while it is easy to say that calves should receive a certain amount of colostrum, the veterinarian in the field who encounters an outbreak of acute diarrhea in beef calves, for example, cannot usually determine easily whether in fact the calves possess protective levels of immunoglobulins.

In outbreaks of diarrhea in neonatal piglets, the enteropathogens which are commonly present in the feces include the transmissible gastroenteritis (TGE) virus, enterotoxigenic *E. coli*, *Isospora* sp., rotavirus, *Clostridium perfringens* type C, and the adenovirus (15). In diarrheic piglets, the TGE virus occurs in piglets under 15 days of age, enterotoxigenic *E. coli* under 5 days of age, *Isospora* sp. between 5 and 15 days of age and the rotavirus in piglets over 10 days of age (15). In outbreaks of diarrhea in litters of piglets, while individual piglets may be infected by a single pathogen it is common for more than one pathogen to be present in the litter. This stresses the importance of submitting to the diagnostic laboratory piglets which are representative of the problem. A seasonal occurrence of the common enteropathogens has also been observed (15). The prevalence of the TGE virus may be highest during the fall, winter and spring months, and the coccidia and *E. coli* are more common during the summer, fall and early winter with the lowest prevalence in the spring.

Diarrhea in foals is common but most cases are mild, transient, and not caused by infectious agents (17). The most common cause of diarrhea in foals is 'foal heat' diarrhea. The rotavirus is thought to be an important enteropathogen. Other pathogens which have been isolated from foals with diarrhea include *Campylobacter jejuni*, *Clostridium perfringens* and *Corynebacterium (Rhodococcus) equi*.

Many interrelated epidemiological factors have been associated with a high incidence of calf diarrhea and have added to the difficulty of understanding the complexity of the disease. The effects of nutrition of the pregnant dam on the quantity and quality of colostrum and the vigor of the calf are thought to be important but there is little supporting evidence. Changes in weather and wet, windy and cold weather are thought to precipitate outbreaks of the disease in beef calves raised outdoors (3). Increases in population density in calf houses, and on calving grounds, resulting in a high infection rate may in part explain the high incidence in large intensified operations. Some studies have shown that the major contributing factor to dairy calf mortality is the care provided by the calf attendant. Not infrequently, however, outbreaks can occur in herds in which the management is excellent and not uncommonly an etiological diagnosis cannot be made.

Thus the disease is considered complex because one or any combination of more than one of the specific etiological agents may be the cause of the disease; or epidemiological influences may precipitate the disease in calves which might not normally get the disease, even though they are infected with a specific enteropathogen. The term acute undifferentiated diarrhea of newborn calves is useful to encompass cases of diarrhea in calves in which the etiological diagnosis is not immediately obvious and may not be determined even after exhaustive diagnostic work.

When a clinician is faced with an outbreak of acute diarrhea in newborn calves in which there is profuse watery diarrhea, progressive dehydration and death in a few days or earlier, the following steps are recommended:

- All affected calves should be identified, isolated and treated immediately with oral and parenteral fluid therapy as indicated
- Antibacterials may be given orally and parenterally for the treatment of enteric and septicemic colibacillosis. When large numbers of calves are affected at one time it is not usually possible clinically or with the aid of a laboratory to determine which calf is septicemic and thus all acutely affected calves should be treated. Treatment, however, should not be continued beyond 3 days
- Each of the commonly recognized epidemiological factors should be examined for its possible role in the particular outbreak. The common ones include quality of diet, origin of calves, overcrowding, recent changes in climate, recent stress of any kind on the herd, recent introductions into the herd, failure of calves to ingest colostrum and the calving of a disproportionately large percentage of first calf heifers which occurs in herds which are expanding their herd size
- Fecal samples (30–50 g) should be collected from diarrheic calves at the first sign of diarrhea and from normal calves and submitted to a laboratory for the attempted isolation and characterization of enterotoxigenic *E. coli*, rotaviruses and *Salmonella* spp. Blood samples from affected and normal calves and colostral samples if available are useful for immunoglobulin and antibody studies. All moribund calves should be submitted for necropsy before they die naturally
- Pregnant cows which are due to calve shortly should be moved to a new calving area (5). In a dairy herd this means a different clean calving stall, preferably in another barn not previously occupied by cattle; in beef herds it may mean moving a large number of cows to a new uncontaminated calving pasture
- The control of the disease in future calf crops will depend on application of the principles of control which are described under colibacillosis and viral diarrhea of calves.

REVIEW LITERATURE

Radostits, O. M. & Acres, S. D. (1980) The prevention and control of epidemics of acute undifferentiated diarrhea of beef calves in Western Canada. *Can. vet. J.*, *21*, 243–249.

Tzipori, S. (1985) The relative importance of enteric pathogens affecting neonates of domestic animals. *Adv. vet. Sci. comp. Med.*, *29*: 103–206.

REFERENCES

(1) Acres, S. D. et al. (1975) *Can. J. comp. Med.*, *39*, 116.
(2) Acres, S. D. et al. (1977) *Can vet. J.*, *18*, 113.
(3) Acres, S. D. (1976) *Proceedings of Minisymposium on Neonatal Diarrhea of Calves and Pigs*. Saskatoon: Veterinary Infectious Diseases Organization and University of Saskatchewan.
(4) Stott, G. H. et al. (1976) *J. dairy Sci.*, *59*, 1306.
(5) Radostits, O. M. & Acres, S. D. (1980) *Can. vet. J.*, *21*, 243.
(6) Moon, H. W. et al. (1978) *J. Am. vet. med. Assoc.*, *173*, 577.
(7) Morin, M. et al. (1978) *Proc. 2nd int. Symp. Neonatal Diarrhea, Vet. inf. Dis. Org., Univ. of Sask.*, Oct. 1978, pp. 347–369.
(8) Tzipori, S. (1985) *Adv. vet. Sci. comp. Med.*, *29*, 103.
(9) Reynolds, D. J. et al. (1986) *Vet. Rec.*, *119*, 34.
(10) Snodgrass, D. R. et al. (1986) *Vet. Rec.*, *119*, 31.
(11) Myers, L. L. et al. (1984) *Am. J. vet. Res.*, *45*, 1544.
(12) Pohjola, S. et al. (1986) *Prev. vet. Med.*, *3*, 547.
(13) Bulgin, M. S. et al. (1982) *J. Am. vet. med. Assoc.*, *180*, 1222.
(14) Waltner-Toews, D. et al. (1986) *Can. J. vet. Res.*, *50*, 307.
(15) Morin, M. et al. (1983) *Can. J. comp. Med.*, *47*, 11.
(16) Sherwood, D. et al. (1983) *Vet. Rec.*, *113*, 208.
(17) Harbour, D. A. (1985) *Equ. vet. J.*, *17*, 263.

Acute undifferentiated diarrhea of other newborn farm animals

Several different pathogenic agents are now being identified in the feces and intestinal tract of diarrheic piglets, lambs, foals and kids. In principle, the situation is similar to the problem described in calves—it is difficult to know which bacteria, virus or protozoa are responsible for the diarrhea. Mixed infections are now more common than single infections. The clinician must make the most logical diagnosis based on the clinical and epidemiological findings, the microbiological and pathological findings and the response to treatment.

Colibacillosis of newborn calves, piglets, lambs and foals

One of the most common diseases of newborn farm animals is colibacillosis caused by pathogenic *E. coli*. There are at least two different types of the disease:

enteric colibacillosis manifested primarily by varying degrees of diarrhea and septicemic colibacillosis manifested by septicemia and rapid death.

Etiology

Specific serotypes of *E. coli* are the causative agents of colibacillosis. Certain serotypes are associated with septicemia and another different series with the development of diarrhea and dilatation of an isolated loop of intestine (1). Both septicemic and enteric colibacillosis have been produced experimentally by the administration of relevant specific serotypes. Conversely the challenge of experimental animals with specific serotypes has been resisted by the administration of serum or colostrum containing antibodies to those specific serotypes (2).

Epidemiology

Colibacillosis occurs commonly wherever farm animals are maintained and is a significant cause of economic loss in raising livestock. There are many epidemiological factors which influence the disease, each one of which must be considered and evaluated when investigating the cause of an outbreak so that effective clinical management and control of the disease may be achieved. The disease is most common in animals under 3 days of age; but it may occur as early as 12–18 hours after birth and occasionally occurs in calves up to several days of age when there is a mixed infection with viral enteropathogens.

Morbidity and mortality

In *dairy calves* raised under intensified conditions the morbidity may reach 75% but is usually about 30%. The case fatality will vary from 10 to 50%. In *beef calves* the morbidity will vary from 10 to 50% and the case fatality from 5 to 25% or even higher in some years. The population mortality rate in calves can vary from a low of 3% in well-managed herds to a high of 60% in problem herds. Among the main causes of neonatal mortality in *piglets* the gastroenteropathies accounted for 2·8% of the total mortality of all piglets born in 17 herds over a 1-year period (4). Losses due to stillbirths, traumatic injuries, starvation and undersize accounted for a much greater combined total loss of 13%. However, colibacillosis of piglets accounted for approximately 50% of the gastroenteropathies encountered during the preweaning period (5). Prevalence information is not readily available for *foals* and *lambs* but the disease accounts for 25% of septicemias in foals.

The prevalence of colibacillosis has increased in recent years for several possible reasons which include size of herd, shortage of qualified labor, automated livestock rearing systems and increased population density.

Immunity

Newborn farm animals are born agammaglobulinemic and must ingest colostrum and absorb colostral immunoglobulins within hours after birth to obtain protection against septicemic and enteric colibacillosis (6). The mortality rate from enteric colibacillosis is much higher in calves with low levels of serum immunoglobulins than in calves with adequate levels (1, 7). Based on surveys, up to 25% of newborn dairy and beef calves have low levels of serum immunoglobulins because they do not receive sufficient colostrum early enough after birth which makes them very susceptible to neonatal disease especially colibacillosis. Colostral immunoglobulins are absorbed for up to 24 hours after birth in calves and up to 48 hours in piglets. However, in calves maximum efficiency of absorption occurs during the first 6–12 hours after birth and decreases rapidly from 12 to 24 hours after birth. Multiple small intakes of colostrum give significantly greater levels of serum immunoglobulins than a single, large intake and calves with continuous access to their dams are in the most favorable position. Newborn calves should ingest approximately 50 ml/kg body weight within the first 8–12 hours (13). Lambs with low serum immunoglobulin levels are also highly susceptible to colibacillosis.

The maximum level of serum immunoglobulins is reached in the calf at 24 hours after birth and the factors which reduce those levels below an adequate level include the effects of maternal behavior and conformation, the vigor of the calf, and environmental influences (15, 16). First calf heifers do not have as much colostrum or as wide a spectrum of specific antibodies as do mature cows (18). Some first calf heifers do not lick and stimulate their calves to get up and suck immediately after birth as does the mature cow with an ostentatious maternal instinct (15). Others ignore their calves completely. The conformation of the udder and the shape of the teats may be undesirable such that the calf cannot find the teat so easily on badly shaped udders or the teat may be misshapen which makes it difficult for the calf to suck.

Calves which receive their first colostrum by bucket do not acquire the same high levels of serum immunoglobulins as calves which receive their first colostrum by natural sucking of the teat. In both cases the presence of the dam improves the absorption (15). Calves which are weak or have an edematous tongue from a prolonged difficult parturition may not be able to suck for several hours, by which time the ability to absorb colostral immunoglobulins has decreased markedly. Beef calves born outside may be subjected to several influences which affect colostral intake. They may be born during a snowstorm and suffer severe cold exposure; when born they may be dropped in a snow-bank and be unable to get up even with the assistance of the dam, or in crowded calving grounds mismothering due to mistaken identity may occur, resulting in the calf not receiving any or very little colostrum.

Diarrhea caused by enterotoxigenic *E. coli* occurs in calves mainly during the first few days of life, rarely in older calves, and never in adults (8). Epidemiological studies of both beef and dairy calves indicate that more than 80% of clinical cases caused by $K99^+$ enterotoxigenic *E. coli* occur in calves younger than 4 days of age (8). The mechanism of this age-related resistance is not well understood but may be related to development of resistance to colonization of the small intestine as the calf becomes older. This could be associated with the replacement of villous epithelial cells which occurs in the first few days after birth.

The disease is more common in piglets born from gilts than from sows, which suggests that immunity develops with developing age in the sow and is transferred to the piglets. In a survey of approximately 4400 litters of piglets over a period of 4 years in a large piggery, 64% of the litters were treated for diarrhea before weaning, and piglets born to sows under parity 2 were 1·7 times more likely to develop diarrhea before weaning than litters born to sows over parity 3 (133).

Piglets which do not obtain a liberal quantity of colostrum within a few hours after birth are very susceptible to colibacillosis. Prolonged parturition, weak piglets, slippery floors, cold drafty farrowing crates, and the condition of the sow and her colostral supply all influence the amount of colostrum ingested by the newborn piglet. Enteric colibacillosis is the major disease in piglets which are weaned from the sow immediately after birth and reared on milk replacers (19). A crude preparation of porcine immunoglobulin added to the milk replacer of colostrum-deprived pigs provided good protection against enteric colibacillosis when fed for the experimental period of 21 days.

The susceptibility or resistance to *E. coli* diarrhea in piglets may have an inherited basis (3). The cell surface receptor for the $K88^+$ antigen is inherited in a simple Mendelian way with adherence (*S*) dominant over non-adherence (*s*). Homozygous dominants (*SS*) and heterozygotes (*Ss*) possess the receptor and are susceptible, whereas in the homozygous recessives (*ss*) it is absent and the pigs are resistant. The highest incidence of diarrhea occurs in susceptible progeny born from resistant dams and sired by susceptible sires. Most if not all pigs have intestinal receptors for $K99^+$ pili (30) and an inheritance pattern similar to $K88^+$ receptors does not exist for $K99^+$ receptors. Pigs with non-adherent phenotype can be identified using a simple enterotomy technique for the examination of the brush border of the intestine (31). Thus breeding stock replacements could be identified.

Effect of meteorological influences

While little epidemiological data are available to support the claim, many veterinarians have observed a relationship between adverse climatic conditions and colibacillosis in both calves and piglets. During inclement weather, such as a snowstorm, a common practice in beef herds is to confine the calving cows in a small area where they can be fed and watered more easily. The overcrowding is commonly followed by an outbreak of enteric colibacillosis in the calves. There is evidence that cold, wet, windy weather during the winter months and hot dry weather during the summer months has a significant effect on the incidence of dairy calf mortality (16, 20). Experimentally, diarrhea reduces the piglets' ability to maintain its rectal and surface temperatures in a cold environment (10).

Nutrition and feeding methods

Dairy calves fed milk substitutes are more prone to enteric colibacillosis than those fed cow's whole milk. Extreme heat treatment of the liquid skim-milk in the processing of dried skim-milk for use of milk substitutes for calves results in denaturation of the whey protein which interferes with digestibility of the nutrients and destruction of any lactoglobulins which are present and may have a protective effect in the young calf (21). Irregular feeding practices resulting in dietetic diarrhea are considered to contribute to a higher incidence of enteric colibacillosis in calves. The person feeding and caring for the calves has been an important factor influencing calf mortality due to diarrhea. While it is generally believed that general or specific nutritional deficiencies such as a lack of energy, protein or vitamin A in the maternal diet predispose to colibacillosis, particularly in calves and piglets, there is no direct evidence that nutritional deficiencies are involved. They probably are, at least in indirect ways, for example, by having an effect on the amount of colostrum available at the first milking after parturition in first calf heifers underfed during pregnancy.

The experimental administration of iron to newborn piglets may increase their susceptibility to enteric colibacillosis (11).

Standard of housing and hygiene

Housing and hygienic practices are probably the most important epidemiological factors influencing the incidence of colibacillosis in calves and piglets but have received the least amount of research effort compared to other aspects, for example, control of the disease through vaccination. As the size of herds has increased and as livestock production has become more intensified the quality of hygiene and sanitation, particularly in housed animals, assumes major importance. Where calves are run at pasture or are individually tethered, or penned, on grass the disease is much less common.

Source of the organism and its ecology and transmission

In most species the major primary source of the infection is the feces of infected animals, although the organism may be cultured from the vagina or uterus of sows whose litters become affected. In swine herds the total number of organisms on each sow was highest in the farrowing barn, decreased when the sow was returned to the breeding barn and was lowest when the sow was in the gestation barn. Calves obtain the organism from contaminated bedding and calf pails, dirty calf pens, diarrheic calves, overcrowded calving grounds, milk from cows affected with coliform mastitis and from the skin of the perineum and udder of the cow. The organism is spread within a herd through the feces of infected animals and all of the inanimate objects which can be contaminated by feces including bedding, pails, boots, tools, clothing and feed and water supplies. The organism is one of the first encountered by newborn farm animals within minutes after birth (23). The high population density of animals which occurs in overcrowded calving grounds in beef herds, heavily used calving pens in dairy herds and the continuous successive use of farrowing crates without a break for clean up contributes to a large dynamic population of *E. coli* (24). The population of bacteria in an animal barn will continue to increase as the length of time the barn is occupied by animals without depopulation, a clean out, disinfection and a period of vacancy (24). In some countries where lambing must be done in buildings to avoid exposure to cold weather the lambing sheds may become heavily contaminated within a few weeks resulting in outbreaks of septicemic and enteric colibacillosis.

Infected animals are the main reservoir for enterotoxigenic *E. coli* and their feces are the major source of environmental contamination with the bacteria. Passage of the *E. coli* through animals causes a 'multiplier effect', as each infected animal executes many more bacteria than it originally ingested. Diarrheic calves are the most extreme multipliers, because they often pass 1 liter or more of liquid feces containing 10^{10}/g enterotoxigenic *E. coli* within 12 hours, and recovered calves can continue to shed bacteria for several months (14).

Normal calves which are subclinically infected and adult cows can serve as reservoirs of infection and the bacteria can persist in a herd by circulating through animals of all ages. Carrier animals introduced to an uninfected herd are thought to be one of the main causes of natural outbreaks. The duration and amount of shedding probably depends on the degree of confinement, resulting population density, herd immunity, environmental conditions, and perhaps the serotype of the organism (8).

The prevalence of enterotoxigenic *E. coli* in diarrheic calves varies widely geographically, between herds and depending on the age of the animals (17, 22). The prevalence can be as high as 50–60% in diarrheic calves under 30 days of age and only 5–10% in diarrheic calves 8 days of age (17). In some countries the prevalence is only 5–8% in diarrheic calves under 3 days of age (22). Thus enterotoxigenic colibacillosis is a major cause of diarrhea in calves less than 3 days of age and is not associated with outbreaks of diarrhea in calves older than 3 days. Enterotoxigenic *E. coli* infection in calves older than 2–3 days will in most cases be associated with a virus infection (26). The prevalence of the organism is also very low or not present in clinically normal calves in herds which have not had a problem with diarrhea.

The prevalence of enterotoxigenic *E. coli* in diarrheic piglets also varies geographically and with herds (25, 81). In some areas the K99$^+$ pilus was found more frequently than the K88$^+$ or 987P (25) whereas in other regions the K88$^+$ will be more common (81).

Ingestion is the most likely portal of infection in calves, piglets and lambs although infection via the umbilical vessels and nasopharyngeal mucosa can occur. It has been suggested that certain serotypes of *E. coli* may enter by the latter route and lead to the development of meningitis.

Virulence attributes of E. coli

Piglets Most enteropathogenic *E. coli* from neonatal pigs produce either K88$^+$, 987P$^+$, or K99$^+$ pilus antigens which adhere to ileal villi, colonize intensively and cause profuse diarrhea when given to newborn pigs (81). However, there are also some enterotoxigenic strains which produce none of the three antigens. The K88$^+$ produces heat-liable enterotoxin (LT), the 987P$^+$ and the K99$^+$ do not produce LT, and all three types produce heat-stable enterotoxin (STa) in infant mice. Some isolates produce neither LT or STa but produce enterotoxin in ligated intestinal loops of pigs (STb).

The porcine enterotoxigenic *E. coli* strains which induce fluid secretion in the intestine of piglets less than 2 weeks of age but not in older pigs are designated class 2, whereas those strains which induce fluid secretion in the intestines of older pigs are class 1 enterotoxigenic *E. coli* (27). The bovine strains of enterotoxigenic *E. coli* have several features in common with the porcine class 2 organisms which includes the possession of the 0 antigens 8, 9, 20 or 101, characterization as mucoid colonies, possession of K99$^+$ pili and production of heat-stable enterotoxin. Most strains of enterotoxigenic *E. coli* of pigs belong to a restricted number of serogroups (32).

Calves The major virulence attributes of the enterotoxigenic strains of *E. coli* in calves are the K99$^+$ antigen which produces heat-stable enterotoxin (ST) (82). The colonization in the small intestine of calves by K99$^+$ ETEC appears to be site-specific, having a predilection for the ileum. Non-enteropathogenic strains do not adhere (98).

The heat-stable enterotoxin from bovine enterotoxigenic *E. coli* have been purified and characterized (33). There is evidence of a form of heat-stable enterotoxin which is common to bovine, porcine and human strains of enterotoxigenic *E. coli*. A small proportion of calves may be infected with *E. coli* that produce a shiga-like toxin.

Lambs Enterotoxigenic strains of *E. coli* can be isolated from the feces of approximately 35% of diarrheic lambs (83). Enterotoxigenic strains of *E. coli* have also been isolated from the blood or a small percentage of diarrheic lambs. However, the isolates have not been characterized as they have been in calves and piglets.

Pathogenesis

The major factors which are important in the understanding of colibacillosis are the immune status of the animal and the properties of the strain of *E. coli*, particularly its capacity to invade tissues and produce a septicemia, or its capacity to produce an enterotoxin which causes varying degrees of severity of diarrhea (1). In calves, the three common forms of the disease described several years ago were septicemic, enteriotoxemic and enteric colibacillosis (2). Recent work suggests that both enteric forms of the disease are caused primarily by enterotoxigenic strains of *E. coli* which are non-invasive and that the invasive strains of the organism are primarily responsible for the septicemic form of the disease (1).

Septicemic colibacillosis

This occurs in all species but is most common in foals and lambs and results from the invasive strains of *E. coli* invading the tissues and systemic circulation via the intestinal lumen, nasopharyngeal mucosae and tonsillar crypts, or umbilical vessels. Calves and piglets which are deficient in immunoglobulins are most susceptible to septicemia. The intestinal permeability to macromolecules in the newborn piglet may predispose to the invasion of septicemia-inducing *E. coli* (84). Colostrum provides protection against colisepticemia in calves but does not prevent diarrhea (86). The clinical findings and lesions in septicemic colibacillosis are attributed to the effects of endotoxin which causes shock. The infusion of *E. coli* endotoxin into the duodenum of newborn calves reproduces the hypoglycemia and lactic acidosis which develops in calves moribund with colibacillosis (34). Also, colostrum-fed calves are much more resistant to endotoxin than colostrum-deprived calves. Calves, piglets and lambs which have normal levels of serum immunoglobulins are protected from septicemic strains. Animals which recover from septicemia may develop lesions due to localization in other organs. Arthritis is a common sequel in calves, foals and lambs. Meningitis is common in calves and piglets. Polyserositis due to *E. coli* has been recorded in pigs (99).

Enterotoxic colibacillosis

Enterotoxigenic strains of *E. coli* possess the ability to colonize and proliferate in the upper part of the small intestine and to produce enterotoxins which causes an increase in net secretion of fluid and electrolytes from the systemic circulation (36). The adhesion of *E. coli* to the intestinal epithelial cells is mediated by bacterial pili and the mechanism of attachment to the receptors is complex (8, 37). The enterotoxic form of colibacillosis occurs most commonly in calves and piglets and less commonly in foals and lambs. The molecular analysis of several virulence determinants of enterotoxigenic strains of *E. coli* has been elucidated (37).

The factors which allow or control the colonization and proliferation of these strains and their production of enterotoxin are not well understood. There is substantial evidence that the bacterial fimbriae attach to specific receptor sites on villous epithelial cells following which the bacteria multiply and form microcolonies that cover the surface of the villi. The capsular polysaccharide of *E. coli* may also be involved in adhesion and colonization (8). The fimbriae of *E. coli* are strongly immunogenic, a factor which is explored in the production of vaccines (38). Some calf bacterial strains produce high levels of shiga-like toxin and cause attachment and effacement lesions in the colonic epithelium (39). Neutrophil emigration into the intestinal lumen of piglets can occur in response to $K88^+$ *E. coli* infection and is due to the ingestion of immune colostrum and absorption of antibody by the piglet (87).

The production of enterotoxin by the *E. coli* results in net secretion of fluid and electrolytes from the systemic circulation into the lumen of the gut resulting in varying degrees of dehydration, electrolyte imbalances, acidosis, hyperkalemia when the acidosis is severe, circulatory failure, shock and death. The response to *E. coli* enterotoxin in calves and piglets is similar to cholera enterotoxin in man (1) and takes place through an intact mucosa. Enterotoxin stimulates mucosal adenylcyclase activity which leads to an increased cyclic AMP which in turn is thought to increase intestinal fluid secretion (8). The secretion originates primarily in the intestinal crypts but the villous epithelium also has a secretory function (88). The fluids secreted are alkaline, and in comparison to serum, isotonic, low in protein, and high in sodium and bicarbonate ions (1). When the disease is confined to the intestine, it responds reasonably well to treatment in the early stages. If death occurs, it is due to acidosis, electrolyte imbalance and dehydration. The acid–base and electrolyte changes in piglets 1–3 days of age infected naturally and experimentally with enterotoxigenic *E. coli* reveal a severe dehydration and metabolic acidosis (42).

Severe metabolic changes may occur in calves with diarrhea. If the disease is progressive, the acidosis becomes more severe, lactic acidosis develops because of a reduced ability to utilize lactic acid and severe hypoglycemia may occur because of a reduced rate of conversion of lactic acid to glucose (48). If extensive fluids are lost, hypovolemia and shock occur. These metabolic changes may in part be due to terminal endotoxemia which may be a sequel to acute diarrheal disease (92).

Metabolic acidosis without clinical evidence of dehydration occurs in some calves which had a history of diarrhea in the previous several days (43). The pathogenesis is unknown. The severity and nature of the acidosis in diarrheic calves varies with the age of the calf. Diarrheic calves under 1 week of age often have a lactic acidosis, while those over 1 week of age have a non-lactic acidosis (131). Younger calves tend to dehydrate more rapidly and severely than older calves which may be related to the greater incidence of enterotoxigenic colibacillosis in the young age group.

An adequate level of serum immunoglobulins will protect calves from death due to diarrhea but not necessarily from diarrhea (6). Best protection is provided if both the serum levels and the levels in the colostrum and the milk of the first week are high. The immunoglobulin subclasses in the plasma of calves which have received sufficient colostrum are IgG, IgM (and IgM is probably the more important of the two for the prevention of septicemia) and IgA. The serum IgG, concentrations of calves under 3 weeks of age, and dying from infectious disease, were much lower than in normal calves. Of the dead calves 50% had serum IgG levels that were more than two standard deviations below the normal mean, and an additional 35% had concentrations greater than one standard deviation below the normal mean (7). In the intestine, no single subclass of immunoglobulin is known to be responsible for protection against the fatal effects of diarrhea. Individually, each immunoglobulin subclass can prevent death from diarrhea even though calves may be affected with varying degrees of diarrhea. In contrast to the pig, IgA appears to be least effective. In pigs, IgA becomes the dominant immunoglobulin in sow colostrum after the first few days of lactation, and this is the immunoglobulin which is not absorbed but is retained in, and reaches a high level in, the gut and plays a major role in providing local protection against enteric colibacillosis in piglets (4). Porcine colostral IgA is more resistant to gastrointestinal proteolytic enzymes than IgG_2 and IgM (85). On the other hand, IgG is at a peak concentration in colostrum in the first day after parturition, is readily absorbed by the newborn piglet and is vital in providing protection against septicemia. Lysozyme in sows' milk may assist in the control of bacterial population in the gut of the unweaned piglet (40).

In general, the enterotoxigenic *E. coli* exert their effects by the enterotoxin causing hypersecretion through an intact intestinal epithelium. However, the enterotoxigenic *E. coli* induce consistent pathological changes in the jejunum and ileum of experimentally infected colostrum-fed calves. The intraluminal exposure of the jejunum of 3-week-old pigs to sterile crude culture filtrates from strains of *E. coli* known to produce two types of heat-stable enterotoxin will induce microscopic alterations of the villous epithelium (28). Focal emigration of neutrophils, especially through the epithelium above aggregated lymphatic follicles, stunting of jejunal and ileal villi and adherence of bacteria to jejunal and ileal mucosae are the most consistent findings (12, 29). These changes are helpful in making the diagnosis of enterotoxigenic colibacillosis in calves. While enterotoxigenic strains are considered to be non-invasive this does not preclude the possibility that invasion into the systemic circulation may occur, resulting in septicemia, or that septicemic strains may not occur together.

Enzyme histochemistry studies of the small intestinal mucosa in experimental infections of calves with rotavirus and enterotoxigenic *E. coli* indicate a marked decrease in enzyme activity in dual infections and a lesser decrease in monoinfections (44). Increased enzyme activity occurred in parts of the intestinal mucosa which were not affected or only slightly affected by the enteropathogens which may be an adaptation of the mucosa to maintain absorptive function (44).

Some atypical *E. coli* can apparently cause naturally occurring diarrhea and dysentery in calves at 18–21 days (45, 49). These are enteropathogenic *E. coli* which do not produce enterotoxin but they adhere to the surface of the enterocytes of the large intestine. Affected calves pass bright red blood in the diarrheic feces. The lesions in experimentally infected calves are indistinguishable from those produced by some *E. coli* which are enteropathogenic for man, rabbits and pigs (49). They do not produce enterotoxin.

Fat and carbohydrate malabsorption frequently occurs in diarrheic calves over 5 days of age and may contribute to the death of these animals in cold weather (61).

Synergistic interaction between enteropathogens
Enterotoxigenic colibacillosis occurs naturally and can be reproduced experimentally in calves under 2 days of age using enterotoxigenic *E. coli*, but not in calves 1 week of age. Diarrheic calves older than 3 days of age may be infected with enterotoxigenic $K99^+$ *E. coli* and rotavirus. There is evidence that prior or simultaneous infection of the intestine with rotavirus will enable the *E. coli* to colonize in older calves (100,102). Thus, there may be synergism between rotavirus and enterotoxigenic *E. coli* in calves older than 2 days which may explain the fatal diarrhea which can occur in calves at 1 week of age which normally would not be fatal with a single infection (120). The rotavirus may enhance colonization of the *E. coli*.

The simultaneous experimental infection of neonatal gnotobiotic calves at 24 hours of age with rotavirus and enterotoxigenic *E. coli* results in a severe diarrheal disease (101). However, the effect was considered to be additive rather than synergistic.

In summary, septicemic colibacillosis occurs in newborn animals which are agammaglobulinemic because they have not ingested sufficient colostrum early enough, and absorbed sufficient immunoglobulins, thus rendering them highly susceptible. Enteric colibacillosis on the other hand occurs in colostrum-fed animals and is caused by the colonization and proliferation of enteropathogenic *E. coli* which produce enterotoxin and cause varying degrees of diarrhea and acidosis and dehydration. While single infections occur commonly, as in piglet diarrhea, and what was previously described as enteric–toxemic colibacillosis in calves, multiple infections with enteropathogenic *E. coli* and viruses and other agents are more common.

Clinical findings

Calves

Septicemic colibacillosis This is most common in calves during the first 4 days of life. The illness is acute, the course varying from 24 to 96 hours. There are no diagnostic clinical signs. Affected animals are depressed and weak, anorexia is complete, there is marked tachycardia and, although the temperature may be high initially, it falls rapidly to subnormal levels when the calf becomes weak and moribund. Diarrhea and dysentery may occur but are uncommon. If the calf survives the septicemic state, clinical evidence of postsepticemic localization may appear in about 1 week. This includes arthritis, meningitis, panophthalmitis and, less commonly, pneumonia.

Enterotoxic colibacillosis This is the most common form of colibacillosis in newborn calves primarily from 3 to 5 days of age. It may occur in calves as early as 1 day of age and only rarely up to 3 weeks. The clinical severity will vary dependent upon the number and kind of organisms causing the disease. The presence of a single enterotoxigenic strain of *E. coli* may cause a state of collapse usually designated as *enteric toxemia*. In this form of the disease the outstanding clinical signs include severe weakness, coma, subnormal temperature, a cold clammy skin, pale mucosae, wetness around the mouth, collapse of superficial veins, slowness and irregularity of the heart, mild convulsive movements and periodic apnea. Diarrhea is usually not evident although the abdomen may be slightly distended and succussion and auscultation may reveal fluid splashing sounds suggesting a fluid-filled intestine. The prognosis for these calves is poor and they commonly die in 2–6 hours after the onset of signs.

In the more common form of the disease in calves, the enteric form of colibacillosis, the calves are affected with a diarrhea in which the feces are profuse and watery to pasty, usually pale yellow to white in color, and occasionally streaked with blood flecks and very foul smelling. The dry matter content of the feces is commonly below 10%. Defecation is frequent and effortless and the tail and buttocks are soiled. The temperature is usually normal in the initial stages but becomes subnormal as the disease worsens. Affected calves may or may not suck or drink depending on the degrees of acidosis, dehydration and weakness. The abdomen may be slightly distended in the early stages when the intestines are fluid-filled which may be detectable on succussion and auscultation. When many calves are affected within a few days in an outbreak some calves when examined early will have a distended abdomen without obvious diarrhea which usually occurs and is profuse a few hours later. Mild-to-moderately affected calves may be diarrheic for a few days and recover spontaneously with or without treatment. However 15–20% of calves with enteric colibacillosis become progressively worse over a period of 3–5 days, gradually become more weak, completely anorexic and progressively more obviously clinically dehydrated. Throughout the course of the diarrhea the degree of dehydration will vary from just barely detectable clinically (4–6% of body weight) up to 10–16% of body weight. It is best assessed by 'tenting' the skin of the upper eyelid or the neck and measuring the time required for the skin-fold to return to normal. In calves with 8% of dehydration, 5–10 seconds will be required for the skin-fold to return to normal; in 10–12% dehydration, up to 30 seconds. Recession of the eyeball is also a useful measure of the degree of dehydration. Slight sinking of the eyeball without an obvious space between the eyeball and the orbit represents 6–8% dehydration; moderate separation of the eyeball from the orbit represents 9–12% dehydration; and marked separation of the eyeball from the orbit represents over 12% and up to 16% dehydration. Death usually occurs in 3–5 days. Affected calves can lose 10–16% of their original body weight during the first 24–48 hours of the diarrhea. In the terminal stages there may be bradycardia with arrhythmia associated with terminal hyperkalemia (1). Outbreaks of the disease in beef calves may last for up to 3 weeks and in epidemics almost every calf will be affected.

In some calves between 10 and 20 days of age with a history of diarrhea in the previous several days, from which they have recovered, there will be metabolic acidosis without clinical signs of dehydration (43). Affected calves are depressed, weak, ataxic and sometimes recumbent and appear comatose (43). Affected calves respond quickly to treatment with intravenous sodium bicarbonate.

Lambs

Although some cases manifest enteric signs, and chronic cases may occur, colibacillosis in lambs is almost always septicemic and peracute. Two age groups appear to be susceptible, lambs of 1–2 days of age and lambs 3–8 weeks old. Peracute cases are found dead without premonitory signs. Acute cases show collapse, and occasionally signs of acute meningitis manifested by a stiff gait in the early stages, followed by recumbency with hyperesthesia and tetanic convulsions. Chronic cases are usually manifested by arthritis.

Piglets

Septicemic colibacillosis is uncommon but occurs in piglets within 24–48 hours of age. Some are found dead without any premonitory signs. Usually more than one, and sometimes the entire litter, are affected. Severely affected piglets seen clinically are weak, almost comatose, appear cyanotic, and feel cold and clammy and have a subnormal temperature. Usually there is no diarrhea. The prognosis for these is unsatisfactory and most will die in spite of therapy.

Enterotoxic colibacillosis (or baby pig diarrhea) is the most common form of colibacillosis in piglets and occurs in anywhere from 12 hours of age up to several days of age with a peak incidence at 3 days of age. As with the septicemic form usually more than one pig or the entire litter is affected. The first sign usually noticed is the fecal puddles on the floor. Affected piglets may still nurse in the early stages but gradually lose their appetite as the disease progresses. The feces vary from a pasty to watery consistency and are usually yellow to brown in color. When the diarrhea is profuse and watery there will be no obvious staining of the buttocks with feces but the tails of the piglets will be straight and wet. The temperature is usually normal or subnormal. The disease is progressive; diarrhea and dehydration continues, the piglets become very weak and lie in lateral recumbency and make weak paddling movements. Within several hours they appear very dehydrated and shrunken, and commonly die within 24 hours after the onset of signs. In severe outbreaks the entire litter may be affected and die within a few hours of birth. The prognosis for these is favorable if treatment is started early before significant dehydration and acidosis occur.

Clinical pathology

If septicemia is suspected, blood should be submitted for isolation of the organism and determination of its drug sensitivity.

The definitive etiological diagnosis of enteric colibacillosis will depend on the isolation and characterization of the *E. coli* from the intestines and the feces of affected animals. The best opportunity of making a diagnosis is when untreated representative affected animals are killed and submitted for pathological and microbiological examination. The distribution of the organism in the intestine and determination of the presence of $K88^+$, $K99^+$ or 987P antigens, the demonstration of enterotoxin by infant mouse test or ligated intestinal loops and the histopathological appearance of the mucosa all contribute to the diagnosis.

The routine culture of feces and intestinal contents for *E. coli* without determining their virulence determinants is of limited value. The laboratory tests used to identify enterotoxigenic $K99^+$ *E. coli* include a direct fluorescent antibody technique with conventional culturing methods (90) and the enzyme-linked immunosorbent assay (ELISA) tests with or without monoclonal antibody to detect the organism or the enterotoxin in the feces (55, 102–104).

The determination of drug sensitivity of the *E. coli* isolated from the feces of diarrheic calves and piglets is commonly done but is of limited value without determining which isolate is enteropathogenic.

A total and differential leukocyte count may indicate the presence of a septicemia or severe intestinal infection. The packed cell volume and the total solids concentration of the blood will indicate the degree of dehydration, and the blood urea nitrogen may be increased in severe cases due to inadequate renal perfusion. The blood bicarbonate values are markedly reduced, blood pH values represent acidosis and the other serum electrolytes are variable (50). The acid–base status of calves can be determined in the field using a simple total carbon dioxide apparatus which provides values close to blood bicarbonate concentrations (129). There is usually a decrease in serum sodium, chloride and potassium but potassium may be elevated in severe cases of acidosis. The total plasma osmolality is decreased and fecal osmolality increased (51).

The determination of the level of serum immunoglobulins of diarrheic calves is considered valuable in assessing prognosis and to determine the intensity of the therapy required for survival. However, the level of serum immunoglobulins as a measure of susceptibility or prognosis is most accurate at 24 hours after birth (52). After this period, it is unreliable because the serum immunoglobulins may be increased in response to septicemia, increased spuriously in dehydration, and decreased in enteric disease (51). A zinc sulfate turbidity test is available for an estimation of the level of serum immunoglobulins and can be used as an aid in surveillance of the colostral intake of calves (53). There is an increase in the excretion of fecal globulins, primarily IgG, which suggests an intraluminal leak of serum globulins (51).

Necropsy findings

In septicemic colibacillosis there may be no gross lesions and the diagnosis may depend upon the isolation of the organism from the abdominal viscera and heart blood. In less severe cases, there may be subserous and submucosal petechial hemorrhages, and a degree of enteritis and gastritis may be present. Occasionally fibrinous exudates may be present in the joints and serous cavities, and there may be omphalophlebitis, pneumonia, peritonitis and meningitis.

In enteric colibacillosis in piglets the flaccidity of the gut is evident and although the tissues may be dehydrated the intestines are usually distended with fluid and clotted milk may be present in the stomach. The intestinal mucosae may appear normal or hyperemic; in prolonged cases there may be edema of the mesenteric lymph nodes. Villous atrophy similar to that in transmissible gastroenteritis has been described and the pathology of the experimental disease in gnotobiotic piglets has been described (54). Attempts should be made to culture the organism from the gut, the mesenteric lymph nodes, spleen, heart blood and cerebrospinal fluid.

The enterotoxigenic *E. coli* may be identified by several tests which include the indirect fluorescent antibody tests (IFA) specific for $K88^+$, $K99^+$ and 987P pilus antigens. The IFA test can be performed on impression smears or frozen sections of ileal tissue and the results are available within a few hours (47) and is more advantageous than histologic examination or seroagglutination testing. The indirect immunoperoxidase technique is also useful (48).

In enteric colibacillosis of calves there is dehydration, the intestinal tract is distended by yellow watery contents and gas, the abomasum is usually grossly distended with fluid and may or may not contain a milk clot. There is usually no milk clot in the abomasum of calves fed poor quality milk replacers. The abomasal mucosae may contain numerous small hemorrhages. The villi in the jejunum and ileum are stunted and may be fused together, there is neutrophil infiltration into the intestinal mucosa and a layer of Gram-negative bacteria adhere to the mucosa (29, 95). The ETEC can be seen adherent to the mucosal surface of the jejunum and ileum of infected calves (98). The ultrastructural changes in the small intestine reveal some increases in epithelial cell loss from the villus about 12 hours after experimental inoculation of calves with an ETEC (78). When a definitive etiological diagnosis is desirable, as in outbreaks of the disease, it is necessary to conduct the necropsy examination on diarrheic calves which are killed specifically for that purpose and the necropsy done on the fresh carcass. Postmortem autolysis of the intestinal mucosae and invasion of the tissues by intestinal microflora occurs within minutes after death, thus making evaluation of results difficult. Samples should be submitted for isolation of bacteria, demonstration and isolation of rotaviruses, and tissues for examination.

Diagnosis

The definitive etiological diagnosis of *septicemic colibacillosis* is dependent on the laboratory isolation of the causative agent, which is usually a single species of organism. The septicemias of the newborn cannot be distinguished from each other clinically. The definitive etiological diagnosis of *enteric colibacillosis* in newborn calves and piglets may be difficult and often inconclusive because the significance of other organisms in the intestinal tract and feces of diarrheic animals cannot be easily determined. Table 51 lists the possible causative agents of diarrhea and septicemia in newborn farm animals. Every effort which is economically possible should be made to obtain an etiological diagnosis. This is especially important when outbreaks of diarrhea occur in a herd or where the disease appears to be endemic. The use of an interdisciplinary team will increase the success of diagnosis.

This includes making a visit to the farm or herd and making a detailed epidemiological investigation of the problem. The diagnosis depends heavily on the epidemiological findings, and the microbiological and pathological findings and sometimes on the results of treatment.

The major difficulty is to determine whether or not the diarrhea is infectious in origin and to differentiate it from dietetic diarrhea which is most common in hand-fed calves and in all newborn species which are sucking high-producing dams. In dietetic diarrhea the feces are voluminous, pasty to gelatinous in consistency, the animal is bright and alert and is usually still sucking but some may be inappetent.

Treatment

The considerations for treatment of acute neonatal diarrhea include: alteration of the diet, fluid and electrolyte replacement, antimicrobial therapy, the possible use of antiparasympathomimetics and intestinal protectants and management of outbreaks. A review of the clinical management and control of neonatal enteric infection of calves is available (50).

The major factor which influences survival of calves with diarrhea is the level of colostral immunity in the calf at the onset of the diarrhea (60). The prognosis is unfavorable if the level of immunoglobulins is low, regardless of intensive fluid and antimicrobial therapy.

Table 51. Possible causes of septicemia and acute neonatal diarrhea in farm animals

Septicemia			
Calves	*Piglets*	*Lambs*	*Foals*
E. coli *Salmonella* spp. *Listeria monocytogenes* *Pasteurella* spp. *Streptococcus* spp. *Pneumonococcus* spp.	*E. coli* *Streptococcus* *Listeria monocytogenes*	*E. coli* *Salmonella* spp. *Listeria monocytogenes* *Erysipelas insidiosa*	*E. coli* *Actinobacillus equuli* *Salmonella abortivoequina* *Salmonella typhimurium* *Strep. pyogenes* *Listeria monocytogenes*
Acute neonatal diarrhea			
Calves	*Piglets*	*Lambs*	*Foals*
Enteropathogenic and enterotoxigenic *E. coli* Rotavirus Coronavirus *Cryptosporidium* *Salmonella* spp. *Eimeria* spp. (calves at least 3 weeks of age) *Clostridium perfringens* type C	Enteropathogenic *E. coli* *Salmonella* spp. Transmissible gastroenteritis virus *Cl. perfringens* type C Rotavirus *Isospora* spp.	*Cl. perfringens* type C Rotavirus	Foal-heat diarrhea Rotavirus *Cl. perfringens* type B

Alteration of the diet

The question of whether or not diarrheic newborn animals should be starved from milk during the period of diarrhea is still debatable. Certainly diarrheic piglets are usually treated and left free to nurse on the sow and diarrheic beef calves are commonly treated and left with the cow. However, it is a common practice to starve for 24 hours diarrheic calves which are being handfed milk replacer or whole milk. In one study it was shown that the offering of milk to diarrheic calves when they were willing to drink following hydration therapy in a clinic resulted in a higher but insignificant improvement in survival rate than calves which were starved from milk for 24 hours (56). Balance studies in diarrheic calves have shown that continued milk intake helped to maintain plasma volume which suggests that calves should continue to receive a source of oral fluid during the periods of diarrhea (79). Because of reduced digestibility in enteric disease, it would appear logical not to feed the animal with nutriments such as milk which must be digested but rather to provide readily absorbable substances such as oral glucose–electrolyte mixtures (57). These are used commonly during the period of diarrhea as a source of energy, fluids and electrolytes. Such mixtures are inexpensive, easy to use, readily available and, if used by the farmer when diarrhea is first noticed, will usually successfully treat existing dehydration and prevent further dehydration and acidosis.

Following recovery, calves should be offered reduced quantities of whole milk three times daily (no more than total daily intake equivalent to 8% of body weight) on the first day and increased to the normal daily allowance in the next few days. Milk should not be diluted with water as this may interfere with the clothing mechanism in the abomasum.

Fluid and electrolyte replacement

The dehydration, acidosis and electrolyte imbalance are corrected by the parenteral and oral use of simple or balanced electrolyte solutions.

Parenteral fluid therapy In severe dehydration and acidosis, solutions containing the bicarbonate ion are indicated. Solutions containing lactates are undesirable as they must be converted to the bicarbonate ion by the liver, which may not be functioning normally and the plasma lactates may already be increased.

An equal mixture of isotonic saline (0·85%), isotonic sodium bicarbonate (1·3%), and isotonic dextrose (5%) is a simple effective solution for parenteral use. The use of sodium bicarbonate, sodium L-lactate, and sodium acetate for the treatment of acidosis in diarrheic calves has been evaluated (80). The use of sodium bicarbonate as an alkalinizing compound in the parenteral fluids is superior to the use of compounds such as sodium acetate or sodium lactate which must be metabolized by the liver, myocardium and other tissues in order to have an alkalinizing effect. Nevertheless, sodium acetate and sodium lactate have merit in treating diarrheic calves with metabolic acidosis. The simple replacement of fluid losses using saline or fluids without alkalinizing compounds is likewise not as effective as sodium bicarbonate. The bicarbonate requirements can be calculated using the equation: weight (kg) × base deficit (mmol/l) × 0·3. The base deficit will range from 5 to 20 mmol/l with an arbitrary average of about 15 mmol/l. Thus, an estimate of the bicarbonate requirements for a 45 kg calf are 45 × 15 × 0·3 = 205 mmol/l; 1 g of sodium bicarbonate will yield 12 mmol of bicarbonate and therefore 16·8 g of sodium bicarbonate are needed. This would mean 1·3 liters of isotonic (1·3%) sodium bicarbonate. This amount of bicarbonate may be an underestimate because the size of the extracellular fluid space may be closer to 0·6 than 0·3. Using a value of 0·6 for the size of the extracellular fluid space, the bicarbonate requirements for a 45 kg calf with a base deficit of 15 mmol/l, are 45 × 15 × 0·6 = 405 mmol, which requires 33·75 g of sodium bicarbonate which could be delivered in 2·5 liters of 1·3% isotonic solution.

Some calves from 10 to 20 days of age with a history of diarrhea in the previous several days may be affected with metabolic acidosis without obvious clinical evidence of dehydration (43). These calves are ataxic, weak, sometimes recumbent and may appear comatose. The intravenous administration of 2–3 liters of isotonic (1·3%) sodium bicarbonate results in recovery within an hour.

For severe dehydration (10–12% of body weight) fluids should be replaced as follows: hydration therapy 100 ml/kg body weight intravenously in the first 1–2 hours at the rate of 50–80 ml/kg body weight/hour followed by maintenance therapy at 140 ml/kg body weight over the next 8–10 hours at the rate of about 20 ml/kg body weight/hour. For example, a 45 kg calf which is 10% dehydrated should receive 4·5 liters of fluid in the first 1–2 hours as hydration therapy followed by 6–8 liters of fluid over the next 8–10 hours. Initially, both the acidosis and the dehydration can be treated by the use of isotonic sodium bicarbonate followed by the use of a combined mixture of isotonic saline and isotonic sodium bicarbonate or multiple electrolyte solutions for maintenance therapy. For moderate dehydration (6–8% of body weight) fluids should be replaced as follows: hydration therapy 50 ml/kg body weight intravenously in the first 1–2 hours at the rate of 50–80 ml/kg body weight/hour followed by maintenance therapy as described above. Maintenance therapy may be provided using oral fluids and electrolytes if the calf is well enough to suck from a nipple bottle or drink from a pail. The techniques for long-term intravenous administration of fluids to the calf have been described (58).

The use of solutions containing potassium chloride is sometimes recommended on the basis that total potassium stores may be depleted in severely affected calves (92). However, they should be used with caution because a severe hyperkalemia may be present when there is a severe acidosis. If the acidosis and hypoglycemia are corrected with glucose and bicarbonate, the administration of potassium may be beneficial in restoring total potassium stores. However, solutions containing potassium can be cardiotoxic particularly if renal function is not restored.

Oral fluid and electrolyte therapy Oral and fluid electrolyte therapy are indicated for animals in the early stages of diarrhea or after they have been successfully hydrated following parenteral fluid therapy. Severely dehydrated or moribund calves may not respond favorably to oral fluid therapy alone. Veterinarians should encourage owners to provide oral fluid and electrolyte therapy to diarrheic neonatal farm animals as soon as possible after the onset of diarrhea. Almost all of the information available on oral fluids has been developed following clinical studies in diarrheic calves and the recommendations here reflect those studies (105, 106).

Oral fluid and electrolyte therapy is beneficial in enteric colibacillosis of neonatal farm animals presumably because molecules of glucose continue to be absorbed by the small intestine by an active transport mechanism accompanied by glucose-coupled sodium absorption and absorption of water. In enterotoxigenic colibacillosis while there is net hypersecretion caused by the enterotoxin, the intestinal mucosa is sufficiently intact so that water and sodium will be absorbed in the presence of glucose. Most oral electrolytes intended for the treatment of dehydration and acidosis in diarrheic calves contain sodium chloride and sodium bicarbonate with one or some of the following substances: glucose, acetates and citrates, phosphates, potassium salts, glycine and amino acids. Several commercial oral preparations are available (91). These preparations are not intended to support normal growth rates (106). Diarrheic calves must receive sufficient fluid therapy to compensate for fluid and electrolyte losses which occurred and for maintenance and contemporary losses during the period of clinical diarrhea and convalescence. However, the calf must be returned to a milk diet within a few days in order to avoid the effects of malnutrition. Oral fluid and electrolyte formulas cannot provide the daily maintenance requirements for energy, protein and fat. Some formulas contain a large quantity of glucose, and are supplemented with glycine, sodium acetate and citric acid, thus making it a calorie-dense partially nitrogen-balanced hyperosmolal solution (106). The acetate, as a partial substitute for chloride, may stimulate sodium and water absorption by the jejunum. Citric acid may contribute to sodium and water absorption as a preferred energy substrate for intestinal mucosal cells. The inclusion of glycine is intended to enhance sodium and water absorption and may improve nitrogen balance.

A hyperosmotic oral fluid and electrolyte replacement for diarrheic calves is available and has been subjected to some preliminary clinical trials (107).

There are marked variations in the alkalinizing abilities of the oral electrolyte solutions which are available commercially (105). Those which contain at least 80 mmol/l of bicarbonate are much more effective for the rapid correction of acidosis and depression in diarrheic calves than administration of rehydrating electrolyte solutions alone. The bicarbonate-rich preparations have the best alkalinizing response when given to calves affected with acidosis from experimentally induced diarrhea (132). Those oral electrolyte solutions containing acid phosphate salts are undesirable because they cause net acidification of the blood with a fall in blood pH. However, there is some evidence that an alkaline electrolyte solution may prolong the clotting of milk by rennin in the abomasum which could cause diarrhea especially if the oral fluids and electrolytes are diluted 1:1 with whole milk.

The compositions of oral fluids are set out below.

Formula no. 1 This is a glucose–glycine–electrolyte mixture in powder form: glucose 67·53%, sodium chloride 14·34%, glycine 10·3%, citric acid 0·81%, potassium citrate 0·21% and potassium dihydrogen phosphate 6·8%. A 64 g amount of the above is dissolved in 2 liters of water to produce an isotonic solution (57). The presence of the glycine and glucose enhances the absorption of water.

This solution has a pH of 4·3 which may enhance the rennet clotting of milk. Other solutions such as Formula no. 2 contain sodium bicarbonate, which is an effective alkalinizing agent. A commercial preparation known as *Lifeguard* (Norden Laboratories) contains the following: glucose monohydrate 152 g, sodium bicarbonate 12·75 g, glycine 4.72 g, potassium chloride 3.6 g, sodium chloride 2.84 g, calcium phosphate 1.33 g and magnesium sulfate 0.76 g. When added to water at the recommended proportions, it will contain 80 mmol/liter of bicarbonate.

The oral fluids and electrolytes should not be mixed with milk but fed or offered between feedings of milk. The oral fluids should be given by nipple bottle if the animal will suck but the use of a stomach tube is satisfactory. Fluids can be administered to the dehydrated calf using an esophageal feeder tube, even though the reticular groove does not close. At least 2 liters of fluid should be given which results in a transfer of fluids to the abomasum (130). If larger doses are required they should be divided and given at intervals of 2 hours or more to avoid abdominal discomfort from the distention.

Calves which respond and recover usually show marked improvement from intravenous and/or oral fluid therapy within 24–36 hours. Calves which are likely to recover will respond to the hydration therapy within 6–10 hours, begin to urinate within an hour after fluid administration was begun, and maintain hydration. Calves which do not respond will not hydrate normally; they may not begin to urinate because of irreversible renal failure, their feces remain watery, they remain depressed and not strong enough to suck or drink and continued fluid therapy beyond 3 days is usually futile.

Antimicrobial and immunoglobulin therapy

Antibiotics, sulfonamides, and other chemotherapeutics have been used extensively for many years for the specific treatment of colibacillosis in calves. These were used because it was assumed that in calves affected with enteric colibacillosis there was an infectious enteritis which had the potential of developing into a bacteremia or septicemia. However, there is a notable lack of well-conducted clinical trials designed to show the efficacy of antibacterials in enteric colibacillosis. Conversely there is no information which indicates that they are not useful. In one study which evaluated the efficacy of antimicrobial agents given orally and parenterally to newborn calves with acute neonatal undifferentiated diarrhea, there was a slight but insignificant improvement in survival rate when chloramphenicol was given parenterally combined with nifuraldezone orally (56).

Experimentally, the attachment of $K88^+$ porcine enterotoxigenic *E. coli* was decreased following growth in the presence of concentrations of oxytetracycline below the minimal inhibitory concentrations (108). There was still a decrease in adhesion when the drug resistance was induced in the bacterial strains. These observations may justify the use of oral antimicrobials for the treatment of enterotoxigenic colibacillosis in neonatal farm animals.

Experimentally, several antibiotics given orally at therapeutic levels to normal calves may cause intestinal mucosal alterations, interference with absorption and diarrhea. Chloramphenicol, neomycin, oxytetracycline and ampicillin have caused varying degrees of reductions in the height of villous epithelium, malabsorption and diarrhea (109). However, these observations have not been made in naturally occurring cases of diarrheic calves. The use of iron chelators and competitors for the treatment of bacterial diarrhea in calves has been suggested as an alternative to antimicrobials (134). However, there is no validated information available to support their recommendation.

One of the major difficulties confronting the veterinarian in the field is deciding if calves or piglets affected with enteric colibacillosis are bacteremic or septicemic. As a result, more animals than necessary are treated systemically to avoid deaths from septicemia. Time does not usually permit pretreatment culture of the organism and determination of the drug sensitivity, so that broad-spectrum antibiotics and selected chemotherapeutics based on previously successful experience are used. Some of the commonly used ones are chloramphenicol, ampicillin and trimethoprim–sulfonamide combinations. The dosages of these drugs for maximum effectiveness for the treatment of coliform septicemia in newborn calves and piglets have not been determined but the adult dose based on body weight appears to be successful and without toxicity. Neonates may be unable to metabolize drugs as effectively as adults. The advantage of parenterally administered antibiotics in colibacillosis in calves and piglets is the enterohepatic circulation which provides a level of the drug in the intestinal lumen which may not require the oral administration of the drug.

Many oral preparations are available and used for the treatment of enteric colibacillosis in calves and piglets. Some consist of a single drug, while others are mixtures with or without absorbents, astringents and electrolytes. They have been used on an empirical basis since controlled trials have not been conducted. Chloramphenicol, neomycin sulfate, tetracyclines, sulfonamides, trimethoprim–sulfonamide mixtures, nifuraldezone and ampicillin are in common use in different mixtures too numerous to discuss here. Any of these drugs may be used but should be discontinued after 3 successive days of treatment to avoid elimination of too many species of drug-sensitive intestinal flora and their replacement by pathogenic fungi (59) or bacteria such as *Candida* spp., *Proteus* spp. and *Pseudomonas* spp. If possible, particularly in outbreaks of enteric colibacillosis in calves and piglets, the causative organism should be isolated from feces or tissues and a drug sensitivity obtained even though there are some limitations on the results unless the organism is more critically characterized as discussed under clinical pathology.

In some countries it may be illegal to use some of the antimicrobials mentioned here because of the regulations regarding their use in food-producing animals. Some are available to farmers on a prescription-only basis, which makes examination of the animals and a diagnosis necessary before recommendations are made. The indiscriminate use of antibiotics in milk replacers or for treatment of newborn calves and piglets is widespread and must be viewed with concern when the problem of drug resistance transfer from animal to animal and to man are considered.

Multiple antimicrobial drug resistance does occur in *E. coli* and other enterobacteria when the drugs are used on a continuous prophylactic basis (93). There is evidence that *E. coli* isolated from the feces of young farm animals with diarrhea have developed resistance to trimethoprim-containing antimicrobial products which have been used widely for the treatment of diarrhea (110). In some studies of the antimicrobial drug resistance in porcine enterotoxigenic *E. coli*, the frequencies of the different drug resistance correlate well with the total amount of active substance of each drug used in farm animals in that geographical area (111).

One of the important factors determining whether or not calves survive enteric colibacillosis is the serum immunoglobulin status of the animal before it develops the disease. Most of the literature on therapy omits this information and is therefore difficult to assess (60). There is ample evidence that the mortality rate will be high in diarrheic calves which are deficient in serum immunoglobulins, particularly IgG, in spite of exhaustive antimicrobial and fluid therapy (7, 60). This has stimulated interest in the possible use of purified solutions of bovine gammaglobulin in diarrheic calves which are hypogammaglobulinemic. However, they must be given by the intravenous route and in large amounts, the cost of which would be prohibitive. In addition, they are unlikely to be of value once the calf is affected with diarrhea; they are protective and probably not curative. Whole blood transfusion to severely affected calves may be used as a source of gammaglobulins but unless given in large quantities would not significantly elevate the serum immunoglobulin levels in deficient calves. Limited controlled trials indicate that there is no significant difference in the survival rate of diarrheic calves treated with either a blood transfusion daily for 3 days; fluid therapy given orally, subcutaneously or intravenously depending on the severity of the dehydration; or fluid therapy with antibiotics (94). Those calves which survived regardless of the type of therapy had high levels of immunoglobulins before they developed diarrhea. This again emphasizes the importance of the calf ingesting liberal quantities of colostrum within the first few hours after birth.

Antiparasympathomimetics and intestinal protectants

Benzetimide has been used for its anticholinergic and antisecretory effect in the treatment of diarrhea in newborn farm animals (62). Chlorpromazine, a potent *in vitro* antagonist to enterotoxin in a cell system, will shorten the duration of experimentally induced and naturally occurring diarrhea in piglets infected with enterotoxigenic *E. coli* (96). Attapulgate and peptobismal are also effective in preventing fluid accumulation in ligated segments of pig intestine infected with enteropathogenic *E. coli* (97). Acetylsalicylic acid and methylprednisolone also reduce fluid accumulation (97). Experimentally, the intravenous infusion of sodium salicylate may be beneficial in treating enterotoxigenic colibacillosis in calves (112). These drugs which inhibit secretion may play an important role in the treatment of enterotoxigenic diarrhea in newborn animals but there is only limited clinical and scientific data available to make a recommendation. However, the rationale is logical. Intestinal protectants such as kaolin and pectin are in general use for diarrheic animals but likewise their beneficial value is difficult to evaluate.

Management of outbreaks

When outbreaks of colibacillosis occur, every effort should be made to isolate affected animals from other susceptible calves and piglets. Recently born calves should be housed or pastured away from affected calves. Beef calves with the disease should be moved out of the calving grounds to an isolation pasture. All new cases should be treated immediately and deaths submitted to necropsy for examination.

Control

Because of the complex nature of the disease, it is unrealistic to expect total prevention, and control at an economical level should be the major goal. Effective control of colibacillosis can be accomplished by application of three principles:

- Reduce the degree of exposure of newborn calves and piglets to the infectious agents
- Provide maximum non-specific resistance with adequate colostrum and optimum animal husbandry
- Increase the specific resistance of the newborn by vaccination of the dam or the newborn.

Reduction of the degree of exposure of newborn calves and piglets to pathogenic E. coli

Dairy calves These comments are directed particularly at calves born inside where contamination is higher than outside.

- Calves should be born in well-bedded box stalls which were previously cleaned out
- The perineum and udder of the dairy cow should be washed shortly before calving
- Immediately after birth the navel of the calf should be swabbed with 2% iodine. Tying off the navel at the level of the abdominal wall with cotton thread is also practiced
- Calves affected with diarrhea should be removed from the main calf barn if possible and treated in isolation.

Beef calves These are usually born outside on pasture or on confined calving grounds.

- Calving grounds should have been free of animals previous to the calving period; the grounds should be well drained, dry and scraped free of snow if possible. A top dressing of the calving grounds with straw or wood shavings will provide a comfortable calving environment
- In a few days following birth when the calf is nursing successfully, the cow–calf pair should be moved to a nursery pasture to avoid overcrowding in the calving grounds.

Veal calves These calves are usually obtained from several different sources and 25–30% or higher may be deficient in serum immunoglobulin.

- On arrival, calves should be placed in their individual calf pens which were previously cleaned, disinfected and left vacant to dry
- Feeding utensils are a frequent source of pathogenic *E. coli* and should be cleaned and air-dried daily
- Calves affected with diarrhea should be removed and isolated immediately.

Piglets Piglets born in a total-confinement system may be exposed to a high infection rate.

- The all in/all-out system of batch farrowing, in which groups of sows farrow within a week, is recommended. This system will allow the herdsman to wean the piglets from a group of sows in a day or two and clean, disinfect and leave vacant a battery of farrowing crates for the next group of sows. This system will reduce the total occupation time and the infection rate. The continuous farrowing system without regular breaks is not recommended
- Before being placed in the farrowing crate, sows should be washed with a suitable disinfectant to reduce the bacterial population of the skin.

Provision of maximum non-specific resistance
This begins with the provision of optimal nutrition to the pregnant dam which will result in a vigorous newborn animal and adequate quantities of colostrum. The next most important control measure is to ensure that colostrum is ingested in liberal quantities within minutes and no later than a few hours after birth. While the optimum amount of colostrum which should be ingested by a certain time after birth is well known, the major difficulty with all species under practical conditions is to know how much colostrum a particular animal has consumed. Because modern livestock production has become so intensive, it is becoming more important for the herdsman to make every effort to ensure that sufficient colostrum is ingested by that particular species. In one study, in large dairy herds, 42% of calves left with their dams for one day following birth had failed either to suck sufficient colostrum or to absorb sufficient colostral immunoglobulins (63). This problem can be alleviated by bottle feeding 1 liter of pooled colostrum to all calves at approximately 1 day after birth (63). Encouraging and assisting the calf to suck within 1 hour after birth is also effective. The provision of early assisted sucking of colostrum to satiation within 1 hour after birth will result in high concentrations of absorbed immunoglobulins in the majority of calves (113). In fact, the ingestion of 80–100 g of colostral immunoglobulins within a few hours after birth is so effective in achieving high levels of colostral immunoglobulins in calves that either leaving the calf with the cow for the next 12–24 hours or encouraging the calf to suck again at 12 hours will not result in a significant increase in absorbed immunoglobulins (113).

Despite early assisted sucking, a small proportion of calves will remain hypogammaglobulinemic because of low concentrations of immunoglobulins in their dams' colostrum, usually associated with leakage of colostrum from the udder before calving (113).

The routine force-feeding of pooled colostrum immediately after birth results in high serum levels of colostrum immunoglobulins in calves (63). However, in some situations there may be no apparent benefit from such a practice (114).

The other factors which influence the ingestion of colostrum and the absorption of immunoglobulin are presented in the section on epidemiology of colibacillosis and in Chapter 3 on diseases of the newborn.

In large herds where economics permit, a laboratory surveillance system may be used on batches of calves to determine the serum levels of immunoglobulin acquired. An accurate analysis may be done by electrophoresis or an estimation using the zinc sulfate turbidity test (53). Blood should be collected from calves at 24 hours of age. Samples taken a few days later may not be a true reflection of the original serum immunoglobulin levels. The information obtained from determination of serum immunoglobulins in calves at 24 hours of age can be used to improve management practices, particularly the early ingestion of colostrum.

The administration of purified bovine gammaglobulin to calves which are deficient appears to be a logical approach but the results have been unsuccessful. Large doses (30–50 g) of gammaglobulin given intravenously would be required to increase the level of serum gammaglobulin from 0·5 g/dl to 1·5 g/dl of serum which is considered an adequate level. The cost would be prohibitive. The administration of gammaglobulins by any parenteral route other than the intravenous route does not result in a significant increase in serum levels of the immunoglobulin.

Some guidelines for ensuring that newborn farm animals ingest sufficient quantities of colostrum and absorb adequate amounts of colostral immunoglobulins are summarized here. Additional details are presented in Chapter 3.

Dairy calves The following should be implemented:

- Immediately after birth, unless the calf is a vigorous sucker, colostrum should be removed from the cow and fed by nipple-bottle or by stomach tube at the rate of at least 50 ml/kg body weight in the first 2 hours. Encouragement and assistance to suck to satiation within the first hour after birth is also highly effective in achieving high levels of colostral immunoglobulins in the serum of the calf (113)
- The calf should be left with the cow for at least 2 days. This contact will improve the absorption of immunoglobulin
- Following the colostral feeding period, dairy calves are usually placed in individual stalls until weaning. A recent development is the feeding of fermented colostrum to newborn calves for up to 3 weeks after birth. This provides a source of lactoglobulins in the intestinal tract and reduces the incidence of neonatal diarrhea of calves due to a wide variety of pathogens
- Calves should be fed regularly and preferably by the same person. One of the most important factors affecting dairy calf mortality is the concern and care provided by the calf rearer (64)

- The housing and ventilation must be adequate to avoid stress.

Lambs Lambs require between 180 and 210 ml of colostrum/kg body weight during the first 18 hours after birth to provide sufficient energy for heat production (117). Such intakes will usually also provide enough colostral immunoglobulins. Early encouragement and assistance of the lambs to suck the ewe is important. Well-fed ewes usually have sufficient colostrum for singletons or twins. Underfed ewes may not have sufficient colostrum for one or more lambs and supplementation from stored colostrum obtained by milking other high-producing ewes is a useful practice (117).

Beef calves The following should be implemented:

- Beef calves should be assisted at birth, if necessary, to avoid exhaustion and weakness from a prolonged parturition
- Normally beef calves will make attempts to get up and suck within 20 minutes after birth but this may be delayed for up to 8 hours or longer. Beef calves which do not suck within 2 hours should be fed colostrum by nipple bottle or stomach tube. Whenever possible they should be encouraged and assisted to suck to satiation within 1 hour after birth (113). The mean volume of colostrum and colostral, immunoglobulins produced in beef cows and the absorption of colostral immunoglobulins by their calves can vary widely (115). Beef calves deserted by indifferent dams need special attention
- Constant surveillance of the calving grounds is necessary to avoid overcrowding, to detect diarrheic calves which should be removed, to avoid mismothering, and to ensure that every calf is seen to nurse its dam. Although up to 25% of beef calves may not have sufficient serum levels of immunoglobulins, the provision of excellent management will minimize the incidence of colibacillosis (65). The recently developed practice of corticosteroid-induced parturition in cattle may result in a major mismothering problem if too many calves are born too quickly in a confined space. Every management effort must be used to establish the cow–calf herd, as soon as possible after birth (65). This will require high quality management to reduce even further the infection rate and minimize any stressors in the environment.

Piglets The following should be implemented:

- Every possible economical effort must be made to ensure that each newborn piglet obtains a liberal supply of colostrum within minutes of birth. The farrowing floor must be well drained and it must be slip-proof to allow the piglets to move easily to the sow's udder. Some herdsmen provide assistance at farrowing, drying off every piglet as it is born and placing it immediately onto a teat
- The washing of the sow's udder immediately before farrowing with warm water and soap will reduce the bacterial population and may provide relief in cases of congested and edematous udders
- The piglet creep area must be dry, appropriately heated for the first week, and free from drafts. During farrowing, colostrum is released in discrete ejections possibly by discrete release of oxytocin associated with parturition (116). Therefore, as the piglets are born they must be as close to the udder as possible in order to take advantage of these discrete ejections.

Increasing specific resistance of the newborn by vaccinating the pregnant dam or the newborn

The immunization of calves and piglets against colibacillosis by vaccination of the pregnant dam or by vaccination of the fetus or the neonate has received considerable research attention in recent years and the results appear promising. The pregnant dam is vaccinated 2–4 weeks before parturition to stimulate specific antibodies to particular strains of enteropathogenic *E. coli*, and the antibodies are then passed on to the newborn. The mechanism of protection is now considered to be the production of antibodies against the pilus antigens which are responsible for colonization of the *E. coli* in the intestine (69).

It must be emphasized that vaccination is an aid to good management and not replacement for inadequate management.

Calves Vaccination of pregnant cattle with either purified *E. coli* $K99^+$ pili or whole cell preparation containing sufficient $K99^+$ antigen can significantly reduce the incidence of enterotoxigenic colibacillosis in calves (8, 66, 67). Good protection is also possible when the dams are vaccinated with a four-strain *E. coli* whole cell bacterin containing sufficient $K99^+$ pilus antigen and the polysaccharide capsular K antigen (68). Colostral antibodies specific for $K99^+$ pilus antigen and the polysaccharide capsular K antigen on the surface of the challenge exposure strain of enterotoxigenic *E. coli* are protective. There is a highly significant correlation between the lacteal immunity to the $K99^+$ antigen and the prevention of severe diarrhea or death in calves challenged with enterotoxigenic *E. coli* (66). The colostral levels of $K99^+$ antibody are highest during the first 2 days after parturition which is the most susceptible period for enterotoxigenic colibacillosis to occur in the newborn calf. The continuous presence of the $K99^+$ antibody in the lumen of the intestine prevents adherence of the bacteria to the intestinal epithelium. The $K99^+$ antibody is also absorbed during the period of immunoglobulin absorption and may be excreted into the intestine during diarrhea. This may be one of the reasons that mortality is inversely proportional to serum immunoglobulin levels. The pregnant dams are vaccinated twice in the first year, 6 and 2 weeks prior to parturition. Each year thereafter they are given a single booster vaccination (71).

Oral vaccination of pregnant cows with live or dead *E. coli* of the $K99^+$ pilus antigen type is not an effective means of stimulating the production of $K99^+$ antibody in serum or colostrum (72).

The oral administration of a $K99^+$-specific monoclonal antibody to calves during the first 12 hours after birth may be an effective method of reducing the incidence of fatal enterotoxigenic colibacillosis particularly when outbreaks of the disease occur in unvaccinated herds (73).

Clinical trials indicate that the severity of dehydration, depression, weight loss and duration of diarrhea were significantly reduced in calves which had received the $K99^+$-specific monoclonal antibody. In experimentally challenged calves the mortality was 29% in the treated calves and 82% in the control calves (73).

Vaccines containing both the $K99^+$ antigen of enterotoxigenic *E. coli* and the rotavirus, and in some cases the coronavirus, have been evaluated with variable results. The colostral antibodies to the $K99^+$ antigen are higher in vaccinated than unvaccinated dams but the colostral antibodies to rotavirus and coronavirus may not be significantly different between vaccinated and unvaccinated dams (118). In these field trials vaccination had no effect on the prevalence of diarrhea, calf mortality or the presence of the three enteropathogens (118). In other field trials the combined vaccine did provide some protection against outbreaks of calf diarrhea (119). To be effective the rotavirus and coronavirus antibodies must be present in the postcolostral milk for several days after parturition during the period when calves are most susceptible to the viral infection.

The decision to vaccinate in any particular year will depend on the recognition of risk factors which have not yet been well defined. However, risk factors include the following: a definitive diagnosis of enteropathogenic $K99^+$ *E. coli* in the previous year, a population density in the calving grounds which is conducive to the disease, calving during the year when the environmental conditions are wet and uncomfortable for the calves, and a large percentage of primiparous dams which do not have protective levels of $K99^+$ antibody in their colostrum.

These favorable results suggest that vaccination may become a valuable method of control of enteric colibacillosis of calves, especially in problem herds. At the present time it appears that the autogenous bacterins will provide protection against only the homologous bacteria used in the bacterin and if heterologous strains should appear there will be no protection. In some studies in which autogenous vaccines did not provide protection against diarrhea in newborn calves, the precise cause of the diarrhea was not determined (70). The other problem is that calves must still ingest colostrum in sufficient quantities soon enough to acquire the protection afforded by the vaccine.

The antibody response of newborn calves to a vaccine depends on their colostral antibody status. There is a marked failure of the colostrum-fed calf to respond to injected antigens, not because of the relatively immature lymphoid system, but rather the presence of maternal antibody to the antigens used interferes with specific antibody stimulation (72).

Piglets Field experience has shown that the piglets born from gilts are more susceptible than those from mature sows, which suggests that immunity improves with parity. On a practical basis this suggests that gilts should be mixed with older sows which have been resident on the premises for some time. The length of time required for such natural immunization to occur is unknown but 1 month during late gestation seems logical.

Naturally occurring enteric colibacillosis in newborn piglets can be effectively controlled by vaccination of the pregnant dam. Three antigen types of pili, designated $K88^+$, $K99^+$, and 987P are now implicated in colonization of the small intestine of newborn piglets by enterotoxigenic *E. coli*. The vaccination of pregnant sows with oral or parenteral vaccines containing these antigens will provide protection against enterotoxigenic colibacillosis caused by *E. coli*-bearing pili homologous to those in the vaccines (76, 121, 124). The parenteral vaccines are cell-free preparations of pili and the oral vaccines contain live enteropathogenic *E. coli*. The oral vaccine is given 2 weeks before farrowing and is administered in the feed daily for 3 days as 200 ml of a broth culture containing 10^{11} *E. coli*/day (76). A simple and effective method of immunization of pregnant sows is by feeding of live cultures of enterotoxigenic *E. coli* isolated from piglets affected with neonatal colibacillosis on the same farm (122). The oral vaccine can be given in the feed beginning about 8 weeks after breeding and continued to parturition. The oral vaccine results in the stimulation of IgA antibody in the intestinal tract which is then transferred to the mammary gland and into the colostrum. A combination of oral and parenteral vaccination is superior to either route alone. The parenteral vaccine is given about 2 weeks after breeding and repeated 2–4 weeks before parturition. The parenteral vaccination results in the production of high levels of IgM antibody for protection against both experimental and naturally occurring enterotoxigenic colibacillosis (75). This vaccination also reduces the number of *E. coli* excreted in the feces of vaccinated sows which are major sources of the organism. Immunization of pregnant sows with an *E. coli* bacterin, enriched with the $K88^+$ antigen results in the secretion of milk capable of preventing adhesion of $K88^+$ *E. coli* to the gut for at least 5 weeks after birth at which time the piglet becomes naturally resistant to adhesion by the organism.

The use of toxoids are currently under investigation for the prevention. A procholeragenoid preparation made from the cholera toxin is highly immunogenic and when given to pregnant sows 5 and 2 weeks before parturition will provide protection against experimental colibacillosis in piglets (123, 125).

The possibility of selecting and breeding from pigs that may be resistant genetically to the disease is being explored (3). The highest incidence of diarrhea occurs in progeny of resistant dams and sired by susceptible sires. The homozygous dominants (SS) and the heterozygotes (Ss) possess the receptor and are susceptible whereas in the homozygous recessives (ss) it is absent and the pigs are resistant. Sows which are genetically resistant may not be able to mount an immune response to the $K88^+$ antigen because of the inability of the organism to colonize in the intestinal tract (126).

The use of abattoir porcine serum-derived immunoglobulins as milk replacer additives for the artificial rearing of colostrum-deprived piglets in a farm environment may have a place under certain special circumstances (77).

Lambs Vaccination of pregnant ewes with $K99^+$ antigen will confer colostral immunity to lambs challenged with homologous enteropathogenic *E. coli* (127, 128).

The pregnant ewes are vaccinated twice in the first year, at 8–10 weeks and 2–4 weeks before lambing, and in the second year one vaccination 2–4 weeks before lambing is adequate (128).

REVIEW LITERATURE

Acres, S. D. (1985) Enterotoxigenic *Escherichia coli* infections in newborn calves: a review. *J. dairy Sci.*, *68*, 229–256.

Bywater, R. J. (1975) Functional pathology of neonatal diarrhoea in calves and piglets. *Vet. Ann.*, *15*, 425.

Chidlow, J. W. & Porter, P. (1979) Intestinal defence of the neonatal pig: interrelationships of gut and mammary function providing surface immunity against colibacillosis. *Vet. Rec.*, *104*, 496–500.

Colloquium on Selected Diarrheal Diseases of the Young (1978) *J. Am. vet. med. Assoc.*, *173*, Part 2, No. 5, pp. 511–576.

Dougan, G. & Morrissey, P. (1985) Molecular analysis of the virulence determinants of enterotoxigenic *Escherichia coli* isolated from domestic animals: application for vaccine development. *Vet. Microbiol.*, *10*, 241–257.

Okerman, L. (1981) Enteric infections by non-enterotoxigenic *Escherichia coli* in animals: occurrence and pathogenicity mechanisms. A review. *Vet. Microbiol.*, *14*, 33–46.

Hinton, M. (1986) The ecology of *E. coli* in animals including man with particular reference to drug resistance. *Vet. Rec.*, *119*, 420–426.

Klemm, P. (1985) Fimbrial adhesions of *Escherichia coli*. *Rev. Infect. Dis.*, 7, 321–340.

Logan, E. F. (1974) Colostral immunity to colibacillosis in the neonatal calf. *Br. vet. J.*, *130*, 405.

Moon, H. W. (1974) Pathogenesis of enteric diseases caused by *Escherichia coli*. *Adv. vet. Sci. comp. Med.*, *18*, 1979.

Porter, P. (1973) Intestinal defence in the young pig. A review of the secretory antibody systems and their possible role in oral immunization. *Vet. Rec.*, *92*, 658.

Proceedings of the Second International Symposium on Neonatal Diarrhoea (1978). *Vet. Infect. Dis. Org.*, University of Sask., Oct. 3–5, pp. 1–551. Saskatoon, Canada.

Rutter, J. M. (1975) *Escherichia coli* infections in piglets: pathogenesis, virulence and vaccination. *Vet. Rec.*, *96*, 171.

Selman, I. E. (1972) The absorption of colostral globulins by newborn dairy calves, *Vet. Ann.*, *13*, 1.

Tennant, B., Ward, D. E., Braun, R. K. Hunt, E. L. & Baldwin, B. H. (1978) Clinical management and control of neonatal enteric infection of calves. *J. Am. vet. med. Assoc.*, *173*, 654–661.

REFERENCES

(1) Moon, H. W. (1974) *Adv. vet. Sci. comp. Med.*, *18*, 179.
(2) Gay, C. C. (1965) *Bacteriol. Rev.*, *29*, 75.
(3) Sellwood, R. (1983) *Ann. richer. Vet.*, *14*, 512.
(4) Nielsen, N. C. et al. (1975) *Nord. VetMed.*, *26*, 137.
(5) Svendsen, J. et al. (1975) *Nord. VetMed.*, *27*, 85.
(6) Logan, E. F. (1974) *Br. vet. J.*, *130*, 405.
(7) McGuire, T. C. et al. (1976) *J. Am. vet. Assoc.*, *169*, 713.
(8) Acres, S. D. (1985) *J. dairy Sci.*, *68*, 229.
(9) Wray, C. & Morris, J. A. (1985) *J. Hyg. Camb.*, *95*, 577.
(10) Balsbaugh, R. K. et al. (1986) *J. anim. Sci.*, *62*, 315.
(11) Kadis, S. et al. (1984) *Am. J. vet. Res.*, *45*, 255.
(12) Pearson, G. R. & Logan, E. F. (1979) *Vet. Rec.*, *105*, 159.
(13) Kruse, V. (1970) *Anim. Prod.*, *12*, 661.
(14) van Zijderveld, A. et al. (1982) *Proc. XII World Cong. Dis. Cattle.*, *The Netherlands*, p. 258.
(15) Selman, I. E. (1972) *Vet. Ann.*, *13*, 1.
(16) Stott, G. H. et al. (1976) *J. dairy Sci.*, *59*, 1306.
(17) Krogh, H. V. (1983) *Nord. VetMed.*, *35*, 346.
(18) Kruse, V. (1970) *Anim. Prod.*, *12*, 619.
(19) Scoot, A. et al. (1972) *J. anim. Sci.*, *35*, 1201.
(20) Martin, S. W. et al. (1975) *Am. J. vet. Res.*, *36*, 1105.
(21) Roy, J. H. B. & Ternouth, J. H. (1972) *Proc. Nutr. Soc.*, *31*, 53.
(22) Sherwood, D. et al. (1983) *Vet. Rec.*, *113*, 208.
(23) Smith, H. W. (1965) *J. Pathol. Bacteriol.*, *90*, 495.
(24) Roy, J. H. B. et al. (1955) *Br. J. Nutr.*, *9*, 11.
(25) Evans, M. G. et al. (1986) *Am. J. vet. Res.*, *47*, 2431.
(26) Snodgrass, D. R. et al. (1982) *Vet. Microbiol.*, 7, 51.
(27) Harnett, N. M. & Gyles, C. L. (1983) *Am. J. vet. Res.*, *44*, 1210.
(28) Rose, R. et al. (1987) *Vet. Pathol.*, *24*, 71.
(29) Bellamy, J. E. C. & Acres, S. D. (1979) *Am. J. vet. Res.*, *40*, 1391.
(30) Grimes, S. D. et al. (1986) *Am. J. vet. Res.*, *47*, 385.
(31) Snodgrass, D. R. et al. (1981) *Vet. Rec.*, *109*, 461.
(32) Wilson, R. A. & Francis, D. H. (1986) *Am. J. vet. Res.*, *47*, 213.
(33) Saeed, A. M. K. et al. (1983) *Infect. Immun.* *40*, 701.
(34) Johnson, B. D. et al. (1979) *Fed. Proc.*, *38* (3, II), 1261.
(35) Sherwood, D. et al. (1985) *Vet. Rec.*, *116*, 217.
(36) Smith, H. W. & Halls, S. J. (1967) *Pathology*, *93*, 531.
(37) Dougan, G. & Morrissey, P. (1985) *Vet. Microbiol.*, *10*, 241.
(38) Klemm, P. (1985) *Rev. infect. Dis.*, 7, 321.
(39) Moxley, R. A. & Francis, D. H. (1986) *Infect. Immun.*, *53*, 339.
(40) Schultze, F. & Muller, G. (1980) *Arch. exp. VetMed.*, *34*, 317.
(41) Porter, P. (1973) *Vet. Rec.*, *92*, 658.
(42) Andren, B. & Persson, S. (1983) *Acta vet. Scand.*, *24*, 84.
(43) Kasari, T. R. & Naylor, J. M. (1984) *Can. vet. J.*, *25*, 394.
(44) Stiglmair-Herb, M. T. et al. (1986) *Vet. Pathol.*, *23*, 125.
(45) Chanter, N. et al. (1986) *Vet. Microbiol.*, *12*, 241.
(46) Larivriere, S. et. al. (1979) *Am. J. vet. Res.*, *40*, 130.
(47) Francis, D. H. (1983) *Am. J. Vet. Res.*, *44*, 1884.
(48) Morris, J. A. et al. (1985) *Br. vet. J.*, *141*, 484.
(49) Hall, G. A. (1985) *Vet. Pathol.*, *22*, 156.
(50) Tennant, B. et al. (1978) *J. Am. vet. med. Assoc.*, *173*, 654.
(51) Fisher, E. W. et al. (1975) *Br. vet J.*, *131*, 402.
(52) Logan, E. F. et al. (1974) *Vet. Rec.*, *94*, 367.
(53) Mullen, P. A. (1975) *Vet. Ann.*, *15*, 451.
(54) Christie, B. R. & Waxler, G. L. (1973) *Can. J. comp. Med.*, *37*, 271.
(55) Ronnberg, B. et al. (1985) *J. clin. Microbiol.*, *22*, 893.
(56) Radostits, O. M. (1975) *Can. vet. J.*, *16*, 219.
(57) Bywater, R. J. (1980) *Vet. Rec.*, *107*, 549.
(58) Sherman, D. M. et al. (1976) *J. Am. vet. med. Assoc.*, *169*, 1310.
(59) Neitzke, J. P. & Schiefer, B. (1974) *Can. vet. J.*, *15*, 139.
(60) Fisher, E. W. & de la Feunte, G. H. (1971) *Vet. Rec.*, *89*, 579.
(61) Youanes, Y. D. & Herdt, T. H. (1987) *Am. J. vet. Res.*, *48*, 719.
(62) Symoens, J. et al. (1974) *Vet. Rec.*, *94*, 180.
(63) Brignole, T. J. & Stott, G. H. (1980) *J. dairy Sci.*, *63*, 451.
(64) Speicher, J. A. & Hepp, R. E. (1973) *J. Am. vet. med. Assoc.*, *162*, 463.
(65) Radostits, O. M. & Acres, S. D. (1980) *Can. vet. J.*, *21*, 243.
(66) Acres, S. D. et al. (1979) *Infect. Immun.*, *25*, 121.
(67) Nagy, B. (1980) *Infect. Immun.*, *27*, 21.
(68) Myers, L. L. (1980) *Am. J. vet. Res.*, *41*, 1952.
(69) Moon, H. W. (1978) *Proc. Second int. Symp. Neonatal Diarrhea. Vet. Inf. Dis. Org.*, Univ. of Saskatchewan, Oct. 1978, pp. 393–410.
(70) Acres, S. D. & Radostits, O. M. (1976) *Can. vet. J.*, *17*, 197.
(71) Haggard, D. L. et al. (1982) *Vet. Med. small Anim. Clin.*, 77, 1391, 1525.
(72) Moon, H. W. & McDonald, J. S. (1983) *Am. J. vet. Res.*, *44*, 493.
(73) Sherman, D. M. et al. (1983) *Infect. Immun.*, *42*, 653.
(74) Nagy, L. K. et al. (1979) *Res. vet. Sci.*, *27*, 289.
(75) Allen, W. D. & Porter, P. (1983) *Dev. Biol. Standard*, *53*, 147.
(76) Moon, H. W. (1981) *Am. J. vet. Res.*, *42*, 173.
(77) McCallum, I. M. et al. (1977) *Can. J. anim. Sci.*, *57*, 151.
(78) Pearson, G. R. & Logan, E. F. (1982) *Vet. Pathol.*, *19*, 190.
(79) Fisher, E. W. & Martinez, A. A. (1970) *Res. vet. Sci.*, *20*, 302.
(80) Kasari, T. R. & Naylor, J. M. (1985) *J. Am. vet. med. Assoc.*, *187*, 392.
(81) Moon, H. W. et al. (1980) *Infect. Immun.*, *27*, 222.
(82) Isaacson, R. E. et al. (1978) *Am. J. vet. Res.*, *39*, 1750.
(83) Ansari, M. M. et al. (1978) *Am. J. vet. Res.* , *39*, 11.
(84) Murata, H. et al. (1979) *Infect. Immun.*, *26*, 339.
(85) Stone, S. S. et al. (1979) *Infect. Immun.*, *40*, 607.
(86) Johnston, N. E. et al. (1977) *Am. J. vet. Res.* , *38*, 1323.
(87) Sellwood, R. et al. (1986) *Res. vet. Sci.*, *40*, 128.
(88) Whipp, S. C. & Moon, H. W. (1985) *Am. J. vet. Res.*, *46*, 637.
(89) Hadad, J. J. & Gyles, L. L. (1978) *Am. J. vet. Res.*, 39, 1651.
(90) Lintermans, P. & Pohl, P. (1984) *Br. vet. J.*, *140*, 44.

(91) Cleek, J. L. & Phillips, R. W. (1981) *J. Am. vet. med. Assoc.*, *178*, 977.
(92) Phillips, R. W. & Case, G. L. (1980) *Am. J. vet. Res.*, *41*, 1039.
(93) Farris, A. S. et al. (1979) *Nord. VetMed.*, *31*, 20.
(94) Buntain, B. J. & Selman, I. E. (1980) *Vet. Rec.*, *107*, 245.
(95) Pearson, G. R. et al. (1978) *Vet. Pathol.*, *15*, 92 & 400.
(96) Lonnroth, I. et al. (1979) *Infect. Immun.*, *24*, 900.
(97) Gyles, C. L. & Zigler, M. (1978) *Can. J. comp. Med. Res.*, *43*, 42.
(98) Hadad, J. J. & Gyles, C. L. (1982) *Am. J. vet. Res.*, *43*, 41.
(99) Wilkie, I. W. (1981) *Can. vet. J.*, *22*, 171.
(100) Snodgrass, D. R. et al. (1982) *Vet. Microbiol.*, *7*, 51.
(101) Torres-Medina, A. (1984) *Am. J. vet. Res.*, *45*, 643, 652.
(102) Mills, K. W. & Tietze, K. L. (1984) *J. clin. Microbiol.*, *19*, 498.
(103) Holley, D. L. et al. (1984) *Am. J. vet. Res.*, *45*, 2613.
(104) Mills, K. W. et al. (1983) *Am. J. vet. Res.*, *44*, 2188.
(105) Naylor, J. M. (1986) *Proc. 14th World Congr. Dis. Cattle*. Vol. 1, pp. 362–367.
(106) Fettman, M. J. & Brooks, P. A. (1986) *J. Am. vet. med. Assoc.*, *184*, 1501.
(107) Jones, R. et al. (1984) *J. Am. vet. med. Assoc.*, *184*, 1501.
(108) Deneke, C. F. et al. (1985) *J. infect. Dis.*, *152*, 1032.
(109) Rollin, R. E. et al. (1986) *Am. J. vet. Res.*, *47*, 987.
(110) Wise, P. J. et al. (1985) *J. appl. Bacteriol.*, *58*, 555.
(111) Franklin, A. (1984) *Vet. Microbiol.*, *9*, 467.
(112) Wise, C. M. et al. (1983) *Am. J. vet. Res.*, *44*, 2221.
(113) Petrie, L. (1984) *Vet. Rec.*, *114*, 157.
(114) Bradley, J. A. & Niilo, L. (1985) *Can. J. comp. Med.*, *49*, 152.
(115) Petrie, L. et al. (1984) *Can. vet. J.*, *25*, 273.
(116) Fraser, D. (1984) *Anim. Prod.*, *39*, 115.
(117) Mellor, D. J. & Murray, L. (1986) *Vet. Rec.*, *118*, 351.
(118) Waltner-Toews, D. et al. (1985) *Can. J. comp. Med.*, *49*, 1.
(119) Snodgrass, D. R. et al. (1982) *Infect. Immun.*, *37*, 586.
(120) Runnels, P. L. et al. (1982) *Am. J. vet. Res.*, *47*, 1542.
(121) Isaacson, R. E. et al. (1980) *Infect. Immun.* *29*, 824.
(122) Kohler, E. M. (1978) *J. Am. Vet. Med. Assoc.* *173*, 588.
(123) Furer, E. et al. (1983) *Dev. Biol. Standard*, *53*, 161.
(124) Nagy, L. K. et al. (1985) *Vet. Rec.*, *117*, 408.
(125) Nagy, L. K. et al. (1985) *Vet. Rec.*, *116*, 123.
(126) Sellwood, R. (1984) *Vet. Microbiol.*, *9*, 477.
(127) Pugh, C. A. & Wells, P. W. (1985) *Res. vet. Sci.*, *38*, 255.
(128) Gregory, D. W. et al. (1983) *Am. J. vet. Res.*, *44*, 2073.
(129) Naylor, J. M. (1986) *Can. vet. J.*, *28*, 45.
(130) Chapman, H. W. et al. (1986) *Can. J. vet. Res.*, *50*, 84.
(131) Naylor, J. M. (1987) *Can. vet. J.*, *28*, 168.
(132) Booth, A. J. & Naylor, J. M. (1987) *J. Am. vet. med. Assoc.*, *191*, 62.
(133) Chapman, H. W. et al. (1986) *Can. J. vet. Res.*, *50*, 84.
(134) Fettman, M. J. & Rollin, R. E. (1985) *J. Am. vet. med. Assoc.*, *187*, 746.
(135) Urcelay, S. et al. (1984) *Can. J. comp. Med.*, *45*, 394.

Escherichia coli infections in weaned pigs

Enteric *E. coli* infection in weaned pigs is a significant cause of mortality between weaning and market. In many herds it is the major cause. Edema disease and coliform gastroenteritis are the two major manifestations. Although the clinical signs in these two conditions are quite different they occur in similar age groups and the same type of management change may precede their occurrence. Both are associated with the proliferation of predominantly hemolytic serotypes of *E. coli* within the small intestine; however, it is rare to encounter both diseases concurrently on the same farm. In coliform gastroenteritis the serotypes are enterotoxigenic and the major manifestation is diarrhea resulting from enterotoxin activity at the time of proliferation. In edema disease non-enterotoxigenic strains produce a vasotoxin which after a period of time indirectly produces the neurological syndrome characteristic of this disease.

In many countries the prevalence of edema disease has decreased markedly during the past decade whereas that of coliform gastroenteritis has increased. It is possible that this change reflects the trend to earlier weaning of pigs although the emergence and spread of new enterotoxigenic strains may also be a factor. More recently a third condition, cerebrospinal angiopathy, has been attributed to the effects of infection with *E. coli*. Although there are some similarities in the etiology and epidemiology of these diseases they are sufficiently different to warrant a separate description.

Edema disease (bowel edema, gut edema, enterotoxemia)

Edema disease occurs in weaner and grower pigs and is characterized by subcutaneous and subserosal edema, a progressive ataxia, paralysis and a high mortality.

Etiology

Edema disease is associated with the proliferation of predominantly hemolytic *E. coli* in the intestine. Most commonly the associated *E. coli* belong to serogroups 0138, 0139 or 0141 (1). The disease is believed to be an enterotoxemia. It has been reproduced by intravenous inoculation with bowel supernatant fluid from affected pigs (2, 3) and with extracts of edema disease-producing *E. coli* strains (4, 5). The toxic factor which is heat-labile and closely related to hemolysin has been partially purified (5, 6) and it is known as *edema disease principle*. There is still some argument for the role of endotoxin in contributing to the lesions (4, 8).

Epidemiology

The specific serotypes of *E. coli* which are capable of causing the disease are introduced into a piggery and become part of the normal intestinal flora. They may not cause trouble until a particular set of environmental conditions arise when they proliferate excessively within the intestine to produce toxin. The disease occurs predominantly in pigs between 6 and 14 weeks of age. It may occur sporadically but more commonly occurs as an outbreak affecting up to 50% of the pigs within the group. Characteristically the larger and faster-growing pigs within the group are affected. The disease is not common in runt or poorly thriving pigs. It frequently occurs within one week following a change in diet or *ad libitum* feeding but may also follow such factors as weaning, vaccination, pen change or regrouping.

The outbreak is sudden in onset but shortlived, averaging 8 days and seldom exceeding 15 days. The epidemiology of the disease in affected herds is not characteristic of a highly contagious disease (9) and it does not usually spread to involve other pens of pigs on the same farm.

The disease follows proliferation of the relevant serotypes within the intestine. Serotypes of *E. coli* associated with gut edema may be isolated from the feces of healthy pigs (10). The factors initiating proliferation are largely unknown but they appear nutritional (10–12) and related to a change of food or a sudden increase in intake of nutritious food especially following a minor check. Management factors that potentiate oral–fecal cycling of these organisms are likely to be of importance in spread within the group.

Pathogenesis

Nutritional factors and possibly gastrointestinal stasis leads to proliferation of hemolytic strains of *E. coli* within the small intestine (10, 13) and toxin production. There is generally a delay between the initial period of maximal intestinal proliferation of the organism and the onset of clinical signs. In the experimental disease, clinical signs occur 5–7 days following initial oral challenge with bacteria (11) and up to 36 hours following intravenous inoculation with toxin (6, 11). The delay appears related to the development of vascular lesions with increased vascular permeability leading to edema formation and encephalomalacia (4, 6). The experimental oral inoculation of the edema disease producing *E. coli* results in colonization of the organisms in the small intestine and lesions of the vessels of the intestinal mucosa are detectable in as early as 2 days after infection (7, 17). Alternate hypotheses proposed are that edema disease is the result of an anaphylactic reaction to the polysaccharides of *E. coli* in previously sensitized pigs (14, 15) and that the disease is the effect of a specific neurotoxin elaborated by gut edema strains (3).

Clinical findings

The disease strikes suddenly in a group, often affecting a number of pigs within a few hours, and shows no tendency to spread from group to group. The thriftiest pigs are most likely to be affected and once the diagnosis is made, all pigs in the pen should be examined in an attempt to detect other animals in the early stages of the disease. The incidence in a litter will vary up to 50% or more.

The earliest and most obvious sign is incoordination of the hindlimbs, although this may be preceded by an attack of diarrhea. The pig has difficulty in standing and sways and sags in the hindquarters. There is difficulty in getting up and in getting the legs past each other when walking because of a stiff, stringhalt-like action affecting either the forelegs or hindlegs. In some cases there are obvious signs of nervous irritation manifested by muscle tremor, aimless wandering and clonic convulsions. Complete flaccid paralysis follows.

On close examination, edema of the eyelids and conjunctiva may be visible. This may also involve the front of the face and ears but cannot usually be seen until necropsy. The voice is often hoarse and may become almost inaudible. Blindness may be apparent. The feces are usually firm and rectal temperatures are almost always below normal. The course of the disease may be very short with some pigs being found dead without signs having been observed. In most cases, illness is observed for 6–36 hours, with a few cases being more prolonged. Recovery does sometimes occur but some degree of incoordination may persist.

Clinical pathology

As an aid to diagnosis, while affected animals are still alive, fecal samples should be cultured to determine the presence of hemolytic *E. coli*. Knowledge of the drug sensitivity of the organism may be important in prescribing control measures. The edema disease principle is cytotoxic to Vero cells and may be useful in an assay system for diagnosis (19).

Necropsy findings

The pig is well grown for its age and the stomach is full of feed. Edema of the eyelids, forehead, belly, elbow and hock joints, throat and ears is accompanied by edema of the stomach wall and colonic mesentery in classical cases. Excess pleural, peritoneal and pericardial fluid are also characteristic and the skeletal muscles are paler than normal. The edema may often be slight and quite localized so that examination of suspected areas should be carried out carefully, using multiple incisions especially along the greater curvature of the stomach near the cardia. The characteristic lesions are more easily detected in pigs that have just died. Hemolytic *E. coli* can be cultured in almost pure culture from the intestine, particularly the colon and the rectum (13) and in some cases from the mesenteric lymph nodes. Histopathologically, the important lesions are mural edema, hyaline degeneration and fibrinoid necrosis in arteries and arterioles, and encephalomalacia (4, 6). A panarteritis is present in more chronic cases (16).

Diagnosis

Although there are a number of diseases of pigs in the susceptible age group in which nervous signs predominate, gut edema is usually easy to diagnose because of the rapidity with which the disease strikes, the number of pigs affected at one time, the short duration of the outbreak and edema of tissues. Affected pigs are usually in prime condition. Rather than attempt to differentiate them here, the reader is referred to the section on diseases of the brain for a list of nervous diseases of pigs. Mulberry heart disease and infection with encephalomyocarditis virus can produce similar signs, and differentiation on postmortem findings and histopathology is frequently necessary. In poisoning by *Amaranthus* spp. and *Chenopodium album*, the signs may be roughly similar but the edema is limited to the perirenal tissues.

Treatment

Many treatments have been tried, recommended and discarded and many veterinarians find that treatment has little effect on the outcome of the disease. When cases are showing nervous signs, little response can be expected. Melperone at a dose rate of 4–6 mg/kg body weight has been recommended for treatment in the early stages of the disease (20). Elimination of the toxin-producing bacteria may be attempted by an antibiotic or oral purgative. Neomycin, nitrofurazone, ampicillin or trimethoprim-potentiated sulfonamides can be added to feed or water supplies and the choice of antimicrobial will vary depending on area variations of the drug sensitivies of *E. coli*. The feed consumption of the unaffected pigs in the group should be reduced immediately, either by reducing the amount fed or, if the pigs are on self-feeders, by mixing more roughage, such as shorts or bran, with the ration in the ratio of 1:1 or 1:2. Slight purgation of the alimentary tract may be achieved by the use of mineral oil in the drinking water or feeding Epsom salts in thin gruel.

Control

Pigs should be kept on the same creep feed for at least 2 weeks after weaning and the change in feed should be made gradually over a 3–5 day period. Food restriction through the critical period is frequently practiced and may reduce the occurrence of gut edema. Similarly an increase in crude fiber and decrease in nutrient quality of the diet through this period may reduce the incidence. However, it is evident that a severe restriction and marked decrease in nutrient quality is required to fully achieve this effect and this is not compatible with the purpose of growing pigs (11). It is essential that pigs on restricted intakes be provided with adequate trough space to allow an even intake of food among the group. For similar reasons, litters of pigs that are batched at or after weaning should be divided into groups of approximately even body weights.

The strategic incorporation of an antibiotic into the feed during the risk period may be necessary on some farms. A reduction in the potential for oral–fecal cycling of organisms in the group may reduce the incidence of gut edema. A reduction in the age of weaning may also reduce the incidence.

No vaccine is available. Parenteral vaccination appears of little value but experimentally oral vaccination has shown some promise (18).

REFERENCES

(1) Sojka, W. J. (1965) *Escherichia coli in Domestic Animals and Poultry*. Farnham Royal: Commonwealth Agricultural Bureaux.
(2) Gitter, M. & Lloyd, M. K. (1957) *Br. vet. J.*, *113*, 212.
(3) Schimmelpfenning, H. (1970) *Vet. Med.*, *13*, 1.
(4) Kurtz, H. J. & Short, E. C. (1976) *Am. J. vet Res.*, *37*, 15.
(5) Nielsen, N. O. & Clugston, R. E. (1971) *Ann. NY Acad. Sci.*, *176*, 176.
(6) Clugston, R. E. et al. (1974) *Can. J. comp. Med.*, *38*, 22, 29, 34.
(7) Methiyapun, S. et al. (1984) *Vet. Pathol.*, *21*, 516.
(8) Johannsen, U. & Schappmeyer, K. (1975) *Arch. exp. Vet. Med.*, *29*, 33, 47.
(9) Kernkamp, H. C. H. et al. (1965) *J. Am. vet. med. Assoc.*, *146*, 353.
(10) Barnum, D. A. et al. (1987) *Colibacillosis*, CIBA Monograph.
(11) Smith, H. W. & Halls, S. (1968) *J. gen. Microbiol.*, *1*, 45.
(12) Varenius, H. (1969) *Nord. VetMed.*, *21*, 524, 535.
(13) Campbell, S. G. (1959) *Vet. Rec.*, *79*, 901.
(14) Buxton, A. & Thomlinson, J. R. (1961) *Res. vet. Sci.*, *1*, 17.
(15) Thomlinson, J. R. & Buxton, A. (1963) *Immunology*, *6*, 126.
(16) Kurtz, H. J. et al. (1969) *Am. J. vet. Res.*, *30*, 791.
(17) Bertschinger, H. U. & Pohlenz, J. (1983) *Vet. Pathol.*, *20*, 99.
(18) Illes, J. (1975) *Zentralbl. Bakteriol.*, *232A*, 477.
(19) Dobrescu, L. (1983) *Am. J. vet. Res.*, *44*, 31.
(20) Alsson, T. & Alsson, S. O. (1982) *Proc. 7th int. Congr. Pig Vet. Soc. Mexico City*, p. 26.

Postweaning diarrhea of pigs (coliform gastroenteritis)

Postweaning diarrhea occurs commonly within several days after weaning and is characterized by reduced growth rate associated with alterations in the mucosa of the small intestine and in some pigs by acute coliform gastroenteritis characterized by sudden death, or severe diarrhea, dehydration and toxemia. It is a major cause of economic loss from both mortality and inferior growth rate for several days to 2 weeks following weaning.

Etiology

The etiology is complex and multifactorial. Following weaning at 3 weeks of age there are marked changes in the mucosa of the small intestine which are thought to be due to changes in the diet at weaning. A transient hypersensitivity of the intestine may occur if piglets are primed by small amounts of dietary antigen before weaning followed by ingestion of greater quantities of the diet after weaning (1, 3).

Coliform gastroenteritis in weaned pigs is associated with the proliferation of specific serotypes of *E. coli* in the small intestines (4–6). These serotypes produce enterotoxin (7) and are usually, but not necessarily, hemolytic (4, 8). More than one serotype may be associated with outbreaks of coliform gastroenteritis on the same farm (9) and there is considerable area-to-area variation in the prevalence of the associated serotypes (10). Most commonly, 0 groups 8, 138, 139, 141 and 149 are associated with the disease.

Although there is an etiological similarity between coliform gastroenteritis in weaned pigs and neonatal enteric colibacillosis in sucking piglets the relationship is not exact. Strains associated with neonatal enteric colibacillosis may not have the ability to produce coliform gastroenteritis (11) and many strains isolated from coliform gastroenteritis lack $K88^+$ antigen (12, 13). It is rare to encounter the two conditions concurrently in the one herd.

Infection with rotavirus may be an etiological factor (14, 15). The rotavirus may infect and destroy villous epithelial cells of the small intestine which may allow colonization of the *E. coli*. Experimentally a high nutrient intake fed three times daily to piglets weaned at 3 weeks of age produced the most prolonged diarrhea, colonization of the intestine by hemolytic enteropathogenic *E. coli*, and persistent shedding of rotavirus (15). However, other observations cast doubt on the importance of rotaviruses as a cause of the diarrhea because rotaviruses may be found in the feces of pigs a few days after weaning without diarrhea (16).

Epidemiology

The weaning of piglets at 3 weeks of age is commonly followed in a few days by a postweaning reduction in growth rate, variations in total dietary intake and the development of diarrhea 3–4 weeks of age into an uncomfortable unsanitary environment appear especially susceptible.

The nature and the amount of the diet which the piglet consumes before and after weaning has been a subject of investigation. In general, weaning at 3 weeks of age is associated with alterations in the villous epithelium of the small intestine which results in varying degrees of malabsorption and a reduction in daily growth rate which may last for 2 weeks (22). Weaning at 3 weeks of age results in large rapid reductions in intestinal lactase activity which coincides with reductions in growth rate and a reduced ability to absorb xylose (17). There is a reduction in villous height and an increase in crypt depth in the small intestine (18) and these alterations are not necessarily associated with the consumption of creep feed before weaning (18) which does not support the hypothesis that hypersensitivity to a dietary antigen caused by priming prior to weaning is a factor (1).

Dietary manipulation can modify several changes which normally occur in the small intestine of the piglet after weaning (19). Feeding a sow milk replacer or a diet based on hydrolyzed casein reduces the increases in crypt depth and the reductions in brush border enzymes (19). The use of an antibiotic to suppress the microbial activity does not alter the changes in the mucosa after weaning (19).

A major factor predisposing to postweaning diarrhea may be the overconsumption of feed immediately after weaning (16). Pigs which develop diarrhea tend to be those which consume more diet after weaning than their contemporaries.

The ecology of *E. coli* and rotavirus in the stomach and intestines of healthy unweaned pigs and pigs after weaning has been examined (20, 21). After weaning, the hemolytic enterotoxigenic *E. coli* serotype 0149:K91, K88a, c (Abbotstown strain) commonly colonizes the anterior small intestine from lower down the intestinal tract (20). This serotype was also never found in the gastric contents of weaned pigs. When this serotype is present it tends to dominate the *E. coli* flora at all levels of the intestine. Rotaviruses are also more common in the intestinal contents of weaned than unweaned pigs. The presence of either or both of these potentially enteropathogens may not induce diarrhea.

The loss of lactogenic immunity at weaning may be an epidemiological determinant. Milk from sows whose progeny develop postweaning diarrhea contain antibodies capable of neutralizing the enterotoxigenic effect of the homologous *E. coli* (32). This suggests that the presence of antibody-mediated activity against enteropathogenic *E. coli* may be important in preventing the disease during the nursing period. At weaning this protection is removed and the piglet is unable to produce its own antibodies rapidly enough to prevent the disease.

The weaning of piglets at birth or 1 day old is associated with a high mortality rate due to diarrhea and septicemia (23). The high mortality rate is associated with a lack of colostral antibodies and the strict hygienic conditions required for the artificial rearing of pigs weaned at birth.

The stress of weaning does not appear to affect immune mechanisms of the pig (24).

Postweaning diarrhea occurs predominantly in pigs 3–10 days after they are weaned. Most commonly, pigs are first observed sick or dead on the 4th or 5th day. The spread within affected groups is rapid and a morbidity rate of 80–90% of the group within 2–3 days is not uncommon. Frequently, other pens of susceptible pigs within the same area will also develop the disease within a short period of the initial outbreak. The problem may persist within a herd affecting successive groups of weaned pigs over a period of weeks or months. The onset of the problem may be associated with the introduction of a different batch or formulation of the creep feed. The case fatality rate may be as high as 30% and survivors may subsequently show a reduced growth rate.

Pathogenesis

Within a few days after weaning pigs at 3 weeks of age there are alterations in the mucosa of the small intestine. There is a reduction in the length of the villi, a marked reduction in intestinal disaccharidase activity and an increase in the depth and activity of the intestinal crypts (17, 18, 25, 26). These changes are maximal at 3–7 days following weaning and persist until the 2nd week and coincide with the reduced growth rate.

The colonization and proliferation of *E. coli* in the small intestine originates from organisms in the lower part of the intestinal tract (20). Serotypes of *E. coli* associated with coliform gastroenteritis may be found in the feces of healthy pigs (27, 28). Following weaning their numbers in feces normally increase markedly even in pigs that remain healthy (8). The *E. coli* proliferate in the small intestine and produce an enterotoxin which causes a net loss of fluid and electrolytes to the lumen and subsequent diarrhea (29). The number of hemolytic *E. coli* present in the proximal portion of the jejunum may be 10^3–10^5 times higher in affected pigs than in weaned pigs of the same age which do not show signs of disease (12). The susceptibility of the small intestine to the enterotoxin varies according to the area, the upper small intestine is highly susceptible and susceptibility decreases through the more distal portions (30). Unlike many other species, the weanling pig depends largely on its large intestine for absorption of fluid and electrolytes with only small changes in net fluid movement occurring along the jejunal and ileal segments (31).

The role of the rotavirus in the pathogenesis of postweaning diarrhea is uncertain. The rotavirus can be found in the feces of healthy unweaned and weaned pigs (14–16). The virus is capable of infecting and destroying villous epithelial cells which could contribute to the partial villous atrophy, loss of digestive enzyme activity, malabsorption and reduced growth rate. Experimental inoculation of an enteropathogenic *E. coli* and the rotavirus causes a more severe disease than either agent does alone (33).

Death results from the combined effects of dehydration and acidosis resulting from fluid and electrolyte losses.

Clinical findings

The postweaning reduction in growth rate may affect 50–100% of the pigs within a few days after weaning and persist for up to 2 weeks. In some situations diarrhea may not develop in any of the pigs in the group. A reduction in feed intake, gaunt abdomens and lusterless hair coats are characteristic findings of piglets with postweaning '*check*'! They may appear unthrifty for 10 days to 2 weeks by which time they will improve remarkably.

Most commonly one or two pigs, in good nutritional condition, are found dead with little having been seen in the way of premonitory signs. At this time the others within the group may appear normal but closer examination will reveal several pigs showing mild depression and moderate pyrexia. A postmortem examination of dead pigs should be conducted early in the examination. A proportion of the group will develop diarrhea within 6–24 hours and by 3 days after the initial onset the morbidity may approach 100%. Feed consumption falls precipitously at the early stages of the outbreak but affected pigs will still drink. Affected pigs may show a pink discoloration of the skin of the ears, ventral neck and belly in the terminal stages. Diarrhea is the cardinal sign, the feces are very watery and yellow in color but may be passed without staining of the buttocks and tail. Pyrexia is not a feature in individual pigs once diarrhea is evident. Affected pigs show a dramatic loss of condition and luster and become progressively dehydrated. Voice changes and staggering incoordinated movements may be observed in the terminal stage in some pigs (7). The course of an outbreak within a group is generally 7–10 days and the majority of pigs that die do so within the initial 5 days. Surviving pigs show poor growth rate for a further 2–3 weeks and some individuals show permanent retardation in growth. In outbreaks in early weaned pigs diarrhea is usually evident before death occurs.

Necropsy findings

Pigs dying early in the course of the outbreak are in good nutritional condition but those dying later show loss of luster with dehydration and sunken eyes. A mild skin discoloration of the ears, ventral areas of the head, neck and abdomen is usually present. In pigs found dead at the onset of the outbreak there is a moderate increase in peritoneal fluid and barely perceptible fibrinous tags between loops of the small intestine may be present. This is not a feature in pigs dying later in the course of the outbreak. The vessels of the mesentery are congested and occasionally petechial hemorrhages and edema are present. The mucosa of the stomach shows mild hyperemia and the small intestines are dilated and contain yellow liquid or occasionally bloodstained material. The mucosa of the small intestine is congested and occasionally there are hemorrhagic areas. There are no lesions in the large intestine but a mild edema may be seen interspersed between the coils of the colon. Hemolytic *E. coli* are isolated in large numbers from the small intestinal contents and mesenteric lymph nodes. In some pigs they may also be isolated from the peritoneal fluid, spleen, and other internal organs.

The histological appearance and enzymological status of the intestinal mucosa of recently weaned pigs has been described (22, 25, 26).

Diagnosis

Coliform gastroenteritis must always be the prime consideration in pigs that are scouring or dying within a 3–10 day period of some feed or management change. Swine dysentery and salmonellosis are manifested by diarrhea and death but they are not necessarily related to weaning or feed change and both are more common in older growing pigs. Salmonellosis poses the greatest difficulty in initial diagnosis from coliform gastroenteritis. In salmonellosis, the feces are generally more fetid with more mucus, mucosal shreds and occasionally blood, and the skin discoloration is more dramatic. On postmortem examination enlarged hemorrhagic peripheral and abdominal lymph nodes and an enlarged pulpy spleen are more suggestive of salmonellosis; however, cultural differentiation is frequently required. If there is doubt the pigs should be treated to cover both conditions until a final decision is obtained. The onset of swine dysentery is comparatively more insidious than that of coliform gastroenteritis and the characteristic feces, clinical and epidemiological pattern and postmortem lesions differentiate these two conditions. Swine fever should always be a consideration in outbreaks in pigs manifested by diarrhea and death. However, the epidemiological and postmortem features are different. Other common causes of acute death in growing pigs such as erysipelas, pasteurellosis, and *Haemophilus parahaemolyticus* infection are easily differentiated on necropsy examination. Edema disease occurs under similar circumstances to coliform gastroenteritis but the clinical manifestation and postmortem findings are entirely different.

Treatment

It is imperative that treatment of all pigs within the group be instigated at the initial signs of the onset of coliform gastroenteritis, even though at that time the majority of pigs may appear clinically normal. Delay will result in high mortality rates. Any pig within the group that shows fever, depression or diarrhea should be initially treated individually both parenterally and orally and the whole group should then be placed on oral antibacterial medication. Water medication (see Chapter 4 on antibiotic medication) is preferable to medication through the feed as it is easier to institute and affected pigs will generally drink even if they do not eat. Neomycin, nitrofurans, tetracyclines, sulfonamides or trimethoprim-potentiated sulfonamides and ampicillin are the usual drugs of choice. In herds with problems with coliform gastroenteritis, prior sensitivity testing will guide the choice of the antibacterial to be used. Antibiotic medication should be continued for a further 2 days after diarrhea is no longer evident and is generally required for a period of 5–7 days. Consideration should be given to the medication of at-risk equivalent groups of pigs within the same environment. Intraperitoneal fluid and electrolyte replacement for severely dehydrated pigs and electrolytes in the drinking water should also be considered.

Control

Recommendations for effective and economical control of postweaning reduced growth rate and coliform gastroenteritis in pigs weaned at 3 weeks of age are currently not possible because the etiology and pathogenesis of this complex disease are not well understood. Epidemiologically the disease is associated with weaning and the effects of the diet consumed before and after weaning.

It has been traditionally accepted, without reliable evidence, that the sudden transition in diet at weaning was the major predisposing factor. However, as presented under epidemiology the experimental observations are conflicting. One set of observations indicates that if pigs eat a small quantity of creep feed before weaning, they are then 'primed' and develop an intestinal hypersensitivity which following the ingestion of the same diet after weaning results in the disease (1). It has been suggested that piglets should consume at least 600 g of creep feed before weaning in order to develop a mature digestive system (1). Another set of observations indicates that those pigs which consumed an excessive quantity of feed after weaning developed the disease (16).

The complete withholding of creep feed followed by abrupt weaning at 3 weeks of age seemed to have a protective effect possibly associated with a low dietary intake (6).

The recommendations set out here are based on the hypothesis that the consumption of adequate quantities of creep feed prior to weaning is the most effective and economical practice.

Every effort should be made to minimize the stress associated with weaning. In order to avoid a sudden transition in diet at weaning creep feed should be introduced to the suckling piglets by at least 10 days of age. It is important that the creep feed and feeder area be kept fresh to maintain palatability. The same feed should be fed for at least 2 weeks following weaning and all feed changes subsequently should be made gradually over a 3–5 day period. Feed restriction in the immediate 2-week period following weaning may reduce the incidence but generally is not successful. It is a common field observation that the incidence of diarrhea varies with different sources of feed but experimental studies to confirm this relationship are not available.

Where possible, at weaning the sow should be removed and the pigs should be kept as single litters in the same pen for the immediate postweaning period. If grouping of litters is practiced at this time, or later, the pigs should be grouped in equivalent sizes. Multiple suckling in the preweaning period may reduce stress associated with grouping of partweaned pigs. With all pigs but especially those weaned earlier than 6 weeks the pen construction should be such as to encourage proper eliminative patterns by the pigs and good pen hygiene (see salmonellosis) so as to minimize oral–fecal cycling of hemolytic *E. coli*. The environment also appears especially important in this group and draft-free pen construction should be such as to encourage proper ventilation. It is preferable to wean pigs on weight rather than age and in many piggeries a weaning weight of less than 6 kg is associated with a high incidence of postweaning enteric disease.

The inclusion of an antibiotic in the feed or water to cover the critical period of susceptibility (generally for 7–10 days after weaning) can be used as a preventive measure. Apramycin at the rate of 150 g/tonne of feed for 2 weeks after weaning may be associated with improved growth rates and a reduction in mortality (35). The high incidence of drug resistance in isolates of *E. coli* makes prior sensitivity testing mandatory and the antibiotic may need to be changed if new strains gain access to the herd. The routine use of prophylactic antibiotics for this purpose needs to be considered in relation to the problem of genetically transmitted drug resistance. However, is is currently often necessary for short-term control of a problem (34).

Vaccination may offer an alternative method of control. Parenteral vaccination for the control of coliform gastroenteritis has proved of variable value (36). Oral immunization by the incorporation of *E. coli* antigens into creep feed has been shown to reduce the incidence and severity of postweaning coliform gastroenteritis (37). Rearing early weaned piglets artificially for the purposes of increasing the efficiency of the sow is an attractive management concept. However, high death losses from diarrhea have slowed progress in this new development. The incorporation of antibodies in the diet of such piglets as a prophylactic measure should be possible and is being explored (38).

REVIEW LITERATURE

Lecce, J. G. (1986) Diarrhea: the nemesis of the artificially reared, early weaned piglet and a strategy for defense. *J. anim. Sci.*, *63*, 1307.

REFERENCES

(1) Miller, B. G. et al. (1984) *Res. vet. Sci.*, *36*, 187.
(2) Miller, B. G. et al. (1984) *Vet. Rec.*, *114*, 296.
(3) Miller, B. G. et al. (1984) *Am J. vet. Res.*, *45*, 730.
(4) Sojka, W. J. (1965) *Escherichia coli in Domestic Animals and Poultry*. Farnham Royal: Commonwealth Agricultural Bureaux.
(5) Smith, H. W. (1971) *Ann. NY Acad. Sci.*, *176*, 110.
(6) Richards, W. P. C. & Fraser, C. M. (1961) *Cornell Vet.*, *51*, 245.
(7) Gyles, C. L. (1971) *Ann. NY Acad. Sci.*, *176*, 314.
(8) Tzipori, S. et al. (1980) *Aust. vet. J.*, *56* 274.
(9) Svendsen, J. et al (1974) *Nord. VetMed..*, 26, 314.
(10) Dam, A. & Knox, B. (1974) *Nord. VetMed.*, *26*, 219.
(11) Moon, H. W. & Whipps, S. C. (1970) *J. infect. Dis.*, *122*, 1220.
(12) Svendsen, J. et al. (1977) *Nord. VetMed.*, *29*, 212.
(13) Larsen, J. L. (1976) *Nord. VetMed.*, *28*, 417.
(14) Lecce, J. G. et al. (1982) *J. clin. Microbiol.*, *16*, 715.
(15) Lecce, J. G. et al. (1983) *J. clin. Microbiol.*, *17*, 689.
(16) Hampson, D. J. & Smith, W. C. (1986) *Res. vet. Sci.*, *41*, 63.
(17) Hampson, D. J. & Kidder, D. E. (1986) *Res. vet. Sci.*, *40*, 32.
(18) Hampson, D. J. (1986) *Res. vet. Sci.*, *40*, 32.
(19) Hampson, D. J. et al. (1985) *Res. vet. Sci.*, *40*, 313.
(20) Hampson, D. J. et al. (1985) *J. comp. Pathol.*, *95*, 353.
(21) Hinton, M. et al. (1985) *J. appl. Bacteriol.*, *58*, 471.
(22) Hall, G. A. et al. (1983) *Res. vet. Sci.*, *34*, 167.
(23) Varley, M. A. et al. (1986) *Livestock Prod. Sci.*, *15*, 83.
(24) Blecha, F. et al. (1985) *Am. J. vet. Res.*, *46*, 1934.
(25) Kenworthy, R. (1976) *Res. vet. Sci.*, *24*, 69.
(26) Gay, C. C. et al. (1976) *Proc. 4th int. Congr. Pig Vet. Soc.*, VII.
(27) Miniats, O. P. & Roe, C. K. (1968) *Can. vet. J.*, *9*, 210.
(28) Craven, J. A. & Barnum, D. A. (1971) *Can. J. comp. Med.*, *35*, 274, 324.
(29) Stevens, J. B. et al. (1972) *Am. J. vet. Res.*, *33*, 2511.
(30) Moon, H. W. & Whipps, S. C. (1971) *Ann. NY Acad. Sci.*, *176*, 107.
(31) Hamilton, D. L. & Roe, W. E. (1977) *Can. J. comp. Med.*, *41*, 241.
(32) Svendsen, J. & Larson, J. L. (1977) *Nord. VetMed.* 29, 533.
(33) Tzipori, S. et al. (1980) *Aust. vet. J.*, 56, 279.
(34) Dawson, K. A. et al. (1983) *J. anim. Sci.*, 57, 1225.
(35) Muller, R. D. (1986) *Agric. Pract.*, 7, 47.
(36) Schipper, I. A. & Killing, C. L. (1974) *Am. J. vet. Res.*, *35*, 1365.
(37) Porter, P. et al. (1974) *Vet. Rec.*, *95*, 99.
(38) Lecce, J. G. (1986) *J. anim. Sci.*, *63*, 1307

Cerebrospinal angiopathy

Cerebrospinal angiopathy is a sporadic disease of recently weaned pigs manifested primarily by neurological signs. In some areas the disease is the more common cause of central nervous system disorders in this age group of pigs (1). The disease affects only one or a few pigs within a litter of a group occurring up to 5 weeks after weaning (1, 2), although a similar condition has been reported in fattening and adult pigs (3). The disease is characterized by the variety of neurological signs that it presents. Incoordination and a decreased central awareness are common presenting signs but abnormal head position, aimless wandering and persistent circling may also be observed. There is usually apparent impairment of vision. Fever is not a feature and the clinical course may last for several days. Affected animals may die but more commonly are destroyed because of their emaciated condition (2, 4). Wasting without neurological disorder may also occur (5). They are also prone to savaging by unaffected pen mates.

Histologically the disease is characterized by an angiopathy that is not restricted to the central nervous system. The similarity of the angiopathy to that seen in chronic edema disease (6) has led to the postulation (1, 2, 4) that this disease is a sequel to subclinical edema disease. The disease has been reported occurring in pigs 15–27 days after experimental *E. coli* infection (5).

The main differential diagnosis is that of spinal or brain abscess and the porcine viral encephalomyelitides. Affected pigs should be housed separately as soon as clinical signs are observed. In view of the nature of the lesion, therapy is unlikely to be of value; however, recovery following treatment with oxytetracycline has been reported (1).

REFERENCES

(1) Hartigan, P. J. & Baker, K. P. (1974) *Irish vet. J.*, *28*, 197.
(2) Harding, J. D. J. (1966) *Pathol. vet.*, *3*, 83.
(3) Szecky, A. & Szabo, I. (1972) *Acta vet. Hung.*, *22*, 283.
(4) Freere, K. & von Sanderslebe, J. (1968) *Berl. Munch. Tierarztl. Wochenschr.*, *81*, 197.
(5) Berlschinger, H. U. & Pohlenz, J. (1974) *Schweiz. Arch. Tierheilkd.*, *116*, 543.
(6) Kurtz, H. J. et al. (1969) *Am. J. vet. Res.*, *30*, 791.

DISEASES CAUSED BY *SALMONELLA* spp.

Salmonellosis (paratyphoid)

Salmonellosis is a disease of all animal species caused by a number of different species of salmonellae and manifested clinically by one of three major syndromes: a peracute septicemia, an acute enteritis or a chronic enteritis.

Etiology

Except in the newborn, especially foals, infection with a salmonella is usually not a single cause of the disease salmonellosis. The response to infection with a *Salmonella* sp. varies depending on the size of the challenge dose, the immunological status of the animal, itself dependent on colostrum intake in neonates, previous exposure to infection and exposure to stress in older animals. It is generally accepted that the intervention of some precipitating factor such as transport, intercurrent disease, anesthesia and surgery, dosing with antibiotics or anthelmintics, acute deprivation of food, or parturition is usually necessary to cause the disease, salmonellosis, as distinct from infection with *Salmonella* spp.

Many species of salmonellae are capable of causing salmonellosis in animals (1). The following list includes only the common ones:

Cattle: *S. typhimurium*, *S. dublin*, *S. newport*
Sheep and goats: *S. typhimurium*, *S. dublin*, *S. anatum*
Pigs: *S. typhimurium*, *S. choleraesuis*
Horse: *S. typhimurium*, *S. anatum*, *S. newport*, *S. enteriditis*, *S. heidelberg*, *S. arizona*, *S. angona* (75).

Unusual or 'exotic' species of *Salmonella* are becoming much more common especially in pigs and poultry but there is also a spillover into the other species, e. g., *S. newport* in cattle (2). This increase appears to result from the greater use of animal and fish byproducts, many of them unsterilized, in the feed. The greater use of such 'junk' feeds to poultry and pigs results in a greater occurrence of the infections in those species. Veterinary teaching hospitals have also become repositories for unusual salmonellae, one reporting a high prevalence of *S. krefeld* and *S. saint-paul* (80).

Epidemiology

Salmonellosis occurs universally and in all species. Its occurrence seems to have increased greatly over the past 30 years, but has declined in recent times. At first this was a major disease of pigs, but the prevalence in that species has declined enormously due to better hygiene, less selling in and out of sale yards, a withdrawal from garbage feeding and the eradication of hog cholera. Latterly the surge of prevalence has been in cattle, in which intensification of husbandry has played a large part, but the emergence of *Salmonella dublin* as the important pathogen has been most important. Horses have also demonstrated a major increase in occurrence of the disease although many of the unidentified enteritides of horses of 40 years ago may well have been caused by *Salmonella* sp. In recent years there has also been an enormous increase in notifications of exotic species of *Salmonella* such as *S. angona* and *S. newport*, which have mostly originated from the use of unusual food materials of animal and fish origin.

General prevalence

Survey data from various countries include a 13–15% infection rate in dairy cows in New Zealand, with similar rates in calves and sheep, and a 4% infection rate in beef cattle. Netherlands data show 25% infection in healthy pigs at abattoirs but similar investigations elsewhere record 10% (New Zealand) and 6% (United Kingdom). American figures indicate a 10–13% infection rate. These data are based on abattoir material and should be viewed with caution because of the very rapid increase in infection rate which occurs when animals are held over in yards for several days.

The morbidity rate in outbreaks of salmonellosis in pigs, sheep and calves is usually high, often reaching 50% or more. In all species the case fatality rate often reaches 100% if treatment is not provided.

The geographical distribution of the serotypes differs: *S. typhimurium* has a universal distribution; *S. dublin* has a more patchy habitat. In the United States it is limited in its occurrence to the western states. In Canada it is unknown. Australia has had little *S. dublin* but there have been many isolations in recent years. South Africa, South America, Great Britain and Europe have had *S. dublin* as the principal pathogen for cattle for some time. It has also come to surpass *S. abortus ovis* as a cause of absorption in sheep. The distribution of the various species also varies with time. A great deal of work and literature is devoted to charting these changes but interested readers will have to consult local publications for details.

Factors affecting spread of infection

Species of Salmonella In any discussion about salmonellosis in large animals there is likely to be a significant difference of opinion about its clinical behavior, particularly with respect to the ease with which it spreads and the ease with which it can be controlled. Part of the difference is probably related to the different ways in which animals are managed, particularly the intensity of stocking, and whether or not the animals are housed. But another, and probably greater, part of the difference is because of the different epidemiological characteristics of the *Salmonella* species. Thus, salmonellosis in cattle is a very serious and continuing disease in areas where it is caused principally by *S. dublin*. But where it is caused by *S. typhimurium* the disease is sporadic and even though it is highly fatal to individual animals it is not really a serious disease. Although there are probably similar differences with the other species they are not particularly well defined. The difference between the diseases caused by *S. dublin* and *S. typhimurium* is the marked tendency for *S. dublin* to persist in cattle and create a significant reservoir of carrier animals. *S. typhimurium* does not do so as much, so that the disease is likely to subside after an initial exposure, and to recur only when the source of infection, from rodents or feedstuffs, or sewage or slurry, reappears. This does not of course preclude the disease from persisting in a flock or herd for long periods (5).

The carrier state When an animal is infected with *S. dublin* it may become a clinical case or an active carrier, passing organisms constantly or intermittently in the feces. It may also become a latent carrier with infection persisting in lymph nodes or tonsils but no salmonellae in the feces, or even a passive carrier which is constantly picking up infection from pasture or the calf-pen floor, but is not invaded so that when it is removed from the environment the infection disappears. These animals probably multiply the salmonellae without becoming permanent carriers. The importance of the latent carriers is that they can become active carriers or even clinical cases under stress, especially at calving time. The cattle themselves then become the means by which the infection is retained in the herd for long periods (6). For *S. typhimurium* the donor can be any domestic animal species, including man, or any wild animal or bird. Although all infected adults become carriers it is rarely for any length of time, and calves rarely become carriers. In sheep and cattle the carrier state may persist for as long as 10 weeks, and in horses up to 14 months (7).

Farming practice generally Intensification of husbandry in all species is recognized as a factor contributing significantly to an increase in the new infection rate. A typical example is the carrier rate of 54% observed in intensive piggeries in New Guinea compared to the 9% in village pigs.

Intensive pasture utilization The means of infection is principally ingestion of feed, especially pasture, contaminated by the feces of an infected animal, so that the new infection rate is dependent on all those factors which govern the bacterial population in the environment. Temperature and wetness are most important as salmonellae are susceptible to drying and sunlight. *S. typhimurium* can remain viable on pasture and in soil, still water and feces for up to 7 months. Survival times of the bacteria in soil are influenced by too many variables to make any overall statement meaningful (23). As well as infection of pasture by cattle or other domestic animal species, the use of 'slurry' as a means of disposal of animal manure from cow housing or zero grazing areas has led to a highly efficient means of spreading *Salmonella* infections. The chances of cows becoming infected increases considerably if they are grazed soon after the slurry is applied (8), and is less likely during dry, sunny periods, and when there is sufficient pasture growth to avoid it being eaten right down to the ground surface. The survival time of *Salmonella* sp. in cold liquid manure depends on several factors including pH of the slurry and the serotype of the organism. It can be as long as 28 weeks (21). Pasture contaminated by human sewage, especially septic tank or sewage plant effluent or sludge (33) is also credited with being a potential source of *Salmonella* infection for cattle, but there are a number of reports (see, for example, reference (78)) which do not support this view. Drinking water can remain infected for long periods, as long as 9 months, and in cattle at extensive pasture infected drinking water in stagnant ponds is a significant source of infection.

Housed animals In housed animals the same factors apply to the spread of infection as apply to pastured animals. Thus, infection can be introduced by infected domestic animal carriers. For example in large-scale calf-rearing units where the disease is often of diabolical severity, many of the calves are infected when they are picked up from their home farms and, if they are penned in groups, all calves in the group are soon infected.

However, because of the failure of most calves to continue as carriers, they are usually free of infection within 6 weeks of arrival (12). The premixing of food into a liquid form for pumping to feeding stations in piggeries and calf rearing units is an effective way of spreading salmonellosis if infection is present in the feedstuffs and the mix is allowed to stand before feeding.

Contaminated feedstuffs Housed animals generally are more susceptible to infection from purchased feeds containing animal byproducts than are pastured animals, which are again more susceptible to animal product-based fertilizers. Organic feedstuffs, including bone meal, are being increasingly incriminated in the spread of salmonellosis and although the usual figure, for example in the United Kingdom, is 23% of consignments being infected (14) the figure may be as high as 70%. Most of the contamination of meat and bone meal occurs after heat sterilization, especially if the material is left in digester tanks (17). Fishmeals are one of the most frequently and badly contaminated feedstuffs. For example, most of a recent increase in reported isolations of salmonellae in the United States was due to *S. angona* introduced in Peruvian fish meal. These feed meals need to be heated at 82°C (180°F) for an hour to be sterilized. The infection of these materials may derive from antemortem infections in the animals used to make the byproduct, but soiling of the material at the preparation plant or abattoir or during storage may also occur. Stored feed not of animal origin, especially grain, is also commonly contaminated by the droppings of rodents which infest it and this can lead to sharp outbreaks of salmonellosis due to *S. typhimurium* (18). Of special importance is colostrum stored without refrigeration, a new development in recent years. If the milk is contaminated in the first place there is a significant chance of multiplication of salmonellae and transmission of the disease (19). On the other hand dried milk products appear to be relatively safe.

Introduction of the infection to a farm Contaminated feedstuffs, carrier animals, infected clothing of visitors and casual workers are the obvious ways. Less obvious as vectors are free-flying birds such as the herring gull (16) and nematode larvae which are already infected with the salmonellae (15).

Factors affecting the development of the disease
The portal of infection in salmonellosis is almost always via the mouth so that the severity of the disease in an individual, or of an outbreak in a group, depends to an extent on the degree of contamination which occurs and the environmental conditions of temperature and dryness which determine the survival time of the salmonellae. But there is also the influence of the host on the outcome of the infection. Many animals become infected naturally and are passive carriers in that they pass salmonellae in their feces without showing clinical signs but only for the duration of their cohabitation with other infected animals. On the other hand it is possible to produce salmonellosis experimentally in most animals provided that a sufficiently large dose of a sufficiently virulent strain of organism is used. There still remains the common occurrence of the animal which is a symptomless carrier of the disease, but which comes down with clinical salmonellosis when it is exposed to some sort of stress such as transport, hospitalization, severe food deprivation or parturition.

Epidemiology in the animal species

Cattle In calves, the disease is usually endemic on a particular farm, although explosive outbreaks can occur. In adult cattle at pasture the picture is about the same although the disease is less common. This is particularly so with *S. typhimurium* infections, but *S. dublin* affects young and old equally readily. Spread between calves in communal pens is by fecal–oral contamination. Infection of the newborn calf may be from the dam because many cows which are latent shedders become active shedders at parturition. The calves are not infected at birth, but become infected soon afterwards from the environment (25). In adult cattle, *S. dublin* is the common infection and occurs sporadically, but also as outbreaks when nutritional stress occurs. It has become much more common during the last two decades. Spread is mostly by the oral route and in cattle at pasture is greatly enhanced by very wet conditions (42).

In cattle, deprivation of food and water is the most common predisposing cause, usually as a result of transportation, but recent calving, vaccination with a living vaccine which produces a systemic reaction, treatment with irritant compounds such as carbon tetrachloride for fluke and fluke infestation can precipitate clinical attacks. In some herds there are sporadic cases in cows as they calve, usually within 1 week afterwards. In calves, the disease is common up to 3 months of age, and on some farms the case rate may be high enough to suggest colibacillosis. In grazing cattle there is a distinct seasonal incidence in late summer, autumn and early winter, due probably to greater exposure to infection at pasture. A greater prevalence in housed cattle in loose housing, compared with cattle which are tied in, is suspected but not invariable.

The pH of rumen contents has been shown to significantly affect the number of salmonellae surviving passage through the rumen. Thus, a high volatile fatty acid content and a low pH, such as prevails when a ruminant is on full feed, would be inimical to salmonellae passing through the forestomachs (50). Concurrent infection with *Fasciola hepatica* may predispose cattle to infection, but is unlikely to be a significant factor affecting the prevalence of the disease (67).

Sheep and beef cattle In range sheep the commonest occurrence of the disease is during drought time when sheep are concentrated onto small areas of surviving grass which are heavily contaminated by droppings. Other occurrences in sheep are when they pass through holding yards or transport vehicles which have been contaminated by previous groups of sheep. This is most likely to happen when they drink from puddles of water, especially in heavily contaminated yards or when they are exposed to recycled dip wash. The modern development of pen-lambing in which ewes about to lamb are brought into small pens is also a means of potentiating spread from a chronic shedder. In all of these situations feed stress by deprivation is likely to contribute to susceptibility. Field outbreaks in range sheep and beef cattle have been recorded. In some instances they have been caused by the use of unsterilized bone meal as a phosphorus supplement. Outbreaks occurring in sheep on a number of farms in the same area at the same time have been ascribed to contamination of drinking water by birds eating carrion. Heavy dosing with zinc oxide as a prophylaxis against facial eczema is also credited with precipitating outbreaks of salmonellosis in young sheep (74).

Goats Outbreaks in goats occur in the same circumstances as in other ruminant species. Transportation and capture are additional stresses in feral goats used for embryo transplantation (26).

Pigs The epidemiology of *S. choleraesuis* infection in pigs has been well documented and has changed greatly since the mid-1960s. In those days there were explosive outbreaks which could easily be mistaken for hog cholera. The morbidity and mortality rates were high and the disease spread very rapidly through a piggery. In place of those outbreaks which regularly devastated commercial pig-fattening units, there are nowadays relatively few outbreaks and these are small in scope. Much of this is due to the restriction of swill or garbage feeding, to restriction of pig movement and sale by auction at public saleyards, and to the positive approaches adopted by the pig industry including the development of a supply of specific pathogen-free pigs, an all-in-all-out policy in commercial fattening units and most important of all the vertical integration of pig enterprises. This ensures a constant supply of disease free growing hogs to fatteners and the assumption of a pyramidal-type responsibility at all levels of the enterprise. The marked decline in prevalence of swine salmonellosis had coincided with the decline and eradication of hog cholera.

In those herds where the disease does occur, introduction is usually effected by the entry of an infected carrier pig. However, it is possible for the infection to be spread by flies and the movement of inanimate objects such as cleaning gear and utensils. Feedstuffs do not provide a favorable environment for *S. choleraesuis* so that foodborne infection is not common. Survival in soil and water approximates 6 months and in slurry up to 5 weeks. Persistence in streams fouled by piggery effluent is unlikely. Susceptibility to salmonellosis in pigs is thought to be increased by intercurrent disease, especially hog cholera, nutritional deficiency of nicotinic acid and other nutritional stress such as a sudden change in diet.

Horses In adult horses, most cases occur after the stress of transport (73) and mostly in horses which are overfed before shipment, receive little or no food or water for the duration of a protracted journey, and are fed excessively on arrival, cases appearing 1–4 days later. Drafts of horses which have been exposed to a contaminated environment, such as saleyards or railroad yards may experience outbreaks in which up to 50% are affected. As with other species, the presence of an asymptomatic carrier in a group of horses is often credited with initiating an outbreak, but the search for the carrier is always laborious and often fruitless. At least five negative cultural examinations of feces should be made before acquitting a suspected donor (11). On the other hand, the cultural examination of large numbers of horses often reveals up to 50% of the population to be carriers. In the light of the high carrier rate in this species it is surprising that not more outbreaks occur.

The occurrence of salmonellosis in horses hospitalized for another disease has become a major problem for hospital administrators (22). In these circumstances there is a constant reintroduction of carriers of the disease, a persisting contamination of the environment, and a large population of horses all of which are under physiological stress because of anesthesia, surgical invasion or intercurrent disease, and many of which are exposed to oral and parenteral treatment with antibiotics which appears to greatly increase their chances of acquiring salmonellosis (76). Other risk factors in these horses are having a nasogastric tube passed and being admitted for treatment of colic. Occasionally outbreaks do occur in young horses at pasture when they are heavily infested with worms. Salmonellosis is also one of the common neonatal septicemias of foals and the disease may occur as an endemic one on particular studs or there may be outbreaks with many foals being affected at the one time (10). The common management on 'visiting studs' of bringing mares and newborn foals onto communal studs and then bringing them daily to a central point for observation and teasing is also likely to facilitate spread of an infection through a group of foals.

Salmonellosis as a zoonosis

As a zoonosis the disease has assumed increasing importance in recent years because of the much more frequent occurrence of human salmonellosis, with animal salmonellosis as the principal reservoir. Although transmission to man does occur via contaminated drinking water, raw milk and meat, particularly sausage, the important pathway today has become that through pigs and poultry. In most instances the increase in human infections is with 'exotic' serotypes other than *S. typhimurium* which come by animal feeding stuffs to pigs and chicken, and then to man through pork and chicken products. The most serious risk is that the transmitted bacteria will have acquired resistance to specific antibiotics because the animals from which they originate have been treated with the particular antibiotics (5) repeatedly or over a long period. One such possible occurrence has been recorded (4).

Contamination of milk usually occurs after the milk leaves the cow, even though the organism can be excreted into the milk during the acute phase of the disease, and occasionally by carrier animals. There is also the chance that contact between animals and man in agriculture, and in a companion animal relationship, especially with horses, can cause interspecies spread. An unusual but predictable transmission from lambs to humans is when sick lambs are foster-fed, especially by children (41).

Pathogenesis

After oral infection with *Salmonella dublin* invasion of the host takes place through the intestinal wall in the terminal ileum and cecum and progresses as far only as the mesenteric lymph nodes. Progress beyond this point, and the development of the disease, salmonellosis, is determined by factors such as immune status, and age of the host, whether or not it is exposed to stress, and the virulence of the strain of organism. A number of characteristics of the bacteria influence their virulence, including the presence of adhesin-pili and flagellae, cytotoxin, enterotoxin, lipopolysaccharide and the inflammatory response that they initiate in the intestinal wall. The effects of some of these factors are not limited to the intestinal tract and contribute also to the systemic complications of salmonellosis (83).

Infection

In young animals, and adults whose resistance has been lowered, spread beyond the mesenteric lymph nodes occurs and the infection is established in the reticulo-endothelial cells of the liver and from there invades the bloodstream. These steps in the infection process can occur very rapidly. For example, in newborn calves, *S. dublin* when taken by mouth can be found in the bloodstream 15 minutes later. And in older calves the bacteria can be isolated from the intestinal lymph nodes 18 hours after their oral administration (27). Provided a sufficient number of a sufficiently pathogenic serotype is used the disease is reproducible with pure cultures, for example of *S. typhimurium* in lambs (28), *S. choleraesuis* in pigs (26), *S. dublin* (46), *S. typhimurium* (47) and *S. enteriditis* in calves and *S. typhimurium* in horses (9, 13). Once systemic infection has been established salmonellosis as a disease can develop. Its principal manifestations are as septicemia, enteritis, abortion and a group of localizations in various tissues as a result of bacteremia.

Septicemia, bacteremia and the carrier state

After invasion of the bloodstream occurs a febrile reaction follows in 24–48 hours, and the acute phase of the disease, similar to that seen in natural cases, is present 3–9 days later. The early septicemia may be rapidly fatal. If the systemic invasion is sufficient to cause only a bacteremia, acute enteritis may develop, and abortion is a common final sequel in sheep and cattle. Many animals survive this stage of the disease but localization of the salmonellae occurs in mesenteric lymph, nodes, liver, spleen, and particularly the gallbladder. In healthy adults there may be no clinical illness when infection first occurs but there may be localization in abdominal viscera. In either instance the animals become chronic carriers and discharge salmonellae intermittently from the gallbladder and foci of infection in the intestinal wall into the feces and occasionally into the milk. For this reason they are important sources of infection for other animals and for humans. Carrier animals may also develop an acute septicemia or enteritis if their resistance is lowered by environmental stresses or intercurrent infection.

Enteritis

Enteritis may develop at the time of first infection or at some other time in carrier animals. The best information available on the pathogenesis of enteritis is derived from the experimentally produced disease. In most instances the disease is produced by the administration of massive doses of bacteria, and this may result in the production of a different syndrome to that which occurs naturally. The clinical response mirrors the natural disease very closely as follows.

In the pig the development of enteritis caused by *S. choleraesuis* begins 36 hours after infection with the appearance of erosions and edema of the cecal mucosa. At 64 hours the wall is thickened and there is diffuse caseation overlying the erosions. The necrotic membrane sloughs at 96 hours and at 128 hours all function is lost and the entire intestinal wall is involved in the inflammatory process, the muscular coat being obliterated by 176 hours (26).

Salmonella dublin infections in calves have been used to create the disease experimentally, resulting in enteritis in the small and large intestines, but the exact chronology of the lesions has not been described. In sheep, the experimental disease produced by oral dosing with *S. typhimurium* (52) includes an early acute enteritis of the small intestine at 24 hours. At 5–8 days there is hemorrhagic and necrotic typhilitis and the infection is established in mesenteric lymph nodes and the liver.

In *ponies* (9) experimental infection with *S. typhimurium* administered orally, there was much variation in the time after infection that the various signs appeared. Pyrexia, neutropenia and high fecal salmonella counts coincided on the second and fourth days, but diarrhea occurred in only some ponies and then on the 3rd to 11th day after inoculation. Positive agglutination tests were recorded from day 1 but were mostly during the period 6–12 days postinoculation. The neutropenia of the early stages of the disease is transient and may have given way to a neutrophilia by the time diarrhea commences.

Although there is sufficient obvious enteritis to account for the diarrhea which characterizes the disease there appear to be other factors involved. For example, it has been shown experimentally that in *Salmonella* enteritis there is stimulation of active chloride secretion combined with inhibition of sodium absorption, but invasion of the mucosa is not essential for these changes to occur (29). These observations are of interest in the light of the known hyponatremia which characterizes the disease. Studies of *calves* with salmonellosis have shown that the fluid loss associated with the diarrhea of this disease is much greater than in other calf diarrheas. This, together with a large solid matter output, contributes to the very significant weight loss which occurs in salmonellosis (30). In *pigs* and to a less extent in *cattle*, ulcerative lesions may develop in the intestinal mucosa, and these may be of sufficient size to cause chronic intermittent diarrhea. In *pigs* it has also been observed that villous atrophy is a sequel to infection with *S. choleraesuis* (31).

Abortion

Abortion is a common manifestation in salmonellosis in cattle. Its pathogenesis when caused by *S. dublin* is based on the growth of the bacteria in the placenta, having been seeded there from a primary lesion in other maternal tissues. Fetal death has already occurred in many cases due to its invasion by bacteria, but live calves also occur suggesting that the placental lesion is the critical one. *Salmonella montevideo* has been associated with a significant number of outbreaks of abortion in ewes (51).

Other forms of salmonellosis

Localization in joints with the subsequent development of polyarthritis is not uncommon in newborn animals that survive a neonatal septicemia caused by *Salmonella* sp.

Clinical findings

The disease is most satisfactorily described as three syndromes classified arbitrarily according to severity as septicemia, acute enteritis, and chronic enteritis. These are described first but the differences between the animal species are sufficiently great to justify describing the disease separately in each of them. There are no significant differences between infections caused by the different *Salmonella* sp.

Septicemia

This is the characteristic form of the disease in newborn foals and calves and young pigs up to 4 months old especially in the early stages of an outbreak. Affected animals show profound depression, dullness, prostration, high fever (40·5–42°C, 105–107°F) and death within 24–48 hours.

Acute enteritis

This is the common form in adult animals of all species. There is a high fever (40–41°C, 104–106°F) with severe, fluid diarrhea, sometimes dysentery, and with tenesmus occasionally. The fever often subsides precipitously with the onset of diarrhea. The feces have a putrid smell and contain mucus, sometimes blood, fibrinous casts which may appear as complete tubular casts of intestine, and intestinal mucosa in sheets or casts. There is complete anorexia, but in some cases increased thirst. The pulse rate is rapid, the respirations rapid and shallow and the mucosae are congested. Pregnant animals commonly abort. The case fatality rate without early treatment may reach 75%. In all species, severe dehydration and toxemia occur, the animal loses weight and strength rapidly, becomes recumbent and dies in 2–5 days. Newborn animals that survive the septicemic state usually develop severe enteritis with diarrhea becoming evident at 12–24 hours after the illness commences. If they survive this stage of the illness, residual polyarthritis or pneumonia may complicate the recovery phase.

Chronic enteritis

Otherwise known as subacute enteritis, this is a common syndrome in pigs and occurs occasionally in cattle and adult horses. In calves there is intermittent or persistent diarrhea, with the occasional passage of spots of blood, mucus and firm fibrinous casts, intermittent moderate fever (39°C, 102°F), and loss of weight leading to emaciation. Although chronic enteritis may occur initially it usually succeeds an acute episode.

Bovine salmonellosis

The disease caused by *Salmonella dublin* is usually endemic on a particular farm with sporadic cases occurring when individual animals are exposed to stress. Severe outbreaks are rare but do occur when there is severe stress, usually acute nutritional deprivation, applied to the whole herd. When *S. typhimurium* is the cause, it is usual to have a single animal or a small number of animals affected at one time. When the disease is in the calf population it is usual for it to be much more severe and with many affected, either as a point outbreak or when there is a succession of calves, a continuing occurrence of the disease. The emphasis, therefore, is generally on the occurrence of individual, sporadic cases in newborn calves and recently calved cows (20).

The septicemic form of the disease is the common one in newborn calves, and in addition to depression and fever may show nervous signs including incoordination and nystagmus. Calves older than a week, and adults, are usually affected by acute enteritis followed in survivors by abortion in pregnant cows and polyarthritis in calves. In severe cases of enteritis, there is often dysentery with whole blood being passed in large clots, and complete agalactia in lactating cows. Abdominal pain, with kicking at the abdomen, rolling, crouching, groaning, and looking at the flanks, is common in adult cattle. Rectal examination at this stage usually causes severe distress.

Chronic enteritis with inappetence, reduced weight gains and unthriftiness may follow an attack of acute enteritis or be the only manifestation of the disease. Abortion is a common sequel in pregnant cows that survive an attack of acute enteritis. However, infection with *S. dublin* is also a significant cause of abortion in cattle without there having been any other clinical signs (34). A sequel to some cases of apparent enteric salmonellosis is the development of *dry gangrene of the extremities* including eartips, tailtip, and the limbs from the fetlock down (37).

The experimental disease produced by infecting adult cattle with *S. dublin* by mouth varies from no clinical illness to fatal dysentery. Abortion occurs in some pregnant females. Many suffer pyrexia, anorexia, and mild diarrhea (46). Experimental infection of calves with *S. typhimurium* has the same general effect (47) with more severe syndromes occurring in younger calves. Chronic cases may develop bone lesions including osteoperiostitis and osteomyelitis, sometimes with epiphyseal separation (48). Experimental infection with *S. enteriditis* causes profuse yellow diarrhea, fever, dehydration, frequent cough, and a mucopurulent nasal discharge (49).

Ovine and caprine salmonellosis

The only recognized form of the disease in sheep is acute enteritis on a flock scale. However, in the early stages of the outbreak there may be some cases of the septicemic form. After experimental infection of sheep with *S. dublin*, fever and diarrhea are followed in pregnant ewes by abortion (35). Abortion is also common in the naturally occurring disease and has come to exceed *S. abortusovis* as a cause of abortion in sheep in the United Kingdom. Some ewes die after abortion and many of the lambs born alive die subsequently. Fever and diarrhea, followed by abortion, have also been produced experimentally in sheep by the administration of *S. dublin* (35).

In goats, naturally occurring cases are not reported often. *S. dublin* is the usual pathogen in those countries where it is a resident, but *S. typhimurium* is also recorded as a cause (68). Peracute septicemia in newborn animals, and acute enteritis occur with signs and lesions similar to those in cattle.

Porcine salmonellosis

In pigs, the disease varies widely and, although all forms occur in this species, there is often a tendency for one form to be more common in any particular outbreak. In the septicemic form in pigs affected by *S. choleraesuis* a dark red to purple discoloration of the skin is evident, especially on the abdomen and ears, and subcutaneous petechial hemorrhages may also be visible. Nervous signs, including tremor, weakness, paralysis and convulsions, may be prominent and occur in a large proportion of affected pigs. The case fatality rate in this form is usually 100%. A semispecific entity occurring in pigs up to 4 weeks old is manifested by meningitis and clinical signs of prostration and clonic convulsions.

In the acute form there is also a tendency for pulmonary involvement to occur, but the main feature of the disease is enteritis, with pneumonia and occasionally encephalitis present as only secondary signs. In some situations pigs dying of septicemia more commonly yield *S. choleraesuis*, while those with acute enteritis are usually infected with *S. typhimurium* (38). Acute pneumonia is a common accompaniment of this form of the disease in swine, and nervous signs and cutaneous discoloration as described in the septicemic form may also be present.

A syndrome of *rectal stricture* occurs in feeder pigs as a sequel to enteric salmonellosis caused by *S. typhimurium* and is described under that heading.

Equine salmonellosis

The disease in horses usually occurs in a single animal and sporadically. However, outbreaks do occur in newborn foals, and in groups of horses recently transported, and horses hospitalized in veterinary clinics. Experimental infection of horses by oral administration of *S. typhimurium* produces a disease similar to the natural disease (62, 65). The incubation period may be as short as 24 hours. Four syndromes occur:

- Asymptomatic shedding of *S. typhimurium* in feces intermittently or continuously for short periods of 4–6 days
- A subacute enteric form in adult horses on farms where the disease is endemic, with fever, depression, anorexia, but without severe diarrhea, although the feces may have the consistency of soft bovine feces. There is no other obvious intestinal abnormality. There may be a neutropenia with a left shift
- Severe, acute fulminating enteritis with diarrhea, fever, dehydration and neutropenia. There is abdominal pain which may be sufficiently severe to stimulate violent actions. This is the common form of the disease, occurring commonly in adults which are exposed to stress in one form or another. Newborn and young foals also often have this form of the disease
- In foals up to about 2 days of age there is a highly fatal septicemia. Localization in survivors includes lesions in the brain causing meningoencephalitis, polyarthritis and many other sites.

Clinical pathology

The three aspects of cases of salmonellosis that profit by clinicopathological support are:

- Diagnosis in the individual animal, when its treatment and prognosis depend on a definitive diagnosis
- Diagnosis of a herd problem to ensure that expensive herd-wide control measures are not implemented unnecessarily
- Monitoring the biochemical status of a sick animal in order to determine most accurately its requirements for supportive therapy, especially fluid and electrolytes.

The diagnostic techniques available are:

- *Bacterial culture*. This is the only way of making a definitive etiological diagnosis of salmonellosis and of exactly determining the serotype. The principal difficulty is that most laboratories have difficulty in isolating the bacteria from the blood or the feces of animals shown subsequently at necropsy to have salmonellosis. The difficulty varies. In cattle with *S. dublin* infections, the bacteria are present in the blood, and milk, for a very brief period during the bacteremic phase and before diarrhea commences
- *Serial blood culture* in the very early stages of the disease when the animal is likely to be bacteremic is not really a practicable technique because of the need to collect serial samples, and the cost of blood cultures
- *Fecal cultures* may be negative in the intensely diarrheic stage of acute salmonellosis and for a period of up to 2 weeks after the onset of illness. This difficulty is noticeable with *S. dublin* infection in cattle (71) and *S. choleraesuis* infections in pigs (26) and *S. typhimurium* infection in horses. The discrepancy in *S. dublin* infections in calves may be as great as 55% accuracy only (39) and in horses only 50% (9). The difficulties relate to dilution by diarrhea and the heavily contaminated nature of the sample; a sample of fluid feces collected in a container is superior to a fecal swab. Selective media must be used, but the results are still not completely satisfying (26). Simultaneous culture of a pinch biopsy of rectal mucosa significantly increases the number of isolations of salmonellae in cattle and horses (79)
- *Serological tests*. Species-specific agglutinins are detectable in the serum of infected animals and have uses as diagnostic aids. However, they do not appear in the serum until about 2 weeks after infection and many animals in cattle and pig populations carry moderate titers against *Salmonella* sp. although they are not infected, so that a positive serological test cannot be depended on to identify individual infected animals

- *Cutaneous delayed hypersensitivity* tests are practicable but fail to identify infected as against recovered animals (36)
- *Indirect tests* include a total and differential white cell count. A leukopenia, neutropenia and a severe degenerative left shift are highly suggestive. There is also a marked hyponatremia and a mild hypokalemia (44). These tests are well established in horses, and the leukopenia has been observed in acute salmonellosis in cattle (45). The fecal leukocyte count is also a worthwhile supportive test in the search for salmonellosis. A high count is strongly suggestive, but many horses with acute or severe diarrhea have high fecal leukocyte counts in the absence of salmonellae in the feces (32).

Laboratory diagnosis in a suspected sick animal
Positive diagnosis has to be culture of the organism, usually from feces, but possibly from blood in the septicemic stage. If serological diagnosis is available a serum sample should also be submitted. Indirect tests are very valuable and if laboratory availability is good, a total white cell count and estimation of serum sodium levels should be undertaken urgently. A presumptive diagnosis is often all that can be stated, and this may be supported by a herd diagnosis—a diagnosis that the disease or infection is present in the herd and that it is presumed that the subject case is one of the group.

Herd diagnosis
A serological examination of a sample of animals is a first step. A completely negative serological test would indicate that the infection is not present. Positive results indicate a need for further examination and periodic fecal cultures at 15-day intervals using enriching media should be undertaken. When *S. typhimurium* is the causative bacteria, the feces of other species of animals on the farm should be examined, because ducks, dogs, horses, pigs, sheep and cattle may be sources of infection for each other. It is always advisable to examine the drinking water and feed for evidence of infection.

Detection of clinically normal carrier animals
The most difficult clinicopathological problem in salmonellosis is the detection of the clinically normal carrier animal. The recommended procedure (43) is to do fecal cultures on all cows at 14–day intervals for three examinations, and repeat the examination on the day of calving. At that time, swabs are taken from feces and the vagina of the cow, and the feces of the calf. The sampling should preferably be done when the cows are tied in stanchions and not grazing pasture, because of the large number of passive carriers of the infection in the latter circumstance.

The reliability of diagnosis based solely on culture of fecal swabs is not very high and represents the principal difficulty in detecting carriers. A combination of fecal culture and serological tests offers some improvement in accuracy, but even with the agglutination or complement fixation tests accuracy is insufficient (40).

Necropsy findings

Septicemic form
There may be an absence of gross lesions in animals which have died peracutely but there is usually evidence of septicemia in the form of extensive submucosal and subserous petechial hemorrhages. In cases that survive for one or more days, the necropsy findings may include those of the acute form.

Acute enteric form
Gross lesions are most prominent in the large and small intestines. Inflammation is evident and varies from a mucoenteritis with submucosal petechiation to diffuse hemorrhagic enteritis. Similar lesions may be present in the abomasum, and in *S. dublin* infections in calves multiple mucosal erosions and petechiation of the abomasal wall may be accompanied by abomasitis. Infections with *S. typhimurium* are characterized by severe necrotic enteritis in the ileum and large intestine. The intestinal contents are watery, have a putrid odor and contain mucus, and are blood-tinged or contain whole blood. In cases which have survived for longer periods, superficial necrosis may proceed to the development of an extensive diphtheritic pseudomembrane. The mesenteric lymph nodes are enlarged, edematous and hemorrhagic. The wall of the gallbladder may be thickened and inflamed. Enlargement and fatty degeneration of the liver occur and the serous cavities may contain bloodstained fluid. Variable degrees of subserous petechiation occur but are always present under the epicardium.

In pigs, the petechiae are very prominent and may give the kidney the 'turkey-egg' appearance usually associated with hog cholera. Congestion and hepatization of lung tissue may be present especially in pigs. Skin discoloration is marked in pigs and, depending on the severity of the case, this varies from extreme erythema with hemorrhages, to plaques and circumscribed scabby lesions similar to those of swine pox.

Chronic form
In cattle, the chronic form is usually manifested by discrete areas of necrosis of the wall of the cecum and colon. The wall is thickened and covered with a yellow-gray necrotic material overlying a red, granular surface. In pigs the lesion is similar but usually more diffuse. Less commonly the lesions are discrete in the form of button ulcers, occurring most commonly in the cecum around the ileocecal valve. Button ulcers commonly occur in chronic hog cholera but there is some doubt as to whether the lesions are caused by the hog cholera virus or by secondary invasion by salmonellae. The mesenteric lymph nodes and the spleen are swollen. Chronic pneumonia may also be present.

Salmonellae are present in the heart blood, spleen, liver, bile, mesenteric lymph nodes and intestinal contents in both septicemic and acute enteric forms. In the chronic form, the bacteria may be isolated from the intestinal lesions and less commonly from other viscera. The most satisfactory method for immediate examination is a thick smear from the lining of the gallbladder. Surveys which set out to determine the percentage of carriers in animal populations by examining abattoir material show that by far the largest number of isolations are made from lymph nodes draining the cecum and lower small intestine.

Diagnosis

The diagnosis of salmonellosis presents considerable difficulty in the living animal largely because of the variety of clinical syndromes which may occur and the variations in clinical pathology outlined above. At necropsy the isolation of salmonellae from tissues and intestinal contents, although suggestive of the presence of salmonellosis, does not of itself confirm the diagnosis and care must be taken to ascertain whether other disease is present.

Cattle

The septicemic form in calves resembles septicemia due to *E. coli* so closely that differentiation is possible only by bacteriological examination. There is a strong tendency for salmonellosis to occur in calves during the second and third weeks of life rather than in the first week, a more common characteristic in colibacillosis. The acute enteric form may be confused with coccidiosis especially if the fever has subsided. The acute abdominal pain may suggest acute intestinal obstruction but profuse diarrhea and dysentery are unlikely to occur in the latter. Winter dysentery occurs in explosive outbreaks and is self-limiting; mucosal disease is characterized by typical mucosal lesions and epizootiology; bracken fern poisoning has considerable resemblance to salmonellosis but a history of access to bracken is usually available. Other poisonings, especially arsenic and to a less extent lead, and a number of miscellaneous weeds may cause a similar acute enteritis. Chronic cases may resemble Johne's disease or chronic molybdenum poisoning but dysentery and epithelial casts do not occur in these diseases. Massive stomach fluke infestations may also cause diarrhea and dysentery.

Sheep

Diarrhea caused by infections with coccidia or *Campylobacter* sp., or by parasitic infestation may be confused with that caused by *Salmonella* spp. but the latter is usually more acute and more highly fatal.

Horses

The acute form in foals may resemble the acute infections caused by *E. coli* and *Actinobacillus equuli*. A history of recent transport often helps in suggesting diagnosis of salmonellosis in adult horses, in which colitis-X is the important differential diagnosis.

Pigs

Septicemic salmonellosis can resemble hog cholera, coliform gastroenteritis and pasteurellosis very closely and laboratory examination is usually necessary for identification. Acute erysipelas, in those cases where characteristic skin lesions have not appeared, is usually indicated at necropsy by the larger, subserous ecchymoses but again laboratory examination may be necessary if doubt exists. The lesions of swine dysentery are confined to the alimentary tract. *Salmonella* meningitis in young pigs is clinically indistinguishable from streptococcal meningitis.

Treatment

There are differences of opinion amongst veterinarians about the probity of treating cases of salmonellosis with antibiotics (70). This difference of opinion depends on two parts of the response to treatment, and which view is taken depends to a large extent on the experience one has with respect to them. The first issue is that of the success of treatment in saving the lives of animals. It is our experience and that of most clinicians that early treatment with broad-spectrum antibiotics and with sulfonamides is highly efficient in preventing deaths and returning animals to normal function but it is also generally agreed that treatment must be early, because delay means loss of the integrity of intestinal mucosa to the point where repair cannot occur. A common pattern of response to treatment in a herd is that the first one or two cases are regarded lightly by the owner and they are treated 24–48 hours after diarrhea begins. When these cases die, a more prompt regimen is instituted in which the farmer has the approved drug on-hand and begins treatment as soon as diarrhea with fever is observed. The cure rate is then likely to be of the order of 100% except in the case of foals and calves in which a fulminating septicemia is apt to defeat even the best treatment program.

The second issue in the debate about antibacterial therapy for salmonellosis is the risk entailed in producing 'carrier' animals. In man and in animals there is evidence that treatment can prolong the duration of the period after clinical recovery during which the causative bacteria can be isolated from the gut. It has to be accepted that this can happen and that the use of antibacterial treatment can theoretically contribute to the spread of disease. However, because of the way in which animals are kept, and because they constantly eat contaminated pasture or other feed, there is an almost universal carrier segment in animal populations, and to regard another survivor from salmonellosis as a significant contributor to the carrier frequency seems an exaggeration. In many situations this appears to be the correct view. But in other situations an animal can contract infection in, for example, a veterinary hospital or an exhibition or show, recover clinically with treatment and on being sent back to its parent herd initiates a devastating outbreak of fatal and debilitating salmonellosis. Both epidemiological patterns occur, and they seem to occur in different places, so that the most appropriate attitude to take seems to be the one that fits local circumstance. In an area where only sporadic cases of the disease occur in herds it would be professionally negligent not to treat infected animals with appropriate antibacterial agents. In areas where epidemicity is the rule recovered animals should not be sent into herds until they are known not to be carriers.

Other related issues in the debate on the treatment of salmonellosis are the creation of drug-resistant strains of the bacteria, and the effect on the normal gut flora which results from oral medication. The problem with resistant strains would not have become a significant one if only individual animals had been treated, but mass medication of in-contact animals and prophylactic treatments generally have resulted in a very large population of resistant strains. The resistance has usually been to streptomycin and sulfonamides. Gentamicin and chloramphenicol-resistant strains have also caused disease in animals (24). A survey of strain susceptibility in the United States showed that 12% of 249 strains of *S. typhimurium* were sensitive to all six of a panel of common antibiotics (55). United Kingdom figures (81) suggest that the position there is the same as that in the United States. The spread of this antibacterial resistance to other serotypes of the organism is likely and most other pathogenic salmonellae now have formidable resistance to many antibiotics (56). Most of these reports about the seriousness of this problem emanate from the United Kingdom and multiresistant strains of salmonella are reported to have migrated from there to Europe (61). Resistance of salmonellae to antibiotics is much less in Australia, a significant resistance being observed only to chloramphenicol and tetracycline (82).

Oral treatment in cattle and pigs is well recognized as being a satisfactory treatment, but it is not recommended in horses in which an immediate worsening of the diarrhea, or its prolongation as a persisting chronic diarrhea, may be encountered. It is thought that both sequels result from a distortion of the normal population of gut microflora resulting from the eight to ten times greater concentration of drug which occurs in the intestine after oral treatment, compared to the concentration resulting from systemic injection.

Thus treatment is recommended for all sick animals using antibacterial agents as set out below but some veterinarians will not use these drugs and will depend solely on what are generally considered to be only supportive treatments, particularly the administration of fluids parenterally.

The choice of drugs to be used depends on a test of drug sensitivity in each case or outbreak but failing this the following generalizations can be applied; a summary is provided in Table 52. In calves with *S. dublin* infections the descending order of preference is chloramphenicol, or a combination of trimethoprim and sulfadiazine, furazolidone, sulfamethylphenazole and neomycin. Ampicillin and amoxycillin (58) are also highly regarded, but they should be administered parenterally. Oral dosing is satisfactory in preruminant calves, but it is much less effective when given to grazing ruminants. Trimethoprim and sulfadiazine are very effective for the treatment of experimental salmonellosis in calves with *S. dublin* (72). There is marked synergism of the two drugs and both parenteral and oral therapy is effective. Sulfadimidine and framomycin are also widely used and recommended. Many veterinarians use a combination of two drugs, e.g. chloramphenicol by injection and nitrofurazone by mouth. One of the advantages of nitrofurazone is its adaptability to large-scale medication via the drinking water. The use of chloramphenicol in food animals is banned in some countries and discouraged in most others.

Foals with septicemic salmonellosis are usually treated both systemically and orally with antibiotics, sometimes a different one by each route. Treatment must be given at least 6-hourly and be accompanied by a supportive fluid therapy. Favored antibiotics are gentamicin (250 mg intravenously, twice-daily) (66), ampicillin (1 g, 6-hourly) and chloramphenicol (20 mg/kg body weight intravenously, 6-hourly). Care needs to be exercised when treating adult horses for salmonellosis because of the tendency for treatment with antibiotics, especially tetracyclines, to precipitate attacks of diarrhea. Parenteral treatment with ampicillin or sulfonamide combinations is recommended.

For pigs, the same list of drugs is available but treatment of individual pigs is usually by ampicillin, chloramphenicol or neomycin and mass treatment by nitrofurazone, or a combination of chlortetracycline and sulfamethazine (75 mg of each per liter of water). Where large numbers of pigs are affected mass medication via the feed or drinking water is usually practiced. Because sick pigs do not eat, water treatment is necessary and if drugs are unpalatable individual treatment is the last recourse. Drugs that dissolve readily and are palatable are therefore in demand.

Ancillary treatment, by providing demulcent and astringent preparations for oral use and fluids, either orally or parenterally, to replace lost electrolytes and fluids will help animals to survive the period of acute dehydration and toxemia.

In adult horses affected with acute salmonellosis, the dehydration, acidosis and loss of electrolytes are severe. The loss of sodium is most serious, followed by potassium and chloride in that order. A solution of 5% sodium bicarbonate at the rate of 5–8 liters/400 kg body weight given intravenously over a period of 2 hours as the initial electrolyte replacement therapy will usually help to convert the hyponatremia and acidosis. The hypertonic solution is considered necessary to correct the severe loss of sodium. Following this initial therapy equal mixtures of isotonic saline (0·9%) and isotonic sodium bicarbonate (1·3%) may be given as maintenance fluid and electrolyte therapy in amounts as indicated. The hypokalemia may be severe in some horses and is recognized clinically by muscular weakness and trembling. It may be corrected by adding potassium chloride to the saline and bicarbonate solution at the rate of 1–2 g/liter for a total of 4–6 g of potassium chloride given over 2–4 hours. Concentrated solutions of potassium must be given slowly and the heart monitored for evidence of arrhythmia. However, provided that renal function has been restored, the hyperkalemia which may result from electrolyte therapy or that which could occur following correction of the acidosis should not be hazardous since the kidney will excrete excess potassium. A safer method would be the oral administration of 30 g of potassium chloride in 8 liters of water given twice daily.

Under practical conditions, with the aid of a laboratory for serial evaluation of serum electrolytes, the field veterinarian is faced with using hypertonic solutions as described above or balanced electrolyte solutions and careful clinical monitoring for evidence of overhydration or electrolyte imbalances.

The administration of electrolyte solutions by the oral route is gaining popularity because of the ease of administration and relative safety. Large quantities of fluids

(10–30 liters) can be administered orally, either all at once, for example in a mature cow, or in smaller quantities (5–10 liters) three to four times daily in mature horses. This has been discussed in more detail under enteritis.

Control

Prevention of introduction

This would be ideal but it is an objective not easily achieved. The principal sources of infection are carrier animals and contaminated foodstuffs containing feeds of animal origin. A closed herd removes half the risk, but is not a practicable procedure for the types of animal producer for which salmonellosis is a major problem—the calf-rearer and the commercial pig fattener. For such people the following rules apply:

- Introduce the animals directly from the farm of origin. Avoid dealers' yards, saleyards and public transport, all of which are likely to be contaminated. Determine that the farm of origin is free of salmonellosis. This is not an attractive proposition to many pig and calf fatteners because the gamble with high stakes in their enterprise rests on the speculative purchase of large groups of animals where and when the local market is depressed
- If possible purchase animals when they are older, say 6 weeks for calves, to give an opportunity for specific and non-specific immunity to develop. If these animals can come from vaccinated herds so much the better
- Dealers' premises, saleyards, and transport vehicles should be under close surveillance and the need for frequent vigorous disinfection stressed. An interesting figure is the observation that the infection rate in calves delivered to calf-dealers' yards in the United Kingdom was less than 1% but the infection rate rose to 36% if the calves were kept on the premises over the weekend (4)
- Introduce only those animals guaranteed not to be carriers. Unfortunately the detection of carriers is inaccurate and expensive. To have any confidence in the results one must submit serum samples for agglutination tests and fecal samples for culture on at least three occasions. Even then, occasional carriers with lesions in the gallbladder or tonsils will escape the net and be capable of reviving the disease on the farm or transferring it to another one (53).

Limitation of spread within a herd

When an outbreak occurs, procedures for limiting spread, as set out below, need to be strictly enforced, and medication of affected groups, and of susceptible groups at high risk, carried out. The drugs to be used are those listed under treatment, the choice of the individual drug depending on its efficiency and cost. In an endemic herd the procedure is the same but the tempo can be more leisurely.

- Identify the carrier animals and either cull them or isolate and treat them vigorously. Treated animals should be rechecked subsequently to determine whether a 'clean' status has been achieved. Our personal experience is that much can be achieved by this measure in well-managed herds whose individual animals are valuable, but experience in the elimination of carrier foals by the administration of nitrofurazone and neomycin, and in pigs by full doses of chloramphenicol, nitrofurazone or ampicillin, has been disappointing
- The prophylactic use of antibiotics such as oxytetracycline in the feed at the rate of 10 g/tonne, or chlortetracycline in the drinking water at the rate of 55 mg/liter is used but not recommended because results are poor and there is a risk of developing resistant strains (54)
- Restrict the movement of animals around the farm and limit the infection to the smallest group. Pasture and permanent buildings are both important although the major source of infection in most cases is the drinking water
- The water supply should be provided in troughs which should not be susceptible to fecal contamination. Static drinking water or pasture may remain infected for as long as 7 months
- Vigorous disinfection of buildings is important. An all-in/all-out policy should be adopted and steam cleaning and chemical sterilization performed after each batch. If economics permit, individual pens for calves are of tremendous value. Where calves

Table 52. Schedule of antibacterials for possible use in the treatment of salmonellosis

Species	*Parenteral*	*Oral*
Cattle and sheep	Chloramphenicol 20 mg/kg body weight intravenously 6-hourly for 3 days where allowed by legislation Trimethoprim and sulfadoxine mixture is highly effective	Nitrofurazone 20 mg/kg body weight daily for 5 days mixed in water and given as drench or via stomach tube. In outbreaks mass medication of water supply of all in-contact animals may be indicated
Horses	Trimethoprim and sulfadoxine mixture Ampicillin Chloramphenicol	Nitrofurazone 20 mg/kg body weight daily mixed in water and given via stomach tube. Give for 3–5 days
Pigs	Chloramphenicol 20 mg/kg body weight intramuscularly twice daily for 2 days Ampicillin	Nitrofurazone 20 mg/kg body weight daily in water supply for 6 days

NB: Parenteral *or* oral treatment alone may be sufficient if cases are detected early, but in all circumstances parenteral *and* oral treatment combined is superior and is recommended. Oral medication may not be necessary if drug used parenterally is secreted into intestinal lumen via enterohepatic circulation.

are reared indoors they are common and economical. Pig houses need especially careful treatment. Dirt yards present a problem, especially those used for sheep and calves, but provided they can be kept dry and empty two sprayings, one month apart, with 5% formalin is recommended

- Suitable construction of housing is important. Impervious walls to stop spread from pen to pen, pen design to permit feeding without entering the pen, avoidance of any communal activity and slatted floors to provide escape routes for manure, all assist in limiting the spread of enteric diseases. Deep litter systems appear to be hazardous but satisfactory provided they are kept very dry and plenty of bedding is available. With pigs the opportunity for oral–fecal cycling of the organism and build-up and spread of infection within and between groups should be kept to a minimum. Pen design and the environment should be such as to encourage proper eliminative behavior and good pen hygiene. Drinkers should be sited at one end of the pen, preferably on a narrow end with oblong pens, to encourage defecation in this area. Wet or damp areas of the floor in other parts of the pen will encourage defecation and urination there should be eliminated. Drinkers of the nipple type rather than bowls are preferable for hygienic reasons. Communal dunging alleys increase the possibility of spread, especially during the cleaning procedure, and the trend is to slatted or meshed areas over a channel. A totally slatted or mesh floor for pigs for weaning until 10–12 weeks of age will markedly reduce the opportunity of oral–fecal cycling or organisms in this age group which is especially susceptible to enteric disease. Feeders should allow the ingress of the pig's head and should be constructed to avoid fecal and other contamination of food and the trough from feces deposited or carried on the feet need to be examined. Pigs need to be grouped according to size, and overcrowding, which may result in improper pen hygiene, must be avoided. Space requirements vary according to pen and housing design but generally fall in the region of $0{\cdot}3\ m^2$ for recently weaned piglets to $0{\cdot}6–1\ m^2$ for market size pigs. In conventionally floored or partially slatted floored pens approximately two-sevenths of the area should be available for the dunging area. The construction of the pen should allow for easy and efficient cleaning. In problem herds an especial vigilance for the occurrence of enteric disease is needed following the breakdown of pen hygiene on very hot days
- Heat treatment of feed is an effective procedure for pigs. Heating during pelleting greatly reduces the bacterial content of feed and special treatment is worthwhile because of the very high proportion of animal derived feeds which are infected. The availability of such feeds guaranteed to be salmonellae-free would be an advantage
- Disposal of infective material should be carried out with great care. Carcasses should be burnt, or better still sent to an institution for diagnosis, rather than to a knackery to be converted into still more contaminated bone meal. Slurry and manure for disposal should be placed on crops rather than on pasture. Slurry does not constitute a danger via hay, and salmonellae do not survive silage making. When slurry is used on pasture it should be stored for at least a month beforehand and even longer if silo effluent is included. Slurried pasture should not be grazed for 1 month and for young animals a 6-month delay is recommended. Pig slurry is most dangerous and should always be avoided
- All persons working on infected premises should be warned of the hazards to their own health. Other peripatetic species, especially dogs, should be kept under close restraint
- Vaccination is an active subject of discussion in salmonellosis control. The reaction of research workers and field workers is mixed. If viewed in a conservative light it must be evident that it is a most valuable procedure but that it is not a complete answer to the problem on its own. If it is combined with the hygienic precautions listed above so that the immune barrier is not assaulted too heavily or too frequently, it is a valuable auxiliary weapon (62). Two methods are available, a killed bacterin and a live attenuated vaccine. Either can be used as prenatal vaccines to provide passive immunization of the newborn. The following generalizations apply. An autogenous bacterin, made from bacteria collected on the farm, has advantages, especially if a killed vaccine of low antigenicity is to be used. Its principal disadvantage is cost.

Cattle In cattle, *S. dublin* is the infection likely to be endemic in a herd and commercial vaccine, to be effective, must have a strong *S. dublin* component. The vaccine strain 51, produced in the United Kingdom from a rough, variant strain of this organism, has been found to be very efficient and safe and to provide good protection against *S. typhimurium* as well as *S. dublin*. It has the disadvantages of a living vaccine but calves can be vaccinated successfully at 2–4 weeks of age. In limited experiments other living, attenuated and killed, adjuvanted vaccines have given calves protection, and a comprehensive program of vaccination, hygiene and adoption of a closed herd policy has been successful in eradicating the disease (71). Reports on killed *S. typhimurium* vaccines used in calves indicated good results provided the antigenic mass in the vaccine is kept high (69), but commercial, killed vaccines are of doubtful value (71).

Attenuated *S. typhimurium* (strain SL 1479) given orally or intramuscularly has shown good efficiency, and attenuated *S. dublin* (strain SL 1438) has been similarly effective (65). The *S. typhimurium* vaccine also gives some protection against *S. dublin* (77).

The autogenous bacterin, which must be precipitated on aluminum hydroxide to have any significant effect, is given as two injections 2 weeks apart. Good immunity is produced but calves and pigs less than 6 weeks of age are refractory, and anaphylactic reactions may cause the loss of a significant number of animals. To protect young calves the best program is to vaccinate the cows during late pregnancy. This will give passive protection to the calves for 6 weeks, provided they take sufficient colostrum, and the calves can be vaccinated at that time if danger still exists. Reports of results have not been enthusiastic (57) but if proper attention is given to the detail of the program it has been sufficient, in our hands, to provide almost complete protection. In foals an autogenous *S. typhimurium* bacterin has been used in several bad field situations and has been credited with preventing further clinical cases and with reducing environmental contamination, in spite of continued poor hygiene and management practices (3, 10). A similar observation has been made with respect of vaccination of calves against *S. typhimurium* (59).

Pigs, horses, sheep A commercial vaccine containing living, attenuated *S. choleraesuis* has also been shown to protect neonatal pigs after vaccination of sows (63) and weaned pigs (64).

Because of the early age at which pigs need to be immune, it is recommended that sows be vaccinated 3 times at 7–14-day intervals. The young pigs are vaccinated at 3 weeks of age.

In horses a similar regimen with a booster dose for all mares in late pregnancy appears to be effective.

Results in sheep have been unconvincing. There has been a report of a commercial adjuvant vaccine containing *S. bovismorbificans* and *S. typhimurium* and of its successful use in sheep (60).

Animals being transported These are a special case. They should be unloaded or exercised at least once every 24 hours and given water and food, the feed being provided first and at least 2 hours before watering. Hay or chopped hay is preferred to succulent feeds. All railroad cars, and feeding and watering troughs should be properly cleaned and disinfected between shipments. Horses which are to be transported should be yarded and handfed on hard feed for 4–5 days beforehand. If the disease is likely to occur, prophylactic feeding with sulfonamides or antibiotics has been shown to decrease the incidence in all species. Apart from the risk that this practice will produce resistant bacteria, there has been a suggestion that it may so change the normal bacterial flora of the gut as to encourage the proliferation of salmonellae and lead to the development of the clinical disease.

REVIEW LITERATURE

Jones, P. W. (1980) Disease hazards associated with slurry disposal. *Br. vet. J.*, *136*, 529 (see also 1980 *Vet. Rec.*, *106*, 4).
Linton, A. H. (1979) Salmonellosis in pigs. *Br. vet. J.*, *135*, 109.
Smith, B. P. (1981) Equine salmonellosis: a contemporary view. *Equ. vet. J.*, *13*, 147.
Williams, B. M. (1980) Bovine salmonellosis. *Bov. Pract.*, *15*, 122.
Wray, C. (1985) Is salmonellosis still a serious problem in veterinary practice? *Vet. Rec.*, *116*, 485.
Wray, C. & Sojka, W. J. (1977) Reviews of the progress of dairy science: bovine salmonellosis. *J. dairy Res.*, *44*, 383.

REFERENCES

(1) Wray, C. (1985) *Vet. Rec.*, *116*, 485.
(2) Richardson, A. (1975) *J. Hyg., Camb.*, *74*, 195.
(3) Carter, M. E. et al. (1979) *J. equ. Med. Surg.*, *3*, 78.
(4) Holmberg, S. D. et al. (1984) *New Engl. J. Med.*, *311*, 617.
(5) Hunter, A. G. et al. (1976) *Vet. Rec.*, *98*, 126.
(6) Richardson, A. (1975) *Vet. Rec.*, *96*, 329.
(7) Morse, E. V. et al. (1976) *Cornell Vet.*, *66*, 198.
(8) Jones, B. W. (1976) *Br. vet. J.*, *132*, 284.
(9) Owen, R. et al. (1979) *Can. J. comp. Med.*, *43*, 247.
(10) Peet, R. L. et al. (1980) *Aust. vet. J.*, *56*, 613.
(11) Smith, B. P. et al. (1980) *J. Am. vet. med. Assoc.*, *176*, 215.
(12) Osborne, A. D. (1974) *Vet. Rec.*, *94*, 604.
(13) Smith, B. P. et al. (1979) *Am. J. vet. Res.*, *40*, 1072.
(14) Skovgaard, N. & Nielsen, B. B. (1972) *J. Hyg., Camb.*, *70*, 127.
(15) Bottjer, K. P. et al. (1978) *Am. J. vet. Res.*, *39*, 151.
(16) Butterfield, J. et al. (1983) *J. Hyg., Camb.*, *91*, 429, 437.
(17) Bensink, J. C. & Bohland, P. H. (1979) *Aust. vet. J.*, *55*, 13 & 521.
(18) Hunter, A. G. et al. (1976) *Vet. Rec.*, *99*, 145.
(19) Wray, C. & Callow, R. J. (1974) *Vet. Rec.*, *94*, 407.
(20) Counter, D. E. & Gibson, E. A. (1980) *Vet. Rec.*, *107*, 191.
(21) Kovacs, F. & Tamasi, G. (1979) *Vet. Acad. Sci. Hung.*, *27*, 47.
(22) Carter, J. D. et al. (1986) *J. Am. vet. med. Assoc.*, *188*, 163, 173.
(23) Zibilske, L. M. & Weaver, R. W. (1978) *J. environ. Qual.*, *7*, 593.
(24) Benson, C. E. et al. (1985) *Can. J. comp. Med.*, *49*, 125.
(25) Wray, C. & Sojka, W. J. (1981) *J. Hyg., Camb.*, *87*, 501.
(26) McOrist, S. et al. (1981) *Aust. vet. J.*, *57*, 389.
(27) Hartman, H. et al. (1974) *Mh. VetMed.*, *29*, 824.
(28) Brown, D. D. et al (1976) *Res. vet. Sci.*, *21*, 335.
(29) Fromm, D. et al. (1974) *Gastroenterology*, *66*, 215.
(30) Fisher, E. W. & Martinez, A. A. (1975) *Br. vet. J.*, *131*, 643.
(31) Arbuckle, T. B. R. (1975) *Res. vet. Sci.*, *18*, 322.
(32) Morris, D. D. et al. (1983) *Cornell Vet.*, *73*, 265.
(33) Johnston, W. S. et al. (1986) *Vet. Rec.*, *119*, 201.
(34) Hinton, M. (1974) *Br. vet. J.*, *130*, 556; *131*, 94.
(35) Thomas, G. W. & Harbourne, J. F. (1974) *Vet. Rec.*, *94*, 414.
(36) Aitken, M. M. et al. (1978) *Res. vet. Sci.*, *24*, 370.
(37) O'Connor, P. J. et al. (1972) *Vet. Rec.*, *91*, 459.
(38) Wilcock, B. P. et al. (1976) *Can. J. comp. Med.*, *40*, 80.
(39) Richardson, A. & Fawcett, A. R. (1973) *Br. vet. J.*, *129*, 151.
(40) Wray, C. & Sojka, W. J. (1976) *Res. vet. Sci.*, *21*, 184.
(41) Findlay, C. R. (1978) *Vet. Rec.*, *103*, 114.
(42) Vandegraaff, R. S. & Malmo, J. (1977) *Aust. vet. J.*, *53*, 453.
(43) Richardson, A. (1974) *Aust. vet. J.*, *50*, 463.
(44) Merritt, A. M. et al. (1975) *J. S. Afr. vet. med. Assoc.*, *46*, 73.
(45) Hall, G. A. et al. (1980) *Br. vet. J.*, *136*, 182.
(46) Hall, G. A. & Jones, P. W. (1979) *Br. vet. J.*, *135*, 75.
(47) Smith, B. P. et al. (1979) *Am. J. vet. Res.*, *40*, 1510.
(48) Gitter, M. et al. (1978) *Br. vet. J.*, *134*, 113.
(49) Petrie, L. et al. (1977) *Vet. Rec.*, *101*, 398.
(50) Chambers, P. G. & Lyons, R. J. (1979) *Res. vet. Sci.*, *26*, 273.
(51) Linklater, K. A. (1983) *Vet. Rec.*, *112*, 372.
(52) Orr, M. B. et al. (1977) *Vet. Sci. Commun.*, *1*, 191.
(53) Lawson, G. H. K. et al. (1974) *J. Hyg., Camb.*, *72*, 311, 329.
(54) Finlayson, M. & Barnum, D. A. (1973) *Can. J. comp. Med.*, *37*, 139.
(55) Timoney, J. F. (1978) *J. infect. Dis.*, *137*, 67.
(56) Blackburn, B. O. et al. (1984) *Am. J. vet. Res.*, *45*, 1245.
(57) Rankin, J. D. & Taylor, R. J. (1970) *Vet. Rec.*, *86*, 254.
(58) Osborne, A. D. et al. (1978) *Vet. Rec.*, *103*, 233.
(59) Bairey, M. H. (1978) *J. Am. vet. med. Assoc.*, *173*, 610.
(60) Cooper, B. S. & McFarlane, D. J. (1974) *NZ vet. J.*, *22*, 95.
(61) Rowe, B. et al. (1979) *Vet. Rec.*, *105*, 468.
(62) Roberts, M. C. & O'Boyle, D. A. (1982) *Aust. vet. J.*, *58*, 232.
(63) Hanna, J. et al. (1979) *Vet. Microbiol.*, *3*, 303.
(64) Hanna, J. et al. (1979) *Res. vet. Sci.*, *26*, 216.
(65) Smith, B. P. et al. (1983) *Proc. US Anim. Hlth Assoc.*, *87*, 492.
(66) Hamm, D. H. & Jones, E. W. (1979) *J. equ. Med. Surg.*, *3*, 159.
(67) Aitken, M. M. et al. (1981) *Res. vet. Sci.*, *31*, 120.
(68) Bulgin, M. S. & Anderson, B. C. (1981) *J. Am. vet. med. Assoc.*, *178*, 720.
(69) Bairey, M. J. (1980) *J. Am. vet. med. Assoc.*, *173*, 610.
(70) Whitlock, R. H. (1984) *J. Am. vet. Med. Assoc.*, *185*, 1210.
(71) Hahn, L. & Scholl, W. (1984) *Mh. VetMed.*, *39*, 208.
(72) White, G. et al. (1981) *Res. vet. Sci.*, *31*, 19 & 27.
(73) Owen, R. R. et al. (1983) *Am. J. vet. Res.*, *44*, 46.
(74) Allworth, M. B. et al. (1985) *NZ vet. J.*, *33*, 171.
(75) Donahue, J. D. (1986) *J. Am. vet. med. Assoc.*, *188*, 592.

(76) Hird, D. W. et al. (1984) *J. Am. vet. med. Assoc.*, *188*, 173.
(77) Smith, B. P. et al. (1984) *Am. J. vet. Res.*, *45*, 1858.
(78) Clegg, F. G. et al. (1986) *J. Hyg., Camb.*, *97*, 237.
(79) Palmer, J. E. et al. (1985) *Am. J. vet. Res.*, *46*, 697.
(80) Ikeda, J. S. et al. (1986) *Am. J. vet. Res.*, *47*, 232.
(81) Sojka, W. J. et al. (1986) *Br. vet. J.*, *142*, 371.
(82) Murray, C. J. et al. (1986) *Aust. vet. J.*, *63*, 286.
(83) Murray, M. J. (1986) *J. Am. vet. med. Assoc.*, *189*, 145.

Abortion in mares and septicemia in foals caused by *Salmonella abortivoequina*

This is a specific disease of equidae characterized by abortion in females, testicular lesions in males and septicemia in the newborn.

Etiology

Salmonella abortivoequina can be isolated from affected animals and cultures of the organism are capable of causing the disease. However, in some outbreaks in which the organism is isolated from aborted material, a filterable agent capable of causing abortion is also found and the salmonellae are judged to be secondary invaders. In the absence of viral infections other predisposing causes are thought to increase the chances of infection and of abortion (1).

Epidemiology

The infection appears to be limited to horses and donkeys (2). Natural infection may be due to the ingestion of foodstuffs contaminated by uterine discharges from carriers or mares which have recently aborted. Transmission from the stallion at the time of service is also thought to occur. The infection may persist in the uterus and cause repeated abortion or infection of subsequent foals.

Although widely reported in the early 1900s, this disease is rarely encountered nowadays and it is one of the less common causes of either abortion or septicemia in horses (3, 4).

Pathogenesis

When infection occurs by ingestion, a transient bacteremia without marked systemic signs is followed by localization in the placenta, resulting in placentitis and abortion. Foals which are carried to term probably become infected *in utero* or soon after birth by ingestion from the contaminated teat surface or through the umbilicus.

Clinical findings

Abortion usually occurs about the 7th to 8th month of pregnancy. The mare may show signs of impending abortion followed by difficult parturition but other evidence of illness is usually lacking. Retention of the placenta and metritis are common sequels and may cause serious illness but subsequent sterility is unusual. A foal which is carried to term by an infected mare may develop an acute septicemia during the first few days of life or survive to develop polyarthritis 7–14 days later. Polyarthritis has also been observed in foals from vaccinated mares who showed no signs of the disease (5).

Infection in the stallion has also been reported, clinical signs including fever, edematous swelling of the prepuce and scrotum, and arthritis. Hydrocele, epididymitis and inflammation of the tunica vaginalis are followed by orchitis and testicular atrophy.

Clinical pathology

The organism can be isolated from the placenta, the uterine discharge, the aborted foal and from the joints of foals with polyarthritis. A high titer of salmonella agglutinins in the mare develops about 2 weeks after abortion. Vaccinated mares will give a positive reaction for up to a year.

Necropsy findings

The placenta of the aborted foal is edematous and hemorrhagic and may show areas of necrosis. Acute septicemia will be manifested in foals dying soon after birth and polyarthritis in those dying at a later stage.

Diagnosis

Abortion in mares may be caused by the viruses of equine viral rhinopneumonitis and equine viral arteritis and by *Streptococcus genitalium*. Septicemia and polyarthritis of foals is also caused by this latter organism, and by *E. coli*, *S. typhimurium* and *Actinobacillus equuli*. Identification of the disease must depend upon isolation of the organism and the positive agglutination test in the mare.

Treatment

The same drugs which have been recommended in the treatment of salmonellosis should also be effective in this disease.

Control

Careful hygiene, including isolation of infected mares and disposal of aborted material, should be practiced to avoid spread of the infection. Infected stallions should not be used for breeding. In the past, when this disease was much more common than it is now, great reliance was placed on vaccination as a control measure. An autogenous or commercial bacterin, composed of killed *S. abortivoequina* organisms, was injected on three occasions at weekly intervals to all mares on farms where the disease was enzootic, commencing 2–3 months after the close of the breeding season. A formol-killed, alum-precipitated vaccine is considered to be superior to a heat-killed, phenolized vaccine (6). In China a virulent strain vaccine is credited with effective protection after two injections 6 months apart (3). The widespread use of vaccines and hyperimmune sera is credited with the almost complete eradication of the disease in developed countries.

REFERENCES

(1) Muranyi, F. & Vanyi, A. (1963) *Magy. Allatorv. Lap.*, *18*, 239.
(2) Singh, I. P. et al. (1971) *Br. vet. J.*, *127*, 378.
(3) Winkinwerder, W. (1967) *Zentralbl. Bakteriol.*, *203*, 69.
(4) Morse, E. V. (1976) *Mod. vet. Pract.*, *57*, 47.
(5) Garbers, G. V. & Monteverde, J. J. (1964) *Revta Med. vet., Buenos Aires*, *45*, 305.
(6) Dhanda, M. R. et al. (1955) *Ind. J. vet. Sci.*, *25*, 245.

Abortion in ewes caused by *Salmonella abortusovis*

Salmonella abortusovis is a relatively uncommon cause of abortion in ewes but appears to be enzootic in particular areas (1). Spread of the disease may occur after the introduction of carrier animals. The reservoir of infection is infected animals which do not abort. In these carriers the organisms persist in internal organs for up to 6 months, and are excreted in the feces and vaginal mucus for periods up to 4 months (2). Ingestion is thought to be the main mode of infection although experimental infection is not easily established by oral dosing, subcutaneous injection being much more effective. Venereal spread has been postulated, and rams certainly become infected but all the evidence is against spread at coitus. Experimental induction of the disease in ewes is more successful after the 3rd month of pregnancy (5). Intrapreputial inoculation results in infection of rams and the passage of infected semen for up to 15 days (6). Abortion 'storms', with up to 10% of ewes aborting, occur about 6 weeks before lambing, and septic metritis and peritonitis subsequently cause a few deaths among the ewes. Mortality in lambs is common due either to death of weak lambs, or to the development of acute pneumonia in previously healthy lambs up to 2 weeks old. Identification of the disease depends upon isolation of the organism which is present in large numbers in the fetus, placenta and uterine discharges and the presence of a strong positive agglutination test in the ewe for 8–10 weeks after abortion. Several vaccines have been developed against *S. abortusovis* and although they are generally well regarded (6, 7) convincing evidence is not readily available.

The clinical and serological findings in *S. dublin* infections in ewes are very similar (4), and that infection has become more important as a cause of abortion in ewes in the United Kingdom than *S. abortusovis*. A strong immunity develops after an attack and an autogenous vaccine has given good results in the control of the disease. The results of vaccination need to be very carefully appraised because flock immunity develops readily and the disease tends to subside naturally in the second year (1).

Salmonella ruiru has also been recorded as a cause of abortion in ewes, and ewes with salmonellosis caused by *S. typhimurium* may also lose their lambs. The administration of broad-spectrum antibiotics may aid in controlling an outbreak but available reports (1) are not generally encouraging. Chloramphenicol is reported to be effective (3) and the trimethoprim and sulfadiazine combination is well regarded for this purpose.

REVIEW LITERATURE

Jack, E. J. (1971) Salmonella abortion in sheep. *Vet. Ann.*, *12*, 57.

REFERENCES

(1) Jack, E. J. (1968) *Vet. Rec.*, *82*, 558.
(2) Tradjebakhche, H. et al. (1974) *Rev. Med. vet.*, *125*, 387, 711.
(3) Boss, P. H. et al. (1977) *Schweiz Arch. Tierheilkd.*, *119*, 395.
(4) Baker, J. R. (1971) *Vet. Rec.*, *88*, 270.
(5) Sanchis, R. & Pardon, P. G. (1984) *Ann. rech. Vét.*, *15*, 97.
(6) Sanchis, R. & Pardon, P. (1986) *Ann. rech. Vét.*, *17*, 387.
(7) Nicolas, J. A. et al. (1981) *Rev. med. Vet.*, *132*, 359.

DISEASES CAUSED BY *PASTEURELLA* spp.

Pasteurellae occur in many animal diseases and, although in some instances they act as primary causes, the number of conditions in which they appear to play only a secondary role is gradually increasing. This is not to say that their importance is any the less. A primary viral pneumonia may be an insignificant disease until the intervention of a secondary pasteurellosis converts it into an outbreak of pneumonia of major economic importance. The common diseases in which *Pasteurella* spp. play an important etiological role are dealt with in this section with due regard to their possible secondary nature. Mastitis caused by *Pasteurella* spp. is dealt with in the section on mastitis. Pasteurellae may also play an important role in atrophic rhinitis of pigs and in calf pneumonia.

Other isolated instances of disease caused by *Past. multocida* are meningoencephalitis of calves (1) and yearling cattle (2), manifested by muscle tremor, opisthotonus, rotation of the eyeballs, collapse, coma and death within a few hours, and lymphadenitis in lambs which show enlargement of the submandibular, cranial, cervical and prescapular lymph nodes (3). An epidemic of meningoencephalitis in horses, donkeys and mules has been reported from Mexico. The causative agent was *Past. hemolytica*. Clinical findings included incoordination, paralysis of the tongue, tremor and blindness. Death occurred 1–7 days after the commencement of the illness (4). There is also a report of a fatal septicemia in horses and donkeys in India in which *Past. multocida* appeared to be implicated as a causative agent (5).

Pasteurella (Yersinia) pseudotuberculosis is a common cause of epizootic disease in birds and rodents and occasionally causes disease in domestic animals. It is dealt under a separate heading in this chapter (p. 676).

REFERENCES

(1) Shand, A. & Markson, L. M. (1953) *Br. vet. J.*, *109*, 491.
(2) Rose, W. K. & Rac, R. (1957) *Aust. vet. J.*, *33*, 124.
(3) Madeyski, S. et al. (1957) *Med. vet. Varsovie*, *13*, 75 cited in (1957) *Vet. Bull.*, *27*, 394.
(4) Valdes Ornelas, O. (1963) *Bull. Off. int. Epizootol.*, *60*, 1059.
(5) Pavri, K. M. & Apte, V. H. (1967) *Vet. Rec.*, *80*, 437.

Pasteurellosis

The nomenclature of the diseases caused by infections with *Pasteurella* spp. in farm animals has been indefinite and confusing. A suggested nomenclature is set out below which is based on the clinical findings and on the bacteria which are commonly associated with each entity (1).

Septicemic pasteurellosis of cattle (hemorrhagic septicemia or barbone), commonly associated with infection by *Past. multocida* type 1 or B, is the classical disease of southern Asia characterized by a peracute septicemia and a high mortality rate.

Pneumonic pasteurellosis of cattle, commonly associated with infection by *Past. multocida* type 2 or A and *Past. hemolytica*, is a common disease in Europe and the western hemisphere. It is characterized by bronchopneumonia, a longer course and a lower mortality rate than is the case in septicemic pasteurellosis.

Pasteurellosis of swine, sheep and goats: in swine this is usually associated with infection by *Past. multocida* and is mainly pneumonic in form. Pasteurellosis of sheep and goats is usually associated with infection by *Past. hemolytica* and although it is often pneumonic in form, a septicemic form of the disease is not unusual, especially in lambs.

There are a number of immunologically distinct types of the common causative organism, *Past. multocida*. These have been classified as types 1 (or B), 2 (or A), 3 (or C), and 4 (or D) and there is a loose relationship between the serotype and the host species (2, 3). There is also some relationship between the serotype and the disease produced. Septicemic pasteurellosis is caused only by type 1 (4) and as this type does not occur in the United Kingdom and is uncommon in North America, it is not surprising to find that this form of the disease does not occur there (5).

The position with *Past. hemolytica* is more obscure but preliminary work suggests that a number of serotypes occur and that there may be biological differences in virulence between them (6, 7).

REFERENCES

(1) Carter, G. R. & Bain, R. V. S. (1960) *Vet. Rev. Annot.*, *6*, 105.
(2) Roberts, R. S. (1947) *J. comp. Pathol.*, *57*, 261.
(3) Carter, G. R. & Rowsell, H. C. (1958) *J. Am. vet. med. Assoc.*, *132*, 187.
(4) Bain, R. V. S. (1954) *Bull. Off. int. Epizootol.*, *42*, 256.
(5) Kyaw, M. H. (1942) *Vet. J.*, *98*, 3.
(6) Biberstein, E. L. et al. (1960) *Cornell Vet.*, *50*, 283.
(7) Smith, G. R. (1961) *J. comp. Pathol.*, *71*, 194.

Septicemic pasteurellosis of cattle (hemorrhagic septicemia barbone)

Septicemic pasteurellosis of cattle, yaks, camels and water buffalo and, to a much smaller extent, of pigs and horses, is recorded chiefly from southern Asia where it causes very heavy death losses, particularly in low-lying areas, and when the animals are exposed to wet, chilly weather or exhausted by heavy work (1). It is also recorded in bison and cattle in the United States (2, 3) and the causative bacteria and its endotoxin have been used to produce the disease experimentally (4). Antibiotics against *P. multocida* capsular types B and E were demonstrated in a high percentage of serum samples from a group of domestic feeder calves in the United States (16). Since capsular E organisms have been isolated only in Africa and there is only one report of capsular B isolation from cattle in the United States, these organisms were not considered likely sources of the antigenic stimulation that provoked production of these antibodies. Both morbidity and mortality rates vary between 50 and 100% and animals that recover require a long convalescence. The overall mean case fatality for buffaloes is nearly three times as high as in cattle (17). The disease is presumed to be a primary pasteurellosis caused by *Past. multocida* type 1 (or B) and occasionally type 4 (D), and type E (12, 13).

Septicemic pasteurellosis occurs in outbreaks during periods of environmental stress, the causative organism in the intervening periods persisting on the tonsillar and nasopharyngeal mucosae of carrier animals. Approximately 45% of healthy cattle in herds associated with the disease harbor the organism in comparison to 3–5% in cattle from herds unassociated with the disease (11). Spread occurs by the ingestion of contaminated foodstuffs, the infection originating from clinically normal carriers or clinical cases, or possibly by ticks (5) and biting insects. The saliva of affected animals contains large numbers of pasteurellae during the early stages of the disease. Although infection occurs by ingestion, the organism does not survive on pasture for more than 24 hours (1).

The disease is an acute septicemia and clinically it is characterized by a sudden onset of fever (41–42°C, 106–107°F), profuse salivation, submucosal petechiation, severe depression and death in about 24 hours. Localization may occur in subcutaneous tissue, resulting in the development of warm, painful swellings about the throat, dewlap, brisket or perineum, and severe dyspnea may occur if the respiration is obstructed. In the later stages of an outbreak, some affected animals develop signs of pulmonary or alimentary involvement. Pasteurellae may be isolated from the saliva and the bloodstream. The disease in pigs is identical with that in cattle (6).

At necropsy, the gross findings are usually limited to generalized petechial hemorrhages, particularly under the serosae, and edema of the lungs and lymph nodes. Subcutaneous infiltrations of gelatinous fluid may be present and in a few animals there are lesions of early pneumonia and a hemorrhagic gastroenteritis. Isolation of the causative bacteria is best attempted from heart blood and spleen.

Apart from its regional distribution, septicemic pasteurellosis presents little in the way of diagnostic, clinical and necropsy findings and it can only be differentiated from anthrax, some cases of blackleg and acute leptospirosis by bacteriological examination.

The disease occurs chiefly in areas where veterinary assistance is not readily available and no detailed reports of the efficiency of various forms of treatment have been published. Oxytetracycline has been shown to be highly effective in pigs (6) and sulfadimidine in cattle (7) and the other treatments listed under pneumonic pasteurellosis of cattle should also be effective in this disease. Vaccines have been used for many years to protect cattle during the danger periods but the method was only moderately effective until the recent introduction of a stable vaccine composed of killed organisms in an adjuvant base containing paraffin and lanolin. This vaccine has been highly effective, especially when used prophylactically, although vaccination in the face of an outbreak may also reduce losses (1). Immunity after vaccination appears to be solid for at least 12 months and the only apparent disadvantage is the development of persistent subcutaneous swellings when the vaccine is improperly administered (8). Anaphylactic shock may occur in up to 1% of animals after the injection of some batches of vaccine. A satisfactory dried vaccine is also in use (9). A potential refinement in the vaccine used is suggested by the finding that endotoxin-free capsular antigen of *Past. multocida* types B and E is capable of immunizing cattle against challenge (10). A live streptomycin-dependent mutant *Past. multocida* vaccine provides good protection (14, 15).

REFERENCES

(1) Bain, R. V. S. (1963) *Hemmorhagic Septicemia*, p. 78, Agricultural Studies, No. 62. Rome: Food and Agriculture Organization.
(2) Heddleston, K. L. & Gallagher, J. E. (1969) *Bull. Wildl. Dis. Assoc.*, *5*, 206.
(3) Kradel, D. C. et al. (1969) *Vet. Med. small Anim. Clin.*, *64*, 145.
(4) Rhoades, K. R. et al. (1967) *Can. J. comp. Med.*, *31*, 226.
(5) Macadam, I. (1962) *Vet. Rec.*, *74*, 689.
(6) Murty, D. K. & Kaushik, R. K. (1965) *Vet. Rec.*, *77*, 411.
(7) Ilahi, A. & Afzal, H. (1965) *W. Pak. J. agric. Res.*, *3*, 1.
(8) Thomas, J. et al. (1969) *Kajian Vet. Malaysia-Singapore*, *2*, 4.
(9) Dhanda, M. R. (1960) *Bull. Off. int. Epizootol.*, *53*, 128.
(10) Nagy, L. K. & Penn, C. W. (1976) *Res. vet. Sci.*, *20*, 249.
(11) Mustafa, A. A. et al. (1978) *Br. vet. J.*, *134*, 375.
(12) Francis, B. K. et al. (1980) *Vet. Rec.*, *107*, 135.
(13) Shigidi, M. T. A. & Mustafa, A. A. (1979) *Cornell Vet.*, *69*, 77.
(14) Wei, B. D. & Carter, G. R. (1978) *Am. J. vet. Res.*, *39*, 1534.
(15) De Alwis, M. C. L. & Carter, G. R. (1980) *Vet. Rec.*, *106*, 435.
(16) Sawada, T. et al. (1985) *Am. J. vet. Res.*, *46*, 1247.
(17) Alwis, M. C. L. De (1981) *Trop. anim. Hlth Prod.*, *13*, 195.

Bovine respiratory disease (BRD)

A major problem which large animal clinicians commonly encounter is a group of cattle which are affected with an acute respiratory disease of uncertain etiology. The clinical findings may include some unexpected deaths, dyspnea, coughing, nasal discharge, inappetence or anorexia, a fever ranging from 40 to 41·5°C (104 to 106°F), evidence of pneumonia on auscultation of the lungs and a variable response to treatment. The affected group may be recently weaned beef calves; feeder cattle which have recently arrived in a feedlot; young growing cattle on summer pasture or mature cows which have recently been placed on a lush pasture; yearling or mature dairy cattle; or a group of veal calves.

The major difficulty facing the clinician is to make an etiological diagnosis based on clinical and epidemiologic findings. Specific treatment and control depend on an etiologic diagnosis, but differentiation between the diseases based on clinical findings can be so difficult and inaccurate that it is necessary to take provisional steps which will include most of the common pathogens until such time as the specific cause can be determined by laboratory examination. In many instances, of course, the specific etiology will not be determined. It is necessary at such a time to think in terms of an 'acute undifferentiated respiratory disease of cattle'; hence the need for the term bovine respiratory disease and the prescription of the recommended control program for it.

It will be apparent to the older generation that the thrust in recent years to get away from the non-specific diagnosis of 'shipping fever' and to aim for specific diagnosis of pneumonic pasteurellosis, infectious bovine rhinotracheitis and so on, has now come full circle and where they used to say 'shipping fever' we now say 'bovine respiratory disease' (BRD).

The common causes of BRD are set out in Table 53 which demonstrates that some of the diseases are not readily differentiable from each other. However, the infectious diseases caused by either viruses or bacteria alone or in combination are often difficult to distinguish from each other on a clinical basis and create the most difficult problems. These include diseases such as pneumonic pasteurellosis and the viral diseases of the respiratory tract. In addition, these infectious diseases must be differentiated from acute interstitial pneumonia which often overlaps in terms of clinical and laboratory findings.

Seroepidemiological surveys indicate the feedlot cattle commonly seroconvert to the viruses of infectious bovine rhinotracheitis, parainfluenza-3, bovine virus diarrhea (BVD) and bovine respiratory syncytial virus (2), and to *Mycoplasma bovis* and *M. dispar* (3) within the first month after arrival. These observations suggest a relationship between the respiratory viruses and *Mycoplasma* spp. and acute bovine respiratory disease but a direct cause and effect link cannot yet be concluded.

The risk factors that have been identified in outbreaks of respiratory disease in feedlot cattle include the purchase of cattle from auction markets whereby cattle arrive at the feedlot over an extended period of time, and mixing of cattle from many different sources (5). Cattle purchased from auction markets and started on high levels of grain were 6·3 times more likely to be treated for any disease, 4·9 times more likely to be treated for respiratory disease, 12·7 times more likely to die, and 6·7 times more likely to die with respiratory disease than groups made up primarily of farm-assembled cattle (5).

Path analysis of the factors affecting morbidity and mortality in Ontario feedlot calves identified the following risk factors: large groups, mixing different groups, feeding silage on arrival, the use of medicated water, supplies and vaccination against respiratory diseases during the first 2 weeks after arrival (6).

A number of important factors contribute to the difficulty of unravelling the etiologies in field outbreaks of respiratory disease.

A review of the literature on the morbidity and mortality rates and disease occurrence in North American feedlots reveals that there are differences in the definition of the terms used that makes the reports difficult to compare (1). In addition, the case-definition or the clinical diagnosis is invariably inadequately defined. In feedlots, the morbidity rate will range from 15 to 45% of cattle within 3 weeks after arrival and the population mortality rate varies from 1 to 5% (1). Respiratory diseases account for about 75% of the diseases.

The course of the disease, especially when animals have been treated, alters the gross and microscopic appearance of tissues, and the microbiological (bacteriological, virological) and serological findings so that the animal's status is impossible to determine.

The length of time that is usually required to work up the material to any sort of conclusion means that the procedure is expensive and to an extent inconclusive because the results are available only when the outbreak is over.

Table 53. Differential diagnosis of bovine respiratory disease (BRD)*

Disease	*Epidemiology*	*Clinical and laboratory findings*	*Response to treatment*
Pneumonic pasteurellosis (shipping fever)	Very common disease in North America. Young cattle recently stressed by weaning or transportation, many animals affected, some found dead, common in feedlots	Acute toxemic bronchopneumonia, moderate dyspnea, fever, increased breath sounds over ventral aspects of lungs, moist crackles, cough, pleuritis. Leukopenia and neutropenia in severe cases	Good response to treatment in early stages
Infectious bovine rhinotracheitis (IBR)	Common disease. All age groups but mostly young feedlot cattle, outbreaks common, occurrence unpredictable	Acute rhinotracheitis with discrete nasal lesions, inspiratory dyspnea, explosive loud coughing, ocular and nasal discharge, high fever 3–5 days. 1% die of secondary bacterial pneumonia. Virus isolation from nasal swabs. Acute and convalescent serology	Gradual recovery occurs in 3–5 days in spite of treatment. Treat secondary pneumonia
Viral interstitial pneumonia (adenovirus, parainfluenza-3 virus respiratory syncytial virus)	Yearling and adult cattle indoors or outdoors, young cows in closed dairy herd, may occur following addition to herd, high morbidity, low mortality	Sudden onset of acute pneumonia, moderate dyspnea and toxemia, loud breath sounds and wheezes due to bronchiolitis, no moist crackles unless secondary pneumonia. Leukopenia and lymphopenia	Gradual recovery occurs in 3–5 days. Treat secondary complications
Enzootic pneumonia of calves	Common disease in housed dairy calves, occasionally in pastured beef calves 2–6 months of age	Acute, subacute and chronic pneumonia, moderate fever, loud breath sounds ventrally, crackles and wheezes	Respond favorably to treatment for uncomplicated secondary bacterial bronchopneumonia
Bovine respiratory syncytial virus (RSV) infection	Young cattle 6–8 months of age, occasionally adult cattle, herd outbreaks are characteristic; case fatality rate varies from 1 to 30%	Inappetence, fever, coughing, dyspnea and abnormal lung sounds suggestive of interstitial pneumonia. Death common in those with severe respiratory distress. Four-fold or greater seroconversion to RSV. Immunofluorescence of nasopharyngeal smears and virus isolation. Acute bronchiolitis and alveolitis	Treat secondary complications
Allergic rhinitis (summer sniffles)	Mostly late summer, autumn when pasture in flower. Sporadic cases. Mostly Channel Island breeds. Cows may have disease each year	Sudden onset, dyspnea, stertor, mucopurulent then caseous yellow to orange nasal discharge. Sneeze, rub muzzle in bushes, twigs up nose, bleed	Into housing, antihistamines, excellent response if early. Older cases stertor persists till nasal mucosa sloughs
Epidemic acute interstitial pneumonia (acute pulmonary emphysema and edema, fog fever)	Occurs 4–10 days after adult cattle turned into lush autumn pasture. Outbreaks usual, sudden onset, high case fatality. Common in beef cattle in North America	Sudden and rapid death, severe loud dyspnea with grunting expiration, loud breath sounds over ventral aspects, crackles, subcutaneous emphysema, severe cases die, laboratory data not helpful, confirm at necropsy	Most severe cases die, moderate to mild cases recover, treatment difficult to evaluate
Acute or chronic interstitial pneumonia (bovine farmer's lung). Extrinsic allergic alveolitis	Not common. Mature cattle housed during winter months and exposed to moldy or dusty feeds. Several animals over period of time	Chronic coughing, dyspnea, weight loss, reduced milk yield, loud breath sounds, crackles, dull but not toxemic, abnormal nasal discharge	No response to treatment
Chronic interstitial pneumonia (diffuse fibrosing alveolitis)	Single animals only. May be chronic form of epidemic acute interstitial pneumonia	Chronic onset of coughing, dyspnea, weight loss, reduced milk yield, decreased breath sounds, no toxemia, cor pulmonale	No response to treatment
Verminous pneumonia (*Dictyocaulus viviparus*)	All ages susceptible, usually young cattle 6–12 months on pasture, wet warm seasons, outbreaks common, enzootic area	Moderate to severe dyspnea, coughing, fever, loud breath sounds, crackles over *dorsal half of lung*, eosinophilia may occur, larvae in feces 3 weeks after infection	No response to antibiotics. Responds to anthelmintics

Table 53. (cont.)

Disease	*Epidemiology*	*Clinical and laboratory findings*	*Response to treatment*
Ascaris suis pneumonia	Not common. All ages. On pasture previously occupied by pigs	Sudden onset, severe dyspnea, rapid deaths, loud breath sounds, crackles over entire lung. Will recover gradually if not too severe	No specific treatment response
Pulmonary abscess	Single animal affected. History of pneumonia with no response to treatment. Occasionally several cases are seen in feedlot	Chronic coughing with epistaxis and hemoptysis, chronic toxemia, mild fever, crackles and wheezes distributed randomly. Neutrophilia	Nil
Calf diphtheria	Occurs universally in young calves, dirty conditions or on rough dry pasture. Usually only few affected	Acute toxemia, fever, inspiratory and stertor, necrotic lesions visible in larynx and oral cavity	Responds to antibacterial and topical treatment
Enzootic nasal granuloma	In enzootic area up to 30% morbidity in a herd, up to 75% of herds. Coastal regions, autumn is worst, Channel Island breeds most affected. Loss is due to continuous loss of production. A chronic debilitating disease. All ages, mostly adults	May be acute 'summer sniffles' early. Then chronic dyspnea with stertor, eat indifferently, lose condition, have to be culled. Chronic nasal discharge. Smear nodules on nasal cavity mucosa palpable through nostril	Nil
Contagious bovine pleuropneumonia	Outbreak in susceptible cattle—morbidity up to 100%, mortality up to 50% if cattle stressed, travelling. Aerogenous spread, no mediate contagion. Outbreaks due to introduction cattle often inapparent 'carriers' which are detectable by CF test. Incubation period 3–6 weeks	Acute fibrinous pneumonia and pleurisy. Dyspnea, fever 40·5°C (104·5°F), deep cough, shallow, fast, elbows out, grunting respiration. Pain on chest percussion. Pleuristic friction rub early, moist crackles. Course 3 days to 3 weeks	Not to be treated. Eradication is urgent. Is treated in enzootic areas where control is not attempted
Aspiration pneumonia	History is important. Following faulty drenching techniques or regurgitation and aspiration in weak cows (i.e. milk fever)	Acute bronchopneumonia with toxemia. 24–48 hours following aspiration. Loud breath sounds ventral half, moist crackles. Marked leukopenia and neutropenia	May respond to treatment if treated early
Dusty feed rhinotracheitis	Few days following introduction of finely chopped dry feed. Feed contains high concentrations of 'fines'	Outbreak of coughing, rhinitis with copious serous nasal discharge, conjunctivitis and ocular discharge. Bright and alert	Recover in few days following removal of dusty feed
Embolic pneumonia due to ruptured vena caval abscess	1–8 years of age. History of respiratory disease with hemoptysis and poor response to treatment	Dullness, polypnea, hyperpnea, thoracic pain, frequent coughing with hemoptysis, temperature variable, anemia. Common, widespread foci of moist crackles and wheezes with increased breath sounds. May die rapidly following massive hemorrhage. Hepatomegaly and congestive heart failure may occur too. Neutrophilia and hypergammaglobulinemia	No response to treatment

* The emphasis is on diseases in which the major lesions are in the respiratory tract. Diseases such as bovine virus diarrhea (BVD), malignant catarrhal fever and *Haemophilus* septicemia in which respiratory lesions may occur as part of the disease are discussed elsewhere.

The practicing veterinarian is limited in most situations to correlating clinical, epidemiological and necropsy findings in making his diagnosis. Diagnostic laboratories may not be readily available and their resources for sophisticated microbiological and serological investigations may be much less than is needed for an acute determination of causes.

In the past, investigations of outbreaks of BRD have been incomplete and the interpretation of the findings almost impossible because one or more pieces of information were missing. A voluminous body of information has been generated on the biology of specific etiologic entities but the information is difficult to use.

Insufficient effort has been directed towards putting it all together to effectively control respiratory disease on the farm. Ideally, future investigations of outbreaks of respiratory disease should consist of in-depth examinations of a representative sample of the affected group using a multidisciplinary approach involving clinical, epidemiologic and laboratory investigation. These procedures, especially those requiring detailed virologic and serologic examinations, are expensive and in the light of the economic status of cattle industries not likely to be lightly borne. But it will only be when such a multidisciplinary approach is brought to bear on BRD that we will improve our position with respect to knowing what actually occurs in outbreaks of the disease.

Treatment

The principles of the clinical management of outbreaks of acute undifferentiated bovine respiratory diseases are:

- Unless otherwise determined, when toxemia and fever are present it is assumed that a primary bacterial pneumonia is present, or if a viral interstitial pneumonia is suspected then a secondary bacterial pneumonia may occur. Therefore, antimicrobial therapy is of prime importance
- New cases must be identified as soon as possible. This will require increased surveillance of the group to detect affected animals as soon as clinical abnormalities such as depression, nasal discharge, dyspnea are noticeable
- New cases must be treated as soon as they are detected. Each treated animal should be suitably identified and a record kept of the initial body temperature and the treatment administered. If the outbreak is due to pneumonic pasteurellosis, failure to respond favorably to antimicrobial therapy or relapses which occur a few days after an initial apparent recovery is usually due to late treatment. Delaying treatment until 48 hours after an experimental aerosol infection of *Past. hemolytica* can prolong the course of the disease and increase mortality (7)
- Any of the common antimicrobials must be administered parenterally daily for at least 3 days. For lactating dairy cows, antimicrobials with the shortest milk withdrawal times commensurate with effectiveness should be used. Milk from treated cows must be kept from the bulk milk supply until the stated withdrawal time has elapsed.

The response to treatment, or lack of it, is valuable information in making a final decision on cause. Animals which do not respond to treatment should be submitted to intensive necropsy examination and culture of affected lungs. One of the emerging problems inherent in such broad policies in treatment is public health concern with the amount of antibiotic residue in meat. Pressure is now being applied to use antibiotics only when necessary, which necessitates a more accurate diagnosis. A good example of this problem is when cattle are treated with antibiotics for BRD but the diagnosis is then refined in a day or two to be interstitial pneumonia and emergency slaughter is then the appropriate course of action. The cattle cannot be slaughtered until the withdrawal period for the specific antibody used has expired, by which time many of the cattle will have died anyway. The regular use of a particular antimicrobial in feedlots may increase the level of resistance to *Past. hemolytica* (9).

When confronted with an outbreak one of the major decisions to be made is whether or not to recommend mass medication of the water or feed supplies for several days or to administer an antimicrobial to all in-contact animals in an attempt to treat cases in the preclinical stage. Veterinarians commonly recommend the use of medicated water supplies as an aid in the treatment of outbreaks of acute respiratory disease and field observations claim beneficial results. However, there is no validated information available to support a recommendation for a medicated water supply for treatment or prophylaxis in the face of an outbreak (8). Depending on the water supply system it can be difficult to deliver and maintain a constant concentration of a drug in the water supply and palatability of certain drugs can be a problem. The medication of the water or feed supplies can also create a false sense of security in the animal attendants who may not be as efficient in the selection of affected animals in the early stages of the disease.

There are no validated reports of the use of medicated feed as an aid to treatment for outbreaks of acute respiratory disease in cattle.

In an outbreak of acute respiratory disease in feedlot cattle when the daily morbidity rate reaches 6–10% the parenteral administration of long-acting oxytetracycline to all in-contact cattle at a dose of 20 mg/kg body weight intramuscularly is recommended (4).

Control

The control of outbreaks of acute bovine respiratory disease will depend on minimizing the effects of the predisposing causes, and in some situations vaccination with vaccines which contain one or more antigens. While vaccines are available for the control of acute respiratory disease caused by infectious bovine rhinotracheitis, parainfluenza-3 virus and *Pasteurella* sp., there are almost no reports available of their efficacy determined under scientifically designed field trials. Based on current immunological technology, efficacious vaccines are considered to be feasible (12). The vaccines have been evaluated by experimental challenge of vaccinated animals with specific pathogens in a laboratory environment. However, there is little scientific evidence available that the vaccines are protective against acute undifferentiated respiratory disease as it occurs in the 'real world' situation (12, 13). Preshipment vaccination of beef calves 3 weeks prior to weaning with vaccines containing infectious bovine rhinotracheitis (IBR) parainfluenza-3, *Pasteurella* sp. and *Hemophilus somnus* did not reduce the incidence of undifferentiated respiratory disease compared to those unvaccinated (16).

The mass medication of feed supplies of newly arrived feedlot cattle has been investigated as a method of reducing the morbidity and mortality due to respiratory disease. The provision of chloretetracycline in the feed at a rate of 1, 2 or 4 g per head daily during the 2 week period after arrival reduced the number of calves that required treatment for respiratory disease (10).

The parenteral administration of antimicrobials to each animal as a form of mass medication may assist in the reduction of morbidity and mortality rates due to respiratory disease. The use of longacting oxytetracycline at a dose of 20 mg/kg body weight intramuscularly to feedlot cattle on arrival significantly reduced morbidity and mortality rates (18). The combined use of longacting oxytetracycline at a dose of 20 mg/kg body weight intramuscularly on arrival followed by the oral administration of 25 g of sustained release sulfadimethoxine on day 3 resulted in a 90% reduction in treatment days per calf purchased (11). Similar results were obtained in other studies (19, 20).

Immunomodulators which may enhance the effectiveness of the immune response to infection are now being evaluated as possible aids in the prevention of BRD in recently arrived feedlot cattle (17).

As a general outline for the control of BRD the following factors are considered as contributing to disease and their effects must be minimized with suitable management and disease prevention techniques.

- Young growing cattle are more susceptible than mature cattle because of a lack of sufficient immunity. Vaccination of calves at strategic times may be necessary
- Cattle purchased from various sources and mingled in a feedlot are more likely to develop BRD than cattle which have originated from one source. Some cattle will be highly susceptible and others relatively resistant because of differences in nasal flora, immunological, genetic and nutritional backgrounds. A high level of management and constant surveillance are necessary to recognize, isolate and treat clinical cases early in order to minimize morbidity and case mortality
- Rapid fluctuations in environmental temperatures and relative humidity, not only during the fall and winter months but also during warm seasons, will commonly precede outbreaks of respiratory diseases. Every practical and economical management technique must be used to provide as much comfort as possible and to avoid overcrowding
- Inadequate ventilation is a major predisposing cause of respiratory disease of cattle raised indoors
- The weaning of beef calves during inclement weather may exacerbate the stress of weaning and commonly results in an outbreak of respiratory disease
- The stress associated with the marketing of cattle is a major factor. The movement of cattle through saleyards—where they may be overcrowded, deprived of adequate feed and water, handled roughly while being sorted, weighed, tagged, blood sampled, vaccinated or injected with antibiotics and/or vitamins and then loaded onto uncomfortable vehicles and transported long distances without adequate rest stops—is stressful. The practice of preconditioning cattle before they enter the feedlot must continue to be examined to determine which aspects are most profitable. In some situations vaccination of non-preconditioned calves is more economical than preconditioned calves (15).

REVIEW LITERATURE

Martin, S. W. (1983) Vaccination: is it effective in preventing respiratory disease or influencing weight gains in feedlot calves. *Can. vet. J.*, *24*, 10–19.

Symposium on Bovine Respiratory Disease (1985) *Vet. Clin. N. Am. food anim. Pract.* Vol. 1, (2) July, Philadelphia: W. B. Saunders.

Yates, W. D. G. (1982) A review of infectious bovine rhinotracheitis, shipping fever pneumonia and viral-bacterial synergism in respiratory disease of cattle. *Can. J. comp. Med.*, *46*, 225–263.

REFERENCES

(1) Kelly, A. P. & Jansen, E. D. (1986) *Can. vet. J.*, *27*, 496.
(2) Martin, S. W. & Bohac, J. G. (1986) *Can. J. vet. Res.*, *50*, 351.
(3) Rosendal, S. & Martin, S. W. (1986) *Can. J. vet. Res.*, *50*, 179.
(4) Jansen, E. D. & McManus, R. F. (1980) *Bov. Pract.*, *15*, 87.
(5) Wilson, S. H. et al. (1985) *Can. vet. J.*, *26*, 335.
(6) Martin, S. W. & Meek, A. H. (1986) *Can. J. vet. Res.*, *50*, 15.
(7) Janzen, E. D. et al. (1984) *Can. vet. J.*, *25*, 78.
(8) Martin, S. W. (1985) *Can. J. comp. Med.*, *49*, 15.
(9) Martin, S. W. et al. (1983) *Can. J. comp. Med.*, *47*, 6.
(10) Perry, T. W. et al. (1986) *J. anim. Sci.*, *62*, 1215.
(11) Lofgreen, P. (1983) *J. anim. Sci.*, *56*, 529.
(12) Wilkie, B. N. (1984) *Can. vet. J.*, *25*, 48.
(13) Martin, S. W. (1983) *Can. vet. J.*, *24*, 10.
(14) Myers, L. L. (1984) *J. Am. vet. med. Assoc.*, *184*, 5.
(15) Kadel, W. L. et al. (1985) *Am. J. vet. Res.*, *46*, 1944.
(16) Martin, S. W. et al. (1984) *Can. vet. J.*, *25*, 145.
(17) Larsson, B. et al. (1985) *Acta. vet. Scand.*, *26*, 262.
(18) Albak, C. et al. (1986) *Bov. Pract.*, *21*, 192.
(19) Smith, R. A. et al. (1986) *Anim. Sci. Res. Report. misc. Publ,. Oklahoma Agric. exp. Station*, *118*, 269.
(20) Gill, D. R. et al. (1986) *Anim. Sci. Res. Report. misc. Publ. Oklahoma Agric. exp. Station*, *118*, 260.

Pneumonic pasteurellosis of cattle (shipping fever pneumonia)

This form of pasteurellosis in cattle is usually associated with infection by *Pasteurella hemolytica* and occasionally *Past. multocida*. Shipping fever is an entity within the bovine respiratory disease complex, characterized clinically by acute bronchopneumonia with toxemia and pathologically by lobar, anteroventrally distributed, exudative pneumonia in which fibrin is usually a prominent part of the exudate and fibrinous pleuritis is common (1, 2).

Etiology

Pasteurella hemolytica biotype A serotype 1 is considered to be the most common cause of the lesion (1). In some cases biotype T strains have been isolated from cases of pneumonic pasteurellosis (7, 8). *Pasteurella multocida* is isolated occasionally. The *Pasteurella* spp. are considered to be the final cause of the pneumonia, but the mechanisms by which the bacteria get into the lung and produce the lesions has not yet been determined. Other pathogens like viruses or mycoplasma may act synergistically to allow the bacteria to be pathogenic.

Epidemiology

Pneumonic pasteurellosis is a common disease of cattle in Europe, the United Kingdom and North America. In Canada and the United States the disease occurs most commonly in beef calves after weaning in the fall of the year and is the most important disease in cattle that have been recently introduced into feedlots. The morbidity may reach 35%, the case fatality rate may range from 5 to 10% and the population mortality rate may vary from 0·75 to 1%.

However, these morbidity and mortality data may not be reliable because of wide variations in the methods used to calculate disease incidence and prevalence. A review of the literature of morbidity and mortality rates and disease occurrence in feedlot cattle in North American revealed deficiencies in the epidemiological data available from feedlots (78). Case-definitions of clinical cases are often poorly defined. The incidence of morbidity ranged from 0 to 69% with most reports between 15 and 45%. The population mortality rate ranged from 0 to 15% with most reports between 1 and 5%. The peak incidence of disease was within the first 3 weeks after arrival of the calves in the feedlot. The most common clinical and pathological diagnoses were respiratory disease often described as shipping fever.

Records from feedlots in North America indicate that up to 50% of all deaths from pneumonic pasteurellosis may be found dead without any premonitory signs having been noted by the animal attendant (3, 4).

Pneumonic pasteurellosis is a major cause of economic loss in the feedlot industry. It is responsible for the largest cause of mortality in feedlots in North America. In addition to the death losses, the costs of treatment (which includes the personnel involved in the detection and actual treatment and the drugs used, and the vaccines) are considerable. While it has been assumed that there is a loss of production following the illness, this has not been documented. In fact, because of compensatory regrowth in animals which have recovered there may be no correlation between average daily gain, feed conversion and treatment (5).

The disease occurs most commonly in young growing cattle from 6 months to 2 years of age but all age groups are susceptible. Beef calves may develop the disease before weaning if subjected to the stress of an early snowstorm in the late fall in Canada. Similar observations in single-suckled calves have been made in the United Kingdom (6). The disease occurs commonly in outbreaks 7–10 days after cattle have arrived in the feedlot following stressful transportation. This forms a major part of the 'shipping fever' complex which is a major hazard in the practice of rearing beef cattle on range country and then transporting them long distances to other centers for growing and finishing. Although the disease occurs most commonly in young beef cattle soon after their introduction to feedlots it is not uncommon in dairy herds, especially when recent introductions have been made or cattle are returned to their home farms after summer grazing on community pastures or exhibition at fairs.

The Bruce County Beef Cattle Project in Canada identified some of the epidemiological factors associated with mortality in cattle shipped from western Canada to small Ontario feedlots over a period of 3 successive years (9, 10). The most common cause of mortality was fibrinous pneumonia. Feeding corn silage as the major roughage in the first month after arrival was associated with increased mortality. Mixing of cattle from different sources and vaccinating cattle against respiratory disease on arrival appeared to be the most important additional factors that increased mortality rates. Path analysis of the factors influencing morbidity and mortality supported the original findings (11). An epidemiologic analysis of the influence of feedlot management on the occurrence of bovine respiratory disease (BRD) revealed that cattle purchased from the auction marts and started on high levels of grain in their rations were 6·3 times more likely to be treated for any disease, 4·9 times more likely to be treated for respiratory disease, 12·7 times more likely to die, and 6·7 times more likely to die with respiratory disease than the group consisting primarily of farm-assembled heifers and started on 10% grain ration with time for adjustment to grain (14). These results indicate the importance of management factors predisposing to the disease. The role of stress as an epidemiologic determinant in shipping fever pneumonia has been examined experimentally. Experimental transportation and handling to mimic stress followed by an aerosol of *Pasteurella hemolytica* did not result in significant lesions of pneumonia but did make the animals susceptible to bovine herpes-1-virus (15). The transportation and assembling of yearling beef calves can result in an increase in the levels of plasma fibrinogen which is an indication of some stress (16). Deprivation of feed and water followed by confinement in unfamiliar surroundings also results in an increase in fibrinogen. The response of the animals was also dependent upon the previous environment and management applied to them before assembly and transportation.

Epidemiological studies have shown that the frequency of isolation of *Pasteurella* spp. from the nasal passages of normal healthy unstressed calves is low and that the frequency increases as the animals are moved to an auction mart and then to a feedlot (12). The prevalence of *Pasteurella hemolytica* serotype 1 in the nasal cavity and tracheas can be low in beef calves from a closed herd that is maintained on range pastures, and serum antibody levels are also low. With time there may be an increase in the frequency of isolation of the bacteria from healthy calves which were moved to pens, held in low population densities, and maintained under low stress conditions (20). In some cases serotype 2 predominates while the calves are on the farm, and serotype 1 predominates when the calves are in the feedlot and affected with pneumonia (12). There also are relationships between the numbers of bacteria in the nasopharynx and the ambient temperature and humidity (13). In calves kept at a constant temperature of 16°C (60°F), the bacterial populations in the nasopharynx were at a minimum between 65 and 75% relative humidity and tended to rise at humidities outside that range.

The incidence of pneumonia in feedlot cattle on feed from 16 to 30 days after arrival may be related to an increase in the concentration of airborne particles 2·0–3·3 μm in diameter, the season of the year and fluctuations in daily ambient temperatures (101).

The possibility that infection with several different viruses and mycoplasma may predispose to pneumonic pasteurellosis has been a subject of intense research activity and is presented in more detail under pathogenesis. Seroepidemiological surveys of cattle in feedlots reveals that the viruses of infectious bovine rhinotracheitis (IBR) and parainfluenza-3, and bovine virus diarrhea (BVD) and bovine respiratory syncytial viruses (RSV) were present, active and associated with respiratory disease (17). The presence of antibody indicates current or recent exposure to the virus but does not indicate resistance. Cattle with low titers to infectious bovine rhinotracheitis and/or bovine respiratory syncytial viruses on arrival were at increased risk of subsequent treatment for bovine respiratory disease. Treated cattle also had greater increases to parainfluenza-3 and/or bovine virus diarrhea viruses than control calves. Serologically there is also evidence of a high prevalence of *Mycoplasma bovis* and *M. dispar* in feedlot calves which may be a risk factor for respiratory disease (18). Calves with low serological titers to *M. dispar* on arrival in the feedlot were at increased risk of respiratory disease. The viral-bacterial synergism in respiratory disease has been reviewed in detail (1).

Prior natural exposure to *Past. hemolytica* appears to enhance the resistance of calves to both natural and experimental pneumonic pasteurellosis (23). Indirect bacterial agglutination titers to *Past. hemolytica* A (1) were low in cattle entering the feedlot and lower levels were also present in cattle which died due to fibrinous pneumonia (21). This illustrates that seroconversion occurs naturally after arrival in the feedlot. Resistance to experimental pneumonic pasteurellosis has been correlated directly with the presence of serum cytotoxin neutralizing titers (19). Animals which were exposed to live organisms resulted in the production of antibodies to both cell surface antigens and cytotoxin, whereas exposures to the killed vaccine resulted in the production of antibodies primarily to cell surface antigens. There does not seem to be any protection associated with serum antibodies to the polysaccharide of the organism (22). Isolates of *Past. hemolytica* and *Past. multocida* from clinical cases may be serum-resistant whereas those from asymptomatic carriers vary in serum-susceptibility (103).

Drafty or humid and poorly ventilated barns, exposure to inclement weather, transport, fatigue and deprivation from feed and water are commonly followed by outbreaks of the disease in cattle. An increase in virulence of the bacteria is often evident after animal passage; at the commencement of an outbreak only those animals which have been subjected to devitalizing influences are affected but the disease may subsequently spread to other animals in the group. There is little tendency for the disease to become an area problem, sporadic outbreaks occurring with the appearance of conditions favorable to the development of the disease.

Transmission of pasteurellae probably occurs by the inhalation of infected droplets coughed up or exhaled by infected animals which may be clinical cases or recovered carriers in which the infection persists in the upper respiratory tract. *Past. hemolytica* and *Past. multocida* are highly susceptible to environmental influences and it is unlikely that mediate contagion is an important factor in the spread of the disease. When conditions are optimum, particularly when cattle are closely confined in inadequately ventilated barns, or when overcrowded in trucks and trains or held for long periods in holding pens in feedlots, the disease may spread very quickly and affect a high proportion of the herd within 48 hours. In animals at pasture, the rate of spread may be much slower.

Pathogenesis

The pathogenesis of shipping fever pneumonia is complex and has been the subject of intense research activity by several groups (1, 2). The relative roles of the etiologic agents and stress factors in causing the disease is not fully understood but tremendous progress has been made in the last 10 years. Considerable research has centered on determining how the pasturellae, which are part of the normal flora of the upper respiratory tract, get down into the terminal bronchioles and alveoli, and when they are in these locations how they produce the lesions. Under normal conditions the bovine lung is relatively free of pasturellae due to an effective lung clearance mechanism (24). The current hypothesis is that a combination of viral infection of the respiratory tract and devitalizing influences from transportation, temporary starvation, weaning, rapid fluctuations in ambient temperature, the mixing of cattle from different origins and the excessive handling of cattle after arrival in a feedlot can all collectively promote an increase in the total numbers and virulence of pasturellae in the nasopharynx which are then inhaled into the alveoli and not effectively cleared. Under normal conditions, alveolar macrophages will effectively clear pasturellae from the alveoli by phagocytic mechanisms (24). Bovine pulmonary macrophages release superoxide anion when exposed to *Past. hemolytica* and the response is dependent on the presence of opsonizing antibody and the quantity of organisms presented to the phagocyte (45). This is an important mechanism by which this phagocyte can initiate microbiocidal activity and may provide clues to further study the defense mechanisms of the lung. The exposure of non-stressed calves to an aerosol of *Past. hemolytica* usually does not result in an acute pneumonia. Such calves usually clear the bacterium within hours (39).

In an attempt to understand the pathogenesis of shipping fever pneumonia the experimental disease has been reproduced using several different methods, the most commonly used being the sequential aerosol infection of calves with either parainfluenza-3 (PI-3) virus or the bovine herpes virus-1 followed by *Past. hemolytica* 3 days or more later. It is suggested that viral-bacterial synergism is an important part of the pathogenesis. The exposure of calves to aerosols of parainfluenza-virus followed by *Past. hemolytica* at intervals of 3–13 days later will result in a purulent bronchopneumonia (25). The virus interferes with the lung clearance of *Past. hemolytica* when an aerosol of the bacteria is given at 7 days following the viral infection, there is little interference after only 3 days and a moderate degree at 11 days (33). Other similar experiments with this combination of pathogens did not result in severe pulmonary lesions (27).

Pneumonic pasteurellosis similar to the naturally occurring disease can be reproduced experimentally by exposing calves sequentially to aerosols of bovine herpes virus-1 and *Past. hemolytica* 4 days apart (1). In this experimental model, vaccination of the animal against the virus before challenge with the viral bacterial aerosol sequence is protective (32). Experimentally, the greater the viral or the bacterial dose the more severe the pneumonia (28, 29). The duration of the interaction between bovine herpes virus-1 and *Past. hemolytica* can persist for up to 30 days after infection with the virus (30). A sequential aerosol infection of bovine herpes virus-1 and *Past. multocida*, or *Past. multocida* alone, can also result in pneumonia (31).

Pneumonic pasteurellosis similar to the natural disease can also be reproduced by transthoracic intrapulmonic infection of unstressed, conventional calves with only *Past. hemolytica* or *Past. multocida* (34), endobronchial inoculation (34), intratracheal challenge (35) or intranasal inoculation (36) of calves with the organism. A certain number of bacteria are necessary to yield consistent results (34), and the 4-hour long phase cultures of *Past. hemolytica* produce more severe pneumonia than the corresponding stationary phase cultures (35). *Past. hemolytica* can be phagocytosed by alveolar macrophages in the declining phase of growth of the organisms but not in the long phase.

Pasteurella hemolytica produces an exotoxin which is a cytotoxin and leukotoxin highly toxic to bovine neutrophils and macrophages (37, 38). The bacteria produces the cytotoxin with maximum production occurring during the long phase of growth peaking after 6 hours of incubation (37, 38). Following the inhalation of *Past. hemolytica* into the lung there is an accumulation of neutrophils (42) which when destroyed by leukotoxin results in the release of proteolytic enzymes, oxidant products, and basic proteins which degrade cellular membranes, increasing capillary permeability which results in fluid accumulation in the interstitium of the alveolar wall, alveolar wall necrosis and pulmonary edema (40). The importance of the neutrophil is supported by experimental evidence that depletion of blood neutrophils in calves made the animals much less susceptible to pulmonary injury following intratracheal inoculation of *Past. hemolytica* (41). The cytotoxin has been purified and partially characterized; it is a protein which is highly immunogenic, is common to all serotypes of *Past. hemolytica* and may be an effective agent for immunization against pneumonic pasteurellosis in cattle (48). Assay tests for determination of cytotoxin neutralizing antibody titers in cattle sera are described (49, 50). There is positive correlation between ELISA titers to cytotoxin and protection to experimental pneumonic pasturellosis (49).

The possible role of stress in the induction of pneumonic pasteurellosis has been examined (15). Experimental transportation and handling were not sufficient to make calves susceptible to an aerosol of *Past. hemolytica* but did make them susceptible to bovine herpes virus-1 (15).

The immunological response of calves to natural and experimental pneumonic pasteurellosis has been examined. Complement-fixing antibody is not correlated with protection (43). Calves which have recovered from the experimental disease are resistant to naturally occurring disease (44). Resistance to experimental challenge with the organism correlates directly with serum cytotoxin neutralizing titers (19). Cattle dying from pneumonic pasteurellosis may have lower levels of cytotoxin neutralizing antibody than animals from the same group dying from other causes (46, 50). Aerosol exposure of calves with *Past. hemolytica* results in the development of toxin-neutralizing antibodies in pulmonary lavage samples and an accompanying increase in serum neutralizing titer (50). Since aerosol exposure of calves to viable *Past. hemolytica* elicits a protective immune response characterized by enhanced clearance of the organism from the lung and by protection against fibrinous pneumonia, it is possible that the presence of preexisting antibodies to the leukotoxin in the lungs may provide immunity by protecting phagocytic leukocytes from the leukotoxin and by promoting phagocytosis and intracellular killing of the organism.

Experimentally, synergism may occur between *Past. hemolytica* and *Mycoplasma bovis* in producing pneumonia in gnotobiotic calves (51) and not in conventional calves (52).

The role of the bovine virus diarrhea (BVD) virus in outbreaks of pneumonic pasteurellosis is unknown. In one study the BVD virus did not impair the pulmonary clearance of *Past. hemolytica* (52). In a different study the endobronchial inoculation of calves with the BVD virus and *Past. hemolytica* sequentially 5 days apart resulted in a severe fibrinopurulent bronchopneumonia and pleuritis involving up to 75% of the total lung volume (53). Endobronchial inoculation of the organism only caused a localized non-invasive lesion in the lungs (39).

The terminal lesion is a fibrinous bronchopneumonia with varying degrees of fibrinous pleuritis. The ventral aspects of the apical and cardiac lobes of the lungs are most commonly affected; in advanced cases a greater portion of the lung becomes affected and other lobes of the lung become involved. Consolidation of affected lobes results in loud breath sounds (bronchial tones and the exudative nature of the lesion causes crackles. The pleuritis causes severe thoracic pain and pleuritic function rubs may be audible. Death occurs as a result of hypoxemia and toxemia. Complications in affected animals which do not fully recover include pulmonary abscessation, chronic pleuritis with or without pleural effusion, bronchiectasis, pericarditis and congestive heart failure due to cor pulmonale.

Clinical findings

The disease usually develops in cattle within 10 to 14 days after they have been stressed. Sudden deaths (54) without any previous warning signs may be the first sign of an outbreak in which many calves are obviously affected and some are in the incubation stages of the disease.

Viewed from a distance affected cattle are usually depressed and the respirations are shallow and rapid. There is a weak protective cough which may become more pronounced and frequent if they are urged to walk. Animals which have been ill for a few days will appear gaunt in the abdomen because of anorexia. A mucopurulent nasal discharge, a crusty nose and an ocular discharge are common. Although affected cattle are anorexic, they may continue to drink maintenance amounts of water which may be useful in mass medication of the water supplies.

In an outbreak of the disease the animals in the earliest stages of the disease are not obviously ill when examined from a distance. If every animal in the affected group is examined closely, up to 10% of apparently normal animals will have a fever ranging from 40 to 41°C (104–106°F) and no other clinical abnormalities. Auscultation of the thorax of some of these subclinical cases will reveal rapid shallow respirations and an increase in breath sounds. Close examination of the nostrils will reveal an excess of serous nasal discharge. These animals respond remarkably well to treatment; if not treated at this stage, they commonly progress to clinical cases within a few days.

Close examination reveals a fever of 40–41°C (104–106°F) and evidence of bronchopneumonia. In the early stages there are loud breath sounds (bronchial tones) audible over the anterior and ventral parts of the lungs. As the disease progresses the loud breath sounds become louder and extend over a greater area and crackles become audible followed by squeaky and musical wheezes in a few days especially in chronic cases which are ill for several days. Pleuritic friction rubs may be audible although their absence does not preclude the presence of extensive pleuritis with adherence together of the affected pleurae. In severe cases or those of several days duration the dyspnea is marked, commonly with an expiratory grunt, although the respiratory rate may not be elevated.

The course of the disease is usually short, 2–4 days. If treated early affected cattle recover in 24–48 hours, but severe cases and those which have been ill for a few days before being treated may die or become chronically affected in spite of prolonged therapy. In outbreaks it appears that some cattle recover spontaneously without treatment. Outbreaks of the disease in feedlots may last for 2–3 weeks or longer after the first index case, dependent on the condition of the cattle when first affected. Outbreaks can be prolonged in feedlots which add groups of newly arrived cattle to an existing pen of cattle every few days in order to fill the pen to optimum capacity. The disease then occurs in each new group of cattle and may spread to previously resident cattle which perpetuates the disease for several weeks.

The origin of the cattle also influences the severity and length of outbreaks. In well-nourished thrifty cattle originating from one ranch and maintained as a single group the morbidity may be less than 5% and the mortality nil. The outbreak will last only a few days and the cattle return to normal quickly. In cattle which have originated from a variety of sources and moved through saleyards and then comingled in the feedlot, the disease may persist for several weeks. Some cattle will develop complications, never fully recover and will need to be culled later.

A mild diarrhea may be present in some cases but is usually of no consequence. On an affected farm, calves may be affected with pneumonia but very young calves may die of septicemia without having shown previous signs of illness.

Clinical pathology

Nasal swabs taken from clinical cases before treatment often yield an almost pure culture of pasteurellae but *Past. hemolytica* biotype A serotype is the most common isolate obtained from cattle with acute pneumonic pasteurellosis (55). The same serotype can usually be isolated from in-contact and apparently healthy calves. The antimicrobial sensitivity of the pasteurellae isolated can be done, but interpretation of the results is often difficult because it is not known if the isolates from nasal swabs represent those causing the pulmonary lesions. Significant differences may exist between the antimicrobial sensitivities of isolates from nasopharyngeal swabs and those from the lung tissues (55). Thus at the present time it is not possible to recommend routine culturing and antimicrobial sensitivity determination of pasteurellae from nasal cavity or nasopharyngeal mucus from cattle with acute shipping fever pneumonia. There is a need to do some correlated clinical, microbiological and immunological monitoring of healthy cattle and those affected with acute pneumonia in order to determine the relationships between the nasal and pulmonary flora. In healthy calves followed from the farm to the feedlot there was no relationship between the nasal flora and pulmonary lesions (56). There is some evidence that antimicrobial resistance is emerging among field isolates of *Past. hemolytica* and plasmid-mediated antimicrobial resistance is now known to occur (57). The levels of plasma fibrinogen are elevated and parallel the increase in body temperature and is a more reliable indication of the presence of the lesion than clinical assessment (58). Young cattle with clinical signs of acute respiratory disease and a fibrinogen concentration greater than 0·7 g/dl and a temperature greater than 40°C (104°F) are likely to have pneumonia pasteurellosis. Hematological examinations are of little value, as a leukocytosis and neutrophilia occur in some animals but in others there may be a neutropenia or no significant change.

Necropsy findings

Pneumonic pasteurellosis is manifested grossly by marked consolidation involving a third or more of the lungs, and most commonly affecting the anteroventral aspects (1, 2). The stage of pneumonia varies from area to area in the lung, commencing with congestion and edema and passing through various stages of consolidation with accumulation of serofibrinous exudate in the interlobular spaces. A catarrhal bronchitis and bronchiolitis, and a serofibrinous pleurisy are usually present and may be accompanied by a fibrinous pericarditis. The bronchi may contain fibrin, mucus, blood clots, and pus. The cut surface usually consists of several colors due to hemorrhage, necrosis and red and gray consolidation. The pleurisy is characterized by the accumulation of large amounts of effusion. In chronic cases there are residual lesions of bronchopneumonia with overlying pleural adhesions. A review of the pathology is available (2).

The sequential gross and microscopic lesions of experimental bovine pneumonic pasteurellosis have been described and may provide guidelines for aging the lesions in naturally occurring cases (59). On days 2–3 after infection the lesion is characterized by soft gray-purple consolidation, on day 6 the affected areas are firm and nodular; on days 9–10 the nodular lesions are more prominent and fibrous tissue encapsulates the lesions and becomes obvious. The microscopic changes consist of acute inflammation with flooding of the alveoli with edema, fibrin and congestion. Large numbers of neutrophils and macrophages move into the alveoli by day 2. By day 4 the classical lesions consist of edema and hemorrhage, with much of the necrotic tissue being surrounded by a dark zone of inflammatory cells. During the phase of resolution in cases which are not fatal a walling-off reaction by fibrous tissue occurs.

The correlation of gross, microscopic and microbiological findings of the lungs of cattle with pneumonic pasteurellosis suggests that *Past. hemolytica* causes a fibrinous pleuropneumonia with extensive thrombosis of interstitial lymph vessels and limited evidence of bronchitis and bronchiolitis. *Past. multocida*, however, is associated with bronchopneumonia, with little fibrin exudation, some interstitial lymph vessel thrombosis and suppurative bronchitis (60).

Isolation of the organism from the affected lung may be attempted and an impression smear may be of value if a rapid diagnosis is required. In chronic cases, species of bacteria other than pasteurellae are commonly found in residual lesions of the lung. Anaerobic bacteria can be isolated from cases of pneumonia in cattle but their significance is difficult to interpret (63).

The lesions in the respiratory tract of calves exposed to sequential aerosol infections of bovine herpes virus-1 and *Past. hemolytica* results in necrosis and purulent inflammatory changes in the upper and lower respiratory tract which are due to a synergistic viral-bacterial effect (61).

Diagnosis

The differential clinical diagnosis of pneumonic pasteurellosis is summarized in Table 53.

Pneumonic pasteurellosis of cattle is an acute, toxemic bronchopneumonia with a high fever and a good response to treatment in the early stages. In infectious bovine rhinotracheitis there is rhinitis usually with discrete lesions in the nares, tracheitis, loud coughing, high fever and no toxemia unless secondary bacterial pneumonia is present. Recovery usually occurs gradually over 4–7 days. Epidemic acute interstitial pneumonia (fog fever) usually occurs in outbreaks in pastured cattle that have been moved from a dry to lush pasture (or just a different species of pasture or onto a recently harvested cereal grain field); the onset is sudden, many cattle may be found dead, while others are in severe respiratory distress with an expiratory grunt. In viral interstitial pneumonia of calves, young and adult cattle there is dyspnea, a moderate fever, only a mild toxemia, loud breath sounds over the ventral aspects of the lungs followed by crackles and wheezes in a few days and recovery may take several days. Pneumonia due to bovine respiratory syncytial virus may be mild with uneventful recovery or severe with dyspnea and subcutaneous emphysema and high case fatality rate. Lungworm pneumonia occurs most commonly in young pastured cattle and is characterized by dyspnea, coughing, only mild toxemia and a moderate or normal temperature and the course may last several days. Usually many cattle are affected. Crackles and wheezes are usually audible over the dorsal aspects of the lungs and the treatment response is usually favorable if treated early when signs are first noticed. Less common causes of acute pneumonia in calves and young cattle include infection with *Klebsiella pneumoniae*, *Streptococcus* spp., and *Fusobacterium necrophorum*, all of which are characterized by a bronchopneumonia indistinguishable clinically from pneumonic pasteurellosis.

Contagious bovine pleuropneumonia resembles pneumonic pasteurellosis but occurs in plague form, there is severe, painful, toxemic pleuropneumonia, and the case fatality rate is high.

As a general guideline the common pneumonias of cattle may be divided into bronchial, interstitial and metastatic. The bronchial pneumonias include pneumonic pasteurellosis and other less common bacterial pneumonias characterized by toxemia and shallow respirations and a good response to early treatment. The interstitial pneumonias include the viral and parasitic pneumonias, and acute interstitial pneumonias characterized by *marked* respiratory distress and a slow response or no response to treatment. The viral pneumonias may die acutely in a few days or recover over a period of several days. The metastatic pneumonias are associated with vena caval thrombosis and pulmonary aneurysm and are characterized by acute respiratory distress and hemoptysis and no response to treatment (62).

Treatment

The recommendations for the treatment of bovine pneumonic pasteurellosis are based on clinical experience because there is no published information available based on clinical field trials. There is some limited information on the efficacy of certain antimicrobials in the experimentally induced disease.

About 85–90% of affected cattle will recover within 24 hours if treated with almost any of the common antimicrobials such as oxytetracycline (65), trimethoprim–sulfonamides, chloramphenicol, penicillin and sulfonamides. One treatment is usually adequate and most economical for most cases but severely affected cattle or those which relapse require treatment daily, or even two to three times daily dependent upon the drug used, for up to 3–5 days.

The choice of antimicrobial agent will depend on the economics and the previous success rate expected with a particular product in a certain area. The antimicrobials and their dosage schedule in Table 54 are recommended as a guideline. The antimicrobial sensitivity of *Past. hemolytica* will vary dependent on the source of the animals, the geographic region and the previous usage of the drug in the herd or the feedlot. In a recent study in the United Kingdom, the degree of sensitivity of *Past. hemolytica* isolated from outbreaks of pneumonia were as follows: chloramphenicol 100%, trimethoprim–sulfamethoxazole 98%, oxytetracycline 80%, ampicillin 85%, penicillin 82%, streptomycin 3%, and lincomycin 1% (55). The isolates from the lungs had greater sensitivity than those from nasopharyngeal swabs. In some regions there may be evidence that the antimicrobial resistance of pasteurellae isolated from cattle with respiratory disease may be increasing associated with continuous use (64). An epidemiological analysis of antimicrobial use in feedlot calves revealed that treatment with a particular drug in the week prior to death of the animal increased the level of resistance in *Past. hemolytica* to that antimicrobial (70). The joint resistance to penicillin and tetracycline suggested that the resistance was probably plasmid-mediated.

In a large feedlot enterprise where large numbers of animals are being treated daily during the period of filling the feedlot, the success rate of particular antimicrobial agents can be assessed almost daily by the use of records and computer analysis. Historical data such as clinical response from previously treated cattle, the results of necropsy and the antimicrobial sensitivities of isolates from the lungs can be used to predict the antimicrobial resistance patterns and the response rate. The odds ratio technique has been suggested for this purpose (89).

The choice of antimicrobial will also depend on the concentrations of the drug which can be achieved in the lung tissues of affected animals. The concentrations of oxytetracyclines are higher in pneumonic lung than in normal lung (66). Pharmacokinetic studies of oxytetracycline in experimental pneumonic pasteurellosis indicates the need for observance of 12-hour dose intervals (67). Pharmacokinetic studies for chloramphenicol and lincomycin indicate that the presence of pneumonia does not change the dose regimen determined in normal calves (67). Because of the increased rate of elimination of erythromycin from the serum of pneumonic calves it may be advisable to use shorter dosage intervals in calves with respiratory disease (68). Similarly, the kinetics of tylosin but not gentamicin are sufficiently altered in pneumonic calves to require increased frequency of administration (69).

In a feedlot situation where large numbers of cattle may be involved, one important step in the treatment is the positive early identification of affected animals. They should be removed from their pen, examined, treated, identified with a suitable tag for reference purposes and placed in a hospital pen until recovered. This avoids confusion in deciding which animal requires treatment the next day. Each clinically affected animal should be treated individually. The duration of treatment will depend on the severity of the individual case, the response achieved in the first few days, the economic worth of the animal, the extent of complications which may be present such as pleurisy, pulmonary abscesses and bronchiectasis and the results which the veterinarian may expect from prolonged therapy in difficult cases.

There is much interest in mass medication of the drinking water and/or feed supply. The rationale is that the medication of the feed or water would successfully abort an outbreak by treating those that are incubating the disease, provide convalescent therapy to those that have already been treated individually, and for the treatment of mild cases before they become acutely ill and need individual treatment. However, there are problems. The amount of water that cattle drink is directly proportional to feed consumption. If they are inappetent or anorexic, water consumption will decline to only maintenance requirements and therapeutic levels of drug will not be achieved if the concentration in the water is provided at a level for normal consumption. The other major problem is the provision of a uniform concentration of drug in the water supply either through automatic water proportioners in the waterline or placing the drug directly into water tanks. Both can be unreliable. There is a need for the development of reliable methods of mass medication of the feed and water supplies of cattle.

The individual treatment of all in-contact animals in

Table 54. Antimicrobials for treatment of bovine pneumonic pasteurellosis

Antimicrobial	*Dosage and route of administration*
INDIVIDUAL TREATMENT	
Oxytetracycline	10 mg/kg body weight, intravenously or intramuscularly daily for 3 days; can also use longacting at 20 mg/kg body weight, intramuscularly
Trimethoprim–sulfamethoxazole	3–5 ml/45 kg body weight, intravenously or intramuscularly daily for 3 days
Chloramphenicol (where allowed)	20 mg/kg body weight, intravenously or intramuscularly three times daily for up to 3 days
Penicillin	20 000–30 000 IU/kg body weight intramuscularly or subcutaneously daily for 3 days
Sulfamethazine (liquid preparation)	150 mg/kg body weight, intravenously or orally daily for 3 days
Sulfamethazine (sustained-release bolus)	250 mg/kg body weight/72 hours; severely affected cattle need to be treated parenterally initially with a rapidly acting sulfonamide because of rumen stasis due to toxemia
Erythromycin	11 mg/kg body weight intramuscularly twice daily
MASS MEDICATION (FEED AND WATER)	
Sulfamethazine	100 mg/kg body weight in drinking water daily for 5–7 days
Oxytetracycline	3–5 mg/kg body weight in feed for 7 days
MASS MEDICATION (INDIVIDUAL)	
Longacting oxytetracycline	20 mg/kg body weight intramuscularly to all in-contact animals

an affected group may be useful in controlling an outbreak of the disease. If the rate of new cases each day ranges from 5 to 10% of the group, each animal in the remainder of the group may be treated with a long-acting preparation of oxytetracycline at the rate of 20 mg/kg body weight intramuscularly (71,100). This form of group medication will treat cases during the subclinical stages and may prevent new infections. Long-acting oxytetracycline at the same dose rate is also effective for the treatment of clinical cases and reduces the labor and the stress of handling associated with daily treatment which may be required in severe cases (72).

Corticosteroids are used widely as ancillary treatment for severe cases of pneumonic pasteurellosis. The rationale is their anti-inflammatory effect but no data are available to support the field experience of some veterinarians that it is beneficial. Dexamethazone at 1 mg/5 kg body weight is used with no apparent adverse effects. Some preliminary work indicates that the use of the non-steroidal anti-inflammatory drug (NSAID), flunixin meglumine, in combination with oxytetracycline reduced mortality rate in calves with experimentally induced pneumonic pasteurellosis (102). However, no data are available on its efficacy in naturally occurring cases.

The causes of failure to respond to therapy include advanced pneumonia, pulmonary abscess, bronchiectasis, pleurisy, inadequate therapy and antibiotic resistance.

Control

Satisfactory economical control of the disease will depend on the successful integration of management and perhaps the use of biologicals and antimicrobials prophylactically. It is unrealistic to depend on a vaccine, an antibiotic or a single management technique to control the disease. Successful control begins with the adoption of good management techniques when the calves are still on the range, the judicious use of efficacious vaccines and care in handling and transportation of cattle.

Because of the common occurrence of the disease at the time of shipment from range to the feedlot, much attention has been given to reducing the incidence of disease at this time. This led to the development of the concept of preconditioning in North America (73). The objective of preconditioning was to prepare the weaned calf for the feedlot environment by vaccinating it for all of the commonly anticipated diseases before weaning and distributing all stressful procedures such as castration, dehorning, branding, deworming over a period of time rather than concentrating these at weaning time. Weaning at least 2 weeks before shipment was also considered a desirable practice. This was to result in a weaned calf which could be moved into a feedlot in which the feed troughs and water tanks would not be strange but familiar and the calf would adjust quickly. Preconditioning has not been widely accepted because its economic value has not been proven. In one study there was no significant difference in either the incidence of shipping fever or weight gains between preconditioned and control calves (74). Nevertheless, these are procedures which logically appear to positively promote health and they can be recommended in that light, even though their economic value remains to be determined (97).

Management

Beef calves should be weaned well in advance of anticipated inclement weather. This is especially true in North America where the fall months can be cold and windy, and snowstorms can occur. A common successful practice is to begin feeding hay and providing water to calves at least 2 weeks before weaning in the same corral or paddock into which they will subsequently be weaned. Following such a weaning program the calves require only a minimum of adjustment: the only adjustment necessary should be the loss of their dams. Recently weaned calves should be observed at least twice daily for evidence of respiratory disease and treated promptly if necessary. They should not be transported long distances until they appear healthy and are eating liberal quantities of hay and drinking water normally. During transportation liberal quantities of bedding are necessary and cattle should not be without feed and water for more than 24–30 hours. For long trips calves should be rested for 8–12 hours and fed water and hay at intervals of 24 hours. This will minimize the considerable loss of body weight due to shrinkage and the effects of temporary starvation.

The use of creep feed for calves for several weeks prior to weaning has been successful but may not be always economical. A high energy ration containing cereal grains, a protein supplement and the necessary vitamins and minerals is provided for the calves in a creep arrangement to which the dams do not have access. At weaning time the dams are removed from the calves and the stress on the calves is minimal. This program has been very successful for purebred herds where it may be economic, but in commercial herds it is only economic when the market value of the calves warrants it.

In the transfer of cattle from one owner to another the ideal situation would be to avoid public saleyards and move the cattle directly from the ranch to the feedlot. This avoids the stress of handling, overcrowding, temporary starvation, exposure to aerosol infection from other cattle and the unnecessary delays associated with buying and selling cattle. However, large intensified feedlots are unable to buy cattle directly from the herd of origin according to their needs at a particular time and thus inevitably purchase large groups of cattle of different backgrounds. This has necessitated the development of conditioning procedures in which, after arrival, the cattle are individually identified, injected with a mixture of vitamins A, D and E, treated with a residual insecticide, perhaps given an anthelmintic, injected with a longacting antimicrobial and vaccinated for clostridial and respiratory diseases. The issue of whether the cattle should be processed immediately after arrival or after a rest period of 2–3 weeks remains unresolved because there is little data to support one time over the other.

The feeding and nutritional status of newly arrived cattle must assume some importance but there is little scientific data to formulate a sound economic feeding program which will promote rapid recovery from shipping stress. In one study, increasing the concentration of energy in the ration up to a level of 72% improved performance of calves during the first 2 days following arrival in the feedlot (75). There is now considerable use of orally administered electrolyte and protein concentration fluid mixtures designed for use in feeder cattle which have been subjected to long transportation and temporary starvation. These mixtures provide an immediate source of nutrients to aid in the restoration of the ruminal microflora.

Biological
Pasteurella bacterins and respiratory viral vaccines have been used extensively in an attempt to control pneumonic pasteurellosis in cattle but only with limited or no success thus far. A review of the literature on the efficacy of the vaccines available for the control of bovine respiratory disease concluded that there is to date little documented data to support the use of vaccines against respiratory disease under feedlot conditions (79, 81).

Based on the immunological and microbiological observations of both naturally occurring and experimentally induced pneumonic pasteurellosis it appears that artificial immunization of cattle is possible (80). High levels of naturally acquired antibody to *Past. hemolytica* have been associated with protection against the disease (23, 46, 50).

Calves which recover from experimentally induced pneumonic pasteurellosis possess increased resistance to subsequent experimental challenge. Calves which were naturally exposed to *Past. hemolytica* or exposed by vaccination subcutaneously, or intradermally to the live organisms developed some resistance to experimental challenge and developed antibodies to all surface antigens and cytotoxin (19). Resistance to experimental challenge with the organism correlated directly with serum cytotoxin neutralizing titers (83). This supports the hypothesis that protection against experimental challenge with *Past. hemolytica* may require an immune response to cytotoxin (82). This is supported by the observation that cattle which died from fibrinous pneumonia due to *Past. hemolytica* had lower cytotoxin neutralizing activity in their sera than cattle from the same group which died from other causes (46). Vaccination of calves with a leukotoxic culture supernatant from pathogenic *Past. hemolytica* provided some protection against experimental challenge with *Past. hemolytica* A1 (104).

The challenge in the development of an efficacious vaccine against pneumonic pasteurellosis is to determine the protective antigen of the organism.

Experimental vaccination of calves with live *Past. hemolytica* or *Past. multocida* by aerosol or subcutaneous route effectively reduced the severity of subsequent experimental disease (84). Vaccinated calves developed high serum antibody titers to the somatic antigens of the homologous organism. Aerosol vaccination using 6-hour cultures of the organism may have provided better protection than did vaccination with 20–22-hour cultures (85). The use of live *Past. hemolytica* enhances resistance to experimental challenge but killed bacterins do not (86). The use of bacterins in an oil adjuvant may enhance resistance (88).

A commercially available live *Past. hemolytica* vaccine for intradermal use did not have any significant effect on performance, morbidity or mortality in one field trial (90) but in another field trial vaccination reduced morbidity and mortality (91). However, there was no indication that the causes of mortality were determined. The vaccine was also evaluated in combination with a *Hemophilus somnus* bacterin and an infectious bovine rhinotracheitis–parainfluenza-3 vaccine administered 3 weeks prior to weaning and shipment and was not beneficial (95). A streptomycin-dependent *Past. hemolytica* live vaccine appeared to provide better protection than a commercial bacterin (92). The same vaccine used in preconditioned and non-preconditioned calves resulted in a marked economic advantage when given to non-preconditioned calves (93), and there was no economic advantage for preconditioning. A potassium thiocyanate extract of *Past. hemolytica* can induce resistance to subsequent experimental challenge (94).

Based on the observation that prior infection of the respiratory tract with either the infectious bovine rhinotracheitis (IBR) or parainfluenza-3 virus may predispose to pneumonic pasteurellosis, the vaccination of beef calves 2–3 weeks before weaning and feedlot cattle 2 weeks before shipment to a feedlot has been recommended as part of a preconditioning program (97). Vaccination of calves at 3–6 months of age with an intranasal modified–liver infectious bovine rhinotracheitis and parainfluenza-3 vaccine has provided protection against experimental pneumonic pasteurellosis induced by aerosol challenge with the IBR virus followed 4 days later by an aerosol of *Past. hemolytica* (96). It is important to vaccinate the calves at least 2 weeks before they are weaned, stressed or transported to a feedlot. Vaccination on arrival, while commonly done, is not reliable and may be associated with increased mortality (98).

Calves vaccinated with formalin-killed *Past. hemolytica* given by the subcutaneous route are adversely affected when compared with controls upon intrabronchial exposure with relatively small doses of the organism (87). The adverse reactions may be due to serum-opsonizing antibody which may enhance bacterial-induced macrophage cytotoxicity. Thus certain systemic immunization procedures with *Past. hemolytica* can result in more severe pneumonia upon challenge or experimentally, than that seen in non-vaccinated cattle. Immunization by the aerosol route is not associated with adverse reactions to challenge exposure and may induce minor protection.

Chemoprophylaxis
Antibiotics and sulfonamides have been used extensively for many years for the control of pneumonic pasteurellosis particularly in cattle which have just been introduced into a feedlot. On a practical basis it is difficult to synchronize the injection of an antibiotic with the expected onset of pneumonia, which probably accounts for some of the failures.

The administration of sustained-release sulfamethazine orally, or a mixture of benzathine and procaine penicillin, or a longacting oxytetracycline 24 hours prior to experimental pneumonic pasteurellosis in calves may reduce mortality, but there is insufficient evidence based on field trials to make a recommendation (65).

Oxytetracycline at a dose rate of 11 mg/kg body weight intramuscularly daily for 3 days followed by the oral administration of sulfadimethoxine orally at a dose of 150 mg/kg body weight on the third injection day reduced the number of treatment days per calf by about 80% compared to controls (76). The use of longacting oxytetracycline reduced the treatment days per calf by 90% (76). The administration of a longacting preparation of oxytetracycline at a dose rate of 20 mg/kg body weight intramuscularly to feedlot cattle on arrival can reduce the morbidity and mortality from respiratory disease (100).

Medication of the feed and water supplies has given variable results because of the difficulties in obtaining adequate levels of the drugs in those cattle which most need them. In normal weaned beef calves, 6–8 months of age, blood levels of sulfamethazine of 5 mg/dl or greater can be achieved in 15–24 hours by providing medicated water at a dose rate of approximately 150 mg/kg body weight; at 75 mg/kg body weight the same blood levels are achieved by 72–84 hours. A standard recommendation is to provide 150 mg/kg body weight for the first 24 hours and reduce the level to 75 mg/kg body weight for the duration of the medication period which may last from 5 to 10 days. However, there is almost no documented clinical evidence from field trials that medication of the water supplies will prevent or reduce the incidence of naturally occurring pneumonic pasteurellosis. There are no data available on the blood levels of sulfamethazine achieved in cattle which have recently arrived in a feedlot and may be incubating the disease and are receiving sulfanamide-medicated water. The animals must be observed at least twice daily for evidence of new clinical cases.

The inclusion of chlortetracycline in the feed at from 1 to 4 g per head daily during the first 2 weeks after arrival in the feedlot may provide some protection against respiratory disease and improve weight gains (77).

A mail survey of the efficacy of prophylactic medication in the feed and/or water of feedlot calves revealed that medicated feed decreased the mortality rate but had no effect on morbidity rate. The use of medicated water appeared to be associated with increased case fatality and overall mortality rates which may be associated with decreased water intake because of a palatability problem or a false sense of security (99).

Medication of the feed and water supplies can result in a false sense of security and the number of advanced cases of disease can actually increase.

REVIEW LITERATURE

Khadom, N. J., Dedieu, J. F. & Viso, M. (1985) Bovine alveolar macrophage: a review. *Ann. réch. vét.*, *16*, 175–183.

Yates, W. D. G. (1982) A review of infectious bovine rhinotracheitis, shipping fever pneumonia and viral-bacterial synergism in respiratory disease of cattle. *Can. J. comp. Med.*, *46*, 225–263.

REFERENCES

(1) Yates, W. D. G. (1982) *Can. J. comp. Med.*, *46*, 225.
(2) Rehmtulla, A. J. & Thomson, R. G. (1981) *Can. vet. J.*, *22*, 1.
(3) Jensen, R. et al. (1976) *J. am. vet. med. Assoc.*, *169*, 497, 500.
(4) Lillie, L. E. (1974) *Can. vet. J.*, *15*, 233.
(5) Andrews, A. H. et al. (1981) *Vet. Rec.*, *108*, 139.
(6) Wiseman, A. et al. (1976) *Vet. Rec.*, *98*, 192.
(7) Allan, E. M. et al. (1985) *Vet. Rec.*, *117*, 629.
(8) Quirie, M. et al. (1986) *Vet. Rec.*, *119*, 93.
(9) Martin, S. W. et al. (1980) *Can. J. comp. Med.*, *44*, 1.
(10) Martin S. W. et al. (1981) *Can. J. comp. Med.*, *45*, 103.
(11) Martin, S. W. & Meek, A. H. (1986) *Can. J. vet. Res.*, *50*, 15.
(12) Frank, G. H. & Smith, P. C. (1983) *Am. J. vet. Res.*, *44*, 981.
(13) Jones, C. D. R. & Webster, A. J. F. (1984) *Res. vet. Sci.*, *37*, 132.
(14) Wilson, S. H. et al. (1985) *Can. vet. J.*, *26*, 335.
(15) Filion, L. G. et al. (1984) *Can. J. comp. Med.*, *48*, 268.
(16) Phillips, W. A. (1984) *Can. J. comp. Med.*, *48*, 35.
(17) Martin, S. W. & Bohac, J. G. (1986) *Can. J. vet. Res.*, *50*, 351.
(18) Rosendal, S. & Martin, S. W. (1986) *Can. J. vet. Res.*, *50*, 179.
(19) Gentry, M. J. et al. (1985) *Vet. Immunol. Immunopathol.*, *9*, 239.
(20) Confer, A. W. et al. (1983) *Vet. Microbiol.*, *8*, 601.
(21) Shewen, P. E. & Wilkie, B. N. (1982) *Can. J. comp. Med.*, *46*, 354.
(22) Confer, A. W. et al. (1986) *Am. J. vet. Res.*, *47*, 1134.
(23) Confer, A. W. et al. (1984) *Am. J. vet. Res.*, *45*, 2622.
(24) Gilka, F. et al. (1974) *Can. J. comp. Med.*, *38*, 251.
(25) Jericho, K. W. F. et al. (1982) *Can. J. comp. Med.*, *46*, 293.
(26) Khadom, N. J. et al. (1985) *Ann. réch. vét.*, *16*, 175.
(27) Carriere, P. D. et al. (1983) *Can. J. comp. Med.*, *47*, 422.
(28) Yates, W. D. G. et al. (1983) *Can. J. comp. Med.*, *47*, 57.
(29) Yates, W. D. G. et al. (1983) *Am. J. vet. Res.*, *44*, 238.
(30) Yates, W. D. G. et al. (1983) *Can. J. comp. Med.*, *47*, 257.
(31) Jericho, K. W. F. & Carter, G. R. (1985) *Can. J. comp. Med.*, *49*, 138.
(32) Stockdale, P. H. G. et al. (1979) *Can. J. comp. Med.*, *43*, 272.
(33) Lopez, A. et al. (1976) *Can. J. comp. Med.*, *40*, 385.
(34) Panciera, R. J. & Corstvet, R. E. (1984) *Am. J. vet. Res.*, *45*, 2532.
(35) Ames, T. R. et al. (1985) *Can. J. comp. Med.*, *49*, 395.
(36) Gibbs, H. A. et al. (1984) *Res. vet. Sci.*, *37*, 154.
(37) Baluyut, C. S. et al. (1981) *Am. J. vet. Res.*, *42*, 1920.
(38) Shewen, P. E. & Wilkie, B. N. (1985) *Am. J. vet. Res.*, *46*,
(39) Potgier, L. N. D. et al. (1984) *Am. J. vet. Res.*, *45*, 1015.
(40) Martin, W. V. II (1984) *Am. Rev. respir. Dis.*, *130*, 209.
(41) Slocombe, R. F. et al. (1985) *Am. J. vet. Res.*, *46*, 2235.
(42) Walker, R. D. et al. (1985) *Am. J. vet. Res.*, *46*, 2429.
(43) Jericho, K. W. F. et al. (1985) *Am. J. vet. Res.*, *46*, 2457.
(44) Hilwig, R. W. et al. (1985) *Am. J. vet. Res.*, *46*, 2585.
(45) Dyer, R. M. et al. (1985) *Am. J. vet. Res.*, *46*, 336.
(46) Shewen, P. E. & Wilkie, B. N. (1983) *Can. J. comp. Med.*, *47*, 497.
(47) Moore, R. N. et al. (1985) *Am. J. vet. Res.*, *46*, 1949.
(48) Himmel, M. E. et al. (1982) *Am. J. vet. Res.*, *43*, 164.
(49) Mosier, D. A. et al. (1986) *J. clin. Microbiol.*, *24*, 218.
(50) Cho, H. J. et al. (1984) *Can. J. comp. Med.*, *48*, 151.
(51) Gourlay, R. N. & Houghton, S. B. (1985) *Res. vet. Sci.*, *38*, 377.
(52) Lopez, A. et al. (1982) *Can. J. comp. Med.*, *46*, 302.
(53) Potgieter, L. N. D. et al. (1985) *Am. J. vet. Res.*, *46*, 151.
(54) Pierson, R. E. et al. (1976) *J. Am. vet. med. Assoc.*, *169*, 527.
(55) Allan, E. M. et al. (1985) *Vet. Rec.*, *117*, 629.
(56) Yates, W. D. G. et al. (1983) *Can. J. comp. Med.*, *47*, 375.
(57) Chang, Y. F. et al. (1987) *Am. J. vet. Res.*, *48*, 378.
(58) Thomson, R. G. et al. (1969) *Can. J. comp. Med.*, *33*, 194.
(59) Allan, E. M. et al. (1985) *Vet. Rec.*, *117*, 438.
(60) Schiefer, B. et al. (1978) *Vet. Pathol.*, *15*, 313.
(61) Jericho, K. W. F. (1983) *J. comp. Pathol.*, *93*, 73.
(62) Pierson, R. E. & Kainer, R. A. (1980) *Bov. Pract.*, *15*, 87.
(63) Chirino-Trejo, J. M. & Prescott, J. F. (1983) *Can. J. comp. Med.*, *47*, 270.
(64) Fales, W. H. et al. (1982) *J. Am. vet. med. Assoc.*, *181*, 477.
(65) Janzen, E. D. et al. (1984) *Can. vet. J.*, *25*, 78.
(66) Ames, T. R. & Patterson, E. B. (1985) *Am. J. vet. Res.*, *46*, 2471.

(67) Burrows, G. E. et al. (1986) *J. vet. Pharmacol. Therap.*, *9*, 213.
(68) Burrows, G. E. (1985) *Am. J. vet. Res.*, *46*, 798.
(69) Burrows, G. E. et al. (1986) *Can. J. vet. Res.*, *50*, 193.
(70) Martin, S. W. et al. (1983) *Can. J. comp. Med.*, *47*, 6.
(71) Janzen, E. D. & McManus, R. F. (1980) *Bov. Pract.*, *15*, 87.
(72) Breeze, R. G. et al. (1980) *Bov. Pract.*, *15*, 96.
(73) Hoerlein, A. B. (1973) *J. Am. vet. med. Assoc.*, *163*, 825.
(74) Wieringa, F. L. et al. (1976) *Can. vet. J.*, *17*, 280.
(75) Lofgreen, G. P. et al. (1975) *J. anim. Sci.*, *41*, 1256.
(76) Lofgreen, G. P. (1983) *J. anim. Sci.*, *56*, 529.
(77) Perry, T. W. et al. (1986) *J. anim. Sci.*, *62*, 1215.
(78) Kelly, A. P. & Janzen, E. D. (1986) *Can. vet. J.*, *27*, 496.
(79) Martin, S. W. (1983) *Can. vet. J.*, *24*, 10.
(80) Wilkie, B. N. (1984) *Can. vet. J.*, *25*, 48.
(81) Myers, L. L. (1984) *J. Am. vet. med. Assoc.*, *184*, 5.
(82) Wilkie, B. N. (1982) *J. Am. vet. med. Assoc.*, *181*, 1024.
(83) Cho, H. J. & Jericho, K. W. F. (1986) *Can. J. vet. Res.*, *50*, 27.
(84) Panciera, R. J. et al. (1984) *Am. J. vet. Res.*, *45*, 2538.
(85) Confer, A. W. et al. (1984) *Am. J. vet. Res.*, *45*, 2543.
(86) Confer, A. W. et al. (1985) *Am. J. vet. Res.*, *46*, 342.
(87) Wilkie, B. N. et al. (1980) *Am. J. vet. Res.*, *41*, 1773.
(88) Confer, A. W. et al. (1987) *Am. J. vet. Res.*, *48*, 163.
(89) Davidson, J. N. & Babish, J. G. (1982) *Am. J. vet. Res.*, *43*, 922.
(90) Purdy, C. W. et al. (1986) *J. Am. vet. med. Assoc.*, *188*, 978.
(91) Smith, R. A. et al. (1986) *Vet. Med.*, *81*, 978.
(92) Blanchard-Channell, M. T. et al. (1987) *Am. J. vet. Res.*, *48*, 637.
(93) Kadel, W. L. et al. (1985) *Am. J. vet. Res.*, *46*, 1944.
(94) Yates, W. D. G. et al. (1983) *Can. J. comp. Med.*, *47*, 550.
(95) Martin, S. W. et al. (1984) *Can. vet. J.*, *25*, 145.
(96) Jericho, K. W. F. et al. (1982) *Am. J. vet. Res.*, *43*, 1776.
(97) Harris, B. & Church, T. (1987) Alberta certified preconditioned feeder program. *Annual Report (1986)*. Edmonton, Alberta: Alberta Agriculture.
(98) Martin, S. W. et al. (1986) *Can. J. comp. Med.*, *45*, 103.
(99) Martin, S. W. (1985) *Can. J. comp. Med.*, *49*, 15.
(100) Albak, C. et al. (1986) *Bov. Pract.*, *21*, 192.
(101) MacVean, D. et al. (1986) *Am. J. vet. Res.*, *47*, 2676.
(102) Selman, I. et al. (1986) *Proc. 14th World Congr. Dis. Cattle, Dublin, 1986*, 1, pp. 606–610.
(103) Blau, K. A. et al. (1987) *Can. J. vet. Res.*, *51*, 157.
(104) Shewen, P. E. & Wilkie, B. N. (1988) *Can. J. vet. Res.*, *52*, 30.

Pasteurellosis of swine, sheep and goats

Pasteurellosis of swine, sheep and goats is usually pneumonic in form although a septicemic form is not uncommon in lambs.

Etiology

Pasteurellosis in swine is usually a complication of enzootic pneumonia of pigs, *Past. multocida* (types A and D) acting as a secondary invader. *Past. multocida* (type B) is a common pathogen in cattle but has been isolated only rarely in pigs (1). This infection causes hemorrhagic septicemia rather than pneumonia.

Pasteurellosis in sheep occurs principally in two forms: a pneumonic form, caused by *Past. hemolytica* biotype A, and a systemic form caused by biotype T (2, 3). The disease has been reproduced experimentally by the aerosol administration of *Past. hemolytica* biotype A(4) which is also the predominant organism recovered from septicemias of young lambs and pneumonias of older sheep while the T biotype is recovered from the majority of septicemias of adult sheep. Within biotype A there are serotypes 1, 2, 5, 6, 7, 8, 9, 11 and 12 and biotype T comprises serotypes 3, 4, and 10. These serotypes differ in their geographic distribution and may be of significance in the formulation of vaccines.

Epidemiology

The overall picture of the epidemiology of the disease in sheep indicates that it is caused by the spread through the flock of a particular bacterial serotype. In some flocks the development of the disease appears to occur in carrier animals which are already infected. The *Pasteurella* spp. involved are normal inhabitants of the upper respiratory tract of sheep. *Past. hemolytica* can be isolated from 95% of the tonsils and 64% of nasopharyngeal swabs from normal sheep (3). Approximately 65% of the tonsillar isolates are of the T biotype, but only 6% of the strains from the nasopharynx are of the T biotype. Based on serological evidence of concurrent infection with the parainfluenza-3 virus during outbreaks of pasteurellosis in sheep, and the experimental production of the disease with the virus and *Past. hemolytica*, it is possible that the virus may be an important predisposing factor to pneumonic pasteurellosis (3, 5). However, outbreaks of the disease in sheep occur without the intervention of the parainfluenza-3 virus (7). Very young lambs and goats are much more susceptible to *Past. hemolytica* than adults and the organism is presumed to be a primary pathogen in kids (8). *Past. multocida* is an uncommon pathogen in sheep (9).

The relationship of the enzootic pneumonia–pleurisy complex in sheep and lambs with pasteurellosis is not clear (25). The cause is not well understood, but viral, mycoplasmal and chlamydial organisms may be important. In the subclinical form the lung lesions are small and may not affect performance of lambs to slaughter. Secondary infection with *Pasteurella* spp. causes severe clinical pneumonia. Enzootic pneumonia-pleurisy is a cause of major economic loss to the sheep industry because of deaths, reduced growth rate, slaughterhouse wastage and the drug and labor costs associated with treatment.

Deleterious changes in environment, similar to those which are thought to precipitate the disease in cattle, also appear to be important in the species, under discussion. Drafty or poorly ventilated barns, exposure to bad weather, transport and malnutrition are often associated with severe outbreaks of the disease. In range sheep, confinement for shearing, mating or supplementary feeding may precipitate an outbreak, and severe parasitism may also increase susceptibility.

As in pneumonic pasteurellosis of cattle, transmission occurs probably by the inhalation or ingestion of infected material, the infection deriving from carrier animals and clinical cases rather than inanimate objects. Another method of spread of the disease is by lambs sucking ewes with mastitis caused by *Past. hemolytica*. The reverse can also happen.

Pasteurellosis causes heavy losses in pigs and sheep in most parts of the world, through both deaths and depression of body weight gains. Morbidity and mortality rates up to 40% and 5% respectively are usual in both species. In sheep at pasture, the disease tends to spread slowly and the morbidity rate is lower than in feeder lambs and pigs maintained in small areas. Death losses in feeder lambs are usually of the order of 5% (10), but may be as high as 20% (11). A mortality rate of 20% has been recorded in goats kept in confined quarters after collection from a number of centers.

Pathogenesis

The development of pasteurellosis in swine, sheep and goats is in general the same as in pneumonic pasteurellosis of cattle. Necrotic lesions in tonsils and pharynx are infected and are the source of systemic or pulmonary infection by the liberation of infected emboli into the bloodstream or via the respiratory passages (6). An acute fibrinous bronchopneumonia is accompanied by pleurisy. An acute septicemia occurs less commonly. Infection with the parainfluenza-3 virus may affect the lung clearance mechanism and allow the pneumonia to develop. Experimental infection of specific pathogen-free lambs with this virus followed 4 or 7 days later with *Past. hemolytica* biotype A results in pneumonic pasteurellosis which resembles the naturally occurring disease (5). Pulmonary disease can also be produced by the administration of emboli containing biotype T (12).

The pathogenesis of the septicemic form is not clear. The organism proliferates in the upper alimentary tract, thorax and liver and produces a fatal quantity of endotoxin. Caseous lymphadenitis caused by *Past. multocida* has also been observed in lambs.

Clinical findings

Pigs

An acute bronchopneumonia, accompanied by fever and toxemia, causes a clinical syndrome similar to that of pneumonic pasteurellosis. There is a marked tendency for the disease to become chronic resulting in reduced weight gains and frequent relapses. A more acute disease with death occurring within 12 hours and without signs of pneumonia has been observed in baby pigs (13).

Sheep and goats

In these animals, outbreaks often commence with sudden deaths in the absence of premonitory clinical signs. In groups of lambs this occurrence of sudden death without prior illness may continue throughout the outbreak (14), but in older sheep some will show signs of respiratory embarrassment which can be accentuated by driving. As the outbreak progresses, respiratory involvement becomes more evident, signs including dyspnea, slight frothing at the mouth, cough and nasal discharge. Death may occur as soon as 12 hours after the first signs of illness but the course in most cases is about 3 days. In cases produced experimentally, arthritis, pericarditis and meningitis occur in lambs that survive the acute stages of the disease, but these are not often observed in natural cases.

Clinical pathology and necropsy findings

The organism can be found in very large numbers in nasal mucus and in one area a bimodal curve of nasal carriage of *Past. hemolytica* in sheep has been observed with the peaks of the carrier rates in spring and autumn coinciding with the seasonal peaks of enzootic pneumonia in the area (16).

In sheep which have died from peracute pneumonic pasteurellosis there is a greenish gelatinous exudate over the pericardium and large quantities of straw-colored pleural exudate. The lungs are enlarged, edematous and hemorrhagic. Histologically, there is diffuse alveolar necrosis, edema of interlobular septa, sloughing of bronchial mucosa, and in sheep which survive the peracute phase of the disease there are so-called oat cells in zones surrounding the necrotic alveoli (5). In the generalized form the principal lesions are in the upper alimentary tract, thorax and liver. Subcutaneous hemorrhages over the neck and thorax are common. The lungs are edematous, there are subpleural ecchymoses, but no pneumonia. The tonsils and pharyngeal lymph nodes are enlarged and there is ulceration and necrosis of the pharynx and esophagus. Histologically there is acute inflammation and emboli in small arterioles and capillaries.

In pneumonic pasteurellosis the organism is present in large numbers in lung lesions and exudates. In generalized infections in young lambs the organism can be recovered from the liver, spleen, kidney and heart blood. The pulmonary lesions may be relatively minor if only virus is present, but are larger if the usual bacterial infections, *Past. hemolytica* or *Mycoplasma* spp., are present also (18). In septicemic pasteurellosis, *Past. hemolytica* biotype T can be isolated in large numbers from the tonsils, lungs, liver and mucosal lesions of the pharynx and esophagus.

Diagnosis

Enzootic pneumonia of pigs, unless accompanied by pasteurellosis, is not manifested by a marked systemic or pulmonary involvement. Dyspnea is a prominent sign in Glasser's disease, but there is obvious arthritis, and at necropsy the disease is characterized by arthritis, a general serositis and meningitis. Pleuropneumonia caused by *Actinobacillus* (*Hemophilus*) *pleuropneumoniae* causes a severe pneumonia with rapid death, and differentiation from pasteurellosis is necessary at necropsy. The septicemic and acute enteric forms of salmonellosis in swine are often accompanied by pulmonary involvement but these usually are overshadowed by signs of septicemia or enteritis. Chronic pasteurellosis has to be differentiated from lungworm infestations and ascariasis.

The common enzootic pneumonia of sheep is of minor clinical importance but it may be accompanied by a secondary bacterial pneumonia which may be caused by *Past. hemolytica* or *Corynebacterium* (*Actinomyces*) *pyogenes*. Its identity in terms of specific cause is poorly defined but the following pattern is suggested (17). A group of primary non-bacterial pneumonias which are largely subclinical are caused by *Mycoplasma ovipneumoniae*, *Myxovirus parainfluenza*-3 virus, and *Chlamydia* spp. Then there is a group of chronic bacterial pneumonias; the bacteria involved include pasteurellae, corynebacteria, *Escherichia*, *Actinobacillus*, *K lebsiella*, *Fusiformis* and *Neisseria*. Parasitic pneumonia is commonly caused by *Dictyocaulus filaria*. Atypical interstitial pneumonia is also recorded.

Parasitic pneumonia, jaagsiekte and maedi are the common chronic clinical pneumonias of sheep, but these should not be confused with pasteurellosis because of their longer course. When deaths occur in lambs without prior clinical illness the disease may be mistaken for septicemia caused by *Hemophilus agni*, especially because of the necropsy findings, but in pasteurellosis the rate of spread in the flock is much slower and the flock mortality rate much less.

Treatment
The treatments prescribed for pneumonic pasteurellosis of cattle are used with similar results in swine, sheep and goats. Penicillin is also a successful treatment in goats. Not all strains of biotype A are sensitive to penicillin, but almost all strains are sensitive to oxytetracycline which may be the drug of choice especially now that longacting preparations are available (15). Medication of the water supplies with oxytetracycline for 7–10 days may be beneficial.

Control
The general recommendations for the control of the disease in cattle apply equally in sheep. Environmental and managerial factors which may precipitate outbreaks of the disease should be controlled where possible.

There has been considerable activity in the development of vaccines for the control of pasteurellosis in sheep (19). The major problems have included the ineffective immunity from pasteurella vaccines, the lack of crossprotection between serotypes and the tissue reactions associated with adjuvants which have been used to improve immunogenicity.

Two different approaches have been explored. One is the use of pasteurella vaccines containing the serotypes most common in the geographical area. The other is the vaccination of lambs with parainfluenza-3 virus vaccines in an attempt to immunize lambs against challenge exposure with both this virus and *Past. hemolytica* which can result in pneumonic pasteurellosis. Vaccines containing various serotypes of *Past. hemolytica* will stimulate antibody production in pregnant ewes and the lambs receive colostral antibody which does interfere with the production of antibody by the lambs if they are vaccinated at an early age (20). Thus, vaccination of the ewes and the lambs at an early age would provide protection for the lambs during the critical first weeks of life.

The use of adjuvants in vaccines containing *Past. hemolytica* will improve the immunological response. A combination of aluminum hydroxide gel and incomplete Freund's adjuvant is superior to the use of the gel alone and the local reaction at the vaccination site is not severe and usually not detectable 1 month after vaccination in most sheep (21). In general terms the vaccines available are not very effective and are unlikely to be so until an aberrant strain can be used in a live vaccine (19).

The experimental vaccination of specific pathogen-free lambs with an inactivated parainfluenza-3 virus vaccine provides protection against the combined effect of an experimental challenge with parainfluenza-3 virus and *Past. hemolytica* (23). The humoral response alone is incapable of affording protection against experimental pasteurellosis; cell-mediated immunity is considered to play an important part in resistance to this disease (22). Intranasal vaccination with a parainfluenza-3 vaccine may provide better protection than by the intramuscular route (24).

Vaccination of swine has had limited success.

The feeding of broad-spectrum antibiotics, especially tetracyclines, to lambs in feedlots is a common method of preventing pneumonia in recently weaned lambs. However, there is no documented evidence of its efficiency.

REVIEW LITERATURE

Gilmour, N. J. L. (1980) Pasteurellosis in sheep. *Vet. Ann.*, *20*, 234–240.
Gilmour, N. J. L. (1978) Pasteurellosis in sheep. *Vet. Rec.*, *102*, 100–102.

REFERENCES

(1) L'Ecuyer, C. et al. (1961) *Am. J. vet. Res.*, *22*, 1020.
(2) Thompson, D. A. et al. (1977) *Res. vet. Sci.*, *22*, 130.
(3) Davies, D. H. et al. (1981) *Vet. Microbiol.*, *6*, 173.
(4) Gilmour, N. J. L. et al. (1982) *Vet. Rec.*, *110*, 406.
(5) Rushton, B. et al. (1979) *J. comp. Pathol.*, *89*, 321.
(6) Dyson, D. A. et al. (1981) *J. med. Microbiol.*, *14*, 89.
(7) Biberstein, E. L. et al. (1971) *J. comp. Pathol.*, *81*, 339.
(8) Gourlay, R. V. & Barber, L. (1960) *J. comp. Pathol.*, *70*, 211.
(9) Palit, N. & Rao, C. C. P. (1969) *Ind. vet. J.*, *46*, 459.
(10) Biberstein, E. L. & Kennedy, P. C. (1959) *Am. J. vet. Res.*, *20*, 94.
(11) Stamp, J. T. et al. (1955) *J. comp. Pathol.*, *65*, 183.
(12) Gilmour, N. J. et al. (1980) *Vet. Rec.*, *106*, 507.
(13) Edwards, B. L. (1959) *Vet. Rec.*, *71*, 208.
(14) Biberstein, E. L. et al. (1959) *J. Am. vet. med. Assoc.*, *135*, 61.
(15) Gilmour, N. J. L. et al. (1982) *Vet. Rec.*, *111*, 97.
(16) Biberstein, E. L. et al. (1970) *J. comp. Pathol.*, *80*, 499.
(17) St. George, T. D. & Sullivan, N. D. (1973) Pneumonia of sheep in Australia, *Vet. Rec.*, *13*, p. 22. Sydney: University of Sydney Postgraduate Foundation in Veterinary Science.
(18) Pfeffer, A. et al. (1983) *NZ vet. J.*, *31*, 196.
(19) Cameron, C. M. & Bester, F. J. (1983) *Onderstepoort J. vet. Res.*, *50*, 101.
(20) Gilmour, N. J. L. et al. (1980) *Vet. Rec.*, *107*, 505.
(21) Wells, P. W. et al. (1979) *Res. vet. Sci.*, *27*, 248.
(22) Wells, P. W. et al. (1979) *Infect. Immun.*, *26*, 25.
(23) Wells, P. W. et al. (1978) *J. comp. Pathol.*, *88*, 253.
(24) Davies, D. H. et al. (1980) *NZ vet. J.*, *28*, 201.
(25) McGowan, B. et al. (1978) *NZ vet. J.*, *26*, 169.

Tularemia

Tularemia is a highly contagious disease of rodents which may spread to farm animals, causing a severe septicemia and a high mortality rate. A number of strains of varying virulence have been identified (1).

Etiology
Pasteurella (*Francisella*) *tularensis* is the causative organism. It is a Gram-negative organism which does not form spores, and gives partial cross-agglutination with *Brucella* spp.

Epidemiology
The organism persists for long periods in mud and water and may proliferate in these media. It does not appear to survive in carcasses for more than 24 hours unless they are frozen when persistence for 60–120 days has been recorded (2). The natural hosts are rodents but almost all animals and birds are susceptible (3), the disease being recorded among farm animals, most commonly in sheep and pigs and to a lesser extent in calves. Sheep and pigs of all ages are susceptible but most losses occur in lambs, and in swine clinical illness occurs only in piglets. There is a sharp seasonal incidence, the bulk of cases occurring during the spring months.

Pasteurella tularensis has remarkable invasive powers

and infection in man can occur through the unbroken skin but many infections arise from bites of the deer fly (*Chrysops discalis*) (5). In sheep, transmission occurs chiefly by the bites of the wood tick, *Dermacentor andersoni*, and the organism has also been isolated from this tick (4) and from *Haemaphysalis otophila*, the ticks becoming infected in the early part of their life cycle when they feed on rodents. The adult ticks infest sheep, and pastures bearing low shrubs and brush are particularly favorable to infestation. The ticks are found in greatest numbers on the sheep around the base of the ears, the top of the neck, the throat, axillae and udder. It is assumed that sheep are relatively resistant to tularemia but become clinically affected when the infection is massive and continuous. Transmission to pigs and horses is thought to occur chiefly by tick bites.

The causative organism persists in mud and water for at least 16 months (1) and this may be the reason for the high incidence in such rodents as beaver and muskrat.

Tularemia is restricted in its occurrences to countries in the northern hemisphere and occurs in most of them. In North America the disease is most prevalent in farm animals in the northwestern states of the United States and the adjoining areas of Canada. The morbidity rate in affected flocks of sheep is usually about 20% but may be as high as 40% and the mortality rate may reach 50% especially in young animals. Man is highly susceptible and the disease is an occupational hazard to workers in the sheep industry in areas where the disease occurs. Serological surveys in this group have indicated a high incidence of positive reactors (6). Spread of the disease to man may also occur in abattoir workers who handle infected sheep carcasses. Shearers are susceptible because outbreaks often occur at shearing time.

Pathogenesis

Tularemia is an acute septicemia but localization occurs, mainly in the parenchymatous organs, with the production of granulomatous lesions.

Clinical findings

Sheep

The incubation period has not been determined. A heavy tick infestation is usually evident. The onset of the disease is slow with a gradually increasing stiffness of gait, dorsiflexion of the head and a hunching of the hindquarters, and affected animals lag behind the group. The pulse and respiratory rates are increased, the temperature is elevated up to 42°C (107°F) and a cough may develop. There is diarrhea, the feces being dark and fetid, and urination occurs frequently with the passage of small amounts of urine. Body weight is lost rapidly, and progressive weakness and recumbency develop after several days, but there is no evidence of paralysis, the animal continuing to struggle while down. Death occurs usually within a few days but a fatal course may be as long as 2 weeks. Animals that recover commonly shed part or all of the fleece but are solidly immune for long periods.

Swine

The disease is latent in adult pigs but young piglets show fever up to 42°C (107°F), accompanied by depression, profuse sweating and dyspnea. The course of the disease is about 7–10 days.

Horses

In horses, fever (up to 42°C, 107°F) and stiffness and edema of the limbs occur. Foals are more seriously affected and may show dyspnea and incoordination in addition to the above signs (7).

Clinical pathology

An agglutination test is available for the diagnosis of tularemia, a titer of 1:50 being regarded as a positive test in swine. Serum from pigs affected with brucellosis does not agglutinate tularemia antigen, but serum from pigs affected with tularemia agglutinates brucellosis antigen. Cross-agglutination between *Past. tularensis* and *Brucella abortus* is less common in sheep and an accurate diagnosis can be made on serological grounds because of the much greater agglutination which occurs with the homologous organism. Titers of agglutinins in affected sheep range from 1:640 to 1:5000 and may persist at levels of 1:320 for up to 7 months. A titer of 1:200 is classed as positive in sheep. In horses the titers revert to normal levels in 14–21 days (7).

An intradermal sensitivity test using 'tularin' is suggested as being more reliable as a diagnostic aid in pigs than the agglutination test but is unreliable in sheep (4).

Necropsy findings

Great care should be exercised when a necropsy examination is made of a suspected case because of the danger of human infection. In sheep, large numbers of ticks may be present on the hides of fresh carcasses. In animals that have been dead for some time, dark red areas of congestion up to 3 cm in diameter are found on the underneath surface of the skin and may be accompanied by local swelling or necrosis of tissues. These lesions mark the attachment sites of ticks. Enlargement and congestion of the lymph nodes draining the sites of heaviest tick infestation are often noted. Congestion and hepatization of the lung and severe pulmonary edema are inconstant findings.

In swine the characteristic lesions are pleurisy, pneumonia and abscessation of submaxillary and parotid lymph nodes. The organisms can be isolated from lymph nodes and spleen and from infected ticks. Isolation can also be effected by experimental transmission to guinea-pigs which are highly susceptible.

Diagnosis

The occurrence of a highly fatal septicemia in sheep during spring months when the sheep are heavily infested with *Dermacentor andersoni* should suggest the possibility of tularemia, especially if the outbreak occurs in an enzootic area. Tick paralysis, which commonly occurs in the same area, and at the same time of the year as tularemia, is not accompanied by fever and there is marked flaccid paralysis. Recovery from tick paralysis occurs commonly if the ticks are removed. Other septicemias of sheep in the age group in which tularemia occurs are unusual. *Past. hemolytica*, *E. coli* and *H. agni* may cause fatal septicemia without diagnostic lesions in very young lambs, but these diseases are not associated with heavy tick infestations. Tickborne fever has a limited and different geographical distribution and rickettsiae can be detected in the lymphocytes.

Treatment

Streptomycin, the tetracyclines and chloramphenicol are effective treatments in man. Oxytetracycline (6–10 mg/kg body weight) has been highly effective in the treatment of lambs and much more effective than penicillin and streptomycin (4).

Control

An outbreak of tularemia in sheep can be rapidly halted by spraying or dipping with an insecticide to kill the vector ticks. In areas where ticks are enzootic, sheep should be kept away from shrubby, infested pasture or sprayed regularly during the months when the tick population is greatest. An experimental live attenuated vaccine has been tested, but results are inconclusive because of the difficulty of monitoring an effective challenge (1).

REVIEW LITERATURE

Hopla, C. E. (1974) The ecology of tularaemia. *Adv. vet. Sci.*, *18*, 25.

REFERENCES

(1) Bell, J. F. et al. (1978) *Can. J. comp. Med.*, *42*, 310.
(2) Airapetyan, V. G. et al. (1957) *J. Microbiol. Epidemiol. Immunobiol.*, *28*, 21.
(3) McKeever, S. et al. (1958) *J. infect. Dis.*, *103*, 120.
(4) Gordon, J. R. (1983) *Can. J. comp. Med.*, *47*, 408.
(5) Klock, L. E. et al. (1973) *J. Am. vet. med. Assoc.*, *226*, 149.
(6) Jellison, W. L. & Kohls, G. M. (1955) *Publ. Hlth Monogr.*, *28*, 17.
(7) Klaus, K. D. et al. (1959) *J. Bacteriol.*, *78*, 294.

Yersiniosis

These are the rare diseases caused by *Yersinia* spp. bacteria which were at one time included in the genus *Pasteurella*. The bacteria are ubiquitous in the environment, but do not tend to concentrate on particular farms or in particular areas of ground. They cause sporadic disease incidents in special circumstances such as cold wet weather.

Caused by Yersinia enterocolitica

This causes acute enteritis manifested by diarrhea, and a high mortality rate, especially in sheep, goats and pigs. Death is due to dehydration and toxemia, and there is sometimes a septicemia. In the outbreaks in sheep the severe, sometimes fatal diarrhea is accompanied by suppurative lesions in the intestinal wall (4, 7).

Caused by Yersinia M. pseudotuberculosis

This is a common inhabitant of the intestines of domestic animals and a common cause of epizootic disease in birds and rodents. Under conditions of stress, notably cold, wet weather, systemic invasion occurs, causing multiple abscesses in the liver and spleen. There may also be enteric lesions and diarrhea, but most cases are simply found dead without obvious prior illness. *Yersinia pseudotuberculosis* may also cause sporadic abortion in cattle and sheep (6, 8), occasional cases of caprine mastitis (1, 2), epididymitis and orchitis in rams, and it may also be found in sporadic cases of abscessation and lymphangitis in ruminants. It is a common isolate in and apparent cause of disease in zoo animals (9) and in farmed and feral deer (3). Clinically the disease in deer is manifested by diarrhea for several days then death. Stress such as yarding or capture commonly precedes the attack.

The diagnosis of yersiniosis in diarrheic cows, based on isolation of the organism in the feces, has become fashionable but is subject to the error that similar isolations can be made from the feces of healthy cows (5).

There are three serotypes of *Y. pseudotuberculosis* found in diseased animals, I, II and III, in that order of frequency.

REFERENCES

(1) Cappucci, D. T. et al. (1978) *J. Am. vet. med. Assoc.*, *173*, 1589.
(2) Jones, T. O. et al. (1982) *Vet. Rec.*, *112*, 231.
(3) Henderson, T. G. (1983) *NZ vet. J.*, *31*, 221.
(4) McSporran, K. D. et al. (1984) *NZ vet. J.*, *32*, 38.
(5) Hodges, R. T. & Carman, M. G. (1985) *NZ vet. J.*, *33*, 175.
(6) White, S. T. et al. (1985) *J. Am. vet. med. Assoc.*, *187*, 834.
(7) Yu, E. S. et al. (1983) *Clin. J. vet. Med.*, *9*, 5.
(8) Karbe, E. & Erickson, E. D. (1984) *Vet. Pathol.*, *21*, 601.
(9) Obwolo, M. J. (1976) *Vet. Bull.*, *46*, 147.

DISEASES CAUSED BY *BRUCELLA* spp.

The important diseases of animals caused by *Brucella* spp. are those caused by *Br. abortus, Br. suis* and *Br. melitensis*, their host preference in order being cattle, swine and sheep and goats. Although *Brucella* have a wide host range, they are not readily transmitted from preferential to dissimilar hosts and, when this occurs, they usually localize in the mammary gland and reticuloendothelial system rather than in the uterus and fetal membranes (1). *Bordetella bronchiseptica* is also not uncommonly present in the lungs of calves and pigs with chronic pneumonia. This organism is also suspected of being a primary cause of pneumonia in baby pigs (2, 3). In affected herds the incidence may be as high as 100% and signs and necropsy lesions characteristic of pneumonia are observed. The pulmonary lesions are scattered areas of bronchopneumonia different in their appearance and distribution from those of enzootic pneumonia. Treatment with tetracyclines, chloramphenicol or sulfonamides is recommended. The disease is likely to persist on the premises, recurring in successive crops of baby pigs. In these circumstances the use of an autogenous bacterin in the pregnant sows is recommended.

REFERENCES

(1) Meyer, M. E. (1964) *Am. J. vet. Res.*, *25*, 553.
(2) L'Ecuyer, C. et al. (1961) *Vet. Med.*, *56*, 420.
(3) Dunne, H. W. et al. (1961) *J. Am. vet. med. Assoc.*, *139*, 897.

Brucellosis caused by *Brucella abortus* (Bang's disease)

The disease of cattle caused by infection with *Br. abortus* is characterized by abortion late in pregnancy and a subsequent high rate of infertility.

Etiology

Brucella abortus is the causative organism and is identifiable as several biotypes (1). Approximately 85% of infections are from biotype 1. In the United States biotypes 1–4 are found.

Epidemiology

Brucellosis is widespread and of major economic importance in most countries of the world, particularly amongst dairy cattle. The incidence varies considerably between herds, between areas and between countries, and details of the percentage of animals affected are of little value for this reason.

From the viewpoint of human health, the disease is important because the causative organism can cause undulant fever in man. The possibility of infection occurring by the drinking of infected milk necessitates the pasteurization of milk. Officially approved methods of commercial pasteurization render naturally *Brucella*-contaminated raw milk safe for consumption (73). However, most cases in humans are occupational and occur in farmers, veterinarians and butchers. The organism can be isolated from many organs other than the udder and uterus, and the handling of a carcass of an infected animal may represent severe exposure. The importance of the disease in humans is an important justification for its eradication. Between the years 1965–74 the incidence of brucellosis in man in the United States increased (1). Most cases occur in people employed in the meat processing industry while other sources include the domestic pig, cattle and unpasteurized dairy products.

Losses in animal production due to this disease can be of major importance, primarily because of the decreased milk production by aborting cows. The common sequel of infertility increases the period between lactations, and in an infected herd the average intercalving period may be prolonged by several months. In addition to the loss of milk production, there is the loss of calves and interference with the breeding program. This is of greatest importance in beef herds where the calves represent the sole source of income. A high incidence of temporary and permanent infertility results in heavy culling of valuable cows and some deaths occur as a result of acute metritis following retention of the placenta.

Infection occurs in cattle of all ages but persists most commonly in sexually mature animals. Congenital infection may occur in calves born from infected dams. The infection occurs *in utero* and may remain latent in the calf throughout its early life and the animal may remain serologically negative until its first parturition at which time it may begin to shed the organism (2). Calves born from reactor dams are usually serologically positive for up to 4–6 months due to colostral antibodies and later usually become serologically negative even though a latent infection may exist in a small proportion of these calves (3). These latent infections in serologically negative animals are of major concern because they remain unnoticed and can potentially serve as a source of infection some time later. In one report a heifer from a herd affected with widespread infection with *Br. abortus* biotype 2 was moved to a brucellosis-free herd, and remained apparently free from brucellosis until 9 years later when the same animal produced a strongly positive serological reaction and the same biotype was isolated from its milk (3). Such observations have resulted in the recommendation that calves from seropositive dams should not be used for breeding (10). Even vaccinated heifers from seropositive dams can harbor a latent infection (2). There is a risk of 2·52% of heifer calves, born from serologically positive dams, reacting in early adulthood and constituting a threat to a reestablished herd (49). The half-life of colostral antibodies to *Br. abortus* in calves which have received colostrum from either vaccinated non-infected or infected dams is about 22 days (58).

The organism can be recovered from naturally infected pigs and, although not normally pathogenic in this species, may occasionally cause abortion. The disease occurs naturally in sheep exposed to infected cattle and can be produced experimentally in sheep (4). The natural occurrence of the disease in sheep in association with infected cattle has significant implications for brucellosis eradication (5). In horses the organism is often found in chronic bursal enlargements but is probably present as a secondary invader rather than a primary pathogen. It is commonly present with *Actinomyces bovis* in fistulous withers and poll evil. It has also been identified as a cause of abortion in mares (6).

The infection is recorded in bison (56), elk (7), deer (8), coyotes (52), wild opossums and raccoons (53), moose (54), camels (55), and other wild and domesticated ruminants (9, 10) but there is no direct evidence that these species are a source of infection for cattle. Experimental inoculation of the organism into badgers resulted in the development of antibodies and elimination of the organism; this indicated that the badger is relatively resistant to infection and unlikely to be a reservoir of the organism (70).

Bison and elk are potential reservoirs of brucellosis and because they are the species of choice for game farming, which is a recent development in North America and elsewhere, they could serve as a source of infection for cattle (100).

A serological survey of horses over a period of 8 years revealed that 8–16% of serum samples were positive (71). However, experimentally infected horses do not excrete the organism in sufficient numbers to infect susceptible cattle with which they were in close contact.

While farm dogs are not generally considered to be a major reservoir of *Br. abortus*, the organism has been isolated from dogs on a farm where several cattle were serologically positive for brucellosis and should be included in any investigation and eradication of the disease (11).

Brucella abortus achieves its greatest concentration in the contents of the pregnant uterus, the fetus and the fetal membranes, and these must be considered as major sources of infection. The numbers of organisms in the tissues of two naturally infected cows and their fetuses were as follows: umbilicus $2{\cdot}4 \times 10^8 - 4{\cdot}3 \times 10^9$/g$-1{\cdot}4 \times 10^{13}$/g (57). This emphasizes the large numbers of organisms which are shed and to which other animals and man are potentially exposed.

The methods by which the disease is transmitted are ingestion, penetration of the intact skin and conjunctiva and contamination of the udder during milking. Grazing on infected pasture or consuming other feedstuffs and water supplies contaminated by discharges and fetal membranes from infected cows and contact with aborted fetuses and infected newborn calves is considered to be the most common method of spread. Intra-herd spread occurs by both vertical and horizontal transmission. Congenital infection due to *in utero* infection does occur but its importance has not yet been defined. Horizontal transmission is usually by direct contamination and, although the possibility of introduction of infection by flies, dogs, rats, ticks, infected boots, fodder and other inanimate objects exists, it is not considered to be of great importance in relation to control measures. The organism can survive on grass for variable periods depending on environmental conditions. In temperate climates, infectivity may persist for 100 days in winter and 30 days in summer. The organism is susceptible to heat, sunlight and standard disinfectants but freezing permits almost indefinite survival. The activity of several disinfectants against *Br. abortus* has been examined, and representatives of the phenolic, halogen, quaternary ammonium and aldehyde groups of disinfectants at 0·5 or 1·0% concentrations in the absence of serum generally inhibited a high concentration of the organism (72).

A cow's tail heavily contaminated with infected uterine discharges may spread infection if it comes into contact with the conjunctiva or the intact skin of other animals. In the same way as the more common forms of mastitis can be spread during milking, *Br. abortus* infection can be spread from a cow whose milk contains the organism to an uninfected cow. This may have little significance in terms of causing abortion, but it is of particular importance in its effects on agglutination tests on milk and the presence of the organism in milk used for human consumption.

Bulls do not usually transmit infection from infected to non-infected cows mechanically. Bulls that are themselves infected and discharge semen containing organisms are most unlikely to transmit the disease but the chance of spread from the bull is very great if the semen is used for artificial insemination (12). Some infected bulls give negative blood agglutination tests and can only be detected by the isolation of organisms from the semen or agglutination tests on seminal plasma. Excretion of *Br. abortus* in the semen of a stallion has also been observed (13).

Few infected cows ever recover completely and therefore it is safest to consider them all as permanent carriers of infection whether or not abortion actually occurs. Excretion of the organism in the milk is usually intermittent but appears to be more common during late lactation and can continue for several years. In cattle vaccinated before infection the degree of excretion of *Br. abortus* in the milk is less than in non-vaccinated animals. Embryo transfer from infected donors may be achieved without transfer of infection and superovulation unlikely to reactivate the release of brucellae into the uterus during the project when embryos are normally collected (74).

Naturally infected animals and those vaccinated as adults with strain 19 remain positive to the serum, and other agglutination tests for long periods. Most animals vaccinated between 4 and 8 months of age return to a negative status to the test within a year. All are considered to have a relative immunity to infection. Calves from cows which are positive reactors to the test are passively immunized via the colostrum. It is possible that some calves remain immune for sufficiently long to interfere with vaccination.

The spread of the disease from one herd to another and from one area to another is almost always due to the movement of an infected animal from an infected herd into a non-infected susceptible herd. The unregulated movement of cattle from infected herds or areas to brucellosis-free herds or areas is the major cause of breakdowns in brucellosis eradication programs. A case control study of brucellosis in Canada indicated that herds located close to other infected herds and those herds whose owners made frequent purchases of cattle had an increased risk of acquiring brucellosis (14). Once infected, the time required to become free of brucellosis was increased by large herd size, by active abortion and by loose housing. The factors of importance in the epidemiology of brucellosis have been summarized (14).

The herd characteristics and the results of the first herd test may be used as predictors of the potential presence or absence of *Br. abortus* in herds with reactors to the tube agglutination test. The presence of only single suspicious reactors on the first test is a good predictor of lack of infection. The presence of one or more positive reactors on the first herd test is a good predictor of the presence of infection (59).

The epidemiological variables which are considered to affect the initiation, spread, maintenance and/or control of bovine brucellosis can be categorized into those related to the animal population, to management, or to the biology of disease (12). The variables which contribute significantly to seropositive animals are size of farm premises, percentage of animals on a premises that are inseminated artificially, size of investment in livestock, whether or not dairying is the major agricultural activity of the premises, and the policy of the owner with regard to disposal of reactor animals (16). In a defined geographic area in northern Mexico where a brucellosis control program did not exist the greatest percentage of seropositive animals were related to larger farms, poor artificial insemination technique, and small financial investment in the farm (16).

Pathogenesis

Brucella abortus has a predilection for the pregnant uterus, udder, testicle and accessory male sex glands, lymph nodes, joint capsules and bursae. After the initial invasion of the body, localization occurs initially in the lymph nodes draining the area and spreads to other lymphoid tissues including the spleen and the mammary and iliac lymph nodes. Congenital infection can occur in newborn calves as a result of *in utero* infection and the infection may persist in a small proportion of calves which may also be serologically negative until after their first parturition or abortion (2, 3). Virgin and other non-pregnant cattle can become infected but lose their humoral antibody to the organism much more quickly than cattle infected while pregnant. In the adult, non-pregnant cow, localization occurs in the udder, and the uterus, if it becomes gravid, is infected from periodic bacteremic phases originating in the udder. Infected udders are clinically normal but they are important as a source of reinfection of the uterus, as a source of infection for calves or humans drinking the milk, and because they are the basis for the agglutination tests on milk and whey. Erythritol, a substance produced by the fetus and capable of stimulating the growth of *Br. abortus*, occurs naturally in greatest concentration in the placental and fetal fluids and is probably responsible for localization of the infection in these tissues. When invasion of the gravid uterus occurs the initial lesion is in the wall of the uterus but spread to the lumen of the uterus soon follows, leading to a severe ulcerative endometritis of the intercotyledonary spaces. The allantochorion, fetal fluids and placental cotyledons are next invaded and the villi destroyed.

In fetuses naturally and experimentally infected with *Br. abortus* the tissue changes include lymphoid hyperplasia in multiple lymph nodes, lymphoid depletion in the thymic cortex, adrenal cortical hyperplasia, and disseminated inflammatory foci composed mainly of large mononuclear leukocytes (75). The fetal pneumonia is probably due to localization of perivascular foci in the interlobular septae of the lung indicative of hematogenous spread in the fetus rather than to aspiration of contaminated fetal fluids. Fetuses inoculated with sufficient numbers of *Br. abortus* will abort from 7 to 19 days postinoculation (75). Goats are susceptible to a bovine pathogenic strain of *Br. abortus* and are considered to be a suitable model for the study of bovine brucellosis (103).

Abortion occurs principally in the last 3 months of pregnancy, the incubation period being inversely proportional to the stage of development of the fetus at the time of infection.

Brucellus abortus is an intracellular organism which is probably an important factor in its survival in the host and may explain both the transitory titers occurring in some animals following isolated episodes of bacteremia and the disappearance of titers in animals with latent infection.

Clinical findings

The clinical findings are dependent upon the immune status of the herd. In highly susceptible non-vaccinated pregnant cattle, abortion after the 5th month of pregnancy is the cardinal feature of the disease in cows. In subsequent pregnancies the fetus is usually carried to full term although second or even third abortions may occur in the same cow. Retention of the placenta and metritis are common sequels to abortion. Mixed infections are usually the cause of the metritis which may be acute, with septicemia and death following, or chronic, leading to sterility.

In the bull, orchitis and epididymitis occur occasionally. One or both scrotal sacs may be affected with acute, painful swelling to twice normal size, although the testes may not be grossly enlarged. The swelling persists for a considerable time and the testis undergoes liquefaction necrosis and is eventually destroyed. The seminal vesicles may be affected and their enlargement can be detected on rectal palpation. Affected bulls are usually sterile when the orchitis is acute but may regain normal fertility if one testicle is undamaged. Such bulls are potential spreaders of the disease if they are used for artificial insemination.

Br. abortus can often be isolated from lesions of non-suppurative synovitis in cattle. Hygromatous swellings, especially of the knees, should be viewed with suspicion. There are reports of progressive and erosive non-suppurative arthritis of the stifle joints occurring in young cattle, from brucellosis-free herds, which had been vaccinated with strain 19 vaccine (50). The calves may or may not be serologically positive, but synovial fluid and joint tissue samples contain immunological evidence of strain 19 *Br. abortus* antigenic material.

The history of the disease in a susceptible herd can usually be traced to the introduction of an infected cow. Less common sources are infected bulls or horses with fistulous withers. In the past in such a susceptible herd it was common for the infection to spread rapidly and for an abortion 'storm' to occur. The 'storm' might last for a year or more, at the end of which time most of the susceptible cows were infected and had aborted and proceeded to carry their calves to full term. Retained placentae and metritis could be expected to be common at this time. As the abortion rate subsided, the abortions were largely restricted to first-calf heifers and new additions because other animals of the herd reached a stage of partial resistance.

In recent years, particularly in areas where vaccination is extensively practiced, there has been a tendency for the development of a more insidious form of the disease which spreads much more slowly and in which abortion is much less common.

In horses, the common association of *Br. abortus* is with chronic bursal enlargements of the neck and withers, or with the navicular bursa causing intermittent lameness and the organism has been isolated from mares which have aborted (6). When horses are run with infected cattle, a relatively high proportion can become infected and develop a positive reaction to the serum agglutination test without showing clinical illness (15). Some horses appear to suffer a generalized infection with clinical signs including general stiffness, fluctuating temperature and lethargy (71).

Clinical pathology

The major objective in the laboratory diagnosis of brucellosis is to identify animals which are infected and potentially shedding the organism and spreading the disease. Most infected animals are identifiable using the standard serological tests but latent infection occurs in some animals which are serologically negative. Furthermore, vaccinated animals may be serologically positive and uninfected, and transitory titers occur sporadically in a small percentage of animals for which there is no clear explanation. These diagnostic problems make control and eradication programs difficult to administer and difficult to explain to animal owners.

Laboratory tests used in the diagnosis of brucellosis include isolation of the organism, and tests for the presence of antibodies of *Br. abortus* in blood, milk, whey, vaginal mucus and seminal plasma. The organism may be present in the cervical mucus, uterine flushings, and udder secretions of experimentally infected cows for up to 36 days after abortion (76). An ELISA test is available for the detection of the organism in vaginal secretions (77).

Isolation of the organism by culture or guinea-pig inoculation is attempted from the organs and lymph nodes of the fetus, the placenta, milk, vaginal mucus or uterine exudate.

Serological tests

In the absence of a positive culture of *Br. abortus* a presumptive diagnosis is usually made based on the presence of antibodies in serum, milk, whey, vaginal mucus, or seminal plasma.

The antibody response following infection depends on whether or not the animal is pregnant and on the stage of gestation. On the average, the agglutinins and complement fixation antibodies become positive 4 weeks following experimental infection during the 4th to 6th month of gestation and not until about 10 weeks if experimental infection occurs 2 months before or after insemination. The serological diagnosis is considered to be unreliable when applied during the period of 2–3 weeks before and after abortion or calving.

Any of the currently available serological tests or combination of tests measures the response of a single animal at one point in time and does not describe the status of the herd. When the tests are used in recommended sequence, and in combination, along with a consideration of accurate epidemiological data the limitations of each test can be minimized. None of the tests is absolutely accurate and there are varying degrees of sensitivity. The result has been the development of a very extensive range of tests, each of which has its own special applicability. It is not possible to provide all the details here and they have been extensively reviewed (17). The salient features are as follows.

The serum tube agglutination test is one of the traditional standard tests which is widely used, but its limitations include the following:

- The test detects non-specific antibodies as well as specific antibodies from *Br. abortus* infection and vaccination
- During the incubation stage of the disease the test is often the last to reach diagnostically significant levels
- After abortion due to *Br. abortus* it is often the last test to reach diagnostically significant levels
- In the chronic stage of the disease, the serum agglutinins tend to wane, often becoming negative when the results of some other tests may be positive.

The rose bengal test (buffered antigen or card test) is a simple, rapid test which detects early infection and can be used as an initial screening test. 'Overkill' using the test is estimated to vary from 1 to 3%, depending on the level of infection and vaccination history in the herd. False-positive reactions are due to residual antibody activity from vaccination, colostral antibody in calves, cross-reaction with certain bacteria and laboratory error. False-negative reactions are observed during early incubation of disease and immediately after abortion. However, the rose bengal test is an excellent test for the large-scale screening of sera.

For beef cattle, screening of herds can be achieved by the collection of blood at abattoirs and submitting it to the rose bengal test or the tube agglutination test. Reactors are traced back to the herd of origin and the herd is tested. In badly infected herds it is probably best to remove all cows positive to the rose bengal test even though the test is highly sensitive and a small percentage of false-positive cows will result. In herds where the prevalence of infection is low and where vaccination has been carried out, this procedure would eliminate too many false-positive cows. In this situation the sera positive to the rose bengal test are submitted to a more definite confirmatory test such as the complement fixation test and only those animals reacting to the test are discarded.

The complement fixation test (CFT) rarely exhibits non-specific reactions and is useful in differentiating the titers of calfhood vaccination from those due to infection. The CFT titers do not wane as the disease becomes chronic and often the CFT reaches diagnostic levels sooner than the serum tube agglutination test following natural infection. In addition, recent technical laboratory advances have allowed much greater speed and accuracy in doing the CFT and it is now considered to be the nearest approach to a definitive test for infection.

The sensitivity and specificity of several serological tests for the diagnosis of brucellosis in Canada have been compared (78, 79). It is recommended that either the buffered plate antigen test or indirect enzyme immunoassay test be used as a screening test. Either the complement fixation test or the indirect enzyme immunoassay is appropriate for use as a confirmatory test in situations requiring a high specificity (78). In brucellosis-free herds, the specificity of tests was 98·9% for buffered plate antigen test (BPAT), 99·2% and 99·3% for the standard tube and plate agglutination tests (STAT and SPAT), respectively, and 99·8% for the 2-mercapto-ethanol test (2 MET). The rose bengal plate test (RBPT), the card test (CARD) and the complement fixation test (CFT) correctly classified all sera as negative (79). On a sample of culture-positive cattle, the sensitivities of the tests were complement fixation 79·0%, buffered plate antigen test 75·4%, rose bengal plate test 74·9%, card test 74·3%, standard plate agglutination test 73·1%, standard tube agglutination test 68·9% and 2-mercapto-ethanol 59·9% (79). All tests combined detected only 82% of infected cattle (79). Analysis of the relative sensitivity of the six agglutination tests gave the following ranking from highest to lowest: BPAT, RBPT, CARD, SPAT, STAT. The 2 MET ranked between BPAT and RBPT or between the RBPT and CARD depending on the analysis used. The BPAT is recommended as a screening test followed by the CFT (79).

The application of the rose bengal test as a screening test followed by a confirmatory complement fixation test along with the indirect hemolysis test can markedly increase the proportion of infected cattle which are positive (80). This combination can be useful during the latter stages of an eradication program.

The enzyme-linked immunosorbent assay (ELISA) test may be useful during an eradication program, after vaccination has ceased, for screening or as a supplementary test to the complement fixation test (81). Preliminary evaluations of the ELISA test alone, or in combination with the complement fixation test and monoclonal antibodies, indicate some comparative advantages over other serological tests (82–86). A 'dipstick' enzyme immunoassay is also available and being evaluated (87).

The anamnestic response has been used to identify the serologically negative but infected animals (24, 26). The use of one injection of K45/20A vaccine results in high titers of complement fixation antibodies, and the test has been highly effective for the detection of latent carriers.

The *milk ring* test is a satisfactory inexpensive test for the surveillance of dairy herds for brucellosis (25). A small sample of pooled fresh milk or cream, from no more than 25 cows, is tested and the herd is classified only as suspicious or negative. Final determination of the status of a suspicious herd and each animal in it is accomplished by blood testing. The more frequently a herd is tested with the milk ring test, the more effective the test becomes as a method to detect early infections and thereby prevent serious outbreaks in susceptible herds. At least three tests done annually are now required by some regulatory agencies. The major limitation of the test is the dilution factor which occurs in large dairy herds where large quantities of milk are stored in bulk tanks. The Bruc ELISA test is a sensitive, specific and inexpensive method for screening large numbers of individual or bulk milk samples for antibody to *Br. abortus* (23).

A major problem in brucellosis eradication programs has been the false-positive animals or *singleton* reactor which may remain persistently suspicious or positive in a herd which is otherwise considered to be free of brucellosis. It is of some concern because of the unnecessary slaughter of uninfected animals. Serological cross-reactions have been demonstrated between smooth *Brucella* sp. and *E. coli* 0:116 and 0:157, *Francisella tularensis*, *Salmonella* serotypes of Kauffman-White group N, *Pseudomonas matophilia*, *Vibrio cholerae* and *Yersinia enterocolitica* serotype 0:9 (18).

Other causes include a *Br. abortus* infected animal, strain 19 residual vaccination titer and naturally occurring non-specific agglutinins which may occur in some cattle populations. These agglutinins are EDTA-labile and can be differentiated from agglutinating antibodies by the addition of EDTA to the diluent used in the standard serum agglutination test (18). The serological cross-reactions are of major significance when the prevalence of infection has decreased to a very low level. At this stage it becomes much more important to correctly identify the status of animals reacting to the serological tests for brucellosis.

The incorrect attributes of such reactions to factors other than brucella infection is likely to result in herd breakdowns and failure to control the disease. On the other hand, the misinterpretation of cross-reactions as evidence of brucellosis results in the imposition of unnecessary restrictions and waste of resources (18). The problem of serological cross-reactions has resulted in considerable research and investigation to find laboratory tests which will accurately distinguish positive infected animals from positive non-infected difficult to achieve, especially in the case of *Yersinia enterocolitica* 0:9 antigen, but immunodiffusion, immunoelectrophoresis and primary binding tests and cross-absorption procedures are useful (18).

Levamisole given 7 days after vaccination with strain 19 vaccine enhanced the antibody response to the vaccine (19).

The culture of the tissues of problem animals and the determination of the specific biotypes of *Br. abortus* may also assist in determining the source of the organism and differentiating it between the field strains as a vaccine particularly in adult vaccinated cattle.

Necropsy findings

Necropsy findings in adults are of no importance in diagnosis. In some fetuses, a primary pneumonia is found. Not all fetuses which abort because of brucellosis have pneumonia, and the lung lesions which are present in some fetuses are non-specific with regard to etiology (20). The placenta is usually edematous, there may be leathery plaques on the external surface of the chorion and there is necrosis of the cotyledons.

Diagnosis

The diagnosis of the cause of abortion in a single animal or in a group of cattle is difficult because of the multiplicity of causes which may be involved. When an abortion problem is under investigation a systemic approach should be used (35). This includes a complete laboratory evaluation and follow-up enquiries into each herd. The radiographic examination of fetuses may often reveal skeletal growth arrest. The following procedure is recommended: ascertain the age of the fetus by inspection and from the breeding records; take blood samples for serological tests for brucellosis, listeriosis and leptospirosis; examine uterine fluids and the contents of the fetal abomasum at the earliest opportunity for trichomonads, and subsequently by cultural methods for *Br. abortus*, *Campylobacter fetus*, trichomonads, listeria and fungi; supplement these tests by examination of urine for leptospirae, and of the placenta or uterine fluid for bacteria and fungi, especially if the fetus is not available; examine placenta fixed in formalin for evidence of placentitis. It is most important that all examinations be carried out in all cases because coincident infections with more than one agent are not uncommon. Major problems exist in the diagnosis of brucellosis in bulls (27). Infected bulls may be serologically positive or negative, their semen may be culturally positive or negative but the organism may be isolated at slaughter. Clinical examination may reveal the presence of epididymitis, orchitis, seminal vesiculitis and ampullitis. Therefore all bulls from known infected herds should be considered as suspicious regardless of their serological status (27) and not be used for artificial insemination.

In the early stages of the investigation, the herd history may be of value in suggesting the possible etiological agent. For example, in brucellosis, abortion at 6 months or later is the major complaint, whereas in trichomoniasis and vibriosis, failure to conceive and prolongation of the diestral period is the usual history. A summary of the differential diagnosis of contagious abortion in cattle is provided in Table 55. Of special interest is epizootic bovine abortion, a major disease of rangeland cattle in western United States (28). A spirochete has been isolated from the soft tick *Ornithodoros coriaceus* and from the blood of fetuses with lesions of epizootic bovine abortion (29). The disease occurs at a very high level of incidence but only in cattle introduced to a certain area; resident cattle are usually unaffected. Cattle returned to the area each winter are unaffected after the first abortion. The cows are unaffected systemically. Aborted fetuses show characteristic multiple petechiae in the skin, conjunctiva and mucosae, enlargement of lymph nodes, anasarca and nodular involvement of the liver.

In most countries where brucellosis is well under control and artificial insemination limits the spread of vibriosis and trichomoniasis, leptospirosis may be the commonest cause of abortion in cattle. However, surveys in such countries reveal the disquieting fact that in about two-thirds of the abortions which occur no causative agent is detectable with routine laboratory techniques. The virus of infectious bovine rhinotracheitis has now assumed major importance as a cause of abortion in cattle. A recent survey of bovine abortions and stillbirths in the United States has shown that 16% of cases examined were caused by the infectious bovine rhinotracheitis virus, 3·5% were mycotic abortions and 3% were caused by vibriosis. In only 35% of cases was the cause determined. Brucellosis accounted for less than 1% of the total (32). In an Australian experience the cause of abortion was determined in only 37% of cases in spite of the submission of the fetus, placenta and maternal serum (101). The general procedures for submission of specimens to the laboratory and laboratory methods are available (31).

Treatment

Treatment is not usually undertaken. Trials using bovine plasma, sulfadiazine, streptomycin and chlortetracycline given parenterally, and the latter two as udder infusions, have been unsuccessful in eliminating the infection. The use of long-acting oxytetracycline at 20 mg/kg body weight intramuscularly at 3–4 day intervals for five treatments in combination with streptomycin at 25 mg/kg body weight intramuscularly or intravenously daily for 7 consecutive days was partially successful in the treatment of infected cows (33). The administration of oxytetracycline concurrently with vaccination may reduce the antibody response (88).

Horses with fistulous withers and positive serum agglutination tests are commonly treated by vaccination with *Br. abortus* strain 19. Three injections of the vaccine are given with 10 days between injections. In the United Kingdom an equine brucellosis vaccine is used for this purpose. Chloramphenicol (1 g/100 kg body weight daily for 12–20 days) is reported as a successful treatment in infected horses (16).

Control and eradication

Bovine brucellosis may be controlled with an effective vaccination program or eradicated using a test and slaughter program. Vaccination using strain 19 will markedly reduce the prevalence of abortion but the level of infection will not be reduced at a corresponding rate. Even with a widespread vaccination program there will be foci of infection which are perpetuated indefinitely. Complete eradication is the alternative to control by vaccination and some countries have already achieved this status and others are currently engaged in eradication programs (69). Apart from the question of human exposure to infection the cost and economic benefits of an eradication program must be assessed against the costs and benefits from a vaccination control program. Computer-simulated modeling is now available to analyze the cost effectiveness of certain eradication programs (51).

Certain basic considerations apply to all programs aimed at the eradication of brucellosis.

- The control programs indigenous to any given area must receive primary recognition, and any plan or plans must be adapted to that area
- Cooperation at all levels of government from the local to the national is absolutely essential for the success of a program. Such cooperation is attained only after an intensive program of education has been carried out. The individual owner of an infected herd must come to recognize the problem of brucellosis and express a willingness to cooperate. Experience has revealed that the owner must be impressed with the hazards of the disease for human health and with the economic losses which may be incurred because of infected animals
- A reliable and uniform diagnostic procedure must be generally available
- If disease is detected in a herd, established procedures should be available for handling the disease. If immunization is to be carried out, a standardized and effective immunization agent should be readily available. The disposal of infected animals may create a serious economic threat for the owner and the possibilities of indemnity must be explored
- Finally, and of major importance, the movement of animals from one area to another must be controlled at a high level, since a rigid eradication program in one area may be nullified by neglect in a neighboring area (34).

Sufficient information exists about bovine brucellosis so that it can be eradicated. The Channel Islands (United Kingdom) succeeded in 1935, Norway in 1952, Sweden in 1957, Finland in 1960, Denmark in 1962, Czechoslovakia in 1964, and the Netherlands in 1967. Australia, New Zealand, the United Kingdom, and the United States are engaged in eradication programs. Canada declared itself brucellosis-free in 1986.

Table 55. Diagnostic summary of causes of abortion in cattle

Disease	*Epidemiology*			*Field examination*		*Laboratory diagnosis*	
	Clinical features	*Abortion rate*	*Time of abortion*	*Placenta*	*Fetus*	*Isolation of agent*	*Serology*
Brucellosis (*Br. abortus*)	Abortion	High, up to 90% in susceptible herds	6 months +	Necrosis of cotyledons. Leathery, opaque placenta with edema	May be pneumonia	Culture of fetal stomach, placenta, uterine fluid, milk and semen	Serum and blood agglutination test, milk ring test, whole milk plate agglutination test. Whey plate agglutination, semen plasma and vaginal mucous agglutination test
Trichomoniasis (*Trichomonas fetus*)	Infertility—return to heat at 4–5 months, abortion and pyometra	Moderate, 5–30%	2–4 months	Flocculent material and clear, serous fluid in uterine exudate	Fetal maceration and pyometra common	Hanging drop or culture examination of fetal stomach and uterine exudate within 24 hours of abortion	Cervical mucous agglutination test
Vibriosis (*Campylobacter fetus*)	Infertility, irregular, moderately prolonged diestrus	Low, up to 5%, may be up to 20%	5–6 months	Semi-opaque, little thickening. Petechiae, localized avascularity and edema	Flakes of pus on visceral peritoneum	Culture of fetal stomach, placenta and uterine exudate	Blood agglutination after abortion (at 3 weeks). Cervical mucous agglutination test at 40 days after infected service
Leptospirosis (*L. pomona* and *L. hardjo*)	Abortion may occur at acute febrile stage, later or unassociated with illness	25–30%	Late, 6 months +	Avascular placenta, atonic yellow-brown cotyledons, brown gelatinous edema between allantois and amnion	Fetal death common	Isolation from pleural fluid, kidney and liver of fetus. Direct examination of urine of cow is best	Positive serum agglutination test 14–21 days after febrile illness
Infectious bovine rhinotracheitis (IBR)	Uneventful	25–50%	Late, 6 months	—	Autolyzed	Culture of placenta and fetus	Acute and convalescent sera
Mycoses (*Aspergillus, Absidia*)	—	Unknown. 6–7% of all abortions encountered	3–7 months	Necrosis of maternal cotyledon, adherence of necrotic material to chorionic cotyledon causes soft, yellow, cushion-like structure. Small yellow, raised, leathery lesions on intercotyledonary areas	May be small raised, gray-buff, soft lesions, or diffuse white areas on skin. Resemble ringworm	Direct examination of cotyledon and fetal stomach for hyphae, suitable cultural examination	—
Listeriosis (*Listeria monocytogenes*)	May be an associated septicemia	Low	About 7 months	—	No abnormality	Organisms in fetal stomach, placenta and uterine fluid	Agglutination titers higher than 1 : 400 in contact animals classed as positive
Epizootic viral abortion	Mainly winter. Herd immunity develops	High, 30–40%	6–8 months	Negative	Subcutis edema, ascites, esophageal and tracheal petechiae, degenerative lesions in liver	Spirochete isolated (28)	No accurate test
Nutritional	Ingestion of excessive amounts of preformed estrogens in the diet may cause abortion. There are usually accompanying signs due to increased vascularity of the udder and vulva. Possibly dietary factor in so-called 'lowlands abortion'						

Table 55. (cont.)

Disease	Epidemiology: Clinical features	Epidemiology: Abortion rate	Epidemiology: Time of abortion	Field examination: Placenta	Field examination: Fetus	Laboratory diagnosis: Isolation of agent	Laboratory diagnosis: Serology
ɔimmunization pregnancy	Has not been observed to occur naturally in cattle. It has been produced experimentally by repeated intravenous injections of blood from the one bull. Intravascular hemolysis occurs in the calves						
ɪknown	From 30 to 75% of most series of abortions examined are undiagnosed. The ingestion of large quantities of pine needles is suspected as a cause of abortion in range cattle in the United States (45). Infection with the viruses of infectious bovine rhinotracheitis and mucosal disease and *Mycoplasma* spp. are other causes of undetermined relative importance						

Control by vaccination

Vaccination with *Br. abortus* strain 19 live vaccine is a valuable aid in brucellosis control. Its main value is that it protects uninfected animals living in a contaminated environment, enabling infected animals to be disposed of gradually. This overcomes the main disadvantage of the test and disposal method of eradication in which infected animals must be discarded immediately to avoid spread of infection. Vaccination cannot eradicate brucellosis but can be used to lay the groundwork for eradication. Eradication requires that the infected animal be identified and eliminated from the herd as a source of infection.

Strain 19 *Br. abortus* has a low virulence and is incapable of causing abortion except in a proportion of cows vaccinated in late pregnancy, although it can cause undulant fever in man. Its two other weaknesses are its failure to completely prevent infection, especially infection of the udder, and the persistence of vaccinal titers in some animals. The optimum age for vaccination is between 4 to 8 months and there is no significant difference between the immunity conferred at 4 or 8 months of age. In calves vaccinated between these ages the serum agglutination test returns to negative by the time the animals are of breeding age, except in a small percentage (6%) of cases. Calves vaccinated with strain 19 at 2 months of age have resistance comparable to those vaccinated at 4–8 months of age (36). Vaccination of calves with a single dose at 3–5 weeks of age does not provide protection compared to vaccination at 5 months of age (65). In most control programs, vaccination is usually permitted up to 12 months of age, but the proportion of persistent postvaccinal serum and whey reactions increases with increasing age of the vaccinates. Such persistent reactors may have to be culled in an eradication program unless the reaction can be proved to be the result of vaccination and not due to virulent infection. Vaccination of adult cattle is usually not permitted if an eradication program is contemplated but it may be of value in reducing the effects of an abortion 'storm'. There is no evidence that vaccination of bulls has any value in protecting them against infection, and vaccination has resulted in the development of orchitis and the presence of *Br. abortus* strain 19 in the semen (37). For these reasons the vaccination of bulls should be actively discouraged. Strain 19 has been isolated from vaccinated cattle; it is estimated that the organism can be recovered from less than 1:100 000, excluding hypersensitivity cases (62).

Efficiency of strain 19 vaccine

This can be assessed by its effect on both the incidence of abortion and of infection as determined by laboratory examination. Field tests show a marked reduction in the number of abortions which occur although the increased resistance to infection, as indicated by the presence of *Br. abortus* in milk, may be less marked. Vaccinated animals have a high degree of protection against abortion and 65–75% are resistant to most kinds of exposure. The remaining 25–35% of vaccinated animals may become infected but usually do not abort (34). Experimentally, 25% of cattle vaccinated with strain 19 will become infected following challenge. With the K45/20 vaccine, 70% of the vaccinated cattle and 83% of the controls (23) will become infected following challenge. Vaccinated animals continually exposed to virulent infection may eventually become infected and act as carriers without showing clinical evidence of the disease. In summary, the position is that vaccination with a single 5 ml dose of *Br. abortus* strain 19 vaccine given subcutaneously at from 2 to 6 months of age confers adequate immunity against abortion for five or more subsequent lactations under conditions of field exposure. Oral vaccination is also effective (99). Multiple or late vaccinations have no appreciable advantage and increase the incidence of postvaccinal positive agglutination reactions. When breakdowns occur, they are due to excessive exposure to infection and not to enhanced virulence of the organism.

The use of strain 19 vaccine in adult cows is highly successful in reducing the number of infected cows in large dairy herds in which it is impossible to institute management procedures for the ideal control of brucellosis (39). The difficulty of eliminating brucellosis from large dairy herds by test and slaughter methods alone is well documented (67, 68). Large numbers of animals are concentrated in relatively small areas, few or no replacements are raised in the herd and the numbers of lactating animals are kept relatively constant by purchase of mature replacements. The infection rate is high and the acutely affected herd experiences abortion and rapidly spreading disease. In the United States this problem resulted in the evaluation and adoption of vaccination of adult cattle with strain 19 *Br. abortus* vaccine. The vaccination of adult cattle with a reduced dose of vaccine is now permitted and efficacious (39, 43, 64). The use of about 1/20th of the standard subcutaneous dose of vaccine results in an agglutinin response which declines more rapidly after vaccination than when the full dose is used. The reduced dose also provides protection comparable to the standard dose (39). The experimental challenge of pregnant adult cattle and sexually mature non-pregnant heifers which had been vaccinated with 1/400 of the standard calf dose of strain 19 revealed that although immunity was incomplete, the increase in resistance to infection was greater than that achieved by standard calfhood vaccination (92, 97). The serological response to vaccination was greatly reduced and there was no adverse effect on pregnancy. Vaccination practically eliminates clinical disease and reduces exposure of infection to susceptible cattle. The reduction of infected adult cattle may vary from 60 to 80% in 6–9 months following vaccination. The complement fixation test becomes negative sooner than the standard tube agglutination test following vaccination and can be used to distinguish postvaccine titers from culture-positive cows. The use of reduced doses of strain 19 vaccine in adult cows will also help to eliminate the problem of postvaccine titers.

The subcutaneous and conjunctival routes of vaccination of adult cattle with strain 19 *Br. abortus* vaccine have been compared (61). The protection provided is the same regardless of the route of administration. However, the subcutaneous route provided a prolonged serological response which required complement fixation testing and milk culture to identify infected animals.

The principal advantages of adult vaccination include: it provides an effective method of control of abortion, it reduces the reactor losses in herds and reduces the number of tests required to eliminate brucellosis from infected herds.

The major disadvantages of adult vaccination are: residual vaccine titers, persistent positive milk ring test, persistent strain 19 infection in a small percentage of adult vaccinates, and the stigma attached to adult vaccinates which identifies them with infected herds, even though brucellosis has been eliminated and the herd released from quarantine. *Brucella abortus* strain 19 has been recovered from the supramammary lymph nodes of cattle at slaughter which were vaccinated with a low dose of the vaccine 9–12 months previously and which had persistent titers to the complement fixation test (96).

The results to be expected following adult vaccination depend on the disease situation. In herds vaccinated in the acute phase of the disease, abortion may continue for 60–90 days, but the incidence should begin to decline by 45–60 days. A large number of serological reactors will be present for the first 120 days following vaccination and testing is usually not done for the first 60 days. The rate of reactors usually declines rapidly after 120 days and with good infected herd management most adult vaccinated herds can be free of brucellosis 18–24 months following vaccination (43). The prevalence of strain 19 *Br. abortus* infection in adult vaccinated cattle is low and often is not permanent (63). The prevalence is lower among cattle given the reduced dose of the vaccine subcutaneously. Bacteriological examination of the milk and serological examination of the infected cattle are necessary to identify strain 19 infected cattle which can be retained for milk production because the infections are temporary. Adult vaccination even with a low dose should not be used in uninfected herds because of persistent titers which may last for more than 12 months in up to 15% of vaccinated animals, and because of the potential of abortion (98). The illegal or unintentional use of the standard dose of strain 19 vaccine in adult cattle will result in a sudden steep antibody titer response in the complement fixation test which will decline in 6–11 months (21).

Systemic reactions to vaccination with strain 19

These occur rarely in both calves and adults, and seem to be more severe in Jersey calves than in other breeds. A local swelling occurs particularly in adult cattle and there may be a severe systemic reaction manifested by high fever (40·5–42°C, 105–108°F) lasting for 2–3 days, anorexia, listlessness and temporary drop in milk production. An occasional animal goes completely dry. The local swellings are sterile and do not rupture but a solid, fibrous mass may persist for many months. Deaths within 48 hours of vaccination have been recorded in calves after the use of lyophilized vaccine. Septicemia due to *Br. abortus* may cause some deaths but in most cases the reaction is thought to be anaphylactic, and vaccinated calves should be kept under close observation. Immediate treatment with adrenalin hydrochloride (1 ml of 1:1000 solution subcutaneously) or antihistamine drugs is recommended and is effective provided it can be administered in time.

Cows in advanced pregnancy may abort if vaccinated, but the abortion rate is only about 1% (38) and although *Br. abortus* strain 19 organisms can be recovered from the fetus and placenta, their virulence is unchanged and they do not cause further spread of infection. Vaccination with strain 19 does not have a deleterious effect on the subsequent conception rate.

Vaccination technique

This is of vital importance; the vaccine is a living agent and must be handled with care if satisfactory results are to be obtained. Lyophilized vaccine is superior to liquid vaccine because of its greater stability and greater longevity but it must be kept under refrigeration at all times, be reconstituted only when required, and unusual material is discarded. It must be used in an aseptic manner to avoid its contamination with other bacteria.

Other vaccines

To overcome the disadvantages of the severe systemic reaction and the persistent agglutination titer which occurs after vaccination with strain 19 vaccine a search is being made for a killed non-agglutinogenic vaccine. The only one with any currency is strain 45/20 in adjuvant. Because it is a dead vaccine it has obvious attractions for vaccination of adult cows and males. For calves up to 8–9 months, strain 19 is significantly more effective. Beyond that age, some consideration should be given to 45/20 in adjuvant because of the lesser tendency to produce persistent high antibody levels. It has proven efficiency in increasing the number of viable calves produced, and the economic benefit conferred in a high risk situation is considerable (40). The vaccine is not completely non-agglutinogenic but titers in serum rarely reach inconclusive levels (41). Complement fixation antibodies are unaffected and no agglutinins appear in the milk (42). There are difficulties with the vaccine. The official vaccine K45/20A has a standard adjuvant but the characteristics of the vaccine can vary from batch to batch and need to be checked in animals. Two vaccinations are necessary. It is ineffective when given before 6 months of age and some batches of vaccine produce severe reactions up to 8 cm in diameter at the injection site. These may persist as severe granulomas. It is expensive, but it has the advantage that it can be used to identify in the chronic inconclusive cow using the anamnestic response as described earlier. The advantages and disadvantages of strain 19 and K45/20A vaccines have been compared and reviewed (91). The efficacy of commercial S45/30 bacterins is variable, even though they have been used with success in some countries for many years. In general, they are less efficacious than strain 19 vaccines (93–95). However, some studies reveal that one vaccination may provide adequate protection, a dosage regimen which would be desirable because two vaccinations often stimulate a serological response causing difficulties in diagnosis (94).

Control programs on a herd basis

These vary with the incidence of infection. Scandinavian countries were the first to achieve eradication by using control programs which could be modified to suit particular sets of conditions. The following recommendations are based on the need for flexibility depending on the existent level of infection and the susceptibility of the herd and the disease regulations in effect at the time.

(a) During an abortion storm Here test and disposal of reactors may be unsatisfactory because spread occurs faster than eradication is possible. In these circumstances, the vaccination of all non-reactors is recommended in some countries or, if testing is impracticable, vaccination of all cattle. Strain K45/20A vaccine may be used and must be given in two doses at 6-month intervals. It is preferable to retest the herd before the second vaccination and to discard cows with a three or more dilution rise in agglutination titer. However, strain 19 vaccine is a superior vaccine even for use in adult pregnant cattle even though it may cause abortion in a small percentage of animals.

(b) Heavily infected herds in which few abortions are occurring These do not present such an urgent problem because a degree of herd resistance has been reached. All calves should be vaccinated with strain 19 immediately and positive reactors among the remainder should be culled as soon as possible. Periodic milk ring tests (preferably at 2-month, no more than 3-month, intervals) on individual cows are supplemented by complement fixation and culture tests. One year after the first herd test, retest by agglutination test and revaccinate with K45/20A. This will result in serological reactions.

(c) Lightly infected herds These present a special problem. If they are situated in an area where infection is likely to be introduced, vaccination of the calves and immediate culling of positive reactors should be carried out. If eradication is the goal in the area the culling of reactors will suffice, but special market demands for vaccinated cattle may dictate a calfhood vaccination policy. When a herd is declared to be free of brucellosis on the basis of serum agglutination tests, its status can be maintained by introducing only negative-reacting animals from brucellosis-free herds, and annual blood-testing.

In areas where dairying predominates, semiannual testing by the milk tests may be substituted for blood testing. In all of the above programs the careful laboratory examination of all aborted fetuses is an important and necessary corollary to routine testing. There are many difficulties in the way of achieving control and eventual eradication on a herd basis. These relate mainly to the failure of owners to realize the highly infectious nature of the disease and to cooperate fully in the details of the program. Particularly they may fail to recognize the recently calved cow as the principal source of infection. In a herd control program such cows should be isolated at calving and blood tested at 14 days, since prior to that time false-negative reactions are not uncommon.

(d) Hygienic measures

These include the isolation or disposal of infected animals, disposal of aborted fetuses, placentas and uterine discharges, and disinfection of contaminated areas. It is particularly important that infected cows be isolated at parturition. All cattle, horses and pigs brought on to the farm should be tested, isolated for 30 days and retested. Introduced cows which are in advanced pregnancy should be kept in isolation until after parturition, since occasional infected cows may not show a positive serum reaction until after calving or abortion. Chlorhexidine gluconate is an effective antiseptic against *Br. abortus* and is recommended for washing the arms and hands of animal attendants and veterinarians who come into contact with contaminated tissues and materials (66).

Eradication on an area basis by test and slaughter and cessation of calfhood vaccination

Following a successful calfhood vaccination program the eradication of brucellosis on an area basis can be considered when the level of infection is below about 4% of the cattle population. Brucellosis-control areas must be established and testing and disposal of reactors and their calves-at-foot are carried out. Financial compensation for disposal of reactors is paid. Infected herds are quarantined and retested at intervals until negative, or in heavily infected herds complete depopulation is often necessary. Brucellosis-free areas are established when the level of infection is sufficiently low, and the movement of cattle between areas is controlled to avoid the spread of infection.

Farms with low incidence may find it possible to

engage in an eradication program immediately provided the incidence on surrounding farms is low. Disastrous breakdowns may occur if there are accidental introductions from nearby farms, and in these circumstances it is hazardous to have a herd which is not completely vaccinated. When the area incidence is judged to be low enough (about 5%) that replacements can be found within the area or adjoining free areas, and that immediate culling of reactors can be carried out without crippling financial loss, compulsory eradication by testing and disposal of reactors for meat purposes can be instituted. Compensation for culled animals should be provided to encourage full participation in the program.

The work of testing can be greatly reduced by using screening tests to select herds for more intensive epidemiological and laboratory investigation. In dairy herds the milk ring test is useful. In beef herds, the most favored procedure is the collection of blood from drafts of cattle at the abattoir and using the rose bengal test (44). The same technique has also been used to screen shipments of beef destined for countries with an aversion to meat infected with *Br. abortus* (45). An additional means of reducing labor costs in an eradication program is the use of automated laboratory systems such as the one available for the rose bengal agglutination test (46) and the one based on the agglutination and complement fixation test (47). An educational program to promote herd owners to voluntarily submit all aborted fetuses to a laboratory for bacteriological examination is also deemed necessary in any eradication scheme. When an area or country is freed of the disease, testing of all or part of the population need be carried out only at intervals of 2–3 years although regular testing of bulk milk samples and of culled beef cows in abattoirs and examination of fetuses should be maintained as checks on the eradication status. Such a program has achieved virtual eradication of the disease in Switzerland, Sweden and Northern Ireland.

However, difficulty has arisen in the United States, Canada, and the United Kingdom in achieving this status. Virtual eradication in the United States was predicted by 1971 (48), but most recent reports indicate a rise in prevalence (60). In that country and in Canada the problem seems to have arisen because of the susceptibility of the national herd now that strain 19 vaccination has been deemphasized, and the uncontrolled movement of cattle of unknown health status. Reintroduction of strain 19 vaccination is being actively promoted as the answer to the problem but regulatory agencies are understandably reluctant to take what is regarded as a retrograde step because of interference with the testing procedure and masking of infection. In all eradication programs some problem herds will be encountered in which testing and disposal does not eliminate the infection. Usually about 5% of such herds are encountered and are best handled by a 'problem herd' program; 50% of these herds have difficulty because of failure to follow directions. The other half usually contain infected animals that do not respond to standard tests. Supplementary bacteriological and serological tests as set out above may occasionally help these spreader animals to be identified and the disease to be eradicated.

The Cooperative State–Federal Brucellosis Eradication program is making progress (102). The numbers of infected herds and the market cattle reactor rate have continued to decline since the introduction of an accelerated program instituted a few years earlier. The declining infection rate made funds available for the complete depopulation of problem herds. The federal involvement will phase out in the near future and more responsibility will be placed on individual states to improve their eradication programs. The federal government will limit itself to such activities as enforcement of interstate regulation, disease surveillance and dissemination of information from the program database (102).

In the last decade the primary surveillance methods for test eligible cattle in the United States have been the market cattle identification (MCI) program in the beef industry and the brucellosis ring test (BRT) in the dairy industry (30). Epidemiological studies have shown a distinct herd size bias in the MSI surveillance system. For example, the probability of detection in a nine-cow herd is 24% compared to 85% for a 645 cow herd 1 year after infection. This herd size bias implies that secondary testing may be efficiently used by concentrating testing in smaller herds when funds for secondary testing are limited (30).

Under range conditions in Australia considerable progress towards eradication of brucellosis in large beef herds has been possible. Management must be motivated and confident that the disease can be permanently eradicated. All cattle should be permanently identified, security between subherds must be good, vaccination histories must be accurate and accurate round-up (mustering) of cattle must be possible. Quarantine facilities for infected subherds must be strict and absolutely reliable and fence lines must be impenetrable. The development of a two-herd system, based on segregation of weaned heifer calves from adult cows and maintenance of testing pressure on the adults, will reduce the chance of infection of heifers. All calves from reactor dams are discarded which necessitates positive identification. Only bulls or semen from brucellosis-free herds should be used in clean herds. In some situations, a laboratory is established on the ranch and equipped to do the rose bengal and complement fixation tests. This increases the efficiency of the testing program and creates an excellent team effort between management, laboratory personnel and the field veterinarian.

An active bovine brucellosis eradication program has been in effect in Canada since 1950 at which time the national infection rate was about 9%. A cooperative Federal–Provincial Calfhood Vaccination Program began in 1950, and by 1956 the infection rate was reduced to 4·5%. In 1957, a test and slaughter program was begun in which brucellosis control areas were established and mandatory testing of all cattle was done using the tube agglutination test. Reactors were identified, ordered slaughtered and compensation paid. Infected herds were quarantined and retested until negative or in some cases completely depopulated. When the infection rate was reduced to below 1% of the cattle population and 5% of the herds, the area was certified for a period of 3 years. When the infection rate was reduced to below 0·2% of the cattle in the area and 1% of the herds, the area was designated as brucellosis-free and certified for a period of 5 years. In the 1960s the milk ring test and the market cattle testing programs were introduced as surveillance procedures. These are done on a continuing basis and are effective in locating infected herds and have reduced the volume of on-farm testing required to recertify areas. When the level of national infection was reduced to below 0·2%, calfhood vaccination was de-emphasized to overcome the problem of distinguishing between persistent vaccinational titers and titers due to natural infection. Thus all positive animals could be disposed of and no vaccination privileges allowed. In 1973 an increase in the incidence of brucellosis occurred which necessitated some modifications in the eradication program. The intensity of milk ring testing was increased, herds adjacent to infected herds are being tested, the length of time of quarantine of infected herds was increased, and calves from reactor dams are ordered slaughtered. In heavily infected herds and in those in which it is not possible to maintain effective quarantine, it may be preferable to completely depopulate a herd rather than conduct tests and successive retests. In the Canadian experience, brucellosis-free herds usually become infected when the owner unknowingly buys a brucellosis-infected animal. The uncontrolled movement of infected animals from infected herds to brucellosis-free herds is considered to be a major obstacle in the final stages of the eradication.

The rate of progress in a brucellosis eradication program is determined mainly by the rate at which herds which are accredited free of the infection have become reinfected. The severity of reinfection (or *breakdown*) is dependent upon the proportion of the herd which has been vaccinated as calves. The cessation of compulsory calfhood vaccination results in a large proportion of cattle which are fully susceptible to *Br. abortus* infection (22). The prevention of reinfection requires a constant surveillance system.

In Canada, three major issues are concerns following eradication of brucellosis in 1986. The first is the need for continuous surveillance to identify hidden foci of infection which might be present but not become apparent until a full generation of cattle has passed, and to detect infection which might be imported with livestock brought into the country (89). A related concern could be the presence of infection in Canadian wildlife, particularly bison and elk which are the species of choice in game farming (100).

The second concern is the dilemma faced by livestock owners to use the vaccine, when normally they do not use it, to vaccinate cattle intended for export to importing states or countries which require vaccination. The continued use of the vaccine in a brucellosis-free area or country perpetuates the diagnostic problem. The third concern is the importance of cattle from countries or regions which have not eradicated brucellosis.

The importance of unknown infected or latent carriers which may be seronegative is a major concern because it can result in herd epidemics of abortion in unvaccinated cattle. The risk can be minimized by pre-entry and post-entry testing combined with certification of the animals on the basis of the regional and herd health status. Limiting the importation of cattle from areas where brucellosis persists and the use of embryo transfer technology can also reduce the risk of introducing infection (89).

Vaccination of adult cattle in Canada was not permitted.

REVIEW LITERATURE

Corbel, M. J. (1985) Recent advances in the study of brucella antigens and their serological cross reactions. *Vet. Bull.*, *55*, 927–942.

Nicoletti, P. (1980) The epidemiology of bovine brucellosis. *Adv. vet. Sci. comp. Med.*, *24*, 69–98.

Pietz, D. E. & Canart, W. O. (1980) Use of epidemiologic data and serologic tests in bovine bruccelosis. *J. Am. vet. med. Assoc.*, *177*, 1221–1226.

Sutherland, S. S. (1980) Immunology of bovine brucellosis. *Vet. Bull.*, *50*, 359–368.

Tessaro, S. V. (1986) The existing and potential importance of brucellosis and tuberculosis in Canadian wildlife: a review. *Can. vet. J.*, *27*, 119–124.

World Health Organization (1986) Joint FAO/WHO Expert Committee, 6th Report. *Tech. Rep. Series*, WHO *740*, 132 pp.

REFERENCES

(1) Jones, R. L. et al. (1982) *J. clin. Microbiol.*, *16*, 641.
(2) Crawford, R. P. et al. (1986) *J. Am. vet. med. Assoc.*, *189*, 547.
(3) Lapraik, R. D. & Moffat, R. (1982) *Vet. Rec.*, *111*, 578.
(4) Shaw, W. B. (1977) *Br. vet. J.*, *132*, 18 & 143.
(5) Luchsinger, D. W. & Anderson, R. K. (1979) *Am. J. vet. Res.*, *40*, 1307.
(6) Hinton, M. et al. (1977) *Vet. Rec.*, *101*, 526.
(7) Thorne, E. T. et al. (1978) *J. Wild. Dis.*, *14*, 74, 280.
(8) Boeer, W. J. et al. (1980) *J. Wild. Dis.*, *16*, 9.
(9) Meyer, M. E. (1974) *Adv. vet. Sci.*, *18*, 231.
(10) Catlin, J. E. & Sheehan, E. J. (1986) *J. Am. vet. med. Assoc.*, *188*, 867.
(11) Prior, M. G. (1976) *Can. J. comp. Med.*, *40*, 117.
(12) Salman, M. D. & Meyer, M. E. (1984) *Am. J. vet. Res.*, *45*, 1557.
(13) Vandeplassche, M. & Devos, A. (1960) *Vlaams Diergeneeskd. Tijdschr.*, *29*, 199.
(14) Kellar, J. et al. (1976) *Can. J. comp. Med.*, *40*, 119.
(15) McCaughey, W. J. & Kerr, W. R. (1967) *Vet. Rec.*, *80*, 186.
(16) Salman, M. D. et al. (1984) *Am. J. vet. Res.*, *45*, 1561 & 1567.
(17) Sutherland, S. S. (1980) *Vet. Bull.*, *50*, 359.
(18) Corbel, M. J. (1985) *Vet. Bull.*, *55*, 927.
(19) Confer, A. W. et al. (1985) *Am J. vet. Res.*, *46*, 2440.
(20) Lopez, A. et al. (1984) *Can. J. comp. Med.*, *48*, 275.
(21) Herr, S. et al. (1985) *J. S. Afr. vet. Assoc.*, *56*, 93.
(22) Hellstrom, J. S. (1982) *NZ vet. J.*, *30*, 33.
(23) Thoen, C. I. et al. (1983) *Am. J. vet. Res.*, *44*, 306.
(24) Sutherland, S. S. (1983) *Vet. Microbiol.*, *8*, 405.
(25) Gray, M. D. & Martin, S. W. (1980) *Can. J. comp. Med.*, *44*, 52.
(26) Corner, L. A. et al. (1983) *Aust. vet. J.*, *60*, 1.
(27) Plant, J. W. et al. (1973) *Aust. vet. J.*, *52*, 17.
(28) Lane, R. S. et al. (1985) *Science*, *230*, 85.
(29) Osebold, J. et al. (1986) *J. Am. vet. med. Assoc.*, *188*, 371.
(30) Omosson, S. H. & Dietrich, R. A. (1984) *Prev. vet. Med.*, *3*, 53.
(31) Kirkbride, C. A. (1984) *Laboratory Diagnosis of Abortion in Food Animals.* A special report of the Committee on Fetal and Placental Diseases of the Am. Assoc. Vet. Lab. Diagnost., 176 pp.
(32) Kirkbride, C. A. et al. (1973) *J. Am. vet. med. Assoc.*, *162*, 556.
(33) Nicoletti, P. et al. (1985) *J. Am. vet. med. Assoc.*, *187*, 493.
(34) National Research Council (1977) *Brucellosis Research: An Evaluation.* Washington, DC: National Academy of Sciences.

(35) Morgan, G. & Richardson, C. (1983) In: *Proc. Third Int. Symp. World Assoc. Vet. Lab. Diag.* June 13–15, 1983, pp. 75–81.
(36) Redman, D. R. et al. (1967) *J. Am. vet. med. Assoc.*, *150*, 403.
(37) Lambert, G. et al. (1964) *J. Am. vet. med. Assoc.*, *145*, 409.
(38) Nicoletti, P. (1977) In: *Bovine Brucellosis. An International Symposium*, ed. R. P. Crawford & R. J. Hidalgo. Texas: A & M University Press.
(39) Nicoletti, P. et al. (1978) *J. Am. vet. med. Assoc.*, *173*, 1445.
(40) Hall, W. T. K. et al. (1976) *Aust. vet. J.*, *52*, 409.
(41) Cunningham, B. & O'Reilly, D. J. (1968) *Vet. Rec.*, *82*, 678.
(42) Cunningham, B. (1970) *Vet. Rec.*, *86*, 2.
(43) Barton, C. E. & Lomme, J. R. (1980) *J. Am. vet. med. Assoc.*, *177*, 1218.
(44) Browne, E. N. (1974) *Aust. vet. J.*, *50*, 127.
(45) Wells, F. D. et al. (1974) *Aust. vet. J.*, *50*, 128.
(46) Gower, S. G. M. et al. (1974) *Vet. Rec.*, *95*, 544.
(47) Miller, J. K. et al. (1973) *Vet. Rec.*, *92*, 492.
(48) Schilf, E. A. (1972) *J. Am. vet. med. Assoc.*, *161*, 1525.
(49) Wilesmith, J. W. (1978) *Vet. Rec.*, *103*, 149.
(50) Wyn-Jones, G. et al. (1980) *Vet. Rec.*, *107*, 5.
(51) Beck, A. C. (1977) *Aust. vet. J.*, *53*, 485.
(52) Davis, D. S. et al. (1979) *J. Wild. Dis.*, *15*, 367.
(53) Swann, A. I. et al. (1980) *Vet. Rec.*, *106*, 57.
(54) Hudson, M. et al. (1980) *Can. vet. J.*, *21*, 47.
(55) Kagunya, D. K. J. & Waiyaki, P. G. (1978) *Kenya Vet.*, *2*, 35.
(56) Choqueete, L. P. E. et al. (1978) *J. Wild. Dis.*, *14*, 329.
(57) Alexander, B. et al. (1981) *Vet. Rec.*, *108*, 500.
(58) Cunningham, B. (1978) *Vet. Rec.*, *102*, 500.
(59) Martin, S. W. & Gerrow, A. F. (1978) *Can. J. comp. Med.*, *42*, 16.
(60) Gue, C. S. et al. (1981) *J. Am. vet. med. Assoc.*, *178*, 839.
(61) Nicoletti, P. et al. (1978) *J. Am. vet. med. Assoc.*, *173*, 1450.
(62) Thomas, E. L. et al. (1981) *Vet. Rec.*, *108*, 1981.
(63) Nicoletti, P. (1981) *J. Am. vet. med. Assoc.*, *178*, 143.
(64) Alton, G. G. et al. (1980) *Aust. vet. J.*, *56*, 369.
(65) Plackett, P. et al. (1980) *Aust. vet. J.*, *56*, 409.
(66) Hall, R. (1979) *Vet. Rec.*, *105*, 305.
(67) Vanderwagen, L. C. et al. (1978) *Proc. US Anim. Hlth Assoc.*, *82*, 70.
(68) Nicoletti, P. (1980) *Adv. vet. Sci. comp. Med.*, *24*, 69.
(69) New Zealand Brucellosis Eradication Scheme (1978) *NZ vet. J.*, *26*, 41–84.
(70) Corbel, M. J. et al. (1983) *Res. vet. Sci.*, *34*, 296.
(71) MacMillan, A. P. (1985) *Vet. Rec.*, *117*, 638.
(72) Quinn, P. J. (1984) *Irish vet. J.*, *38*, 86.
(73) Heever, L. W. Van Den et al. (1982) *J. S. Afr. vet. Assoc.*, *53*, 233.
(74) Stringfellow, D. A. et al. (1985) *Theriogenology*, *23*, 701.
(75) Enright, F. M. et al. (1984) *Am. J. vet. Res.*, *45*, 424.
(76) Stringfellow, D. A. et al. (1983) *Theriogenology*, *20*, 77.
(77) Chen, I-Ming, et al. (1984) *Am. J. vet. Res.*, *45*, 32.
(78) Dohoo, I. R. et al. (1986) *Can J. vet Res.*, *50*, 485.
(79) Stemshorn, B. W. et al. (1985) *Can. J. comp. Med.*, *49*, 391.
(80) Sutherland, S. S. & MacKenzie, R. M. (1983) *Aust. vet. J.*, *60*, 240.
(81) Sutherland, S. S. (1985) *J. clin. Microbiol.*, *22*, 44.
(82) Sutherland, S. S. (1984) *Vet. Microbiol.*, *10*, 23.
(83) Sutherland S. S. & Den Hollander, L. (1986) *Vet. Microbiol.*, *12*, 55.
(84) Sutherland, S. (1985) *Aust. vet. J.*, *62*, 264.
(85) Hobbs, I. F. (1985) *NZ vet. J.*, *33*, 112.
(86) Cargill, C. et al (1985) *Aust. vet. J.*, *62*, 49.
(87) Nielsen, K. et al. (1985) *Can. J. comp. Med.*, *49*, 298.
(88) Smith, R. A. et al. (1983) *J. Am. vet. med. Assoc.*, *183*, 70.
(89) Stemshorn, B. W. (1985) *Can. vet. J.*, *26*, 35.
(90) Worthington, R. W. et al. (1974) *J. S. Afr. vet. med. Assoc.*, *45*, 87.
(91) Dolan, L. A. (1980) *Vet. Rec.*, *106*, 241.
(92) Alton, G. G. & Corner, L. A. (1981) *Aust. vet. J.*, *57*, 548.
(93) Woodard, L. F. & Jasman, R. L. (1983) *Am. J. vet. Res.*, *44*, 907.
(94) Alton G. G. et al. (1983) *Aust. vet. J.*, *60*, 175.
(95) Sutherland, S. et al. (1981) *Aust. vet. J.*, *57*, 470.
(96) Duffield, B. J. et al. (1984) *Aust. vet. J.*, *61*, 411.
(97) Alton, G. G. et al. (1980) *Aust. vet. J.*, *56*, 369.
(98) Beckett, F. W. & MacDarmid, S. C. (1985) *Br. vet. J.*, *141*, 507.
(99) Nicoletti, P. & Milward, F. W. (1983) *Am. J. vet. Res.*, *44*, 1641.
(100) Tessaro, S. V. (1986) *Can. vet. J.*, *27*, 119.
(101) Jerrett, I. V. et al. (1984) *Cornell Vet.*, *74*, 8.
(102) Nelson, C. J. et al. (1986) *Proc. 90th Ann. Mtg US Anim. Hlth Assoc.*, pp. 177–190.
(103) Meador, V. P. & Deyoe, B. L. (1986) *Am. J. vet. Res.*, *47*, 2337.

Brucellosis caused by *Brucella ovis*

The disease caused by the infection of sheep with *Br. ovis* is characterized by infertility in rams due to epididymitis. Abortion and neonatal mortality are thought to be caused by the infection.

Etiology

The causative organism has been designated as *Br. ovis* (1).

Epidemiology

In nature only sheep are affected and most laboratory animals are refractory to the infection. Goats (25) and white-tailed deer (2) can be infected experimentally leading to the development of an epididymitis. Amongst sheep Merinos show a much lower incidence of the disease than do British breeds and crossbreeds. The disease occurs more commonly in adult rams, due probably to greater exposure to infection (2). The organism can survive on pasture for several months but transmission from ram to ram via the ewe's vagina seems to be the most common method.

Complete details of the method of spread of infection are not yet available. Experimentally rams can be infected by the intravenous, subcutaneous, intratesticular, oral, and conjunctival and preputial instillation routes. Ewes in early pregnancy can also be infected by the oral and intravenous routes. Under natural conditions, spread from ram to ram occurs during the breeding season and when the rams are run together. However, spread from rams to ewes during mating does not occur readily, and spread between ewes by ingestion of contaminated pasture has not been observed. The exact means by which the disease spreads in a flock of ewes is not understood.

The infection in ewes is shortlived and persists in only a few animals but the organism is present in the placenta, vaginal discharges and milk after abortion. In most rams the active excretion of the bacteria in semen probably persists indefinitely. Lambs born from infected ewes and drinking infected milk do not become infected.

Brucellosis of sheep caused by *Br. ovis* has been reported in Australia, New Zealand, the United States, South Africa, and Europe. The incidence has been very high in some areas, and there was much economic loss at one time. In California 30–40% of rams were thought to be affected and annual loss of $2 million was estimated. In one survey of a large number of rams conducted in Australia, the incidence of clinical epididymitis was 5·3% and the incidence on individual farms was a high as 50% (2). If the number of affected rams in a flock is greater than about 10% the fertility of the flock is appreciably decreased.

Pathogenesis

An initial bacteremia, often with a mild systemic reaction is followed by localization in the epididymis of the ram, usually in the tail and unilaterally, causing a spermatocele and therefore infertility. Experimental infection of rams (5, 15) results in a chronological development of the disease which is important in the diagnosis of the disease. The first observable abnormality is the presence of inflammatory cells in the semen which appear at 2–8 weeks. The organism *Brucella ovis* appears in semen smears at 3 weeks, but is intermittent in its appearance so that from 4 weeks postinfection onwards only 52% of infected rams give a positive test. Culture of semen is more definitive and all infected rams are positive from 5 weeks onwards. Testicular and epididymal lesions can be palpated at about 9 weeks after infection. The severity of the lesions varies with the immunological status of the ram, the larger lesions appearing in vaccinated rams and those which are positive serologically.

In ewes, abortion due to placentitis has been produced experimentally and has been observed in natural cases in New Zealand and the United States (23), but has not been observed in other countries. Intrauterine infection produced experimentally also causes lesions in and death of the fetus but the significance of this in natural cases is undertermined. In general, the evidence is that *Br. ovis* has low pathogenicity for ewes (8): the primary effect of infection is a placentitis which interferes with fetal nutrition, sometimes to the point of causing its death but more commonly producing lambs of low birth weight and poor viability (1).

Clinical findings

The first reaction in rams is a marked deterioration in the quality of the semen together with the presence of leukocytes and brucellae. Acute edema and inflammation of the scrotum may follow. A systemic reaction, including fever, depression and increased respiratory rate accompanies the local reaction. Regression of the acute syndrome is followed, after a long, latent period, by the development of palpable lesions in the epididymis and tunicae of one or both testicles. Palpation of both testicles simultaneously from behind is the best method of examination. The epididymis is enlarged and hard, more commonly at the tail, the scrotal tunics are thickened and hardened and the testicles usually atrophic. The groove between the testis and epididymis may be obliterated. The abnormalities are often detectable by palpation but many affected rams show no acute inflammatory stage and others may be actively secreting brucellae and poor quality semen in the chronic stage in the absence of palpable abnormalities.

Abortion in ewes is a characteristic of the disease as it occurs in New Zealand but not elsewhere. In the ewe, abortion, or the birth of weak or stillborn lambs, is accompanied by macroscopic placentitis. The placental lesion varies from a superficial purulent exudate on an intact chorion to a marked edema of the allantois, with necrosis of the uterine surface and the fetal cotyledons.

In spite of the seminal changes in affected rams, the fertility of their flock is often relatively unimpaired provided the proportion of affected rams is less than 10%.

Clinical pathology

In the ram, semen examination is essential. Semen quality should be determined, smears made for examination of inflammatory cells and culture for the organism undertaken. Virgin rams support a varied population of fastidious Gram-negative rods including *Actinobacillus*, *Hemophilus*, *Moraxella* and *Pasteurella* spp. (10). In affected animals the findings include the isolation of *B. ovis* in the semen and a reduction in semen quality generally, a reduced total sperm output, poor motility, and a high proportion of spermatozoa with morphological abnormalities. Bacteriological examination of the placenta and fetus should be carried out on aborted material. Complement fixation is now used routinely to detect serum antibodies to *Br. ovis* and a gel diffusion test, a hemagglutination inhibition test and an ELISA (9, 11) are also available. The serological tests available are quite accurate and are suitable for testing individual animals, with the complement fixation test being the standard one (15). There may be an unexpectedly high prevalence of false-positive reactors in some flocks because of the relatively common circumstance of a ram being exposed to infection and developing a positive reaction to a serological test but not developing the disease (26). The ELISA test promises to be able to avoid this error. A highly sensitive microtiter complement fixation test (CFT) has also become available (6).

Necropsy findings

In the acute stage, there is inflammatory edema in the loose scrotal fascia, exudate in the tunica vaginalis and early granulation tissue formation. In the chronic stage, the tunics of the testes become thickened and fibrous and adhesions develop between them. There are circumscribed indurations in the epididymis and these granulomata may also be present in the testicle. In advanced stages they undergo caseation necrosis. As the epididymis enlarges the testicle becomes atrophied. *Brucella ovis* can usually be isolated from the genital organs, especially the tail of the epididymis, and rarely from internal organs and lymph nodes (14).

The abortus is characterized by thickening and edema, sometimes restricted to only a part of the placenta, firm, elevated yellow-white plaques in the intercotyledonary areas and varying degrees of abnormality of the cotyledons which in the acute stages are much enlarged, firm and yellow-white in color. When abortion occurs the organism can be isolated from the placenta and the stomach and lungs of the lamb.

Diagnosis

The diagnosis of brucellosis in rams is based on three examinations: a complement fixation test on serum, physical palpation of the contents of the scrotum, and cultural examination of semen or aborted material. The complement fixation, or other serological test is by far the most important; many infected rams have palpably normal scrotal contents and microbiologically negative semen (12). Many rams with abnormalities of intrascrotal tissues do not have brucellosis (13). Most are cases of epididymitis and need to be differentiated. Suppurative epididymitis of rams is a specific, transmissible disease caused by *Cor. pseudotuberculosis* or by infection with

Actinobacillus seminis (3, 13). Of the lesions in the scrotal sac it is the tail or the head of the epididymis that are the best indicators of the presence of ovine brucellosis (27). Abortion in ewes may be caused by a number of infectious diseases summarized in Table 56. A severe infection with Q fever in sheep can be a cause of abortion (2).

Treatment

Treatment of naturally occurring cases is not undertaken as far as we know. In experimentally infected rams, the combined administration of chlortetracycline (800 mg intravenously) and streptomycin (1 g subcutaneously), injected daily for 21 days, eliminated infection. Streptomycin alone and streptomycin plus sulfadimidine were not satisfactory (14). Treatment is economically practicable only in valuable rams and must be instituted before irreparable damage to the epididymis has occurred.

Control

The primary objective in control programs directed against brucellosis in sheep is to prevent the spread of infection between rams. Thus the basis of any such program is the rigid isolation of young rams from old rams which are likely to be affected and from ewe flocks which have been mated to these older rams. To further reduce the chances of spread to young rams vaccination or test and slaughter programs are recommended. Neither strategy is without problems and it is not uncommon for both to be used, especially when the disease is spreading rapidly, and test and slaughter is unlikely to stem the tide. In a chronic situation where the disease has been present for a long time, a test and slaughter policy should be implemented, provided the risk of invasion from the outside can be neutralized. Eradication is achievable fairly readily in individual flocks, and provided regulatory control is efficient and the test and slaughter program is vigorously practiced the disease can be eradicated from an area in as short a period as 2 or 3 years (4).

Vaccination

Vaccination is carried out on all yearling rams at least 2–3 months before they are used for mating (16). A number of vaccines are in use. The most common one is a single injection of a combination of killed *Br. ovis* in an adjuvant base and *Br. abortus* strain 19. Although a high level, durable immunity is produced, the vaccine has several disadvantages; if used within 2 months of mating the fertility of the rams is likely to be reduced; a high titer of antibodies against *Br. ovis* as detected by the tube agglutination test persists for up to 3 years (17), which may confuse diagnosis and hinder eradication; some severe outbreaks of osteomyelitis have been recorded 10–20 days after vaccination in which affected rams are lame and weak in one or all limbs, many become recumbent and although recovery is usual the illness is a long one and affected animals are badly stunted in growth (18). An epiphysitis affecting the distal epiphysis of either the radius or the tibia has also occurred in a number of rams after vaccination with this vaccine (16). A satisfactory alternative to the above procedure is two injections of killed *Br. ovis* adsorbed on aluminum hydroxide, the vaccinations to be 3–6 weeks apart (7, 19).

In all vaccination programs there should be a concurrent program of culling of clinically abnormal rams as detected by palpation of the scrotal contents. Vaccine and examination should be carried out annually. All ram replacements should be yearlings vaccinated at 4–5 months of age with two injections 3–6 weeks apart.

In South Africa, a vaccine containing live attenuated *Br. melitensis* (referred to as Elberg Rev 1) has been found to be highly effective and is generally recommended (20). It too suffers from the disadvantage that vaccinated animals become positive to the complement fixation tests, but the titers produced are very low (28). In China, a vaccination strain of *Br. suis* (strain 2) or strain 19 *Br. abortus* are used to vaccinate sheep and goats with apparent success (24).

If venereal transmission is the only means by which the disease is spread, effective vaccination and control of the rams is all that should be necessary. There is no evidence that vaccination of the ewes is of value in reducing spread but where it has been carried out vaccination has increased the percentage of lambs weaned (16).

Test and slaughter

In some countries vaccination is not permitted and eradication by test and slaughter is attempted and provides an effective solution if the threshold for culling is set at suspicious reactors in the initial tests (21). The identification of animals to be culled must depend on laboratory testing. Culling based on physical palpation can achieve only temporary improvement in a flock. The program of testing used has varied and depends largely on the incidence and rate of spread of the disease. In static situations where the new infection rate is low, semiannual testing is satisfactory, but when the disease has been recently introduced testing at monthly intervals may be necessary.

In both instances the rate of spread of infection is highest during the mating season and it is not recommended that eradication should be attempted until after the rams are taken out of the flock. Any policy which does not permit vaccination is likely to be hazardous in areas where the disease is not under control and infected replacements are likely to be introduced.

REVIEW LITERATURE

Afzal, M. & Kimberling, C. V. (1986) How to control *Brucella ovis*-induced epididymitis in rams. *Vet. Med.*, *81*, 364–370.

Moule, G. R. (1969) *The Management of Breeding Sheep in Australia*, Veterinary Review No. 6. Sydney: University of Sydney Postgraduate Foundation in Veterinary Science.

Rahaley, R. S. (1986) Ovine brucellosis; recent advances. *Aust. Adv. Vet. Sci.*, pp. 90–92.

REFERENCES

(1) Meyer, M. E. (1974) *Adv. vet. Sci. comp. Med.*, *18*, 231.
(2) Barron, S. J. et al. (1985) *Am. J. vet. Res.*, *46*, 1762.
(3) Tonder, E. M. van (1979) *Onderstepoort J. vet. Res.*, *46*, 129.
(4) Prokofev, A. G. et al. (1977) *Veterinariya, Moscow*, *7*, 54.
(5) Rahaley, R. S. & Dennis, S. M. (1984) *Aust. vet. J.*, *61*, 353.

Table 56. Diagnostic summary of infectious abortion in ewes

Disease	*Epidemiology*			*Laboratory findings*		
	Transmission	*Time of abortion*	*Clinical data*	*Fetus*	*Serology*	*Vaccination*
Brucellosis (*Br. ovis*)	Probably coitus	Late or stillbirth	Epididymitis in rams. In ewes abortion only. Not in United States	Organisms in fetal stomach and placenta	Complement fixation test (CFT)	Simultaneous strain 19 *Br. abortus* and killed *Br. ovis* adjuvant vaccine
Vibriosis (*Campylobacter fetus*)	Ingestion	2 months	Metritis in ewes after abortion	Vibrios in stomach	Agglutination test, flock only	—
Enzootic abortion of ewes	Ingestion	Last 2–3 weeks	Illness before. Retained placenta and metritis after	*Chlamydia* sp. in fetal cotyledons. Degenerative changes in placenta	Complement fixation test	Killed vaccine. Gives good immunity to 30 months (22)
Listeriosis (*Listeria monocytogenes*)	Probably ingestion, possibly coitus	After 3 months	Retained placenta and metritis. Septicemia in some ewes	Organisms in fetal stomach	Agglutination test of doubtful value	—
Salmonellosis (*Salmonella abortusovis*)	Probably ingestion	Last 6 weeks	Metritis after abortion	Organisms in fetal stomach	Agglutination test	—
Salmonellosis (*S. dublin*)	Ingestion	Last month	Abortion: fatal metritis, neonatal mortality	Organisms in stomach	Agglutination test	—
Toxoplasmosis (New Zealand type 2)	Not known	Late or stillbirths	Abortion, stillbirths and neonatal mortality	Multiple small necrotic foci in fetal cotyledons. Toxoplasma in cells of trophoblast epithelium	Dye tests for toxoplasmosis appear efficient	Nil
Rift valley fever	Insects	—	Important cause of abortion in all species Central Africa. Heavy mortality in young animals	Acidophilic inclusions hepatic cells	Fluorescent antibody and other available	Available

(6) Searson, J. E. (1982) *Aust. vet. J.*, *58*, 5.
(7) McGowan, B. (1979) *Cornell Vet.*, *69*, 67 & 73.
(8) Hughes, K. L. (1972) *Aust. vet. J.*, *48*, 12, 18.
(9) Rahaley, R. S. et al. (1983) *Vet. Rec.*, *113*, 467.
(10) Bulgin, M. S. & Anderson, B. S. (1983) *J. Am. vet. med. Assoc.*, *182*, 372.
(11) Lee, K. et al. (1985) *Aust. vet. J.*, *62*, 3.
(12) Hughes, K. L. & Claxton, P. (1976) *Aust. vet J.*, *44*, 41.
(13) Rothwell, J. T. et al. (1986) *Aust. vet. J.*, *63*, 209.
(14) Searson, J. E. (1986) *Aust. vet. J.*, *63*, 30.
(15) Worthington, R. W. (1983) *NZ vet. J.*, *32*, 58.
(16) West, D. M. et al. (1978) *NZ vet. J.*, *26*, 133.
(17) Ris, D. R. (1967) *NZ vet. J.*, *15*, 94.
(18) Kater, J. C. & Hartley, W. J. (1963) *NZ vet. J.*, *11*, 65.
(19) Buddle, M. B. et al. (1963) *NZ vet. J.*, *11*, 90.
(20) Erasmus, J. A. & Bergh, E. C. (1985) *J. S. Afr. vet. Assoc.*, *56*, 205.
(21) Walker, R. L. et al. (1985) *Am. J. vet. Res.*, *46*, 1642.
(22) Foggie, A. (1973) *Vet. Bull.*, *43*, 587.
(23) Libal, M. C. & Kirkbride, C. A. (1983) *J. Am. vet. med. Assoc.*, *163*, 553.
(24) Xie Xin et al. (1981) *Acta vet. Zootol. Sinica*, *12*, 175.
(25) Burgess, G. W. et al. (1985) *Aust. vet. J.*, *62*, 262.
(26) Plant, J. W. et al. (1986) *Aust. vet. J.*, *63*, 409.
(27) Searson, J. E. (1986) *Aust. vet. J.*, *64*, 108.
(28) Erasmus, J. A. (1986) *J. S. Afr. vet. Assoc.*, *56*, 205.

Brucellosis caused by *Brucella suis*

Brucellosis caused by *Br. suis* is a chronic disease of pigs manifested by sterility and abortion in sows, heavy piglet mortality and orchitis in boars.

Etiology

The disease is caused by *Br. suis*.

Epidemiology

The organism *Br. suis* is more resistant to adverse environmental conditions than *Br. abortus*, although its longevity outside the body has not been fully examined. It is known to survive in feces, urine and water for 4–6 weeks (1). The organism is pathogenic only for pigs and man although other species, including cattle and horses, may be infected, especially if they share a range with feral pigs (6). Isolations have also been made from wild animals including rats (2) and hares (3). An unexpected outbreak in Switzerland where the disease had not appeared since 1946 has been attributed to a spread of infection from horses (4). Amongst pigs, susceptibility varies with age, the incidence of infection being much higher in adults than in young pigs. Although infection before weaning is uncommon, sucking pigs on infected sows may become infected, with maximum agglutinin titers appearing at 8–12 weeks of age but disappearing at 16 weeks. The susceptibility is much greater in the postweaning periods and is the same for both sexes.

No durable immunity develops, and although a stage of herd resistance is apparent after an acute outbreak, the herd is again susceptible within a short time and a further outbreak may occur if infection is reintroduced.

Under field conditions the disease is spread by ingestion and by coitus. Although ingestion of food contaminated by infected semen and urine and discharges from infected sows is probably the commoner method of spread, the localization of infection in the genitalia of the boar makes venereal transmission important in this disease. Introduction into a piggery is usually effected by the introduction of infected pigs. Less commonly the infection may be brought in by other species or on inanimate objects. Wild animals, including hares and rats, may provide a source of infection and ticks are also suspected of transmitting the disease. Spread through a herd is rapid because of the conditions under which pigs are kept. The severe effects of the disease subside quickly as herd resistance is attained, and in herds in which replacements are reared no further trouble may be experienced. When pigs are introduced continuously, further outbreaks are likely to occur.

The disease occurs in most countries but, in spite of its widespread occurrence in the United States, it has not appeared in Canada or Great Britain. Its rate of occurrence in the United States has decreased to the point where it can be considered to be virtually eradicated (5). The disease now achieves its greatest importance as a health hazard for pork butchers. In an enzootic area, the proportion of herds infected is usually high (30–60%) but the number of individual pigs infected may be quite low (5–10%). The disease owes its economic importance to the infertility and reduction in numbers of pigs weaned per litter which occur in infected herds (7). The mortality which occurs during the first month of life may be as high as 80%. The mortality rate is negligible in mature animals but sows and boars may have to be culled because of sterility, and occasional pigs because of posterior paralysis. In addition, eradication involves much financial loss if complete disposal of a registered herd is undertaken.

Br. suis presents a public health hazard particularly to abattoir workers, and to a less extent to farmers and veterinarians. *Br. abortus* and *Br. melitensis* may also be found in pig carcasses and present similar hazards to public health. *Br. suis* may also localize in the mammary gland of cattle without causing clinical abnormality, and where cattle and pigs are run together, the hazard to humans drinking unpasteurized milk may be serious.

Pathogenesis

As in brucellosis caused by *Br. abortus*, there is initial systemic invasion, the organism appearing in the bloodstream for up to 2 months. However, infection with *Br. suis* differs from that caused by *Br. abortus* in that it shows no predilection for localization in the uterus and udder, the organism being found in all body tissues and producing a disease similar to undulant fever in man. The more common manifestations of localization are abortion and infertility due to localization in the uterus; lymphadenitis, especially of the cervical lymph nodes; arthritis and lameness due to bone and joint localization, and posterior paralysis due to osteomyelitis. In boars, involvement of testicles often leads to clinical orchitis (9). It is the widespread involvement of all body tissues which makes handling of the freshly killed carcass such a hazardous procedure and increases the risk of undulant fever in humans eating improperly cooked pork.

A characteristic of the disease is that positive agglutination titers tend to subside with time, especially in sows, although such animals may still be infected and be capable of transmitting the disease.

Clinical findings

The clinical findings in swine brucellosis vary widely, depending upon the site of localization. As in undulant fever in man, the signs are not diagnostic and in many herds a high incidence of reactors is observed with little clinical evidence of disease.

Most prominent are signs of genital tract involvement. In the sow, infertility, which may be temporary, irregular estrus, small litters and abortion occur. The incidence of abortion varies widely between herds but is usually low. Sows abort only once as a rule, and although abortion is most common during the third month, it may occur earlier. Affected sows usually breed normally thereafter. In boars, orchitis with swelling and necrosis of one or both testicles is followed by sterility. Lameness, incoordination and posterior paralysis occur fairly commonly. They are usually gradual in onset and may be caused by arthritis, or more commonly, osteomyelitis of lumbar and sacral vertebral bodies.

A heavy mortality in piglets during the first month of life is sometimes encountered. Most of the losses result from stillbirths and the death of weak piglets within a few hours of birth.

Clinical pathology

Laboratory identification of the disease is difficult. Isolation of the organism should be attempted if suitable material is available. Such material for culture or guinea-pig inoculation includes aborted fetuses, testicular lesions, abscesses and blood. An *agglutination test* carried out on serum is the simplest diagnostic aid but in this disease it has serious limitations. A positive titer does not arise until 8 weeks after infection and many infected pigs have a low titer. For these reasons the test can be used only as a herd test. Herds in which no pigs have titers greater than 1:100 are classified as negative but, in infected herds, any individual pig with a titer greater than 1:25 is classified as positive (10). Because of the limitations of the standard agglutination test, other tests have been under review. Of them the enzyme-linked immunoabsorbent assay (ELISA) appears to be the one most likely to provide a practical answer to the problem (8).

Necropsy findings

Many organs may be involved with chronic changes being most apparent. Chronic metritis manifested by nodular inflammatory thickening and abscessation of the uterine wall is characteristic. Arthritis and necrosis of vertebral bodies in the lumbar region may be found in lame and paralyzed pigs. The clinical orchitis of boars is revealed as testicular necrosis, often accompanied by lesions in the epididymis and seminal vesicles. Pronounced lymphadenopathy, due to reticuloendothelial hyperplasia, and splenic enlargement occur in some cases. Nodular splenitis, in the absence of other lesions, justifies a presumptive diagnosis of brucellosis in pigs (11).

Diagnosis

The protean character of this disease makes it difficult to diagnose unless one is accustomed to including it in a list of diagnostic possibilities. Once this difficulty is overcome, the routine serological examinations of herds soon places the disease in its proper local perspective. It is likely to be confused with brucellosis caused by *Br. melitensis*. Individual animals with posterior paralysis present a major problem in diagnosis since there are so many causes in pigs, including hypovitaminosis A, deficiency of vitamin B complex factors, and fractures of the lumbar vertebrae in osteomalacia. Many poisonings such as organic arsenicals, mercury, rotenone and organophosphatic insecticides may cause posterior paralysis among other things. A summary of the differential diagnosis of posterior paralysis is given in the section on diseases of the spinal cord.

Abortion 'storms' are common in piggeries but in most instances the cause is not determined (12). Known causes include leptospirosis and acute infectious diseases, especially erysipelas. Other bacteria commonly isolated from aborted porcine fetuses include *Listeria monocytogenes*, *Staphylococcus*, *Streptococcus* and *Corynebacterium* spp., and occasionally *Salmonella abortusovis*. Mortality in young sucking pigs is also caused by many agents and the important entities are listed under diseases of the newborn.

Treatment

Exhaustive trials of treatment with a combination of streptomycin parenterally and sulfadiazine orally for long periods failed to reduce the infection rate in pigs (13). Chlortetracycline is also ineffective (14). It is unlikely that the treatments available at present will ever be attempted on a commercial scale.

Control

No suitable vaccine is available. Strain 19 *Br. abortus*, *Br. abortus* 'M' vaccine, and phenol and other extracts of *Br. suis* are all ineffective (15, 16). Control must be by test and disposal. In herds where the incidence of reactors is high, complete disposal of all stock as they reach marketing age is by far the best procedure because of the difficulty in detecting individual infected animals. This is most practicable in commercial pork-producing herds. Restocking the farm should be delayed for 6 months.

The alternative is to commence a two-herd segregation program and this is recommended for pure-bred herds which supply pigs for breeding purposes. Total disposal is not usually economical in these herds. Once a herd diagnosis has been established, all the breeding animals must be considered to be infected; all piglets at weaning are submitted to the serum agglutination test and, if negative, go into new quarters to start the nucleus of a free herd (7). It is probably safer to wean the pigs as young as possible and submit them to the test again at a later stage before mating. If complete protection is desired, these gilts should be allowed to farrow only in isolation, be retested and their piglets used to start the clean herd. A modified scheme based on the above method of weaning and isolating the young pigs as soon as possible but without submitting them to the serum agglutination test has been proposed, but its weakness is that infections may occur and persist in young pigs. Repopulation programs utilizing specific pathogen-free pigs should be effective in eliminating the disease.

After eradication is completed, breakdowns are most likely to occur when infected animals are introduced. All introductions should be from accredited, free herds, should be clinically healthy, and be negative to the serum agglutination test twice at intervals of 3 weeks before introduction.

Eradication of swine brucellosis from an area can only be achieved by developing a nucleus of accredited, free herds and using these as a source of replacements for herds which eradicate by total disposal. Sale of pigs from infected herds for breeding purposes must be prevented.

REFERENCES

(1) Luchsinger, D. W. et al. (1965) *J. Am. vet. med. Assoc.*, *147*, 632.
(2) Cook, I. et al. (1965) *Aust. vet. J.*, *42*, 5.
(3) Bendtsen, H. (1960) *Nord. VetMed.*, *12*, 343
(4) Nicolet, J. et al. (1979) *Schweiz. Arch. Tierheilkd.*, *121*, 231.
(5) Frye, G. H. (1983) *Proc. US Anim. Hlth Assoc.*, *87*, 137.
(6) Cook, D. R. & Noble, J. W. (1984) *Aust. vet. J.*, *61*, 263.
(7) Cameron, H. S. (1957) *Adv. vet. Sci.*, *3*, 275.
(8) Thoen, C. O. et al. (1980) *Can. J. comp. Med.*, *44*, 294.
(9) Retnasabapathy, A. & Chong, S. K. (1967) *Malay vet. J.*, *4*, 130.
(10) Hubbard, E. D. & Hoerlein, A. B. (1952) *J. Am. vet. med. Assoc.*, *120*, 138.
(11) Anderson, W. A. & Davis, C. L. (1957) *J. Am. vet. med. Assoc.*, *131*, 141.
(12) Saunders, C. N. (1958) *Vet. Rec.*, *70*, 965.
(13) Hutchings, L. M. et al. (1950) *Am. J. vet. Res.*, *11*, 388.
(14) Bunnell, D. E. et al. (1953) *Am. J. vet. Res.*, *14*, 160.
(15) Manthei, C. A. (1948) *Am. J. vet. Res.*, *9*, 40.
(16) Bunnel, D. E. et al. (1953) *Am. J. vet. Res.*, *14*, 164.

Brucellosis caused by *Brucella melitensis*

Brucella melitensis causes brucellosis in goats and 'Malta' or 'Mediterranean' fever in man.

Etiology

Brucella melitensis causes brucellosis in goats and is capable of infecting most species of domestic animals. It appears to be increasing in numbers in the cattle population in developing countries.

Epidemiology

Goats are highly susceptible, sheep less so (1). The organism is capable of causing disease in cattle and has been isolated from swine. In Europe the incidence of the infection in cattle appears to be increasing and in Malta about a third of the cattle reacting positively to the brucellosis agglutination test are infected with *Br. melitensis* (2). Accurate identification of the organism can only be carried out by the use of serological tests and many identifications based on cultural and biochemical tests have been invalid (3).

Transmission between species occurs readily and is probably by ingestion as in other forms of brucellosis. Infected does, whether they abort or kid normally, discharge large numbers of brucellae in their uterine exudates. The vaginal exudate of infected virgin or open animals may also contain the bacteria, but transmission between animals is thought to require the massive exposure that only an infected placenta can provide. In sheep the degree of infection of milk and uterine exudate is much less than in goats. Viable kids are infected, and in some cases the disease persists in a latent form until sexual maturity when clinical signs become evident (4). However, if kids are weaned early from their dams and from the infected environment they are usually free from the infection as adults. The same conditions may apply in *Br. melitensis* infection in sheep (2).

This disease was originally observed in southern Europe but has since been found in Central America, the United States and Africa, and probably occurs in most parts of the world where goats are raised except perhaps Britain and Scandinavia. The importance and distribution of this form of brucellosis in animals have not been accurately determined but it has considerable importance because of the role of the organism in the production of 'Malta' or 'Mediterranean' fever in humans drinking infected milk from goats, cattle and sheep. The disease is of special importance in African native communities where goats cohabit with their owners at night (5).

Pathogenesis

As in other forms of brucellosis, the pathogenesis depends upon localization in lymph nodes, udder and uterus after an initial bacteremia. In goats, this bacteremia may be sufficiently severe to produce a systemic reaction, and blood culture may remain positive for a month, often with no detectable agglutinins in the serum. Localization in the placenta leads to the development of placentitis with subsequent abortion (6). After abortion, uterine infection persists for up to 5 months and the mammary gland may remain infected for years. Spontaneous recovery may occur particularly in goats which become infected while not pregnant (2). In sheep the development of the disease is very similar to that in goats (7).

Clinical findings

Abortion during late pregnancy is the most obvious sign in goats and sheep, but as in other species there may be a 'storm' of abortions when the disease is introduced, followed by a period of flock resistance during which abortions do not occur. In experimental infections, a systemic reaction with fever, depression, loss of weight and sometimes diarrhea occurs. These signs may also occur in acute, natural outbreaks in goats and may be accompanied by mastitis, lameness, hygroma and orchitis. Osteoarthritis, synovitis and nervous signs are not uncommon in sheep. In pigs the disease is indistinguishable clinically from brucellosis caused by *Br. suis*. In many instances, *Br. melitensis* infection reaches a high incidence in a group of animals without signs of obvious illness.

Clinical pathology

Positive blood culture soon after the infection occurs, or isolation of the organism from the aborted fetus, vaginal mucus or milk are the common laboratory procedures used in diagnosis. The bacteremia persists for a month after infection, and mammary gland infection may persist for years (8). An agglutination test and a complement fixation test are available (9) but results with the former are likely to be confusing because of the transient rise in titer in some animals. The results with the complement fixation test are more consistent (7). An intradermal allergic test has been described but is of limited value in control of the disease in areas where the disease is enzootic (2). Tests are also conducted on milk. They include the milk ring test, the whey complement fixation tests, whey Coombs or antiglobulin test and whey agglutination tests (10). The milk ring test is less specific than serum agglutination test but is good enough for a screening test. *Br. melitensis* is often present in the milk. Laboratory diagnosis is not easy and for detection of the disease in individual animals a number of tests carried out on several occasions may be necessary (11). If only one test is possible the complement fixation test is recommended (5). The serum agglutination test is thought to be unsatisfactory and the rose bengal plate and agar immunodiffusion tests are reasonable substitutes for the complement fixation test if that is not available (2).

Necropsy findings

There are no lesions characteristic of this form of brucellosis. The causative organism can often be isolated from all tissues but the spleen is the most common site of infection.

Diagnosis

In many instances, a diagnosis of *Br. melitensis* infection in animals is made only because the infection has been diagnosed in human contacts, provoking an examination of the local animal population. The disease varies in its manifestations, and its positive diagnosis can only be made by isolation of the organism.

Treatment

Treatment is unlikely to be undertaken in animals.

Control

Control measures must include hygiene at kidding or lambing and the disposal of infected or reactor animals. Separate pens for kidding does, early weaning of kids from their does, and their environment, and vaccination are recommended. The need to test and cull introduced and resident animals likely to be carriers is recommended, but difficult to effect because of the inaccuracy of the tests. Because of the possibility that kids may be infected at birth and carry the disease for life, it may be more economic to dispose of the entire flock. In developing countries it is often not possible to follow the standard hygienic procedures recommended for use in more closely controlled environments. In those circumstances vaccination may be the only worthwhile procedure available (3). The universally recommended vaccine is Elberg's Rev 1 which is effective in both sheep and goats (3, 13). A high degree of immunity is produced and lasts for more than 4 years in goats (3) and 2½ years in sheep (14). However, vaccination of adult or pregnant does has drawbacks, because of the excretion of living *Br. melitensis* in the milk, the long-term persistence of positive serological tests making eradication by test and slaughter difficult (12), or abortion which may result. Reduction of the number of organisms in the vaccinating dose has made it less likely to cause abortion, be excreted in the milk or interfere with serological tests (15).

A similar degree of immunity is claimed from a formalin killed adjuvant vaccine 53 H 38 which can be used in lactating and pregnant does (16). *Br. abortus* strain 19 has also been used and appears to give protection which is as good as that achieved with the attenuated *Br. melitensis* vaccine (17). *Br. suis* type 2 vaccine is reported to have the same effect (18).

REFERENCES

(1) Renoux, G. et al. (1957) *Vet. Bull.*, *27*, 283 (see also 1957 *Adv. vet. Sci.*, *3*, 241).
(2) Waghela, S. et al. (1980) *Res. vet. Sci.*, *28*, 168.
(3) Kolar, J. (1984) *Prev. vet. Med.*, *2*, 215.
(4) Alton, G. G. (1970) *Br. vet. J.*, *126*, 61.
(5) Philpott, M. & Auko Otieno (1972) *Br. vet. J.*, *128*, 642.
(6) Collier, I. R. & Molello, J. A. (1964) *Am. J. vet. Res.*, *25*, 930.
(7) Shimi, A. & Tabatabayi, A. H. (1981) *Bull. Off. int. Epizootol.*, *93*, 1411.
(8) Meyer, K. F. (1951) *Boln Of. sanit. pan-am.*, *30*, 9.
(9) Unel, S. et al. (1969) *J. comp. Pathol.*, *79*, 155.
(10) Ebadi, A. (1971) *Br. vet. J.*, *127*, 105.
(11) Renoux, G. (1961) *Ann. Zootechnol.*, *10*, 233.
(12) Waghela, S. (1983) *Vet. Rec.*, *112*, 476.
(13) Elberg, S. S. (1981) *Vet. Bull.*, *51*, 67.
(14) Entessor, F. et al. (1967) *J. comp. Pathol.*, *77*, 367.
(15) Alton, G. G. et al. (1974) *Am. J. vet. Res.*, *33*, 1747.
(16) Miereles, M. L. et al. (1974) *Bull. Off. int. Epizootol.*, *82*, 25.
(17) Neeman, L. (1963) *Refuah Vet.*, *20*, 134.
(18) Lu, B. K. et al. (1983) *Acta vet. zootol. Sinica*, *14*, 133.

DISEASES CAUSED BY *HEMOPHILUS* AND *MORAXELLA* spp.

Hemophilus suis plays an important role as a secondary bacterial invader in swine influenza and is dealt with under that heading. The exact identity of the related organism *Histophilus ovis* is still debated and it may be the same genus and species as *Hemophilus agni* and *H. somnus* (1). It is recorded as a cause of epididymitis in rams (2) and of polyarthritis in young lambs and abortion and mastitis in ewes (3).

REFERENCES

(1) Stephen, L. R. et al. (1983) *J. clin. Microbiol.*, *17*, 728.
(2) Low, J. C. & Graham, M. M. (1985) *Vet. Rec.*, *117*, 64.
(3) Webb, R. F. (1983) *Res. vet. Sci.*, *35*, 30.

Infectious keratitis of cattle (pinkeye, blight)

The common infectious keratitis of cattle is caused by *Moraxella* (*Hemophilus*) *bovis*. It is not a fatal disease, but its total economic impact is enormous, its occurrence is worldwide and there is at present no control program of even moderate efficiency.

Etiology

Hemolytic *M. bovis* is known to be an important factor in the development of the disease and it is likely that it is the only infectious agent concerned (1). From the results of experiments to reproduce the disease experimentally in gnotobiotic calves (25) and from studies on corneal tissue culture (23), it seems likely that there is a great deal of variation in virulence between strains of *M. bovis* which can also be distinguished by their pilus antigens (29). There appear to be at least six distinct serogroups. It has also been demonstrated that some of the cultural characteristics of the organisms isolated from the conjunctiva changed markedly as the level of solar ultraviolet radiation changed (3). This may account for previous variations in the results of transmission experiments. It also seems likely that *M. bovis* initiates the disease and that other agents are responsible for some of the severe keratitis which occurs. The infectious bovine rhinotracheitis virus causes a different disease, a conjunctivitis rather than a keratitis, but it may also be involved with *M. bovis* in causing the more severe disease. Other unidentified rickettsiae, chlamydia and viruses have been identified as common participants, and *Neisseria catarrhalis* (6) and *Mycoplasma* sp. especially *M. bovoculi* (11, 19), are also suspected of some etiological involvement. An organism, closely related to *Moraxella bovis*, *Branhamella ovis* (syn. *Neisseria ovis*), has been the cause of a severe conjunctivitis in goats. The importance of *Neisseria* spp. (35) is supported by the observation that a vaccine containing it is highly protective in experimental circumstances in spite of the presence of pathogenic *M. bovis* (35). Because the naturally occurring disease is usually much more severe than that produced experimentally factors other than infectious agents have been examined. Solar radiation has been shown to have an enhancing effect (4) and flies and dust are suspected. On the other hand, the introduction of pure cultures of *M. bovis* into the conjunctival sac of cattle causes the disease, mild though it may be, even when the conjunctiva is uninjured (5). A microbiological model of the disease in cattle has been produced in a specific strain of mice (32). Also the organism is not usually found in the conjunctival sacs of cattle with no history of 'pinkeye'.

Epidemiology

Only cattle are affected, the young being most susceptible. Previous infection appears to confirm a significant immunity which lasts through to the next season when further reinfection confers further immunity (8).

There is no mortality, and cases in which there is permanent blindness or loss of an eye are rare. However, the morbidity rate can be as high as 80% with the peak infection rate at the 3rd to 4th week of the outbreak. It is commonly observed that there is a much higher prevalence of the disease in *Bos taurus* (British breed) cattle as distinct from *Bos indicus* (hump-backed Zebu type) cattle (7, 22). The severity and proportion of bilateral infections is much greater in *Bos taurus* cattle than in crossbreds, and the disease can be considered not to occur in pure-bred Zebus. In British-bred cattle there was also a relationship between rate and severity of infection and the degree of eyelid pigmentation, eyes with complete pigmentation being less affected. The variation in susceptibility was reflected in body weights, differences being as high as 10%. This effect of pigmentation on susceptibility may be the basis of an apparent inherited resistance of some families of Hereford cattle (37).

Because the disease is most common in summer and autumn, and reaches epizootic proportions when flies and dust are abundant and grass is long, transmission is thought to be by means of these agents contaminated by the ocular discharges of infected cattle. The face fly (*Musca autumnalis*), because of its preference for the area around the eyes, is thought to be an important vector of the infection and is known to remain infected for periods of up to 3 days. Under experimental conditions, transmission is unusual in the absence of flies (10) and occurs generally in their presence (30). *M. bovis* can be isolated from the crops of *Musca autumnalis* that have fed on the eyes of infected cattle (38). The conjunctiva is the probable portal of infection. Persistence of the disease from year to year is by means of infected animals which can act as carriers for periods exceeding 1 year. In herds in which the disease is enzootic the prevalence will vary from year to year but it will always be most common in young cattle during their first summer. When the disease invades a susceptible population, cattle of all ages are likely to be affected.

The disease occurs in most countries of the world and is most common in summer and autumn. The incidence and severity of the disease both affect the degree of wastage which results, and both vary greatly from year to year and may reach epizootic proportions in feedlots and in cattle running at pasture. Loss of milk production or bodily condition may be caused by the discomfort, failure to feed and temporary blindness. The mean body weight of affected calves at weaning time may be reduced by as much as 10% (9). Such differences are common and are an indication of the severity of the disease (12). Occasionally animals become completely blind and those at pasture may die of starvation.

Although summer and autumn are the seasons in which the disease occurs most commonly, severe outbreaks can be experienced in winter time especially if the cattle are confined in close quarters such as barns or intensive feedlots.

Pathogenesis

A dermonecrotic endotoxin is produced by the organism and is capable of causing typical lesions in calves and rabbits when injected intracorneally. In natural cases the lesions are localized in the eye, the organism not reaching the bloodstream of the affected animal. Serum agglutinins to *M. bovis* are detectable and immunity after an attack is usually good for up to a year although recurrent attacks may occur in the one animal. The immunity has been shown to be a general one (24) and not one confined to the conjunctival sac.

Clinical findings

An incubation period of 2–3 days is usual although longer intervals, up to 3 weeks, have been observed after experimental introduction of the bacteria. Injection of the corneal vessels and edema of the conjunctiva are the earliest signs and are accompanied by a copious water lacrimation, blepharospasm, photophobia and, in some cases, a slight to moderate fever with fall in milk yield and depression of appetite. In 1–2 days, a small opacity appears in the center of the cornea and this may become elevated and ulcerated during the next 2 days although spontaneous recovery at this stage is quite common. This opacity becomes quite extensive and at the peak of the inflammation, about 6 days after signs first appear, it may cover the entire cornea. The color of the opacity varies from white to deep yellow. As the acute inflammation subsides, the ocular discharge becomes purulent and the opacity begins to shrink, complete recovery occurring after a total course of 3–5 weeks.

One or both eyes may be affected. The degree of ulceration in the early stages can be readily determined by the infusion of a 2% fluorescein solution into the conjunctival sac, the ulcerated area retaining the stain.

About 2% of eyes have complete residual opacity but most heal completely with a small, white scar persisting in some. In severe cases the cornea becomes conical in shape, there is marked vascularization of the cornea, and ulceration at the tip of the swelling leads to underrunning of the cornea with bright yellow pus surrounded by a zone of erythema. These eyes may rupture and result in complete blindness.

Clinical pathology

Swabs should be taken from the conjunctival sac and the sensitivity of cultured organisms determined. *M. bovis* has rather exacting requirements in culture media and special care is needed if the organism is to be identified. The hemolytic form of the bacterium is noticeably more pathogenic than the non-hemolytic form.

Serum agglutinins (1:80 to 1:640) are present 2–3 weeks after clinical signs commence and a modified gel diffusion precipitin test is capable of detecting *M. bovis* antibodies. A fluorescent antibody technique for identification of *M. bovis* is available also (24). Necropsy examinations are not usually carried out and the paucity of pathological information contributes to the poor definition of the disease.

Diagnosis

Traumatic conjunctivitis is usually easily diagnosed because of the presence of foreign matter in the eye or evidence of a physical injury. The infectious nature of keratitis caused by *M. bovis* presents difficulties in differentiation between it and the conjunctivitis of infectious bovine rhinotracheitis (IBR) and the keratitis of bovine malignant catarrh, rinderpest and bovine viral diarrhea (mucosal disease). All of these diseases have other obvious signs and their ocular lesions and development are quite different. Photosensitive keratitis and thelaziasis are other diseases requiring to be differentiated.

Pasteurella multocida (capsular type A) has also been isolated from the eyes of housed heifers which experienced outbreaks of severe keratitis. The lesions are different from the typical ones caused by *Moraxella bovis* because there is no conjunctivitis until the late stages of the disease. It is marked by a severe loss of corneal stroma within 72 hours of onset. The lesion is a severe interstitial keratitis with deep ulceration. Intensive topical treatment with gentamicin plus autogenous vaccination gives good response quickly (2).

Treatment

Early, acute cases respond well to treatment with ophthalmic ointments and solutions containing antibiotics such as chloramphenicol, oxytetracycline, penicillin–streptomycin mixtures and other common antibiotics. For best results with most medications the preparation should be instilled in the conjunctival sacs at least three times daily but under field conditions one treatment is usually all that is practicable and economical. An exception to this rule is benzathine cloxacillin which appears to have an affinity for corneal and conjunctival tissues and persists in the conjunctival sac for 2–3 days, longer than the duration of subconjunctivally injected antibiotics (36). Severe cases should be placed in a dark shelter out of direct sunlight. If housing is not possible, eye flap-patches are now available and effective. They are glued on above the eye and can be flipped up like a flap for medication of the eye. Animal attendants must be instructed on the importance of carefully instilling the ophthalmic ointment under both the upper and lower conjunctival sacs to ensure diffuse medication.

When corneal vascularization is extensive the injection of a mixture of corticosteroid and antibiotic under the *bulbar* conjunctivae is recommended to promote healing and the more rapid local absorption and distribution of the drug and to minimize the rapid loss of topically administered preparations. Injection of the penicillin through the skin rather than through the conjunctiva confers a significantly longer presence of penicillin in the conjunctival sac (27). Dexamethasone (1 mg) with 2 ml of a mixture of penicillin–streptomycin is a satisfactory subconjunctival injection but many other preparations are also suitable. Often one injection is sufficient but a repeated one may be necessary daily for a few days in advanced cases. Recovery may require 3–4 weeks and daily examination of the eye should be made to detect any complication which might occur. Another technique for prolonging the maintenance of high levels of antibiotic in the conjunctival sac is the use of collagen inserts which are impregnated with an antibiotic (33).

Because of the short period of effectiveness of medicaments applied topically it is sometimes expedient to treat affected animals systemically if blood levels of an antibacterial can be maintained. At therapeutic levels for 12–24 hours the levels in tears may be similar to those in serum and provide a constant source to the affected eye. For example, sulfadimidine at the normal dose rate of 100 mg/kg body weight is an effective parenteral treatment, and a longacting oxytetracycline (20 mg/kg intramuscularly) appears to be effective with one injection (31).

When corneal ulceration has occurred recovery is always protracted and daily medication with ophthalmic antibiotic ointment is necessary. The use of topical ophthalmic anesthetics combined with atropine administration may also be indicated to minimize ciliary spasm and pain. Severe cases may require that the third eyelid be temporarily sutured across the globe of the eye for several days to promote healing. A modified membrana nictitans flap technique was successful in the treatment of 96% of 1845 cattle affected with ulcerative keratitis (15). The flap was held in place for 7–10 days.

The injection of an autogenous bacterin repeated several times at weekly intervals may aid in the resolution of existing ocular lesions (14).

Control

Eradication or prevention of the disease does not seem possible under extensive range conditions, because of the method of spread but if fly control can be fitted into the farm's management program this should significantly reduce the infection rate. In many herds the best that can be done is to keep animals under close surveillance and isolate and treat any cattle that show excessive lacrimation and blepharospasm. The fact that affected animals are immune for up to 12 months suggests that vaccination may be efficient in control. However, the commercial bacterins, although available, have given inconsistent results, providing at best limited protection from subsequent infection and clinical disease (16, 18). They are killed, whole-cell vaccines injected intramuscularly. Their disadvantages include the need to give at least three injections 14 days apart, to allow a sufficient period of about 40 days before the disease is expected for the vaccination program to begin, and the not infrequent occurrence of anaphylaxis after injection of the vaccine made from suspensions of whole culture. To avoid the need for repeated injections an adjuvant vaccine has been tested but without apparent benefit (26). It is possible that the variation in virulence and antigenicity between strains of *M. bovis* may affect the efficacy of available bacterins (25). Autogenous vaccines have also been tried and appear to exert little influence on the occurrence of the disease (16). Vaccination of cattle with a vaccine made from sonicated pili of *Moraxella bovis* may induce protective immunity against homologous strain challenge exposure (18). This appears to be the most effective vaccination technique so far. However, field results are not uniformly favorable (28) and it does not reduce the duration of the infected state in calves vaccinated during the course of the disease (13).

Weekly treatment of both eyes of calves, but not the cows, with a furazolidone eye spray has been shown to be a more effective prophylaxis than vaccination with a commercial bacterin (16).

Total eyelid pigmentation may reduce the incidence of this disease but the recorded differences (20, 21, 37) are unlikely to arouse enthusiasm for a genetic approach to the problem.

REVIEW LITERATURE

Cox, P. J. (1984) Infectious bovine keratoconjunctivitis; *recent progress. Vet. Ann.*, 75–79.
George, L. W. (1984) Clinical infectious bovine keratoconjunctivitis. *Comp. cont. Educ.*, 6, S712.
George, L. W. (1984) Antibiotic treatment of *Moraxella bovis* infection of cattle. *J. Am. vet. med. Assoc.*, *185*, 1206.
Punch, P. I. & Slatter, D. H. (1984) A review of infectious bovine keratoconjunctivitis. *Vet. Bull.*, *54*, 193–207.

REFERENCES

(1) Pugh, G. W. et al. (1976) *Am. J. vet. Res.*, *37*, 57, 493.
(2) van Damme, D. et al. (1980) *Bov. Pract.*, *1*, 35.
(3) Lepper, A. V. D. & Barton, I. J. (1987) *Aust. vet. J.*, *64*, 33.
(4) Kopecky, K. E. et al. (1980) *Am. J. vet. Res.*, *41*, 1412.
(5) Weech, G. M. et al. (1983) *Comp. Immunol. Microbiol. infect. Dis.*, *6*, 81.
(6) Wilcox, G. E. (1970) *Aust. vet. J.*, *46*, 253.
(7) Makinde, A. A. et al. (1985) *Br. vet. J.*, *141*, 643.
(8) Pugh, G. W. & Hughes, D. E. (1975) *J. Am. vet. med. Assoc.*, *167*, 310.
(9) Killenger, A. H. et al. (1977) *Vet. Med.*, *72*, 618.
(10) Kopecky, K. E. et al. (1986) *Am. J. vet. Res.*, *47*, 622.
(11) Kelly, J. I. et al. (1983) *Vet. Rec.*, *112*, 482.
(12) Thrift, F. A. & Overfield, J. R. (1974) *J. anim. Sci.*, *38*, 1179.
(13) Pugh, G. W. et al. (1980) *Am. J. vet. Res.*, *41*, 264.
(14) Storey, R. C. et al. (1977) *Vet. Med. SAC*, *72*, 1050.
(15) Anderson, J. F. et al. (1976) *J. Am. vet. med. Assoc.*, *168*, 706.
(16) Pugh, G. W. et al. (1982) *Am. J. vet. Res.*, *43*, 1081
(17) Bulgin, M. S. & Dubose, D. A. (1982) *Vet. Med.*, *77*, 1791.
(18) Lehr, C. et al. (1985) *Cornell Vet.*, *75*, 484.
(19) Rosenbusch, R. F. (1983) *Am. J. vet. Res.*, *44*, 1621.
(20) Caspari, E. L. et al. (1980) *Br. vet. J.*, *136*, 210.
(21) Ward, J. K. & Nelson, M. K. (1979) *J. anim. Sci.*, *49*, 361.
(22) Dodt, R. M. (1977) *Aust. vet. J.*, *53*, 128.
(23) Chandler, R. L. et al. (1985) *J. comp. Pathol.*, *95*, 415.
(24) Kopecky, K. E. et al. (1983) *Am. J. vet. Res.*, *44*, 260.
(25) Pugh, G. E. et al. (1978) *Am. J. vet. Res.*, *39*, 55.
(26) Hughes, D. E. et al. (1977) *Am. J. vet. Res.*, *38*, 1905.
(27) Abeynayake, P. & Cooper, B. S. (1985) *NZ vet. J.*, *33*, 6.
(28) Bateman, K. G. et al. (1986) *Can. vet. J.*, *27*, 23.
(29) Lepper, A. W. D. & Hermans, L. R. (1986) *Aust. vet. J.*, *63*, 401.
(30) Arends, J. J. et al. (1984) *J. econ. Entomol.*, *77*, 394 & 399.
(31) George, L. W. & Smith, J. A. (1985) *J. vet. Pharmacol. Therap.*, *8*, 55.
(32) Chandler, R. L. et al. (1982) *Res. vet. Sci.*, *32*, 128.
(33) Slatter, D. H. et al. (1982) *Aust. vet J.*, *59*, 14.
(34) Kopecky, K. E. et al. (1983) *Am. J. vet. Res.*, *44*, 260.
(35) Gwin, R. M. et al. (1984) *Proc. 16th Ann. Conv. Am. Assoc. Bov. Practnrs*, pp. 198–203.
(36) Buswell, J. F. & Hewett, G. R. (1983) *Vet. Rec.*, *113*, 621.
(37) Pugh, G. W. et al. (1986) *Am. J. vet Res.*, *47*, 885.
(38) Glass, H. W. & Gerhardt, R. R. (1983) *J. econ. Entomol.*, *76*, 532.

Septicemia caused by *Hemophilus agni*

An acute, highly fatal septicemia caused by *H. agni* has occurred in lambs aged 4–7 months (1, 4). Depression, high fever (42°C, 107°F) and disinclination to move due to muscle stiffness are the obvious clinical signs and affected lambs may die within 12 hours of becoming ill. Lambs which survive more than 24 hours develop a severe arthritis. The method of transmission is unknown but the disease does not appear to spread by pen contact nor can it be produced by oral, nasal or conjunctival exposure to the organism. At necropsy the most striking feature is the presence of multiple hemorrhages throughout the carcass. Focal hepatic necrosis surrounded by a zone of hemorrhage is also a constant finding. Lambs which die in the early stages of the disease show minimal joint changes but those that survive for more than 24 hours develop a fibrinopurulent arthritis. A basilar meningitis also develops in the more protracted cases. Death appears to result from asphyxia due to pulmonary congestion and edema. Histologically the disease is basically a disseminated bacterial thrombosis leading to a severe focal vasculitis. This change is most apparent in the liver and skeletal muscles.

The characteristic hepatic lesions and histology serve to identify the disease, and final diagnosis depends on isolation of the organism. A complement fixation test is available (2), detectable antibodies persisting for about 3 months. The disease is likely to be confused with acute septicemia caused by *E. coli* or *Past. hemolytica*, and enterotoxemia.

The morbidity rate is undetermined but the mortality rate is likely to be 100% unless treatment is undertaken. Streptomycin is effective if given early. Because of the acute nature of the disease, vaccination is likely to be the only satisfactory method of control. Although a satisfactory vaccine has not been developed, immunity after a field attack seems to be solid.

A similar disease has been observed in baby pigs of 1–2 weeks of age and from which an organism of the *H. parainfluenzae* group has been isolated (3). Treatment of in-contact pigs with streptomycin after the first death prevented further losses in subsequent episodes.

REFERENCES

(1) Kennedy, P. C. et al. (1958) *Am. J. vet. Res.*, *19*, 645.
(2) Biberstein, D. L. et al. (1959) *J. Am. vet. med. Assoc.*, *135*, 61.
(3) Thomson, R. G. & Ruhnke, H. L. (1963) *Can. vet. J.*, *4*, 271.
(4) Lundberg, M. S. (1986) *Can. vet. J.*, *27*, 501.

Hemophilus septicemia of cattle

This is a septicemia caused by *Hemophilus somnus* which results in localization in several tissues and organs causing meningoencephalitis, synovitis, pleuritis and pneumonia.

Etiology

Hemophilus somnus is considered as the causative agent although the correct taxonomic position of the organism has been a point of concern because of serological cross-reaction with other *Hemophilus* spp. (1).

Examination of a large number of strains of the organism reveals that most are antigenically identical (1). A commercially available API ZYM system can be used to distinguish isolates of *H. somnus* from different anatomical locations and from bacteria which are similar, namely, *Histophilus ovis* and *Hemophilus agni* (17). There is, however, considerable heterogeneity among *H. somnus* cultures (22). There are at least three sets of antigen in *H. somnus*—American, Swiss, and common—and they reflect the geographical origin of the respective strains and not the pathological or anatomical origin (22). The ultrastructure of the organism has been described (10).

Epidemiology

The disease occurs most commonly in feedlot cattle in North America after they have been comingled from different sources. The disease also occurs in nursing beef calves and young cows on pasture and in young dairy cattle, but to a much lesser extent. The disease has also been recognized in the United Kingdom, Germany and Switzerland (1). The incidence of inapparent infection is much greater than the rate of clinical disease. Serological surveys indicate that about 25% of normal cattle have antibody to the organism. Among those which have had the disease and survived, the serological reactor rate varies from 56 to 100%. Some surveys indicate more positive reactors in beef cattle and dairy cattle from infected herds than in dairy cattle from clinically normal herds (21). The percentage of cattle which seroconvert may be higher in dairy herds of more than 100 cows than in smaller herds (19). One of the perplexing questions about this disease is why only a small percentage of animals (usually less than 2%) in a population will develop meningoencephalitis when almost 100% of the animals have seroconverted to the organism. The morbidity in a herd is low and averages about 2%, but may be up to 10% in some outbreaks. The case fatality rate, however, is 90% if affected animals are not identified and treated early in the course of the disease.

The disease occurs most commonly in feedlot cattle from 4 to 12 months of age during the fall and winter months, which may be a reflection of stress associated with crowding and cold and changing weather. In Canadian studies the disease occurs most commonly in cattle about 4 weeks after arrival in the feedlot with a range from 1 week to 7 months (2). A history of respiratory tract disease preceding the outbreak is common and in some cases the hemophilus meningoencephalitis had occurred in the same herd in the previous year.

The method of transmission and portal of entry are unclear. The organism can be isolated from the respiratory and reproductive tracts from 3 to 10% of normal animals (9). In bulls, the organism has been isolated from semen (12, 13) and the preputial orifice, preputial cavity, urinary bladder, accessory sex glands, ampulla of the ductus deferens, and the preputial washings of steers (14). Thus, the potential for venereal transmission of *H. somnus*, for lateral spread from the genital tract, and for environmental contamination by the organism is possible. The organism has also been isolated from the vagina, vestibular gland, cervix, uterus and bladder of cows (15). The organism can colonize the vagina of cows without causing disease and it is thought to have a primary etiological role in vaginitis and cervicitis in cows (41, 42). The role of *H. somnus* in diseases of the bovine reproductive tract has been reviewed (16). The organism has been isolated from the udder secretions of cattle with naturally occurring mastitis (43, 44).

Urine is also a source of the organism. The young beef calf in a cow-calf herd can become infected as early as a month of age and become a nasal carrier of the organism without showing any signs of clinical disease. The mature cow is considered to be a major source of the organism for the calf. The method of transmission is presumed to be by contact with infective respiratory and reproductive secretions or by aerosol transmission especially in close-contact feedlots.

The organism can survive more than 70 days when it is mixed with cerebrospinal fluid, whole blood, blood plasma, vaginal mucus and milk and frozen at $-70°C$ ($-94°F$) (18). At 23·5°C (73·5°F) the organism can survive beyond 70 days when mixed with whole blood and nasal mucus. The viability of the organism urine at all temperatures is less than 24 hours and less than 15 minutes at 20°C (68°F) and 37°C (98°F).

Serum antibody tests measured by several serological tests do not correlate with susceptibility to clinical disease (4). Naturally acquired humoral immunity does not influence the outcome of experimental intravenous inoculation of the organism. The role of naturally occurring antibodies in protecting cattle from naturally occurring disease is not known. The levels of naturally occurring serum bactericidal activity to *H. somnus* are low or absent in calves at 4–6 months of age, when they are most susceptible to the nervous form of the disease (20). The levels increase with age and are high in mature cows; yearlings have intermediate levels. Vaccinated animals also develop high serum concentrations of bactericidal activity.

Certain suppressive components in *H. somnus* have been identified which inhibit the function of polymorphonuclear leukocytes (23, 24).

Pathogenesis

The disease is now considered to be a septicemia with localization in many tissues and organs, causing a vasculitis. The sequence of events in the genesis of the lesions may be adhesion of the organism to vascular endothelial cells. Contraction and desquamation of cells with exposure of subendothelial collagen, thrombosis, and vasculitis is followed by ischemic necrosis of adjacent parenchyma (3). The common site of localization is the brain, causing a thrombomeningoencephalitis. The meningoencephalitis is characterized by multifocal areas of hemorrhagic necrosis throughout the brain resulting in the major clinical findings of depression, paresis and recumbency. Other sites include the synovia, causing synovitis and arthritis, and the pleura and lungs, causing pleuritis and pneumonia. Fibrin thrombi occur in the small vessels and capillaries of the liver, spleen, kidney, lung, heart and brain which suggests that disseminated intravascular coagulation may be a feature of the pathogenesis of hemophilus septicemia (25). Although *H. sommus* has been isolated from cattle with bronchopneumonia and fibrinous pneumonia in pure culture and in combination with *Pasteurella* spp., the lungs of cattle dying with thrombomeningoencephalitis are not usually affected with a fibrinous pneumonia. The microscopic lesions in the lungs of cattle with pneumonia from which *H. somnus* was isolated consists of suppurative to necrotizing bronchiolitis, particularly in calves with subacute to chronic pneumonia (26). There may be hemorrhagic interstitial pneumonia, with thrombosis and neutrophil infiltration. Laryngitis and polypoid tracheitis have been attributed to *H. somnus*, but the evidence is limited (8).

Hemorrhagic necrotic lesions also occur in the spinal cord which contributes to the paralysis. Lesions in the esophagus, forestomachs and intestines may account for the bloat and alimentary tract stasis which occurs in the experimental disease (1).

The septicemia usually causes a marked leukopenia, neutropenia and degenerative left shift.

Cattle dying of experimentally induced and naturally occurring disease have high levels of agglutinating anti-*H. somnus* antibody, but not of complement-fixing antibody (4). Because septicemia can occur even with high levels of serum antibody it is hypothesized that the formation of antigen–antibody complexes may contribute to the development of the vasculitis. It is possible that previous exposure to *H. somnus* infection is necessary for typical thrombomeningoencephalitis to occur. Inoculation of colostrum-deprived calves with *H. somnus* causes septicemia but does not produce lesions typical of thrombomeningoencephalitis (6). This suggests that the disease may be an example of a type III hypersensitivity reaction or serum sickness (4).

Following experimental inoculation the organism will produce lesions in developing chick embryos (27), epididymitis in hamsters (28), a suppurative vaginitis followed by a severe placentitis and metritis when the organism invades the uterus at the time of parturition (29), death of fetuses with a placentitis with vascular lesions when injected into the amniotic cavity (30) and chronic or gangrenous mastitis when injected into the mammary gland of lactating cows (31).

Clinical findings

It is common for several animals to be affected within a few days or at one time, but single cases do occur. In the peracute form of the disease cattle may be found dead without any premonitory signs and often this may be the first sign of disease. The organism has been isolated from a 5-month-old ram which died suddenly with pathological evidence of septicemia (32).

In the more common acute form, in which there is usually neurological involvement, cattle may be found down in lateral or sternal recumbency and may or may not be able to get up. The temperature is usually increased up to 41–42°C (105·8–107·6°F) but in some cases it may be normal. There is usually depression, the eyes are usually partially or fully closed and, while blindness may be present in both eyes, it is usually confined to one eye, or the eyes may be normal. Some cattle which attempt to rise from the recumbent position have considerable difficulty and exhibit obvious ataxia and weakness. Others which are able to stand, when attempting to walk, will knuckle over on the hind fetlocks, are grossly ataxic and usually fall down after walking a short distance. In the recumbent position opisthotonus, nystagmus, muscular tremors, hyperesthesia and occasionally convulsions will occur, but the emphasis is on muscular weakness and paralysis rather than signs of irritation. Otitis media with concurrent meningitis has been described in an 8-month-old heifer (35).

The ocular lesions consist of foci of retinal hemorrhages and accumulations of exudate which appear like 'cotton tufts'. While these fundic lesions are not present in all cattle affected with *Hemophilus somnus*, they are considered a valuable aid to clinical diagnosis. The organism has been isolated from the conjunctival sacs of feedlot cattle affected with conjunctivitis (33).

The synovitis is characterized by distension of the joint capsules, usually of the major movable joints such as the hock and stifle joints, but any joint may be involved. Pain and lameness are only mild and in animals which are treated early the synovitis usually resolves in a few days. In a few cases there is marked lameness and a preference for recumbency associated with hemorrhages in muscle. Laryngitis, tracheitis, pleuritis and pneumonia occur alone or in combination with the acute neurological form of the disease. Dyspnea is common in all of these and the respirations are usually rapid and shallow. Chronic suppurative orchiepididymitis in a calf from which *H. somnus* was isolated has been described (34).

The disease is rapidly fatal in 8–12 hours if not treated when signs are first noticed. Affected cattle which are treated before they become recumbent will commonly recover within 6–12 hours, which is an important clinical characteristic of the disease. Once recumbent, particularly with obvious neurological involvement, they will either die in spite of treatment or remain recumbent and fail to improve or get worse for several days. Secondary complications, such as pneumonia and decubitus ulcers usually result.

Chronic free-gas bloat is not an uncommon finding in naturally occurring cases and occurs frequently in the experimental disease.

Clinical pathology

In most cases there are changes in the total and differential leukocyte count. Leukopenia and neutropenia may be present in severe cases while in less severe cases a neutrophilia with a left shift is more common. In the cerebrospinal fluid the total cell count is markedly increased and neutrophils predominate. The Pandy globulin test on CSF is usually strongly positive. In the synovial fluid the total cell count is also increased and neutrophils predominate. The organism can be cultured from blood, CSF, synovial fluid, urine and brain, kidney and liver, less commonly from pleuritic fluid and tracheal washings. The laboratory isolation of *H. somnus* from swabs, tissues, and body fluids requires special transport media and selective culture media to ensure reliable recovery (36, 37). Serologically, cattle with experimental or naturally occurring disease have high levels of agglutinating anti-*H. somnus* antibody (4). Recovered animals are positive to the complement-fixation test within 10 days following infection and titers begin to decline to low levels 30 days after infection. Acute and convalescent sera are required for accurate interpretation of results.

Necropsy findings

The characteristic lesions of the nervous system are hemorrhagic infarcts in any part of the brain and spinal cord. These are usually multiple and vary in color from bright red to brown and in diameter from 0.5 to 3 cm. Cerebral meningitis may be focal or diffuse and the cerebrospinal fluid is usually cloudy and slightly yellow tinged, frequently containing flocculent debris. Hemorrhages may also be present in the myocardium, skeletal muscles, kidneys, serosal surfaces of the forestomach, abomasum and intestines.

In the joints the synovial membranes may be edematous with small petechial hemorrhages. There is an excessive quantity of synovial fluid which is usually cloudy and may contain fibrinous flecks. The articular cartilage is usually not affected. Fibrinous or serofibrinous inflammation of the peritoneum, pericardium, or pleura is common in more than 50% of cases. In the larynx there may be focal ulceration and pseudodiphtheritic membranous inflammation extending from the pharynx down into the trachea. Polypoid tracheitis has also been reported (8).

Histologically, vasculitis and thrombosis with or without infarctions and a cellular exudate composed almost entirely of neutrophils are common in all tissues and organs in which there is localization of the organism. There is no histological evidence of embolic pneumonia.

Diagnosis

The sudden onset in a number of young cattle of weakness with obvious neurological signs, with respiratory tract and joint involvement and a fever, with marked changes in the cell count of the CSF and the leukocyte count should suggest hemophilus septicemia. There is a rapid response to treatment in the early stages. In polioencephalomalacia, blindness, normal temperature, nystagmus, opisthotonus and convulsions are common. In listeria meningoencephalitis there is unilateral facial paralysis with deviation of the head and neck and a normal or slightly increased temperature. The CSF in listeriosis usually contains an increased number of mononuclear cells. Hypovitaminosis A in young cattle of 6–12 months of age is usually characterized by sudden onset of short-term convulsions and syncope lasting 10–30 seconds, during which they may die but from which they more commonly recover to appear normal. Exercise will commonly precipitate the seizures. Eyesight may be slightly impaired but the menace reflex is usually present. The differential diagnosis of diseases of the brain of cattle has been summarized in Table 88.

Treatment

Affected cattle must be treated immediately with antibiotics. Oxytetracycline at 20 mg/kg body weight intravenously daily for 3 days is usually effective when treatment is begun within a few hours after the onset of clinical signs. The prognosis in recumbent cattle is unfavorable but treatment for 2–4 days may be attempted. A failure to respond after 3 days of treatment usually indicates the presence of advanced irreversible lesions. Penicillin–streptomycin, chloramphenicol and sulfonamides are also effective. The minimal inhibitory concentrations (MIC) of 33 antimicrobial agents for *H. somnus* indicated that they were highly susceptible to penicillin G, ampicillin, colistin and novobiocin (38). Oxytetracycline and chloramphenicol also showed high activity. Once the disease has been recognized, all in-contact animals should be examined closely from a distance every 6 hours for the next 7–10 days to detect new cases during the initial stages for early treatment. Failure to do this may result in many cases developing beyond the curable stage. Mass medication of the feed and water supplies may be indicated but benefit–cost data are not available to recommend it.

Control

Satisfactory control procedures are not available because the pathogenesis and epidemiology of the disease are not well understood. When an outbreak is encountered the provision of constant surveillance and early treatment is probably the most economical and effective means of control.

A killed bacterin containing whole bacteria in aluminum hydroxide adjuvant has been available for use in North America. Experimental studies indicate that the bacterin is immunogenic and will protect vaccinated cattle against intravenous and intracisternal inoculation of the organism (7). Two injections of the bacterin given subcutaneously 2–3 weeks apart are necessary. Controlled field trials indicate that the bacterin reduces the morbidity and mortality rates of clinical disease in vaccinated cattle compared to non-vaccinated animals. Seroconversion rates occur in more than 80% of cattle vaccinated twice (5). However, the efficacy of the bacterin has been difficult to evaluate because the incidence of naturally occurring disease in non-vaccinated control animals is usually low and may not be significantly greater than in vaccinated animals. Furthermore, the disease has occurred in young cattle which have been vaccinated according to the prescribed recommendations. However, the protection is not complete; in one experiment three of 18 twice-vaccinated animals died from the disease which was produced by intravenous inoculation of the organism (39). Serum antibody titers were unrelated to the outcome of challenge infection regardless of vaccination status.

The bacterin may be used in the face of an outbreak along with improved surveillance and treatment of new cases. There is some limited evidence that vaccination of all in-contact animals in the face of an outbreak will reduce the incidence of new cases (1).

When the disease has been confirmed in a cow–calf herd, the disease can be expected to occur in subsequent years. A vaccination program would include vaccination of the calves beginning at least 3 weeks before weaning.

An economic decision analysis can be used to determine the most economical method of controlling the disease in a feedlot (11). Three alternative programs are compared: no preventive measures; vaccination of all incoming cattle and mass medication with an antibiotic in the face of an outbreak. The methods used to prevent the disease (vaccination) or to control an outbreak (mass medication) will depend on the expected morbidity and case fatality rates, and the costs of vaccination and treatment. The choice of the most economical method will change depending on changes in the variables which must be indentified as accurately as possible in each case.

There is some preliminary evidence that resistance to experimental hemophilus meningoencephalitis is dependent on the use of specific antigens of the organism in a vaccine (40). Antigenic warrants of *H. somnus* have been described and vaccine failures may be due to infection with serotypes of the organism not present in vaccine stocks.

REVIEW LITERATURE

Cobeil, L. B., Widders, P. R., Gogolewski, R., Arthur, J., Inzana, T. J. & Ward, A. C. S. (1986) *Haemophilus somnus*: bovine reproductive and respiratory disease. *Can. vet. J.*, *27*, 90–93.

Humphrey, J. D. & Stephens, L. R. (1983) *Haemophilus somnus:* a review. *Vet. Bull.*, *53*, 987–1004.

Little, P. B. (1986) *Haemophilus somnus* complex: pathogenesis of the septicemic thrombotic meningoencephalitis. *Can. vet. J.*, *27*, 94–96.

Miller, R. B., Lein, D. H., McEntee, K. E., Hall, C. E. & Shin, S. (1983) *Haemophilus somnus* infection of the reproductive tract: a review. *J. Am vet. med. Assoc.*, *182*, 1390–1392.

Stephens, L. R., Little, P. B., Wilkie, B. N. & Barnum, D. A. (1981) Infectious thromboembolic meningoencephalitis in cattle: a review. *J. Am vet. med. Assoc.*, *178*, 378–384.

REFERENCES

(1) Humphrey, J. D. & Stephens, L. R. (1983) *Vet. Bull.* *53*, 987.
(2) Saunders, J. R. et al. (1980) *Can. vet. J.*, *21*, 119.
(3) Thompson, K. G. et al. (1981) *Am. J. vet. Res.*, *42*, 748.
(4) Stephens, L. R. et al. (1981) *Am. J. vet. Res.*, *42*, 468.
(5) Saunders, J. R. & Janzen, E. D. (1980) *Can vet. J.*, *21*, 219.
(6) Pritchard, D. G. et al. (1979) *Res. vet. Sci.*, *26*, 7.
(7) Williams, J. M. et al. (1978) *Am. J. vet. Res.*, *39*, 1756.
(8) Jensen, R. et al. (1980) *Vet. Pathol.*, *17*, 667.
(9) Janzen, E. D. et al. (1981) *Can. vet. J.*, *22*, 361.
(10) Stephens, L. R. & Little, P. B. (1981) *Am. J. vet. Res.*, *42*, 1638.
(11) Davidson, J. N. et al. (1981) *Cornell Vet.*, *71*, 383.
(12) Humphrey, J. D. et al. (1982) *Can. J. comp. Med.*, *46*, 215.
(13) Krogh, H. V. et al. (1983) *Vet. Rec.*, *112*, 460.
(14) Humphrey, J. D. et al. (1982) *Am. J. vet. Res.*, *43*, 791.
(15) Miller, R. B. et al. (1983) *Vet. Pathol.*, *20*, 515.
(16) Miller, R. B. et al. (1985) *J. Am. vet. med. Assoc.*, *182*, 1390.
(17) Groom, S. C. et al. (1986) *Can. J. vet. Res.*, *50*, 238.
(18) Dewey, K. J. & Little, P. B. (1984) *Can. J. comp. Med.*, *48*, 23.
(19) Sanfacon, D. & Higgins, R. (1983) *Can. J. comp. Med.*, *47*, 456.
(20) Simonson, R. R. & Maheswaran, S. K. (1982) *Am. J. vet. Res.*, *43*, 1160.
(21) Sanfacon, D. et al. (1983) *Can. J. comp. Med.*, *47*, 304.
(22) Canto, G. J. & Biberstein, E. L. (1982) *J. clin. Microbiol.*, *15*, 1009.
(23) Chiang, Y. W. et al. (1986) *Infect. Immun.*, *52*, 792.
(24) Hubbard, R. D. et al. (1986) *Vet. Microbiol.*, *12*, 77.
(25) Momotani, E. et al. (1985) *J. comp. Pathol.*, *95*, 15.
(26) Andrews, J. J. et al. (1985 *Vet. Pathol.*, *22*, 131.
(27) Nivard, J. L. et al. (1982) *Am. J. vet. Res.*, *43*, 1790.
(28) Dewey, K. J. & Little P. B. (1984) *Can. J. comp. Med.*, *48*, 27.
(29) Miller, R. B. & Barnum, D. A. (1983) *Vet. Pathol.*, *20*, 584.
(30) Miller, R. B. et al. (1983) *Vet. Pathol.*, *20*, 574.
(31) Hazlett, M. J. et al (1985) *Am J. vet. Res.*, *46*, 2229.
(32) Groom, S. G. et al. (1984) *Can. vet. J.*, *25*, 409.
(33) Lamont, H. H. & Hunt, B. W. (1982) *Vet. Rec.*, *111*, 21.
(34) Metz, A. L. et al. (1984) *J. Am. vet. med. Assoc.*, *184*, 1507.
(35) McEwen, S. A. & Hulland, T. J. (1985) *Can. vet. J.*, *26*, 7.
(36) Brewer, R. A. et al. (1985) *Res. vet. Sci.*, *39*, 299.
(37) Slee, K. J. & Stephens, L. R. (1985) *Vet. Rec.*, *116*, 215.
(38) Sugimoto, C. et al. (1983) *Antimicrob. Agents Chemotherap.*, *23*, 163.
(39) Stephens, L. R. et al. (1982) *Am. J. vet. Res.*, *43*, 1339.
(40) Stephens, L. R. et al. (1984) *Am. J. vet. Res.*, *45*, 234.
(41) Patterson, R. M. et al. (1986) *Aust. vet. J.*, *63*, 163.
(42) Stephens, L. R. et al. (1986) *Aust. vet. J.*, *63*, 182.
(43) Higgins, R. & Martin, J. R. (1987) *Can. vet. J.*, *28*, 117.
(44) Armstrong, K. R. et al. (1986) *Can. vet. J.*, *27*, 211.

Infectious polyarthritis (Glasser's disease, porcine polyserositis)

This disease of young pigs caused by *Hemophilus* spp. occurs in outbreaks and is manifested by acute polyarthritis, pleurisy, pericarditis and peritonitis.

Traditionally, Glasser's disease is associated with infection by *H. suis* (1, 2) but more recently it has been observed that the majority of outbreaks are associated with an X factor independent species *H. parasuis* (3, 4). The disease has been reproduced with both species (5, 2) which have an affinity for serous surfaces. It is also probable that some strains of *H. parainfluenzae* can cause a similar syndrome (6). *Actinobacillus pleuropneumoniae* produces pleuropneumonia in pigs and is described separately.

Epidemiology

Although the disease has probable worldwide occurrence, reports are rare and come mainly from Europe (1). The disease has also been observed in Australia (7, 8), the United States (9), Canada (10) and the United Kingdom (11). The disease occurs as sporadic outbreaks usually in weanling to 4-month-old pigs which have been recently chilled, transported, weaned or moved to different pens. The onset is sudden with several pigs in the group affected and occurs within 2–7 days of the initiating stress. The mortality rate is high if the pigs are not treated.

Little is known of the method of transmission of the disease. The causative organisms are facultative pathogens and can be frequently isolated from pig lungs diseased from other causes even though they are generally not present in normal lungs (11). There are at least five pathogenic serovars of *H. parasuis* (15). It is probable that a respiratory carrier state does exist and that invasion with subsequent septicemia and polyserositis is initiated by stress situations in young pigs that have lost maternal immunity but not yet gained an active immunity. It has been suggested that the causative bacteria are common in most herds and that the disease arises only when pigs from uninfected herds are introduced to a contaminated environment, especially if they have been exposed to environmental stress during transport (12). When infection is introduced into a previously non-infected herd the disease may act as a contagious disease until herd immunity is developed or the infection eliminated (12).

Pathogenesis

Glasser's disease is a fibrinous meningitis, polyserositis and polyarthritis. A fatal septicemia can occur spontaneously (13) or following the intraperitoneal inoculation of pigs with *Hemophilus parasuis* (14).

Clinical findings

The onset is sudden with a moderate to high fever (40–42°C, 104–107°F), complete anorexia, an unusual, rapid, shallow dyspnea with an anxious expression, extension of the head, and mouth-breathing. Coughing may occur. The animals are very lame, stand up on their toes and move with a short, shuffling gait. All the joints are swollen and painful on palpation and fluid swelling of the tendon sheaths may also be clinically evident. A red to blue discoloration of the skin appears near death. Most cases die 2–5 days after the onset of illness. Animals which survive the acute stage of the disease may develop chronic arthritis and some cases of intestinal obstruction caused by peritoneal adhesions occur. Meningitis occurs in some pigs and is manifested by muscle tremor, paralysis and convulsions (6). Although Glasser's disease can occur in pigs of any age, weanling pigs are most commonly and most seriously affected.

Clinical pathology

Few details are available but the organism is recoverable from joint fluid and pleural exudate. The disease can be diagnosed serologically on the presence of precipitins in the serum of recovered pigs (1) and complement-fixing antibody can be detected following infection (4).

Necropsy findings

A fibrinous pleurisy, pericarditis and peritonitis are constantly present. Pneumonia may also be apparent. The joint fluid is turbid, there is inflammation and edema of the periarticular tissues and the joint cavities contain flattened, discoid deposits of yellowish green fibrin. A fibrinopurulent meningitis is common and often extends to involve the superficial layers of the brain.

Diagnosis

As a rule the unusual combination of arthritis, fibrinous serositis and meningitis is sufficient to make a diagnosis of Glasser's disease, but differentiation from the many similar disease entities apparently caused by other agents can only be confirmed by bacteriological examination (1).

The disease may be confused with erysipelas, mycoplasma arthritis and streptococcal arthritis on clinical examination. Mycoplasmosis is a much milder disease and is manifested principally by the presence of a few unthrifty or lame pigs in the litter just before weaning, rather than an acute outbreak with a high mortality (8). Differentiation between cases of Glasser's disease with meningitis and the other diseases of the nervous system in young pigs, especially streptococcal meningitis and Teschen disease, may not be possible without necropsy examination.

Treatment

Sulfadimidine and streptomycin appear to be highly effective in clinical cases provided they are given early in the course of the disease, but the tetracyclines, either by injection or administration in drinking water, are preferred.

Control

Avoidance of undue exposure to adverse environmental conditions at weaning is recommended. Prophylactic dosing at the time of shipping or medication of feed or drinking water on arrival with the above-mentioned drugs may be of value in preventing outbreaks. A formalin-killed bacterin administered before weaning with two injections at 5 and 7 weeks of age has proved highly effective in preventing the disease (4, 12).

REFERENCES

(1) Hjarre, A. (1958) *Adv. vet. Sci.*, *4*, 235.
(2) Neil, D. H. et al. (1969) *Can. J. comp. Med.*, *33*, 187.
(3) Biberstein, E. L. & White, D. C. (1969) *J. med. Microbiol.*, *2*, 75.
(4) Nielsen, R. & Danielsen, V. (1975) *Nord. VetMed.*, *27*, 20.
(5) Little, T. W. A. & Harding, J. D. J. (1971) *Vet. Rec.*, *88*, 540.
(6) Radostits, O. M. et al. (1963) *Can. vet. J.*, *4*, 265.
(7) Sutherland, A. K. & Simmons, G. C. (1947) *Aust. vet. J.*, *23*, 91.
(8) King, S. J. (1968) *Aust. vet. J.*, *44*, 227.
(9) Willigan, D. A. & Beamer, P. D. (1955) *J. Am. vet. med. Assoc.*, *126*, 118.
(10) Carter, G. R. & Schroder, J. D. (1956) *Cornell Vet.*, *46*, 344.
(11) Little, T. W. A. (1970) *Vet. Rec.*, *87*, 399.
(12) Riising, H. J. (1981) *Zentralbl. VetMed. B.*, *28*, 630.
(13) Peet, R. L. et al. (1983) *Aust. vet. J.*, *60*, 187.
(14) Morozumi, T. et al. (1981) *Nat Inst. Anim. Hlth Q.*, *21*, 121.
(15) Morozumi, T. & Nicolet, J. (1986) *J. clin. Microbiol.*, *23*, 1022.

Pleuropneumonia of pigs caused by *Actinobacillus (Hemophilus) pleuropneumoniae*

Actinobacillus pleuropneumoniae causes a highly contagious pleuropneumonia in pigs characterized by a rapid onset and a short course with severe dyspnea, the passage of bloodstained foam from the mouth and nose and a high case fatality rate. Subclinical infection and the carrier state following recovery are common.

Etiology

Actinobacillus pleuropneumoniae formerly known as *Hemophilus pleuropneumoniae* (50) is the causative organism and requires factor V for growth (9).

Epidemiology

The disease has worldwide occurrence and appears to be increasing in prevalence as swine herds become more intensified (1, 9). An abattoir survey in eastern England revealed that the lungs from pigs from approximately 50% of herds monitored for several months had lesions attributable to *A. pleuropneumoniae* (14). A seroepidemiological survey in Iowa swine revealed that about 70% of the herds had swine with antibodies to one or more of the five recognized serotypes of the organism (15). The prevalence of infection has increased in the last 15–20 years presumably due to confinement rearing, crowding, inadequate ventilation, close contact and comingling of pigs of various age groups. The incidence of clinical disease is much less than the prevalence of infection. The disease affects predominantly growing pigs from 2 to 6 months of age with rapid spread both within the initially affected group and subsequently to other older or younger pigs within the herd (6). The morbidity rate varies from 30 to 50% and the case fatality rate may be as high as 50%. Severe outbreaks may occur unexpectedly in susceptible breeding herds with no previous history of the disease (5) or in intensive feeder pig operations in which pigs are introduced on a regular basis from a variety of sources (1). Herds which continuously introduce replacement stock are highly susceptible to an outbreak (4). Following the initial outbreak a general herd immunity develops, but the infection persists and sporadic cases may continue to occur. The organism is not readily isolated from normal respiratory tissues, but persists in chronic lesions within the lungs of recovered and apparently clinically healthy pigs. These pigs provide a source of infection especially in finishing herd buying from diverse sources.

The economic losses associated with the disease are considered to be due to peracute deaths, the costs of treatment of individually affected pigs and mass medication of the feed and water, and chronic disease which delays the marketing of finishing pigs (57, 58). However, other observations and investigations indicate that average daily gain is not significantly affected by infection with *A. pleuropneumoniae* (56). Undoubtedly, there are major economic losses associated with the endemic nature of the disease which is characterized by peracute deaths which recur sporadically and sometimes punctuated by outbreaks.

Transmission is by the respiratory route and overcrowding and inadequate ventilation may facilitate spread. Experimental intranasal challenge has been followed by death in a period as short as 24 hours (3). Following natural infection serum antibody titers persist for several months, but may be transient and much shorter in some pigs (4). Outbreaks of the disease appear to occur in pigs which lack immunity and are overcrowded or have been subjected to recent stressors such as marked changes in ambient temperature or a failure in the ventilation system. Outbreaks may occur in breeding herds following transportation to and from livestock shows and sales. Presumably, the infection was contacted by comingling with clinically healthy but infected pigs. The highest risk is associated with the introduction of pigs from salesbarns and the lowest risk from stock of health status known to the purchaser (16).

There is some limited evidence that *A. pleuropneumoniae* may interact with *Past. multocida* to produce a severe pneumonia (12), whereas *Past. multocida* alone was relatively non-pathogenic.

There are currently at least nine serotypes of *A. pleuropneumoniae* involved in the disease but only five are common (17, 44). The prevalence of serotypes of *A. pleuropneumoniae* varies considerably between geographical location (9, 17–19). In North American surveys, serotype 1 is most common in eastern Canada (21) accounting for 66–83% of the isolates, and the second most prevalent isolate in western Canada and the United States (20). Serotype 2 is of low frequency in Canada, not reported in the United States but is the dominant isolate in Sweden, Switzerland and Denmark (2). Serotype 3 has a low incidence in Canada (9) and the United States and has been reported in Ireland (21). A single isolate of serotype 4 has been reported in the United States. Serotype 5 isolations are common in Canada (9, 17–19) and the United States (20, 24). Serotype 6 has not been reported in North America but occurs in Denmark (23). Serotype 7 is found in Canada (17) and the United States, and a serotype 8 has recently been identified in outbreaks of pleuropneumonia in pigs in Ireland and Denmark (23). The most common serotypes isolated in Quebec were 1, 5, 2, and 7 in that order (25).

The serotyping of isolated strains is important in the epidemiologic and immunologic studies of *A. pleuropneumoniae* infection. It is also important when comparing or analyzing the effectiveness of different treatments to know precisely the virulence of the strains involved as well as their sensitivity to antimicrobials. The development of an effective immunization program will depend on consideration of the multiplicity of immunogenic types which occur in a particular area or country.

There is considerable cross-immunity between the various serotypes of the organism following natural infection (1). Active immunity to pleuropneumonia usually follows experimentally induced and naturally occurring infections as well as vaccinations. The antibody response to *A. pleuropneumoniae* infections or vaccination is demonstrated by the complement fixation test or other serological tests. There is a good correlation between a CF titer and resistance to infection, and the organism usually cannot be isolated from seropositive animals. However, the organism may persist in necrotic foci in the lungs or tonsils of pigs considered immune to the infection. Natural infection with one serotype of *A. pleuropneumoniae* confers a strong immunity to all serotypes (44). Within 2–3 weeks after an acute outbreak of disease the morbidity decreases owing to the development of immunity. Clinical disease is unlikely in adult immune animals, and immune sows confer passive immunity to their piglets which provides protection for the first several weeks of life. However, acute disease may occur in piglets 3–8 weeks of age if colostral immunity is initially low and wanes to below protective levels. Also, severe cases can occur in non-immune gilts and boars introduced into infected herds.

Pigs infected with hemolytic *Actinobacillus* spp. may become false-positive reactors against *A. pleuropneumoniae* (26). Such pigs may also be less susceptible to pleuropneumonia caused by *A. pleuropneumoniae*.

The difference in virulence between the serotypes has been examined experimentally (27). The differences between serotypes 1, 2 and 7 is low. Serotype 3 seems less virulent than 1 (27). The differences in capsular structure and biochemical composition between virulent and avirulent isolates may contribute to virulence (28). A smooth-type lipopolysaccharide and a roughtype lipopolysaccharide have been isolated and characterized from serotype 5 (51). The intrabronchial infusion of the preparations into pigs induces lesions typical of those in pigs which die from acute pleuropneumonia.

Pathogenesis

In growing pigs the disease appears to be a simple respiratory infection without septicemia producing a fibrinous necrotizing hemorrhagic pleuropneumonia with pleuritis. Experimentally, by aerosol exposure of pigs to *A. pleuropneumoniae* a severe fibrinous hemorrhagic necrotizing pleuropneumonia occurs which simulates that seen in natural infections (10). The lesion is particularly marked in the dorsocaudal regions of the lung. The ability of *A. pleuropneumoniae* hemolysin to debilitate pulmonary macrophages may enhance the multiplication of the organism (30). In the acute stages there are marked vascular changes in the lungs. There are many necrotic foci which serve as reservoirs of the organism in pigs which recover. The ultrastructural changes in the lungs of experimentally induced pleuropneumonia have been described (29). There was marked capillary dilatation, mild degeneration of endothelial cells and fibrin thrombi. Inflammatory cells were primarily macrophages and few neutrophils.

Clinical findings

The onset is sudden. Several pigs which were not seen ill may be found dead and others show severe respiratory distress. Affected pigs are disinclined to move and are anorexic. A fever of up to 41°C (105·8°F) is common and labored respirations with an exaggerated abdominal component ('thumps'), cyanosis, and frequently a bloodstained frothy discharge from the nose and mouth are characteristic. In peracute cases the clinical course may be as short as a few hours, but in the majority of pigs it is 1–2 days. Chronic cases are febrile and anorexic initially, but respiratory distress is less severe and a persistent cough may develop. If affected pigs are not treated there will be a high case fatality rate.

The course of the disease in a herd may last for several weeks during which time new acute cases develop and chronic cases become obvious by an unthrifty appearance and chronic coughing.

Abortions may occur (1, 11) and the disease may cause sudden deaths in adult pigs, particularly those which are kept outdoors during the summer months and exposed to very warm weather.

Clinical pathology

In the face of an outbreak, the diagnosis is preferably made by culture at necropsy. A selective medium for the culture of the organism from the airways of slaughtered pigs may increase the isolation rate because of the high degree of contamination (31). Tests to determine the serotype include slide agglutination (18), immunodiffusion (32), ring precipitation (18), indirect hemagglutination (23), immunofluorescence (17), coagglutination (33) and counterimmunoelectrophoresis (34). The latter is quicker, more sensitive and more easily performed than direct immunofluorescence and immunodiffusion procedures. The coagglutination test is simple and rapid (35), the immunodiffusion test is considered to be the most serotype-specific (32), and there is a good correlation between the rapid slide agglutination test and the indirect fluorescent antibody tests (24). The rapid slide agglutination test is the method of choice of some workers (18) but the coagglutination test is serotype-specific, sensitive, simple, rapid, reproducible and easier to read and interpret than the rapid slide or tube agglutination tests (18).

For the serological diagnosis of infection in live animals the complement fixation is reliable (36) but an enzyme-linked immunosorbent assay (ELISA) test is highly specific and more sensitive than the complement fixation test (37). A 2-mercaptoethanol tube agglutination test is an alternative to the complement fixation test and easier to perform (38). The detection of antibodies to *A. pleuropneumoniae* is an essential feature in the epidemiological study and control of pleuropneumonia in pigs. None of these serological tests is completely reliable and in certain situations a combination of two tests is needed for interpretation of low titers in some pigs. In most instances serological diagnosis is type-specific and protection obtained by vaccination is type-specific and will protect only against the serotype contained in the vaccine. Thus it is important to determine the serotype(s) which are causing disease in the herd.

A major challenge with this disease is to detect the infected pig in a herd or to exlude infected pigs from being imported into a herd. Because there is no reliable method for the detection of every infected pig, the effectiveness of this barrier is reduced whenever pigs, such as breeding stock or weanlings, are allowed into a herd. There is a need for a highly sensitive and specific test for the identification of infected pigs. While bacteriological culture is specific it is not sensitive (55). The ELISA test may be a useful test for the antemortem diagnosis of infected herds (55).

Necropsy findings

Characteristic lesions are confined to the thoracic cavity and consist of pleuropneumonia with a tendency to sequestration in the chronic form. In peracute cases the lungs are swollen, firm, dark red in color, and fluid and blood oozes from the cut surface. There may be marked edema of the interglobular septa due to interalveolar septal capillary permeability (39). In pigs which die less acutely, focal black or red raised areas of pneumonia are present which in chronic cases become encapsulated. Lesions are distributed throughout the lung and may occur in the diaphragmatic and apical and cardiac lobes. A fibrinous pleurisy with adhesions overlies the affected lung tissue. A fibrinous pericarditis may also be present. The organism can be isolated from affected lung tissue, but generally not from other internal organs. The quantitative morphology of peracute pulmonary lesions induced by the organism has been described (39). The remarkable interalveolar septal edema may be associated with platelet aggregation in interalveolar septal capillaries, neutrophil accumulation on endothelial cells and infiltration into the interalveolar septa and endothelial cell swelling (39).

In a chronically infected herd chronic pleuritic adhesions may be present in a large proportion of the pigs at market as a result of infection several months earlier.

Diagnosis

The rapidity of onset and spread with fever, anorexia, severe dyspnea and high mortality differentiates *A.*

pleuropneumoniae pleuropneumonia from the majority of respiratory diseases in pigs. Enzootic pneumonia is more insidious in its occurrence and has distinctively different epidemiologic, clinical and pathologic features. Pasteurellosis is characterized by a necrotizing bronchopneumonia. Swine influenza is characterized by an explosive outbreak of respiratory disease. However, this is not restricted to growing pigs and the mortality is low. There is a distinct difference in the respiratory lesion on necropsy examination. Glasser's disease is characterized by serositis, arthritis and meningitis, and occurs in younger pigs. Mulberry heart disease may present with similar clinical findings but there is no pneumonia on necropsy examination.

Treatment

The results of treatment are often disappointing because of the severity of the acute disease and the persistence of infection in recovered pigs. Affected and in-contact pigs should be treated parenterally with antibiotics. Tetracycline, spectinomycin and penicillin are effective and have been recommended. Lincomycin at a dose rate of 10 mg/kg body weight intramuscularly daily for 3 days followed by medication of the feed with oxytetracycline at a dose of 500 g/tonne is credited with good results (6). In finishing units where outbreaks of the disease have been confirmed, the twice-daily intramuscular injection of pigs early in the course of the disease with antimicrobials, based on drug sensitivity tests, daily until clinical recovery occurred, was superior to the mass medication of feed and water (56). A considerable amount of labor is required but it is considered to be the most cost-effective method. Tetracycline should be administered through the feed or drinking water of all in-contact pigs during the outbreak, but the persistence of the organism in chronically affected pigs may result in clinical disease when the medication is withdrawn. Sulfathiazole at the rate of 28 g/3·8 l of drinking water for 12 days has also been successful (5). Tiamulin in the drinking water at a concentration to deliver 23 mg/kg body weight for 5 days after an initial individual treatment of affected pigs has also been recommended.

The antimicrobial sensitivities of isolates of *A. pleuropneumoniae* have been monitored and there is some variation in the sensitivities based on geographical location (40, 41). Thus, it is necessary to determine antimicrobial sensitivity on a herd basis when recommending therapy. Plasmid-mediated antimicrobial resistance is also a possibility (42).

The therapeutic efficiency of some commonly used antibiotics has been evaluated for the treatment of experimentally induced pleuropneumonia using serotype 1 *A. pleuropneumoniae* (43). Longacting oxytetracycline at a dose of 20 mg/kg body weight intramuscularly one day before experimental challenge prevented all manifestations of disease. When treatment commenced immediately after the first signs of disease, each of the injected antibiotics (penicillin-chloramphenicol and long-acting oxytetracycline) reduced the case fatality rate but did not improve average daily gain nor reduce the incidence of infection or incidence of lung lesions. Oxytetracycline in the water at 222 mg/l for 7 days beginning 24 hours before experimental challenge reduced the case fatality rate, lung lesions and the isolation of the organism compared to the unmedicated group. Treatment of chronically affected pigs did not improve rate or gain nor eliminate the infection.

Control

There are no effective control measures for this disease. Pigs which recover are likely to provide a source of future infection and finishing operations which purchase all of their introductions should depopulate their finished stock prior to new introduction. The all-in, all-out system of purchasing, feeding and marketing pigs in a finishing operation should be adopted. The disease is highly contagious and control measures must be directed towards identifying and eliminating infected pigs into uninfected herds and the possible use of vaccines. Every economical effort must be made to identify and isolate infected pigs and to exclude the importation of clinically normal but infected pigs into herds in which the infection is not present. This is a major challenge which is dependent on the availability of a highly sensitive and specific laboratory test. The acquisition of new breeding stock for herds free of the infection should include a period of quarantine and two serological tests 3 weeks apart. Only seronegative animals should be introduced into the herds. A seropositive animal should be considered a potential carrier.

Management practices must emphasize the rearing of weaned pigs in pens separate from older stock which are carriers of the organism. Large breeding herds and finishing units should subdivide the total herd into separate units which minimizes the spread of infection. Early weaning and segregation of gilts from infected stock have been used to develop a seronegative herd.

Natural infection with a serotype of *A. pleuropneumoniae* confers a strong immunity to all serotypes. Nasal inoculation of one serotype of live *A. pleuropneumoniae* induces a strong immunity to both homologous and heterologous serotypes (44). Vaccination has been attempted to prevent pleuropneumonia in pigs. However, the protection obtained by parenteral vaccination is serotype-specific and vaccines must therefore contain the serotype existing in the swine population. Serotype 8 is closely related to serotypes 3 and 6, and parenteral revaccination using a capsular extract or killed *A. pleuropneumoniae* serotype 8 provides a high degree of protection against challenge with serotypes 3 or 6 (45). This suggests that the serological and cross-protective properties of *A. pleuropneumoniae* serotypes should be identified before they are used as antigen in the complement fixation test and in vaccines. The vaccines which have been evaluated are killed vaccines with an adjuvant. In one experimental trial, two and three vaccinations using a bacterin containing serotypes 1 and 5 prevented mortality following an aerosol challenge with the same serotypes as present in the vaccine (46). However, all vaccinated pigs had severe signs of respiratory disease and the vaccine did not prevent the development of lung lesions (44). The use of a formalin-inactivated alum-precipitated vaccine containing serotype 1 was effective in decreasing the morbidity and mortality rates from naturally occurring pleuropneumonia (47). The adjuvanted vaccines have caused considerable tissue reaction resulting in abscesses and granulomas (48). The mineral oil adjuvants are highly irritant and cause granulomas which are present 8 weeks after vaccination, the aluminum hydroxide adjuvants are less irritant, while the peanut oil did not produce significant lesions (48).

The immunization of pigs with crossreacting core antigens of the lipopolysaccharide of an *Rc* mutant of *E. coli* 0111:B4 (strain J5) protected against a lethal challenge with *A. pleuropneumoniae* under laboratory conditions (49). Vaccination of pigs with the *E. coli* J5 in commercial swine herds endemically infected with *A. pleuropneumoniae* did lower mortality compared to controls (54). The use of a commercial bacterin also lowered mortality. The serum titers against *E. coli* J5 increased following vaccination with the *E. coli* J5 bacterin and in pigs which were naturally infected with *A. pleuropneumoniae*, but not in pigs vaccinated with the *A. pleuropneumoniae* bacterin. The capsular antigens of *A. pleuropneumoniae* have some protective immunogenic efficacy in pigs and mice but it is not sufficient to warrant field use of these preparations (53).

REVIEW LITERATURE

Sebunya, T. N. K. & Saunders, J. R. (1983) *Hemophilus pleuropneumoniae* infection in swine: a review. *J. Am. vet. med. Assoc.*, *182*, 1331–1337.

REFERENCES

(1) Sanford, S. E. & Josephson, G. K. A. (1981) *Can. J. comp. Med.*, *45*, 2.
(2) Nielsen, R. (1979) *Nord. VetMed.*, *31*, 401.
(3) Nielsen, R. (1979) *Nord. VetMed.*, *31*, 407.
(4) Nielsen, R. & Mandrup, M. (1977) *Nord. VetMed.*, *29*, 465
(5) Davidson, J. N. & King, J. M. (1980) *Nord. VetMed.*, *70*, 360.
(6) Cameron, R. D. A. & Kelly, W. R. (1979) *Aust. vet. J.*, *55*, 389.
(7) Gunnarsson, A. (1979) *Am. J. vet. Res.*, *40*, 1564.
(8) Greenway, J. A. (1981) *Can. vet. J.*, *22*, 21
(9) Sebunya, T. N. K. & Saunders, J. R. (1983) *J. Am. vet. med. Assoc.*, *182*, 1331.
(10) Sebunya, T. N. K. et al. (1983) *Can. J. comp. Med.*, *47*, 48.
(11) Wilson, R. W. & Kierstead, M. (1976) *Can. vet. J.*, *17*, 222.
(12) Little, T. W. A. & Harding, J. D. J. (1980) *Br. vet. J.*, *136*, 371.
(13) Rosendal, S. et al. (1981) *Can. vet. J.*, *22* 34.
(14) Brandreth, S. R. & Smith, I. M. (1985) *Vet. Rec.*, *117*, 143.
(15) Schultz, P. A. et al. (1982) *Am. J. vet. Res.*, *43*, 1848.
(16) Rosendal, S. & Mitchell, W. R. (1983) *Can. J. comp. Med.*, *47*, 1.
(17) Rosendal, S. & Boyd, D. A. (1982) *J. clin. Microbiol.*, *16*, 840.
(18) Mittal, K. R. et al. (1982) *J. clin. Microbiol.*, *15*, 1019.
(19) Rosendal, S. et al. (1981) *Can. J. comp. Med.*, *45*, 271.
(20) Schultz, R. A. et al. (1983) *Vet. Med. SAC*, *78*, 1451.
(21) Power, S. B. et al. (1983) *Vet. Rec.*, *113*, 113.
(22) Desrosiers, R. et al. (1984) *Vet. Rec.*, *115*, 628.
(23) Nielsen, R. & O'Connor, P. J. (1984) *Acta vet. Scand.*, *25*, 96.
(24) Rapp, V. J. (1985) *Am. J. vet. Res.*, *46*, 185.
(25) Mittal, K. R. et al. (1983) *J. clin. Microbiol.*, *18*, 1351.
(26) Rosendal, S. et al. (1985) *Can. J. comp. Med.*, *49*, 164.
(27) Rosendal, S. et al (1985) *Can. J. comp. Med.*, *49*, 68.
(28) Jensen, A. E. & Bertram, T. A. (1986) *Infect. Immun.*, *51*, 419.
(29) Perfumo, C. J. et al. (1983) *Zentralbl. VetMed. B.*, *30*, 678.
(30) Kume, K. et al. (1986) *Infect. Immun.*, *51*, 419.
(31) Gilride, K. A. & Rosendale, S. (1983) *Can. J. comp. Med.*, *47*, 445.
(32) Lombin, L. H. et al. (1985) *Vet. Microbiol.*, *10*, 393.
(33) Mittal, K. R. et al. (1983) *J. clin. Microbiol.*, *18*, 351.
(34) Piffer, I. A. et al. (1986) *Vet. Rec.*, *118*, 292.
(35) Hunter, D. & Livingstone, J. (1986) *Vet. Rec.*, *118*, 129.
(36) Lombin, L. H. et al. (1982) *Can. J. comp. Med.*, *46*, 109.
(37) Nicolet, J. et al. (1981) *Am. J. vet. Res.*, *42*, 2139.
(38) Mittal, K. R. et al. (1984) *Am. J. vet. Res.*, *45*, 715.
(39) Bertram, T. A. (1985) *Vet. Pathol.*, *22*, 598.
(40) Gilbride, K. A. & Rosendal, S. (1984) *Can. J. comp. Med.*, *48*, 47.
(41) Didier, P. J. et al. (1984) *J. Am. vet. med. Assoc.*, *184*, 716.
(42) Hirsh, D. C. et al. (1982) *Am. J. vet. Res.*, *43*, 269.
(43) Willson, P. J. & Osborne, A. D. (1985) *Can. vet. J.*, *26*, 312.
(44) Nielsen, R. (1984) *Nord. VetMed.*, *36*, 221.
(45) Nielsen, R. (1985) *Nord. VetMed.*, *37*, 217.
(46) Higgins, R. et al. (1985) *Can. vet. J.*, *261*, 86.
(47) Mason, R. W. et al. (1982) *Aust. vet. J.*, *58*, 108.
(48) Straw, B. E. et al. (1985) *Can. J. comp. Med.*, *49*, 149.
(49) Fenwick, B. W. et al. (1986) *Infect. Immun.*, *53*, 298.
(50) Pohl, S. et al. (1983) *Int. J. syst. Bacteriol.*, *33*, 510.
(51) Fenwick, B. W. et al. (1986) *Am. J. vet. Res.*, *47*, 1433.
(52) Desrosiers, R. (1986) *Vet. Rec.*, *119*, 89.
(53) Rosendal, S. et al. (1986) *Vet. Microbiol.*, *12*, 229.
(54) Fenwick, B. W. et al. (1986) *Am. J. vet. Res.*, *47*, 1888.
(55) Willson, P. J. et al. (1987) *Can. vet. J.*, *28*, 111.
(56) Desrosiers, R. (1986) *Vet. Rec.*, *119*, 89.
(57) Willson, M. R. et al. (1986) *Can. J. vet. Res.*, *50*, 209.
(58) Friendship, R. M. et al. (1984) *Proc. int. pig vet. Soc.*, 97.

19

Diseases Caused by Bacteria—IV

DISEASES CAUSED BY *MYCOBACTERIUM* spp.

TUBERCULOSIS, Johne's disease and skin tuberculosis are described in this section. Mastitis due to *Mycobacterium lacticola* is described in Chapter 15 on mastitis.

Tuberculosis caused by *Mycobacterium bovis*

The disease caused by *M. bovis* is characterized by the progressive development of tubercles in any of the organs in most species.

Etiology

M. bovis is the common cause of tuberculosis in cattle. In the other animal species, *M. avium* may account for a considerable proportion of cases of tuberculosis especially in pigs kept in close association with infected birds (1). In these circumstances many of the infections are caused by *M. avium*-like bacteria rather than *M. avium* itself. Infection seems to occur via the alimentary tract and there is a great tendency for self-cure of gross lesions to occur. The subject is discussed elsewhere under the heading of tuberculosis caused by atypical mycobacteria (p. 721). The human strain (*M. tuberculosis*) may account for a small proportion of cases in animals.

Epidemiology

Tuberculosis occurs in every country of the world and is of major importance in dairy cattle. The disease can occur in all species including man and is of importance for public health reasons as well as for its detrimental effects on animal production. The causative organism does not form spores but it is moderately resistant to heat, desiccation and many disinfectants. It is readily destroyed by direct sunlight unless it is in a moist environment. In warm, moist, protected positions, it may remain viable for some weeks.

Cattle

The infected animal is the main source of infection, although mediate contagion can occur. Organisms are excreted in the exhaled air, in sputum, feces (from both intestinal lesions and swallowed sputum, from pulmonary lesions), milk, urine, vaginal and uterine discharges and discharges from open peripheral lymph nodes. Animals with gross lesions that communicate with airways, skin or intestinal lumen are obvious disseminators of infection. It has also been shown that cattle in the early stages of the disease before any lesions are visible, may also excrete viable mycobacteria in nasal and tracheal mucus (46). Commonly, entry is effected by inhalation or ingestion. Inhalation is the almost invariable portal of entry in housed cattle, and even in those at pasture it is considered to be the principal mode of transmission. Infection by ingestion is obviously more likely at pasture when feces contaminate the feed and communal drinking water and feed troughs. Under natural conditions, stagnant drinking water may cause infection up to 18 days after its last use by a tuberculous animal, whereas a running stream does not represent an important source of infection to cattle in downstream fields. It is difficult to give details of the persistence of infectivity of pasture and other inanimate objects because of the varying conditions under which experiments have been carried out. Viable *M. tuberculosis* can be isolated from the feces of infected cattle and from ground in contact with the feces for 6–8 weeks after the feces are dropped but the duration of the infectivity of the pasture to susceptible cattle varies widely. The period may be as short as 1 week if the weather is dry and pastures are harrowed but will be much longer in wet weather. Separation of infected and susceptible animals by a fence provides practical protection against spread of the disease.

The drinking of infected milk by young animals is one of the commonest methods by which tuberculosis is spread. Less common routes of infection include intrauterine infection at coitus, by the use of infected semen or of infected insemination or uterine pipettes, and intramammary infection by the use of contaminated teat siphons or by way of infected cups of milking machines. The feeding of tuberculous cattle carcasses to pigs has also caused a severe outbreak of the disease. Unusual sources of infection are infected cats, goats or even human caretakers.

Housing predisposes to the disease, as does zero grazing, so that the disease is more common and serious where these forms of husbandry are practiced. In spite of the low overall incidence in countries where cattle are at pasture all the year round, individual herds with 60–70% morbidity may be encountered. Amongst beef cattle the degree of infection is usually much lower because of the open range conditions under which they are kept. However, individual beef herds may suffer a high morbidity if infected animals are introduced and large numbers of animals have to drink from stagnant water holes, especially during dry seasons. It is difficult to assess the economic importance of the disease in cattle. Apart from actual deaths, it is estimated that infected animals lose 10–25% of their productive efficiency (4).

Zebu (Brahman) type cattle are thought to be much more resistant to tuberculosis than European cattle, and the effects on these cattle are described as being much less severe (3). However, under intensive feedlot conditions a morbidity rate of 60% and a depression of weight gain can be experienced in tuberculous Zebu cattle (4).

Pigs

In pigs the incidence is usually much lower but reflects the incidence in the local cattle population from which the infection derives either by the ingestion of dairy products or by grazing over the same pasture as cattle. The lower relative incidence in pigs is due to a number of factors, particularly the tendency of the disease to remain localized in this species and the early age of slaughter. The incidence is higher in older pigs. When the disease is common among dairy cattle in an area, 10–20% of the local pigs are likely to be infected. A high incidence has been observed in pigs bedded on shavings already infected with *M. bovis* before purchase. In countries where bovine tuberculosis is uncommon mycobacteriosis in pigs is usually caused by *Mycobacterium avium*, *M. intracellulare* or *M. scrofulaceum* and the lesions are restricted to the cervical lymph nodes (42). Feral pigs in Australia have a very high prevalence of tuberculoid lesions, with 18% of the affected pigs yielding *M. bovis*. *M. intracellulare* is also common. However the disease is likely to be inconsequential in domestic pigs, the feral pig being an end host (43). Because the disease is relatively benign in pigs, major financial loss does not occur. Some losses are experienced due to the rejection of carcasses or parts at the abattoir.

Other species

Sheep have always been considered to be resistant, but recent experience in New Zealand has shown that the disease can be quite prevalent in this species with up to 5% of flocks being infected (41). The particular circumstances seem to be a high prevalence in local cattle and possums.

In horses the disease occurs rarely, largely due to limited exposure to infection but natural resistance also appears to play a part.

Spread of tuberculosis from animals to man makes this an important zoonosis. Infection in man occurs largely through consumption of infected milk by children but spread can also occur by inhalation. Transmission to man can be almost completely eliminated by pasteurization of milk but only complete eradication of the disease can protect the farmer and his family. Transmission from cattle to humans is an unlikely event nowadays but still occurs (45).

All species and age groups are susceptible to *M. bovis*, with cattle, goats and pigs most susceptible and sheep and horses showing a high natural resistance. Goats are quite susceptible and if they are maintained in association with infected herds of cattle the incidence may be as high as 70% (16). Tuberculosis may also be encountered in elk (47), wild deer (10), water buffaloes (44), camels, deer, bison and other wild fauna (22), and birds and these animals may act as a source of infection for cattle. A high prevalence rate has been demonstrated in wild badgers in the United Kingdom and they appear to be important in the epidemiology of tuberculosis in cattle (6, 7), so much so that a badger eradication program has been undertaken in some areas. The brush-tailed possum (*Trichosurus vulpecula*) occupies the same relative position in New Zealand. This animal is very susceptible to *M. bovis* and fulminating infections develop and provide a ready source of infection for cattle. Much of New Zealand's residual problem with bovine tuberculosis is in cattle running on the pasture–bush margin where there is ample opportunity for cattle–possum contact (26). Affected possums contaminate their environment heavily because of the many discharging sinuses which they develop. The possums also have been the means of causing a significant prevalence of tuberculosis in local sheep flocks (41). The widespread occurrence of tuberculosis in exotic animals maintained in captivity emphasizes the public health importance of these infections (9).

Pathogenesis

Tuberculosis spreads in the body by two stages, the primary complex and postprimary dissemination. The primary complex consists of the lesion at the point of entry and in the local lymph node. A lesion at the point of entry is common when infection is by inhalation. When infection occurs via the alimentary tract, a lesion at the site of entry is unusual although tonsillar and intestinal ulcers may occur. More commonly the only observable lesion is in the pharyngeal or mesenteric lymph nodes. A visible primary focus develops within 8 days of entry being effected by the bacteria. Calcification of the lesions commences about 2 weeks later. The developing necrotic focus is soon surrounded by granulation tissue and lymphocytes and the pathognomonic 'tubercle' is established. Bacteria are transmitted from this primary focus, which is in the respiratory tract in 90–95% of cases in cattle, to a regional lymph node and cause the development of a similar lesion there. In calves fed tuberculous milk the primary focus is likely to be in the pharyngeal or mesenteric lymph nodes, with hepatic lesions as the major manifestation of postprimary spread.

Postprimary dissemination from the primary complex varies considerably in rate and route. It may take the form of acute miliary tuberculosis, discrete nodular lesions in various organs, or chronic organ tuberculosis caused by endogenous or exogenous reinfection of tissues rendered allergic to tuberculoprotein. In the latter case there may be no involvement of the local lymph node. Depending upon the sites of localization of infection, clinical signs vary but, because the disease is always progressive, there is the constant underlying toxemia which causes weakness, debility and the eventual death of the animal.

In cattle, horses, sheep and goats, the disease is a progressive one and, although generalized tuberculosis is not uncommon in pigs, localization as non-progressive abscesses in the lymph nodes of the head and neck is the most common finding. Tuberculosis produced experimentally in pigs by the oral administration of *M. avium* is generalized provided the inoculation dose is sufficiently large. Transmission from these pigs to contact pigs occurs readily (8). In cattle experimental tuberculosis has been produced by the intravenous injection of *M. tuberculosis* resulting in a range of syndromes from peracute tuberculous pneumonia to chronic progressive generalized tuberculosis (12).

Clinical findings

Cattle

Although signs referable to localization in a particular organ usually attract attention to the possible occurrence of tuberculosis, some general signs are also evident. Some cows with extensive miliary tubercular lesions are clinically normal but progressive emaciation unassociated with other signs should always arouse suspicion of tuberculosis. A capricious appetite and fluctuating temperature are also commonly associated with the disease. The condition of the hair-coat is variable; it may be rough or sleek. Affected animals tend to become more docile and sluggish but the eyes remain bright and alert. These general signs often become more pronounced after calving.

Pulmonary involvement is characterized by a chronic cough due to bronchopneumonia. The cough is never loud or paroxysmal, occurring only once or twice at a time and is low, suppressed and moist. It is easily stimulated by squeezing the pharynx or by exercise and is most common in the morning or in cold weather. In the advanced stages when much lung has been destroyed, dyspnea with increased rate and depth of respiration becomes apparent. At this stage, abnormalities may be detected by auscultation and percussion of the chest. Areas with no breath sounds and dullness on percussion are accompanied by areas in which squeaky crackles are audible. Tuberculous pleurisy may occur but is usually symptomless and there is no effusion. Involvement of the bronchial lymph nodes may cause dyspnea because of constriction of air passages, and enlargement of the mediastinal lymph node is commonly associated with recurrent and then persistent ruminal tympany.

The most common signs of alimentary involvement are caused by pressure of enlarged lymph nodes on surrounding organs. Rarely tuberculous ulcers of the small intestine cause diarrhea. Retropharyngeal lymph node enlargement causes dysphagia and noisy breathing due to pharyngeal obstruction. Such lymph node enlargements may be part of a primary complex or be due to postprimary dissemination. Pharyngeal palpation with the aid of a speculum reveals a large, firm, rounded swelling in the dorsum of the pharynx.

Chronic, painless swelling of the submaxillary, prescapular, precrural and supramammary lymph nodes is relatively rare. Uterine tuberculosis is uncommon with bovine strains except in advanced cases. It may occur as a result of coitus or the use of contaminated uterine catheters, or by contiguity from tuberculous peritonitis, but in most cases it results from generalized hematogenous spread. In the case of spread by contiguity from peritonitis, bursitis and salpingitis are common, the lesions in the salpinx taking the form of small enlargements containing a few drops of yellow fluid. Similar lesions may occur by upward spread from the uterus to the peritoneum. In tuberculous metritis, there may be interference with conception, or conception may be followed by recurrent abortion late in pregnancy, or a live calf is produced which in most cases dies quickly of generalized tuberculosis. Lesions similar to those of brucellosis occur on the placenta. In cows which fail to conceive, there may be a chronic purulent discharge heavily infected with the organism and the condition is very resistant to treatment. A number of cows will have an associated tuberculous vaginitis affecting chiefly the ducts of Gartner. Rare cases of tuberculous orchitis are characterized by the development of large, indurated, painless testicles.

Tuberculous mastitis is of major importance because of the danger to public health, and of spread of the disease to calves and the difficulty of differentiating it from other forms of mastitis. Its characteristic feature is a marked induration and hypertrophy which usually develops first in the upper part of the udder, particularly in the rear quarters. Palpation of the supramammary lymph nodes is essential in all cases of suspected tuberculous mastitis. Enlargement of the nodes with fibrosis of the quarter does not necessarily indicate tuberculosis but enlargement without udder induration suggests either tuberculosis or lymphomatosis. In the early stages, the milk is not macroscopically abnormal but later very fine floccules appear which settle after the milk stands leaving a clear, amber fluid. Later still the secretion may be an amber fluid only.

Pigs

Tuberculous lesions in cervical lymph nodes usually cause no clinical abnormality unless they rupture to the exterior. Generalized cases present a syndrome similar to that seen in cattle although tuberculous involvement of the meninges and joints is rather more common.

Horses

The commonest syndrome in horses is caused by involvement of the cervical vertebrae in which a painful osteomyelitis causes stiffness of the neck and inability to eat off the ground. Less common signs include polyuria, coughing due to pulmonary lesions, lymph node enlargement, nasal discharge and a fluctuating temperature.

Sheep and goats

Bronchopneumonia is the commonest form of the disease in these species and is manifested by cough and terminal respiratory embarrassment. In some goats intestinal ulceration, with diarrhea, and enlargement of the lymph nodes of the alimentary tract occurs. In both species the disease is only slowly progressive, and in affected flocks many more reactors and necropsy-positive cases are often found than would be expected from the clinical cases which are evident. In kids the disease may be more rapidly progressive and cause early death.

Clinical pathology
Because of the universal dependence on the tuberculin test for diagnosis and the policy of slaughtering all positive reactors whether they are open cases or not, few clinicopathological tests are now carried out. Sputum or discharges may be examined by inoculation into guinea-pigs but improved cultural techniques make animal injection tests unnecessary.

The basis of all tuberculosis eradication schemes is the tuberculin test and a knowledge of the various tests used, their deficiencies and advantages is essential. It should be remembered, however, that clinical examination is still of value particularly in seeking out the occasional advanced cases which do not give a positive reaction to a tuberculin test. Much attention is being directed to devising tests to detect such animals but the eye of an observant clinician can still be the most important factor in problem herds where positive reactors keep recurring. The application of control measures based on a knowledge of the epidemiology of the disease is too often neglected when such measures may considerably reduce the time necessary to eradicate the disease from a herd.

Single intradermal (SID) test
This test is applied by the intradermal injection of 0·05 ml of tuberculin into a skin fold. The tuberculin is prepared from cultures of *M. tuberculosis* or *M. bovis* grown on synthetic media. The former is more potent than the latter, particularly when used on poorly sensitized animals, the latter is more specific. The reaction is read between 48 and 96 hours after injection with a preference for 48–72 hours for maximum sensitivity (17) and at 96 hours for maximum specificity, and a positive reaction constitutes a diffuse swelling at the injection site. In some countries the injection is made into an anal or caudal fold at the base of the tail. In others it is made into a cervical fold, a fold of skin picked up in the centre of the lateral aspect of the neck. The cervical fold test is thought to provide greater sensitivity, the caudal fold providing the greater specificity. In the caudal fold test comparison with the opposite fold by palpation and inspection is desirable when making a decision. In the United States, an additional injection is made into the lip of the vulva at the mucocutaneous junction.

In England the injection is made into the skin of the neck and measurement of the injection site with calipers in an attempt to achieve more accuracy in measuring reactions. However, the use of calipers is very time-consuming, and the subjective method of simple palpation has been shown to be more accurate (17). It also permits a decision to be shaded by the nature of the lesion. The skin of the neck area is much more sensitive than that of the tail area but the test suffers from the necessity to restrain each animal and measure all reactions carefully. Varying dose rates of tuberculin have been recommended and, with increasing demands for standardization of the test to increase its accuracy, the exact dose for the particular tuberculin should be strictly adhered to when the cervical skin test in used. In the United States, 0·1 ml is recommended for herds of unknown status and 0·2 ml in known infected herds when cases with low sensitivity are to be carefully sought. The method of injection of tuberculin also has some importance when the cervical site is used. A careful intradermal injection produces the largest swelling and a quick thrust the least. Variations in technique appear to have little effect on the size of reaction when the caudal fold is used.

The main disadvantage of the SID test is its lack of specificity and the number of no-visible-lesion reactors (NVLs) which occur. Mammalian tuberculin is not sufficiently specific to differentiate between reactions due to infection with *M. bovis* and infection with *M. avium*, *M. tuberculosis*, *M. paratuberculosis* (including vaccination) or *Nocardia farcinicus*. The maximum permissible rate of NVL reactors is 10% and when this rate is exceeded, tests other than the SID test should be used. Other disadvantages of the SID test include failure to detect cases of minimal sensitivity such as may occur in the early or late stages of the disease, in old cows and in cows which have recently calved. This failure to detect tuberculous animals can be of considerable importance and must receive close attention when reactors are detected at an initial test. Serological tests to detect these cases of minimal sensitivity have been devised but are not sufficiently accurate for use in individual animals. The available tests devised to overcome these deficiencies of the SID test are the short thermal, Stormont and comparative tests. The use of diluted tuberculins does not increase the specificity of the tuberculin test (11).

Short thermal test
Intradermal tuberculin (4 ml) is injected subcutaneously into the neck of cattle with a rectal temperature of not more than 39°C (102°F) at the time of injection and for 2 hours later. If the temperature at 4, 6 and 8 hours after injection rises above 40°C (104°F), the animal is classed as a positive reactor. The temperature peak is usually at 6–8 hours and is generally over 41°C (105·8°F (48)). Preliminary evidence indicates a high efficiency of the test in detecting 'spreader' cases giving negative intradermal tests. Occasional deaths due to anaphylaxis occur at the peak of the reaction, and there is one report of recumbency, which responded to intravenous therapy with calcium salts, in a large number of tuberculous cows submitted to this test.

Intravenous tuberculin test
Such a test has been used experimentally but requires a special research tuberculin. As in the previous test a positive reaction is a febrile one at 4–6 hours after injection, continuing for at least 8 hours and the elevation of temperature to exceed 1·7°C (35°F). There is difficulty in interpreting the test and hematological changes such as a transient lymphopenia (13) may have to be considered to avoid false negative tests (13).

Stormont test
This test has been devised to select those animals which are poorly sensitized for any reason. The test is performed similarly to the single intradermal test in the neck with a further injection at the same site 7 days later. An increase in skin thickness of 5 mm or more, 24 hours after this second injection is a positive result. The increased sensitivity is thought to be due to the attrac-

tion of antibodies to the site by the first injection. The increased sensitivity begins at the 5th day, is at its peak at the 7th and ends on the 12th day after the injection. Preliminary trials indicate very high efficiency in detecting the poorly sensitized animal but extensive field trials have not as yet been reported. Cattle infected with *M. avium* do not give a positive reaction but 'skin tuberculosis' cases do. It is more accurate than the single intradermal test and has been adopted as the official test in Northern Ireland, although a practical difficulty is the necessity for three visits to the farm. Special purified protein derivative (PPD) tuberculin of a specified potency must be used to fulfil the requirements of the test.

Comparative test
Where the presence of Johne's disease or avian tuberculosis is suspected or 'skin tuberculosis' is apparent, non-specific sensitization must be considered, and a comparative test used. Transitory sensitization may occur in cattle due to the presence of human tuberculosis in their attendants but the comparative test will not differentiate the sensitivity from that due to bovine strain infection.

The comparative test depends on the greater sensitivity to homologous tuberculin. Avian and mammalian tuberculin are injected simultaneously into two separate sites on the same side of the neck, 12 cm apart and one above the other, and the test is read 72 hours later. Care must be taken in placing the injections as sensitivity varies from place to place in the skin. The greater of the two reactions indicates the organism responsible for the sensitization. The test is not generally intended for primary use in detecting reactors but only to follow up known reactors to determine the infecting organism. However, the single intradermal comparative test has been used in the highly successful eradication program in Great Britain. Its use as a primary test is recommended when a high incidence of avian tuberculosis or Johne's disease is anticipated, or when vaccination against Johne's disease has been carried out. The comparative test is adequate to differentiate between vaccination against Johne's disease and tuberculosis and the distinction is easier the longer ago the vaccination was performed (14).

Special aspects of sensitivity to tuberculin

Site of injection
Sensitivity to tuberculin injected intradermally varies considerably from site to site on the body. In cattle the relative sensitivities of different areas to tuberculin and to johnin have been determined as follows: back 1, upper side 1·75, lower side 2·5, neck 2·75–3. The cervical area is also much more sensitive than the anal fold, and has the advantages that reactions are more pronounced, animals can be retested immediately and the area is more sanitary. Its disadvantages are that restraint of each animal is necessary and the proportion of NVL reactors increases.

Potency of tuberculins
In the search for more specific and potent allergens, bovine and human types have been used to prepare tuberculins for comparison, the latter being the more potent. However, for maximum specificity tuberculin prepared from *M. bovis* is recommended, and for preference it should be a purified protein derivative (PPD). PPDs are in general use because of their greater specificity and the greater ease with which they can be standardized. One of the important problems in tuberculin testing is deciding the optimum amount of tuberculin to be used to get maximum specificity. More accurate determination of the amount to be used could dispel many of the difficulties of non-specific reactions. A dose rate between 5000 and 10 000 tuberculin units (0·1 ml tuberculin containing 0·1 or 0·2 mg of bovine PPD) is considered to be most suitable. The 0·2 mg dose is preferred as detecting more infected animals (17). A dose of 0·4 mg does not seem to be more advantageous (21). For Australian conditions a dose of 0·3 mg is recommended (28). For farmed deer a special tuberculin is used which contains 2 mg tuberculin/ml and gives an 0·1 ml dose containing 0·2 mg tuberculin.

Desensitization during tuberculin testing
When a suspicious reactor is encountered, the question of when to retest is complicated by the phenomenon of desensitization. When tuberculin is absorbed into the body, desensitization occurs and its degree increases in general terms with the amount of tuberculin and the amount of other foreign proteins absorbed. Thus desensitization is more marked and of longer duration after a subcutaneous than after an intradermal injection. One of the characteristics of the allergic reaction is the variation in differential white cell count of the blood which occurs. Polymorphonuclear cells increase and lymphocytes decrease and there is a suggestion that the greater the variation in cell count the longer the duration of desensitization. After a single intradermal injection, the leukocytic reaction is of a minor degree and is not a very reliable guide to the diagnosis of tuberculosis. Moreover, the period of desensitization is short and the animal can be retested within a few days. However, after a Stormont test the leukocyte reaction is very marked in sensitive animals and is of diagnostic significance. Although the period of desensitization after this test is not definitely known, it is of relatively long duration although not more than 6 months. The diagnostic value of this leukocyte reaction is vitiated to some extent by the variation in the time at which it occurs (6–24 hours) and by the fact that other factors such as parturition, injection of adrenal cortical hormone and infective processes produce a similar reaction.

One further aspect of the desensitization phenomenon is that use can be made of it to obscure a positive reaction. If tuberculin is injected so that the test is made in the desensitized period, no reaction will occur in infected animals.

Postparturient desensitization
Tuberculous cattle go through a period of desensitization immediately before and after calving and as many as 30% give false-negative reactions returning to a positive status 4–6 weeks later. The loss of sensitivity is probably due to the removal of fixed cell antibodies from the skin into the general circulation and subsequent drainage into the colostrum. Calves drinking this colostrum give positive reactions for up to 3 weeks after birth even though they are not infected.

Anergy generally
Anergic animals are those with visible lesions of tuberculosis but which do not react to a cutaneous delayed hypersensitivity test. The number of these can be reduced by being careful to inject sufficient tuberculin (0·2 mg) at the right site, and to read the test at 48–72 hours. There is still a residuum of cases which do not respond, especially those with extensive pulmonary involvement (17).

Summary of testing procedures in cattle
In summary it is usual to use the single intradermal test as a routine procedure but the test is not completely accurate and the following deficiencies may occur.

False-positive reactions (no gross lesion reactors) may be given by:

- Animals sensitized to other mycobacterial allergens. These may include animals infected with human or avian tuberculosis or with Johne's disease. Animals with minimal local lesions caused by relatively non-pathogenic mycobacteria, e.g. skin tuberculosis, also react to tuberculin. It is also possible that animals infected with, or which perhaps only ingest, nonpathogenic mycobacteria can also become sensitized and react to the test. For example, atypical mycobacteria in permanent waters inhabited by birds are thought to be the cause of the very high incidence of non-specific reactors in Kenyan cattle. Stagnant water is one of the most potent sources of saprophytic mycobacteria and some attention should be given to it when non-specific reactors occur. Another source is poultry litter fed to cattle when the birds are infected with *M. avium*. Experimentally it is possible to stimulate hypersensitivity by the injection of atypical mycobacteria from feral pigs, trough water, soil and many other sources.
- Animals sensitized to other allergens which may be bacterial, e.g. *Nocardia farcinicus* in bovine farcy (18), or not.

False-negative reactions may be given by:

- Advanced cases of tuberculosis
- Early cases until 6 weeks after infection
- Cows which have calved within the preceding 6 weeks
- Animals desensitized by tuberculin administration during the preceding 8–60 days
- Old cattle.

A summary of the tests available and their recommended use is set out in Table 57.

Reactors which are thought to be non-specific should be retested by the comparative test in the cervical region 7 days after the response to the caudal fold test (20). For greater accuracy sensitins prepared from other mycobacteria, e.g. the poorly pathogenic Runyon IV (1), can be included in the test agents.

Tuberculin testing in pigs
The most generally used method is the SID test, injecting 0·1 ml of standard potency mammalian tuberculin

Table 57. Tuberculin tests and when to use them

Circumstances	*Tests to be used*	*Comments*
Initial test in unknown herd	SID	Preferred because only two visits required and period of desensitization short. Considerable error with non-specific reactors and animals with reduced sensitivity, e.g. recent calving, advanced cases and animals tested with tuberculin during the preceding 60 days (19).
	Stormont	Three trips required and long period of desensitization preventing frequent retests
	SID comparative	As below if the presence of avian tuberculosis or Johne's disease is suspected, i.e. in the United Kingdom generally (40)
Probable advanced cases in heavily infected herd	Stormont	Accurate
	Short thermal	Time-consuming but useful to sort out reactors to SID test soon after that test (48)
Cows calved within preceding 6 weeks	Stormont	Accuracy of short thermal test unknown in this group
Suspicious reactors	Stormont	SID easily converted to Stormont with two more visits and answer obtained quickly
	Isolate and retest with SID in 1 month	Long wait for answer
	Immediate SID in other fold	During desensitization period and animal may not react
	Comparative cervical SID 7 days later (15)	Previous recommendation was to delay 60–90 days before retest
In herds where avian tuberculosis or Johne's disease suspected	SID comparative Stormont	Relative merits uncertain. Stormont does not react with Johne's or avian tuberculosis
Introduction to free herd or recently assembled herd	SID and repeat in 1 or 2 months	Stormont would prevent quick retest and early cases may be missed for too long

into a fold of skin at the base of the ear, but the test is relatively inaccurate in this species (5). The test is read 24–48 hours later and an increase in skin thickness of 5 mm or more constitutes a positive reaction. In positive animals the reactions are quite marked, the skin thickening often exceeding 10 mm and showing superficial necrosis and sloughing. If the animal is infected with *M. avium*, the maximum skin thickening may not occur until 48 hours after injection. When no attempt is being made to determine the type of infection, mixed avian and mammalian tuberculins may be used and the test read at 24–48 hours. If avian tuberculin alone is used, the test should be read at 48–72 hours and an increase in skin thickness of 4 mm is classed as positive.

Many suspicious reactions occur in pigs because of the tendency of lesions to regress and the sensitivity to tuberculin to diminish, maximum sensitivity occurring 3–9 weeks after infection. A retest in 6–8 weeks should determine whether or not the disease is progressing. Although positive reactors may in time revert to a negative status, there may be macroscopic lesions in these animals at necropsy. However, viable organisms are not usually recoverable from the lesion, the infection apparently having been overcome.

The Stormont test is unlikely to have any application in pigs because there is no local increase in skin sensitivity after one injection. Some decrease in skin sensitivity after parturition occurs in sows affected with *M. bovis* but may not occur when the infection is caused by *M. avium*. Comparative tests work efficiently in this species with little or no reaction to heterologous tuberculin. Hematological changes in pigs during the period of reaction to tuberculin are comparable to those which occur in cattle.

Tuberculin testing in other species

In the horse the results obtained with subcutaneous and intradermal tuberculin tests are very erratic and must be assessed with caution especially when the test is positive as many false-positives occur (24). The horse appears to be much more sensitive than cattle to tuberculin and much smaller doses of standardized tuberculin are required than in cattle. As little as 0·1 ml of PPD tuberculin is sufficient to elicit a positive reaction and a normal dose may provoke an anaphylactic reaction. No safe recommendations can be made on tests in this species because of lack of detailed information, but the occurrence of a systemic reaction with a positive cutaneous test can be accepted as indicating the presence of infection.

The single intradermal test has been used in sheep and goats but is relatively inaccurate, some tuberculous animals giving negative reactions. The SID test appears to be satisfactory on the basis of results achieved in experimentally infected goats (15). This test has also proved satisfactory when applied to the skin of the inside of the thigh of sheep (41). The test injection is usually given in the caudal fold as in cattle and an increase in thickness of 5 mm in the fold constitutes a positive reaction.

Serological tests for diagnosis of tuberculosis

In the final stages of a tuberculosis eradication program the percentage of reactors which are not in fact tuberculous increases to the point where a more discerning test than the one based on cutaneous hypersensitivity is required. Most of the tests tried so far have been serological ones. Their aim is to identify early cases, cases which are anergic because of the advanced stage of the disease, and cases which are sensitized by some other bacteria, e.g. *Corynebacterium* sp. (23).

Serological tests including complement fixation, fluorescent antibody (27), direct bacterial agglutination, precipitin and hemagglutination tests are under review but seem to have little potential value for the routine diagnosis of tuberculosis (29). The fluorescent antibody test can detect sensitivity to *M. avium* in calves, but is unable to distinguish between that antigen and *M. paratuberculosis*. Cattle experimentally infected with *M. tuberculosis* also react poorly to the indirect fluorescent antibody test (12). The complement fixation test response to both antigens is poor. An enzyme-linked immunoabsorbent assay (ELISA) has also been tested in pigs (5) and cattle (30). In spite of these efforts, the single intradermal test read at 72 hours in a caudal fold and using an 0·3 ml dose of PPD tuberculin is still the preferred method of detecting carriers of tuberculosis.

Necropsy findings

Cattle, sheep and goats

These show identical lesions with a standard distribution. Tuberculous granulomas may be found in any of the lymph nodes, but particularly in bronchial and mediastinal nodes, and many organs. In the lung, miliary abscesses may extend to cause a suppurative bronchopneumonia. The pus has a characteristic cream to orange color and varies in consistency from thick cream to thick, crumbly cheese. Small nodules may appear on the pleura and peritoneum. These also contain tuberculous pus but are not accompanied by effusion.

All localized lesions of tuberculosis tend to stimulate an enveloping fibrous capsule but the degree of encapsulation varies with the rate of development of the lesion. Apart from the value of a necropsy examination in making a diagnosis, a close study of the lesions may indicate the importance of the subject animal as a spreader of the disease to others. Active or 'open' cases are the dangerous spreaders and these are denoted by the presence of miliary tuberculosis with small, transparent, shot-like lesions in many organs, or by pulmonary lesions which are not well encapsulated and caseated. The presence of bronchopneumonia or hyperemia around pulmonary lesions is highly suggestive of active disease. Cases with tuberculous mastitis or discharging tuberculous metritis must also be considered as open cases.

'Closed' lesions are characteristically discrete and nodular and contain thick, yellow to orange, caseous material, often calcified and surrounded by a thick, fibrous capsule. Although such lesions are less likely to cause heavy contamination of the environment than open lesions, affected animals may still be important as sources of infection.

Pigs

Some cases of generalized tuberculosis, with miliary tubercles in most organs, are found in pigs. The common finding is localization in the tonsils, submaxillary, cervical, hepatic, bronchial, mediastinal and mesenteric lymph nodes. The nodes are markedly enlarged and consist of masses of white, caseous, sometimes calcified, material, surrounded by a strong, fibrous capsule and interlaced by strands of fibrous tissue. Because of the regressive nature of the disease in pigs, these lesions are often negative on culture and guinea-pig inoculation.

Horses

Although the lesions in horses have a characteristic distribution in the intestinal wall, mesenteric lymph nodes and spleen, the lesions themselves have a distinctive appearance which is peculiar to this species. Chronic lesions are firm to the touch and on cutting have an appearance similar to that of neoplastic tissue. In the horse, too, there is a tendency for lesions to develop in the skeleton, particularly the cervical vertebrae.

Diagnosis

Because of the chronic nature of the disease and the multiplicity of signs caused by the variable localization of the infection, tuberculosis is difficult to diagnose on clinical examination. If the disease occurs in an area, it must be considered in the differential diagnosis of many diseases of cattle. In pigs the disease is usually so benign that cases do not present themselves as clinical problems and are found only at necropsy. The rarity of the disease in horses, sheep and goats makes it an unlikely diagnostic risk except in groups which have had abnormally high exposure to infected cattle.

In cattle other chronic pulmonary diseases which may be confused with tuberculous pneumonia are lung abscess due to aspiration pneumonia, pleurisy and pericarditis following traumatic reticulitis and chronic contagious bovine pleuropneumonia. A few animals survive the acute stages of aspiration pneumonia, and show emaciation, chronic cough and changes at auscultation and percussion identical with those of tuberculosis. A history of previous parturient paresis or inefficient drenching are the only points short of tuberculin testing on which to base a differentiation. Sequels of traumatic reticulitis can produce a clinical picture indistinguishable from tuberculosis but there is usually a history of a severe attack of illness some time previously with gradual but incomplete recovery. Chronic contagious bovine pleuropneumonia is to be suspected in an enzootic area and the complement fixation test provides a suitable diagnostic method. Simultaneous infection with both diseases is not uncommon.

Snoring respiration is relatively common in cattle and some differentiation of the cause is necessary and practicable. In true 'snoring' due to pharyngeal obstruction, the noise produced in guttural and nasal airflow is unobstructed. Enlarged pharyngeal lymph nodes and granulomatous lesions can be detected on internal palpation of the pharynx. Lymph node enlargement may be due to tuberculosis or actinobacillosis but granulomatous lesions are usually caused by the latter. A tuberculin test is usually necessary to differentiate between these diseases.

Nasal snoring is more common and is a higher-pitched, wheezing noise often audible from a distance. It is usually accompanied by nasal discharge and partial or complete obstruction to nasal airflow. Pharyngeal palpation is negative and mouth-breathing may be evident. The common causes of nasal obstruction in cattle are allergic rhinitis, mucous polyps in the posterior nares and nodular thickening of the nasal mucosa.

In tuberculous mastitis, fibrosis begins at the base of the gland instead of about the cistern as in most other forms of mastitis, and abnormal milk commonly comes at the end of milking instead of the first few streams and is not marked until the late stages of the disease. Avian tuberculosis may localize in the udder on rare occasions. Tuberculous metritis is characterized by the continued discharge of large quantities of yellow pus. The pus has the appearance of curdled milk and is unlike that in any other form of metritis.

Peripheral lymph node enlargements should be suspected of having a tuberculous origin, but abscesses caused by mixed infections or infection with *Actinobacillus lignieresii or Corynebacterium* (*Rhodococcus*) *equi* (34) of the lymph nodes of the head are much more common. Bacteriological examination of pus obtained by needle puncture is a simple method of differentiation. Lymphomatosis may be confused with tuberculous lymphadenitis but it is usually characterized by simultaneous, bilateral enlargement of several lymph nodes. The enlarged nodes are softer and smoother than tuberculous nodes and do not usually contain pus.

At necropsy the lesions of tuberculosis in cattle are characteristic, but differentiation from lesions caused by actinobacillus, *Corynebacterium* (*Rhodococcus*) *equi* coccidioidomycosis and mucormycosis requires some care. Accurate identification may necessitate laboratory examination. In horses, tuberculous lesions closely resemble neoplastic tissue and in pigs, confusion with a number of other diseases is likely to occur. In meat inspection surveys, as many as 50% of suspected tuberculous lesions in pigs are non-tuberculous (22). Opinions differ on the ease with which infections with *Cor.* (*Rhodococcus*) *equi* can be distinguished from those caused by mycobacteria on macroscopic or histological grounds (31). Lesions caused by *M. avium* are characterized by an absence of necrosis, the lesions being firm and homogeneous with rare foci of calcification.

Treatment

Because of the progress being made in the treatment of human tuberculosis with such drugs as isoniazid, combinations of streptomycin and *para*-aminosalicylic and other acids, the treatment of animals with tuberculosis has undergone some examination and claims have been made for the efficiency of longterm oral medication with isoniazid both as treatment and as prophylaxis (32).

Control

Eradication of bovine tuberculosis has been virtually achieved in many countries. The methods used have depended on a number of factors but ultimately the test and slaughter policy has been the only one by which effective eradication had been achieved.

Control on a herd basis

Control in a herd rests on removal of the infected animals, prevention of spread of infection and avoidance of further introduction of the disease. All three points are of equal importance and neglect of one may result in breakdown of the eradication program.

Detection of infected animals depends largely upon the use of the tuberculin test. The single intradermal test is widely used but other tests are available (see Table 57) and should be used where they are indicated. All animals over 3 months of age should be tested and positive reactors disposed of according to local legislation. Suspicious reactors may be dealt with in several ways as indicated in Table 57. At the initial test, a careful clinical examination should be conducted on all animals to ensure that there are no advanced clinical cases which will give negative reactions to the test. Doubtful cases and animals likely to have reduced sensitivity, particularly old cows and those that have calved within the previous 6 weeks, may be tested by one of the special tests described above or retested subsequently. The comparative test should be used where infection with *M. paratuberculosis* or *M. avium* is anticipated or where a high incidence of reactors occurs in a herd not showing clinical evidence of the disease.

If the incidence of reactors is high at the first test or if 'open' lesions are found at necropsy in culled animals, emphasis must be placed on repeat testing at short intervals or the spread of the disease may overtake the culling rate. Tests should be conducted at 2-monthly intervals if the incidence is high. Other herds may be retested at 3-monthly intervals until a negative test is obtained. A further test is conducted 6 months later and if the herd is again negative, it may be classed as free of the disease. Subsequent check tests should be carried out annually.

Hygienic measures to prevent the spread of infection should be instituted as soon as the first group of reactors is removed. Feed troughs should be cleaned and thoroughly disinfected with hot, 5% phenol or equivalent cresol disinfectant. Water troughs and drinking cups should be emptied and similarly disinfected. Suspicious reactors being held for retesting should be isolated from the remainder of the herd. If a number of reactors are culled, attention must be given to the possibility of infection being reintroduced with replacements which should come from accredited herds. Failing this, the animals should be tested immediately, isolated and retested in 60 days.

It is most important that calves being reared as herd replacements be fed on tuberculosis-free milk, either from known free animals or pasteurized. Rearing calves on skim milk from a communal source is a particularly dangerous practice unless the skim milk is properly sterilized. All other classes of livestock on the farm should be examined for evidence of tuberculosis. Farm attendants should be checked as they may provide a source of *M. tuberculosis* infection, resulting in transient positive reactions in the cattle. Humans may also act as a source of *M. bovis* infection.

Steps should be taken to ensure that reinfection does not occur by testing all introductions, preventing communal use of watering facilities or pasture, and maintaining adequate boundary fences. A special problem is created when tuberculosis occurs in cattle run on extensive range country with little manpower and few fences. It is inadvisable to attempt a control program until it can be guaranteed that all animals can be gathered, identified, tested and segregated. In some areas it is uneconomic to do this.

Control on an area basis

The method used to eradicate bovine tuberculosis from large areas will depend on the incidence of the disease, methods of husbandry, attitude of the farming community and the economic capacity of the country to stand losses from a test and slaughter program.

An essential first step in the inauguration of an eradication program is the prior education of the farming community. Livestock owners must be apprised of the economic and public health significance of the disease, its manifestations and the necessity for the various steps in the eradication program. Eradication must also be compulsory since voluntary schemes have never achieved more than limited control and always leave foci of infection. Adequate compensation must be paid to encourage full cooperation. This may take the form of compensation for animals destroyed or bonuses for disease-free herds or their milk or beef.

It is essential at the beginning of a program to determine the incidence and distribution of the disease by tuberculin testing of samples of the cattle population and a meat inspection service. Information collected in this way indicates the herds and areas which are free of tuberculosis or which have a low incidence. The disease can be readily eradicated from these latter areas, thus providing a nucleus of tuberculosis-free cattle which can supply replacements for further areas as they are brought into the eradication scheme. Finally, the eradication program can be extended to the residual area.

When the incidence of tuberculosis is high, a routine test and slaughter program may be economically impossible. Two herd schemes have been used in Europe and elsewhere but are now of historical interest only.

Vaccination may be considered under certain circumstances, particularly when an eradication program cannot be instituted for some time but it is desired to reduce the incidence of the disease in preparation for eradication. BCG vaccination is the only method available for field use, the vole acid-fast vaccine varying too much in virulence. BCG vaccine has many disadvantages. Vaccination is carried out by the subcutaneous injection of 50–100 ml vaccine and large and unsightly lumps appear at the injection site. Injection by the alternative intravenous route is attended by risk of severe systemic reactions. Vaccination must be repeated annually and the vaccinated animal remains positive to the tuberculin test. Calves must be vaccinated as soon after birth as possible and do not achieve immunity for 6 weeks. The immunity is not strong and vaccinated animals must not be submitted to severe exposure. In field circumstances where the disease is prevalent only modest results, if any, can be expected (33).

When the overall incidence of tuberculosis is 5% or less, compulsory testing and the slaughter of reactors is the only satisfactory method of eradication. A combination of lines of attack is usually employed. Accredited areas are set up by legislation, and all cattle within these areas are tested and reactors removed. Voluntary accreditation of individual herds is encouraged outside these areas. In some countries, focal points of extensive infection outside accredited areas have been attacked under special legislation. The usual method of encouraging herd accreditation and then introducing compulsory eradication has resulted in the virtual eradication of the disease in the United States. When an area or country has been freed from the disease, quarantine barriers must be set up to avoid its reintroduction. Within the area, the recurrent cost of testing can be lessened by gradually increasing the intertest period to 2 and then to 3 or even 6 years as the amount of residual infection diminishes. Meat inspection services provide a good observation point should any increase in incidence of the disease occur. Amongst range beef cattle it is usual to check samples of animals at intervals rather than the entire cattle population.

Problems in tuberculosis eradication

Complete eradication of tuberculosis has not really been achieved in any country. In many a state of virtual eradication has been in existence for years but minor recrudescences occur. The major problems which arise are as follows.

In the final stages of an eradication program a number of problems achieve much greater importance than in the early stages of the campaign (36). The percentage of no gross lesion reactors which occurs rises steeply and creates administrative and public relations difficulties. Individual herds which have been accredited after a number of free tests are found to have the disease again, often with a very high incidence. Another major problem is that of 'traceback' of infected animals at packing plants, or as a result of area testing, to their herds of origin—even with vigorous effort it is often impossible to determine the origin of many affected animals (25). The answer to the first problem must await the definition of a test or tests which will differentiate between tuberculosis and sensitivity to other agents, particularly other mycobacteria. There is as yet no highly reliable test to detect the poorly sensitized animals in the early or late stages of the disease which are the usual cause of recrudescence in herds that have been classified as being free of the disease. 'Traceback' becomes the principal source of information on the location of infected herds in the final stages of a program (37), and a major advance would be a suitable method of identifying individual animals which could be utilized up to the killing floor (36).

The two most popular methods are fabric labels stuck on the rump with skin contact glue which are not removable but messy to handle, and wraparound plastic or metal tail-tags. These have an identification number for the property or farm of origin. They have two problems: they can be removed at the abattoir and reused; and they do fall off if the tail is docked, a popular practice in some areas.

Another area of difficulty in eradication is where cattle are run under very extensive conditions on large ranches or stations as in Canada, South America and Australia. It is necessary in these circumstances to develop special management systems (35) and there is a great need for a test that does not require that cattle be held in a mustering site for 3 days before the test is read (38).

Control of tuberculosis in pigs

In pigs, because of the non-progressive nature of the disease, transmission from pig to pig is unlikely to occur to a significant extent except perhaps in breeding animals. Pigs serve mostly as a repository for tuberculosis from other species and elimination of the source of infection is usually sufficient to eradicate the disease from previously affected groups. When tuberculosis is positively diagnosed, every effort should be made to type the organism as this gives some indication of the species from which the infection has been derived. Human type (*M. tuberculosis*) infections are usually the result of feeding offal from a tubercular household or contact with a tuberculous attendant. Avian type (*M. avium*) infections occur when tuberculous chickens are allowed to run freely with the pigs. *M. bovis* infection in pigs usually results from the feeding of infected milk, skim milk or whey to pigs or allowing cattle and pigs to graze the same pasture. The first step in the control of tuberculosis in a pig herd is to remove the source of infection, and then to test and remove the reacting animals. This second step is made less efficient by the relative inaccuracy of the tuberculin test in this species (39).

REVIEW LITERATURE

Alhaji, I. (1976) Bovine tuberculosis: a general review with special reference to Nigeria. *Vet. Bull.*, 46, 829.

Collins, C. H. & Grange, J. M. (1983) A review: the bovine tubercle bacillus. *J. appl. Bacteriol.*, 55, 13–29.

Lepper, A. W. D. & Corner, L. A. (1983) Naturally occurring mycobacteriosis of animals. In: *The Biology of Mycobacteria*, Vol. 2. London: Academic Press.

REFERENCES

(1) Songer, J. G. et al (1980) *Can. J. comp. med.*, *44*, 115.
(2) Duffied, B. J. & Young, D. A. (1985) *Vet. Microbiol.*, *10*, 193.
(3) Dalchow, W. & Nassal, J. (1979) *Tierärztl. Umschau*, *34*, 253.
(4) Blancou, J. M. & Cheneau, Y. (1974) *Rev. Élev. Méd. vét. Pays trop.*, *27*, 75.
(5) Thoen, C. O. et al. (1983) *Proc. US Anim. Hlth Assoc.*, *87*, 582.
(6) Wilesmith, J. W. et al. (1986) *J. Hyg., Camb.*, 97, 11.
(7) Pritchard, D. G. et al. (1986) *J. Hyg., Camb.*, 97, 27.
(8) Jorgensen, J. B. (1978) *Acta vet. Scand.*, *19*, 49.
(9) Thoen, C. O. & Richards, W. D. (1977) *J. Am. vet. med. Assoc.*, *170*, 987.
(10) Dodd, K. (1984) *Vet. Rec.*, *115*, 592.
(11) Lesslie, I. W. & Hebert, C. N. (1965) *Br. vet. J.*, *121*, 427.
(12) Lepper, A. W. D. et al. (1977) *Aust. vet. J.*, *53*, 301.
(13) Miller, L. D. (1984) *Proc. Ann. Mtg Am. Assoc. vet. Lab. Diag.*, *26*, 39.
(14) Larsen, A. B. et al. (1969) *Am. J. vet. Res.*, *30*, 2167.
(15) Duffied, B. J. et al. (1985) *Aust. Vet. J.*, *62*, 424.
(16) Perrin, G. et al. (1984) *Point Vét.*, *16*, 59.
(17) Lepper, A. W. D. et al. (1977) *Aust. vet J.*, *53*, 208 & 214.
(18) Awad, F. I. (1963) *Proc. 17th Wld vet. Congr., Hanover*, *1*, 465.
(19) Radunz, B. L. & Lepper, A. W. D. (1985) *Aust. vet. J.*, *62*, 191.
(20) Roswurm, J. D. & Konyha, L. D. (1974) *Proc. US Anim. Hlth Assoc.*, *77*, 368.
(21) Lepper, A. W. D. et al. (1979) *Aust. vet. J.*, *55*, 251.
(22) Wilesmith, J. W. et al. (1986) *J. Hyg., Camb.*, 97, 37.

(23) Mackenzie, R. W. & Donald. B. A. (1979) *J. comp. Pathol.*, *89*, 31.
(24) Konhya, L. D. & Kreter, J. P. (1971) *Rev. resp. Dis.*, *103*, 91.
(25) Bennett, R. W. & Konyha, L. D. (1978) *Proc. US Anim. Hlth Assoc.*, *82*, 474.
(26) Adlam, G. H. (1977) *NZ vet. J.*, *55*, 507.
(27) Lepper, A. W. D. & Pearson, C. W. (1975) *Aust. vet. J.*, *51*, 250.
(28) Lepper, A. W. D. et al. (1979) *Aust. vet. J.*, *55*, 507.
(29) Alhan, I. (1976) *Vet. Bull.*, *46*, 829.
(30) Thoen, C. O. et al. (1984) *Proc. US Ann. Hlth Assoc.*, *87*, 603.
(31) Lesslie, I. W. et al. (1968) *Vet. Rec.*, *83*, 647.
(32) Kleeberg, H. H. et al. (1966) *J. S. Afr. vet. med. Assoc.*, *37*, 219.
(33) Berggren, S. A. (1977) *Br. vet. J.*, *133*, 490.
(34) McKenzie, R. A. et al. (1981) *J. comp. Pathol.*, *91*, 347.
(35) Mitchell, V. (1984) *Proc. No. 68 Univ. Syd. Postgrad. Com. Vet. Sci.*, Refresher Course 'Beef Cattle Production', p. 249.
(36) Roswurm, J. D. & Ranney, A. F. (1973) *Am. J. publ. Hlth*, *63*, 884.
(37) Johnson, D. C. et al. (1975) *J. Am. vet. med. Assoc.*, *167*, 833.
(38) Andrews, L. (1984) *Proc. No. 68 Univ. Syd. Postgrad. Com. Vet. Sci.*, Refresher Course 'Beef Cattle Production', p. 229.
(39) Mallinan, W. L. et al. (1962) *Proc. US livestk sanit. Assoc.*, *180*, 184.
(40) Cordes, D. O. et al. (1981) *NZ vet. J.*, *29*, 60.
(41) Davidson, R. M. et al. (1981) *NZ vet. J.*, *29*, 1.
(42) Payeur, J. B. et al. (1983) *Proc. 85th Ann. Mtg US Anim. Hlth Assoc.*, p. 475.
(43) Corner, L. A. et al. (1981) *Aust. vet. J.*, *57*, 537.
(44) Hein, W. R. & Tomasovic, A. A. (1981) *Aust. vet. J.*, *57*, 543.
(45) Jorgensen, J. B. et al. (1985) *Dansk vet. Tidskr.*, *68*, 793.
(46) McKroy, S. G. et al. (1986) *Vet. Rec.*, *118*, 718.
(47) Stumpff, C. D. (1982) *Proc. Am. Ann. Hlth Assoc.*, *86*, 524.
(48) Radunz, B. L. (1984) *Aust. vet. J.*, *61*, 195.

Mycobacteriosis caused by *Mycobacterium avium*

Tuberculosis caused by the avian tubercle bacillus is not a major disease problem in cattle but can cause much difficulty in tuberculosis eradication programs in cattle and pigs since infected animals are sensitive to mammalian tuberculin and many valuable animals may be slaughtered as positive reactors. In the United Kingdom where the situation has been carefully examined it is apparent that in recent years the proportion of positive reactors to tuberculin in pigs which are due to *M. avium* has increased to the point where 80–90% of cases are caused by *M. avium* (1). Infected cattle and pigs are now considered to be sources of infection for the increasing number of *M. avium* infections in man. Although the infection is commonly contracted from domestic poultry, there is the possibility that infection is transmitted between mammals, especially pigs. Outbreaks in pig herds can cause heavy losses because of carcass condemnation (3). The use of a comparative tuberculin test to differentiate between infections with the two bacterial species has already been discussed.

In cattle, sensitivity to tuberculin may disappear soon after they are removed from contact with infected birds. Local lesions may persist in the mesenteric lymph nodes, the meninges and in the uterus and udder, and occasional cases of open pulmonary tuberculosis, caused by *M. avium*, have been observed. The uterus is a common predilection site for avian tuberculosis and recurrent abortion may occur. Mammary localization is common and induration and involvement of lymph nodes, as in infection with *M. bovis*, do occur (5). Generalized tuberculosis can occur in up to 50% of cases (6).

In pigs the naturally occurring disease is nonprogressive and usually restricted to the lymph nodes of the head and neck (7). Occasional generalized cases occur and an outbreak of pulmonary tuberculosis caused by *M. avium* has been recorded in pigs (8). The lesions are characteristically free of suppuration and resemble neoplastic tissue rather than tuberculous lesions. Similar lesions are caused by atypical mycobacteria and other species, e.g. *Corynebacterium* (*Rhodococcus*) *equi* (15). The experimentally produced disease in pigs is generalized provided the oral dose is sufficiently large (4). Granulomatous and caseous lesions in lymph nodes are characteristic and in some studies (4) granulomatous lesions which develop in the tonsils and intestinal wall result in the passage of *M. avium* in the feces for at least 55 days (17) making the animals infective for this period. Transmission from these to in-contact pigs occurs readily. Subcutaneous injection into calves also causes the development of a generalized disease consisting of disseminated granulomas (9). Vaccination of pigs with BCG vaccine provides partial protection against experimental infection with *M. avium* (16). Horses are resistant to infection with *M. avium*, although rare, generalized cases of avian tuberculosis have been recorded in this species (10). Two cases have been recorded in which the lesions in the cervical lymph nodes were accompanied by lesions in cervical vertebrae. The lesions were similar to those seen in cervical vertebral osteomyelitis caused by *M. bovis* (11). Goats and sheep appear to have a strong natural resistance to infection with *M. avium* but their relative freedom from the disease may be due to lack of contact with infected birds. A high incidence of avian tuberculosis has been observed in a flock of goats (12) and although the disease progresses slowly in this species goats may act as spreaders for other species. Infection in wild deer has been observed and it is postulated that deer may serve as a source of infection for carrion-eating birds (13). Humans associated with infected animals and birds also develop positive reactions to avian tuberculin (14).

REVIEW LITERATURE

Boughton, E. (1969) *Vet. Bull.*, *39*, 757.

REFERENCES

(1) Prichard, W. D. et al. (1977) *Am. J. Epidemiol.*, *106*, 222.
(2) Acland, H. M. & Whitlock, R. H. (1986) *J. comp. Pathol.*, *96*, 247.
(3) Windsor, R. S. et al. (1984) *J. Hyg., Camb.*, *92*, 129.
(4) Jorgensen, J. B. (1977–78) *Acta vet. Scand.*, *18*, 545 & *19*, 49.
(5) Cassidy, D. R. et al. (1968) *Am. J. vet Res.*, *29*, 405.
(6) Lesslie, I. W. & Birn, K. J. (1967) *Vet. Rec.*, *80*, 559.
(7) Szabo, I. et al. (1975) *Acta vet. Hung.*, *25*, 67, 77.
(8) Jorgensen, J. B. et al. (1972) *Acta vet. Scand.*, *13*, 56, 68.
(9) McGavin, M. D. (1977) *Vet. Pathol.*, *14*, 56.
(10) Baker, J. R. (1973) *Vet. Rec.*, *93*, 105.
(11) Binkhorst, G. J. et al. (1972) *Tijdschr. Diergeneeskd.*, *97*, 1268.
(12) Lesslie, I. W. (1960) *Vet. Rec.*, *72*, 25.
(13) Hopkinson, F. & McDiarmid, A. (1964) *Vet. Rec.*, *76*, 1521.
(14) Bader, A. et al. (1975) *Tierärztl. Umschau*, *30*, 373.
(15) Flesja, K. I. et al. (1978) *Nord VetMed.*, *30*, 61.
(16) Jorgensen, J. B. (1978) *Acta vet. Scand.*, *19*, 430.
(17) Ellsworth, S. et al. (1980) *Am. J. vet. Res.*, *41*, 1526.

Mycobacteriosis caused by atypical mycobacteria

An extensive literature has accumulated about the subject of infections, especially of pigs, caused by the atypical group of mycobacteria. This includes *M. intracellulare, M. kansasii, M. fortuitum, M. aquae* and *M. scrofulaceum* and other identified species (2, 3). Many of them produce microgranulomas in the lymph nodes of calves (11). *M. fortuitum* is recorded as a cause of chronic arthritis in pigs (12). There are a number of serotypes of *M. intracellulare*. Some of them are quite virulent, producing extensive lesions in mesenteric lymph nodes in calves (11) and pigs (5). It is not intended to review that literature completely but it is necessary to point out that these infections can cause macroscopic lesions visible at necropsy examination and cause false-positive reactions to the tuberculin test especially when the single intradermal test (SID) is used. These lesions and sensitivities have been produced experimentally in cattle (4), and the sensitivity produced has been compared to the sensitivity to avian and bovine tuberculin. Sensitivity occurs to both but is greater to avian tuberculin (6). In general the response to bovine tuberculin is significant only with mycobacteria of bovine origin (7). The response is also shortlived, significant changes in sensitivity occurring between successive tests (13). The comparative tuberculin test is becoming more widely used because of the growing importance of these infections. It is not uncommon for there to be more than one species of mycobacteria causing disease in a herd at the one time.

The use of peat as bedding for cattle has led to infection with atypical mycobacteria, the peat being contaminated before use.

In pigs the use of deep litter, rather than bare concrete, enhances the prospects of infection with *M. intracellulare* and the development of macroscopic lymphadenitis in the majority of the pigs (8). The length of time that pigs are kept on the litter is important and severe outbreaks can occur in pigs kept on litter for the entire period from weaning to the baconer stage (9). Of the materials used for pig litter, sawdust, straw and wood shavings have all been found to be highly infected (1, 14) and bedding must be considered to be a common source of infection.

In pigs the lesions are restricted to lymph nodes, none is found in the lungs or liver. The lesions are essentially non-progressive and become calcified. Although not clinically ill, human workers have been found to be infected on farms when the disease occurred in pigs (10). Drinking water is also commonly identified as a source of infection of atypical mycobacteria.

There is an important zoonotic aspect of these diseases. Infections with atypical mycobacteria are not uncommon in man and their differential diagnosis can present difficulties. It is likely that infections in man and animals on the one farm come from the one source, but it is also possible that spread from animals to man occurs (4).

REFERENCES

(1) Pavlas, M. & Patlokova, V. (1985) *Acta vet. Brno.*, *54*, 85.
(2) Yochida, S. & Shimizu, K. (1973) *Jap. J. vet. Sci.*, *35*, 459.
(3) Ray, J. A. et al. (1972) *Am. J. vet. Res.*, *33*, 1333.
(4) Corner, L. A. & Person, C. W. (1979) *Aust. vet. J.*, *55*, 6.
(5) Tuffley, R. E. et al. (1973) *J. comp. Pathol.*, *83*, 467.
(6) Pearson, C. W. et al. (1977) *Aust. vet. J.*, *53*, 67.
(7) Corner, L. A. & Pearson, C. W. (1978) *Aust. vet. J.*, *54*, 280 & 379.
(8) Szabo, I. et al. (1974) *Magy. Allatorv. Lap.*, *29*, 511, 515.
(9) Brooks, I. H. (1971) *Aust. vet. J.*, *47*, 424.
(10) Reznikov, M. & Robinson, E. (1971) *Aust. vet. J.*, *46*, 606.
(11) Jorgensen, J. B. (1981) *Rev. infect. Dis.*, *3*, 979.
(12) Chengappa, M. M. et al. (1983) *Vet. Med. SAC*, *78*, 1273.
(13) Corner, L. A. (1987) *Aust. vet. J.*, *57*, 216.
(14) Windsor, R. S. et al. (1984) *Vet. Rec.*, *114*, 497.

Tuberculosis caused by *Mycobacterium tuberculosis*

Most cases of tuberculosis in animals caused by *M. tuberculosis* of human origin are transitory and without lesions. Removal of tuberculous humans from the environment usually results in the disappearance of positive reactors in cattle. In cattle herds the reactors and necropsy lesions are most common in the young stock (1). Many reactors have no visible lesions: those which do occur are small and confined to the lymph nodes of the digestive and respiratory systems. Pigs may develop minor lesions in lymph nodes, but sheep, goats and horses appear to be resistant. A high incidence of sensitivity to tuberculin due to exposure of cattle to tuberculous attendants has been recorded in Kenya (2).

REFERENCES

(1) Lesslie, I. W. (1960) *Vet. Rec.*, *72*, 218.
(2) Waddington, J. G. (1965) *Br. vet. J.*, *121*, 319.

'Skin tuberculosis'

Chronic indurative lesions of the skin in cattle, occurring usually on the lower limbs, are called 'skin tuberculosis' because they frequently sensitize affected animals to tuberculin. They are not caused by pathogenic mycobacteria.

Etiology

Acid-fast organisms can often be found in the lesions in small numbers. They have not been identified and are probably not true pathogens (1). The similarity between this disease and cattle farcy can cause confusion, especially now that *Mycobacterium farcinogenes* has been identified as a cause of farcy (2). Iatrogenic lesions appear to have been caused by the use of aluminum adsorbed vaccines. These produced subcutaneous gra nulomas which were colonized by acid-fast bacteria (3).

Epidemiology

The frequent occurrence of lesions on the lower extremities suggests cutaneous abrasions as the probable portal of entry of the causative organism.

The disease occurs in most countries of the world, particularly where animals are housed. The lesions cause little inconvenience but they are unsightly and affected animals may give a suspicious or positive reaction to the tuberculin test when they are in fact free of tuberculosis. This becomes important when herds and areas are undergoing eradication and attention is focussed on any condition which complicates the tuberculin test.

Pathogenesis

Tuberculoid granulomas occur at the site of infection with spread along local lymphatics but without involvement of lymph nodes.

Clinical findings

Small (1–2 cm diameter) lumps appear under the skin. The lower limbs are the most common site, particularly the forelimbs, and spread to the thighs and forearms and even to the shoulder and abdomen may occur. The lesions may be single or multiple and often occur in chains connected by thin, radiating cords of tissue. The nodules are attached to the skin, may rupture and discharge thick, cream to yellow pus. Ulcers do not persist. Individual lesions may disappear but complete recovery to the point of disappearance of all lesions is unlikely if the lesions are large and multiple.

Clinical pathology

Affected animals may react to the tuberculin test. Bacteriological examination of smears of pus may reveal the presence of acid-fast bacteria.

Necropsy findings

The lesions comprise much fibrous tissue, usually containing foci of pasty or inspissated pus, and are sometimes calcified.

Diagnosis

The lesions of cattle farcy and ulcerative lymphangitis have a similar distribution but chronic ulcers and lymph node involvement occur. Bacteriological examination may be necessary to confirm the diagnosis. In herds with tuberculosis, reactors which have lesions of skin tuberculosis are disposed of in the usual way. In herds free of tuberculosis a positive reaction to the tuberculin test in animals with skin tuberculosis is usually taken to be non-specific and the affected animal is retained provided it is negative on retest (4).

Treatment and control

Treatment or control measures are not usually instituted although surgical removal may be undertaken for cosmetic reasons.

REFERENCES

(1) Thomann, H. (1949) *Schweiz. Arch. Tierheilkd.*, *91*, 237.
(2) Chamoiseau, G. (1974) *Revue Élev. Med. vét. Pays trop.*, *27*, 61.
(3) Lami, G. et al. (1970) *Magy. Állatorv. Lap.*, *25*, 151.
(4) Anonymous (1948) *So-called Skin Tuberculosis of Bovines and Its Relation to the Tuberculin Test*, p. 16. National Vet. Med. Assoc. Gr. Britain & Ireland.

Paratuberculosis (Johne's disease)

Johne's disease is a specific, infectious enteritis of cattle, sheep and goats. It is characterized by progressive emaciation in all species affected, and in cattle by chronic diarrhea and a thickening and corrugation of the wall of the intestine.

Etiology

Three strains of *M. paratuberculosis* are capable of causing the disease in cattle, the usual bovine strain and two sheep strains. The two sheep strains include the one which causes Johne's disease of sheep in Iceland (31) and a highly pigmented strain which occurs only in the United Kingdom. There are several additional variants. There is a pigmented one which causes orange-colored lesions in the intestines and mesenteric lymph nodes when introduced experimentally into calves (1), and a Norwegian strain which is pathogenic for goats.

Epidemiology

The disease occurs throughout the world and the prevalance seems to be increasing in some countries. It is most common in cattle and to a lesser extent in sheep and goats. It is widespread in cattle in Europe and has been spread to many countries by the export of infected clinically normal purebred stock. It is of major importance in cattle and sheep in temperate climates and some humid, tropical areas. The incidence is greatest in animals kept intensively under climatic and husbandry conditions which are conducive to the spread of infection. The disease is common in sheep, particularly in Iceland where it was introduced by a small shipment of stud rams from Germany. The disease has recently been recognized in sheep in Australia and the source of the infection was not determined (40). The disease is being recognized with increased frequency in goats (43, 44) and when it becomes established in goat flocks it can cause large losses and immunization may be advisable. Sheep are easily infected experimentally (7) and excrete large numbers of the organism but many recover spontaneously. In some instances the disease can cause significant financial losses to the sheep farmer. For example, the disease has become established in sheep flocks in Cyprus where sheep are farmed semi-intensively for milk production for cheese and losses can be as high as 4% per year (9). The infection also occurs in many different wildlife and exotic species. Water buffalo, captive and freeliving wild ruminants including deer, bighorn sheep, Rocky Mountain goats, aoudads, mouflon sheep, camels, mountains goats, reindeer, antelopes, llamas and yaks are all susceptible. Mice and hamsters are also susceptible and are used extensively in experimental work. The epidemiological implications of cattle and wildlife comingling on the same pasture are not known. The rate of infection can be the same in both species and it seems that both share a common source, which might well be a common herd of deer and cattle (37). The organism has been isolated from the intestinal tract tissues of Eastern white-tailed deer which were killed on a farm that had a history of bovine paratuberculosis (49). Pigs running with infected cattle may develop enlargement of the mesenteric lymph nodes suggestive of tuberculosis and from which the causative organism can be isolated. Pigs infected experimentally develop granulomatous enteritis and lymphadenitis (10), as do horses (11).

A distinguishing characteristic of Johne's disease is that infection occurs in animals at a very early age, usually under 30 days of age, and clinical disease does not occur until 3–5 years of age (45, 46). This age limit should not be used as a reliable diagnostic criterion; in extreme circumstances, for example, calves reared on infected nurse cows, clinical disease can occur at 12–18 months of age (30). Exact details of the effect of exposure to infection in adults are not available, but it is probable that some animals exposed for the first time as adults develop clinical disease while others develop only a sensitivity to johnin for short periods although they may become carriers of the organism without manifesting clinical signs (2).

There has been some controversy about breed incidence. Field observations indicate a much higher incidence in the Channel Island and Shorthorn breeds of cattle, but this may be related to increased exposure rather than to increased susceptibility. The frequency of disease in any particular breed is proportional to the abundance of that breed and paratuberculosis will be observed with highest frequency in the most predominant breed. In comparison to dairy breeds, beef cattle generally range over greater areas and have less exposure to other cattle and their feces. Thus, the prevalence is usually lower in beef than in the dairy breeds. Since Holstein cattle are the predominant dairy breed in the United States, paratuberculosis is seen with a greater frequency in that breed than in any other breed (45). The possibility that there may be some cross-protection between tuberculosis and paratuberculosis has given rise to the suggestion that eradication of tuberculosis may make the cattle population generally more susceptible to Johne's disease, but this has not been borne out by field experience in North America.

Under field conditions the disease is transmitted principally by the ingestion of feed and water contaminated by the feces of infected animals which are excreting the organism. Because of the normally long incubation period, infected animals may excrete organisms in the feces for 15–18 months before clinical signs appear. Also, animals reared in a contaminated environment may become permanent or temporary excretors of the organism without becoming clinically affected. The organism has been isolated from the genitalia and the semen of infected bulls, survives antibiotic addition and freezing (3), and as a result intrauterine infection occurs commonly. However, the experimental inoculation of small numbers of the organism into the uterus of cattle at the time of insemination are probably destroyed and do not lead to systemic infection of the dam or to persistent hypersensitivity (47). Although the organism can be isolated from up to 85% of fetuses from dams which are infected and affected with severe clinical illness, intrauterine transmission of paratuberculosis does not appear to be a significant cause of natural infection. The organism can be cultured from the milk of cows with clinical Johne's disease which makes it possible that calves could become infected by consuming such milk (48). Infection has been produced experimentally by infusion of the organism into the udder but this is an unlikely portal of entry in nature (36).

Mycobacterium paratuberculosis persists without multiplication in pasture for long periods and such pastures are infective for up to 1 year. The organism is relatively susceptible to sunlight and drying, to a high calcium content and high pH of the soil and continuous contact with urine and feces reduces the longevity of the bacteria. However, in slurry stored in tanks the organism can survive for 98–287 days depending on the composition and alkalinity of the slurry (4). The alkalinity of the soil may also influence the severity of the clinical signs. Herds raised on alkaline soils, particularly in limestone areas, may have a high incidence of infection but little clinical disease. A high prevalence of infection is recorded in the United States on acid soils in contrast to alkaline soils (33). Adult cattle moved from herds where the soil is alkaline to areas where the soil is acid often develop severe fatal clinical disease. This observation may have some practical value in the control of the disease, but it is probable that factors other than the dietary intake of calcium or the pH of the soil will also influence susceptibility to infection. Experimental work in goats did not reveal any significant difference in susceptibility between goats on normal or calcium-deficient rations. Other factors which affect susceptibility to infection include size of infective dose, age, stress, and immunosuppressive agents such as bovine virus diarrhea (BVD) virus. These factors may affect the probability of development of clinical disease (19) but they have not been well documented. Field observations indicate that stress, including parturition, transportation and nutritional deficiencies or excesses may influence the development of clinical disease. Housed animals are subjected to a high risk of infection because of the heavy contamination by feces and the long survival of the bacteria in protected sites.

The prevalence rate in an area is difficult to estimate because of the uncertainty of the diagnosis and the failure to report cases unless a specific survey or eradication program is undertaken. The prevalence of the organism in the ileocecal lymph nodes of cattle culled in the United States was 1·6% overall, with 2·9% in dairy culls and 0·8% in beef culls (42). Abattoir surveys in Wisconsin revealed a prevalence of 10·8% and in Connecticut 18% (51, 61). The population mortality rate in infected herds is usually less than 1% per year. In exceptional circumstances it can be as high as 10% although death losses are not high; when these are added to the losses caused by long periods of ill-health and reduced productivity, the disease may cause severe economic losses in affected herds. The salvage value of clinically affected animals is usually negligible because of severe emaciation. Johne's disease in not a dramatic disease, the slow spread and chronic course resulting in a recurrent rather than an acute economic loss. Infected cattle also have a significantly higher mastitis and infertility rates than non-infected cattle (5). The principal losses are through shorter life expectancy and reduced milk production. Cost benefit analysis of a modest control program has shown a net gain of 450 kg per cow per year (32).

Pathogenesis

Following oral ingestion, the organism localizes in the mucosa of the small intestine, its associated lymph nodes and, to a lesser extent, in the tonsils and suprapharyngeal lymph nodes. The primary site of bacterial multiplication is the terminal part of the small intestine and the large intestine. At least three different groups of animals can occur depending on the host–bacteria relationship which becomes established. In the first group, animals develop resistance quickly, control the infection and do not become shedders (*infected-resistant*). In the second group, the infection is not completely controlled; some animals will partially control the infection and will shed the organism intermittently, others will become *intermediate* cases which are incubating the disease and will be heavy shedders of the organism.

Table 58. The relationship between the stages in the pathogenesis of Johne's disease, the presence of clinical disease and the results of diagnostic tests (adapted from Duncan et al. (30))

	Resistant animals	*Intermediate (incubation period)*	*Advanced clinical disease*
Clinical signs present	–	+	+++
Fecal shedding	+(–)	++	+++
Antibody response	–	++	+++
Skin test	+(–)	+(–)	+(–)
Lymphocyte transformation	+++	+++	+(–)

In the third group, the organism persists in the intestinal mucosa and from among these animals the *clinical* cases develop. The different possibilities are summarized in Table 58. The organism is phagocytosed by macrophages which in turn proliferate in large numbers and infiltrate the intestinal submucosa which results in decreased absorption, chronic diarrhea and resulting malabsorption. There is a reduction in protein absorption and leakage of protein into the lumen of the jejunum. In cattle, the loss of protein results in muscle wasting, hypoproteinemia and edema. In sheep, a compensatory increase in protein production in the liver masks the protein loss and clinical signs appear only when this compensatory mechanism fails (12). Within the macrophages, the bacteria remain viable and protected from humoral factors. *In vitro* studies indicate that blood-derived macrophages from clinically normal cows or cows infected with *M. paratuberculosis* were incapable of destroying the organism (50).

In summary, there appears to be an immune spectrum and no serologic or cellular immunity test will identify all animals in the spectrum. There are infected resistant animals which control their infection but are unable to completely eliminate the organism. These animals do not react in antibody assays, only rarely or never shed organisms and respond to the lymphocyte transformation test because their circulating lymphocytes are sensitized. In the intermediate stage, the animal fails to control the infection, antibodies appear in the serum and organisms are shed in the feces. In the stage of clinical disease, the organisms are shed in the feces and the antibody responses and skin tests are variable.

The immunological response following infection is variable and depends on the stage of the infection and whether or not clinical disease develops. In general, infected animals initially develop a cell-mediated response, followed by a humoral response initiated by the release of bacteria by dying macrophages as the disease progresses. In the late stages of clinical disease anergy may occur and neither cell-mediated or humoral immunity may be detectable (49). These immunologic features occur independent of the stages of clinical disease and may appear at any time during the clinical course.

The bacteria are carried by macrophages to other sites particularly the uterus, the fetus and the mammary gland, and the testes and semen of bulls. The postprimary dissemination of the lesions is more widespread in adult animals than in calves and the early lesions are more severe in the former but the organisms do not persist. In calves, the organism proliferates slowly, particularly in the small intestinal site, which results in a massive cellular infiltration of the intestinal submucosa. In adult cows, infection may penetrate to the fetus and cause prenatal infection. Uterine infection occurs more frequently than is commonly thought, and often in animals which are clinically normal (34). There is evidence also that intrauterine infection occurs in sheep (35). From experimental observations in sheep and calves it appears that vaccination against Johne's disease does not prevent infection but restricts the cellular response to the intestinal wall and thus prevents the onset of clinical disease.

Important features of the natural history of the disease are the long incubation period of 2 years or more and the development of sensitization to johnin and to mammalian and avian tuberculin. This sensitivity develops in the preclinical stage but has disappeared in most cases by the time clinical signs are evident. On the other hand, complement fixing antibodies appear late in the disease and in general increase with increasing severity of the lesions. This suggests that two independent antibodies are involved in the two reactions.

Clinical findings

In cattle, clinical signs do not appear before 2 years of age and are commonest in the 2–6-year age group. Emaciation is the most obvious abnormality and is usually accompanied by submandibular edema which has a tendency to disappear as diarrhea develops. A fall in milk yield and absence of fever and toxemia are apparent, the fall in milk yield often being apparent in the lactation before diarrhea commences. The animal eats well throughout but thirst is excessive. The feces are soft and thin, like thick pea soup, homogeneous and without offensive odor. There is marked absence of blood, epithelial debris and mucus. Diarrhea may be continuous or intermittent with a marked tendency to improve in late pregnancy only to reappear in a severe form soon after parturition. A temporary improvement may also occur when animals are taken off pasture and placed on dry feed. The course of the disease varies from weeks to months but always terminates in severe dehydration, emaciation and weakness necessitating destruction. Cases occur only sporadically because of the slow rate of spread of the disease.

In sheep and goats the disease is manifested principally by emaciation although shedding of wool may occur in sheep. Diarrhea is not severe although the feces may be sufficiently soft to lose their usual pelleted form in both species. Affected sheep may lose weight for up to 4 months, be partially anorexic and their feces may appear normal until the terminal stages when the feces may become soft and pasty (57). Depression and dyspnea are evident in goats but are less obvious in sheep.

Clinical pathology

In an infected herd, animals may be divided into four categories:

(1) Animals with clinical disease
(2) Asymptomatic carriers (intermediate and incubating)
(3) Infected, but neither ill nor shedding enough bacteria to be culturally detectable (infected-resistant)
(4) Uninfected cattle.

For successful eradication and control of the disease the diagnostic tests must be able to identify the intermediate group.

The clinicopathological tests used to help in the diagnosis of Johne's disease are listed below for each of the animal species involved. They have always been difficult to interpret and control of the disease has been correspondingly delayed. What follows is a summary of the position at the present time and it is apparent that many questions still remain to be answered.

False-positive reactions are due to crossreactivity and resistant animals which have recovered. Crossreactivity can occur as a consequence of infection with other *Mycobacterium* spp., *Actinomyces* spp., *Dermatophilus* spp., *Nocardia* spp., *Streptomyces* spp., and *Corynebacterium* spp., *M. avium* and *M. paratuberculosis* cannot be distinguished by immunologic methods.

False-negative responses occur as a result of tolerance and anergy which occurs most often during the terminal stages of clinical disease, but it may occur at any stage of chronic infection.

Cattle

Because of the very long incubation period during which infected animals shed very large numbers of *M. paratuberculosis* to contaminate the environment, the control of Johne's disease cannot be contemplated without a test to detect the clinically normal carrier. This need has dominated recent research into the disease and although finality has not been achieved a reasonable attempt can now be made. However, no single test will suffice. It is necessary to use at least three tests in a diagnostic profile. These need to match the stages of pathogenesis of the disease as set down in Table 58. The serological tests are in general too inaccurate although the complement fixation test is still required by many statutory agencies. The most promising profile of tests is:

- A lymphocyte immunostimulation test to detect the early infections
- A serological test, preferably a fluorescent antibody or an enzyme test or a labelled antibody test for greater specification. The agar gel immunodiffusion test is most reliable for clinical cases (52)
- Stained fecal smear or rectal pinch biopsy (13)
- Fecal culture as the final definitive diagnosis
- A combination of diagnostic techniques such as the complement fixation test, intravenous johnin, microscopic examination of the feces and a biopsy examination of the rectal mucosa is considered to be 96% sensitive in clinically suspect cases (53).

Deer

Deer and other wild species present a special problem because their capture and restraint are so hazardous. A single capture technique is required and this eliminates any delayed hypersensitivity skin tests. Fecal culture, complement fixation and lymphocyte immunostimulation tests are satisfactory, with a preference for the latter as being most accurate (23).

Goats

Approximately the same tests are applicable to goats. However, the intradermal johnin test is generally inconclusive and the complement fixation test is accurate for only a short time in the early stages of the clinical illness. Microscopic examination of feces or rectal scrapings is an effective test; so is fecal culture (3).

Clinicopathological tests

Cutaneous delayed hypersensitivity tests These are still in wide use even though all three available tests suffer from the deficiences that preclinical and advanced cases have minimal skin sensitivity and animals with bovine or avian tuberculosis and animals vaccinated against Johne's disease may give suspicious or positive reactions. The latter problem may be overcome by the use of a comparative tuberculin test, but in general terms the tests are of value only as herd tests. There is little to choose in efficiency between the single intradermal johnin, the double intradermal avian tuberculin and the intravenous avian tuberculin tests, although severe systemic reaction may occur after the intravenous injection of avian tuberculin into infected cattle. The single intradermal johnin test is most popular and is reasonably accurate although not sufficiently so as to be a dependable diagnostic method in individual animals because of the poor sensitivity which the infection produces. The test is performed by injecting 0·2 ml of johnin or its PPD fraction intradermally in the cervical area. This area is more sensitive than the caudal fold which also suffers from its lack of availability if further tests are to be performed. For a period of over 3 months after an injection of johnin there is local desensitization of the skin at the site of injection and if further tests are required, the neck offers a greater choice of sites than the caudal fold. The test should be read at 48 hours as most significant reactions occur at that time. The development of an appreciable edematous swelling signifies a positive reaction. In the United States the official criterion of a positive reaction is an increase of skin thickness of 3 mm or more. Failure to pick out early clinical cases can be overcome by repeated testing. The intradermal avian tuberculin test is carried out in the same way as a double intradermal tuberculin test.

The intravenous test using avian tuberculin is performed by injecting 10 ml of avian tuberculin intravenously. A rise in temperature of 1°C (33·8°F) at 5–8 hours after injection is a positive reaction. A systemic reaction, including anorexia, depression, dyspnea, erection of the hair coat and severe scouring may accompany the temperature rise. An intravenous johnin test has also been devised. A temperature rise to over 39·5°C (103·2°F) (an elevation of over 1°C, 33·8°F) within 3 and 7½ hours after the intravenous injection of 2–4 ml johnin is considered to be a positive reaction. The sensitivity of intravenous johnin was found to be 84% in clinically suspect cattle (53). A general systemic reaction accompanied the temperature rise. The sensitivity in non-clinically suspect cattle ranged from 22 to 57%.

Bacteriological examination of the feces This is a valuable diagnostic aid for detecting infection in clinically diseased animals and to some extent in apparently healthy cattle in known infected herds. Fecal culture is considered to be both 100% specific and 100% sensitive on a herd basis, assuming herds of about 50 or more animals and an infection rate of 20% or more within the herds (51). Newly developed laboratory techniques using growth factors in the culture medium has decreased the time required to visualize colonies from 12 to 3 weeks (51). Current techniques also allow the recovery of one organism per gram of feces and primary identification can be done in about 8 weeks.

Direct examination of stained fecal smears is also valuable when diarrhea is present in cows in known infected herds. It may be difficult to distinguish the Johne's bacillus from other acid-fast organisms which are frequent in feces. Also it may be necessary to examine smears on several occasions to obtain a positive result. Of the infected animals some are non-shedders, some are light shedders (less than 100 organisms/g of feces) and some are heavy shedders and, of these, the heavy shedders develop clinical disease. Clumps of acid-fast bacteria in epithelial cells are diagnostic and are more likely to be observed during a diarrheic phase than in a period when feces are normal, as epithelial cells are more likely to be shed at the former time. A pinch biopsy collected with the fingernails, or scrapings of rectal mucosa are of no great advantage compared to fecal smears, as it is probably only in the late clinical stages that the rectal mucosa is invaded. If rectal scrapings or rectal pinch biopsy are used a positive finding is clumps of acid-fast bacilli in epithelial cells or macrophages (19).

Serological tests Complement fixation and microcomplement fixation tests are available for cattle and small stock. They reflect severity of lesions rather than severity of the clinical abnormality, but early cases and non-clinical carriers fail to give positive reactions and a number of non-specific, transient, positive reactions do occur. The same criticism applies to the other serological test available, the agar gel immunodiffusion test, although good results are recorded with this test in goats (41). The test is probably about 90% accurate in clinically affected animals and 25% accurate in infected but clinically unaffected animals. The sensitivity of the agar gel immunodiffusion (AGID) test for the diagnosis of clinical paratuberculosis was 96% (52) with a specificity of 94%. The AGID test is considered to be the most appropriate available for the diagnosis of clinical disease. The test is rapid, inexpensive, and accurate and the results are available within 48 hours. Because positive reactions are given by tuberculous animals, the test is limited to use in tuberculosis-free herds. A fluorescent antibody test is available but is unable to distinguish between the antigens of *M. avium* and *M. paratuberculosis*. It does distinguish between *M. paratuberculosis* and *Cor. renale* which are easily confused by the complement fixation test. Combined with the complement fixation test the fluorescent antibody test is used to detect early, subclinical cases, but the results are far from accurate (20). A refinement of the conventional fluorescent antibody test which gives greater accuracy in identifying specific mycobacterial antigens is the observation of the uptake by macrophages of fluorescein-coated insoluble spheres (19). The trouble with all of these serological tests is the failure to detect early cases. An enzyme linked immunoabsorbent assay (ELISA) test is being assessed (14). The use of purified antigens may improve the sensitivity and specificity of an ELISA test (55). The latter has been used to determine the presence of paratuberculosis in white-tailed deer (62).

After experimental infection in sheep, sensitivity to avian tuberculin and johnin appears at 8 weeks and disappears at 6–8 months, with 50% of the sheep dying before 2 years (7).

Tests measuring cell-mediated responses These have greatly improved the efficiency of diagnosis in the early stages of the infection. They include several lymphocyte immunostimulation tests. Of these the lymphocyte stimulation test is highly accurate and recommended (18, 17). There is also a leukocyte migration agarose test (16). A combination of lymphocyte blastogenesis, complement fixation and fecal culture for the diagnosis of paratuberculosis in North American wild ruminants and domestic sheep yielded high sensitivity and specificity rates (56).

Surgical biopsy Surgical biopsy of the terminal ileum or ileocecal lymph node is recommended as a method of making a positive diagnosis of Johne's disease (21, 38). The biopsy sample is submitted for histopathological examination and culture.

Necropsy findings

In cattle, lesions are confined to the posterior part of the alimentary tract and its associated lymph nodes. The terminal part of the small intestine, the cecum and the first part of the colon are usually affected. In advanced cases the lesions may reach from the rectum to the duodenum. Thickening of the intestinal wall up to three or four times normal thickness, with corrugation of the mucosa, is characteristic. The ileocecal valve is always involved, the lesion varying from reddening of the lips of the valve in the early stages to edema with gross thickening and corrugation later. A high incidence of arteriosclerosis has been observed in advanced cases of Johne's disease, with a distinct correlation between the vascular lesions and macroscopic changes in the intestine. In sheep there may be a deep yellow pigmentation of the intestinal wall and, although corrugation of the mucosa is not a common finding, the wall may be thickened. No ulceration or discontinuity of the mucosal surface occurs. The mesenteric and ileocecal lymph nodes are enlarged and edematous in cattle, and in sheep there may be necrosis, caseation and calcification in these nodes. Gross necropsy lesions are often minimal in animals that showed severe clinical signs during life. In these animals the presence of lymphadenitis of the intestinal lymph vessels and characteristic histological findings provide satisfactory confirmation of the diagnosis. No lesions occur in an infected fetus but the organism can be isolated from its viscera and from the placenta and uterus. The lesions in goats are similar to those in cattle (22). Although it is generally agreed that the most accurate postmortem identification of the presence of *M. paratuberculosis* is achieved by the culture of the organism rather than by histopathology (29), it is still possible for infected animals to be missed at necropsy unless both culture and histopathology are used (39).

Diagnosis

The characteristic features of clinical Johne's disease includes chronic diarrhea which does not respond to therapy, progressive weight loss and emaciation in a single animal. The definitive etiological diagnosis can be obtained by using a combination of serological tests, fecal culture and biopsy of intestine. In cattle the clinical disease must be differentiated from diseases which cause chronic diarrhea in adult cattle. The chronic nature of Johne's disease is usually sufficient to differentiate it from the other common enteritis of cattle. Salmonellosis, coccidiosis and parasitism are usually acute and the latter two occur principally in younger animals and are distinguishable on fecal examination for oocysts and helminth eggs. Secondary copper deficiency (chronic molybdenum poisoning) is likely to be confused with Johne's disease in cattle, but is usually an area problem affecting large numbers of animals and responds well to the administration of copper. Other debilitating diseases in which diarrhea is not an important clinical finding are malnutrition, chronic reticuloperitonitis, hepatic abscess, pyelonephritis, lymphosarcoma and amyloidosis.

The characteristic features of clinical Johne's disease in sheep and goats are emaciation, weakness and normal feces with intermittent bouts of mild diarrhea. The other causes of unexplained weight loss in sheep and goats include caseous lymphadenitis, internal abscesses, gastrointestinal parasitism, caprine arthritis-encephalitis, ovine progressive pneumonia, dietary deficiencies and dental disease. A guide to the differential diagnosis, therapy, and management of unexplained weight loss in sheep and goats is available (59).

The major difficulty encountered in the diagnosis of paratuberculosis is the accurate identification of animals which are resistant and not infected but may be positive to one of the skin or serological tests, and those which are in the intermediate stage and excreting the organism in their feces and may be negative to a serological test. It is a major difficulty in an individual animal. On a herd basis the serological tests will usually indicate if the infection is present or absent in the herd and this can then be followed up by fecal culture to identify animals which are shedders. A combination of a highly sensitive and specific serological test, with fecal culture should improve the accuracy of diagnosis.

Treatment

Mycobacterium paratuberculosis is more resistant to chemotherapeutic agents *in vitro* than *M. tuberculosis* so that prospects for suitable treatment are poor. Streptomycin has most activity against the organism but treatment of affected cattle with daily doses of 50 mg/kg body weight causes only a transient improvement in clinical signs. Isoniazid has a minor degree of activity against the organism but has failed to cure clinical cases of Johne's disease. Clofazimine, a phenazine dye, shows some activity against early infections in sheep, and causes transitory but obvious clinical improvement in cattle (24). The use of a combination of 500 mg dihydrostreptomycin intramuscularly, and 300 mg rifampin with 300 mg isoniazid orally twice daily provided some clinical improvement in a goat with the disease (58).

Control

The lack of accurate tests and the long incubation period of the disease combine to make Johne's disease difficult to control. Because of the inaccuracy of the diagnostic tests available it is impossible to eradicate the disease, other than by completely clearing a farm and then restocking, and to prevent the subsequent reintroduction of infected animals. The other factor which greatly impedes the control and eradication of Johne's disease is the low level of clinical cases. A 5% population mortality rate per year is probably a reflection of a 50% infection rate at any one time. The remainder of the animals are either infected-resistant or incubating cases. In the usual plan for containing the disease without eradicating it, the separation of the infected-resistant animals from the early developing clinical cases is of paramount importance financially.

On a herd basis

This depends upon eradication of infected animals, hygiene to prevent further spread and, in some instances, vaccination to increase the resistance of the residual population.

The conservative method of eradication depends upon the identification of carrier animals by the tests described above, and their immediate sale for slaughter. The farm is quarantined and residual animals are retested at 6-month intervals until two consecutive negative herd tests are achieved. Unfortunately the method rarely succeeds in eradicating the disease. If the individual animals are of such value that complete disposal of all stock is impracticable, the above method may keep losses at a low level. A variant of this method is the 'culture and cull' method (25). Cultures are made of feces from all adult cows every 6 months. Culturally positive cows and their offspring are slaughtered. The disease can be greatly reduced by this method but results depend largely on the degree of contamination of the environment. The method has the virtue that many heavy fecal shedders are detected early, and the contamination of pastures is reduced. Eradication programs based on skin sensitivity and serological tests are accompanied by the needless loss of many uninfected cattle because of the many false-positive reactions to the test (8). The culture and cull method is much more accurate (15), but still has the deficiency that resistant intermittent shedders are likely to escape detection. A further alternative is to maintain infected and non-infected herds separately. The progeny of the infected cows are raised separately from their dams, but any suggestion that they be returned to the uninfected herd should be treated with great caution. Finally, the attempt to eradicate can be made by depopulating the farm of all cattle and sheep, and leaving it unstocked for 1–3 years. This strategy is not usually applicable for obvious economic reasons.

If one has to live with the disease, a number of hygienic precautions can be taken to limit the spread of infection. Avoidance of fecal pollution of drinking water and feed by providing troughs in high positions, fencing of marshes and ponds, and closing up of contaminated pastures for up to 3 years are worthwhile measures. Strip grazing should be avoided as fecal contamination of pasture is likely to be intense. The provision of piped water supplies to cattle on pasture rather than the use of ponds and ditches has been associated with a decline in the incidence of Johne's disease in Britain (60). Frequent harrowing of pasture fields to disseminate dung pats facilitates destruction of the bacteria by exposing them to sun and drying. Yard and barn manure should be spread only on cultivated fields. Although congenital infection may occur, it is still advisable to rear calves away from infected cows, and if possible in individual pens to prevent spread among the calves. If it is appreciated how commonly crossinfection occurs between cattle, and especially between very young cattle, there is a great deal of point in separating parturient cows and newborn calves from the rest of the herd (26). Cows coming up to calving should be kept separately from the milking herd and their calves fed colostrum for 1 day only, and reared in individual pens. Calves from cows which are clinically affected should not be reared as herd replacements. Sucking on dams and nurse cows should not be permitted. Milk for bucket feedings should be collected hygienically and rearing on milk substitutes should be encouraged. In infected herds, any animal which shows mild signs suggestive of the disease should be isolated until its status has been determined. Adoption of these hygienic precautions has been shown to greatly reduce the prevalence of the disease, down to a third, and of sensitivity to johnin, reduced by 90%.

If local legislation permits it, vaccination will provide protection against clinical disease and reduce the rate of spread of infection (28). Vallée's vaccine of live *M. paratuberculosis* organisms in a paraffin oil-pumice stone vehicle, or the Sigrudsson vaccine which contains killed organisms, are the vaccines in common use, although a microvaccine prepared by grinding the bacteria in a ball mill and suspending them in a paraffin oil vehicle has been used in sheep. There is less local reaction than with the usual ovine vaccine of live or killed organisms in oil, but the resulting antibody titer, and probably the immunity, wanes more quickly than with the other vaccines. Vaccines which contain killed whole bacterial cells have superior immunizing power in cattle compared to vaccines made up of fractionated cells (27).

In cattle, vaccination is carried out only in calves less than 1 month of age. Contrary to previous recommendations, revaccination is not carried out because the degree of protection appears to diminish as a result and because of the unsightly nodules which sometimes develop. The vaccine is of no benefit to infected animals, but it is incapable of causing the disease or of producing carriers. A major complication is that vaccinated animals are positive to the johnin test and to the tuberculin test, using both avian and mammalian tuberculin, but the reaction is much less to the mammalian tuberculin. The positive test to tuberculin is maximum at 5 weeks after vaccination and has completely disappeared at 18 months (6). In general terms, vaccination can be recommended in heavily infected, tuberculosis-free herds, but only in areas where tuberculosis eradication is neither under way nor projected (28). It is possible that the vaccine gives some protection against tuberculosis. The comparative tuberculin test can be used to detect tuberculosis in Johne's vaccinated herds (28).

During a 10-year period the use of a live attenuated vaccine in herds of cattle in Britain was associated with freedom from clinical disease an average of 4 years after vaccination was initiated in calves up to 1 month of age (60). The culling of progeny of clinical cases and the provision of piped water supplies to cattle on pasture were considered to be beneficial management practices along with the vaccination. Clinical cases occurred in 9·7% of the herds in the 10th year following the start of vaccination. Before the start of vaccination the mean annual herd incidence of clinical disease was 10·6% (range 0·75–50%). In the first year following vaccination the incidence was reported to have declined 3·6% (60). Contemporary unvaccinated control herds were not studied and thus the efficacy of the vaccine cannot be adequately evaluated. Nevertheless, field observations indicate that the vaccine is of value, and controlled trials should be conducted.

In sheep, vaccination with Sigurdsson vaccine of heat-killed *M. paratuberculosis* in mineral oil has given excellent results, reducing the disease to negligible proportions. The use of vaccination in sheep is not impeded by interference with tuberculin testing.

On an area basis

Eradication on an area basis has seldom been attempted because of the lack of dependability of available diagnostic tests and the relative unimportance of Johne's disease in the past. Two general lines of approach to the eradication problem can be followed. If the incidence is sufficiently low, a test and slaughter program on a herd basis could be instituted with all cattle being cleared from infected farms and the farms being left unoccupied by ruminants for at least 1 year. A great deal of public support would be necessary for such a program to succeed. If the incidence is high and tuberculosis eradication has been completed or is not projected, vaccination may be advisable, and is at present undergoing trials in European countries. If the disease is eradicated, the prevention of reinfection becomes a problem. The tests used to detect infected animals are not sufficiently accurate and quarantine of introductions is impossible because of the long incubation period. A guarantee of freedom from disease in the place of origin is the best recommendation but is still subject to error.

A proposed method of qualifying individual herds as *M. paratuberculosis*-free includes freedom from clinical cases for 3 years, negative intradermal johnin tests on all cattle 6 months or older on two tests 6 months apart, negative fecal cultures on all cattle over 2 years of age, with these to be repeated on skin test positive cattle. Continued qualification is planned to depend on negative fecal culture tests every 6 months (15).

At the present time, in most countries the incidence of Johne's disease is not sufficiently high to necessitate an intensive area eradication program, nor are the available diagnostic tests sufficiently accurate to form the basis for such a program. In these circumstances, the owners of affected farms should be encouraged to adopt the general procedures outlined under herd control, preferably with technical and financial assistance from government authorities.

REVIEW LITERATURE

Chiodini, R. J., Van Kruiningen, H. J. & Merkal, R. S. (1984). Ruminant paratuberculosis (Johne's disease): the current status and future prospects. *Cornell Vet.*, *74*, 218–262.

Duncan, J. R., Hall, C. E. & de Lisle, C. (1978) Johne's disease and the practitioner. *Cornell Vet.*, *68*, supp. 179.

Gilmour, N. J. L. (1979) The pathogenesis, diagnosis and control of Johne's disease. *Vet. Rec.*, *99*, 433.

Jorgensen, J. B. & Aalund, O. (1984). Agriculture. Paratuberculosis, diagnostic methods, their practical application and experience with vaccination. *Workshop in the CEC Prog. Coord. Res. Anim. Pathol.*, Copenhagen Nov. 22–23, 1983, pp. 159. Commission of the European Communities.

Riemann, H. P. & Abbas, B. (1983) Diagnosis and control of bovine paratuberculosis (Johne's disease). *Adv. vet. Sci. comp. Med.*, *27*, 481–506.

Thoen, C. D. & Muscoplat, C. C. (1979) Recent developments in diagnosis of paratuberculosis. *J. Am. vet. med. Assoc.*, *174*, 838.

REFERENCES

(1) Stuart, P. (1976) *Br. vet. J.*, *121, 332.*
(2) Larsen, A. B. et al. (1975) *Am. J. vet. Res.*, *36*, 255.
(3) West, G. et al. (1979) *Calif. Vet.*, *33*, 28.
(4) Jorgensen, J. B. (1977) *Nord. VetMed.*, *29*, 267.
(5) Merkal, R. S. et al. (1975) *Am. J. vet. Res.*, *36*, 837.
(6) Moodie, P. A. (1977) *Br. vet. J.*, *133*, 642.
(7) Karpinski, T. & Zorawski, C. (1975) *Bull. vet. Inst. Pulawy*, *19*, 59.
(8) Lisle, G. W. de et al. (1980) *Can. J. comp. Med.*, *44*, 177 & 183.
(9) Crowther, R. W. et al. (1976) *Vet. Rec.*, *98*, 463.
(10) Larsen, A. B. et al. (1971) *Am. J. vet. Res.*, *32*, 539.
(11) Larsen, A. B. et al. (1972) *Am. J. vet. Res.*, *33*, 2185.
(12) Allen, W. M. et al. (1974) *J. comp. Pathol.*, *84*, 381, 385, 391.
(13) Jorgensen, J. B. (1980) *Dansk vet. Tidschr.*, *63*, 151.
(14) Yokomizo, Y. et al. (1983) *Am. J. vet. Res.*, *44*, 2205.
(15) Merkal, R. S. (1973) *J. Am. vet. med. Assoc.*, *163*, 1100.
(16) Bendisen, P. H. (1977) *Am. J. vet. Res.*, *38*, 2023.
(17) Johnson, D. W. et al. (1977) *Am. J. vet. Res.*, *38*, 2023.
(18) Buergelt, C. D. et al. (1978) *Am. J. vet. Res.*, *39*, 591.
(19) Thoen, C. D. & Muscoplat, C. C. (1979) *J. Am vet. med. Assoc.*, *174*, 838.
(20) Gilmour, N. J. L. & Angus, K. W. (1976) *Res. vet. Sci.*, *20*, 6, 10.
(21) Julian, R. J. (1975) *Can. vet. J.*, *16*, 33.
(22) Alisbasoglu, M. et al. (1973) *Vet. Fak. Derg. Anka Univ.*, *20*, 43.
(23) Temple, R. M. S. et al. (1979) *J. Am. vet. med. Assoc.*, *175*, 914.
(24) Merkal, R. S. & Larsen, A. B. (1973) *Am. J. vet. Res.*, *34*, 27.
(25) Moyle, A. I. (1975) *J. Am. vet. med. Assoc.*, *166*, 689.
(26) Merkal, R. S. et al. (1975) *Am. J. vet. Res.*, *36*, 837.
(27) Larsen, A. B. et al. (1978) *Am. J. vet. Res.*, *39*, 65.
(28) Gilmour, N. J. L. et al. (1977) *Vet. Rec.*, *100*, 434, 460.
(29) Fodstad, F. H. & Gunnarson, E. (1979) *Acta vet. Scand.*, *20*, 157.
(30) Duncan, J. R. et al. (1978) *Cornell Vet.*, *68*, supp. 179.
(31) Gunnarson, E. (1979) *Acta vet Scand.*, *20*, 191.
(32) Buergelt, C. D. & Duncan, J. R. (1978) *J. Am. vet. med. Assoc.*, *173*, 478.
(33) Kopecky, K. E. (1977) *J. Am. vet. med. Assoc.*, *170*, 320.
(34) McQueen, D. S. & Russell, E. G. (1979) *Aust. vet. J.*, *55*, 203.
(35) Muhammed, S. I. & Eliasson, E. C. (1979) *Vet. Rec.*, *105*, 11.
(36) Larsen, A. B & Miller, J. M. (1978) *Am. J. vet. Res.*, *39*, 1972.
(37) Riemann, H. et al. (1979) *J. Am. vet. med. Assoc.*, *174*, 841.
(38) Pemberton, D. H. (1979) *Aust. vet. J.*, *55*, 217.
(39) Summers, B. A. (1981) *Vet. Rec.*, *108*, 166.
(40) Seaman, J. T. & Thompson, D. R. (1984) *Aust. vet. J.*, *61*, 227.
(41) Sherman, D. M. & Gezon, H. M. (1980) *Am. vet. med. Assoc.*, *177*, 1208.
(42) Merkal, R. S. et al. (1987) *J. Am. vet. med. Assoc.*, *190*, 676.
(43) Morin, M. (1982) *Can. vet. J.*, *23*, 55.
(44) Moser, C. L. (1982) *Can. vet. J.*, *23*, 63.
(45) Chiodini, R. J. et al. (1984) *Cornell Vet.*, *74*, 218.
(46) Riemann, H. P. & Abbas, B. (1983) *Adv. vet. Sci. comp. Med.*, *27*, 481.
(47) Merkal, R. S. et al. (1982) *Am. J. vet. Res.*, *43*, 676.
(48) Taylor, T. K. et al. (1981) *Vet. Rec.*, *109*, 532.
(49) Chiodini, R. J. & Van Kruiningen, H. J. (1983) *J. Am. vet. med. Assoc.*, *182*, 168.
(50) Bendixen, P. H. et al. (1981) *Am. J. vet. Res.*, *42*, 109.
(51) Merkal, R. S. (1984) *J. Am. vet. med. Assoc.*, *184*, 939.
(52) Sherman, D. M. et al. (1984) *J. Am. vet. med. Assoc.*, *185*, 179.
(53) Benedictus, G. & Bosma, J. (1985) *Vet. Q.*, *7*, 139.
(54) Muhammed, S. I. & Ivoghli, B. (1983) *Trop. Anim. Hlth Prod.*, *15*, 53.
(55) Abbas, B. et al. (1983) *Am. J. vet. Res.*, *44*, 2229.
(56) Williams, E. S. et al. (1985) *Am. J. vet. Res.*, *46*, 2317.
(57) Sweeney, R. W. et al. (1984) *J. Am. vet. med. Assoc.*, *185*, 444.
(58) Slocombe, F. (1982) *Can. vet. J.*, *23*, 100.
(59) Sherman, D. M. (1983) *Vet. Clin. N. Am. large Anim. Pract.*, *5*, 571.
(60) Wilesmith, J. W. (1982) *Br. vet. J.*, *138*, 321.
(61) Chiodini, R. J. & Van Kruiningen, H. J. *Cornell Vet.*, *76*, 91.
(62) Shulaw, W. P. et al. (1986) *Am. J. vet. Res.*, *47*, 2539.

DISEASES CAUSED BY *ACTINOMYCES* spp., *ACTINOBACILLUS* spp., *NOCARDIA* spp. AND *DERMATOPHILUS* spp.

This group of infectious diseases includes actinomycosis, actinobacillosis, mycotic dermatitis, strawberry footrot of sheep, bovine farcy, glanders and shigellosis of foals. Painless, granulomatous lesions of the skin (mycetoma) occur naturally, especially in horses, and have been produced experimentally by infection with *Nocardia brasiliensis* and with *Actinomadura* spp. (2). Nocardial mastitis in cattle has been dealt with in

Chapter 15 on mastitis. Other infections by *Nocardia* spp. are rare (2).

Less common occurrences of infection with this group of organisms include *Actinomyces actinoides* as a secondary bacterial invader in enzootic pneumonia of calves (1) and seminal vesiculitis in bulls, *Actinomyces bovis* in a large proportion of unopened lesions of fistulous withers and poll evil, and *Actinomyces* spp. in an abscess in a mandibular lymph node in a horse. A septicemic disease of newborn and young pigs has been attributed to *Actinomyces suis* (5, 6). Non-specific signs of illness may be observed for 24 hours before death but most pigs are found dead. *Actinobacillus equuli* has also been identified as a cause of abortion (7) and of septicemia in newborn pigs (8). Fever and cutaneous petechiation are observed in living pigs, and petechiation in the kidney and excessive pleural fluid at necropsy. A series of five cases of peritonitis in horses had *Actinobacillus equuli* as the cause (3). Two syndromes appeared. In one there was acute abdominal pain, intestinal stasis, pain and tenseness on palpation of the abdominal wall, fever up to 40·5°C (104·5°F) and colic in one. The other syndrome comprised chronic weight loss, ventral edema, pleurisy, and pallor of the mucosae. There was no fever. In all horses, paracentesis provided ample amber fluid with a high white cell count, up to 270 000/μl, and a marked neutrophilia. Treatment with ampicillin or penicillin/streptomycin gave excellent responses. Some horses showed evidence of verminous arteritis and were also treated for this. *Actinobacillus suis* has been isolated from young pigs with septicemia and arthritis (9) and from the horse (10). *Act. equuli* has also been linked with field outbreaks of diarrhea in calves (11). *Actinobacillus seminis* has been isolated from the joints of lambs affected by purulent polyarthritis (12) and from the semen of rams with epididymitis (4, 14) in Australia, South Africa and New Zealand.

A bacterium with some justification for classification in the genus *Actinobacillus* is *Histophilus ovis*. It has many similarities to *Actinobacillus seminis*. The organism has been recovered from specimens from a series of outbreaks in young lambs of septicemia, synovitis and abscessation in various sites. There have also been several outbreaks of neonatal mortality (13).

REFERENCES

(1) Allen, J. G. (1976) *Aust. vet. J.*, *52*, 100.
(2) Gumaa, S. A. & Abu-saura, M. T. (1981) *J. comp. Pathol.*, *91*, 341.
(3) Gay, C. C. & Lording, P. M. (1980) *Aust. vet. J.*, *56*, 296.
(4) Bruere, A. N. et al. (1977) *NZ vet. J.*, *25*, 191.
(5) Mair, N. S. (1974) *J. comp. Pathol.*, *84*, 113.
(6) Cutlip, R. C. et al. (1972) *Am J. vet. Res.*, *33*, 1621.
(7) Werdin, R. E. et al. (1976) *J. Am. vet. med. Assoc.*, *169*, 704.
(8) Windsor, R. S. (1973) *Vet. Rec.*, *92*, 178.
(9) MacDonald, D. W. et al. (1976) *Can. vet. J.*, *17*, 251.
(10) Kim, B. H. et al. (1976) *Vet. Rec.*, *98*, 239.
(11) Osbaldistone, G. & Walker, R. D. (1972) *Cornell Vet.*, *62*, 364.
(12) Watt, D. A. et al. (1970) *Aust. vet. J.*, *46*, 515.
(13) Rahaley, R. S. & White, W. E. (1977) *Aust. vet, J.*, *53*, 124.
(14) Tonder, E. M. van (1979) *Onderstepoort J. vet. Res.*, *46*, 129.

Actinomycosis (lumpy jaw)

The most common manifestation of this disease in cattle is a rarefying osteomyelitis of the bones of the head, particularly the mandible and maxilla. On rare occasions it involves soft tissues, particularly the alimentary tract.

Etiology

Actinomyces bovis is the primary cause but other bacteria may be present in extensive lesions.

Epidemiology

The disease is common only in cattle where a tendency towards inherited susceptibility has been observed (1). Occasional cases occur in pigs and horses (2).

Act. bovis is a common inhabitant of the bovine mouth and infection is presumed to occur through wounds to the buccal mucosa caused by sharp pieces of feed or foreign material. Infection may also occur through dental alveoli, and may account for the more common occurrence of the disease in young cattle when the teeth are erupting. Infection of the alimentary tract wall is probably related to laceration by sharp foreign bodies.

Although actinomycosis occurs only sporadically in affected herds, it is of importance because of its widespread occurrence and poor response to treatment. It is recorded from most countries of the world.

Pathogenesis

In the jawbones a rarefying osteomyelitis is produced. The lesion is characteristically granulomatous both in this site and where visceral involvement occurs. The effects on the animal are purely physical. Involvement of the jaw causes interference with prehension and mastication, and when the alimentary tract is involved there is physical interference with ruminal movement and digestion, both resulting in partial starvation. Rarely localization occurs in other organs, caused apparently by hematogenous spread from these primary lesions.

Clinical findings

Cattle

Actinomycosis of the jaw commences as a painless, bony swelling which appears on the mandible or maxilla, usually at the level of the central molar teeth. The enlargement may be diffuse or discrete and in the case of the mandible may appear only as a thickening of the lower edge of the bone with most of the enlargement in the intermandibular space. Such lesions are often not detected until they are too extensive for treatment to be effective. The more common, discrete lesions on the lateral surfaces of the bones are more readily observed. Some lesions enlarge rapidly within a few weeks, others slowly over a period of months. The swellings are very hard, are immovable and, in the later stages, painful to the touch. They usually break through the skin and discharge through one or more openings. The discharge of pus is small in amount and consists of sticky, honey-like fluid containing minute, hard, yellow-white granules. There is a tendency for the sinuses to heal and for fresh ones to develop periodically. Teeth embedded in the affected bone become malaligned and painful and cause difficult mastication with consequent loss of condition. In severe cases, spread to contiguous soft tissues may be extensive and involve the muscles and fascia of the throat. Excessive swelling of the maxilla may cause dyspnea. Involvement of the local lymph nodes does not occur. Eventually the animal becomes so emaciated that destruction is necessary although the time required to reach this stage varies from several months to a year or more.

The most common form of actinomycosis of soft tissues is involvement of the esophageal groove region, with spread to the lower esophagus and the anterior wall of the reticulum. The syndrome is one of impaired digestion (3, 4). There is periodic diarrhea with the passage of undigested food material, chronic bloat and allotriophagia. Less common lesions of soft tissue include orchitis in bulls (5), the trachea causing partial obstruction (12) and abscess in the brain (6–8) or lungs (9).

Pigs

Rare cases of wasting occur due to visceral actinomycosis (10) but extensive granulomatous lesions on the skin, particularly over the udder, are more common.

Clinical pathology

Smears of the discharging pus stained with Gram's stain provide an effective simple method of confirming the diagnosis. Gram-positive filaments of the organism are most readily found in the centers of the crushed granules.

Necropsy findings

Rarefaction of the bone and the presence of loculi and sinuses containing thin, whey-like pus with small, gritty granules is usual. An extensive fibrous tissue reaction around the lesion is constant, and there may be contiguous spread to surrounding soft tissues. The presence of 'club' colonies containing the typical, thread-like bacteria is characteristic of the disease. These formations may be seen on microscopic examination of smears made from crushed granules in pus or on histological examination of sections. Granulomatous lesions containing pockets of pus may be found in the esophageal groove, the lower esophagus and the anterior wall of the reticulum. Spread from these lesions may cause a chronic, local peritonitis. There may be evidence of deranged digestion with the rumen contents sloppier than usual, an empty abomasum and a mild abomasitis and enteritis. Involvement of local lymph nodes does not occur, irrespective of the site of the primary lesion.

Diagnosis

Abscesses of the cheek muscles and throat region are quite common when spiny grass-awns occur in the diet. They are characterized by their movability and localization in soft tissues compared to the immovability of an actinomycotic lesion. Needle puncture reveals the presence of pus, which may be thin and fetid or caseous depending on the duration of the abscess. Prompt recovery follows opening and drainage. Foreign bodies or accumulations of dry feed jammed between the teeth and cheek commonly cause a clinical picture which resembles that caused by actinomycosis and the inside of the mouth should be inspected if the enlargement has occurred suddenly.

The syndrome of indigestion caused by visceral actinomycotic lesions resembles that caused by chronic peritonitis.

Cutaneous and mammary lesions in sows closely resemble necrotic ulcers caused by *Borrelia suilla*.

Treatment and control

The treatment and control of actinomycosis dealt with under actinobacillosis applies. Additional treatment recorded as being effective include isoniazid given orally at the rate of 10–20 mg/kg body weight daily for about 30 days. Cessation of the growth of the lesion should occur (11).

REFERENCES

(1) Becker, R. B. et al. (1964) *Bull. Fla agric. Exp. Stn*, *670*, 24.
(2) Tritschler, L. G. & Romach, F. E. (1965) *Vet. Med.*, *60*, 605.
(3) Bruere, A. N. (1955) *NZ vet. J.*, *3*, 121.
(4) Begg, H. (1950) *Vet. Rec.*, *62*, 797.
(5) Kimball, A. (1954) *Am. J. vet. Res.*, *15*, 551.
(6) Trevisan, G. (1957) *Veterinaria, Milano*, 6, 122.
(7) Fankhauser, R. (1950) *Schweiz. Arch. Tierheilkd.*, *92*, 82
(8) Ryff, J. F. (1953) *J. Am. vet. med. Assoc.*, *122*, 78.
(9) Gill, B. S. & Singh, B. (1977) *Orissa vet. J.*, *11*, 104.
(10) Vawter, L. R. (1946) *J. Am. vet. med. Assoc.*, *109*, 198.
(11) Watts, T. C. et al. (1973) *Can. vet. J.*, *14*, 223.
(12) Bertone, A. L. & Rebhun, W. C. (1984) *J. Am. vet. med. Assoc.*, *185*, 221.

Actinobacillosis (wooden tongue)

Actinobacillosis is a specific infectious disease, and in cattle it is characterized by inflammation of the tongue, less commonly the pharyngeal lymph nodes and esophageal groove. In sheep the lesions are restricted to the soft tissues of the head and neck and occasionally the nasal cavities. Involvement of the tongue does not usually occur.

Etiology

Actinobacillus lignieresii may be recovered in pure culture from the lesions but other pyogenic organisms may also be present.

Epidemiology

Act. lignieresii is susceptible to ordinary environmental influences and does not survive for more than 5 days on hay or straw (1).

Infected discharges are the source of the infection and transmission is effected by the ingestion of contaminated pasture or feed. As in actinomycosis, injury to the buccal mucosa permits easy entry of the infection and a high incidence is recorded in cattle grazing 'burnt-over' peat pastures in New Zealand (2). These pastures contain much gravel and ash likely to cause oral injury. A similar high incidence has been observed in sheep fed prickly pear (*Opuntia* spp.). A severe outbreak has also been reported in heifers fed on very dry, stemmy, tough haylage. It was thought that the infection was introduced via lacerations of the oral mucosa caused by the feed (8).

The disease in cattle is worldwide in distribution and, like actinomycosis, it is usually of sporadic occurrence on particular farms. However, it is amenable to treatment and causes only minor losses. In sheep, the disease is common in Scotland (3) and is recorded in most sheep-raising countries (4, 5, 6). In most instances, only occasional cases occur but in some flocks a morbidity rate of up to 25% may be encountered. A single case of lingual actinobacillosis is recorded in a horse (16).

Pathogenesis

Local infection by the organism causes an acute inflammatory reaction and the subsequent development of granulomatous lesions in which necrosis and suppuration occur, often with the discharge of pus to the exterior. Spread to regional lymph nodes is usual. Lingual involvement in cattle causes interference with prehension and mastication due to acute inflammation in the early stages and distortion of the tongue at a later stage. Visceral involvement is recorded and is identical with that described under actinomycosis.

Clinical findings

Cattle

The onset of glossal actinobacillosis is usually acute, the affected animal being unable to eat for a period of about 48 hours. There is excessive salivation and gentle chewing of the tongue as though a foreign body were present in the mouth. On examination the tongue is swollen and hard, particularly at the base, the tip often appearing to be normal. Manipulation of the tongue causes pain and resentment. Nodules and ulcers are present on the side of the tongue and there may be an ulcer at the anterior edge of the dorsum. In the later stages when the acute inflammation is replaced by fibrous tissue, the tongue becomes shrunken and immobile and there is considerable interference with prehension. Lymphadenitis is common and is often independent of lesions in the tongue. There may be visible and palpable enlargement of the submaxillary and parotid nodes. Local, firm swellings develop and often rupture with the discharge of thin, non-odorous pus. Healing is slow and relapse is common. Enlargement of the retropharyngeal nodes causes interference with swallowing and loud snoring respiration.

An unusual occurrence of cutaneous actinobacillosis has been recorded in cattle (7). Lesions occurred in the mouth, but not on the tongue, on the head, chest wall, flanks and thighs and were in the form of large ulcers which exuded yellow pus, or nodules of various shapes and sizes (up to 15 cm) often obviously on lymphatics. Local lymph nodes were always involved but were firm, cold and painless. *Act. lignieresii* was isolated and although treatment with chloramphenicol or streptomycin was effective, spontaneous recovery occurred in other animals which were not treated.

Sheep

In sheep the tongue is not usually affected. Lesions up to 8 cm in diameter occur on the lower jaw, face and nose, or in the skin folds from the lower jaw to the sternum. They may be superficial or deep and usually extend to the cranial or cervical lymph nodes. Viscid, yellow-green pus containing granules is discharged through a number of small openings. Extensive lesions cause the formation of much fibrous tissue which may physically impede prehension or respiration. Thickening and scabbiness of the lips may also be observed. Involvement of the nasal cavities may cause persistent bilateral nasal discharge. Affected sheep have difficulty in eating and many die of starvation. *Act. lignieresii* has been incriminated as an occasional cause of mastitis in ewes (9).

Clinical pathology

Examination of smears or culture of pus for the presence of *Act. lignieresii* is advisable.

Necropsy findings

Necropsy examination is not usually carried out in cattle affected by the disease. In sheep, lymphangitis and abscesses containing thick, tenacious, yellow-green pus occur around the local lesion. Typical club colonies are visible on staining sections of affected tissue. Culture of material from lesions usually detects the presence of *Act. lignieresii*.

Diagnosis

The salivation, chewing and anorexia of the lingual form in cattle may resemble early rabies or foreign bodies in the mouth, particularly bones jammed between the molars. Enlargement of the lymph nodes, particularly when the tongue is unaffected, requires careful consideration. A tuberculin test may be necessary to differentiate this form of the disease from tuberculosis. Treatment with iodine effects considerable reduction in the size of the nodes in both diseases. Lymphomatosis usually affects multiple nodes. Abscesses of the throat region of cattle may be caused by a number of non-specific pyogenic infections following trauma. They usually consist of a single cavity containing thin pus and heal readily after draining.

In sheep, mandibular abscesses due to grass seed penetration of alveoli cause large, bony swellings on the mandible. The lesion is usually on the anterior part of the mandible, causing displacement of the incisor teeth. It is an osteomyelitis, and grayish, fluid, foul-smelling pus is present (10). Actinobacillosis of the nasal cavities bears some resemblance to melioidosis in this species.

Treatment

Iodides are still a standard treatment for both actinomycosis and actinobacillosis. In the former the results are relatively inefficient, but in actinobacillosis response is usually dramatic and permanent. Laboratory studies suggest that iodides have little bactericidal effect against *Act. lignieresii* and that the sulfonamides are of greater value (11). It is probable that iodides exert their effect by reducing the severity of the fibrous tissue reaction. The sulfonamides, penicillin, streptomycin and the broad-spectrum antibiotics are now in general use for both diseases. *In vitro* sensitivity tests of a large series of strains have shown the organism to be sensitive to streptomycin, the tetracyclines, chloramphenicol and erythromycin but not to other antibiotics (1). Treatment of any sort is more likely to be of value in actinobacillosis than in actinomycosis and surgical treatment may be necessary in the latter. Roentgenological treatment has been used extensively but is of doubtful permanent value.

Oral or intravenous dosing of iodides may be used. Potassium iodide, 6–10 g/day for 7–10 days, given orally as a drench to cattle, is a time-consuming treatment but effective. Treatment may be continued until iodism develops. Lacrimation, anorexia, coughing and the appearance of dandruff indicate that maximum systemic levels of iodine have been reached. Sodium iodide (1 g/12 kg body weight) can be given intravenously as a 10% solution in one dose to both cattle and sheep. One course of potassium iodide or one injection of sodium iodide is usually sufficient for soft tissue lesions, the acute signs in actinobacillosis disappearing in 24–48 hours after treatment. At least one or preferably two further treatments at 10–14-day intervals are required for bony lesions.

The most that can be expected with bony lesions is the arrest of further development. With time, the lesion may subside but rarely disappears completely. Occasional animals show distress, including restlessness, dyspnea, tachycardia and staggering during injections of sodium iodide. Although abortion has been recorded in heavily pregnant cows after injection (12), this does not appear to be a common occurrence. Subcutaneous injections of sodium iodide have also been recommended (13). The injection causes severe irritation and local swelling immediately. The irritation disappears within an hour or two but the swelling persists for some days. Subcutaneous injection is the standard route of administration for sheep, the dose rate of sodium iodide being 20 ml of a 10% solution weekly for 4–5 weeks.

Sulfanilamide, sulfapyridine and sulfathiazole effect rapid cures in human actinomycosis and have been used in the disease in cattle: 1 g/7 kg body weight per day for 4–5 days is suggested as a course of treatment.

Streptomycin, given by intramuscular injection (5 g/day for 3 days) and repeated if necessary, has given good results in actinomycosis in cattle when combined with iodides and local surgical treatment (14). Isoniazid has been used as a treatment for actinomycotic infections in man and it has been reported on favorably as an adjunct to antibiotic or iodide therapy in cattle. The daily dose rate recommended is 10 mg/kg body weight orally or intramuscularly, continued for 3–4 weeks (15). Surgical treatment usually consists of the opening of the bony tumor to provide drainage, and packing, usually with gauze soaked in tincture of iodine.

Control

Restriction of the spread of both diseases is best implemented by quick treatment of affected animals and the prevention of contamination of pasture and feed troughs. Isolation or disposal of animals with discharging lesions is essential, although the disease does not spread readily unless predisposing environmental factors cause a high incidence of oral lacerations.

REFERENCES

(1) Till, D. H. & Palmer, F. P. (1960) *Vet. Rec.*, *72*, 527.
(2) Gerring, J. C. (1947) *Aust. vet. J.*, *23*, 122.
(3) Taylor, A. W. (1944) *J. comp. Pathol.*, *54*, 228.
(4) Hayston, J. T. (1948) *Aust. vet. J.*, *24*, 64.
(5) Johnston, K. G. (1954) *Aust. vet. J.*, *30*, 105.
(6) Marsh, H. & Wilkins, H. W. (1939) *J. Am. vet. med. Assoc.*, *94*, 363.
(7) Hebeler, H. F. et al. (1961) *Vet. Rec.*, *73*, 517.
(8) Campbell, S. G. et al. (1975) *J. Am. vet. med. Assoc.*, *166*, 604.
(9) Laws, L. & Elder, J. K. (1969) *Aust. vet. J.*, *45*, 401.
(10) Edgar, G. (1935) *Aust. vet. J.*, *11*, 19.
(11) Smith, H. W. (1951) *Vet. Rec.*, *63*, 674.
(12) Miller, H. V. & Drost, M. (1978) *J. Am. vet. med. Assoc.*, *172*, 466.
(13) Linton, J. A. (1946) *NZ J. Agric.*, *73*, 25.
(14) Kingman, H. E. & Palen, J. S. (1951) *J. Am. vet. med. Assoc.*, *118*, 28.
(15) Watts, T. C. et al. (1973) *Can. vet. J.*, *14*, 223.
(16) Baum, K. H. et al. (1984) *J. Am. vet. med. Assoc.*, *185*, 792.

Glanders

Glanders is a contagious disease of solipeds, occurring in either acute or chronic form, and characterized by nodules or ulcers in the respiratory tract and on the skin. The disease is highly fatal and of major importance in any affected horse population.

Etiology

Actinobacillus (*Malleomyces*) *mallei* is the causative organism.

Epidemiology

Act. mallei is readily destroyed by light, heat and the usual disinfectants and is unlikely to survive in a contaminated environment for more than 6 weeks. Horses, mules and donkeys are the species usually affected. Horses tend to develop the chronic form, mules and donkeys the acute form. Man is susceptible and the infection is usually fatal. Cases usually occur in persons working with the organism in the laboratory or in close contact with affected animals. Animals which are badly fed and kept in a poor environment are more susceptible.

Infected animals or carriers that have made an apparent recovery from the disease are the important sources of infection. Spread to other animals occurs mostly by ingestion, the infection spreading on fodder and utensils, particularly communal watering troughs, contaminated by nasal discharge or sputum. Rarely the cutaneous form appears to arise through contamination of skin abrasions by direct contact or from harness or grooming tools. Spread by inhalation can also occur but this mode of infection is probably rare under natural conditions.

Glanders is restricted geographically to eastern Europe, Asia Minor, Asia and North Africa. It has been virtually eradicated from North America. Since the elimination of large concentrations of horses in cities, the disease is of major importance only when there is extensive movement of horses. In such circumstances, heavy mortality rates occur and in the few animals that recover, there is a long convalescence with the frequent development of the ‘carrier’ state. Rarely animals make a complete recovery. Carnivores, including lions (5), may be infected by eating infected meat, and infections have been observed in sheep and goats.

Pathogenesis

Invasion occurs mostly through the intestinal wall and a septicemia (acute form) or bacteremia (chronic form) is set up. Localization always occurs in the lungs but the skin and nasal mucosa are also common sites. Other viscera may become the site of the typical nodules. Terminal signs are in the main those of bronchopneumonia, and deaths in typical cases are caused by anoxic anoxia.

Clinical findings
In the acute form there is a high fever, cough and nasal discharge with rapidly spreading ulcers appearing on the nasal mucosa, and nodules on the skin of the lower limbs or abdomen. Death due to septicemia occurs in a few days. In the chronic form, the signs may be related to the lesions which occur in one or more of the prediction sites. When the localization is chiefly pulmonary, there is a chronic cough, frequent epistaxis and labored respiration. The chronic nasal and skin forms commonly occur together. Nasal lesions appear on the lower parts of the turbinates and the cartilaginous nasal septum. They commence as nodules (1 cm in diameter) which ulcerate and may become confluent. In the early stages there is a serous nasal discharge which may be unilateral and which later becomes purulent and bloodstained. Enlargement of the submaxillary lymph nodes is a common accompaniment. On healing, the ulcers are replaced by a characteristic stellate scar. The skin form is characterized by the appearance of subcutaneous nodules (1–2 cm in diameter) which soon ulcerate and discharge pus of the color and consistency of dark honey. In some cases the lesions are more deeply situated and discharge through fistulous tracts. Thickened fibrous lymph vessels radiate from the lesions and connect one to the other. Lymph nodes draining the area become involved and may discharge to the exterior. The predilection site for cutaneous lesions is the medial aspect of the hock but they can occur on any part of the body. Animals affected with the chronic form are usually ill for some months, frequently showing improvement but eventually either dying or making an apparent recovery to persist as occult cases.

Clinical pathology
The principal tests used in the diagnosis of glanders are the mallein test, the complement fixation test on serum, and the injection of pus from lesions into guinea-pigs. Other tests used are an indirect hemagglutination test using mallein as the antigen (2) and the conglutinin complement absorption test (3).

The disease is accompanied by an anemia including a low hemoglobin content of the blood, a low erythrocyte count and packed cell volume and a moderate leukocytosis and neutrophilia.

Mallein test
The intradermopalpebral test has largely displaced the ophthalmic and subcutaneous tests. Mallein (0.1 ml) is injected intradermally into the lower eyelid with a tuberculin syringe. The test is read at 48 hours, a positive reaction comprising marked edema of the lid with blepharospasm and a severe, purulent conjunctivitis.

Serological tests
The complement fixation test (CFT) is the most accurate of the serological tests available but some strains of *Act. mallei* give crossreactions with *Pseudomonas pseudomallei*. The accuracy of the test is improved by the simultaneous application of an indirect hemagglutination test (1). If pus is available, from either open ulcers or necropsy material, the organism can be cultured or the pus injected intraperitoneally into male guinea-pigs to attempt to elicit the Strauss reaction. This is a severe orchitis and inflammation of the scrotal sac but it is not highly specific for *Act. mallei*.

Necropsy findings
In the acute form there are multiple petechial hemorrhages throughout the body and a severe catarrhal bronchopneumonia with enlargement of the bronchial lymph nodes. In the more common chronic form, the lesions in the lungs take the form of miliary nodules, similar to those of miliary tuberculosis, scattered throughout the lung tissue. Ulcers are present on the mucosa of the upper respiratory tract, especially the nasal mucosa and to a lesser extent that of the larynx, trachea and bronchi. Nodules and ulcers may be present in the skin and subcutis of the limbs which may be greatly enlarged. Local lymph nodes receiving drainage from affected parts usually contain foci of pus and the lymphatic vessels have similar lesions. Necrotic foci may also be present in other internal organs. *Actinobacillus mallei*, and sometimes *Corynebacterium (Actinomyces) pyogenes*, are isolatable from infected tissues.

Diagnosis
In advanced clinical cases, the typical lymphangitis in the cutaneous form and the nasal ulcers in the pneumonic form immediately attract attention. Epizootic lymphangitis is very similar, especially as it occurs in outbreaks like glanders. However, the lesions on the nasal mucosa derive from nibbling of the leg lesions and do not penetrate into the nasal cavity to the septum, nor is pneumonia present as in glanders. Gram-positive, double-walled spores are present in the pus. Other forms of lymphangitis and skin ulceration, e.g. sporotrichosis and ulcerative lymphangitis, occur sporadically only, and there is no lymph node or systemic involvement. A horse with an infected tooth may show a unilateral nasal discharge but the discharge is odorous and no ulceration of the mucous membrane occurs. The acute pneumonic form may be confused with other pneumonias of the horse, particularly infectious equine pneumonia and severe strangles. Clinically they may be difficult to distinguish, and the area in which the disease occurs and necropsy and cultural findings may have to be considered in making a definite diagnosis. The mallein or complement fixation tests must be used to detect the occult, carrier cases which are the chief problem in the control of the disease.

Treatment
Penicillin and streptomycin have no detectable effect on the progress of the disease but sodium sulfadiazine has been highly effective in the treatment of experimental glanders and melioidosis in hamsters (4). Treatment for a period of 20 days was necessary to effect 100% recovery. Combinations of a formolized preparation of *Actinobacillus (Malleomyces) mallei* and sulfadiazine, or mallein and sulfadimidine, are reported to be effective in the treatment of affected horses.

Control
Although clinical and serological recovery from glanders occurs occasionally, it has been observed that recovered animals are not solidly immune and attempts to produce artificial immunity have been uniformly unsuccessful.

Complete quarantine of affected premises is necessary. Clinical cases should be destroyed and the remainder subjected to the mallein test at intervals of 3 weeks until all reactors have been removed. A vigorous disinfection program for food and water troughs and premises generally should be instituted to prevent spread while eradication is being carried out. Restriction of the movement of horses should be instituted and the mallein test carried out in horses which may have had contact with the infected group (6).

REFERENCES

(1) Zhang, W. D. & Lu, Z. B. (1983) *Chin. J. vet. Med.*, *9*, 8.
(2) Gangulee, P. C. et al. (1966) *Ind. vet. J.*, *43*, 386.
(3) Sen, G. P. et al. (1968) *Ind. vet. J.*, *45*, 286.
(4) Miller, W. R. et al. (1948) *Am. J. Hyg.*, *47*, 205.
(5) Alibasoglu, M. et al. (1986) *Biol. Munch. Tierärztl. Wochenschr.*, *99*, 57.
(6) Hickman, J. (1970) *Equ. vet. J.*, *2*, 153.

Bovine farcy (mycotic lymphangitis, bovine nocardiosis)

This disease of cattle occurs principally in tropical countries. The specific cause is thought to be *Nocardia farcinicus* (1) but *Mycobacterium farcinogenes* has also been proposed as the causative agent (2). The disease has been produced experimentally by the intravenous injection of *M. farcinogenes* (4). It is characterized by purulent lymphangitis and lymphadenitis, and the common occurrence of lesions on the lower limbs suggests that the causative organisms are soil-borne and gain entry through minor injuries. Initially there is a chronic, painless, localized subcutaneous cellulitis which spreads along lymphatics to involve local lymph nodes. Further spread to the lungs may occur.

Typical lesions include chronic indurated, subcutaneous swellings, and enlargement and thickening of local lymphatics and lymph nodes. Discrete swellings develop along the affected lymphatic vessels and these may rupture and discharge pus through sinuses or from indolent ulcers. The general health of affected animals is not impaired unless the lesions are extensive or pulmonary involvement occurs. The lesions may occur at the prescapular, precrural or head lymph nodes, in front of the shoulder joint, along the lymphatics in all four legs, at the base of the ear, in the cheeks or on the mandible or in the parotid area (3). Farcy nodules may also be present at favored points of tick attachment, on the perineum, in the axilla or the crutch. The lesions may rupture to discharge odorless thick gray or yellow pus which is often granular or cheesy. Healing and redischarging is common. The causative organism can be isolated from the purulent discharges by the examination of smears or by culture. In fatal cases there are usually multiple, small nodules throughout the lungs.

The disease may be confused with 'skin tuberculosis' but ulcers and sinuses do not usually develop in the latter. Ulcerative lymphangitis caused by *Cor. paratuberculosis* is a rare occurrence in cattle but is manifested by involvement of local lymph nodes and lymphatics as well as cutaneous lesions. Cases of bovine farcy with pulmonary involvement bear some clinical and pathological resemblance to tuberculosis and may give transient positive reactions to the tuberculin test (5). Although smears from pus may be sufficient to establish a diagnosis (6) inoculation of material into guinea-pigs may be necessary in some cases (7). An antigen prepared from *N. asteroides* has been used to detect cutaneous hypersensitivity and the presence of complement-fixing antibodies in the serum of affected animals. The resulting tests have diagnostic value (8).

The parenteral administration of sodium iodide is recommended as a treatment. Early disinfection of cutaneous abrasions in cattle on affected farms is recommended to reduce the incidence of the disease.

REFERENCES

(1) Mostafa, I. E. (1966) *Vet. Bull.*, *36*, 189.
(2) Chamoiseau, G. (1974) *Rev. Élev. Med. vet. Pays trop.*, *27*, 61.
(3) Mostafa, I. E. (1967) *J. comp. Pathol.*, *77*, 223, 231.
(4) el Sanousi, S. M. & Salih, M. A. M. (1979) *Vet. Pathol.*, *16*, 372.
(5) Mostafa, I. E. (1967) *Vet. Rec.*, *81*, 74.
(6) El Nasri, M. (1961) *Vet. Rec.*, *73*, 370.
(7) Awad, F. I. (1961) *Vet. Rec.*, *73*, 515 (corresp.).
(8) Pier, A. C. et al. (1968) *Am. J. vet. Res.*, *29*, 397.

Mycotic dermatitis (cutaneous streptotrichosis, Senkobo disease of cattle, lumpy wool of sheep, cutaneous actinomycosis)

This is a dermatitis occurring in all species and is caused by infection with organisms of the genus, *Dermatophilus* Van Saceghem. It has been suggested that the disease in cattle be called cutaneous streptotrichosis and the disease in sheep, mycotic dermatitis.

Etiology

The nomenclature of the causative organisms has not been finalized and we have used that suggested by Roberts (1). The previous nomenclature of *D. congolensis* in cattle, *D. dermatonomus* and *D. pedis* in sheep has been discarded and *D. congolensis* is the officially approved name. The *Dermatophilus* spp. infecting horses has also been identified as *D. congolensis* (2). The difficulty encountered in reproducing the disease experimentally has led to the proposal that serious disease is caused only when there is a predisposing mechanism, for example, infection with contagious ecthyma virus (23), application of a contact-sensitizing agent, for example, developed at the site of an insect bite (24) and exposure to *Brassica* spp. crops (27). In Africa the disease is often combined with demodicosis to produce 'Senkobo disease' a more severe and often fatal combination.

Epidemiology

Animals of all ages are susceptible, including sucklings a few weeks old. In these young animals, infection commences on the muzzle, probably from contact with the infected udder or because of scalding by milk in bucket-fed calves. Cool, wet weather conditions predispose to the disease. From observations on fleece rot of sheep it seems probable that continued wetting of the skin causes softening and swelling of the cornified epithelium leading to a mild dermatitis and increasing the chances of infection. Increased environmental humidity, and temperature as distinct from wetting of the skin, does not appear to promote the development of lesions (8). Maceration or slight trauma of the skin appear to be the critical predisposing factors. A low wax and high suint content of wool on a sheep is also conducive to infection, but removal of skin surface lipids in cattle does not alter their susceptibility to infection with *D. congolensis* (15). The introduction of infection into the skin through cuts made at shearing time is thought to be an important portal of entry. The dried spore form of the causative organism is relatively resistant and may be the form by which the infection persists from year to year. The infective form is a motile zoospore which has a much shorter life, probably only a few hours. It is activated from the dried spore by wetting. The usual source of infection is thought to be active cases or inapparent carriers in sheep and in cattle (5). Mycotic dermatitis has been observed in deer in the United States (3) taking the form of a chronic dermatitis on the lower parts of the legs, flanks, back, neck and around the nostrils. The disease spread to four persons who handled the deer. The organism isolated closely resembled *D. congolensis*. This disease in cattle and horses has not been observed to infect man in spite of ample opportunity (4).

Contact with infected animals leads to spread of the disease. In beef cattle there is a particular tendency for lesions to occur on the rump in young males and females probably due to the introduction of the infection through minor skin abrasions caused by mounting. In cattle, the role of ticks in transmission may be important in some areas and under these conditions tick control reduces the incidence of the disease. In horses, biting flies (*Stomoxys calcitrans*) are thought to act as mechanical vectors of the infection (2) and the house fly (*Musca domestica*) has also been shown to act as a carrier. In sheep, the infection appears to exist in a mild form in many animals and is manifested by a few, small scabs on the hair-covered face and ears. In these animals the disease spreads to the wool-covered areas under the influence of climatic factors. Between sheep, the disease is spread by contact for periods as short as 15 seconds, especially in wet conditions. Thus dipping, showering or yarding wet sheep are conducive to spread. Dipping fluids may become contaminated and further aid spread.

Mycotic dermatitis has been recorded in cattle, sheep, goats, horses and donkeys, and it has been transmitted experimentally to additional species including camels and rabbits (10). The disease appears to be most common under warm, moist climatic conditions but has been reported as far north as Canada, northern United States and Great Britain. Large numbers of animals may become affected. In sheep, damage to the fleece causes severe losses, up to 30% loss of value of wool and 40% loss of skin value (12, 31), and may be so extensive in lambs that spring lambing has to be abandoned. Other losses in sheep are caused by interference with shearing and a very great increase in susceptibility to blowfly infestation (9). In most countries the disease is enzootic but in tropical Africa the disease in cattle causes great losses and many death (13). Goats in the same area also suffer a high incidence (33). In temperate climates deaths are uncommon but cows that fail to respond to treatment and have to be culled are not infrequent. Reproductive inefficiency is a common accompaniment in severe cases (25, 29).

Pathogenesis

The organism invades cutaneous abrasions and sets up a bacterial dermatitis. Exudate, epithelial debris and the mycelial forms of the organism produce characteristic crusts not unlike those of ringworm. Secondary bacterial invasion may occur and gives rise to extensive suppuration and severe toxemia. In most cases the lesion appears to be self-limiting and the scab separates from the healed lesion but is still held loosely in place by hair or wool fibers. There are three stages in development of the lesions (4). At first the hair is erect and in tufts with greasy exudate forming crumbly crusts which are hard to remove. Next come dirty yellow scabs which are greasy and fissure at flexion points. In the third stage the scabs are hard, horny and confluent and there is alopecia. In some animals the disease is acute, developing quickly, responding well to treatment or disappearing spontaneously in a matter of weeks. In others the disease is chronic and persists for months, resisting all efforts to completely cure it. The sequence of histological changes in the skin has been described (5). The disease in cattle in Africa is much more serious than in other countries. The lesions are more extensive and less responsive to treatment and the disease is often fatal. This may be due to hypersensitivity to the bites of the insects that transmit this infection (28).

The natural skin and wool waxes act as effective barriers to infection and coarse-wooled sheep and Merino lambs, being deficient in wax, are most susceptible to the disease. Factors such as continuous wetting of the face or injury by shearing blades predispose to infection. In cattle, the extension of lesions on the body appears to be largely through the agency of ectoparasites (2).

Clinical findings

In cattle, lesions occur on the neck, body, or back of the udder and may extend over the sides and down the legs and the ventral surface of the body. Commonly they commence along the back from the withers to the rump and extend halfway down the rib cages. In some animals the only site affected is the flexor aspect of the limb joints. In adult cattle the characteristic lesions are thick, horny crusts, varying in color from cream to brown. They are 2–5 cm in diameter and are often in such close opposition that they give the appearance of a mosaic. In the early stages the crusts are very tenacious and attempts to lift them cause pain. Beneath the crusts there is granulation tissue and some pus. In the later stages, the dermatitis heals and the crusts separate from the skin but are held in place by penetrating hairs or wool fibers and are easily removed.

In young calves, plaque and crust formation does not occur. There is extensive hair loss with tufting of the fibers, heavy dandruff and thickening and folding of the skin in later stages. Vesicular and pustular lesions 1 cm in diameter have also been described in the early stages of the disease. In calves lesions usually commence on the muzzle and spread over the head and neck.

In goats, lesions appear first on the lips and muzzle and then spread, possibly by biting, to the feet and scrotum. In sheep, the distribution of lesions is chiefly over the dorsal parts of the body, spreading laterally and ventrally. The muzzle, face and ears may also be involved.

Lesions in horses may appear on the head, beginning at the muzzle and spreading up the face to the eyes, and if sufficiently extensive they may be accompanied by lacrimation and a profuse, mucopurulent nasal discharge. In other horses the lesions are confined to the lower limbs, with a few on the belly. In very bad environmental conditions the lesions may be widespread and cover virtually the whole of the back and sides (16). The lesions on lower limbs are most common behind the pastern, around the coronet and on the anterior aspect of the hind cannon bones. If the underlying skin cracks, the horse can become very lame (17). This variable distribution of lesions may depend upon the origin of the cutaneous wounds which act as portals of entry. No itching or irritation is apparent although in horses the sores are tender to the touch. The hairs are matted together over the lesion and an exudative dermatitis produces a firm mat of hairs and debris just above the skin surface. If this hair is plucked the entire structure may lift off leaving a characteristic ovoid, slightly bleeding skin area.

The crusts are often pyramidal in a sheep fleece because of the spread of the lesion as the crust is formed. In this animal, too, the crusts are much thicker, up to 3 cm, roughly circular and often pigmented. The value of an affected fleece is much reduced. Part of the damage is the secondary discoloration which is commonly present. These bacterial discolorations of wool have been reviewed (18).

Heavy mortalities can occur in very young lambs but in general the health of the animal is unaffected unless the lesions are widespread. Such animals are covered with scabs and are in poor condition and may die. Many develop cutaneous blowfly myiasis and in occasional cases a secondary pneumonia due to the organism may cause the death of the animal. In the average case, healing of skin lesions occurs in about 3 weeks. The lesions in goats commence on the external ear where heavy crust formations may block the ear canal and on the external nares (32). They may extend to all parts of the body especially the dorsal midline and inside the thighs (33).

Clinical pathology

The causative organism may be isolated from scrapings or a biopsy section and is much easier to isolate from an acute case than a chronic one (4). An impression smear, made directly from the ventral surface of a thick scab and pressed firmly on to a slide, may also be of value, suitable staining techniques demonstrating the presence of typical branching organisms. Because of the motility of the zoospores in water the technique of chopping up a scab and making a suspension in water before examining the material is recommended (1). Fluorescent antibody (30), ELISA (10) and counterimmunoelectrophoresis (26) techniques have also been used to detect serological evidence of infection with *D. congolensis*. The immunofluorescent antibodies are potential causes of error in the interpretation of immunofluorescence tests.

Necropsy findings

In the occasional animals that die, there is extensive dermatitis, sometimes a secondary pneumonia, and often evidence of intercurrent disease.

Diagnosis

Diagnosis depends upon the detection of the mycelia-like organisms in scrapings or biopsy sections, and culture of suspected tissues, using polymyxin B sulfate to suppress contaminants (11). In the early stages, the disease may be confused with photosensitization because of the dorsal distribution of the lesions but they are not selectively distributed on unpigmented areas. Fleece rot is a very similar condition and occurs under the same circumstances, but the thick scabs of mycotic dermatitis are absent. A disease known as 'cockle' occurs in sheep in New Zealand and may be confused with mycotic dermatitis (19). Lesions begin on the neck and shoulders and may extend over the entire body. The lesions, which are worst in unshorn sheep, are inflammatory nodules, possibly allergic in origin, and possibly an allergic reaction to molds. In calves, involvement of the muzzle and face may arouse suspicion of bovine malignant catarrh or mucosal disease. The thick scabs of mycotic dermatitis are characteristic and there is no diarrhea or stomatitis. Congenital ichthyosis of calves is present at birth but the mosaic of scabs may resemble that of mycotic dermatitis.

Treatment

There is no completely satisfactory treatment for cases which show very extensive involvement, or those being constantly reinfected or exposed to predisposing causes. In general terms, better results are obtained during dry hot weather and in dry climates. In tropical Africa treatments which are reasonably effective elsewhere are of little or no value (2). Topical applications are not generally recommended because of the impossibility of introducing them into infected layers of skin. If these are applied to acute cases where spontaneous recovery is about to occur the recovery rate will be attractive.

For adult beef cattle which are difficult to handle, some of the treatments set out below for sheep may be suitable. Adult dairy cows are treated individually and parenterally with antibiotics which are the only rational treatment and have been found to be effective. Tetracycline (5 mg/kg body weight) repeated weekly as required is recommended, and longacting tetracycline (20 mg/kg body weight) in one injection has been reported to give excellent results in cattle (16) and sheep, even in wet weather (14). Penicillin and streptomycin at very heavy dose rates (70 mg streptomycin and procaine penicillin G 70 000 units/kg body weight) is recommended as being 100% effective in heavily infected sheep.

Affected sheep should be shorn as soon as the scabs lift sufficiently. For large numbers it is best to treat immediately by dipping or spraying with 0·2–0·5% zinc sulfate. A solution containing 0·2% copper sulfate has also been used but causes staining of the wool. Its use should be limited to hand application to individual lesions. For this purpose quaternary ammonium compounds in a 1 in 200 dilution have been reported to be even more effective. *In vitro* studies indicate that a dilute solution of alum (potassium aluminum sulfate) should be highly effective and significant improvement has been observed in natural and artificial cases in sheep. The alum was administered as a 1% dip or 57% dust in an inert carrier (22). Dipping fluids may become contaminated and act as carriers of infection. This can be prevented by the use of alum, zinc sulfate or magnesium fluosilicate in the dip solution (7). The removal of scabs and exudate prior to topical treatment is recommended when practicable.

It should be remembered that one could not expect a dramatic response to the treatment of establishing or established cases with the above topical applications if weather conditions are suitable for spread of the disease (8).

To overcome the problem of shearing infected sheep, chemical defleecing has been used and is reported to be highly effective (20). Cyclophosphamide administered orally at a dose rate of 25 mg/kg body weight alone was an effective treatment in 77% of cases. Severely affected sheep were not cured. When the treatment was combined with parenteral penicillin and streptomycin the cure rate was raised to 93%.

Although horses generally respond well, in bad weather even they can be recalcitrant to treatment. Topical applications are of limited value but are preferred when horses are racing. Chloramphenicol as a 25% solution, brushed on daily for several days, is well recommended (21). Daily treatment for 2–3 days by injection with penicillin with or without streptomycin is the recommended treatment in bad cases (16).

Control

The disease usually disappears in dry weather. Isolation of infected animals and avoidance of contact with infected materials such as grooming tools appears desirable. Many farmers find it simplest to cull affected sheep or sheep that do not respond to simple treatment. In tropical areas, tick control is thought to be of considerable importance. A satisfactory control measure in sheep is spraying or dipping in 0·2–0·5% solution of zinc sulfate or a solution of magnesium fluosilicate. The prophylactic use of alum as set out under treatment is recommended after shearing as a means of controlling the disease without eradication. Attempts at prophylaxis by vaccination have been unsuccessful, but investigations are proceeding (16). Dipping of sheep right after shearing is the principal inciter of the disease, so that its severity can be reduced by delaying dipping, for example, from the 1st to the 10th day after shearing. Dips containing arsenic produce less lesions and less severe lesions than those which occur after dipping in a fluid containing only organophosphorus insecticides (6).

REVIEW LITERATURE

Bida, S. A. & Dennis, S. M. (1976) Dermatophilosis in Northern Nigeria. *Vet. Bull.*, *46*, 471, 478

Lloyd, D. H. & Sellers, K. C. (1976) *Dermatophilus Infections in Man and Animals. Proceedings of a Conference held at the University of Ibadan, Nigeria.* New York: Academic Press.

Scanlan, C. M., Garrett, P. D. & Geiger, D. B. (1984) *Dermatophilus congolensis* infections of cattle and sheep. *Comp. cont. Educ.*, 6, S4–S9.

REFERENCES

(1) Lloyd, D. H. (1981) *Vet. Rec.*, *109*, 429.
(2) Macadam, I. (1964) *Vet. Rec.*, 76, 194, 354, 420.
(3) Gordon, M. A. et al. (1977) *J. Wild. Dis.*, *13*, 184.
(4) Searcy, G. P. & Hulland, T. J. (1967) *Can. vet. J.*, 9, 716.
(5) Bida, S. A. & Dennis, S. M. (1977) *Res. vet. Sci.*, *22*, 18.
(6) Wilkinson, F. C. (1979) *Aust. vet. J.*, *55*, 74.
(7) Le Riche, P. D. (1968) *Aust. vet. J.*, *44*, 64.
(8) Lloyd, D. H. (1984) *Prev. vet. Med.*, *2*, 93.
(9) Gherardi, S. G. et al. (1983) *Aust. vet. J.*, *60*, 27.
(10) Abu-Samra, M. T. et al. (1976) *J. comp. Pathol.*, *86*, 157.
(11) Abu-Samra, M. T. (1978) *Zentralbl. VetMed.*, *25B*, 641.
(12) Lefevre, E. et al. (1978) *Rec. Med. Vet.*, *154*, 913.
(13) Oduye, O. O. & Lloyd, D. H. (1971) *Br. vet. J.*, *127*, 505.
(14) Gyang, E. O. et al. (1980) *Vet. Rec.*, *106*, 106.
(15) Adekeye, J. D. & Timoszyk, J. (1983) *Bull. Anim. Hlth Prod. Afr.*, *31*, 21.
(16) Ilemobade, A. A. (1984) *Prev. vet. Med.*, *2*, 83.
(17) Pascoe, R. R. (1972) *Aust. vet. J.*, *48*, 32.
(18) Mulcock, A. P. (1965) *NZ vet. J. B.*, *13*, 87.
(19) Dempsey, M. et al. (1972) *NZ J. agric. Res.*, *15*, 741.
(20) McIntosh, G. H. et al. (1971) *Aust. vet. J.*, *47*, 542.
(21) Pascoe, R. R. (1973) *Aust. vet. J.*, 49, 35.
(22) Hart, C. B. & Tyszkiewiczk, K. (1968) *Vet. Rec.*, *82*, 272.
(23) Abu-Samra, M. T. & Walton, G. S. (1981) *J. comp. Pathol.*, *91*, 317.
(24) Davis, D. (1984) *J. comp. Pathol.*, *94*, 25.
(25) Ogwu, D. et al. (1981) *Theriogenology*, *15*, 469.
(26) Makinde, A. A. & Majiyagbe, K. A. (1982) *Res. vet. Sci.*, *33*, 265.
(27) Allworth, M. B. et al. (1985) *NZ vet. J.*, *33*, 210.
(28) Davis, D. (1984) *J. comp. Pathol.*, *94*, 25.
(29) Huffman, E. M. & Cowen, P. (1984) *Theriogenology*, *21*, 941.
(30) Scott, D. W. et al. (1984) *Cornell Vet.*, *74*, 305.
(31) Edwards, J. R. (1985) *Aust. vet. J.*, *62*, 173.
(32) Larsen, J. W. A. (1987) *Aust. vet. J.*, *64*, 160.
(33) Scott, D. W. et al. (1984) *Comp. cont. Educ.*, 6, S190.

Strawberry footrot (proliferative dermatitis)

This is a proliferative dermatitis of the lower limbs of sheep.

Etiology

The causative agent is *Dermatophilus congolensis* (*D. pedis*) (1).

Epidemiology

All ages and breeds appear susceptible but under natural conditions lambs are more commonly affected. Most outbreaks occur during the summer months and lesions tend to disappear in cold weather. Although the disease is recorded naturally only in sheep, it can be transmitted experimentally to man, goats, guinea-pigs and to rabbits. Complete immunity does not develop after an attack and there is no cross-immunity against sheep pox (2), although sheep recently recovered from contagious ecthyma may show a transient resistance (3).

The natural method of transmission is unknown but the frequency of occurrence of lesions at the knee and coronet suggests infection from the ground through cutaneous injuries. Dried crusts containing the causative agent are infective for long periods and ground contamination by infected animals is the probable source of infection.

The disease is recorded only from the United Kingdom (4) and occurs extensively in some parts of Scotland and in Australia. It is not fatal but severely affected animals do not make normal weight gains. Up to 100% of affected flocks may show the clinical disease.

Pathogenesis

Histologically the lesions are those of a superficial epidermitis similar to that of contagious ecthyma.

Clinical findings

Most cases appear 2–4 weeks after sheep have been moved on to affected pasture but incubation periods of 3–4 months have been observed. Small heaped-up scabs appear on the leg from the coronet to the knee or hock. These enlarge to 3–5 cm in diameter and become thick and wart-like. The hair is lost and the lesions may coalesce. Removal of the scabs reveals a bleeding, fleshy mass resembling a fresh strawberry, surrounded by a shallow ulcer. In later stages the ulcer is deep and pus is present. There is no itching or lameness unless lesions occur in the interdigital space. Most lesions heal in 5–6 weeks but chronic cases may persist for 6 months.

Clinical pathology

Swabs and scrapings should be examined carefully for the causative organism.

Diagnosis

Lesions of strawberry footrot closely resemble those of contagious ecthyma but are restricted in their distribution to the lower limbs whereas lesions of contagious ecthyma occur mostly on the face and rarely on the legs. Sheep which have recovered from the disease are still susceptible. The absence of a systemic reaction and the wart-like character of the lesions differentiate it from sheep pox. A final diagnosis must depend on the isolation of the organism or the experimental transmission of the disease.

Treatment

No specific treatment is available but iodides by mouth or parenterally may be of value.

Control

In the light of present knowledge, isolation of infected sheep and the resting of infected fields are the only measures which can be recommended.

REFERENCES

(1) Austwick, P. K. C. (1984) *Vet. Rev. Annot.*, *4*, 33.
(2) Horgan, E. S. & Haseeb, M. A. (1948) *J. comp. Pathol.*, *58*, 329.
(3) Abdussalam, M. & Blakemore, F. (1948) *J. comp. Pathol.*, *58*, 333.
(4) Harriss, S. T. (1948) *J. comp. Pathol.*, *58*, 314.

Shigellosis of foals (sleepy foal disease)

Shigellosis is an acute, highly fatal septicemia of newborn foals. Foals that survive for a few days show evidence of localization in various organs.

Etiology

The causative organism, *Actinobacillus equuli (Shigella equirulis)*, is often found in the intestine and tissue of normal horses.

Epidemiology

Shigellosis is limited to horses and although newborn foals are the most susceptible age group, there have been reports of the septicemic form of the disease in older animals (1) especially when their resistance is lowered by concurrent infection.

Although foals may become infected *in utero*, it is probable that postnatal infection, usually via the navel, is more frequent. The mare is not clinically affected and the organism does not persist in the uterus for long periods. The method of spread between mares is unknown but intrauterine infection appears to occur in the same mare in successive years, possibly from a focus in some other organ. Some foals are immunodeficient because of colostrum deficiency or failure of transfer of immunoglobulins from the mare's colostrum (2).

Shigellosis is an important cause of neonatal deaths in foals in most countries of the world and may represent as high a proportion as 25% of all infections in newborn foals (3–8). Successive foals on a particular farm may be affected with a mortality rate approaching 100%.

Pathogenesis

In foals, the disease is an acute septicemia, in many cases causing death before specific lesions are produced. In such cases adrenal cortical deficiency may be a major factor in causing death (9). Foals which survive the illness for more than 24 hours develop suppurative lesions in the renal cortex, in joints and intestines. In older animals it has been postulated that the infection may be carried to various organs by migrating strongyle larvae.

Clinical findings

The foal may be sick at birth or show signs from within a few hours of birth up to 3 days of age. There is a sudden onset of fever, prostration, diarrhea, occasionally dysentery and rapid respiration, and the foal ceases to suck. Foals which are sleepy or comatose at birth or soon afterwards occur commonly. These so called sleepers may be aroused but quickly revert to a comatose state. Death within 24 hours is usual. Occasional foals show severe abdominal pain in the early stages of the disease. Foals that survive the acute, febrile phase develop arthritis with swollen joints and lameness within 1–2 days. Death usually occurs in these more protracted cases during the period between the 2nd and 7th days.

Clinical pathology

Cervical swabs from the mare should be examined bacteriologically for the presence of the organism.

Necropsy findings

Foals that die within 24 hours of the onset of illness show septicemia and severe enteritis but there may be no pinpoint abscesses in the kidney. The adrenals are enlarged and dark red in color (9). Foals dying after a longer interval show tenosynovitis and arthritis. In the early stages the synovial fluids are sanguineous and turbid but soon become purulent. In these foals it is also usual to find the diagnostic pinpoint abscesses in the renal cortices. Shigella are recoverable from the bloodstream in acute cases and from joints and other organs in cases of longer duration.

Diagnosis

The presence of minute abscesses in the renal cortices and *Act. equuli* in the fetal tissues is diagnostic. Other than the high proportion of sleeper foals in shigellosis, there is little to go on in the differentiation of this disease from septicemias caused by *Escherichia coli, Salmonella typhimurium* and *S. abortivoequina*. Other conditions to be considered in arriving at a diagnosis include congenital heart anomalies, ruptured bladder and isoimmune hemolytic anemia as set out in Table 59.

Other diseases which occur in this age group, but are unlikely to be confused with those listed in Table 59, are neonatal maladjustment syndrome (barkers and wanderers) and idiopathic myopathy.

Treatment

In foals, streptomycin gives excellent results when administered parenterally, early and in sufficiently large and frequent doses (1 g 6-hourly). Chlortetracycline (10 mg/kg body weight) given intravenously for 5 days gives good results also, although *in vitro* tests of blood levels reached with this drug suggest that the dose rate should be 20 mg/kg body weight once daily (10). Chloramphenicol (20 mg/kg body weight) intramuscularly daily, is also highly effective and can be supplemented by oral administration of the same drug at the same dose rate (11). Supportive treatment by blood transfusions is also of value and is described in diseases of the newborn.

Control

Control of the disease depends upon elimination of the infection by culling or treating infected mares, preventing spread by hygienic precautions at foaling time, and by treating susceptible foals prophylactically at birth with one of the drugs prescribed for treatment.

REFERENCES

(1) Stricker, F. & Gouvert, Z. (1956) *Vet. Cas.*, *5*, 260.
(2) Kamada, M. et al. (1985) *Bull. equ. Res. Inst. No. 22*, pp. 38–42.
(3) Gunning, O. V. (1947) *Vet. J.*, *103*. 47.
(4) Cottew, G. S. & Ryley, J. W. (1952) *Aust. vet. J.*, *28*, 302.
(5) Dimock, W. W. et al. (1947) *Cornell Vet.*, *37*, 89.
(6) Flatla, J. L. (1942) *Norsk Vet. Tidsskr.*, *54*, 249, 322.
(7) Harms, F. (1942) *Dtsch Tierärztl. Wochenschr.*, *50*, 408.
(8) Leader, G. H. (1952) *Vet. Rec.*, *64*, 241.
(9) Du Plesis, J. L. (1963) *J. S. Afr. vet. med. Assoc.*, *34*, 25.
(10) McCollum, W. H. & Doll, E. R. (1951) *Vet. Med.*, *46*, 84.
(11) Littlejohn, A. (1959) *J. S. Afr. vet. med. Assoc.*, 30, 143.

Table 59. Differential diagnosis of 'sleeper' newborn foals

Disease	*Epidemiology*	*Clinical findings*	*Clinical pathology*	*Necropsy findings*	*Treatment and response*
Shigellosis	Enzootic to particular farms. In foals up to 3 months. Recurs in foals from same mare	Sudden onset, recumbency, anorexia, fever, diarrhea, comatose, peripheral circulatory collapse. Death in 24 hours	Blood culture. Cervical swabs of mare	Pinpoint abscesses in kidney. Septicemia, enteritis. Longstanding cases have joint lesions	Excellent if early. Chloramphenicol, fluids, blood transfusion possibly
Other septicemias	*E. coli, S. typhimurium, Str. pyogenes equi.* Enzootic to a farm	As above	Blood culture	Septicemia and enteritis. Longstanding cases have arthritis	Fortunate to save them in spite of early vigorous treatment, broad-spectrum antibiotic plus fluids
Isoimmune hemolytic anemia	May recur with identical matings. Rare. Confused with icterus neonatorum	Acute early cases, anemia, hemoglobinuria. Later cases, jaundice, plus anemia	*Essential* to prove anemia and agglutination response of foal erythrocytes to dam serum	Anemia, jaundice. May be faulty placentation in mare	Blood transfusion from compatible donor. Prevent sucking of mare for first 48 hours
Ruptured bladder	Colt foals mostly. Probably inherited	Frequent straining, small amount urine passed, abdominal swelling	Paracentesis, heat fluid for urine odor. Pass catheter, put dye into bladder, collect via paracentesis	Incomplete closure of dorsal bladder wall	Excellent response to surgical repair
Retained meconium	Colt foals mostly. Worst in dry years	Frequent straining. Meconium palpable on rectal. May be severe pain and tympany of large bowel	Nil	Not usually fatal	Medical with lubricants and fecal softener mostly sufficient. Enterotomy rarely
Congenital cardiac defect	Sporadic	Dyspnea, heart murmur and thrill. Cyanosis. Exercise tolerance poor	Polycythemia. Pressure shunt demonstrable with intracardiac catheter	Patent ductus arteriosus, interventricular septum, tetralogy of Fallot	Intrepid surgeons only. Success rate poor

20

Diseases Caused by Bacteria—V

DISEASES CAUSED BY *FUSOBACTERIUM* AND *BACTEROIDES* spp.

INFECTION by *Fusobacterium* spp., especially *F. necrophorum*, is common in all species of farm animals. In many instances the organism is present as a secondary invader rather than as a primary cause of disease. The specific diseases dealt with here as being caused by primary infection with *Fusobacterium* spp. are footrot of cattle, oral necrobacillosis, footrot of sheep and pigs and foot abscess of sheep. In footrot of sheep the causative organism (*Bacteroides nodosus*) occurs in association with *Spirochaeta penortha* and in footrot of pigs a species of *Fusobacterium* and spirochetal organisms are commonly found together.

Some of the common conditions in which *Fusobacterium* spp. are found as secondary invaders are navel ill and hepatic necrobacillosis in sheep and cattle, in pneumonia of calves and in the secondary infections of covering epithelium. These include necrotic enteritis caused by *Salmonella* spp. in pigs, necrotic rhinitis and atrophic rhinitis of pigs, most diseases in which vesicular eruption and erosive lesions of the buccal mucosa and coronary skin of cattle and sheep occur, and in vulvitis, vaginitis and metritis.

Fusobacterium spp. have been associated with stomatitis, enteritis and granulocytopenia in a calf (1), hematogenous metaphyseal osteomyelitis in a 6-month-old calf (2), and endocarditis of swine examined at slaughter (3).

The factors which contribute to the pathogenicity of *F. necrophorum* include a potent endotoxin, a polysaccharide capsule, an exotoxin (a leukocidin) and a hemolysin. The biochemical and functional properties of a leukocidin produced by afferent strains of *F. necrophorum* have been described (8, 9). Extensive studies have been directed towards the immunity of the organism and the possibility of vaccination against the several diseases caused by *F. necrophorum*. However, the main virulence factors of *F. necrophorum* are only weakly immunogenic and the experiments give little encouragement for an effective necrobacillosis vaccine (4, 5).

The susceptibility of *Bacteroides* spp. isolated from swine abscesses to several antimicrobials has been examined (7).

An enzyme-linked immunosorbent assay (ELISA) for the detection of *F. necrophorum* antibodies in the serum of cattle and sheep has been developed (6).

REVIEW LITERATURE

Langworth, B. F. (1977) *Fusobacterium necrophorum*. Its characteristics and role as an animal pathogen. *Bacteriol. Rev.*, *41*, 373.

REFERENCES

(1) Nimmo-Wilke, J. S. & Radostits, O. M. (1981) *Can. vet. J.*, *22*, 166.
(2) Rudman, J. et al. (1982) *J. Am. vet. med. Assoc.*, *180*, 944.
(3) Narushima, T. et al. (1986) *J. Jap. vet. med. Assoc.*, *56*, *39*, 221.
(4) Smith, G. R. et al. (1985) *J. Hyg., Camb.*, *95*, 59.
(5) Emery, D. L. & Vaughan, J. A. (1986) *Vet. Microbiol.*, *12*, 255.
(6) Evans, J. W. & Berg, J. N. (1985) *Am. J. vet. Res.*, *46*, 132.
(7) Benno, Y. & Mitsuoka, T. (1984) *Am. J. vet. Res.*, *45*, 2631.
(8) Emery, D. L. et al. (1984) *Aust. vet. J.*, *61*, 382.
(9) Scanlan, C. M. et al. (1982) *Am. J. vet. Res.*, *43*, 1339.

Necrobacillosis of the liver

This disease of cattle and lambs is caused by localization in the liver of an infection originating in the navel or rumen. In many cases the animal's health is unaffected and the abscesses are discovered only at necropsy. There may be acute, fatal toxemia or chronic ill-health without localizing signs.

Etiology

Fusobacterium (Sphaerophorus) necrophorum is commonly found in pure culture in hepatic abscesses in ruminants. The disease can be produced experimentally in cattle and sheep by the intraportal injection of cultures of the organism (1). *Actinomyces (Corynebacterium) pyogenes* and streptococci are also often present in the lesions (2).

Epidemiology

The organism is a common inhabitant of the environment of farm animals and the existence of a predisposing injury may be all that is required for the disease to occur. In lambs, infection usually occurs through the navel at birth or through ruminal ulcers, the infection originating from infected bedding grounds or barns (4). *F. necrophorum* is not capable of prolonged survival outside the animal body, 1 month being the probable maximum period under favorable conditions, and constant reinfection is probably necessary to render soil or surroundings highly infective (5). The organism is a common inhabitant of the intestine and rumen in normal cattle.

Of the three biotypes of *F. necrophorum*, A, B, and C, only biotypes A and B have been implicated in liver abscesses (2). Type B is the predominant biotype isolated from ruminal lesions, and type A the predominant biotype isolated from liver abscesses. Type A is usually found in pure culture in the liver abscesses, whereas type B is usually found in mixed culture with either type A or with other bacterial species (2). *Actinomyces (Corynebacterium) pyogenes*, *Streptococcus* spp., *Staphylococcus* spp., and *Bacteroides* spp. are the most prevalent bacteria recovered from mixed cultures. *Actinomyces (Corynebacterium) pyogenes* is the most common species isolated and can cause disease synergistically with type B isolates.

The disease is of greatest importance in feeder cattle where it occurs secondarily to rumenitis. In these animals there is considerable financial loss due to condemnation of livers in abattoirs. An incidence of 22% has been observed in 'barley beef' cattle in the United Kingdom (6) and about 5% of bovine livers in the United States are rejected because of hepatic abscess. In lambs, occasional losses are recorded in housed and range flocks.

Pathogenesis

Vascular drainage from the primary lesion, omphalitis or rumenitis, leads to localization in the liver. It is commonly held that in cattle the sudden change from pasture to high grain diets causes rumenitis due to the development of acidity in the rumen, and *F. necrophorum* invades the erosive lesion produced (1). Doubt has been thrown on this as being the only pathogenesis by the absence of ruminal lesions in cattle on heavy grain diets that show a very high incidence of hepatic abscess (6).

It is postulated that the ruminal wall in rumenitis is colonized by the bacteria in the rumen including both type A and type B strains of *F. necrophorum*. Most of the ruminal wall lesions would heal without penetration especially if they contained only the less virulent type B strains. The more virulent type A strains would persist longer and possibly penetrate the portal system with the help of leukotoxin. The lower virulence of type B would require helper organisms to penetrate the defense mechanisms and lead to a mixed infection. This may explain why type A strains predominate in the liver and type B strains may predominate in the rumen (14).

The experimental inoculation of viable cultures of *F. necrophorum* into the hepatic portal veins of cattle results in the development of diffusely distributed microabscesses within 30 minutes up to 2 hours (1). Gross abscesses develop from 3 to 36 hours. Neutrophils are the predominant phagocyte in lesions of 8 hours or less, and macrophages are the predominant phagocyte in lesions of 12 hours duration or more. The leukotoxin is postulated to be responsible for allowing the bacteria to withstand the phagocyte cell response and enable the infection to persist. If there is sufficient hepatic involvement a toxemia develops from the bacterial infection causing a chronic or acute illness. An endotoxic lipopolysaccharide has been isolated from *F. necrophorum* (7) and probably contributes to the toxemia. However, in most instances the lesions are too small to produce clinical signs. Hematogenous spread from hepatic lesions, including rupture into the caudal vena cava, may result in multiple lesions in many organs and rapidly fatal termination.

Clinical findings

In most cases of hepatic abscessation in feeder cattle there are no clinical signs unless the abscesses are very large when they may result in an acute or chronic illness. In acute cases there is fever, anorexia, depression, fall in milk production and weakness. Abdominal pain is evidenced on percussion over the posterior ribs on the right side and affected cattle show arching of the back, and reluctance to move or lie down. The liver may be so enlarged that it is readily palpable behind the costal arch. The abdominal pain may be sufficiently severe to cause grunting with each breath. In chronic cases there are no localizing signs but anorexia, emaciation and intermittent diarrhea and constipation occur. Animals affected at birth show signs at about 7 days of age and omphalophlebitis is usually present.

Clinical pathology

A high leukocytosis with a marked neutrophilia may be present with large or multiple abscesses. Liver function tests are valuable when the disease is suspected.

Necropsy findings

In rumenitis in cattle the anterior, ventral sac is most commonly affected. There are local or diffuse lesions of rumenitis with thickening of the wall, superficial necrosis and the subsequent development of ulcers. Multiple hepatic abscesses are present, and in lambs there may be lesions at the cardial end of the esophagus. The hepatic lesions may be deep in the parenchyma or under the capsule, especially on the diaphragmatic surface. Extension to the diaphragm or perirenal tissues is not unusual.

Diagnosis

The diagnosis of non-specific liver abscess is discussed elsewhere. Bacillary hemoglobinuria is characterized clinically by fever, jaundice and hemoglobinuria and at necropsy by hepatic infarcts instead of abscesses. Acute cases in cattle resemble cases of traumatic reticuloperitonitis and differentiation can only be made on localization of the pain and by exploratory rumenotomy. The latter is essential if traumatic hepatitis is a possible diagnosis.

Treatment

A course of sulfadimidine or tetracyclines causes a transitory response but relapse is common because of incomplete control of the localized infection. The antimicrobial susceptibility of the organism has been determined by the disc method (8).

However, to achieve the minimum inhibitory concentration (MIC) in the serum of affected animals would require much higher dose rates than are currently used and for which claims are made (3).

Control

The high incidence of hepatic abscesses in feedlot cattle can be reduced by the feeding of a lower proportion of grain in the ration and by a gradual changeover from pasture to fattening rations when the animals first come into the lot (1). Feeding chlortetracycline (75 mg/day) throughout the fattening period may reduce the number of hepatic abscesses which occur but the incidence may still be as high as 70% (9, 10). In sheep, the disease can be controlled by disinfection of the navel at birth and providing clean bedding or bedding grounds.

Vaccination of young cattle before they enter feedlots has been under intensive investigation, and good results have been claimed for a toxoid (11, 12). The continuous administration of 70 mg tylosin daily to young cattle can reduce the occurrence of liver abscess and improve weight gain and feed conversion (13).

REVIEW LITERATURE

Scanlan, C. M. & Hathcock, T. L. (1983) Bovine rumenitis—liver abscess complex: A bacteriological review. *Cornell Vet.*, *73*, 288–297.

REFERENCES

(1) Scanlan, C. M. & Berg. J. N. (1983) *Cornell Vet.*, *73*, 117.
(2) Scanlan, C. M. & Hathcock, T. L. (1983) *Cornell Vet.*, *73*, 288.
(3) Berg, J. N. & Scanlan, C. M. (1982) *Am. J. vet. Res.*, *43*, 1580.
(4) Harris, A. N. A. (1947) *Aust. vet. J.*, *23*, 152.
(5) Smith, L. D. S. (1963) *Bull. Off. int. Epizootol.*, *59*, 1517.
(6) Rowland, A. C. (1966) *Vet. Rec.*, *78*, 713.
(7) Warner, J. F. et al. (1975) *Am. J. vet. Res.*, *36*, 1015.
(8) Simon, P. C. (1977) *Can. J. comp. Med.*, *41*, 166.
(9) Flint, J. C. & Jensen, R. (1958) *Am. J. vet. Res.*, *19*, 830.
(10) Avery, R. J. (1962) *Can. vet. J.*, *3*, 15.
(11) Katic, R. et al. (1974) *Vet. Glasn.*, *28*, 947.
(12) Garcia, M. M. et al. (1947) *Can. J. comp. Med.*, *38*, 222.
(13) Brown, H. (1975) *J. anim. Sci.*, *40*, 207.
(14) Nakajima, Y. et al. (1986) *Jap. J. vet. Sci.*, *48*, 509.

Interdigital necrobacillosis (foul in the foot, footrot)

This is an infectious disease of cattle characterized by inflammation of the sensitive tissues of the feet and severe lameness.

Etiology

Footrot is usually described as being caused by *Fusobacterium necrophorum* but there is lack of conclusive evidence on this point. Other bacteria such as *Bacteroides melaninogenicus* (3) have also been named as possible causes. Experimentally, the subcutaneous inoculation of only *F. necrophorum* into the interdigital skin of cattle will result in typical lesions of interdigital necrobacillosis (13) and the inclusion of *Bacteroides melaninogenicus* was not necessary to produce the lesion. There is also an increasing number of reports of recovery of *Bacteroides nodosus*, the causative organism of ovine footrot, from lesions in the feet of cattle (1, 2). To date the isolates have been capable, with one exception only, of producing benign footrot in sheep. So that although there may be an etiological relationship between the footrots of the two species it seems at present as though the relationship is restricted to cattle acting as carriers of the sheep disease. The possibility still exists that the mild interdigital dermatitis caused by *B. nodosus* in cattle could provide the starting point of the much more severe dermatitis that characterizes infectious bovine footrot (8).

Epidemiology

The disease appears to be contagious and the incidence is much higher during wet humid weather or when conditions are wet underfoot. Stony ground, lanes filled with sharp gravel and pasturing on coarse stubble also predispose to the condition. The observation that the disease is common on some farms and does not occur at all on others suggests that there may be factors which limit the persistence of infectivity in certain soils. Introduction of the infection to a farm by transient cattle is often observed but again the disease may not develop on some farms in spite of the introduction of the infection. Cattle of all ages, including young calves, may be affected but the disease is much more common in adults. A field observation is that *Bos indicus* (Zebu-type, Brahman) cattle are much more resistant to infectious footrot than *Bos taurus* breeds (5).

Discharges from the feet of infected animals are the probable source of infection. Duration of the infectivity of pasture or bedding is unknown. Infection gains entrance through abrasions to the skin on the lower part of the foot. Abrasions are more likely to occur when the skin is swollen and soft due to continual wetting. The increased incidence in wet summer and autumn months may be so explained in part although wet conditions may also favor persistence of the infection in pasture.

The disease is common in most countries. It is of greatest economic importance in dairy cattle, in which it reaches the highest level of incidence, because of the intensive conditions under which they are kept. In beef cattle at range the incidence is usually low but many cases may occur in purebred herds and in feedlot cattle. Loss of production occurs in affected cattle and an occasional animal may suffer a serious involvement of the joint and other deep structures of the foot necessitating amputation of a claw. Under favorable conditions as many as 25% of a group may be affected at one time but the usual picture is for the disease to occur sporadically on affected farms. The disease is not fatal but some cases may have to be slaughtered because of joint involvement.

An epidemiological study of footrot in pastured cattle in Denmark over a 12-year period revealed that incidence rates annually ranged from 0·1% to 4·8% but in most years it was below 1% (16). The incidence rates were higher in some breeds than others, higher in some geographical areas than others (usually where the fields were smaller and soil pH higher), and 4–8 weeks after periods of high rainfall. The majority of isolates of *F. necrophorum* obtained from the feet of cattle and sheep belong to biotypes AB, produce a soluble exotoxin, a leukocidin, and are pathogenic experimentally in cattle and mice (14). The isolates of *F. necrophorum* obtained from lesions which are not classified as interdigital necrobacillosis and from clinically normal feet are predominantly of the B biotype, cause few experimental lesions and produce little or no leukocidin (14).

Pathogenesis

The pathogenesis is not completely understood, but with the experimental subcutaneous inoculation of the virulent biotype of *F. necrophorum* into the interdigital skin of cattle the typical lesion of footrot develops in approximately 5 days (13). This suggests that any injury or constant wetting of the skin of the cleft which interferes with its integrity will allow the organism to invade the tissues. There is acute swelling and necrosis of the skin and subcutaneous tissues which may spread to adjacent tendon sheaths, joint capsules and bone if treatment is delayed or ineffective.

Clinical findings

Severe foot lameness appears suddenly, usually in one limb only and may be accompanied by a moderate systemic reaction with a fever of 39–40°C (103–104°F). There is temporary depression of milk yield in cows and affected bulls may show temporary infertility. The animal puts little weight on the leg although the limb is carried only when severe joint involvement occurs. Swelling of the coronet and spreading of the claws are obvious.

The typical lesion occurs in the skin at the top of the interdigital cleft and takes the form of a fissure with swollen, protruding edges which may extend along the length of the cleft or be confined to the anterior part or that part between the heel bulbs. Pus is never present in large amounts but the edges of the fissure are covered with necrotic material and the lesion has a characteristic odor. Occasionally in early cases no external lesion may be visible but there is lameness and swelling of the coronet. Such cases are usually designated 'blind fouls' and respond well to parenteral treatment.

Spontaneous recovery is not uncommon but if the disease is left untreated the lameness usually persists for several weeks with adverse effects on milk production and condition. The incidence of complications is also higher if treatment is delayed and some animals may have to be destroyed because of local involvement of joints and tendon sheaths. In such cases the lameness is severe, the leg usually being carried and the animal strongly resenting handling of the foot. Swelling is usually more obvious and extends up the back of the leg. There is poor response to medical treatment and surgical measures are necessary to permit drainage. Radiological examination may be of value in determining the exact degree of involvement of bony tissue. Long continued irritation may result in the development of a wart-like mass of fibrous tissue, the interdigital fibroma, in the anterior part of the cleft and chronic mild lameness. Interdigital fibroma occurs commonly without the intervention of footrot, the important cause being inherited defects in foot conformation in heavy animals.

Clinical pathology

Bacteriological examination is not usually necessary for diagnosis but direct smears of the lesion will usually reveal large numbers of a mixture of *Fusobacterium and Bacteroides* spp. Routine differentiation between virulent and non-virulent bovine isolates of *F. necrophorum* can be done by assessment of the cultural characteristics of the colonies grown on blood agar (14).

Necropsy findings

Necropsy examinations are rarely carried out in cases of footrot but details of the pathology are available (1). Dermatitis is followed by necrosis of the skin and subcutaneous tissues. In complicated cases there may be suppuration in joints and tendon sheaths.

Diagnosis

The characteristic site, nature and smell of the lesion, the pattern of the disease in the group and the season and climate are usually sufficient to indicate the presence of true footrot. Traumatic injury to bones and joints, puncture by foreign bodies, bruising of the heels and gross overgrowth of the hoof can usually be distinguished by careful examination of the foot. Laminitis may cause lameness but there are no local foot lesions. Young cattle maintained wholly on slatted floors over manure storage pits may develop severe lameness due to constant abrasion of the sole of the foot, or the lateral and medial aspects of the limb joints when lying down, if the slats have rough edges or the gaps between them are too great. The sole of the foot is worn flat and the wall is separated at the lateral edge. Similar lesions can be found in cows using new milking parlors where steep ramps have been surfaced with very abrasive non-slip concrete surface. Animals which spend a long time in concrete yards at milking time are also susceptible to excessive sole wear. They are likely to be the timid ones, and especially heifers which are likely to be chased around a good deal, increasing the wear problem still further (9). Another form of lameness seen in housed cattle is manifested by hard painful swelling of the fetlock joints with knuckling of the joint caused by contracture of the flexor tendons. It is thought to result from continuous strain of the collateral ligaments of the joints because of the discontinuity of the surface of the gratings.

Stable footrot is a disease which occurs commonly in cattle which are housed for long periods. Although the condition occurs most commonly when the cattle are kept under insanitary conditions it is also seen in well-managed herds. The causative agent has not been established but *B. nodosus* has been isolated in outbreaks which were clinically and pathologically similar (6, 7). The initial lesion is an outpouring of sebaceous exudate at the skin–horn junction, particularly at the bulbs of the heel. There is a penetrating foul odor, the lesion is painful to touch but there is little swelling and no systemic reaction. More than one foot is commonly affected. In longstanding cases there is separation of the horn at the heel-bulb and this is followed by secondary bacterial infection of the sensitive structures of the foot. Often there is a purulent dermatitis of the interdigital space. Stable footrot does not respond satisfactorily to the standard parenteral treatments used in footrot but local treatments as set out below are effective. Verrucose dermatitis is a proliferative inflammatory lesion of the skin of the plantar surface of the foot extending from the bulb of the heels to the fetlock joint. The condition is seen particularly in feedlot cattle which are overcrowded in wet muddy conditions and may occur in outbreaks. All four feet may be affected, there is considerable pain and lameness and, on smear of the lesion, *Fusobacterium necrophorum* is present in large numbers.

Treatment

Parenteral administration of antibiotics or sulfonamides and local treatment of the foot lesion are necessary for best results. Immediate treatment as soon as possible after the onset of swelling and lameness will give excellent recovery in 2–4 days. When treatment was delayed for a few days after the onset of signs in the experimental disease (3) severe lesions developed and recovery was extended. Under field conditions the disease may have been present in cattle at pasture for several days before being recognized, making it necessary to confine them for daily treatment until recovery is apparent. Sodium sulfadimidine (150–200 mg/kg body weight) solution given by intravenous or intraperitoneal injection is highly effective. Procaine penicillin G at a dose rate of 22 000 IU/kg body weight intramuscularly twice daily has been recommended (4). Oxytetracycline at a dose rate of 10 mg/kg body weight intravenously may also be used. When a high incidence of footrot is experienced in a herd treatment of all animals simultaneously has been carried out (11). Sulfabromomethazine at the rate of 30 g/kg grain was given for 2 consecutive days to calves weighing 150 kg and results were excellent.

Local treatment necessitates casting, slinging the affected leg to an overhead beam or, if the veterinarian's physique and stamina are appropriate, restraining the animal properly and holding the foot up by hand. This procedure is greatly facilitated by the intravenous injection of a very small dose of xylazine. The foot is scrubbed, all necrotic tissue curetted away and a local dressing applied under a pad or bandage. Any antibacterial, and preferably astringent, dressing appears to be satisfactory. A wet pack of 5% copper sulfate solution is cheap and effective. Any suitable antibacterial ointment preparation may be applied and secured with a bandage which may be left on for several days. The main advantage of local treatment is that the foot is cleaned and kept clean. The clinical management of bovine foot problems with emphasis on local treatment of the affected foot has been described (4). If conditions underfoot are wet the animal should be kept stabled in a dry stall. In cattle running at pasture, or in the case of large numbers of feedlot cattle, examination of the foot and local treatment are often omitted because of the time and inconvenience involved. However, identification of the animal with a marker is considered necessary in outbreaks to avoid unnecessary confusion in the days following, and examination of the foot is deemed necessary to ensure that foreign bodies are not involved. Local treatment may not be necessary in the early stages of the disease if the animal can be prevented from gaining access to wet, muddy areas.

In cases where the lesion has remained superficial but has become chronic with separation of the horn from the coronary band, the horn should be trimmed back and the area cleaned and painted daily with a 5% copper sulfate solution or less frequently with a mixture of 10% copper sulfate in wood tar. In refractory cases or when complications with spread to deeper tissues have occurred, surgical drainage may be necessary and the techniques have been described (12).

Control

Prevention of foot injuries by filling in muddy and stony patches in barnyards and lanes will reduce the incidence of the disease. Provision of a footbath containing a 5–10% solution of formaldehyde copper sulfate, in a doorway so that cattle have to walk through it twice daily, will practically eliminate the disease on dairy farms. A mixture of 10% copper sulfate in slaked lime is often used in the same manner. Similar measures can be adopted for small groups of beef animals.

For young cattle on feed and which stand inside on litter, a method of disinfecting the litter with paraformaldehyde has been used with apparent good results (17). Feeding chlortetracycline to feedlot cattle 500 mg/ per head/day for 28 days, followed by 75 mg/day throughout the finishing period has been recommended but controlled comparative trials have not been done. The feeding of organic iodides (200–400 mg) of ethylenediamine dihydriodide (EDDI) daily in the feed has been used for many years as a preventive against the disease in feedlot cattle. The daily oral administration or feeding of EDDI at a dose of 50–200 mg/head/day for 2 weeks will reduce the incidence and severity of experimentally induced footrot lesions (18). There was a direct relationship between dosage levels of EDDI and serum iodine levels. At the dose level of 200 mg/head/day some animals were unable to adequately metabolize and excrete the iodine. The use of EDDI in an *ad libitum* salt mixture at a level of 0·156% EDDI (0·125% iodine) was efficacious in reducing the incidence rate of footrot from 20·8% in the controls, fed 0·0025% iodine, to 8·3% in the treated group (19).

Commercial vaccines against bovine interdigital necrobacillosis are available but their efficacy has not been established in controlled comparative trials (10). A mineral-oil adjuvant vaccine containing whole cells or fractions of *F. necrophorum* provided about 60% protection from experimentally induced interdigital necrobacillosis (10). A similar vaccine containing *Bacteroides nodosus* appeared to reduce the severity of lesions but not the incidence rate compared to non-vaccinates (20). The protection may be closely associated with the exotoxins of the organism (21).

The treatment of verrucose dermatitis consists of washing the affected skin with a disinfectant soap followed by daily applications of 5% copper sulfate solution. When many animals are affected a daily walk through and soaking in a foot bath containing the copper sulfate solution is very effective.

REVIEW LITERATURE

Weaver, A. D. (1974) Lameness in cattle. The interdigital space. *Vet. Rec.*, *95*, 115.

REFERENCES

(1) Egerton, J. R. & Laing, E. A. (1979) *Vet. Microbiol.*, *3*, 269.
(2) Richards, R. B. et al. (1980) *Aust. vet. J.*, *56*, 517.

(3) Berg, J. N. & Loan, R. W. (1975) *Am. J. vet. Res.*, *36*, 1115.
(4) Rebhun, W. C. & Pearson, E. G. (1982) *J. Am. vet. Med. Assoc.*, *181*, 572.
(5) Frisch, J. E. (1976) *Aust. vet. J.*, *52*, 228.
(6) Egerton, J. R. & Parsonson, I. M. (1966) *Aust. vet. J.*, *42*, 425.
(7) Raven, E. T. & Cornelisse, J. L. (1971) *Vet. med. Rev.*, *213*, 223.
(8) Laing, E. A. & Egerton, J. R. (1978) *Res. vet. Sci.*, *24*, 300.
(9) Dewes, H. F. (1978) *NZ vet. J.*, *26*, 147.
(10) Clark, B. L. et al. (1986) In: *Footrot in Ruminants. Proceedings of a workshop, Melbourne, 1985.* eds D. J. Stewart, J. E. Peterson, N. M. McKern & D. L. Emery. CSIRO Australia, pp. 275–278.
(11) Breen, H. & Ryff, J. F. (1961) *J. Am.vet. med. Assoc.*, *138*, 548.
(12) Greenough, P. R. et al. (1972) *Lameness in Cattle*. Edinburgh: Oliver & Boyd.
(13) Clark, B. L. et al. (1985) *Aust. vet. J.*, *62*, 47.
(14) Emery, D. L. et al. (1985) *Aust. vet. J.*, *62*, 43.
(15) Berg, J. N. et al. (1976) *Am. J. vet. Res.*, *37*, 509.
(16) Monrad, J. et al. (1983) *Acta vet. Scand.*, *24*, 403.
(17) Greenfield, J. et al. (1972) *Br. vet. J.*, *128*, 578.
(18) Berg, J. N. et al. (1984) *Am. J. vet. Res.*, *45*, 1073.
(19) Maas, J. et al. (1984) *Am. J. vet. Res.*, *45*, 2347.
(20) Clark, B. L. et al. (1986) *Aust. vet. J.*, *63*, 61.
(21) Clark, B. L. et al. (1986) *Aust. vet. J.*, *63*, 107.

Infectious footrot of sheep

Infectious footrot is a disease of sheep characterized by inflammation of the skin at the skin–horn junction, under-running of the horn and inflammation of the sensitive laminae of the foot, and severe lameness.

Etiology

The lesions of footrot are caused by infection with *Bacteroides* (*Fusobacterium*) *nodosus*. Although two other bacteria, *Spirochaeta* (*Treponema*) *penortha* and a motile fusiform bacillus, are commonly present and were thought to have etiological importance, the disease can occur in their absence (1). On the basis of agglutination tests for K (surface) antigens three serotypes of *B. nodosus* have been isolated. Serotypes A and B are sufficiently similar antigenically to protect against each other, but C is antigenically quite distinct (2). A fourth serotype has also been suggested in Australia (11). In the United States ten serotypes are identified (15).

It is also evident that there are a number of strains of *B. nodosus* with varying virulence and they have been subdivided into benign, intermediate and virulent strains (24) to conform with the types of clinical footrot observed in the field. The level of virulence of each strain of bacteria depends on its keratolytic capacity and this can be measured in the laboratory (18, 27).

Epidemiology

Sheep and goats are the species principally affected and they are susceptible at all ages over 2 months; the disease has also been identified in farmed red deer (8). Sheep of the Merino type are most susceptible. British breeds, particularly Romney Marsh, are less susceptible and suffer from a milder form of the disease (10), respond better to vaccination by suffering less subsequent attacks of footrot but have worse reactions to the vaccination than merinos (30). In an uncontrolled situation some animals never become infected, a few become infected but recover and many persist as chronic cases (16).

The great variation in the incidence of the disease is due principally to variations in climate, particularly moistness of pasture, and environmental temperature. Most serious outbreaks in sheep at pasture occur in the spring when the weather is warm and wet and the wetness has to be of considerable duration; short, heavy rainfalls are not significant, persistent rain over several months is. The climate must provide continued free water on the ground for transmission to occur. But free surface water in winter exerts no effect on footrot—the daily mean temperature must be above 10°C (50°F). Housed sheep are also most commonly affected when conditions underfoot are wet. Any factor which concentrates sheep in small areas will favor spread of the disease. Improved pasture, especially when irrigated, is particularly conducive to a high incidence of footrot. The feet of the sheep become soft and the bacteria are protected in a moist, warm environment. Skin penetration by larvae of the nematode *Strongyloides* spp. may also be a predisposing cause. The severity of the disease once the sheep are injected is probably dependent on the virulence of the strain of *B. nodosus* involved.

Discharge from infected feet is the source of infection. Many affected sheep recover spontaneously but about 10% persist as non-clinical, chronic 'carriers' for several years. Infection can persist for years in the feet of sheep but is eliminated within a few days in pasture, a point of great importance in the control of the disease. Conditions of wetness and warmth favor persistence of the bacteria in pasture and increase susceptibility of the feet to injury and dermatitis, thus facilitating spread of the disease from carrier sheep. Hot, dry conditions aid healing of the feet and are inimical to persistence of the bacteria on pasture. Spread of footrot occurs for very short periods but the infection rate may be very high so that a lot of acute cases occur together creating 'outbreak' conditions. Infected cattle may on occasions serve as a source of infection for sheep.

Footrot of sheep is common in most countries where there are large numbers of sheep except that it does not occur in arid and semi-arid areas. The incidence is highest on good, improved pastures during warm, moist periods. In these circumstances as many as 75% of a flock may be affected at one time and lameness be so severe that many sheep are forced to walk on their knees. In such circumstances loss of bodily condition is extreme and this, combined with a moderate mortality rate and the expense of labor and materials to treat the disease adequately, makes footrot one of the most costly of sheep diseases. In experimentally infected sheep it has been shown that moderate to severe footrot causes 10% reduction in wool yield and a significant but lesser decrease in body weight (3). Little other quantitative pathology has been done so that an accurate estimate of total wastage is impossible.

Pathogenesis

An initial local dermatitis, caused by infection with *F. necrophorum* at the skin–horn junction, may progress no further (6) or it may be complicated by invasion with *B.*

nodosus and the development of clinical footrot, or by extension of the original infection into the bulbar soft tissues of the heel. This preliminary dermatitis is sometimes dignified by the title 'ovine interdigital dermatitis' because it may affect as many as 30% of a flock but it rarely causes lameness, and largely goes undetected unless it leads to infectious footrot or to foot abscess. It resolves spontaneously when the pasture dries up. At least part of the capacity of *B. nodosus* to invade horny tissue lies in its characteristic of producing keratolytic enzymes which digest horn.

Clinical findings

It is now conceded that ovine footrot may be *virulent* or *intermediate* but that both of these are different from *benign* footrot or footscald. The earliest sign of virulent footrot is swelling and moistness of the skin of the interdigital cleft. This inflammation is accompanied by slight lameness which increases as necrosis underruns the horn in the cleft. When extensive under-running has occurred lameness is severe, the animal may carry the leg, and if more than one foot is affected, may walk on its knees or remain recumbent. At this stage there is a foul-smelling discharge, which is always small in amount. The detached horn can be lifted up and pared off in large pieces. Abscessation does not occur. A systemic reaction, manifested by anorexia and fever, may occur in severe cases. Recumbent animals become emaciated and may die of starvation. Secondary bacterial invasion may result in the spread of inflammation up the legs and in severe cases the hoof may slough off. Rams appear to be more severely affected than ewes or wethers, possibly because of their greater weight.

Intermediate footrot is characterized by less severe under-running than in virulent footrot and by a lesser tendency to develop chronic lesions. There is much difficulty in specifying exactly the characteristics of these clinical forms, the more so because the severity of the lesions also varies with the climatic conditions.

There is a significant fall in body weight and wool production during the period of lameness but these appear to be completely compensated soon afterwards. The severity of the losses is greatest with infections by the virulent strains of *B. nodosus* (32).

Symptomless 'carriers' may be affected for periods of up to 3 years. Most such animals have a misshapen foot and a pocket of infection beneath underrun horn can be found if the foot is pared. A less common form of the chronic disease is an area of moist skin between the claws without involvement of the claw. With either form acute footrot may develop when warm, moist climatic conditions occur.

Footrot caused by *B. nodosus* in goats is manifested by severe interdigital dermatitis; rarely is there any under-running of the horn (21).

Clinical pathology and necropsy findings

No clinicopathological tests are usually performed although bacteriological examination of swabs of pus is necessary for accurate identification of the disease. With the identification of benign footrot and ovine interdigital dermatitis the prognosis in a flock with foot lesions depends largely on the identity of the organisms isolated and particularly the proteolytic/keratolytic index of any *B. nodosus* present (18, 27). Identification of *B. nodosus* is made in most laboratories by examining a smear made of exudate from underneath some underrun horn, and stained with Gram stain. This is potentially inaccurate and to increase the validity of a decision a fluorescein-stained antibody is used. Because of the non-fatal nature of footrot necropsy examinations are not usually performed.

Diagnosis

Because of the rigorous control measures required sometimes by law to control or eradicate infectious footrot of sheep, it is imperative that the diagnosis be made with great care. Positive identification should only be made if the clinical signs, *and* the epidemiological facts, *and* the laboratory findings are all positive. There are a number of conditions which may be confused with footrot, especially when they occur in the same environment conditions (Table 60). Foot abscess, affecting usually only one foot, is not so highly contagious and is characterized by extensive suppuration. Cases of contagious ecthyma and bluetongue may have foot lesions but typical lesions are always present around the mouth. Ulcerative dermatosis is characterized by lesions on the feet and on the external genitalia. Strawberry footrot has characteristic lesions distributed on the skin of the lower limb and not between the claws. Dermatitis causing local irritation and perhaps lameness may also be caused by infestations with *Strongyloides papillosus* or with trombiculid mites.

Benign footrot, or footscald, is very similar to early virulent footrot and like it occurs under very wet conditions but often on farms where footrot is not known to occur and where there is no history of the recent introduction of sheep. It is caused by infection with strains of *B. nodosus* with low keratolytic capacity and is capable of being converted to virulent footrot by the introduction of virulent strains of *B. nodosus*. The interdigital skin becomes inflamed and covered by a thin film of moist necrotic material; the horn is pitted and blanched. Maceration and necrosis occur at the skin–horn junction and although there is an odor, it lacks the rancidity of footrot. There is separation of the horn at the heel but the dermis is normal and there is no suppuration. Under-running of the horn is limited to the heel. The extensive under-running of the horn of the wall and sole and the accumulation of foul-smelling exudate which are characteristic of footrot do not occur in footscald.

Laminitis, after engorgement on grain, may cause lameness and recumbency, but although the feet may be hot and painful there are no superficial lesions. Laminitis caused by *E. insidiosa*, and occurring after dipping, is similarly lacking in externally visible lesions. Suppurative cellulitis, caused by *F. necrophorum*, commences as an ulcerative dermatitis of the pastern above the bulb of the heel, and extends up the leg to the knee or the hock and more deeply into subcutaneous tissues. Separation of the wall of the foot (shelly hoof) occurs commonly in Merino sheep on improved pasture. The abaxial wall of the hoof separates from the sole near the toe and the crevice formed becomes packed with mud and manure. The hoof in the region is dry and crumbly.

Table 60. Differential diagnosis of lameness accompanied by foot lesions in sheep

Disease	*Epidemiology*	*Foot lesions*	*Other lesions*	*Other clinical signs*	*Response to treatment*	*Diagnostic microbiology*
Infectious footrot	Serious outbreaks in wet warm weather. High morbidity. Few chronic lame sheep in dry seasons	Interdigital dermatitis, under-running of horn medial aspect of claw. Strong smell of necrotic horn	Nil	Very severe lameness. Walk on knees	To penicillin excellent	*Bacteroides nodosus* on smear, or fluorescent antibody test
Benign footrot (scald)	High morbidity in wet warm weather. Disappears with dry weather	Interdigital dermatitis, no smell, almost no underrunning of horn	Nil	Mild lameness	Not treated	*B. nodosus* but avirulent strains not distinguishable microbiologically
Infectious bulbar necrosis	Adult sheep, usually less than 10% affected. Serious in wet seasons	Toe abscess usually in front feet. Heel abscess in hind feet. Swelling, pain, discharge of pus	Nil	Very severe lameness	Good to sulfonamides or penicillin—streptomycin	*F. necrophorum* and *Actinomyces* (*Corynebacterium*) *pyogenes*
Contagious ecthyma	Lambs mostly or non-immune adults. Dry summer	Raised proliferative lesions with tenacious scabs on coronet skin	Lesions around mouth almost always	Rarely lambs have septicemia. Lameness mild only	Nil	Nil
Ulcerative dermatosis	Spread by physical contact at mating. Morbidity usually 20%	Raw granulating ulcers in interdigital space and on coronet. No pus	Around mouth and genitalia usually	Moderate lameness	Nil	Nil
Bluetongue	Insect-borne exotic disease. Variable morbidity	Coronitis, separation of horn. Are late in syndrome	Severe erosions around mouth and nasal cavities	High fever, salivation. Severe lameness and recumbency	Nil	Nil
Strawberry footrot	In summer, high morbidity, carrier sheep infect	Proliferative dermatitis, piled up scabs. Heal in 5–6 weeks. Coronet to kneehock	Nil	No itching or lameness	Nil	*Dermatophilus congolensis*
Infestation with *Strongyloides* or trombiculid mites	Wet summer conditions. Local distribution only	Non-specific dermatitis of skin of lower legs	Nil	Nil	Organophosphates for trombiculids	Parasites in scrapings

Treatment

Bacteroides nodosus is susceptible *in vitro* to penicillin, cefamandole, clindamycin, tetracycline, chloramphenicol, erythromycin, sodium cefoxitin, tylosin tartrate, nitrofurazone, tinidazole and dihydromycin sulfate and, in order of reducing effectiveness, copper sulfate, zinc sulfate and formalin (12). A high rate of recovery (96%) can be achieved by a single intramuscular injection of penicillin and streptomycin (70 000 units procaine penicillin G and 70 mg streptomycin per kg body weight) without paring the feet (13). As with most other treatments for footrot the treatment is much more effective in dry weather (14). In wet conditions the concentrations of antibiotic at the tissue level is much reduced. Treatment can be carried out in wet weather but treated sheep should be kept indoors for 24 hours after treatment. The method is expensive but reduces labor costs and removes the need for ruthless, severe hoof paring.

Vaccination of affected sheep with a bacterin composed of *Bacteroides nodosus* cells in an oil adjuvant has shown significant improvement in the recovery rate. The improvement seems to be due to accelerated healing of the lesions. The response is greatest with oil-based vaccines as compared to aqueous ones, and in unvaccinated sheep (7). It is also much less apparent during dry climatic conditions when conditions for transmission of the disease are unfavorable (35). Two injections of the vaccine do not enhance the recovery rate.

Although parenteral treatment alone may be sufficient, the result can be significantly improved by trimming, not paring, the feet and foot bathing in 5% formalin. The following comments apply to that circumstance and to those circumstances in which only local treatment is used. Because of the labor required for topical treatments an intensive search has been carried out to determine the most satisfactory treatment based on the proportion of permanent cures, keeping in mind the varying environmental circumstances in which the disease occurs. This is most important during wet weather when topical applications are likely to be washed off the feet. Irrespective of the local medicament used one principle of treatment is inescapable. All underrun horn must be carefully removed so that the antibacterial agent to be applied can come into contact with infective material. This necessitates painstaking and careful examination and paring of all feet. When only a few sheep are affected, bandaging heavily pared feet may hasten recovery. Very sharp instruments including a knife and hoof secateurs are necessary to do the job properly and they should be disinfected after each use. The parings should be collected and burned.

The local preparation to be used will depend on a number of factors. Some of the less efficient may be adequate in dry seasons when natural recovery is likely to occur. They may be applied by brush, by spray or aerosol or in a foot bath. Preparations suitable for foot baths include 10% zinc sulfate with or without a surfactant to aid wetting of tissues, 5% formalin, which does not deteriorate with pollution, and 5% copper sulfate solution which does, and has the added disadvantage of coloring the wool. Farmers can be neglectful in maintaining proper concentrations of formalin in foot baths, and frequent use of the bath combined with hot weather can result in a concentration of 30% formalin. Such concentrations cause extensive cellulitis around the coronets, and a high proportion of animals may be so badly affected that they need to be destroyed. The safest precaution is to empty the vat and prepare a new mixture each day. The local application of formalin to normal feet after all treatments and examinations for footrot reduces the chance of spread of infection by material left on the hooves. Regardless of the agent used, it is recommended that the sheep be kept standing on concrete or dry ground for a few hours after treatment.

The relative merits and disadvantages of the various preparations used are: copper sulfate solutions (5%) colors the wool, deteriorates with pollution and may cause excessive contamination of the environment with copper; zinc sulfate 10% solution applied by brush is reported to give excellent results but has had no extensive field trial (4); a footbath of 10% zinc sulfate is also recommended in a control program (22); so is zinc sulfate in the drinking water (19), but feeding of $ZnSO_4$ appears to be ineffective (17); formalin solution (5%) must be applied weekly for 4 weeks and delayed relapses are likely to occur about 3 weeks later. This is a major disadvantage as sheep may be classified as cured and subsequently become active spreaders of the disease. The use of solutions containing more than 5% formalin or dipping at intervals of less than 1 week may cause irritation of the skin. Local applications include chloramphenicol (10% tincture in methylated spirits or propylene glycol), oxytetracycline (5% tincture in methylated spirits) and cetyltrimethyl ammonium bromide or Cetavlon (20% alcoholic tincture); dichlorophen as a 10% solution in diacetone alcohol or ethyl alcohol give comparable results with single treatments. Chloramphenicol is expensive but efficient, provided the 10% tincture is used, and is probably as good as any other preparation under both wet and dry conditions. Oxytetracycline must be used as a 5% tincture for optimum results and is not as efficient as chloramphenicol under wet conditions, but gives excellent results when the weather is dry. Delayed relapses occur with this drug as well as with formalin. Cetavlon is a relatively cheap product and appears to be as effective as chloramphenicol under all conditions. It is possible that in different countries with different climates and environmental conditions the efficiency of particular treatments will vary. Thus, English experience is that about the same results are achieved by the use of a 10% formalin foot bath as by the application of a 10% tincture of chloramphenicol or oxytetracycline, whereas under Australian conditions treatment with antibiotics is much superior.

With all of these treatments the treated feet must be examined subsequently and feet showing inflammation retreated. In dry summer months 90–100% cures can be anticipated with one treatment but in wet seasons 75% is the maximum rate of cure with one treatment. Animals showing persistent inflammation should be treated until cured or culled.

Control

Eradication of ovine footrot is a feasible objective. Area eradication is a much more daunting task. It is being attempted in Victoria, Australia and is proceeding satisfactorily.

The eradication can be accomplished with relative ease in many areas, but where rainfall is heavy and the ground moist most of the year, much greater difficulty may be encountered. Control programs are based on the fact that the causative bacteria do not usually persist in pasture for long periods and if fields are kept free of sheep for 14 days they can be considered to be clean. Thus if all infected animals are culled or cured and infection removed from the pasture eradication is achieved. The program must take into account the fact that *B. nodosus* can be carried on the feet of cattle (3).

Eradication of the disease should be undertaken during a dry summer season, but active measures must be taken. Simply exposing infected animals to dry conditions will not cure the lesions (5). All feet of sheep are examined and affected or suspicious sheep are segregated. Clean sheep are run through a foot bath (5% formalin) and put into fresh fields, while the affected are isolated and treated, either parenterally with antibiotics, or locally with one of the preparations described above, or by vaccination with an effective vaccine. Local treatments must be repeated weekly. Sheep which do not respond may be treated intensively, for example 2 × 1 hour soaks in 10% zinc sulfate (29) or be culled. If the incidence of carriers is high the clean flock should be re-examined 1 month later. When examinations are carried out during dry weather the feet are likely to be hard and the disease at a quiescent stage. In such circumstances minor lesions may be missed, necessitating an extremely careful trimming and examination of all feet. Most breakdowns in eradication occur because of inefficient examination and treatment or the introduction of affected sheep without first ensuring that they are free from the disease. In areas where flocks are small and there are insufficient fields to carry out this program completely, it has been found to be sufficient to treat all affected sheep weekly but to put all affected sheep back in the flock and the flock back onto the infective pasture.

During a major outbreak new infections are occurring too rapidly to make eradication practicable at that time. The objective should be to limit the spread as much as possible so that the mess to be cleared up later is manageable. Foot bathing and isolation of infected flocks are the two important procedures at this time.

Vaccination has become one of the most effective weapons in the control of ovine footrot, especially in circumstances where climate and management practices make other strategies difficult to apply (33). Until recent years results were very disappointing because of poor antigenicity of the vaccines and poor protection in the field. There have been several important innovations. The use of an oily adjuvant in the vaccine has improved its antigenicity but has the disadvantage of usually causing a lesion at the site of the injection (23). It is also expensive. The introduction of vaccines made of the pili of the bacterial cells of *B. nodosus* has also greatly increased the antigenicity of the vaccine. The specificity of the protection is to the serotypes from which the pili were harvested although there is some cross-protection to some other serotypes but none at all to some others (31). This makes it necessary to include material from all eight of the antigenically distinct serotypes of the bacterium and as much pilus antigen as possible in the vaccine (9, 11). Whole cell vaccines do not suffer from this deficiency of specificity of protection (34). It is also necessary to preserve the structural integrity of the pili in the vaccine for it to be effective (20). Field reports on this type of vaccine indicate that it is effective (25, 28). Its superiority over non-depiliated vaccines is apparent when the challenge is severe as in penned sheep but it may not be significant in sheep at pasture (30). The choice of an adjuvant which will maintain the vaccine's antigenicity but will reduce the reaction at the injection site is a current preoccupation of workers in the field. Incomplete Freund's adjuvant appears to be best (26) and the further addition of alum adds to the antigenicity (31). A still more advanced vaccine with good therapeutic and prophylactic effect is one made from the pili of *Pseudomonas aeruginosa*. Early results are most promising (7).

REVIEW LITERATURE

Boundy, T. (1979) Footrot in sheep. *Vet. Rec. In Pract.*, *1(3)*, 28.
Egerton, J. R. & Graham, N. P. H. (1969) Diseases causing lameness in sheep, *Vet. Rev.*, 5, 22, University of Sydney Postgraduate Foundation in Veterinary Science.
Scalan, C. M. et al. (1985) Ovine contagious footrot. *Comp. cont. Educ.*, *7 (1)*, S15.

REFERENCES

(1) Beveridge, W. I. B. (1934) *Aust. vet. J.*, *10*, 43.
(2) Egerton, J. R. (1974) *Aust. vet. J.*, *50*, 59.
(3) Symons, L. E. A. (1978) *Aust. vet. J.*, *54*, 362.
(4) Cross, R. F. (1978) *J. Am. vet. med. Assoc.*, *173*, 1567 & 1569.
(5) Egerton, J. R. (1983) *Aust. vet. J.*, *60*, 315.
(6) Parsonson, I. M. et al. (1967) *J. comp. Pathol.*, 77, 309; 79, 207, 217.
(7) Stewart, D. J. & Elleman, T. C. (1987) *Aust. vet. J.*, *64*, 79.
(8) Skerman, T. M. (1983) *NZ vet. J.*, *31*, 102.
(9) Cameron, C. M. & Fuls, W. J. P. (1978) *Onderstepoort J. vet. Res.*, *45*, 143.
(10) Emery, D. L. et al. (1984) *Aust. vet. J.*, *60*, 10.
(11) Stewart, D. J. et al. (1980) *Vict. vet. Proc. J.*, *38*, 10.
(12) Gradin, J. L. & Schmitz, J. A. (1983) *J. Am. vet. med. Assoc.*, 183, 434.
(13) Egerton, J. R. & Parsonson, I. M. (1966) *Aust. vet. J.*, *42*, 97.
(14) Egerton, J. R. et al. (1968) *Aust. vet. J.*, *44*, 275.
(15) Schmitz, J. A. & Gradin, J. L. (1977) *Proc. Ann. Mtg US Anim. Hlth Assoc.*, *81*, 401.
(16) Egerton, J. R. et al. (1983) *Aust. vet. J.*, *60*, 334.
(17) Skerman, T. M. et al. (1983) *NZ vet. J.*, *31*, 54.
(18) Green, R. S. (1985) *NZ vet. J.*, *33*, 11.
(19) Golikov, A. V. & Melnikova, K. V. (1982) *Veterinariya, Moscow*, 9, 41.
(20) Emery, D. L. et al. (1984) *Aust. vet. J.*, *61*, 237.
(21) Claxton, P. O. & O'Grady, K. C. (1986) *Proc. CSIRO Workshop, Footrot of Ruminants, Melbourne, 1985.*
(22) Skerman, T. M. et al. (1983) *NZ vet. J.*, *31*, 91.
(23) Ross, A. D. & Titterington, D. M. (1984) *NZ vet. J.*, *32*, 6.
(24) Stewart, D. J. et al. (1982) *Aust. Adv. vet. Sci.*, p. 219.
(25) Bulgin, M. S. et al. (1985) *Vet. Med.*, *80(2)*, 105.
(26) Stewart, D. J. et al. (1983) *Res. vet. Sci.*, *35*, 130.
(27) Kortt, A. A. et al. (1983) *Res. vet. Sci.*, *35*, 171.
(28) Glenn, J. et al. (1985) *J. Am. vet. med. Assoc.*, *187*, 1009.
(29) Bulgin, M. S. et al. (1986) *J. Am. vet. med. Assoc.*, *189*, 194.
(30) Stewart, D. J. et al. (1985) *Aust. vet. J.*, *62*, 116.
(31) Stewart, D. J. et al. (1985) *Aust. vet. J.*, *62*, 153.
(32) Stewart, D. J. et al. (1984) *Aust. vet. J.*, *61*, 348.
(33) Lambell, R. G. (1986) *Aust. vet. J.*, *63*, 415.
(34) Stewart, D. J. et al. (1986) *Aust. vet. J.*, *63*, 101.
(35) Kennedy, D. J. (1985) *Aust. vet. J.*, *62*, 249.

Foot abscess of sheep

Foot abscess occurs most commonly during very wet seasons as does footrot but the former is limited largely to adult sheep, especially ewes heavy in lamb, or rams (1) and does not cause such a high morbidity as footrot. An increased prevalence in a flock of young rams may be due to close flocking and to increased muddying of pasture due to this high concentration of livestock (3). Usually only one foot and one claw is involved, although in severe outbreaks all four feet may become affected (2). *F. necrophorum* is the cause of the disease although *Actinomyces* (*Corynebacterium*) *pyogenes* and *Escherichia coli* are commonly found in chronic lesions. 'Foot abscess' really includes two diseases (3). Toe abscess is a lamellar suppuration with purulent underrunning of the horn, particularly at the toe. There is severe lameness, swelling of the coronet with pain and heat apparent, and usually rupture and purulent discharge at the coronet between the toes. Penetration to deeper structures may also occur.

The other common lesion is 'heel abscess' or infectious bulbar necrosis. It results as an extension from ovine interdigital dermatitis into the soft tissues of the heel and is therefore caused by *F. necrophorum* and *Actinomyces* (*Corynebacterium*) *pyogenes* (4). When the phalangeal joints are involved there is severe swelling at the back of the feet. Rupture of the swellings is followed by a profuse discharge of pus which does not occur in footrot. Treatment by surgical drainage, parenteral treatment with sodium sulfadimidine solution (1 g/8 kg body weight) and the application of a local dressing, is usually adequate (1). Sulfonamide therapy may need to be continued for several days. Because of the frequent involvement of the distal interphalangeal joints (5) treatment with antibiotics without surgical intervention is unlikely to be successful.

REFERENCES

(1) Thomas, J. H. (1962) *Aust. vet. J.*, *38*, 159.
(2) Goodner, D. E. (1961) *NZ vet. J.*, *9*, 59.
(3) West, D. M. (1983) *NZ vet. J. 31*, 71.
(4) Roberts, D. S. (1969) *J. infect. Dis.*, *120*, 720.
(5) West, D. M. (1983) *NZ vet. J.*, *31*, 152.

Footrot of pigs

Footrot in pigs bears some clinical resemblance to footrot in other species and is included here for this reason although the cause of the disease appears different and in most instances the disease is more analogous to foot abscess.

Etiology

In the majority of cases the disease appears to result from secondary infection of lesions that are traumatic in origin. The most common traumatic lesions are erosions of the sole and wall of the claw that occur in pigs reared on rough abrasive flooring. By themselves these lesions do not usually produce lameness, unless they are extensive, but when pigs are also reared in dirty conditions infection and subsequent lameness may occur. Wet conditions underfoot may cause maceration of the horn and exacerbate the abrasive effect of the flooring. Dietary deficiency, especially biotin deficiency, may also result in foot lesions that predispose to secondary infection. *F. necrophorum*, *Actinomyces* (*Corynebacterium*) *pyogenes*, staphylococci and an unidentified spirochete may be found in affected feet. The possibility of a specific primary keratinolytic infection in footrot in pigs has not been eliminated.

Epidemiology

The disease has been reported from several countries and is probably universal in occurrence. Erosive lesions on the foot are common and have been reported at an incidence as high as 65% (1). They have been reproduced experimentally and the nature of the flooring has a marked influence on claw wear in pigs (2–4). Recently poured alkaline concrete and poorly laid concrete with constituents leading to a rough abrasive surface lead to a high incidence. A slope inadequate to allow proper drainage may also be an important predisposing factor. All ages of pigs are susceptible, but clinical lameness is uncommon. In individual herds where the unfavorable predisposing factors prevail, a high incidence of infection and clinical lameness can occur. The disease may cause reproductive inefficiency due to reluctance to stand or mount for mating.

Pathogenesis

Perforation of the horn leads to infection of the sensitive laminae. The infection may track up the sensitive laminae to the coronary band and discharge to the exterior.

Clinical findings

Where the disease is due to abrasion of the horn by rough concrete surfaces a number of characteristic lesions occur. These include erosion of the sole at either the toe or the heel, bruising of the sole with hemorrhagic streaks in the horn, separation of the hard horny wall from the heel or sole to produce a fissure at the white line, or a false sand crack in the posterior third of the lateral wall of the claw. In the majority of cases these do not produce lameness nor do they have any apparent effect on productivity (2); however, when they are extensive or where infection has occurred severe lameness is apparent. In most cases only the lateral digit of one foot is affected. Heat and obvious pain with only moderate pressure being applied to the affected claw are constant findings. Necrosis extends up between the sole and sensitive laminae and may discharge at the coronet causing the development of a granulomatous lesion, or it may extend to deeper structures of the foot with multiple sinuses discharging to the exterior. Very little pus is present. Productivity is affected with this type of lesion. With deeply infected feet the recovery rate is only fair with treatment. A permanently deformed foot may result and destruction may be necessary in severe cases. Secondary abscessation in other parts of the body is an occasional sequel and may result in partial carcass condemnation.

Clinical pathology

Bacteriological examination of discharges from the lesions may aid in deciding the treatment to be used.

Necropsy findings

Necrosis of the laminar tissue with indications of progression from an infected sole are the usual findings.

Diagnosis

Most other causes of lameness in pigs are not manifested by foot lesions. In adult pigs housed indoors an overgrowth of the hoof may occur and be followed by underrunning of the sole, necrosis and the protrusion of granulation tissue causing severe lameness and often persistent recumbency (5). The general appearance of these feet is not unlike that of canker in horses. Swelling of the hoof is caused by an extensive fibrous tissue reaction. Vesicular exanthema and foot-and-mouth disease are characterized by the presence of vesicular lesions on the coronets and snout.

Treatment

Parenteral injection of sodium salts of sulfonamides (6), or penicillin (7), have given inconsistent results and topical applications of copper sulfate or formalin (5–10%) have been more successful. Surgical removal of the affected digit is feasible.

Control

Prevention of excessive wear of the feet by the use of adequate bedding and less abrasive flooring in pig pens is suggested as a reasonable control measure. The use of a footbath containing 5–10% formalin, or twice weekly use of one containing 10% copper sulfate, delays but does not prevent the development of lesions (2). Any existing dietary deficiency should be corrected. Of particular interest is the response to biotin supplementation of the diet of pigs in the prevention of foot lesions of various kinds. The subject is discussed under the heading of biotin deficiency.

REFERENCES

(1) Penny, R. H. C. et al. (1983) *Vet. Rec.*, *75*, 1225.
(2) Wright, A. I. et al. (1972) *Vet. Rec.*, *90*, 93.
(3) Klatt, G. et al. (1973) *Mh. Vet Med.*, *28*, 608.
(4) Penny, R. H. C. (1977) *Vet. Ann.*, *17*, 111.
(5) Hogg, A. H. (1952) *Vet. Rec.*, *64*, 39.
(6) Bishop, W. H. (1948) *Aust. vet. J.*, *24*, 256.
(7) Osborne, H. G. & Ensor, C. R. (1953) *NZ vet. J.*, *3*, 91.

Oral and laryngeal necrobacillosis

The term oral necrobacillosis is applied to infections of the mouth and larynx with *Fusobacterium necrophorum*. It includes *calf diphtheria*, in which the lesions are largely confined to the larynx and pharynx, and *necrotic stomatitis*, in which the lesions are restricted to the oral cavity. They are considered together because the essential lesion and infection are the same in both instances.

Etiology

Fusobacterium necrophorum is present in large numbers in the lesions and is considered to be the causative agent, probably aided by prior injury to the mucosa. In the case of the laryngeal disease the point of entry is thought to be contact ulcers in the mucosa caused by repeated closure of the larynx (2).

Epidemiology

Oral infection occurs principally in calves less than 3 months old whereas laryngeal involvement is more common in older animals up to 18 months of age. The disease is seen commonly only in cattle but has been observed in sheep (1). Animals suffering from intercurrent disease or nutritional deficiency are most susceptible and the incidence is highest in groups kept in confined quarters under unsanitary conditions.

The causative bacterium is a common inhabitant of the environment of cattle and under unsanitary conditions the infection may be spread on dirty milk pails and feeding troughs. Entry through the mucosa is probably effected through abrasions caused by rough feed and erupting teeth. The difficulty of reproducing the disease and the irregularity of its occurrence even when *F. necrophorum* is known to be present suggests the possibility of etiological factors presently unknown.

The disease has no geographical limitations but is more common in countries where animals are housed in winter or maintained in feedlots. In the United States, infections involving the pharynx and larynx appear to be more prevalent in the western states than in other sections of the country. It is a common disease in feedlots in yearling cattle, often in company with papillomatosis of the larynx (2). There is also a difference in age incidence, necrotic stomatitis occurring mainly in calves 2 weeks to 3 months of age while laryngeal infections commonly affect older calves and yearlings. Although the disease is more common in housed or penned animals it can occur in animals running at pasture (3–5).

Laryngeal chondritis has been described in Texel sheep which may be predisposed to the disease because of anatomical factors, namely the short head of the breed (7). This may affect the shape of the larynx or its relationship to adjacent tissues.

Pathogenesis

Fusobacterium necrophorum is a normal inhabitant of the oral cavity and causes inflammation and necrosis following injury of the mucosa of the oral cavity, pharynx and larynx. Edema and inflammation of the mucosa of the larynx results in varying degrees of closure of the rima glottidis and inspiratory dyspnea and stridor. The presence of the lesion causes discomfort, painful swallowing and toxemia. Extension of the lesion to the arytenoid cartilages will result in laryngeal chondritis (7). Involvement of the cartilage will usually result in delayed healing or failure to recover completely.

Clinical findings

In describing the clinical findings a distinction must be made between calf diphtheria characterized by involvement of the larynx and the more common necrotic stomatitis. In the former a moist painful cough, accompanied by severe inspiratory dyspnea, salivation, painful swallowing movements, complete anorexia and severe depression are the characteristic signs. The temperature is high (41°C, 106°F), the pharyngeal region may be swollen and is painful on external palpation and there is salivation and nasal discharge. The breath has a most foul rancid smell.

Examination of the pharynx and larynx by visual inspection through the oral cavity with the aid of a speculum positioned over the base of the tongue will often reveal the lesions. The mucosa of the larynx and glottis are usually edematous, inflamed and a necrotic lesion is usually present and visible on one or both arytenoid cartilages. The opening of the larynx is commonly reduced due to the edema and inflammation. Careful visual inspection of the larynx during inspiration may reveal that the lesion extends into one or both vocal cords. The examination usually causes considerable discomfort, anxiety and the production of purulent or bloodstained saliva.

Death is likely to occur from toxemia or obstruction to the respiratory passages on the 2nd to 7th day. Most affected calves die without treatment but only a small proportion of calves in a group are usually affected. Spread to the lungs may cause a severe, suppurative bronchopneumonia.

In calves affected with necrotic stomatitis there is usually a moderate increase in temperature (39·5–40°C, 103–104°F), depression and anorexia. The breath is foul and saliva, often mixed with straw, hangs from the mouth. A characteristic swelling of the cheeks may be observed posterior to the lip commissures. On opening the mouth this is found to be due to a deep ulcer in the mucosa of the cheek. The ulcer is usually filled with a mixture of necrotic material and food particles. An ulcer may also be present on the adjacent side of the tongue and cause severe swelling and protrusion of the tongue. In severe cases the lesions may spread to the tissues of the face and throat and into the orbital cavity. Similar lesions may be present on the vulva and around the coronets, and spread to the lungs may cause fatal pneumonia. In other cases death appears to be due to toxemia.

Clinical pathology

Bacteriological examination of swabs from lesions may assist in confirming the diagnosis.

Necropsy findings

Severe swelling, due to edema and inflammation of the tissues surrounding the ulcer, is accompanied by the presence of large masses of cheesy, purulent material. Similar lesions to those in the mouth, pharynx and larynx may be found in the lungs and in the abomasum.

Diagnosis

Necrotic laryngitis is characterized by inspiratory dyspnea and stridor, toxemia, fever, and edema, inflammation and necrotic lesions of the laryngeal mucosa. Neoplasms of the larynx occur only rarely, usually in mature cattle and cause chronic inspiratory dyspnea. Traumatic pharyngitis may resemble laryngitis but the lesions are obvious on visual inspection of the pharynx. In chronic cases of traumatic pharyngitis there may be perisophageal cavities containing rumen contents. Foreign bodies such as pieces of wire and small wooden sticks may become lodged in the mucosa of the arytenoid cartilages and cause clinical signs similar to necrotic laryngitis.

Visual inspection of the larynx is relatively easy and simple with the aid of a cylindrical plastic speculum placed over the base of the tongue in calves and adult cattle. The larynx can be viewed directly and illuminated with a strong source of light. A flexible fiberoptiscope is also useful when available and is necessary for examination of the equine larynx.

Treatment

The lesions of necrotic stomatitis will usually heal in a few days following debridement of the ulcers, the application of a solution of tincture of iodine, and the parenteral administration of sulfamethazine at a dose of 150 mg/kg body weight daily for 3–5 days (6). Parenteral administration initially followed by oral therapy is recommended. Other broad-spectrum antimicrobials can also be used and daily therapy for up to 3 weeks or more may be necessary.

Successful treatment of necrotic laryngitis is dependent on early recognition and prompt therapy with antimicrobials daily for several days. Corticosteroids may be a beneficial adjunctive therapy especially to reduce the edema. Tracheostomy may be necessary in some cases to relieve dyspnea. Failure to respond is usually associated with chronic suppurative chondritis which requires subtotal arytenoidectomy.

Control

Proper hygienic precautions in calf pens or feeding and drinking places together with avoidance of rough feed should prevent the spread of the disease. When the incidence is high prophylactic antibiotic feeding may keep the disease in check.

REFERENCES

(1) Diplock, P. T. (1958) *Vet. Insp. NSW*, *51*, 53.
(2) Jensen, R. et al. (1981) *Vet. Pathol.*, *18*, 143.
(3) Kingman, H. E. & Stansbury, W. M. (1944) *N. Am. Vet.*, *25*, 671.
(4) Lovell, R. (1945) *Vet. Rec.*, *57*, 179.
(5) Sutherland, A. K. (1950) *Aust. vet. J.*, *26*, 238.
(6) Hayes, A. J. & Wright, G. M. (1949) *J. Am. vet. med. Assoc.*, *114*, 80.
(7) Lane, J. G. et al. (1987) *Vet. Rec.*, *121*, 81.

Necrotic rhinitis (bullnose)

Necrotic rhinitis is often confused with atrophic rhinitis. It occurs in young growing pigs and may occur in herds where atrophic rhinitis is present and even in the same pig but there appears to be no relationship between the two diseases. The common occurrence of *Fusiformis necrophorus* in the lesions suggest that any injury to the face or nasal or oral cavities may lead to invasion especially if the environment is dirty and heavily contaminated. The incidence of the disease has diminished in recent years, due probably to a general improvement in hygiene in piggeries.

The lesions develop as a necrotic cellulitis of the soft tissues of the nose and face but may spread to involve bone. Local swelling is obvious and extensive lesions may interfere with respiration and mastication. Depression of food intake and toxemia result in poor growth and some deaths. Treatment by the local application of antibacterial drugs and the oral administration of sulfonamides is satisfactory in early cases. Oral dosing with sulfadimidine has been effective in young pigs (1). Improvement of sanitation, elimination of injuries and disinfection of pens usually result in a reduction of incidence.

The disease differs from atrophic rhinitis by the presence of oral and facial lesions. Necrotic ulcer of pigs may involve the mouth and face but the lesions are erosive rather than necrotic.

REFERENCES

(1) Eieland, E. & Faanes, T. (1950) *Nord. VetMed.*, *2*, 204.

DISEASES CAUSED BY *PSEUDOMONAS* spp.

Occasional cases of generalized infection with *Pseudomonas aeruginosa* have been described, usually following an attack of mastitis caused by this organism (1, 2). Systematic invasion is manifested by fibrinous pericarditis and pleurisy and chronic pyelonephritis. An acute, fatal pneumonia has also been recorded in pigs in contact with infected cows (3) and in calves (4). Infections with *Pseudomonas* spp. are notoriously difficult to treat. But the antibiotic carbenicillin (Pyopen) on its own, or in combination with gentamicin, is effective against these bacteria (5).

REVIEW LITERATURE

Lusis, P. I. & Soltys, M. A. (1971) *Pseudomonas aeruginosa*. *Vet. Bull.*, *41*, 169.

REFERENCES

(1) Winter, H. & O'Connor, R. F. (1957) *Aust. vet. J.*, *33*, 83.
(2) Gardiner, M. R. & Craig, J. (1961) *Vet. Rec.*, *73*, 372.
(3) Baker, W. L. (1962) *Vet. Med.*, *57*, 232.
(4) Prasad, B. M. et al. (1967) *Acta vet. Hung.*, *17*, 363.
(5) Rolinson, G. N. & Sutherland, R. (1968) *Antimicrob. Agents Chemotherap.*, 609.

Melioidosis

Melioidosis is primarily a disease of rodents with an occasional case occurring in humans but the disease has been observed in farm animals. Clinical and necropsy findings are similar to those of glanders in the horse.

Etiology

Pseudomonas (*Malleomyces*) *pseudomallei* is the sole cause, and occurs in strains with varying pathogenicity.

Epidemiology

Pseudomonas pseudomallei is relatively susceptible to environmental influences and disinfectants although it can survive in water at room temperature for up to 8 weeks, and muddy water for up to 7 months (1), and in soil in the laboratory for up to 30 months (12). In tropical and subtropical areas water-borne infection is probably an important source of infection. Cases have occurred in rodents, rabbits, pigeons, humans, animals in zoological gardens including sika deer (2) and in dogs, cats, horses, cattle, pigs, sheep and goats. The disease can also be produced experimentally in rats, mice and hamsters. Varying degrees of virulence are observed in different strains of the organism but starvation or other conditions of stress appear to increase the susceptibility of experimental animals to infection.

The source of infection is infected animals which pass the organism in their feces. The disease in rodents runs a protracted course, making these animals important reservoirs of infection for man and possibly other species. Infection can be spread by ingestion of contaminated food or water, by insect bites, cutaneous abrasions and possibly by inhalation.

Amongst rodents and humans, the disease occurs almost exclusively in tropical countries. In domestic animals the disease has occurred in outbreak form in pigs, goats and sheep in Australia (3), in the Caribbean area (6) and in Cambodia, in horses in Malaya (8) and Iran (9), in pigs and cattle in Papua–New Guinea (10) and Australia (11), and in horses in France in 1976–78 (4). Most cases occur during the wet season and in low-lying swampy areas. Its chief importance in farm animals has been in sheep in which heavy mortalities have occurred. The fatal nature of this disease in man makes melioidosis an important zoonosis.

Pathogenesis

The development of the natural disease is presumed to be the same as in glanders with an initial septicemia or bacteremia and subsequent localization in various organs. Experimentally induced melioidosis in goats is characterized by septicemia with widely scattered microabscesses after intraperitoneal injection, and a chronic disease with abscesses in the lungs and spleen when the infection is administered subcutaneously (7).

Clinical findings

In humans the disease is highly fatal, an acute septicemia terminating after an illness of about 10 days. Melioidosis in rodents is also highly fatal and is characterized by weakness, fever and ocular and nasal discharge. In these animals the course may be as long as 2–3 months. Signs in sheep consist mainly of weakness and recumbency with death occurring in 1–7 days. In experimentally infected sheep, a severe febrile reaction occurs and is accompanied by anorexia, lameness and a thick, yellow exudate from the nose and eyes. Some animals show evidence of central nervous system involvement including abnormal gait, deviation of the head and walking in circles, nystagmus, blindness, hyperesthesia and mild tetanic convulsions. The disease is usually fatal. Skin involvement is not recorded. In horses the syndrome is one of an acute metastatic pneumonia with high fever and a short course. Cough and nasal discharge are minimal and there is a lack of response to treatment with most drugs. In goats, the syndrome may resemble the acute form as seen in sheep, but more commonly runs a chronic course. The disease in pigs is usually chronic and manifested by cervical lymphadenitis but in some outbreaks there are signs similar to those in other species. In such outbreaks slight posterior paresis, mild fever, coughing, nasal and ocular discharge, anorexia, abortion and some deaths may occur.

Clinical signs in horse include septicemia, hyperthermia, edema, colic diarrhea and lymphangitis of the legs. Subacute cases become debilitated, emaciated and develop edema (4). Affected horses may survive for several months. A case of acute meningoencephalitis is described in a horse. The onset was sudden and the only sign was violent convulsions (5).

Clinical pathology

The organism is easily cultured and may be isolated from nasal discharges. Injection into guinea-pigs and rabbits produces the typical disease. An allergic skin test using melioidin as an antigen (4), a complement fixation test (13), and an indirect hemagglutination test (14) are available but have not had extensive trials. Affected horses may give a positive reaction to the mallein test (15).

Necropsy findings

Multiple abscesses in most organs, particularly in the lungs, spleen and liver, but also in the subcutis and the associated lymph nodes, are characteristic of the disease in all species. In sheep these abscesses contain thick or caseous, green-tinged pus similar to that found in *Corynebacterium pseudotuberculosis* lesions. Lesions in the nasal mucosa proceed to rupture with the development of ragged ulcers. An acute polyarthritis, with distension of the joint capsules by fluid containing large masses of greenish pus, and acute meningoencephalitis have been observed in experimental cases.

Diagnosis

The fatal nature of the disease and the multiple abscessation in various organs serve to differentiate it from caseous lymphadenitis in sheep. The lesions offf nasal actinobacillosis of sheep may also resemble those of melioidosis but this disease is relatively non-fatal and isolation of the organism provides a positive diagnosis. In horses the disease may be confused with strangles or glanders, but there is no enlargement of lymph nodes or involvement of the nasal mucosae or skin.

Treatment

Little information is available on satisfactory treatments of melioidosis. Penicillin, streptomycin, chlortetracycline and polymyxin are ineffective but *in vitro* tests suggests that oxytetracycline, novobiocin, chloramphenicol and sulfadiazine (16) are most likely to be valuable with oxytetracycline preferred. In horses chloromycetin has been shown to be an effective treatment (4). Treatment is unlikely to be undertaken because of the nature of the disease and the risk of exposure to humans.

Control

The elimination of infected animals and the disinfection of premises should be the basis of control procedures.

REFERENCES

(1) Laws, L. & Hall, W. T. K. (1964) *Aust. vet. J.*, *40*, 309.
(2) Sheikh-Omar, A. R. & Muda, H. (1986) *Aust. vet. J.*, *63*, 168.
(3) Thomas, A. D. (1981) *Aust. vet. J.*, *57*, 146.
(4) Loganathan, P. & Tan, S. H. (1983) *Kajian vet. Malaysia*, *15*, 74.
(5) Ladds, P. W. et al. (1981) *Aust. vet. J.*, *57*, 36.
(6) Sutmoller, P. et al. (1957) *J. Am. vet. med. Assoc.*, *130*, 415.
(7) Narita, M. et al. (1981) *Natl Inst. Anim. Hlth Q. (Japan)*, *22*, 170.
(8) Davie, J. & Wells, C. W. (1952) *Br. vet. J.*, *108*, 161.
(9) Baharsefat, M. & Amjadi, A. R. (1970) *Arch. Inst. Razi*, *22*, 209.
(10) Rampling, A. (1964) *Aust. vet. J.*, *40*, 241.
(11) Ketterer, P. J. et al. (1975) *Aust. vet. J.*, *51*, 345.
(12) Thomas, A. D. et al. (1981) *Aust. vet. J.*, *57*, 535.
(13) Laws, L. (1967) *Q. J. agric. Anim. Sci.*, *24*, 207.
(14) Ileri, S. Z. (1965) *Br. vet. J.*, *121*, 164.
(15) Zhang, W. D. & Lu, Z. B. (1983) *Clin. J. vet. Med.*, *9*, 8.
(16) Eickhoff, T. C. et al. (1970) *J. infect. Dis.*, *121*, 95.

DISEASES CAUSED BY *CAMPYLOBACTER* spp.

Several species of the genus *Campylobacter* are known to cause disease in farm animals; some are potentially zoonotic and the role of some is uncertain. *Campylobacter fetus* var. *venerealis* is the cause of infertility and abortion in cattle and will not be presented here. *Campylobacter fetus* subsp. *fetus* causes sporadic abortion in cattle and enzootic abortion in sheep and has been associated with bacteremia in man (1). The organism has also been isolated from the intestines of healthy sheep and cattle and from enteric lesions in cattle with enteritis, but its significance as the causative agent is uncertain. *Campylobacter sputorum* subsp. *mucosalis* is considered to be the cause of intestinal adenomatosis in swine and is presented under that heading. A closely related species, *Campylobacter hyointestinalis*, has been isolated from pigs affected with proliferative ileitis.

Campylobacter jejuni and *C. coli* can be isolated from the intestines of healthy farm animals, poultry, pets, zoo animals and wild birds. Raw milk contaminated by infected cows is a major cause of foodborne human campylobacteriosis in the United States (2, 10). Only rarely can the organism be isolated directly from the milk of cows during an outbreak of disease in humans (12, 15). Fecal contamination, rather than udder infection, is considered to be the means by which campylobacters enter milk and thereby infect man (14). *C. jejuni* has been isolated from the bulk milk supply of goats whose milk was associated with campylobacter infection in a human (13).

The organism may be present in about 15% of cattle at the time of slaughter (9). Approximately 60% of the specimens of healthy slaughter pigs may yield the organism (22). The details of surveys of the incidence of campylobacters from the tissues of cattle at slaughter and from fresh and frozen meat and poultry collected at slaughter are available (17–19). An adaptation of the ELISA test is available for the detection of antibodies to *Campylobacter* sp. for use in seroepidemiological studies in herds of cattle and sheep (29). Wild birds probably constitute the main natural reservoir of infection (20).

Campylobacter fecalis has been isolated from intestinal lesions of cattle and experimentally will cause a diarrhea and dysentery in calves (23).

Campylobacter coli (formerly *Vibrio coli*) has been isolated from the small intestines of diarrheic piglets and experimentally can cause colitis in young piglets (21). The organism may be the cause of naturally occurring diarrhea in nursing piglets and weaned pigs in certain circumstances.

The role of *C. jejuni* as primary pathogens in farm animals is uncertain. The organism was originally thought to be the causative agent of winter dysentery in cattle but reliable evidence for this relationship has not found. Experimentally, the organism will cause a mucoid diarrhea, often with dysentery and a fever in calves (4). The disease may be so mild as to be inapparent, without fever, and may be manifested only by mild depression and soft feces with occasional strands of mucus. At necropsy, there may be a diffuse catarrhal to severe hemorrhagic enteritis of the jejunum and ileum. *C. jejuni* or *C. coli* can cause a mild self-limiting enteritis and bacteremia when inoculated orally into newborn calves (7). The organism has been isolated from the feces of diarrheic calves and lambs which suggests that it may be a causative agent in some outbreaks of diarrhea but this has not yet been substantiated (5, 16). The oral inoculation of pure cultures of *Campylobacter fetus* subsp. *intestinalis* into young calves will also result in an enteritis (6) similar to that caused by *C. jejuni*. A *Campylobacter*-like organism has been isolated from young sheep about 1–2 months after weaning, when they were about 6 months of age, affected with weaner colitis (8). The morbidity rates in flocks ranged from 20 to 75% and the case fatality rate was about 3%. Outbreaks of severe gastroenteritis in fattening lambs have been attributed to *C. jejuni* which were treated successfully with daily injections of erythromycin followed by a single injection of longacting oxytetracycline (11).

Campylobacter jejuni has been isolated from an aborted fetus from a goat (27) and the fetus of a heifer which aborted (28).

The pathogenicity of *C. jejuni* and *C. coli* can be examined in guinea-pigs (24).

The antimicrobial sensitivities of campylobacters from pigs indicate that carbadox, furazolidone, nitrofurantoin, gentamicin and dimetridazole were the most active drugs (25) and clavulanate-potentiated amoxycillin is most effective against isolates from cattle (26).

REVIEW LITERATURE

Garcia, M. M., Eaglesome, M. D. & Rigby, C. (1983) Campylobacters important in veterinary medicine. *Vet. Bull.*, *53*, 793–818.
Lander, K. P. (1985) *Campylobacter. Proc. Conf. Brussels. Jan. 17–18, 1985*. Commission of the European Communities.

REFERENCES

(1) Garcia, M. M. et al. (1983) *Vet. Bull.*, *53*, 793.
(2) Kornblatt, A. N. et al. (1985) *Am. J. Epidemiol.*, *122*, 884.
(3) Prescott, J. F. & Munroe, D. L. (1982). *J. Am. vet. med. Assoc.*, *181*, 1524.
(4) Al-Mashat, R. R. & Taylor, D. J. (1980) *Vet. Rec.*, *107*, 459.
(5) Firehammer, B. D. & Myers, L. L. (1981) *Am. J. vet. Res.*, *42*, 918.
(6) Al-Mashat, R. R. & Taylor D. J. (1983) *Vet. Rec.*, *112*, 54.
(7) Warner, D. P. & Bryner, J. H. (1984) *Am. J. vet. Res.*, *45*, 1822.
(8) Stephens, L. R. et al. (1984) *Aust. vet. J.*, *61*, 183.
(9) Warner, D. P. et al. (1986) *Am. J. vet. Res.*, *47*, 254.
(10) Finch, M. J. & Blake, P. A. (1985). *Am. J. Epidemiol.*, *122*, 262.
(11) Stansfield, D. G. et al. (1986) *Vet. Rec.*, *118*, 210.
(12) Hudson, P. J. et al. (1984) *J. infect. Dis.*, *150*, 789.
(13) Hutchinson, D. N. et al. (1985) *Lancet*, *1*, 1037.
(14) Waterman, S. C. et al. (1984) *J. Hyg. Camb.*, *93*, 333.
(15) Hutchinson, D. N. et al. (1985) *J. Hyg. Camb.*, *94*, 205.
(16) Morgan, J. H. et al. (1986) *Proc. 14th World Congr. Dis. Cattle, Dublin*, Vol. 1, 325.
(17) Garcia, M. M. et al. (1985) *Appl. environ. Microbiol.*, *49*, 667.
(18) Manser, P. A. & Dalziel, R. W. (1985). *J. Hyg., Camb.*, *95*, 15.
(19) Stern, N. J. et al. (1984) *J. Food Protect.*, *47*, 372.
(20) Skirrow, M. B. (1982) *J. Hyg., Camb.*, *89*, 175.
(21) Olubunmi, P. A. & Taylor, D. J. (1982) *Vet. Rec.*, *111*, 197.
(22) Sticht-Groh, V. (1982) *Vet. Rec.*, *110*, 104.
(23) Al-Mashat, R. R. & Taylor, D. J. (1981) *Vet. Rec.*, *109*, 97.
(24) SultanDosa, A. B. et al. (1983) *Am. J. vet. Res.*, *44*, 2175.
(25) Gebhart, C. J. et al. (1985) *Antimicrob. Agents Chemotherap.*, *27*, 55.
(26) Corbel, M. J. et al. (1984) *Vet. Rec.*, *115*, 465.
(27) Anderson, K. L. et al. (1983) *J. Am. vet. med. Assoc.*, *183*, 90.
(28) Welsh, R. D. (1984) *J. Am. vet. med. Assoc.*, *185*, 549.
(29) Grohn, K. & Genigeorgis, C. (1985) *Acta vet. Scand.*, *26*, 30.

Winter dysentery of cattle

Winter dysentery is a highly contagious disease of cattle characterized by a brief attack of severe diarrhea and sometimes dysentery.

Etiology

In cattle, *Campylobacter fetus* var. *jejuni* has been proposed as the causative agent but there is a strong possibility that this organism plays a secondary role in the disease. Considerable difficulty is experienced in transmitting the disease from some outbreaks but not from others. This suggests that a precipitating cause, either environmental or infectious, may operate or that cattle used in transmission experiments have been immune as a result of previous attacks (1). The possibility of a primary virus infection being the precipitating cause is suggested by work in Canada (2) and Israel (3), but the viruses of infectious bovine rhinotracheitis (IBR) and bovine virus diarrhea (BVD) have been exonerated as well as parvoviruses, enteroviruses, and other cytopathogenic viruses (4–6). A similar disease has been described in Sweden in which no vibrios were detected in the feces (7), and in Australia a disease similar to winter dysentery has been observed as a large-scale epidemic (8). At least winter dysentery and mucosal disease of cattle are not the same disease (1).

With the recent observation that the calf rotavirus may be the cause of a transient diarrhea in mature cattle (9), the possibility that winter dysentery may be caused by this virus deserves consideration and investigation. A coronavirus-like agent was present in the feces of cows affected with a herd outbreak in New Zealand (10) and in several outbreaks in France (15).

The vibrio organisms isolated from sheep with dysentery have not been identified but closely resemble *Campylobacter fetus* var. *jejuni*.

Epidemiology

Winter dysentery in cattle is most serious in adult milking cows, particularly those which have recently calved. Young stock may be affected but show only mild clinical signs. The disease is most common in cattle when they are housed. A moderate immunity, which persists for about 6 months, develops after a natural attack, and recurrent attacks in the one animal or herd seldom occur in less than 2–3 years.

Feces from clinical cases, or clinically normal carriers, are the source of infection, and contamination of feed or drinking water is the method of spread. The disease is highly contagious and appears to be brought on to farms by human visitors, carrier animals and on inert objects. Details of the viability of the organisms are not available but oral ingestion is the method by which infection occurs.

Winter dysentery occurs commonly in cattle in North America, and possibly in Britain (11), Sweden (7) and Australia (12). Its similarity to other diseases, particularly mucosal disease, makes its positive identification difficult to establish. The disease is a serious one in dairy herds because, although few animals die, there may be serious loss of condition and milk flow. From 10 to 100% of the herd may show clinical signs.

Pathogenesis

The disease appears to be a simple enteritis affecting chiefly the small intestine. Attempts to reproduce the disease with *Campylobacter fetus* var. *jejuni* have been equivocal (14).

Clinical findings

Cattle

After an incubation period of 3–7 days, there is an explosive herd outbreak of diarrhea which, in the course of the next 4–7 days, affects the majority of adult cattle. Young stock in the group may show mild signs of the disease. A transient febrile period (39·5–40·5°C, 103–105°F) may precede the attack of diarrhea but when clinical signs are evident, the temperature is usually normal. At this time there is a precipitate fall in milk yield which lasts for about a week, anorexia of short duration, and some loss of condition. The feces are very thin, watery and homogeneous without much odor and with no mucous or epithelial shreds, and are dark green to almost black in color. They are often passed with little warning and with considerable velocity. A harsh cough occurs in some outbreaks and may be accompanied by the explosive expulsion of feces. In most animals the course is short and the feces return to normal consistency in 2–3 days. In occasional cases the syndrome is more severe, dehydration and weakness are apparent, and dysentery, either with feces flecked with blood or the passage of whole blood, occurs. The disease in the herd usually subsides in 1–2 weeks.

Sheep

Little information is available but scouring and emaciation have been reported (12).

Clinical pathology

A smear of feces from a clinical case may reveal evidence of *Campylobacter* spp., but a recent investigation of a typical outbreak failed to demonstrate any bacteria from 22 out of 23 fecal samples from affected cows (16). However, *Campylobacter fetus* subsp. *jejuni* and a *Shigella* sp. were recovered from the feces and the intestines of one cow which died after clinical signs of winter dysentery (16).

Necropsy findings

Necropsy material is not usually available but in experimentally infected cattle the changes are limited to the alimentary canal and comprise hyperemia of the abomasal mucosa and a mild catarrhal inflammation of the small intestine. There may be focal degeneration and necrosis of crypt epithelium in the colon which may be virus-induced (16). There may be some hyperemia of the cecal and colonic mucosae. More severe changes have been recorded in some outbreaks of a disease which resembles winter dysentery in cattle but which also has some similarity to mucosal disease (2).

Diagnosis

The disease in cattle is characterized by the explosive nature of the outbreaks that occur. Similar outbreaks may occur in mucosal disease but lesions of the oral mucosa are evident and the clinical signs are more severe. Individual cases of winter dysentery may resemble coccidiosis or salmonellosis, but both of these diseases are more severe and usually affect only one or two animals at a time. Final differentiation depends upon examination of fecal material for the causative agent. A variety of toxic agents may also cause outbreaks of diarrhea in cattle. The more common of these are listed under the etiology of enteritis.

Treatment

The treatment of winter dysentery is of doubtful value because affected cattle usually respond spontaneously in 24–36 hours (1). Copper sulfate (30 ml of 5% solution), sulfonamides and nitrofurazone have been given orally. Occasionally dehydration will become severe and is best treated with fluids and balanced electrolytes as indicated.

Control

Because of the explosive nature of the disease and the lack of information on possible precipitating causes, effective control measures cannot be recommended. Every effort must be made to avoid the spread of infection on inanimate objects such as boots, feeding utensils and bedding but even the greatest care does not appear to prevent the spread of the disease within a herd.

REVIEW LITERATURE

Campbell, S. G. & Cookingham, C. S. (1978) The enigma of winter dysentery. *Cornell Vet. 68*, 423.

VanKruiningen, H. J., Hiestad, L., Hill, D. L., Tilton, R. C. & Ryan, R. W. (1985) Winter dysentery in dairy cattle: recent findings. *Comp. cont. Educ. Pract. Vet.*, 7, S591–S599.

REFERENCES

(1) Kahrs, R. F. (1965) *Cornell Vet.*, *55*, 505.
(2) McPherson, L. W. (1957) *Can. J. comp. Med.*, *21*, 184.
(3) Komarov, A. et al. (1959) *Refuah Vet.*, *16*, 111.
(4) Kahrs, R. F. et al. (1973) *Bov. Pract.*, *8*, 36.
(5) Scott, F. W. et al. (1973) *Bov. Pract.*, *8*, 40.
(6) Anderson, A. A. & Scott, F. W. (1976) *Cornell Vet.*, *66*, 232.
(7) Hedstrom, H. & Isaacson, A. (1951) *Cornell Vet.*, *41*, 251.
(8) Edwards, M. J. & Sier, A. M. (1960) *Aust. vet. J.*, *36*, 402.
(9) Woode, G. N. (1976) *Vet Ann.*, *16*, 30.
(10) Horner, G. W. et al. (1975) *NZ vet. J.*, *23*, 98.
(11) Rollinson, D. H. L. (1948) *Vet. Rec.*, *60*, 191.
(12) Hutchins, D. R. (1958) *Aust. vet. J.*, *34*, 300.
(13) Russells, R. R. (1955) *NZ vet J.*, *3*, 60.
(14) Firehammer, B. D. & Myers, L. L. (1981) *Am. J. vet. Res.*, *42*, 918.
(15) Espinasse, J. et al. (1982) *Vet. Rec.*, *110*, 385.
(16) VanKruiningen, H. J. et al. (1985) *Comp. cont. Educ. Pract. Vet.*, 7, S591.

DISEASES CAUSED BY *LEPTOSPIRA* spp.

Leptospirosis

Leptospirosis occurs in all farm animal species and is an important zoonosis. It causes septicemia, interstitial nephritis, hemolytic anemia and abortion in most species, mastitis in cattle and it may be the cause of equine periodic ophthalmia.

Etiology

All leptospires are now classified into one species *Leptospira interrogans* containing over 100 serotypes, for exam ple, *L. interrogans* serovar *pomona*.

Epidemiology

For most leptospiral serotypes the important carrier hosts are rodents but *L. interrogans* serovars *pomona*, *tarassovi* and *hardjo* are adapted to agricultural animals as carrier hosts, with obvious epidemiological implications. Freeliving animals that are predators for rodents do not appear to be a natural route of transmission for the infection (3).

In some countries, leptospirosis is endemic and infection is much more common than clinical disease. Financial losses due to it are correspondingly less and the disease then achieves its greatest importance as a zoonosis (7). The international distribution of *L. interrogans* serovar *pomona* is also erratic; it had not been present in the United Kingdom until recent years and then only very sporadically (59). *Leptospira interrogans* serovar *pomona* is the commonest infection in all animals. Its survival in the environment depends largely upon variations in soil and water conditions in the contaminated area; it is particularly susceptible to drying, and to changes in pH away from neutrality or mild alkalinity. A pH lower than 6 or greater than 8 is inhibitory. Temperatures lower than 7–10°C (44·6–50°F) or higher than 34–36°C (93–96°F) are detrimental to its survival. Moisture is the most important factor governing the persistence of the organism in bedding or soil: it can persist for as long as 183 days in water-saturated soil but survives for only 30 minutes when the soil is air-dried. In soil under average conditions survival is likely to be at least 42 days for *L. interrogans* serovar *pomona* (10). The organism survives in free, surface water for very long periods, the survival period being longer in stagnant than in flowing water although persistence in the latter for as long as 15 days has been recorded.

L. interrogans serovar *pomona* infection has been recorded in cattle, pigs and horses, and the ovine infection has been provisionally identified as *L. interrogans* serovar *pomona*; the disease has been produced experimentally in this latter species by injection of bovine and porcine strains of the organism. *L. interrogans* serovar *hardjo* has become a very common infection in Australia and the United Kingdom (1) and in many areas outranks *L. interrogans* serovar *pomona* in cattle. It is now the commonest serological finding in cattle in some parts of Australia (42), New Zealand (48) and the United States (49). Cattle are the maintenance host for *L. interrogans* serovar *hardjo* and are considered to be the only reservoir. It is not a significant infection in sheep (30) although it occurs in them. *L. interrogans* serovar *hardjo* is an important cause of bovine abortion (42), but there is difficulty reproducing the abortion form of the disease experimentally (69). In Australia at least 86% of herds have serological evidence of exposure to *Leptospira* sp. It is also the commonest leptospiral infection in man, and is a very common infection in Australian sheep (44) and may affect up to 40% of the population. The position of leptospirosis in pigs in the United Kingdom is an interesting one because there appears to be no host-adapted endemic serotype in this species. The serotypes known to be present are all chance invaders which are endemic in other species especially rodents. They include *L. interrogans* serovars *copenhageni*, *ballum*, *muenchen*, *icterohaemorrhagiae* (60).

Because of the severity of the systemic disease, the high rate of abortions and abnormalities of milk, its importance is greater even than its prevalence. *L. interrogans* serovar *canicola* infection has been recorded in cattle and in pigs and specific antibodies have been detected in horses. *L. interrogans* serovar *icterohaemorrhagiae* is a rare isolation in large animals but has been reported in cattle and pigs, and serological evidence of infection has been found in the horse. *L. interrogans* serovar *hyos* (*L. interrogans* serovar *mitis*) has been isolated from cattle and pigs, *L. interrogans* serovar *grippotyphosa* from cattle and goats, and positive serological tests have been obtained in horses. *L. sejroe*, *L. interrogans* serovar *hebdomadis* and *L. interrogans* serovar *australis* infection have been observed in cattle. *L. interrogans* serovar *szwajizak* is thought to be the predominant serotype in Israel (8). One of the more interesting serotypes is *L. interrogans* serovar *balcanicus* which is a common inhabitant of brush-tailed possums (34). It was thought at one time that it might produce false positive serological reactions for *L. interrogans* serovar *hardjo* (37), although it is not a natural parasite for sheep (35) and is unlikely to be endemic in, or cause disease in, sheep or cattle (58). Its status in cattle is uncertain, but sporadic small outbreaks have occurred (46) and vaccination against *L. interrogans* serovar *hardjo* protects against it. More detailed lists of leptospiral serotypes and their hosts are available.

Calves and lambs are highly susceptible and are likely to develop the septicemic form of the disease. Strong immunity after an attack may occur and a reduced susceptibility has been observed in pigs which is probably sufficient to produce a state of herd immunity. Passive transfer of antibodies to newborn calves occurs via the colostrum and the antibodies persist in the calves for 2–6 months.

The source of infection is usually an infected animal which contaminates pasture, drinking water and feed by infected urine, aborted fetuses and infected uterine discharges. All of the leptospiral types are transmitted in this way and can pass between the animal species although the importance of sheep and horses in the epizootiology of leptospirosis is uncertain. A viable infected fetus can carry the infection for as long as 7 weeks after birth (68). The semen of an infected bull may carry leptospirae and transmission from such a bull to heifers by coitus and artificial insemination has been observed. In rams the semen is likely to be infective for only a few days during the period of leptospiremia and in boars there is no evidence of coital transmission. For most leptospiral serotypes the most important carrier hosts are rodents but *L. interrogans* serovars *pomona*, *tarassovi* and *hardjo* are adapted to agricultural animals as carrier hosts, with obvious epidemiological implications.

Because of the rapidly accumulating evidence of a high rate of infection with *Leptospira* spp. in wildlife these animals are suspected of playing a significant role in the spread of the disease to domestic animals. For example, feral pigs have been shown to have a very high incidence of infection (9), rats are known to be a source of *L. interrogans* serovar *icterohaemorrhagiae*, *L. interrogans* serovar *canicola* is known to spread from domestic dogs and jackals to cattle and, when hygiene is poor, even from humans to cattle. Although surveys of the incidence of leptospirosis in wildlife have been conducted and the pathogenic effects of *L. interrogans* serovar *pomona* on some species, particularly deer, have been determined, the real significance of feral leptospirosis as a source of infection for domestic animals has not been determined. There seems little doubt, from experimental evidence and from observations on field outbreaks, that many wild species (6) including skunks (5) do act as carriers of the disease.

Entrance of the organism into the body occurs most probably through cutaneous or mucosal abrasions. Transplacental transmission is not common but neonatal infection, probably contracted *in utero*, has been recorded (13). Oral dosing is an unsatisfactory method for experimental transmission as compared to injection and installation into the nasal cavities, conjunctival sac and vagina. Contamination of the environment and capacity of the organism to survive for long periods under favorable conditions of dampness lead to a high incidence of the disease on heavily irrigated pastures, in areas with high rainfall and temperate climate, in fields with drinking water supplies in the form of easily contaminated surface ponds, and in marshy fields and muddy paddocks or feedlots. Because of the importance of water as a means of spreading infection new cases are most likely to occur in wet seasons and low lying areas, especially when contamination and susceptibility are high (8). A differential distribution has been observed in the prevalence of seropositives in cattle in Australia. *L. interrogans* serovar *hardjo* antibodies have a high prevalence through all rainfall areas, but *L. interrogans* serovar *pomona* is much more common in low rainfall areas (9).

Urine is the chief source of contamination because animals, particularly pigs, even after clinical recovery, may pass leptospirae in the urine for long periods. For example, young pigs may act as carriers for a year and adult sows for 2 months. Because of the high intensity and long duration of the infection in pigs they play an important role in the epidemiology of leptospirosis. They are considered to be a common source of infection in calves which run with them.

Cattle have been shown to have leptospiruria for a mean period of 36 days (10–118 days) with the highest excretion rate in the first half of this period. Sheep do not appear to be a ready source of infection for other species, probably because of their intermittent and low grade leptospiruria, although this may persist for 9 months in natural cases of the disease. Horses are also a dubious source of infection because the leptospiruria is of slight degree although it may persist for up to 4 months. In goats, leptospiruria persists for at least a month after infection. The leptospirae may persist in the kidney for much longer periods than they can be recovered from the urine by routine laboratory methods. It is probable that apparently recovered animals intermittently pass the organisms in the urine and thus act as 'carriers'. Urine drinking is not an uncommon form of pica in some dairy herds and can be a means of spreading leptospirosis actively. *L. interrogans* serovar *hardjo* is excreted from the genital tract of aborting cows for as long as 8 days after abortion or calving and is detectable in the oviducts and uterus for up to 90 days after experimental infection (21) and in naturally infected cows (45). It is also commonly found in the genital tract of bulls and venereal spread of the infection is thought to occur in cattle (61).

Leptospirosis in the large domestic animals has come into prominence only during relatively recent years and details of its incidence are only now becoming available. The disease appears to be worldwide in its distribution. In general terms the disease is most common in areas or seasons when the climate is warm and humid, soils are alkaline and there is an abundance of surface water.

Cattle

Although the mortality rate is low (5%) in this species, the morbidity rate is usually high as determined clinically and serologically and may approach 100% of in-contact animals. In calves the mortality rate is much higher than in adult cattle. A high rate of abortions (up to 30%) and loss of milk production are the major causes of loss but deaths in calves may also be significant. As a measure of the loss caused by *L. interrogans* serovar *hardjo* in beef cattle, the percentage of cows which are serologically positive has been related to the proportion of the herd which suffer lactation failure; there is a significantly greater wastage in the reactor cows (11). High herd level of seroprevalence for *L. interrogans* serovar *pomona* are related to low relative humidity, a particular soil type and the presence of feral pigs. For *L. interrogans* serovar *hardjo* the etiological determinants are a particular series of soil types and the presence of other cattle.

Pigs

In infected herds the incidence of positive reactors to serological tests is high, and in large affected pig populations averages about 20%. Economic losses are about equally divided between abortions and deaths of weak and unthrifty newborn pigs. *L. interrogans* serovar *pomona* has been the predominant infection in pigs but with the widespread use of bacterins against it other infections are assuming new importance. *Leptospira interrogans* serovars *tarassovi*, *copenhageni*, *ballum*, *bratislava*, *muenchen* and *hardjo* are being isolated more frequently. Pigs in intensive housing present a different problem from those in more conventional housing or at pasture. In these large pig units the possibility for cross-infection is very great because of the concentration of the population. The movement of pigs from pen to pen, and access to effluent from other pens are the critical means of spread in these circumstances (33). Introduction onto a farm may be via an imported boar who frequently will be found to harbor *Leptospira* in his genital tract (47). A significant difference between genetic strains of pigs of susceptibility to leptospirosis is recorded (20).

Sheep and goats

The disease in sheep has been reported from many countries and the disease in goats is reported from Israel. Deaths of animals and loss of condition in mildly affected animals are the main causes of loss. Although few outbreaks are recorded, a morbidity rate of 100% is not uncommon in sheep and mortality rates usually average about 20% in this species and up to 45% in goats. *L. interrogans* serovar *pomona* is the common infection. Infection with *L. interrogans* serovar *hardjo* occurs but is unlikely to a source of infection for cattle herds (58).

Horses

The disease is relatively mild in horses, and losses, except for blindness due to associated periodic ophthalmia, are negligible. When groups of horses are known to be infected, an average of up to 30% of the adult horses can be expected to give positive serological tests. Surveys generally show the disease to be endemic in most horse populations (24), with a higher prevalence in tropical areas (71). The dominant serovar of *Leptospira interrogans* varies widely between localities (72, 73).

Humans

One of the important features of leptospirosis is its transmissibility to man and it represents an occupational hazard to butchers, farmers and veterinarians. The incidence of positive agglutination tests in humans in contact with infected cattle is surprisingly low and clinical cases in man in which the infection is acquired from animals are not common. Human infection is most likely to occur by contamination with infected urine or uterine contents. Although leptospirae may be present in the milk for a few days at the peak of fever in an acute case the bacteria does not survive for long in the milk and does not withstand pasteurization. However, farm workers who actually milk cows are highly susceptible to *L. interrogans* serovar *hardjo* infection and one New Zealand survey has shown 34% of milkers to be seropositive, most to *L. interrogans* serovar *hardjo*, but a high proportion also to *L. interrogans* serovar *pomona*. This has aroused alarm to the point where leptospirosis is referred to as 'New Zealand's No. 1 dairy occupational disease' (62) and bovine vaccines are being specifically tested for their efficacy in preventing leptospiruria in cattle.

Pathogenesis

Leptospirosis manifests itself as a disease in a number of ways. There are acute and subacute forms, a so-called chronic or abortion form and an occult form in which there is no clinical illness. Which form of the disease occurs depends largely on the species of the host as set out in Table 61. Variations between serotypes of *L. interrogans* in their pathogenicity also affects the nature of the signs which appear. For example, in *L. interrogans* serovar *pomona* infections intravascular hemolysis and interstitial nephritis are important parts of the disease. However, *L. interrogans* serovar *hardjo* produce no hemolysin and cause no interstitial nephritis. It is capable of growing only in the pregnant uterus and lactating mammary gland so that it produces septicemia and then mastitis and/or abortion. The pathogenesis of the disease caused by *L. interrogans* serovar *pomona* is set out below.

Table 61. Forms of leptospirosis (*L. interrogans* serovar *pomona*) in the animal species

	Acute form	*Subacute form*	*Chronic form*
Cattle	+ (calves only)	+	+ (abortion)
Sheep and goat	+ (includes abortion)	–	–
Pig	+ (rarely and only in piglets)	–	+ (abortion)
Horse	–	+	+ (abortion and periodic ophthalmia)

Acute form

After penetration of the skin or mucosa the organisms multiply rapidly in the liver and then migrate to, and can be isolated from, the peripheral blood for several days and until the accompanying fever subsides. At this time antibodies begin to appear in the bloodstream and organisms in the urine.

Septicemia, capillary damage, hemolysis and interstitial nephritis

During the early period of septicemia sufficient hemolysin may be produced to cause overt hemaglobinuria as a result of extensive intravascular hemolysis. This is an unlikely event in adult cattle, but common in young calves. If the animal survives this phase of the disease, localization of the infection may occur in the kidney. Whether or not hemolysis occurs depends on whether the particular serotype produces a hemolysin. The effects of the toxin on the erythrocyte are visible microscopically (79). Capillary damage is common to all serotypes and during the septicemic phase, petechial hemorrhages in mucosae are a common expression of this. The vascular damage occurs also in the kidney and if the hemolysis is sufficiently severe, anemic anoxia and hemoglobinuric nephrosis are added to this basic vascular lesion. The infection localizes in the renal parenchyma and causes an interstitial nephritis and persistence of the leptospirae in these lesions leads to a prolonged leptospiruria. The renal lesion develops because the infection persists there long after it has been cleared from other tissue sites. In the acute phase of the disease, therefore, the animal may die of septicemia or hemolytic anemia or a combination of the two. Subsequently, the animal may die of uremia caused by interstitial nephritis.

Abortion
A common sequel after the initial systemic invasion is abortion which is caused by the death of the fetus, with or without placental degeneration, both effects resulting from invasion of the conceptus during the septicemic stage of the disease. Abortion always occurs several weeks after septicemia because of the time required to produce the changes in the fetus, which is usually degenerated at birth, and has obviously been dead for more than 24 hours. Abortion occurs most commonly in the second half of pregnancy, due probably to the greater ease of invasion of the placenta at this stage, but may occur at any time from 4 months on. Although abortion occurs commonly in both cattle and horses after either the acute or the subacute form of the disease, abortion without prior clinical illness is also common. This is particularly the case in sows and occurs to a less extent in cows and mares, and may be due to degenerative changes in the placental epithelium. Leptospirae are rarely present in the aborted fetuses. However, if the aborted fetus has survived the infection long enough to produce antibodies these may be detectable.

Encephalitis
Localization of leptospirae in nervous tissue is common in sheep and goats and may result in the appearance of signs of encephalitis.

Subacute and occult forms of leptospirosis
In the subacute form, the pathogenesis is similar to that of the acute septicemic form except that the reaction is less severe. It occurs in all species, but is the common one in adult cattle and horses. Occult cases, with no clinical illness but with rising antibody titers, are common in all animals. These are difficult to explain epidemiologically unless it is conceded that there are strains of varying pathogenicity. On the other hand numerical differences between groups are usually explainable in terms of prior immune status, or of environmental conditions, or of number of carriers in relation to severity of exposure.

Periodic ophthalmia in the horse
Although final proof is lacking that there is a direct causal relationship between leptospiral infection and periodic ophthalmia in the horse, there is strong presumptive evidence linking the two (18, 82). There is a much higher incidence of positive reactors to serum agglutination tests for leptospiral antibodies in groups of horses affected with periodic ophthalmia than in normal animals. Agglutinins are present in the aqueous humor in greater concentration than in the serum. The absence of leptospirae from affected eyes and the fact that ophthalmia may not occur for 1–2 years after systemic infection has given rise to the suggestion that the ophthalmia may be due to an allergic reaction to spirochetal protein. Many other factors including a nutritional deficiency of riboflavin and invasion of the eye by microfilariae of *Onchocerca cervicalis* have been considered as causes of the disease.

Experimental leptospirosis
A large part of the knowledge of pathogenesis of leptospirosis comes from extensive studies of the experimentally produced disease. A summary of the clinical and pathological findings of this work is set down below.

In calves Experimental production of leptospirosis with *L. interrogans* serovar *pomona* in calves (12) causes a febrile reaction, accompanied by leptospiremia, after a 4–9 day incubation period. The disappearance of organisms from the bloodstream 2–4 days later coincides with a fall in temperature and is followed by leptospiruria and albuminuria coinciding with active infection of the kidney. During the febrile period, there is a leukocytosis, and transitory anemia, hemoglobinuria and jaundice due to intravascular hemolysis. Although focal interstitial nephritis and hepatic necrosis occur during the experimental disease, no biochemical indications of renal or hepatic insufficiency have been observed. Experimental production of leptospirosis with *L. interrogans* serovars *hebdomadis* and *hardjo* in heifers causes fever, but infection with *L. interrogans* serovar *hardjo* alone causes no clinical illness (56). *L. interrogans* serovar *canicola* produces a syndrome similar to that produced by *L. interrogans* serovar *pomona* except that there is no hemoglobinuria or jaundice and there is no significant renal or hepatic impairment. There is a mild anemia.

In sheep and goats In sheep, the experimental disease caused by *L. interrogans* serovar *pomona* is manifested by high fever, and significant pathological changes in the uterine endometrium. Although abortion may not be a common field sequel of leptospiral infection in sheep it can be produced experimentally, the pathogenesis consisting of fetal death with a degree of autolysis of the fetus and placenta preceding abortion. Death due to acute hemolytic anemia, such as occurs in calves, also occurs in lambs (16). Experimental infection with *L. interrogans* serovars *pomona* or *hardjo* in goats causes no apparent illness. *L. interrogans* serovar *hardjo* infection in sheep causes mild fever and loss of appetite (67). *L. interrogans* serovar *balcanica* causes transient hyperthermia on experimental inoculation in sheep.

In pigs Leptospirosis produced experimentally in pigs is manifested by practically no clinical illness other than a slight fever, and in pregnant sows abortion or stillbirths. Maximum leptospiruria occurs 20–30 days after exposure, and although the urine is virtually clear of infection in most pigs 3 weeks later the leptospiruria may persist for much longer. The most severe lesion is an interstitial nephritis and the leptospirae persist longer in the kidney (more than 45 days) than in any other organ.

In horses The experimental disease in horses is similar to that seen in calves except that hemoglobinuria is exceptional. A moderate fever occurs on the 7th to 10th day after exposure at which time leptospirae can be cultured from the blood. Leptospirae subsequently appear in the urine and may persist for up to 120 days. Agglutinating antibodies appear at 9 days after exposure and ocular lesions of periodic ophthalmia are present in most horses up to 15 months later (17).

Clinical findings

The clinical findings in leptospirosis are similar in each animal species and do not vary greatly with the species of *Leptospira* except that infection with *L. interrogans* serovar *icterohaemorrhagiae* usually causes a severe septicemia. For convenience the various forms of the disease are described as they occur in cattle, and comparisons are made with the disease in other species. In all animals the incubation period is from 3 to 7 days.

Cattle

Leptospirosis in cattle may appear as acute subacute or chronic forms and is usually caused by *L. interrogans* serovars *pomona* or *hardjo*.

Acute leptospirosis caused by L. interrogans *serovar* pomona Calves up to a month old are most susceptible. The disease is manifested by septicemia, with high fever (40·5–41·5°C, 105–107°F), anorexia, petechiation of mucosae, depression, and by acute hemolytic anemia with hemoglobinuria, jaundice and pallor of the mucosae. Because of the anemia there is a marked increase in heart rate, an increase in the absolute intensity of the heart sounds and a more readily palpable apex beat. Dyspnea is also prominent. The mortality rate is high and if recovery occurs, convalescence is prolonged. Abortion, due to the systemic reaction, is likely to occur at the acute stage of the disease. Additional signs in cattle are related to the udder and milk flow. Milk flow almost ceases and the secretion is red-colored or contains blood clots, and the udder is limp and soft. Mastitis, as part of leptospirosis, has often been described in cattle and the presence of many leukocytes in the grossly abnormal milk does suggest this diagnosis, but these changes are due to a general vascular lesion rather than local injury to mammary tissue. Severe lameness due to synovitis is recorded in some animals and a necrotic dermatitis, probably due to photosensitization, in others.

Subacute leptospirosis caused by L. interrogans *serovar* pomona This differs from the acute form only in degree, approximately the same signs being observed in a number of affected animals but not all of the signs necessarily being present in the one animal. Fever is milder (39–40·5°C, 102–105°F), depression, anorexia, dyspnea and a degree of hemoglobinuria are constant but jaundice may or may not be present. Abortion may occur 3–4 weeks later. In addition, one of the characteristic signs is the fall in the milk yield and the appearance of bloodstained or yellow-orange, thick milk in all four quarters without apparent physical change in the udder.

Chronic leptospirosis caused by L. interrogans *serovar* pomona This is manifested by mild clinical signs which may be restricted to abortion. Severe 'storms' of abortions occur most commonly in groups of cattle which are at the same stage of pregnancy when exposed to infection. The abortions usually occur during the last third of pregnancy. Apart from the production of abortion there appears to be no significant depression of reproductive efficiency in cattle affected by leptospirosis. Many animals in the group develop positive agglutination titers without clinical illness.

There are occasional reports of leptospiral meningitis in cattle. Incoordination, excessive salivation, conjunctivitis and muscular rigidity are the common signs.

Leptospirosis caused by L. interrogans *serovar* hardjo This occurs only in pregnant or lactating cows because the organism is restricted to growing in the pregnant uterus and the lactating mammary gland. There is a sudden onset of fever, anorexia, immobility and agalactia. The milk is yellow to orange and may contain clots. The udder is flabby, has no heat or pain, and all four quarters are equally affected (19). This mastitis can occur in outbreak form affecting up to 50% of cows at one time and causing a precipitate fall in the herd's milk yield, also known as the milk drop syndrome, a name more commonly given to fescue toxicosis (29). The milk has a high leukocyte count which subsides over a period of about 14 days as milk production returns.

Abortion may occur several weeks later, may also occur as the only evidence of the disease (75) and in some areas or circumstances it is the principal clinical manifestation of leptospirosis due to *L. interrogans* serovar *hardjo* (2), and the principal cause of abortion in cattle (66). In others it is thought to be an uncommon cause of abortion (63). This may be related to different strains of the serotype, or to the degree to which the disease has become enzootic. Thus outbreaks of mastitis and systemic illness appear to be the characteristic clinical picture when the disease first appears in an area, but as natural immunity develops in adult cows, only heifers become newly infected, and they show abortion only. Also many cows have subclinical infections with *L. interrogans* serovar *hardjo* in which only a fall in milk yield may be detectable.

Leptospirosis caused by *L. interrogans* serovar *szwajizak*, produced experimentally, is characterized by a short bout of fever, listlessness and anorexia, and diarrhea in some. The illness lasts for 24 hours.

Pigs

L. interrogans serovar *pomona* is the common infection, *L. interrogans* serovar *tarassovi* being the other common infection, and chronic leptospirosis is the commonest form of the disease in pigs. It is characterized by the occurrence of abortion and a high incidence of stillbirths. Failure to conceive is not usually observed in leptospirosis but has been reported in infections with *L. interrogans* serovar *canicola*. In an infected herd the rearing rate may fall as low as 10–30%. An abortion 'storm' may occur when the disease first appears in a herd but abortions diminish as herd immunity develops. Most abortions occur 2–4 weeks before term. Piglets produced at term may be dead or weak and die soon after birth. *L. interrogans* serovar *hardjo* may be a sporadic cause of reproductive disease (70) and *L. interrogans* serovar *muenchen* and *bratislava* are occasional isolations during investigations of porcine abortion and stillbirths (74).

Rarely the acute form as it occurs in calves also occurs in piglets in both natural field outbreaks and in experimentally produced cases. *L. interrogans* serovar *icterohaemorrhagiae* infection causes septicemic leptospirosis with a high mortality rate.

Sheep and goats
The disease is rare in these species so that good descriptions of the naturally occurring disease in them are lacking, most affected animals being found dead, apparently from septicemia (15). Affected animals are febrile, dyspneic, snuffle, and hang their heads down; a proportion show hemoglobinuria, pallor of mucosae and jaundice, and most die within 12 hours. Lambs, especially those in poor condition, are most susceptible. The chronic form may occur and is manifested by loss of bodily condition, but abortion seems to be almost entirely a manifestation of the acute form when the infection is *L. interrogans* serovar *pomona*. With *L. interrogans* serovar *hardjo*, abortion has been recorded as the only clinical sign (22), and oligolactia and agalactia, similar to the bovine milk drop syndrome, have been observed in lactating ewes (32).

Horses
The subacute form as described for cattle occurs commonly but the illness is mild and shortlived (23). Icterus and a degree of depression are common signs. Abortion and periodic ophthalmia may follow. The chronic form, with abortion (55) at the 7th to 10th month of pregnancy, has also been reported. Periodic ophthalmia is characterized clinically by recurrent attacks of ocular signs including photophobia, lacrimation, conjunctivitis, keratitis, a pericorneal corona of blood vessels, hypopyon and iridocyclitis. Recurrent attacks usually terminate in blindness in both eyes (18). The disease has been produced experimentally by producing infection with *L. interrogans* serovar *pomona*. Infection with *L. interrogans* serovar *pomona* in foals has been observed in association with *Corynebacterium* (*Rhodococcus*) *equi* to cause a very heavy mortality. The foals died of a combination of interstitial nephritis and uremia and pulmonary abscessation and chronic enteritis (25).

Clinical pathology
Laboratory procedures are most important in the diagnosis of the disease and include cultural isolation of the organism, serological tests, a hamster inoculation test and a growth inhibition test. During the septicemic stage, leptospirae are present only in the blood. There is laboratory evidence of acute hemolytic anemia and increased erythrocyte fragility and often hemoglobinuria. A leukopenia has been observed in cattle while in other species there is a mild leukocytosis. However, the only positive diagnostic measure at this stage of the disease is culture of the blood. If abortion occurs, the kidney, lung and pleural fluid of the aborted fetuses should be examined for the presence of the organism. Serological testing at the time of abortion may be seriously inaccurate (65). In the stage immediately after the subsidence of the fever, antibodies begin to develop and the leptospirae disappear from the blood and appear in the urine. The leptospiruria is accompanied by albuminuria of varying degrees and persists for varying lengths of time in the different species.

Demonstration or culture of the organism
Of all the laboratory diagnostic tests for leptospirosis, the examination of urine samples for the organism probably offers the most profitable opportunity of demonstrating the presence of infection. Urine samples should be obtained from as many affected and non-affected (in-contact) animals as possible. For maximum efficiency, one-half of each urine sample should be submitted with added formalin (1 drop to 20–30 ml of urine) and the other half submitted in the fresh state. The formalin prevents bacterial overgrowth and the fresh urine sample may be used for culture. Examination of the centrifuged urine using dark-field illumination is considered to be a very useful diagnostic test.

Culture of the organism from blood, urine and milk may be attempted by injection of fresh samples directly into hamsters or guinea-pigs on the farm or using special media. There are a number of difficulties associated with injecting urine into guinea-pigs or hamsters, especially on the farm, and a transport medium should be used so that these examinations can now be carried out in the laboratory. The medium is suitable for use with a midstream sample. Culture of the organism from blood and milk is difficult even under ideal conditions, and is a technique usually used in experimental work.

Serological and related tests
These include the ELISA-antiglobulin test, the microscopic agglutination test (MAT) (formerly known as the agglutination–lysis test), and the macroscopic agglutination test. The ELISA test is much more accurate than the others and has many advantages from the point of view of laboratory practice (28). Some difficulty is encountered in interpreting the significance of titers of antibody in serum. For a diagnosis of leptospiral abortion in cattle a reciprocal titer of 3000 is proposed as the threshold for *L. interrogans* serovar *pomona* but no similar critical figure is available for *L. interrogans* serovar *hardjo* (76). For a herd diagnosis of leptospirosis due to *L. interrogans* serovar *hardjo* ten animals from each of the yearling, first calf heifer, second calf heifer and adult cow groups should be tested (78).

Fluorescent staining of antibody in urine or cultures is a fast and accurate diagnostic method for detecting the presence of leptospirae (26) and for identifying serotypes. Antibodies also appear in urine and milk and their measurement may have some significance in special circumstances. A semiautomated complement fixation test is available and is comparable in efficiency with the MAT (23).

Serological examination in pigs has proved to be difficult especially when it is desired to test individual pigs. An enzymatic radioimmunoassay is available for the detection of leptospiral antigen in urine and an enzyme immunoassay for the detection of antibody in serum (39). An enzymatic immunoassay test has had successful trials in sheep (14).

Necropsy findings
In the acute form, anemia, jaundice, hemoglobinuria and subserous and submucosal hemorrhages are con-

stant. There may be ulcers and hemorrhages in the abomasal mucosa in cattle, and if hemoglobinuria has been severe there may be associated pulmonary edema and emphysema. Histologically there is focal or diffuse interstitial nephritis and centrilobular hepatic necrosis and in some cases vascular lesions in the meninges and brain. Leptospirae may be visible in sections and attempts should be made to isolate them from the kidney.

In the later stages the characteristic finding is a progressive interstitial nephritis manifested by small, white, raised areas in the renal cortex. Many clinically normal cattle presented to abattoirs have these lesions of interstitial nephritis. Aborted bovine fetuses are usually autolyzed to the point where no lesions or bacteria can be demonstrated. Even in a fresh fetus the positive identification of leptospirae in lesions is very difficult, especially with *L. interrogans* serovar *hardjo* which is very fastidious in its cultural requirements. The use of a fluorescent antibody technique makes the identification very much simpler. In some but not all aborted fetuses leptospiral antibodies are detectable in their serum (13).

A characteristic focal hepatitis has been observed in aborted piglets. The necrotic foci are 1–4 mm in diameter, irregular in outline and are found in the liver in 40% of aborted fetuses. The fetal membranes are thick, edematous, brown and necrotic. Leptospirae can be isolated from the kidney and genital tract of aborted porcine fetuses (77).

Diagnosis

Positive diagnosis of leptospirosis in individual animals is often difficult because of the variation in the nature of the disease, the rapidity with which the organism dies in specimens once they are collected and their transient appearance in various tissues.

Acute and convalescent sera taken 7–10 days apart should be submitted from each clinically affected animal, or from those with a history of abortion, and sera should also be taken from 15–25% of apparently normal animals. If possible wildlife or rodents which are known to inhabit the farm and use nearby water supplies should be captured and laboratory examinations of their tissues and blood carried out and the results compared with those obtained in the farm animals.

The diagnosis of leptospirosis is much easier on a herd basis than in a single animal because in an infected herd some animals are certain to have high titers and the chances of demonstrating or isolating the organism in urine or milk are increased with samples being taken from many animals; whereas in a single animal, depending on when the infection occurred, the titer may have declined to a low level and be difficult to interpret. This becomes particularly important for the clinician confronted with a diagnosis of abortion due to leptospirosis in which the infection may have occurred several weeks previously and the serum may be negative or the titers too low for an accurate interpretation. Examination of the urine may be useful in these cases.

The differential clinical diagnosis of the common forms of leptospirosis in each species is given below.

Cattle

The acute and subacute forms in this species need to be differentiated from babesiosis, anaplasmosis, rape and kale poisoning, postparturient hemoglobinuria, bacillary hemoglobinuria, and the acute hemolytic anemia which occurs in calves after drinking large quantities of water (Table 62). The discoloration or presence of blood in the milk is the principal abnormality which differentiates leptospirosis clinically from the other infectious hemolytic diseases, which as a group are differentiated from the non-infectious group by the occurrence of fever. The absence of swelling of the udder is sufficient to differentiate this abnormality from mastitis. The chronic form can be differentiated from abortion due to other causes by laboratory examination.

Pigs

Abortion in the last trimester is the common manifestation of leptospirosis in pigs and can be distinguished from brucellosis only by laboratory examination, although hepatic necrosis in fetuses aborted due to leptospiral infection may help in presumptive diagnosis. The herd history of brucellosis, with infertility, orchitis in the boar and high neonatal mortality, may also give a general idea of the causative infection. Severe systemic reactions caused by many bacterial infections including erysipelas may also cause abortion in sows. Parvovirus infection can cause outbreaks of abortion involving all ages of sows with the concurrent occurrence of early embryonic death and infertility, or the subsequent occurrence at term of stillborn and mummified fetuses and small litter size when the infection gains access to SPF or other herds for the first time. The virus is present in feces and spreads rapidly to produce immunity within the sow herd where managemental conditions allow. In endemically affected herds problems may persist in gilts due to infection in early pregnancy after loss of their maternal immunity and this permits the development of a problem of infertility, stillborn pigs and low litter size. Diagnosis is by the detection of virus or hemagglutinating antigen in fetuses of less than 70 days of age and antibody in stillborn or colostrum-deprived piglets and the sow. Current knowledge suggests that gilts should be exposed to the sow herd prior to mating in order to allow infection to occur and subsequent natural immunity to develop prior to the susceptible period in early pregnancy. Pigs may not lose maternal immunity for some months after birth and are resistant to infection during this period. There is evidence that incomplete herd immunity develops where sows are individually housed. The differential diagnosis of abortion, mummification and stillbirth in pigs is summarized in Table 63. *L. interrogans* serovar *icterohaemorrhagiae* infection may be confused with eperythrozoonosis because of the severe hemolytic anemia which is common to both diseases. Examination of blood smears reveals the presence of protozoa in erythrocytes in the latter.

Sheep and goats

Chronic copper poisoning and poisoning caused by rape in sheep may present a clinical picture similar to that in leptospirosis but there will be no febrile reaction. Anaplasmosis caused by *Anaplasma ovis* may be accompa-

Table 62. Differential diagnosis of diseases of cattle characterized by acute hemolytic anemia with or without hemoglobinuria

Disease	*Epidemiology*	*Clinical findings*	*Laboratory findings*
Leptospirosis	All ages, cattle on pasture	Acute fever, red-colored milk. Abortion. May die in 24–48 hours	Leptospira titers
Postparturient hemoglobinuria	High-producing lactating cows 4-6 weeks postpartum	Acute. No changes in milk. No fever. Die in 12–48 hours. Marked hemoglobinuria	Hypophosphatemia
Bacillary hemoglobinuria	Usually mature cattle on summer pasture in enzootic area	Acute fever, abdominal pain. May die in 2–4 days. Hemoglobinuria	Leukopenia or leukocytosis
Babesiosis	Enzootic areas, tick-borne, young animals	Acute fever, jaundice, abortion, course of 2–3 weeks. Marked hemoglobinuria	Blood smear, complement fixation test, transmission tests
Anaplasmosis	Yearling and mature cattle, common in summer, insect-borne, common in feedlots	*No* hemoglobinuria, jaundice common, fever	Anaplasms on blood smear, complement fixation test
Chronic copper poisoning	Follows longterm oral administration of medicines or feeds containing copper	Severe jaundice. No fever. Hemoglobinuria	Toxic levels of copper in blood, liver and feces
Cold-water hemolytic anemia of calves	Following consumption of large quantities of cold water after period of limited intake	Sudden onset within 1 hour after ingestion. No fever. May die in few hours. Hemoglobinuria	Acute hemolytic anemia
Rape and kale poisoning	All ages of cattle on rape crop grown for fodder in fall	Peracute hemolytic anemia, may die in few hours after onset. No fever. Hemoglobinuria	Acute hemolytic anemia
Drug-induced	Some drug preparations when given intravenously	Mild hemoglobinuria. No hemolytic anemia	Nil
Blood transfusion reaction	Using blood from same donor more than 1 week after initial transfusion	Sudden onset, dyspnea, hiccoughs, trembling, responds to adrenalin	Nil

The common causes of *hematuria* in cattle are pyelonephritis and cystitis due to *Corynebacterium renale*, non-specific cystitis and enzootic hematuria.

Myoglobinuria occurs occasionally in young cattle affected with enzootic-nutritional muscular dystrophy and may be confused with hemoglobinuria.

nied by fever and hemoglobinuria but is more commonly a chronic, emaciating disease.

Horses

Leptospirosis does not appear to occur commonly in newborn foals so that isoimmunization hemolytic anemia in this group is a much more likely cause of acute hemolytic disease. Infectious equine anemia, especially the peracute form, has clinical similarity to leptospirosis except that the latter is much milder and unlikely to be fatal. The myoglobinuria of azoturia must not be mistaken for the hemoglobinuria of leptospirosis. Abortion in mares is an important problem and although leptospirosis may be a cause, infection with the viruses of equine viral rhinopneumonitis and equine viral arteritis and with *Streptococcus genitalium* and *Salmonella abortusequi* are more common. Periodic ophthalmia is characterized by periodic attacks of panophthalmitis and blindness. Hypopyon due to other causes, for example, in foal septicemia due to *Str. genitalium*, is restricted to the anterior chamber. Conjunctivitis, keratitis and hypopyon may also occur in equine viral arteritis.

Treatment

The primary aim of treatment in all leptospiral infections is to control the infection before irreparable damage to the liver and kidneys occurs. This is best effected by treatment with streptomycin preferably, or one of the tetracyclines, as soon as possible after signs appear. The results of treatment are often disappointing because in most instances animals are presented for treatment only when the septicemia has subsided. The secondary aim of treatment is to control the leptospiruria of 'carrier' animals and render them safe to remain in the group. In this instance the shedding of leptospirae in the urine can be controlled but the microscopic agglutination titer is not affected.

Blood transfusions (5–10 liters/450 kg body weight) are indicated as treatment for the hemolytic anemia in acute leptospirosis in cattle. The clinical indications for a blood transfusion include obvious pallor of the mucous membranes, weakness and tachycardia.

For *L. interrogans* serovar *pomona* streptomycin (12 mg/kg body weight twice daily for 3 days) injected intramuscularly is effective in the treatment of the sys-

Table 63. Diagnostic summary of common causes of abortion, mummification and stillbirths in swine

Disease	*Epidemiology*	*Clinical features*	*Laboratory diagnosis*	
			Isolation of agent	*Serology*
Leptospirosis (*L. interrogans* serovar *pomona*)	Abortion last 2–3 weeks of gestation. Follows introduction of infected boar or sow or contamination of water supply	Abortion, sow systemically normal. Weak piglets sometimes	Fetal tissues and *urine of sow*	Positive or rising titers in aborting sows
Brucellosis (*Br. suis*)	Abortion may occur any time during gestation. Spread by coitus	Embryonic death, infertility, abortion. Orchitis in boars	Fetal injuries	Positive titers in herd
Porcine parvovirus infection	Herd outbreak when introduced for first time. Subsequently herd immunity develops and problem sporadic, affecting primarily gilts. May be continual low-grade problem in piggeries where sows are stalled. Due to incomplete spread	Abortion outbreaks possible. Mainly mummification, stillbirth and infertility. Sow clinically normal	Virus detectable by hemagglutinating antibody or fluorescent antibody in fetuses less than 16 cm crown–rump (C–R) length	Antibody present in fetuses greater than 16 cm C–R length. Antibody in high titer in sow
SMEDI virus	Poorly defined. Similar to parvovirus. Sporadic, affecting gilts primarily	Small litter size, uneven pigs and poor piglet viability, stillbirth and mummification. Infertility	Virus difficult to isolate from affected fetuses	Antibody in fetus, greater than 16 cm C–R length, and sow
Aujeszky's disease (pseudorabies)	Abortion usually 10–20 days after clinical illness. At any time but especially first 2 months of pregnancy. Concurrent or preceding clinical disease in young pigs in herd	Sows may show mild clinical disease at time of infection, anorexia, depression, transient pyrexia. Abortion or stillborn or mummified fetuses at term	Difficult. CNS and lungs of fetus and vaginal swab sow	Positive titers in herdmates
Hog cholera (swine fever)	Usually signs of clinical disease within piggery. Low virulence strains may produce reproductive/teratogenic effects only	Abortion of sows during or following acute clinical disease. Also embryonic death, small litter size, stillbirth and mummification. 'Trembling pigs' at birth may be only manifestation.	Fetal pigs and affected pigs within herd. Transmission studies	Positive titers in herds and resistant to challenge

Other agents such as *Erysipelothrix*, Japanese encephalitis virus, Japanese hemagglutinating virus, fungi, nutritional deficiency may produce abortion or reproductive inefficiency. Many outbreaks of abortion in sows remain undiagnosed and there must be important agents as yet unrecognized producing this syndrome.

temic infection. For the elimination of leptospiruria in cattle and pigs a single injection of streptomycin (25 mg/kg body weight) is recommended. In an outbreak of the disease in cattle the simultaneous treatment of all animals with dihydrostreptomycin at 25 mg/kg body weight and vaccination with the causative serotype bacterins has been successful in preventing new cases, and especially abortion when many pregnant cattle are involved. A similar approach is recommended for outbreaks in swine. Annual revaccination and regular serological testing for new infections, combined with controlling the source of new infections, will usually successfully control further outbreaks. A surveillance system in the area is necessary, however, to detect the introduction of new serotypes. In groups of pigs, the feeding of antibiotics provides a much simpler method of treatment than individual dosing. The feeding of oxytetracycline (800 g/tonne of feed for 8–11 days) is claimed to eliminate carriers (3). Antibiotic feeding should begin 1 month before farrowing to avoid the occurrence of abortion. Other experimental trials using long-acting tetracycline (31) by injection or tetracycline in the feed have been inconclusive and the use of mass feeding techniques as control programs should not be recommended lightly. Antibiotic feeding has also been suggested as a preventive measure in calves. The feeding of small amounts of tetracyclines (3 mg/kg body weight per day) for 7 days before and 14 days after exposure prevents the appearance of clinical signs but not infection as measured by the agglutination–lysis reaction.

Dihydrostreptomycin is not an effective treatment for *L. interrogans* serovar *hardjo*, failing to clear leptospirae from cattle (25 mg/kg body weight) genital tracts (81).

The treatment of periodic ophthalmia has undergone many changes in recent years and most recommended treatments have little effect on the course of the disease. A course of a suitable antibiotic systemically, and the administration of a corticosteroid, either parenterally in an acute episode, or subconjunctivally in a chronic case is most likely to be satisfactory. Atropine eye ointment is also usually applied three times daily to maintain dilatation of the pupil.

Control

The control of leptospirosis on an individual farm can take the form of eradication or of limitation of occurrence. Because of the development of serological methods of diagnosis, of vaccination, and pharmaceutical elimination of the carrier state, it is now reasonable to attempt eradication of the disease from individual herds, and possibly from areas. The principal hazard in such a scheme is the introduction of carrier animals of any species, or by reintroduction of the infection by rodents or other wildlife. It is because of this hazard that most programs aim at containment rather than eradication. In these circumstances where only sporadic cases occur, it might be more profitable to attempt to dispose of reactors or treat them to ensure that they no longer act as carriers.

A degree of immunity is likely to occur in pigs after natural infection, and when the disease is enzootic, 'herd immunity' may significantly decrease the ravages of the disease. This must be taken into account when assessing the results of vaccination.

Eradication

Detection and elimination of carrier animals presents some difficulties. Positive reactors to the microscopic agglutination test may not void infected urine and to determine their status as carriers necessitates repeated examination of their urine by culture and guinea-pig or hamster inoculation. For practical purposes, suspicious and positive reactors to the serum test should be considered as carriers and be culled or treated as described above unless examination of the urine can be carried out. In groups of pigs, it is probably advisable to consider the infection to be herd-wide and to treat all pigs as though they were carriers. In these circumstances the feeding of antibiotics, as described above, provides some protection although it is not guaranteed to eliminate the carrier state from the herd. Leptospirosis has been eradicated from commercial pig herds by injecting streptomycin at the rate of 25 mg/kg body weight intramuscularly into all pigs at the one time (36). However, if the pigs have been exposed to heavy infection not all of them are completely cleared of leptospiruria, and further injections of a heavier dose rate will be required to complete the elimination (50). Treatment of infected cows at this dose rate does not clear affected animals of the infection (21).

In cattle herds the procedure might seem simpler because of the easier identification of carriers. However, an eradication program is rarely if ever adopted. Some consideration must be given to the bulls because if they are infected they should not be used naturally or for artificial insemination even though the standard concentration of penicillin and streptomycin in the semen diluent is sufficient to ensure that no spread occurs.

If eradication is attempted and completed introduced animals should be required to pass a serological test on two occasions at least 2 weeks apart before allowing them to enter the herd. Urine examination for leptospirae should be carried out if practicable.

Containment

A program aimed at limiting the prevalence rate to a financially acceptable level is based on hygiene and vaccination.

Hygiene If the mediate source of infection is identifiable, in the form of yards, marshes and damp calf pens, every attempt must be made to avoid animal contact with the infected surroundings. Damp areas should be drained or fenced and pens disinfected after use by infected animals. The possibility that rats and other wild animals may act as a source of infection suggests that contact between them and farm animals should be controlled.

Vaccination Vaccination against leptospirosis in cattle and swine is now in general use and an effective method for control of the disease. The majority of vaccines are formalin-inactivated bacterins which contain one or more serotypes (37, 48, 51) and contains aluminum hydroxide. Vaccines containing Freund's complete adjuvant stimulate much higher serological responses, but do not provide additional protection (52). The immune response provided by the bacterins is serotype-specific and protection is dependent on the use of bacterins containing serotypes prevalent in the area. The bacterins stimulate the production of a low titer to the microscopic agglutination test which appears early and declines after several weeks, but protective immunity against the disease and renal infection has been demonstrated to last at least 12 months in cattle (38). Regular serological testing in herds which are being vaccinated annually can be used successfully to monitor new infections since these will stimulate a titer to the microscopic agglutination test. Vaccination as part of a herd health program should start with the calves at 4–6 months of age, followed by revaccination annually. Such programs should provide significant rises in calving rates, but have little or no effect on perinatal or postnatal losses. Vaccination of sows and gilts at the time of breeding with a bivalent vaccine, usually containing *L. interrogans* serovars *pomona* and *tarassovi*, protects them against infection and the development of leptospiruria (53) and is widely practiced, especially in large intensive piggeries (43).

There is no cross-immunity between *L. interrogans* serovars *pomona* and *hardjo*, and in areas where both diseases occur a bivalent vaccine is used routinely. If separate vaccines are used the *L. interrogans* serovar *pomona* vaccine should be administered at least once annually, but the *L. interrogans* serovar *hardjo* vaccine provides some protection against *L. interrogans* serovar *szwajizak*. There is a need to keep foreign proteins out of vaccines and special precautions are necessary in the production of *L. interrogans* serovar *hardjo* vaccines because of the organism's cultural requirements (27).

Vaccination of animals less than 3 months of age is unlikely to be effective and is not recommended (41), but vaccination of cows in late pregnancy gives effective immunity to their calves. This procedure appears to be less effective in sows although moderately good results are possible with an adjuvant vaccine (40).

The question of whether or not to vaccinate depends largely upon the cost of the procedure relative to the losses which can be anticipated. If the disease is spreading rapidly, as evidenced by the frequent appearance of clinical cases, a high range of titers or rising titers in a number of animals, all clinical cases and positive reactors should be treated, the negative animals vaccinated and the herd moved on the first day of treatment to a clean field. Retesting a group to determine the rate of spread would be an informative procedure but active measures must usually be commenced before this information is available. Another variation of this program, and a highly practical one, is the vaccination of all cattle in the herd, and the treatment with one injection of dihydrostreptomycin (25 mg/kg body weight) of all pregnant cows (54). In beef herds and dairy herds which calve seasonally this means treatment of the entire herd. The administration of streptomycin is with the objective of eliminating carriers of leptospira. This is not assured in the case of *L. interrogans* serovar *hardjo* (43). A still further circumstance in which vaccination is recommended, and has been shown to be very effective, is in the protection of animals continuously exposed to infection from wild-life, other domestic species, and particularly rodents. Surveys of the serological status of these groups are necessary before a decision to vaccinate can be made authoritatively.

If only sporadic cases occur, it might be more profitable to attempt to dispose of reactors or treat them to ensure that they no longer act as carriers. A degree of immunity is likely to occur in pigs after natural infection, and when the disease is enzootic, 'herd immunity' may significantly decrease the ravages of the disease. This must be taken into account when assessing the results of vaccination.

One of the theoretical disadvantages of vaccination against leptospirosis is the possible development of renal carrier animals which are sufficiently immune to resist systemic invasion but not colonization of the kidney, leading to the development of a carrier animal showing transient leptospiruria. It is accepted that this does occur but not sufficiently frequently to invalidate the vaccination as a procedure, but it would need to be kept in mind when considering breakdowns in vaccination programs. For example, this is recorded in pigs vaccinated with a bivalent *L. interrogans* serovars *pomona* and *tarassovi* vaccine which gave very good protection against abortion (57); it is also recorded in cattle (64), but the number of animals with leptospiruria is greatly reduced.

REVIEW LITERATURE

Armatredjo, A. & Campbell, R. S. F. (1975) Bovine leptospirosis. *Vet. Bull.*, *45*, 875.

Ellis, W. A. (1984) Bovine leptospirosis in the tropics; prevalence, pathogenesis and control. *Prev. vet. Med.*, *2*, 411–421.

Hanson, L. E. (1982) Leptospirosis in domestic animals: the public health perspective. *J. Am. vet. med. Assoc.*, *181*, 1505–1509.

Sullivan, N. D. (1974) Leptospirosis in animals and man. *Aust. vet. J.*, *50*, 216.

Thiermann, A. B. (1984) Leptospirosis. Current developments and trends. *J. Am. vet. med. Assoc.*, *184*, 722–725.

REFERENCES

(1) Ellis, W. A. & Michna, S. W. (1976) *Vet. Rec.*, *99*, 368, 387, 409, 430, 458.
(2) Sullivan, N. D. (1970) *Aust. vet. J.*, *46*, 121, 123, 125.
(3) Hathaway, S. C. & Blackmore, D. K. (1981) *NZ vet. J.*, *29*, 115.
(4) Smith, R. E. et al. (1965) *Cornell Vet.*, *55*, 412.
(5) Schowalter, D. B. et al. (1981) *Can. vet. J.*, *22*, 321.
(6) Salt, G. F. H. & Little, T. W. A. (1977) *Res. vet. Sci.*, *22*, 126.
(7) Cordes, D. D. et al. (1982) *NZ vet. J.*, *30*, 122.
(8) Nervig, R. M. et al. (1978) *Am. J. vet. Res.*, *39*, 523.
(9) Elder, J. & Ward, W. H. (1978) *Aust. vet. J.*, *54*, 297.
(10) Hellstrom, J. S. & Marshall, R. B. (1978) *Res. vet. Sci.*, *25*, 29.
(11) Holroyd, R. G. & Smith, P. C. (1976) *Aust. vet. J.*, *52*, 258.
(12) Spradbrow, R. B. & Seawright, A. A. (1963) *Aust. vet. J.*, *39*, 423.
(13) Ellis, W. A. et al. (1978) *Vet. Rec.*, *103*, 237.
(14) Cousins, D. V. & Robertson, G. M. (1986) *Aust. vet. J.*, *63*, 36.
(15) Davidson, J. & Hirsh, D. C. (1980) *J. Am. vet. med. Assoc.*, *176*, 124.
(16) Smith, R. E. & Armstrong, J. M. (1975) *J. Am. vet. med. Assoc.*, *167*, 739.
(17) Blackmore, D. N. et al. (1982) *NZ vet. J.*, *30*, 38.
(18) Hathaway, S. C. et al. (1981) *Vet. Rec.*, *108*, 396.
(19) Tripathy, D. N. et al. (1985) *Am. J. vet. Res.*, *46*, 2512 & 2515.
(20) Przytulski, T. & Porzcezkowska, D. (1980) *Br. vet. J.*, *136*, 25.
(21) Ellis, W. A. et al. (1985) *Res. vet. Sci.*, *39*, 292, 296.
(22) Andreani, E. et al. (1975) *Ann. Fac. Med. Vet. Univ. Pisa*, *27*, 33.
(23) Hodges, R. T. et al. (1979) *NZ vet. J.*, *27*, 101.
(24) Carpio, M. M. & Iverson, J. O. (1979) *Can. vet. J.*, *20*, 127.
(25) Hogg, G. A. (1974) *Aust. vet. J.*, *50*, 326.
(26) Hirschberg, N. & Vaughan, J. (1973) *Vet. Med. small Anim. Clin.*, *68*, 67.
(27) Broughton, E. S. et al. (1984) *Prev. vet. Med.*, *12*, 423.
(28) Thiermann, A. B. & Garrett, L. A. (1983) *Am. J. vet. Res.*, *44*, 884.
(29) Higgins, R. J. et al. (1980) *Vet. Rec.*, *107*, 307.
(30) Ellis, W. A. (1983) *Vet. Rec.*, *112*, 291.
(31) Ketterer, P. J. & Dunster, P. J. (1985) *Aust. vet. J.*, *62*, 348.
(32) McKeown, J. D. & Ellis, W. A. (1986) *Vet. Rec.*, *118*, 482.
(33) Breddle, J. R. & Hodges, R. T. (1977) *NZ vet. J.*, *25*, 56 & 65.
(34) Hathaway, S. C. et al. (1978) *J. Wild. Dis.*, *14*, 345.
(35) Hathaway, S. C. (1981) *NZ vet. J.*, 29, 121, 147.
(36) Dobson, K. J. (1950) *Aust. vet. J.*, *50*, 471.
(37) Durfee, P. T. & Presidente, P. J. A. (1977) *Aust. vet. J.*, *53*, 508.
(38) Killinger, A. H. et al. (1976) *Am. J. vet. Res.*, *37*, 93.
(39) Chappel, R. J. et al. (1985) *Aust. Adv. vet. Sci.*, p. 113.
(40) Chaudhary, R. K. et al. (1966) *Can. vet. J.*, *7*, 106, 121.
(41) Schollum, L. M. & Marshall, R. B. (1985) *NZ vet. J.*, *33*, 146.
(42) Slee, K. J. et al. (1983) *Aust. vet. J.*, *60*, 204.
(43) Ellis, W. A. et al. (1985) *Res. vet. Sci.*, *39*, 292.
(44) Gordon, L. M. (1980) *Aust. vet. J.*, *56*, 348.
(45) Ellis, W. A. et al. (1986) *Vet. Rec.*, *118*, 11.
(46) Blackmore, D. K. et al. (1981) *NZ vet. J.*, *29*, 19.
(47) Ellis, W. A. et al. (1986) *Vet. Rec.*, *118*, 563.
(48) Marshall, R. B. (1979) *NZ vet. J.*, *27*, 114.
(49) Stoenner, H. G. (1975) *Proc. 79th Ann. Mtg US Anim. Hlth Assoc.*, *79*, 145.
(50) Hodges, R. T. et al. (1979) *NZ vet. J.*, *27*, 124.
(51) Marshall, R. B. et al. (1979) *NZ vet. J.*, *27*, 169.
(52) Ris, D. R. & Hamel, K. L. (1979) *NZ vet. J.*, 27, 169.
(53) Hodges, R. T. et al. (1985) *NZ vet. J.*, *33*, 31.
(54) South, P. J. & Stoenner, H. G. (1974) *Proc. 78th Ann. Mtg US Anim. Hlth Assoc.*, *78*, 126.
(55) Tyndel, P. E. (1977) *NZ vet. J.*, *25*, 401.
(56) Thiermann, A. B. & Handsaker, A. L. (1985) *Am. J. vet. Res.*, *46*, 329.
(57) Whyte, P. B. D. et al. (1982) *Aust. vet. J.*, *59*, 41.
(58) Hathaway, S. C. et al. (1984) *Vet. Rec.*, *114*, 428.
(59) Hathaway, S. C. et al. (1984) *Vet. Rec.*, *115*, 623.
(60) Hathaway, S. C. et al. (1983) *Br. vet. J.*, *139*, 393.
(61) Ellis, W. A. et al. (1986) *Vet. Rec.*, *118*, 333.
(62) Flint, S. H. & Liardet, D. M. (1980) *NZ vet. J.*, *28*, 263.

(63) Dixon, R. J. (1983) *NZ vet. J.*, *31*, 107.
(64) Hancock, G. A. et al. (1984) *Aust. vet. J.*, *61*, 54.
(65) Ellis, W. A. et al. (1982) *Vet. Rec.*, *110*, 178.
(66) Ellis, W. A. et al. (1982) *Vet. Rec.*, *110*, 147, 193.
(67) Andreani, F. et al. (1983) *Br. vet. J.*, *139*, 165.
(68) Giles, N. et al. (1983) *Vet. Rec.*, *113*, 174.
(69) Thiermann, A. B. (1982) *Am. J. vet. Res.*, *43*, 780.
(70) Hathaway, S. C. et al. (1983) *Vet. Rec.*, *113*, 153.
(71) Slatter, D. H. & Hawkins, C. D. (1982) *Aust. vet. J.*, *59*, 84.
(72) Ellis, W. A. et al. (1983) *Equ. vet. J.*, *15*, 317.
(73) Swart, K. S. et al. (1982) *Aust. vet. J.*, *59*, 25.
(74) Ellis, W. A. et al. (1986) *Vet. Rec.*, *118*, 63.
(75) Ellis, W. A. et al. (1986) *Vet. Rec.*, *117*, 101.
(76) Elder, J. K. et al. (1985) *Aust. vet. J.*, *62*, 258.
(77) Ellis, W. A. et al. (1986) *Vet. Rec.*, *118*, 294.
(78) Hathaway, S. C. et al. (1980) *Vet. Rec.*, *119*, 84.
(79) Thompson, J. C. (1986) *J. comp. Pathol.*, *96*, 517 & 529.
(80) Elder, J. K. et al. (1986) *Prev. vet. Med.*, *3*, 501.
(81) Ellis, W. A. et al. (1985) *Res. vet. Sci.*, *39*, 292.
(82) Davidson, M. G. et al. (1987) *Equ. vet. J.*, *19*, 155.

Swine dysentery

Swine dysentery is a contagious disease of pigs caused by *Treponema hyodysenteriae* and characterized clinically and pathologically by a mucohemorrhagic colitis.

Etiology

Treponema hyodysenteriae, a large strongly beta-hemolytic spirochete, is considered the principal causative agent (3). The morphological characteristics of the pathogenic and non-pathogenic spirochetes from the feces from normal and infected pigs have been described (2). Since the original description of this organism, it has been identified from cases of swine dysentery from several countries and the isolates appear identical (4). The disease has been reproduced with pure cultures of *T. hyodysenteriae* in conventional and specific-pathogen-free (SPF) pigs. Challenge of gnotobiotic pigs with pure cultures results in colonization of the organism (1) but disease does not occur until other intestinal organisms are given which suggests that the disease is the result of a mixed synergistic infection of the spirochete and other intestinal anerobic organisms (3, 4). Experimentally, the oral inoculation of gnotobiotic pigs with a combination of *T. hyodysenteriae* and *Bacteroides vulgatus* or *Fusobacterium necrophorum* will result in the development of the characteristic clinical signs and lesions of swine dysentery (3). These results and others (15) are consistent with the concept that *T. hyodysenteriae* is the primary causative agent of swine dysentery and that the presence of one or more other anaerobes is a prerequisite for expression of pathogenicity of *T. hyodysenteriae*. This prerequisite can be met by a variety of anaerobes. Other spirochetes which are antigenically and biochemically distinct from *T. hyodysenteriae* may cause diarrhea and dysentery in pigs similar to that associated with swine dysentery (5).

Non-pathogenic isolates of *T. hyodysenteriae* have been isolated from the feces of swine and dogs and an isolated colonic loop challenge has been described as a test for pathogenicity (6, 16). Pathogenic strains may also be differentiated on the basis of the type of hemolysis they produce on blood agar (7).

Epidemiology

Swine dysentery has been reported from most major pig-producing countries (14) and it is one of the most important and prevalent diseases in pigs. The disease can cause heavy mortality in growing pigs but it is also equally important for its effect on production efficiency (15, 16). The subclinical economic losses from decreased feed efficiency are estimated at four times the cost of medication. The infection tends to be persistent within a herd and may have a cyclic occurrence (18), which poses a problem in intensive pig-rearing enterprises and frequently control can be achieved only by costly continuous prophylactic medication. It is most prevalent in the 7–16-week-old age group but may affect older and occasionally adult pigs and rarely suckling piglets. Clinical disease may initially be precipitated by stress but it subsequently spreads by direct contract. The organism is present in the feces of affected pigs and an asymptomatic carrier status with shedding during a period of stress has been demonstrated.

Pigs which have recovered from clinical disease with or without treatment may become carriers and shed the organism and infect in-contact animals for 50–90 days (9, 10). The frequency of shedding varies with time and only a small proportion of a convalescent population may be expected to be carriers. The feeding of sodium arsanilate to pigs previously exposed to and treated for swine dysentery can induce non-diarrheic carrier animals into developing a swine dysentery diarrhea. This has the potential of identifying carrier pigs (8).

Treated and untreated convalescent pigs develop elevated serum agglutinin titers that are maintained as long as 150 days after infection (10). Carrier pigs shed *T. hyodysenteriae* while elevated agglutination titers against the organism are present. The relationship between the magnitude of the agglutinin titers and protective immunity is not clear.

Untreated pigs which recover from swine dysentery are resistant to experimental challenge for up to 16–17 weeks (11). In herds affected with swine dysentery the disease may reappear at 3–4 week intervals following therapeutic treatment. Treatment with the more efficacious drugs may inhibit the development of immunity. It is presumed that infection is perpetuated within piggeries and spread between piggeries by carrier pigs but it is unknown if other species are involved. Epidemiological evidence indicates that most outbreaks occur in herds which have purchased infected animals from herds known to have the disease (49). Following experimental transmission the incubation period is generally between 10 and 16 days, but outbreaks following the introduction of presumed carrier pigs into a herd may have a considerably longer delay period.

The organism has been isolated from a dog on a swine farm where swine dysentery was present (12). Experimentally, mice are susceptible to the infection and may be a potential source of infection in a piggery (18). They are capable of carrying the organism for up to 180 days after inoculation.

The factors that affect the survival of the organism in the feces of affected pigs have been examined (13). The organism can survive for up to 48 days in dysenteric feces at 0–10°C (32–50°F); survival was reduced to 7 days at 25°C (77°F) and to less than 24 hours at 37°C (98·6°F). Dilution of dysenteric feces with tap water

1:10 enhanced survival to 61 days at 5°C (41°F). Drying and disinfection rapidly eliminated the organism from the environment. Phenolic and sodium hypochlorite disinfectants are most effective. The organism has been isolated from the lagoon of a waste-handling system of a swine farm which could be partially responsible for maintenance of swine dysentery within a herd (12).

The influence of diet on experimental swine dysentery has been examined. A deficiency of vitamin E and selenium will decrease the resistance of pigs to the experimental disease (17). Pigs fed a diet deficient in selenium may be more susceptible to the effects of experimental swine dysentery than pigs given a daily supplement of 0·4 mg of selenium (17).

Infection is by ingestion and it is enhanced by conditions leading to oral–fecal cycling. The spread within a group is slow, taking up to 7–14 days, and the disease may spread to involve adjacent or other pens of pigs over a 2–3-week period. The morbidity within a group of pigs may approach 100% and if the disease is untreated a case fatality rate of up to 50% is not uncommon.

Pathogenesis

Multiplication of the organism and invasion of the colonic crypts leads to the production of the disease. The experimental inoculation of a pure culture of, or colonic contents containing, *T. hyodysenteriae* into the pigs with intact colons or into ligated colonic segments leads to an acute erosive colitis (19). There is progressive erosion of superficial epithelium, excess mucus production, edema and hemorrhage of the lamina propria and pseudomembrane production. It is not clear how the organism produces the lesion; a cytotoxin was not present in cell-free filtrates of spirochetal broth cultures or colonic content from pigs with swine dysentery (19). The erosive colitis is the cause of the diarrhea, dysentery and excessive quantities of mucus in the feces.

The large absorptive capacity of the colon is abolished while that of the small intestine remains intact (20). Swine dysentery is a colonic malabsorption syndrome (20). Up to 50% of the extracellular fluid volume of the pig is presented daily to the colon; the colon of the 40 kg pig is capable of an absorptive capacity of 1.5 mol/day of sodium ion and 8.6 l/day of water (20).

Death usually results from chronic dehydration and bacterial toxemia. In some animals an acute shock syndrome results in rapid and sudden death.

Clinical findings

Most commonly the disease initially affects only a few pigs within the group but spreads over a period of a few days to 2 weeks to involve the majority. Affected pigs show moderate fever, slight depression and some reduction in appetite. The feces are characteristic. They are only partially formed, usually of a porridge-like consistency and are passed without apparent conscious effort and splatter on contact with the pen floor. Affected pigs commonly defecate almost anywhere and on anything in the pen. The feces are light gray to black and on close inspection much mucus is present and flecks of blood and epithelial casts may be seen. In some pigs the presence of larger amounts of blood will discolor the feces accordingly. The occurrence of blood in the feces generally occurs 2–3 days after the initial onset of diarrhea. Affected pigs become progressively dehydrated and their abdomens appear gaunt and sunken. Death usually occurs some days to weeks after the initial onset of signs and results primarily from dehydration and toxemia. Pigs with a severe hemorrhagic diarrhea die more quickly. Skin discoloration is not a feature except in the terminal stages. In untreated pigs the disease may persist for 3–4 weeks before clinical recovery. Less commonly an outbreak may start with the sudden death of one or two pigs with no evidence of premonitory signs or a terminal hemorrhagic diarrhea. This occurs more commonly in market age pigs and adults in herds where swine dysentery has been introduced for the first time. It also is a rare cause of sporadic death of gilts and sows in conventional herds. The disease responds well to treatment but following withdrawal of treatment the disease may recur within the same group of pigs. A chronic form of the disease with persistent diarrhea and failure to grow occurs in some pigs with irreversible lesions of the colonic mucosa.

Clinical pathology

The organism may be demonstrated in the feces of affected pigs by dark-field microscopy as highly motile organisms with a characteristic serpentine motility or in dried smears with Giemsa or Victoria blue 4R staining (21, 25). Fecal samples submitted for laboratory examination should be diluted 1:10 in phosphate buffered saline or rectal swabs placed in Amies medium to avoid death of the organisms which will occur when the samples are stored at room temperature or sent in the post (50). It may be difficult to culture the organism from pigs which have been on medication and the direct fluorescent antibody test may be more reliable (23). The use of selective culture techniques is more sensitive than the fluorescenct techniques when the pigs have not been medicated.

Fluorescent antibody staining aids considerably in its demonstration, but may not distinguish non-pathogenic strains (7). This presumptive diagnosis can be supplemented with a variety of laboratory tests which serve to identify the spirochetes as pathogenic. A rapid slide agglutination test is available which will identify and distinguish the organism from other spirochetes (22). An enzymatic reaction testing system can be used to differentiate between strains related to swine dysentery and those unrelated (24). A disk growth-inhibition test for differentiating *T. hyodysenteriae* from other intestinal spirochetes has been described (28).

A major diagnostic problem has been the identification of carrier pigs which are infected with the organism and are a potential source of infection to other pigs. Indirect and direct fluorescent antibody tests used to examine feces and colonic material from pigs for *T. hyodysenteriae* have not been sensitive or specific enough to identify individual infected pigs (30).

Several serologic tests have been developed and used to assist in the identification of carrier pigs infected with the organism. The enzyme-linked immunosorbent assay (ELISA) test and the microtitration agglutination test (MAT) have been compared and the ELISA is considered to give the highest sensitivity for the detection of herds affected with swine dysentery (30). The microtitration serum agglutination test is useful for diagnosis on a herd basis but lacks sensitivity for diagnosis in individual pigs. In individual pigs the ELISA titer is detectable 1–2 weeks after infection, peaks at 3 weeks and remains at a high level for up to 19 weeks (51). An indirect fluorescent antibody test for the measurement of serum anti-*T. hyodysenteriae* antibodies is also available (52).

Biological tests may be used to test the enteropathogenicity of isolates of *T. hyodysenteriae*. A multiple-ligated swine-colonic-loop system is a rapid, economical method (27). A mouse test will differentiate between *T. hyodysenteriae* and *T. innocens* (26).

Necropsy findings

Colitis, typhlitis and usually hyperemia of the fundus of the stomach are present in pigs that die from swine dysentery. The colitis is initially present in the coils of the colon in the region of the apex but subsequently spreads to involve the whole colon and the cecum (9). In the early stages there is inflammation and necrosis with varying degrees of hemorrhage into the lumen. The submucosal glands are enlarged and frequently visible through the serosa of the colon as opaque spots. In advanced cases there is a fibrinonecrotic diphtheritic membrane and a rough reddened granular appearance at the mucosal surface. Intestinal contents may be adherent. The draining lymph nodes are enlarged and congested. There is no abnormality in the small intestine except for the terminal ileum in advanced cases. Spirochetes may be demonstrated in large numbers in smears from the mucosal surface of these lesions, especially in early cases, but there is no systemic invasion.

Electron microscopic examination of the colon of pigs with swine dysentery revealed changes indicative of stasis in the microcirculatory vessels of the lamina propria (29). The earliest colonic lesion consists of superficial vascular congestion and dilatation, edema of the lamina propria and intracellular separation of the epithelial cells at the crypt shoulders. This lesion progresses to epithelial cell necrosis and extrusion and extravasation of red blood cells into the lumen. Degeneration, necrosis and extrusion of superficial colonic enterocytes follows progressively. The spirochetes also penetrate into the superficial colonic enterocytes. The characteristic lesion of swine dystentery is necrosis of the superficial epithelium of the colon.

Large spirochetes are present in the crypts, free in the cytoplasm of damaged epithelial cells and in cavities around vessels of the lamina propria. The necrosis of the colonic mucosa may be due to disturbances in the microcirculation of the lamina propria.

Pigs which do not fully recover following the use of drugs for the treatment of swine dysentery may develop chronic colonic lesions consisting of enlarged lymphoid nodules adjacent to the submucosal glands in the colon which are enlarged and visible on the serosal surface as 'white spots' (44). These lesions often contain the organism which, following withdrawal of medication, may proliferate and produce clinical disease.

Diagnosis

Swine dysentery must be differentiated from other diseases in which there is diarrhea in growing pigs. These include coliform gastroenteritis, salmonellosis and hog cholera. With all of these diseases the onset and spread within a group is much more sudden and rapid than with swine dysentery and death occurs earlier. With coliform gastroenteritis and salmonellosis the initial sign of disease may be the finding of dead or severely sick pigs with fever, skin discoloration, anorexia and a profuse watery diarrhea. Swine dysentery is more insidious in onset, the appetite is rarely completely lost and the feces are soft and mucohemorrhagic. There are also epidemiological differences in the occurrence of hog cholera and coliform gastroenteritis and swine dysentery. Coliform gastroenteritis has a close association with weaning whereas hog cholera occurs in all ages of pig. At necropsy the lesions of swine dysentery are confined to the large intestine whereas in coliform gastroenteritis, salmonellosis and hog cholera lesions are also present in the small intestine and other organs. Other diseases may result in the passage of bloody feces. The intestinal hemorrhage syndrome generally persists as a severe hemorrhagic diarrhea with rapid death rather than as a chronic syndrome but pathological differentiation may be necessary. Chronic hemorrhage due to an esophagastric ulcer results in melena, the epidemiological findings are different, and the necropsy findings are characteristic.

Treatment

Treatment for swine dysentery is usually administered to all pigs within the group. Treatment by water medication rather than feed medication is preferable in that it is generally easier and faster to institute. On the other hand feed medication is suitable for prophylaxis. When outbreaks of the disease occur the usual course of action is to treat severely affected pigs individually, medicate the drinking water or feed (preferably the water) for several days at therapeutic levels and continue medication in the feed for up to 3 weeks or longer at prophylactic levels. Pigs with severe hemorrhagic diarrhea and toxemia may not drink sufficient medicated water and should be treated initially by parenteral injection.

Several antimicrobials are suitable for the treatment and control of swine dysentery and the choice is largely dependent on availability, cost, efficacy and the regional individual withdrawal regulations. The concentrations recommended for feed and water are shown in Table 64.

Organic arsenicals are the least expensive and are recommended as the first drug of choice. When given in either the feed or water there is a risk of toxicity. The general recommendation is to administer the medication for a 7-day period and then withdraw it for a 7-day period before reintroduction. However, this is frequently impractical and continuous medication at 250 ppm in the feed is often used as follow-up therapy. Poisoning does not usually occur below levels of 500 ppm but it has occurred at levels as low as 200 ppm where continuous medication is practiced, and constant surveillance for signs of toxicity is necessary. While resistance to organic arsenicals has been suspected it has not been documented.

Table 64. Suggested dose rates of drugs for treatment and control of swine dysentery

Drug	*Treatment*		*Control*
	Water (mg/4 liters)	*Feed* (mg/kg)	*Feed* (mg/kg)
Organic arsenicals			
Sodium arsanilate	700	—	—
Arsanilic acid	—	150–250	90–150
3-Nitro-4-hydroxyphenyl-arsonate	540	—	—
Tiamulin (31)	240	—	40
Tylosin (37)	500–1000	—	100
3-Acetyl-4″-isovaleryltylosin (61)	—	—	55 or 110
Virginiamycin (32)	—	100	25–100
Lincomycin–spectinomycin (33, 39)	264	110	44
Carbadox (38)	—	50	50
Nitroimidazoles			
Dimetridazole (41)	1000	300–500	100–250
Ipronidazole (35, 36)	200–400	1000	100
Ronidazole	240	120	60–120

N.B.: All water treatment should be given for 5–7 days. Feed medication for treatment should continue for at least 14 days and preferably 21 days. Drug withdrawal periods and legality should be determined according to local regulation. Prophylactic levels may be permitted on a continuous basis until shortly before the pigs are sent to slaughter.

Feeding sodium arsanilate at 200 ppm for 21 days to non-diarrheic swine previously exposed to and treated for swine dysentery can result in the development of clinical swine dysentery (8). This technique may be useful for the identification of carrier pigs in a herd. Tiamulin given once at a dose of 10–15 mg/kg body weight intramuscularly is effective for the treatment of acute cases, recovery often occurring within 24 hours (53). Tiamulin in the drinking water of clinically affected pigs at a dose of 45 or 60 mg/l of water for 5 days is efficacious (54). Treated pigs improved clinically and returned to normal and the average daily gains and feed efficiency were significantly better than untreated controls (54). There was also evidence that the organism could not be found in the feces of treated pigs after the treatment period. Tiamulin at a dose rate of 20 ppm in the feed for 4–6 weeks is reported to be effective for the control and prevention of the naturally occurring disease (57).

There appear to be some differences in the efficacy of different drugs and there is evidence that the duration of diarrhea following the start of medication with nitroimidazole compounds or lincomycin–spectinomycin is less than that with drugs such as carbadox or the organic arsenicals. Also, relapses immediately following the withdrawal of treatment may be less common.

The evaluation of the efficacy of drugs for the treatment and control of swine dysentery has been a major problem because of variations in experimental designs. An experimental model has been recommended which provides a critical evaluation of the prophylactic efficacy of drugs under the most severe conditions, comparable with those frequently found in commercial pig production facilities (42). The model is a combination of a single oral infection plus pen contamination each day for 25 days which produces consistent, homogeneous, and severe swine dysentery with 100% morbidity and 92% case fatality (42).

Using this system, carbadox alone at 50 mg/kg of feed for 30 days or carbadox combined with sulfamethazine at 100 mg/kg of feed for 30 days is effective in preventing swine dysentery during the infection plus medication period and during the postmedication period (43). Other drugs are less successful in preventing the disease during infection or during the postmedication period (43). Lincomycin at 11 mg/kg body weight or tylosin at 8·8 mg/kg body weight intramuscularly daily for 3 days for both drugs and up to 7 days for lincomycin are effective (34). A 1:1 mixture of lincomycin–spectinomycin given orally at a dose of 66 ppm in the feed for 8 days followed by a level of 44 ppm for 20 days was successful for the treatment of the disease in adult swine (56).

The major problems with the treatment of swine dysentery are the failure of some outbreaks of the disease to respond favorably to treatment, and relapses or new cases which may occur following withdrawal of medication of the feed or water. Several drug-related problems have been postulated to explain these problems (44). *Drug-delayed* swine dysentery occurs several days after withdrawal of medicated feed. It may be due to either an ineffective drug or inadequate dosage of an effective drug and failure to eliminate the causative organism from the colon. However, reinfection from other swine must also be considered. The nitroimidazoles at high levels will apparently prevent the delay or recurrence of dysentery (44).

In experimentally induced swine dysentery using colon from affected pigs as the oral inoculums, tiamulin in the drinking water at 45 or 60 mg/l for 5 days was also effective in treating clinical disease. However, diarrhea commonly recurred 2–10 days after withdrawal of the drug and repeated medication of the water with tiamulin was necessary to reduce the severity of diarrhea and prevent deaths. After one to three retreatments, the pigs were immune to experimental exposure and there was a significant increase in their serum anti-*Treponema hyodysenteriae* antibodies (55). This supports the observation that when certain antimicrobial agents such as dimetridazole, which are highly effective in preventing the development of diarrhea, after being withdrawn, the affected pigs do not become immune.

Drug-diminished swine dysentery occurs when suboptimal levels of the drug are used. The severity of the diarrhea is reduced; deaths do not occur, but the disease is not eliminated. However, severe disease may follow withdrawal of medication.

The feeding of ronidazole at 60 ppm for 10 weeks, or carbadox at 55 ppm or lincomycin at 110 ppm for 6 weeks eliminated an experimental infection, and swine dysentery did not recur during a 9-week period after withdrawal of the medication (58). The feeding of sodium arsanilate at a level of 220 ppm for 3 weeks to pigs which had been fed ronidazole for only 6 weeks did cause the development of swine dysentery.

In both drug-delayed and drug-diminished swine dysentery there are chronic lesions in colon. In *drug-resistant* swine dysentery, medication of the feed is not effective and diarrhea and deaths occur. Certain outbreaks of the disease may be resistant to both tylosin and sodium arsanilate. Selection of an effective drug is necessary. The sensitivity of *T. hyodysenteriae* to dimetridazole has not decreased significantly following use of the drug over several years (46).

A more severe form of the drug-resistant disease is *drug-augmented* swine dysentery in which affected pigs are more severely affected than non-medicated controls. The cause is unknown. In *drug-delayed–augmented* swine dysentery the disease occurs in a severe form several days or weeks following withdrawal of successful medication for a previous outbreak of the disease. This form appears to occur most commonly in pigs which did not have clinical disease during an earlier outbreak, but received medication. The concentration of drug administered was sufficient to prevent diarrhea, but not sufficient to eliminate the spirochetes from the colon. During the delay of the initial diarrhea by the drug, there may have been intraglandular recolonization of spirochetes throughout the colon. After withdrawal of medication rapid intraglandular multiplication of the large spirochetes may occur and result in clinical disease. Drug-delayed–augmented dysentery usually occurs only in those pigs which have been infected but did not develop clinical disease which usually results in immunity. The occurrence of diarrhea is necessary for its development which occurs 4–13 weeks after infection (45). Treatment of swine dysentery with the more efficacious drugs has been shown to inhibit the development of this immunity and serum antibody to *T. hyodysenteriae* (46). However, the clinical significance of this is undermined and at present it is suggested that outbreaks of swine dysentery be treated vigorously.

It should be possible to minimize these drug-related problems of swine dysentery by the use of therapeutic levels of effective drugs in the drinking water for short periods followed by prophylactic levels in the feed for 3 or more weeks. This must be combined with proper management techniques and waste disposal systems which minimize or prevent reexposure.

Regardless of the drug used many pigs are reinfected following withdrawal of medication because of the continual presence of the organism in the environment. The sources of the organism include in-contact carrier pigs which are shedding the organism and survival of the organism in waste materials, which was presented under epidemiology.

After the institution of treatment thorough cleansing of the contaminated pen should be instituted. This is usually done after 3–6 days when all diarrhea has ceased. The decision to continue with prophylactic medication depends upon the hygiene and a knowledge of past patterns of the disease on the farm. It is generally wise to continue prophylaxis for at least 2 weeks.

Control

Effective control of swine dysentery is dependent on elimination of the source of the organism from affected pigs, the prevention of reinfection and avoidance of the introduction of carrier animals into herds considered free of the disease. The reduction of the stress of transportation and overcrowding is also necessary. The prevention of a build-up of fecal wastes is also of paramount importance.

Elimination of the organism from a group of affected pigs is accomplished by early treatment with adequate levels of drugs for a sufficient length of time. This must be combined with adequate removal of fecal wastes to prevent reinfection. Pigs destined for market should be moved out as a group and their pens cleaned, disinfected and allowed to dry for a few days before restocking with pigs. Where possible the purchase of feeder pigs should be restricted to private sales from herds with no history of the disease. Communal trucks should not be used for transport. Where this is not possible pigs should be placed in isolation pens for 3 weeks and provided with medicated feed or water to eliminate the carrier state in infected pigs. Every effort should be made to avoid potential oral–fecal cycles and contamination by feces between pens. Pigs from different source farms should not be grouped in the same pen.

In farrowing-to-market enterprises where the disease is always a threat, routine prophylactic medication may also be necessary. This is commonly done following weaning and during the early growing phase. In countries where withdrawal periods are in force the use of drugs such as carbadox is precluded for this purpose.

Eradication of swine dysentery from closed swine herds may be possible (48). Lincomycin at 4 mg/kg body weight as a top-dressing to feed is given to the sows and gilts for 3–6 weeks. The weaned pigs are given lincomycin at 110 g/tonne of feed between 18 days and 6 weeks of age. Following the use of lincomycin, dimetridazole was used at the rate of 200 ppm in the feed for 6 months.

The feeding of tiamulin at a dose of 20 mg/kg body weight to pregnant sows beginning 10 days before farrowing and continued until 5 days after farrowing when the piglets are weaned and transferred to an isolation unit has been successful in the prevention of infection of newborn piglets (59). This is known as the *barrier method* which can be an efficient method of eradicating endemic infections. To reduce the risk of postnatal infection of the progeny, the piglets should stay with the latently infected sows for the shortest possible time. Thus early weaning is necessary and strict isolation is an important condition of success. *T. hyodysenteriae* is spread primarily by carrier pigs, and contact between infected and uninfected pigs must be avoided.

With the proper use of drugs, effective sanitation, serial depopulation of possible carrier animals and the introduction of non-infected animals, it should be possible to virtually eradicate the infection from a herd.

The disease is eliminated by SPF (specific-pathogen-free) techniques and herds established in this manner and maintained closed should remain free of the disease, but breakdowns do occur without known cause. A major problem exists where it is necessary to introduce new genetic material into a herd which is free of the disease. Serious consideration should be given to the use of semen for this purpose because of the risk of breakdown with the introduction of live pigs. There is need for a test to identify the asymptomatic carrier of the cause of swine dysentery.

A control scheme for swine dysentery has been supervised by the Pig Health Control Association in Britain (60). To qualify, there must not be any clinical signs of swine dysentery or, if any suspicious signs are noticed, laboratory tests for *T. hyodysenteriae* must be negative. In addition, a list of pharmaceutical compounds which might mask the disease or its laboratory diagnosis may not be used routinely after weaning, either for treatment or control. Qualifying herds can import pigs only from other qualifying herds or by hysterectomy/hysterotomy or embryo transfer methods. Artificial insemination is also permitted; over a period of 6 years the scheme has been highly successful.

There is as yet no available vaccine for swine dysentery. Pigs which have recovered from clinical swine dysentery may be protected against subsequent challenge (10, 45), but attempts to immunize pigs with *Treponema hyodysenteriae* revealed incomplete protection (47) and have involved complex procedures which may have limited practical value (46). The serum from pigs which have recovered from swine dysentery will protect intestinal loops from experimental inoculating with *T. hyodysenteriae* (62). The immunization of pigs with formolized *T. hyodysenteriae* in an oil adjuvant reduced the incidence, severity and duration of swine dysentery and also weight loss compared to control groups (62).

REVIEW LITERATURE

Fernie, D. S. (1983) A review of swine dysentery vaccines. *Pig vet. Soc. Proc.*, *110*, 63–74.

Lysons, R. J. (1979) Swine dysentery. *Br. vet. J.*, *135*, 395.

Meyer, R. C. (1978) Swine dysentery: a perspective. *Adv. vet. Sci. comp. Med.*, *22*, 133–158.

Taylor, D. (1979) Swine dysentery. *In Practice*, *1*, No. 2, 4–9.

Windsor, R. S. (1979) Swine dysentery. *Vet. Ann.*, *19*, 89–96.

REFERENCES

(1) Brandenburg, A. C. et al. (1977) *Can. J. comp Med.*, *41*, 294.
(2) Elazhary, M. A. S. Y. et al. (1978) *Can. J. comp. Med.*, *42*, 302.
(3) Harris, D. L. et al. (1978) *J. Am. vet. med. Assoc.*, *172*, 468.
(4) Harris, D. L. (1974) *J. Am. vet. med. Assoc.*, *164*, 809.
(5) Taylor, D. J. et al. (1980) *Vet. Rec.*, *106*, 326.
(6) Lysons, R. J. (1979) *Br. vet. J.*, *135*, 395.
(7) Kenyon, J. M. et al. (1977) *Infect. Immun.*, *15*, 638.
(8) Olson, L. D. & Rodabaugh, D. E. (1986) *Can. J. vet. Res.*, *50*, 359.
(9) Griffin, R. M. & Hutchings, D. A. (1980) *Vet. Rec.*, *107*, 559.
(10) Fisher, L. F. & Olander, H. J. (1981) *Am. J. vet. Res.*, *42*, 450.
(11) Joens, L. A. et al. (1979) *Am. J. vet. Res.*, *40*, 1352.
(12) Sanger, J. G. et al. (1978) *J. Am. vet. med. Assoc.*, *172*, 464.
(13) Chia, S. P. & Taylor, D. J. (1978) *Vet. Rec.*, *103*, 68.
(14) Meyer, R. C. (1978) *Adv. vet. Sci. comp. Med.*, *22*, 133.
(15) Whipp, S. C. et al. (1979) *Infect. Immun.*, *26*, 1042.
(16) Kenyon, J. M. & Harris, D. L. (1979) *Int. J. syst. Bacteriol.*, *29*, 102.
(17) Teige, J. Jr. et al. (1984) *Acta vet. Scand.*, *25*, 1.
(18) Joens, L. A. (1980) *Am. J. vet. Res.*, *41*, 1225.
(19) Wilcock, B. P. & Olander, H. J. (1979) *Vet. Pathol.*, *16*, 450.
(20) Schmall, L. M. et al. (1983) *Am. J. vet. Res.*, *44*, 1309.
(21) Harris, D. L. (1974) *J. Am. vet. med. Assoc.*, *164*, 809.
(22) Burrows, M. R. & Lemcke, R. M. (1981) *Vet. Rec.*, *108*, 187.
(23) Smith, H. F. et al. (1985) *Vet. Q.*, 7, 150.
(24) Hunter, D. & Wood, T. (1979) *Vet. Rec.*, *104*, 383.
(25) Olson, L. D. (1978) *Vet. med. SAC*, *73*, 80.
(26) Joens, L. A. et al. (1980) *Vet. Rec.*, *107*, 527.
(27) Whipp, S. C. et al. (1978) *Am. J. vet. Res.*, *39*, 1293.
(28) Lemcke, R. M. & Burrows, M. R. (1979) *Vet. Rec.*, *104*, 548.
(29) Albassam, M. A. et al. (1985) *Can. J. comp. Med.*, *49*. 384.
(30) Egan, I. T. et al. (1983) *Am. J. vet. Res.*, *44*, 1323.
(31) Taylor, D. J. (1980) *Vet. Rec.*, *106*, 526.
(32) Olson, L. D. & Rodabaugh, D. E. (1977) *Am. J. vet. Res.*, *38*, 1485.
(33) Hambdy, A. H. (1978) *Am. J. vet. Res.*, *39*, 1175.
(34) Hambdy, A. H. & Kratza, D. D. (1981) *Am. J. vet. Res.*, *42*, 178.
(35) Messersmith, R. E. et al. (1976) *Vet med. small Anim. Clin.*, *71*, 343.
(36) Olson, L. D. & Rodabaugh, D. E. (1977) *Am. J. vet. Res.*, 38, 1289.
(37) Miller, C. R. et al. (1972) *Vet. Med. small Anim. Clin.*, *67*, 1246.
(38) Rainier, R. H. et al. (1980) *Am. J. vet. Res.*, *41*, 1349.
(39) Coulson, A. (1981) *Vet. Rec.*, 108, 503.
(40) Griffin, R. M. (1979) *Vet. Rec.*, *104*, 73.
(41) Windsor, R. S. (1979) *Vet. Ann.*, *19*, 89.
(42) Raynaud, J. P. et al. (1981) *Am. J. vet. Res.*, *42*, 49.
(43) Raynaud, J. P. et al. (1981) *Am. J. vet. Res.*, *42*, 51.
(44) Olson, L. D. & Rodabough, D. E. (1978) *J. Am. vet. med. Assoc.*, *173*, 843.
(45) Olson, L. D. & Rodabough, D. E. (1976) *Am. J. vet. Res.*, *37*, 757, 763, 769.
(46) Fernie, D. S. (1983) *Pig vet. Soc. Proc.*, *10*, 63.
(47) Fernie, D. S. et al. (1983) *Res. vet. Sci.*, *35*, 217.
(48) Tasker, J. B. et al. (1981) *Vet. Rec.*, *108*, 382.
(49) Windsor, R. S. & Simmons, J. R. (1981) *Vet. Rec.*, *109*, 482.
(50) Taylor, D. J. et al. (1985) *Vet Rec.*, *116*, 48.
(51) Joens, L. A. et al. (1982) *J. clin. Microbiol.*, *15*, 249.
(52) Schlink, G. T. & Olson, L. D. (1983) *Can. J. comp. Med.*, *47*, 320.
(53) Burch, D. G. S. et al. (1983) *Vet. Rec.*, *113*, 236.
(54) Pickles, R. W. (1982) *Vet. Rec.*, *110*, 403.
(55) Olson, L. D. (1986) *J. Am. vet. med. Assoc.*, *188*, 1165.
(56) van Leengoed, L. A, M. G. et al. (1985) *Vet. Q.*, 7, 146.
(57) Burch, D. G. S. (1982) *Vet. Rec.*, *110*, 244.
(58) Olson, L. D. (1986) *Can. J. vet. Res.*, *50*, 365.
(59) Meszaros, J. et al. (1985) *Vet. Rec.*, *116*, 8.
(60) Goodwin, R. F. W. & Whittlestone, P. (1984) *Vet. Rec.*, *115*, 240.
(61) Jacks, T. M. et al. (1986) *Am. J. vet. Res.*, *47*, 2325.
(62) Joens, L. A. et al. (1985) *Am. J. vet. Res.*, *46*, 2369.

Ulcerative granuloma (necrotic ulcer)

Ulcerative granuloma is an infectious disease of pigs caused by the spirochete, *Borrelia suilla* (1), and characterized by the development of chronic ulcers of the skin and subcutaneous tissues.

It occurs most commonly under conditions of poor hygiene in Australia and New Zealand and is recorded in the United Kingdom (2, 3).

Lesions occur on the central abdomen of sows and on the face of sucking pigs, suggesting infection of cutaneous or mucosal abrasions as the portal of entry.

Initially the lesions are small, hard, fibrous swellings which ulcerate in 2–3 weeks to form a persistent ulcer with raised edges and a center of excessive granulation tissue covered with sticky, gray pus. The lesions expand, often to 20–30 cm in diameter, on the belly of the sow. They are usually single or in small numbers. In young pigs whole litters may be affected. The lesions commence about the lips and erode the cheeks, sometimes the jawbone, and often cause shedding of the teeth. The disease has also been described in weaned pigs, affecting the lower margin of both ears close to the junction with the neck, with extensive tissue destruction and sloughing.

In adult animals there is considerable inconvenience if the lesions are permitted to develop. In young pigs there may be heavy losses due to severe damage to the face.

In growing pigs, the lesions need to be differentiated from necrotic lesions resulting from the vices of snout rubbing in colored pigs and ear-biting and those resulting from excessive self-trauma with mange infestation. Necrotic ulcers on the udders of sows may be mistaken for lesions of actinomycosis and swabs should be taken from the ulcers for bacteriological examination. A course of potassium iodide given orally, or a single injection of penicillin provide a method of treatment. Topical tetracycline spray has been used effectively with early lesions (3). Dusting with sulfanilamide, arsenic trioxide or tartar emetic has also been recommended. The injection of 0·2 ml of a 5% solution of sodium arsenite into the substance of the lesion is reported to give good results. Improvement in hygiene and disinfection of skin wounds should reduce the incidence in affected piggeries.

REFERENCES

(1) Mullowney, P. C. & Baldwin, E. W. (1984) *Vet. Clin. N. Am.*, *6(1)*, 113.
(2) Blandford, T. B. et al. (1972) *Vet. Rec.*, *90*, 15.
(3) Harcourt, R. A. (1973) *Vet. Rec.*, *92*, 647.

DISEASES CAUSED BY *MYCOPLASMA* spp.

The relatively late arrival of mycoplasmas on the diagnostic scene has meant that their role in the production of disease is still uncertain. This is compounded by the difficulty of their culture in the laboratory and confusions about their nomenclature. There is uncertainty also about the real importance of mycoplasmas in many diseases from which they are consistently isolated. A common finding is that mycoplasmas are apparently imitative of disease processes which are mild and subclinical unless a more pathogenic agent such as another mycoplasma or *Corynebacterium* or *Fusobacterium* spp. is added.

Those diseases in which mycoplasmas have been positively identified as the causative agent are described separately. They are contagious bovine pleuropneumonia, bovine arthritis, bovine mastitis, caprine pleuropneumonia and enzootic pneumonia of pigs. Other diseases in which mycoplasmas also appear to play a contributory part are set out below. There is a summary in Table 65 (27). In general the antibiotic sensitivity of mycoplasmas and ureaplasmas is greatest to tiamulin, then tylosin and least to oxytetracycline, but individual sensitivities vary sufficiently for it to be necessary to carry out laboratory tests of sensitivity on each isolate (35).

Diseases of the genital tract

Vulvovaginitis in cattle, sheep and goats may be caused by *M. agalactia* var. *bovis* (1). The same infection when introduced with semen into the uterus can cause endometritis and salpingitis resulting in a temporary infertility and failure to conceive.

Persistent infection in the genital tract of bulls has also been produced experimentally (4). To counter this, some work has been done looking for an antibiotic additive for semen used in artificial insemination without any recommendation being made so far. Ureaplasmas have been isolated from the vulva of ewes with granular vulvitis and the disease was transmitted experimentally. However, the same organisms are present in the vulva of normal ewes. Similar findings are reported with cows (5) including the observation that *Ureaplasma* spp. are usually limited in their distribution to the vestibule and vulva of normal cows (3). This specific infection has been shown to adversely affect reproduction when either acute or chronic. It is also evident that it is capable of producing granular vaginitis and that some strains can, if introduced to the upper reproductive tract, cause transitory endometritis and salpingitis (30). A combination of lincomycin–spectinomycin–tylosin has been shown to be most effective in the treatment of *Ureaplasma* spp. in bull semen (46).

Attempts to produce abortion in cows by the injection of mycoplasmas isolated from aborted fetuses and from weak calves has had varying success (6) and *Acholeplasma* spp. have been isolated from aborted equine fetuses (7). *M. bovigenitalium* has been a frequent isolate from bovine genital tracts for many years, but its role in genital disease is still uncertain. It has been isolated from frozen bull semen (41, 42) and poses a threat to cows inseminated with infected semen. *M. capricolum* has been isolated from ewes with severe vulvovaginitis that appeared to have been transmitted by a ram (40). Thus in general terms, the mycoplasmas cannot be ignored as causes of reproductive disease, but their full importance is yet to be determined and they do not create great anxiety.

Diseases of the respiratory tract

A number of mycoplasmas has been isolated from pneumonic and non-pneumonic lungs of cattle, sheep and goats, but attempts to reproduce respiratory tract disease with them has resulted in inconclusive findings. In general, they are capable of causing a subclinical, mild pneumonia in gnotobiotic animals, but in combination with unidentified agents in lung homogenates administered intranasally 'enzootic' or chronic progressive pneumonia is produced in sheep. For example, *M. dispar* has a cytopathogenic effect and stops ciliary motility, and also destroys ciliated epithelial cells in organ cultures (11). *M. ovipneumoniae* also has the capacity to colonize the sheep lung and produce mild pneumonic lesions (16), but in combination with pasteurellae in sheep a proliferative exudative pneumonia appears (17, 31). *M. ovipneumoniae* has also been credited with causing pneumonia in goats (19, 28).

A more serious pneumonia, a naturally occurring proliferative interstitial pneumonia, similar morphologically to enzootic pneumonia of pigs and lambs, has been reproduced by the administration of a culture of a mycoplasma isolated from field cases (14). The lambs have obvious clinical signs including intolerance to exercise, dyspnea at rest, poor growth and a moderate mortality. The naturally occurring disease affects lambs primarily at 5–10 weeks of age. There is obvious pneumonia with coughing, sneezing, a copious mucoid, nasal discharge and loud dry crackles are audible on auscultation. A similar disease in Icelandic sheep (*Kregda*) has been identified as being caused by *M. ovipneumoniae* (15). In Switzerland a similar disease, from which *M. ovipneumoniae* is a common isolate, causes a great deal of economic loss (17).

Although contagious caprine pleuropneumonia has not been observed in Australia, a non-fatal respiratory disease of goats characterized by coughing, fever and extensive pleurisy and pneumonia has occurred. A variety of mycoplasmas, including *M. agalactia* and also *M. mycoides* and *M. mycoides* var. *capri* (2), have also been found in goats. The caprine *M. mycoides* var. *mycoides* (large colony type) is not pathogenic for cattle and has been associated with a variety of syndromes in goats including fibrinous peritonitis, pneumonia, arthritis, mastitis and abortion.

The most common syndrome in goats caused by mycoplasma is a chronic interstitial pneumonia with cough, unthriftiness proceeding to extreme emaciation, chronic non-painful bony enlargement of joints and chronic indurative mastitis. The pneumonia in some cases progresses to the point where cor pulmonale develops with a subsequent appearance of the signs of congestive heart failure.

In calves, mycoplasmas are involved in the causation of enzootic pneumonia. *M. arginini*, *M. ovipneumoniae* (8) and *Acholeplasma laidlawii* are common findings of doubtful significance in the lungs of both calves and goats (9). *M. dispar* is capable of producing a pneumonia without clinical signs in gnotobiotic calves, and in conjunction with *Ureaplasma* spp. it has been found commonly in 'cuffing' pneumonia of calves (10). It could, therefore, be a significant precursor to other infections causing development of 'enzootic pneumonia' in calves or with pasteurellae producing progressive clinical pneumonia of calves (11). *M. bovis* has a similar reputation (47). *M. agalactia* var. *bovis* has also been isolated from pneumonic calf lung (12) and produced subclinical cuffing pneumonia in gnotobiotic calves (13). Vaccination by intramuscular inoculation and intratracheal infusion with killed organisms appear to offer some protection against this infection. The common finding of a variety of mycoplasmas in the lungs of pneumonic calves (29) suggests that either they are a common precursor, or secondary invaders or that they are normal inhabitants with very little pathogenicity. This is probably the relationship between *Mycoplasma bovis* and *Pasteurella hemolytica* in the pneumonia produced experimentally in calves (45).

In horses, *M. felis* has been isolated from the pleural exudate in cases of pleurisy (48) and a causal relationship seems likely.

Diseases of the eyes

Mycoplasma bovoculi (*Acholeplasma oculosis*) has been associated with, without necessarily being the cause in the field of, outbreaks of infectious keratoconjunctivitis of cattle (18), sheep and goats (20, 32). The mycoplasmas are capable of producing keratitis experimentally. The naturally occurring disease in goats (24) is manifested by rapid spread and development with intense lacrimation, conjunctival hyperemia, corneal opacity and vascularization. A concurrent respiratory illness occurs in some. Response to treatment with oxytetracycline and polymyxin B is good. The disease is reproducible experimentally.

Diseases of the joints

Mycoplasma (*M. hyorhinis*, *M. hyosynoviae*) are associated with arthritis and polyarthritis in pigs (22) and the disease is reproducible experimentally. Both organisms are carried in the respiratory tract. *M. hyorhinis* most commonly affects sucking and young pigs, especially after weaning or some stress, and may produce a polyserositis in addition to arthritis. The case fatality rate is generally low, but residual fibrinous pericardial and pleural adhesions may occur and the pigs may fail to thrive.

Disease associated with *M. hyosynoviae* is more common in older growing pigs and presents principally as arthritis. The disease is endemic in some herds and may affect up to 15% of the herd. Clinically there is an acute episode of fever, lameness and swelling of the joint. The pathological lesion is a serofibrinous arthritis. Most cases recover, but some may be affected chronically. The case fatality rate is low and never exceeds 10%. Tylosin and lincomycin are indicated and give good results in practice.

In goats, *M. capricolum* is a cause of arthritis (26). The infection is transmissible experimentally via infected milk administered orally. The infection results in septicemia with following pneumonia and arthritis (37, 39).

M. mycoides var. *mycoides* (large colony type) has been isolated from goats with arthritis (36), 38). In particular it has caused acute arthritis in 3–8 week old kids manifested by lameness, recumbency, diarrhea and fever (24). The infection may originate from infected milk from does that have experienced acute mastitis due to *M. mycoides* var. *mycoides*. It may also be transmitted by ear mites, *Psoroptes cuniculi* (43). A similar disease is observed in sheep (44). At necropsy the kids have polyarthritis, pneumonia and pleurisy. *M. putrefaciens* has caused major losses due to mastitis and arthritis in a large goat herd (49). Abortion was common in some groups.

M. capricolum is also a cause of arthritis in sheep (25). The well-identified mycoplasmal arthritis of cattle is dealt with separately.

Diseases in horses

There are few records of mycoplasmosis in horses. What records there are relate to the isolation of mycoplasmas, usually from respiratory and female genital tracts, and almost always without any associated lesions (23). One such organism is *M. equirhinis*, thought to be a specific parasite of horses, but without any apparent pathogenicity (21).

Table 65. Summary of systemic mycoplasmoses of sheep and goats (27)

Bacterial species	*Animals affected*	*Disease caused*	*Pathogenicity*
M. agalactiae	Sheep/goats	Contagious agalactia, arthritis, pneumonia, granular vaginitis, pinkeye	High
M. arginini	Sheep/goats	Pneumonia, arthritis, vaginitis, pinkeye, mastitis	Low
M. capricolum	Sheep/goats	Arthritis, mastitis, pneumonia	High
M. mycoides subsp. *capri*	Goats	Contagious caprine pleuropneumonia, pneumonia, arthritis	Moderate
M. mycoides subsp. *mycoides* (large colony type)	Sheep/goats	Contagious caprine pleuropneumonia, mastitis, arthritis, high mortality in young kids	Moderate
M. ovipneumoniae	Sheep/goats	Pneumonia	Commonly precursor to pneumonic pasteurellosis
M. putrefaciens	Goats	Mastitis and arthritis	High
Acholeplasma laidlawii	Sheep/goats	Bacteria found in lungs	Non-pathogenic
Ureaplasma sp.		Vaginitis	
Mycoplasma strain F38	Sheep/goats	Contagious caprine	Low
	Goats	pleuropneumonia	High pathogenicity

Diseases in sheep and goats

The moderately well-identified syndromes of these species are dealt with separately. There are many other reports of mycoplasmal diseases in these species in which the mycoplasma is not identified, and a number of diseases as set out above in which the etiological significance of the mycoplasmas is in doubt. For example, the three main clinical syndromes of these species are serositis-arthritis, pleuropneumonia and agalactia, as set out in subsequent sections. However, the signs and lesions of more than one of these 'specific' diseases and the infections themselves can be encountered in the one animal (33, 34). See Table 65.

REVIEW LITERATURE

Gourlay, R. N. (1976) Current situation on mycoplasma infections in cattle. *Vet. Ann.*, *16*, 48.
Jones, G. E. (1983) Mycoplasmas of sheep and goats: a synopsis. *Vet. Rec.*, *113*, 619–620.
St George, T. D. & Sullivan, N. D. (1973) Pneumonias of sheep in Australia. University of Sydney, Post Graduate Foundation, *Vet. Rev.* No. 13.
Whittlestone, P. (1975) Mycoplasmas in diseases of domestic mammals. *Vet. Ann.*, *15*, 432.

REFERENCES

(1) Afshar, A. (1975) *Vet. Bull.*, *45*, 211.
(2) Baas, E. J. et al. (1977) *Infect. Immun.* *18*, 806 & 916.
(3) Ball, H. J. & McCaughey, W. J. (1979) *Vet. Rec.*, *104*, 482.
(4) Lein, D. H. & Nielsen, S. W. (1975) *Lab. Invest.*, *32*, 450.
(5) Ruhnke, H. L. et al. (1978) *Can. J. comp. Med.*, *42*, 151.
(6) Stalheim, O. H. V. & Proctor, S. J. (1976) *Am. J. vet. Res.*, *37*, 879.
(7) Kirchoff, H. (1978) *Int. J. syst. Bacteriol.*, *28*, 76.
(8) Orning, A. P. et al. (1979) *Am J. vet. Res.*, *39*, 1169.
(9) Livingston, C. W. & Gauer, B. B. (1979) *Am. J. vet. Res.*, *40*, 407.
(10) Pirie, H. M. & Allan, E. M. (1975) *Vet. Rec.*, *175*, 812.
(11) Tinant, M. K. et al. (1975) *J. Am. vet. med. Assoc.*, 55.
(12) Thomas, L. H. et al. (1976) *Vet. Rec.*, *97*, 55.
(13) Howard, C. J. et al. (1976) *Res. vet. Sci.*, *21*, 227.
(14) Sullivan, N. D. et al. (1973) *Aust. vet. J.*, *49*, 63.
(15) Friis, N. F. et al. (1976) *Acta vet. Scand.*, *17*, 255.
(16) Alley, M. R. & Clarke, J. K. (1979) *NZ vet. J.*, *27*, 217.
(17) Hu, J. S. et al. (1982) *Chin. J. vet. Med.*, *8*, 2.
(18) Nicolet, J. & Buttiker, W. (1974) *Vet. Rec.*, *95*, 442.
(19) Jones, G. E. at al. (1979) *Vet. Microbiol.*, *4*, 47.
(20) Al-Aubaidi, J. M. et al. (1973) *Cornell Vet.*, *63*, 117.
(21) Hooker, J. M. et al. (1977) *J. comp. Pathol.*, *87*, 281.
(22) Duncan, J. R. & Ross, R. F. (1973) *Am. J. vet. Res.*, *34*, 363, 367.
(23) Moorthy, A. R. S. & Spradbrow, P. B. (1976) *Vet. Rec.*, *98*, 233.
(24) East, N. E. et al. (1983) *J. Am. vet. med. Assoc.*, *182*, 1338.
(25) Swanepoel, R. et al. (1977) *Vet. Rec.*, *101*, 446.
(26) Perreau, P. & Beard, A. (1979) *Comp. Immunol., Microbiol. infect. Dis.*, *2*, 87.
(27) Jones, G. E. (1983) *Vet. Rec.*, *113*, 619.
(28) Masiga, W. N. & Rurangirwa, F. R. (1979) *Bull. Anim. Hlth Prod. in Africa*, *27*, 287.
(29) Muenster, O. A. et al. (1978) *Can. J. comp. Med.*, *43*, 392.
(30) Ruhnke, H. L. et al. (1984) *Theriogenology*, *21*, 295.
(31) Jones, G. E. et al. (1982) *J. comp. Pathol.*, *92*, 261, 267.
(32) Arbuckle, J. B. & Bonson, M. D. (1980) *Vet. Rec.*, *106*, 15.
(33) Barton, M. B. & Cottew, G. S. (1980) *Aust. vet. J.*, *56*, 614.
(34) Bar-Moshe, B. & Rappaport, E. (1979) *Refuah Vet.*, *36*, 53 & 117.
(35) Allan, E. M. & Pirie, H. M. (1981) *Res. vet. Sci.*, *31*, 174.
(36) Ruhnke, H. L. et al. (1983) *Can. vet. J.*, *24*, 54.
(37) DaMassa, A. J. et al. (1983) *Aust. vet. J.*, *60*, 125.
(38) DaMassa, A. J. et al. (1983) *Am. J. vet. Res.*, *44*, 322.
(39) Cordy, D. R. (1984) *Aust. vet. J.*, *61*, 201.
(40) Jones, G. E. et al. (1983) *Vet. Rec.*, *113*, 540.
(41) Harbi, M. S. M. A. et al. (1983) *Vet. Rec.*, *113*, 114.
(42) Jurmanova, K. et al. (1983) *Arch. exp. vet. Med.*, *37*, 421.
(43) Hazell, S. L. et al. (1985) *Aust. vet. J.*, *62*, 421.
(44) Okoh, A. E. & Ocholi, R. A. (1986) *Vet. Rec.*, *118*, 212.

(45) Gourlay, R. N. & Houghton, S. B. (1985) *Res. vet. Sci.*, *38*, 377.
(46) Truscott, R. B. & Ruhnke, H. L. (1984) *Can. J. comp. Med.*, *48*, 171.
(47) Rosendal, S. & Martin, S. W. (1986) *Can. J. vet. Res.*, *50*, 179.
(48) Rosendal, S. et al. (1986) *J. Am. vet. med. Assoc.*, *188*, 292.
(49) Damassa, A. J. et al. (1987) *Vet. Rec.*, *120*, 409.

Contagious bovine pleuropneumonia

Contagious bovine pleuropneumonia is a highly infectious septicemia characterized by localization in the lungs and pleura. It is one of the major plagues in cattle causing heavy losses in many parts of the world.

Etiology

Mycoplasma mycoides var. *mycoides* (small colony type) is the cause of the disease in cattle. The causative organisms of contagious pleuropneumonia in cattle and in goats are very similar culturally and antigenically but they can be differentiated culturally and biochemically (9). Large colony types are pathogenic for sheep and goats, but not for cattle. Small colony types include the contagious bovine pleuropneumonia agent, and also affect goats and are potentially pathogenic for sheep. Infection does not spread between the two species (1). It is extremely pleomorphic and some of its forms are filtrable.

Epidemiology

The organisms *M. mycoides* var. *mycoides* are sensitive to all environmental influences, including disinfectants, heat and drying and do not survive outside the animal body for more than a few hours, although they can be maintained readily in special culture media and in embryonated hens' eggs. The disease occurs commonly only in cattle although rare natural cases have been observed in buffalo, yak, bison, reindeer and antelopes. The disease has been produced experimentally in captive Africa buffalo (2) and white-tailed deer (8), but was not detectable in eight species of wildlife (3). A local cellulitis without pulmonary involvement occurs in sheep and goats after injection of cultures. A strong immunity develops after an attack of the natural disease in cattle and vaccination plays an important part in control. The exact nature of the immunity conferred by vaccination or by naturally occurring disease is not understood although it can be transferred by the administration of serum from an immune animal (4). There is no difference in the susceptibility of *Bos taurus* and *Bos indicus* cattle and both races respond equally to vaccination (5).

The principal method of spread of this disease is by the inhalation of infective droplets from active or carrier cases of the disease. Mediate infection by contamination of inanimate objects is an unlikely means of transmission under natural conditions, but it has been effected experimentally, the infected hay remaining infective up to 144 hours (13). Other inanimate objects such as placenta and urine can also remain infective for long periods (26).

Because of the method of spread, outbreaks tend to be more extensive in housed animals and in those in transit by train or on foot. The focus of infection is often provided by recovered 'carrier' animals in which a pulmonary sequestrum preserves a potential source of organisms for periods as long as 3 years. It has long been thought that conditions of stress due to starvation, exhaustion or intercurrent disease can cause the sequestrum to break down and convert the animal into an active case. Experimental evidence (13) throws some doubt on this assumption. However, droplet infection is usually associated with a donor lesion in the lungs. Renal lesions are not uncommon in this disease and large numbers of viable *M. mycoides* are passed in the urine in infected animals, leading to the suggestion that the inhalation of urine droplets may be a route of infection (6).

A low incidence can be anticipated in arid regions because of the rapid destruction of the organism in exhaled droplets. Although 6 m is usually considered to be sufficient separation between animals, transmission over distances as great as 45 m has been suspected to occur. Spread of the disease may also occur by discharges from local tail lesions resulting from vaccination with virulent culture. Cattle may be exposed to infection for periods of up to 8 months before the disease becomes established and this necessitates a long period of quarantine before a herd can be declared to be free of the disease.

Contagious bovine pleuropneumonia is still endemic in many large areas throughout eastern Europe, Asia, Africa, and the Iberian Peninsula. The disease was eradicated from the United States in 1892, South Africa in 1916, and Australia in 1972. The disease recurred in France in the recent past but was successfully eradicated. In the affected countries enormous losses are experienced each year from the deaths of animals and the loss of production during convalescence. The highly fatal nature of the disease, the ease of spread and the difficulty of detecting carriers also mean that close restriction must be placed on the movement of animals from enzootic areas. For example, in Australia many feeder cattle are reared on range country where the disease was endemic and it was necessary to move these animals for fattening into more closely settled areas which were free of the disease. In spite of strict quarantine measures to prevent the movement of infected animals, periodic outbreaks occurred in these free areas with heavy losses of cattle and major expense for eradication programs. In groups of susceptible cattle the case morbidity approaches 90% and the case mortality may be as high as 50%.

Pathogenesis

Contagious bovine pleuropneumonia is an acute lobar pneumonia and pleurisy developing by localization from an initial septicemia. An essential part of the pathogenesis of the disease is thrombosis in the pulmonary vessels, probably prior to the development of pneumonic lesions. The mechanism of development of the thrombosis is not understood, but there is no general increase in coagulability, and no generalized tendency to spontaneous thrombosis (7). Death results from anoxia and presumably from toxemia. Under natural conditions a number of animals in a group do not become infected, either because of natural immunity or because they are not exposed to a sufficiently large infective dose. These animals may show a transient positive reaction to the complement fixation test. Approximately 50% of the animals that do not become infected go through a mild form of the disease and are often recognized as clinical cases.

Clinical findings

After an incubation period of 3–6 weeks (in occasional instances up to 6 months) there is a sudden onset of high fever (40°C, 105°F), a fall in milk yield, anorexia and cessation of rumination. There is severe depression and the animals stand apart or lag behind a travelling group. Coughing, at first only on exercise, and chest pain are evident, affected animals being disinclined to move, standing with the elbows out, the back arched and head extended. Respirations are shallow, rapid and accompanied by expiratory grunting. Pain is evidenced on percussion of the chest. Auscultation reveals pleuritic friction sounds in the early stages of acute inflammation, and dullness, fluid sounds and moist gurgling crackles in the later stages of effusion. Dullness of areas of the lung may be detectable on percussion. Inconstantly, edematous swellings of the throat and dewlap occur.

Recovered animals may be clinically normal but in some an inactive sequestrum forms in the lung, with a necrotic center of sufficient size to produce a toxemia causing unthriftiness and mild respiratory distress on exercise. These sequestra commonly break down when the animal is exposed to environmental stress and cause an acute attack of the disease. A chronic cough is also common. Approximately 50% of the affected animals die acutely and 25% remain as recovered carriers with or without clinical signs. In fatal cases death occurs after a variable course of from several days to 3 weeks.

Clinical pathology

The complement fixation (CF) test on serum is the most useful method of detecting infection. In a small proportion of animals the results may be deceptive. Early cases may give a negative reaction and some positive reactors show no lesions on necropsy. The test is particularly effective in detecting carriers. Animals recovering from the disease gradually become negative and vaccinated animals give a positive reaction for about 6 weeks although this period may be much longer if severe vaccination reactions occur. A slide flocculation test and a rapid slide agglutination test (10) have been used but their sensitivity is lower than that of the complement fixation test and they are recommended for herd diagnosis rather than for use in individual animals. However, the plate agglutination test has been very accurate and efficient in Australia and has made eradication of the disease a possibility (11). A modified complement fixation test, the 'plate CF test', has been introduced (12). It is more accurate than the standard CF test and is much more economical of time and equipment. With all of these tests there is a progressive loss of reliability if testing is delayed for very long after the clinical disease has passed.

A major development in the tests available for the diagnosis of contagious bovine pleuropneumonia is the single comparative intradermal allergic test similar to the tuberculin test (14). It has the advantages of speed, and of requiring no laboratory facilities. There are disadvantages to the test, for example animals with acute infections are negative. Its particular value is in identifying animals, and more importantly herds, which have been exposed to the disease, and particularly those animals with chronic lesions.

Necropsy findings

Lesions are confined to the chest cavity. There is thickening and inflammation of the pleura often with heavy deposits of fibrin and large amounts of clear, serous effusion containing shreds of fibrin. One or both lungs may be completely or partially affected with marked consolidation. Affected lobules show various stages of gray and red hepatization and the interlobular septa are greatly distended with serofibrinous exudate—the classical 'marbled' lung of this disease. In recovered cases careful section of the lung tissue is necessary to detect the presence of foci and necrotic tissue surrounded by a fibrous capsule—the sequestra of carrier cases. Adhesions between pleural surfaces are also a constant finding in such cases. The postmortem diagnosis can be confirmed by examination of freshly collected effusion fluid for the presence of the organism or by culture from lung or fluid. In a few cases only edematous lesions may be found in the lymph nodes of the chest or in the tonsillar tissue.

Diagnosis

A diagnosis based on a history of contact with infected animals, clinical findings, a complement fixation test, necropsy findings and cultural examination leaves little room for error. Pneumonic pasteurellosis may be very similar clinically and at necropsy but is differentiated bacteriologically by the presence of pasteurellae in the tissues and by the complement fixation test. Other severe pulmonary disorders of cattle include fog fever and enzootic and parasitic pneumonia of calves.

Treatment

Treatment is usually undertaken only in areas where the disease is endemic, eradication being the more logical practice when the disease breaks out in a new area. Sulfadimidine and organic arsenicals are used extensively and appear to reduce the mortality rate. Penicillin is of little value, streptomycin has some curative effect, and oxytetracycline and chloramphenicol have some value. Tylosin is highly effective in the control of excessive vaccination reactions and should be of value in the treatment of clinical cases (15). The dose rate of tylosin tartrate recommended for intramuscular injection is 10 mg/kg body weight every 12 hours for 6 injections. Daily injections are not effective. Erythromycin is effective against some mycoplasmas. Spiramycin (10 mg/kg body weight, up to 20 or even 50 mg/kg) is highly effective in treating reactions to vaccination. In severe cases the treatment may need to be given on three consecutive days (16).

Control

On a herd basis

When the disease becomes established in a herd the

following measures may be adopted to prevent its spread.

Hygiene Any procedure which brings the animals together should be avoided if possible, especially in the early stages of the disease. Passage through the milking shed, collecting for inspection, bleeding and vaccination all facilitate the spread of the disease. It should be remembered that droplet infection is more likely to occur in humid conditions. Strict quarantine of the infected and in-contact herds must be maintained until all residual infection has been eliminated; usually 12 weeks after the removal of the last reactor and/or clinical case is sufficient time. Animals in quarantine should be kept under constant surveillance so that clinical cases may be observed.

Removal of sources of infection Infected animals should be removed from the herd as soon as possible. The complement fixation test is adequate to identify the infected animals and if possible it should be carried out in conjunction with clinical examination. Because animals in the incubative and early stages of the disease may give negative reactions it is necessary to have two completely negative tests 2 months apart before the herd can be classified as clean. After vaccination a positive reaction occurs but it usually disappears within 2 months although in rare cases it may persist for as long as 5 months. All positive and suspicious reactors and clinical cases are destroyed or transported under close control to abattoirs. Where this cannot be done without a chance of spread to animals along the route destruction on the property is necessary. Animals which are eventually to go to abattoirs should be kept under quarantine until slaughter, irrespective of their status.

In circumstances where a minimum of handling is desired the herd may be blood tested and examined for clinical signs, and vaccinated all in the one visit. Animals which react to the test are then destroyed even though they have been vaccinated. The only difficulty that arises with this method is that cattle in the incubative stages of the disease may give a negative reaction to the test and because of the serological reaction resulting from vaccination retesting cannot be performed until 2 months later.

Vaccination Vaccination is an effective procedure in the control of bovine pleuropneumonia but its application is usually controlled by local legislation. All the vaccines in use are living preparations, and their use is always subject to the suspicion that they may spread the disease. When tail vaccination with organisms of reduced virulence is practiced the possibility of spreading the disease is remote but, because the possibility exists, vaccination is usually only permitted in herds or areas where the disease is known to be present. The value of calfhood vaccination is limited, because although calves give sufficient serological reactions arthritis, myocarditis and valvular endocarditis occur 3–4 weeks after vaccination of calves less than 2 months old. Vaccination of calves after this age is recommended because it avoids the occasional deaths which occur after vaccination of adults.

The vaccines available include pleural exudate from natural cases (natural lymph), cultured organisms of reduced virulence, and an avianized vaccine of low virulence. Vaccination is usually carried out by injection into the tough connective tissue at the tip of the tail with a high-pressure syringe. 'Natural lymph' is unsatisfactory because of the possibility of spreading this and other diseases and because of the severe lesions which commonly result. Severe reactions with this type of vaccine may cause sloughing of the tail and extensive cellulitis of the hindquarters necessitating destruction or causing death of the animal. An intranasal vaccine avoids these sequels and appears to give satisfactory results. If animals which develop a severe local lesion after vaccination are treated with a mycoplasmocidal drug, such as tylosin, the treatment will interfere with the development of immunity and animals treated in this way should be revaccinated (18).

In general, vaccines made from *M. mycoides* grown in broth-culture produce less severe reactions but a correspondingly briefer immunity of about 6–10 months and require annual revaccination (19). The T1 strain broth-culture vaccine is the one in most general use in the nomadic cattle herds of Africa. It has the virtue of long-term immunity, of at least 2 years duration (20). Avianized vaccines were developed which overcame the brevity of the immunity, increasing its duration to 3–4 years (21). These vaccines are the major ones in use now and are capable of great variation in their virulence. In spite of increasing the attenuation the use of these vaccines was followed on occasions by severe local reactions and pulmonary lesions. This led to an investigation of the KH3J strain which is less virulent than the standard V5 strain (1, 22) and the production of a vaccine attenuated by egg culture but grown in its last passage in broth (23). This latter procedure eliminated the egg proteins from the vaccine which were thought to produce some of the local reactions. However, the more virulent vaccines are still in use and, provided tylosin is available to control undesirably severe reactions, are generally preferred (24, 25).

Difficulty has been experienced in the preparation of a dried vaccine for field use. A dried vaccine is available but it must be reconstituted in agar and used within 2 hours (27). It has the advantage of requiring a very small dose and of retaining its potency for well over a year (28). Another vaccine containing a virulent strain KH3J plus 20% brain suspension is an efficient immunizing agent and is stable and freeze dries easily (29). All vaccines against CBPP are susceptible to light and should be kept in a dark place.

On an area basis

The prevention of entry of contagious bovine pleuropneumonia into a free area is a difficult task. Only the following classes of cattle should be permitted to enter:

- Cattle which have not been in an infected area nor in contact with infected animals for at least 6 months. This may be relaxed to permit entry of cattle going to immediate slaughter after a clinical examination and a period of 1 month in a free area
- Cattle which have given negative reactions to the complement fixation test on two occasions within the preceding 2 months and have not been in contact with infected animals during this period.

These animals may or may not have been vaccinated. Less rigid measures than these will permit introduction of the disease.

When the disease is already present in an area, two methods of control are possible, vaccination, and eradication by test and slaughter of reactors. The method chosen will depend largely on the economy of the cattle industry in the affected area. A vaccination program may be the first step to reduce the incidence of the disease to the point where eradication becomes possible.

In areas where properties are large, fencing is poor and the collection of every animal cannot be guaranteed, eradication of the disease by test and slaughter is impractical. Vaccination with culture vaccine can be practiced whenever the cattle are brought together. Animals moving from infected areas or into infected areas, and groups of cattle which contain active cases, must be vaccinated. Moving cattle which develop the disease should be halted, clinical cases slaughtered and the remainder vaccinated. Results are usually good provided the vaccination is carried out carefully but some further cases due to prevaccination infection are to be expected. Extensive vaccination in Australia reduced the incidence of the disease to an extremely low level (30) and complete eradication of the disease was achieved shortly afterwards. The residual problems were largely geographical and an annoying but low proportion of false-positive reactors to the complement fixation test. Eradication was greatly facilitated by the use of the Huddart plate test in a mobile laboratory and autopsy of reactors 24 hours later. Of great help also was the appointment of special meat inspectors to local abattoirs during the eradication program.

In countries where the cattle population is nomadic the control and eradication of contagious bovine pleuropneumonia seems impossible by the conventional means described above. Annual vaccination of as many cattle as can be found does have the capacity to reduce the occurrence of the disease to negligible proportions (10).

When outbreaks occur in small areas where herds can be adequately controlled, complete eradication should be attempted by periodic testing and the destruction of reactors, and in-contact animals should be vaccinated. To avoid unnecessary contact between cattle, retesting is delayed until 5–6 months after the first test when vaccination reactions have usually subsided. Under most circumstances all non-reactors should be vaccinated. This practice is particularly applicable in feeder cattle which will be slaughtered subsequently and when extensive outbreaks occur in closely settled areas where the chances of spread are great. Simple test and slaughter in these latter circumstances will be too slow to control the rate of spread. In either case the herd should not be released from quarantine until two tests at an interval of more than 2 months are completely negative.

REVIEW LITERATURE

Lindley, E. P. (1979) Control of contagious bovine pleuropneumonia with special reference to the Central African Empire. *World Anim. Rev.*, *30*, 18.

Windsor, R. S. (1977) The diagnosis of contagious bovine pleuropneumonia. *Vet. Ann.*, *17*, 59.

REFERENCES

(1) Hudson, J. R. & Leaver, D. D. (1965) *Aust. vet. J.*, *41*, 29, 36, 43.
(2) Shifrine, M. et al. (1970) *Bull. epizoot. Dis. Afr.*, *18*, 201.
(3) Shifrine, M. & Domermuth, C. H. (1967) *Bull. epizoot. Dis. Afr.*, *15*, 319.
(4) Masiga, W. N. & Windsor, R. S. (1975) *Vet. Rec.*, *97*, 350.
(5) Masiga, W. N. & Read, W. C. S. (1972) *Vet. Rec.*, *90*, 499 (see also (1974) *Vet. Rec.*, *95*, 87).
(6) Scudamore, J. M. (1976) *Res. vet. Sci.*, *20*, 330.
(7) Lloyd, I. C. et al. (1975) *J. comp. Pathol.*, *85*, 583.
(8) Yedloutschnig, R. J. & Dardiri, A. H. (1976) *Proc. Ann. Mtg US Anim. Hlth Assoc.*, *80*, 262.
(9) Cottew, G. S. (1979) *Zentralbl. Bakteriol.*, *Parasitol.*, *Infektionskr. Hyg.* (Erste Abteilung Originale), *245A*, 164.
(10) Lindley, F. P. (1979) *World Anim. Rev.*, *30*, 18.
(11) Ladds, P. W. (1969) *Aust. vet. J.*, *45*, 1.
(12) Karst, D. (1970) *Bull. epizoot. Dis. Afr.*, *18*, 5.
(13) Windsor, R. S. & Masiga, W. N. (1977) *Res. vet. Sci.*, *23*, 224 & 230.
(14) Windsor, R. S. et al. (1978) *Br. vet. J.*, *134*, 162.
(15) Hudson, J. R. & Etheridge, J. R. (1965) *Aust. vet. J.*, *41*, 130.
(16) Provost, A. (1974) *Cah. Med. vet.*, *43*, 140.
(17) Karst, O. & Mitchel, S. (1972) *J. comp. Pathol.*, *82*, 171.
(18) Windsor, R. S. & Masiga, W. N. (1976) *J. comp. Pathol.*, *86*, 173.
(19) Gilbert, F. R. et al. (1970) *Vet. Rec.*, *86*, 29.
(20) Masiga, W. N. & Windsor, R. S. (1974) *Bull. epizoot. Dis.Afr.*, *22*, 27.
(21) Hyslop, N. St. G. (1956) *Br. vet. J.*, *112*, 519.
(22) Hudson, J. R. & Turner, A. W. (1963) *Aust. vet. J.*, *39*, 373.
(23) Davies, G. et al. (1968) *Vet. Rec.*, *83*, 239.
(24) Hyslop, N. St. G. (1968) *Bull. Off. int. Epizootol.*, *69*, 695.
(25) Hudson, J. R. (1968) *Aust. vet. J.*, *44*, 83, 123.
(26) Windsor, R. S. & Masiga, W. N. (1977) *Bull. Anim. Hlth Prod. Afr.*, *25*, 357.
(27) Webster, W. (1945) *Aust. vet. J.*, *21*, 64.
(28) Priestley, F. W. & Dafalla, E. N. (1957) *Bull. epizoot. Dis. Afr.*, *5*, 177.
(29) Hudson, J. R. (1968) *Bull. epizoot. Dis. Afr.*, *16*, 165.
(30) Lloyd, L. C. (1960) *Aust. vet. J.*, *45*, 147.

Serositis–arthritis of goats

A disease observed in California and Australia in goats is characterized by a diffuse, fibrinous peritonitis, pleurisy, pericarditis and arthritis, and in some cases a leptomeningitis. An unnamed mycoplasma, antigenically unrelated to *M. mycoides* var. *capri* or *M. agalactiae*, has been identified as the cause of the disease. There is high fever, pain and swelling of limb joints and suppression of lactation. Neither mammary nor pulmonary involvement has been observed. Although the organism can be isolated from pneumonic lungs it is not capable of causing a primary pneumonia. In California the disease has been found to occur most commonly in very young kids and yearling does at parturition and weaning time. Cellulitis occurs after local inoculation of the organism and secondary eye involvement may occur if the eye is injured. The disease is transmissible experimentally to goats, sheep and pigs but not to calves, and the organism is present in the feces and urine of infected animals. Complement fixation antibodies to *M. mycoides* are present in the serum 15 days after experimental inoculation. *In vitro* the organism is only slightly susceptible to streptomycin and chloramphenicol but highly sensitive to oxytetracycline and erythromycin. Sensitivity to organic arsenicals and other tetracyclines is variable.

Contagious caprine pleuropneumonia (CCPP)

This classical disease of goats is commonly confused with other serious pneumonias of goats and sheep. It is caused by *Mycoplasma* strain F38 (7). The disease has many similarities clinically and at necropsy to contagious bovine pleuropneumonia, but is not transmissible to cattle. The clinical picture includes an incubation period of 6–10 days, extreme infectivity with a morbidity of 100%, and an acute severe illness with a case mortality of 60–100%. This represents the response to the introduction of infection into a susceptible flock. What the epidemiological picture would be in a naturally immunized flock receiving constant invasions of infected animals is not clear. Signs include cough, dyspnea, lagging, lying down a lot, but the animal can stand and walk, fever (40·5–41·5°C; 104·5–106°F) and in the terminal stages, mouth breathing, tongue protrusion and frothy salivation with death in 2 or more days. Under adverse climatic conditions the disease may occur in a septicemic form with little clinical or postmortem evidence of pneumonia. The more usual necropsy findings are similar to those of contagious bovine pleuropneumonia except that sequestra are not formed in the lungs and the reaction of the interlobular tissue is much less. The lesions may be confined to one lung.

There is still confusion about the exact cause of the disease, but a specific mycoplasma (strain F38) is the cause of the highly contagious lethal disease which is not the clinical or epidemiological picture produced by infections with other mycoplasmas (2–4). It is more generally accepted that *M. mycoides* var. *capri* is the cause (5, 9, 12). Reports of the disease come mostly from North Africa, Spain and the Mediterranean littoral, Asia Minor and India. The disease *Abu Nini* of the Sudan is probably the same disease, but may be complicated by the presence of other organisms.

The disease is readily transmitted by inhalation (6), but the organism does not survive for long outside the animal body so that infection is brought into the flock by a carrier or infected animal. The disease is not transmissible experimentally or naturally, to cattle or sheep. Control depends on isolation of affected flocks, vaccination and revaccination at intervals of 6 months. A characteristic of the disease is the failure to cause local inflammation reaction when infectious material is injected subcutaneously.

It is emphasized that this description does not fit most current descriptions of the disease. It is customary in them to include other serious pneumonias of goats caused by *M. mycoides* var. *capri* and *M. mycoides*.

Treatment of cases of CCPP with tylosin tartrate (10 mg/kg body weight) or oxytetracycline (15 mg/kg daily) is highly successful (10) and vaccination with an aluminum hydroxide terpene vaccine has given good results. The severity of the disease is reduced but treated animals are still sources of infection (20). A vaccine consisting of sonicated antigens of F38 strains in incomplete Freund's adjuvant also appears effective (18).

Contagious agalactia of goats and sheep

The disease has approximately the same geographical distribution as contagious pleuropneumonia of goats and sheep. There is usually an acute onset of mastitis, ophthalmitis and arthritis with painful swelling of affected joints. The mortality rate is high (10–30%) and the udder is permanently damaged. Kids are more seriously affected than adults. Abortion occurs commonly and there is a long period of illness of from one to several months (10).

Herd diagnosis is possible by the isolation of the organism (*M. agalactiae*) from the bloodstream and mammary tissue and by a complement fixation test which becomes positive soon after a clinical attack. There is also an ELISA test which has comparable sensitivity to the complement fixation test (16). If recovery occurs a solid immunity persists. Three types of causative organism have been identified (11). One is non-pathogenic, another causes most outbreaks of the disease, but the third is associated with severe udder edema and a high mortality in goats. *M. mycoides* var. *mycoides* is also thought to be a possible cause of caprine agalactia (1). *M. arginini* (21) and *M. putrefaciens* (19) are also recognized as causes of caprine mastitis. The results of intramammary infusion with mycoplasma and allied bacteria in sheep and goats do not coincide well with isolates from natural cases (8). This may be related to variations in virulence between serotypes of the one bacterial species.

Vaccination of sheep and goats with either an attenuated live vaccine or a killed adjuvant vaccine gives mixed results; in late pregnant ewes the former was rather too virulent, and the latter insufficiently so and in ewes before mating good efficiency was observed (12). Treatment of affected goats with tylosin or erythromycin was found to be effective in 80% of cases provided treatment was given early (13). Oxytetracycline was thought to limit the severity of the disease without reducing the excretion of mycoplasmas in the milk (11). The extensive use of a live, attenuated vaccine and a killed, adjuvant vaccine over a period of 13 years has resulted in almost complete disappearance of the disease from Romania (14). Comparison between three commercial vaccines has shown that a saponized vaccine gave better results than an egg-cultured vaccine (15). Vaccination against *M. mycoides* var. *mycoides* with a formol-killed vaccine is also thought to be effective (17).

REVIEW LITERATURE

McMartin, D. A. et al. (1980) A century of classical contagious caprine pleuropneumonia. *Br. vet. J.*, *136*, 507.

Stalheim, O. H. V. (1983) Mycoplasmal respiratory disease of ruminants: a review and update. *J. Am. vet. med. Assoc.*, *182*, 403.

REFERENCES

(1) Bar-Moshe, B. & Rappaport, E. (1978) *Refuah Vet.*, *35*, 75.
(2) McMartin, D. A. et al. (1980) *Br. vet. J.*, *136*, 507.
(3) Kalnier, G. & MacOwan, K. J. (1976) *Zentralbl. VetMed.*, *23B*, 652.
(4) MacOwan, K. J. & Minette, J. E. (1977) *Trop. Anim. Hlth Prod.*, *9*, 185.
(5) Barber, T. L. & Yedloutschnig, R. J. (1970) *Cornell Vet.*, *60*, 297.
(6) Ojo, M. O. (1976) *J. comp. Pathol.*, *86*, 519.
(7) MacOwan, K. J. & Minette, J. E. (1977) *Vet. Rec.*, *101*, 380.
(8) Jones, G. E. (1985) *J. comp. Pathol.*, *95*, 305.
(9) Littlejohns, I. R. & Cottew, G. W. (1977) *Aust. vet. J.*, *53*, 297.

(10) Foggie, A. et al. (1971) *J. comp. Pathol.*, *81*, 165 & 393.
(11) Arisoy, F. et al. (1967) *Türk vet. Hekim. Dern. Derg.*, *37*, 11.
(12) Gee, R. W. (1977) *Aust. vet. J.*, *53*, 298.
(13) Spais, A. G. et al. (1970) *Hellen. Kten. Thessaloniki*, *13*, 113.
(14) Popovici, I. & de Simon, M. (1966) *Arch. vet.*, *1*, 21.
(15) Baharsefat, M. et al. (1971) *Arch. Inst. Razi*, *23*, 113.
(16) Schaeren, W. & Nicholer, J. (1982) *Schweiz. Arch. Tierheilkd.*, *124*, 163.
(17) Bar-Moshe, B. et al. (1982) *Refuah Vet.*, *39*, 77 & 85.
(18) Rurangirwa, F. R. et al (1984) *Res. vet. Sci.*, *36*, 174.
(19) Abegunde, T. O. et al. (1981) *Am. J. vet. Res.*, *42*, 1798.
(20) El Hassan, S. M. et al. (1984) *Theriogenology*, *8*, 65.
(21) Prasad, L. N. et al. (1985) *Aust. vet. J.*, *62*, 341.
(22) Jones, G. E. (1985) *J. comp. Pathol.*, *95*, 305.

Mycoplasmal arthritis of cattle

A synovitis and arthritis in feedlot cattle caused by *Mycoplasma agalactiae* subsp. *bovis* has been recognized with increasing frequency in recent years. The disease has been reported in Canada (2), United States, Europe (3), and the United Kingdom (4, 5). It has been recognized most commonly in young feedlot cattle and usually affects many animals a few weeks after arrival and mingling in the lot. During 14 outbreaks in feedlot cattle the morbidity ranged from 18 to 85% and the case mortality from 3 to 50%. In Canada the disease has been seen commonly in young cattle (6–8 months of age) following shipment from western rangelands to eastern feedlots, which suggests that long transportation and mixing of cattle of different origins may be important epidemiological characteristics. Calves sucking cows with experimental mastitis due to this organism developed mycoplasmal arthritis (6), and a high incidence is recorded in calves in dairy herds where mycoplasmal mastitis was occurring (7).

Mycoplasma alkalescens has been isolated from three-week-old calves affected with polyarthritis (10) and a group 7 mycoplasma has been recovered from a calf with polyarthritis (9). *Mycoplasma bovis* may be found in calves with polyarthritis and enzootic pneumonia which may suggest a pneumonia–arthritis syndrome (12, 14, 15).

The intra-articular injection of *Mycoplasma bovis* into calves results in a severe arthritis characterized by fibrinosuppurative synovitis and tenosynovitis (13), erosion of cartilage and its replacement by polypoid granulation tissue. Erosion of the cartilage is accompanied by chronic osteomyelitis and formation of pannus tissue (11). Histologically there is extensive ulceration of synovial membranes of leukocytic infiltration of the subsynovium, congestion, hyperemia, and thrombosis of the subsynovial vessels (11).

Clinical findings

Clinical findings include stiffness of gait, lameness, inappetence, moderate fever, and progressive loss of weight. Swelling of the large movable limb joints and distension of tendon sheaths, associated with fibrinous synovitis and synovial fluid effusions, are characteristic (3). Pneumonia is a common finding in the affected group. Some affected cattle spend considerable time in recumbency and lose weight and develop decubitus ulcers and must be destroyed. Mildly affected cases recover spontaneously in 10–14 days, while severe ones become progressively worse and must be culled. At necropsy, the fibrinous synovitis is remarkable. There is severe thickening and edema of the synovial membranes and large quantities of fibrinopurulent synovial fluid. The tendon sheaths are similarly affected. There may also be pneumonia, pleuritis and pericarditis (2, 5).

Differential diagnosis

The disease must be differentiated from other causes of joint swelling and lameness in feedlot cattle. There are usually several animals affected in a short period of time, which serves to distinguish it from other sporadic causes of arthritis in feedlot cattle. A diagnosis of infection by *Mycoplasma agalactiae* subsp. *bovis* should be considered when pneumonia and arthritis and synovitis occur at about the same time. For a definitive diagnosis, joint fluid must be placed immediately into laboratory media specially prepared for *Mycoplasma* spp. The failure to isolate the mycoplasma from the joint fluid of joints which have been affected for more than 14 days does not exclude a diagnosis of mycoplasma arthritis. The pathogenesis of the arthritis may be similar to an allergic response, either systemically or locally, and the organisms may have been eliminated from the joint (5).

Treatment

Treatment is usually ineffective. Several antibiotics, including tylosin, oxytetracycline, lincomycin and oleandomycin, have been used in natural and experimental cases and while the organism is sensitive to these antibiotics *in vitro*, the response in affected animals has been unsatisfactory (8). A good response is reported to the intra-articular injection of a combination of corticosteroid and antibiotic (1).

Control

Effective control of the disease is not yet possible. However, a formalinized *M. bovis* vaccine gives good protection against experimentally induced mycoplasmal arthritis and may offer a practicable control method (16, 17). Long-term oral administration of tiamulin hydrogen fumarate is claimed to prevent the disease (1). The disease usually disappears from an affected group, which suggests that herd immunity may develop.

REFERENCES

(1) Keller, H. et al. (1980) *Schweiz. Arch. Tierheilkd.*, *122*, 15.
(2) Langford, E. V. (1977) *Can. J. comp. Med.*, *41*, 89.
(3) Romvary, J. et al. (1977) *Magy. Allatorvo. Lap.*, *32*, 801.
(4) Gourlay, R. N. et al. (1976) *J. Am. vet. med. Assoc.*, *98*, 506.
(5) Thomas, L. H. et al. (1975) *Vet. Rec.*, *97*, 55.
(6) Stalheim, O. H. V. & Page, L. A. (1975) *J. clin. Microbiol.*, *2*, 165.
(7) Pfutzner, H. et al. (1980) *Mh VetMed.*, *35*, 499.
(8) Stalheim, O. H. V. (1976) *J. Am. vet. med. Assoc.*, *169*, 1096.
(9) Shiel, M. J. et al. (1982) *Aust. vet. J.*, *59*, 192.
(10) Whithear, K. G. (1983) *Aust. vet. J.*, *60*, 191.
(11) Ryan, M. J. et al. (1983) *Vet. Pathol.*, *20*, 472.
(12) Bocklisch, H. et al. (1983) *Arch. exp. vet. Med.*, *37*, 435.
(13) Pfutzner, H. et al. (1983) *Arch. exp. vet. Med.*, *37*, 445.
(14) Rosendal, S. & Martin, S. W. (1986) *Can. J. vet. Res.*, *50*, 179.
(15) Howard, C. J. (1983) *Yale J. Biol. & Med.*, *56*, 789.
(16) Chima, J. C. et al. (1980) *Vet. Microbiol.*, *5*, 113.
(17) Chima, J. C. et al. (1981) *Can. J. comp. Med.*, *45*, 92.

Enzootic pneumonia of pigs

This is a highly contagious disease of pigs manifested clinically by a pneumonia of moderate severity and failure to grow at a normal rate.

Etiology

The search for the causative agent in this disease was prolonged and exhaustive (1). It is now known to be *Mycoplasma hyopneumoniae* (syn. *suipneumoniae*) (1, 12). The organism inhabits the respiratory tract of pigs and appears to be host-specific. It survives in the environment for only a very short period of time (4). The disease has been reproduced with pure cultures and the organism demonstrated directly or indirectly from pigs with enzootic pneumonia from most areas of the world. Many laboratories have had difficulties in growing the causal agent and a diagnosis of enzootic pneumonia has often been made on clinical and pathological grounds. Other agents can produce similar pathological changes (5) but current evidence suggests that *M. hyopneumoniae* is the primary cause of enzootic pneumonia.

Epidemiology

Enzootic pneumonia occurs in pigs throughout the world and the incidence is high in intensive pig rearing enterprises. It is not uncommon to find lesions in 40–80% of lungs at abattoirs (1). In an abattoir survey, 75% of the pigs may have lesions of enzootic pneumonia, approximately 60% may have atrophic rhinitis and 11% may have pleuropneumonia and pleuritis (58). The organism is an inhabitant of the respiratory tract of pigs and transmission occurs by direct pig-to-pig contact. Air-borne transmission has been demonstrated. There is no other known host for the organism although infection and breakdown of closed pneumonia-free herds has occurred without any pig introductions. The number of organisms required for infection is very small and the possibility of wind-borne infection has been raised (4).

There is considerable variation in the severity of the lung lesions following experimental infection (6) and both host and environmental factors are influential. The extent of the lesions produced by *M. hyopneumoniae* may be markedly influenced by other contributing factors. Concurrent infection with lungworm, migrating ascarids and an adenovirus has resulted in lesions of greater severity and secondary invasion of pneumonic lesions by pasteurellae, streptococci, mycoplasmas, *Bord. bronchiseptica* and *Klebsiella pneumoniae* is very common and largely influences the outcome of the disease in individual pigs. In some abattoir surveys of the lungs, *Past. multocida* can be cultured from 16% of normal lungs and from 55% of lungs with lesions resembling those of enzootic pneumonia (2). *Pasteurella multocida* and *Haemophilus* spp. may also be found in conjunction with *Mycoplasma hyopneumoniae* in the lungs of slaughter weight swine affected with pneumonia and examined at the abattoir (39). Those lungs with both *Mycoplasma pneumoniae* and *Pasteurella multocida* had the most macroscopic pneumonia and those lungs with either of the agents alone had much less pneumonia (39). Along with *Mycoplasma suipneumoniae*, other mycoplasma species such as *M. hyorhinis*, *Acholeplasma granularum* and *Acholeplasma laidlawii* have been isolated from the lungs of pigs at slaughter (3), but their significance is unclear. *Mycoplasma hyopneumoniae* and *Mycoplasma hyorhinis* have been isolated from 30% and 50% of pneumonic lungs, respectively, from pigs examined at slaughter (40). *M. hyopneumoniae* was also isolated from 12% of lungs with no gross lesions of pneumonia.

In many countries and herds, atrophic rhinitis is also present along with enzootic pneumonia and the two diseases in concert may have a greater economic effect than either disease alone. When outbreaks of respiratory disease in pigs occur they are frequently the result of complex interactions between many agents. The importance of *M. hyopneumoniae* is not only its effect as a primary pathogen but also its ability to act synergistically with other infecting agents to produce significant respiratory disease.

Transmission is by the respiratory route (12) and in infected herds occurs primarily from the sow to the suckling piglets. The disease is also transmitted and exacerbated during the grouping and stress of pigs that occurs at weaning. The highest clinical and pathological incidence occurs in the postweaning and growing period and in most herds this is maintained through the growing period to market age. Frequent coughing by infected, intensively reared pigs suggests that repeated aerosol exposure occurs and is an important natural mode of transmission of respiratory pathogens (60). There is general agreement that management and environmental conditions considerably influence the severity of the disease.

In South Australia, in small herds, the factors commonly associated with a high prevalence of enzootic pneumonia were larger numbers of pigs per pen section, larger group sizes and drafty farrowing and weaner accommodation. In large herds, factors associated with a high prevalence were higher pen stocking rate and air-space stocking rate, and a trend toward higher atmospheric ammonia levels in the summer months (41). The trend to increased herd size has not been accompanied by the satisfactory control of pneumonia (42).

A computer-based guide has been developed to study how the prevalence of the disease can be influenced by the combined effect of risk factors (46). The expected prevalence is estimated by consideration of 11 risk factors which include the following: the number of pigs in the same room, all-in/all-out versus continuous flow of pigs, type of partitions separating adjacent pens, presence or absence of diarrhea as a clinical problem, liquid versus solid manure disposal, ascarid control efficiency, and the presence or absence of active Aujeszky's disease (46).

The temperature and humidity influence the penetration into the lungs of both primary and secondary pathogens by influencing the size of infected aerosol particles and the protective mechanism in the respiratory tract. Temperature and humidity also influence the sedimentation of infected particles in the air, and the ventilation and stocking density their concentration (13, 14). Pigs kept at high stocking densities and subjected to environmental temperature fluctuations, cold drafty conditions and poor nutrition are more likely to suffer greater adverse effects from this disease.

In infected herds the morbidity rate is high during

the growing period but the case fatality rate is usually low. There is, however, an increase in the number of treatments of sick pigs in comparison with herds free of the disease (15, 16) and secondary bacterial pneumonia can be a significant cause of mortality in the weaning-to-market period. The morbidity rate falls markedly with increasing age and there is a much lower incidence of pneumonic lesions in sows even though they may still harbor the organism (1, 12). However, when enzootic pneumonia gains entry into a herd which has been previously free of the disease all ages of pigs are affected and mortality, even in adults, can occur. Experimentally, there are no differences in susceptibility of pigs between 3 and 12 weeks of age (47).

The reinfection of enzootic-pneumonia free herds, so-called breakdowns, occurs at a rate of about 3% of herds every 6 months (48). In a study of swine herds which had participated in the Pig Health Control Association Scheme in the United Kingdom, the close proximity of the uninfected herds to infected herds appeared to be the most important risk factor which could explain the introduction of the infection (49). There was little evidence to indicate that unexplained breakdowns occurred in association with long-term latent infection in other herds from which animals had been imported (48). Clinical signs of enzootic pneumonia in these herds commonly did not occur for several months after the introduction of infected pigs.

The prime importance of enzootic pneumonia is in its economic effects on pig-rearing. The disease adversely affects feed conversion efficiency and daily rate of gain. The extent to which it does this is very much dependent upon the conditions in which the pigs are reared and has been a subject of much controversy (16). An accurate assessment of the economic effect has not been possible because of the difficulty of conducting a controlled experiment in which pigs of equivalent genetic merit both free of the disease and infected are raised in an identical manner. In addition, studies on the association between performance parameters and the presence of lesions of enzootic pneumonia have yielded widely variable results dependent on the management and environmental conditions and the different research design and techniques used (43). These problems have been reviewed (43). Experiences in temperature climates such as Australia have shown that, where pigs are under good management, infection of herds previously free of the disease has resulted in no adverse economic effect other than during the initial period of acute infection in the herd. There is no doubt, however, that in other situations adverse economic effects are associated with the disease and these effects have been reviewed elsewhere (16). An early study (17) estimated a reduction of feed conversion efficiency as high as 22% and although the effect of the disease is probably not this severe in most piggeries, a significant economic reduction can occur even under good management conditions (15).

A recent evaluation of the effect of enzootic pneumonia on growth performance revealed a reduction in growth rate of about 13% when pigs were infected between 50 and 85 kg body weight and about 16% from weaning to slaughter when the piglets were infected by the dam (44). The feed conversion rate was depressed by about 14% between 10 and 25 kg body weight. At slaughter, there was evidence of gross lesions of enzootic pneumonia in 40% of the lungs which were free of secondary bacteria. Because there is no universally accepted method of measuring the extent or prevalence of pneumonia in pigs at slaughter the results of studies of correlations between the lesions and performance have been difficult to compare (45). Some methods have been compared and the most informative procedure is assessing the percentage of lung involved and calculating a mean value for the herd sample (45). Assessing the prevalence of affected lungs, or evaluating the maximally affected lung is equally as informative for a herd-based indicator, as scoring the percentage of each lung and calculating a mean value (45). Because the prevalence of pneumonia peaks at about 60–65 kg body weight and then declines steadily to a very low level in pigs that are 125 kg or more, the age and weight at slaughter must be considered when evaluating the effects of the lesions on performance and when comparing results between different observations (43).

Pathogenesis

The experimental inoculation of the J strain of *M. suipneumoniae* into piglets results in gross pneumonic lesions which can usually be detected 7–10 days later. Moderately extensive pneumonia is present 6 weeks after inoculation, progressive recovery can be observed after 10 weeks and residual lung lesions are detectable in a few pigs up to 37 weeks after inoculation (12). Pigs which recover from experimentally induced enzootic pneumonia are resistant to subsequent challenge. The nature of the immunity, whether serum or local antibody-mediated, T-cell mediated, or a combination of these factors, is not understood. Based on lymphocyte transformation tests of experimentally infected pigs, it is possible that cell-mediated immunity correlates with protective immunity (7). Immunity is not conferred through colostral immunoglobulins and thus piglets born from immune dams are susceptible to infection and clinical disease. However, while pigs vaccinated with inactivated *M. hyopneumoniae* organisms develop both a cell-mediated and humoral immune response, the animals are not protected from challenge exposure by natural infection (11). Local immunity, particularly secretory IgA, is considered to be important in protection against mycoplasma infection (19).

M. suipneumoniae causes peribronchiolar lymphoreticular hyperplasia and mononuclear accumulation in the lamina propria which causes obliteration of the bronchial lumina. There is also perivascular lymphoid hyperplasia. The bronchial mucous glands undergo hypertrophy, there are increased numbers of polymorphonuclear cells in the bronchial lumina and macrophages in the alveoli. Lymphocytes, together with plasma cells and macrophages (8) are responsible for the increase in the thickness of the interlobular septa as the disease progresses. Hyperplasia of type II alveolar epithelial cells is progressive as the disease becomes worse. Affected pigs cough persistently, show labored respiration and reduced exercise tolerance. The lesions are similar to those of chronic bronchitis. The effects of *M. suipneumoniae* on the trachea and bronchi of gnotobiotic pigs have been examined (10). The mycoplasmas localize on the tracheal and bronchial mucosae and gradually there is extensive loss of cilia (10). There is a significant increase in the gland/wall ratio and a decrease in the ratio of respiratory to expiratory resistance (9).

The effects of this chronic pulmonary lesion have been the subject of considerable investigation. It is thought that the presence of mycoplasmal lesions uncomplicated by secondary bacterial infections has minimal effect on the production of the pig if the environmental conditions are suitable. The lesions will heal and any loss in production from the initial infection will be regained by compensatory regrowth. Severe lesions or those accompanied by secondary bacterial bronchopneumonia and pleuritis will usually cause a significant decrease in average daily gain and feed efficiency. Secondary infection with *Pasteurella* spp. results in acute episodes of toxemic bronchopneumonia and pleuritis.

The pulmonary and hematologic changes in pigs with experimental *Mycoplasma hyopneumoniae* pneumonia indicate no significant changes in heart rate, respiratory rate, and rectal temperature, even though at necropsy well-demarcated pulmonary lesions were present (50). There were several measurable changes in respiratory functions due to the atelectasis, partial occlusion of the bronchioles with exudate, localized pulmonary edema and a reduction in oxygen perfusion to the alveoli leading to a decrease in the partial pressure of oxygen in the arterial blood (50). There were no remarkable changes in the hematology. The body weight gains were decreased compared to the control animals.

The distribution of lesions is characteristic. They occur in the right cardiac lobe, the right apical and left cardiac lobes, the left apical and the diaphragmatic lobes in that order of frequence. It has been suggested that their distribution is in part due to the more commonly affected lobes (18).

Clinical findings

A natural incubation period of 10–16 days is shortened to 5–12 days by experimental transmission. Two forms of the disease are described. In the relatively rare acute form a severe outbreak may occur in a susceptible herd when the infection is first introduced. In such herds pigs of all ages are susceptible and a morbidity of 100% may be experienced. Sucking piglets as young as 10 days of age have been infected. Acute respiratory distress with or without fever is characteristic and mortality may occur. The usual course of this form of the disease within a herd is usually about 3 months after which it subsides to the more common chronic form.

The chronic form of the disease is much more common and is the pattern seen in endemically infected herds. Young piglets are usually infected when they are 3–10 weeks of age and clinical signs may be seen in suckling piglets. More commonly the disease shows greatest clinical manifestation after weaning and in the growing period. The onset of clinical abnormality is insidious and coughing is the major manifestation. Initially only a few pigs within the group may show clinical abnormality but then the incidence generally increases until coughing may be elicited from most pigs. It may disappear in 2–3 weeks or persist throughout the growing period. In affected herds individual pigs may be heard to cough at any time but coughing is most obvious at initial activity in the morning and at feeding time. Coughing may also be elicited by exercising the pigs around the pen and it occurs with greater frequency in the period immediately following the exercise. A dry or crackling, hacking cough, which is usually repetitive, is characteristic. Respiratory embarrassment is rare and there is no fever or obvious inappetence. Subsequently there is retardation of growth which varies in severity between individuals so that uneven group size is common. Some pigs affected with the chronic form of the disease may later develop acute pneumonia due to secondary invasion with pasteurellae or other organisms.

Clinical disease becomes less obvious with increasing age and is rarely detected in the sow herd though gilts and young sows frequently harbor *M. hyopneumoniae*.

Clinical pathology

The serological tests available for the detection of *M. hyopneumoniae* infection include the complement fixation test (22), latex agglutination test (20), an indirect hemagglutination test (21) and an enzyme-linked immunosorbent assay (ELISA) test (23). The serological tests are more reliable for the detection of infection in a herd than in the individual animal. As these tests were developed they yielded promising results, but are known to have limitations of sensitivity and specificity in routine diagnosis. The complement fixation test is a good predictor of the presence of gross lesions in pigs sent to slaughter (24). However, complement fixation titers may not be detectable by 24 weeks after experimental infection. Latex agglutination titers may persist for 48 weeks after experimental infection and is considered more reliable as a predictor of the presence of microscopic lesions typical of enzootic pneumonia (20). The ELISA test is highly sensitive and specific and antibodies can be detected several weeks before the clinical manifestation of enzootic pneumonia (27).

The indirect hemagglutination test is now considered to have limited value (51). The ELISA test is a very sensitive test for the detection of antibodies to *M. hyopneumoniae*; however, it is not sufficiently specific due to the antigenic relationships between other porcine mycoplasmas such as *M. flocculare* (52–54). The ELISA test could be made more specific if crossreactive antibodies could be removed from the test sera, or crossreactive determinants removed from the test antigen. The ELISA test may also remain positive for up to 1 year after experimental exposure even when pulmonary lesions are absent and the lungs are culturally and immunofluorescent negative for *M. hyopneumoniae* (53). An immunoblotting procedure to characterize the sequential antibody response to *M. hyopneumoniae* infection is currently being examined (62).

Necropsy findings

Lesions are confined almost entirely to the apical and cardiac lobes and are clearly demarcated from the normal lung tissue. The lesions are commonly more severe in the right than in the left lung. Plum-colored or grayish areas of consolidation resembling lymphoid tissue are scattered along the ventral borders of the lobes. Liquefaction of the pneumonic tissue, pericarditis and pleurisy are unusual in the pure infection. Enlarged edematous bronchial lymph nodes are characteristic. In acute cases there is intense edema and congestion of the lung and frothy exudate in the bronchi. When secondary invasion occurs, pleurisy and pericarditis are common and there may be severe hepatization and congestion with necrotizing bronchopneumonia.

A definitive diagnosis of mycoplasmal pneumonia of swine requires that *M. hyopneumoniae* be demonstrated in indirect immunofluorescent stained lung sections or that it be recovered culturally (55). Up to 19% of grossly normal lungs may be infected with *M. hyopneumoniae*. About 33% of the lungs of pigs from herds thought to be affected with mycoplasma pneumonia may have lesions which appear to be typical of mycoplasma pneumonia, but *M. hyopneumoniae* could not be demonstrated by immunofluorescence or by culture techniques, the sensitivity of which may also be a problem (55). In experimentally induced pneumonia of piglets with *M. hyopneumoniae* the organism was detected by immunofluorescence primarily on bronchial and bronchiolar epithelial surfaces of lungs with gross lesions of pneumonia (61). Fluorescence was most intense 4–6 weeks after infection and began to decrease at 8–12 weeks. This suggests a decrease in the number of *M. hyopneumoniae* in the more advanced stages of the disease.

Diagnosis

There are two major problems in the diagnosis of pneumonia in swine. One is the differential clinical diagnosis of pneumonia when the clinical findings suggest pneumonia. Elective necropsy and routine laboratory examination will usually yield a diagnosis. The other more difficult problem is making a definitive etiological diagnosis of the presence of the subclinical form of enzootic pneumonia caused by *M. hyopneumoniae* or, more difficult, certifying the absence of infection in a group or herd of pigs.

Enzootic pneumonia of pigs, with or without secondary bacterial invasion, is the commonest respiratory infection in this species. An acute outbreak may be confused with swine influenza, but this disease is much less common and is characterized by a short course in which sneezing and muscle pain are prominent and the signs are in general more indicative of an upper respiratory infection than of pneumonia. In swine influenza, *Hemophilus suis* is always present and lungworm infestation is an integral part of the disease. Uncomplicated lungworm (*Metastrongylus* spp.) infestation may also cause respiratory signs in pigs. However, at necropsy, patchy bronchopneumonia is most marked in the dorsal part of the diaphragmatic lobes and worms can be demonstrated. Contagious pleuropneumonia of pigs caused by *Actinobacillus* (*Hemophilus*) *pleuropneumoniae* is a much more acute and highly fatal disease.

Ascaris lumbricoides infestations are commonly cited as a cause of chronic swine pneumonia, but experimental ascariasis produces mainly hepatic damage by migrating larvae. In the lungs some hemorrhage occurs and there may be a mild febrile reaction and a soft moist cough lasting for up to 5 days during the stage of larval migration, but the respiratory signs do not persist. Occasional fatal cases of pulmonary ascariasis occur. Under field conditions coughing is never marked in ascariasis, while it is the major sign in enzootic pneumonia.

The determination of the presence or absence of enzootic pneumonia within a herd for certification purposes can be difficult and should be approached with caution. It should not be based on a single examination procedure. It requires a surveillance system which combines regular farm visits and serological, cultural and tissue examination of selected pigs and of those sent to slaughter. The herd should be examined clinically for evidence of the disease and the lungs from several shipments of pigs should be examined at the abattoir and subsequently histologically. There can be seasonal variation in the severity of lung lesions (25) and at certain times market-age pigs may not have any visible gross lesions even though infection may be present in the herd. If doubt exists, the lungs of younger pigs, preferably clinically suspect pigs, or recently weaned pigs, should be examined after elective slaughter. The herd should also be examined for the presence of antibody to *M. hyopneumoniae*. There is evidence that infection can exist within a herd for a period of time without the presence of positive serological, clinical or pathological manifestations (26).

The gross and histological findings in the lungs of pigs with enzootic pneumonia are not pathognomonic for this infection alone and a positive diagnosis relies on the identification of *M. hyopneumoniae*, a technique which can be difficult. The organism is difficult to grow and is easily supplanted in cultures by other organisms, especially *M. hyorhinis*, which may be present. A negative culture does not indicate freedom from infection and there is evidence that the exposure of susceptible pigs to suspect lung tissue is a much more sensitive test system (12). The organisms may also be demonstrated by fluorescent antibody techniques on touch preparations of lung tissue (12) or by the enzyme-linked immunoperoxidase technique (27).

The radiological examination of pigs for the presence of lesions of enzootic pneumonia has limitations because foci of consolidation less than 2 cm^3 may not be detected (38).

Treatment

There is no effective treatment that will eliminate infection with *M. hyopneumoniae* although the severity of the clinical disease may be reduced. A mixture of tylosin tartrate at a dose of 50 mg/kg body weight and tiamutilin at 10 mg/kg body weight administered orally daily for 10 days can significantly reduce the pulmonary lesions caused by the experimental inoculation of *M. hyopneumoniae* (56). Tetracyclines will either prevent transmission or suppress lesion formation in experimental pigs (28) but the levels required are high and in an infected herd continuous administration would be necessary which would be uneconomic. Treatment is generally restricted to individual pigs showing acute respiratory distress as a result of a severe infection or secondary invaders. Broad-spectrum antibiotics are used, usually tetracyclines, but the response is only moderately good. The occurrence of severe signs within a group of pigs may necessitate treatment. Tetracyclines, tylosin or spiramycin fed at 200 mg/kg feed for 5–10 days are recommended (29). Preliminary studies of treatment with tiamulin at 200 mg/kg feed for 10 days are promising (30).

Control

M. hyopneumoniae infects only pigs and transmission requires close pig-to-pig contact. If transmission can be prevented it is possible to limit or even eradicate the disease from a herd. There are thus two levels at which control can be practiced: complete eradication, or keeping the disease and its effects at a low level.

Control by eradication

This method of control is the most satisfactory and it is probably mandatory for large breeding companies and herds supplying replacement stock to other herds and for large intensive farrow-to-finish enterprises. There have been several ways in which eradication has been attempted but the most satisfactory is by repopulation with specific-pathogen-free (SPF) pigs. The principle behind this method is that the piglet *in utero* is free of infection with *M. hyopneumoniae*. If it is taken from the uterus at term by suitable sterile hysterectomy or hysterotomy techniques and reared artificially in an environment free of pigs it will remain free of this infection. In practice this has been done in special units and the piglets have been subsequently used to repopulate existing farms where all pigs have been removed 30 days prior to the introduction of the SPF pigs and a thorough cleansing program completed. This method was initially developed for the control of enzootic pneumonia and atrophic rhinitis. Moreover, if suitable precautions are taken and if the piglets are used to populate new units that have had no previous exposure to pigs, then freedom from other important diseases such as internal and external parasitism, leptospirosis, brucellosis, swine dysentery and others can be achieved. The progeny of these primary SPF herds can subsequently be used to repopulate other or secondary SPF herds. The details of these procedures have been reviewed elsewhere (31).

In view of the cost and technical difficulty of this method, other methods of eradicating enzootic pneumonia have been attempted but they are generally less satisfactory and have a higher failure rate. These include 'snatching' of pigs at birth and isolated farrowing. In the former the piglets are caught and removed from the sow immediately at birth and reared as previously described or foster-suckled on SPF sows in another environment. Although enzootic pneumonia may be eliminated by this method, fecal contamination during parturition of the vulva and vagina and consequently of the piglet is common and this method is less satisfactory for disease control than removal by hysterectomy.

Isolated farrowing techniques have proved successful in small herds but have a high failure rate when practiced on a large scale. Briefly, with this method, older sows believed to be free of infection are farrowed in isolation in individual pens erected outside on pasture and each sow and litter is kept as a separate unit. The litter is inspected clinically at regular intervals and subsequently a proportion of the litter, usually excess males and gilts undesirable for breeding, are examined at slaughter for evidence of pneumonia. Any litters that show clinical, pathological or laboratory evidence of pneumonia are eliminated from the program. Litters that pass inspection are kept for repopulation of the herd. Because of the difficulties in detecting carrier pigs without lesions (32) eradication by methods using these principles frequently fails.

Eradication has also been attempted by antibiotic treatment of newborn piglets with subsequent removal to clean premises (33) and by serological testing of the breeding herd and culling of positive reactors (34). None of these methods has proved as satisfactory as eradication by SPF pig repopulation (31, 35, 36), and if eradication is to be attempted this is the method of choice.

SPF herds have been established in most countries with significant pig populations either by breeding companies or private purebred breeders often with government supervision and assistance (31, 36). As a result there is, in most countries, a nucleus of enzootic pneumonia-free stock. The establishment of primary SPF herds is technically difficult and very costly and should not be undertaken lightly. There is also a considerable delay in cash flow between the time of initial population and build-up of herd numbers to the time when significant numbers of pigs are available for sale. Because of this, if eradication by repopulation is intended, it is preferable to purchase pregnant gilts from established primary SPF herds unless the maintenance of existing genetic lines dictates otherwise. Before recommending eradication by this method it is essential that the pig owner understands the principles of this method of control and the restrictions that will need to apply if it is to be successful. Farrow-to-finish enterprises established by this method should be run as closed herds and if further genetic material is required it should be introduced by hysterectomy techniques, or by purchase from the initial source herd. The use of semen is an alternate method; however, isolation of *M. hyopneumoniae* from semen is recorded (37).

The problem of certifying and maintaining herds free of enzootic pneumonia is a major task and is probably best done by governmental agencies.

Reinfection of enzootic pneumonia-free pig herds occurs despite high standards of isolation and strict precautions whereby complete protective clothing and showering routines are required for all visitors entering the unit (48, 49). Time rules are also in effect whereby all visitors were debarred entry if they had been to a possible source of infection during the previous 48 hours and even up to 7 days. Also, the majority of breakdowns occur in herds which have not imported infected stock recently. In reinfected herds which imported stock there was no concurrent evidence of breakdown in the parent herds, which supported the contention that the importation of infected pigs was an unlikely source of the infection (48). An epidemiological investigation of these reinfections suggests that close proximity of uninfected herds to infected herds may be an important factor. The organism does not survive for more than a few days under dry conditions; however, it can survive in diluted tapwater and rainwater for 2–3 weeks and it has been suggested that the organism may be transported in moist air and that air-borne infection between piggeries is a possible method of transmission (49). Some preliminary estimates of risk indices based on the proximity of other pig units has indicated that the most important factor was the reciprocal of the square of distance to the nearest other unit. The crucial distance for maximum survival was about 3·2 km (49).

Low level disease

The second level of control is to attempt to limit the effects of the disease in those herds where eradication is either not desirable or feasible. The effects of the disease are generally less severe in non-intensive rearing situations and in small herds where individual litters are reared separately and where litters from older sows can be reared separately from other pigs. Where litters are grouped at weaning, a low stocking density with less than 25 pigs in initial pen groups and 100 pigs in a common airspace may also reduce the severity. Temperature, humidity and ventilation also have an important influence on the disease (1). They are interrelated with stocking density and housing. The subject is too broad for treatment here and the requirements for pigs at different ages and under different housing situations may be found in standard texts on pig housing and production.

Where possible the purchase of weaners or pigs for fattening should be from herds free of the disease or from a single source. Purchase through sale yards or the purchase of coughing or uneven litters is not advisable. When pigs from infected herds are purchased it may be necessary to medicate the feed prophylactically with one of the tetracycline group of antibiotics or tylosin or spiramycin at 100–200 mg/kg of feed for a 2-week period after introduction. Medication of the feed of finishing pigs with tiamulin at 20 and 30 mg/kg of feed over an 8-week period on farms with histories of severe complicated enzootic pneumonia resulted in improved weight gains and feed efficiency, but the extent and severity of the lung lesions did not change (57). The level of 30 mg/kg in the feed was superior to the level of 20 mg/kg. Tiamulin at 100 mg/kg combined with chlortetracycline at 300 mg/kg of feed for 7 days was effective in herds with a history of enzootic pneumonia complicated by the presence of *Past. multocida* and *A. pleuropneumoniae* (59).

Introduced pigs should be isolated from the rest of the herd and preferably they should be reared as a batch through a house on the all-in, all-out system. A high stocking density should be avoided and internal parasites should be controlled (36).

Immunization

Vaccination with killed *M. hyopneumoniae* induces protection in pigs against experimental challenge exposure with the organism (63). However, vaccination with the same preparations are not protected against mycoplasma pneumonia when placed in herds with the naturally occurring disease (11). The failure of the vaccine to protect against naturally occurring disease may be due to the presence of heterologous mycoplasma or factors other than infectious agents (60). A method for assessing induced resistance to enzootic pneumonia has been evaluated and recommended (64).

REVIEW LITERATURE

Huhn, R. G. (1970) Enzootic pneumonia of pigs: a review of the literature. *Vet. Bull.*, *40*, 249.

Morrison, R. B., Pijoan, C. & Leman, A. D. (1986) Association between enzootic pneumonia and performance. *Pig News Inf.*, *7*, 23–31.

Whittlestone, P. (1973) Enzootic pneumonia of pigs (EPP). *Adv. vet. Sci.*, *17*, 1.

REFERENCES

(1) Huhn, R. G. (1970) *Vet. Bull.*, *40*, 249.
(2) Osborne, A. D. et al. (1981) *Can. vet. J.*, *22*, 82.
(3) Tiong, S. K. & Sing, K. Y. (1981) *Vet. Rec.*, *108*, 75.
(4) Goodwin, R. F. W. (1972) *Res. vet. Sci.*, *13*, 257, 263.
(5) Jericho, K. (1977) *Vet. Bull.*, *47*, 887.
(6) Roberts, D. H. (1974) *Br. vet. J.*, *130*, 68.
(7) Adegboye, D. S. (1978) *Res. vet. Sci.*, *25*, 323.
(8) Baskerville, A. (1972) *Res. vet. Sci.*, *13*, 570.
(9) Marshall, P. W. et al. (1980) *Br. vet. J.*, *136*, 388.
(10) Mebus, C. A. & Underdahl, N. R. (1977) *Am. J. vet. Res.*, *38*, 1249.
(11) Kristensen, B. et al. (1981) *Am. J. vet. Res.*, *42*, 784.
(12) Whittlestone, P. (1973) *Adv. vet. Sci.*, *17*, 2.
(13) Jericho, K. W. (1967) *Vet. Rec.*, *80*, *clin. Suppl.* 9, VII.
(14) Gordon, W. A. M. (1963) *Br. vet. J.*, *119*, 263, 307.
(15) Braude, R. & Planka, S. (1975) *Vet. Res.*, *96*, 359.
(16) Jericho, K. W. F. et al. (1975) *Can. vet. J.*, *16*, 44.
(17) Betts, A. O. et al. (1955) *Vet. Rec.*, *69*, 661.
(18) Edwards, M. J. et al. (1971) *Aust. vet. J.*, *47*, 477.
(19) Whittlestone, P. (1976) *Adv. vet. Sci. comp. Med.*, *20*, 227.
(20) Slavik, M. F. & Switzer, W. P. (1981) *Am. J. vet. Res.*, *42*, 862.
(21) Holmgren, N. (1974) *Res. vet. Sci.*, *17*, 145.
(22) Blackburn, B. O. et al. (1975) *Am. J. vet. Res.*, *36*, 1381.
(23) Nicolet, J. et al. (1980) *Res. vet. Sci.*, *29*, 305.
(24) McKean, J. D. (1979) *J. Am. vet. med. Assoc.*, *174*, 1979.
(25) Penny, R. H. C. (1976) *Vet. Ann.*, *17*, 111.
(26) Keller, H. (1976) *Proc. 4th int. Congr. Pig vet. Soc.*, PP11.
(27) Bruggman, S. et al. (1977) *Vet. Rec.*, *101*, 109.
(28) Huhn, R. G. (1971) *Can J. comp. Med.*, *35*, 77.
(29) Taillandier J. J. (1973) *Rec. med. Vet.*, *149*, 1393.
(30) Goodwin, R. F. W. (1979) *Vet. Rec.*, *104*, 194.
(31) Twiehaus, M. J. & Underdahl, N. R. (1975) In *Diseases of Swine*, eds H. W. Dunne & A. D. Leman, pp. 1163–1179. Ames, Iowa: Iowa State University Press.
(32) Goodwin, R. F. W. & Whittlestone, P. (1967) *Vet. Rec.*, *81*, 643.
(33) Glawischnig, E. & Schuller, W. (1972) *Dtsch Tierärztl. Wochenschr.*, 79, 261.
(34) Preston, K. S. (1976) *Proc. 4th int. Congr. Pig vet. Soc.*, PP7.
(35) McDermid, K. A. (1964) *Can. vet. J.*, 5, 95.
(36) Rapports 2 (1974) La pneumonie enzootique du porc. *Bull. Off. int. Epizootol.*, *82*, 175.
(37) Schulman, A. & Estola T. (1974) *Vet. Rec.*, *94*, 330.
(38) Wood, A. K. W. & Lloyd, L. C. (1980) *Res. vet. Sci.*, *29*, 8.
(39) Morrison, R. B. et al. (1985) *Can. J. comp. Med.*, 49, 129.
(40) MacPherson, M. R. & Hodges, R. T. (1985) *NZ vet. J.*, *33*, 194.
(41) Pointon, A. M. et al. (1985) *Aust. vet. J.*, 62, 98.
(42) Pointon, A. M. & Sloane, M. (1984) *Aust. vet. J.*, 61, 408.
(43) Morrison, R. B. et al. (1986) *Pigs News Inf.*, 7, 23.
(44) Pointon, A. M. et al. (1985) *Aust. vet. J.*, *62*, 13.
(45) Morrison, R. B. et al. (1985) *Can. vet. J.*, *26*, 381.
(46) Morrison, R. B. & Morris, R. S. (1985) *Vet. Rec.*, *117*, 268.
(47) Piffer, I. A. & Ross, R. F. (1984) *Am. J. vet. Res.*, *45*, 478.
(48) Goodwin, R. F. W. (1984) *Vet. Rec.*, *115*, 320.
(49) Goodwin, R. F. W. (1985) *Vet. Rec.*, *116*, 690.
(50) Intraraksa, Y. et al. (1984) *Am. J. vet. Res.*, *45*, 474.
(51) Freeman, M. J. et al. (1984) *Vet. Microbiol.*, *9*, 259.
(52) Freeman, M. J. et al. (1984) *Can. J. comp. Med.*, *48*, 202.
(53) Armstrong, C. H. et al. (1983) *Can. J. comp. Med.*, *47*, 464.
(54) Piffer, I. A. et al. (1984) *Am. J. vet. Res.*, *45*, 1122.
(55) Armstrong, C. H. et al. (1984) *Can. J. comp. Med.*, *48*, 278.
(56) Hannan, P. C. T. et al. (1982) *Res. vet. Sci.*, *33*, 76.
(57) Burch, D. G. S. (1984) *Vet. Rec.*, *114*, 209.

(58) Wilson, M. R. et al. (1986) *Can. J. vet. Res.*, *50*, 209.
(59) Burch, D. G. S. et al. (1986) *Vet. Rec.*, *119*, 108.
(60) Jericho, K. W. F. (1986) *Can. J. vet. Res.*, *50*, 136.
(61) Amanfu, W. et al. (1984) *Am. J. vet. Res.*, *45*, 1349.
(62) Young, T. F. & Ross, R. F. (1987) *Am. J. vet. Res.*, *48*, 651.
(63) Ross, R. F. et al. (1984) *Am. J. vet. Res.*, *45*, 1899.
(64) Etheridge, J. R. & Lloyd, L. C. (1982) *Res. vet. Sci.*, *33*, 188.

Mycoplasmal arthritis in pigs

Mycoplasmal arthritis occurs in suckling and growing pigs.

Etiology

There are two species of mycoplasma associated with arthritis in pigs: *M. hyorhinis* which produces arthritis and polyserositis predominantly in young pigs, and *M. hyosynoviae* which produces arthritis in growing pigs. The respective conditions have been reproduced experimentally (1–3). An isolate named *M. hyoarthrinosa* (4) has been associated with a syndrome similar to that produced by *M. hyosynoviae*. However, these organisms may be the same species. Other mycoplasmas including *M. flocculare* (5) and *Acholeplasma* spp. (6) have been isolated from pigs but appear to have no propensity to produce arthritis.

Epidemiology

M. hyorhinis is an inhabitant of the respiratory tract and conjunctivae of pigs and is a common secondary infection in pre-existing respiratory disease. It colonizes the mucosa of suckling piglets within the first few weeks of life (7) and may invade spontaneously to produce bacteremia with subsequent polyserositis and arthritis but more commonly does so following stress. Disease is essentially restricted to pigs between 3 and 10 weeks of age and occurs in older suckling pigs and following weaning, but may occur occasionally in older pigs. Disease occurs sporadically in most herds and is a significant cause of sporadic runting in young pigs. Outbreaks can occur with multiple cases within and between litters. The case fatality rate seldom exceeds 10% but chronically affected pigs fail to grow and become runts.

M. hyosynoviae is carried on the pharyngeal mucosa and tonsil. Shedding is less frequent than with *M. hyorhinis* and the organism cannot usually be isolated from the pharynx of piglets prior to 7 weeks of age (8). There is some variation in virulence between strains (6, 9). With virulent strains, bacteremia with subsequent arthritis follows within a few days of minor stress such as vaccination, movement, regrouping or a change in weather (10, 11). The overall prevalence of clinical disease appears to be low but it achieves significance in certain herds which experience a persistent problem. Clinical disease occurs primarily in pigs over 3 months of age and in replacement stock brought into these problem herds (10, 11). It is more prevalent in heavily muscled pigs with straight-legged conformation and there is variation in breed susceptibility (6). Morbidity in problem herds is generally 5–15% but may reach 50%. Mortality is rare but 2–15% may become chronically affected.

Transmission of infection is by direct contact or possibly by aerosol infection. *M. hyosynoviae* can survive drying for up to 4 weeks (12) and may be capable of survival in the environment for longer periods than most mycoplasmas. A further consideration of the importance of these diseases must be given to their possible contribution to the occurrence of carcass condemnation from arthritis.

Pathogenesis

Invasion with clinically undetectable bacteremia may follow stress. Clinical disease is manifest if localization occurs but this is probably the exception rather than the rule. In the experimental disease the incubation period varies from 4 to 10 days (1–3). The reason for the variation in age susceptibility between the two diseases is unknown. *M. hyorhinis* produces a polyserositis in which fibrinous pericarditis, pleuritis and occasionally pneumonia, or polyarthritis, may be the predominant feature (1, 2). *M. hyosynoviae* produces synovitis with some arthritis, especially in the larger joints of the hindlimbs (3).

Clinical findings

Pigs affected with *M. hyorhinis* show initial transient fever, depression and inappetence. Dyspnea with abdominal breathing and a pleural friction rub may be present. There is polyarthritis with lameness, reluctance to rise and moderate swelling and heat in affected joints. Pigs may recover spontaneously in 1–2 weeks but more commonly become unthrifty. Acute outbreaks may occur in suckling pigs 3–8 weeks of age but more commonly the disease is more sporadic and insidious, producing moderate illthrift in a proportion of the sucklers which then show severe runting following weaning. With *M. hyosynoviae* infection there is a sudden onset of acute lameness in one or more limbs, usually without fever. Lameness may be referable to one or more joints and the stifle, hock and elbow joints are most commonly affected. The lameness is severe although clinical swelling of the affected joint may be minimal. In the majority of affected pigs clinical recovery occurs after 3–10 days but some may become permanently recumbent.

Clinical pathology

Blood cell counts remain within the normal range but there is an increase in leukocytes and protein in synovial fluid (13). The organisms may be detected by immunofluorescent techniques, and complement fixing antibody develops following infection (6, 8).

Necropsy findings

A serofibrinous pleuritis, pericarditis and peritonitis are present with *M. hyorhinis* infections. Chronic cases show fibrous pleural and pleural–pericardial adhesions. Synovial hypertrophy with an increased amount of serosanguineous synovial fluid occurs in affected joints with both mycoplasmal species. Chronic cases show thickening of the joint capsule with a varying degree of articular erosion and pannus formation (1–3). With both infections the organism is more easily demonstrated during the acute stage of the disease.

Diagnosis

The initial diagnosis and differentiation from other conditions is most commonly made following postmortem and laboratory examination. Streptococci are the most common cause of polyarthritis in pigs but the disease usually occurs in younger piglets and produces a more purulent arthritis with marked swelling of joints. Glasser's disease is very similar to infection with *M. hyorhinis*. The onset of the former is usually more dramatic and the swelling of joints and tendon sheaths more severe but cultural differentiation is frequently necessary. Erysipelas, arthritis and osteochondrosis are common in the same age group as arthritis due to *M. hyosynoviae* and apart from epidemiological considerations frequently require laboratory differentiation.

Treatment

Treatment with injectable tylosin at 1–2 mg/kg body weight or lincomycin at 2·5 mg/kg has been recommended (10). Early treatment of *M. hyosynoviae* arthritis with 8 mg of betamethasone intramuscularly has been found to reduce the occurrence of chronic lameness (11). Tiamulin at both 10 and 15 mg/kg body weight intramuscularly daily for 3 days is effective for treatment of pigs affected with arthritis caused by *M. hyosynoviae* and is as effective as lincomycin (14).

Control

The control of both diseases rests largely in the avoidance of stress situations. The administration of tylosin or tetracyclines in the drinking water or feed during unavoidable stress such as weaning can reduce the incidence. Early weaning at 3–5 weeks of age has been recommended as a method of preventing infection of pigs with *M. hyosynoviae* and thus of reducing the occurrence of the disease in growing pigs (8).

REFERENCES

(1) Roberts, E. D. et al. (1963) *Am. J. vet. Res.*, *24*, 9, 19.
(2) Ennis, R. S. et al. (1971) *Arthritis Rheum.*, *14*, 202.
(3) Ross, R. F. et al. (1971) *Am. J. vet. Res.*, *32*, 1743.
(4) Robinson, F. R. et al. (1967) *Am. J. vet Res.*, *28*, 483.
(5) Friis, N. F. (1976) *Proc. 4th int. Congr. Pig vet. Soc.*, 15.
(6) Ross, R. F. (1973) *Ann. NY Acad. Sci.*, *225*, 347.
(7) Gios, M. M. et al. (1969) *Zentralbl. VetMed.*, *B16*, 253.
(8) Ross, R. F. & Spear, M. L. (1973) *Am. J. vet. Res.*, *34*, 373.
(9) Furlong, S. L. & Turner, A. J. (1975) *Aust. vet. J.*, *51*, 291.
(10) Bailey, J. H. (1972) *Vet. Med. small Anim. Clin.*, *67*, 197.
(11) Roberts, D. H. et al. (1972) *Vet. Rec.*, *90*, 307.
(12) Friis, N. F. (1973) *Acta vet. Scand.*, *14*, 489.
(13) Barden, J. A. & Decker, J. L. (1971) *Arthritis Rheum.*, *14*, 193.
(14) Birch, D. G. S. & Goodwin, R. F. W. (1984) *Vet. Rec.*, *115*, 594.

21

Diseases Caused by Viruses and Chlamydia—I

THE comments made earlier about diseases caused by bacteria and their importance as infectious diseases to agriculture apply also to diseases caused by viruses, which are presented in this chapter and Chapter 22. However, there are in addition other factors which have made viral diseases even more important.

- Viruses have a much greater capability for surviving independently of their host. Spore-forming bacteria live for much longer periods, but in general terms viruses are more viable at large than are bacteria
- Viruses also have a greater capacity for living in harmony with the host, without destroying it. This has concentrated attention on the so-called 'slow viruses', those of equine infectious anemia, maedi and scrapie
- Viruses have a much greater capacity of changing antigenically, either as mutations or as antigenic drift in response to mounting defense pressures
- Because of their structure viruses are much less susceptible to cleaning and disinfectant agents than bacteria
- Many of the viruses are insect-borne and have reservoir hosts in other species, especially wildlife.

These properties pose very real problems in infectious diseases, in diagnosis and therefore in control and eradication, and in the development of suitable vaccines. In terms of exotic disease threats they represent a much more significant challenge than bacterial diseases did, and always have the capacity for escaping beyond standard prophylactic barriers and set out on a path of global disease. In recent times African swine fever, bluetongue and African horse sickness have made territorial gains in this way, while the vesicular diseases and the insect-borne encephalitides are constantly on the move into new territory. Perhaps the biggest threat, because of its zoonotic potential, is Rift Valley fever.

The role of the field veterinarian is made very much more onerous by the presence of these diseases. Because of the speed with which they spread, for example when foot-and-mouth disease virus is airborne, or when ephemeral fever is carried by *Culicoides* sp., they can appear for the first time in an outbreak some distance from their point of entry and in places where an imported exotic disease would not be expected to appear for the first time. The field veterinarian has to be on the alert at all times for the appearance of a new disease in his/her practice area, and be aware of the implications of their presence, and the sort of emergency action necessary when they are recognized.

There is no way to prepare oneself for an encounter with an exotic viral disease other than becoming familiar with their clinical and clinicopathological findings and their epidemiological behavior. This chapter and Chapter 22 attempt to fill that need.

A summary of relevant viral diseases is given in Table 66.

VIRAL DISEASES WITH MANIFESTATIONS ATTRIBUTABLE TO INVOLVEMENT OF THE BODY AS A WHOLE

Hog cholera (swine fever)

Hog cholera is a highly infectious, viral septicemia affecting only pigs. Its former characterization as an acute, fatal disease with a clinical and postmortem picture of septicemia and hemorrhage has been expanded to include a chronic illness, recovery when supportive treatment is given to older pigs, and the appearance of newborn pigs with congenital defects (1). This expansive definition has led to the suggestion that the disease should be defined as 'any disease associated with a swine fever virus' (2).

Table 66. Summary of the viral diseases of food animals and horses.

Disease	*Syndrome*	*Species affected*	*Identification* *Family*	*Genus/subfamily*	*Serotypes*
Equine viral *abortion*	Abortion	Horse	Herpesviridae	Alphaherpesvirinae	1
Ovine pulmonary *adenomatosis*	Pneumonia	Sheep	Retroviridae	Oncovirinae	1
Equine *adenovirus* infection	Upper respiratory tract infection	Horse	Adenoviridae	Mastadenovirus	?
African horse sickness	(1) Cardiac edema (2) Pulmonary edema	Horse, dog	Reoviridae	Orbivirus	9
African swine fever	Septicemia	Pig	Unclassified	Unclassified	?
Akabane disease	Congenital arthrogryposis hydranencephaly	Cattle, sheep, pig	Bunyaviridae	Bunyavirus	1
Infectious equine *anemia*	Anemia, incoordination	Horse	Retroviridae	Lentivirinae	1
Equine viral *arteritis*	Upper respiratory trait infection, edema, abortion	Horse	Togaviridae	Arterivirus	1
Caprine *arthritis-encephalitis*	Encephalitis, arthritis pneumonia, mastitis	Goat	Retroviridae	Lentivirinae	1
Bluetongue	Stomatitis, coronitis	Sheep, cattle, goat	Reoviridae	Orbivirus	24
Border disease	Congenital tremor, hairy fleece	Sheep	Togaviridae	Pestivirus (the BVD virus)	1
Borna disease	Encephalomyelitis	Horse	Unclassified	Unclassified	1
CAE	*See caprine arthritis-encephalitis*				
Hog cholera	Septicemia	Pig	Togaviridae	Pestivirus	1
Equine *coital* exanthema	Vaginitis, posthitis	Horse	Herpesviridae	Alphaherpesvirinae	1
Bovine *coronavirus* diarrhea	Diarrhea	Cattle	Coronaviridae	Coronavirus	1
Equine *coronavirus* diarrhea	Diarrhea	Horse	Coronaviridae	Coronavirus	1
Cowpox	Dermatitis	Cattle	Poxviridae	Orthopoxvirus	1
Bovine virus *diarrhea*	Diarrhea, congenital disease, nervous system	Cattle	Togaviridae	Pestivirus (*see* border disease)	1
Contagious *ecthyma*	Dermatitis, stomatitis	Sheep, goat	Poxviridae	Parapoxvirus	1
Eastern equine *encephalomyelitis*	Encephalitis	Horse	Togaviridae	Alphavirus	1
Venezuelan equine *encephalomyelitis*	Encephalitis	Horse	Togaviridae	Alphavirus	7
Western equine *encephalomyelitis*	Encephalitis	Horse	Togaviridae	Alphavirus	1
Encephalomyocarditis	Heart failure, encephalitis	Pig	Piconaviridae	Cardiovirus	1
Bovine *ephemeral* fever	Septicemia	Cattle	Rhabdoviridae	Not named	1
Vesicular *exanthema* swine	Stomatitis/coronitis	Pig	Caliciviridae	Calicivirus	Multiple
Foot and mouth disease	Stomatitis/coronitis	Cattle, sheep, goat, pig	Picornaviridae	Aphthovirus	7
Goatpox	Dermatitis	Cattle	Poxviridae	Capripoxvirus	1
Porcine *hemagglutinating* encephalomyelitis	Encephalitis	Pig	Coronaviridae	Coronavirus	1
Porcine cytomegalic *inclusion* body disease	Rhinitis	Pig	Herpesviridae	Betaherpesvirinae	1
Equine infectious *influenza*	Upper respiratory tract infection	Horse	Orthomyxoviridae	Influenzavirus	2
Swine *influenza*	Upper respiratory tract infection	Pig	Orthomyxoviridae	Influenzavirus	Multiple
Japanese encephalitis	Abortion, neonatal death	Pig	Flaviviridae	Flavivirus	1
Bovine viral *leukosis*	Lymph node enlargement etc.	Cattle	Retroviridae	Oncovirinae	1
Porcine *lymphosarcoma*	Lymph node enlargement	Pig	Retroviridae	Oncovirinae	1
Louping ill	Encephalitis	Sheep	Flaviviridae	Flavivirus	1
Lumpy skin disease	Dermatitis	Cattle	Poxviridae	Capripoxviridae	1
Maedi visna	Pneumonia	Sheep	Retroviridae	Lentivirinae	1
Bovine *malignant* catarrh	Stomatitis, coronitis	Cattle	Herpesviridae	Gammaherpesvirinae	1
Bovine *mammillitis*	Teat dermatitis	Cattle, *see* pseudolumpy skin disease	Herpesviridae	Alphaherpesvirinae (bovine herpesvirus 2)	1
Mucosal disease	Stomatitis	Cattle, *see* BVD	Togavirus	Pestivirus	1
Nairobi sheep disease	Enteritis, abortion	Sheep, goat	Bunyaviridae	Nairovirus	1
Orf	*see* ecthyma				
Papillomatosis	Skin growth	Cattle, horse	Papoviridae	Papillomavirus	6
Bovine *papular* stomatitis	Stomatitis	Cattle	Poxviridae	Parapoxvirus	1
Parainfluenza-3	Pneumonia	Cattle, sheep	Paramyxoviridae	Paramyxovirus	1
Porcine *parvovirus* disease	Reproductive insufficiency (SMEDI)	Pig	Parvoviridae	Parvovirus	1
Peste des petits ruminants	Stomatitis, enteritis	Sheep, goat	Paramyxoviridae	Morbillivirus	1
Porcine *polioencephalomyelitis*	Encephalitis	Pig	Picornaviridae	Enterovirus	1
Ovine *progressive* pneumonia	Pneumonia	Sheep	*see* maedi	*see* maedi	—
Pseudocowpox	Teat dermatitis	Cattle	Poxviridae	Parapoxvirus	1
Pseudorabies	Encephalitis, neonatal deaths	Pig	Herpesviridae	Alphaherpesvirinae	1
Pseudolumpy skin disease	Dermatitis	Cattle, *see* bovine mammillitis	Herpesviridae	Alphaherpesvirinae	—

Table 66 (cont'd)

Disease	*Syndrome*	*Species affected*	*Identification* *Family*	*Genus/subfamily*	*Serotypes*
Ovine *pustular* dermatitis	*see* ecthyma		*see* ecthyma		
Rabies	Encephalitis	Cattle, horse, sheep, goat, pig, man	Rhabdoviridae	Lyssavirus	1
Equine viral *rhinopneumonitis*	Upper respiratory tract infection, pneumonia	Horse	Herpesviridae	Alphaherpesvirinae	2
Infectious bovine *rhinotracheitis*	Upper respiratory tract infection, pneumonia	Cattle	Herpesviridae	(Bovine herpesvirus 1) Alphaherpesvirus	1
Rift Valley fever	Hepatitis, abortion	Cattle, sheep, goat, man	Bunyaviridae	Phlebovirus	1
Rinderpest	Stomatitis, enteritis	Cattle, sheep, goat	Paramyxoviridae	Morbillivirus	1
Bovine *rotavirus* diarrhea	Calf diarrhea	Cattle	Reoviridae	Rotavirus	Multiple
Equine *rotavirus* diarrhea	Foal diarrhea	Horse	Reoviridae	Rotavirus	1
Porcine *rotavirus* diarrhea	Piglet diarrhea	Pig	Reoviridae	Rotavirus	Multiple
Sarcoidosis	Skin neoplasia	Horse	*see* papillomatosis	*see* papillomatosis	
Scrapie	Encephalitis	Sheep	Unknown	Unknown	
Sheeppox	Dermatitis	Sheep	Poxviridae	Capripoxvirus	1
Swine fever	Septicemia	Pig	*see* hog cholera	*see* hog cholera	
Bovine respiratory *syncytial* virus disease	Pneumonia	Cattle	Paramyxoviridae	Pneumovirus	1
Swinepox	Dermatitis	Pig	Poxviridae	Suipoxvirus	1
Transmissible gastroenteritis	Enteritis	Pig	Coronaviridae	Coronavirus	1
Vesicular exanthema of swine	Stomatitis	Pig	Caliciviridae	Calicivirus	Multiple
Swine *vesicular* disease	Stomatitis	Pig	Picornaviridae	Enterovirus	1
Vesicular stomatitis	Stomatitis	Pig, horse, cattle, sheep	Rhabdoviridae	Vesiculovirus	7
Visna	Encephalitis	Sheep	*see* maedi		—
Infectious pustular *vulvovaginitis*	Vaginitis, posthitis	Cattle	Herpesviridae	Bovine herpesvirus 1 Alphaherpesvirus	1
Wesselbron virus disease	Hepatitis, abortion	Sheep	Flaviviridae	Flavivirus	1

Etiology

The disease is caused by a pestivirus (family Togaviridae). There is only one antigenic type (3) but there are a number of strains of variable virulence and antigenicity. The most virulent produce clinical disease in pigs of all ages. The less virulent strains may produce little clinical disease or disease restricted primarily to fetal and newborn piglets. It is probable that this variance has always occurred in field strains of the virus but the use of inadequately attenuated live virus vaccines is also a contributory factor. The occurrence of variation in virulence and antigenicity has been recognized as a cause of failure of vaccination and 'vaccine breakdowns'. It is equally important in causing problems with the diagnosis of hog cholera in eradication programs when infection is manifest in patterns not traditionally associated with this disease.

Swine appear to be the only animals naturally infected with the virus although it can be experimentally transmitted and passaged through laboratory animals. The virus of hog cholera has an antigenic relationship to that causing bovine virus diarrhea (BVD). In Denmark, BVD antibodies were found in 6·4% of the sera pigs while all sera were found to be free from antibodies to the hog cholera virus (8).

The virus of hog cholera is destroyed by boiling, by 5% cresol, or 3% sodium hydroxide (4) and by sunlight but it persists in meat which is preserved by salting, smoking and particularly by freezing. The virus can be inactivated in at least 80% of pork hams after exposure to a flash temperature of 71°C (159°F) (6). Survival for 1 month in the meat, and 2 months in the bone marrow of saltcured pork is recorded. Persistence in frozen meat has been observed after 4½ years. The virus persists for 3–4 days in decomposing organs and for 15 days in decomposing blood and bone marrow.

Epidemiology

Although hog cholera appears to have originated in the United States it is now virtually worldwide in distribution. In the past, the important free areas have been Canada, Australia, New Zealand and South Africa, which has not experienced the disease since it was eradicated in 1918. Swine fever was eradicated from the United Kingdom during the period 1963–67 (2, 5) and an eradication program in the United States appears to be successful. Outbreaks have occurred in these countries from time to time but have been quickly controlled by a rigorous policy of slaughter and quarantine. Usually the disease occurs in severe outbreak form, often with a morbidity of 100% and a mortality rate approaching this. This is especially true when a virulent virus gains access to a susceptible population. Between 1982 and 1984 epidemics of the disease have occurred in the Federal Republic of Germany, the Netherlands, Belgium, France, Italy, Greece and in the Iberian peninsula (7). As of 1985, six countries in Europe were free of classical swine fever: Denmark, Ireland (including Northern Ireland), Norway, Sweden, Finland and Switzerland (7). However, in recent years outbreaks of a relatively slowly spreading, mild form of the disease have caused great concern in many countries (9). Hog cholera is undoubtedly the most costly disease affecting swine. Losses due to the death of pigs are aggravated by the high cost of vaccination programs in enzootic areas and by the problem that vaccination may not be completely effective in controlling epidemics (10). Recovered or partially recovered pigs are very susceptible to secondary infections, and exacerbation of existing chronic infections such as enzootic pneumonia are likely to occur during the convalescent period.

The resistance and high infectivity of the virus make spread of the disease by inert materials, especially uncooked meat, a major problem. The source of virus is always an infected pig and its products and the infection is usually acquired by ingestion but inhalation is also a possible portal. With infections with virulent virus all excretions, secretions and body tissues of affected pigs contain the virus and it is excreted in the urine for some days before clinical illness appears and for 2–3 weeks after clinical recovery. Outside pens, in warm weather and exposed to sunlight, lose their infectivity within 1–2 days. The ability of the virus to survive in the environment in more favorable situations is uncertain. However, it is probable that it can survive for considerable periods as the virus is quite resistant to chemical and physical influences. Survival periods in meat are given above.

In areas free of the disease, introduction is usually effected by the importation of infected pigs or the feeding of garbage containing uncooked pork scraps. Birds and humans may also act as physical carriers for the virus. In enzootic areas transmission to new farms can occur in feeder pigs purchased for fattening, or indirectly by flies and mosquitoes (11, 12), or on bedding, feed, boots, automobile tires or transport vehicles. The most common cause of dissemination occurs through the movement and sale of infected or carrier pigs through communal sale yards when there is ample opportunity for infection of primary and secondary contacts.

In the past it has been thought that infection with hog cholera virus rapidly resulted in the occurrence of severe clinical disease. It is now recognized that with less virulent strains a carrier state can occur, at least for a period of time. Following exposure to these strains, pigs may become infected without showing overt signs of the disease and although they may eventually develop clinical disease this latent period is of importance in dissemination of infection when such pigs are sold and come in contact with others (13). Susceptible pregnant sows if exposed to less virulent strains of hog cholera virus may remain clinically healthy but infection of the fetuses *in utero* is common and virus may be introduced into susceptible herds by way of these infected offspring. Fully virulent virus may also be transmitted in this manner if the sows are treated with inadequate amounts of antiserum at the time of exposure or if they are exposed following inadequate vaccination (16, 17). Piglets infected *in utero*, if they survive, may support a viremia for long periods after birth (14–17).

When the disease is introduced into a susceptible population an epidemic usually develops rapidly because of the resistance of the virus and the short incubation period. In recent years outbreaks have been observed in which the rate of spread is much reduced and this has delayed field diagnosis (9).

Pathogenesis

Passage of the virus through the mucosa of the upper part of the digestive or respiratory tracts is followed by septicemia and invasion of vascular endothelium. Most of the lesions are produced by hydropic degeneration and proliferation of vascular endothelium which results in the occlusion of blood vessels. Atrophy of the thymus, depletion of lymphocytes and germinal follicles in peripheral lymphoid tissues, renal glomerular changes and splenitis are characteristic (18). In many cases secondary bacterial infection occurs and plays an important part in the development of lesions and clinical signs.

The experimental disease is characterized by a biphasic temperature elevation at the second and sixth day after inoculation, a profound leukopenia and an appreciable anemia 24 hours after inoculation, diarrhea at the seventh day, and anorexia and death on the 4th to 15th day (13).

The experimental production of congenital persistent hog cholera infection is described (15–17). The inoculation of pregnant sows with a low-virulent field strain of hog cholera virus at various stages of pregnancy results in prenatal mortality in litters from sows infected at 40 days pregnancy and postnatal death at 65 days. The later that infection occurs in pregnancy the greater the number of uninfected piglets born in infected litters. The earlier the infection occurs in pregnancy the greater the number of persistent infections in piglets born alive with immunological tolerance (16). The immunological tolerance is specific to the virus because affected piglets respond to other selected antigens (16).

Clinical findings

Clinical signs usually appear 5–10 days after infection, although longer incubation periods of 35 days or more are recorded. At the beginning of an outbreak young pigs may die peracutely without clinical signs having been evident. Acute cases are the most common. Affected pigs are depressed, do not eat, and stand in a drooped attitude with the tail hanging. They are disinclined to move and, when forced, do so with a swaying movement of the hindquarters. They tend to lie down and burrow into the bedding, often piled one on top of the other. Prior to the appearance of other signs a high temperature (40·5–41·5°C, 105–107°F) is usual. Other early signs include constipation followed by diarrhea and vomiting. Later a diffuse purplish discoloration of the abdominal skin occurs. Small areas of necrosis are sometimes seen on the edges of the ears, on the tail, and lips of the vulva. A degree of conjunctivitis is usual and in some pigs the eyelids are stuck together by dried, purulent exudate. Nervous signs are often observed even in the early stages of illness. Circling, incoordination, muscle tremor and convulsions are the commonest manifestations. Death can be expected 5–7 days after the commencement of illness. Infection with *Salmonella choleraesuis* may also be potentiated by hog cholera infection and the two diseases in combination can result in high mortality.

A form of the disease in which nervous signs predominate has been described and attributed to a variant strain of the virus. The incubation period is often shorter and the course of the disease more acute than usual. Pigs in lateral recumbency show a tetanic convulsion for 10–15 seconds followed by a clonic convulsion of 30–40 seconds. The convulsion may be accompanied by loud squealing and may occur constantly or at intervals of several hours, often being followed by a period of terminal coma. In some cases convulsions do not occur but nervous involvement is manifested by coarse tremor of the body and limb muscles. Apparent blindness, stumbling and allotriophagia have also been observed.

With the recognition of low virulence strains of virus, less dramatic syndromes have been recognized. A chronic form occurs in field outbreaks and occasionally after serum–virus simultaneous vaccination (19). The incubation period is longer than normal and there is emaciation and the appearance of characteristic skin lesions including alopecia, dermatitis, blotching of the ears and a terminal, deep purple coloration of the abdominal skin. Pigs may apparently recover following a short period of illness but subsequently redevelop clinical disease and die if stressed.

Pigs infected with low virulence strains of hog cholera virus appear more susceptible to intercurrent bacterial disease. The protean nature of this combination is such that hog cholera should be suspected in a herd, or area, where there is an increase in mortality from any apparent infectious cause that either does not respond, or responds only temporarily, to therapeutic ploys that are usually effective.

Reproductive failure can be a significant feature of infection with hog cholera virus and may occur without other signs of disease within the herd. It may occur when inadequately protected pregnant sows are exposed to virulent virus, or when susceptible pregnant sows are vaccinated with live attenuated vaccines or exposed to low virulent field strains. Infection of the sow may result in no clinical signs other than a mild pyrexia but it may be followed by a high incidence of abortion, low litter size, mummification, stillbirth and anomalies of piglets (16, 17, 20–22). Liveborn pigs, although carriers, may be weak or clinically normal. A congenital hog cholera infection is described (14). The infection is characterized by persistent viremia, continuous virus excretion and late onset of disease, with death occurring 2–11 months after birth. No antibodies to the virus are present in spite of the persistent infection; affected pigs have a normal immune response to other antigens, but do not respond to the hog cholera virus (15). Cell mediated immunity appears to be normal. A high incidence of myoclonia congenita (congenital trembles) associated with cerebellar hypoplasia has been observed in some outbreaks where prenatal infection with hog cholera virus has occurred and this syndrome has been reproduced experimentally (23). The prevalence of any one of these manifestations appears to vary with the strain of the virus and the stage of gestation at the time of infection (17, 20, 21, 24).

Clinical pathology

A valuable antemortem laboratory examination is the total and differential leukocyte count. Pigs in the early stages of hog cholera show a pronounced leukopenia, the total count falling from a normal range of 14 000–24 000/μl to 4000–9000/μl. This can be of value in differentiation from bacterial septicemias but it should not be used as the sole method of differentiation. In the late stages of hog cholera a leukocytosis, due to secondary bacterial invasion, may develop. Baby pigs less than 5 weeks old normally have low leukocyte counts. Negative cultural examination of feces may help to eliminate other diseases as diagnostic possibilities. When hog cholera is suspected material should be taken for serological and other diagnostic tests. These are discussed later under diagnosis.

Necropsy findings

In peracute cases there may be no gross changes at necropsy. In the common, acute form there are many submucosal and subserosal petechial hemorrhages but these are inconstant and to find them it may be necessary to examine two or more cadavers from an outbreak. The hemorrhages are most noticeable under the capsule of the kidney, about the ileocecal valve, in the cortical sinuses of the lymph nodes and in the bladder and larynx. The hemorrhages are usually petechial and rarely ecchymotic. Enlargement of the lymph nodes is constant and the spleen may contain marginal infarcts. Infarction in the mucosa of the gallbladder is a common but not constant finding and appears to be an almost pathognomonic lesion. There is congestion of the liver and bone marrow and often of the lungs. Circular, raised button ulcers in the colonic mucosa are highly suggestive but are now seldom seen. Although these gross necropsy findings are fairly general in cases of hog cholera, they cannot be considered as diagnostic unless accompanied by the clinical and epizootological evidence of the disease. They can occur in other diseases, particularly salmonellosis.

There are characteristic, microscopic lesions of a nonsuppurative encephalitis in most cases and a presumptive diagnosis of hog cholera can be made if they are present. Histologically, the main site of tissue injury in hog cholera is the reticuloendothelial system where hydropic degeneration and proliferation of the vascular endothelium cause occlusion of blood vessels. The more virulent 'neurotropic' strains produce lesions of similar nature but greater severity.

In the chronic form of the disease, necrotic ulceration of the mucosa of the large intestine is usual and histologically there is transverse calcification of the distal portion of the rib. Secondary pneumonia and enteritis commonly accompany the primary lesions of hog cholera.

Infection of the fetus produces a persistent immunologically tolerant non-cytolytic infection often with little evidence of cell necrosis or inflammatory reaction to suggest the presence of a virus. Aborted fetuses show non-diagnostic changes of petechial hemorrhage and ascites. Malformations such as microcephaly, cerebellar hypoplasia, pulmonary hypogenesis and joint deformity appear due to inhibition of cell division and function in these areas (20, 22, 23). Antibody is not detected in fetal blood (22, 24) when infection occurs early in fetal life. In pigs showing signs of myoclonia congenita, cerebellar hypoplasia is highly suggestive of hog cholera infection (23).

Diagnosis

A positive diagnosis of hog cholera is always difficult to make without laboratory confirmation. This is particularly true of the chronic, less dramatic forms of the disease. A highly infectious, fatal disease of pigs with a course of 5–7 days in a group of unvaccinated animals should arouse suspicion of hog cholera, especially if there are no signs indicative of localization in particular organs. Nervous signs are probably the one exception. The gross necropsy findings are also non-specific and reliance must be placed on the leukopenia in the early stages and the non-suppurative encephalitis visible on histological examination. Both of these features may be obscured if a coincident bacterial infection, particularly salmonellosis, is present.

With the advent of eradication programs there has been considerable work on the development of accurate diagnostic tests for hog cholera. The available tests have been reviewed (19). There is, in general, a need for these tests to be accurate and rapid so that control measures can be rapidly instituted or lifted as the case may be. Diagnosis by virus isolation is slow, cytopathic effect may be minimal and some strains have low infectivity and limited growth in tissue culture. This method is seldom used as a primary diagnostic method. Animal inoculation tests still provide an excellent method for the diagnosis of hog cholera and involve the challenge of susceptible and immune pigs with suspect material followed by subsequent challenge at a later date with fully virulent hog cholera virus. However, this test is time-consuming and costly and, although it is used for the final confirmatory test for the presence of hog cholera infection in various situations, it is not satisfactory for a rapid diagnostic test.

The more rapid tests rely on the detection of antigen in infected pig tissues or the detection of antibody following infection. Fluorescent antibody techniques (19, 25) allow the rapid detection of antigen in frozen sections of tissue or impression smears and in infected tissue cultures and these methods have been adopted as a primary test in the eradication program in the United States. Antigen can be detected up to 2 days after death and this method has been considered more reliable than the agar gel precipitation test. The method is capable of detecting virus carriers among vaccinated pigs (26).

The agar gel precipitation test detects antigen in tissues by means of a precipitin formed with immune sera. Usually pancreas from suspect pigs is tested. This test was used widely in the United Kingdom eradication program and is the standard primary test in many countries.

Antibody can be detected by the fluorescent antibody neutralization test, tissue culture serum neutralization test or an indirect enzyme-labelled antibody test (27) which uses enzyme labelled antiporcine gammaglobulin to detect antigen–antibody combination. Serological tests are less satisfactory for detection of hog cholera in the acute phase and are of limited value in vaccinated animals. They are of value in the detection in sows of the subclinical infection of hog cholera associated with reproductive failure and for survey studies to determine the prevalence of hog cholera infection. BVD virus may infect pigs, especially those in close contact with cattle, and may give false positive serological reactions. The incidence of these false positive reactions may be quite high and they pose a problem for hog cholera identification in eradication programs. The neutralizing peroxidase-linked antibody assay is a highly sensitive and specific test for hog cholera and will distinguish between pigs infected with different strains of the hog cholera virus and the bovine virus diarrhea virus (33). The enzyme-linked immunosorbent assay test (ELISA) is useful for large-scale testing of sera in eradication programs (28).

When hog cholera is suspected, tissues submitted for examination should include the brain and sections of intestine and other internal organs in formalin, and pancreas, lymph node and tonsil unpreserved in sealed containers. Local regulations and requirements should be followed.

The major diseases which resemble hog cholera include salmonellosis which is usually accompanied by enteritis and dyspnea, acute erysipelas in which the subserous hemorrhages are likely to be ecchymotic rather than petechial, and acute pasteurellosis. Epidemiological considerations and hematological and bacteriological examination will usually differentiate these conditions. Other encephalitides, particularly viral encephalomyelitis and salmonellosis produce similar nervous signs. African swine fever, apart from its greater severity, is almost impossible to differentiate from hog cholera without serological tests.

Treatment

Hyperimmune serum is the only available treatment and may be of value in the very early stages of the illness if given in doses of 50–150 ml. It has more general use in the protection of in-contact animals. A concentrated serum permitting the use of much smaller doses is now available.

Control

The methods used in the control of the disease include eradication and control by vaccination. In areas where effective barriers to reintroduction of the disease can be established, eradication of the disease by slaughter methods is feasible and usually desirable. In contrast, in areas where the structure and economics of the pig industry requires considerable within-country and across-border movement of pigs it may not be practical or economically feasible to institute a slaughter eradication program. The establishment of a highly susceptible population in a high risk area is unwise. If repeated breakdowns occur, the restriction of movement of pigs within the quarantine areas creates considerable managemental problems for pig owners and they may, as a result, eventually become non-cooperative in the program. In these areas, control and possibly even eradication by vaccination is the approach of choice and this method is in force in many European countries (29). General control procedures are dealt with first and are followed by a description of the immunizing products available.

Outbreak control in hog cholera-free areas

In areas where the disease does not normally occur complete eradication by slaughter of all in-contact and infected pigs is possible and should be practiced. The pigs are slaughtered and disposed of, preferably by burning. All piggeries in the area should be quarantined and no movement of pigs permitted unless for immediate slaughter. Hyperimmune hog cholera antiserum may be used to protect pigs on farms in the quarantine area but this method is expensive. All vehicles used for the transport of pigs, all pens and premises and utensils must be disinfected with strong chemical disinfectant such as 5% cresylic acid. Contaminated clothing should be boiled. Entry to and departure from infected premises must be carefully controlled to avoid spread of the disease on footwear, clothes and automobile tires. Legislation prohibiting the feeding of garbage or commanding the boiling of all garbage before feeding must be enforced. This eradication procedure has controlled outbreaks which have occurred in Canada and Australia and has served to maintain these countries free from the disease.

Control where hog cholera is enzootic

In enzootic areas control is largely a problem of choosing the best vaccine and using it intelligently. Much can also be done to keep the incidence of the disease low by the education of farmers whose cooperation can be best assured by a demonstration that eradication is both desirable and practicable. Once farmer enthusiasm is aroused the greatest stumbling block to control, failure to notify outbreaks, is eliminated. Education of the farmer should emphasize the highly infectious nature of the disease and the ease with which it can be spread by the feeding of uncooked garbage and the purchase and sale of infected or in-contact pigs. The common practice of sending pigs to market as soon as illness appears in a group is one of the major methods by which hog cholera is spread.

Of the vaccines available those containing killed or attenuated virus are to be preferred. Live, virulent virus vaccines produce a solid immunity but are capable of introducing the infection and of actually causing the disease when vaccination 'breaks' occur. The reaction to live virus vaccine may be severe and the susceptibility of pigs to other disease may be increased. Eradication of the disease is impossible while the use of this type of vaccine is permitted.

When an outbreak occurs in a herd the immediate need is to prevent infection from spreading further. This can be best achieved by removing the source of infection and increasing the resistance of in-contact animals by the injection of hyperimmune serum or one of the available vaccines. Removal of the source of infection necessitates isolation of infected animals, suitable hygienic precautions to prevent the spread of infections on boots, clothing and utensils, disposal of carcasses by burning and disinfection of pens. The pens should be scraped, hosed and sprayed with 5% cresylic acid solution or other suitable disinfectant. The choice of serum or vaccine may depend on local legislation and will depend upon circumstances. Pigs in the affected pen should receive serum (20–75 ml depending on size) and pigs in unaffected pens should be vaccinated. Pigs receiving only serum will require active vaccination at a later date if a strong immunity is to be achieved. Routine vaccination of all pigs is desirable.

Hog cholera eradication

The elimination of hog cholera from a country where it is well established presents a formidable problem. Before the final stage of eradication can be attempted, the incidence of the disease must be reduced to a low level by widespread use of vaccination and enforcement of garbage cooking regulations.

One of the most important problems encountered in eradication programs is the clinically normal 'carrier' animal (14, 15, 30) and steps need to be taken to avoid the sale of all pigs from infected premises. A procedure which has been particularly effective in the control of this and other diseases of pigs is the complete prohibition of all community sales of feeder pigs. There are obvious political difficulties in such a prohibition but, despite their usefulness as marketing agencies, community sales continue to be a major source of swine infections. When the occurrence of virulent hog cholera has been eliminated further necessary steps include the prohibition of use of any vaccine and serological studies to detect low virulence carrier states.

The eradication of swine fever in the United Kingdom during a 4-year campaign ending in 1966 has been a very important achievement and the salient features of the campaign have been recorded (2, 5). Control was radical in that all herds in which the disease was diagnosed were slaughtered and all carcasses burned or buried to avoid missing atypical cases and recurrence through the swill cycle. The two focal points which became apparent were the need to avoid vaccination and the need to diagnose accurately. Vaccination was not permitted because it was not completely effective, because it produced 'carriers', and because it encouraged the development of mild and chronic forms of the disease. The need to diagnose accurately led to changes in diagnostic procedure as the campaign progressed. As the proportion of textbook outbreaks lessened there was increasing dependence on serological and antigen detection tests. The program in the United States, which currently appears complete, is an equivalent achievement and the details are recorded (6, 7).

Immunization methods

Very few pigs possess natural immunity to hog cholera and, until the introduction of the serum–virus method of vaccination, an outbreak of the disease in a herd meant virtually that the herd would be eliminated. The situation changed rapidly thereafter and it can be safely claimed that the development of the swine industry in the United States would have been impossible without the protection which serum and virus afforded. On the other hand, the dangers inherent in the use of fully virulent or partially avirulent virus do not recommend their use and they have led to a continuing search for safe methods of immunization. The ideal vaccine should retain strong immunogenicity but should be completely avirulent, even for pregnant sows, the fetus and young or stressed pigs. It should be stable in the degree of attenuation and should not persist in the vaccinate nor transmit from the vaccinate to in-contact pigs. Killed vaccines are safe and do not directly spread virus, but in general, they engender only a limited immunity. Live vaccines provide a longer lasting immunity but frequently have not met the criteria listed above.

Serum–virus vaccination

This produces an immediate, solid and lasting immunity when properly administered to healthy swine. The virus, produced by collecting blood 6–7 days after artificial infection, is injected subcutaneously in 2 ml doses followed immediately by serum in doses graduated to the size of the pigs and varying from 20 ml for suckling pigs to 75 ml for adults. Overdosing with serum will not prevent the development of immunity. Vaccination is performed at any age after 4 weeks. Because of the availability of safer vaccines this method is not recommended.

Attenuated vaccines
These include tissue culture vaccines attenuated by repeated passage through tissue culture of porcine or other origin, lapinized vaccines produced by repeated rabbit passage, and vaccines from mutant strains. Many of the early vaccines of this type were not stable and could cause disease when not used in conjunction with serum (3, 19). Furthermore, transmission to in-contact pigs, especially with porcine origin vaccines, and fetal disease following vaccination of pregnant sows have been problems. Attenuated vaccines are in wide use in Europe and Asia and include the Chinese or LPC and GPE strains. Highly passaged preparations are antigenically stable and show no evidence of reversion. They produce a very limited viremia, or none, and no leukopenia or clinical illness. Protection is evident within 5–10 days of vaccination. Piglets from non-immune sows can be vaccinated within the first 2 weeks of life. Because the presence of maternal immunity can interfere with effective immunization, the vaccination of piglets from immune sows should be delayed until at least the second month (32). The French Thiverval strain (3, 31) is a cold mutant strain which has lost its virulence but retained good immunogenicity. Vaccination of piglets even with ten times the regular dose produced no clinical illness and virtually no viremia. A single intramuscular vaccination will produce resistance to challenge by 5–10 days and immunity persists for 3 years. Colostral immunity will protect piglets for periods up to 2 months after birth. When given to pregnant sows even the highly attenuated strains have the ability to cross the placenta and produce fetal infection even though no clinical evidence of this may be manifest. Consequently it is recommended that replacement gilts be vaccinated at least 2 weeks prior to mating and that recently vaccinated animals be kept separate from susceptible pregnant sows.

In the Netherlands, the control of swine fever has relied on a slaughter policy on affected farms plus an emergency vaccination program in which all pigs over 2 weeks of age in areas of risk are vaccinated (34). The mass vaccination program is followed by supplementary vaccination of pigs at 7–9 weeks of age and revaccination of breeding gilts when 6–7 months of age. The serological response of piglets born from vaccinated sows is best at 9–10 weeks of age rather than at 5–6 weeks of age (34).

Inactivated vaccines
These are usually prepared from the blood or tissues of infected pigs. Crystal violet vaccine has been the one most widely used of this type and was used in the United Kingdom prior to eradication but never gained full acceptance in the United States (19). It is completely safe but its immunogenicity is poor. Immunity does not develop until 12 days after vaccination. Its duration is short and booster injections are required for maintenance. Vaccinated sows may still develop fetal infection when exposed to virulent virus (17) and there is a danger that the use of this vaccine in enzootic areas may in this way induce virus carriers. The production of immune antibodies to the blood components of the vaccine may result in the occurrence of isoimmune hemolytic anemia in some breeds. For these reasons inactivated vaccines are not in common use.

REVIEW LITERATURE

Harkness, J. W. (1985) Classical swine fever and its diagnosis: a current review. *Vet. Rec.*, *116*, 288–293.

REFERENCES

(1) Carbrey, E. A. et al. (1966) *J. Am. vet. med. Assoc.*, *149*, 1720.
(2) Done, J. T. (1969) *Br. vet. J.*, *125*, 349.
(3) Aynaud, J. M. & Corthier, G. (1976) *Wld Anim. Rev.*, *20*, 17.
(4) Torrey, J. P. & Amtower, W. C. (1964) *Proc. US live Stk sanit. Assoc.*, 287.
(5) Beynon, A. G. (1969) *Vet. Rec.*, *84*, 623.
(6) Stewart, W. C. et al. (1979) *Am. J. vet. Res.*, *40*, 739.
(7) Harkness, J. W. (1985) *Vet. Rec.*, *116*, 288.
(8) Jensen, M.H. (1985) *Acta vet. Scand.*, *26*, 72.
(9) Keast, J. C. & Golding, N. K. (1964) *Aust. vet. J.*, *40*, 137.
(10) Schlegel, H. L. (1976) *Berl. Munch. Tierärztl. Wochenschr.*, *89*, 237.
(11) Tidwell, M. A. et al. (1972) *Am. J. vet. Res.*, *33*, 615.
(12) Stewart, W. C. et al. (1975) *Am. J. vet. Res.*, *36*, 611.
(13) Carbrey, E. A. et al. (1980) *Am. J. vet. Res.*, *41*, 946.
(14) Van Oirschot, J. T. & Terpstra, C. (1977) *Vet. Microbiol.*, *2*, 121.
(15) Van Oirschot, J. T. (1977) *Vet. Microbiol.*, *2*, 133.
(16) Van Oirschot, J. T. (1979) *Vet. Microbiol.*, *4*, 177 & 133.
(17) Plateau, E. et al. (1980) *Am. J. vet. Res.*, *41*, 2012.
(18) Cheville, N. F. & Mengeling, W.L. (1969) *Lab. Invest.*, *20*, 261.
(19) Dunne, H. W. (1973) *Adv. vet. Sci.*, *17*, 315.
(20) Johnson, K. P. et al. (1974) *Lab. Invest.*, *30*, 608.
(21) Brack, M. (1971) *Zentralbl. VetMed.*, 18B, 749.
(22) Johnson, K. P. & Byington, D. P. (1972) *Teratology*, 5, 259.
(23) Done, J. T. (1976) *Vet. Ann.*, *16*, 98.
(24) Trautwein, G. et al. (1976) *Proc. 4th int. Congr. Pig vet. Soc.*, H8.
(25) Carbrey, E. A. et al. (1971) *Proc. 74th ann. Meet. US Anim. Hlth Assoc.*, 502.
(26) Engler, E. et al. (1972) *Arch. exp. VetMed.*, *26*, 661.
(27) Saunders, G. C. (1977) *Am. J. vet. Res.*, *38*, 21.
(28) Have, P. (1984) *Acta vet. Scand.*, *25*, 463.
(29) Terpstra, C. & Robijins, K. G. (1977) *Tijdschr. Diergeneeskd.*, *102*, 106.
(30) Huck, R. A. & Alston, F. W. (1964) *Vet. Rec.*, *76*, 1151.
(31) Aynaud, J. M. et al. (1976) *Proc. 4th int. Congr. Pig vet. Soc.*, H1, H2.
(32) Precausta, P. et al. (1983) *Comp. Immunol. Microbiol. inf. Dis.*, *6*, 281.
(33) Terpstra, C. et al. (1984) *Vet. Microbiol.*, 9, 113.
(34) Terpstra, C. & Wensvoort, G. (1987) *Vet. Microbiol.*, *13*, 143.

African swine fever (African pig disease, warthog disease)

African swine fever is a peracute, highly fatal, highly contagious disease of pigs caused by a virus which is antigenically distinct from that of hog cholera. Clinically and at necropsy the disease resembles hog cholera closely but is even more severe. The disease poses a considerable threat to pig-producing countries. It causes high mortality and in pigs which survive a persistent viral infection. The only effective method of control is slaughter eradication.

Etiology
The disease is caused by a specific virus that is physically, chemically and antigenically distinct from that causing hog cholera but is otherwise unclassified (1). Pigs artificially immunized against hog cholera are still fully susceptible to the virus of African swine fever.

Epidemiology
African swine fever is indigenous to the African continent where warthogs, bushpigs and forest hogs act as reservoirs of the virus. Wild pigs in some areas are free of infection and consequently the disease is not endemic in all areas (5). Infection of wild pigs produces no clinical disease but with virulent strains infection in the domestic pig is almost always fatal, the morbidity rate approaches 100% and no effective method of vaccination is available. Since its recognition, the disease in South Africa has shown a cyclic occurrence with periods of 10–12 years of clinical disease and then absence (5). Until 1957 African swine fever had not occurred outside the African continent. To the rest of the world it represented the most formidable of the exotic diseases of swine, a disease which had to be kept within its existing boundaries at all costs. However, African swine fever broke out of Africa, appearing in Portugal in 1957 and Spain in 1960, resulting in the death and slaughter of thousands of pigs. Subsequently the disease appeared in France and then Italy and in 1971 occurred in Cuba. It was successfully eradicated from these latter three countries by extensive slaughter and quarantine programs. In 1978 outbreaks occurred in Malta (4), Sardinia, Brazil, Dominican Republic and Haiti. The disease in Malta resulted in the death or slaughter of the entire population of 80 000 pigs within 12 months of the diagnosis (4). This is one of the few examples of a country having to slaughter an entire species of domestic animal in order to eliminate a disease.

The African swine fever virus appears to consist of a multiclonal population of viruses in which all combinations of at least four markers (hemabsorption, virulence, plaque size, and antigenicity) may be found (2). This may explain the epidemiological observation that when the disease was confined to Africa and the Iberian peninsula in the early 1960s, the viruses isolated were highly virulent to swine, but in subsequent years mortality decreased and subacute and chronic infection became more common (3). The Malta 78 isolate of the virus experimentally produces a clinical syndrome similar to the African isolates of the virus (6).

The virus is highly resistant to putrefaction, heat and dryness and survives in chilled carcasses for up to 6 months (1).

Only pigs are affected, domestic pigs of all ages and breeds being highly susceptible, but the virus can be passaged in tissue cultures, rabbits, goats and embryonated hen eggs.

Until recent years the occurrence of African swine fever in Africa was limited to explosive outbreaks in European pigs which came in contact with indigenous African pigs. These outbreaks tended to be self-limiting because all pigs in affected herds died or were destroyed, but after a number of years the disease became enzootic in domestic herds. The virus which was introduced to Europe in 1957 was quite capable of persisting in European pigs and after a period of several years in which the disease was epizootic a change to an enzootic character occurred (3). The outbreak in Cuba was of a comparatively virulent form (7).

When the disease was present in the Caribbean region it posed a major threat to the large swine industry of the United States principally because of the possible spread of the virus to the federal swine population in Florida (9). The federal swine population in Florida is the largest in the United States and is of major recreational and economic importance to hunters, trappers, taxidermists and to dealers who sell federal swine to hunting clubs. The federal swine in Florida are descendants of domestic swine which were allowed to run wild. Experimental inoculation of these pigs with virulent isolates of the virus will cause fatal disease (8).

In Africa the method of transmission of the disease from the reservoir in wild pigs to the domestic pig has been the subject of considerable interest (5). Available evidence suggests that infection is primarily transmitted to domestic pigs via the argasid tick *Ornithodoros moubata*. The viremic warthog provides a source of infection for the ticks. The virus can be maintained in warthog-associated argasid ticks by transtadial, transovarial and sexual (male to female, but usually not vice versa) transmission mechanism (10). The tick is relatively restricted in its habitat and if contact between domestic pigs and wild pigs and their burrows is prevented transmission can be prevented (4). The virus can be maintained in these ticks for long periods in the absence of fresh sources of infection, so that they act as a reservoir as well as vectors of infection. Sporadic outbreaks may thus occur in endemic areas when the virus spreads from infected ticks or warthogs to domestic pigs. In some areas where infected warthogs are common but where *O. moubata* is apparently absent, *O. savignyi* may be a natural field vector of the virus (32).

The long-held belief that the source of the virus in primary epidemics of African swine fever in southern and East Africa is the carrier, wild pig, appears not to be tenable (10). It is postulated that infected ticks are transported to the vicinity of domestic pigs either by warthogs or on the carcasses of warthogs.

The literature on the persistence of African swine fever in African and the Mediterranean has been reviewed (4). In Africa the virus is maintained primarily by a cycle of infection between warthogs and soft ticks (*Ornithodoros moubata*). The virus does not have any apparent effect on either warthogs or ticks and it is only when infection of domestic pigs occurs that the virus produces disease. The tick has a wide distribution in Africa south of the Sahara and its main habitat is in burrows which are inhabited by the warthog. There is a good correlation between antibodies in warthogs and the presence of ticks. Newborn warthogs can become infected soon after birth if bitten by infected ticks and the consequent viremia would be high enough to infect previously uninfected ticks feeding on them. In Spain and Portugal the most important methods of spread are by contact between neighboring farms and the introduction of infected pigs either during the incubation period or as persistently infected virus carriers. During the last 20 years an increasing number of outbreaks occurred in which clinical disease was not readily recognized. The mortality rates decreased and a wide range of clinical disease occurred ranging from acute to chronic and including apparent recovery to normal health. The major consequence of the emergence of these less virulent forms of the virus was the development of persistently viremic carriers and a large population of pigs with inapparent infection. Thus the African swine fever virus may persist in the pig population by persistent infection in recovered pigs for several months during which time the virus must be reactivated before transmission can occur and also by reinfection of recovered pigs in which virus replicates without producing clinical disease and transmission occurs by excretion and by infected blood and tissues. The presence of the tick *Ornithodoros erraticus* in the region can also act as a vector of the virus (4).

In Sardinia, the major factors involved in the spread of the disease are related to the mountainous terrain in which pigs may range freely in previously infected areas, the movement of pigs which may survive infection and mingle with other herds, the introduction of infected pigs from unknown sources into healthy herds because of the uncontrolled movement of pigs, and the feeding of waste food containing meat from infected pigs (4).

The virus has been experimentally transmitted to healthy swine by *Ornithodoros coriaceus*, an argasid tick indigenous to the United States (25). Other possible methods of transmission from wild to domestic pigs have been examined (5).

Once established in domestic pigs the disease can spread rapidly. Virus is present in high titer in nasopharyngeal excretions at the onset of clinical signs and is present in all organs and excretions in acutely sick pigs. In experimentally inoculated domestic pigs the virus is present in substantial amounts in secretions and excretions of acutely infected pigs for only 7–10 days after the onset of fever and is present in the greatest amount in the feces (33). The virus can persist in the blood of some recovered pigs for 8 weeks and in the lymphoid tissues for 12 weeks. Feces are the environmental contaminant most likely to spread the infection, but blood is also highly infective and transmission could occur by contamination of wounds created by fighting. Infection occurs via oral and nasal routes and with the short incubation period once the disease is established in a herd it spreads rapidly by direct contact. Infection amongst domestic pigs can also reputedly spread by indirect contact by infected pens, the ingestion of contaminated feed and water and by feeding uncooked garbage containing infected pig material. Transmission via the hog louse *Haematopinus suis* is also probable (11). An important source of infection is the recovered pig which may remain persistently infected and a carrier indefinitely. Pigs which have recovered from the western hemisphere isolates (Brazilian and Dominican Republic) may be persistently infected and are resistant to experimental challenge (24).

Antibodies against the African swine fever virus occur in the colostrum of sows previously infected with the virus and are transferred passively to nursing pigs (26). Passively acquired antibodies are partially protective against an experimental challenge (26).

Pigs infected with virulent or attenuated African swine fever virus may recover and resist challenge exposure with virulent homologous and, under certain conditions, heterologous viruses (30). Although pigs develop antibodies which are detectable by different tests, virus-neutralizing antibodies have not been demonstrated. The sera from pigs which have been infected and are resistant will inhibit virus replication but the nature of the inhibition is not understood (30).

Pathogenesis

The virus invades through the tonsils and respiratory tract and replicates in the draining lymph nodes prior to the occurrence of a generalized viremia which can occur within 48–72 hours of infection (15). Infectivity and contact transmission develops at this time and continues for at least 7 days. Pigs inoculated with field isolates of the virus from the western hemisphere develop thrombocytopenia with a characteristic pattern (12). Infected pigs become thrombocytopenic over a 48-hour period after 3–4 days of illness. After several days of thrombocytopenia, the platelet count returns to baseline level even with a continuing viremia. Tissue necrosis and generalized endothelial cell infection are not features of the disease caused by isolates of moderate virulence. Early in the infection there is prolongation of coagulation times due to inhibition of fibrin formation and later thrombocytopenia develops (12, 13). The thrombocytopenia is now considered to be immune-mediated (14). The thrombocytopenia and coagulation defects leads to the development of hemorrhages, serous exudates, infarction, local edema and engorgement of tissues. All clinical forms of the disease are characterized by extensive hemorrhages at necropsy and it is this feature which often establishes a presumptive diagnosis in the field (14). The lymphopenia is largely due to the massive destruction of lymphocytes, a characteristic result of infection with the African swine fever virus. The virus infects macrophages and reticular cells.

The virus can cross the placenta, replicate in fetal tissues and cause abortion (16).

Clinical findings

The incubation period after contact exposure varies from 5 to 15 days. A high fever (40·5°C, 105°F) appears abruptly and persists, without other apparent signs, for about 4 days. The fever then subsides and the pigs show marked cyanotic blotching of the skin, depression, anorexia, huddling together, disinclination to move, weakness and incoordination. Extreme weakness of the hindquarters with difficulty in walking is an early and characteristic sign. Coordination remains in the front legs and affected pigs may walk on them, dragging the hindlegs. A rapid pulse rate, and serous to mucopurulent nasal and ocular discharges occur and dyspnea and cough are present in some pigs. Diarrhea, sometimes dysentery, and vomiting occur in some outbreaks and pregnant sows usually abort. Purple discoloration of the skin may be present on the limbs, snout, abdomen and ears. Death usually occurs within a day or two after the appearance of obvious signs of illness, and is often preceded by convulsions.

Early in its history, African swine fever was an acute to peracute disease with a case fatality rate of almost 100%. However, later, subacute and chronic diseases were observed. More recently, an even less virulent form of the disease has evolved (17). High fever and varying degrees of depression and lethargy are observed during the acute phase but some pigs continue to eat, case fatality rate is usually less than 5%, the fever subsides in 2–3 weeks and the pigs return to full feed and grow at a normal rate. Recovered pigs have no lesions suggestive of the disease but may be viremic for several weeks. These persistently infected pigs would pass routine antemortem inspection at slaughter and potentially infectious offal and carcass trimming could be fed unknowingly to other pigs. Chronic cases are intermittently febrile, become emaciated and develop soft edematous swellings over limb joints and under the mandible.

Clinical pathology

As in hog cholera there is a fall in the total leukocyte count to about 40–50% of normal by the fourth day of fever. There is a pronounced lymphopenia and an increase in immature neutrophils. Chronic cases show hypergammaglobulinemia. Antigen can be detected by the fluorescent antibody technique in tonsil and mandibular lymph node within 24–48 hours of infection and elsewhere once generalization has occurred. Antibody to the virus may be detected within 7 days of infection. The enzyme-linked immunosorbent assay (ELISA) is highly sensitive and specific and can be automated for screening large numbers of sera (18).

Necropsy findings

Gross changes at necropsy resemble closely those found in hog cholera except that in the acute cases the lesions are more severe. In chronic cases the lesions are essentially the same but there are, in addition, pericarditis, interstitial pneumonia and lymphadenitis (19). Petechial hemorrhages are present under all serous surfaces and in lymph nodes, and under the epicardium and endocardium, and there is severe, submucosal congestion in the colon and edema and congestion of the lungs. Button ulcers in the cecum and colon and splenic infarcts and the petechial hemorrhages in the renal cortex and bladder are less common than in hog cholera. Histologically the lesions are more diagnostic. There is severe damage to vascular endothelium and marked karyorrhexis of lymphocytes in both normal lymphoid deposits and in infiltrations in parenchymatous organs. An encephalitis comparable in type to that of hog cholera is present.

Diagnosis

The disease is easily confused with hog cholera and very careful examination is required to differentiate the two. Clinically the illness is much shorter (2 days as against 7 days) than in hog cholera. Gross necropsy changes are similar to but more severe than those of hog cholera. The marked karyorrhexis of lymphocytes characteristic of African swine fever is not observed in hog cholera. Differential diagnosis must rely on laboratory testing. In the past, differentiation has been achieved by the challenge of hog cholera-susceptible and immune pigs with suspect material. More recently reliance has been placed on the demonstration of hemadsorbing activity with virus from suspected outbreaks grown on pig leukocyte tissue cultures. But hemadsorbing activity may be weak, delayed or even absent and there is sometimes difficulty in isolating virus from subacute or chronic cases in enzootic areas. Demonstration of antigen by fluorescent antibody staining will allow diagnosis of acute cases. For chronic cases serological testing has been recommended and with the use of more than one test a high degree of accuracy can be achieved. Several sensitive laboratory tests for detection of the virus in tissues, and serum antibody are now available. Enzyme-linked immunosorbent assay (ELISA) tests are highly sensitive (18). Radioimmunoassay tests are also sensitive (28, 31) and isolates of the virus may be titrated in swine monocyte cultures using a microtechnique (27). In the lymphocyte response test to virus infection, there is a cytolytic effect on the lymphocytes, the effect is greater on the B-lymphocytes than on the T-lymphocytes (29). Pigs with demonstrable antibody should be considered as chronic carriers of the virus as it is doubtful that true recovery ever occurs.

Treatment and control

No effective treatment has been described. The control and eradication of African swine fever is difficult because of: the lack of an effective vaccine; the transmission of the virus in fresh meat and cured pork products; the recognition of persistent infection in some pigs; the clinical similarity of hog cholera and African swine fever; and the recognition that in some parts of the world soft ticks of the genus *Ornithodoros* are involved in the biological transmission of the disease. Prevention of introduction of the disease to free countries is based on the prohibition of importation of live pigs or pig products from countries where African swine fever occurs. Strict application of the prohibition has prevented the spread of the disease from enzootic areas within South Africa. If a breakdown does occur control must consist of prevention of spread by quarantine, slaughter of infected and contact animals and suitable hygienic precautions. The need for close contact between pigs for the disease to spread and the ease with which this can be prevented by the erection of pig-proof fences facilitates control. Conversely, the disease is virtually uncontrollable when pigs from a number of farms have access to communal grazing (4). The virus is highly resistant to external influences including chemical agents and the most practicable disinfectant to use against the virus is a strong solution of caustic soda. Contaminated sties can remain infective for periods exceeding 3 months. These factors and the persistence of the virus in recovered pigs probably contributed to the difficulties encountered in the eradication program in Portugal where the disease was stamped out but reappeared in 1960 (20). However the most important factor appears to have been the indiscriminate use of attenuated vaccines which fostered the development of carrier pigs.

The immunology of African swine fever is poorly

understood. Pigs that survive virulent infection are usually resistant to subsequent challenge exposure with the homologous strain. However, neutralizing antibody cannot be demonstrated and recovered pigs may be chronically infected and act as carriers even though both humoral and cellular immune systems are functional (21). Several vaccines have been used including an ineffective killed virus vaccine (22) and vaccines composed of virus attenuated by passage through eggs, rabbits and tissue culture (17, 23). Although the latter have some protective properties, results following their use have been neither satisfactory nor safe and they have the two disadvantages of confounding laboratory tests and producing 'carrier' pigs.

REVIEW LITERATURE

Commission of the European Communities (1983) *African Swine Fever.*

Hess, W. R. (1981) African swine fever: a reassessment. *Adv. vet. Sci. comp. Med.*, *25*, 39–69.

Thomson, G. R. (1985) The epidemiology of African swine fever: the role of free-living hosts in Africa. *Onderstepoort J. vet. Res.*, *52*, 201–209.

Wardley, R. C., Andrade, Cde, M., Black, D. N. et al. (1983) African swine fever virus. *Arch. Virol.*, *76*, 73–90.

Wilkinson, P. J. (1980) African swine fever. *Pig News Inf.*, *1*, 17–20.

Wilkinson, P. J. (1984) The persistence of African swine fever in African and the Mediterranean. *Prev. vet. Med.*, *2*, 71–82.

REFERENCES

(1) Wardley, R. C. et al. (1983) *Arch. Virol.*, *76*, 73.
(2) Pan, I. C. & Hess, W. R. (1985) *Am. J. vet. Res.*, *46*, 314.
(3) Pan, I. C. & Hess, W.R. (1984) *Am. J. vet. Res.*, *45*, 361.
(4) Wilkinson, P. J. (1984) *Prev. vet. Med*, *2*, 71.
(5) Pini, A. & Hunter, L. R. (1975) *J. S. Afr. vet. med. Assoc.*, *46*, 227.
(6) Wilkinson, P. J. et al (1981) *J. comp. Pathol.*, *91.*, 277.
(7) Rodriguez, O. N. et al. (1972) *Revta cub. Cienc. vet.*, *3*, 1.
(8) Degner, R. L. et al. (1982/1983) *Prev. vet. Med.*, *1*, 371.
(9) Gibbs, E. P. J. & Butler, J. F. (1984) *J. Am. vet. Med. Assoc.*, *184*, 644.
(10) Thomson, G.R. (1985) *Onderstepoort J. vet. Res.*, *52*, 201.
(11) Sanchez Botija, C. & Badiola, C. (1966) *Bull. Off. int. Epizoot.*, *66*, 699.
(12) Edwards, J. F. et al. (1984) *Am. J. vet. Res.*, *45*, 2414.
(13) Edwards, J. F. & Dodds, W. J. (1985) *Am. J. vet. Res.*, *46*, 181.
(14) Edwards, J. F. et al (1985) *Am. J. vet. Res.*, *46*, 2058.
(15) Hamdy, F. M. & Dardini, A. H. (1984) *Am. J. vet. Res. 45*, 711.
(16) Schlafer, D. H. & Mebus, C. A. (1987) *Am. J. vet. Res.*, *48*, 246.
(17) De Boer, C. J. et al. (1972) *J. Am. vet. med. Assoc.*, *160*, 528.
(18) Hamdy, F. M. et al. (1981) *Am. J. vet. Res.*, *42*, 1441.
(19) Moulton, J. & Coggins, L. (1968) *Cornell Vet.*, *58*, 364.
(20) Ribiero, M. J. & Azevedo, R. J. (1961) *Bull. Off. int. Epizoot.*, *55*, 88.
(21) Shimuzu, M. et al. (1977) *Am. J. vet. Res.*, *38*, 27.
(22) Stone, S. S. & Hess, W. R. (1967) *Am. J. vet. Res.*, *28*, 475.
(23) Coggins, L. et al. (1968) *Cornell Vet.*, *58*, 525.
(24) Mebus, C. A. & Dardini, A. H. (1980) *Am. J. vet. Res.*, *41*, 1867.
(25) Groocock, C. M. et al. (1980) *Am. J. vet. Res.*, *41*, 591.
(26) Schlafer, D. H. et al. (1984) *Am. J. vet. Res.*, *45*, 1361, 1367.
(27) Wardley, R. C. & Wilkinson, P. J. (1980) *Arch. Virol.*, *64*, 93.
(28) Wardley, R. C. & Wilkinson, P. J. (1980) *Vet. Microbiol.*, *5*, 169.
(29) Wardley, R. C. & Wilkinson, P. J. (1980) *Res. vet. Sci.*, *28*, 185.
(30) Gonzalvo, F. R. et al. (1986) *Am. J. vet. Res.*, *47*, 1249, 1858.
(31) Crowther, J. R. et al. (1979) *J. Hyg.*, *Camb.*, *83*, 353.
(32) Mellor, P. S. & Wilkinson, P. J. (1985) *Res. vet. Sci.*, *39*, 353.
(33) McVicar, J. W. (1984) *Am. J. vet. Res.*, *45*, 1535.

Equine infectious anemia (swamp fever)

Equine infectious anemia (EIA) is a contagious disease of horses caused by a virus and characterized by a long, relapsing illness after an initial acute attack. Periodic replication of the virus in macrophages causes an immunologically mediated acute anemia.

Etiology

The virus of equine infectious anemia is a lentivirus (family Retroviridae) (1, 22). It has been used to produce the disease experimentally in horses and possibly in pigs and sheep, but the disease occurs naturally only in Equidae. Although a number for antigenically different, serologically identifiable serotypes have been identified by the virus neutralization test (2), there is so much variation by way of antigenic drift in the virus that a finite number of serotypes does not seem to fit the observed data (22). The virus can be cultivated on equine leukocytes and tissue culture.

Epidemiology

The disease has been diagnosed on all continents (1). In Europe it is most prevalent in the northern and central regions. It has appeared in most of the states of the United States and the provinces of Canada but the principal enzootic areas are the Gulf Coast region and the northern wooded sections of Canada. Diagnosis of the disease was made in Australia in 1959 but how long the disease had been present there and its distribution have not been determined. The incidence appears to be very low (3). Although statistics of prevalence of the disease are unreliable because of failure to diagnose and report the disease, it is of major importance and appears to be increasing in incidence. The morbidity varies considerably and may approach 100% in small areas where the populations of carrier horses and insect vectors are particularly dense, for example in Hong Kong (5). Extensive serological surveys over large areas, using the Coggins (agar gel immunodiffusion, AGID) test, have shown morbidity rates of 1·5–2·5% in the United States, 6% in Canada, a low level in France, 1.6% in West Germany (5) and 15–25% in Argentina (13). The case mortality rate is usually about 50% although true recovery in the sense that the animal no longer carries the virus seldom, if ever, occurs, so that horses, once infected, must be considered to be infected for life (14). The difficulty of diagnosis and the persistence of the 'carrier' state for periods of many years have resulted in embargoes on the introduction of horses into free countries, resulting in recent years not so much in economic embarrassment as in interference with sporting events. Large-scale movements of horses during wartime have been responsible for extensive dissemination of the disease. At the present time there is another surge of infection, or possibly of detection because of obligatory testing. It is suggested that the rapid expansion of 'pleasure horse' activity in affluent countries leads to more movement, and opportunities for spread of the infection (14).

All breeds and age groups of Equidae are susceptible.

The indigenous Criollo horses of Argentina are reported to be much more resistant to infection and only mildly affected by the disease (6). The virus is relatively resistant to most environmental influences such as boiling for up to 15 minutes and disinfectants but is destroyed by sunlight. It persists for several months at room temperature in urine, feces, dried blood and serum. Whether or not true immunity to EIA develops is uncertain, but most animals in which the virus persists for long periods and yet are clinically normal, are resistant to reinfection. It appears probable that there are marked differences in virulence between different strains of the virus.

There is a marked seasonal incidence of the disease, most cases occurring in the summer and autumn. It has been associated with low-lying and newly settled bush areas due to the greater number of insect vectors in such areas. Undernourished, parasitized and debilitated animals are most susceptible.

The virus is present in all tissues, secretions and excretions and may persist in the body for up to 18 years, preventing reinfection but providing a source of infection for most of the animal's life. These clinically normal 'carriers' are the usual means by which the disease is introduced into clean areas, although its failure to become established permanently after introduction to some areas is a feature of EIA. Short-term contact is usually insufficient to cause spread but continued, close association with susceptible animals usually results in infection. Spread within a group is slow although occasionally fairly rapid spread is observed in large groups of horses assembled at racetracks or army depots.

The disease can be readily transmitted by the injection of small quantities of infected blood intravenously, subcutaneously, intramuscularly or intracerebrally. Biting flies, particularly Tabanidae, and mosquitoes can transmit the infection and this, together with the observation that the disease spreads most actively in summer and in marshy or wooded areas, suggests that bites by insects may be the most important method of spread. It is probable that transmission is mechanical only so that spread by this means will be over short distances and require a heavy fly population (4). *Stomoxys calcitrans* (8) and *Chrysops flavidus* (deerfly) (29) have been shown to be vectors. Intrauterine infection can occur but is uncommon (9) and foals have become infected through the milk of infected dams, but relatively large amounts of virus must be ingested to cause infection and the digestive tract is not a major portal of entry. Foals of infected dams are less susceptible to natural infection than adults possibly due partly to persistence of colostral antibodies (26). The opposite can also happen and the passively immune foal develops a fatal case of the acute disease (28). Transmission via migrating strongyle larvae has been mooted because of the isolation of the virus from the worm. However, the virus has not been found in the worm eggs.

Infection can be readily achieved by the use of contaminated surgical instruments or needles or by the injection of minute quantities of virus, and the use of a common needle when injecting groups of horses may cause a serious outbreak of the disease. The increasing use of injections by non-veterinarians, particularly at racetracks, increases the chance of spread of the disease because of the frequent neglect of asepsis. In enzootic areas outbreaks have been caused by the use of untreated biological preparations of equine origin. In such circumstances all biological preparations produced in horses can be sterilized by the addition of 0·5% phenol and storage for 3 months before use.

The virus is also capable of invasion through intact oral and nasal mucosae, wounds and even unbroken skin, but these portals are probably of minor importance in field outbreaks. Transmission of infection from horse to horse seems possible via swabbing instruments used in collecting saliva for doping tests. It can also be transmitted in the semen of an infected stallion.

Pathogenesis

The virus is present in the blood 2–5 days after experimental inoculation but a febrile reaction does not occur until the 10th–29th day. The virus localizes in many organs, especially spleen, liver, kidney and lymph nodes, and can be detected there in greatest quantity when a severe clinical attack is evident. It disappears from tissues during periods between attacks. Although there is a persistent viremia, probably for the duration of the horse's life, the level is low except during periods of clinical activity, so that it is at these times that the animal is most infective.

Damage to the intima of the small blood vessels, reticuloendothelial involvement, and excessive destruction of erythrocytes follow invasion by the virus. Damage to the vascular endothelium is followed by inflammatory changes in the parenchymatous organs, particularly the liver. Similar changes occur in nervous tissue and result in the ataxia and spinal leptomeningitis and encephalomyelitis which are characteristic of the disease (7, 21). The acute disease is thought to be associated with massive virus replication in and destruction of macrophages, but the actual cause of death is unknown. There is good evidence that the vascular lesions and the erythrocyte fragility are part of an immune reaction. The hemolysis, which is both intravascular and extravascular, is characterized by shorter lifespans of erythrocytes. The virus can pass the placental barrier and infect the fetal foal.

Much about the pathogenesis of equine infectious anemia is not understood. However, it is generally assumed that the anemia and the glomerulonephritis result from the deposition of complexes composed of viral antigen and antibody (19). The hepatitis and lymphadenopathy probably have the same basis. Also, in some way which is not understood the complexity of the host's immunological response permits the survival of the virus while at the same time producing a hypergammaglobulinemia (15).

An eminently plausible scheme of pathogenetic events (22) includes:

- Primary entry and infection of macrophages
- Destruction of macrophages and release of virus and components
- Production of antibodies to antigenic components
- Formation of antigen–antibody complexes, which

induce fever, glomerulitis and complement depletion
- Specific complexes cause hemolysis or phagocytosis by activating the reticuloendothelial system
- Delayed release of iron from macrophages causes temporary iron-deficient erythropoiesis
- Pathological processes subside as virus neutralizing antibody restrains viral multiplication in macrophages
- A new antigenic variant of the virus appears, a new cycle of viral replication in macrophages and a new clinical episode commence. The antigenic variation is due to changes in the surface glycoprotein of the EIA virus (30)
- Recurrence of these episodes becomes less frequent and the horse becomes permanently asymptomatic. The animal can be said to have achieved an appropriate level of immune response sufficient to protect it against antigenic epitopes that are common to all EIA virus strains (30).

Clinical findings

An incubation period of 2–4 weeks is usual in natural outbreaks of equine infectious anemia. Outbreaks usually follow a pattern of slow spread to susceptible horses after the introduction of an infected animal. On first exposure to infection, horses manifest signs of varying degree, classified as acute or subacute. Occasionally the initial attack is mild and may be followed by rapid clinical recovery. As a rule there is initial depression, profound weakness, and loss of condition. Ataxia is a prominent sign in many cases (7) and in some is recorded as the only clinical abnormality (21). There is intermittent fever (up to 41°C, 105°F) which may rise and fall rapidly, sometimes varying as much as 1°C within 1 hour. Jaundice, edema of the ventral abdomen, the prepuce and legs, and petechial hemorrhages in the mucosae, especially under the tongue and in the conjunctivae, may be observed. Pallor of the mucosae does not occur in this early stage and they tend to be congested and edematous. There is a characteristic increase in rate and intensity of the heart sounds which are greatly exacerbated by moderate exercise. Myocarditis, manifested by tachycardia and arrhythmia, is described as being diagnostic. Respiratory signs are not marked, there is no dyspnea until the terminal stages, but there may be a thin serosanguineous nasal discharge. There is considerable enlargement of the spleen which may be detectable per rectum. Pregnant mares may abort. Many animals show temporary recovery from this acute stage, after a course of 3 days to 3 weeks. Others become progressively weak, recumbent and die after a course of 10–14 days of illness.

Animals showing temporary recovery may appear normal for 2–3 weeks and then relapse with similar but usually less severe signs, although death may occur during such a relapse. Relapses continue to occur often coinciding with periods of stress, and are characterized by recurrent febrile episodes, increasing emaciation, weakness and cardiac insufficiency and the development of pallor of the mucosae, a late sign of this disease. In this chronic stage the appetite is usually good although allotriophagia may be observed. Some affected animals appear to make a complete recovery although they may remain infected and suffer relapses in later years. Prolonged therapy with corticosteroids can cause such a relapse (20). Even in the absence of clinical illness infected animals perform less efficiently than the uninfected (5). Most deaths occur within a year of infection.

Alimentary involvement is not commonly recorded in equine infectious anemia but a fetid, watery diarrhea has been observed as a prominent sign. In such cases secondary infection is probably involved.

Clinical pathology

The marked fall in erythrocytes which is characteristic of the disease is not usually seen during the initial attack. When it occurs during subsequent episodes its degree varies with the severity of the signs. In the acute form, the packed cell volume (PCV) is low (14–20%), there is a leukopenia (down to 2000/μl) with a marked neutropenia and a lymphopenia. Also, some horses show a marked drop in blood platelet count at each febrile episode. The anemia is normocytic and normochromic. The horse rarely releases immature erythrocytes (reticulocytes and nucleated erythrocytes) to the circulation in response to severe hemolytic or blood loss anemias. In the subacute form, the changes are essentially similar, with a progressive anemia produced by episodes of hemolytic disease. The total serum proteins are reduced and the albumin–globulin ratio is below normal. A single hematological examination is of less value in diagnosis than serial tests matched with a temperature curve because the blood picture gradually returns to near normal between attacks.

The only available *in vitro* assay for field strains of the virus is a cumbersome leukocyte culture system. The horse is the only experimental animal available. So that the level of infectivity of an animal is very difficult to measure. It is relatively simple, however, to determine that a horse has been exposed to infection.

At the present time an agar gel immunodiffusion (AGID) test, which depends on the presence of precipitins in the sera of infected horses, is in general use as a diagnostic tool (18). Several different antigens have been used in the past but tissue culture virus is now used for this purpose. The precipitating antibodies appear early, at the same time as the CF antibody, but persist longer, for as long as neutralizing antibody persists. The period between inoculation and the appearance of the positive reaction may be as long as 45 days. Foals become passively immunized, and react positively if they absorb antibodies in the dam's colostrum. Their serum levels become negative at 65–182 days old. The AGID test has proved to be very accurate and is suitable as a basis for an eradication program. Except in foals, a positive AGID test is accepted as being synonymous with being infected and infective. The only identifiable limitation of the test is its inability to identify cases which are still in the period of incubation, which are not yet showing clinical signs and which may even die during this period (10). In newborn foals a positive reaction may indicate that the foal has acquired passive immunity via its dam's colostrum.

Other serological tests are also available. An indirect immunofluorescence test is being used to detect the presence of virus in tissue. In the CF test there is a measurable titer for as long as 2 or 3 months after an attack with the titer peak occurring within 10–20 days. Its rapid disappearance limits its practical value in diagnosis. Neutralizing antibody is detectable about a month later than the first febrile period and persists indefinitely. An indirect hemagglutination test is as accurate as the immunodiffusion test (10). An enzyme-linked immunoabsorbent assay (ELISA) has also produced results which replicate those of the other tests (16), and at an early stage of development of the disease (27), but will identify some false positive animals (12). Counterimmunoelectrophoresis has been recommended as being much faster and more sensitive than the AGID test (31). Experimental transmission of the disease to susceptible horses by the subcutaneous injection of 20 ml whole blood or Seitz-filtered plasma is also used as a diagnostic test and is a valuable, although expensive, supplement to other tests. For example, a final diagnosis in one horse was made only after a transmission experiment. The AGID test had proved negative (3). The donor blood should be collected during a febrile episode when the viremia is most pronounced. The recipient animals are checked for increases in body temperature twice daily. Liver biopsy has been used in diagnosis but is unreliable. Some significance is attached to changes in the albumin–globulin ratio of affected horses, all having a significant hypergammaglobulinemia. Albuminuria is usually present during clinical episodes.

Necropsy findings

In the acute stages there may be subcutaneous edema, jaundice and petechial or ecchymotic subserous hemorrhages. There is considerable enlargement, with swelling of the edges, of the liver and spleen and their local lymph nodes. In the chronic stages emaciation and pallor of tissues are the only gross findings. Histological examination is helpful in diagnosis even in asymptomatic chronic carriers. Characteristic lesions include extensive proliferation of the reticuloendothelial system and vascular intima, perivascular round cell infiltrations, especially in the liver, hemosiderosis, and a glomerulitis, caused probably by the deposition of virus–antibody complexes on glomerular epithelium. Virus is present in greatest concentration in the spleen, liver, bone marrow and abdominal lymph nodes.

Diagnosis

Laboratory diagnosis is now satisfactorily provided for with the agar gel immunodiffusion test—the Coggins test (AGID). Clinical diagnosis is still difficult irrespective of whether the disease is in the acute or chronic stage. Continuous observations are necessary, particularly as recurrent fever and hemolytic crises are important features of the disease. Transmission experiments are still relevant and should always be carried out when the disease is suspected in a new area. The identification of the transmitted disease depends upon the clinical, clinicopathological and necropsy findings listed above. The administration of corticosteroids to horses with the chronic disease may result in the development of the acute clinical form of the disease (20). In individual animals the disease may be confused with purpura hemorrhagica, babesiosis, ehrlichiosis, leptospirosis, severe strongylosis or fascioliasis, and with anemia caused by suppression of hemopoiesis by chronic suppurative processes. Of these purpura hemorrhagica is the most likely cause of confusion because of the presence of mucosal hemorrhages and subcutaneous aggregations of fluid. Leptospirosis is a much milder disease and affected horses usually recover spontaneously within a few days.

Treatment

No specific treatment is available. Supportive treatment including blood transfusions, and hematinic drugs may facilitate clinical recovery.

Control

The control of equine infectious anemia is still universally based on the eradication of the disease by identifying the infected, clinically normal animals with a serological test and then destroying them—in fact, a test-and-slaughter policy. The test used is the Coggins (AGID) test, and eradication on a one-farm or small area (17) basis has been carried out in this way, and results in Kentucky, USA, point to the effectiveness of the program (25). In most countries the probability of reinfection by insect vectors would discourage such a program. Canada has an intensive voluntary control program for equine infectious anemia. Horses positive to the Coggins test are quarantined, in-contact horses are searched out and tested and euthanasia is recommended for horses having positive reactions. Owners are compensated for their loss.

Restriction of introduction of infected horses into clean herds or areas is desirable, but the insect-borne character of the disease is likely to result in its recrudescence. If suspect horses are to be introduced they should be kept under close surveillance for at least 6 months before being admitted and then submitted to the AGID test at intervals afterwards. Operators of open stud farms, and rest farms can also insist on a negative Coggins test before admitting each horse. One deficiency of this policy is the long period of 'incubation' of up to 45 days between infection and the appearance of a positive test.

Control programs based on this test-and-slaughter policy are under fire because of the view of horse owners that many asymptomatic horses, with very low infectivity, are being destroyed unnecessarily (18). A decision on the matter really depends on whether the objective is eradication or containment, and if the latter, at what level. Until now the policy has been eradication and it is obvious that another attitude is possible. The record of an infective horse which was negative to the AGID test adds fuel to the fire (24).

Draining of marshy areas and the control of biting insects may aid in limiting spread of the disease. A degree of protection may be obtained by the use of insect repellents and by stabling in screened stables. Great care must be taken to avoid transmission of the disease on surgical instruments and hypodermic needles which can only be satisfactorily sterilized by boiling for 15 minutes or by autoclaving at 6·6 kg pressure for a similar period. Chemical disinfection of instruments and tattoo equipment requires their immersion for 10 minutes in one of the less corrosive phenolic disinfectants. All materials to be disinfected need to be cleaned of organic matter first. For personal disinfection sodium hypochlorite, ethanol or iodine compounds are safe, and for materials where organic matter is not removable, agents such as chlorhexidine or phenolic compounds combined with a detergent are satisfactory (11).

Although the immune response in recovered animals is poor and there seems to be little possibility of producing a satisfactory vaccine (21) the practicability of this approach is still being explored (23).

REVIEW LITERATURE

Issel, C. J. & Coggins, L. (1979) Equine infectious anemia. Current knowledge. *J. Am. vet. med. Assoc.*, *174*, 727.

Johnson, A. W. (1976) Equine infectious anaemia. Review. *Vet. Bull.*, *46*, 559.

Kemen, M. J. (1977) Equine infectious anemia. *Cornell Vet.*, *67*, 177.

McGuire, T. C. & Crawford, T. B. (1979) Immunology of a persistent retrovirus infection. Equine infectious anemia. *Adv. vet. Sci.*, *23*, 137.

Tashjian, R. J. (1984) Transmission and clinical evaluation of an equine infectious anemia herd and their offspring over a 13-year period. *J. Am. vet. Med. Assoc.*, *184*, 282–288.

REFERENCES

(1) Ishii, S. & Ishitani, R. (1976) *Adv. vet. Sci. comp. Med.*, *19*, *195*.
(2) Johnson, A. W. (1976) *Vet. Bull.*, *46*, 559.
(3) Lepherd, E. E. (1981) *Aust. vet. J.*, *57*, 435.
(4) Issel, C. J. & Foil, L. D. (1984) *J. Am. vet. med. Assoc.*, *184*, 293.
(5) Coggins, L. & Auchnie, J. A. (1977) *J. Am. vet. med. Assoc.*, *170*, 1299.
(6) Mettler, N. E. et al. (1981) *Gac. Vet.*, *43*, 49.
(7) McClure, J. J. et al. (1982) *J. Am. vet. med. Assoc.*, *180*, 279.
(8) Cupp, E. W. & Kemen, W. J. (1980) *Proc. 84th Ann. Mtg US Anim. Hlth Assoc.*, p. 362.
(9) Tashjian, R. J. & Kittelson, S. L. (1976) *Vet. Med. small Anim. Clin.*, *71*, 333, 335.
(10) Sugiura, T. & Nakajima, H. (1982) *Can. J. comp. Med.*, *46*, 60.
(11) Shen, D. T. et al. (1977) *Am. J. vet. Res.*, *38*, 1217.
(12) Evans, K.S. et al. (1984) *Am. J. vet. Res.*, *45*, 20.
(13) Pauli, R. et al. (1978) *Gac. Vet.*, *40*, 169.
(14) Coggins, L. (1984) *J. Am. vet. med. Assoc.*, *184*, 279.
(15) Coggins, L. (1975) *Cornell Vet.*, *65*, 143.
(16) Suzuki, T. et al. (1982) *Vet. Microbiol.*, *7*, 307.
(17) Burki, F. et al. (1979) *Tierärztl. Monatschr.*, *66*, 3.
(18) Pearson, J. E. & Knowles, R. C. (1984) *J. Am. vet. med. Assoc.*, *184*, 798.
(19) Gorham, J. R. et al. (1977) *J. equ. med. Surg.*, *1*, 71.
(20) McConnell, S. et al. (1983) *Equ. Pract.*, *5(7)*, 32.
(21) Held, J. P. et al. (1983) *J. Am. vet. med. Assoc.*, *183*, 324.
(22) McGuire, T. C. & Crawford, T. B. (1979) *Adv. vet. Sci.*, *23*, 137.
(23) Toma, B. (1975) *Contribution à l'Etude Immunologique de l'Anemie Infectieuse des Equides*, p. 262. Maisons-Alfort, France.
(24) McConnell, S. & Katada, M. (1981) *Equ. vet. J.*, *13*, 123.
(25) Cornell, W. D. (1981) *Vet. med SAC*, *76*, 485.
(26) Issel, C. J. et al. (1985) *Am. J. vet. Res.*, *46*, 1114.
(27) Shen, D. T. et al. (1984) *Am. J. vet. Res.*, *45*, 1542.
(28) Tashjian, R. J. (1984) *J. Am. vet. med. Assoc.*, *184*, 282.
(29) Foil, L. D. et al. (1983) *Am. J. vet. Res.*, *44*, 155.
(30) Cheevers, W. P. & McGuire, T. C. (1985) *Rev. infect. Dis.*, *7*, 83.
(31) Sun, H. M. (1986) *Chin. J. vet. Med.*, *12*, 12.

Bovine ephemeral fever (BEF)

Ephemeral fever is an infectious disease of cattle characterized by inflammation of mesodermal tissues as evidenced by muscular shivering, stiffness, lameness and enlargement of the peripheral lymph nodes. The disease is caused by a virus which is transmitted by insect vectors.

Etiology

Ephemeral fever is caused by an insect-borne, unnamed rhabdovirus. There are four serotypes: DDP63 (13), CSIRO368 (6), DDP61 (22) and FUK-11 (19). It is closely associated with the leukocyte–platelet fraction of the blood, and can be maintained on tissue culture and chick embryos. The disease can also be transmitted by the injection of whole blood or the leukocyte fraction of it. Repeated intracerebral passages in sucking mice produce strains that are pathogenic for adult mice on intracerebral injection. Adult rats, guinea-pigs and lambs are similarly susceptible (18).

Epidemiology

Ephemeral fever occurs enzootically on the African continent, in most of Asia and the East Indies. It has occurred sporadically in Australia. Although it is of minor importance, considerable loss occurs in dairy herds due to the depression of milk flow. The reduction may be as great as 80% in cows in late lactation. There is also a lowered resistance to mastitis and a significant delay in the occurrence of estrus. Occasional animals die of intercurrent infection or prolonged recumbency. The morbidity rate in outbreaks is usually about 35%, but if the population is highly susceptible and environmental conditions favor the spread of the disease, the morbidity rate may reach 100%. In enzootic areas only 5–10% will be affected.

After experimental infection of cattle there is solid immunity against homologous strains for up to 2 years. Immunity against heterologous strains is much less durable which probably accounts for the apparent variations in immunity following field exposure. Among domestic animals, only cattle are known to be naturally affected and although all age groups are susceptible the disease is more common in adults. However, calves as young as 3 months are as susceptible as adults to experimental infection. Newborn colostrum-deprived calves are susceptible. It appears very unlikely that the BEF virus, in its virulent field form, will act as a fetal pathogen, but vaccine strains have not been examined in this respect. In Africa, based on serological results, the virus is thought to be cycling in populations of wild ruminants between epidemics in domestic cattle (5). Buffalo (*Bubalus bubalis*) are susceptible to experimental infection, but the resulting viremia is very shortlived so that it is unlikely that they will play any part as a reservoir host (1). Experimental animals are in general not susceptible but the infection is transmissible to unweaned hamsters and mice.

The source of infection is the animal affected with the clinical disease. Spread occurs via insect vectors of which the sandfly, Ceratopogonidae family, is probably the most important. A great deal of work in recent years has not clearly defined the vector list which probably includes the mosquitoes *Aedes* spp. (15), *Culex annulirostris* and *Anopheles bancroftii* and the sandfly *Culicoides brevitarsis* (7), and in many countries the reservoir host, other than cattle, has not been identified. This is of particular importance when the epidemiological pattern of occurrence of the disease changes as it has done in Australia. The disease now occurs annually in areas where it used to occur only once each decade, probably because of establishment of the virus in a new vector (9).

Spread is largely independent of cattle movement and transmission does not occur through contact with infected animals or their saliva or ocular discharge. The disease is not spread through semen, nor is intrauterine administration of the virus a suitable route of transmission (8). The disease occurs in the summer months and spread depends largely on the insect vector population and the force and direction of prevailing winds. When strong winds prevail the vectors may be carried over large tracts of land or water. Cyclical development of the virus in insect vectors is suspected. The disease tends to disappear for long periods to return in epizootic form when the resistance of the population is diminished. Recurrence depends primarily on suitable environmental conditions for increase and dissemination of the insect vector (15). During periods of quiescence the disease is still present but the morbidity is reputed to be very low. However, in the usual sorts of enzootic areas the degree of surveillance is less than intense, and clinical cases may occur without being observed. The reason why an epizootic develops out of an enzootic herd, or area population, may be due to a change in virulence, or in the vector population (10).

Pathogenesis

After an incubation period of 2–10 days a viral septicemia develops with localization and inflammation in mesodermal tissues particularly joints, lymph nodes and muscles. A febrile reaction, lasting 2 days, increased respiratory rate, dyspnea, limb stiffness and pain are characteristic at this time. The virus is thought to grow principally in the reticuloendothelial cells in the lungs, spleen, and lymph nodes and not in vascular endothelium or lymphoid cells (4). Experimental intravenous injection of the virus causes serofibrinous inflammation in serous cavities and the virus can be detected in the serosal and synovial fluids and in the mesothelial cells of synovial membrane and epicardium and in neutrophils in the fluids (23).

Clinical findings

Calves are least affected, those less than 6 months of age showing no clinical signs. Fat cows and bulls are worst affected.

In most cases the disease is acute. There is a sudden onset of fever (40·5–41°C, 105–106°F), sometimes with morning remissions. Anorexia and a sharp fall in milk yield occur. There is severe constipation in some animals and diarrhea in others. Respiratory and cardiac rates are increased and stringy, nasal and watery ocular discharges are evident. The animals shake their heads constantly and muscle shivering and weakness are observed. There may be swellings about the shoulders, neck and back. Muscular signs become more evident on the second day with severe stiffness, clonic muscle movements and weakness in one or more limbs. A posture similar to that of acute laminitis, with all four feet bunched under the body, is often adopted. About the third day the animal begins eating and ruminating, and the febrile reaction disappears, but lameness and weakness may persist for 2–3 more days. Some animals remain standing during the acute stages but the majority go down and assume a position reminiscent of parturient paresis with the hindlegs sticking out and the head turned into the flank. Occasional animals adopt a posture of lateral recumbency. Some develop clinically detectable pulmonary and subcutaneous emphysema (2). In most cases recovery is rapid and complete after an illness of 3–5 days unless there is exposure to severe weather, or unless aspiration of a misdirected drench or ruminal contents occurs. Occasional cases show persistent recumbency and have to be destroyed and abortion occurs in a small proportion of cases (24). Milder cases may occur at the end of an epizootic with signs restricted to pyrexia and lack of appetite.

Clinical pathology

A leukocytosis with a relative increase in neutrophils occurs during the acute stage of the disease. There is a shift to the left and a lymphopenia. Plasma fibrinogen levels are elevated for about 7 days and there is also a significant hypocalcemia (11). Available serological tests include a complement fixation serum neutralization, a fluorescent antibody test, and an agar gel immunodiffusion test (AGID) which is used successfully as a diagnostic aid (20).

Necropsy findings

Postmortem lesions are not dramatic. All lymph nodes are usually enlarged and edematous and the serous membranes show patchy congestion with some effusion and occasionally petechiation. Congestion of the abomasal mucosa is usual and may also be apparent in the nasal cavities, the small intestine and the kidneys. Pulmonary emphysema and bronchiolitis are standard findings. The joints show degenerative changes in synovial membranes and an increase in synovial fluid. Pathological examinations of animals that develop persistent recumbency have shown severe degenerative changes in the spinal cord similar to those produced by physical compression (12). The possibility exists that there has been trauma to the cord during violent movements while attempting to rise. In experimentally produced cases a serofibrinous polysynovitis, tendovaginitis and periarthritis are obvious lesions. Identification of the virus in most tissues can be done by demonstrating specific bovine ephemeral fever (BEF) viral antigen immunofluorescence or by isolation in mice (4).

Diagnosis

The diagnosis of ephemeral fever in a cattle population is not difficult on the basis of its transient nature and its rapidity of spread. It may present a problem in individual animals in which it may resemble traumatic reticulitis, acute laminitis, or parturient paresis. In the case of traumatic reticulitis differentiation is almost impossible unless a metal detector test is negative or a rumenotomy is performed. Laminitis is accompanied by local pain in the feet and usually occurs after overfeeding. The response to injected calcium solutions is a good diagnostic test to differentiate the disease from parturient paresis.

Treatment
Palliative treatment with salicylates or Butazolidin may benefit the muscle stiffness but drenching should be avoided because of the risk of aspiration pneumonia. Proper nursing of the recumbent animal is all that is required.

Control
Control of the vectors is not possible. Because of the immunity that develops after the natural disease and because the virus becomes attenuated by passage through mice and hamsters strong efforts have been made to produce vaccines. There are no commercially available vaccines which have been extensively tested in the field. Killed vaccines are generally considered to have low efficiency. Even attenuated viruses need to be used in an adjuvant base, for example, Quil A, a saponin derivative, and two injections are required (3, 21). The worry about their use is the possibility of their transmission by insects from vaccinated animals to the general population, and subsequent interference with a test and eradication program. There is, too, the possibility that they may assume full virulence while undergoing natural passage. These factors combined with uncertainty about the host range, especially the fetus and neonates (13) are inhibiting the immediate development of vaccines.

The establishment of sentinel cattle herds in northern Australia allows constant virological surveillance against the entry of bovine ephemeral fever which is repeatedly epizootic in the area (16, 17). Laboratory techniques used in this monitoring program are mainly serological, but some tissue culture work is possible.

REVIEW LITERATURE

Burgess, G. W. (1971) Bovine ephemeral fever, a review. *Vet. Bull.*, *41*, 887.
Combs, G. P. (1978) Bovine ephemeral fever. *Proc. 82nd ann. Mtg US Anim. Hlth Assoc.*, *82*, 29.

REFERENCES

(1) Young, P. L. (1979) *Aust. vet. J.*, *55*, 349.
(2) Theodoridis, A. & Coetzer, J. A. W. (1979) *Onderstepoort J. vet. Res.*, *46*, 125.
(3) Vanselow, B. A. (1986) *Aust. Adv. vet. Sci.*, p. 48.
(4) Burgess, G. W. & Spradbrow, P. B. (1977) *Aust. vet. J.*, *53*, 363.
(5) Davies, F. G. et al. (1975) *J. Hyg., Camb.*, *75*, 231.
(6) Cybinski, D. H. & Zaktzewski, H. (1983) *Vet. Microbiol.*, *8*, 221.
(7) Standfast, H. A. & Miller, M. J. (1985) *Veterinary Viral Diseases*, ed. A. J. Della-Porta, Academic Press, p. 394.
(8) Parsonson, I. M. & Snowdon, W. A. (1974) *Aust. vet. J.*, *50*, 329, 335.
(9) Kirkland, P. D. (1982) Arbovirus research in Australia, *Proc. 3rd Symp.*, p. 65–75.
(10) St. George, T. D. et al. (1977) *Aust. vet. J.*, *53*, 17.
(11) Uren, M. F. & Murphy, G. M. (1985) *Vet. Microbiol.*, *10*, 493, 505.
(12) Hall, M. W. M. & Schultz, K. (1977) *Aust. vet. J*, *53*, 217.
(13) Gard, G. P. et al. (1983) *Aust. vet. J.*, *60*, 89.
(14) Elamin, M. A. G. & Spradbrow, P. B. (1978) *J. Hyg., Camb.*, *81*, 1.
(15) Davies, E. G. et al. (1985) *Bull. WHO*, *63*, 941.
(16) Doherty, R. L. (1977) *Aust. J. exp. Biol. med. Sci.*, *55*, 103.
(17) St. George, T. D. (1980) *Vet. sci. Comm.*, *4*, 39.
(18) Elamin, M. A. G. & Spradbrow, P. B. (1978) *Zentralbl. VetMed.*, *25B*, 425.
(19) Kaneko, N. et al. (1986) *Aust. vet. J.*, *63*, 29.
(20) Gard, G. P. & Melville, L. F. (1985) *Aust. adv. vet. Sci.*, p. 152.
(21) Vanselow, B. A. et al. (1985) *Vet. Rec.*, *117*, 37.
(22) Gard, G. P. et al. (1984) *Aust. vet. J.*, *61*, 332.
(23) Young, P. L. & Spradbrow, P. B. (1985) *Vet. Microbiol.*, *10*, 199.
(24) Li, X. Q. et al. (1985) *Chin. J. vet. Med.*, *11*, 26.

African horse sickness

African horse sickness is a highly fatal, infectious disease of horses, mules and donkeys. It is caused by a number of strains of a virus spread by insect vectors. Acute, subacute and mild forms of the disease occur. Its spread from the African continent in recent times presents a potential threat to the horse industry in countries of the western world.

Etiology
African horse sickness is caused by an orbivirus (family Retroviridae). A number of antigenic strains of the virus exist (42 at present) and although there is evidence of some cross-immunity between strains it is essential in large-scale vaccination programs to include a number of strains in the vaccine. The vaccine currently in use contains seven strains and is effective in most areas. The current strain in the Middle East is not related to known African strains (2).

Epidemiology
African horse sickness was confined to the African continent until World War II when serious outbreaks occurred in the Middle East (3). The disease came into prominence again in 1959 when it spread to Iran and Pakistan (3). In 1960 further spread occurred, in the east to India and to the west through the Middle East, including Turkey, to the eastern Mediterranean, Cyprus, and Spain. Much of this continental spread is now attributed to long-range carriage of vector midges on spells of unusual wind (1). The disease continues as an enzootic disease in Africa, recurring annually in most of southern, equatorial and eastern Africa, south of the Sahara. In enzootic areas it is virtually impossible to raise horses. In areas where outbreaks occur the morbidity rate varies with the number of insect vectors present; the mortality rate in susceptible horses is about 90%. Mules (50%) and donkeys do not suffer such a high mortality rate but the disease is a crippling one in these species because of gross debility.

The serious nature of the disease itself is compounded by the tremendous problem of eradication. Vaccination reduces the ravages of horse sickness but even when practiced on a wide scale cannot eradicate it because the infection is insect-borne, and uncontrolled hosts provide a reservoir of infection.

The virus is present in all body fluids and tissues of affected animals from the onset of fever until recovery. It is moderately resistant to external environmental influences such as drying and heating and it can survive in putrid blood for 2 years.

Natural infection occurs in the equine species, the

most severe disease occurring in horses, with mules and donkeys showing lesser degrees of susceptibility in that order. Dogs also contract the infection usually by eating the raw flesh of an animal with the disease (17). Natural insect-borne infection is very rare in dogs, and may never occur. Zebras are highly resistant and there is one record of the disease in dogs (4). Dogs, goats, ferrets, mice, guinea-pigs and rats can be infected experimentally; the virus can be isolated from street dogs (13), causes clinical diseases in dogs (17), and can be grown in tissue culture (5, 6), chick embryos and the brains of mice. Rabbits are not susceptible. Immunity after natural infection or vaccination by an homologous strain is solid but can be overcome by strong challenge by another strain. The development of immunity is slow and may require 3 weeks to be appreciable: titers may continue to rise for 6 months after infection. Foals from immune dams appear to derive passive immunity from the colostrum and are immune until 5–6 months of age.

The incidence of the disease is often seasonal because of the seasonal variations in the number of *Culicoides* spp. present. New cases of the disease do not appear more than 10 days after a killing frost causes disappearance of the insects, and extensive outbreaks are always preceded by a period of heavy rain. Even in Africa the disease has a geographical distribution, the areas most severely affected being low lying and swampy, and most cases occur after midsummer.

The ecology of African horse sickness is not properly understood. Spread by insects is a 'fact of life', but it has not been possible to transmit the disease experimentally. Nor has the basic reservoir been identified although it is almost certain that it is not the horse (9). The disease is spread by the passive transfer of very small quantities of blood by biting insects. Spread does not occur between animals in direct contact unless the requisite insect vectors are present. The tick *Hyalomma dromedarii* has been shown to transmit the virus between horses (12). Biting midges or gnats, *Culicoides* spp., are the most probable other vectors and climatic conditions which govern the breeding status and movement of these insects also govern the spread and morbidity rate of horse sickness. These insects have almost worldwide distribution. Many other biting insects have been named as vectors but there is a lack of satisfactory evidence in many reports. The mosquitoes *Aedes aegypti*, *Anopheles stephensi* and *Culex pipiens* have been shown to be true biological carriers (10).

Although clinically affected Equidae are the major source of virus during an outbreak the current view is that in enzootic areas there must be a silent, non-equine reservoir host which perpetuates the virus between seasons when no insects are present. It is possible that dogs may act as silent hosts. It has been shown that they can be infected naturally by the ingestion of infected meat (4). Elephants and zebra, in spite of their known resistance to infection, have been proposed as reservoir hosts (2). However, in some countries the disease has been introduced but has died out in the succeeding winter, presumably because no reservoir hosts were available. In those new countries to which the disease has now been introduced, presumably through air travel, a silent host is not necessary because the mild winters permit the persistence of the insects and the constant infection of fresh horses.

Artificially the disease is readily transmitted by the intravenous injection of very small amounts of blood. Transmission can also be effected by subcutaneous injection or oral dosing but larger amounts of blood are required, particularly with oral dosing.

In areas where the disease is enzootic outbreaks still occur, often cyclically at intervals of 10–20 years. This is a common enough pattern in diseases carried by insects and is caused by periodic elevations in immunity, seasonal and yearly variations in the vector population and periodic redistribution of new strains of the virus.

Pathogenesis

African horse sickness is a disease of vascular endothelium, with virus clones affecting endothelium in different organs, resulting in a variety of 'forms' of the disease (9).

The virus is present in the bloodstream from the first day of clinical illness and persists for about 30 days and up to 90 days. It can be recovered from defibrinated blood by intracerebral inoculation into infant mice.

Clinical findings

The incubation period in natural infections is about 5–7 days; in artificially produced infections it varies from 2 to 21 days. Three clinical forms of the disease occur, an acute or pulmonary form, a cardiac or subacute form and a mild form known as horse sickness fever. An intermittent fever of 40–41°C (105–106°F) is characteristic of all forms.

Acute (pulmonary) horse sickness

This is the most common form in acute outbreaks in susceptible animals. Initially there is fever followed by very labored breathing and severe paroxysms of coughing. There is a profuse nasal discharge of yellowish serous fluid and froth. Profuse sweating commences and the horse becomes very weak, develops a staggery gait and becomes recumbent. At this time the nasal discharge is usually voluminous. The appetite may be good until the breathing becomes so labored that the animal is unable to eat. Death follows within a few hours after a total course of 4–5 days. In the few animals which recover severe dyspnea persists for many weeks. This is the form of the disease which has been reported as occurring naturally in dogs.

Subacute (cardiac) horse sickness

This is most common in horses in enzootic areas. The incubation period may be longer, up to 3 weeks, and the fever develops more slowly and persists for longer than in the acute disease. The most obvious sign is edema in the head region, particularly in the temporal fossa, the eyelids and the lips, and this may spread to the chest. This may not develop until the horse has been febrile for a week. The oral mucosa is bluish in color and petechiae may develop under the tongue. Restlessness and mild abdominal pain are often evident. Auscultation of the heart and lungs reveals evidence of hydropericardium, endocarditis and pulmonary edema. Paralysis of the esophagus with inability to swallow and regurgitation of food and water through the nose is not uncommon. The mortality rate is not as high as in the acute disease but recovery is prolonged. A fatal course may be as long as 2 weeks.

A mixed form is described in which both pulmonary and cardiac signs appear. A horse with an initial subacute cardiac syndrome may suddenly develop acute pulmonary signs; a primary pulmonary syndrome may subside but cardiac involvement causes death. This mixed form is not common in field outbreaks.

Horse sickness fever

This presents no diagnostic signs and may go unrecognized except that it usually occurs in areas in which the disease is enzootic. It occurs most commonly as an immunization reaction or when an existing immunity is partially overcome and it is the only form of the disease which can be produced artificially in donkeys and Angora goats. The temperature rises to 40·5°C (105°F) over a period of 1–3 days but returns to normal about 3 days later. The appetite is poor, there is slight conjunctivitis and moderate dyspnea.

Clinical pathology

A complement fixation (CF) test is available but requires convalescent serum and the test is suitable only for rough diagnosis. A fluorescent antibody test shows promise (11). For accurate detection of the virus strain, the homotypic neutralization test, the neutralization in the mouse of the suspected viral material by known horse sickness immune serum is recommended (12).

Necropsy findings

Gross findings in acute cases include severe hydrothorax and pulmonary edema and moderate ascites. The liver is acutely congested and there is edema of the bowel wall. The pharynx, trachea and bronchi are filled with yellow serous fluid and froth. In cases of cardiac horse sickness there is marked hydropericardium, endocardial hemorrhage, myocardial degeneration and anasarca, especially of the supraorbital fossa.

Diagnosis

The possibility that this disease may spread to and become permanently established in very large areas which have been free hitherto makes accurate diagnosis of great importance. The complement fixation and serum neutralization tests are adequate for this purpose, the latter being necessary for strain identification.

Pulmonary horse sickness resembles equine infectious pneumonia, but the latter is rare nowadays and is restricted in its occurrence almost entirely to large groups of horses in confined quarters and under poor hygienic and management conditions. Cardiac horse sickness has much in common with equine infectious anemia, babesiosis and purpura hemorrhagica. Equine viral arteritis also has a passing resemblance to this form of the disease. The paucity of diagnostic signs in horse sickness fever would make it difficult to differentiate from many mild, sporadic diseases were it not for the rare occurrence of the disease separate from obvious clinical cases of the other forms of horse sickness.

Treatment

No treatment has been shown to have any effect on the course of the disease but careful nursing and symptomatic treatment is not without value.

Control

This disease can be introduced into new areas by the spread of infected *Culicoides* spp., either blown by strong winds or carried in fast-moving air transport. Provided the carrier insects can persist in the environment, the disease is then permanently established. It is possible that infected horses may introduce the disease, again especially if they are shipped by air. This eventuality can be prevented by restricting the importation of horses from countries known to have the disease, by vaccinating and quarantining horses at the point of embarkation, by quarantining them in insect-proof enclosures at the point of entry, and by vaccinating all horses within a 9·6 km (10 mile) radius of where horses are permitted to enter from abroad. At the present time there is a 30-day quarantine period for horses brought into the United States from Asia, Africa and the Mediterranean countries.

To prevent the spread of the disease across large land masses, vaccination of all Equidae in a wide buffer zone is the only effective measure. Vaccination of horses in the infected area with polyvalent virus attenuated by adaptation to mouse brain tissue (neurotropic virus) should be instituted, but the individual protection obtained is not absolute and this measure alone will not prevent spread. Some of the vaccine 'breaks' observed in enzootic areas are attributed to the poor antigenicity of some of the component viruses used in the vaccines (8). The vaccine in use in the Middle East and India is the one developed by African workers. It contains seven strains of attenuated virus and has proved to be effective in the 1960 outbreak (14). Immunity after vaccination is solid for at least a year but annual revaccination of all horses, mules and donkeys is recommended. Vaccination of foals from immune mares is without effect and should be delayed until they are at least 8 months old. Live tissue culture, formalized tissue culture and egg-attenuated vaccines are also produced (8, 15). The formalin-killed aluminum-precipitated vaccine, injected twice 1 month apart, gave protection for at least 6 months (16).

In enzootic areas the vector insect cannot be controlled but some protection of horses against being bitten can be obtained by stabling indoors in insect-proof stables, not permitting horses outside except in broad daylight, using fly repellents when risk is high and by keeping horses and stables on high, insect-free ground as much as possible. None of these measures is more than mildly effective.

With the use of attenuated living vaccines an eradication program could be possible, provided some control of vectors was available. Attempts at control by slaughter without the use of vaccination have had disastrous results (2).

REFERENCES

(1) Sellers, R. F. et al. (1977) *J. Hyg., Camb.*, *79*, 279.
(2) Davies, F. G. & Otieno, S. (1977) *Vet. Rec.*, *100*, 291.
(3) Reid, N. R. (1961) *Br. vet. J.*, *118*, 137.
(4) Piercy, S. E. (1951) *E. Afr. agric. J.*, *17*, 1.

(5) Mirchamsy, H. & Taslimi, H. (1962) *C. r. hebd. Séanc. Acad. Sci., Paris 255*, 424.
(6) Erasmus, B. J. (1963) *Nature, Lond.*, *200*, 716.
(7) Rafyi, A. (1961) *Bull. Off. int. Epizoot.*, *56*, 216.
(8) Howell, P. G. & Erasmus, B. J. (1963) *Bull. Off. int. Epizoot.*, *60*, 883.
(9) Erasmus, B. J. (1972) *Proc. 3rd int. Conf. equ. infect. Dis., Paris*, 1, 12, 31, 38, 45, 58, 69, 81, 88, 97.
(10) Ozawa, Y. et al. (1970) *Arch. Inst. Razi*, *22*, 113.
(11) Tessler, J. (1972) *Can. J. comp. Med.*, *36*, 167.
(12) Amad, F. I. et al. (1981) *Bull. Anim. Hlth Prod. Afr.*, *29*, 337.
(13) Salama, S. A. et al. (1981) *Can. J. comp. Med.*, *45*, 392.
(14) Maurer, F. D. (1960) *J. Am. vet. med. Assoc.*, *138*, 15.
(15) Rwevemamu, M. M. (1970) *Vet. Bull.*, *40*, 73.
(16) Mirchamsy, H. et al. (1970) *Arch. Inst. Razi*, *22*, 11, 103; (1970) *Proc. 2nd int. Conf. equ. infect. Dis., Paris*, 212.
(17) van Rensburg, I. B. J. (1981) *J.S. Afr. vet. Assoc.*, *52*, 323.

Encephalomyocarditis virus disease of pigs

Encephalomyocarditis virus may produce sporadic disease in pigs which is manifested primarily as sudden death. The cause is a cardiovirus (family Picornaviridae) that is primarily a pathogen of rodents but which has the ability to produce disease in other species including man. Infected rodents may excrete virus for a long period, and disease in pigs is probably a reflection of the close association of these two species. The virus is relatively resistant to heat and chemical influences but is sensitive to desiccation (1) and outbreaks are frequently associated with rodent plagues in the piggery or area, or with rodent infestation of feed stores (2). A recent epidemic in Australia was associated with a plague of mice which were present in all piggeries reporting the disease (7, 8).

The disease has been recorded in North and South America (3) and in Australia (1, 3) but serological studies suggest that infection, possibly by low virulence virus and without clinical disease, may be more widespread. Serological studies on pigs in the United Kingdom, where the disease has not yet been recorded, show that approximately 30% possess antibody to this virus (4). There is serological evidence of the infection in swine in Canada (5). The disease has been observed in very young sucking pigs to grower pigs up to 4 months of age but not in adults. It may occur as a sporadic disease or as an outbreak involving several litters of pigs, or pigs within a group. Mortality is variable but it may approach 50% in younger pigs. The virus can cause fetal death if the pregnant sow is infected in late pregnancy (6).

The clinical course is short and manifested by inappetence, depression, trembling, incoordination and dyspnea. Most frequently pigs are found dead. Death appears to result from cardiac failure and clinical signs referable to encephalitis are rare.

Dead pigs show patchy reddening of the skin, excess peritoneal, pleural and pericardial fluid, frequently with fibrinous strands and edema of the omentum and mesentery. Characteristically there is diffuse or focal myocardial pallor involving the ventricles and associated with myocardial necrosis. In acute cases virus may be isolated from the heart muscle and also from the brain, spleen and other tissues. Neutralizing antibody becomes detectable 5–7 days after infection.

Encephalomyocarditis virus infection must be differentiated from gut edema and mulberry heart disease in growing pigs and the peracute bacterial septicemias in sucking pigs. The myocardial lesion in sucking pigs has similarities to that produced by foot-and-mouth disease in this age group. There is no treatment and the control of the disease currently rests with rodent control and eradication in the piggery.

REFERENCES

(1) Littlejohns, I. R. & Acland, H. M. (1976) *Proc. 53rd ann. Conf. Aust. vet. Assoc.*, 148.
(2) Acland, H. M. & Littlejohns, I. R. (1975) *Aust. vet. J.*, *51*, 409, 416.
(3) Gainer, J. H. et al. (1968) *Cornell Vet.*, *58*, 31.
(4) Sanger, D. V. et al. (1977) *Vet. Rec*, *100*, 240.
(5) Sanford, J. T. et al. (1985) *Can. vet. J.*, *26*, 228.
(6) Love, R. J. & Grewal, A. S. (1986) *Aust. vet. J.*, *63*, 128.
(7) Seaman, J. T. et al. (1986) *Aust. vet. J.*, *63*, 292.
(8) Hiel, B. D. et al. (1985) *Aust. vet. J.*, *62*, 433.

Rift Valley fever

Rift Valley fever is an acute, febrile disease of cattle, sheep and man characterized in lambs and calves by hepatitis and high mortality, in adult sheep and in cattle by abortion and in man by an influenza-like disease. Transmission of the infection between animals is by biting insects, chiefly mosquitoes.

Etiology

The causative phlebovirus (family Bunyaviridae), of which there appear to be at least three strains (9), can be grown on embryonating hen eggs and tissue culture and can be attenuated by serial passage through mouse brains.

Epidemiology

Although Rift Valley fever is still confined to the African continent it has great potential for spread to other countries (14). The main occurrence of the disease is in epizootics observed in southern and central Africa, the first thoroughly investigated epizootic being in 1930. Losses are due mainly to deaths in young lambs and calves although there may be a high incidence of abortions, and some deaths, in adult sheep and cattle.

A particular point of interest is the ability of the virus to infect humans. The groups exposed to greatest risk are laboratory workers handling the virus and those working amongst infected animals or their products. In massive outbreaks in Egypt in 1977 and 1978 the occurrence rate in man was very high (more than 20 000) cases in 1977 with 600 deaths). This was the first occurrence of the disease in Egypt, and its appearance presents a major epidemiological problem for human and animal health authorities (11).

Cattle, sheep, camels, domestic buffalo, monkeys, man, mice, rats, ferrets and hamsters are highly susceptible and goats moderately so, but pigs, rabbits, guinea-pigs and poultry are not. The virus is transmissible to African buffalo (*Syncerus caffer*) but there is no serological evidence of natural infection (13). There is a report of viral isolation from one horse (10). Mice and other rodents may provide a means of supporting the virus during periods between epidemics. The real means by which the virus persists between epizootics is not known. In regions where epizootics occur the majority of the cattle population remains seronegative for as long as 5 years beween outbreaks. A small number of seroconversions occur in forest and edge-of-forest areas (4) suggesting a faunal reservoir.

A pronounced viremia occurs for about a week and facilitates the spread of the disease by biting insects. Other than milk and aborted fetuses no body secretions or excretions contain the virus. The incidence of the disease varies with the size of the vector population and is greatest in warm, moist seasons. Eight species of mosquitoes have been identified as vectors, and other blood-sucking insects are likely to be implicated (5). Experimental transmission can be effected by most routes including the inhalation of aerosols. In man infection is most likely to occur via skin abrasions in persons handling infective material.

Pathogenesis

The disease appears to be an acute hepatic insufficiency caused by destruction of liver cells by the rapidly multiplying virus (7).

Clinical findings

In lambs and calves after an incubation period of about 12 hours there is a sudden onset of high fever and incoordination followed by collapse and sudden death within 36 hours in 95–100% of affected lambs and 70% of young calves.

In adult sheep and cattle, abortion is the outstanding sign but the mortality rate in adult sheep may be as high as 20–30% and 10% in cattle. In fatal cases sudden death is preceded by a high fever for 1–2 days. Goats show a febrile reaction but few other clinical signs.

In man there is an abrupt onset of anorexia, chills, fever, headache and muscular and joint pains. Deaths from the disease are rare, but some patients suffer temporary or permanent impairment of vision due to retinal hemorrhage.

Clinical pathology

Severe leukopenia is a common finding. Antibodies appear in the serum about 1 week after infection and persist for long periods. Efficient serum-neutralization, enzyme-linked immunosorbent assay (ELISA) (15), hemagglutination, gel diffusion precipitation and CF tests are available and a fluorescent antibody technique has been developed (8). Transmission tests to white Swiss mice and sheep are also used.

Necropsy findings

Extensive hepatic necrosis is the characteristic lesion in Rift Valley fever. Other non-specific lesions include venous congestion and petechiation in the heart, lymph nodes and alimentary tract. Microscopically there is focal or diffuse necrosis of the liver and in young lambs there are usually acidophilic inclusion bodies in hepatic cells. The lesions are much more extensive in newborn lambs and calves than in older animals (12).

Diagnosis

Rift Valley fever is unlikely to be confused with other diseases because of its characteristic hepatic lesions. Its seasonal limitation may lead to confusion with bluetongue in sheep and ephemeral fever in cattle and its capacity to kill large numbers of lambs quickly may suggest a diagnosis of enterotoxemia. In adult animals other causes of abortion, including infection with the Wesselbron and other flaviviruses which cause abortions and neonatal deaths associated with brain deformities in sheep (16), would need to be considered. A tentative diagnosis can be based on the clinical, epidemiological and necropsy findings but a definitive diagnosis must depend on the laboratory tests listed above.

Treatment

Little attention has been given to this aspect of the disease and no known treatment of any value.

Control

To prevent introduction of Rift Valley fever into countries free of the disease the importation of all susceptible species from Africa should be prohibited and all necessary steps to prevent the introduction of infective insects and infected biological materials should be taken. The possibility of human beings carrying the infection from country to country is a very real one and international travellers should be made aware of the clinical symptoms of the disease and of the importance of the disease to other humans and to domestic animals.

Mosquito control suggests itself as an essential first step in any attempt to reduce the ravages of the disease in endemic areas. Mosquitoes are much easier to control than other insect vectors, and because of the need to protect human life, funds for clearing water breeding grounds are likely to be available. Intensive mosquito control and cold weather can terminate an outbreak. In an enzootic area control of the disease depends largely on the use of vaccines. Both killed (6) and living attenuated virus vaccines are available. The latter are not recommended for pregnant ewes because they are abortigenic, causing fetal death and some anomalies. The recorded problems (1) include hydrops amnii, arthrogryposis, hydranencephaly and microencephaly. The attenuated vaccine has also provided good protection for cattle which lasted for at least 28 months (2). The annual vaccination of all dairy cattle is recommended as the most cost-effective control program in endemic countries (3).

REVIEW LITERATURE

Shimshony, A. & Barzilai, R. (1983) Rift Valley fever. *Adv. vet. Sci.*, *21*, 347–425

REFERENCES

(1) Coetzer, J. A. W. & Barnard, B. J. H. (1977) *Onderstepoort J. vet. Res.*, *44*, 119 & 205.
(2) Barnard, B. J. H. (1979) *J. S. Afr. vet. Assoc.*, *50*, 155.
(3) Van-Ham, M. & Spharim, I. (1982) *Refuah Vet.*, *39*, 179.
(4) Davies, F. G. (1975) *J. Hyg., Camb.*, *75*, 219.
(5) McIntosh, B. M. (1972) *J. S. Afr. vet. med. Assoc.*, *43*, 391.
(6) Harrington, D. G. et al. (1980) *Am. J. vet. Res.*, *41*, 1559.
(7) Easterday, B. C. et al. (1962) *Am. J. vet. Res.*, *23*, 470.
(8) Davies, F. G. & Lung, L. J. (1974) *Res. vet. Sci.*, *17*, 128.
(9) Tomori, O. (1979) *Res. vet. Sci.*, *26*, 152 & 160.
(10) Imam, I. Z. E. et al. (1979) *Bull. WHO*, *57*, 441.
(11) Meegan, J. M. et al. (1979) *Vet. Rec.*, *105*, 124.
(12) Coetzer, J. A. W. (1982) *Onderstepoort J. vet. Res.*, *49*, 11.

(13) Davies, F. G. & Karstad, L. (1981) *Trop. Anim. Hlth Prod.*, *13*, 185.
(14) Lupton, H. W. et al. (1982) *Proc. US Anim. Hlth Assoc.*, *86*, 261.
(15) Niklasson, B. S. & Gargan, R. T. (1985) *Am. J. trop. Med. Hyg.*, *34*, 400.
(16) Barnard, B. J. H. & Voges, S. F. (1986) *Onderstepoort J. vet. Res.*, *53*, 235.

Akabane virus diseases of cattle (enzootic bovine arthrogryposis and hydranencephaly)

Infection of cattle during early pregnancy with the Akabane virus results in the production of calves, lambs, and kids with congenital arthrogryposis (deformities of the limbs and vertebral column, caused by fixation of joints) or hydranencephaly (a deficiency of cerebral cortex and of intelligence). Abortion and stillbirth are other manifestations of the infection.

Etiology

There is substantial circumstantial evidence that the disease is caused by infection of the dam by the Akabane virus (a bunyavirus) capable of cultivation in chicken embryos (28), during early pregnancy (1, 2). The dam is not affected clinically. The evidence comprises a high prevalence of high titers of antibodies to the Akabane virus in calves (2, 4); precolostral serum from affected calves has high antibody titers compared to normal calves (4, 5). Confirmation of the relationship between the virus and the disease has now been established by experimental production of the disease in cattle (11). The virus has also been inoculated into pregnant sheep and goats and affected young have resulted (8, 21). Virus has been isolated from naturally occurring cases in calves and has also been isolated from affected lambs born in the same enzootic area in which the calves are born (10).

Another virus, the Aino virus, is also credited with causing the disease in Australia (26) and Japan (27). It appears to be much less frequent in its occurrence in cattle, and no antibodies to it have been found in camels, dogs or horses, although they do occur in buffalo and sheep. Akabane antibodies occur in all of these species and in goats (3), but no Akabane or Aino viral antibodies have been observed in man (29), pigs, chickens (16) or wallabies (13). This differentiation may be due to differences in susceptibility between the species, or to failure of the vector insect to attack them. The Akabane virus has been transmitted to mice, producing a non-purulent encephalitis (18), and to hamsters (9).

Antibodies to the related, but as far as is known non-pathogenic, viruses Douglas, Tinaroo and Peaton, have been detected in cattle, sheep, goat, buffalo and deer (9).

Epidemiology

The disease has been recorded as an enzootic, or more exactly as recurring epizootics, in cattle in Australia, Israel, Japan, Korea (6) and Kenya (25) and is the probable cause of the 'rigid lamb syndrome' in Zimbabwe (24). Transmission by *Culicoides brevitarsis* has been demonstrated but other vectors may exist. Serological data in Australia shows that all identified infections are carried within the known range of *C. brevitarsis* (29). Introduction of the virus into the bovine uterus in semen causes no developmental defects (32). Abortions and premature births commence in autumn, with clinical cases of arthrogryposis and hydranencephaly occurring in midwinter. The offspring of sheep and goats are also affected. The disease in cattle is likely to disappear for intervals of 5–10 years until there is a combination of a susceptible population and a heavy vector population. Occurrences of the disease are also dependent on the presence of early pregnant females at the time that the vectors are plentiful.

Pathogenesis

From observations in naturally occurring infections (12) it is thought that a viremia occurs in the dam for at least 3 or 4 days, with an antibody peak 4–5 days after the viremia, but with a subsequent secondary rise.

The virus passes from the dam, which is unaffected, to the fetus, and causes cessation of differentiation in its growing neural tube. Which part of the tube is most affected depends on the stage of its development, and therefore its fetal age. Usually three forms, or principal manifestations, of the disease are described. The first ones to appear are calves with arthrogryposis; they are therefore at an older fetal age when infected than others. The next groups are those with arthrogryposis accompanied by hydranencephaly. The third group is those with hydranencephaly only. With arthrogryposis there is almost complete absence of ventral horn cells in the spinal cord and an accompanying neurotropic failure of muscle development. Contracture of the joints results. The hydranencephaly is manifested by a complete failure of development of cerebral cortex and its replacement by a fluid-filled sac. The brainstem and cerebellum are normal.

Several other manifestations have been described (14). They include prearthrogryposis groups of calves with incoordination and a mild to moderate non-suppurative encephalitis, another group with flaccid paralysis and active secondary demyelination in motor areas of the spinal cord. A posthydranencephaly group of calves were unable to stand and had thickened dorsal cranial bones and hydranencephaly involving anterior and midbrain stem, and a diminutive cerebellum. The infection with Akabane virus is also credited with causing abortion, stillbirth, and premature birth (30). Which manifestation appears probably depends on the age of the fetus when infection occurs. Lesions in other tissues include absence of ventral horn cells in the spinal cord, and lesions in the thymus (31).

Lesions produced in lambs by experimental inoculation of the ewes during early pregnancy (32nd–36th day) include skeletal muscle atrophy and degeneration, inflammatory and degenerative lesions in the cerebrum; the lesions in the nervous system vary from porencephaly to hydranencephaly. There are also brachygnathism, scoliosis, hypoplasia of the lungs, agenesis or hypoplasia of the spinal cord, and arthrogyposis (8).

Clinical findings

The cow is unaffected. The two syndromes, arthrogryposis and hydranencephaly, occur separately: arthrogryposis in the early stages of the outbreak and hydranencephaly at the end (15). Calves with both defects occur in the middle of the outbreak. The two diseases represent cows which were at different stages of their pregnancies when the Akabane virus infected the population. Estimated fetal ages are 3–4 months for hydranencephaly, 5–6 months for arthrogryposis and late pregnancy for abortion.

Calves with arthrogryposis, almost always, are the subjects of difficult birth requiring physical assistance. They are small and significantly underweight but they are fully mature in terms of teeth eruption and hair coat and hoof development. They are unable to rise, stand or walk. One or more limbs is fixed at the joints : there is a congenital articular rigidity. The limb is usually fixed in flexion but it may be in extension, and the joint becomes freely movable if the tendons around it are severed; that is, there is no abnormality of the articular surface. The muscles of affected limbs are severely wasted. Severe deformity of the vertical column, as kyphosis or scoliosis, is common. Calves with hydranencephaly have no difficulty rising and walking. The major defect is a lack of intelligence and blindness. They will suck if put onto the teat but if this is not done they stand and bleat and have no apparent dam-seeking reflex. A few calves have micrencephaly and are more severely affected still. They are dummies, very uncoordinated in gait, unable to stand properly and move erratically when stimulated. These calves appear at the very end of the outbreak.

As well as the skeletal and neurological diseases, cases of abortion, stillbirth and premature birth are also recorded as a result of Akabane virus infection in cows (2). They are usually recorded at the beginning of the outbreak before the neurological defects occur.

Clinical pathology

Antibodies to Akabane virus should be detected at high titer in the dam, and in the surviving calves. The latter could also be expected to have high levels of gammaglobulin in their precolostral sera (17). Affected calves are also reported to have high creatinine phosphokinase levels (19) whereas calves with inherited arthrogryposis are reported to have normal such levels.

Necropsy findings

In calves with arthrogryposis there is severe muscle atrophy, fixation of joints by tendon contracture and normal articular surfaces. The joints are easily released by cutting the surrounding tendons. Histologically there is almost complete absence of ventral horn cells in the spinal cord. This lesion may be localized to one segment of the cord. In calves with hydranencephaly the cerebral hemispheres are completely absent and the vacant space is filled with fluid enclosed by the normal meninges. In most cases the brainstem and cerebellum are normal (20) but diminution of their size is also recorded (14).

Although the virus has been isolated from affected newborn lambs and calves it is often difficult because of the presence of neutralizing antibodies in the full-term fetus.

Diagnosis

Akabane virus disease, as it is manifested in cattle, is a well defined and easily recognizable entity. It can be confused with other forms of congenital articular rigidity (CAR) which are dealt with elsewhere under that heading. These include inherited CAR, usually accompanied in cattle by cleft palate, and in pigs by thick forelimbs (the thick-leg syndrome). Environmentally induced cases are caused by vitamin A deficiency in pigs, and by manganese deficiency in cattle and an inherited arthrogryposis of most breeds of cattle; the most recent recognition is in Charolais cattle, although the limb abnormalities are usually accompanied by cleft palate. Similar arthrogrypotic defects are found in Devon and Murray Grey cattle. Other inherited congenital defects often accompany these joint fixations, especially deformities of the spinal column including kyphosis, scoliosis and spina bifida. These abnormalities also occur in Akabane virus disease. Small epidemics of defective development of pectoral muscles accompanied by arthrogryposis occur in Japanese Shorthorn calves. The cause is not determined (22).

In sheep, an inherited arthrogryposis has been recorded. Small epidemics of micrencephaly also occur but the cause is not determined (23). Congenital arthrogryposis appears to be inherited in goats and may be the result of a defect in storage in lysozymes. Poisonings known to cause arthrogryposis include tobacco, Jimson weed (*Datura stramonium*) and lupins.

Treatment and control

No treatment would be contemplated because affected calves are not viable. Because the disease is transmitted by insect bites vaccination would be the only control method likely to be effective. A killed vaccine has been produced and has proved very effective against natural exposure (7).

REVIEW LITERATURE

Konno, S. et al. (1982) Akabane disease in cattle: congenital abnormalities caused by viral infection. Spontaneous disease. *Vet. Pathol.*, *19*, 246–266.

Shepherd, N. C. et al. (1978) Congenital bovine epizootic arthrogryposis and hydranencephaly. *Aust. vet. J.*, *54*, 171.

Swatland, H. J. (1974) Developmental disorders of skeletal muscle in cattle, pigs and sheep. *Vet. Bull.*, *44*, 179.

REFERENCES

(1) Hartley, W. J. et al. (1975) *Aust. vet. J.*, *51*, 103.
(2) Inaba, Y. et al. (1975) *Aust. vet. J.*, *51*, 584.
(3) Furuya, Y. et al. (1980) *Vet. Microbiol.*, *5*, 239.
(4) Della-Porta, A. J. et al. (1976) *Proc. 53rd ann. Conf. Aust. vet. Assoc.*, 89; (1976) *Aust. vet. J.*, *52*, 496, 594.
(5) Kurogi, H. et al. (1975) *Arch. Virol.*, *47*, 71.
(6) Bak, U. B. et al. (1980) *Kor. J. vet. Res.*, *20*, 65.
(7) Kirkland, P. D. et al. (1984) *Aust. Adv. vet. Sci.*, p. 47.
(8) Parsonson, I. M. et al. (1981) *Vet. Microbiol.*, *6*, 197 & 209.
(9) Cybinski, D. H. (1984) *Aust. J. biol. Sci.*, *37*, 91.
(10) Della-Porta, A. J. et al. (1977) *Aust. vet. J.*, *53*, 51.
(11) Kurogi, H. et al. (1977) *Infect. Immun.*, *17*, 338.
(12) St. George, T. D. et al. (1978) *Aust. vet. J.*, *54*, 558.
(13) Cybinski, D. H. et al. (1978) *Aust. vet. J.*, *54*, 1.
(14) Hartley, W. J. et al. (1977) *Aust. vet. J.*, *53*, 319.
(15) Blood, D. C. (1956) *Aust. vet J.*, *12*, 125.
(16) Furuya, Y. et al. (1977) *J. Jap. vet. med. Assoc.*, *30*, 440.
(17) Wanner, R. A. & Husband, A. J. (1974) *Aust. vet. J.*, *50*, 560.
(18) Nakajima, Y. et al. (1979) *Nat. Inst. Anim. Hlth O., Jpn.*, *19*, 47.
(19) Hamana, T. (1974) *Vet. Rec.*, *95*, 441.
(20) Whittem, J. H. (1957) *J. Pathol. Bacteriol.*, *73*, 375.

(21) Narita, M. et al. (1979) *J. comp. Pathol.*, *89*, 229.
(22) Ohshima, K. et al. (1974) *J. Fac. Agric. Iwate Univ.*, *12*, 1.
(23) Hartley, W. J. & Haughey, K. G. (1974) *Aust. vet. J.*, *50*, 323.
(24) Rudert, C. P. et al. (1978) *Vet. Rec.*, *102*, 374.
(25) Metselar, D. & Robin, Y. (1976) *Vet. Rec.*, *99*, 86.
(26) Coverdale, D. R. et al. (1978) *Aust. vet. J.*, *54*, 152.
(27) Miura, Y. et al. (1974) *Arch. ges. Virusforsch.*, *46*, 377.
(28) Miah, A. H. & Spradbrow, P. B. (1978) *Res. vet. Sci.*, *25*, 253.
(29) Cybinski, D. H. & St. George, T. D. (1978) *Aust. vet. J.*, *54*, 371.
(30) Inaba, Y. (1979) *Jap. agr. Res. Q.*, *13*, 123.
(31) Parsonson, I. M. et al. (1977) *Infect. Immun.*, *15*, 254.
(32) Parsonson, I. M. et al. (1981) *J. comp. Pathol.*, 91, 611.

BOVINE VIRAL LEUKOSIS (BVL) (BOVINE LYMPHOSARCOMA, ENZOOTIC BOVINE LEUKOSIS)

This is a highly fatal, systemic, malignant neoplasia of the reticuloendothelial system of cattle, characterized by the development of aggregations of neoplastic lymphocytes in almost any organ, with a corresponding variety of clinical signs. There are a number of forms taken by the disease:

- Enzootic bovine viral leukosis—the common form of adults
- Sporadic—affecting animals under 3 years of age and including:
  - juvenile form in calves less than 6 months old, characterized by multiple lymph node enlargement
  - thymic form in yearlings less than 2 years old, characterized by a swelling in the neck causing bloat and edema
  - cutaneous form in cattle 1–3 years old, characterized by the development of nodes and plaques in the skin
- Persistent lymphocytosis—a benign lymphoproliferative process.

Etiology

Enzootic bovine viral leukosis and persistent lymphocytosis
The causative virus is a retrovirus of the genus Oncovirinae (1) and the disease is most aptly entitled bovine viral leukosis (BVL). The virus is identified as the bovine leukemia virus and is morphologically similar to the leukemia viruses of other species. It has leukemogenic activity, can be grown in tissue culture and produces specific antibodies in calves (2) and sheep.

Infection with the virus is not synonymous with being affected by the disease lymphosarcoma which is characterized by neoplasms of the reticuloendothelial system. Most animals which become infected with the virus do not in fact develop the neoplastic disease. Those that do so are predisposed by their genetic constitution. This interaction between the causative agents reconciles the previously opposed views of infection versus inheritance.

Persistent lymphocytosis which is another benign reaction to infection with the BVL virus is similarly influenced in its expression by genetic susceptibility in the host.

Sporadic bovine leukosis
Similar detailed information is not available about this disease. However, the virus cannot be cultured from nor antibodies to the virus be detected in animals affected with the juvenile, thymus or cutaneous forms of the disease. There is incidental suggestive information from transmission experiments with sheep and goats that the BVL virus may be present in these forms of the disease, but transmission experiments in cattle do not support this. Without direct evidence it is not possible to be sure, but the available evidence seems to be against the involvement of BVL virus in the sporadic disease (3).

Epidemiology
The disease does not spread rapidly and the number of herds containing positive reactors to the AGID test is usually small. However, in infected herds the number of reactions is often high, of the order of 80%. The effect is that eradication by test and cull is usually achieved rapidly.

Source of the BVL virus
Cattle are the only animals infected naturally, although sheep and goats can be infected experimentally. The infection does not spread from cattle to comingled sheep, nor between experimentally infected and non-infected sheep. However, horizontal transmission of a naturally occurring lymphosarcoma in sheep is caused by an antigenically similar virus to the BVL virus. It is assumed that horizontal spread of the BVL virus from cattle to sheep will not occur (34). The experimental transfer of infection from cattle to sheep is effected so readily that it has become a preferred technique for testing for the presence of virus.

In cattle, infection with the virus is permanent, and spontaneous recovery has not been demonstrated. This is probably the result of the virus location in lymphocytes in a covert non-productive state, resulting in an inability of developed antibodies to arrest the infection. In any case, multiplication of the virus is not necessary for survival or transmission. In addition to its location, the virus is capable of undergoing periodic antigenic change, thus circumventing control by immunity mechanisms. Therefore, the infected animal remains a source of infection for long periods, probably for life, regardless of the simultaneous presence in the animal of specific antibodies. This virus–host system is the same as that of other retroviruses especially equine infectious anemia (EIA) and visna-maedi of sheep. In most circumstances infection occurs when animals are in close physical contact and are more than 12 months old (66). Infection is established readily by subcutaneous and intradermal injection and by intratracheal infusion, but it does not occur after oral administration (67).

Genetic predisposition
There is a marked familial tendency to the disease (4, 5) and although the mechanism is not completely clear there is preliminary evidence that resistance to infection with the BVL virus is genetically determined. There is

also firm evidence that once infection has occurred the subsequent development of just antibody response, or antibody plus persistent lymphocytosis or antibody plus lymphosarcoma, with or without persistent lymphocytosis, is determined by the host's genetic makeup. However, it seems probable that genetic resistance to any one of these developments can be overcome by stress, a period of immunological inadequacy or a large infective dose of the virus. The previous concept, that the spread of the disease depended largely on the vertical transmission from dam to offspring through the ovum, is no longer tenable.

Transmission of the virus
The virus is present mostly in lymphocytes and can be found in the blood and the milk and in tumor masses. Most workers have failed to find it in semen and artificial insemination is not thought to be a method of spread (56), nor is embryo transplantation using zona-intact embryos (57), and fertilized embryos from donors infected with BVL virus have been transferred without infection of the fetus having occurred (10). However, the virus has been found in semen collected by the massage technique (6). Transmission experiments suggest that the virus is not present in saliva but that it does appear intermittently in urine (7). It is present in nasal and tracheal washings but only in cells not as free virus (11).

Experimental transmission of the infection using tumor material or tissue culture virus can be effected successfully in cattle, sheep, goats and with some doubts to chimpanzees (8) but the tumors are produced only in the three ruminants.

Natural transmission occurs mostly in cattle more than 1·5 years of age, usually during the summer months between in-contact animals and possibly by insect or bat transmission of infected lymphocytes in whole blood. Iatrogenic transmission also occurs via infected blood which contaminates surgical instruments (62), such as dehorning gouges (55), ear tattooing pliers (63) and hypodermic needles (12), used on infected and then susceptible animals without disinfection and also in blood transfusions and vaccines containing blood such as those for babesiosis and anaplasmosis. Amounts of blood as small as 0·1 ml are capable of transmitting the infection (9). Thus the infection can be transmitted via the tuberculin intradermal test (65). Transmission via infected milk is possible by the passage of infected lymphocytes through intestinal mucosal epithelium during the first few hours of life. However, infection via this route appears to occur very rarely, if at all, possibly because of the presence of maternal antibodies in the milk (68).

Up to 20% of cases may derive from infections which occur *in utero*, apparently from invasion of and passage through the placenta. There is no evidence that infection occurs via germinative material, either through the egg or spermatozoa. The long-held view that the common mode of transmission was vertical from the dam through the egg, appears to be unfounded.

Very few calves are serologically positive at birth because of the low infection rate *in utero* (13), but they passively acquire maternal antibodies in their colostrum. The rate of new infections is then low until the young animals return to the adult herd and start to mingle with a large population of infected animals (14, 15). The method of spread between animals, although probably by insects (16), does depend on close physical contact between animals, as though the virus does not survive for long in or on the vector.

Population statistics
Infection with BVL virus is estimated to be at least 20% in the adult dairy cow population of the United States, 6–11% in Canada, 27% in France, 37% in Venezuela, and almost no reactors in the United Kingdom, New Zealand and Australia. The prevalence of lymphosarcoma in countries where the infection occurs is of the order of 1 per 1000 per annum and in free countries probably 1 per 50 000 per annum. All of these figures are subject to serious error because of the very spotted nature of occurrence of the disease and until much larger surveys of unselected samples are conducted it will not be possible to give accurate figures. Even in countries or areas where the infection and the disease are common there are many herds that remain uninfected. Dairy cattle are much more commonly infected than beef cattle, and have a much higher prevalence of lymphosarcoma. In badly affected dairy herds an annual mortality rate of 2% is unremarkable and it may be as high as 5%.

All breeds of cattle are susceptible to BVL. It occurs rarely in animals less than 2 years of age and increases in incidence with increasing age (7). The incidence appears to be much greater in large herds than in smaller herds. The greater prevalence in dairy herds is probably due to their closer confinement and the higher average age of the herds.

Other species
Lymphosarcoma occurs sporadically in all species, but natural infection with the BVL virus has been demonstrated only in sheep and capybaras (1). The possibility of transmission of the virus from cattle to man is a real one; the virus is commonly present in the milk of infected cows (17) and the disease has been transmitted to chimpanzees in this way. However, in spite of exhaustive, but certainly not complete, studies there is no evidence that transmission occurs from cattle to man (59). There is one report of a high positive correlation between high prevalence dairy herds and the prevalence of leukemia in a special group of patients (18). Other surveys have shown that there were no significant differences between farms that did have and farms that did not have the disease with respect to death rate and cancer and leukemia–lymphoma occurrence in humans (19). The measurement of occurrence in persons living on farms is the critical measurement because short-term pasteurization procedures destroy the infective agent in milk (64); farm dwellers who take their milk from the supply before the pasteurization points are thus exposed (20).

Although there is no evidence of a relationship between bovine viral leukosis and any disease of pigs, there is a record of enzootic leukosis in that species (21) which is inherited. The inheritance is conditioned by an autosomal recessive character (22).

Sources of wastage

Lymphosarcoma resulting from BVL viral infection kills very few cows overall so that as a cause of loss on a national basis it does not rate very highly. However, for individual farms that have a high incidence of it the effect can be disastrous. This is especially so in high-producing dairy herds where pedigreed livestock are sold. Individual animals are kept to a much older age than in the average commercial herd and, because of the increased prevalence of lymphosarcoma in cows over 5 years of age, the death losses are likely to be very severe in exactly the group of cows which is critical to the success of the stud's operation. In addition, there is the severe downgrading effect on the saleability of stock from a herd known to have a disease in which genetic susceptibility is an important causative factor.

Loss may also result from lymphosarcoma by way of reduced production during the developmental stages of the disease. The course of the disease is usually sufficiently brief to make this a relatively unimportant consideration. Similarly, the immunosuppressive effect of infection with the virus appears not to have influence on the prevalence of other diseases.

Probably more important potentially than any of the above wastage modes is the deleterious effect that would result if it were shown that the BVL virus was transmissible from animals to man. A similar effect is one which is already operating. It is the practice, particularly in countries that do not have the disease, to require proof of freedom from infection with the virus from animals about to be imported into the country. This trend has been increased by the introduction of the infection into the United Kingdom in cattle imported from Canada. This is a matter of major importance when the cattle are purebred and are sold at high prices as breeding animals. Some countries are already demanding a negative blood test for all cattle and meat to be imported, and this could represent a loss of export markets for others.

Transmission of the infection by artificial insemination has not been demonstrated and this is not considered to be a means of spread. However, it is possible that if the semen contained infected lymphocytes transmission could occur. Therefore, it is likely in the future that bulls standing at AI centers will be required to be negative serologically to BVL virus.

Pathogenesis

The virus and the lesion

As set down graphically in Fig. 23, there are four possible outcomes after exposure of cattle to BVL virus. They are:

- Failure of the animal to become infected, probably because of genetic resistance
- Establishment of a permanent infection and the development of detectable levels of antibodies. These animals are latent carriers of infection
- Establishment of a permanent infection, plus the animal becomes seropositive, and also develops a persistent lymphocytosis, a benign lymphoproliferative process. It is not a preclinical stage of lymphosarcoma (23)
- Infected, seropositive animals, which may or may not have been through a stage of persistent lymphocytosis, who develop neoplastic malignant tumors—lymphosarcoma.

Whether or not the animal becomes infected or develops any of the other forms of the disease depends principally on the recipient's genetic constitution (24). The outcome may also be influenced by the animal's immune status and the size of the infective dose of virus. About 80% of animals with the adult form of the disease have a severe and significant depression of IgM globulins (25). The immunological responsiveness of leukotic cattle to administered antigens is significantly depressed overall, but particularly with respect to IgM, resulting from a deficiency in its production in the spleen and lymph nodes (25).

Lymphomatosis is a neoplasm of the whole lymphoreticular system. It is never benign, the lesions developing at varying rates in different animals so that the course may be quite short or protracted over several months.

The pathogenesis of the experimentally induced disease begins by the infection quickly becoming established in the spleen and the virus is recoverable from

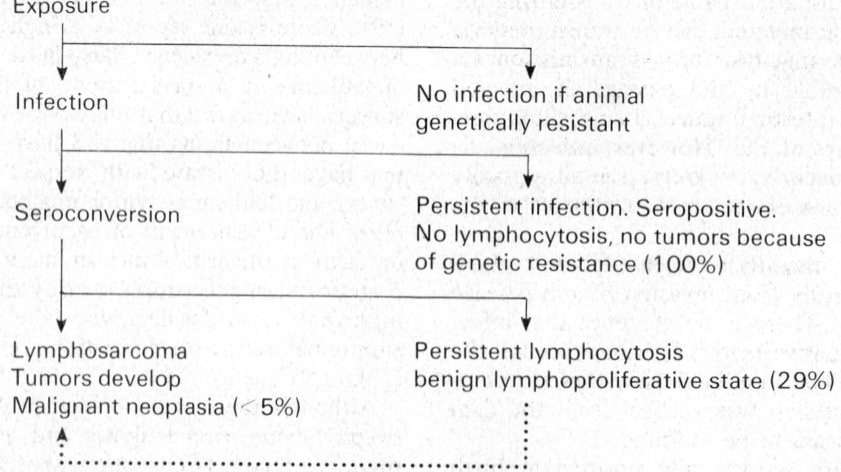

Fig. 23. Possible pathways after exposure to BVL virus (percentage figures indicate proportion of seroconverted animals that develop the particular form referred to) (23).

that organ 8 days after infection. After this initial splenic phase the virus appears in peripheral blood leukocytes a week later and antibodies are detectable in serum 6 weeks after infection (26).

The lesion and the clinical disease
In adult cattle, almost any organ may be the site of lesions, but the abomasum, heart, and visceral and peripheral lymph nodes are the organs most commonly affected. In calves, the visceral lymph nodes and spleen and liver are the common sites. Depending upon the organ which is most involved, a number of clinical syndromes occur. With major involvement of the abomasal wall, the syndrome is one of impaired digestion resulting in persistent diarrhea. When the atrial wall is affected, congestive heart failure may supervene. Involvement of the spinal meninges and nerves is followed by the gradual onset of posterior paralysis. In nervous tissue, the primary lesion is in the roots of peripheral nerves and spreads along the nerve to involve meninges and cord. Other common localizations of the diseases are in the skin, genitalia and periorbital tissues. In the cutaneous form, intradermal thickenings develop which persist but do not cause discontinuity of the epithelium. They are composed of aggregations of neoplastic lymphocytes. Esophageal obstruction may result from mediastinal lymph node involvement in calves.

The exact nature of the tumor is open to question. The tumors consist of aggregations of neoplastic lymphocytes, but in many cases they may be more accurately described as reticulosarcoma. Certainly, they are highly malignant and metastasize widely. The blood picture is variable and, although there may be an accompanying lymphocytosis, the presence of large numbers of immature lymphocytes in the blood smear is a more reliable indication of the presence of the disease. Some degree of anemia is almost always present.

Clinical findings
Because there are in general two patterns of development of the disease in adult cattle as suggested in the discussion of etiology they are described as separate entities here.

Enzootic (adult) bovine viral leukosis (bovine lymphosarcoma)

This disease is characterized by the occurrence of multiple cases of *adult multicentric lymphosarcoma*, with tumors developing rapidly in many sites with an accompanying great variation in clinical signs and syndromes. An approximate indication of the frequency with which individual signs appear is set out in Fig. 24.

The usual incubation period is 4–5 years with most occurring 4–5 years after the original case was introduced or a blood transfusion from an outside herd was given. This form is rarely seen in animals under 2 years of age and is most common in the 4–8 years age group. Lymphocytosis without clinical signs occurs earlier, but again rarely before 2 years of age . Many cows remain in the preclinical stage for years, often for their complete productive lifetime, and without any apparent reduction in performance, but in a proportion clinical disease appears. The clinical signs and the duration of the illness vary with the number and importance of the sites involved and the speed with which the tumor masses grow.

A proportion (5–10%) run a peracute course and the affected animals often die without showing prior signs of illness. Involvement of the adrenal glands, rupture of an abomasal ulcer or an affected spleen followed by acute internal hemorrhage are known causes of such terminations. Such animals are often in good bodily condition.

Most cases run a subacute (up to 7 days) to chronic (several months) course and are initiated by loss of condition and appetite, anemia and muscular weakness. The heart rate is not increased unless the myocardium is involved and the temperature is normal unless tumor growth is rapid and extensive when it rises to 39·5–40°C (103–104°F). Although the following specific

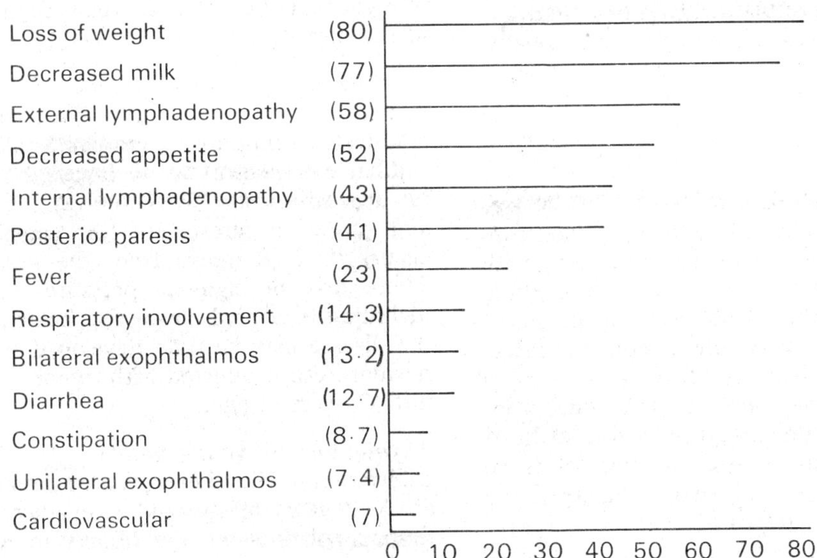

Fig. 24. Clinical diagnosis: frequency of predominant signs of bovine leukemia—1100 field cases. (By courtesy of *Canadian Veterinary Journal* (53).)

forms of the disease are described separately, in any one animal any combination of them may occur. In many cases clinical illness sufficient to warrant the attention of the veterinarian is not observed until extensive involvement has occurred and the possibility of slaughter of the animal for meat purposes cannot be considered. On the other hand many cases are examined at a time when diagnostic clinical signs are not yet evident. Once signs of clinical illness and tumor development are detectable the course is rapid and death is usually only 2–3 weeks away.

Enlargement of the superficial lymph nodes
This is common (75–90% of cases show it) and is often an early sign. This is usually accompanied by small (1 cm in diameter) subcutaneous lesions, often in the flanks and on the perineum. These skin lesions are probably enlarged hemolymph nodes and are of no diagnostic significance, often occurring in the absence of other signs of the disease. In many cases with serious visceral involvement peripheral lesions may be completely absent. Enlargement of visceral lymph nodes is common, but these are usually subclinical unless they press on other organs such as intestine or nerves. However, they may be detected on rectal examination. Special attention should be given to the deep inguinal and iliac nodes. In advanced cases extensive spread to the peritoneum and pelvic viscera makes diagnosis easy.

Although the enlargement of lymph nodes is often generalized many cows have only a proportion of their nodes involved. Thus, the enlargements may be confined to the pelvic nodes or to one or more subcutaneous nodes. Involvement of the symphysis of the mandible and the nodes of the head is sometimes observed. The affected nodes are smooth and resilient and in dairy cows are easily seen. Their presence may be marked by local edema. Occasional cases are seen in which the entire body surface is covered with tumor masses 5–11 cm in diameter in the subcutaneous tissue.

Digestive tract lesions
These are common. With involvement of the abomasal wall there is a capricious appetite, persistent diarrhea, not unlike that of Johne's disease and occasionally, melena due to bleeding from the not infrequent abomasal ulcer. Tumors of the mediastinal nodes may cause chronic, moderate bloat.

Cardiac lesions
Lesions in the heart usually invade the right atrial wall primarily and the signs are referable to right-sided congestive heart failure. There is hydropericardium with muffling of the heart sounds, hydrothorax with resulting dyspnea, engorgement of the jugular veins and edema of the brisket and sometimes of the intermandibular space. The heart sounds, besides being muffled, show a variety of abnormalities. There may be tachycardia due to insufficiency and there is often irregularity due to heart block. A systolic murmur is also common as is an associated jugular pulse. The liver may be enlarged and portal stasis may lead to diarrhea.

Nervous system involvement
Neural lymphomatosis is usually manifested by the gradual onset over several weeks of posterior paralysis. The cow begins to knuckle at the hind fetlocks while walking; sometimes one leg is affected more than the other. She then has difficulty getting up and is finally unable to do so. At this stage, sensation is retained, but movement is limited or absent. There may be a zone of hyperesthesia at the site of the lesion which is usually at the last lumbar or first sacral vertebra. Appetite and other functions, apart from the effects of recumbency, are usually normal. Metastases in the cranial meninges produce signs of space-occupying lesions with localizing signs referable to the site of the lesion.

Less common lesions
These include enlargement of the retropharyngeal lymph nodes which may cause snoring and dyspnea. Sometimes clinically detectable lesions occur in the periorbital tissues causing protrusion of the eyeball (70), and in limb muscles, ureter, kidney and genitalia. Involvement of the uterus may be detectable as multiple nodular enlargement on rectal examination. Periureteral lesions may lead to hydronephrosis with diffuse enlargement of the kidneys while tumors in renal tissue cause nodular enlargements. In either case terminal uremia develops.

Sporadic bovine leukosis

There are three forms.

Cutaneous form
This is commonest in cattle less than 3 years of age. It is very rare and manifested by cutaneous plaques (1–5 cm diameter) which appear on the neck, back, croup and thighs. The plaque becomes covered with a thick gray-white scab and the hair is shed; then the center becomes depressed and the nodule commences to shrink. After a period of weeks or months hair grows again and the nodules disappear as does the enlargement of the peripheral lymph nodes. Relapse may occur in 1–2 years with reappearance of cutaneous lesions and signs of involvement of internal organs as in the enzootic form of the disease.

Juvenile or calf lymphosarcoma
This disease of calves of 2 weeks to 6 months of age is manifested primarily by gradual loss of weight and the sudden enlargement of all lymph nodes, accompanied by depression and weakness (27). Fever, tachycardia and posterior paresis are less constant signs. Death occurs in 2–8 weeks from the first obvious illness. There may be signs of pressure on internal organs, including bloat and congestive heart failure. Unusually the disease may be fully developed *in utero* so that the newborn calf is affected with tumors (28), or be delayed until 2 years of age.

Thymic form of young cattle
Infiltration of the thymus is a common finding in animals 1–2 years of age and is characterized by massive thymic enlargement and lesions in bone marrow and regional lymph nodes. Jugular engorgement, respiratory obstruction and local edema usually result (29). This form is more common in beef than in dairy cattle.

Other species
Outbreaks in sheep have been observed with clinical, epidemiological, hematological and necropsy findings similar to those of enzootic bovine leukosis (30).

Infection of other species with BVL virus has not been demonstrated, but epizootic occurrences of lymphosarcoma have been observed in pigs, but only sporadic cases in horses. Details are as follows: the clinical picture in pigs is poorly defined, non-specific emaciation, limb weakness and anorexia being most commonly observed. Sporadic cases in this species are unlikely to be recorded, and although outbreaks have occurred, they (46) and the enzootic form are not commonly encountered. In one herd with the enzootic disease all cases encountered were in pigs less than 6 months of age. There was stunting of growth, development of a pot belly, enlargement of peripheral lymph nodes, and a lymphocytosis, including the presence of immature cells (21). In horses, the disease occurs most commonly in animals over 6 years of age. The chief clinical manifestations are subcutaneous enlargements which may ulcerate, enlargement of internal and external lymph nodes, jugular vein engorgement, cardiac irregularity, exophthalmia and anasarca. The course varies from acute to chronic, but most affected horses die within a month of first showing signs (31).

Clinical pathology
A definitive antemortem diagnosis depends on the clinicopathological examination of the animal. A great variety of techniques are available and it is important to make the appropriate selection for the particular stage of the disease that is being considered. Thus:

- Diagnosis of the viral infection is by virological or serological techniques
- Persistent lymphocytosis is diagnosed with hematological techniques
- Neoplastic tumors are identified by histological examination of a biopsy specimen.

Diagnosis of the presence of infection with BVL virus
A definitive diagnosis is based on a system using tissue culture on lamb spleen cells inoculated with leukocytes from the suspect animal. An alternative is transmission of the infection from suspect cattle to seronegative sheep. If growth is established the virus is identified by electron microscopy, or by a fluorescent antibody technique (FAT), an enzyme-linked immunoabsorbent assay (ELISA) (32), a radioimmunoassay (RIA) or a syncytial infectivity assay (33,34). Because of the expense of tissue culture work, a presumptive diagnosis, using a serological test, is all that is attempted. This should not be used if it is possible that the animal is seropositive for a reason other than infection, e.g., a young calf still seropositive from maternal antibodies acquired from colostrum. Of the many serological tests available including virus neutralization and immunofluorescence tests, the preferred ones are:

- Agar gel immunodiffusion (AGID) test which has particular attractions as a screening test to establish a diagnosis of the presence of infection in a herd, but is not accurate enough to be used to decide the status of an individual animal because of the large number of false positive reactions it produces. This is the test recognized by most governments as the official test for purposes of imports.
- Radioimmunoassay (RIA) which is suitable for individual cow identification because of its accuracy. There are several versions of this and the one using the virion gp antigen is preferred (35).
- ELISA is claimed to be more sensitive than other tests, can be used on milk, but is more difficult to set up (32,38).
- A protein immunoblot test has also been developed for the detection of antibodies in cattle and sheep serum. It is claimed to be more sensitive than the agar gel immunodiffusion (AGID) test (71).

For specimens likely to have low antibody titres, for example pooled serum samples, the RIA and the ELISA tests are recommended (36); they appear to be about equally accurate (72).

The chronology of seroconversion is important. Calves from infected dams have a 20% chance of being infected *in utero* and seropositive at birth. If they are serologically negative at birth they seroconvert at their first sucking and this passively acquired immunity persists for 2–7 months. These calves, and calves from uninfected mothers become positive at varying ages depending on when they come into contact with infection, usually when they are put back with the infected adult herd. This can be as early as 9 months of age, but as a general rule positive reactions are uncommon in cattle which are less than 2 years of age. Seroconversion usually takes place 3–4 months after the negative animals are placed in the infective group, although the interval is longer in the winter than in the summer. Infected animals are seropositive, and infected, for long periods, usually for life (39).

Diagnosis of persistent lymphocytosis
The major pathological change on which this diagnosis is based is the leukocyte count of the blood. In affected animals there is a marked increase in the number of lymphocytes present, especially immature cells. The total count is raised from a normal of 6000 to as high as 15 000 μl. The percentage of lymphocytes in the total white blood cell count will be increased from the normal of 50%, and 65% is considered to be a positive result. The presence of 25% or more of the total lymphocyte count as atypical immature cells is also considered to be a significant aberration.

If animals affected by the persistent lymphocytosis form of the disease subsequently develop lymphosarcoma, the lymphocytosis has usually subsided (40). Careful examination of the lymphocytes by electron microscopy may reveal the presence of blood lymphocyte nuclear pockets (NPs), a specific morphological marker for bovine viral leukosis, and an indication of the presence of virus within the lymphocytes (41). There are alternative views about the significance of NPs (69).

Diagnosis of lymphosarcoma
This can only be done by histopathological examination of a section of tumor material obtained by biopsy or

necropsy. Enlarged lymph nodes or hemolymph nodes are the usual sources, but when the genital tract is involved an exploratory laparotomy is usually performed so that a sample can be obtained. Chromosomal changes may be detectable in cells from lymph nodes or in leukocytes from peripheral blood of affected animals (42, 43). When there is myocardial involvement there may be obvious changes in the electrocardiogram (44), but these are unlikely to be of value in differential diagnosis.

Necropsy findings

In cattle, firm white tumor masses may be found in any organ although two rather different patterns of distribution are apparent. In newborn and young animals, the common sites are kidneys, thymus, liver, spleen and peripheral and internal lymph nodes (45). This may or may not be a characteristic of the 'sporadic' form of the disease. In adults, the heart, abomasum and spinal cord are often involved. In the heart, the tumor masses invade particularly the right atrium, though they may occur generally throughout the myocardium and extend to the pericardium. The frequency of early changes in the subepicardial tissue of the right atrium suggests that this is an area from which tissues should be selected in latent or doubtful cases. The abomasal wall, when involved, shows a gross, uneven thickening with tumor material in the submucosa, particularly in the pyloric region. Similar lesions occur commonly in the intestinal wall. Deep ulcerations in the affected area are not uncommon. Involvement of the nervous system usually includes thickening of the peripheral nerves coming from the last lumbar or first sacral cord segment or more rarely in a cranial cervical site. This may be associated with one or more circumscribed thickenings in the spinal meninges. Affected lymph nodes may be enormously enlarged and be composed of both normal and neoplastic tissue. The latter is firmer and whiter than normal lymphoid tissue and often surrounds foci of bright yellow necrosis. Less common sites include the kidney, the ureters, usually near the renal pelvis, the uterus, either as nodular masses or diffuse infiltration, mediastinal, sternal, mesenteric and other internal lymph nodes, and mandibular ramus. Histologically, the tumor masses are composed of lymphocytic cells. In Indian buffalo the lesions predominantly affect serous surfaces and produce large volumes of fluid, usually turbid, in the relevant body cavity.

Diagnosis

Because of the very wide range of signs, a positive diagnosis of BVL is often difficult. Enlargement of peripheral lymph nodes without fever or lymphangitis is unusual in other diseases, with the exception of tuberculosis which can be differentiated by the tuberculin test. In the absence of these enlargements, the digestive form may easily be confused with Johne's disease or even mucosal disease. In BVL there are no oral lesions and the johnin test and examination of fecal smears for typical acid-fast bacilli are negative. The cardiac form closely resembles traumatic pericarditis and endocarditis, but there is absence of fever and toxemia, and the characteristic neutrophilia of these two diseases is usually absent. Involvement of the spinal nerves of meninges may be confused with spinal cord abscess or with the dumb form of rabies. An examination of cerebrospinal fluid may be of value in determining the presence of an abscess and rabies has a much shorter course and other diagnostic signs. Multiple lymph node enlargements in the abdominal cavity, and nodular lesions in the uterine wall may be confused with fat necrosis, but the nature of the lesion can usually be determined by careful rectal palpation. Snoring caused by enlargement of the retropharyngeal lymph nodes is also commonly caused by tuberculosis and actinobacillosis.

Treatment

Treatment has not been attempted in large numbers of animals. The use of nitrogen mustard (30–40 mg daily for 3–4 days) has resulted in temporary remissions of signs in affected cattle. Triethylenemelamine has also been reported to cause some improvements.

Control

Because of uncertainty about the real cause of the disease, control programs based firmly on good epidemiological knowledge have not been extensively examined. Slaughtering of infected herds and slaughtering of clinical and early cases based on hematological examination have been unsuccessful techniques. Now that the virus is identifiable it is thought that the disease is amenable to complete eradication. This judgement is based on:

- The exogenous nature of the virus
- The slow spread from herd to herd, provided trade between herds is minimal or prohibited altogether; artificial insemination provides a means of infusing new blood into a herd without risking the introduction of leukosis (49)
- The apparent absence of natural reservoirs of the virus (48)
- Avoidance of genetically susceptible cattle would reduce the chances of reinfection occurring.

The strategies likely to be employed to control the disease are eradication and limitation of spread as set down below. Measures to prevent the introduction of the disease into known free areas could be based on the eradication strategy.

Eradication

Enzootic bovine leukosis (or bovine viral leukosis, BVL) can only be eradicated by:

- Test and slaughter of cattle infected with the virus of BVL
- Programs based on the culling of seropositive cows appear to be highly effective (47, 50, 51)
- The maintenance of a closed herd which permits the entry of only those animals that are free of the infection.

The efficiency of such a program depends on the accuracy of the test used to identify the infected animals, and the repetition of the test at an appropriate interval so that animals that were in the incubation stages of the disease at the time of the first test will have had time to seroconvert. The recommended procedure (1) is:

- Identify the infected carriers by the use of the radioimmunoassay technique
- Repeat the test 3 months later (the animals having been kept in isolation meanwhile).

Other tests could be used, but are usually insufficiently accurate. For example, the AGID test has been extensively used and, although it is less valuable than the RIA test, a program based on its use, either by testing animals quarterly or at 6-week intervals, has been found to be practicable and successful (51). The reactors are removed immediately and testing is continued until the herd has a clean test. When the herd is clean, testing is carried out every 6 months and the herd declared free when there have been no positive reactors for 2 years (50). Future importations into the herd are managed most safely by artificial insemination or fertilized ovum transfer (49).

In herds where the prevalence is very high a two-herd scheme can be successful. The calves, mostly from infected cows, are isolated from them and raised on the milk from their dams. They are tested periodically for virus and antibodies and positive animals culled. The parent herd is eventually disposed of as negative replacement animals become available (51). Only those bulls which are seronegative may be used and they must be tested every 3 months.

Limitation of spread

When eradication is not practicable it may be appropriate to take some measures to limit the spread of the disease within a herd. The removal of clinically affected animals has almost no effect on prevalence. Nor does the culling of cattle on the basis of abnormal hematological findings. Attempts to eradicate by this means have been well tried in Europe, but with no success.

Some reduction in the transmission rate can possibly be effected by:

- Control of insect vectors
- Special care to avoid iatrogenic transmission on veterinary equipment, especially dehorning, castrating, drawing blood samples and vaccination. Blood transfusions and vaccines containing blood, such as those used for babesiosis and anaplasmosis are particulary potent means of spreading the disease, and donors must be carefully screened to ensure that they are free of the disease
- Vaccination is a tempting goal as an alternative to test and slaughter, but the risk of actually spreading the disease is a very real one. It seems unlikely that vaccination could be an effective prophylaxis because of the very reasons which make the virus invulnerable to the animals' already well-developed immune systems. However, one killed vaccine has protected sheep (58), and sheep and cattle (60), against experimental challenge. A similar vaccine has been ineffective (61)
- Selection of cattle for inclusion in the herd from animals known to have inherent resistance to infection and to the development of lymphosarcoma. In the light of the successful results of test and slaughter programs it seems likely that genetic selection would be important only in long-term programs (52)
- Calves from infected dams have about 20% chance of being infected, transmission occurring *in utero*
- Removal of fertilized ova to an uninfected environment in another uterus may aid in reducing the prenatal transmission. Even in these herds participating voluntarily in a test and slaughter eradication program, the cattle would need to be valuable if the operation were to be financially viable (54).

Insemination is not a method of transmission so that artificial breeding programs are not disrupted.

Although eradication is biologically feasible, it is unlikely that area eradication programs will be implemented on an extensive scale because losses from the disease are not sufficiently high, and there is a high risk of insect vectors reintroducing it which poses a real threat to maintenance of a BVL-free herd. The cost effectiveness of an eradication program on a national basis would be poor. For an individual herd it is feasible provided some steps were taken to increase genetic resistance of the residual stock and to reduce the chances of in-contact infection occurring.

REVIEW LITERATURE

Burny, A. et al. (1978) Bovine leukaemia virus involvement in enzootic bovine leucosis. *Adv. Cancer Res.*, *28*, 251.

Ferrer, J. F. et al. (1979) Bovine leucosis. Natural transmission and principles control. *J. Am. vet. med. Assoc.*, *175*, 1281.

Ferrer, J. F. (1980) Bovine lymphosarcoma. *Adv. vet. Sci.*, *24*, 2.

Grimshaw, W. R. et al. (1979) Bovine leucosis (lymphosarcoma). A clinical study of 60 confirmed cases. *Vet. Rec.*, *105*, 267.

Maaten, M. van der & Miller, J. M. (1979) Appraisal of control measures for bovine leucosis. *J. Am. vet. med. Assoc.*, *175*, 1287.

Parodi, A. L. (Ed.) (1978) Commission of European Communities third international symposium on bovine leucosis. *Ann. rech. vét.*, *9*, 601.

Reed, V. I. (1981) Enzootic bovine leucosis. *Can. vet. J.*, *22*, 95.

Stober, M. (1981) The clinical picture of the enzootic and sporadic forms of bovine leucosis. *Bov. Practnr*, *16*, 119–129.

REFERENCES

(1) Ferrer, J. F. (1980) *Adv. vet. Sci.*, *24*, 2.
(2) Schmidt, F. W. et al. (1976) *Vet. Microbiol.*, *1*, 231.
(3) Mammerickx, M. et al. (1980) *Zentralbl. VetMed.*, *27B*, 291.
(4) Nachmanson, V. M. (1973) *Veterinariya, Moscow*, *11*, 52.
(5) Cypess, R. H. et al. (1974) *Am. J. Epidemiol.*, 99, 37.
(6) Lucas, M. H. et al. (1980) *Vet. Rec.*, *106*, 128.
(7) Gupta, P. & Ferrer, J. F. (1980) *Int. J. Cancer*, *25*, 663.
(8) Gentile, G. et al. (1980) *Clin. vet.*, *103*, 143.
(9) Evermann, J. F. et al. (1986) *Am. J. vet. Res.*, *47*, 1885.
(10) Eaglesome, M. D. et al. (1982) *Vet. Rec.*, *111*, 122.
(11) Roberts, D. H et al. (1982) *Vet. Rec.*, *111*, 501.
(12) Brightling, P. & Radostits, O. M. (1983) *Can. vet. J.*, *24*, 362.
(13) Jacobsen, K. L. et al. (1982) *Prev. vet. Med.*, *1*, 265.
(14) Piper, C. E. et al. (1979) *J. Natl Cancer Inst.*, *62* 165.
(15) Straub, O. C. (1978) *Ann. rech. vét.*, *9*, 809.
(16) Bech-Nielsen, S. et al. (1978) *Am. J. vet Res.*, *39*, 1089.
(17) Ferrer, J. F. et al. (1981) *Science, USA*, *213*, 1014.
(18) Donhem, K. J. et al. (1980) *Am. J. Epidemiol.*, *112*, 80.
(19) Priester, W. A. et al. (1970) *Lancet*, *i*, 367.
(20) Rubino, M. J. & Donham, K. J. (1984) *Am. J. vet. Res.*, *45*, 1553.
(21) Head, K. W. et al. (1974) *Vet. Rec.*, *523*, 527.
(22) McTaggart, H. S. et al. (1979) *Vet. Rec.*, *105*, 36.
(23) Ferrer, J. F. et al. (1979) *J. Am. vet. med. Assoc.*, *175*, 705.

(24) Karlipov, D. V. & Korolev, N. I. (1977) *Veterinariya, Moscow*, 6, 56.
(25) Trainin, Z. et al. (1976) *J. comp. Pathol.*, *86*, 571.
(26) Maaten, M. J. van der & Miller, J. M. (1978) *Ann. réch. vét.*, *9*, 831.
(27) Richards, A. B. et al. (1981) *Cornell Vet.*, *71*, 214.
(28) Sheriff, D. & Newlands, R. W. (1976) *Vet. Rec.*, *98*, 174.
(29) Dungworth, D. L. et al. (1964) *Pathol. vet.*, *1*, 323.
(30) Boyt, W. P. et al. (1976) *Vet. Rec.*, *98*, 112.
(31) Theilen, G. H. & Fowler, M. E. (1962) *J. Am. vet. med. Assoc.*, *140*, 923.
(32) Mammerickx, M. et al. (1984) *Zentralbl. VetMed.*, *31*, 210.
(33) Ferrer, J. F. et al. (1977) *Am. J. vet. Res.*, *38*, 1977.
(34) Rogers, R. J. et al. (1984) *Aust. vet. J.*, *61*, 196.
(35) Gupta, P. & Ferrer, J. F. (1981) *Int. J. Cancer*, *28* 179.
(36) Mammerickx, M. et al. (1985) *Comp. Immunol. Microbiol. infect. Dis.*, *8*, 305.
(37) Shettigara, P. T. et al. (1986) *Can. J. vet. Res.*, *50*, 221.
(38) Takahashi, K. & Kono, Y. (1985) *Jap. J. vet. Sci.*, *47*, 193.
(39) Chander, S. et al. (1978) *Ann. rech. vét.*, *9*, 797.
(40) Ferrer, J. F. et al. (1978) *Prakt. Tierärztl.*, *59*, 589.
(41) Weber, A. et al. (1980) *Am. J. vet. Res.*, *44*, 1912.
(42) Marshak, R. R. et al. (1964) *Can. vet. J.*, *5*, 180.
(43) Hare, W. C. D. & McFeely, R. A. (1966) *Nature, Lond.*, *209*, 108.
(44) Horvath, Z. & Szekeres, T. (1980) *Acta vet. Acad. Sci. hung.*, *28*, 109.
(45) Theilen, G. H. & Dungworth, D. O. (1965) *Am. J. vet. Res.*, *26*, 696.
(46) Slanina, L. et al. (1976) *Veterinarstvi*, *26*, 245.
(47) Ruppaner, R. et al. (1983) *Can. vet. J.*, *24*, 192.
(48) Burny, A. et al. (1978) *Adv. Cancer Res.*, *28*, 251.
(49) Kaja, R. W. et al. (1984) *J. Am. vet. med. Assoc.*, *184*, 184.
(50) Mammerickx, M. (1982) *Ann. med. Vet.*, *126*, 227.
(51) Ferrer, J. F. (1982) *J. Am. vet. med. Assoc.*, *180*, 890.
(52) Przytulski, T. et al. (1981) *Acta vet. Brno*, *50*, 61.
(53) Reed, V. I. (1981) *Can. vet. J.*, *22*, 95.
(54) Hugoson, G. & Wald-Troell, M. (1983) *Nord. VetMed.*, 35, 1.
(55) DiGiacomo, R. F. et al. (1985) *Can. J. comp. Med.*, *49*, 340.
(56) Monke, D. R. (1986) *J. Am. vet. med. Assoc.*, *188*, 823.
(57) Hare, W. C. D. et al. (1985) *Can. vet. J.*, *26*, 231.
(58) Kono, Y. et al. (1986) *Jap. J. vet. Sci.*, *48*, 117.
(59) Burridge, M. J. (1981) *Vet. Res. Commun.*, *5*, 117.
(60) Parfanovich, M. I. et al. (1983) *Br. vet. J.*, *139*, 137.
(61) Miller, J. M. et al. (1983) *Am. J. vet. Res.*, *44*, 64.
(62) Romero, C. H. et al. (1984) *Vet. Rec.*, *115*, 440.
(63) Lucas, M. H. et al. (1985) *Br. vet. J.*, *141*, 647.
(64) Chung, Y. S. et al. (1986) *Aust. vet. J.*, *63*, 379.
(65) Roberts, D. H. et al. (1981) *Vet. Res. Commun.*, *4*, 301.
(66) Thurmond, M. C. et al. (1982) *J. Am. vet. med. Assoc.*, *181*,1530.
(67) Roberts, D. H. et al. (1982) *Vet. Rec.*, *110*, 222.
(68) Romero, C. H. et al. (1983) *Trop. Anim. Hlth Prod.*, *15*, 215.
(69) Kim, D. H. et al. (1983) *Jap. J. vet. Sci.*, *45*, 407.
(70) Rebhun, W. C. (1982) *J. Am. vet. med. Assoc.*, *180*, 149.
(71) Walker, P. J. et al. (1987) *J. Virol. Meth.*, *15*, 201.
(72) Perrin, B. et al. (1986) *Rev. med. Vet.*, *137*, 839.

VIRAL DISEASES CHARACTERIZED BY ALIMENTARY TRACT SIGNS

Foot-and-mouth disease (FMD)

Foot-and-mouth disease is an extremely contagious, acute disease of all cloven-footed animals, caused by a virus and characterized by fever and vesicular eruption in the mouth and on the feet.

Etiology

Three major strains of the causative aphthovirus (family Picornaviridae) occur—A, O and C—but there are a number of immunologically and serologically distinct serotypes with different degrees of virulence within each of these strains. Three additional strains, SAT1, SAT2 and SAT3, have been isolated in Africa and a further strain, ASIA-1, from the Far East. Unfortunately the virus seems to be capable of infinite mutation so that new, antigenically different, subtypes (serotypes) are constantly appearing; more than 60 of these have been identified. The difficulties presented to vaccination programs are obvious—not only may there be great changes in antigenicity between developing serotypes, but the virulence may also change dramatically. There may also be biotypical strains, strains which become adapted to particular species, and then infect other species only with difficulty. Thus there are strains that are much more virulent for pigs, some for buffalo, and some even for *Bos indicus* cattle.

Of the three standard strains, O appears to be the most common and C the least common. There is no crossimmunity between strains and substrains.

Epidemiology: basic data

Foot-and-mouth disease is enzootic in Africa, Europe, Asia, Japan, the Philippines and South America. Many countries in Europe, for example, the Scandinavian countries, Albania, Ireland, and Luxembourg, have not had FMD for 20 years. Eastern Europe is generally free except for the German Democratic Republic (GDR) and the USSR. In modern times the most important new territories invaded by the disease have been Mexico, where it followed the introduction of cattle from Brazil, and Canada, where the virus was apparently introduced in the baggage of a European immigrant. In both instances the disease was promptly controlled and eradicated but the movement of cattle and cattle products between the affected countries and the United States was brought to a standstill. Outbreaks also occur from time to time in Britain and in the Channel Islands being introduced from Europe and South America. There was a massive outbreak in 1967–68 which lasted for 8 months and looked at one time as though it could not be contained. It was, and the only outbreak since then, in 1980, quickly controlled. Australia and New Zealand have never experienced the disease and the United States has not had an outbreak since 1929. The eradication of foot-and-mouth disease from Mexico in 1954 restored North America to its previous status of being free from the disease. The importance of the Darien Gap in maintaining this freedom from the disease is well known. This tract of impassable territory between Colombia and Panama prevents any chance of direct contact between cattle populations in North and South America. The threat to open the Gap by constructing a highway through it is recognized as a very significant threat to North America's continuing freedom from foot-and-mouth disease (26).

Losses due to the disease occur in many ways although loss of production, the expense of eradication and the interference with movement of livestock and meat between countries are the most important economic effects. Although the disease is not a killing one (the mortality rate in adults is only 2% and in young stock 20%) animals are so severely affected during the acute stages of the disease and the period of convalescence is so prolonged that production, both of meat and milk, is seriously impaired. When the disease breaks out in susceptible cattle it spreads very rapidly and the morbidity approximates 100%. Although the mortality is usually low severe outbreaks of a more violent form sometimes occur with a mortality of up to 50%.

The virus is resistant to external influences including common disinfectants and the usual storage-practices of the meat trade. It may persist for over a year in infected premises, for 10–12 weeks on clothing and feed, and up to a month on hair. It is particularly susceptible to changes in pH away from neutral. Sunlight destroys the virus quickly but it may persist on pasture for long periods at low temperatures. Boiling effectively destroys the virus if it is free of tissue but autoclaving under pressure is the safest procedure when heat disinfection is used. The virus can survive for at least a month in bull semen frozen to −79°C (−110°F). In general, the virus is relatively susceptible to heat and insensitive to cold. Most common disinfectants exert practically no effect, but sodium hydroxide or formalin (1–2%) or sodium carbonate (4%) destroy the virus within a few minutes.

Elephants (5), capybara (6), hedgehogs, coypu, many rodents and wild ruminants are susceptible and may provide reservoirs of infection for domestic animals (6). In the United Kingdom it is thought that, although all five species of deer which reside there are susceptible, they play little part in the epidemiology of the disease. This is principally because of the limited contacts between the two species (7). Experimental transmission by direct contact from cattle to deer, and deer to cattle and sheep have been effected. Roe deer and muntjac showed typical severe clinical signs, sika deer had a less severe form of foot-and-mouth disease, and fallow and red deer were affected only subclinically. Water buffalo (*Bubalus bubalis*) in Brazil become infected but may show no clinical signs and there may be no cross-infection to comingled cattle (35). Indian reports indicate a high prevalence of typical clinical disease and spread from buffalo to other species.

Of the wild ungulates in Africa many can become infected (22) but very few harbor the virus sufficiently long, nor an immunity to it, to have any significant effect on the epidemiology of foot-and-mouth disease. Only the buffalo (*Syncercus caffer*) appears to be a significant host (9), although interspecies transmission from the buffalo to domestic animals is probably rare because of the transient contacts between them. The disease in buffalo is much milder than in cattle (25).

The disease is most important in cattle but pigs, goats and sheep are also affected, some strains of the virus being limited in their infectivity to particular species. The importance of these small stock is largely as carriers of the disease to cattle. Sheep may remain as carriers for up to 5 months maintaining a continuous low-level multiplication of virus, principally in the pharyngeal area. An examination of the importance of sheep and goats as carriers of foot-and-mouth disease in Kenya showed that goats were infrequent carriers, and sheep did not act in this way at all (13). Immature animals and those in good condition are relatively more susceptible, and hereditary differences in susceptibility have also been observed. The typical disease occurs rarely in man.

In enzootic areas periodic outbreaks occur which sweep through the animal populations and then subside. This is probably due to the disappearance of immunity which develops during an epizootic and the sudden flaring up from small foci of infection when the population becomes susceptible again. In cattle the immunity which develops after natural infection varies between 1 year and more than 4 years. In pigs the duration of this immunity is abour 30 weeks. When outbreaks follow each other in quick succession the presence of more than one strain of the virus should be suspected. The same explanation usually applies when epidemics occur in vaccinated cattle. In countries when general vaccination is practiced every year, outbreaks are usually caused by the importation of carrier animals, or infected meat. The emphasis in control in these countries is to prevent importation, and when outbreaks do occur to eradicate by slaughter.

Foot-and-mouth disease has different epidemiological characteristics in the different animal species. For example, a common pattern is the importation of the virus into a country in sheep meat, from sheep which showed no illness. There is an initial infection in pigs and then spread to cattle. It is suggested that the roles are those of maintenance of the infection, then multiplication of the virus, and finally the major clinical manifestations of the presence of the virus.

Epidemiology: patterns of spread

Foot-and-mouth disease is spread both by inhalation and by ingestion. In cattle, the first introduction to a new area is often via pigs which contract infection by ingestion of meat scraps which are infected. Spread from these pigs to cattle is via movement of people, abattoir waste, or animals, in which case ingestion is the likely method of spread. Further spread to cattle and between cattle is more likely to be by airborne means, and inhalation is the portal of entry. The virus can persist in aerosol form for long periods. The speed and direction of the wind are important factors in determining the rate of airborne spread. Humidity is also important but rain as such appears not to be. In the most favorable circumstances it is now estimated that sufficient virus to initiate an infection can be windborne as far as 100 km (62 miles) and possibly across expanses of sea (29). There are peaks of spread at dawn and dusk. It seems probable that the portal of infection with aerogenous spread is the respiratory tract (15). The quantitative aspects of foot-and-mouth disease virus, the yield of virus, its movement and the infective dose required, have been examined and throw light on the probable relative importance of each mode of transmission (16). In pigs, the most sensitive and initial route of infection is by inhalation in which the virus multiplies in the lung but the disease spreads within a group by the oral route (17).

In cattle the first site of infection and of subsequent rapid multiplication of the virus is the pharynx (28). Subsequent to infection the virus appears in the blood and milk soon after infection and in the saliva before the appearance of vesicles in the mouths. All excretions including the urine, milk, feces and semen may be infective before the animal is clinically ill and for a short period after signs have disappeared. However, the period of maximum infectivity is when vesicles in the mouth and on the feet are discharging, the vesicular fluid containing the virus in maximum concentration. Although it is generally conceded that affected animals are seldom infective for more than 4 days after the rupture of vesicles, except in so far as the virus may persist on the skin or hair, the possibility exists that some animals may remain as carriers for very long periods, and the intermittent passage of small amounts of virus may lead to the establishment of new outbreaks. In cattle, carriers may develop during convalescence from the natural disease, or more importantly in vaccinated animals which are exposed to infection. Up to 50% of cattle, sheep and goats may become carriers, but pigs do not. The actual importance of carriers is debated. They appear not to transmit infection naturally, but the virus can be recovered from them and the infection transmitted experimentally for periods of up to 6 months (35). The nasopharynx is the common site for persistence of the virus. Mammary gland is another tissue in which persistence can take place, the virus living in this tissue for 3–7 weeks. Wild fauna may also serve as a reservoir of the disease, as may ticks. Man may also be a vehicle for transmission of foot-and-mouth disease virus. It has been recovered from the nasal mucosa of persons working with infected cattle for up to 28 hours after contact. Nose-blowing did not eliminate the virus nor cotton face-masks prevent the infection.

All meat tissues, including bone, are likely to remain infective for long periods, especially if quick-frozen and to a less extent meat chilled or frozen by a slow process. The survival of the virus is closely associated with the pH of the medium. The development of acidity in rigor mortis inactivates the virus but quick freezing suspends acid formation and the virus is likely to survive. However, on thawing, the suspended acid formation recommences and the virus may be destroyed. Prolonged survival is more likely in viscera, bone marrow and in blood vessels and lymph nodes where acid production is not so great. Meat pickled in brine, or salted by dry methods may also remain infective. Fomites, including bedding, mangers, clothing, motor tires, harness, feedstuffs and hides may also remain a source of infection for long periods.

The disease is spread from herd to herd either directly by the movement of infected animals, or possibly even infected humans, or indirectly by the transportation of the virus on inanimate objects, particularly uncooked and unprocessed meat products and animal products other than meat. Milk is now recognized as an important vehicle by which the virus may be spread (21). The pH and the temperature of the milk significantly affect survival which may be as long as 18 hours. Flash pasteurization procedures, as distinct from the holding method, do not inactivate foot-and-mouth disease virus in milk; neither does evaporation to milk powder (23). Butter, butter oil, casein and casein products, and cheese, can also act as vehicles for the virus (2, 48, 49). Introduction of the disease into a herd or country as a result of the use of infected cattle semen for artificial insemination is possible. Virus has also been detected in the semen of boars affected by the disease, but it has not been a means of transmitting it (30). The virus can pass unchanged through the alimentary tracts of birds which may thus act as carriers and transport infection for long distances and over natural topographical barriers such as mountain ranges and sea.

Epizootics in free areas occur intermittently and from a number of sources. In England it is estimated that outbreaks arise in the following manner—transportation by birds 16%, by meat products used as pig food 40%, contact with meat and bones other than swill 9%, unknown causes (probably swill) 7%, and completely obscure 28%. The greatest danger appears to be from uncooked meat scraps fed to pigs. However, more unusual methods of introduction must not be disregarded. Infected smallpox vaccine has been the cause of some outbreaks. With modern methods of transport it is possible that farm workers may carry the virus long distances in their clothing and that frozen bull semen could be a source of infection.

During the latter months of 1967 the United Kingdom experienced a very bad outbreak of foot-and-mouth disease. Control measures which had been effective in many hundreds of outbreaks for many years failed to halt the spread of the disease. As a result a great deal of investigational work was carried out, especially with respect to methods of spread. A committee, the Northumberland Committee, considered the control programs being used and made recommendations about future policies (27). The most important decision was that a basic choice existed—either introduce vaccination and admit the disease was endemic in the United Kingdom. or prevent the importation of meat and offal from countries in which foot-and-mouth disease exists. The decision was for the latter option. The outbreak is thought to have originated from frozen Argentine lamb fed to pigs.

Pathogenesis

Irrespective of the portal of entry, once infection gains access to the bloodstream, the virus shows a predilection for the epithelium of the mouth and feet and, to a less extent, the teats. Characteristic lesions develop at these sites after an incubation period of 1–21 (usually 3–8) days. Predilection for lesions to occur on the oral mucosa is attributed to the hyperplastic state of the epithelium caused by persistent local irritation. The initial phase of viral septicemia is often unnoticed and it is only when localization in the mouth and on the feet occurs that the animal is found to be clinically abnormal. The experimental disease in sheep is characterized by an incubation period of 4–9 days after contact. After inoculation the period is 1–3 days, viremia occurs at 17–74 hours, hyperthermia from the 17th to 96th hour. Clinical signs are serous nasal discharge, salivation and buccal lesions in 75% and foot lesions in 25% of cases.

Clinical findings

In typical field cases in cattle there is an incubation period of 3–6 days, but it may vary between 1 and 7 days. The onset is heralded by a precipitate fall in milk yield and a high fever (40–41°C, 104–106°F), accompanied by severe dejection, and anorexia, followed by the appearance of an acute painful stomatitis. At this stage the temperature reaction is subsiding. There is abundant salivation, the saliva hanging in long, ropey strings, a characteristic smacking of the lips, and the animal chews carefully. Vesicles and bullae (1–2 cm in diameter) appear on the buccal mucosa, and on the dental pad and the tongue. These rupture within 24 hours leaving a raw painful surface which heals in about a week. The vesicles are thin-walled, easily ruptured and contain a thin, straw-colored fluid. Concurrently with the oral lesions, vesicles appear on the feet particularly in the clefts and on the coronet. Rupture of the vesicles causes acute discomfort and the animal is grossly lame, often recumbent, with a marked, painful swelling of the coronet. Secondary bacterial invasion of the lesions may interfere with healing and lead to severe involvement of the deep structures of the foot. Vesicles may occur on the teats and when the teat orifice is involved severe mastitis often follows. Abortion and subsequent infertility are common sequels. Very rapid loss of condition and fall in milk yield occur during the acute period and these signs are much more severe than would be anticipated from the extent of the lesions. Eating is resumed in 2–3 days as the lesions heal but the period of convalescence may be as long as 6 months. Young calves are rather more susceptible than adults and heavy mortality may occur during an outbreak without typical lesions being present.

In most outbreaks of foot-and-mouth disease the rate of spread is high and the clinical signs are as described above but there is a great deal of variation in the virulence of the infection and this may lead to difficulty in field diagnosis. For example, there is a malignant form of the disease in which acute myocardial failure occurs. There is a typical course initially but a sudden relapse occurs on the 5th–6th day with dyspnea, a weak and irregular heart action, and death during convulsions. Occasional cases show localization in the alimentary tract with dysentery or diarrhea indicating the presence of enteritis. Ascending posterior paralysis may also occur.

A sequel to foot-and-mouth disease in cattle, due probably to endocrine damage, is a chronic syndrome of dyspnea, anemia, overgrowth of hair and lack of heat tolerance described colloquially as 'panting'. Diabetes mellitus has also been observed as a sequel in cattle.

In sheep, goats and pigs the disease is usually mild and is important mainly because of the danger of transmission of the disease to cattle. Rarely sheep develop a syndrome identical with that of cattle so that it becomes a crippling disease with a high mortality in lambs due to myocardial and skeletal muscle necrosis. An acute syndrome can also occur in goats and pigs, but experimental transmission of the infection to cattle causes only a mild disease. After experimental infection piglets often die without showing signs of vesication, death being due to myocarditis (20). The more common syndrome in these species is the appearance of a few, small lesions, but with more severe involvement of the feet, often causing severe lameness in all four.

Clinical pathology

Exhaustive laboratory studies are needed for diagnosis, for determination of the strain of virus involved and to differentiate the disease from vesicular stomatitis and vesicular exanthema. The major methods available are tissue culture, the complement fixation test and experimental transmission in test animals; a rapid ELISA test is available for examination of fresh epithelial tissues (12).

Tissue culture

The foot-and-mouth disease virus is cultivable on tissue culture and in hen eggs, and use is made of this in the preparation of live, attenuated vaccines. In diagnosis, neutralization of virus by known antisera is highly efficient.

Complement fixation (CF) test

The direct complement fixation test on the original epithelial suspension is the fastest method of making a positive diagnosis, within a few hours. But negative samples must be checked in tissue cultures because of the number of false negatives which occur with the CF test, especially in poorly collected and packaged samples when they are sent over long distances (31). Type-specific and strain-specific complement-fixing antisera can be prepared which permit the typing of strains in an outbreak. Diagnostic antisera can also be prepared for differentiation from vesicular stomatitis. The test can take the place of large animal inoculation for the differentiation of the two diseases but large animal inoculation is still necessary to determine the presence of a mixed infection.

The virus infection associated (VIA) test

A non-viral antibody is detectable serologically in infected and recovered animals. The use of this VIA test simplifies the testing of imported animals. A decision about whether the animal is infected can be made quickly without the need to include a large number of serotypes in a test screen (35).

Other serological tests

Plaque-reduction neutralization radial immunodiffusion and serum neutralization tests are available. With these tests some confusions are created by serological cross-reactions with unrelated viruses (24).

Experimental transmission in unweaned white mice

The propagation of the virus in unweaned white mice can be used to detect the presence of virus in suspect material, the presence of antibodies in serum and for investigations into the transmission of immunity and the pathogenesis of the disease.

Guinea-pig inoculation

The presence of virus in suspected material can be detected by the intradermal injection of fresh vesicular fluid into the plantar pads of guinea-pigs. Vesicles appear on the pads in 1–7 days and secondary vesicles in the mouth 1–2 days later.

Large animal inoculation

This may be used for the differentiation of foot-and-mouth disease, vesicular stomatitis and vesicular exanthema based on the different species susceptibilities to the three viruses.

Necropsy findings

The lesions of foot-and-mouth disease are relatively mild except for those in the mouth and on the feet and udder. These lesions may be extensive if secondary bacterial infection has occurred. In some cases the vesicles may extend to the pharynx, esophagus, forestomachs and intestines. The trachea and bronchi may also be involved. In the malignant form of the disease there is extensive myocarditis. If the animal survives there is replacement fibrosis and the heart is enlarged and flabby. On section the heart muscle appears streaked with patches of yellow tissue interspersed with apparently normal myocardium.

Diagnosis

The need to identify foot-and-mouth disease is of paramount importance in all countries even in those countries where it occurs enzootically. It is of particular importance in those countries which do not experience the disease because of the need to introduce control measures quickly. The field veterinarian must be able to recognize suspicious cases, and laboratory facilities must be available to confirm the diagnosis. In countries where the disease is enzootic there are special difficulties in clinical recognition because of the frequently subdued severity of the oral and digital lesions (1). In countries where the other vesicular diseases do not occur suspicions will be readily aroused, but in North America the presence of vesicular stomatitis and vesicular exanthema may result in misdiagnosis. Vesicular stomatitis of horses, cattle and swine, vesicular exanthema of swine and swine vesicular disease resemble foot-and-mouth disease closely. There are three other unclassified vesiculoviruses, Piry (8), Chandipura and Isfahan, that are usually bracketed with the virus of vesicular stomatitis (13) but are much less virulent. The observation that white-skinned pigs fed on parsnips or celery and exposed to sunlight will develop vesicles on the snout and feet (32) is a further confounding factor in the differentiation of the vesicular diseases in this species.

Bluetongue of sheep may also present a problem in differentiation. Details of these diseases are provided separately but a summary of the differential points is given in Table 67.

Rapid differentiation and diagnosis of these diseases may also be achieved by fluorescent antibody staining or complement fixation of antigen in vesicular epithelium, virus morphology, complement fixation or virus neutralization of antigen in tissue culture or embryonated hens eggs. Less rapid differentiation involves serology on affected animals.

Mucosal-type diseases and rinderpest are easily differentiated by the lesions which develop in the mucosa and sometimes on the feet. The lesions are never vesicular, commencing as superficial erosions and proceeding to the development of ulcers.

Treatment

Treatment with mild disinfectant and protective dressings to inflamed areas to prevent secondary infection is recommended. A good symptomatic response is reported to the administration of flunixin meglumine (33).

Control

Many factors govern the control procedure in a given area. The procedures commonly used are control by eradication and control by vaccination or a combination of the two. In countries where the disease is enzootic, eradication is seldom practicable. In areas where the disease occurs only as occasional epizootics, slaughter of all infected and in-contact animals is usually carried out. It must be remembered that vaccination is costly and

Table 67. Differentiation of acute vesicular diseases.

Animal species	*Route of inoculation*	*Foot-and-mouth disease*	*Vesicular stomatitis*	*Vesicular exanthema of swine*	*Swine vesicular disease*	*Bluetongue*
NATURAL INFECTION						
Cattle		+	+	−	−	+ (rarely occurs)
Pig*		+	+	+	+	−
Sheep and goat		+	±	−	−	+
Horse		−	+	−	−	−
EXPERIMENTAL TRANSMISSION						
Cattle	Intradermal in tongue, gums, lips	+	+	−	−	
	Intramuscular	+	−	−	−	+
Pig*	Intradermal in snout, lips	+	+	+	+	
	Intravenous	+	+	+	+	
	Intramuscular	+	−	−	+	
Sheep and goat	Various	+	+	−	(+) (no lesions)	+
Horse	Intradermal in tongue	−	+	+ (some strains)	−	
	Intramuscular			+ (some strains)	−	
Guinea-pig	Intradermal in footpad	+	+	−	−	−
UWW mice		+	+	−	+	+ (hamsters also)
Adult chicken	Intradermal in tongue	+	+	−	−	

* White-skinned pigs fed on parsnips or celery and exposed to sunlight develop vesicles.

sometimes ineffective and that eradication is the logical objective in all countries. It seems evident that this is not achievable in countries in large continents such as Europe, unless international cooperation is achieved.

As in the control of all epidemic infectious diseases, the problems posed for its administrators are complex and continually changing. For example, the prospect of making a wrong decision about when to switch from an eradication-by-slaughter program to a containment-by-vaccination program, when a foot-and-mouth disease outbreak is raging and public sentiments are running high, is a daunting one. A wrong decision may cost a cattle industry many millions of dollars. To avoid making such errors it is customary nowadays to develop a mathematical model which simulates the progress of an outbreak in terms of numbers of animals infected, affected and dead, and how these numbers will change under pressure from control procedures, management practices and weather prevailing. Such a model is described for use in the United States (42) and one for South America (50). An essential aspect of such an analysis is the economic effect of the various control programs and their outcomes. The cost-benefit aspects of a computer simulation model of foot-and-mouth disease is also available and provides some of these answers (43).

Control by eradication

The success of an eradication program depends on the thoroughness with which it is applied. As soon as the diagnosis is established all cloven-footed animals in the exposed groups should be immediately slaughtered and burned or buried. No reclamation of meat should be permitted and milk must be regarded as infected. Inert materials which may be contaminated must not leave infected premises without proper disinfection. This applies particularly to human clothing, motor vehicles and farm machinery. Bedding, feed, feeding utensils, animal products and other articles which cannot be adequately disinfected must be burned. Barns and small yards must be cleaned and disinfected with 1–2% sodium hydroxide or formalin or 4% sodium carbonate solution. Acids and alkalis are the best inactivators of foot-and-mouth disease virus and their activity is greatly enhanced by the presence of a detergent. The effective pH at a disinfection surface may be grossly altered by the presence of organic matter and needs to be adequately maintained. When all possible sources of infection are destroyed the farm should be left unstocked for 6 months and restocking permitted only when 'sentinel' test animals are introduced and remain uninfected. Recommendations for outdoor sites are difficult to make. Observations in Argentina suggest that contaminated pastures and unsheltered yards are clear of infection if left unstocked for 8–10 days. Human movement to and from infected premises must be reduced to minimum. Persons working on the farm should wear waterproof clothing which can be easily disinfected by spraying and subsequently removed as the person leaves the farm. Clothing not suitable for chemical disinfection must be boiled. Because of the rapidity with which the disease may spread immediate quarantine must be imposed on all farms within a radius of 16–24 km (10–15 miles) of the outbreak. No animal movement can be permitted and human and motor traffic must be reduced to a minimum.

Although the eradication method of control is favored when the incidence is low, it imposes severe losses on the cattle industry in affected areas and is economically impracticable in many countries. However, it must be regarded as the final stage in any control program when vaccination has reduced the incidence of the disease to a suitably low level. The standard strategy is the containment of the disease by ringing the outbreak with a zone of vaccinated animals and setting about reducing the infection rate within the ringed area and eventually eradicating remaining hotspots by slaughter. Containment of an outbreak in a country free of foot-and-mouth disease is a difficult task with high rewards. A cost-benefit analysis foot-and-mouth disease control in the United Kingdom (34) revealed that both slaughter and general vaccination policies are highly profitable and vaccination is less profitable.

The United Kingdom has always been the leader in the controversy about whether to eradicate or vaccinate, and has been the strongest proponent of immediate eradication by test and slaughter. However, the 1967–68 epizootic was so damaging financially that it was arranged for vaccination to be available should there be a recurrence of such an epizootic (20). Part of the increased concern about the disease in the United Kingdom derives from the greatly increased size of the herds in recent times and the risks involved if infection is introduced. On the other hand, hygiene at these large herd premises is usually very good and chance infections are much less likely to enter.

Vaccination

Regular vaccination against foot-and-mouth disease is a way of life for most of the world. Europe, Asia, Africa, South America, and South-east Asia are heavily infected with the disease and eradication of it does not seem possible within the foreseeable future. Even in those countries which are free of the disease a fallback position to regional vaccination is usually maintained.

Killed trivalent (containing O, A and C strains) vaccines are in general use, but because of the increasing occurrence of antigenically dissimilar substrains the production of vaccines from locally isolated virus is becoming a more common practice. The virus is obtained from infected tongue tissue, a tissue culture of bovine tongue epithelium or other tissue culture (28). Baby hamster kidney (BHK) is a favored viral cultural medium and BHK vaccine is fast coming into general use. Its principal virtue is its adaptability to deep suspension culture in contrast with its growth on monolayer culture, enabling large-scale production of virus to be carried out within practicable space limits. Inactivation of the virus to produce a killed vaccine used to be done with formalin but there are disadvantages with its use and more sophisticated agents, especially acetylethyleneimine are now used. Serviceable immunity after a single vaccination can be relied on for only 6–8 months, vaccines produced from 'natural' virus giving longer immunity than those produced from 'culture' virus. Oil-adjuvanted, inactivated vaccines offer promise of providing longer immunity, and requiring only annual vaccination in adult cattle and twice yearly for young stock (4). A general vaccination program for an area must be planned for that area. Thus in Europe the program includes once-a-year vaccination of all adults with an additional campaign every 6 months to vaccinate the calves as they reach about 4 months of age. In South America, the only satisfactory strategy is the vaccination of all cattle every 4 months. The specific recommendations are that calves from unvaccinated dams should be vaccinated at 4 and revaccinated at 8 months of age, but calves from vaccinated cows should be done twice, the first at 6 and the second at 10 months of age (36). The important consideration in calves is to avoid vaccination while the calf is still carrying the maternal antibodies derived from colostrum. Calves as young as 1 week respond as actively to vaccination as adult animals provided they are free of maternally derived antibody (18). Immunity is present 7–20 days after vaccination, the time interval varying with the antigenicity of the vaccine. It is not usual to include sheep and pigs in a general vaccination program unless the species is suffering outbreaks of foot-and-mouth disease.

Because of the short duration of the immunity produced by killed vaccines, attention has been focused on the production of an attenuated living virus vaccine. The major difficulty encountered so far has been the narrow margin between loss of virulence and loss of immunogenicity. Attenuated vaccines have been produced by passage through white mice, embryonated hen eggs, rabbits and tissue culture (6). Their use in South Africa has contributed to the eradication of the disease and in Venezuela has proved effective where killed virus vaccines failed to stem a major outbreak. Provided constant surveillance can be maintained over vaccinated animals, their value in such circumstances cannot be denied. However, their early promise has not been fulfilled, and improved killed vaccines are most generally favored. In spite of the uncertain stability of the lapinized virus, control of the disease in Russia has been reported after the use of a rabbit-passaged vaccine. In those countries where vaccination of very large numbers of animals is carried out annually one of the emerging problems is the quality control of the vaccines with respect to innocuity and to immunizing capacity or potency. The techniques to monitor these characteristics are available, but they do add to the costs of the vaccine, and if commercial competition is keen this aspect of production may be skimped. If a regular vaccination program is not being highly effective in depressing the rate of occurrence of the disease, one of the most important investigations to conduct is that of the quality of the vaccine used.

A great deal has been written about genetically engineered FMD vaccine produced by biotechnological manipulation of *Escherichia coli*, but the chances of any practical vaccine production by this technique seems remote (19).

General vaccination as a means of control is recommended for countries where the disease is enzootic, or where the threat of introduction is very great, e.g. Switzerland and Israel. If an outbreak occurs, a booster vaccination with the relevant serotype will greatly increase the resistance of the population. However, the strategy of general vaccination has many difficulties. The following disadvantages are suggested:

- To be effective, the program should consist of vaccination against a number of strains three times yearly. More frequent vaccination may be necessary in the face of outbreaks during optimum conditions for spread
- Vaccination of sheep and pigs is also used in control programs. In pigs a trivalent, inactivated, adjuvant vaccine gives strong immunity for 6 months and some resistance for 12 months. Severe local reactions occur at vaccination sites, but these can be reduced by the inclusion of emulsifying agents in the vaccine. This eliminates the development of granuloma and abscess formation (39). In a large-scale field trial, 95% protection has been claimed after use of a bivalent vaccine in oil adjuvant (40). The problem in vaccinating pigs is the severity of the local reaction, and the high rate of abortions and stillbirths when pregnant sows are vaccinated (41). In sheep, monovalent or trivalent vaccines give immunity for 5–6 months but the sheep may act as inapparent carriers
- Inapparent infections may occur in animals whose susceptibility has been reduced by vaccination permitting the existence of 'carrier' foci. It has become generally recognized that the number of carrier animals produced by vaccination is very much greater than previously thought. Apart from the fact that these animals are a potent method of spreading the disease, they also provide an excellent medium for the mutation of existing virus strains, because the hosts are immune (31). The carrier state in vaccinated and unvaccinated cattle may persist for as long as 6 months and be capable of causing new outbreaks in all species. But the problem needs to be kept in perspective. The number of carriers produced in this way is directly related to the rate of occurrence of the disease in the population, and if this is kept to a minimum by an assiduous vaccination program and a strict limitation on the movement of infected animals into the population the rate of occurrence of carriers can be very small (44)
- Importation of vaccinated animals is often prohibited. An additional disadvantage is the production of sensitivity resulting in anaphylaxis in 0·005% of cattle vaccinated repeatedly, especially when the vaccines contain antibiotics or the vaccine contains foreign protein not associated with the antigen, or the virus has been killed with formalin which has also denatured the protein in the vaccine. Edema, urticaria, dermatitis, abortion and fatal anaphylaxis all occur (45). There does not appear to be any practical means of detecting the hypersensitive animals before revaccinating them (46). Some batches of vaccine also appear to cause a significant number of premature births and abortions if cows are vaccinated during the last 4 months of pregnancy (47). Satisfactory purification and standardization of the vaccine can eliminate many of the problems because

the hypersensitivity is to the culture medium, and the agent used to kill the virus, rather than to the virus itself (3). Calves from immune cows are passively immunized by antibodies passed to them by the colostrum and do not respond to vaccination.

Alternatives to general vaccination are modified programs including 'ring' vaccination to contain outbreaks, 'frontier' vaccination to produce a buffer area between infected and free countries and vaccination of selected herds on a voluntary basis when an outbreak is threatened. It is generally conceded that vaccination of an entire population may be necessary when eradication is incapable of preventing the spread of the disease.

Prevention of entry of the disease into free areas is an ever-increasing problem because of modern developments in communications. The following prohibitions are necessary if the disease is to be excluded:

- There must be a complete embargo on the importation of animals and animal products from countries where the disease is enzootic. The embargo should include hay, straw and vegetables. Where the disease occurs only as occasional outbreaks the importation of animals can be permitted provided they are subjected to a satisfactory period of quarantine
- Particular attention should be given to preventing the entry of uncooked meats from ships, airplanes and other forms of transport and in parcels originating in infected areas. In danger areas all swill fed to pigs must be cooked and all food waste satisfactorily disposed of
- The personal clothing and other effects of people arriving from infected areas should be suitably disinfected
- Of particular importance are semen and fertilized ova. The virus can survive in frozen bull semen and in some fertilized ova, for example, zona pellucida-free bovine embryos but not in others, for example, zona pellucida-intact bovine embryos (51).

REVIEW LITERATURE

Blackwell, J. H. (1980) Internationalism and survival of foot-and-mouth disease virus in cattle and foot products. *J. dairy Sci.*, *63*, 1019.

Brown, F. (1986) Review literature. Foot-and-mouth disease—one of the remaining great plagues. *Proc. Roy. Soc. Lond. B*, *229*, 215–226.

Donaldson, A. I. (1979) Air-borne foot and mouth disease. *Vet. Bull.*, *49*, 653.

Pay, T. W. F. (1984) Control of footrot by vaccination. *Proc. 13th World Cong. Cattle Dis.*, 353–358.

Rweyemamu, M. M. et al. (1982) The control of foot and mouth disease by vaccination. *Vet. Ann.*, *22*, 63–80.

Sard, D.M. et al. (1978) Foot-and-mouth diseases. Clinical aspects, control in Great Britain, etc. *Vet. Rec.*, *102*, 184, etc. (6 papers).

REFERENCES

(1) Kennedy, D. J. et al. (1984) *Aust. vet. J.*, *61*, 163.
(2) Blackwell, J. H. (1980) *J. dairy Sci.*, *63*, 1019.
(3) Pappous, C. & Verbelis, P. (1977) *Proc. Int. Symp. FMD, Lyon, France*, Oct. 1976, p. 97.
(4) Sutmoller, P. (1977) *Proc. Int. Symp. FMD, Lyon, France*, Oct. 1976, p. 135.
(5) Bengis, R. G. et al. (1984) *Proc. 13th World Cong. Cattle Dis.*, p.39.
(6) Gomes, I. & Rosenberg, F. J. (1984) *Prev. vet. Med.*, *3*, 197.
(7) Gibbs, E. P. J. et al. (1975) *Vet. Rec.*, *96*, 558; *J.comp.Pathol.*, *85*, 361.
(8) Wilks, C. R. & House, J. A. (1984) *J. Hyg., Camb.*, *93*, 147.
(9) Gainaru, M. D. et al. (1986) *Onderstepoort J. vet. Res.*, *53*, 69 & 75.
(10) Hedger, R. S. (1972) *J. comp. Pathol.*, *82*, 19.
(11) Young, E. at al. (1972) *Onderstepoort J. vet. Res.*, *39*, 181.
(12) Hamblin, C. et al. (1984) *Vet. Microbiol.*, *9*, 435.
(13) House, J. A. & Wilks, C. R. (1983) *Proc. 8th Ann. Mtg US, AHA*, p. 276.
(14) Dutta, P. K. et al. (1983) *Vet. Rec.*, *113*, 134.
(15) Norris, K. P. & Harper, G. J. (1970) *Nature, Lond.*, *225*, 98.
(16) Sellers, R. F. (1971) *Vet. Bull.*, *41*, 431.
(17) Terpstra, C. (1972) *Bull. Off. int. Epizoot.*, *77*, 359.
(18) Nicholls, M. J. et al. (1985) *Br. vet. J.*, *141*, 17.
(19) Della-Porta, A. J. (1983) *Aust. vet. J.*, *60*, 129.
(20) Donaldson, A. I. (1984) *Vet. Rec.*, *115*, 509.
(21) Callis, J. J. et al. (1975) *Bull. Off. int. Epizoot.*, *83*, 183.
(22) Paling, R. W. et al. (1979) *J. Wildlife Dis.*, *15*, 351.
(23) Blackwell, J. H. & Hyde, J. L. (1976) *J. Hyg., Camb.*, *77*, 77.
(24) Andersen, A. A. (1978) *Am. J. vet. Res.*, *39*, 59.
(25) Thomson, G. R. et al. (1984) *Proc. 13th World Cong. Cattle Dis.*, p. 33.
(26) Poppensieck, G. C. (1977) *J. Am. vet. med. Assoc.*, *170*, 838.
(27) Northumberland Committee Report (1970) *Vet. Rec.*, *86*, 11.
(28) Burrows, R. et al. (1981) *J. comp. Pathol.*, *91*, 599.
(29) Gloster, J. et al. (1982) *Vet. Rec.*, *108*, 371; *110*, 47; *111*, 290.
(30) McVicar, J. W. & Eisner, R. J. (1977) *Proc. ann Mtg US Anim. Hlth Assoc.*, *81*, 221.
(31) Buckley, L.S. et al. (1975) *Bull. Off. int. Epizoot.*, *83*, 123.
(32) Montgomery, J. F. et al. (1987) *NZ vet. J.*, *35*, 21, 27.
(33) Benitz, A. M. et al. (1984) *Proc. 13th World Cong. Dis. Cattle*, p. 71.
(34) Power, A. P. & Harris, S. A. (1973) *J. agric. Econ.*, *24*, 573.
(35) Samara, S. I. & Pinto, A. A. (1983) *Vet. Rec.*, *113*, 472.
(36) Condert, M. et al. (1975) *Bull. Off. int. Epizoot.* *83*, 263.
(37) McKercher, P. D. & Bachrach, H. L. (1976) *Can. J. comp. Med.*, *40*, 67.
(38) Morgan, D. O. & McKercher, P. D. (1977) *Proc. ann. Mtg US Anim. Hlth Assoc.*, *81*, 224.
(39) Dhennin, L. (1976) *Rec. Med. Vet.*, *152*, 183.
(40) Zanny, E. et al. (1974) *Proc. 3rd Congr. int. Pig vet. Soc., Lyon*, 1974, FA3, 1–2.
(41) Garcia Ferrero, J. L. et al. (1971) *Bull. Off. int. Epizoot.*, *76*, 679.
(42) Miller, W. M. (1978) In: *New Techniques in Veterinary Epidemiology and Economics*, eds P. R. Ellis et al. Dept. Agric., Univ. of Reading, U.K.
(43) McCauley, H. et al. (1978) In: *New Techniques in Veterinary Epidemiology and Economics*, eds. P. R. Ellis et al. Dept. Agric., Univ. of Reading, UK.
(44) Anderson, E. C. et al. (1974) *J. Hyg., Camb.*, *73*, 229.
(45) Eyal, J. & Meyer, E. (1971) *Refuah vet.*, *28*, 62.
(46) Black, L. & Pay, T. W. F. (1975) *J. Hyg., Camb*, *74*, 169.
(47) Baljer, G. & Mayr, A. (1971) *Zentralbl. VetMed.*, *18B*, 293.
(48) Cunliffe, H. R. & Blackwell, J. H. (1977) *J. Food Prot.*, *40*, 389.
(49) Blackwell, J. H. (1978) *J. dairy Res.*, *45*, 283.
(50) Carpenter, I. E. & Thieme, A. (1980) *Proc. 2nd Int. Symp. Vet. Epidemiol.*, May 1979, Canberra, Australia, 511.
(51) Singh, E. L. et al. (1986) *Theriogenology*, *26*, 587.

Swine vesicular disease

Swine vesicular disease is an apparently new disease of pigs that is spreading rapidly throughout the world. Although its primary economic effects are minor it is of considerable significance as it is clinically indistinguishable from foot-and-mouth disease.

Etiology

The disease is caused by an enterovirus (family Picornaviridae) that is related to human coxsackie B5 virus and it has been postulated that the disease may have arisen from a variant of this virus that has become adapted to swine (1, 2). Human isolates of coxsackie B5 virus have not been shown to produce disease in pigs (1, 3) although swine vesicular disease virus may infect man (2). In animals the disease is restricted to pigs although experimental challenge of sheep has produced subclinical infection (4). There are minor antigenic differences and variation in virulence between some isolates of swine vesicular disease virus from different countries and it would appear that several variants of the virus are now in existence (5, 6). There are differences in the polypeptide structures between isolates from the United Kingdom and those from Hong Kong (29). Swine vesicular disease virus can be grown in tissue culture and has characteristics distinguishing it from the viruses associated with foot-and-mouth disease, vesicular stomatitis and vesicular exanthema (7). The virus is extremely resistant to chemical and physical influences. These properties have made control of the disease very difficult. It is inactivated only at extremes of pH and it may remain infective in the environment and in manure for periods of at least 6 months (1). It is resistant to the action of many disinfectants, and recommendations for disinfectants which should be used include 2% sodium hydroxide, 8% formaldehyde and also 0·04% sodium hypochlorite if organic material is not present (8). The virus survives the processing of pork and pork products except heating at greater than 68°C (154°F) and can persist in these products indefinitely (9, 10).

Epidemiology

The disease was first recognized as a limited outbreak in Italy in 1966 and was eradicated by slaughter. Following this it appeared in Hong Kong (1970), England (1972), many countries in Europe (1972–74), Japan (1973) and Malta (1975). There is no serological evidence of the disease in Denmark (30). Eradication programs based on slaughter of affected and in-contact pigs were instituted in most of these outbreaks and in most cases have been effective in controlling the disease (11–13). Serological surveys have not detected any evidence of widespread undetected evidence of infection in England, Scotland and Wales (32). There has been some variation in virulence and epidemiological pattern of the disease in the various outbreaks due presumably to different strains of the virus and this has influenced the effectiveness of control programs (4, 5, 12).

Although the economic effects of the primary disease are minor, the cost of the slaughter method for eradication is high (31). Although the morbidity rate with most strains is high the disease generally runs its course in 2–3 weeks and produces a negligible mortality and only a minor setback to production. The major importance of the disease is its close clinical similarity to other vesicular diseases. The necessity for immediate differentiation of an outbreak from foot-and-mouth disease and the problem of having such a similar clinical entity present in the pig population has made eradication of the disease desirable. In most countries this has proved extremely expensive.

Infection generally occurs through minor abrasions on the feet but may occur through other routes. The incubation period is 2–14 days and virus may be excreted prior to the onset of clinical signs. During and for a short period following the viremic phase, virus is excreted in oral and nasal secretions. It is excreted in feces for periods up to 3 weeks, and vesicular fluid and shed vesicular epithelium are potent sources of infection (4). A chronic infection with shedding of virus for periods up to 3 months has been described (14).

As a consequence large amounts of virus are shed in the immediate vicinity of infected pigs. Transmission occurs by direct contact or contact with infected food or water or infected feces and the disease spreads rapidly between pigs within the same group. Airborne transmission of the virus is not a feature and the spread between groups of pigs is less rapid than that which occurs with foot-and-mouth disease (4). The resistance of the virus and its persistence within the environment allows spread by mechanical methods such as trucks and contaminated boots. Areas which have housed infected pigs may remain infective for a considerable period of time. The potential for contaminated communal livestock trucks and markets to spread infection is considerable due to the occurrence of minor foot abrasions that occur during the movement of pigs.

The disease may be sufficiently mild to escape clinical detection. This plus the occurrence of subclinical infection and the reluctance of farmers to report suspicions of its occurrence facilitates spread by the movement of infected pigs to other farms or through markets. Vertical transmission has not been demonstrated (15).

The disease may also be spread by the feeding of uncooked garbage. Pigs killed during the incubation period of the disease or with subclinical infection possess a considerable amount of virus in body tissues. There is little reduction in infectivity with cold storage and the virus can persist in pork and pork products indefinitely (4, 10). Recycling of the virus through garbage feeding with subsequent spread to other piggeries has been a major source of new outbreaks of swine vesicular disease in England and along with spread by direct movement of infected pigs to other piggeries or infection following movement through contaminated markets or livestock trucks accounts for the majority of outbreaks investigated (12).

Pathogenesis

There is variation in the susceptibility of different sites of the body to invasion by swine vesicular disease virus (16, 17) and in natural outbreaks initial infection is most likely through damaged skin. Once infection is established in a pig, virus excretion is so massive as to result in infection of others in the group through the tonsil and gastrointestinal tract as well as through skin abrasions. Experimentally the disease can be reproduced by intravenous, intramuscular, subcutaneous and intradermal inoculation of virus. Infection is followed by viremia and the virus has an especial affinity for epithelium of the coronary band, tongue, lip and snout and for myocardium (18). Lesions in the brain, especially the brainstem (18–20) are seen histologically but nervous signs are not a common clinical finding.

Clinical findings

The incubation period varies from 2 to 14 days. The

disease is usually mild in its manifestation. The morbidity rate varies from 25 to 65% and up to 100% of pigs within a pen may be affected. A transient fever (40–41°C, 104–105°F) and temporary mild inappetence may be seen. Lameness, arching of the back and other signs of foot discomfort are evident but are less severe than with foot-and-mouth disease. Both the incidence of lameness and of foot lesions are influenced by management and are less severe on bedding or with soft conditions underfoot (17). Characteristic vesicles occur at predilection sites frequently associated with trauma. They occur most commonly on the coronary band of the claws, especially at the heel, and of the supernumerary digits. They start as areas of blanching and swelling and progress in 1–2 days to thick-walled vesicles which rupture to give the appearance of an ulcer. In severely affected pigs the lesions will encircle the coronary band and the horn may be shed as in foot-and-mouth disease. Lesions also occur on the tongue, lips and snout and the skin of the legs and belly. They are much less frequent in these areas and frequently do not progress to typical vesicles. An examination of the feet of other apparently normal pigs within the group will often reveal the presence of minor lesions, and the extent of involvement of pigs within the group may be underestimated without careful examination (17, 21). In some outbreaks the incidence of clinical lesions has been minimal and even a single vesicle on the pig's foot should be treated as suspect. Some pigs show no clinical signs but develop significant titers of neutralizing antibody (22). The course of the disease within a group is generally 2–3 weeks, mortality is very uncommon and there is only a minor setback to production unless complete separation of the horny foot occurs. Nervous signs with ataxia, circling, headpressing and convulsions and paralysis have been observed rarely.

Clinical pathology

Tests for the identification of swine vesicular disease include the demonstration of antigen in tissue and the detection of antibody. Vesicular epithelium provides the best material for direct antigen demonstration and it may be present even in the remnants of 10-day-old lesions (4). With fluorescent antibody or direct complement fixation a result may be obtained within 8–12 hours. Virus can also be grown on tissue culture and identified. Specific antibody is produced within 4–6 days and may be demonstrable before clinical disease is evident (4). Antibody may be detected by virus neutralization, double immunodiffusion, counterimmunoelectrophoresis (23) or the enzyme-linked immunosorbent assay (ELISA) for the diagnosis and surveillance of the disease (24). The latter test has been stated to be more sensitive than virus neutralization (23). The counterimmunoelectrophoresis test is rapid, economical and is suggested as an initial large-scale screening test (33).

Necropsy findings

There are no gross or histological findings that differentiate swine vesicular disease from foot-and-mouth disease. Lesions in the skin consist of areas of coagulative necrosis with intraepithelial vesicle formation. Additional necrotic foci are present in the tonsils, renal pelvis, bladder, salivary glands, pancreas and myocardium (25). There is also non-purulent meningoencephalitis (19, 20). Intranuclear inclusions are present in the ganglion amphicytes (34).

Diagnosis

The occurrence of vesicles differentiates this disease from other non-vesicular diseases of pigs. So-called foot-rot in pigs is associated with lesions on the sole and horn of the claw rather than the epithelial area of the coronary band. The differentiation of swine vesicular disease from other vesicular diseases relies on laboratory examination and virus identification as detailed above.

Treatment and control

No treatment is described and none is warranted. In most countries where outbreaks have occurred control has been attempted or achieved by slaughter eradication (11, 12). Depopulation is followed by thorough cleansing and disinfection and limited repopulation effected after a period of 2–3 months. The disposal of infected carcasses can be important as the disposal site may remain infective (26).

The detection of infected herds can prove a problem. The mild nature of the disease means that it can easily escape detection, especially in darkened pig houses or where conditions underfoot obscure observation of the feet. Mild infections may produce little clinical disease and any vesicular lesions should be treated with suspicion. The reluctance of some farmers to report suspicious lesions can also be important and it is essential to institute educational programs emphasizing the necessity for early detection and diagnosis of outbreaks. Serological surveys to identify present or past infections have proved of value in aiding detection of the disease (27).

The three most important methods of spread are the feeding of garbage containing infected pig meat, the movement of pigs from infected farms either directly from farm to farm or indirectly through markets, and the movement of pigs in contaminated transport vehicles. Control of these methods of spread needs to include strict enforcement of garbage-cooking regulations, the closing of markets except perhaps for holding areas for pigs going directly to slaughter, strict control of movement and sale of pigs and adequate cleansing and sanitation of infected areas and transport vehicles. Transmission through feeding of infected meat in garbage appears the most difficult to control and the latent period of this cycle means that outbreaks can recur at a time when eradication was thought to be complete. Control measures that have been used for this disease have been published (11, 12).

Vaccination has not been used for control in most countries; however, an inactivated vaccine is reported to provide significant protection in France (14, 28).

REVIEW LITERATURE

Watson, W. A. (1981) Swine vesicular disease in Great Britain. *Can. vet. J.*, *22*, 195–200.

REFERENCES

(1) Groves, J. H. (1973) *Nature, Lond.*, *245*, 314.
(2) Brown, F. et al. (1976) *J. comp. Pathol.*, *86*, 409.

(3) Garland, A. J. M. (1974) *J. Hyg., Camb.*, *73*, 85.
(4) Burrows, R. (1975) *Adv. vet. Sci.*, *15*, 111.
(5) Burrows, R. et al. (1974) *J. Hyg., Camb.*, *73*, 109.
(6) Brown, F. et al. (1973) *Nature, Lond.*, *245*, 315.
(7) Liebermann, H. C. et al. (1976) *Arch. exp. VetMed.*, *30*, 433.
(8) Blackwell, J. H. et al. (1975) *Br. vet. J.*, *131*, 317.
(9) Cunliffe, H. R. (1975) *Proc. 78th ann. Mtg US Anim. Hlth Assoc.*, 200.
(10) McKercher, P. D. et al. (1975) *Proc. 78th ann. Mtg US Anim. Hlth Assoc.*, 213.
(11) Ford, G. W. (1976) *World Anim. Rev.*, *20*, 42.
(12) Anon (1974) *Vet. Rec.*, *95*, 306.
(13) Tokui, T. et al. (1975) *Natl Inst. Anim. Hlth Q., Tokyo*, *15*, 165.
(14) Gourreau, J. M. et al. (1975) *Rec. Med. vét.*, *151*, 85, 283.
(15) Burrows, R. et al. (1977) *Zentralbl. VetMed.*, *B24*, 177.
(16) Burrows, R. et al. (1974) *J. Hyg., Camb.*, *72*, 135.
(17) Mann, J. A. & Hutchings, G. H. (1980) *J. Hyg., Camb.*, *84*, 355.
(18) Chu, R. M. et al. (1979) *Can. J. comp. Med.*, *43*, 29.
(19) Monlux, W. S. et al. (1975) *Am. J. vet. Res.*, *36*, 1745.
(20) Lai, S. S. et al. (1979) *Am. J. vet. Res.*, *40*, 463.
(21) Groves, J. H. & McKercher, P. D. (1974) *Proc. 77th ann. Mtg US Anim. Hlth Assoc.*, 155.
(22) Mann, J. A. et al. (1976) *Proc. 4th int. Cong. Pig vet. Soc.*, F6.
(23) Bellhouse, R. et al. (1982) *Vet. Rec.*, *110*, 357.
(24) Hamblin, C. & Crowther, J. R. (1982) *Br. vet. J.*, *138*, 247.
(25) Lenghaus, C. & Mann, J. A. (1976) *Vet. Pathol.*, *13*, 186.
(26) Coombs, G. P. (1974) *Proc. 77th ann. Mtg US Anim. Hlth Assoc.* 332.
(27) Hendrie, E. W. et al. (1977) *Vet. Rec.*, *100*, 363.
(28) Gourreau, J. M. et al. (1975) *Rev. Med. Vet.*, *126*, 357.
(29) Harris, T. J. R. et al. (1979) *Infect. Immunol.*, *24*, 593.
(30) Sorensen, K. J. (1980) *Acta vet. Scand.*, *21*, 324.
(31) UK Ministry of Agriculture, Fisheries and Food (1980) *Anim. Dis. Rep.*, *3*, 3–6.
(32) Hendrie, E. W. et al. (1978) *Vet. Rec.*, *102*, 126.
(33) Sorensen, K. J. (1980) *Acta vet. Scand.*, *21*, 318.
(34) Wells, G. A. H. et al. (1979) *Vet. Rec.*, *104*, 552.

Vesicular stomatitis

Vesicular stomatitis (VS) is an infectious disease caused by a virus and characterized clinically by the development of vesicles on the mouth and feet. While primarily a disease of horses, it has come to assume major importance as a disease of cattle and pigs.

Etiology

The causative virus is a vesiculovirus (family Rhabdoviridae). There are two antigenically distinct types, New Jersey and Indiana, with three subtypes of Indiana, Fort Lupton, Alagar (Brazil) and Cocal (Trinidad). The New Jersey strain is the most virulent and the one most commonly found. The virus is much less resistant to environmental influences than the virus of foot-and-mouth disease and it is more readily destroyed by boiling.

Cattle, horses, donkeys and pigs are susceptible, with pigs least so. Goats and sheep are resistant. Outbreaks of the disease are most common in cattle and to a less extent in pigs. Calves are much more resistant to infection than adult cattle. Large numbers of free-living pronghorn antelope in the United States have been found to be seropositive (12). Humans are susceptible, infection causing an influenza-like disease and the development of high antibody titers in man often accompanies outbreaks in cattle (2). Experimentally the disease can be produced in swine by intradermal injection in the snout and by intravenous injection but not by intramuscular injection. In horses and cattle transmission can also be effected by intradermal and intramucosal injection but not by intramuscular injection. Guinea-pigs can be infected by intradermal injection in the foot pads or by intralingual injection. The susceptibility of rabbits varies depending upon the strain of virus used. Passage can also be effected in unweaned white mice and embryonated hen eggs. There is considerable evidence that natural infection in deer, raccoon and feral swine can occur. The importance of these animals in the epidemiology of the disease is doubtful except that deer, because of their liberation of large quantites of virus from oral vesicles, can act as an amplifier host (3). Immunity after a natural attack is solid but lasts for only about 6 months (4).

Epidemiology

Geographically the disease is limited to the western hemisphere and is enzootic in parts of North, Central and South America. The first major occurrence of the disease was in military horses in the United States during the 1914–18 war but in recent years it has come to assume greater importance in cattle and pig herds. The disease itself causes little permanent harm but the losses on large dairy farms due to disruption of continuity of milk supplies may cause severe financial loss (5, 6). There is also much inconvenience and temporary inability to feed. The morbidity rate varies considerably (5–10% is usual but in dairy herds it may be as high as 80%) and there is usually no mortality. Outbreaks are not usually extensive but the disease closely resembles foot-and-mouth disease and has achieved considerable importance for this reason. Occasional human infections give the disase some public health significance.

The saliva and vesicular fluid from clinically affected animals are highly infective but infectivity diminishes rapidly and may be lost within a week after the vesicles rupture. Although mediate or immediate contagion can occur by ingestion of contaminated materials the disease appears to be spread in this way only in large intensive dairies where there is much communal use of water and feed troughs. The transmission of the infection over large distances is by bites of insect vectors but transmission by the ingestion of contaminated pasture occurs also (5). In fed cattle the use of coarse roughage or hard pellets encourages the spread of the infection (10).

Spread within dairy herds also appears to be aided by milking procedures (6). There is a marked seasonal incidence of the disease, cases decreasing sharply with the onset of cold weather. The disease is enzootic in low-lying coastal countries with tropical climates, heavy rainfall and high insect populations. There is also a greater prevalence in geographically protected areas with heavy rainfall, such as valleys in the mountains and foothills (4). Areas of low incidence are protected by natural barriers to insect migration. These observations have given rise to the view that insects, including biting flies and mosquitoes, play a large part in the spread of the disease both locally and from infected to clean areas. The virus has been isolated from *Phlebotomus* spp. sandflies (1) and from *Aedes* spp. mosquitoes (7) and has been shown to multiply in the mosquito *Aedes aegypti* and it is therefore a true arthropod-borne virus. The phlebotomine sandfly *Lutzomyia trapidoi* is also a true vector of the virus (8). It is thought that biting insects carry infection in from Mexico, where the disease is enzootic, to the United States, giving rise to periodic outbreaks (6). In Columbia where the disease is endemic (4) the clinical disease occurs in epidemics about every 4 years. Between these waves the occurrence rate is endemic. Native fauna may similarly provide a reservoir of infection and by their uncontrolled movement act as a means of spread of the disease. It has also been suggested that the infection may persist from year to year in cold-blooded animals such as frogs. Although the causative virus is resistant to environmental influences, its infectivity is not high and outbreaks are not so extensive as in foot-and-mouth disease. For the same reason control of the disease is readily achieved by standard hygienic precautions.

Pathogenesis

As in foot-and-mouth disease there is a primary viremia with subsequent localization in the mucous membrane of the mouth and the skin around the mouth and coronets. The frequent absence of classical vesicles on the oral mucosa of affected animals in field outbreaks has led to careful examination of the pathogenesis of the mucosal lesions. Even in experimentally produced cases only 30% of lesions develop as vesicles, the remainder dehydrating by seepage during development and terminating by eroding as a dry necrotic lesion.

Clinical findings

In cattle after a short incubation period of several days there is a sudden appearance of mild fever and the development of vesicles on the dorsum of the tongue, dental pad, lips and the buccal mucosa. The vesicles rupture quickly and the resultant irritation causes profuse, ropey salivation and anorexia. Confusion often arises in field outbreaks of the disease because of failure to find vesicles. In some outbreaks with thousands of cattle affected, vesicles have been almost completely absent. They are most likely to be found on the cheeks and tongue where soft tissues are abraded by the teeth. At other sites there is an erosive, necrotic lesion. In milking cows there is a marked decrease in milk yield. Lesions on the feet and udder occur only rarely except in milking cows where teat lesions may be extensive and lead to the development of mastitis (13). Recovery is rapid, affected animals being clinically normal in 3–4 days, and secondary complications are relatively rare. In horses the signs are broadly similar but not infrequently the lesions are limited to the dorsum of the tongue or the lips. Other less common sites include the udder of the mare and the prepuce of males. In pigs vesicles develop on or behind the snout or on the feet and lameness is more frequent than in other animals.

Clinical pathology

Animal transmission experiments and culture on embryonated hen eggs as set out in Table 67 may be attempted using fluid collected from unruptured vesicles. Typical vesicles develop after inoculation. A complement fixation test is available which is capable of differentiating the virus from that of foot-and-mouth disease and between the two strains of vesicular stomatitis virus. A resin agglutination inhibition and a serum neutralization test are also used in diagnosis, titers to the latter persisting for much longer than the CF test, often well beyond the point at which the animal has again become susceptible to experimental challenge (9).

Necropsy findings

Necropsy examinations are not usually undertaken for diagnostic purposes but the pathology of the disease has been adequately described.

Diagnosis

Because of its case-for-case similarity to foot-and-mouth disease, prompt and accurate diagnosis of the disease is essential. Foot-and-mouth disease does not occur in horses and vesicular exanthema occurs naturally only in pigs. The morbidity with vesicular stomatitis is much lower and more sporadic than with foot-and-mouth disease. Apart from these species susceptibilities, differentiation on clinical and epizootiological grounds is hazardous. To ensure accurate diagnosis material must be sent to a laboratory for examination as set out in Table 67. Other forms of stomatitis in which lesions occur on the feet, including mucosal disease and bovine malignant catarrh are not characterized by vesicle formation and can be differentiated on this and other clinical grounds. The frequent absence of vesicles in vesicular stomatitis has already been pointed out. Failure to recognize this feature of the disease may unnecessarily delay a correct diagnosis. Similar necrotic lesions occur in necrotic glossitis of steers but this disease can be differentiated serologically from vesicular stomatitis.

Treatment

Treatment is seldom undertaken but mild antiseptic mouthwashes may contribute to the comfort of the animal and the rapidity of recovery.

Control

Hygienic and quarantine precautions to contain the infection within a herd are sufficient control, the disease usually dying out of its own accord. Immunity after an attack appears to be of very short duration, probably not more than 6 months. A live virus vaccination procedure appears to have given good results (11).

REVIEW LITERATURE

Knight, A. P. & Messer, N. T. (1983) Vesicular stomatitis. *Comp. cont. Educ.*, *5*, S517–S522.

Mason, J. et al. (1976) Vesicular stomatitis in Mexico. *Proc. 80th ann. Mtg US Anim. Hlth Assoc.*, p. 234.

REFERENCES

(1) Orrego, U.A. et al. (1978) *Rev. Inst. Colombiano Agropecuoric*, *13*, 321.
(2) Fields, B. N. & Hawkins, K. (1967) *New Engl. J. Med.*, *277*, 989.
(3) Karstad, L. H. (1963) *Proc.1st int. Conf. Wildlife Dis., New York, 1962*, 298.
(4) Mason, J. et al. (1976) *Proc. 80th ann. Mtg US Anim. Hlth Assoc.*, p. 234.
(5) Goodger, W. J. et al. (1985) *J. Am. vet. med. Assoc.*, *186*, 370.
(6) Leder, R. R. et al. (1983) *Bov. Practnr*, *18*, 45.
(7) Sudia, W. D. et al. (1967) *Am. J. Epidemiol.*, *86*, 598.
(8) Tesh, R. B. et al. (1972) *Science, NY*, *175*, 1477.

(9) Geleta, J. N. & Holbrook, A. A. (1961) *Am. J. vet. Res.*, *22*, 713.
(10) Hansen, D. E. et al. (1985) *Am. J. vet. Res.*, *46*, 789.
(11) Lauerman, L. H. &. Hanson, R. P. (1964) *Proc. US live Stk sanit. Assoc.*, *473*, 483.
(12) Thorne, E. T. et al. (1984) *Proc. US Anim. Hlth Assoc.*, *87*, 638.
(13) Alderink, F. J. (1984) *Prev. vet. Med.*, *3*, 29.

Vesicular exanthema of swine

Vesicular exanthema of swine is an acute, febrile, infectious disease of swine caused by a virus. It is indistinguishable clinically from foot-and-mouth disease in swine, vesicular stomatitis and swine vesicular disease.

Etiology

The causative virus is classified as a calicivirus and 13 antigenic strains have been isolated (1–3). There is some variation in virulence between the strains. Only pigs are susceptible although experimental transmission to horses can be effected with some strains of the virus. No experimental animals are susceptible but the virus can be grown in tissue culture. All ages and breeds of pigs are susceptible to infection. The virus is resistant to environmental influences and persists in frozen and chilled meats. It is readily destroyed by several different commonly used disinfectants including sodium hypochlorite, sodium hydroxide, and phenol (4). A good immunity develops after an attack and persists for about 20 months. There is no appreciable crossimmunity between the strains of the virus and a series of outbreaks, each caused by a different strain of the virus, may occur in the one herd of pigs.

A similar if not identical virus, San Miguel sealion virus, has been isolated from sealions and fur seals off the coast of California. It is physically, chemically and morphologically identical to vesicular exanthema virus although the same antigenic types have not been found (5). The virus produces an identical disease to vesicular exanthema when inoculated into pigs and appears to have a similar host range (6). The vesicular exanthema of swine virus is infective for the harp seal but the disease is inapparent and self-limiting (9). The intradermal inoculation of the vesicular exanthema of swine virus into otrarid (fur) seal pups will result in plaque-like lesions (10). Feeding swine the seal tissues from the inoculation experiments will result in seroconversion in swine which were fed tissues from seals infected with the vesicular exanthema of swine virus but not in those which were fed tissues from seals infected with San Miguel sealion virus (10). Antibody to this virus has also been detected in California gray whales and in feral swine inhabiting coastal areas (3, 5).

Epidemiology

Except for isolated outbreaks in Hawaii and Iceland the disease has occurred only in the United States. It is important because of its direct effect and because of the confusion it causes in the diagnosis of foot-and-mouth disease. Although vesicular exanthema is a mild disease with a low mortality rate (usually less than 5% although there may be many deaths in unweaned pigs) affected animals may suffer a severe loss of body weight and convalescence may require several weeks. Pregnant sows may abort and lactating sows may go dry with resultant heavy losses in baby pigs. The disease was eradicated from the United States in 1959, 27 years after its initial appearance (7).

The sources of infection are infected live pigs and infected pork. Infected pigs excrete the virus in saliva and feces but not in the urine for 12 hours before vesicles develop and for 1–5 days afterwards. Raw garbage containing infected pork scraps is the most common medium of spread from farm to farm. On infected premises the disease is spread by direct contact and, although the virus is resistant to environmental influences, spread by indirect means does not occur readily (7). Pigs frequently become infected, as evidenced by the development of immunity, without showing clinical signs of the disease. Ingestion of infected material is sufficient to produce infection.

The isolation from marine animals of an identical virus, which is capable of producing a disease identical to vesicular exanthema when inoculated into pigs, has led to the hypothesis that the primary reservoir for vesicular exanthema is in marine animals. Epizootics in pigs may have been initiated by the feeding of marine meat or garbage containing marine animal products.

Pathogenesis

As in other vesicular diseases there is a viremia, lasting for 72–84 hours and commencing 48 hours before vesication, with localization occurring in the buccal mucosa and the skin above the hooves. The intradermal inoculation of the vesicular exanthema of swine virus and the San Miguel sealion virus into swine results in fluid-filled vesicles at the sites of inoculation in the snout, coronary band, and tongue (11). Lesions are usually limited to the non-haired portions of the integument and tongue. A mild viral encephalitis occurs in pigs inoculated with the swine virus and the sealion virus can be recovered from the brain tissue of pigs infected with the virus (11).

Clinical findings

The incubation period varies with the virulence of the causative strain of virus but is usually 1–3 days. There is an initial high fever (40·5–41°C, 105–106°F) followed by the development of vesicles in the mouth, on the snout, on the teats and udder and on the coronary skin, the sole, the heel bulbs and between the claws, and accompanied by extreme lassitude and complete anorexia. The initial lesion is a blanched area which soon develops into a vesicle full of clear fluid. The vesicles rupture easily leaving raw, eroded areas. This usually occurs about 24–48 hours after they appear and is accompanied by a rapid fall of temperature. Secondary crops of vesicles often follow and may cause local swelling of the face and tongue. Lesions on the feet may predominate in some outbreaks whereas in others they may be of little significance. The affected feet are very sensitive and there is severe lameness. Healing of the oral vesicles occurs rapidly although secondary bacterial infection often exacerbates the lesions on the feet. Recovery in uncomplicated cases is usually complete in 1–2 weeks. When sows become infected late in pregnancy abortion frequently occurs and lactating sows may go dry.

Clinical pathology
Fluid from the vesicles is used in transmission experiments and for tissue culture. Blood serum is used for the complement fixation, viral neutralization in cell culture and gel diffusion precipitin tests (7).

Necropsy findings
Postmortem examinations are not of much value in the diagnosis of vesicular exanthema but the pathology of the disease has been defined (4).

Diagnosis
Vesicular exanthema in pigs cannot be differentiated from foot-and-mouth disease, vesicular stomatitis or swine vesicular disease by clinical or necropsy examination and a definite diagnosis can only be made on transmission experiments or by use of the serological tests (see Table 67). All cases of lameness in pigs in which a number of animals are affected should be examined for the presence of vesicular lesions. Footrot of pigs is readily distinguishable by the absence of vesicles and by the typical underrunning of the hoof wall.

Treatment
No treatment appears to be of value but hyperimmune sera against strains A and B appear to have prophylactic efficiency even in pigs exposed to infection 24 hours previously.

Control
Eradication of the disease should be attempted whenever practicable. The first step is to quarantine infected premises and restrict movement of pigs in the area. Infected animals should be slaughtered but the carcasses may be salvaged for human consumption provided the meat undergoes special treatment to ensure destruction of the virus. Normal freezing and chilling procedures are not sufficient to destroy it. All garbage fed to pigs must be boiled. Infected premises should be thoroughly cleaned and disinfected with a 2% sodium hydroxide solution before restocking. The implementation of these measures was eminently successful in eradicating the disease from the United States (8).

In view of the reservoir of virus in marine animals and apparent infection in feral swine in the coastal areas of California it is possible that the disease could recur in domestic swine in the United States. Possible methods of reintroduction that need to be guarded against have been described (3).

Active immunization may be practicable if the disease reappears and other control measures fail. A formalin-killed virus preparation produces an immunity lasting for at least 6 months. Multivalent vaccines may be required if more than one strain of virus is involved (4).

REVIEW LITERATURE

Smith, A. W. & Akers, T. G. (1976) Vesicular exanthema of swine. *J. Am. vet. med. Assoc.*, *169*, 700.

REFERENCES

(1) Bankowski, R. A. et al. (1957) *Proc. US live Stk sanit. Assoc.*, 302
(2) Shahan, M. S. (1960) *Can. vet. J.*, *1*, 427.
(3) Smith, A. W. & Akers, T. G. (1976) *J. Am. vet. med. Assoc.*, *169*, 700.
(4) Blackwell, J. H. (1978) *Res. vet. Sci.*, *25*, 25.
(5) Sawyer, J. C. (1976) *J. Am. vet. med. Assoc.*, *169*, 707.
(6) Smith, A. W. et al. (1977) *Am. J. vet. Res.*, *38*, 101.
(7) Bankowski, R. A. (1965) *Adv. vet. Sci.*, *10*, 23.
(8) Henderson, W. M. (1960) *Adv. vet. Sci.*, *6*, 19.
(9) Gelberg, H. B. et al. (1982) *Vet. Pathol.*, *19*, 406.
(10) Gelberg, H. B. et al. (1982) *Vet. Pathol.*, *19*, 413.
(11) Gelberg, H. B. & Lewis, R. M. (1982) *Vet. Pathol.*, *19*, 424.

Rinderpest

Rinderpest is an acute, highly contagious disease of ruminants and swine caused by a virus and characterized by high fever and focal, erosive lesions confined largely to the mucosa of the alimentary tract. The disease occurs in plague form and is highly fatal.

Etiology
The causative morbillivirus (family Paramyxoviridae) occurs as many strains with considerable variation in virulence between them but all are immunologically identical. The virus seems to have some antigenic relationship to the viruses of distemper (1) and measles (9) and to a virus of sheep and goats which appears to be a strain of rinderpest virus which has become adapted to these species but which has lost its ability to infect cattle by contact (2). There are two related diseases that need to be noted. They are *peste des petits ruminants* (PPR) of sheep and goats, and *kata*, a stomatitis pneumoenteritis of Nigerian dwarf goats. Although there is some confusion about the causative viruses they do appear to be very closely related biologically and antigenically (3, 4). In goats, *peste des petits ruminants* is a disease which spreads very rapidly like rinderpest in cattle, and large amounts of virus are excreted in all body excretions, especially diarrheic feces (14). Morbidity rates of 40% and mortality rates of 85% are not unusual (22). Although sheep are easily infected and become seropositive the development of severe clinical disease is unusual in this species (6). These diseases represent a formidable barrier to the eradication of rinderpest from the African continent.

Epidemiology
Historically rinderpest (cattle plague) has been among the most devastating of cattle diseases. It is capable of complete eradication but the disruptions of war and civil strife in which disease controls disappear have caused the disease to be undiminished. It was eradicated from China in 1955 and has not recurred there since, an extraordinary achievement. The disease was almost cleared from East Africa in the 1960s, but because of failure to maintain vaccination programs it is undergoing a dangerous resurgence (8). It still occurs enzootically in equatorial and northeast Africa and in parts of Asia and epizootics of major importance occur from time to time in free countries, such as eastern Europe, when diseased cattle are introduced. The disease has never appeared in North America but there have been single outbreaks which were quickly eradicated in South America and Australia. Rinderpest still has more influence on the world's food supply than any other animal disease and has tremendous destructive potential in such high-risk areas as central and southern Africa.

When epizootics occur in highly susceptible populations the morbidity and mortality rates are high and large numbers of in-contact animals must be destroyed if eradication is undertaken. In enzootic areas most of the cattle population have some degree of immunity and major outbreaks are rare although subacute cases are common. In outbreaks which occur as a result of spread from these areas to areas with highly susceptible populations morbidity rates approximating 100% and mortality rates of 50% (25–90%) are to be anticipated (7).

The rinderpest virus is very sensitive to environmental influences and is readily destroyed by heat, drying and most disinfectants. It is relatively resistant to cold and may survive for as long as a month in blood kept under refrigeration. It survives in premises for a few days only.

All ruminants and pigs are susceptible to infection with rinderpest virus. Natural infection occurs commonly only in cattle and buffalo but in some outbreaks, sheep and goats do become infected, and in some cases are the primary target of the infection, subsequently spreading the infection to cattle. Indian buffalo develop typical signs of the disease and are protected against infection by vaccination with tissue-culture vaccine. European pigs are susceptible to infection but a mild transient fever is the only clinical sign ; however, spread from pig to pig does not occur and the species is considered to be unimportant in the epidemiology of the disease (11). Pigs indigenous to Thailand and Malaysia are highly susceptible and natural spread of the clinical disease occurs commonly. Goats and sheep in India, Ceylon and Africa contract the disease in the field although they are relatively resistant to infection. Egyptian sheep and goats develop antibodies when inoculated with virulent virus but show no clinical signs and are not a source of infection for other animals (10). Wild ruminants are a common source of infection and are a very great hindrance to an eradication program. Those most commonly affected are the water and shade-loving species, the buffalo, bushbuck, waterbuck and warthogs. Amongst the races of cattle the zebus are most resistant. Rabbits can be artificially infected and this is made use of in the production of lapinized virus. One-humped camels become infected, but show no clinical signs and are considered not to be a source of infection for other animals.

Immunity after a natural infection is long but does not always persist for life. Immunity after vaccination varies in duration, generally in proportion to the severity of the clinical response obtained.

The virus is present in the blood, tissues, secretions and excretions of infected animals, reaching its peak of concentration at about the height of the temperature reaction and subsiding gradually to disappear about a week after the temperature returns to normal in those animals that recover. The virus is very susceptible to external influences and does not persist outside the animal body for more than a few hours at normal temperatures and dies in cadavers within 24 hours. Close contact between infected and non-infected animals is usually necessary for spread of the disease to occur. Although the precise site of entry of field strains of the virus in natural infections is not known, the bulk of evidence indicates that infection occurs principally by inhalation (2, 12). Aerosol inhalation has been demonstrated (5) with survival of the virus in this form depending particularly on humidity, the period being longer at relatively low humidity, sometimes lasting more than 30 minutes. Ingestion of food contaminated by the discharges of clinical cases or animals in the incubation stage, or animals with subclinical infections, may also be an important mode of infection, especially in pigs. Insects, many of which have been shown to contain the virus, are unlikely to act as vectors. Other species including European breeds of pigs in particular, and sheep, goats, camels and wild ruminants may serve as a source of the virus for cattle. Although there may be rare exceptions (13), it is doubtful that recovered animals act as carriers for more than a few days. Because of the failure of the virus to persist outside the body rinderpest is relatively easy to control provided wild animals do not serve as a reservoir of infection.

Pathogenesis

The virus of rinderpest has a high degree of affinity for lymphoid tissue and alimentary mucosa. There is a striking destruction of lymphocytes in tissues, and although this has little or no effect on the clinical or gross necropsy findings it is the cause of the leukopenia which occurs. The virus is intimately associated with the leukocytes, only a small proportion being free in the plasma and thus filterable. The focal, necrotic stomatitis and enteritis which are characteristic of the disease are the direct result of the viral infection (13).

Clinical findings

The following descriptions present the principal clinical signs of rinderpest but it must be remembered that an almost unlimited series of variations in syndromes may be encountered depending upon the virulence of the strain of virus, the susceptibility of the host and the presence of other diseases which may occur concurrently or be aggravated by the occurrence of the clinical illness of rinderpest.

An incubation period of 6–9 days is usual in field cases but it may be only 2–3 days after experimental administration of the virus. The first stage of the disease is a period of several days in which there is high fever (40·5–41·5°C, 105–107°F), without localizing signs. Anorexia, a fall in milk yield, lacrimation and a harsh, staring coat accompany the fever. Inflammation of the buccal and nasal mucosae and the conjunctivae follows and there may be hyperemia of the vaginal mucosa and swelling of the vulva. The lacrimation becomes more profuse and then purulent and is accompanied by blepharospasm. Bubbly salivation of clear bloodstained saliva is followed by purulent saliva as mouth lesions develop. A serous nasal discharge similarly becomes purulent. Discrete, necrotic lesions (1–5 mm in diameter) develop, appearing in the first instance on the inside of the lower lip and the adjacent gum, on the cheek mucosa at the commissures and the lower surface of the tongue. Later they become general in the mouth, including the dorsum of the tongue, and may become so extensive that they coalesce. Similar lesions are common on the nasal, vulval and vaginal mucosae. The lesions are grayish in color, slightly raised and obviously necrotic. The necrotic material sloughs leaving a raw, red area with sharp edges. Vesicles are not present at any stage. Skin lesions affecting the perineum, scrotum, flanks, the inner aspects of the thighs and the neck occur in some cases. The skin becomes moist and reddened and later covered with scabs. Severe diarrhea, and sometimes dysentery with tenesmus, appear as lesions developing in the abomasum and intestines.

After a period of illness lasting from 3 to 5 days there is a sudden fall in temperature accompanied by exacerbation of the mucosal lesions, dyspnea, cough, severe dehydration and sometimes abdominal pain. Prostration and a further fall in body temperature to subnormal occur on the 6th–12th day after which death usually occurs within 24 hours.

In enzootic areas where resistance to the infection is high both a subacute form and a skin form occur. In the subacute form the temperature reaction is mild and the accompanying anorexia and malaise are not marked. The inflammation of the mucosae is catarrhal only and there is no dysentery. Ulcers may develop in the abomasum without causing clinical signs. In the skin form the systemic reaction is absent and small pustules develop on the neck and over the withers, inside the thighs and on the scrotum.

Signs and lesions similar to those which occur in cattle develop in sheep and goats but the disease does not appear to spread readily from these species to cattle. European pigs are susceptible but the disease is clinically inapparent, whereas Asian pigs develop the typical clinical disease and suffer a high mortality. Spread from pigs to cattle occurs sufficiently frequently to make them a dangerous source of infection for cattle. In some areas rinderpest is featured by pneumonia, the disease closely resembling contagious pleuropneumonia.

The clinical syndrome in *peste des petits ruminants* is very similar to that of rinderpest (17). Affected goats show fever, oral mucosal erosions, diarrhea and pneumonia. There may be erosions of the vulva or prepuce and abortions occur in some.

Clinical pathology

A marked leukopenia occurs at the height of the infection and after vaccination in cattle and in experimentally infected sheep and pigs even though these animals may show minimal clinical illness. The total count usually falls to below 4000/μl with a marked neutrophilia a few days later.

A complement fixation test suitable for diagnostic purposes on a herd basis is available. Antibodies in serum reach peak levels about 14 days after the development of the clinical disease. In animals which have recovered for longer periods the antibody level may be so low that the test is unsatisfactory and the serum neutralization test is used. The test is unlikely to be used in countries where outbreaks occur for the first time. In these circumstances material is likely to be submitted for examination at earlier stages of the disease and virus recovery and identification are more applicable. Other available serological tests include those based on the detection of fluorescent antibody and immunoperoxidase (13), an ELISA which is accurate and easy to perform (10), and a rapid dot-immunoassay test suitable for field use (24).

Confirmation by the experimental transmission of the disease is expensive and dangerous unless isolation facilities with maximum security are available. The recipient group should include one or more animals immune to rinderpest, an unlikely facility in a country free of the disease. The intravenous injection of 5 ml of blood from an affected animal at the height of the disease into susceptible cattle is followed by the development of signs in 3–10 days. Sheep can be used as recipients but there may be only a mild febrile reaction and erosions may not appear.

A technique suitable for laboratory use is the agar gel diffusion (AGID) technique using needle biopsy samples of lymph node as antigen. Provided samples are taken at the optimum time, 3–5 days after fever commences, a high proportion of correct diagnoses is obtained. The proportion of positive reactors to the test falls sharply after diarrhea commences. Other satisfactory methods of detecting rinderpest antigen in feces, buccal scrapings, and ocular and nasal discharges in the early stages of the disease are the agar gel precipitation test and the counterimmunoelectrophoresis techniques (15).

The isolation of the virus and its identification is now practicable in tissue culture. Irrespective of the method used, the optimum tissue for the detection of antigen or the isolation of virus is fresh lymph node and the optimum time of collection is the 3rd–6th day of fever (13).

Necropsy findings

The important necropsy findings are observed in the alimentary tract. Small, discrete, necrotic areas develop on the mucosa and separation of the necrotic material leaves sharply walled, deep erosions with a red floor which may coalesce to form large erosions. They are present in the mouth, pharynx and first third of the esophagus and may extend into the nasal cavities. Similar lesions are present on the mucosa of the abomasum which is characteristically red and swollen and shows multiple small, submucosal hemorrhages. These changes are most marked in the pyloric region. There are no lesions in the forestomachs. In severe cases the lesions extend into the first and last parts of the small intestine and into the large intestines particularly at the cecocolic junction. Zones of hemorrhage and erythema running transversely across the colonic mucosa produce a characteristic striped appearance. Congestion, swelling and erosion of the vulval and vaginal mucosae may occur. The histology of rinderpest is characterized by the massive destruction of lymphocytes, particularly noticeable in lymph nodes and material sent for laboratory examination should include fixed sections of lymph node and alimentary tract lesions as well as fresh spleen, blood and alimentary tract for transmission experiments.

Lesions in *peste des petits ruminants* include erosions of the vulval and preputial skin and mucosa and of the alimentary tract, and a giant-cell pneumonia (17).

Diagnosis

Rinderpest should be suspected when a number of animals are affected by a febrile, fatal, highly infectious disease characterized by erosion and inflammation of the alimentary tract mucosa and by diarrhea. Salivation, nasal discharge and lacrimation are also characteristic. Confirmation of the diagnosis requires transmission experiments or suitable laboratory tests. Because the disease spreads so rapidly and because animals are capable of discharging infective virus before signs appear an early provisional diagnosis is essential.

Foot-and-mouth disease and hemorrhagic septicemia are other diseases which occur in epizootics but are sufficiently dissimilar to present no difficulty in differentiation. Jembrana disease and the mucosal type diseases, including bovine malignant catarrh and mucosal disease present the major difficulty in diagnosis. Bovine malignant catarrh rarely affects many animals in one herd and is characterized by specific eye lesions and nervous signs. Mucosal disease either occurs in explosive outbreaks like rinderpest but the mortality rate is low, or it occurs sporadically, but is uniformly fatal. In sheep and goats bluetongue and sheep and goat pox may present problems in differentiation.

Treatment

Treatment is ineffective and should not be undertaken because of the danger of disseminating the disease. Caprinized vaccine is of no value in treatment and animals in the incubation stage or infected up to 48 hours after vaccination are not protected by use of the vaccine.

Control

Rinderpest is a simple disease and should be easy to eradicate. Theoretically its complete elimination awaits only the development of sufficient veterinary personnel and suitable facilities and the control of freeliving animals of susceptible species. For example, the prevalence in India had been reduced to less than 10 per 100 000 head before 1963, but complete eradication remains an elusive goal, the prevalence remaining at 5–7·5 per 100 000 cattle for the past 10 years in spite of great expansion of numbers of vaccinated cattle (16).

Although the introduction of rinderpest to a previously uninfected country is most likely to occur by the importation of infected animals, particularly to zoological gardens, the possibility does exist that carcass meat infected with the virus could be a portal of entry. Uncooked, infected garbage has been shown to be capable of infecting pigs which subsequently spread the infection to other pigs and to cattle. Prevention of the introduction of ruminants and pigs from known infected areas is routinely practiced in countries which do not have the disease. Countries with land borders to enzootic areas can usually be adequately protected by satisfactory quarantine at the border and the erection of immune barrier zones.

When epizootics occur in normally free areas it is necessary to prevent movement of both living animals and fresh animal products. All susceptible animals in infected and in-contact groups must be slaughtered and disposed of on the respective farms. All ruminants and pigs must be considered susceptible and special attention should be given to native fauna. Infected premises should be disinfected as an additional precaution. When outbreaks are threatened or when an outbreak is extensive and likely to get out of control, all ruminants and pigs in the danger area should be vaccinated with an attenuated virus vaccine. This includes wild ruminants, all of whom are likely to be susceptible and potential carriers of the infection (19).

In enzootic areas control depends upon the use of an efficient vaccination procedure. Periodic vaccination of all susceptible livestock, especially yearling cattle, is generally practiced. When outbreaks occur all affected and in-contact animals are vaccinated. Suitable legal and administrative powers are necessary for the proper use of control by vaccination. The choice of vaccine depends upon the availability of livestock for repeated vaccinations, a necessary step if attenuated vaccines are used. Failing this, lapinized virus is preferred. Eradication can be contemplated in an enzootic area if wild ruminants can be eliminated as a source of infection and if the incidence in domestic species can be reduced to a suitable level by vaccination. The greatest problem in a vaccination program is the selection of a vaccine which will produce adequate immunity without causing a severe reaction in the vaccinated animals. Susceptibility to the rinderpest virus varies greatly between different classes of stock. In general young animals and British breeds of cattle are much more susceptible than indigenous native stock although some local African breeds are highly susceptible. A standard vaccine capable of producing an immune reaction in susceptible cattle may fail to produce a satisfactory immune response in native cattle. Conversely, a standard vaccine capable of producing immunity in native cattle often produces severe reactions in susceptible cattle. The ideal vaccine is one which can be produced with varying degrees of attenuation suitable for safe and effective vaccination of cattle with different levels of susceptibility.

The second most important problem associated with rinderpest vaccination is the activation of existing latent infections in vaccinated animals. In general the problem is greater after the use of less attenuated vaccines. Although protozoal infections present the greatest risk, bacterial and viral diseases may also be activated (2). Vaccination of cattle with ears heavily infested with the tick *Rhiphicephalus appendiculatus* should be avoided. Calves present a special problem. If they receive no antibodies in the colostrum they can be successfully vaccinated at 1 day of age, but if they are from immune cows the vaccination will be ineffective if carried out before about 9 months of age. Correspondingly colostrum-fed calves from immune cows are passively immune for periods of 4–8 months, the duration depending upon the immune status of the dam. The possibility that vaccinated animals can be infected and become active carriers of the virus is unresolved. Vaccinated calves or calves with colostral antibody are susceptible to experimental intranasal infection with the rinderpest virus and will subsequently excrete the virus to susceptible in-contact animals (18). A number of vaccination procedures is available (2). Preparation of the vaccines is simplified by the common antigenicity of all known strains of the rinderpest virus. Thus a vaccine prepared from one strain will protect against all other strains. The simultaneous serum–virus vaccine has been virtually discarded because of the danger of spreading the disease. An inactivated virus vaccine has been used but produces immunity for short periods only unless multiple vaccination is practiced. An adjuvant vaccine containing formalinized, rinderpest-infected bovine spleen in a mixture of mineral oil and freeze-dried, heat-killed myobacteria is an effective immunizing agent but is not practicable because of the severe local reaction produced. Rinderpest vaccine protects goats against infection with the virus of *peste des petits ruminants* for at least 12 months although the two viruses are antigenically different (3). Although the rinderpest virus has no serological similarity to that of mucosal disease, immunity to the latter provides some protection against infection with the former.

Although attenuated virus vaccines have universally replaced killed vaccines in rinderpest control in enzootic countries, there is still a need for a killed vaccine for use in countries where rinderpest does not occur but the risk of its introduction is high. For this purpose a killed vaccine prepared from tissue culture virus is available (20). A dual vaccine against rinderpest and contagious bovine pleuropneumonia is in use in Africa but its efficiency against contagious bovine pleuropneumonia (CBPP) is less than maximal and it is not generally recommended (26).

The following attenuated viruses are in general use.

Goat-adapted virus
This produces lifelong immunity and is satisfactory for use in zebu-type cattle and in some areas where a degree of natural immunity is to be anticipated. It is still sufficiently virulent to cause undesirably severe reactions in susceptible animals, particularly calves, buffalo and British breeds of cattle. Pyrexia, severe gastroenteritis and agalactia result. The reaction can be prevented by the use of hyperimmune serum but this is too costly for general use.

Rabbit-adapted virus
Lapinized virus vaccine can be sufficiently attenuated to avoid severe reactions in susceptible animals but it is then too attenuated for use in zebu-type animals. There is doubt also as to the stability of the attenuation of vaccine. The immunity produced is solid for about 2 years. A particular advantage claimed for the lapinized virus is that it can be transported and maintained in rabbits where no refrigeration facilities are available.

Chicken embryo-adapted virus
Adaptation of the rinderpest virus to grow on hen eggs is achieved with some difficulty but the vaccine produced is cheap, stable, and capable of varying degrees of attenuation so as to be safe for highly susceptible and partially resistant cattle. The vaccine has not undergone extensive field trials and its efficiency is variable (21). Until the vaccine has been proved under all field conditions it is unlikely to supplant the goat-adapted virus which is in general use in enzootic areas. The immunity produced persists for at least 16 months.

Cell culture vaccine
The adaptation of the rinderpest virus to tissue culture has led to the development of cell culture vaccines (22, 23) which have almost completely supplanted the other attenuated virus vaccines. They are easy and cheap to produce, can be freeze-dried and therefore have a long shelf-life, are capable of varying degrees of attenuation, and are thus safer in all situations, and appear to produce an immunity of up to 10 years duration. The attenuated virus does not spread from vaccinated to in-contact cattle (12). The vaccine used for cattle is suitable for use in sheep and goats.

Measles vaccine
This protects calves against rinderpest at an age when ordinary rinderpest vaccines are ineffective. It is also an efficient vaccine for use in adult cattle (25).

REVIEW LITERATURE

DeTray, D. E. (1980) Rinderpest. *Bov. Practnr*, *15*, 181.
Plowright, W. (1986) *Rinderpest Virus*, Virology Monographs. Vienna and New York: Springer Verlag.
Saouma, E. (1983) Rinderpest. *World Anim. Rev.*, *Spec. Suppl. Issue.*

REFERENCES

(1) Delay, P. D. et al. (1965) *Am. J. vet. Res.*, *26*, 1359.
(2) Scott, G. R. (1964) *Adv. vet. Sci.*, *9*, 114.
(3) Taylor, W. P. (1980) *Res. vet. Sci.*, *27*, 321.
(4) Taylor, W. P. & Abegunde, A. (1979) *Res. vet. Sci.*, *26*, 94.
(5) Hyslop, N. St. G. (1979) *Int. J. Biometeorol.*, *23*, 1.
(6) Obi, T. U. et al. (1983) *Trop. Vet.*, *1*, 209.
(7) Abraham, A. et al. (1984) *Refuah Vet.*, *41*, 112.
(8) Rossiter, P. B. et al. (1983) *Vet. Rec.*, *120*, 59.
(9) Dardiri, A. H. et al. (1976) *Proc. 19th ann. Mtg Am. Assoc. Vet. Lab. Diagnosticians*, p. 337.
(10) Sharma, B. et al. (1983) *Ind. J. anim. Sci.*, *53*, 292.
(11) Nawathe, D. R. & Taylor, W. P. (1979) *Trop. Anim. Hlth Prod.*, *11*, 120.
(12) Taylor, W. P. & Plowright, W. (1965) *J. Hyg.*, *Camb.*, *63*, *263*, 497.
(13) Joshi, R. C. et al. (1984) *Trop. Anim. Hlth Prod.*, *16*, 67.
(14) Shanthikumar, S. R. et al. (1985) *Vet. Rec.*, *117*, 469.
(15) Obi, T. U. & Patrick, D. (1984) *J. Hyg.*, *Camb.*, *93*, 579.
(16) Scott, G. R. & Ramachandran, S. (1974) *Trans. R. Soc. trop. Med. Hyg.*, *68*, 276.
(17) Obi, T. U. et al. (1983) *Zentralbl. VetMed.*, *30*, 751.
(18) Provost, A. (1972) *Rev. Elev. Med. vet. Pays trop.*, *25*, 155.
(19) Paling, R. W. et al. (1979) *J. Wildlife Dis.*, *15*, 351.
(20) Mirchamsy, H. et al. (1974) *Res. vet. Sci.*, *17*, 242.
(21) Provost, A. et al. (1961) *Rev. Elev. Med. vet. Pays trop.*, *14*, 375, 385.
(22) Opasina, B. A. et al. (1985) *Trop. Anim. Hlth Prod.*, *17*, 219.
(23) Plowright, W. (1984) *J. Hyg.*, *Camb.*, *92*, 285.
(24) Afshar, A. & Myers, D. J. (1986) *Trop. Anim. Hlth Prod.*, *18*, 209.
(25) Provost, A. et al. (1986) *Rev. Elev. Med. vet. Pays trop.*, *21*, 145.
(26) Jeggo M. H. et al. (1987) *Vet. Rec.*, *120*, 131.

Bovine malignant catarrh (malignant head catarrh, malignant catarrhal fever)

Bovine malignant catarrh (BMC) is an acute, highly fatal, infectious disease of cattle and farmed deer caused by a virus. It is characterized by the development of an erosive stomatitis and gastroenteritis, and erosions in the upper respiratory tract, keratoconjunctivitis, encephalitis, cutaneous exanthema and lymph node enlargement. It may occur sporadically or in explosive outbreaks.

Etiology
The identified virus which causes bovine malignant catarrh is the alcelaphine herpesvirus-1 derived from wildebeeste. The agent which originates from and

causes the same disease in cattle is assumed to be identical or very similar to the wildebeeste virus but it has not yet been isolated and identified. The causative herpesvirus is difficult to isolate from the blood because of its close association with either red or white blood cells, particularly the latter. It is very fragile and the usual methods of storage, including freezing, destroy it quickly. Material collected for transmission experiments must be used within 24 hours. The exact definition of the virus may not be complete and it has been suggested that it may be a morbillivirus and be related to the rinderpest virus (19).

There appear to be a number of strains of the virus which may be antigenically different. Some strains can be transmitted with difficulty by intracerebral inoculation in rabbits (1) and, in general, the European and American virus, the so-called 'sheep-associated bovine malignant catarrh', is difficult to transmit experimentally to cattle; the virus isolated from a red deer or an infected rabbit has been passed to fetal lambs (37). On the other hand the African virus, the 'wildebeeste associated' virus, can be readily transmitted by several routes. This virus, identified also as the alcelaphine herpesvirus-1, or AHV-1, has been adapted to grow on egg yolk-sac and transmission to rabbits, to yolk-sac, to cattle has been achieved (2). The African bovine malignant catarrh virus isolated from blue wildebeeste has been cultivated successfully in tissue culture (3). The African virus is identified as bovid herpesvirus-3; the European–US virus is not yet identified but has been transmitted, with great irregularity, from cattle to other cattle, to rabbits and Syrian hamsters (18). Neither of the viruses cause any disease in their principal host, the wildebeeste and the sheep.

Epidemiology

Bovine malignant catarrh in Africa appears to be an infection of wildebeeste and hartebeest which causes them no harm, but when the infection spills over into abnormal hosts, specifically cattle, a highly fatal disease results. In North America, Europe and Australia a similar epidemiological pattern appears to exist, with sheep as the normal inapparent host, and cattle again the recipient of a highly fatal infection. Sheep are not always the donors and there may be other viruses in other hosts, possibly goats, which play the same epidemiological war game (4).

Bovine malignant catarrh occurs in most countries but is probably of most importance in Africa. The disease has also been recorded in the United States, Canada, Australia, New Zealand, Europe, Scandinavia and the East Indies. The disease is almost invariably fatal, although a recovery rate of 38% is recorded (4). The morbidity rate varies. In most instances the disease occurs as an isolated case in individual herds but a high morbidity (up to 50% in a herd) occurs occasionally in North America (5) and Scandinavia (4) and even higher morbidity rates have been observed in Africa. A severe outbreak in a feedlot in the United States resulted in the death of 87 of 231 cattle over a period of 68 days (6) and in drylot dairy cattle 166 of 1000 cows were affected (22). Similar outbreaks occur in Australia, New Zealand (7) and Malaysia (25).

Amongst domestic animals the clinical disease occurs only in cattle and buffalo, but sheep and goats develop inapparent infections. The causative virus has been isolated from clinically normal blue wildebeeste in Africa. A presumptive diagnosis has been made in white-tailed deer in which a serious outbreak occurred. The disease has also occurred in housed red deer. Buffalo, American bison and European bison are also affected (23, 31). In Africa assorted wild ruminants contract the disease and suffer a severe illness and a high mortality. Similar species in zoos are also commonly affected, e.g. Pere David's deer and Greater kudus (10). Captive sika deer exposed to wildebeeste or sheep have developed the head and eye form of the peracute form of bovine malignant catarrh (17). One of the forms of this disease which is of increasing importance is the disease of cultivated deer (8, 30). The clinical signs and necropsy findings closely resemble those of bovine malignant catarrh in cattle (24) and the morbidity and mortality are disastrously high resulting in heavy losses for the deer farmer. There are frightening implications for nearby cattle farms, but there are no reports of cross-infection, and attempted experimental transmission has not been successful. All ages, races and breeds of cattle are equally susceptible but Banteng (5), buffalo (*Bubalus bubalis*) (9) and deer (8) are more susceptible and suffer a more severe form of the disease then do commercial cattle. The disease shows the greatest incidence in late winter, spring and summer months.

Transmission can be effected experimentally at the height of the febrile reaction by the transfusion of uncoagulated blood but the difficulty of obtaining infective blood causes many failures in transmission, especially with the European virus. The inoculation of lymph node material into lymph node is a satisfactory technique for the African virus.

The method by which bovine malignant catarrh spreads naturally is uncertain. Spread by direct contact between cattle does not seem to occur but it may do so. The slow rate of spread in most instances and the seasonal incidence in the warmer months suggests spread by an insect vector of an infection that is available from the donor for a short period only. However, the occurrence of outbreaks in which large numbers of cattle become affected within a short period and during the winter months suggests that infection can occur by other routes.

Most records show a close association between outbreaks of bovine malignant catarrh and communal raising of cattle and sheep (4). This is particularly true in Europe and North America where affected cattle usually have a history of close contact with sheep and there is no doubt that sheep and probably goats can carry the virus as an inapparent infection. Cattle-to-sheep-to-cattle transmission has been effected on a number of occasions. In North America outbreaks of bovine malignant catarrh most commonly occur when cattle are housed with the sheep, the outbreak usually occurring soon after lambing (5). This is not a prerequisite, one outbreak having occurred when cattle comingled with rams (25). Spread from lambing ewes supports the view that congenital infection can occur and may be an important method of transmission, especially in carrier species. A report is on record of a cow giving birth to four infected calves during an 80-month period following an inapparent infection (11).

In Africa, outbreaks in cattle occur commonly where they have access to wild ruminants, particularly blue wildebeeste when they are calving and transmission from this species to cattle has been observed when they are housed together. A continuous viremia of up to 10 weeks' duration, during which they are infective to cattle, makes the young blue wildebeeste an important source of infection (3). The virus is present in a cell-free form in the nasal and ocular secretions, rendering them infective, a situation not duplicated in cattle (12). The proportion of sheep in a wildebeeste area which are serologically positive and presumably infected with the wildebeeste-associated virus is very high (36).

The persistence of the infection in a particular feedlot, or on a particular farm, from year to year when no contact with these carrier species exists, is unexplained. Persistence of the virus on inanimate fomites has been suggested but the virus is a most fragile one and this seems unlikely. The observation that some recovered cattle show a persistent viremia for many months suggests that carrier animals may be the source of these carryover infections (13, 14). Sheep running over the same paddocks or housed in the same barn are an obvious source of infection (15). A reservoir of infection in wild rabbits has also been suggested.

Pathogenesis

Bovine malignant catarrh is a fatal, multisystemic disease characterized by lymphoid hyperplasia, and widespread vascular epithelial and mesothelial lesions which are morphologically associated with lymphoid cells (28). Involvement of the vascular adventitia (13) accounts for the development of gross lesions, including the epithelial erosions and keratoconjunctivitis. The lymph node enlargement is due to atypical proliferation of sinusoidal cells, and the cerebromeningeal changes, usually referred to as encephalitis, are in fact a form of vasculitis. There is commonly a synovitis, especially involving tibiotarsal joints. This is associated with a lymphoid vasculitis. The disease is essentially an immunological dysfunction in which a subset of T-lymphocytes is the target. Subsequent changes result in widespread lymphoid cell hypoplasia and tissue necrosis, the characteristic lesions of BMC (19).

Clinical findings

The incubation period in natural infection varies from 3 to 8 weeks, and after artificial infection averages 22 days (14–37 days). Bovine malignant catarrh is described as occurring in a number of forms, the peracute, the alimentary tract form, the common 'head and eye' form and the mild form, but these are all gradations, cases being classified on the predominant clinical signs. In serial transmissions with one strain of the virus all of these forms may be produced.

The 'head and eye' form

In the 'head and eye' form there is a sudden onset of extreme dejection, anorexia, agalactia, high fever (41–41·5°C, 106–107°F), rapid pulse rate (100–120 /min), a profuse mucopurulent nasal discharge, severe dyspnea with stertor due to obstruction of the nasal cavities with exudate, ocular discharge, with variable degrees of edema of the eyelids, blepharospasm, and congestion of scleral vessels. Superficial necrosis is evident in the anterior nasal mucosa and on the buccal mucosa. This begins as a diffuse reddening of the mucosa, and is a consistent finding about the 19th or 20th day after infection. Discrete local areas of necrosis appear on the hard palate, gums and gingivae. The mouth is painful at this time and the animal moves its jaws carefully, painfully and with a smacking sound. The mucosa as a whole is fragile and splits easily. The mouth and tongue are slippery and the mouth is hard to open. The erosive mucosal lesions may be localized or diffuse. They may occur on the hard palate, the dorsum of the tongue, the gums below the incisors, the commissures of the mouth, or inside the lips. The cheek papillae inside the mouth are hemorrhagic, especially at the tips which are later eroded. At this stage there is excessive salivation with saliva, which is ropey and bubbly, hanging from the lips. The skin of the muzzle is extensively involved commencing with discrete patches of necrosis at the nostrils which soon coalesce causing the entire muzzle to be covered by tenacious scabs. Similar lesions may occur at the skin–horn junction of the feet especially at the back of the pastern. The skin of the teats, vulva and scrotum in acute cases may slough off entirely on touching or become covered with dry, tenacious scabs. Nervous signs, particularly weakness in one leg, incoordination, a demented appearance and muscle tremor may develop very early, and with nystagmus are common in the late stages. Head-pushing, paralysis and convulsions may occur in the final stages. Trismus has been described in affected cattle in one outbreak (25), but it was probably due to pain in the mouth rather than a neuromuscular spasm. In natural cases the superficial lymph nodes are often visibly and usually palpably enlarged. Lymphadenopathy is also one of the earliest, most consistent, and persistent signs of the experimental disease (33).

The consistency of the feces varies from constipation to profuse diarrhea with dysentery. In some cases there is gross hematuria with the red coloration most marked at the end of urination. Opacity of the cornea is always present in some degree, commencing as a narrow, gray ring at the corneoscleral junction and spreading centripetally. Hypopyon is observed in some cases. The ocular discharge and the nasal discharge may become profuse and purulent if the animal survives for more than a few days. With the development of oral lesions, continual chewing movements and bubbly salivation occur. In cases of longer duration, skin changes, including local papule formation with clumping of the hair into tufts over the loins and withers, may occur and eczematous weeping may result in crust formation particularly on the perineum, around the prepuce, in the axillae and inside the thighs. Infection of the cranial sinuses may occur with pain on percussion over the area. The horns and rarely the hooves may be shed. Persistence of the fever is a characteristic of bovine malignant catarrh, even cases that persist for several weeks having a fluctuating temperature, usually exceeding 39·5°C (103°F).

During some outbreaks an occasional animal makes an apparent recovery but usually dies 7–10 days later of acute encephalitis. In the more typical cases the illness lasts for 3–7 and rarely up to 14 days.

The peracute form

In the peracute form the disease runs a short course of 1–3 days and characteristic signs and lesions of the 'head and eye' form do not appear. There is usually a high fever, dyspnea and an acute gastroenteritis. The alimentary tract form resembles the 'head and eye' form except that there is marked diarrhea and only minor eye changes consisting of conjunctivitis rather than ophthalmia. This form of the disease has been encountered in outbreak form in cattle in large dairy herds in drylots, with only indirect contact with sheep (22), and in cattle to which transmission was attempted and in farmed deer (33). A feature of this form of the disease is reported to be a brief period of slight illness followed by the final fulminating disease (21). The mild form occurs most commonly in experimental animals. There is a transient fever and mild erosions appear on the oral and nasal mucosae. Recovery is usual.

Clinical pathology

A leukopenia, commencing at first illness and progressing to a level of 3000–6000/µl has been recorded but is not a general observation. The leukopenia recorded was due mainly to an agranulocytosis. In our experience a moderate leukocytosis is more common.

Transmission experiments are commonly used in identifying the presence of bovine malignant catarrh virus—with histological lesions in the recipient rabbits or calves as the criterion. All such attempted transmission, including the use of tissues from necropsy material, should be carried out with minimal delay after collection of the material. Material for transmission experiments should include whole blood (500 ml), nasal swabs or washings and preferably lymph node collected by biopsy, and should be used immediately after collection (1). The wildebeeste-associated virus is present in the nasal and ocular discharges of some affected animals and transmission experiments using this material may be attempted to cattle, rabbit or tissue culture as recipients (2).

Until recently the virus neutralization test has been the only serological test available for the presumptive diagnosis of bovine malignant catarrh, and its use was limited to the detection of the African (wildebeeste-associated) virus. The position has changed only in that tests for the detection of immunofluorescent antibodies and complement-fixing antibodies have now been developed (1), but their field application is not well defined. All of this work is related to the African virus. The 'sheep-associated', or European virus is still undetectable serologically.

Necropsy findings

Lesions in the mouth, nasal cavities and pharynx vary from minor degrees of hemorrhage and erythema, through extensive, severe inflammation to discrete erosions. These may be shallow and almost imperceptible or deeper and covered by cheesy diphtheritic deposits. Erosion of the tips of the cheek papillae, especially at the commissures, is common. Longitudinal, shallow erosions are present in the esophagus. The mucosa of the forestomachs is not grossly abnormal. There may be some erythema, or sparse hemorrhages or erosions. Similar lesions occur in the abomasum and are more marked than in forestomachs. Catarrhal enteritis of moderate degree and swelling and ulceration of the Peyer's patches are constant. The feces may be loose and bloodstained.

Similar lesions to those in the mouth and nasal cavities are present in the trachea and sometimes in the bronchi but the lungs are not usually involved except for occasional emphysema or secondary pneumonia. The liver is swollen and shows evidence of degeneration. All lymph nodes are swollen, edematous and often hemorrhagic. The ocular lesions are as described clinically. Petechial hemorrhages may be visible in brain and meninges as well as congestion and cloudiness of the meninges especially over the cerebellum and occipital poles.

Histologically bovine malignant catarrh is characterized by perivascular, mononuclear cell cuffing in most organs and by degeneration and erosion of affected epithelium. The pathognomonic lesions are a necrotizing vasculitis, thrombosis, infiltration of tissue with dividing lymphocytes and macrophages and an intense inflammatory reaction with hyperemia and exudation of fluid pointing to a hypersensitivity-like reaction (15). Acidophilic, intracytoplasmic inclusion bodies in neurons have been described by one author (4) but the identity of these as viral inclusions has not been established. Inclusion bodies have been recorded in nasal epithelium by some authors but others regard these as being degenerate cytoplasmic droplets. Large numbers of inclusion bodies have been observed in the tissue of artificially infected rabbits (6).

Both the wildebeeste and sheep-associated viruses (32) can be transmitted to rabbits in which infection causes an acute, fatal, lymphoproliferative disorder (27), but a minimum of time must be allowed to elapse after collection of the material to be used in the transmission attempt. There is a disappointing lack of viral antigens capable of detection by immunofluorescent techniques in infected tissues (20) and electron microscopy does not demonstrate the presence of virus particles (26). Material for histological examination should include brain, lymph node, alimentary tract mucosa, liver, adrenal gland and kidney.

Diagnosis

A definitive diagnosis of bovine malignant catarrh is very difficult because of the absence of a suitable virological technique. A very detailed clinical and pathological examination is an essential first step in diagnosis (15). Clinically, a presumptive diagnosis of bovine malignant catarrh can be made when the nasal, oral and ocular lesions are observed, with a persistent high temperature, enlargement of the peripheral lymph nodes and terminal encephalitis. The histological findings of perivascular, mononuclear cell aggregations in most organs can be accepted as confirmatory evidence. Difficulties involved in isolating the virus have so far prevented the use of serological tests.

Mucosal disease, rinderpest and the infectious stomatitides are not accompanied by typical ocular lesions, lymph node enlargement or encephalitis and they each have a distinctive histopathology. Infectious bovine rhinotracheitis (IBR) is not usually fatal, recovery is rapid, the lesions are restricted to the upper respiratory tract and the disease is readily transmitted. Rinderpest may resemble bovine malignant catarrh but there is primarily inflammation of the alimentary tract, rapid spread of the disease, a high mortality rate and karyorrhexis of lymphocytes visible on histological examination. Pneumonic pasteurellosis is not accompanied by oral, nasal or ocular lesions and responds well to treatment. In younger animals, calf diphtheria may show many of the characteristics of bovine malignant catarrh but there is no involvement of the eye and the buccal ulcers are usually much deeper, have a strong smell and are covered by thick, caseous pus. The poor response to treatment in chronic cases of calf diphtheria may arouse suspicion of bovine malignant catarrh.

The other important viral encephalitis of cattle is sporadic bovine encephalomyelitis in which there are no epithelial lesions. Mycotic dermatitis may cause lesions on the muzzle, particularly in sucking animals, but extensive cutaneous lesions are usually present and there are no oral lesions. Photosensitive dermatitis causes skin lesions with a similar distribution to those of bovine malignant catarrh but again there is no spread of lesions to the mucosae.

Treatment

Treatment of affected animals is unlikely to influence the course of the disease. Most antibiotics, including oxytetracyline, have been used without effect.

Control

Isolation of affected cattle is usually recommended but its value is questioned because of the slow rate of spread and the uncertainty regarding the mode of transmission. Because of the field observation that sheep are important in the spread of the disease, separation of cattle and sheep herds is recommended and has resulted in the disappearance of the disease in some instances. The introduction of sheep from areas where the disease has occurred should be avoided.

Recovered animals are immune to further infection with an homologous strain for 4–8 months.

Attempts to immunize cattle with liver or inactivated culture vaccines with Freund's incomplete adjuvant did not provide protection against experimental challenge or natural challenge by exposure to wildebeeste herds (16). High and persistent levels of virus-neutralizing antibody are demonstrable following vaccination but humoral mechanisms are probably not important in determining resistance to infection with the virulent virus. An inactivated African bovine malignant catarrh virus vaccine has protected against challenge with virulent viruses (34).

REVIEW LITERATURE

Reid, H. W. et al. (1984) Malignant catarrhal fever. *Vet. Rec.*, *114*, 581–583.

Selman, I. E. (1987) The epidemiology of malignant catarrhal fever *Vet. Ann.*, 27, 98–102.

REFERENCES

(1) Rossiter, P. B. et al. (1980) *Res. vet. Sci.*, *29*, 235.
(2) Kalunela, M. et al. (1981) *Can. J. comp. Med.*, *45*, 70.
(3) Plowright, W. (1968) *J. Am. vet. med. Assoc.*, *152*, 795.
(4) Mare, C. J. (1977) *Proc. 81st ann. Mtg US Anim. Hlth Assoc.*, p. 151.
(5) Hutkin, J. (1980) *J. Wildlife Dis.*, *16*, 439.
(6) Pierson, R. E. et al. (1975) *NZ vet. J.*, *23*, 9.
(7) James, M. P. et al. (1975) *NZ vet. J.*, *23*, 9.
(8) Pierson, R. E. et al. (1974) *Am. J. vet. Res.*, *35*, 523.
(9) Hoffman, D. et al. (1984) *Aust. vet. J.*, *61*, 113 & 108.
(10) Boever, W. J. & Kurka, B. (1974) *J. Am. vet. med. Assoc.*, *165*, 817.
(11) Plowright, W. et al. (1972) *Res. vet. Sci.*, *13*, 37.
(12) Mushi, E. Z. & Rurangirwa, F. R. (1981) *Vet. res. Commun.*, *5*, 127.
(13) Liggitt, H. D. & Dernating, J. C. (1980) *Vet. Pathol.*, *17*, 59 & 74.
(14) Reweyemamu, M. M. et al. (1976) *Br. vet. J.*, *132*, 393.
(15) Selman, I. E. et al. (1974) *Vet. Rec.*, *94*, 483.
(16) Plowright, W. et al. (1975) *Res. vet. Sci.*, *19*, 159.
(17) Sanford, S. E. et al. (1977) *J. Wildlife Dis.*, *13*, 29.
(18) Reid, H. W. et al. (1986) *Res. vet. Sci.*, *41*, 76.
(19) Reid, H. W. et al. (1984) *Vet. Rec.*, *114*, 581.
(20) Lassiter, P. B. (1980) *Br. vet. J.*, *136*, 478.
(21) Pierson, R. E. et al. (1978) *Am. J. vet. med. Assoc.*, *173*, 833.
(22) Weaver, L. D. (1979) *Bov. Practnr*, *14*, 121.
(23) Mebus, C. A. et al. (1979) *Bov. Practnr*, *14*, 130.
(24) Denholm, L. J. & Westbury, H. A. (1982) *Aust. vet. J.*, *58*, 81.
(25) Vanselow, B. A. (1980) *Vet. Rec.*, *107*, 15.
(26) Liggitt, H. D. (1979) *Dissert. Abs. Int.*, *39B*, 5854.
(27) Patel, J. R. & Edington, N. (1980) *J. gen. Virol.*, *48*, 437.
(28) Liggitt, H. D. et al. (1980) *J. comp. Pathol.*, *90*, 519.
(29) Liggitt, H. D. et al. (1978) *Am. J. vet. Res.*, *39*, 1249.
(30) Reid, H. W. et al. (1979) *Vet. Rec.*, *104*, 120.
(31) Strover, P. J. & Beckeem van, J. G. (1979) *Res. vet. Sci.*, *26*, 165.
(32) Buxton, D. & Reid, H. W. (1980) *Vet. Rec.*, *106*, 243.
(33) Oliver, R. E. et al. (1983) *NZ vet. J.*, *31*, 209.
(34) Russell, P. H. (1980) *Vet. Microbiol.*, *5*, 161.
(35) Mushi, E. Z. et al. (1980) *Res. vet. Sci.*, *29*, 168.
(36) Rossiter, P. B. (1981) *J. comp. Pathol.*, *91*, 303.
(37) Burton, D. et al. (1982) *Res. vet. Sci.*, *38*, 22.

Bovine virus diarrhea (BVD), mucosal disease (MD)

The bovine virus diarrhea virus (BVDV) causes several different diseases including: the benign infection of bovine virus diarrhea which is usually subclinical, mucosal disease which is usually fatal and occurs in animals which are persistently viremic and specifically immunotolerant as a result of a congenital infection acquired in early fetal life; and congenital abnormalities in calves as a result of infection of the fetus in mid-gestation. The virus may also cause reproductive failure and be immunosuppressive.

Remarkable progress has been made in the last several years in elucidating the epidemiology and pathogenesis of this disease complex. From 1946 to 1960, bovine virus diarrhea and mucosal disease were regarded as distinct entities with many clinical features in common but with epidemiological differences. BVD was described as being of high morbidity (80–100%) and low case fatality rate (0–20%), whereas MD was of low morbidity (5–10%) and high case fatality (90–100%) (1). In the early 1960s, evidence was accumulating that both diseases were a manifestation of infection caused by viruses that were antigenically related or identical (2).

Mucosal disease was first recognized in 1946 (3) and for approximately the next 25 years it was assumed that the disease was the result of an infection just prior to the onset of illness. There is now substantial evidence to support the pathogenetic mechanism that mucosal disease occurs only in animals which are persistently viremic as a result of a congenital infection with a non-cytopathic strain of the virus acquired in early fetal life. These animals remain specifically immunotolerant to the homologous strain of the BVDV throughout postnatal life, and fatal mucosal disease is precipitated by a superinfection with a cytopathic strain of the virus (or some other mechanism) which occurs usually from 6 to 24 months of age or older. *There is no evidence that postnatal infection alone will cause mucosal disease in an immunocompetent animal.*

Etiology

The bovine virus diarrhea virus is a pestivirus within the family Togaviridae (4). It is closely related to the viruses causing border disease in sheep and hog cholera (swine fever) in pigs. Several isolates have been identified that are antigenically related, but there may be antigenic variants that are immunologically distinct (5). There are non-cytopathic and cytopathic strains of the virus which reflect the activity of the virus in tissue culture not necessarily the pathogenicity of the virus in the animal. Differentiation of cytopathic and non-cytopathic isolates of the BVDV has been attempted by virus neutralization (84). The morphology of the virus has been examined (86).

Epidemiology

Diseases caused by the BVDV have been recorded in most countries where cattle are produced. Serological surveys indicate that 60–80% of cattle over 1 year of age may have serum neutralizing antibodies to the virus (6, 7). Much of the information on the prevalence of infection based on seroepidemiological surveys must now be re-examined in the light of the new information on the existence of persistently viremic animals which excrete the virus and are probably responsible for the serologically positive animals in a herd. The absence of persistently viremic animals in a herd could result in a serologically negative herd. Thus the virus is not necessarily ubiquitous. Seroepidemiological surveys of feedlot cattle reveal that animals seroconvert to the BVDV during the first several weeks following arrival in the feedlot (88).

The mean prevalence of persistently viremic animals in herds is about 1–2% (7–10). In Denmark, the prevalence of persistent infection in cattle going to slaughter is about 1% (9); in 66 selected herds in the United States the mean frequency of persistent infection was 1·9% from six herds and none from 60 herds (7). However, in two of the six herds the prevalence of persistently viremic animals was 27% and 18% (7), and in one herd all persistently viremic animals died of mucosal disease within 5 months of the initial sampling (7).

The incidence of clinical mucosal disease in a herd is usually less than 5% of the animals up to 2 years of age. Occasionally, epidemics have been observed in which up to 25% or more of the animals of the most commonly affected age group will develop mucosal disease.

Cattle are the only species which develop mucosal disease. There is serological evidence of BVDV infection in exotic ruminants (12). Serological surveys of some populations of sheep and goats revealed that 11% of sheep and 16% of goats had neutralizing antibodies to the virus (13, 14). A pestivirus which crossreacts with the BVDV causes border disease in lambs following *in utero* infection of pregnant ewes (15, 16). Sheep can be infected naturally and transmission of the virus from cattle to sheep has been demonstrated. Some strains of the BVDV when inoculated into pigs cause false-positive reactions to tests for swine fever antibodies and may protect against subsequent challenge with swine fever virus (17). The importance of these and other species as a source of infection for cattle is unknown.

The BVDV is transmitted by direct contact between animals and by transplacental transmission. The virus can be isolated from nasal discharge, saliva, semen, feces, urine, tears and milk, each of which would allow wide dissemination of the virus. Animals with persistent BVDV infection are the major source of the virus to infect non-immune animals (18, 19).

Transmission of the virus between healthy immunocompetent animals is probably insignificant because they produce antibodies and eliminate the virus. Susceptible animals introduced into a herd, typically heifers, become infected by contact with persistently viremic animals and major economic losses can occur if they are at a vulnerable stage of pregnancy. The introduction of an unknown persistently infected cow or heifer into a susceptible herd can also cause major economic losses (19, 20).

The fetus can be infected by transplacental transmission of the virus from the infected dam, whether the dam is transiently or persistently infected (19, 20). Fetal infection has been produced by inoculation of non-immune pregnant dams (21–23). Epidemics of abortion and congenital defects of calves have occurred when transplacental virus infection of the fetuses of cows in the first trimester, in previously virus-free herds, has followed the introduction of BVDV-infected animals (24, 25).

Persistently viremic females can remain clinically normal for several years during which time they may breed successfully and their progeny may also be apparently normal but are invariably also persistently viremic (26, 27). In this way a maternal viremic family can be established which can persist for several generations and provides one of the major mechanisms for maintenance of the virus as endemic in the herd (28).

A persistently viremic bull can shed the virus in the semen for a long period (29, 31), and if introduced into a susceptible herd could have immediate undesirable effects on reproductive performance. Previously unexposed heifers have been shown not to conceive to service by a persistently infected bull until they have seroconverted (30).

The economic losses associated with the introduction of the BVDV into a susceptible herd of pregnant cattle are due to abortion, congenital defects, stillbirths, increased neonatal mortality, prenatal and postnatal growth retardation, suboptimal reproductive performance due to infertility deaths from mucosal disease, and the early disposal of persistently infected animals (19, 32).

The magnitude of the losses in an infected herd may be expected to fluctuate, being relatively large, with the occurrence of disease on an epidemic scale, after initial horizontal transmission to non-immune pregnant cows but considerably lower when endemic infection is maintained in the herd through the presence of viremic families. However, a further phase of high losses may occur should management allow heifers to reach breeding age without being exposed to infection or vaccinated.

A recent report of an investigation of BVDV infection in a dairy herd of 200 milking cows indicated that 16% of the calves died of pneumonia in the year following the introduction of the infection into the herd with purchased suckler calves (20). A non-cytopathic isolate of the virus was recovered from 55% of the calves which died from pneumonia and it was concluded that calves may have been persistently viremic from early prenatal infection. Over a period of 2 years following the introduction of the infection, the herd also experienced an increased incidence of diarrhea in adult cattle, abortions, congenital defects and mucosal disease. A cytopathic isolate of the virus was recovered from the calves with mucosal disease.

Pathogenesis

The pathogenesis of disease due to infection with the BVDV is governed by several features of the infection. These include the occurrence of viremia, the ability of the virus to compromise, the immune system, the occurrence of transplacental infection, the induction of immune tolerance, and the emergence of fetal immune competence at about 180 days of gestation. Apart from those infected with the virus *in utero*, most cattle are immunocompetent to the virus and will successfully control a natural infection, develop antibodies and eliminate the virus so that latency and shedding does not occur. Accordingly, infection may result in any of the following.

Postnatal infections

Bovine virus diarrhea This is usually a clinically unrecognizable infection with the development of serum neutralizing antibodies and elimination of the virus from normal immunocompetent animals. This accounts for the high percentage of normal animals that are serologically positive (6). A mild transient clinical disease characterized by inappetence for a few days, depression, fever, mild diarrhea, transient leukopenia and recovery in a few days may occur occasionally.

Immunosuppression Experimentally, the virus can impair the immune response of cattle and enhance the pathogenicity of other agents. Experimentally, the virus can also alter neutrophil function (33), impair immunoglobulin secretion by peripheral lymphocytes, allow infectious bovine rhinotracheitis (IBR) virus to be more widely distributed in various tissues (34) and infect tissue culture cells and cause the release of substances which can suppress the proliferative response of bovine mononuclear cells to blastogenic substances (35). Impairment of neutrophil function in cattle persistently infected with the BVDV differs from impairment of neutrophil function in healthy cattle mounting an immune response to the infection (33). A modified live-virus vaccine strain of the BVDV can experimentally have a detrimental effect on lymphocyte and neutrophil function (36). This suggests that stressed cattle should not be vaccinated with a modified live-virus mucosal disease vaccine because impairment of lymphocyte or neutrophil function could potentiate other viral or bacterial infections. This impairment may be potentiated by increased plasma cortisol.

The evidence incriminating the virus as a predisposing pathogen in naturally occurring cases of bovine respiratory disease is largely circumstantial. The presence of the virus in the respiratory tract tissues of cattle affected with pneumonia is difficult to interpret. Several different viruses have been incriminated in the cause of acute bovine respiratory disease but experimental evidence to support their involvement has centered on the IBR and parainfluenza-3 (PI-3) viruses (40). Experimentally the BVDV can facilitate the colonization of *Pasteurella hemolytica* in the lungs resulting in severe pulmonary lesions (3). Severe fibrinopurulent bronchopneumonia and pleuritis involving 40–75% of lung volume developed in calves experimentally inoculated sequentially with the BVDV and *P. hemolytica* (38). However, in some experiments the BVDV has no effect (39). BVDV may be present with other pathogens, such as those viruses or *Pasteurella* sp. and this may indicate that synergism occurs. However, it is also possible that the virus may casually present in some animals and have no significant adverse effect.

Diarrhea of neonatal calves Experimental neonatal calves with the BVDV has resulted in enteric disease, occasionally fatal, and the virus has been recoverable for up to 103 days (41). However, if the virus causes clinical diarrhea naturally in newborn calves it is difficult to explain in the light of the new information. Calves born from cows free of the infection are not likely to be exposed to the infection. Further immunocompetent cows in contact with a virus shedding carrier will have antibody which they will pass on to their calves and which should be protective. Conceivably, calf diarrhea associated with pestivirus infection might occur either as a form of BVDV or, alternatively, through immunosuppressive enhancement of other enteric disease. However, naturally occurring cases of acute neonatal diarrhea in calves due to the BVDV have not yet been documented.

Reproductive failure Infection at the time of breeding may interfere with conception. Of five susceptible heifers which were mated to a viremic bull, all seroconverted within 2 weeks, and of these three did not hold to service until serum virus neutralization titers rose to 1:128, while a fourth aborted at 6 months (30). Experimentally, the intrauterine infusion of virus into cattle at the time of insemination has prevented conception and has been attributed to prevention of fertilization (43) or simply recognized as an empty uterus at 5 weeks after breeding (44). It seems that intrauterine infection at the time of breeding may have some effects on the very early stages of reproduction in addition to those that could be attributed to infection by other contact routes (45). Experimentally there is no indication of impairment of *in vitro* development of bovine embryos when they are exposed to the BVDV (42). The zona pellucida appears to prevent the virus from gaining access to the embryonic cells.

Numerous reports describe abortion as a result of infection of susceptible cows in early pregnancy. In one study experimental infection of pregnant cows with the BVDV during the first 100 days of gestation caused abortion or mummification, but inoculation of fetuses or pregnant cows in the second and third trimester failed to cause abortion, although fetuses were infected and developed virus neutralization antibody (46).

Fetal infections

Following the infection of a non-immune pregnant animal the virus is capable of crossing the placental barrier and invading the fetus. The congenital infection can result in a wide spectrum of abnormalities from death of the fetus to congenital defects, to a persistent lifelong infection without clinical signs. The results are mainly dependent on the stage of fetal development at which infection takes place (25). In general, the risk for the fetus is highest during early pregnancy.

The bovine fetus gains immune competence to the BVDV around day 180 of gestation (47). However, it can produce immunoglobulins without detectable specificity in response to a BVDV infection before attaining immune competence to the virus (48).

No fetal disease is recognized to occur after full immunocompetence has been acquired and antibody to the virus is demonstrable at birth, before colostral intake has occurred.

Persistent viremia and mucosal disease Following infection of the fetus with a non-cytopathic isolate of the virus before about 125 days of gestation, it will not develop serum virus neutralization and may be carried normally to term and be born with a persistent infection with the virus. Mucosal disease will develop in a proportion of these, and only in these, persistently viremic animals. From birth to the time of clinical disease, which is most likely at between 6 and 24 months of age, these animals are specifically immunotolerant and persistently viremic, and may appear clinically normal or unthrifty. During this postnatal period, superinfection with a cytopathic isolate of the virus may precipitate fatal clinical mucosal disease in these animals (19, 21, 49, 50). Persistently viremic calves have been reproduced experimentally by the inoculation of fetuses with a non-cytopathic isolate of the BVDV from 42 to 125 days of gestation (23). Fatal mucosal disease has been reproduced by the inoculation of persistently viremic specifically immunotolerant calves with a homologous cytopathic isolate of the virus (21, 50).

The pathogenesis of the lesions of mucosal disease remains obscure (61). The viral antigen can be detected in many tissues including lymph nodes, Peyer's patches in the ileum and lymphoid tissue in the proximal colon, the palatine tonsils, spleen, bronchiolar epithelial cells, the crypts of the intestinal mucosa, the salivary glands, the tongue, esophagus and skin. The pathological changes which characterize the disease involve the integument and the epithelia of the respiratory and alimentary tracts as well as lymphoid tissues.

The basic lesion is a small vesicle-ulcer, which affects only epithelial cells. The erosions occur throughout the oral cavity, esophagus, forestomachs, abomasum, small intestine, cecum and colon. Vascular injury leading to vasculitis is a characteristic feature of disease due to the pestiviruses which may explain the type and distribution of the lesions which occur in fatal mucosal disease. The vascular injury may be initiated by degenerative changes of the endothelial cells which may lead to thrombus formation, which can detach and circulate as emboli, resulting in generalized vasculitis.

Death from acute mucosal disease usually occurs within 2 weeks of the onset of clinical signs and both cytopathic and non-cytopathic isolates of the virus can be recovered from the tissues of affected cattle (49).

Animals that are immunotolerant to the BVDV are immunocompetent to other antigens since they develop neutralizing serotiters to the IBR and PI-3 viruses and agglutinating titers to *Pasteurella haemolytica* (23). They will also produce virus neutralization, following the administration of commercial live BVDV vaccine, against the vaccine virus as well as other laboratory strains (51). Furthermore, in spite of this antibody formation, the original virus will persist.

Because maternal colostral antibodies to the BVDV persist for about 6–8 months (52, 53), it is interesting to speculate if those antibodies protect the persistently viremic calf from clinical mucosal disease. This is not known. They do subsequently remain seronegative to, and do not respond to experimental infection with, the *homologous* non-cytopathic virus (23).

In spite of the new information on the pathogenesis of mucosal disease, some important unresolved questions remain. What is the source of the cytopathic isolate of the virus? It has been suggested that a mutation of the non-cytopathic virus within the animal is a possibility and more likely than the introduction of the cytopathic virus by way of an infected animal introduced into the herd (54). Although mucosal disease as a consequence of superinfection by a cytopathic pestivirus has been convincingly demonstrated separately in Britain (21) and the United States (23) and the mechanism is undoubtedly effective in the field as one of the triggers to manifest mucosal disease, it seems not to be the complete answer to the questions of etiology and pathogenesis. Disease is not always induced or not by all cytopathic strains (55), and serotypic identity between original and superinfecting viruses, presumably a condition for persistence of infection by the latter, was not thought to be necessary (5). An alternative hypothesis suggested that a defective infectious agent, which is incapable of independent replication but uses pestivirus as a helper, may contribute, in some cases, to both the cytopathogenicity in cell culture and the pathogenicity for the animal (28).

Recent work has shown that typical mucosal disease occurs within 2–3 weeks following superinfection of persistently viremic calves with the antigenically homologous cytopathic virus (54). The affected cattle do not respond serologically to the homologous cytopathic virus. Superinfection with an antigenically heterologous cytopathic virus does not result in mucosal disease within 2–3 weeks. Such infected animals develop atypical mucosal disease several months later, or not at all, and respond serologically to the heterologous cytopathic virus (54).

It has also been noted that there are a number of pathological facets to mucosal disease and that it may be necessary to consider different pathogenetic mechanisms for those different facets (28). Some lesions may be caused by direct cytolytic effects of the virus, especially when cytopathic strains are involved, but glomerulonephritis (56), and other evidence of immune complex disease (57), present something of a paradox in a disease which is generally dominated by immune tolerance. The presence of these lesions suggests that at least this aspect of mucosal disease, like many other late pathological consequences of various virus infections recognized these days, is due to an inappropriate immune response rather than to any direct effect of the virus. A superinfecting virus which is serologically similar to the persistent virus, and hence is also able to persist, may differ from the original virus in regard to other antigens, that is antigens that are not involved in neutralization or the determination of serotype. This could conceivably provide a basis for immune complex disease as the host's tolerance is strictly limited to the antigens of the original virus strain.

Congenital disease Congenital defects of newborn calves can result from infection of the fetus with the virus between approximately 125 and 180 days of gestation (58). Cerebellar hypoplasia occurs and ocular abnormalities consist of retinal atrophy, optic neuritis, cataract, and microphthalmia with retinal dysplasia (59). Calves with cerebellar hypoplasia are unable to stand and walk normally immediately after birth. Defects of the eyes result in varying degrees of blindness; the cataracts are obvious when they occur.

Congenital morphological defects follow infections which occur somewhat later in gestation than do infections which result in persistent viremia and may be due, in part, to the emerging immunological capability. The presence of either persistent infection or antibody is variable.

Border disease Border disease of sheep is caused by an *in utero* infection with a related pestivirus which crossreacts with the BVD virus (15). Ewes are clinically normal, but affected newborn lambs have a hairy fleece, clonic rhythmic tremors, and are unthrifty. The lesions consist of hypomyelination and abnormal cells in the central nervous system. The hairy birthcoats have been attributed to hypertrophy of primary follicles and medullation of wool fibers. Surviving lambs are also persistently infected with the virus. The virus can be isolated in cell culture and detected by immunofluorescent staining of the peripheral leukocytes, cellular debris in urine, and cerebrospinal fluid of lambs for up to 1 year of age. Affected lambs, like calves, have no detectable serum neutralizing antibody. Adult sheep, after recovery from infection by the virus, have no detectable virus in the leukocytes and have serum neutralizing antibodies. Pestivirus of sheep and cattle will readily infect the alternative species, both naturally and experimentally, but the role that such crossreaction plays in causing the respective diseases has not been determined.

Clinical findings

Inapparent or subclinical infection (bovine virus diarrhea)

The most frequent form of BVDV infection in cattle is non-clinical or a mild disease of high morbidity and low case fatality characterized by a mild fever, leukopenia, inappetence and mild diarrhea followed by rapid recovery in a few days and the production of virus neutralizing antibodies. This form occurs in cattle which are infected after birth and presumably accounts for the high proportion of adult animals which possess serum neutralizing antibodies to the virus (6). The literature commonly refers to this subclinical infection as bovine virus diarrhea. Similar infection, with no long-term consequences other than the development of antibody, occurs in fetuses over about 150–180 days of gestation.

Acute mucosal disease

This form is characterized by the sudden onset of clinical disease in animals from 6 to 24 months of age which were infected during early fetal life. The morbidity is low and the case fatality rate is high (over 90%). Within herds, from 5 to 25% of animals in this age group may develop the disease over a period of several days or sporadic cases may occur over several weeks or months. Well-nourished, thrifty and clinically normal animals can be affected.

Affected animals are depressed, anorexic and slobber saliva, wetting hair around the mouth. The body temperatures are elevated up to 40–41°C (104–105°F) and tachycardia and polypnea are common. Ruminal movements are usually absent and a profuse and watery diarrhea occurs 2–4 days after the onset of clinical illness. The feces are foul-smelling and may contain mucus and variable quantities of blood. Occasionally, small tags of fibrinous intestinal casts are present. Straining at defecation is common and the perineum is usually stained and smeared with feces.

The lesions of the buccal mucosa consist of discrete, shallow erosions which become confluent, resulting in large areas of necrotic epithelium becoming separated from the mucosa. These erosions occur inside the lips, on the gums and dental pad, on the posterior part of the hard palate, at the commissures of the mouth and on the tongue. The entire oral cavity has a cooked appearance with the grayish colored necrotic epithelium covering the deep pink raw base. Similar lesions occur on the muzzle and may become confluent and covered with scabs and debris. Although the oral lesions are highly significant in the identification of the disease, they may be absent or difficult to appreciate visually in up to 20% of the affected animals, particularly in the latter part of an outbreak.

There is usually a mucopurulent nasal discharge associated with some minor erosions on the external nares and similar lesions in the pharynx. Lacrimation and corneal edema are sometimes observed. Lameness occurs in some animals and appears to be due to laminitis, coronitis and erosive lesions of the skin of the interdigital cleft, which commonly affect all four feet.

Dehydration and weakness are usually progressive and death occurs 5–7 days after the onset of signs. Occasionally, in peracute cases, which die within a few days after the onset of illness, the diarrhea is not evident even though the intestines are distended with excessive fluid. Presumably, there is paralytic ileus and the intestinal fluid is not being moved down the intestinal tract.

Chronic mucosal disease
Some acute cases of mucosal disease do not die within the expected time of several days and become chronically ill. There may be intermittent bouts of diarrhea, inappetence, progressive emaciation, rough dry hair coat, chronic bloat, hoof deformities and chronic erosions in the oral cavity and on the skin. Shallow erosive lesions covered with scabs can be found on the perineum, around the scrotum, preputial orifice and vulva, between the legs and at the skin–horn junction around the dew-claws, in the interdigital cleft and at the heels, and there may be extensive scurfiness of the skin. The failure of these skin lesions to heal is an important clinical finding suggesting chronic mucosal disease. Chronic cases will sometimes survive for up to 18 months during which time they are unthrifty and ultimately die from chronic inanition.

The chronic clinical form of the disease described above must be distinguished from the unthrifty persistently viremic animal described next.

Unthrifty persistently viremic calves
Calves which are born persistently viremic may be smaller in body size than their contemporaries and may fail to grow normally. They may survive and appear unthrifty for several months or more until they develop fatal mucosal disease or some other infectious disease such as pneumonia (22, 25). While these calves are stunted and unthrifty in appearance they do not have detectable clinical evidence of mucosal disease and they are seronegative to the BVDV (32).

Congenital defects in calves
These include cerebellar-ocular agenesis, ocular defects, cerebellar agenesis, brachygnathism, musculoskeletal deformities, alopecia and intrauterine growth retardation (22, 24).

Clinical pathology
The diagnosis of mucosal disease is usually made on the basis of the presence of characteristic clinical and pathologic findings. A severe leukopenia is characteristic of acute mucosal disease. The decrease is commonly to below 50% of normal and total leukocyte counts of 1000–3000/μl are common and may persist for weeks.

Virus isolation can be attempted by inoculation of nasopharyngeal swabs, ocular swabs, intestinal tissues, spleen, or most other tissues, or any fraction of blood to cell cultures. Recovery of virus from feces is generally difficult. Isolation of virus, from any source, in cell culture may require more than one passage before it is detectable. It is then recognized by cytopathic effects or, in the case of non-cytopathic strains, various serological methods may be used to demonstrate the presence of virus or virus-associated antigens. Both cytopathic and non-cytopathic pestivirus have been isolated from spleen (21) or blood (50) of individual cattle with mucosal disease. The serological methods used to detect non-cytopathic virus in cell culture, or virus or antigen in tissues, such as intestine, kidney, spleen from affected animals, or aborted fetal tissue, include direct or indirect immunofluorescent or enzyme-linked antibody staining (62, 63) or immunodiffusion (64). Nasal epithelial cells collected on cotton swabs were stained by fluorescent antibody for the diagnosis of field cases of BVDV in calves (65) and, using a similar technique, the detection of virus antigen in cells, obtained from the nasopharynx using Belmont brush swabs, was shown to be a rapid and efficient method for identifying persistently infected cattle, agreeing perfectly with virus isolation from leukocytes and clotted blood (19).

Serological techniques are also used to detect antibody. According to the range of antibody specificities detected they fall into two groups: those that are serotype-specific; and those that are group-specific, or serotype-common.

Virus neutralization tests are serotype-specific, although varying degrees of crossreactivity occur between many strains. However, the virus neutralization test may be of limited value if a field isolate is encountered which is serotypically remote from the laboratory strain in use.

The gel diffusion precipitation (GDP) test is based on a virus-associated soluble antigen. As comparable antigens, associated with different pestiviruses, and including all known strains of BVDV are, by techniques used to date, indistinguishable, a GDP test based on one such antigen will recognize antibody responses to all serotypes of BVDV and the test is said to be group-specific. Other serological techniques, including complement fixation (CF), immunofluorescent (IF) staining or enzyme-linked immunosorbent assays (ELISA), may, according to how the antigen is prepared, detect antibody to an indeterminate number of antigens. They do, however, generally appear to react with all serotypes, implying that serotype-common or group-specific antigens or determinants are dominant in these reactions. Two recently described ELISA tests are of high serological sensitivity and appear likely to be group-specific (66, 67).

In the past, the virus neutralization test has sometimes been used to determine the occurrence of a rising titer between acute and convalescent sera. It is now apparent that this is only a valid procedure in the uncommon case where clinical BVDV is under consideration. It is not valid for the diagnosis of mucosal disease because the specific immune tolerance precludes the development of virus neutralization antibody. In the specific case in which immune complex disease is a component of the pathology, antibody (usually weak) to a soluble virus-associated antigen, may be demonstrable by the GDP test. Development of this reaction in a persistently viremic animal would presage clinical deterioration.

Precolostral serum from calves infected *in utero* as immunocompetent fetuses may have virus-specific neutralizing antibodies (26) and their demonstration is meaningful for the diagnosis of past infection.

The pathological criteria for the diagnosis of the BVDV as a cause of abortion have not been established (68). Finding antibody in a fetus, as in an unsuckled neonate, indicates that intrauterine infection had occurred but its diagnostic significance in regard to the abortion is not clear. The recovery of virus from, or the serological identification of virus or viral antigen in, fetal tissues is strongly suggestive of a diagnosis of pestiviral abortion. Experimentally it has been found that viral antigen was demonstrable by immunocytochemical methods in secretions of several fetal organs, primarily lymphoid tissues, even though virus was not recoverable (69). These observations were made on viable fetuses, recovered surgically 3 weeks after direct fetal inoculation with a large dose of virus, so the relevance of the finding to the diagnosis of natural fatal fetal infection is not certain.

Necropsy findings

The lesions found at necropsy are in general the same for most recorded forms of the disease. The gross abnormalities are confined to the alimentary tract (89). Characteristic shallow erosions with very little inflammation around them and with a raw, red base are present on the muzzle, in the mouth, to a less extent in the pharynx, larynx and posterior nares, but in large numbers in the esophagus where they are linear in shape and lie in the direction of the folds of the esophageal mucosa. Similar lesions may be present in the forestomachs, but are usually confined to the pillars of the rumen and the leaves of the omasum. Histologically the lesions of the squamous cell mucosa of the alimentary tract begin with necrosis of individual cells and groups of cells. These foci enlarge and result in areas of necrosis with little or no inflammation of the lamina propria. If the necrotic foci are abraded erosions and ulcers develop, ulcerations of the squamous epithelium are accompanied by inflammation in the lamina propria. In the abomasum there is a marked erythema of the mucosa accompanied by multiple submucosal hemorrhages and gross edema of the wall. Erosions and ulcers are common on the sides of the rugae of the abomasum and may be punctate to 1.0 cm or more in diameter. The lesions have raised margins with a distinct pale halo. Histologically there is epithelial necrosis of the deep parts of the glandular epithelium. The mucosa of the small intestine often appears normal with the unusual exceptions of patchy or diffuse congestion and edema in some cases. In acute cases it is common to find coagulated blood and fibrin overlying and outlining Peyer's patches, the covering of which is eroded. This is a very distinctive lesion which is paralleled only on rinderpest. Severely affected Peyer's patches may be obvious through the serosa as red-black oval areas up to 10–12 cm long on the antimesenteric border of the intestine. In the large intestine the mucosa may be congested often in a 'tiger stripe' pattern following colonic folds. The characteristic lesion in the intestinal mucosa is destruction of the epithelial lining of the crypts of Lieberkuhn. The microscopic lesion of Peyer's patches are distinctive and consist of complete destruction of the underlying glands, collapse of the lamina propria and lysis of the follicular lymphoid tissues.

In chronic bovine virus diarrhea, the necrotic epithelium may not be eroded by alimentary movements but instead remain *in situ* as slightly elevated, yellow, friable plaques, especially between the villi on the tongue and in the rumen. Subacute cases with a very prolonged course may show very few lesions in the mouth, some in the esophagus and none in the stomachs and intestines.

The congenital defects in calves consist of cerebellar hypoplasia, cataracts, retinal degeneration, and hypoplasia and neuritis of the optic nerves (24).

Diagnosis

The differentiation of the diseases causing erosive lesions of the buccal mucosa can be perplexing both clinically and at necropsy. The similarity between them is the more important because rinderpest and foot-and-mouth disease are major plague diseases. The situation is so dangerous that if there is any doubt as to the identity of the disease under examination, samples should be submitted for laboratory examination.

There are many diseases of the alimentary tract of cattle which can be grouped according to the presence or absence of oral lesions with or without diarrhea. These have been summarized in Table 68. An erosive stomatitis and gastroenteritis are characteristic of rinderpest, bovine virus diarrhea and bovine malignant catarrh. The stomatitis and hyperemia are remarkably severe in bovine malignant catarrh along with a corneoscleral opacity, lymph node enlargement, hematuria and terminal encephalitis. Rinderpest is characterized by a high morbidity and mortality and knowledge of the disease in the area.

The vesicular diseases are characterized by the presence of vesicles on the tongue and buccal mucosa, tests and coronets and should be distinguishable from erosions.

Diseases causing diarrhea with no oral lesions include winter dysentery, salmonellosis, Johne's disease, molybdenum poisoning (conditioned copper deficiency), parasitism (ostertagiasis), and arsenic poisoning.

A definitive diagnosis depends on isolation of BVDV from the buffy coat or serum of blood and other tissues. Calves with congenital defects can be provisionally identified as bovine virus diarrhea by detection of specific antibodies in calves which have not sucked; this is not an easy specimen to obtain in beef cattle running at pasture.

Although bovine virus diarrhea is not a disease of the respiratory tract it is not uncommon for respiratory signs to be evident and confusion in diagnosis between it and infectious bovine rhinotracheitis (IBR), and even pneumonic pasteurellosis, does arise. It is necessary to depend on a careful clinical examination of oral and nasal mucosae to ensure that there are no mucosal lesions. It is also necessary to include bovine virus diarrhea in the list of diagnostic possibilities when considering the causes of abortion and stillbirth in cattle. Immunoglobulin determinations in aborted fetuses may be of diagnostic value (70).

The definitive diagnosis of chronic bovine virus diarrhea presents problems because often the affected

Table 68. Differential diagnosis of diseases of cattle in which there are either oral lesions or diarrhea alone or together in the same animal.

Disease	*Epidemiology*	*Clinical findings*	*Clinical pathology and pathology*	*Response to treatment*
DISEASES WITH ORAL LESIONS AND DIARRHEA	*N.B.*: Rinderpest, mucosal disease and bovine malignant catarrh closely resemble each other clinically. The erosive stomatitis and gastroenteritis are common to all three and in outbreaks of mucosal disease or bovine malignant catarrh it may be impossible to distinguish either disease from rinderpest on clinical grounds. This necessitates notification of regulatory authorities and confirmation of the diagnosis by transmission tests or suitable laboratory tests			
Rinderpest	Occurs most commonly in rinderpest areas, young and mature cattle, outbreaks common, rapid spread, up to 90% of susceptible cattle affected and mortality may reach 90%. Subacute and chronic forms occur in relatively resistant populations	Severe erosive stomatitis, bloodstained saliva, blepharospasm, high fever, severe diarrhea and dysentery, many cattle affected and many die	Marked leukopenia, lymphopenia, karyorrhexis (submit lymph nodes)	Nil
Bovine virus diarrhea (BVD) (mucosal disease, MD)	Young cattle (8 months to 2 years). Low incidence (5%) of acute clinical disease but high case mortality. Sporadic cases of chronic form. Acute clinical disease rare in cattle over 2 years of age	*Acute*: Diffuse erosive stomatitis, moderate fever for few days, profuse diarrhea and severe dehydration, lymph nodes not usually enlarged, skin lesions common, die in 7–10 days *Chronic*: Inappetence, scant soft feces, normal temperature, small rumen, intermittent bloat, chronic skin lesions which do not heal (especially interdigital space)	Leukopenia, neutropenia and lymphopenia. Seronegative. Nasal and fecal swabs. Erosions throughout gastrointestinal tract	Almost all die
Bovine malignant catarrh (BMC)	Usually sporadic in single animals. Affects mature and young animals. In North America outbreaks occur commonly after contact with sheep. In Africa outbreaks after contact with wildebeeste. Varying forms: peracute, alimentary tract, head and eye, and mild	Severe diffuse intensely hyperemic, erosive stomatitis; persistent high fever, severe dejection, severe conjunctivitis, corneoscleral opacity, hematuria, enlarged lymph nodes, prominent skin lesions, horn coverings shed, terminal encephalitis, diarrhea and dysentery. Peracute die in 3 days, acute in 7–10 days and chronic form may live few weeks	Leukopenia and neutropenia early. Leukocytosis later. Transmission tests. Vasculitis	Nil
Alimentary form of infectious bovine rhinotracheitis in newborn calves	Outbreaks in newborn calves (25–50% morbidity). Recent herd introduction of carrier. Case mortality high (90–100%)	Small pin-point gray pustules on soft palate, rhinotracheitis, conjunctivitis, persistent mild fever, usually die from secondary tracheitis and pneumonia	Virus isolation from feces and nasal swabs. Lesions in turbinates, rumen and abomasum	Unlikely to respond
DISEASES WITH ORAL LESIONS AND NO DIARRHEA				
Foot-and-mouth disease	High morbidity (100%), low mortality. Spreads quickly. Occurs in enzootic areas	High fever, severe dejection, painful stomatitis, ropey saliva, large vesicles in mouth, vesicles on teats and coronets, recovery in 3–5 days, deaths in myocardial form	Animal transmission tests. Serology rapid and accurate	No specific treatment

Table 68 (cont'd)

Disease	*Epidemiology*	*Clinical findings*	*Clinical pathology and pathology*	*Response to treatment*
Vesicular stomatitis	In certain geographical areas, variable morbidity and mortality, insect-borne	Mild fever, anorexia, vesicles in oral cavity, less commonly on teats and feet. Recover in few days	Animal transmission tests. Serology rapid and accurate	Usually not indicated
Bluetongue	Clinical disease not common in cattle, insect vector, seasonal	Fever, stiffness, laminitis, coronitis, erosive lesions in oral cavity, edema of lips, drool saliva, nasal and ocular discharge, most cattle recover	Animal transmission tests. Serology rapid and accurate	No specific treatment
Bovine papular stomatitis	Worldwide, common in young cattle (2 weeks to 2 years), morbidity may reach 100%, nil mortality, may occur coincidentally with ostertagiasis	Round, dark red, raised papules on muzzle, in oral cavity. Heal in 4–7 days but remnants of lesion persist for several weeks. No significant effect on animal. In same age group as, and often associated with, severe ostertagiasis	Clinical diagnosis obvious	Spontaneous recovery
Necrotic stomatitis	Young calves. In dirty conditions or on dry rough pasture	Painful stomatitis with large deep necrotic foul-smelling ulcers on tongue, cheek and pharyngeal mucosa	Clinical diagnosis. Necrotic esophagitis	Respond in few days to parenteral antibiotics or sulfonamides
DISEASES WITH DIARRHEA AND NO ORAL LESIONS (does not include diarrhea of calves)				
Salmonellosis	All ages. Outbreaks occur, case mortality may be high. Stress-induced. Contaminated feed supplies. Veal calves. Auction mart problem	*Acute*: High fever, diarrhea, dysentery, feces foul-smelling, fibrinous cast, abdominal pain, die in 24 to 48 hours. *Subacute* and *chronic*: diarrhea occurs too	Leukopenia, neutropenia. Fecal culture. Fibrinohemorrhagic enteritis	Favorable response in early stage. Later many cases die or become chronically ill
Winter dysentery	Housed dairy cattle, winter, explosive outbreak, 100% morbidity, no mortality	Acute profuse watery diarrhea and dysentery, mild fever, inappetence and drop in milk yield for 24 hours, recover spontaneously	Nil	Recovery is spontaneous
Johne's disease	Single animal, 2 years and older, low morbidity, long course of several months	Chronic diarrhea, feces homogeneous, progressive loss of weight, normal temperature, appetite usually normal, hydration almost normal	Rectal scraping, intestinal biopsy, Johnin test, culture feces. Chronic granulomatous-like enteritis	No response to treatment
Secondary copper deficiency (molybdenosis)	Enzootic to farm/area. Young cattle particularly. Marginally copper-deficient areas, especially spring	Chronic diarrhea without smell, mucus or blood. Black coats are gray-flecked; red coats are rusty yellow. Very thin	Plasma copper below 0.5 μg/ml, liver copper below 20 mg/kg dry matter	Excellent response in body weight and resolution of diarrhea to copper, by injection, drench, pasture dressing
Ostertagiasis	Mostly young cattle 6 months to 2 years, can be adults. Many in group affected	Persistent diarrhea, without smell, mucus or blood. Decreased appetite, bottle jaw, very thin	May be heavy egg count, not if larvae inhibited but plasma pepsinogen level then greater than 5000 units	Several treatments with fenbendazole. Good results. But lesion may be irreversible
Coccidiosis	Young cattle, when overcrowded, fed on ground, gather at water source	Subacute dysentery, mild fever, 2–3 days, appetite and hydration remain normal. About 20% develop 'nervous signs' and die	Feces for oocysts. Hemorrhagic cecitis and colitis	Self-limiting disease. Amprolium and sulfonamides

Table 68 (cont'd)

Disease	*Epidemiology*	*Clinical findings*	*Clinical pathology and pathology*	*Response to treatment*
Arsenic poisoning	Access to source of arsenic	Sudden and rapid death. Acute abdominal pain, bellowing, regurgitation, diarrhea, muscular tremors, convulsions, die 4–8 hours after onset of signs	Feces and tissues and feed supplies for analysis. Edema of abomasum	Unfavorable response. Difficult to treat
Carbohydrate engorgement	One to several animals. History of access to grain.	Anorexia, depression, ataxia, recumbency, dehydration, profuse, foul-smelling diarrhea, grain-kernels in feces, rumen static with fluid-splashing sounds, no rumen protozoal activity	Rumen pH below 5, lactic acidosis, hemoconcentration	Respond favorably if ruminal and systemic acidosis; may need rumen lavage or rumenotomy
Renal amyloidosis	Single animal, mature cow	Profuse chronic diarrhea, anasarca, inappetence, decreased milk production, enlarged kidney	Proteinuria, hypoalbuminemia, grossly enlarged kidneys	Nil

Some additional causes of diarrhea in adult cattle include ragwort poisoning, squamous cell carcinoma of the upper alimentary tract of cattle in Scotland and England, and abdominal fat necrosis.

animal has no specific neutralizing antibody because of immunosuppression or the inability to secrete antibody. A presumptive diagnosis can be made on the basis of the clinical characteristics of the acute disease, the absence of other lesions to account for the chronic form of the disease and the presence of pancytopenia. Virus isolation must be attempted along with detailed pathological examination.

Treatment

There is no specific treatment for mucosal disease.

The prognosis for severe cases with profuse watery diarrhea and marked oral lesions is unfavorable and slaughter for salvage or euthanasia should be considered. Animals with chronic bovine virus diarrhea should be culled and destroyed. No reports of successful treatment of these are available.

Control and prevention

The successful control and prevention of the bovine virus diarrhea–mucosal disease complex will depend on the identification and eradication of persistently viremic animals and immunization of breeding animals before breeding.

Detection and elimination of persistently viremic animals

The basic strategy here is to detect and eliminate virus carriers.

In investigating a herd prior to eliminating infection it may not always be practicable to attempt virus isolation from individual animals on the scale necessary to identify carriers directly. Under those circumstances, useful information, on which a control strategy can be based, may be obtained from a careful analysis of serological tests for antibody. With an understanding of the epidemiology of BVDV infection, the best use of diagnostic tests, and management and background of the particular herd, the control strategy is best designed individually for that herd. The following provides a general guide.

The first step is to take plain blood samples, which are allowed to clot, from all animals over 6 months of age. Sera are removed from the samples and tested for antibody, preferably using a group-specific test so that all serotypes are equally represented. The clot residues should be retained frozen for later attempts at virus isolation should this be necessary. The overall prevalence of antibody, and its distribution within recognizable subgroups within the herd, for example by age, management or origin, should be carefully considered before further action is decided.

If the incidence of seronegative animals is in the range of 10%, then in the absence of any explanation for their negative status they should be regarded as likely carriers and culled immediately. They may be examined for virus, but since this operation may be less than 100% efficient they will never be free of suspicion and so it is largely a waste of time and effort. Note however that in other circumstances—for example, if a controlled exposure program is to be contemplated—it may be useful, of even necessary, to confirm the status of these animals.

If there are marginally more negatives, of the order of 5–10%, too many to willingly cull, then either they should all be examined for virus or, if this is not feasible, the serological results should be analyzed in an attempt to deduce the status of the negatives, that is, whether they are viremic or unexposed. Subgroups within the herd, defined by age, origin or location, should be considered separately. Small numbers of negative animals within subgroups that are otherwise positive come under suspicion and should be eliminated on that basis if opportunity for confirmation of their status by virus isolation is not available. In some cases the proper interpretation of serological results may be clarified, and immunotolerant carriers identified, by further testing after some tactic to promote seroconversions. Suitable tactics for this purpose might include vaccination or simply intensive management of the group to maximize intimate contacts with any unrecognized carrier animal that may be present, followed by serological retesting in 2 weeks. Although it is obviously impossible to forecast precise transmission rates for all situations, interpretation of data for single groups should be made in the knowledge that transmission rates are likely to be relatively low under extensive grazing conditions but greatly increased by any handling or intensive husbandry. Progeny of suspect virus carriers will also be under suspicion.

As the endemic presence of the virus appears to depend almost entirely on the presence of one or more persistently infected carriers, and these animals are at a survival disadvantage compared to normal animals, it can be expected that the infection will be ultimately naturally eliminated from some herds following which, barring reintroduction of infection, reactors will be confined to those animals which were present in the herd prior to the elimination of the infection. If a substantial part of a herd, which has been of stable composition for some time, is serologically negative, and reactors can be recognized to be confined to groups defined by either age or origin, this may indicate that the virus has been active in those groups in the past but is no longer active in the herd. In these cases no further investigatory action is necessary before vaccination and precautions against the reintroduction of infection are employed. Calves present a special case and testing should be deferred until they are over 6 months of age and are likely to have lost maternal antibody.

A final scenario which should be considered is the herd which has already been comprehensively vaccinated. As in a herd with a very high natural antibody prevalence, the viremic animals might be recognized as those that are still lacking antibody. However, in the case of the vaccinated herd there is a further complication, in that viremic animals may respond to the vaccine strain, if it differs serotypically from the persistent virus, and produce antibody that will be recognized in a virus neutralization test if there is a serotypic relationship between the strains used in the vaccine and the test. A group-specific test may be more informative than the virus neutralization test because the group antigen, shared by all serotypes, is included in the carrier's spectrum of immune tolerance and so the carrier is more likely to remain seronegative. On theoretical grounds, the GDP test would be preferred, as it involves only the single common antigen whereas those of the serotype may also contribute to reactivity in other tests, even though those tests may normally be dominated by the group antigen. The use of a group-specific test may avoid this problem and expose the carrier because of its negative status to the serotype-common antigen. Animals which are purchased for introduction into a virus-free herd, and bulls entering artificial insemination centers, should be tested for the presence of virus (86).

After the persistently viremic animals have been eliminated the new virus-free status of the herd should be maintained by a program of vaccination of all animals before puberty and testing of all introduced animals for freedom from infection. The testing of introduced animals is important because the efficacy of vaccination against serotypes which differ from those contained in the vaccine is open to question. As far as the vaccinate is concerned it can be expected to be effective, if only through a heterotypic response, but this may not be sufficient to prevent transplacental infection in a pregnant animal (71). In many cases introductions can be guaranteed, as far as is reasonably possible, to be free of infection by selecting animals which have convincing titers of serum antibody or are negative *and* are derived from a totally negative herd or stable subherd. According to the period over which the herd of origin has been established and has been free from introductions, its free status may be established by testing an adequate sample of animals. In other cases, antibody negative introductions should be examined for virus or held for a period of on-property quarantine in close contact with a few serologically negative test animals which are subsequently examined for antibody.

Immunization of breeding females

The prevention of mucosal disease in young cattle from 6 to 24 months of age has been unreliable, up until recently, because the pathogenesis was not understood. Conventional wisdom suggested that calves should be vaccinated with the vaccine at or around weaning time when the level of colostral antibody had declined to a level where it did not interfere with the vaccine. Modified BVD live virus vaccines have been available for the past 20 years and were used with varying degrees of apparent success. However, few clinical trials, if any, examined the efficacy of the vaccines under field conditions. When outbreaks of mucosal disease occurred, vaccination of the in-contact animals to prevent further occurrence of the disease was commonly practiced. However, the results were difficult to evaluate. In some herds no further cases occurred and success was attributed to the vaccine. In other herds, outbreaks of clinical disease occurred about 10–14 days following vaccination (72). The possible causes postulated for these so-called *'vaccination breaks'* included the following: the vaccine virus may not have been sufficiently attenuated and actually caused the disease; the calves may have been incubating the disease when vaccinated; and some calves were immunologically tolerant because of infection during fetal life allowing the vaccine virus to cause the disease. These vaccination breaks gave the vaccines a poor reputation and as a result they have not been used on a regular basis. Also, veterinarians began to make regular reports that the vaccine was ineffective against mucosal disease, but the reasons were unknown (73).

The new information on the pathogenesis of mucosal disease explains why vaccination of calves at about 6 months of age may not provide protection in all cases. If mucosal disease is a late sequel to fetal infection, then some calves will be persistently infected, specifically immunotolerant, will not be cured of that original infection, and may eventually develop mucosal disease whether they respond to the vaccine virus or not. Thus they could become affected with clinical disease regardless of vaccination (55). Also, new cases of mucosal disease may occur in 5–10% calves within a few weeks following vaccination with a live-virus vaccine. It has been postulated that this is likely to be due to the vaccine virus fulfilling the role of a superinfecting virus to precipitate clinical disease. However, it is a relatively infrequent occurrence and it did not occur on one occasion when known persistently viremic cattle were vaccinated with a cytopathic live-virus vaccine, but clinical disease was subsequently induced following experimental infection with a different cytopathic strain (55).

It is now clear that testing the efficacy of BVDV vaccines by vaccinating calves at 4–6 months of age followed by experimental challenge a few weeks after vaccination is of limited value. Immunocompetent calves whether vaccinated or not, will not develop mucosal disease following experimental or natural infection. The key to successful control is vaccination of the breeding female at least several weeks before breeding (74). Experimental exposure of pubertal heifers to the virus 6 weeks before breeding stimulated the production of serum neutralizing antibodies which protected against transplacental infection of the fetuses when the pregnant dams were challenged with homologous virus at 100 days of gestation. A high incidence of fetal death and intrauterine growth retardation occurred in the non-immune dams. Thus the presence of maternal immunity protected the fetus from homologous infection (74). These observations provide justification for the use of BVDV vaccines in females before breeding in an attempt to stimulate maternal immunity to provide protection of the fetus. However, immunization, in terms of protecting the fetus, may not be effective against serotypes which are different from that contained in the vaccine and the ultimate precaution is to prevent cows or heifers from making new contacts shortly before or during the first half of pregnancy. It should also be emphasized that control of the infection, and of mucosal disease, depends entirely on control among the breeding stock. Infection among non-breeders is of no long-term consequence except in so far as they may be a source of infection to breeders and compromise the continuing freedom from infection of that group.

The emphasis must be on the vaccination of immunocompetent animals which do not have persistent viral infection. This should provide at least partial if not complete protection against fetal infection, abortion, stillbirth, intrauterine growth retardation, congenital defects, and persistent viral infection of the newborn calf. The aim of a vaccination program is, therefore, to ensure that all breeding females have antibodies to the virus before they become pregnant. It is important to emphasize that vaccination be done at least 3 weeks before breeding so that the breeding females become seropositive to the virus before conception. This is necessary regardless of the type of vaccine used. The suppliers of inactivated virus vaccines commonly promote their vaccines on the basis that they can be given safely to pregnant cows. While it is true that the inactivated virus vaccines are not fetopathogenic, only successful vaccination *before* conception will protect the fetus from natural infection for the entire gestational period. Vaccination of pregnant cows cannot be recommended at this time in spite of published advice (75).

The inoculation of pregnant cattle, without detectable neutralizing antibodies to the virus, between 51 and 190 days of gestation with a commercial modified BVD live vaccine can result in transplacental transmission of the vaccine virus (76). The possible effects of such vaccination are variable and dependent on the stage of gestation when the vaccination occurs. Abortions, congenital abnormalities of the nervous and musculoskeletal systems, perinatal deaths, growth retardation, persistent viral infection and the late onset of mucosal disease are all possible outcomes of vaccinating pregnant cattle with a modified live vaccine before 120 days of gestation (76). Between 120 and 190 days of gestation the fetus can be expected to become immunocompetent and produce serum neutralizing antibodies which can be detected in the precolostral serum of the calf at birth (76). The vaccination of pregnant cattle without neutralizing antibodies to the virus between 190 and 265 days of gestation will also result in transplacental transmission of the virus and the presence of neutralizing antibodies in the precolostral serum of calves at birth (77). Calves derived from dams vaccinated between 90 and 118 days of gestation showed ataxia, torticollis, opisthotonus and/or growth retardation (85).

Both modified live virus and inactivated virus vaccines are available. The modified live-virus vaccines are potentially fetopathogenic and should not be used in pregnant cows. Some other modified live-virus vaccines (not specifically BVDV vaccines) have been contaminated with pathogenic isolates of the BVDV and their use has been followed by serious economic losses due to abortions, chronic wasting in dams, severe growth retardation in the calves and high neonatal mortality with thymic atrophy (78). The inactivated virus vaccines are safe but must be given twice, 10 days to 2 weeks apart (79). More research and field experience are necessary to more accurately assess the relative value of each vaccine. At the present time it is not possible, on the basis of scientific information, to recommend the use of one form of the vaccine over any other. A temperature-sensitive vaccine will cause seroconversion, produces no clinical signs of disease or leukopenia and, when used experimentally in pregnant cows, does not result in fetal infection as evidenced by lack of virus isolation and absence of precolostral antibodies in the calves which are born healthy (80).

Some workers have cautioned against the widespread adoption and use of BVDV vaccines which have not been tested for efficacy (81). An inactivated quadrivalent vaccine, which induced a serological response in cows before insemination, failed to protect about one-third of the fetuses against transplacental infection from a multiple heterologous strain challenge. This indicates a need for additional understanding of the antigenic relationships between the many isolates of the virus.

With the present state of knowledge a rational vaccination program, for both beef breeding herds and dairy herds, would consist of vaccinating all of the cows and heifer replacements at from 3 to 6 weeks before breeding. Each year thereafter, all heifer replacements are vaccinated at least 3 weeks before breeding. Colostral immunity is present for up to 6 months of age in calves born from immune cows. Calves with even high titers of colostral BVDV antibody may have an active response to vaccination (52) but it is questionable whether this is of any useful purpose. If vaccination of the dam before conception is the vital part of the program, the vaccination of calves born from immune cows may be unnecessary until they approach breeding age. There is no evidence that postnatal primary infection with BVDV will cause acute fatal mucosal disease in immunocompetent calves born from immune cows.

There is no substantive evidence to warrant the vaccination of feedlot cattle. In a population of feedlot cattle originating from several sources, there will be present some animals which are immunotolerant and persistently infected. As noted previously, they are likely to develop mucosal disease, either in the short term as a result of superinfection, or in the long term because the vaccination cannot be expected to eliminate persistent infection.

In the Bruce County Beef Cattle Project, the use of modified BVD live-virus vaccines in feedlot calves on arrival in the lot after transportation of 3200 km (2000 miles) increased the risk of mortality (82). The risk declined following decreased use of the live-virus vaccine (83). This observation may support the experimental work that the field isolates of the virus and live-virus vaccines may cause immunosuppression.

REVIEW LITERATURE

Ames, T. R. (1986) The causative agent of BVD: its epidemiology and pathogenesis. *Vet. Med.*, *81*, 848–870.

Baker, J. C. (1978) Bovine viral diarrhea virus: a review. *J. Am. vet. med. Assoc.*, *190*, 1449–1458.

Duffell, S. J. & Harkness, J. W. (1985) Bovine virus diarrhea—mucosal disease infection in cattle. *Vet. Rec.*, *117*, 240–245.

Perdrizet, J. A., Rebhun, W. C., Dubovi, E. J. & Dovis, R. O. (1987) Bovine virus diarrhea—clinical syndromes in dairy herds. *Cornell Vet.*, *77*, 46–74.

REFERENCES

(1) Pritchard, W. R. (1963) *Adv. vet. Sci.*, pp. 1–47.
(2) Thomson, R. G. & Savan, M. (1963) *Can. J. comp. Med..*, *21*, 207.
(3) Childs, T. (1946) *Can. J. comp. Med*, *10*, 316.
(4) Westaway, E. G. et al. (1985) *Intervirology*, *24*, 125.
(5) Steck, F. et al. (1980) *Zentralbl. VetMed. B*, *27*, 429.
(6) Harkness, J. W. et al. (1978) *Res. vet. Sci.*, *24*, 98.
(7) Bolin, S. R. et al (1985) *Am. J. vet. Res.*, *46*, BC2385.
(8) Alenius, S. et al. (1986) *Proc. 14th World Cong. Dis. Cattle*, *1*, 204.
(9) Meyling, A. (1984) In: *Recent Advances in Virus Diagnosis*; eds, M. S. McNulty & J. B. MacFerran. Boston: Martinus Nijhoff, pp. 37–46.
(10) Howard, C. J. et al. (1986) *Vet. Rec.*, *119*, 628.
(11) Perdrizet, J. A. et al. (1987) *Cornell Vet.*, *77*, 46.
(12) Doyle, L. G. & Heuschele, W. P. (1983) *J. Am. vet. med. Assoc.*, *183*, 1257.
(13) Lamontagne, L. & Roy, R. (1984) *Can. J. comp. Med.*, *48*, 225.
(14) Elazhary, M. A. S. Y. et al. (1984) *Am. J. vet. Res.*, *45*, 1660.
(15) Ames, T. R. et al. (1982) *J. Am. vet. med. Assoc.*, *180*, 619.
(16) Barlow, R. M. & Patterson, D. S. P. (1982) *Adv. vet. Med.*, *36*, 1.
(17) Stewart, W. C. et al. (1980) *Am. J. vet. Res.*, *41*, 459.
(18) Duffell, S. J. & Harkness, J. W. (1985) *Vet. Rec.*, *117*, 240.
(19) Roeder, P. L. & Drew, T. W. (1984) *Vet. Rec.*, *114*, 309.
(20) Barber, D. M. L. et al. (1985) *Vet. Rec.*, *117*, 459.
(21) Brownlie, J. et al. (1984) *Vet. Rec.*, *114*, 535.
(22) Done, J. T. et al. (1980) *Vet. Rec.*, *106*, 473.
(23) McClurkin, A. W. et al. (1984) *Can. J. comp. Med.*, *48*, 156.
(24) Ohmann, H. B. (1984) *Acta vet. Scand.*, *25*, 36.
(25) Roeder, P. L. et al. (1986) *Vet. Rec.*, *118*, 44.
(26) Binkhorst, G. J. et al. (1983) *Vet. Q..*, *5*, 145.
(27) Strauer, P. J. et al. (1983) *Vet. Q..*, *5*, 156.
(28) Littlejohns, I. R. & Walker, K. H. (1985) *Aust. vet. J.*, *62*, 101.
(29) Coria, M. F. & McClurkin, A. W. (1978) *J. Am. vet. med. Assoc.*, *172*, 449.
(30) McClurkin, A. W. et al. (1979) *J. Am. vet med. Assoc.*, *174*, 1116.
(31) Barlow, R. M. et al. (1986) *Vet. Rec. 118*, 321.
(32) Duffell, S. J. et al. (1986) *Vet. Rec.*, *118*, 38.
(33) Roth, J. A. et al. (1986) *Am. J. vet. Res.*, *47*, 1139.
(34) Potgieter, L. N. D. et al. (1984) *Am. J. vet. Res.*, *45*, 687.
(35) Markham, R. J. F. & Ramnaraine, M. L. (1985) *Am. J. vet. Res.*, *46*, 879.
(36) Roth, J. A. & Kaeberle, M. L. (1983) *Am. J. vet. Res.*, *44*, 2366.
(37) Potgieter, L. N. D. et al. (1984) *Am. J. vet. Res.*, *45*, 1582.
(38) Potgieter, L. N. D. et al. (1985) *Am. J. vet. Res.*, *46*, 151.
(39) Lopez, A. et al. (1986) *Am. J. vet. Res.*, *47*, BC1283.
(40) Yates, W. D. G. (1982) *Can. J. comp. Med.*, *46*, 225.
(41) Lambert, G. et al. (1974) *J. Am. vet. med. Assoc.*, *164*, 287.
(42) Potter, M. L. et al. (1984) *Am. J. vet. Res.*, *45*, 1778.
(43) Grahn, T. C. et al. (1984) *J. Am. vet. med. Assoc.*, *185*, 429.
(44) Whitmore, H. L. et al. (1981) *J. Am. vet. med. Assoc.*, *178*, 1065.
(45) Archbald, L. F. et al. (1979) *Theriogenology*, *11*, 81.
(46) Kendrick, J. W. (1971) *Am. J. vet. Res.*, *32*, 533.
(47) Brown, T. T. et al, (1979) *Infect. Immun.*, *25*, 93.
(48) Braun, K. et al. (1973) *Am. J. vet. Res.*, *34*, 1127.
(49) McClurkin, A. W. et al. (1985) *Am. vet. med. Assoc.*, *186*, 568.
(50) Bolin, S. R. et al (1985) *Am. J. vet Res.*, *46*, 573.
(51) Liess, B. et al. (1983) *Dtsch Tierärztl. Wochenschr.*, *90*, 261.
(52) Menanteau-Horta, A. M. et al. (1985) *Can. J. comp. Med.*, *49*, 10.
(53) Coria, M. F. & McClurkin, A. W. (1978) *Can. J. comp. Med.*, *42*, 239.
(54) Brownlie, J. et al. (1986) *Proc. EEC Conf. Pestivirus Infect. Ruminants*, Brussels, Sept. 1985.
(55) Bolin, S. R. et al (1985) *Am. J. vet. Res.*, *46*, 2467.
(56) Winter, H. & Majid, N. H. (1984) *Vet. Bull.*, *54*, 327.
(57) Cutlip, R. C. et al. (1976) *Am. J. vet. Res. 41*, 1938.
(58) Wilson, T. M. et al. (1983) *J. Am. vet. med. Assoc.*, *183*, 544.
(59) Ohmann, H. B. (1984) *Acta vet. Scand.*, *25*, 36.
(60) Sawyer, M. M. et al. (1986) *J. Am. vet. med. Assoc.*, *189*, 61.
(61) Ohmann, H. B. (1983) *Res. vet. Sci.*, *34*, 5.
(62) Ward, A. C. S. & Kaeberle, M. L. (1984) *Am. J. vet. Res.*, *45*, 165.
(63) Ohmann, H. B. et al. (1981) *Acta Pathol. Microbiol. Scand.*, *89*, 281.
(64) Hopkinson, M. F. et al. (1981) *Am. J. vet. Res.*, *40*, 1189.
(65) Silim, A. & Elazhary, M. A. S. Y. (1983) *Can. J. comp. Med.*, *47*, 18.
(66) Chu, H. J. et al. (1985) *Vet. Microbiol.*, *10*, 325.
(67) Howard, C. J. et al. (1985) *Vet. Microbiol.*, *10*, 359.
(68) Jerrett, I. V. et al. (1984) *Cornell Vet.*, *74*, 8.
(69) Ohmann, H. B. et al. (1982) *Can. J. comp. Med.*, *46*, 357, 363.
(70) Miller, R. B. & Quinn, P. J. (1975) *Can. J. comp. Med.*, *39*, 270.
(71) Roeder, P. L. & Harkness, J. W. (1986) *Vet. Rec.*, *118*, 143.
(72) Peter, C. P. et al. (1967) *J. Am. vet. med. Assoc.*, *150*, 46.
(73) Ernst, P. B. & Butler, D. G. (1983) *Can. J. comp. Med.*, *47*, 118.
(74) Duffell, S. J. et al. (1984) *Vet. Rec.*, *114*, 558.
(75) Sanders, D. E. et al. (1983) *Agri-Practice.*, *4*, 30.
(76) Leiss, B. et al. (1984) *Zentralbl. VetMed.*, B31, 669.
(77) Orban, S. et al. (1983) *Zentralbl. VetMed.*, B30, 619.
(78) Lohr, C. H. et al. (1983) *Vet. Med. SAC*, *78*, 1263.
(79) McClurkin, A. W. & Coria, M. F. (1980) *Proc. US Anim. Hlth Assoc.*, *84*, 223.
(80) Lobmann, M. et al. (1986) *Am.J. vet. Res.*, *47*, 557.
(81) Roeder, P. L. et al. (1984) *Vet. Rec.*, *115*, 525.
(82) Martin, S. W. et al. (1980) *Can. J. comp. Med.*, *44*, 1.
(83) Martin, S. W. et al. (1981) *Can. J. comp. Med.*, *45*, 103.
(84) Coria, M. F. et al. (1984) *Am. J. vet. Res.*, *45*, 2129.
(85) Trautwein, G. et al. (1986) *J. vet. Med.*, B33, 260.
(86) Chu, H. J. & Zee, Y. C. (1984) *Am. J. vet. Res.*, *45*, 845.
(87) Lucas, M. H. (1986) *Vet. Rec.*, *119*, 15.
(88) Martin, S. W. & Bohac, J. G. (1986) *Can. J. vet Res.*, *50*, 351.
(89) Jubb, K. V. P., Kennedy, P. C. & Palmer, N. (1985) *Pathology of Domestic Animals*, 3rd edn, vol. 2, pp. 95–100. London: Academic Press.

Bovine papular stomatitis

A disease of little importance in its own right, although it may cause mild illness and serve as a portal of entry for secondary bacterial infection, bovine papular stomatitis is of importance chiefly because of the confusion it may cause in the diagnosis of those diseases of cattle in which erosive and vesicular lesions of the mouth are an important diagnostic feature. Bovine papular stomatitis has been known for very many years but has only achieved importance in recent years because of increased interest in viral diseases of the bovine alimentary tract. It has been reported in Africa, the United States, Australia, New Zealand, Canada, Great Britain and Europe.

The causative parapoxvirus has many of the characteristics of the pox group and is classed as a 'paravaccinia virus'. There is good evidence that the papular stomatitis and the pseudocowpox virus are identical (1, 2). It occurs in several closely related strains and can be grown on tissue culture. Clinical cases are encountered in young animals from 2 weeks up to 2 years of age and in a group the morbidity often approximates 100%. A high incidence occurred in neonatal calves following neonatal thymectomy for experimental purposes (11). There may be transient anorexia, weight loss, ptyalism (11), and a slight fever (39·5°C, 103°F) but in most instances the disease goes unnoticed unless a careful examination of the mouth is made. Lesions are confined to the muzzle, just inside the nostrils and on the buccal mucosa. Occasional cases occur in which the only lesions are in the esophageal mucosa (3). They commence as small (0·5–1 cm) papules which become dark red in color, develop a roughening of the surface and expand peripherally so that the lesions are always round or nearly so. Confluence of several lesions may cause the development of a large irregularly shaped area. As the lesion expands the periphery becomes reddened and the center depressed, gray-brown in color and rough on the surface, and eventually covered with necrotic tissue, or on external lesions by a scab. Those on the muzzle may be difficult to see if the area is pigmented. In the mouth the lesions occur on all mucosal surfaces except the dorsum of the tongue, and are most common inside the lips and in close proximity to the teeth. Individual lesions heal quickly, sometimes in as short a time as 4–7 days, but evidence of healed lesions, in the form of circular areas of dark pink mucosa, usually surrounded by a slightly paler raised zone, may persist for weeks. In the one animal there may be successive crops of lesions so that they can be found continuously or intermittently over a period of months. It is suggested that no immunity occurs and the virus may only cause lesions when intercurrent disease causes lowering of the animal's resistance (4).

Histological examination shows a characteristic ballooning degeneration and the presence of cytoplasmic inclusions in affected cells. The infection can be transmitted by the inoculation of scrapings from lesions into the oral mucosa of susceptible calves and by submucosal inoculation of undiluted tissue culture virus. Diagnosis of the presence of the virus can be made by electron microscopy of the saliva. It can also be grown in cell culture (9, 12) and a virus neutralization test is available for positive identification (10). Indirect immunofluorescence can be used on cattle sera to distinguish antigenic differences between bovine papular stomatitis, milker's nodules and contagious ecthyma (13).

Bovine papular stomatitis resembles endemic erosive stomatitis of cattle recorded in Africa (5). Spread of the disease from calves to man (6) and from man to calves (7) is recorded.

The disease known as 'rat-tail syndrome' in young cattle in feedlots is probably a manifestation of sarcocytosis. However, there is also a high prevalence of bovine papular stomatitis lesions and virus in these cattle and it is possible that it may contribute to the development of the disease (8). A concurrent infection of bovine papular stomatitis and bovine virus diarrhea has been described in a calf (14).

REFERENCES

(1) Nagington, J. et al. (1967) *Vet. Rec.*, *81*, 306.
(2) Liebermann, H. (1967) *Arch. exp. Vet. Med.*, *21*, 1337, 1353, 1391, 1399.
(3) Crandall, R. A. & Gosser, H.S. (1974) *J. Am. vet. med. Assoc.*, *165*, 282.
(4) Plowright, W. & Ferris, R. D. (1959) *Vet. Rec.*, *71*, 718, 828.
(5) Schaaf, J. (1955) *Arch. exp. VetMed.*, 9, 194.
(6) Schnurrenberger, P. R. et al. (1980) *Can. J. comp. Med.*, *44*, 239.
(7) Carson, C. A. et al. (1968) *Am. J. vet. Res.*, *29*, 1783.
(8) Brown, L. N. et al. (1976) *Proc. 19th Ann. Mtg Am. Assoc. Vet. Diagnosticians*, p. 405.
(9) Aguilar-Setien, A. et al. (1978) *Ann. Méd. vét.*, *122*, 555.
(10) Aguilar-Setien, A. et al. (1980) *Cornell Vet.*, *70*, 10.
(11) Snider, T. G. (III) et al. (1982) *Arch. Virol.*, *71*, 251.
(12) Abraham, A. et al. (1985) *Vet. Rec.*, *116*, 379.
(13) Rosenbusch, R. F. & Reed, D. E. (1983) *Am. J. vet. Res.*, *44*, 875.
(14) Bohac, J. G. & Yates, W. D. G. (1980) *Can. vet. J.*, *21*, 310.

Transmissible gastroenteritis of pigs

Transmissible gastroenteritis of pigs (TGE) is a highly infectious disease of pigs caused by a virus and is manifested clinically by vomiting, diarrhea, dehydration and a high mortality rate in very young pigs.

Etiology

The disease is caused by a coronavirus which is relatively host-specific for pigs. Laboratory animals cannot be infected but the virus will replicate in dogs without the production of clinical disease and is shed in the feces for periods up to 2 weeks (1). The virus can be grown in tissue culture but repeated passage generally results in lowered pathogenicity for piglets (51) and greater cytopathogenic effect. There is variation in virulence between isolates but they appear to be of one antigenic type (2).

Epidemiology

During the past three decades transmissible gastroenteritis has changed from a sporadic disease occurring in the mid-west of the United States to a major economic disease endemic in most countries of the northern hemisphere. An analysis of the economic losses due to the disease in swine farms in Missouri over a 2 year period estimated the average loss between 13 and 18%

of the average return earned above total production costs (57). Climatic factors appear to be of considerable importance in the occurrence and establishment of the disease. It does not yet have significance in the tropics or southern hemisphere and there is evidence that its spread is limited in hot climates. In endemic areas it has a distinct seasonal occurrence with the majority of outbreaks occurring from midwinter to spring, and cyclic occurrence is recorded (4). Experimentally, a decrease and fluctuation in the environmental temperature will result in a more severe clinical disease than when the climate is warm (40). The disease tends to occur in area outbreaks. The epidemiology of the disease in the United States (5), Europe (6) and the United Kingdom (4) has been described.

With the classic form of the disease an outbreak in a herd is explosive and dramatic. There is rapid spread and high morbidity of pigs of all ages within 2–3 days but major clinical disease is restricted to pigs prior to weaning and to lactating sows. Case fatality rates may approach 100% in pigs under 10–14 days of age but fall dramatically with increasing age and mortality is low in postweaned and adult pigs. The outbreak terminates in 3–5 weeks with the loss of young susceptible pigs and the development of herd immunity and the disease generally does not recur again for a 3–6 year period.

The exact mode of transmission of transmissible gastroenteritis is uncertain. Virus shedding in the feces of infected pigs usually ends at or within a few weeks of recovery although recovered pigs may harbor virus in pulmonary or intestinal tissue for periods over 100 days. Feeder pigs which may show no clinical signs can be an important reservoir of the virus (7). The virus has also been isolated from pharyngeal swabs taken from farm-raised sows sent to slaughter (8). Outbreaks commonly follow the introduction of pigs into a herd and the carrier pig is probably the major source of infection and transmission of the disease. Frequently the disease first appears in older pigs in the herd and then subsequently spreads to newborn pigs and sows in the farrowing area. Visitors, transport vehicles and starlings have also been incriminated in the transfer of infection to new locations (4, 5, 9). It is postulated that starlings may act as vectors to spread adjacent farms (52). The virus can also multiply in house flies (*Musca domestica* Linneaus) and they may be a vector (56). Details of the resistance of the virus are incomplete but it does not persist in infected premises for more than a few weeks and is readily destroyed by standard solutions of phenol and formalin, by boiling and by drying. It is not destroyed by freezing. The virus is photosensitive and this may account for the more frequent occurrence of the disease during the winter and spring months (3). The virus can survive freezing, and infected pork scraps or offal may provide a source of infection either directly through feeding of uncooked garbage or possibly indirectly via dogs. Purposeful infection by the feeding of frozen infected piglet intestine to sows to induce immunity may also be a significant source of continued infection of a herd or area (5).

Once infection has gained access to a herd, transmission probably occurs by both oral and respiratory routes. The speed of spread without direct contact indicates that virus can be spread by aerosol. Respiratory transmission appears significant in adults and replication in the respiratory tract is followed by excretion in nasal secretions, and milk within 1 day of infection and also in feces (11). Excretion in milk results in rapid transmission to suckling piglets which in turn may excrete large quantities of virus within 2 days of infection.

Immunity to clinical disease in newborn piglets is dependent on the level of secretory IgA antibody in the colostrum of the sow. Only after stimulation of the intestinal tract of the sow following oral or natural infection with virulent transmissible gastroenteritis virus are IgA antibodies produced in the milk (41). The parenteral administration of the modified live virus will not provide protective immunity which explains the failure of parenteral vaccines to be effective. Serum antibody does not provide immunity for protection of pigs from reinfection. Following oral inoculation of pigs with the virus, IgA antibody develops in the small intestine and serum, and active immunity to the disease can be evaluated by a quantitative determination of the IgA in the serum (42). Another mechanism which may be involved in active immunity in recovered pigs is the local cell-mediated immunity in the small intestine (44). Following intestinal stimulation the IgA and IgM-producing cells leave the intestinal mucosa and are trapped by distant secretory epithelia.

Suckling pigs are protected from infection by continued ingestion of antibody of the IgA class secreted in milk. The IgA antibody occurs in milk of sows only after oral exposure to virulent transmissible gastroenteritis virus, but not after intramuscular or intramammary introduction. It has been proposed that this secretory antibody is produced by cells whose precursors are stimulated by transmissible gastroenteritis viral antigen in the intestinal mucosa and then enter the circulation and localize in other secretory sites such as the mammary and salivary glands (43). The level of serum IgA antibody as an indicator of immunity to transmissible gastroenteritis can be measured using the indirect immunoperoxidase antibody test (45). Young pigs, 6 weeks of age, which are exposed to experimental infection with the virus develop both a humoral and cellular immunity (55) which reach peaks at 21 and 28 days respectively.

In recent years, less typical forms of the disease have been observed. With continuous farrowing and the continual introduction of susceptible pigs into an infective environment, outbreaks may be considerably prolonged and this or recrudescence is more likely than when pregnant sows are kept in relative isolation on pasture or elsewhere. Atypical enzootic forms of the disease with a low morbidity and mortality and frequently with the onset of clinical disease delayed until piglets are 2–4 weeks of age have been observed (4, 7, 12) and may go unrecognized because of the atypical clinical picture. They are more likely to occur in large continuous farrowing units and may be associated with partial herd immunity and low virulence virus (4, 7). Some sows do not develop a significant immunity following a single infection and in large herds there may be a sufficient number of these to allow the disease to perpetuate in a low incidence endemic form.

A recrudescence of the disease may occur after a period of up to 11 months and is thought to be due to inadequate exposure and immunity of some pigs, particularly dry stock, during the intial outbreak, followed by reinfection from a carrier pig (10). Recrudescence of clinical disease is usually of much shorter duration than the primary outbreak and commonly lasts only 6–10 days. The periods of recrudescence are commonly precipitated by the simultaneous farrowing of several susceptible gilts in the same farrowing room. Of greater longterm concern is that some large herds continue to experience clinical recrudescences for almost 2 years or more. In some prospective epidemiological surveys the endemic infection remained clinically mild or inapparent in about 50% of the herds for 2 years or more (58). The endemic form of the disease appears to be correlated with herds of more than 100 sows and in herds where finishing pigs were kept. In large herds the virus may spread more slowly and replacement gilts entering the herd may take several months to become infected and to seroconvert. In large herds the rapid turnover of breeding stock and continuous farrowing and early weaning also contributes to perpetuate an endemic infection (59). Thus endemic transmissible gastroenteritis can maintain itself by the slow and incomplete spread of the virus among adult pigs, particularly herd replacements.

Pathogenesis

The virus infects the upper respiratory tract and the intestine but the major clinical signs are associated with the intestinal infection. Following oral challenge of susceptible piglets the incubation period may be as short as 24 hours. The virus infects mature differentiated columnar epithelial cells of the intestinal villi but not the undifferentiated cells of the crypts. Replication occurs within 4–5 hours with sloughing of the infected cell and release of virus, and after several replication cycles there is a marked reduction in villous size with villous atrophy. The loss of epithelial cells results in increased migration of undifferentiated cells from the crypts to line the shortened villi. With virulent virus, epithelial cells at all levels of the small intestine are infected with major lesions occurring at the proximal jejunum and to a lesser extent the ileum (14). The lesser virulence of attenuated strains of virus may be associated with their inability to infect and produce lesions in the villi of the more cranial portions of the jejunum (17).

Diarrhea results from a combination of malabsorption and osmotic effects subsequent to the loss of intestinal surface area and disaccharidase activity, and impaired lumen-to-extracellular fluid flux of sodium consequent on the occurrence of undifferentiated cells lining the stunted villi (14). The virus invades the villus, but not the crypt epithelium of the small intestine within hours after experimental administration. The infected villus cells are quickly shed and replaced by relatively undifferentiated enterocytes. As infected cells are shed, the epithelium proliferates and migration of cells from the crypts accelerates (14). There are marked abnormalities in ion transport function in the jejunum and ileum at the height of the diarrhea. There is failure of the intestine to actively transport sodium and chloride and there is a defect of the glucose-mediated sodium ion transport (13). Experimentally induced infection of 3-week-old pigs with the virus results in villous atrophy and crypt hyperplasia and marked decrease in the secretory response of the villous epithelium to *Escherichia coli* enterotoxins (15). The disease is more severe in gnotobiotic pigs that are infected with *E. coli* in addition to transmissible gastroenteritis virus, suggesting that bacterial factors also influence the severity of the diarrhea.

In the experimental disease in 2 day-old pigs, vomiting and diarrhea occur 12–24 hours after oral inoculation of the virus and affected piglets are moribund 1 or 2 days later (16). Before becoming moribund most piglets become lethargic and comatose. In addition to dehydration and metabolic acidosis there is a severe hypoglycemia due to a combination of inadequate glucose metabolism inherent to neonatal piglets and the acute maldigestion and malabsorption from the diffuse and severe villous atrophy (16). Thus the high mortality may be due to a combination of dehydration, acidosis and severe hypoglycemia.

The age dependent resistance to transmissible gastroenteritis can be explained, in part, by a decreased susceptibility of the epithelial cells of older pigs to infection and by an increased proliferative capacity of crypt cells with much more rapid regeneration of atrophic villi in pigs over 2 weeks of age (19).

Clinical findings

In a primary or epidemic outbreak the clinical findings of classical acute transmissible gastroenteritis are characteristic.

After an incubation period of 24–48 hours there is a sudden onset of vomiting and diarrhea but some affected piglets may continue to suck to within a few hours of death. The diarrhea is profuse and violent, the feces being watery and usually yellow-green in color. They may contain clots of white undigested milk and have an offensive odor. There may be a transitory fever but in most cases the temperature is normal. Depression and dehydration are pronounced, the hair coat is ruffled, and weakness and emaciation progress with death occurring on the 2nd–5th day. Affected piglets which survive are severely emaciated and gain weight slowly. The illness may commence as soon as 24 hours after birth. It is not uncommon on an individual farm for the disease to become less severe and to spread more slowly with the passage of time.

In older pigs there may be signs similar to those which occur in piglets but many animals become infected without showing clinical abnormality. In clinically affected older pigs recovery is much more likely to occur, the illness lasting for up to 10 days. Lactating sows may or may not show clinical signs of infection. Fever and inappetence, with or without diarrhea, are seen and agalactia is a common complication in sows showing clinical illness. In endemically affected herds with continuous farrowing and partial sow immunity the disease usually manifests itself in a milder form of diarrhea affecting piglets about 6 days of age or older, diarrhea in weaner pigs; brief periods of overt clinical recrudescence in part of the herd mortality is low, but affected pigs subsequently grow poorly.

Clinical pathology

A severe dehydration, metabolic acidosis and a marked hypoglycemia occur (16, 18).

The virus can be detected in the fresh tissue and feces by an enzyme-linked immunosorbent assay (ELISA) test (20), immune electron microscopy (21), fluorescent antibody staining or by the immunoperoxidase test (24). A reversed passive hemagglutination test for detection of the virus in feces is also available (60).

Several serological tests for the detection and measurement of antibody to the transmissible gastroenteritis virus infection in live animals are available. The serum neutralization test is sensitive and reliable, but is time-consuming and requires facilities for cell culture techniques. Neutralizing antibodies appear in the serum as soon as 7–8 days after infection and persist for at least 18 months (23). An ELISA test has been developed and is more sensitive than the virus neutralization test (47).

Necropsy findings

Except for pallor of the renal cortex and congestion of the renal medullary rays, the major necropsy lesions are confined to the intestine and stomach. In many field outbreaks and in the experimental disease the lesions may be minor. The intestinal wall is thin and translucent and the intestine is distended with fluid ingesta. Despite the presence of milk in the intestine there is little evidence of fat absorption in the draining lymphatics. In the stomach there may be engorgement of vessels, and necrosis of the epithelium deep in mucosal crypts. No inclusion bodies are detectable. The important histopathological change is villous atrophy with failure of epithelial cell differentiation in the small intestine. The atrophy is evident 24 hours after infection and regeneration occurs 5 –7 days later. The marked reduction in villous size may be detected at low magnification on a stereomicroscope. Examination of frozen sections of jejunum from acutely ill piglets by the fluorescent antibody technique is a rapid and effective method for the detection of virus in tissues (46). A simple test for the presence of intestinal lactase in intestinal washings may assist in the laboratory diagnosis (50). When secondary pathogens contribute to the disease there may be inflammatory lesions present in the intestines. In chronic cases a thickening of the intestinal wall identical with that seen in terminal (regional) ileitis has been described.

The disease, as it occurs in Europe, is characterized by more severe intestinal lesions, often to the point of diphtheresis of the mucosa. There is also degeneration of heart muscle and, in some cases, of the skeletal muscle.

Diagnosis

The epidemiological and clinical characteristics of transmissible gastroenteritis should make possible a presumptive diagnosis, but confirmation must depend upon the finding of compatible histological lesions, the detection of antigen, transmission experiments and evidence of seroconversion. It is not unusual to encounter outbreaks of diarrhea in piglets which appear to be typical of transmissible gastroenteritis, and either the virus can be demonstrated in the tissues by fluorescent antibody test but serum antibodies cannot be detected in the breeding animals (48), or serum antibodies can be detected in the adults but the virus cannot be demonstrated in the tissues by either immunofluorescence or tissue culture (27).

Villous atrophy is not pathognomonic for transmissible gastroenteritis, since it occurs in 3-week-old piglets affected with diarrhea and steatorrhea (25), in rotavirus infections of piglets (26), and in some herds for undetermined causes immediately following weaning (28, 29). Rotavirus infection has been associated with diarrhea in suckling and weaned piglets. Due to its recent recognition and the extreme difficulty in growing this virus its importance in diarrheal syndromes of pigs has yet to be determined. However, it is probable that its main significance lies in inducing changes following the removal of lactogenic immunity following weaning and in predisposing to subsequent coliform gastroenteritis.

Two types of porcine epidemic diarrhea of unknown etiology, but with marked epidemiological and clinical similarities to transmissible gastroenteritis, have recently been described in the United Kingdom (30). Type I is associated with profuse diarrhea in all ages of pigs except suckling pigs, whereas type II produces a syndrome identical to transmissible gastroenteritis except that mortality in suckling pigs under 1 week of age is generally less than 30%. Severe villous atrophy may not be present and antigen and serological tests are negative. A coronavirus antigenically distinct from the transmissible gastroenterology virus can cause an outbreak of diarrhea in piglets similar to the usual outbreak of the disease (54).

Hog cholera in its early stages may present a similar clinical picture to that of transmissible gastroenteritis, but its severity in pigs of all ages is an important point of difference. Vomiting and wasting disease has much in common with transmissible gastroenteritis in the manner in which it occurs and the age groups affected. Diarrhea is not a feature and laboratory differentiation is available. Enteritis due to *Escherichia coli* is a common disease, especially in very young pigs in which it may cause a very high mortality, but it is usually enzootic in a piggery, there is no vomiting and the causative bacteria can easily be isolated from the gut and the mesenteric lymph nodes and there is usually good response to treatment.

Treatment

There is no specific treatment for the disease. Because dehydration and metabolic acidosis are severe and hypoglycemia occurs, treatment with fluids and electrolytes containing glucose is indicated. Because there is loss of intestinal villi and the enzyme lactase, the ideal treatment would be to reduce the intake of milk for up to 5 days and administer a glucose–glycine–electrolyte solution orally every few hours to maintain hydration. However, removal of affected piglets from the sow is impractical and not recommended. Oral fluid therapy should improve the survival rate, affected piglets recovering in a few days following treatment (49). In experimentally induced transmissible gastroenteritis, removal of the milk diet and the use of an oral glucose–glycine–electrolyte solution plus a 5% dextrose solution given intraperitoneally at the rate of 25 ml/kg body weight once daily decreased the severity of the diarrhea, dehydration and metabolic acidosis but did not prevent or improve significantly the renal failure and severe hypoglycemia (18). A newborn piglet weighing 1·25 kg has an energy expenditure of about 170 kcal (711 kJ) per day if maintained at 30°C (86°F); 30 ml of a 5% dextrose solution supplies 1·5 g of glucose for a total of about 5·6 kcal per day (the gross energy of glucose being 3·74 kcal/g. Because the volume of 5% dextrose solution injected daily into piglets should not exceed 8% of their body weight it is unlikely that the hypoglycemia can be prevented or treated.

Control

The highly contagious nature of the disease makes the immediate control of an outbreak in a herd difficult and almost impossible. There are two approaches. One involves an attempt to avoid any further infection of newborn piglets by the individual isolation of farrowing sows under strict hygienic precautions. This is impractical in intensive swine production enterprises where isolation facilities are usually not available. The other approach attempts to minimize the duration of the outbreak by the purposeful infection of all pregnant sows either by mixing them with infected animals, or by using diarrheic feces on feed for oral challenge and the development of immunity in the sows (54). The use of immune serum for protection of piglets during an outbreak is of limited value (4). To be effective it must be given orally and not parenterally.

Sows which have recovered from oral infection with the virus, at least 2 weeks before farrowing will produce specific IgA antibody in the intestine which is then transferred to the mammary gland by immunocytes (31). In the mammary gland specific transmissible gastroenteritis secretory IgA is produced and transferred to both colostrum and milk which provides intestinal immunity to the suckling piglet. Piglets sucking such sows are resistant to infection while sucking, but become fully susceptible if transferred to a non-immune sow. The protective antibodies in the milk are associated primarily with immunoglobulins of the IgA class (32).

Effective vaccination of the sow with subsequent protection of piglets is achieved by purposeful infection of sows with virulent virus in infected material prior to farrowing. This, however, has the disadvantage of perpetuating infection within a herd and may lead to further spread of the disease within an area.

Because of the effectiveness of acquired immunity following natural infection, vaccination of the pregnant sow would appear to be the method of choice for control of the disease. However, the development of an effective vaccine has been a problem. Circulating antibodies either actively or passively acquired, provide little immunity to the disease, and parenterally administered vaccines have proven of no value. Protection against the disease requires the presence of antibody in the intestine, either actively or passively acquired.

The vaccination of pregnant sows with attenuated strains of the virus by either the parenteral or oral routes does not provide sufficient lactogenic immunity to protect their piglets against the virulent transmissible gastroenteritis virus (53). The virulent virus appears to lose its capacity to replicate sufficiently in the intestine of sows after it has undergone passages in cell cultures. There is a need to develop an attenuated virus strain which is completely avirulent for pigs, but which at the same time can replicate sufficiently in the small intestine of sows after oral administration and produce a lactogenic immunity. It appears that there are no strains of the virus available which are sufficiently attenuated and safe for pigs while yet able to provide a sufficient immune stimulus in the intestine of the sow (53). A double-protease resistant variant of the transmissible gastroenteritis virus used as a vaccine experimentally was able to induce some protective passive lactogenic immunity for newborn pigs (38). A subunit vaccine prepared from the virus was able to provide lactogenic immunity of short duration (39). Because of the close antigenic relationship between the transmissible gastroenteritis virus and other coronaviruses the revaccination of pregnant sows with tissue-cultured adapted feline infectious peritonitis virus (36) and canine coronavirus to stimulate lactogenic immunity against the transmissible gastroenteritis virus are being explored (37).

If vaccines are used, it is generally recommended that the two vaccinations, 14 days apart, be given during the last trimester of pregnancy. The antibody subsequently found in the milk following the use of these vaccines is largely in the IgA class of immunoglobulin and protection against experimental challenge is not complete (32–34). Intramammary vaccination may result in secretory IgA antibody in milk and more effective protection (35).

REVIEW LITERATURE

Ferris, D. H. (1973) Epizootiology of transmissible gastroenteritis. *Adv. vet. Sci.*, *17*, 57.

Haelterman, E. O. (1972) On the pathogenesis of transmissible gastroenteritis of swine. *J. Am. vet. med. Assoc.*, *160*, 534.

Pritchard, G. C. (1983) Transmissible gastroenteritis of pigs. *Pig News Inf.*, *4*, 145–149.

Woode, G. N. (1969) Transmissible gastroenteritis of swine. *Vet. Bull.*, *39*, 239.

REFERENCES

(1) Larson, D. J. et al. (1979) *Am. J. vet. Res.*, *40*, 477.
(2) Ritchie, A. E. (1976) *Proc. 4th int. Cong. Pig. vet. Soc.*, K15.
(3) Cartwright, S. F. et al. (1964) *Vet. Rec.*, *76*, 1332.
(4) Giles, N. (1976) *Vet. Ann.*, *16*, 111.
(5) Ferris, D. H. (1973) *Adv. vet. Sci.*, *17*, 57.
(6) Leopoldt, D. et al. (1974) *Mh. VetMed.*, *30*, 641.
(7) Morin, M. et al. (1978) *Can. J. comp. Med.*, *42*, 379.
(8) Kemeny, L. J. (1978) *Am. J. vet. Res.*, *39*, 703.
(9) Giles, N. (1977) *Vet. Rec.*, *100*, 92.
(10) Pritchard, G. C. (1982) *Vet. Rec.*, *110*, 465.
(11) Kemeny, L. J. & Woods, R. D. (1977) *Am. J. vet. Res.*, *38*, 507.
(12) Larson, D. J. et al. (1980) *J. Am. vet. med. Assoc.*, *176*, 539.
(13) Shepherd, R. W. et al. (1979) *Gastroenterology*, *76*, 20.
(14) Shepherd, R. W. et al. (1979) *Gastroenterology*, *76*, 770.
(15) Whipp, S. C. et al. (1985) *Am. J. vet. Res.*, *46*, 637.
(16) Drolet , R. et al. (1984) *Can. J. comp. Med.*, *48*, 282.
(17) Frederick, G. T. et al. (1976) *Am. J. vet. Res.*, *37*, 165.
(18) Drolet, R. et al. (1985) *Can. J. comp. Med.*, *49*, 357.

(19) Moon, H. W. et al. (1975) *Vet. Pathol.*, *12*, 434.
(20) Bernard, S. et al. (1986) *Am. J. vet. Res.*, *47*, 2441.
(21) Saif, L. J. et al. (1977) *Am. J.vet. Res.*, *38*, 13.
(22) Bohac, J. et al. (1975) *Can. J. comp. Med.*, *39*, 67.
(23) Cartwright, S. F. (1969)*Br. vet. J.*, *125*, 410.
(24) Chu, R. M. et al. (1982) *Am. J.vet. Res.*, *43*, 77.
(25) Mouwen, J. M. U. M. (1971) *Vet. Pathol.*, *8*, 364.
(26) Woode, G.N. et al. (1976) *J. med. Microbiol.*, *9*, 203
(27) Bauck, S. (1983) *Can. vet. J.*, *24*, 137.
(28) Gay, C. C. et al. (1976) *Proc. 4th int. Cong. Pig vet. Soc.*, VII.
(29) Kenworthy, R. et al. (1976) *Res. vet. Sci.*, *21*, 69.
(30) Bollwahn, W. (1983) *Pig News Inf.*, *4*, 141.
(31) Sprino, P. J. et al. (1976) *Am. J. vet. Res.*, *37*, 171.
(32) Bohl, E. H. & Saif, L. J. (1975) *Infect. Immun.*, *11*, 23.
(33) Bohl, E. H. et al. (1975) *Am. J. vet. Res.*, *36*, 267.
(34) Tamaglia, T. W. (1972) *J. Am. vet. med. Assoc.*, *160*, 554.
(35) Saif, L. J. & Bohl, E. H. (1983) *Ann. NY Acad. Sci.*, *409*, 708.
(36) Woods, R. D. (1984) *Am. J. vet. Res.*, *45*, 1726.
(37) Woods, R. D. & Wesley, R. D. (1986) *Am. J. vet. Res.*, *47*, 1239.
(38) Chen, K.-S. & Kahn, D. E. (1985) *Am. J. vet. Res.*, *46*, 1632.
(39) Gough, P. M. et al. (1983) *Vaccine*, *1*, 37.
(40) Shimizu, M. et al. (1978) *Infect. Immun.*, *21*, 747.
(41) Saif, L. J. & Bohl, E. H. (1979) *Am. J. vet. Res.*, *40*, 115.
(42) Kodama, Y. et al. (1980) *Am. J. vet. Res.*, *41*, 740.
(43) DeBuysscher, E. V. & Berman, D. T. (1980) *Am. J. vet. Res.*, *41*, 1214.
(44) Shimizu, M. & Shimizu, Y. (1979) *Am. J. vet. Res.*, *40*, 208.
(45) Kodama, Y. et al. (1981) *Am. J. vet. Res.*, *42*, 437
(46) Solorzano, R. F. et al. (1978) *Can. J. comp. Med.*, *42*, 385.
(47) Nelson, L. D. & Kelling, C. L. (1984) *Am. J. vet. Res.*, *45*, 1654.
(48) Bauck, S. & Stone, M. W. (1985) *Can. vet. J.*, *26*, 230.
(49) Marriott, D. W. et al. (1981) *Vet. Rec.*, *108*, 264.
(50) Giles, N. et al. (1977) *Vet. Res.*, *100*, 336.
(51) Laude, H. et al. (1981) *Am. J. vet. Res.*, *42*, 445.
(52) Pritchard, G. C. (1983) *Pig News Inf.*, *4*, 145.
(53) Voets, M. T. et al. (1980) *Vet. Q.*, *2*, 211.
(54) Dea, S. et al. (1985) *Can. vet. J.*, *26*, 108.
(55) Woods, R. D. (1979) *Am. J. vet. Res.*, *40*, 108.
(56) Gough, P. M. & Jorgensen, R. D. (1983) *Am. J. vet. Res.*, *44*, 2078.
(57) Miller, G. Y. & Kliebenstein, J. B. (1985) *Prev. vet. Med.*, *3*, 475.
(58) Pritchard, G. C. (1987) *Vet. Rec.*, *120*, 226.
(59) Hogg, A. (1982) *Mod. vet. Pract.*, *63*, 489.
(60) Asagi, M. et al. (1986) *Am. J. vet. Res.*, *47*, 2161.

Vomiting and wasting disease of pigs (hemagglutinating encephalomyelitis virus disease of pigs)

Vomiting and wasting disease occurs in suckling piglets and is characterized by vomition and constipation with subsequent illthrift. An acute encephalomyelitis may also occur following infection with the same virus.

Etiology

A coronavirus with hemagglutinating properties is the cause of both vomiting and wasting disease and an encephalomyelitis of piglets. The physical properties of the virus have been described (1, 2). The same isolate may be capable of causing either syndrome following experimental infection (3).

Epidemiology

Vomiting and wasting disease was reported from Canada in 1958 (4) and subsequently from the United Kingdom (5), Europe (6–8) and Australia (15). Following its occurrence in Canada a hemagglutinating virus was isolated from suckling piglets showing encephalomyelitis (9) and it has been subsequently demonstrated that both syndromes are caused by the same agent (3, 5). The encephalitic form has subsequently been reported in the United States (10). Although clinical disease is comparatively rare, serological surveys suggest that infection is widespread even in countries that have not experienced the disease or where it has been absent for some years (5, 10–12). The infection is widespread in breeding swine herds (16). Piglets suckled by immune sows will obtain maternal antibodies which disappear by 15 weeks of age. Active immunity begins between 8 and 16 weeks of age. Disease presumably occurs when the virus gains access to a susceptible herd but the reason for the age limitation is unknown. Transmission is by the oral or respiratory route (3).

Both syndromes tend to occur in outbreak form affecting several litters within a short period of time. Morbidity approaches 100% and case fatality is high. The disease occurs in suckling pigs as early as 2 days of age but generally not in pigs older than 3 weeks of age. The encephalitic form tends to involve younger piglets than the gastroenteric form. The clinical course of the encephalitic form is usually 2–3 days whereas pigs with vomiting and wasting may survive several days to several weeks. The course of the outbreak is usually 2–3 weeks and subsequent litters are not affected. Area outbreaks may occur.

Pathogenesis

The pathogenesis is uncertain. Vomiting and wasting disease and the encephalomyelitis are probably two clinical extremes of the same disease, and both syndromes may be observed in the same outbreak (3, 10). Differences in pathogenicity of the strain of virus, and age and litter susceptibility may influence the form that the disease takes. Virus may be isolated from the brain of pigs with acute encephalomyelitis but in cases of chronic vomiting and wasting disease neither virus nor encephalomyelitis is demonstrable. It is possible that the vomiting and wasting syndrome is centrally mediated but that during the course of chronic illness the virus is eliminated and the inflammatory lesions resolved (3). Localization of antigen in the stomach wall has been demonstrated in vomiting and wasting syndromes (13). After experimental oral inoculation the virus replicates preferentially in the tonsils, lungs and small intestines (13). This is followed by spread to the central nervous system via the ganglia of the peripheral nervous system. The cause of the vomition is unknown.

Clinical findings

Vomition of yellow-green vomitus is the first sign and is accompanied by anorexia and thirst. Ineffective attempts to drink are characteristic. The temperature is usually normal or slightly elevated except for transient febrile reactions (up to 40·5°C, 105°F) for 24 hours in the early stages in some pigs, and the feces are usually hard and dry. Diarrhea may occur but is not severe and occurs mostly in the older piglets. Vomiting may continue for some days but, in all affected pigs, there is severe, rapid emaciation and dehydration. They may continue in this state for some weeks and eventually die, apparently of starvation, or they are destroyed by the owner.

The encephalitic form is manifest initially by depression. Piglets continue to suck for the first day but rapidly become inappetent and there is rapid loss of condition. Hyperesthesia, incoordination and muscle tremor with occasional vomiting is followed in 48–72 hours by an acute encephalitis with paddling convulsions and death.

Sows may show inappetence and mild fever for 1–2 days at the onset of the outbreak.

Clinical pathology

Infection may be demonstrated by the detection of antigen in tissues or tissue culture by hemagglutination, fluorescent antibody or electron microscopic techniques. The demonstration of rising antibody titers in surviving piglets is also satisfactory for diagnosis. Virus neutralization and hemagglutination inhibition tests are more sensitive than agar gel immunodiffusion (14).

Necropsy findings

Gross necropsy findings are generally negative. Nonsuppurative encephalomyelitis with perivascular cuffing, gliosis and neuronal death are present in pigs dying with clinical signs of encephalitis but not necessarily in pigs with vomiting and wasting disease.

Treatment and control

There is no effective treatment. The control of the disease must depend on prior exposure of sows to infection at least 10 days before farrowing, if necessary by purposeful exposure. The piglets will be protected by colostral antibody. Sows that have had affected litters will be immune to the disease and should not be discarded from the herd.

REFERENCES

(1) Garwes, D. J. et al.(1975) *Nature, Lond.*, *275*, 508.
(2) Pensaert, M. B. & Callebout, P. E. (1974) *Arch. ges. Virusforsch.*, *44*, 35.
(3) Mengeling, W. L. & Cutlip, R. C. (1976) *J. Am. vet. med. Assoc.*, *168*, 236.
(4) Roe, C. K. & Alexander, T. J. L. (1958) *Can. J. comp. Med.*, *22*, 305.
(5) Cartwright, S. F. & Lucas, M. (1970) *Vet. Rec.*, *86*, 278.
(6) Steinicke, O. & Nielsen, A. (1959) *Nord. VetMed.*, *11*, 399.
(7) Bugnowski, H. & Lange, S. (1978) *Mh. VetMed.*, *33*, 607.
(8) Hess, R. G. & Bachmann, P. A. (1978) *Tierärztl. Umschau*, *33*, 571.
(9) Grieg, A. S. et al. (1962) *Can. J. comp. Med.*, *26*, 49.
(10) Werdin, R. E. et al. (1976) *J. Am. vet. med. Assoc.*, *168*, 240.
(11) Hirai, K. et al. (1974) *Jap. J. vet. Sci.*, *36*, 375.
(12) Sorenson, K. J. (1975) *Nord. VetMed.*, *27*, 208.
(13) Andries, K. & Pensaert, M. B. (1980) *Am. J. vet. Res.*, *41*, 1372.
(14) Mengeling, W. L. (1974) *Am. J. vet. Res.*, *35*, 1429.
(15) Forman, A. J. et al. (1979) *Aust. vet. J.*, *55*, 503.
(16) Pansaert, M. B. et al. (1980) *Vet. Q.*, *2*, 142.

Viral diarrhea of calves, lambs, kids, piglets and foals

There is now firm evidence that some viruses can be the primary cause of acute diarrhea in any of the newborn farm animal species. The rotavirus and coronavirus are most commonly involved, but other viruses have also been isolated from young diarrheic farm animals.

Etiology

Rotaviruses have been isolated from calves (97), lambs (1), piglets (1), and foals (1) and are considered to be primary causes of diarrhea in those species (1). All members of this group share a common morphology and were previously known as the reovirus-like viruses (7). Details of the virological aspects of the rotaviruses are available (7, 20). Comparative studies have confirmed that the rotaviruses of human infants, calves, pigs and foals are morphologically indistinguishable from each other and from the virus of infant mice. In addition, the lamb rotavirus is similar to both calf and pig viruses (20).

Some atypical rotaviruses known as *pararotaviruses* have been isolated from pigs and cattle (2, 3) and lambs (4). They are morphologically similar to rotaviruses but do not possess the common group antigen and are therefore characterized by their failure to be detected in serological tests, such as immunofluorescence or enzyme-linked immunosorbent assay (ELISA) which are based on the presence of the common group antigen (2, 3).

There are at least four separate groups of rotaviruses definable by serology and electrophoretype (19).

Coronavirus-like viruses are also considered as causative agents of acute diarrhea in calves (122, 123) and piglets (124). The coronavirus-like virus in pigs is similar to, but distinct from, the virus of transmissible gastroenteritis (TGE) and is thought to be the cause of porcine epidemic diarrhea type II (10, 11). A coronavirus has been isolated from adult cows with diarrhea which may suggest a causative agent for winter dysentery (12, 13). The physicochemical and biological properties of some neonatal calf coronaviruses have been compared (82).

While the rotavirus and coronavirus are considered to be the most important causes of viral diarrhea in newborn farm animals (other than transmissible gastroenteritis of piglets) an adenovirus (15, 16) and a parvovirus (107, 108) have also been isolated from the feces of diarrheic calves, but their etiological significance is not yet clear. Small viruses resembling astroviruses (6, 9) and caliciviruses (6, 8), and the Breda virus (5, 9), have also been isolated from diarrheic calves and piglets with acute enteritis (16), but their relative etiological and economic significance is not fully known. A fringed virus-like particle has been isolated from the feces of diarrheic calves and dogs (17).

Multiple mixed viral infections are being recognized more frequently as diagnostic techniques are improved. Both rotavirus and coronavirus may occur in the same diarrheic calf with or without the presence of enteropathogenic *E. coli* (24, 27). A concurrent rotaviral and transmissible gastroenteritis infection has occurred in a newborn piglet (35) and calicivirus-like particles have been isolated along with the rotavirus from young pigs with diarrhea (36).

Epidemiology

Rotavirus infections occur characteristically in young animals. The rotavirus is ubiquitous in the environment of domestic animals and has been isolated in outbreaks of diarrhea in calves (97), pigs (125), lambs (126) and foals (127). Serological surveys indicate that up to 90%

and more of adult cattle (128, 129), sheep (126), horses (127) and pigs (125) have antiviral antibody. Antibody to typical and atypical rotaviruses is widespread in pigs in both the United Kingdom and the United States (18).

The intestinal tract is the site of multiplication of rotavirus and virus is excreted only in the feces. Infected feces may contain as many as 10^{10}/g virus particles. Because rotaviruses are stable in feces and relatively resistant to commonly used disinfectants it is extremely difficult to prevent gross contamination of animal housing once infection has been introduced. The mature animal is considered to be the source of infection for the neonate (97).

The factors which influence rotavirus infection and its clinical severity include the age of the animal, immune status of the dam and absorption of colostral antibody, ambient temperature, degree of viral exposure, the occurrence of weaning, and the presence of other enteropathogens (79). The mortality is highest in the youngest animals which have received insufficient colostrum and are subjected to severe weather conditions. Under experimental conditions, the mortality rate in gnotobiotic piglets inoculated with the rotavirus is 100% at birth, 5–30% at 7 days and only a mild disease at 3–4 weeks of age.

An important epidemiological characteristic of rotavirus infection in newborn farm animals is that protection against disease is dependent on the presence of specific rotavirus colostral antibody in the lumen of the intestine of the newborn. Colostral serum antibody in the newborn does not protect animals against clinical disease. The protective effect of colostrum depends on its antibody titer and on the amount ingested. The daily oral administration of colostrum containing specific antibody or hyperimmune serum to lambs will protect them against experimental challenge (75). The protection is against clinical disease and not necessarily infection. Calves, lambs and piglets may still excrete virus in the feces while they are protected against clinical disease by the presence of colostral antibody in the intestinal lumen (20). The protection lasts only as long as colostral antibody is present which explains why rotaviral diarrhea occurs commonly after 5–7 days of age. Survival from rotavirus diarrhea in calves may be dependent on a high level of serum colostral immunoglobulin (97).

The rotaviruses from one species can infect members only of some other species. Experimental infection of pigs, calves and lambs with human rotavirus have been described (20). The calf rotavirus can infect pigs. However, the significance of interspecies infection under field conditions has not been evaluated. Cross-infection between species is not a property shared by all rotaviruses (29).

There are at least four different group of rotaviruses definable by serology and electrophoretype (19). The most clinically significant strains in the animal and human populations belong to group A. Those strains which belong to groups B and C and possibly others are known as atypical rotaviruses (1). There are differences in virulence among the bovine rotaviruses which may explain the variability in the severity of disease in natural outbreaks and must be considered when developing vaccines (95).

The susceptibility of the lamb rotavirus to disinfectants has been examined. An iodophore preparation at 4% will partially inactivate virus in feces-contaminated material (31). Lysol at 5% and formol saline at 10% are more effective, while a 3% solution of sodium hypochlorite with 11% available chlorine is ineffective (31).

Calves

Many of the epidemiological characteristics of neonatal calf diarrhea caused by the rotavirus and coronavirus which have been reported must be considered in the context of 'acute undifferentiated diarrhea of newborn calves' because rarely would an outbreak of diarrhea in newborn calves be caused by the virus alone.

The reovirus-like virus (rotavirus) was first isolated in the United States in 1969 (21) and thought to be the cause of outbreaks of diarrhea in beef calves in Nebraska. Since then the virus has been recovered from calves affected with diarrhea in many countries, including Canada, the United Kingdom and Australia, which suggests that it may have a worldwide distribution (20).

While the rotavirus has been most commonly associated with outbreaks of diarrhea in beef calves raised in groups outdoors, it has also been recovered from dairy calves raised together in large groups in large dairy herds (22). The morbidity rate in beef herds has varied from herd to herd and from one year to another. In some herds the disease started at a low rate of 5–10% in the first year, increased to 20–50% in the second, and to 50–80% in the third year. In other herds, explosive outbreaks affecting 80% of the calves have occurred in the first year. The case fatality rate has also been variable, in some herds as low as 5%, while in others it has been as high as 60%. The mortality rate probably depends upon the level of colostral immunity in the calves, the incidence of enteric colibacillosis, and the level of animal husbandry and clinical management provided in the herd.

A unique epidemiological characteristic of rotavirus infection in calves is the short-term nature of the immunity provided by colostrum. Newborn calves are protected from the effects of the rotavirus only during the first few days after parturition, during which time the colostrum contains specific rotavirus antibody which is active in the lumen of the intestine (97). The serum immunoglobulins acquired by the calf from the colostrum do not provide protection against infection in the intestine. This correlates well with the peak incidence of rotavirus diarrhea which is 5–7 days of age, which would coincide with a marked drop in colostral immunoglobulins by the third day after parturition and allow for an incubation period of 18–24 hours for the disease to occur. The levels of serum and colostral antibody are lower in first-calf heifers which may explain the higher morbidity and mortality in their calves.

The virus is excreted by both calves and adult cattle in large numbers (up to 10^{10}/g of feces) and excretion may last for several weeks. Even under open-range conditions, there is a rapid spread of the virus throughout calves which come in frequent contact with each other, particularly during the calving season (20). It would appear that calves are contaminated after birth from the dam's feces or from other infected diarrheic calves.

There is no evidence that the virus crosses the placental barrier and infects fetuses *in utero* (24).

There is evidence that subclinical infection is common. Antibody to rotavirus and coronavirus can be found in the serum of 90–100% of young adults, and clinically normal calves with high serum antibody may excrete the virus (97). The explanations include: (*a*) calves may be protected from disease but excrete the virus during the colostral feeding period; (*b*) calves may be infected at a subclinical level but still excrete the virus although they may have been denied colostral antibody. The excretion of the virus by adult cattle may serve as a source of the virus for calves.

The prevalence of subclinical infection may be greater than that indicated by isolation of the virus from feces. Rotavirus–immunoglobulin and coronavirus–immunoglobulin complexes may be present in the feces of 44% and 70% of adult cattle, respectively, while the free rotavirus and coronavirus may be absent or in only 6% of fecal samples, respectively (47). Clinically normal cows can shed the virus for several weeks in the presence of fecal and serum antibody (92). Repeated bovine rotavirus infection and re-excretion can occur in calves several months of age even in the presence of serum antibodies (93). Clinically normal calves may also shed the virus and there may be histological evidence of lesions of the small intestine due to rotavirus infection (111, 112).

In a longitudinal survey of calves in a herd over two successive calving periods, the rotavirus was first detected in calves at about 6 days of age (112). Diarrhea or excretion of abnormal feces was associated with rotavirus infection in 58% of infected calves while in the remaining 42% infection was subclinical (112).

The calf rotavirus can be experimentally transmitted to piglets and has been isolated from natural outbreaks of diarrhea in piglets. The isolation of a rotavirus from neonatal deer affected with diarrhea in a zoo in Australia raises some interesting epidemiological possibilities (30). The bovine rotavirus has been found in the feces of dogs, and dogs have been experimentally infected (91) which suggests that they may play a role in the dissemination of the virus (91).

The occurrence and distribution of the virus in diarrheic and normal calves have been studied. The rotavirus has been found before, during and after the onset of diarrhea (26). It has been found along with the coronavirus and adenovirus in diarrheic calves (25, 27). This serves to emphasize that while the virus can be considered as a primary pathogen in calves the results of field and laboratory investigations indicate that multiple mixed pathogen infections are probably more common than single pathogen infections. There may also be differences in the virulence between isolates (23). Earlier work suggested that most cases of naturally occurring rotavirus diarrhea in calves were also infected with *E. coli*. However, no attempt was made to determine if the *E. coli* possessed the virulence characteristics described under colibacillosis.

The coronavirus has been isolated from field outbreaks of diarrhea in calves in the United States, Canada (8), the United Kingdom and Denmark (47). The enteric coronavirus can be shed by adult cows (129). The shedding peaks during the winter months and at parturition and can be found in up to 60% of adult cows. Vaccination of the cows with modified-live rotavirus–coronavirus *E. coli* combination vaccine did not influence seasonal shedding but in vaccinated cows the incidence of shedding did not increase at parturition as it did in non-vaccinated cows. The morphological and antigenic characteristics of the viruses from the United Kingdom, the United States and Denmark have been compared and cultivated in tissue culture. The viruses have been serially passed in gnotobiotic calves which developed diarrhea (47), and there is some evidence that bovine coronaviruses have a dual tropism for the intestinal and respiratory mucosa (94). There are also antigenic differences between isolates of bovine coronaviruses (96). The physicochemical and biological properties of some coronaviruses isolated from calves are described (28).

The parvovirus has been associated with outbreaks of postweaning diarrhea in beef calves (107). Seroconversion to the virus occurred following weaning which may have been the stressor which precipitated clinical disease. The presence of subclinical coccidiosis may also be associated with the onset of postweaning diarrhea and parvovirus infection (108).

Lambs

The rotavirus has been isolated from the feces of lambs with diarrhea under 3 weeks of age (76). The disease appears to be sporadic in lambs and no particular epidemiological characteristics have been described. The experimental disease in lambs is mild and characterized by mild diarrhea, abdominal discomfort and recovery in a few days (62). The mortality in lambs is much higher when both the rotavirus and enteropathogenic *E. coli* are used (87).

Pigs

In piglets, rotaviral diarrhea occurs from 1 to 8 weeks of age, but is most common in pigs which are weaned under intensive management conditions at 3 weeks of age (32). The disease resembles what has been referred to as *milk-scours*, or 3-week scours of piglets. The morbidity may reach 80% and the case fatality rate ranges from 5 to 20% depending on the level of sanitation. Rotavirus infection under Venezuelan conditions occurs in piglets from 2 to 6 weeks of age, rarely in younger animals, and appears to be associated with the decline of passive immunity (98).

The sow is the source of infection. Seropositive sows can shed rotavirus from 5 days before to 2 weeks after farrowing when piglets are most susceptible to infection (101). The early weaning of piglets at a few days of age (33, 34) or at 3 weeks of age results in the removal of the antibody supplied by the sow's milk (32).

There are different serotypes of porcine rotavirus which must be considered when developing vaccines (99). Most isolates from outbreaks of diarrhea belong to group A while a small percentage are atypical rotaviruses (100).

Outbreaks of diarrhea caused by a coronavirus-like virus may occur in pigs of all ages (11). The mortality is high in piglets under 7 days of age while most of the adult pigs recover.

Diarrhea in unweaned piglets 1–3 weeks of age has

been associated with a combined infection of rotavirus and *Isospora suis* (88).

Foals

Rotaviral diarrhea occurs in foals from 5 to 35 days of age (1). Outbreaks of the disease occur on horse farms with a large number of young foals where the population density is high (1). Serological surveys indicate the presence of the rotavirus antibody in almost all of the mares whose foals are infected with the virus (1). The available evidence suggests that the rotavirus is a major cause of diarrhea in foals. The rotavirus has been isolated from foals affected with salmonellosis which suggests the possibility that the virus may have precipitated the bacterial disease (89).

Pathogenesis

The rotavirus infects mature brush border villous epithelial cells in the small intestine, and to lesser extent in the large intestine (37). The infected cells are sloughed leading to partial villous atrophy and the atrophic villi are rapidly recovered with relatively undifferentiated crypt cells which mature over a few days and lead to healing of the lesion. The activity of the mucosal beta-galactosidase (lactase) in the brush border of the villous epithelium is less than in normal animals which results in decreased utilization of lactose. This reduction in enzymes is associated with immature enterocytes on the villi during rotavirus infection. *In vitro* studies have suggested that lactase may be the receptor and uncoating enzyme for rotavirus which may explain the high degree of susceptibility of the newborn with high levels of lactase. The net effect of the morphological and functional changes in the intestine is malabsorption resulting in diarrhea, dehydration, loss of electrolytes and acidosis. The diarrhea in milk-fed calves with the experimental disease can be stopped if the milk is withdrawn and replaced with glucose and water which is similar to transmissible gastroenteritis. The D-xylose absorption test can be used to measure the degree of malabsorption in calves infected with rotavirus (43).

While it has been generally accepted that lactose malabsorption is an important factor in the pathogenesis of diarrhea the experimental infection of gnotobiotic lambs with rotavirus did not result in lactose intolerance as assessed by the measurement of reducing substances in the feces or by the clinical effects and blood glucose levels after a lactose load (102). Lactose intolerance could be demonstrated by using extremely high doses of lactose, three to four times the normal dietary intake. Thus, lactose-containing feed such as milk are not necessarily contraindicated in rotavirus diarrhea (102).

The pathogenesis of rotaviral infection is similar in calves (37), lambs, pigs (39, 40, 42) and foals. The lesions occur within 24 hours after infection, villous epithelial cells of the small intestine are infected and become detached and regeneration occurs within 4–6 days after the onset of the diarrhea. The intestinal villi usually returns to near normal within about 7 days after recovery from the diarrhea. However, calves and pigs may require 10–21 days to fully recover to a normal growth rate following rotavirus infection (43).

A combined infection with rotavirus and enterotoxigenic *E. coli* may result in a more severe disease than produced by rotavirus infection alone, particularly in calves several days of age when normally the rotavirus produces a mild disease and when calves are resistant to enterotoxigenic colibacillosis (104). The intestinal lesions of villous atrophy are also more severe and extend into the colon in dual infections (104). Naturally occurring cases of the dual infection in calves are considered to be more severe than single infections (103). Under field conditions more than one enteropathogen is likely to be involved in the pathogenesis of the diarrhea (41).

The pathogenesis of coronaviral enteritis in calves is similar to the rotavirus infection (45, 46). The villous epithelial cells of the small and large intestines are commonly affected (47). The crypt epithelium is also affected which makes regeneration of villous epithelial cells much longer, which results in persistent diarrhea for several days and death from dehydration and malnutrition. The pathophysiological changes due to coronavirus-induced diarrhea in the calf have been described (74) and are similar to the changes which occur in acute diarrheal disease in the calf caused by other enteropathogens.

The porcine coronavirus, CV777, replicates in the villous epithelial cells of both the small and large intestine and clinically resembles transmissible gastroenteritis of piglets (44).

A major factor in the pathogenesis of rotavirus and coronavirus infection in newborn farm animals is the amount of colostrum-derived antibody present in the intestinal lumen at the time of viral challenge. The protective effect of colostrum against rotavirus infection of the intestine is dependent upon both the volume and the antibody titers of the ingested colostrum (75). To be effective the colostrum must be ingested within a few hours after birth. Low levels of intestinal antibody may allow viral replication and result in clinical disease.

The calicivirus-like (Newbury) agent causes degeneration of the villous epithelial cells of the proximal part of the small intestine leading to villous atrophy, a reduction in disaccharidase activity and xylose malabsorption (105). In gnotobiotic calves experimentally infected with the Breda virus the villous epithelial cells of the ileum and colon are affected including the dome epithelial cells (106).

Experimental infection of calves with parvovirus results in lymphopenia and viremia and damage to the small intestinal crypt epithelium and the associated mitotically active lymphoid tissues (107). This results in villous atrophy because of failure of replacement of villous epithelial cells by the crypts and those cells which are replaced are immature for a longer than normal period. By 5 days after inoculation there was evidence of repair of the intestinal lesions. Following experimental challenge the tonsillar tissues, intestinal mucosa and mesenteric lymph nodes all become infected. Subsequent spread also results in greater involvement in the large intestine and the upper jejunum, Peyer's patches and mesenteric lymph nodes (107).

Clinical findings

Calves

In experimental rotavirus infection in newborn colostrum-deprived gnotobiotic calves a profuse liquid diarrhea may occur by 10–14 hours after oral inoculation. Affected calves are mildly depressed, anorexic and may have a mild fever.

The naturally occurring disease usually occurs in calves over 4 days of age and is characterized by a sudden onset of a profuse liquid diarrhea (22). The feces are pale yellow, mucoid and may contain flecks of blood. Recovery usually occurs in a few days. Explosive outbreaks occur and up to 50% of calves from 5 to 14 days of age in the affected population may develop the disease. If enterotoxigenic *E. coli* are present the disease may be acute; dehydration is severe and deaths may occur. Multiple mixed infection with *E. coli* and coronavirus are common in calves over 4 days of age and thus it may be impossible to describe a typical case of uncomplicated naturally occurring rotavirus or coronavirus-like diarrhea. There is a tendency for viral diarrhea in newborn calves to occur in explosive outbreaks, the calves are usually not toxemic, but the character of the diarrhea cannot be differentiated clinically from that caused by the other common enteric pathogens of newborn calves.

A coronaviral enteritis affecting calves from 1 to 7 days of age has been described (83), but there are no distinguishing clinical characteristics. The diarrhea may be persistent for several days, followed by death in spite of fluid therapy and careful realimentation with milk. The feces are voluminous, mucoid and slimy and may be dark-green or light-brown in color.

Lambs

Experimentally, newborn gnotobiotic lambs develop diarrhea 15–20 hours following oral inoculation and show dullness and mild abdominal discomfort. There are only a few documented descriptions of naturally occurring rotaviral diarrhea in newborn lambs (76). Affected lambs under 3 weeks of age develop a profuse diarrhea and the case fatality rate is high. It is not clear if outbreaks of uncomplicated rotaviral diarrhea occur in newborn lambs.

Pigs

Rotaviral diarrhea may occur in nursing piglets from 1 to 4 weeks of age and in pigs following weaning (3,4). The disease in nursing piglets resembles milk-scours or 3-week scours. Most of the pigs in the litter are affected with a profuse liquid to soft diarrhea with varying degrees of dehydration. Recovery usually occurs in a few days unless complicated by enterotoxigenic *E. coli* or unsatisfactory sanitation, overcrowding and poor management. The disease is often most severe in herds in which there is continuous farrowing with no period of vacancy for cleaning and disinfection in the farrowing barn. The disease may also occur in pigs a few days after weaning and may be a major factor in postweaning diarrhea of piglets weaned at 3 weeks of age or earlier in the case of weaning pigs at 1–2 days of age (3, 4).

Epidemic diarrhea type II, associated with coronavirus-like particles, causes a profuse fluid diarrhea in pigs of all ages, including nursing piglets. Explosive outbreaks may occur and the morbidity may reach 100%. Mortality is usually restricted to piglets under 3 weeks of age (48).

Experimental rotavirus infection in newborn colostrum-deprived gnotobiotic piglets results in a profuse liquid diarrhea in 16–24 hours following inoculation. The feces are yellow and vomiting may occur. Dehydration and death may occur in 2–4 days.

Foals

Affected foals appear depressed, fail to suck and become recumbent. The temperature ranges from 39·5 to 41·0°C (103–106°F) and the respiration may be rapid and shallow. A profuse, foul-smelling fluid diarrhea commences 4–12 hours after the onset of depression and affected foals become markedly dehydrated. Recovery following treatment usually occurs within 2–4 days. Death may occur within 24 hours after the onset of diarrhea.

Clinical pathology

Fecal samples (20–30 g) should be collected from affected animals as soon after the onset of diarrhea as possible and submitted to the laboratory in a chilled state. Samples of intestinal mucosa from several sections of the small and large intestine should be submitted chilled for virus detection and possible isolation.

Because multiple mixed viral and bacterial infections are common, the request for a laboratory diagnosis must include consideration of all of the common pathogens. The viruses are much more difficult to detect than enteropathogenic *E. coli*. In herd outbreaks, fecal samples from several affected animals and some normal animals should be submitted. The rotavirus may be present in both normal and diarrheic animals which presents problems in interpretation (77) and requires identification of the epidemiological factors which may have precipitated the disease in animals in which the viruses are ubiquitous (78).

Several laboratory tests are available for detection of rotaviruses and coronaviruses in the feces and intestinal contents and tissues. The particular test used will depend on the facilities and equipment available. Electron-microscopic examination of fecal material has been a standard diagnostic technique. It is easier to see the virus if it has been concentrated by ultracentrifugation or clumped by immune electron microscopy using specific antiserum. However, since the equipment and expertise necessary for electron microscopy are not available in many laboratories, alternative diagnostic techniques have been developed.

Several tests are based on immunofluorescence. These include immunofluorescent staining of fecal smears and of cell cultures infected with fecal preparations. The immunofluorescent staining of a fecal smear would appear to be a more convenient test for diagnostic laboratories because a diagnosis can be made in a few hours and it eliminates the need for electron microscopy. However, the immunofluorescence tests may not be as reliable as some other tests. The fluorescent antibody technique will only detect virus within epithelial cells which are present in the feces for 4–6 hours after the onset of diarrhea. With electron microscopy the virus can be detected for up to 6–10 days after the onset of diarrhea (52). In some studies the fluorescent antibody technique detected the virus in only 20% of samples while electron microscopy detected the virus in about 60% of the samples. The immunodiffusion test and electron microscopy are superior to the fluorescent antibody technique. Treatment of the feces with chymotrypsin improves the detection rate (52).

Some of the methods for the detection of rotavirus antigens in calf feces have been compared (50). The enzyme-linked immunosorbent assay (ELISA) is more sensitive and simple than immunoelectro-osmophoresis, complement fixation, immunofluorescence on inoculated cell cultures or electron microscopy. A counterimmunoelectrophoresis test is also available and compares favorably with the ELISA test (54), which utilizes reagents that are both stable and non-radioactive and is ideal for handling large numbers of specimens. The test can also be read with the naked eye or a simple colorimeter and there is no need for sophisticated equipment.

The ELISA test and electron microscopy of feces are considered to be equally reliable in detecting the rotavirus and coronavirus in the feces of experimentally infected calves (51). The agreement between the two tests was 95% for coronavirus and 84% for rotavirus (51). There will always be borderline samples containing antigen in quantities near the detection limit for each test. Some samples will be positive for one test and negative by the other, and vice versa. This problem can be minimized if several individual samples from a disease outbreak are examined. The morphological identification of rotavirus is usually straightforward but the pleomorphism of bovine coronavirus can present problems. The ELISA test may also fail to detect viral antigen in feces which also contain antibody. The test can provide diagnostic results within 24 hours after collection of the fecal samples (110). Three techniques for the detection of rotavirus in fecal samples from diarrheic calves have been compared (130). The reverse passive hemagglutination (RPHA) was at least as sensitive as the ELISA test, and both were compared with the polyacrylamide gel electrophoresis (PAGE). The overall agreement between RPHA and PAGE was 96%; the ELISA was not as sensitive (130).

A field enzyme immunoassay test (Rotazyme test) is highly accurate and reliable for the detection of rotavirus in the feces of horses with and without diarrhea (109). The test is a simple, rapid and specific procedure which can take the place of the more expensive and slower procedure such as electron microscopy.

Solid-phase radioimmunoassay gives comparable results to electron microscopy, but requires the need for radioactive unstable reagents and expensive counting equipment.

The isolation of rotavirus from the feces of calves can be improved by treatment of the feces with trypsin which enhances the infectivity of the virus for tissue culture (56). Normally replication of the virus in tissue culture using conventional methods is limited.

Immunofluorescent sections of spiral colon is the diagnostic method of choice for the detection of coronavirus in calves; fecal samples are unreliable (49). Isolation of coronavirus in tracheal organ culture is the most sensitive *in vitro* culture technique (47). A hemadsorption–elution–hemagglutination assay test for the detection of coronavirus in feces of calves is a simple and rapid procedure (53). A counterimmunoelectrophoresis test is available for the detection of coronavirus in calves (55). Continuous cell live culture techniques for the isolation of bovine coronavirus have been described (81).

Several serological tests are available for the detection and measurement of rotaviral antibody in serum and lacteal secretions. The radioimmunoassay is the most sensitive test compared to the agar gel immunodiffusion, complement fixation, hemagglutination and hemagglutination inhibition tests (57, 58).

Pathology

The pathology of experimentally induced rotavirus and coronavirus diarrhea in colostrum-deprived and gnotobiotic calves (60, 61, 85), lambs (62), and piglets (42, 63) has been described. Grossly, the changes are unremarkable and consist of dehydration, fluid-filled intestinal tract and distension of the abomasum. The microscopic changes consist of shortening of the length of the villi and replacement of the tall columnar villous epithelial cells by cuboidal and squamous cells. Segments of the small intestine may reveal villous fusion, rounded absorptive cells, villous atrophy and exposure of lamina propria. Crypt hyperplasia occurs in response to the loss of columnar epithelial cells from the villi. Histological lesions due to previous rotavirus infection may be present in the small intestine of clinically normal calves (111). In coronavirus enteritis in calves there is commonly villous atrophy of both the small and large intestines and destruction of the crypt epithelium, which destruction does not occur in rotavirus enteritis. The changes are more severe in field cases of acute diarrhea in calves in which both viruses and enteropathogenic *E. coli* can be isolated (41, 86).

The histological appearance of the intestinal lesions of experimental infection of calves with Breda virus (106), calicivirus-like agent (105), and parvovirus (107) have been described. In general, the lesions are similar to those caused by rotavirus and coronavirus infection.

Diagnosis

The cause of acute diarrhea in newborn farm animals cannot usually be determined on clinical grounds. All of the common bacterial and viral enteropathogens of calves can cause an acute profuse fluid diarrhea with progressive dehydration and death in a few days.

When outbreaks of diarrhea are encountered, a detailed examination of the possible epidemiological factors should be made and the appropriate fecal samples and tissues from affected animals submitted to the laboratory. The most reliable specimens include fecal samples obtained from animals within a few hours after the onset of diarrhea, and untreated affected animals which are submitted for necropsy and microbiological examination within a few hours after the onset of diarrhea.

The common clinical and epidemiological characteristics of the acute diarrheas of neonatal farm animals are as follows.

Calves

Enteric colibacillosis occurs primarily in calves under 4 days of age and is characterized clinically by an acute, profuse liquid diarrhea. Recovery following treatment usually occurs in 2 days. Outbreaks occur in beef and dairy calves. *Rotavirus* and *coronavirus* diarrhea usually occurs in calves over 5–10 days of age and up to 3 weeks of age. Explosive outbreaks occur characterized by an acute profuse liquid diarrhea with recovery in 2–4 days. Recovery is assisted by oral fluid therapy. *Cryptosporidiosis* occurs in calves from 5 to 15 days of age and is characterized by a persistent diarrhea which may last for several days. The cryptosporidia may be detected by Giemsa stain of fecal smears or by fecal flotation.

Whether or not the BVD virus causes clinically significant diarrhea with lesions of the small intestine of calves 3–6 weeks of age is unknown. Diagnostic laboratories report the presence of intestinal lesions such as villous atrophy and crypt cell destruction in calves 3–6 weeks of age which have been affected with an intractable diarrhea and from which the BVD virus was isolated from the feces. However, to date there is no evidence of a cause and effect relationship.

Piglets
Transmissible gastroenteritis occurs most commonly in piglets under 1 week of age and explosive outbreaks are common. There is acute profuse diarrhea and vomiting. Affected piglets may continue to nurse for several hours after the onset of the diarrhea. The case fatality rate is high in piglets under 7 days of age; older pigs commonly survive. *Enteric colibacillosis* usually occurs in piglets under 3 days of age. There is acute diarrhea, dehydration and rapid death. Pigs with coliform septicemia may die without obvious diarrhea and usually appear cyanotic. Entire litters may be affected and the case fatality rate may be 100%. Early treatment with antibiotics and subcutaneous fluids will result in recovery. *Coccidiosis* occurs in piglets from 5 to 10 days of age and is characterized by an acute diarrhea in which the feces are foul-smelling and vary in consistency from being cottage cheese-like to liquid, and gray or yellow and frothy. The diarrhea is persistent for several days and non-responsive to antibiotics. Some pigs recover spontaneously, others die in 2–4 days. Coccidial oocysts can be detected in the feces. The morbidity rate varies from 50 to 75% and the case fatality rate from 10 to 20%. *Hemorrhagic enterotoxemia* due to *Clostridium perfringens* type C affects entire litters of pigs under 1 week of age, is characterized clinically by severe toxemia, dysentery and rapid death, and at necropsy there is a hemorrhagic enteritis.

Lambs
Enteric colibacillosis occurs in lambs most commonly under 1 week of age and is characterized by dullness, failure to suck and acute diarrhea which responds to antibiotic and fluid therapy. *Coliform septicemia* affects lambs under a few days of age and usually causes sudden deaths. *Lamb dysentery* occurs most commonly in lambs under 10 days of age and there may be sudden death or acute toxemia, tucked-up abdomen and a severe diarrhea and dysentery. At necropsy the characteristic findings are hemorrhagic enteritis.

Foals
Rotaviral diarrhea occurs in foals from 5 to 35 days of age, but most commonly in foals under 2 weeks of age. There is acute profuse watery diarrhea, failure to suck, recumbency, dehydration; recovery is common within 1 week. A mild fever is common. Less common causes of diarrhea in foals include salmonellosis, *Clostridium perfringens* type B and dietary diarrhea.

Treatment
The treatment of viral diarrheas in newborn farm animals is essentially the same as described for colibacillosis. There is no specific therapy for viral diarrhea, but antimicrobial agents are used both orally and parenterally to treat the possible presence or occurrence of enteric and systemic bacterial infections. In the absence of complications, recovery from viral enteritis usually occurs without specific treatment in 2–5 days which parallels the replacement of the villous epithelial cells. Complete replacement and maturation probably requires several days after the cessation of diarrhea.

The withholding of milk for 24–48 hours is beneficial, but often not possible or practical when nursing beef calves or litters of pigs are involved. Milk can be withheld from hand-fed calves easily and replaced with oral fluids and electrolytes.

Oral and parenteral fluid therapy as indicated is essential. A glucose–glycine electrolyte formulation is an effective fluid therapy for pigs affected with experimental rotaviral diarrhea (64). The formula is: glucose 67·53%, sodium chloride 14·34%, glycine 10·3%, citric acid 0·8%, potassium citrate 0·2% and potassium dihydrogen phosphate 6·8%. A weight of 64 g of the above is dissolved in 2 liters of water to produce an isotonic solution.

When possible, affected animals, particularly calves, should be isolated from calving grounds and other newborn calves which are highly susceptible up to 3 weeks of age. When outbreaks of the disease occur in any species, the principles of good sanitation and hygiene should be emphasized to minimize the spread of infection.

Control
The principles of control of viral diarrhea are similar to those described for colibacillosis. The management of pregnant animals at the time of parturition must ensure that the degree of exposure of the newborn to infectious agents is minimized. Control of population density to avoid overcrowding, and sanitation and hygiene are important.

Because infected calves excrete large numbers of viral particles for several weeks, effective control may in part be dependent on management of the environment of the calf with particular emphasis on hygiene.

Two major approaches have been used to control rotavirus and coronavirus diarrhea in calves. One is the stimulation of active immunity by vaccinating the newborn calf with an oral vaccine containing the modified live viruses. The other is the stimulation of lactogenic immunity by vaccinating the dam during pregnancy.

A modified live virus rotavirus vaccine designed for oral administration to calves immediately after birth has been available commercially for many years and good results were claimed. However, the field trials did not include contemporary controls and the efficacy of the vaccine has been in doubt. The incidence of diarrhea in herds not vaccinated in the previous year was compared with the incidence during the year of vaccination which cannot adequately assess the efficacy of the vaccine. In one study in which the double-blind technique was used to evaluate the efficacy of the rotavirus vaccine given orally to the calves after birth and an *E. coli* bacterin given to the dams in late pregnancy, there was no difference in the incidence of diarrhea in vaccinated or non-vaccinated calves (67). In sequential field trials in which calves were vaccinated for an uninterrupted period of time, the morbidity and mortality rates were significantly lower than during the control periods before and after vaccination (68). In the double-blind trial, the morbidity and mortality rates in vaccinated and placebo calves were comparable. This suggests that the double-blind techniques may not be satisfactory for testing the efficacy of a vaccine when vaccinated and non-vaccinated animals are allowed to comingle. Recent controlled evaluations of the oral vaccine indicate a failure of protection of calves against rotavirus infection (65, 69) and rotavirus coronavirus infection (66). Effective oral vaccination of calves in the field against diarrhea caused by rotavirus or coronavirus is hindered by the presence of specific antibodies in the colostrum—*the colostrum barrier*. This may explain the failure of the vaccine under field conditions. Most of the efficacy trials with the vaccine were done on colostrum-deprived gnotobiotic calves which were vaccinated orally at birth and experimentally challenged a few days after birth. It is probably futile to vaccinate calves orally immediately after birth, particularly in herds where the disease is endemic. The colostrum of cows will contain high levels of specific antibodies.

The second approach to control relies on lactogenic immunity to provide passive protection against enteric viral infection of newborn farm animals. The success of this method depends on the presence of a sufficient amount of specific antibody to the rotavirus and coronavirus in the colostrum and milk of the dam which will neutralize the infection in the intestine of the newborn (116, 117). However, a major problem with this method of control is the rapid decline in colostral antibodies, commonly to below protective levels, which occurs within 24–48 hours following parturition. The circulating antibody which the newborn calf acquires in the first 24 hours of life is not protective against intestinal viral infection. This makes control in calves difficult under even ideal conditions.

In outbreaks of rotavirus or coronavirus diarrhea in calves, the daily feeding of stored colostrum from cows of the affected herd will reduce the incidence of clinical disease in the calves. In affected herds the colostral antiviral antibody may be sufficient to prevent the disease if colostrum is fed daily for up to 30 days (113, 114). If a large number of cows are calving over a short period of time, the colostrum can be pooled and fed to the calves daily. Even small amounts of colostrum from immunized cows are efficacious if mixed with cows' whole milk or milk replacer (113, 114).

The parenteral vaccination of the pregnant dam before parturition with a rotavirus and coronavirus vaccine may increase the level and duration of specific antibody in the colostrum (70). The major problem has been to develop a vaccine which when given to pregnant cattle will result in protective levels of specific antibody to the rotavirus and coronavirus in the colostrum initially, and then in the milk for a sufficient period such as 10 days to 3 weeks, the period most susceptible to these viral diarrheas. The use of a modified live rotavirus–coronavirus vaccine may stimulate a small but insignificant increase in colostral and milk antibodies (118). By 3 days after parturition the rotavirus and coronavirus antibody titers in the milk of vaccinated heifers had declined to low or undetectable levels. The use of an inactivated rotavirus vaccine resulted in significantly increased antirotavirus antibody in colostrum and milk from vaccinated dams compared to controls but the severity of diarrhea was the same in calves from both groups (70). The increased milk antibody delayed the establishment of infection but did not reduce the severity of clinical disease which was experimentally induced. It is possible that a natural infection may have been less severe and protection may have been provided. The use of an adjuvanted rotavirus vaccine given simultaneously intramuscularly and by the intramammary route can significantly enhance serum, colostrum and milk rotavirus antibody titers, whereas intramuscular vaccination with a commercial modified live rotavirus–coronavirus vaccine may not (115). Colostrum supplements, from the cows vaccinated by the intramammary and intramuscular routes, fed to rotavirus-challenged calves at a rate of 1% of the total daily intake of milk provided protection against both diarrhea and shedding (115, 119). The 30-day milk antibody titers from these cows were also considered to be protective when by which time calves should have developed a high degree of age-specific resistance to rotavirus infection. The use of an inactivated rotavirus vaccine in an oil adjuvant given to pregnant cows 60–90 days before calving and repeated on the day of calving resulted in a significant increase and prolongation of colostral antibodies up to 28 days after calving (121). Diarrhea in calves from vaccinated cows was less common and less serious. Similar results were obtained with a combined inactivated adjuvanted rotavirus and *E. coli* vaccine (59). Similar results have been achieved by vaccination of pregnant ewes (71, 72). Vaccination of ewes can result in an elevation of specific colostral antibody and prolong the period over which the antibody is present in the lumen of the intestines of the lambs. The antirotavirus activity is in the IgG fraction (73). The vaccination of cows with a monovalent vaccine results in a heterotypic response to all serotypes of rotavirus to which the animals have been previously exposed which suggests that single serotype vaccination may be sufficient (120).

In utero vaccination of the fetus with a rotavirus vaccine may offer an effective method for protection (80). The bovine fetus from 63 to 190 days of gestation is able to respond immunologically to the rotavirus. Infection *in utero* with the rotavirus induces resistance to experimental disease caused by both the human and bovine viruses (90). The calf rotavirus is ineffective as an antigen for the protection of experimental rotaviral diarrhea of piglets (84).

REVIEW LITERATURE

Bohl, E. H. (1979) Rotaviral diarrhea in pigs. Brief review. *J. Am. vet. med. Assoc.*, *174*, 613–615.

Bridger, J. C. (1980) Rotavirus: the present situation in farm animals. *Vet. Ann.*, *20*, 172–179.

Cilli, V. & Castrucci, G. (1981) Viral diarrhea of young animals. A review. *Comp. Immun. Microbiol. infect. Dis.*, *4*, 229–242.

Colloquium on selected diarrheal diseases of the young (1978) *J. Am. vet. med. Assoc.*, *173*, 509–676.

Dea, S., Roy, R. S. & Elizhary, M. A. S. Y. (1981) Calf coronavirus neonatal diarrhea. A literature review. *Can. vet. J.*, *22*, 51–58.

Flewett, T. H. & Woode, G. N. (1978) The rotaviruses. Brief review. *Arch. Virol.*, *57*, 1–23.

McNulty, M. S. (1978) Rotaviruses. A review article. *J. gen. Virol.*, *40*, 1–18.

Proceedings Second International Symposium on Neonatal Diarrhea. Veterinary Infectious Disease Organization, 3–5 October 1978. University of Saskatchewan, Saskatoon, Sask., pp. 1–551.

Saif, L. J. & Smith, K. L. (1985) Enteric viral infections of calves and passive immunity. *J. dairy Sci.*, *68*, 206–228.

Tzipori, S. (1985) The relative importance of enteric pathogen affecting neonates of domestic animals. *Adv. vet. Sci. comp. Med.*, *29*, 103–206.

Woode, G. N. (1978) Epizootiology of bovine rotavirus infection. *Vet. Rec.*, *103*, 44–46.

REFERENCES

(1) Tzipori, S. (1985) *Adv. vet. Sci. comp. Med.*, *29*, 103.
(2) Chasey, D. & Davies, P. (1984) *Vet. Rec.*, *114*, 16.
(3) Chasey, D. et al. (1986) *Arch. Virol.*, *89*, 235.
(4) Chasey, D. & Banks, J. *Vet. Rec.*, *115*, 386.
(5) Woode, G. N. et al. (1985) *Am. J. vet. Res.*, *46*, 1003.
(6) Bridger, J. C. et al. (1984) *Infect. Immun.*, *43*, 133.
(7) Flewett, T. H. & Woode, G. N. (1978) *Arch. Virol.*, *57*, 1
(8) Smith, A. W. et al. (1983) *Am. J. vet. Res.*, *44*, 851.
(9) Woode, G. N. et al. (1984) *J. clin. Microbiol.*, *19*, 623.
(10) Chasey, D. & Cartwright, S.F. (1978) *Res. vet. Sci.*, *25*, 255.
(11) Ducatelle, R. et al. (1981) *Arch. Virol.*, *68*, 35.
(12) Takahashi, E. et al. (1980) *Vet. Microbiol.*, *5*, 151.
(13) Shiraishi, T. et al. (1980) *J. Jap. vet. med. Assoc.*, *33*, 70.
(14) Storz, J. et al. (1978) *J. Am. vet. med. Assoc.*, *173*, 624.
(15) Orr, J. P. (1984) *Can. vet. J.*, *25*, 72.
(16) Abid, H. N. et al. (1984) *Vet. Med. SAC*, *79*, 105.
(17) Timoney, P. J. et al. (1983) *Vet. Rec.*, *113*, 318.
(18) Bridger, J. C. & Brown, J.F. (1985) *Vet. Rec.*, *116*, 50.
(19) Snodgrass, D. R. et al. (1984) *J. gen. Virol.*, *65*, 909.
(20) McNulty, M. S. (1978) *J. gen. Virol.*, *40*, 1.
(21) Mebus, C. A. et al. (1969) *Res. Bull. Univ. Neb.*, *233*, 1.
(22) De Leeuw, P. W. et al. (1980) *Res. vet. Sci.*, *29*, 135.
(23) Carpio, M. et al. (1981) *Can. J. comp. Med.*, *45*, 38.
(24) Dagenais, L. et al.(1981) *Vet. Rec.*, *108*, 11.
(25) Durham, P. J. K. et al. (1979) *NZ vet. J.*, *27*, 266, 271 & 272.
(26) Acres, S. D. et al. (1975) *Can. J. comp. Med.*, *39*, 116.
(27) Morin, M. et al. (1974) *Can. J. comp. Med.*, *38*, 236.
(28) Dea, S. et al. (1980) *Am. J. vet. Res.*, *41*, 23.
(29) Tzipori, S. R. et al. (1980) *Aust. J. exp. Biol. Med.*, *58*, 309.
(30) Turner, A. J. et al. (1976) *Aust. vet. J.*, *49*, 544.
(31) Snodgrass, D. R. & Herring, J. A. (1977) *Vet. Rec.*, *101*, 81.
(32) Leece, J. G. & King, M. W. (1978) *J. clin. Microbiol.*, *8*, 454.
(33) Tzipori, S. & Williams, I. H. (1978) *Aust. vet. J.*, *54*, 188.
(34) Barrow, P. A. et al. (1979) *Res. vet. Sci.*, *27*, 52.
(35) Theil, K. W. et al. (1979) *Am. J. vet. Res.*, *40*, 719.
(36) Saif, L. J. et al. (1980) *J. clin. Microbiol.*, *12*, 105.
(37) Woode, G. N. & Crouch, C. F. (1978) *J. Am. vet. med. Assoc.*, *173*, 522.
(38) Thiel, K. W. et al. (1978) *Am. J. vet.*, *39*, 213.
(39) Torres-Medina, A. & Underdahl, N. R. (1980) *Can. J. comp. Med.*, *44*, 403.
(40) Pearson, G. R. & McNulty, M. S. (1979) *Arch. Virol.*, *59*, 127.
(41) Morin, M. et al. (1976) *Can. J. comp. Med.*, *40*, 228.
(42) McAdaragh, J. P. et al. (1980) *Am. J. vet. Res.*, *41*, 1572.
(43) Woode, G. N. et al. (1978) *Vet. Rec.*, *102*, 340.
(44) Debouck, P. et al. (1981) *Vet. Microbiol.*, *6*, 157.
(45) Storz, J. et al. (1978) *J. Am. vet. med. Assoc.*, *173*, 633.
(46) Mebus, C. A. (1978) *J. Am. vet. med. Assoc.*, *173*, 631.
(47) Crouch, C. F. & Acres, S. D. (1984) *Can. J. comp. Med.*, *48*, 340.
(48) Wood, E. N. (1979) *Br. vet. J.*, *135*, 305.
(49) Woode, G. N. et al. (1978) *Vet. Rec.*, *102*, 15.
(50) Ellens, D. J. et al. (1978) *Med. Microbiol. Immunol.*, *166*, 157.
(51) Reynolds, D. J. et al. (1984) *Vet. Rec.*, *114*, 397.
(52) Rhodes, M. B. et al. (1979) *Can. J. comp. Med.*, *43*, 84.
(53) Van Balken, J. A. M. et al. (1979) *Vet. Microbiol.*, *3*, 205.
(54) Ekern, L. J. et al. (1981) *Can. J. comp. Med.*, *45*, 135.
(55) Dea, S. et al. (1979) *J. Clin. Microbiol.*, *10*, 240.
(56) Babiuk, L. A. et al. (1978) *J. clin. Microbiol.*, *6*, 610.
(57) Mohammed, K. A. et al. (1978) *Vet. Microbiol.*, *3*, 115.
(58) Acres, S. D. & Babiuk, L. A. (1978) *J. Am. vet. med. Assoc.*, *173*, 555.
(59) McNulty, M. S. & Logan, E. F. (1987) *Vet. Rec.*, *120*, 250.
(60) Mebus, C. A. et al. (1971) *Vet. Pathol.*, *8*, 490.
(61) Mebus, C. A. et al. (1973) *Vet. Pathol.*, *10*, 45.
(62) Snodgrass, D. R. et al. (1977) *Arch. Virol.*, *55*, 263.
(63) Pearson, G. R. & McNulty, M. S. (1977) *J. comp. Pathol.*, *87*, 363.
(64) Bywater, R. J. & Woode, G. N. (1980) *Vet. Rec.*, *106*, 75.
(65) Van Zaane, D. et al. (1986) *Vet. Immunol. Immunopathol.*, *11*, 45.
(66) DeLeeuw, P. W. & Tiessink, J. W. A. (1985) *Zentralbl. VetMed. B.*, *32*, 55.
(67) Acres, S. D. & Radostits, O. M. (1976) *Can. vet. J.*, *17*, 197.
(68) Thurber, E. T. et al. (1977) *Can. J. comp. Med.*, *41*, 131.
(69) Burki, F. et al. (1983) *Zentralbl. VetMed. B.*, *30*, 237.
(70) Snodgrass, D. R. et al. (1980) *Infect. Immun.*, *28*, 344.
(71) Wells, P. W. et al. (1978) *Vet. Rec.*, *103*, 46.
(72) Snodgrass, D. R. & Wells, P. W. (1978) *Vet. Rec.*, *102*, 146.
(73) Fahey, K. J. et al. (1981) *Vet. Immunol. Immunopathol.*, *2*, 27.
(74) Lewis, L. D. & Phillips, R. W. (1978) *J. Am. vet. med. Assoc.*, *173*, 636.
(75) Snodgrass, D. R. & Wells, P. W. (1978) *J. Am. vet. med. Assoc.*, *173*, 565.
(76) Snodgrass, D. R. et al. (1976) *Res. vet. Sci.*, *20*, 113.
(77) Begin, M. E. et al. (1978) In: *Proc. 2nd Int. Symp. Neonatal Diarrhea.* Oct., 1978. *Vet. Inf. Dis. Org., Saskatoon*, pp. 273–284.
(78) Morin, M. et al. (1979) In:*Proc. 2nd Int. Symp. Neonatal Diarrhea.* Oct., 1978. *Vet. Inf. Dis. Org., Saskatoon*, pp. 347–369.
(79) Woode, G. N. (1979) In: *Proc. 2nd Int. Symp. Neonatal Diarrhea.* Oct., 1978. *Vet. Inf. Dis. Org., Saskatoon*, pp. 205–223.
(80) Schalfer, D. H. et al. (1979) *Can. J. comp. Med.*, *43*, 405.
(81) Dea, S. et al. (1980) *Am. J. vet. Res.*, *41*, 30.
(82) Dea, S. et al. (1980) *Am. J. vet. Res.*, *41*, 23.
(83) Langpap, T. J. et al. (1979) *Am. J. vet. Res.*, *40*, 1476.
(84) Leece, J. G. & King, M. W. (1979) *Can. J. comp. Med.*, *43*, 90.
(85) Logan, E. F. et al. (1979) *Vet. Rec.*, *104*, 206.
(86) Pearson, G. R. et al. (1978) *Vet. Rec.*, *102*, 454.
(87) Wray, C. et al. (1981) *Res. vet. Sci.*, *30*, 379.
(88) Nilsson, O. et al. (1984) *Nord. VetMed.*, *36*, 103.
(89) Eugster, A. K. & Whitford, H. W. (1978) *J. Am. vet. med. Assoc.*, *173*, 857.
(90) Wyatt, R. G. et al. (1979) *Science*, *203*, 548.
(91) Schwers, A. et al. (1983) *J. comp. Pathol.*, *93*, 135.
(92) Crouch, C. F. et al. (1985) *J. gen. Virol.*, *66*, 1489.
(93) Schwers, A. et al. (1984) *Vet. Rec.*, *114*, 411.
(94) Reynolds, D. J. et al. (1985) *Arch. Virol.*, *85*, 71.
(95) Castrucci, G. et al. (1983) *Comp. Immunol. Microbiol. Infect. Dis.*, *6*, 321.
(96) Dea, S. et al. (1982) *Ann. rech. vét.*, *13*, 351.
(97) Woode, G.N. (1978) *Vet. Rec.*, *103*, 44.
(98) Utrera, V. et al. (1984) *Res. vet. Sci.*, *36*, 310.
(99) Dea, S. et al. (1986) *Can. J. vet. Res.*, *50*, 130.
(100) De San Juan, C. S. et al. (1986) *Res. vet. Sci.*, *41*, 270.
(101) Benfield, D. A. et al. (1982) *J. clin. Microbiol.*, *16*, 186.
(102) Ferguson, A. et al. (1981) *Gut*, *22*, 114.
(103) Sihvonen, L. & Miettinen, P. (1985) *Acta vet. Scand.*, *26*, 205.
(104) Hess, R. G. et al. (1984) *Zentralbl. VetMed. B*, *31*, 585.
(105) Hall, G. A. et al. (1984) *Vet. Pathol.*, *21*, 208.
(106) Pohlenz, J. F. L. et al. (1984) *Vet. Pathol.*, *21*, 407.
(107) Durham, P. J. K. et al. (1985) *Res. vet. Sci.*, *38*, 209, 234.
(108) Durham, P. J. K. et al. (1985) *Res. vet. Sci.*, *39*, 16.

(109) Conner, M. E. et al. (1983) *Cornell Vet.*, *73*, 280.
(110) McGuire, S. J. & Castro, A. E. (1982) *Bov. Practnr*, *17*, 66.
(111) Reynolds, D. J. et al. (1985) *Res. vet. Sci.*, *38*, 264.
(112) McNulty, M. S. & Logan, E.F. (1983) *Vet. Rec.*, *113*, 333.
(113) Castrucci, G. et al. (1984) *Comp. Immun. Microbiol. infect. Dis.*, *7*, 11.
(114) Snodgrass, D. R. et al. (1982) *Res. vet. Sci.*, *32*, 70.
(115) Saif, L. J. et al. (1984) *Am. J. vet. Res.*, *45*, 49.
(116) Leece, J. G. & King, M. W. (1982) *Can. J. comp. Med.*, *46*, 434.
(117) Saif, L. J. & Smith, K. L. (1985) *J. dairy Sci.*, *68*, 206.
(118) Myers, L. L. & Snodgrass, D. R. (1982) *J. Am. vet. med. Assoc.*, *181*, 486.
(119) Saif, L. J. et al. (1983) *Infect. Immun.*, *41*, 1118.
(120) Snodgrass, D. R. et al. (1984) *J. clin. Microbiol.*, *20*, 342.
(121) Dauvergne, M. et al. (1983) *Dev. Biol. Standard*, *53*, 245.
(122) Dea, S. et al. (1981) *Can. vet. J.*, *22*, 51.
(123) Bridger, J. C. et al. (1978) *Vet. Microbiol.*, *3*, 10.
(124) Morin, M. et al. (1980) *Can. vet. J.*, *21*, 100.
(125) Bohl, E. H. (1979) *J. Am. vet. med. Assoc.*, *174*, 613.
(126) Bridger, J. C. (1980) *Vet.Ann.*, *20*, 172.
(127) Conner, M. E. and Darlington, R. W. (1980) *Am. J. vet. Res.*, *41*, 1699.
(128) Schlafer, D. H. & Scott, F. W. (1979) *Cornell Vet.*, *69*, 262.
(129) Collins, J. K. et al. (1987) *Am. J. vet. Res.*, *48*, 361.
(130) Edwards, S. et al. (1987) *Vet. Microbiol.*, *13*, 19.

Bluetongue

Bluetongue is a disease of sheep and occasionally cattle, caused by an orbivirus and transmitted by insect vectors. It is characterized by catarrhal stomatitis, rhinitis and enteritis and lameness due to inflammation of the coronary bands and sensitive laminae of the feet.

Etiology

A provisional antigenic classification of the causative reovirus (genus *Orbivirus*) indicates that in Africa there are at least 20 serotypes. In the United States there are four serotypes of the bluetongue virus (45) and two serotypes of the closely related epizootic hemorrhagic disease virus of deer (2). Four bluetongue serotypes have been identified in Australia, and although no clinical bluetongue disease occurs in that country experimental infection with these serotypes causes very mild buccal hyperaemia and pyrexia with three of the serotypes and nasal excoriations and coronitis with the fourth (17). Outbreaks caused by different serotypes may follow one another in quick succession in a sheep population. The serotypes vary widely in their virulence with a corresponding variation in the severity of the disease produced.

A bluetongue-like disease of cattle in Japan and Korea (18) is caused by a related virus, the Ibaraki virus. It is not related antigenically to bluetongue virus, but is antigenically similar to the virus of epizootic hemorrhagic disease of deer (30). The viral diseases of deer and other wild fauna are listed in this book when they impinge on the study of the diseases of domestic animals, but they are not dealt with in detail.

The bluetongue viruses are stable and resistant to decomposition and to some standard viricidal agents including sodium carbonate. They are susceptible to 3% sodium hydroxide solution, and to Wescodyne, a complex organic iodide.

Epidemiology

The causative virus of bluetongue is well adapted to survive in some wild African ruminants and cattle in which it produces little clinical illness. However, when the infection spills over into sheep, and other unusual hosts, outbreaks of serious disease can occur. Under natural conditions the viral infection is common in sheep and cattle, but it is also recorded in elk, white-tailed deer, pronghorn antelope, camels and other wild ruminants (50). Neither the infection nor the disease are recorded as occurring naturally in goats. It is necessary to remember when investigating outbreaks of disease in deer that either bluetongue or epizootic hemorrhagic disease of deer, or both, can be present in the one animal. Both viruses have also been isolated from cattle (36). The diseases are very similar and the viruses are also similar, but distinguishable serologically and in culture in chick embryos (5). Amongst sheep, sucking lambs are relatively resistant, and if the ewes are resistant, solid passive immunity, lasting for about 2 months, is transmitted via the colostrum. Young sheep about a year old are most susceptible and British breeds and Merinos are more susceptible than native African sheep. Bluetongue virus is infective for cattle and has been isolated from this species as long as 81 days after infection. Clinical illness is not common in cattle, but it does occur naturally and may cause fatalities among a highly susceptible population. On the basis of serological surveys the infection rate in cattle populations may be as high as 48% (41). The situation in goats is similar to that in cattle. Natural infection rarely occurs but the infection can be transmitted experimentally (4, 9). Exposure to solar irradiation appears to increase the severity of the disease and other forms of environmental stress are likely to be contributory. Such factors may account for the difficulty encountered in producing the clinical disease in cattle kept under experimental conditions.

The infection is widespread on the African continent and has also occurred in India, Papua-New Guinea, Australia, the West Indies, Brazil, Cyprus, West Pakistan, Japan, Israel, Turkey, the United States and Portugal and Spain, but the clinical disease is not recorded in some of them, for example, Australia, the West Indies, Brazil, and Canada (15). Bluetongue has been diagnosed in many states in the United States and appears to have spread widely since its first identification in 1952. The prevalence of seropositive cattle varies from low in the northern states to high in the southern and western states, and with a national average of 18% (48). A new serotype has recently been isolated in the United States, a potentially dangerous one previously located in South Africa (4). In Canada there have been serological identifications of infection in animals in quarantine stations, but no virus has been isolated. Serologically positive animals have also been found at large, but only in one locality (23), and the prevalence of serological reactors has reduced greatly since the first detection of the infection (51). In Australia four serotypes of the bluetongue virus have been isolated. One of them, BT20, came from an insect vector, the other two from healthy sentinel cattle posted along the country's northern coastline.

The morbidity rate varies with the size of the insect population and the immune status of the sheep. When the disease occurs in a flock for the first time the morbidity may reach 50–75% and the mortality 20–50%.

In subsequent years when herd immunity is present and the insect population is low the morbidity may be as low as 1–2%. Although the mortality rate is low in adult sheep, severe losses may occur in young sheep (6). Usually 2–5% of affected animals die but in the Spanish outbreak the mortality rate was 60–80%. However, as in foot-and-mouth disease in cattle, the indirect losses are of greatest importance. Adults either lose their fleece or develop a break in the staple and pregnant ewes commonly abort. There is a severe loss of condition and convalescence is prolonged, particularly in lambs.

All common ruminants are susceptible to experimental infection and the virus will infect hamsters, unweaned white mice and developing chick embryos. It has also been grown in tissue culture and after suitable attenuation is capable of immunizing sheep without producing ill effects. After a clinical attack of the disease sheep have a solid immunity to the particular serotype virus involved but there is no crossimmunity to other serotypes.

Athough the infection is readily transmitted experimentally by the inoculation of infective blood into susceptible sheep, under natural conditions it appears to be spread only by insect bites. In the United States the vectors are sandflies (*Culicoides* spp.) especially *C. pallidipennis* and *C. variipennis*. *C. brevitarsis*, *C. actoni* and *C. schultzei* are the vectors in Australia. *Culicoides pallidipennis* (syn. *C. imicola*) is also the principal vector in Africa, and the Middle East. *Aedes lineatopennis* and *Melophagus ovinus* are the only other known vectors. The argasid tick *Ornithodoros coriaeceus* has been shown experimentally to be capable of transmitting the virus and being a potential vector (13). Culicoid flies do not become infective until about 10 days after ingesting infective blood. The sheep ked (*Melophagus ovinus*) ingests the virus when sucking the blood of infected sheep and can transmit the infection in a mechanical manner. It is not spread by contact and there is a marked seasonal incidence, most clinical cases occurring in the late summer and early autumn when the vector population is highest. The disease is most prevalent in wet seasons and in low-lying areas, conditions which favor insect multiplication (41).

The reason for the persistence of the infection from season to season has not been found. Virus has been isolated from recovered sheep 4 months after an attack of bluetongue and in some cases for longer periods. The infection may thus persist in carrier animals which may be cattle or wild ruminants. There is also the possibility of the virus overwintering in the insect vector (14). Cattle appear to be much more attractive to *Culicoides* spp. and this may enhance the importance of cattle as carriers. The virus may be spread to new areas by the transport of infected vectors or more frequently by the introduction of infected sheep or cattle. It is thought that an outbreak in Cyprus in 1977 was caused by infected insects being blown from the mainland across the sea. The distance could have been covered by insect flight time of 5–20 hours (38). A similar proposal has been made to account for the 1956 outbreak in Portugal (34). Serological data also shows that the infection is limited to northern cattle areas of Australia and its incidence varies widely from year to year (16). This suggests that the infection is introduced into the country periodically from countries to the north by migrating *Culicoides* spp. Similar wind-borne migrations of infected midges have been credited with the movement of bluetongue to western Turkey from Cyprus (3).

The duration of infectivity in cattle is uncertain, although it has been described as being as long as 49 days. However, there is a record of recovery of the virus from one bull on a number of occasions over a period of 4 years. Multiple feedings by the vector were necessary (44). The bluetongue virus has been found in the semen of infected bulls, the infection transmitted by insemination from an infected bull (37) and this has resulted in the prohibition of importation into free countries of bovine semen from countries where bluetongue exists. However, transplanted embryos from infected services are free of the virus and this is regarded as a suitable technique for obtaining clean offspring from infected parents (4). Infection of the fetus via the placenta does not appear to occur (54). To prevent the introduction of bluetongue very stringent regulations preventing the importation of ruminants from infected areas have been adopted in Australia and New Zealand.

Pathogenesis

A viremia occurs in the early stages of the disease and localization of the virus in vascular endothelium follows. Destruction of the vessel walls produces the characteristic epithelial lesions of bluetongue. The virus of bluetongue is largely confined within the erythrocytes suggesting that bovine marrow stem cells are a site of replication for the virus. This hypothesis also explains how the virus coexists with virus neutralizing (VN) antibodies in nature (10). The severe clinical disease that occurs in only a few infected cattle has been identified as a hypersensitivity reaction (22, 42).

The presence of the bluetongue virus in the semen of bulls is accompanied by structural abnormalities of the spermatozoa and by the presence of virus particles in them (7). After experimental inoculation in cattle a viremia occurs with a peak about 7 days later and a positive reaction to the gel diffusion test after the 21st day.

The virus penetrates the placental barrier and congenital infection occurs readily with both wild and culture viruses. The congenital defects of the nervous system of lambs which result are common with attenuated vaccine virus, but occur rarely with natural infection. These have been produced experimentally in lambs in early pregnancy (11). The location and the nature of the lesions may be related to the level of maturation and migration of nerve cells at the time infection occurs (19). The degenerative nature of the lesions results from the presence of immature neural cells with enhanced viral susceptibility combined with an inability to mobilize an effective immunological response. In older fetuses, a typical inflammatory response develops (20) and there is also a generalized retardation of growth and lymphoreticular activity (20).

Experimental inoculation of pregnant ewes is more likely to lead to invasion of the fetus and to its death. The invasion of the fetus occurs after 6–7 days and in the fetus there is a generalized hepatic necrosis and suppressed hepatic hematopoiesis (40). Infection of the ewe in mid-pregnancy can result in infection of the lamb which is unaffected and born normally, but viremic so that it may remain as a source of infection for a further 2 months (32), but such lambs are not expected to have a major role in the spread of the disease. Vertical transmission also occurs in cattle, thus prolonging the availability of the virus (11, 12). Experimental inoculation of pregnant cows at 60–120 days of pregnancy with virulent viruses can cause congenital defects including excessive gingival tissue, agnathia (tilted mandible), arthrogryposis, ataxia and head pressing (11). Hydranencephaly may also be a sequel (12). Experimental infection of gnotobiotic newborn lambs and kids appears to have no deleterious affects (46).

Clinical findings

There is a classical syndrome, set out below, which occurs when virulent serotypes infect susceptible sheep exposed to infection for the first time. The syndrome is not easily reproducible experimentally; on inoculation the localizing, identifying lesions are often minimal, with erythema of the coronary bands as the only visible abnormality in some cases.

Naturally occurring, florid bluetongue in sheep has the following clinical characteristics. After an incubation period of less than a week (2–4 days experimentally), a severe febrile reaction with a maximum temperature of 40·5–41°C (105–106°F) is usual, although afebrile cases may occur. The fever continues for 5 or 6 days. About 48 hours after the temperature rise, nasal discharge and salivation, with reddening of the buccal and nasal mucosae are apparent. The nasal discharge is mucopurulent and often bloodstained and the saliva is frothy. Swelling and edema of the lips, gums, dental pad and tongue occur and there may be involuntary movement of the lips. Excoriation of the buccal mucosa follows and the saliva becomes bloodstained and the mouth has an offensive odor. Lenticular, necrotic ulcers develop, particularly on the lateral aspects of the tongue, which is swollen and purple in color. Swallowing is often difficult. Respiration is obstructed and stertorous and is increased in rate up to 100/min. Diarrhea and dysentery may occur. Foot lesions, including laminitis and coronitis and manifested by lameness and recumbency, appear only in some animals, usually when the mouth lesions begin to heal. The appearance of a dark red to purple band in the skin just above the coronet, due to coronitis, is an important diagnostic sign. Wryneck, with twisting of the head and neck to one side, occurs in a few cases, appearing suddenly about the 12th day. This is apparently due to the direct action of the virus on muscle tissue as is the pronounced muscle stiffness and weakness which is severe enough to prevent eating. There is a marked, rapid loss of condition. The lower parts of the face, the ears and jaws are edematous and hyperemia of the woolless skin may be present. Some affected sheep show severe conjunctivitis, accompanied by profuse lacrimation. A break occurs in the staple of the fleece. Vomiting and secondary aspiration pneumonia may also occur. Death in most fatal cases occurs about 6 days after the appearance of signs.

In animals that recover there is a long convalescence and a return to normal may take several months. Partial or complete loss of the fleece is common and causes great financial loss. Other signs during convalescence include separation or cracking of the hooves and wrinkling and cracking of the skin around the lips and muzzle. Although the subsequent birth of lambs with porencephaly and cerebral necrosis is usually recorded after vaccination with attenuated virus, it also occurs rarely after natural infections (21).

In sheep in enzootic areas the disease is much less severe and often inapparent. Two syndromes occur. There is an abortive form in which the febrile reaction is not followed by local lesions. In the subacute type the local lesions are minimal, but emaciation, weakness and extended convalescence are severe. A similar syndrome occurs in lambs which become infected when colostral immunity is on the wane.

In cattle, most infections are inapparent although a few animals may develop a clinical syndrome not unlike that seen in severely affected sheep. Authenticated clinical signs which have been recorded include fever (40–41°C, 104–106°F), stiffness and laminitis in all four limbs, excessive salivation, edema of the lips, inappetence, nasal discharge and fetid breath. Some affected cattle also have ulcerative lesions on the tongue, dental pad, and muzzle. A severe coronitis, sometimes with sloughing of the hoof, may occur. Serosanguineous exudate may appear in the nostrils and a discharge from the eyes. This florid form of the disease in cattle appears to be a hypersensitivity reaction in a previously infected animal (22). Sheep do not seem to develop the same hypersensitivity (25). Contraction of the infection during early pregnancy may cause abortion or congenital deformities (24). These include hydranencephaly, microcephaly, curvature of the limbs, blindness and deformity of the jaw (53).

Infected goats show very little clinically. There is a mild to moderate fever, and hyperemia of the mucosae and conjunctivae. Bluetongue in deer is clinically identical to bluetongue in sheep. Epizootic hemorrhagic disease of deer is also very acute in most cases and is characterized by multiple hemorrhages throughout the body.

Infection of pregnant cows with bluetongue virus needs to be included in the list of diagnostic possibilities when examining outbreaks of congenital defects in calves.

Clinical pathology

Diagnosis can be confirmed by inoculation of blood into susceptible sheep, unweaned white mice or hamsters or culture in tissue culture or in developing chick embryos. It is recommended that blood be subinoculated from the first to a second recipient sheep when even a slight fever peak occurs in the first 14 days in the first sheep. A number of serological tests are available including a modified direct complement fixation test, a microprecipitation test on agar gel, a fluorescent antibody technique and a plaque reduction neutralization test (27). The tests are of approximately equal value, but the plaque neutralization test is most sensitive (28). The more recently developed tests, including enzyme-linked immunoabsorbent assay (ELISA), immunodiffusion, radioimmunoassay, and a hemolysis-in-gel assay (1) have been developed to encompass large-scale testing for eradication programs. A genetic probe technique has also been developed for identification of bluetongue viral DNA in fluids and tissues (26). The skeletal myopathy which occurs in this disease is reflected by a rise in serum enzymes including creatinine phosphokinase. The slight leukocytosis which occurs in the early stages of the disease is commonly followed by a marked leukopenia, due largely to lymphopenia. Infected cattle show a similar leukopenia.

Necropsy findings

The mucosal and skin lesions have already been described. Other consistent lesions include generalized edema, hyperemia and hemorrhage and necrosis of skeletal and cardiac muscles and aspiration pneumonia. There is a most distinctive hemorrhage at the base of the pulmonary artery. Hyperemia and edema of the abomasal mucosa are sometimes accompanied by ecchymoses and ulceration. Muscle lesions include hemorrhages and hyaline degeneration.

Diagnosis

Although bluetongue is not a vesicular disease, and its epidemiology is characteristic of an insect-borne disease, it is not uncommon to confuse it, in the field, with foot-and-mouth disease in both cattle and sheep. Bluetongue has a seasonal incidence, disappearing when the insect vectors diminish. The serological tests make it possible to detect that exposure to bluetongue virus has occurred, and the virus can be identified in a number of ways as set out above. One of the most satisfactory tests is the inoculation of blood from suspected animals into susceptible sheep. A positive test depends on the appearance of diagnostic clinical signs and resistance to subsequent challenge with bluetongue virus, or a significant increase in virus neutralizing (VN) antibodies in the recipient sheep (16).

Because of the great variations in epidemiology and symptomatology of the disease, diagnosis, except in the classical severe form of the disease, can be greatly delayed by failure to recognize the possibility of bluetongue at a field examination.

Contagious ecthyma and ulcerative dermatosis have characteristic lesions, and sheeppox is a highly fatal disease with typical pox lesions. An epizootic disease of cattle, Ibaraki disease, resembling bluetongue has been identified in Japan. The causative virus is antigenically different from that of bluetongue (29). Clinically the disease is characterized by fever, ulcerative stomatitis and dysphagia. Hyperemia and edema of the mucosae are accompanied by hemorrhages, as in bluetongue in cattle. Epizootic hemorrhagic disease of white-tailed deer has much in common with bluetongue in that species (31). Very heavy mortality rates are recorded in deer herds. All ages and types of animals are susceptible. Morbidity can be as high as 90% and mortality as high as 60%. Although all deer species can be affected, by far the most commonly affected is the white-tailed deer (33). The orbivirus of epizootic hemorrhagic disease of deer produces low level viremia in various species of deer and in sheep and cattle, but not in goats or pigs (39). Cattle and sheep may play a part in the epidemiology of the disease.

Treatment

Local irrigations with mild disinfectant solutions may afford some relief. Affected sheep should be housed and protected from weather, particularly hot sun, and treatment to control secondary infection may be desirable.

Control

Prevention of entry of the disease into a country which has effective natural barriers against uncontrolled livestock entry depends on quarantine measures to prevent the introduction of any ruminant animals from countries where the disease occurs and adequate treatment of aircraft to prevent the accidental introduction of infective insects. Because of resentment by livestock owners to the complete prohibition of international movement of ruminants, several procedures aimed at permitting limited movement are being examined. The introduction of bovine semen from low-risk areas after suitable tests of donors and a prolonged storage period is already in limited use. The importation of live cattle which have passed a test of not causing serological reactions to bluetongue in sheep after repeated blood transfusions is projected in some countries. Although these procedures provide minimum risks, the drastic consequences of an introduction of bluetongue make their use inadvisable unless there is very great need for the introduction of new genetic material. A specific protocol for the certification of bulls as being free of bluetongue has been produced. It includes the injection of the donor's semen and blood into sheep and the serological testing of the donor bull and the sheep (49).

In enzootic areas any measure which prevents exposure to nightflying insect vectors will reduce spread. Spraying with repellents, housing at night, and avoidance of low, marshy areas are recommended prophylactic measures. Because of vector preference for cattle as a feeding object they have been used as decoys to reduce parasitization of nearby sheep. Vaccination is the only satisfactory control procedure once the disease has been introduced into an area. Periodic revaccination of all sheep is now practiced in such areas and although the practice will not eradicate the disease it has been highly successful in keeping losses to a very low level provided immunity to all local strains of the virus is attained. It is therefore necessary to continually monitor the identity and prevalence of the serotypes in infected countries. The principal difficulty in control programs is the way in which the virus persists in inapparent carriers in wild ruminants. Attempts to vaccinate these animals by putting lyophilized vaccine out in food have been unsuccessful, and only vaccination by injection is satisfactory (35).

An egg-attenuated living virus is in current use in South Africa as a vaccine. The vaccine is polyvalent and contains a number of strains of virus with wide antigenicity. Reactions to vaccination are slight but ewes should not be vaccinated within 3 weeks of mating as anestrus often results. Annual revaccination 1 month before the expected occurrence of the disease is recommended. Immunity is present 10 days after vaccination so that early vaccination during an outbreak may substantially reduce losses. Lambs from immune mothers may be able to neutralize the attenuated virus and fail to be immunized, whereas field strains may overcome their passive immunity. In enzootic areas it may therefore be necessary to postpone lambing until major danger from the disease is passed and lambs should not be vaccinated until 2 weeks after weaning. A modified live virus vaccine has also given good results in the United States with a strong immunity lasting for 12 months (47). Vaccination of cattle is not usually recommended, but there are obvious reasons why this should be done in enzootic areas, so that the matter may need attention.

American workers have reported that vaccination of pregnant ewes is attended by risk of deformity in the lambs. The danger period is between the 4th and 8th weeks of pregnancy with the greatest incidence of deformities occurring when vaccination is carried out in ewes pregnant for 5–6 weeks. The incidence of deformities may be as high as 13%, with an average of 5%. Abortions do not occur although some lambs are stillborn. The deformities include retinal dysplasia, spasticity and edema of the limbs and a 'dummy' syndrome. At necropsy there is no evidence of bacterial or viral infection. The cranial cavity is filled with fluid and the brain is hypoplastic with evident degenerative changes. Similar lesions occur in calves as a result of natural infection with virulent virus (11).

As a matter of principle it is not recommended that living vaccines be used to control insect-borne diseases because of the risk of the vaccine strain being transmitted, and being exalted in virulence by passage. Even without any change in virulence, the vaccine strain of bluetongue virus could cause a great deal of loss from congenital defects if it became widespread in occurrence. However, living vaccines are used for practical reasons including the fact that inactivated vaccines do not provide protection against infection (25, 43). In experimental work a neutralizing, monoclonal antibody has prevented bluetongue (52).

REVIEW LITERATURE

Erasmus, B. J. (1975) Symposium on Bluetongue. Australian Veterinary Association Annual General Meeting, Adelaide 1975. *Aust. vet. J.*, *51*, 185.

Gibbs, E. P. J. (1983) Bluetongue: an analysis of current problems, with particular reference to importation of ruminants to the USA *J. Am. vet. med. Assoc.*, *182*, 1190–1194.

Osburn, B. I. et al. (1983) A review of bovine bluetongue. *Proc. Am. Assoc. Bov. Practnrs*, *15*, 23–28.

REFERENCES

(1) Jochim, M. M. & Jones, S. C. (1980) *Am. J. vet. Res.*, *41*, 595.
(2) Barber, T. L. & Jochim, M. M. (1974) *Proc. 77th ann. Mtg US Anim. Hlth Assoc.*, *77*, 352.
(3) Sellers, R. F. & Pedgley, D. E. (1985) *J. Hyg., Camb.*, *95*, 149.
(4) Barber, T. L. & Collison, E. W. (1983) *Proc. US Anim. Hlth Assoc.*, *87*, 90.
(5) Thomas, F. C. et al. (1974) *J. Wildlife Dis.*, *10*, 187.
(6) Esai, M. et al. (1980) *Vet. Rec.*, *106*, 481.
(7) Foster, N. M. et al. (1980) *Am. J. vet. Res.*, *41*, 1045.
(8) Hubbert, W. T. et al. (1972) *Am. J. vet. Res.*, *33*, 1879.
(9) Luedke, A. J. & Anakwenze, E.I. (1972) *Am. J. vet. Res.*, *33*, 1739.
(10) Alstad, A. P. et al. (1977) *Proc. Am. Assoc. Vet.Lab. Diagnosticians*, *20*, 273.
(11) Thomas, F. C. et al. (1986) *Can. J. vet. Res.*, *50*, 280.
(12) MacLachlan, N. J. & Osburn, B. I. (1983) *Vet. Pathol.*, *20*, 563.
(13) Stott, J. L. et al. (1985) *Am. J. vet. Res.*, *46*, 1197.
(14) Nevill, E. M. (1971) *Onderstepoort. J. vet. Res.*, *38*, 65.
(15) Gibbs, E. P. J. (1985) *Bov. Practnr*, *20*, 155.
(16) Coackley, W. et al. (1980) *Aust. vet. J. Res.*, *56*, 487.
(17) Uren, M. F. & St. George, T. D. (1985) *Aust. vet. J.*, *62*, 175.
(18) Bak, B. et al. (1983) *Korean J. vet. Res.*, *23*, 81.
(19) Narayan, O. & Johnston, R. T. (1972) *Am. J. Pathol.*, *68*, 1.
(20) Richardson, C. et al. (1985) *Am. J. vet. Res.*, *46*, 1912.
(21) Schmidt, R. E. & Panciera, R. J. (1973) *J. Am. vet. med. Assoc.*, *162*, 567.
(22) Stott, J. L. et al. (1984) *Proc. 13th World Cong. Dis. Cattle.*, p. 126.
(23) Goltz, J. (1978) *Can. vet. J.*, *19*, 95.
(24) Luedke, A. J. et al. (1970) *J. Am. vet. med. Assoc.*, *156*, 1871.
(25) Mahrt, C. R. & Osborne, B. I. (1986) *Ann. J. vet. Res.*, *47*, 1191 & 1198.
(26) Roy, P. et al. (1985) *J. gen. Virol.*, *66*, 613.
(27) Boulanger, P. & Frank, J. F. (1975) *Aust. vet. J.*, *51*, 185.
(28) Thomas, F. C. et al. (1976) *Can. J. comp. Med.*, *40*, 291.
(29) Inaba, Y. (1976) *Aust. vet. J.*, *51*, 178.
(30) Campbell, C. H. et al. (1978) *Vet. Microbiol.*, *3*, 15.
(31) Frank, J. F. & Willis, N. G. (1975) *Aust. vet. J.*, *51*, 174.
(32) MacLachlan, N. J. et al. (1984) *Am. J. vet. Res.*, *45*, 1469.
(33) Roughton, R. D. (1975) *J. Wildlife Dis.*, *11*, 177.
(34) Sellers, R. F. (1978) *J. Hyg., Camb.*, *81*, 189.
(35) Robinson, R. M. et al. (1974) *J. Wildlife Dis.*, *10*, 228.
(36) Foster, N. M. et al. (1980) *J. Am. vet. med. Assoc.*, *176*, 126.
(37) Bowen, R. A. & Howard, T. H. (1984) *Am. J. vet. Res.*, *45*, 1386.
(38) Sellers, R. F. et al. (1979) *J. Hyg., Camb.*, *83*, 547.
(39) Gibbs, E. P. J. & Lawman, M. J. P. (1977) *J. comp. Pathol.*, *81*, 335.
(40) Bwangamoi, O. (1978) *Bull. Anim. Hlth Prod., Africa*, *26*, 79.
(41) Thomas, F. C. et al. (1985) *Theriogenology*, *24*, 345.
(42) Emau, P. et al. (1984) *Am. J. vet. Res.*, *45*, 1852.
(43) Stott, J. L. et al. (1985) *Am. J. vet. Res.*, *46*, 1043.
(44) Luedke, A. J. et al. (1977) *Am. J. trop. Med. Hyg.*, *26*, 313.
(45) Barber, T. L. (1979) *Am. J. vet. Res.*, *40*, 1654.
(46) Livingston, C. W. et al. (1983) *Am. J. vet. Res.*, *44*, 129.
(47) McConnell, S. & Livingstone, C. W. (1982) *Proc. US Anim. Hlth Assoc.*, *86*, 103.
(48) Metcalf, H. E. et al. (1981) *Am. J. vet. Res.*, *42*, 1057.
(49) Osburn, B. L. et al. (1983) *Proc. US Anim Hlth Assoc.*, *87*, 105.
(50) Jessup, D. A. et al. (1984) *Proc. US Anim. Hlth Assoc.*, *88*, 616.
(51) Thomas, J. C. et al (1982) *Can. J. comp. Med.*, *46*, 350.
(52) Letchworth, G. J. & Appleton, J. A. (1983) *Infect. Immun.*, *39*, 208.
(53) Sharma, M. M. et al. (1986) *Ind. J. anim. Sci.*, *56*, 1055.
(54) Parsonson, I. M. et al. (1987) *Aust. vet. J.*, *64*, 14.

Nairobi sheep disease

This is a disease of East African goats and sheep caused by a bunyavirus and transmitted transstadially and transovarially by the tick *Rhipicephalus appendiculatus* (1). It is characterized clinically by fever, anorexia, nasal discharge, dyspnea and a severe diarrhea, sometimes with dysentery, and abortion in pregnant ewes. At necropsy there is serositis, lymphadenopathy and hyperemia of the abomasal and intestinal mucosa. The disease is a severe one and the mortality rate may be as high as 70%. A number of serological tests are suitable for diagnostic purposes including hemagglutination, indirect immunofluorescence and an enzyme-linked immunoabsorbent test (2).

REFERENCES

(1) Davies, F. G. & Mwakima, F. (1982) *J. comp. Pathol.*, *92*, 15.
(2) Munz, E. et al. (1983) *Zentralbl.VetMed.*, *30*, 473.

22

Diseases Caused by Viruses and Chlamydia—II

VIRAL DISEASES CHARACTERIZED BY RESPIRATORY SIGNS

Viral infections of the upper respiratory tract of horses

Until relatively recent years the infectious diseases of the respiratory tract of horses, apart from strangles, were differentiated largely on clinical grounds and the specific causative agents were unknown. The picture is still confused, but the identification of a number of viruses including those of equine viral arteritis, equine rhinopneumonitis and equine influenza and the definition of the syndromes they produce has done much to reduce the confusion.

The specific diseases dealt with in detail are equine viral rhinopneumonitis, equine viral arteritis and equine influenza. Other viral infection of the equine upper respiratory tract are set down below.

Infection with a *rhinovirus*, equine rhinovirus 1 (ERV 1), is recorded (1). There is an equine rhinovirus 2, but is appears to have little significance. The disease ERV 1 is characterized by an incubation period of 3–8 days, fever, pharyngitis, pharyngeal lymphadenitis, and a copious nasal discharge which is serous early and becomes mucopurulent later. A cough persists for 2–3 weeks. The uncomplicated disease is mild and self-limiting. Epidemiologically there is rapid spread and high morbidity. For example, in Australian horses there may be 100% of seropositive horses in some groups, and as many as 70% of a large population may have antibodies to a rhinovirus (2). Immunity after natural infection is solid and long-lasting (3). Diagnosis is based on serological testing and tissue culture of the virus. There is no commercial vaccine available but production is feasible because there are only a few serotypes. Alternatively a planned exposure of young horses to infection is recommended (4).

Epizootic cough or 'Hoppengarten' cough is a disease with a long history in Germany, but its etiology is still not determined. It is manifested by transient fever, serous nasal discharge, lacrimation, pharyngeal lymphadenitis and a persistent dry, painful cough (5).

Infections with equine herpesviruses 2 and 3 are dealt with briefly under equine viral rhinopneumonitis. *Equine coital exanthema*, caused by equine herpesvirus 3, is not dealt with in detail here because of its common inclusion in textbooks of diseases of the reproductive system. It is a venereal disease manifested by papular, then pustular, and finally ulcerative lesions of the vaginal mucosa which is generally reddened. The ulcers may be as large as 2 cm in diameter and 0·5 cm deep and are surrounded by a zone of hyperemia. In severe cases the lesions extend onto the vulva, and the perineal skin to surround the anus. In the male similar lesions are found on the penis and prepuce. Many mild cases are unobserved because there is no systemic disease and affected horses eat well and behave normally.The effect on fertility is equivocal although there may be a loss of libido during the active stage of the disease in stallions (9). The infection appears to be spread by clinically normal carrier mares (7). The incubation period is 2–10 days and the course up to complete healing of ulcers is about 14 days. Secondary bacterial infection may lead to suppurative discharge and a longer course. In some outbreaks lesions occur on the skin of the lips and around the nostrils and on the conjunctiva. They may also be present on the muzzle of the foal (7). Ulcerative lesions of the pharyngeal mucosa also occur in infections with equine herpesvirus 2 (6) and with equine adenovirus.

Ulcerative lesions of the oral mucosa are of great importance because of the necessity to diagnose vesicular stomatitis early. Elongated shallow erosions (2 × 0·5 cm) can occur in profusion in the mouths of a large proportion of a band of horses grazing pasture infested with hairy caterpillars or pastures containing grass with bristly seedheads.

Upper respiratory tract infection with *equine parainfluenza 3* (PI-3) virus appears to have been recorded only once and is of doubtful importance (8). The clinical record is of a mild self-limiting disease of the upper respiratory tract which is not clinically distinguishable from the others in the group. Mild respiratory signs and transient softness of the feces in adult horses are related to serological evidence of infection with an *adenovirus* (4). In foals, equine adenovirus also causes a mild respiratory disease but in some cases, and on experimental infection, a severe, non-fatal pneumonia follows. The full scope of lesions includes conjunctivitis, upper respiratory tract disease with rhinitis, tracheitis and bronchopneumonia and interstitial pneumonia (13). In Arab foals with *inherited combined immunodeficiency*, the adenoviral pneumonia is usually fatal. Adenovirus infection is common in horses; in the United Kingdom 35% of adult horses are seropositive (2). Experimental infection of the adenovirus into pregnant mares can cause abortion without illness in the dam. Diagnosis can be by serum neutralization, hemagglutination inhibition, complement fixation, or precipitating antibody tests. The serum neutralization test is most accurate, but the hemagglutination inhibition test is most suitable for a screening test (14). An inactivated vaccine with high immunogenic potency has been produced against adenovirus infection, but has not had extensive exposure in the field (12).

A *reovirus*, or a series of serotypes, has also been added to the list of viruses suspected of causing upper respiratory tract disease of horses (16).

The clinical and epidemiological features of all of the diseases in this section, and of strangles which is dealt with elsewhere, are sufficiently similar to make differential diagnosis between them in the field virtually impossible. However, many field situations demand a presumptive diagnosis, at least in the first instance. Strangles will need treatment with antibiotics, impending abortions in a stud may necessitate immediate quarantine, and so on. Strangles is usually easily identifiable by its profuse nasal discharge, lymphadenitis and abscessation. The severe conjunctivitis, dyspnea, anasarca and abortion of equine viral arteritis are of diagnostic importance. Unfortunately both strangles and equine viral arteritis can be mild and lack outstanding clinical signs, thus closely resembling equine viral rhinopneumonitis, and infections with adenovirus, rhinovirus, parainfluenza virus and equine influenza virus. In these circumstances a positive diagnosis can be made only by isolation and identification of the virus concerned, although serological examination of paired—acute and convalescent phase—sera is often used for presumptive identification before virus isolation is attempted. For positive identification on the basis of paired sera a fourfold increase in titer over a 3-week interval is recommended.

Fortunately most of the respiratory viruses can be isolated from nasal swabs or washings, preferably collected in the early stages of the disease and presented to the laboratory in a frozen state. When pharyngitis is a prominent clinical sign, swabs of the pharyngeal area are superior to nasal swabs (5). It is also of importance in comparative medical studies to record the occurrence of upper respiratory tract infections in stable attendants and to submit specimens from affected persons. The position with respect to transmissibility of influenza viruses and rhinoviruses between the two species requires further clarification.

When the occurrence of these virus diseases is being monitored it is particularly important to maintain diagnostic surveillance over all aborted fetuses. Detection of inclusion bodies in nasal and pharyngeal mucosal smears is of some value in identifying adenovirus infection in foals, and in infections with equine herpes viruses (8).

The relative importance of the viruses is identified in surveys in the United Kingdom (rhinovirus type 1 in 64–75% of horses in training with equine influenza virus at a low level, and adenovirus and rhinopneumonitis viruses present in a high proportion) (2, 10) and Germany (79% of cavalry horses having a respiratory disease during a 3-month period of mingling; the viruses identified were equine herpesvirus 1, influenza A equine 1 and 2 and a high prevalence of rhinovirus 1; strangles occurred in 5% and purpura hemorrhagica in 0·8%; parainfluenza 3 virus was not identified) (11).

Stud farms

Two epidemiological factors which significantly affect the occurrence of the disease at the present day are air transport, which provides optimum opportunity for spread of new infections, and the increasing tendency to maintain closed bands of horses, especially in studs, so that when infection is introduced the outbreaks are likely to be severe. In more usual circumstances where the movement of horses between bands is common the diseases are usually a problem in yearlings and 2-year-olds. Young foals acquire a passive immunity, and adults have acquired a permanent immunity. All of the diseases are transmitted by droplet infection, and over long distances so that limitation of their spread is possible only by rigid isolation and intensive sanitary precautions so that even the best protected studs are likely to be invaded from time to time.

Racetracks

At racetracks serious outbreaks of upper respiratory tract disease can ruin a racing season and racing administrators have become increasingly authoritative about requirements for vaccination. Most of these outbreaks are caused by equine viral influenza and this subject is dealt with in detail under that heading. The problem is greatest where the horses are housed semipermanently in accommodation provided at the racetrack. In other circumstances where horses are in respiratory contact only on the day of racing the outbreaks are much less serious. The same general comments apply to all forms of horse management, and dressage and other pleasure horses are at great risk from these diseases.

The most serious outbreaks in racing horses occur in the winter and spring (15) with equine viral rhinopneumonitis being commonest in winter and influenza causing most of the outbreaks at the track in the summer; 2 and 3-year-old horses are the most frequent sufferers, as most horses over 4 years of age appear to have developed resistance to the infections. In a horse population it is the average age and the mix of ages which largely determine its herd resistance, and when 30–40% of that population has not previously been exposed to infection then major outbreaks are likely.

REVIEW LITERATURE

Coggins, L. (1979) Viral respiratory disease. *Vet. Clin. N. Am. large Anim. Pract.*, *1*, 59.

Reif, J. S. (1979) Epidemiology of equine infection respiratory disease. *Vet. Clin. N. Am. large. Anim. Pract.*, *1*, 3.

REFERENCES

(1) Burrows, R. (1970) *Proc. 2nd int. Conf. equ. infect. Dis, Paris*, 154.
(2) Harden, T. J. et al. (1974) *Aust, vet. J.*, *50*, 477. 488.
(3) Kelier, H. (1974) *Berl. Münch. Tierärztl. Wochenschr.*, *87*, 251.
(4) Powell, D. G. (1975) *Vet. Rec.*, *96*, 30
(5) Erasmus, B. J. (1965) *J. S. Afr vet. met. Assoc.*, *36*, 209.
(6) Studdert, M. J. (1974) *Cornell Vet.*, *64*, 94.
(7) Crandell, R. A. & Davis, E. R. (1985) *J. Am. vet. med. Assoc.*, *187*, 503.
(8) Coggins, L. & Kemen, M. J. (1975). *J. Am vet. met. Assoc.*, *166*, 80.
(9) Pascoe, R. R. (1981) *Aust. vet. J.*, *57*, 111.
(10) Rose, M. A. et al. (1974) *Vet. Rec.*, *95*, 484.
(11) Hofer, B. et al. (1973) In: *Equine Diseases*, eds J. T. Bryans & H. Gerber, vol. 3. Basel: Karger.
(12) Lew, A. M. (1979) *Am. J. vet. Res.*, *40*, 1707.
(13) Gleeson, L. J. et al. (1978) *Am. J. vet. Res.*, *39*, 1636.
(14) Kamada, M. (1978) *Exp. Rpt. Equ. Hlth Lab.*, *15*, 91.
(15) Sherman, J. et al. (1979) *Can. J. comp. Med.*, *43*, 1.
(16) Thein, P. & Hartle, G. (1977) *Prakt. Tierärztl.*, *58*, 24 & 30.

Equine viral rhinopneumonitis (EVR)

This is a mild disease of the upper respiratory tract of horses caused by a specific virus which also commonly causes abortion.

Etiology

Equine viral rhinopneumonitis is caused by a herpesvirus, equine herpesvirus 4 (EHV 4). It can be grown in tissue culture and has been adapted to embryonated eggs and hamsters.The virus has 20% homology with EHV 1, the cause of viral abortion in horses (8) and until recently the two were considered to be serotypes of EHV 1. Both are respiratory pathogens, the disease caused by EHV 4 being much milder (39). EHV 1 is the only significant abortifacient (30). There are some antigenic similarities between EVH 4 and the bovine herpesvirus (33). Virus of fetal origin is more infective, grows better on tissue culture, is more likely to cause abortion, and be excreted into the environment more generally than the subtype of virus isolated from the respiratory tract.

Two other related viruses are EHV 2 and EHV 3. EHV 2 (or equine cytomegalovirus or slow-growing herpesvirus) is the cause of a common infection commencing at birth and continuing for very long periods in foals. Some of the infected ones develop clinical signs of purulent nasal discharge, fever and lymphadenopathy in a syndrome which lasts about 1 week; rarely affected animals die (7). EHV 3 (the equine coital exanthema virus) is the cause of the venereal infection of skin of genitalia and perineum.

Epidemiology

Infection with the virus EHV 1 is universally common; a recent survey of Australian horses showed that 82% had been exposed to infection. The upper respiratory tract disease, which is the principal clinical manifestation of the disease, is also universally common, but abortion has a patchy distribution. It is common in the United States, has occurred but very rarely in the United Kingdom and Australia and New Zealand (36). Before 1977 the respiratory infection was common in both countries for many years.

Mild infection of the respiratory tract of horses, characterized by coughing and nasal discharge, are of widespread occurrence particularly when horses are congregated in the colder months. The initial identification of the virus was made in the United States and its presence is now known or suspected in most countries. The association between viral abortion and upper respiratory tract infection was originally suggested by European observers. It seems clearly established that equine viral rhinopneumonitis is mild in character and fatalities in uncomplicated cases are unlikely. Affected animals are unable to work, racehorses have to break their training, and 'storms' of abortions occur in bands of brood mares. The infection is widespread.

Although horses of all ages become infected, signs of upper respiratory tract disease are usually limited to young horses. On breeding farms outbreaks occur in foals, the mares showing only abortion. Most outbreaks of abortion are associated directly with outbreaks of the respiratory disease in 6–10 week old foals and yearlings several weeks earlier. These latter outbreaks occur most commonly in autumn and winter months. Recovery is followed by an immunity lasting for 6–12 months. In recent years there has been an extension of these syndromes to include septicemia and heavy mortality in newborn foals.

Mares with serum antibodies to the equine viral rhinopneumonitis virus secrete the antibodies in their colostrum and these create a passive immunity in their foals with the antibodies reaching zero in them on the average at 180 days of age (32). Unfortunately, virus neutralizing (VN) antibodies are not necessarily an indication of resistance to infection. Cell-mediated immunity is an important feature of resistance to herpesviruses and the lymphocyte transformation test is available to measure this. Cell-mediated immunity is significantly depressed by pregnancy and this may account for the occurrence of abortion in the presence of high titers of virus neutralizing antibodies (35).

The disease is highly infectious and transmission probably occurs by the inhalation of infected droplets or by the ingestion of material contaminated by nasal discharges or aborted fetuses. Mediate infection may occur, the virus surviving for 14–45 days outside the animal. The duration of the infectivity of animals is unknown, but is probably some weeks and possibly longer because carrier animals seem to be necessary for persistence of the disease from year to year. The observation that the infection may persist in a latent state and be reactivated subsequently, for example by treatment with corticosteroids (31), will assist in the understanding of the epidemiology.

Pathogenesis

Although equine herpesvirus 1 (EVH 1) is a respiratory pathogen there are at least four identifiable syndromes attributable to it in the horse. These are:

- Upper respiratory tract infections especially in young horses
- Abortions in bands of stud mares; infection is not always associated with abortion
- Highly fatal septicemia and viremia in neonatal foals less than 1 week old
- Encephalomyelopathy—the paralysis syndrome in adult horses
- There is also a suggestion that the 'poor performance syndrome' of racing horses may be important due to the effects of the respiratory infection (9).

In the respiratory tract there is an initial phase after infection in which there is rapid proliferation of the virus in the nasal, pharyngeal and tonsillar mucosae, resulting in rhinitis, pyrexia and associated clinical respiratory signs. This is followed by a systemic, viremic phase in which the virus is closely associated with the lymphocytes, from which it can be isolated. It is from this point that the invasion of lungs, placenta, fetus and nervous tissue occur.

Damage to the placenta is in the form of local edema at the fetomaternal junction so that the chorioallantois separates from the endometrium. The fetus is infected and tissues are damaged so that there are diagnostic lesions present in many aborted foals. Part of the disease process in these foals is massive destruction of lymphocytes in the spleen and the thymus (22).

Foals which are infected *in utero* but survive without abortion may be stillborn or weak and die soon after birth as a result of pulmonary or hepatic lesions (2). Other foals may be normal at birth, but are agammaglobulinemic, highly susceptible to viral and bacterial infections, and die quickly after a brief period of normality.

The pathogenesis of the nervous form of the disease is complex. Because of its relationship to reinfection, it has been suggested that it may be an immunological reaction (11) and immune complexes are detectable in the circulation. In the experimentally produced neurological disease there is a disseminated vasculitis and thrombus formation resulting in degeneration of nervous and many other tissues. The vasculitis may have an immunological basis or be the result of invasion of endothelium (12). In experimental production of the neurological disease only mares pregnant for early and midpregnant terms could become affected—late mares escape. The mechanism is unknown (12).

Clinical findings

Respiratory disease

In the classical respiratory tract form of the disease there is an incubation period of 2–20 days. Fever, conjunctivitis, coughing and mild inflammation of the upper respiratory tract are the cardinal manifestation of the disease, but inapparent infection is common. The temperature varies from 39 to 40·5°C (102·5 to 105·5°F). In most clinical cases there is only limited involvement of the respiratory system and the appetite is unimpaired. There may be slight enlargement of the lymph nodes of the throat. These signs are more likely to occur in young horses or when horses are assembled in sale barns. Edema of the limbs and diarrhea occur rarely. The length of the illness is usually 2–5 days, although the nasal discharge and cough may persist for 1–3 weeks. Secondary bacterial invasion, usually streptococcal, may result in pneumonia. Young foals may develop primary pneumonia.

Abortion

A heavy outbreak of abortions (up to 90%) in mares may occur up to 4 months after the respiratory phase, and in many instances the latter is so mild that it is not observed. Abortion occurs without premonitory signs and the placenta is not retained. There is frequently no mammary development. The incidence of abortion is highest in the last third of pregnancy—particularly in the 8–10 month period—but can occur as early as the 5th month. Some foals are stillborn; others are weak and die soon after birth.

Neonatal viremia and septicemia

Some of the infected foals are normal at birth, but become weak and die within 3 days of birth with signs of respiratory distress (38) and severe mental depression (sleepy foals). Secondary bacterial infection with *Escherichia coli* or *Actinobacillus equuli* may follow.

Paralytic syndrome

This nervous system involvement can occur in an outbreak in which abortion and respiratory system involvement also occur (24, 37). Recently reported outbreaks (27) have been massive with 90% of mares on a stud being affected. Foals and stallions are also affected. It is most common in horses being reinfected with the virus. The standard vaccine is not preventive and it has been suggested that the vaccine virus may be causative because the disease occurs soon (8–11 days) after vaccination (28) or experimental or natural infection (1, 11, 16). The clinical signs vary from slight, transient ataxia to severe ataxia followed by paresis and recumbency, leading to death or euthanasia (18). Urinary incontinence occurs in some (20).

The ataxia and paresis lasts for up to several weeks and is followed by recumbency. Some die after an illness of only 2 days. All have to be euthanized within a month. In one outbreak 14 of 24 horses exposed to the respiratory form of the disease developed nervous signs. The disease was reproduced experimentally and was characterized by an incubation period of 7 days (18).

Clinical pathology

Hematological findings include a pronounced leukopenia, due largely to depression of neutrophils. This is marked in young foals. The tests of critical importance are serological. Of those available the immunofluorescent test is most sensitive and most broadly reactive (21). Complement-fixing antibody is present, appearing on the 10th–12th day after experimental infection but persists for only a limited period. However, the virus neutralizing antibodies persist for over a year and testing for them is a more reliable means of determining that previous infection with the virus has occurred. The virus can be isolated in tissue culture, chick embryos and hamsters, from either nasal washings or aborted fetuses. Bacteriological examination of nasal discharges and aborted fetuses is negative unless secondary bacterial invasion has occurred. *Streptococcus equi* and *Salmonella abortivoequina* are the common secondary invaders in the respective sites.

Necropsy findings

The major necropsy manifestations are rhinitis and pneumonitis. Aborted fetuses show severe pulmonary congestion and focal hepatic necrosis with acidophilic intranuclear inclusion bodies in the bronchial and alveolar epithelium and in hepatic parenchyma. The focal necroses in the liver appear grossly as grayish-white, subcapsular spots up to 5 mm in diameter, and there is slight icterus. Petechial and ecchymotic hemorrhages are common especially beneath the respiratory mucosae of aborted fetuses and the most consistent macroscopic lesion is an excess of clear yellow fluid in the pleural and peritoneal cavities. In foals that are alive at birth and die soon afterwards there is usually massive pulmonary congestion and edema, and collapse of lung with hyaline membrane development in those that survive longer (30, 38).

In the nervous form of the disease in which paresis is the principal clinical sign, there is an acute disseminated encephalomyelopathy (18). Disseminated vasculitis occurs in the experimental disease (12, 34) and the malacic lesions present in nervous tissue are the result of leakage fron these damaged vessels.The virus can be isolated from the brain (23).

For laboratory examination of a fetus it is necessary to send liver and lung tissue in formalin for rapid presumptive diagnosis on the basis of examination of a frozen section; the same tissues plus thymus in formalin are necessary for histological examination of paraffin blocks, plus deeply frozen similar tissues for virus isolation. Forwarding of these latter specimens in various transport media is preferred. The laboratory examination should include a search for virus by tissue culture and immunofluorescent techniques, and histological examination of lung and liver for the presence of inclusion bodies.

Diagnosis

The clinical picture of a mild upper respiratory infection in young and adult horses, with a high incidence of abortions in convalescent mares, and characteristic lesions in the aborted fetuses are virtually diagnostic of equine viral rhinopneumonitis. As an upper respiratory tract infection it must be differentiated from strangles, with its catarrhal rhinitis and lymph node abscessation, from the more severe equine viral arteritis in which there are no lesions in aborted fetuses, and from equine influenza. It may also be confused with purpura hemorrhagica in which subcutaneous edema of the legs is severe.

Experimentally the rhinopneumonitis virus has been shown to cause vaginitis in mares. This is not to be confused with coital vesicular exanthema which is also caused by equine herpesvirus 3 (EHV 3).

Until proved to be otherwise all abortions in mares should be considered as being caused by this disease, equine herpesvirus 1. A tabular description of its differential diagnosis is set out in Table 46.

Confirmation of the diagnosis requires isolation of the virus in chick embryos or hamsters, the demonstration of the pathognomonic lesions in the aborted fetuses and production of the disease by injection into susceptible horses. The complement fixation tests are of value in detecting previous infection, but should not be used to determine the cause of abortion. The occurrence of a rise in antibody titer in paired sera collected several weeks apart is of more value, but isolation of the virus from the aborted fetus is the only definitive diagnostic procedure.

Treatment

No specific treatment is likely to modify the action of the virus, but it is usual to provide antibiotics to horses with equine viral rhinopneumonitis to prevent and treat infection with secondary bacterial invaders.The treatment should be continued over 4–6 days. Warm, draft-free, isolated quarters should be provided if possible, with laxative foods and a constant supply of fresh drinking water.

Control

Standard hygienic procedures should be adopted to avoid spread of the disease, with particular attention being given to the isolation of introduced horses and brood mares.This may be impossible in boarding studs where mares are brought in from many places for breeding. Mares which abort should be rigidly isolated and the contaminated area thoroughly cleaned and disinfected. Aborted fetuses should be completely disposed of, preferably to a laboratory for diagnosis. Attendants need to avoid indirectly infecting other pregnant mares by carrying virus on clothing and equipment.

Vaccination against equine rhinopneumonitis has been the subject of investigation for a long time but without significant gains. The main impetus has been the need to protect mares against abortion. Protection against the upper respiratory tract disease would be a distinct advantage but the disease is sufficiently mild and infrequent to make the need less than pressing. Although the need is to vaccinate mares, vaccination of sucklings and yearlings is also carried out because they are running with the mares, or on the same farms at the critical part of pregnancy and when the disease is likely to occur.

Two living vaccines have been used (26). A hamster-adapted live virus is applied by intranasal administration. The vaccine is so little attenuated that it provides the equivalent of a planned infection and can cause abortion in a small percentage of pregnant mares. The immunity is of short duration and the vaccine virus can spread to other horses and cause abortion or respiratory disease in them. All horses on the farm, therefore, need to be vaccinated at the same time and kept isolated from others for several weeks. This vaccine should not be used on farms where the disease is not known to occur.

Cell-culture adapted modified live virus vaccines have been developed in Europe and the United States (29) and are generally accepted and widely used in the United States, so much so that most herd health programs for breeding farms include its routine use. It has the virtue of not spreading between horses and does not cause respiratory disease or abortion (14). A disadvantage is the brevity of the immunity. It is poorly protective for yearlings (4) and fails to protect foals of less than 2 weeks of age (13). The level of protection against fetal and foal deaths is so low (5) that other forms of protection, especially by management, must be provided. These should be directed towards reducing exposure to infection and the amount of nutritional and other stress to which the mares are subjected. The foals of vaccinated mares should be vaccinated at 3 months, 2 weeks, before weaning and at 12 months of age (6). It is generally accepted that the vaccines available are of limited usefulness and they are recommended only when the disease is a serious enzootic problem, as it is in the United States. They should contain, for convenience, viruses EHV 1 and EHV 4 even though some cross-protection appears to occur (10). The need for a clear understanding of the different roles of the two viruses is paramount (29).

An inactivated, adjuvanted vaccine has been developed which appears to be highly antigenic (15). Its effectiveness under field conditions has not been determined, but the level of protection achieved against viral challenge is only moderate (10, 25).

The biggest problem created by equine viral rhinopneumonitis is on the standard commercial stud where one or more stallions and a band of mares are kept by the owner, but there are a large number of visiting mares which foal on the stud and are bred very soon afterwards. They move back to their own home farms when they are diagnosed pregnant. The owners of the studs 'visited' by mares are understandably anxious to avoid disease occurring, or being caught, on their farms, and the owners of the mares are not anxious to take mares which have become infected back to their home farms to infect the other mares there. So that the management of open or 'visiting' studs in areas where the disease occurs commonly needs to include prophylactic husbandry tactics in their management strategies (1). The same need does not arise in private studs where there is no traffic in and out. The recommendations include:

- When an abortion occurs on the stud no mares should be allowed to enter or leave it until the possibility of equine herpesvirus 1 infection is excluded. Except that maiden and barren mares, that is mares which have foaled normally at home but which are not in foal, and come from home studs where no signs of the disease are occurring, are admitted without question, because they are considered to be not infected
- If equine herpesvirus 1 infection is identified on the stud, pregnant mares are assumed to be not infected and are allowed to go home, provided they have been rigidly isolated from aborting mares for 1 month after the last abortion. As a final precaution they should be kept isolated from in-foal mares at the home stud for 2 months
- Mares from the infected stud can go out to other studs provided the limitations on movement as set down in the second paragraph above are observed (22). Mares returning from an infected visiting stud to their home stud must be kept in isolation until they have foaled.

The main problem that arises in this program is in deciding what to do with mares which come into contact with the respiratory disease but not the abortion disease. This may occur very early in pregnancy, and to isolate them would mean a very long period indeed. If the abortion disease does not occur in the area the inclination will be to chance the development of abortion. The decision usually depends on the owner's risk aversion and the availability of facilities to maintain long-term isolation.

REVIEW LITERATURE

Bagust, T. J. (1971) The equine herpesviruses. *Vet. Bull.*, *41*, 79.

Campbell, T. M. & Studdert, M. J. (1983) Equine herpesvirus type 1 (EHV 1). *Vet. Bull.*, *53*, 135.

Coggins, L. (1979) Viral respiratory disease. *Vet. Clin. N. Am. large Anim. Pract.* *1*, 59.

Jeffcott, L. B. (1976) The practical aspects of equine virus abortion in the U.K. *Vet. Rec.*, *98*, 153.

Martin, W. B. (1976) The herpesviruses. *Vet. Rec.*, *99*, 352.

Rossdale, P. D. & Ricketts, S. W. (1976) Equine abortion. *Vet. Ann.*, *16*, 133.

REFERENCES

(1) Jeffcott, L. B. (1976) *Vet. Rec.*, *98*,153.
(2) Jain, N. C. & Ram, G. C. (1980) *Haryana vet.*, *19*, 51.
(3) Horner, G. W. (1981) *NZ vet. J.*, *29*, 7.
(4) Neely, D. P. & Hawkins, D. L. (1978) *J. equ. med. Surg.*, *2*, 532.
(5) Fu, Z. F. et al. (1986) *NZ vet. J.*, *34*, 14.
(6) Eaglesome, M. D. et al. (1979) *J. Reprod. Fertil.*, Suppl. *27*, 607.
(7) Fu, Z. F. et al. (1986) *NZ vet. J.*, *34*, 152.
(8) Fitzpatrick, D. R. & Studdert, M. J. (1984) *Am. J. vet. Res.*, *45*, 1947.
(9) Mumford, J. A. & Rossdale, P. D. (1980) *Equ. vet. J.*, *12*, 3.
(10) Mumford, J. A. & Bates, J. (1984) *Vet. Rec.*, *114*, 375.
(11) Edington, N. et al. (1986) *Arch. Virol.*, *90*, 111.
(12) Jackson, T. A. et al. (1977) *Am. J. vet. Res.*, *38*, 709.
(13) Purdy, C. W. et al. (1978) *Am. J. vet. Res.*, *39*, 745.
(14) Crandell, R. A. et al. (1980) *Am. J. vet. Res.*, *41*, 994.
(15) Bryans, J. T. (1980) *Am. J. vet. Res.*, *41*, 1743.
(16) Bitsch, V. & Dam, A. (1971) *Acta vet. Scand.*, *12*, 134.
(17) Dalsgaard, H. (1970) *Medlemsbl. danske Dyrlaegeforen*, *53*, 71.
(18) Little, P. B. & Thorsen, J. (1976) *Vet. Pathol.*, *13*, 161.
(19) Jackson, T. A. & Kendrick, J. W. (1971) *J. Am. vet. med. Assoc.*, *158*, 1351.
(20) Greenwood, R. E. S. (1979) *Vet. Rec.*, *104*, 534.
(21) Thomas, G. R. et al. (1976) *Equ. vet. J.*, *8*, 58.
(22) Bryans, J. T. et al. (1977) *J. equ. med. Surg.*, *1*, 20.
(23) Carroll, C. L. & Westbury, H. A. (1985) *Aust. vet. J.*, *62*, 345.
(24) Coignoul, F. L. et al. (1984) *Am. J. vet. Res.*, *45*, 1972.
(25) Burrows, R. et al. (1984) *Vet. Rec.*, *114*, 375.
(26) Kemen, M. J. (1975) *J. Am. vet. med. Assoc.*, *166*, 85.
(27) Greenwood, R. E. S. & Simson, A. R. B. (1980) *Equ. vet. J.*, *12*, 113.
(28) Lui, K. M. & Castleman, W. (1977) *J. equ. Med. Surg.*, *1*, 397 & 400.
(29) Studdert, M. J. (1983) *Vet. Rec.*, *112*, 334.
(30) Studdert, M. J. et al. (1984) *Aust. vet. J.*, *61*, 345.
(31) Edington, N. et al. (1985) *Equ. vet. J.*, *17*, 369.
(32) Kendrick, J. W. & Stevenson, W. (1979) *J. Reprod. Fertil.*, Suppl. *27*, p. 615.
(33) Crandell, R. A. et al. (1979) *Can. J. comp. Med.*, *43*, 94.
(34) Platt, H. et al. (1980) *Equ. vet. J.*, *12*, 118.
(35) Gerber, J. D. et al. (1977) *Can. J. comp. Med.*, *41*, 471.
(36) Hutton, J. B. & Durham, P. J. K. (1977) *NZ vet. J.*, *25*, 42.
(37) Crowhurst, F. A. et al. (1981) *Vet. Rec.*, *109*, 527

(38) Hartley, W. J. & Dixon, R. J. (1979) *Equ. vet. J.*, *11*, 215.
(39) Coignoul, F. L. et al. (1984) *Vet. Microbiol.*, *9*, 533.

Equine viral arteritis (EVA)

This disease of horses is caused by a specific virus and is manifested clinically by an acute, upper respiratory tract infection and by abortion in mares. It is characterized by specific lesions in the small arteries.

Etiology

An arterivirus (family Togaviridae) is the cause of the disease. It cannot be grown on egg embryos or be propagated in experimental animals, nor does it cause hemagglutination. It can be attenuated by serial passage through tissue culture and the resulting virus is capable of causing strong immunity in vaccinated horses. The virus resists freezing but not heat. It has no relationship to human or porcine influenza viruses and only one antigenic type of the virus is known to occur.

Epidemiology

Although information about equine viral arteritis comes largely from the United States, it has been identified in Europe (1). The occurrence in the United States is principally in standardbreds (56% of mares) with a low level in thoroughbreds. The disease appears to be widespread. In the United Kingdom the level is only 2%, in Switzerland 11%, and no cases have been identified in Japan or Australia. On serological evidence higher infection rates have been described—France 15%, other European countries 28%, African countries 37% (with the highest rates in older age groups)—up to 80% at 20 years of age (3). In natural outbreaks it occurs most commonly in mares in breeding studs and, although the illness is a severe one, the mortality rate is low, the chief cause of loss being the high rate of abortions (3). In 1977 outbreaks occurred in standardbred horses at racetracks in the United States (5). This was the first recorded occurrence in horses at the track. A subsequent outbreak in 1984 caused serious losses on Kentucky thoroughbred farms (2). The virus appeared to be unusually pathogenic.

Although the mortality rate is very low in natural outbreaks, it may be as high as 33% in the experimental disease. The abortion rate is commonly 50% in natural and experimental cases. Horses of all age groups are susceptible. The disease spreads rapidly in a group of susceptible horses, and although the course is short, an outbreak in a group of horses may persist for a number of weeks.

The proportion of the cases diagnosed clinically as influenza in horses which are caused by the equine viral arteritis virus is unknown, although equine viral rhinopneumonitis appears to be the more common cause of both upper respiratory tract infection and of abortion in mares.

Details of transmission in field outbreaks are not available but it is presumed that infection in racing stables occurs by ingestion of contaminated material or by inhalation of droplets derived from the nasal exudate of infected horses which remain infective for 8–10 days.

The virus is also shed in urine and in semen. Infected stallions are commonly short-term, convalescent carriers, but a number of them are also long-term carriers and continue to shed virus for up to 2 years (11). This may be the major method of spread on stud farms. The tissues and fluids of infected aborted fetuses contain large quantities of virus. Foals of immune mares are resistant to infection, and viral neutralization antibodies are present in mare's milk and foal's serum after sucking, with persistence of the antibodies to the age of 2–6 months in the foals (4).

Pathogenesis

The necropsy findings suggest that this is a viral septicemia causing severe vascular damage, especially in the small arteries and in the intestinal tract, the visceral lymph modes, and the adrenals. A hemorrhagic enteritis results and causes diarrhea and abdominal pain. Pulmonary edema and pleural effusion occur and are manifested by severe dyspnea. Petechiation of the mucosae and the conjunctiva, and edema of the limbs also occur. Death, when it occurs, is due to a combination of dehydration and anoxia. Viral arteritis has been produced experimentally and the development of vascular lesions accurately defined (6). The abortion is caused by a severe necrotizing myometritis; the fetus is unaffected but contains virus. The disease as described below is as it occurred in the early 1950s. Since then many strains of low virulence have been described and the disease has assumed a milder form with many infections being subclinical.

Clinical findings

An incubation period of 1–6 days is followed by the appearance of fever (39–41°C, 102–106°F), a serous nasal discharge which may become purulent and be accompanied in some horses by congestion and petechiation of the nasal mucosa, conjunctivitis, excessive lacrimation developing to purulent discharge, keratitis, palpebral edema and blepharospasm. Opacity of the aqueous humor and petechiation of the conjunctiva may also occur. Cough and dyspnea develop and the latter is extreme in severely affected animals in which pulmonary edema and congestion occur. The appetite is reduced or absent and in severe cases abdominal pain and diarrhea occur due to enteritis. In these animals there may be jaundice. Edema of the limbs is common and more marked in stabled horses than those at pasture. In stallions, edema of the belly wall may extend to involve the prepuce and scrotum (7). Depression is usual and varies in degree with the severity of the syndrome. The disease is acute and severe and deaths may occur without secondary bacterial invasion. In these cases dehydration, muscle weakness and prostration develop quickly. The course in non-fatal cases is usually within the range of 3–8 days. Secondary bacterial invasion is usually manifested by a catarrhal rhinitis and infection of the respiratory tract. In stallions there is often edema of the prepuce and scrotum. Abortion occurs within a few days of the onset of clinical illness, as distinct from the much later abortions which occur in equine viral rhinopneumonitis, and is recorded between the 160th and 300th day of pregnancy and 12–30 days after exposure. The abortion is not foreshadowed by premonitory signs, and the placenta is not retained.

The overt clinical disease is rare nowadays and many infections result in a subclinical state with sporadic abortions (3). However, outbreaks of the classical disease can still occur (4).

Clinical pathology

Complement fixation and serum neutralization tests are available for serological diagnosis and tissue culture techniques are available for isolation of the virus.

There is a pronounced leukopenia due to depression of the lymphocytes and to a less extent of the neutrophils, occurring usually 1–3 days after the onset of fever. The virus is present in the blood during the febrile period and the disease can be transmitted to susceptible horses.

Necropsy findings

Gross lesions include edema of the eyelids, congestion and petechiation of the upper respiratory tract, edema of the lungs and mediastinum, pleural and peritoneal effusion, petechiae on the serous surfaces, edema of viscera, catarrhal and hemorrhagic inflammation of the intestinal mucosa, hemorrhage and infarction in the spleen and degeneration in the liver and kidneys. There are characteristic histological changes in the small arteries.

The virus can be isolated from the lung and spleen of aborted fetuses and from the spleen of dead animals, but there are no inclusion bodies or specific lesions in the fetus.

Diagnosis

The disease is much more severe than equine viral rhinopneumonitis and equine influenza, but in individual animals differentiation may be difficult except by laboratory examination using complement fixation or serum protection tests. The histological lesion of arteritis is characteristic of this disease and serves to differentiate it from equine infectious anemia, which is also accompanied by petechiation of the mucosae and jaundice in acute cases. Another viral respiratory disease which needs to be differentiated from equine viral arteritis is the Getah virus infection identified in Japan (8, 10). The disease does not affect the respiratory system, but does cause fever, exanthema of mucosae and edema of limbs. It has a high infectivity, can replicate in the mosquito *Aedes vexans* (8) and possibly in pigs (13) but causes little permanent damage. Leptospirosis may present a rather similar clinical picture also. In purpura hemorrhagica the subcutaneous effusions contain blood and serum, are not confined to the limbs, and histologically there are septic thrombi in local veins. Clinical signs and lesions are similar to African horse sickness but the diseases have not occurred in the same area and can be distinguished serologically.

It is a significant cause of abortion in mares and may present a diagnostic dilemma if the respiratory signs are minimal (14). The known bacterial causes of equine abortion, *Salm. abortivoequina* and *Str. genitalium* should be eliminated by cultural examination, and equine viral rhinopneumonitis should be eliminated as far as is possible by histological examination of the fetus and isolation of the virus.

Treatment and control

The same general principles of treatment and control as apply to EVR can be applied in this disease. An effective, live, attenuated vaccine is regarded as being without risk although there is a mild fever and a leukopenia and other evidence that the vaccine virus replicates in the vaccinates (9). Vaccination of foals from non-immune mares results in good protection, but foals from immune mares have been found to be non-immune at 6 months of age (4). Vaccination of stallions with attenuated virus vaccines is recommended. The virus does not appear to pass via the semen to mares bred by the stallions and there are no vaccination reactions in the stallions (12).

REFERENCES

(1) Moraillon, R. & Moraillon, A. (1974) *Rec. Méd. vét.*, *150*, 1015.
(2) Scoggins, R. D. (1986) *Equ. Pract.*, *8* (*5*), 30.
(3) Moraillon, A. & Moraillon, R.(1978) *Ann. rech. vét.*, *9*, 43.
(4) McCollum, W. H. (1976) *Vet. Microbiol.*, *1*, 45.
(5) McCollum, W. H. & Swerczek, T. W. (1978) *J. Equ. med. Surg.*, *2*, 293.
(6) Coignoul, F. L. & Cheville, N. F. (1984) *Vet. Pathol.*, *21*, 333.
(7) Jaksch, W. et al. (1973) *Dtsch Tierärztl. Wochenschr.*, *80*, 317.
(8) Kumanomido, T. et al. (1982) *Bull. equ. Res. Inst. Japan.*, *19*, 93.
(9) Harry, T. O. & McCollum, W. H. (1981) *Am. J. vet. Res.*, *42*, 1501.
(10) Wada, R. et al. (1982) *Jap. J. vet. Sci.*, *44*, 411.
(11) Timoney, P. J. et al. (1986) *Res. vet. Sci.*, *41*, 279.
(12) McKinnon, A. O. et al. (1986) *J. equ. vet. Sci.*, *6*, 66.
(13) Kumanomido, T. et al. (1982) *Bull. equ. Res. Inst. Japan.*, *19*, 89.
(14) Cole, J. R. et al. (1986) *J. Am. vet. med. Assoc.*, *189*, 769.

Equine influenza (infectious equine bronchitis, laryngotracheobronchitis, Newmarket cough, infectious equine cough)

This is an infectious respiratory disease caused by a virus and characterized by mild fever and a severe, persistent cough. The name equine influenza is now restricted to those respiratory infections of horses caused by viruses belonging to the influenza family. Whether it will include all the clinically similar diseases which are recorded, and listed as alternate names in this section, is undecided.

Etiology

The two identified causative myxovirus type A influenza viruses IA/E1 and IA/E2 are serologically distinct. There are also differences between the two diseases caused by these viruses, that caused by IA/E2 being rather more severe especially with respect to pulmonary involvement in the form of a non-bacterial pneumonitis especially in foals (13). All age groups of horses including newborn foals are susceptible. The virus is capable of growing on embryonated eggs and has been adapted to grow on tissue culture (12). There is some evidence that human strains of influenza virus can infect horses, but the exact relationship is not defined (18).

Epidemiology

The disease is reported from most countries and, although it is not serious in itself, it causes much inconvenience in racing stables because it occurs in explosive outbreaks and affected horses have to break training. One of the more annoying aspects of the disease is its poor response to most forms of treatment.

Although clinically similar diseases have occurred as explosive outbreaks in most countries for many years, equine influenza was not recognized as a specific disease entity until the mid-1950s. In 1963 major epidemics of respiratory disease, affecting 50–90% of horses in some areas, occurred in the United Kingdom and the United States. The causative viruses were identified as myxovirus influenza A/equi 1 (IA/E1) in the United Kingdom and this virus and influenza A/equi 2 (IA/E2) in the United States. At the time investigations failed to reveal the presence of IA/E2 in the United Kingdom, but in 1965 a new outbreak due to this virus did occur. In 1979 another outbreak occurred in the United Kingdom. It appeared to begin at an equestrian event attended by horses from several European countries. The outbreak was due to infection with IA/E2 virus, the predominant virus in the outbreak in France the year before (2).

The disease occurred for the first time in Japan in 1971 when explosive outbreaks occurred; in one such outbreak 168 of a group of 171 horses were affected within 6 days. The usual occurrence rate of serologically positive horses in Japan since then has been from 70 to 75% (8) and in Germany from 50 to 65% (6).

A major outbreak due to an unidentified virus occurred in Germany in 1961 and positive serological evidence of infection with influenza virus was obtained in France and Poland in 1963. The magnitude of these outbreaks might have suggested that the equine population in which they occurred was being exposed to a new virus for the first time. However, outbreaks of a clinically similar disease have occurred at intervals in the preceding years and antibodies to the viruses have been detected in the sera of horses collected 15 years earlier (16). In eastern Canada viral influenza is the commonest cause of epidemics, the IA/E1 virus being the commonest infection (7). In western Canada equine influenza and equine viral rhinopneumonitis appear to be of approximately equal importance (3). Both influenza viruses are known to have infected horses in the United States for many years, and major outbreaks which cause suspension of racing programs still occur (23).

Nowadays most cases of the disease occur in 2-year old or younger horses, probably because horses of 3 years of age or older are immune (17). The greatest risk appears to be between the ages of 2 and 6 months (1). It is probable that the outbreaks occur as a result of a natural accumulation of young animals which have not been previously exposed, the comingling of these susceptible animals with older infected ones at race and show meetings, and to the significant level of antigenic 'drift' which occurs in this virus, especially IA/E2. This capacity to change slightly and continuously in antigenic composition leads to the frequent appearance of new strains which are likely to breach existing natural and induced immunological barriers.

Most outbreaks occur during the summer months, possibly due to greater movement at this time. There is no difference in prevalence between the sexes, but quarter horses appear to be significantly more susceptible to the clinical disease than do thoroughbreds. There appears to be a high incidence of infection without clinical signs (19). In horses the mortality rate, in the absence of complications, is nil. Rare deaths result from a viral pneumonitis in foals, and occasional deaths due to secondary pneumonia. After infection immunity to the homologous subtype of the virus is present, and persists for 1 year, possibly up to 2 years (20).

By analogy with the human disease the transmission of equine influenza is thought to occur by droplet inhalation over short distances, but spread via infected fomites may also occur. In aerosol form, the equine influenza virus survives longer (24–36 hours) than human or porcine strains (15 hours) (21). The duration of infectivity of affected horses is 3–8 days and with the short incubation period of 2–3 days and frequent coughing combine to produce a very rapid new infection rate and a characteristic explosive outbreak.

Pathogenesis

The disease is principally one of inflammation of the upper respiratory tract. The virus is inhaled, multiplies in the epithelial cells of the respiratory mucosa, especially in the upper part of the tract, and causes erythema, edema and focal erosions. Bacterial secondary invasion may occur at these sites. Viremia, if it occurs, is mild and brief. It seems to be the likely explanation of the myocarditis which has been nominated as a sequel to influenza. Infection with IA/E2 causes a more severe clinical syndrome than the other virus and a non-bacterial pneumonitis may occur, especially in foals. Repeated infections or concurrent stress or illness may also lead to lung damage (22).

Clinical findings

Clinically the disease starts with a fever (38·5–41°C, 101–106°F) after an incubation period of 2–3 days. The dominating sign is cough, which is dry and hacking in the beginning and moist later, and which commences soon after the temperature rise and lasts for 1–3 weeks. It is easily stimulated by manual compression of the upper trachea. Nasal discharge is not a prominent sign and, if it occurs, is watery only. There is no marked swelling of the submaxillary lymph nodes but they may be painful on palpation in the early stages of the disease. Lassitude, immobility and anorexia are inconstant accompaniments, and stiffness and difficulty or clumsiness in rising or lying also occur. Horses that are protected against environmental stress pursue an uncomplicated course, but horses that are worked or transported or exposed to adverse climatic conditions may experience a worsening of the cough, and severe bronchitis, pneumonia and edema of the legs may develop. Guttural pouch empyema and chronic pharyngitis are also thought to be common sequels.

Young foals, especially those which are foaled while the mare is clinically affected, may develop a severe bronchopneumonia with streptococci and *Escherichia coli* present in the lungs at necropsy. The foal is normal until the 4th–5th day and then develops a high fever (45·5°C, 105°F), severe dyspnea with signs of bronchopneumonia on auscultation, and a respiratory rate of 80–90 per minute. Death is usual after a course of about 4 days.

The epidemiology is characteristic. In a susceptible population spread is very rapid with most of the horses showing clinical signs within a few days.

Clinical pathology

Isolation of the virus is desirable for a definitive diagnosis, but a rise in antibody titer in paired sera collected 3 weeks apart is acceptable as evidence of infection provided there is a fourfold increase in titer. The serological tests available include the complement fixation test, the hemagglutination inhibition test, and the serum neutralization test (14). A test using a fluorescent antibody technique is available and isolation of the virus in chick embryo is a good diagnostic aid (25). Material for viral culture should be collected as early as possible during the illness and inoculated into the transport medium quickly.

Necropsy findings

The characteristic lesion is a bronchiolitis which is accompanied by a profuse serous discharge which later becomes mucoid and tends to accumulate in bronchioles.

Diagnosis

Equine influenza resembles equine viral rhinopneumonitis and equine viral arteritis sufficiently to require laboratory assistance in diagnosis. However, some situations demand a presumptive diagnosis. The important features of this differentiation are included in Table 46, the important similar diseases being equine viral rhinopneumonitism, influenza, rhinovirus and adenovirus infections. Strangles and equine viral arteritis are usually much more serious diseases. Strangles is marked by abscessation and profuse purulent nasal discharge. Equine viral arteritis is characterized by severe conjunctivitis, dyspnea, edema and abortion. The other three diseases are very similar. The incubation period is the same, the fever is moderate, there is a moderate cough, the appetite is poor and the course of the illness is about a week in each disease. In those countries where the abortigenic strain of equine viral rhinopneumonitis does not occur not even this aid to diagnosis is available, so that a laboratory diagnosis is the only option if an etiologically specific diagnosis is required. For laboratory satisfaction samples should include deep nasal or pharyngeal swabs for culture, early and late paired sera, and a hematological sample so that leukopenia can be identified. Smears of nasal mucosa are desirable for detection of the inclusion bodies of adenovirus infection and herpesvirus infection. Laboratory examination is also necessary to ensure that any vaccines used in control programs contain the local virus.

Treatment and control

Little information is available on methods of treatment. Hyperimmune serum appears to have some therapeutic efficiency and may also be of value in prophylaxis, especially in foals which are unlikely to have received passive immunity via their dam's colostrum. Heavy doses of broad-spectrum antibiotics seem logical as prophylaxis against secondary bacterial infections in foals.

Hygienic precautions

These can be of value in limiting the spread of the disease. Vehicles used for the transport of horses are thought to play a large part in transmission and should be thoroughly disinfected between shipments. The massive movement of horses from place to place for many purposes encourages the rapid spread of the disease, and the isolation of introduced animals is an essential precaution, especially when an outbreak is in progress. The degree of isolation required cannot be specified because of lack of basic information, but it is suggested that droplet infection can occur over a distance of 32 m and that maximum security with regard to clothing, utensils and personnel must be practiced.

Vaccination

Vaccination against equine influenza is now in general use, but is not without its problems. All the vaccines are killed ones and in aqueous suspension. The antibody and protection responses are satisfactory, but oil adjuvants are being tested to improve antigenicity without increasing the already worrisome reactions that occur. The standard vaccine contains elements of both IA/E1 and IA/E2 viruses and are for parenteral injection. The objective of the program is to immunize the young horses before they go to training establishments. Delaying vaccination until the foals are 6 months of age has the advantage that the immunity resulting from the vaccination is much better; this may leave foals unprotected because passively acquired immunity is shortlived and most foals of recently vaccinated dams are seronegative by 4 weeks of age (16). Vaccinations are carried out at 6–12 weeks (preferably 12) intervals for at least two injections. Subsequently, booster injections are given at least once a year. However, in bad outbreaks this is insufficient and for complete protection the booster injections should be administered at intervals of 6, or even 4, months. Vaccination during the racing season is disliked by trainers because of the local and sometimes systemic reactions which occur. These include a local reaction of a transitory swelling at the injection site and a systemic reaction, comprising a cough 48 hours after vaccination (9). Vaccination appears to have no adverse affect on performance (10).

On breeding farms all horses should be vaccinated similarly in the first instance; in subsequent years only the foals are vaccinated just before weaning. The vaccine should contain the virus or viruses which occur in the area as crossimmunity between the serotypes does not occur.

An epidemic of the disease in Sweden in 1979, with a disease incidence of 37% in regularly vaccinated horses, 77% in irregularly vaccinated ones, and 98% in unvaccinated groups was thought to be due largely to antigenic drift (15). The vaccination program in France, which had been giving very good results for years, broke down in 1978–79, with large epidemics occurring particularly in horses vaccinated recently. An inadequate antigenicity of the vaccine is thought to have been the cause. There had been no drift in antigenicity (11). The outbreak, which was due to IA/E2, subsequently spread to the United Kingdom where similar problems were encountered with breaks in vaccination. The pandemic was thought to have been due principally to an inadequate vaccination program and a tighter schedule was proposed:

- Mandatory vaccination for all horses entering racing premises
- Horses not to race in the 10 day period following vaccination
- Horses coming from international locations must be vaccinated before departure
- All horse events, including shows, sales, gymkhanas should apply the same restrictions.

The recommended vaccination program is:

- Vaccinate foals at 6 months of age
- Two vaccinations initially at 21 days apart and not more than 92 days
- A booster vaccination 5–7 months later
- Annual boosters subsequently. In bad years or when risk is high these should be at 6-month or even 4-month intervals
- When vaccination schedules break down and a horse goes longer than 12 months without a booster, recommence with a two-vaccination schedule.

North American experience is that severe epidemics occur annually during the summer racing season, but that these can be prevented by using a proper vaccination program. Only horses that have not been vaccinated during the preceding 6 months develop a clinical illness (5). Recommended vaccines contain both viruses. Yearlings are vaccinated in October, repeated in November and a booster in April 2–4 weeks before the expected recurrence of the disease at the race track (4). Older horses are vaccinated twice annually in mid-April and mid-October.

REVIEW LITERATURE

Coggins, L. (1979) Viral respiratory diseases. *Vet. Clin. N. Am., large Anim. Pract.*, *1*, 59.

REFERENCES

(1) Nyaga, P. N. et al. (1980) *Comp. Immun. Microbiol. inf. Dis.*, *3*, 67.
(2) Fontaine, M. et. al. (1980) *Comp. Immun. Microbiol. inf. Dis.*, *3*, 75.
(3) Fretz, P. B. et al. (1979) *Can. vet. J.*, *20*, 58.
(4) Sherman, J. et al. (1977) *Can. vet. J.*, *18*, 154.
(5) Higgins, W. P. et al. (1986) *J. equ. Vet. Sci.*, *6*, 15.
(6) Thein, P. & Hartl, G. (1977) *Prakt. Tierärztl.*, *58*, 24.
(7) Sherman, J. et al. (1977) *J. clin. Microbiol.*, *5*, 285.
(8) Goto, H. et al. (1978) *Jap. J. vet. Sci.*, *40*, 367.
(9) Eagles, B. W. & Higgins, A. J. (1985) *Vet. Rec.*, *116*, 478.
(10) Hugoson, G. et al. (1984) *Prev. vet. Med.*, *3*, 93.
(11) Fontaine, M. & Moraillon, A. (1980) *Rec. Med. Vet.*, *156*, 139.
(12) Archibald, J. M. et al. (1978) *Rev. Milit. Vet.*, *25*, 302.
(13) Smith, B. P. (1979) *J. Am. vet. med. Assoc.*, *174*, 289.
(14) Thomson, G. R. et al. (1977) *Vet. Rec.*, *100*, 405.
(15) Klingeborn, B. et al. (1980) *Vet. Rec.*, *106*, 363.
(16) Liu, I. K. M. et al. (1985) *Am. J. vet. Res.*, *46*, 2078.
(17) Bryans J. T. et al. (1967) *Am. J. vet. Res.*, *28*, 9.
(18) Coggins, L. & Kemen, M. J. (1975) *J. Am. vet. med. Assoc.*, *166*, 80.
(19) Lief, F. S. & Cohen, D. (1965) *Am. J. Epidemiol.*, *82*, 225.
(20) Beveridge, W. I. B. & Rose, M. A. (1967) *Br. vet. J.*, *123*, 8.
(21) Mitchell, C. A. B. & Guerin, L. F. (1972) *Can. J. comp. Med.*, *36*, 9.
(22) Kroneman, J. & Sasse, H. H. L. (1972) *Tijdschr. Diergeneeskd.*, *97*, 1229.
(23) Kemen, M. J. et al. (1985) *Cornell Vet.*, *75*, 277.
(24) Fontaine, M. P. et al. (1970) *Proc. 2nd int. Conf. equ. infect. Dis., Paris, 1969*, 99.
(25) Masurel, N. et al. (1968) *Tijdschr. Diergeneeskd.*, *93*, 1019.
(26) Estola, T. & Neuvonen, E. (1976) *Nord. Vet Med.*, *28*, 353.
(27) Pressler, K. (1970) *Zentrabl. VetMed.*, *17B*, 1003.

Swine influenza

Swine influenza is a specific, highly contagious disease of pigs characterized clinically by fever and signs of repiratory involvement. The disease is not usually fatal.

Etiology

Swine influenza is caused by the type A influenza virus of the orthomyxovirus group. Molecular microbiology has now revealed the antigenic diversity of the virus (1). Several different H and N antigens have been identified and grouped on the basis of serological tests which refines the diagnosis and reveals more about the epidemiological relationships. The viral infection is commonly complicated by bacterial infection due to *Hemophilus parasuis*, *Hemophilus pleuropneumoniae* and possibly other opportunists of the upper respiratory tract of the pig.

Epidemiology

Swine influenza first appeared in the United States immediately following the 1918 pandemic of human influenza, and it was generally believed that it was caused by adaptation of the human influenza virus to swine. The disease still occurs in the United States, but apparently with decreasing frequency. It has also been reported from the United Kingdom, and a number of European countries as *ferkelgrippe*, although in the latter instance the virus has not been identified as identical with that causing swine influenza in the United States. The epidemiological characteristics of swine influenza in Hawaii are described (15). Epidemics of swine influenza have been reported recently from Japan (2), Quebec (3), Ontario (4), Belgium (13) and France (19). Serological surveys indicate that the infection is widespread in the swine populations in some countries (4, 6).

The disease occurs in the form of explosive outbreaks with a high morbidity rate but with a low mortality rate of less than 4%. Loss of condition is marked and ordinarily this is the principal cause of financial loss, although on occasions death losses may be extensive if the pigs are kept under bad husbandry conditions or if secondary bacterial infections develop. Abortions and deaths of newborn pigs have also been reported as causes of loss in this disease.

Although pigs of all ages may be affected, the disease is often confined to young pigs. Outbreaks occur mainly during the cold months of the year, commencing in the late autumn or early winter and terminating with a few outbreaks in early spring. Several days of inclement weather often precede an outbreak.

When an outbreak occurs, most of the pigs in the herd are affected within a few days, which suggests that all animals are previously infected and the interference of some external factor, probably inclement weather, precipitates the outbreak. The very rapid spread of infection from pig to pig is via the inhalation of infected droplets. The disease may appear almost simultaneously in several herds within an area following the first cold period in late autumn. The virus can persist in infected swine which can act as convalescent carriers and be the reservoir of the virus between epidemics (7, 8). However, the experimental inoculation of a swine influenza virus into specific pathogen-free (SPF) pigs resulted in a mild disease and the period of viral shedding was less than 4 weeks (20).

Contrary to widespread belief there is no evidence that the virus carries reproductive failure in swine. The experimental inoculation of seronegative pregnant gilts did not reveal any evidence of transplacental transmission of the virus to the fetus (16).

The influenza viruses may be transmissible between man and pigs (18). Swine may become infected with related type A human influenza strains during epidemics of human influenza, but show no clinical signs of infection (1). The human strains have been isolated from pigs in Hong Kong and pigs may serve as a reservoir for pandemics in man as well as a source of genetic information for recombination between human and porcine strains. In Japan, a new influenza virus is thought to be due to recombination of human and porcine strains. In Czechoslovakia, influenza A viruses are brought into pig herds by carrier people (14). There is one report which claims that outbreaks of influenza in turkeys followed outbreaks of swine influenza in pigs from nearby swine herds (19). Swine and other influenza viruses have also been isolated from cattle and experimental inoculation of calves has been successful. The swine influenza virus may cause natural infection in cattle and the virus can be transferred to uninoculated calves (21).

Pathogenesis

Swine influenza is primarily a disease of the upper respiratory tract, the trachea and bronchi being particularly involved, but secondary lesions may develop in the lung because of the drainage of copious exudate from the bronchi. These lesions disappear rapidly, leaving little or no residual damage. This is in contradistinction to the lesions of enzootic pneumonia of pigs which persist for very long periods. Secondary pneumonia, usually due to infection with *Pasteurella multocida*, occurs in some cases and is the cause of most fatalities. Experimental intrafetal infection can result in congenital pulmonary hypoplasia (17).

Clinical findings

After an incubation period of 2–7 days the disease appears suddenly with a high proportion of the herd showing fever (up to 41·5°C, 107°F), anorexia and severe prostration. The animal is disinclined to move or rise because of muscle stiffness and pain. Labored jerky breathing ('thumps') is accompanied by sneezing and a deep, painful cough which often occurs in paroxysms. There is congestion of the conjunctivae with a watery ocular and nasal discharge. In general the severity of the illness appears greater than in fact it is and after a course of 4–6 days signs disappear rapidly depending, in part, on the level of colostral antibody (9). However, there is much loss of weight which is slowly regained. Clonic convulsions are common in the terminal stages in fatal cases.

Clinical pathology

A moderate leukopenia develops in the early stages and recovered animals can be identified by a virus neutralization and a hemagglutination inhibition test. A lymphopenia and acute inflammatory cellular response with neutrophilia and a left shift, hyperfibrinogenemia and a decreased plasma protein: fibrinogen ratio have been reported in some outbreaks (4).

Necropsy findings

The outstanding lesions are in the upper respiratory tract. Swelling and marked edema of cervical and mediastinal lymph nodes are evident. There is congestion of the mucosae of the pharynx, larynx, trachea and bronchi, and much tenacious, colorless, frothy exudate is present in the air passages. Copious exudate in the bronchi is accompanied by collapse of the ventral parts of the lungs. This atelectasis is extensive and often irregularly distributed, although the apical and cardiac lobes are most affected, and the right lung more so than the left. The lesions are clearly demarcated, dark red to purple in color and leathery in consistency. Surrounding the atelectatic areas the lung is often emphysematous and may show many petechial hemorrhages. The gross pulmonary lesions are very similar to those of enzootic pneumonia of pigs, but there is a great deal of difference in the histological lesions in the two diseases. Histologically in swine influenza there is a necrotizing bronchitis and bronchiolitis with a neutrophilic cellular exudate (4). *Pasteurella multocida* is frequently isolated from affected lungs. There is often moderate to severe engorgement of the spleen and severe hyperemia of the gastric mucosa, especially along the greater curvature. Patchy congestion and mild catarrhal exudation occurs in the large intestine, but there are no erosions of the mucosa. The virus can be isolated by intra-allantoic inoculation of embryonated hen's eggs and demonstration of hemagglutination in the allantoic fluids.

Diagnosis

The explosive appearance of an upper respiratory syndrome, including conjunctivitis, sneezing and coughing with a low mortality rate, serves to differentiate swine influenza from the other common respiratory diseases of swine. Of these enzootic pneumonia of pigs is most commonly confused with swine influenza, but it is more insidious in its onset and chronic in its course. Hog cholera is manifested by less respiratory involvement and a high mortality rate. Outbreaks of inclusion body rhinitis in piglets may resemble swine influenza quite closely, but atrophic rhinitis has a much longer course and is accompanied by characteristic distortion of the facial bones.

Treatment

No specific treatment is available. Treatment with penicillin, sulfadimidine, or preferably a wide-spectrum antibiotic, may be of value in controlling possible secondary invaders. The provision of comfortable, well-bedded quarters, free from dust, is of major importance. Clean drinking water should be available, but feed should be limited during the first few days of convalescence. Medication of the feed or water supplies with a broad-spectrum antibiotic for several days is a rational approach to minimizing secondary bacterial pneumonia.

Control

Control is difficult because of the lack of exact information on the mechanism of perpetuation and activation of infection within a herd. Good housing and protection from inclement weather help to prevent the occurrence of severe outbreaks. Once the disease has appeared little can be done to prevent spread to other pigs. Recovered animals are immune to subsequent infection for up to 3 months (9). An inactivated, formolized, avianized vaccine with adjuvant has been produced (10). However, the antigenic diversity of the influenza virus must be considered in the development and use of any vaccine. Vaccines should contain those strains of the virus which are prevalent in the affected area. A method of eradication similar to that used in the control of enzootic pneumonia and atrophic rhinitis has been recorded as giving good results in the eradication of swine influenza (11).

REVIEW LITERATURE

Ada, G. L.& Jones, P. D. (1986) The immune response to influenza virus. *Curr. Top. Microbiol. Immunol.*, *128*, 1–54.

Kaplan, M. M. (1982) The epidemiology of influenza as a zoonosis. *Vet. Rec.*, *110*, 395–399.

Lopez, J. W. & Woods, G. T. (1984) Influenza virus in ruminants:a review. *Res. Commun. Chem. Pathol. Pharmacol.*, *45*, 445–462.

REFERENCES

(1) Kaplan, M. M. (1982) *Vet. Rec.*, *110*, 395.
(2) Sugimura, T. et al. (1981) *Res. vet. Sci.*, *31*, 345.
(3) Morin, M. et al. (1981) *Can. vet. J.*, *22*, 204.
(4) Sanford, S. E. et al. (1983) *Can. vet. J.*, *24*, 167.
(5) Hjärre, A. (1958) *Adv. vet. Sci.*, *4* 235.
(6) Elazhary, M. A. S. Y. et al. (1985) *Can. vet. J.*, *26*, 190.
(7) Wallace, G. W. (1977) *J. infect. Dis.*, *132*, 490.
(8) Nakamura, R. M. et al. (1972) *Bull. World Hlth Org.*, *47*, 481.
(9) Easterday, B. C. (1972) *J. Am. vet. med. Assoc.*, *160*, 645.
(10) Rweyemamu, M. M. (1970) *Vet. Bull.*, *40*, 73.
(11) Kubin, G. (1953) *Wien Tierärztl. Monatschr.*, *40*, 332.
(12) Shortridge, K. F. et al. (1977) *Science*, *196*, 1454.
(13) Haesebrouck, F. et. al. (1985) *Am. J. vet. Res.*, *46*, 1926.
(14) Tumova, B. et al. (1980) *Zentralbl. VetMed.*, *27B*, 517 & 601.
(15) Wallace, G. D. (1979) *Am. J. vet. Res.*, *40*, 1159 & 1165.
(16) Brown, T. T. Jr. et al. (1982) *Am. J. vet. Res.*, *43*, 817.
(17) Brown, T. T. et al. (1980) *Vet. Pathol.*, *17*, 455.
(18) Kendal, A. P. et al. (1977) *Virology*, *82*, 111.
(19) Andral, B. et al. (1985) *Vet. Rec.*, *116*, 617.
(20) Vannier, P. et al. (1985) *Can. vet. J.*, *26*, 138.
(21) Lopez, J. W. & Woods, G. T. (1984) *Res. Commun. Chem. Pathol. Pharmacol.*, *45*, 445.

Inclusion body rhinitis (generalized cytomegalic inclusion body disease of swine)

Inclusion body rhinitis, caused by a beta herpesvirus (family Herpesviridae), is an extremely common but generally minor disease in young pigs. The disease has probable worldwide occurrence (1–4) and clinical and serological (5, 6) observations suggest that it is present in most pig herds. SPF herds established by hysterectomy techniques are not necessarily exempt and congenital transmission of the virus has been demonstrated (7).

The virus is present in the upper respiratory tract of pigs and high excretion occurs predominantly in the 2–4-week period after infection (5). Transmission is via the respiratory route through direct contact and aerosol infection and possibly also via urine. The virus invades epithelial cells, especially those of the nasal mucous glands, to produce destruction of acinar cells and metaplasia of the overlying epithelium and the major clinical manifestation is that of upper respiratory disease. Following infection the virus may become generalized. In older pigs generalization is restricted to epithelial cells of other organ systems, especially those of the renal tubules, and is clinically inapparent. However, in very young pigs the virus also shows a predilection for reticuloendothelial cells and generalization may result in further clinical abnormality (8).

Clinically the disease affects piglets up to approximately 10 weeks of age but the age at manifestation in any herd can depend upon the method of husbandry. A wide age spectrum of involvement may be seen initially when the disease is introduced into the herd for the first time. In most herds the disease affects pigs in the late suckler and early weaner stage. Sneezing is the most prominent sign and frequently occurs in paroxysms and following play fighting. There is a minor serous nasal discharge which rarely may be bloodstained and a brown or black exudation around the eyes. The clinical course varies from approximately 2–4 weeks. All pigs within the group are affected but there is usually no mortality.

Generalized cytomegalic inclusion body disease may occur in pigs exposed to infection and usually occurs as an outbreak involving several litters. The syndrome is characterized by sudden death and anemia. There is often a history of scouring within the group within the first week of life and affected pigs show skin pallor and often superficially appear plump and well-developed due to edema, especially in the neck and forequarter regions. Death, resulting primarily from anemia, occurs during the 2nd and 3rd week of life, and mortality within the group may approach 50%. Petechial hemorrhages have been a feature of the experimentally produced disease in gnotobiotic pigs (8) but do not necessarily occur in field outbreaks. A moderate anemia producing a check to growth but without significant mortality may also be seen in recently weaned pigs experiencing the disease.

More serious effects from generalized infection are seen when piglets are exposed to heavy infection at a very young age. This commonly occurs in large herds with high density continual throughput farrowing to weaning houses. In addition to upper respiratory disease infection at this age may result in enteric disease, sudden death, anemia and wasting with a marked unevenness of growth within the litters.

Inclusion body rhinitis is not a primary cause of atrophic rhinitis. However, it is probably contributory in lowering local resistance to infection and in predisposing to more severe infection with *Bordetella bronchiseptica* and other respiratory pathogens.

The diagnosis of inclusion body rhinitis is commonly

made following the demonstration of typical intranuclear inclusion bodies in histological sections from electively slaughtered piglets. Inclusion bodies may also be demonstrated in exfoliated cells obtained via nasal swabs from live pigs. These are best taken at the height of clinical infection from several pigs. Diagnosis by virus isolation is uncommon as the virus has proved difficult to grow but it will establish in porcine lung macrophage cultures (9). Antibody to infection may be detected by indirect immunofluorescent techniques (5, 6). An enzyme-linked immunosorbent assay (ELISA) is also a sensitive reproducible and practical test (10).

There is no effective treatment and in most herds none is warranted. With severe rhinitis antibiotics may temporarily reduce the severity of secondary bacterial infection. Control of severe disease rests with managemental procedures that avoid severe challenge to very young piglets.

REFERENCES

(1) Done, J. T. (1955) *Vet. Rec.*, *67*, 525.
(2) Cohrs, P. (1959) *Dtsch Tierärztl. Wochenschr.*, *66*, 605.
(3) Corner, A. H. et al. (1964) *J. comp. Pathol.*, *74*, 192.
(4) Cameron-Stephens, I. D (1961) *Aust. vet. J.*, *37*, 87, 91.
(5) Plowright, W. et al. (1976) *J. Hyg., Camb.*, *76*, 125.
(6) Kanitz, C. L. & Woodruff, M. E. (1976) *Proc. 4th int. Cong. Pig. vet. Soc.*, P9.
(7) L'Ecuyer, C. et al. (1972) *Proc. 2nd int. Cong. Pig. vet. Soc.*, 99.
(8) Edington, N. et al. (1976) *J. comp. Pathol.*, *86*, 191.
(9) Watt, R. W. et al. (1973) *Res. vet. Sci.*, *14*, 119.
(10) Assaf, R. et al. (1982) *Can. J. comp. Med.*, *46*, 183.

Enzootic pneumonia of calves (viral pneumonia of calves)

Enzootic pneumonia of calves is an infectious disease primarily of housed calves, characterized clinically by varying degrees of severity of viral pneumonia with or without secondary bacterial bronchopneumonia. The disease also occurs occasionally in beef calves on pasture.

Etiology

Enzootic pneumonia is a disease complex caused by a combination of one or more respiratory viruses commonly complicated by secondary bacterial invasion and predisposed to by environmental factors, usually inadequate ventilation and housing.

The evidence for viruses as primary etiological agents is based on virus isolation, serological evidence of active infection and pathological lesions of viral pneumonia. The parainfluenza-3 (PI-3) paramyxovirus virus has been isolated most commonly from affected calves (1, 2). However, the role of the PI-3 virus is still uncertain because the virus does not consistently result in disease. Experimental inoculation of the PI-3 virus into colostrum-deprived calves results in a pneumonia which resembles the naturally occurring disease (23). A survey of virus infections of the respiratory tract of calves over a 3-year period revealed that only the bovine respiratory syncytial virus (BRSV), the PI-3 virus and the bovine virus diarrhea virus (BVDV) were significantly associated with disease (28). The rhinoviruses, adenoviruses, reoviruses and enteroviruses were also isolated but in much lower frequency and were considered not to be important.

The bovine respiratory syncytial virus (BRSV) is known to cause a fatal viral pneumonia (3, 4) and is now considered to be an important causative agent of viral pneumonia of both dairy and beef cattle of all ages but primarily in young growing calves.

The secondary causative agents which are being recovered from the lungs of calves with pneumonia include *Mycoplasma bovirhinis* most frequently, and *Mycoplasma dispar*, *Mycoplasma bovis* and *Ureaplasma* spp., less frequently and *Pasteurella haemolytica* (27). *Pasteurella haemolytica* is associated more often with fatal cases than subclinical cases (29). The experimental disease produced in gnotobiotic calves by the intratracheal inoculation of unpassed respiratory material, closely resembles the naturally occurring disease (27). *Mycoplasma* spp. are being recovered more frequently from calves with respiratory disease and some species of mycoplasmas can cause pulmonary lesions in calves experimentally (5). *Chlamydia* spp. have also been associated with respiratory disease in calves and usually as part of a mixed infection with viruses and bacteria (7).

Epidemiology

Enzootic pneumonia occurs most commonly in calves from 2 to 5 months of age, but it can occur in calves during the first week of life and in young growing cattle up to 8–12 months of age. The age incidence may coincide with the decline of colostral immunity at about 2 months of age and the development of acquired immunity from 3 to 5 months of age (1). The peak onset of pneumonia in housed calves may be between 2 and 4 weeks of age when the concentration of serum IgG_1, IgG_2 and IgA are lowest (8). When the concentrations of serum IgG_2 begin to increase, the incidence rate of new cases of pneumonia may decline.

The disease occurs most commonly in calves being raised indoors as herd replacements (1). The disease is also common in veal calves raised indoors under intensified conditions (9). The calves are purchased at about 10 days of age, assembled into large groups of 25–50 per group and fed a milk substitute diet for about 16 weeks at which time they are sent to slaughter (9). In these calves the peak incidence of disease occurs about 5 weeks after arrival in the calf house. In a sero-epidemiological survey of veal calves the incidence of respiratory disease appeared at 5–6 weeks of age, lasted for a few weeks and the PI-3 and BRSV viruses were recovered most often (30).

The major factors which influence the occurrence and severity of the disease are the *infectious agents*, the *environment* and the *immune status* of the calf.

Infectious agents

The infectious agents are ubiquitous but probably more numerous in crowded poorly ventilated conditions. The spectrum of infectious agents which are present and acting in a calf population and the severity of clinical disease will vary between farms, between countries and from season to season. It has been assumed that the older calves and mature animals in a herd are the source of infection for the young calves. This assumes major importance in control measures which are commonly designed to rear calves separate from older animals. Parainfluenza-3 virus infection is worldwide (24) and is commonly subclinical in a group of calves and clinical disease may not occur until other pathogens are present or when adverse environmental conditions precipitate clinical disease (25). Following natural infection of young calves the PI-3 virus may persist for several weeks (55). However, the presence of PI-3 infection may predispose to respiratory disease by interfering with normal pulmonary clearance mechanisms and allowing secondary invasion by bacteria or mycoplasmas (26). Similarly, infection with the BRSV may be subclinical, mildly clinical or highly fatal (4). Raising calves in close proximity to older cattle may result in constant exposure to infectious agents to which the mature animals are immune. The disease may be endemic on particular farms in which almost every calf experiences clinical disease. Herd epidemics may occur following the introduction of a different virus such as the BRSV or following a breakdown in the ventilation system. The disease occurs specifically in nursing beef calves from 1 to 4 months of age while on pasture.

While a mixed flora of viruses, mycoplasma and bacteria can be isolated from the respiratory tract of calves with pneumonia, and the unpassaged respiratory material can cause disease similar to the naturally occurring disease, the inoculation of pure cultures of *M. dispar*, *M. bovis* and *Ureaplasma* spp. or pure cultures of BRSV PI-3 into calves does not produce the severe clinical disease seen in the field (27). The failure of pure cultures of a pathogen to produce a severe pneumonia may be for one of three reasons:

- Combinations of organisms are required for disease
- Laboratory passage of the pathogens, necessary for purification causes their attenuation
- Material in the respiratory secretion other than the pathogens identified is required for disease which may include agents that were not detected by routine culture techniques.

Aerosol infection and direct contact are thought to be the methods of transmission and both of these are accentuated in crowded inadequately ventilated conditions.

The morbidity and mortality will vary considerably depending on the condition of housing, the quality of the management provided and the kind and number of viruses and bacteria which predominate at any one time. The morbidity rate may reach 100% and the case fatality rate is usually less than 5% (1). In acute respiratory syncytial viral pneumonia of calves there may be an unexpected acute onset of respiratory disease in which 80–90% of calves are affected, with a case fatality rate which may reach 30% or higher. The economic losses associated with enzootic pneumonia may be considerable. One estimate reports that the disease accounts for 50% of all calf mortality and a reduction of 7·2% in liveweight gain (11). In commercial veal units, the presence of enzootic pneumonia may be associated with a prolonged time in the unit because of reduced daily liveweight gain (9).

The role of antibody in the protection of calves from enzootic pneumonia is becoming more clear (8). The peak incidence of calf pneumonia occurs when the serum Ig concentrations are at their lowest levels between 2 and 4 weeks of age (8). The peak onset of pneumonia may also be correlated with the lowest IgG and IgA concentrations in the nasal secretions (8). Most calves which recover from clinical enzootic pneumonia appear to be resistant to further attacks of the disease caused by the same infectious agents. Nasal and serum antibodies develop following infection, but the role of these antibodies in providing protection from clinical disease is uncertain. The spectrum of colostral antibodies present in home-raised calves will depend on the spectrum of infection in the adult cows. Herd immunity to one or more viruses probably develops and severe outbreaks of disease usually occur following the introduction of animals which may be carriers of infectious agents to which the resident animals are non-immune. In commercial veal calf units where market-purchased calves are being introduced on a regular basis, there is commonly a succession of minor epidemics of enzootic pneumonia. The incidence is highest in the recently introduced calves and the disease will occur in a small percentage of resident calves.

Environment

The environmental conditions are considered to be important predisposing factors. Crowding results in close contact and promotes spread of infection, and also results in excess moisture which, in the presence of inadequate ventilation (movement of air) and supplemental heat, causes a high relative humidity and chilling of calves. Many calf barns are old adapted barns which are occupied for several months without depopulation and disinfection. In commercial veal units, the longer the disinfection and vacancy break, up to 6–7 days, the lower the incidence of disease in new calf crops entering the unit (9). Ventilation is commonly inadequate because of poor design of the building. Rapid changes in weather, particularly during the winter months, are often followed by outbreaks of acute pneumonia because of inadequate ventilation. A common practice during cold weather is to close the air inlets and turn off the ventilating fans in an attempt to maintain the inside temperature at a comfortable level. This usually leads to increased relative humidity, condensation of moisture on walls and on the calves leading to wet conditions, and the reduced ventilation results in an increase in the concentration of droplet infection (32). Attempts to correlate meteorological data with the daily morbidity rate have not yet provided evidence for the hypothesis that climatic factors have an influence on incidence (9). This may be due to the difficulties associated with accurately monitoring meteorological data and the lack of a direct relationship between the environment outside of a calf barn and the microclimate of the calf inside the barn. The disease appears to be most common during the winter months when calves are housed continuously and when ventilation is commonly inadequate.

An examination of the weather-induced changes on airborne bacteria in calf barns reveals that humid weather results in a marked increase in the percentage of bacterial colony forming particles of less than 4–7 μm in size (33). This provides the beginnings of a sound physical framework for the explanation of this and other, as yet, empirical relationships between the microenvironment in calf barns and the etiology and epidemiology of calf pneumonia.

In an epidemiological study of a large commercial veal calf unit there was transient synchronization of epidemics of enzootic pneumonia in separate pens throughout the unit which were preceded by periods in which there was relatively little disease in the unit (9). This suggests that there may be important, as yet unidentified, environmental or managemental factors which predispose to the disease.

Immune status

The bovine respiratory syncytial virus (BRSV) appears to have assumed major importance as a causative agent of herd epidemics of pneumonia in housed dairy calves, weaned beef calves and even adult cows (6); serological surveys indicate that the prevalence of infection is high and varies from 60 to 80% of the cattle populations examined (6, 38). Most mature cattle in some populations have seroconverted to the virus (51). However, the incidence of clinical respiratory disease associated with the BRSV is much lower. Respiratory disease in weaned beef calves 6–8 months of age in North America has also been attributed to the BRSV and is characterized by a sudden onset commonly after the cold weather begins in the fall of the year (34–36). Affected animals are commonly in good bodily condition and are well nourished (37). The BRSV was the most common isolated viral agent in a series of 14 epidemics of pneumonia in housed dairy calves (10). The disease may be mild, moderate, or severe. In infected herds, newborn calves acquire colostral antibodies to the BRSV which declines to undetectable levels in an average of about 100 days with a range of 30–200 days (36). It appears that colostral immunity does not protect calves from experimental (47) or naturally occurring clinical disease, but active immunity from natural infection with or without evidence of clinical disease will protect the animals from clinical disease but not from reinfection upon later exposures to the BRSV. Because field observations suggest that outbreaks of pneumonia due to the BRSV are commonly preceded by a mild respiratory disease several days previous to the acute fatal form of the disease, a hypersensitivity to the virus similar to the sequence of events in infants with a similar disease has been proposed in calves (6).

In dairy herds, clinical disease attributed to the BRSV may appear initially in the youngest calves from 2 to 8 weeks of age in which the mortality will be highest followed by disease in the mature lactating cows in which milk production will drop (39).

Seroepidemiological surveys in feedlot calves indicate that seroconversion to the BRSV may occur in up to 71% of animals within 1 month after arrival (40). The animals with low titers to the BRSV on arrival were at increased risk of subsequent treatment for respiratory disease which suggests that the BRSV may have been a factor in bovine respiratory disease.

Pathogenesis

The respiratory viruses are capable of causing a viral interstitial pneumonia affecting the cranial lobes of the lung which may be subclinical, mildly clinical or severe and highly fatal. Subclinical viral pneumonia associated with the PI-3 virus uncomplicated by secondary bacterial invasion is usually of minor importance (25). In subclinical PI-3 infection in calves, seroconversion will occur and at necropsy there are microscopic lesions consisting of bronchiolitis, bronchial and bronchiolar epithelial hyperplasia, alveolar epithelialization and giant cell syncytial formation (25). In the mild form there are slight clinical signs such as coughing and polypnea. In the severe form of viral pneumonia, such as in respiratory syncytial viral infection, there is severe dyspnea, with mouth breathing and an expiratory grunt, but a marked absence of toxemia compared with a bacterial pneumonia (4). Death can occur without secondary bacterial bronchopneumonia. Atelectasis and consolidation of the anterior lobes of the lungs are characteristic and account for the loud bronchial tones audible on auscultation over the anterior ventral aspect of the thorax.

The experimental intranasal inoculation of the PI-3 virus into colostrum-deprived calves results in a pneumonia which is grossly and histologically similar to the naturally occurring disease. Within 2–4 days following infection there is bronchiolitis and bronchitis and cellular exudate in the bronchiolar lumina. These lesions become more severe and are accompanied by alveolar cell thickening and hyperplasia. Beginning at about 14 days following infection there is healing of the bronchiolar and alveolar lesions. The bronchiolar exudate becomes organized by fibroblasts and mononuclear cells predominate in the alveolar exudate (23). Bronchiolitis obliterans is widespread but re-epithelialization of damaged bronchiolar mucosa and alveoli occur.

Experimentally, the PI-3 virus can affect alveolar macrophages which may impair the lung clearance mechanisms and allow *Past. hemolytica* to produce a secondary bacterial bronchopneumonia (41, 42). However, aerosols of PI-3 followed by *Past. hemolytica* 7 days later does not necessarily result in significant pulmonary disease (43).

After the primary viral pneumonia is established, bacterial invasion may occur and the resulting pneumonia will vary with the species of bacteria which are present. Secondary bacterial pneumonias usually respond to treatment, although relapses are common if the viral pneumonia is extensive. Viruses are capable of reducing the resistance of mucous nembranes, allowing bacteria such as pasteurellae to invade tissues. They are also capable of destroying the cilia on the bronchial mucosa which act as an escalator and help to keep the lower respiratory tract free of potential pathogens. In animals where there is an uncomplicated viral pneumonia with very extensive lesions there may be minimal clinical signs and almost complete resolution.

Infection with the BRSV in calves causes rhinitis, tracheitis, bronchitis, proliferative and exudative bronchiolitis with accompanying alveolar collapse and multinucleated syncytial giant cell formation in the epithelial lining and in the lumen of the bronchioles and alveoli (12, 13). The pulmonary function changes observed during the acute phase of the disease are consistent with a diffuse obstructive disease (44). This lesion could impair the lung clearance mechanism and predispose to bacterial bronchopneumonia. Experimental inoculation of gnotobiotic calves with BRSV produces macroscopic lesions of the lungs without clinical signs (58). The lesions consist of proliferative and exudative bronchiolitis with accompanying alveolar collapse and mononuclear cellular infiltration of the peribronchiolar tissue and alveolar walls. Infected calves respond serologically by 11 days after inoculation. The experimentally induced lesions are commonly resolved by about 30 days after inoculation (12). The acute fatal disease which has been attributed to the BRSV has not been reproduced experimentally.

The pathogenesis of acute fatal pneumonia due to the BRSV is not well understood. The characteristic lesions are exudative or necrotizing bronchiolitis, atelectasis, interstitial edema and emphysema (45). Field observations have recorded that the acute fatal disease is commonly preceded by a mild respiratory disease several days previously which suggests that hypersensitivity may be an important pathogenetic machanism causing lung injury (35, 37). The second stage may follow initial improvement or recovery from the first stage and is associated with the onset of extreme respiratory distress (6). However, these observations have not yet been validated.

The effects of the BRSV on bovine pulmonary alveolar macrophage function have been studied and there is only limited impairment at the *in vitro* level (46). In experimentally infected calves the virus can be detected in the epithelial cells of bronchioli and alveoli by immunofluorescence (47).

The virus can replicate and induce cytopathologic changes in airway epithelial cells which include bronchial ciliated and mucous cells and bronchiolar ciliated and non-ciliated epithelial (Clara) cells (48). Syncytial epithelial cells may be observed in bronchi, bronchioles, alveoli, and in alveolar macrophages. However, syncytial cell formation is not unique to infection with the BRSV since it may also occur in other viral infections of the lung. Whether or not the BRSV can predispose to bacterial pneumonia is unknown. The experimental inoculation of lambs with the respiratory syncytial virus and *Past. hemolytica* results in a more severe acute respiratory disease than that produced by either agent alone and the severity of the disease may be a result of synergistic action of the two agents (49).

Clinical findings

Regardless of the identity of the causative virus, the clinical findings in all viral pneumonias of calves are similar. In the experimental disease, a febrile reaction occurs about the 5th day and is followed by the appearance of rhinitis, pneumonia and mild diarrhea. The fever is moderate only (40–45·5°C, 104–105°F). A harsh, hacking cough, easily stimulated by pinching the trachea, is characteristic.

In field cases, the clinical findings are similar although the temperature tends to be higher. This may be due to bacterial invasion in the early stages. The nasal discharge is only moderate in amount and is mucopurulent. On auscultation of the thorax the major abnormalities can be detected over the ventral aspects of the apical and cardiac lobes. The breath sounds are loud and harsh and represent bronchial tones transmitted through consolidated lung. The intensity of the heart may be audible more clearly than usual because of shrinkage of lung tissue in the cardiac area. Some peracute cases of uncomplicated viral pneumonia die within a few hours, although cases of average severity usually recover in 4–7 days. Infections with the PI-3 virus generally cause mild respiratory disease characterized by coughing, nasal discharge, slight fever and recovery in a few days.

In outbreaks of BRSV infection in young dairy cattle under 16 months of age the first clinical abnormalities usually noticed by the owner are coughing and a mild nasal discharge in 50–75% of the animals (50). A general illness of anorexia and a fever of 40°C (104°F) or higher lasted less than 3 days, in most cases followed by recovery. Coughing, nasal discharge and conjunctivitis commonly persists for several days or weeks in 10–30% of the animals. Abdominal breathing and loud and abnormal lung sounds may occur in about 50% of the animals but commonly resolves within 10 days (50).

In respiratory syncytial viral pneumonia there may be a sudden onset of acute pneumonia in 80–90% of a group of calves (4).The clinical findings are characteristic of a severe viral pneumonia. Affected calves are usually mentally alert and there is only a mild fever. There is polypnea and dyspnea which in a few days became worse with mouth breathing and an expiratory grunt. Loud bronchial tones indicating consolidation are audible over the anterior lobes of the lung. Squeaky wheezing sounds due to the bronchiolitis are also commonly audible over the periphery of the consolidated areas. Loud crackling sounds due to interstitial emphysema may also be audible over the dorsal aspects of the lungs. Death may occur in 2–4 days in spite of intensive therapy.

The clinical findings of BRSV infection of the respiratory tract of recently weaned beef calves 6–8 months of age include nasal and lacrimal discharge, polypnea, fever of 40–42°C (104–108°F) decreased feed intake, coughing and lethargy. Within a few days the dyspnea becomes marked with mouth breathing and the production of frothy saliva created by the labored respirations. Subcutaneous emphysema over the winters due to severe, intestinal emphysema has been recorded (35, 37). Loud breath sounds and wheezing and crackling sounds are audible over the ventral aspects of the lungs and indicates atelectasis or consolidation and bronchiolitis. Secondary bacterial bronchopneumonia may be present. Death may occur within a few days after the onset of the dyspnea.

When secondary bacterial bronchopneumonia occurs, the fever, the dyspnea and the toxemia are usually more severe. When secondary infection with *Pasteurella* spp. occurs the temperature rises to 41–41·5°C (106–107°F), the area of lung affected is much increased, and loud harsh breath sounds due to congenital and edema are followed by crackles and a pleuritic friction rub. These cases usually respond rapidly to adequate treatment. When *Actinomyces* (*Corynebacterium*) *pyogenes* is the secondary invader, consolidation is marked, there is a profound toxemia and loud breath sounds. In cases where *Fusobacterium necrophorum* is present the clinical findings are similar and pulmonary abscesses are likely to develop. Necrotic lesions are often present in the mouth and pharynx in these cases and the pulmonary infection probably originates from here. With both of these latter infections there may be some response to antibiotic treatment, but there is a predisposition to relapse soon after treatment is terminated. Coughing, dyspnea, anorexia and emaciation continue and the animal eventually has to be destroyed.

Clinical pathology

Nasopharyngeal swabs, transtracheal aspirates and lung lavage samples (59) may be taken for isolation of viruses, mycoplasmas and bacteria. Determination of drug sensitivity to the bacteria may be valuable particularly when a number of calves are involved in an outbreak. The isolation of the BRSV from natural infections is difficult due to the labile nature of the virus. A fluorescent antibody technique is available for the detection of the BRSV in nasopharyngeal epithelial cells in both natural and experimental infections (14). However, this diagnostic technique has not proven entirely satisfactory because of the subjectivity of assessing the degree of fluorescence and the variations due to the strain of the virus involved and non-specific fluorescence (51). Serological tests have been more extensively used for confirmation of suspected BRSV infections and include a modified indirect fluorescent antibody test (51), indirect hemagglutination (52) and an ELISA test (53, 54) the latter of which is considered to be sensitive and specific and has the advantage of giving test results within several hours whereas the virus neutralization test requires 5–6 days for completion. The complement-fixation test is less specific and less sensitive than the ELISA test (54).

Necropsy findings

In uncomplicated viral pneumonia, irrespective of the specific cause, there are areas of collapse with little bronchiolar reaction, accompanied by emphysema in the apical lobes and to a less extent in the cardiac lobes, and with little involvement of the diaphragmatic lobes. In the later stages a dark red consolidation with little or no fluid present in the lung and a hobnail appearance of the pleural surface affects most of the ventral portions of the apical and cardiac lobes. The lesions are always bilateral. Histologically there is interstitial pneumonia. The remainder of the lungs reveals congestion and occasionally a few hemorrhages. Acute inflammation of the nasal mucosa, particularly on the turbinate and ethmoid bones, is usually accompanied by a marked, mucopurulent exudation. A catarrhal enteritis is present occasionally and myocarditis has also been observed. In the PI-3 infection intracytoplasmic inclusion bodies are widespread in the lungs; and after experimental infection, are present on the 5th day, but have disappeared by the 7th day after infection (15).

In respiratory syncytial viral pneumonia there is severe interstitial pneumonia and interstitial emphysema. Histopathologically there is severe bronchiolitis, alveolitis with multinucleated syncytia, which often contain eosinophilic intracytoplasmic inclusion bodies and alveolar epithelial cell hyperplasia.

When bacterial invasion has occurred the lesions vary with the bacteria present. Extensive hepatization with mottled red and gray lobules and considerable interlobular aggregations of serofibrinous fluid, and often accompanied by a fibrinous pleurisy, is characteristic of *Past. multocida* infection. Extensive consolidation and suppuration occur with *Actinomyces (Corynebacterium) pyogenes* and *Fusobacterium necrophorus* infections. In the latter case there may be necrotic lesions in the mouth and upper respiratory tract.

Diagnosis

The diagnosis of pneumonia is usually not difficult to make; but determination of the cause of the pneumonia is much more difficult. Young calves raised indoors and affected with a cough, nasal discharge and pneumonia are usually affected with a viral pneumonia which may be complicated by a bacterial bronchopneumonia. It is usually assumed that the causative agents may be the PI-3 virus and/or the BRSV. Lungworm pneumonia usually occurs in young calves at pasture, and marked dyspnea, coughing and a few deaths are characteristic. A fever is common in lungworm pneumonia and there are loud breath sounds over the ventral aspects of the lungs and loud and moist crackles over the dorsal aspects.

A primary acute bacterial pneumonia due to *Past. hemolytica* or *Klebsiella pneumoniae* may occur in young calves and is characterized by severe toxemia, fever, dyspnea and grunting and a poor responsible therapy. *Str. pneumoniae* may cause a similar pneumonia.

Chronic cases of enzootic pneumonia are affected by bronchiectasis and pulmonary abscessation and may be confused with congenital cardiac defects. Acute myocardial dystrophy is characterized by tachycardia, arrhythmias, pulmonary edema and perhaps some evidence of skeletal muscular weakness. Aspiration pneumonia occurs occasionally in calves which have been force-fed colostrum or milk. There is a sudden onset of marked dyspnea, anxiety and distress and death may occur within a few minutes. However, some calves survive and there is marked dyspnea with abdominal breathing and loud breath sounds and crackles over the dorsal and ventral aspects of both lungs. Some calves will recover completely in a few days.

The differential diagnosis of the viral pneumonia, caused by the BRSV in weaned beef calves must include acute interstitial pneumonia and pneumonic pasteurellosis. The so-called hypersensitivity form of acute interstitial pneumonia occurs in cattle from 6 to 18 months of age and is characterized by a sudden onset of marked dyspnea, fever, loud breath sounds over the ventral aspects of the lungs and failure to respond to treatment with antimicrobials. The case fatality rate is usually over 75%. In pneumonic pasteurellosis, depression, toxemia, fever, loud breath sounds over the ventral aspects of the lungs and a favorable response to treatment are characteristic.

In weaned beef calves with bovine respiratory syncytial virus pneumonia there is a sudden onset of marked dyspnea, fever, anxiety but not toxemia, mouth breathing in advanced cases, loud bronchial sounds and crackles over both lung fields especially over the ventral the aspects, subcutaneous emphysema and several animals are usually involved. There may be a history of mild respiratory disease in the affected group about 10 days previously.

Treatment

Uncomplicated viral pneumonia is unlikely to respond to treatment but antibacterial therapy is necessary because of the high probability of secondary bacterial pneumonia. A broad spectrum antimicrobial should be used. Sulfadimidine (sulfamethazine) 150 mg/kg body weight parenterally or orally gives good results. A mixture of penicillin and streptomycin is often adequate and is inexpensive and easy to administer when large numbers of uncontrolled, young animals have to be treated. The short-acting or long-acting oxytetracyclines, chloramphenicol or trimethoprim-potentiated sulfonamides, are also efficacious and are recommended. Drug legislation may prohibit the use of chloramphenicol. Early treatment is necessary to avoid the development of incurable secondary complication such as pulmonary abscesses, pleuritis, bronchiectasis and suppurative pneumonia. In commercial veal calf units, the case fatality rate can be kept to a low level by early and adequate treatment (9). In some cases it may be sufficient to treat animals once only, but a proportion of cases are likely to relapse after an initial response. Such cases require repeated daily therapy for 3 to 5 days. If the number of relapses in an area or on a farm is excessive, all cases should receive multiple treatments. Following treatment of individual animals, medicated feed containing tetracycline at a level of 10–20 mg/kg body weight/day for 3 weeks may be used to improve convalescent performance.

The use of bronchodilators and non-steroidal anti-inflammatory drugs (NSAIDs) as adjunctive therapy for viral pneumonia in calves is being evaluated. Clenbuterol hydrochloride, a beta$_2$ receptor sympathomimetic agent, a bronchodilator, had no beneficial effect on clinical signs in naturally occurring cases of bovine respiratory syncytial virus infection in calves (55). Flunixin meglumine, a prostaglandin synthetase inhibitor with anti-inflammatory, analgesic and antipyretic activities appeared to have some beneficial effect in experimentally induced PI-3 pneumonia in conventional 10–12-week-old calves (56). The drug controlled the coughing, reduced the fevers and lowered the respiratory rates of affected calves. There was a reduction in extent of the pulmonary consolidation. Flunixin meglumine had no overall beneficial effect when given at a rate of 2 mg/kg body weight intravenously to calves 3–8 months of age affected with field cases of BRSV (57). Mean body temperatures were reduced significantly in treated calves.

Any treatment of an outbreak of enzootic pneumonia in calves must include correction of adverse environmental conditions which may have precipitated the disease.

Control

Control of the diseases in housed calves is dependent on good husbandry. Overcrowding, drafty or inadequately ventilated housing, exposure to inclement weather, and sudden changes in environmental temperatures all predispose calves to the disease and should be avoided if possible. Newly purchased calves should be isolated for several weeks before being introduced to the group. The control of enzootic pneumonia of calves is particularly difficult and expensive in countries where the animals are housed for up to 6 months' duration during the winter months. The most comfortable temperature for young calves ranges from 13 to 21°C (55 to 70°F) with a relative humidity of 70%. To achieve these environmental conditions requires a suitable insulation material in the walls and ceilings, ample bedding to absorb moisture from feces and urine, and adequate movement of air to remove aerosol particles which may be infectious. This requires an adequate air inlet and outlet system, adequate capacity fans and supplemental heat during very cold periods. The installation of recirculating air filter units can lead to a substantial reduction in the concentration of airborne bacteria to which calves are exposed (32). Field studies in veal calf units indicate that mean aerial bacteria concentration in filtered barns can be reduced by 45%, the number of calves requiring treatment reduced by 19%, the number of repeat courses of treatment and the total antibiotic usage reduced by 29% and 35%, respectively. At slaughter the average area of lung consolidation in calves from filtered barns can be reduced by 35%. In general, air filtration can result in a reduction in both the incidence and severity of clinical and subclinical pneumonia in calves and in improved weight gain. Where economics permit, the ideal situation is to construct a calf barn completely removed from the main adult cow barn to minimize the spread of infection from adults which may be symptomless carriers. After the colostral feeding period calves are removed from the calving barn and placed in individual pens in the calf barn. The raising of young calves outdoors in calf 'hutches' or 'igloos' has been satisfactory and economical even in countries where the outside temperatures go well below freezing. With adequate bedding, protection from the prevailing winds and adequate nutrition, calves will grow satisfactorily. Dairy herds which have had difficulty controlling enzootic pneumonia of calves have found this system to be an excellent alternative to the construction of a completely air-conditioned calf house. Nutritional deficiencies, usually of energy and protein, are common in young calves and often accentuate the severity of the pneumonia. Young calves should receive a balanced calf starter grain ration supplemented with essential vitamins and minerals, and good quality hay beginning by at least 3 weeks of age.

However, in spite of the very best hygiene and management it may not be possible to prevent the development of new cases if the infection already exists in a herd, or if cattle from other herds are moved into the herd. Those situations require a vaccine but an effective vaccine is not available and seems unlikely. At the present time it is feasible only to be vigilant and treat new cases urgently and vigorously, because a strict hygiene program may not be feasible in the average commercial herd. If management is inadequate and the general resistance of the animals is low, losses due to calf pneumonia with significant bacterial or mycoplasmal invasion can be sufficient to make a farming venture unprofitable.

The concern is usually with young dairy or beef calves which are raised indoors. Calves reared as herd replacements may be born inside and raised indoors until they are about 6 months of age and then turned out to pasture for the summer. In the case of veal calf-rearing units, the calves are kept and fed indoors under intensive conditions from a few days of age until they reach 150 kg body weight at 12 weeks of age. In the barley-beef units, the calves are fed indoors on an intensive basis from weaning until they reach market weight at 10–12 months of age. In all of these situations, young growing calves are raised together under confined conditions which promotes the spread of bovine respiratory disease caused by several viruses, *Mycoplasma* and *Pasteurella* spp. Based on serological surveys, most calves raised in close confinement will have become infected by several viruses which include the PI-3 virus, adenoviruses, bovine respiratory syncytial virus, infectious bovine rhinotracheitis and bovine viral diarrhea (16). If natural exposure to these viruses, *Mycoplasma* spp. and bacteria is so widespread and inevitable, it raises serious questions about the rationale for vaccination. In most cases the effects of the viruses and *Mycoplasma* spp. are minimal. The stress factors associated with inadequate ventilation, high relative humidity, and chilling and the secondary bacterial complications are responsible for the onset of clinical disease.

There is insufficient information available from field trials to make recommendations for the use of vaccines for the control of enzootic pneumonia in calves. It is difficult to evaluate the results of vaccination trials because investigators use so many combinations of vaccine, programs of vaccination, combinations with management variable and differences in methods of evaluation. In addition, and probably of major importance, most vaccination trials are not randomized controlled trials. Any successful vaccine would have to be multivalent and would have to be effective when given before 2 months of age or earlier to coincide with the decline in immunity and the occurrence of enzootic pneumonia in calves. Vaccination of calves in a commercial calf-rearing unit which compared the use of no vaccine, intranasal IBR, intranasal IBR PI-3, and intranasal IBR—PI-3 plus BRSV on three occasions at 7,10 and 16 weeks did not have a significant effect on growth rates during a 10-month period to slaughter (19). There is good field evidence that the colostral immunological status of the calf has a significant effect on the susceptibility of the calf to pneumonia (8). There is a clear association between low levels of IgG_1, IgG_2, and IgA of calves at 2½ weeks of age and subsequent susceptibility to pneumonia at 2½ months of age. Calves with signs of pneumonia had low levels of IgG_1 compared with non-pneumonic calves which had relatively higher levels. This again seems to emphasize the importance of colostrum in the control of infectious diseases of young calves. In addition, calves with high levels of serum immunoglobulin do not respond normally to vaccine and any vaccine for enzootic pneumonia would have to be administered during this relatively refractory period. However, for veal calves which are purchased at a few days of age and with low levels of immunoglobulin this may not be a problem.

The intranasal inoculation of calves with virulent or a modified strain of PI-3 virus stimulates the development of both serum antibody and nasal secretion antibody (20). The nasal secretion antibody is dose-dependent. Challenge exposure of these calves provides protection against clinical disease. These factors should be considered in the development and administration of PI-3 viral vaccines if the objective is to establish an optimal concentration of antibody in the nasal secretion. The parenteral administration of two sequential doses, 2 weeks apart, of an inactivated PI-3 virus vaccine with adjuvant will induce high levels of serum antibody and prevent virus excretion in nasopharyngeal secretions after challenge (17). Successful immunization of calves against PI-3 infection may be useful for protection against pneumonic pasteurellosis if PI-3 precedes the bacterial infection. This is presented in greater detail in the section on pneumonic pasteurellosis (p. 663).

An inactivated vaccine containing five viral antigens has been used in the United Kingdom in an attempt to control the disease (5). The vaccine stimulates the production of systemic antibody, mainly IgG, and local antibody IgA in the nasal secretions. The use of the vaccine intranasally stimulates only a small amount of IgA.

The evaluations of the BRSV vaccines are currently in progress and the preliminary results are inconclusive. Some claims are made for the efficacy of a modified live BRSV vaccine for protection of BRSV pneumonia in weaned beef calves (16) but randomized controlled trials were not done (16, 22).

An inactivated BRSV vaccine provided protection against infection from an experimental challenge (18). Two live vaccines did not provide protection. The nature of the protection has not been determined. An inactivated vaccine did not cause exacerbation of a mild respiratory tract disease after challenge infection (31).

A double-blind field trial using live attenuated BRSV vaccine appeared to provide some protection against lower respiratory tract disease due to the virus in vaccinated groups compared to unvaccinated groups (21).

REVIEW LITERATURE

Baker, J. C. (1986) Bovine respiratory syncytial virus: pathogenesis, clinical signs, diagnosis, treatment and prevention. *Comp. cont. Educ. Pract. Vet.*, *8*, F31–F38.

Baker, J. C. & Frey, M. L. (1985) Bovine respiratory syncytial virus. *Vet. Clin. N. Am. Food Anim. Pract.*, *1*, 259–275.

REFERENCES

(1) Bryson, D. G. et al. (1978) *Vet. Rec.*, *103*, 485.
(2) Bryson, D. G. et al. (1978) *Vet. Rec.*, *103*, 503.
(3) Bryson, D. G. et al. (1979) *Vet. Rec.*, *104*, 45.
(4) Pirie, H. M. et al. (1981) *Vet. Rec.*, *108*, 441.
(5) Gourlay, R. N. (1976) *Vet. Ann.*, *16*, 48.
(6) Baker, J. C. (1986) *Comp. cont. Educ. Pract. Vet.*, *8*, f F31.
(7) Ronsholt, L. (1978) *Acta Pathol. Microbiol. scand. Sect. B.*, *86*, 291.
(8) Corbeil, L. B. et al. (1984). *Am. J. vet. Res.*, *45*, 773.
(9) Miller, W. M. et al. (1980) *Res. vet. Sci.*, *28*, 267.

(10) Baker, J. C. et al. (1986) *J. Am. vet. med. Assoc.*, *189*, 66.
(11) Thomas, L. H. (1978) *Vet. Ann.*, *18*, 73.
(12) Castleman, W. L. et al. (1985) *Am. J. vet. Res.*, *46*, 547.
(13) Bryson, D. G. et al. (1983) *Am. J. vet. Res.*, *44*, 1648.
(14) Thomas, L. H. & Stott, E. J. (1981) *Vet. Rec.*, *108*, 432.
(15) Betts, A. O. et al. (1964) *Vet. Rec.*, *76*, 382.
(16) Bohlender, R. E. (1984) *Mod. vet. Pract.*, *65*, 606.
(17) Probert, M. et al. (1978) *Res. Vet. Sci.*, *24*, 222.
(18) Stott, E. J. et al. (1984) *J. Hyg., Camb.*, *93*, 251.
(19) Thomson, J. R. et al. (1986) *Vet. Rec.*, *119*, 450.
(20) Marshall, R. G. (1981) *Am. J. vet. Res.*, *42*, 907.
(21) Verhoeff, J. & van Nieuwstadt, A. P. K. M. I. (1984) *Vet. Rec.*, *115*,488.
(22) Kucera, C. J. et al. (1983) *Vet. Med. SAC*, *78*, 1599.
(23) Bryson, D. G. et al. (1983) *J. comp. Pathol.*, *93*, 397.
(24) Eisa, M. et al. (1979) *Br. vet. J.*, *135*, 192.
(25) Allan, E. M. et al. (1978) *Res. vet. Sci.*, *24*, 339.
(26) Lopez, A. et al. (1976) *Can. J. comp. Med.*, *40*, 385.
(27) Thomas, L. H. et al. (1982) *Res. vet. Sci.*, *33*,170.
(28) Stott, E. J. et al. (1980) *J. Hyg., Camb.*, *85*, 257.
(29) Houghton, S. B. & Gourlay, R. N. (1984) *Res. vet. Sci.*, *37*, 194.
(30) Wellemans, G. et al. (1985) *Vlaams Diergeneeskd. Tijdschr.*, *54*, 392.
(31) Mohanty, S. B. et al. (1981) *Am. J. vet. Res.*, *42*, 881.
(32) Pritchard, D. G. et al. (1981) *Vet. Rec.*, *109*,5.
(33) Jones, C. R. & Webster, A. J. F. (1981) *Vet. Rec.*, *109*, 493.
(34) Baker, J. C. et al. (1986) *Am. J. vet. res.*, *47*, 246.
(35) Bohlender, R. E. et al. (1982) *Mod. vet. Pract.*, *63*, 613.
(36) Baker, J. C. et al. (1986) *Am. J. vet. Res.*, *47*, 240.
(37) Frey, M. L. (1983) *Bovine Pract.*, 18, 73–78.
(38) Baker, J. C. et al. (1985) *Am. J. vet. Res.*, *46*, 891.
(39) Harrison, L. R. & Pursell, A. R. (1985) *J. Am. vet. med. Assoc.*, *187*, 716.
(40) Martin, S. W. & Bohac, J. G. (1986) *Can. J. vet. Res.*, *50*, 351.
(41) Hesse, R. A. & Toth, T.E. (1983) *Am. J. vet. Res.*, *44*, 1901.
(42) Liggitt, D. et al. (1985) *Am. J. vet. Res.*, *46*, 1740.
(43) Carriere, P. D. et al. (1983) *Can. J. comp. Med.*, *47*, 422.
(44) LeKeux, P. et al. (1985) *Res. vet. Sci.*, *39*, 324.
(45) Van Den, Ingh, T. S. G. A. M. et al. (1982) *Res. vet. Sci.*, *33*, 152.
(46) Trigo, E. et al. (1985) *Am. J. vet. Res.*, *46*, 1098.
(47) McNulty, M. S. et al. (1983) *Am. J. vet. Res.*, *44*, 1656.
(48) Castleman, W. L. et al. (1985) *Am. J. vet. Res.*, *46*, 554.
(49) Al-Darraji, A. M. et al. (1982) *Am. J. vet. Res.*, *43*, 236.
(50) Verhoeff, J. et al. (1984) *Vet. Rec.*, *114*, 9.
(51) Lynch, J. A. & Derbyshire, J. B. (1986) *Can. J. vet. Res.*, *50*, 384.
(52) Martin, H. T. (1983) *Vet. Rec.*, *113*, 290.
(53) Westenbrink, F. et al. (1985) *Res. vet. Sci.*, *38*, 334.
(54) Gillette, K. G. (1983) *Am. J. vet. Res.*, *44*, 2251.
(55) Verhoeff, J. et al. (1986) *Vet. Rec.*, *119*, 105.
(56) Selman, I. E. et al. (1984) *Vet. Rec.*, *115*, 101.
(57) Verhoeff, J. et al. (1986) *Vet. Rec.*, *118*, *14*.
(58) Thomas, L. H. et al. (1984) *Br. J. exp. Pathol.*, *65*, 19.
(59) Kimman, T. G. et al. (1986) *Am. J. vet. Res.*, *47*, 143.

Viral pneumonia in older calves, yearlings and adult cattle

In addition to enzootic pneumonia which is a viral pneumonia of housed calves, acute viral interstitial pneumonia may occur in calves 3–8 months of age which are reared outside, and in yearlings and adult cattle raised indoors or outdoors (1, 2). The viruses isolated include PI-3, adenoviruses and the bovine respiratory syncytial virus (BRSV) (a pneumovirus in the family Paramyxoviridae (3, 4). The prevalence of BRSV infection in the cattle population is high but the incidence rate of clinical disease is much lower (12). Several viruses including the PI-3 virus, BRSV, rhinovirus and enteroviruses occur in young cattle from 1 to 8 months of age (7). However, the presence of these viruses in the respiratory tract and evidence of seroconversion to the viruses in young cattle is not always associated with clinical disease. A high percentage (71%) of cattle entering feedlots may seroconvert to the BRSV which may also be correlated with an increased risk to subsequent treatment for respiratory disease (8). The factors which predispose some cattle to develop acute and often fatal pneumonia are not understood, but the stressors associated with acute bovine respiratory disease are considered important.

The disease occurs in beef calves 3–6 months of age running at pasture with their dams without any history of previous stress. In dairy herds, recent introductions of young cattle purchased from a public saleyard are thought to have introduced the infection to home-farm cattle which had no previous exposure to the viruses or their immunity had declined. Adult dairy cows may be affected (10). A common occurrence is in beef calves 6–8 months of age within 2–3 weeks following weaning and comingling in confinement. Yearling cattle in feedlots are also susceptible.

The pathogenesis is not clearly understood. The PI-3 virus, adenovirus, BRSV are ubiquitous and capable of producing a viral interstitial pneumonia. Normally, however, these viruses are relatively innocuous and experimentally produce a transient respiratory disease. The factors that result in acute fatal pneumonia in 1–2% of animals at risk have not been described.

The characteristic features include a sharp outbreak of acute respiratory disease in a group of animals. The morbidity will vary from 25 to 50%, but the case fatality is usually below 5%. Many animals are coughing, there is dyspnea, serous and nasal discharges, agalactia in lactating dairy cows and a fever is usually present. The fever usually persists for 3–5 days in spite of therapy with antibiotics. Toxemia is not a feature unless there is secondary bacterial pneumonia. On auscultation of the lungs there are loud breath sounds over the ventral aspects indicating consolidation and wheezes indicating bronchiolitis. These are the findings of a viral interstitial pneumonia. Most animals recover within 5–7 days. About 1–2% of affected animals will develop a fatal viral pneumonia characterized by severe dyspnea, persistent fever, severe respiratory insufficiency with mouth breathing in a few days and death 2–5 days after onset. Loud bronchial tones are audible over the ventral two-thirds of both lung fields indicating extensive consolidation.

Acute respiratory disease due to BRSV infection in weaned beef calves is characterized by marked dyspnea, anorexia, mouth breathing, fever, subcutaneous emphysema, loud breath sounds and death in a few days or less (5, 6). In some cases there may be a history of respiratory disease in the affected group several days previously (9).

It is not usually possible to make a definitive etiological diagnosis based on the clinical findings. However, the combination of the epidemiological and clinical findings are usually suggestive of an acute viral respiratory disease. It is usually not possible to be more specific than making a clinical diagnosis of acute undifferentiated respiratory viruses. The disease must be differentiated clinically from infectious bovine rhinotracheitis in which nasal lesions are common and pneumonia is not common, and from pneumonia pasteurellosis in which there is a toxemic bacterial bronchopneumonia.

A leukopenia and neutropenia are common and an aid to diagnosis.

Nasopharyngeal swabs for virus isolation and paired serum samples are necessary to make a definitive etiological diagnosis. Direct staining of nasopharyngeal swabs with immunofluorescent hyperimmune serum is useful for the diagnosis of bovine respiratory syncytial virus infection (11). The indirect fluorescent antibody test is also available for the detection of bovine respiratory syncytial virus (12, 13).

At necropsy the gross findings are those of interstitial pneumonia and histologically there is alveolar edema, alveolar cell proliferation and the presence of inclusion of bodies. In bovine respiratory syncytial virus infection there is acute bronchiolitis and alveolitis, and eosinophilic intracytoplasmic inclusion bodies in bronchiolar and alveolar cells (3, 11). There are also multinucleate giant cell syncytia in the alveoli. There may be evidence of secondary bacterial pneumonia.

Broad-spectrum antibodies given daily for 3–5 days for secondary bacterial pneumonia are usually indicated. Recovery usually occurs gradually over a period of 3–5 days. Severely affected animals will become worse in spite of therapy.

Control depends on minimizing the stressors associated with bovine respiratory disease in young cattle.

REFERENCES

(1) Bartha, A. & Koves, B. (1976) *Acta vet. Hung.*, *25*, 349.
(2) Welch, D. C. & Dellers, R. W. (1973) *J. Am. vet. med. Assoc.*, *163*, 741.
(3) Bryson, D. G. & McFerran, J. B. (1978) *Vet. Rec.*, *102*, 45.
(4) Holzhauer, C. (1978) *Curr. Top. vet. Med.*, *3*, 216.
(5) Bohlendar, R. E. et al. (1982) *Mod. vet. Pract.*, *63*, 613.
(6) Frey, M. L. (1983) *Bov. Pract.*, *18*, 73.
(7) Stott, E. J. et al. (1980) *J. Hyg., Camb.*, *85*, 257.
(8) Martin, S. W. & Bohac, J. G. (1986) *Can. J. vet. Res.*, *50*, 351.
(9) Baker, J. C. et al. (1986) *Am. J. vet. Res.*, *47*, 246.
(10) Castleman, W. L. et al. (1985) *Cornell Vet.*, *75*, 473.
(11) Thomas, L. H. & Stott, E. J. (1981) *Vet. Rec.*, *108*, 432.
(12) Barker, J. C. (1986) *Comp. Cont. educ. Pract. Vet.*, *8*, F31.
(13) Elazhary, M. A. S. Y. et al. (1981) *Am. J. vet. Res. 42*, 1378.

Infectious bovine rhinotracheitis (red nose)

Infectious bovine rhinotracheitis (IBR), or bovine herpesvirus 1 infection, is a highly infectious disease caused by a virus. Rhinotracheitis, conjunctivitis, fever and a short course with a high recovery rate is the most commonly observed syndrome. Encephalitis, the systemic form of the disease in newborn calves and infectious pustular vulvovaginitis (IPV) are other syndromes also all caused by the same virus.

Etiology

An alphaherpesvirus known as *bovid herpesvirus* 1 (1) has been isolated from affected animals and is capable of growth on tissue culture and of producing the respiratory disease (2), abortion, and conjunctivitis and, after intracerebral inoculation, encephalitis. Minor strain differences occur but do not clearly offer an explanation for the diverse epidemiological and pathological patterns of behavior of this herpesvirus.

The virus of infectious bovine rhinotracheitis is similar to the virus of infectious pustular vulvovaginitis (IPV) of cows and balanoposthitis of bulls. Manifestations which occur suggest that strains with differing tissue affinities may exist in the field, and slight differences can be detected by immunological and biochemical means (1). Only rarely do the respiratory and genital forms of the disease occur together. However, by routine methodology it is difficult and usually impossible to distinguish between isolates obtained from the reproductive tract and the respiratory mucosa. Likewise, with the exception of temperature-sensitive mutants, vaccine strains cannot be distinguished from field isolates (2). Using DNA restriction endonuclease and polyacrylamide gel electrophoresis (PAGE) it is now possible to compare the antigenic differences between isolates obtained from different clinical syndromes and tissues (6). Five major biotypes of herpesvirus of cattle have been defined in the United States, one of which is the IBR-IPV virus (BHV 1) (8).

Epidemiology

All ages and breeds of cattle are susceptible on experimental challenge, but the disease occurs naturally mostly in animals over 6 months of age, probably because of their greater exposure. There is no seasonal variation in incidence, except possibly a higher occurrence in feedlot cattle in the fall and winter months when large numbers of susceptible animals are assembled. Although seldom reported, the disease can affect swine naturally in both the respiratory and genital form (2). Mule deer are susceptible to infection, the disease has occurred naturally in a goat (2), and antibodies to the virus have been found in pronghorn antelope in western Canada (9), and in Tanzania in game animals and cattle (1). Based on serological surveys the virus is widespread in African wildlife, particularly the buffalo which may play an important role in the maintenance of the infection among the wildlife population (4). The virus has been recovered from the wildebeeste in Africa (11), all of which may suggest that wildlife may serve as reservoirs for the virus.

There is epidemiological evidence that the virulence of the virus or its host tissue specificity changes due to unknown factors. It has been suggested that the infectious pustular vulvovaginitis virus was carried to North America from Europe in infected cattle, but continued to cause lesions in only the genital tract until its introduction into dense populations of cattle in feedlots encouraged rapid passage through many hosts and thus encouraged adaptation to the respiratory tract (5). The sudden occurrence of outbreaks of infectious bovine rhinotracheitis in countries where previously mild disease occurred may be due to the importation of cattle infected with a virulent strain of the virus or the emergence of a more virulent strain following mutation of a domestic strain (5).

A comparison of the virulence of three strains of the virus indicate that the recent epidemic of severe respiratory disease in Britain was the result of the importation of a new strain of the virus (5). The Colorado and

Strichen strains produced the characteristic clinical signs, whereas the Oxford strain produced a mild clinical response with minimal pathological lesions (5). Restriction endonuclease DNA fingerprints of herpesviruses isolated from unrelated epidemics of bovine encephalitis have revealed that they are similar to each other and totally different from bovine herpesvirus 1 and other ruminant herpesviruses (17). A BHV 1 type 3 has been isolated from naturally occurring cases of non-suppurative meningoencephalitis in calves (81).

Infectious bovine rhinotracheitis has been identified in the United States (2), Australia (12), the United Kingdom (6), Canada (7), New Zealand, South Africa and Zimbabwe, and Europe. The disease occurs most commonly in large groups of cattle confined in feedlots and dairy farms. In beef herds in northern Australia up to 96% of bulls and 52% of cows have serological evidence of infection (13), presumably venereal since respiratory infectious bovine rhinotracheitis is uncommon in cattle on extensive range conditions. The genital carrier state is considered to be an important factor in the maintenance of venereal IBR virus and in the occurrence of sporadic vulvovaginitis (IPV) and infectious pustular balanoposthitis in these herds (14).

The disease is not highly fatal, losses are due mainly to secondary bacterial bronchopneumonia, abortion, loss of newborn calves and a temporary reduction in body condition and milk yield. The morbidity and case fatality rates in dairy cattle are about 8% and 3% respectively while in feedlot cattle the morbidity rate is usually 20–30% in unvaccinated cattle and may rarely reach 100%. The case fatality rate in feedlot cattle is invariably due to secondary bacterial tracheitis and bronchopneumonia and may reach 10%, but is usually no more than 1%. Morbidity and mortality are higher in feedlot cattle than in dairy herds because of the frequent introduction of susceptible animals into an enzootic situation.

The main sources of infection are the nasal exudate and coughed-up droplets, genital secretions, semen and fetal fluids and tissues. Aerosol infection is considered to be the method of spread of the respiratory disease; venereal transmission is the method of spread of the genital diseases. The infectious bovine rhinotracheitis virus may survive for up to 1 year in semen frozen at −196°C (−321°F) (16). Introduction of animals into a group often precedes an outbreak of the disease. However, it can arise simultaneously in a number of dairy farms in an area and spread from these to adjacent farms until the entire area is affected. The same pattern of occurrence simultaneously in a number of foci is seen in feedlots, and from these foci infection spreads to other pens in the lot. An outbreak usually reaches its peak in the 2nd or 3rd week and ends by the 4th–6th week.

One of the remarkable features of the BHV 1 is its ability to become latent following primary infection with a mild strain of the virus or following vaccination with an attenuated strain (3). The virus may remain latent indefinitely and recrudescence, reactivation and shedding of the virus may be achieved by the use of large doses of corticosteroids which mimic the effects of stress (2, 3). Attenuated vaccine strains can remain in a latent stage and vaccination with attenuated strains does not provide protection against the establishment of latent infection with a wild strain. Vaccination also does not inhibit re-excretion of a wild strain which was in the latent form at the time of vaccination (3). The vaccine virus and the field strain of the virus can be excreted after live virus vaccination and subsequent field virus challenge (42).

The actual site of latency of BHV 1 is not yet known but the latent virus remains localized near the site of its first multiplication and during recrudescence will be re-excreted by the tissue primarily infected. The BHV 1 can be isolated from the trigeminal ganglion of clinically normal cattle during the latent period, and trigeminal ganglionitis can be observed during recrudescence.

Latent infection with virulent BHV 1 virus may occur in the trigeminal ganglion of calves previously vaccinated with the modified live vaccine (25). The virulent virus may spread along the trigeminal peripheral nerve despite the presence of humoral antibodies in vaccinated calves. Recrudescence of the virus from the trigeminal ganglion and spread along the peripheral nerves by intra-axonal flow to the nasal mucosa can occur in calves treated with corticosteroids and presumably may occur following stress (25). The virus has been isolated from the trigeminal ganglia of 10% of clinically normal cattle at slaughter, 40% of which had serum neutralization antibody to the virus (2).

The practical significance of these findings is that all cattle from endemic herds or areas must be considered as potential sources of BHV 1 virus and capable of spreading infection to previously unexposed animals (42). A combined serological and clinical surveillance of 20 dairy herds over 3 consecutive years revealed wide variations in the circulation of the virus (84). In some herds there was no identification of active infection while in others one or two cycles of infection occurred in calves and yearlings, often without any clinical evidence of disease (84). Reactivation and shedding of the BHV 1 can occur in known carrier bulls at the time of mating (18) which may explain the higher incidence of titers in bulls than cows in some beef herds. Breeding bulls in an artificial insemination center which were vaccinated with a modified-like BHV 1 vaccine were found to shed the vaccine virus in the semen and the virus could be recovered from preputial washings (66) 2–3 months after the last immunization. However, the frequency of recurrent infections and the amount of virus excreted are reduced after vaccination. Parturition may also be a stimulus for reactivation and shedding of a thermosensitive vaccine strain of the virus in vaccinated animals (19). Reactivation and shedding of the virus has also been observed in cattle which recovered from the respiratory form of the disease and 5 months later were experimentally infected with *Dictyocaulus viviparus* (57). The placenta may harbor the virus in a latent stage for up to 90 days without transmitting the virus to the fetus. Recrudescence may be differentiated from primary infection and reexposure by the intranasal route based on the distribution of antiviral antibody activity among serum IgM, IgG_1, and IgG_2 isotypes (56).

Immunity to infectious bovine rhinotracheitis is complex and consists of relationships between local and systemic antibody and cell-mediated immunity. Following natural infection or vaccination with the modified live virus vaccines, both cell-mediated and humoral components of the immune system are activated. The level of humoral immunity has been used as an indicator of previous infection and an indirect measure of resistance to clinical disease. However, the level of serum neutralizing antibody is not a reliable indicator of resistance to clinical respiratory disease. Animals with low levels of antibody may be immune because of cell-mediated immunity. Following intranasal infection or the use of a modified live infectious bovine rhinotracheitis virus vaccine intranasally, local secretory antibody and interferon are produced (15). The interferon appears in 3 days and persists for 10 days. The presence of the interferon does not protect calves against experimental challenge 3 days after vaccination (15). However, the presence of even low levels of antibody in the serum or nasal secretion, which appears by day 7 following vaccination, does provide varying degrees of resistance to clinical disease for 9 months (15).

Calves acquire colostral antibodies from dams with humoral antibody. The duration of the colostral immunity varies from 1 to 6 months of age and is dependent on the initial level transferred to the calf. The presence of maternal antibody in the calf may interfere with the successful vaccination of calves before 6 months of age.

Pathogenesis

In the respiratory disease the virus multiplies in the nasal cavities and upper respiratory tract resulting in rhinitis, laryngitis and tracheitis. There is extensive loss of cilia in the trachea leaving the tracheal epithelium covered by microvilli (20). Intratracheal administration of the virus results in almost complete denudation of tracheal columnar cells which presumably has an adverse effect on the defense mechanisms of the respiratory tract (26). The virus causes varying degrees of obstructive lung disease resulting in increased resistance to breathing, retention of carbon dioxide and increased resting lung volume (21). A severe fatal infectious bovine rhinotracheitis virus pneumonia can occur (28). Spread from the nasal cavities to the ocular tissues probably occurs by way of the lacrimal ducts and causes conjunctivitis with edema and swelling of the conjunctiva, multifocal plaque formation on the conjunctivae, and peripheral corneal edema and deep vascularization (22). Spread from the nasal mucosa via the trigeminal peripheral nerve to the trigeminal ganglion may occur resulting in a non-suppurative encephalitis (1). Intranasal inoculation of young calves and adult cows with the BHV 1 can result in non-fatal trigeminal ganglionitis and encephalitis which may be an important mechanism for latent infection (48).

Systemic invasion by the virus is followed by localization of the virus in several different tissues. The virus may be transported by peripheral leukocytes to the placenta and transferred to the fetus to cause abortion (23). The fetus is highly susceptible to the infectious bovine rhinotracheitis virus and experiences a peracute infection which is usually fatal. There is a report in which 78% of a group of 200 pregnant heifers aborted between the 5th and 9th month of pregnancy (61). Recently hatched bovine embryos can be infected with any of several strains of BHV 1 and such infection *in vitro* is embryocidal (62). Infection in the last trimester of gestation may result in mummification, abortion, stillbirth, or weak calves with the usual lesions of infectious bovine rhinotracheitis as well as the lesions of the stomachs and intestines which have been produced by experimental administration of the virulent virus to newborn calves (29). The systemic form of the infection in newborn calves is characterized by severe inflammation and necrosis of the respiratory and alimentary tracts, including the pharynx, esophagus, lungs, larynx, lymph nodes, liver, and nephritis and encephalitis (24, 59). There is severe laryngeal edema and respiratory distress which results in difficulty in swallowing and aspiration pneumonia. A severe highly fatal syndrome characterized by diffuse erosion and ulceration of the upper alimentary tract including the oral cavity has occurred in beef feedlot cattle (8).

The rabbit (30) and the English ferret (39) are good laboratory animals for the study of experimental infection with the infectious bovine rhinotracheitis virus.

The role of the BHV 1 in affecting the lung clearance mechanism of cattle in the pathogenesis of pneumonic pasteurellosis has been reviewed (60) and is presented in the section on shipping fever pneumonia in cattle. Experimental aerosol exposure of calves with the BHV 1 virus can impair the function of alveolar macrophages which allows *Pasteurella hemolytica* to persist and proliferate in the lung and produce the characteristic lesion.

The intranasal administration of an avirulent vaccine virus results in peak levels of local interferon in 3–4 days and local nasal and serum antibody in 7 days. The interferon is not, however, effective against the infectious bovine rhinotracheitis virus in cell cultures (15). A local and serum antibody and the cell-mediated immunity are considered to be important in resistance to clinical disease. Earlier work (27) indicated that the production of nasal interferon was responsible for the resistance to challenge exposure 60–72 hours after vaccination with an intranasal vaccine.

The intrauterine inoculation of the BHV 1 into cattle results in an acute necrotizing endometritis in the uterine body and caudal portions of the uterine horns but minimal lesions in the anterior parts of the horns (63). Experimental inoculation of the virus into heifers on the day after estrus and insemination can result in lesions of the ovaries consisting of focal necrosis and cellular infiltration (64). Commercially available vaccinal strains of the BHV 1 virus can produce similar lesions (65). The ovarian lesions have marked effects on luteal function and plasma progesterone values in the first estrus after inoculation are markedly lower than those in subsequent normal cycles. Whether the BHV 1 virus causes reproductive failure as a result of necrosis of the corpus luteum or embryonic infection remains to be determined. Experimentally induced infection during early pregnancy (7–28 days) will cause oophoritis and in some cases embryonic mortality (83).

The effects of the virus on the genital tract and on reproductive performance in cattle has been reviewed (1, 2).

Clinical findings

After experimental infection there is an incubation period of 3–7 days (2), but in infected feedlots the disease occurs 10–20 days after the introduction of susceptible cattle. A longer incubation period has been recorded by some authors.

There is considerable variation in the severity of clinical signs following natural infection with the infectious bovine rhinotracheitis virus. Presumably this is dependent upon the strain of the virus, the age susceptibility and environmental factors (5). In North America where the disease is endemic, the clinical disease is usually mild in dairy cattle and in range cattle. A severe form of the disease can occur in feedlots where crowding and comingling from several sources occur.

There is sudden onset of severe signs including anorexia, fever (up to 42°C, 108°F), severe hyperemia of the nasal mucosa with numerous clusters of grayish foci of necrosis on the mucous membranes of the nasal septum visible just inside the external nares, a serous discharge from the eyes and nose, increased salivation and a degree of hyperexcitability. A drastic fall in milk yield may be the earliest sign in dairy cattle. The respirations are increased in rate and are shallow, but the lungs are normal on auscultation. Respiratory distress is evident on exercise. A short, explosive cough has been characteristic of some outbreaks but is not recorded in others. Sudden death within 24 hours after first signs appear can result from extensive obstructive bronchiolitis (28).

In dairy cattle, in which the disease assumes its mildest form, signs may not increase beyond this stage, the temperature returning to normal in a day or two and recovery being complete in 10–14 days. In feeder cattle the illness is often more prolonged, the febrile period is longer, the nasal discharge becomes more profuse and purulent, and the convalescent period is longer. Some deaths may occur in the acute febrile period, but most fatalities are due to a secondary bronchopneumonia and occur after a prolonged illness of up to 4 months in which severe dyspnea, complete anorexia and final recumbency are obvious signs. Some recovered cows have a persistent snoring respiration and a grossly thickened, rough nasal mucosa accompanied by nasal discharge (18).

Conjunctivitis is a common but not constant sign and, in some outbreaks of infectious bovine rhinotracheitis, is the only sign of abnormality (22). It may affect one or both eyes and is easily mistaken for infectious keratoconjunctivitis caused by *Moraxella bovis*. However, the lesions are confined to the conjunctiva and there is no invasion of the cornea. Thus, the conjunctiva is red and swollen, there is profuse, primarily serous, ocular discharge but no corneal ulceration, but there may be corneal edema which may last for a few days. Calves less than 6 months of age may develop encephalitis, which is marked by incoordination, excitement alternating with depression and a high mortality rate. Salivation, bellowing, convulsions and blindness are also recorded (1).

In newborn calves, the systemic form of the disease is severe and highly fatal (24, 59). Clinical findings include sudden anorexia, fever, excessive salivation and rhinitis often accompanied by unilateral or bilateral conjunctivitis. The oral mucous membranes are usually hyperemic, erosions of the soft palate covered by tenacious mucus are common, and an acute pharyngitis covered by tenacious mucopurulent exudate is characteristic. The larynx is usually edematous and respiratory distress is common. Bronchopneumonia is also common and loud breath sounds, crackles and wheezes associated with consolidation and pulmonary edema are common. Outbreaks of the disease may occur in newborn calves in susceptible herds where the herd immunity has declined, the dams are not vaccinated and there is minimal if any specific colostral immunity. Some affected calves will have diarrhea and moderate dehydration which has been referred to as the alimentary form of BHV 1 infection. The cause of the diarrhea is uncertain but it may be related to the ruminal lesions.

Abortion is a common sequel and occurs some weeks after the clinical illness or vaccination of non-immune pregnant cows with the modified live-virus vaccine of bovine tissue culture origin. Abortion may occur as long as 90 days following vaccination if the virus becomes latent in the placenta and infects the fetus much later than usual (19). This raises the possibility that vaccination even with the safe vaccine may appear to be the cause of abortion if natural infection preceded vaccination. It is most common in cows which are 6–8 months pregnant. Retention of the placenta often follows, but residual infertility is unimportant. However, endometritis, poor conception and short estrus can occur after insemination with infected semen (31). The infectious bovine rhinotracheitis virus has been isolated from semen 12 months after storage.

Clinical pathology

Isolation of the virus from nasal swabs using tissue culture combined with a rise in antibody titers between acute and convalescent phase sera are desirable for positive diagnosis of the disease. Cotton and polyester swabs are recommended rather than calcium alginate swabs which are viricidal within 2 hours (32). A modified nasopharyngeal swab with nylon bristles has certain advantages for sampling the bovine respiratory tract for viruses when compared with the cotton-tipped swab (29). The virus can be detected in nasal swabs by the use of an enzyme-linked immunosorbent assay (ELISA) test (10), direct and indirect immunofluorescence techniques (33, 34) immunoperoxidase (35) and by electron microscopic examination which may reveal herpes-like viral particles (1). The sensitivity of the direct immunofluorescence techniques is comparable to the cell culture technique (33). The ELISA is considered to be highly sensitive (10). A combination of the indirect immunofluorescence test and virus isolation from both ocular and nasal swabs of several animals will increase the recovery rate (34). In experimentally infected calves virus isolation in cell culture was the most sensitive and successful for up to 11 days after inoculation. The direct immunofluorescence test, the immunoperoxidase test and the ELISA test were highly sensitive during the pyrexic phase but less reliable in the later stages of the disease (35).

Several serological tests are available for the detection of antibody and a rise in titer between the acute and convalescent phases of the infection. The virus neutralization (VN) test has been widely used and is the standard by which other techniques have been evaluated. An evaluation of five serological tests for the detection of antibody to BHV 1 in vaccinated and experimentally infected animals indicated a high correlation between the ELISA test, the indirect or passive hemagglutination test and the virus neutralization test (36). The sensitivities of ELISA and the 24-hour neutralization tests were similar in contrast to passive hemagglutination and 1 hour neutralization which failed to detect BHV 1 antibodies in some low titer sera. The ELISA is a specific, sensitive and practical test for detection of BHV 1 antibodies and has advantages over the serum neutralization test (67, 68). A micro-ELISA test is being used for the control program of BHV 1 infection in Switzerland (70). The test is simple, rapid and convenient compared to the serum neutralization test which requires cell culture facilities and is time-consuming.

The primary immune response to BHV 1 experimental inoculation of cattle is characterized by the formation of IgM and IgG antibodies, primarily IgG_1, by postinoculation day 7. Secondary immune responses are characterized primarily by the formation of IgG_2 antibody. A secondary immune response resulting from abortion induced by intra-amniotic virus inoculation is characterized by a substantial increase in IgM antibody. A secondary BHV 1 exposure by the intranasal route does not result in secondary IgM antibody formation (40). Thus the serologic diagnosis of BHV 1 infection is possible without the acute and convalescent phase serum samples which traditionally have been used to demonstrate seroconversion.

Specific antibody against BHV 1 may be detectable in fetal fluids and increases the rate of diagnosis of abortion (37).

Using restriction endonuclease analysis of viral DNA it is now possible to distinguish field isolates of the virus from vaccine strains which may be useful in the investigation of vaccine-induced epidemics of the disease (82).

A definitive etiological diagnosis of infectious bovine rhinotracheitis is difficult and has created serious problems for those concerned with an exact diagnosis. Following infection with the infectious bovine rhinotracheitis/infectious pustular vulvovaginitis virus the development of serum neutralizing antibodies may be slow (up to 18 days) and the duration of demonstrable titer is extremely variable between animals thus making serum antibody titers an unreliable method of diagnosis (38) when used alone. A definitive diagnosis can be made only by combining clinical findings with serological results and the isolation of the virus. Isolation of the virus from semen requires special laboratory techniques (69).

Necropsy findings

Gross lesions are restricted to the muzzle, nasal cavities, pharynx, larynx and trachea, and terminate in the large bronchi. There may be pulmonary emphysema or secondary bronchopneumonia, but for the most part the lungs are normal. In the upper respiratory tract there are variable degrees of inflammation, but the lesions are essentially the same in all anatomical regions. In mild cases there is swelling and congestion of the mucosae, petechiae may be present and there is a moderate amount of catarrhal exudate. In severe cases the inflammation is more severe and the exudate is profuse and fibrinopurulent. When the exudate is removed, the mucosa is intact except for small numbers of necrotic foci in the nasal mucosa and diffuse denudation of epithelium in the upper part of the trachea. Lymph nodes in the throat and neck region are usually swollen and edematous. Histologically there is acute, catarrhal inflammation of the mucosa. Inclusion bodies are not recorded in natural cases but do occur transiently in respiratory epithelial cells in experimentally infected animals. Secondary bacterial invasion will cause a more severe necrotic reaction which is usually followed by the development of bronchopneumonia.

In the systemic form in neonatal calves a severe epithelial necrosis has been observed in the esophagus and rumen, the adherent necrotic epithelium having the pultaceous quality of milk curd. The laryngeal mucosa is congested and edematous with multiple focal lesions in the mucosa (59). Bronchopneumonia is common with milk-like material which coats the tracheal lumen and extends into the bronchial lumen. Histologically, there is necrosis of the pharynx, larynx, associated lymph nodes, esophagus and liver (24). Inclusion bodies were evident in many surviving epithelial cells (24).

Aborted fetuses show moderately severe autolysis and focal necrotizing hepatitis (2). The encephalitis is characterized by typical viral lesions located particularly in the cerebral cortex and the internal capsule (1).

Diagnosis

Acute rhinotracheitis with characteristic nasal lesions, bilateral conjunctivitis, fever and a gradual recovery in a few days should suggest the respiratory form of infectious bovine rhinotracheitis. In pneumonic pasteurellosis there is toxemia, lung involvement and a good response to therapy. In bovine virus diarrhea and bovine malignant catarrh there are erosive lesions in the oral cavity in addition to those in the nares. The alimentary tract form of the disease in calves in which there are oral lesions may present problems in differentiation from the viral diseases of the alimentary tract of cattle. Calf diphtheria may resemble infectious bovine rhinotracheitis because of the inspiratory dyspnea, but the oral and laryngeal lesions and the severe toxemia are typical. In viral pneumonia of calves and shipping fever there is obvious pulmonary involvement, while in bovine malignant catarrh and the mucosal diseases lesions in the digestive tract are evident. Allergic rhinitis may resemble infectious bovine rhinotracheitis but is characterized by sneezing and wheezing with inspiratory dyspnea, the temperature is usually normal and the nasal discharge is characteristically thickened, sometimes caseous and greenish-orange in color. In infectious bovine rhinotracheitis the nasal discharge is copious, serous to mucopurulent, and discrete lesions are commonly present on the nasal septum. A summary of the differential diagnosis of bovine respiratory disease appears in Table 53.

Treatment

Although they are unlikely to have any effect on the virus, broad-spectrum antibiotics should be administered to avoid losses caused by secondary bacterial invaders. Affected cattle should be identified, isolated and monitored frequently for evidence of secondary bacterial tracheitis and pneumonia accompanied by anorexia and toxemia and treated accordingly. The tracheitis is particularly difficult to treat; antibiotics daily for several days are necessary and often slaughter for salvage is the most economical course.

Control

The methods and vaccines available for the effective control of IBR have not been entirely satisfactory. The disease may occur unpredictably at any time and even closed herds with no introductions may remain free of the disease for several years and suddenly experience an acute outbreak. Eradication of the bovine herpesvirus 1 virus from a single herd or the cattle population in a country can be considered as an alternative to vaccination. In a preliminary study in one closed beef herd in which there was latent BHV 1 infection, following weaning the calves were raised in isolation separate from the cows. All of the maternally derived BHV 1 titers in the calves decayed to zero at weaning time and remained seronegative while raised in isolation (71). Serologically positive animals are removed or culled and only seronegative animals introduced into the herd.

Switzerland has declared BHV 1 virus infection as a notifiable disease and has begun a control program which prohibits the use of vaccination and identifies and culls infected animals (70).

The alternative to an eradication program is control of the infection by the development of immunity following natural exposure or vaccination. Cattle which have recovered from a natural infection with the BHV 1 virus are protected against clinical disease after experimental infection with a virulent virus.

Based on the effectiveness of active immunization following natural exposure, vaccines have been available for the control of the disease. Modified live-virus and inactivated vaccines have been available. There are two types of modified live-virus vaccines. One is the intramuscular vaccine, made usually with bovine fetal kidney tissue culture, and the other is an intranasal vaccine of rabbit tissue culture origin (27). An intranasal vaccines of bovine tissue culture origin containing a temperature-sensitive mutant is also available (52).

Both vaccines stimulate the production of humoral antibody, the intranasal vaccine stimulates the production of local interferon and local antibody in the nasal and mucous membranes and is safe for use in pregnant cows. The intranasal vaccine is very effective for the prevention of abortion due to infectious bovine rhinotracheitis (54). The intramuscular vaccine of bovine origin can be abortigenic, especially in non-immune cows (41). The intranasal vaccine provides protection against respiratory disease induced by experimental challenge 72 hours after vaccination (27). Such rapid protection is attributed to the production of local interferon but no direct proof for this is available. *In vitro* studies have shown that the interferon stimulated by the intranasal infectious bovine rhinotracheitis vaccine is not effective against the disease (15). The vaccinated calves were not resistant to challenge 3 days after vaccination, but were resistant 3 weeks, 3 months or 9 months after intranasal vaccination (15). Thus, there are some conflicting results with respect to the degree of protection present 3 days after intranasal vaccination. Based on experimental work the advantages of the intranasal vaccine are that it can be used safely in pregnant cattle and it provides rapid and effective protection against the respiratory form of the disease. Immunity to infectious bovine rhinotracheitis is not well understood and a combination of humoral, local and cell-mediated immunity may be operative. However, there appears to be sufficient data to support the claim that modified live-virus vaccines provide immunity if properly used (2). The intranasal vaccines have been used in the face of an outbreak in an attempt to reduce the number of new cases. The vaccine produces almost no systemic reaction and all in-contact animals in an outbreak can be safely vaccinated (7).

A major requirement of the intranasal vaccine is that the vaccine virus must multiply on the nasal mucous membranes. If the vaccine is not administrated into the nasal cavities carefully or if the animal is difficult to handle or sneezes out the vaccine, vaccination will not occur. The careful administration of a temperature-sensitive vaccine in 2 ml of diluent into one nostril is as effective as a two-nostril vaccination method using a total of 5 ml of diluent (80). The pre-existence of some local antibody from natural exposure or coinfection with a virulent strain of the virus may also restrict the multiplication of the vaccine virus, especially the temperature-sensitive mutants (77).

An intranasal IBR vaccine containing a modified live-virus strain whose growth is restricted to the upper respiratory tract has been developed in Europe. The vaccine strain is chemically treated to produce a temperature-sensitive (TS) characteristic, so that it cannot replicate at the body temperature of the animal (52). The vaccine is efficacious and safe for use in pregnant cattle. Intranasal vaccination with a temperature-sensitive infectious bovine rhinotracheitis virus vaccine stimulates both systemic and local cell-mediated immunity and antibody. The intramuscular vaccine stimulates leukocytes in the nasal mucosa to produce a local antibody response and inhibit infectious bovine rhinotracheitis viral cytopathological changes (53).

There is some concern that vaccinated calves may shed the vaccine virus which could spread to pregnant cattle resulting in abortion (44). Calves vaccinated with a live temperature-sensitive mutant of infectious bovine rhinotracheitis virus vaccine were protected against clinical illness from experimental challenge, but excreted the virus 2 months later following treatment with corticosteroid (42). This emphasizes the general principle that the use of a modified live-virus vaccine implies a continuing commitment to vaccination which may reduce the incidence of disease but is unlikely to eradicate the infection (42). However, the development of subunit vaccines may alleviate shedding problems. Subunit vaccines do not contain live virus, are very effective experimentally and could be used in young calves with colostral antibody (55). However, some work has shown subunit vaccines did not protect calves against experimental respiratory disease. The results indicate that the calves were in a refractory state when immunized

(46) and may explain why similar vaccine failures occur in the field. In some cases there is minimal or no detectable evidence of seroconversion following vaccination and the calves are not protected against natural or experimental infection.

Inactivated vaccines are generally ineffective (73) unless prepared with an adjuvant (72).

Both the aerosol and intramuscular administration of a virulent strain of infectious bovine rhinotracheitis virus to colostrum-deprived seronegative cattle (6–12 months of age) results in comparable levels of serum antibody but no measurable nasal secretory antibody (45). When these same cattle are challenged later by aerosol exposure they are protected from clinical disease and nasal secretory antibodies will develop.

The justification for the use of infectious bovine rhinotracheitis vaccine is based on the following: the virus is ubiquitous and the occurrence of the disease unpredictable, and economic losses from abortion, neonatal disease and respiratory disease can be high; colostral immunity in calves wanes by 4–6 months of age; the vaccine will prevent abortions due to the infectious bovine rhinotracheitis virus and provide protection against respiratory disease if given at least 10 days before natural exposure.

Beef calves should be vaccinated 2–3 weeks before weaning as part of a preweaning preconditioning program (2). Calves vaccinated with the intramuscular modified live-virus vaccine before colostral infectious bovine rhinotracheitis antibody titers reached low levels do not develop an immediate, active serological response, as indicated by serological titers, but are sensitized to the infectious bovine rhinotracheitis virus. Revaccination at a later date when maternal antibodies have decreased to undetectable levels results in a marked serological response (43). Heifer and bull replacements are vaccinated at least 2 weeks before breeding. When outbreaks of the disease occur in unvaccinated beef herds all cattle in the herd may be vaccinated with the intranasal vaccine. Whether or nor beef herds should be vaccinated annually following the initial vaccination is uncertain. There are field reports of outbreaks of abortion due to infectious bovine rhinotracheitis in beef cattle which were vaccinated 3 years previously, which suggests that revaccination of breeding females every 2 years may be indicated. Since both natural infection and vaccination results in latent infection it may be that the persistence of the virus combined with natural exposure may result in persistence of antibody. There is an urgent need for some long-term immunological studies to determine the length of protective immunity following vaccination. Antibodies last for at least 5½ years in heifers following experimental infection and complete isolation during that time (47).

Feeder cattle should be vaccinated at least 10 days before being placed in the lot, especially one in which the disease may be enzootic (48). If this is not done a high incidence of infectious bovine rhinotracheitis may occur in recent arrivals. If vaccination before arrival is not possible, the next best procedure is to vaccinate the cattle on arrival and place them in an isolation starting pen for 7–10 days during which time immunity will develop.

A field trial of preshipment vaccination of cattle with a combination BHV 1 and PI-3 vaccine administered intranasally 3 weeks before shipment from western Canada to Ontario did not have a significant effect on treatment rates of the animals for pneumonia after their arrival in the feedlot (74). The vaccination trial was designed to examine the hypothesis that vaccination with a BHV 1 virus vaccine prior to the stress of shipment would decrease the incidence of bovine respiratory disease. Vaccination of cattle with the BHV 1 virus vaccine prior to experimental induction of pneumonic pasteurellosis with an aerosol BHV 1 virus followed later by an aerosol of *Past. hemolytica* will provide protection against the bacterial pneumonia (75). A commercially available modified live-virus intranasal vaccine has been used in a group of veal calves (76). There was no significant difference between vaccinated and non-vaccinated animals in terms of liveweight gains and incidence rate of subclinical disease.

The necessity of vaccinating dairy cattle will depend on the prevalence of the disease in the area and in the herd and the movement of cattle in and out of the herd. A closed herd may remain free of infectious bovine rhinotracheitis indefinitely and vaccination may not be indicated. But to avoid unpredictable abortion storms due to infectious bovine rhinotracheitis in dairy herds, heifer replacements should be vaccinated for the disease 2–3 weeks before breeding. Vaccination of a large dairy herd with a persistent infectious bovine rhinotracheitis problem was successful in controlling the disease (49). The intranasal vaccine has been used extensively in newborn calves in problem herds but its efficacy at such an age is unknown. If the disease poses a threat to a potential calf crop, the pregnant cows could be vaccinated with the intranasal vaccine in late pregnancy; this will increase the level of colostral antibody available to the newborn calf (54) and will provide newborn calves with protection against the highly fatal systemic form of the disease (85).

Bulls intended for use in artificial insemination centers present a special problem of disease control because the virus in semen can have severe consequences on reproductive performance (31). Bulls which are seropositive to infectious bovine rhinotracheitis must be considered as carriers and potential shedders of the virus and should not be allowed entry to these centers. Not all bulls which are seronegative can necessarily be considered free of the virus and regular attempts at the isolation of the virus must be made from preputial washings and semen. Bulls which become infected while at the centers should be kept isolated and culled and replaced with clean bulls (50). Bulls from herds which routinely vaccinate for infectious bovine rhinotracheitis should not be vaccinated if destined for an AI center. Cattle destined for export should not be vaccinated in case importing countries prohibit the introduction of seropositive cattle (51). This will not guarantee that such animals will not become positive from natural infection.

Some preliminary results indicate that the administration of human leukocyte A interferon daily for 1 week and inoculated with the BHV 1 virus on the first day of interferon treatment reduced the severity of clinical disease (78). Production of disease was considered dependent on the amount of virus and interferon given, since calves given a large inoculum of virus and a reduced amount of interferon were not protected against infection. The intranasal administration of interferon into calves 48 hours before exposure to an aerosol of BHV 1 virus provided some protection against the experimentally induced pneumonic pasteurellosis (79).

REVIEW LITERATURE

Gibbs, E. P. J. & Reweyemamu, M. M. (1977) Bovine herpesvirus. Part I, Bovine herpesvirus I. *Vet. Bull.*, *47*, 317.

Kahrs, R. F. (1977) Infectious bovine rhinotracheitis: a review and update. *J. Am. vet. med. Assoc.*, *171*, 1055.

Pastoret, P. P., Thiry, E., Borchier, B. & Derboven, G. (1982) Bovid herpes virus-1 infection of cattle: pathogenesis, latency, consequences of latency. *Ann. rech. vét.*, 13, 221–235.

Wittman, G., Gaskell, R. M. & Rziha, H. J. (1984) *Latent Herpesvirus in Veterinary Medicine*. Boston, The Hague, Dordrecht, Lancaster: Martinus Nijhoff.

Yates, W. D. G. (1982) A review of infectious bovine rhinotracheitis, shipping fever pneumonia and viral-bacterial synergism in respiratory diseases of cattle. *Can. J. comp. Med.*, *46*, 225–263.

REFERENCES

(1) Gibbs, E. P. J. & Rweyemamu, M. M. (1977) *Vet. Bull.*, *47*, 317.
(2) Kahrs, R. F. (1977) *J. Am. vet. Assoc.*, *171*, 1055.
(3) Pastoret, P. P. et al. (1982) *Ann. rech. vét.*, *13*, 221.
(4) Hedger, R. S. & Hamblin, C. (1978) *J. comp. Pathol.*, *88*, 211.
(5) Msolla, P. M. et al. (1983) *Vet. Microbiol.*, *8*, 129.
(6) Misra, V. et al. (1983) *Arch. Virol.*, *76*, 341.
(7) Janzen, E. D. et al. (1980) *Can. vet. J.*, *21*, 24.
(8) Osorio, F. A. et al. (1985) *Am. J. vet. Res.*, *46*, 2104.
(9) Barrett, M. W. et al. (1975) *J. Wildlife Dis.*, *11*, 157.
(10) Collins, J. K. et al. (1985) *J. clin. Microbiol.*, *21*, 375.
(11) Karstad, L. et al. (1974) *J. Wildlife Dis.*, *10*, 392.
(12) Rogers, R. J. et al. (1980) *Aust. vet. J.*, *56*, 147.
(13) Zyambo, G. C. N. et al. (1973) *Aust. vet. J.*, *49*, 413.
(14) Bennett, D. P. et al. (1976) *Res. vet. Sci.*, *20*, 77.
(15) Savan, M. et al. (1979) *Can. vet. J.*, *20*, 207.
(16) Chapman, M. S. et al. (1979) *Vet. Sci. Commun.*, *3*, 137.
(17) Brake, F. & Studdert, M. J. (1985) *Aust. vet. J.*, 62, 331.
(18) Allan, P. J. et al. (1975) *Aust. vet. J.*, *51*, 370.
(19) Thiry, E. et al. (1985) *Vet. Rec.*, *116*, 599.
(20) Allan, E. M. & Msolla, P. M. (1980) *Res. vet. Sci.*, *29*, 325.
(21) Kiorpes, A. L. et al. (1978) *Am. J. vet. Res.*, *39*, 779.
(22) Rebhun, W. C. et al (1978) *Cornell Vet.*, *68*, 297.
(23) Nyaga, P. N. & McKercher, D. G. (1979) *Comp. Immunol., Microbiol. Infect. Dis.*, *2*, 587.
(24) Higgins, R. J. & Edwards, S. (1986) *Vet. Rec.*, *119*, 177.
(25) Narita, M. et al. (1980) *Am. J. vet. Res.*, *41*, 1995.
(26) Nelson, R. D. (1974) *Am. J. vet. Res.*, *35*, 831.
(27) Todd, J. D. et al. (1972) *Infect. Immun.*, *5*, 699.
(28) Curtis, R. A. et al. (1966) *Can. vet. J.*, *7*, 208.
(29) Miller, R. B. et al. (1978) *Can. J. comp. Med.*, *42*, 438.
(30) Lupton, H. W. et al. (1980) *Cornell Vet.*, *70*, 77.
(31) Parsonson, I. M. & Snowdon, W. A. (1975) *Aust. vet. J.*, *51*, 365.
(32) Hanson, B. R. & Schipper, I. A. (1976) *Am. J. vet. Res.*, *37*, 707.
(33) Silim, A. & Elazhary, M. A. S. Y. (1983) *Can. J. comp. Med.*, *47*, 18.
(34) Nettleton, P. F. et al. (1983) *Vet. Rec.*, *112*, 298.
(35) Edwards, S. et al. (1983) *Res. vet. Sci.*, *34*, 42.
(36) Edwards, S. et al. (1986) *Res. Vet. Sci.*, *41*, 378.
(37) Miller, R. B. & Quinn, P. J. (1975) *Can. J. comp. Med.*, *39*, 270.
(38) Hurk, R. A. et al. (1973) *J. comp. Pathol.*, *83*, 271.
(39) Smith, P. C. (1978) *Am. J. vet. Res.*, *39*, 1369.
(40) Guy, J. S. & Potgieter, L. N. D. (1985) *Am. J. vet. Res.*, *46*, 893.
(41) Mitchell, D. (1974) *Can. vet. J.*, *15*, 148.
(42) Nettleton, P. F. et al. (1984) In: G. Wittman et al. (1984) *Latent Herpesvirus Infections in Veterinary Medicine*, pp. 191–209. Boston, The Hague, Dordrecht, Lancaster: Martinus Nijhoff.
(43) Brar, J. S. et al. (1978) *Am. J. vet. Res.*, *39*, 241.
(44) Keeling, C. L. et al. (1973) *Cornell Vet.*, *63*, 383.
(45) Frank, G. H. et al. (1977) *Am. J. vet. Res.*, *38*, 1497.
(46) Darcel, C. leQ. & Jericho, K. W. F. (1981) *Can. J. comp. Med.*, *45*, 87.
(47) Chow, T. L. (1972) *J. Am. vet. med. Assoc.*, *160*, 151.
(48) Curtis, R. A. & Angulo, A. (1974) *Can. vet. J.*, *15*, 327.
(49) Straub, O. C. et al. (1973) *Dtsch Tierärztl. Wochenschr.*, *80*, 73.
(50) Abshagen, H. & Kokles, R. (1973) *Mh. VetMed.*, *28*, 579.
(51) Magwood, S. E. (1974) *Can. vet. J.*, *15*, 260
(52) Kucera, C. J. et al. (1978) *Am. J. vet. Res.*, *39*, 607.
(53) Gerber, J. D. et al. (1978) *Am. J. vet. Res.*, *39*, 753.
(54) Smith, M. W. et al. (1978) *Can. vet. J.*, *19*, 63.
(55) Lupton, H. W. & Reed, D. E. (1980) *Am. J. vet. Res.*, *41*, 383.
(56) Guy, J. S. & Potgieter, L. N. D. (1985) *Am. J. vet. Res.*, *46*, 899.
(57) Msolla, P. M. et al. (1983) *J. comp. Pathol.*, *93*, 271.
(58) Narita, M. et al. (1982) *J. comp. Pathol.*, *92*, 41.
(59) Ross, H. M. et al. (1983) *Vet. Rec.*, *113*, 271.
(60) Yates, W. D. G. (1982) *Can. J. comp. Med.*, *46*, 225.
(61) Tanyi, J. et al. (1983) *Acta vet. Hung.*, *31*, 135.
(62) Bowen, R. A. et al. (1985) *Am. J. vet. Res.*, *46*, 1095.
(63) Miller, J. M. et al. (1984) *Am. J. vet. Res.*, *45*, 790.
(64) Van Der Maaten, M. J. & Miller, J. M. (1985) *Vet. Microbiol.*, *10*, 155.
(65) Van Der Maaten, M. J. et al. (1985) *Am. J. vet. Res.*, *46*, 1996.
(66) Gregersen, J. P. & Wagner, K. (1985) *Zentralbl. VetMed. B.*, *32*, 354.
(67) Durham, P. J. K. & Sillars, H. M. (1986) *NZ vet. J.*, *34*, 27.
(68) Cho, H. J. & Bohac, J. G. (1985) *Can. J. comp. Med.*, *49*, 189.
(69) Loewen, K. G. & Darcel, C. Le Q (1985) *Theriogenology*, *23*, 935.
(70) Bommlli, W. & Kihm, U. (1982) In: *The ELISA Enzyme-linked Immunosorbent Assay in Veterinary Research and Diagnosis*, pp. 242–251. Boston, the Hague, Dordrecht, Lancaster:Martinus Nijhoff.
(71) Bradley, J. A. (1985) *Can. vet. J.*, 26, 195.
(72) Zuffa, A. et al. (1983) *Zentralbl. VetMed.*, B32, 724.
(73) Frerichs, G. N. et al. (1982) *Vet. Rec.*, *111*, 116.
(74) Martin, W. et al. (1983) *Can. J. comp. Med.*, 47, 245.
(75) Jericho, K. W. F. & Babiuk, L. A. (1983) *Can. J. comp. Med.*, *47*, 133.
(76) Lucas, M. H. et al. (1982) *Br. vet. J.*, *138*, 23.
(77) Thiry, E. et al. (1985) *Vet. Microbiol.*, *10* 371.
(78) Roney, C. S. et al. (1985) *Am. J. vet. Res.*, *46*, 1251.
(79) Babiuk, L. A. et al. (1985) *J. gen. Virol.*, *66*, 2383.
(80) Burns, P. M. & Lloyd-Evans, L. P. (1981) *Vet. Rec.*, *109*, 515.
(81) Schudel, A. A. et al. (1986) *J. vet. Med. B.*, *33*, 303.
(82) Whetstone, C. A. et al. (1986) *Am. J. vet. Res.*, *47*, 1789.
(83) Miller, J. M. & Van Der Maaten, M.J. (1986) *Am. J. vet. Res.*, *47*, 223.
(84) Nieuwstadt, A. P. Van & Verhoeff, J. (1983) *J. Hyg., Camb.*, *91*, 309.
(85) Meckor, S. et al. (1981) *Can. J. Vet. Res.*, *51*, 542.

Enzootic pneumonia of sheep

Enzootic pneumonia is defined here as the common, lowly pathogenic disease of sheep, particularly lambs, which is common in all sheep populations. It can be differentiated from the acute fibrinous pneumonia and pleurisy caused by *Pasteurella hemolytica*, and from the chronic progressive pneumonias, maedi and jaagsiekte.

Although the disease is well known it is not commonly identified in terms of cause. This is partly due to its non-fatal character, which leads to incomplete examination of early cases; most of those submitted are distorted by the addition of secondary bacterial invaders. Chlamydia, parainfluenza-3 virus, adenovirus, a respiratory syncytial virus, reovirus and mycoplasmas are commonly nominated as causes (1). The disease, which might be most accurately identified as chronic undifferentiated enzootic pneumonia of sheep, is therefore a collection of etiologically specific diseases.

In many affected flocks 80% of 4–5-month-old lambs have lesions and the disease is credited with causing a significant depression in growth rate after weaning in lamb flocks with a high prevalence (3). The weight loss is greatest soon after the disease commences and is not so apparent several months later (2). There are virtually no death losses. The situation is reminiscent of that in enzootic pneumonia of pigs. Serious losses do occur when secondary bacterial pathogens invade lungs already compromised by the chronic pneumonia under discussion. An example is the severe pneumonia recorded in lambs brought into California for fattening. *Actinomyces (Corynebacterium) pyogenes* is commonly present in the lungs of the large numbers of lambs that are fatally affected. Cases commence within 1–3 weeks after transport. Something similar occurs in New Zealand (13) where enzootic pneumonia occurs commonly in lambs as young as 6 weeks, but becomes less prevalent as the lamb grows, the pneumonia being supplanted by pleurisy. The experimental production of a viral PI-3 *Pasteurella hemolytica* pneumonia of lambs (16) demonstrates the preparatory role of the virus, and the resulting highly damaging effects of the pasteurellae.

Attempts to reproduce pneumonia in lambs by the administration of chlamydiae, mycoplasmas or pasteurellae is usually not successful unless some form of stress is also provided. With chlamydiae and most of the viruses the introduction of the agent into the lung by nebulization or intratracheal injection results in the development of lesions, but no clinical illness. Chlamydiae may cause fever, anorexia and dyspnea in newborn lambs, and macroscopic lesions of pneumonia of varying degrees of severity are present. The chlamydia may be related to the one which causes enzootic abortion of ewes. *Mycoplasma ovipneumoniae* (5) and *M. argini* are respiratory strains which cause pneumonia in sheep but perhaps only when associated with parainfluenza-3 or other virus (1). Lungworms, especially *Dictyocaulus filaria*, must be considered as a cause of chronic pneumonia in sheep but they cause only a small section of the total pneumonias observed in the species.

In the United Kingdom, Europe and Australia parainfluenza-3 virus remains the favored principal cause of undifferentiated pneumonia (2). In New Zealand (7), antibodies to PI-3 and adenovirus are present in lambs soon after birth, but the titers fade so quickly that the lambs become susceptible and infections with the two viruses subsequently spread amongst them. The disease is clinically mild and marked by the presence of interstitial pneumonia (14). In the experimentally produced disease in lambs (15) there is a slight seromucosal nasal discharge, coughing, increased sensitivity to tracheal compression and fever of 40–41°C (104–106°F). At necropsy there is obvious hyperemia of the upper respiratory mucosa, including the trachea, the bronchial lymph nodes are enlarged and there are small foci of catarrhal inflammation of pulmonary parenchyma of the apical and cardiac lobes. The usual outcome of experimental infection with PI-3 virus is the production of subclinical disease, but there are also reports of clinical illness caused by the virus (4). Similar variations occur with the adenoviruses. Experimental infection with an ovine adenovirus also produced a mild respiratory and enteric disease. Other lesions, including nephrosis and interstitial nephritis resulted when particular isolates of the same serotypes were used as pathogens (17). Methods of vaccination against PI-3 virus infection are constantly being developed, but results are consistently unexciting (7). Intranasal vaccination appears to be much superior to systemic administration.

An adenovirus (9, 12) and a type 3 reovirus (10) have been used experimentally to produce pneumonic lesions and a vaccine has been produced to protect lambs against the adenovirus infection (11).

The pneumonia produced experimentally in sheep with a bovine respiratory syncytial virus (RSV) was evidenced clinically by fever and hyperpnea, and pathologically by multifocal pulmonary consolidation, and necrosis of epithelial cells in airways (8). Similar clinical signs and necropsy lesions resulted from experimental infection with an ovine RSV (6). The cause of the residuum of undifferentiated pneumonias, the bulk of them, remains to be determined.

REVIEW LITERATURE

Shewen, P. E. (1980) Chlamydial infection in animals. A review. *Can. vet. J.*, *21*, 2.

St George, T. D. & Sullivan, N. D. (1973) Pneumonias of sheep in Australia. Univ. of Sydney. *Post. Grad. Found. Vet. Sci.*, *Vet. Rev.*, No. 13.

REFERENCES

(1) Hore, D. E. (1976) *Aust. vet. J.*, *52*, 502.
(2) Jones, G. E. et al. (1982) *Vet. Rec.*, *110*, 168.
(3) Kirton, A. H. et al. (1976) *NZ vet. J.*, *24*, 59.
(4) Singh, V. P. Phathak, R. C. (1979) *Ind. J. exp. Biol.*, *17*, 221.
(5) Sullivan, N. D. et al. (1973) *Aust. vet. J.*, *49*, 57, 63.
(6) Lehmkuhl, H. D. & Cutlip, R. C. (1979) *Am. J. vet. Res.*, *40*, 412. & 1729.
(7) Davies, D. H. et al. (1983) *NZ vet. J.*, *31*, 87.
(8) Al-Darraji, A. M. et al. (1982) *Am. J. vet. Res.*, *42*, 224, 230 & 236.
(9) Cutlip, R. C. & Lehmkuhl, H. D. (1986) *Vet. Pathol.*, *23*, 589.
(10) McFarran, J. B. et al. (1974) *Res. vet. Sci.*, *17*, 356.
(11) Palfi, V. & Belak, S. (1979) *Vet. Microbiol.*, *3*, 191.
(12) Pavlov, N. (1979) *Arch. exp. VetMed.*, *33*, 253.
(13) McGowan, B. (1978) *NZ vet. J.*, *26*, 169.
(14) Singh, V. P. et al. (1977) *Ind. J. anim. Sci.*, *47*, 804.
(15) Cutlip, R. C. & Lehmkuhl, H. D. (1982) *Am. J. vet. Res.*, *43*, 2101.
(16) Rushton, B. et al. (1979) *J. comp. Pathol.*, *89*, 321.
(17) Belak, S. et al. (1980) *J. comp. Pathol.*, *90*, 169.

Ovine progressive interstitial pneumonia (maedi, maedi-visna)

Maedi is primarily a chronic pneumonia of sheep which is caused by a virus, which also causes visna when it invades the brains of sheep. 'Maedi' is Icelandic for dyspnea. Additional manifestations of infection with the virus are arthritis, indurative mastitis and illthrift.

Etiology

The causative lentivirus (family Retroviridae) of maedi (and visna) has been well defined (2). It has a strong serological relationship to the viruses of progressive interstitial pneumonia in Holland and Montana, United States. Transmission experiments using culture virus have been satisfactorily concluded, and show that the same virus is capable of causing both maedi and visna. Although maedi and visna do not usually occur together in the one animal there is a record of this occurring in one sheep (22). The incubation period after experimental transmission is 24–36 months.

Epidemiology

The disease occurs in Canada, Italy, France, Iceland, Germany, Holland, Denmark, Sweden, Norway and the United States. However, in the United Kingdom the virus has been isolated from imported and indigenous sheep (20), but clinical disease has been recorded in only one case (14). Neither the virus nor the disease has been recorded in New Zealand or Australia. *La bouhite* and *Graff-Reinet* disease are local names for maedi in France and South Africa respectively. Montana progressive pneumonia appears to be identical to maedi. In Holland, under the name of *zwoergerziekte*, it has been found in 80% of flocks and 28% of sheep over 1 year old (5). Very similar diseases are recorded in Kenya (9) and India (10).

At one time maedi was enzootic in Iceland and approximately 150 000 sheep are believed to have died of the disease during a 13-year period. A high morbidity and mortality of 10–20% per year occurred and complete destruction of all sheep in the area was necessary to eradicate the disease, which has since reappeared in sporadic form (8).

The disease occurs principally in sheep but it has been observed in goats. Among sheep only those 2 years old or over are affected. The clinical disease is likely to appear after prolonged physical exertion or exposure to bad weather in sheep that have been infected and seropositive for years. In the United Kingdom there are many flocks with a high prevalence of seropositive sheep but the clinical disease has not been observed. The clinical disease is more likely to appear when the infection prevalence exceeds 50% (5). The causes of loss are reproductive inefficiency and significantly reduced longevity—the case fatality rate is 100%. Accurate data on wastage are not available, but in some flocks in western United States up to 64% of ewes are seropositive, varying from 25% in yearlings to 85% in 7 year olds (1).

The natural mode of spread is not known, but from field observations direct contact between affected and unaffected sheep seems to be necessary. Much transmission appears to occur soon after birth, probably via the milk of infected ewes, but some does occur before birth (16). Lambs taken from infected ewes at birth remain unaffected, but if they are left on the ewes for periods as short as 10 hours 28% of them can eventually become affected. The longer the period of contact with the ewes the greater the spread of the disease (16).

Successful transmission with cultured virus has been effected using intrapulmonic and intracerebral inoculation; an incubation period of at least 2 years follows. There is no evidence of prenatal transmission but the virus is present in ewe's milk.

Pathogenesis

Experimentally infected sheep remain viremic with virus present in the blood for long periods, often without the appearance of clinical signs. In heavily infected flocks the clinical syndromes of illthrift, chronic pneumonia, arthritis and indurative mastitis develop (2). The virus replicates principally in tissue macrophages and to a less extent in circulating monocytes. The infected macrophages in the various tissues are surrounded by an inflammatory response creating a focus of mononuclear cell aggregation.

In the lung there is a gradual development of an interstitial pneumonia without any evidence of healing or shrinkage of tissue, so that the lungs continue to increase in size and weight. The alveolar spaces are gradually filled so that anoxia develops. Many of the features of the lesions in the brain (visna) are reminiscent of an allergic encephalitis, and it is apparent that an unconventional immune response occurs and that although antibodies are produced the virus survives for the duration of the long course of the disease (22). The pathological lesions develop very slowly during the preclinical and clinical stages of the disease so that they are very widespread and uncompensatable when clinical signs appear (12).

Clinical findings

There is a very long incubation period of at least 2 years. Early signs of the disease include a slow advance of listlessness, emaciation and dyspnea. There is no evidence of excess fluid in the lungs. The respiratory rate is increased to 80–120/min at rest. There may be coughing and some nasal discharge. Natural cases may also have mammary lesions characterized by firmness of the udder and a lymphoplasmacytic mastitis (13, 21). The udder is enlarged and very firm but full of milk which cannot pass through the ductal system because of the lymphocytic accumulation. It is called colloquially, 'hard udder'. The lambs of these ewes suffer growth retardation. The body temperature is in the high normal range. Clinical illness lasts for 3–6 months in most cases but may persist for several years.

Clinical pathology

The virus can be isolated from leukocytes on cell culture and complement fixation and virus neutralizing antibodies are measurable. An agar gel immunodiffusion test, an immunosorbent assay, and an ELISA serological test are all used in various countries and have approximately equal accuracy (4). Together with histopathological examination these tests make the diagnosis of the disease possible.

There is a progressive, moderate hypochromic anemia, with hemoglobin levels falling from 12–14 g/dl down to 7–8 g/dl and some depression of the red cell count. There is a tendency to leukocytosis, and in experimental cases this is observed to be quite marked in the period between exposure and the onset of clinical disease, but the count returns to normal when signs appear.

Necropsy findings

Gross abnormalities occur in lungs, brain, joints and mammary glands but most seriously in the lungs. They are larger and two to four times as heavy as normal lungs. They collapse much less than normal when the chest is open and are gray-blue to gray-yellow in color. There is a diffuse thickening of the entire bulk of both lungs and the abnormal color and consistency are generalized and unvarying in all lobes. Enlargement of the bronchial and mediastinal lymph nodes is constant. Histopathological changes are characteristic of a chronic interstitial pneumonia and the bulk of the alveolar space is replaced by thickened alveolar walls. The air passages are unaffected. There is a complete absence of healing, suggesting that the disease is a progressive one and never reaches a healing stage. A vasculitis is often a significant lesion (6).

There are frequently associated lesions of arthritis, encephalitis, pneumonitis (11) and mastitis (12). The mastitic lesion comprises an interstitial accumulation of lymphocytes which cause periductal lymphoid nodules some of which are necrotic.

Diagnosis

There are several chronic pneumonias which require to be differentiated from maedi, including jaagsiekte, in which the histological picture is quite different, profuse nasal discharge is a common sign and there is a shorter course. Epizootic adenomatosis appears to be identical with jaagsiekte. Maedi and jaagsiekte have occurred in the one flock, creating a major differential diagnostic problem (15, 18). Parasitic pneumonia causes a persistent chronic cough and dyspnea, but there are pronounced bronchial crackles on auscultation over the diaphragmatic lobes. It does not run a course as prolonged as in maedi but is more chronic than pasteurella pneumonia. The morbidity rate is usually higher than in either of these diseases. Melioidosis may resemble maedi clinically, but there are typical abscesses in lung tissue at necropsy. 'Laikipia' lung disease of sheep in Kenya is a progressive enzootic pneumonia resembling maedi and jaagsiekte and may, indeed, include both. One form is caused by a virus capable of producing the disease in lambs after an incubation period of 4–6 months, and which can be grown on eggs. A vaccine composed of formalin-killed virus is highly effective in preventing the disease. The indurative mastitis associated with maedi also occurs in caprine arthritis encephalitis.

Treatment

No treatment has been successful.

Control

In the past the only control attempted has been eradication of the disease by complete destruction of all sheep in the area and subsequently restocking it. However, it is possible to greatly reduce the prevalence by either of two methods. A management system of separating the lambs from the ewes at birth, giving them no colostrum and rearing them quite separately works well (3, 17). The detection of seropositive animals by an ELISA or immunodiffusion test (1, 17, 19) and eliminating them and all of their progeny by slaughter or separate domiciling is also effective. Shed lambing is thought to be very conducive to spread of the disease and its discontinuance is recommended in infected flocks.

In countries where the disease is enzootic there is often a great deal of movement, especially of rams, between farms, and close cohabitation of the sheep is the rule in winter. Severe restriction of interfarm movement, and outdoor housing are obvious aids to limiting the spread of the disease. The popularity of the Texel breed as a fat lamb sire has made its importation into other countries an issue of some political importance. The breed is known to be badly infected with maedi-visna (7), making the formulation of import certification most difficult.

REVIEW LITERATURE

Dawson, M. & Spence, J. B. (1982) Maedi/visna virus in sheep. *Vet. Ann.*, *22*, 122.

Martin, W. B. & Stamp, J. T. (1980) Slow virus infections of sheep. *Br. vet. J.*, *136*, 290.

Sharp, J. M. (1981) Slow virus infections of the respiratory tract of sheep. *Vet. Res.*, *108*, 391.

Watson, W. A. et al. (1978) Viral diseases of sheep caused by slow viruses. *Bull. Off. int. Epizoot.*, *89*, 429, etc. (6 papers).

REFERENCES

(1) Huffman, E. M. et al. (1981) *J. Am. vet. med. Assoc.*, *178*, 708.
(2) Dawson, M. (1987) *Vet. Rec.*, *120*, 451.
(3) Light, M. R. et al. (1979) *J. anim. Sci.*, *49*, 1157.
(4) Dawson, M. et al. (1982) *Vet. Rec.*, *111*, 432.
(5) Lamontagne, L. et al. (1983) *Can. J. comp. Med.*, *47*, 309.
(6) Cutlip, R. C. et al. (1985) *Am. J. vet. Res.*, *46*, 61.
(7) Sheffield, W. D. et al. (1980) *Vet. Pathol.*, *17*, 544.
(8) Cutlip, R. et al. (1977) *Am. J. vet. Res.*, *38*, 1081.
(9) Wandera, J. G. (1970) *Vet. Rec.*, *86*, 434.
(10) Chauhan, H. V. S. & Singh, C. M. (1970) *Br. vet. J.*, *126*, 364.
(11) Cutlip, R. C. et al. (1985) *Am. J. vet. Res.*, *46*, 65.
(12) Cutlip, R. C. et al. (1985) *Am. J. vet. Res.*, *46*, 326.
(13) Deng, P. et al. (1986) *Vet. Pathol.*, *23*, 184.
(14) Jones, T. O. et al. (1982) *Vet. Rec.*, *110*, 252.
(15) Snyder, S. P. et al. (1983) *Am. J. vet. Res.*, *44*, 1334.
(16) Cutlip, R. C. et al. (1981) *Am. J. vet. Res.*, *42*, 1795.
(17) Cutlip, R. C. & Lehmkuhl, H. D. (1986) *J. Am. vet. med. Assoc.*, *188*, 1026.
(18) Houwers, D. J. & Terpstra, C. (1984) *Vet. Rec.*, *114*, 23.
(19) Houwers, D. J. et al. (1984) *Vet. Microbiol.*, *9*, 445.
(20) Pritchard, G. C. et al. (1984) *Vet. Rec.*, *115*, 427.
(21) Anderson, B. C. et al. (1985) *J. Am. vet. med. Assoc.*, *186*, 391.

Pulmonary adenomatosis (jaagsiekte)

Jaagsiekte is Afrikaans for 'driving disease' because of the tendency for affected sheep to show clinical signs when driven. The disease is a chronic, progressive pneumonia, with the development of typical adenomatous ingrowths of the alveolar walls.

Etiology

Jaagsiekte is caused by a retrovirus (1, 7, 10) which cannot be cultivated *in vitro*. It is morphologically distinct from all known retroviruses (2) and has not been further identified.

Epidemiology

Only sheep are affected, but the disease has been transmitted experimentally to goat kids (8). The disease is recorded in Britain, the United States (3), Canada (4), Europe, South Africa, Israel, Asia and Iceland. North America is otherwise clear, and Australia and New Zealand do not appear to have the disease although its presence has been suspected. In Britain, Scotland appears to be the focus of infection from which other outbreaks arise. European and English figures quote an annual flock mortality of about 2–8%, but a high morbidity has been observed in Iceland. The disease is uniformly fatal. Because of the method of spread the disease is likely to assume more importance as sheep husbandry becomes intensified.

Close housing during the winter is a potent predisposing cause and probably accounts for the occurrence of the disease in epizootic form in Iceland. However, the disease occurs commonly in range sheep in other countries. There is no seasonal variation in incidence and only mature sheep are affected. A genetic susceptiblity to the disease has been suggested.

Experimental transmission has been effected by pulmonary or intravenous injection or by insufflation of infected lung material (5). The disease has also been transmitted by inhalation of infected droplets when sheep are kept in close contact, and it is assumed that this is the natural mode of transmission. Vertical transmission by passing into the fetus from the pregnant ewe has been shown not to occur naturally (6).

Pathogenesis

The adenomatous ingrowths of alveolar epithelium encroach gradually upon alveolar air space so that anoxic anoxia occurs. There is no inflammation and no toxemia. The lesions produced by experimental inoculation are identical with those of the naturally occurring disease (5).

Clinical findings

The incubation period in natural cases is 1–3 years, but may be as short as 5–12 months after experimental transmission. Occasional coughing and some panting after exercise are the earliest signs but coughing is not a prominent sign in this disease. Emaciation, dyspnea, lacrimation and a profuse watery discharge from the nose follow. Death occurs 6 weeks to 4 months later. A diagnostic test in this disease is to hold the sheep up by the hindlegs: in affected animals a quantity of watery mucus (up to about 200 ml) runs from the nostrils. Moist crackles are audible over the affected lung areas and may be heard at a distance so that a group of affected animals are said to produce a sound like slowly boiling porridge. There is no elevation of body temperature and the appetite is normal.

Clinical pathology

A complement fixation test is available and has limited use, but there is no practicable laboratory means of identifying infected animals. Nasal exudate from affected animals may show clusters of epithelial cells with the hyperplastic adenomatous epithelium typical of pulmonary lesions (9).

Necropsy findings

Lesions are restricted to the thoracic cavity. As in maedi the lungs are grossly increased in size and in weight (up to three times normal). Extensive areas of consolidation, particularly of the ventral parts of the apical lobes and excess frothy fluid in the bronchi, are characteristic. Secondary pulmonary abscesses and pleurisy may develop. Histologically there are characteristic adenomatous ingrowths of alveolar epithelium into the alveolar spaces.

Diagnosis

Other chronic pneumonias in sheep are described under maedi (p. 907).

Treatment

No treatment has been attempted.

Control

In Iceland, where the disease assumed epizootic proportions, eradication was effected by complete slaughter of all sheep in the affected areas. In areas where the incidence is lower the disease can be satisfactorily controlled by slaughter of the clinically affected sheep. A formolized vaccine prepared from the lungs of diseased sheep has undergone an extensive trial in Kenya and appears to have greatly reduced the incidence of the disease.

REVIEW LITERATURE

Martin, W. B. et al. (1979). The herpes virus of sheep pulmonary adenomatosis. *Comp. Immun. Microbiol. infect. Dis.*, *2*, 313.

Wandera, J. G. (1971). Sheep pulmonary adenomatosis (jaagsiekte). *Adv. vet. Sci.*, *15*, 251.

REFERENCES

(1) Verwoerd, D. W. et al. (1983) *Onderstepoort J. vet. Res.*, *50*, 309.
(2) Payne, A. L. et al. (1983) *Onderstepoort J. vet. Res.*, *50*, 317.
(3) Cutlip, R. C. & Young, S. (1982) *Am. J. vet. Res.*, *43*, 2108.
(4) Stevenson, R. G. et al. (1982) *Can. vet. J.*, *23*, 147.
(5) Wandera, J. C. (1970) *Br. vet. J.*, *126*, 185.
(6) Cross, R. F. et al. (1975) *Am. J. vet. Res.*, *36*, 465.
(7) Payne, A. et al. (1986) *Onderstepoort J. vet. Res.*, *53*, 55.
(8) Sharp, J. M. et al. (1986) *Vet. Rec.*, *119*, 245.
(9) Nobel, T. A. et al. (1970) *Zentralbl. VetMed.*, *17B*, 958.
(10) Herring, A. J. et al. (1983) *Vet. Microbiol.*, *8*, 237.

VIRUS DISEASES CHARACTERIZED BY NERVOUS SIGNS

Viral encephalomyelitis of horses

Viral encephalomyelitis is an infectious disease affecting horses and characterized clinically by signs of deranged consciousness, motor irritation and paralysis.

Etiology

Three known strains of the causative alphavirus (family Togaviridae) exist, the eastern (EE), western (WE), and Venezuelan (VE) strains. They are immunologically distinct and vary in their virulence, although the clinical disease produced is similar with all three viruses. The molecular basis for the antigenic differences between the western and eastern strains are described (47). Although there is some degree of cross-protection between WE and EE and between EE and VE there is none between WE and VE. In the Venezuelan virus there are a number of subtypes. Subtype 1 causes the epidemic disease of horses and man, the other subtypes cause endemic disease of wild rodents and although they rarely affect man and horses the disease is subclinical. No subtypes are identified in WE and EE. The virus can be grown on embryonated hen eggs and in tissue culture. It is extremely fragile and disappears from infected tissues within a few hours of death.

Epidemiology

The disease is restricted to the Americas; the United States, Canada, Venezuela, Brazil and Argentina all record its occurrence. Most states of the United States have experienced the disease and, although the incidence has fallen considerably in recent years, an appreciable number of horses are fatally affected each year.

Morbidity varies widely depending upon seasonal conditions and the prevalence of insect vectors; and cases may occur sporadically or in the form of severe outbreaks affecting 20% or more of a group. The prevalence of infections as judged by serological examination is much higher than the clinical morbidity. The mortality rate differs with the strain of the virus; in infection with the western strain it is usually 20–30% and with the eastern and Venezuelan strains it is usually between 40 and 80% and it may be as high as 90%. The disease is more severe and mortality is higher in unvaccinated horses than in vaccinated horses (50). The mortality in young foals from non-immune mares, and infected with western encephalomyelitis virus, is always high, often as high as 100%. The western strain is the least virulent for horses, man and experimental animals and occurs chiefly in the western states of the United States and western Canada, extending eastwards to the Appalachian mountain region. The ecology of WE in the eastern United States has been reviewed (1). Epidemics of WE in the eastern United States are uncommon because of the lack of abundance of the primary vector, *Culex tarsalis*. In Florida, the western strain is considered to be of minor importance for man and the horse, is transmitted in a continuous cycle throughout the year by *Culiseta melanura* mosquitoes, and is restricted to freshwater swamps and waterways (46). The eastern strain is more virulent for all species and, in the United States, occurs chiefly in the eastern and southern states but overlaps the western strain to some extent, extending as far west as the midwestern states.

Eastern equine encephalomyelitis continues to cause significant death losses in horses in Florida, primarily in unvaccinated horses (4). It is suggested that the incidence of clinical disease due to EE in Florida is much higher than reported and there is a need to increase public awareness about the importance of vaccination particularly in foals (4). Unexpected epizootics occur in inland states of the United States after absence for many years and frequently the source of the infection is undetermined (62). An outbreak of EE occurred in the Dominican Republic in 1978 and was successfully controlled approximately 40 days after a vaccinated program was begun (64). In fact, diagnostic data indicates that EE in the eastern United States is considerably more common than previous surveillance data have suggested (63).

It has also been recognized in Jamaica, Brazil, and in Panama (52). Both strains occur in Argentina. The Venezuelan strain (VE) was originally observed in Venezuela and has since occurred in much of northern South America (2). An outbreak of VE occurred in Guatemala in 1969 and in 1971 an extensive outbreak occurred in the southern United States, Mexico, and Costa Rica. The virus has spread its geographical range greatly and causes a great deal of alarm because of the high rate of clinical disease occurrence in man and the very large numbers of horses which die of the disease. The possibility exists that migratory birds can transmit the VE strain from South to Central America (49).

The susceptibility of man to the causative virus gives the disease great public health importance. The infection in man is a mild, influenza-like illness in which recovery occurs spontaneously. When clinical encephalitis does occur it is usually in very young or older people. Occurrence of the disease in man can be limited by the use of a vaccine in horses which limits the occurrence of the disease in horses in the area (3). There is a strong relationship between the mosquito population and the incidence of the disease in horses and in man (51). The occurrence of the disease in man may be predicted by an unusually high activity of virus in mosquitoes. There are usually widespread mortalities in horses before the disease occurs in man (51).

The EE and WE viruses

Under natural conditions the disease caused by the WE and EE viruses is a disease of birds and only accidental infections occur in horses, mules, donkeys, man and possibly monkeys. Many species of wild and captive birds become infected and, although many escape any serious effects, a fatal encephalitis occurs in others. Antibodies to WE and EE have been found in pronghorn antelope in western Canada (5). The natural disease has been observed in turkey poults. Experimentally the disease can be produced by intracerebral inoculation in calves, dogs, white mice, guinea-pigs and many species of birds. Snakes are highly susceptible to experimental infection. Pigs have a high natural susceptibility and may carry high levels of neutralizing antibodies, but the disease has been considered non-clinical. The recent recording of the VE virus from a suckling pig with a nervous disturbance, and the subsequent transmission of the disease, may lead to a revision of this opinion (6). The same comment applies to cattle now that two naturally occurring cases of EE have been detected in calves (7). Transmission between horses and other mammals is rare because the viremia in them is usually insufficient to infect mosquitoes.

The disease has a marked seasonal incidence, with the great majority of cases occurring in mid and late summer when the insect population is highest. In warm climates the seasonal variation may be less evident. Young horses are most susceptible. Immunity after natural infection persists for about 2 years.

Spread occurs by insect bite, chiefly from mosquitoes but also from ticks, blood-sucking bugs, and chicken mites and lice. Mosquitoes of the *Aedes*, *Culex* (8) and *Mansonia* genera have been identified as vectors, the virus persisting in them for a number of generations and passing through all stages of their lifecycles. Spread may occur occasionally from horse to horse by direct contact or by insect transmission, but the major route of spread appears to be from birds through insects to horses and man. The wild bird population acts as a reservoir of infection in an area and probably serves to maintain the persistence of the virus from summer to summer and may be a factor in the spread of the disease to new areas. Migratory birds appear not to be involved in distributing the virus (21). Small wild vertebrates can also serve as reservoirs for VE and EE during the non-epidemic period (66). In Jamaica, the domestic chicken is considered to be a reservoir for the eastern strain (45). Under experimental conditions, snakes and turtles have been shown to act as overwintering reservoirs (9) and there is evidence that the infection occurs naturally in snakes and frogs (10), but the importance of these species in maintaining the infection over long insect-free periods is undetermined.

The VE virus

Because the level of the viremia produced in horses by the VE virus is very high, they act as amplifiers of the virus and the disease has a much different host range, a difference which is very important in understanding the epidemiology of the disease. Subtype 1 is principally a disease of horses and the virus cannot usually be isolated from other farm animals. However, experimental subcutaneous inoculation of it into cattle, pigs and goats is followed by infection and the development of antibodies. But the viremia produced is so low in level that the animals are not considered to be amplifiers of the virus; they are, however, suitable as sentinel animals (11–13). Infection does occur in many other small vertebrates, e.g.possums (3), rodents (14), deer, feral swine and peccaries (15) and rabbits (16). The position of dogs is not clear but they do appear to be able to multiply the virus and must be considered to act as donor hosts (17). The mosquito vectors include *Aedes, Psorophora* and *Deinocerites* species. The cliff swallow bug, *Oeciacus vicarius*, may be an overwintering reservoir for the western strain (48).

In examining the epidemiological status of VE in an animal community, the presence of the endemic virus, subtypes which are not pathogenic for horses and man must be taken into account. The viruses maintain a continuous low level cycle between small rodents and mosquitoes (18, 19). Spread of the disease on a broad front is readily explained by the movement of insect vectors and of donor hosts including horses, birds and other wildlife. The sudden appearance of unfamiliar strains of virus in far-distant areas is not so readily explainable unless the accidental carriage of mosquitoes in aircraft is accepted as a real possibility (20). The development of subtyping techniques now makes it possible to investigate more precisely outbreaks of equine encephalomyelitis in order to correlate the antigenic diversity of the viruses with the epidemiological observation (64).

Pathogenesis

Inapparent infection is the mildest form of the disease and may be characterized by only a transient fever. A more severe form of the disease is manifested by tachycardia, depression, anorexia, occasional diarrhea, and fever.

A transitory viremia occurs at the height of the fever in the North American disease but in the Venezuelan disease the viremia persists throughout the course and the blood provides a source of infection for biting insects. Transplacental transmission of the VE strain can occur in pregnant mares infected near term (53). The virus is present in saliva and nasal discharge, and this material can be used to transmit the disease experimentally by intranasal instillation. Penetration of the virus into the brain does not occur in all cases and the infection does not produce signs, other than fever, unless involvement of the central nervous system occurs, although antibodies to the virus do appear in the blood. The lesions produced in nervous tissue are typical of a viral infection and are localized particularly in the gray matter of the cerebral cortex, thalamus and hypothalamus, with minor involvement of the medulla and spinal cord. It is this distribution of lesions which is responsible for the characteristic signs of mental derangement followed at a later stage by paralysis. The early apparent blindness and failure to eat or drink appear to be cortical in origin. True blindness and pharyngeal paralysis occur only in the late stages. Much has been written of the pathogenesis of this disease in mice but the extent to which this information can be extrapolated to the horse is problematical (22). Experimental Venezuelan equine encephalomyelitis has been produced by inoculation of the virus peripherally or by the intrathecal route (54).

Clinical findings

The diseases caused by the different viruses are clinically indistinguishable. The incubation period is 1–3 weeks. In the initial viremic stage there is fever which may be accompanied by anorexia and depression, but the reaction is usually so mild that it goes unobserved. In the experimental disease the temperature may reach 41°C (106°F) persisting for only 24–48 hours, with nervous signs appearing at the peak of the fever. Animals that have shown nervous signs for more than 24 hours may then have a temperature within the normal range.

Early nervous signs include hypersensitivity to sound and touch and in some cases transient periods of excitement and restlessness with apparent blindness. Affected horses may walk blindly into objects or walk in circles. Involuntary muscle movements occur, especially tremor of shoulder and facial muscles and erection of the penis. A stage of severe mental depression follows. Affected horses stand with the head hung low; they appear to be asleep and may have a half-chewed mouthful of feed hanging from the lips. At this stage the horse may eat and drink if food is placed in its mouth. The pupillary light reflex is still present. The animal can be aroused but soon relapses into a state of somnolence.

A stage of paralysis follows. There is inability to hold up the head, and it is often rested on a solid support. The lower lip is pendulous and the tongue may hang out. Unnatural postures are adopted, the horse often standing with the weight balanced on the forelegs or with the legs crossed. Head-pressing or leaning back on a halter are often seen. On walking there is obvious incoordination, particularly in the hindlegs, and circling is common. Defecation and urination are suppressed and the horse is unable to swallow. Complete paralysis is the terminal stage. The horse goes down, is unable to rise and usually dies within 2–4 days from the first signs of illness. A proportion of affected horses do not develop paralysis and survive but are often deficient mentally and are of little use because of their inability to respond satisfactorily to stimuli.

In the experimental infection of horses with the endemic strain of the VE virus a fever and mild leukopenia occurs (18). Following infection with the epidemic strain of the virus a high fever, severe leukopenia are common, and a high level of neutralizing antibodies develop at about 5–6 days after infection. Clinical findings include profound depression, accompanied by flaccidity of lips, partially closed eyelids, drooped ears, and some horses chew continuously and froth at the mouth. In the terminal stages there is recumbency and nystagmus.

Clinical pathology

Acute and convalescent sera taken 10–14 days apart for the presence of neutralizing, or hemagglutination inhibiting, or complement fixing antibodies in the serum of affected or in contact horses is of value in detecting the presence of the virus in the group or in the area. A fourfold increase in CF antibodies is considered positive.

The presence of a high hemagglutination-inhibition, complement fixation and neutralizing antibody in a single serum sample obtained from a horse during the acute phase of illness caused by the WE virus can be used as presumptive evidence of infection with this virus (23). However, these antibodies against WE can persist for years, are produced after vaccination with WE or WE/EE bivalent vaccines and in foals may be due to colostral immunity. Therefore, a single serum sample cannot be used to make a confirmed diagnosis of WE using the hemagglutination-inhibition, complement fixation or neutralization tests. Horses infected experimentally or naturally with either the WE or the EE virus do not produce detectable hemagglutination-inhibition or neutralizing antibody for 5–10 days after infection. Circulating antibody appears on or near the day of onset of clinical illness. Infection with the WE virus results in the production of serum IgM specific to WE, and the ELISA test is a rapid, sensitive and specific test for IgM against WE and EE viruses (60).

Isolation of the western strain of the virus can be achieved by inoculation of suspected brain into infant mice. The inoculation of brain suspension into embryonated chicken eggs followed by inoculation of a suspension of the infected embryos into cell culture and examination for cytopathic effect and examination for typical alphavirus particles will provide a rapid preliminary diagnosis (55). Blood may be taken in the early febrile stages and attempts made to passage the virus to sucking mice or to culture it on duck embryo. The VE virus is likely to be present in detectable quantities but the other two viruses are often not. The growing virus is identified by one of a number of tests including a plaque reduction neutralization test and a hemagglutination-inhibition test. A modification of a microtiter hemagglutination-inhibition test is also available which can provide results within 48 hours after inoculation of field samples (24). A modified hemagglutination-reduction test can provide reliable diagnosis of EE as early as 24 hours after receipt of field specimens (56). The presence of neutralizing, or hemagglutination-inhibiting, or complement fixing antibodies in the serum of recovered or in-contact animals may be of value in detecting the presence of the virus in the group or in the area. Identification of the WE strain of the virus has been achieved by the use of a complement fixation test on virus grown on chick embryos. A leukopenia occurs.

Necropsy findings

There are no gross changes. Histological examination of brain reveals perivascular accumulations of leukocytes and damage to neurons (25). No inclusion bodies are present. In VE, liquefactive necrosis and hemorrhage are prominent lesions in the cerebral cortex (26). The lesions are midway in severity between the severe lesions caused by the EE strain and those of the WE strain which are the least extensive and severe (27). Sections for histological examination should be taken from the cerebral cortex and mid-brain. Transmission experiments after death are carried out using the brain as a source of virus. The brain should be removed within an hour of death or preferably after euthanasia when the animal is in extremis. Transmission is by intracerebral inoculation of brain tissue into sucking mice or duck embryo tissue culture. A more rapid and sufficiently accurate test for the presence of VE virus in tissues is the fluorescent antibody test (28). A fluorescent antibody test on brain tissue is also available for the rapid diagnosis of EE (61).

Diagnosis

When cases of central nervous system disease occur in groups of horses in North America in the summer time the diagnosis is not usually in doubt, only the identity of the strain. Clinically the disease has very great similarity to the other viral encephalomyelitides, and to the hepatic encephalopathies and to a number of other diseases set down bellow, and in Table 69.

The epidemic equine encephalomyelitides (WE, EE and VE) affects horses principally in the western hemisphere. Borna occurs primarily in Germany and the incubation period and the course are considerably longer. Inclusion bodies are present in Borna disease but not in WE, EE or VE. The seasonal incidence of WE, EE and VE is also an epidemiological feature. Japanese encephalitis is an important cause of abortion and stillbirth of swine in Asia, where it is also associated with epidemics of encephalomyelitis of horses. Another arbovirus causing meningoencephalitis in horses in the French Mediterranean littoral is the West Nile arbovirus (29).

Nervous signs resembling those of an encephalomyelitis occur in a number of poisonings in horses. Botulism is rare in this species and the syndrome is specifically one of paralysis. There is no derangement of consciousness and signs of motor irritation are absent. At necropsy there is no histological evidence of encephalitis. Poisoning caused by *Crotalaria*, *Senecio*, and *Amsinckia* spp. produces a syndrome with all the signs of an encephalomyelitis except fever. Histologically there is no

Table 69. Differential diagnosis of diseases of the nervous system of the horse.

Disease	*Etiology and epidemiology*	*Clinical and laboratory findings*	*Treatment and control*
Viral encephalomyelitis (western, eastern, Venezuelan WE, EE, VE)	Summer season. Insect vector. Young non-vaccinated horses, outbreaks may occur	Stage of slight hyperexcitability and mild fever initially, impaired eyesight, circling and walking. Stage of mental depression, somnolence, leaning, feed hanging from mouth, unsteady. Stage of paralysis, unable to swallow, weakness, recumbency; dies 2–4 days after onset. Serology for diagnosis	Supportive therapy, thick bedding. Recovery rate 60–75%. Vaccinate foals at 6 months of age and other horses for the first time, twice 2 weeks apart and once or twice annually thereafter
Rabies	All age groups, knowledge of disease in area, wildlife. Usually single animal affected. Not common	Ascending paralysis, hypersalivation, will bite. Incoordination followed by sensory and motor paralysis and recumbency in 2–4 days. Dies in 1 week. Brain for positive diagnosis	No treatment. All die. Vaccinate horses if anticipate outbreak
Herpesvirus paralysis (equine viral rhinopneumonitis)	Usually follows upper respiratory tract disease. Experimentally 7 days after inoculation of virus into pregnant mares	Symmetrical ataxia and paresis, bladder paralysis, recumbency may occur, spontaneous recovery possible, CSF (hemorrhage or xanthochromia). Necrotizing arteritis and focal malacia in gray and white matter of brain and spinal cord	No specific therapy. Recovery may occur spontaneously
Liver–brain disease (hepatoencephalopathy) caused by hepatotoxic plants (*Crotalaria*, *Senecio* and *Amsinckia*)	Horses on inadequate pasture forced to eat poisonous plants. More than one animal may be affected. Geographical distribution	Develops slowly, commonly ill for 2–3 weeks previously, depression, pushing, ataxia, hypertonic face and lips, yawning, compulsive walking, loss of weight, icterus, photosensitization occasionally. Serum liver enzymes elevated and liver function tests abnormal. Hyperammonemia. Gross and histopathological liver lesions	No treatment. Prevent access to poisonous plants
Yellow-star thistle poisoning (nigropallidal encephalomalacia of horses)	Ingestion of yellow-star thistle in California and Australia. Summer months on weedy pasture	Difficult prehension, fixed facial expression with mouth held half open, hypertonic face and lips, persistent chewing movements and rhythmic protrusion of tongue, yawning and somnolence but easily aroused, aimless walking, slight stiffness of gait, high mortality. Malacia of globus pallidus and substantia nigra	No treatment. Prevent access to poisonous plants
Cerebrospinal nematodiasis (verminous encephalitis)	Migration of *Strongylus vulgaris*. Not common	Clinical signs referable to gray matter lesions are common. Hypalgesia, hyporeflexia, hypotonia, muscle atrophy and cerebral, cerebellar and cranial nerve involvement. Progressive encephalitis, incoordination, sensory deficits, blindness in one or both eyes, course of several days. Pleocytosis of CSF. Hemorrhage and malacia of thalamus, brain stem, cerebellum	No treatment. Parasite control
Cerebellar hypoplasia of Arabian and Swedish Gotland foals	Inherited. Signs noticeable from 2 to 6 months of age	Defective eye blinks, ataxia, headnodding, slight tremor of head and neck, intention tremor of the head, high-stepping gait, difficulty in rising, legs wide apart, difficulty in jumping over obstacles, fall backwards if dorsiflex head and neck. Cerebellar hypoplasia grossly or histologically	Eliminate carrier animals

Table 69 (cont.)

Disease	*Etiology and epidemiology*	*Clinical and laboratory findings*	*Treatment and control*
Barkers and wanderers of newborn foals (neonatal maladjustment syndrome)	Premature clamping of umbilical cord, birth asphyxia, increased intracranial pressure during birth. Usually in thoroughbred foals following easy birth. Signs occur within few minutes to 24 hours after birth	Jerking movements of head, inability to stand, erection of tail, collapse of external nares, inspiratory dyspnea and barking sound. Clonus, convulsions, loss of sucking reflex and affinity for mare, apparent blindness, opisthotonus, extension rigidity, chewing, wandering dummy-like behavior, asymmetric pupils, respiratory distress, cardiac irregularities. Pulmonary atelectasis, hyaline membrane, cerebral necrosis and hemorrhage	Supportive therapy. Recovery may occur in about 50 hours and is usually complete
Traumatic injury to the brain	History of traumatic injury (falling, rearing-up)	Sudden onset of collapse, lateral recumbency, nystagmus, tremors and recovery in few minutes or lapse into coma lasting several days, areflexia. Intracranial hemorrhage and cerebral edema	Mannitol, dexamethazone. Unfavorable prognosis
Facial nerve paralysis	Associated with prolonged surgical recumbency and compression of facial nerve	Facial nerve paralysis lasting several days. Paralysis of ear, eyelid, lip, nostril on one side	Supportive
Equine degenerative myeloencephalopathy	Young horses. Etiology is unknown. May be due to vitamin E deficiency and may be familial (65).	Signs noticeable before 12 months of age, abnormal gait and posture of thoracic and pelvic limbs, hypermetria, fall while backing	Nil
'Wobblers'	Focal contusive lesion in cervical spinal cord due to anatomical or functional narrowing, or both, of the C2 to C7 foramina that is not the result of gross external injury to the vertebral bodies	Most cases have history of previous fall or violent activity followed by incoordination, clumsiness when turned, lurching and swaying when walking. Special radiographic techniques of cervical vertebra	Nil
Protozoal encephalomyelitis (toxoplasmosis)	Single animal affected. Source of infection in horses usually unknown. Not common	Incoordination becoming progressively worse over few weeks, some circling, dysphagia, hypermetria, serology, histology and isolation	Nil
Spinal cord compression and contusion (equine myelopathy)	Atlanto-occipital malformation of Arabian foals, cervical vertebral fracture or luxation, neoplasia, epidural abscess, vertebral osteomyelitis	Abnormal posture and gait of pelvic and thoracic limbs. General proprioceptive defects and upper motor neurone dysfunction. Thoracic limbs base wide hypermetria, dragging toes, fall backwards when pushed, progressive. Flaccid paralysis of hindlimbs when lumbar vertebrae affected	Nil
Neuritis of the cauda equina	Single animal affected. Etiology unknown	Difficult defecation and urination, inability to move the tail. Anus and tail flaccid, areflexic and analgesic, bladder atonic. Fibrous tissue proliferation and demyelination and axonal degeneration of neurones of cauda equina	Unfavorable prognosis. No treatment
Horsetail poisoning (*Equisetum arvense*)	Ingestion of plants mixed with hay. Not common	Incoordination, swaying from side to side, muscle tremor, recumbency, bradycardia, cardiac arrhythmia	Thiamine parenterally. Good response
Lead poisoning	Grazing on pastures contaminated by atmospheric lead from nearby factories, not common now	Usually a chronic disease. Inspiratory dyspnea due to paralysis of recurrent laryngeal nerve. Pharyngeal paralysis, dysphagia, aspiration pneumonia, paralysis of lips, weakness and recumbency. Ingestion of large amounts causes subacute form similar to that seen in cattle	Calcium versenate

Table 69 (cont.)

Disease	*Etiology and epidemiology*	*Clinical and laboratory findings*	*Treatment and control*
Borna	Virus. Direct transmission. Germany. Low morbidity, high case fatality rate	Pharyngeal paralysis, muscle tremor, flaccid paralysis, course 1–3 weeks. Viral encephalomyelitis with inclusion bodies	No treatment. Vaccination in endemic areas
Japanese encephalitis	Sporadic. Malaya. Infection from humans	Fever, lethargy, jaundice, dysphagia, incoordination, staggering, recovery in 1 week. Serology	Spontaneous recovery. Vaccination in endemic areas
Tetanus	Wounds infected with *Cl. tetani*. Sporadic	Generalized tetany of all skeletal muscles. Fever, hyperesthesia, protrusion of third eyelid, trismus, recumbency followed by tetanic convulsions, profuse sweating, die in 5–10 days	Prognosis unfavorable. Dark stall, penicillin, muscle relaxants, supportive therapy and antitoxin parenterally or into subarachnoid space. Toxoid vaccination
Lactation tetany	Lactating mares, suckling foals. Hypocalcemia	Acute onset of generalized stiffness, trismus, no hyperesthesia, no prolapse of third eyelid, diaphragmatic flutter, soft heart sounds. Serum hypocalcemia	Rapid response to calcium borogluconate intravenously
Botulism	Ingestion of preformed toxin of *Cl. botulinum* in decaying grass or spoiled silage, hay or grain. Sporadic in horses	Flaccid paralysis of skeletal muscles leading to weakness, stumbling and recumbency. Skin sensation normal. Paralysis of tongue and thoracic muscles. Die in 2–4 days. Some recover. Filtrates of intestinal tract into laboratory animals	Supportive therapy, antitoxins. Purgatives. Vaccination in enzootic areas. Provide good feed
Idiopathic epilepsy	Single horse. First noticed from shortly after birth up to 6 months of age. Etiology unknown	Recurrent episodes of typical clonictonic convulsions lasting 10–15 minutes, loss of consciousness, sweating, tachycardia, spontaneous defecation. No lesions	General anesthesia. Euthanasia commonly recommended

NOTE: Other less common diseases affecting the nervous system of horses include: space-occupying lesions (cholesteatomas of old horses, tumors), intracranial myiasis due to migration of *Hypoderma bovis*, hydrocephalus in young horses, the accidental injection of an ataractic drug into the carotid artery and bacterial meningitis in young horses as a sequel to streptococcal infection.

encephalitis and gross abnormality of the liver is a prominent feature. These diseases are, of course, not transmissible. Poisoning by yellow star thistle and moldy corn causes an encephalomalacia. Sporadic cases of brain tumor, hydrocephalus and cholesteatoma usually run a long course, often with intermittent periods of normal behavior. There is no fever and there are often localizing signs.

Treatment

Supportive treatment should be undertaken, as it may enable the animal to survive the danger period. Horses able to bear some weight should be supported in stocks and fed a nutritious, laxative diet, if necessary by nasal tube. All horses should be kept in the shade and protected from flies and heat. Recumbent animals should be provided with ample bedding and turned frequently. The disease occurs in the summertime and affected horses can be nursed outside. This is most advantageous if a grassy paddock is available. This will ensure a good footing and encourage the horse to get to its feet, and at the same time minimize the chances of self injury.

Control

Control of viral encephalomyelitis of horses is based on a five-point program of accurate clinical and laboratory diagnosis of the disease in horses, the use of sentinel animals to monitor the presence of the virus in the region, the quarantine of infected horses to stop movement of virus donors, insect abatement when deemed necessary and vaccination of all horses (23, 30, 31). Control of the disease in man in areas where the disease may occur is dependent on insect control and a monitoring and surveillance early warning system is necessary to decide whether or not to take control measures (23, 32). In areas where WE occurs, clinical cases of the disease in unvaccinated horses usually precede the occurrence of the disease in man (32). The establishment of a reporting system whereby practicing veterinarians report all clinical cases of the disease in horses will also assist in predicting potential epidemics of WE virus infection in the human population (33). Serological surveys of wildlife may also serve as good indicators of the geographical distribution and seasonality of circulation of these viruses and provide an early warning system prior to the detection of human cases (34, 35).

Housing of horses indoors at night, especially in flyproofed stables, and the use of insect repellents may restrain the spread of the virus. Complete eradication appears to be impossible because of the method of spread and high incidence of the infection in wild birds.

For the control of WE and EE formalin inactivated vaccines are currently available which are highly effective (36). Horses should be vaccinated well in advance of the anticipated encephalomyelitis season in a given area. Vaccination against both strains of the virus is advisable in areas where the strain has not been identified or where both strains exist. The currently recommended vaccination schedule consists of two doses of the vaccine initially, 10 days apart, followed by annual revaccination using two doses. Annual revaccination is currently recommended because the duration of effective immunity beyond 1 year is not known. It is probable that the initial two-dose vaccination lasts for up to 3–4 years. The emphasis in a vaccination program should be on the young horses. Colostral antibody can be detected in the blood of foals from vaccinated dams for up to 6–7 months after which time it declines rapidly. Foals from vaccinated dams should be vaccinated at 6–8 months of age and revaccinated at 1 year of age. Foals from unvaccinated dams may be vaccinated at 2–3 months of age and again at 1 year of age. Colostral antibodies in the foal will prevent the development of autogenous antibodies, and foals vaccinated when less than 6 months should be revaccinated when they are 1 year old (57). A postvaccinal hepatitis has been recorded in horses after vaccination but is uncommon, and it is described under that heading.

One of the most important aspects of the control of Venezuelan encephalomyelitis is the vaccination of the horse population to minimize the number of horses which are viremic and serve as amplifying hosts. A tissue culture-attenuated virus vaccine, TC83, is available for immunization of horses against Venezuelan encephalomyelitis. A highly effective immunity is produced within a few days following vaccination and serum neutralizing antibodies persist for 20–30 months (37, 38). The vaccine causes a mild fever, leukopenia and a viremia (39) and there are conflicting reports about its capacity to cause abortion (40). The persistence of antibodies following vaccination with the TC83 vaccine is dependent on whether or not the horse was previously vaccinated with WE and EE vaccines (41). The levels of serum antibody obtained following vaccination with TC83 are not as high nor do they persist as long in horses which are vaccinated annually for WE and EE as in horses with no record of WE and EE vaccination. Antibodies to the heterologous alphaviruses, WE and EE, existing at the time of TC83 vaccination, may suppress the VE antibody response to the vaccine. However, the response to the vaccine is adequate to provide protection against VE and the interference is not considered significant (58). The vaccine is considered to be safe and efficacious (59). The presence of prevaccination antibodies to VE virus vaccine, TC83, has no influence on antibody stimulation by WE or EE vaccines (42). There is inconclusive evidence that WE and EE antibodies protect horses against infection with virulent VE virus, or conversely that VE antibodies protect against infection with WE and EE viruses (42). Simultaneous vaccination using all three strains of the virus is effective and recommended in areas where all three viruses may be present (43). The CT83 vaccine appears to have stable virulence and is not passaged by insects. The vaccine was used extensively in an outbreak of Venezuelan encephalomyelitis in the United States in 1971, and was augmented by large-scale aerial spraying to reduce vector population (16). The failure of the disease to recur in 1972 is credited to the immunogenicity of the vaccine and to the highly organized vaccination program carried out in the southern United States in 1971 combined with quarantine regulations and one of the largest spray operations ever conducted (44).

REVIEW LITERATURE

Johnson, K. M. & Martin, D. H. (1974) Venezuelan equine encephalitis. *Adv. vet. Sci. comp. Med.*, *18*, 79

Monath, T. P. & Trent, D. W. (1981) Togaviral diseases of domestic animals.*Comp. Diag. Viral Dis.*, *4*, 332–440.

REFERENCES

(1) Hayes, C. G. & Wallis, R. C. (1977) *Adv. Virus Res.*, *21*, 37.
(2) Walton, T. E. & Johnson, K. M. (1971) *J. Am. vet. med. Assoc.*, *161*, 1509.
(3) Parker, R. L. et al. (1973) *J. Am. vet. med. Assoc.*, *162*, 777.
(4) Wilson, J. H. et al. (1986) *Prev. vet. Med. 4*, 261.
(5) Barrett, M. W. & Chalmers, G. A. (1975) *J. Wildlife Dis.*, *11*, 157.
(6) Pursell, A. R. et al. (1972) *J. Am. vet. med. Assoc.*, *161*, 1143.
(7) Pursell, A. R. et al. (1976) *J. Am. vet. med. Assoc.*, *169*, 1101.
(8) Galindo, P. & Grayson, M. A. (1971) *Science, NY*, *172*, 594.
(9) Hayes, R. O. et al. (1964) *Am. J. trop. Med. Hyg.*, *13*, 595.
(10) Spalatin, J. et al. (1964) *Can. J. comp. Med.*, *28*, 131.
(11) Walton, T. E. & Johnson, K. M. (1972) *Infect. Immun.*, *5*, 155.
(12) Erickson, G. A. et al. (1974) *Am. J. vet. Res.*, *35*, 1533.
(13) Dickerman, R. W. et al. (1975) *Am. J. vet. Res.*, *34*, 357.
(14) Bigler, W. J. et al. (1974) *Am. J. trop. Med. Hyg.*, *23*, 513.
(15) Smart, D. L. et al. (1975) *J. Wildlife Dis.*, *11*, 195.
(16) Sudia, W. D. & Newhouse, V. F. (1975) *Am. J. Epidemiol.*, *101*, 1, 17.
(17) Dickerman, R. W. et al. (1973) *Am. J. Epidemiol.*, *98*, 311.
(18) Walton, T. E. et al. (1973) *J. infect. Dis.*, *128*, 271.
(19) Sudia, W. D. & Newhouse, V. F. (1975) *Am. J. Epidemiol.*, *101*, 1, 36.
(20) Franck, P. T. & Johnson, K. M. (1971) *Am. J. Epidemiol.*, *94*, 487.
(21) Emord, D. E. & Morris, C. D. (1984) *J. med. Entomol.*, *21*, 395.
(22) Calisher, C. H. et al. (1982) *Am. J. trop. Med. Hyg.*, *31*, 1260.
(23) Calisher, C. H. et al. (1983) *J. Am. vet. med. Assoc.*, *183*, 438.
(24) Kirk, L. J. & Holden, P. (1974) *Can. J. Microbiol.*, *20*, 215.
(25) Roberts, E. D. et al. (1970) *Am. J. vet. Res.*, *31*, 1223.
(26) Monlux, W. S. & Luedke, A. J. (1973) *Am. J. vet. Res.*, *34*, 465.
(27) Miller, L. D. et al. (1974) *Proc. 77th ann. Mtg. US. Anim. Hlth Assoc.*, 77, 629.
(28) Erickson, G. A. & Mare, C. J. (1975) *Am. J. vet. Res.*, *36*, 167.
(29) Joubert, L. et al. (1974) *Bull. Soc. Sci. vét. Med. comp. Lyon*, *76*, 255.
(30) Omohundro, R. E. (1971) *J. Am. vet. med. Assoc.*, *161* 1516.
(31) Wong, F. C. & Lillie, L. E. (1976) *Can. J. publ. Hlth*, *67*, Suppl. 1, 15.
(32) McLintock, J. (1976) *Can. J. publ. Hlth*, 67 Suppl. 1, 8.
(33) Potter, M. E. et al. (1977) *J. Am. vet. med. Assoc.*, *170*, 1396.
(34) Bigier, W. J. et al. (1975) *J. Wildlife Dis.*, *11*, 348.
(35) Smart, D. L. et al. (1975) *J. Wildlife Dis.*, *11*, 195.
(36) Bryne, R. J. (1973) *Proc. 3rd int. Conf. equ. infect. Dis.*, 115.
(37) Walton, T. E. et al. (1974) *Proc. 77th ann. Mtg. US Anim. Hlth Assoc.*, 77, 196.
(38) Sampson, G. R. et al. (1973) *Mod. vet. Pract.*, *54*, No. 8, 19.
(39) Walton, T. E. et al. (1972) *Am. J. Epidemiol.*, *95*, 247
(40) Anon (1973) *J. Am. vet.med. Assoc.*, *162*, 226.
(41) Vanderwagen, L. C. et al. (1975) *Am. J. vet. Res.*, *36*, 1567.
(42) Ferguson, J. A. et al. (1977) *Am. J. vet. Res.*, *38*, 425.
(43) Barber, T. L. et al. (1978) *Am. J. vet. Res.*, *39*, 621.

(44) Spears, J. F. (1972) *Agric. Chem.*, *27*, 12.
(45) Griffiths, B. B. et al. (1978) *Res. ves. Sci.*, *25*, 200.
(46) Hoff, G. L. et al. (1978) *J. Am. vet. med. Assoc.*, *172*, 351.
(47) Trent, D. W. & Grant, J. A. (1980) *J. gen. Virol.*, *47*, 261.
(48) Hayes, R. O. et al. (1977) *J. med. Entomol.*, *14*, 257.
(49) Dickerman, R. W. et al. (1980) *Am. J. trop. Med. Hyg.*, *29*, 269.
(50) Neufeld, J. L. & Nayar, G. P. S. (1982) In: *Western Equine Encephalitis in Manitoba.*, L. Sekla. Dept. of Health, Winnipeg, Manitoba, pp. 62–79.
(51) Grady, G. F. et al. (1978) *Am. J. Epidemiol*, *107*, 170.
(52) Dietz, W. H. Jr. et al. (1980) *Am. J. trop. Med. Hyg.*, *29*, 133.
(53) Justines, G. et al. (1980) *Am. J. trop. Med. Hyg.*, *29*, 653.
(54) Dietz, W. H. Jr. et al. (1978) *J. infect. Dis.*, *137*, 227.
(55) Pantekoek, J. F. C. A. (1979) *Proc. Am. Assoc. vet. Lab. Diag.*, *21*, 507.
(56) Srihongse, S. et al. (1978) *Am. J. trop. Med. Hyg.*, *27*, 1240.
(57) Ferguson, J. A. et al. (1979) *Am. J. vet. Res.*, *40*, 5.
(58) Ferguson, J. A. et al. (1978) *Am. J. vet. Res.*, *39*, 371.
(59) Baker, E. F. et al. (1978) *Am. J. vet. Res.*, *39*, 1627.
(60) Calisher, C. H. et al. (1986) *Am. J. vet. Res.*, *47*, 1296.
(61) Monath, T. P. et al. (1981) *Am. J. vet. Res.*, *42*, 1418.
(62) McLean, R. G. et al. (1985) *Am. J. trop. Med. Hyg.*, *34*, 1190.
(63) Maness, K. S. C. & Calisher, C. H. (1981) *Curr. Microbiol.*, *5*, 311.
(64) Calisher, C. H. et al. (1979) *Bull. Pan. Am. Hlth Org.*, *13*, 380.
(65) Mayhew, I. G. et al. (1987) *J. vet. int. Med.*, *1*, 45.
(66) Waldner, R. et al. (1984) *Am. J. trop. Med. Hyg.*, *33*, 699.

Japanese encephalitis

Japanese encephalitis is primarily a disease of humans who provide the source of infection for animals in most instances. Sporadic cases of encephalitis in racehorses have been observed in Malaysia (1) and serum neutralization tests have indicated the presence of Japanese encephalitis in affected horses.

The clinical manifestations of the disease in horses vary widely in severity. Mild cases show fever up to 39·5°C (103°F), anorexia, sluggish movements and sometimes jaundice for 2–3 days only. More severe cases show pronounced lethargy, mild fever and somnolence. Jaundice and petechiation of the nasal mucosa are usual. There is difficulty in swallowing, incoordination, and staggering and falling, although little difficulty may be experienced in getting up. Transient signs which persist for about 36 hours include neck rigidity, radial and labial paralysis, and blindness. In the most severe cases there is high fever (40·5–41·5°C, 105–107°F), hyperexcitability, profuse sweating and muscular tremor. Violent, uncontrollable activity may occur for a short period. This severe type of the disease is uncommon, representing only about 5% of the total cases, but is more likely to terminate fatally. In most cases complete recovery follows an illness lasting from 4 to 9 days. An enzyme-linked immunosorbent assay (ELISA) test is available for the diagnosis of active or recent infection in swine (9).

Transmission can be effected by the subcutaneous injection of whole blood from a clinically affected to a normal horse. Mosquitoes are the natural vectors and a human–mosquito–pig cycle maintains the infection throughout the year. The period of greatest prevalence is when vectors are most prevalent. The mosquito *Culex tritaeniorhyncus* is the principal vector and the virus can overwinter in it (2). The disease can be differentiated from viral encephalomyelitis of horses by serological and by virus neutralization tests (3).

The disease in cattle, sheep and goats is largely symptomless (4) and of little overall significance. Widespread losses, however, have been reported in swine, particularly in Japan, and these animals are thought to be a major natural source of the virus. The disease occurs as a non-suppurative encephalitis in pigs under 6 months of age. Sows abort or produce dead pigs at term. Formolized vaccines afford excellent protection against the encephalitis produced experimentally or occurring naturally in pigs and horses (5), but are not effective in preventing stillbirths in pigs (6). Living vaccines containing attenuated strains of the virus (6, 8) do fulfill this requirement.

REFERENCES

(1) Kheng, C. S. et al. (1968) *Aust. vet. J.*, *.44*, 23.
(2) Fukumi, H. et al. (1975) *Trop. Med.*, *17*, 97, 129.
(3) Gould, D. J. et al. (1964) *Am. J. trop. Med. Hyg.*, *13*, 742.
(4) Spradbrow, P. (1966) *Vet. Bull.*, *36*, 55.
(5) Goto, H. (1976) *Equ. vet. J.*, *8*, 126.
(6) Kawakubo, A. et al. (1971) *J. Jap. vet. Med. Assoc.*, *24*. 237.
(7) Kwon, H. J. et al. (1978) Research reports. Office of rural development, Korea, *Veterinary Seniculture*, *20*, 11.
(8) Ito, H. et al. (1974) *J. Jap. vet. med. Assoc.*, *27*, 331.
(9) Burke, D. S. et al. (1985) *Am. J. vet. Res.*, *46*, 2054.

Borna disease

Borna disease is an infectious encephalomyelitis of horses first recorded in Germany. It is caused by an unclassified virus which is more resistant to environmental influences than other equine encephalomyelitis viruses. The disease and the virus are indistinguishable from near eastern equine encephalomyelitis (NEEE) (1). The method of transmission is unknown, but it is thought to be by inhalation or ingestion (2), both sheep and horses being susceptible to intranasal infection (3). The NEEE virus is thought to be transmitted by a tick, probably *Hyalomma anatolicum* and the infection of horses to be accidental and outside a normal tick-bird cycle. It is possible that the viruses are the same and that the German disease is created by the periodic transfer of the virus from the Near East to Europe by migratory birds (4).

The morbidity in Borna disease is not high, but most affected animals die. As a rule only horses are susceptible, but occasional cases (6), and rarely outbreaks (1) occur also in sheep. Goats are susceptible to experimental infection. Rabbits can be infected by all routes, but other experimental animals are less susceptible. Continued passage of the virus through rabbits causes its attenuation, and a lapinized vaccine has been used to give satisfactory immunity to horses.

In field outbreaks the incubation period is about 4 weeks, and possibly up to 6 months (6). There is moderate fever, pharyngeal paralysis, lack of food intake, muscle tremor and hyperesthesia. Lethargy, somnolence and flaccid paralysis are seen in the terminal stages and death occurs 1–3 weeks after the first appearance of clinical signs. Infection without detectable clinical signs is thought to be common on infected premises. Clinicopathological identification is possible with complement fixation and fluorescent antibody tests. Antibody titers in CSF exceed those in serum (5), and CSF or brain tissue are suitable for diagnosis of the disease (2). At necropsy there are no gross findings, but histologically there is a typical viral encephalitis, affecting chiefly the brainstem, and a lesser degree of myelitis. Diagnostic intranuclear inclusion bodies are present in nerve cells of the hippocampus and olfactory lobes of the cerebral cortex. The virus can be grown on tissue culture (7). The immunohistological and ultrastructural aspects of the brain tissue of naturally infected horses has been examined (8).

REFERENCES

(1) Metzler, A. et al. (1976) *Schweiz. Arch. Tierheilkd.*, *118*, 483.
(2) Danner, K. (1976) *Zentralbl. VetMed.*, *23B*, 865.
(3) Heinig, A. (1964) *Arch. exp. VetMed.*, *18*, 753.
(4) Gibbs, E. P. J. (1976) *Equ. vet. J.*, *8*, 66.
(5) Ludwig, H. & Thein, P. (1977) *Med. Microbiol. Immunol.*, *163*, 215.
(6) Metzler, A. et al. (1979) *Schweiz. Arch. Tierheilkd.*, *121*, 37 & 207.
(7) Mayr, A. & Danner, K. (1974) *Zentralbl. VetMed.*, *21B*, 131.
(8) Gosztonyi, G. & Ludwig, H. (1984) *Acta Neuropathol.*, *64*, 213.

Other equine encephalomyelitides

The three North American encephalomyelitides (EE, WE and VE), Japanese encephalitis, Borna disease and near eastern equine encephalomyelitis are dealt with above. The equine herpesvirus 1 is attracting a good deal of attention as a cause of encephalomyelitis in horses and is dealt with under the heading of equine viral rhinopneumonitis. Rabies in horses is not uncommon in countries where that disease occurs; it is dealt with in the next section. There are still a number of other viral infections recorded as causes of encephalomyelitis of horses (1).

West Nile virus meningoencephalitis occurs in horses in the French Mediterranean littoral. Benign infection occurs in man and only serological evidence has been demonstrated in sheep, pigs, wild pigs and birds. *Culex modestus* is the vector. As in equine viral encephalomyelitis there is a biphasic fever, a course of 2–3 weeks, and a succession of signs from incoordination to paresis and eventually paralysis (2). Austria reports an outbreak of unidentified, but probably viral, hemorrhagic encephalomyelitis in 1974 (3, 4). Horses imported into Malaysia from Australia are sometimes found to have antibody titers against Murray Valley encephalitis, a disease of man, but the virus of this disease is not thought to infect wildlife or domestic animals. During an outbreak of Murray Valley encephalitis in man in Australia in 1974 (5) horses were found with titers against Murray Valley encephalitis and against Ross River encephalitis, another human disease, and two horses with histological evidence of viral encephalitis were also observed (6). Experimental infection with the Murray Valley encephalitis virus has been attempted in several different vertebrates including pigs, cattle and sheep; pigs developed antibody while cattle and sheep were non-responsive (8). The louping-ill virus has been isolated from cases of nervous disease in the horse (7).

The Powassan virus is capable of producing a non-suppurative, focal necrotizing meningoencephalitis in horses (9). The Powassan virus, a member of the flavivirus genus of the family Togaviridae is relatively common in Ontario and eastern United States (9). The virus is active in a forest animal tick cycle including *Ixodes cookei*, *I. marxi*, *Dermacentor andersoni*, groundhogs, snowshoe hares and the striped skunk. Infection in man has occurred following bites by infected ticks. Approximately 13% of horses sampled across Ontario in 1983 were serologically positive to the virus.

Experimental intracerebral inoculation of the Powassan virus into horses resulted in a neurological syndrome within 8 days. Clinical findings included a 'tucked-up' abdomen, tremors of the head and neck, slobbering and chewing movements resulting in foamy saliva, stiff gait, staggering and recumbency. Pathologically there was a non-suppurative encephalomyelitis, neuronal necrosis, and focal parenchymal necrosis. The virus could not be isolated from the brain. The lesions must be distinguished from those in rabies, equine viral rhinopneumonitic encephalitis, and western (WE), eastern EE and Venezuelan (VE) equine encephalomyelitides.

The California serogroup of viruses can also cause acute encephalitis in horses (10). In one case reported the horse recovered completely within 1 week and there was seroconversion to the snowshoe hare serotype of the California serogroup of viruses.

The Main Drain virus has been isolated from a horse with severe encephalitis in California (11). Clinical findings included incoordination, ataxia, stiffness of the neck, head-pressing, inability to swallow, fever and tachycardia. The virus is transmitted by rabbits and rodents and by its natural vector *Culicoides varipennis*.

An unusual incidence of neurological disease affecting 12 unrelated horses, over a period of several months during a drought, has been recorded (12). The clinical findings were dissimilar but the pathological findings were similar. However, the etiology was undetermined. It is postulated that a toxicosis may have been involved because of the unusually long dry period.

REFERENCES

(1) Gibb, E. P. J. (1976) *Equ. vet. J.*, *8*, 66.
(2) Joubert, L. & Oudar, J. (1974) *Bull. Soc. Sci. vet. Med. comp. Lyon*, *76*, 255.
(3) Jaksch, W. & Oulehla, J. (1974) *Wien. Tierärztl. Monatschr.*, *61*, 153.
(4) Burtscher, H. (1974) *Wien. Tierärztl. Monatschr.*, *61*, 157.
(5) Campbell, J. & Hore, D. E. (1975) *Aust. vet. J.*, *51*, 1.
(6) Gard, G. P. et al. (1976) *Aust. vet. J.*, *53*, 61.
(7) Timoney, P. J. et al. (1976) *Equ. vet. J.*, *8*, 113.
(8) Kay, B. H. et al. (1985) *Aust. J. exp. Biol. med. Sci.*, *63*, 109.
(9) Little, P. B. et al. (1985) *Vet. Pathol.*, *22*, 500.
(10) Lynch, J. A. et al. (1985) *J. Am. vet. med. Assoc.*, *186*, 389.
(11) Emmons, R. W. et al. (1983) *J. Am. vet. med. Assoc.*, *183*, 555.
(12) Robertson-Smith, R. G. et al. (1985) *Aust. vet. J.*, *62*, 6.

Rabies

Rabies is a highly fatal viral infection of the central nervous system, which occurs in all warm-blooded animals, and is transmitted by the bites of affected animals. It is manifested by motor irritation with clinical signs of mania and an attack complex, and by an ascending paralysis.

Etiology

The rhabdovirus (genus lyssavirus) of rabies is truly neurotropic and causes lesions only in nervous tissue. It is one of the larger viruses and is relatively fragile. It is susceptible to most standard disinfectants and dies in dried saliva in a few hours. The virus can be propagated in tissue culture and chick embryos.

On a worldwide basis there are minor and major antigenic variants of rabies virus (1). As measured by monoclonal nucleocapsid antibodies, old and new world rabies viruses as well as those from Asia may differ slightly but significantly from each other. Major antigenic determinants allow the grouping of viruses and minor determinants the differentiation of virus strains. Certain antigenic variants exist in nature against which conventional vaccines do not fully protect. In Canadian studies two major antigenic groups can be distinguished among the rabies virus isolates examined (2). One group is found in Ontario, Quebec and the Northwest Territories and is represented in the wild by endemic red fox and striped skunk rabies which originated in northern Canada. The second group is found in Manitoba where striped skunk rabies is endemic (2).

The term 'fixed' rabies virus refers to those strains which have been adapted to secondary hosts for experimental use and whose biological behavior is reproducible and characteristic of the strain. The 'street' viruses are those strains which are isolated from naturally infected warm-blooded animals.

Although the virus of classical rabies is a single antigenic entity it has become apparent that there are antigenically similar rabies-like viruses including the Makola and Lagos bat rabies which are found principally in small vertebrates (3). These strains appear to be limited in their geographical distribution to regions in Africa, unlike rabies virus which is distributed worldwide (3).

Epidemiology

Rabies occurs in most countries of the world except the island countries which are able to exclude it by rigid quarantine measures or prohibition of the entry of dogs. Australia and New Zealand have never had the disease, and Britain, Hawaii and Scandinavia are currently free. Britain had two minor outbreaks each involving one dog in 1969–70 but the disease was controlled successfully on each occasion. The disease is enzootic in Yugoslavia, Turkey and much of the United States, particularly the eastern and southern states. Vampire bat transmitted bovine paralytic rabies is endemic in the tropical regions extending from northern Mexico to northern Argentina and on the island of Trinidad (42). A recent outbreak in cattle in Guyana was epidemiologically associated with a large number of bats which had inhabited a large culvert which was not cleaned regularly because of excessive rainfall (42). It has become an important problem in Canada only in recent years, being carried down from the north to the populated areas largely by the migration of foxes, and has recently been diagnosed for the first time in dogs and foxes in Greenland. Sylvatic rabies is now the major problem in much of Europe. The disease is still spreading from a focal point which developed in Poland in the mid-1930s. The disease has spread westward to East and West Germany, Denmark, Belgium, Czechoslovakia, Austria, Switzerland and France (4) and spread continues at the rate of about 30–60 km (18–37 miles) per year and the threat to the United Kingdom increases each year. Foxes are the principal vectors and, as in Canada, cattle are the principal receptors. In North America skunks are the common vectors (6). In Western Canada, the main reservoirs of infection are skunks, bats and foxes (33).

There appears to be a difference in role between vectors. For example, in Europe it is thought that foxes carry the infection into a new area, but it is other species which disseminate it within an area (8). This would have important repercussions for control programs based on wildlife surveillance. Rabies occurs in most countries in the African continent, but the reported incidence is surprisingly low for an area with such a high population of wild carnivores. A number of wildlife hosts has been identified, including wild dogs, jackals and mongoose (34). Because of dislocation of civilian life rabies in Zimbabwe has increased in prevalence and geographical distribution in recent years (37).

Rabies is not of major economic importance in farm animals, although individual herds and flocks may suffer many fatalities. The disease is *always* fatal. The prime importance of rabies is its transmissibility to humans with veterinarians being at special risk. European data indicate that by far the greatest proportion of humans requiring pretreatment for rabies have been exposed to a rabid *domestic* animal, not a wild one (10). The disease is a major occupational hazard for veterinarians who should receive preexposure prophylaxis (5).

All warm-blooded animals, with the possible exception of opossums, are susceptible, and there is no variation in susceptibility with age, pigs 1 day old having contracted the disease. Variation in susceptibility between species is noticeable. Foxes, cotton rats, and coyotes are extremely susceptible; cattle, rabbits and cats are highly susceptible; dogs, sheep and goats are moderately susceptible, and opossums little if at all. The question of immunity after natural infection does not arise, but immunity can be produced artificially by vaccination.

Because of rapid developments in virological techniques, especially serological screening of animal populations to obtain presumptive diagnoses of the presence of a virus in the population, the question of latent infection and inapparent carriers of rabies has assumed some importance. The presence of rabies antibodies in animals in a supposed rabies-free area is likely to arouse concern. Inapparent carriers do occur in bats and there is some evidence that latent infections can occur in other species.

The source of infection is always an infected animal, and the method of spread is almost always by the bite of an infected animal, although contamination of skin wounds by fresh saliva may result in infection. Because of the natural occurrence of rabies in animals in caves inhabited by infected insectivorous bats, inhalation as a route of infection came under suspicion. It is now accepted that interbat spread, and spread from bats to other species is principally by bites, but that infection by inhalation also occurs. Ingestion of virus can also lead to infection if the dose is large enough (18).

The knowledge that infection can be transferred by ingestion has been put to use in devising systems of vaccinating wildlife by baiting them with virus-laden baits. The knowledge also has implications for epidemiological study generally. For example, attenuated viruses used in baits could be taken by other than the target species thus creating an unexpected seropositive segment of the animal population. It is also considered likely that outbreaks occurring naturally amongst carnivores may originate by them eating bats which have died of rabies (9).

Traditionally, the dog, and to a minor extent the cat, have been considered to be the main source animals. However, native fauna, including foxes, skunks, wolves, coyotes, vampire, insectivorous and fruit-eating bats, raccoons, mongoose, and squirrels may provide the major source of infection in countries where domestic carnivora are well controlled. Bats are the important species in which symptomless carriers are known to occur. Multiplication of the virus without invasion of the nervous system is known to occur in fatty tissues in bats and may be the basis of the 'reservoiring' mechanism known to occur in this species. Violent behavior is rare in rabid animals of this species, but has been observed. They represent a serious threat of spread of rabies in bats because of their migratory habits. Most spread is within the species, but the threat to humans and animal species by bats cannot be completely disregarded (15). Although rodents can be infected with the rabies virus they are not thought to play any part in the epidemiology of rabies, either as multipliers or simply as physical carriers of the virus. Many of the viruses they carry are rabies-like rather than classical rabies. A list of North American bats species from which rabies virus has been isolated is available (38). Surveys of the prevalence of rabies in different species of bats in certain geographical areas have been recorded (32). Rabies is enzootic in northern insectivorous bats in western Canada (49). The geographical and seasonal distribution of rabies in skunks, foxes and bats in Texas has been described (50). In some areas, skunks may account for up to 90% of the rabies diagnosed in animals over a period of a few years (51).

Domestic livestock are rarely a source of infection although chance transmission to man may occur if the mouth of a rabid animal is manipulated during treatment or examination. The virus may be present in the saliva for periods up to 5 days before signs are evident.

Spread of the disease is quite often seasonal with the highest incidence in the late summer and autumn because of large-scale movements of wild animals at mating time and in pursuit of food. Rabies has occurred in several swine herds in southern Saskatchewan where the skunk population is high, and where farms were settled from rough terrain resulting in considerable interface between wildlife and domestic animals, and in which the management system allows the pigs to run free on the premises (40). The disease has also occurred in pigs reared in a closed feeder barn where access by wildlife was very unlikely (41). In general, foxes are less dangerous than dogs, foxes tending to bite only one or two animals in a group, while dogs will often bite a large proportion of a herd or flock. Not all bites from rabid animals result in infection because the virus is not always present in the saliva and moreover may not gain entrance to the wound if the saliva is wiped from the teeth by clothing or the coat of the animal. The virus may appear in the milk of affected animals but spread by this means is unlikely as infection through ingestion is not known to occur.

Pathogenesis

Following the deep introduction of rabies virus by the bite of a rabid animal, initial virus multiplication occurs in striated muscle cells at the site. The second tissues to become infected are the neuromuscular spindles which provides an important site of virus entry into the nervous system (43). The virus may also enter the nervous system at motor end plates. In the olfactory end organ in the nares, neuroepithelial cells are in direct contact with the body surface and these cells extend without interruption into the olfactory bulb of the brain. Following entry of the virus into nerve findings there is invasion of the brain by passive movement of the virus within axons first into the spinal cord then into the brain. The immune response during this phase of the infection is minimal and explains why neutralizing antibody and inflammatory infiltration are usually absent at the time of onset of encephalitic signs. Antibody titers reach substantial levels only in the terminal stages of the disease. Following entry of rabies virus to the central nervous system, usually in the spinal cord, an ascending wave of neuronal infection and neuronal dysfunction occurs.

The only lesions produced are in the central nervous system, and spread from the site of infection occurs only by way of the peripheral nerves. This method of spread accounts for the extremely variable incubation period which varies to a large extent with the site of the bite. Bites on the head usually result in a shorter incubation period than bites on the extremities. The severity and the site of the lesions will govern to a large extent whether the clinical picture is primarily one of irritative or paralytic phenomena. The two extremes of the paralytic or dumb form and the furious form are accompanied by many cases which lie somewhere between the two. It might be expected that when irritation phenomena do occur they will be followed by paralysis as the stimulated nerve cells are subsequently destroyed. This is not always the case. Gradually ascending paralysis of the hindquarters may be followed by quite severe signs of mania which persist almost until death. In these cases it is probable that destruction of spinal neurons results in paralysis, but when the virus invades the brain, irritation of higher centers produces manias, excitement and convulsions. Death is usually due to respiratory paralysis. The clinical signs of salivation, indigestion and pica, paralysis of bladder and anus and increased libido all suggest involvement of the autonomic nervous system, including endocrine glands. At death there are viral inclusions and particles in virtually every neuron in the brain, spinal cord and ganglia, but none in the supportive cells of the CNS (12). Electron microscopic examination also shows the presence of the virus in the cornea, which it reaches centrifugally along the peripheral nerves. Virus reaches the salivary glands and many other organs in the same way but the highly infective nature of saliva arises from passage of the virus along the olfactory nerve to taste buds and other sensory end organs in the oropharynx, rather than from the salivary glands. The virus may be found in milk, in some organs and in fetuses, but the virus cannot be demonstrated in the blood at any time.

Variations in the major manifestations as mania or paralysis may depend in part upon the source of the virus. Virus from vampire bats almost always causes the paralysis form of the disease. Certainly, 'fixed' virus which has been modified by serial intracerebral passage causes ascending paralysis in contrast to 'street' virus, which more commonly causes the furious form of the disease. The site of infection and the size of the inoculum may also influence the clinical course. There is also an apparent geographical difference in the proportion of animals affected by the furious or paralytic form of the disease. In the Americas a preponderance of cases are paralytic. In Africa and India most farm animals suffer the furious form (27, 29).

For all practical purposes the disease can be considered to be always fatal. But infrequently an experimentally infected animal shows clinical signs of the disease but recovers. There are two recent records of spontaneous recovery in man (13), and the occurrence of non-fatal rabies in all species has been reviewed (31). There appears to be no field occurrence in domestic animals of the finding in experimentally infected mice that some strains of virus invade only peripheral nerves and spinal ganglia leaving a number of survivors with permanent nervous disability. The pathogenesis of recovery from rabies is of great importance in relation to vaccination and to serological testing to determine the incidence and prevalence of the disease.

Clinical findings

Among farm animals, cattle are most commonly affected. The incubation period is usually about 3 weeks, but varies from 2 weeks to several months in most species, although incubation periods of 5 and 6 months have been observed in cattle and dogs. In one large-scale outbreak in sheep deaths occurred 17–111 days after exposure.

In the paralytic form, knuckling of the hind fetlocks, sagging and swaying of the hindquarters while walking, often deviation or flaccidity of the tail to one side, are common early signs. Decreased sensation always accompanies this weakness and is one of the best diagnostic criteria in the detection of rabies. It is most evident over the hindquarters. Tenesmus, with paralysis of the anus, resulting in the sucking in and blowing out of air usually occurs late in the incoordination stages just before the animal goes down. This again is a characteristic sign but it may be transient or absent. Drooling of saliva is one of the most constant signs. The so-called yawning movements are more accurately described as voiceless attempts to bellow. Paralysis follows, the animal goes down and is unable to rise. Bulls in this stage often have paralysis of the penis. Death usually occurs 48 hours after recumbency develops and after a total course of 6–7 days. This clinical picture has been produced experimentally by the intramuscular injection of brain tissue from naturally occurring cases of paralytic rabies ('derriengue') in cattle in Mexico.

In furious rabies the animal has a tense, alert appearance, is hypersensitive to sounds and movement and is attracted by them so that it may look intently or approach as though about to attack. In some cases they will violently attack other animals or inanimate objects. These attacks are often badly directed and are impeded by the incoordination of gait. Frequently, loud bellowing is usual at this stage. The sound is characteristically hoarse and the actions are exaggerated. Sexual excitement is also common, bulls often attempting to mount inanimate objects. Multiple collections of semen for artificial insemination have been made during very short periods from bulls which later proved to be rabid. With this violent form of the disease the termination is characteristically sudden. Severe signs may be evident for 24–48 hours and the animal then collapses suddenly in a paralyzed state, dying usually within a few hours.

There is no constant pattern in either the development or the range of signs. Body temperatures are usually normal but may be elevated to 39·5–40·5°C (103–105°F) in the early stages by muscular activity. Appetite varies also. Some animals do not eat or drink, although they take food into the mouth. There is apparent inability to swallow. Others eat normally until the terminal stages. The course may vary from 1 to 6 days. So great is the variation in clinical picture that any animal known to be exposed and showing signs of spinal cord or brain involvement should be considered rabid until proved otherwise.

In sheep, rabies often occurs in a number of animals at one time due to the ease with which a number can be bitten by a dog or fox. Clinically the picture is very similar to that seen in cattle. The minority show sexual excitement, attacking humans or each other, and vigorous wool pulling, sudden falling after violent exertion, muscle tremor and salivation are characteristic. Excessive bleating does not occur. Most sheep are quiet and anorectic. Goats are commonly aggressive, and continuous bleating is common (29).

Most recorded cases in horses are lacking in distinctive nervous signs initially, but incline to the paralytic form of the disease (44). The initial clinical findings may include abnormal postures, frequent whinnying, unexplained aggressiveness and kicking, biting, colic, sudden onset of lameness in one limb followed by recumbency the next day, high-stepping gait, ataxia, apparent blindness and violent head-tossing (44). Lameness or weakness in one leg may be the first sign observed but the usual pattern of development starts with lassitude, then passes to sternal recumbency and lateral recumbency, followed by paddling convulsions and terminal paralysis. Horses which develop the furious form show excitement, become vicious and bite and kick. Their uncontrolled actions are often violent and dangerous and include blind changes, sudden falling and rolling and chewing of foreign material on their own skin. Hyperesthesia and muscular twitching of the hindlimbs followed by crouching and weakness are also recorded in the horse (45).

Pigs also show excitement and a tendency attack, or dullness and incoordination. Affected sows show twitching of the nose, rapid chewing movements, excessive salivation and clonic convulsions (16). They may walk backwards. Terminally there is paralysis and death occurs 12–48 hours after the onset of signs. The clinical findings in pigs are extremely variable, and individual cases may present in a variety of ways and only one or two of the classical findings may occur (40).

Clinical pathology

No antemortem laboratory examination has proved to be of diagnostic value, but tests for lead on blood, urine and feces may help to eliminate lead poisoning as a possible diagnosis. Virus neutralization tests are available, but the presence of neutralizing antibodies is not necessarily diagnostic of rabies. Other available tests are passive hemagglutination, complement fixation, radioimmunoassay, indirect fluorescent antibody staining. But these are used more to determine immune status than as a diagnostic aid to detect the presence of the disease. However, the virus has been identified in experimentally infected living dogs by direct immunofluorescence, and by intracerebral injection into mice, utilizing corneal smears and saliva as test materials. The results were much better when the test materials were collected during the clinical rather than preclinical stages (19).

Necropsy findings

Confirmation of a diagnosis of rabies depends on careful laboratory examination of fresh brain. Dogs or other species, which are suspected of having rabies because of abnormal behavior, should be kept in isolation where they cannot bite others, for 10 days. The animal can be classified as non-rabid if it is alive at the end of that time: of course it may still be desirable to carry out a postmortem examination. Dogs which die during the surveillance are submitted to laboratory tests aimed at completing the diagnosis. Also if any doubt exists that an animal has survived clinical rabies some attempt should be made to determine this: it would be the first natural case known to recover (13).

The recommended laboratory procedure (17) includes the following three tests and it is recommended that at least two of them be used on all specimens (22).

- A fluorescent antibody (FA) test on impression smears from the brain—preferably hippocampus, medulla oblongata, cerebellum or gasserian ganglion. The test can be completed in approximately 2 hours and is highly accurate when done routinely by experienced personnel (7). The reliability of the fluorescent antibody test confirmed by the mouse inoculation test is over 99% (33, 39)
- A histological search for Negri bodies in tissue sections with results available in 48 hours. Because of false positive diagnoses the technique is in some disrepute (24)
- Intracerebral inoculation of weaned mice with brain tissue with results in 3 weeks or less. The incubation period in mice before clinical signs are seen averages 11–12 days (range of 4–18 days), and death occurs in 7–21 days. The mouse brain is harvested as soon as signs appear and is submitted to the same tests described above. Thus a positive result can be obtained as soon as 4–7 days after inoculation. Some mice must be left for the full 21 days because only a negative result at that time can give a complete negative to the test.

Although brain is recommended as a source of virus for testing, spinal cord is just as satisfactory, and salivary gland is also a dependable source of virus. Fluorescent antibody staining is a satisfactory way of demonstrating its presence there (35). This provides an accurate and practical method of making a positive diagnosis when brain is not available (26).

Diagnosis

The diagnosis of rabies is one of the most difficult and important duties that a veterinarian is called upon to perform. Since in most cases there is a probability of human exposure, failure to recognize the disease may place human life in jeopardy. It is not even sufficient to say that if rabies occurs in the area one will classify every animal showing nervous signs as rabid, because nervous signs may not be evident for some days after the illness commences. In addition, many animals suffering from other diseases will be left untreated. The safest attitude to adopt is to handle all suspect animals with extreme care but continue to treat them for other diseases if such treatment appears to be indicated. If the animal is rabid, it will die and the diagnosis can then be confirmed by laboratory examination.

There are many diseases which are manifested by signs of abnormal mental state or paralysis or a combination of both (see page 914). In cattle with acute and subacute lead poisoning the clinical findings are similar to those of furious and dumb rabies. In acute lead poisoning the common clinical findings are blindness, convulsions, champing of the jaws with the production of frothy saliva and twitching of the eyelids and ears. In subacute lead poisoning in cattle there is blindness, stupor, head-pressing, grinding of the teeth and almost no response to treatment. Rabid cattle are usually not blind and signs of motor irritation such as convulsions and twitching of the facial muscles usually do not occur. However, there are signs of bizarre mental behavior, such as wild gazing, bellowing, yawning, attacking and compulsive walking. Lactation tetany and avitaminosis A are commonly more convulsive than maniacal. Polioencephalomalacia is accompanied by obvious cerebral involvement including blindness, nystagmus, opisthotonus and convulsions in sheep and cattle but salivation, bawling, anesthesia and tenesmus do not occur. Listeriosis in cattle and sheep is usually manifested by localizing signs of circling and facial nerve paralysis. In sheep, enterotoxemia is usually confined to lambs on heavy carbohydrate diets, pregnancy toxemia is entirely a disease of pregnant ewes and is readily differentiated by the presence of ketonuria, and louping-ill is transmitted by insects, has a seasonal occurrence and a localized geographical distribution. In pigs rabies must be differentiated from pseudorabies, Teschen's disease, and involvement of the brain in several other diseases of the pigs such as hog and African swine fever, meningitis caused by *Streptococcus suis* type II, *Hemophilus* spp., Glasser's disease, *E. coli* septicemia and erysipelas.

In horses, rabies must be differentiated from many different encephalomyelitides which are summarized in Table 69.

Treatment

No treatment should be attempted after clinical signs are evident. Immediately after exposure irrigation of the wound with 20% soft soap solution or a solution of Zephiran may prevent the establishment of the infection (9). Post-exposure vaccination is unlikely to be of value in animals, as death usually occurs before appreciable immunity has had time to develop. Euthanasia of suspect animals must be prevented, particularly if human exposure has occurred, since the development of the disease in the animals is necessary to establish a diagnosis. Antirabies serum may become available for animal treatment at some future date.

Control

It is not possible to give complete details of programs for rabies control here. Such programs include control of the disease in dogs, other domestic animals, wildlife and bats, and have been reviewed in detail (9).

For farm animals there are two useful control techniques: the prevention of exposure and vaccination. The former can be achieved to a degree by destruction of wild fauna, muzzling, restraint and vaccination of all cats and dogs, and keeping farm animals indoors.

Foxes account for a very large proportion (85% in Europe) of wildlife rabies and a control program aimed at reducing their population is capable of controlling the spread of rabies; the disease dies out for want of sufficient multiplying hosts (20). However, the difficulty of limiting their population size without eliminating them altogether has led to a search for ways of vaccinating them. It is now known that foxes can be protected by orally administered ERA vaccine (21) which is more effective than the inactivated vaccine (46). As stated earlier there is some risk that rodents will eat the baits that are set out for foxes and become rabid, and even bite and infect other rodents (23) or foxes. But rats and mice are generally considered to play no part in rabies epidemiology, possibly because they die quietly and without biting (25). However, intensive measures necessary for controlling the size of fox populations are unlikely to be applied consistently in a variety of countries (36). For this and other similar reasons (8) there is no practical, effective way of reducing a fox population other than by gassing them in their earths, a technique unlikely to be acceptable to the population at large (14). However, mass oral vaccination of terrestrial wild animals is a rabies control method which is feasible, effective and internationally accepted (52).

Both inactivated and attenuated live virus vaccines are used but only the attenuated ones are acceptable. Often the high egg passage (HEP) Flury strain produced in chick embryo and the ERA strain virus propagated in tissue culture are in general use with better results deriving from the latter (28). The field duration of immunity with the ERA vaccine is 3 years in cattle and 2 years in horses and dogs. With the HEP Flury vaccine the duration of the immunity is 6–12 months. Vaccine produced from the Kelev strain also has a modest reputation (21). An inactivated vaccine used in Italy appears to stimulate serum antibody almost equivalent to that provided by the live vaccine (47). A vaccine inactivated with binary-ethylenimine and containing aluminum hydroxide adjuvant will provide excellent protection for up to 3 years and is very useful for the control of rabies in cattle in Latin America where the vampire bat is the main vector (48).

Vaccinal antibodies are present in the colostrum of vaccinated cows and it is recommended that, where annual vaccination of all cattle is carried out, calves be vaccinated at 4 months of age and again when 10 months old. Calves from unvaccinated dams can be protected by vaccinating them at 17 days of age. Post-vaccinal paralysis does not occur after its use. The value of post-exposure vaccination is unknown although in our own experience vaccination of a heifer with living, attenuated virus after exposure has been followed by death from rabies 30 days later. The vaccine must be administered intramuscularly and be kept in a viable state until used. Low passage virus intended for use in dogs has caused heavy mortality when used in cattle and the tendency has been to use high egg passage vaccine for all species. Occasional cases of anaphylaxis occur, presumably due to sensitivity to egg protein, but are preventable by the use of antihistamines. In man a single-dose, inactivated, highly concentrated vaccine is now available and seems likely to supplement the attenuated, multiple dose vaccines at present in use. There is a massive literature on human vaccination and it is not reviewed here.

The most effective method of preventing the entry of rabies into a country free of the disease is the imposition of a quarantine period of 4–6 months on all imported dogs. This system has successfully prevented the entry of the disease into island countries, but has obvious limitation in countries which have land borders. The occurrence of the disease in two dogs in the United Kingdom in 1969–70 in which the incubation period appeared to last 7–9 months suggests that the more usual period of 6 months may give incomplete protection and vaccination on two occasions with an inactivated vaccine while the animal is still in quarantine for 6 months is the current recommendation. To require a longer period of quarantine would encourage evasion of the law by smuggling. The situation in the United Kingdom and in any country where the disease does not occur, is a vexed one. It is possible to rely chiefly on quarantine and act swiftly to stamp the disease out if it occurs. The shock eradication program would include quarantine of and vaccination in a risk area, ring vaccination around it, and destruction of all wildlife. This procedure is likely to be adopted in countries where the risk is small, such as Australia. (Details of the recommended administrative procedures are available (30).) Where the risk is great consideration must be given to mass vaccination of wildlife by baits, because wildlife are the cracks in the defense armor. The use of combined vaccines containing rabies vaccine in a lot of other vaccines used in dogs would be an effective and panic-free way of increasing the immune status of the pet population (6).

REVIEW LITERATURE

Baer, G. M. (1984) Control of rabies infection in animals and humans. In: *Control of Virus Diseases*, eds Kurstak, E. & Marusyk, R. G. New York: Marcel Dekker.

Charlton, K. M., Webster, W. A., Casey, G. A., Rhodes, A. J., MacInnes, C. D. & Lawson, K. F. (1986). Recent advances in rabies diagnosis and research. *Can. vet. J.*, *27*, 85–96, 1986.

Kaplan, C., Turner, G. S. & Warrell, D. A. (1986) *Rabies, the Facts*, 2nd edn, 126 pp. Oxford:Oxford University Press.

WHO Expert Committee on rabies (1984) *WHO Tech Report Series*, *709*. Geneva: WHO.

Pilet, C. (1982) Special issue on animal rabies. *Comp. Immunol. Microbiol. infect. Dis.*, *5*, 1–395.

Tabel, H. et al. (1974) History and epizootiology of rabies in Canada. *Can. vet. J.*, *15*, 271.

Taylor, D. et al. (1976) Rabies; epizootic aspects, diagnosis, vaccines. *Vet. Rec.*, *99*, 157.

REFERENCES

(1) Schneider, L. G. (1982) *Comp. Immunol. Microbiol. infect. Dis.*, *5*, 101.
(2) Webster, W. A. et al. (1985) *Can. J. comp. Med.*, *49*, 186.
(3) Wunner, W. H. (1985) In: *World's Debit to Pasteur. The Wistar Symp. Series*, Vol. 3, pp. 171–186.
(4) Schneider, L. G. & Jackson, A. C. (1980) *Rabies Bull. Eur.*, *3*. 7.
(5) Martin, R. J. et al. (1982) *Can. vet. J.*, *23*, 317.
(6) Taylor, D. (1976) *Vet. Rec.*, *99*, 157.
(7) Charlton, K. M. et al. (1986) *Can. vet. J.*, *27*, 85.
(8) Steck, F. & Wandeler, A. (1980) *Epidemiol., Rev.*, *2*, 71.
(9) Lord, R. D. et al. (1975) *J. Wildlife Dis.*, *11*, 210.
(10) Thillerot, M. (1980) *Bull. Mens. Soc. Vet. Prat. France*, *64*, 485.
(11) Dubreuil, M. et al. (1979) *Ann. Rêch. vét.*, *10*, 9.
(12) Murphy, F. A. et al. (1973) *Lab. Invest.*, *29*, 1.
(13) Fischman, H. R. & Strandberg, J. D. (1973) *J. Am. vet. med., Assoc.*, *163*, 1050.
(14) Wachendorfer, G. (1976) *Prakt. Tierarztl.*, *57*, 80.
(15) Schowalter, D. B. (1980) *Can. J. comp. Med.*, *44*, 70.
(16) Morehouse, L. G. et al. (1968) *J. Am. vet. med. Assoc.*, *153*, 57.
(17) Done, J. T. et al. (1976) *Vet. Rec.*, *99*, 259.
(18) Afshar, A. (1979) *Br. vet. J.*, *135*, 142.
(19) Vasoncellos, A. A. et al. (1978) *Rev. Fac. Med. Vet. Zootech., Univ. São Paulo*, *15*, 75 & 143.
(20) Wandeler, A. et al. (1974) *Zentralbl. VetMed.*, *21B*, 735, 765.
(21) Black, J. G. & Lawson, K. F. (1980) *Can. J. comp. Med.*, *44*, 169.
(22) Germano, P. M. L. et al. (1977) *Rev. Fac. Med. Vet. Zootech., Univ. São Paulo*, *14*, 133.
(23) Winkler, W. G. et al. (1976) *Am. J. Epidemiol.*, *104*, 294.
(24) Derakhshan, I. et al. (1978) *Lancet*, *1* (8059), 302.
(25) Macadam, I. (1972) *Trop. Anim. Hlth Prod.*, *4*, 90.
(26) Howard, D. R. (1977) *Proc. 19th Ann. Mtg Am. Assoc. Vet. Lab. Diagnosticians*, p. 265.
(27) Parthasarathy, G. et al. (1978) *Ind. vet. J.*, *5*, 744.
(28) Abelseth, M. K. (1975) In: *The Natural History of Rabies*, ed. G. M. Baer, vol. 2, p. 206. New York:Academic Press.
(29) Barnard, B. J. H. (1979) *J. S. Afr. Vet. Assoc.*, *50*, 109.
(30) Anon. (1976) *Vet. Rec.*, *99*, 169.
(31) Afshar, A. & Bahmanyar, M. (1978) *Vet. Bull.*, *48*, 553.
(32) Rosatte, R. C. (1985) *Can. vet. J.*, *26*, 81.
(33) Prins, L. & Yates, W. D. G. (1986) *Can. vet. J.*, *27*, 164.
(34) Barnard, B. J. H. (1979) *Onderstepoort J. vet. Res.*, *46*, 155.
(35) Samol, S. (1976) *Bull. Off. int. Epizoot.*, *86*, 259.
(36) Toma, B. & Andral, L. (1977) *Adv. Virus Res.*, *21*.
(37) Foggin, C. M. & Swanepoel, R. (1979) *Cent. Afr. J. of Med.*, *25*, 98.
(38) Constantine, D. G. (1979) *J. Wildlife Dis.*, *15*, 343.
(39) Bradley, J. A. (1979) *Can. vet. J.*, *20*, 186.
(40) Yates, W. D. G. et al. (1983) *Can. vet. J.*, *24*, 162.
(41) Hazlett, M. J. & Koller, M. A. (1986) *Can. vet. J.*, *27*, 116.
(42) World Health Organization (1984) Control of rabies in wildlife. WHO Expert Committee on Rabies. *Technical Report Series*, 709, p. 64.
(43) Murphy, F. A. (1985) *The Wistar Symposium Series*, Vol. 3, pp. 153–169.
(44) West, G. P. (1985) *Equ. vet. J.*, *17*, 280.
(45) Meyer, E. E. et al. (1986) *J. Am. vet. med. Assoc.*, *188*, 629.
(46) Lawson, K. F. et al. (1982) *Can. J. comp. Med.*, *46*, 382.
(47) Prosperi, S. et al. (1984) *Vet. Res. Commun.*, *8*, 181.
(48) Larghi, O. P. & Nebel, A. E. (1985) *Zentralbl. VetMed. B.*, *32*, 609.
(49) Pybus, M. J. (1986) *J. Wildlife Dis.*, *22*, 307.
(50) Pool, G. E. & Hacker, C. S. (1982) *J. Wildlife Dis.*, *18*, 405.
(51) Heidt, G. A. et al. (1982) *J. Wildlife Dis.*, *18*, 269.
(52) Baer, G. M. (1985) In: *World's Debit to Pasteur. The Wistar Symp. Series*, Vol. 3, pp. 235–247.

Pseudorabies (Aujeszky's disease)

Pseudorabies is a viral disease affecting primarily pigs but occurring incidentally in most other species. In pigs the disease affects the respiratory, nervous and reproduction systems and its main manifestations are encephalitis and reproductive failure. In the other species there is both encephalitis and marked local pruritis.

Etiology

The disease is caused by an alphaherpesvirus, porcine herpesvirus 1 (PHV 1). The virus may survive for 2–7 weeks in an infected environment dependent on temperature fluctuations and pH level (3) and for up to 5 weeks in meat. The virus is lipophilic and sensitive to several commonly used disinfectants (44). Sodium hypochlorite (5·25%) is probably the most desirable and practical disinfectant to use in most instances. The virus grows in tissue culture and produces cytopathic change, and can also be passaged in rabbits and day-old chickens. Strain variation in virulence has been observed in field isolates and produced by laboratory attenuation (1, 2). There are numerous genomically different strains in the United States and restriction endonuclease analysis and DNA hybridization can be used to provide epidemiological information (83).

Epidemiology

Pseudorabies has a wide geographical distribution including the United States, Britain, Europe, North Africa, Asia and South America. There are also recent reports of its occurrence in New Zealand (4) and Ireland (5). Within affected countries there is a tendency for the disease to have a high prevalence in certain areas and in many countries there has been a marked increase in the prevalence of the disease over the past 5–10 years (6). There has been a marked increase in the number of recorded cases in most affected countries and rapid escalation to epidemic proportions in Holland, France, Belgium and the United States. In 1982 there was a sharp increase in the number of previous cases newly affected with the disease (62). The clinical disease has not been recorded in Canada and there is no serological evidence of infection in native cows (8).

Clinical disease occurs primarily in pigs. Naturally occurring cases in other species are rare and are usually fatal. Cases in cattle occur only sporadically, but a number of animals may be affected when cattle and pigs are comingled. The disease has occurred in goats which have been housed with swine (7).

Typically the disease spreads rapidly in infected piggeries over a period of 1–2 weeks and the acute stage of the outbreak lasts 1–2 months. In young, sucking pigs the morbidity and mortality rates approach 100%, but in mature swine the disease may produce no clinical signs, and animals that are affected usually recover. In herds of pigs the highest morbidity occurs initially in unweaned piglets, but as the outbreak continues and piglets become passively immunized through the sow's colostrum, the major incidence may move to weaners.

However, in recent years there has also been an increase in the morbidity and case fatality rates in older pigs associated with the intensification of pig rearing and the dominance of more virulent strains (12). In large breeding herds or finishing herds with the continual influx of susceptible pigs, the disease may become endemic. Pseudorabies may also be a significant cause of reproductive inefficiency in pig herds, and infection within the herd may be initially manifest by abortions in the sow herd, followed after a period by the more typical occurrence of neurological disease in suckling and growing pigs. The economic losses due to the disease can be very high because of mortality in young pigs, decreased reproductive performance and the necessity to depopulate to eradicate the disease from a herd (10). An economic assessment of an epidemic of pseudorabies in 150-sow farrow to finish operation on selected production and economic variables has been made (32). The mean litter size remained the same throughout the period of observation but there was a 2-fold increase in suckling pig mortality and 3·5-fold increase in stillbirths during the months of the epidemic compared with the period before the epidemic. Following the epidemic suckling pig mortality was 14% greater and stillbirth rate was 71% greater than during the months preceding the outbreak. The major economic losses (88% of the total loss) were related to breeding herd removal/depopulation and production downtime (32).

Following a natural infection with pseudorabies, sows build up an immunity which is transferred to their piglets in the colostrum. Maternal antibodies persist in piglets until 5–7 weeks of age. The colostral antibodies are almost entirely of the IgG type with small amounts of IgM. Following intranasal challenge, piglets with colostral immunity from naturally infected sows are protected from clinical disease, but not against subclinical infection. Vaccination of pregnant sows will induce a maternal immunity which will protect first litter piglets from experimental challenge exposure to the virus until about 24 days of age (56).

Pigs and possibly rodents appear to be the primary host for the virus. Pigs that recover from infection may be latent carriers of the virus and may convert to active shedders following stress such as transport or farrowing (1). The latent virus can be reactivated experimentally by the administration of corticosteroids (10). Latent infection with the virus can also be established in pigs vaccinated with an inactivated vaccine. The virus can be recorded from tissue fragments of pigs clinically recovered from disease for up to 13 months (12) and followed by a challenge with the live virus (67) which may be shed by sows for up to 19 months after initial infection (14). The disease may spread from normal or clinically affected pigs to animals of other species, but does not usually spread between animals of the other species. For example, sheep and calves can be infected experimentally, but there is no evidence that they excrete the virus. The virus was not transmitted horizontally from experimentally infected calves to control calves kept in close contact (9). The disease may occur in pigs, sheep and cattle on the same farm (13). Brown rats may be a minor source of infection but are unlikely to be an important reservoir. They are capable of spreading the disease to dogs. The wild Norway rat is thought to have only a minor role in the transmission of the disease to farm animals (41). The virus causes fatal disease in dogs which are usually infected from close association with infected pigs (42). The raccoon can be infected experimentally, but is not considered to be a long-term subclinical carrier of the virus (43). The possible role of wild animals in transmission of pseudorabies in swine has been examined with inconclusive results (58).

The virus is present in the nasal discharge and in the mouth of affected pigs on the first day of illness and for up to 17 days after infection (12). Transmission is primarily by direct contact but can also occur via contaminated drinking water and feed, and spread of the virus within and between farms can occur mechanically (12). Airborne transmission of the virus is now considered to be a possibility (62, 66). The virus has been recovered from air samples taken from boxes containing groups of pigs infected with the virus (66). It is postulated that sneezing infected pigs may generate the airborne virus which can spread by the airborne route between adjacent loose boxes under experimental conditions (66). The greatest recovery of the virus was aerosol which suggests that dust particles may be an important method of transmission.

An analysis of a series of outbreaks of Aujeszky's disease in Britain suggests that airborne spread is between pig premises 2–9 km apart (62). Virus is also excreted in the milk of infected sows and *in utero* infection occurs. The virus is inactivated in meat after 35 days of storage at −18°C (0·5°F) (11). Meat from infected pigs may cause infection when fed to dogs. Venereal transmission of latent infection in sows and boars has been suspected, but no direct evidence of venereal transmission has been presented (60). The effects of pseudorabies infection in adult boars appears to be related to the effects of the clinical disease rather than any direct effect on semen quality (20). The virus cannot usually be isolated from the urine or semen from infected boars and therefore the preputial secretions and the ejaculate are unlikely vehicles for shedding of the virus (60). The rarity of spread to other species is due to the scanty nasal discharge and the improbability of the discharge coming into contact with abraded skin or nasal mucosa of animals other than pigs. The disease has occurred in sheep and cattle following the use of a multiple-dose syringe previously used in infected swine (59).

The portal entry is through abraded skin or via the intact nasal mucosa. Experimentally the disease can be transmitted by these routes and by intracerebral injection. Although the virus is detectable in the blood in the early stages of the disease, there is no evidence that biting insects act as vectors. Care should be exercised during necropsy examination, as infection of humans may occur through skin wounds.

Pathogenesis

The virus is pantropic and affects tissues derived from all embryonic layers. In the pig there is a short and ill-defined period of viremia with localization of the virus in many viscera, but with multiplication occurring primarily in the respiratory tract. Spread to the brain is thought to occur by way of the olfactory, glossopharyngeal or trigeminal nerves. Virus disappears from the brain by the 8th day, coinciding with the appearance of neutralizing antibody in the blood (15). When the virus gains entry through a skin abrasion, it quickly invades the local peripheral nerves, passing along them centripetally and causing damage to nerve cells (16). It is this form of progression which causes local pruritis in the early stages of the disease and encephalomyelitis at a later stage when the virus has invaded the central nervous system. In pigs, pruritis does not develop after intramuscular injection, but a local paralysis indicative of damage to low motor neurons occurs prior to invasion of the central nervous system in some pigs. In cattle, pruritis of the head and neck is usually associated with respiratory tract infection, while perianal pruritis is usually due to vaginal infection (17).

When the virus is instilled into nasal cavities or inoculated into the brain, signs of encephalitis rather than local pruritus predominate. With oral inoculation there is an initial stage of viral proliferation in the tonsillar mucosa (19). Systemic invasion occurs and, as with intravenous injection, is followed by localization and invasion of the central nervous system along peripheral and autonomic nerve trunks and fibers. Localization in the lower part of the small intestine can result in necrotizing enteritis (18). The virus may be present in the trigeminal ganglion of a naturally infected sow without any history of clinical disease (45).

The virus can invade the uterus and infect preimplantation embryos which can lead to degeneration of the embryo and reproductive failure (69). Through the use of embryo transfer procedures, infected embryos may disseminate the virus from donors to recipients (68).

Clinical findings

The incubation period in natural outbreaks is about a week, whereas it may be as short as 2 days following experimental inoculation.

Pigs

The major signs are referable to infection of the respiratory, nervous and reproductive systems. However, there is considerable variation in the clinical manifestation depending on the virulence and tropism of the infecting strain. Nervous system disease is the major manifestation, but with some strains respiratory disease may be the initial and prime presenting feature. There is also strain variation in the pattern of age susceptibility.

Young pigs a few days to a month old show the greatest susceptibility. Very young sucklings develop an indistinct syndrome, but prominent nervous signs occur in older piglets. A febrile reaction, with temperatures up to 41·5°C (107°F), occurs prior to the onset of nervous signs. Incoordination of the hindlimbs causing sideways progression is followed by recumbency, fine and coarse muscle tremors and paddling movements. Lateral deviation of the head, frothing at the mouth, nystagmus, slight ocular discharge and convulsive episodes appear in a few animals. A snoring respiration with marked abdominal movement occurs in many, and vomiting and diarrhea in some affected pigs. Deaths occur about 12 hours after the first signs appear. In California a consistent sign has been blindness due to extensive retinal degeneration (22).

The disease in growing and adult pigs is generally much less severe but there is considerable variation depending upon the virulence of the infecting strain. In growing pigs the mortality falls with increasing age and is generally less than 5% in pigs at 4–6 months of age. With some strains, fever is a prominent sign with depression, and vomition and sometimes marked respiratory signs including sneezing, nasal discharge, coughing and severe dyspnea are common. Trembling, incoordination and paralysis and convulsions follow and precede death. With others, the disease may be manifest at this age by mild signs of posterior incoordination and leg weakness. In adults, fever may not be present and the infection may cause only a mild syndrome of anorexia, dullness, agalactia and constipation. However, virulent strains may produce acute disease in adults characterized by fever, sneezing, nasal pruritus, vomition, incoordination and convulsions and death (23). Infection in early pregnancy may result in embryonic death or abortion and early return to heat. An abundant vaginal discharge may occur. Infection in late pregnancy may result in abortion or in the subsequent birth of mummified fetuses which may involve all or only part of the litter (23, 24). Abortion may result from the effects of fever or from viral infection of the fetus (23). The virus has also been incriminated as a cause of an outbreak of myoclonia congenita in pigs (25).

Cattle and goats

There may be sudden death without obvious signs of illness. More commonly there is intense, local pruritus with violent licking, chewing and rubbing of the part. Itching may be localized to any part of the body surface, but is most common about the head, the flanks or the feet, the sites most likely to be contaminated by virus. There is intense excitement during this stage and convulsions and constant bellowing may occur. Maniacal behavior, circling, spasm of the diaphragm and opisthotonus are often evident. A stage of paralysis follows in which salivation, respiratory distress and ataxia occur. The temperature is usually increased, sometimes to as high as 41–41·5°C (106–107°F). Final paralysis is followed by death in 6–48 hours after the first appearance of illness. A case of non-fatal pseudorabies in a cow is recorded (54). There is also a report of pseudorabies occurring in feedlot cattle in which there were nervous signs, bloat, acute death, but no pruritus (61). The disease is recorded in young calves and is characterized clinically by encephalitis, no pruritus, erosion in the oral cavity and esophagus and a high case fatality rate (26). In goats, rapid deaths, unrest, lying down and rising frequently, crying plaintively, profuse sweating and spasms and paralysis terminally are characteristic. There may be no pruritus (27).

The clinical picture in dogs and cats is similar to that in cattle, with death occurring in about 24 hours (28).

Clinical pathology

In infected pigs the virus is usually present in nasal secretions for up to 10 days. A common method for the diagnosis of pseudorabies in sows is to take swabs from the nasal mucosa and vagina. Polyester and wire swabs shipped in 199 tissue culture medium supplemented with 2% fetal bovine serum (FBS) buffered with 0·1% sodium bicarbonate and HEPES will yield optimum recovery of the virus (45). Wooden applicator sticks with cottonwool have antiviral activity and recovery of the virus may not be possible after 2 days, which is of practical importance if the samples are shipped by mail (46).

Specific virus neutralizing antibodies are detectable in the serum of recovered pigs and this test is in routine use for herd diagnosis and survey purposes. Antibody is detectable on the 7th day after infection, reaches a peak about the 35th day and persists for many months (1). Paired serum samples taken as early as possible and about 3 weeks later show a marked antibody rise. The serological tests available include the serum neutralization test, countercurrent immunoelectrophoresis test, microimmunodiffusion test and the enzyme-linked immunosorbent assay (ELISA) test (29). The ELISA is most suitable based on sensitivity specificity, speed and cost (29). It does not depend on a continuous supply of cell cultures and can be automated (30). The radial immunodiffusion enzyme assay is a useful field test where cell cultures or ELISA equipment are not available (31). The dot enzyme immunoassay test is a rapid and economical field test with relative sensitivity of specificity in the order of 98–99% (47). A skin test is currently being evaluated (48).

Necropsy findings

There are no gross lesions typical and constant for the disease and diagnosis must rely on laboratory examination. When pruritus has occurred there is considerable damage to local areas of skin and extensive subcutaneous edema. The lungs show congestion, edema and some hemorrhages. Hemorrhages may be present under the endocardium and excess fluid is often present in the pericardial sac. In pigs there are additional lesions of visceral involvement. Slight splenomegaly, meningitis and excess pericardial fluid are observed and there may be small necrotic foci in the spleen and liver. Necrotic foci in the liver may also be seen in aborted fetuses. Histologically, in all species, there is severe and extensive neuronal damage in the spinal cord and brain. Perivascular cuffing and focal necrosis are present in the gray matter, particularly in the cerebellar cortex. Intranuclear inclusion bodies occur infrequently in the degenerating neurons particularly in cerebral cortex in the pig. These are of considerable importance in differential diagnosis. The presence of the characteristic necrotizing lesions with inclusion-body formation in the upper respiratory tract and lungs is specific for pseudorabies and the changes in the lung are readily distinguishable from other forms of pneumonia in pigs (1). Virus may be detected by direct fluorescent antibody examination or by growth in tissue culture. Virus may be detected in tissues such as impression smears of brain and pharynx by direct immunofluorescence (49). The immunoperoxidase test can be used to study the distribution of the virus in different tissues (50). The tissues of the head and neck regions of non-immune pigs yield most consistently and in the highest concentration after challenge (66). Latent virus can be detected using a DNA hybridization dot blot assay (84). Where possible, whole carcasses and fetuses should be submitted for laboratory examination. The placental lesions in pregnant sows which have aborted from natural infection with pseudorabies consist of necrotizing placentitis and the presence of intranuclear inclusions (52). The laboratory diagnosis of the disease has been reviewed (1).

Diagnosis

In pigs the protean nature of the disease warrants its inclusion in the differential diagnosis of many syndromes. The pattern of occurrence within a herd is similar to that of transmissible gastroenteritis but the clinical features are dissimilar. Pseudorabies presents a similar clinical picture to viral encephalomyelitis (Teschen disease). The inclusion bodies of pseudorabies, serological tests and particularly the isolation of virus in tissue culture are of help in diagnosis. Rabies is rare in pigs and is usually accompanied by pruritus at the site of the bite. Streptococcal meningitis is restricted in occurrence to sucking pigs of 2–6 weeks of age and the causative organism is readily cultured from the meninges. The response to treatment with penicillin is good and is of value as a diagnostic test. Hypoglycemia of baby pigs has a very similar clinical picture.

In enzootic areas louping-ill and Japanese encephalitis may have to be considered as possible causes of encephalitis in pigs. Involvement of the nervous system with the development of encephalitis may occur in outbreaks of hog cholera and African swine fever, but there are other diagnostic features in these outbreaks. In a number of bacterial infections there may be similar involvement of the central nervous system. These include salmonellosis, Glasser's disease, *E.coli* septicemia and erysipelas. Gut edema and salt poisoning produce obvious nervous signs, as does organophosphate toxicity, and the disease may closely mimic these syndromes when it occurs in weaner pigs. Pseudorabies should also be considered in any outbreak of respiratory disease that is poorly responsive to usually effective therapeutic measures.

Reproductive inefficiency associated with enterovirus (SMEDI) and parvovirus infections closely resembles that associated with pseudorabies and requires laboratory differentiation by virus isolation and serological testing.

In cattle the local pruritus is distinctive but the disease may be confused with the nervous form of acetonemia in which paresthesia may lead to excitement. The rapid recovery which ordinarily occurs in this form of acetonemia is an important diagnostic point. The furious form of rabies and acute lead poisoning cause signs of mania but pruritus does not occur.

Treatment

There is no effective treatment. The administration of hyperimmune serum to piglets at the time of infection will result in a significant reduction in mortality but it does not prevent infection occurring. The subcutaneous administration of 5 ml of hyperimmune serum to sucking piglets in a herd in which the disease has been confirmed will markedly reduce the mortality rate (53). The effect of the serum is greatest in piglets born from sows with serum antibody to the virus. Wet fed growers should be provided with water as inappetence may significantly reduce intake.

Control

The control of pseudorabies is difficult and currently unreliable because normal healthy pigs may be infected and shed or harbor the virus for up to several months (1, 2). The selection of a strategy for the control or elimination of the disease will depend on factors such as the source of the herd infection, the method of transmission of the virus, the survival of the virus in the environment, the sensitivity and specificity of the diagnostic test and the epidemiological determinants of the herd which include the type of operation, the degree of herd isolation, the prevalence of infection, the value of the genetic material, the level of management expertise and the availability of suitable virus-free replacement swine if depopulation and repopulation is chosen as a strategy (6).

The methods of control or eradication include depopulation and repopulation, test and removal, and segregation of progeny (6). Vaccination is also used to reduce clinical disease when outbreaks occur or when the disease is endemic in the herd.

When the prevalence of infection in the herd is over 50% eradication can be achieved by depopulation and repopulation with virus-free breeding stock (6). However, depopulation is the most expensive method and not compatible with the retention of valuable pedigree stock. The entire herd should be depopulated over a period of months as the animals reach market weight. After removal of the animals the entire premises must be cleaned and disinfected. Repopulation should be delayed at least 30 days after the final disinfection, and swine should originate from a pseudorabies-free qualified herd and be isolated on the premises and retested 30 days after introduction. All herd additions should likewise be isolated and tested 30 days after introduction.

The test and removal program is recommended when the prevalence of infection in the herd is below 50%. This method requires serologic testing of the entire breeding herd and immediate removal of all seropositive animals; 30 days after removal of seropositive animals, the herd is retested and if necessary at 30-day intervals until the entire herd tests are negative. Following a second negative test, the testing regimen may be changed to test only 25% of the herd every 4 months. Seropositive animals are identified and culled. The test and removal method is superior to the vaccination system as a method of control (85). Valuable genetic material may be salvaged from breeding stock which are seropositive using embryo transfer techniques. Embryos may be transferred safely to susceptible recipient gilts from sows that have recovered from infection (63), but not from sows that are in the active stages of infection. The virus does not penetrate the outer covering of the embryo, but it can become attached to it so that it may physically transfer to the uterus of the recipent. This transfer of infection may occur if the donor sow is in the active phase of infection (6).

An Aujeszky's disease control program was introduced in Great Britain in 1983 when the infection was spreading rapidly (55). New legislation imposed restrictions on the movement of pigs where clinical signs of the disease were present in the herd. The first part of the eradication scheme involved testing all of those herds previously known to have Aujeszky's disease (86). Within several months after the beginning of the eradication campaign 417 herds had been slaughtered, involving 342 275 pigs of which 72·5% were salvaged. Only 121 herds had been known to be previously infected, while the remaining 296 herds had been identified through tracebacks and reports of new cases. By 1985 it was concluded that the disease was well controlled in England with only 10–14 infected herds remaining. Farmers were compensated for all animals slaughtered and also for consequential loss associated with the loss of stock. The cost of the eradication program was financed by a levy on all pigs normally marketed for slaughter in England. The program has been very expensive and as of 1987 a cost-benefit analysis is not yet available. In Northern Ireland, Aujeszky's disease is more widespread than it ever was in Britain before the eradication program. Because the infection rate is over 50%, an eradication program based on slaughter of infected herds would destroy the swine industry. Thus the control program in Northern Ireland is based on the use of vaccination, the culling of seropositive animals and the gradual introduction of seronegative animals.

The strategy of segregation of progeny involves rearing piglets in isolation from the infected sow. This is used when the prevalence rate is about 50% and there is no clinical disease. After weaning the sow is culled and sent to slaughter and the piglets are reared in isolation facilities. The pigs are tested at 16 weeks, and the entire pen or litter of pigs is culled if any pig is seropositive. Groups of seronegative pigs are identified and combined into larger groups to establish a new herd. The original herd is gradually depopulated and the premises cleaned and disinfected. The new herd is then monitored on a regular basis.

The Pig Health Control Association in Britain has supervised a control scheme for Aujeszky's disease (51). Clinical disease due to the virus must not occur and the herd must be tested every 6 months and be seronegative. Importations are allowed only from other listed herds or by artificial insemination.

Vaccination can be useful in infected herds to reduce clinical disease and death losses. An effective immunity develops after natural infection or vaccination and piglets from immune sows are generally protected from clinical disease during the nursing period by colostral immunity (35). However, the presence of circulating antibody does not prevent infection with the virus, the development of latency and subsequent activation and excretion of the virus.

When an outbreak of the disease occurs in a susceptible herd the mortality may be very high, and the first consideration must be to prevent spread to uninfected sows and litters and pregnant sows from infected pigs. They should be attended by separate personnel or adequate barriers to mechanical transmission of infection should be arranged. On affected premises, cattle should be separated from pigs, and dogs and cats should be kept from the area. The affected herd should be quarantined and all pigs sold off the farm should be for slaughter only. On farms in which the disease is endemic or outbreaks have occurred, the use of hyperimmune serum in the suckling piglets, vaccination of the sows and management procedures to reduce the spread of infection have markedly reduced preweaning mortality and reproductive failures (40).

It is often virtually impossible to prevent the spread of infection in a susceptible herd and vaccination of all pigs at risk, especially pregnant sows, may be indicated. The vaccine will reduce losses in infected herds, limit the spread of infection and decrease the incidence in endemic areas (24). With a properly controlled and monitored vaccination and culling program in a breeding herd it is possible to control clinical disease and reduce the infection pressure (24). All breeding stock present during an outbreak are subsequently vaccinated regularly until they are all culled which removes the major sources of virulent virus. Following this phase, newly introduced gilts and boars are tested, and monitored regularly. This is considered to be less costly than the test and slaughter policy.

However, in vaccinated herds the virus continues to circulate and an accurate epidemiological analysis is not possible because titers caused by vaccination cannot be distinguished from those caused by natural infections (85).

Modified live virus and inactivated virus vaccines are available. Both vaccines will reduce the incidence rate and severity of clinical disease in an infected herd. Pigs are vaccinated by the intranasal or parenteral routes (39). In general, intranasal vaccination confers a more effective immunity to experimental infection than parenteral vaccination. All of the vaccines are based on experimental challenge of vaccinated animals. There appears to be no information available on field testing of the vaccine under controlled conditions. However, the vaccines will not prevent new infections in vaccinated animals nor latency and possible subsequent reactivation and shedding of the virus. Thus vaccinated swine can serve as reservoirs of infection.

The mechanism of protection provided by vaccination is not understood (57). The functional antibody tests, including virus neutralizing activity of serum, antibody-dependent cellular cytotoxicity and complement-mediated lysis did not correlate with protection (57). Cell-mediated immunity may be more important than humoral immunity in this disease which is characteristic of herpesvirus infections. Neither the modified live virus vaccine nor the inactivated vaccine will prevent infection or the development of microscopic lesions in vaccinated pigs which are challenge exposed to a virulent strain of the virus (70). Protection against clinical signs and microscopic lesions may be absent by 10 months after vaccination. The levels of cellular and humoral immunity following challenge are similar (71).

The presence of maternally derived colostral immunity in piglets interferes with the effectiveness of the vaccines (36). Intranasal vaccination confers better immunity in pigs with colostral antibody than does parenteral vaccination with either inactivated or attenuated vaccines. However, the efficacy of intranasal vaccination decreases with increasing levels of colostral immunity at the time of vaccination (38).

Vaccination of pregnant sows stimulates neutralizing antibodies which are transferred to the newborn piglets and provide protection against contact and experimental intranasal infection.

Newborn pigs rely on antibodies from colostrum and milk for protection against pseudorabies. The vaccination of piglets born from vaccinated sows does not produce a significant serological response until the piglets are about 12 weeks of age. Earlier vaccination of piglets from infected or vaccinated sows is ineffective because high levels of maternal antibodies interfere with a serological response stimulated by the vaccine (36). The parenteral vaccination of weaned pigs at 8 weeks of age with an inactivated oil adjuvanted vaccine did not provide full protection against experimental challenge when the pigs were 22–27 weeks of age (64). However, the severity and duration of clinical disease decreased with increasing seroneutralizing titers. Challenge resulted in severe disease and weight loss in control pigs. Maternal immunity appears to interfere markedly with the development of active immunity from vaccination until at least 15 weeks of age even when the serum neutralizing titers are low (64). Thus in a situation in which the majority of sows have been infected or vaccinated, vaccination of weaned pigs may not yield desirable results (64). Both inactivated virus and attenuated live virus vaccines provide similar results when piglets born from vaccinated sows are vaccinated before colostral immunity has weaned (65). The intranasal vaccination of 10-week-old pigs with low levels of maternal antibody with an attenuated live virus vaccine conferred much better protection than parenteral vaccination with two inactivated vaccines followed by experimental challenge 2 months later (80).

The parenteral vaccination of fattening pigs (35–45 kg body weight) with either a modified live or inactivated vaccine did not prevent infection or clinical disease following experimental challenge with the field strain of the cows (79). However, the duration and severity of the clinical syndrome was reduced and vaccinated pigs did not suffer the severe weight loss and high mortality experienced by non-vaccinated pigs in the acute phase of the disease (66). Vaccination reduced the range of tissues in which the virus replicated and shedding of the virus was also reduced. The efficacy of the attenuated live virus and inactivated vaccines has been evaluated under experimental conditions using both the intranasal and parenteral routes (81, 82).

Although attenuated live virus vaccines are non-pathogenic for adult swine they may have residual virulence for newborn pigs and may not be entirely safe for pregnant swine. Vaccine-induced Aujeszky's disease in lambs has also been recorded (72). Lambs were reactivated using a syringe previously used to vaccinate pigs with a modified live virus vaccine (72). The subcutaneous vaccination of lambs with a modified live vaccine can cause fatal encephalitis within 1 week (78). Thymidine kinase-deficient mutants of the virus are avirulent and immunogenic and are currently being evaluated (73, 74). Pigs inoculated with this mutant are resistant to experimental challenge with the virulent virus and the virulent virus cannot be recovered from the ganglia which suggests that vaccination reduced colonization of the ganglia (73, 74). The ideal vaccine strain should prevent clinical disease and mortality, should not be transmitted to non-immunized animals, should prevent colonization of the ganglia by a potential superinfecting virulent virus and thereby reduce the natural reservoir of the virus. The thymidine kinase deficient mutant virus possesses these desirable characteristics. A subunit vaccine can prevent clinical disease and shedding of virus and latent infection following experimental challenge of vaccinated pigs (75). Pigs vaccinated with the subunit vaccine and subsequently exposed to the virulent virus can be identified by a diagnostic test (76). A genetically engineered second generation Aujeszky's disease virus has been developed for possible vaccine use (77). Pigs immunized with the virus resisted challenge with a large dose of virulent virus, and it was possible to distinguish pigs vaccinated with the virus from pigs infected or vaccinated with other strains.

Vaccination of cattle with an inactivated vaccine is recommended where they are in close contact with swine and where a low level of exposure is likely (33). Vaccination of cattle with inactivated or attenuated vaccines did not provide protection against an experimental challenge (21).

REVIEW LITERATURE

Basinger, D. (1979) A brief description of Aujeszky's disease in Great Britain and its relative importance. *Br. vet. J.*, *135*, 215–224.

Baskerville, A. et al. (1973) Aujeszky's disease in pigs. *Vet. Bull.*, *43*, 465.

Lee, J. Y. S. & Wilson, M. R. (1979) A review of pseudorabies (Aujeszky's disease) in pigs. *Can. vet. J.*, *20*, 65–69.

Nara, P. L. (1985) Porcine herpes virus 1. In: *Comparative Pathobiology of Viral Diseases*. Vol. 1. Edited by R. G. Olsen, et al. pp. 89–113.

Thawley, D. G., Gustafson, D. P. & Beran, G. W. (1982) Procedures for the elimination of pseudorabies virus from herds of swine. *J. Am. vet. med. Assoc.*, *181*, 1513–1518.

Whittman, G. & Hall, S.A. (1982) Aujeszky's disease. *Curr. Top. Vet. Med. Anim. Sci.*, *17*.

REFERENCES

(1) Baskerville, A. (1983) *Vet. Bull.*, *43*, 465.
(2) Nara, P. L. (1985) In: *Comparative Pathobiology of Viral Diseases*, Vol. 1. Ed. R. G. Olsen et al., pp. 89–113.
(3) Davies, E. B. & Beran, G. W. (1981) *Res. vet. Sci.*, *31*, 32.
(4) Durham, P. J. K. & O'Hara, P. J. (1980) *NZ vet. J.*, *28*, 179.
(5) McRory, F. J. & McParland, P. J. (1975) *Irish vet. J.*, *29*, 103.
(6) Thawley, D. G. et al. (1982) *J. Am. vet. med. Assoc.*, *181*, 1513.
(7) Baker, J. C. et al. (1982) *J. Am. vet. med. Assoc.*, *181*, 607.
(8) Dulac, G. C. & Binns, M. (1979)*Can. Vet. J.*, *20*, 318.
(9) Crandell, R. A. et al. (1982) *Am. J. vet. Res.*, *43*, 326.
(10) Thawley, D. G. et al. (1985) *Am. J. vet. Res.*, *45*, 981.
(11) Durham, P. J. K. et al. (1980). *Res. vet. Sci.*, *28*, 256.
(12) Beran, G. W. et al. (1980) *J. Am. vet. med. Assoc.*, *176*, 998.
(13) Thawley, D. G. et al. (1980) *J. Am. vet. med. Assoc.*, *176*, 1001.
(14) Davies, E. B. & Beran, G. W. (1980) *J. Am. vet. med. Assoc.*, *176*, 1345.
(15) McFerran, J. B. & Dow, C. (1965) *Am. J. vet. Res.*, *26*, 631.
(16) McCracken, R. M. et al. (1973) *J. gen. Virol.*, *20*, 17.
(17) Bitsch, V. (1975) *Acta vet. Scand.*, *16*, 420, 434, 449.
(18) Narita, M. et al. (1984) *Vet. Pathol.*, *21*, 450.
(19) Narita, M. et al. (1984) *Am. J. vet. Res.*, *45*, 247.
(20) Hall, L. B. et al. (1984) *Can. J. comp. Med.*, *48*, 192, 303.
(21) Biront, P. et al. (1982) *Am. J. vet. Res.*, *43*, 760.
(22) Howarth, J. A. & dePaolsi, A. (1968) *J. Am. vet. med. Assoc.*, *152*, 1114.
(23) Wohlgemuth, K. et al. (1978) *J. Am. vet. med. Assoc.*, *172*, 478.
(24) McCraken, R. M. et al. (1984) *Vet. Rec.*, *115*, 348.
(25) Mare, C. J. & Kluge, J. P. (1974) *J. Am. vet. med. Assoc.*, *164*, 309.
(26) Wellemans, G. et al. (1976) *Ann. Méd. vét.*, *120*, 196.
(27) Herweijer, C. H. & Jonge, W. K., de (1977) *Tijdschr. Diergeneeskd.*, *102*. 425.
(28) Dow, C. & McFerran, J. B. (1963) *Vet. Rec.*, *75*, 1099.
(29) Bank, M. & Cartwright, S. (1983) *Vet. Rec.*, *113*, 38.
(30) Durham, P. J. K. et al. (1985) *NZ vet. J.*, *33*. 132.
(31) Thawley, D. G. et al. (1985) *J. Am. vet. med. Assoc.*, *186*, 1080.
(32) Hoblet, K. H. et al. (1987) *J. Am. vet. med. Assoc.*, *190*, 405
(33) Van Oirschot, J. T. et al. (1985) *Zentralbl. VetMed. B.*, *32*, 173.
(34) Kanitz, C. L. (1977) *J. Am. vet. med. Assoc.*, *170*, 889.
(35) McFerran, J. B. & Dow, C. (1973) *Res. vet. Sci.*, *15*, 208.
(36) Wright, J. C. et al. (1984) *Can. J. comp. Med.*, *48*, 184.
(37) Zuffa, A. et al. (1975) *Zentralbl. VetMed.*, *22B*, 89.
(38) Van Oirschot, J. T. (1987) *Res. vet. Sci.*, *42*, 12.
(39) Martin, S. & Wardley, R. C. (1986) *Rev. Sci Techn. Off. int. Epizoot.*, *5*, 379.
(40) Hsu, F. S. & Lee, R. C. T. (1984) *J. Am. vet. med. Assoc.*, *184*, 1463.
(41) Maes, R. K. et al. (1979) *Am. J. vet. Res.*, *40*, 393.
(42) Shell, L. G. et al. (1981) *J. Am. vet. med. Assoc.*, *178*, 1159.
(43) Wright, J. C. & Thawley, D. G. (1980) *Am. J. vet. Res.*, *41*, 581.
(44) Brown, T. T. (1981) *Am. J. vet. Res.*, *42*, 1033.
(45) Gutenkunst, D. E. et al. (1980) *Am. J. vet. Res.*, *41*, 1315.
(46) Lloyd, G. & Baskerville, A. (1978) *Res. vet. Sci.*, *25*, 257.
(47) Afshar, A. et al. (1986) *J. clin. Microbiol.*, *23*, 563.
(48) Crandell, R. A. et al. (1984) *J. Am. vet. med. Assoc.*, *184*, 692.
(49) Allan, G. M. et al. (1984) *Res. vet. Sci.*, *36*, 235.
(50) Ducatelle, R. et al. (1982) *Res. vet. Sci.*, *32*, 294.
(51) Goodwin, R. F. W. & Whittlestone, P. (1986) *Vet. Rec.*, *119*, 493.
(52) Hsu, F. S. et al. (1980) *J. Am. vet. med. Assoc.*, *177*, 636.
(53) Crandell, R. A. et al. (1977) *J. Am. vet. med. Assoc.*, *171*, 59.
(54) Hagemoser, W. A. (1978) *J. Am. vet. med. Assoc.*, *173*, 205.
(55) Watson, W.A. (1986) *Rev. Sci. Techn, Off. int. Epizoot.*, *5*, 363.
(56) Andries, K. et al. (1978) *Am. J. vet. Res.*, *39*, 1282.
(57) Martin, S. et al. (1986) *Res. vet. Sci.*, *41*, 331.
(58) Kirkpatrick, C. M. et al. (1980) *J. Wildlife Dis.*, *16*, 601.
(59) Centraal Diergeneeskundig Instituut (1978) *Tijdschr. Diergeneeskd.*, *103*, 1187.
(60) Larsen, R. E. et al. (1980) *Am. J. vet. Res.*, *41*, 733.
(61) Beasley, V. T. et al. (1980) *Vet. Res. Commun.*, *4*, 125.
(62) Gloster, J. et al. (1984) *Vet. Res.*, *114*, 234.
(63) James, J. E. et al. (1983) *J. Am. vet. med. Assoc.*, *183*, 525.
(64) Pensaert, M. B. et al. (1982) *Res. vet. Sci.*, *32*, 12.
(65) Vannier, P. (1985) *Am. J. vet. Res.*, *46*, 1498.
(66) Donaldson, A. I. et al. (1983) *Vet. Rec.*, *113*, 490.
(67) Wittman, G. et al. (1983) *Archiv. Virol.*, *75*, 29.
(68) Bolin, S. R. & Bolin, C. A. (1984) *Theriogenology.*, *22*, 101.
(69) Bolin, C. A. et al. (1985) *Am. J. vet. Res.*, *46*, 1039.
(70) Alva-Valdes, R. et al. (1983) *Am. J. vet. Res.*, *44*, 588.
(71) Alva-Valdes, R. et al. (1983) *Can. J. comp. Med.*, *47*, 451.
(72) Van Alstine, W. G, & Anderson, T. D. (1984) *J. Am. vet. med. Assoc.*, *185*, 409.
(73) Kit, S. et al. (1985) *Am. J. vet. Res.*, *46*.
(74) McGregor, S. et al. (1985) *Am. J. vet. Res.*, *46*, 1494.
(75) Maes, R. K. & Schutz, J. C. (1983) *Am. J. vet. Res.*, *44*, 123.
(76) Platt, K. B. et al. (1986) *Vet. Microbiol.*, *11*, 25.
(77) Kit, S. et al. (1986) *Vet. Rec.*, *118*, 310.
(78) Clark, L. K. et al. (1984) *J. Am. vet. med. Assoc.*, *185*, 1535.
(79) Donaldson, A. I. et al. (1984) *Vet. Rec.*, *115*, 121.
(80) DeLeeuw, P. W. & Van Oirschot, J. T. (1985) *Res. vet. Sci.*, *39*, 34.
(81) DeLeeuw, P. W. & Van Oirschot, J. T. (1985) *Vet. Q.*, *7*, 191.

(82) Van Oirschot, J. T. & DeLeeuw, P. W. (1985) *Vet. Microbiol.*, *10*, 401.
(83) Pirtle, E. C. et al. (1984) *Am. J. vet. Res.*, *45*, 1906.
(84) McFarlane, R. G. et al. (1986) *Am. J. vet. Res.*, *47*, 2329.
(85) Wright, J. C. et al. (1982) *Can. J. comp. Med.*, *46*, 420.
(86) Anonymous (1985) *Vet. Rec.*, *117*, 401.

Viral encephalomyelitis of pigs (Teschen disease, Talfan disease, poliomyelitis suum)

This encephalomyelitis occurs only in pigs and is characterized by hyperesthesia, tremor, paresis and convulsions.

Etiology

A number of closely related but antigenically different enteroviruses, capable of growth in tissue culture, are known to be causes of encephalomyelitis in pigs (1–4). Some have been given names. Teschen virus, initially isolated in Czechoslovakia, appears to be the most virulent and there have been a number of independent isolates such as the Konratice and Reporyje strains. Talfan virus, isolated from England, and other unnamed isolates appear less virulent. There have been several attempts at classification of the isolates from encephalomyelitis of pigs and of strains of enterovirus isolated from normal pigs and pigs with diarrhea or reproductive inefficiency, and on the basis of crossneutralization tests they can be broadly divided into eight subgroups (5). Teschen and Talfan virus occur in subgroup 1 but isolates from encephalomyelitis are also associated with other subgroups. Within subgroups strains may be further differentiated using a complement fixation test (2), and monospecific sera for differentiation have been prepared (6). There is variation in virulence between strains and virulence may also be increased or decreased by passage depending upon the strain (7). With many strains clinical encephalitis following infection appears to be the exception rather than the rule.

Epidemiology

Prior to the early 1940s the incidence of known porcine viral encephalomyelitis was restricted to certain districts in Czechoslovakia. Since then reports of the disease have come from many countries and there is serological evidence that the disease occurs throughout the world (4, 8). The most severe form of the disease—Teschen disease—appears to be limited to Europe and Madagascar but the milder forms—Talfan disease, poliomyelitis suum and viral encephalomyelitis—are known to occur extensively in Europe, Scandinavia and North America. Losses due to the disease result primarily from deaths although there may be some crippling. The morbidity is usually about 50% and the mortality rate 70–90% in Teschen disease as it is described in eastern Europe. The disease in Denmark and the United Kingdom is much milder and the morbidity rate approximately only 6%. Serological surveys in areas where the disease occurs indicate that a high proportion of the pig population is infected without showing clinical evidence of the disease. In the majority of field occurrences porcine encephalomyelitis is a sporadic disease affecting either one or a few litters or a small number of weaned pigs.

The causative viruses will infect only pigs and are not related to any of the viruses which cause encephalomyelitis in other species. They are resistant to environmental conditions, including drying, and are present principally in the central nervous system and intestine of affected pigs.

Experimentally the disease is transmissible by ingestion, intranasal instillation and by intramuscular and intracerebral injection. It is presumed that in natural outbreaks the first two routes are of first importance.

The virus replicates primarily in the intestinal tract but also in the respiratory tract. When infection first gains access to a herd the spread is rapid and all ages of pigs may excrete virus in feces. Depending upon the virulence of the infecting strain clinical disease affecting primarily young pigs but occurring in older pigs may also occur at this stage. As infection becomes endemic and herd immunity develops, excretion of the virus is largely restricted to weaned and early grower pigs. Adults generally have high levels of circulating antibody and suckling piglets are generally protected from infection by colostral and milk antibody (9, 10). Sporadic disease in suckling pigs may occur in these circumstances in the litters of non-immune or low antibody sows and may also occur in weaned pigs as they become susceptible to infection.

Pathogenesis

The virus multiplies in the intestinal and respiratory tracts and may invade to produce viremia. Invasion of the central nervous system may follow depending upon the virulence of the strains and the age of the pig at the time of infection (17).There is some strain difference in the areas of the central nervous system primarily affected which accounts for variations in the clinical syndrome and it is possible for histopathological evidence of encephalitis to be present in pigs that have shown no clinical signs of the disease (7). This may also occur with adenovirus infection (11).

Clinical findings

Acute viral encephalomyelitis (Teschen disease)

The experimental disease, which closely resembles the natural disease (12), commences with an incubation period of 10–12 days followed by several days of fever (40–41°C, 104–106°F). Signs of encephalitis follow, although these are more extensive and acute after intracerebral inoculation. They include stiffness of the extremities, and inability to stand, with falling to one side followed by tremor, nystagmus and violent clonic convulsions. Anorexia is usually complete and vomiting has been observed. There may be partial or complete loss of voice due to laryngeal paralysis. Facial paralysis may also occur. Stiffness and opisthotonus are often persistent between convulsions, which are easily stimulated by noise and often accompanied by loud squealing. The convulsive period lasts for 24–36 hours. A sharp temperature fall may be followed by coma and death on the 3rd–4th day, but in cases of longer duration the convulsive stage may be followed by flaccid paralysis affecting particularly the hindlimbs. In milder cases early stiffness and weakness are followed by flaccid paralysis without the irritation phenomena of convulsions and tremor.

Subacute viral encephalomyelitis

This is called Talfan disease in the United Kingdom, viral encephalomyelitis in North America and Australia, poliomyelitis suum in Denmark. The clinical findings in the subacute disease are much milder than in the acute disease and the morbidity and mortality rates are lower. The disease is most common and severe in pigs less than 2 weeks of age. Older sucking pigs are affected also but less severely and many recover completely. Sows suckling affected litters may be mildly and transiently ill. The morbidity rate in very young litters is often 100% and nearly all the affected piglets die. In litters over 3 weeks old there may be only a small proportion of the pigs affected. The disease often strikes very suddenly—all litters in a piggery being affected within a few days—but disappears as suddenly, subsequent litters being unaffected. Clinically the syndrome includes anorexia, rapid loss of condition, constipation, frequent vomiting of minor degree and a normal or slightly elevated temperature. In some outbreaks diarrhea may precede the onset of nervous signs. Nervous signs appear several days after the illness commences. Piglets up to 2 weeks of age show hyperesthesia, muscle tremor, knuckling of the fetlocks, ataxia, walking backwards, a dog-sitting posture and terminally lateral recumbency, with paddling convulsions, nystagmus, blindness and dyspnea. Older pigs (4–6 weeks of age) show transient anorexia and posterior paresis, manifested by a swaying drunken gait, and usually recover completely and quickly.

Individual instances or small outbreaks of 'leg weakness' with posterior paresis and paralysis in gilts and sows may also occur with this disease.

Clinical pathology

A virus neutralization test in tissue and a complement fixation test have been utilized in the diagnosis of the disease. The antibodies are detectable in the early stages and persist for a considerable time after recovery. Challenge of previously hyperimmunized pigs by the intracerebral injection of the suspect material is also a satisfactory diagnostic technique. Virus is present in the blood of affected pigs in the early stages of the disease and in the feces in very small amounts in the incubation period before signs of illness appear, but brain tissue is usually used as a source of virus in transmission experiments.

Necropsy findings

There is a diffuse non-suppurative encephalomyelitis of viral type with involvement of gray matter predominating. The brain stem and spinal cord show the most extensive lesions. Meningitis affecting particularly the meninges over the cerebellum is an early manifestation of the disease. Virus can be isolated from brain, from gastric mucosa and feces in very small amounts, or from the blood during the incubation period. However, routine isolation of the virus can be difficult and elusive and biochemical and biophysical procedures may be necessary in order to make a diagnosis (18). No inclusion bodies are present in neurones as there are in cases of pseudorabies.

Diagnosis

The diagnosis of diseases causing signs of acute cerebral involvement in pigs is extremely difficult and a confirmatory diagnosis usually depends on exhaustive laboratory work. Pseudorabies and hemagglutinating encephalomyelitis virus disease may present with very similar clinical syndromes. In general, viral diseases, bacterial diseases and intoxications must be considered as possible groups of causes and careful selection of material for laboratory examination is essential. The differentiation of the possible causes of diseases resembling viral encephalomyelitis is described under pseudorabies and in general medicine under diseases of the nervous system.

Treatment

None is recommended.

Control

The sporadic occurrence of viral encephalomyelitis in a herd is usually an indication that infection is endemic. When outbreaks occur the possibility that introduction of a new strain has occurred should be considered. However, by the time clinical disease is evident it is likely that infection will be widespread and isolation of affected animals may be of little value. A closed herd policy will markedly reduce the risk of introduction of new strains into a herd but there is evidence that they can gain access by indirect means (13). The sporadic nature of the occurrence of most incidents of porcine encephalomyelitis does not warrant a specific control program. However, Teschen disease is a different problem.

Vaccines prepared by formalin inactivation of infective spinal cord and adsorption onto aluminum hydroxide have been used extensively in Europe. Two or three injections are given at 10–14-day intervals and immunity persists for about 6 months (14). A modified live virus vaccine is also available (15).

In the event of its appearance in a previously free country eradication of the disease by slaughter and quarantine should be attempted if practicable. Austria reported eradication of the disease which had been present in that country for many years (16). A slaughter policy was supplemented by ring vaccination around infected premises.

REVIEW LITERATURE

Long, J. F. (1985) Pathogenesis of porcine polioencephalomyelitis. In: *Comparative Pathobiology of Viral Diseases*, Vol. 1. Eds R. G. Olsen et al., pp. 179–197.

REFERENCES

(1) Done, J. T. (1961) *Bull. Off. int. Epizoot.*, *56*, 177.
(2) Darbyshire, J. H. & Dawson, P. S. (1963) *Res. vet. Sci.*, *4*, 48.
(3) Mason, R. W. (1970) *Br. vet. J.*, *126*, xix.
(4) Mill, J. H. & Nielsen, S. W. (1968) *Adv. vet. Sci.*, *12*, 33.
(5) Dunne, H. W. et al. (1971) *Infect. Immunol.*, *4*, 619.
(6) Christofnis. G. J. et al. (1972) *Am. J. vet. Res.*, *33*, 1915.
(7) Edington, N. et al. (1972) *J. comp. Pathol.*, *82*, 393.
(8) Paterson, A. B. (1962) *Bull. Off. int. Epizoot.*, 57, 1569.
(9) Alexander, T. J. L. (1962) *Am. J. vet. Res.*, *23*, 756.
(10) Derbyshire, J. B. & Collins, A. P. (1972) *J. comp. Pathol.*, *82*, 315.
(11) Edington, N. et al. (1972) *Res. vet. Sci.*, *13*, 289.
(12) Dardiri, A. H. et al. (1966) *Can. J. comp. Med.*, *30*, 71.
(13) Derbyshire, J. B. et al. (1971) *Br. vet. J.*, *127*, 436.

(14) Lalonne, O. (1958) *Bull. Off. int. Epizoot.*, *50*, 439.
(15) Korych, B. & Patocka, F. (1967) *Cslka Epidemiol. Mikrobiol. Immunol.*, *16*, 257.
(16) Schaupp, W. (1968) *Wien. Tierärztl. Wochenschr.*, *55*, 346.
(17) Long, J. F. (1985) In: *Comparative Pathobiology of Viral Diseases*, vol. 1, eds Olsen, R. G. et al., pp. 179–197.
(18) Lynch, J. A. et al. (1984) *Can. J. comp. Med.*, *48*, 233.

Sporadic bovine encephalomyelitis (SBE, Buss disease, transmissible serositis)

Sporadic bovine encephalomyelitis is caused by a chlamydia and characterized by inflammation of vascular endothelium and mesenchymal tissue. There is secondary involvement of the nervous system, with nervous signs, in some cases.

Etiology

The disease is caused by a chlamydia (1). It resists freezing but is highly susceptible to sodium hydroxide, cresol and quaternary ammonium compounds in standard concentrations. The chlamydia can be passaged in guinea-pigs and hamsters and adapted to grow in the yolk sac of developing chick embryos.

Epidemiology

The disease has been reported only from the United States, Japan and Israel but a provisional diagnosis has been made in Australia, where it is thought that the disease may have been present for some time, and in Canada, South Africa and Hungary. In the United States it occurs most commonly in the midwestern and western states. Sporadic cases or outbreaks occur in individual herds. Although the disease has not reached serious economic proportions in the enzootic areas, there is some serological evidence that widespread subclinical infections occur (2). As a rule only sporadic cases occur, but in some outbreaks there may be severe loss due to both deaths of animals and loss of condition (2). There is considerable variation in morbidity and mortality rates from herd to herd. Morbidity rates average 12·5% (5–50%), being highest in calves (25%) and lowest in animals over a year old (5%). Mortality rates average about 31% and are higher in adults than in calves. In affected herds a stage of herd immunity is reached when only introduced animals and newborn calves are susceptible.

Only cattle and buffalo (3) are affected and calves less than 6 months of age are most susceptible. Other domestic and experimental species appear to be resistant. There is no seasonal incidence, cases appearing at any time of the year. A strong and apparently persistent immunity develops after an attack of the disease.

Intracerebral inoculation of the virus in calves produces fever, anorexia, weight loss, inactivity, lacrimation and stiffness of gait, with histological but no clinical signs of encephalitis. Intraperitoneal inoculation results in peritonitis, perisplenitis, and perihepatitis. The virus can be isolated from many organs, including liver, spleen and central nervous system and from the blood, feces, urine, nasal discharges and milk in the early stages of the disease. There is some evidence that the virus is eliminated in the feces for several weeks after infection.

The method of spread under natural conditions is not known. The pattern of incidence is variable. Spread from farm to farm does not occur readily. On some farms only sporadic cases may occur, but on others one or two cases occur every year. In still other herds the disease occurs in outbreak form, with a number of animals becoming affected within a period of about 4 weeks. The epizootiology of sporadic bovine encephalomyelitis resembles in many ways that of bovine malignant catarrh (BMC).

Pathogenesis

The virus is not specifically neurotropic and attacks principally the mesenchymal tissues and the endothelial lining of the vascular system, with particular involvement of the serous membranes. Encephalomyelitis occurs secondarily to the vascular damage.

Clinical findings

In field cases the incubation period varies between 4 days and 4 weeks. Affected calves show depression and inactivity but the appetite may be unaffected for several days. Nasal discharge and salivation with drooling are frequently observed. Temperatures are raised (40·5–41·5°C, 105–107°F), and remain high for the course of the disease. About half of the animals have dyspnea and cough and mild catarrhal nasal discharge and diarrhea may occur. During the ensuing 2 weeks difficulty in walking and lack of desire to stand may appear. Stiffness with knuckling at the fetlocks is evident at first, followed by staggering, circling and falling. Opisthotonus may be present but there is no excitement or head-pressing. The course of the disease varies between 3 days and 3 weeks. Animals that recover show marked loss of condition and are slow to regain the lost weight.

Clinical pathology

In experimental cases leukopenia occurs in the acute clinical stage. There is a relative lymphocytosis and depression of polymorphonuclear cells. Virus can be isolated from the blood in the early clinical phase and can be used for transmission experiments in calves and guinea pigs and for culture in eggs. Elementary bodies are present in the guinea-pig tissues and yolk-sac preparations. Serological methods, including a complement fixation test for the detection of circulating antibody, are available although there is difficuly in differentiating antibodies to the virus from those to the typical psittacosis virus.

Necropsy findings

A fibrinous peritonitis, pleurisy and pericarditis accompanied by congestion and petechiation are characteristic. In the early stages thin serous fluid is present in the cavities, but in the later stages this has progressed to a thin fibrinous net covering the affected organs or even to flattened plaques or irregularly shaped masses of fibrin lying free in the cavity. Histologically there is fibrinous serositis involving the serosa of the peritoneal, pleural and pericardial cavities. A diffuse encephalomyelitis involving particularly the medulla and cerebellum and a meningitis in the same area are also present. Minute elementary bodies are present in infected tissues and in very small numbers in exudate.

Diagnosis

The necropsy findings are diagnostic for sporadic bovine encephalomyelitis (SBE) and confirmation can be obtained by the complement fixation test or virus neutralization tests. Clinically the disease resembles other encephalitides of cattle. The epizootiology and pathogenesis resemble those of bovine malignant catarrh (BMC), but the mortality rate is much lower, there are no ocular or mucosal lesions and the serositis of SBE does not occur in bovine malignant catarrh. A viral encephalomyelitis of calves (Kunjin virus) has been identified but has not been associated with clinical signs of disease of the nervous system (4). An encephalomyocarditis virus, a primary infection of rodents which also occurs in primates, and causes myocarditis in pigs (5) has been transmitted experimentally to calves but without causing significant signs of disease (6). Listeriosis is usually sporadic and is accompanied by more localizing signs, especially facial paralysis and circling. Rabies may present a very similar clinical picture, but the initial febrile reaction and the characteristic necropsy findings as well as the epizootiological history of SBE should enable a diagnosis to be made. Lead poisoning can be differentiated by the absence of fever, the more severe signs of motor irritation and the shorter course of the disease. Because of the respiratory tract involvement SBE may be easily confused with pneumonic pasteurellosis, especially if outbreaks occur, but in the latter disease nervous signs are unusual and the response to treatment is good.

Treatment

Broad-spectrum antibiotics control the virus *in vitro*. Clinical results with chlortetracycline and oxytetracycline have been irregular (3), but they are likely to be effective if used in the early stages of the disease.

Control

Control measures are difficult to prescribe because of lack of knowledge of the method of transmission. It is advisable to isolate affected animals. No vaccine is available.

REFERENCES

(1) Harshfield, G. S. (1970) *J. Am. vet. med. Assoc.*, *156*, 466.
(2) Harshfield, G. S. (1957) *Sporadic Bovine Encephalomyelitis*, Technical Bulletin 8. Agriculture Experiment Station. Brookings, SD: South Dakota State College of Agriculture.
(3) Ognyanov, D. et al. (1974) *Vet. Med. Nauki, Sofia*, *11*, 3.
(4) Spradbrow, P. B. & Clark, L. (1966) *Aust. vet. J.*, *42*, 65.
(5) Gainer, J. H. (1967) *J. Am. vet. med. Assoc.*, *151*, 421.
(6) Spradbrow, P. B. et al. (1970) *Aust. vet. J.*, *46*, 373.

Ovine encephalomyelitis (louping-ill)

Louping-ill is an acute encephalomyelitis affecting chiefly sheep, but occurring occasionally in other animals and man. The causative virus is transmitted by the bite of an infective tick. Clinically the disease is characterized by fever, abnormality of gait, convulsions and paralysis.

Etiology

The causative flavivirus can be cultivated in all sites of the developing chick embryo and tissue culture and, after experimental injection, causes encephalitis in mice.

Epidemiology

Louping-ill is recorded only in Scotland, the border counties of England and Ireland, although a similar and probably identical disease, Russian spring–summer encephalitis, occurs in Russia and central Europe. The distribution of these diseases is probably limited by the bionomics of the vector ticks. The morbidity rate of louping-ill in Britain is low in areas where the disease is enzootic, only 1–4% of adult sheep becoming infected. In lambs the morbidity rate may be as high as 60%, although lambs born to immune ewes may resist infection for about 3 months. The death rate in lambs is low so that overall losses are low in spite of the large number of lambs which become infected (1). It would appear that in enzootic areas inapparent infection followed by immunity must be common, since the morbidity rate may be considerably higher in introduced mature sheep. The mortality rate is of the order of 10–15%.

The virus is not very resistant to environmental influences and is readily destroyed by disinfectants. Immunity after an attack persists for life. Sheep are the only animals commonly infected, but occasional cases occur in all other domestic species, especially goats, and occasionally cattle (19), various rodents and man. Up to 10% of a population of horses in Eire has been shown to be seropositive, and deaths have occurred and virus has been isolated from brain (2). Experimental infection in horses produces a viremia of sufficient magnitude to infect mosquitoes which are feeding at the time (3). Pigs fed the carcasses of sheep which had died of louping-ill become infected with the louping-ill virus (6). Pigs are also susceptible to experimental infection by the virus by all routes. Rodents may act as reservoirs and amplifiers of the virus, especially in years of peak population. Red deer (*Cervus elaphus*) and roe deer (*Capreolus capreolus*) are alternative hosts of the virus in Scotland (18) and the elk (*Alces a. alces*) may be in Sweden (5). The virus has also been isolated from birds (7), especially red grouse in which it can cause heavy mortalities (8). Grouse probably play a significant role in the epidemiology of the disease and they should be regarded as temporary multipliers of the virus (4). Red deer and roe deer are considered to be tangential hosts of the virus and of little epidemiological importance in the maintenance of the viral population. However, when these animals are subjected to the stress of captivity, clinical illness is more likely to occur. This may be important to commercial deer farmers as well as in the spread of the disease in sheep (12). Cases in man occur principally in laboratory workers, and the incidence in the human population does not vary with change in the incidence in local sheep.

Although the major method of spread is by the bites of infected ticks, spread by droplet infection may be of some importance. The vector ticks in the United Kingdom are *Ixodes ricinus* and *Rhipicephalus appendiculatus*, and in the USSR, *I. ricinus* and *I. persulcatus*. Only adult *I. ricinus* are infective; the virus persists in individual ticks for long periods, but whether it is transmitted through the egg is uncertain. Other ectoparasites, especially fleas, are suspected as vectors of the virus. The virus is actively excreted in the milk of experimentally infected female goats and ewes but is unlikely to be important in the transmission of the infection to lambs (15) nor to humans. Because of the frequent consumption of new goat milk by humans the presence of the virus in the milk of goats is a greater threat (17). The disease has a seasonal occurrence during spring and summer when the ticks are active.

Pathogenesis

After infection a viremia occurs, concurrent with pyrexia. If entrance to nervous tissue is effected across the blood–brain barrier, a secondary febrile reaction occurs at the time of appearance of the nervous signs. In those animals in which invasion of nervous tissue does not occur, recovery is rapid and uneventful and there is immunity to subsequent infection. The virus persists for some time in the blood of these animals, whereas it disappears immediately if the blood–brain barrier is passed. Because invasion of brain occurs in only a proportion of naturally or artificially infected animals, it has been suggested that a concurrent tick-borne fever infection may reduce the resistance of the blood–brain barrier to the louping-ill virus. Invasion of the central nervous system may occur in most if not all experimentally infected animals, although the lesions may be small and isolated (9). Hemagglutination-inhibition antibodies are detectable 5–10 days after experimental infection provided the inoculation was not given intracerebrally (9). The development of the disease in the brain is associated with the replication of the virus in nerve cells so that the majority of neurons come to contain virus, and the animal dies (10).

Clinical findings

In sheep there is an incubation period of 6–18 days followed by a sudden onset of high fever (up to 41·5°C, 107°F) followed by a return to normal and then a second febrile phase starting about the 5th day during which nervous signs appear. Affected animals stand apart, often with the head held high. There is marked tremor of muscle groups and rigidity of the musculature, particularly in the neck and limbs. This is manifested by jerky, stiff movements and a bounding gait which gives rise to the name—louping-ill. Incoordination is most marked in the hindlimbs. The sheep walks into objects and may stand with the head pressed against them. Hypersensitivity to noise and touch may be apparent. The increased muscle tone is succeeded by paralysis and recumbency. In fatal cases death follows after a course of 7–10 days, although young lambs may die suddenly after an illness of 1–4 days with no specifically nervous signs (11). The clinical picture in cattle is very similar to that observed in sheep although convulsions are more likely to occur in cattle, and in the occasional animals which recover from the encephalitis there is usually persistence of signs of impairment of the central nervous system. In humans an influenza-like disease followed by meningoencephalitis occurs after an incubation period of 6–18 days. Complete recovery is usual.

Clinical pathology

The virus can be isolated from the blood of infected animals at the height of the initial viremia, and for an indeterminate period afterwards in those which show no nervous signs. Intracerebral injection into mice produces a fatal encephalomyelitis. Neutralizing antibodies can be detected in the serum of recovered animals. Complement fixing antibodies are also detectable but are so transient that the test lacks dependability as a diagnostic tool. Mice immunized by the injection of serum are protected against experimental infection.

Necropsy findings

No gross changes are observed. Histologically there are perivascular accumulations of cells in the meninges, brain and spinal cord with neuronal damage most evident in cerebellar Purkinje cells and to a less extent in the cerebral cortex. No pathognomonic inclusion bodies are present. For laboratory examination tissue fixed in formalin should be sent for histological examination and fresh tissue, unrefrigerated, in 30% glycerol for virus isolation. The louping-ill virus can be consistently demonstrated in nervous tissue by the use of fluorescent antibody (13).

Diagnosis

The histological findings are not specific and transmission of the disease to mice and serum neutralization tests are required to confirm the diagnosis. Clinically the disease in sheep bears resemblance to some stages of scrapie, to incoordination due to plant poisons, to tetanus and to hypocalcemia and pregnancy toxemia. The short course and high fever differentiate it from scrapie and from plant poisonings. Tetanus is characterized by tetany of the limbs and occurs usually after skin wounds or minor surgery. Pregnancy toxemia and hypocalcemia are usually related to lambing and show no febrile reaction. There is a similar disease of lactating ewes in New Zealand and the United Kingdom (16) characterized by a polyneuropathy which selectively affects the radial nerves. Affected ewes are unable to move their front legs normally and advance with a bounding gait like that of a kangaroo. The syndrome disappears at the end of lactation.

Treatment

An antiserum has been used and affords protection if given within 48 hours of exposure, but is of no value once the febrile reaction has begun.

Control

A formalinized tissue vaccine derived from brain, spinal cord and spleen provides excellent immunity and in enzootic areas vaccination of all animals over 4 months of age is recommended. The vaccine is not without risk for persons manufacturing it and it has been largely replaced by a new killed vaccine, prepared by growing the virus in tissue culture and mixing it with an adjuvant. This vaccine has been shown to give excellent results in field trials (14). Vaccination of ewes in late pregnancy is recommended to provide passive immunity to the lambs via the colostrum. Serial cultivation in hen eggs causes attenuation of the virus, but the potency of the avianized virus diminishes rapidly on storage. Control of ticks by frequent dipping helps to control tick-borne fever and lamb pyemia as well as louping-ill.

REFERENCES

(1) Reid, H. W. & Boyce, J. B. (1976) *J. Hyg., Camb.*, *77*, 349.
(2) Timoney, P. J. et al. (1976) *Equ. vet. J.*, *8*, 113.
(3) Timoney, P. J. (1980) *J. comp. Pathol.*, *90*, 73.
(4) Reid, H. W. (1978) *Proc. int. conf. tickborne diseases and their vectors*, Edinburgh, UK.
(5) Svedmyr, A. et al. (1965) *Acta pathol. microbiol. Scand.*, *65*, 613.
(6) Bannatyne, C. C. et al. (1980) *Vet. Rec.*, *106*, 13.
(7) Timoney, P. J. (1972) *Br. vet. J.*, *128*, 19.
(8) Reid, H. W. et al. (1980) *J. comp. Pathol.*, *90*, 257.
(9) Reid, H. W. & Doherty, P. C. (1971) *J. comp. Pathol.*, *81*, 291, 331.
(10) Doherty, P. C. et al. (1972) *J. comp. Pathol.*, *82*, 337.
(11) Ulvund, M. J. et al. (1983) *Norsk. vet. Tidsskr.*, *95*, 639.
(12) Reid, H. W. et al. (1987) *Vet. Rec.*, *102*, 463.
(13) Doherty, P. C. & Reid, H. W. (1971) *J. comp. Pathol.*, *81*, 531.
(14) Brotherston, J. G. et al. (1971) *J. Hyg., Camb.*, *69*, 479.
(15) Reid, H. W. & Pow, I. (1985) *Vet. Rec.*, *117*, 470.
(16) Duffell, S. J. et al. (1986) *Vet. Rec.*, *118*, 296.
(17) Reid, H. W. et al. (1984) *Vet. Rec.*, *114*, 163.
(18) Reid, H. W. et al. (1982) *Vet. Rec.*, *111*, 61.
(19) Reid, H. W. et al. (1981) *Vet. Rec.*, *108*, 497.

Caprine arthritis encephalitis (CAE)

This is a viral disease of goats characterized by either acute encephalitis, chronic arthritis especially of the carpal joints (big knee), severe enlargement and firmness of the udder (hard udder or indurative mastitis) or chronic pneumonia.

Etiology

The cause is a lentivirus of the family Retroviridae which crossreacts with, and has significant genome homology with, the virus of maedi-visna (15). It also seems that there are two antigenically different isolates which cause approximately the same disease (23).

Epidemiology

The infection is recorded in the United Kingdom (15), United States (4, 7), Canada (6), Australia (8), and Switzerland (9). The prevalence of the infection, as distinct from the clinical disease, varies widely and may be as high as 80% of a large goat population but the average is probably 25%. The prevalence is noticeably less in developing countries that have not had importations of goats from North America or Europe. Other countries such as New Zealand have a low prevalence with a distribution related to exotic importations (16). The disease is common in dairy breeds but rare in Angoras.

The mode of transmission is principally through the colostrum and milk, and newborn kids can be reared free from infection by removing them from the dam immediately after birth and rearing them on pasteurized milk. Prolonged direct contact between infected and non-infected older goats can result in a few crossinfections and the rate is increased if the female goats share milking facilities (20).

The infection has been transferred experimentally to lambs by feeding them infected colostrum (14) or by injection (24) and kids have been similarly infected with the maedi virus (19). The arthritic form of the disease has been produced experimentally in caesarean-derived kids injected with virus isolated from the joints of infected goats (4).

Pathogenesis

The virus causes a multisystem disease syndrome which primarily involves synovial-lined connective tissue causing chronic arthritis, the central nervous system causing leukoencephalitis (2), the udder causing swelling and hardening of the glands, with or without mastitis (17), and the lungs causing a chronic interstitial pneumonia. All of the lesions are lymphoproliferative (21) and result from continuous stimulation by the virus which is not eliminated. The arthritis is thought to be part of an immune response to the CAE virus, including the vaccine virus (26).

Clinical findings

The arthritis is a chronic hyperplastic synovitis which occurs primarily in adult goats and is noticeable only in the carpal joints, giving rise to the lay term of big-knee. The onset may be insidious or sudden, and unilateral or bilateral. If the goat is lame in the leg lameness is not severe. Affected goats lose weight gradually and develop poor hair coats and swollen joints. They are recumbent most of the time and decubitus ulcers are common as a result. Dilatation of the atlantal and supraspinous bursae occurs in some cases. The course of the disease is long, lasting several months. The arthritis may be accompanied by enlargement and hardening of the udder and by interstitial pneumonia.

The leukoencephalitis form of the disease occurs primarily in kids from 2 to 4 months of age. The syndrome is characterized by unilateral or bilateral posterior paresis and ataxia. In the early stages the gait is short and choppy, followed by weakness and eventually recumbency. In animals that are still able to stand there may be a marked lack of proprioception in one hindlimb. Brain involvement is manifested by head tilt, torticollis and circling (18). Affected kids are bright and alert and drink normally. Kids with unilateral posterior paresis usually progress to bilateral posterior paresis in 5–10 days. The paresis usually extends to involve the forelimbs so that tetraparesis follows. Most kids are euthanized. The interstitial pneumonia which commonly accompanies the nervous form of the disease is usually not sufficiently severe to be obvious clinically.

Indurative mastitis or hard udder, which is not necessarily caused by the CAE virus, develops a few days after kidding. The udder is firm and hard but no milk can be expressed. There is no systemic illness and no bacterial mastitis. Recovery is never complete but there may be some gradual improvement.

Clinical pathology

The synovial fluid from affected joints is usually brown to red-tinged and the cell count is increased up to 20000/μl with 90% mononuclear cells. The cerebrospinal fluid may contain an increased cell count and protein concentration (7). Radiographically there are soft tissue swellings in the early stages and calcification of periarticular tissues and osteophyte production in the later stages (4).

An agar gel immunodiffusion test (AGID) is widely used and an ELISA of high accuracy has been established (34). Identification of the presence of CAE is usually provided by isolation of the virus from tissue explants into tissue culture (1).

Necropsy findings

At necropsy of a case of the arthritic form there is emaciation and chronic polysynovitis. There is evidence of degenerative joint disease in almost all of the joints. The local lymph nodes are grossly enlarged and a diffuse interstitial pneumonia is usually present. In the neural form the diagnostic lesions are in the nervous system and involve the white matter especially of the cervical spinal cord and sometimes the cerebellum and the brainstem. The lesion is a bilateral, non-suppurative demyelinating encephalomyelitis (5). There is usually also a mild, diffuse, interstitial pneumonia.

Diagnosis

The differential diagnosis of the arthritic form of the disease includes the other infectious arthritides such as those caused by mycoplasma, chlamydia and corynebacteria. The nervous form must be differentiated from swayback due to copper deficiency, listeriosis, polioencephalomalacia and toxoplasmosis.

Treatment and control

There is no treatment likely to be of value for any form of the disease. Control of it is dependent on the identification of the infected animals and on maintaining them physically separated from the non-infected animals. Newborn kids may be raised free of the infection by removing them from the dam immediately they are born, rearing them on pasteurized milk and testing them serologically at regular intervals to ensure their continued freedom from infection. The common practice of feeding kids on pooled colostrum must not be allowed. The colostrum of infected females contains antibodies but the infectivity of the virus which is also present is not restrained (22). Continued contact between infected adults will encourage horizontal transmission and may reduce the efficiency of an eradication program based on control of vertical transmission in the young (27). A suitable protocol for the voluntary eradication of CAE from goat flocks is available (13).

REVIEW LITERATURE

Al-Ani, F. K. & Vestweber, J. G. E. (1984) Caprine arthritis–encephalitis syndrome (CAE). *Vet. Res. Commun.*, *8*, 243–353.

Dawson, M. (1978) Caprine arthritis–encephalitis. *In Pract.*, *9(1)*, 8.

Robinson, W. F. & Ellis, T. M. (1986) Caprine arthritis–encephalitis virus infection; from recognition to eradication. *Aust. vet. J.*, *63*, 237–241.

REFERENCES

(1) Crawford, T. B. et al. (1980) *Science*, *207*, 997.
(2) Adams, D. S. et al. (1980) *Am. J. Pathol.*, *99*, 257.
(3) Schroeder, B. A. et al. (1985) *NZ vet. J.*, *33*, 213.
(4) Crawford, T. B. & Adams, D. S. (1981) *J. Am. med. vet. Assoc.*, *178*, 713.
(5) Cordy, D. R. et al. (1984) *Vet. Pathol.*, *21*, 269.
(6) Thomson, R. G. (1981) *Can. vet. J.*, *22*, 358.
(7) Summers, B. A. et al. (1980) *Cornell Vet.*, *70*, 372.
(8) O'Sullivan, B. M. et al. (1978) *Aust. vet. J.*, *54*, 479.
(9) Fatzer, R. (1979) *Schweiz. Arch. Tierheilk.*, *121*, 329.
(10) Cork, L. C. & Narayan, O. (1980) *Lab. Invest.*, *42*, 596.
(11) Clements, J. E. et al. (1980) *J. gen. Virol.*, *50*, 423.
(12) Cheevers, W. P. et al. (1981) *Arch. Virol.*, *67*, 111.
(13) MacDiarmid, S. C. (1984) *NZ vet. J.*, *32*, 165 & 166.
(14) Oliver, R. et al. (1984) *NZ vet. J.*, *32*, 199.
(15) Dawson, M. & Wilesmith, J. W. (1985) *Vet. Rec.*, *117*, 86.
(16) Adams, D. S. et al. (1984) *Vet. Rec.*, *115*, 493.
(17) Kennedy-Stoskopf, S. et al. (1985) *J. comp. Pathol.*, *95*, 609.
(18) Norman, S. & Smith, M. C. (1983) *J. Am. vet. med. Assoc.*, *182*, 1342.
(19) Banks, K. L. et al. (1983) *Am. J. vet. Res.*, *44*, 2307.
(20) Adams, D. S et al. (1983) *Am. J. vet. Res.*, *44*, 1670.
(21) DeMartini, J. C. et al. (1983) *Am. J. vet. Res.*, *44*, 2064.
(22) Ellis, A. S. et al. (1986) *Aust. vet. J.*, *63*, 242.
(24) Grewal, A. S. et al. (1986) *Aust. vet. J.*, *63*, 341.
(25) Smith, V. W. et al. (1985) *Vet. Rec.*, *117*, 61.
(26) McGuire, T. C. et al. (1986) *Am. J. vet. Res.*, *47*, 537.
(27) East, N. E. et al. (1987) *J. Am. vet. med. Assoc.*, *190*, 182.

Scrapie

Scrapie is a non-febrile, fatal, chronic disease of adult sheep and goats characterized clinically by pruritus and abnormalities of gait, and by a very long incubation period.

Etiology

The present view is that scrapie is caused by a particle which can be transmitted from one animal to another and which multiplies itself within these hosts. Although it is often referred to as virus-like, or a provirus, it has few of the characteristics of a virus. It is capable of withstanding the usual viricidal procedures and is not destroyed by boiling for 30 minutes, by rapid freezing and thawing or by exposure to ether or 20% formalin, although infectivity is greatly reduced by heating at 100°C (212°F) for 1 hour. There are opposing views on the nature of the agent (26) which include the opinion that the agent is a virus and is susceptible to viricidal materials (6). At present it is assumed that the scrapie transmitting agent is a small basic protein, or is associated with one, and may not contain nucleic acid (3). It is generally referred to currently as a viroid, and it is known that there are differences in virulence between strains of the viroid. The agent is not antigenic so that there are no antibodies and no serotypes, and the agent cannot be cultured in *in vitro* media. Nor is there any evidence of development of immunity in infected animals. The viral agent is probably identical with that of transmissible milk encephalopathy (TME) (28).

Epidemiology

Scrapie occurs enzootically in the United Kingdom and Europe. Small outbreaks have been reported in Australia, New Zealand, India, the Middle East, Japan, Scandinavia, Canada and the United States, principally in sheep imported from enzootic areas. The flock morbidity ranges up to 20% and on occasions up to 40%. A mortality rate of 100% is usual although the possibility of recovery cannot be disregarded. The death loss is added to by the slaughter of infected and in-contact animals when eradication is undertaken. The disease is of major importance because of the embargos maintained by several countries against sheep from enzootic areas. A similar disease to scrapie has been recorded in Iceland under the name of Rida, and there has been a positive identification of scrapie in a nondescript breed of mountain sheep in the foothills of the Himalayas (4). The disease is thought to have been introduced by Rambouillet rams imported into the flocks 20 years ago.

Experimentally, transmission of the disease to sheep

is effected readily, and accidental transmission has been recorded in sheep vaccinated with louping-ill vaccine prepared by formalinization of brain tissue infected with the scrapie agent. Under natural conditions scrapie occurs in sheep and occasionally spontaneously in goats. Under experimental conditions scrapie has been observed to spread from sheep to goats by contact (7). Experimental transmission to goats is readily effected, the percentage of positive transmission being greater than in sheep (100% as against 60%). Only sheep over 18 months of age show clinical evidence of the disease in natural circumstances. Transmission of scrapie agent from sheep and goats to mice can be effected by intracerebral inoculation and force feeding and material from these mice can be used to produce scrapie in goats.

All breeds of sheep are thought to be equally susceptible, but the disease does appear to occur more commonly in some breeds, and this has formed the basis for an hypothesis that the disease is inherited (10). There is no doubt that the occurrence of the clinical disease is strongly conditioned by inheritance. The controversy that has existed about the etiology and epidemiology of scrapie relates to the relative importance of infection and inheritance and the means of their interaction. With increasing knowledge of the epidemiology and pathogenesis of 'slow virus' infections, it is possible to reconcile the opposing views in a hypothesis based on an inherited susceptibility to the infective agent expressing itself in the form of clinical disease (2). A very similar situation exists with current views on the etiology of bovine viral leukosis. Inheritance of susceptibility to scrapie has been firmy established in sheep (11), largely under the control of a single allele, the dominant allele conferring susceptibility. Practical expression of this mechanism has been given by the manipulation of the breeding program of 40 000 ewes which has eliminated scrapie from amongst them (1). Under laboratory conditions a flock of Swaledale sheep with a much lower susceptibility to scrapie has been developed by selecting against the progeny of scrapie-infected ewes (13).

An important corollary to the hypothesis of inheritance of susceptibility to the rabies viroid is whether resistant sheep can become infected and act as inapparent carriers of the infection. Information is not available on the subject.

The agent is present in the brain, spinal cord, lymph nodes and spleen of infected sheep and has been extracted from sheep and goat brain. Experimental transmission can be effected by subcutaneous, intraocular and intracerebral injection with incubation periods of 20, 15 and 12 months respectively, and by oral dosing with scrapie brain suspension in sheep and goats. Transmission of the disease to sheep has also been effected by the oral or intracerebral administration with fetal membrane material from known infected ewes. Vaccination against louping-ill with vaccine contaminated by the agent of scrapie has in the one instance referred to above resulted in widespread dissemination of the disease.

Under natural conditions the method of spread is uncertain and there are unexplained regional differences in the ease with which it spreads. Most transmissions are thought to occur by ingestion or by infection prenatally (15). Scrapie appears to have been transmitted by mediate contagion of pasture (14) and is often restricted to particular farms and even to certain fields on these farms. The duration of infectivity of inanimate materials such as pasture has not been defined, but field observations indicate that it is a long time, probably in excess of 3 years. Congenital infection deriving from either the ram or ewe is also thought to occur, even though neither parent may at any time show evidence of the disease. Most of these apparently unexplained observations can be rationalized about the new information that infection can arise from ingestion of infected placenta. Unfortunately the long incubation period of scrapie means that it may be some years before the epidemiology is fully explained.

For the present it is reasonable to assume the following as a basis for understanding the epidemiology and for devising control programs (16). There is considerable evidence that:

- Transfer of infection occurs laterally by contact and possibly by mediate contagion. At least one of the methods is the ingestion of material contaminated by placenta from infected sheep
- Vertical transmission of infection occurs from the dam, and possibly the sire, in sheep but not in goats.
- Susceptibility to scrapie is inherited.

The present views on the transmission of scrapie have been best summarized (15) as follows: 'that field control of the disease and maintenance of animals under experiment should have regard to the considerable evidence that: (*a*) contact transfer of the agent from affected to healthy animals can occur in certain rare circumstances, that possibly involve ingestion of the agent; (*b*) hereditary or congenital transmission is important in sheep, but much less so, if at all, in goats.' The little evidence available on the natural disease in goats is consistent with the view that the scrapie virus can be maintained by contagion in a herd of goats living apart from infected sheep (20).

Pathogenesis

In mice, and probably in sheep, the virus shows a predilection first for lymphocytic tissues, especially the spleen, where it replicates during the incubation period before invading other tissues, including the nervous system. In nervous tissue there is firstly a period of replication in the spinal cord, followed by a stage of replication in the brain. The onset of clinical signs depends upon the concentration of infectious agent in the brain, itself dependent on the site of infection and the size of the original infective dose (12). How the scrapie viroid reaches the central nervous system from a peripheral site is unexplained, but there is evidence that the major route may be via sympathetic nervous system tissues (22). The essential lesion in scrapie is the vacuolation of neurones in the spinal cord, medulla, pons and midbrain and the consequential wallerian degeneration in dorsal, ventral and ventrolateral columns of the spinal cord and in nerve fibers in the cerebellar peduncles and the optic nerve (18). In addition there is degeneration of the cerebellar and hypothalamoneurohypophyseal systems (19). The lesions in the brain, which are non-inflammatory, bilateral, and the only pathognomonic lesion, are suggestive of autoimmunity.

It has been suggested that there may be several forms of scrapie, e.g. the itching form and the muscle tremor form, and that these may be caused by different strains of the agent (21). There are some biological differences between the types but whether there are other differences is unknown. The distribution of the lesions in the brain are, within the limits imposed by lack of knowledge of the neuroanatomy of the sheep and goat, easily reconciled with the clinical signs observed.

Clinical findings

The incubation period varies from several months up to 3 years and a course of 4 years and 11 months has been recorded in a goat infected experimentally (23). The course is protracted, varying from 2 to 12 months, but lasting in most cases for about 6 months. The earliest signs are transient nervous phenomena occurring at intervals of several weeks or under conditions of stress. These episodes include sudden collapse and sudden changes of behavior, with sheep charging at dogs or closed gates. Rubbing and biting at the fleece then begin but are often unobserved because of their infrequent occurrence. The apparent pruritus is manifested chiefly over the rump, thighs and tail base. The poll and dorsum of the neck may also be involved and, less commonly, the neck in front of the shoulder and the ribs behind the elbow. In all cases the affected areas are bilaterally symmetrical. In this early stage a stilted gait is often observed. A general loss of condition may also be observed as an early sign although the appetite may not be severely affected.

The stage of gross clinical signs is manifested by intense pruritus, muscle tremor and marked abnormalities of gait, and severe emaciation. Persistent rubbing causes loss of wool over the areas mentioned above. Scratching with the hindfeet and biting at the extremities also occur. Hematoma of the ears and swelling of the face may result from rubbing. Light or deep pressure, pinpricking and application of heat or cold may elicit the characteristic 'nibbling' reaction, during which the animal elevates the head and makes nibbling movements of the lips and licking movements with the tongue. The sheep's expression suggests that the sensations evoked are pleasant ones. The reaction may not be observed consistently, often disappearing when the sheep is excited or in new surroundings.

Simultaneously with the development of pruritus there is serious impairment of locomotion. Hindlimb abnormalities appear first. There is incomplete flexion of the hock, shortening of the step, weakness and lack of balance. The sense of spatial relationship appears to be lost and the sheep is slow to correct abnormal postures. Adduction occurs during extension and abduction during flexion. When the animal is attempting to evade capture, gross incoordination of head and leg movements is likely and the animal often falls. Convulsions, usually transient but occasionally fatal, may occur at this time. General hyperexcitability is evident. In the animal at rest an intermittent nodding and jerking of the head and fine tremor of superficial muscles may also be observed. In some cases nystagmus can be produced by rotating the head sideways. Other nervous signs include inability to swallow, although prehension is unaffected, vomiting, loss of bleat and blindness. A change of voice to a trembling note is often most noticeable. Anorexia is not evident until the last 4–5 weeks and results in rapid loss of body weight. Pregnancy toxemia may occur as a complication in pregnant ewes during this stage of scrapie. Finally the sheep reaches a stage of extreme emaciation and inability to move without becoming readily fatigued. Sternal recumbency follows and lateral recumbency with hyperextension of the limbs is the final stage. Pyrexia is not evident at any time.

The experimentally produced disease in goats differs clinically from that of sheep in that pruritus is rare, the tail is always cocked up over the back and there is a characteristic posture of the hindlegs.

Clinical pathology

Antemortem laboratory examinations are not of positive value in diagnosis, but the examination of skin scrapings may help in the elimination of other diseases.

Necropsy findings

Significant gross findings are restricted to traumatic lesions caused by rubbing and to emaciation and loss of wool; gross distension of the abomasum has been recorded in some natural cases (27). Histologically the characteristic lesions are in the gray matter of the brain and include vacuolation and degeneration of the neurons, particularly in the medulla, astrocytosis, and a spongy appearance in the neuroparenchyma. Although vacuolation of neurons does occur apart from cases of scrapie, the much higher incidence of vacuoles in the brains of animals affected with scrapie permits a positive diagnosis to be made on this basis. Supporting evidence is the presence of cytoplasmic enzymic inclusions in brain cells (24), and cerebrovascular amyloidosis (25) and scrapie-associated fibrils (SAF) in extracts of infected brain (26) and of infected brain, and visible by electron microscopy. Some diagnostic use may be made of the development of clinical scrapie in white mice as early as the 96th day after intracerebral inoculation of brain emulsion from affected sheep. Although brain tissue is usually used as a source of virus in transmission experiments, almost every tissue, other than blood, is capable of causing the disease. The significance of the muscle lesions seen in some cases of scrapie is unknown, but it is probable that they are caused by a coincident disease.

Diagnosis

A final diagnosis can be made on the basis of positive necropsy findings or transmission experiments. The characteristic signs of pruritus, incoordination and terminal paralysis occurring during a period of prolonged illness should suggest the possibility of this disease. The long incubation period, slow spread and high mortality rate should also be considered when making a diagnosis. Differentiation from louping-ill, pseudorabies, photosensitization, pregnancy toxemia and external parasitism is necessary. Louping-ill occurs in sheep of all ages, has characteristic nervous signs and a short, acute course. Pseudorabies is very rare in sheep and is also characterized by an acute course. Photosensitive dermatitis may cause scratching but there are marked skin lesions which are distributed over the woolless part of the body. Pregnancy toxemia has a seasonal incidence and a short course, there is ketonuria and pruritus is absent. External parasitism can usually be detected by simple examination of the skin. Visna (see below) has distinctive lesions.

Treatment

No treatment has proved capable of changing the course of the disease.

Control

Vaccines are not available. All clinical cases should be slaughtered. In herds and areas where the disease is not enzootic all in-contact animals should also be destroyed, and land on which the flock has run should be left unstocked for at least 2 months. Barns and shelter sheds should be cleaned and disinfected with a 2% lye (caustic soda) solution. Special care should be taken to avoid contact between susceptible animals and the placenta of a possibly infected one.

In the United States and Canada the disease is under official control, and in those countries and the United Kingdom the disease has largely disappeared. In the United States the original eradication program was as follows. Affected flocks were destroyed and animals transferred from them during the preceding 2 months traced, and they and their immediate progeny slaughtered. The recipient flock was placed under long-term surveillance. Currently a flock is destroyed if more than one family bears infected animals. Otherwise only the infected family is destroyed. The exposed unrelated sheep are quarantined and inspected. There is particular interest in the possibility of eradicating the disease simply by selection. Such programs are based on the belief that the disease is inherited and that the inheritance is conditioned by a single recessive gene (2). Scrapie-resistant sheep have been selected from amongst those who have resisted artificial challenge. The selected survivors produced scrapie-resistant offspring (5). Such results need to be assessed over a very long period because of the long incubation period of the disease and the known great variation in incubation periods between strains of the scrapie infective agent (9). It is possible, for example, that genetically resistant sheep may not be resistant to all strains of the scrapie viroid.

REVIEW LITERATURE

Bruere, A. N. (1977) Scrapie. A point of view. *NZ vet. J.*, *25*, 259, 399 & 400 and *26*, 36, 37, 190 & 217.

Hourrigan, J. L. et al. (1979) In: *Slow Transmissible Diseases of the Nervous System*, eds Prusiner S. B & Hadlow W. J, vol. 1, p. 331. New York: Academic Press.

Kimberlin, R. H. (1981) Scrapie. *Wellcome Veterinary Series, Br. vet. J.*, *137*, 105.

Klingsporn, A. L. & Hourrigan, J. L. (1976) Progress in the scrapie eradication program. *Proc. 80th ann. Mtg US Anim. Hlth Assoc.*, p. 376.

Parry, H. B. (1983) *Scrapie Disease in Sheep*. London: Academic Press.

REFERENCES

(1) Kimberlin, R. H. (1979) *Nature, Lond.*, *278*, 303.
(2) Parry, H. B. (1979) *Nature, Lond.*, *277*, 127.
(3) Pattison, I. H. & Jones, K. M. (1967) *Vet. Rec.*, *80*, 2.
(4) Zlotnik, I. &. Katiyar, A. D. (1961) *Vet. Rec.*, *73*, 542.
(5) Hoare, M. et al. (1977) *Vet. Rec.*, *101*, 482.
(6) Rohwer, R.G. (1984) *Nature, London*, *308*, 658.
(7) Pattison, I. H. & Jones, K. M. (1968) *Res. vet. Sci.*, *9*, 408.
(8) Zlotnik, I. & Stamp. J. T. (1966) *Vet. Rec.*, *78*, 222.
(9) Martin, W. B. & Stamp, J. T. (1980) *Br. vet. J.*, *136*, 290.
(10) Parry, H. B. (1962) *Heredity*, *17*, 75.
(11) Nussbaum, R. E. et al. (1975) *Res. vet. Sci.*, *18*, 49.
(12) Kimberlin, R. H. et al. (1983) *J. neurol. Sci.*, *61*, 315.
(13) Davies, D. C. & Kimberlin, R. H. (1985) *Vet. Rec.*, *116*, 211.
(14) Gordon, W. S. (1964) *Vet. Rec.*, *58*, 516.
(15) Hadlow, W. J. et al. (1982) *J. infect. Dis.*, *146*, 657.
(16) Dickinson, A. G. et al. (1974) *J. comp. Pathol.*, *84*, 19.
(17) Eklund, C. M. et al. (1964) *Report of Scrapie Seminar, Washington DC*, pp. 288–91.
(18) Palmer, A. C. (1968) *Vet. Rec.*, *82*, 729.
(19) Beck, E. et al. (1964) *Brain*, *87*, 153.
(20) Hadlow, W. J. et al. (1980) *Vet. Pathol.*, *17*, 187.
(21) Brotherston, J. G. et al. (1968) *J. comp. Pathol.*, *78*, 9.
(22) Kimberlin, R. H. & Walker, C. A. (1980) *J. gen. Virol.*, *51*, 183.
(23) Pattison, I. H. (1965) *Vet. Rec.*, *77*, 1388.
(24) Mackenzie, A. (1984) *J. comp. Pathol.*, *94*, 9.
(25) Gilmour, J. S. & Bruce, M. E. (1986) *Neuropathol. Appl. Neurobiol.*, *12*, 434.
(26) Gibson, P. H. et al. (1987) *Vet. Rec.*, *120*, 125.
(27) Sharp, M. W. & Collings, D. F. (1987) *Vet. Rec.*, *120*, 125.
(28) Hadlow, W. J. & Rose, R. E. (1986) *Vet. Pathol.*, *23*, 543.

Visna

Visna is a meningoencephalitis of sheep recorded principally in Iceland. It can be transmitted by intracerebral injection of cell-free filtrates of brain tissue and by intrapulmonary inoculation (2) but its mode of transmission in the field is unknown. The causative lentivirus (a retrovirus) has been cultivated in tissue culture (3) and is identical with the virus of maedi, or zwoergersiekte (4). Another related virus is that of caprine encephalomyelitis.

The pathogenesis of visna depends on the antigen–antibody relationship which usually exists between a slow virus and the tissues of the host. Although age has little effect on the development of disease, fetal and neonatal lambs have slightly greater permissiveness for replication of the virus. However, free infectious virus is present only in small quantities, but over very long periods. The genotype of the host is important and all breeds of sheep do not react to the same degree. Thus, Icelandic sheep react much more severely than English breeds (9). Experimental transmission of the infection and the disease is effected by intracerebral inoculation and spread occurs from these to comingled sheep (10). There are two basic lesions, an inflammatory lesion which is not related to the occurrence of nervous signs, and a focal demyelination in the spinal cord, the occurrence of which is related to the appearance of paresis (11). Most observations of the pathology of visna point to the disease being an immunopathological process (6). For example, experimental immunosuppression greatly reduces the severity of lesions, by suppressing the cellular proliferative response without suppressing the growth of the virus (3). Antigenic drift occurs to a significant degree during the prolonged period of infection (1). This may help to account for the slow and uneven progress of the disease with severity depending largely on the amount of virus present (5).

The characteristic histological lesion is an inflammation of the glial and ependymal cells, followed by demyelination, in the white matter of the cerebrum and cerebellum. Lymphocytic meningitis, choroiditis and leukoencephalitis are present in some sheep (8). There is an increased cell count in cerebrospinal fluid and neutralizing antibodies to the virus are present in the sera of affected sheep.

The incubation period and the course of the disease are very long; clinical signs may not appear for 2 years after experimental inoculation and affected animals may show clinical signs for 1–2 years before final paralysis necessitates slaughter. The early clinical signs include lagging behind the flock because of ataxia and body wasting. A normal appetite and consciousness are retained. Additional signs include severe tremor of the facial muscles, and knuckling of the distal limbs so that the animal stands on the flexed tarsi. The clinical picture is not unlike that of scrapie without the pruritus. During the course of the disease periods of relative normality may occur but the disease is usually fatal. Visna has been successfully eradicated from Iceland. The disease also occurs rarely in goats (7). The clinical syndrome is the same as that for sheep. This should be read in conjunction with the section on caprine encephalomyelitis with which visna is closely related. A similar disease of adult sheep in Australia (Murrurrundi disease) is characterized by progressive ataxia and paresis and histopathologically by widespread neuronal vacuolation in the white matter (12).

REFERENCES

(1) Lutley, R. et al. (1983) *J. gen. Virol.*, *64*, 1433.
(2) Gudnadottir, M. & Palsson, P. A. (1965) *J. int. Dis.*, *115*, 217.
(3) Nathanson, N. et al. (1976) *Lab. Inv.*, *35*, 444.
(4) Ressang, A. A. et al. (1966) *Pathol. Vet.*, *3*, 401.
(5) Petursson, G. et al. (1976) *Lab. Inv.*, *35*, 402.
(6) Georgeson, G. et al. (1979) *Acta Neuropathol.*, *48*, 39.
(7) Sundquist, B. et al. (1981) *Acta vet. Scand.*, *22*, 315.
(8) Cutlip, R. C. et al. (1979) *Am. J. vet. Res.*, *40*, 1370.
(9) Georgeson, G. et al. (1978) *J. comp. Pathol.*, *88*, 597.
(10) Palsson, P. A. et al. (1977) *Acta vet. Scand.*, *18*, 122.
(11) Georgeson, G. et al. (1982) *Acta Neuropathol.*, *57*, 171.
(12) Hartley, W. J. & Loomis, L. N. (1981) *Aust. vet. J.*, *57*, 399.

Border disease (hairy shaker disease of lambs, hairy shakers, *Hypomyelinogenesis congenita*)

This congenital disease of lambs is characterized by an abnormally hairy birth coat, gross tremor of skeletal muscles, defective myelination of the central nervous system, inferior growth of lambs and variable degree of skeletal deformity.

Etiology

The cause of the disease is a pestivirus of the family Togaviridae which is now known as the border disease (BD) virus which is closely related to the bovine virus diarrhea virus (BVDV) and to the swine fever/hog cholera virus (1). There is more than one strain of the virus with differing pathogenicities between the strains (2). Variations also result from interactions between the virus and different host genotypes, specifically between different breeds of sheep. The virus is capable of passing the placenta and is transmissible from dam to offspring, as well as horizontally between ewes (3). The disease has been reproduced by the inoculation of ewes with the bovine virus diarrhea virus (BVDV), the ewes being pregnant 8–9 weeks (4, 5) and by inoculation of cell-free homogenates of border disease brains, but a comparison of these experimentally produced similar diseases is reported to show significant histologic differences (6). The causal virus has also been isolated from the brains of natural cases of border disease by culture on tissue culture and the disease has been reproduced in lambs with this culture by inoculating it into their dams (7), and the intracerebral inoculation of the BD virus into lambs (34).

Epidemiology

Border disease has been recognized in the United Kingdom (12), New Zealand (13), Australia (14), the United States (15, 16), Switzerland (17), Greece (18) and Norway (19). The prevalence of infection varies between countries and is much higher than the incidence of clinical disease. Seroepidemiological surveys in England and Wales revealed a prevalence of 11% with a very patchy distribution (20). In Canada, a serological survey revealed that 10% and 16% of sheep and goats respectively were positive, but clinical disease has not yet been recognized (21). Up to 43% of goats in a flock may be seropositive (32).

The disease occurs naturally primarily in sheep and occasionally in goats. The disease has also been produced experimentally in goat kids by inoculation of female goats but there are no abnormalities of haircoat and there are more abortions than in ewes (8). Injection of brain tissue from affected lambs into pregnant heifers also causes many of them to abort. Some fetuses also have cavitation of the cerebrum (9) and the heifers develop antibodies to the bovine virus diarrhea virus. Experimental infection of sows causes in their piglets a striped effect in the haircoat and some cerebellar hypoplasia (10) and other minor lesions in nervous tissue (11).

The natural spread of the disease is both vertical and horizontal. How the virus is transmitted horizontally in nature is not known. However, congenitally infected lambs are persistently infected for up to 2·5 years and the virus is present in most tissues and organs and is excreted in saliva, feces and urine (22). Persistently infected lambs may be born apparently clinically normal and are usually immunotolerant and seronegative for the border disease virus. It is probable that persistently infected lambs which survive to breeding age will infect their progeny and this is probably the principal source of the virus (23), and lateral spread between these and comingled sheep is common (2). Some sheep remain persistently infected indefinitely.

An assessment of the economic losses due to infertility, abortion, neonatal losses and low carcass weight indicate that an outbreak of border disease can result in a potential reduction of income in excess of 20% (24).

Pathogenesis

Following infection of the pregnant ewe with the border disease virus there is maternal viremia and *in utero* and fetal infection. Prenatal death, in particular early embryonic death and abortion, is more common when maternal infection occurs in early pregnancy such as from 45 to 72 days (25). Early embryonic death with subsequent resorption may occur in up to 40% of experimentally infected ewes. Abortion occurs as a result of infection up to midpregnancy in about 50% of infected ewes. Fetal death and abortion are also common in goats. Fetuses which die in early pregnancy may become mummified in up to 20% of infected ewes. Stillbirth is the consequence of infection in the last third of pregnancy and may occur in up to 11% of animals. The effect of the virus of the immunocompetent ewe is usually subclinical but may be manifested by barrenness or abortion.

There are different strains of the pestivirus which, when inoculated into ewes at susceptible stages of pregnancy, can produce clinical border disease with a range of effects on the fetus (25).

The ultimate outcome of the infection depends on the age of the fetus, the properties of the strain of the fetus, the dose of the virus, the genotype of the host and the ability of the fetus to respond to the virus (30). In general, the fetus is most vulnerable in the first 10 weeks of gestation before the onset of immune competence. Infection after 80 days of gestation is likely to be controlled or eliminated. The consequences of infection can be divided into general effects and organ-specific alterations. Examples of the former are intrauterine growth retardation, the failure of lambs to thrive and their increased susceptibility to parasitic diseases and pneumonia. The organ-specific consequences of infection are related to the interference of virus replication with the growth, maturation and differentiation of fetal tissues.

The effects of the BVDV in pregnant sheep and, conversely, the BDV in pregnant cows have been examined. Experimental infections of pregnant ewes with the BVDV produces placental lesions, abortions, mummified fetuses and congenital malformations, including hydrocephalus, porencephaly, cerebellar hypoplasia and dysplasia and arthrogryposis (26). In addition, fetal growth retardation, hypomyelinogenesis, the birth of weak lambs with nervous signs and a hairy birth coat have been described which are consistent with the clinical and pathological features of both natural and experimental infection of BDV infection in sheep. Experimental infections of pregnant cows with the BDV results in placental necrosis, mummification and abortion of fetuses, intrauterine growth retardation with abnormal osteogenesis and hypomyelinogenesis all of which occur in congenitally infected sheep. Thus the defects produced by the BDV and the BVDV in the two host species have several characteristics in common (30).

The intramuscular inoculation of a cytopathic strain of BVDV into pregnant goats results in embryonic mortality and abortion and histological lesions of the nervous system of the kids (36).

The BDV and the BVDV can cause a wide range of congenital defects in fetuses which survive the infection. The fetal infection is often chronic and may persist into postnatal life. The congenital defects of the nervous system include hypomyelinogenesis (35), nodular periarteritis and necrosis and inflammation of the germinal layers of the central nervous system resulting in gross malformation such as hydranencephaly and cerebellar dysplasia. Most of these lambs exhibit nervous signs at birth which vary from a continuous light tremor to tonic–clonic contraction of the skeletal muscles involving the whole body and head (*shakers*). In some cases there are no nervous signs or abnormalities of the fleece (37). The major lesion in the skin is an enlargement of the primary hair follicles and a concurrent reduction in the number of secondary follicles. The resulting hairiness, which is due to the presence of medullated primary fibers, only becomes manifest in normally smooth-coated breeds. The BDV appears to have no effect on the skin and hairy birth coat of coarse-fleeced breeds of sheep or on goats. Intrauterine growth retardation is a common feature of infection with the BVD. Deformities of the skeleton include abnormally shortened long bones, a reduction in crown–anus length and the long axis of the skull which results in lambs appearing more compact and short-legged than normal. In the long bones there is evidence of growth arrest lines and disturbed osteogenesis and ossification.

Infection of the fetus during the first half of gestation is usually chronic and persists into postnatal life. The infection may persist for up to 2·5 years in clinically normal animals, for up to 2·5 years or less in unthrifty lambs.

The BD virus can persist in the central nervous system, cerebrospinal fluid and peripheral leukocytes for up to 12 months after birth (31). In such persistently infected animals serum neutralizing antibody to the BD virus is not detectable. In contrast, sheep exposed to the BD virus as adults have no detectable virus in the same tissues but develop serum neutralizing antibodies. However, some lambs appear to eliminate the virus during prenatal or postnatal life and thrive as normal healthy individuals. The intramuscular inoculation of immunocompetent lambs with the BD virus results in a mild transient disease and a subsequent reduction in growth rate but no gross or microscopic lesions (33).

Experimental inoculation of a homologous strain of the BD virus into persistently infected but clinically recovered lambs results in a severe clinical syndrome characterized by persistent diarrhea and respiratory distress associated with an inflammatory lymphoproliferative response in the central nervous system, intestines, lungs, heart and kidney (28, 29). This syndrome resembles certain aspects of mucosal disease in cattle in which it is postulated that superinfection of persistently viremic immunotolerant cattle with a homologous strain of the BVD virus results in fatal mucosal disease. In such animals a specific and dynamic equilibrium exists between an attenuated form of the virus and the immunotolerant host. Disturbance of this equilibrium either by injection of the homologous strain of the BD virus or some other factor results in fatal disease (29).

Clinical findings

The most obvious and characteristic features of border disease are evident at birth and relate to conformation, fleece type and locomotor activity of the limbs (30).

Affected lambs are usually smaller than is normal for the breed. The long bones are shorter than normal and the head may be narrow and the cranium slightly domed. The characteristic nervous signs consist of rhythmic tremors most commonly of the muscles of the pelvis and upper parts of the hindlimbs, resulting in a characteristic jerking movement. Involvement of the trunk muscles leaves the appearance of the lamb continually jerking to free itself from some imaginary object. Affected lambs have difficulty in rising, and if able to stand with assistance exhibit an erratic gait especially of the hindquarters. Paralysis does not occur. Affected lambs are often unable to nurse the ewe because they cannot hold onto the teat. A flock severely affected with border disease is a picture of despair. Affected lambs appear languid and lie around listlessly. They do not suck as they should and bloat continuously and the ewes' udders become engorged with milk (30). In some less severe cases only fine tremors of the ears are evident. The tremors usually decline in severity as the lamb matures and may seem to disappear unless the animal is stressed.

When dry, the fleece appears hairy and rough due to long hairs rising above the fleece to form a halo especially over the nape, back, flanks and rump. This feature is most evident in normally smooth-coated breeds and is not observed in the coarse kempy fleeced breeds such as the Scottish Blackface.

Affected lambs are unthrifty and the majority will die before or at weaning time from parasitism or pneumonia. With good nursing care they can be reared but not normally. Puberty is reduced. In males, the testes do not develop normally. Many are persistently infected and are a source of the virus.

On a flock basis, there is poor performance because of low fertility, abortion and poor viability. However, these abnormalities are much more commonly recorded in experimental rather than natural cases. The clinical effects of the virus on the immunocompetent pregnant ewe are limited to a mild fever for a few days. However, the fetal death and embryonic resorption, abortion and mummification do occur which affects the reproductive performance of the flock and may explain the cause of unexpected barren ewes.

Clinical pathology

Serum neutralization tests on paired samples taken 4 weeks apart can be used to detect antibodies in immunocompetent animals which have been recently infected. Where abortion has occurred, paired serum samples taken 4 weeks apart may reveal significant changes in antibody status and indicate an active infection. Absence of serum antibody in a single ewe does not preclude border disease because the animal may be persistently infected, immunotolerant and seronegative. The absence of antibody in affected lambs is of no significance but the presence of antibody in precolostral serum indicates fetal infection.

After natural infection or inoculation of BD virus-containing samples, seronegative sheep, goats, calves and pigs develop antibody against bovine virus diarrhea virus which can be detected by virus neutralization tests.

Necropsy findings

The details of the pathology have been reported (30). Gross findings include an abnormally small size of brain and spinal cord. Arthrogryposis, hydranencephaly, porencephaly and cerebellar ataxia may also be present (30). Histologically, there is a deficiency of stainable central myelin and with neurochemical and histochemical evidence of demyelination or myelin dysmorphogenesis (30). The myelin defect resolves substantially during the first few months of life. The brain which has been very small, returns to normal weight, and chemical composition and degree of myelination. However, there is a recent report in which dysmyelination and glial proliferation in the central nervous system and microencephaly were noted in lambs with BD and these lesions appeared to remain the same over a year (31).

The immunofluorescent staining of cryostat sections of tissues from affected lambs provides the best approach to diagnosis (30). Virus titers reach high levels in the placentomes, and caruncles or cotyledons should be cultured for virus. Most isolates are non-cytopathic and the presence of viral antigens must be demonstrated by direct or indirect immunofluorescence or immune peroxidase techniques.

In sheep experimentally infected with the BD virus following recovery from naturally congenitally acquired border disease there is evidence of severe inflammatory lymphoproliferative lesions in several organs especially the central nervous system and the intestines (28).

The histological lesions of the skin consist of primary follicle enlargement, increased primary fiber size and an increased number of medullated primary fibers (30).

Diagnosis

Diagnosis is based on clinical epidemiological and histopathological evidence. Serological tests may be of assistance in immunocompetent animals. The immunofluorescent staining of cryostat sections of tissues from affected lambs is a reliable diagnostic aid (30). The abortion form of the disease must be differentiated from Rift Valley fever, Wesselbron tick-borne fever, chlamydiosis, toxoplasmosis and leptospirosis. In lambs with nervous signs, swayback due to copper deficiency, and caprine encephalomyelitis of kids must be considered.

Treatment

There is no treatment.

Control

Severely affected lambs are a continuous source of infection and should be culled. Eradication is only possible by complete depopulation and repopulation from virus-free flocks. The disease may be controlled at a tolerable level by maintaining groups of lambing ewes suspected of being infected and therefore capable of transmitting the virus separate from other ewes during the period between joining and the 3rd week of pregnancy.

REVIEW LITERATURE

Barlow, R. M. & Patterson, D. S. P. (1982) Border disease of sheep: a virus induced teratogenic disorder. *Adv. vet. Sci. Supp. J. vet. Med. No, 36*, 1–90.

Terpstra, C. (1985) Border disease: a congenital infection of small ruminants. *Prog. Vet. Microbiol. Immunol.*, *1*, 175–198.

REFERENCES

(1) Terpstra, C. (1985) *Prog. vet. Microbiol. Immunol.*, *1*, 175.
(2) Vantsis, J. T. et al. (1980) *J.comp. Pathol.*, *90*, 39, 57, & 67.
(3) Harkness, J. W. et al. (1977) *Vet. Rec.*, *100*, 71.
(4) Orr, M. B. et al. (1976) *Res. vet. Sci.*, *22*, 56.
(5) Richardson, C. et al. (1976) *Br. vet. J.*, *132*, 202.
(6) Weavers, E. D. et al. (1975) *Irish vet. J.*, *29*, 161.
(7) Potts, B. J. et al. (1982) *Am. J. vet. Res.*, *43*, 1460, 1464.
(8) Barlow, R. M. et al. (1975) *J. comp. Pathol.*, 85, 291.
(9) Gibbons, D. F. et al. (1974) *Br. vet. J.*, *130*, 357.
(10) Terlecki, S. (1977) *Vet. Ann.*, *17*, 74.
(11) Wrathall, A. E. et al. (1978) *Zentralbl. VetMed.*, 25 B, 62.
(12) Gardiner, A. C. & Barlow, R. M. (1972) *J. comp. Pathol.*, *82*, 29.
(13) Porter. W. L. et al. (1972) *NZ vet. J.*, *20*, *1*, 4.
(14) Plant, J. W. et al. (1983) *Vet. Rec.*, *113*, 58.
(15) Sawyer, M. M. et al. (1986) *J. Am. vet. med. Assoc.*, *189*, 61.
(16) Ames, T. R. et al. (1982) *J. Am. vet. med. Assoc.*, *180*, 619.
(17) Cravero, G. C. et al. (1975) *Schweiz. Arch. Tierheilkd.*, *117*, 119.
(18) Spais, A. G. et al. (1975) *Proc. 20th World Vet. Congr.*, *Thessaloniki*, p. 622.
(19) Loken, T. et al. (1982) *Acta vet. Scand.*, *23*, 46.
(20) Sands, J. J. & Harkness, J. W. (1978) *Res. vet. Sci.*, *25*, 241.
(21) Lamontagne, L. & Roy, R. (1984) *Can. J. comp. Med.*, *48*, 225.
(22) Terpstra, C. (1981) *Res. vet. Sci.*, *30*, 185.
(23) Barlow, R. M. (1980) *J.comp. Pathol.*, *90*, 87.
(24) Sharp, M. W. & Rawson, B. C. (1986) *Vet. Rec.*, *119*, 128.
(25) Plant, J. W. et al. (1983) *Aust. vet. J.*, *60*, 137.
(26) Barlow, R. M. et al. (1980) *J. comp. Pathol.*, *90*, 67.
(27) Terlecki, S. et al. (1973) *Res. vet. Sci.*, *15*, 310.
(28) Barlow, R. M. et al. (1983) *J. comp. Pathol.*, *93*, 451.
(29) Gardiner, A. C. et al. (1983) *J. comp. Pathol.*, *93*, 463.
(30) Barlow, R. M. & Patterson, D. S. P. (1982) *Adv. vet. Sci. Suppl. J. vet. Med.*, *No. 36*, 1.
(31) Potts, B. J. et al. (1985) *J. infect. Dis.*, *151*, 337.
(32) Loken, T. et al. (1982) *Res. vet. Sci.*, *33*, 130.
(33) Roeder, P. L. et al. (1983) *Br. vet. J.*, *139*, 129.
(34) Terlecki, S. & Roeder, P. L. (1983) *J. comp. Pathol.*, *93*, 243.
(35) Anderson, C. A. et al. (1987) *Am. J. vet. Res.*, *48*, 499.
(36) Loken, T. (1987) *J. comp. Pathol.*, *97*, 85.
(37) Bonniwell, M. A. et al. (1987) *Vet. Rec.*, *120*, 246.

VIRAL DISEASES CHARACTERIZED BY SKIN LESIONS

Contagious ecthyma (contagious pustular dermatitis, orf, soremouth)

Contagious ecthyma is a highly infectious viral disease of sheep and goats characterized by the development of pustular and scabby lesions on the muzzle and lips. The virus can also produce lesions on the teats of cattle.

Etiology

A parapoxvirus (family Poxviridae), composed of at least six immunological strains, is the cause of the disease (1). The virus is immunologically distinct from vaccinia, but very similar to the causative agent of pseudocowpox, and has antigenic similarity to goat pox virus (5), but not to sheeppox virus (2).

Epidemiology

The disease occurs wherever sheep are raised and causes unthriftiness and some economic loss. The incidence within a flock may be as high as 90%. The few deaths which occur are due to the extension of lesions in the respiratory tract, but the mortality rate may reach 15% if lambs are badly cared for or if secondary infection and cutaneous myiasis are allowed to occur. In the rare outbreaks where systemic invasion occurs the mortality rate averages 25% and may be as high as 75%.

The virus withstands drying and is capable of surviving at room temperature for at least 15 years. Among farm animals, sheep, goats and cattle are affected naturally, and a few cases have occurred in humans working among sheep. In abattoir workers it is commonest in those handling wool and skins (13). The disease has also been observed in musk ox (6) in which it causes heavy losses, reindeer (9), mountain goats and bighorn sheep (4), chamois, caribou, Dall sheep (11), buffalo (18) and wild thar goats. The disease is also recorded as occurring in camels (12). The virus can be passaged in rabbits if large doses are placed on scarified skin or injected intradermally. Mild lesions develop on the chorioallantois of the 9–12-day chick embryo. Guinea-pigs and mice are not susceptible.

The disease is commonest in lambs 3–6 months of age although lambs 10–12 days of age and adult animals can be severely affected. Outbreaks occur at any time but they are most common in dry conditions when the sheep are at pasture. Recovered animals are solidly immune for 2–3 years, but no antibodies appear to be passed in the colostrum and newborn lambs of immune ewes are susceptible (1). In man typical lesions occur at the site of infection, usually an abrasion infected while handling diseased sheep or milking affected cows or by accidental means when vaccinating. The lesions are very itchy and respond poorly to local treatment.

Spread in a flock is very rapid and occurs by contact with other affected animals or inanimate objects such as ear-tagging pliers (17), emasculators, resulting in an outbreak of lesions on the tails (15). The common occurrence in dry seasons suggests that abrasion of the skin by dry feed may provide a ready portal of entry for infection. The scabs remain highly infective for long periods, but survival of the disease in a flock may be the result of chronic lesions which survive for long periods on individual animals (16).

Pathogenesis

Identical diseases occur in sheep and goats (8). Histologically the changes in the skin closely resemble those which occur in the pox diseases and the development of the diseases is very similar. That there is some relationship between the viruses of goat pox and contagious ecthyma is indicated by the finding that goat pox antiserum neutralizes the ecthyma virus, although the reverse does not hold.

Clinical findings

Lesions develop initially as papules and then pustules, stages which are not usually observed, then as thick, tenacious scabs covering a raised area of ulceration, granulation and inflammation. The first lesions develop at the oral mucocutaneous junction, usually at the oral commissures. From here they spread on to the muzzle and nostrils, the surrounding haired skin and, to a lesser extent, on to the buccal mucosa. They may appear as discrete, thick scabs 0·5 cm in diameter, or be packed close together as a continuous plaque. Fissuring occurs and the scabs are sore to the touch. They crumble easily but are difficult to remove from the underlying granulation. Affected lambs suffer a severe setback because of restricted suckling and grazing. Rarely systemic invasion occurs and lesions appear on the coronets and ears, around the anus and vulva or prepuce, and on the nasal and buccal mucosae. There is a severe systemic reaction and extension down the alimentary tract may lead to a severe gastroenteritis, and extension down the trachea may be followed by bronchopneumonia.

A malignant form of the disease has also been observed. It begins with an acute episode manifested by oral vesicles, and extension of these lesions down the gastrointestinal tract, followed later by granulomatous lesions and shedding of hooves (3). In rams, lesions on the scrotum may be accompanied by fluid accumulation in the scrotal sac. In benign cases the scabs dry and fall off, and recovery is complete in about 3 weeks. Affected lambs sucking ewes may cause spread of the disease to the udder. Secondary infection of the lesions by *Fusobacterium necrophorus* occurs in some cases.

Clinical pathology

Laboratory examination is not usually undertaken for diagnostic purposes, but a definitive diagnosis requires transmission experiments to susceptible sheep or rabbits and the demonstration of resistance in previously immunized animals. Recovered animals have a high level of neutralizing antibodies in their serum and this is detectable by a gel diffusion test. Techniques for a complement fixation test and tissue culture on lamb testicular tissue are also available. Electron microscopic identification of the virus is the quickest and most reliable method.

Necropsy findings

In malignant cases there are typical ulcerative lesions in the nasal cavities and the upper respiratory tract, and in some cases erosion in the mucosae of the esophagus, abomasum and small intestine.

Diagnosis

In most outbreaks of ecthyma, the cases are sufficiently mild to cause no real concern about losses or about diagnosis. Violent outbreaks of a very severe form of the disease may occur, however, and are likely to be confused with bluetongue. Very severe cases are also commonly seen in housed experimental sheep especially colostrum-free lambs.

Ulcerative dermatosis, and its causative agent, are sufficiently similar to cause confusion in diagnosis. Mycotic dermatitis usually occurs on woolled skin. Facial eczema is distinguished by diffuse dermatitis and severe edema and damage to the ears.

The lesions of proliferative dermatitis (strawberry footrot) are confined to the lower limbs. Bluetongue is always accompanied by a high mortality rate, a severe systemic reaction, and lesions occur on the muzzle and on the coronets and extensively on the buccal mucosa. It is more common in adults than sucking lambs. Because it is transmitted by insect vectors, the morbidity rate is usually much less than the 90% commonly seen in contagious ecthyma. Sheeppox may present a rather similar clinical picture, but the scabs are typical hard crusts and there is a severe systemic reaction and heavy mortality rate.

Treatment

There is no specific treatment. Removal of the scabs and the application of ointments or astringent lotions are practiced but delay healing in most cases. The provision of soft, palatable food is recommended.

Control

In the early stages of an outbreak, the affected animals should be isolated and the remainder vaccinated. Vaccination is of little value when a large number of animals are already affected. Persistence of the disease in a flock from year to year is common and in such circumstances the lambs should be vaccinated at 6–8 weeks of age. Vaccination when a few days old evokes a protective response but prelambing vaccination of the ewe does not and is not recommended (10). The vaccine is prepared from a suspension of scabs in glycerol saline and is painted on to a small area of scarified skin inside the thigh or by pricking the ear with an icepick dipped in the vaccine. Vaccination is completely effective for at least 2 years, but the lambs should be inspected 1 week after vaccination to ensure that local reactions have resulted. Absence of a local reaction signifies lack of viability of the vaccine or the existence of a prior immunity. The immunity is not solid until 3 weeks after vaccination. A small proportion of vaccinated lambs may develop mild lesions about the mouth because of nibbling at the vaccination site. The efficiency of this vaccine is much greater (14) than that of the standard commercial vaccine containing live attenuated virus (7). As a further protective measure, removal of abrasive material from the environment is recommended but is not usually practicable.

REVIEW LITERATURE

Robinson, A. J. & Balassu, T. C. (1981) Contagious pustular dermatitis (orf). *Vet. Bull.*, *51*, 771.

REFERENCES

(1) Hardy, W. T. (1964) *Proc. US live Stk sanit. Assoc.* 293.
(2) Rao, M. V. S. & Malik, B. S. (1979) *Acta virol.*, *23*, 165.
(3) Valder, W. A. et al. (1979) *Tierärztl. Umschau*, *34*, 828.
(4) Samuel, W. M. et al. (1975) *J. Wildlife Dis.*, *11*, 26.
(5) Dubey, S. C. & Sawhney, A. N. (1979) *Ind. J. anim. Sci.*, *49*, 135.
(6) Mathieson, S. D. et al. (1985) *Acta vet. Scand.*, *26*, 120.
(7) Mayr, A. et al. (1981) *Zentralbl. VetMed.*, *28*, 535.
(8) Ott, R. S. & Nelson, D. R. (1978) *J. Am. vet. med. Assoc.*, *173*, 81.
(9) Kummeneje, K. & Krogsrud, J. (1979) *Vet. Res.*, *105*, 60.
(10) Buddle, B. M. & Pulford, H. D. (1984) *Vet. Microbiol.*, *9*, 515.
(11) Zarnke, R. L. et al. (1983) *J. Wildlife Dis.*, *19*, 170.
(12) Munz, E. et al. (1986) *J. vet. Med.*, B, *33*, 73.
(13) Robinson, A. J. & Petersen, G. V. (1983) *NZ med. J.*, *96*, 81.
(14) Buddle, B. M. et al. (1984) *Am. J. vet. Res.*, *45*, 263.
(15) Ames, T. et al. (1984) *J. Am. vet. med. Assoc.*, *184*, 88.
(16) McKeever, D. J. & Reid, H. W. (1986) *Vet. Rec.*, *118*, 613.
(17) Allworth, M. B. et al. (1987) *Aust. vet. J.*, *64*, 61.
(18) Huang, Y. X. & Li, N. J. (1986) *Chin. J. vet. Med.*, *12*, 2.

Papillomatosis

The common wart of cattle and horses is transmissible by intradermal injection and is caused by a virus with considerable host specificity.

Etiology

A series of papillomaviruses in the family Papovaviridae are the cause of cutaneous warts in cattle and horses.

In cattle, warts occur on almost any part of the body, but when a number of animals in a group is affected it is common to find them all affected in the same part of the body. It is known that some of these topographically specific warts, which are often characterized by a particular structure grossly and microscopically, hence morphologically specific warts, are caused by distinct viruses; so that immunity to one of them does not necessarily confer immunity to others. Some of these viral isolates have been demonstrated to have different antigen reactions and DNA composition (6). Six of these viruses have been identified, as follows: subgroup A including BVP1, BVP2 and BVP5 which cause fibropapillomas; and subgroup B which includes BVP3, BVP4 and BVP6 which cause true epithelial papillomas (4). Their detailed roles are:

- Rice grain lesions on the teat skin—the BVP5 virus
- Frond epithelial papillomas of the bovine udder—BVP6
- Frond fibropapillomas of teat skin—BVP1
- Typical fibropapilloma of the skin of the anteroventral part of the body including the forehead, neck and back—the BVP2 virus
- Cauliflower-like fibropapillomas of the anogenital and ventral abdominal skin—the BVP2 virus
- Squamous papilloma of the esophagus, esophageal groove, forestomachs and small intestine; this has been identified as BVP4 (7) and is capable of becoming malignant
- Other cutaneous papilloma—BVP3.

Other papilloma of cattle which have regional distribution and may have separate antigenic identity are:

- Oral papillomas, mostly in adult cattle and apparently reaching a high incidence, up to 16% in some areas (15); these are probably BVP4
- Papilloma of the larynx in steers
- Interdigital fibropapillomata have not been positively identified as having a viral etiology
- Papillomavirus has been observed in squamous cell carcinomata of bovine eyes (14), but is absent from similar equine lesions (21).

In horses, papillomata occur mostly on the lower face, but they also occur on the penis and vulva, in the mouth, on the conjunctiva (21), and they can occur in the newborn. The bovine papilloma virus injected intradermally into horses causes a lesion indistinguishable from those of bovine papillomatosis (9).

Epidemiology

Warts are quite common in young cattle, especially when they are housed, but ordinarily they cause little harm and disappear spontaneously. In pure-bred animals they may interfere with sales because of their unsightly appearance and in such groups the incidence may be as high as 25%. Animals with extensive lesions may lose condition and secondary bacterial invasion of traumatized warts may cause concern. Warts on the teats of dairy cows often cause interference with milking. Several outbreaks have been recorded in sheep (8) and a similar condition is described in goats (18). In pigs papillomatosis commonly affects the genitalia and in wildlife it occurs in white-tailed deer (*Odocoileus virginianus*) and mule deer (*O. hemionus*) (20).

In horses the lesions are usually small and cause little inconvenience. They usually occur sporadically, although there is one report of five cases appearing within a 6-week period in a relatively small group, four of them occurring in a single inbred family (5).

The lack of susceptibility of adults to natural infection with warts is thought to be due to immunity acquired by apparent or inapparent infection when young. Immunity after an attack is solid and persists for at least 2 years. The transmissibility of the sheep disease was proven, and the presence of virus in the lesions was detected by electron microscopy (8). In deer the lesions are commonly in the form of cutaneous fibromas (20).

The method of spread is probably by direct contact with infected animals, infection gaining entry through cutaneous abrasions. Crops of warts sometimes occur around eartags or along scratches made by barbed wire and can be spread by tattooing implements and dehorning shears. An extensive outbreak of perianal warts is recorded in beef heifers, the infection having been spread by rectal examination for pregnancy (16). A high prevalence of papillomas on the larynx of feedlot steers is ascribed to implantation of the virus in contact ulcers which are also entry sites for *Fusobacterium nodosum* which causes calf diphtheria (17). Warts can be spread experimentally by the intradermal injection of a suspension of wart tissue in both horses and cattle. The rare occurrence of congenital papillomatosis is difficult to explain other than by transmission of the infection across the placenta (11). It has been recorded only in horses.

Pathogenesis

The virus infects the basal cells of the epithelium causing the excessive growth which is characteristic of wart formation. The tumor contains epithelial and connective tissues and is a fibropapilloma. Similar lesions include papillomata, with very little connective tissue content, and fibromata which are mostly fibrous tissue, with very little epithelial tissue.

Clinical findings

The incubation period after experimental inoculation in cattle is 3–8 weeks but is usually somewhat longer after natural exposure. Warts are solid outgrowths of epidermis and may be sessile or pedunculated. In young cattle and goats, they occur most commonly on the head, especially around the eyes, and on the neck and shoulders (19), and may spread to other parts of the body. They vary in size from 1 cm upwards and their dry, horny, cauliflower-like appearance is characteristic. Cutaneous warts are common in older animals and warts on the teats show an increasing frequency with age (15).

These teat warts appear in several forms. There is a frond type, a flat round type and an elongated rice grain structure. They are usually multiple, always sessile and are up to 2 cm in diameter. The frond form have filiform projections on them and appear to have been drawn out into an elongated shape of about 1 cm in length by milking machine action. If sharp traction is used they can often be pulled out by the roots.

Perianal warts are esthetically unattractive, but do not appear to reduce activity or productivity. Genital warts on the vulva and penis make mating impracticable because the lesions are of large size and crumble and bleed easily. They commonly become infected and flyblown.

Interdigital fibropapillomas (not to be confused with interdigital fibromas as described under footrot) are round, flat, sessile lesions located on the skin of the fleshy pad behind the pastern and just above the heel bulbs (10). Enlargement of them leads to the development of finger-like projections and cauliflower-like excrescences. These are painful and lameness may be so severe that animals lie down a lot and lose much condition. Mostly they are sporadic in occurrence, but a high prevalence rate may occur in some herds.

Less common manifestations of papillomatosis in cattle include lesions in the urinary bladder which cause no clinical signs. Sporadic cases occur in the esophageal groove and in the reticulum causing chronic ruminal tympany. The concurrent occurrence of papillomata and squamous cell carcinomas of the bovine alimentary tract is recorded (1). The causative agents were thought to be the papilloma virus and the carcinogen in bracken. Direct transformation of papilloma to carcinoma was observed. Lesions were present on the lateral and dorsal aspects of the tongue, the soft palate, oropharynx, esophagus, esophageal groove and rumen.

In goats (18) the papillomas may be on the udder or on the skin generally, especially on unpigmented skin. Most completely regress, others regress and recur and occasional lesions progress to carcinomas.

In horses, warts are confined to the muzzle, nose and lips and are usually sessile and quite small, rarely exceeding 1 cm in diameter. The lesions produced in horses by the intradermal injection of the bovine papilloma virus is very much like a sarcoid. Horses resistant to infection with sarcoid material are still susceptible to the papilloma virus (3). In both species spontaneous recovery is usual, but the warts may persist for 5–6 months and in some cases for as long as 18 months. In such cases there may be serious loss of condition. Persistence of papillomas may be due to immunodeficiency in an animal.

Clinical pathology

Biopsy of a lesion is rarely necessary to confirm a diagnosis, but it may be advisable when large growths are found on horses, particularly on the lower limbs, to determine whether or not they are sarcoids. The need to identify the specific virus in a crop of warts creates a requirement for serological and histological examinations. An ELISA is available (2).

Diagnosis

Clinically there is little difficulty in making a diagnosis of papillomatosis with the possible exception of atypical papillomas of cattle. These lesions are characterized by an absence of dermal fibroplasia, the lesion is a true papilloma rather than a fibropapilloma. The tumors contain a virus which is morphologically similar to fibropapilloma virus but the disease is not transferable. Nor does commercial wart vaccine have any effect in preventing it. All ages of animals are affected and the lesions persist for long periods. They are characteristically discrete, low, flat and circular. They do not form stalks and often coalesce to form large masses. They do not protrude like regular warts and the external fronds are much finer and more delicate. Differentiation from sarcoids in the horse may necessitate biopsy and histological examination. Carcinoma of the eye (cancer–eye) affects only eyelids or cornea.

Treatment

For cattle, autogenous vaccines prepared from wart tissues of the affected animal are effective. The vaccine may be fully virulent or inactivated with formalin, and suspended in saline, buffered glycerol, bovine serum, or saline merthiolate, with added antibiotics. The virus may be obtained directly from a wart or by tissue culture. Because of the multiplicity of viruses care is required in the selection of the tissues. In general terms they can be selected on tumor type, location and histological composition. The stage of development is also important because of variation in the amount of virus which is replicating (7). The alternative is to use many types of tissue in the vaccine. It can be injected subcutaneously, but better results are claimed for intradermal injection. Two injections 1–2 weeks apart are recommended. Recovery in 3–6 weeks is recorded in 80–85% of cases where the warts are on the body surface or penis of cattle, but in only 33% when the warts are on the teats. The response of low, flat, sessile warts to vaccination has always been poor, and has been thought to be due to their low content of epithelial tissue, as distinct from fibrous tissue. It may be a difference between antigenically different viruses. The live virus remains fully viable at room temperature for at least 3 weeks.

Other treatments include the injection of proprietary preparations containing antimony and bismuth and removal by traction or ligation, but results with these treatments have been very poor. In all cases the tendency for spontaneous recovery to occur makes assessment of the results of treatment very difficult. Surgical removal is sometimes necessary and removal of one or two warts in cattle may be followed by the rapid disappearance of the remainder. Partial resection of a wart or warts in a horse does not promote resolution of the residue (12). On the other hand surgical intervention, and even vaccination, in the early stages of wart development may increase the size of residual warts and prolong the course of the disease. The causative virus is present in much greater concentration in the epithelial tissue of older warts than young ones, and this may have some effect on the efficiency of autogenous vaccines.

In horses, surgical removal may be indicated followed immediately by the administration of an autogenous vaccine, repeated with increasing dosage at 4-day intervals for about a month (13). However, in young horses warts usually resolve spontaneously in 4–6 weeks and treatment is usually unnecessary. When the course is long, local treatment by topical application or systemic treatment by vaccination or medication, as recommended for cattle, may be used. Topical treatments include cauterization with trichloracetic acid or 20% tincture of salicylic acid. The surrounding skin needs to be protected with petroleum jelly, and horses must be prevented from nibbling the treated site.

Control

Specific control procedures are usually not instituted or warranted because of the unpredictable nature of the disease and its minor economic importance.

Vaccination has been used to prevent the occurrence of the disease. Vaccines prepared from tissues produce satisfactory immunity but those prepared from egg-adapted virus are of dubious value. Tissue vaccines are capable of producing an immunity in epidermal tissues, but not in connective tissue, so that mild connective tissue outgrowths may occur after infection. The now apparent multiplicity of antigenic variants of the virus points up the difficulties likely to be encountered in a vaccination program, even when an autogenous vaccine is used. Avoidance of close contact between infected and uninfected animals should be encouraged.

REVIEW LITERATURE

Hunt, E. (1984) Fibropapillomatosis and papillomatosis. *Vet. Clin. N. Am. large Anim. Pract.*, *6 (1)*, 163–167.

REFERENCES

(1) Jarrett, W. F. H. et al. (1978) *Nature*, *274*, 215.
(2) Shazly, M. O. et al. (1985) *Am. J. vet. Res.*, *46*, 1737.
(3) Ragland, W. L. et al. (1970) *Equ. vet. J.*, *2*, 168.
(4) Jarrett, W. F. H. et al. (1984) *Virology*, *136*, p. 225.
(5) Ragland, W. L. et al. (1966) *Nature, Lond.*, *210*, 1399.
(6) Lancaster, W. D. & Olson, C. (1978) *Virology*, *89*, 372.
(7) Jarrett, W. F. H. et al. (1984) *J. Natl Career Inst.*, *73*, 499.
(8) Gibbs, E. P. J. et al. (1975) *J. comp. Pathol.*, *85*, 327.
(9) Olson, R. O. et al. (1982) *Am. J. vet. Res.*, *43*, 2250.
(10) Rebhun, W. C. et al. (1980) *J. Am. vet. med. Assoc.*, *177*, 437.
(11) Atwell, R. B. & Summers, P. M. (1977) *Aust. vet. J.*, *53*, 299.
(12) Sundberg, J. P. et al. (1985) *Vet. Med. SAC*, *80*, 71.
(13) Page, E. H. et al. (1967) *J. Am. vet. med. Assoc.*, *150*, 177.
(14) Ford, J. N. et al. (1982) *Res. vet. Sci.*, *32*, 257.
(15) Samuel, J. L. et al. (1985) *Zentralbl. VetMed.*, *32*, 706.
(16) Tweddle, N. E. & White, W. E. (1977) *Aust. vet. J.*, *53*, 492.
(17) Jensen, R. et al. (1981) *Vet. Pathol.*, *18*, 143.
(18) Theilin, G. et al. (1985) *Am. J. vet. Res.*, *46*, 2519.
(19) Nooruddin, M. (1984) *Agri-Practice*, *5 (10)*, 33.
(20) Sundberg, J. P. et al. (1985) *Am. J. vet. Res.*, *46*, 1145 & 1150.
(21) Junge, R. E. et al. (1984) *J. Am. vet. med. Assoc.*, *185*, 656.

Sarcoid

This is a locally invasive cutaneous tumor of equids caused by a virus which has not been definitely identified. It is characterized by the presence of cutaneous lumps of all sizes and located anywhere on the body.

Etiology

Equine sarcoid is the commonest neoplasm in horses. It is transplantable and is obviously caused by a virus, possibly BPV1 and BPV2 as described under papillomatosis. These are suspected because papillomaviral DNA has been detected in sarcoid tumors (1, 2) and because similar tumors can be produced by the intradermal injection of bovine papillomavirus in horses. A retrovirus would be a logical cause and one has been isolated from a tumor (3). It is possible that there is a genetic susceptibility to the disease (4).

Epidemiology

Horses, donkeys and mules are affected. There may be a familial predilection and there is a tendency for the disease to occur more frequently in animals less than 6 years of age.

Pathogenesis

Sarcoids are localized proliferations of epidermal and dermal tissue which may remain small and dormant for many years and then undergo a stage of rapid cancer-like growth. The lesions show moderate malignancy but do not metastasize to other sites although there may be multiple cutaneous lesions.

Clinical findings

Lesions occur singly or in groups and have the general appearance of rather large warts. They are hairless, and large ones commonly ulcerate. Four clinical types of lesion are described (5). They include a verrucous or wart-like type which is dry, flat and horny and may be sessile or pedunculated, a fibroplastic or proud-flesh type which commence as small (5 mm) hard nodules which ulcerate and spread laterally to become large ulcers which may be more than 20 cm diameter, and mixtures of these two types. The fourth type is a slow-growing slight thickening of the skin with a roughened surface. It is an almost insignificant lesion but is likely to be stimulated into fibroblastic activity by surgical interference.

The lesions occur most commonly on the lower limbs but also on the lips, eyelids, eye, penile sheath and around the base of the ears.

Clinical pathology

The lesions are obvious and characteristic but confirmation of the diagnosis requires histological evidence and a biopsy specimen is required for this purpose. The tumor has some features in common with papillomas and also those of sarcoma.

Diagnosis

Sarcoids resemble papilloma but do not regress with time as papillomas almost always do. Sarcoids must also be differentiated from fibromas, fibrosarcomas, granulation tissue, squamous cell carcinomas and other less common tumors by histopathological examination. Cutaneous habronemiasis and phycomycosis have some similarity to equine sarcoids and are differentiated on the basis of microscopic identification of the larvae or fungal elements in the lesions.

Treatment

Radiotherapy is an effective treatment (6) and local hyperthermia induced by a radiofrequency current of 2 MHz is also reported to be effective (7). Excellent results are recorded after the intralesional injection of vaccine (8); similar injections of cell-wall fractions in oil have given good results in periocular lesions but sarcoids of the axilla did not react favorably (11), and immunotherapy using mycobacterial cell wall skeleton combined with trehalose dimycolate has resulted in total tumor regression (10). The most favoured treatment is cryosurgery but great care is required to ensure that the lesion is completely removed, otherwise it will recur (9). This is also likely if there are multiple lesions.

REVIEW LITERATURE

Tarwid, J. N. (1985) Equine sarcoid: a study with emphasis on pathologic diagnosis. *Comp. cont. Educ.*, 7, S293–300.

REFERENCES

(1) Trenfield, K. et al. (1985) *Equ. vet. J*, *17*, 449.
(2) Gorman, N. T. (1985) *Equ. vet. J.*, *17*, 412.
(3) Cheevers, W. P. et al. (1982) *Am. J. vet. Res.*, *43*, 804.
(4) Lazary S. et al. (1985) *Equ. vet. J.*, *17*, 283.
(5) Pascoe, R. R. (1984) *Vet. Clin. N. Am. large Anim. Pract.*, *6 (1)*, 39.
(6) Wyn-Jones, G. (1983) *Equ. vet. J.*, *15*, 361.
(7) Hoffman, K. D. et al. (1983) *Equ. Pract.*, *5 (7)*, 24.
(8) Lavach, J. D. et al. (1985) *Equ. vet. J.*, *17*, 445.
(9) Cookerell, G. L. & MacCoy, D. M. (1978) *Cornell Vet.*, *68*, *(Suppl. 7)*, 133.
(10) Schwartzman, S. M. et al. (1984) *Equ. Pract.*, *6 (8)*, 13.
(11) Owen, R. R. & Jagger, D. W. (1987) *Vet. Rec.*, *120*, 548.

Lumpy skin disease (knopvelsiekte)

Lumpy skin disease is a highly infectious skin disease of cattle caused by a virus. It is characterized by the sudden appearance of nodules on all parts of the skin.

Etiology

Lumpy skin disease is really two diseases: the severe form is caused by the Neethling poxvirus: the mild form in the United Kingdom is caused by the Allerton herpesvirus, and in the United States it is caused by the dermatotrophic bovine herpesvirus (2), both of which appear to be identical with the virus of bovine mammillitis. The Neethling virus has similar cultural characteristics in tissue culture to sheeppox and goatpox viruses and all three are classified as capripoxviruses. Although prior infection with sheeppox virus confers immunity against the Neethling virus infection, it is not considered that the two viruses are identical; at least no cases of pox occur in mingled sheep during lumpy skin disease outbreaks in cattle and *vice versa* (4). There is a possibility that the Neethling virus is originally a pox virus of some wild species (4).

Epidemiology

The disease used to be confined to South Africa and Kenya. It is now on the move to the north and west so that Sudan, Chad, Niger and the Central African Republic are now infected (5). A related but much milder disease, pseudolumpy skin disease, occurs in the United Kingdom.

Although the mortality rate is low (less than 10%), the economic loss caused is high due to loss of milk production, damage to hides and loss of bodily condition during the long course of the disease. In South Africa the morbidity in a group is high (5–50%) and many animals may be affected at one time. Spread to neighboring farms may be similarly rapid. In Kenya the disease is characterized by a much lower morbidity rate and the disease is much milder.

All ages and types of cattle are susceptible to the causative virus except animals recently recovered from an attack, in which case there is a solid immunity lasting for about 3 months. The disease has been produced experimentally with Neethling virus in giraffe and impala, but wildebeeste were resistant (6). There is serological evidence of infection in African buffalo *(Syncerus caffer)* (11).

Although the method of spread under natural conditions is not known, the rapid spread of the disease and the ease with which it traverses long distances suggest an insect vector. Experimental transmission can be accomplished using ground-up nodular tissue and blood.

Pathogenesis

After an initial viremia accompanied by a febrile reaction, localization in the skin occurs with development of inflammatory nodules.

Clinical findings

An incubation period of 2–4 weeks is common in field outbreaks. In severe cases there is an initial rise of temperature, sometimes accompanied by lacrimation, nasal discharge, salivation and lameness. Multiple nodules appear suddenly about a week later, the first ones usually appearing in the perineum. They are round and firm, varying from 1 to 4 cm in diameter, and are flattened and the hair on them stands on end. They vary in number from a few to hundreds; they are intradermal and, in most cases, are confined to the skin area. In severe cases the lesions may also be present in the nostrils and on the turbinates, causing respiratory obstruction and snoring. They may also be in the mouth. Oral and nasal lesions tend to be present as plaques, which later ulcerate. Nodules may develop on the conjunctiva, causing severe lacrimation. Lesions on the prepuce or vulva may spread to nearby mucosal surfaces. In most cases the nodules disappear rapidly, but they may persist as hard lumps or become moist, necrotic and slough. Lymph nodes draining the affected area become enlarged and there may be local edema. When sloughing of the yellow center of nodules occurs there is often exposure of underlying tissues, e.g. testicles or tendons, especially if the nodules have coalesced. A convalescence of 4–12 weeks is usual. Pregnant cows may abort.

Clinical pathology

Biopsy of lesions caused by the Neethling virus reveals a granulomatous reaction in the dermis and hypodermis. In the earlier acute stages, there are intracellular, eosinophilic inclusion bodies (10).

Necropsy findings

The cutaneous lesions are described under clinical pathology. Similar lesions are present in the mouth, pharynx, trachea, skeletal muscle, bronchi and stomachs, and there may be accompanying pneumonia. Animals in which extension to the mucosae of the digestive and respiratory tracts occur often die. There is obstruction to respiration by the necrotic ulcers and surrounding inflammation in the nasal cavities.

Diagnosis

The rapid spread of the disease and the sudden appearance of lumps in the skin after an initial fever make this disease quite unlike any other affliction of cattle. Diagnosis depends on recognition of inclusion bodies in sections of skin lesions, and in tissue cultures of the virus. Electron microscopy and fluorescent antibody tests are applicable (7). An intradermal test has been described and may be of value in herd diagnosis (8).

The disease identified as 'generalized infection of cattle with bovine herpesvirus 2' (1) is thought to be the same disease as the Allerton form of lumpy skin disease. However, the lesions described in the former are quite unlike those of the latter. They are described as being like a ringworm, circular, up to 2 cm in diameter, some with an intact central area and raised edges. Only the superficial layers of skin appear to be involved. This is in contrast to the lesions of lumpy skin disease which are often deep enough to expose underlying tissues.

Treatment

No specific treatment is available, but prevention of secondary infection is essential. The use of antibiotics or sulfonamides is recommended.

Control

A safe vaccine against the Neethling virus, and produced by 60 passages of the virus through lamb kidney culture, is effective. It is administered to all animals over 6 months of age (9). A freeze-dried, living attenuated virus vaccine is also available (3). Vaccination of cattle with sheeppox virus, also attenuated by passage through tissue culture, is effective in preventing infection with the Neethling virus (4). A small percentage of cattle show local reactions but there is no spread of the sheep pox to sheep running with the cattle. The method has the obvious disadvantage that it can be used only in those countries where sheeppox exists.

REVIEW LITERATURE

Weiss, K. E. (1968) *Virol. Monogr.*, *3*, 111.

REFERENCES

(1) St. George, T. D. et al. (1980) *Aust. vet. J.*, *56*, 47.
(2) Gigstad, D. C. et al. (1972) *Proc. 75th ann. gen. Mtg US Anim. Hlth Assoc.*, 201.
(3) Lefevre, P. C. (1979) *Rev. L'Elevage Med. Vet. Pays trop.*, *32*, 233.
(4) Ai, B. H. & Obeid, H. M. (1977) *Br. vet. J.*, *133*, 184.
(5) Woods, J. A. (1974) *Vet. Rec.*, *95*, 326.
(6) Young, E. et al. (1970) *Onderstepoort J. vet. Res.*, *37*, 79.
(7) Nawathe, D. R. & Osagka, M. O. (1977) *Bull. Anim. Hlth Prod., Afr.*, *25*, 313.
(8) Capstick, P. B. & Coackley, W. (1962) *Res. vet. Sci.*, *3*, 287.
(9) Jansen, B. C. (1966) *Aust. vet. J.*, *42*, 471.
(10) Prozesky, L. & Barnard, B. J. H. (1982) *Onderstepoort J. vet. Res.*, *49*, 167.
(11) Davies, F. G. (1982) *J. Hyg., Camb.*, *88*, 95.

Viral papular dermatitis

This disease of horses occurs in the United States (1), United Kingdom and Australia. It is characterized by cutaneous lesions in the form of firm papules 0·5–2 cm in diameter. No vesicles or pustules are formed but after 7–10 days a dry crust is detached leaving small circumscribed areas of alopecia. The lesions are not itchy, there is no systemic disease and the distribution of the lesions, and the way in which they can develop simultaneously in large numbers in introduced horses, is suggestive of an insect-borne disease. The course of the disease varies between 10 days and 6 weeks. An unidentified virus has been isolated from lesions and cultured on eggs. A febrile reaction, up to 40·2°C (104·5°F), precedes the appearance of skin lesions by about 24 hours. Recovery is usually complete and uncomplicated.

REFERENCE

(1) McIntyre, R. W. (1949) *Am. J. vet. Res.*, *10*, 229.

Cowpox and buffalopox

Cowpox is a benign, contagious skin disease of cattle characterized by the appearance of typical pox lesions on the teats and udder.

Etiology

The causative orthopoxvirus of true cowpox is closely related to the viruses of horsepox and that of smallpox. Probably the three are variants of the one virus produced by adaptation to the various animal species. Buffalo pox virus is also closely related (6). Experimental infection of buffalo calves with buffalo pox virus causes larger lesions and a shorter course of the disease than when bovine pox virus is injected. There is also a cultural difference, but cross-protection tests show the two viruses to be antigenically identical (5).

Epidemiology

The clinical syndrome of cowpox occurs sporadically in most countries of the world but the incidence of true cowpox appears to have diminished to the point of being rare. (1). Most outbreaks of diseases manifested principally by teat lesions are outbreaks of the clinically similar pseudocowpox and bovine ulcerative mammillitis. In an affected herd most cows become infected unless there is immunity from previous attacks or suitable preventive measures are adopted. Losses result from inconvenience at milking time because of the soreness of the teats and from occasional cases of mastitis which develop when lesions involve teat sphincters. Milk from affected cows is suitable for human consumption.

Spread from cow to cow within a herd is effected by milkers' hands or teat cups. Spread from herd to herd is probably effected by the introduction of infected animals, by carriage on milkers' hands, and in the absence of either of the above methods, transport by biting insects is possible. In a herd in which the disease is enzootic only heifers and new introductions may develop lesions. The virus of horsepox can be transmitted to cattle and causes typical cowpox. Milkers recently vaccinated against smallpox may serve as a source of infection for cattle (2) although the smallpox vaccine virus, or vaccinia virus, is different from the cowpox virus (3).

It is generally assumed that the virus gains access to tissues through injuries to teat skin. Therefore extensive outbreaks of cowpox, and even pseudocowpox are likely to occur when there are circumstances conducive to teat injuries such as grazing in long millet and so on. Spread is rapid within a herd and immunity is solid so that the disease tends to occur in sharp outbreaks of several months' duration with subsequent immunity protecting the cattle for at least several years.

Pathogenesis

In true cowpox, the five stages of a typical pox eruption can be observed. After an incubation period of 3–6 days, a roseolar erythema is followed by firm, raised papules light in color but with a zone of hyperemia around the base. Vesiculation follows, a yellow blister with a pitted center being characteristic. The pustular stage, which develops soon afterwards, is followed by the development of a thick, red, tenacious scab.

In experimentally produced vaccinia virus mammillitis (produced by inoculation of smallpox vaccine) the lesions have three zones, a central brown crusty area of necrosis, surrounded by a gray-white zone of microvesicle formation, again surrounded by a red border due to congestion (3). The lesions are essentially hyperplastic.

Clinical findings

Typical lesions in both species may be seen at any stage of development, but are mostly observed during the scab stage, the vesicle commonly having been ruptured during milking. True cowpox scabs are 1–2 cm in diameter and are thick, tenacious and yellow-brown to red in color. In cows being milked, scab formation is uncommon, the scab being replaced by a deep ulceration.

Distribution of the lesions is usually confined to the teats and lower part of the udder. Soreness of the teats develops and milk letdown may be interfered with; the cow usually resents being milked. Secondary mastitis occurs in a few cases. Individual lesions heal quite quickly, within 2 weeks, but in some animals fresh crops of lesions may cause the disease to persist for a month or more. In severe cases lesions may spread to the insides of the thighs and rarely to the perineum, vulva and mouth. Sucking calves may develop lesions about the mouth. In bulls lesions usually appear on the scrotum.

Clinical pathology

Differentiation is possible by electron microscopy (2, 4). The virus is also generally capable of propagation in tissue culture (1).

Diagnosis

A number of skin diseases may be accompanied by lesions on the udder, but should not be confused with true cowpox. It is easy to do so especially if the lesions are advanced in age. The differential points are listed in Table 70. Cowpox is quite uncommon. Individual lesions are small and few, but severe. They are quite painful, but heal quickly in 2–3 weeks. Most of the outbreaks of disease of teat skin which clinically resemble classical cowpox are in fact almost always caused by vaccinia virus (*Poxvirus officinalis*) the laboratory virus used to vaccinate humans against smallpox. It is a laboratory-generated virus antigenically related to the cowpox virus, and infection usually arises from contact with a recently vaccinated person. Pseudocowpox lesions are larger, more numerous, less painful and more prolonged. Bovine ulcerative mammillitis is a much more severe disease and has characteristic plaques and ulceration of the skin of the teat. The differentiation of these diseases is not always easy on clinical grounds. It is not infrequent that two or all three of the diseases are present in the one herd. Udder impetigo begins as thin-walled pustules and the lesions are variable in size and occur only on the udder, usually at the base of the teat. It spreads in a manner similar to cowpox and is often mistaken for this disease by farmers. Staphylococci can usually be isolated from unbroken lesions. The relationship between udder impetigo and 'mammary pustular dermatitis' is obscure. The latter appears to be an infection with bovine herpesvirus DN599 which is usually associated with respiratory tract disease (7). A vesicular eruption may also occur on the udder in severe cases of foot-and-mouth disease, but always in conjunction with lesions on the buccal mucosa and coronet. Diffuse erythema and exfoliation with severe irritation may occur on the lateral aspects of the teats in photosensitized animals, but there are no discrete lesions. Mycotic dermatitis not infrequently affects the udder, although lesions are more usual on the dorsal aspect of the body. These are characteristic crusts usually with pus and a raw ulcerating surface beneath. The lesions in so-called 'black pox' are confined to the teats as crater-shaped ulcers with raised edges and a black spot in the pitted center. Most frequently the tip of the teat is involved and spread to the sphincter leads to the development of mastitis. Warts and chronic pseudocowpox have much in common, but lesions in various stages of development are usually present in the latter.

Treatment

Only palliative treatment is practicable. The application of a soft emollient cream before milking and an astringent lotion after milking facilitates recovery. Whitfield's ointment and 10% sulfathiazole ointment are also used. A similar ointment (5% sulfathiazole, 5% salicylic acid) is recommended for 'black pox'.

Control

Prevention of spread is difficult, since the virus responsible for the disease is readily transmitted by direct or indirect contact. Udder cloths, milking machines and hands should be disinfected after contact with infected animals. Dipping of the teats in an alcoholic tincture of a suitable disinfectant, such as quaternary ammonium compound, is usually satisfactory in preventing immediate spread. Control by vaccination has been attempted but is of dubious value (2). The most important factor limiting the value of all pox vaccinations is the lack of definition of many of the strains of the virus that have been isolated. Many of them overlap each other in their genetic composition and there is a significant amount of recombination between them (4).

Table 70. Differential diagnosis of diseases characterized by lesions of the teat skin only.

Disease	Epidemiology: Method of spread	Epidemiology: Course of disease	Lesions	Clinical pathology	Treatment and/or control
Cowpox (usually vaccinia) virus	Very rare. More commonly vaccinia from recently vaccinated people. Contact spread via teat injuries	2–4 weeks. In immune herd heifers only	Vesicle to pustule to scab (ulcers if cows milking) 1–2 cm diameter thick red brown scabs on teats and lower udder. Mastitis in few. Rarely to perineum, vulva mouth of calves. Scrotum of bull	Electron microscopy of swab from lesion. Tissue culture	Bland ointment for dry lesions. Astringent lotion for wet ones. Disinfection hands, cloths
Pseudocowpox	Very common. Morbidity 5–10% at one time, affects whole herd in time. Little immunity and recurs quickly. Spread by contact, hand, cloth, teat cups. On milker's hands as nodule	Relatively slow spread, long healing time, and cyclical recurrence in individual cows, disease lasts up to 18 months in herd	Erythema, vesicle, pustule scab in ring or horseshoe pattern. Usually three up to eight lesion complexes per teat. Elevated due to granulation tissue. 0·5–2·5 cm in diameter. Heal in 7–10 days. Rare—lesions in mouth	Electron microscopy of vesicle fluid. Tissue culture on teat skin culture. A poxvirus of orf group	As above, try to reduce teat abrasions
Bovine ulcerative mammillitis	Affects 20–100% (average 50%). Insect transmission into herd. Seasonal autumn. Unknown transmission mode within herd. Milking machine spread *plus* teat injury. Recurs in herd after 13 months	Self-limiting. Persists 6–14 weeks. Many cows culled because of bad ulcers and mastitis; subsequently heifers only affected—only milking cows affected	Teat swollen, painful, exudes serum, skin sloughs, leaving raw ulcer covering most of teat. Milder cases show smaller less severe lesions 0·5–2 cm in diameter. Mild lesions may be ring-like erythema around nodule or ulcer. Lesions heal 10 days to 2 months. Recently calved cows have very extensive sloughing lesions on udder. Rare cases lesions in mouth especially calves sucking cows	Tissue culture of herpes virus from *early* lesion. High antibody titer	Symptomatic. Iodophors or chlorhexidine teat dip
Udder impetigo	Spread during milking by contact. Pustules on milker's hands	Disappears quickly from each cow but recurs within 6 months and may persist in herd	Small 2–4 mm diameter pustules (may be large boils) at teat base, spread to teat and udder skin	Microbiological culture of swab of pus: *Staphylococcus aureus*. Tissue culture of herpesvirus DN599	Symptomatic, good teat dip (e.g.chlorhexidine) and teat cup disinfection. Autogenous killed vaccine effective
Black pox	Sporadic only. Thought due to poor milking machine technique	Intractable to treatment	Deep crater-shaped ulcer with black spot in center. At teat tip, involve sphincter. Mastitis commonly follows	Culture of *Staph. aureus*	Salicylic 5% ointment, iodophors teat dip and ointment. Check milking machine vacuum pressure and technique
Teat fibropapilloma	Contact at milking time via teat cups, hands etc. To abrasions of teat skin. May be 20% of herd affected	Disappear spontaneously 2–3 up to 5 months	Two forms; small white slightly elevated nodules 0.3 cm in diameter or elongated to tags 1 cm long removable by traction. Annoying only	—	Vaccine very little benefit—33% respond

REFERENCES

(1) Gibbs, E. P. J. et al. (1973) *Vet. Rec.*, *92*, 56.
(2) Gibbs, E. P. J. et al. (1970) *Vet. Rec.*, *87*, 602.
(3) Lauder, I. M. et al. (1971) *Vet. Rec.*, *89*, 571.
(4) Kitching, R. P. (1987) *Vet. Ann.*, *27*, 109.
(5) Tantawi, H. H. et al. (1979) *Bull. anim. Hlth Prod., Afr.*, *27*, 101.
(6) Iwad, F. I. et al. (1981) *Acta Vet. Yugo.*, *31*, 47.
(7) Reed, D. E. et al. (1977) *Am. J. vet. Res.*, *38*, 1631.

Pseudocowpox (milkers' nodule)

Pseudocowpox of cattle and 'milkers' nodule' of man are both caused by the same virus and are manifested by similar cutaneous lesions, on the teats in the former, on the hands in the latter.

Etiology

The causative agent of pseudocowpox in cattle and milkers' nodule in man is parapoxvirus with some similarity to the virus of infectious papular stomatitis and to that of contagious ecthyma (1–5). The virus can be propagated in tissue culture.

Epidemiology

Pseudocowpox has been a common disease of cattle for many years and has been reported from most countries. It is a relatively benign disease, most losses occurring as a result of difficulty in milking and an increase in the incidence of mastitis. In an affected herd the rate of spread is relatively slow and this, together with the prolonged healing time in individual cows, may result in the disease being present in the herd for up to a year. The morbidity rate approximates 100%, but at any given time varies between 5 and 10%, and occasionally up to 5% (1). The disease is transmissible to man, infection usually resulting in the development of milkers' nodule on the hand. Little immunity develops and the disease is likely to recur in the herd within a short time (6). In most countries it is benign and endemic and most herds experience a bad outbreak of it at one time or another.

Freshly calved and recently introduced cattle are most susceptible, but all adult cattle in a herd, including dry cows, are likely to be affected. The disease does not appear to occur in animals less than 2 years of age unless they have calved. However, the virus has been isolated from the mouth of a calf sucking an affected cow (7). It has also been isolated from the semen of two infertile bulls (8). There is no seasonal variation in incidence.

The methods of spread of the disease have not been defined, but physical transport by means of contaminated milkers' hands, wash cloths and teat cups is considered to be the logical route. The virus cannot penetrate mucosa, and a pre-existing discontinuity of it is necessary for the virus to gain entry. Transmission by biting insects seems likely.

Pathogenesis

The production of typical lesions by the introduction of the virus onto scarified areas of skin suggests that the lesions produced are the result of the local action of the virus. The lesions are characterized by hyperplasia of squamous epithelium.

Clinical findings

Acute and chronic lesions occur and there may be up to ten on one teat.

Acute lesions commence as erythema followed by the development of a vesicle or pustule which ruptures after about 48 hours resulting in the formation of a thick scab. Pain is moderate and present only in the prescab stage. The scab, varying in size from 0·5 to 2·5 cm in diameter, becomes markedly elevated by developing granulating tissue beneath it; 7–10 days after lesions appear the scabs drop off, leaving a horseshoe-shaped ring of small scabs surrounding a small, wart-like granuloma which may persist for months. The disease tends to disappear from a herd after 18–21 days but may recur cyclically about 1 month later (9). There are reports of lesions occurring occasionally in cows' mouths.

Chronic lesions also commence as erythema, but progress to a stage in which yellow-gray, soft, scurfy scabs develop. The scabs are readily rubbed off at milking leaving the skin corrugated and prone to chapping. There is no pain and the lesions may persist for months.

Milkers' nodules are clinically indistinguishable from human lesions caused by ecthyma virus. The lesions vary from multiple vesicles to a single, indurated nodule.

Clinical pathology and necropsy findings

Material for examination by tissue culture or electron microscopic examination, the latter being highly recommended as a diagnostic procedure (10), should include fluid from a vesicle. The virus is also capable of propagation in tissue culture of bovine teat skin (11).

Diagnosis

Differentiation of those diseases in which lesions of the teat are prominent is dealt with in the section on cowpox (p. 951)

Treatment

Locally applied ointments of various kinds appear to have little effect on the lesions. The recommended treatment includes the removal of the scabs, which should be burned to avoid contaminating the environment, application of an astringent preparation, such as triple dye, after milking and an emollient ointment just before milking.

Control

Recommended measures such as treatment and isolation of affected cows, or milking them last, the use of disposable paper towels for udder washing and disinfection of teat cups appear to have little effect on the spread of the disease. An iodophor teat dip is recommended as the most effective control measure (12). An effort should be made to reduce teat trauma because infection is facilitated by discontinuity of the skin.

REVIEW LITERATURE

Gibbs, E. P. J. (1984) Viral diseases of the skin of the bovine teat and udder, *Vet. Clin. N. Am. large Anim. Pract.*, *6 (1)*, 187–202.
Tripathy, D. N. et al. (1981) Poxvirus of veterinary importance. In: *Comparative Diagnosis of Viral Diseases*, vol. 3. New York: Academic Press.

REFERENCES

(1) Nagington, J. et al. (1967) *Vet. Rec.*, *81*, 306.
(2) Lauder, I. M. et al. (1966) *Vet. Rec.*, *78*, 926.
(3) Friedman-Kein, A. E. et al. (1963) *Science, NY*, *140*, 1335.
(4) Liebermann, H. et al. (1967) *Arch. exp. VetMed.*, *21*, 625.
(5) Huck, R. A. (1966) *Vet. Rec.*, *78*, 503.
(6) Gibbs, E. P. J. & Osborne, A. D. (1974) *Br. vet. J.*, *130*, 150.
(7) Moscovici, C. et al. (1963) *Science, NY*, *141*, 915.
(8) Johnston, W. S. (1971) *Vet. Rec.*, *89*, 450.
(9) Cheville, N. F. & Shey, D. J. (1967) *J. Am. vet. med. Assoc.*, *150*, 855.
(10) Gibbs, E. P. J. et al. (1970) *Vet. Rec.*, *87*, 602.
(11) James, Z. H. & Povey, R. C. (1973) *Res. vet. Sci.*, *15*, 40.
(12) Puddle, B. M. et al. (1986) *NZ vet. J.*, *34*, 16.

Bovine ulcerative mammillitis

Bovine ulcerative mammillitis is a viral disease manifested by severe ulceration of the skin of the teats and udder.

Etiology

The causative virus, bovine herpesvirus 2 (BVH2), is an alphaherpesvirus and is identical with the Allerton virus of lumpy skin disease, and with dermatotrophic bovine herpesvirus (9). The difference in clinical manifestations between the two diseases may be due to the strain of the virus, or the method of infection. The virus has been maintained in tissue culture and transmitted to rabbits and guinea-pigs, and to day-old rats, mice and Chinese hamsters. Sheep and pigs show mild reactions and man, mice and rats appear to be refractory. The virus has no apparent relationship to other herpesviruses—infectious bovine rhinotracheitis or feline viral rhinotracheitis viruses. However, a second herpesvirus (DN599 strain) which is usually associated with respiratory disease in cattle is also capable of causing mammary pustular dermatitis (14).

Epidemiology

Cowpox and pseudocowpox have been recognized diseases of cattle for many years. The description, for the first time, of bovine ulcerative mammillitis (2) may record the appearance of a new disease or the identification of one which has been present in the cattle population for some time. The morbidity rate varies between 18 and 96% (average 50%) and, although the mortality rate is negligible, losses due to the disease may be severe. Forms of loss include a much higher incidence of mastitis, reduction in milk in affected herds by up to 20%, the culling of some cows because of severe mastitis and intractable ulcers, and a great deal of interference with normal milking procedure.

The disease is self-limiting, persisting in a herd for 6–15 weeks, the severity of the lesions decreasing as the outbreak progresses. An incidence of 19% of serologically positive cattle has been observed in the United Kingdom. The disease has also been identified in Australia, where extensive outbreaks have occurred, and the United States. Only cows in milk appear to be affected, heifers more severely than adult cows. Whether appreciable immunity occurs after natural infection has not been determined, but the disease has recurred in herds 13 months after an initial attack. Herds infected for the first time have a high morbidity rate. Subsequently the incidence is low and is limited to fresh heifers. A suggested nomenclature is that herds with more than 30% affected are classified as susceptible, herds with less than 30% of cases are partially immune, and herds where only the heifers are affected are immune (5). A high seasonal incidence in autumn and early winter has been noted in the United Kingdom. There is no obvious explanation for it (4).

Introduction of bovine ulcerative mammillitis into a herd may occur with the introduction of infected animals, but outbreaks have been observed in self-contained herds and because of the seasonal incidence in autumn, insect transmission suggests itself; a careful examination of a good deal of epidemiological data in the United Kingdom points to insect transmission as the method of spread between herds. Spread within the herd can occur in the same way but the standard picture of high morbidity and rapid spread suggests a more assured vector such as physical contact. For example, calves sucking infected dams often develop mouth lesions. But the milking machine appears to be an unlikely vehicle, because the virus must be deposited in the deep layers of the skin, and even rubbing it into pseudocowpox lesions is not an efficient way of transmitting the disease (7). Nevertheless, milking machine liners, and hands and udder cloths, may act as carriers of virus when a large amount of it is being released (8). It would require another mechanism to deposit the virus in the wall of the teat. Survival of the virus for long periods within the host is known and it is thought that this may be the means of survival of the virus within a herd which has become immune (1).

Pathogenesis

Typical clinical lesions and histopathological changes can be produced locally by introduction of the virus into scarifications of the skin of the teat and the oral mucosa and by intradermal and intravenous injection (10). In contrast to the poxes, the characteristic lesion in mammillitis is destructive. The higher incidence of the disease and the greater severity of the lesions close to calving are thought to be due to the immunosuppression caused by parturition (4).

Clinical findings

In this disease there is an incubation period of 5–10 days. There is no systemic illness and lesions are confined to the teats and udder. When the disease occurs in a herd for the first time the first case is usually in a cow which has calved during the previous 2–3 days (4). Rapid lateral spread then occurs to other cows.

In cows calved for more than a few weeks the characteristic lesions are almost entirely confined to the skin of the teats; in recently calved cows they are restricted to the skin of the udder. The severity of the disease in recently calved cows appears to be directly proportional to the degree of postparturient edema which is present. Vesication occurs, commencing at the base of the teat and spreading over much of the udder surface, but rupture and confluence of the vesicles leads to weeping and extensive sloughing of the skin.

The severity of lesions on the teats on longer-calved cows varies, but in all cases the lesions are sufficiently painful to make milking difficult. In the most severe cases the entire teat is swollen and painful, the skin is bluish in color, exudes serum and sloughs leaving a raw ulcer covering most of the teat. In less severe cases there are raised deep red to blue, circular plaques, 0·5–2 cm in diameter, which develop shallow ulcers. In most cases scab formation follows but machine milking causes frequent disruption of them, resulting in frequent bleeding. The least severe lesions are in the form of lines of erythema, often in circles and enclosing dry skin or slightly elevated papules, which occasionally show ulceration. Mild lesions tend to heal in about 10 days but severe ulcers may persist for 2 or 3 months.

Vesicles occur but are not commonly seen. They are characteristically thin-walled, 1–2 cm in diameter, variable in outline and easily ruptured during milking. Ulcers in the mouth of affected cows have been observed rarely and calves sucking affected cows develop lesions on their oral mucosae and muzzles (5). Ulcerative lesions on the vaginal mucosa have been recorded in one experimentally produced case (11). During the recovery phase there is obvious scar formation and depigmentation. Lesions on the skin of the udder are similar to those on the teats but are usually less severe and heal more rapidly because of the absence of trauma.

The disease identified as 'general infection of cattle with bovine herpesvirus 2' (6) is discussed under the heading of lumpy skin disease (p. 950).

Clinical pathology and necropsy findings

Material for tissue culture or cutaneous transmission tests is best obtained by syringe from early vesicles. Swabs from early ulcers or oral lesions may also be used. Recovered animals show a high titer of antibodies which persist for at least 2 years (1). The virus is cultivable in bovine kidney cell cultures but may be difficult to find if the lesions are as old as 7 days, and if there has been intensive application of teat disinfectants such as iodophors (8). No necropsy reports of cases of bovine ulcerative mammillitis are available.

Diagnosis

Differentiation of other diseases of the skin of the teat and udder is dealt with in the section on cowpox (p. 951).

Treatment

There is no specific treatment and the aim should be to develop scabs which can withstand machine milking. This is most easily effected by the application of a water-miscible antiseptic ointment just before putting the cups on, followed by an astringent lotion, such as triple dye, immediately after milking. Crystal violet dyes have an excellent reputation as treatment.

Control

Isolation of affected animals and strict hygiene in the milking parlor are practiced but have little effect on the spread of the disease. An iodophor disinfectant is recommended for use in the dairy to prevent spread (12). Inoculation of the natural virus away from the teats produces a local lesion and good immunity, and the method has been tested as a control procedure (13). A cell culture virus vaccine with different adjuvants is reported to be effective against experimental challenge (3).

REVIEW LITERATURE

Gibbs, E. P. J. & Rweyemamu, M. M. (1977) Bovine herpesvirus 2 & 3. *Vet. Bull.*, *47*, 411.

Martin, W. B. (1973) Bovine mammillitis: epizootiologic and immunologic features. *J. Am. vet. med. Assoc.*, *163*, 915.

REFERENCES

(1) Martin, W. B. & Scott, F. M. M. (1979) *Arch. Virol.*, *60*, 51.
(2) Martin, W. B. et al. (1970) *Vet. Rec.*, *86*, 661.
(3) Dilovski, M. et al. (1977) *VetMed Nauki*, *14*, 68.
(4) Martin, W. B. et al. (1976) *Proc. 20th World Vet. Cong.*, *2*, 1307.
(5) Gibbs, E. P. J. & Collings, D. F. (1972) *Vet. Rec.*, *90*, 66.
(6) St George, T. D. et al. (1980) *Aust. vet. J.*, *56*, 47.
(7) Gibbs, E. P. J. et al. (1973) *Res. vet. Sci.*, *14*, 139, 145.
(8) Turner, A. J. et al. (1976) *Aust. vet. J.*, *52*, 166, 170.
(9) Gigstad, D. C. & Stone, S. S. (1977) *Am. J. vet. Res.*, *38*, 753.
(10) Martin, W. B. et al. (1969) *Am. J. vet. Res.*, *30*, 2151.
(11) Povey, R. C. & James, Z. H. (1973) *Vet. Rec.*, *92*, 231.
(12) Martin, W. B. & Jaines, Z. H. (1969) *Vet. Rec.*, *85*, 100.
(13) Rweyemamu, M. M. & Johnson, R. H. (1969) *J. comp. Pathol.*, *79*, 419.
(14) Reed, D. E. et al. (1977) *Am. J. Vet. Res.*, *38*, 1631.

Sheeppox and goatpox

In sheeppox, typical pox lesions occur particularly under the tail. A malignant form with a general distribution of lesions occurs in lambs.

Etiology

The causative capripoxvirus (family Poxviridae) affects only sheep, and animals of all ages are susceptible. A highly contagious pox occurs also in goats and is also caused by a capripox virus which is antigenically distinct from sheeppox virus (1), although it is transmissible experimentally and naturally to both goats and sheep (1). Both the sheeppox and goatpox viruses are classified as capripoxvirus. A third virus, identified in Kenya (2), is not species-specific as the goatpox and sheeppox viruses are.

Epidemiology

Sheeppox is restricted in its distribution to the Middle East countries, south-eastern Europe, Scandinavia, North Africa, China, India and Russia. It is the most serious of all the pox diseases in animals, often causing death in 50% of affected animals. Major losses may occur in each new crop of lambs.

Goatpox in sheep is more severe than sheeppox, and lesions occur on the lips and oral mucosa, the teats and udder. The goatpox virus affords solid protection in sheep against both goatpox and sheeppoxes but sheeppox vaccine does not protect goats against goatpox. The goatpox virus can be propagated in the developing hen's egg and egg-adapted virus can be used as a prophylactic. In areas where sheeppox is enzootic imported breeds may show greater susceptibility than the native stock. The virus has been cultivated on chick embryos and in tissue culture.

Sheeppox is highly contagious and, although in most cases spread appears to occur by contact with infected animals and contaminated articles, spread by inhalation also occurs. Capripox has been shown to spread via *Stomoxys calcitrans* (11).

Pathogenesis

After an incubation period of 7–8 days a viremia occurs with virus being lodged in most tissues including the skin. The development of typical pox lesions, as in vaccinia, is characteristic of the disease. Because of the close relationship between sheeppox and lumpy skin disease virus, a close study of the pathogenesis of sheeppox lesions has been made (5). The virus is present in greatest quantities between the 7th and 14th day after inoculation.

Clinical findings

There is an incubation period of 2–14 days. In lambs, the malignant form is the more common type. There is marked depression and prostration, a high fever and discharges from the eyes and nose. Affected lambs may die during this stage before typical pox lesions develop. They commence as papules, then become nodular, vesicular, pustular and finally scabs. Some of them progress from nodules to tumor-like masses (12). Skin lesions reappear on unwoolled skin and on the buccal, respiratory, digestive and urogenital tract mucosae. The mortality rate in this type may reach 50%. In the benign form, which is the common one in adults, only skin lesions occur, particularly under the tail, and there is no systemic reaction. The mortality rate is low, usually about 5%. In ewes severe losses may occur if the udder is invaded because of the secondary occurrence of acute mastitis. In some outbreaks adult sheep are affected with the more severe form of the disease (9).

The clinical disease in goats is very similar to that of sheeppox in sheep. A morbidity of 90% and mortality of 4% occur in susceptible goat flocks. Young kids suffer a systemic disease with lesions spread generally over the skin, and on the respiratory and alimentary mucosae. In adult goats the disease is mild and lesions are occasional only (4).

Clinical pathology

Direct fluorescent antibody test is used to detect the presence of pox virus in the edema fluid. The virus can be cultured in tissue culture. Serological testing, using an indirect fluorescent antibody test (FAT) will determine the antibody status of a flock (10).

Necropsy findings

In the malignant form pox lesions extend into the mouth, pharynx, larynx and vagina. Lesions may also appear in the trachea with an accompanying catarrhal pneumonia. Lesions occasionally reach the abomasum and are accompanied by a hemorrhagic enteritis.

Diagnosis

The disease occurs in enzootic areas and the lesions are characteristic of a pox disease. Confusion with bluetongue and contagious ecthyma may occur, but differentiation on the basis of clinical signs and lesions is ordinarily not difficult. An immunodiffusion technique for the identification of the sheeppox and goatpox viruses has been described (6). Attention has been drawn to the ease with which lesions of bovine skin can be diagnosed by electron microscopy (7). Characteristic 'sheeppox cell' containing inclusion bodies are present in large numbers in the skin (5).

Treatment

No specific treatment is advised, but palliative treatment may be necessary in severely affected animals.

Control

Control in free countries necessitates prohibition of importation from infected areas, and if the infection is introduced, the destruction of affected flocks and the quarantine of infected premises should be instituted. Vaccination with natural lymph is still practiced in affected areas but is capable of spreading the disease. A large variety of commercial vaccines is now available. Some are favored in one country, others in another, and there is no easy basis for comparison. Most of them, including killed vaccines with adjuvants, or living attenuated vaccines, appear to give excellent protection for periods greater than 1 year (3, 8, 9). Vaccination in the face of outbreak is unlikely to prevent deaths during the subsequent 2 weeks.

REVIEW LITERATURE

Singh, I. P. & Srivastava, R. N. (1979) Sheeppox. A review. *Vet. Bull.*, *49*, 145.

REFERENCES

(1) Kitching, R. P. & Taylor, W. P. (1985) *Res. vet. Sci.*, *39*, 196.
(2) Davies, F. G. (1976) *J. Hyg., Camb.*, *76*, 163.
(3) Kitching, R. P. et al. (1987) *Res. vet. Sci.*, *42*, 53.
(4) Tantawi, H. H. et al. (1979) *Trop. Anim. Hlth Prod.*, *11*, 208.
(5) Murray, M. et al. (1973) *Res. vet. Sci.*, *15*, 201.
(6) Bhambani, B. D. & Krishnamurty, D. (1963) *J. comp. Pathol.*, *73*, 349.
(7) Gibbs, E. P. J. et al. (1970) *J. comp. Pathol.*, *80*, 455.
(8) El-Zein, A. et al. (1983) *Zentralbl. VetMed.*, *30*, 341.
(9) Solyom, F. et al. (1980) *Acta vet. Acad. Sci. Hung*, *28*, 389.
(10) Sarkar, P. et al. (1980) *Ind. J. anim. Sci.*, *50*, 428.
(11) Kitching, R. P. & Mellor, P. S. (1986) *Res. vet. Sci.*, *40*, 255.
(12) Afshar, A. et al. (1986) *Can. vet. J.*, *27*, 301.

Camelpox

A specific orthopoxvirus capable of transmission only to camels and rabbits, appears to be the cause of pox in camels. Sheeppox and vaccinia viruses are non-pathogenic for camels. There seem to be several distinct antigenic strains of camelpox virus (1, 2). The disease attacks young camels and has an incubation period of 3–15 days. The typically pox lesions are confined to the hairless parts of the body, and the disease runs a benign course of 2–3 weeks for the most part, but the case fatality rate may be as high as 5·4% in young camels (3). It does not appear to be pathogenic for humans (4). Dromedaries are also susceptible to infection with the contagious ecthyma virus and differentiation between camelpox and ecthyma requires serological and virological examination.

REFERENCES

(1) Tantawi, K. H. (1974) *Acta virol.*, *18*, 347.
(2) Mahnel, H. & Bartenbach, G. (1973) *Zentralbl. VetMed.*, *20B*, 572.

(3) Kriz, R. (1982) *J. comp. Pathol.*, *92*, 1.
(4) Jezek, Z. et al. (1983) *J. Hyg. Microbiol. Immunol.*, *27*, 29.

Swinepox

Swinepox is usually a benign disease characterized by the appearance of typical pox lesions on the ventral abdomen.

Etiology
The primary cause is a swinepox virus, the suipoxvirus of the family Poxviridae.

Epidemiology
Swinepox occurs in most countries where swine are raised and, although the incidence in individual herds may be high, the disease is not usually widespread through an area. In some outbreaks the mortality rate in young sucking pigs may be heavy, but older animals seem to suffer little ill effect. An important feature of the disease is that its presence may increase the hazard of breaks occurring after hog cholera vaccination.

Solid immunity appears to persist after infection with either virus. The disease may occur only in pigs brought into a herd in which the indigenous pigs are immune carriers and will spread the virus to the new animals (5). Swinepox virus has been cultured in tissue culture (1, 2).

Outbreaks usually accompany infestation with the pig louse (*Hematopinus suis*) and transmission is usually effected by bites of this louse (3), although there is some evidence that flies and other insects may also act as transmitting agents. Young sucking pigs may have lesions on the face with similar lesions on the udder of the sow, and spread by direct contact may occur in these circumstances. A pustular dermatitis associated with a poxvirus has been reported in a stillborn pig which suggests that intrauterine infection is possible (6).

Pathogenesis
In field cases, the lesions do not proceed past the vesicle stage as a rule. Rupture of the vesicles and the formation of scabs which heal and drop off are the final stages.

Clinical findings
Small 1 cm diameter papules develop first and may pass through the vesicular stage very quickly with the formation of red-brown, round scabs. In neonatal pigs the rupture of many vesicles at one time may cause wetting and scab formation over the cheeks, and conjunctivitis and keratitis are present in many affected animals (4). In most cases the lesions are restricted to the belly and inside the upper limbs, but may involve the back and sides and sometimes spread to the face. A slight febrile reaction may occur in the early stages in young animals and in sucking pigs some deaths are observed.

Diagnosis
The distribution of the pox-like lesions and the association of the disease with louse infestations suggest the diagnosis. Lesions caused by *Tyroglyphid* spp. mites are usually larger and occur anywhere on the body, and like those of sarcoptic mange, are usually accompanied by itching. The causative mites are detectable in skin scrapings. Ringworm and pityriasis rosea have characteristic lesions which do not itch and fungal spores are present in scrapings in the former disease.

Treatment
No specific treatment is available and lesions cause so little concern to the pig, and heal so rapidly, that none is attempted.

Control
Vaccination is not usually practiced and control of the pig lice is the principal prophylactic measure attempted in most outbreaks (3).

REFERENCES

(1) Kasza, L. & Griesemer, R. A. (1962) *Am. J. vet. Res.*, *23*, 443.
(2) Datt, N. S. (1964) *J. comp. Pathol.*, *74*, 62, 70.
(3) Schang, P. J. (1952) *Rep. 14th int. vet. Congr.*, *2*, 421.
(4) Doman, I. (1962) *Magy. Allatorv. Lap.*, *17*, 121, 365.
(5) Olufemi, B. E. et al. (1981) *Vet. Rec.*, *109*, 278.
(6) Neufeld, J. L. (1981) *Can. vet. J.*, *22*, 156.

Horsepox

Horsepox is a benign disease characterized by the development of typical pox lesions either on the limbs or on the lips and buccal mucosa.

Etiology
The causative ungulate poxvirus is identical antigenically with the virus of true cowpox and is transferable to cattle and to man.

Epidemiology
Horsepox occurs only in Europe and appears to be quite rare. In general it is a benign disease, but badly affected horses become debilitated and occasionally young animals may die.

Immunity after an attack is solid. Horsepox may be spread by contact with infected grooming tools, harness and by handling.

Clinical findings
Typical pox lesions develop either on the back of the pastern, the so-called 'leg form', or in the mouth, the 'buccal form'. In the 'leg form' nodules, vesicles, pustules and scabs develop in that order on the back of the pastern and cause pain and lameness. There may be a slight systemic reaction with elevation of temperature. In the 'buccal' form similar lesions appear first on the insides of the lips and spread over the entire buccal mucosa, sometimes to the pharynx and larynx and occasionally into the nostrils. In very severe cases lesions may appear on the conjunctiva, the vulva and sometimes over the entire body. The buccal lesions cause a painful stomatitis with salivation and anorexia as prominent signs. Most cases recover with lesions healing in 2–4 weeks.

Diagnosis
The leg form may be confused with greasy heel, but no nodules, vesicles or pustules occur in the latter disease. Vesicular stomatitis occurs in horses but the lesions are much larger, rupture very readily and do not go through the typical stages of a pox lesion. Differentiation from viral papular dermatitis, which is insect-borne, and a

Table 71. Differential diagnosis of diseases of horses characterized by discrete lesions of the skin only.

Disease	*Epidemiology*		*Lesions*	*Clinical pathology*	*Treatment and/or control*
	Method of spread	*Behavior in herd*			
Horsepox	Rare, benign. Spread by contact, rugs, grooming tools	Solid immunity after attack. No recurrence. Lesions heal 2–4 weeks	Typical pox lesions. 'Buccal' form, lesions in mouth. 'Leg' form lesions behind pasterns. Rare cases have lesions in mouth, nostrils, vulva	Electron microscopy of swab from lesion—ungulate poxvirus present	Rigid isolation, hygiene. Treat symptomatically
Vesicular stomatitis	Occurs horses, cattle, pigs. Insect spread, geographical and climatic distribution. Within herd spread, likely by contact	Lesions last only 3–4 days. Solid immunity for 6 months	Often only on tongue and lips. Uncommon on udder or prepuce. Vesicles up to 2 cm diameter rupture leaving raw area, profuse ropey saliva. Heal quickly	Tissue culture on hen eggs. Transmission to laboratory animals. CF and virus neutralization tests available	Nil
Viral papular dermatitis	Insect vector. May affect many horses at one time. Local horses immune. Summer and autumn	Recovered in 10 days. Rare cases 6 weeks. Benign—disappears without trace	Cutaneous papules (no pustules or vesicles) 0·5–2 cm in diameter, develop dry crust at 7–10 days, falls off, leaving spot of alopecia and generalized over body. Mild fever at beginning	Virus in lesions culturable in eggs	Nil
Staphylococcal dermatitis	Sporadic. Lesions under harness suggest pressure or spread by contact. A common disease	No information, does not spread much. But very difficult to cure in individual	Small (up to 5 mm diameter) nodules then pustules, slough taking small scab and hair. Very painful to touch. Horse will not work under harness	*Staphylococcus aureus* culturable from swab of lesion	10-day course of penicillin or ampicillin. Results poor. Autogenous bacterin effective
Deep ringworm	Diffuse ringworm more common. Spread easily by direct contact or harness or tools	Sporadic usually. Difficult to cure	Follicular nodule, hair lost over top leaving 3 mm diameter bald patch. No extensive lesions. Sore to touch, itchy. Over axilla first, spreads	*Trichophyton* or *Microsporum* spp. on swab	Systemic fungistatic required: sodium iodide or griseofulvin
Canadian horsepox	Rare. Contact with grooming kit	Lesions heal 1 week, but successive crops for about 4 weeks	In groups under harness. Painful to touch. Papules to pustules 1–2·5 cm in diameter. Greenish pus	*Corynebacterium pseudotuberculosis* in smear and culture	Parenteral penicillin or sulfonamide
Demodectic mange	Spread via grooming tools and rugs. Rare	Slow spread	Lesions around face and eyes initially	*Demodex* spp. in scraping	Systemic and local organophosphate (O/P) insecticide

pox-like disease of horses recorded in Africa (1), is necessary. Other similar diseases are Uasin gishu skin disease which is a poxvirus infection characterized by verrucous papillomatous lesions (2) in Kenyan horses, and molluscum contagiosum, characterized by a large number of 2–3 mm diameter papules with a smooth pale surface on the prepuce and muzzle. The histopathological findings include typical molluscum bodies in the skin sections (3). Uasin gishu has a poxvirus associated with it, and both diseases have a pathology similar to that of human molluscum contagiosum. The diseases are set out in tabular form in Tables 71, 72 and 73.

Treatment

Local astringent treatment, as in the other forms of pox, may facilitate healing.

Control

Because of the contagious nature of the disease rigid isolation and hygiene in the handling of infected horses is essential.

REFERENCES

(1) Kaminjolo, J. S. et al. (1974) *Zentralbl. VetMed.*, *21B*, 592.
(2) Kaminjolo, J. S. et al. (1983) *Bull Anim. Hlth Prod. Afr.*, *31*, 17.
(3) Rahaley, R. S. & Mueller, R. E. (1983) *Vet. Pathol.*, *20* 274.

Table 72. Differential diagnosis of diseases of horses characterized by diffuse lesions of the skin only.

Disease	Epidemiology: Method of spread	Epidemiology: Behavior in herd	Lesions	Clinical pathology	Treatment and/or control
Mycotic dermatitis	Wet humid weather predisposes. Mud leads to foot lesions. Biting flies may spread other forms	May be number affected if weather conditions suitable	Commence on head at muzzle, around eyes, may be lacrimation and mucopurulent nasal discharge. May also be on lower legs—or all over. Not itchy, may be sore. Matted hair and scab can be lifted off an ovoid, slightly bleeding area	Branching filamentous *Dermatophilus congolensis* on smear of lesion	Penicillin–streptomycin systemically for 2–3 days. Chloramphenicol 2–5% solution topically
Tyroglyphosis	When horses fed on recently harvested infested grain. Autumn. Also at pasture	Transient self-limiting disease	On muzzle and face. Lower limbs at flexures. Dermatitis, itchy, scaly with rubbing get alopecia and scab formation	Larvae of chigger mites *Pediculoides* and *Trombicula* spp. in scraping	Topical parasiticide
Photosensitization	Rare in horses. Feeding on St John's wort or liver damage producing plants or cholangitis	Occurs only in sunlight. Disappears on removal from damaging feed and sun	Extensive edema, weeping dermatitis or skin sloughing on white parts. May also be signs of hepatic insufficiency	Nil	Remove from sun and change pasture. Treat cholangiohepatitis
Queensland itch	Sporadic. During insect season. Only in horses outdoors	Only hypersensitive horses affected. Disease persists as long as insects present	Intense itching interferes with work and grazing. Lesions at tail butt, along back, withers,crest, poll, ears. Down sides. Discrete papules, hair rubs off. Pachydermia, no weeping	Hypersensitivity indicated by eosinophilia in skin biopsy	Keep insects away. Topical and systemic antihistamines
Ringworm	Ready transmission by contact and with equipment and premises. Most serious in winter	Chance of spontaneous recovery in about 3 months in individual. Spread in herd can be very rapid	Thick crusts of dry crumbly scab, 2–3 cm in diameter, or diffuse alopecia with scaliness of skin. Lesions begin at girth or under head stall	*Trichophyton* and *Microsporum* spp. on scraping. Send to laboratory dry in envelope	Fungistatic topically. Rigid isolation of affected horse and equipment

Note: See also cutaneous globidiosis, multiple abscess caused by *Cor. pseudotuberculosis*, anhidrosis, congenital absence of skin.

Ulcerative dermatosis of sheep

Ulcerative dermatosis of sheep is an infectious disease characterized by the destruction of epidermal and subcutaneous tisssues, the development of raw, granulating ulcers on the skin of the lips, nares, feet, legs and external genital organs. The lesions on the lips occur between the lip and the nostril, those on the feet occur in the interdigital space and above the coronet, and the genital lesions occur on the glans and the external opening of the prepuce of rams and the vulva of ewes.

A virus, very similar but antigenically different to the ecthyma virus, is the cause of the disease (1, 2) which is likely to be confused with contagious ecthyma. However, the lesions are ulcerative and destructive rather than proliferative as in ecthyma. It is not highly infectious like bluetongue or sheeppox and the 'lip-and-leg' distribution of the lesions differentiates it from balanoposthitis of wethers, strawberry footrot, footrot and interdigital abscess. The presence of lesions on the glans penis and their absence from mucosae, the typical ulcerative form of the lesion, the absence of pus and the susceptibility of recovered animals to infection with ecthyma virus are diagnostic features of ulcerative dermatosis.

A morbidity rate of 15–20% is usual, but up to 60% of a flock may be affected. Mortality is low if the sheep are in good condition and the lesions are treated. Physical contact at breeding time seems to be the most probable method of spread.

REFERENCES

(1) Tunnicliffe, E. A. (1949) *Am. J. vet. Res.*, *10*, 240.
(2) Trueblood, M. S. (1966) *Cornell Vet.*, *56*, 521.

Table 73. Differential diagnosis of diseases of horses characterized by lesions of the skin of the lower limbs only.

	Epidemiology				
Disease	*Method of spread*	*Behavior in herd*	*Lesions*	*Clinical pathology*	*Treatment and/or control*
Glanders	Contact with infected horses. Ingestion from contaminated environment	This is chronic form. Other cases of classical glanders with pulmonary and nasal mucosal involvement	Nasal lesions include nodules and ulcers on nasal mucosa, purulent discharge. Stellate scars on septum. Limb lesions mostly at hock (medial aspect): nodules 1–2 cm, discharge honey-like pus	Mallein test. Complement fixation tests on serum. Transmission to guinea-pigs. *Actinobacillus mallei* in smears	Sulfadiazine or potentiated sulfonamide
Epizootic lymphangitis (equine blastomycosis)	Occurs in outbreaks. Spread by spores on contaminated bedding. May survive in soil. Entry through skin abrasions	Great inconvenience. Horses cannot be worked. Common in large groups, e.g. military horses	Mostly at hocks. Chiefly ulcers, lymph nodes swell and rupture. Lymphangitis. All sites have thick creamy pus. Some cases generalized with pulmonary abscesses	*Histoplasma farciminosum* in smears of pus	Iodides parenterally
Sporotrichosis	Slow spread, mainly sporadic cases. Spread by contact and contamination of environment	Lesions heal 3–4 weeks but new crops keep disease going	Nodules around fetlocks. Lymphangitis in some animals but not marked. Nodules ulcerate then heal. Painless	*Sporotrichum schenkii* on smear	Systemic and local iodide
Swamp cancer	Sporadic. Infection or invasion of wound	Does not spread	On lower limbs, or ventral abdomen, or below medial canthus of eye, lips. Papules to large plaques 1 cm thick, hard connective tissue with deep ulcerated center up to 20 cm in diameter. May have inspissated pus in pockets	Biopsy and scrapings for hyphae of *Hyphomyces destruens*, larvae of *Habronema megastoma*, hyphae of *Entomophthora coronata*	Systemic organophosphates for *Habronema*. Iodide for fungi
Greasy heel	Currently thought to be virus infection. Sporadic cases only. Horses standing in manure and urine	Not contagious. But can be chronic and incapacitating	Horizontal cracks and fissures behind pastern, very lame, carries leg. Soon see break out of sebaceous exudate. May develop secondary cellulitis	Nil	Wash with warm water and detergent. Dry. Apply white lotion frequently
Ulcerative lymphangitis	Infection of skin wounds in dirty stable	Lesions heal 1–2 weeks. New lesions develop for up to 12 months	Lesions around pastern. Swelling, pain, lame, nodules rupture, creamy green pus. Lymphangitis with ulcers but not usually lymph node involvement	*Corynebacterium pseudotuberculosis* in pus. In foals may be *Str. zooepidemicus*	Long course penicillin or sulfonamides
Chorioptic mange	Widespread. Mostly draft and other working horses	Most horses in group affected	Violent stamping, rubs back of pasterns, swollen, scabby, cracked, greasy, painful to touch	Scrapings reveal mites *Chorioptes equi*	Clip and treat as for greasy heel. Add topical insecticide

Note: See also Canadian horsepox, and horsepox (Table 71).

CHLAMYDIAL DISEASES CHARACTERIZED BY MUSCULOSKELETAL LESIONS

Polyarthritis

A virulent chlamydia has been isolated from the joints of calves (1, 2), sheep (3, 4) and a foal (5) clinically affected by polyarthritis. The disease has also been produced experimentally and is characterized in calves by a chlamydemia with subsequent localization in joints (6). In calves the disease has a high mortality; in lambs there is a high morbidity but deaths are few. The causative agent in calves is related to the chlamydia which causes sporadic bovine encephalomyelitis in that species. All diseases of animals caused by chlamydia are thought to be infections with *Chlamydia psittaci*.

In lambs it is one of the commonest, non-fatal diseases in feedlots in the United States, but also occurs in unweaned lambs at pasture (7). The morbidity rate in affected flocks ranges up to 80% (8) but deaths are usually restricted to less than 1%.

In lambs the clinical signs include stiffness, lameness, unwillingness to move, recumbency, depression, fever of 39–42°C (102–108°F) and conjunctivitis. The clinical disease in calves is similar to that in lambs. The joints are often grossly swollen and the navel is unaffected. There may be clinical signs relating to lesions which occur in other tissues, e.g. pneumonia, encephalomyelitis and interstitial focal nephritis (2). Focal pneumonitis is a common lesion in lambs (9). Laboratory diagnosis is by complement fixation test and culture on chicken egg embryos. The disease is likely to be confused with polyarthritis caused by *Hemophilus* and *Mycoplasma* spp. Early treatment with tylosin and penicillin is recommended. In the newborn foal mentioned above there was severe polyarthritis, fever, leukocytosis, and conjunctivitis (5).

REVIEW LITERATURE

Shewen, P. E. (1980) Chlamydial infection in animals. A review. *Can. vet. J.*, *21*, 2.

REFERENCES

(1) Storz, J. et al. (1966) *Am. J. vet. Res.*, *27*, 633, 987.
(2) Kolbl, O. & Psota, A. (1968) *Wien. Tierärztl. Monatschr.*, *55*, 443.
(3) Mendlowski, B. & Segre, D. (1960) *Am. J. vet. Res.*, *21*, 68, 74.
(4) Tammemagi, L. & Simmons, G. C. (1968) *Aust. vet. J.*, *44*, 585.
(5) McChesney, A. E. et al. (1974) *Am. vet. med. Assoc.*, *165*, 259.
(6) Eugster, A. K. & Storz, J. (1971) *J. infect. Dis.*, *123*, 41.
(7) Pierson, R. E. (1967) *J. Am. vet. med. Assoc.*, *150*, 1487.
(8) Cutlip, R. C. et al. (1972) *J. Am. vet. med. Assoc.*, *161*, 1213.
(9) Page, L. A. & Cutlip, R. C. (1968) *Iowa Vet.*, *39*, 10, 14.

23

Diseases Caused by Rickettsia

Ovine and caprine contagious ophthalmia

CONTAGIOUS ophthalmia is a disease of sheep and goats characterized by conjunctivitis and keratitis.

Etiology

Rickettsia (Colesiota) conjunctivae can be isolated from affected eyes and is capable of causing the disease in sheep and goats. The occurrence of rickettsial ophthalmitis in cattle is open to doubt, most cases of ophthalmia in this species being caused by *Moraxella bovis*. A rickettsia isolated from cases of keratoconjunctivitis in pigs less than 2 months of age is capable of causing the disease in piglets and can be passaged through chick embryos and mice.

In sheep a bacterium—*Neisseria catarrhalis (ovis)*—is commonly present in affected eyes but its etiological significance is doubtful. It may be capable of causing disease when the resistance of the conjunctiva is lowered from other causes. All breeds of sheep are equally affected but the disease in lambs is less severe than in adults, and recently weaned animals are most severely affected. *Mycoplasma* spp. are frequently identified in the eyes of ewes with pinkeye and many, especially *M. conjunctivae*, are currently identified as etiological agents of the disease (1–3). *Acholeplasma oculi* may be present, but positive pathogenicity has not been proposed (1). *Mycoplasma* spp. have also been found in association with keratoconjunctivitis in goats (4). The evidence available suggests strongly that mycoplasmas play an etiological role in pinkeye of sheep but proof that they can initiate the disease is lacking. The disease is not transmissible experimentally to cattle, guinea-pigs or rabbits.

Epidemiology

The disease in sheep is widespread in most countries including Africa, Australia, the United States, the United Kingdom and Europe. It causes only minor inconvenience by interfering with grazing for a few days in pastured animals. The disease occurs as widespread outbreaks in some years and in such circumstances may cause appreciable losses in weight gains. Outbreaks during the mating season can reduce the incidence of twinning. The morbidity rate varies widely depending on seasonal conditions. It is usually about 10–15% but may be as high as 50%.

After a clinical attack recurrence of the disease is unusual before the following summer probably because of the persistence of the infection in the eye—a state of premunity. Resistance to infection seems to be reduced by concurrent diseases, poor nutrition and adverse weather.

The disease is spread indirectly by flies, long grass and dust contaminated by the tears of infected sheep, or directly by means of exhaled droplets or immediate contact. The incidence is highest during the warm, summer months and when conditions are dry and dusty, and the fly population is heavy. Experimentally the disease can be transmitted by instillation of infected tears into the conjunctival sac but not by parenteral injection. Infection persists in the eye for periods up to 250 days and carrier animals are a source of reinfection in subsequent years (5). A degree of flock immunity appears to develop which may be sufficient to prevent the occurrence of acute outbreaks of the disease for 2 or 3 years.

Pathogenesis

Contagious ophthalmia commences as a conjunctivitis with frequent spread to the cornea.

Clinical findings

Initially in sheep there is lacrimation and blepharospasm followed by keratitis with cloudiness of the cornea and some increase in vascularity. The watery discharge later becomes purulent but recovery commences in 3–4 days and is complete at about 10 days. In some animals the cloudiness of the cornea may persist for several weeks or even permanently. Local ulceration of the cornea may cause collapse of the eyeball. Both eyes are affected in many cases and spread through the flock is rapid. In goats the disease is milder with little apparent ophthalmia or keratitis. Conjunctivitis is followed by the development of granular lesions on the palpebral conjunctiva.

Clinical pathology

Swabs or scrapings from the affected conjunctiva should be examined for the presence of rickettsiae in the epithelial cells.

Diagnosis

This is the most common contagious ophthalmia known to occur in sheep. In goats *R. conjunctivae* causes only a mild conjunctivitis. Chlamydial agents have also been found to be common accompaniments of ovine conjunctivitis in feedlots, either alone or in combination with polyarthritis. The lesions are often bilateral, and include conjunctival hyperemia and edema, epiphora, vascularization, pannus formation, follicular conjunctivitis and keratitis (6, 7). The agent is probably *Chlamydia psittaci*.

A more severe conjunctivitis and keratitis occurs in goats but its cause has not been established (3). All age groups are affected and although the morbidity is usually 12–20% it may reach 50%. Direct contact between animals appears to be necessary for spread of the infection, but the disease has not been transmitted experimentally. Conjunctivitis, opacity, vascularization and sometimes ulceration of the cornea are accompanied by an ocular discharge and blepharospasm. Recovery begins in 4–7 days but in severe cases healing may not be complete for 2–4 weeks.

In cattle *Mor. bovis* is the cause of most outbreaks of ophthalmia. Phenothiazine may also cause photosensitization of the cornea, but the resulting opacity is limited to the lateral half of the cornea.

Treatment

Local irrigation with astringent collyria, such as a 2·5% solution of zinc sulfate, is usually used to allay the discomfort, but treated animals are more likely to relapse or become reinfected than the untreated. Chloramphenicol has appeared to have some beneficial effect in field studies but in controlled experiments aureomycin (0·5% collyria) was much more effective, although relapses occurred quickly after the use of the latter. Ethidium bromide (0·5% ointment or 0·5–1.0% lotion once or twice daily for 3–4 days) and oxytetracycline (8) are also effective. Neither of these drugs appears to prevent the subsequent development of immunity after natural infection but they do reduce the severity of the ocular lesion when they are applied. Clinically affected animals may require supplementary feeding if their sight is impaired.

Control

Complete eradication of the disease is not attempted but isolation of affected sheep, and removal to grassier, less dusty pasture may reduce the rate of spread. Confinement of affected sheep should also be avoided.

REFERENCES

(1) Arbuckle, J. B. R. & Bonson, M. D. (1980) *Vet. Rec.*, *106*, 15.
(2) Langford, E. V. (1971) *Can. J. comp. Med.*, *35*, 8.
(3) Jones, G. E. et al. (1976) *Vet. Rec.* , *99*, 137.
(4) McCauley, E. H. et al. (1971) *Am. J. vet. Res.*, *32*, 861.
(5) Beveridge, W. I. B (1942) *Aust. vet. J.*, *18*, 155.
(6) Hopkins, J. P. et al. (1973). *J. Am. vet. med. Assoc.*, *163*, 1157.
(7) Stephenson, E. H. et al. (1974) *Am. J. vet. Res.*, *35*, 177.
(8) Hofland, G. et al. (1969) *Tijdschr. Diergeneeskd.*, *94*, 353.

Anaplasmosis

Anaplasmosis of cattle, sheep and goats is caused by infection with *Anaplasma* spp. In cattle severe debility, emaciation, anemia and jaundice are the major clinical signs. The disease is usually subclinical in sheep and goats.

Etiology

The rickettsia *Anaplasma marginale* is the causative agent in cattle and wild ruminants, and *A. ovis* in sheep and goats. Crossinfection and crossimmunity do not occur with *A. ovis* but subclinical infections with *A. marginale* can occur in sheep and goats. There may be a relationship between *A. marginale* and *Eperythrozoon wenyoni*, the latter interfering with the establishment of experimental anaplasmosis in splenectomized calves. *Anaplasma* sp. can now be maintained in and replicate themselves in suspensions of bovine erythrocytes, which need to be replenished repeatedly (13). There are antigenic variants of *A. marginale*, but they are sufficiently similar to avoid the need for the separate isolates to be included in a vaccine (31).

Epidemiology

Anaplasmosis in cattle is common in South Africa, Australia, the USSR, South America and the United States. Its spread is largely determined by the presence of suitable insect vectors and the incidence of the disease depends on the same factors, particularly the introduction of susceptible animals and sudden expansion of the vector population into previously free areas, which govern the incidence of babesiosis. Losses in enzootic areas may not be great because of widespread immunity. In general the disease has the same distribution as babesiosis but in both the United States and Australia it has spread beyond the boundaries of tick-infested areas. The disease is now present in 40 of the 50 states of America and is reputed to cost that country $100 million annually (1). Such estimates of wastage are usually gross underestimates because occurrences of the disease are underreported. However, the value of these losses due to anaplasmosis is thought to be much less than previously because of the adoption of suitable control measures. Nevertheless, the disease is thought to be the second most important in the United States.

The morbidity rate is usually high in outbreaks but the mortality rate varies widely depending on susceptibility, and may be 50% or more in introduced cattle. Recovered animals are emaciated and there is a prolonged convalescence.

Anaplasmosis of sheep and goats occurs in Africa, the Mediterranean countries, the USSR and the United States.

Young animals are relatively resistant to the disease and to *A. centrale* vaccine although they develop good levels of antibodies (19). They are susceptible to infection and remain permanently infected but immune. Animals over 3 years of age are usually affected by a peracute fatal form of the disease. The observed resistance to infection in very young calves is due to passive immunization as a result of the passage of antibodies from the dam to the calf in the colostrum. The average age at which calves in enzootic areas become infected is 11 (4–24) weeks and the clinical and pathological changes in them are mild and brief. Animals in an infected environment which have become seronegative for whatever reason are fully susceptible to infection (36).

Zebu-type cattle are as susceptible as British breeds but under field conditions are not as commonly affected probably because of their relative resistance to heavy tick infestation. However, the effects of the infection on body weight and clinicopathological parameters are the same for the two races of cattle (30). Deer can become infected and possibly act as reservoirs of infection for cattle but their epidemiological importance to cattle is still debated (3). If they are important there seems to be little point in establishing anaplasmosis-free herds when the cattle share pasture with roaming deer. American bison (*Bison bison*) appear to be naturally resistant to infection (4) but *A. marginale* can be transmitted to them experimentally (27). There is serological evidence of infection in elk and bighorn sheep but anaplasms have not been demonstrated in these animals. In Africa a large number of wild ruminants are considered to be susceptible to natural infection.

Exposure of infected, clinically normals animals to devitalizing environmental influences, particularly shortage of feed, and the presence of other diseases, may result in the development of acute anaplasmosis. For example, cattle introduced into feedlots are highly susceptible and outbreaks among them are not uncommon 2–3 weeks after entry. On the other hand thin, hungry cattle are less susceptible than fat well-fed ones.

The source of infection is always the blood of an infected animal. Once infected the animal remains a carrier for many years, probably for life, even though the parasite may not be always demonstrable in the blood. Spread from animal to animal occurs chiefly by insect vectors. In Australia the ticks *Boophilus microplus* and *Rhipicephalus sanguineus* (40) are the vectors, but in the United States *Boophilus annulatus*, *Dermacentor andersoni*, *D. variabilis*, *Argas persicus* and biting flies of *Tabanis* spp. and eye gnats (*Hippelates pusio*) (29) also act as vectors (5) and many others are thought to do so. Ticks, at least in some areas, are much the more important group of vectors (28). The male ticks of *Dermacentor albipictus* and *D. occidentalis* (the Pacific Coast tick of the United States) parasitize both deer and cattle and probably act as vectors (29). The organisms survive for long periods in *Dermacentor andersoni* and *D. variabilis* (25), but in *B. microplus* anaplasms do not pass to succeeding generations of tick (6), but transmission occurs as the ticks move from one host to another while they are engorging. There appears to be no developmental sequence of *Anaplasma* sp. in flying insects such as eye gnats. In sheep and goats a variety of ticks are known to spread the disease. Bovine anaplasmosis may also be spread mechanically by infected hypodermic needles and castrating, spaying and dehorning instruments and by blood transfusions and embryo transplants. The ease with which the infection is spread mechanically may vary with the virulence of the protozoan strain and this method of spread may be more important in some countries than others. Anaplasmosis may also be spread when cattle, used as donors of infected blood for immunization against babesiosis, are infected with *A. marginale*, the reaction occurring some 3 weeks later than that due to the babesiae. Intrauterine infection also occurs in cattle but much less frequently in field cases than in experimental ones (26). Abortion or neonatal infection may result. In ewes intrauterine infection appears to occur with ease in experimental cases provided the ewe is exposed during the latter two-thirds of pregnancy (37).

Pathogenesis

Anaplasmosis is primarily an anemia, the degree of anemia varying with the proportion of erythrocytes which are parasitized. The first appearance of the protozoa in the blood coincides with a fall in the hematocrit and erythrocyte levels, and the appearance of immature erythrocytes in blood smears and the development of fever. Acutely affected animals may die shortly after this phase is reached. If the animal recovers from the initial acute attack, periodic attacks of parasitic invasion of mature erythrocytes occur regularly, but with diminishing intensity. The degree of anemia varies widely in young cattle up to 3 years of age but is always severe in adults and in splenectomized animals.

Clinical findings

In cattle the incubation period varies with the amount of infected material injected but is usually recognized to be longer than in babesiosis, being about 3–4 weeks or more after tick-borne infection and 1–5 weeks after the inoculation of blood. In most cases the disease is subacute, especially in young animals. The temperature rises rather slowly and rarely to above 40·5°C (105°F) It may remain elevated or fluctuate with irregular periods of fever and normal temperature for from several days up to 2 weeks. Anorexia is seldom complete. The animal may die at this stage but many survive in an emaciated condition, and their fertility may be impaired. The mucous membranes are jaundiced and show marked pallor, particularly after the acute stage is passed, but hemoglobinuria is absent. Peracute cases, with a sudden onset of high fever, anemia, icterus, severe dyspnea and death often within 24 hours, are not uncommon in adult dairy cows. Affected animals are often hyperexcitable and tend to attack attendants just before death. Pregnant cows frequently abort. In convalescent bulls there may be depressed testicular function for several months.

In sheep and goats the disease is usually subclinical but in some cases, particularly in goats, a severe anemia may occur and a clinical picture similar to that found in cattle may be seen. Severe reactions of this type in goats are most frequent when the animals are suffering from concurrent disease. The experimental disease in lambs includes fever, constipation or diarrhea, pale, icteric conjunctivae and severe anemia 15–20 days after inoculation. The anemia is not completely repaired in 3–4 months.

Clinical pathology

Hemolysis may be so severe that the erythrocyte count is reduced to 1·5 million/μl. Immature red cells are common at this stage and their presence is considered to be a favorable sign. The small dot-like protozoa are discernible at the periphery of up to 10% of the red cells in subacute cases, but in peracute cases more than 50% of the cells may be parasitized. *A. ovis* are usually situated at the periphery of erythrocytes but as many as 40% of infested cells may show submarginal protozoa. Transmission experiments are best carried out on splenectomized animals and carriers can be detected by the same technique, severe relapses occurring after splenectomy. Calves often show anemia without clinical signs after inoculation. There are no significant clinical chemistry findings (1).

For the detection of carrier animals the most accurate test is the complement fixation (CF) test. It is satisfactory for use in cattle, goats and sheep but the antibody titer is highest during the active phase of the disease and sufficiently low in carrier animals to give a proportion of false-negative results. For unexplained reasons a small percentage of false-positive reactions to the test also occur. A capillary tube agglutination test of comparable efficiency is available, is more economical and faster than the CF test (10) and is particularly suited to testing in extensive field situations. A rapid card agglutination test, which tests serum or plasma for antibodies against *A. marginale*, is cheap and quick, and sufficiently accurate to be used as a herd test. An indirect fluorescent antibody test is also accurate (11) and has a particularly suitability for testing blood which has been dried onto paper for passage through the mails (15). It is also the most accurate test for selecting recently affected animals (9). Vaccinated animals react to all of the serological tests for periods of over 1 year.

Necropsy findings

At necropsy the most obvious findings are emaciation, jaundice and pallor of the tissues, and thin, watery blood. The liver is enlarged and deep orange in color, the kidneys congested, the spleen enlarged with soft pulp and there may be hemorrhages in the myocardium. Postmortem indentification of *A. marginale* can be established by staining blood smears with Giemsa and direct fluorescent stains. Peripheral blood is superior to organ smears, and brain smears are unsatisfactory (32). The technique is applicable to fetuses suspected of being aborted as a result of infection with *Anaplasma* sp. (20).

Diagnosis

A positive diagnosis of anaplasmosis depends upon positive transmission and complement-fixation tests. The history of the outbreak, experience of the occurrence of the disease in the area and the presence of insect vectors or other means of spread of the disease may suggest the possible presence of anaplasmosis. Babesiosis is clinically much more acute, is accompanied by hemoglobinuria and can be distinguished on examination of smears of peripheral blood. *Borrelia theileri* is another organism associated with the development of anemia, fever and petechiation of mucosae (5). The differential diagnosis of other causes of hemolytic anemia has been discussed in detail elsewhere. The possible occurrence of more than one cause of hemolytic anemia in the same group of animals should not be overlooked.

Treatment

In the treatment of clinical disease, tetracycline 6–10 mg/kg body weight given in a single injection is effective, although it is more usual to give three such daily injections, but the parasite is not eliminated and immunity persists. Supportive treatment should include massive blood transfusions administered slowly to avoid cardiac embarrassment. Rough handling should be avoided at all cost. During treatment care must be taken to ensure sterilization of equipment between cases. A number of methods have been recommended for the treatment of carrier animals. Parenteral treatment with a tetracycline 10–30 mg/kg body weight daily for 10–16 days, or intravenous injection of 22 mg/kg body weight daily for 5 days (12) are effective in sterilizing carriers, but have obvious disadvantages for large numbers of animals. Oral administration of chlortetracycline (10 mg/kg body weight for 30–60 days), or 1 mg/kg body weight for 120 days is effective in eliminating the carrier state. When infected animals are sterilized by this treatment their immunity persists for 6 months, an important feature in herd management (14).

The recent advent of a long-acting tetracycline preparation has made treatment easier still. The L-200 or T-200 product injected at the rate of 20 mg/kg body weight intramuscularly every 7 days for two to four injections sterilized cattle of their parasitemia (24). A single injection is an effective treatment, but does not sterilize the patient (21, 22). The treatment is about as effective as imidocarb.

Imidocarb (3 mg/kg body weight) is an effective treatment for clinical cases but sterility is not easily achieved, requiring two injections of 5 mg/kg body weight (17). It has the advantage that it does not interfere with the development of acquired immunity to *A. marginale* (38). Amicarbalide (20 mg/kg body weight subcutaneously divided into two equal daily doses) has the same disadvantage (16). A problem with imidocarb is the tolerance for it that *B. argentina* can develop when exposed to the above-mentioned therapeutic level (3 mg/kg body weight on four occasions) (18).

Control

The eradication of anaplasmosis is not in most countries a practicable procedure at the present time because of the wide range of insects which are capable of carrying the disease, the long period of infectivity of carrier animals, the inability to detect satisfactorily infected animals and, in some areas, the presence of carriers in the wild animal population. In enzootic areas some benefit is derived from the control or eradication of ticks, and the control of other vectors. Attention should also be given to preventing artificial transmission by instruments used for injections or surgical operations by disinfection after use on each animal. This is particularly important in feedlots where introduced groups are often subjected to multiple vaccinations and implantations at a time when their resistance is lowered by transport and change of feed. Some advantage can be gained when introducing animals into an enzootic area by limiting the introductions to animals of less than 2 years of age and by bringing them in when the insect populations is least numerous.

Most control programs in enzootic areas are based on increasing the resistance of the population by immunization. Four forms of vaccination are used:

- Living *A. marginale* is used as a vaccine but its administration is limited to the relatively resistant age group below 1 year of age, to the winter months when vectors are sufficiently rare to avoid the chance of spread to other age groups, and to circumstances where animals which react severely can be restrained and treated adequately. The method has the serious disadvantage of creating a large population of carrier animals which may subsequently spread the disease

- Attenuated vaccines are available for testing. They include a naturally avirulent strain and a virulent strain adapted for growth in sheep (23). The immunity established with the latter is as effective as that provided by a fully virulent infection. A frozen *A. marginale* vaccine is available (39)
- Living *A. centrale* which causes a mild, inapparent disease, does cause severe reactions in occasional animals. *A. centrale* is used extensively in Australia but not in the United States and there is some reluctance to introduce it into areas where it does not already occur. Vaccination with *A. centrale* reduces the severity of the reaction when infection with *A. marginale* occurs, vaccination with *A. marginale* eliminates the reaction
- Killed *A. marginale*, usually in an adjuvant vehicle, is receiving most attention as a vaccine at the present time. Its most serious disadvantage is that the immune response to one injection is poor and two vaccinations at least 6 weeks apart are required. The vaccine does not completely protect against infection but does significantly reduce the severity of the disease, thus permitting the development of a large population of carrier animals. It does have the advantage over the other vaccines of having a relatively short postvaccination period (1–2 months) when animals remain positive to serological tests. The duration of the immunity is at least 5 months (14). Its use has been reduced because of the increased incidence of neonatal isoerythrolysis which results. This can be avoided by vaccinating only empty cows and avoiding unnecessary booster injections (2). Another possible solution is the development of purified *A. marginale* material from which the contaminating host cell antigens have been removed by lysis (35). Anaplasma particles can also be obtained from ticks feeding on infected cattle.

One of the problems with the living vaccines, the need to maintain a supply of living 'donor' animals at all times, may have been overcome by the observation that infective blood used as vaccine can be stored for up to $4\frac{1}{2}$ years by deep freezing. Whenever living vaccines are used, vaccinated animals should be carefully observed to ensure that infection does in fact take place and that animals which suffer severe reactions are treated. Another suggested method of reducing the severity of reactions which occur after preimmunization with *A. marginale* is that of injecting a minimum infective dose (0·01 ml of infective blood) rather than the regular 5 ml dose. As with any whole-blood vaccine there is a risk of transmitting unsuspected viruses such as that of bovine viral leukosis.

In any vaccination program particular attention should be paid to the animals in high-risk situations, particularly animals brought in from non-enzootic areas, those in surrounding similar areas to which infection may be spread by expansion of the vector population under the influence of suitable climatic conditions, and animals within the area which are likely to be exposed to climatic or nutritional stress.

The introduction of the disease into areas by carrier animals can be prevented by the use of the complement fixation test or the capillary tube agglutination test. Vaccination with a killed vaccine in the area may be necessary when the risk of introduction by vector insects is high.

If an outbreak does occur affected animals should be treated vigorously as described above and in-contact animals put onto a daily intake of 1–2 mg/kg body weight oxytetracycline for at least 10 days, or alternatively one injection of the longacting tetracycline (8), to prevent infection. The results generally are good except when the cattle are exposed to infection during the 14 days prior to the treatment (33). Another favored technique when an outbreak develops is to treat all cattle with a tetracycline and repeat this 4–6 weeks later. This should protect the cattle over a good part of the season when vectors are bad (2). Subsequently all exposed animals should be submitted to a suitable test and the reactors treated or preferably salvaged. An unfortunate sequel to vaccination is the high incidence of positive reactors to serological tests used in diagnosis (7). These reactors persist for as long as 15 months. These chronic carriers are important causes of breakdowns in eradication programs. They can be eliminated as carriers by a series of four injections at 3-day intervals of longacting tetracycline (34).

REVIEW LITERATURE.

McHardy, N. (1984) Immunization against anaplasmosis:a review. *Prev. vet. Med.*, *2*, 135.

Ristic, M. (1977) Bovine anaplasmosis. In: *Parasitic Protozoa*, vol. IV, ed. J. Kreier, pp. 235–249. New York: Academic Press.

Wilde, J. K. H. (1976) Tick-borne diseases and their vectors. *Proc. Int. Conf., Edinburgh*, 1976.

REFERENCES

(1) Allen, P. C. et al. (1981) *Am. J. vet. Res.*, *42*, 322 & 326.
(2) Searl, R. C. (1980) *Vet. Med. SAC*, *75*, 101.
(3) Dalgliesh, R. J. & Stewart, N. P. (1977) *Aust. vet. J.*, *53*, 176.
(4) Peterson, K. J. & Roby, T. O. (1975) *J. Wildlife Dis.*, *11*, 395.
(5) Kiptoon, J. C. et al. (1979) *Kenya Vet.*, *3*, 11.
(6) Connell, M. L. (1974) *Q. J. agric. Anim. Sci.*, *31*, 185.
(7) Luther, D. G. et al. (1980) *Am. J. vet. Res.*, *41*, 2085.
(8) Howarth, J. A. et al. (1982) *Cal. Vet.*, *36*, 12.
(9) Gonzalez, E. F. et al. (1978) *Am. J. vet. Res.*, *39*, 1538.
(10) Akinboade, O. A (1984) *Prev. vet. Med.*, *3*, 317.
(11) Kuttler, K. L. et al. (1977) *Am. J. vet. Res.*, *38*, 153.
(12) Magonigle, R. A. et al. (1975) *J. Am. vet. med. Assoc.*, *167*, 1080.
(13) Kessler, R. H. et al. (1979) *Am. J. vet. Res.*, *40*, 1767 & 1774.
(14) Richey, E. J. et al. (1977) *Am. J. vet. Res.*, *38*, 169.
(15) Wilson, A. J. et al. (1978) *Aust. vet. J.*, *54* 383.
(16) de Vos, A. J. et al. (1978) *Onderstepoort J. vet. Res.*, *45*, 203.
(17) Kuttler, K. L. (1975) *SW Vet.*, *28*, 47.
(18) Dalgliesh, R. J. & Stewart, N. P. (1977) *Aust. vet. J.*, *53*, 176.
(19) Pipano, E. et al. (1985) *Br. vet. J.*, *141*, 174.
(20) Correa, W. M. et al. (1978) *Can. J. comp. Med.*, *42*, 227.
(21) Stewart, C. G. et al. (1979) *J. S. Afr. vet. Assoc.*, *50*, 83.
(22) Corrier, D. E. et al. (1980) *Am. J. vet. Res.*, *141*, 1062 &1066.
(23) Wilson, A. J. et al. (1979) *Aust. vet. J.*, *55*, 71.
(24) Roby, T. O. et al. (1978) *Am. J. vet. Res.*, *39*, 1115.
(25) Kocan, K. M. et al. (1983) *Am. J. vet. Res.*, *44*, 1617.
(26) Zaugg, J. L. (1985) *Am. J. vet. Res.*, *46*, 570.
(27) Zaugg, J. L. (1985) *Am. J. vet. Res.*, *46*, 438.

(28) Peterson, K. J. et al. (1977) *Am. J. vet. Res.*, *38*, 351.
(29) Stiller, D. et al. (1983) *Proc. US Anim. Hlth Assoc.*, *87*, 59.
(30) Otim, C. et al. (1980) *Aust. vet. J.*, *56*, 262.
(31) Kuttler, K. L. et al. (1984) *Am. J. vet. Res.*, *45*, 2229.
(32) Johnston, L. A. Y. et al. (1980) *Aust. vet. J.*, *56*, 116.
(33) Kuttler, K. L. (1983) *Am. J. vet. Res.*, *44*, 882.
(34) Magonigle, R. A. & Newby, T. J. (1982) *Am. J. vet. Res.*, *43*, 2170.
(35) Hart, L. T. et al. (1981) *Curr. Microbiol.*, *5*, 95.
(36) Lincoln, S. D. et al. (1987) *J. Am. vet. med. Assoc.*, *190*, 171.
(37) Zaugg, J. L. (1987) *Am. J. vet. Res.*, *48*, 100.
(38) Vos, A. J. de (1987) *Aust. vet. J.*, *64*, 81.
(39) Pipano, E. et al. (1986) *Br. vet. J.*, *142*, 553.
(40) Partner, R. J. (1982) *Aust. vet. J.*, *58*, 47.

Tick-borne fever

Tick-borne fever is a disease of cattle and sheep caused by rickettsiae, and characterized clinically by a mild fever and a short course.

Etiology

The causative agents, *Rickettsia bovina* and *R. ovina* (also known as *Cytoecetes phagocytophila* and *Erlichia phagocytophila*) (1), resemble each other very closely and the disease produced experimentally in cattle by the ovine strain is almost identical with that produced by the bovine strain although slightly less severe. There is considerable cross-immunity between the two strains, the main difference between the two being the difficulty of establishing the bovine strain in sheep and vice versa. Attempts to grow the rickettsiae on hen eggs have not been successful.

Epidemiology

The disease recorded in the United Kingdom, Scandinavia and India (sheep only) is of minor importance because of its mild nature. It causes some loss of weight in lambs. It may recur each year on affected farms. One of the indirect effects of the disease is that it increases the susceptibility of lambs to staphylococcal pyemia (3), staphylococcal pneumonia, and louping-ill and possibly to other diseases. The mortality rate is negligible in cattle but may be higher in sheep.

Cattle, deer, goats and sheep are susceptible and newborn calves and lambs are much more susceptible than adults. The rickettsia has been adapted to grow in mice and guinea-pigs but is still infective for sheep after 90 serial passages. Information on immunity is scanty but under natural conditions the disease commonly recurs in the one animal in successive years. A state of low-grade premunity due to the presence of the rickettsia in the blood develops after infection and provides partial resistance to subsequent infections, the disease manifesting itself in a less severe form. Challenge of previously affected sheep did not produce any reaction during the next 3 months. Deep freezing of blood at −74°C (−101°F) preserves its infectivity for 8 months (4).

Experimentally in cattle the disease significantly reduces body weight gain (5). Clinical signs are restricted to fever for 3–8 days after an incubation period of 4–8 days. Detectable parasitemia persists for a slightly lesser period. The necropsy lesions in cattle which die of tick-borne fever are very similar to those of bovine petechial fever (Ondiri disease) which occurs only in Kenya and is caused by a rickettsia closely related to that of tick-borne fever (5).

The disease is transmitted by ticks, including *Ixodes ricinus* in Great Britain and *Rhipicephalus hemaphysaloides* in India and although the rickettsia persists in the tick through its stages of development, persistence to further tick generations has not been shown to occur. The rickettsiae persist in the bloodstream of animals for a considerable period, up to 2 years in sheep, and this represents the major source of infection in an enzootic area.

Pathogenesis

The presence of the rickettsia in the leukocytes, and the emptied lymphoid deposits which are characteristic of the disease suggest that the disease is primarily leukolytic. The leukopenia combined with thrombocytopenia suggests myeloid inhibition and a similarity to other radiomimetic diseases such as bracken poisoning (6). This similarity is increased by the appearance in adult sheep of a hemorrhagic syndrome, with lesions particularly evident on the alimentary mucosa. It is not known whether the abortion which occurs in sheep, and less commonly in cattle, is due to the fever or to a specific effect of the rickettsia (5).

A severe clinical syndrome, including severe diarrhea and dysentery and a high mortality rate results from a combined infection of *C. phagocytophila* and louping-ill virus (8). Similarly, a concurrent experimental infection in sheep of the rickettsia and *Chlamydia psittaci* resulted in chlamydial pneumonia (7) possibly as a result of the reduced resistance created by the rickettsia (4). A similar situation results after the simultaneous infection with the rickettsia of tick-borne fever and parainfluenza-3 (PI-3) virus (11), *Listeria monocytogenes* or *Pasteurella hemolytica*.

Clinical findings

In cattle there is an incubation period of 6–7 days after experimental infection followed by a rise in temperature to about 40·5°C (105°F) which persists for 2–8 days. The temperature falls gradually and is followed by a secondary febrile period and, in some cases, further attacks of pyrexia occur. During each febrile period there is a marked fall in milk yield, lethargy and polypnea and in experimentally produced cases, a mild cough. Cattle affected during the last 2 months of pregnancy commonly abort and occasionally animals die suddenly. The abortions occur shortly after the systemic disease.

In sheep the syndrome is similar to that observed in cattle except that respiratory distress is not observed. The reaction in young lambs is quite mild and manifested only by a moderate rise in temperature. Ewes exposed to the disease for the first time commonly experience outbreaks of abortion and affected rams are temporarily infertile. A hemorrhagic syndrome, affecting the intestinal mucosa, has been observed in experimentally infected adult sheep (6).

Tick-borne fever in goats is characterized by high fever, dullness and tachycardia (10).

Clinical pathology

Serological diagnosis is possible with the development of an accurate specific complement fixation test.

The rickettsiae are present in the neutrophils and monocytes during each febrile period and for a few days afterwards in cattle and for several weeks in sheep, and can be detected in suitably stained blood smears. An unusually pathogenic strain of *E. phagocytophila* has been recorded in the United Kingdom (2). It is characterized by a greater than usual tendency to invade monocytes. At the peak of the fever there is a marked leukopenia (4000–5000/mm^3), due largely to a depression first of lymphocytes and then of the neutrophils. This is soon followed by a leukocytosis with a marked increase in immature neutrophils. At the commencement of the fever in the experimentally induced disease there is a severe but transient thrombocytopenia (6). Transmission of the disease may be effected by the intravenous injection of blood taken at the height of the fever.

Necropsy findings

There are no gross changes other than splenomegaly in sheep, and histologically the only characteristic lesion is an apparent draining of lymphocytes from lymphoid tissue.

Diagnosis

The diagnosis is not difficult if the disease is suspected because of the ease with which the rickettsiae are found in leukocytes. The strict geographical restriction of the disease and its relation to tick infestation are diagnostic features but the clinical signs are quite non-specific. The disease in cattle has some similarity to bovine petechial fever (Ondiri disease), caused by *Cytoectes ondiri*, which occurs only in Kenya (9). It is characterized by lymphadenopathy, mucosal petechiation and sometimes dysentery.

Treatment

The best results are claimed for treatment with tetracyclines or sulfadimidine. In dwarf goats good results are provided by single doses of oxytetracycline (10 mg/kg body weight intravenously) or a potentiated sulfonamide containing trimethoprim and sulfadimidine and sulfamethylphenazole (20, 50 and 50 mg/kg body weight respectively); ampicillin is ineffective (12). The rickettsiae persist in treated animals which may subsequently suffer a relapse.

Control

Control of tick-borne fever depends upon control of the tick population. The circumstance of greatest danger is when pregnant ewes are moved onto new tick-infested pasture; the lambs are very susceptible.

REVIEW LITERATURE

Brodie, T. A. et al. (1986) Some aspects of tick-borne disease of British sheep. *Vet. Rec.*, *118*, 415.

Scott, G. R. (1984) Tick-borne fever in sheep. *Vet. Ann.*, *24*, 100–106.

REFERENCES

(1) Foggie, A. et al. (1966) *J. comp. Pathol.*, *76*, 413.
(2) Purnell, R. E. & Brocklesby, D. W.(1978) *Vet. Rec.*, *102*, 552.
(3) Foster, W. N. M. & Cameron, A. E. (1970) *J. comp. Pathol.*, *80*, 429.
(4) Batungbacal, M. R. & Scott, G. R (1982) *J. comp. Pathol.*, *92*, 409.
(5) Taylor, S. M. & Kenny, J. (1980) *Br. vet. J.*, *136*, 364.
(6) Batungbacal, M. R. et al. (1982) *J. comp. Pathol.*, 92, 403.
(7) Munro, R. et al. (1982) *J. comp. Pathol.*, *92*, 117.
(8) Reid, H. W. et al. (1986) *Res. vet. Sci.*, *41*, 56.
(9) Mugera, G. M. & Kiptoon, J. (1978) *Bull. Anim. Hlth Prod., Afr.*, *26*, 99.
(10) van Miert, ASJPAM et al. (1984) *Vet. Parasitol.*, *16*, 225.
(11) Batungbacal, M. R. & Scott, G. R. (1982) *J. comp. Pathol.*, *92*, 415.
(12) Anika, S. M. et al. (1986) *Res. vet. Sci.*, *41*, 386.

Heartwater

This is a tick-borne disease of wild and domestic cattle, sheep and goats caused by *Cowdria ruminantium* and characterized by fever, nervous signs, edema of the body cavities and diarrhea.

Etiology

The rickettsia *Cowdria* (syn. *Rickettsia*) *ruminantium* is the cause. It can be cultivated on a calf endothelial cell-line (3) and maintained in mice, rats and ferrets. It is a member of the tribe Ehrlichiae and crossreacts strongly with *Ehrlichia equi*, the cause of equine ehrlichiosis (5).

Epidemiology

Heartwater affects imported breeds of cattle, sheep and goats in southern Africa and is regarded as the most important tick-borne disease in the region (1). It is also found in many related game animals, many of which may die of the disease. Others become symptomless carriers. Young animals have an innate resistance, not due to passive immunity derived from their dams. Goats are more susceptible than cattle (8).

The disease is limited in its occurrence to Africa, Madagascar and some of the West Indies (4, 7). It is transmitted by many ticks of the *Amblyomma* genus, especially *A. variegatum*. Because of the large number of *Amblyomma* spp. that are capable of acting as vectors it is feared that the disease will spread much farther than it has. In the ticks the infection is transmitted transstadially but not transovarially. The most serious losses caused by heartwater are in exotic, susceptible cattle, sheep and goats that are imported into areas in which the disease is enzootic and at times when the vector population is high. The incubation period is 1–3 weeks.

Pathogenesis

The infection is introduced by the bite of an infected tick, multiplies in the local lymph node and then invades the endothelial cells of blood vessels in all organs where they cause vascular damage. One of the endpoints of this damage in goats is renal ischemia and a resulting nephrosis (9).

Clinical signs

Peracute cases show only high fever, prostration and death with terminal convulsions. Acute cases have a course of about 6 days and show the classical nervous syndrome which is characteristic of heartwater. It comprises ataxia, chewing movements, twitching of the eyelids, circling, aggression, apparent blindness, recumbency, convulsions and death. In less severe cases the principal sign may be diarrhea. The case mortality rate in peracute cases is 100%, in acute cases 50–90%, and in mild cases most animals recover.

Clinical pathology
Originally the diagnosis was based on being able to identify the rickettsia in a stained, squash preparation of tissue at postmortem. Transmission of the disease by injection of blood into a merino sheep was also used as a diagnostic procedure. Available serological tests now include an indirect fluorescent antibody test which has limited value (1), but an ELISA is credited with good sensitivity and reliability (6). The close antigenic relationship with *Ehrlichia equi* makes serious diagnostic errors possible with these serological tests (5).

Necropsy findings
Standard lesions are ascites, hydrothorax and hydropericardium. There may be pulmonary edema and subserosal hemorrhages in most cavities and there is splenomegaly and lymphadenopathy. Histopathological findings include perivascular infiltrations in most organs and encephalitis with rickettsia visible in the brain tissue.

Diagnosis
In enzootic areas a diagnosis of heartwater is the first choice for animals with a fever of unknown origin. The clinical and pathological findings are not specific and the diagnosis must be based on clinicopathological tests. Differentiation from other diseases characterized by fever, septicemia and nervous signs, such as sporadic bovine encephalomyelitis, may be difficult.

Treatment and control
Tetracyclines are the standard treatment and may be used, combined with natural or contrived infection, as a prophylactic measure. For treatment 1 ml of long-acting tetracycline/10 kg body weight given to sheep at the first peak of fever is effective (13). The exposure of calves of 2–4 weeks of age is considered to be the optimum natural exposure. Contrived exposure can be effected in several ways, the most common of which is the intravenous injection of heartwater infected blood or ground-up, infected ticks. Vaccination by these methods is very effective in terms of the protection provided but it is hazardous because of the deaths that may occur in spite of the treatment (2, 12). Its use is usually confined to imported cattle which can be kept under close surveillance and treated intensively. Longacting tetracycline administered to calves weekly for 4 weeks when they enter an enzootic zone has been an effective preventive strategy against heartwater (11) and appears to exert an immunostimulant effect (12). Control by eradication of the tick population is not usually a practical option but regular dipping of cattle and other livestock at 3–7 day intervals is a common practice in enzootic areas and serves to keep the disease in check.

REVIEW LITERATURE

Uilenberg, G. (1983) Heartwater. *Adv Vet. Sci.* , *27*, 427.

REFERENCES

(1) Bezuidenhout, J. D. (1985) *Onderstepoort J. vet. Res.*, *52*, 211.
(2) Bezuidenhout, J. D. & Spickett, A. M. (1985) *Onderstepoort J. vet. Res.*, *52*, 269.
(3) Bezuidenhout, J. D. et al. (1985) *Onderstepoort J. vet. Res.*, *52*, 113.
(4) Uilenberg, G. (1983) *Adv. vet. Sci.*, *27*, 427.
(5) Logan, L. et al. (1986) *Vet. Rec.*, *119*, 458.
(6) Neitz, A. W. H. et.al. (1986) *Onderstepoort J. vet. Res.*, *52*, 39, 205.
(7) Birnie, E. F. et al. (1985) *Vet. Rec.*, *116*, 121.
(8) Gruss, B. (1983) *J. S. Afr. vet. Assoc.*, *54*, 67.
(9) Gueye, A. et al. (1984) *Rev. Elev. Med. Vet. Pays trop*, *37*, 268.
(10) Purnell, R. E & Schroder, J. (1984) *Proc. 13th World Cong. Dis. Cattle*, *1*, 488.
(11) Uilenberg, G. et al. (1984) *Prev. vet. Med.*, *2*, 255.
(12) Simpson, B. C. et al. (1987) *Vet. Rec.*, *120*, 135.
(13) Gueye, A. & Vassilides, G. (1985) *Rev. Elev. Med. Vet. Pays trop.*, *38*, 428.

Equine ehrlichiosis

Equine ehrlichiosis caused by *Ehrlichia equi* has been recorded in the United States (1, 2). It is caused by a rickettsia and can be transmitted experimentally by the injection of blood collected from the donor at the peak of a febrile period. There are specific rickettsiae for each species. Positive identification of the disease is made on the presence of inclusion bodies in neutrophil leukocytes. Clinically there is high fever 40–42°C (104–107°F) followed by mucosal pallor, jaundice, anorexia, depression, increased respiratory movement, incoordination and reluctance to move, and after 3 or 4 days edema and heat of the extremities. The edema persists for 7–10 days. On laboratory examination there is a transient mild anemia due to intravascular hemolysis. There is a marked, transient leukopenia and a thrombocytopenia. At necropsy there are petechiae and edema of the legs and at histological examination there is a vasculitis. The disease must be distinguished from equine infectious anemia. It bears no similarity to equine ehrlichial colitis caused by *E. risticii*.

Treatment with tetracycline effects a complete and rapid recovery (2). Recovery from the disease is followed by a long period (more than 300 days) of positive serological testing. An indirect fluorescent antibody test is available (3).

REFERENCES

(1) Stannard, A. A. et al. (1969) *Vet. Rec.*, *84*, 149.
(2) Madigan, T. E. & Gribble, D. (1987) *J. Am. vet. med. Assoc.*, *190*, 445.
(3) Nyindo, M. B. A. et al. (1978) *Am. J. vet. Res.*, *39*, 15.

Equine ehrlichial colitis (equine monocytic ehrlichiosis, Potomac horse fever)

This is an acute, infectious colitis and typhlitis of horses caused by *Ehrlichia risticii* and probably transmitted by ticks.

Etiology
The rickettsia *Ehrlichia risticii* is the cause of the disease. It is cultivable in tissue culture (5) and is transmissible to mice (6).

Epidemiology
Equine ehrlichial colitis is infectious but not contagious between horses (2). It is recorded in the United States

and Europe (1, 3) and occurs only in the summer months. The highest incidence is near large rivers but the disease can occur elsewhere. It is sporadic in occurrence so that its presence may not be suspected on farms where there are only a few animals. It is uncommon in young horses and does not require stress as a predisposing cause, occurring in robust animals. The case fatality rate varies between 5% and 30% (3). The method of spread has not been determined but transmission by insects, especially ticks, is the favoured explanation. It fits the epidemiological pattern (2) and is compatible with the known capacity of the infection to occur via the intradermal route (7). Preliminary evidence suggested that the vector might be *Dermacentor variabilis* but this now seems unlikely (9). Small rodents, especially mice (6), are thought to be reservoir hosts. Infected horses may be infective for at least as long as 8 months. The incubation period in experimentally infected horses is 9–15 days (8).

Pathogenesis

The colitis and typhlitis cause loss of fluid into the intestinal lumen and the profuse, watery diarrhea which is characteristic of this disease.

Clinical findings

The basic syndrome includes fever, paralytic ileus and profuse watery diarrhea which may be projectile in character. Colic, laminitis and anasarca are common accompaniments. Severe cases are in a state of hypovolemic shock.

Clinical pathology

An indirect fluorescent antibody test (4) and an ELISA (5) are available. Seroconversion to *Ehrlichia risticii* is accepted as evidence of infection but is not always accompanied by illness. The disease is marked by a significant leukopenia in the early stages and a leukocytosis subsequently. Other findings are those of hemoconcentration and match the diarrhea-originated dehydration.

Necropsy findings

Congestion, hemorrhage, and mucosal erosion or ulceration occur throughout the alimentary tract but are concentrated in the colon and cecum. The mesenteric lymph nodes are swollen and edematous and there is subcutaneous edema of the ventral abdominal wall. There may be lesions of laminitis. Experimentally induced cases reflect the lesions of naturally occurring cases (10).

Diagnosis

Ehrlichial colitis is clinically indistinguishable from salmonellosis or colitis-X in horses.

Treatment and control

Tetracyclines are the drugs of choice for this disease but the choice is not without hazard because of the tendency of these drugs to cause fatal enteritis in their own right. In most cases the response is quick and complete.

REVIEW LITERATURE

Robl, M. G. (1985) Potomac horse fever; closing in on an unknown killer. *Vet. Med.*, *80(10)*, 49.

REFERENCES

(1) Palmer, J. E. et al. (1986) *J. Am. vet. med. Assoc.*, *189*, 197.
(2) Perry, B. D. et al. (1986) *Prev. vet. Med.*, *4*, 69.
(3) Holland, C. J. et al. (1985) *Science, USA*, *227(4686)*, 522.
(4) Ristic, M. et al. (1986) *J. Am. vet. med. Assoc.*, *189*, 39.
(5) Dutta, S. K. et al. (1985) *J. clin. Microbiol.*, *22*, 265.
(6) Jenkins, S. K. et al. (1985) *Vet. Rec.*, *117*, 556.
(7) Perry, B. D. et al. (1985) *Vet. Rec.*, *116*, 246.
(8) Ziemer, E. L. et al. (1987) *Am. J. vet. Res.*, *48*, 63.
(9) Schmidtmann, E. T. et al. (1986) *Am. J. vet. Res.*, *47*, 2393.
(10) Cordes, D. O. et al. (1986) *Vet. Pathol.*, *23*, 531.

Jembrana disease

This highly fatal and infectious, rinderpest-like disease occurred in cattle in Bali during the period 1964–67 (1). Clinical signs included fever (40–42°C, 104–107°F), anorexia, generalized lymphadenopathy, nasal discharge, increased salivation and anemia. Diarrhea was followed by dysentery; mucosal erosions were rare. Hemorrhages were present in the vagina, mouth and occasionally the anterior chamber of the eye. Necropsy lesions included generalized lymphadenopathy, with enlargements up to 20-fold, and generalized hemorrhages. The spleen was enlarged to three to four times normal size. Vasculitis and perivasculitis were marked histologically, mucosal lesions were present only occasionally. Intracellular organisms resembling rickettsiae were present in smears from hepatic lymph nodes. Intraperitoneal injections of spleen and lymph tissue into guinea-pigs caused peritonitis and orchitis.

Subsequent to the initial outbreaks the disease has been much less widespread, but is still enzootic in Bali. Clinically, the disease, Bali disease (3), is similar to tick-borne fever. A rickettsia has been isolated from affected animals and the disease is generally considered to be a rickettsiosis. The rickettsia has a predilection for lymphocytes and can be found concentrated in them. The probable vector is the tick *Boophilus microplus*. Transmission to buffalo and Bali cattle can be effected, but not to sheep or goats (2).

REFERENCES

(1) Budiarso, I. T. & Hardjosworo, S. (1976) *Aust. vet. J.*, *52*, 97.
(2) Johnson, R. H. (1979) *Aust. Adv. vet. Sci.*, 18.
(3) Teuscher, E. et al. (1982) *Zentralbl. VetMed.*, *29*, 547 & *28*, 608.

'Q' fever

This well-known disease of man caused by *Coxiella burnetii* is reputed to be non-pathogenic for domestic livestock but there are several records of very heavy infections causing abortion in sheep and goats (1, 2, 8). In the experimental disease produced in cattle (3) a few abortions resulted. Anorexia was the only consistent clinical finding. Interest in the organism as a cause of abortion has increased and it is credited with causing placentitis and abortion in dairy goats (6) and sheep. In cattle the position is unclear, but there is no real evidence that this infection is a cause of abortion in that species (7). A vaccine has been developed which is effective in preventing cattle from acting as shedders of the rickettsiae in their milk (4), and has greatly reduced the volume of rickettsia that are shed in the placenta in ewes (9). Because of the current upsurge of use of goats as a source of private milk supply to individual households, attention has been focused on goats as a source of the zoonosis. One survey has shown 24% of goats serologically positive and 7% of them excreting rickettsiae in the milk (5). Infected sheep and goats may communicate the disease to humans especially at parturition (1). Abattoir workers are most exposed and a high rate of crossinfection is recorded in persons killing feral goats (10).

REVIEW LITERATURE

Polydorou, K. (1981) Q fever in Cyprus. *Br. vet. J.*, *137*, 470.

REFERENCES

(1) Hall, C. J. (1982) *Lancet*, *1*, *8279*, 1004.
(2) Crowther, R. W. & Spicer, A. J. (1976) *Vet. Rec.*, *99*, 29.
(3) Plommet, M. et al. (1973) *Ann. Réch. vét.*, *14*, 325.
(4) Biberstein, E. L. et al. (1977) *Am. J. vet. Res.*, *38*, 189.
(5) Ruppanner, R. et al. (1978) *Am. J. vet. Res.*, *39*, 867.
(6) Palmer, N. C. et al. (1983) *Can. vet. J.*, *24*, 60.
(7) Schutte, A. P. et al. (1976) *Onderstepoort J. vet. Res.*, *43*, 129.
(8) Rady, M. et al. (1985) *Acta Vet. Hung.*, *33*, 169.
(9) Brooks, D. L. et al. (1986) *Am. J. vet. Res.*, *47*, 1235.
(10) Rich, G. et al. (1982) *Aust. Adv. vet. Sci.*, 257.

24

Diseases Caused by Fungi

SYSTEMIC AND MISCELLANEOUS MYCOSES

SYSTEMIC mycoses in animals are usually sporadic infections which occur by chance and cause non-specific syndromes because of variation in the organs in which they localize. Their epidemiology is based on the failure of the diseases to be transmitted from one host to another, all the infections deriving from sources in the environment. The causative fungi exist as saprophytes in organic matter, and the portal of entry is by inhalation of dust containing fungal elements, with a primary focus developing in a lung. Another less common site of infection is the forestomachs and abomasa of ruminants, the abomasa of young calves being the commonest site (6).

A necrohemorrhagic mastitis accompanied by pneumonia is also recorded in adult cows (13).

An important development has been the observation that a proportion of bovine abortions, unrelated to other known infectious agents, are caused by infections with fungi and yeasts (14). Mycotic abortions have also been observed in ewes (1) and sows. The incidence of mycotic abortions is much greater in the winter months in housed cows than in any other group and the disease occurs rarely in cows running at pasture all the year round. The general impression is that cows confined to indoor housing are exposed to an environment which is likely to be heavily contaminated with spores from moldy hay and ensilage. In these circumstances mycotic abortion may represent a high proportion (10–15%) of all abortions that occur in the population. An incidence of 30% has been observed in cattle housed in sheds all the year round (2). A strong positive correlation has been shown to exist between the incidence of mycotic abortion and the rainfall in the haymaking season prior to conception (3). Because of the common occurrence of fungal infections where antibiotics are used extensively, it has been suggested that the increasing incidence of mycotic placentitis may be related to the general use of antibiotic-treated semen in artificial insemination programs. However, the incidence of the disease does not seem to be higher in artificially bred cows than in those mated naturally. It is more likely that infection occurs by inhalation or via abomasal ulcers (4) with subsequent localization in the pregnant uterus, and sometimes in other organs. The lesions produced by the infection include lobar pneumonia, pneumonic granuloma and placentitis with abortion.

The infections most commonly recorded in mycotic abortion are mucormycosis and aspergillosis (12) but infections with *Mortierella wolfii* are also common in cattle in New Zealand (7). This fungus is normally saprophytic and its preferential habitat is overheated, dark-colored, wet, rotting plant material of pH 8–9 (8). It has caused abortion, encephalitis in newborn calves and pneumonia (5) and mastitis (15) in adult cows. *Petriellidium boydii (Allescheria boydii)* also causes mycotic abortion in cattle; it is a significant pathogen in man. It has been found as a dominant denizen of feces in feedlots (9).

Algae

There is a need to record algal infections somewhere in this book even though they are extremely rare. Systemic infections with *Prototheca* sp. (10) and mastitis caused by algae (11) are recorded in cattle and unidentified algae in sheep (16). Poisoning by algae is discussed under that heading.

REVIEW LITERATURE

Kaplan, W. (1973) Epidemiology of the principal systemic mycoses of man and lower animals, and the ecology of their aetiologic agents. *J. Am. vet. med. Assoc.*, *163*, 1043.

Williams, B. M. et al. (1977) Bovine mycotic abortion: some epidemiological aspects. *Vet. Rec.*, *100*, 382.

REFERENCES

(1) Gardner, D. E. (1967) *NZ vet. J.*, *15*, 85.
(2) Turner, P. D. (1965) *Vet. Rec.*, 77, 273.
(3) Hugh-Jones, M. E. & Austwick, P. K. C. (1967) *Vet. Rec.*, *81*, 273.
(4) Cordes, D. O. et al. (1964). *NZ vet.J.*, *12*, 95, 101.
(5) Neilan, M. C. et al. (1982) *Aust. vet. J.*, *59*, 48.
(6) Sheridan, J. J. (1981) *Vet. Res. Commun.*, *5*, 1.
(7) Carter, M. E. et al. (1973) *Res. vet. Sci.*, *14*, 29.
(8) Austwick, P. K. C. (1976) *NZ J. agric. Res.*, *19*, 25.
(9) Bell, R. G. (1976) *Can. J. Microbiol.*, *22*, 552.
(10) Rogers, R. J. (1974) *Aust. vet. J.*, *50*, 281.
(11) Frank, N. et al. (1969) *Am. J. vet. Res.*, *30*, 1785.
(12) Stuker, G. et al. (1979) *Zentralbl. VetMed.*, *26B*, 184.

(13) Werdin, R. E. et al. (1980) *Proc. Ann. Mtg Am. Assoc. Vet. Lab. Diagnosticians*, *23*, 293.
(14) Stuker, G. & Ehrensperger, F. M. (1983) *3rd Int. Symp. World Assoc. Vet. Lab. Diagnosticians*, p. 91.
(15) MacDonald, S. M. & Corbel, M. J. (1981) *Vet. Rec.*, *109*, 419.
(16) Kaplan, W. et al. (1983) *Am. J. trop. Med. Hyg.*, *32*, 405.

Coccidioidomycosis

Coccidioidomycosis is a comparatively benign disease of farm animals, usually causing no apparent illness. Sporadic cases are recorded in all species but are most common in dogs (1) and in cattle (2) and to a much less extent in pigs, sheep and horses (3). The disease is enzootic in the southwestern United States and up to 20% of cattle fattened in feedlots in the area may be affected (3). The incidence of the disease in humans in the area provides a major problem in public health (4, 5).

Coccidioides immitis is the cause of the disease in all species including man but the infection does not spread readily from animals to man, nor from animal to animal. Infection occurs by inhalation of spores of the fungus which grows in the soil, and possibly by ingestion and through cutaneous abrasions (6). The lesions produced in cattle and pigs (7) are granulomatous, contain a cream-colored pus and are sometimes calcified. They are usually observed at necropsy or in abattoirs, and because of their appearance and location in the bronchial, mediastinal and rarely the mesenteric, pharyngeal and submaxillary lymph nodes and in the lungs, they may be mistaken for tuberculosis (8). Similar lesions in sheep bear some similarity to those of caseous lymphadenitis. Microscopic or cultural examination may be required to differentiate these diseases.

Two clinical cases have been recorded in horses (9, 10). In one there was severe emaciation, a fluctuating temperature, edema of the legs, anemia and a leukocytosis. Rupture of the liver caused death. In the other case intermittent colic also occurred and there were peritoneal adhesions at necropsy. Typical lesions were present in the lung, liver and spleen. The clinical disease has been recorded in sheep with fever and abscesses in peripheral lymph nodes. In diagnosis, an extract of the fungus, coccidioidin, has been used in an intradermal sensitivity test, and complement fixation and immunodiffusion tests are used diagnostically in humans (4). Isolation of the organism is preferred as evidence because of the non-specificity of coccidioidin (3). No effective treatment is available. Because infection occurs by the inhalation of soil-borne spores, control of dust in feedlots may help to prevent the spread of the disease. Dust control is a major factor in prevention of human coccidioidomycosis because there is no vaccine or effective therapeutic agent available and the eradication of *C. immitis* from the soil seems highly impracticable (4).

REFERENCES

(1) Maddy, K. T. (1958) *J. Am. vet. med. Assoc.*, *132*, 483.
(2) Prchal, C. J. (1948) *J. Am. vet. Assoc.*, *112*, 461.
(3) Shibatani, M. et al. (1986) *Jap. J. vet. Sci.*, *48*, 155.
(4) Drutz, D. J. (1986) *New Engl. J. Med.*, *314(2)*, 115.
(5) Kaplan, W. (1973) *J. Am. vet. med. Assoc.*, *163*, 1043.
(6) Stiles, G. W. & Davis, C. L. (1942) *J. Am. vet. med. Assoc.*, *119*, 765.
(7) Prchal, C. J. & Crecelius, H. G. (1966) *J. Am. vet. med. Assoc.*, *148*, 1168.
(8) Maddy, K. T. (1954) *J. Am. vet. med. Assoc.*, *124*, 456.
(9) Zontine, W. J. (1958) *J. Am. vet. med. Assoc.*, *132*, 490.
(10) Rehkemper, J. A. (1959) *Cornell Vet.*, *49*, 198.

Mucormycosis (zygomycosis)

Infections of animals with fungi of the family Mucoraceae include infections with the genera *Rhizopus*, *Absidia*, and *Mucor*. Fungal placentitis resulting in abortion has been recorded in cattle (1, 2). Abortions usually occur at 3–7 months. There is necrosis of the maternal cotyledons and the adherent necrotic material gives the placental cotyledon the appearance of a soft, yellow, cushion-like structure, and there are small yellow, raised leathery lesions on the intercotyledonary areas. Corresponding lesions occur on the endometrium and ringworm-like lesions occur on the fetal skin. Hyphae can be seen on examination of direct smears of cotyledons, fetal stomach and skin. If mycotic abortion is suspected the placental cotyledons offer the best source of material. Every effort should be made to obtain the entire placenta as the infection may be patchy and involve only a few cotyledons. The fungi can be cultured on suitable media. Preputial catarrh accompanied by slowness of service and masturbation has been associated with infection in bulls by an *Absidia* spp. fungus thought to be transmitted at coitus.

Granulomatous lesions, typical of those produced by fungal infections, may occur in the mesenteric lymph nodes and intestinal wall in pigs and in submandibular lymph nodes (3). Granulomatous lesions also occur in the mesenteric and mediastinal lymph nodes and other organs of cattle (4). The lesions closely resemble those of tuberculosis and require laboratory examination for accurate differentiation; they usually cause no apparent illness.

Mucormycosis of the alimentary tract occurs relatively commonly in pigs and also in young calves. It is often associated with prolonged antibiotic therapy. In pigs it may be manifested by gastroenteritis with vomiting and diarrhea, or gastritis and gastric ulcer, again manifested by diarrhea and edema, hemorrhage and ulceration at necropsy (5). Esophageal lesions are a common accompaniment (6). Similar outbreaks occur in calves (7, 8) and abomasal infection and ulceration are common lesions. Copper sulfate administered in the drinking water has been an effective agent in controlling the infection.

Primary rumenitis due to lactic acid fermentation after overloading of the rumen with concentrate is often complicated by invasion of the ruminal wall by the *Rhizopus* spp. fungi. The wall becomes much thickened, edematous and black. The lesions may be diffuse or patchy and are usually located in the ventral sac of the rumen. There is necrosis of the cornified epithelium and an extensive peritonitis. Metastases may be present in the liver. Clinically the animal may respond to treatment for acute indigestion but relapses with the development of complete anorexia and ruminal atony and dies 3–4 days later.

Cutaneous candidiasis causing dermatitis has been recorded as a severe outbreak in pigs kept in moist conditions (9).

REFERENCES

(1) Austwick, P. K. C. & Venn, J. A. J.(1962) *Proc. 4th int. Congr. Anim. Reprod., The Hague*, *3*, 562.
(2) Munday, B. L. (1967) *NZ vet. J.*, *15*, 149.
(3) Sanford, S. F. et al. (1985) *J. Am. vet. med. Assoc.*, *186*, 171.
(4) Cordes, D. O. et al. (1967) *NZ vet. J.*, *15*, 143.
(5) Gitter, M. & Austwick, P. K. C. (1959) *Vet. Rec.*, *71*, 6.
(6) Baker, E. D. & Cadman, L. P. (1963) *J. Am. vet. med. Assoc.*, *147*, 763.
(7) Mills, J. H. L. & Hirth, R. S. (1967) *J. vet. med. Assoc.*, *150*, 862.
(8) Smith, J. M. B. (1967) *Sabouraudia*, *5*, 220.
(9) Reynolds, I. M. et al. (1968) *J. Am. vet. med. Assoc.*, *152*, 182.

Aspergillosis

Systemic aspergillosis is uncommon in large animals although *Aspergillus* spp. appears to be a relatively common cause of abortions in cattle (1, 2) and has also been reported in mares (3) and sows (4). In cattle a placentitis, identical to that caused by infection with *Mucor* spp., is a characteristic feature and hyphae can be seen on examination of direct smears of the cotyledon or the fetal stomach, preferably the former. Most abortions occur during the 6th–8th months of pregnancy. Material should be submitted for culture. A dermatomycosis occurs rarely in the aborted fetal calves, with discrete patches of alopecia, covered by a raised, grayish, felted covering occurring all over the body (5). Congenital infection may also accur, granulomatous lesions containing the fungus having been found in the lungs of a day-old lamb (6).

Infection of the placenta is thought to originate from abomasal ulcers or from the respiratory tract which becomes infected by the inhalation of spores from moldy hay or straw or other moist feeds such as beet pulp or brewers' grains which are allowed to go moldy. Infection of the placenta and uterus can be established by intravenous injection during pregnancy (5) but not by intrauterine inoculation before fertilization. Only a proportion of infected animals develop placentitis and this proportion can be increased by increasing the dose of spores injected (7). Mycotic granulomas in the liver and lungs can also be produced experimentally by intravenous injection of the fungus (8).

Invasion of the alimentary tract occurs and is similar to candidiasis. In calves there is a severe fatal gastroenteritis. Areas of necrosis and ulceration occur in the esophagus and forestomachs (9). Although pulmonary aspergillosis is uncommon in animals occasional cases have been recorded in all species, sometimes with generalization (10–12). A high prevalence, 20–80%, has been recorded in calves kept indoors in intensive rearing units. The calves were 4–6 weeks old and subject to the stress of diarrhea, and poor ventilation and temperature control; hypogammaglobulinemia predisposed to the disease (13). A similar experience is recorded in lambs (14). The pulmonary form of the disease appears as a chronic, subacute or acute pneumonia. The acute, fibrinous pneumonia is of very short duration and is accompanied by fever and dyspnea. All forms are usually fatal (15). Occasional cutaneous granulomata, causing lesions similar to those of cutaneous tuberculosis, also occur in cattle. At necropsy the lungs have multiple discrete granulomata often with necrotic centers, giving a superficial resemblance to tuberculosis. In lambs the granulomata appear as very small nodules (1–3 mm diameter) and resemble those caused by infestation with *Muellerius capillaris*. A persistent diarrhea, which responded to treatment with nystatin, has been associated with *Aspergillus fumigatus* infection in foals (16). Response to treatment with nystatin is also recorded in calves with mycotic gastroenteritis (17).

REFERENCES

(1) Dijkstra, R. G. (1963) *Tijdschr. Diergeneeskd.*, *88*, 563.
(2) Austwick, P. K. C. & Venn, J. A. J. (1961) *Proc. 4th int. Congr. Anim. Reprod., The Hague*, *3*, 452.
(3) Mahaffey, L. W. & Adam, N. M. (1964). *J. Am. vet. med. Assoc.*, *144*, 24.
(4) Mason, R. W. (1971) *Aust. vet. J.*, *47*, 18.
(5) Pier, A. C. et al. (1972) *Am. J. vet. Res.*, *33*, 349.
(6) Nobel, T. A. & Shamir, A. (1956) *Refuah Vet.*, *13*, 23.
(7) Day, C. A. & Corbel, M. J. (1974) *Br. J. exp. Pathol.*, *55*, 352.
(8) Whiteman, C. E. et al. (1972) *Vet. Pathol.*, *9*, 408.
(9) Neitzke, J. P. & Schiefer, B. (1974) *Can. vet. J.*, *15*, 139.
(10) Oksanen, A. (1972) *Nord. VetMed.*, *24*, 281.
(11) Gracey, J. F. & Baxter, J. T. (1961) *Br. vet. J.*, *117*, 11.
(12) Chauhan, K. V. S. & Dwivedi, P. (1974) *Vet. Rec.*, *95*, 58.
(13) Praisler, P. & Lupascu, I. (1973) *Rev. Zootech. Med. vet.*, *23*, 69.
(14) Shreeve, B. J. (1976) *Vet. Ann.*, *16*, 78.
(15) Cordes, D. O. et al. (1964) *NZ vet. J.*, *12*, 101.
(16) Lundvall, R. L. & Romberg, P. F. (1960) *J. Am. vet. med. Assoc.*, *137*, 481.
(17) Barinov, V. N. (1971) *Veterinariya, Moscow*, *12*, 70.

Histoplasmosis

Histoplasmosis caused by infection with *Histoplasma capsulatum* is rare in farm animals compared to dogs and is unusual amongst fungal infections in that granulomatous lesions are not produced. Invasion of the cells of the reticuloendothelial system is characteristic of the disease and the lesions consist of groups of macrophages packed with fungal cells. The fungus is able to survive for periods as long as 4 months in soil and water (2). Infection occurs by the inhalation of contaminated dust and primary invasion usually takes place in the lung. The disease may spread from animals to man. Attempts at experimental infection in cattle, sheep, horses and pigs have resulted in non-fatal infections, unless the agent is given intravenously, but the animals become positive to the histoplasmin test (1).

Cases have been recorded in horses, cattle and pigs (3). An affected cow showed chronic emaciation, dyspnea, diarrhea and anasarca. At necropsy there was ascites, enlargement of the liver, considerable edematous thickening of the wall of the large intestine and moderate, pulmonary, interstitial emphysema. Histologically, typical eosinophilic round bodies were seen in endothelial cells in the portal triads. The incidence of hypersensitivity to the cutaneous histoplasmin test was high in other animals in the vicinity. The affected foal showed emaciation, dyspnea and jaundice at 6 months of age. At death there was extensive consolidation of the lungs and gross enlargement of the bronchial lymph nodes. An aborted foal (4) had necrotic foci in the liver and lungs. *Histoplasma* sp. were present and the abortion was thought to be caused by the fungus.

As a diagnostic aid for herd or area use the histoplasmin skin test appears to be satisfactory.

The disease caused by infection with *H. farciminosum* is dealt with under the heading of epizootic lymphangitis (p. 980).

REFERENCES

(1) Saslaw, S. et al. (1960) *Proc. Soc. exp. Biol.*, *105*, 76.
(2) Gabal, M. A. et al. (1983) *Mykosen*, *26*, 481.
(3) Kaplan, W. (1973) *J. Am. vet. med. Assoc.*, *163*, 1043.
(4) Saunders, J. R. et al. (1983) *J. Am. vet. med. Assoc.*, *183*, 1097.

Rhinosporidiosis

Rhinosporidiosis is a chronic disease of the nasal mucosa in cattle and horses causing formation of large polyps in the posterior nares and interference with respiration. The causative fungus, *Rhinosporidia seeberi*, can be found in large sporangia in the polyps.

Nasal granuloma which are thought to be fungal in origin also cause obstruction to respiration in cattle. In these cases the lesions consist of small (0·5–2 cm diameter) nodules, limited in distribution to the mucosa of the anterior third of the nasal cavity. Histologically there is a marked eosinophilic reaction and yeast-like bodies are present in cells or free in the tissue spaces. The fungi have not been positively identified but resemble *Rhinosporidia* spp. Clinically there is severe dyspnea with a mucopurulent nasal discharge, sometimes blood-stained, from both nostrils. The lesions can be easily seen and palpated. The respiration is stertorous and can be heard from quite a distance. A high incidence of the disease may occur on some farms and in particular areas. Rhinosporidiosis of this type has been recorded in the United States (1), Australia (2), India and South America (3).

Clinically the disease resembles nasal obstruction caused by the blood fluke, *Schistosoma nasalis* (4, 5), and chronic allergic rhinitis seen in cattle and sheep. Lesions may also occur on the vaginal and oral mucosae, usually close to the mucocutaneous junction.

REFERENCES

(1) Robinson, V. B. (1951) *Am. J. vet. Res.*, *12*, 85.
(2) Albiston, H. E. & Gorrie, C. J. R. (1935) *Aust. vet. J.*, *11*, 72.
(3) Saunders, L. Z. (1948) *Cornell Vet.*, *38*, 213.
(4) Choudhury, B. (1955) *Ind. vet. J.*, *31*, 403.
(5) Biswal, G. & Das, L. N. (1956) *Ind. vet. J.*, *33*, 204.

Cryptococcosis (European blastomycosis, torulosis)

Infection with the yeast *Cryptococcus neoformans* occurs in most species either as a generalized disease or as a granulomatous meningoencephalitis (1, 2). Several cases of meningitis have been recorded in horses which showed stiffness and hyperesthesia or blindness and incoordination (4, 5). Myxomatous lesions of the nasal mucosa caused by *Crypt. neoformans* infection have been observed in horses and cattle, and pulmonary abscess in horses and goats (6, 7), extensive pneumonia in horses (3, 8), a jejunal granuloma in a horse leading to intussusception (10), and lymphadenitis in cattle have also been recorded. Mastitis caused by *Crypt. neoformans* is described elsewhere. Minute, focal lung lesions developing as metastases from cryptococcal mastitis have been observed in a cow (3) and abortion in a mare and pneumonia in her foal are also recorded (9). In humans an accurate serological test is used in diagnosis.

REFERENCES

(1) Cho, D. Y. et al. (1986) *Vet. Pathol.*, *23*, 207.
(2) Drutz, D. J. (1986) *New Engl. J. Med.*, *314*(2), 115.
(3) Pearson, E. G. et al. (1983) *J. Am. vet. med. Assoc.*, *183*, 577.
(4) Steebel, R. G. et al. (1982) *J. Am. vet. med. Assoc.* *180*, 1085.
(5) Barton, M. D. & Knight, I. (1972) *Aust. vet. J.*, *48*, 534.
(6) Sutmoller, P. & Poelma, F. G. (1957) *W. Ind. med. J.*, *6*, 225.
(7) Dickson, J. & Meyer, E. P. (1970) *Aust. vet. J.*, *46*, 558.
(8) Hibert, B. J. et al. (1980) *Aust. vet. J.*, *56*, 391.
(9) Ryan, M. J. & Wyand, D. S. (1981) *Vet. Pathol*, *18*, 270.
(10) Boulton, C. H. & Williamson, L. (1984) *Equ. vet. J.*, *16*, 548.

Moniliasis (candidiasis)

Moniliasis, caused by infection with the mycelial yeast *Candida albicans*, occurs in malnourished human infants as mycosis of the oral mucosa (thrush). Cases of a similar disease have been observed in baby pigs reared on an artificial diet (1–3). Frequent vomiting and emaciation develop at 2 weeks of age. A white pseudomembrane covers the back of the tongue and extends down the esophagus to the cardia of the stomach. The contents of the stomach and intestines are fluid. The fungus has been isolated from the bedding in pens in which the infection occurred, but it is thought that the fungus is not a primary pathogen, invasion of the mucosa occurring either in association with *E. coli* infection or because of the high sugar content of the artificial diet (4). Treatment of affected piglets with nystatin appears to effect little improvement.

A chronic pneumonia caused by *C. albicans* has been observed at a relatively high level of incidence in cattle in a feedlot (5). Clinical signs are those of pneumonia with a characteristically severe dyspnea which may cause mouth-breathing but only a moderate febrile reaction. Profuse, stringy salivation and a mucopurulent, often brown-streaked, nasal discharge appear. A profuse diarrhea may occur and there may be crusting of the muzzle with dried exudate but there are no discrete ulcerative, erosive or vesicular lesions on the muzzle, nor in the nostrils or mouth. A profuse lacrimal discharge often mats the facial hair but there is no conjunctivitis. The disease is slowly progressive and the animal eventually dies or is slaughtered. At necropsy there is consolidation of the lungs, which may be extreme in advanced cases, and small caseated abscesses are present in the pneumonic tissue. Local lesions may also be present in intestinal wall. The fungus can be seen in smears and sections and can be cultured on special media. *C. parapsilosis* has been implicated as the probable cause of abortion in a cow (6).

REFERENCES

(1) Adamesteanu, I. et al. (1974) *Berl. Münch. Tierärztl. Wochenschr.*, *87*, 28.
(2) Saunders, L. Z. (1984) *Cornell Vet.*, *38*, 213.
(3) Gitter, M. & Austwick, P. K. C. (1959) *Vet. Rec.*, *71*, 6.
(4) Osborne, A. D. et al. (1960) *Vet. Rec.* *72*, 237.
(5) McCarty, R. T. (1956) *Vet. Med.*, *51*, 562.
(6) Bisping, W. et al. (1964) *Berl. Münch. Tierärztl. Wochenschr.*, *77*, 260.

North American blastomycosis

This disease is relatively common in dogs (1) but appears to have been recorded only once in large animals (2). In the affected horse the appearance of a series of abscesses in the perineal region was followed by emaciation and death. In man and in dogs the disease usually takes the form of granulomatous lesions in the lung or on the skin. No effective treatment is available and the disease is an important zoonosis. The causative fungus is *Blastomyces dermatiditis*.

REFERENCES

(1) Kaplan, W. (1973) *J. Am. vet. med. Assoc.*, *163*, 1043.
(2) Benbrook, E. A. et al. (1948) *J. Am. vet. med. Assoc.*, *112*, 475.

DERMATOMYCOSES

Ringworm

Ringworm of the skin is caused by the invasion of the keratinized epithelial cells and hair fibers by dermatophytes.

Etiology

The causative agents are fungi which grow on the hair or skin or both. The common fungi which occur in each species are:

Horse: *Trichophyton equinum*, *Tr. quinckeanum*, *Tr. mentagrophytes*, *Tr. verrucosum*, *Microsporum equinum*, *M. gypseum*
Donkey: *Tr. mentagrophytes* (2)
Cattle: *Tr. verrucosum*, *Tr. mentagrophytes*, *Tr. megnini*, *Tr. verrucosum* var. *album*, *Tr. verrucosum* var. *discoides*
Pig: *Tr. mentagrophytes*, *M. canis*, *Tr. verrucosum* var. *discoides*, *M. nanum*, *Tr. rubrum*
Sheep: *Tr. verrucosum* var. *ochraceum*, *Tr. quinckeanum*, *Tr. mentagrophytes*, *Tr. gypseum*, *M. canis*
Goat: *Tr. verrucosum* (9) commonly with many other sporadic isolations (27).

Trichophyton spp. produce spores in long chains, *Microsporum* spp. produce a mosaic pattern of spores, and both are capable of growth on hair.

Mycotic keratitis occurs rarely in horses. *Aspergillus* and *Fusarium* spp. are recorded in them (26).

Epidemiology

Ringworm occurs in animals in all countries but more commonly where animals are housed in close proximity to each other for long periods. It is relatively rare in sheep and quite rare in goats. Injury to affected animals is of a minor nature and little economic loss occurs. A high incidence of clinical cases in the winter and of spontaneous recovery in the spring is commonly reported. However, outbreaks often occur during the summer months and close confinement and possibly nutrition seem to be more important in the spread of the disease than other environmental factors such as temperature and sunlight. Humidity is known to be important, a high humidity being conducive to multiplication of the fungus. Animal susceptibility is determined largely by immunological status so that young animals are most susceptible (1).

Transmission between species occurs readily and in rural areas 80% of human ringworm may derive from animals. *Trichophyton* spp. infections are commonly contracted from horses and cattle and *M. canis* infections from dogs. Ringworm of animal origin affects adult humans as well as children and diagnosis and treatment are often very difficult.

Largely because of the developing interest in comparative mycology and the transmission of dermatomycoses from animals to man, an increasing number of previously unidentified fungi are being found in cutaneous lesions in animals. Three such fungi are *M. gypseum* in horses, *Keratinomyces allejoi* in horses and *Scopulariopsis brevicaulis* in cattle. Of particular interest is the observation of a widespread infection of pigs with *M. nanum* in which the lesions are often so mild as to go unnoticed by the farmer. The disease occurs chiefly in adult pigs.

Direct contact with infected animals is a common method of spread of ringworm and licking with the tongue undoubtedly aids spread of the fungus (8). However, indirect contact with any inanimate objects, particularly bedding, harness, grooming kits and horse blankets, is probably more important. Spores can exist on the skin without causing lesions, and 'carrier animals' of this type may act as important sources of infection. Premises and harness may remain infective for long periods because fungal spores can remain viable for years provided they are kept dry and cool. Moderate heat and desiccation destroy them (4).

M. gypseum, *K. allejoi* and *M. nanum* are soil saprophytes and the reasons for their assumption of pathogenicity are not understood.

Pathogenesis

Ringworm fungi attack chiefly keratinized tissues, particularly the stratum corneum and hair fibers resulting in autolysis of the fiber structure, breaking off of the hair and alopecia. Exudation from invaded epithelial layers, epithelial debris and fungal hyphae produce the dry crusts characteristic of the disease. The lesions progress if suitable environmental conditions for mycelial growth exist, including a warm humid atmosphere, and a slightly alkaline pH of the skin. Ringworm fungi are all strict aerobes and the fungi die out under the crust in the center of most lesions leaving only the periphery active. It is this mode of growth which produces the centrifugal progression and the characteristic ring form of the lesions.

The significance of skin pH in the development of ringworm is widely known. The susceptibility of humans to ringworm infection is much greater before puberty than afterwards when the skin pH falls from about 6·5 to about 4·0. This change is largely due to excretion of fatty acids in the sebum and these fatty acids are often highly fungistatic. For this reason some treatments for human ringworm are based on ointments containing propionic and undecylenic acids. Calves are more commonly infected than adult cattle but whether this is due to increased susceptibility in calves or the development of immunity in adults has not been determined.

Secondary bacterial invasion of hair follicles is common. The period after experimental infection before distinct lesions appear is about 4 weeks in calves, but considerably less in horses. Spontaneous recovery occurs in calves in 2–4 months, the duration and severity of the disease often depending upon the nutritional status of the host. A resistance to reinfection occurs after recovery from experimental or natural infection even though a local mycotic dermatitis may occur at the reinfection site. The immunity is specific to the fungal species concerned, and in horses lasts up to 2 years (6). The development of immunity and allergic dermatitis due to ringworm fungi has been reviewed (2).

Clinical findings

Cattle

The typical lesion is a heavy, gray-white crust raised perceptibly above the skin. The lesions are roughly circular and about 3 cm in diameter. In the early stages the surface below the crust is moist, in older lesions the scab becomes detached and pityriasis and alopecia may be the only obvious abnormalities. Lesions are most commonly found on the neck, head and perineum but a general distribution over the entire body may occur, particularly in calves, and in severe cases the lesions may coalesce. Itching does not occur and secondary acne is unusual.

Horses

The lesions may be superficial or deep. Superficial infections are more common. Lesions due to *T. equinum* commence as round patches of raised hair and soreness of the lesions to touch. This stage is followed about 7 days later by matting of the hair, which becomes detached leaving a bald, gray, shining area about 3 cm in diameter. Fine scabs appear and recovery with regrowth of hair commences in 25–30 days. Heavier scabs and larger lesions are usually due to rubbing by harness. Lesions caused by *M. gypseum* are smaller, about 10 mm in diameter (3), and are manifested either by the development of thick crusts, or more generally a diffuse moth-eaten appearance with desquamation and alopecia. Less commonly, deeper structures are infected through the hair follicles causing small foci of inflammation and suppuration. A small scab forms over the follicle and the hair is lost but extensive alopecia and crust formation do not occur. Some irritation and itching may be caused by this type. The distribution of lesions in the horse differs from that in cows, lesions usually appearing first on the axillary girth area and spreading generally over the trunk and over the rump and may spread to the neck, head and limbs.

Pigs

Ringworm lesions in pigs develop as a centrifugally progressing ring of inflammation surrounding a scabby, alopecic center. The cutaneous lesion produced in pigs by *M. nanum* differs from the standard lesions of ringworm in this species. There is an absence of pruritus and alopecia and a minimal cutaneous reaction due to the superficial nature of the lesion. There is a characteristic centrifugal enlargement of each lesion which may reach an enormous size. Superficial, dry, brown crusts cover the affected area but are not obviously raised except at the edges in some cases. The crusts are formed of flakes or dust composed of epithelial debris. Most lesions occur on the back and sides. Spontaneous recovery does not occur in adult pigs.

Sheep

In sheep the lesions occur on the head and although they usually disappear in 4–5 weeks the disease may persist in the flock for some months. The lesions are discrete, round, almost bald patches covered with a grayish crust (21). Similar lesions occur in goats, but they are distributed generally over all parts of the body.

Clinical pathology

Laboratory diagnosis depends upon the examination of skin scrapings for spores and mycelia by direct microscopic means and by culture. Skin scrapings should be made after defatting the skin with ether or alcohol if greasy dressings have been used. Scrapings are warmed gently in a 20% solution of either potassium or sodium hydroxide. Spores are the diagnostic feature and appear as round or polyhedral, highly refractile bodies in chains (*Trichophyton* spp.) or mosaics (*Microsporum* spp.) in hair follicles, epithelial scales, and in or on the surface of hair fibers.

Examination of the skin of infected animals to detect the fluorescence caused by some fungal infections can also be a useful clinical aid. A source of possible error in this test is that many trichophyton fungi do not fluoresce, whereas petroleum jelly and other oily skin dressings may do so. The examination is made with a Wood's filter in front of a source of short-wave, ultraviolet light. A green fluorescence indicates hairs infected with ringworm fungi. Hairs which fluoresce should be selected for laboratory examination. A home laboratory technique has been developed for the cultural diagnosis of ringworm infection. It incorporates an easily read color change of the medium as a positive diagnosis. It has some limitations in animal work and should not be depended on for a final decision (20).

Specimens to be sent for laboratory examination should be packed in envelopes, as airtight jars and cans favor the growth of non-pathogenic fungi.

Diagnosis

The diagnosis of ringworm depends on evidence of infectivity, the appearance of characteristic lesions and the presence of fungal mycelia and spores. Clinically it may be confused with mycotic dermatitis in cattle, and in pigs with pityriasis rosea, exudative epidermitis and dermatitis caused by infestations with *Tyroglyphus* spp. mites. The two former diseases are common only in young pigs; *M. nanum* infection is rare in pigs of this age. Examination of skin scrapings may be necessary to differentiate ringworm from mange and miscellaneous cutaneous infections.

A rare but similar disease is tinea versicolor dermatomycosis reported in goats (22). The lesions are circular, discrete, slightly thickened and scaly at the edges but not painful. They are characterized by an alteration in the color of the surrounding skin, either darker or lighter (24).

Treatment

Experimental work suggests that the treatments in current use have little effect on individual lesions and that most recorded cures are due to strategic treatment just prior to spontaneous recovery (3). However, treatment is still widely practiced and has the advantage that the contamination of the environment by infected animals is greatly reduced. Local or systemic treatments are used, the latter when lesions are widespread.

For local application the crusts should be removed by scraping or brushing with a soft wire brush and the medicament brushed or rubbed in vigorously. Care should be taken that the scrapings are removed and burnt. Suitable topical applications include a weak solution of iodine, Whitfield's ointment, 10% ammoniated mercury ointment, and solutions of quaternary ammonium compounds (1 in 200 to 1 in 1000). Ointments containing propionic and undecylenic acids and their esters are effective, non-irritant and control secondary bacterial invasion. Rapid and effective cure of affected cattle, horses and pigs is claimed with two to three applications at 3–4 day intervals of 0·25% hexadecamethylene-1:16-*bis*, isoquinolinium chloride (Tinevet). The preparation is best applied with a stiff brush and removal of thin scabs may not be necessary. Hexetidine (*bis*-1,3 beta-ethyl-hexyl-5-methyl 5 amino-hexa-hydropyrimidine), is reputed to be highly successful in young calves following one treatment. Borotannic complex is also an effective fungicide and has given good results in the treatment of equine ringworm. It has the particular advantage of being in a solvent—ethyl acetate and alcohol—which is a strong skin penetrant. Thiabendazole ointment, two to four applications of a 2–4% ointment or as a suspension in glycerine, 3–5 days apart, gives excellent results (23). Local aqueous preparations and oral dosing with the anthelmintic are ineffectual. Failure of the preparation to combat new infections may account for some of the bad results reported (5). An antibiotic with antifungal capacity, natamycin, has been used successfully for topical application to horses with ringworm (19). The material was sponged on twice at 4-day intervals and at a concentration of 100 ppm (0·01%). The preparation is odorless and non-irritant. Spraying of cattle with 0·1% solution also gave excellent results using 0·75–1·51 per spraying for two sprayings at 3–4 day intervals (17). A similar protocol using 0·01% suspension is also successful. Ketoconazole, a product used orally in the treatment of cutaneous fungal infections in humans, should be effective in animals (14).

The above topical treatments are probably of greater value in the early stages of an outbreak when the lesions are small and few in number. When infection in a group is widespread, washes or sprays which can be applied over the entire body surface of all animals are preferred. For example agricultural Bordeaux mixture has given good results in the control of ringworm in large groups of horses. Copper sulfate 2 kg and unslaked lime 2 kg should be dissolved in separate solutions and mixed in a wooden or earthenware container and made up to 180 liters. Spraying with a handspray at weekly intervals gives good results. Similarly a spray of 5% lime sulfur (20% w/v polysulfides diluted 1 in 20) is applied daily for 5 days, and harness and gear are soaked in it after defatting with soap and hot water. Captan (N-trichloromethyl-mercapto-4-cyclo-hexene-1,2-dicarboxamide) in a concentration of 1 in 300 to 1 in 400 has been used successfully in the control of ringworm in cattle when applied at the rate of 4–7 liters per animal on two occasions 2 weeks apart. Another preparation which has given good results when used as a spray for affected horses and their harness is N-trichloromethylthico-tetrahydrophthalamide; 60 g of a 45% solution of this compound are mixed with 13 liters of water and applied daily as a spray or wash to the horses and the harness scrubbed with it. One study of topical treatments in horses showed that washes of any sort were ineffective and some ointments, including 10% nystatin, and some lotions such as 10% iodine fortis, 10% Medol, were also ineffective. Povidone-iodine, and thiabendazole and captan ointments were effective (3).

A systemic treatment in common use in farm animals is the intravenous injection of sodium iodide (1 g/14 kg body weight) as a 10% solution. More than one injection is often required and should be accompanied by topical application of fungistatic agents. Another systemic approach to the treatment of ringworm is the oral administration of griseofulvin. The original recommendation for calves of 0·25 g/kg body weight daily for 7–10 days was economically impracticable but a good response has subsequently been obtained from much smaller doses (5–7·5 mg/kg body weight daily for 7 days (12) and a similar regimen for horses (11). A dose rate of 1 g/100 kg body weight has been recommended for pigs with a 30–40 day course of treatment (7). A fine particle preparation is used which can be given by drench or in the feed. It is highly effective and is now marketed as a premix of crude mycelia which is economically attractive. Another griseofulvin-like antibiotic, tricothecin, is on trial.

Spontaneous recovery is common in individual animals and careful appraisal of results in clinical trials is necessary. Carefully controlled trials suggest that the main virtue of topical applications with any fungicide to ringworm lesions in calves is 'to curtail the extension of recent lesions and limit the dissemination of infective material'. Many farmers overtreat their animals with irritant preparations administered daily for long periods. A crusty dermatitis, or even a neoplastic acanthosis may result which is not unlike ringworm.

Control

Failure to control an outbreak of ringworm is usually due to the widespread contamination of the environment before treatment is attempted. Isolation and treatment of infected animals, the provision of separate grooming tools, horse blankets and feeding utensils, and disinfection of the items after use on affected animals are necessary if the disease is to be controlled. Cleaning and disinfection of stables with a commercial detergent or a strong solution (2·5–5%) of phenolic disinfectant or sodium hypochlorite (0·25% solution) is advisable where practicable. Good results are also claimed for the disinfection of buildings with a spray containing 2·0% formaldehyde and 1·0% caustic soda. In a control program this is combined with spraying of all cattle in the herd, using a similar solution (0·4% formaldehyde plus 0·5% caustic soda), twice at intervals of a week.

There is an increasing interest in the use of vaccines against bovine ringworm. A Russian vaccine LTF-130 has achieved a great deal of success in most countries of Europe and Scandinavia (16, 18). Vaccination of all animals in the group is recommended. A live vaccine prepared from a highly immunogenic strain of *Tr. faviforme* is favorably reported (13). Only moderately good results are recorded with a killed vaccine. All round best results are achieved when vaccination is carried out in newly infected herds with few clinical cases. Herds with a longstanding problem usually react disappointingly.

The vaccine is almost totally without side-effects except for very rare deaths due to anaphylaxis apparently related to keeping reconstituted vaccine for too long a period. Existing cases of ringworm may be exacerbated (16). A live vaccine of *Trichophyton equinum* has also produced good results in prophylaxis in horses (15). Oral administration to calves of 7·5 mg/kg body weight of griseofulvin/kg, gave moderately good protection against infection with *T. verrucosum* (25).

Although ringworm occurs in well-nourished as well as poorly fed animals, there does seem to be a tendency for the latter to become infected more readily and to develop more extensive lesions. Supplementation of the diet, particularly with vitamin A to young housed animals, should be encouraged as a preventive measure.

REFERENCES

(1) Pascoe, R. R. (1979) *Aust. vet. J.*, *55*, 403.
(2) Ali, K. E. M. et al. (1981) *Ann. trop. Med. Parasitol.*, *75*, 623.
(3) Pascoe, R. R. (1984) *Aust. vet. J.*, *61*, 231.
(4) Hashimoto, T. & Blumenthal, H. J. (1978) *Appl. envir. Microbiol.*, 35, 274.
(5) Pascoe, R. R. (1974) *Aust. vet. J.*, *50*, 380.
(6) Petrovich, S. V. & Andryushin, V. V. (1979) *Veterinariya, Moscow*, *10*, 67.
(7) Kielstein, P. & Gottschalk, C. (1970) *Mh. VetMed.*, *25*, 127, 130.
(8) Edwardson, J. & Andrews, A. H. (1979) *Vet. Rec.*, *104*, 474.
(9) Philpot, C. M. & Arbuckle, J. B. R. (1983) *Vet. Rec.*, *112*, 550.
(10) Andryushin, V. V. (1980) *Veterinariya, Moscow*, 6, 40.
(11) Reuss, U. (1978) *Dtsch Tierärztl. Wochenschr.*, *85*, 231.
(12) Reuss, U. (1978) *Tierärztl. Umschau*, *33*, 85.
(13) Tornquist, M. et al. (1985) *Acta. vet. Scand.*, *26*, 21.
(14) Gabal, M. A. (1986) *Am. J. vet. Res.*, *47*, 1229.
(15) Petrovich, S. V. & Sarkisov, A. K. (1981) *Veterinariya, Moscow*, No. 9, 40.
(16) Gudding, R. & Naess, B. (1986) *Am. J. vet. Res.*, *47*, 2415.
(17) Oldenkamp, E. P. (1982) *Proc. 12th World Cong. Dis. Cattle*, vol. 2, p. 922.
(18) Naess, B. & Sandvik, O. (1981) *Vet. Rec.*, *109*, 199.
(19) Oldenkamp, E. P. (1979) *Equ. vet. J.*, *11*, 36.
(20) Dion, W. M. (1978) *Can. vet. J.*, *19*, 203.
(21) Kuttin, E. S. et al. (1974) *Refuah Vet.*, *31*, 190.
(22) Bliss, E. L. (1984) *J. Am. vet. med. Assoc.*, *184*, 1512.
(23) Pandey, V. S. (1979) *Trop. Anim. Hlth Prod.*, *11*, 175.
(24) Wolfe, D. F. et al. (1984) *J. Am. vet. med. Assoc.*, *184*, 1511.
(25) Andrews, A. H. & Edwardson, J. (1981) *Vet. Rec.*, *108*, 498.
(26) Kern, T. J. et al. (1983) *Equ. vet. J.*, Suppl 2, p. 33.
(27) Scott, D. W. et al. (1984) *Comp. cont. Educ.*, 6, S190.

Epizootic lymphangitis (pseudoglanders, equine blastomycosis, equine histoplasmosis)

Epizootic lymphangitis is a chronic, contagious disease of horses characterized by suppurative lymphangitis, lymphadenitis and ulcers of the skin and by keratitis or pneumonia. The disease is of importance both in its own right and because of its similarity to glanders.

Etiology

A fungus *Histoplasma* (or *Zymonema*, *Cryptococcus*, *Saccharomyces*, *Blastomyces*) *farciminosum* is the cause of the disease.

Epidemiology

The disease occurs chiefly in Asia, Africa and the Mediterranean littoral. It occurs in outbreaks rather than as an enzootic disease and although not highly fatal (the mortality rate is 10–15%), the course is prolonged and loss of function of affected animals can cause serious economic loss. Most outbreaks occur when large numbers of horses are gathered together for military or other purposes.

Horses and rarely cattle and man are the species affected, horses under 6 years of age being most susceptible. In enzootic areas most cases occur during the autumn and winter.

Fungal spores are carried from infected animals by direct contact or on inanimate objects such as bedding, grooming utensils, horse blankets or harness, and gain entry through cutaneous abrasions. A saprophytic stage in the soil has been suggested to account for the difficulty experienced in eradicating the disease. Because of the frequent occurrence of abrasions on the lower limbs lesions are most commonly seen in this area. The organism has been isolated from the alimentary tract of biting flies and their possible role in the transmission of the disease has been suggested (1).

Pathogenesis

There has always been a question about the pathogenesis of this disease. Is it a systemic disease or a disease of many forms, the cutaneous being one? The latter seems the more likely on the evidence and the disease might be best defined as 'being associated with *H. farciminosum* infection', and named equine histoplasmosis.

The fungus invades subcutaneous tissue, sets up a local granuloma or ulcer and spreads along the lymphatic vessels (3).

Clinical findings
In the cutaneous form of the disease an indolent ulcer develops at the portal of entry, making its appearance several weeks to 3 months after infection occurs. Lymphatic vessels leaving the ulcer become thickened and enlarged and develop nodules along their course. These nodules rupture discharging a thick creamy pus. Local lymph nodes also enlarge and may rupture. Thickening of the skin in the area and general swelling of the whole limb are common. The lesions are quite painless.

In most cases the lesions develop on the limbs particularly about the hocks but may also be present on the back, sides, neck, vulva and scrotum. Occasionally lesions appear on the nasal mucosa, due usually to nibbling of lesions on the trunk and limbs, but are situated just inside the nostrils and do not involve the nasal septum. Ocular involvement, manifested by keratitis and conjunctivitis, and sinusitis and primary pneumonia occur in other forms of the disease.

The disease is chronic, persisting for 3–12 months, and affected animals lose much condition and cannot be worked. Spontaneous recovery occurs and immunity is solid after an attack but many animals are destroyed because of the chronic nature of the disease.

Clinical pathology
Gram-positive, yeast-like cells, with a characteristic double-walled capsule are easily found in discharges but this is not a sure diagnostic method. The agent can be cultured on special media but the fungus dies quickly in specimens unless these are collected in antibiotic solutions, refrigerated and cultured promptly. The specimen should be collected into a solution containing 500 units/ml penicillin. The mallein test is negative but a sterile filtrate of a culture of *H. farciminosum* has been used in a cutaneous sensitivity test (8) and several serological tests, including a fluorescent antibody test (4) are available (2).

Necropsy findings
Lesions are usually confined to the skin, subcutaneous tissues, and lymph vessels and nodes. In some cases granulomatous lesions may be found in the lungs, liver and spleen (5).

Diagnosis
Because of its characteristic clinical picture including cutaneous ulceration, lymphadenitis and lymphangitis, the disease may be confused with glanders. However, there is no systemic reaction, and rarely pulmonary involvement, lesions do not occur on the nasal septum and the pus is creamy. In ulcerative lymphangitis the pus is greenish, the lesions usually occur about the fetlocks and heal quickly. In sporotrichosis only small amounts of pus are discharged from the lesions and there is often no lymphatic involvement, but differentiation should be made only on the basis of laboratory examinations.

Treatment
Many treatments have been tried, largely without success. Early cases can be cured by extensive excision of affected parts followed by frequent local applications of silver nitrate or tincture of iodine. Parenteral iodides have been reported as effective in some cases (6).

Control
Strict hygienic precautions must be observed. Outbreaks in uninfected areas are probably best controlled by slaughter of affected animals. In enzootic areas severe cases should be destroyed and less severe cases kept in strict quarantine while undergoing treatment. All infected bedding, harness and utensils should be destroyed or vigorously disinfected. A formolized aluminum hydroxide adsorbed vaccine has been reported to give serviceable immunity (7).

REFERENCES

(1) Singh, T. et al. (1965) *Ind. J. vet. Sci.*, *35*, 102, 111.
(2) Abou-Gabal, M. & Khalifa, D. (1983) *Mykosen*, *26*, 89.
(3) Khater, A. R. et al. (1968) *J.Egypt. vet. med. Assoc.*, *28*, 165.
(4) Abou-Gagal, M. et al. (1983) *Zentralbl. VetMed.*, *30*, 283.
(5) Fawi, M. T. (1971) *Sabouraudia*, 9, 123.
(6) Singh, S. (1956) *Ind. vet.J.*, *32*, 260.
(7) Noskov, A. I. (1960) *Trudӯ vses. Inst. Vet. Sanit.*, *16*, 368.
(8) Soliman, R. et al. (1985) *Mykosen*, *28*, 457.

Sporotrichosis

Sporotrichosis is a contagious disease of horses characterized by the development of cutaneous nodules and ulcers on the limbs and may or may not be accompanied by lymphangitis.

Etiology
The cause of the disease, *Sporotrichum schencki* (*Sporothrix beurmannii*, *S. schencki*, *S. equi*), is a Gram-positive fungus, which forms single-walled spores.

Epidemiology
The disease is reported to occur in Europe, India and the United States. Economic loss caused by sporotrichosis is not great because the disease spreads slowly, the mortality rate is low, and treatment is effective. Rare cases have been reported in man. Horses are the only species commonly affected but cases have been recorded in man, dogs, cats, camels and cattle (1).

The causative agent persists in organic matter and contamination of cutaneous wounds can occur either by direct contact with discharges from infected animals, or directly from contaminated surroundings. The disease spreads slowly and only sporadic cases occur in a group.

Pathogenesis
Local invasion through cutaneous wounds results in the development of abscesses and discharging ulcers.

Clinical findings
Multiple,small, cutaneous nodules develop on the lower parts of the legs, usually about the fetlock. The nodules are painless, develop a scab on the summit, discharge a small amount of pus and heal in 3–4 weeks. Succeeding crops of lesions may cause the disease to persist in the animal for months. Lymphangitis, causing cording of

the lymphatics, occurs in some outbreaks and not in others.

Clinical pathology
Gram-positive spores are present in the discharges but they may be few in number and difficult to find, and diagnosis by culture of pus is preferred. The hyphal stage is rare in tissues. Injection of pus into rats or hamsters produces a local lesion containing large numbers of the yeast-like cells. This may be of value when organisms are scarce in the pus from natural lesions.

Diagnosis
The disease occurs only sporadically in affected groups of animals and this helps to differentiate it from glanders, epizootic lymphangitis and ulcerative lymphangitis. In cases where there is lymphangitis identification of the yeast-like cells is necessary to complete the diagnosis. Maduromycotic mycetoma, in which small (0·5–1·0 cm in diameter) nodules are present in the skin over most of the body has been reported in the horse (2). A few lesions discharge exudate; section of the nodules shows dark brown specks in pale pink tissue. The causative fungus has been identified as *Brachycladium spiciferum* Bainier.

Treatment
Systemic treatment with iodides (potassium iodide orally or sodium iodide intravenously) is the most effective treatment. Local application of tincture of iodine daily to ulcers may suffice in mild cases. A good response has been recorded in one case in a horse, which did not respond to iodine therapy, after the oral administration of griseofulvin (3). Natamycin therapy as described under ringworm should be effective.

Control
Prophylactic treatment of all cuts and abrasions, isolation and treatment of clinical cases, and disinfection of bedding, harness and gear will prevent spread of the disease in enzootic areas.

REFERENCES

(1) Saunders, L. Z. (1948) *Cornell Vet.*, *38*, 213.
(2) Bridges, C. H. & Beazley, J. N. (1960) *J. Am vet. med. Assoc.*, *137*, 192.
(3) Davis, H. H. & Worthington, W. E. (1964) *J. Am. vet. med. Assoc.*, *145*, 692.

Swamp cancer (equine phycomycosis, cutaneous pithyosis, hyphomycosis destruens, Florida horse leech, bursattee)

This is a common lesion of the skin and mucosae of horses and rarely cattle in tropical climates and caused by a variety of agents, chiefly fungi.

Etiology
The causes include infestation with *Habronema megastoma* larvae, or fungi including especially *Pythium* spp. (syn. *Hyphomyces destruens*), *Basidiobolus haptosporus* (6) (syn. *B. haptosporus* var. *minor*) (4), *Conidiobolus coronatus* (syn. *Entomophthora coronata*). Unidentified fungi also cause lesions containing black-colored granules or grains, the so-called 'black-grain mycetomas' (5). *B. haptosporus* is a terrestrial fungus which lives in decaying vegetation but it can parasitize the alimentary tract of wild animals including kangaroos (8).

Epidemiology
The disease occurs only in tropical and semitropical climates and the incidence is highest in summer and when the insect population is heaviest. The lesions caused by *H. megastoma* tend to regress in cold weather. In particular areas the local cause of the disease may be one or a combination of those listed. A survey in tropical northern Australia showed the prevalence as: *H. destruens* 77%, *B. haptosporus* 18%, *C. coronatus* 5% (11). Although the disease is recorded most commonly in horses it does occur in young cattle (9). The lesions occur on the limbs and lower abdomen and resemble the lesions in horses except that grains are infrequent.

Pathogenesis
The lesions are phycomycoses or chronic granulomas with masses of yellow-gray necrotic tissue containing hyphae or larvae and many eosinophils located in fistulae in dense connective tissue. These grains, leeches, kunkurs or bursattee are easily removable intact and may be calcified. They are more frequent in the lesions caused by *Pythium* spp.

Clinical findings
The lesions are granulomas with a raised edge and a raw granulating center. Initially they appear as small intracutaneous nodules and subsequently enlarge peripherally and develop into ulcerating, subcutaneous granulomas which are itchy and may be further traumatized. The enlargement may be very rapid and reach 20 cm in diameter within a few weeks. The lesions are most common on the limbs and lower abdomen, below the medial canthus of the eye, on the alae nasi, lips and the neck. The fungal lesions are not commonly found on the legs, but the parasitic ones are found there commonly. Lesions caused by *C. coronatus* are most common on the skin around the nostrils, on the nasal mucosa, and on the lips. They contain small grains.

Clinical pathology
Culture of the causative fungus is a laborious task and other diagnostic tests are being developed. Horses infected with *H. destruens* show a positive reaction to an agar gel double diffusion test, and complement fixation and intradermal hypersensitivity tests are also of diagnostic value (10). Examination of a biopsy specimen is also of value but care is needed to include a portion of necrotic tissue in which either the larvae or hyphae are most likely to be found.

Diagnosis
The disease is easily diagnosed from its physical appearance but differentiation into its etiological entities presents difficulties unless laboratory services are available.

Treatment
The simplest and most satisfactory treatment is surgical excision when the lesion is small (2) although recurrence is common unless the excision is complete (3). Larger lesions are usually treated medically. Treatment of the

parasitic lesion is described in the section on cutaneous habronemiasis. Fungal lesions respond to treatment intravenously with sodium iodide (1 g/13 kg body weight) or orally with potassium iodide (6–10 g daily for 7 days). Amphotericin also gives good results as a systemic treatment (intravenously 0·4 mg/kg body weight increasing to 1·5 mg/kg/day for 10–40 days) combined with local infiltration and after surgical excision in extensive lesions (1).

A vaccine composed of elements of the fungus has been used in the treatment of horses with lesions caused by *H. destruens*. It causes recovery or improvement in most cases, but also causes a severe reaction, sometimes a cold abscess, at the injection site. Other complications include osteitis and laminitis which necessitate euthanasia (7). Surgical excision results in a higher proportion of recoveries (12).

REVIEW LITERATURE

Miller, R. I. & Campbell, R. S. F. (1984) The comparative pathology of equine cutaneous phycomycosis. *Vet. Pathol.*, *21*, 325–332.

REFERENCES

(1) McMullan, W. C. et al. (1977) *J. Am. vet. med. Assoc.*, *170*, 1293.
(2) Hutchins, D. R. & Johnston, K. G. (1972) *Aust. vet. J.*, *48*, 269.
(3) Chauhan, H. V. S. (1973) *Vet. Rec.*, *92*, 425.
(4) Connole, M. D. (1973) *Aust. vet. J.*, *49*, 214.
(5) Boomker, J. et al. (1977) *Onderstepoort J. vet. Res.*, *44*, 249.
(6) Owens, W. R. et al. (1985) *J. Am. vet. med. Assoc.*, *186*, 703.
(7) Miller, R. I. (1983) *J. Am. vet. med. Assoc.*, *182*, 1227.
(8) Speare, R. & Thomas, A. D. (1985) *Aust. vet. J.*, *62*, 209.
(9) Miller, R. I. et al. (1985) *J. Am. vet. med. Assoc.*, *186*, 984.
(10) Miller, R. I. & Campbell, R. S. F. (1982) *Aust. vet. J.*, *58*, 227.
(11) Miller, R. I. & Campbell, R. S. F. (1982) *Aust. vet. J.*, *58*, 221.
(12) Miller, R. I. (1981) *Aust. vet. J.*, *57*, 377.

Maduromycosis

This is a skin disease of horses characterized by cutaneous granuloma caused by a variety of fungi including *Helminthosporium spiciferum*, *Brachycladium spiciferum*, *Curvularia geniculata*, *Monosporium apiospermum*. There are one or more lesions 1–2·5 cm diameter anywhere on the skin but with a special frequency at the coronet. The incised lesion has a mottled appearance and drains pus which contains the fungus.

25

Diseases Caused by Protozoa

Babesiosis (Texas fever, redwater fever, cattle tick fever)

BABESIOSIS includes those diseases caused by *Babesia* spp. in cattle, sheep, pigs and horses. They are all characterized by fever and intravascular hemolysis causing a syndrome of anemia, hemoglobinemia and hemoglobinuria, and are transmitted by blood-sucking ticks.

Etiology

The nomenclature of these intraerythrocytic parasites is still subject to change, but the following list represents the classification in general use at the present time:

Cattle: *Babesia bovis* (includes *B. argentina*, *B. berbera*), *B. bigemina*, *B. major*, *B. divergens*
Water buffaloes: (*Bubalis bubalis*), *B. bovis*, *B. bigemina*
Sheep and goats: *B. motasi*, *B. ovis*
Pigs: *B. trautmanni*, *B. perroncitoi*
Horses: *B. equi*, *B. caballi*.

There are some serological relationships between these species which suggest that the distinctions between them are not complete. There are also some antigenic variant strains within the species. These discrepancies in identification and in antigenicity may raise some problems when vaccines are being prepared (4). Preservation of live protozoa is difficult. Cryopreservation has been achieved by using tick nymphs as a source of babesia (58). Also, *B. bovis* has been cultured in a medium containing infected bovine erythrocytes (18, 45).

Epidemiology

Geographical distribution

The distribution of the causative protozoa is governed by the geographical distribution of the insect vectors that transmit them.

Bovine babesiosis In general terms *B. bigemina* and *B. bovis* are infections of the tropics and subtropics. *B. major* and *B. divergens* are denizens of temperate regions. More detailed information includes the following: *B. bigemina* occurs in South America, the West Indies, Australia and Africa; *B. bovis* (*argentina*) in the tropics including South and Central America, Australia, Asia and southern Europe. *B. divergens* occurs in north-west Europe, Spain, Eire, and it is the principal cause of babesiosis in the United Kingdom. *B. bovis* occurs in Europe, South America and Africa; *B. berbera* in mediterranean Europe and north Africa; *B. major* in the United Kingdom and Europe.

Ovine babesiosis This is caused by *B. motasi* and by *B. ovis* and occurs in south-eastern Europe, Africa and South America. The babesiosis in sheep in the United Kingdom has not been identified (6).

Porcine babesiosis This is caused by *B. trautmanni* and *B. perroncitoi* and occurs in south-eastern Europe and Africa.

Equine babesiosis This is caused by *B. equi* and *B. caballi* and occurs in Asia and the Americas.

Wild animals Serological surveys show that red deer can be infected with babesia (47), and American bison in a fauna park in the United Kingdom have been found to be infected with *B. major* (59).

Transmission

Ticks are the natural vectors of babesiosis and the causative parasites persist and pass through part of their lifecycle in the invertebrate host. Both *B. bovis* (*argentina*) and *B. bigemina* pass part of their lifecycle in the tick *Boophilus microplus* which is the only vector in Australia. In Africa, *B. decoloratus* is the vector. *Boophilus* (*Margaropus*) *annulatus* and *B. microplus* are the major vectors of babesiosis, but other *Boophilus*, *Rhipicephalus* and *Haemaphysalis* spp. also act as vectors. *Ixodes ricinus* is the common carrier of *B. divergens* in the United Kingdom (16). There is an extensive literature on tick vectors of babesiosis and it is not reviewed here. *Rhipicephalus* spp. are the vectors in sheep; *Dermacentor*, *Rhipicephalus*, and *Hyalomma* spp. are the vectors in horses; and *Rhipicephalus* and *Boophilus* spp. are the vectors in pigs.

A knowledge of the life-history of the tick is most important in applied control. Those ticks which parasitize only one host are easier to eradicate and cause less spread of the disease than those which parasitize two or three hosts. Control of ticks which are capable of surviving on both domestic and wild animals presents a major problem.

For many years tick control as a tool for redwater control has been based on the assumption that *Babesia* sp. survive in insect vectors for several generations of those insects, without the need of a vertebrate host in the cycle. This may occur with some species of *Babesia*, but the important parasite, *B. bovis*, does not persist in *B. microplus* as an infectious agent beyond the larval stage (57). Transovarial passage does occur from the engorged adult to the larvae, but does not persist beyond that stage. This persistence, or lack of it, is an important characteristic and must be determined for each *Babesia* sp. and each insect vector if control programs are to be soundly based.

B. bigemina and *B. caballi* do persist through several generations of ticks, in *Boophilus microplus* and *Dermacentor nitens* (19) respectively, and *B. bigemina* and *B. bovis (berbera)* are transmitted transovarially in *Boophilus annulatus* (11).

Contaminated needles and surgical instruments can transmit the infection physically. The ease with which infection can be transmitted in this way depends largely on the degree of parasitemia which occurs with each species. Thus, the chances of physical transmission are slight with *B. bovis* and high with *B. equi* and *B. bigemina*.

Susceptibility to infection

Strong immunity occurs after natural infection with most *Babesia* sp. If the infection recurs repeatedly the immunity is permanent. If it is treated urgently and efficiently and the protozoa are killed before antibodies are produced, no immunity occurs. If the infection is not repeated the protozoa survive in the host for a variable time, usually about 6 months, and then disappear. A sterile immunity persists for a further 6 months and the host is susceptible again about a year after infection occurred. These periods of latent infection and resistance to reinfection are subject to significant variation and to different responses between races of cattle and the species of *Babesia* (1). Thus, all races of cattle are equally susceptible to *B. bigemina*, but zebu and Afrikander cattle have a higher resistance to *B. bovis* than British and European breeds, Santa Gertrudis cattle occupying an intermediate position. Zebu-type cattle also enjoy a relative freedom from the disease because of their resistance to heavy infestations with ticks (10). Although the infection rate need not reflect the rate of occurrence of the clinical disease, there appears to be a variation in susceptibility to infection according to age in cattle. The greatest infection rate is in animals in the 6–12 month age group and infection is uncommon in animals over 5 years of age. Animals under 1 year of age are infected predominantly with *B. bigemina* and those over 2 years of age by *B. bovis*. The resistance of calves and foals below 6 months of age is much more protracted than would seem to be explicable by the acquisition of maternal antibodies via the colostrum. But it has been observed that such antibodies are still detectable in the calves for 150–170 days (13). After 6 months of age the number of infected animals in enzootic areas increases (14). The average age at which calves in enzootic areas become infected is 11 weeks (2–34 weeks). Clinical signs and pathological changes are mild and shortlived. Foals from infected mares receive antibodies via the colostrum and this passive immunity persists for 3–4 months after birth (50). Experimental infection of buffalo yearlings with *B. bigemina* elicits no clinical response and parasites are not present in the erythrocytes (53).

Occurrence of disease outbreaks

In enzootic areas the animals most commonly affected are susceptible cattle introduced for breeding purposes, for slaughter, or in transit. Cattle indigenous to these areas are rarely affected because the natural resistance of the very young and passive immunity via colostrum from immune dams is gradually replaced by a state of immunity. Severe clinical cases which occur in these cattle are usually caused by exposure to some stress such as parturition, starvation or intercurrent disease. Such breakdowns in immunity are most likely to occur if there is a superimposed infection with a different parasite, especially *Anaplasma marginale*.

Heaviest losses occur in marginal areas where the tick population is highly variable depending on the environmental conditions. In seasons when the tick population decreases, infection may die out and immunity be lost. Then in favorable seasons when ticks multiply, the disease spreads quickly amongst what has become a susceptible population. Comparable circumstances may be created artificially by an inefficient dipping program which reduces the tick population to a low level and is subsequently unable to keep it under control. The morbidity rate in such circumstances is often 90% and the mortality may be of the same order. There is also a seasonal variation in the prevalence of clinical babesiosis, the greatest incidence occurring soon after the peak of the tick population.

The disease may have a seasonal incidence if the tick population varies with climate. For example, in England babesiosis is largely a disease of spring, summer and autumn for this reason. The climatic factors which could have an important effect on seasonal prevalence are temperature, humidity and rainfall. Of these, air temperature is the most important because of its effect on tick activity, higher temperatures increasing it. Humidity and rainfall have little effect, and even with temperature the effect is limited once a threshold of 7–10°C (44–50°F) minimum temperature is exceeded (56).

Causes of wastage

Bovine babesiosis is of the greatest economic importance both because of direct losses and because of restriction of movement by quarantine laws. Many animals die or undergo a long period of convalescence entailing loss of meat and milk production. Incidental costs of immunization and treatment add to the economic burden created by the disease. With early, effective treatment the mortality rate can be reduced to 5%. The morbidity and mortality rates and the losses caused by babesiosis in other animal species are difficult to determine because they exist as enzootic diseases in areas where they occur.

The relative importance of the several species of bovine babesia is of interest. For example, in Australia over a 10-year period, in terms of outbreaks of redwater caused by each of them, the order of importance was *B.*

bovis (*argentina*) 73%; *B. bigemina* 6%, *Anaplasma marginale* accounted for the other 21% (51).

Although the mortality rate in the outbreak of equine babesiosis in Florida in 1961 was 10% and actual losses were high, the big losses in this species result from the interference with racing and pleasure horse meetings and competitions. At one time it appeared to be an emerging disease which threatened to be of major importance to the horse industry. For example, until 1961 equine babesiosis was thought to occur only in southeastern Europe, Africa, Asia, the Philippines and South and Central America. However, at that time there was an unexpected occurrence of the disease with heavy losses in Florida, United States. The disease was thought to have been introduced in horses imported from Cuba. Only one case of babesiosis due to *B. equi* has since been detected in Florida. Several cases caused by *B. equi* were also identified in Australia in 1976 (60) with no cases since then, and seropositive horses have also been identified in the United Kingdom. The prevalence of the disease in India as indicated by serological survey has been 50% (55).

Pathogenesis

The principal pathogenic effect of infection with *Babesia* spp. is intravascular hemolysis. In *B. bovis* infections there is also a profound hypotension which results from stimulation of production of vasoactive substances (41). The vasodilatation is accompanied by increased vascular permeability, leading to circulatory stasis and shock. A further pathogenetic effect of *B. bovis* is intravascular coagulation. Disseminated intravascular coagulation (DIC) and subsequent, fatal pulmonary thrombosis has been demonstrated in calves infected with *B. bovis* (21). *B. bigemina* is an uncomplicated hemolytic agent and does not exert these additional effects. The effect of the hemolysis is to produce a hemolytic anemia which may be acutely fatal due to anoxia. In longer surviving animals there are ischemic changes in skeletal and heart muscle.

When an animal becomes infected, multiplication of the protozoa in the peripheral vessels (*B. bigemina*, *B. ovis*), or in the visceral vessels (*B. bovis*), reaches a peak with the development of clinically detectable hemolysis after an incubation period of 7–20 days. The hemolysis results in profound anemia, jaundice and hemoglobinuria. Death is presumably due to anemic anoxia. If the animal survives it becomes a carrier in which a harmless, subclinical infection is maintained by a delicate immunological balance between protozoa and antibodies. This balance is readily disturbed by environmental stress, especially transport and deprivation of food, and intercurrent disease. In this carrier state the animal is resistant to infection and it persists for about a year. With constant reinfection such as occurs in an enzootic situation the protection is constant. Even though the infection persists, the virulence of the blood in transmission experiments is lost periodically due to disappearance of infective forms of the parasite from the peripheral blood.

A detailed study of the natural history in individual animals has been conducted in cattle run in a tick-free environment and after a single infective episode. With *B. bovis* recurrences of parasitemia occurred for up to 2 years. With *B. bigemina* there were fewer, shorter recurrences. The ability of cattle to infect ticks was much longer (1 year) with *B. bovis* than *B. bigemina* (4–7 weeks). Similarly, the peak incidence was at a younger age and the reinfection rate was faster with *B. bigemina*.

Experimental transmission of *B. ovis* infection in sheep produces an acute attack of clinical illness, parasitemia and the subsequent development of immunity, as in cattle (54).

When cows become infected during pregnancy there is no apparent infection of the calf *in utero*, but there is an apparent transfer of passive immunity via colostrum to the newborn calf.

Although the susceptibility of cattle to infection with *Babesia* sp. decreases with age, their susceptibility to the pathogenic effects of the parasite appears to increase. With *B. bovis* this effect has been demonstrated by showing that calves up to 5–6 months of age show little effect, aged cows have a severe, often fatal, clinical disease, and cattle of 1–2 years of age have a moderately severe disease (48).

Specific antibodies to the parasites are produced and are used in serological diagnosis. The highest titers are obtained in the sera of cows which have had a series of infections and reinfections. The degree of immunity in the animal is not related to the complement fixing antibody titer. The antibodies can be passively transferred via serum or colostrum, but their exact nature is uncertain (52). There are a number of strains of *B. bovis*, and the immunity to each is specific. However, when an infection occurs the host's immune system is primed so that subsequent infection with a heterologous strain soon afterwards elicits a heightened response.

Clinical findings

Cattle

In field infections the incubation period is 2–3 weeks. Subclinical infections occur fairly commonly, especially in young cattle. *B. bigemina* and *B. bovis* produce syndromes which are clinically indistinguishable, and are characterized by an acute onset of high fever (41°C, 106°F), anorexia, depression, weakness, cessation of rumination and a fall in milk yield. Respiratory and heart rates are increased and the brick-red conjunctivae and mucous membranes soon change to the extreme pallor of severe anemia. In the terminal stages there is severe jaundice, and the urine is dark red to brown in color and produces a very stable froth. Many severely affected animals die precipitately at this point, after an illness of only 24 hours. In those that survive, the febrile stage usually lasts for about a week and the total course about 3 weeks. Pregnant animals often abort. Animals that survive recover gradually from the severe emaciation and anemia which are inevitable sequelae. A subacute syndrome also occurs, especially in young animals, in which the fever is mild and hemoglobinuria is absent. Occasional animals infected with *B. bigemina* show cerebral babesiosis manifested by incoordination followed by posterior paralysis or by mania, convulsions and coma. The mortality rate in these cases is high in spite of treatment.

The syndrome in infection with *B. divergens* is similar to the above, except that in addition there is spasm of the anal sphincter causing the passage of 'pipe stem' feces. The feces are evacuated with great force in a long, thin stream, even in the absence of diarrhea.

Horses
The incubation period is 8–10 days. In adults there is a sudden onset of immobility and reluctance to move; some are in lateral recumbency and do not respond to stimuli. There is complete anorexia and fever at 40°C (104°F), although the fever often subsides after one day. Edema of the fetlocks occurs and may also be present on the head and ventral abdomen. Feces are mucus-covered and colic occurs frequently. Often there is no hemoglobinuria; bronchitis occurs occasionally. The mucosae are pale pink and tinged with jaundice. In young horses the signs are more severe, jaundice and weakness are marked, and mucosal petechiae are evident. The course is 8–10 days. Afflicted horses may die within 24–48 hours of the first signs appearing. Chronic cases may survive for months and 'carriers' may persist for as long as 4 years. The experimental disease produced by *B. equi* is mild. A high percentage of erythrocytes are parasitized by the protozoa and the horses are anemic, but there is no clinical evidence of anemia (22).

Other species
In all other species the syndrome observed is clinically similar to that described for cattle.

Clinical pathology
The detection of these diseases by laboratory methods presents some difficulties. Examination of smears of peripheral blood is the simplest diagnostic method. There is no exact correlation between the percentage of erythrocytes which contain protozoa and the severity of the clinical signs, but this form of measurement is of value in estimating the stage of development and the severity of the disease. Although *B. bigemina* is numerous in peripheral capillaries, *B. bovis* is much less readily found, but the difficulty can be largely overcome by the use of thick blood smears. A positive smear in all cases confirms the diagnosis but a negative smear does not eliminate it and for accurate diagnosis in these circumstances transmission tests are essential. *B. equi* are usually found quite readily in the erythrocytes of affected horses.

For a transmission test the animals to be inoculated must be susceptible and this can be ensured only by using animals from tick-free areas. To overcome the difficulty of subinfective numbers of the organism in donor blood it may be necessary to increase the susceptibility of the recipient by splenectomy. This technique is particularly necessary when infection with *B. argentina* is suspected. In transmission experiments 50–100 ml of blood are injected into the recipient either subcutaneously or intravenously. In the latter case the incubation period will be shorter. The recipients are examined daily and the blood examined for protozoa at the peak of the febrile reaction.

Because of the difficulty in finding protozoa in smears in animals during the subclinical stages of the disease much attention has been directed to serological tests, but although these are now well-established none of them enjoys a completely satisfactory reputation (17). They are accurate enough for *B. bovis*, but lack specificity for *B. bigemina* (15). The tests which are being used in bovine babesiosis include a complement fixation test (14), a passive agglutination test, an indirect fluorescent antibody test (IFAT) (19), an indirect hemagglutination test, an enzyme-linked immunoabsorbent assay (ELISA) (2), a microplate enzyme immunoassay (EIA) (8), a latex agglutination test (3), a capillary agglutination and a slide and a card agglutination test (23). All of the tests have good reputations with the EIA being probably the most sensitive.

In horse, the tests used include the widely used complement fixation test, a passive hemagglutination test, a fluorescent antibody inhibition test, a card agglutination test (1), a leukocyte migration inhibition test, an intradermal skin test (5), and an indirect fluorescent antibody test (62). An important aspect of serological testing in horses is its application in deciding whether or not a horse known to be a carrier previously has been rendered non-infective by a course of treatment, and thus eligible to be let out of quarantine. In the past this decision has been made on the basis of a transmission test, an expensive and largely impractical test. It is considered that the complement fixation test is sufficiently accurate to be used for this purpose (26).

Severe anemia with erythrocyte counts as low as 2 million/μl and hemoglobin levels down to 3 g/dl is present in most clinical cases. In cattle and horses the anemia peaks 9–16 days after infection occurs (27). Also in both species there is a significant fall in platelet counts and a depression in the fibrinogen content of the blood (27).

Necropsy findings
In acute cases jaundice is marked, the spleen is enlarged, swollen and of a soft, pulpy consistency, the liver is grossly enlarged and dark brown in color, and the gallbladder is distended with thick, granular bile. The kidneys are enlarged and dark and the bladder contains red-brown urine. Ecchymotic hemorrhages are present under the epicardium and endocardium and the pericardial sac contains an increased quantity of blood-stained fluid. A characteristic lesion in both cattle and horses which have died from the acute disease is severe intravascular clotting. In cases of fairly long duration the carcase is emaciated but hemoglobinuria is absent and the other changes observed in acute cases are present but less pronounced. Smears for direct examination should be taken from peripheral blood, from kidney and heart muscle and, in the case of suspected *B. bovis* infection, from the brain.

B. bovis parasites are detectable in smears of heart, lung and kidney, when stained by Giemsa, and are still detectable up to 8 hours after death, and up to 28 hours afterwards in brain (7). Brain smears are used extensively in postmortem diagnosis (30). Using direct fluorescent antibody staining slightly later identifications can be made. With *B. bigemina* the morphology of the parasite changes quickly after the host's death so that they resemble *B. bovis*. Organ smears are still usable 5 days after collection provided they are kept stored at 22°C

(72°F). Blood serum collected after death can also be used for detection of antibodies in serological tests.

Diagnosis

The presence of the insect vector must be verified before the diagnosis can be made unless the animal has left an enzootic area within the preceding month. Clinically, jaundice with hemoglobinuria and fever are suggestive but confirmation by examination of blood smears or by transmission experiments is essential. A necropsy which shows splenomegaly, jaundice, hemoglobinuria, swollen dark kidneys and liver, and myocardial ecchymoses, while highly suggestive, should also be confirmed by laboratory examination.

Differentiation from other diseases which are characterized by hemolytic anemia may be difficult in cattle. Anaplasmosis is usually less acute, relapses are more common and hemoglobinuria is a rare occurrence. Eperythrozoonosis is less severe and the clinical findings are largely limited to those of anemia. Theileriasis caused by *Theileria annulata* is commonly manifested by hemoglobinuria. The protozoa are readily identifiable in a blood smear and serological diagnosis is available. Leptospirosis has a much shorter course and is more severe in young calves than in adults, the reverse of the picture in babesiosis and anaplasmosis. Equine babesiosis can be so similar to equine infectious anemia that laboratory differentiation is usually necessary. Other causes of hemolytic anemia in horses are discussed in detail elsewhere and in summary form in Table 74. A similar table for diseases of cattle is Table 75.

Treatment

Effective drugs are available for the treatment of these diseases in cattle but two important factors must always be kept in mind, especially when the drugs are being used to control a reaction produced artificially for purposes of vaccination. The initial phase of the disease is acute and if treatment is delayed for too long the animal may succumb to the anemia in spite of sterilization of the blood. Care must also be taken to avoid complete sterilization of the blood before sufficient antibody is produced to provide a durable immunity. There is one other important aspect of treatment; it has no suppressing effect on the protozoa that are residing in the ticks which are parasitizing the cattle at the time. There is therefore no effect on the rate of transmission (33). A summary of the recommended drugs follows, but diminazene aceturate, imidocarb dipropionate and amicarbalide diisethionate are most often used (35).

Table 74. Differential diagnosis of diseases of horses characterized by anemia and anasarca.

Disease	*Epidemiology*	*Clinical findings*	*Clinical pathology*	*Response to treatment*
Babesiosis (*B. equi*, *B. caballi*)	In recent years *B. equi* in the United States, United Kingdom, and Australia. Foals younger than 6 months not affected. Transmission by ticks, possibly other insects or needles or instruments	Incubation period 8–10 days. Immobility, sometimes recumbency, anoxia, 40°C (104°F) briefly. Dependent edema. Frequent colic. Mild jaundice. Course 8–10 days. Young horses more severe jaundice and mucosal petechiae	Often no hemoglobinuria. *B. equi* easily found in erythrocytes. Complement fixation and other serological tests available. Anemia	Pattern not well-established. Many drugs used with good clinical response but no efficient sterilant identified for *B. equi*. Imidocarb best
Equine infectious anemia	Insect-borne (*Tabanus* sp. and mosquitoes). Also needles, surgical instruments, doping swabs, vaccines, sera. Many inapparent carriers. Slow spread in a population	Very prolonged disease; may be years. Recurrent fever, anemia, mucosal petechiation, dependent edema, jaundice. Periods of normality (3 weeks) between periods of illness (3 weeks)	Episodes of anemia. Increased sedimentation rate. Slight leukopenia. Diagnostic agar gel immunodiffusion test	No specific treatment
Purpura hemorrhagica	Sporadic. Usually sequel to respiratory tract infection	Several subcutaneous swellings, cold edema. Mostly face and muzzle, also ventrally, not necessarily symmetrical or dependent. Skin normal. Mucosal petechiation always. HR 100, mild fever. Most die within a few days	Anemia mild, leukocytosis, neutrophilia, no depression platelet count	Recovery rate very poor. Blood transfusion, broad-spectrum antibiotic, corticosteroid
Equine viral arteritis	Rapid spread in susceptible population. All ages. Spread by ingestion/inhalation	High fever. Severe illness, serous nasal discharge, mucosal engorgement and petechiation. Edema of limbs, prepuce, scrotum but not extensive, nor dependent. Abortion in mares	No anemia. Serum neutralization, tissue culture. Severe leukopenia	No specific treatment
Angioneurotic edema	Sporadic. Response to injection, e.g. penicillin, insect bite, or allergy by contact or ingestion	Acute onset, restless, moderate fever. Edematous plaques and bullae, often very large, mostly around head, also body. Very rapid recovery 24–48 hours	Nil. Maybe transitory eosinophilia very early	Antihistamines. Adrenaline. Rapid spontaneous recovery the rule
Strongylosis	All pastured horses are infected. Disease occurs in horses where control not practiced especially neglected young horses and brood mares	Weak, thin, anemic. Some severe cases scour, ventral edema. Verminous aneurysm colic, thromboembolic colic common sequels	Fecal examination for worm eggs. More than 1000 eggs/g is significant. Hematology shows anemia and hypoproteinemia	Excellent to modern, broad-spectrum anthelmintics

Table 75. Differential diagnosis of diseases of cattle in which red urine is a principal manifestation.

Disease	*Epidemiology*	*Clinical findings* *General*	*Urinary*	*Clinical pathology*	*Treatment and/or control*
DISEASES WITH HEMATURIA					
Enzootic hematuria	Subjects older than 1 year. Endemic to specific areas with access to bracken mostly	Severe hemorrhagic anemia, acute or chronic. Rectal in acute cases nil; chronic cases have local or diffuse thickening. Long course, death by anemia	Persistent, intermittent hematuria	Urine has no pus, leukocytes or bacteria	Blood transfusion to save life. Cull. Eradicate bracken. Soil dressing with gypsum
Enzootic bovine pyelonephritis	Adults only. Sporadic cases usually. May be a series suggesting origin in one bull and relationship to mating events	Mild fever. Frequent painful urination, toxemia. Late cases, rectal examination shows cystitis, ureters thickened and enlarged, kidney the same. Pain on palpation. Long course, death by uremia	Intermittent hematuria and pyuria	Urine has pus, erythrocytes, leukocytes, *Cor. renale* on culture catheter sample	Response to penicillin excellent. Chronic cases may recur. Breed cows by artificial insemination
Non-specific diseases	Sporadic cases hematuria are caused by acute glomerulonephritis, embolic nephritis and renal infarction, embolism of the renal artery, cystitis and urolithiasis				
Other specific diseases	Hematuria also occurs incidentally in other specific diseases but is not the principal presenting sign, e.g. any case of hemorrhagic disease or severe septicemia				
DISEASES WITH HEMOGLOBINURIA					
Babesiosis (*B. bigemina* and *B. bovis*)	Most likely outbreaks in marginal areas in seasons when tick population explodes. Outbreaks, not in calves. Incubation 2–3 weeks. 90% morbidity and mortality	High fever 41°C (105°F), pallor general signs of toxemia. Severe jaundice terminally	Red urine. Low level *Babesia bovis* in smears. Transmission to splenectomized calf. Serological tests efficient	Babesia in red cells in smear—inaccurate. Transmission test. Indirect agglutination or indirect fluorescent antibody test	Effective anti-protozoal drugs. Prevent by effective vaccination. Tick control
Theileriosis (*Theileria annulata*)	Transmitted only by ticks *Hyalomma anatolicum*	Fever, anorexia, lymph node enlargement	Hemoglobinuria	Piroplasms in erythrocytes. Serological tests	Tetracyclines. Immunotherapy as control
Postparturient hemoglobinuria	Postcalving 2–4 weeks. Adult dairy cows in 3rd–6th lactation. Sporadic but tends to endemicity on individual farms. Low phosphorus or low copper diet	Acute onset, weakness, tremor, pallor, bounding pulse, loud heart sounds, tachycardia. No jaundice. Mortality 50%. Long convalescence. Die of anemia, especially if stressed	Deep brown to black frothy	No cells in urine but good deposit on standing. Severe hemolytic anemia. Serum inorganic P < 1·5 mg/dl and down to 0·1 mg/dl	Respond well to parenteral plus oral administration of phosphorus. Blood transfusion in emergency
Bacillary hemoglobinuria	Summer time on irrigated pasture. Sporadic. Very few cases. Endemic to particular farms. Mortality 100%	Often found dead. Very acute onset, hemolytic anemia plus toxemia. Fever 41°C (105°F). Abdominal pain, pain on percussion right anterior abdomen. Diarrhea. Shallow, rapid respiration due to diaphragmatic pain	Deep red brown, no cells	Hemolytic anemia, increased serum bilirubin	Penicillin tetracycline, blood transfusion. Vaccinate *Cl. novyi* type D
Leptospirosis (*L. interrogans pomona* only, not *L. hardjo*)	Calves high mortality 50%. Adults low mortality <5%. Abortion storm more common is adults. Many subclinical infections in adults	Hemolytic disease mostly in young calves. Sudden onset septicemia with red urine. Severe toxemia, fever 40·5–41·5°C (104·5–106°F). Mucosal petechiae, pallor and jaundice. Adults have thick orange milk all quarters	Red urine, hemoglobinuria	Initially leptospiruria 3 days. Leptospiruria by intraperitoneal injection into guinea-pigs. Rising titer leptospira antibodies with peak 4 weeks after infection	Streptomycin for clinical cases and to stop shedding in urine. Vaccination with bivalent *L. interrogans pomona* and *L. hardjo*
Chronic copper poisoning	Rarely if ever at pasture. Feeding of copper supplement in diet, use of a swine copper-supplemented diet by mistake	Sudden onset, weakness, pallor, jaundice, death usually in 24–48 hours	Hemoglobinuria, some methemoglobinuria	High liver copper on biopsy 2000 ppm dry material. High plasma ceruloplasmin and copper	Acute cases, blood transfusion and calcium versenate. Chronic, try molybdate

Cattle

Quinuronium derivatives Acaprin, Babesan, Piveran, Piroparv, Piroplasmin are closely related drugs and are of most value against the larger babesiae, especially *B. bigemina*. They can be given subcutaneously without causing sloughing, but they are relatively toxic and can produce alarming reactions including salivation, sweating, diarrhea, panting, collapse and occasional deaths; adrenaline is the antidote. Acaprin is the most widely used and is universally accepted as an efficient safe drug. The recommended dose rate is 1 ml/50 kg body weight with a maximum dose of 6 ml. At a similar dose rate quinuronium sulfate is effective when given early in the clinical disease but relapse is likely 2 weeks later (17).

Acridine derivatives Acriflavine, gonacrine and euflavine—the latter is the only drug with a significant use and was the drug of choice against *B. equi* and *B. argentina* until imidocarb became available.

Aromatic diamidines Stilbamidine, Propamidine, Phenamidine, diminazene aceturate, Diampron have all been well received and are in general good drugs of use in treatment of clinical cases. But they are inclined to incompletely sterilize the patient. This may be a desirable result. The drugs are well tolerated and safe for intramuscular or subcutaneous injection.

Imidocarb (Imizol) This, and the allied drug amidocarb are effective babesiocides for cattle at the dose rate of 1 mg/kg body weight. At 2 mg/kg body weight it completely eliminates the parasites from the host and maintains some residual activity; non-infected cattle derive a month's resistance to clinical infection but can be infected subclinically. It can therefore be used to protect cattle when vaccination is undesirable, e.g. pregnancy, or when exposure to infection is shortlived and as a temporary protection while awaiting vaccination. The drug can be given subcutaneously but the hydrochloride is inclined to be irritant; the propionate is less so.

Horses

The treatment of equine babesiosis is not well established. Many drugs including amicarbalide isothionate (Phenamidine), diminazene, Pirevan, Berenil, euflavine (36), Diampron and oxytetracycline have been used. But the consensus of opinion is that there is no efficient sterilant for *B. equi* and, although *B. caballi* is more susceptible, it is expected to develop resistance quickly. Imidocarb is currently the most favored drug even though there are significantly different opinions about its efficiency. It does appear that it is effective against *B. equi* provided a strict treatment regimen is followed (four intramuscular injections of 10% solution at a dose of 4 mg/kg body weight at intervals of 72 hours) (40). *B. caballi* is more susceptible to the drug and a regimen of 2 mg/kg body weight on two occasions 24 hours apart is sufficient (6). The hydrochloride salt of imidocarb is strongly acid and may provoke severe local reactions in horses so that the dipropionate is being used more. A note of warning is necessary about the treatment of donkeys which are very susceptible to imidocarb (the LD_{50} is less than 2 mg/kg body weight).

Sheep

Diminazene aceturate is effective as a treatment in sheep (3·5 mg/kg body weight on two successive days or 12 mg/kg body weight as a single dose). The recommended dose rate for sheep is 3 mg/kg body weight.

In all species ancillary treatment in severely affected cases should include blood transfusions, and hematinics during convalescence.

Control

Eradication of bovine babesiosis from an area depends upon eradicating the vector tick—a problem in applied entomology. Eradication has been achieved in the United States by this technique.

Cattle

A number of important factors govern when and how a control program should be put into operation. The principal ones are the tick, the host and the control measures. These have been incorporated in a computer simulation model (39) so that a control program can be managed to most effectively reduce losses.

In control not aimed at eradication two principles operate. One is that indigenous cattle must maintain a sufficient population of vector ticks to ensure that all animals become infected and reinfected sufficiently early and often to maintain a constant state of immunity-infection. Too rigorous a program of tick control may lead to losses caused by babesiosis in non-immune animals. From another point of view it can be observed that good tick control reduces the infection rate with *Babesia* spp. but increases the risk of outbreaks (10, 46). The other principle to be followed is that cattle introduced into enzootic areas and in marginal tick belts should be exposed to artificial infection by vaccination with living protozoa. Three other programs have been suggested for these marginal areas. They are vaccination with a killed vaccine, usually incorporating an incomplete Freund adjuvant, or chemoprophylaxis with a drug such as imidocarb which has a residual effect and therefore allows the animal to become infected gradually while the chemotherapeutic influence is fading, and chemo-immunization. The latter technique is universally applied and includes vaccination with virulent organisms and the simultaneous or subsequent administration of an appropriate chemical babesicide (20). Using imidocarb, with its prolonged effect, it is possible to give the vaccine and the chemotherapeutic agent simultaneously, or with the vaccine before or after the chemical, with very similar results (12). It is preferred to the first two techniques because it has the positive effect of vaccination with a living parasite. However there is the danger that the imidocarb treatment will completely suppress the vaccine and leave the animal unprotected (42). A fourth and least-tried technique is the use of attenuated vaccines. These are produced by passaging the babesiae through susceptible, splenectomized calves. The babesiae become attenuated, less virulent and no longer infective for tick vectors. The parasitized erythrocytes are suspended in cell-free plasma as a diluent. The results are excellent, the level of immunity equalling that achieved by natural or artificially induced infection with, for example, *B. bovis* (25). A similar effective vaccine has been produced with *B. bigemina* (24). Several vaccines can be put together so that vaccination against *B. bovis* and *Anaplasma marginale* are carried out simultaneously (43). Although vaccination with *B. bigemina* may confer some immunity to *B. bovis* both protozoa must be included in a vaccine, if immunity against both is required. Some of the difficulties of maintaining infected animals as permanent donors of vaccine are overcome by the technique of storing infective blood by deep freezing. Virulence of the blood is maintained for at least 2 years. The 'vaccine' used is stored at 1–5°C (34–41°F), contains 10^5 *B. bovis* organisms per dose as the minimum infecting dose. Reaction occurs 7–14 days after the vaccination. Treatment of cattle with excessive reactions, indicated by fever at greater than 40·5°C (105°F), with quinuronium sulfate at half the normal dose rate is effective. Pentamidine (0·5–1·0 mg/kg body weight as a single dose) is also effective and has the advantage that the sterilizing dose is five times greater than the therapeutic dose, allowing the animal to be protected without loss of immunity (9).

The demand for effective and error-proof vaccines has been greatly increased because of the needs of developing countries. Many technical advances have been made in recent years due largely to an active research program in Australia. A quite novel addition to vaccines has been the one composed of irradiated infected blood (37). Results in small trials with these vaccines against *B. major* (31) and *B. divergens* (32) have been excellent. The biggest attraction is that of preparing an antigen capable of stimulating a sterile immunity without depending on the replication of the infection. They also have the advantage that the irradiated babesia are probably not transmitted transovarially through the cattle tick (20). Cattle that have been treated with prophylactic drugs such as imidocarb dipropionate are not susceptible to vaccination for at least 4 weeks after the treatment. Some of these 'blood-origin non-viable' vaccines have been given limited trials. In general their effect is one of reducing the severity of the reactions produced by subsequent infection without completely preventing it (28, 34, 44).

Vaccinated cattle should be housed or kept under close observation for a month in case excessive reactions occur. Greater care is taken with pure-bred cattle vaccinated at centers en route to infected areas. It is most important that such animals be vaccinated before they are exposed to tick infestation. The efficiency of the vaccine is excellent, the clinical disease prevalence rate of 18% being reduced to 1·2% in one trial (14).

One of the major problems in vaccination is the occasional apparent failure to transmit the protozoa. This may be due to the absence of the protozoa from the bloodstream of the donor at the time that the blood is drawn to the presence of a prophylactic drug, for example, imidocarb dipropionate, in the animal's tissues, or to failure of individual animals in a group to become infected due possibly to a low-grade natural immunity. In all instances a reaction does not occur after injection and the animals are still susceptible to natural infection. Revaccination is necessary in these circumstances, preferably with blood from a donor which is undergoing a severe reaction at the time.

Another problem has recently been described with the vaccination of pregnant cows using whole blood particularly when repeated vaccinations are made. Antibodies to the donor red cells may be produced, absorbed from the colostrum, and produce isoimmune hemolytic anemia in the calves. As a safety precaution cows should not be vaccinated in the last 6 months of pregnancy.

Whole blood vaccines also have the disadvantage that they may transmit other pathogens, for example, bovine leukosis virus. In order to avoid this the culture of babesia *in vitro* has been attempted successfully and the cultured protozoa used in vaccines (2) but their effectiveness is much less than that of conventional whole blood vaccines (29).

Babesiosis of other species

These are controlled similarly to the disease in cattle with attention focused on eradicating the vector tick, selecting infected and carrier animals by the complement fixation test and sterilizing the positive reactors by appropriate treatments. Control of ticks in pleasure horses by periodic spraying and inspection is a practical proposition when the animals are in constant use. An attenuated vaccine produced by rapid passage through splenectomized lambs has produced solid immunity in sheep (38).

The prevention of introduction of the disease into an area depends on effective quarantine and other measures to prevent the introduction of the vector tick. The international movement of animals has become a very important matter to the horse industry where teams of pleasure horses attend competitions in other countries, and where valuable stallions move to another country for a brief period to stand at stud. There is a tendency for some countries to be very restrictive in their quarantine procedures for horses and international relations would be enhanced if more information was available on the relationship between a positive complement fixation test and infectivity for other horses (49).

REVIEW LITERATURE

Aliu, Y. O. (1983) Tick-borne diseases of domestic animals in Nigeria: current treatment procedures. *Vet. Bull.*, *53*, 233–251.

Callow L. L. & Dalgleish, R. J. (1982) *Immunity and Immunopathology in Babesiosis in Immunology of Parasitic Infections*. Oxford: Blackwell Scientific Publications, pp. 475–526.

Mahoney, D. E. (1977) Babesia of domestic animals. In: *Parasitic Protozoa*, vol. 4, ed. J. P. Kreier, pp. 1–52. New York:Academic Press.

Mahoney, D. E. et al. (1984) Immunization against babesiosis: current studies and future outlook. *Prev. vet. Med.*, *2*, 401–408.

Purnell, R. E. (1981) Tick-borne disease. *Br. vet. J.*, *137*, 221.

REFERENCES

(1) Amerault, T. E. et al. (1979) *Am. J. vet. Res.*, *40*, 529.
(2) Levy, M. G. & Ristic, M. (1982) *Am. J. vet. Res.*, *207*, 1218.
(3) Montenegro, S. et al. (1981) *Vet. Parasitol.*, *8*, 291.
(4) Purnell, R. E. et al. (1976) *J. comp. Pathol.*, *86*, 609.
(5) Banerjee, D. P. et al. (1977) *Trop. Anim. Hlth Prod.*, *9*, 153.
(6) Reid, J. F. et al. (1976) *Vet. Rec.*, *99*, 419.
(7) Johnston, L. A. Y. et al. (1977) *Aust. vet. J.*, *53*, 222.
(8) Barry, D. N. et al. (1982) *Aust. vet. J.*, *59*, 136.
(9) Pipano, E. et al. (1979) *Trop. Anim. Hlth Prod.*, *11*, 13.
(10) Mahoney, D. F. et al. (1981) *Aust. vet. J.*, *57*, 461.
(11) Aadami, A. et al. (1974) *Refuah Vet.*, *31*, 149.

(12) Taylor, R. J. & McHardy, N. (1979) *J. S. Afr. vet. Assoc.*, *50*, 326.
(13) Weisman, J. et al. (1974) *Refuah Vet.*, *31*, 108.
(14) Callow, L. L. et al. (1976) *Aust. vet. J.*, *52*, 446, 451.
(15) Callow, L. L. (1979) *J. S. Afr. vet. Assoc.*, *50*, 353.
(16) Donnelly, J. & Pierce, M. A. (1975) *Int. J. Parasitol.*, *5*, 363.
(17) Purnell, R. E. et al. (1981) *Vet. Rec.*, *108*, 538.
(18) Erp, E. E. et al. (1980) *Am. J. vet. Res.*, *41*, 1141.
(19) Morzaria, S. P. et al. (1977) *Vet. Rec.*, *100*, 484.
(20) Wright, I. G. et al. (1983) *Res. vet. Sci.*, *34*, 124.
(21) Dalgleish, R. J. et al. (1977) *Res. vet. Sci.*, *23*, 105.
(22) Kuttler, K. L. et al. (1986) *Am. J. vet. Res.*, *47*, 1668.
(23) Todorovic, R. A. & Kuttler, K. L. (1974) *Am. J. vet. Res.*, *35*, 1347.
(24) Dalgleish, R. J. et al. (1981) *Aust. vet. J.*, *57*, 8.
(25) DeVos, A. J. et al. (1982) *Onderstepoort J. vet. Res.*, *49*, 133 & 155.
(26) Frerichs, W. M. (1974) *Vet. Rec.*, *95*, 188.
(27) Allen, P. C. et al. (1975) *Exp. Parasitol.*, *37*, 67, 373.
(28) Wright, I. G. et al. (1985) *Infect. Immun.*, *48*, 109.
(29) Kuttler, K. L. et al. (1982) *Am. J. vet. Res.*, *43*, 281.
(30) Hadani, A. et al. (1983) *Br. vet. J.*, *139*, 208.
(31) Purnell, R. E. et al. (1978) *Res. vet. Sci.*, *25*, 388.
(32) Taylor, S. M. et al. (1980) *Vet. Rec.*, *106*, 385.
(33) DeVos, A. J. et al. (1984) *Int. J. Parasitol.*, *14*, 249.
(34) Mahoney, D. F. et al. (1981) *Vet. Immunol. Immunopathol.*, *2*, 145.
(35) Aliu, Y. O. (1983) *Vet. Bull.*, *53*, 233.
(36) Kirkham, W. W. (1969) *J. Am. vet. med. Assoc.*, *155*, 457.
(37) Purnell, R. E. et al. (1981) *Vet. Rec.*, *108*, 28.
(38) Kyurtov, N. (1977) *Veterinarnomiditinski*, *14*, 25.
(39) Smith, R. D. (1983) *Exp. Parasitol.*, *56*, 27.
(40) Frerichs, W. M. et al. (1973) *Vet. Rec.*, *93*, 73.
(41) Goodger, B. V. et al. (1981) *J. exp. Biol. med. Sci.*, *59*, 531.
(42) DeVos, A. J. et al. (1986) *Aust. vet. J.*, *63*, 174
(43) Mellors, L. T. et al. (1982) *Res. vet. Sci.*, *32*, 194.
(44) Timms, P. et al. (1983) *Aust. vet. J.*, *60*, 75.
(45) Levy, M. G. & Ristic, M. (1980) *Science, USA*, *207*, 1218.
(46) DeVos, A. J. & Potgieter, F. T. (1983) *Onderstepoort J. vet. Res.*, *50*, 3.
(47) Adam, K. M. G. et al. (1977) *Res. vet. Sci.*, *23*, 133.
(48) Trueman, K. F. & Blight, G. W. (1978) *Aust. vet. J.*, *54*, 301.
(49) Barnett, S. F. (1974) *Vet. Rec.*, *95*, 346.
(50) Donnelly, J. et al. (1982) *Equ. vet. J.*, *14*, 126.
(51) Copeman, D. B. et al. (1976) In: Tick-borne disease and their vectors. *Proc. Int. Conf., Edinburgh*, 1976.
(52) Mahoney, D. F. et al. (1979) *Int. J. Parasitol.*, *9*, 297.
(53) Roychoudhury, G. K. & Gautam, O. P. (1979) *Trop. Anim. Hlth Prod.*, *11*, 91.
(54) Khalacheva, M. (1979) *Vet. med. Nauki*, *16*, 78.
(55) Malhotra, D. V. et al. (1978) *Equ. vet. J.*, *10*, 24.
(56) Gray, J. S. (1980) *Br. vet. J.*, *136*, 427.
(57) Mahoney, D. F. & Mirre, G. B. (1979) *Res. vet. Sci.*, *26*, 253.
(58) Morzaria, S. P. et al. (1977) *Res. vet. Sci.*, *22*, 190.
(59) Findlay, C. R. & Begg, T. B. (1977) *Vet. Rec.*, *100*, 406.
(60) Mahoney, D. F. et al. (1977) *Aust. vet. J.*, *53*, 461.
(61) Johnston, L. A. Y. et al. (1978) *Aust. vet. J.*, *54*, 14.
(62) Callow, L. L. et al. (1979) *Aust. vet. J.*, *55*, 555.

Eperythrozoonosis

The causative agent, *Eperythrozoon* sp. is a member of the *Bartonella* group and therefore a rickettsia.

The disease occurs in swine, sheep and cattle, and is of particular importance in the former in which it is recorded in the midwestern and southern states of America. Latent eperythrozoonosis also occurs in mule deer, elk and goats.

The method of spread of the infection is probably via biting insects. In an infected flock or herd the disease persists by passing from dam to offspring, and the development of a state of infection with immunity with the infectious agent persisting in the host at a low level (9).

Pigs

The causative agent in swine is *Ep. suis*. The classical syndrome is one of acute icteroanemia of stressed feeder pigs. The pathogenesis is one of an acquired autoimmune hemolytic anemia due to cold antibodies (6). It is characterized by weakness of the hindlegs, mild fever (40°C, 104°F), increased pulse rate, pallor of the mucosae and emaciation. Jaundice is a frequent but inconstant feature of the disease. Hematological examination reveals extreme anemia and the bartonellae are present in the erythrocytes. However, there are other manifestations in pigs (7) including reproductive failure, anemia and weakness in newborn pigs, and failure of feeder pigs to gain weight at the expected rate. Subclinical infections are also common. At necropsy there is apparent anemia, and in sheep at the height of the parasitemia the spleen is grossly enlarged by up to 250% by weight.

A more acute form of the disease can be produced by the injection of infective blood into splenectomized pigs, death usually occurring on the 12–30th day after injection.

A single intramuscular injection of tetracyline or oxytetracycline (3 mg/kg body weight or more) is an effective treatment, with clinical improvement occurring in 24 hours. Neoarsphenamine given as a single intravenous injection (14–40 mg/kg body weight) has also been shown to be effective.

Cattle and sheep

Eperythrozoonosis of cattle caused by *Ep. wenyoni* occurs in Africa and of sheep caused by *Ep. ovis* occurs in Africa, the United States, France, Iran, Great Britain, Norway and Australia. The disease in these species is similar to that described above for pigs, but in both species it is often subclinical and appears to require the presence of some other debilitating disease to manifest itself. In some areas it may be the principal cause of illthrift in lambs. Reduced wool yield and exercise tolerance are also evident (4). In the experimental disease in lambs at pasture a retardation of growth of up to 2 kg has been recorded 5 weeks after infection (12). Lambs suckled by infected ewes are passively immunized via the colostrum until weaning (10). The classical clinical form of the disease may be more common than is generally believed in adult commercial dairy cattle (3). It is manifested by lassitude, stiffness, diarrhea, pyrexia and a severe macrocytic anemia (8). Hemoglobinuria is not a feature because the hemolysis occurs at extravascular sites—the erythrocytes are very fragile as a result of incomplete antibody formation (1).

Treatment of affected lambs with neoarsphenamine (30 mg/kg body weight) or Antimosan (6 mg/kg body weight antimony) is effective in relieving clinical illness, but does not cause complete sterilization of the host. Imidocarb dipropionate apparently sterilizes sheep of their infection but recrudescence at 2–4 weeks is common (11). In enzootic areas, that is to say in most places, reinfection occurs so quickly that control by treatment seems an unwarranted expenditure.

A complement fixation test (3) and an indirect fluorescent antibody test (IFA) (2, 13) similar to those used in anaplasmosis can be used in diagnosis (3). Sera from affected animals give positive reactions on the 3rd day of clinical illness, remain positive for 2–3 weeks, and then gradually revert to negative. Chronic carriers of the disease are usually negative reactors. For pigs the indirect hemagglutination test is recommended (7) and for sheep the indirect immunofluorescent antibody test is used (5). The presence of the organism can also be established by examination of a blood smear taken preferably during a clinical episode. Lowered values for hemoglobin and packed cell volume (PCV) are evident on hematological examination.

REFERENCES

(1) Sheriff, D. (1978) *NZ vet. J.*, *26*, 315.
(2) Hung, A. L. & Lloyd, S. (1985) *Res. vet. Sci.*, *39*, 275.
(3) Daddow, K. N. (1977) *Aust. vet. J.*, *53*, 139.
(4) Daddow, K. N. (1979) *Aust. vet. J.*, *55*, 433.
(5) Ilemobade, A. A. & Blotkamp, C. (1978) *TropMed. Parasitol.*, *29*, 307.
(6) Hoffman, R. et al. (1981) *Vet. Immunol. Immunopathol.*, *2*, 111.
(7) Henry, S. C. (1979) *J. Am. vet. med. Assoc.*, *174*, 601.
(8) Sonoda, M. et al. (1977) *J. Jap. vet. med. Assoc.*, *30*, 374.
(9) Daddow, K. N. & Dunlop, L. B. (1976) *Q. J. Agric. Anim. Sci.*, *33*, 233.
(10) Daddow, K. N. (1982) *Vet. Parasitol.*, *10*, 41.
(11) Hung Cho, A. L. (1986) *Trop. Anim. Hlth Prod.*, *18*, 97.
(12) Sutton, R. H. & Jolly, R. D. (1973) *NZ vet. J.*, *21*, 160.
(13) Nicholls, T. J. & Veale, P. I (1986) *Aust. vet. J.*, *63*, 157.

Coccidiosis

Coccidiosis is a contagious enteritis caused by infection with both *Eimeria* and *Isospora* spp. and occurs in all domestic animals. A high rate of subclinical infection may occur or there may be diarrhea and dysentery. In some cases there is anemia and the chronic form of the disease is characterized by inferior growth rates and production.

Etiology

The coccidial species which are considered to be pathogenic are as follows:

Cattle: *Eimeria zuernii*, *E. bovis (smithii)* and *E. ellipsoidalis*.
Sheep: *E. arloingi A (ovina)*, *E. weybridgenis (E. arloingi B)*, *E. crandallis* (1), *E. ahsata* and *E. ovinoidalis* (previously known as *E. ninakohlyakimovae*) (1) and *E. gilruthi*.
Goats: *E. arloingi*, *E. faurei* and *E. gilruthi*, *E. caprovina*, *E. ninakohlyakimovae* (2) and *E. christenseni* (3).
Pigs: *Isospora suis* (4), *E. debliecki*, *E. scabra* and *E. perminuta*.
Horses and donkeys: *E. leuckarti* (5).

Epidemiology

Coccidiosis occurs universally but is of most importance where animals are housed or confined in small areas. All domestic animals are susceptible but the coccidia are in general host-specific and infection does not pass readily from one animal species to another nor does cross-immunity between species of coccidia occur. Clinical disease is most common in cattle and sheep in which outbreaks occur. Porcine coccidiosis is now recognized as a major problem in the swine industry because of outbreaks in diarrhea in newborn piglets (6). The incidence of clinical disease is less common in horses but sporadic clinical cases and death do occur particularly in weaning age foals (5). Coccidiosis is considered to be sufficiently important economically in calves to warrant control measures. One estimate suggests that the economic losses from coccidiosis in calves amounts to US$1·00 per animal less than 1 year of age annually (7).

Most animals in a group become infected but only a minority develop clinical disease. Thus the infection rate is high, but the rate of clinical disease is usually low (10–15%) although outbreaks affecting up to 80% may occur (12). The mortality rate is also usually low, with the exception of the high mortality rate which may occur in bovine winter coccidiosis accompanied by nervous signs (12). The mortality rate may also be high in calves or lambs with no previous exposure to coccidia after suddenly being introduced to a high level of infection. In calves, body weight gains and feed consumption were severely affected for many weeks after acute clinical coccidiosis and affected calves did not regain losses in body weight compared to controls (13). In lambs on pasture, subclinical infections are common but there is no good evidence that growth rate is affected even with high levels of infection (14). While medication with a coccidiostat may lower the infection rate, there is no difference in performance between the medicated and non-medicated groups. In lambs raised under crowded conditions indoors, the acquisition of a natural multiple species infection had no effect on growth rate but an artificial infection with *E. ninakohlyakimovae* resulted in severe clinical disease and a mortality rate of 50% (15). Piglets infected with *Isospora suis* have significantly reduced body weight at 7, 14 and 21 days of age (11). The reduction in 21-day-old weight is economically important because this weight is a component of the sow productivity index which is used as a management aid to help producers quantitatively determine the potential value of gilts as replacement animals.

Coccidiosis occurs most commonly in young animals at particular times of the year. The seasonal incidence may in part be a reflection of the time of year at which young calves and lambs are brought together for weaning or moved into confinement fattening units or fed in small areas for the winter months. In North America the disease occurs most commonly in beef calves after they are weaned in the fall of the year and confined and fed in small overcrowded areas (16). The disease also occurs in the middle of the winter usually following a prolonged period of cold weather (12). Infection occurs commonly when weaned calves are fed hay on the ground and there is continuous fecal contamination of the feed. The prevalence of infection in calves in the northwestern and midwestern part of the United States is highest in summer, fall and spring compared to midwinter (January) and early summer (June) (18). In North America, the incidence of clinical coccidiosis is highest in late fall and winter. Bovine winter coccidiosis occurs most commonly following a prolonged cold period or a sudden change from a moderate winter to severely cold temperatures (12) which suggests that cold may act as a stressor to precipitate clinical disease in animals previously infected. Experimentally, acute clinical coccidiosis and a marked increase in the numbers of oocysts discharged will occur following the treatment of infected calves with a corticosteroid on the 20th day after infection when clinical signs are apparent (20) or from the 12th to 15th day after infection (21).

Occasional outbreaks occur in beef calves on pasture which gather together near sources of water supply. Coccidiosis may be important in postweaning diarrhea of beef calves in dry tropical regions possibly associated with environmental and dietary stressors and concurrent infections with the parvovirus (19). Coccidiosis can be more severe in dry years which suggests that oocyst challenge was less important than possibly the immunosuppressive effect of weaning and dietary stress in precipitating clinical disease (75). In dairy calves, the disease occurs when calves are overcrowded in dirty wet conditions and when fecal contamination of the feed is common. Lambs may become infected soon after birth (before 4 weeks of age) from three possible sources of infective oocysts: (*a*) oocysts surviving in old fecal contamination of the lambing area arising from previous occupation; (*b*) fresh oocysts constantly passed by the ewes; and (*c*) fresh oocysts passed out by other lambs (22). The fecal oocyst burden is high at 4 weeks of age but gradually declines so that by 5 months of age the fecal oocyst count is similar to that of their parent ewes.

Acute coccidiosis in intensively grazed lambs in Britain, occurs at about 6 weeks of age when the oocyst output is very high in healthy as well as in clinically affected lambs (22). There is no periparturient rise in oocyst output by the ewes. The oocyst output by grazing lambs is very large compared to the output by ewes. Infection also occurs commonly in lambs following their introduction into a feedlot situation where overcrowding and other stressors are operative (24). Often such lambs come directly off range and have very little if any previous exposure to coccidia, making them highly susceptible to infection and outbreaks of clinical disease (25). Acute coccidiosis may occur in animals of any age when their resistance is affected by intercurrent disease or inclement weather (12).

In piglets the disease occurs between 5 and 15 days of age with the highest frequency between 7 and 10 days of age (9). The disease occurs most commonly during the warm summer months when high temperatures favor the sporulation of the oocysts (72). The reported morbidity rates are variable and the case fatality rates may be up to 20%. Rotavirus infection may occur concurrently with *Isospora suis* infection in piglets 1–3 weeks of age and may be important causes of steatorrhea, or unspecified diarrhea known as milk scour, white scour or 3-week diarrhea (67, 69). Coccidiosis caused by *Eimeria scabra* has also occurred in a 40 kg finishing pig affected with severe diarrhea and weight loss (27). An outbreak of severe enteritis with dysentery in grower pigs from 7 to 16 weeks of age, due to a mixture of *Eimeria* spp. including *E. porci* has been recorded (65).

The factors which suggest the presence of neonatal porcine coccidiosis include: repeated outbreaks of neonatal diarrhea in piglets 5–15 days of age; no response to therapy with antimicrobials; and failure of vaccination of the pregnant sow with *E. coli* bacterins to control neonatal piglet diarrhea (10).

Multiple infections comprising more than a single species of coccidia are the rule in natural infections (19). A single species of coccidia may be the major pathogen but others probably contribute to the disease. In some surveys, clinical coccidiosis in cattle occurred only when *E. bovis* and *E. zuernii* occurred together (84). In fecal surveys in sheep and goats, the prevalence of multiple species can be as high as 95% and 85% respectively (26, 70). Similar results have been obtained in surveys done in feeder cattle brought from different geographical locations in the United States to a feedlot (16). While *Eimeria bovis* and *E. zuernii* are the species most commonly associated with bovine coccidiosis, as many as 11 different species may be present in the cows and calves of one beef herd (23). This provides evidence that coccidia have a widespread distribution wherever animals kept.

Specific immunity to each coccidial species develops after infection so that young animals exposed for the first time are often more susceptible to a severe infection and clinical disease than other animals. In lambs, natural infection acquired at pasture and artificial infections acquired by experimental inoculation result in immunity to challenge (27). A single initial infection of as few as 50 oocysts will provoke a solid immunity to reinfection with the same species, and oocyst production ceases after about 10 days. Under field conditions lambs are probably continually ingesting oocysts from pastures which become increasingly contaminated as the season progresses. Thus, immunity to a range of species of coccidia is boosted by frequent reinfection. Resistance to *E. zuernii* infection in calves occurs after chemotherapy, of experimental infection, with monensin or amprolium (17). Both drugs suppress the development of the experimental disease during which time immunity develops. An effective immunity develops in piglets following natural or experimental infection with *Isospora suis* which is the most immunogenic species of swine coccidium (4). Susceptible piglets are exposed to this species of infection in older swine. Piglets develop a more severe clinical disease when infected with *Isospora suis* at 1–3 days of age than when infected at 2 weeks of age (63).

The source of infection is the feces of clinically affected or carrier animals, and infection is acquired by ingestion of contaminated feed and water or by licking the hair coat contaminated with infected feces. Oocysts passed in the feces require suitable environmental conditions if they are to become sporulated. Moist, temperate or cool conditions favor sporulation whereas high temperatures and dryness impede it. In general, oocysts sporulate at a range of 12–32°C (53·5–89·5°F) and require oxygen. They resist freezing down to about −7 to −8°C (19·5–17·5°F) for 2 months but −30°C (−22°F) is usually lethal (19). It has been suggested that oocysts might sporulate in the winter months on the hair coats of animals contaminated with feces. This may explain the continual production of several different species of coccidia during the cold winter months when sporulation on the ground was not possible (19). Dry conditions and high temperatures also destroy sporulated oocysts within a few weeks but the oocysts may survive for up to 2 years under favorable conditions. Ingestion of the sporulated oocysts results in infection but very large numbers must be taken in before clinical disease results. This level of ingestion usually comes about by continual reinfection and building up the degree of environmental contamination. This most commonly occurs when calves or lambs are crowded into small pens or confined in feedlots. Lambs may become infected within a few weeks after birth from a heavily contaminated lambing ground (22). Overcrowding of pastured animals on irrigated pasture or around surface water holes in drought conditions may also cause heavy infestations. Feeder lambs and calves brought into feedlots from sparse grazing may carry a few oocysts which build up into heavy infestations in the lots, especially if conditions are moist. In such situations, clinical signs of the disease usually appear about a month after the animals are confined. Young calves and lambs on pasture may shed large numbers of oocysts for long periods which may be a factor in the development of large coccidial populations.

The origin of the oocysts of *Isospora suis* which infect newborn piglets is uncertain (8). Oocysts of *Isospora suis* cannot usually be found in the feces of sows on swine farms where neonatal coccidiosis occurs. In one survey, no oocysts of *I. suis* were found in sows on farms with a history of neonatal coccidiosis due to *I. suis* but 82% of the sows were infected with *Eimeria* spp. (8). On farms without a history of neonatal coccidiosis the prevalence of *I. suis* in the sows was 0·6% (8). In a survey in Papua-New Guinea 83% of sows raised on concrete were infected with *Isospora suis* (70). In another study, the authors claim that in two swine herds where neonatal coccidiosis due to *I. suis* occurred, the sows either began to excrete oocysts, or oocyst excretion rose to a detectable level from 5 days before to 3 days after farrowing (67). It is possible that sows on problem farms may be shedding oocysts in such low numbers which are not detectable using standard fecal flotation techniques. The oocysts of *Isospora suis* can sporulate and become infected within 12–16 hours at temperature ranges of 32–35°C (89·5–95°F) which are common in modern farrowing units (68).

In confined pigs, infection is much less extensive if they are housed on concrete floors than if they are housed on dirt floors or pasture (28).

The effects of nutrition and nutritional status of the animal as predisposing factors in precipitating clinical coccidiosis have been examined. Early weaning of lambs at 21 days of age followed by experimental infection results in a failure in growth (29). Field observations have shown that early weaned lambs are more susceptible to coccidiosis than those weaned at a later date. This may be a reflection of lack of immunity in the younger lambs but dietary stress in early weaned lambs may contribute to the disease.

Pathogenesis

The coccidia of domestic animals pass through all stages of their life cycle in the alimentary mucosa and do not invade other organs although schizonts have been found in the mesenteric lymph nodes of sheep and goats. The different species of coccidia manifest a tendency to localize in different parts of the intestine. *Eimeria zuernii* and *E. bovis* occur chiefly in the cecum, colon and last part of the ileum whereas *E. ellipsoidalis* and *E. arloingi* parasitize the small intestine.

The coccidial life cycle is self-limiting. Sporozoites are released from the ingested oocysts and invade the endothelial cells of the lacteals in the villi of the posterior half of the small intestine and develop into asexual schizonts. After the schizont matures, the merozoites are released by rupture of the epithelial cell. New epithelial cells are again invaded and second generation schizogony occurs in the large intestine. This is followed by the release of another generation of merozoites which invade epithelial cells and produce the sexual stages, the macrogametocyte and the microgametocyte. The second generation schizogony and fertilization of the macrogametocyte by the microgametocyte (gametogony) are the stages of the lifecycle which cause functional and structural lesions of the large intestine. As the second generation schizonts or gamonts mature, the cells containing them slough from the basement membrane and cause hemorrhage and destruction of the cecum and colon. The oocysts are the result of fertilization of the gametocytes and are discharged at the time of rupture of the cells which usually coincides with the onset of clinical signs of dysentery. The prepatent period varies with the species of coccidia; with *E. bovis* it is 15–20 days and with *E. zuernii*, 15–17 days. Oocyst production in calves infected with *E. zuernii* reaches peak numbers on the 19th and 20th day after experimental infection (21).

The two species of coccidia which are considered most pathogenic to cattle are *E. zuernii* and *E. bovis* and their lifecycles are similar (53). In calves experimentally infected with *E. zuernii*, first generation schizogony occurs in the lower ileum and second generation schizogony and gametogony occurs in the cecum and proximal colon (31). The gametocytes are the pathogenic stages and cause rupture of the cells they invade with consequent exfoliation of the epithelial lining of the intestine. It is notable that the oocyst count is often low when the disease is at its peak as the oocysts have not yet formed. Exfoliation of the mucosa causes diarrhea, and in severe cases, hemorrhage into the intestinal lumen, and the resulting hemorrhagic anemia may be fatal. If the animal survives this stage, the lifecycle of the coccidia terminates without further damage and the intestinal mucosa will regenerate and return to normal. The patent period for *E. bovis* and *E. zuernii* varies from 5 to 12 days depending on the infecting dose of oocysts.

The treatment of calves with a corticosteroid can convert subclinical infection in calves into a peracute clinical form of the disease which suggests that environmental, nutritional and management factors may also act as stressors in producing clinical disease (20, 21). The pathophysiological changes associated with experimental infection of calves with *E. zuernii* include a decrease in packed cell volume and reduction in plasma sodium and chloride levels (18). However, these are not remarkable; in naturally occurring cases the changes are not significant (53). Experimental *E. bovis* infection in calves is reported (66).

In lambs, most natural infections are composed of a number of different species of coccidia and there is a wide range of values in the production of oocysts from individual lambs, either in the feces from the same lamb over a period of time or in the feces from a number of lambs on any one occasion (32). Under practical conditions, constant reinfection occurs and waves of pathogenic stages succeed each other. The occurrence of villous atrophy in the intestinal mucosa of lambs affected by coccidiosis is probably related to the recurrence of diarrhea and loss of body weight (33).

However, in lambs at least, there is some doubt about the effects of coccidial infection on growth rate, feed consumption and clinical signs in the experimental disease. There may be no obvious relationship between infective dose, the fecal oocyst production and clinical disease. This suggests that in lambs, the mere presence of large numbers of fecal oocysts does not constitute a diagnosis of coccidiosis and that other pathogenetic factors may be involved in conversion to clinical disease (29). However, the large number of oocysts present may represent non-pathogenic coccidia.

Severely affected calves which survive the acute phase of the disease do not regain losses in body weight unless they are fed for an additional 3–4 weeks (13) which indicates that bovine coccidia can have a marked effect on performance. A subclinical coccidial infection superimposed on an established, low-grade, subclinical nematode infection in the small intestine may have a marked effect on the mineralization of the skeletal matrix in young adult ruminants (30) and predisposing these animals to osteodystrophy.

The fact that multiple infections are so common may explain the variations in oocyst discharge from infected animals (34) but more importantly in groups of animals; new cases may develop every few days for a few weeks because of the variations in the length of the prepatent period between species of coccidia.

The pathogenesis of the nervous signs of coccidiosis in calves has not been determined (35). Based on the detailed examination of a series of cases the following abnormalities have been tentatively excluded as possible explanations: alternations in serum sodium, potassium, calcium, phosphorus or magnesium concentrations; and vitamin A and thiamin deficiencies; lead poisoning; uremia, *Hemophilus somnus* meningoencephalitis; severity of clinical disease; and gross alteration in intestinal bacterial flora and hepatopathy (83). A labile neurotoxin in the serum of calves with 'nervous coccidiosis' has been identified and characterized but its significance is unknown (83).

The pathogenesis of bovine winter coccidiosis which occurs during or following very cold weather in Canada and the northern United States is not well understood. In January, February and March, the outside temperatures may reach −40°C (−40°F) with daily mean temperatures of −10 to −15°C (14–5°F) for several days consecutively, which should be too cold for sporulation of oocysts in feces on the ground. Sporulation may occur on the moist hair coats of the animals or the endogenous stages of *E. zuernii* may be in a latent phase and reactivated by the stress of cold weather (66).

Isospora suis has at least three asexual and one sexual intraintestinal multiplication cycles (61). All stages are most prominent in the distal half of the small intestine but also occur in the proximal small intestine and cecum and spiral colon. The prepatent period is 5 days and the patent period is biphasic at 5–9 days and 11–14 days postinoculation (61). This biphasic disease course results in diarrhea, villous atrophy and necrosis of intestinal epithelium at 4–6 and 8–10 days after infection. The feces may also be negative for oocysts between the biphasic peaks (64). Under temperature ranges of 32–35°C (89·5–95°F) the oocysts of *Isospora suis* can sporulate and become infective within 12–16 hours (68). An extraintestinal stage of the lifecycle related to the second patent period is postulated. The lesions are most pronounced in the small intestine and consist of villous atrophy and focal ulceration from the destruction of villous epithelial cells principally during the peak of asexual reproduction (62). A fibrinonecrotic pseudomembrane may develop in severe cases (9, 62).

Clinical findings

The incubation period after experimental dosing varies between species of coccidia and animals infected. It ranges from 16 to 30 days in cattle infected with *E. zuernii* and *E. bovis*, from 14 to 18 days in sheep, and as short as 5 days in piglets. The clinical syndromes caused by the various coccidia are similar in all animal species. A mild fever may occur in the early stages but in most clinical cases the temperature is normal or subnormal. The first sign of clinical coccidiosis is usually the sudden onset of severe diarrhea with foul smelling, fluid feces containing mucus and blood. The blood may appear as a dark tarry staining of the feces or as streaks or clots, or the evacuation may consist entirely of large clots of fresh, red blood. The perineum and tail are commonly smudged with bloodstained feces. Severe straining is characteristic, often accompanied by the passage of feces, and rectal prolapse may occur. The degree of hemorrhagic anemia is variable depending on the amount of blood lost. In most naturally acquired cases in calves and lambs anemia is not a feature. In experimental cases of coccidiosis in lambs, due to *E. ninakohlyakimovae*, although 50% of the animals died, there was no evidence of blood loss but there was significant hemoconcentration (15). However, in exceptional cases anemia is severe with pale mucosa, weakness, staggering and dyspnea. Dehydration is common but is not usually severe if affected animals continue to drink water.

There is a decrease in the appetite of most animals with clinical coccidiosis and in exceptional cases there is complete anorexia. The course of the disease is usually 5–6 days but some animals undergo a long convalescent period during which feed consumption and body weight gains are subnormal (13). Severely affected calves do not quickly regain the body weight losses which occurred during the clinical phase of the disease. In mild cases there is diarrhea and reduced growth rate but not necessarily dysentery too. Subclinical cases show inferior growth rate and chronic anemia only.

Nervous signs consisting of muscular tremors, hyperesthesia, clonic–tonic convulsions with ventroflexion of the head and neck and nystagmus and high mortality rate (80–90%) have been reported in calves with acute clinical coccidiosis (12, 35). Outbreaks of this 'nervous form' have occurred in which 30–50% of all susceptible calves are affected. The problem has occurred most commonly during or following severely cold weather in midwinter in Canada and the northern United States. Affected calves may die within 24 hours after the onset of dysentery and the nervous signs, or they may live for several days, commonly in a laterally recumbent position with a mild degree of opisthotonus. In spite of intensive supportive therapy the mortality is high. Nervous signs have not been reported in experimental clinical coccidiosis in calves which suggests that the nervous signs may be unrelated to the dysentery or, indeed, even to coccidiosis.

Coccidiosis in lambs is generally similar to that in calves but with much less dysentery. In groups of lambs raised and fed under intensified conditions the major clinical finding may be inferior growth rate, gradual onset of weakness, inappetence, recumbency, emaciation and death with a course of 1–3 weeks. The diarrhea may escape cursory examination of the animals, but clinical examination of affected lambs reveals a perineum smudged with feces, and soft feces in the rectum. Lambs which have been brought off range with little or no previous exposure to coccidia when mingled in a feedlot may develop the acute disease and the case mortality rate may reach 50%. However, there is some doubt that coccidial infections are the cause of such acute diarrheic outbreaks in lambs even though large numbers of oocysts can be found in the feces (36). It has been suggested that these outbreaks are due to nutritional disorders or concurrent bacterial and helminth infections. Normal, apparently healthy lambs will not uncommonly discharge large numbers of oocysts with no demonstrable effect on growth rate (14). There is evidence that these lambs have developed a solid immunity from naturally acquired infection beginning soon after birth (15). Thus outbreaks of diarrhea and dysentery in lambs must be examined for causes other than coccidia even when large numbers of oocysts are present.

In the horse, while there is some doubt about the pathogenicity of *E. leuckarti*, diarrhea of several days duration, and acute massive intestinal hemorrhage leading to rapid death has been described in foals and young horses (5, 55).

In piglets, severe outbreaks of coccidiosis occur between 5 and 15 days of age (9, 10). Anorexia and depression are common. There is profuse diarrhea and the feces are yellow, watery and sometimes appear foamy. The diarrhea may persist for several days when dehydration and unthriftiness are obvious. Although affected piglets continue to suck they become dehydrated and lose weight. Vomition may occur. Entire litters may be affected and the case fatality rate may reach 20%. The disease may persist in a herd for several weeks or months particularly where a continuous farrowing program is used.

Clinical pathology

Affected animals subjected to a massive infestation of oocysts may develop severe dysentery a few days before occysts appear in the feces. However, this is not commonly observed when the feces from several affected animals are examined, and usually within 2–4 days after the onset of dysentery the oocysts will appear in the feces. The period during which oocysts are discharged in significant numbers (patent period) will vary between species of coccidia, the age of the animal and the degree of immunity, which often makes it necessary to examine a number of animals in a group or herd rather than rely on the results from a single animal. For example, in lambs at pasture, oocysts first appear in the feces at about 2 weeks of age. The oocyst count continues to rise in the lambs until about 8–12 weeks when the counts will be 10^5-10^6/g of feces. Thereafter, the count declines to about 500/g when the lambs are 6–12 months of age. There is also considerable variation, both between lambs and in day-to-day samples from individuals, in the numbers and species of oocysts present in the feces. Hence the need for examination of several samples over a period of several days to assess the burden. In piglets, the prepatent period varies from 4 to 7 days (most commonly 5 days) and oocysts are shed in the feces for 5–8 days after the onset of clinical signs (62, 63). Piglets may develop the disease at 5 days of age and oocysts may not be present in the feces until 3 days later.

A count of over 5000 oocysts/g of feces of ruminants is considered significant. Although counts below 5000/g of feces do not ordinarily suggest clinical infestation, they may indicate a potential source of severe infestation if environmental conditions for spread become favorable. Oocyst counts of over 100 000/g are common in severe outbreaks although similar counts may also be encountered in normal sheep. The output of oocysts following an acute infection falls sharply after the peak which may result in a critically affected animal with dysentery and low oocyst count (71). If oocysts are not found and the disease is suspected, merozoites can be looked for in direct smears; they do not float on the conventional concentrated sugar or salt solutions used for flotation of oocysts. The several species of coccidia can be differentiated up to a point by the characteristics of the oocysts.

Necropsy findings

Congestion, hemorrhagic enteritis and thickening of the mucosa of the cecum, colon, rectum and ileum are the characteristic gross changes at necropsy. The thickening may be severe enough to produce ridges in the mucosa. Small white cyst-like bodies, formed by large schizonts, may be visible on the tips of the villi of the terminal ileum. Ulceration or sloughing of the mucosa may occur in severe cases. The lesions caused by experimental *E. bovis* infection in the small and large intestines are characterized by a diphtheritic typhlitis and colitis (19). Whole-blood or bloodstained feces may be present in the lumen of the large intestine, and the carcass may show profound anemia. Histologically there is denudation of the epithelium, and merozoites may be observed in some cells. Smears of the mucosa or intestinal contents should be examined for the various developmental stages. The necropsy findings in sheep are marked by more severe involvement of the small intestine than in cattle. Villous atrophy of the proximal ileum occurs in both natural and experimental infection in lambs (33). In piglets, the characteristic lesions are villous atrophy and a fibronecrotic enteritis often with a diphtheritic membrane (9, 62). The pathology of acute intestinal coccidiosis in goats is described (57).

Diagnosis

In calves, clinical coccidiosis is characterized by dysentery, tenesmus, mild systemic involvement and dehydration. The presence of large numbers of oocysts supports the diagnosis and necropsy findings are usually characteristic. Differentiation from other diseases of the alimentary tract of cattle is summarized in Table 68. When nervous signs occur in calves which appear to have coccidiosis, differentiation from other diseases causing brain dysfunction must be made. The important points are summarized in Table 95.

In sheep, the diagnosis is dependent on the clinical findings of diarrhea and dysentery, the presence of large numbers of oocysts in the feces and the intestinal lesions at necropsy. Large numbers (100 000/g) of oocysts may occur in the feces of normal lambs and thus the observation of large numbers of oocysts in the feces of lambs affected with diarrhea and/or dysentery may not, in itself, constitute a diagnosis of coccidiosis (36). In lambs which have had previous contact with coccidia and which may be relatively immune, other causes of diarrhea such as *Escherichia coli*, *Salmonella* spp., *Clostridium perfringens* Type C and helminthiasis should be considered.

In piglets, diarrhea due to coccidiosis must be differentiated from enteric colibacillosis, transmissible gastroenteritis, rotavirus infection, *Strongyloides ransomi* and *Clostridium perfringens* type C. Necropsy examination of selected untreated clinical cases is often necessary to make the diagnosis. The disease should be suspected when piglets 5–8 days of age develop a diarrhea which responds poorly to treatment. Outbreaks of diarrhea in piglets under 5 days of age are usually caused by *E. coli* or transmissible gastroenteritis. However, mixed infections are being recognized more frequently and extensive laboratory investigations are often necessary to isolate the causative agents. The diagnosis often requires a combination of consideration of the history of diarrhea in piglets 5–15 days of age, gross and microscopic lesions, the presence of coccidial stages in mucosal smears and histological sections and identification of oocysts in intestinal contents and feces (72). In heavy infections, piglets may die before the sexual stages of the parasite develop and the diagnosis is dependent upon finding lesions, schizonts and merozoites of *Isospora suis* in the middle jejunum and ileum (72). The developmental stages can be detected by the mucosal smear technique (72). A rapid field diagnostic procedure consists of staining glass slide impression smears of the mucosa of the ileum and jejunum (73).

Treatment

Coccidiosis is a self-limiting disease and clinical signs subside spontaneously when the multiplication stage of the parasite has passed. Many treatments have been recommended without taking this into account and it is unlikely that any of the chemotherapeutic agents which are in common use for the treatment of clinical coccidiosis will have any significant effect on the late stages of the coccidia. Most of the drugs used in control (coccidiostats) have a depressant effect on the early first stage schizonts (37). In an outbreak, the clinically affected animals should be isolated and treated if possible. An attempt should be made to reduce the stocking rate of the animals in affected pens or corrals. Overcrowding is a common occurrence in epidemics of coccidiosis. All feed and water should be high enough off the ground to avoid fecal contamination. For severe cases, oral and parenteral fluid therapy is indicated. Mass medication of the feed and water supplies may be indicated in an attempt to abort an outbreak and to minimize the rate of development of new cases. Cattle affected with coccidiosis accompanied with nervous signs should be brought indoors, kept well bedded and warm, and given fluid therapy orally and parenterally. However, the case fatality is high in spite of intensive supportive therapy. Sulfonamide therapy parenterally may be indicated to control the development of secondary bacterial enteritis or pneumonia which may occur in calves subjected to coccidiosis during very cold weather. Corticosteroids are contraindicated in the treatment of acute coccidiosis because they appear to aggravate the lesions and increase the case fatality rate (20).

The chemotherapeutic agents which have been recommended for treatment and control of coccidiosis in calves and lambs have been summarized in Table 76. There is insufficient information available to make reliable recommendations for the specific treatment of acute clinical coccidiosis. None of these chemotherapeutic agents has been adequately tested in clinical trials. Sulfadimidine is used widely for the treatment of acute clinical coccidiosis in calves (37). Amprolium is also used for treatment, and in one trial there was a beneficial effect in terms of increased body weight gains and increased feed consumption compared to affected controls which were allowed to recover spontaneously (13, 38).

For the treatment of coccidiosis in piglets, 2 ml of 9·6% amprolium solution given orally daily for 5 days is recommended (49).

Some preliminary results are available on the use of salinomycin for the treatment of experimental coccidiosis in calves (56).

Control

The control of coccidiosis assumes greatest importance in calves and lambs and has been difficult to achieve with reliability. Successful economical control will depend on avoiding the overcrowding of animals while they develop an immunity to the coccidial species in the environment (47). Only small numbers (50/day) of oocysts are required for the development of solid immunity in lambs. Lambing and calving grounds should be well drained and kept as dry as possible. Lambing pens should be kept dry, cleaned out frequently and bedding disposed of so that oocysts do not have time to sporulate and become infective. All measures which minimize the amount of fecal contamination of hair coats and fleece should be practiced regularly. Feed and water troughs should be high enough to avoid heavy fecal contamination. Feeding cattle on the ground should be avoided if possible, particularly when overcrowding is a problem.

In groups of lambs at pasture, the frequent rotation of

pastures for parasite control will also assist in the controls of coccidial infection. However, when lambs are exposed to infection early in life as a result of infection from the ewe and a contaminated lambing ground, a solid immunity usually develops and only when the stocking density is extremely high will a problem develop.

The control of coccidiosis in feeder calves and lambs brought into a crowded feedlot will again depend on management or chemotherapeutic measures which will control the numbers of oocysts ingested by the animals while effective immunity develops. Management procedures include establishing the optimum stocking density for which there is no scientific information available. However, when animals are overcrowded they usually become dirty, there is excessive competition for feed supplies and growth rate is affected. These can usually be assessed by visual inspection.

Recycling manure into cattle diets poses a problem because of the continual reintroduction of oocysts. Sporulation can be inhibited by proper ensiling to ensure that 25–35°C (77–95°F) is maintained over a 3-week storage period (60). Many chemotherapeutics have been examined for the control of both experimental and naturally occurring coccidiosis in calves and lambs. The ideal coccidiostat will suppress the full development of the lifecycle of the coccidia, allow immunity to develop and not interfere with production performance (78, 79). Those which have been used are summarized in Table 76.

To be effective, cocciostats must be given beginning early in the lifecycle of the coccidia (48). In any group of animals, there will be several different species of coccidia at different stages of the cycle: some at the drug-susceptible stage (before 13–15 days in calves) and some beyond the drug-susceptible stage (after 16–17 days) which explains why coccidiostats appear to be effective in some animals and ineffective in others. In an outbreak in calves, new cases may develop for up to 12–15 days after the commencement of feeding of an effective coccidiostat to in-contact calves. However, there is no method of knowing the stage of the prepatent period in the animals and the most that can be done is to medicate the feed and water supplies with the chemotherapeutic of choice, treat new cases which develop and avoid the stresses of overcrowding and nutritional disorders which may make clinical cases more severe than usual.

Routine prophylactic medication of the feed and water supplies of feeder calves and lambs with the most economical coccidiostat will usually control the disease and allow the development of effective immunity.

The control of coccidiosis in newborn piglets infected with *Isospora suis* has been unreliable. The use of coccidiosis in the feed of the sow for several days or a few weeks prior to and following farrowing has been recommended and used in the field but the results are variable (46). The coccidiostats for coccidiosis due to *Isospora suis* have not been evaluated using well-designed clinical trials (46). A control program designed to decrease the number of oocysts has been recommended and consists of proper cleaning, disinfection and steam cleaning of the farrowing housing (46). Amprolium (25% feed grade) at the rate of 10 kg/tonne of sows' feed beginning 1 week before farrowing and continued until the piglets are 3 weeks of age is also recommended (49).

Some comments about some of the coccidiostats are made here. *Sulfonamides* in the feed at a level of 25–35 mg/kg body weight for at least 15 days have been effective for the control of coccidiosis in calves and lambs. Sulfadimidine at 55 g/tonne is also effective in goats. A combination of chlortetracycline and a sulfonamide has provided protection in calves and lambs (43).

Ionophorous antibiotics

Monensin This is an effective coccidiostat and growth promotant in cattle (38, 39), sheep (40) and goats (74). The recommended levels are 16–33 g/tonne feed for calves (40) and 20 g/tonne of feed for lambs (40). Levels

Table 76. Chemotherapeutics which have been recommended for the treatment and control of coccidiosis in calves and lambs

Chemotherapeutic agent	*Treatment*	*Prevention*
Sulfadimidine (sulfamethazine)	*Calves and lambs*: 140 mg/kg body weight orally daily for 3 days individually	*Calves*: in feed 35 mg/kg body weight for 15 days *Lambs*: daily dose 25 mg/kg body weight for 1 week (14)
Nitrofurazone	*Calves and lambs*: 15mg/kg body weight daily for 7 days or 0·04% in feed for 7 days. In water at 0·0133% for 7 days	*Calves*: in feed at 33 mg/kg body weight for 2 weeks (49) *Lambs*: in feed at 0·04% for 21 days
Amprolium	*Calves*: individual dose at 10 mg/kg body weight daily for 5 days (50) or 65 mg/kg body weight one dose (51) *Lambs*: individual dose 50 mg/kg body weight for 4 days (52) *Piglets*: 2 ml 9·6% amprolium solution orally each day for 5 days	*Calves*: in feed at 5 mg/kg body weight for 21 days (50) *Lambs*: in feed, 50 mg/kg body weight for 21 days (24, 52) *Piglets*: in sows fed at a rate of 10 kg/tonne (25% amprolium feed grade) feed beginning 1 week before farrowing and continue until piglets 3 weeks of age
Monensin	*Lambs*: 2 mg/kg body weight daily for 20 days beginning on 13th day following experimental inoculation (41)	*Lambs*: 20 mg/kg feed fed continuously *Calves*: 16·5 or 33 g/tonne for 31 days
Lasalocid		*Lambs*: 25–100 mg/kg feed from weaning until market. Also, in ewe's diet from 2 weeks before and until 60 days after lambing

of 11 g/tonne feed are not as reliable as the higher dose for calves (77). The recommended level for goats is 16 g/tonne of feed (74). A concentrated ration containing monensin at 15 ppm can be fed to ewes from 4 weeks before lambing until weaning and to lambs from 4 to 20 weeks of age (76). Monensin can markedly reduce the oocyst output of ewes and lambs when fed before and after lambing (22). Withdrawal of the monensin may be followed by the development of fatal coccidiosis in some animals presumably because the drug suppressed the development of immunity. Postweaning coccidiosis in beef calves has been controlled using monensin from intraluminal continuous release devices (75). The toxic level of monensin for lambs is 4 mg/kg body weight (59).

Lasalocid This is an ionophore related to monensin and is also an effective coccidiostat for ruminants. For maximum benefit, lasalocid should be used daily in the feed of coccidia-susceptible lambs for as long as possible. An effective method of control is to medicate the feed of the ewes beginning about 2 weeks before lambing and continue the medication until the lambs are weaned. The lambs begin to receive lasalocid in their creep ration and later in their rations from weaning until market (42). For maximum control of coccidiosis and improved feedlot performance, lasalocid should be given before and during the time that coccidia-naive lambs are first exposed to the natural occurrence of oocysts. A level as low as 25 mg/kg of feed will control coccidiosis and improve performance when fed to lambs in early life. Similar improvements in feedlot performance do not occur in heavier lambs which are already passing oocysts and being fed lasalocid at 25 mg/kg feed (42). Lasalocid is also effective as a coccidiostat when fed free-choice in salt at a level of 0·75% of the total salt mixture (42). Lasalocid at levels from 0·75 to 3 mg/kg body weight are effective in preventing experimental coccidiosis in calves (58). The level of 1 mg/kg body weight is the most effective and rapid and is recommended when outbreaks of coccidiosis are imminent in cattle (80). Monensin, lasalocid and decoquinate at the manufacturer's recommended levels are equally effective (80). A combination of monensin and lasalocid at 22 and 100 mg/kg of diet, respectively, is an effective prophylactic against naturally occurring coccidiosis in early weaned lambs under feedlot conditions (41). The ionophorous compounds are used in the feed continuously from weaning to market and provide control of coccidiosis and improve feedlot performance. The continuous feeding of lasalocid, decoquinate or monensin will effectively control coccidiosis, cessation of medication may result in the appearance of oocysts in the feces and diarrhea (81). Monensin and aureomycin used together for the control of coccidiosis in lambs appears to have detrimental effects on performance and is not recommended (44).

Other coccidiostats

Decoquinate in the feed at levels of 0·5–1·0 mg/kg body weight suppressed oocyst production in experimentally induced coccidiosis of calves (45). A level of 0·5 mg/kg body weight is effective in goats (82).

REVIEW LITERATURE

Gregory, M. W. & Joyner, L. P. (1985) Ovine coccidiosis. *Vet. Ann.*, *25*, 112–119.

McDougald, L. P. (1982) Chemotherapy of coccidiosis. In: *The Biology of the Coccidia*, ed. P. L. Long, pp. 373–427.

Gregory, M. W., Joyner, L. P. & Catchpole, J. (1982) Medication against ovine coccidiosis—a review. *Vet. Res. Commun.*, *5*, 307–325.

Schillhorn van Veen, T. W. (1986) Coccidiosis in ruminants. *Comp. cont. Educ. pract. Vet.*, *8*, F52–F58.

Tubbs, R. C. (1986) A review of porcine neonatal coccidiosis. *Mod. vet. Pract.*, *67*, 899–903.

REFERENCES

(1) Gregory, M. W. & Joyner, L. P. (1985) *Vet. Ann.*, *25*, 112.
(2) Schillorn van Veen, T. W. (1986) *Comp. cont. Educ. pract. Vet.*, *8*, F52.
(3) Lima, J. D. (1981) *J. Protozool.*, *28*, 59.
(4) Stuart, B. P. et al. (1982) *Vet. Parasitol.*, *9*, 185.
(5) Eugster, A. K. & Jones, L. P. (1985) *Southwestern Vet.*, *36*, 197.
(6) Tubbs, R. C. (1986) *Mod. vet. Pract.*, *67*, 899.
(7) Fitzgerald, P. R. (1980) *Adv. vet. Sci.comp. Med.*, *24*, 121.
(8) Lindsay, D. S. et al. (1984) *J. Am. vet. med. Assoc.*, *185*, 419.
(9) Robinson, Y. & Morin, M. (1982) *Can. vet. J.*, *23*, 212.
(10) Sanford, S. E. & Josephon, G. K. A. (1981) *Can. vet. J.*, *22*, 282.
(11) Lindsay, D. S. et al. (1985) *Am. J. vet. Res.*, *46*, 1511.
(12) Nillo, L. (1970) *Can. vet. J.*, *11*, 91.
(13) Fitzgerald, P. R. & Mansfield, M. E. (1972) *Am. J. vet. Res.*, *33*, 1391.
(14) Chapman, H. D. et al. (1973) *Res. vet. Sci.*, *14*, 369.
(15) Chapman, H. D. (1974) *Res. vet. Sci.*, *16*, 1, 7.
(16) Rutz, A. V. (1973) *Zentralbl. VetMed.*, *20B*, 392, 405 & 594.
(17) Stockdale, P. H. G. & Yates, W. D. G. (1978) *Vet. Parasitol.*, *4*, 209.
(18) Stockdale, P. H. G. et al. (1981) *Can. J. comp. Med.*, *45*, 34.
(19) Parker, R. J. et al. (1984) *Aust. vet. J.*, *61*, 181.
(20) Niilo, L. (1970) *Can. J. comp. Med.*, *34*, 325.
(21) Stockdale, P. H. G. & Niilo, L. (1976) *Can. vet. J.*, *17*, 35.
(22) Gregory, M. W. et al. (1983) *Parasitology*, *87*, 421.
(23) Ernst, J. V. et al. (1984) *Vet. Parasitol.*, *15*, 213.
(24) Baker, N. F. et al. (1972) *Am. J. vet. Res.*, *33*, 83.
(25) Pout, D. D. (1969) *Vet. Bull.*, *39*, 609.
(26) Vercruysee, J. (1982) *Vet. Parasitol.*, *10*, 297.
(27) Hill, J. E. et al. (1985) *J. Am. vet. med. Assoc.*, *186*, 981.
(28) Vetterling, J. M. (1966) *Cornell Vet.*, *56*, 155.
(29) Pout, D. D. (1974) *Br. vet. J.*, *130*, 54.
(30) Frandsen, J. C. (1982) *Am. J. vet. Res.*, *43*, 1951.
(31) Stockdale, P. H. G. (1976) *Vet. Parasitol.*, *1*, 367.
(32) Pout, D. D. et al. (1973) *Br. vet. J.*, *129*, 568.
(33) Pout, D. D. (1974) *Br. vet. J.*, *130*, 45.
(34) Catchpole, J. et al. (1976) *Parasitology*, *72*, 137.
(35) Fanelli, H. H. (1983) *Bov. Pract.*, *18*, 50.
(36) Pout, D. D. (1976) *Vet. Rec.*, *98*, 340.
(37) McDougald, L. R. (1982) In: *The Biology of the Coccidia.*, ed. P. L. Long, pp. 373–427.
(38) Gregory, M. W. et al. (1982) *Vet. Res. Commun.*, *5*, 307.
(39) Fitzgerald, P. R. & Mansfield, M. E. (1978) *Am. J. vet. Res.*, *39*, 7.
(40) McDougald, L. R. & Dunn, W. J. (1978) *Am. J. vet. Res.*, *39*, 1459 & 1748.
(41) Horton, G. M. J. & Stockdale, P. H. G. (1981) *Am. J. vet. Res.*, *42*, 433.
(42) Foreyt, W. et al. (1981) *Am. J. vet. Res.*, *42*, 54 & 57.
(43) Ajayi, J. A. (1976) *J. Parasitol.*, *72*, 335.
(44) Samizadeh-Yazd, A. et al. (1979) *Am. J. vet. Res.*, *40*, 1107.
(45) Fitzgerald, P. R. (1986) *Am. J. vet. Res.*, *47*, 130.
(46) Ernst, J. V. et al. (1985) *Am. J. vet. Res.*, *46*, 643.
(47) Rose, M. E. (1976) *Vet. Rec.*, *98*, 481.
(48) Hammond, D. M. (1964) *Coccidiosis of Cattle. Some Unsolved Problems*. 30th Faculty Honour Lecture. The Faculty Association, Utah State University, Logan, Utah.
(49) Coussement, W. et al. (1981) *Vet. Q.*, *3*, 57.

(50) Norcross, M. A. et al. (1984) *Vet. Med. small Anim. Clin.*, *69*, 459, 462.
(51) Newman, A. J. et al. (1968) *Irish vet. J.*, *22*, 142.
(52) Horak, I. G. et al. (1969) *J. S. Afr. vet. med. Assoc.*, *50*, 293.
(53) Radostits, O. M. & Stockdale, P. H. G. (1980) *Can. vet. J.*, *21*, 227.
(54) Morin, M. et al. (1980) *Can. vet. J.*, *21*, 65.
(55) Wheeldon, E. B. & Greig, W. A. (1977) *Vet. Rec.*, *100*, 102.
(56) Benz, G. W. & Ernst, J. V. (1979) *Am. J. vet. Res.*, *40*, 1180.
(57) Opoku-Pare, G. A. & Chineme, C. N. (1979) *Bull. Anim. Hlth Prod. Afr.*, *27*, 269.
(58) Stromberg, B. E. et al. (1982) *Am. J. vet. Res.*, *43*, 583.
(59) Bergstrom, R. C. & Jolley, W. R. (1977) *Vet. Med. small Anim. Clin.*, *72*, 1052.
(60) Farquhar, A. S. et al. (1979) *J. anim. Sci.*, *49*, 1331.
(61) Harleman, J. H. & Meyer, R. C. (1984/85) *Vet. Parasitol.*, *17*, 27.
(62) Robinson, Y. et al. (1983) *Can. J. comp. Med.*, *47*, 401.
(63) Stuart, B. P. et al. (1982) *Can. J. comp. Med.*, *46*, 317.
(64) Harleman, J. H. & Meyer, R. C. (1985) *Vet. Rec.*, *116*, 561.
(65) Jones, G. W. et al. (1985) *Aust. vet. J.*, *62*, 319.
(66) Friend, S. C. E. & Stockdale, P. H. G. (1980) *Can. J. comp. Med.*, *11*, 129.
(67) Roberts, L. & Walker, E. J. (1982) *Vet. Rec.* , *110*, 11.
(68) Ernst, J. V. et al. (1986) *Vet. Parasitol.*, *22*, 1.
(69) Nilsson, O. et al. (1984) *Nord. VetMed.*, *36*, 103.
(70) Varghese, T. (1986) *Vet. Parasitol.*, *21*, 11.
(71) Gregory, M. W. et al. (1980) *Vet. Rec.*, *106*, 161.
(72) Lindsay, D. S. et al. (1983) *Vet. Med. small Anim. Clin.*, *78*, 89.
(73) Cunningham, J. M. (1984) *Agri-Practice.*, *5*, 24.
(74) Shelton, M. et al. (1982) *Southwestern Vet.*, *35*, 27.
(75) Parker, R. J. et al. (1986) *Trop. Anim. Hlth Prod.*, *18*, 198.
(76) Catchpole, J. et al. (1986) *Vet. Rec.*, *118*, 75.
(77) Stromberg, B. E. et al. (1986) *Vet. Parasitol.*, *22*, 135.
(78) Stockdale, P. H. G. & Sheard, A. (1982) *Vet. Parasitol.*, *9*, 171.
(79) Fitzgerald, P. R. & Mansfield, M. E. (1984) *Am. J. vet. Res.*, *45*, 1984.
(80) Foreyt, W. J. et al. (1986) *Am. J. vet. Res.*, *47*, 2031.
(81) Conlogue, G. et al. (1984) *Am. J. vet. Res.*, *45*, 863.
(82) Foreyt, W. J. et al. (1986) *Am. J. vet. Res.*, *47*, 333.
(83) Isler, C. M. et al. (1987) *Can. J. vet. Res.*, *51*, 253, 261, 271.
(84) Kennedy, M. J. & Kralka, A. (1987) *Can. vet. J.*, *28*, 124.

Sarcocystosis (sarcosporidiosis)

The commonest occurrence of this disease is as a lesion encountered during meat inspection—sarcosporidiosis. However, there is an increasing incidence of systemic clinical disease—sarcocystosis—in ruminants and pigs, arising from infestation with sarcocysts of dogs. The causative protozoa pass part of their lifecycle in dogs and cats from which they are transmitted to ruminants causing lesions in all tissues and organs, but especially in skeletal muscle.

Etiology

There are a number of species, each specific to a final host, e.g. *Sarcocystis bovicanis* (cattle as a final host, dog as intermediate host), *S. bovifelis*, *S. porcifelis*. This is the type of terminology which is in common use. It ignores the correct taxonomy, for example, *S. bovifelis* = *S. hirsuta*, *S. ovicanis* = *S. tenella.*

Epidemiology

Sarcocystis is a sporozoan parasite with an obligatory intermediate host. The definitive hosts of the various *Sarcocystis* spp. infecting sheep, cattle, pigs and horses are dogs, cat and man (18). Each definitive host may have several species of *Sarcocystis*, each one being specific for a particular intermediate host, and similarly, each intermediate host may be infected with several species of *Sarcocystis* from different definitive hosts. Thus, *Sarcocystis ovicanis* has a lifecycle from dogs to sheep, *S. porcifelis* from cats to pigs, etc. The nomenclature has recently been revised (1). The *Sarcocystis* spp. undergo an enteric cycle in the intermediate host: the oocysts form in the cells of the intestine and sporocysts are passed in the feces which either contaminate the food directly or indirectly after drying and being blown as dust. The sporocysts from the cat have low pathogenicity, but form large cysts in the esophagus and muscles throughout the body. Those from the dog, when ingested, are converted to sporozoites which invade tissues and undergo two schizogonous phases in the endothelial cells of the arterioles and capillaries respectively of the intermediate host, before passing to the muscles where they form microscopic cysts.

The infections are very widespread and the macroscopic cysts are a cause of meat condemnation. More than 75% of cattle in the United States have cysts in skeletal or cardiac muscles (20). It is also known that infection depresses the growth rate (10, 15). Norwegian data indicates an infection rate of 80% (12). The species from dogs are very pathogenic in experimental work, but rarely cause disease naturally. However, Dalmeny disease (3) is now thought to be due to *Sarcocystis* infection. An outbreak of clinical sarcocystosis is also recorded in cattle, with the infection stemming from dogs housed in the same shed (9, 25). Other similar outbreaks have been reviewed (1). Asymptomatic infection is very common. For example, in animals continually at pasture, the ingestion of a few sporocysts when they commence grazing probably provokes a strong immunity to later challenge. When groups of animals that have not been exposed to infection previously are suddenly brought into contact with heavy contamination, especially from dogs and cats, outbreaks of clinical disease are likely to occur.

Pathogenesis

Sarcocystis spp. are organisms with a two-host cycle, a prey–predator system. The species from the dog undergo schizogony in the endothelial cells of the arterioles and capillaries of the intermediate host causing widespread hemorrhage and anemia, and the disease has been transmitted by blood transfusion from acutely affected donors (16). Experimental sarcocystosis produced in goats by oral dosing with *S. capricanis* is characterized by vasculitis, interstitial pneumonia and necrosis of mesenteric lymph nodes (5). The species from man that infects pigs has also been found to be pathogenic (4). The vascular lesion appears to be an essential part of the disease's pathogenesis. The species from cats produces large sarcocysts that cause rejection at meat inspection but they do not have a schizogony stage and are not pathogenic.

The severity of the illness and the degree of infection of tissues at postmortem in experimentally induced cases increase with the size of the infective dose. In natural infections very heavy contamination of feed with fecal oocysts has been encountered, but how closely naturally occurring cases resemble experimentally induced ones still remains to be clarified.

Clinical findings

Laboratory and natural infections of sheep, goats (5), buffalo calves (6) and cattle (24) and calves have been characterized by anorexia, fever, emaciation, nervousness, hypersalivation, lameness, loss of tail switch creating a 'rat-tail' appearance, anemia and abortion (19). Obvious illness commences 23–26 days (7) after infection and a rise in temperature and heart rate is noticed first. The course of the disease depends on the dose rate of sporocysts and less serious forms of the disease occur. For example, in sheep a reduction in growth rate may be the only manifestation (10). Abortion in cows associated with a non-suppurative, multifocal encephalitis in the fetuses is reputed to have been a manifestation of sarcosporidiosis (22). A non-suppurative encephalomyelitis of lambs has also been suspected to be caused by sarcosporidia (23). Affected lambs showed ataxia then flaccid paralysis (26). Experimental transmission in pregnant ewes can cause abortion as a major manifestation of the severe form of the disease (17). The experimental disease in horses is characterized by fever, apathy, inappetence and motor disturbances related to a myopathy (2). *Sarcocystis* sp. have also been identified in the spinal cord of horses with protozoal myeloencephalitis (13). Sarcocystosis produced experimentally in pigs is manifested by cutaneous purpura on the snout, ears and buttocks, and dyspnea, tremor and weakness or recumbency (5).

Clinical pathology

Characteristic laboratory findings in the systemic disease include a responsive anemia and high titers of anti-sarcocystis antibodies and serum levels of creatine phosphokinase, lactic dehydrogenase and aspartate aminotransferase are significantly elevated (27). An indirect hemagglutination test (IHA) is the commonly used test but an indirect fluorescent antibody test is also available. Titers of antibodies are not high at the time of an acute illness but are at diagnostic levels 1 week to 3 months afterwards (14).

Necropsy findings

Emaciation, lymphadenopathy, laminitis, anemia and ascites are present, but the most obvious feature is the petechial and ecchymotic hemorrhages throughout the body (7). There are also erosions and ulcerations in the oral cavity and esophagus (7). Microscopically, schizonts are found in endothelial cells throughout the body and hemorrhages, lymphocytic infiltration and edema are seen in heart, brain, liver, lung, kidney and striated muscle (7). Death is probably a result of the severe necrotizing myocarditis that occurs.

Diagnosis

Diagnosis in clinical cases would be very difficult because of the non-specific signs observed. At necropsy it would be necessary to differentiate the disease from septicemia of any kind and from those other diseases such as bracken poisoning which are characterized by extensive hemorrhage in serosa.

Treatment

No effective treatment is available but amprolium or salinomycin may relieve the signs. Amprolium 100 mg/kg given daily from the time of inoculation was shown to reduce the severity of infection in experimentally infected calves (8), but treatment of naturally occurring cases has not been recorded. Treatment of experimentally infected calves with salinomycin (4 mg/kg body weight daily in divided doses for 30 days) reduced the severity of the illness (3). Monensin may have a similar ameliorating effect (9).

Control

Control is difficult as it involves the separation of dogs and stock which is not possible on most farms. However, infection in dogs could be avoided if all meat was thoroughly cooked (2). Prior exposure to small numbers of pathogenic sarcocysts produces a strong immunity and there have been preliminary examinations of possible vaccination procedures (11).

REVIEW LITERATURE

Briggs, M. & Foreyt, W. (1985) Sarcocystosis in cattle. *Comp. cont. Educ.*, 7, S396.
Dubey, J. P. & Fayer, R. (1983) Sarcocystosis. *Br. vet. J.*, *139*, 371.
Markus, M. B. (1978) Sarcocystis and sarcocystosis in domestic animals and man. *Adv. vet. Sci.*, *22*, 159.

REFERENCES

(1) Dubey, J. P. (1976) *J. Am. vet. med. Assoc.*, *169*, 1061.
(2) Schnieder, T. et al. (1985) *Zentralbl. VetMed. B*, *32*, 29.
(3) McDaniel, H. T. et al. (1983) *Ann. Mtg Am. Assoc. Swine Pract.*, p. 17.
(4) Heydorn, A. O. (1977) *Berl. Münch. Tierärztl. Wochenschr.*, *11*, 218.
(5) Barrows, P. L. et al. (1982) *Am. J. vet. Res.*, *43*, 1409.
(6) Achuthan, H. N. (1983) *Ind. vet. J.*, *60*, 344.
(7) Johnson, A. J. et al. (1975) *Am. J. vet. Res.*, *36*, 995.
(8) Fayer, R. & Johnson, A. J. (1975) *J. Parasitol.*, *61*, 932.
(9) Foreyt, W. J. (1986) *Am. J. vet. Res.*, *47* 1674.
(10) Munday, B. L. (1986) *Vet. Parasitol.*, *21*, 21.
(11) Fayer, R. & Dubey, J. P. (1984) *Vet. Parasitol.*, *15*, 187.
(12) Bratberg, B. & Landsverk, T. (1980) *Acta vet. Scand.*, *21*, 395.
(13) Simpson, C. R. & Mayhew, I. G. (1980) *J. Protozool.*, *27*, 288.
(14) Fayer, R. (1982) *Proc. 14th Ann. Conf. AABP*, p. 117.
(15) Erber, M. (1981) *Prakt. Tierärztl*, *62* 422.
(16) Fayer, R. & Leek, R. G. (1979) *J. Parasitol.*, *65*, 890.
(17) Leek, R. G. & Fayer, R. (1978) *Cornell Vet.*, *68*, 108.
(18) Ford, G. E. (1975) *Aust. vet. J.*, *51*, 407.
(19) Collins, G. H. et al. (1980) *NZ vet. J.*, *28*, 156.
(20) Stalheim, O. H. V. (1980) *J. Am vet. med. Assoc.*, *176*, 299.
(21) Foreyt, W. J. et al. (1986) *Vet. Med.*, *81*, 275.
(22) McCausland, I. P. et al. (1984) *Cornell Vet.*, *74*, 146.
(23) Morgan, G. et al. (1984) *Br. vet. J.*, *140*, 64.
(24) Fayer, R. et al. (1983) *J. dairy Sci.*, *66*, 904.
(25) Carrigan, M. J. (1986) *Aust. vet. J.*, *63*, 22.
(26) Stubbings, D. P. & Jeffrey, M. (1985) *Vet. Rec.*, *116*, 373.
(27) Prasse, K. W. & Fayer, R. (1981) *Vet. Pathol.*, *18*, 351 & 358.

Cryptosporidiosis

Cryptosporidiosis is a protozoan disease of the intestinal tract primarily of neonatal farm animals, especially calves, characterized clinically by varying degrees of diarrhea for which there is no specific therapy. It is a zoonosis and can cause severe clinical disease in immunologically comprised people.

Etiology

Crytosporidiosis is caused by the genus *Cryptosporidium*. *Cryptosporidium parvum* and *Cryptosporidium muris* are distinct species (24).

Cryptosporidium parvum is the most common species found in calves and man, and is transmitted readily to several newborn species of mammals. *Cryptosporidium muris* infects the stomach of mice and is more host and tissue specific than *C. parvum* (4).

There has been much controversy about the role of *Cryptosporidium* as a causative agent of diarrhea in animals and man because the protozoan parasite can be found in normal healthy animals. However, it is now considered that the parasite is a significant cause of varying degrees of naturally occurring diarrhea in neonatal farm animals and the disease has been produced experimentally although it is not completely certain that only cryptosporidia were present in the experimental inoculum.

Epidemiology

Cryptosporidiosis has been recognized worldwide primarily in neonatal calves (1–4), but also in lambs (8, 9), goat kids (10), foals (11) and piglets (36). The protozoan can be found in the feces of calves without clinical signs of diarrhea which has created some doubt about the cause and effect relationship (5). The infection is most common in young animals which develop immunity and recover from the infection (4).

The current range of known hosts includes seven orders of mammals, four orders of birds, one order of reptiles and two orders of fish (23). Various isolates from mammals and birds have been successfully transmitted to both homologous and heterologous host species. Because the parasite can cross host species barriers, infections in domestic animals, wildlife species and companion animals must be regarded as possible reservoirs of infection. Surveys of neonatal calves on dairy farms have revealed that concurrent diarrhea was present in only about 50% of calves which were shedding oocysts of *Cryptosporidium* (7). In a survey of fecal samples from dairy calves in Idaho 45–67% of the participating herdsmen had one or more calves infected with cryptosporidia (13). Cryptosporidium were detected in 70% of 1–3-week-old dairy calves based on a single examination of feces (14). The parasite could not be found in the feces of the dams of infected calves. The source of the cryptosporidia is unknown. One survey failed to demonstrate cryptosporidium oocysts in the feces of 1600 clinically normal adult cows on premises where the prevalence of infection with cryptosporidia in the calves was high (41). In a retrospective study of adult cattle in Canada approximately 40% had serum antibody to *Cryptosporidium* (27).

In most naturally occurring cases of diarrhea in calves in which cryptosporidia are present in the feces, other enteropathogens such as the rotavirus and the coronavirus are also present as a mixed infection (12). About 25% of diarrheic calves 5 days to 1 month of age are infected with *C. parvum*.

In dairy herds ranging from 60 to 250 cows in size, calves may begin excreting oocysts at 10–12 days of age and even as early as 5 days of age, usually continues for up to 1 week and may be excreted in up to 85 of calves (22).

Cryptosporidium is considered to be a relatively common non-viral cause of self-limiting diarrhea in immunocompetent persons, particularly in children during the late summer and fall (6). In immunologically compromised persons, clinical disease may be severe (29). This is particularly serious in human patients with acquired immune deficiency syndrome (29). In a laboratory survey of fecal samples from humans affected with diarrhea, oocysts of *Cryptosporidium* were found in 1% of the samples (19). Oocysts were found in 25% of the fecal samples from diarrheic beef calves and no epidemiological association between the infection in man and cattle could be established (19).

Animal handlers on a calf farm can be at high risk of diarrhea due to cryptosporidiosis transmitted from infected calves (27, 28).

Diarrhea associated with cryptosporidia has occurred in calves primarily from 5 to 15 days of age (8), in lambs from 4 to 10 days of age (9, 15), goat kids from 5 to 21 days of age (10), and in foals from 5 days to 6 weeks of age (11). The oocysts were not present in the feces of neonatal foals all of which had diarrhea between 7 and 22 days of age (42). In a retrospective study of piglets submitted to a diagnostic laboratory over a 4 year period, cryptosporidia were detected histologically in 5·3% of about 3500 piglets (50). Infected pigs were primarily from 6 to 12 weeks of age and only 26% of cryptosporidia-infected pigs had diarrhea and most of those with the protozoan had other enteropathogens capable of causing diarrhea.

The method of transmission is considered to be by oocysts that are fully sporulated and infective when they are passed in the feces (16, 30).

The thick-walled oocysts are resistant to most disinfectants and can survive for several months in cool and moist conditions. The infectivity of the oocysts can be destroyed by ammonia, formalin, freeze-drying and exposure to temperatures below 0°C (32°F) and above 65°C (149°F) (1). Only 10% formol saline and 5% ammonia are effective in destroying the infectivity of the oocysts (20). The infectivity of oocysts in calf feces is reduced after 1–4 days of drying (21).

The factors which make animals susceptible to infection or which predispose infected animals to develop clinical disease are not well understood. Concurrent infections with other enteropathogens especially rotavirus and coronavirus in calves are common (12, 18). In a study of diarrheic calves submitted to a diagnostic laboratory, in 55% of the cases cryptosporidia were the only pathogens isolated, while in 39% the protozoan agent was found in combination with rotavirus and/or coronavirus (18). Immunologically comprised animals may be more susceptible to clinical disease than immunocompetent animals but this has not been substantiated. In one series of observations there was a tendency for the prevalence of infection to be higher during the winter months of the year when the calves were confined which suggests a build-up of contamination (17). The disease has been a cause of chronic diarrhea and cachexia in veal calves (39).

There is only limited information available on the case fatality rate in calves affected with diarrhea due to *Cryptosporidium*. Case fatality rates of about 15% in diarrheic beef calves and 35–60% in dairy and mixed herds have been recorded (19).

The inoculation of cryptosporidia isolated from calves into different host species such as the calf, lamb (31), pig, rat, mouse, guinea-pig and chicken will result in infection (23). Thus cryptosporidia are non-host specific parasites (23). Because the parasite can cross host species barriers, infections in domestic animals and pets may be regarded as reservoirs of infection for susceptible humans. Oocysts from the feces of wild mice are infective for calves which may develop non-fatal clinical cryptosporidiosis (25). Some strains of *Cryptosporidium* such as those infective for guinea pigs are host specific and may be used as experimental models for the study of immunity and therapy (26).

Pathogenesis

The lifecycle of *Cryptosporidium* consists of six major developmental events. Following ingestion of the oocyst there is excystation (release of infective sporozoites), merogony (asexual multiplication), gametogony (gamete formation), fertilization, oocyst wall formation, and sporogony (sporozoite formation) (3). Thus the oocysts of *Cryptosporidia* spp. can sporulate within the host cell, in contrast to the oocysts of *Eimeria* and *Isospora* sp. which do not sporulate until they are passed from the host, and they are infective when passed in the feces (3). Sporulated oocysts can excyst in the intestine before being excreted in the feces and the infection can persist until the immune response of the animal eliminates the parasite. In naturally occurring cases in calves the cryptosporidia are most numerous in the lower part of the small intestine and occasionally in the cecum and colon (34). The middle and lower portions of the jejunum and ileum have the largest numbers of organisms following experimental infections in newborn calves (32). In the initial stages of the experimental disease the infection predominates in the small intestine but later the large intestine is also affected (38). The prepatent period is 4–6 days and oocysts may be passed in the feces of calves as early as 5–12 days of age and continue for 3–12 days. Calves which recover from the infection are not chronic carriers and do not recrudesce when treated with corticosteroids (4). The complete development of *Cryptosporidium* in cell culture has been achieved and allows a means of studying its behaviour, development, metabolism and the effect of therapeutic agents (29).

The intracellular stages of the organism are within a parasitophorous vacuole which is confined to the microvillous region of the host cell (3). The cryptosporidia appear free in the lumen of the intestine and attached to the microvilli of the villous epithelial cells. The parasitophorous envelope of the trophozoites and schizonts are derived from the microvilli, and the intracellular location of the organism is confined to fusion of the organism with the apical cytoplasm of the epithelial cells and their enclosure by host membranes (33). Thus the organism is intracellular but extracytoplasmic. The pathogenesis of the diarrhea is unknown but the varying degrees of villous atrophy suggests that digestion and absorption may be impaired resulting in diarrhea. The experimental inoculation of gnotobiotic calves with a monoinfection of *Cryptosporidium* species which were treated with peracetic acid to destroy other possible enteropathogens results in lesions of villous atrophy and diarrhea which indicates that the organism can cause intestinal lesions (35) without concurrent infection with other enteropathogens. There is also evidence of hyperplastic crypt epithelium which along with damaged villous epithelium and atrophic villi indicates that the lesions develop as a result of accelerated destruction or loss rather than decreased production of epithelial cells (35).

Experimentally, inoculation of oocysts into the trachea and conjunctival sacs of pigs will result in focal destruction and loss of epithelial cells (37) which is similar to naturally occurring infections of birds.

Clinical findings

There are no clinical findings which are characteristic of diarrhea due to infection with *Cryptosporidium* in calves. In general, calves are usually 5–15 days of age and have usually had a mild to moderate diarrhea for a few days which for several days seems to persist with or without treatment with fluids and electrolytes and the usual treatments for diarrhea. In fact, the persistence of the diarrhea usually suggests the presence of cryptosporidiosis. Some descriptions include the observation of yellow, watery feces containing mucus (40). The persistent diarrhea results in marked loss of body weight and an appearance of emaciation in some cases. However, in most cases the diarrhea is self-limiting after several days. Varying degrees of apathy, reduced feed intake and dehydration are present. Only rarely does severe dehydration, weakness and collapse occur as in other causes of acute diarrhea in neonatal calves.

In the experimental disease in calves, depression and anorexia are the earliest and most consistent clinical findings. Feed intake is reduced and combined with the persistent diarrhea over several days may cause emaciation. However, recovery may occur between 6 and 10 days after the onset of diarrhea (38). Both the incubation period and the clinical course of diarrhea in calves affected with cryptosporidiosis tends to be a few days longer than the diarrheas caused by rotavirus, coronavirus or enterotoxigenic *E. coli* (38). Varying degrees of dehydration occurs but severe dehydration is not a constant feature.

In the experimental disease in lambs, depression, diarrhea and reduced feed intake are common and recovery occurs within a few days.

Clinical pathology

The oocysts can be detected in the feces by examination of fecal smears with certain stains or by fecal flotation. It has been suggested that if the diarrhea is caused by cryptosporidia the feces should contain 10^5-10^7 oocysts per ml of feces (4). The oocysts are small (5–6 μm in diameter), difficult to see and often confused with yeast bodies because of their similar size and color. The oocysts are relatively non-refractile and difficult to detect by normal light microscopy. They are readily detected by phase-contrast microscopy. The demonstration of oocysts concentrated from fecal samples is by centrifugal flotation in high specific-gravity salt solutions (23). The Giemsa stain has been used but oocysts have a poor affinity for the stain and tend to fade into the background of protein and other debris present in fecal smears and may be missed when present in low numbers. The dichromate solution flotation technique is simple, rapid and inexpensive and more sensitive than fecal smears stained with Wright–Giemsa stain (43). The staining of fecal smears with a methylene blue–eosin stain is also highly sensitive (44). The dimethylsulfoxide–Ziehl-Neilsen is a simple and rapid procedure well suited for large-scale routine diagnosis of cryptosporidia (45). An immunofluorescence technique on fecal smears is also available (46).

Necropsy findings

Varying degrees of dehydration, emaciation and serous atrophy, are present in calves which have had persistent diarrhea for several days. In the intestine there is villous atrophy in the ileum, cecum and colon. Histologically, the cryptosporidia are associated with the microvilli of the villous epithelial cells. Large numbers of the parasite are embedded in the microvilli of jejunal and ileal absorptive enterocytes (40). In low-grade infections only a few parasites are present, with no apparent histological changes in the intestine. The scanning and transmission electron microscopic appearances of the intestine of calves with cryptosporidiosis are recorded (33). The villi are shorter than normal and there is crypt hyperplasia and infiltration with a mixture of inflammatory cells (35).

Diagnosis

Cryptosporidiosis occurs primarily in calves from 5 to 15 days of age and is characterized by a mild to moderate self-limiting diarrhea which usually lasts for 4–6 days unless concurrent infections or possibly immune deficiency are present in which case the diarrhea may persist indefinitely and the prognosis is unfavorable. The disease must be differentiated from other common infectious diarrheas in calves. On a clinical basis some differentiation may be possible based on the age occurrence of the diarrhea. Acute enterotoxigenic colibacillosis occurs in calves under 3 days of age, and rotavirus and coronavirus diarrhea occurs in calves 5 to 10 days of age from 3 to 6 weeks of age and is characterized by a fibrinous enteritis.

A presumptive diagnosis of cryptosporidiosis can be made by finding the oocysts in the feces of diarrheic calves.

Treatment

There is no known specific treatment for cryptosporidiosis in neonatal farm animals. Several different types of antiprotozoal drugs (47) and antimicrobials (48) have been evaluated with no therapeutic effect. The prophylactic effects of anticoccidial drugs in experimental murine cryptosporidiosis has been examined but with insignificant success (49). Affected calves should be treated with fluids and electrolytes both orally and parenterally as necessary until spontaneous recovery occurs. Cow's whole milk should be given in small quantities several times daily to optimize digestion and to minimize loss of body weight. Several days of intensive care and feeding may be required before recovery is apparent. Parenteral nutrition could be considered for valuable calves.

Control

The disease is difficult to control because the original source of the organism in a herd is unknown.

The rational approach to prevention is to minimize the fecal–oral transmission between the source of the organism and neonatal farm animals and between the animals. Reducing the number of oocysts ingested may reduce the severity of infection and allow immunity to develop. Mature oocysts are strongly resistant to many disinfectants but their infectivity can be destroyed by exposure to 5% ammonia or 10% formol saline. Calves should be born in a clean environment. Diarrheic calves should always be isolated from healthy calves during the course of the diarrhea and for several days after recovery. Calf-rearing houses should be vacated and cleaned out on a regular basis; an all-in all-out management system, with thorough cleaning and several weeks of drying between batches of calves, should be used. Rats and mice should be controlled where possible.

REVIEW LITERATURE

Anderson, B. C. (1982) Cryptosporidiosis: a review. *J. Am. vet. med. Assoc.*, *180*, 1455–1456.

Angus, K. W. (1983) Cryptosporidiosis in man, domestic animals and birds: a review. *J. Roy. Soc. Med.*, *76*, 62–70.

Current, W. L. (1985) Cryptosporidiosis. *J. Am. vet. med. Assoc.*, *187*, 1334–1338.

Levine, N. D. (1984) Toxonomy and review of the coccidian genus *Cryptosporidium* (Protozoa: Apicomplexa). *J. Protozool.*, *31*, 94–98.

Moon, H. W. & Woodmansee, D. B. (1986) Cryptosporidiosis. *J. Am. vet. med. Assoc.*, *189*, 643–646.

Tzipori, S. (1983) Cryptosporidiosis in animals and humans. *Microbiol. Rev.*, *47*, 84–96.

REFERENCES

(1) Tzipori, S. (1983) *Microbiol. Rev.*, *47*, 84.
(2) Anderson, B. C. (1982) *J. Am. vet. med. Assoc.*, *180*, 1455.
(3) Current, W. L. (1985) *J. Am. vet. med. Assoc.*, *187*, 1334.
(4) Moon, H. W. & Woodmansee, D. B. (1986) *J. Am. vet. med. Assoc.*, *189*, 643.
(5) Fayer, R. et al. (1985) *Proc. Helminthol. Soc. Wash.*, *52*, 64.
(6) Wolfson, J. S. et al. (1985) *New Engl. J. Med.*, *312*, 1278.
(7) Leek, R. G. & Fayer, R. (1984) *Proc. Helminthol. Soc. Wash.*, *51*, 360.
(8) Anderson, B. C. (1982) *J. Am. vet. med. Assoc.*, *181*, 151.
(9) Ahourai, P. et al. (1985) *Trop. Anim. Hlth Prod.*, *17*, 6.
(10) Tzipori, S. et al. (1982) *Vet. Rec.*, *111*, 35.
(11) Gajadhar, A. A. et al. (1985) *Can. vet. J.*, *26*, 132.
(12) Morin, M. et al. (1976) *Can. J. comp. Med.*, *40*, 228.
(13) Anderson, B. C. & Hall, R. F. (1982) *J. Am. vet. med. Assoc.*, *181*, 484.
(14) Markovics, A. et al. (1984) *Refuah Vet.*, *41*, 134.
(15) Angus, K. W. et al. (1982) *Vet. Rec.*, *110*, 129.
(16) Angus, K. W. (1983) *J. Roy. Soc. Med.*, *76*, 62.
(17) Henriksen, S. A. & Krogh, H. V. (1985) *Nord. VetMed.*, *37*, 34.
(18) Krogh, H. V. & Henriksen, S. A. (1985) *Nord. VetMed.*, *37*, 42.
(19) Mann, E. D. et al. (1986) *Can. J. vet. Res.*, *50*:174.
(20) Campbell, I. et al. (1983) *Vet. Rec.*, *111*, 414.
(21) Anderson, B. C. (1986) *Am. J. vet. Res.*, *47*, 2272.
(22) Leeuw, P. W. De, et al. (1984) *Proc. 13th World Congr. Dis. Cattle*, *1*, 104.
(23) O'Donoghue, P. J. (1985) *Aust. vet. J.*, *62*, 253.
(24) Upton, S. J. & Current, W. L. (1985) *J. Parasitol.*, *71*, 625.
(25) Klesius, P. H. et al. (1986) *J. Am. med. vet. Assoc. 189*, 192.
(26) Angus, K. W. et al. (1985) *J. comp. Pathol.*, *95*, 151.
(27) Mann, E. D. et al. (1987) *Can. vet. J.*, *28*, 126.
(28) Rahaman, A. S. M. H. et al. (1984) *Lancet*, *2*, (8396) 221.
(29) Current, W. L. & Haynes, T. B. (1984) *Science*, USA, *224* (4649) 603.

(30) Moon, H. W. & Bemrick, W. J. (1981) *Vet. Pathol.*, *18*, 248.
(31) Snodgrass, D. R. et al. (1984) *J. comp. Pathol.*, *94*, 141.
(32) Anderson, B. C. (1984) *Am. J. vet. Res.*, *45*, 1474.
(33) Pearson, G. R. & Logan, E. F. (1983) *Res. vet. Sci.*, *34*, 149.
(34) Pearson, G. R. et al. (1982) *Res. vet. Sci.*, *33*, 228.
(35) Heine, J. et al. (1984) *J. Infect. Dis.*, *150*, 768.
(36) Tzipori, S. et al. (1981) *Res. vet. Sci.*, *31*, 358.
(37) Heine, J. et al. (1984/85) *Vet. Parasitol.*, *17*, 17.
(38) Tzipori, S. et al. (1983) *Vet. Rec.*, *112*, 116.
(39) Hage-Noordam, A. W. et al. (1982) *Tijdschr. Diergeneeskd.*, *107*, 497.
(40) Sanford, S. E. & Josephson, G. K. A. (1982) *Can. vet. J.*, *23*, 343.
(41) Anderson, B. C. (1982) *Proc. 11th Ann. Mtg Am. Assoc. Bov. Pract.*, pp. 92–94.
(42) Reinemeyer, C. R. et al. (1984) *Equ. vet. J.*, *16*, 217.
(43) Willson, P. J. & Acres, S. D. (1982) *Can. vet. J.*, *23*, 240.
(44) Redman, D. R. et al. (1983) *Proc. 26th Ann. Mtg Am. Assoc. Vet. Lab. Diag.*, pp. 231–240.
(45) Pohjola, S. et al. (1985) *Vet. Rec.*, *116*, 442.
(46) Stibbs, H. H. & Ongerth, J. E. (1986) *J. clin. Microbiol.*, *24*, 517.
(47) Moon, H. W. et al. (1982) *Vet. Rec.*, *110*, 181.
(48) Tzipori, S. R. et al. (1982) *Aust. J. Exp. Biol. Med. Sci.*, *60*, 187.
(49) Angus, K. W. et al. (1984) *Vet. Rec.*, *114*, 166.
(50) Sanford, S. E. (1987) *J. Am. vet. med. Assoc.*, *190*, 695.

Giardiasis

Many infections with the protozoa *Giardia* spp. (such as *G. bovis*, *G. caprae*, *G. equi*) are subclinical and the evidence in calves (1), goats (2) and horses (3) that they are pathogens is unconvincing. Suspected cases and outbreaks are very rare and other more common pathogenic protozoa are often present also. The disease ascribed to *Giardia* spp. is a chronic, mucoid intermittent diarrhea, suggestive of malabsorption. The diagnosis is made on the presence of typical cysts in a flotation specimen made over a zinc sulfate solution. Atabrine (1) and metronidazole (2) have been used as treatment with apparent success.

REFERENCES

(1) Willson, P. J. (1983) *Can. vet. J.*, *23*, 83.
(2) Sutherland, R. J. & Clarkson, A. R. (1984) *NZ vet. J.*, *32*, 34.
(3) Kirkpatrick, C. E. & Skand, D. L. (1985) *J. Am. vet. med. Assoc.*, *187*, 163.

Besnoitiosis

Cutaneous besnoitiosis is restricted in its distribution to south-western Europe and the African continent. *Besnoitia besnoiti* has been isolated from cutaneous lesions in cattle and horses and *B. bennetti* from burros in the United States (1) and cattle, especially beef bulls in Israel (11).

Infection is thought to occur by ingestion of feed contaminated by the feces of an infected cat (5). Cats become infected by eating cysts in the tissues of infected intermediate hosts. The development of the disease in the cat is confined to the intestine. In cattle, infections of the teat skin may result in lesions around the mouth in suckled calves. In cattle in the early stages there is high fever, an increase in pulse and respiratory rates, and warm, painful swellings appear on the ventral aspects of the body, interfering with movement. The superficial lymph nodes are swollen, diarrhea may occur and pregnant cows may abort. Affected bulls often become sterile for long periods, especially if the scrotal skin is affected (12). Cystic stages of the besnoitia have been found in the testes of a male burro, and in the uterus and vagina of two cows (3). Lacrimation and an increased nasal discharge are evident and small, whitish, elevated macules may be observed on the conjunctiva and nasal mucosa. Cysts on the scleral conjunctiva are considered to be of particular diagnostic significance. The nasal discharge is serous initially but becomes mucopurulent later and may contain blood. Subsequently the skin becomes grossly thickened and the hair falls out. A severe dermatitis is present over most of the body surface. The mortality rate is about 10% and the convalescence in survivors is protracted over a period of months. Necropsy lesions in cattle with the severe form of the disease are characterized by widespread vascular lesions and secondary lesions in skeletal and heart muscle, and lungs. Sarcocystis-like schizonts are present in some lesions (9).

In wild goats and domesticated family goats besnoitiosis is recorded in Iran, New Zealand (7) and Kenya (4). The principal lesions are on the skin and the genital tract. The cutaneous lesion is a chronic dermatitis of the legs and ventral surface of the abdomen. The hair is sparse, the skin cracked and oozing. The worst lesions are usually around the fetlock. There are also white, gritty granules subcutaneously over the hindquarters.

Horses are affected in much the same manner but the disease is less severe and the course less protracted. The disease also occurs in many species of wildlife in Australia (8), in impala and blue wildebeeste in Africa and caribou in Canada but on the basis of crossinfection tests the individual isolates are distinct strains.

Clinicopathological diagnosis depends upon detection of the cysts containing a number of spindle-shaped spores in scrapings or sections of skin. Many infected animals show no clinical signs of infection, and laboratory diagnosis using a complement fixation test has been attempted unsuccessfully (4). Serum antibodies to *Besnoitia* sp. are also identifiable by an indirect immunofluorescence technique (2) and by an ELISA (2, 10). No specific treatment is available and affected animals should be treated symptomatically for enteritis or dermatitis.

A vaccine containing *Besnoitia besnoiti*, grown on tissue culture, and originally isolated from blue wildebeeste, has been used to vaccinate cattle. A durable immunity to the clinical form of the disease was produced in 100% of vaccinates, but subclinical infection at a low level did occur (6).

REFERENCES

(1) Terrell, T. G. & Stookey, J. L. (1973) *Vet. Pathol.*, *10*, 177.
(2) Janitschke, K. et al. (1984) *Onderstepoort J. vet. Res.*, *51*, 239.
(3) Nobel, T. A. et al. (1977) *Bull. Acad. vet. Franç.*, *50*, 569.
(4) Cheema, A. H. et al. (1979) *Cornell Vet.*, *69*, 159.
(5) Dubey, J. P. (1977) Toxoplasma, hammondia, besnoitia and sarcocystis. In: *Parasitic Protozoa*, *vol. 3*, ed. J. Kreier, pp. 102–238. New York: Academic Press.
(6) Bigalke, R. D. et al. (1974) *J.S. Afr. vet. med. Assoc.*, *45*, 207.
(7) Collins, G. H. & Crawford, S. J. S. (1970) *NZ vet. J.*, *26*, 288.

(8) Munday, B. L. et al. (1981) *J. Wildlife Dis.*, *14*, 417.
(9) Landsverk, T. (1979) *Acta vet. Scand.*, *20*, 238.
(10) Shkap, V. et al. (1984) *Trop. Anim. Hlth Prod.*, *16*, 233.
(11) Goldman, M. & Pipano, E. (1983) *Trop. Anim. Hlth Prod.*, *15*, 32.
(12) Kumi-Diaka, J. et al. (1981) *Theriogenology*, *16*, 523.

Toxoplasmosis

Toxoplasmosis is a contagious disease of all species, including man. Clinically it is manifested chiefly by abortion and stillbirths in ewes, and in all species by encephalitis, pneumonia and neonatal mortality.

Etiology

The causative agent *Toxoplasma gondii* is a systemic coccidian, a universal parasite, a sporozoan, and a member of the suborder *Eimeria*. It is a specific parasite of the definitive host (members of the Felidae family), but has a wide range of intermediate hosts. Cats acquire infection by eating meat containing bradyzoites in tissue cysts or by ingesting infective oocysts. In the small intestine of the cat the parasites go through a typical coccidian lifecycle resulting in the shedding of unsporulated oocysts in feces. After several days the oocysts sporulate and are then infective, and often in large numbers and for long periods, exceeding a year. When ingested by the intermediate host the oocysts multiply in reticuloendothelial cells for 2 or 3 weeks then invade tissues and become tissue cysts. The invasion can include the fetus in a pregnant female. It is the tissue cysts in the intermediate host which cause damage to the nervous system, the myocardium, lung tissue and placenta.

There appear to be a number of strains which differ appreciably in their virulence, an inoculum containing as few as ten oocysts can be infective for goats (1). This needs to be taken into account when evaluating the results of transmission experiments.

Epidemiology

Toxoplasmosis is a true zoonosis occurring naturally in man, and in domesticated and wild animals and birds. It occurs in most parts of the world and surveys of its distribution indicate that a high incidence may occur in particular areas. In the United States, survey data based on serological findings include an incidence of 34–59% in dogs, 34% in cats, 47% in cattle, 30% in pigs and 48% in goats. Similar data are available for Denmark (3). A US survey of horses showed 10–20% positive reactors, the number varying from 0 to 67% between farms (26). Canadian data (25) includes 17% cattle, 65% sheep, 45% pigs, 9% horses, 33% dogs and 20% cats as seropositive. An Australian survey shows 41% of all sheep farms to be infected (5). A high prevalence rate is also recorded in Canadian wildlife (24). Positive serological tests were found in 53% of red foxes, 56% of striped skunks, 78% coyotes, 33% black bears, 18% shrews, and no voles. Other Canadian data (25) showed 11% mice, 5% deer, 3% rats and less than 2% sparrows as seropositive. Short-tailed field mice, squirrels, chipmunks, meadow jumping mice and starlings were all negative.

Toxoplasmosis is one of the common causes of abortion in sheep and neonatal lamb deaths. Apart from these, animal losses, other than in dogs, appear to be small and the importance of the disease is in its potential threat to humans. In man and animals the proportion of latent cases is very high, especially in adults, and one of the major risks associated with the disease is its elevation to the clinical level when the host's resistance is reduced. Conversely toxoplasmosis is thought to lower the resistance of the infected animal and this may lead to more serious attacks of louping-ill (41). The disease in man is likely to be occupational (28) but may occur sporadically after the ingestion of infected milk and meat. The latter is unlikely as very light cooking kills the toxoplasma and most human cases arise from eating raw or rare meat. Extensive outbreaks in mink have been considered to result from the ingestion of carcasses of animals dying of toxoplasmosis.

Ovine abortion and neonatal mortality have been observed in New Zealand, Australia, Canada, United States (1) and the United Kingdom. Perinatal mortality rates (including abortions and neonatal deaths) in affected flocks may be high as 50%. Abortion, with associated mummification of fetuses and perinatal deaths (17), due to toxoplasmosis is also recorded in goats (1, 7), and a high rate of occurrence of seropositive milking goats (27) or ewes (1) may be encountered in flocks where abortion is a problem. Because of the increasing use of milk goats as sources of raw milk to homes, the possibility of a public health risk has been raised. The chances of human infection occurring in this way is thought to be infinitesimal, but the issue is still debated (34). A clearer view will be possible when the proportion of the goat population which is infected is determined (1).

The organism is readily destroyed by heating, drying and freezing and thawing, and dies quickly in the carcasses of affected animals. The tissue cysts formed in the tissues of chronically sick animals are more resistant and may provide the most effective means of perpetuating the disease. Most species of animals and birds become infected and there is some variation in virulence of strains, those isolated from ovine abortions being of reduced pathogenicity. In sheep, a high rate of infection has been shown to be related to a high rainfall which allows longer survival of oocysts on pasture. Wild animals, especially water rats, and ravens may be infected and some viable infections do occur in wild ruminants (2); excluding wildlife from grazing land and buildings may be an important factor in a control program (40).

The common method of spread in ruminants is the ingestion of feed contaminated by cat feces which contain infective oocysts. This is well established as the means of transmission in sheep. There is the interesting observation that sheep raised in cat-free populations have almost no toxoplasmosis whereas sheep raised in similar environments with cats can have an infection rate as high as 32% (6). In many recorded outbreaks with high prevalence rates in sheep and goats there has been serious exposure to stored feed containing cat feces. It is also possible that outbreaks are the result of a recrudescence of a previously acquired infection which has been latent, but is now active because of a decline in the animal's resistance (30). Direct sheep-to-sheep transmission might occur by close contact with grossly infected placenta, but this proposal is contested (16). Transmission via the semen of infected rams is discounted as a possible portal (8).

Sheep are naturally rather resistant to toxoplasmosis and the occurrence of abortion as the most common clinical manifestation of the disease in this species suggests that the placenta and fetus are the most vulnerable tissues. In pigs transmission may be effected by cannibalism of pen mates (31).

Pathogenesis

Toxoplasma gondii is an intracellular parasite which attacks most organs with predilection for the reticuloendothelial and central nervous systems. After invasion of a cell the parasite multiplies and eventually fills and destroys the cells. Liberated toxoplasms reach other organs via the bloodstream after release from their development site. The clinical character of the disease varies with the organs attacked, which itself varies depending on whether the disease is congenital or acquired. In general the development of the disease in animals is the same as it is in man. The commonest syndromes are encephalitis when infection is congenital, and febrile exanthema with pneumonitis and enterocolitis when the disease is acquired postnatally. One or more tissue cysts can be found in many animals and appear to cause no harm. When the immunity of the animal falls because of stress, disease or immunosuppression therapy, tissue cysts rupture and large numbers of inflammatory cells invade surrounding tissue. The characteristic granulomatous lesions are thought to be the result of a hypersensitivity reaction.

In pregnant sheep and goats (1) the fetus is commonly invaded via an initial placentitis. The placentitis may result in fetal resorption or abortion and if the fetus is carried to term it is commonly born dead or affected with congenital toxoplasmosis. Maceration of fetuses is common and histological examination of fetuses may be necessary to demonstrate the presence of toxoplasma.

In latent infections there will be little or no antibody detectable in the bloodstream. If a recrudescence occurs, or in a new case, the antibody titer rises sharply at the time that the parasite is circulating in the blood stream, but this may have subsided by the time clinical signs, for example abortion, appear. For this reason changes in antibody titers are important as absolute levels.

A great deal of work has been done on experimental production of the disease in various animal species. Summaries are set down below, but caution is counseled in transposing the results to natural incidents largely because of the variation in the size of the experimental inoculum—in most cases it is very much larger than is likely to be encountered in nature.

Sheep

These are naturally rather resistant to toxoplasmosis and the occurrence of abortion as the most common clinical manifestation of the disease in this species suggests that the placenta and fetus are the most vulnerable tissues. Although transmission has been effected experimentally by the intravenous and subcutaneous injection of vegetative forms of the parasite injestion of cyst forms is though to be the common mode of infection in sheep. Only those sheep which become infected during pregnancy abort, those becoming infected at other times of the year developing sufficient immunity to prevent abortion. This probability is supported by the known higher incidence of abortion in young ewes.

Cattle

Oocysts of *Toxoplasma gondii* are slightly to moderately pathogenic when fed to calves (29). Diarrhea, anorexia, poor weight gain, depression, weakness, fever and dyspnea result. With strains of low virulence there is a mild fever and lymphadenopathy, and the organisms are detectable only in the lymph nodes and for only a few weeks (35). Adult cows are relatively insusceptible also and it is apparent that cattle do not readily acquire persistent *T. gondii* infections, probably because of rapid elimination of parasites from the tissues (34, 37).

Other ruminants

The reaction in buffalo calves is described as peracute with pulmonary consolidation, necrotic foci in all organs, and fluid accumulations in body cavities (36). Large doses of oocysts fed to goats cause a febrile, anorectic, fatal illness, and pregnant does abort (34).

Pigs

In pigs experimental infections can be set up by intramuscular injection or by inhalation. Piglets below the age of 12 weeks are much more susceptible than older animals. With a mild strain and pigs of 8–10 days of age the reaction is minor, but day-old pigs may have a high mortality rate (23).

Horses

These appear to be relatively non-susceptible to the development of the disease or the persistence of infection. Attempts at experimental transmission are rarely successful (32).

Clinical findings

The clinical syndrome and the course of toxoplasmosis vary a great deal between species and between age groups. The only clinical syndrome recognized with any regularity in field work is the abortion/neonatal mortality form in sheep. The other, less common, syndromes are as follows.

Cattle

In cattle the disease usually runs an acute course with fever, dyspnea, and nervous signs, including ataxia and hyperexcitability, in the early stages, followed by extreme lethargy. Stillborn or weak calves which die soon after birth may also be observed. Toxoplasmosis appears to play no significant role in bovine abortion (33). Congenitally affected calves show fever, dyspnea, coughing, sneezing, nasal discharge, clonic convulsions, grinding of the teeth and tremor of the head and neck. Death occurs after a course of 2–6 days.

Pigs

Pigs are highly susceptible, and in outbreaks pigs of all ages are affected. In adult pigs there is debility, weakness, incoordination, cough, tremor and diarrhea, but no fever. Young pigs are often acutely ill with a high fever of 40–42°C (104–107°F) and develop diarrhea and die after a course of several weeks (17, 19). Pigs of 2–4 weeks of age have additional signs including wasting, dyspnea, coughing, nervous signs, especially ataxia. Pregnant sows commonly abort, piglets are premature or stillborn, or survive and develop the above syndrome at 1–3 weeks of age. Toxoplasmosis may also be the cause of a resident problem of abortions and stillbirths in a pig herd (20).

Sheep
In sheep although a syndrome of fever, dyspnea, generalized tremor, abortions and stillbirths can occur, the systemic disease is rare. The common finding is one of abortion and neonatal deaths only (15). Abortion occurs during the last 4 weeks of pregnancy and the rate may be as high as 50%. Full-term lambs from infected ewes may be born dead or alive but weak, with death occurring within 3–4 days of birth. Lambs affected after birth show fever and dyspnea but a fatal outcome is uncommon. Fetal resorption can occur in ewes infected in early pregnancy but the significance of this is uncertain.

Goats
In goats caprine toxoplasmosis is manifested by perinatal deaths, including abortions and stillbirths (12). However, the systemic disease, with a high case fatality rate, is more common, especially in young goats (39).

Horses
Progressive neurological signs have been observed in horses with toxoplasmosis (10). Clinical signs include ataxia, circling, paresis and apparent blindness.

Equine protozoal myeloencephalitis, as an identifiable part of spinal cord disease in the horse, and as a likely component of the wobbler syndrome, is a probable manifestation of equine toxoplasmosis (13).

Clinical pathology
Serological tests are commonly used to determine the presence of toxoplasmosis but the results are apt to be equivocal. Results in paired sera are most informative, remembering that positive titers tend to remain static for years, except perhaps in pigs where they are fairly shortlived and have disappeared within several months. A complement fixation test is adequate but a positive titer develops only late in the disease and the test has been largely discarded because of risks to laboratory workers who are using live protozoa. The Sabin–Feldman dye test becomes positive at an earlier stage but is of limited value in the acute stages when titers are minimal. In these circumstances two tests are required, with the first one taken early to maximize any rise in titer. Titers of 1 in 256 or greater in the Sabin–Feldman test are taken to indicate a recently acquired or activated infection. An indirect fluorescent antibody test is now widely used for the serological diagnosis of toxoplasmosis. An indirect hemagglutination test is also available, but a lack of specificity, resulting in crossreactions with other protozoan parasites such as *Besnoitia* and *Sarcocystis* spp., mars its accuracy (4). An ELISA is used (14), and a modified direct agglutination test (MAT) is the most useful for serological surveys (26). Serological examination of fluids from unautolysed sheep fetuses can be used to diagnose congenital toxoplasmosis (9).

Necropsy findings
Multiple, proliferative and necrotic granulomata are characteristic of toxoplasmosis and in cattle the lesions may undergo calcification. The lesions occur most commonly in the nervous system and lungs. When there is visceral involvement, pneumonitis, hydrothorax, ascites, lymphadenitis, intestinal ulceration and necrotic foci in the liver, spleen and kidneys may be observed.

In toxoplasmosis of the horse with neurological involvement the characteristic lesions are hemorrhagic malacic lesions in brain and spinal cord associated with toxoplasma-like protozoan bodies. Similar lesions restricted to the spinal cord have been observed in sheep with toxoplasmosis (18). In sheep but not in the other species, there may be involvement of the uterine wall, the placenta and the fetus. The lesions in the fetal lambs are usually limited to focal necrotic lesions in brain, liver and lungs (42). Similar lesions are present in the fetal membranes.

On histological examination, granulomatous, necrotic lesions can be found in the viscera and in the brain. Toxoplasma can be found in the cells of most organs, particularly the lungs and brain. Material for transmission experiments should include brain and lung if there is evidence of visceral involvement. If it is necessary to differentiate between *Toxoplasma* and *Hammondia* spp. oocysts intracerebral and intraperitoneal injection of aseptically collected material into mice is accepted as a suitable procedure. Feeding the material to mice is also practiced and is thought to be quicker and more accurate. Brain or diaphragm tissue is used as the donor material, with the highest recovery rate coming from the latter. A positive diagnosis depends upon the presence of toxoplasma cysts in the brains of the mice 8 weeks after the injection.

Diagnosis
The reciprocal dye test and complement fixation tests are the only satisfactory method of diagnosing toxoplasmosis in the living animal. Histological examination of tissues, particularly lung and brain, can also be used as a basis for diagnosis, but if a dead animal is available the preferred test is to inject tissue emulsions into mice. An incubation period of 8 weeks is necessary for the disease to manifest itself in mice. Toxoplasmosis is clinically such a protean disease that it is likely to go unsuspected until detected by an observant pathologist. It should be considered particularly when there is a high incidence of unidentified abortions and stillbirths in sheep. The differential diagnosis of abortion in cattle is dealt with under brucellosis (p. 678), in sheep under brucellosis (p. 690), and in pigs under leptospirosis (p. 758). The causes of encephalitis in animals are listed under that heading (p. 437), and of pneumonitis under pneumonia (p. 367). Similar clinical syndromes of encephalopathy in newborn animals occur in vitamin A deficiency and as congenital defects after vaccination of pregnant dams with attenuated virus vaccines against hog cholera and bluetongue.

Treatment

Pyrimethamine (Daraprim) or sulfadiazine have limited value in treatment, curing less than 50% of affected animals when used alone. Administration of both drugs together, however, is highly effective in mice and humans. Of the sulfonamides, the sulfapyrimidines (sulfadimidine, sulfamerazine and sulfadiazine) and sulfapyrazine are the most effective. Best results are obtained when they are combined with pyrimethamine. The drugs are effective against the proliferating parasites and not against the pseudocysts. SDDS (2-sulfamoyl–4,4′-diaminodiphenyl sulfon) has also been shown to completely prevent experimental infection in pigs. A dose rate of 5 mg/kg per day was necessary to achieve this (21).

Control

The need for a specific prophylactic agent is not great and no program is available. A killed vaccine might suffice but initial experiments have had no success (44). At present a preventive program would have to depend on a low-level administration of a suitable antibiotic in the feed (43). To effect any limitation on the occurrence of toxoplasmosis it is essential to eliminate comingling of cats with farm animals, or the contamination of the food of farm animals by cat feces. Neither is an easy task whether domestic or feral cats are involved, but public health authorities will probably insist that proper measures be taken to protect the human food chain. The risk for humans is not in meat containing cysts, but in eating food contaminated by cat feces. The carcasses of infected or suspect animals should be totally destroyed, or at least be made inaccessible to carnivores. The oocysts are destroyed by exposure to temperatures between 90°C (194°F) for 30 seconds and 50°C (122°F) for 2·5 minutes (22). Because of the risk of transmission to humans, consideration should be given to the complete disposal of groups of animals in which the disease appears. Exclusion of feral animals from the domains of domestic animals may also be desirable (40). A proposal has been advanced to protect goats against clinical toxoplasmosis by vaccinating them with live *Hammondia hammondi*, the related, innocuous coccidian (38).

REVIEW LITERATURE

Blewett, D. A. (1984) The epidemiology of ovine toxoplasmosis. *Vet. Ann.*, *25*, 120.

Dubey, J. P. (1986) Toxoplasmosis. *J. Am. vet. med. Assoc.*, *189*, 166–170.

Stalheim, O. H. V. (1980) Update on bovine toxoplasmosis and sarcocystosis with emphasis on their role in bovine abortions. *J. Am. vet. med. Assoc.*, *176*, 299.

REFERENCES

(1) Dubey, J. P. (1981) *J. Am. vet. med. Assoc.*, *178*, 661 et seq. (4 papers).
(2) Dubey, J. P. (1981) *Am. vet. Res.*, *42*, 126.
(3) Work, K. (1971) *Acta pathol. microbiol. Scand.*, *Suppl. 221B*, 51.
(4) Stalheim, O. H. V. (1980) *J. Am. vet. med. Assoc.*, *176*, 299.
(5) Plant, J. W. (1980) *Aust. adv. vet. Sci.*, p. 65.
(6) Munday, B. L. (1972) *Res. vet. Sci.*, *13*, 100.
(7) Dubey, J. P. et al. (1986) *J. Am. vet. med. Assoc.*, *188*, 159.
(8) Teale, A. J. et al.(1982) *Am. J. vet. Res.*, *111*, 53.
(9) Dubey, J. P. et al. (1985) *Am. J. vet. Res.*, *46* 1137.
(10) Beech, J. & Dodd, D. C. (1974) *Vet. Pathol.*, *11*, 87.
(11) Munday, B. L. & Dubey, J. P. (1986) *Aust. vet. J.*, *63*, 353.
(12) Plant, J. W. et al. (1978) *Aust. vet. J.*, *56*, 254.
(13) Mayhew, I. G. et al. (1978) *Cornell Vet.*, *68*, Suppl. 6, p. 207.
(14) Berdale, B. P. et al. (1983) *Acta. vet. Scand.*, *24*, 65.
(15) Waldeland, H. (1976) *Acta vet. Scand.*, *17*, 412, & 432.
(16) Waldeland, H. (1977) *Acta vet. Scand.*, *18*, 91, 227, 227, 237 & 248.
(17) Nurse, G. H. & Lenghaus, C. (1986) *Aust. vet. J.*, *63*, 27.
(18) McErlean, B. A. (1974) *Vet. Rec.*, *94*, 264.
(19) Dubey, J. P. et al. (1979) *J. Am. vet. med. Assoc.*, *174*, 604.
(20) Moriwaki, M. et al. (1976) *Jap. J. vet. Sci.*, *38*, 377.
(21) Ohshima, S. et al. (1970) *Am. J. trop. Med. Hyg.*, *19*, 422.
(22) Ito, S. et al. (1975) *Natl. Inst. Anim. Hlth Q., Tokyo*, *15*, 128.
(23) Beverley, J. K. A. et al. (1978) *Res. vet. Sci.*, *24*, 139.
(24) Quinn, P. J. et al. (1976) *J. Wildlife Dis.*, *12*, 504.
(25) Tizard, I. R. et al. (1978) *Can. J. comp. Med.*, *42*, 177.
(26) Dubey, J. P. et al. (1985) *Am. J. Vet. Res.*, *46*, 1085.
(27) Tizard, I. R. et al. (1977) *Can. vet. J.*, *18*, 274.
(28) Behymer, D. E. et al. (1985) *Am. J. vet. Res.*, *46*, 1141.
(29) Fayer, R. & Frenkel, J. K. (1979) *J. Parasitol.*, *65*, 756.
(30) Perry, B. D. et al. (1979) *Vet. Rec.*, *104*, 231.
(31) Dubey, J. P. et al. (1986) *J. Am. vet. med. Assoc.*, *189*, 55.
(32) Al-Khalidi, N. W. et al. (1980) *Am. J. vet Res.*, *41*, 1549.
(33) Stalheim, O. H. V. et al. (1980) *Am. J. vet Res.*, *41*, 10.
(34) Dubey, J. P. et al. (1980) *Am. J. vet Res.*, *177*, 1203.
(35) Beverley, J. K. A. et al. (1977) *Res. vet. Sci.*, *23*, 33.
(36) Kalita, C. C. et al. (1978) *Ind. J. Public Hlth*, *22*, 325.
(37) Munday, B. L. (1978) *Int. J. Parasitol.*, *8*, 285.
(38) Dubey, J. P. (1981) *Am. J. vet. Res.*, *42*, 2068 & 2155.
(39) Mehdi, N. A. P. et al. (1983) *J. Am. vet. med. Assoc.*, *183*, 115.
(40) Lubroth, J. et al. (1983) *Prev. vet. Med.*, *1*, 169.
(41) Reid, H. W. et al. (1982) *J. comp. Pathol.*, *92*, 181.
(42) Buxton, D. et al. (1982) *Res. vet. Sci.*, *32*, 170.
(43) Blewett, D. A. & Trees, A. J. (1987) *Br. vet. J.*, *143*, 128.
(44) Wilkins, M. F. et al. (1987) *NZ vet. J.*, *35*, 31.

Theilerioses

The principal disease caused by *Theileria* is East Coast fever which is dealt with separately below. Other minor theilerioses are those caused by *T. annulata*. In cattle this causes a disease like East Coast fever but has the additional signs of pallor due to anemia, hemoglobinuria and jaundice. There may be subcutaneous nodules containing schizonts (4). Transmission is by the ticks *Hyalomma anatolicum excavatum* and *H. a. anatolicum*.

T. mutans causes a usually innocuous disease but it may be manifested by fever, anorexia and anemia. Transmission is by the ticks *Amblyomma variegatum* and *Haemaphysalis* spp.

T. hirci and *T. ovis* occur in sheep and goats and cause a syndrome similar to that of East Coast fever. *T. hirci* causes a disease of usually moderate severity but may cause severe losses. It is transmitted by *Rhipicephalus* spp. and *Hyalomma anatolicum*. *T. ovis* causes a mild disease and is transmitted by *Rhipicephalus evertsi* and *Haemaphysalis punctata*.

T. orientalis causes sereve anemia in heavily parasitized cattle but is otherwise relatively benign. *Haemaphysalis longicornis* and *H. punctata* (5) are the probable vectors. It is recorded in New Zealand (2) and Malaysia (3). British breeds are more susceptible than zebu breeds.

T. sergenti is a benign parasite recorded in Japan and transmitted by *H. longicornis*. *T. buffeli* is the benign theileria observed in Australia (1). It is transmitted by *Haemaphysalis longicornis* and *H. humerosa*, the latter being the major vector.

REFERENCES

(1) Stewart, N. P. et al. (1987) *Aust. vet. J.*, *64*, 81.
(2) James, M. P. et al. (1984) *NZ vet. J.*, *32*, 154.
(3) Fadzil, M. & Ragavan, K. (1986) *Kajian vet.*, *18*, 65.
(4) Manickam, R. et al. (1984) *Ind. vet. J.*, *61*, 13.
(5) Uilenberg, G. et al. (1985) *Res. vet. Sci.*, *38*, 352.

East Coast fever (ECF)

An acute disease of cattle caused by *Theileria parva*, transmitted by ticks and characterized by fever, lymph node enlargement, weakness, emaciation and a high death rate.

Etiology

The protozoan parasite *Theileria parva* is the cause of East Coast fever but there is a variability in the manifestation of the disease and in the antigenic makeup of the causes of the individual forms of the disease. Accordingly *T. lawrencei* is also listed as a cause. Cattle and buffalo are the usual hosts with zebu cattle being more resistant than British breeds. There also appears to be a great deal of variation in virulence between the antigenically distinct strains of the parasite.

Epidemiology

Transmission is by one of the ticks of the *Hyalomma* or *Rhipicephalus* spp. The principal vector is probably *Rhipicephalus appendiculatus*. Developmental stages of the parasite occur in the tick and these pass transstadially through the stages of larva, nymph and adult but there is no transovarial transmission. The epidemiology of the disease is completely dependent on the distribution of the vector tick, and in tick-infested areas all animals become infected. The serious losses occur when exotic animals are introduced from outside. Many wild members of the family Bovidae act as reservoir hosts for *Theileria* spp. and are implicated in the epidemiology of theilerial disease.

The disease has a high case fatality rate and those that survive have a solid and sterile immunity.

Pathogenesis

Infective particles, usually nucleated sporozoites of *T. parva*, are injected by the vector tick in its saliva when it is feeding. The particles pass to the local lymph nodes, develop into macroschizonts and are disseminated through the lymphoid system. In the lymphoblastoid cells they develop to merozoites which migrate to erythrocytes and become piroplasms. The dominating pathological lesion is the damage caused to the lymphoid organs, with erythrocyte damage as a contributing factor in some cases.

The incubation period is 1–3 weeks depending on the virulence of the strain and the size of the infecting dose. The mortality rate in calves is 5–50% and in adults it is usually fatal; the mortality rate is about 95% in adult zebus.

Clinical findings

The basic syndrome caused by *T. parva* infection has no distinctive indicants. There is fever, depression and anorexia plus, in the later stages, a nasal and ocular discharge, dyspnea, lymph node enlargement and splenomegaly. There may also be pica (4). In severe cases there is diarrhea, sometimes with dysentery, but usually only late in the course of the disease. Emaciation, weakness and recumbency lead to death after 7–10 days. Terminally there may be a frothy nasal discharge. Occasional cases of brain involvement occur characterized by circling, hence 'circling disease' or cerebral theileriosis. There are localizing nervous signs and convulsions, tremor, profuse salivation and head pressing.

T. lawrencei infection causes a similar acute syndrome with the additional lesion of keratitis and an accompanying blepharospasm.

Clinical pathology

The piroplasms are easily visible in erythrocytes in a blood smear but are difficult to differentiate from other piroplasms. The protozoa can be grown on a tissue culture of lymphoblastoid cells. A range of serological tests is available including indirect immunofluorescence, complement fixation and indirect agglutination tests.

Necropsy findings

Gross findings are not very informative. They include enlargement of the liver, lymph nodes and spleen, and ulceration of the abomasum. In acute cases there is pulmonary edema, hydrothorax and hydropericardium.

Diagnosis

Comparable diseases which may confuse the diagnosis include theileriosis due to *T. annulata* which is similar to ECF but with the addition of anemia, hemoglobinuria and jaundice.

Treatment

Tetracyclines have been the recommended treatment for many years but have only moderate efficacy especially if the disease has been present for a few days. Two more recently introduced treatments have had a much higher success rate: halofuginone lactate is an effective treatment for the acute syndrome, but recrudescence is common unless the correct dose rate (two doses × 1·2 mg/kg body weight) is used (17); parvaquone (10 mg/kg body weight × two doses 48 hours apart) is effective in most cases but recovered animals may be carriers (2, 3).

Control

Premunity is established early in cattle located in enzootic areas and this provides lifelong immunity if reinfection continues. There is some cross immunity between *T. parva* and *T. lawrencei* and between antigenically different strains of the one parasite. Nutritional or climatic stress may seriously reduce the animal's premunity. In enzootic areas reasonable control is maintained by avoiding nutritional stress and controlling the tick population. For more positive control programs vaccination has obvious advantages especially for exotic animals entering a danger area. The technique used is immunotherapy in which protozoa which have been grown on tissue culture are injected into the patient and the infection that they cause is controlled by the administration of longacting oxytetracycline (20 mg/kg body weight) given at the same time so that premunity is established similar to that induced against babesiosis with the aid of babesicides (5). It is usually successful provided local strains of theileria are used. A similar procedure using parvaquone instead of tetracycline has given better results. The virulence of the tissue culture organisms can be reduced by repeated passages. Vaccination with irradiated sporozoites is undergoing trial. Such a vaccine could avoid the inevitable breakdowns which occur with any immunotherapeutic technique (8).

REFERENCES

(1) Dolan, T. T. (1986) *Acta. Trop*, *43*, 165.
(2) Chema, S. et al. (1986) *Vet. Rec.*, *118*, 165.
(3) Dolan, T. T. (1986) *J. comp. Pathol*, *96*, 137.
(4) Kiptoon, J. C. (1983) *Kenya Vet*, 7, 9.
(5) Aliu, Y. O. (1983) *Vet. Bull*, *53*, 233.
(6) Dolan, T. T. et al. (1984) *Res. vet. Sci.*, *37*, 175.
(7) Chema, S. et al. (1987) *Vet. Rec.*, *120*, 575.
(8) Groocock, C. M. (1982) *Proc. 86 Ann Mtg US Anim. Hlth Assoc.*, 202.

DISEASES CAUSED BY TRYPANOSOMES

The diseases caused by these protozoan parasites are dealt with as follows:

- The tsetse-transmitted trypanosomiases: *Nagana* caused by *Trypanosoma brucei*, *T. congolense* (syn. *T. dimorphon*), *T. vivax* and *T. simiae*; *dourine*, caused by *T. equiperdum*, transmitted venereally; *surra*, caused by *T. evansi* in horses and camels, transmitted by a variety of biting flies.
- Trypanosomiasis caused by *T. theileri*. This is usually a non-pathogenic trypanosome transmitted by many biting fly species and with a very wide distribution on most continents. Occasional cases of illness are recorded, usually in cattle that are severely stressed or in newborn calves after transplacental transmission. The latter causes death of the neonate (1).

Nagana

The tsetse-transmitted trypanomiasis group of diseases is caused by the salivarian trypanosomes and characterized by an acute or chronic course, fever, anemia, emaciation and a heavy mortality rate, and transmitted principally by *Glossina* spp., the tsetse fly.

Etiology

These trypanosomiases are diseases of all species but of major importance in cattle because of their dominance of animal populations in the areas in which the disease occur. They are all members of the *Salivaria* group of trypanosomes and are transmitted via the mouthparts of their vector flies hence the name salivarian trypanosomes. They are all transmitted by the tsetse fly, in which they undergo part of their lifecycle and are mostly limited in their occurrence to Africa. *T. vivax* is also transmitted mechanically by biting flies and occurs also in Central and South America. The important trypanosomes are *Trypanosoma brucei*, *T. congolense*, *T. dimorphon* (a dimorphic form of *T. congolense*) and *T. vivax*, probably the most important of the three and one which also occurs in Central and South America in the absence of tsetse flies. *T. simiae* causes a very acute and highly fatal disease in pigs, camels and sheep, death occurring within a few hours of the parasites appearing in the blood.

Epidemiology

The trypanosomes are insect-borne and their epidemiology is determined by the ecology of their insect vectors. The tsetse flies *Glossina fusca*, the brush fly, *G. morsitans*, which inhabits principally savannah areas, and *G. palpalis*, a riverine species, effectively prevent the raising of cattle over large areas of Africa. The other flies known to be vectors are *G. austeni*, *G. brevipalpis*, *G. longipennis*, *G. pallidipes*, *G. swynnertoni*, and *G. tachinoides*. Reservoirs of infection of the trypanosomes are found in many wild animals and in domestic ones that are affected by the chronic disease.

The lifecycle of the trypanosome once it is taken up by the tsetse fly after feeding on an infected animal is to undergo a phase of further development in the fly which then remains infective for the remainder of its life. In the mammalian host the effect of the infection varies with the host in that most wild animals and some domestic ones establish a balance with the parasite and remain as clinically normal carriers for long periods. Also some breeds of cattle indigenous to Africa, such as the N'Dama, are resistant to the infection and also act as reservoirs of the infection. A spinoff of this phenomenon is that African native humpless cattle which are naturally immunotolerant are being used to develop cattle industries in enzootic areas (13). Even within these breeds and races of resistant animals there are significant differences, for example, the N'Dama and Baoule being more resistant than the West African zebu (6), and amongst zebu cattle the Orma Boran has superior resistance (3). The resistance may also be restricted to individual cows within a breed (12). In goats there appears to be no difference in susceptibility between the Toggenburg, British Alpine, Saanen and Anglo-Nubian breeds (4).

Pathogenesis

Nagana in all species is a progressive and usually fatal disease. The trypanosomes exert their effect by multiplying rapidly in the bloodstream, causing disseminated intravascular coagulation and then entering and blocking capillaries causing ischemia and anemia. *T. brucei* has the added capability of passing out of the capillaries into the tissues and causing injury to all organs. It also passes through the placenta and into the fetus in pregnant cows. As a result some cows abort and some calves are born prematurely (5). A cerebral form of trypanosomiasis occurs with mixed infections (9) or as a relapse after an apparently successful treatment (2, 9). The latter is thought to be due to the protection of the trypanosomes against the chemotherapeutic agent by the blood–brain barrier (2).

Clinical findings

The syndrome is not diagnostic. There are no pathognomonic signs and a clinical examination is of little help in pinpointing a diagnosis. The general clinical picture in these trypanosomiases is as follows but there are many variations on this central theme determined by the size of the inoculating dose, the strain of the pathogen and the nature of the host. There may be an acute episode lasting for a few days from which the animal dies or lapses into a chronic stage or the illness may be chronic from the beginning. Chronic cases may run a steady course, may be interrupted by periodic incidents of severe illness or undergo a spontaneous recovery. The basic clinical syndrome appears after an incubation period of 5–10 days. There is fever, which is likely to be intermittent and to last for a long period. Affected animals are dull, anorexic, apathetic, have an ocular discharge and lose condition. The lymph nodes become visibly swollen, occasional cases have diarrhea and some have edema of the throat and underline. The quality of the seminal ejaculate of rams is severely affected (14). The animal becomes very emaciated and dies within 2–4 months. The disease caused by *T. vivax* is milder in most cases. Some outbreaks are of a more severe kind with animals showing mucosal petechiation and a shorter course, dying after an illness of only a few weeks. Many animals will have mixed infections and these are usually severe cases. The cerebral form of the disease is manifested by ataxia, circling and paralysis (11).

Clinical findings peculiar to the individual trypanosome are as follows. *T. congolense* affects all species usually with an acute disease lasting 4–6 weeks but some chronic cases occur.

T. simiae affects pigs especially, sometimes sheep with a fulminating infection in which the animal dies within a few hours of first appearing ill. In pigs there is fever, stiff gait, dyspnea and cutaneous hyperemia.

T. vivax affects all agricultural species except pigs. Acute outbreaks occur in some areas with extensive mucosal hemorrhages, rhinorrhagia and dysentery. A less acute form of the disease is more usual.

T. brucei affects all species with a chronic disease. In cattle the disease is mild and may be asymptomatic.

Clinical pathology

The classical method of confirming the diagnosis is to demonstrate the parasites in a blood smear. This is easiest if the animal is in the early stages of the disease and is febrile. At other times the number of trypanosomes in the peripheral blood may be very small. Special techniques for the detection of parasites are recommended in preference to the standard thick smears and include a darkground/phase contrast, buffy coat method of concentrating and viewing the parasites, and a hematocrit centrifuge method of concentrating them into the buffy layer (13). The efficiency of the several tests varies with the species. The alternatives to parasite detection needed in the less active and chronic stages of the disease are the transmission of the disease to experimental animals, unsatisfactory because of the difficulty of quantifying the result, and a series of serological tests. These include complement fixation and passive hemagglutination tests and other tests using live trypanosomes, which have the disadvantage that they indicate past as well as present infections.

Necropsy findings

The postmortem lesions are, like the clinical findings, not definitive. The carcass is marked by anemia, emaciation, anasarca and enlargement of the liver, spleen and lymph nodes. Severe cases show a general congestion of the viscera and extensive hemorrhages in all tissues. Smears from tissues, usually the cut surface of a lymph node, are examined for the trypanosomes.

Diagnosis

Nagana is difficult to diagnose without laboratory services because it resembles any other chronic disease and has no characteristic clinical signs or postmortem lesions. It is necessary to depend on clinicopathological findings of parasites in the blood or on serological tests in the affected animals or in the experimental animals to which the disease has been passaged.

Treatment

There is a wide range of trypanocidal drugs available. They are extraordinarily effective but the circumstances in which they are used are likely to create all sorts of difficulties and inadequacies. They are used prophylactically as well as for curative purposes so that they are likely to be used a number of times in the one animal. The development of drug resistance in the trypanosomes is common and special techniques are necessary to combat the trend. One of them is to establish the use of a group of sanative drugs which are to be used as a break in a course of one of the more common drugs and which will provide moderate prophylaxis and avoid the development of resistance of the prime drug. The range of therapeutic safety of the drugs is small and many of them cause severe local reactions. Relapses are common if the commencement of treatment is delayed or the dose rate is inadequate.

The common drugs in use against trypanosomes are set out below. There is an extensive literature (10, 11) which should be consulted for specific dose rates to be used in individual animal species against specific trypanosomes for specific (curative, prophylactic or sanative) purposes.

Diminazene aceturate (Berenil) is used against *T. brucei* as curative.

Homidium bromide is used against *T. congolense* and *T. vivax* as curative and sanative.

Isometamidium (Samorin) is used against *T. congolense*, *T. vivax* as curative and prophylactic.

Prothidium bromide is used against *T. congolense*, *T. vivax* as curative and prophylactic.

Quinapyramine dimethylsulfate (Antrycide) is used against *T. congolense* and *T. vivax* as curative.

Suramin is used against *T. brucei* as curative and prophylactic.

Control

Control of the tsetse fly has been successfully attempted but relapses are frequent. It requires a strict regimen of regular spraying of animals, spraying of foliage likely to harbour the fly, destruction of brush and fly trapping. Most attempts at control have been directed to prophylactic dosing with chemicals such as suramin, prothidium and isometamidium (Samorin). This may be the only possible strategy in areas where there is a heavy population of trypanosome-infested tsetse flies, especially areas that are invaded by the flies in a particularly favourable season for fly propagation. The duration of the prophylactic effect of each drug is supplemented by the development of antibodies and the total period of protection may be as long as 5 months. However it is customary in practice to give four or five treatments per year and the productivity response to this pattern of treatment in goats (11) and cattle is excellent.

Dourine

Dourine is a contagious trypanosomiasis of horses transmitted by coitus and characterized clinically by inflammation of the external genitalia, cutaneous lesions and paralysis.

Etiology

One strain of the causative protozoon, *Trypanosoma equiperdum*, has been passaged in guinea-pigs (1).

Epidemiology

Dourine is enzootic in Africa (2), Asia, southeastern Europe, South America and a small area in the southern United States. It has been eradicated from Canada and the greater part of the United States and strict control measures have reduced the incidence to a low level in most parts of Europe (6). The mortality rate varies; in Europe it may be as high as 50–75% but in other areas the milder form of the disease is much less fatal although many animals may have to be destroyed (3).

The causative protozoon, *Trypanosoma equiperdum*, is incapable of surviving outside the host and dies quickly in cadavers. All equidae are susceptible but the disease is transmitted to ruminants only with great difficulty.

Natural transmission occurs only by coitus but infection can be introduced artificially through other intact mucosae and the conjunctiva. The source of infection may be an infected male actively discharging trypanosomes from the urethra, or an uninfected male acting as a physical carrier after serving an infected mare. The trypanosomes inhabit the urethra and vagina but disappear periodically so that only a proportion of potentially infective matings result in infection. Invasion occurs through intact mucosa, no abrasion being necessary. Some animals may be clinically normal but act as carriers of the infection.

Pathogenesis

The trypanosomes multiply locally and produce an edematous swelling. Subsequent systemic invasion occurs and localization in other tissues causes vascular injury and edema, manifested clinically by subcutaneous edema and paralysis.

Clinical findings

The severity of the clinical syndrome varies depending either on the strain of the trypanosome or the general health of the horse population. The disease in Africa and North America is much more chronic than the disease in Europe (3, 4) and may persist for many years, often without clinical signs, although these may develop when the animals' resistance is lowered by other disease or malnutrition.

The incubation period varies between 1 and 4 weeks with much longer periods in occasional animals. In the stallion the initial signs are swelling and edema of the penis, scrotum, prepuce and surrounding skin extending as far forward as the chest. Paraphimosis may occur and the inguinal lymph nodes are swollen. There is a moderate mucopurulent urethral discharge. In mares the edema commences in the vulva and is accompanied by a profuse fluid discharge, hyperemia and sometimes ulceration of the vaginal mucosa. The edema spreads to the perineum, udder and abdominal floor.

Nervous signs appear at a variable time after genital involvement. Stiffness and weakness of the limbs are evident and incoordination develops. Marked atrophy of the hindquarters is common and in all animals there is loss of condition, in some to the point where extreme emaciation necessitates destruction.

In Europe the disease is more severe, genital tract involvement often being accompanied by sexual excitement and more severe swelling. Cutaneous urticaria-like plaques 2–5 cm in diameter, develop on the body and neck and disappear within a few hours up to a few days. Succeeding crops of plaques may result in persistence of the cutaneous involvement for several weeks.

The course is variable. In Europe death occurs commonly and within a few weeks of the onset, but in the milder form of the disease the course may be as long as several years with recurrent mild attacks, or the disease may be subclinical, infected animals remaining spreaders of the disease for many years.

Clinical pathology

The trypanosomes can be detected in edema fluid and in the vaginal or urethral washings in the early stages of the disease. In the European disease the trypanosomes can also be found in the blood between the 2nd and 5th weeks after infection. An efficient complement fixation test is available and was the basis for a successful eradication program in Canada (3).

Necropsy findings

Emaciation, anemia and subcutaneous edema are always present and edema of the genitalia may be still evident. There is softening of the spinal cord, particularly in the lumbosacral area.

Diagnosis

The syndrome is diagnostic, no other disease having the clinical and epizootiological characteristics of dourine.

Treatment

Many trypanocidal drugs have been used in the treatment of dourine but results are variable, chronic cases in particular being unresponsive to treatment. Recommended treatments are Berenil (diminazene) at a dose rate of 7 mg/kg body weight as a 5% solution injected intramuscularly, with a second injection of half the dose 24 hours later (5), or suramin (10 mg/kg intravenously for two to three treatments at weekly intervals). Treatment should not be attempted if eradication is contemplated as many treated animals are likely to remain inapparent 'carriers' of the disease.

Control

In dourine-free countries an embargo should be placed on the importation of horses from countries where the disease is enzootic. In enzootic areas the disease can be eradicated on an area or herd basis by the application of the complement-fixation test. Positive reactors are disposed of and two negative tests not less than a month apart can be accepted as evidence that the disease is no longer present. The same measures can be applied when the disease occurs in a country for the first time. When the disease is enzootic and eradication is not contemplated it is customary to treat all mares with an effective treatment, for example Berenil, at the time of mating.

REFERENCES

(1) Pavlov, P. & Christoforov, L. (1966) *Proc. 1st int. Congr. Parasitol., Roma, 1964*, 323.
(2) Williamson, C. C. & Herr, S. (1986) *J. S. Afr. vet. Assoc.*, *57*, 163.
(3) Watson, E. A. (1920) *Dourine in Canada, 1904–1920. History, Research and Suppression*. Ottawa: Health of Animals Branch, the King's Printer.
(4) Parkin, B. S. (1948) *Onderstepoort J. vet. Sci.*, *23*, 41.
(5) Vecherkin, S. S. et al. (1975) *Veterinariya, Moscow*, *2*, 70.
(6) Caporale, V. P. et al. (1980) *Zentralbl. VetMed.*, *27B*, 489.

Surra

This disease affects all animal species but is most important in camels and horses. It has a wide distribution in North Africa, the Middle East, Asia and Central and South America. It is caused by *Trypanosoma evansi* and is transmitted by biting flies. Feral animals and domestic animals other than dogs, camels and horses, which are the species that develop the clinical disease, can become infected and act as reservoirs. Clinically the disease is similar to that caused by *T. brucei*. There may be an acute or chronic illness. The chronic disease in horses in South America affects the central nervous system and is called *mal de caderas* or *murrina*. Preferred treatments are suramin, isometamidium (used also as a prophylactic), quinapyramine dimethylsulfate and diminazene aceturate (Berenil).

REVIEW LITERATURE

Losos, G. (1986) *Infectious Tropical Diseases of Domestic Animals*. Chapter 3, Trypanosomiases, pp. 182–318. London: Longman.
Wandera, J. G. (1979) Diseases caused by protozoa trypanomiasis. In *Diseases of Cattle in Tropical Africa* (eds Mugera, G. M. et al.) Nairobi, Kenya: Kenya Literature Bureau.

REFERENCES

(1) Liggett, A. D. & Goldsmith, S. W. (1986) *Agri-Practice*, *7*, 29.
(2) Moulton, J. E. (1986) *Vet. Pathol.*, *23*, 21.
(3) Njogu, A. R. et al. (1985) *Vet. Rec.*, *117*, 632.
(4) McGuire, T. G. et al. (1985) *Res. vet. Sci.*, *39*, 252.
(5) Ogwu, D. et al. (1986) *Theriogenology*, *25*, 383.
(6) Akol, G. W. O. et al. (1986) *Vet. Immunol. Immunopathol.*, *11*, 361.
(7) Whitelaw, D. D. et al. (1986) *Vet. Rec.*, *118*, 722.
(8) Whitelaw, D. D. et al. (1985) *Parasitology.*, *90*, 255.
(9) Masake, R. A. et al. (1984) *Acta Trop.*, *41*, 237.
(10) Chabeuf, N. (1983) *J. St. Afr. vet. Assoc.*, *54*, 165.
(11) Kanyari, P. W. N. et al. (1983) *Trop. Anim. Hlth Prod.*, *15*, 153.
(12) Roelants, G. E. et al. (1983) *Acta Trop.*, *40*, 99.
(13) Paris, J. et al. (1982) *Acta Trop.*, *39*, 307.
(14) Akpavie, S. O. et al. (1987) *Res. vet. Sci.*, *42*, 1.

26

Diseases Caused by Helminth Parasites

INTRODUCTION

It is impossible to give an accurate estimate of the economic importance of parasitic disease because it varies so greatly between countries and between regions, depending both on climate and on the intensiveness of farming in the area. It is probably fair to say that the countries which have suffered most in the past have been those in which exploitative agriculture has been practiced. In these countries periods of malnutrition are common and the effects of parasitic disease are exacerbated. The position seems to have changed, however, so that now the principal problem has moved to those areas of highly productive land on which large numbers of animals have been concentrated. As a result there has been a great increase in interest in the epidemiology of parasitic diseases, a rapidly expanding field of investigation, and in the control and treatment of parasitism by treatment with highly effective compounds during the season most adverse to the freeliving forms.

Etiology of parasitic diseases

The incidence of parasitic diseases varies greatly between areas depending on the relative importance of many of the factors listed below. In most instances the importance of these individual factors is related to the level of agriculture in the area; nutritional deficiency, for example, achieves major importance in poorly developed countries where extensive grazing on native pastures is widely practiced. Where agriculture is more intensive and land more productive, pasture management tends to dominate other factors. Although a great deal of work has been, and is being, done on the bionomics of helminth larvae it is not yet possible to reliably predict the potential transmissibility of a particular parasite at a particular place and time for more than a few regions. The micro-climate and macroclimate of the environment, the shade characters, volume and height of the pasture, the grazing habits and the immunological and nutritional status of the host, the presence of intermediate hosts and vectors and the numbers of infective larvae and eggs in the environment present a meshwork of interacting variables which greatly confound even an understanding of epidemiological dynamics (1).

At our present state of knowledge of causes of parasitic disease it is difficult and even dangerous to lay down rigid rules for their control which are applicable to all regions. For example, a program for the control of haemonchosis in sheep in Australia may be ineffective in Scotland. For this reason a study of the epidemiology of each parasitic disease should be carried out on a regional basis and recommended control measures should be similarly limited.

Nutrition

General nutritional status

It is a well-established principle that poorly fed animals are more susceptible to the effects of internal parasites and are more inclined to carry heavy worm burdens because of their failure to throw off infestations quickly. However, optimum nutrition does not offer complete protection against overwhelming numbers of some kinds of worms. Thus in general terms trichostrongylosis achieves its greatest importance in sheep when nutrition is poor; on the other hand haemonchosis causes most losses when nutrition is excellent but environmental conditions are such that massive infestations occur. In calves both ostertagiosis and haemonchosis can be significant in either set of circumstances. Verminous pneumonia also is commonly thought of as a secondary disease which is likely to exacerbate the effects of poor nutrition and gastrointestinal helminthiasis, but it can be a major disease in its own right when fat calves on an excellent diet are exposed to large numbers of larvae. Although it has become fashionable, in terms of the above discussion, to categorize worms as primary or secondary, depending upon their ability to cause disease in the absence of nutritional or other stress, the concept is not a particularly valuable one because so many species can be primary or secondary depending on circumstances.

It has become evident that a number of factors, of which nutrition is only one, can have marked effects on the resistance of animals to helminths. Specific immunity, hypersensitivity (self-cure) which may or may not be accompanied by immunity, and age are some of these. It is often very difficult to separate the effects of these factors which may be acting in concert and it is particularly important to differentiate between resistance to the establishment of an infestation, such as occurs in an immune animal, and resistance to the effects of the established infestation, such as may occur in a well-nourished animal.

Specific nutritional deficiencies
A dietary deficiency of a specific nutrient such as cobalt, copper, phosphorus or protein can lead to a reduction in the animal's resistance in much the same way as does general malnutrition. The anemia, poor growth and condition associated with these deficiencies are generally accepted as predisposing to heavy worm burdens. There is an apparent contradiction to this in that *Haemonchus contortus* develops better in sheep fed a cobalt supplement than in sheep on cobalt-deficient diet. This and similar observations suggest that there may be some profit to be obtained from an examination of the dietary requirements of the helminths themselves.

Pasture management
One of the important reasons for the increasing importance of parasitic diseases is the increase in productivity of pasture. By the introduction of new plants, new strains of existing plants, irrigation and improved fertilization, heavier stocking rates are being maintained. As a result the fecal contamination of pasture is greater, the pasture is of greater length and bulk and provides more protection for eggs and larvae from sunlight and desiccation, and the manure of animals grazing the pasture is more fluid so that it spreads farther and the eggs or larvae are much more likely to develop and be available to the grazing animal than if they are imprisoned in a firm pat of manure. Further, the animals may be forced to graze over fecal contamination that they would normally avoid. In these circumstances it is imperative to know the lifecycles of the parasites in the area, the source and timing of contamination, the time interval between contamination and larval availability for eggs deposited throughout the year, the availability of infective stages throughout the year and the ability of larvae to survive different seasonal climatic conditions; all of these are under the pastoral conditions in question.

A heavy concentration of animals can also occur on extensive range, especially in bad seasons, when the only feed available is restricted to watercourses, around bores, wells and dugouts and in swampy areas. The opportunities for parasitic multiplication in such circumstances can be as great as on irrigated pasture and there is usually the added insult of malnutrition. Draining such areas, or fencing them to prevent access, may necessitate supplementary feeding but this may be more economic in the long run.

Although rotational grazing has been strongly recommended in the past, further investigation has shown that no practical system of rotational grazings has any relevance to the control of parasites (5). Pastures cannot be spelled until practically all larvae have died off without damaging the pasture. Further, if sheep are returned to pastures spelled for only a few weeks, their return could coincide with the maximum occurrence of larvae on the herbage (3). Sufficient evidence is now available to suggest that 'set-stocking' may be a safer method in many circumstances. Two agronomic reasons put forward for rotating pasture grazings are increased productivity of feed and preservation of some desirable plant species, but there is little evidence to support this (25). For complete elimination of infestation of pasture an interval of 1 year between grazing is necessary but is not usually practicable. Zero grazing with suitable hygiene provides the complete answer, especially if lambs are weaned early. Eventually it may be possible to create an artificial immunity by vaccination but this work is in its infancy.

The problem of how animal droppings on pasture should be handled has some interesting aspects, especially in cattle and sheep. Dung pats, and presumably fecal balls, act as incubators by trapping heat but they also prevent migration of larvae unless their hard outer covering is softened by rain. Under relatively dry conditions and on short pasture, dung pats can act as reservoirs of larvae for up to 5 months in summer and 7–8 months in winter, only releasing larvae after constant heavy rain which softens the covering and aids release of the larvae by splashing. It is probably advisable to break up dung pats frequently by the use of a chain harrow in those seasons when survival of larvae is short. The introduction of suitable dung beetles can also play a role in worm control.

Some parasites of domestic animals are also able to survive in wild animals, and some may even be primary to them, so that when both groups have access to the one pasture crossinfestation can occur. The same applies to transfer of infestation from one domestic species to another. There is a great deal of confusion on this particular aspect of parasitic diseases and the degree of crossinfestation which actually occurs is uncertain. In many instances parasites of one species may be able to survive in another but not to the point of laying eggs or, if patency is achieved, the period of egg-laying is much reduced and the importance of the infestation, in terms of perpetuating itself in the environment is negligible. The alternation of grazing animals or mixed grazing reduces parasite burdens and may play an important part in parasite control. A great deal of work has been done on the zoological identification of parasitic species but little on the biological identification. The early phases of this work, such as has been carried out on *H. contortus* and *H. placei*, have been highly significant and further work in the same field will be watched with interest.

Barn management
Most parasitic diseases affect animals at pasture but animals kept indoors may be affected if management is inadequate. For example, if fecal contamination of feed can occur when animals are fed on the floor or in very low troughs or the animals are so overcrowded that defecation into raised troughs occurs frequently, infestation can develop. If insufficient bedding is provided the entry of hookworm larvae through the skin is facilitated, and the coats of animals may be so contaminated with infective larvae of other worms that normal licking may result in infestation.

Inadequate nutrition is a constant hazard in animals housed for long periods. Young animals are most susceptible to parasitic infestation and if, when they are turned out to pasture, they are in poor condition because of poor feeding the stage is set for a serious outbreak. Animals reared indoors and turned on to an infected pasture may, even if in good condition, acquire large burdens of parasites, such as *D. viviparus*, and succumb before an immunity can develop. In the same way animals coming off pasture in good condition but carrying a heavy burden of worms may suddenly succumb to the effects of the worms when their diet is restricted during the stabling period. Some of these animals may have low fecal egg counts because they carry large burdens of dormant larvae. Subsequently the larval population matures en masse for reasons which are not understood.

Because of the possibility of crossinfestation between animal species and the untoward results of infestation by a worm of an unnatural host, housing of different animal species in the one pen or substitution of a different species without proper cleaning of the pen is not recommended. For example, cattle may suffer a massive pulmonary invasion by *Ascaris suum* if penned on pig litter containing infective eggs.

Climate

The most suitable conditions for the translation of eggs to larvae in the majority of helminth parasites are provided by warm, wet weather and under these conditions larvae can remain alive for 6–8 weeks. Few species can withstand desiccation and high temperatures, although *Nematodirus*, which is protected within the egg and by two larval sheaths, may survive the summer to infect the next season's lambs, and *Trichuris* spp. are of greatest importance in Australia in times of drought. On the other hand, many larvae appear to be resistant to cold and many species, particularly *Ostertagia* and *Nematodirus*, can survive through a Canadian winter (11). In areas with less severe winters where animals graze throughout the year, the survival of the larvae in the winter together with very short pasture in a period of little or no pasture growth, can lead to very heavy parasite burdens. Factors which are detrimental to larval survival may, if applied in lesser degree, prolong the rate of development. For example, a mild winter instead of killing heavy infestations of larvae on pasture may so delay their development that when sheep are turned on to the pasture in the spring they are immediately exposed to a gross infestation (12). Another effect of climate is to vary the severity of infestations from year to year. Thus in areas with a severe winter and dry summer the parasite burden of the local livestock may be light in most years, but in those years when the winter is mild and the summer is wet the normally light burdens are rapidly multiplied so that severe outbreaks of parasitic diseases occur.

Insect vectors are important in some helmintic diseases, especially those caused by members of the superfamily Filarioidea. The population of these vectors is dependent largely on climatic conditions and the incidence of the diseases is similarly subject to the vagaries of the climate. The same variations are implicit in those diseases in which snails, beetles and earthworms act as intermediate hosts.

Immunity

It is not easy to generalize on this aspect of parasitic disease as our understanding is far from complete. A great deal of the work has been done on inbred strains of laboratory animals and it may be dangerous to extrapolate this directly to domestic animals. Evidence from this work suggests that damage and expulsion of worms in an immune animal result from a sequential interaction between antibodies and the cell-mediated immune response together with non-specific inflammatory changes due to biogenic amines and prostaglandins (13). In domestic animals, antibodies are produced by the host against antigens in the exsheathing fluid and against enzymes secreted by the worms. Antibody or sensitized small lymphocytes may damage the worms and biogenic amines or prostaglandins may cause their expulsion (13).

There are some serological crossreactions between nematodes but the antigens responsible for the production of these antibodies are apparently not the antigens which produce the preventive immune reactions.

Helmintic immunity is usually less efficient and more transient than the immunity to microorganisms, possibly because they do not reproduce in the host as do bacteria, viruses and protozoa. Further, the immunity produced by helminths that migrate in the host appears to provoke a greater immunological response than those confined to the lumen of the intestine. Larvae acquired by immune animals may become established but are later destroyed. Inhibition of larvae during their development (hypobiosis) was first thought to be related to the development of immunity but it now appears that this is an adaptation process similar to diapause in insects. It is probable, however, that the maintenance of large numbers of larvae in an inhibited state in the presence of an adult worm burden and the maturation of these inhibited larvae when the adults are removed, may be related to immunity. An important feature of parasitic disease is that the young are much more susceptible than adults. While this is usually due to an acquired resistance such as in trichostrongylosis, an immunity due to age may play some part, e.g. in *Nematodirus* infections.

The periparturient rise in the nematode egg output by the ewe is of complex etiology but a reduction in resistance of the ewe is involved. This reduction in resistance allows increased fecundity of the worms present during pregnancy, maturation of inhibited larvae and the development of newly acquired infection. The phenomenon is of great importance in the epidemiology of parasitic gastroenteritis in sheep and provides a large number of larvae at a time when highly susceptible lambs are present (14). A related phenomenon is the restriction by the immune response of the number of eggs laid by mature worms. Thus the fecal egg count in an immune animal may be a grossly inefficient measure of the actual worm burden.

Hypersensitivity to helminths also occurs, the two commonest manifestations being the allergic response of a sensitized animal to a massive pulmonary invasion by lungworm larvae and the 'self-cure' phenomenon in parasitic gastroenteritis in sheep. In the latter there is a sudden evacuation of a heavy, adult, parasite load apparently because of a local hypersensitivity reaction in the stomach and intestine provoked by a second larval infestation. The larvae themselves are not necessarily affected and may reach maturity, sometimes in sufficient numbers to be fatal. Animals which evidence this phenomenon are not necessarily immune subsequently and the greatest practical importance of 'self-cure' other than a temporary remission, is in the misleading effect it may have on the assessment of control programs.

The practical aspects of parasitic immunity are pertinent to the question of a planned immunity. The two obvious channels by which such immunity could be produced are by vaccination with antigenic material derived from helminths, or by animal husbandry maneuvers by which the animals are exposed to planned larval infestations on pasture, the latter practice being fraught with obvious dangers. Vaccination, apart from vaccination against *D. viviparus*, is still not a practicable procedure and because of the many difficulties involved is unlikely to be so in the immediate future. However, it has recently been found that within a group of sheep there are some sheep that can respond to vaccination with irradiated *T. colubriformis* larvae and that the ability to respond is genetically controlled (26). The possibility of building up a flock of 'responders' so that vaccination becomes a useful tool is one of the exciting advances in parasite control. The development of efficient vaccines against larval cestodes in sheep and cattle, by using excretory antigens derived from larvae cultivated *in vitro*, has recently opened up a new method of approach (15).

The question is often raised of the possibility of removing the stimulus to immunity, and hence the immunity, by overzealous use of anthelmintics. At least with respect to *T. colubriformis* this seems unlikely unless the sheep are drenched at intervals of 1 week or less (16) for long periods.

The development of immunity also has some relationship to the serological diagnosis of helminthiasis. Some serological techniques are in use, particularly in those diseases in which helminths invade tissues, but no reaction has been shown to detect protective antibody so that determination of a state of protective immunity is not presently possible. There is also a great deal of crossreaction between many antigen–antibody systems, and serological reactions decline in titer quickly unless there is further stimulation (17).

Principles of control of parasitic diseases

'The fundamental ecological concepts of helmintic parasitism in general and especially of grazing animals are that every animal is infected and that contamination of the environment is continuous. The epidemiological factors which explain why outbreaks of helminthosis are not more numerous and more severe are the destruction of freeliving stages and the development of resistance and immunity by the host' (18). This concept of helminthiasis includes two principles which are nowadays accepted as axioms: first, there is sufficient potential in most grazing animals to permit the development of a major outbreak of helminthosis whenever the correct circumstances are provided; second, the appearance of clinical helminthosis indicates that proportionate losses due to subclinical levels of infestation are also occurring in the same group. Although the following principles of control are aimed at preventing both forms of loss it is necessary to remember that the objective of a parasite control program must be the achievement of a maximum economic gain and this may not be synonymous with total control of infection. The objective may be different with different classes of stock. For example, in fat lambs any restraint on speed and degree of growth is expensive and control of parasitism justifies a greater degree of control than in ewe lambs that are going to be flock replacements where mild infections are desirable to stimulate resistance (19). Maintaining these infestations at moderate levels, below the point at which they adversely affect future productivity is one of the challenges of preventive veterinary medicine. The principles of a control program are as follows.

The unit is the herd of flock and its environment

The presence of one clinically affected animal suggests the presence of other developing clinical cases in the group. Treatment and control measures must be directed at the group together with its pasture or housing.

Nutritional status

In general a good nutritional status and freedom from specific nutritional deficiencies increase the resistance of livestock to the effects of helminth parasites but are insufficient protection against more than a moderate infestation.

Pasture management

It is possible to manage pasture so that animals are raised virtually free of worms but this is seldom practical. The trend in recent years has been to more intensive agriculture with large numbers of animals set stocked on pasture. While set-stocking is potentially more dangerous, it works well if combined with anthelmintic treatments given at times suggested by epidemiological studies and aimed at maintaining a low level of pasture contamination. It must be realized that a management program is specific for a particular area and, if adopted without alteration by another area where climate is different, it may not only fail but actually further the development of parasitosis. The concentration of animals, their state of nutrition and the suitability of climate and herbage cover to the survival of larvae all influence the choice of which method of control is best in particular circumstances. Pasture which is short in length, besides being poor nutritionally, encourages infestation because larval concentration will be at a maximum—the distance they have to travel to get onto pasture is less and larvae, which are concentrated in pasture litter, will be taken in with roots and soil. On the other hand, very short, dry pasture encourages desiccation and destruction of larvae because of the removal of leaf cover. Animals on range pasture should be denied access to marshes, wet areas around troughs and where surface water collects. In circumstances of very high risk, e.g. where flood-irrigated pastures are heavily stocked with ewes and lambs, satisfactory control may be possible only by the regular use of an efficient anthelmintic, or in some cases by the use of zero-grazing—maintaining the animals in a dry lot and cutting and carrying the pasture to them.

Barn management
The important recommendations for housed animals are to avoid overcrowding, remove manure frequently, provide plenty of bedding, have feed and water troughs high enough off the floor to avoid fecal contamination and, probably most important of all, maintain the plane of nutrition. The provision of adequate feeding space so that all animals have access to feed at the same time is essential to avoid a 'tail' of poorly nourished individuals.

Utilization of immunity to helminths
Vaccines against *Dictyocaulus* spp. are available. Stimulation of immunity by controlling pastoral exposure to natural infestation is too hazardous to attempt on a practical scale with existing knowledge, and so low levels of parasite burdens must be maintained in the grazing animals until an adequate immunity has developed. This will vary from area to area depending on the severity of the parasite challenge and the time over which it occurs. In general terms cattle are resistant by 12–15 months and sheep by about 18 months. Because immunity is basically an acquired state it is dangerous to bring animals from areas where a particular parasitic disease does not occur and expose them to heavy infestations in areas where it does.

Avoidance of interspecies transmission
Existing knowledge of the transmission of helminths from one animal species to another suggests that the running of sheep and cattle together (10) or successively (9) on the one pasture can be a successful control procedure. While some parasites are species-specific, others will cross to other hosts but may not remain patent as long as in their normal host. It is of interest that the establishment of *H. contortus* infection in sheep is greatly reduced when given with, or superimposed upon, a *T. axei* infection. Access to domestic pastures by wild fauna may lead to spread and multiplication of helminth parasites.

Protection of young animals
Control measures should be aimed primarily at protecting the most susceptible group—young animals up to 18 months of age which are exposed to infestation for the first time. Thus one of the major principles in the control of helminths is the regular treatment of breeding females, especially of ewes before or about the time of lambing to avoid the effect of the 'periparturient rise' in worm egg production at 4–8 weeks after lambing. For the lamb the ewe is usually more important as a source of infection than is pasture contamination. Thus early weaning may be an important control measure in some circumstances, and lambing at different times of the year may reduce the importance of the ewe. Ewes should be treated before lambing and placed onto a clean pasture. If allowed to remain on the same paddock the prelambing treatment will have little effect on the periparturient rise but will kill those adult and hypobiotic larvae in the ewe and prevent the early expression of the rise in fecal egg count. This delays the larval challenge to the lambs which may be weaned before gaining pathogenic burdens. Ewes remain cleaner and may produce more milk. If clean pastures are not available then another treatment can be given 3–4 weeks after lambing. However, for this to be meaningful the ewes must be divided into groups lambing over a short interval; this can be done most conveniently by the use of ram raddles at joining. The use of two treatments, prelambing and postlambing, gives the best response but may not be possible on all farms (27). As lambs do not suffer from parasitic disease before 10–12 weeks of age, as long as the ewe has adequate milk good results can be obtained by the use of prelambing treatment combined with early weaning. The lambs should be treated at weaning and placed onto the safest pasture available (14). The treatment system adopted will vary with the type of sheep enterprise. In wool sheep, a prelambing treatment may not be necessary if the lambs are weaned at 10–12 weeks of age, treated and moved to a clean paddock. On a prime lamb farm where early weaning is not possible, anthelmintic treatment will be more intensive. It is particularly important that young sheep should not be run on the lambing paddock, which will be heavily infected (20), until it has been spelled for long periods and preferably passed through the season most inimical to the larvae.

Although most work on the 'periparturient rise' has been done on ewes, the phenomenon is not restricted to that species. It occurs in sows, at least with respect to *Oesophagostomum* spp. and *Hyostrongylus rubidus*. The rise begins 1–2 weeks before farrowing, peaks 6 weeks after that and ends abruptly when the pigs are weaned. The most satisfactory control measure to prevent infestation of the young pigs is to treat the sow at farrowing, confine the young pigs on concrete and remove the dung frequently. A small rise has also been reported in the fecal egg count of beef cattle calving in the spring.

Control by protective treatments
Protective dosing with anthelmintics has become an important part of most preventive programs against clinical or subclinical parasitic disease. Two classes of treatment are usually programmed: strategic treatments carried out at the same time each year, or at the same stage in the management program, with the specific purpose of reducing contamination; and tactical treatments which are added to the strategic program, particularly in pastured animals, to abort outbreaks when abnormal climatic or nutritional conditions arise.

A good deal of controversy revolves around the question of how frequently and when strategic and tactical treatments need be applied. A management program should not rely solely on the use of anthelmintics, but this approach is often accepted by farmers who lack the managerial skills to adopt an integrated approach to worm control. Reliance on frequent treatment is unnecessarily expensive and leads to the development of anthelmintic resistance. A moderate approach to the problem based upon a critical prediction of danger periods, usually results in an optimum use of preventive treatment programs. Because there are such great differences between areas in the frequency and severity of danger periods, control programs can also be expected to vary widely and still be optimum for the particular farm or area.

Strategic treatments
Strategic treatments are usually administered two to four times a year depending on the climate and management procedures. Because of the much greater susceptibility of young animals the most important strategic treatments are those planned to provide maximum protection until weaning and at weaning when the young animals suffer their greatest nutritional stress. The former can be accomplished in sheep by controlling the periparturient rise in the ewe, treating the lambs at weaning and regular use through their early growth period. In older animals, strategic treatments are usually given to eliminate contamination at a time when the pastures will be cleansed by adverse weather conditions, e.g. hot dry summers (14). Strategic treatment in horses is given at regular intervals throughout the year to prevent contamination of the pastures, but epidemiological studies have shown that contamination is mainly in the late spring and summer (29). Several treatments at that time, preferably using compounds effective against hypobiotic or migrating larvae, may be equally effective.

When animals are housed for part of the year, young animals are often exposed to a falling plane of nutrition when they leave the pasture and it is customary to provide a strategic treatment at this time.

Tactical treatments
Tactical treatments are provided on an ad hoc basis, usually in periods of abnormally heavy rainfall and mild temperatures but also occasionally when nutrition is unusually poor or when animals from a worm-free environment, and thus lacking in acquired immunity, are introduced to a danger area. For proper use of tactical treatments the diagnosis of critical levels of infestation at which treatment is warranted becomes an important procedure. The emphasis has shifted in recent years from the need to prevent outbreaks to include the need to reduce losses caused by subclinical infestations.

Computer modeling of the lifecycle and epidemiology of the principal parasites in an area can predict optimum times for anthelmintic treatments for that area, and if climatic conditions are regularly recorded and used in the model, the need for further treatments can be predicted (2). The effect of suppressive treatments on quantity and quality of wool produced has been measured and compared with that obtained in flocks with less intensive treatment programs (22).

The diagnosis of significant levels of infestation
Many of the epidemiological studies of helminths have been directed to determining optimum conditions of climate and pasture for parasitic multiplication and to determine the availability of larvae throughout the year. Where suitable local data are available it is possible to institute strategic programs and to recognize abnormal climatic conditions that require tactical treatments. In the absence of this information there are other methods of assessing the helminth status of a group of animals. Visual appraisal of body weight and clinical evidence of parasitism is the time-honored method but lacks sufficient definition for most situations. Assessment by fecal egg count has limitations in all but very young animals as egg counts are modified by immunity, the species present, the consistency of the feces, stage of maturity of the worms and the occurrence of the parturient rise. They do, however, give a direct measurement of the degree of contamination (23) and they correlate sufficiently well with worm burden to allow their use as a diagnostic tool in young weaners (30).

The total worm count, which has with modern methods become an accurate and simple field technique, is superior to a fecal egg count as a measure of the severity of an infestation but does not take into account whether or not the worms are in a high contaminative phase. The method is often preempted by the unavailability of a sufficient number of guts for examination; there should be at least two. Because of the increasing availability of broad-spectrum anthelmintics, there is an increasing tendency to avoid accurate diagnosis and to use the rate of body weight gain after dosing as a measure of the degree of parasitic infestation. However, it should be clearly understood that in a well-managed worm control program, animals are treated to avoid contamination of the pasture and the acquisition of larvae by young susceptible animals. If animals respond visibly after treatment this is evidence that the program has failed and needs modification. Further, farmers who rely on treatments to salvage animals already heavily parasitized, should realize that considerable production losses have occurred before treatment was instituted.

Choice of treatments, dose rates and dose frequency
Most naturally acquired helminth infestations are multiple, the incidence of individual species depending largely on the suitability of the climate and on the presence of other suitable primary and intermediate hosts. The emphasis on research into better anthelmintics has thus been directed towards the development of broad-spectrum anthelmintics to avoid the use of mixtures.

Although recommendations on the choice of drugs for each helminth species are made in the sections which follow, it is not possible to lay down rigid rules of their order of preference. The range of parasites to be controlled may affect the selection, as may cost, the severity of the infestation, the presence of anthelmintic resistances and the physical status of the animals relative to possible toxic effects of the drug. In some circumstances, for example when large numbers of young, wild cattle are to be treated, the use of an injectable preparation may be essential.

To avoid injury to treated animals and to conserve costly drugs, the current tendency is to quote dose rates in terms of body weight and to adhere as strictly as possible to the recommendations. In an effort to standardize dose recommendations we have used the most favored calibration of mg/kg body weight. The dose rates recommended in the text are based largely on published work but because of the large amount of high quality adaptive research carried out by the manufactures their dose rates are more generally to be preferred. It is important that when estimating the dose rate for a group of animals, it should be calculated on the weight of the heaviest animal in the group. This ensures that the optimal dose is given to all animals and reduces the likelihood of anthelmintic resistance emerging.

Because a diagnosis of parasitic disease is a diagnosis of a herd or flock problem it is customary to treat all animals in the group to reduce environmental contamination to a minimum. The animals should then be moved to a pasture that has been spelled for an appropriate period depending on the climate or to a paddock that has been grazed by a different host.

It is necessary in many instances to repeat the treatment after several weeks to remove recently matured worms which were in an immature, more resistant stage at the first treatment. Modern anthelmintics appear to remove such stages in sheep but fenbendazole, oxfendazole, albendazole, febantel and ivermectin are the only products that will remove dormant *Ostertagia* in cattle, and oxfendazole and ivermectin are the only products that at normal dose rates and in a single treatment will remove immature dormant strongyles from horses. Frequent dosing is to be avoided as it is one of the major factors leading to the development of anthelmintic resistance (6, 7). An integrated management approach should be adopted whenever possible, with greater reliance being placed on management procedures and anthelmintics being used to reduce pasture contamination.

Continuous or intermittent treatment

In situations of very high risk, continuous or intermittent dosing at low levels calculated to inhibit egg production may be a suitable alternative to frequent repeated dosing at therapeutic levels. The method is used in the control of strongylosis in horses but has severe limitations for other species (see under haemonchosis, p. 1056). In general it is satisfactory only for animals that are fed individually or at least in troughs in dry lots. This technique has been used to provide anthelmintics in supplementary feed blocks, e.g. molasses or urea blocks, or in the water supply. Medicated blocks give a variable intake and cannot be relied upon to provide a therapeutic dose over a short period. Water medication should be avoided where non-medicated water is also available. In intensively farmed animals such as poultry of pigs or in species such as deer where handling is difficult, water medication may be acceptable, but efficiency is never as good as individual treatment and a compromise must be reached between efficiency and ease of administration (31). Metering equipment has been devised to medicate water and its use in cattle has been monitored (32). An extension of continuous treatment is the use of products such as closantel and dinitrophenol which persist for long periods in the body and kill for extended periods.

Techniques that provide continuous low level dosage and adequate efficiency have been devised and commercial preparations are now available. A morantel slow-release bolus relies on diffusion through a semipermeable membrane and contains sufficient morantel tartrate to give continuous release over 60 days (34). Another system is a dissolution-controlled release device in which the choice of carrier matrix determines the rate of dissolution (35). A different system is the pulse release bolus which releases a series of full anthelmintic doses at predetermined intervals which may cover the grazing period after cattle are released from their winter quarters.

Assessment of treatment response

The efficiency of treatment used to be measured in terms of changes in egg counts or total worm burdens. It is becoming more common to accept a level of infection that does not interfere with economic performance. It then becomes rational to assess the result of treatment in terms of increased productivity related to the value of treatment (24).

Causes of breakdown in control programs

Most of the principles laid down above, although they are implicit in any control program, are applicable to the treatment of clinically affected animals. The need to treat such animals is usually an admission that the control program has broken down. Breakdowns are usually due to:

- Failure to reduce contamination in periods when climatic conditions are unfavorable for the survival of the free-living stages
- Failure to use tactical treatment when weather conditions are conducive to the buildup of heavy pasture infection
- Failure to move treated animals to an uncontaminated environment
- Use of an insufficient dose or incorrect anthelmintic
- Failure to repeat treatment or repeating at overlong intervals in times of high risk
- Failure to appreciate the relative resistance of the immature stages of most parasites, in some instances by virtue of their inaccessibility while migrating through tissue
- The introduction of non-immune sheep from a worm-free environment into a danger area
- Failure to adequately protect young animals
- A very common inclination on the part of farmers to dose only that portion of the group which is not doing well or which is showing clinical signs of parasitic disease.

Anthelmintic resistance has been reported from a number of areas. It is particularly important in the control of *Haemonchus contortus* in sheep and the small strongyles in horses, but other resistant species have been reported particularly in sheep and goats, and care should be taken that anthelmintics are used at the correct time and dose rate so that the emergence of resistant strains is minimized.

A full discussion of anthelmintic resistance cannot be given here but all advisers should be aware of the dangers of (*a*) the overuse of anthelmintics; (*b*) underdosing whether as single doses or in mass medication; (*c*) the use of persistent anthelmintics whether given as boluses or as a single dose; and (*d*) the role of some management procedures in the development of resistance (36). Most field reports of resistance are incorrect, the problem being one of reinfestation, and the steps to be taken to investigate suspected anthelmintic resistance have been outlined (33).

If anthelmintic resistance is proved, then a drug with a different mode of action should be used, and thought should be given to the use of narrow-spectrum drugs at appropriate times to reduce the selection pressure in the broad-spectrum compounds. A series of papers on anthelmintic resistance is given as a review reference.

REVIEW LITERATURE

Anderson, N. & Waller, P. J. (1985) *Resistance in Nematodes to Anthelmintic Drugs* Publ. CSIRO Australia.

Armour, J. (1980) The epidemiology of helminth disease in farm animals. *Vet. Parasitol.*, *6*, 7.

Brunsdon, R. V. (1980) Principles of helminth control. *Vet. Parasitol.*, *6*, 185.

Morley, F. H. W. & Donald, A. D. (1980) Farm management and systems of helminth control. *Vet. Parasitol.*, 6, 105.

REFERENCES

(1) Levine, N. D. (1963) *Adv. vet. Sci.*, *8*, 215.
(2) Callinan, A. P. L. et al. (1982) *Agric. Syst.*, 9, 199
(3) Donald, A. D. (1968) *Aust. vet. J.*, *44*, 139.
(4) O'Sullivan, B. M. & Donald, A. D. (1970) *Parasitology*, *61*, 301.
(5) Michel, J. F. (1969) *Adv. Parasitol.*, 7, 211.
(6) Martin, P. J. et al. (1984) *Int. J. Parasitol.*, *14*, 177.
(7) Barton, N. J. (1983) *Int. J. Parasitol.*, *13*, 125.
(8) McBeath, D. G. et al. (1979) *Br. vet. J.*, *135*, 271.
(9) Southcott, W. H. & Barger, I. A. (1975) *Int. J. Parasitol.*, 5, 45.
(10) Arundel, J. H. & Hamilton, D. (1975) *Aust. vet. J.*, *51*, 436.
(11) Smith, H. J. & Archibald, R. McG. (1965) *Can. vet. J.* , 6, 257.
(12) Rose, J. H. (1965) *Vet. Rec.*, 77, 749.
(13) Kelly, J. D.(1973) *NZ vet. J.*, *21*, 183.
(14) Arundel, J. H. (1971) *Aust. vet. J.*, *47*, 275.
(15) Rickard, M. D. et al. (1981) *Res. vet. Sci.*, *30*, 104.
(16) Gibson, T. E. et al. (1970) *Res. vet. Sci.*, *11*, 138.
(17) Castelino, J. B. (1970) *Vet. Bull.*, *40*, 751.
(18) Gordon, H. McL. (1957) *Adv. vet. Sci.*, *3*, 287.
(19) Southcott, W. H. (1971) *Aust. vet. J.*, *47*, 170.
(20) Salisbury, J. R. & Arundel, J. H. (1970) *Aust. vet. J.*, *46*, 523.
(21) Connan, R. M. et al. (1967) *Vet. Rec.*, *80*, 424.
(22) Johnstone, I. L. (1976) *Proceedings of the International Sheep Breeding Congrees*, ed. Tomes, G. L. West Australia Institute of Technology.
(23) Michel, J. F. (1968) *Vet. Rec.*, *82*, 132.
(24) Morris, R. S. et al. (1977) *Vet. Parasitol.*, *3*, 349.
(25) Morley, F. H. W. (1978) Animal production studies on grassland. In: *Measurement of Grassland Productivity*, ed. t'Mannetje, pp. 103–162. London: CAB.
(26) Windon, R. G. & Dineen, J. K. (1981) *Int. J. Parasitol.*, *11*, 11.
(27) Darvill, F. M. et al. (1978) *Aust. vet. J.*, *54*, 575.
(28) Hammerberg, B. & Lamm, W. D. (1980) *Am. J. vet. Res.*, *41*, 1686.
(29) Herd R. P. (1987) *Mod. vet. Pract.*, *67*, 895.
(30) McKenna, P. B. (1981) *NZ vet. Res.*, *29*, 129.
(31) Neilsen, P. et al. (1983) *Res. vet. Sci.*, *35*, 122.
(32) Downey, N. E. & O'Shea, J. (1985) *Vet. Rec.*, *116*, 42.
(33) Pritchard, R. K. et al. (1980) *Aust. vet. J.*, *56*, 239.
(34) Jones, R. M. (1983) *Vet. Parasitol.*, *12*, 223.
(35) Anderson, N. & Laby, R. H. (1979) *Aust. vet. J.*, *55*, 244.
(36) Martin, P. J. (1986) *Proc. 6th Int. Congr. Parasitol., Brisbane, Australia*, ed. M. J. Howell. Australian Academy of Sciences, p. 493.

HEPATIC FASCIOLIASIS (LIVER FLUKE DISEASE)

Liver fluke disease is caused by members of the genera *Fasciola*, *Fascioloides*, and *Dicrocoelium*. With the first two genera, acute or chronic hepatic insufficiency may result. Infectious necrotic hepatitis may develop as a result of infestation by any of the three genera and this is considered to represent the only pathogenic effect of flukes of the genus *Dicroelium*. The term hepatic fascioliasis is reserved for infestation with *Fasciola hepatica*.

Etiology

Fasciola hepatica is the most common and important liver fluke and has a cosmopolitan distribution. It is of economic importance only in sheep or cattle but it may infest all domestic animals and many wildlife species. A high incidence has been reported in donkeys in the United Kingdom (1) but horses are less commonly infected (2). Other species may provide a source of infection for sheep and cattle. Human cases occur not infrequently and are usually associated with the ingestion of marsh plants such as watercress.

Fasciola gigantica is more common in Africa and India, where it occurs commonly in goats and buffalo, and in southern United States, while *Fascioloides magna* is found mainly in North America and Europe. In Canada *F. magna* is widely distributed in elk, deer and moose and has caused isolated outbreaks of fascioliasis in cattle and sheep. Sheep and goats are particularly susceptible to infestation with *F. magna*, especially when they share pasture with deer. The prevalence of infestation in cattle may be very high but only in rare cases are these animals affected clinically. In the United States *Fasciola hepatica*, *F. gigantica* and *Fascioloides magna* may all occur. *Dicrocoelium dendriticum* has a restricted distribution in North America but is widespread in Europe and Asia and in those countries is causally related to infectious necrotic hepatitis.

The spread of hepatic fascioliasis to new areas depends upon the spread of the host snail or of infested ruminants. The snails themselves may be infected and spread the disease without any movement of the host. Important host snails for *F. hepatica* are *Lymnaea truncatula* in Great Britain and Europe and *Galba bulimoides*, *G. b. techella* and others in the United States. *L. columella* has been identified as an intermediate host in Canada (4). In New Zealand *L. tomentosa* and *L. truncatula* have occurred without fascioliasis becoming a major disease but the recent introduction of *L. columella* has markedly increased the range and severity of the disease (3). *L. tomentosa* is the major host snail in Australia although *L. columella* has been reported to be present in non-farming areas, and *L. viridis* has recently been found. For *Fascioloides magna* they are *G.b. techella* and at least five other lymnaeid snails. Intermediate hosts for *D. dendriticum* in the *United States* are the land snail *Cionella lubrica* and the ant *Formica fusca*.

Lifecycle and epidemiology

All of the above parasites, with the exception of *Fascioloides magna* in cattle and in sheep, mature in the bile ducts of the host and their eggs pass down the bile ducts and are excreted with the feces. The eggs may hatch miracidia which actively invade the host snails (*Fasciola and Fascioloides* spp.) or be eaten by the snails and hatch in their gut (*D. dendriticum*). In either instance sporocysts develop in the tissue of the snail. Temperatures above 5–6°C (41–43°F) are necessary if the miracidia are to reach the snail, the optimal temperatures being 15–24°C (59–75°F) (8). Miracidia must find a suitable snail within 24–30 hours or they die.

Temperatures above 10°C (50°F) are necessary before the snails will breed or before *F. hepatica* can develop within the snail. No development therefore takes place during the winter in most countries, and in spring the eggs that have accumulated over winter hatch. The miracidia infect snails and cercariae emerge some 5–8 weeks later depending on the temperature. For any area the emergence of the cercariae is a fairly regular occurrence with only minor changes depending on climatic variations. A separate cycle may occur with snails being infected in the autumn. Development ceases in the snail in the winter but is resumed as temperatures rise in the spring and early summer. This winter infection is less important than the spring infection, possibly due to the mass mortality of snails in the winter and the preferential mortality of infected snails (5). The cercariae encyst on herbage and are ingested by the final host. The survival of metacercariae will vary depending on the climate of the area. In general, availability of metacercariae is greatest in the late summer and autumn particularly when animals are forced to feed in swampy areas. In areas with dry winters, infection may occur in the winter when stock graze wet areas to obtain green feed. Some infections may occur in early spring from overwintering metacercariae. These may be sufficiently numerous to cause losses or may simply infest animals and cause contamination of the area.

The snails that act as intermediate hosts for *F. hepatica* prefer low lying swampy areas with slowly moving water, but land with small streams or springs must also be considered dangerous. Land frequently irrigated is also highly suitable, the snails burrowing into the soil between irrigations and releasing large numbers of cercariae when free water is present.

Under severe winter conditions metacercariae do not survive. Housed animals will be protected against the disease unless they are fed hay with sufficient moisture to enable the metacercariae to survive. Hay harvested in moist conditions and not properly dried may remain infective for up to 8 months but the cercariae are killed by ensiling the cut material. In hot dry regions metacercariae die quickly and so in Australia infections are usually due to recent contaminations (6) while in the United Kingdom and Europe massive levels of metacercariae can accumulate (7).

Those metacercariae which reach the alimentary tract of a ruminant escape from their cysts, invade the intestinal wall and, in the case of *Fasciola* and *Fascioloides* spp., migrate through the peritoneal cavity to the liver. The migration is often misdirected and many ectopic flukes can be found in the lungs, particularly in cattle. After invasion of the liver the young fluke follows a definite pattern of free migration in the parenchyma before following a more localized migratory pattern prior to entering the bile duct (14). Young *Fasciola hepatica* migrate through the hepatic parenchyma for about 4–5 weeks before they reach the bile ducts. Here they remain fixed and commence laying eggs about 10–12 weeks after infestation. Adult sheep and cattle may remain as carriers of *F. hepatica* for many years because of the longevity of the individual mature flukes in bile ducts.

Sheep and goats do not develop a strong immune reaction to *F. hepatica* (10, 11), although fluke from challenge infections may be reduced in size and produce less eggs. The severe reaction in cattle, which results in hepatic fibrosis, and hyperplasia and calcification of the bile ducts, appears to hinder the establishment and feeding of challenge infections and adds to the immune reaction (22) in reducing numbers of fluke in previously affected cattle. Immature *F. hepatica* release a proteolytic enzyme that can cleave immunoglobulins (Ig) of the mouse, rabbit, rat and sheep and this may also play some part in preventing the development of an immunity (12).

Prenatal infections occur in cattle and to a lesser extent in sheep, foals and man. It has been suggested that these infections may impair the ability of cattle to develop resistance and that these animals may play an important epidemiological role (15).

A special exception to this general life history is the passage of *D. dendriticum* through a snail and then through an ant before it is infective for sheep. This species also differs in that it reaches the liver via the common bile duct and so does not migrate in the parenchyma. *Fascioloides magna* also differs from this pattern. It is essentially a parasite of elk and deer. In its normal hosts after wandering in the peritoneal cavity for 3–4 weeks, it then enters the liver and migrates in the parenchyma until it eventually forms a thin-walled cyst which has connections with the bile ducts. In cattle and pigs, the cyst wall is much thicker and there is no connection with the bile ducts through which eggs may escape, while in sheep and goats the fluke continually migrates, never becoming encapsulated, and the damage is so severe that one or two flukes can kill the sheep.

Pathogenesis

Acute and chronic hepatic fascioliasis are caused by different stages of *Fasciola hepatica* in the liver. Acute hepatic fascioliasis occurs 5–6 weeks after the ingestion of large numbers of metacercariae and is due to the sudden invasion of the liver by masses of young flukes. Sufficient parenchyma may be destroyed to cause acute hepatic insufficiency and to this may be added the effects of hemorrhage into the peritoneal cavity (16–18). Hypoalbuminemia occurs due to reduced albumin synthesis and plasma volume expansion caused by liver damage (9). Immature flukes are tissue feeders but may accidentally ingest some blood and the minor degree of anemia that develops in the first 4–5 weeks of infection probably reflects the loss of blood into the migratory track of the young fluke (5). Migration occurs more rapidly in pregnant sheep and it has been suggested that this may be analogous to the periparturient rise in egg count that occurs in *Ostertagia* and *Haemonchus* infection (13).

Chronic fascioliasis develops slowly and is due to the activity of the adult flukes in the bile ducts. These cause cholangitis, biliary obstruction, destruction of hepatic tissue and fibrosis, and anemia. The cause of the anemia seen in chronic fascioliasis can be explained by the blood-sucking activity of the flukes and the continuous drain on iron reserves that this imposes (5), but recent work suggests that a substance produced by the worms, possibly proline, may contribute to the development of anemia (32). Hypoalbuminemia is more marked in the chronic disease and is due mainly to the increased protein plasma leakage into the gut. It is more severe in sheep with anorexia or in those on a low plane of nutrition (9). Chronic infection has been shown to limit growth rate and feed conversion in growing heifers (26) and to reduce growth rate in beef cattle (43). *F. hepatica* infection has been reported to increase the susceptibility of cattle to *Salmonella dublin* and predispose to prolonged infection and fecal excretion (64). Infected ewes have reduced fertility (45) and body growth rate and wool weight is proportional to the number of fluke present (54). Food intake is reduced and this leads to a reduction in efficiency of utilization of metabolizable energy and reduction in calcium and protein deposition in the carcass (55). *Fascioloides magna* infestations in cattle are usually inapparent but may cause a syndrome similar to chronic hepatic fascioliasis, *F. gigantica* in cattle can cause severe anemia and acute liver damage (19), and *F. magna* and *F. gigantica* in sheep (20) cause a syndrome similar to acute hepatic fascioliasis. *D.dendriticum* is of low pathogenicity.

As might be expected the number of metacercariae ingested governs to a large extent the way in which fascioliasis is manifested. For example, the prepatent period is shorter with smaller numbers, with larger numbers hepatic fibrosis and damage retards migration (18). The number of metacercariae ingested at any one time is probably not the only factor which determines whether acute or chronic fascioliasis occurs, or whether the pathogenesis is related chiefly to hepatic parenchymal damage or to biliary tract obstruction. Previous exposure to infection appears to reduce bile duct populations and to inhibit migration (21), but a significant degree of immunity has not been demonstrated in sheep and it is not possible to protect them by vaccination. Cattle are more resistant to infection than sheep. Both horses and pigs are generally highly resistant to infection with *F. hepatica* but differ in their mode of resistance. Horses overcome the migrating fluke at an early stage so that few reach the liver, while in the pig the resistance mechanism operates in the liver parenchyma (23).

Migration of the young *Fasciola hepatica* through hepatic tissue containing quiescent spores of *Clostridium novyi* may cause the development of infectious necrotic hepatitis in sheep and cattle. This migration has also been thought to stimulate the development of occasional cases of bacillary hemoglobinuria in cattle.

Clinical findings

Acute fascioliasis

Acute fascioliasis in sheep is often a syndrome of death without other apparent clinical abnormality (24). It usually occurs in the summer and autumn but its timing is influenced by the release of cercariae in a particular district and the opportunity for sheep to obtain large numbers. If the disease is observed clinically in sheep it is manifested by dullness, weakness, lack of appetite, pallor and edema of mucosae and conjunctivae, and pain when pressure is exerted over the area of the liver. Death occurs quickly, usually less than 48 hours, and may be accompanied by the passage of bloodstained discharges from the nostrils and anus. Outbreaks are most common and severe in young sheep and are of relatively short duration, most deaths occurring within a period of 2–3 weeks.

Subacute fascioliasis

A subacute fascioliasis is also described in sheep and results from the ingestion of large numbers of metacercariae over a longer period of time. The major clinical signs are weight loss and pallor of the mucous membranes. Submandibular edema will be seen in only a few cases, but many animals will resent palpation over the region of the liver.

Chronic fascioliasis

Chronic fascioliasis occurs when small numbers of metacercariae are ingested over a long period. Infected sheep lose weight, develop submandibular edema (bottle-jaw) and pallor of the mucosae over a period of weeks. Shedding of the wool may occur. The course of the disease is often as long as 2–3 months in those which die; many survive but are emaciated for longer periods. Cattle also lose weight, especially when there is the added drain of lactation, milk production falls and anemia and chronic diarrhea develop (56).

The clinical findings in black disease (necrotic hepatitis) and bacillary hemoglobinuria are described under those headings (pp. 608 and 610). The disease in cattle is usually chronic but an acute or subacute disease does occur in dairy calves in heavily infected areas. The clinical findings are similar to those in sheep.

Clinical pathology

In acute fascioliasis there is a severe normochromic anemia, eosinophilia and a severe hypoalbuminemia. Eggs will not be present in the feces. In the subacute and chronic diseases, rapid weight loss with a severe hypochromic, macrocytic anemia and hypoalbuminemia will be seen. Submandibular edema and ascites is seen in only a few cases in the subacute condition but is a constant finding in the chronic disease (5). Serum levels of enzymes show high levels while the young flukes are migrating through the liver but fall after the flukes enter the bile ducts usually reaching base levels by 8–10 weeks after infection (25). SGOT levels have been used in the past but plasma glutamate dehydrogenase and gamma-glutamyl transpeptidase are more sensitive indicators of liver cell damage, while serum sorbitol dehydrogenase can also be used as an indicator of the development of fascioliasis in sheep (57). Increases in aspartate aminotransferase (ASP) can be measured from 4 weeks and are useful as a measure of immature infection (63).

A diagnosis of chronic hepatic fascioliasis can be confirmed by the detection of large numbers of characteristic, operculated fluke eggs in the feces. The eggs are thin-walled and stained yellow-brown by biliary pigments but are not suspended satisfactorily by all flotation solutions. Sedimentation tests are more accurate (27) and it has been suggested that treatment may cause improvement if any eggs are present (28). Operculated fluke eggs are also characteristic of paramphistomiasis but in this latter disease the eggs are somewhat larger, are not stained yellow, have a transparent shell, a much more distinct operculum and well-defined embryonic cells. Anemia is characteristic of fascioliasis. Hyperimmunoglobulinemia occurs but total proteins are normal. Liver function tests are not significantly affected.

Necropsy findings

Acute hepatic fascioliasis
This is characterized by a badly damaged, swollen liver. The capsule shows many small perforations and subcapsular hemorrhages and the parenchyma shows tracts of damaged tissue and is much more friable than normal. The immature flukes are often so small that they are not readily discernible. They are most easily demonstrated by slicing a piece of liver thinly and shaking in water, permitting the flukes to settle to the bottom. The peritoneal cavity may contain an excess of bloodstained serum (24).

Chronic hepatic fascioliasis
This is characterized by the presence of the large, leaf-like flukes in grossly enlarged and thickened bile ducts, particularly in the ventral lobe of the liver. The bile ducts may protrude above the surface of the liver and cysts may be seen due to blockage of ducts with flukes and desquamated epithelial cells. Calcification of the bile duct walls is a common finding in cattle but not in sheep. The hepatic parenchyma is extensively fibrosed and the hepatic parenchyma is extensively fibrosed and the hepatic lymph nodes are dark brown in color. Anemia, edema and emaciation are attendant abnormalities.

One of the important facets of a necropsy examination is to estimate the duration of the infection from the length of the flukes. This may help locate the habitat of the snail and be an important factor in a control program. In infestations with *D. dendriticum* the lesions are much less marked and comprise fibrosis of the parenchyma and thickening of the smaller bile ducts. The flukes are smaller and lanceolate in shape. In *Fascioloides magna* infestations in sheep the lesions are large, black tracts and in cattle the liver shows dark, black cysts up to 4 cm in diameter and elevated slightly above the surface, and tracts of necrotic hepatic tissue in the parenchyma.

Diagnosis

In an area where liver flukes occur every case of chronic ill-health in sheep must be considered as a possible case of fascioliasis. To support the diagnosis there should be fluke eggs in the feces and hepatic lesions characteristic of the disease in the liver at necropsy. In a flock where fluke is present probably every adult sheep will show the characteristic necropsy lesions and it is necessary to estimate the severity of the lesions to determine whether or not they could be the sole or main contributing factor to the ill-health or death of the animal. The infestation may be the main cause of disease or may occur with another debilitating disease such as nutritional deficiencies of copper or cobalt, other internal parasitisms or Johne's disease. In cattle the common presence of fascioliasis and ostertagiasis has caused diagnostic problems, resolved in a general sense by the preponderance of anemia in the former and diarrhea in the latter. Serological tests have shown promise, the ELISA being the best test for routine diagnosis of fascioliasis in cattle and sheep. A rise in antibody could be detected by 2 weeks after infection but was not sufficiently high to be diagnostic until 6–8 weeks (58).

Acute fascioliasis of sheep is most difficult to differentiate from infectious necrotic hepatitis because of the small lesions which may, in the latter disease, require histological examination for identification. In general, acute fluke disease occurs only in young animals whereas black disease is usually confined to animals in the 2–4-year age group. If vaccination against black disease has been carried out, the disease can be rejected as a possible cause of mortality. The friable, badly damaged liver of acute fascioliasis and the presence of immature parasites are usually sufficient to differentiate the disease from other causes of acute, heavy mortality, especially haemonchosis, eperythrozoonosis, anthrax and enterotoxemia. There are also characteristic necropsy findings which help to identify these latter diseases.

Treatment

Little work has been done on the treatment of liver fluke other than on that caused by *Fasciola hepatica* and the bulk of the following information refers specifically to that disease. The optimum treatment of hepatic fascioliasis must destroy the migrating immature flukes as well as the adult flukes fixed in the bile ducts. Relative lack of toxicity is also essential because of the already impaired efficiency of hepatic detoxicating mechanisms.

Carbon tetrachloride is still used by many farmers to treat fascioliasis in sheep because of its low cost. It is basically effective against mature *F. hepatica* only but the recommended dose rate of 1 ml/9 kg will kill some 6-week-old and 8-week-old flukes. While mortalities are rare, heavy mortality has occurred on occasions and is unpredictable. The drug is not effective against *D. dendriticum* and is regarded as being too toxic to use in cattle. However intramuscular injections of the pure drug (i.e. not diluted with paraffin) have been used in cattle with good results. It should be given in a site of low economic values as considerable muscle necrosis occurs and the carcass should not be sold for at least 3 months after treatment. The milk will be tainted for several days.

Hexachlorethane, given orally, has been used for many years in cattle and is generally regarded as being less toxic than carbon tetrachloride. However, there is very little evidence to support this and mortalities do occur on occasions. Hexachlorophene is another old compound which has now been largely superseded. It had higher efficiency against immature flukes than the other compounds but toxicity occurred at normal dose rates.

In recent years a variety of new compounds that have high efficiency against adult and immature fluke have been introduced. Rafoxanide is an efficient compound in sheep and cattle and will kill the majority of flukes older than 4 weeks in sheep and over 8 weeks in cattle. It has low toxicity and like many of the newer compounds is active against *Haemonchus contortus*. Closantel 7·5 mg/kg has a similar spectrum to rafoxanide against *F. hepatica*, and has a residual effect of up to 2 months against *H. contortus*. Brotianide is used routinely against *F. hepatica* in sheep at 5 mg/kg while a higher dose of

7·5 mg/kg will remove more than 90% of 6-week-old fluke. No claims are made for the use of this compound in cattle. Diamphenethide has excellent efficacy against all immature stages from 1 week old but the dose rate has to be increased to remove stages over 8 weeks of age. It is too expensive to use in most countries.

Triclabendazole is a specific, highly efficient compound for use against *F. hepatica* in sheep and cattle (65–67). Doses of 10 mg/kg in sheep and 12 mg/kg in cattle are highly effective against all stages of fluke from 1 day old. It is the drug of choice in outbreaks of acute fluke disease and its use in control programs allows a longer period between treatments. If used in lactating dairy cattle, the milk should be withheld from human consumption.

Clorsulon has recently been introduced for liver fluke control and at the recommended dose rate of 20 mg/kg is effective against fluke 2 weeks and older and has a 10-fold safety margin (68). It will also be a valuable tool for treatment of outbreaks and for use in control programs.

Clioxanide is a useful compound against immature and mature forms but its efficiency is reduced markedly if the drug passes directly to the abomasum (38). Niclopholan has the same deficiency (39). Nitroxynil is given subcutaneously at 10 mg/kg in cattle (40) and has good efficiency. It is also effective in sheep (41) but spillage from subcutaneous injection stains the fleece yellow. It cannot be given orally as the rumen microflora reduce the compound to an inactive metabolite.

Only two compounds are known that do not significantly taint the milk. Oxyclozanide is used only in cattle. It has a significant effect against adult fluke but is inactive against in immature forms (42). This compound has been combined with levamisole to provide activity against fluke and gastrointestinal nematodes. Bromsalans, a mixture of isomers of bromsalicylanilids, has also been widely used in cattle and activity against flukes from 8 weeks of age has been claimed. The combination of bromsalans and the broad-spectrum anthelmintics fenbendazole, oxfendazole or febantel have proved to be toxic. Albendazole, a broad-spectrum compound, is effective against nematodes and cestodes and has some effect against adult *F. hepatica* (59) and at doses of 15 mg/kg and above is effective against *D. dendriticum* (60) and against natural infections of *F. magna* (61). Rafoxanide at 10 and 15 mg/kg is highly efficient against *F. magna* (62) but may show some toxicity at those dose rates. Triclabendazole is also effective against *F. magna* (66), as is closantel orally at 15 mg/kg or by intramuscular injection at 7·5 mg/kg (69), and clorsulon 25 mg/kg (61).

Many of the newer compounds do not appear to have been tested against *F. gigantica* but rafoxanide and triclabendazole (62) are known to be active.

Control

In general, adult and well-nourished animals are less susceptible to the effects of the disease and maintenance of a good plane of nutrition may help to reduce its severity. Disruption of the lifecycle of the liver fluke, with the eventual aim of control or eradication, can be effected by a combined attack on the egg-laying adult flukes in sheep and on the host snails in the pasture. However, because of the extreme 'efficiency' of this parasite and the way in which it takes advantage of environmental conditions to multiply enormously, careful study of its ecology is necessary to predict periods of danger and initiate strategic attacks on both snails and flukes. The most dangerous times are when wet seasons, which allow snail multiplication, are followed immediately by dry seasons which force sheep to graze on small, heavily infested areas. In temperate winter rainfall climates the period of maximum infestation is in summer but in summer rainfall areas the infestation period of pasture may occur during the winter months, thus necessitating a variation in the times at which control measures are carried out.

With the advent of the new highly efficient compounds, control is now based on anthelmintic treatment at times decided by epidemiological studies. Work in the United Kingdom has directed attention to the use of climatic data to forecast the escalation of metacercariae (44) and this knowledge aids greatly in timing treatments.

In general, a treatment should be given towards the end of winter to remove egg laying flukes and reduce contamination, and in those areas where overwintering cercariae are important another treatment in the spring, given when the flukes are large enough to be susceptible but before they are egg laying, may be desirable. Further treatments should be given in the autumn to remove flukes before they contaminate the pasture. The use of modern compounds, such as rafoxanide or closantel at 5–6-week intervals (45) will almost completely suppress the passage of fluke eggs. However, this allows fluke to migrate through the liver and cause considerable damage and production loss before treatment. Triclabendazole given at 8–11 week intervals can be used to reduce this early damage, and if given consistently at less than the prepatent period for 1 year will reduce contamination to such low levels that treatment in subsequent years can be markedly reduced (65). Diamphenethide given at 4–5-week intervals should prevent the productivity depression associated with the migrating flukes and may be economically justified. An intensive program, such as outlined above, may be necessary in a bad fluke year but once the contamination has been reduced by such a program then the number of treatments may be reduced. It is usually not necessary to treat lambs, but other hosts that may be contaminating the pasture should be treated and access of wild animals should be prevented.

Dairy cattle may suffer a loss of production and as compounds other than oxyclozanide and bromsalans taint the milk and prevent it being marketed for some days, it is usual to treat cattle as they are dried off. If other treatments are to be given an autumn treatment is recommended.

Snail control

Eradication of the host snails from the environment has been a major facet of fluke control for many years, but this eradication may be extremely difficult, some times impossible, in lowlying, wet areas with a temperate climate. Multiplication of the snails is extremely rapid and incomplete eradication achieves only a temporary reduction in their population.

Because of the poor practicability of snail control and its high cost the emphasis on it has decreased in recent years and its implementation is probably best restricted to farms which have a small localized area suitable for snail growth. These small areas are best neutralized in a permanent manner by drainage or being fenced off.

In areas where control of the snail is necessary a molluscicide should be applied, preferably on a warm sunny day when the snails are active and before the breeding season in that area. This may be in late winter in mild temperate areas or spring and early summer when conditions are more severe. Copper sulfate at 22·5 kg/ha of 0·5% solution has been recommended. However, this may be dangerous in areas where chronic copper poisoning or hepatitis due to plant poisoning occurs, and drainage into streams will kill edible fish. Further, the copper ions are quickly inactivated by organic matter.

Copper pentachlorphenate has been found to be much more effective as a molluscicide than copper sulfate (49). When applied at the rate of 11·2 kg/ha in a high volume spray 4500 liters/ha it has the advantage of not being inactivated by organic matter. The nitrogenous fertilizer calcium cyanamide has been given a preliminary trial as a molluscicide and has significantly reduced the new infection rate (50). *N*-Tritylmorpholene (Frescon) is a very effective molluscicide which has been shown to reduce the new infection rate of sheep with fluke, after administration to the pasture (51). It is most effective in small, low density snail habitats. When it is used on large high snail density areas the infestation rate of lambs can be dangerously high (52). The application of any molluscicide is made more efficient if the area to be treated is surveyed and marked beforehand and a dye marker included in the material applied. Where irrigation is the principal hazard it may be possible to add the molluscicide to the water by means of a mechanical device such as is used in streams.

Various biological methods for control of snails have been suggested (46) and an unsuccessful attempt at control has been made by using larvae of the sciomyzid fly *Dichetophora biroi* (47). It has been shown that the presence of non-susceptible snails reduces the infection rate in *L. truncatula* (48).

Because of the habits of snails in sheltering under foliage beside water, a control measure of great importance is the cleaning of the banks of streams and water reservoirs. Herbage cleared from these areas should not be available to animals as it may be heavily infested with cercariae. Cattle are more inclined to graze in marshy areas than sheep and may serve as a means of carrying infection to sheep on the same pasture. Separation of cattle from sheep, especially during warm periods when infestation of snails is more likely, is particularly desirable. Many livestock owners do not appreciate that cattle can carry the parasite.

The implementation of control measures against *D. dendriticum* is complicated by the existence of two intermediate hosts, a land snail and an ant. Infestation with *Fascioloides magna* can be avoided by keeping wild ruminants, particularly elk and deer, off the pasture.

REVIEW LITERATURE

Boray, J. C. (1969) Experimental fascioliasis in Australia. *Adv. Parasitol.*, 7, 95.

Brunsdon, R. V. (1977) *Bull. Off. int. Epizootol.*, 87, 665.

REFERENCES

(1) Pankhurst, J. W. (1963) *Vet. Rec.*, *75*, 434.
(2) Owen, J. M. (1977) *Equ. vet. J.*, *9*, 29.
(3) Harris, R. E. & Charleston, W. A. G. (1980) *Vet. Parasitol.*, 7, 39.
(4) Whitney, H. et al. (1981) *Can. vet. J.*, *22*, 334.
(5) Reid, J. et al. (1973) *Helminth Diseases of Cattle, Sheep and Horses in Europe*, eds G. M. Urquhart & J. Armour, p. 81. Glasgow: Robert MacLehose.
(6) Meek, A. H. & Morris, R. S. (1979) *Aust. vet. J.*, *55*, 58.
(7) Ross, J. G. & Todd, J. R. (1968) *Vet. Rec.*, *82*, 695.
(8) Christiansen, N. O. et al. (1976) *J. Parasitol.*, *62*, 698.
(9) Dargie, J. D. & Berry, C. I. (1979) *Int. J. Parasitol.*, *9*, 17.
(10) Reddington, J. J. et al. (1986) *Vet. Parasitol.*, *19*, 145.
(11) Haroun, El. T. M. & Hillyer, G. V. (1986) *Vet. Parasitol.*, *20*, 63.
(12) Chapman, C. B. & Mitchell, G. F. (1982) *Vet. Parasitol.*, *11*, 65.
(13) Sinclair, K. B. (1972) *Br. vet. J.*, *138*, 249.
(14) Dow, C. et al. (1968) *Parasitology*, *58*, 129.
(15) Rees, J. B. et al. (1975) *Aust. vet. J.*, *51*, 497.
(16) Ross, J. G. et al. (1966) *J. comp. Pathol.*, *76*, 67.
(17) Roberts, H. E. (1968) *Br. vet. J.*, *124*, 433.
(18) Boray, J. C. (1967) *Ann. trop. Med. Parasitol.*, *61*, 439.
(19) Bitakaramire, P. K. & Bwangamoi, O. (1970) *Bull. epizoot. Dis. Afr.*, *18*, 149.
(20) Alibasoglu, M. & Guralp, N. (1969) *Vet. Fak. Derg. Ankara Üniv.*, *16*, 110.
(21) Ross, J. G. (1967) *J. Helminth.*, *41*, 217, 223.
(22) Doyle, J. J. (1973) *Res. vet. Sci.*, *14*, 97.
(23) Nansen, P. et al. (1975) *Exp. Parasitol.*, *37*, 15.
(24) Ross, J. G. et al. (1967) *Vet. Rec.*, *80*, 543.
(25) Thorpe, E. & Ford, E. J. H. (1969) *J. Pathol.*, 97, 619.
(26) Oakley, G. A. et al. (1978) *Vet. Rec.*, *104*, 503.
(27) Boray, J. C. & Pearson, I. G. (1960) *Aust. vet. J.*, *36*, 331.
(28) Happich, F. A. & Boray, J. C. (1969) *Aust. vet. J.*, *45*, 326.
(29) Somesen, M. et al. (1968) *Nord. VetMed.*, *20*, 638, 651.
(30) Ross, J. G. (1968) *Irish vet. J.*, *22*, 62.
(31) Reid, J. F. S. et al. (1967) *Vet. Rec.*, *80*, 371.
(32) Spengler, C. B. & Isseroff, H. (1981) *J. Parasitol.*, *67*, 886.
(33) Guilhon, J. et al.(1970) *Bull. Acad. Vét. Franç.*, *43*, 419.
(34) Presidente, P. J. A. & Knapp, S. E. (1972) *Am. J. vet. Res.*, *33*, 1603.
(35) Egerton, J. R. et al. (1970) *Res. vet. Sci.*, *11*, 382.
(36) Corba, J. et al. (1976) *Vet. Med. Rev.*, *2*, 181.
(37) Kendall, S. B. & Parfitt, J. W. (1973) *Res. vet. Sci.*, *15*, 37.
(38) Boray, J. C. & Roseby, F. B. (1969) *Aust. vet. J.*, *45*, 363.
(39) Boray, J. C. et al. (1969) *Aust. vet. J.*, *45*, 94.
(40) Reid, J. S. F. et al. (1970) *Vet. Rec.*, *86*, 41.
(41) Colegrave, A. J. (1968) *Vet. Rec.*, *82*, 343, 373.
(42) Froyd, G. (1969) *Vet. Rec.*, *85*, 705.
(43) Chick, B. F. et al. (1980) *Aust. vet. J.*, *56*, 588.
(44) Ollerenshaw, C. B. & Smith, L. P. (1969) *Adv. Parasitol.*, 7, 283.
(45) Cawdery, M. J. H. (1976) *Br. vet. J.*, *132*, 568.
(46) Gordon, H. McL. & Boray, J. C. (1970) *Vet. Rec.*, *86*, 289.
(47) Fontana, P. G. (1972) *Parasitology*, *64*, 89.
(48) Christensen, N. O. & Nansen, P. (1976) *Parasitology*, *73*, 161.
(49) Gordon, H. McL. et al. (1959) *Aust. vet. J.*, *35*, 465.
(50) Ross, J. G. (1970) *Vet. Rec.*, *87*, 373.
(51) Crossland, N. D. (1976) *Vet. Rec.*, *98*, 45.
(52) Ross, J. G. et al. (1970) *Br. vet. J.*, *126*, 283.
(53) Whitelaw, A. & Fawcett, A. R. (1981) *Vet. Rec.*, *109*, 118.
(54) Meek, A. H. & Morris, R. S. (1979) *Aust. vet. J.*, *55*, 61.
(55) Sykes, A. R. et al. (1980) *Res. vet. Sci.*, *28*, 63.
(56) Eckert, J. et al. (1977) *Schweiz. Arch. Tierheilkd*, *199*, 135.
(57) Hawkins, C. D. (1984) *Vet. Parasitol.*, *15* , 117.
(58) Zimmermann, G. L. et al. (1982) *Am. J. vet. Res.*, *43*, 2097.
(59) Theodorides, V. J. & Freeman, J. F. (1980) *Vet. Rec.*, *106*, 78.
(60) Himonas, C. A. & Liakos, V. (1980) *Vet. Rec.*, *107*, 288.

(61) Foreyt, W. J. & Drawe, D. L. (1985) *J. Am. vet. Med. Assoc.*, *187*, 1187.
(62) Hymen, W. B. et al. (1984) *XIII Wld Congr. Dis. Cattle, Durban, Rep. S. Afr.*, p. 422.
(63) Wyckoff, J. H. & Bradley, R. E. (1985) *Am. J. vet. Res.*, *46*, 1015.
(64) Aitken, M. M. et al. (1978) *J. comp. Pathol.*, *88*, 75.
(65) Boray, J. C. et al. (1985) *NZ vet. J.*, *33*, 182.
(66) Craig, T. M. & Huey, R. L. (1984) *Am. J. vet. Res.*, *45*, 1644.
(67) Owen, I. L. (1987) *Aust. vet. J.*, *64*, 59.
(68) Boray, J. C. (1986) *6th Int. Congr. Parasitol. Brisbane, Australia*, Abstract 79.
(69) Stromberg, B. E. et al. (1985) *Am. J. vet. Res.*, *46*, 2527.

PARAMPHISTOMIASIS (STOMACH FLUKE DISEASE)

The intestinal phase of amphistomiasis is a common parasitic disease of cattle, and to a lesser extent sheep, caused by paramphistome flukes and characterized by a severe enteritis.

Etiology

Paramphistomum cervi, *P. microbothrioides*, *P. liorchis*, *P. ichikawai*, *P. microbothrium*, *Calicophoron calicophorum*, *Ceylonocotyle streptocoelium*, *Calicophoron ijimai*, and *Cotylophoron cotylophorum* are the commonly recorded species in sheep and cattle.

Epidemiology

As a serious disease, intestinal amphistomiasis has been recorded in cattle in the United States, Australia and India, in sheep in the United States, South Africa, New Zealand, Australia and India and in goats in India. Cattle are most commonly affected and the mortality rate in groups of heavily infested animals may be as high as 96%. The mortality rate in sheep has been as high as 90%. Acute mortalities appear to be the only manifestation of the disease.

Most outbreaks occur during the late summer, autumn and early winter when pastures have become heavily contaminated with encysted cercariae. All ages of cattle, sheep, goats and wild ruminants may be affected but young cattle in the yearling class are the usual subjects. It is possible that some degree of immunity develops; this is suggested by the uncommon occurrence of the disease in adults.

Lifecycle

All these flukes have as intermediate hosts, aquatic planorbid snails which are much more adaptable and occupy more diverse habitats than the lymnaeid snails, thus leading to different geographical distribution of the stomach and liver fluke. The immature flukes excyst in the duodenum and as they mature migrate through the abomasum to the rumen and reticulum. The period required for maturation varies from 6 weeks to 4 months and the factors which cause this variation have not been determined (2, 3).

Pathogenesis

Clinical illness is produced only when there are enormous numbers of the immature flukes in the duodenum and abomasum, the migrating flukes setting up an acute enteritis. Mature flukes in the forestomachs appear to cause little harm.

Clinical findings

Infestation by immature flukes cause a persistent fetid diarrhea which is characteristic, and is accompanied by weakness, depression, dehydration and anorexia. There may also be submaxillary edema and obvious pallor of the mucosae. Death usually occurs 15–20 days after the first signs appear.

A syndrome has also been ascribed to heavy infestations with adult flukes (4). The disease is chronic and signs include loss of weight, anemia, rough dry coat and a drop in production.

Clinical pathology

Because the acute disease is caused by immature forms, eggs are not usually present in the feces, although they may be detectable in older animals in the same herd. A sedimentation method is preferred to detect eggs and it may be advisable to use a sedimentation and decanting technique to find immature flukes which have been passed. The latter is in fact a more common basis for diagnosis than identification of the eggs. The larvae are characterized by their round shape and the presence of anterior and posterior suckers. The eggs have a distinct operculum, the shell is thin and colorless and the embryonic cells are clearly outlined. There is a knob at the posterior pole. There is a marked drop in total plasma protein, due largely to a fall in plasma albumin (5).

Necropsy findings

There is muscular atrophy, subcutaneous edema and accumulations of fluid in the body cavities, and the fat depôts are gelatinous. In the upper part of the duodenum the mucosa is thickened, covered with blood-stained mucus and there are patches of hemorrhage under the serosa. Large numbers of small, flesh-colored-flukes (3–4 mm long and 1–2 mm wide) are present in this area but decrease in number towards the ileum. There may be none in the abomasum and forestomachs. There may be a few in the peritoneal cavity and on histological examination the young flukes are present not only on the mucosal surface but are also embedded in the mucosa and deeper layers (5).

Diagnosis

Intestinal amphistomiasis may be easily missed because, although intestinal parasitism is often suspected in animals of this age group, immature flukes, which usually cause illness, will not be laying eggs and even at necropsy the small parasites may be missed. The occurrence in yearling cattle of a severe enteritis, unaccompanied by fever, in environmental conditions suitable for the propagation of flukes and where host snails can be found should arouse suspicion of the disease. A nutritional deficiency of copper and infestation with liver flukes or intestinal roundworms are the diseases with which it is most likely to be confused. The infectious enteritides, including the viral and bacterial infections, are usually accompanied by fever and other diagnostic signs. Johne's disease in adult animals is a much more chronic disease. Poisonings, including many weeds, inorganic arsenic and lead, can only be differentiated by their detection in the environment and in tissues at necropsy.

Treatment

Most of the newer trematocides do not appear to have been tested against paramphistomes and many of the early compounds have not been evaluated critically. Two doses of oxyclozanide 18·7 mg/kg days apart, or a single dose of hexachlorophene 20 mg/kg, give consistent results against immature paramphistomes in cattle, but hexachlorophene may show toxicity at this dose rate (1). Niclosamide 160 mg/kg as a single dose or as two doses 3 days apart is effective but somewhat variable (1); however it has good activity at 90 mg/kg against immature paramphistomes in sheep (6). Resorantel also has high efficiency against the migrating forms in sheep and at 65 mg/kg removes 84% of adults in cattle (9). Bithionol 15 mg/kg, carbon tetrachloride and hexachlorethane are effective against adults but not against the immature forms, and are toxic. Brotianide 15 mg/kg is also effective against adult but not immature stages (7). Triclabendazole, diamphenathide and clorsulon have high activity against immature *F. hepatica* but do not appear to have been tested against paramphistomes. Treatment with intestinal sedatives to control the enteritis and parenteral fluids to repair the dehydration are recommended. During an outbreak it is essential to remove animals from the infected pasture.

Control

Routine treatments to control paramphistomes are rarely given but in areas where a regular problem occurs, routine treatment to eliminate adults before they mature and contaminate the pasture should be given. Drainage of lowlying areas and destruction of host snails by the use of molluscicides should be considered. Small scale experiments have shown that vaccination with irradiated larvae of *P. microbothrium* is an efficient procedure in sheep, goats and cattle (8).

REVIEW LITERATURE

Dinnik, J. A. (1964) *Bull. epizoot. Dis. Afr.*, *12*, 439.
Horak, I. G. (1971) *Adv. Parasitol.*, *9*, 33.

REFERENCES

(1) Rolfe, P. F. & Boray, J. C. (1986) *6th Int. Congr. Parasitol., Brisbane, Australia*, Abstract 557.
(2) Dinnik, J. A. & Dinnik, N. N. (1962) *Bull. epizoot. Dis. Afr.*, *10*, 27.
(3) Durie, P. H. (1953) *Aust. J. Zool.*, *1*, 192.
(4) McFadden, G. M. (1968/69) *Vict. vet. Proc.*, *27*, 69.
(5) Boray, J. C. et al. (1969) *Aust. vet. J.*, *45*, 133.
(6) Boray, J. C. (1969) *Vet. med. Rev.*, *4*, 290.
(7) Corba, J. et al. (1976) *Vet. med. Rev.*, *2*, 181.
(8) Horak, I. G. (1966) *J. S. Afr. vet. med. Assoc.*, *37*, 428.
(9) Chowanlec, W. et al. (1976) *Med. Weterynaryma*, *32*, 739.

TAPEWORM INFESTATION

Tapeworm infestations have little apparent effect on the health of farm livestock but heavy infestation in young animals may cause failure to thrive. Disease caused by infestation with the intermediate stages of tapeworms is not dealt with because of its lack of applicability to clinical disease. Coenurosis is dealt with under diseases of the nervous system (p. 437).

Etiology and epidemiology

The common tapeworms of ruminants, *Moniezia expansa*, *M. benedini* and *Helictometra (Thysaniezia) giardi*, have cosmopolitan distribution, while *Avitellina* spp. (Mediterranean countries and India), *S. hepatica* (Africa) and *Thysanosoma actinioides* (North America) are less widely distributed. In horses *Anoplocephala magna*, *A. perfoliata* and *Paranoplocephala mamillana* are cosmopolitan in their distribution.

Although tapeworms may infest animals of any age they appear to have little if any deleterious effects on adults and heavy infestations are necessary to cause clinical illness in the young.

Lifecycle

The eggs of mature tapeworms pass in the feces of the host to the exterior, either singly or protected by the tapeworm segment or in egg capsules or parauterine organs. At this time the eggs contain developed embryos. All of the above tapeworms require an intermediate host which ingests the eggs and in which the intermediate stage is produced. Mature tapeworms develop only when the primary host ingests the intermediate stage. As far as is known the intermediate hosts of the worms under consideration are oribatid mites.

Pathogenesis

Tapeworms, according to their species, are either confined to the small intestine or invade its associated organs, the biliary and pancreatic ducts (*T. actinioides* and *S. hepatica*). In the former instance the mechanisms by which the worms affect the host are by competing for nutrients, by the excretion of toxic materials and, because of their length, by interfering with the motility of the gut. Infestation of pancreatic and biliary ducts appears to cause little harm and the most serious effect is the rejection of damaged livers at meat inspection. Some interference with the flow of digestive juices and with digestion is to be expected and very heavy infestations with *M. expansa* in lambs have been associated with outbreaks of enterotoxemia (1). In horses, *A. perfoliata* localizes near the ileocecal valve and causes inflammation and ulceration. This may cause interference with passage of ingesta and also intermittent low grade colic. The feces may be covered with bloodstained mucus and rupture of the cecum has been known to occur.

In general, the gastrointestinal signs commonly attributed to tapeworm infestation occur in very young animals when the diet is inadequate and the infestation is gross (2).

Clinical findings

There is disagreement over the importance of tapeworms in causing disease in ruminants, farmers usually overemphasizing their importance while veterinarians underestimate it. Most infestations do not cause clinical signs but, on occasions, heavy infestations may result in unthriftiness, poor coat, vague digestive disturbances including constipation, mild diarrhea and dysentery and sometimes anemia. These signs are restricted chiefly to animals less than 6 months of age, which may also show stunting and become pot-bellied. In infestations with *T. actinioides* signs may be delayed to a later age. Infested animals may be more susceptible to the effects of other internal parasites and to other diseases or adverse environmental conditions. In horses, mild colic, unthriftiness and diarrhea may be seen in heavily infested animals.

Clinical pathology

Segments of the tapeworms may be visible macroscopically in the feces. On microscopic examination of flotation specimens the thickwalled, embryonated eggs may be present singly or in egg capsules.

Necropsy findings

Most commonly, tapeworms are present in the small intestine. The site of attachment may be indicated by the presence of an ulcer. Secondary, non-specific lesions include emaciation and anemia. In the case of infestations with *T. actinioides* and *S. hepatica* the immature worms may be present in the biliary and pancreatic ducts and be accompanied by fibroses and thickening of the duct walls.

Diagnosis

A diagnosis of tapeworm infestation as a cause of illness is made rarely except on necropsy because of the general view that the worms are of low pathogenicity. Young lambs up to 6 months of age and young horses are the only groups in which the diagnosis needs to be seriously entertained. Other causes of stunting and emaciation in these groups include many diseases but the two common ones are heavy infestations with nematodes and malnutrition. A positive diagnosis depends upon finding large numbers of eggs or proglottides in the feces or large numbers of worms in the intestine at necropsy.

Treatment

In ruminants, lead arsenate (0·5 g for lambs, 1 g for adult sheep, 0·5–1·5 g for young cattle) is effective against all tapeworms and is often administered combined with thiabendazole to control other parasites. The toxic dose of lead arsenate for adult sheep is about 4 g, although debilitated animals may be more susceptible. Niclosamide (Yomesan, Lintex, Mansonil) has proved to be highly effective against *Moniezia*, *Helictometra* and *Avitellina* spp. in lambs and calves (4). The recommended dose rate is 100 mg/kg body weight except for very young lambs which require 1 g irrespective of their weight. Bunamidine hydroxynaphthoate is highly effective against *M. expansa* in sheep at a dose rate of 50 mg/kg (6). Some of the newer benzimidazoles used against nematodes have cesticidal activity. Cambendazole 20 mg/kg (8), oxfendazole (3), fenbendazole (5), and albendazole (7) at 5 mg/kg are highly effective against intestinal cestodes in sheep and cattle, while albendazole 7·5 mg/kg is effective against cestodes in the bile ducts (9). Praziquantel (Droncit) 10 mg/kg is also effective against the bile duct parasites (10) but is too expensive for general use. In horses niclosamide 200 mg/kg or pyrantel pamoate 13·2 mg/kg should be used (11).

Control

Control of the mites which act as intermediate hosts is impractical, and in areas where infestation is sufficiently heavy to retard the growth of lambs periodic dosing, particularly during the summer and autumn, with one of the above taeniacides may be necessary.

REVIEW LITERATURE

Rickard, M. D. and Arundel, J. H. (1985) Chemotherapy of tapeworm infections. In: *Handbook of Experimental Pharmacology—Chemotherapy of Intestinal Helminths*, vol. 77, ed, H. Van den Bossche & D. Thienpont. Berlin:Springer.

REFERENCES

(1) Thomas, P. L. et al. (1956) *NZ vet. J.*, *4*, 161.
(2) Rees, G. (1967) *Helminth. Abstr.*, *36*, 1.
(3) Michael, S. A. et al. (1979) *Vet. Rec.*, *104*, 338.
(4) Allen, R. W. et al. (1967) *Proc. helminth. Soc. Wash.*, *34*, 195.
(5) Malan, F. S. (1980) *J. S. Afr. vet. Assoc.*, *51*, 25.
(6) Czipri, D. et al. (1968) *Vet. Rec.*, *82*, 505.
(7) van Schalkwyk, P. C. et al. (1979) *J. S. Afr. vet. Assoc.*, *50*, 31.
(8) Horak, I. G. & Snijders, A. J. (1975) *J. S. Afr. vet. Assoc.*, *46*, 271.
(9) Craig, T. M. & Shepherd, E. (1980) *Am. J. vet. Res.*, *41*, 425.
(10) Bankov, D. (1976) *Vet. Med. Nauki*, *13*, 28. (*Vet. Bull.*, *47*, 5050, 1977.
(11) Slocombe, J. O. D. (1979) *Can. vet. J.*, *20*, 136.

ASCARIASIS

Heavy infestations of the intestine with adult ascarid worms can cause digestive disturbances and poor growth in young animals and this is the major source of economic loss caused by the worm, but in individual animals more acute signs are caused by migration of the immature worms through the liver and lungs and occasionally other organs, by migration into the bile ducts, or by perforation or blockage of the small intestine.

Etiology

Each species has its specific ascarid, *Ascaris suum* in pigs, *Parascaris equorum* in horses and *Toxocara vitulorum* in cattle and buffalo. Sheep do not have a specific ascarid but may rarely become infected with *A. lumbricoides* (1). *A. suum* of the pig has only minor morphological differences from *A. lumbricoides* of man, but each is host-specific and although cross-infections may occur, the infestations do not mature. Infections of an atypical host can be produced experimentally (2) but there is no evidence that such cross-infections occur naturally in large animals other than with *A. suum*.

Lifecycle and epidemiology

Ascarids occur generally throughout the world but the occurrence of ascariasis is limited largely to farms on which the concentration of horses or pigs is high, where the animals run at pasture and on the same pasture year after year. The incidence may also be high in penned pigs when they are fed on the floor in pens which are seldom or never cleaned.

The lifecycles of all *Ascaris* spp. are very similar, with the exception of *T. vitulorum* in which infestation occurs via the colostrum. Adult worms live in the small intestine and lay very large numbers of eggs. Because the eggs have very thick walls the infective stage is very resistant to deleterious environmental influences. The eggs are very resistant to cold and survive most readily in cool, moist surroundings. Periods of survival of up to 5 years have been recorded. When the egg is passed it is not infective but under suitable environmental conditions, particularly high humidity, a first, then a second and third stage larva develops within the egg which, after a period of several weeks, is infective. In the United Kingdom, *A. suum* eggs shed from September to May become infective more or less synchronously in July and the number of eggs becoming infective then falls away rapidly. This corresponds to the prevalence of milk spot liver lesions which peak in July and August (3). However, as the eggs are very resistant, pigs may, in the absence of good hygiene, become infected at all periods of the year. These infective eggs hatch quickly in the intestine of the host and the larvae migrate through the intestinal wall, reach the portal vein and are transported to the liver, sometimes within 24 hours of being swallowed. They again enter blood vessels and move to the lungs, are passed up the bronchi and trachea to the pharynx, are swallowed and come to rest again in the intestine where they mature. The total period required for re-entry into the intestine after infestation is 3–4 weeks and the worms are mature and commence laying eggs about 5 weeks later, or 8–9 weeks after infestation.

Parascaris equorum has a similar lifecycle. After artificial infection, larvae can be found in the liver by 48 hours, in the lungs from 7–14 days and they return to the small intestine by day 33. Patent infections develop from 101 days (14). Under field conditions eggs are passed by foals from 12–13 weeks of age and spontaneous expulsion of worms occurs in animals 9–12 months. Occasionally eggs are seen in the feces of very young foals and this is thought to be due to the ingestion of uninfective eggs during coprophagia.

The adult worms are long (20–50 cm), cylindrical, pointed at both ends and have a thick, glistening, yellow-white cuticle.

T. vitulorum are acquired by the calf by transfer of larvae in colostrum (4). Thus infections are seen early in calfhood, mature worms being present by 10 days and eggs are passed within 2–3 weeks of birth. Worms are expelled by 5 months of age. *T. vitulorum* is an important cause of mortality in buffalo calves in India and South-east Asia.

Pathogenesis

In experimental infections, lesions due to migrating larvae can be seen in the intestinal wall, liver and lungs. However, in natural infections, which are caused by the ingestion of lower doses of eggs over longer periods and which are mediated by immunity, lesions are not seen in the intestine. Migration of larvae through the liver results in hemorrhage and fibrosis appearing as white spots under the capsule. In heavy infection diffuse fibrosis may occur. The most serious damage occurs in the lungs where they provoke alveolar injury with edema and consolidation. Sensitization to antigens prepared from ascarids can be produced experimentally in pigs and a second administration 11–20 days after the first can cause fatal anaphylaxis. Immunity to migrating larvae is acquired and can be transferred through colostrum or immune serum (5).

In infestations by *A. suum* in animals other than pigs, larval migration and development occur but the worms do not reach the small intestine. During larval migration severe clinical signs of pulmonary involvement may appear. The disease has been produced experimentally in lambs (6) and calves (2, 7) and has also been observed as a field occurrence in yearling cattle (8, 9).

Foals infected with *P. equorum* have reduced gut motility, an increase in the ratio of body water to body solids and a lowering of the body pool of albumin (18).

Clinical findings

In all animal species only the young are seriously affected. In pigs up to 4–5 months old, the important clinical signs are poor growth and lowered resistance to other disease. Enzootic pneumonia of pigs and swine influenza are reported to be much more serious diseases when accompanied by ascariasis, and breaks in hog cholera vaccination with live virus are often attributed to this cause. There may be cough but this is not marked and there is seldom sufficient damage to the lungs to cause a noticeable increase in respiratory rate or depth. In rare cases the infestation may be so severe that pigs manifest severe dyspnea or die of acute hepatic insufficiency. Adult worms may be vomited up and occasional cases of obstructive jaundice and intestinal obstruction or rupture occur.

The effects in calves due to infestation with *T. vitulorum* and foals up to about 8 months of age with *P. equorum* are similar to those observed in young pigs and include poor coat, diarrhea and occasionally colic. In addition, in foals, convulsions, intestinal obstruction and perforation may occur. In calves reduced weight gains, anemia and steatorrhea are additional signs (10).

In older animals no clinical signs are observed but infested animals, particularly adult sows and yearling horses, continue to contaminate the surroundings and are an important link in the chain of infection. With infestation by *A. suum* in other species fever, dyspnea and anorexia occur about the 8th day after infestation (6).

Clinical pathology

Ascarid eggs have thick walls with a pitted surface. The eggs are usually present in very large numbers in the feces of clinically affected animals. A marked eosinophilia often accompanies the early stages of infestation in pigs and in other species and has been shown to persist in calves for at least one year (2). In experimentally infested pigs there is an appreciable rise in serum transaminase levels, the peak being reached about the 2nd and 3rd day after infestation, presumably due to damage to the liver during larval migration. Egg counts in excess of 1000 epg are considered to be indicative of significant infections. Some attention has been given to serological examination for antibodies as a diagnostic tool but no practical techniques have transpired (11).

Necropsy findings

Necropsy findings vary with the stage of development of the disease. In the early stages of a massive infestation the liver is enlarged and congested and there may be hemorrhages under the capsule. Microscopically, necrotic tracts and sections of larvae are observed. There are subpleural hemorrhages, and edema and cyanosis of the lungs. The larvae are too small to be observed by the naked eye and should be looked for by microscopic examination of scrapings of bronchial mucus. The pleural cavity may contain bloodstained fluid.

In chronic cases the capsule of the liver is marked with white spots of small diameter which may, in severe cases, be confluent and constitute a network of connective tissue. Histologically, the necrotic tracts have been replaced by fibrous tissue. The carcass is usually in poor condition and may be jaundiced. Large numbers of mature worms may almost fill the lumen of the small intestine. In species other than the pig infestation with *A. suum* is accompanied by emphysema, alveolar wall thickening with fibrin, eosinophils and hemorrhage in the lungs and necrotic tracts in the liver.

Diagnosis

Ascariasis in all species is a disease of the young animals, causing less than optimal growth and an afebrile diarrhea. Older animals do not show symptoms although they may be infected and be an important source of contamination.

In young pigs, chronic cough and increased rate and depth of respiration are caused much more commonly by enzootic pneumonia and there are many other causes of debilitation including malnutrition and chronic enteritis due to infections with *Salmonella* and *Treponema* spp. In young foals the chronic form of corynebacterial pneumonia may be mistaken for ascariasis but auscultation of the lungs reveals gross abnormality of the lung sounds. Ascariasis of calves must be differentiated from the many other causes of enteritis.

Treatment

In pigs the piperazine salts (at 200 mg/kg body weight) are effective and economical. Sodium fluoride administered in the feed has several disadvantages but is cheap and efficient and is still used in many areas. Dichlorvos 30–40 mg/kg and levamisole 5–8 mg/kg have broad-spectrum activity against *A. suum* and other important pig nematodes, while haloxon 30–50 mg/kg has high efficiency against *Ascaris* and *Oesophagostomum*. Morantel 5 mg/kg is highly effective against *A. suum*, but is used at high dose rates (7·5–12 mg/kg) to include other nematodes in its spectrum of activity. At 30 ppm in the feed it will prevent migration of *A. suum* larvae. Parbendazole 20 mg/kg (14) and pyrantel tartrate 22 mg/kg (15) mixed in the feed and fed continuously are effective as broad-spectrum wormers, as is mebendazole 30 ppm for 5 days, oxibendazole 100 ppm or febantel 15–30 ppm, or flubendazole 30 ppm for 6–10 days (12). Dichlorvos at normal dose rates kills fourth larval stages of *A. suum* and morantel 30 ppm in the feed kills many migrating stages.

Ivermectin is active against *A. suum* and most other nematodes other than *Trichuris suis*, but in pigs is used at 0·3 mg/kg (13).

A number of satisfactory treatments are available for horses and the choice depends on cost, formulation to allow dosing by paste, by stomach tube or in the feed and the spectrum of susceptible parasites. Piperazine salts 200 mg/kg, cambendazole 20 mg/kg, parbendazole 20 mg/kg, mebendazole 8·8 mg/kg, pyrantel 12·5 mg/kg, morantel 10–12·5 mg/kg, fenbendazole 10 mg/kg, oxfendazole 10 mg/kg, febantel 6 mg/kg, oxibendazole 10 mg/kg and albendazole 5 mg/kg are all effective. Haloxon 60 mg/kg is effective but is somewhat toxic (20). Levamisole 8–10 mg/kg is active but has a low safety margin. It is rarely used in horses. Thiabendazole is inactive against *P. equorum* at normal dose rates, and piperazine is usually added to thiabendazole or to any of the benzimidazoles to give added activity against *P. equorum* and to remove benzimidazole-resistant small strongyles. Calves should be treated with piperazine 88 mg base/kg (21) at 2 weeks of age to expel worms before they are mature.

Control

The important features of the ascarid lifecycle which must be taken into account when devising a control program are that the worms are prolific egg-layers, the infective eggs are very long-lived and resistant to damaging influences and young animals are most susceptible. Emphasis must be placed on avoiding exposure of young pigs and foals to infested adults and soil contaminated by them and on periodic treatment of the young animals. In pigs these principles are laid down in more detail in the 'McLean County System' of control of ascariasis. In this system the sow is washed with soap and warm water and placed in a farrowing pen which has been thoroughly cleaned with boiling lye solution 4 g/140 liters water 3–4 days before her due date. It is not imperative that the sow be treated by an ascaricide at this time but such a treatment should still further lessen the chances of infection of the piglets. If the litter and sow are turned out to pasture they must not walk over infested ground but be drawn in an enclosed vehicle and the pasture should preferably be one on which pigs have not previously been grazed or has been rested for at least 2 years. This exacting control of the young pigs must be maintained until they are at least 4 months old.

If the pigs are kept in houses and allowed access to small earthern yards, these must be kept well drained and the manure moved frequently to an area to which neither pigs nor cattle have access. The eggs do not become infective until about 4 weeks after deposition and deep burial of contaminated soil should prevent their maturation. With modern pig-raising methods of keeping pigs confined at all times in concrete pens the risk of ascarid infestation is very greatly reduced if normal hygienic precautions are maintained. Epidemiological studies in the United Kingdom resulted in the recommendation that all bedding should be removed at the end of June to remove eggs that have accumulated in the preceding months before they become infective, and again at the end of August to remove the eggs deposited in the summer and which would become infective in the same season (3).

If sows are treated prior to being placed in the farrowing pen which has been cleaned with high pressure water, this may be sufficient to produce weaners without anthelmintic treatment (22). If this is impractical then prefarrowing treatment with a broad-spectrum compound combined with treatment of the piglets at 3–4 weeks of age is recommended. Periodic treatments or continuous low-level treatment with compounds listed above will eliminate ascarids in growing pigs. If large quantities of skim milk or whey are fed ascarids will be kept at a low level (19).

Young foals present more of a problem, especially as concurrent infestations with ascarids, strongyles and botfly larvae are not uncommon. The foals run with the mares which act as a source of infestation, and they almost always run at pasture on which foals have run the previous year and which can become very heavily contaminated with eggs. Because of their curiosity the foals often nibble at foreign material, including feces. Recommendations for control include thorough cleaning and disinfection of the maternity stall after each foaling, the use of small paddocks for exercise which have been rested from occupation by horses for a year if possible, and weekly removal of manure from the pasture (16). The foals should be routinely treated at about 10–12 weeks of age when the worms are first becoming mature and the treatment repeated bimonthly. In this way heavy egg contamination of the pasture can be avoided. Piperazine or dichlorvos gel are easily administered. Piperazine will also remove the small strongyles that may be present while dichlorvos gel will also remove first instar bots that cause mouth soreness and reduced growth rate (17).

REFERENCES

(1) Gunn, A. (1980) *Vet. Rec.*, *107*, 581.
(2) McCraw, B. M. (1973) *Can. J. comp. Med.*, *37*, 21.
(3) Connan, R. M. (1977) *Vet. Rec.*, *100*, 421.
(4) Warren, E. G. (1971) *Int. J. Parasitol.*, *1*, 85.
(5) Kelley, P. W. & Nayak, D. P. (1965) *Cornell Vet.*, *55*, 607.
(6) Fitzgerald, P. R. (1962) *Am. J. vet. Res.*, *23*, 731.
(7) Greenway, J. A. & McCraw, B. M. (1970) *Can. J. comp. Med.*, *34*, 227, 247.
(8) Morrow, D. A. (1968) *J. Am. vet. med. Assoc.*, *153*, 184.
(9) McCraw, B. M. & Lautenslager, J. P. (1971) *Can. vet. J.*, *12*, 87.
(10) Enyenihi, U. K. (1969) *Bull. epizoot. Dis. Afr.*, *17*, 171.
(11) Castelino, J. B. (1970) *Vet. Bull.*, *40*, 751.
(12) Rochette, F. (1985) *Handb. exp. Pharmacol.*, *77*, 463.
(13) Campbell, W. C. & Benz, G. W. (1984) *J. vet. Pharmacol. Therap.*, *7*, 1.
(14) Clayton, H. M. & Duncan, J. L. (1979) *Int. J. Parasitol.*, *9*, 285.
(15) Arakana, A. et al. (1971) *Vet. Med.*, *66*, 108.
(16) Herd, R. P. (1986) *Mod. vet. Pract.*, *67*, 893.
(17) Hass, D. K. et al. (1973) *Am. J. vet. Res.*, *34*, 41.
(18) Clayton, H. M. et al. (1980) *Equ. vet. J.*, *12*, 23.
(19) Alfredsen, S. A. (1980) *Vet. Rec.*, *197*, 179.
(20) Rose, R. J. et al. (1981) *Equ. vet. J.*, *13*, 171.
(21) Akhtar, M. S. et al. (1982) *J. vet. Pharmacol. Therap.*, *5*, 71.
(22) Nilsson, O. (1982) *Acta vet. Scand.*, Suppl. 79.

STRONGYLOSIS OF HORSES (REDWORM INFESTATION)

Strongylus vulgaris, the most important parasite in the horse, causes verminous arteritis and colic and in common with others of the genera *Strongylus*, *Triodontophorus* and members of the subfamily Cyathostominae (1) causes debility and anemia.

Etiology

The common nematodes found in the large intestine of the horse are *Strongylus vulgaris*, *S. edentatus* and *S. equinus*, *Triodontophorus* sp. and some members of the genera *Cylicostephanus*, *Cyathostomum* and *Cylicocyclus*. Other species within these genera and the genera *Cylicodontophorus*, *Poteriostomum*, *Gyalocephalus*, *Cylindropharynx* and *Oesophagodontus* are much less common. The *Strongylus* spp., or large strongyles, are 2–5 cm long. They suck blood and the presence of blood in their alimentary tracts is responsible for the common name of redworms. *Triodontophorus* spp. and *Oesophagodontus robustus* also suck blood but are smaller, up to 2 cm. These two species along with the *Strongylus* spp. comprise the subfamily Strongylinae or large strongyles. The other species, the small strongyles, have smaller buccal capsules, lack teeth and do not suck blood. In natural infestations most species may be represented and the clinical picture seen represents the net effects of a mixed infestation.

Lifecycle and epidemiology

Strongylosis is a common disease of horses throughout the world and causes deaths when control measures are neglected. However, the greatest losses are probably the failure of young horses to grow properly and the less efficient performance of working horses that are moderately parasitized.

The lifecycle of all species is direct. Eggs are passed in the feces and under suitable climatic conditions produce infective third stage larvae from 7 days onwards. As in other parasitic conditions the survival of eggs and larvae is favored by shade, moisture and moderate temperature. Desiccation is particularly unfavorable and hot dry summers will cleanse a pasture. Some eggs and larvae may withstand freezing but development ceases below 7·5°C (46°F) (2) but may be resumed when temperatures increase. Optimum chances for infection of the host occur in the early morning or evening when dew produces a moisture film on plants, or after rain, both of which give conditions that encourage larvae to migrate on to pasture.

The epidemiology of infection depends on the time of deposition of eggs and the temperature and moisture conditions at that time. In most areas with cold winters and mild summers, egg deposition peaks in spring and remains high over summer (12). At this time temperatures are suitable for larval development, and massive contamination may occur in late summer and early autumn when young susceptible horses are present. If the summers are hot and dry, only a small proportion of the eggs may develop to larvae and the larvae may be short-lived, but the continual reinfestation keeps pasture contamination high.

In subtropical regions eggs can hatch throughout the

year and larval availability is influenced more by rainfall than temperature (25). For example, in Florida, fecal egg counts remain high throughout the year, and there is an autumn rise in infective larvae which arises from those eggs deposited in the autumn (13). This has important implications in the timing of treatments. *S. vulgaris* larvae can overwinter in considerable numbers in Europe and become available as infective larvae from May to July (20).

The timing of the clinical condition resulting from ingestion of larvae depends on the prepatent period of the parasite and whether the immature or adult stages are pathogenic. Outbreaks of scouring due to heavy small strongyle infection (winter cyathostomosis) is commonly seen in Europe from November to May (27) while arterial lesions due to larval *S. vulgaris* are first seen in late summer and reach a maximum by midwinter.

The parasitic lifecycle varies depending on the species. The small strongyles do not migrate through the body. After ingestion the larvae exsheath, enter the walls of the cecum and colon, where they remain in small subserous nodules for some time depending on the species and probably the degree of immunity of the host. Their prepatent periods vary from 6 to 10 weeks of age (3) but eggs of these species appear in the feces from about 12–18 weeks onward depending on the species (4).

Larvae of *S. edentatus* penetrate the intestine and travel via the portal vessels to the liver where larvae remain and produce hemorrhagic tracts for a month or so. They then migrate via the hepatorenal ligament to the connective tissue under the peritoneum and form hemorrhagic nodules. After about 3 months they return via the root of the mesentery to the large bowel wall and again form hemorrhagic nodules which finally rupture and release the worms into the lumen. Adult egg-laying females are present from 40 weeks (5). Many larvae may be found in other organs, e.g. they are not uncommon in the testes (6), but these larvae do not return to the intestine. The migratory route of *S. equinus* is via the liver to the pancreas and peritoneal cavity but how they return to the intestine is not certain (7).

The migratory route of *S. vulgaris* was in dispute for many years but has now been clarified (8,9). The exsheathed larvae penetrate the intestinal wall, molt to the fourth stage larvae in the submucosa and then pass into small arteries. By 14 days they have reached the cranial mesenteric artery by migration in the lumen or on the intima of the arteries. Here they develop to the late fourth stage larvae, in 3–4 months they molt and the young adults then return to the intestine via the lumina of the arteries. Nodules are formed in the intestine wall and later rupture, releasing adults into the lumen of the intestine. The prepatent period is 6 months.

Although young horses are most susceptible, adult horses carry appreciable burdens and mares are the main source of infection for the younger horses (10). Horses do gain some acquired immunity to infection (11) and the possibilities for vaccination are being investigated (5) but are not promising.

The epidemiology of the small strongyles is similar to that of *S. vulgaris*. The availability of the larvae is seasonal and large numbers of third stage larvae accumulate in the gut wall as hypobiotic forms, and emerge in the winter (17). Synchronous emergence can cause severe diarrhea and death.

Pathogenesis

The disease processes produced by the strongyles can be divided into those produced by the migrating larvae and those produced by the adult worms. The larvae of *S. vulgaris* are the most pathogenic, causing arteritis and thrombosis and thickening of the artery walls. It has been accepted that emboli may break away and lodge in smaller blood vessels, leading to partial or complete ischemia in part of the intestine, thus producing colic. The result of this depends on the length of the segment of intestine infected and the ability of the collateral blood supply to become established before necrosis and gangrene occurs.

Recent findings do not support the hypothesis that thromboembolism is the major cause of infarction (31, 32). Experimental occlusion of mesenteric vessels does not produce colic or any change in physiological values (28). However, experimental embolism of the intramural vessel network causes local ischaemia, colic and other signs (28). It is suggested that the rich vascular network in the gut wall will overcome blockage of a number of vessels, and that the vascular injury may be multiple microthrombi and emboli which are difficult to find, or may be a hypersensitivity reaction to the migrating parasites producing a diffuse intravenous coagulation and/or vasoconstriction. It has been suggested that thromboxane, a prostaglandin-like substance produced by platelets, which is a potent vasoconstrictor, may be involved. While the hypothesis has not yet been directly tested in horses, the clinical response of horses with verminous arteritis to the non-steroidal anti-inflammatory agent flunixine meglumine support this view (33). The pathogenesis of thromboembolic colic has been reviewed (33). Greatly enhanced mobility proximal to the lesion follows ischaemia and can cause volvulus or torsion. Intussusception or aneurysms are seen occasionally. Lesions may be seen in many other blood vessels and these are caused by larvae migrating beyond the cranial mesenteric artery. Multiple lesions may be seen in the cecal and colic arteries. These may completely occlude the lumen and gangrene of parts of the bowel may follow. Smaller lesions are occasionally seen in iliac, renal, splenic, hepatic and coronary arteries. Lesions due to *S. vulgaris* have been reported from a variety of other locations and these have been reviewed in one of the review references. The aortic and iliac thrombosis resulting in hindlimb lameness has recently been proven to be due to *S. vulgaris* (37). Colic may also be caused by pressure of the thickened artery on the mesenteric plexus. Motility of the intestinal musculature may be deranged by reduced blood flow, and changes in ileal myoelectrical activity have been related to mucosal penetration and early migration of *S. vulgaris* larvae (36).

Clinical descriptions of these disorders are presented in Chapter 5, on diseases of the alimentary tract. Larvae of *S. edentatus* cause hemorrhagic tracts in the liver and adhesions and disruptions of the omental architecture.

Hemorrhagic nodules 1–3 cm in diameter are produced in the subperitoneal region and these are reported to cause colic and anemia. Larvae of all the large strongyles may be found in any organ and may cause an inflammatory response. Field and experimental cases of cerebrospinal nematodiasis due to *S. vulgaris* invasion of the central nervous system have been reported (14). The larvae of most large and small strongyles may cause nodules in the wall of the cecum and colon and when these rupture releasing larvae, considerable bleeding may follow. In very heavy burdens sufficient bleeding to cause death can occur.

The adult strongylids can be divided into those that are bloodsuckers and those that are tissue feeders. The large strongyles, *Strongylus* spp., *Triodontophorus* spp. and *Oes. robustus* all cause anemia by direct bloodsucking and by blood loss from feeding points once the worm detaches. *Triodontophorus tenuicollis* tend to attach in groups in the right dorsal colon and can cause ulceration. The small strongyles cause superficial damage and large numbers of adults usually cause little harm. Larval stages in the mucosa may be associated with localized changes and, in heavy infections, the emergence of large numbers of larvae over a short period causes an inflammation of the cecum or ventral colon, with small ulcers where larvae have emerged, hemorrhages of varying sizes and excess mucus production. Affected animals may have a diffuse diarrhea (27).

Clinical findings

It is only in recent years that attention has been drawn to the association between performance in racehorses and their hemoglobin levels. There are a number of factors that may cause anemia and although the importance of strongylosis compared to dietary deficiency and the effect of racing for long periods has not been determined, it is generally accepted that strongylosis is probably the most important of these causes.

In natural infestations it is impossible to quantify the effects of individual species as mixed infections are always present. In artificial infections of *S. vulgaris*, in foals, weakness, poor coat and loss of condition are common sequelae of infection. Pyrexia is a constant finding in artificial infections of low numbers of larvae and infected foals are anorexic, dull and have intermittent colic (15). Doses of 2500–5000 larvae to foals 2–12 months old produce marked increase in body temperature, anorexia, rapid loss of body condition, depression, colic, diarrhea or constipation and death in 14–22 days (16).

Adult mares, late in pregnancy and carrying heavy infections, may become very weak to the point of recumbency. On clinical examination the mucosae are pale, the heart rapid and loud and respiration moderately increased. Intestinal sounds are increased to the point where enteritis may be suspected although the feces are normal. Abortion may occur and the mare usually dies.

The clinical syndromes caused by arteritis in the cranial mesenteric artery, aorta and iliac artery are described elsewhere.

The small strongyles cause winter cyathostomosis, due to the simultaneous maturation of large numbers of hypobiotic larvae in stressed horses. It almost always occurs in the winter and is characterized by severe diarrhea, and rapid loss of condition.

Clinical pathology

Examination of feces for strongylid eggs is used commonly in most laboratories. It is difficult to interpret as it does not differentiate between the different strongylid genera nor from *Trichostrongylus axei*. Larval cultures are necessary for this, but these delay results by 10 days. Egg counts taken after treatment may be relatively low but may consist solely of the more pathogenic large strongyle eggs as these are more difficult to kill or of eggs from small strongyles that are resistant to the anthelmintic in use. The levels of eggs/g (epg) may have little correlation with the worm burden as epg is influenced by immunity and the species present as well as the number of worms present. In foals, eggs may be passed in the first few weeks of life and these are eggs obtained by coprophagia and which are passing through the intestine unchanged. However, egg counts are important as they are a direct measure of contamination which must be minimized in a control program and regular egg counts are necessary to monitor the efficiency of worm control.

Estimations of hemoglobin levels, erythrocyte counts and packed cell volumes of the blood are often taken as an indication of the degree of infestation with strongyles, but a number of other factors including dosing with phenothiazine, excitement, dietary deficiency, continued racing over long periods, toxic depression of bone marrow by infectious processes and a number of infectious diseases may cause depression of these values. Appreciable differences have been noted between normal horses in different countries and between different breeds (e.g. thoroughbreds and standardbreds) but it can be assumed that any horse with a hemoglobin level of less than 12 g/dl, an erythrocyte count of less than 8 million/μl or a packed cell volume less than 35% will profit by treatment for anemia and this may include treatment for strongylosis.

Indirect tests are important when one is attempting to assess the burden of migrating larvae. The most important measurement for this is serum analysis, a marked increase in beta-globulins particularly IgG(T), and a fall in albumin being consistent in equine strongylosis (18). However, these changes may be related to helminth infection in general, to tissue injury or to other factors and may not be of value as a specific guide to verminous arteritis. Further, changes occur mainly in young ponies and may reflect a response to *T. axei* rather than to the strongyles (38). It must be concluded that serum protein and IgG(T) responses are of limited value because of the difficulties of interpretation (38), and results of these tests must be used together with other laboratory findings, clinical signs and the history of the property. Similarly eosinophilia may reflect invasion by larvae other than *S. vulgaris*. However, while serum analysis and a total and differential white cell count will provide a safer diagnostic tool than a fecal egg count or a hemoglobin estimation, there is a great need for a precise diagnostic test in verminous arteritis in the horse. Arteriography in ponies has shown promise (19).

Necropsy findings

Because most cases of strongylosis are caused by mixed infestations with all genera, necropsy findings usually include most of the lesions characteristic of each worm.

In cases dying of anemia and enteritis, the basic disease in strongylosis, very large numbers of adult worms will be found in the cecum and colon: there may be so many that they appear to form a living cover to the contents of these organs. Catarrhal, hemorrhagic or fibrinous inflammation of the cecum and ventral colon associated with widespread disruption of the mucosa from which larvae have emerged leaving small ulcers is the main finding in cyathostomosis. There may be edema with excessive mucus production or numerous punctate hemorrhages. *Triodontophorus tenuicollis* are often found in large numbers in the right dorsal colon in association with small circular hemorrhages, and they are sometimes attached in groups at the base of deep mucosal ulcers.

There may be larvae in many subserous sites, especially in nodules in the intestinal wall, and the body cavities may contain an excess of bloodstained fluid. Verminous arteritis lesions of varying size are common at the root of the cranial mesenteric artery and occasionally in the iliac artery. The affected arterial wall is greatly thickened and contains loculi on its internal surface, many of which contain living larvae. Lamellated thrombi are also common at this site and these are sometimes infected. The thickening of the arterial wall often extends along the cecal and colic arteries and complete occlusion of these may be followed by gangrene of a segment of intestine. Similar lesions of arteritis may be present at the base of the aorta. Spontaneous rupture of the vessel may occur. A highly significant correlation has been reported between lesions in the proximal aorta and the presence of focal ischemic lesions in the myocardium (29). These were thought to be caused by microembolization causing arteriosclerotic lesions in the myocardial arterioles.

Diagnosis

A diagnosis of strongylid infestation should be considered when poor growth, inappetence, diarrhea and some degree of anemia are the presenting signs. Ascariasis is another cause of poor growth and debility in foals but anemia is not a prominent sign. These conditions can be differentiated by examining the feces for ascarid eggs. A gross nutritional deficiency, or agalactia in the mare, may have the same effect but these causes are usually evident. Specific nutritional deficiencies in foals and adults are not commonly recorded as causes of anemia and are unlikely in horses running at pasture, but horses fed stored feeds in stables may require dietary supplementation with a mineral containing iron and copper. Of the infectious causes of anemia, babesiosis and equine infectious anemia are usually accompanied by other clinical signs of diagnostic significance.

The diagnosis of verminous arteritis presents difficulty. The thickening of the cranial mesenteric artery may be palpable per rectum, the artery being situated below the aorta at the level of the posterior pole of the kidneys. Experimentally, pyrexia, inappetence, depression, leukocytosis and intermittent or continuous colic is seen in the migratory phase of *S. vulgaris* infection (15). In more chronic cases there is a persistent low grade fever, poor appetite, intermittent colic and poor weight gain. Diarrhea may be present. Low serum albumin and increased beta-globulins particularly IgG(T) are the best laboratory tests while arteriography may demonstrate lesions in a number of arteries (19).

In cases of winter cyathostomosis, due to the emergence of hypobiotic small strongyle larvae, diarrhea, marked weight loss, leukocytosis and hypoalbuminemia are seen. Egg counts may be negative. All cases of diarrhea, colic or wasting should be regarded as being of parasitic origin and should be treated with a compound effective against hypobiotic larvae.

Treatment

Many of the newer broad-spectrum anthelmintics have high efficiency against the large and small strongyles and a choice of drug can now be made not only on the criteria of efficiency and toxicity but also on the route of application as many are available for use in the feed, as pastes or by tubing. Ivermectin paste is available for use at 0·2 mg/kg, and is effective against adult and immature strongyles, including migrating larvae and hypobiotic larvae, as well as many other nematodes and some external parasites (39). Phenothiazine plus piperazine is still used as a synergistic mixture with high efficiency against both large and small strongyles, *Oxyuris equi* and ascarids. Thiabendazole 44 mg/kg, mebendazole 10 mg/kg (21), cambendazole 25 mg/kg (22), fenbendazole 5 mg/kg (23), oxibendazole 10 mg/kg (24), pyrantel pamoate 12·5 mg/kg (30), febantel 6 mg/kg and oxfendazole 10 mg/kg (31) have all proved to be efficient and safe. Thiabendazole can be used with a piperazine salt to give efficiency against ascarids while the other broad-spectrum compounds are active against both ascarids and strongyles. However, piperazine is often added to benzimidazoles to remove the benzimidazole-resistant small strongyles that are now common in most countries. The strongyles do not appear to have become resistant to oxibendazole and this compound can be used to remove parasites resistant to other benzimidazoles (40). Dichlorvos also is active against the small and large strongyles and oxyurids and also has high efficiency against bots particularly if the horses are deprived of water for a few hours before dosing (26). Because of the variation in dose rate obtained in foals due to erratic consumption of concentrate feed, the slow release dichlorvos is not recommended for use in foals. Trichlorphon can be used with the above broad-spectrum compounds to give efficiency against bots with the one treatment.

A major clinical problem is the treatment of animals with verminous arteritis. Ivermectin 0·2 mg/kg (41) and oxfendazole 10 mg/kg (44) as single doses are highly effective against migrating *S. vulgaris*. Fenbendazole at an increased dose rate of 60 mg/kg as a single dose is effective (42), but five daily doses of 7·5 or 10 mg/kg are more effective against migrating *S. vulgaris* and *S. edentatus* (43). Thiabendazole at the high dose rate of 440 mg/kg on two successive days is effective and safe (15), but this compound has now been superseded by the compounds given above.

Hypobiotic small strongyles can be removed by ivermectin 0·2 mg/kg or oxfendazole 10 mg/kg. High doses of fenbendazole, 30 or 60 mg/kg, are also effective. Benzimidazole-resistant small strongyles are now widespread. They can be removed by adding piperazine 20–40 mg base/kg to the benzimidazole or by using ivermectin or pyrantel which act on nematodes in a different manner. A resistant population may be slow to revert, as parasites were still resistant after 3 years of use of non-benzimidazole compounds (45).

Control

As in most parasitic infestations adequate control measures depend upon an accurate knowledge of the lifecycle of the worms. Because of the heavy egg-laying capacity of adult strongyles, the heavy worm burdens carried by older animals, especially yearlings, and the longevity of the larvae on pasture, the control of strongylosis by management alone is impossible. Foals are the group which are most seriously affected and because of the universal practice of running them at pasture with their dams they are easily exposed to gross infestation.

Although on some breeding farms, routine collections of feces are made twice weekly in an effort to remove the eggs and early larval forms before they become infective, on most farms control of parasitism by management is impractical. However, manure removal has been shown to be highly effective. The use of commercial equipment twice weekly increased the grazing area by 50% and allowed treatments to be reduced to once a year (46). Another technique that has been used to reduce pasture contamination is to use small doses (1–2 g) of phenothiazine in the feed daily on alternate months or on the first 21 days of each month to reduce egg output of the strongyles and the fertility of those eggs that are laid, although this regimen does not remove the adult worms.

It is more common today to rely on regular treatments with compounds to remove the adult worms. Parasitism is a herd problem and all horses should be treated. After treatment, fecal egg counts are generally reduced to zero for about 6–8 weeks. This appears to be the time taken for larvae to emerge from nodules in the bowel wall and develop to egg-laying females. As the mare is the main source of contamination for the foal, she should be treated about 2 months before foaling, again at foaling and regularly thereafter. Six to eight treatments per year, depending on the compound, are recommended on the breeding farm where maximum reduction of contamination is required. Where ivermectin is used, the interval between treatments can be increased to 10 weeks. On properties of lower stocking intensities or where horses are run with other stock, less frequent dosing may be necessary. Treatment of foals should commence at 10 weeks of age to remove small strongyles before they become patent, and should be repeated at intervals of 6–10 weeks depending on the choice of drug. If a drug that removes migrating and hypobiotic larvae is used and the treatments are continued to cover the period during which freeliving larvae are killed, then the pastures can be substantially cleansed. Once the contamination of a property has been reduced then fewer treatments per year may be given.

As most eggs are deposited on the pasture in spring and summer, concentration of treatments at this time should reduce contamination and give much lower pasture larvae counts in the following autumn and winter (12). Treatment with a compound highly effective against all lifecycle stages and movement of horses of clean pastures has been shown to be effective in keeping parasites low for some months (47).

All horses introduced onto a property must be isolated and treated to prevent contamination of clean pastures. Regular fecal examination of a sample of horses to monitor the success of a control program is recommended.

Resistance to some anthelmintics has been reported. This is particularly prevalent in the benzimidazole group with side resistance to related compounds (34). Techniques to measure resistance are available (35) and when resistance is confirmed then an anthelmintic not chemically related to the one previously used should be tried. Benzimidazole resistance is particularly seen in the small strongyles but this can easily be overcome by the addition of piperazine, or by the use of non-related compounds.

REVIEW LITERATURE

Arundel, J. H. (1985) Parasitic diseases of the horse. Veterinary Review 28. Postgraduate foundation in veterinary science, University of Sydney, Australia.

Ogbourne, C. P. & Duncan, J. L. (1984) *Strongylus vulgaris in the Horse: Its Biology and Veterinary Importance*. Farnham Royal, Bucks, UK: Commonwealth Agricultural Bureaux.

Ogbourne, C. P. (1978) *Pathogenesis of Cyathostome (Trichonema) Infections of the Horse. A Review.* Farnham Royal, UK: Commonwealth Agricultural Bureaux.

REFERENCES

(1) Lichtenfels, J. R. (1975) *Proc. helminth. Soc. Wash.*, *42* (Special issue on helminths of domestic equids).
(2) Ogbourne, C. P. (1972) *Parasitology*, *64*, 461.
(3) Round, M. C. (1969) *J. Helminth.*, *43*, 185.
(4) Russell, A. F. (1948) *J. comp. Pathol.*, *58*, 107.
(5) McCraw, B. M. & Slocombe, J. O. D. (1978) *Can. J. comp. Med.*, *42*, 320.
(6) Smith, J. A. (1973) *Vet. Rec.*, *93*, 604.
(7) Wetsel, R. (1972) *Dtsch Tierärztl. Wochenschr.*, *50*, 443.
(8) Georgi, J. R. (1973) *Cornell Vet.*, *63*, 220.
(9) Duncan, J. L. & Pirie, H. M. (1972) *Res. vet. Sci.*, *13*, 374.
(10) Duncan, J. L. (1974) *Vet. Rec.*, *94*, 337.
(11) Duncan, J. L. (1976) *Equ. vet. J.*, 7, 192.
(12) Herd, R. P. et al. (1985) *Equ. vet. J.*, *17*, 202.
(13) Courtney, C. H. & Asquith, R. L. (1985) *Equ. vet. J.*, *17*, 240.
(14) Little, P. B. et al. (1974) *Am. J. vet. Res.*, *35*, 1501.
(15) Duncan, J. L. (1973) *Equ. vet. J.*, *5*, 20.
(16) Drudge, J. H. et al.(1966) In: *Biology of Parasites*, ed. E. J. L. Soulsby, p. 199. New York: Academic Press.
(17) Eysker, M. & Jansen, J. (1984) *Res. vet. Sci.*, *37*, 355.
(18) Patton, S. et al. (1978) *Am. J. vet. Res.*, *39*, 19.
(19) Slocombe, J. O. D. et al. (1977) *Can. J. comp. Med.*, *41*, 137.
(20) Eysker, M. & Wemmenhove, R. (1987) *Vet. Parasitol.*, *87*, 69.
(21) Drudge, J. H. et al. (1974) *Am. J. vet. Res.*, *35*, 1409.
(22) Bello, T. R. et al. (1973) *Am. J. vet. Res.*, *34*, 771.
(23) Urch, D. L. & Allen, W. R. (1980) *Equ. vet. J.*, *12*, 74.
(24) Nawalinski, T. & Theodorides, V. J. (1976) *Am. J. vet. Res.*, *37*, 469.
(25) English, A. W. (1979) *Aust. vet. J.*, *55*, 299.
(26) Drudge, J. H. & Lyons, E. T. (1972) *Am. J. vet. Res.*, *33*, 1365.

(27) Mirck, M. H. (1977) *Tijdschr. Diergeneeskd.*, *102*, 876.
(28) Davies, J. V. & Gerring, E. L. (1985) *Equ. vet. J.*, *17*, 219.
(29) Cranley, J. J. & McCullagh, K. G. (1981) *Equ. vet. J.*, *13*, 35.
(30) Slocombe, J. O. D. & Smart, J. (1975) *Can. vet. J.*, *16*, 310.
(31) White, N. A. (1981) *J. Am. vet. med. Assoc.*, *178*, 259.
(32) Sellers, A. F. et al. (1982) *Am. J. vet. Res.*, *43*, 390.
(33) White, N. A. (1985) *Comp. cont. Educ. pract. Vet.*, *7*, S156.
(34) Slocombe, J. O. D. & Cote, J. F. (1977) *Can. vet. J.*, *18*, 212.
(35) Whitlock, H. V. et al. (1980) *Vet. Parasitol*, *7*, 215.
(36) Berry, C. R. et al. (1986) *Am. J. vet. Res.*, *47*, 27.
(37) Maxie, M. G. & Physick-Sheard, P. W. (1985) *Vet. Pathol.*, *22*, 238.
(38) Herd, R. P. & Kent, J. E. (1986) *Equ. vet. J.*, *18*, 453.
(39) Craig, T. M. & Kunde, J. M. (1981) *Am. J. vet. Res.*, *42*, 1442.
(40) Drudge, J. H. et al. (1984) *Am. J. vet. Res.*, *45*, 804.
(41) Slocombe, J. O. D. & McCraw, B. M. (1984) *Can. J. comp. Med.*, *48*, 343.
(42) Duncan, J. L. et al. (1977) *Equ. vet. J.*, *9*, 146.
(43) Lyons, E. T. et al. (1983) *Am. J. vet. Res.*, *44*, 1058.
(44) Slocombe, J. O. D. & McCraw, B. M. (1983) *10th Int. Congr. Parasitol. Perth, Australia*, p. 108.
(45) Uhlinger, C. & Johnstone, C. (1984) *J. equ. vet. Sci.*, *4*, 7.
(46) Herd, R. P. (1986) *Mod. vet. Pract.*, *67*, 893.
(47) Dunsmore, J. D. (1985) *Equ. vet. J.*, *17*, 191.

LUNGWORM INFESTATION IN CATTLE (VERMINOUS PNEUMONIA, VERMINOUS BRONCHITIS)

Invasion of the lungs of cattle by *Dictyocaulus vipiparus* results in the development of any one of several disease states including verminous pneumonia, acute interstitial pneumonia and secondary bacterial pneumonia. All are serious diseases which must be differentiated from pneumonia caused by infectious agents because they do not respond satisfactorily to treatment and control measures used for pneumonias caused by bacteria or viruses. Lungworm infestations in pigs, sheep and horses are dealt with in a separate section (p. 1043).

Etiology

D. viviparus is the only lungworm of cattle. All lungworm species are host-specific and cross-infections to other hosts do not occur. It primarily affects dairy calves that have been reared indoors until 4–5 months of age and then placed on a paddock grazed each year by successive calf crops. However, beef calves at grass may also be affected particularly after weaning in the autumn. Yearlings and adults may be affected on rare occasions.

Lifecycle and epidemiology

Infestation of cattle with lungworm has a very wide distribution through temperate and cold areas and, depending on climatic conditions and season, can cause serious losses. The disease reaches its greatest importance in Great Britain and parts of western Europe. The disease is often restricted to particular areas and to particular farms where it is likely to recur each autumn.

The mature lungworm live in the bronchi and their eggs are coughed up and swallowed by the host. The eggs hatch in the air passages or alimentary canal and only larvae are passed in the feces. The first stage larvae of *D. viviparus* develop in the external environment into second and then third stage infective larvae, provided conditions are suitable. The third stage larvae are protected by both of the shed cuticles from the first and second molts which are retained. The worm is a heavy egg producer and it has been estimated that a single infested calf may contaminate a pasture with 33 million larvae. Moisture is essential for the survival and development of the larvae and a moderate temperature of 18–21°C (65–70°F) permits their full development to the infective state in 3–7 days. Under optimum conditions the larvae may survive in the pasture for over a year. They are quite resistant to cold although it greatly delays their maturation. They can withstand temperatures of 4.5°C (40°F) for a year. Larvae can overwinter in climates as cold as Canada (1) and Germany (2).

The infective larvae are quite inactive, few migrate from the fecal pad and most of these remain within 5 cm of the pad. Factors that help spread the larvae on the pasture are therefore important and include diarrhea, mechanical spreading and a high concentration of animals. Fungi (*Pilobolus* spp.) are important in spreading *D. viviparus* larvae; up to 50 larvae may be found on the sporangium and its explosive discharge may propel larvae for up to 3 m. The presence of *Pilobolus* spp. in dung pads can result in a 19-fold increase in larvae from the surrounding herbage (3). Larvae survive best in cool damp surroundings especially when the environment is stabilized by the presence of long herbage or free water.

The third stage larvae must be ingested to infest the primary host. On entering the intestine they migrate through its wall and reach the mesenteric lymph nodes where they become fourth stage larvae. From here they enter the lymphatics and pass eventually to the venous bloodstream, through the heart and reach the lungs where they escape into the alveoli; 3–6 weeks after infestation they have migrated to the bronchi and are mature and laying eggs. Adult worms survive in the bronchi for about 7 weeks at which time immunity has developed and the 'self-cure' process causes death and discharge of a high proportion of the worms. The approximate timing of these phases in *D. viviparus* infestations in calves is: penetration phase (ingestion to arrival of larvae in lung), days 1–7; prepatent phase (larvae in lung), days 7–25; patent phase (mature worm in lung) days 25–55; postpatent phase (lungworm disappearing from lung), days 55–70 (4).

A number of factors affect the epidemiology of lungworm disease. The larvae resist cold and some will overwinter even in extreme climates. In older animals many larvae remain hypobiotic over the winter and resume their development in the spring, further contaminating the pasture. If susceptible calves are introduced to heavily contaminated paddocks early in the spring an acute disease may follow in a week or so. However, clinical disease usually occurs 2–4 months after the introduction of the calves. This delay may be due to the need for the overwintered larvae to pass through one or more generations before the pasture are sufficiently contaminated to cause clinical disease, the numbers of parasites affecting calves in each generation being insufficient to provoke protective immunity. However, it has been suggested that large numbers of larvae may suddenly emerge from the soil in mid-spring to early summer and that some may even survive until cattle are grazed on the hay aftermath (9). Management plays an important role in control of this disease and even a short delay in placing calves on pasture may have a profound effect on the development of disease (25).

In Denmark, larvae that have survived the winter disappear from late April to early May (28), and a delay in the time of grazing in England is an effective means of control (25). However, this alone may not be reliable as larvae may in some circumstances survive to infect hay aftermath, and larvae may be transmitted by *Pilobolus* from adjoining paddocks or may emerge from the soil later in the season.

Immunity to reinfestation with *D. viviparus* occurs after an initial infestation but is variable in degree and duration. Yearling and adult cattle removed from infected pastures for long periods can suffer clinical disease when exposed, and clinical disease may occur in housed cattle when a population of dormant larvae mature synchronously (19). However, the immunity developed from natural infection or vaccination appears to provide protection during the first grazing season and the overwintered larvae boosts this immunity at the beginning of each grazing season. A highly effective vaccination procedure against this parasite is based on the known immunological data.

Pathogenesis

The migrating larvae cause little damage until they reach the lungs and all of the effects of the worms, except possibly for minor irritation of the intestinal mucosa during migration, are centered there. However, the response of the lung varies widely depending largely on the number of larvae which are ingested but also on the nutritional status and age of the host and whether or not it is being exposed for the first time.

Although the severity of the clinical disease is not directly proportional to the number of larvae ingested it is generally accepted that there is an acute and a subacute syndrome depending on the degree of infestation. A massive invasion of the lungs of calves with a very large number of larvae causes an acute, general involvement of the parenchyma. Moderate infestations usually lead to the subacute form of the disease and with light infestations no clinical signs may be apparent.

In the acute form of the disease the reaction of pulmonary tissue to a massive invasion of larvae is initially one of areas of collapse throughout all lobes, edema of the septa, interstitial emphysema and the accumulation of eosinophils. This is followed by alveolar epithelialization, edema and hyaline membrane formation. The lesions are widespread and irreversible and cause severe dyspnea, cough and usually a fatal outcome. Frothy fluid containing many larvae is present in the air passages terminally but death usually occurs before adult worms are present.

In the chronic form of the disease the areas of collapse are widespread but initially are much fewer than in the acute disease. There is a more marked bronchiolar reaction and the bronchi are soon filled with mucus, pus and larvae. The collapsed portion of the lung becomes much more extensive, particularly in the diaphragmatic lobes, and although many adult worms may be present in the bronchi, the lesions persist for long periods after the worms have died. Secondary bacterial bronchopneumonia is a common sequel.

It is evident that the presence of adult worms and exudate in the air passages contributes little to the severity of the acute form of the disease. Collapse of the alveoli, and in acute cases edema, hyaline membrane formation and emphysema, are the major causes of the anoxic dyspnea and death of the animals. It is notable that alveolar epithelialization, a major cause of collapse and consolidation in this disease, is most marked in the later stages and often reaches its greatest magnitude when no larvae or adult worms are present. It is also worthy of mention that treatments which kill the worms, especially adults, will not affect the lesions already present. If, as has been suggested, the epithelialization is a reaction to lungworm tissue this may explain the continued development of the lesion after the worms are dead (5).

Although it is common to find a combined infestation of lungworms and gastrointestinal helminths in which the latter appear to play the more important role, and although poorly nourished animals appear less able to throw off an infestation of lungworms, it is not unusual, provided the right environmental conditions exist, for severe lungworm infestations to be fatal to well-fed calves. This refers not only to the hypersensitivity reaction in the lungs of cattle sensitized to lungworm tissue by previous infestation but also to primary infestations with large numbers of larvae as described above. That a hypersensitivity reaction, particularly in yearlings, can occur and cause acute interstitial pneumonia seems highly probable. However, very many cases of interstial pneumonia can occur without lungworms being present and it must be considered to be a hypersensitivity caused by one of a number of sensitizing agents. Animals recovered from a natural infestation are partially immune for about 7 months but are also in a sensitized state which may result in atypical pneumonia as described above (6, 7). Larvae may invade the tissues of immune animals but appear to be destroyed in lymph vessels and mesenteric lymph nodes. Immunity appears to be related to the numbers of lymphoreticular broncho-occlusive lesions present in the lungs but these may not be the only site of the immunological reaction (8). One would expect the molt that takes place in the mesenteric nodes to provide excellent opportunities for the immune mechanisms to be exposed to exsheathing fluid, a potent antigen, and for this system to be important in the developments of immunity.

Clinical findings

The disease in cattle is almost entirely confined to those running at pasture and occurs most frequently in young animals in their first year on grass but severe outbreaks of the acute form are occurring more commonly in adults. Outbreaks of disease follow sudden exposure to large numbers of larvae on the pasture rather than a slow build-up of infection following ingestion of smaller numbers. Whether the calves develop the acute or subacute disease pattern depends largely on the degree of pasture infestation. Disease may also occur in housed cattle due to the maturation of hypobiotic larvae (19).

Acute verminous pneumonia

The first sign in experimentally produced cases (10) is diarrhea preceding the onset of respiratory signs but this is often not noticed in natural cases. There is a sudden onset of rapid shallow breathing which is largely abdominal in type and often reaches a rate of 100/min. There is a frequent bronchial cough, a slight nasal discharge and a high temperature of 40–41°C (104–105°F). The heart rate is increased to 100–120/min. On auscultation all parts of the lungs are involved approximately equally, the abnormalities including a markedly increased vesicular murmur and bronchial tones. The animal is bright and active and will attempt to eat although the severe respiratory distress often prevents this. Progress of the disease is rapid and within 24 hours dyspnea may become very severe and be accompanied by mouth breathing, a violent respiratory heave and grunt, cyanosis and recumbency. Changes in the sounds heard on auscultation are also evident. Consolidation is evidenced by loud bronchial tones and moist rales are heard over the bronchial tree. The crackling of interstitial emphysema commences over the dorsal two-thirds of the lung but is never as evident as in subacute cases. Fever persists until just before death, which usually occurs in 3–14 days and is greatly hastened by exercise or excitement. The case fatality rate in this form of the disease is high, probably of the order of 75–80%. As a rule a number of animals are affected at one time and the calves have often been moved on to the pasture 7–12 days previously.

Subacute verminous pneumonia

This is more common in calves than the acute form. The onset is usually sudden, there is evidence of recent diarrhea, the temperature is normal or slightly elevated and there is an increase in the rate (60–70/min) and depth of respiration. An expiratory grunt is heard in severe cases and expiration may be relatively prolonged. There are frequent paroxysms of coughing. The course of the disease is long, 3–4 weeks, and auscultation findings vary widely with the duration of the illness and the area of lung involved. In general, there is consolidation and bronchitis ventrally, and marked emphysema dorsally. Affected animals lose weight very quickly and although the mortality rate is much less than in the acute form, many of the surviving calves have severely affected lungs and may have labored breathing for several months, are very susceptible to secondary bacterial bronchopneumonia and remain stunted for long periods. A proportion of the surviving calves may show a sudden exacerbation of the dyspnea during the 7th and 8th weeks and many of these animals die, the important lesion appearing to be the development of a proliferative pneumonia which is probably allergic in origin.

Clinical pathology

The important observation to be made in *D. viviparus* infestation is the presence of larvae in the feces. These may not be present in the early stages of clinical illness because the worms in the bronchi are not yet mature. In general, larvae can be found about 12 days after signs appear, that is to say 24 days after infestation occurs. They may be few in number at first but may be as numerous as 500–1500/g of feces 3–4 weeks after the illness commences. A common but not diagnostic finding is that of eosinophilia which is apparent in subacute cases from the first day of illness but is most marked about 3 weeks later. A detectable level of complement fixing antibodies against *D.viviparus* antigen occurs in calves on the 30th–35th day after infestation with this worm and rises to a peak about the 75th day but this is unlikely to be used as a diagnostic procedure. An intradermal sensitivity test is being investigated.

If the disease is suspected but the lungworms are still in the prepatent stage, and confirmation of the diagnosis by necropsy is impracticable, examination of pasture clippings for larvae may be necessary. This is a laborious procedure because large amounts of herbage must be used and the yield of larvae is low. Counts of less than one larva per 500 g indicate a non-fatal level of infestation, a count of one to three larvae per 500 g indicates a lethal level and counts of over three larvae per 500 g are associated with the acute syndrome and heavy mortalities. Attention must also be given to the fact that the number of larvae on pasture will vary from day to day and at different times during the day depending on the humidity and temperature in the pasture. A technique which effectively separates larvae from plant debris by migration through agar gel has been reported (26).

Necropsy findings

The wide variation in necropsy findings in this disease necessitates caution during the examination (5). In subacute cases the total number of adult worms in the bronchi may be as high as 3000 and counts of 10 000–20 000 are not uncommon. However, if the case is of sufficient duration and self-cure has been completed, no worms may be visible and careful microscopic examination of bronchial mucus is necessary to find larvae.

The morphological changes in the lung in acute cases include enlargement of the lungs due to edema and emphysema, widespread areas of collapsed tissue of a dark pink color, hemorrhagic bronchitis with much fluid filling all the air passages and enlargement of the regional lymph nodes. Histologically the characteristic lesions are edema, eosinophilic infiltration, dilatation of lymphatics, filling of the alveoli and bronchi with inflammatory debris and larvae in the bronchioles and alveoli.

In subacute cases interstitial emphysema is usually gross, areas of dark pink consolidation are present in all lobes but particularly in the diaphragmatic lobe and occupy about two-thirds of the lung volume and tend to be gathered around the bronchi. There is froth in the bronchi and the lymph nodes are enlarged. Histologically, eggs and larvae can be seen in the air passages, the bronchial epithelium is much thickened, the bronchioles are obstructed with exudate and the alveoli show epithelialization and foreign-body giant-cell reaction.

Diagnosis

Verminous pneumonia in calves can be easily confused clinically with bacterial bronchopneumonia, with acute and chronic interstitial pneumonia and with viral pneumonia. Antemortem, the factors that suggest lungworm infestation are a history of exposure to pasture previously grazed by animals of the same species, and of the presence of the disease in the area, failure to respond to standard treatments for bacterial or viral pneumonia and the occurrence of the disease in outbreak form in summer and autumn. The presence of fever, cough and auscultation findings suggesting a consolidation of the lungs and interstitial emphysema are common to all of these diseases, and, although absence of bronchial involvement characterizes early cases of viral and interstitial pneumonia, secondary bacterial bronchopneumonia occurs sufficiently commonly to make this an undependable criterion. One clinical feature which may be of some value in differentiation is the relative softness and paroxysmal nature of the cough in parasitic pneumonia as compared to viral pneumonia. The cough in the latter is harsher and drier. The presence of larvae in the feces supports the diagnosis but it must be remembered that there is a prepatent period of 3 weeks and affected animals may be ill for as long as 2 weeks before larvae appear and may still show obvious clinical signs for some weeks after larvae disappear from the feces. Fecal samples should be collected from all of the animals in the group and for a complete examination samples of pasture, preferably selected from wet low-lying areas, should also be checked for larvae. Deaths are sufficiently frequent to make necropsy diagnosis a common practice.

In adult cattle the major problem in diagnosis is to differentiate the acute form of the disease from acute interstitial pneumonia due to other causes. Clinically the diseases are indistinguishable, and a history of movement on to a new pasture 1–2 weeks before the onset of the disease is common to both. Careful examination of the pasture for larvae and of the feces of the young cattle for evidence of infestation and of necropsy material should make definition possible. That all cases of interstitial pneumonia are not due to lungworm infestation is shown by the persistence of the disease on farms on which lungworm disease is controlled by vaccination (8). Heavy infestations with ascarid larvae in young and adult cattle occur rarely but should be suspected when cattle and infested pigs run together.

Treatment

Most of the modern broad-spectrum drugs are active against *D. viviparus*. Ivermectin is particularly effective against immature and mature stages, doses as low as 0.05 mg/kg being effective. At the commercial dose rate a residual protection of up to 21 days is obtained after subcutaneous injection (11) and intervals between treatments can be increased. Oxfendazole 2·5 mg/kg, fenbendazole 5 mg/kg, albendazole 7·5 mg/kg, febantel 10 mg/kg and levamisole 8 mg/kg are also active against all stages of the parasite. Diethylcarbamazine 22 mg/kg daily for 3 days or 44 mg/kg as a single dose is effective against the immature stages, but not the adult worms.

For the veterinarian in the field the effects of treatment are often unpredictable. If the infestation is massive and much damage has been done by larvae, treatment will effect no clinical improvement. If, however, treatment is administered in the early patent stages, when much of the damage is being caused by adults in the bronchi, clinical improvement is often dramatic but it must be recognized that treatment may exacerbate the clinical signs to a fatal termination in some animals (27).

Because the disease in calves depends for its severity on the number of larvae which invade the lungs, treatment of early clinical cases is recommended in a control program to reduce pasture contamination.

Because acute verminous pneumonia is so highly fatal, a combined treatment with an anthelmintic, an antihistamine to reduce the severity of the reaction to the larvae and an antibiotic or sulfonamide to prevent secondary bacterial infection is often given.

Control

The factor governing the severity of the disease is the concentration of larvae on the pasture on which susceptible cattle are grazed. Control methods must be aimed at reducing the concentration of larvae on the pasture and this may be combined with protecting the calves by vaccination. Exposure to a few larvae will not result in clinical disease but results in the development of immunity. Calves should not be run with older animals and lush wet pastures or paddocks with swampy areas should be avoided. Control of gastrointestinal parasites to control diarrhea should be maintained. Deer may contaminate paddocks although they are clinically not affected. Where animals are housed during winter, yearling cattle, which are the main carriers, should be treated before being released. In problem areas manure from barns should be heaped and turned several times to destroy larvae before being spread on pastures.

Because of the solidity of the immunity which occurs after natural infestation a great deal of attention has been given to preventing infestation by the use of vaccines prepared from irradiated third-stage larvae (4, 5, 16, 17). An effective method of preventing *D. viviparus* infestation in calves has been shown to be two oral vaccinations with 1000 irradiated larvae on two occasions. Under field conditions it is recommended that the calves be 8 weeks old when given the first dose and there is 4 weeks between treatments. Earlier vaccination has not been as successful under conditions of heavy challenge (30). Infective larvae attenuated by exposure to triethylene melamine have also been used to make a vaccine which is as effective as the irradiated larvae (18). It is recommended that calves be confined indoors until at least 2 weeks after the second vaccination. Although vaccinated calves can act as carriers and cause clinical verminous pneumonia in non-vaccinated calves running with them, the vaccination is claimed to be 98% effective in preventing clinical lungworm disease in average conditions (8). There are some limitations. For example, it is recommended that vaccinated calves should not be exposed to grossly infested pastures nor be mixed with heavily infested calves and that on problem farms they be allowed only gradual access to pasture. In both naturally and artificially immunized animals, subsequent infestations of larvae migrate to the lungs where their further development is suppressed, but not before the occasional appearance of mild signs of the disease and death in some cases (20).

The vaccine has a relatively short shelf-life and is rather expensive. The requirement to house cattle during vaccination is most inconvenient and it is possible, by avoiding periods when massive pasture contamination is likely, to vaccinate at pasture (21). Recent work has shown that young milk-fed calves in the field may be immunized at 3 weeks of age. This will be useful in beef calves. Also, dairy calves may be vaccinated earlier than the present recommended age of 8 weeks and thus allow spring-born calves to graze during late summer and autumn (22). Provided satisfactory control procedures are maintained during production of the vaccine this vaccination procedure offers the most efficient method of controlling verminous pneumonia in calves. Although natural immunity can achieve the same effect it can never be accurately measured nor predetermined and systems of control that rely on therapy and reinfection are unpredictable (29). Vaccination provides a known and calibrated weapon. The development of a satisfactory immunity as a result of natural exposure probably occurs in a significant number of beef calves sucking cows. Other methods of vaccination which have been investigated include the parenteral injection of living fourth-stage *D. viviparus* larvae (23) and oral dosing with *D. filaria* larvae (24).

Calves released from barns and not vaccinated should be treated at regular intervals to remove the lungworms before they become patent and increase the pasture contamination.

Ivermectin given subcutaneously 3, 8 and 13 weeks after turnout (four treatments are given if the cattle are turned out before May 1) prevents clinical disease and pasture contamination, and the cattle are resistant in their second season (12). Cattle treated with ivermectin in this way compare favourably with vaccinated cattle (13). If other compounds, effective against mature and immature lungworms are used to treat cattle, they must be used at least every 3 weeks and this should be continued untill the following winter. An oxfendazole pulse release intraruminal device is now available and will release a full therapeutic dose every 3 weeks. Preliminary studies have shown it has great efficacy in removing worms and preventing pasture contamination and yet allowing the development of immunity (31). Such intensive treatment may provoke anthelmintic resistance. Vaccination is probably a safer alternative at this time (14). If the turnout can be delayed until early May, pasture contamination will be reduced and the challenge to vaccinated or treated calves will be minimized.

In areas where enzootic pneumonia of calves and verminous pneumonia both occur a difficult decision may have to be made—whether to have the calves out on pasture to avoid spread of enzootic pneumonia or to keep them housed to avoid lungworm infestation. In such a situation it is preferable to run them at pasture and treat periodically as suggested above or confine them in outdoor pens without access to infested pasture.

REFERENCES

(1) Gupta, R. P. & Gibbs, H.C. (1970) *Can. vet. J.*, *11*, 149.
(2) Supperer, R. & Pfeiffer, H. (1971) *Berl. Munch. Tierarztl. Wochenschr.*, *84*, 386.
(3) Somers, C. J. et al. (1985) *Vet. Rec.*, *116*, 657.
(4) Jarrett, W. F. H. et al. (1961) *Am. J. vet. Res.*, *22*, 492.
(5) Jarrett, W. F. H. et al. (1959) *Am. J. vet. Res.*, *20*, 522.
(6) Michel, J. F. (1958) *Vet. Rec.*, *70*, 554.
(7) Weisman, J. (1970) *Proefschrift, Fac. Diergeneeskd. Rijksuniv. Utrecht*, p. 123.
(8) Poynter, D. et al. (1970) *Vet. Rec.*, *86*, 148.
(9) Duncan, J. L. et al. (1979) *Vet. Rec.*, *104*, 274.
(10) Urquhart, G. M. et al. (1973) In: *Helminth Diseases of Cattle, Sheep and Horses in Europe*. Glasgow: University Press.
(11) Amour, J. et al. (1985) *Vet. Rec.*, *116*, 151.
(12) Ryan, W. G. (1987) *Vet. Rec.*, *120*, 351.
(13) Taylor, S. M. et al. (1986) *Vet. Rec.*, *119*, 370–372.
(14) Bain, R. K. & Urquhart, G. M. (1986) *Vet. Rec.*, *118*, 82.
(15) Chalmers, K. (1979) *NZ vet. J.*, 27, 8.
(16) Jarrett, W. F. H. et al. (1962) *Am. J. vet. Res.*, *23*, 1183.
(17) Edds, G. T. et al. (1963) *Am. J. vet. Res.*, *24*, 139.
(18) Cornwell, R. L. & Jones, R. M. (1970) *Res. vet. Sci.*, *11*, 533.
(19) Oakley, G. A. (1979) *Vet. Rec.*, *104*, 460.
(20) Downey, N. E. (1965) *Vet. Rec.*, *77*, 890.
(21) Downey, N. E. (1968) *Vet. Rec.*, *82*, 338.
(22) Benitez-Usher, C. et al. (1976) *Vet. Parasitol.*, *2*, 209.
(23) Cornwell, R. L. (1962) *J. comp. Pathol.*, *77*, 181.
(24) Lucker, J. T. et al. (1964) *Proc. helminth. Soc. Wash.*, *31*, 153.
(25) Jacobs, D. E. & Fox. M. T. (1985) *Vet. Rec.*, *116*, 75.
(26) Jorgensen, R. J. (1975) *Vet. Parasitol.*, *1*, 61.
(27) Jarrett, W. F. H. et al. (1980) *Vet. Rec.*, *106*, 135.
(28) Jorgensen R. J. et al. (1987) *Vet. Parasitol.*, *10*, 331.
(29) Urquhart, G. M. et al. (1981) *Vet. Rec.*, *108*, 180.
(30) Downey, N. E. (1984) *Vet. Rec.*, *114*, 29.
(31) Jacobs, D. E. et al. (1987) *J. vet. Pharmacol. Therap.*, *9*, 337.

LUNGWORM INFESTATION IN OTHER SPECIES

Sheep and goats

Infestations with *Dictyocaulus filaria*, *Muellerius capillaris* and *Protostrongylus rufescens*, are all encountered. Lambs 4–6 months of age are most severely affected but sheep of all ages are susceptible. Lungworm infestation in sheep needs to be differentiated from maedi and jaagsiekte. Infestations with *Cystocaulus ocreatus* and *Neostrongylus linearis*, the latter similar in most of its characters to *M. capillaris*, have also been observed in sheep in Great Britain (1) and Iran (2) but their economic significance has not been defined.

D. filaria infestations in sheep appear to follow the same pattern as those of *D. viviparus* in calves; the lifecycle is direct and the third-stage larvae are longlived in damp, cool surroundings. The lambs of one season are the main source of infection for the next season's lambs, but overwintering larvae passed by ewes and yearlings also contribute to pasture contamination (3). The prevalence of infection is low in spring and summer but rises rapidly in the autumn and winter when most clinical cases are seen (3). Warm, wet summers give rise to heavier burdens in the following autumn and winter (3, 4). Acute cases, caused by massive infestations with larvae, do not appear to occur. Adult worms live in the bronchi and cause alveolar and bronchiolar damage. The resulting blockage of bronchioles by exudate leads to the collapse of portions of lung. The area of lung damaged is usually not sufficiently extensive to cause severe dyspnea. Clinically the emphasis is on bronchial irritation and its resulting cough, on moderate dyspnea and loss of condition. There may be added fever and evidence of toxemia if secondary bacterial infection occurs. Laboratory diagnosis depends upon the detection of first-stage larvae in the feces of infested animals. Although *D. filaria* is primarily a lungworm of sheep it can infest and grow to maturity in cattle and can, after experimental infestation, cause the death of calves (5). It is highly pathogenic to young goats.

At necropsy the lesions are similar to those of the subacute disease in calves with exudate in the bronchioles and scattered patches of consolidation.

Ivermectin 0·2 mg/kg, oxfendazole 5 mg/kg, fenbendazole 5 mg/kg (7), levamisole 7·5 mg/kg (6), albendazole 3·8 mg/kg and febantel 5 mg/kg have high activity against mature and immature stages as well as against gastrointestinal parasites. Control by vaccination with irradiated larvae of *D. filaria* has been examined in sheep (8) and goats (17), but this disease is rarely sufficiently pathogenic to justify vaccination. Vaccination with viable *D. viviparus* larvae reduced the number of worms and the severity of lesions in sheep later challenged with *D. filaria* larvae (9). Inmmunity after natural exposure is strong and durable (at least 46 months) in sheep but less so in goats (10).

Infestations with *Muellerius capillaris* in sheep has been recorded from most parts of the world, and although the worm appears to be relatively innocuous it may constitute a limiting factor in the production of choice market lambs. Massive invasion with larvae is uncommon because the intermediate host snails and slugs are usually not ingested in large numbers nor are they grossly infested with larvae. Those larvae which reach the lungs of sheep remain in the parenchyma and become encysted in fibrous nodules and because such nodules may not contain adults of both sexes, fertile eggs may not be deposited in the air passages. For this reason the number of larvae in the feces is often no indication of the degree of infestation. Also, in many animals the infestation is carried over from one year to the next. Massive infestations with this worm do not develop acutely and heavy infestations, when they occur, appear to develop over a long period of time (11).

At necropsy the worms are found in small fibrous nodules up to 5 mm in diameter. Most of the nodules are in the parenchyma of the lung immediately under the pleura. Many of them are calcified and they often contain only one live or dead worm. Infestation of goats leads to a diffuse infection quite different to the nodular reaction in sheep and to the production of an interstitial pneumonia (18). Whether this is due solely to *Muellerius* infection or whether a chlamydial or viral agent needs to be present has not been determined. It is doubtful whether treatment of sheep is ever justified. In goats one or two doses of ivermectin 0·2 mg/kg, fenbendazole 15 mg/kg, or albendazole destroys the adult worms but not the immature stage (20, 21), but regular doses of fenbendazole at 1·25, 2·5 or 5·0 mg/kg in the feed for 1–2 weeks or albendazole 1·0 mg/kg for 2 weeks is highly effective against all stages (21). Single doses of fenbendazole as high as 30 mg/kg or cambendazole at 60 mg/kg are ineffective (22).

P. rufescens infestations in sheep and goats cause clinical signs similar to those of *D. filaria*. The adult worms live in the bronchi, causing verminous bronchitis and pneumonia. Only lambs and kids show serious clinical involvement. Because the lifecycle is indirect, requiring a land snail for completion of the second stage larval development, massive infestations are unlikely to occur. Few modern anthelmintics have been tested against *P. rufescens*, but compounds effective against *Dictyocaulus* spp. should be active. In preliminary experiments fenbendazole has been shown to be active against *C. ocreatus*.

Pigs

The lungworms which infest pigs are *Metastrongylus apri* (*M. elongatus*), *M. salmi* and *M. pudendodectus*; *M. apri* is the most common species but mixed infestations are not uncommon. They have an indirect life history, passing their intermediate stages in earthworms. Eggs laid by adult worms in the lungs are coughed up and swallowed and, passing out with the manure in an embryonated stage do not hatch until they reach the exterior. The eggs first appear in the feces 3–4 weeks after infestation and at their peak reach levels of 25–50 epg. The embryonated eggs or first-stage larvae are either eaten by the earthworms or migrate actively into the worms. Here they develop successively into second and third stage larvae in about 2 weeks. Details of the ability of the first stage larvae to survive before they infest the intermediate host are lacking but they appear to be fairly resistant. The larvae of *M. apri* may survive for as long as a year after hatching. The primary host must ingest an intermediate host to become infested and this is an important factor influencing the spread of the disease. Once ingested the infective larvae migrate to the lungs in much the same manner as do *D. viviparus* larvae.

In natural cases bronchitis accompanied by sporadic bouts of a barking cough which is easily stimulated by exercise, pneumonia in severe cases, poor growth and debility are the obvious signs but minimal clinical signs are apparent after experimental production of the disease (12). These worms are suggested as vectors in the transmission of swine influenza virus, and possibly hog cholera virus, from pig to pig.

At necropsy the lesions in early cases comprise small areas of consolidation due to verminous pneumonia. More chronic cases have bronchitis, emphysema, peribronchial lymphoid hyperplasia and bronchiolar muscular hypertrophy. The lesions are small and discrete, appearing as grayish nodules up to 1 cm in diameter and are present particularly at the ventral border of the diaphragmatic lobes (12). In more severe experimental cases acute and chronic lesions are more widely disseminated and often involve the anterior lobes.

Levamisole 8 mg/kg given in the water or levamisole resinate, given as 0·08% levamisole hydrochloride equivalent, in the feed has high efficiency in pigs (13) and has broad-spectrum activity against other parasites of the pig. Mebendazole when given at 15 mg/kg on two successive days showed activity but when given in pelleted feed no effect was noted (14). A single dose of ivermectin is highly effective (24), while fenbendazole 3 mg/kg for 3 days or febantel given in the feed for 5 days can also be used.

Horses

Infestations with *D. arnfieldi* are recorded more commonly in donkeys than in horses and the former are considered to be the more normal host. Heavy infestations in donkeys do not cause clinical illness while horse foals may also be symptomless but some show clinical signs. Experimental infections produce an afebrile condition with coughing, increased respiratory rates and forced expiration being most intense during the 3rd–5th weeks after infection. Thereafter the signs decrease in severity but coughing may persist for several months (15). At necropsy both horses and donkeys show discrete areas of overinflation surrounding bronchi blocked with worms and a greenish mucus (19). In horses the worms usually do not mature and therefore infection cannot be made by fecal examination, but the presence of eosinophils in the tracheobronchial washings is a helpful diagnostic aid (19). *D. arnfieldi* has been reported only rarely from many countries but is probably overlooked because of the mild symptoms usually exhibited. Ivermectin 0·2 mg/kg has high efficiency against immature and mature stages (23), while fenbendazole at the higher dose of 30 mg/kg is also effective (19).

Control of miscellaneous lungworm infestations

Those worms with direct lifecycles, *D. filaria* and *D. arnfieldi*, can be controlled by methods set out in the beginning of this chapter. Lungworms are specific but infections of other hosts may occur and while the worms do not become patent, they may cause some degree of immunity (5, 9). Concurrent or alternate grazing of different species may therefore be beneficial in controlling lungworm as well as gastrointestinal parasites. Combined infections of lungworms and intestinal nematodes are normal and the control program placed on a property for intestinal parasites will also control lungworms provided a broad-spectrum compound is used.

In those worm species which have indirect lifecycles, *Muellerius capillaris*, *Protostrongylus rufescens* and *Metastrongylus* spp., the control measures must include avoidance of the intermediate hosts. Snails and slugs are most active in wet weather and in the early morning or evening. Pasturing of animals on wet, undrained areas at those times of the day should be avoided where possible. Little can be done to control earthworm populations, and pigs which run in dirt yards or at pasture should be moved at short intervals to prevent ingestion of infested worms. Rooting by pigs can be discouraged by providing adequate feed and by the insertion of nose rings. Pastures which are known to be contaminated should be left for at least 6 months before restocking, although infested earthworms may persist in hog lots for up to 4 years.

REVIEW LITERATURE

Poynter, D. & Selway, S. (1966) *Vet. Bull.*, *36*, 539.
Rose, J. H. (1973) *Adv. Parasitol.*, *11*, 559.

REFERENCES

(1) Rose, J. H. (1965) *Res. vet. Sci.*, *6*, 189.
(2) Eslami, A. H. & Anwar, M. (1976) *Vet. Rec.*, *99*, 129.
(3) Gallie, G. J. et al. (1977) *Res. vet. Sci.*, *22*, 251.
(4) Ayalew, L. et al. (1974) *Can. J. comp. Med.*, *38*, 448.
(5) Parfitt, J. W. (1963) *Vet. Rec.*, *75*, 124.
(6) Turton, J. A. (1973) *Vet. Rec.*, *93*, 108.
(7) Malan, F. S. & Roper, N. A. (1983) *J. S. Afr. vet. Assoc.*, *54*, 92.
(8) Movsesijan, M. (1973) In: *Helminth Diseases of Cattle, Sheep and Horses in Europe*. Glasgow: University Press.
(9) Wilson, G. I. (1970) *Proc. helminth. Soc. Wash.*, *37*, 24.
(10) Wilson, G. I. (1970) *Res. vet. Sci.*, *11*, 7.
(11) Rose, J. H. (1959) *J. comp. Pathol.*, *69*, 414.
(12) Kruse, G. O. W. & Ferguson, D. J. (1980) *Vet. Med. Rev.*, *2*, 113.
(13) Poeschl, G. P. & Omro, J. E. (1972) *J. Am. vet. med. Assoc.*, *160*, 1637.
(14) Kutzer, E. et al. (1975) *Wien. Tierärztl. Monatschr.*, *62*, 61.
(15) Mackay, R. J. & Urquhart, K. A. (1979) *Equ. vet. J.*, *11*, 110.
(16) Britt, D. P. & Preston, J. M. (1985) *Vet. Rec.*, *16*, 343.
(17) Dhar, D. W. & Sharma, R. L. (1978) *Ind. J. anim. Sci.*, *48*, 762.
(18) Nimmo, J. S. (1979) *Can. vet. J.*, *20*, 49.
(19) Clayton, H. & Murphy, J. (1980) *Vet. Rec: In Practice*, *2*, 25.
(20) McCraw, B. M. et al. (1981) *Can. vet. J.*, *22*, 205.
(21) Helle, O. (1986) *Vet. Parasitol.*, *22*, 293.
(22) Bliss, E. L. & Greiner, E. C. (1985) *Am. J. vet. Res.*, *46*, 1923.
(23) Lyons, E. T. et al. (1985) *Vet. Med.*, *80*, 58.
(24) Stewart, T. B. et al. (1981) *Am. J. vet. Res.*, *42*, 1425.

ESOPHAGOSTOMIASIS (NODULE WORM DISEASE, PIMPLY GUT)

Infestations with worms of *Oesophagostomum* spp. occur in all farm animals except horses. The disease produced is characterized clinically by emaciation and the passage of soft droppings containing more than normal amounts of mucus and in most species at necropsy by the presence of necrotic nodules in the wall of the intestine. Although deaths may occur the major losses are caused by failure to thrive. The damage done to intestines renders them unsuitable for use as sausage casings.

Etiology

All of the species of the genus *Oesophagostomum* are thick, white roundworms (0·5–2·5 cm long, except the species in the pig which reach 1·5 cm) which inhabit the large intestine. The important species are:

Sheep and goats: *Oesophagostomum columbianum*; *Oe. venulosum*; *Oe. asperum*

Cattle: *Oe. radiatum*; *Oe. venulosum*

Pig: *Oe. dentatum*; *Oe. quadrispinulatum*; *Oe. brevicaudum*

Although there is obvious species specificity, some cross-infection occurs. Thus *Oe. venulosum* is found in both sheep and cattle, while *Oe. columbianum* can develop in cattle to the point of penetrating the mucosa and producing lesions similar to those in lambs, but without any apparent effect on health (1). The infection does not confer any resistance against infection with *Oe. radiatum*.

Lifecycle and epidemiology

Infections with *Oesophagostomum* spp. occur most commonly in temperate or subtropical climates with summer rainfall and cause economic loss in sheep, cattle and pigs. Infections are gained mostly in the summer months and if sufficient are ingested an acute condition may occur. Lighter infestations or infestations in older animals give rise to a chronic condition that is mainly seen in the following winter months and which results from the effects of worms in a time of limited feed availability and the presence of nodules in the intestinal wall. In spite of the predilection of the worms for warm, moist conditions the more chronic form of the disease is quite common in eastern Canada and the New England states of America.

The lifecycle is direct. Eggs passed in the feces hatch and, after undergoing two molts, become infective third stage larvae; under optimum conditions this takes 6–7 days. The requirements of the freeliving larvae are quite strict, both eggs and larvae of *Oe. columbianum* being susceptible to cold and dryness. Infestation occurs only by ingestion. The larvae of all species, except perhaps those of *Oe. venulosum*, invade the intestinal wall at any level. In young sheep exposed to *Oe. columbianum* for the first time, the larvae enter the intestinal wall, mainly in the anterior small intestine, and stay there for about 5 days. The larvae then re-enter the lumen and move to the large intestine where some of them enter a second histotrophic stage while others develop directly to adults and commence egg-laying about 6 weeks after infection. In second infections few larvae develop directly to adults and most are arrested in either the first or second histotrophic stages (1). Persistence of the larvae in the intestinal wall for long periods is usually taken to indicate immunity on the part of the host and is followed by nodule formation. Thus in older sheep nodules develop in the intestinal wall at any level and occasional nodules may also be present in nearby organs. In these animals the larvae may remain alive in the nodules for periods up to a year. When the resistance of the animal is lowered, due for example to poor nutrition, the larvae leave the nodules, re-enter the intestinal lumen and pass down to the colon, where they complete their development and become adults. The adults attach themselves to the colonic mucosa and commence egg-laying. In animals with some immunity many larvae never re-enter the bowel from the nodules, being destroyed by the host reaction. This is the probable explanation for the three common findings at necropsy: young sheep with many adult worms and no nodules, adult sheep with many nodules and no adult worms, and adults with both.

The lifecycles of the *Oesophagostomum* spp. in cattle and pigs are similar to that of *Oe. columbianum*. The species in pigs has a periparturient rise in fecal egg counts which is closely related to lactation and which is terminated when the piglets are weaned. This is the most important source of eggs for the young pigs (2). The persistent reappearance of *Oesophagostomum* spp. in pigs may result from ingestion of larvae contained in rats and other rodents or from larvae carried on dipterans of the genus *Psychoda* (3).

Pathogenesis

Oesophagostomum spp. exert serious effects in the migratory phase by the adult worms and by the nodules produced as a host reaction. In general, young susceptible animals suffer from the effect of the adult worms, whereas in older immune animals the nodules play a more important role. *Oe. radiatum* and *Oe. columbianum* cause anorexia, severe and persistent diarrhea, loss of weight, anemia, hypoproteinemia and death. The hypoproteinemia follows edema of the cecum and colon and is caused by loss of albumin into the lumen (4). Anemia is produced as a result of blood loss when histotrophic larvae re-enter the lumen and the fall in plasma fibrinogen levels and platelet numbers that occurs 6–7 days after primary infection of calves probably aggravates this loss (5). Adult worms also cause intestinal bleeding by a direct action (6).

Emergence of the larvae from the intestinal wall causes a catarrhal colitis and this, together with the increased number of mucus cells associated with an adult infection and the loss of albumin into the bowel, causes a diarrhea with an increased mucus content. Nodules eventually caseate and calcify and may cause interference with intestinal motility or local peritonitis and adhesion formation leading to intussusception or stenosis. In sheep the nodules cause considerable pain and an arched back (humpy back) and a stilted gait may develop.

The lesions produced experimentally in pigs have been well defined (7). Edema and marked thickening of the colon and cecum develop. With heavy infestation, outbreaks of necrotic enteritis may be activated in pigs carrying *Salmonella* spp. populations (8). *Oe. quadrispinulatum* rarely caused nodules in minimal disease pigs following challenge with a single larval dose but these were common when *Oe. dentatum* was included (11).

Clinical findings

In heavy infestations in young sheep there may be severe persistent diarrhea but in the more common syndrome observed in older sheep in the winter months there is an intermittent passage of semi-soft droppings containing more than normal amounts of mucus, and occasionally blood. There is rapid loss of condition, hollowing of the back, stiffness of gait and elevation of the tail. Nodules may be palpated on rectal examination. Anemia is not characteristic and is never marked. Severe outbreaks of intussusception sometimes occur in young sheep and esophagostomiasis is often implicated as a primary cause.

Young calves may show clinical signs of anorexia, diarrhea, emaciation and anemia. Initially the diarrhea may alternate with constipation but later it is continuous and is dark and fetid. In pigs, although loss of condition and diarrhea have been attributed to this infection, it is unusual for *Oesophagostomum* spp. to be the primary cause of death.

Clinical pathology

The severity of the disease may bear no relation to the number of eggs in the feces, counts varying widely with the season of the year and the stage of development of the disease. In the early stages of a massive infestation, signs may be evident but there may be no eggs in the droppings. After the prepatent period in young sheep, eggs are usually present in large numbers and may be accompanied by living adult worms. However, in chronic cases there may be very few eggs in the droppings. The eggs cannot be readily distinguished from those of other strongylid worms.

Necropsy findings

In early acute cases there is a mild catarrhal enteritis and larvae may be detectable in scrapings of intestinal mucosa. In the later, more chronic stage there are adult worms in the colon. The adult worms are usually lying in thick mucus overlying a chronic catarrhal colitis. Nodules, when they are present, may be found at all levels of the intestine. They are up to 6 mm in diameter and, depending on their age, contain a green, pasty material or yellow-brown, crumbly, partly calcified material. There may be a great deal of thickening of the intestinal wall and local peritonitis.

The number of worms in the lumen of the colon is usually quite small and 200 *Oe. columbianum* adult females is considered to be a heavy infestation.

Diagnosis

A definite diagnosis of esophagostomiasis can only be made by necropsy examination or identification of larvae from a fecal culture. The diseases with which it is most likely to be confused are trichostrongylosis, which is also at its peak during the winter but in which diarrhea is more evident, and malnutrition, especially when sheep are housed and poorly fed. The disease has a relatively restricted geographical distribution and this should be taken into account.

Both *Oesophagostomum* spp. and *Hyostrongylus rubidus* have been associated with the 'thin sow syndrome'. The sows rapidly lose condition late in pregnancy and while they are lactating. In many herds a high proportion of sows have to be culled. Although emaciated, the sows usually eat well and rear their litters satisfactorily. Parasitism is probably a minor cause of this condition; insufficient energy content of the diet is the most important cause and bullying of timid sows may occasionally result in a similar condition.

Treatment

All of the modern broad-spectrum compounds are effective against *Oesophagostomum* spp. In pigs, none of these compounds has high activity against the larval stages, but fenbendazole 5 mg/kg and flubendazole 4 mg/kg given as a single dose or in the feed for 1–2 weeks are probably the most effective. Other benzimidazoles, including the probenzimidazoles, thiophanate and febantel, are active against the adult stages but vary in their effectiveness against immature forms. Levamisole and dichlorvos are often used in pigs because they have broad-spectrum activity including *H. rubidus* and *A. suum*, while dichlorvos also removes *T. suis*. Pyrantel pamoate can also be used as a single dose, but if given in the feed at 510 mg base/kg will also remove *H. rubidus* and *A. suum*. Ivermectin has been shown to be variable against *Oesophagostomum* spp.

In ruminants any of the newer broad-spectrum anthelmintics is efficient against the adult worms although efficiency is reduced against the immature forms.

Control

To keep infestation at a minimum level in sheep flocks and at pasture all the year round, three strategic dosings with an efficient anthelmintic in early spring, midsummer and late autumn are recommended. The flock should be moved to a clean pasture after each drenching. The aim should be to treat the flock immediately after a period when climatic conditions, particularly a dry summer or a cold winter, are likely to have destroyed the majority of larvae on the pasture. Sheep which are housed in the winter months and suffer greatest damage at this time are usually dosed only once a year, preferably 1–2 months before lambing. The observation that grazing sheep on a field of green oats is highly effective in removing *Oe. columbianum* from the colon may have some significance as a control measure. In grazing pigs the ability of the eggs and larvae to survive on the pasture must be considered. In the United Kingdom eggs deposited in the winter and early spring do not reach the infective stages but infective larvae can survive for a year in feces or on pasture (13). Under these conditions pigs should be treated twice in the autumn and then moved to clean pasture so that contamination of pastures in the late spring and early summer is markedly reduced (13). In Canada the colder winter kills all freeliving stages and it is important that all pigs are treated before being placed on pasture (14).

The control program in pigs must also take the 'periparturient rise' into account. Dosing of the sow before farrowing is recommended and the piglets should be treated at 5–6 weeks of age and again about 30 days later. Boars should be treated once a year (12). Housing is not a protection unless there is an absence of litter and manure is removed frequently.

REFERENCES

(1) Dash, K. M. (1973) *Int. J. Parasitol.*, *3*, 843.
(2) Jacobs, D. E. & Dunn, A. M. (1968) *Nord.VetMed.*, *20*, 258.
(3) Jacobs, D. E. et al. (1968) *Vet. Rec.*, *82*, 57.
(4) Bremner, K. C. (1969) *Exp. Parasitol.*, *24*, 364.
(5) Bremner, K. C. & Fridemanis, R. (1975) *J. comp. Pathol.*, *85*, 383.
(6) Bremner, K. C. & Keith, R. K. (1970) *Exp. Parasitol.*, *28*, 416.
(7) McCracken, R. M. & Ross, J. G. (1970) *J. comp. Pathol.*, *80*, 619.
(8) Stockdale, P. H. G. (1970) *Br. vet. J.*, *126*, 526.
(9) Martinsson, K. & Nilsson, O. (1986) *Nord. VetMed.*, *38*, 156.
(10) Barnes, D. M. et al. (1979) *Vet. Rec*, *105*, 81.
(11) Kendall, S. B. et al. (1977) *J. comp. Pathol.*, *87*, 223.
(12) Batte, E. G. (1977) *J. Am. vet. med. Assoc.*, *170*, 343.
(13) Rose, J. H. & Small, A. J. (1980) *Vet. Rec.*, *107*, 223.
(14) Smith, H. J. (1979) *Can. vet. J.*, *20*, 184.

STEPHANURIASIS (KIDNEY WORM DISEASE)

Stephanuriasis is a disease of swine caused by the migration of larvae and young adults of *Stephanurus dentatus* through the body. Poor growth and feed utilization is characteristic in mildly affected animals whereas badly affected animals become emaciated and develop ascites and muscle stiffness.

Etiology

Stephanurus dentatus are large (2–5 cm) thick roundworms which inhabit the perirenal tissues, and less commonly the other abdominal organs and spinal canal of the pig. They have been observed rarely in cattle. Experimentally dosed calves develop severe hepatic injury similar to that which occurs in pigs but the lifecycle is not completed and no perirenal lesions develop.

Lifecycle and epidemiology

Kidney worms occur commonly in most tropical and subtropical countries such as Africa, the East and West Indies, Brazil, Hawaii, Philippines, southern United States and Australia where the climate is sufficiently mild to permit the survival of eggs and larvae. The mortality rate is not high, the important causes of loss being poor growth and condemnation of parts or all of the infested carcass.

Adult worms inhabit cysts around the renal pelvis and the wall of the ureter. The cysts communicate with the urinary passages and the eggs are passed out into the urine of the host. They are very heavy egg layers and an infective adult sow may void as many as a million eggs in a day. Under suitable environmental conditions the eggs hatch and, after undergoing two molts, the non-infective larvae develop into the infective third stage in about 4 days. The eggs and larvae are very sensitive to cold and desiccation, eggs in a dry situation dying within an hour. Exposure to temperatures below 10°C (50°F) is damaging and 4°C (40°F) is lethal. Most larvae in optimum conditions of moisture, warmth and shelter from sunlight survive for about 3 months, some for as long as 5 months. Larvae may survive for long periods as facultative parasites in earthworms and this may enable the larvae to survive even though the microclimate of the soil is adverse.

Larvae may penetrate the skin or be ingested. Larvae that are ingested pass through the stomach, or more commonly the small intestine, and reach the liver via the portal vessels; from the skin the larvae reach the systemic circulation and pass to the liver via the lungs in 1–6 weeks (2). In the liver the larvae migrate from the blood vessels through the parenchyma and eventually, about 3 months after infestation, having undergone a fourth molt, penetrate the capsule of the liver and reach the perirenal tissues to establish themselves as adults. Egg-laying usually commences about 6 months after infestation but the prepatent period may be very much longer and individual worms appear to live as long as 2 years (9).

During their migration the larvae often follow an erratic path and cause the development of atypical lesions and clinical signs. These larvae often reach maturity in these aberrant sites and prenatal infection can occur in this way (3).

Pathogenesis

The principal effect of these worms is the damage caused by the migrating larvae and young adults. The migrating worms cause a great deal of necrosis, fibrosis and occasional abscess formation along the path of their migration and this is most marked in the perirenal tissues and the liver. Many apparently unrelated clinical signs are produced by aberrant larvae which may invade the spinal cord, causing paralysis, or blood vessels, particularly portal veins, hepatic artery and posterior vena cava, causing thrombus formation, and psoas muscles, causing the local pain and stiffness so marked in some badly affected pigs. Passage through the peritoneum and pleura causes the formation of adhesions and many larvae become encysted in the lung. Body weight gain is depressed in infected animals and feed conversion is increased (10).

Clinical findings

Poor growth in spite of a good appetite may be the only sign in mild cases. Severely affected pigs are emaciated and may have ascites. Stiffness and lameness of the hindlegs followed by weakness and eventually paralysis occur in a number of pigs. In the early stages nodules in the skin of the belly wall and enlargement and soreness of the peripheral lymph nodes may be evident (3).

Clinical pathology

The large, thin-walled, embryonated eggs are present in the urine when adult worms are present in the ureteral wall. An eosinophilia is seen 2–3 weeks after infection, peaks at 6–7 weeks and is still elevated at 20 weeks (4). However this has little diagnostic significance. Anemia does not occur. Only a transient rise in aspartate aminotransferase is seen and serum enzymes seem to be of little value in diagnosis (4).

Necropsy findings

The common findings include fibrosis and abscess formation in perirenal tissues with large adult worms present here and occasionally in the pelvis of the kidney and ureter, infarcts and scars in the kidney and enlargement and scarring of the liver, sometimes accompanied by ascites. The hepatic lesions include irregular whitish tracks in the parenchyma, extensive fibrosis, hemorrhage and eosinophilic abscess formation. The liver may be covered with a diphtheritic membrane. Larvae may also be present in peripheral lymph nodes and cutaneous nodules, in small abscesses in the lung and pancreas and in thrombi of blood vessels, particularly in the liver and lungs. Pleurisy and peritonitis if they are present are usually manifested by adhesions.

Diagnosis

Poor growth and emaciation in pigs is commonly associated with poor nutrition and sporadically with a number of chronic bacterial diseases. Most of the latter, including necrotic enteritis and swine dysentery, affect the alimentary tract and are accompanied by intermittent diarrhea. Other parasitic diseases such as ascariasis and hyostrongylosis may cause similar clinical syndromes. Posterior weakness in pigs may be caused by stephanuriasis but is more commonly caused by vitamin A deficiency, osteodystrophia, sometimes by fracture of a lumbar vertebra, brucellosis, erysipelas when intervertebral joints are involved, or by spinal cord abscess or lymphoma. Experimental visceral larval migrans, caused by infestations of pigs with larvae of *Toxocara canis*, can also cause a syndrome of ataxia and posterior paralysis (5) but the natural occurrence of this disease does not seem to have been observed.

A definite diagnosis of stephanuriasis may be made by finding eggs in the urine but necropsy examination is preferred. Young pigs with a heavy infestation of larvae may present a problem in diagnosis because adult worms and characteristic renal lesions may not yet be present. An ELISA test can detect infection from 2 weeks after infection (11), but serological tests are not likely to become a routine diagnostic procedure.

Treatment

Ivermectin 0·3 mg/kg subcutaneously (8), fenbendazole 10 mg/kg orally or 3 mg/kg in the feed for 3 days (1), or flubendazole 1·5 mg/kg for 5 days (12) are effective against migrating and adult stages, while levamisole 8 mg/kg orally or subcutaneously removes the adults and reduces egg counts to zero for 5 weeks (6).

Control

Regular anthelmintic treatment of all pigs with fenbendazole or ivermectin at 4-month intervals should eliminate contamination and the free-living stages should then die out. Treatments would have to continue for some time as infected earthworms may survive for at least 1 year. Similar results would be achieved with levamisole if used monthly.

Management techniques were devised to control kidney worm when effective treatments were not available. The principles used in these programs are important and could still be used on many farms. One method is to breed entirely from gilts until control is achieved. Under this system the gilts are raised, allowed to farrow and sent to market as soon as the litter is weaned. This is before the parasites achieve patency. The boars are confined on concrete to prevent contamination of the soil by eggs in their urine (7). This technique has the advantage of maintaining a fully stocked farm while control is being achieved but has economic penalties associated with breeding from gilts only.

Other management techniques have been derived which depend on the provision of bare ground. Sleeping shelters should be placed on high ground, preferably bare of vegetation, so that the infectivity of the urine is reduced. Because pigs in yards commonly urinate against the fences it is recommended that a 2–3 m strip of earth inside the fence be kept free of pasture and preferably packed hard. Muddy spots and water holes must be filled in and drainage provided. Water and feed troughs should be on a concrete apron. Young animals should be segregated from adults and fields rested for 3–6 months after the adults are removed. Results are excellent if the program is carried out diligently and intelligently but the extra work involved has militated against the general acceptance of the program.

Indoor pens should be constructed with a good slope to the floor to avoid dampness. A recommended control measure is weekly spraying of the pens with 10% copper sulfate solution or a 5% solution of Kerol. These sprays are also recommended for the spraying of dirt yards, the latter being particularly effective when applied at the rate of 5 liters/10 m^2, maintaining the toxicity of mud for larvae for a period of at least 66 days. Neither spray is toxic for pigs kept in the treated yards. Because of the importance of mature animals as sources of infestation, early replacement of breeding stock is recommended in problem herds.

Vaccination did not prevent liver lesions or migration of worms to the perirenal region but did reduce the adult worm burdens by up to 92% (9). However, more efficient reduction of both mature and immature worms can now be achieved with anthelmintic treatment.

REFERENCES

(1) Becker, H. N. & Bradley, R. E. (1981) *Vet. Parasitol.* 9, 111.
(2) Waddell, A. H. (1969) *Aust. J. Zool.*, *17*, 607.
(3) Batte, E. G. et al. (1966) *J. Am. vet. med. Assoc.*, *149*, 758.
(4) Hutchinson G. W. et al. (1983) *Aust. vet. J.*, *60*, 171.
(5) Done, J. T. et al. (1960) *Res. vet. Sci.*, *1*, 133.
(6) Batte, E. G. et al. (1975) *Vet. Med.*, *70*, 809.
(7) Stewart, T. B. et al. (1964) *Am. J. vet. Res.*, *25*, 1141.
(8) Becker, H. N. (1986) *Am. J. vet. Res.*, *47*, 1622.
(9) Tromba, F. G. & Romanowski, R. D. (1976) *J. Parasitol.*, *62*, 250.
(10) Hale, O. M. & Marti, O. G. (1983) *J. anim. Sci.*, *56*, 616.
(11) Partoutomo, S. et al. (1983) *Int. J. Parasitol.*, *13*, 45.
(12) Bradley, R. E. et al. (1983) *Am. J. vet. Res.*, *44*, 1329.

BUNOSTOMIASIS (HOOKWORM DISEASE)

Infestations with hookworms (*Bunostomum* spp.) cause poor growth and blood loss manifested by anemia and anasarca.

Etiology

Hookworms are small (1–2·5 cm), reddish roundworms which inhabit the small intestine of their hosts. The important species are:

Cattle: *Bunostomum phlebotomum* is the important hookworm but *Agriostomum vryburgi* may occur in cattle in India and Sumatra

Sheep: *Bunostomum trigonocephalum* and in India, Indonesia and Africa *Gaigeria pachyscelis*

Pigs: Infestations with some species of hookworms occur but are rarely important.

Immunity to *B. phlebotomum* in cattle appears to develop with age (1) and calves affected one year appear to be completely immune the next. Calves 4–12 months of age are most commonly affected and the degree of infestation is always greatest in the winter months.

Lifecycle and epidemiology

The lifecycle of all the hookworms is direct. The eggs hatch and a parasitic larva is produced in about a week. There are two free-living, non-parasitic larval stages which are very susceptible to desiccation, and an infective larva which is capable of entering the body of the host through the skin. Larvae of *G. pachyscelis* enter only in this way; *Bunostomum* spp. larvae enter by this route and via the mouth. Percutaneous entry greatly enhances the chances of infestation when the surroundings are wet, and this, together with the susceptibility of the larvae to desiccation, leads to the higher incidence of the disease in humid subtropical countries.

The larvae, after cutaneous penetration, enter the bloodstream, are carried to the heart and lungs, enter the alveoli where the fourth stage larvae develop, pass up the air passages to the pharynx, are swallowed and reach the small intestine. Ingested larvae penetrate the intestinal wall and return to its lumen without further migration. In *B. trigonocephalum* infestations the fourth stage larvae reach the intestine in about 11 days and egg-laying adults are present about 7 weeks after infestation. The prepatent period in *B. phlebotomum* infestations is about 8 weeks and in *G. pachyscelis* 10 weeks.

Hookworm infestations are most common and cause greatest losses in subtropical and temperate countries including the southern United States, Africa, Australia and Europe where climatic conditions are most suited for completion of the worms' lifecycles. However, the disease is encountered in such countries as Scotland and Canada, especially when animals are housed during the winter in dirty surroundings with insufficient bedding.

Pathogenesis

Hookworms are active bloodsuckers and cause severe anemia in all animal species. Total worm numbers as low as 100 may cause clinical illness and 2000 may cause death in young cattle. There is a loss of whole blood and hypoproteinemic edema may result. Some irritation to the intestinal mucosa is inevitable and mild or intermittent diarrhea follows. Penetration of the skin by larvae may cause signs of irritation and lead to the introduction of pathogenic bacteria.

In experimental disease in lambs (2) sheep with less than 100 worms showed no obvious effect, but some degree of anemia may be measured. More than 500 worms quickly produced anemia and hypoproteinemia. Anorexia was not noted.

Clinical findings

In mild infestations in stabled cattle fidgeting, stamping and licking of the feet may be observed. Constipation, accompanied by mild abdominal pain, is seen in the early stages and is followed by bouts of diarrhea. The cattle are unthrifty and anemic. In severe infestations there is obvious pallor of mucosae, weakness, anasarca under the jaw and along the belly, prostration and death in 2–3 days. Signs in sheep are similar to those in cattle. The convalescent period, even after treatment, is prolonged unless the diet is supplemented to stimulate erythrocyte production.

Clinical pathology

The blunt ends and deeply pigmented embryonic cells of hookworm eggs enable them to be differentiated fairly accurately from the eggs of other strongylid worms. Egg counts of 400–500 epg are usually associated with fatal infestations. The adult worms are heavy egg-layers and both they and the immature worms are strong bloodsuckers. Clinical signs are often evident in the prepatent period before eggs appear in the feces (3). The presence of severe anemia and occult blood in the feces are only contributory evidence but can be used as a measure of the severity of the infestation.

Necropsy findings

The number of worms present may be quite small. In calves total worm counts of 100 or more suggest a significant level of infestation, counts of over 2000 worms indicate a degree of infestation likely to be fatal. In sheep and goats 24 adult *G. pachyscelis* have been reported to be fatal, but the usual fatal figure is probably closer to 100. Most of the worms are found in the first few feet of the small intestine and the intestinal contents nearby are often deeply bloodstained. Some of the worms may have been washed down into the colon and are likely to be mistaken for *Oesophagostomum* spp.

Diagnosis

Hookworm infestations in young animals may be confused with many diseases in which anemia, diarrhea and anasarca occur. Haemonchosis is probably the most similar disease and mixed infestations of these two worms are not uncommon in some countries. Hepatic fascioliasis may also be manifested by a similar clinical picture and as both diseases usually occur in the winter, this constitutes the most important differential diagnosis. The anemia and diarrhea of coccidiosis and the anemia caused by *Eperythrozoon ovis* or heavy louse infestation may also cause difficulty in diagnosis. A dietary deficiency of cobalt or copper, and chronic molybdenosis should also be considered in the differential diagnosis of bunostomiasis in lambs and calves.

Treatment

Most of the newer benzimidazoles, levamisole and morantel are effective against adult *Bunostomum* spp. in sheep and cattle. Nitroxynil and rafoxanide, which bind to blood protein and are ingested by bloodsucking worms, are effective, and presumably closantel which acts in a similar fashion would also be active. The newer benzimidazoles—oxfendazole, fenbendazole and albendazole —are also active against the immature stages (4). Fenbendazole 5 mg/kg is highly efficient against adult and larval *G. pachyscelis* in sheep (5).

Supportive treatment is essential in this disease because of the severe anemia which occurs. The provision of a mineral mixture containing iron, copper and cobalt is recommended and a general improvement in the quality of the diet, particularly in respect of protein, may shorten the convalescent period.

Control

Wet surroundings, in pastures, in yards and in barns, should be avoided to reduce the chances of percutaneous infestation and reduce the viability of the freeliving larvae. Pens should be cleaned frequently and ample bedding provided. Heavy stocking of sheep or calves in small pens should be avoided. Under conditions of heavy risk periodic treatment should be administered. *B. trigonocephalum* is known to occur in Scottish red deer and these animals may provide a source of infestation for sheep grazing the same pasture. The hookworms of cattle and sheep are not host-transferable, and it is often suggested that rotation of the two animal species on a pasture may tend to clear up the infestation.

REFERENCES

(1) Roberts, F. H. S. (1951) *Aust. vet. J.*, 27, 274.
(2) Graham, J. M. & Charleston, W. A. G. (1971) *Vet. med. Rev.*, 4, 452.
(3) Soulsby, E. J. L. et al. (1955) *Vet. Rec.*, 67, 1124.
(4) Boersema, J. H. (1985) *Handb. exp. Pharmacol.*, 77, 407.
(5) Tiefenbach, B. (1977) *Hoechst Blue Book*, 27, 256.

TRICHOSTRONGYLIASIS, OSTERTAGIASIS, COOPERIASIS, NEMATODIRIASIS (SCOUR WORMS, HAIR WORMS)

Although infestations with the worms *Trichostrongylus*, *Ostertagia*, *Cooperia*, and *Nematodirus* spp. are specific diseases they commonly occur together in the abomasum and small intestine of sheep and cattle and have similar effects. These infestations are probably the most important single cause of losses, in both deaths and poor growth, in countries where ruminants are run at pasture the whole year and the disease they cause is characterized by persistent diarrhea and wasting.

Etiology

The anatomical predilection sites are indicated in Table 77.

In most natural infestations a mixture of genera and species is found but in most districts one species will be of greater importance. In sheep and cattle, *Ostertagia* tends to be the most important parasite in the winter rainfall areas while *Haemonchus* is more important in the summer rainfall zones. However, other genera may assume dominance in some areas or under certain management practices. Although the same species may occur in both sheep and cattle, there is a degree of host-specificity and thus those species specific for sheep are reduced if mixed grazing is used, while those species normally found in cattle are found in increasing numbers in sheep as the proportion of cattle in the stocking ratio rises (1).

These worms are predominantly parasites of young animals. In sheep the two age groups most commonly affected are weaner lambs and yearlings. Failure to reduce contamination at critical periods, malnutrition and overcrowding are important predisposing causes. Sheep over 18 months of age are less commonly affected because of immunity resulting from previous infestation.

In all species the disease is of most importance when the plane of nutrition is low but massive infestations can overwhelm well-fed animals. Moderate infestations can be borne by animals on good feed while poorly nourished animals may succumb. In weaner lambs the reduction of food intake because of weaning increases the susceptibility, while in yearlings in the winter months it is the general reduction in available feed combined with increased availability of infective larvae. In dairy cattle the disease is most common in calves of 3–6 months while in beef cattle it can be seen in animals up to 2 years of age and occasionally in adults.

Clinically, trichostrongyliasis is favored by cool, wet weather so that in Australia and South Africa this is a disease of the winter months in those areas where the rainfull occurs chiefly at this time of the year. In arid areas the disease is of little significance except in years of unusually heavy precipitation. Although the eggs and larvae of *Trichostrongylus* spp. are resistant to cold they are not resistant to freezing and in cold climates trichostrongyliasis may be more common in the late summer and autumn when rainfall is heavy and temperatures generally cool. However, the disease under these conditions is rarely as severe as in winters in temperate climates. Thus it is much less important in Canada than in Australia. The eggs and larvae of *Ostertagia* and *Nematodirus* spp. are much more resistant to cold and can survive the coldest winter. In the United Kingdom *N. battus* can develop throughout the year and greatest numbers of infective larvae are available in spring following the mass hatch of eggs containing infective third stage larvae (4). The larvae of *Cooperia* spp. are less affected by high temperatures and the disease occurs in all seasons in temperate climates.

Table 77. Anatomical distribution of trichostrongylid worms in ruminants*.

	Cattle		*Sheep and goats*	
Parasite	*Abomasum*	*Small intestine*	*Abomasum*	*Small intestine*
Trichostrongylus spp.				
T. axei	×		×	
T. colubriformis, *T. longispicularis*		×		×
T. falculatus, *T. vitrinus*, *T. capricola*, *T. rugatus*, *T. probolurus*				×
Ostertagia spp.				
O. ostertagi	×		×	
O. circumcincta			×	
O. trifurcata			×	
Cooperia spp.				
C. punctata, *C. oncophora*		×		×
C. pectinata		×		
C. curticei				×
Nematodirus spp.				
N. spathiger, *N. battus*, *N. filicollis*, *N. abnormalis*		×		×
N. helvetianus		×		

* *Trichostrongylus axei* occurs in the stomach of horses.

Lifecycle and epidemiology

The lifecycle in all of these genera is direct. The eggs are passed in the feces and under suitable environmental conditions hatch, producing two successive non-parasitic larval stages and then the third or infective larva. The eggs of *Nematodirus* spp. do not hatch and the infective larvae are retained within the egg, thus gaining greater resistance to environmental conditions. When the infective larva is ingested by the host, it exsheathes, usually in the organ before that in which the adult form lives, and may enter the mucosa. Here it molts, returns to the lumen and after a fourth molt matures to the adult worm. The uncomplicated parasitic lifecycle from ingestion of larvae to egg-laying females takes about 3 weeks except with *Nematodirus* which takes a week or so more. However, in some species the fourth stage larvae may become hypobiotic and the lifecycle can be prolonged for some months.

The eggs and free-living larvae of most of these species can survive and develop at much lower temperatures than *Haemonchus* and *Oesophagostomum* spp. Upper temperature limits for survival are, however, lower. Although the eggs and larvae of all the worms under discussion can survive through a moderate winter, the bulk of the infective larvae of *Trichostrongylus* spp. disappear quickly in hot dry weather and reinfection is low in the absence of dew or rain which is necessary before infective larvae can ascend grass blades. Under these conditions the perpetuation of infestation is due largely to carrier animals. This is not so with *Nematodirus* spp., the eggs of which may survive in large numbers on the pasture from one year to the next. In areas where the summers are not so hot and dry, sufficient eggs or larvae may persist on the pasture to initiate infections after the autumn rains, while in colder climates, such as Scotland, larvae of *O. ostertagi* and *C. oncophora* can survive for 18 months or more (14).

The behavior of infective strongyle larvae in pats of cattle manure can have an appreciable effect on persistence of the disease. In hot dry areas few eggs develop to infective larvae in pats deposited in the summer but these may remain alive for 4–5 months and emerge to contaminate the paddock after the autumn rains. During the summer, migration of larvae from pats may occur after heavy rain which softens the hard crust of the pat and allows larvae to escape. This may occur intermittently with the crust forming between storms. In temperate areas a much greater proportion of the eggs deposited in the autumn and winter will develop and these larvae quickly become available and remain alive until the following summer.

Minimum prepatent periods are quite short; in *Trichostrongylus* spp. infestations in sheep 2–3 weeks with maximum egg production 4 weeks later; *T. axei* in the horse 25 days; *O. ostertagi* in calves 3–4 weeks; *C. punctata* in calves 12–15 days; and *C. oncophora* in this species 17–22 days; *Nematodirus spathiger* in sheep 3–4 weeks; and *N. helvetianus* in 21 days. However, these periods may be much longer in animals with an acquired immunity. Further, many larvae, particularly *O. ostertagi* in cattle, may become hypobiotic when picked up and may not emerge until some 4–5 months later. This is thought to be due to an adaptation phenomenon similar to diapause in insects and allows the larvae to avoid adverse pasture conditions (2), winter in Canada and Britain, and summer in Australia and New Zealand. The stimulus for *O. ostertagi* to become hypobiotic in Europe appears to be exposure to low temperatures, while in Australia this is not an effective stimulus for inhibition (20). There is evidence for a genetic basis for inhibition and inhibiting and non-inhibiting strains with different abilities to survive over the summer have been reported (22).

Increased resistance to infestation develops and the immunity decreases the number of worms in the animal and the number of eggs laid. The development of resistance depends on the larval intake. Lambs can develop a high resistance to *Trichostrongylus* spp. by about 6 months when larval intake is high, but this is extended when intake is low (23). While resistance does build up it can be overcome in times of stress and is generally much poorer than the immunity built up against *Dictyocaulus viviparus*. The response of lambs to vaccination is influenced by nutrition, those on good feed produce more antibody and have less worms on challenge (24). Vaccination against gastrointestinal nematodes has not been successful (3). However, it has been shown that a group of animals can be divided into those that respond to vaccination and those that do not and that the capacity to respond is genetically determined (3). If a simple test can be devised to determine which are likely to respond to vaccination, this may lead to flocks capable of being protected by vaccination being developed. A degree of age resistance can be seen with *Nematodirus* sp.

For each region it is important that the animals providing the source of the major contamination are identified, the period of development from egg to infective larvae is known and the availability of infective larvae throughout the year is plotted so that a program can be devised to reduce contamination and protect the susceptible animals in time of greatest danger. Such work has been done for sheep and cattle in several areas (6–9).

In considering the epidemiology of the infection, it is important to consider any special factor such as the periparturient rise of fecal egg count in ewes. This occurs before or at the time of lambing and reaches a peak 6–8 weeks after lambing. It is the most serious source of contamination for the lamb (11) and steps should be taken to control the rise or to protect the lamb in some other fashion (12).

Nematodirus spp. in sheep follow a different pattern from other infection in this group as the young lambs of one season provide contamination which survives to infect the next season's lambs (13). *Trichostrongylus* spp. should also be considered separately as they also do not undergo hypobiosis to any significant degree and disease is usually the result of self-augmentation of infection. *T. axei* is primarily a disease of cattle and is usually only seen in horses when they are run with cattle.

The epidemiology of *Ostertagia* in cattle is complex and several forms of ostertagiasis have been described. In dairy calves, ostertagiasis type I is seen with high stocking rates on permanent calf paddocks. In this form the lifecycle proceeds from infective larvae to adult form in about 3 weeks and the majority of worms found are adults. Egg counts will be high. In areas with mild climates, type I disease may be seen in almost any season but is particularly important in winter and spring. In areas with more severe winters, such as Scotland, sufficient larvae overwinter to infect calves in the spring and further contaminate the pasture, so that disease usually occurs from mid-July to the end of the grazing season (2). Type I ostertagiasis also occurs in beef cattle particularly if they are placed on heavily infected pastures immediately after weaning.

When hypobiosis occurs, many fourth stage larvae of *O. ostertagi* enter the gastric glands and remain there, causing little or no pathological findings. This form, called pre-type II ostertagiasis, does not cause clinical symptoms, and occurs at a definite time each year which varies depending on the area. This is autumn in Britain and spring in Australia. Type II disease occurs mainly in beef cattle, when the hypobiotic larvae emerge from the parasitized glands some 4–5 months later when the cattle may be 18–24 months of age. A similar condition is seen in cows calving for the first or second time and in some seasons cows of all ages and the bulls may be affected. Ostertagiasis occurs occasionally in dairy cattle calving for the first time (25).

Pathogenesis

While the effects of infestation will depend on the species present, their location and numbers, anorexia is an important feature of all of these diseases. Local effects on digestion, absorption and protein loss will depend on the organ affected and will interact with loss of appetite. Intestinal trichostrongylosis in sheep causes villous atrophy and plasma loss into the intestine from increased vascular permeability and discontinuity of the epithelium. This is most important in the extremely atrophic type O mucosa where erosion of the epithelium is observed (15). Observations on guinea-pigs infected with *T. colubriformis* show that hepatic synthesis of plasma protein and catabolism of muscle protein are increased in the presence of plasma protein loss into the intestine and this plays a part in loss of productive body functions (16). Part of dietary ill-effects may be due to the loss of enzymes normally found on the microvilli and which are lost when villous atrophy occurs (10). *T. colubriformis* infection of lambs reduces the absorption of phosphorus and increases the loss of endogenous phosphorus, thus leading to a phosphorus deficiency (26). This parasite causes reduced acid production and a rise in abomasal pH to 4 or above (27). Parasitic infestation can cause the loss of copper from the bowel and exacerbate a marginal copper deficiency (28).

T. axei causes gastritis with superficial erosion of the mucosa, hyperemia, edema and diarrhea. Anorexia, with its resultant reduction of dietary protein, and plasma loss from the damaged mucosa appear to be the main causes for the hypoproteinemia that occurs. *Nematodirus* spp. also causes villous atrophy, reduction in disaccharase and alkaline phosphatase activity in the mucosa, inappetence, weight loss and diarrhea (17).

Modes of pathogenesis in ostertagiasis

In type I ostertagiasis the penetration of the larvae into the glands causes white, raised, umbilicate nodules which surround the parasitized gland. This is due to hyperplasia of the mucus-secreting cells and the nodules may be discrete or confluent forming a morocco-leather appearance. Severe epithelial cytosis occurs when the larvae emerge and may result in a diphtheritic appearance of the abomasum. Edema of the folds and protein leakage may occur.

In the pre-type II stage when large numbers of larvae may be found in the abomasal glands there are no biochemical changes in the abomasal fluid or in the blood and almost no reaction in the cells. When the larvae emerge the type II syndrome is seen. Marked cellular changes occur with hyperplasia and loss of cell differentiation of the cells lining the glands and in adjacent glands. There is a loss of parietal cells and the pH of the abomasum rises to 6–7. Consequently pepsinogen is not converted to pepsin, there is a failure of peptic digestion and the number of bacteria in the abomasum rises. Epithelial sloughing can be severe and diphtheresis, inflammation and congestion may occur. Because pepsinogen accumulates, some leaks back to the blood vessels and plasma pepsinogen rises. Plasma protein leakage occurs and this, combined with anorexia and poor conversion of dietary protein, produces hypoproteinemia. Moderate anemia also occurs. Diarrhea is constant and weight loss is rapid.

Clinical findings

In all species the onset is insidious and the young animals start to lose weight and fail to grow. They are unthrifty and lack vitality and bloom. If they are observed sufficiently closely their food intake can be seen to be reduced. This may be the full clinical picture in many flocks which are considered to have 'weaner illthrift' (18). More severely affected sheep pass dark green, almost black, soft feces which foul the wool of the breech. Lamb and yearling flocks are most seriously affected and a constant mortality begins, a few animals dying each day. The losses are not acute but may eventually exceed 35%. A rather more dramatic picture may occur with heavy infestations of *Nematodirus* spp. in young lambs, especially those in the 6–12-week age group. Clinical signs are similar to those described above but deaths may start within 2 days of the first observed illness.

Calves show the same clinical signs as lambs but being kept under closer observation more details of signs are available. They lose weight, pass soft feces which eventually becomes very thin and dark green to yellow in color, develop a long, dry hair coat and become dehydrated with sinking of the eyes in the terminal stages. Until the last they continue to eat although the amount of food taken is much below normal. Gross anemia is not evident but the mucosae are pale and dry. Submandibular edema is common, especially in the type II disease. The temperature may be elevated (39·5°C, 103°F) and the heart rate increased (120/minute) in calves showing dehydration. In the terminal stages the calves become so weak and emaciated that they are unable to stand but they may persist in this recumbent state for several weeks if they are provided with a good diet. A characteristic of the disease is that the diarrhea often continues after treatment in severely affected calves if the treatment only removed the adult worms. Standard treatments for diarrhea are also unsuccessful. Clinical differentiation between types I and II ostertagiasis in calves is not easy, although the signs generally are more severe in the latter and the prognosis is a great deal poorer. The absence of eggs from the feces and the poor response to treatment are the diagnostic features of type II. Although parasitism generally, and ostertagiasis in particular, is a disease principaly affecting the young, it can be encountered, especially the type II disease, in adults and is relatively common in cattle of 2–3 years of age.

In horses, *Trichostrongylus* may be present in the stomach in very large numbers, often associated with localized thickening and irritation of the mucosa, but it is impossible to define the signs caused by this infestation because it always occurs concurrently with infestations of other, more pathogenic, strongylid worms.

Clinical pathology

Except in young animals, there is little correlation between fecal egg count and worm burden and this should not be used as the only diagnostic test (19). However, in type I ostertagiasis in cattle, egg counts, which are usually over 1000 epg, are a valuable guide in differentiation of type I and type II diseases. A necropsy including a total worm count should be done preferably with a peptic digest of the mucosa. The eggs of the different species, other than *Nematodirus*, cannot be differentiated and cultures must be made if one wishes to determine the species present. Plasma pepsinogen estimations are now done as a routine test to aid in the diagnosis of ostertagiasis. The test must be standardized so that results from different laboratories can be compared. Levels higher than 3000 i.u. tyrosine are considered to be positive, but because levels remain high after the worms have been removed (5), and some animals with long-standing infections have low values, the plasma pepsinogen test alone should not be used to establish categorically whether or not an animal is suffering from ostertagiasis (5). We have found it a valuable herd test but individual animals may give false-negative results. An examination of the changes in biochemical and serological values during the development of types I and II ostertagiasis, show that 3000 i.u. may be too low as levels of 2000–3000 occur in normal cattle and 6000 i.u. may be a more realistic level at which to diagnose abomasal damage due to types I or II ostertagiasis (29). Gastrin level and pH may also be used as indicators of abomasal damage.

Hemoglobin levels are usually in the vicinity of 6–8 mg/dl and serum protein levels 4–5 mg/dl with a marked reduction in serum albumin levels. Anemia is more evident in *Cooperia* and *Ostertagia* spp. infestations, whereas in trichostrongyliasis there may be polycythemia.

Necropsy findings

The adult worms are found in the abomasum or small intestine depending on the predilection site of the individual species. A total worm count is the critical measure of the degree of infestation. Counts less than 2000 mixed species in sheep are considered to be light, while counts over 10 000 are heavy, but massive counts of 50 000 and more are often seen. In cattle, burdens of 40 000 and above are seen in type I ostertagiasis outbreaks with the majority being adults, while in type II outbreaks worm numbers may be 100 000–200 000 with occasional animals harboring a million or more. In these cases about 90% are in the fourth larval stage.

Most of these worms are sufficiently small to evade detection by the naked eye. A method of demonstrating the worms is to roll a loop of duodenum inside out on a test tube or piece of glass rod and immerse this in aqueous iodine solution (iodine 30 g, potassium iodide 40 g, water 100 ml) for several minutes and then into a 5% solution of sodium thiosulfate for a few seconds. The mucosa is decolorized but the brown-stained worms retain their color and are easily seen. This method has been satisfactorily adapted as an efficient, rapid field technique for performing a total worm count (21).

Gross pathological findings are often not apparent, that is apart from the non-specific lesions of emaciation, dehydration, moderate anemia and evidence of scouring. The mucosa of the abomasum and upper duodenum may be hyperemic and swollen in severe cases, and on histological examination there is a fibrinocatarrhal gastritis. In chronic cases of type II ostertagiasis there are diagnostic lesions including a morocco-leather-like appearance of the mucosa with some umbilicated nodules present, epithelial cytolysis and a putrid smell resulting from the growth of bacteria in the lowered acid medium. Estimation of the pH is a worthwhile procedure. Ringworm-like lesions of hyperplastic gastritis have been described in chronic cases of trichostrongyliasis in lambs, calves and horses.

Diagnosis

In most outbreaks of gastrointestinal helminthiasis in sheep, and to a less extent in calves, the two factors of malnutrition and parasitism are probably of equal importance and to place undue emphasis on one may lead to neglect of the other when treatment and control programs are outlined.

Parasitic gastroenteritis should not be diagnosed on the basis of a fecal egg count alone. A total worm count should be done whenever possible and the results considered together with the clinical signs, the age of the animal and the season of the year. The critical test in an outbreak of disease is the response to treatment. However, in a control program, infection rates in animals should always be kept low and no response will be seen following routine treatments. Because the epidemiology of the various species differ it is important that the main contributing species be determined so that adequate control measures can be taken.

Other common causes of emaciation and diarrhea in group of young animals include secondary copper deficiency in calves and coccidiosis. In adults Johne's disease, secondary copper deficiency and chronic fascioliasis are the common causes of a similar syndrome.

Treatment

Many broad-spectrum anthelmintics are now available that have high efficiency and low toxicity in sheep and cattle. Most of these are benzimidazoles, but levamisole, morantel and ivermectin are also used. The use of different combinations of substituents on the benzimidazole ring has provided a large number of compounds with broader-spectrum activity, some being active against cestodes and one, albendazole, is also active against mature *F. hepatica*.

Dose rates and other pharmacological data are available from the manufacturers and are not repeated here. The range of benzimidazoles used in sheep and cattle includes thiabendazole, parbendazole, mebendazole, fenbendazole, oxibendazole, oxfendazole, albendazole and the probenzimidazole, febantel. A choice between these and other available drugs will depend on price, safety, ease of administration and spectrum of activity. Mebendazole, albendazole, fenbendazole and oxfendazole have activity against cestodes. Parbenzole has been shown to have teratogenic effects in sheep when used at three times the normal dose rate in ewes early in pregnancy (31); albendazole (32) also has teratogenic effects at higher dose rates. Activity against lungworms is provided by fenbendazole, albendazole, mebendazole, oxfendazole and febantel. Resistance of *Trichostrongylus* spp. and *O. circumcincta* to the benzimidazoles has been reported but appears to be at a low level in field populations in most countries. Field strains have been selected in laboratory tests that are resistant against the benzimidazoles, morantel and levamisole (19). The modern anthelmintics are divided into the benzimidazoles and pro-benzimidazoles, i.e. compounds that are metabolized to benzimidazoles, compounds such as morantel and levamisole which act on ganglions, and ivermectin. Where resistance to one class of compound appears then a change should be made away from that group. If anthelmintics are to be rotated the interval between changes should be not less than 1 year.

Levamisole has wide usage, particularly in cattle, because it is injectable and has efficiency against lungworms as well as gastrointestinal parasites. Morantel is an efficient compound against intestinal parasites and has been combined with diethylcarbamazine to provide a mixture effective against lungworms and intestinal worms. Ivermectin is now available in most countries. It represents a new class of compound and acts by potentiating the effect of the nerve transmitter gamma-aminobutyric acid (GABA) in nematodes. It has a very broad spectrum of activity being highly efficient against adult and larval stages of all gastrointestinal parasites, lungworms and many arthropods. The organophosphates are too narrow in their spectrum and are not sufficiently active against *Nematodirus* or in the large intestine to be recommended. Type II ostertagiasis has been a difficult therapeutic problem. The compounds available only removed the lifecycle stages in the lumen of the abomasum and these were quickly replaced from the store of hypobiotic larvae. The constant emergence of hypobiotic larvae produced massive abomasal damage. Many compounds claimed activity against early stages of *O. ostertagi* and these were often confused and thought to be claims against hypobiotic larval stages. Fenbendazole was the first compound to show high activity against dormant *O. ostertagi* but oxfendazole, albendazole, febantel and ivermectin are also effective.

Irrespective of the drug used it is important that animals should be removed after treatment to a clean paddock. The benzimidazoles inhibit the development of eggs in the lumen of the bowel and this ovicidal action may be useful if animals are being placed on very clean areas such as cereal stubble. However, it is probably of little importance on many farms where a residual pasture contamination is always present. Supplementation of the diet, particularly the provision of minerals, may be important.

Control

The general principles of the control of these helminthoses have been dealt with at the beginning of this chapter. Specific recommendations are difficult to make because the epidemiology of the diseases varies so much from area to area.

The aim of control measures is to prevent outbreaks and allow optimal growth rates. The benefits obtained must be justified on economic grounds of increased production above the cost of treatments. In some areas where individual animals are valuable, then regular treatments throughout the year may be justified or animals may be treated whenever they are brought in for any other management procedure. Regular treatments for long periods may aid the development of resistant strains and in most circumstances, control programs should be integrated into the epidemiology of the particular parasite. Strategic drenching to reduce contamination and to prevent the young susceptible animals from being challenged with large number of larvae should be introduced and management techniques may have to be adjusted to aid control. For ostertagiasis and trichostrongyliasis in areas with hot dry summers, all sheep should be treated once or twice in early to midsummer to reduce contamination on the paddock and to allow those lifecycle stages on the paddock to be destroyed by climatic conditions.

In Europe, calves should be treated regularly from 3 weeks after turnout to prevent contamination of the pasture. If ivermectin is used by subcutaneous injection the interval between treatments can be extended to 5 weeks from the 3 weeks used with the benzimidazoles, morantel and levamisoles. Two treatments with ivermectin 3 and 8 weeks after turnout may be all that is necessary (30). The treatment of ewes housed during the last 10 weeks of pregnancy may improve the lambing percentage (34).

The contamination arising from the periparturient rise should be controlled. In ewes producing lambs for meat, prelambing and postlambing treatment may be necessary (35), but in wool sheep the lambs should be weaned at 12 weeks, treated and placed on the cleanest available pasture. Techniques for the use of clean grazing and strategic dosing have been described (39).

Weaners may need regular treatments at 4–6-week intervals throughout the winter and spring period. Such a program also controls *Cooperia* spp. Where fat lambs are being produced and early weaning is not possible, then treatment of the ewes and lambs at 10–12 weeks after lambing, combined with removal to cattle paddocks or to pastures rested for long periods, should control parasitism. Such programs limit the number of treatments to ewes and wethers and it is only the weaners, about one-fifth of the total flock, that are receiving more frequent treatments. Such treatments not only give optimal economic control but also aid in preventing the development of resistance. Simulation models have been devised for parasitic infections and can be used to predict the timing of treatment (40, 41).

Nematodirus infection of sheep has a lamb-to-lamb transmission, i.e. the lambs of one season contaminate the ground for the lambs of the following season. To control this infection, alternation of lambing paddocks may be all that is necessary or lambs may be treated regularly at 3-weekly intervals.

Type I *Ostertagia* infection and trichostrongyliasis of dairy calves can be controlled by treating with any of the modern available drugs and moving the animals to a clean pasture. If other pastures are not available, regular treatments at short intervals of 2–4 weeks may be necessary to allow adequate growth of the calves. In beef calves, treatment is not usually justified until weaning, but in the first season at pasture, care must be taken to control type I ostertagiasis and *T. axei* by regular treatment early in the season to limit contamination and later challenge. Strategies for nematode control in cattle in the United States have been described (42).

The method of control of type II ostertagiasis in most areas has now been assessed but in many areas practical difficulties arise in achieving control. When possible the susceptible age group should be treated before the time when ingested larvae will become hypobiotic and should then be moved to clean pastures. If clean pastures are not available the cattle should be treated once or twice with a compound efficient against dormant larvae, fenbendazole, albendazole, febantel, oxfendazole or ivermectin, before the emergence of the dormant larvae. A bolus containing morantel tartrate and designed to release small quantities over a period of 90 days has been released and shown to be effective. Administration to calves before turnout of spring pasture in the United Kingdom markedly reduced contamination later in the season and allowed greater weight gains (33). In New Zealand, prophylactic use also gave greater weight gains (36) but in both trials it was not as effective when used therapeutically. Its high cost will preclude its widespread use. Administration of oxfendazole in pulse-release systems immediately before the calves are placed on pasture provides five therapeutic doses at 3-week intervals and protects throughout the growing period.

On those farms with suitable ratios of sheep and cattle, alternation of sheep and cattle will aid considerably in achieving control. Concurrent grazing also effectively lowers the stocking rate of each host species and has benefits in pasture control.

When experiments are done using control methods based on the principles outlined above, remarkable results may be obtained. Gains of 300% total live weight production and 1000% return on investment are recorded in the treatment of ostertagiasis in calves (37) while a 538% return has been achieved in sheep (38).

REVIEW LITERATURE

Anderson, N. & Waller, P. J. (1985) *Resistance in Nematodes to Anthelmintic Drugs*. Publ. CSIRO, Australia.

Armour, J. (1980) The epidemiology of helminth disease in farm animals. *Vet. Parasitol.*, *6*, 7.

Brunsdon, R. V. (1980) Principles of helminth control. *Vet. Parasitol.*, *6*, 185.

Morley, F. H. W. & Donald, A. D. (1980) Farm management and systems of helminth control. *Vet. Parasitol.*, *6*, 105.

REFERENCES

(1) Arundel, J. H. & Hamilton, D. (1975) *Aust. vet. J.*, *51*, 436.
(2) Armour, J. et al. (1973) *Helminth Diseases of Cattle, Sheep and Horses in Europe*, eds G. M. Urquhart & J. Armour. Glasgow: Robert MacLehose.
(3) Windon, R. G. & Dineen, J. K. (1981) *Int. J. Parasitol.*, *11*, 11.
(4) Mitchell, G. B. B. et al (1985) *Res. vet. Sci*, *38*, 197.
(5) Michel, J. F. (1978) *Vet. Rec.*, *103*, 370.
(6) Anderson, N. (1973) *Aust. J. agric. Res.*, *24*, 599.
(7) Herd, R. P. (1984) *Comp. cont. Educ. pract. Vet.*, 6, S67.
(8) Brunsdon, R. V. (1969) *NZ vet. J.*, *17*, 161.
(9) Michel, J. F. et al. (1970) *Res. vet. Sci.*, *11*, 255.
(10) Coop, R. L. et al. (1984) *Res. vet. Sci.*, *36*, 71.
(11) Salisbury, J. R. & Arundel, J. H. (1970) *Aust. vet. J.*, *46*, 523.
(12) Arundel, J. H. (1971) *Aust. vet. J.*, *47*, 275.
(13) Gibson, T. E. (1959) *Vet. Rec.* , *71*, 362.
(14) Bairden, K. et al. (1985) *Res. vet. Sci.*, *39*, 116.
(15) Barker, I. K. & Beveridge, I. (1983) *Vet. Parasitol.*, *13*, 67.
(16) Symons, L. E. A. & Jones, W. O. (1971) *Exp. Parasitol.*, *29*, 230.
(17) Coop, R. L. et al. (1973) *Int. J. Parasitol.*, *3*, 349.
(18) Ritchie, J. D. S. et al. (1966) *Am. J vet. Res.*, *26*, 659.
(19) LeJambre, L. F. et al. (1978) *Int. J. Parasitol.*, *8*, 443.
(20) Smeal, M. G. & Donald, A. D. (1982) *Parasitology.*, *85*, 27.
(21) Arundel, J. H. (1967) *Aust. vet. J.*, *43*, 592.
(22) Smeal, M. G. & Donald, A. D. (1984) *Parasitology*, *89*, 577.
(23) Waller, P. J. & Thomas, R. J. (1981) *Vet. Parasitol.*, *9*, 47.
(24) Wagland, B. M. et al. (1984) *Int. J. Parasitol.* *14*, 39.
(25) Petrie, L. et al. (1984) *Vet. Rec.*, *114*, 168.
(26) Poppi, D. P. et al. (1985) *J. comp. Pathol.*, *95*, 453.
(27) Barker, I. K. & Titchen, D. A. (1982) *Int. J. Parasitol.*, *12*, 345.
(28) Hucker, D. A. & Yong, W. K. (1986) *Vet. Parasitol.*, *19*, 67.
(29) Entrocasso, C. et al. (1986) *Vet. Parasitol.*, *21*,173.
(30) Jacobs, D. E. et al. (1987) *Vet. Rec.*, *120*, 29.
(31) Saunders, L. Z. et al. (1974) *Cornell Vet.*, *64*, Suppl. 4, 7.
(32) Johns, J. D. & Philip, J. R. (1977) *Proc. 8th int. Conf. World Assoc. Adv. vet. Parasitol., Sydney*, 58.
(33) Armour, J. et al. (1981) *Vet. Rec.*, *108*, 532.
(34) Brown, D. C. et al. (1984) *Vet. Rec.*, *114*, 58.
(35) Darvill, F. M. et al. (1978) *Aust. vet. J.*, *54*, 575.
(36) Brunsdon, R. V. & Vlassof, A. (1981). *NZ vet J.*, *29*, 139.
(37) Brunsdon, R. V. (1968) *NZ vet. J.*, *16*, 176.
(38) Anderson, N. et al. (1976) *Aust. vet. J.*, *52*, 174.
(39) Mitchell, G. B. B. & Fitzsimmons, J. (1983) *Res. vet. Sci.*, *35*, 100.
(40) Callinan, A. P. L. et al. (1982) *Agric. Syst.*, *9*, 199.
(41) Thomas, R. J. et al. (1986) *Vet. Parasitol.*, *21*, 127.
(42) Herd, R. P. (1985) *Mod. vet. Pract.*, *66*, 741.

HAEMONCHOSIS (BARBER'S POLE WORM)

Haemonchosis is an important disease of sheep, goats and cattle wherever they are kept but the disease exerts its greatest economic effect in sheep in temperate and tropical countries especially where there is a good summer rainfall. It is not uncommon for serious outbreaks to occur in colder climates such as those of Canada and the United States when humidity is high in summer. The disease is uncommon in semi-arid regions. Haemonchosis causes heavy death losses and poor growth and production. In sheep, losses occur mostly in lambs, especially those recently weaned, but yearlings and mature sheep may also be affected. Poor growth in lambs results when their ewes' milk production is restricted by a heavy infestation. Dairy calves are the most commonly affected group amongst cattle but steers and other young cattle up to 3 years of age may also be affected. The disease is characterized clinically by severe anemia and anasarca. A chronic wasting disease has also been described (1).

Etiology

Sheep, cattle and goats are all affected by haemonchosis. *Haemonchus contortus* is the species most commonly found in sheep and goats. It inhabits the abomasum and is easily seen, being 1–2·5 cm long and relatively thick. Adult males are homogeneously red, the females are a spiral red and white. *H. placei* also develops well in sheep and causes clinical haemonchosis but of less severity than that caused by *H. contortus*. *H. placei* is the usual *Haemonchus* spp. in cattle, and also inhabits the abomasum. *H. contortus* may also be present but usually only when the cattle are grazing the same pasture as sheep or goats.The infestations are usually not as heavy and are eliminated sooner than *H. placei* infestations. In goats, *Trypanosoma congolense* infection has been shown to increase the susceptibility to *H. contortus* (15). Infestations with *Mecistocirrus digitatus* occur in the Orient and in Central America. Adults of this species inhabit the abomasum of sheep, cattle and buffalo and cause a disease very similar to haemonchosis.

Haemonchosis is for the most part a primary parasitosis, predisposing causes for infestation including overcrowding, lush pasture and hot, humid climatic conditions. However, development of clinical illness is favored by a fall in the plane of nutrition particularly in calves. This infestation can occur in several ways. Lambs in excellent condition and running on the very best pasture may be suddenly overcome by a massive infestation. In sheep this is by far the most important occurrence of the disease but sheep in poor condition may become clinically affected by a worm burden which would not bother a fat sheep. Under excellent nutritional conditions cattle may develop a subclinical infestation but when the pasture subsequently fails the disease appears.

The importance of diet as a predisposing cause has been debated but there is good evidence that lambs on a low protein diet are less able to withstand the pathogenic effects of infection (5) than with a normal diet; the worms become established more readily and persist for longer periods. Diets as low as this in protein are commonly encountered in range sheep and cattle. Sudden depression of the protein content of the diet can cause a serious fall of resistance in an animal and permit progression of a latent infestation. It will also exacerbate the disease which causes serious hypoproteinemia due to the blood loss caused by the worm. This may be why the epizootiology in calves differs somewhat from that in sheep, heavy infestations occurring in summer but clinical signs not appearing until winter when the plane of nutrition declines. The cobalt status of sheep is also important in haemonchosis, animals on a cobalt-deficient diet being less susceptible to the effects of infestation with *H.contortus* (2). Hayfree rations have been shown to inhibit fertile egg production, the inhibition being overcome by the addition of 5% alfalfa (3).

Lifecycle and epidemiology

As in other trichostrongylid worms the lifecycle is direct, infestation of the host occurring by the ingestion of food contaminated by infective larvae. Adult *H. contortus* are prolific egg-layers, individual females laying up to 10 000 eggs per day for several months and under optimum climatic conditions gross contamination of the pasture can occur in a very short time. Several geographical strains of *H.contortus* have been reported, each with different hatching requirements. The egg hatches and passes through two non-infective larval stages in 4 days under optimal conditions but in less suitable environments this may be prolonged. For example, in Scotland the shortest period required for development from egg to third stage larva is 2 weeks and may be a great deal longer. Preinfective larvae are susceptible to desiccation while the infective larvae withstand desiccation better than those of *T. colubriformis* but do not withstand winter temperatures as well (4). Infective larvae migrate best in hot moist conditions. Some larvae can be found 90 cm from fecal pellets in 24 hours but more than 90% are found within 10 cm of the feces and the number decreases logarithmically as the distance from the feces increases (16). After ingestion the larvae migrate into the abomasal mucosa and develop into fourth stage larvae. They may become hypobiotic or develop through to maturity and commence egg laying in about 18 days depending on seasonal conditions. Egg production increases until maximum egg output is reached at 25–30 days. The lifecycle of *H. placei* is similar except that in cattle the first eggs do not appear in the feces until the 26th day after infestation, rising to a peak at 6–7 weeks and declining rapidly to low levels by 11–14 weeks.

A great deal of effort has been devoted to determining the conditions in which haemonchosis occurs in sheep so that outbreaks can be predicted and preventive measures taken. Bioclimatographs have been produced for different geographic areas and it has been accepted that months which have a mean maximum temperature of 18°C (64°F) with rainfall over 5·25 cm are those in which outbreaks may occur. This has been shown to refer particularly to areas with narrow diurnal temperature fluctuations and where wide fluctuations occur the best temperature criterion may be a mean minimum temperature of 10°C (50°F) (6). Thus outbreaks are more likely to occur in wet hot conditions where cold nights are not encountered.

Hypobiosis occurs with *H. contortus* and outbreaks of disease may occur in sheep that have been placed inside (7). Under field conditions larvae may become hypobiotic in the autumn and winter and remain so until spring, when they mature and commence egg-laying (8). This is an important means by which this shortlived worm survives the winter months (9). In areas with regular summer rainfall, larval availability increases from late spring to reach maximum levels by late summer to early autumn and quickly declines in winter. A similar pattern occurs in areas with more variable rainfall, but the pattern is influenced markedly by rainfall. It is not clear whether the etiology of hypobiosis of this species is due to environmental conditions acting on the larvae (8, 10) or whether a host effect is important (9). Other factors such as blood group of the sheep (11) and breed (12) may also play a part. In some areas where climatic conditions are not adverse to the freeliving stages, hypobiosis may not occur and intake of larvae is related to rainfall.

Development of a strong sensitivity to *H. contortus* has been demonstrated in sheep and self-cure occurs under natural conditions. Classically, self-cure occurs in sheep when a dose of infective larvae is superimposed on an established worm burden in a sensitized animal. This results in expulsion of the adult worms and may also, although not invariably, eliminate the incoming larvae. Self-cure may also expel existing *O. circumcincta* and *T. axei* from the abomasum and *Trichostrongylus* spp. from the small intestine. Investigation of the self-cure reaction has been hindered by the lack of a predictable system for reproducing the phenomenon (24). Recent evidence suggests a relationship between blood type and resistance and the ability to mount a self-cure reaction (11). It has been suggested that climatic or pastoral changes are themselves sufficient stimulus for a self-cure (13). Strain or breed differences occur (17) and a genetic resistance operating primarily against worm establishment and probably controlled by the immune response has been reported (18). Prior infection with *T. axei* but not *O. circumcincta* or *H. placei* has been shown to protect against *H. contortus* in sheep (19). A complete self-cure, due to *H. placei*, does not occur in calves but after an initial infection there is a rapid decline in egg-laying, adults are expelled and larval development is retarded. Immunity is much stronger than in sheep.

Pathogenesis

Both fourth stage larvae and adults are vigorous blood suckers and by passing large amounts of the host's blood through their alimentary tracts cause loss of all blood components including erythrocytes and plasma protein. Anemia and hypoproteinemia result. There is no evidence that any factor other than simple blood loss causes the anemia, although intravascular hemolysis and depression of bone marrow activity have both been suggested as accessory causes (23). The migration of the larvae into the pits of the gastric glands in the abomasal wall and the physical injury caused to the mucosa by the attachment of adults cause abomasitis. The presence of *H. contortus* in the abomasum appears to interfere with the digestibility and absorption of protein, calcium and phosphorus. There is a significant rise of abomasal pH soon after infection due to loss of gastric acidity and plasma pepsinogen levels rise at the same time (14), but never reach the levels seen in ostertagiasis. In continuing infections, the increased rate of red cell production is maintained at the expense of the animals' iron stores and a state of iron deficiency occurs. Death may be acute and result purely from blood loss or may be more gradual, be accompanied by weight loss and result from exhaustion of iron and protein stores (1).

Clinical findings

Lambs and young sheep are commonly affected by the acute form of the disease in which animals are found dead without premonitory signs having been observed. The mucosae and conjunctivae of such sheep are always extremely pale. More chronic cases show lethargy and muscular weakness, pallor of the mucosae and conjunctivae, and anasarca, particularly under the lower jaw and to a less extent along the ventral abdomen. Affected sheep are often noticed for the first time when the flock is being driven: they lag behind, breathe faster, have a staggery gait and often go down; some may die as a result of exercise but most can rise and walk a little further after rest. Grazing animals lie down a good deal of the time, often around the water troughs; the energy needed to walk and eat appears to be lacking. Most cases show constipation rather than diarrhea. There is a loss of body weight but this may not be noticeable and the effects on wool growth may extend for weeks before the period of infection. In the chronic condition there is extreme weight loss during the dry season when larval uptake is negligible. Sheep not fatally affected develop a break in the wool and the fleece may be lost at a later date. Calves show a similar syndrome.

Clinical pathology

In pure infections of *H. contortus* there is a strong correlation between egg counts and worm numbers (20) but counts have a negative binomial distribution. In field outbreaks the level of variance remains high as egg counts increase and this suggests that, in outbreaks of acute haemonchosis, only a small proportion of the flock may become seriously affected (26). However, in very severe outbreaks a large proportion of the flock may become affected if not treated. In mixed infections, eggs of *Haemonchus* spp. cannot be easily differentiated from those of *Oesophagostomum*, *Trichostrongylus*, *Ostertagia*, and *Cooperia* spp., and identification and quantification depends on counting larvae in fecal cultures, a procedure not readily applicable in routine diagnosis. Although egg counts of the above worms in the range of 500 epg in cattle and 5000 epg in sheep are considered to be pathogenic, it must be remembered that low counts of eggs may be encountered in gross haemonchosis when the bulk of the pathogenic worms are in the larval stage. Severe infestations, usually mixed, are accompanied by egg counts of about 10 000 epg.

Necropsy findings

Gross necropsy findings include severe anemia, gelatinization of fat depôts, general anasarca and the presence of large numbers of readily visible *H. contortus* or *H. placei* in the abomasum. If the cadaver is fresh the worms may still be attached or swimming actively in the ingesta but a careful search may be necessary if the animal has been dead for some time. There is a positive correlation between worm counts and hemoglobin levels but the number of worms required to depress hemoglobin levels varies with the weight of the sheep. In Merino sheep up to 20 kg, hemoglobin levels of 10·5 g/% is associated with 112 worms and levels of 8·0 g/% with 355 worms. However in sheep over 50 kg 355 and 1259 worms were required to give similar values (25). Counts of 3000 in lambs and 9000 in adult sheep are usually associated with heavy mortalities. The abomasal wall is hyperemic and blood clots may be present in the mucosa where larvae have migrated. Small ulcerations may be present where adult worms have been attached. The abomasal contents usually have a distinct brownish color due to the presence of free blood.

Diagnosis

In sheep other causes of sudden death, such as lightning stroke, snakebite, anthrax or enterotoxemia are often suggested by the farmer and can only be differentiated by necropsy. The other common causes of acute anemia in sheep include coccidiosis, in which diarrhea and dysentery are usually present, acute hepatic fascioliasis in which hepatic damage is characteristic, and eperythrozoonosis. Less acute cases have to be differentiated from nutritional deficiencies of copper and cobalt and chronic hepatic fascioliasis in which anasarca is more evident than anemia. Other parasitic infestations, particularly trichostrongyliasis, are characterized by diarrhea rather than anemia but infestations with *Haemonchus* and *Oesophagostomum* spp. commonly coexist and the soft manure caused by the latter infestation may be confusing.

In calves, coccidiosis, heavy infestations with *Bunostomum* spp. and sucking lice, hemolytic anemia caused by drinking large quantities of cold water, the ingestion of rape, kale and chou moellier, bacillary hemoglobinuria, leptospirosis, babesiosis and anaplasmosis are characterized by acute anemia.

Treatment

Many compounds are effective in sheep including all the newer broad-spectrum anthelmintics. Some strains of *H. contortus* are now showing considerable resistance to the benzimidazoles, and some strains have been shown to have multiple resistance to benzimidazoles, levamisole, morantel and naphthalophos (21). A strain partially resistant to rafoxanide has also been reported (22). Where benzimidazole resistance occurs the newer compounds such as oxfendazole and albendazole may still be active because they give higher tissue levels for longer periods than the earlier benzimidazoles. However, it is probably safer to change to ivermectin, levamisole or morantel which are chemically unrelated and act in a different manner. Where specific action against *H. contortus* is required at low cost, then the organophosphates may be used. Naphthalophos and haloxon have been used at a single dose rate for all classes of sheep but their poor activity against nematodes in the large intestine limits their wider use. Some of the new trematocides such as closantel, clioxanide, rafoxanide and nitroxynil have high effciency against *H. contortus* and may be used where *F. hepatica* is also a problem. Closantel and disophenol bind to blood protein and exert an effect against *H. contortus* for up to 2 months (27). Clioxanide is less effective when it enters the abomasum rather than the rumen and erratic results may be obtained with this compound.

In cattle where an injectable treatment is of practical advantage ivermectin, and levamisole or trichlorphon may be used, but ivermectin and levamisole have a much wider spectrum of activity and are preferred.

Control

Apart from the general recommendations for control of parasitic gastroenteritis as set out in the first part of this chapter, especially as they apply to the epidemiology of this disease, the important control measure in haemonchosis is strategic dosing to keep the worm population at a minimum.

In sheep flocks, treatment should be given at the end of winter to remove inhibited larvae before they emerge and contaminate the paddock. In those areas with severe winters which would kill most of the free-living stages, this single drench may be sufficient to remove the risk of an outbreak, but in areas where larvae overwinter on pasture and infest lambs in early spring, other treatments may be needed in spring and early summer to maintain low levels of infection in the sheep and prevent a build-up of pasture contamination.

As frequent treatments lead to the build-up of anthelmintic resistance, a program has been devised to control *H. contortus* by using closantel which has a sustained action against this species. Treatment in late winter to kill the hypobiotic larvae and those larvae overwintering on the pasture as they are ingested, with further treatments in late spring and late summer, gives excellent control in ewes lambing in early spring. Strategic treatment with a broad-spectrum compound must also be given prelambing and again in late spring to control *O. circumcincta* and *Trichostrongylus* spp. The lambs are treated with closantel and a broad-spectrum compound when they are about 12 weeks of age and again 12 weeks later. This procedure has been designated the 'Wormkill' program and has been widely accepted in parts of Australia where benzimidazole-resistant *H. contortus* are widespread (28). Disophenol which also has a sustained action has been used in other areas (29).

If no routine control is practiced and pasture contamination becomes high, the use of a sustained acting compound or the regular use of a broad-spectrum compound at 2–4 week intervals will be necessary.

The anthelmintic of choice will depend on the spectrum of activity required, the presence of resistant strains, cost and route of administration.

Although a number of investigations have been conducted on the efficiency of vaccination against *H. contortus* with X-irradiated larvae, the results have been disappointing. Parenteral vaccination of large amounts of worm homogenates plus infective larvae emulsified in Freund's adjuvant has also given poor results (30).

REFERENCES

(1) Allonby, E. W. & Dargie, J. D. (1973) In: *Helminth Diseases of Cattle, Sheep and Horses in Europe*, eds G. M. Urquhart & J. Armour. Glasgow:Robert MacLehose.
(2) Downey, N. E. (1965) *Br. vet. J.*, *121*, 362.
(3) Theuer, R. C. et al. (1965) *Am. J. vet. Res.*, *26*, 123.
(4) Levine, N. D. et al. (1974) *Am. J. vet. Res.*, *35* 1413.
(5) Abbott, E. M. et al. (1986) *Vet. Parasitol.* *20*, 291.
(6) Swan, R. A. (1970) *Aust. vet. J.*, *46*, 485.
(7) Field, A. C. et al. (1960) *Parasitology*, *50*, 387.
(8) Southcott, W. H. et al. (1976) *Aust. J. agric. Res.*, *27*, 277.
(9) Coadwell, W. J. & Ward, P. F. V. (1977) *Parasitology*, *74*, 121.
(10) McKenna, P. B. (1973) *Res. vet. Sci.*, *14*, 312.
(11) Luffau, G. et al. (1981) *Vet. Parasitol.*, *9*, 57.
(12) Knight, R. A. et al. (1973) *Am. J. vet. Res.*, *34*, 323.

(13) Allonby, E. W. & Urquhart, G. M. (1973) *Parasitology*, *66*, 43.
(14) Shoo, M. K. & Wiseman, A. (1986) *Res. vet. Sci.*, *41*, 124.
(15) Griffin, L. et al. (1981) *J. comp. Pathol.*, *91*, 85.
(16) Skinner, W. D. & Todd, K. S. Jnr. (1980) *Am. J. vet. Res.*, *41*, 395.
(17) Preston, J. M. & Allonby, E. W. (1978) *Vet. Rec.*, *103*, 509.
(18) Altaif, K. I. & Dargie, J. D. (1978) *Parasitology*, *77*, 161.
(19) Reinecke, R. K. et al. (1984) *Onderstepoort J. vet. Res.*, *51*, 25.
(20) Roberts, J. L. & Swan, R. A. (1981) *Vet. Parasitol.*, *8*, 168.
(21) Green, P. E. et al. (1981) *Aust. vet. J.*, 57, 79.
(22) Schroder, J. (1981) *J. S. Afr. vet. Assoc.*, *52*, 338.
(23) Hunter, A. R. & MacKenzie, G. (1982) *J. Helminthol.*, 56, 135.
(24) Adams, D. B. (1983) *Int. J. Parasitol.*, *13*, 571.
(25) Roberts, J. L. & Swan, R. A. (1982) *Vet. Parasitol.*, *9*, 201.
(26) Roberts, J. L. & Swan, R. A. (1982) *Vet. Parasitol.*, *9*, 211.
(27) Hall, C. A. et al. (1981) *Res. vet. Sci.*, *31*, 104.
(28) Dash, K. M. et al. (1985) In: *Resistance in Nematodes to Anthelmintic Drugs*, eds N. Anderson & P. J. Waller, CSIRO, Australia.
(29) Schillhorn van Veen, T. W. (1981) *Bull Anim. Hlth Prod. Afr.*, 29, 279.
(30) Adams, D. B. et al. (1982) *Int. J. Parasitol.*, *12*, 445.

PARASITIC GASTRITIS OF PIGS

The parasites present in the stomach of the pig are found in most countries but clinical illness is unusual and deaths and poor growth are only rarely recorded.

Etiology

Hyostrongylus rubidus occurs in most countries where pigs are kept; *Ollulanus tricuspis* is seldom recorded; *Ascarops strongylina*, *A. dentata*, and *Physocephalus sexalatus* occur in pigs in the United States, the Malayan peninsula, the East Indies and Australia; *Simondsia paradoxa* occurs in Europe and India. *Hyostrongylus rubidus* is a small (0·5–1·25 cm) thin, red worm, and *Ascarops*, *Physocephalus*, and *Simondsia* spp. are thick white worms 1–2·5 cm long. Young pigs are most susceptible but adult sows especially when lactating may also be affected. Although, among farm animals, pigs are the only common host for these worms, *H. rubidus* has been propagated in a calf and the larvae of this worm have been found in the intestinal wall of fowls, ducks and geese. In some birds they were present in very large numbers. It is possible that such larvae could complete their lifecycles in pigs fed on the intestines of infected birds.

Lifecycle and epidemiology

H. rubidus has a direct lifecycle similar to that of most strongylid worms. Eggs develop at temperatures between 10 and 27°C (50 and 80°F). In the United Kingdom, eggs deposited from May to October develop to infective larvae, and larvae can survive on pasture for up to 10 months. However the larvae are rapidly killed by desiccation and by freezing (3). Infestation occurs by ingestion of the infective larvae which enter the mucosa for 13–14 days during which time they undergo both molts. They then return to the lumen and the first eggs are passed 20–25 days after infection. In some circumstances larvae become hypobiotic and remain in the gastric glands for some months. *Ascarops* and *Physocephalus* spp. have indirect lifecycles; eggs passed in the feces of the pig are eaten by dung beetles in which hatching and development to infective larvae occur. Infestation of the final host occurs when they eat infested beetles.

A postparturient rise in fecal egg count of *H. rubidus* has been reported (1) but has proved difficult to reproduce experimentally (2). All reported cases have been due to a mixed burden of *H. rubidus* and *Oesophagostomum* spp. and it has been shown to occur only during lactation. It is not clear whether the postparturient rise is an important source of infection for the young pigs. There is a seasonal incidence of inhibited *H. rubidus* larvae but there is little evidence that synchronous maturation occurs.

Pathogenesis

All of these worms burrow into the gastric mucosa and cause some irritation but there is little evidence of clinical illness unless the resistance of the animal is reduced by poor nutrition or other diseases. Even then, infestations, with the exception of *H. rubidus*, are usually quite light. *H. rubidus*, having a direct lifecycle, may be present in very large numbers and, besides burrowing into the gastric mucosa and causing ulceration and nodules may suck large amounts of blood. Its effect on young pigs is not usually clinically apparent (4) although massive experimental infestation produce fever, listlessness, lack of appetite, diarrhea and reduced weight gains (5). The effect of *H. rubidus* on sows is still uncertain, particularly its role in the 'thin-sow syndrome'. If sows become debilitated the normal self-cure mechanism, that eliminates burdens at weaning, fails and thus parasitic gastritis may become a factor in the syndrome. In chronic adult infections, the mucosa is covered with a thick tenacious mucus and the rugae may be hyperemic.

Clinical findings

Young pigs infested with *H. rubidus* may show anemia, unthriftiness, poor growth and diarrhea (6). The appetite is poor but there is marked thirst. In adult sows there is emaciation, pallor due to anemia and often a depraved appetite. Poor reproductive performance often results and if the disease is not controlled, unnecessary heavy culling may result (7). Adult sows may carry heavy infestations without clinical illness but sudden death due to hemorrhage from gastric ulcers or to peritonitis by ulcerative perforation has been observed (6, 8).

As discussed under pathogenesis there are doubts about the practical importance of *H. rubidus* infections and the clinical pictures described above may subsequently need to be modified.

Clinical pathology

The eggs of *H. rubidus* are typical strongylid eggs and in the pig are indistinguishable from those of *Oesophagostomum* spp.; those of *Physocephalus* and *Ascarops* spp. are small and thick-shelled, and contain larvae when laid. Examination of larvae which develop in fecal cultures may enable an antemortem diagnosis of hyostrongylosis to be made if it is not possible to obtain a clinically affected animal for necropsy. Fecal counts of 300–1200 epg are recorded in *H. rubidus* infestations in adults and counts greater than 500 epg must be considered significant, but fecal egg count at the day of slaughter does not correlate with worm burden nor does the absence of eggs in the feces indicate that there are no egg-bearing worms in the stomach (10).

In spite of the pallor observed clinically in adult infested sows, there is no evidence of anemia in experimentally infected young pigs (9).

Necropsy findings

Adult *Physocephalus*, *Ascarops* and *Simondsia* spp. are readily visible but a total worm count should be done and an aliquot stained with iodine to determine the presence and number of *H. rubidus*. There may be several thousand of the latter worms present in the one pig. In moderate cases there is hyperemia of the mucosa which is covered with an excess of thick mucus beneath which the worms lie. In severe cases the mucosa may be thickened and edematous and covered with a diphtheritic pseudomembrane. Deep, extensive ulcers may also be present.

Diagnosis

The clinical picture of unthriftiness, weakness, emaciation and anemia of young pigs may also be the result of vibrionic dysentery, necrotic enteritis caused by *Salmonella* spp., coccidiosis, infestation with *Oe. dentatum* and malnutrition. A satisfactory definitive diagnosis can only be made on a necropsy specimen.

Treatment

Levamisole and dichlorvos, which have been widely used in the treament of pig nematodes, are active at their usual dose rates, while fenbendazole 5 mg/kg is also effective (12). Oxfendazole 4·5–6·0 mg/kg given in the feed is effective against all lifecycle stages in the pig (12).

Control

Standard hygienic precautions including frequent removal of manure, the provision of drainage in outside pens and rotation of pastures will reduce environmental contamination. Control of dung beetles, the intermediate hosts of *Physocephalus* and *Ascaris* spp., is impracticable.

To avoid the effects of the postparturient rise on young and old the pigs should be housed on concrete with an absence of deep litter and the frequent removal of manure (1, 7).

The sows should be treated just before farrowing to remove those worms that will contaminate the area for the young pigs and to eliminate a possible postparturient rise. Young pigs should be treated about 8 weeks of age.

A management system for an extensive piggery, which relies on the movement of treated sows in autumn and spring, gives good worm control and minimizes the number of treatments (11). In such a system it is important that a compound with high activity against both mature and immature worms in the gut wall is used.

REFERENCES

(1) Connan, R. M. (1967) *Vet. Rec.*, *80*, 424.
(2) Burden, D. J. & Kendall, S. B. (1973) *J. comp. Pathol.* *83*, 71.
(3) Rose, J. H. & Small, A. J. (1982) *Parasitology*, *85*, 33.
(4) Baskerville, A. & Ross, J. G. (1970) *Br. vet. J.*, *126*, 538.
(5) Castelino, J. B. et al. (1970) *Br. vet. J.*, *126*, 579.
(6) Dodd, D. C. (1960) *NZ vet. J.*, *8*, 100.
(7) Davidson, J. B. et al. (1986) *Vet. Rec.*, *83*, 582.
(8) Mouwen, J. M. V. M. et al. (1986) *Tijdschr. Diergeneeskd.*, *93*, 211.
(9) Stockdale, P. H. G. (1974) *Br. vet. J.*, *130* 366.
(10) Masaba, S. & Herbert, I. V. (1978) *J. comp. Pathol.*, *88*, 575.
(11) Rose, J. H. & Small, A. J. (1983) *J. Helminthol.*, *57*, 1.
(12) Enigk, K. A et al. (1974) *Dtsch Tierärztl. Wochenschr.*, *81*, 177.

HABRONEMIASIS (SUMMER SORES, SWAMP CANCER, BURSATTEE)

Habronema spp. cause a chronic catarrhal gastritis while *Draschia megastoma* produces gastric tumors. The larvae of both genera invade wounds and produce granulomatous lesions of the skin particularly on the lower limbs, the abdomen, glans penis or the eye. Massive larval invasion of the lungs causes pulmonary habronemiasis.

Etiology

There are three species, *Habronema muscae*, *H. majus* (*microstoma*) and *Draschia megastoma*, all of which infest the stomach of horses. Adults of the first two species are larger (1–2·5 cm); those of *D. megastoma* rarely exceed 1·25 cm in length. Gastric granulomas and most cutaneous lesions appear to be caused by *D. megastoma* although typical cutaneous lesions do occur naturally and have been produced experimentally in horses by the cutaneous implantation of *H. majus* or *H. muscae* larvae, but the latter only causes a transitory reaction. Horses of all ages are susceptible but the disease is most common in adults.

Lifecycle and epidemiology

The lifecycles are indirect, all species using flies as their intermediate hosts. *H. muscae* and *D. megastoma* mainly use the house fly (*Musca domestica*) but can use other muscid species, while *H. majus* usually passes through the stable fly (*Stomoxys calcitrans*) but *Haematobia irritans exigua*, *Sarcophaga melanura* and the house fly can also act as intermediate hosts. The eggs hatch in the manure and are ingested by maggots in which they develop. The infective form is reached about the time the adult fly emerges from the puparium. Horses become infected by taking in dead flies with feed or water or larval forms may pass through the proboscis of the fly when it is feeding on the lips or on wounds. Larvae that are swallowed reach maturity in the stomach while those deposited in wounds cause cutaneous habronemiasis. Stray larvae may be found anywhere throughout the body but occasionally massive invasion of the lungs is seen (2).

These worms have a worldwide distribution but are of importance only in warmer climates and especially in wetter areas where the intermediate hosts are common.

Gastric habronemiasis is relatively common and although it may cause sporadic deaths most affected horses show no signs of illness. Cutaneous and conjunctival habronemiasis are rarely fatal but may cause considerable inconvenience.

Pathogenesis

Gastric habronemiasis
The larvae of *D. megastoma* invade the gastric mucosa and cause the development of large granulomatous masses. These 'tumors' contain adult worms and have a central orifice through which eggs and larvae escape into the lumen. In many horses, the lesions cause only a mild chronic gastritis but in rare cases perforation may occur and is followed by a local peritonitis which may involve the intestine causing constriction, or the spleen causing abscesses. *H. majus* and *H. muscae* do not cause 'tumors' but may penetrate the stomach glands and cause a catarrhal gastritis with the production of a thick tenacious mucus. Heavy burdens may cause ulceration.

Cutaneous habronemiasis
Habronema spp. larvae deposited in wounds cause local inflammation and the development of extensive granulation tissue. Secondary bacterial or mycotic invasion may occur.

Conjunctival habronemiasis
Small granulomatous lesions up to 3–5 mm, similar histologically to the cutaneous lesions, form on the inner canthus, the nictitating membrane or even the skin of the eyelid (1). These can cause profuse lacrymation and other signs of local irritation.

Clinical findings

Gastric habronemiasis
There are usually no clinical signs, but affected animals may, on occasions, have a poor coat and a variable appetite. Large tumors may cause pyloric obstruction and gastric distension. When perforation occurs there is depression, a fever of 39·5–40·5°C (103–105°F) and pain and heat on the left side just behind the costal arch. Mild to moderate colic may be evidenced when intestinal stenosis is present. If the spleen is involved there is marked anemia and a gross increase in the total leukocyte count with a shift to the left.

Cutaneous habronemiasis
Otherwise known as swamp cancer, summer sores, and bursattee, this is manifested by the appearance of lesions on those parts of the body where skin wounds or excoriations are most likely to occur and where the horse cannot remove the vector flies. Thus they are most common on the face below the medial canthus of the eye and on the midline of the abdomen, extending in males onto the prepuce and penis. Less commonly, lesions may be found on the legs and withers but those occurring in the region of the fetlocks and coronary band are especially serious. The cutaneous lesions commence as small papules with eroded, scab-covered centers. Development is rapid and individual lesions may increase to 30 cm in diameter in a few months. The center is depressed and composed of coarse, red granulation tissue covered with a grayish necrotic membrane and the edges are raised and thickened. Although the lesions do not usually heal spontaneously, they may regress in colder weather and recur the following summer. There is little discharge. The sores are unsightly and inconvenient and cause some irritation.

Conjunctival habronemiasis
Lesions on the nictitating membrane may be as large as 5 mm diameter. The conjunctivitis is manifested by small, yellow, necrotic masses about 1 mm diameter under the conjunctiva (1). It is accompanied by soreness and lacrimation and does not respond to standard treatments for bacterial conjunctivitis. In conditions conducive to the development of flies extensive outbreaks with acute severe signs may occur.

Clinical pathology
Diagnosis is difficult in the gastric form of the disease because the larvae are not easy to find in the feces. Biopsy of a cutaneous lesion reveals connective tissue containing small, yellow caseous areas up to 5 mm in diameter. Larvae may be found in skin scrapings or biopsies and in ocular lesions can be found in the conjunctival sac or discharges. A marked local eosinophilia occurs.

Necropsy findings
Granulomatous lesions may be found in all the sites mentioned in the description of clinical signs, and although varying in size are of essentially the same composition as described under biopsy above. Horses which have had the cutaneous form of the disease may have small nodules in the parenchyma of the lung. These are hard, yellowish and contain inspissated pus and larvae.

Diagnosis
Infestations with *Habronema* spp. are strongly associated with infestations of both *Strongylus* and *Gasterophilus* spp. and it is difficult to differentiate the gastric form of the disease from these infestations. Cutaneous habronemiasis may be confused with fungal granulomata caused by *Hyphomyces destruens*. Both cause a proliferative inflammatory reaction containing masses of yellow to gray necrotic tissue. Other differential diagnoses are an overgrowth of granulation tissue and equine sarcoids. There is no other communicable conjunctivitis of horses.

Treatment
Ivermectin 0·2 mg/kg has high efficiency against adult and immature *Habronema* and *D. megastoma* and is the only compound that will remove these species at a single treatment (3). Fenbendazole used at 10 mg/kg for 5 days has high efficiency against *D.megastoma* and possibly *Habronema* spp. (5). Older treatments such as carbon bisulfide 2·5 ml/45 kg body weight have been superseded. Cutaneous habronemiasis is effectively treated by ivermectin 0·2 mg/kg, but some horses may require a second dose (6).

Control
Interruption of the lifecycle by careful disposal of horse manure and control of the fly population are obvious measures. In enzootic areas all skin wounds and excoriations should be treated to promote healing and protect them against flies.

REFERENCES

(1) Rebhun, W. C. et al. (1981) *J. Am. vet. Med. Assoc.*, *179*, 469.
(2) Bain, A. M. et al. (1969) *Aust. vet. J.*, *45*, 101.
(3) Drudge, J. H. et al. (1984) *Am. J. vet. Res.*, *45*, 2267.
(4) Wheat, J. D. (1961) *Vet. med.*, *56*, 477.
(5) Lyons, E. T. et al. (1983) *Am. J. vet. Res.*, *44*, 1058.
(6) Herd, R. P. & Donham, J. C. (1981) *Am. J. vet. Res.*, *42*, 1953.

MISCELLANEOUS HELMINTH INFESTATIONS

Oxyuriasis

Infestation of the horse by the worm *Oxyuris equi* is a disease of stabled horses. It is not a serious disease, but its major manifestation, that of intense irritation of the perianal region, is annoying and may cause disfigurement of valuable animals. Affected horses rub and bite their tails, causing loss of hair at the base and sometimes physical damage to the tissues of the area. The mature worms are gray in color and inhabit the cecum and colon. The male worm is about 1·2 cm long, but the female is much longer, up to 15 cm, and has a long thread-like tail.

The lifecycle is simple. Mature females migrate down the gut and crawl onto the perianal area where they lay their eggs in yellow patches of egg clusters. An embryo develops in the egg in about 3 days under favorable conditions and is then infective. Infestation occurs by ingestion of these eggs either by biting at the area or by feeding on contaminated material. The eggs resist desiccation, may be airborne in dust and remain viable in stables for long periods. Diagnosis is by detection of the operculated eggs, which may be flattened on one side, in scrapings from around the anus, or by the presence of worms in the feces.

Treatment comprises the application of a mild disinfectant ointment to the perianal region and the administration of a piperazine compound (200 mg/kg body weight up to a maximum of 80 g) or thiabendazole (44 mg/kg body weight), the latter being more effective. Cambendazole, mebendazole, oxibendazole, febantel, fenbendazole, pyrantel, oxfendazole, ivermectin and dichlorvos are also effective.

Strongyloidosis

Infestations of farm animals with *Strongyloides* spp. are recorded from most countries and although their overall economic importance does not appear to be very great, individual outbreaks occur in pigs, foals, calves and lambs. *Strongyloides papillosus* occurs in sheep and cattle, *S. ransomi* in pigs, and *S. westeri* in horses. All are parasites of the small intestine. Mature females lay their shelled eggs containing embryos, and these may hatch in the intestine. The larvae may be parasitic or nonparasitic and the latter forms lead to male and female adults and a freeliving cycle. Eventually, parasitic forms are produced and these infect the hosts either orally or by skin penetration. Young animals are infected via the milk (1, 2) and mature egg-laying females may be present from about a week after birth. After skin penetration, the larvae travel via the capillaries to the lungs where they break into the alveoli, travel via the air passages to the pharynx and are then swallowed. During their migration through the skin heavy infestations may cause dermatitis and, in bulls, balanoposthitis may be seen. It has been suggested that the larvae of *S. westeri* disrupt skin integrity of the foal and allow the entry of *Corynebacterium* (*Rhodococcus*) *equi* and the development of a lymphangitis (3).

In young animals diarrhea is the most common sign of infestation. Experimental infections in calves cause pallor and coughing (4) and in lambs dermatitis, pulmonary hemorrhage and enteritis occur. Sheep may also develop lameness or be more susceptible to footrot when subject to heavy infestations. Pigs may show anorexia, listlessness and anemia but diarrhea is the principal clinical sign. Infestation in pigs has been shown to reduce intestinal enzyme activity, to increase intestinal plasma and blood loss and to reduce protein synthesis in the liver (5). In foals diarrhea occurs and no relationship could be found between this diarrhea and the first heat of the mare.

Thiabendazole, levamisole and probably most of the modern broad-spectrum anthelmintics are effective in eliminating this parasite. Thiabendazole, ivermectin (10), oxibendazole and cambendazole are preferred in foals (9) while these and levamisole, febantel or fenbendazole (6) are used in sheep. Levamisole and thiabendazole are effective in pigs. Control can be achieved in foals and pigs by continuous administration of cambendazole or mebendazole in the feed to the mare (7) or pig (8) respectively. The treatment of mares with ivermectin on the day of parturition did not prevent mammary transmission to the foals but markedly reduced egg counts in the foal. Treatment of infected sows was effective in removing arrested third stage larvae from the subventral fat (11). Control depends on the elimination of warm, moist areas such as damp litter or bedding, suitable for parasite multiplication.

REFERENCES

(1) Lyon, E. T. et al. (1973) *J. Parasitol.*, *59*, 780.
(2) Stewart, T. B. et al. (1976) *Am. J. vet. Res.*, *37*, 541.
(3) Etherington, W. C. & Prescott, J. F. (1980) *J. Am. vet. med. Assoc.*, *177*, 1025.
(4) Stewart, T. B. et al. (1968) *Vet. Med.*, *63*, 1145.
(5) Dey-Hazra, A. et al. (1979) *Vet. Parasistol.*, *5*, 339.
(6) Grimbeek, P. & Terblanche, H. J. J. (1980) *J. S. Afr. vet. Assoc.*, *51*, 49.
(7) Lyons, E. T. et al. (1977) *Am. J. vet. Res.*, *38*, 889.
(8) Enigk, K. et al (1974) *Zentralbl. VetMed.*, *21*, 413.
(9) Drudge, J. H. et al. (1983) *Mod. vet. Pract.*, *64*, 414.
(10) Ryan, W. G. & Best, P. J. (1985) *Vet. Rec.*, *117*, 169.
(11) Murrell, K. D. (1981) *Am. J. vet. Res.*, *42*, 1915.

Rhabditis dermatitis

Dermatitis caused by the larvae of the nematode *Peloderma strongyloides* is rare and is recorded most commonly in the dog. Several outbreaks in cattle have been observed (1, 2), and several cases have been seen in horses. Alopecia is marked, particularly on the neck and flanks. In moderate cases the skin on affected areas is thickened, wrinkled and scurfy and some pustules are present on the ventral abdomen and udder (3). The pustules are up to 1 cm in diameter and contain thick yellow caseous material, and larvae or mature worms. In severe cases affected areas are swollen, raw and exude serum, and there is marked irritation. Infestation is encouraged by housing animals on warm, wet bedding conducive to multiplication of the worm, and under highly favorable conditions the disease may spread rapidly (2). In these circumstances the lesions occur most commonly where the skin contacts the bedding.

The worm is a facultative parasite; that is, it can lead a free-living or parasitic existence, and usually lives free in the soil or in decaying organic matter. Only infrequently do the larvae invade the skin of an animal host. The nematodes are easily detected in skin scrapings or biopsy specimens, and in samples of the bedding, preferably taken from the top few centimetres in the pen.

Recommended control measures include frequent removal of manure from the sides of the body, frequent additions of bedding to avoid overheating and keeping the bedding dry. Spontaneous recovery usually occurs if these precautions are taken but local application of a parasiticide should be effective. Control of a dry exfoliative dermatitis in a horse was obtained by giving clean bedding, and treatment with thiabendazole and dimethylsulfoxide (DMSO) applied as a paint over the lesions.

Micronema deletrix is a small free-living parasite 250–430 μm which occasionally infects horses. Enormous numbers may be seen in granulomatous tissue which has been reported in the nares and the maxilla. The lesions in the maxilla may be sufficiently large to cause the hard palate to bulge, displacing the molars and causing difficulty in mastication (6). This infection must also be considered in the differential diagnosis of equine cerebrospinal nematodiasis (4, 5). Lesions in the brain are usually microscopic and consist of discrete granulomata with a vascular orientation. Sections of worms and larvae are frequently seen in the affected areas (5). Clinically it causes lethargy, ataxia, incoordination, recumbency and death (4). Diagnosis is made at autopsy.

REFERENCES

(1) Levine, N. D. et al. (1950) *J. Am. ved. med. Assoc.*, *116*, 294.
(2) Rhode, E. A. et al. (1953) *N. Am. Vet.*, *34*, 634.
(3) Farrington, D. D. et al. (1976) *Vet. Med.*, *71*, 1199.
(4) Alstad, A. D. & Berg, I. F. (1979) *J. Am. vet. med. Assoc.*, *174*, 264.
(5) Pletcher, J. M. & Howerth, E. (1980) *J. Am. vet. med. Assoc.* *177*, 1090.
(6) Cho, D. Y. et al. (1985) *J. Am. vet. med. Assoc.*, *187*, 505.

Trichuriasis (whipworm infestation)

Trichuris spp. infestations in farm livestock are usually considered to be innocuous. They all inhabit the cecum of the host and if they are present in large numbers may cause sufficient irritation to result in diarrhea, sometimes accompanied by the passage of mucus and blood. Experimentally produced trichuriasis in pigs causes a variety of signs depending on the dose rate of infective eggs; acute conditions cause anorexia, dysentery, anemia, incoordination, emaciation and death (1). It is suggested that a microbial component in the gut acts synergistically with *T. suis* to produce the severe clinical syndrome (2). Naturally occurring cases in pigs and lambs are recorded (3, 4), the clinical signs including diarrhea, anorexia, and weight loss. The mortality rate can be high in recently weaned pigs (5). A fatal case has been recorded in a heifer (6). The common species are: ruminants—*Trichuris ovis*, *T. discolor*, *T. globulosa*; pigs—*T. suis*. The life cycle is direct and eggs, which become embryonated, are very resistant to external environmental conditions. *T. suis* eggs can survive for up to 6 years in old pigsties, and for at least 2 years on pasture in the south of England (7). The disease in sheep occurs most commonly after hot dry weather which effectively cleanses the pasture of nematode larvae but the resistant *Trichuris* spp. eggs survive and are ingested when the sheep eat close to the ground to obtain grain given as drought feed. Hatching occurs only after ingestion, infective eggs producing mature adults in about 7 weeks after ingestion in pigs and 12–20 weeks in lambs and goats. Diagnosis depends on detection in the feces of the yellow oval eggs, which have a transparent plug at each end, and possibly adult worms which are 2–5 cm long and shaped characteristically like a whip, the anterior third being much thinner than the handle-like posterior end.

In sheep, fenbendazole (8) and ivermectin (9) are effective, while oxfendazole usually has high efficiency but may be variable (10). In pigs dichlorvos, fenbendazole, pyrantel and levamisole are used, while febantel used in the feed for 5 days is also effective.

REFERENCES

(1) Batte, E. G. (1977) *Am. J. vet. Res.*, *38*, 1075.
(2) Rutter, J. M. & Beer, R. J. S. (1975) *Infect. Immunol.*, *11*, 395.
(3) Beer, R. J. (1971) *Vet. Bull.*, *41*, 343.
(4) Farleigh, E. A. (1966) *Aust. vet. J.*, *12*, 462.
(5) Schoneweis, D. A. & Rapp, W. R. (1970) *Vet. Med.*, *65*, 63.
(6) Georgi, J. R. et al. (1972) *Cornell Vet.*, *62*, 58.
(7) Burden, D. J. & Hammet, N. C. (1979) *Res. vet. Sci.*, *26*, 66.
(8) Malan, F. S. (1981) *J. S. Afr. vet. Assoc.*, *51*, 39.
(9) Armour, J. et al. (1982) *Vet. Rec.*, *111*, 80.
(10) Borgsteede, F. H. M. & Reid, J. F. S. (1982) *Tijdschr. Diergeneeskd.*, *67*, 139.

Chabertiasis

Chabertiasis of sheep, goats and cattle is caused by *Chabertia ovina*, a worm 1–2 cm in length, which inhabits the colon and causes a clinical syndrome similar to that of esophagostomiasis. The lifecycle is direct, and resembles that of other strongylid worms. The non-parasitic larvae are relatively resistant to cold and heavy infestations may occur in mild winters. The infective third stage larvae exsheathes and undergoes an extensive histotrophic stage in the wall of the small intestine before passing to the cecum and then to the colon. About 26 days after infection, the immature adults attach to the colon and eggs are passed in about 7 weeks (1). The larval stages do not cause any clinical signs in natural infections although excessively heavy laboratory infections may cause diarrhea and anemia (2). Clinical signs are seen as soon as the immature adults attach to the colon, and soft feces with excess mucus and flecked with blood are passed. The parasite causes a protein-losing enteropathy with lowered blood albumin and weight loss. Death may occur in heavy infections (3). In heavy burdens clinical signs may be seen before the worms are patent or a sufficiently strong immune response may be provoked that will reduce or eliminate the production of eggs.

Changes seen at necropsy are thickening, edema and petechiation of the wall of the colon, with blood sometimes present in the intestinal contents. The worms are usually confined to the first 25–30 cm of the coiled colon except in very heavy infections. The number of worms present is often surprisingly small and severe morphological changes may be evident with only five to ten worms. More than 100 worms is considered to be a heavy infestation.

Chabertiasis is mainly seen in sheep in the colder areas and in the winter months. Infections can be seen in cattle but they rarely cause symptoms. All the newer broad-spectrum anthelmintics are effective against *C. ovina*.

REFERENCES

(1) Herd, R. P. (1971) *Int. J. Parasitol.*, *1*, 189.
(2) Herd, R. P. & Arundel, J. H. (1969) *Vet. Rec.*, *83*, 487.
(3) Herd, R. P. (1971) *Int. J. Parasitol.*, *1*, 251.

Neurofilariasis

This is a disease of sheep caused by infestation of the brain and spinal cord with the metastrongyloid worm *Parelaphostrongylus tenuis* (*Elaphostrongylus tenuis*, *Pneumostrongylus tenuis*, *Neurofilaria cornellensis*). The worm is primarily a parasite of white-tail deer in eastern North America although it may be spreading into western Canada. In deer the worm is found in the cranial subarachnoid space, cranial venous sinuses and occasionally in the spinal subarachnoid space. Eggs or larvae are carried to the lungs, undergo a tracheal migration and the first-stage larvae are passed in the feces. These are quite resistant and enter slugs or snails where they develop into infective larvae in 3–4 weeks. The lifecycle is complete when infected molluscs are ingested by deer and the larvae penetrate the abomasum, migrate, possibly along spinal nerves, to the spinal cord where they develop into adults and migrate into the subarachnoid space (1).

Infected deer do not show clinical symptoms but in sheep and goats the worm continues to migrate through nervous tissue causing limping and incoordination followed by almost complete paralysis of the hindlimbs or of the neck, body and all four legs (1, 2). There are no signs of cerebral involvement and affected animals remain bright and continue to eat. If given supportive treatment they may survive for at least a month. The worm also transmits to moose and other deer species and is responsible for the nervous signs in 'moose sickness' of these species (3).

The clinical signs in moose includes weakness, incoordination, circling, impaired vision, blindness, abnormal carriage of the head, paralysis, lack of fear of man and aggressiveness (3).

The experimental disease in goats may result in peritonitis, colitis, death within 2 weeks, but kids that survive later show paresis and nervous signs (1). No treatment is available. Ivermectin at dose rates up to 0·4 mg/kg have not affected adult worms in the meninges (5).

A related parasite (*Elaphostrongylus rangifer*) in reindeer causes paralysis and death in deer. Experimental infection of lambs and calves with this species has been described (4).

REFERENCES

(1) Mayhew, I. G. et al. (1976) *Cornell Vet.*, *66*, 56.
(2) Alden, C. et al. (1975) *J. Am. vet. med. Assoc.*, *166*, 784.
(3) Smith, H. J. & Archibald, R. McG. (1967) *Can. vet. J.*, *8*, 173.
(4) Bakken, G. et al. (1975) *Nord. VetMed.*, *27*, 220.
(5) Kohan, A. A. (1985) *J. Wildlife Dis.*, *21*, 454.

Cerebrospinal nematodiasis (lumbar paralysis, kumri)

Filarid worms of the genus *Setaria* are commonly found in the peritoneal cavity of most domestic animals. One of them, *S. labiatopapillosa* (*S. digitata*) of cattle, is reputed to invade the central nervous system and eye of other animal species and to cause paralysis and blindness, while *S. equina*, although of little pathological significance, has occasionally been found in the eye. A high incidence of *S. equina* infestation has been observed in horses in Europe and although no clinical illness was observed there was evidence of recent peritonitis at slaughter (1).

Etiology

S. labiatopapillosa, a long (5–10 cm), threadlike worm, occurs commonly only in the peritoneal cavity of cattle, its natural host. However, it can infest unnatural hosts, especially horses, sheep, goats and man in which it migrates in an abnormal manner, causing epizootic cerebrospinal nematodiasis (2), when it invades the brain and spinal cord. The disease has been produced experimentally in goats, foals and lambs (3).

Lifecycle and epidemiology

Although infestations of cattle with *Setaria* spp. are recorded from many countries the occurrence of cerebrospinal nematodiasis is recorded only from Israel, Japan, Korea, India and Sri Lanka, while a single case has been reported from the United States (4). Ocular filariasis appears to have been observed only in Japan. No details of the incidence of the two diseases are available but they appear to be quite common, the cerebrospinal form sometimes occurring in epidemic proportions, causing death in horses, sheep and goats.

Microfilariae are taken up from the peripheral blood of the infected animal by blood-sucking mosquitoes which transmit the disease to others. The number of microfilariae in capillary blood varies: in horses *S. equina* microfilariae are present in greatest numbers in capillary blood between 8 and 12 pm, at lower temperatures and at higher barometric pressures. All of these factors would probably increase the chances of spread by insect vectors and infective larvae have been shown to develop in *Aedes vittatus* and *Armigeres obturans*, but not *Culex fatigans or Stomoxys calcitrans* (5). In cattle *S. labiatopapillosa* migrates only to the abdominal cavity where it reaches maturity in 8–10 months. An occurrence of congenital infection in a goat has been recorded (6). Cerebrospinal nematodiasis and ocular filariasis are diseases of the summer and autumn when the vectors are most prevalent.

Pathogenesis

In horses, sheep and goats invasion of the eye may cause endophthalmitis (7) and of the nervous system an acute focal encephalomyelomalacia (8). Migration of the adult worm into the oviduct in cattle has been reported (9). The clinical picture which develops depends on the site and severity of the lesions.

Clinical findings

In cerebrospinal nematodiasis the onset may be rapid or it may occur gradually over a few days. There may be acute or subacute paresis with weakness and incoordination or paralysis involving the hindlegs most commonly, but sometimes all four legs. The onset may be sudden with affected animals dying within a few days but many animals may partially recover or show only a mild neurological disorder which may gradually become indiscernible. There are no systemic signs and the animals may continue to eat.

Clinical pathology

Antemortem diagnosis has been accomplished by detection of microfilariae in the bloodstream but false negatives are common, possibly as a result of the immune response suppressing production of microfilariae.

Necropsy findings

There are no macroscopic changes and sections taken from many levels of the spinal cord should be submitted to careful histological examination. Focal areas of malacia or microcavitation are seen and in areas adjacent to the malacic sites there may be loss of myelin, axonal swelling, degeneration and gitter cell formation (4). The tracts of migrating worms are indicated by necrosis of nervous tissue. Occasionally the whole or part of a worm may be found in a case where nervous signs have been present for only a few days.

Diagnosis

There are many diseases which are capable of producing a similar clinical syndrome. A feature of cerebrospinal nematodiasis is its occurrence in the late summer and autumn when insect vectors are most common. In horses enzootic equine ataxia (wobbles) is clinically almost identical, in sheep and goats paralytic rabies must be considered. In all species traumatic injury, spinal cord abscess and migration of other parasites, e.g. warble fly in cattle, may cause similar clinical signs. In horses migration of *S. vulgaris* larvae, infestation with *M. delatrix* or *Hypoderma* spp. must be considered.

Treatment

There is no treatment which could be reasonably expected to have any effect on the lesion but systemic anthelmintics may prevent further damage. Diethylcarbamazine (Caricide) has given encouraging results in early experimental work in sheep and goats, horses and cattle (10).

Control

Control of the vector mosquitoes is usually impracticable in those countries where the disease is common. Diethylcarbamazine (10 mg/kg body weight daily for 10 days by mouth) effectively kills *Setaria* spp. in cattle, and a control program to prevent cerebrospinal nematodiasis in sheep and goats by eliminating the worm from cattle in the area by the use of this drug has been recommended.

REFERENCES

(1) Jirina, K. (1959) *Dtsch Tierärztl. Wochenschr.*, *66*, 439.
(2) Saunders, L. Z. (1959) *Vet. Rec.*, *71*, 631.
(3) Shoho, C. & Nair, V. K. (1960) *Ceylon vet. J.*, *8*, 2.
(4) Frauenfelder, H. C. et al. (1980) *J. Am. vet. med. Assoc.*, *177*, 359.
(5) Varma, A. K. et al. (1971) *Z. ParasitKd.*, *36*, 62.
(6) Patnaik, B. (1966) *Ind. J. anim. Hlth*, *5*, 1.
(7) Ahmed, S. A. & Gupta, B. N. (1965) *Ind. vet. J.*, *42*, 140.
(8) Innes, J. R. M. & Pillai, C. P. (1952) *Br. vet. J.*, *108*, 71.
(9) Manspeaker, J. E. et al. (1983) *Vet. Med. Small. Anim. Clin.*, *78*, 109.
(10) Katiyar, R. D. (1960) *Ind. vet. J.*, *37*, 167.

Thorn-headed worm of pigs (*Macracanthorhyncus hirudinaceus*)

Infestations in pigs with these thick-bodied (0·5–1·25 cm), long (up to 38 cm) transversely wrinkled worms are not usually heavy and cause relatively little loss. They inhabit the small intestine and eggs passed in the pig's feces are very resistant to environmental stress, surviving for up to 2 years in average conditions. The lifecycle is indirect, the intermediate hosts being 'June-bug' or 'Christmas' beetles. The beetle larvae become infested by eating the worm eggs and a new infestation is set up in a pig when it eats an infested grub or adult beetle. Periodic increases in the degree of infestation by this worm have been related to the 3-year lifecycle of these beetles (1). The adult female commences egg-laying in 2–3 months, is a very heavy egg-layer and lives in the host for about a year.

Heavy infestations cause slow growth and loss of body weight and occasional deaths may occur due to perforation of the intestinal wall. The thorny head of the worm penetrates deeply into the mucosa and causes nodules that are clearly visible from the serous surface.

Treatment is rarely given as the condition is usually only diagnosed at necropsy. Sodium fluoride removes some worms and carbon tetrachloride has also been used. Other anthelmintics are either not effective or have not been tested. Suitable disposal of pig manure and avoidance of contact with the beetles that are intermediate hosts are the recommended control measures.

REFERENCE

(1) Swales, W. E. & Gwatkin, R. (1948) *Can. J. comp. Med.*, *12*, 297.

Thelaziasis (eyeworm)

Thelazia spp. occur in the conjunctival sac of mammals throughout the world and may cause excessive lacrimation, photophobia, conjunctivitis, keratitis, corneal ulceration and abscess formation on the eyelids (1–4). In horses it mainly occurs in young animals, up to 3 years old but in Kentucky, USA, 43% of horses up to 4 years old are infected (5). In those species that have been studied the lifecycles are indirect, *Musca* sp., particularly the face fly *M. autumnalis* (6), being the intermediate hosts, depositing larvae on the conjunctiva when feeding on fluid in the eye. The disease is mainly seen in summer and autumn when the flies are active and is usually more common is cattle than horses (4). The condition of cattle must be differentiated from infectious keratitis by finding the adult worm in the conjunctival sac or by microscopic examination of rinsings from the lacrimal duct. Treatments in the past have mainly been 1 in 2000 aqueous iodine solution or a 3% solution of piperazine adipate applied locally or by a catheter inserted into the nasolacrimal duct, or by manual removal with fine forceps. More recently levamisole 5 mg/kg orally or applied as a 1% eye lotion has proved to be highly efficient while 0·2% Lugol's iodine and morantel per os were ineffective (7). None of 15 new compounds tested against *T. lacrymalis* in horses were active (8).

REFERENCES

(1) Vohradsky, F. (1970) *Bull. epizoot. Dis. Afr.*, *18*, 159.
(2) Ladouceur, C. A. & Kazacos, K. R. (1981) *J. Am. vet. Med. Assoc.*, *178*, 385.
(3) Arbuckle, J. B. R. & Khalil, L. F. (1978) *Vet. Rec.*, *102*, 207.
(4) Patton, S. & McCracken, M. D. (1981) *Equ. Pract.*, *3*, 53.
(5) Lyons, E. T. et al. (1986) *Am. J. vet. Res.*, *47*, 315.
(6) Moolenbeck, W. J. & Surgeoner, G. A. (1980) *Can. vet. J.*, *21*, 50.
(7) Vassiliades, G. et al. (1975) *Rev. Élev. Méd. Vét. Pays, trop.*, *28*, 315.
(8) Lyons, E. T. et al. (1981) *Am. J. vet. Res.*, *42*, 1046.

Onchocerciasis (worm nodule disease)

Infestations by the filarid worms of *Onchocerca* spp. cause rejection of meat for human consumption, while their microfilariae have been associated with ocular and skin lesions.

Etiology

In cattle, *Onchocerca gibsoni* infests the subcutaneous tissues, especially the brisket, *O. ochengi* causes a dermatitis resembling demodectic mange and pox (1), *O. gutturosa* infests the ligamentum nuchae and *O. lienalis* is found in the gastrosplenic ligament (4). *O. armillata* is recorded as causing aortitis in cattle, Indian buffalo and goats in India and Iran (2). In horses *O. cervicalis* infests the ligamentum nuchae while *O. reticulata* is found in the connective tissue around the flexor tendons. *O. cervicalis* larvae have also been found in the cornea of large numbers of horses and occasionally in cases of dermatitis. The worms are thin and threadlike and vary in length, those of the horse being 15–18 cm long, but cattle species may be as long 75 cm.

Lifecycle and epidemiology

Microfilariae in the skin and subcutaneous lymph are ingested by midges, sandflies or blackflies (*Culicoides* or *Simulium* spp.) and the infective larvae that develop within them are deposited in the skin of other animals whilst feeding. The larvae migrate to their predilection sites where they become encased in fibrous tissue or, in the case of *O. gibsoni*, in nodules. Microfilariae produced by adult females remain in the skin or subcutaneous lymph but some are carried to the eyes. In man *O. volvulus* is a major cause of blindness in West Africa, while in horses and cattle, microfilariae have been linked with the condition periodic ophthalmia. However, most authors now agree that there is no causal relationship.

Onchocerciasis of cattle, Indian buffalo and horses occurs in a number of tropical and subtropical countries including South Africa, the Malay peninsula, India, Australia, the United States and parts of the USSR. A high incidence of infestation has also been recorded in cattle in Great Britain. In both *O. gibsoni* and *O. gutturosa* infections the prevalence increases with age, and sex differences have been noted (3, 5, 6).

Pathogenesis

Losses caused by *Onchocerca* spp. are slight although *O. gibsoni* in cattle causes unsightly trimming which causes rejection of beef carcasses from the high class meat trade. Hide damage may also be important.

The characteristic nodules of *O. gibsoni* consist of fibrous tissue canalized by the long body of the worms. Other species of *Onchocerca* cause the formation of fibrous tissue without producing nodules.

Skin lesions in horses are caused by a hypersensitivity to microfilaria. *O. armillata* is found in nodules on the aorta of cattle and the inner wall may be corrugated and swollen. *O. reticulata* may cause swelling of the flexor tendons and suspensory ligaments, particularly in the forelegs.

Clinical findings

In cattle there are no specific clinical signs other than the presence of nodules about 3 cm in diameter in the subcutaneous tissue. They are usually freely movable but may be attached to the skin. The brisket is the most common site but nodules are also often found around the stifle and on the lateral surface of the thigh. In infestations with *O. ochengi*, the cutaneous lesions are most common on the scrotum and udder.

In horses, new infections with *O. reticulata* may cause swelling of the suspensory ligament and a hot edematous swelling of the posterior part of the cannon which persists for 3–4 weeks. After the swelling subsides, the suspensory ligament remains thickened and small caseated or calcified nodules may be palpated. Affected animals are lame while the area is edematous and swollen, but many recover when the swelling disappears. *O. cervicalis* causes fibrotic, caseous and calcified lesions in the ligamentum nuchae but clinical signs are not seen. The relationship between microfilariae in the eye of horses and periodic ophthalmia must be regarded as not proven, as the condition occurs in the absence of microfilariae and when present they do not cause any reaction.

Lesions in horses, due to *O. cervicalis* microfilariae hypersensitivity, are characterized by alopecia, scaliness and pruritis particularly along the ventral abdomen. They may extend between the forelegs and backlegs and include the thigh, and in severe cases they may extend up the lower abdominal wall. Some horses have lesions on the face, neck or thorax (7). In mild cases lesions may be confined to the forehead (8).

Clinical pathology

Microfilariae are not detectable in the bloodstream but excision of a subcutaneous nodule will show the presence of an adult worm or debris, and microfilariae may be found in skin snips or in subcutaneous lymph. Large adult worms may be found in the connective tissue around the ligamentum nuchae during surgical operations.

Diagnosis

In cattle 'skin tuberculosis' and demodectic mange cause lesions which may be confused with those of onchocerciasis due to *O. ochengi*.

Control

There is no specific treatment for the adult worms. Ivermectin 0·2 mg/kg is the drug of choice to eliminate microfilariae in horses (7, 8). About 10% of treated horses may develop an edematous reaction restricted to the area of the lesion within 24 hours, and some may develop a ventral edema that is pruritic (7). Control of the insect vector is virtually impossible but valuable horses can be partially protected by housing at night, by the use of insect repellents and by avoidance of areas where the insects are likely to be present in large numbers. In cattle herds animals showing large numbers of nodules should be culled.

REFERENCES

(1) Bwangamoi, O. (1969) *Bull. epizoot. Dis. Afr.*, *17*, 435.
(2) Cheema, A. H. & Ivoghli, B. (1978) *Vet. Pathol.*, *15*, 495.
(3) Ferenc, S. A. et al. (1986) *Am. J. vet. Res.*, *47*, 2266.
(4) Ottley, M. L. & Moorhouse, D. E. (1978) *Aust. vet. J.*, *54*, 528.
(5) Ladds, P. W. et al. (1979) *Aust. vet. J.*, *55*, 445.
(6) Ladds, P. W. et al. (1979) *Aust. vet. J.*, *55*, 455.
(7) Herd, R. P. & Donham, J. C. (1983) *Am. J. vet. Res.*, *44*, 1102.
(8) Pollitt, C. C. et al. (1986) *Aust. vet. J.*, *63*, 152.
(9) Attenburrow, D. P. et al. (1983) *Equ. vet. J.*, *Suppl. 2*, p. 48.

Elaeophoriasis (filarial dermatitis of sheep)

Elaeophoriasis is a chronic disease of sheep characterized by dermatitis, stomatitis, rhinitis and keratitis and caused by the nematode *Elaeophora schneideri*.

Etiology

The disease is produced by microfilariae of *Elaeophora schneideri*. The adult worm, which grows to 120 mm, is primarily an arterial worm of mule deer and is usually found in the common carotid and internal maxillary arteries but has been found in every artery big enough to accommodate it.

Lifecycle and epidemiology

The disease has been recorded in North America (1) and Italy (2). It is seen mainly in sheep 2–6 years old, grazing at high altitudes during the summer months, but is more common in the 4–6-year-old group. Transmission from the natural host, the mule deer, is by the horse flies *Hybomitra* and *Tabanus* spp. (3). Larvae begin development in the sheep in the leptomeningeal arteries where they remain for 4–5 weeks after which they migrate into the carotid arteries and grow to maturity in about 5 months (4). Elk, white-tailed deer and moose also become infected and may act as reservoirs from which transmission to sheep may occur. The incidence in a sheep flock summering at about 1800 m is usually about 1% and losses result from the inconvenience of the disease and the scarred nodules that affect the market value of the skins. However, this figure will vary as management practices change and many affected areas are now grazed by cattle (1).

Pathogenesis

The longer lifecycle in abnormal hosts such as sheep or elk poses difficulties for those hosts. The longer sojourn in the smaller arteries can cause reduced blood flow and result in clinical signs of blindness, deafness, and circling. It also means that the larvae are larger when they pass through the cerebral retina to get to the common carotid or internal maxillary arteries and rupture of a rete artery, hemorrhage and death may follow.

In sheep the lesions are mostly confined to the skin, conjunctivae and the oral nasal mucosae although adult worms can be found in most arteries. This suggests a positive heliotropism or a requirement of a surface membrane for viability (5). The remissions and exacerbations of the itching associated with the disease are probably caused by periodic arrival of new generations of microfilariae.

Clinical findings

Mule deer usually show no detectable effects while sheep usually show a severe dermatitis on the poll, forehead, face and feet. Lesions also occur in the nasal and oral mucosae and on the cornea. Abnormalities of the eye include cataract, iridocyclitis and corneal opacity but sight often remains adequate in sheep but is usually lost in elk. The feet and ventral abdomen are other common sites. Initially the lesions are small, circumscribed areas of dermatitis but the irritation produced by them is so intense that scratching causes the development of extensive areas of bleeding, granular surface containing numerous small abscesses. On the feet the lesions extend from the coronary band to above the fetlock and cause much local swelling. Recurrent periods of quiescence occur and scabs form over the lesions, but 2–3 days later scratching recommences and the lesions are spread further. The course is long, often 7 months and up to 3 years, but recovery may eventually occur. Residual lesions include deformity of the hooves and bare, thickened patches of skin. Elaeophoriasis is a serious disease in young elk as the parasites normally live in the arteries supplying the brain, eye, ears, muzzle and microfilarial invasion of these tissues causes cropping of the ears, necrosis of the muzzle, antler deformity, central nervous damage and blindness.

Clinical pathology

Microfilariae may be detected in a skin biopsy by a maceration technique which may be followed by a peptic digestion (4), or by histological examination. Skin scrapings and examination of blood for microfilariae are not satisfactory. The number of microfilariae in the skin of sheep is always low and negative results may be obtained in known positive sheep.

Necropsy findings

A search for adult worms in arteries supplying affected parts can be supplemented by cutting the sheep's throat and allowing the blood to pass through a wire gauze to trap any free worms. The adult worms are not usually attached and cause no vascular lesions. Lesions, especially those in the oral and nasal mucosae, are often unilateral.

Diagnosis

Other forms of dermatitis, particularly photosensitization, contagious ecthyma, mycotic dermatitis and strawberry footrot, are likely to be confused with elaeophoriasis. The latter two conditions do not have the same distribution on the body, mycotic dermatitis occurring chiefly along the back and strawberry footrot only on the lower legs. No irritation occurs in either of these diseases. Contagious ecthyma lesions are restricted to the lips in most cases and have a characteristic granulomatous structure with a thick scab. Photosensitization lesions may have a very similar distribution and appearance to those caused by the elaeophorid filaria but there is usually marked edema and swelling and a history of access to photosensitizing or hepatotoxic plants.

Treatment

Systemic treatment with arsenic, antimony and bismuth preparations is effective. Most satisfactory results are obtained by the intramuscalar injection of 35 ml of stibophen (Fuadin) or antimony lithium thiomalate (Anthiomaline) (150 mg/g antimony) on two occasions 10 days apart (1). Unfortunately the death of adult parasites in heavily infected sheep may cause the death of the host, presumably by blocking branches of the carotid arteries.

Control

Avoidance of grazing sheep in close proximity to deer seems a logical control procedure.

REFERENCES

(1) Hibler, C. P. & Adlock, J. L. (1971) In: *Parasitic Diseases of Wild Mammals*, eds J. W. Davies & R. C. Anderson, p. 263. Philadelphia: Lea & Febiger.
(2) Micozzi, G. (1956) *Zooprofilassi*, *11*, 441.
(3) Clark, C. G. & Hibler, C. P. (1973) *J. Wildlife Dis.*, 9, 21.
(4) Hibler, C. P. & Metzger, C. J. (1974) *J. Wildlife Dis.*, *10*, 361.
(5) Jensen, R. & Seghetti, L. (1955) *J. Am. vet. med. Assoc.*, *127*, 499.

Miscellaneous filarial dermatidites (cutaneous stephanofilarosis)

A number of filarid worms, other than *Elaeophora schneideri* and *Onchocerca* spp., which are dealt with elsewhere, cause intramuscular subcutaneous and cutaneous lesions in domestic animals.

Parafilaria multipapillosa occurs in eastern countries, Europe, China, South America and North Africa, and in horses causes the development of subcutaneous nodules which ulcerate, bleed, heal and disappear spontaneously. The worm is up to 6 cm long and a blood-sucking fly acts as the intermediate host. The female lives in a nodule in the skin and pierces the skin to lay eggs on the surface. The hemorrhagic exudate from the nodule also passes through this lesion. The condition is relatively benign, occurring in the spring, summer and autumn. Many nodules may occur on a horse but they do no harm unless they interfere with harness straps. *P. bovicola* causes similar lesions in cattle in Sweden, eastern Europe, India, the Philippines, Japan and South Africa, and again the lesions are most common in summer. This parasite has been introduced into Canada in cattle imported from France. *Musca* spp. acts as the intermediate host in South Africa (1) and the prepatent period is more than 8 months.

The majority of lesions are superficial and localized and only require the removal of the affected tissue. Sometimes these superficial lesions cover the whole carcass and such carcasses invariably display intermuscular lesions within the fascia and lesions in adjacent muscles. Subperitoneal, abdominal, subpleural and thoracic lesions also occur although they may be localized. Carcasses with these lesions may be condemned (2).

The only clinical signs are the presence of bleeding points and a diagnosis may be made by examining congealed blood and hair microscopically for the presence of microfilaria-bearing eggs. Nitroxynil 20 mg/kg twice at 72-hour intervals is effective in reducing the number and area of lesions but care must be taken to ensure accuracy of dosing or toxic signs of drug overdose may be seen (6). Levamisole at 12 mg/kg daily for 4 days is active but less effective than nitroxynil (7). *Suifilaria suis* causes similar lesions in the pig in South Africa.

Stephanofilaria spp. also causes connective and subcutaneous tissue lesions. *Stephanofilaria dedoesi* occurs in the East Indies in cattle, causing a dermatitis called 'cascado'; *S. kaeli* and *S. assamensis* cause dermatitis in cattle in Malaya and India known as 'humpsore'; *S. assamensis* has also been recovered from dermatitis in buffalo and goat (3). *S. assamensis* is viviparous and the disease can be produced experimentally only by deposition of the microfilariae in abraded skin (4). The common site for lesions caused by this worm is on the hump which is frequently damaged when the cattle rub against rough objects. Lesions are also produced around the base of the dewclaws, each lesion having a superficial resemblance to a papilloma (5). The insect vector for *S. kaeli and S. assamensis* is the biting fly *Musca conducens*, while the horn fly *H. irritans irritans* is the vector of *S. stilesi* in the United States (8). *S. zaheeri* causes a dermatitis around the ears of buffalo, referred to as 'earsore' or contagious otorrhea. *S. stilesi* causes a dermatitis, mostly on the ventral abdomen of cattle in the United States. An unnamed species is widespread in Queensland, Australia, 38% of cattle in the eastern part of the state being infected. The distribution of the disease closely matches that of the buffalo fly, *Haematobia irritans exigua* which is the probable vector (8). Raised, circumscribed, hairless lesions are found on the head, neck, dewlap and sternum. *S. okinawaensis* causes a pruritic dermatitis on the muzzle of cattle in Japan and in some of these cattle a chronic dermatitis of the teat, characterized by a papule-like swelling with pain, an ulcerating core, hemorrhage, loss of skin pigment and hyperkeratosis occurs (9).

The lesions in cutaneous stephanofilarosis vary from 3 to 15 cm in diameter. Initially there are small papules which later coalesce to form lesions up to 25 cm diameter. The lesions are itchy and a good deal of irritation and rubbing are evident. Part but not all of the hair is lost and dried exudate forms a thick, crumbly scab which may crack with the appearance of bloodstained moisture in the crack. If healing occurs the scab disappears and a scar is left. Worms live in cysts at the base of the hair follicle and parts of them can be found in dry skin scrapings made after scabs are removed. Infection does not affect growth rate, and treatment and control is required only in stud cattle where lesions are esthetically undesirable. Ointments containing 40% trichlorphon (10), 4% Supona-20 twice daily for 15 days or once daily for 30 days, or 4% fenitrothion once daily for 30 days (11) are reported to give control. Oral levamisole 7·5 mg/kg once or twice at 3–4 week intervals was effective against muzzle and teat lesions due to *S. okinawaensis* (12). The disease is spread by flies and projected control measures must consider this.

REFERENCES

(1) Neville, E. M. (1985) *Onderstepoort J. vet. Res.*, *52*, 261.
(2) Kretzmann, P. M. et al. (1984) *J. S. Afr. vet. Assoc.*, *55*, 127.
(3) Patnaik, B. & Roy, S. P. (1968) *Ind. J. vet. Sci.*, *38*, 455.
(4) Srivastava, H. D. & Dutt, S. C. (1963) *Ind. J. vet. Sci.*, *33*, 173.
(5) Pal, A. K. & Sinha, P. K. (1971) *Ind. vet. J.*, *48*, 190.
(6) Wellington, A. C. (1980) *J. S. Afr. vet. Assoc.*, *51*, 243.
(7) Viljoen, J. H. & Boomker, J. D. F. (1977) *Onderstepoort J. vet. Res.*, *44*, 107.
(8) Johnson, S. J. et al. (1986) *Aust. vet. J.*, *63*, 121.
(9) Ueno, H. et al. (1977) *Vet. Parasitol.*, *3*, 41.
(10) Ivashkin, V. M. et al. (1971) *Veterinariya, Moscow*, *3*, 66.
(11) Das, P. K. et al. (1977) *Orissa vet. J.*, *11*, 16.
(12) Ueno, H. & Chibana, T. (1980) *Vet. Parasitol.*, *7*, 59.

27

Diseases Caused by Arthropod Parasites

GASTEROPHILUS spp. INFESTATION (BOTFLY)

INFESTATIONS with larvae of *Gasterophilus* spp. have a general distribution. They cause a chronic gastritis and a loss of condition, and reduced performance is often attributed to them. On rare occasions they cause perforation of the stomach and death.

Etiology

There are five species of flies of veterinary importance, *Gasterophilus nasalis*, *G. intestinalis*, *G. haemorrhoidalis*, *G. pecorum* and *G. inermis*, and their larvae are the parasitic 'bots' of horses. *G. intestinalis* is the most important species. The larvae inhabit the stomach and are thick, fat, segmented and about 5–12 mm long. They are creamy pink in color. The adult fly is brown and hairy, about the size of a bee with two wings and vestigial mouth parts.

Lifecycle and epidemiology

The adult fly does not feed and lives for 7–10 days. It is prevalent during the summer months and the various species may overlap in their periods of activity. In areas with mild winters the flies may be active throughout the year (1) while in colder areas fly activity ceases and the second and third instars remain in the stomach over the winter (2).

Eggs are attached to hairs while the fly hovers close to the horse. Fecundity is correlated to the size of the fly. *G. haemorrhoidalis* matures about 160 eggs, *G. nasalis* 300–500 eggs and *G. intestinalis* 400–700. Eggs of the various species are laid in specific locations and are attached in a specific manner, allowing identification of eggs to species. The eggs are laid on the horse's coat although *G. pecorum* may lay its eggs on inanimate objects in the horse's environment. The eggs of *G. pecorum* and *G. haemorrhoidalis* are dark brown, the eggs of the others are yellow and are readily visible glued to the hairs, usually one to a hair. The eggs of *G. intestinalis*, the most common fly, are laid on the front legs, particularly the lower parts: those of *G. nasalis* in the intermandibular area; the others on the cheeks and lips.

The eggs hatch in about 5–10 days and the first instars enter the mouth either by biting or licking or by migration through the cheeks. The eggs of *G. intestinalis* and *G. pecorum* require friction, which is provided by licking or rubbing, before they will hatch. The larvae are not swallowed directly into the stomach but spend some time migrating in the tissues of the mouth. The larvae of *G. intestinalis* penetrate the anterior end of the tongue and burrow in the buccal mucosa for about 3–4 weeks before invading pockets between the teeth or between the gum and molars (6). *G. nasalis* may also accumulate in pockets alongside the molar teeth and cause mouth irritation. *G. haemorrhoidalis* can penetrate the skin of the cheek and after wandering in the tissues of the mouth may attach in the pharynx. The second instar of *G. intestinalis* may also attach for a few days to the pharynx and the sides of the epiglottis before passing to the stomach. All species eventually reach the stomach where they attach as second instars. Occasional larvae migrate to abnormal sites including the brain, the cranial sinuses, the heart and lungs.

G. intestinalis larvae are found in the cardiac area of the stomach, where they become attached to the mucosa, usually in bunches. *G. nasalis* larvae are found in the pyloric region of the stomach and the duodenum. *G. pecorum* larvae may be found in the pharynx and upper part of the esophagus and in the fundus of the stomach. *G. haemorrhoidalis* larvae are found in the tongue, the pharynx and the gastric fundus.

In the host, two molts are made and the larvae pass out in the droppings 10–12 months after infestation, usually in the spring and early summer. Some larvae may attach temporarily to the rectal mucosa on their way through. The larvae migrate into the ground, pupate and adult flies emerge after 3–5 weeks to recommence the late summer attacks on horses.

Pathogenesis

The adult fly causes considerable annoyance when ovipositing. The droning noise and the sudden attacks to lay eggs causes head tossing and running. *G. nasalis* is particularly troublesome as it darts at the lips and throat.

There is some doubt as to the importance of the lesions caused by the larvae. At the sites where they adhere there is an area of thickening and inflammation and in rare cases gastric perforation occurs. It is probable that there is some chronic gastritis and interference with digestion in most infestations. *G. intestinalis*, the most common species, attaches to the squamous epithelium and this has a relatively slight role in digestion in the horse. However, the ulceration, edema and abscessation caused by this species (5) cannot be overlooked and one must expect some effect from such lesions although it is difficult, in practice, to separate these findings from those caused by a concurrent worm burden. The larvae do not remove sufficient blood to cause anemia, feeding mostly on tissue exudate. In very heavy infestations with *G. pecorum* the presence of large numbers of larvae (100–500) on the soft palate and base of the tongue can cause stomatitis and some deaths. Migration of first instars into pockets adjoining the molars may produce irritation or pain and may prevent foals eating.

Clinical findings

A non-specific syndrome of unthriftiness, poor coat, occasional mild colic and lack of appetite, plus bad temper and unwillingness to work is usually ascribed to bot infestations. Adult flies frighten horses by their hovering, darting flight, especially around the head of the horse, and may be a cause of shying and balking.

Clinical pathology

The eggs on the hairs can be seen by direct inspection but the presence of larvae in the stomach and intestines can only be detected after treatment with a suitable boticide.

Necropsy findings

A few larvae are present in the stomach of most horses at necropsy but clinical illness is usually associated with very large numbers. The areas of attachment of the larvae are pitted and the gastric wall thickened and there may be an adhesive peritonitis and attachment and abscessation of the spleen over such areas.

Diagnosis

The syndrome produced is not sufficiently characteristic to make antemortem diagnosis possible and bot infestations are commonly associated with helminth infestations which produce most of the signs observed.

A tentative diagnosis of infestation of the gums can be made by signs of pain on mastication and the presence of bot fly eggs on the horse at that time.

Treatment

Carbon disulfide 2·5 ml/45 kg body weight was used for many years, although its use requires fasting of the horse for 18 hours before medication and for 4 hours afterwards, and transitory abdominal pain occurred in some horses. This compound is now rarely used. The piperazine–carbon disulfide complex has been recommended but the compound is rarely hydrolyzed sufficiently quickly to provide carbon disulfide in high enough concentration to kill the bot larvae.

Many of the organophosphates are effective. Trichlorphon 40 mg/kg (3) is effective and is usually given with a benzimidazole to control strongyles as a common broad-spectrum mixture in the horse. It can also be used as a paste. Dichlorvos 37 mg/kg as a gel, paste or granule formulation has high efficiency (4). It also has high activity against ascarids when given as the gel or paste and good broad-spectrum activity when used as slow-release granules.

Ivermectin 0·2 mg/kg has high efficacy against *Gasterophilus* larvae as well as all gastrointestinal nematodes, including migrating and hypobiotic strongyles, microfilaria of *Onchocerca cervicalis* and larval stages of *Habronema* spp. and *D. megastoma* in the skin (7) and has gained high acceptance in horse practice.

Control

Treatment should preferably be administered after fly activity has ceased and the larvae have reached the stomach but before gastric damage has occurred (5). In most districts two doses should be given in winter, or in late winter and early spring. In foals showing pain on mastication, treatment with ivermectin paste or dichlorvos should be given as needed throughout the fly season.

The use of repellents or agents to kill the larvae in manure has not been successful, nor has bathing the affected hairs to encourage mass hatching and death of the larvae. The use of fringes, veils and tassels on the head harness helps protect horses against fly worry but is of little use in preventing bot infestation.

REFERENCES

(1) Drudge, J. H. et al. (1975) *Am. J. vet. Res.*, *36*, 1585.
(2) Hatch, C. et al. (1976) *Vet. Rec.*, *98*, 274.
(3) Drudge, J. H. et al. (1975) *Am. J. vet. Res.*, *36*, 251.
(4) Drudge, J. H. et al. (1972) *Am. J. vet. Res.*, *33*, 2191.
(5) Waddell, A. H. (1972) *Aust. vet. J.*, *48*, 332.
(6) Cogley, T. P. et al. (1982) *Int. J. Parasitol.*, *12*, 473.
(7) Campbell, W. C. and Benz, G. W. (1984) *J. vet. Pharmacol. Therap.*, 7, 1.

OESTRUS OVIS INFESTATION (NASAL BOTS)

The adult fly is a stout, dark gray fly about 1 cm long. Its mouth parts are rudimentary and it cannot feed. In North America, flies emerge in the late spring, mate and larviposit. Mature third instars leave the sheep in July or August, pupate and form another generation larviposting in the autumn. These larvae remain dormant as first instars over the winter to emerge the following spring (2). In temperate areas there may be one or two generations per year but several generations may be completed in hot areas. The fly deposits larvae around the nostrils of sheep and occasionally in goats. The larvae migrate to the dorsal turbinates and frontal sinuses where they remain for some weeks to several months before they migrate to the nostrils and are sneezed out to pupate on the ground. *O. ovis* are adapted to the various climates prevailing wherever sheep are kept. When winters are cold, the larvae can overwinter by remaining dormant in the first instar, but in warmer climates development may continue throughout the winter (1). The larvae are thick, yellow-white in color and when mature there is a dark dorsal band on each segment. The ventral surface has rows of small spines on each segment. The adult fly may emerge from the puparium in 4–5 weeks in summer but this may be extended in the winter. *O. ovis* may deposit larvae in the eye, nose or on the lips of man, and in some countries ocular myiasis or infection of the upper respiratory tract is an important zoonosis.

Adult flies attempting to deposit larvae at the nares annoy the sheep and cause them to seek shelter. Stamping of the feet and shaking of the head are common. Sheep may bunch together and press their heads into the fleece of others. In bad seasons the sheep may lose a good deal of grazing time. The spiny surface of the larvae causes irritation of the nasal mucosa resulting in catarrhal rhinitis with sneezing, a mucopurulent discharge, and difficult, snoring respiration. Secondary bacterial infections are uncommon but may cause occasional deaths. The infections are not usually severe enough to necessitate treatment but production losses and mortality have been recorded (3, 4). Control can be obtained by treatment in late summer to prevent the build-up of heavy infestations and in winter to remove the overwintering larvae. Rafoxanide 7·5 mg/kg (1), closantel 7·5 mg/kg, nitroxynil 15–20 mg/kg (5) and ivermectin 0·2 mg/kg (6) are effective and the use of these compounds for fluke or worm control also controls nasal bots.

REFERENCES

(1) Horak, I.G. (1977) *Onderstepoort J. vet. Res.*, *44*, 55.
(2) Rogers, C. E. & Knapp, F. W. (1973) *Envir. Entomol.*, *2*, 11.
(3) Sheherban, N. F. (1973) *Veterinariya, Moscow*, *2*, 71.
(4) Horak, I. G. & Snijders, A. J. (1974) *Vet. Rec.*, *94*, 12.
(5) Bouchet, A. & Dupre, J. J. (1971) *Cah. Méd. vét.*, *43*, 142.
(6) Roncalli, R. A. (1984) *Vet. Med.*, *79*, 1095.

HYPODERMA spp. INFESTATION (WARBLE FLIES)

Infestations of cattle with the larvae of *Hypoderma* spp. cause serious damage to hides, occasional deaths due to anaphylactic shock or toxemia and damage to the central nervous system or esophagus.

Etiology

There are two species which parasitize cattle, *Hypoderma bovis* and *H. lineatum*. The adult flies are heavy-set and hairy, about the size of a bee (12–18 mm long), are yellow-orange in color and have two wings. They are not easily seen because of the rapidity of their flight. Young animals are usually more seriously affected than adults. Occasional cases of warble fly infestation are seen in horses. The losses caused by warble fly have not been estimated recently, but in 1965 the loss was estimated to be $192 million per annum in the United States, and in 1976 approximately $100 million in Canada. In 1982 the cost of warble fly was estimated as £35 million for Great Britain and $85 million for Italy.

H. aeratum and *H. crossi* are similar to the above and parasitize sheep and goats in Cyprus and India respectively. Although the larvae of these two flies migrate through tissues they do not do so as extensively as cattle warbles, the eggs being laid on the sides of the animals and the larvae emerging at almost the same site. *H. silenus* has been reported to cause losses in goats in Russia and Greece.

The larvae of *Dermatobia hominis*, a small (12 mm long) related fly, parasitize man in a manner similar to the way in which warbles parasitize cattle. Infestations may also occur in most other animals. The habitat of the fly is Central and South America where it causes heavy losses in cattle. Larvae have been found on at least two occasions in imported animals in the United States but the fly does not seem to have become established. The larva is about 2·5 cm long and causes a painful cutaneous swelling. The lifecycle is similar in many ways to that of *Hypoderma* spp. except that the eggs are transported by mosquitoes and migration through tissues does not occur. Some strains of cattle in Colombia are completely resistant to *D. hominis* which points to the possibility of control by breeding. Treatment and control measures are the same as for *H. bovis*.

Lifecycle and epidemiology

Warble flies are common parasites of cattle in the northern hemisphere between 25° and 60° from the United States through Europe to China. *H. lineatum* favors a warmer climate and is the only species present in the southern states of America, while in the northern states and Canada both species occur. Infestations south of the equator are rare and are due to imported cattle although endemic cases have occurred in Chile (1).

Adult flies are active in the spring to late summer, *H. lineatum* usually appearing 3–4 weeks before *H. bovis*. *H. lineatum* usually deposits several hundred eggs attached to hairs on the legs or lower parts of the body while *H. bovis* commonly attaches its eggs to the rump and upper parts of the hindleg. Hatching occurs in 4–6 days and the larvae penetrate the skin and migrate through connective tissues to reach the esophagus (*H. lineatum*) or the epidural fat in the spine (*H. bovis*) where they stay, feeding and growing, for 2–4 months. They eventually continue their migration and reach the subdermal tissue of the back in the early spring. Here they make a breathing hole and after 1–2 months, during which time they develop to the second and then third instar, they emerge through this hole, fall to the ground and pupate. Adult flies emerge some 3–5 weeks later. The fully developed larvae are thick and long (25–30 mm), light cream to dark brown depending on age, with small spines on all but the last one or two segments. A single animal may have up to 300 larvae each forming breathing holes in its back.

The timing of the lifecycle, that is the period when grubs are present under the skin of the back and the time at which the flies are present in large numbers, varies with the climate and is of importance in a control program. *H. lineatum* generally is 1–2 months ahead of *H. bovis* and where the two flies are present both 'grub' and 'fly' seasons may be very long. In the southern United States the 'fly season' is February and March, in Canada June to August. The period when grubs are present in the back is December in the south and February to May in Canada. In Europe the larvae begin to move to the back in January to July.

Pathogenesis

Larvae maturing under the skin of the back form holes in the skin and the reaction of the host encloses each grub or group of grubs within a cyst of gelatinous material. On rare occasions an anaphylactic reaction may occur in a sensitized animal due to the death of migrating larvae and chance migration into the brain may occur. Intracranial myiasis due to *H. bovis* has also been recorded in the horse (2). Treatment of animals when the first instars are in the esophagus may cause a massive inflammatory edema which may prevent feeding and swallowing of saliva, eructation may stop and bloating may occur. Treatment of *H. bovis* while it is in the spinal canal may also cause edema and mild to severe paraplegia.

Clinical findings

If the fly population is heavy, cattle at pasture may be worried by their attacks and be prevented from feeding properly. Heavy infestations with larvae are commonly associated with poor growth, condition and production but such heavy infestations are often complicated by other forms of mismanagement including malnutrition and parasitic gastroenteritis. Infected cattle milk poorly and a considerable increase in milk production and milk fat occurs after treatment (1–3).

The presence of the larvae causes obvious swelling with pain on touch. The swellings are usually soft and fluctuating and about 3 cm in diameter. There may be as many as 200–300 such lesions on the back of one animal.

With involvement of the spinal cord there is a sudden onset of posterior paralysis without fever and without other systemic signs. The suddenness of onset and the failure of the disease to progress usually suggest traumatic injury. A similar disease can occur in horses and is reputed to be more common in horses than in cattle (4).

Clinical pathology

An intradermal test, using an antigen derived from first instar *H. lineatum*, has been developed to screen cattle for infection with first instar larvae (5).

Necropsy findings

The larvae are usually found in an area of tissue surrounded by a zone of red or green discoloration. Mature larvae lie in a cyst-like structure surrounded by a yellow, cloudy fluid.

Diagnosis

No other disease causes the characteristic swellings on the back. The differential diagnosis of posterior paralysis and anaphylaxis are discussed in detail under the respective headings of disease of the spinal cord and anaphylaxis. The clinical signs of organophosphate poisoning usually occur within 12–24 hours following application of the compound. Posterior paralysis due to destruction of the larvae in the epidural space usually occurs approximately 72 hours after application of the organophosphate.

Treatment

Systemic insecticides, particularly the organophosphates, have been the only means of destroying migrating warble larvae. These preparations can be applied by spray or a 'pour-on' technique, by individual oral dosing, by mixing in the feed or by attachment of dichlorvos-impregnated slow-release strips to the legs (6). They are highly effective but unless used in strict accordance with the recommendations of the manufacturer toxic effects may occur. Ivermectin, which has high efficacy against all instars, is now available and its use in worm control programs will play a major role in controlling warble flies (7).

There has been so much activity in this field during the past few years that it is impossible to make specific recommendations on the drugs to be used, the most efficient dose rates and the most suitable methods and times of application. Trichlorphon is the most commonly used insecticide in control programs followed by crufomate, fenthion, phosmet, bromophos, coumaphos and fenchlorphos (11). They are usually sprayed on but some can used as feed additives. Fenthion and crufomate have also been used in spot-on applications, i.e. low volumes of high concentration.

The time of administration varies with climate. The emphasis on timing is to provide treatment early in the autumn after all eggs have hatched and larvae are in subcutaneous sites. Later dosing means that the third-stage larvae, which are less susceptible to these drugs, may not be controlled and larvae killed in some sites, especially spinal cord and esophagus may cause serious illness.

All routes of treatment appear to be effective, including feeding in grain for 7 days. Administration in the feed has the advantage that individual dosing, often a problem in young beef cattle, is unnecessary but the method requires at least twice the amount of drug and individual animals may refuse to eat the treated feed, or in free-choice feeding be prevented from eating it, and have very heavy infestations of grubs.

Application in the form of a spray should ensure that the skin is wetted by using a pressure spray (20–30 kg/cm^2; and spraying the flat body surfaces such as the neck, back, shoulders, sides and thighs. Use of a low pressure spray or wash should be followed by vigorous use of a curry comb or brush. Pour-on applications should be made carefully along the midline in a thin stream which penetrates the hair coat. Spot-on applications of crufomate have been shown to be as effective as pour-on formulations (8).

Although these compounds disappear very quickly from tissues, recommendations are that they should not be administered to milking animals, and beef animals should not be slaughtered for at least 60 days after dosing. Milking cattle with back lesions can be treated with derris dust but this must be brushed in vigorously or sprayed under pressure so that the material penetrates to the larvae.

Toxic effects of organophosphates have been described elsewhere. The pitfalls in their use in warble control are related chiefly to the time of administration. If they are administered when the larvae are well grown, severe systemic reactions may occur and the dead larvae may cause severe local inflammatory edematous lesions of the esophagus or in the spinal cord (9). These reactions also occur in cattle treated with ivermectin at this time. These have been discussed earlier. Attempts to pass a stomach tube may cause further damage to the esophagus or even rupture it.

Dosing late in the season may also be accompanied by other signs of toxicity including staggering, mild bloat and salivation. In northern climates this is thought to be due to reduced water intake in cold weather. Severe signs and heavy mortalities, such as occur after accidental administration of large quantities of these compounds, seldom occur if the manufacturers' recommendations are followed accurately. The antidote is atropine sulfate administered subcutaneously, 1 mg/5 kg body weight. The frequency of reactions to organophosphatic treatment is about one in every 10 000 treated.

When small numbers of cattle are affected with relatively few warble grubs, manual removal of the larvae is practiced. Incomplete removal or breaking the larvae during removal may cause a severe systemic reaction. This reaction and the one which sometimes occurs after systemic treatment of cattle infected with warble fly has been ascribed to anaphylaxis. However, there is evidence that it is due directly to toxins liberated from dead warble maggots and that phenylbutazone may control this toxin (13). The clinical signs include dullness, salivation, lacrimation, dyspnea, wrinkling of skin on the side of the neck and edema under the jaw.

Control

While rotenone has been used successfuly to kill the larvae in the subcutaneous tissues in the back, this technique does not prevent damage to the hide and has been largely superseded by the use of systemic organophosphates. The progress in control of warble fly in seven countries is given in the review reference. In general, systemic treatments are given in autumn (between September 15 and November 30) and a spring treatment after March 1. Treatments in the autumn also prevent the buildup of lice.

Warble fly has been eradicated in Norway, Sweden, Denmark and Malta and its prevalence is negligible in Ireland and Cyprus. The control of warble fly in Great Britain and the European community has recently been reviewed (14).

Rotenone to be effective must come in contact with the grub. If the season is extended, treatments must be repeated at 4-week intervals. The material is applied by a power spray (180–270 kg/cm^2 pressure) with the spray held close to the skin so that the material penetrates the breathing holes. Care should be taken not to spray the eyes or a painful keratoconjunctivitis may result. If only small numbers of cattle are to be treated, a wash (2 kg derris powder per 25 liters of water) or a dust (0·5 kg derris per 2 kg talc) can be used but care must be taken to brush them vigorously into the breathing holes.

Vaccination of cattle using crude larval extracts has reduced both the number of warbles in the back and the number of larvae that could pupate (15).

REVIEW LITERATURE

Khan, M. A. (1977) *Vet. Parasitol.* Special issue: Eradication of warble flies, 3, 205–271.

REFERENCES

(1) Andrews, A. H. et al. (1978) *Vet. Rec.*, *103*, 348.
(2) Hadlow, W. J. et al. (1977) *Cornell Vet.*, *67*, 272.
(3) Riha, J. et al. (1978) *Vet. Med.*, *23*, 597.
(4) Olander, H. H. (1967) *Pathol. Vet.*, *4*, 477.
(5) Khan, M. A. (1981) *Can. vet. J.*, *22*, 36.
(6) Hunt, L. M. et al. (1980) *J. econ. Entomol.*, *73*, 32.
(7) Campbell, W. C. & Benz, G. W. (1984) *J. vet. Pharmacol. Therap.*, *7*, 1.
(8) Loomis, E. C. et al. (1973) *J. econ. Entomol.*, *66*, 439.
(9) Nelson, D. L. (1970) *Can. vet. J.*, *11*, 62.
(10) Hiepe, T. et al. (1974) *Angew. Parasitol.*, *15*, 57.
(11) Khan, M. A. et al. (1977) *Vet. Parasitol.*, *3*, 271.
(12) Khan, M. A. (1968) *Vet. Rec.*, *83*, 345.
(13) Eyre, P. et al. (1981) *Am. J. vet. Res.*, *42*, 25.
(14) Wilson, G. W. C. (1986) *Vet. Rec.*, *118*, 653.
(15) Baron, R. W. & Weintraub, J. (1986) *Vet. Parasitol.*, *21*, 43.

SCREW-WORM INFESTATION

Myiasis caused by screw-worms has been a cause of great financial loss in livestock in the western hemisphere, Africa and Asia. Deaths may be heavy in groups of livestock which are at range and seen infrequently.

Etiology

Larvae of the flies *Cochliomya hominivorax* and *Chrysomya bezziana* cause 'screw-worm disease' of animals. The flies are typical blowflies, *C. hominovorax* being blue-green with an orange head; *Ch. bezziana* is of similar coloring. *C. hominovorax* occurs in the Americas, *Ch. bezziana* in Africa and Asia. The occurrence of *Ch. bezziana* in Papua-New Guinea provides a constant threat to livestock on the Australian mainland. A similar fly is *Callitroga (Cochliomyia) macellaria* which is not a true 'screw-fly' in that it infests only cadavers or badly necrotic sores.

Epidemiology

True 'screw-flies' are obligatory parasites of all domestic and wild, warm-blooded animals and birds, laying their eggs only in fresh wounds. The navel of a newborn animal is the most favored site but fresh accidental or surgical wounds, especially those produced by castration, docking and dehorning, are readily infested. Wounds which have already been infested are markedly attractive to the flies because of their odor. In bad seasons the flies will lay eggs on minor wounds such as areas of excoriation, tick bites, running eyes, peeling brands and on the perineum soiled by vaginal and uterine discharges in animals which have recently given birth. Injury is not necessarily a prerequisite for screw-worm strike in sheep, which can be struck in the intact infraorbital fossa and vulva. Wool loss and tenderness may occur and the remaining fleece may be stained.

The development of the fly is favored by hot, humid weather. The optimum temperature range for the adult fly is 20–30°C (68–86°F). Below this the flies become sluggish and at 10°C (50°F) and below the flies will not move. Temperatures above 30°C (86°F) can be tolerated provided shade is available. The disease can be spread either by migration of flies or by shipment of infested cattle or other livestock. *C. bezziana* have been known to travel up to 50 km in wind-assisted flight, but usually flies rest on vegetation in windy conditions. In the new environment the flies may die out if the climate is unsuitable or persist to set up a new enzootic area. Persistence of the fly in an area may depend upon persistence in wild life or in neglected domestic animals, although the latter do not usually survive unattended for more than about 2 weeks. In many enzootic areas it is common for the fly to persist in neighboring warmer areas during winter, returning to its normal summer habitat as the temperature rises. This pattern is exemplified by the introduction of screw-worms into the southeastern United States in 1933 where they had not previously occurred. The flies died out in most areas in winter but persisted in southern Florida. In succeeding summers migrations of flies northwards caused outbreaks. The disease has since been eradicated from the area.

The disease is of importance in tropical and subtropical areas of Africa, Asia, North and South America, especially Central America, the Caribbean islands, Mexico and American states bordering on Mexico. The prevalence of the fly in enzootic areas places severe restriction on the times when prophylactic surgical operations can be carried out.

Lifecycle

The adult female fly lays 150–500 white eggs in shingle-like clusters at the edges of fresh wounds. Larvae hatch in about 12 hours and penetrate the tissues surrounding the wound. They mature in 5–7 days, reaching a length of about 2 cm, and then leave the wound, falling to the ground. The larvae feed as a group and at their time of maturation will have created a cavity 10–12 cm in diameter. Oviposition by other flies is encouraged by the presence of larvae already in the wound. The period of pupation in the ground varies widely depending on climatic conditions. It may be as short as 3 days or as long as 2 months. Emerging flies commence egg-laying in about 1 week, having completed the lifecycle, under optimum environmental conditions, in less than 3 weeks. There may be 15 or more generations per year.

The susceptible point in the lifecycle is the pupal stage which is unable to survive freezing for more than short periods and soil temperatures below 15°C (60°F) inhibit development. Temperatures below this point for more than 2 months cause death of the pupa. Thus the occurrence of the disease is limited to warm climates. Pupae are also affected by the moisture content of the soil. The emergence of adults is reduced when the moisture content is more than 50%, while temporary floods can drown pupae.

Pathogenesis

Following invasion of the wound a cavernous lesion is formed, characterized by progressive liquefaction, necrosis and hemorrhage. Anemia and decreased total serum protein results from hemorrhage into the wound (1).

Secondary bacterial infection, toxemia and fluid loss contribute to the death of the animal. Surviving calves frequently develop infectious polyarthritis.

Clinical findings

The young larvae invade the surrounding tissues vigorously and, unlike other maggots, burrow deeply rather than feed on necrotic superficial tissue. A profuse brownish exudate pours from the wound and an objectionable odor is apparent. This is highly attractive to other flies and multiple infestations of a single wound may occur within a few days. The resulting tissue damage may be so extensive that the animal is virtually eaten alive.

Affected animals show irritation early after infection and by day 3 show pyrexia. Animals do not feed but wander about restlessly, seeking shade and shelter.

Clinical pathology

It is imperative to differentiate screw-worm infestation from infestation with other fly larvae. The appearance and smell of the wound are significant but careful examination of the larvae is necessary to confirm the diagnosis. Mature larvae are 1–2 cm long and pink in color; they are pointed anteriorly and blunt posteriorly; two dark lines are visible reaching from the blunt posterior to the middle of the body and they have rows of dark fine spines on the anterior part of each segment. Specimens forwarded to a laboratory for identification should be preserved in 70% alcohol.

Necropsy findings

Superficial examination of infested wounds is usually sufficient to indicate the cause of death.

Diagnosis

The presence of maggots in the wound is usually apparent. It is important to differentiate them from blowfly larvae as described above.

Treatment

Affected wounds should be treated with a dressing containing an efficient larvicide and preferably an antiseptic. The larvicide should be capable of persisting in the wound for some time to prevent reinfestation. A number of proprietary preparations containing 5% lindane or an organophosphate are available; 3% coumaphos is as efficient as lindane and gives a longer period of protection against *Ch. bezziana* (2). Stirophos (15%) and dichlorvos (20%) give season-long protection in the ears of cattle against *C. hominovorax* and *Amblyomma maculatum* (3). An ointment or gel base is preferred so that as much of the medicament as possible is left in the site. It should be liberally and vigorously applied with a paint brush to ensure that larvae in the depths of the wound are destroyed. To avoid reinfestation in extensive lesions or in bad seasons the treatment should be repeated twice weekly.

When large numbers of animals are affected and individual treatment is impractical, spraying with a 0·25% solution of coumaphos, chlorfenvinphos or fenchlorphos, using a power sprayer, is recommended (4). The spray is directed forcibly into wounds and, except for young calves, applied generally over the body to provide protection for about 2 weeks. Young calves may show signs of toxicity if sprayed too liberally and application should be restricted to the belly. These sprays can be used to protect animals which are not infested but are exposed to considerable risk or are to be shipped to free areas. In the latter situation dusts are also available if spraying is undesirable in cold weather. A pyrophyllite dust containing 5% coumaphos and 2% mineral oil is effective as a protectant if applied at the rate of 60–180 g per animal. Residual protection lasts for 3–7 days.

Thirteen acaricides, commonly used for *Boophilus microplus* control, have been tested against *C. bezziana* larvae (6). The organophosphorus, carbamate and organophosphorus-synthetic pyrethroid products showed moderate activity, and while they are not sufficiently active to use as a primary treatment, their continued use for tick control would reduce screw-worm populations.

Ivermectin 0·2 mg/kg given subcutaneously kills all *C. bezziana* larvae up to 2 days old and many older larvae. It provides residual protection for 16–20 days. Bull calves treated with ivermectin at the time of castration were completely protected against strike (7).

Control

In an enzootic area the incidence of the disease can be kept at a low level by the general institution of measures designed to break the lifecycle of the fly. Surgical procedures should be postponed where possible until cold weather. In the warm months all wounds including shearing cuts must be immediately dressed with one of the preparations described under treatment. All range animals should be inspected twice weekly and affected animals treated promptly. Infestation of fresh navels is common and newborn animals should be treated prophylactically. If possible the breeding program should be arranged so that parturition occurs in the cool months. The routine use of ivermectin for internal parasite control provides protection for about 2 weeks (7).

In the United States an eradication program has been successfully carried out. Cultured pupae were exposed to the sterilizing effects of cobalt 60 and the resulting sterile male flies competed with natural males for available females which mate only once. *C. hominovorax* has now been eliminated from the United States and from most of Mexico where the program is to eliminate the fly north of the isthmus of Tehuantepec in southern Mexico (5).

Attractants may also be used to reduce the fly population. A chemical bait has been developed, and when combined with an insecticide forms a screw-worm adult suppression system (SWASS) which reduces the fly population and the incidence of strikes (8).

REFERENCES

(1) Humphries, J. D. et al. (1980) *Exp. Parasitol.*, *49*, 381.
(2) Spradbery, J. P. (1976) *Aust. vet. J.*, *52*, 280.
(3) Gladney, W. J. (1976) *J. econ. Entomol.*, *69*, 757.
(4) Drummond, R. O. et al. (1966) *J. econ. Entomol.*, *59*, 395.
(5) Anon (1988) *S. West Vet.*, *35*, 67.
(6) Spradbery, J. P. et al. (1983) *Aust. vet. J.*, *60*, 57.
(7) Spradbery, J. P. et al. (1985) *Aust. vet J.*, *62*, 311.
(8) Coppedge, J. R. et al. (1978) *J. econ. Entomol.*, *71*, 579.

CUTANEOUS MYIASIS (BLOWFLY STRIKE)

Cutaneous infestation by blowfly maggots causes serious loss of sheep and wool in many countries. The disease is sufficiently important that the term 'cutaneous myiasis' should be reserved for this condition and diseases caused by other members of the Calliphoridae, such as screw-worm flies, should be given other names. The cost of blowfly control and production losses in Australia for 1985 have been estimated as $200 million. A review of blowfly strike in Australia has been published and is given here as a review reference.

Etiology

There are a large number of species capable of causing the disease and they are grouped geographically below:

North America: *Phormia regina*, *P. terrae-novae*
Britain : *Calliphora erythrocephala*, *C. vomitoria*, *P. terrae-novae*, *Lucilia cuprina*, *L. sericata*
New Zealand: *L. sericata*, *Calliphora stygia*
Australia: *L. cuprina*, *L. sericata*, *C. stygia*, *C. nociva*, *C. augur*, *C. hilli*, *C. albifrontalis*, *Chrysomya rufifacies*, *Ch. varipes*

Lifecycle and epidemiology

Cutaneous myiasis can be a very important cause of losses in sheep in most countries where large numbers are kept. In bad years many sheep may die (up to 30% of a flock) and the expense of controlling the flies and failure of wool to grow after recovery may be a serious strain on the local sheep economy. Merino sheep, especially those with heavy skin wrinkles, are by far the most susceptible breed. *L. cuprina* is overwhelmingly important in the initiation of strike. Accordingly Australia and South Africa are the greatest sufferers from this disease. The problem is milder in Great Britain, New Zealand, India and the United States where *L. cuprina* does not occur or is less common because of climatic conditions.

In sheep, the incidence varies widely depending largely on the climate, warm humid weather being most conducive to a high incidence. In summer rainfall areas fly strike may be seen most of the year, being limited only by dry winter conditions, while in winter rainfall areas it is usually too cold in the winter and too dry in the summer for outbreaks to occur. Under these conditions abnormally heavy summer or autumn rains may be necessary before an outbreak will occur.

Two factors operate to encourage the development of the disease, a large fly population and the presence of susceptible sheep.

The fly population

Primary flies are of particular importance as these initiate the strike and provide suitable conditions for subsequent invasion by secondary flies. Tertiary flies are not of economic importance but may infest wool matted with dried exudate or feed on a healing strike. In warm areas pupae may hatch throughout the year but as soil temperatures fall an increasing number of larvae fail to pupate and larvae may overwinter until the following spring. In the spring adult flies emerge and numbers will build up to a peak in summer. Numbers may remain high if climatic conditions are suitable, moisture being of prime importance, but may fall dramatically in hot dry conditions. An increase in numbers may occur again in the autumn. Adult flies require carbohydrate and water to sustain life and, in addition, they require protein which is necessary for the development of the ovaries. The flies are attracted to sheep that have undergone prolonged wetting so that bacterial decomposition of the skin has occurred. The association of fly strike with fleece rot, mycotic dermatitis, diarrhea, urine staining and footrot is related to the excessive moisture deposited on the skin or to the production of serous exudates. Fractions of *Pseudomonas aeruginosa* infected fleece have been shown to stimulate oviposition (1).

Adult *L. cuprina* produce eggs in batches of up to 300, the actual number depending on its size and its ability to locate sufficient protein for egg development. The average life expectancy in the field in Australia is about 2 weeks and females rarely live long enough to mature more than two or three batches of eggs. The larvae mature in 12–24 hours and feed on the protein-rich serous exudate that has been provoked by bacterial damage or some other irritation. The second and third instars can damage the skin and their activity in extending the lesion ensures a continuing supply of food. When fully grown they are 6–12 mm long, thick, yellow and white in color and move actively. When mature, the larvae on the sheep fall to the ground, burrow into the earth and pupate, while those on carrion usually leave the carcass to pupate. The lifecycle can be completed in as little as 8 days in hot moist conditions but this is prolonged in colder weather. They survive adverse conditions as larvae or pupae (10). Primary flies breed mainly on sheep but will also breed in carrion, arriving soon after the death of an animal and depositing their eggs usually in the nostrils, mouth and anus. Many of the *Lucilia* larvae on carrion are eaten by predaceous beetles or by the carnivorous larvae of *Ch. rufifacies* which arrive later. Few *L. cuprina* result from breeding in carrion and this fly can be considered an obligate parasite.

Several generations of primary flies are necessary before numbers are high enough to cause severe outbreaks and therefore warm humid weather must persist for some time before severe outbreaks occur. Other primary flies are not as effective as *L. cuprina* in initiating a strike, and in Australia at least 85–90% of all primary strikes are due to *L. cuprina*. Primary flies, other than *L. cuprina*, and secondary flies breed in carrion or in rotting vegetation and their main role is to invade and extend the primary strike. *Ch. rufifacies* is the most important secondary fly in Australia. It requires higher temperatures than the other flies, is found later in the season and is the first to disappear as temperatures fall.

Lucilia cuprinais is the most important primary fly but *L. sericata*, *Calliphora stygia*, *C. augur*, *C. novica* and *C. hilli* may occasionally initiate strikes. The *Calliphora* spp. plus *Chrysomya rufifacies* and *Ch. varipes* act as secondary flies. The species responsible for strike in eastern Australia has not varied significantly in recent years.

Susceptibility of sheep

By far the most common site is the breech: infestation occurs here because of soiling and excoriation by soft feces and the urine of ewes. Lush pasture and parasitic gastroenteritis are predisposing factors but individual sheep are predisposed because of the conformation of this part of their anatomy. Excessive wrinkling of the skin on the back of the thighs and the perineum, a narrow perineum and crutch and an excessively long or short tail favor continuous soiling of the area and encourage 'crutch or breech strike' or 'tail strike'. Less common sites for infestation are around the prepuce ('pizzle strike'), on the dorsum of the head when there is excessive folding of the skin ('poll strike') and along the dorsum of the body ('body strike') in wet seasons when fleece rot is common. Sheep grazing on tall, dense pasture are commonly affected by body strike because of the way in which the wet plants keep the fleece on the lower part of the body wet (2). Wounds, especially castration incisions, docking wounds and head wounds on rams caused by fighting, are likely to provide good sites for blowfly strike. Young sheep are more susceptible. Ewe weaners are usually the most susceptible group and losses up to 30% may occur. Ewes which have recently lambed may be struck on the back of the udder where it is soiled with uterine discharges. In bad fly years the total number of sheep affected at these less common sites may reach alarming proportions.

Pathogenesis

Gravid flies are continually searching for oviposition sites. Odors emanating from moist skin exudate attract gravid flies in the vicinity. Searching and ovipositing flies give off pheromonal stimuli that attract other gravid flies. Eggs are laid in moist areas which provide the high humidity necessary for the eggs to hatch. The first instars feed on the exudate present, but later instars can cause severe skin damage to provide themselves with food.

The larvae shun light and burrow into the fleece surrounding the struck area. They also prefer an alkaline medium and prosper in decomposing fleece and tissues. From here the larvae burrow into normal skin and often undermine it, thus spreading the original lesion. They may also migrate from the original area of strike, along the surface of skin to set up another focus of damage. Many primary strikes remain small and may never be noticed by the farmer. Such covert strikes may outnumber overt strikes and are important as a source of future generations of flies. Once the initial strike is made, the site becomes suitable for the secondary flies that now invade and extend the lesion. The effects of strike include toxemia due to absorption of toxic products of tissue decomposition, loss of skin and subsequent fluid loss, and secondary bacterial invasion.

Clinical findings

Individual sheep may be 'struck' at any time from spring to autumn provided they are in a susceptible condition. Massive oubreaks tend to be confined to periods of humid, warm weather and are therefore usually limited in length to relatively short periods of 2–3 weeks.

The clinical effects of 'blowfly' strike vary with the site affected but all struck sheep have a basic pattern of behavior caused by the irritation of the larvae. The sheep are restless, sometimes markedly so, will not feed, and move about from place to place with their heads held close to the ground. They tend to bite or kick at the 'struck' area and continually wriggle their tails. If the area is large there is an obvious odor and the wool can be seen to be slightly lifted above normal surrounding wool. The affected wool is moist and usually brown in color although in wet seasons when fleece rot is prevalent other colors may be evident. In very early cases the maggots may still be in pockets in the wool and not yet in contact with the skin. When they have reached the skin it is inflamed and then ulcerated and the maggots begin burrowing into the subcutaneous tissue. Three days after egg deposition feed intake is reduced, rectal temperature rises to about 42°C (108°F) and pulse and respiratory rates increase. Some sheep may die. The wool may be too hot to handle as a result of the inflammation caused by the swarm of maggots that can be seen when the wool over the strike is opened. When primary strikes are invaded by secondary flies, particularly *Ch. rufifacies*, the affected area is extended and the maggots may burrow deeply into the tissues. Affected sheep may lose their fleece over the affected area and may suffer a break in the remaining fleece. Tracts of discolored wool may lead to other affected areas of skin. As the struck area extends a scab forms over the center, the wool falls out and the maggots are active only at the periphery.

Blowfly strike in sheep is commonly classified according to the site involved. This has more than casual significance because the site of strike is usually closely related to predisposing conditions which can, in some instances, be corrected.

Clinical pathology and necropsy findings

A clinical examination is all that is necessary to make the diagnosis but identification of the flies responsible may be important if epidemiology is being considered. Identification of larvae should be done by a specialist. Fly trapping may not correlate with larval findings as not all flies are equally attracted by commonly used baits.

Diagnosis

Attention will be drawn to affected sheep by their foot stamping, tail twitching and biting at the affected part. Affected sheep can easily be diagnosed by finding the moist, malodorous, maggot-infested area. Many covert strikes may be present without producing clinical signs.

Predisposing diseases such as footrot, wound infections and diarrhea due to parasitic gastroenteritis are usually easily detected and fleece rot is indicated by matting of the wool and discoloration.

Treatment

A local dressing containing a larvicide and an antiseptic is applied. The prevention of reinfestations is also an important aim and as repellents have been largely unsatisfactory, it has become apparent that the larvicide in a suitable dressing must be one with maximum retention in the treated area. Efficient older type dressings are BTB (boric acid, tar oil, bentonite mixture) and BKB (boric acid, kerosene, bentonite mixture). When these older type dressings are used affected areas should be clipped as closely as possible, ensuring that all tracts are followed and pockets of maggots and secondary strike areas are exposed. These compounds have been largely superseded in fly dressings by the organophosphates which are listed under control measures. They give a complete kill of maggots within about 12 hours and have the advantage that the wool need not be clipped. Powder and liquid dressings containing diazinon and chlorfenvinphos (Supona) are most generally favored.

Cyromazine is now widely used. It is particularly active against second and third instars, but is slow-acting and so live larvae may be seen in the fleece for some days after treatment.

Control

Practical control of crutch strike in extensive farming areas depends on the use of the Mules operation to extend the bare areas around the perineum and tail, good worm control to prevent contamination of the perineal region, correct tail length and a mid-season crutching. Control of strike in other situations is based on insecticidal treatment and treatment of wounds as they occur. Under conditions of extensive sheep raising, such as occur in Australia and South Africa and where climatic conditions are conducive to the development of the disease, the control of blowfly strike is a major undertaking and an extensive bibliography on the subject is available; the most recent collection and review are given as review references. Only a summary can be presented here.

The subject can be divided into three phases: reduction in fly numbers; prediction of fly waves followed by prophylactic crutching and application of larvicides; and reduction in susceptibility of sheep.

Reduction of fly numbers

Reducing the fly population has been of limited value as there are usually enough flies present to strike all susceptible sheep if suitable conditions are present. However if the primary fly responsible for initiating strikes can be controlled the importance of secondary flies is greatly reduced. The measures used include trapping, early treatment of clinical cases and the disposal of carcasses and wool waste. Biological control by the use of insects parasitizing blowflies has been generally unsuccessful. Trapping, provided the traps are carefully looked after and satisfactory baits are used, can reduce the number of blowflies in a small area but they are not efficient in reducing the primary fly population. For example, *L. cuprina* is almost impervious to trapping. Destruction of carcasses must be prompt. Burying is adequate provided the carcasses are either poisoned with a larvicide or buried at least 60 cm below the surface. However, often it is counterproductive to bury carcasses as it is rarely done properly, and may prevent invasion by maggots of the secondary flies which reduce the primary fly maggots by predation. Burning is more effective and is preferred if there is no fire hazard. In either instance disposal must take place within 72 hours or many primary larvae will have left the carcase. Clippings (crutchings) from infested sheep should be disposed of similarly. Clinically affected sheep, particularly those affected early in the season, must be detected before larvae have had time to mature. If these early season strikes are not treated they serve to multiply the fly population and outbreaks will occur later in the season. When affected areas are clipped, the clippings should be disposed of and larvae on the sheep destroyed with a suitable dressing.

Control by genetic means offers promise for long-term control. Chromosome translocation to produce reduced fertility in male flies and lethal mutants, such as yellow or white eyes, in subsequent generations, which will be blind under field conditions and die, has been reported (4). This technique is logistically and economically feasible and more cost effective than the irradiated male technique used for screw-worm control, as only two or three early-season releases of males would be required rather than continuous release.

However, where eradication is the final aim, the sterile male technique should be used, but suppression of the fly population by genetic means followed by release of sterile males would be cheaper than complete reliance on the sterile male technique.

Prediction of fly waves

Sporadic cases of body strike may occur in sheep at any time and cannot reasonably be prevented, but if the environmental circumstances conducive to high fly populations and high susceptibility of sheep are recognized fly 'waves' can be predicted and short-term prophylactic measures taken. Warm, showery weather extending over several weeks allows several generations to be completed and sufficient flies to be available to cause an outbreak of strike. Once sufficient flies are present, an outbreak of cutaneous myiasis may occur whenever the sheep become susceptible. Warm humid weather, rain over 2 or 3 days, or grazing in long wet grass, may provide suitable conditions for the sheep to become susceptible to body strike. Sheep with yellow fleece, i.e. high suint content, comprised of pointed, thin staples less tightly packed and with a low wax content, would be most susceptible. Sheep with long fleeces are more susceptible and the time at which shearing is carried out may exert an influence on the frequency and severity of outbreaks.

Outbreaks of breech strike will occur if the sheep have diarrhea, or if ewes have urine splashing on to the breech area because the tails are too long. If an outbreak is predicted or has begun, 'crutching' and the prophylactic application of larvicides will reduce the severity of the infestation. 'Crutching' refers to clipping of the wool around the breech or crutch of the sheep to avoid it becoming wet with urine and feces and providing a focus of attraction for flies. It is carried out routinely before lambing and immediately prior to a strike wave but provides protection for no more than 6 weeks. All the wool from above the tail, to the posterior aspect of the thighs and down to the hocks, must be removed. Because of the labor and loss of wool involved most sheep farmers depend on prophylactic dressing with a larvicide.

Prophylactic dressing with a larvicide has been a major part of blowfly control for many years but the preparations used and the methods of their administration have undergone many important changes. The triazine, Vetrazin, gives 8–10 weeks protection (11). Its action is specific to dipteran larvae. It should be noted that it is slow to kill as it affects the development of the subsequent lifecycle stage. Diazinon, chlorfenvinphos (Supona), fenthion ethyl, coumaphos and other organophosphorous insecticides are widely used (5), but the period of protection gained by their use has markedly declined as the flies have built up resistance (6). (Table 82 gives common names of insecticides.)

Further, the organophosphorous insecticides may be degraded by *Pseudomonas aeruginosa* (14). However most fly waves are of short duration, and if the insecticide is applied thoroughly at the time an outbreak commences, these compounds may still give sufficient protection to minimize losses.

The methods of application include dipping, jetting and tip spraying. Dipping has the advantage of thorough wetting but requires high equipment and labor costs. Jetting is still recommended for crutch strike and if the jetting piece is combed through the wool from the poll to the rump with the solution at high pressure (392–589 kPa), good control of body strike will also be achieved. Tip spraying, which is the deposition of a higher concentration of insecticide onto the tip of the fleece, is only of use with dieldrin or aldrin as it relies on the ability of these compounds to diffuse down the wool fibers. The compounds are now banned in most countries. Tip spraying is not effective with organophosphates. If insecticides are applied prophylactically to all sheep early in the season, the level of insecticide in the fleece may decline by the time the flies are active and the heterozygote-resistant flies may survive, thus aiding the development of a resistant population (12). Further, if a fly wave does not occur, the treatment is then seen to be wasteful. However, if the approach is to hand-treat early season strikes and only treat the flock when a fly wave occurs, many early season covert strikes will be missed and many sheep may be lost because of the inability of the farmer to muster and treat sheep sufficiently quickly.

Reduction in susceptibility of sheep

Breech strike should not occur if proper management practices are followed. Sheep should be mulesed at marking (castration and tailing), their tails should be cut to just cover the vulva or to the corresponding length in males and an effective worm control program instituted. Almost total control will be gained if a mid-season crutching is also given. Because of the prevalence of myiasis in Merino sheep with a heavily wrinkled skin, most attempts have been directed towards removing the wrinkles. A breeding program aimed at the selection of plain-bodied animals suggests itself as a suitable control measure, but because wrinkliness is not inherited in a simple manner a genetic approach to the problem has not been well accepted. The easiest method of reducing wrinkliness in the crutch area is by the Mules operation (3). Originally the important folds of skin in the breech area were removed with sharp sheep-shears after shearing or crutching. The method has been modified and is applied to all sheep in the flock. Rather than removing the wrinkles the aim is to increase the width of the woolless area in the crutch or breech region by removing a crescentic strip of skin on both sides starting just above and to the side of the butt of the tail, continuing down the back of the thigh to just above and inside the beginning of the gastrocnemius tendon. Only woolled skin is removed, the strip terminating at a point at either end and being widest (5–6 cm) opposite the vulva. The operation is best done at marking (tailing and castration) as the lambs heal more quickly and suffer little, if any, setback in growth. Further, minimum death rates due to fly strike and maximum wool weights are obtained when sheep are mulesed as lambs. However, sheep of any age can be mulesed. The technique has been developed extensively in Australia and is not described in detail here. In the hands of an experienced technician the time required to improve the perineal topography need be no longer than 1–2 minutes. The improvement is permanent and reduces crutch strike by 80–90% (7). However, if sheep are grazed on lush pasture or fresh crops and scouring is prevalent, this protection may be overcome (8). Mulesing is accompanied by some pain, but current data unequivocally establishes the positive health and welfare benefits conferred upon sheep in the Australian environment. The protection gained by mulesing surpasses that afforded by breeding and is immediate and permanent.

The Mules operation is often supplemented by including a tail-strip operation in which a thin strip of woolled skin is removed from each side of the tail to above its butt. This results in a reduction of the amount of wool on the tail and less chance of fecal and urinary contamination. Since the introduction of elastic rings for castration and removal of the tail, a tendency has developed to remove the tail at the butt. This allows wool to grow in around the anus where it may become soiled and struck and, when combined with the Mules operation which slightly everts the vulva, has caused a dramatic increase in carcinomas of the mucocutaneous junction in the vulva (9). Tail stripping is important when tails are left at the longer recommended length, that is to the tip of the vulva. Docking so that the tail is of the correct length and so that a flap of ventral woolless skin is left to seal over the stump is important. The latter can be effected by pushing the skin back with the back of the docking knife before severing the tail.

Removal of the wool and skin wrinkles from the breech of sheep by surgical means or by selective breeding reduces the susceptibility of sheep to crutch strike and when combined with good worm control to prevent scouring, tails cut to the correct length and a midseason crutching, crutch strike will be minimized (13). Pizzle strike will be reduced by the use of testosterone implants and by pizzle dropping (surgical separation of the preputial sheath from the belly) although this procedure may cause some difficulty at shearing unless the shearers are warned. Ringing (shearing of the pizzle area) will give 6–8 weeks protection. Fleece rot occurs most commonly on the withers of sheep, and the conformation that allows accumulation of moisture and the development of fleece rot and fly strike have been shown to be hereditary. Sheep with these faults should be culled. Although control is mainly a matter of management, in periods particularly suitable for fly strike the periodic application of an insecticide is still essential.

Sheep may gain a resistance by repeated larval infestation (15) but immunization with extracts from third stage instars did not protect (16). Vaccination against *P. aeruginosa* to protect against fleece rot and the likelihood of body strike has given encouraging results (17).

REVIEW LITERATURE

Arundel, J. H. & Sutherland, A. K. (1988) *Ectoparasitic Diseases of Sheep, Cattle, Goats and Horses*, vol. 10. *Animal Health in Australia*. Canberra: Australian Government Publishing Service.

National Symposium on the Sheep Blowfly and Flystrike in Sheep (1983) Dept. Agriculture, NSW, Australia.

REFERENCES

(1) Watts, J. E. et al. (1981) *Aust. vet. J.*, *57*, 450
(2) Axelsen, A. & Willoughby, W. M. (1968) *Aust. vet. J.*, *44*, 15.
(3) Morley, F. H. W. & Johnstone, I. L. (1984) *J. Aust. Inst. Agric. Sci.*, *50*, 86.
(4) Whitten, M. J. et al. (1976) *Proc. 15th int. Congr. Entomol., Washington*.
(5) Wood, J. C. et al. (1965) *Vet. Rec.*, 77, 896.
(6) Shanahan, C. J. & Roxburgh, N. A. (1974) *Aust. vet. J.*, *50*, 177.
(7) Morley, F. H. W. et al. (1976) *Aust. vet. J.*, *52*, 325.
(8) Watts, J. E. & Perry, D. A. (1975) *Aust. vet. J.*, *51*, 586.
(9) Vandegraaff, R. (1976) *Aust. vet. J.*, *52*, 21.
(10) Callinan, A. P. L. (1980) *Aust. J. Zool.*, *28*, 679.
(11) Shanahan, G. J. & Hughes, P. B. (1980) *Vet. Rec.*, *106*, 306.
(12) Whitten, M. J. et al. (1980) *Aust. J. biol. Sci.*, *33*, 725.
(13) Watts, J. E. et al. (1979) *Aust. vet. J.*, *55*, 325.
(14) Merritt, G. L. et al. (1981) *Aust. vet. J.*, *57*, 531.
(15) Sandeman, R. M. et al. (1986) *Int. J. Parasitol.*, *16*, 69.
(16) O'Donnell, I. J. et al. (1981) *Aust. J. biol. Sci.*, *34*, 411.
(17) Burrell, D. H. (1985) *Aust. vet. J.*, *62*, 55.

KED AND LOUSE INFESTATIONS

Infestations with these insects cause irritation resulting in skin or wool damage. Blood loss may occur with some species.

Sheep ked (*Melophagus ovinus*)

This flat brown wingless fly, about 6–7 mm in length, is an important parasite of sheep throughout the world. It is a bloodsucker and although the degrees of infestation usually encountered cause only irritation with resulting scratching, biting and damage to the fleece, very heavy infestations may cause severe anemia. The ked may transmit *Trypanosoma melophagium* and *Rickettsia melophagi*, harmless blood parasites of the sheep. Staining of the wool by the feces of the ked reduces its value and gives it a peculiar musty odor. Heavy infestations cause skin blemishes which are costly to the leather industry. Sheep in poor condition suffer most from infestations. Goats may also be infested.

Keds live their entire lifecycle on the host and spread for the most part is by direct contact between hosts. Single larvae are deposited on the host and pupate within a few hours. The female ked lives for 4–5 months and lays 10–15 larvae in this time, so buildup of infection is slow. The larvae are attached to the wool fiber some distance above the skin and many larvae and pupae are removed at shearing. The young ked usually emerges in 20–22 days but this period may be prolonged for up to 35 days in winter. The complete lifecycle takes 5–6 weeks in optimum warm conditions. Heavy infestations usually occur in winter months and they decline in the summer. The parasite is mainly seen in colder, wetter areas and infestations may be lost when sheep are moved to hot dry districts. Resistance is acquired in time and resistant sheep grow better and produce more wool (1).

A seasonal pattern of infestation occurs. Keds are sensitive to hot, dry weather and numbers decrease markedly over the summer. Populations increase slowly over the autumn and winter. While keds that have been dislodged from the host can live for up to 2 weeks if in mild moist conditions, most die in 3–4 days and probably do not play a part in reinfesting sheep. At shearing 80–90% of adults and almost all the pupal cases will be removed, and the combination of hot conditions and a short fleece kills many of the remaining ked. However some remain alive in protected places such as the ventral neck and breech regions. If dipping is carried out within the next 2–4 weeks eradication will be achieved as long as all sheep are dipped and the insecticide used has a residual protection longer than the time taken for the last pupae to hatch. Keds are particularly susceptible to organophosphates and most of those used to eliminate lice will also remove ked. They can also be used in higher dose rates in pour-on applications. Diazinon 42 mg/kg given in this manner eradicated an infestation (3), while the application of undiluted diazinon concentrate (48%) to the belly of sheep from a single nozzle at delivery rates of 4·8 and 9·0 ml/second eliminated infestation from sheep passing through the race at 60 sheep/minute (2).

The synthetic pyrethroids are also active against ked; deltamethrin, cyhalothrin and cypermethrin are used. Amitraz will kill adult keds but has little residual action and is therefore usually combined with another compound to provide sufficient residual action to eliminate infections. Ivermectin given at the standard anthelmintic dose will also eliminate ked.

Arsenic will not persist long enough to eliminate keds in a single dipping and rotenone may be added to improve efficiency, but as rotenone strips badly when used on long woolled sheep it should be used as soon as possible after shearing. The chlorinated hydrocarbons are also efficient but are banned in most countries. Power dusting can also be used, coumaphos 1% giving good results, but diazinon can also be used.

Louse infestations (pediculosis)

Lice infestations are common throughout the world. The species are host-specific and are divided into biting and sucking lice.

The important species are:

Cattle: *Linognathus vituli* (long-nosed sucking louse), *Solenopotes capillatus* (small blue sucking louse), *Haematopinus eurysternus* (short-nosed sucking louse), *H. quadripertusus* (tail louse), *H. tuberculatus* (buffalo louse), *Damalinia bovis* (biting louse).

Sheep: *Linognathus ovillus* (sucking face louse), *L. africanus*, *L. stenopsis* (sucking goat louse), *L. pedalis* (sucking foot louse), *Damalinia ovis* (biting louse).

Goats: *Linognathus stenopsis* (sucking blue louse), *L. africanus*, *Damalinia caprae* (biting louse), *D. limbata*, *D. crassipes*.

Pigs: *Haematopinus suis* (sucking louse).

Horses: *Haematopinus asini* (sucking louse), *Damalinia equi* (biting louse).

All species cause irritation of the skin and stimulate scratching, rubbing and licking leading to restlessness, damage to fleece and hides and loss of milk production. It is commonly believed that lice cause weight loss but experimental evidence does not support this. The coat of affected animals is rough and shaggy and there is usually marked pityriasis.

The effect of lice on cattle is controversial, but it is usually believed that infestation has little or no effect on weight gains and haematological values (5, 6) except where *H. eurysternus* is present in significant numbers as, in contrast to other species, this louse is stated to increase in numbers as the cattle get older and cause a progressive anemia sufficiently severe on occasions to cause death (4). Treatment, however, may be warranted to reduce the damage to hides and prevent damage to fences and other fixtures. Hairballs may be present in infested calves due to continual licking.

The pig louse spreads swinepox and while weight loss may not occur, even with heavy burdens, some pigs develop an allergic dermatitis and the consequent rubbing leads to skin lesions (9).

Sheep body lice causes irritation and rubbing. The wool loses its brightness and becomes more yellow (9).

The quantity and quality of the fleece is reduced (9, 11) and losses up to $3·20 Australian per infested sheep have been measured (12). Foot lice are believed to live on blood. Light infestations may not cause clinical signs, but moderate to severe infestations cause stamping and biting the affected parts. Lice cause goats to rub or to bite their coat, which becomes matted and damaged. Angora goats can damage the hair shaft and lose their coats. Signs of infestation are restlessness, hair loss and decreased milk production. In horses *H. asini* is the more serious species as it removes blood and may cause some anemia.

In searching for lice on cattle and horses special attention should be paid to the back, the sides of the neck, escutcheon and tail switch. Biting lice tend to congregate on the dorsal surface and flanks, while sucking lice are found on the head and in the long hair of the mane and tail but, in heavy winter infestations, lice may be found on any part of the body. In sheep with long wool, greatest numbers of *D. ovis* may be seen on the midside, particularly the shoulders, from where they spread to the back and rump. After shearing, small residual infestations may be found on the ventral neck. Foot lice are usually found in clusters on those parts covered with hair, mainly on the lower limbs, but in heavy infestations they can be found in clusters above the hock, on the scrotum, in the belly wool and more rarely on the face.

While there is some disagreement as to the effect of lice on weight gain, animals in poor condition, improperly fed and exposed to cold and debilitating disease carry heaviest infestations. Such animals will probably benefit from the removal of lice while animals in good condition and well fed may not show increased weight agains after treatment. Young cattle are more heavily infected and numbers decrease as the animal matures, even when self-grooming is prevented (13). Biting lice of cattle, sheep and horses are small and pale-colored and are not readily visible unless seen in a strong light, although the eggs can usually be detected fixed to dark hair of cattle or horses. Sucking lice remain fixed particularly in the long hair of the mane and at the base of the tail in horses and cattle and on the haired parts of sheep. They are blue-gray in color and may be difficult to see in dark hair.

Lifecycles of all lice are similar and are confined to the host, although some species, such as the foot lice of sheep, may survive away from the host for up to 2 weeks. The eggs are laid, attached to coat fibers, and there are three nymphal stages before mature lice appear. The lifecycle of most species varies from 2 to 4 weeks under optimum conditions. Lice breed within a narrow temperature range: when temperatures are cooler than optimum, eggs do not develop, while hotter temperatures prevent egg-laying and kill the lice (7). Lice therefore show a seasonal periodicity with very low numbers in the summer when conditions are hot. Breeding commences in the autumn and maximum numbers are reached in the spring (8).

Shearing is the most important factor in reducing body lice populations on sheep. Between 30 and 50% of the population is removed with the fleece and those remaining are subjected to a more variable microclimate. Populations are at their lowest 30–60 days after shearing. Reversing temperature gradients as sheep move in and out of shade, and very wet conditions, will also reduce lice numbers. The population dynamics of *D. ovis* have been determined (8). The loss of the winter coat in cattle and horses is most important in reducing populations in those species.

Transmission is effected by direct contact but inert objects such as blankets, grooming tools and harness may remain infective for several days and the foot-louse of sheep may gain infection from the pasture. Young pigs may become infected some 10 hours after birth (10).

Body lice of sheep are relatively easy to eradicate if a clean muster is achieved if the sheep are thoroughly treated and reinfestation is avoided. Treatment should be given by plunge or shower dipping, by jetting or by pour-on application. Sheep should not be plunge-dipped or shower-dipped until cuts have healed, otherwise infections with *Erysipelas rhusiopathiae*, *Dermatophilus congolensis* or *Clostridium* spp. may cause lameness, fleece lesions or deaths.

Affected animals can be effectively treated with sodium arsenite or magnesium fluosilicate in a dip or with sprays, dips or dusts containing chlorinated hydrocarbon insecticides (e.g. lindane, toxaphene, methoxychlor, dieldrin), organophosphate insecticides (diazinon, coumaphos, chlorfenvinphos, carbophenothion, propetamphos) or carbamates. Synthetic pyrethroids, cypermethrin and cyhalothrin, have been shown to be effective in sheep and give good residual protection (16) while cypermethrin, alphamethrin and decamethrin are marketed as pour-ons for sheep. They must be used immediately after shearing. A small proportion of sheep show irritation after application and some may show fleece damage.

The distribution of synthetic pyrethroid following backline treatment is very uneven and is less satisfactory than dipping. However, the ease of application, low capital outlay required and the need for only one muster has lead to rapid acceptance of backline treatments. Failures to eradicate occur if the sheep are not cleanly shorn, and in large-bodied sheep with extensive neck folds which are difficult to shear cleanly. The presence of unshorn lambs, cotted or *Dermatophilus*-affected fleeces, wrinkly sheep or inexpert shearers make backline pour-on application an inappropriate method. Heavy rain following application may also cause failure.

The manufacturer's recommendations should be accurately followed particularly when using shower dips, dust or surface sprays. Sprays are only efficient when used with chlorinated hydrocarbons because of the ability of these compounds to translocate and because of their stability.

However, because of their persistence their use is now banned in many countries. In infested long-woolled sheep it has been usual to recommend jetting to reduce the population until the sheep can be shorn and dipped. Cyhalothrin has been shown to eradicate body lice from long-woolled sheep when applied by jetting at 20 ppm (17). Phoxim 125 mg/l has also been reported to eliminate lice in long-woolled sheep, while 250 mg/l gave at least 4 months protection against reinfestation (18).

High concentrations of cyhalothrin (1500 ppm) and diazinon 36 000 (ppm) in 100 ml applied to sheep has also proved effective (19) but requires a practical method of application. Following treatment of foot lice, sheep should be moved to a paddock that has been free of sheep for a month.

Fenthion, famfur, chlorpyriphos, temephos, methidathion, phosmet, deltamethrin and fenchlorphos have been used in pour-on application on cattle (14), and 20% fenthion has been claimed to be as efficient when used as a spot-on or as 2% used as a pour-on (15). While pour-on applications are easy to use none will kill all lice, they are expensive compared with sprays if large numbers are to be treated, and in many countries they should not be used on lactating cows (14). Diazinon, coumaphos, ethion, and cypermethrin or bromophos-ethyl combined with chlorfenvinphos are used as sprays or dips in cattle. Fenthion 2% has been widely used on horses in Australia with good results although coat color changes and, rarely, hair loss does occur (see Table 82).

Lice develop resistance to insecticides quite rapidly and strains of *D. ovis* which are resistant to the chlorinated hydrocarbon insecticides are common in the United Kingdom.

Treatment of all animals and spraying of housing should be done in the autumn when numbers are at a minimum and before lice breeding has commenced. All compounds recommended for use in sheep can eradicate lice in a single dipping if used correctly, with the exception of sodium arsenite and magnesium fluosilicate against the sheep sucking lice, and failure to eradicate is usually a management problem. In cattle and horses the residual protection obtained is only 3–4 days and animals must be retreated in 14–16 days if eradication is attempted. Eradication is a practicable procedure but should not be undertaken unless reinfestation can be prevented.

REFERENCES

(1) Nelson, W. A. & Slen, S. B. (1968) *Exp. Parasitol.*, *22*, 223.
(2) Lloyd, J. E. et al. (1978) *J. econ. Entomol.* *71*, 548.
(3) Lloyd, J. E. et al. (1982) *J. econ. Entomol.*, *75*, 5
(4) Nelson, W. A. (1970) *Exp. Parasitol.*, *28*, 263
(5) Bailey, P. J. et al. (1984) *Aust. J. exp. Agri. Anim. Husb.*, *24*, 140.
(6) Cumings, L. J. & Graham. J. F. (1980) *Aust. vet. J.*, *58*. 194.
(7) Murray, M. D. (1968) *Aust. J. Zool.*, *16*, 725.
(8) Murray, M. D. & Gordon, G. (1969) *Aust. J. Zool.*, *17* 179.
(9) Kettle, P. R. & Lukies, J. M. (1982) *NZ J. Agric. Res.*, *25*, 531.
(10) Hiepe, T. & Ribbeck, R. (1975) *Angew. Parasitol.*, *16*, Suppl. 2.
(11) Wilkinson, F. C. et al. (1982) *Vet. Parasitol.*, *9*, 243.
(12) Niven, D. R. & Pritchard, D. A. (1985) *Aust. J. exp. Agric.*, *25*, 37.
(13) Callinan, A. P. L. (1980) *Aust. vet. J.*, *56*, 484.
(14) Kettle, P. R. & Lukies, J. M. (1979) *NZ vet. J.* *27*, 78.
(15) Neuhauser, H. (1974) *Vet. med. Rev.*, *4*, 348.
(16) Hall, C. A. (1978) *Aust. vet. J.*, *54*, 471.
(17) Rundle, J. C. & Forsyth, B. A. (1984) *Aust. vet. J.*, *61*, 396.
(18) Hopkins, T. J. & Lindsay, G. D. (1982) *Vet. med. Rev.*, *1*, 59.
(19) Wilkinson, F. C. (1986) *Aust. adv. Vet. Sci.*, p. 130.

TICK INFESTATIONS

Tick infestations are of great importance in the production of diseases of animals. Apart from their role as vectors and potential reservoirs of infectious diseases, as outlined below, heavy infestations can cause direct losses. Many are active bloodsuckers and may cause death from anemia. Some species cause tick paralysis and it is possible that other ticks may elaborate toxins other than those causing paralysis (4). Heavy tick burdens cause sufficient worry to interfere with feeding which may lead to loss of production and weight gain (2).

The lifecyles of the ticks vary widely. Some species pass their entire life on the one host, others pass different stages of the cycle on successive hosts, and others are parasitic only at certain stages. The eggs are laid in the soil and larvae attach themselves to a passing host on which they may develop through one on more nymphal stages before becoming adults. Adult females engorge on blood or lymph and drop to the ground to lay their eggs. One-host ticks are more easily controlled than those which pass part of their lifecycles away from the host. A list of the single and multiple host ticks is shown in Table 78.

Although many ticks favor a particular host they are usually not completely host-specific and many parasitize a wide variety of animals. In the limited space available here the species are listed according to whether they cause worry only or transmit infectious diseases of large-domestic animals.

For more detailed information on transmission of infectious diseases and the biology and distribution of ticks the papers by Neitz (3) and Theiler (4) should be consulted.

Table 78. Single and multiple host ticks.

ONE-HOST TICKS

Boophilus spp.
Margaropus winthemi
Otobius megnini (adults are not parasitic)

TWO-HOST TICKS

Rhipicephalus evertsi
R. bursa
Hyalomma spp. (most have two or three hosts)

THREE-HOST TICKS

Ixodes spp.
Rhipicephalus spp. (except *R. evertsi* and *R. bursa*)
Haemaphysalis spp.
Amblyomma spp.
Hyalomma spp. (most have two or three hosts)
Ornithodorus spp.—many hosts
Dermacentor spp.

Ticks causing paralysis

Paralysis is not uncommon in young domestic animals which are heavily infested with the ticks. A recent review lists 31 species in seven genera of ixodid ticks and seven species of three genera of argasid ticks as being implicated in tick paralysis (20) and the most important species are given in Table 79. Details of the clinical syndrome are provided in Chapter 32. Recovery is usual in early mild cases if the ticks are removed but antiserum against some (e.g. *I. holocyclus*) is available.

Ticks which transmit protozoan diseases

Ticks are the most important vectors of many protozoan diseases, the protozoan in most instances surviving from generation to generation of ticks by infecting their eggs. Where control of these diseases is to be undertaken it is necessary to know which ticks are vectors, how many hosts the tick parasitizes during a lifecycle and which animals can act as hosts. Much of the information on these points is fragmentary and only a summary is presented in Table 80.

Bacterial, viral and rickettsial diseases transmitted by ticks

The transmission of diseases caused by these agents may be effected by means other than ticks. *Anaplasma marginale* can be spread by biting flies if large numbers are present when the animals are experiencing a heavy parasitemia. Outbreaks of anaplasmosis can also occur following the use of unclean instruments for dehorning, vaccination, castration or blood sampling, and is easily caused by blood transfusions. The ticks involved more commonly in transmitting bacteria, viruses and rickettsia are given in Table 81. Transmission of *Anaplasma* may be transovarially, from one stage becoming infected and a subsequent stage passing the infection to a new host, or ticks may transmit infection within the one stage if they detach and reach a new host.

Ticks which cause worry

Ticks cause damage to hides and loss of production, and anemia and death when they are present in large numbers. They also cause greater morbidity and mortality during periods of drought, and delays in fattening so that animals are held longer before they can be sold. A list of ticks which have this effect but are not known to cause paralysis or transmit infectious diseases in farm animals is given below.

Otobius megnini, the 'spinose ear tick' of the United States and Canada
Amblyomma americanum, the 'Lone Star tick' of the United States
A. maculatum, the 'Gulf Coast tick' of the United States
Margaropus winthemi of South America and Africa
Ornithodorus moubata of Africa and southeast Asia
O.savignyi of Africa and southeast Asia
Haemaphysalis longicornis of Australia and New Zealand.

Table 79. Ticks reported to cause paralysis.

Animal	*Tick*	*Country*
Sheep, calves, goats	*Dermacentor andersoni* *D. occidentalis* (17)	United States United States
Calves, lambs, foals, goats	*Ixodes holocyclus*	Australia (16)
Sheep, goats, calves	*I. pilosus*	South Africa
Sheep, goats, calves, antelopes	*I. rubicundus*	South Africa
Lambs	*Rhipicephalus evertsi*	South Africa
Calves, sheep, goats	*Haemaphysalis punctata*	South Africa, Europe, Japan
Sheep	*Ornithodorus lahorensis*	Central Asia
Sheep	*Hyalomma aegyptium*	Yugoslavia
Sheep, goats	*Ixodes ricinus*	Crete, Israel (18)

Treatment and control of tick infestations

Three methods have been used to control ticks: treating with acaricidal agents; pasture spelling; and the use of resistant cattle. Vaccination against ticks has been shown to be possible, although the response is variable (5). Vaccinated animals show damage to the gut cells, possibly induced by antibody, and rupture of the gut allows antibody to enter the hemocele and attack other tissues. Males are also affected (6). Certain *Stylosanthes* spp., tropical legumes, can kill or immobilize larval ticks and the use of these plants may simultaneously improve pasture quality and reduce the pasture contamination of larval ticks (10).

Choice of insecticide

Individual animals can be effectively treated by the application of any one of a number of insecticides applied either as a spray or by dipping. The choice of insecticides depends largely on three factors: the persistence of the compound on the skin and hair coat; the likelihood of residues of insecticide toxic to man appearing in the milk or meat; and whether or not the ticks in the area have developed resistance to the particular insecticide. The more modern insecticides have the advantage over arsenical preparations, which have served so well for so long, of ease of administration and persistence on the skin, but resistance to chlorinated hydrocarbons, organophosphates and carbamates appears to develop quite rapidly. Resistance to arsenic also occurs and although it develops much more slowly than, for example, resistance to benzene hexachloride it may make its use unwarranted over large areas. The problem of resistance of ticks to insecticide is increasing rapidly and emphasizes the need to use resistant cattle and better management procedures.

The same criteria apply in control as in treatment except that cost becomes a limiting factor when large numbers of animals require frequent treatments and it is obvious in some circumstances that the effect of tick infestation on Brahman-cross steers is insufficiently great to warrant treating them. It is impossible to make specific recommendations on methods of application and the most efficient insecticide to use because these vary widely between species of ticks. However, whenever possible, treatment should be given systematically in a program based on the lifecycle and epidemiology of the tick. A number of treatments may be used early in the tick season to prevent the increase in tick numbers. Care must be taken in areas where tick fevers also occur, not

Table 80. Ticks reported to transmit protozoan diseases (17).

Disease	*Protozoan*	*Vector ticks*	*Country*
BABESIOSIS			
Cattle	*Babesia bigemina*	*Boophilus annulatus*	N. America
		B. microplus	Australia and S. America
		B. (annulatus) calcaratus, B. decoloratus, Rhipicephalus appendiculatus, R. bursa, R. evertsi, Ixodes ricinus	Africa
		Haemaphysalis punctata	Europe
	Babesia bovis	*Ixodes persulcatus*	USSR
		I. ricinus	Europe
		Boophilus annulatus	Iran
		B. microplus	Australia
	Babesia berbera	*B. annulatus (calcaratus), Rhipicephalus bursa*	Africa
Sheep and goats	*Babesia motasi*	*Dermacentor silvarum, Rhipicephalus bursa, Haemaphysalis punctata, Ixodes rinicus*	Europe
	Babesia ovis	*Rhipicephalus bursa*	USSR
		Haemaphysalis bispinosa	India
Horses	*Babesia caballi*	*Hyalomma dromedarii*	Africa
		Dermacentor (reticulata) marginatus, D. pictus, D. silvarum, Hyalomma (excavatum) anatolicum, H. marginatum, H. volgense, Rhipicephalus bursa, R. sanguineus	USSR and the Balkans, S. America and Florida, United States
	Babesia equi	*Hyalomma dromedarii, Rhipicephalus evertsi, R. sanguineus, Dermacentor marginatus, D. pictus, Hyalomma anatolicum, H. marginatum, H. uralense, Rhipicephalus bursa, R. sanguineus*	Africa, the Balkans, S. America, Australia
Pigs	*Babesia trautmanni*	*R. sanguineus (turanicus)*	USSR
ANAPLASMOSIS			
Cattle	*Anaplasma marginale*	*Boophilus annulatus, Argas persicus, Dermacentor albipictus, D. andersoni, D. occidentalis, D. variabilis, Ixodes scapularis, Rhipicephalus sanguineus*	North America
		Boophilus microplus	Australia and S. America
		B. decoloratus, Hyalomma excavatum, Rhipicephalus bursa, R. simus	Africa
		Haemaphysalis punctata, Ixodes ricinus	Europe
		Boophilus (annulatus) calcaratus	USSR
Sheep and goats	*Anaplasma ovis*	*Dermacentor silvarum, Rhipicephalus bursa, Ornithodorus lahorensis*	USSR
THEILERIOSIS			
Cattle	*Theileria parva*	*Rhipicephalus appendiculatus*	Africa
	Theileria annulata	*Hyalomma anaticolicum*	Africa, Asia, USSR, Europe, China, India
	Theileria mutans	*Amblyoma variegatum*	Africa, Asia,
		Haemaphysalis spp.	Europe, USSR, North America
	Theileria buffeli	*Haemaphysalis* spp.	Australia
Sheep	*Theileria ovis*	*Rhipicephalus bursa*	Africa, Asia,
		Rhipicephalus evertsi	Europe
		Hyalomma spp.	
		Rhipicephalus spp.	Africa, Middle
	Theileria hirci	*Hyalomma anaticolicum*	East, USSR

to disrupt the transmission of the tick fever organisms and leave the cattle susceptible to later infection.

Arsenic was usually used as a dip containing 0·1–0·2% arsenic trioxide. The proportion of arsenic used varied depending on the frequency of dipping. Arsenic preparations are used only as dips because of the danger of contaminating surroundings with sprays. As in all dips the concentration of insecticide is likely to be gradually reduced by repeated use and this 'stripping' must be repaired by periodic replenishment of the dip. Arsenic is no longer used in most countries.

Amitraz, a formamidine, and the synthetic pyrethroids have been used widely in Australia and have proved to be efficient, active against organophosphate resistant strains and safe. Ticks resistant to DDT are also resistant to the synthetic pyrethroids, and to overcome this the pyrethroids can be combined with an organophosphate. Successful combinations in Australia, cypyermethrin plus chlorfenvinphos and deltamethrin plus ethion. One synthetic pyrethoid, flumethrin, has been marketed by itself at higher use concentrations for both plunge dipping and as a pour-on treatment. Cyhalothrin also controls multiresistant strains in Australia and is used in plunge dips.

The organophosphates as a group are effective but strains resistant to many of them have appeared. Other drugs in current use include dioxathion, diazinon, carbophenothion, coumaphos, ethion, bromophos ethyl, chlorpyriphos, and phosmet (see Table 82 for common names). Pour-on applications of chlorpyriphos and

Table 81. Diseases caused by bacteria, viruses and rickettsia and reported to be transmitted by ticks (7).

Disease	*Causative agent*	*Vector ticks*	*Country*
Tick pyemia (lambs)	*Staphylococcus aureus*	*Ixodes ricinus*	Great Britain
Tularemia (sheep)	*Pasteurella tularense*	*Haemaphysalis leporispalustris, H. otophila, Dermacentor andersoni, D. variabilis, D. pictus, D. marginatus, Ixodes luguri*	United States Norway, Europe, USSR
Brucellosis	*Brucella abortus* and *Br. melitensis*	Many ticks may be infected but infection of host appears to occur only if ticks or their feces are eaten	USSR
Encephalomyelitis of horses	Western type virus	*Dermacentor andersoni* *Ixodes ricinus, Dermacentor* spp. (lab. only)	United States USSR
Louping-ill	Virus	*Rhipicephalus appendiculatus* (lab. only) *Ixodes ricinus*	Africa England
Tick-borne fever	*Rickettsia* spp.	*I. ricinus* *Rhipicephalus haemaphysaloides*	Great Britain, Norway India
Caseous lymphadenitis of sheep	*Corynebacterium pseudotuberculosis*	*Dermacentor albipictus*	North America
Epizootic bovine abortion (19)	*Spirochete*	*Ornithodorus coriaceus*	United States

phosmet have been tested but were not as effective as spray applications (8). Addition of acaricides to the feed has also been tried but has not been successful (9), while eartags impregnated with tetrachlorvinphos did not give satisfactory control and increased the risk of resistance developing to the drug (12). Ivermectin given subcutaneously gives satisfactory control of *B. microplus* for 21 days following an initial lag period of 2 days (13). As little as 0·015 mg/kg/day gives complete control and raises the possibility of a slow-release subcutaneous implant (13). Two treatments of 0·2 mg/kg at 4-day intervals is considered satisfactory in cleansing cattle under field conditions (14). However, ivermectin may not be effective against *I. ricinus* (23).

Table 82. Names of commonly used insecticides.

Generic names	*Trade names*
alphamethrin	Duracide
amitraz	Tactic, Triatox
bromophos ethyl	Nexagon, Nexajet
carbaryl	Sevin, Arylan, Seffein
carbophenothion	Trithion
chlorfenvinphos	Supona
chlormethiuron	Dipofene 60
chlorpyriphos	Dursban, Dowco 109
coumaphos	Asuntol, Baymix, Bayer 21/199, Muscatox, Resitox, Co-Ral, Meldane
crotoxyphos	Ciodrin
crufomate	Ruelene, Montrel, Dowco 132
cyhalothrin	Grenade
cypermethrin	Ripcord, Barricade
cyromazine	Vetrazin
deltamethrin	Decis, Clout, Takfly
diazinon	Diazinon
dimethoate	Rogor, Roxion, Cygon, Fostion
dioxathion	Delnav, Navadel
ethion	Nialate
famfur	Warbex, Famaphos
fenchlorphos	Ronnel, Nankor, Korlan, Ectoral
fenthion	Tiguvon, Baytex, Bayer S 1752
fenthion ethyl	Lucijet, S 1751
fenvalerate	Sumifly
flumethrin	Bayticol
methoxychlor	Marlate, Metachlor
phosmet	Imidan, Phthalophos, Prolate
phoxim	Sebacil, Bay 9053, Sarnadip (S. Africa) Sarnacuran (S. America)
promacyl	Promacide
propetamphos	Safrotin, Ectomorph
propoxur	Baygon, Aprocarb, Baygole
temophos	Lypor
tetrachlorvinphos	Stirophos, Gardona, Rabon
trichlorphon	Neguvon, Dylox, Dipterex, chlorophos

Ticks in the ear of horses should be treated by the insertion of a few drops of an oily acaricidal preparation.

These preparations vary in the duration of the protection they afford and local conditions of rainfall and tick population must be taken into account when determining the time intervals between sprayings or dippings.

A special case is that of young lambs which are exposed to tick pyemia. Sprays, dips and ointments are too toxic and the most effective procedure is the application of a liquid emulsion cream containing the insecticide to the woolless parts of the body. Chlorpyriphos 0·48 kg/ha markedly reduces the number of ticks on the pasture (24), but is too expensive for routine use.

Control and eradication

In most countries all that is attempted is reduction of the tick population by periodic dipping or spraying. Complete eradication is extremely difficult because of the persistence of ticks, especially multihost ticks, on wild fauna, and the ability of adult ticks to live for very long periods apart from a host. On the other hand, continuous treatment to restrain the tick population is highly conducive to the development of resistance, a problem which has become apparent in many tick areas. *Boophilus annulatus* was eradicated from the southeastern United States by a program of continuous dipping at short intervals of all livestock in the area. *B. microplus* was also eradicated from Florida by a similar procedure but 20 000 head of deer, the important alternate host in the area, had to be slaughtered (11). Attempts to eradicate other single-host ticks in other countries have not been generally successful. Although both dipping and spraying are recommended for the control of ticks, complete wetting of the animals, which can only be effected by dipping, is essential if eradication is to be undertaken. This adds another impediment to eradication plans because of the cost of constructing proper dips and yards. When one considers that dipping may have to be carried out every 14 days for 15 months, that every animal in the eradication area must be dipped, and that a strict quarantine of the area must be maintained, it is obvious that eradication cannot be undertaken lightly. The use of pour-on applications, which allow a longer period between treatments, and of ivermectin will necessitate a review of control and eradication techniques.

Measures other than the application of insecticides used in the control of tick infestation include burning of pasture, removal of native fauna, plowing of fields, and rotational grazing. So little is known of the bionomics of specific ticks in specific areas that these measure have been largely unsuccessful and it is impossible to provide details for their proper implementation (4).

In those areas where the epidemiology is known it has been shown that in regions with a cold winter the females stop laying eggs, and that the development of eggs is prolonged. This results in few larvae being available in the spring, and if repeated treaments are given at this time, pasture contamination will remain low for some months. In hot tropical areas where the required temperatures for tick breeding are always present, the dry period may cause mortality by desiccation.

Pasture spelling and rotational grazing have been shown to be capable of greatly reducing the tick population on farms in some areas. If cattle are placed on spelled pastures early in winter when the ticks are producing few or no progeny and then alternated at 4-monthly intervals, the tick population can be controlled with a markedly lower number of treatments. The practicability of the procedure depends upon a full-scale financial assessment of the increased weight gains relative to the costs of management. Duration of the spelling period varies between 2 and 3 months in summer to 3–4 months in the winter, but these intervals need to be determined for each district. In practice, pasture spelling is rarely used.

It is possible to reduce the ravages of ticks and tick-borne diseases by the introduction of Brahman and Brahman-cross cattle which are more resistant than British breeds. The resistance has been shown to be largely acquired, and is mainly expressed against the larvae in the first 24 hours after attachment (15). In Australia the possibility that *B. microplus* might escape from its control area because of increased resistance to acaricides has been realized. For this reason a great deal of attention is being paid to the possibility of selecting cattle for tick resistance. In most tick-infested areas, cattle should have up to 50% *B. indicus* blood, as this allows a reduction in the frequency of treatments. Penalties such as reduced live weight gains, late maturity and poor temperament become evident when cattle have more than 50% *B. indicus*. With successive infestations cattle differ in their response to *B. microplus*.Thus there is increased irritation and more licking (15) and a decrease in the number of ticks carried. Resistance to ticks has been shown to be heritable (21) and can be increased by breeding from cows and bulls selected for resistance. Selection for tick resistance does not affect milk production (22).

Other special cases include *Otobius megnini*, the nymphs of which drop off to molt and lay eggs in protected spots, necessitating the spraying of buildings, fence posts, feed troughs and tree trunks in feedlots where heavy infestations are most common. *Ornithodorus* spp. ticks are difficult to control because the nymphs and adults attach to feed for brief periods only. Where ticks which cause paralysis are common it may be necessary to apply an insecticide as a dust and dip at short intervals.

REVIEW LITERATURE

Binnington, K. C. & Kemp, D. H. (1980) Role of tick salivary glands in feeding and disease transmission. *Adv. Parasitol.*, *18*, 316.

Matthewson, M. D. (1984) The future of tick control: a review of the chemical and non-chemical options. In *Impact of Diseases on Livestock Production in the Tropics*, eds H. P. Riemann & M. J. Burridge, pp. 559–568. Amsterdam: Elsevier.

Office Internationale des Épizooties (1974) Special issue on the control of ticks and tick borne protozoal diseases of livestock. *Bull. Off. int. Épizootol.*, *81*, 1.

Sutherst, R. W. et al. (1979) An analysis of management strategies for cattle tick (*Boophilus microplus*) control in Australia. *J. appl. Ecol.*, *16*, 359.

REFERENCES

(1) Riek, R. F. (1965) *Aust. vet. J.*, *41*, 211.
(2) Sutherst, R. W. et al. (1983) *Aust. J. agric. Res.*, *34*, 317.
(3) Neitz, W. D. (1956) *Onderstepoort J. vet. Res.*, *27*, 115.
(4) Theiler, G. (1959) *J. S. Afr. vet. med. Assoc.*, *30*, 195.
(5) Johnston, L. A. Y. et al. (1986) *Int. J. Parasitol.*, *16*, 27.
(6) Agbede, R. I. S. & Kemp, D. H. (1986) *Int. J. Parasitol.*, *16*, 35.
(7) Wharton, R. H. (1976) *World Anim. Rev.*, *20*, 8.
(8) Loomis, E. C. et al. (1972) *J. econ. Entomol.*, *65*, 1638.
(9) Gladney, W. J. et al. (1972) *J. med. Entomol.*, *9*, 439.
(10) Sutherst, R. W. et al. (1982) *Nature (Lond).*, *295*, 320.
(11) Anon. (1959) *Proc. US live Stk sanit. Asoc.*, *1958*, 187.
(12) Owen, L. G. (1985) *Aust. vet. J.*, *62*, 24.
(13) Nolan, J. et al. (1981) *Aust. vet J.*, *57*, 493.
(14) Nolan, J. et al. (1985) *Aust. vet. J.*, *62*. 386.
(15) Wagland, B. M. (1980) In *Ticks and Tick-Borne Diseases, Proc. 56th Ann. gen. Mtg, Aust. Vet. Assoc., Townsville*, p. 55.
(16) Doube, B. M. (1975) *Aust. vet. J.*, *51*, 511.
(17) Loomis, E. C. & Bushnell, R. B. (1968) *Am. J. vet. Res.*, *29*, 1089.
(18) Hadani, A. et al. (1971) *Refuah Vet.*, *28*, 165.
(19) McKercher, D. G. et al. (1980) *Am J. vet. Res.*, *41*, 922.
(20) Murnaghan, M. F. & O'Rourke, F. J. (1978) Tick paralysis in arthropod venoms. In: *Handbook of Experimental Pharmacology*, ed. S. Bettini, *48*, 419. Berlin: Springer-Verlag.
(21) Hewetson, R. W. (1972) *Aust. vet. J.*, *48*, 299.
(22) Utech, K. B. W. & Wharton, R. H. (1982) *Aust. vet. J.*, *58*, 41.
(23) Giles, M. B. deC. (1986) *Vet. Rec.*, *118*, 82.
(24) Bevan, W. J. & Sykes, G. B. (1983) *Vet. Rec.*, *113*, 341.

MISCELLANEOUS FLIES, MIDGES AND MOSQUITOES

Although these insects differ quite markedly they are dealt with together because they exert similar deleterious effects, particularly the worry they cause livestock and the capacity they have for transmitting infectious diseases.

Stable flies

The stable fly, *Stomoxys calcitrans*, occurs in most countries. Other species, including *S. nigra*, occur in South Africa. *S. calcitrans* is about the size of a housefly, is gray in color and sits head upwards. It can readily be recognized by the prominent, forward-directed, pointed proboscis between short palps. It is a bloodsucker attacking particularly horses and cattle and to a lesser extent pigs. Bites from the fly are quite painful and often bleed freely when fresh. The eggs are laid in rotting hay and straw, especially when it is contaminated with urine, and in horse manure. A complete lifecycle may be completed in 2–3 weeks, the larval and pupal stages taking place in the organic matter. Warm, moist conditions favor multiplication of the flies and in bad seasons the large numbers of flies may cause anemia, worry, loss of grazing time and reduction of growth and yield and reduced feed efficiency. A localized sensitivity of the forelimbs of cattle may develop and result in the formation of intradermal blisters which coalesce to form bleeding sores. With very heavy infestations some deaths may occur. Among the important infectious diseases transmitted by *S. calcitrans* are anthrax, infectious equine anemia and surra. The fly is not a true intermediate host but acts as a mechanical vector. The fly also acts as the intermediate host for *Habronema majus* and is reputed to be a cause of allergic dermatitis in horses in Japan.

Control of the fly necessitates removal or close covering of rotting organic matter from the environment. Silage stacks, horse manure and compost heaps are favored breeding spots. Destruction of flies is difficult because they feed for only short periods. Spraying of cattle with repellents such as *o*-diethyl toluamide protects for 3–4 hours but is costly. Spraying of fixtures and walls, particularly sunlit walls where the flies often remain unnoticed, with long-acting compounds such as tetrachlorvinphos, diazinon, crotoxyphos and propoxur reduces infestations for 2 weeks or longer.

Crotoxyphos and methoxychlor can also be sprayed onto cattle giving about 4 days protection. Fenchlorphos can also be used but requires daily spraying or daily or alternate daily wipe-on application for good control. Affected horses can be treated locally with an analgesic cream, and if the irritation is severe, they can be tranquilized with acetyl promazine.

Horse flies, march flies or breeze flies (*Tabanus* spp.); deer flies (*Chrysops, Haematopota* and *Pangonia* spp.)

These large brown robust flies are widespread in many countries and like *S. calcitrans* worry large animals, particularly horses and cattle and being bloodsuckers can cause anemia. They can also act as mechanical vectors of such diseases as infectious equine anemia, surra and anthrax. *Haematopota* spp. are commonly suspected of acting as vectors for corynebacterial mastitis (summer mastitis) of cattle. The lifecycle differs from that of *S. calcitrans* in that the eggs are laid on the leaves of plants growing in or near water. The larval and pupal stages are passed in water or mud and the lifecycle takes 4–5 months to complete. The flies are active in summer and attack animals principally on the legs and ventral abdomen. Control is difficult unless wet areas can be drained or livestock kept away from these areas where the flies are most active. Repellents have been used and are reasonably effective in horses subject to fly-worry. The use of *o*-diethyl toluamide affords protection for only a few days and is costly, but its use in milking cattle gives increased milk yield and butter fat. Permethrin, a synthetic pyrethroid, used as a spray or as a dust on cattle and horses killed 90% of flies for about 2 weeks after treatment.

Buffalo flies; horn flies (*Haematobia* spp.)

These small (6 mm) grayish flies have fairly limited geographical distributions, *H. irritans exigua* in Australia and south-east Asia, *H. irritans irritans* in the continental United States and Hawaii and *H. minuta* in Africa. They have similar lifecycles and habits. Although they are primarily parasites of cattle and water buffalo and are unable to survive apart from these animals, they can be a nuisance to horses and man in bad seasons. They are bloodsuckers but are not known to transmit diseases other than *Stephanofilaria* spp., their chief importance being to worry animals and interfere with their grazing. The irritation and blood loss caused by burdens of 200–500 or more flies will reduce weight gains of beef cattle and milk yield of dairy cows, while very heavy infestations (over 1000 flies) can cause serious loss of condition and deaths. Control of *H. irritans exigua* results in better food intake and conversion (9), 18% better growth rate (10) and better calf weaning weights (11). The flies congregate chiefly on the withers, shoulders and flanks and around the eyes. Zebu cattle are less affected by the flies than British breeds and although they may carry large populations of flies, they show fewer sores. Horses may develop sores around the eyes and under the belly which provide sites for infestation of larvae of *Draschia megastoma*. The flies are easily recognized by the way in which the wings are held at rest, slightly divergent and angled upwards away from the body. Adult flies stay on the host most of the time, only leaving the host as feces are passed to deposit eggs beneath the freshly dropped buffalo or cattle dung. The eggs and larvae have narrow environmental limits in which they can survive: they are very susceptible to drying, requiring 75–85% free moisture; the optimum temperature for development is 26–35°C (78–95°F) higher or lower temperatures arresting development (7). Thus the flies can only persist in warm moist climates, requiring an annual rainfall of at least 50 cm and a mean temperature greater than 22°C (72°F). The larvae live in the fresh manure and pupate in the soil, a complete lifecycle ending in 8 days to 3 weeks under optimal environmental conditions. Adult flies are permanent parasites of cattle and buffalo and rarely leave the host other than to lay eggs. When dislodged they are active only in warm weather and while they may be carried long distances by prevailing strong winds, the main method of spread is by the movement of cattle. Little transmission occurs by free flight but *H. irritans exigua* is known to have colonized an island 7 km off the Australian coast. In hot conditions the flies can only live for 1–2 days off the host. The distribution of *H. irritans exigua* is controlled by environmental factors, particularly temperature and humidity. Below 21°C (70°F) the flies become sluggish and at 5°C (41°C) they become comatose.

Infestations have been controlled by traps, insecticide sprays, back rubbers, dust bags or eartags impregnated with insecticides. Traps have been designed for use with dairy cattle that walk through them on their way to and from the dairy. The flies are dislodged by gauze strips, are retained in the trap and killed when they rest on the insecticide-coated walls. Traps are rarely used today.

Back rubbers consist of absorbent material, impregnated with insecticide or oil, wrapped around a wire suspended a little over a metre above the ground between two posts 4–5 metres apart. Cattle quickly learn to use rubbers to dislodge flies and their coats become smeared with insecticide. Ethion 1% in fuel oil is commonly used against *H. irritans exigua* while coumaphos 1 or 2% has been shown to be effective against horn flies. Insecticidal-impregnated eartags attached to back rubbers and dust bags controlled horn fly for about 6 weeks, while fenvalerate tags were still effective 18 weeks after application (12).

Eartags impregnated with organophosphorus compounds and synthetic pyrethroids have been widely used, but resistance has built up to levels that make this technique ineffective (13). In areas where resistance is not present, eartagging young nursing calves is effective in controlling infestations in cows and calves and more convenient than treating adult cattle (14). Flies can also be controlled by dipping, but this technique is rarely used solely for flies. Organophosphorus compounds have a residual protection of only a few days and products are combined with synthetic pyrethroids to extend the protective period. In areas where cattle ticks require regular treatment adequate control of flies may be gained incidentally, but if treatments are not effective cattle can be oversprayed with pyrethroids.

Ivermectin is a highly effective larvicide against horn fly, face flies, stable flies and house flies; 1 μg/kg B.W./day to cattle kills horn fly larvae in the feces but higher doses are required for other flies (16). The standard anthelmintic dose controls horn flies in the feces for up to 4 weeks, but probably causes severe mortality among most dung-frequenting arthropods, including natural enemies to the buffalo fly. The technique used will vary with the size of the herd and the labor and facilities available.

Horse louse-flies (*Hippobosca equina, H. rufipes* and *H. maculata*)

Hippobosca equina is the common fly and is a parasite of horses and cattle in most countries with a warm climate. It is a flat, glossy, reddish-brown fly, slightly bigger than a housefly. It is a bloodsucker and lives most of the time on the host, particularly on the perineum and between the hindlegs. Female flies deposit individual puparia in dry humus in which they mature to adult flies. The flies appear to cause little annoyance in horses which are accustomed to them but horses experiencing them for the first time manifest fright and fly-worry. Being bloodsuckers they may act as mechanical vectors for infectious diseases. Topical spraying of susceptible areas of the body with chlorinated hydrocarbons appears to keep these parasites in check. Local application of 0·2% coumaphos solution quickly kills flies but only gives protection for 3 days.

Biting midges

These tiny flies are members of the family Ceratopogonidae, the important genera being *Culicoides* spp. They are 1–3 mm long, suck blood and, apart from causing annoyance and worry, can transmit infectious diseases such as bluetongue in sheep, horse sickness, ephemeral fever in cattle and act as intermediate hosts for *Onchocerca* spp. Because of their importance as vectors of arboviruses (31), studies have been done on their feeding habits. Cattle and sheep are the most common hosts attacked but some species also feed on birds or dogs (18, 19). Hypersensitivity to the bites of *Culicoides brevitarsis* is the cause of allergic dermatitis (Queensland itch) in horses in Australia and is discussed elsewhere. Cattle also show considerable irritation during attacks by large numbers of midges. They react with vigorous stamping of the feet, switching of the tail and continuous movement.

The flies are plentiful in the warmer months and are most active at dusk and in the early morning. Because of their small size they are capable of being carried long distances by wind. Control of the flies is virtually impossible and most measures to reduce their importance are based on preventing access of the flies to the animals. Repellents, especially dimethyl phthalate or *o*-diethyl toluamide, are effective on a short-term basis but mosquito screens are insufficient protection. Antihistamines can be used regularly but are too expensive for general use. Keeping horses away from areas where the flies are present in large numbers is advisable.

Black flies, buffalo gnats, sandflies

These small gray to black flies (5 mm) are members of the family Simuliidae and include a number of species and genera. The important flies appear to be *Cnephia pecuarum* which is common in the southern states of the United States, *Simulium arcticum* in northern Canada, *Austrosimulium pestilens* and *A. bancrofti* in Australia, and *Simulium ornatum* in Great Britain. These very small flies occur in most parts of the world and with the exception of *S. arcticum* are troublesome only in warm climates. They are particularly active in the summer months and frequent areas where fresh, surface water and shade-trees are plentiful. Very large numbers of flies are often present after periods of flooding or in areas with many streams. *A. pestilens* has adapted to reach large numbers, mate and oviposit within a very short time to utilize the flood situations that occur in northern Australia (15). The flies congregate in swarms and attack all animals, causing much worry and annoyance. They tend to bite animals around the legs, on the belly and around the head, causing wheals and papules. The annoyance may be so intense that animals stampede or mill about and young animals may be injured or even trampled to death and are frequently separated from their dams. Cattle may spend much of their time wallowing in mud or kicking up dust to keep the flies away. Herding of cattle onto bare areas reduces fly attacks as the flies commonly rest in tall grass but this reduces feeding. Sudden deaths in cattle have also been recorded after attacks by very large numbers of flies. The cause of death is unknown although swelling of the throat causing suffocation, anaphylaxis or direct toxicity are suspected (17). Filarid worms of *Onchocerca* spp. are transmitted by these flies and their role as an intermediate host of nematodes has been discussed (32).

Because the larval stages of these worms are passed in flowing streams, large-scale control measures must be directed at killing the larvae at this stage. Aerial distribution of DDT has been effective when added to streams and water supplies or control can be effected by adding insecticides into rivers and canals. However, rapid reinfestation occurs with increased rate of water flow after heavy rains (19). For less ambitious control programs, efforts should be directed towards keeping flies away from animals by the application of repellents or the use of smudge fires. Repellents are of limited use but alcoholic or aqueous solutions and dusts of permethein, cypermethrin and resmethrin applied to the whole body repelled black flies for some days (20).

Mosquitoes

A number of mosquitoes including *Psorophora*, *Aedes*, *Mansonia*, *Culex* and *Anopheles* spp. are important parasites of domestic animals. When present in large numbers they cause annoyance and worry to animals and have been known to kill young pigs and puppies by the severe anemia they produce. Although such occurrences are rarely recorded this is surprising in the light of the blood loss that can occur in severe infestations. This is apparently sufficient to cause a brake on productivity even in mature large animals. Their most important role is as vectors of disease. *Culex tarsalis*, *Aedes dorsalis*, and *A. nigromaculis* transmit equine encephalomyelitis, *Culex tritaeniorhyncus* is the principal vector of Japanese B encephalitis in Japan (21), *Psorophora confinnis* is instrumental in spreading the eggs of *Dermatobia hominis*, the tropical warble fly, and *Mansonia* spp. transmits Rift Valley fever. The filarid worm *Setaria digitata* is also spread by mosquitoes.

Control over a large area must include drainage of collections of still surface water or destruction of the larvae by the addition of any one of a number of insecticides, particularly DDT or Abate. For small groups of animals protection from the attacks of mosquitoes can only be satisfactorily effected by mosquito-proof screens. Temporary protection by repellents such as dimethyl phthalate is partial only.

Housefly (*Musca domestica*)

The common housefly has a worldwide distribution and achieves veterinary importance because it is capable of transmitting, in a mechanical manner, the causative bacteria of many infectious diseases. It is often cited as a means whereby anthrax, erysipelas and brucellosis are spread but its importance in this regard is largely unproven. It acts as an intermediate host for the larvae of *Habronema muscae* and *D. megastoma*. The eggs are laid in decaying organic matter of any kind but fresh horse manure is preferred. A lifecycle may be completed in 12–14 days in warm weather so that in wet summers the fly population may increase very rapidly causing annoyance to livestock and farm workers.

To reduce the fly population it is necessary to remove all manure and organic matter or spray it *in situ*. In dry weather the manure can be spread thinly on fields but a more dependable method is to place it in a special fly trap, e.g. Baber's fly traps, from which larvae and adult flies cannot escape. Measures to control fly emergence from manure include spraying with diazinon (1 g/m^2) or other insecticides.

To reduce the fly population in buildings is an important procedure in public health work and many measures are recommended. It is not possible to give details of them here because so many factors have to be taken into consideration, including toxicity of the products used for man and animals, development of resistance to the insecticides, and contamination of food products such as milk by the insecticides.

Bush flies (*Musca vetustissima*)

These flies occur commonly in Australia in drier areas and are a cause of much worry to livestock in the summer months. Bush flies die out in southern Australia each winter but breeding continues in the north and the regular northern winds that commence about September each year blow flies southwards and repopulate the areas that are now suitable for breeding. *Musca vetustissima* occur in very large numbers and during the day congregate around the eyes, on the lips, on any visible mucous membrane and on wounds to obtain moisture. They are thought to carry contagious ophthalmia of sheep, infectious keratoconjunctivitis of cattle and contagious ecthyma of sheep, to delay the healing of wounds, to contribute to the lesions produced by buffalo flies (*H. irritans exigua*) and to act as intermediate hosts for the larvae of *Draschia megastoma*, *Habronema muscae* and *Thelazia* spp. Control of the fly population is virtually impossible in the areas where it occurs but individual animals may be protected by repellents such as dimethyl phthalate or *o*-diethyl toluamide. Sprays containing 1% of dichlorvos or crotoxyphos are effective but must be applied daily. Fenvalerate and cypermethrin give excellent relief and lasting protection against the related *Musca autumnalis* and could be tried.

Facefly (*Musca autumnalis*)

This small fly, indigenous to Europe and Asia, first appeared in North America in 1952 and is now present over large areas of eastern Canada and north-eastern and north-central United States. The flies resemble the housefly but are slightly larger. They congregate on the face of cattle, feeding on nasal and lacrimal secretions and saliva. Very large numbers cause a certain amount of fly-worry, cause petechiation in the eye, and they are thought to be instrumental in transmitting infectious keratoconjunctivitis (pink eye) of cattle. Fly numbers are greatest in summer and cattle are worried particularly when outdoors. Repellents have been extensively used but are not highly successful. Syrup baits containing 0·25% dichlorvos applied three times weekly to the forehead of cows or horses may help to eliminate these flies. Self-applied or hand-applied dusts containing organophosphate insecticides are more extensively used. Fenvalerate and cypermethrin give immediate relief, and a lasting reduction in fly numbers when used on fly breeding sites (22). Fresh cattle feces are the only fly breeding grounds, and these may inhibit the larvae if the cattle are fed low levels of organophosphates, but the usefulness of this procedure in the field is limited by the migration of flies from surrounding infested areas.

Several other species of Muscidae, *Musca larvipara*, *M. convexifrons* and *M. amica*, act as intermediate hosts for *Thelazia* spp. worms which infest the conjunctival sacs and lacrimal ducts of domestic animals.

Head fly (*Hydrotaea irritans*)

This small fly, similar in appearance to the housefly but having an olive abdomen and yellow wing bases, is found in the United Kingdom and Europe. It is a non-biting muscid fly that swarms around animals and man from late June to September. Breeding is in soil and litter and there is only one lifecycle per year. The lesions on sheep are self-inflicted trauma in attempts to alleviate fly irritation. Sores are often large, open and may be made more severe by bacterial invasion. The wounds may predispose to blowfly strike by *Lucilia sericata*. The pathogens of summer mastitis of cattle can be spread mechanically by muscid flies, and *Actinomyces (Corynebacterium) pyogenes* has been shown to persist in *H. irritans exigua* for up to 4 days (30). Control is difficult and is similar to that used for the other non-biting muscid fly, *M. autumnalis*. Eartags impregnated with 8·5% cypermethrin or 10% permethrin reduce the severity of fly damage in sheep, and tagged ewes give protection to their lambs (31). However, it is likely that resistance will quickly occur in the same manner as in the facefly. Pour-on applications of synthetic pyrethroids are easier to apply, are cheaper and leave a higher concentration than a spray or an eartag (34). Crotoxyphos cream is effective but at least two applications are needed. Head-caps are most effective but are tedious to apply.

REFERENCES

(1) Moorhouse, D. E. (1972) *Aust. vet. J.*, *48*, 664.
(2) Blume, R. R. et al. (1971) *J. econ. Entomol.*, *64*, 1193.
(3) Campbell, J. B. et al. (1977) *J. econ. Entomol.*, *70*, 592.
(4) Campbell, J. B. & Hermanussen, J. F. (1971) *J. econ. Entomol.*, *64*, 1188.
(5) Schmidt, C. D. et al. (1977) *S. West. Entomol.*, *2*, 144.
(6) Minar, J. et al. (1979) *Fol. Parasitol.*, *26*, 285.
(7) Cook, I. M. & Spain, A. V. (1982) *Aust. J. zool.*, *30*, 923.
(8) Bay, D. E. et al. (1976) *S. West Entomol.*, *1*, 198.
(9) Kinzer, H. G. et al. (1984) *S. West. Entomol.*, *9*, 212.
(10) Haufe, W. O. (1982) *Can. J. anim. Sci.*, *62*, 567.
(11) Campbell, J. B. (1976) *J. econ. Entomol.*, *69*, 711.
(12) Harvey, T. L. et al. (1983) *J. econ. Entomol.*, *76*, 96.
(13) Drummond, R. O. (1984) *Proc. 88th Ann. Mtg US Anim Hlth Assoc., Fort Worth, Texas*, p. 414.
(14) Harvey, T. L. & Brethour, J. R. (1986) *Prev. vet. Med.*, *3*, 537.
(15) Hunter, D. M. & Moorhouse, D. E. (1976) *Bull. entomol. Res*, *66*, 453.
(16) Miller, J. A. et al. (1981) *J. econ. Entomol.*, *74*, 608.
(17) Lukyanov, N. I. & Ivanenko, N. M. (1965) *Veterinariya, Moscow*, *42*, 89.
(18) Muller, M. J. & Murray, M. D. (1977) *Aust. J. Zool.*, *25*, 75.
(19) Kay, B. H. et al. (1978) *J. Aust. entomol. Soc.*, *17*, 145.
(20) Shemanchuk, J. A. (1981) *Pesticide Sci.*, *12*, 412.
(21) Hoffman, R. A. & Roberts, R. H. (1963) *J. econ. Entomol.*, *56*, 258.
(22) Supperer, R. & Heimbucher, J. (1982) *Wien. Tierärztl. Monatsschr.*, *69*, 229.
(23) Poindexter, C. E. & Adkins, T. R., jun. (1970) *J. econ. Entomol.*, *63*, 946.
(24) Treece, R. E. (1964) *J. econ. Entomol.*, *57*, 881, 962.
(25) Tarry, D. W. & Kirkwood, A. C. (1974) *Br. vet. J.*, *130*, 180.
(26) Robinson, J. & Luff, M. L. (1976) *Bull. entomol. Res.*, *65*, 599.
(27) French, N. et al. (1977) *Vet. Rec.*, *100*, 40.
(28) Schmidt, C. D. (1983) *Envir. Entomol.*, *12*, 455.
(29) Muller, M. J. et al. (1984) *Proc. 3rd Symp. Arbovirus Res. Austr.*, p. 43.
(30) Hillerton, J. E. & Bramley, A. J. (1985) *Vet. Parasitol.*, *18*, 223.
(31) Appleyard, W. J. et al. (1984) *Vet. Rec.*, *115*, 463.
(32) Poinar, G. O. Jnr. (1977) *Bull. World Hlth Org.*, *55*, 509.
(33) Shugard, J. I. et al. (1979) *J. econ. Entomol.*, *72*, 633.
(34) Titchener, R. (1984) *Vet. Rec.*, *114*, 386.

HARVEST MITE INFESTATIONS (CHIGGER MITES)

Infestations with trombidiform mites cause dermatitis in all species. Except for *Psorergates ovis*, *P. bos* and *Demodex* spp. they are all harvest or grain mites, primarily attacking harvested grain and infesting animals only secondarily and usually transiently. *P. bos* has no significant pathogenicity.

The larvae of *Pyemotes ventricosus*, *Neotrombicula autumnalis*, *Eutrombicula alfreddugesi*, *E. splendens*, *E. batatas* and some species of *Leptotrombidium* and *Schoengastia* are parasitic on man and most animals causing dermatitis and, in man, transmitting disease. The natural hosts are usually small rodents but nymphs and adults are freeliving predators feeding mainly on arthropods in grain and hay. The larvae are most active in the autumn at harvest time and may cause dermatitis in animals grazing at pasture or those confined in barns and being fed newly harvested grain.

Horses and cattle are usually affected on the face and lips, which, in white-faced horses, may suggest a diagnosis of photosensitization, and about the feet and lower limbs, especially in the flexures. Affected areas are itchy and scaly but, with rubbing, small fragile scabs and absence of hair may become apparent. Infestation of horses with *Trombicula sarcina* causes a severe pruritus and yearlings show irritation by lip-biting their legs and rubbing against stable walls. Stamping is uncommon, and usually occurs when yearlings are stabled on fresh, contaminated bedding (1). Sheep, when first affected, stamp their feet repeatedly and bite their legs. The skin at the heels, coronet and pasterns, and sometimes the shank, becomes erythematous and weeps fluid. The mites detach after 3–5 days and leave a small ulcerated area. In light infestations the mites may be confined to the area between the accessory digits, but in heavy infestations the skin over the whole of the lower limbs may be swollen and thickened. The infestation is self-limiting and treatment is not usually necessary but the legs can be washed in 0·25% maldison. Area control of the mite may be obtained by the use of chlorpyriphos either as 0·5% granules 1·1 kg/ha or the 22·4% spray at 1·6 kg/ha (2).

Infestation with *Tyroglyphus* spp. in pigs appears to be manifested by itchiness and the development of fragile scabs about 3 cm in diameter scattered over the body. Unlike the thick scabs of sarcoptic mange, the skin beneath appears normal. The infestations occur in pigs eating dry ground grain from automatic feeders, lesions appearing several weeks after the dry feeding is begun and disappearing spontaneously about 3 weeks later. No treatment is necessary although spraying with malathion is usually recommended. Affected pigs show no ill-effects but the lesions may be mistaken for those of swine pox or sarcoptic mange. The ingestion of large numbers of mites appears to have no ill-effects.

REFERENCES

(1) Pascoe, R. R. (1981) Equine dermatitis. *Vet. Rev.*, 22. University of Sydney: Postgrad. Found. Vet. Sci.
(2) Mount, G. A. et al. (1978) *J. econ. Entomol.*, *71*, 27.

SHEEP ITCHMITE (*PSORERGATES OVIS*)

The 'itchmite' has been recorded as a parasite of sheep in Australia, New Zealand, South Africa, the United States, Argentina and Chile. The lifecycle comprising eggs, larvae, three nymphal stages and adults, takes 4–5 weeks and is completed entirely on the sheep. Adult mites are extremely small and can be seen only with a microscope. Only the adults are mobile and they effect spread of the disease by direct contact between recently shorn sheep when contact is close and prolonged such as when shorn sheep are packed in yards after shearing, or from ewe to lamb while suckling. All stages occur in the superficial layers of the skin and cause irritation leading to rubbing and biting of the affected parts (principally the sides, flanks and thighs) and raggedness, sometimes shedding, of the fleece. Wool over these areas becomes thready and tufted and contains dry scales (1). The skin shows no gross abnormality but carries more scales than normal and histologically there is hyperkeratosis and desquamation. The irritation appears to be a hypersensitivity and results in biting and chewing of the fleece on the flanks and rump behind a line approximately from the elbow to the hips. In the individual sheep and in flocks the disease spreads slowly so that it may be several years before clinical cases are observed and an appreciable number are visibly affected. The incidence of clinical cases in a neglected flock may be as high as 15%. Affected sheep may become tolerant after 1 or 2 years and show no signs, even though they remain infested. Amongst sheep, Merinos are most commonly affected. The highest incidence is observed in this breed, particularly in areas where the winter is cold and wet. There is a marked seasonal fluctuation in the numbers of mites; the numbers are very low in summer, commence to rise in the autumn and peak numbers are found in the spring. Spring or summer shearing exacerbates the decline in numbers. Clinically, the disease resembles louse infestation, but may be distinguished clinically on the smaller proportion of the flock affected (10–15%), the less severe irritation and tendency of the sheep to bite those areas it can reach. Hence lesions are confined to parts of the flank and the hindquarters and the wool tufts have a chewed appearance.

Diagnosis depends on finding the mites in a skin scraping. The selection of sheep with excess scurf and fleece derangement increases the chance of finding mites and in the absence of lice, ked and grass seed infestation, about 75% of such sheep prove positive for *P. ovis*. The wool should be clipped as close as possible, the skin smeared lightly with oil and scraped over an area of about 25 cm^2. The mites have a seasonal incidence and may be very difficult to find in summer and autumn. For best results the scraping should be made high on the ribs or shoulder in winter or spring. Scrapings are usually teased out in oil and examined microscopically without digestion (2). A number of scrapings may be needed from each sheep before mites can be demonstrated.

There is no compound available that will eradicate itchmite after a single treatment. Arsenic, lime sulfur or finely divided sulfur have been used and markedly reduce the number of mites. Because the mites are slow to build up, dipping every second year will mask the signs of infestation. Finely divided rotenone by itself or mixed with the synergist piperonyl butoxide reduces the mite population. It is usually combined with an organophosphate to include lice and ked control in the one product. Phoxim, an organophosphorus compound, has good activity but two dippings 1 month apart are necessary to eradicate infestations (3). Amitraz causes a marked reduction in mites that will be maintained for some months. Ivermectin also causes a marked reduction for some months and two treatments 1 month apart will eradicate infestations. Dippings are most effective if given within 2 weeks of shearing (4).

REFERENCES

(1) Sinclair, A. N. (1986) *NZ vet. J.*, *24*, 149.
(2) Skerman, K. D. et al. (1962) *Aust. vet. J.*, *38*, 439.
(3) Malan, F. S. & Roper, N. A. (1982) *J. S. Afr. vet. Assoc.*, *53*, 171.
(4) Sinclair, A. N. & Gibson, A. J. F. (1975) *NZ vet. J.*, *23*, 14.

DEMODECTIC MANGE (FOLLICULAR MANGE)

Mites of *Demodex* spp. infest hair follicles of all species of domestic animals. The disease causes little concern but in cattle there may be significant damage to the hide and rarely death due to gross secondary bacterial invasion (1). The disease may also be severe in goats (3).

Etiology

Mites infesting the different host species are considered to be specific and are designated as *Demodex bovis* for cattle, *D. ovis* for sheep, *D. caprae* for goats, *D. equi* for horses and *D. phylloides* for pigs. The alternate nomenclature is *D. folliculorum* var. *bovis*, etc.

Demodicosis may occur in farm animals of any age, especially those in poor condition but most cases in cattle occur in adult dairy cattle in late winter and early spring. This differs from the well-known condition in the dog which occurs in young, immunodeficient animals.

Lifecycle and epidemiology

The entire lifecycle is spent on the host. Adult mites invade the hair follicles and sebaceous glands which become distended with mites and inflammatory material. The lifecycle passes through the egg, larval and two nymphal stages. The disease spreads slowly and transfer of mites is thought to take place by contact, probably early in life. Calves can acquire mites from an infected dam in half a day (4, 8). However, in horses grooming instruments and rugs may transmit infection.

Pathogenesis

Invasion of hair follicles and sebaceous glands leads to chronic inflammation (2), loss of the hair fiber and in many instances the development of secondary staphylococcal pustules or small abscesses. It is these foci of infection which cause the small pinholes in the hide which interfere with its industrial processing and limit its use. In most farm animals the lesions are difficult to see externally and only the advanced ones will be diagnosed (5).

Clinical findings

The important sign is the appearance of small (3 mm diameter) nodules and pustules which may develop into larger abscesses, especially in pigs and goats. The small lesions can be seen quite readily in short-coated animals and on palpation feel like particles of bird-shot in the hide. In severe cases there may be a general hair-loss and thickening of the skin in the area, but usually there is no pruritus and hair-loss is insufficient to attract attention. The contents of the pustules are usually white in color and cheesey in consistency. In large abscesses the pus is more fluid. In cattle and goats the lesions occur most commonly on the brisket, lower neck, forearm and shoulder, but also occur on the dorsal half of the body, particularly behind the withers. Larger lesions are easily visible but very small lesions may only be detected by rolling a fold of skin through the fingers. In horses the face and around the eyes are predilection areas. Demodicosis in pigs usually commences on the face and spreads down the ventral surface of the neck and chest to the belly. There is little irritation and the disease is observed mainly when the skin is scraped at slaughter (6). The disease may be especially severe in goats, spreading extensively before it is suspected and in some instances causing deaths. Severe cases in goats are commonly affected with several skin diseases such as mycotic dermatitis, ringworm, besnoitiosis and myiasis. Demodicosis is rare in sheep. In this species pustules and scabs appear on the coronets, nose, tips of the ears and around the eyes (7), but clinical signs are not usually seen and mites may be found in scrapings from areas of the body not showing lesions.

Clinical pathology

The characteristically elongated mites are usually easy to find in large numbers in the waxy material which can be expressed from the pustular lesions. They are much more difficult to isolate from squamous lesions. Lesions in hides can be detected as dark spots when a fresh hide is viewed against a strong light source (1). However, lesions may not be readily seen until the hair has been removed and the skin has been soaking for some time.

Diagnosis

The commonest error is to diagnose the disease as a non-specific staphylococcal infection. In cattle and goats the disease often passes unnoticed unless the nodules are palpated. Deep-seated ringworm in horses has much in common with demodicosis. A satisfactory diagnosis can only be made by demonstration of the mite.

Treatment and control

Repeated dipping or spraying with the acaricides recommended for other manges is usually carried out but is more to prevent spread than cure existing lesions.

REFERENCES

(1) Smith, H. J. (1961) *Can. J. comp. Med.*, *25*, 165, 201, 243, 307.
(2) Slingenbergh, J. et al. (1980) *Vet. Q.*, *2*, 90.
(3) Das, D. M. & Misra, S. C. (1972) *Ind. vet. J.*, *49*, 96.
(4) Fisher, W. F. (1973) *J. Parasitol.*, *59*, 223.
(5) Murray, M. D. et al. (1976) *Aust. vet. J.*, *52*, 49.
(6) Rapp, J. & Koch, F. (1979) *Vet. med. Rev.*, *1*, 67.
(7) Murray, M. D. (1959) *Aust. vet. J.*, *35*, 93.
(8) Fisher, W. F. et al. (1980) *Vet. Parasitol.*, *7*, 233.

SARCOPTIC MANGE (BARN ITCH)

Sarcoptic mange occurs in all species causing a severe itching dermatitis.

Etiology

The causative mite, *Sarcoptes scabiei*, is usually considered to have a number of subspecies each specific to a particular host and designated *S. scabiei*, var. *bovis*, *S. scabiei*, var. *suis* etc., but this host-specificity is not complete and transference from one host species to another can occur, a point of some importance when attempting to control the disease. Animals in poor condition appear to be most susceptible but conditions, especially overcrowding, in which sarcoptic mange occurs often go hand in hand with poor feeding and general mismanagement. The disease is most active in cold, wet weather and spreads slowly during the summer months.

Lifecycle and epidemiology

The females form shallow burrows in the horny layer of the skin in which to lay their eggs. The larval and nymphal stages may remain in the tunnels or emerge on to the skin. The normal exfoliation of the skin eventually exposes the tunnels and any of the lifecycle stages may transmit by contact to other animals. The lifecycle from egg to egg-laying female takes 10–14 days.

The infestation is spread chiefly by direct contact between hosts, all three stages being capable of migration, but inert materials such as bedding, blankets, grooming tools and clothing may act as carriers. Adult mites do not usually survive for more than a few days away from the host but in optimum laboratory conditions they may remain alive for up to 3 weeks. In pigs adult sows are often the source of infestation for young pigs even though they show no signs of the disease. Large numbers of mites can often be found in the ears of normal sows and the mites are transmitted soon after farrowing. Significant scratching does not occur until a hypersensitivity develops some 8–10 weeks later and may continue until slaughter (1). A small proportion of young pigs do not develop a hypersensitivity and these become chronically affected (1).

Amongst domestic species pigs are most commonly affected, but it is an important disease in cattle and camels and occurs in sheep. It is a notifiable disease in most countries and is important because of its severity.

Pathogenesis

Piglets become infected in the first few weeks of life and develop a hypersensitivity within 8–10 weeks. This allergic phase lasts for 8–9 months (4) and during this time affected animals are constantly itchy. Many infestations have little or no effect on weight gain and feed efficiency (2), but in some loss of condition, production and vitality may be severe, and the appearance of affected animals is esthetically displeasing. Erythema, papules and intense pruritis may be seen. Few mites may be necessary to cause a reaction in a previously sensitized animal. A chronic condition is uncommon but is seen in pigs with an immunodeficiency (3).

It is thought that sarcoptic mange may occur in animals predisposed to infection by stress or disease, yet iron deprivation in young experimentally infected pigs reduced the severity of urticarial and pruritic symptoms. This was thought to be related to the pallor and cooler temperature of the skin in iron-deprived piglets that made them less suitable hosts (4).

In cattle and camels, severe hypersensitivity lesions occur and often lead to death. Sheep initially show an intense pruritus and rub the affected part against fences or bite at the skin. Later papules and vesicles occur and the skin becomes thickened, covered with pale scabs and the hair is lost (5).

Clinical findings

Early lesions are characterized by the presence of small red papules and general erythema of the skin. The affected area is intensely itchy and frequently excoriated by scratching and biting. Loss of hair, thick brown scabs overlying a raw surface, and thickening and wrinkling of surrounding skin soon follow. In pigs the lesions commence on the trunk, in sheep and goats on the face, in cattle on the inner surface of the thighs, the underside of the neck and brisket and around the root of the tail, and in horses and camels on the head and neck. Except in sheep where the lesions do not spread to the woolled skin, lesions become widespread if neglected and such animals may show systemic effects including emaciation, anorexia and weakness, and in neglected cases death may occur.

The course of sarcoptic mange is rather more acute than in the other forms of mange and may involve the entire body surface of cattle in a period as short as 6 weeks.

Clinical pathology

Necropsy examinations are not usually undertaken. Examination of scapings either directly or after digestion in 10% potassium hydroxide may reveal mites. However, very few mites may be present and a number of scrapings may be necessary. Examination of the ear wax of pigs often shows mites when none can be seen in scrapings.

Diagnosis

Sarcoptic mange is the only mange which occurs in pigs. It can be confused with infestation with *Tyroglyphus* spp. mites or lice, or with swinepox, parakeratosis, infectious dermatitis, pityriasis rosea and ringworm. In most of these diseases there are clinical features which are characteristic and final diagnosis can be made on the presence or absence of the mite. The same comments apply to the differentiation in cattle of sarcoptic mange from chorioptic and psoroptic mange and from chlorinated naphthalene poisoning and ringworm. Horses may be affected by psoroptic or chorioptic mange but the lesions are most common at the base of the mane and tail and at the back of the pastern respectively. Infestation with the trombidiform mites and photosensitization may resemble sarcoptic mange. The disease is uncommon in sheep.

Treatment and control

Treatment must be thorough so that all parts of the skin, especially under the tail, in the ears and between the legs are wetted by the acaricide. Although buildings, bedding, and other inert materials do not support the mite for more than a few days they should also be treated unless they can be left in a dry state for 3 weeks.

None of the treatments used can penetrate the burrows in the skin and repeated treatments are necessary. The older treatments, sulfur, dioxide fumigation and spraying or dipping in lime–sulfur dip, were effective but difficult to apply and they have been largely superseded by more modern insecticides, most of which are effective. Sows should be treated three times at 7-day intervals, commencing 3 weeks before farrowing. Special attention should be paid to the ears. Trichlorphon, maldison (0·5%), diazinon (0·02%), coumaphos (0·05–0·1%), fenchlorphos, chlorfenvinphos, amitraz (0·1%) and phoxim (0·025%) have been used (3, 6). All animals should be treated. Phosmet 20% applied as a pour-on at weaning eliminated *Sarcoptes* and allowed 12% increase in live weight gain (7). Ivermectin (0·2 mg/kg) given subcutaneously eliminated *Sarcoptes* from a camel (8) and when given orally eliminated infection in pigs (9).

REFERENCES

(1) Dobson, K. J. & Cargill, C. F. (1979) In *Vet. Epidemiol. Econ. Proc. 2nd Int. Symp. Aust. Bur. Anim. Hlth*, p. 401.
(2) Wooten, E. L. et al. (1986) *Vet. Parasitol.*, *22*, 315.
(3) Liebish, A. et al. (1980) *Vet. med. Rev.*, *1*, 3.
(4) Sheahan, B. J. (1974) *Vet. Rec.*, *94*, 202.
(5) Abu-Samra, M. T. et al. (1981) *Ann. trop. Med. Parasitol.*, *75*, 639.
(6) Palmer, C. R. & Amelsfoort, A. van (1983) *J. S. Afr. vet. Assoc.*, *54*, 99.
(7) Hewett, G. R. (1985) *Vet. Parasitol.*, *18*, 265.
(8) Opferman, R. R. (1985) *J. Am. vet. Med. Assoc.*, *187*, 1240.
(9) Alva-Valdes, R. et al. (1984) *Am. J. vet. Res.*, *45*, 2113.

PSOROPTIC MANGE (SHEEP-SCAB, BODY MANGE, EAR MANGE)

Psoroptic mange is of greatest importance in sheep, in which it causes sheep scab, but it is also responsible for body mange in cattle and horses and ear mange in horses, sheep, goats and rabbits.

Etiology

The various species of *Psoroptes* have now been reduced to four body mites and two ear mites. *P. ovis* is the only mite on sheep but may also occur on cattle, horses and possibly the donkey. However, there is some doubt whether the mites on cattle and sheep are the same (1). *P. equi* occurs on horses, donkeys and mules in Great Britain and *P. natalensis* on cattle and the water buffalo. The ear mites are all *P. cuniculi*. *P. cervinus* assumes a dual role, being an ear mite of the American bighorn and a body mite of the wapiti.

Lifecycle and epidemiology

Psoroptic mange or sheep-scab is a major disease in sheep and has now been virtually eliminated in most progressive countries where wool production is an important industry. The disease in cattle was widespread in the United States but has now largely been brought under control. It can spread rapidly and cause serious losses in cattle if neglected as shown by the serious losses that can occur in feedlots. The ear manges cause irritation and, in horses, a touchiness around the head.

Psoroptic mites feed on tissue fluid and cause the formation of scabs, under which they live. The eggs are laid on the skin at the edge of a scab and hatch in 1–3 days, although this is prolonged if eggs are not in contact with the skin. There is the usual larval and nymphal stages and the whole lifecycle is complete in 10–11 days (2). All stages are capable of survival away from the host for up to 10 days and under optimum conditions adult females may survive for 3 weeks. Optimum conditions for development include moistness and cool temperatures. Thus the disease is most active in autumn and winter months. This is due not only to increased activity of the mites but also to the more rapid development in housed animals and to the tendency for the disease to be most severe in animals in poor condition. If cattle are housed in stanchions that prevent grooming infestation will be more severe (2). Although individual mites survive for only 4–6 weeks the disease is continuous and a very rapid increase in mite numbers may occur (2). When conditions are adverse, as in summer, mites survive in protected parts in the perineum, in the inguinal and interdigital regions, the infraorbital fossae and the scrotum. Spread occurs from sheep to sheep but transmission from infected premises and by passive spread of pieces of wool occurs. Premises left free of sheep for at least 2 weeks can be assumed to be safe (2). The lifecycle of the other species is thought to be similar. Spread of ear mite in horses can occur by grooming or by the use of infected harness.

Pathogenesis

The mite migrates to all parts of the skin and prefers areas covered with hair or wool. The adults puncture the epidermis to feed on lymph and cause local inflammation resulting in itchiness and the exudation of serum which accumulates to form a crust. The mites are most active at the edge of the crust and the lesion spreads peripherally. Infested calves have lower weight gains, lower feed conversion and lower energy retention than non-infested calves (6).

Clinical findings

Sheep

Cutaneous lesions may occur on any part of the body but characteristically in badly affected sheep they are most obvious on the sides. Very early lesions are small (6 mm diameter) papules which ooze serum. Attention may be attracted to the area by raggedness of the wool caused by bitting and scratching. In older lesions thin yellow crusts are present and the wool commences to shed. The wool may contain large masses of scab material which bind the fibers together in a mat.

In a typical outbreak of 'sheep-scab' many animals are affected and show itchiness and shedding of the fleece. Some become markedly emaciated and weak and deaths may occur. However, it is possible to have the disease in a flock at a very low level of incidence and with minimal lesions. This usually occurs when the sheep are highly resistant because of good nutrition, or climatic conditions are adverse for mite development, or treatment has been carried out but has been incomplete. In such cases there may be little or no clinical evidence of the disease and a careful search for latent cases may be necessary. This is facilitated by packing the animals into a confined space, so that the mites become active, and watching for signs of itchiness. Sheep which bite or scratch should be carefully examined by palpating the surface of the skin in search of papules and scabs. Special attention should be paid to the ears, the base of the horns, the infraorbital fossa and the perineal and scrotal areas in rams.

Goats

Lesions can vary from a dry crusty scab on the external ear canal with no clinical signs to severe lesions covering much of the body and causing death. However, it is commonly an ear mite, feeding on whole blood, and causing the production of scabs which vary from a single layer lining the large sulcus at the base of the concha to abundant laminated scab formation occluding the meatus. In severe cases the poll may be affected, and scabs may also be found on the pasterns. Female goats serve as the source of infection for the kid, mites may be found by 10 days and clinical signs are seen by the 3rd week of life (3). *Raillietina manfredi* may also be found in the ear of goats but is easily differentiated microscopically as all legs are on the anterior part of the body (5).

Horses

P. equi causes the production of large, thick crusts on those parts of the body carrying long hair, the base of the mane and the root of the tail, and hairless areas such as the udder, prepuce and axilla. Affected parts are itchy, the hair is lost and with constant rubbing the surrounding skin becomes thickened. *P. cuniculi* infestations in horses cause severe irritation in the ear accompanied by discharge, shaking of the head, rubbing of the head and tenderness of the poll (4).

Cattle

Typical lesions appear first on the withers, neck and around the root of the tail. In severe cases they may spread to the rest of the body. The lesions are intensely itchy. They commence as papules but soon are covered with a scab which enlarges peripherally and coalesces with other lesions so that very large areas of skin may become involved. The hair is lost, the skin becomes thickened, wrinkled and covered with scabs. Badly affected animals become weak and emaciated and may die.

Clinical pathology

The mites can be easily demonstrated in scrapings taken from the edges of the lesions. Examination is facilitated by prior digestion of the scraping in warm, 10% potassium hydroxide solution.

Diagnosis

Severe cases of psoroptic mange in sheep are similar to mycotic dermatitis except that there is no itching in the latter. Disease causing itchiness such as scrapie, ked and louse infestations and infestations with *Psorergates ovis* and harvest mites do not have typical cutaneous lesions and the latter group can usually be detected by examination for the causative parasites. In horses attention is drawn to the condition because of the horse rubbing its head (4), by swelling around the base of the ear or by resentment to the bridle passing over the ears. In some horses the affected ear may droop.

Treatment and control

Psoroptic mange in sheep is a notifiable disease in most countries and local legislation may determine the agents to be used and the methods and frequency of its application. In Britain, where the disease has increased because of the vast increase in the movement of sheep, all sheep are compulsorily dipped within a 4-week period in summer and again in the winter in an effort to eliminate the infestation. It is important to wet the skin thoroughly and pay special attention to severe cases where mites are likely to be present in inaccessible sites on the body. Thus a plunge dip is almost essential and the sheep must be kept immersed in the dipping fluid for 2 minutes. Prior shearing may be advisable but may lead to further spread of the infestation. Care must be taken to ensure that the concentration of the acaricide in the dip is maintained, especially when large numbers of sheep are being treated. Badly affected animals should be set aside and inaccessible sites including ears, horn bases and perineum treated manually with the dipping fluid. Dipped sheep should not be returned to their pastures, nor to the barn unless the latter has been thoroughly cleaned and sprayed with the dipping fluid.

Benzene hexachloride (0·016%), diazinon (0·01%) and propetamphos (0·0125%) will all eliminate *P. ovis* from sheep with a single dipping and will give at least 4 weeks protection (1, 7). Ivermectin 0·2 mg/kg is effective in cattle when given intramuscularly or subcutaneously and protects against reinfestation for 21 days (8, 9). Cattle treated with ivermectin must be separated from non-infested cattle for at least 9 days, otherwise spread may occur (10). Oral administration is not completely effective (8). In sheep variable results have been reported; subcutaneous administration at standard dose rates did not eliminate infestations (1), but higher doses (0·5 and 1·0 mg/kg) given intramuscularly eliminated infections from big-horn sheep (11). Two treatments 1 week apart also eliminated infestations (14). Toxophene (0·5%) will also eliminate infestation from cattle in one dipping (12), but only 8 days residual protection is obtained (8).

Coumaphos (0·1%), phoxim (0·05%) and amitraz (0·05%) require two treatments at 7–10 days intervals to eliminate infestations. The synthetic pyrethroids are variable in their efficacy. Flumethrin, used as a non-stripping dipping compound, eradicated *P. ovis* from sheep when used at 55 ppm and gave at least 7 weeks protection (15). Fenvalerate (0·05%) used twice will also clear infested cattle; but another synthetic pyrethroid, cypermethrin, when used at 150 ppm did not eliminate infestations after three treatments (13).

In horses, affected ears should be cleaned of all wax and ear preparations containing benzene hexachloride should be used at weekly intervals. Local treatment of diazinon or propetamphos could also be used. Benzyl benzoate is a safe and effective treatment when given every 5 days for three treatments (4). Ivermectin is highly effective against *P. equi* (16).

Eradication of 'sheep-scab' on an area basis is usually undertaken by quarantine and compulsory dipping of all susceptible animals in the area at the same time. The necessity to dip all animals in the area during a short period presents difficulties and the cost of construction of dips and lack of desire to dip in cold climates are other obstructing factors. Where it is desired to keep the disease at a low level short of eradication, the disease is made notifiable, movement of stock is restricted and infested farms are quarantined and the sheep dipped until clean.

REFERENCES

(1) Kirkwood A. C. (1985) *Vet. Parasitol.*, *18*, 269.
(2) Guillot, F. S. (1981) *J. med. Entomol.*, *18*, 44.
(3) Williams, J. F. & Williams, C. S. F. (1978) *J. Am. vet. med. Assoc.*, *173*, 1582.
(4) Montali, R. J. (1976) *J. Am. vet. med. Assoc.*, *169*, 630.
(5) Cook, R. W. (1981) *Aust. vet. J.*, *57*, 72.
(6) Cole, N. A. & Guillot, F. S. (1987) *Vet. Parasitol.*, *23*, 285.
(7) Bramley, P. S. & Henderson, D. (1984) *Vet. Rec.*, *115* 460.
(8) Meleney, W. P. et al. (1982) *Am. J. vet. Res.*, *43*, 1767.
(9) Guillot, F. S. et al. (1986) *Am. J. vet. Res*, *47*, 525.
(10) Wright, F. C. & Guillot, F. S. (1984) *Am. J. vet. Res.*, *45*, 228.
(11) Kinzer, H. G. et al. (1983) *J. Wildlife Dis.*, *19*, 52.
(12) Guillot, F. S. et al. (1982) *Prev. vet. Med.*, *1*, 179.
(13) Palmer, C. R. & Amelsfoort, A. van (1983) *J. S. Afr. vet. Assoc.*, *54*, 99.
(14) Wasfi, I. A. & Hashim, N. H. (1986) *World Anim. Rev.*, *59*, 29.
(15) Kirkwood, A. C. & Bates, P. G. (1987) *Vet. Rec.*, *120*, 197.
(16) Mukhtar, T. et al. (1987) *Equ. vet. J.*, *19*, 143.

CHORIOPTIC MANGE (TAIL MANGE, LEG MANGE, SCROTAL MANGE)

Chorioptic mange is the commonest form of mange in cattle and horses. In cattle it usually causes little other than esthetic damage, while in horses leg mange is a source of annoyance and inefficiency at work. In sheep it affects the scrotum and causes a decrease in fertility (1).

Etiology

Chorioptic mites were formerly named according to the host species but those on cattle, horses and sheep are now all thought to be one species, *C. bovis*. Another species, *C. texanus*, has been reported on goats and Canadian reindeer (2). In cattle, the mites are much more active in the latter part of the winter and tend to disappear in cattle at pasture. This diminution in activity is not noted in cattle kept housed in the summer time.

Lifecycle and epidemiology

The lifecycle of *C. bovis* is similar to that of *Psoroptes* and is complete in 3 weeks. The number of parasites is influenced by temperature and humidity; the mites commence breeding on sheep in early autumn, numbers reach a peak in late autumn or early winter and decline in spring (6). In cattle the cycle is longer, peak numbers occurring in late winter and early spring and declining in summer. Transmission is probably effected by direct contact in most instances although in animals housed in barns, grooming tools may be an additional method of spreading the disease. Infestation of bedding is not a common method of transmission.

In horses, the parasites occur almost entirely in the long hair on the lower parts of the legs and are rarely found on other parts of the body. In cattle the disease is most evident in the winter time, lesions occurring most commonly on the perineum, and back of the udder, extending in severe cases to the backs of the legs and over the rump. In the summer months the mites persist in the area above the hooves, particularly the pasterns of the hind leg. In sheep, lesions are confined to the woolless areas, chiefly the lower parts of the hindlegs, and scrotum. Rams are more heavily infected than ewes and probably infect ewes while copulating. Lactating ewes probably act as the source of infection for lambs (6).

Pathogenesis

The mites cause an allergic, exudative dermatitis, the yellowish serous exudate coagulates and breaks as the hair grows so that small scabby lesions are seen on the hair. In horses the mites cause severe irritation and itchiness. The initial lesion in cattle is a small nodule which exudes serum causing matting of the hair. In severe cases these coalesce to form heavy scabs and cause thickening and wrinkling of the skin. Mites can be isolated from many animals which show no clinical evidence of the disease. While most cases do not cause any symptoms, a rapidly spreading syndrome characterized by coronitis, intense irritation and a marked fall in milk production has been reported (3). *C. bovis* is a common parasite of sheep in the United States, New Zealand and Australia, and causes an allergic exudative dermatitis on the scrotum of rams. This may cause a rise in temperature of the scrotal contents and a severe testicular degeneration if the lesion has an area greater than 10 cm^2 (1).

Clinical findings

The first sign in horses is usually violent stamping of the feet and rubbing of the back of the hind pasterns on wire, rails or stumps. This is most evident during periods of rest and at night. Examination of the area is difficult because of the long hair present and the horses may resent manipulation. In cases of long duration the skin is seen to be swollen, scabby, cracked and usually greasy and small amounts of serous exudate may be attached to most hair in the affected area.

Cattle show little evidence of cutaneous irritation but the small crusty scabs (3 mm diameter) on the escutcheon, udder and thighs are unsightly. Although the mites appear to cause little trouble in the summer time, occasional animals are seen which have thick, crusty scabs on the skin, just above the coronets and around the muzzle.

The main lesion in sheep is seen on the scrotum of rams where an allergic dermatitis results in the production of a yellowish serous exudate over areas from a few millimeters to several centimeters (1).

Clinical pathology

Scrapings from the affected areas usually contain large numbers of mites.

Diagnosis

Greasy heel in horses resembles chorioptic mange except that pain is more evident in the former and itchiness in the latter. It has been suggested that the two diseases are etiologically related. The lesions in cattle may go unnoticed but are not likely to be mistaken for those of any other disease with the possible exception of other manges. The presence of chorioptic mites in footrot and mucosal disease lesions may be purely coincidental, but cases of chorioptic mange which have lesions around the coronet and muzzle may be mistaken for one of the erosive disease. Sheep with itchy, scabby legs may be infested with other forms of mange or have contagious ecthyma or strawberry footrot.

Treatment and control

Although control of the mites appears to be effected easily complete eradication from an animal or herd is not, and apparent eradication in a herd is often followed by a reappearance of the disease the following winter, even if multiple treatments are undertaken.

Crotoxyphos 0·25% solution applied once as a spray is claimed to be completely effective and leave no residue in meat or milk (4), while 0·03–0·06% used twice is also effective (5). This compound can also be used as a 2% solution in livestock spray oil. Phoxim 0·05% and 0·1% used twice at 10-day intervals has also eradicated the infection from cattle (7). Other compounds if used repeatedly will reduce mite numbers but recrudescences may occur. Ivermectin 0·2 mg/kg given subcutaneously on two occasions reduced but did not eliminate the infestation on cattle.

REFERENCES

(1) Rhodes, A. P. (1976) *Aust. vet. J.*, *52*, 250.
(2) Sweatman, G. K. (1957) *Can. J. Zool.*, *35*, 641.
(3) Diplock, P. T. & Hyne, R. H. J. (1975) *NSW vet. Proc.*, *11*, 31.
(4) Smith, H. H. (1967) *Can. vet. J.*, *8*, 88.
(5) Matthysse, J. G. et al. (1967) *J. econ. Ent.*, *60*, 1615.
(6) Heath, A. C. G. (1978) *NZ vet. J.*, *26*, 299.
(7) Stendel, W. (1980) *Prakt. Tierärztl.*, *61*, 240.
(8) Sweatman, G. K. (1958) *Can. J. Zool.*, *36*, 391.

28

Metabolic Diseases

INTRODUCTION

AMONGST domestic farm animals the metabolic diseases achieve their greatest importance in dairy cows and pregnant ewes. In the other species these diseases occur only sporadically. The high-producing dairy cow always verges on abnormality and the breeding and feeding of dairy cattle for high milk yields is etiologically related to the diseases of metabolism so common in these animals. In dairy cows, the incidence of metabolic diseases is highest in the period commencing at calving and extending until the peak of lactation is reached, and their susceptibility appears to be related to the extremely high turnover of fluids, salts and soluble organic materials during the early part of lactation. With this rapid rate of exchange of water, sodium, calcium, magnesium, chlorides and phosphates, a sudden variation in their excretion or secretion in the milk or by other routes, or a sudden variation in their intake because of changes in ingestion, digestion or absorption, may cause abrupt, damaging changes in the internal environment of the animal. It is the volume of the changes in intake and secretion and the rapidity with which they can occur that reduce the metabolic stability of the cow. When one considers that the continued nutritional strain of a pregnancy is often exacerbated by an inadequate diet in the dry period this point becomes obvious. The effect of pregnancy is particularly important in ewes, especially those carrying more than one lamb.

In the next phase of the production cycle, parturition is followed by the sudden onset of a profuse lactation which, if the nutrient reserves have already been seriously depleted, may further reduce them to below critical levels and clinical metabolic disease then occurs. The essential metabolite which is reduced below the critical level determines the clinical syndrome which will occur. Most attention has been paid to variations in balances of calcium and inorganic phosphates relative to parturient paresis, of magnesium relative to lactation tetany, of blood sugar and ketones and hepatic glycogen relative to ketosis, and of potassium relative to hyperkalemia on cereal grazing, but it is probable that other imbalances are important in the production of as yet unidentified syndromes.

During the succeeding period of lactation, particularly in cows on test schedules and under the strain of producing large quantities of milk, there is often a variable food intake, especially when pasture is the sole source of food, and instability of the internal environment inevitably follows. The period of early lactation is an unstable one in all species. Hormonal stimulation at this stage is so strong that nutritional deficiency often does not limit milk production and a serious drain on reserves of metabolites may occur.

The fact that some dams are affected much more by these variations than others is probably explainable on the basis of variations in internal metabolism and degree of milk production between species and between individuals. Between groups of cows, variations in susceptibility appear to depend on either genetic or management factors. Certainly Jersey cows are more susceptible to parturient paresis than cows of other breeds, and Guernseys, in our experience, seem to be more susceptible to ketosis. Even within breeds considerable variation is evident in susceptibility between families. Under these circumstances it seems necessary to invoke genetic factors, at least as predisposing causes.

Management practices of most importance are housing and nutrition. In those sections of North America where cattle are housed during the winter, and in poor pasture areas, ketosis is prevalent. In the Channel Islands, local cattle are unaffected by lactation tetany whereas the disease is prevalent in Great Britain. In New Zealand metabolic diseases are complex and the incidence is high, both probably related to the practice of having the cows calve in late winter when feed is poor, to the practice of depending entirely on pasture for feed, and to the high proportion of Jerseys in the cattle population.

A knowledge of these various factors is essential before any reasonable scheme of prevention can be undertaken. It should also indicate that although the more common disease entities are presented in this chapter there is high probability that a disturbance of more than one of the metabolites mentioned may occur simultaneously in the one animal and give rise to complex syndromes which are not described here. The disease entities dealt with must be considered as arbitrary points in a long scale of metabolic disturbances.

Finally, only a knowledge of the etiological factors

involved will help in understanding the incidence of the various syndromes. Largely because of variations in climate the occurrence of metabolic disease varies from season to season and from year to year. In the same manner, variations in the types of disease occur. For example in some seasons most cases of parturient paresis will be tetanic; in others, most cases of ketosis will be complicated by hypocalcemia. Further, the incidence of metabolic disease and the incidence of the different syndromes will vary from region to region. Ketosis may be common in low rainfall areas and on poor pasture. Lactation tetany may be common in colder areas and where natural shelter is poor. Recognition of these factors can make it possible to devise means whereby the incidence of the diseases can be reduced.

The metabolic diseases, because of high prevalence and high mortality rate, are of major importance in some countries, so much so that predictive systems are being set up. Rapid analysis of stored feed samples, pasture and soil is commonly used in Europe and North America but the interesting development has been the recognition of 'production diseases' and the consequent development of metabolic profile tests, particularly in the United Kingdom and in Europe (2, 3).

PRODUCTION DISEASES

The term 'production disease' encompasses those diseases previously known as 'metabolic diseases', such as parturient paresis (milk fever), hypomagnesemia, acetonemia and perhaps some other conditions, all of which are attributable to an imbalance between the rates of 'input' of dietary nutrients and the 'output' of production. When the imbalance is maintained, it may lead to a change in the amount of the body's reserves of certain metabolites, or their 'throughput', and sufficiently large changes in 'throughput' will give rise to signs of production disease (4, 5). The generalization applies principally to the hypoglycemias (ketosis) and hypomagnesemias and partly to the hypocalcemias. In these diseases, output is greater than input either because of the selection of cattle which produce so heavily that no naturally occurring diet can maintain the cow in nutritional balance or because the diet is insufficient in nutrient density or unevenly balanced. For example, a ration may contain sufficient protein for milk production but contains insufficient precursors of glucose to replace the energy excreted in the milk. While agreeing with the generalization on which the term 'production disease' is based, we propose to continue to use the expression metabolic disease because of common usage.

Because of the emphasis being placed on preventive medicine, it is currently popular to explore for methods of predicting the occurrence of disease well in advance, so that preventive measures can be considered. It may be possible to predict the occurrence of production disease in a herd of lactational group by monitoring certain components of the blood on a regular basis. If the level falls below 'normal' it is assumed that intake needs to be increased to compensate for the negative balance created by excessive output.

The Compton metabolic profile test

This metabolic profile is based on the concept that the laboratory measurement of certain components of the blood will reflect the nutritional status of the animal, with or without the presence of clinical abnormalities. For example, a lower than normal mean blood glucose in a group of dairy cows in early lactation may indicate an insufficient intake of energy which may or may not be detectable clinically. On a theoretical basis, the ability of the laboratory to make an objective assessment of the input–output (nutrient–productivity) relationships is an attractive tool for the veterinarian engaged in providing a complete health service to a herd. The test would theoretically be able to detect the qualitative and quantitative adequacy of the diet of cows expected to produce a certain quantity of milk or return to estrus within a desirable length of time following parturition. A reliable test for the early diagnosis of nutritional deficiency or metabolic disease would be a major step forward in attempting to optimize livestock production and obtain maximum yields at minimum costs. There was considerable interest in the test following its earlier descriptions which stimulated considerable field research. The results of the research have thus far indicated that the test may be useful only as an aid in the diagnosis of nutritional imbalance and production diseases. The results of the test are usually difficult to interpret without a careful conventional assessment of the nutritional status and reproductive performance of the herd and it appears doubtful that the test would reveal significant abnormalities which could not be detected using conventional clinical methods. Mixed feelings are expressed about the practical usefulness of the system. European reactions are generally favorable (1), but United Kingdom and New Zealand (6) reactions are not enthusiastic. The test must be carefully planned and is expensive. A regional diagnostic laboratory with automated analytical equipment should be available and this is often a major limiting factor. The test should not be undertaken unless normal values for each laboratory measurement are available from the population within the area. The results from the groups within the herd are compared to local population means. Metabolic profiles have also been suggested as an aid in the selection of superior individuals.

Test procedure

Blood samples are collected from three groups of seven cows each: dry cows, medium-yield lactating cows and high-yield lactating cows. The samples are collected at least three times yearly: summer, autumn and winter or when nutritional imbalance is suspected. The samples must be collected at the same time of day at each collection and should be done with a minimum of excitement. An aliquot (5 ml) of blood is placed in vials containing oxalate-fluoride for glucose and serum inorganic phosphorus, and 20–30 ml in heparinized vials for the determination of the other components. The samples must be dispatched to the laboratory within a few hours and must not be subjected to delays in delivery or to heat or cold. Ideally the samples should be handled similarly each time. In some cases, urine samples are collected from each test lactating cow and tested for the presence of urinary ketones and the results correlated with the blood glucose levels of each cow.

The following laboratory analyses have been done in the Compton metabolic profile test (9).

- Blood glucose
- Packed cell volume
- Hemoglobin
- Blood urea nitrogen
- Serum inorganic phosphate, magnesium, calcium, potassium and sodium
- Total serum protein, albumin, and globulins (calculated by difference)

Others occasionally

- Serum copper
- Serum iron
- Plasma non-esterified free fatty acids

A miniprofile test which measures levels of blood glucose, serum urea nitrogen and albumin in cows between 4 and 10 weeks after calving has been recommended as a sufficient test to assess the adequacy of energy and protein intakes (10, 11). The sampling is done at intervals of 4–6 weeks. The time of sampling can affect the results. The values will change with the season and stage of lactation. In general, sampling should be done when nutritional imbalance and/or the occurrence of metabolism diseases are anticipated which is usually during early lactation as cows approach their peak in the lactation curve. In regions or situations where subclinical metabolic disease may be predictable, based on previous experience (for example, seasonal hypomagnesemia in pregnant beef cattle) the sampling should be done before the probable occurrence of the disease.

At the time of sampling, the following supplementary information should be collected (10):

- Relating to the individual animals sampled
  - Age
  - Exact milk yield and mastitis status
  - Date of calving
  - Weight of concentrate fed per day (on an average basis in the case of loose-housing or the exact amount fed in the milking parlor)
- Relating to the whole herd
  - Estimates of the average daily forage intakes
  - Analyses of forages and grains
  - Total herd production and number of cows in milk
  - The most recent bulk milk quality data
  - The individual daily yield of six cows past their peak on three consecutive occasions. This is used to calculate the rate of decline.

Interpretation of results and causes of variations

The interpretation of the results can be difficult. In dairy cattle the major objective is to demonstrate the interrelationships between the components of the blood, nutrition, productivity and fertility. The mean values for each lactational group of cows for each parameter are calculated and compared with the population mean values which have been predetermined by survey (7). Most of the values of individual cows and the mean values of the lactational groups will fall within the normal ranges for the population. The difficulty has been in deciding when an individual value is abnormal or low normal or high normal compared to the population mean and 'normal' ranges. Animals whose values are 2 SD (standard deviation) or more different from the population means are considered abnormal (12). The percentage of abnormals determines whether the herd or area is to be classified as an abnormal group. However, the threshold percentage has not been determined.

The results should be presented in the form of histograms on graph paper indicating the individual cow levels and for comparison the population means. It is important to present the results to the farmer in a form in which the data can be easily recognized and compared. Scatter diagrams with values plotted from all cows are also useful.

One of the major difficulties with the Compton metabolic profile test has been to identify the common causes of variation. The most consistent variation occurs between herds and next between lactational groups within herds.

There is a direct relationship between protein intake and the concentration of blood urea nitrogen (14). Low concentrations of urea indicate that protein intake is minimal and an early warning that 'low protein status' may develop in lactating cows later if protein intake is not increased (14). Low levels of albumin and hemoglobin are indicative of a long-standing low protein status. Concentrations of albumin were directly related to the number of services required for conception and not to blood glucose in 351 cows which were between 40 and 100 days postcalving in 21 herds (15). Mean values of packed cell volume (PCV), hemoglobin and serum iron are consistently higher in non-lactating cows than in lactating cows (16). Individual animals also possess different patterns of blood chemistry which may change with age (17). Globulin and total protein concentrations increase with age, and concentration of inorganic phosphate, albumin, magnesium, sodium and urea decrease with increasing age (17). These individual patterns exist even in the varied environment of a dairy herd and in spite of changes in the concentrations with season, pregnancy and stage of lactation and tend to be more similar in related than unrelated animals.

Serum inorganic phosphate levels tend to fall following long-term insufficient dietary intake, and hyperphosphatemia may occur in cattle grazing on highly fertilized pasture.

Serum calcium levels vary only within narrow limits and are not sensitive indications of input–output balance. However, abnormally low levels in late pregnancy indicate a dangerous situation. Serum magnesium levels are usually low during the winter months and subclinical hypomagnesemia exists in many herds, especially pregnant beef cattle. This can be converted into clinical hypomagnesemia with a sudden deprivation of feed or a sudden fall in environmental temperature. Supplementation of the diet with magnesium salts is protective.

Low levels of serum sodium occur in early lactation in cows grazing on summer pastures without supplementation with salt. Levels down to 135 mmol/l may be associated with depraved appetite and polydipsia and polyuria.

Serum potassium levels have been difficult to interpret because the levels of the electrolyte in serum are not necessarily indicative of potassium deficiency. Its normal serum concentration is much more variable than sodium and its average concentration in roughages of all kinds is nearly always in excess of requirements; any abnormalities are usually in the direction of excess.

There are significant fluctuations in the blood composition of dairy cows associated with the interaction between the effects of season, milk yield and stage of lactation. Urea and hemoglobin, together with packed cell volume, have consistently been found to increase during the summer months in both lactating and non-lactating cows. In addition, values for hemoglobin and packed cell volume have been found to be inversely related to current milk yield in both summer and winter while magnesium concentrations show a reverse trend, being lower in non-lactating than in lactating cows, particularly in winter.

Blood glucose concentrations are usually lower in early lactation and during the winter months; in early lactation there is a heavy demand for glucose and during the winter the energy intake is likely to be lower than necessary to meet requirements. One major cause of variation in blood glucose may be the major fluctuations in daily feed intake. Investigations of feed intake of dairy cows on commercial farms have shown that concentrate dispensers are commonly incorrectly adjusted and errors of more than 50% in feed intake are sometimes found (9). In situations of marginal energy imbalance, blood glucose concentration levels may be unreliable as an index of the adequacy of energy intake. Several factors may cause short-term changes in blood glucose (9). Blood glucose decreases at the time of milk secretion, which makes sampling time critical. Blood glucose may also be influenced by the chemical nature of the carbohydrate and physical form of the feed and the roughage content of the feet. In addition, elevation of blood glucose has been associated with excitement and low environmental temperature.

There is some conflicting evidence about the relationship between mean values of blood glucose of a lactational group and insufficient energy intake and reproductive inefficiency. In some work there is an expected relationship between low blood glucose and an increased incidence of ketosis. In others, the relationship is not clear (9, 15) but there was a more consistent relationship between the actual energy intake as a percentage of requirement and the plasma non-esterified fatty acids (9, 15) but not sufficiently reliable to be useful. The mean plasma glucose concentrations within 3 days before or after first service of cows which conceived on first service was higher than that of cows which returned, but the difference was only approaching significance at the 5% level and it is doubtful whether it could be of practical value (9). Although free fatty acids are more sensitive than blood glucose as an indicator of energy status of the lactating cow, the excessive variability of this relationship during early lactation limits its usefulness (19). Free fatty acids begin to increase several weeks prepartum, peak at parturition, and decrease gradually to normal levels after several weeks of lactation. Blood glucose levels follow a similar pattern but there may be a period in early lactation when blood metabolite levels, and particularly free fatty acids, are not entirely responsive to energy intake, but are perhaps under additional hormonal regulation (19).

One excellent investigation of the relationship of selected blood components to nutrition and fertility of dairy cows under commercial farm conditions concluded that within the nutritional ranges encountered, the levels of selected blood components did not show a consistent relationship to nutrient balance or potential fertility. The metabolic profile test is more appropriately regarded as an aid to the conventional approach involving the examination of feeding systems and feedstuffs, herd records, management and clinical condition (9). The test is probably useful for diagnosis and prognosis in extreme variations from normalcy. Management procedures should not become unduly dependent on the metabolic profile concept for the evaluation of energy status in early lactation (19).

Metabolic profiles for individual cows

The prediction of whether an individual cow is metabolically sound enough to undergo a stressful lactation at a high level of production would seem to be a useful undertaking. This could be particularly important under management conditions of heavy concentrate feeding, lead feeding or zero grazing or even indoor housing. There are no well-established protocols for conducting such profile tests. The 'parturition syndrome', dealt with later under the 'fat cow syndrome' is considered to be predictable by the estimation of blood levels of total cholesterol and glutamic oxalate transaminase (3). In pastured cattle in New Zealand the test has been found to be ineffective (8). Similar tests conducted on individual cows using many serum enzymes and electrolytes as indicators have not proved to be useful if used on only one occasion (13, 18).

REVIEW LITERATURE

Adams, R. S. et al. (1978) Use and limitations of profiles in assessing health or nutritional status of dairy herds. *J. dairy Sci.*, *61*, 1671.

Lee, A. J. et al. (1978) Blood metabolic profiles:their use and relationship to nutritional status of dairy cows. *J. dairy Sci.*, *61*, 1652.

Littledike, E. T. et al. (1981) Common metabolic diseases of cattle; ketosis, milk fever, grass tetany and downer cow complex. *J. dairy Sci.*, *64*, 1465–1482.

Payne, J. M., Hibbitt, K. G. & Sansom, B. F. (1972) *Production Disease in Farm Animals*. London: Baillière Tindall.

REFERENCES

(1) Michel, M. P. & Perrier, J. M. (1977) *Bull. Group. Tech. Vet.*, *5B*, 109.

(2) Rossow, N. et al. (1976) *Mh VetMed.*, *31*, 486, 497.

(3) Sommer, H. (1975) *Vet. Med. Rev.*, *1/2*, 42.

(4) Manston, R. & Allen, W. M. (1981) *Br. vet. J.*, *137*, 241.

(5) Payne, J. M. et al. (1972) *Production Disease in Farm Animals* London: Baillière Tindall.

(6) Wolff, J. E. et al. (1978) *NZ vet. J.*, *26*, 266.
(7) Rowlands, G. J. et al. (1979) *Br. vet. J.*, *135*, 64.
(8) Sutherland, R. J. (1979) *NZ vet. J.*, *27*, 275.
(9) Parker, B. N. J. & Blowey, R. W. (1976) *Vet. Rec.*, *98*, 394.
(10) Blowey, R. W. (1975) *Vet. Rec.*, *97*, 324.
(11) Collins, J. D. (1979) *Irish vet. J.*, *33*, 26.
(12) Rowlands, G. J. & Pocock, R. M. (1976) *Vet. Rec.*, *98*, 333.
(13) Baumgartner, W. (1979) *Dtsch Tierarztl. Wochenschr.*, *86*, 336.
(14) Manston, R. et al. (1975) *Vet. Rec.*, *96*, 497.
(15) Rowlands, G. J. et al. (1977) *J. dairy Res.*, *44*, 1.
(16) Rowlands, G. J. et al. (1974) *J. agric. Sci.*, *Camb.*, *83*, 27.
(17) Kitchenham, B. A. et al. (1976) *J. agric. Sci.*, *Camb.*, *86*, 171.
(18) Hacker, U. & Siering, W. (1979) *Mh VetMed.*, *34*, 361.
(19) Erfle, J. D. et al. (1974) *Can. J. anim. Sci.*, *54*, 293.

Parturient paresis (milk fever)

Parturient paresis is a metabolic disease occurring most commonly about the time of parturition in adult females and is characterized by hypocalcemia, general muscular weakness, circulatory collapse and depression of consciousness. A similar disease has been dealt with separately as lactation tetany of mares because of its more frequent occurrence during lactation and after transport.

Etiology

It is generally conceded that a depression of the levels of ionized calcium in tissue fluids is the basic biochemical defect in parturient paresis. There is a fall in serum calcium levels in all cows at calving and a significantly greater fall occurs in cows which develop the disease. The importance of the calcium ion in maintaining muscle tone is well known and affected cows respond rapidly to the parenteral administration of calcium solutions. Although total serum calcium levels are used to express the animals' status with regard to calcium, it is possible that differences between the ionized and non-ionized compartments of total calcium may be more important than the total level (64). Little is known of intrinsic factors, such as levels of serum protein and acid–base balances, which influence the proportion of total serum calcium which is ionized, but those observations which have been made on cows with parturient paresis indicate that both total and ionized serum calcium levels fall proportionately (1).

Serum calcium levels fall in all adult cows at calving due to the onset of lactation. This has been satisfactorily demonstrated by comparing the effects of parturition on serum calcium levels in normal and mastectomized cows, and by alternating periods of milking and non-milking (43). In the latter there is an obvious lag time between the stimulus of hypocalcemia, brought on by milking, and the onset of the compensatory hypercalcemia. This delay in the operation of calcium homeostatic mechanisms is probably vital in causing milk fever. The important fact is that the serum calcium levels fall more in some cows than in others and it is this difference which results in the varying susceptibility of animals to parturient paresis. There are three factors which affect calcium homeostasis and variations in one or more of them may be instrumental in causing the disease in any individual. First, it may simply be the excessive loss of calcium in the colostrum beyond the capacity of absorption from the intestines and mobilization from the bones to replace. Variations in susceptibility between cows could be due to variations in the concentraion of calcium in the milk and the volume of milk secreted. Second, there may be an impairment of absorption of calcium from the intestine at parturition and there is evidence suggesting that this does occur (2). The third and probably most important possibility is that mobilization of calcium from storage in the skeleton may not be sufficiently rapid to maintain normal serum levels. Certainly the calcium mobilization rate and the immediately available calcium reserves are sufficiently reduced in cows in later pregnancy to render them incapable of withstanding the expected loss of calcium in the milk. This theory is supported by the reproduction of the clinical disease by the administration of EHDP (a selective bone resorption inhibitor) (4). This deficiency in mobilization and reserves is not a permanent characteristic of cows prone to parturient paresis; in fact their rate of mobilization appears to be better than that of non-susceptible animals except at parturition (5).

Failure to mobilize skeletal calcium could arise because of parathyroid insufficiency, as first suggested by Dryerre and Greig who postulated that the gland was relatively quiescent due to the decreased calcium and phosphorus metabolism of the dry period. There is conflicting evidence on this point and although susceptibility to parturient paresis may be associated with parathyroid dysfunction, it is unlikely that the relationship is a simple one (3, 7, 66, 70). However, parturient paresis can be prevented by the feeding of a ration high in phosphorus and low in calcium during late pregnancy. Such a ration would stimulate parathyroid activity during the dry period and condition the gland for the increased activity required at parturition. Conversely the observation that feeding a diet high in calcium at this time increases the incidence of the disease, probably by depressing the activity of the gland, lends additional support to the hypothesis. The possibility exists that rather than a deficiency of parathormone the presence of excess calcitonin, or thyrocalcitonin, the serum calcium-depressing hormone of the thyroid gland, may be an important factor (8), but the normal function of this hormone tends to be limited to the fine adjustment of calcium homeostasis rather than causing major adjustments like those we are concerned with in parturient paresis. Also, the secretion of calcitonin in response to an injection of calcium salt is the same in clinically normal cows and cows with milk fever, suggesting that there is no impairment of calcitonin function (65). There is no evidence of interference with vitamin D synthesis in affected cows, blood levels of 1·25-dehydroxyvitamin D being high even in affected cows (40). Nor is there any evidence of hormonal aberrations, the levels of parathormone, calcitonin and prolactin being within normal range (55). There is evidence, however, that estrogen levels are raised and may interfere with calcium mobilization from bones (60). Another possible factor is hypomagnesemia which is also known to reduce the rate of calcium mobilization in cattle (7, 77). Chronic hypomagnesemia is therefore likely to predispose a cow to milk fever.

A perplexing situation in dairy practice is the recently calved cow with coliform mastitis which also appears to have some of the clinical signs of milk fever and may require treatment for that condition. It has been shown that the toxin of *Escherichia coli* given intravenously depresses serum calcium and phosphate levels so that coliform mastitis may contribute to the development of milk fever in individual cows (11).

In summary, parturient paresis in *dairy cows* is a hypocalcemia caused by a failure to mobilize calcium reserves, and by a depletion of these reserves caused by the development of a negative calcium balance in late pregnancy. Prevention of the disease therefore seems to depend largely upon the preservation of a positive balance in susceptible cows. The recommended ratio of Ca:P in the diet is 2·3:1 (11).

Hypocalcemic syndromes are also observed at times other than related to parturition. Thus, it can be part of an early or mild overeating of fermentable carbohydrate. The intravenous injection of aminoglycoside antibiotics, especially neomycin, dihydrostreptomycin and gentamycin may cause a reduction in the degree of ionization of serum calcium, and an attack of a syndrome similar to milk fever. Oral dosing with zinc oxide (40 or 120 mg Zn/kg body weight) as a prophylaxis against facial eczema in ewes causes a serious fall in serum calcium levels 24 hours later (25). Caution is recommended with the use of these drugs in parturient cows (25).

In *goats*, a depression in serum levels of calcium and phosphorus occurs similar to that in cows but in *ewes* no such depression occurs at lambing and the intervention of a precipitating factor appears to be necessary to further reduce the serum calcium level below a critical point. For example, in *sheep*, sudden deprivation of feed or forced exercise can cause marked depression of the serum calcium levels. However, ewes are in a susceptible state in early lactation because they are in negative calcium balance. In late lactation a state of positive balance appears due largely to a low rate of bone resorption (13). There is an unexplained occurrence of hypocalcemia in sheep fed on hay when they are supplemented with an energy-rich concentrate which considerably increases their calcium intake (49). Some of the concentrates fed to ewes in feedlots contain supplementary magnesium as a prevention against hypomagnesemia and this appears to have the effect of restraining calcium absorption and may precipitate hypocalcemia in a susceptible ewe (75). Another occurrence in ewes is at the end of a drought when the pasture growth is luxuriant and very low in calcium content. The incidence may be as high as 10% and the case fatality rate 20% in ewe flocks in late pregnancy or early lactation (2).

Epidemiology

In cattle the disease is essentially one of domestication and occurs in high-producing cows in all countries. Few figures are available on the incidence of the disease although annual morbidity rates of 3·5 and 8·8% have been recorded in the United Kingdom. In Sweden 8% of all parturitions are estimated to be accompanied by milk fever. In Australia, about 3·5% of cows are risk and in Finnish Ayrshires the rate is 3·8% (78). Generally the disease is sporadic but on individual farms the incidence may rarely reach 25–30%. With standard treatment relatively few deaths occur in uncomplicated cases but incidental losses due to aspiration pneumonia, mastitis and limb injuries are often quite high. The occurrence of parturient paresis causes some loss by significantly increasing the intercalving period in affected cows (15). Several surveys suggest that 75–85% of those cases clinically diagnosed as parturient paresis are uncomplicated and respond to calcium therapy alone. A proportion of these animals require more than one treatment, either because complete recovery is delayed, or because relapse occurs. The remaining 15–25% are either complicated by other conditions or incorrectly diagnosed. The economic importance of the disease has been minor since the introduction of calcium borogluconate as treatment and depends almost entirely on the cost of veterinary treatment and losses due to intercurrent disease. However, during late years the position appears to have changed in most countries. Simple cases of parturient paresis which respond to treatment with calcium borogluconate seem to have decreased and there has been an increase in cases which are apparently complicated by metabolic factors other than hypocalcemia. The disease also occurs in water buffalo, with clinical findings similar to those in cattle (16).

Parturient paresis is rare in sows but does occur in outbreak form in groups of sheep in which 25% of a flock may be affected at one time. In sheep the disease occurs most commonly in ewes in late pregnancy but also in ewes in early lactation. It also occurs in young sheep up to about a year old, especially when they are grazed on green oats, but also when pasture is short in winter and spring in south–east Australia. The disease is manifested by paresis but in the rest of the flock poor growth, lameness and bone fragility can be detected.

Amongst cattle mature cows are most commonly affected usually in the 5–10-year age group, although rare cases have been observed at the first and second calvings. This age relationship also appears in serum calcium levels, a hypocalcemia occurring at calving in most cows with their third to seventh calves but infrequently in first-calf heifers. There is considerable difference in susceptibility between the breeds. Jerseys are most susceptible, an incidence of 33% having been observed in a sample compared with 9·6% incidence in other breeds. Although there is no definite evidence on the point, the consensus of opinion is that cows are more susceptible if they are heavily fed before and after calving, especially if the protein level of the diet is high. There is no specific seasonal occurrence or relationship to weather conditions.

Individual cows, and to some extent families of cows, are more susceptible than others, the disease tending to recur at successive parturitions. The heritability of susceptibility to milk fever and hypocalcemia has been assessed as insignificant; in several breeds examined it was of the order of 6–12% (18). Complete milking in the first 48 hours after calving, as opposed to normal sucking by a calf, appears to be a precipitating factor.

Parturient paresis in cattle occurs at three main stages in the lactation cycle. Most prepartum cases occur in the last few days of pregnancy and during parturition but rare cases occur several weeks before calving. The great majority of cases occur within the first 48 hours after calving and the danger period extends up to about the 10th day postpartum. Up to 20% of cases can occur subsequent to the 8th day after calving. In such cases the falls in serum calcium and phosphorus levels are smaller and the rises in serum magnesium levels are greater than in parturient cows. The clinical signs are also less severe and there are fewer relapses after treatment (10). Occasional cases occur 6–8 weeks after the commencement of lactation. Such cases are most often recurrences of the disease in highly susceptible cows which were affected at calving. Undue fatigue and excitement may precipitate such attacks and there is a special susceptibility at estrus. In the latter case the depression of appetite by the elevation of blood estrogen levels may be a significant factor (3). Starvation for 48 hours also causes severe depression of serum calcium levels and this may be of importance in the production of hypocalcemic paresis in this species at times other than in the postparturient period. Pregnant beef cattle may develop hypocalcemic paresis during the winter months when they are fed on poor quality roughage (19), and within a group of such cows the less aggressive ones may suffer selective malnutrition (37). As another explanation of the heightened susceptibility of cows at estrus a possible depression of the degree of ionization of calcium under the influence of increased serum estrogens is suggested. However, there were no significant differences in total serum calcium or plasma ionized calcium values in cows from 48 hours before and after estrus (21).

Milking goats become affected mostly during the 4–6-year age group. Cases occur before and after kidding, some later than 3 weeks after parturition. Clinical syndromes are identical with those in cows, including the two stages of ataxia and recumbency. Serum calcium levels are reduced from normal levels for parturient does of 9·4–3·6 mg/dl (2·35–0·9 mmol/l) (67).

In sheep and pigs only sporadic cases occur except under special circumstances. For example, there may be outbreaks in groups of ewes exposed to forced exercise, long-distance transport, sudden deprivation of food, and grazing on oxalate-containing plants or green cereal crops. These circumstances commonly precipitate outbreaks of hypocalcemic paresis in sheep, mature ewes being most susceptible, particularly in the period from 6 weeks before to 10 weeks after lambing.

Pathogenesis

The bulk of evidence points to hypocalcemia as the cause of the signs of classical 'milk fever' with hypophosphatemia and variations in levels of serum magnesium playing subsidiary roles. Skeletal muscle and plain muscle atony are known physiological effects of hypocalcemia. In experimental hypocalcemia in cattle, there is a marked reduction in the stroke volume, cardiac output, a 50% reduction in arterial blood pressure (20), and a reduction in ruminal and abomasal tone and motility (50). If these changes occur in naturally occurring cases they would account for the muscle weakness, hypothermia and depression of consciousness. Serum calcium and serum phosphate levels are significantly lower in clinical cases than in normal, comparable cows and there is some relationship between the severity of the signs and the degree of biochemical change. The complete response to the parenteral administration of calcium salts in most cases, and the occurrence of tetany coincident with hypocalcemia after the intravenous administration of disodium ethylenediamine tetra-acetate is further proof. In addition some signs reminiscent of parathyreoprivic tetany in other species are observed in the initial stages of parturient paresis. Early excitement, muscle twitching, tetany, particularly of the hindlimbs, hypersensitiveness and convulsive movements of the head and limbs fall within this category. The demonstration of failure of neuromuscular transmission of stimuli in cows with parturient paresis is in accord with the clinical signs of the disease (24).

When *hypomagnesemia* coexists these signs continue but where serum magnesium levels are normal or high, relaxation, muscle weakness, depression and coma supervene. It is likely that the hypocalcemic tetany is overcome by the relative hypermagnesemia (the ratio of Ca:Mg may change from 6:1 to 2:1) approximating the ratio at which magnesium narcosis develops. There is normally a rise in serum magnesium levels at calving but in those cases of parturient paresis in which tetany is a feature serum magnesium levels are low. These low levels are in many cases expressions of a seasonal hypomagnesemia.

Low serum phosphorus levels have been observed in clinical cases of parturient paresis and have been credited with an influence on the signs which occur. It has been observed that some cases do not respond to calcium injections even though serum calcium levels return to normal, but do recover when the udder is inflated and serum phosphorus levels rise. In addition there are reports on the efficacy of orally or intraveneously administered sodium acid phosphate in some cases of parturient paresis. There are difficulties in reconciling the biochemical and the clinical findings because of the absence of nervous signs and recumbency in other animals with profound hypophosphatemia for long periods. A possible explanation is that the hypophosphatemia which occurs in milk fever is the result of the hypocalcemia and recumbency rather than being a concurrent event. There is experimental evidence to support this (52) and it also seems probable that the hypophosphatemia could prolong the duration of recumbency.

Experimentally, the intravenous infusion of ethylene diamine tetra-acetate (EDTA) into cows over a period of 4–8 hours results in severe hypocalcemia and paresis (26). Significant increases occur in plasma enzyme (CPK and SGOT) activities and blood glucose levels and decreases in serum phosphorus and potassium levels. A distinct prolongation of the ST interval of the electrocardiogram occurs which may be useful as a diagnostic aid if suitable mini-electrocardiograph recorders could be made available for field use. The increased plasma enzyme activities induced by experimental hypocalcemia suggest that hypocalcemia may alter the permeability of muscle cell membranes and allow an increased outflow of enzymes.

Clinical findings

Cattle

Three arbitrary stages of the disease have been described. *The first stage* is a brief one of excitement and tetany with hypersensitiveness and muscle tremor of the head and limbs. The animal is disinclined to move and does not eat. There may be shaking of the head, protrusion of the tongue and grinding of the teeth. The rectal temperature is usually normal to slightly above normal. Stiffness of the hindlegs is apparent and the animal is ataxic and falls easily and, on going down, the hindlegs are stuck out stiffly.

Careful observations by owners and veterinarians have revealed an even earlier stage than the first one. It is characterized by anorexia, agalactia, rumen stasis, scant feces and a normal temperature, heart rate and respirations. Affected cows may remain in this prodromal stage for several hours, they are perplexing diagnostically and they respond quickly to calcium therapy.

The *second stage* is one of sternal recumbency. Consciousness is usually depressed, the cow having a very drowsy appearance and sitting up, usually with a lateral kink in the neck or the head turned into the flank. Tetany of the limbs has disappeared and the cow is unable to rise. The muzzle is dry, the skin and extremities cold, and the rectal temperature subnormal (36–38°C, 97–101°F). The pupils are dilated and the eyes are dry and staring. There is relaxation of the anus and loss of the anal reflex. Circulatory signs are prominent including a marked decrease in the intensity of the heart sounds and an increase in rate (about 80/minute). Also the pulse is weak, the pressures and amplitude being considerably reduced. Venous pressure is also low and difficulty may be experienced in raising the vein. Ruminal stasis and constipation are characteristic. Respiration is not markedly affected although a forced expiratory grunt may be heard. The pupillary light reflex is incomplete or absent and the diameter of the pupil varies from normal to maximum dilatation.

The *third stage* is that of lateral recumbency. The cow is almost comatose and although the limbs may be stuck out there is complete flaccidity on passive movement and the cow cannot sit up. In general, the depression of temperature and the circulatory signs are more marked. The pulse is, in most cases, impalpable, the heart sounds almost inaudible and increased in rate up to 120/minute, and it may be impossible to raise the jugular vein. Bloat is usual because of the posture.

Without treatment very rare cases recover spontaneously, a few remain unchanged for several hours and most deteriorate rapidly during a period of 12–24 hours, the animal dying imperceptibly from cessation of respiration, or during a convulsion.

A concurrent hypomagnesemia has a modifying effect on the classical syndrome. Tetany and hyperesthesia persist beyond the first stage. There is considerable excitement and fibrillary twitching of the eyelids, and tetanic convulsions are readily precipitated by sound or touch. Trismus may be present. The cardiac and respiratory rates are greatly increased and the heart sounds are much increased in intensity. Without treatment death occurs during a convulsion. The clinical picture when there is a concurrent hypophosphatemia is one of classical parturient paresis which responds to calcium therapy in all respects except that the cow is unable to rise.

Uterine prolapse is an occasional accompaniment of milk fever and it has been established that cows with uterine prolapse have significantly lower serum calcium levels than parturient cows without uterine prolapse (14). It is standard practice to treat cases of uterine prolapse with an injection of a calcium solution. Other problems with a significant association with milk fever (44) are dystocia, retained fetal membranes, ketosis and mastitis and a less significant association with left abomasal displacement.

Sheep and goats

The syndrome in pastured ewes is very similar to that in cattle. Early signs include a stilty, proppy gait and tremor, particularly of the shoulder muscles. Recumbency follows, sometimes with tetany of the limbs but the proportion of ewes with hypocalcemia which are recumbent is much less than in cattle. A similar generalization applies to female goats. The characteristic posture is sternal recumbency, with the legs under the body or stretched out behind. Ruminal movements are absent, the head is rested on the ground, there may be an accumulation of mucous exudate in the nostrils and the respiratory rate is increased. The venous blood pressure is low and the pulse impalpable. Mental depression is evidenced by a drowsy appearance and depression of the corneal reflex. Constipation is usual. Response to parenteral treatment with calcium salts is rapid, the ewe being normal 30 minutes after a subcutaneous injection. Death often occurs within 6–12 hours if treatment is not administered. The syndrome is usually more severe in pregnant than in lactating ewes, possibly because of the simultaneous occurrence of pregnancy toxemia or hypomagnesemia. Fat late pregnant ewes on high grain diets indoors or in feedlots show a similar syndrome accompanied by prolapses of the vagina and intestine (74).

Swine

As in cattle, signs develop within a few hours of farrowing. There is restlessness, a normal temperature, and anorexia followed by inability to rise and later lateral recumbency and coma. Milk flow is decreased.

Clinical pathology

No completely satisfactory field test is available. The Sulkowitch test, based on the detection of calcium in the urine, is not an accurate guide to the calcium status of the animal. A rapid semiquantitative test, based upon the amount of sodium ethylene diamine tetra-acetate (EDTA, Sequestrene) required to prevent clotting of a sample of blood and hence the approximate calcium concentration, seems worthy of a trial as a field test for calcium concentrations in serum. Total serum calcium levels are reduced to below 8 mg/dl (2·0 mmol/l), usually to below 5 mg (1·2 mmol/l) and sometimes to as low as 2 mg (0·5 mmol/l). The reduction is usually, but not always, proportional to the severity of the clinical syndrome. Average figures for total serum calcium levels in the three species are cows 5·2 ± 1·2 mg/dl (1·30 ± 0·30 mmol/l), ewes 4·6 ± 1·5 mg/dl (1·15 ± 0·37 mmol/l), goat does, 3·8 ± 0·6 mg/dl (0·94 ± 0·15 mmol/l) (64). Total serum calcium levels are a basis for comparison; blood levels of ionized calcium are a better indicator of calcium status but their estimation has been too difficult until recent times. Normal levels of ionized calcium (as CaF) in venous whole blood of cows are

4·3–5·1 mg/dl (1·06–1·26 mmol/l) serum, slight hypocalcemia 4·2–3·2 mg/dl (1·05–0·80 mmol/l), moderate 3·2–2·0 mg/dl (0·79–0·50 mmol/l) and severe hypocalcemia <2·0 mg/dl (<0·50 mmol/l) serum (76). Other data have levels higher than these (73). Total serum calcium levels are reduced below normal in all cows at calving whether they have milk fever or not. This is not so in ewes.

Serum levels of magnesium are usually moderately elevated to 4–5 mg/dl (1·65–2·06 mmol/l) but in some areas low levels may be encountered, especially in cows at pasture. Serum inorganic phosphorus levels are usually depressed to 1·5–3·0 mg/dl (0·48–0·97 mmol/l). Blood glucose levels are usually normal although they may be depressed if ketosis occurs concurrently. Higher than normal blood glucose levels are likely to occur in cases of long duration and are therefore an indication of a poorer than normal prognosis.

Increased plasma activity in some tissue enzymes is also described, including fructose-1,6-diphosphate aldolase, glutamate-oxaloacetate transaminase and creatine phosphokinase, and interpreted as resulting from damage to muscle cell membranes. This is thought to result from hypocalcemia and to lead to the outward diffusion of intracellular enzymes into tissue fluids and the circulation (6). Plasma levels of hydroxyproline are interpreted as an indicator of bone resorption and are higher in cows with milk fever than in those without (79).

Changes in the leukocyte count include an eosinopenia, a neutrophilia and a lymphopenia suggestive of adrenal cortical hyperactivity, but similar changes occur at calving in cows which do not develop parturient paresis. High plasma cortisol levels (12) and packed cell volumes (17) occur in cows with milk fever, and are higher still in cows that do not respond to treatment. They are expressions of stress and dehydration. Clinicopathological findings in the other species are not described in detail except for depression of total serum calcium levels.

Necropsy findings

There are no gross or histological changes unless concurrent disease is present.

Diagnosis

A diagnosis of parturient paresis is usually based on the occurrence of paresis and depression of consciousness in animals that have recently given birth to young. The diagnosis is confirmed by a favorable response to treatment with parenteral injections of calcium solutions, and by biochemical examination of the blood. In ewes the history usually contains some reference to recent physical stress and the disease is quite common in the period preceding lambing.

In the immediately postpartum period there are many conditions which cause recumbency in cows and their differentiation is summarized in Table 83. Hypomagnesemia may occur as the sole cause of recumbency or it may accompany a primary hypocalcemia so that the case presented is one of parturient paresis complicated by lactation tetany. Hyperesthesia and tetany are present instead of the classical signs of coma and flaccidity. A complicating hypophosphatemia is suggested as a cause of continued recumbency in cows after partial response to calcium therapy (63). Ketosis may complicate parturient paresis, in which case the animal responds to calcium therapy by rising but continues to manifest the clinical signs of ketosis, including in some cases the nervous signs of licking, circling and abnormal voice.

Toxemia

During the immediate postparturient period this is likely to occur in coliform mastitis, aspiration pneumonia, acute diffuse peritonitis resulting from traumatic perforation of the reticulum or uterus, and acute septic metritis. The depression in these instances may be profound and the animal unable to rise, but careful clinical examination reveals a much more rapid heart rate than is usual in a corresponding stage of parturient paresis, and some localizing signs of abnormality of the milk and udder, of the lungs or of the uterus. Aspiration pneumonia should be suspected if the animal has been lying on its side, especially if there is evidence of regurgitation of ruminal contents from the nostrils, no matter how small the amount, or if there is a history of the animal having been drenched. Abnormal auscultatory findings may not be detectable until the second day. Early diagnosis is imperative if the animal is to be saved and the mortality rate is always high.

Although some elevation of the temperature may be observed in these severe toxemic states it is more usual to find a subnormal temperature. The response to calcium therapy is usually a marked increase in heart rate, and death during the injection is common. Every case of recumbency must be carefully examined as these conditions may occur either independently or as complications of parturient paresis. In our experience about 25% of cases of postparturient recumbency in cows are due primarily to toxemia or injury rather than to hypocalcemia. A few cases occur in which recumbent cows with a degree of hyperactivity suggestive of lactation tetany fail to respond to treatment with calcium and magnesium and have been found to have hemorrhages in the tissue of the midbrain; other have subarachnoid hemorrhages.

Injuries to the hindquarters

These are common at the time of parturition because of the marked relaxation of the ligaments of the pelvic girdle. Fenwick (31) records seven types of leg abnormality in this group at an incidence level of 8·5% in 400 consecutive cases of parturient paresis. The abnormalities included radial paralysis, dislocation of the hips and rupture of gastrocnemius muscle. In most instances the affected animals are down and unable to rise but they eat, drink, urinate and defecate normally, show no rise in temperature or pulse rate and make strong efforts to rise particularly with the forelimbs. Maternal obstetrical paralysis is the most common injury. Although this occurs most frequently in heifers after a difficult parturition it may also occur in adult animals following an easy birth, and occasionally before parturition especially in cows in poor condition. The mildest form is evidenced by a frequent kicking movement of a hindleg as though something was stuck between the claws. All degrees of severity from this, through knuckling and weakness of one or both hindlegs, to complete inability to rise may occur, but sensation in the affected limb is usually normal. The cause of the condition is thought to

Table 83. Differential diagnosis of recumbency in parturient adult cattle.

Disease	*Epidemiology*	*Clinical signs*	*Clinical pathology*	*Response to treatment*
Classical milk fever (parturient paresis)	Mature cows, especially Channel Island breeds, within 48 hours of calving, few outside this period	Early excitement and tetany. Then depression, coma, hypothermia, flaccidity, pupil dilatation, impalpable pulse. No rumen movements. Soft heart sounds. HR 70–80	Hypocalcemia, less than 5 mg/dl (1·25 mmol/l) calcium. High serum magnesium, over 3 mg/dl (1·25 mmol/l) low inorganic phosphate, less than 3 mg/dl (0·9 mmol/l)	Quick, characteristic response (muscle tremor, sweating on muzzle, defecation, urination, pulse amplitude and heart sound intensity improves first) after intravenous injection soluble calcium salt
Hypomagnesemia (lactation, grass tetany)	All classes of cattle, but mostly recently calved females. Age no barrier and cases occur up to several months after calving. May occur in pregnant beef cattle	Excitement, hypersensivity, muscle tremor, tetany. Down with tetanic convulsions, loud heart sounds, rapid rate. Subacute cases remain standing	Low serum magnesium, less than 1·2 mg/dl (0·5 mmol/l)	Even after intravenous injection response in a bad case may take 30 min, much slower than response to calcium in milk fever
Severe toxemia (acute diffuse peritonitis, coliform mastitis)	Sporadic only. Mastitis most common where hygiene poor. Peritonitis due to foreign body perforation of reticulum, rupture of uterus or vagina	Recumbency, depression to coma, sleepy, dry nose, hypothermia, gut stasis, *HR over 100/min*, may be grunting	Profound leukopenia. Serum calcium may be as low as 7–8 mg/dl (1·75–2·0 mmol/l)	Require supportive response for toxemia and shock. Response is poor and temporary. Prognosis very bad. May die if treated intravenously with calcium or magnesium salts
Maternal obstetrical paralysis (MOP)	Prolonged difficult calving. Heifers and young cows or large calves delivered with excessive traction	Bright, alert, eat, drink, defecate, try to rise and cannot quite make it or do splits. TRP and rumen movements normal	Normal. CPK may become high if much muscle damage	Nil to clinical treatments. Need slinging by hip sling or nursing on deep straw with frequent movement. If not recovered by third day prognosis may be unfavorable
Downer cows	Most common in situation where milk fever and lactation tetany common and intensity of treatment is lax, cows are left down too long before treatment	Moderately bright, active, eating. Temp. slightly raised, HR 80–100. Unable to rise but try—'creepers'. When dull and depressed, are 'non-alert downers'. Long course 1–2 weeks	Variable. May be low inorganic phosphate, or potassium, or glucose. Ketonuria, usually proteinuria. CPK and SGOT elevated	Variable response to calcium, phosphorus and potassium salts. Fluid therapy and provision of deep bedding and hourly rolling from side to side are necessary
Physical injuries	Ruptured gastrocnemius, dislocation of hip, etc. Sporadic sequelae to milk fever, may be contributed to by osteoporosis, slippery ground surface, stimulating to rise too early	As for MOP with ruptured gastrocnemius, hock remains on ground when standing. Excessive lateral mobility of limb with hip dislocation	Increase CPK and SGOT	Supportive therapy, deep bedding and frequent rolling
Ephemeral fever	Epidemics at times when insect vectors rife	Transitory fever, lymphadenitis, watery nasal discharge, myositis	High white cell count	Nil. Spontaneous recovery within 3 days. Rare cases that persist are euthanized

be trauma to peripheral nerves during passage of the calf, or in pregnant animals to compression of the sciatic nerve by a calf crammed into the pelvic canal. In many cases of maternal obstetric paralysis there are gross hemorrhages, both deep and superficial, and histopathological degeneration of the sciatic nerves. Individual animals may show involvement of the obturator nerve with defective adduction of the thighs. The position of the hindlimbs is often normal but in severe cases, especially those with extensive hematoma along the sciatic nerve trunk, the leg may be held extended with the toe reaching the elbow as in dislocation of the hip, but in the latter case there is exaggerated lateral mobility of the limb. Additional injuries causing recumbency near parturition include those associated with degenerative myopathy, dislocation of the hip and ventral hernia.

Degenerative myopathy (ischemic muscle necrosis)
Affecting chiefly the heavy muscles of the thighs, this occurs commonly in cattle which are recumbent for more than 48 hours. At necropsy large masses of pale muscle can be found surrounded by muscle of normal color. Clinically the condition is indistinguishable from sciatic nerve paralysis. Markedly increased serum levels of glutamic–oxaloacetic transaminase have been observed in some cows recumbent for long periods after an initial attack of parturient paresis. Such increased SGOT activity may be related to muscle damage of this sort but it is apparent that a dietary deficiency of selenium is not associated with the muscular lesion. Serum levels of creatine phosphokinase and alanine and aspartate aminotransferases are elevated in milk fever cases and are highest in persistently recumbent cows. The muscle damage is probably a result of the recumbency (6). Other conditions which may have their origin in lesser degrees of this myopathy include rupture of the gastrocnemius muscle or separation of its tendon from either the muscle or the tuber calcis. Most of these injuries occur rather commonly in cattle but rarely in other species. Shock at parturition may occur with prolapse or rupture of the uterus but the cause is usually obvious.

'Downer cow' syndrome
One of the major problems in dairy cattle practice is the so-called 'downer cow' syndrome in which the animal goes down during the period of susceptibility to parturient paresis but fails to respond to treatment. Clinically the animal may be normal except for recumbency, or show nervous signs varying from lateral recumbency with opisthotonus to constant clonic convulsions.

Non-parturient hypocalcemia
Paresis with mental depression and associated with low total serum calcium levels can occur in cows at times other than at parturition. The cause is largely unexplained but the syndrome occurs rarely in animals other than ruminants. Hypocalcemia may occur after gorging on grain and may be a significant factor in particular cases. Sudden rumen stasis due to traumatic reticulitis may rarely cause hypocalcemic paresis. Diarrhea, particularly when cattle or sheep are placed on new lush pasture, may also precipitate an attack. Access to plants rich in oxalates may have a similar effect particularly if the animals are unaccustomed to the plants. Affected animals respond well to calcium therapy but relapse is likely unless the primary cause is corrected. The differential diagnosis of diseases of non-parturient cows manifested principally by recumbency is also summarized in Table 83.

Hypocalcemic paresis in sheep
This must be differentiated from pregnancy toxemia in which the course is much longer, the signs indicate cerebral involvement and the disease is restricted to pregnant ewes. There is no response to calcium therapy and a positive test for ketonuria is almost diagnostic of the disease. In horses, transit tetany is virtually identical clinically but occurs in both sexes and is always associated with transport. In sows, the absence of fever may help to differentiate the disease from metritis and mastitis, but in hot weather a temperature of 40–41°C (104–105°F) is not unusual in sows with parturient paresis. At parturition, goats are susceptible to enterotoxemia and hypoglycemia, both of which present clinical signs reminiscent of parturient paresis.

Treatment
Every effort should be made to treat affected cows as soon as possible after clinical signs are obvious. Treatment during the first stage of the disease, before the cow is recumbent, is the ideal situation. Clinical findings of lateral recumbency, low body temperature and a history of occurrence of a relapse after recovery induced by treatment are all indicators of a poor response to treatment. A temperature of greater than 39°C (102°F) is an indication of a higher than average mortality rate (69). The longer the interval between the time the cow first becomes recumbent and treatment, the greater the incidence of the downer cow syndrome due to ischemic muscle necrosis from prolonged recumbency. Cows which are found in lateral recumbency (third stage) should be placed in sternal recumbency until treatment is available. This will reduce the chances of aspiration if the cow regurgitates. Cows that have difficulty finding solid, non-slip footing beneath them, for example, a slippery barn floor or slippery mud, will often not try to rise and develop ischemic myonecrosis as a result. Avoidance of this complication means putting rubber or other mats under the cow or transporting her to a piece of pasture with a dense sward on it.

Standard treatment
The treatment of parturient paresis by the parenteral injection of calcium salts is standard practice. Calcium borogluconate is the preparation of choice. For cattle 100–200 g of the compound as a 20–30% solution is the usual dose (i.e. 400–800 ml of a 25% solution). In goats the recommended amount is 15–20 g intravenously with an optional 5–10 g subcutaneously (67). The dose rate of calcium to be used in treatment is always under discussion. Our own view is that there is a general tendency among veterinarians to underdose with calcium salts, largely because of toxic effects which tend to occur when all of the calcium is given intravenously. As an initial dose a heavy cow (540–590 kg) requires 800–1000 ml of a 25% solution and a small cow (320–360 kg) 400–500 ml. Underdosing increases the chances of incomplete response, with inability of the cow to rise, or of relapse.

There is usually a strong inclination to use smaller doses of calcium, but the overall view is that 12 g of calcium is superior to 8 g, which in turn is superior to 6 g (21). Calcium borogluconate contains 8·3% calcium.

Available injection routes
The intravenous route is preferred. The response is quicker and more apparent. Subcutaneous injections are used when the cow is impossible to restrain in the early stages of the disease, and when she is still standing, or when the effects of the intravenous injection on the heart rate are worrying. The best recommendation is to give as much of the injection as possible intravenously and the remainder subcutaneously. The common practice of giving half the dose intravenously and half sub-

cutaneously is a reasonable compromise (14), and there appear to be less relapses after administration of the calcium preparation in the two sites (22, 35). If a cow has previously been treated subcutaneously by the farmer it should be treated by in intravenous injection only (36), but toxicity may occur if large depôts of subcutaneous calcium are picked up quickly by the improving circulation. This also tends to avoid deaths due to overdosage and too rapid intravenous injection. Subcutaneous or intraperitoneal administration is preferred in cows with severe toxemia due to aspiration pneumonia, metritis and mastitis. Toxemic cows are very susceptible to voluminous intravenous injections and death may occur due to overloading of the circulation. In such cases the heart rate increases markedly (up to 180/minute), there is respiratory distress, trembling and collapse and the cow dies within a few minutes. Sows should receive 100–150 ml of a similar solution intraveneously or subcutaneously.

Cows suffering from hypocalcemic paresis show a definite *pattern of response* to specific therapy. The classical response includes belching, muscle tremor, particularly of the flanks and often extending to the whole body, slowing, and improvement in the amplitude and pressures of the pulse, increase in the intensity of the heart sounds, sweating of the muzzle and defecation. The feces are characteristically in the form of a firm stool with a hard crust and covered with mucus containing a few flecks of blood. Urination usually does not follow until the cow rises. Tetany may also be observed to return transitorily in the limbs.

Unusual reactions

These include a marked increase in heart rate in cows suffering from toxemia and acute heart block in apparently normal animals especially with overdosage, with too rapid injection and in cases in which treatment has been unduly prolonged. In the latter the maximum tolerated dose of calcium borogluconate by intravenous injection is likely to be of the order of 250 ml of 25% solution. Overdosage may occur when farmers treat cases unsuccessfully by multiple subcutaneous injections and these are followed by an intravenous injection. When the peripheral circulation is very poor it is probable that the calcium administered subcutaneously is not absorbed until the circulation improves following the intravenous injection and the massive doses of calcium then absorbed cause acute toxicity. In all cases of intravenous injection close watch should be kept on the circulation. Some degree of irregularity occurs in most cases but if there is gross irregularity or sudden increase in heart rate the injection should be stopped temporarily or continued with great caution. In normal circumstances at least 10 minutes should be taken to introduce the standard dose. The acute toxic effect of calcium salts seems to be exerted specifically on heart muscle with a great variety of defects occurring in cardiac action, the type depending on the specific calcium salt used and the speed of injection. Electrocardiographic changes after induced hypercalcemia show increased ventricular activity and reduced atrial activity. Atropine is capable of abolishing the resulting arrhythmia (39). Sudden death may also occur after calcium injections if the cow is excited or frightened. It has been suggested that these deaths are caused by undue sensitivity to adrenaline. When affected cows are exposed to the sun or a hot, humid atmosphere, heatstroke may be a complicating factor. In such cases an attempt should be made to bring the temperature to below 39·5°C (103°F) before administering calcium. The incidence of cardiac irregularity and other abnormalities as detected by ECG during treatment with calcium salts intravenously is so high that there are doubts expressed about the suitability of this form of treatment (35).

Chronic toxicity may also occur. In rabbits and rats severe uremia due to extensive calcium deposits in the kidney occur after the subcutaneous injection of calcium chloride and borogluconate and similar deposits are often seen at necropsy in cows dying after multiple injections of calcium salts administered at short intervals.

The rate of response to treatment is affected by many factors as set out below and it is dangerous to quote what might be expected as an acceptable rate of recovery after treatment. This is particularly so if many of the cows are treated by farmers, and only difficult cases are presented to the veterinarians. If all cases are considered and there are no exceptional circumstances, recovery can be expected immediately after treatment in about 60% of cases, and in a further 15% after 2 hours; 10% have recoveries complicated by one of the diseases set out above, and 15% can be expected either to die or to require disposal. Of those which recover after one treatment 25–30% can be expected to relapse and require further treatment.

Failure to respond to treatment

This may be due to incorrect or incomplete diagnosis, or inadequate treatment. An inadequate response also includes relapse after a temporary improvement, most such cases occurring within 48 hours of the previous treatment. The same factors which cause poor response apply but relapses are much the most common in middle-aged Jersey cows who may have as many as five or six attacks around one calving. In all cases the incidence of relapse is much higher in cases which occur just before calving than in those which occur afterwards. The needs of individual animals for calcium replacement vary widely, depending on their body weight and the degree of hypocalcemia. In cattle, cows that have very recently calved, and older cows, are likely to show an incomplete response. In the latter instance the poor response is probably an indication of diminished skeletal reserves of calcium and inability of the normal mechanisms to maintain serum calcium levels in the face of excessive drain in the milk. The duration of the illness and the posture of the cow are also important in relation to response. Thus, in an extensive study, there were no downer cows or deaths in cows still standing at treatment, 13% downers and 2% deaths in cows in sternal recumbency and 37% downers and 12% deaths in cows in lateral recumbency at treatment (41). The longer the period from onset of illness to treatment the longer the period of post-treatment recumbency and the more cows lost by destruction or sale for slaughter. In another study (3) 67% recovered after a single treatment, 90%

after two treatments and 92–99% after three treatments. After routine treatment 37% of cases rose unassisted within 10 minutes and 23% required some assistance, 26% recovered after longer periods of recumbency and 14% died, or were destroyed or sold for slaughter. Another interesting relationship is the observation that a low body temperature, due probably to exposure to low environmental temperature, and increased wind velocities, is positively correlated with a high proportion of deaths and poor responses. The best procedure to follow if response does not occur is to revisit the animal at 12-hourly intervals and check the diagnosis. If no other cause of the recumbency can be determined the initial treatment should be repeated on a maximum of three occasions. Beyond this point further calcium therapy is seldom effective.

At the second visit alternative treatments, including inflation of the udder, and the injection of solutions containing either phosphorus, magnesium or dextrose, may also be administered, depending upon the clinical signs presented and the results of available biochemical tests. Glucose is usually administered as 500 ml of a 40% solution, sodium acid phosphate as 200 ml of a 15% solution, and magnesium sulfate as 200–400 ml of a 15% solution. Composite solutions containing calcium, magnesium, phosphorus and glucose are also in common use as initial treatments. There is a great deal of criticism of these so-called 'polypharmacy' preparations and they appear to have little real advantage (22), but they are likely to remain popular in those areas where milk fever cases are usually complicated by metabolic disorders other than hypocalcemia. They have also been shown to have no effect on the relapse rate, when compared with calcium salts on their own (62). Injections of phosphorus compounds alone do not have the same reputation as the composite mixtures. However, it is sometimes desirable to inject phosphorus alone with a calcium preparation. This can be conveniently done by adding 30 g of sodium dihydrogen phosphate in 200 ml water to the injection fluid (61). Calcium glycerophosphate has been found to be a suitable injection material for increasing plasma levels of both calcium and phosphorus (23).

Udder inflation

This has been largely superseded because of the possibility of damage to the udder but it is still a valuable alternative treatment, particularly in cows which do not respond completely to the injections described above. It is recommended as the routine treatment for cows which are likely to relapse. When combined with parenteral treatment with calcium solutions it produces less relapses than either treatment on its own (42). Serum calcium and phosphorus levels are raised but hypercalcemia, such as occurs after injected calcium solutions, is avoided and the depression of homeostatic mechanisms is also avoided. The response is good and often prompt, but may not be apparent for up to 12 hours. Serum magnesium levels are not affected by udder inflation and in view of the high levels of calcium and phosphorus and low level of magnesium in colostrum, it seems probable that udder inflation acts by preventing the further secretion of milk and slowing down the excretion of calcium and phosphorus. Inflation is best carried out with a special hand pump carrying an air filter and teat siphon. The udder is pumped up to a uniform, moderate firmness and the teats taped with broad tape which must be removed, the teats massaged and the tape replaced, at half-hourly intervals. Scrupulous cleanliness is necessary to prevent the introduction of infection into the quarters.

A further aid to parenteral therapy with solutions of calcium salts, especially for the purpose of increasing recovery rates and preventing relapses, is the oral administration of gels containing calcium chloride (45) described under prevention.

General nursing procedures

These are important. The calf should be removed and for the first 48 hours only sufficient milk drawn for its maintenance. A gradual return to full milking can then be permitted. If the cow is down for any length of time she must be kept propped up, since to leave her lying flat is to invite regurgitation and aspiration pneumonia. She should be moved from side to side three or four times a day and the legs and bony prominences massaged. Erection of a shelter over the cow is advisable if she cannot be moved to permanent shelter. If a cow is recumbent for more than 48 hours she should be raised in a hip sling several times daily. However, drastic measures to get cows up should be avoided. Gentle nudging in the ribs or the use of an electric prod are the maximum stimulants advised. The best assistance that can be given to a cow attempting to rise is a good heave at the base of the tail when she is halfway up. In many cases of parturient paresis which fail to rise after treatment it seems that there is no physical reason for the recumbency and that 'tonic immobility' is the cause. The common ways of testing this possibility are to bring on a dog, remove or stimulate the calf, open the door of the pen or cause fright in some way.

Control

Although no completely satisfactory method of prevention is available much attention has been directed to this aspect of the disease.

Calcium intake

The feeding of high calcium diets before calving is contraindicated and may increase the incidence of milk fever especially if the diet is alkaline, so much so that the feeding of either an acid-type diet or a low calcium diet for the last 5 weeks of pregnancy (8) have been recommended as control measures. A natural excess of calcium in the diet may predispose cows to milk fever because it promotes dependence on gastrointestinal absorption and not on skeletal mobilization. It is the efficiency of the latter which governs the cow's ability to maintain calcium homeostasis during periods of additional calcium drain, or when there is temporary gastrointestinal dysfunction, and no absorption. High calcium intakes before parturition in ewes have also been thought to contribute to the development of hypocalcemia in them (48). On the other hand the maintenance of appetite and the avoidance of alimentary tract stasis in late pregnancy appear to be important preventive measures which are likely to ensure an adequate calcium absorption. Testosterone derivatives with anabolic actions are undergoing trials to assess their efficiency as stimulators of appetite in cows near parturition. To improve mobilization the efficiency of prepartum milking and high-phosphate feeding have been examined. If the sudden onset of profuse lactation precipitates the hypocalcemia it might be expected that milking before calving would prevent the sudden drop in serum calcium levels which occurs in all cows. However, prepartum milking does not reduce the incidence of parturient paresis, nor significantly affect the changes in serum which normally occur in cows at parturition.

The administration of large quantities of phosphate in the ration should result in increased phosphate, and concurrently calcium, excretion in the urine. If the ration is also low in calcium the resulting negative balance of calcium can be expected to stimulate activity of the parathyroid gland. Boda and Cole have made use of this physiological mechanism by feeding a high phosphorus/low calcium ration to cows during the last month of pregnancy. With a Ca:P ratio of 6:1 30% of cows developed parturient paresis, at a Ca:P ratio of 1:1 15% developed the disease, and at a ratio of 1:3·3 no cases occurred. Although there is no apparent effect on the subsequent lactation there is the possibility, if the negative balance of calcium is prolonged or repeated frequently, that such a ration may contribute to the development of oesteoporosis. The inclusion of 5% of monosodium phosphate in a concentrate ration is also recommended as a preventive. The phosphate-treated diet is fed continuously.

A ration high in protein, designed to stimulate maximum milk production at calving, is thought to increase the incidence of parturient paresis, although the opposite view is also held. From our own observations, herds which are 'steamed up' or have access to plenty of lush pasture before calving do, as a rule, have a higher incidence of the disease. Restriction of food intake during the dry period is credited with being able to reduce milk fever prevalence by 80% (68). This should be interpreted as meaning to reduce the feed intake to overfed cows. Dietary restriction in cows on normal feed could precipitate acetonemia or pregnancy toxemia. Such a diet that inclines to alkalinity is also promoted as being prophylactic against milk fever. Such a diet may contain calcium chloride, magnesium sulfate and aluminum sulfate (72). Diets low in magnesium reduce the rate of calcium mobilization and such diets may contribute to a high incidence of milk fever (7, 77).

Management practices

The following management practices are suggested. Avoid excessive calcium intake during the dry period; feed adequate phosphorus to meet requirements and limit calcium intake to no more than 100–125 g/day. This appears to be a more practical approach to maintaining calcium homeostasis during the milk fever prone period than establishing a given Ca:P ratio. Since intestinal absorption is a major inflow source of serum calcium during the milk fever prone period, keeping cows on feed is essential. This may also reduce outflow of serum calcium. Avoid overfattening by either reducing the energy concentration of the ration or restricting the intake during the prepartum period. This also appears to stimulate appetite, thus keeping cows on feed. Avoid stresses at the time of parturition. Provide a clean well-bedded box stall with conditions conducive to cow comfort and allow the animal to exercise. Frequent observations of milk fever prone cows from 48 hours before to 48 hours after parturition for evidence of milk fever and immediate treatment will reduce the incidence of the downer cow syndrome associated with milk fever. At calving the cow should receive an oral dose of a calcium salt in a gel, as set out below, followed by a diet with a high calcium content (over 1% dry matter). If hypomagnesemia is a likely concomitant the diet should be supplemented with 60 g magnesium oxide daily. The critical day as far as feeding is concerned is the day of calving, and a sharp increase in calcium intake on this day can significantly reduce the occurrence of milk fever (51).

Calcium gel dosing

The most recent addition to the list of preventive measures is the provision by mouth of supplementary calcium in the form of a calcium gel (53). This is given by drench or in the feed at a level to provide 100 g of calcium daily. Excellent results are claimed provided the dose is raised to 150 g and three doses are given 24 hours before, 1–2 hours before and 10–14 hours after calving. The problem with the technique is that the calcium chloride is bitter and cows will not take it on feed or by drench, so it is given by stomach tube as a solution. The advantage of the gel is that cattle have to swallow it when it is given as a drench.

Administration of vitamin D and its metabolites and analogs

Vitamin D_3 (cholecalciferol) administered parenterally is at present the most popular prophylactic against milk fever. However, there is great interest in the efficiency of its active metabolites. Vitamin D_3 is hydroxylated in the liver and the resulting metabolite is 25-hydroxycholecalciferol. This is metabolized in the kidney to 1·25-dihydroxycholecalciferol. This metabolite has a very active hypercalcemic effect but is difficult to synthesize. One of its analogs, 1-alpha-hydroxycholecalciferol is as active, is easy to prepare and is consequently used pharmacologically.

In an attempt to reverse the negative calcium balance of susceptible cows the administration of vitamin D is now commonly used to increase intestinal absorption of calcium. Oral dosing with vitamin D_2, the intramuscular administration of vitamin D_3 and the intramuscular injection of dihydrotachysterol all have their proponents. Oral dosing with 20 million units of vitamin D_2 per day for 5 days to cows immediately prior to calving greatly reduces the expected incidence of parturient paresis. The exact date of calving is often difficult to determine and if the administration is discontinued for up to 4 days before calving an unusually high incidence of the disease may follow, probably because of the depression of parathyroid activity which follows the administration. The danger of causing metastatic calcification also exists as this has been produced with smaller doses (10–20 million units daily for 10 days). Pregnant cows are more susceptible to calcification than non-pregnant animals. Treatment with larger doses or for longer periods than those recommended above should be avoided because of the danger of toxic effects. Smaller doses reduce the risk of calcification but also reduce the degree of calcium retention.

A single dose of 10 million units intramuscularly given 2–8 days before parturition has been considered as optimal (54). A dose of 1 million units per 45 kg of body weight has given consistently better results. This may explain the variable results (53) and why results have been more favorable in Jersey cattle. If the cow fails to calve after the 8th day, another 10 million units may be administered and repeated every 8 days until the cow calves. Subclinical calcification may occur in vessel walls but this is unlikely if dietary calcium and phosphorus intake is adequate. Single doses of 40 million units can be lethal. One of the disadvantages of the method is the likelihood that cows which do not calve at the anticipated time can be more seriously affected than if they receive no treatment. The hypercalcemic effect of cholecalciferol by injection is very much longer when it is administered by intramuscular injection (up to 25 days) than by intravenous injection (up to 3 days) (56). For this reason and because occasional cases of shock occur after the intravenous injection, especially if more than one injection is given, the intramuscular route is preferred. The injection of vitamin D is preferred to feeding it and a protection rate of up to 80% can be anticipated. It is estimated that 95% of Jersey cattle are protected. To avoid the problems created by cows not calving at the predicted time, a combined regimen including induction of parturition by the administration of corticosteroid with the injection of 1-alpha-hydroxy-cholecalciferol is reported as being successful (57). Injection of cows with the same vitamin D analog plus a prostaglandin (cloprostenol) was unsuccessful in preventing milk fever.

In spite of the very variable results obtained, the injection of vitamin D_3 is still the most commonly used method of prevention, principally because of its simplicity. But there are obvious differences in response between breeds (3) and between workers. Up to 44% of treated cows have subsequently developed the disease in one series (32) and in another the morbidity fell from 50 to 95% down to 2% (33). When combined with management of the calcium and phosphorus content of the diet, restricting them to 0·5% calcium and 0·25% potassium of the total dry matter in the ration, the injection gives better results than the injection or the dietary management alone (34).

Other compounds with vitamin D activity but which avoid the possibility of causing hypervitaminosis D and are therefore useful in the prevention of milk fever are:

- *25-Hydroxycholecalciferol* injected intramuscularly at a dose of 8 mg 3–10 days before calving (47, 58) and repeated at weekly intervals. Single doses of 4 mg are not effective in reducing the occurrence of parturient hypocalcemia or parturient paresis (54).
- *1,25-Dehydroxyvitamin D_3* given in 200 μg doses daily, orally, to calving cows reduces the development of hypocalcemia but does not completely prevent milk fever (28).
- *1-Alpha hydroxyvitamin D_3*; an injection of 350 μg is effective as a preventive to milk fever provided it is given more than 24 hours and less than 100 hours before calving. If calving has not occurred naturally within 100 hours of treatment, parturition is induced (59).

Injection within 24 hours of the onset of milk fever is ineffective, but if it is given more than 24 hours and less than 1 week before the onset of the disease the protection is excellent (29). Single dose rates of 0·1 mg intravenously and 1·0 mg intramuscularly have also been used (38) and although soft tissue calcification is not generally recorded after its use, there are doubts about the safety of all of the synthetic analogs of vitamin D. Dosing is recommended to commence 5 days before anticipated calving date and be repeated at 5-day intervals (46). Successful results are recorded with a combination of the treatment with corticosteroid to ensure that the cow calves (60). With all of these treatments the effects are likely to be enhanced by the cows receiving a ration with a low to normal phosphorus content (27).

Miscellaneous prophylactic measures

These include injections of parathyroid extract which have no apparent effect, incomplete milking after calving which is similarly disappointing, and the prophylactic injection of calcium solutions as soon after calving as possible, which may be effective but is largely impractical. Years ago the administration of ammonium chloride by mouth to produce acidosis and enhance calcium mobilization and ionization was recommended to prevent milk fever. There is some support for its use on the same basis now (59). The ammonium chloride is fed with grain over the last few weeks of pregnancy, commencing with 25 g and increasing to 100 g/day at calving.

The heritability of susceptibility to milk fever is thought by some authorities to be quite high, but there is a notable lack of good evidence to support the view. However, it is probably best that the opinion be taken into account when breeding plans are made. Most attention should be given to the use or deletion of susceptible cows as mothers of bulls to be used in artificial insemination.

In species other than cattle the disease is commonly caused by errors in management, and prevention depends on their avoidance. Pregnant and lactating ewes and cows should not be subjected to unnecessary exercise or excitement. It is good practice to improve the plane of nutrition during late pregnancy in ewes to avoid pregnancy toxemia but changes, particularly to lush pasture, should be made gradually, and sheep moved from wooded pasture to open fields with little natural shelter should be provided with some protection from the weather.

REVIEW LITERATURE

Braithwaite, G. D. (1976) Calcium and phosphorus metabolism in ruminants with special reference to parturient paresis. *J. dairy Res.*, *43*, 501.

Horst, R. L. & Reinhardt, T. A. (1982) Vitamin D metabolism in

ruminants and its relevance to the periparturient cow. *J. dairy Sci.*, *66*, 661–678.
Mosdol, G. & Waage, S. (1981) Hypocalcemia in the ewe. *Nord. VetMed.*, *33*, 310–326.
Jonsson, G. & Simesen, M. G. (1973) Parturient paresis. A review. *Aust. vet. J.*, *49*, 252.
Jonsson, G. (1978) Milk fever prevention. *Vet. Rec.*, *102*, 165.
Stober, M. & Dirksen, G. (1982) The recumbent cow:differential diagnosis and differential therapy, *Vet. Ann.*, *22*, 81–94.

REFERENCES

(1) Carlstrom, G. (1970) *Acta vet. Scand.*, *11*, 89.
(2) Larsen, J. W. A. et al. (1986) *Aust. vet. J.*, *63*, 25.
(3) Robertson, J. A. (1985) *Svensk Vet.*, *38*, 481.
(4) Yarrington, J. T. et al. (1976) *Am. J. Pathol.*, *83*, 569.
(5) Payne, J. M. et al. (1963) *Vet. Rec.*, *75*, 588.
(6) Waage, S. (1984) *Nord. VetMed.*, *36*, 282.
(7) van de Braak, A. E. et al. (1987) *Res. vet. Sci.*, *42*, 101.
(8) Barlet, J. P. & Ross, R. (1984) *Br. vet. J.*, *140*, 392.
(9) Seidel, H. & Schroter, J. (1977) *Monatsschr. VetMed.*, *32*, 137.
(10) Vlahos, N. & Tsakalov, P. (1977) *Hellenic Vet. Med*, *20*, 139 & 189.
(11) Sandstedt, H. et al. (1984) *Nord. VetMed.*, *36*, 406.
(12) Waage, S. et al. (1984) *Res. vet. Sci.*, *36*, 164.
(13) Braithwaite, G. D. et al. (1969) *Br. J. Nutr.*, *23*, 827.
(14) Risco, C. A. et al. (1984) *J. Am. vet. med. Assoc.*, *185*, 1517.
(15) Belonje, P. C. & van der Walt, K. (1971) *J. S. Afr. vet. med. Assoc.*, *42*, 135.
(16) Singh, B. et al. (1974) *Ind. vet. J.*, *51*, 642.
(17) Waage, S. et al. (1984) *Nord. VetMed.*, *36*, 19.
(18) Dyrendahl, L. et al. (1972) *Zentralbl. VetMed.*, *19A*, 621.
(19) Janzen, E. (1976) *Can. vet. J.*, *17*, 298.
(20) Daniel, R. C. W. & Moodie, E. W. (1978) *Res. vet. Sci.*, *24*, 380.
(21) Mullen, P. (1977) *Vet. Rec.*, *101*, 405.
(22) Curtis, R. A. et al. (1978) *Can. vet. J.*, *19*, 155.
(23) Sachs, M. & Hurwitz, S. (1974) *Refuah Vet.*, *31*, 171.
(24) Bowen, J. M. et al. (1970) *Am. J. vet. Res.*, *31*, 831.
(25) Smith, B. L. et al. (1984) *NZ vet. J.*, *32*, 48.
(26) Berger, V. U. & Gerber, H. (1977) *Schweiz. Arch. Tierheilkd.*, *119*, 9.
(27) Jorgenson, N. A. (1978) *Vet. Rec.*, *103*, 136.
(28) Hove, K. & Kristiansen, T. (1984) *Acta vet. Scand.*, *25*, 510.
(29) Davies, D. C. et al. (1978) *Vet. Rec.*, *102*, 440 & 442.
(30) Dauth, J. et al. (1984) *J. S. Afr. vet. Assoc.*, *55*, 71.
(31) Fenwick, D. C. (1969) *Aust. vet. J.*, *45*, 118.
(32) Mosdol, G. & Skeie, A. H. (1978) *Nord. VetMed.*, *30*, 83.
(33) Oetzel, H. et al. (1977) *Monatsschr. VetMed.*, *32*, 661.
(34) Julien, W. E. et al. (1977) *J. dairy Sci.*, *60*, 431.
(35) Kvart, C. (1983) *Br. vet. J.*, *139*, 192.
(36) Mullen, P. (1977) *Vet. Rec.*, *101*, 366.
(37) Church, T. L. et al. (1978) *Can. vet. J.*, *19*, 110.
(38) Gast, D. R. et al. (1977) *J. dairy Sci.*, *60*, 1910.
(39) Littledike, E. T. et al. (1976) *Am. J. vet. Res.*, *37*, 383.
(40) Horst, R. L. et al. (1977) *Science*, *196*, 662.
(41) Fenwick, D. C. (1969) *Aust. vet. J.*, *45*, 111, 454.
(42) Gregorovic, V. et al. (1974) *Proc. 8th int. Mtg Dis. Cattle, Milan*, 408.
(43) Littledike, E. T. (1976) *J. dairy Sci.*, *59*, 1947.
(44) Curtis, C. R. et al. (1983) *J. Am. vet. med. Assoc.*, *183*, 559.
(45) Mayer, G. P. (1972) *Proc. 7th int. Mtg Dis. Cattle, London.*
(46) Gast, D. R. et al. (1979) *J. dairy Sci.*, *62*, 1009.
(47) Hoffsis, G. F. et al. (1978) *Bov. Pract.* No. 13, 88.
(48) Jonsson, G. et al. (1973) *Nord. VetMed.*, *25*, 97.
(49) Jones, B. & Luthman, J. (1978) *Acta vet. Scand.*, *19*, 204.
(50) Daniel, R. C. W. (1983) *Can, J. comp. Med.*, *47*, 276.
(51) Haalstra, R. T. (1973) *Tijdschr. Diergeneeskd.*, *98*, 529.
(52) Daniel, R. C. W. & Moodie, E. W. (1979) *Br. vet. J.*, *135*, 440.
(53) Jonsson, G. & Pehrson, B. (1970) *Vet. Rec.*, *87*, 575, 583.
(54) Allsop, T. F. & Pauli, J. V. (1985) *NZ J. exp. Agric.*, *13*, 19.
(55) Hollis, B. W. & Draper, H. H. (1979) *Fed. Proc.*, *38*, 31.
(56) Boling, J. A. & Evans, J. M. (1979) *Int. J. Vit. Nutr. Res.*, *49*, 29.
(57) McMurray, C. H. et al. (1980) *Vet. Rec.*, *107*, 188 & 431 (and *108*, 20 & 21).
(58) Olson, W. G. et al. (1973) *J. dairy Sci.*, *56*, 889.
(59) Sachs, M. et al. (1987) *Vet. Rec.*, *120*, 39.
(60) Vagg, M. J. et al. (1981) *Vet. Rec.*, *109*, 273.
(61) Lachmann, G. (1980) *Monatsschr. VetMed.*, *35*, 59.
(62) Curtis, R. A. et al. (1979) *Bov. Pract.*, *14*, 56.
(63) Bostedt, H. et al. (1979) *Prakt. Tierärztl.*, *60*, 18.
(64) Mosdol, G. & Waage, S. (1981) *Nord. VetMed.*, *33*, 310.
(65) Furslund, K. et al. (1980) *Acta vet. Scand.*, *21*, 171.
(66) Jonsson, G. et al. (1980) *Zentralbl. VetMed.*, *27A*, 173.
(67) Overby, I. & Odegaard, S. A. (1980) *Norsk Vet. Tidsskr.*, *92*, 21.
(68) Sanstedt, H. (1980) *Svensk Vet.*, *32*, 127 & 495.
(69) Waage, S. (1984) *Nord. VetMed.*, *36*, 346.
(70) Tollman, R. L. & Gantvik, K. M. (1980) *Acta vet. Scand.*, *21*, 457.
(71) Kichura, T. S. et al. (1982) *J. Nutr.*, *112*, 480.
(72) Dishington, I. W. & Bjornstad, J. (1982) *Acta vet. Scand.*, *23*, 336.
(73) Kvart, C. et al. (1982) *Acta vet. Scand.*, *23*, 184.
(74) Tindall, J. R. (1986) *Vet. Rec.*, *118*, 518.
(75) Kemp, J. et al. (1985) *Vet. Rec.*, *117*, 450.
(76) Larsson, L. et al. (1983) *Zentralbl. VetMed.*, *A30*, 401.
(77) Sanson, B. F. et al. (1983) *Vet. Rec.*, *112*, 447.
(78) Grohn, Y. et al. (1986) *Acta vet. Scand.*, *27*, 209.
(79) Hollis, B. W. et al. (1981) *J. Endocrinology*, *88*, 161.

The 'downer cow' syndrome

The 'downer cow' syndrome is a condition which occurs in cattle usually following hypocalcemic parturient paresis. It is characterized clinically by prolonged recumbency even after two successive treatments with calcium. At necropsy there is traumatic injury to limb muscles and nerves, ischemic necrosis of limb muscles, myocarditis, and fatty infiltration and degeneration of the liver.

Etiology

The etiology is not clear but the available evidence and clinical experience suggests that the disease is a complication of hypocalcemic parturient paresis (1). Traumatic injuries of the medial thigh muscles and of the tissues around the hip joint and of the obturator muscles are common in cows which do not recover. The traumatic injuries may be the result of cows 'spreadeagling' their hindlegs if they are unsteady during parturition or if they are forced to get up or walk on a slippery floor immediately before or following parturition. A difficult parturition due to an oversized calf may result in peripelvic traumatic injury with extensive edema of the pelvic tissues and vulva, and failure of the cow to get up following parturition. If these cows develop hypocalcemic parturient paresis, it is unlikely they will get up following treatment with calcium.

The evidence to support traumatic injury to muscle as an important cause is the observation of a marked increase in the SGOT levels in cows affected with hypocalcemic parturient paresis and failure to rise after repeated treatments (1). The SGOT levels increased markedly between the first and second treatments which indicated that muscle damage had occurred and the levels were highest in cows which did not recover.

Traumatic injuries to the nerves of the limbs are present in 25% or more of downer cows (1). In the hindquarters the sciatic and the obturator nerves are vulnerable to injury by pressure from the calf during parturition. Pressure injuries on the superficial nerves (radial and peroneus) of the extremities readily occur in recumbent cows.

Prolonged recumbency after an overlong delay in the treatment of what was an uncomplicated hypocalcemic parturient paresis is considered to be an important cause of the downer cow. Prolonged recumbency (more than 4–6 hours) can result in ischemic necrosis due to obstruction of the blood supply, especially in a heavy cow if she lies on one leg for a long period (8). Cows which develop milk fever while in a standing tie-stall will often slide into the gutter behind the stall with the result that their hindquarters are subjected to extreme pressure leading to ischemic necrosis.

Experimentally, enforced recumbency of cattle for 6, 9, or 12 hours with one hindlimb positioned under the body will result in a downer syndrome (11). Affected cows are unable to stand and the affected limb is swollen and held rigid similar to the injured limbs of human patients with compartmental/crush syndrome.

Serum electrolyte imbalances or deficits have been suggested as the cause of the prolonged recumbency following treatment for parturient paresis. A persistent hypophosphatemia is regarded as a common cause in some regions and in some cases appears to respond to treatment with phosphorus. Persistent hypocalcemia may occur but is unlikely to be the principal cause because treatment with calcium salts does not relieve the signs, even temporarily. However, the use of an insufficient amount of calcium for the treatment of milk fever in large heavy cows may result in an incomplete response and failure of the cow to rise. If these cows are not retreated soon enough, ischemic necrosis of the leg muscles will occur leading to prolonged recumbency even after the cow is subsequently treated with sufficient calcium.

A long-term low-level hypomagnesemia has been suggested as a cause especially when it accompanies hypocalcemia. But it is usually manifested by a tetanic hyperesthetic state which is not part of the downer cow syndrome. Hypokalemia is, with hypophosphatemia, the most commonly quoted cause, especially in the so-called 'creeper' cows which are bright and alert and crawl about, but are unable to rise (3).

One hypothesis is that the hypocalcemic state, or ischemia due to prolonged recumbency, may increase the cell membrane permeability of muscle fibers and allow the loss of potassium from the cell which in turn causes the myotonia which appears to be the basis of the 'downer cow syndrome'. This view is supported by the observed low serum and muscle potassium levels in downer cows (4). Claims are made that potassium salts are successful in treatment (6), but they are highly toxic and opportunities of establishing a response to their use are limited. A response would be difficult to interpret, anyway, since even a reduction in food intake can result in a mild hypokalemia.

However, excellent clinical and laboratory evaluation of the downer cow has demonstrated that there are no differences in the serum biochemistry between cows which have had hypocalcemic parturient paresis and become downers and those which do not become downers (uncomplicated hypocalcemic parturient paresis) (1).

Based on clinical experience and our interpretation of the literature we conclude that the downer cow syndrome is a complication of hypocalcemic parturient paresis. Traumatic injury to leg muscles at the time of parturition or when the cow is unsteady and falls during the first stage of milk fever will result in the inability of the cow to get up quickly following treatment for milk fever. Another plausible complication is an overlong delay (4 hours or more) in the treatment of cows with milk fever (8) which results in ischemic necrosis of the muscles of both the hindlegs and forelegs. There is now experimental evidence to support the clinical and epidemiological observation (11).

Epidemiology

The incidence of the downer cow syndrome is distressingly high, particularly because so many of the affected animals are heavy producers and of great value. It is impossible to give accurate figures on incidence because of variations in nomenclature and in the accuracy of diagnoses. For example, some find that all cases are caused by nerve injury (2). Cases included in this classification by some veterinarians are classified by others as maternal obstetric paralysis, as obturator paralysis or as hypophosphatemia. Because it is a syndrome lacking in definition and comprising the residual cases which cannot be otherwise classified, it varies in size depending largely upon the clinical acuity of the individual veterinarian, and probably also on varying environmental factors in different areas. Nevertheless, the incidence seems to be increasing, particularly in intensive farming areas, although this impression could arise from the increased necessity to effect a cure in valuable animals.

A mail survey of 723 dairy herds in Minnesota revealed an incidence of 21·4/1000 cow years at risk (30). The overall outcome was that 33% recovered, 23% were slaughtered and 44% died. The herd owners perceived that the downer cows were high producers (48%) or average producers (46%), with only 6% being low producers. Approximately 58% occurred within 1 day of parturition and 37% occurred during the first 100 days of lactation. The incidence was highest (39%) during the three coldest months, December, January and February.

The disease occurs most commonly in the first 2 or 3 days after calving in heavy milk producers and in many cases occurs concurrently with parturient paresis.

Pathogenesis

Several different primary factors or diseases like parturient hypocalcemia initially cause recumbency. The recumbency results in pressure damage which occurs secondarily and is a factor common to all cases (2). Traumatic injury to limb muscles and nerves immediately prior to parturition or at the time of parturition can result in prolonged recumbency and subsequent pressure damage (1). An overlong delay in the treatment for hypocalcemic parturient paresis can result in pressure damage and the subsequent inability to rise after treatment for the primary disease (9).

Regardless of the cause, the prolonged recumbency results in varying degrees of ischemic necrosis of major muscles of the hindlimbs particularly the semitendinous and the muscles caudal to the stifle. Prolonged compression of the muscle lead to tissue anoxia, cell damage and inflammation which causes swelling which causes a further increase in pressure which limits tissue perfusion leading to a detrimental cascade of events (11). The thick fascial boundaries of the semitendinous muscle prevents expansion which results in pressure-induced compartmental syndrome. Sciatic nerve damage due to pressure also occurs and may contribute to the downer syndrome. Experimental external compression of the pelvic limb of the goat, to simulate limb compression in recumbent cows, resulted in a marked reduction in nerve condition velocity of the peroneal nerve which was associated with clinically evident limb dysfunction (8). Damage to the peroneal nerve will result in hyperflexion of the fetlock if and when the cow is able to stand. Experimentally induced sternal recumbency with one hindlimb positioned under the body to simulate prolonged recumbency will result in a swollen rigid limb within 6–9 hours (12). Following injury to the muscle cells the serum levels of creatine phosphokinase activity are markedly elevated at about 12 hours after the onset of recumbency. Proteinuria and in some severe cases myoglobinuria occurs between 12 and 36 hours, after the onset of prolonged recumbency, due to the release of myoglobin from damaged muscles. In cows which make efforts to rise but cannot do so, continued struggling will result in rupture of muscle fibers and hemorrhage which may make the condition worse.

Acute focal myocarditis is present in about 10% of cases and explains the tachycardia, arrhythmia and unfavorable response to intravenous calcium salts observed in some cases of downer cows. The cause of the myocardial lesion is unknown but the repeated administration of calcium salts has been suggested (1).

The prolonged recumbency can result in additional complication such as acute mastitis, decubitus ulcers and traumatic injuries of the limbs.

The pathogenesis of the non-alert downer cow is unknown (5). Most have had an initial episode of parturient hypocalcemia but did not respond satisfactorily. Within 1 or 2 days affected cows have a preference for lateral recumbency and exhibit expiratory moaning. They represent about 2% of all cases of milk fever.

Clinical findings

The 'downer cow' syndrome may occur independently, or follow apparent recovery after treatment for parturient paresis, except for the continued recumbency which, in effect, constitutes the disease.

In the typical case, affected cows either make no effort or are unable to rise following treatment for parturient paresis. About 30% of cows treated for parturient paresis will not rise for up to 24 hours following treatment. Those which are unable to rise after 24 hours and after two treatments can be classified as downers. They are usually bright and alert and, although the appetite is reduced, the cow eats and drinks moderately well. The temperature is normal and the heart rate may be normal or elevated to 80–100/min. Tachycardia and arrhythmia occur in some cows especially immediately following the administration of calcium intravenously and sudden death has occurred. Respirations are usually unaffected. Defecation and urination are normal and proteinuria is common. A marked proteinuria may indicate extensive muscle damage.

Some affected cows may make no effort to rise but most will make frequent attempts to rise but are unable to completely extend their hindlegs and to lift their hindquarters more than a few centimeters off the ground. These frequent attempts to rise result in the cow 'crawling' or 'creeping' along the ground with both hindlegs in a partially flexed position and displaced posteriorly—the frogleg attitude. On a non-slippery surface (bare ground or deep bedding) some cows are able to stand with some assistance by lifting on the tail head or with the use of hip slings. Those cows which do not make an effort to rise usually cannot stand with assistance and if supported with hip slings will usually make no effort to bear weight with either the hindlegs or the forelegs. It gives one the impression that their limbs are very painful or numb and therefore they are unable or reluctant to bear weight. Damage to the peroneal nerve is usually present when there is hyperflexion of the fetlock joints which is evident if and when the cow is able to stand and bear weight on the hindlimbs.

In some cases, the hindlegs are extended on each side of the cow and reach up to elbow joints on each side. In this position, the cow is bearing considerable weight on the medial thigh musculature and causing ischemic necrosis. Some of these are due to dislocation of the hip joints and others are associated with traumatic injuries surrounding the hip joints with or without rupture of the ligamentum teres. The cow seems to prefer this position for some unexplainable reason because invariably she will shift the legs back to this abnormal position if they are placed in their normal position.

In some cows the signs may be more marked and include particularly a tendency to be in lateral recumbency with the head drawn back. When lifted and supported, these cows appear almost normal but, when they are left alone, they always revert to the position of lateral recumbency within a short time. Still more severe cases show hyperesthesia and some tetany of the limbs but only when lying in lateral recumbency. These more severe cases do not usually eat or drink. These have been described as 'non-alert downers', and are thought to have brain damage (5).

Complications in the downer cow syndrome are common and often result in death or the need for euthanasia. Coliform mastitis, decubitus ulceration, especially over the prominences of the hock and elbow joint, and traumatic injuries around the tuber coxae caused by the hip slings are common. When these complications occur in the early stages of the disease they commonly interfere with any progress being made and become the centre of concern.

The course of the disease is variable and dependent on the nature and extent of the lesions and the quality of the care and comfort which is provided for the cow during the first few days. About 50% of downer cows will get up within 4 days or less if cared for properly. The prognosis is poor for those which are still recumbent after 7 days, although some affected cows have been down for 10–14 days and subsequently stood up and recovered. Death may occur in 48–72 hours following the onset and is usually associated with myocarditis.

Clinical pathology

The calcium, phosphorus, magnesium and glucose levels of the blood are within the normal range and the results of hematological examinations are usually consistent with those found in normal cows which have recently calved. The levels of creatinine phosphokinase (CPK) and serum glutamic oxaloacetic acid (SGOT) are usually markedly elevated by 18–24 hours after the onset of recumbency and continue to elevate within the next few days. The elevated CPK levels are indicative of muscle damage and their continued elevation suggests continued muscle damage. In experimentally induced recumbency in cows the creatinine phosphokinase activity remained within normal limits for the first 6 hours. However, by 12 hours there was a marked increase to mean values of 12 000 i.u./l rising to 40 000 i.u./l by 24 hours (12). There may be moderate ketonuria. A marked proteinuria is usually evident by 18–24 hours after the onset of recumbency. The proteinuria may persist for several days or be absent within a few days. In severe cases, the urine may be brown and turbid because of severe myoglobinuria. Low arterial blood pressures and abnormal electrocardiograms have been observed in some animals (10).

Necropsy findings

Hemorrhages and edema of the skin traumatic in origin are common. The major pathological changes consist of hemorrhages and degeneration of the medial thigh muscles. Hemorrhages around the hip joint with or without rupture of the ligamentum teres are also common. Local areas of ischemic necrosis of the musculature (gracilis, pectineus and adductor muscles) occur at the anterior edge of the pelvic symphysis (1). Hemorrhages and edema of the nerves of the limbs (obturator, ischiatic, peroneus, radial) are also common and usually associated with severe muscle damage. The heart is dilated and flabby and histologically there is focal myocarditis. There is fatty degeneration of the liver and the adrenal glands are enlarged. Histologically there are also degenerative changes in the glomerular and tubular epithelium of the kidneys.

Diagnosis

The diagnosis of the downer cow syndrome is made after all other known causes of recumbency have been eliminated in a cow which had hypocalcemic parturient paresis and failed to rise within 24 hours following two successive courses of treatment. The other common causes of recumbency are described under the diagnosis of parturient paresis. It can be very difficult to eliminate all other causes of recumbency but only by repeated careful clinical examination will the clinician avoid the embarrassment of failing to detect the presence of coliform mastitis, a fractured leg or a dislocated hip.

Treatment

Many treatments including the injections of magnesium salts, phosphates, corticosteroids, stimulant tonics and vitamin E and selenium have been used without consistent success. Attempts at slinging are usually unsuccessful unless the cow is partially able to get up on her own. The use of solutions containing potassium, calcium, magnesium and phosphorus has been recommended (3) but there is no scientific evidence that these electrolytes, in addition to what was probably given to the cow already, are indicated or are of any beneficial value. Fluid therapy by the oral or parenteral route is indicated for cows which may not be drinking a normal amount of water.

The most important aspect of treatment is to provide the most comfortable bedding possible and to turn the cow from side to side several times daily to minimize the degree of ischemic necrosis and para-analgesia which results from prolonged recumbency. There is a need to develop a field technique for the provision of physiotherapy in the form of muscle massage to restore the normal muscle activity in the affected limbs. With conscientious care and the provision of good bedding, most cows will attempt to rise in a few days and can stand normally a day or two later. If affected cows are left on a slippery ground surface, they will not make an effort to rise and will become progressively worse.

Control

The early detection and treatment of hypocalcemic parturient paresis should reduce the incidence and severity of the downer cow syndrome. Under ideal conditions, cows should be treated during the first stage of parturient paresis before they become recumbent. Once recumbent they should be treated as soon as possible and if treatment is to be delayed, the cow should be well bedded with liberal quantities of straw or moved to a soft-ground surface. Recumbent cows should be coaxed and assisted to stand if possible. If they are unable to stand, they should be rolled from one side to another on an hourly basis if possible. It is usually difficult to get owners to comply with this recommendation but frequent rolling from side to side is necessary to minimize the ischemic necrosis. Dairy cows should be placed in a comfortable well-bedded box stall for calving and should be left in that box stall until at least 48 hours after parturition in the event that parturient paresis develops.

REVIEW LITERATURE

Andrews, T. (1986) The downer cow. *In Practice*, *8*, 187–189.

Cox, V. S. (1981) Understanding the downer cow syndrome. *Comp. cont. Educ. pract. Vet.*, *3*, S472–S478.

Cox, V. S. (1982) Pathogenesis of the downer cow syndrome. *Vet. Rec.*, *111*, 76–79.

REFERENCES

(1) Jonsson, G. & Pehrson, B. (1969) *Zentralbl. VetMed.*, *16A*, 757.
(2) Cox, V. S. et al. (1986) *Prev. vet. Med.*, *4*, 249.
(3) Kronfeld, D. S. (1976) *Mod. vet. Pract.*, *57*, 599.
(4) Kowalczyck, D. F. & Mayer, G.P. (1972) *Am. J. vet. Res.*, *33*, 751.
(5) Fenwick, D. C. et al. (1986) *Vet. Rec.*, *118*, 124.
(6) Johnson, B. L. (1967) *J. Am. vet. med. Assoc.*, *151*, 1681.
(7) Ward, G. M. (1966) *J. Am. vet. med. Assoc.*, *148*, 543.
(8) Fenwick, D. C. (1969) *Aust. vet. J.*, *45*, 184.
(9) Bjorsell. K. A. et al. (1969) *Acta vet. Scand.*, *10*, 36.
(10) Sellers, A. F. et al. (1956) *Proc. 92nd Ann. gen. Mtg Am. vet. med. Assoc.*, *1955*, 35.
(11) Cox, V. S. et al. (1982) *Am. J. vet. Res.*, *43*, 26.

Transit recumbency of ruminants

Transit recumbency (tetany) is a disease which occurs after prolonged transport, usually in cows and ewes in late pregnancy. It is also recorded in lambs transported to feedlots (1), and in cows (2) and sheep (4) delivered to abattoirs. It is characterized by recumbency, alimentary tract stasis and coma and is highly fatal. It has a wide distribution and can be expected to occur in most countries. Most affected animals die and heavy losses are encountered when cows and ewes in late pregnancy are moved long distances by rail or on foot.

Although cows of any age in late pregnancy are most commonly affected the disease has also been recorded in cows recently calved, in bullocks, steers, dry cows and lambs. Precipitating causes include heavy feeding before shipment, deprivation of food and water for more than 24 hours during transit and unrestricted access to water and exercise immediately after unloading. There is an increased incidence during hot weather. The cause is unknown although physical stress is an obvious factor. In lambs there is restlessness, staggering, partial paralysis of hindlegs and the early assumption of lateral recumbency. Death may occur quickly, or after 2–3 days of recumbency. There is a mild hypocalcemia (7–7·5 mg/dl; 1·75–1·87 mmol/l). The recovery rate even with treatment is only fair.

Clinical signs may occur while the cattle are still on the train or up to 48 hours after unloading. In the early stages there may be excitement and restlessness, trismus and grinding of the teeth. A staggering gait with paddling of the hindlegs and recumbency occur, and are accompanied by stasis of the alimentary tract and complete anorexia. Animals that do not recover gradually become comatose and die in 3–4 days. There may be a moderate hypocalcemia and hypophosphatemia in cattle. In sheep of various ages some are hypocalcemic and hypomagnesemic and some are hypoglycemic, but some have no detectable biochemical abnormality (4). There are no lesions at necropsy other than those related to prolonged recumbency. Ischemic muscle necrosis is the most obvious of these. The relationship of the disease to transport or forced exercise is diagnostic.

Some cases respond to treatment with combined calcium, magnesium and glucose injections. Udder inflation, induced abortion and general stimulants, such as strychnine are of no apparent value. Repeated parenteral injections of large volumes of electrolyte solutions are recommended. In lambs the subcutaneous injection of a solution of calcium and magnesium salts is recommened but the response is usually only 50%, due probably to an intercurrent myonecrosis (6).

If prolonged transport of cows or ewes in advanced pregnancy is unavoidable, they should be fed on a moderately restricted diet for several days beforehand and provided with adequate food, water and rest periods during the trip. The administration of an ataractic before loading is highly recommended especially for nervous animals (5). On unloading they should be allowed only limited access to water for 24 hours and should be allowed a minimum of exercise for 2–3 days.

REFERENCES

(1) Pierson, R. E. & Jensen, R. (1975) *J. Am. vet. med. Assoc.*, *166*, 260.
(2) Warnock, J. P. et al. (1978) *Aust. Vet. J.*, *54*, 566.
(3) Lucas, M. J. et al. (1982) *J. Am. vet. med. Assoc.*, *181*, 381.
(4) Shorthose, W. R. & Shaw, F. D. (1977) *Aust. vet. J.*, *53*, 330.
(5) van der Walt, K. (1961) *J.S. Afr. vet. med. Assoc.*, 32, 283.
(6) Lucas, M. J. (1983) *Mod. vet. Pract.*, *64*, 213.

Lactation tetany of mares (eclampsia, transit tetany)

Lactation tetany of mares appears to have been a common occurrence when draught horse breeding was widely practiced but is observed rarely nowadays. The mortality rate is high in untreated animals.

Hypocalcemia occurs constantly, with serum levels in the range of 4–6 mg/dl (1·00–1·50 mmol/l) and response to treatment with injections of calcium salts is excellent. The degree of hypocalcemia has been related to the clinical signs (1). When serum calcium levels are higher than 8 mg/dl (2·00 mmol/l) the only sign is increased excitability. At levels of 5–8 mg/dl (1·25–2·00 mmol/l) there are tetanic spasms and slight incoordination. At levels of less than 5 mg/dl (1·25 mmol/l) there is recumbency and stupor. Hypomagnesemia (with serum magnesium levels of 0·9 mg/dl (0·37 mmol/l) has been observed in some cases (2) but only in association with recent transport. Hypermagnesemia has been reported in other cases (3).

A number of factors appear to predispose to the disease. Most cases occur in lactating mares, either at about the tenth day after foaling or 1–2 days after weaning (4).

Mares which are grazing on lush pasture and have an exceptionally heavy flow of milk appear to be most susceptible and in many instances hard physical work (5), the housing of wild ponies (6), or prolonged transport (3) appears to precipitate an attack. The latter has been a particularly important factor in the etiology of the disease in Britain and has been credited with precipitating it even in stallions and dry mares (6). Occasional cases occur without there being any apparent cause (7, 9).

Many mild cases which recover spontaneously occur after transport but the mortality rate in some shipments may be greater than 60%. Mares affected at the foal heat or at weaning are usually more seriously affected and the mortality rate appears to be higher still.

Severely affected animals sweat profusely and have difficulty in moving because of tetany of the limbs and incoordination. The gait is stiff and the tail is slightly raised. Rapid, violent respirations and wide dilatation of the nostrils are accompanied by a distinct thumping sound from the chest, thought to be due to spasmodic contraction of the diaphragm. Muscular fibrillation, particularly of the masseter and shoulder region, and trismus are evident but there is no prolapse of the membrana nictitans. Affected animals are not hypersensitive to sound but handling may precipitate increased tetany. The temperature is normal or slightly elevated, and, although the pulse is normal in the early stages, it later becomes rapid and irregular. The mare may make many attempts to eat and drink but appears to be unable to swallow and passage of a stomach tube may be impossible. Urination and defecation are in abeyance, and peristalsis is reduced.

Within about 24 hours the animal goes down, tetanic convulsions develop and become more or less continuous, the mare dying about 48 hours after the onset of illness. The tetany and excitement in the early stages may suggest tetanus but there is no prolapse of the third eyelid and there is the usual relationship to recent foaling or weaning and physical exertion. The anxiety and muscle tremor of laminitis may also be confused with those of lactation tetany, especially as it may occur in mares which have foaled and retained the placenta. Pain in the feet is the diagnostic feature of this latter disease. Treatment by intravenous injection of calcium solutions as recommended in the treatment of parturient paresis causes rapid, complete recovery. One of the earliest signs of recovery is the voiding of a large volume of urine. Occasional cases which persist for some days are recorded (8).

REFERENCES

(1) Muylle, E. et al. (1973) *Vlaams Diergeneeskd. Tijdschr.*, *42*, 44.
(2) Green, H. H. et al. (1935) *J. comp. Pathol.*, *48*, 74.
(3) De Gier, C. J. (1935) *Tijdschr. Diergeneeskd.*, *62*, 1186.
(4) Forsyth, H. & Hodgkinson, E. J. (1945) *Vet. Rec.*, *57*, 503.
(5) Kjos-Hanssen, J. (1943) *Norsk VetTidsskr.*, *55*, 116.
(6) Montgomerie, R. F. et al. (1929) *Vet. Rec.*, *9*, 319.
(7) Baird, J. D. (1971) *Aust. vet. J.*, *47*, 402.
(8) Rach, D. J. et al. (1972) *Can. vet. J.*, *13*, 78.
(9) McAllister, F. S. (1977) *J. equ. med. Surg.*, *1*, 230.

Hypomagnesemic tetanies

Tetany associated with depression of serum magnesium levels is a common occurrence in ruminants. The syndrome associated with hypomagnesemia is relatively constant, irrespective of the cause, but the group of diseases in which it occurs has been divided into hypomagnesemic tetany of calves, which appears to be due specifically to a deficiency of magnesium in the diet, and lactation tetany, in which there may be a partial dietary deficiency of magnesium but in which nutritional or metabolic factors reduce the availability, or increase the body's loss, of the element so that serum magnesium levels fall below a critical point. In general, the occurrence of lactation tetany is related to three sets of circumstances. Most common is the occurrence in lactating cows turned out on to lush, grass-dominant pasture in the spring after wintering in closed housing—the classical lactation or grass tetany of Holland. Wheat pasture poisoning may occur when any type of cattle or sheep is grazed on young, green cereal crops. The third occurrence is in beef or dry dairy cattle running at pasture in the winter time, usually when nutrition is inadequate and where no shelter is provided in changeable weather, rather than in severe, prolonged cold. Hypomagnesemia of sheep, although it is less common, occurs in the same general groups of circumstances as the disease in cattle.

Lactation tetany (hypomagnesemic tetany, grass tetany, grass staggers, wheat pasture poisoning)

Lactation tetany is a highly fatal disease of all classes of ruminants but reaches its highest incidence in lactating cows. It is characterized by hypomagnesemia, and usually hypocalcemia, and clinically by tonic–clonic muscular spasms and convulsions, and death due to respiratory failure.

Etiology

The most constant and significant biochemical disturbance reported in lactation tetany in both cattle and sheep is hypomagnesemia. Hypocalcemia is often present concurrently and, although it is of less severe degree than in parturient paresis, there is increasing evidence that the actual onset of clinical tetany may be associated with a rapid fall in serum calcium levels superimposed on a preexisting seasonal hypomagnesemia (1). Most investigations into the causes of lactation tetany are directed at determining the causes of the hypomagnesemia. A short period of starvation (24–48 hours) in lactating cows and ewes is capable of causing a significant sudden depression of calcium and magnesium levels and this may be the important factor in many instances. When the disease occurs in association with transport a similar mechanism may be involved.

Some attention has been given to the high serum levels of potassium which occur in ruminants on lush grass pasture and green cereal crops, and the relationship of this hyperkalemia to the development of tetany. It seems probable that the mechanism is one of competition with magnesium for absorption, a secondary hypomagnesemia then being the cause of tetany (5). A high potassium intake is effective in inducing hypomagnesemia in sheep and cattle only when the dietary intake of magnesium is low. The mechanisms which maintain magnesium homeostasis in ruminants are still very much under review (5) with a general consensus at present that there is no significant, effective mechanism for this purpose in ruminants. These species appear especially vulnerable with regard to magnesium because there is no readily mobilizable large store of magnesium in the body and the delicate balance of serum (or more properly extracellular fluid) magnesium levels depends largely on the daily intake of magnesium in the diet. In lactating animals the daily loss of magnesium in the milk, urine and digestive secretions is high and a marked reduction in intake or availability of ingested magnesium can cause hypomagnesemia. Also, the body does not have efficient homeostatic mechanisms such as those which maintain calcium levels, probably because the depletion of the element does not occur violently, as it does with calcium. The levels are also therefore more likely to be seasonably low over large numbers of animals than is hypocalcemia. Also, if this seasonably low level is suddenly exacerbated by a deprivation due to lack of food intake for one day there is no homeostatic mechanism to retrieve the situation from body stores.

Until relatively recent years the hypomagnesemia, which is characteristic of lactation tetany, was thought to arise because of defects in internal metabolism. This view has been re-examined in the light of work which shows that young, green grass has a lower content of available magnesium than mature grass, that lush grass pasture has a lower content of total magnesium than mature pasture, that grasses have a lower magnesium content than clovers and other dicotyledonous plants, and that heavy applications of potassium-rich and nitrogen-rich fertilizers reduce the availability of soil magnesium (9). As a result it is now generally accepted that cattle and sheep, particularly those in heavy lactation, may be receiving a diet deficient in magnesium when they graze many grass-dominant, lush, heavily fertilized pastures. In view of the estimation that milking cows need to ingest about 20 g and to absorb about 4 g of magnesium daily the observation that cows fed on winter rations usually receive 32–34 g/day and cows on dangerous pasture receive only 10–22 g daily is a significant one. The critical figure for concentration of magnesium in pasture is 0·2% of the dry matter. Pasture with a magnesium content below this level is likely to cause hypomagnesemia, and there is some evidence of a relationship between a low soil content of magnesium and an increased rate of occurrence of clinical lactation tetany in cattle (3).

Apart from the question of the concentration of magnesium in the diet there is the question of the amount of food ingested. A reduction in dry matter intake must reduce the magnesium intake and, in situations where hypomagnesemia is already present, a further depression of serum magnesium levels can be anticipated when complete or partial starvation occurs. Whether hypomagnesemia pre-exists or not, a period of starvation in lactating cows and ewes is sufficient to produce a marked hypomagnesemia and the fall may be sufficiently great to cause clinical tetany. A period of bad weather, yarding, transport or movement to new pastures or the production of unpalatable pastures by heavy top-dressing with nitrogenous fertilizers may provide such a period of partial starvation, and even if the intake of magnesium to the diet is adequate, an insufficient intake of fiber in the winter months can precipitate hypomagnesemia in pastured cows (2) and ewes (45).

A number of factors are thought to reduce the availability of the magnesium which is ingested. Some of these are:

- The production of large quantities of ammonia in the rumen when the diet is very rich in protein may, by a process akin to chelation, reduce the availability of magnesium (11)
- Heavy top-dressing of pasture with ammonia fertilizers leads to reduced uptake of magnesium by plants, and a reduction of availability of ingested magnesium because of the high concentration of ammonia ions in the rumen (12)
- The failure of the disease to develop on legume-dominant pasture suggests that protein intake per se is not the critical factor, although this has to be viewed in the light of the higher magnesium content of clovers
- The presence of chelating agents, e.g. alpha keto-butyric acid, in plants or in the ruminal contents is not unlikely and these would, of course, be inimical to magnesium absorption (5)
- Diarrhea is commonly associated with lactation tetany on spring pasture and by decreasing the alimentary sojourn may also reduce magnesium absorption
- A high potassium content in the diet may also reduce the magnesium absorption from the alimentary tract (8). It has also been observed that grasses with a high ratio of potassium to calcium and magnesium (e.g *Dactylis glomerata, Phalaris arundinacea*) are more likely to cause grass tetany than those with low ratios (e.g. *Bromus inermis, Poa pratensis* etc.) (18). The greater tendency of wheat grazing, contrasted with other cereals to cause hypomagnesemia, is also probably related to its low content of magnesium (44). Other work indicates that wheat pasture poisoning has a much more complicated pathogenesis than this and that the disease is due essentially to hypocalcemia (17). In areas where the disease is common, grass pastures top-dressed with nitrogenous fertilizers are dangerous and their toxicity may be increased by the application of potash
- Potash is known to compete with sodium for absorption by plants and thus interfere with magnesium absorption by them. Experimentally the administration of potassium to sheep diets decreases the apparent absorption of magnesium and seriously increases the hypomagnesemic effect of a low magnesium intake (19). The reduction of magnesium intake of high-producing dairy cows from 25 to 5 g/day produced hypomagnesemia and some clinical cases but the administration, in addition, of disodium hydrogen phosphate or sodium sulfate precipitated acute attacks of the disease (20)
- A high dietary intake of aluminium has been proposed as a cause of poor magnesium absorption. There appears to be such a relationship but it is not consistent (21).

A close association between climatic conditions and serum magnesium levels has also been observed. Reduced levels occur in adult cattle and sheep exposed to cold, wet windy weather with little sunshine and with no access to shelter or to supplementary feed. Supplementary feeding appears to reduce the effect of inclement weather on serum magnesium levels and it is possible that failure to eat during bad weather may be the basic cause of hypomagnesemia. There is also a suggestion that cold weather stress may increase urinary excretion of magnesium (15).

Alternatively, attention has been drawn to the possible role of hyperthyroidism in the production of seasonal hypomagnesemia. Depression of serum magnesium levels and clinical 'grass staggers' have been produced in recently calved cows by reducing the dietary intake or by feeding thyroprotein. This has led to the rather wider concept of a negative energy balance as a possible cause of hypomagnesemia, with increased activity of the thyroid gland as the hormonal mediator. It is likely that hypomagnesemia and hyperthyroidism occur concurrently without there being any cause–effect relationship between them.

In summary, it appears that a number of factors are capable of causing hypomagnesemia in ruminants and that under particular circumstances one or other of them may be of major importance. In lactation tetany of cows and ewes turned on to lush pasture in the spring, a primary dietary deficiency of magnesium or the presence of some factor in the diet which reduces the absorption or internal metabolism of magnesium and calcium appears probable. In wheat pasture poisoning the ingestion of abnormally large amounts of potassium in the diet probably leads to a relative or absolute hypomagnesemia as serum potassium levels rise. Hypomagnesemic tetany occurring in cattle wintered at pasture (1) and exposed to inclement weather may be related to inadequate caloric intake and possibly to the resultant hyperactivity of the thyroid gland. Although the above suggestions as to the most important etiological factors in each set of circumstances in which lactation tetany occurs may be valid, undoubtedly combinations of these and other factors have etiological significance in individual outbreaks of the disease. The worst combination of causative factors, and the most common circumstances in which the disease occurs, is inadequate energy intake (lush pasture) with a low dietary content of magnesium (grass pasture) in recently calved cows during a spell of cold, wet and especially windy weather. One other important factor which must be borne in mind is the variation between individual animals in their susceptibility to hypomagnesemia and to the clinical disease. These variations are quite marked in cattle and in intensively managed, high-producing herds it is probably worth while to identify susceptible animals and give them special treatment.

Epidemiology

Lactation tetany of dairy cows turned out to graze on lush, grass-dominant pasture after winter housing is most common in northern Europe and the United Kingdom and a similar condition occurs in Australia and New Zealand, where the cows are not housed but have access to a phenomenal flush of pasture growth in the spring. In cases where an autumn flush of pasture occur, a high incidence of hypomagnesemic tetany may occur in the autumn or early winter. Wheat pasture poisoning has been recorded in many countries but is most prevalent where young cereal crops are utilized for winter grazing. The southwestern United States has experienced heavy losses of cattle caused by this disease. Hypomagnesemic tetany in cattle wintered in the open causes some losses in Britain, New Zealand, southern Australia and the east-central states of the United States. Although the disease is preeminently one of animals at pasture, it can occur in housed cattle if the total energy intake is low.

In all of these forms of the disease the morbidity rate is highly variable, reaching as high as 12% in individual herds, and up to 2% in particular areas. The incidence varies from year to year depending largely on climatic conditions and management practices, and the disease is often limited in its occurrence to particular farms and even to individual fields.

The disease is a serious one and although an effective treatment is available the mortality rate is high because of the short course. Since animals die before they can be observed to be ill, a mortality rate is difficult to estimate because of inability to determine the cause of death in animals 'found dead', but it is probably of the order of 20%.

Hypomagnesemia has been recognized as a disease of sheep in Australia and Great Britain and although the incidence is not great it appears to be increasing and can cause heavy losses in individual flocks.

The major occurrence of lactation tetany is in cattle and sheep turned out to lush, grass-dominant pasture in the early spring after wintering indoors, and in late autumn. Most cases occur during the first 2 weeks after the animals leave the barn. Pasture which has been heavily top-dressed with fertilizers rich in nitrogen and potash is potentially most dangerous. The disease may also occur on this type of pasture even when the cattle have wintered outdoors.

The high incidence on cereal crops has given rise to the name of wheat pasture poisoning although the disease occurs on all types of cereal, including oats and barley. The pasture is usually dangerous for only a few weeks but heavy losses may occur in all classes of sheep and cattle, particularly when the pasture is in the early stages of growth.

Exposure to bad weather is exacerbated by absence of trees or other shelter in fields and by failure to supply supplementary feed, circumstances particularly likely to arise in stubble fields, or when dry dairy cattle, beef cattle or sheep are not housed in the winter time in moderately cold climates. The disease does not seem to occur in cattle kept outside in prolonged winters where environmental temperature is consistently very low. Although the disease is not specifically related to parturition it is most common in the first 2 months after calving, hence the name 'lactation tetany'. The disease is most common in lactating dairy cattle, may reach a moderate level of incidence in beef cattle and calves and has occurred in dry cows and bulls. Cattle in the 4–7-year age group are most susceptible but adult sheep and calves and lambs may be affected. Ewes which have lambed during the preceding month are by far the most susceptible group. As in cattle the greatest incidence is on cereal grazing and lush grass pasture, losses usually ceasing when the flock is moved onto rough, unimproved pasture. Cases also occur in sheep which are exposed to inclement weather when on a low nutritive intake. Simultaneous hypomagnesemia and ketosis can occur in ewes after lambing if they are exposed to low feed availability. These cases do not respond well to treatment (13).

Pathogenesis

Most evidence points to hypomagnesemia as the cause of the tetanic signs observed but the concurrent hypocalcemia may have a contributory effect and in many instances may even be the dominant factor (1). Most clinical cases of the disease have serum magnesium levels below 1 mg/dl (0·41 mmol/l) compared with the normal levels in cattle of 1·7–3 mg/dl (0·70–1·23 mmol/l) and there is a striking relationship between the incidence of the clinical disease and the occurrence of a seasonal hypomagnesemia. The reduction in serum levels of magnesium is concurrent with a marked fall in the excretion of magnesium in the urine. Unfortunately field outbreaks do not always follow the classical picture. In affected herds many clinically normal cows have low serum magnesium levels and in these circumstances a concurrent hypocalcemia may be the precipitating cause.

In sheep the experimentally induced disease is characterized by hypocalcemia (4·5–6·9 mg/dl; 1·12–1·72 mmol/l) and hypomagnesemia (0·5–0·7 mg/dl; 0·21–0·29 mmol/l) and hypophosphatemia (0·9–1·2 mg/dl;

0·29–0·39 mmol/l). The clinical disease did not occur in ewes with hypophosphatemia and hypomagnesemia if normal calcium levels existed (22).

There has been little investigation of the mechanism by which the tetany and convulsions are produced. In parallel to work in other species it has been shown in calves that the increased, excessive muscular contractions of hypomagnesemic tetany are due to facilitation of transmission of impulses through the neuromuscular system (23). Clinical signs in hypomagnesemic animals, other than nervous signs, are rare. Experimentally induced hypomagnesemia in sheep is attended by reduced gastrointestinal motility, especially with respect to the amplitude of movements (16).

The recent observation that CSF levels of magnesium are greatly reduced in grass tetany leads to the suggestion that the tetany may result from a central effect on the brain. It is also evident that CSF levels of magnesium in hypomagnesemic animals rise significantly after treatment with a magnesium salt (24). The need for this to happen would explain the delay of about 30 minutes after an intravenous injection before recovery occurs.

Clinical findings

For convenience, lactation tetany can be described in acute, subacute and chronic forms.

Acute lactation tetany

The animal may be grazing at the time and suddenly cease to graze, adopt a posture of unusual alertness and appear uncomfortable, and twitching of the muscles and ears is evident. There is severe hyperesthesia and slight disturbances precipitate attacks of continuous bellowing and frenzied galloping. The gait becomes staggering and the animal falls with obvious tetany of the limbs which is rapidly followed by clonic convulsions lasting for about a minute. During these convulsive episodes there is opisthotonus, nystagmus, champing of the jaws, frothing at the mouth, pricking of the ears and retraction of the eyelids. Between episodes the animal lies quietly but a sudden noise or touch may precipitate another attack. The temperature rises to 40–40·5°C (104–105°F) after severe muscle exertion; the pulse and respiratory rates are also high. The absolute intensity of the heart sounds is increased so that they can be heard some distance away from the cow. Death usually occurs within ½–1 hour and the mortality rate is high because many die before treatment can be provided. The response to treatment is generally good.

Subacute lactation tetany

In this form of the disease the onset is more gradual. Over a period of 3–4 days there is slight inappetence, wildness of the facial expression and exaggerated limb movements. The cow often resists being driven and throws her head about as though expecting a blow. Spasmodic urination and frequent defecation are characteristic. The appetite and milk yield are diminished and ruminal movements decrease. Muscle tremor and mild tetany of the hindlegs and tail with an unsteady, straddling gait may be accompanied by retraction of the head and trismus. Sudden movement, noise, the application of restraint or insertion of a needle may precipitate a violent convulsion. Animals with this form of the disease may recover spontaneously within a few days or progress to a stage of recumbency with a similar but rather milder syndrome than in the acute form. Treatment is usually effective but there is a marked tendency to relapse.

Chronic lactation tetany

Many animals in affected herds have low serum magnesium levels but do not show clinical signs. A few animals do evidence a rather vague syndrome including dullness, unthriftiness and indifferent appetite and may subsequently develop one of the more obvious syndromes. The chronic type may also occur in animals which recover from the subacute form of the disease.

Parturient paresis with hypomagnesemia

This syndrome is described under parturient paresis (p. 1104) and consists of paresis and circulatory collapse in an adult cow which has calved within the preceding 48 hours but in which dullness and flaccidity are replaced by hyperesthesia and tetany.

Clinical pathology

Diagnostic clinical pathology depends upon estimation of total calcium and magnesium levels in serum and cerebrospinal fluid. The majority of healthy animals will have a serum magnesium concentration of 1·7–3 mg/dl (0·70–1·23 mmol/l) (5). These levels in cattle are often reduced in seasonal subclinical hypomagnesemia to between 1 and 2 mg/dl (0·41 and 0·82 mmol/l) but tetany is not usually evident until the level falls to below 1·2 mg/dl (0·49 mmol/l). The average level at which signs occur is about 0·5 mg/dl (0·21 mmol/l) and in sheep it is suggested that clinical tetany does not occur until the serum magnesium level is below 0·5 mg/dl (0·21 mmol/l). However, levels may fall as low as 0·4 mg/dl (0·16 mmol/l) without clinical illness. These discrepancies may be explainable in terms of variations between animals in the degree of ionization of the total magnesium. It is also possible that a transitory elevation of the level occurs after violent muscular exercise. Total serum calcium levels are often reduced to 5–8 mg/dl (1·25–2·00 mmol/l) and this may have an important bearing on the development of clinical signs. Serum inorganic phosphate levels may or may not be low. Similar changes occur in lactation tetany in sheep. In wheat pasture poisoning of cattle there is hypocalcemia, hypomagnesemia and hyperkalemia. In acute tetany, serum potassium levels are usually dangerously high and may contribute to the high death rate.

The occurrence of low urine magnesium levels is good presumptive evidence of hypomagnesemia and a field test is available (26). The xylidyl blue test on urine shows promise as a field test for hypomagnesemia. It appears to give results comparable to sophisticated laboratory tests (4). It is based on the colorimetric estimation of urine magnesium which shows a decline in urine magnesium levels in hypomagnesemic cows, but the results are not sufficiently consistent to encourage the diagnostic use of the method (10). Determination of the magnesium status of a herd, relative to a suspected need to supplement the diet to prevent lactation tetany, can be done by examination of serum magnesium levels, urinary magnesium fractional clearance ratio or creatinine-corrected urinary magnesium concentration (25). The latter two are more suited to assessing the need to supplement the diet with magnesium, or having supplemented it, to determine the response.

The use of magnesium levels in CSF as a diagnostic procedure is relatively new (27). The levels in CSF do appear to be better correlated with the severity of signs than do plasma magnesium levels. Fluid collected up to 12 hours after death can be used diagnostically. Levels in CSF of 1·25 mg/dl (0·51 mmol/l) magnesium were found in tetanic cows with hypomagnesemia (serum magnesium levels of 0·54 ± 0·41 mg/dl; 0·22 ± 0·17 mmol/l). In clinically normal cows with hypomagnesemia comparable levels in CSF were 1·84 mg/dl (0·16 mmol/l) and in serum 0·4 mg/dl (0·76 mmol/l). In normal animals CSF levels are the same as in plasma, i.e. 2·0 mg/dl (0·82 mmol/l) and up. The magnesium content of ventricular CSF may be quite different to that of lumbar CSF. It is also more responsive to changes in magnesium levels of the blood and is preferred for pathology purposes (26).

Necropsy findings

Extravasations of blood may be observed in subcutaneous tissues and under the pericardium, endocardium, pleura, peritoneum and intestinal mucosa. Agonal emphysema may also be present. A low magnesium content of heart muscle has attracted attention as providing evidence of hypomagnesemia at necropsy examination (28). The procedure is time-consuming and expensive and is insufficiently accurate to justify its use (29). The magnesium content of the bovine vitreous humor of the eye is an accurate reflection of the blood level of magnesium immediately before death. It is considered to be an accurate estimate of magnesium status for 48 hours after death provided the environmental temperature does not exceed 23°C (73°F) (28). The aqueous humor is not recommended as a source of material for testing in this way (46).

Diagnosis

Incoordination, hyperesthesia and tetany are the major clinical abnormalities which should arouse suspicion of hypomagnesemic tetany especially if they occur in ruminants exposed to bad weather or grazing green cereal crops or lush grass-dominant pasture. Lactating animals are likely to be affected first. There are many other diseases which present a similar clinical picture. Acute lead poisoning is usually accompanied by blindness and mania, sometimes with an attack complex and there is usually a history of access to lead. Rabies may also resemble hypomagnesemic tetany but is characterized by straining, ascending paralysis, anesthesia and an absence of tetany. The nervous form of ketosis is not usually accompanied by convulsions or tetany and there is marked ketonuria. Poisoning caused by *Claviceps paspali* occurs only if there is access to the ergots and the syndrome is typically one of cerebellar ataxia.

In sheep it is almost impossible to differentiate between an uncomplicated hypocalcemia and one which is complicated by hypomagnesemia. The latter is to be expected in recently lambed ewes on lush spring pasture. Failing estimation of serum levels of magnesium and calcium, the response to treatment may be the best indication of the disease state present.

Treatment

Most authors have recorded satisfactory results with solutions containing both calcium and magnesium salts or even calcium salts alone. The former is recommended for general use in all forms of lactation tetany and details are provided under the treatment of parturient paresis. However, solutions containing only magnesium salts are also used and the final choice must depend upon the results of biochemical tests and the response obtained. The efficiency of the various treatments appears to vary from area to area, and even within areas under different conditions of management and climate. The safest general recommendation is to use a combined calcium–magnesium preparation (e.g 500 ml of a solution containing 25% calcium borogluconate and 5% magnesium hypophosphite for cattle, 50 ml for sheep) intravenously followed by a subcutaneous injection of a concentrated solution of a magnesium salt. When magnesium solutions are used 200–300 ml of a 20% solution of magnesium sulfate may be injected intravenously: this is followed by a rapid rise in serum magnesium levels which return to preinjection levels within 3–6 hours. A much slower rise and fall occurs after subcutaneous injection. For optimum results the subcutaneous injection of 200 ml of a 50% solution of magnesium sulfate has been recommended. A rise in serum magnesium of 0·5 mg/dl (0·21 mmol/l) occurs within a few minutes and subsequent levels do not go above 5 mg/dl (2·06 mmol/l). In cases where serum magnesium levels are low because of a seasonal hypomagnesemia, the injection of magnesium salts is followed by a rise and then a return to the subnormal preinjection levels.

The intravenous injection of magnesium salts is not without danger. There may be cardiac embarrassment or medullary depression may be severe enough to cause respiratory failure. If signs of respiratory distress or excessive slowing or increase in heart rate are noticed the injection should be stopped immediately and, if necessary, a calcium solution injected.

The substitution of magnesium lactate for magnesium sulfate has been recommended to provide a more prolonged elevation of serum magnesium levels. A dilute solution (3·3%) causes no tissue injury and can be administered intravenously or subcutaneously. Magnesium gluconate has also been used as a 15% solution and good results were obtained with dose rates of 200–400 ml. High serum magnesium levels are obtained more slowly and are maintained longer than with magnesium sulfate (30). A combination of 12% magnesium adipate and 5% calcium gluconate at a dose rate of 500 ml is also recommended (31). The feeding of magnesium-rich supplements, as described under control below, is recommended after parenteral treatment. Because of the tendency for acute cases to have convulsions during treatment, it is common practice to give a large intramuscular dose of an ataractic drug before commencing specific treatment and to continue this until recovery is apparent.

Control

Feeding of magnesium supplements

The preventive measure which is now universally adopted is the feeding of magnesium salts to cows during the danger period. The feeding of magnesite (containing not less than 87% magnesium oxide) prevents the seasonal fall in serum magnesium levels and daily administration by drenching or in the feed of at least 60 g of magnesium oxide per day is recommended to prevent the disease. This is not always completely effective and in some circumstances large doses may be necessary. Daily feeding of 120 g is safe and effective but 180 g daily may cause diarrhea. The dose for sheep is 7 g daily or 14 g every second day (32). The protection afforded develops within several days of commencing administration and terminates abruptly after administration ceases. Difficulty may be experienced in getting the stock to eat the required amount of magnesite, especially when it is in the powder form. It is not unpalatable but the powdery consistency is unattractive. This can be countered by mixing it with molasses in equal parts and allowing free access to the mixture. The problem with any sort of free supplement that the cattle are not forced to eat to get subsistence, is to ensure that animals take any of it and that all animals take enough, because this disease is sufficiently dangerous that in many circumstances an unprotected animal is a dead one. In field circumstances the provision of magnesium in tasty mixtures for cattle has been disappointing and is not recommended (33). Magnesium acetate–molasses mixtures in ball feeders are satisfactory but are expensive (34). Magnesium phosphate (53 g/d) is also a safe and effective way of ensuring a good intake of magnesium (7). The retention of phosphorus in sheep is similar to that with monocalcium or dicalcium phosphate (14). The more common practice is to mix the magnesite with molasses and dilute with water which is then sprayed on to the hay in the windrows when it is being made, injected into the bales before feeding or sprayed on to the hay at feeding. The preparation may also be used in a granular form, or in a cake or pellets or by mixing in damp feed. Magnesium-rich pellets suggest themselves as a means of supplementation when the additional cost can be borne. The only difficulty is the usual one with magnesium, palatability (35), and care needs to be taken to include palatable material in the pellets, or be prepared to mix them with other grain or molasses when feeding them out.

Heavy magnesium 'bullets' The use of heavy 'bullets' of magnesium to prevent hypomagnesemia has shown early promise in laboratory trials but in field trials the results have varied. The objective is to place a heavy 'bullet' of magnesium in the reticulum from which site it constantly liberates small amounts of magnesium, about 1 g daily. This objective is achieved and the occurrence of the clinical disease is usually greatly reduced (36, 37) but serum magnesium levels are often little altered and it is felt that the animals are still very susceptible. In dangerous situations it is customary to administer up to four 'bullets' at a time. As with all 'bullets' there is a proportion lost by regurgitation and by passage on through the gut. A special sheep-sized 'bullet' is used in ewes with similar results (39).

Top dressing of pasture This, together with magnesium-rich fertilizers raises the level of magnesium in the pasture and decreases the susceptibility of cattle to hypomagnesemia. For top dressing, calcined magnesite (1125 kg/ha) or magnesic limestone (5600 kg/ha) are satisfactory, the former causing the greater increase in pasture magnesium. The duration of the improved magnesium status is unknown, but the degree varies with the type of soil, being greatest on light sandy loams on which a dressing of 560 kg/ha of calcined magnesium can provide protection for 3 years. On heavy soils protection for only 1 year is to be expected (40). To avoid unnecessary expense it may be possible to top dress one field with the magnesium fertilizer and keep this field in reserve for spring grazing.

Spraying The magnesium content of pastures can be raised much more quickly by spraying with a 2% solution of magnesium sulfate at fortnightly intervals (8) or by application of very finely ground magnesium oxide to the pasture (30 kg/ha) before grazing commences (41). The technique is referred to as 'foliar dusting or spraying' and has the advantage over feed supplementation that the intake is standard. It is very effective in cattle in maintaining serum magnesium levels and preventing the occurrence of the clinical disease (42). Magnesium oxide at high levels of intake (2 and 4% of the ration) is toxic to calves, causing diarrhea with much mucus in the feces.

In some high risk situations it may be advisable to provide magnesium in several forms to ensure adequate intake.

Management of pasture fields

The economics of daily farming make it necessary to produce maximum pasture growth, and the development of tetany-prone pastures is unavoidable in many circumstances. It may be possible to reduce the danger of such pastures by encouraging the development of legumes, by restricting the amount of potash added especially in the early spring and by ensuring that ample salt is available during the danger period to counteract the high intake of potassium. The addition of magnesite to the fertilizer, as described above, is strongly recommended.

Whenever magnesium supplements are used in the diet of cattle, attention must be given to the phosphorus intake of the herd. It is strongly suspected that a high magnesium intake reduces the availability of phosphorus (43) and the possibility of provoking clinical hypophosphatemia seems to be a real one.

Provision of shelter

In areas where winter pasturing is practiced the observation that serum magnesium levels fall during the winter and in association with inclement weather suggests that cattle and sheep should be provided with shelter at such times. If complete housing is impractical it may be advisable to erect open access shelters in those fields that have no tree cover or protection from prevailing winds. Fields in which lactating cows are kept should receive special attention in this regard. Unfortunately the disease is most common on highly improved farms where most natural shelter has been removed and it is desired to keep the cows on the highly improved pasture to maintain milk production or fatten calves rapidly.

Time of calving
In areas where the incidence of the disease is high it may be advisable to avoid having the cows calve during the cold winter months when seasonal hypomagnesemia is most likely to develop. Unfortunately it is often important to have cows calve in late winter to take advantage of the flush of spring growth when the cows are at the peak of their lactation.

Feeding on hay and unimproved pasture
Because of the probable importance of lush, improved, grass pasture in producing the disease, the provision of some grain, hay or rough grazing may reduce the incidence. It is most important that the periods of fasting, such as occur when cattle or sheep are yarded, or moved or during bad weather, should be avoided especially in lactating animals and when seasonal hypomagnesemia is likely to be present.

REVIEW LITERATURE

Burns, K. M. & Allcroft, R. (1967) *Br. vet. J.*, *123*, 340, 383.
Rendig, V. V. & Grunes, D. L. (1979) *Grass Tetany. Special Publication No 35*, American Society of Agronomy, Wisconsin.
Rogers, P. A. M. (1979) Hypomagnesemia and its clinical syndromes in cattle: a review. *Irish vet. J.*, *33*, 115.

REFERENCES

(1) Hemingway, R. G. & Ritchie, N. S. (1965) *Proc. Nutr. Soc.*, *24*, 54.
(2) Rogers, G. et al. (1977) *Aust. vet. J.*, *53*, 523.
(3) Haggard, D. L. et al. (1978) *J. Am. vet. med. Assoc.*, *172*, 495.
(4) Simesen, M. G. (1977) *Nord. VetMed.*, *29*, 284.
(5) Wilson, A. A. (1964) *Vet. Rec.* , *76*, 1382.
(6) Turner, M. A. et al. (1978) *NZ J. agric. Res.*, *21*, 583.
(7) Ritchie, N. S. & Fishwick, G. (1977) *J. agric. Sci.*, *88*, 71.
(8) Field, A. C. & Suttle, N. F. (1979) *J. comp. Pathol.*, *89*, 431.
(9) Moodie, E. W. (1965) *Br. vet. J.*, *121*, 338.
(10) Hooker, H. et al. (1979) *Schweiz. Arch. Tierheilkd.*, *121*, 187.
(11) Ashton, W. M. & Sinclair. K. B. (1965) *J. Br. Grassld Soc.*, *20*, 118.
(12) Wilcox, G. B. & Hoff, J. E. (1974) *J. dairy Sci.*, *57*, 1085.
(13) Jopp, A. J. & Quinlivan, T. D. (1981) *NZ Vet. J.*, *29*, 37.
(14) Hemingway, R. G. & McLaughlin, A. M. (1979) *Br. vet. J.*, *135*, 411.
(15) Shiga, A. et al. (1979) *J. Fac. Agric.*, *Iwate Univ.*, *14*, 173.
(16) Bueno, L. et al.(1980) *Can. J. anim. Sci.*, *60*, 293.
(17) Bohman, I. R. et al. (1983) *J. anim. Sci.*, *57*, 1352, 1364.
(18) Thill, J. L. & George, J. R. (1975) *Agronomy J.*, *67*, 89.
(19) Suttle, N. F. & Field, A. C. (1969) *Br. J. Nutr.*, *23*, 81.
(20) Dishington, I. W. & Tollesrud, S. (1967) *Acta vet. Scand.*, *8*, 14.
(21) Kappel, L. C. et al. (1983) *Am. J. vet. Res.*, *44*, 770.
(22) Schuster, N. H. et al. (1969) *Aust. vet. J.*, *45*, 508.
(23) Todd, J. R. & Horvath, D. J. (1970) *Br. vet. J.*, *126*, 333.
(24) Meyer, H. (1977) *Vet. sci. Commum.*, *1*, 43.
(25) Sutherland, R. J. et al. (1986) *NZ vet. J.*, *34*, 133.
(26) Allsop, T. F. & Pauli, J. V. (1985) *Res. vet. Sci.*, *38*, 61.
(27) Meyer, H. & Scholz, H. (1972) *Dtsch Tierärztl. Wochenschr.*, *79*, 55, 615.
(28) Lincoln, S. D. & Lane, V. M. (1985) *Am. J. vet. Res.*, *46*, 160.
(29) Field, A. C. (1969) *Vet. Rec.*, *23*, 591.
(30) Fischer, W. (1968) *Tierärztl. Wochenschr.*, *75*, 8.
(31) Hadlich, M. & Kolb, E. (1975) *Arch. exp. VetMed.*, *29*, 379.
(32) Herd, R. P. (1966) *Aust. vet. J.*, *42*, 160, 369.
(33) Horvath, D. J. et al. (1967) *J. anim. Sci.*, *26*, 875.
(34) Ross, E. J. & Gibson, W. W. C. (1969) *Vet. Rec.*, *84*, 520.
(35) Gurtler, H. et al. (1976) *Mh VetMed.*, *31*, 294, 401, 404, 508, 511.
(36) Davey, L. A. & Gilbert, G. A. (1969) *Vet. Rec.*, *85*, 194.
(37) Foot, A. S. et al. (1969) *Vet. Rec.*, *84*, 467.
(38) Stuedemann, J. A. et al. (1984) *Am. J. vet. Res.*, *45*, 698.
(39) Smyth, P. J. & Egan, D. A. (1971) *Irish vet. J.*, *25*, 4.
(40) Todd, J. R. (1965) *Br. vet. J.*, *121*, 371.
(41) Todd, J. R. & Morrison, N. E. (1964) *J. Br. Grassld Soc.*, *19*, 179.
(42) Rogers, P. A. M. & Poole, D. B. R. (1971) *Irish vet. J.*, *25*, 197.
(43) Mudd, A. (1970) *J. agric. Sci.*, *Camb.*, *74*, 11.
(44) Mayland, H. G. et al. (1976) *Agron. J.*, *68*, 665.
(45) Terashima, Y. et al. (1982) *J. Nutr.*, *112*, 1914.
(46) Whitaker, D. A. et al. (1986) *Vet. Rec.*, *118*, 570.

Hypomagnesemic tetany of calves

Hypomagnesemic tetany of calves is a disease with a close clinical similarity to lactation tetany of adult cows.

Etiology
Hypomagnesemia is a common finding and is accompanied in many cases by hypocalcemia. A condition closely resembling the field syndrome has been produced experimentally by feeding an artificial diet with a very low content of magnesium and the evidence points to the disease being caused by a dietary deficiency of magnesium exacerbated by a high intake of calcium which causes depletion of magnesium stores and lower serum and bone levels of magnesium (2). Milk, in spite of its low magnesium content, is an adequate source of the element for very young calves because their absorptive capacity is good. However, the efficiency of magnesium absorption decreases markedly up to about 3 months of age when maximum susceptibility to the disease occurs. The efficiency of absorption is also decreased by a reduction in transit time in the intestine and this may be related to the occurrence of the disease in scouring calves. A significant loss of magnesium in the feces also occurs in calves allowed to chew fibrous material such as bedding, the chewing stimulating profuse salivation and creating greater loss of endogenous magnesium. Peat and wood shavings are bedding materials known to have this effect (4).

Hypomagnesemic tetany in calves is often complicated in field cases by the coexistence of other diseases, especially enzootic muscular dystrophy.

Epidemiology
The disease is common in some areas, particularly where animals are housed during the winter and are inadequately fed. Cases may occur sporadically or a number of deaths may occur on the one farm within a short period of time. Hypomagnesemia has also been produced experimentally in very young foals by feeding a diet with a very low magnesium content (5). The clinical signs are similar to those in calves, and the calcification found in the walls of vessels of calves also occurs in foals.

Hypomagnesemic tetany occurs in calves 2–4 months of age or older which are fed solely on a diet of whole milk, and calves receiving the greatest quantity of milk and growing most rapidly are more likely to be affected because of their greater need for magnesium for incorporation into developing soft tissues. It is most likely to occur in calves being fattened for veal. Cases have also been reported in calves fed milk replacer diets or milk, concentrates and hay, and in calves running at pasture with their dams. Deaths due to hypomagnesemic tetany are also recorded in 3–4 months old calves whose hay and silage rations were low in magnesium content (6). Those cases which occur on milk replacer appear to be related to chronic scours and low magnesium content of the replacer. It also occurs in young cattle about 6 months of age which are being fattened intensively indoors for the baby beef market. The phosphorus content of their diet is high and a lack of vitamin D is probable. The situation is exacerbated by a shortage of roughage. The hypomagnesemia is accompanied by a hypocalcemia.

Pathogenesis

On affected farms calves are born with normal serum magnesium levels of 2–2·5 mg/dl (0·82–1·03 mol/l) but the levels fall gradually in the succeeding 2–3 months, often to below 0·8 mg/dl (0·33 mmol/l). Tetany does not occur until the serum magnesium falls below this point and is most severe at levels below 0·6 mg/dl (0·25 mmol/l) although calves may have levels even lower than this and show few clinical signs. It seems probable that depression of the serum calcium level precipitates tetany in animals rendered tetany-prone by low serum magnesium levels. It is also apparent that tetanic convulsions can occur in hypocalcemic calves in the absence of hypomagnesemia (7). The disease is not related in any way to enzootic muscular dystrophy although the diseases may occur concurrently. The depletion of body stores of magnesium in the bones by a continued nutritional deficiency of magnesium places calves in a vulnerable position if further deprivation occurs—in such circumstances the serum magnesium in the bones, and the estimation of the calcium: magnesium ratio in bones can be used in the diagnosis of the disease.

Clinical findings

The first sign in the experimental disease is constant movement of the ears. The temperature is normal and the pulse rate accelerated. Hyperesthesia to touch, and grossly exaggerated tendon reflexes with clonus, are present. Shaking of the head, opisthotonus, ataxia without circling, and a droopy, backward carriage of the ears are constant. There is difficulty in drinking due to inability to get to the bucket. The calves are apprehensive, show agitation and retraction of the eyelids when approached, and are hypersensitive to all external stimuli but show no tetany. Later, fine muscle tremors appear, followed by kicking at the belly, frothing at the mouth and spasticity of the limbs. Convulsions follow, beginning with stamping of the feet, head retraction, champing of the jaws and falling. During the convulsions the jaws are clenched, respiratory movements cease and there are tonic and clonic movements of the limbs, and involuntary passage of urine and feces, and cycles of protrusion and retraction of the eyeballs. The pulse rate rises to 200–250/minute and the convulsions disappear terminally. The pulse becomes impalpable and cyanosis appears before death. In field cases the signs are almost identical but are rarely observed until the terminal tetanic stage. Older calves usually die within 20–30 minutes of the onset of convulsions but young calves may recover temporarily only to succcumb to subsequent attacks. Cases which occur in young calves with scours, usually at about 2 weeks of age, show convulsions as the earliest sign. The convulsion is usually continuous and the calves die within an hour.

Clinical pathology

Serum magnesium levels below 0·8 mg/dl (0·33 mmol/l) indicate severe hypomagnesemia and clinical signs occur with levels of 0·3–0·7 mg/dl (0·12–0·29 mmol/l). Normal values are 2·2–2·7 mg/dl (0·91–1·11 mmol/l) (3). Serum calcium levels tend to fall when serum magnesium levels become very low and are below normal in most clinical cases. This concurrent hypocalcemia in hypomagnesemic animals appears to be consequential, but the relationship is not understood. It is not due to an increase in calcitonin secretion nor to a decrease in the secretion of parathyroid hormone (1). The estimation of the magnesium in bone (particularly ribs and vertebrae) is a reliable confirmatory test at necropsy. Values below a ratio of 70:1 for calcium : magnesium may be regarded as normal and above 90:1 are indicative of severe magnesium depletion. Absolute bone calcium values are not decreased and are often slightly elevated. An incidental change is the marked increase in serum creatinine phosphokinase levels observed in calves after an acute attack of hypomagnesemic tetany. SGOT levels are marginally elevated (8).

A field test on urine for hypomagnesemia is the xylidyl blue test which gives good agreement with sophisticated laboratory tests (3).

Necropsy findings

There is a marked difference between the necropsy lesions of some natural and the experimental cases. In some field cases there is calcification of the spleen and diaphragm, and calcified plaques are present in the aorta and endocardium, together with hyaline degeneration and musculature. In other cases necropsy lesions similar to those in enzootic muscular dystrophy occur. In experimentally produced cases these lesions are not evident but there is extensive congestion in all organs, and hemorrhages in unsupported organs, including the gallbladder, ventricular epicardium, pericardial fat, aorta, mesentery and intestinal wall. The lesions are obviously terminal and are associated with a terminal venous necrosis. Some field cases present a picture identical with this and doubtless some factor other than hypomagnesemia is responsible for the calcification of tissues described above.

Diagnosis

Clonic convulsions in calves may occur as a result of acute lead poisoning, tetanus, strychnine poisoning, polioencephalomalacia, enterotoxemia caused by *Clostridium perfringens* type D and avitaminosis A. It may be virtually impossible to distinguish between these diseases clinically and a careful examination of the history with particular reference to feeding, water supply, and possible access to poisons may be the only basis on which a tentative diagnosis can be made. Tetanus has a longer course and is usually accompanied by bloat and prolapse of the third eyelid. Tetany is persistent between convulsions which do not occur until the late stages of the disease. Poisoning by organic arsenical or mercurial compounds is less common but the syndrome is essentially the same as that of hypomagnesemic tetany. Viral encephalitides including rabies and sporadic bovine encephalomyelitis are not restricted to calves and have other signs of diagnostic value, and the signs do not fluctuate as much as in hypomagnesemic tetany; in rabies there is anesthesia and ascending paralysis; and in sporadic bovine encephalomyelitis a high fever and serositis. Bacterial meningitis and encephalitis are usually accompanied by fever.

Treatment

Response to magnesium injections (100 ml of a 10% solution of magnesium sulfate) is only transitory because of the severe depletion of bone reserves of magnesium. This dose provides only a single day's requirements. Follow-up supplementation of the diet with magnesium oxide or carbonate as described below is advisable. Chloral narcosis or tranquilization with an ataractic drug may be essential to avoid death due to respiratory paralysis.

Control

The provision of hay in the diet helps to prevent the disease. Supplementary feeding of magnesium, if begun during the first 10 days of life, will prevent excessive falls of serum magnesium but if begun after the calf is 7 weeks old may not prevent further depression of the levels. Supplementation should continue until at least 10 weeks of age. Daily feeding of the magnesium compound and fairly accurate dosing are necessary to avoid scouring or inefficient protection. Detailed dose schedules are available but for calves of average growth rate appropriate dose rates are 1 g daily for calves to 5 weeks, 2 g for calves 5–10 weeks and 3 g for 10–15 week calves of magnesium oxide or twice this dose of carbonate (3). Supplementation of the diet with magnesium restores serum calcium levels to normal as well as correcting the hypomagnesemia, but hypomagnesemia occurs when administration is stopped (6). Magnesium alloy bullets, two of the sheep size per calf, have shown high efficiency in preventing the clinical disease and also the hypomagnesemia which precedes it (9). Calves kept indoors and fed largely on milk should get adequate mineral supplement and vitamin D (70 000 i. u. vitamin D_3/day). Magnesium utilization will not be affected but calcium absorption, which is often sufficiently reduced to cause a concurrent hypocalcemia, will be improved.

REFERENCES

(1) Rayssiguier, Y. et al. (1977) *Ann. Rech. vét.*, *8*, 267.
(2) Ivins, L. N. & Allcroft, R. (1969) *Br. vet. J.*, *125*, 548.
(3) Simesen, M. G. (1977) *Nord. VetMed.*, *29*, 284.
(4) Ivins, L. N. & Allcroft, R. (1970) *Br. vet. J.*, *126*, 505.
(5) Harrington, D. D. (1974) *J. Am. vet. med. Assoc.*, *35*, 503.
(6) Rayssiguier, P. J. et al. (1977) *Vet. Sci. Commun.*, *1*, 235.
(7) Holtenius, P. et al. (1970) *Nord. VetMed.*, *22*, 463.
(8) Todd, J. R. et al. (1969) *Vet. Rec.*, *84*, 176.
(9) Hemingway, R. G. & Ritchie, N. S. (1969) *Vet. Rec.*, *84*, 465.

Ketosis of ruminants (acetonemia of cattle, pregnancy toxemia of sheep)

Ketosis in ruminants is a disease caused by impaired metabolism of carbohydrate and volatile fatty acids. Biochemically it is characterized by ketonemia, ketonuria, hypoglycemia and low levels of hepatic glycogen. Clinically, the diseases in cattle (acetonemia) and in ewes (pregnancy toxemia) are rather different entities and occur in different parts of the pregnancy–lactation cycle, but the biochemical disturbance is essentially the same and they occur under similar conditions of management, all of which lead to a state of negative nutritional balance. The disease in cattle responds readily to treatment and is self-limiting, but the disease in sheep is highly fatal.

Etiology

Bovine ketosis

It is not unreasonable to view the disease as an extreme degree of a metabolic state which at lower levels is a constant, or at least common occurrence in heavily producing cows in the postcalving period. This is because all high-yielding cows in early lactation are in negative energy balance, and are all subclinically ketotic as a result. It takes only a small additional nutritional or metabolic insult for them to develop clinical ketosis. The rate of occurrence of negative energy status, and therefore the frequency of clinical cases, has undoubtedly increased sharply in the recent past because of the steep increase in individual milk production. Because of the mammary gland's metabolic precedence in the partitioning of nutrients, especially glucose, milk production continues at a high rate causing an energy drain. In many individual cows the need for energy is beyond their capacity for dry matter intake. Clinical ketosis has been produced in recently calved dairy cows by reducing the daily feed intake by 15–20% ad lib intake and supplementing it with 1,3-butanediol, a ketogenic substrate (8, 52). The biochemical characteristics of ketosis including depletion of hepatic glycogen and major increases in hepatic stores of triglycerides and ketone bodies were produced.

The major biochemical manifestation of ketosis in cattle is hypoglycemia, and treatment of affected cattle which returns the blood glucose level to normal is followed by at least a transient recovery. There are many theories on the cause of ketosis and the disease must be considered as one in which there are many significant predisposing causes. This hypothesis is supported by the variety of circumstances in which the disease can occur. As a general statement it is safe to say that clinical ketosis occurs in ruminants at times when they are subjected to heavier demands on their resources of glucose and glycogen than can be met by their digestive and metabolic activity. Most discussion on the causation of the disease centers on the exact manner in which this failure to provide available glucose arises. This failure could be purely relative if the requirement is greater than the maximum carbohydrate intake could physically provide. It would be absolute if an adequate supply of carbohydrate is not provided by the ration. Again it could be a defect of digestion or metabolism in converting what is an adequate dietary supply of carbohydrate into available glucose. Bovine, and to a less extent ovine, ketosis occurs in the field when the failure of supply of available glucose to tissues results from any of the above causes. A direct result of this deficiency is an increase in gluconeogenesis in the liver with a parallel rise in ketone body formation. If the latter rise is beyond the limit of physiological needs clinical ketosis ensues (1).

In more detail, the salient points of the etiology of ketosis can be set out as follows. All carbohydrate ingested is converted in the rumen to acetic and butyric acids which are potentially ketogenic, and to propionic acid, which is glycogenic. These two groups of acids are produced under normal conditions in the ratio of about 4:1. The production of propionic acid and its conversion to glucose in the liver must continue at a normal level if glucose supplies to tissues are to be maintained. If this system is inefficient the alternative pathway of providing glucose by synthesis from amino acids and glycerol increases in volume. The stimulation of this type of energy producing reaction results in a much increased demand for oxaloacetate which is used preferentially for this purpose. As a result the utilization of ketone bodies by tissues, which also requires oxaloacetate, is impeded. The ketone bodies then accumulate to the point where ketosis occurs (Fig. 25).

Ruminants are in a particularly vulnerable position compared to other species with regard to their carbohydrate metabolism because, although very little carbohydrate is absorbed as such, a direct supply of glucose is essential for tissue metabolism, particularly the formation of lactose, and in addition the utilization of volatile fatty acids for energy purposes is also dependent upon a supply of available glucose. This vulnerability is further exacerbated, particularly in the cow, by the tremendous rate of turnover of glucose and the relatively poor reserves of glycogen. In the period from immediately after calving until the peak of lactation is reached in the case of cattle, and the last third of pregnancy in ewes, the demand for glucose is increased and cannot be completely restrained. Even though the milk flow in cows can be reduced by reduction of energy intake, this does not follow automatically nor proportionately in early lactation because hormonal stimuli for mammary activity overcome the effects of reduced food intake. It is this factor which makes the difference between the ketosis of simple starvation and the more severe spontaneous ketosis of high-producing cows in early lactation. In ovine ketosis it is the developing fetuses which cause the unremitting drain on available maternal nutrients although in this species a fall in blood glucose and an elevation of plasma ketones also occur on exposure to inclement weather and it is a combination of undernutrition and stress which leads to the development of most cases of pregnancy toxemia. A combination of cold stress and undernutrition, each alone readily tolerated by ewes in late pregnancy, may together prove fatal.

Most of the investigational work of recent years has been directed towards elucidating the pathogenesis of ketosis in cows that are fed heavily on rations which at first glance appear to contain adequate carbohydrate. However, such a diet need be deficient only in precursors of propionic acid to be ketogenic. A high protein

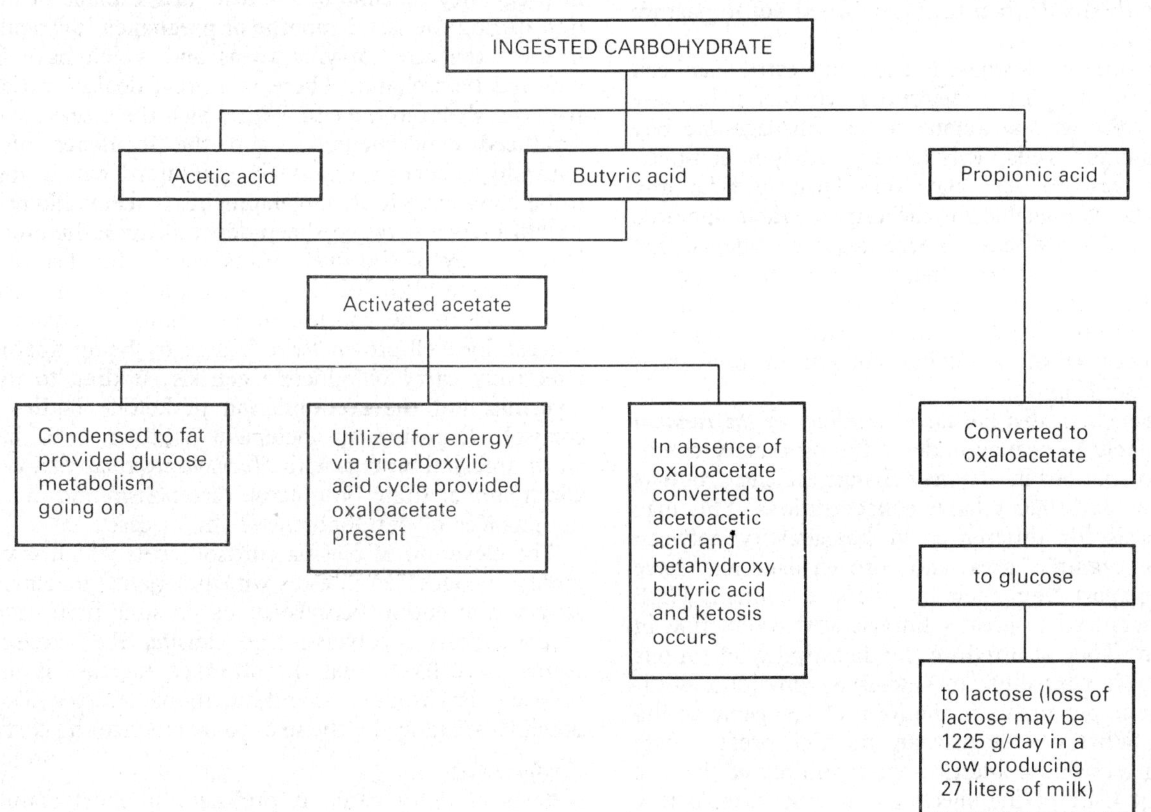

Fig. 25. A schematic representation of carbohydrate metabolism in ruminants.

level in the diet is also contributory. Excess protein will exacerbate an energy deficit because of energy losses resulting from its metabolism and excretion (11).

In the search for causative factors in high-producing animals a number of endocrinal and metabolic mechanisms have been investigated. The claim that *dysfunction of the adrenal gland* is the primary cause of bovine ketosis has not been substantiated. The stress of parturition and lactation in cattle, and of late pregnancy in ewes, must lead to increased adrenocortical activity, and this may be further stimulated by the additional stress of malnutrition. In such circumstances some diminution of the hormonal reserves of the gland may follow, leading to a state of relative adrenocortical insufficiency which exacerbates the metabolic defect inaugurated by the stress factors mentioned. That there is only a relative insufficiency is evidenced by the ability of affected animals to respond to adrenocorticotrophins. It is probable therefore that the endocrinal changes observed are secondary only. The observed changes include normal plasma cortisol levels in preketotic and ketotic cows although levels tended to decline as blood sugar levels fell and ketone levels rose (24).

A relative hypothyroidism has also been suggested as a cause on the basis of low protein-bound iodine levels in the serum of affected cows, because iodine and thyroprotein are preventive and curative in some instances, and because of the tendency for the disease to occur in ewes and cows which get insufficient exercise. That lack of exercise is entirely responsible for the high incidence of the disease in housed animals is unlikely although clinical cases rarely occur in well fed animals at pasture, and plasma ketone levels of lactating dairy cows usually show a marked fall when they are turned out to pasture in the spring.

The composition of rations fed to dairy cattle has been examined in an effort to determine whether it has any effect on their glucose ketone status. Ensilage and hay are the common feeds likely to vary widely in composition from year to year and from farm to farm and therefore be responsible for the unpredictable sporadic occurrence of the disease. There is some evidence that this may be the case. In general, hay is less ketogenic than ensilage, and ensilage made from succulent material may be more highly ketogenic than other types of ensilage because of its higher content of preformed butyric acid (45).

The composition and metabolic activities of the ruminal flora are likely to change under differing dietary conditions and variations in diet may change the end products of digestion and their relative concentrations. This may be the basis for differences in ketogenicity between feeds. For example, grass and corn ensilage may have this effect apart from their butyric acid content. High protein diets lead to greater butyric acid production in the rumen. They also reduce the digestibility of rations and probably contribute to ketosis by providing additional ketone precursors in the form of ketogenic amino acids (5). Whatever the mechanism, high protein diets have been shown to increase susceptibility to ketosis induced by L-thyroxine injections. Starvation leads to a relative lowering of the propionic acid concentration in the rumen and this probably adds to the effects of starvation on internal metabolism, particularly the excessive utilization of fat, in producing ketosis. From quantitative and qualitative estimations on the ketone bodies present in ruminal liquor and body fluids, it appears that abnormal ruminal conditions may play an important part in the production of clinical ketosis.

From time to time, factors other than those mentioned above have come under consideration. Hepatic insufficiency has been shown to occur in bovine (42) and ovine ketosis but whether it occurs in all cases and whether it is primary or a result of ketosis is unknown. As one of the reactions to hypoglycemia is mobilization of fat reserves and deposition of fat in the liver, some degree of hepatic insufficiency is to be expected as a secondary development of the disease. Bovine ketosis has also been described as a result of persistent hypomagnesemia. The two diseases do occur together in herds subjected to a shortage of feed energy during early pregnancy, so that both may have a common cause. On the other hand, the response of ketotic cows to treatment with magnesium is described (7).

Ovine ketosis

Although hypoglycemia and hyperketonemia are the primary metabolic disturbances in ovine ketosis as they are in the bovine disease, and although the precipitating causes are similarly a dietary deficiency of net energy exacerbated by the increased demand for energy in the latter part of pregnancy, there are some biochemical differences between the two diseases, e.g. an elevation of plasma cortisol levels in pregnancy toxemia, and in the terminal stages their pathogenesis appears to be quite dissimilar. The most important etiological factor in pregnancy toxemia is a decline in the plane of nutrition during the last 2 months of pregnancy, particularly in ewes that are carrying twins and which have been well fed beforehand. There is a great deal of variation between sheep in the ease with which the disease can be produced experimentally, and the incidence of the naturally occurring disease in conditions which appear to be conducive to its development. It seems likely that the difference between sheep depends upon the metabolic efficiency of the liver. Ewes which, because of impaired hepatic function, are predisposed to the disease may react to the continued, preferential demands for glucose by well-grown twin fetuses by being unable to effectively carry on gluconeogenesis, leading to hypoglycemia and the accumulation of ketone bodies and cortisol. Exposure to inclement weather or a heavy worm infestation, e.g. with *Haemonchus contortus*, would add a similar drain on glucose metabolism and increase the chances of development of the disease.

The elevation of plasma cortisol levels which is commonly encountered in ewes with pregnancy toxemia has attracted attention because of its possible indication of adrenocortical involvement in causing the disease. It seems more likely that the observed increase is in response to environmental and nutritional stresses (8), and possibly to failure by the liver to metabolize the cortisol.

Epidemiology

Ketosis of dairy cattle is prevalent in most countries where intensive farming is practiced. It occurs mainly in animals housed during the winter months although it is seen occasionally in animals at pasture. The wastage due to the disease is difficult to assess accurately; its high incidence and known effects suggest that it is one of the major causes of loss to the dairy farmer. In rare instances the disease appears to be irreversible and the affected animal dies but the bulk of the economic loss is due to the loss of production while the disease is present and failure to return to full production after recovery. Subclinical ketosis is also common and although it has received little attention it may rank with the clinical disease in its economic effects. The morbidity is very variable and difficult to measure. Its occurrence depends so much on management, nutrition and climate. An occurrence rate of 10.5% has been recorded in one population (9), and in Finnish Ayrshires it is 6% (53), but the estimated occurrence in the national herd in the United Kingdom is only 1–5% (10). The mortality rate is nil. The prevalence of subclinical ketosis may be as high as 10%, and in herds which are undernourished it may be as high as 30% (41).

Ketosis of pregnant ewes, however, is highly fatal, and in individual flocks can reach a level of incidence sufficient to be classed as an outbreak. The disease in cattle may also occur in outbreak form with virtually every cow being affected but this is unusual and most herds suffer only sporadic cases.

Cattle

Bovine ketosis occurs under the following conditions:

- In high-producing, heavily fed dairy cows housed in barns
- In cattle at pasture, and less frequently when housed and fed on rations of inadequate caloric content
- Under conditions of specific nutritional deficiency
- As a complication of another primary disease.

Ketosis of heavily fed, high-producing cows—so-called 'estate acetonemia'—is the most important occurrence of the disease. Genetic susceptibility may be a factor but adequate proof on this point is lacking. The tendency for the disease to recur in individual animals is probably a reflection of variation between cows in digestive capacity or metabolic efficiency but these characters may or may not be inherited. It is more probable that the rations fed cause abnormal internal metabolism or ruminal function and lead to the development of ketosis in these circumstances. Other factors which are known to influence the development of the disease are excessive feeding of ensilage, particularly when it has a high content of butyric acid, inadequate exercise, overfatness at calving time and inadequate energy intake during early lactation.

Specific dietary deficiencies of cobalt and possibly phosphorus may also lead to a high incidence of ketosis. This may be due in part to a reduction in the intake of total digestible nutrients (TDN), but in cobalt deficiency the essential defect is a failure to metabolize propionic acid. It may be necessary to re-evaluate the role of cobalt in view of the observation that blood and liver levels of vitamin B_{12} are significantly reduced during the early stages of lactation in apparently normal cows and may sometimes fall below the critical level necessary for adequate gluconeogenesis from propionic acid.

A secondary ketosis may also develop, due usually to a reduction in appetite as a result of abomasal displacement, traumatic reticulitis, metritis, mastitis or other diseases common to the postparturient period. A high incidence of ketosis has also been observed in herds affected with fluorosis. An extraordinary occurrence has been an outbreak of acetonemia in a dairy herd fed on a ration contaminated by a low level (9·5 ppm) of lincomycin (46). The proportion of cases of acetonemia which are secondary, and their diagnosis as such, are both matters of great interest which are generally neglected in veterinary literature. In one sample of 120 cases 42% of the affected animals had an accompanying disease (13).

Regardless of the specific etiology, bovine ketosis occurs most commonly during the first month of lactation, less commonly in the second month, and only occasionally in late pregnancy. The highest frequency is between 20 and 30 days after calving (14). Cows of any age may be affected but the disease increases from a low prevalence at the first calving to a peak at the fourth.

Sheep

Ovine ketosis occurs only in ewes in late pregnancy, usually during the last month in ewes carrying more than one lamb, although ewes bearing a single, large lamb may be affected. It is primarily a disease of intensive farming systems and is relatively rare in extensive grazing units. Most commonly the precipitating cause is a prolonged and gradual fall in the plane of nutrition followed by sudden, short periods of starvation of up to 48 hours caused by management changes. In ewes on a good plane of nutrition such changes lead more commonly to the development of hypocalcemia. The level of nutrition at which the disease occurs may appear to be good but in such instances the plane of nutrition will usually be found to have fallen recently. This may be an explanation for the common occurrence of the disease in overfat ewes. In some outbreaks the ewes have been moved on to better pasture during late pregnancy to prevent the occurrence of ketosis but it occurs because the ewes are unaccustomed to the type of feed and do not eat well, or because they are more exposed to bad weather and seek shelter rather than graze. Cold, inclement weather and an absence of shelter also appear to markedly increase the incidence. Another common occurrence is when ewes are bred too early and the pasture is not sufficiently advanced to provide a rising plane of nutrition in late pregnancy. The disease occurs in goats during late pregnancy and is identical with ovine ketosis.

Pathogenesis

The principal metabolic disturbances observed, hypoglycemia with a low level of hepatic glycogen, and ketonemia may both exert an effect on the clinical syndrome. In many cases the severity of the clinical syndrome is proportional to the degree of hypoglycemia and this, together with the rapid response to parenterally administered glucose, suggests hypoglycemia as the predominant factor. This hypothesis is supported by the development of prolonged hypoglycemia and a similar clinical syndrome to that of ketosis, after the experimental, intravenous or subcutaneous injection of insulin (2 units/kg body weight). Moreover in the experimentally induced disease in ewes, pregnancy toxemia, the onset of clinical signs was always preceded by hypoglycemia and hyperketonemia although the onset of signs was not related to minimum glucose or maximum ketone levels (15).

The evidence that the irreversible stage of ovine ketosis is a hypoglycemic encephalopathy is further support for hypoglycemia as the important factor, although it has been suggested alternatively that the effects of the hypoglycemia are added to by inhibition of glucose utilization and a resulting depression of cerebral metabolism. This may provide the reason for the irreversible cerebral lesion. In affected ewes there is an abnormally high level of cortisol in plasma—an expected reaction to continued environmental stress and hypoglycemia, especially if hepatic metabolism of cortisol is reduced. Renal dysfunction is also apparent in the terminal stages of ovine ketosis, and may also contribute to the development of clinical signs and the fatal outcome (33). Azotemia and proteinuria should be especially looked for in ewes showing no neurological signs. The observed decline in renal function is comparable to human preeclampsia (19). Those ewes which are carrying only one lamb and have been well fed prior to a short period of undernutrition may develop a subacute syndrome both clinically and biochemically.

However, in most field cases the severity of the clinical syndrome is also roughly proportional to the degree of ketonemia. This is an understandable relationship as ketone bodies are produced in larger quantities as the deficiency of glucose increases. However, the ketone bodies may exert an additional influence on the signs observed. Acetoacetic acid is known to be toxic and probably contributes to the terminal coma in diabetes mellitus in man. The nervous signs which occur in some cases of bovine ketosis are thought to be caused by the production of isopropyl alcohol, a breakdown product of acetoacetic acid in the rumen, although the requirement of nervous tissue for glucose to maintain normal function may also be a factor in these cases.

Spontaneous ketosis in cattle is usually readily reversible by treatment; incomplete or temporary response is usually due to the existence of a primary disease with ketosis present only as a secondary development, although fatty degeneration of the liver in protracted cases may prolong the recovery period. Changes in ruminal flora after a long period of anorexia may also cause continued impairment of digestion.

Clinical findings

In many herds and flocks in which clinical cases occur, biochemical examination of the urine and blood of clinically normal animals may show degrees of hypoglycemia and ketonemia suggestive of early ketosis. It is probable that there is some reduction in milk yield of cattle in this subclinical stage. The disease occurs in goat does and resembles bovine ketosis in most ways (44).

Bovine ketosis

Two major forms of the disease are described, the wasting and the nervous forms, but these are the two extremes of a range of syndromes in which wasting and nervous signs are present in varying degrees of prominence.

The wasting type is the most common of the two and is manifested by a well-known syndrome which has recently been assessed in one of the few statistical appraisals of clinical findings in veterinary literature (13). The syndrome is based primarily on the gradual but moderate decrease in appetite and milk yield over 2–4 days. On the statistical assessment, these were present in 85% and 87% respectively of the cases seen. The pattern of appetite loss is often unusual in that the cow first refuses to eat grain, then ensilage but may continue to eat hay. The appetite may also be depraved. Body weight is lost rapidly, usually at a greater rate than one would expect from the decrease in appetite. Farmers usually describe affected cows as having a 'woody' appearance due to the apparent wasting and loss of cutaneous elasticity due presumably to disappearance of subcutaneous fat. The feces are firm and dry but serious constipation does not occur. The cow is moderately depressed and the hangdog appearance and disinclination to move and to eat may suggest the presence of mild abdominal pain.

The temperature and the pulse and respiratory rates are normal and although the ruminal movements may be decreased in amplitude and number they are within the normal range unless the course is of long duration when they may virtually disappear. A characteristic odor of ketones is detectable on the breath and often in the milk. Very few affected animals die but without treatment the milk yield falls and although spontaneous recovery usually occurs over about a month, as equilibrium between the drain of lactation and food intake is established, the milk yield is never fully regained. The fall in milk yield may be as much as 25% and there is an accompanying sharp drop in the SNF content of the milk (38). In the wasting form, nervous signs may occur in a few cases but rarely comprise more than transient bouts of staggering and partial blindness.

In typical cases of the nervous form the signs are usually bizarre and begin quite suddenly. The syndrome is suggestive of delirium rather than of frenzy and the characteristic signs include walking in circles, straddling or crossing of the legs, head-pushing or leaning into the stanchion, apparent blindness, aimless movements and wandering, vigorous licking of the skin and inanimate objects, depraved appetite and chewing movements with salivation. Hyperesthesia may be evident, the animal bellowing on being pinched or stroked. Moderate tremor and tetany may be present and the gait is usually staggery. The nervous signs usually occur in short episodes which last for 1 or 2 hours and may recur at intervals of about 8–12 hours. Affected cows may injure themselves during the nervous episodes.

Subclinical bovine ketosis Many cows that are in negative energy balance in early pregnancy will have ketonuria but without showing clinical signs that are recognizable by the farmer. Such cows may, however, have diminished productivity including mild depression of milk yield and a reduction in fertility (50). Infertility in this context may appear as an ovarian abnormality or as endometritis. The combined effects of these factors is a reduction in reproductive efficiency so that calving to conception interval is prolonged and the conception rate for insemination may be drastically reduced. In Europe, endometritis itself is thought to be a sequel to a nutritional stress at this time (21), but much of the stress there is due to overfeeding rather than undernutrition. It is thought therefore that both endometritis and acetonemia occur as a result of overfeeding (16).

Subclinical cases may have their milk production reduced by 1–1·5 kg/day (41). Surveys of large populations, using milk samples collected for other purposes, show a declining prevalence of ketosis-positive cows after a peak in the period immediately after calving, and a positive relationship between hyperketonemia and high milk yield (18).

Ovine ketosis

In ewes the syndrome is similar to that of the nervous form of ketosis in cows. The earliest sign is separation from the flock and apparent blindness which is manifested by an alert bearing but a disinclination to move. The ewe will stand still when approached by attendants or dogs and will turn and face them but make no attempt to escape. If it is forced to move it blunders into objects and when an obstacle is encountered, presses against it with the head. Many stand in water troughs all day and lap the water. Constipation is usual, the feces are dry and scanty and there is grinding of the teeth. In later stages marked drowsiness develops and episodes of more severe nervous signs occur but they may be infrequent and are easily missed. In these episodes tremors of the muscles of the head cause twitching of the lips, champing of the jaws and salivation, and these are accompanied by a cog-wheel type of clonic contraction of the cervical muscles causing dorsiflexion or lateral deviation of the head, followed by circling. The muscle tremor usually spreads to involve the whole body, the sheep goes down and has a tonic–clonic convulsion. The ewe lies quietly after each convulsion and rises normally afterwards but is still blind. In the periods between convulsions there is marked drowsiness which may be accompanied by head-pressing, the assumption of abnormal postures including unusual positions of the limbs and elevation of the chin—the 'stargazing' posture—and incoordination and falling when attempting to walk. A smell of ketones may be detectable on the breath.

Affected ewes usually become recumbent in 3–4 days and remain in a state of profound depression or coma for a further 3–4 days. Fetal death occurs commonly and is followed by transient recovery of the ewe, but the toxemia caused by the decomposing fetus soon causes a relapse. Affected ewes commonly have difficulty in lambing. Recovery may ensue if the ewe lambs or the lambs are removed by cesarean section in the early stages of the disease. In an affected flock the disease usually takes the form of a prolonged outbreak, a few ewes becoming affected each day over a period of several weeks.

Clinical pathology

Hypoglycemia, ketonemia and ketonuria are characteristic of the disease and there is an increase in plasma free fatty acids in some cases due probably to accelerated gluconeogenesis from tissues. Blood glucose levels are reduced from the normal of 50 mg/dl to 20–40 mg/dl in cattle and sheep. In cattle, ketosis secondary to other diseases is usually accompanied by blood glucose levels above 40 mg/dl and often above normal. Blood ketone levels in bovine ketosis are elevated from a normal of up to 10 mg/dl to 10–100 mg/dl. The levels are high also in secondary ketosis but are rarely above 50 mg/dl. Quantitative estimation of urinary ketones may be unsatisfactory because of the wide variations that occur depending upon the concentration of the urine. In clinically normal cattle urinary ketones may be as high as 70 mg/dl although usually they are lower than 10 mg/dl. Levels of 80–1300 mg/dl indicate the presence of ketosis which may be primary or secondary. Ketone levels in milk are rather less variable, ranging from a normal of 3 mg/dl up to an average level of 40 mg/dl in cows with ketosis. Liver glycogen levels are low and the glucose tolerance curve is normal. Volatile fatty acid levels in blood and rumen are much higher in ketotic than in normal cows and the ruminal levels of butyric acid are markedly increased relative to acetic and propionic acids. The assessment of energy status and correspondingly the likelihood or otherwise of acetonemia occurring is usually based on blood glucose levels. But blood levels of volatile fatty acids or of beta-hydroxybutyric acid could also be used (2). In terms of metabolic profiles to monitor nutritive balance it is known that herds with a higher than normal prevalence of clinical ketosis are identifiable because they have higher average blood levels of hydroxybutyrate and lower levels of glucose (39, 40). However, the severity and rate of onset of clinical signs are more closely related to blood sugar levels than to plasma acetone-plus-acetoacetate or free fatty acid levels (13).

In many cases of severe ketosis it would be an advantage to prognosis to know the extent of fatty infiltration of the liver. Estimation of serum levels of liver enzymes is not accurate enough to do this and only liver biopsy is suitable (49). There is a small but significant fall in serum calcium levels (down to about 9 mg/dl (2·25 mmol/l)) due probably to increased loss of base in the urine to compensate for the acidosis. Changes in the leukocyte count include eosinophilia, lymphocytosis and neutropenia. The neutrophil count may be as low as 10%, the lymphocytes may be as high as 60–80% and the eosinophils 15–40%. Severe cases show an increase in serum glutamic-oxaloacetic transaminase but the reason for this increase in serum enzyme activity is unexplained.

Field tests to detect ketosis are in general use and may be carried out on urine or milk. They are subject to several minor sources of error. The concentration of ketone bodies in these fluids will depend not only on the ketone level of the blood but also on the amount of urine excreted or on the milk yield. Milk is less variable and suitable laboratory procedures are available but field reagents in general use are only sufficiently sensitive to detect severe cases. The other disadvantage of these tests is that they measure only the acetoacetic acid content of the urine, beta-hydroxybutyric acid giving no reaction and acetone very little. This is not of major importance as the ketone bodies are usually present in approximately the same proportions.

Tests on urine are based on Rothera's reaction and many commercial reagents are now available. A reagent should be used in conjunction with a color chart to give an approximate estimate of the amount of ketones present in the specimen. In most cases the test must be read at a specified time, usually 30 seconds, for accurate appraisal. There is some difference of opinion as to whether primary and secondary ketosis can be differentiated on the basis of the degree of color change in the reagent, but primary cases always give a strong reaction whereas a moderate reaction is more common in secondary cases. Rough quantitative estimations of blood ketones can also be quickly made with some commercial reagents.

Present preoccupation with subclinical ketosis has meant that there is a need to differentiate between clinical and non-clinical hyperketonemia. In one survey the overall prevalence of subclinical ketonuria was 33·8%, that of the clinical disease was 13·1% (47).

In sheep a terminal uremia, indicated by a rise in plasma non-protein nitrogen levels, may occur but may be due to the death and decomposition of the fetuses. Now that estimations of steroid hormones are becoming diagnostically commonplace, the elevation of plasma cortisol which occurs in pregnancy toxemia in ewes has been used as a diagnostic feature; pregnancy toxemia and clinical hypocalcemia can both cause sufficient stress to promote such an elevation.

Necropsy findings

The disease is not usually fatal in cattle but fatty degeneration of the liver and secondary changes in the anterior pituitary gland and adrenal cortex may be present. Pregnancy toxemia in ewes is almost always fatal. At necropsy there is severe fatty degeneration of the liver and there are usually twin lambs and evidence of constipation. Histopathologically there is also a poorly defined renal lesion (19). The lambs may be dead and in varying stages of decomposition. Hepatic glycogen levels are usually very low in both sheep and cattle.

Diagnosis

The clinical picture is usually too indefinite, especially in cattle, to enable a diagnosis to be made solely on clinical grounds. General consideration of the history, with particular reference to the time of calving, the duration of pregnancy in ewes and the feeding program, and biochemical examination to detect the presence of hypoglycemia, ketonemia and ketonuria are necessary to establish a diagnosis.

Subclinical ketosis, diagnosed on the presence of ketonemia in the absence of clinical signs, is poorly defined. In heavily fed and intensively fed cows in Europe ketonuria is a transient phenomenon in recently calved cows. It occurs most commonly in the period 3–6 weeks after calving and it may persist for about 3 weeks. In this subclinical state it is stated that there is a fall in milk yield of approximately 2 kg/day, a mild ketonuria, and a slight fall in body weight, all of them discernible only if these parameters are being monitored routinely.

Cattle

Traumatic reticulitis, bovine pyelonephritis, indigestion and abomasal displacement may be confused with the wasting form of ketosis, and a secondary ketosis, due to these diseases and to metritis and mastitis, often presents a problem in diagnosis. Careful clinical examination of these cases usually reveals a mild fever, an increased heart rate, only a moderate ketonuria and some localizing signs of the primary disease. Traumatic reticulitis does not necessarily have the same relationship to recent calving, the onset of anorexia and fall in milk production is much more acute and severe, and pain can usually be elicited on percussion over the hypogastrium. In the early stages ruminal movements are completely absent. A leukocyte count and blood glucose examination are useful aids in difficult cases. Vagus indigestion may also lead to a secondary ketosis but is usually accompanied by marked stasis of the alimentary tract, abdominal distension and moderate bloat. A diagnosis of indigestion usually depends on a history of improper diet, the presence of ruminal stasis and an absence of other clinical signs. Abomasal displacement occurs usually right at calving, anorexia develops suddenly and persists intermittently, there is a reduction in abdominal size, the feces are pasty and passed in small amounts, and abomasal sounds may be audible over the lower left abdomen. There is incomplete and temporary response to treatment for ketosis. Rare cases of diabetes mellitus have been recorded in cattle (20, 43, 48) and its diagnosis must depend on the detection of a high blood glucose level and reduced glucose tolerance. The response to insulin is good. Clinical signs include anorexia, weight loss, decreased milk production. The syndrome is accompanied by glycosuria and ketonuria.

The nervous form of bovine ketosis is usually distinguished by the marked signs of delirium and the ketonuria. The episodes are transient, unlike those of listeriosis, and there is no fever. Rabies is characterized by mania, ascending paralysis and anesthesia and is always fatal. Convulsions such as occur in lactation tetany, acute lead poisoning and poisoning with *Claviceps paspali* are not observed. The nervous form of bovine ketosis is never fatal and responds quickly to treatment.

Some difficulty may be encountered in cows which have ketosis and parturient paresis concurrently. Cows which show a partial response to treatment for parturient paresis but fail to eat well should be examined for evidence of ketosis. The nervous form of bovine ketosis combined with early parturient paresis is manifested by a reeling, staggery gait and signs of nervous involvement including narcosis and drunken behavior. Later these animals go down and may show hyperesthesia and clonic convulsions.

Sheep

Ovine ketosis is usually suspected in heavily pregnant ewes which show nervous signs and die within 6–7 days. Parturient paresis occurs in pregnant and lactating ewes, is manifested by paralysis, has a much shorter course of 12–24 hours, usually affects a considerable proportion of the flock at one time, and is accompanied by a history of exertion or sudden deprivation of food. Affected animals respond well to treatment with solutions of calcium salts. Listeriosis and rabies are differentiated as in cattle. Local lesions caused by *Coenurus cerebralis* larvae, and cerebral abscess, and otitis media usually affect only one or two sheep, and have a long course and localizing signs. Louping-ill occurs only when the vector ticks are present, is accompanied by fever and has a characteristic histopathology.

Treatment

In cattle a number of effective treatments are available but in some affected animals the response is only transient and in rare cases the disease may persist and cause death or necessitate slaughter of the animals. Most of these cases are secondary and failure to respond satisfactorily to treatment is due to the primary disease.

Although the pathogenesis of the disease in ewes is similar in some ways to that in cows, the response to the same treatments as are used in cattle is variable and in general much less satisfactory. This is probably due to the added biochemical lesions of decreased glucose utilization, hypoglycemic encephalopathy, severe fatty degeneration of the liver, and increased plasma cortisol levels which occur in severe cases. Neither replacement therapy nor hormonal treatments are likely to have any effect in these cases, and the variability of response to treatment in ewes probably depends on the severity of the cases and the duration of the disease. When clinical cases are obvious the rest of the flock should be examined daily for any evidence of ketosis and affected animals treated with propylene glycol or glycerol immediately. Supplementary feeding of the flock should be commenced immediately, particular attention being given to an increase in carbohydrate intake. With timid sheep, especially Merinos, the simple provision of feed may not be enough. It may be necessary to improve the palatability of the ration, and to get the sheep started by pushing some feed into their mouths. With clinical cases an immediate cesarean section to remove the lambs is favored by many but results are not good. If expense is not a great object parenteral treatment with glucocorticoids plus glucose or glycerol is recommended (8).

The only rational treatment in ketosis is to relieve the need for glucose formation from tissues and allow ketone body utilization to continue normally. Theoretically the simplest means of doing this is by the administration of glucose replacement therapy.

Replacement therapy

The intravenous injection of 500 ml of a 50% solution of glucose (dextrose) effects marked improvement in most cows but relapses occur commonly unless repeated treatments are used. This is probably due to the transience of the hyperglycemia, or insufficient dosing, the dose required varying directly with the amount of lactose being lost in the milk. Subcutaneous injections prolong the response but are not recommended as they cause discomfort, and large unsightly swellings, which often become infected, may result. Intraperitoneal injections of 20% solution of dextrose may be used alternatively. Other sugars, especially fructose, either alone or as a mixture of glucose and fructose (invert sugar), have been used in an effort to prolong the response but idiosyncrasy to some preparations, in the form of polypnea, muscle tremor, weakness and collapse, occur rather commonly while the injection is being given. To overcome the necessity for repeated injections, propylene glycol or glycerine (225 g twice daily for 2 days followed by 110 g daily for 2 days to cattle) can be administered as a drench or in the feed and give excellent results; administration in feed is preferred because the dangers of aspiration with drenching are avoided. It is recommended that for best results dosing with these preparations be preceded by an intravenous injection of glucose. Parenteral infusions of glucose solutions and the feeding of glycerol depress the fat content of milk, and the net saving in energy may favorably influence response to these drugs. Glycerol and propylene glycol are not as efficient as glucose because this conversion to glucose does utilize oxaloacetate (1), but they are probably least damaging in this respect of all glucose precursors and for practical reasons their use is justified.

The results of replacement therapy in sheep vary widely. Propylene glycol or glycerine (110 g daily by mouth) have given excellent results for some workers but poor results for others. Parenteral treatment with glucose solutions is not recommended because relapses occur commonly unless the injections are repeated and the glucose is poorly utilized unless accompanied by insulin. One of the common complications in sheep, which seldom occurs in cattle, is severe acidosis. A complete treatment program in sheep should include the intravenous injection of sodium bicarbonate or lactated Ringer's solution.

Because of its glucogenic effect sodium propionate is theoretically a suitable treatment but when administered in 110–225 g doses daily the response in cattle is often very slow. Lactates are also highly glucogenic but both calcium or sodium lactate (1 kg initially, followed by 0·5 kg daily for 7 days) and sodium acetate (110–500 g daily) have given less satisfactory results than those obtained with sodium propionate. Ammonium lactate (200 g daily for 5 days) has, however, been used extensively with reported good results. Sodium ethyloxaloacetate given intravenously is effective in natural and experimental cases in ewes but is unlikely to be a practical form of treatment because of cost.

Hormonal therapy

The efficiency of adrenocortical hormones in the treatment of bovine ketosis has been amply demonstrated in both experimental and field cases. Their chief attractions are their ease of administration and the fact that glucose or its precursors need not be administered concurrently. Many preparations are available and have been used successfully, the newer preparations being more potent, requiring less dosage, and having fewer side-effects. Gluconeogenesis is stimulated for about 48 hours after a single injection of a suitable preparation (22). It is not proposed to review the literature on this subject as the number of preparations is too extensive but in general the recommendations of the manufacturer with regard to dosage should be followed. The major disadvantage of treatment with adrenocortical preparations is that gluconeogenesis is stimulated at the expense of other body tissues and possibly at the expense of oxaloacetate utilization in removing excess ketone bodies. It is also noted that successful treatment with glucocorticoids is often accompanied by a significant depression in milk yield, which may contribute to the recovery rate (23). In sheep the results with standard doses (26) are poor, and the treatment is not recommended. Very large doses (25 mg of dexamethasone) are reported to be effective in ewes still able to stand.

Anabolic steroids are also highly effective in ketosis in dairy cows (25) and are prescribed as the only effective treatment for pregnancy toxemia of cows. Experimentally 60 mg and 120 mg of trenbolone acetate are effective as single injections but no extensive field trials are recorded. Similar experimental work in ketotic sheep indicates little likely effect of anabolic steroids as treatment for pregnancy toxemia (12). However, about 50% recovery rate is achieved with an injection of 30 mg trenbolone acetate. Better results are claimed for a similar injection daily for 1 week accompanied by oral propylene glycol (100 ml twice daily) but the advent of parturition is the critical factor in promoting recovery (27).

A further recommendation is the estimation of beta-hydroxybutyrate levels in the blood of cows in early lactation (51). The criterion used could vary with circumstances but it is suggested that a group mean level of greater than 10.0 mg/100 ml of beta-hydroxybutyrate in serum suggests that subclinical ketosis is present in the herd.

Insulin has been used occasionally in conjunction with glucose or glucocorticoids but does not appear to confer marked therapeutic advantage (22). A depressed blood level of insulin has been demonstrated in bovine ketosis but it is thought to result from the persisting hypoglycemia rather than be a cause of it (3).

Miscellaneous treatments

Chloral hydrate has long been used in the treatment of both forms of bovine ketosis. An initial oral dose of 30 g can be followed by 7 g doses twice daily for several days. The larger dose is usually given in a capsule and subsequent doses as drenches in molasses and water. The method of action of chloral hydrate appears to be its capacity to increase the breakdown of starch in the rumen and stimulate the production and absorption of glucose (28). It is also thought to selectively influence rumen fermentation in the direction of increased production of propionate (29). Vitamin B_{12} and cobalt are sometimes administered either as a sole treatment or in conjunction with more standard therapy. Because of the suspected deficiency of coenzyme A in ketosis of cattle, cysteamine (a biological precursor of coenzyme A) and also sodium fumarate have been used to treat cases of the disease (31). Results reported initially were good but the method has not been generally adopted. The recommended dose rate of cysteamine is 750 mg intravenously for three doses at 1–3 day intervals. There is some limited evidence that nicotinic acid given in the feed (12 g daily) has beneficial effect on the disease in cattle (17), because of its lipolytic action and the known need to remove fat from the liver. Affected animals should be provided with adequate feed and water, and in hot weather sheep at pasture should be driven into the shade to avoid heatstroke. Provided ewes are in the early stages of the disease, removal of the lambs by cesarean section or hormonal induction of parturition is recommended. In later stages the ewe's condition is irreversible and the fetuses are often dead and decomposed. Induction with corticosteroids has been effected with dexamethasone 21-isonicotinate or the sodium phosphate at a dose rate of 10 mg but the trimethylacetate appears to be ineffective.

Control

It is difficult to make general recommendations for the control of the disease because of the many conditions under which it occurs and its probable multiple etiology. A list of the recommended procedures is set out below.

Cattle

- Cows should neither have been starved nor be overfat at calving. An adequate caloric intake should be ensured in the early part of lactation and especially after treatment. In heavy-producing, heavily-fed herds the big problem is to provide enough feed to avoid a deficient caloric intake relative to utilization, but at the same time to avoid imbalance, to avoid ruminal acidosis on a too-high carbohydrate diet and to avoid acetonemia on a diet too high in protein. Careful estimation of diets by reference to feed value tables is recommended and a detailed set of recommendations on diet and management has been provided (10). Points of general advice are that cows should not be too fat nor too thin at the end of lactation, and that feeding in preparation for the next lactation should not begin until about 4 weeks prior to calving. At that time, the silage, or hay, or pasture being used as a maintenance ration should be supplemented with 1 kg/day concentrate and this amount gradually increased to 5 kg daily at calving time. After calving the concentrate ration should be increased gradually as production increases, and be of the order of 3 kg/100 kg body weight hay for maintenance (3 kg ensilage is equivalent to 1 kg hay) and 1 kg grain for each 3 kg milk produced. In general, feeding should be at a slightly higher level than production actually warrants—lead feeding. The protein in the total ration should not exceed 16%, certainly not more than 18%, the carbohydrate be readily digestible, and if oats or maize are used they should be crushed, and the hay or ensilage must be of good quality. In high-producing cows being fed stored feeds it is most commonly poor quality roughage which leads to acetonemia or the 'parturition syndrome' described earlier. Wet ensilage containing much butyrate, and moldy or old and dusty hay, are the main offenders. In concentrates it is the change of source which creates off-feed effects and precipitates attacks of acetonemia
- Ground maize has a particular quality in providing readily available glucose in a ration and is a logical preventive feed. It contains significant quantities of alpha-polymerized glucose which is not fermented in the rumen, but is passed to the intestine and absorbed there (11). The intensity of lead feeding can be reduced after the first 100 days of lactation
- Cows that are housed should get some exercise

each day and in herds where the disease is a particular problem during the stabling period, the cattle should be turned out to pasture as soon as possible in the spring

- Ensure that the ration contains adequate cobalt, phosphorus and iodine
- If there is a high incidence in a herd receiving large quantities of ensilage, reduction of the amount fed for a trial period is indicated
- The prophylactic feeding of sodium propionate may be considered in problem herds (35): 110 g daily for 6 weeks, commencing at calving, has given good results in reducing the incidence of clinical bovine ketosis and improving production. Propylene glycol (350 ml daily for 10 days after calving, or as 6% of a concentrate ration for 8 weeks) has been similarly used with moderately good results (36)
- Theoretically, any procedure which increases the ratio of propionate to acetate production in the rumen would be of assistance in preventing ketosis. Monensin is a growth stimulant which acts in this way and the effective use of the compound in the prevention of ketosis in dairy cows has been reported (37). The dose rate used was 25 mg monensin daily in a grain feed mix. Dose rates need to be monitored carefully because of the risks of toxicity which are described separately.

Experimental observations have tended to reduce the importance of heavy feeding of grass ensilage, failure to provide an adequate mineral mixture and failure to provide grain to stall-fed cows in late pregnancy but, in view of the known multiple-factor etiology of this disease, these experiments do not prove that under particular sets of circumstances one or other of these factors may not be the precipitating cause. In fact, in many field outbreaks adoption of the recommendations made above appears to markedly reduce the incidence of the disease.

Sheep

The same general recommendations apply in the prevention of ovine ketosis as in the prevention of ketosis in cattle. Ensure that the plane of nutrition is rising in the second half of pregnancy even if it means restricting the diet in the early stages. The last 2 months are particularly important. During this period the provision of a concentrate containing 10% protein at the rate of 0·25 kg/day, increasing to 1 kg/day in the last 2 weeks, has provided good protection.

There are managemental difficulties in any nutritional program for sheep because of the way they are husbanded. If there were a satisfactory way of easily determining the stage of pregnancy and whether there are one, two or three fetuses present, or none, and if the sheep could then be divided into a number of subflocks so that the appropriate feeding regime could be provided it would be economical, if separate paddocks and labor were available, to arrange a preventive feeding program. Some account would need to be taken also of those ewes which are timid and for this and other reasons slow feeders. If supplementary feeding is practiced in a confined space, with insufficient troughing for all the flock to eat at one time, and if the feed fed is in small amounts and highly edible, a large proportion of ewes will get little no feed. These difficulties add up to a formidable barrier in large flocks with minimum labor. It is necessary before embarking on a nutritional support program to estimate cost-effectiveness. At the low level of prevalence that pregnancy toxemia usually achieves it is often most profitable to do nothing and to let the disease occur. Two general nutritional principles have been established for this situation (34). One is that recommended energy levels for late pregnancy in ewes are often too low so that lamb birth weight is too low and milk secretion is inadequate. Where it is not possible to provide additional energy, an elevation of protein intake will correct these errors. Similarly, an elevation of protein intake in early lactation will improve milk production and promote better lamb growth, in a cost-effective way.

Sudden changes in type of feed should be avoided and extra feed provided during bad weather. Shelter sheds should be available, and in purely pastoral areas lambing should not occur before the pasture is well grown.

A high incidence is often encountered in small, well-fed flocks where the ewes get insufficient exercise. In such circumstances the ewes should be driven about for half-an-hour twice daily and, if pasture is available, only concentrate should be fed so that they will be encouraged to forage for themselves.

General control

It has been suggested that the control of ketosis may be achieved by manipulation of the ration so that the production of propionate in the rumen is increased relative to that of acetate. Not only is propionate antiketogenic, but its increased production, and a corresponding decrease in acetate production in the rumen, is associated with a reduction in the percentage of fat in the milk and, as a result, a reduction in energy loss. Under experimental conditions the proportion of propionate produced in the rumen has been increased both by feeding a ration of finely ground roughage and cooked grain, and by the feeding of cod liver oil and certain unsaturated fatty acids. If these experimental results could be duplicated under conditions of practical daily cattle feeding a satisfactory method of controlling ketosis by dietary means would be a reality.

With the current emphasis on monitoring to provide early warning of the probable occurrence of a largely subclinical disease it has been suggested that for a herd diagnosis, blood glucose estimations be carried out on a sample of cows in their 2nd–6th weeks of lactation (39). Blood glucose levels of below 35 mg/dl (1·9 mmol/l) should raise the alarm. Regular tests for ketones in urine in the 2nd week after parturition is recommended for early detection of developing cases (6). For individual cows blood glucose estimations should be done at about 14 days after calving and the cow given special treatment if her blood sugar is low.

REVIEW LITERATURE

Baird, G. D. (1982) Primary ketosis in the high-producing dairy cow: clinical and subclinical disorders, treatment, prevention and outlook. *J. dairy Sci.*, 65, 1–10.

Bergman, E. N. (1973) Glucose metabolism in ruminants as related to hypoglycaemia and ketosis. *Cornell Vet.*, *63*, 341.
Brockman, R. P. (1979) Roles for insulin and glucagon in the development of ruminant ketosis. *Can. vet. J.*, *20*, 121.
Hibbitt, K. G. (1979) Bovine ketosis and its prevention. *Vet. Rec.*, *105*, 13.

REFERENCES

(1) Krebs, H. A. (1966) *Vet. Rec.*, *78*, 187.
(2) Kelly, J. M. (1979) *Vet. Rec.*, *101*, 499.
(3) Brockman, R. P. (1979) *Can. vet. J.*, *20*, 121.
(4) Kauppinen, K. (1983) *Acta. vet. Scand.*, *24*, 349.
(5) Hibbitt, K. G. et al. (1969) *Res. vet. Sci.*, *10*, 245.
(6) Markusfeld, O. et al. (1984) *Bov. Practnr*, *19*, 219.
(7) Yoshida, S. (1979) *J. Fac. Fisheries Anim. Husb., Hiroshima Univ.*, *17*, 117.
(8) Mills, S. E. et al. (1986) *J. dairy Sci.*, *69*, 352.
(9) Overby, I. et al. (1974) *Nord. VetMed.*, *26*, 353.
(10) Baird, G. D. et al. (1974) *Br. vet. J.*, *130*, 214, 318.
(11) Hibbitt, K. G. (1979) *Vet. Rec.*, *105*, 13.
(12) Ford, E. J. H. et al. (1979) *J. agric. Sci.*, *92*, 323.
(13) Cote, J. F. et al. (1969) *Can. vet. J.*, *10*, 179.
(14) Halse, K. & Magstad, O. (1975) *Norsk. VetTidsskr.*, *87*, 311.
(15) Procos, J. & Gilchrist, F. M. C. (1966) *Onderstepoort J. vet. Res.*, *33*, 161.
(16) Markusfeld, O. (1985 *Vet. Rec.*, *116*, 489.
(17) Fronk, T. J. & Schultz, L. H. (1979) *J. dairy Sci.*, *62*, 1804.
(18) Anderson, L. & Emanuelson, L. I. (1985) *Prev. vet. Med.*, *3*, 449.
(19) Hill, P. A. et al. (1984) *J. Pathol.*, *144*, 1.
(20) Mostaghni, K. & Ivoghli, B. (1977) *Cornell Vet.*, *67*, 24.
(21) Muller, F. et al. (1980) *Mh VetMed.*, *35*, 55.
(22) Cote, J. F. (1971) *Can. vet. J.*, *12*, 19.
(23) Braun, R. K. et al. (1970) *J. Am. vet. med. Assoc.*, *157*, 941.
(24) Breves, G. et al. (1980) *J. anim. Sci.*, *50*, 503.
(25) Heitzmann, R. J. & Walker, M. S. (1973) *Res. vet. Sci.*, *15*, 70.
(26) Ford, E. J. H. & Evans, J. (1986) *J. agric. Sci.*, *106*, 337.
(27) Weirda, A. et al. (1985) *Vet. Rec.*, *116*, 284.
(28) Quaghebeur, D. & Oyaert, W. (1971). *Zentralbl. VetMed.*, *18A*, 55, 64.
(29) Prins, R. A. & Seekles, L. (1968) *J. dairy Sci.*, *51*, 882.
(30) Heitzmann, R. J. et al. (1977) *Vet. Rec.*, *100*, 317.
(31) Bach, S. J. & Hibbitt, K. G. (1962) *Vet. Rec.*, *74*, 965.
(32) Hunt, E. R. (1976) *Aust. vet. J.*, *52*, 338.
(33) McCausland, I. P. et al. (1979) *J. comp. Pathol.*, *84*, 375.
(34) Robinson, J. J. (1980) *Vet. Rec.*, *106*, 282.
(35) Halse, K. & Moller, O. M. (1976) *Norsk. VetTidsskr.*, *88*, 83, 90.
(36) Moller, O. M. & Halse, K. (1978) *Norsk VetTidsskr.*, *90*, 930 & 945.
(37) Rogers, P. A. M. & Hope-Cawdery, M. J. (1980) *Vet. Rec.*, *106*, 311.
(38) King, J. O. L. (1979) *Br. vet. J.*, *135*, 40.
(39) Rossow, N. et al. (1976) *Mh VetMed.*, *31*, 486.
(40) Herdt, T. H. et al. (1981) *Am. J. vet. Res.*, *42*, 503.
(41) Dohoo, I. R. & Martin, S. W. (1984) *Can. J. comp. Med.*, *48*, 1.
(42) Mills, S. E. et al. (1986) *J. dairy Sci.*, *69*, 362.
(43) Tontis, A. & Wittwer, F. (1986) *Arch. Tierheilkd.*, *128*, 475.
(44) Blaxter, A. (1985) *Goat vet. Soc. J. (UK)*, *6*, 68.
(45) Andersson, L. & Lyndstrom, K. (1985) *Zentralbl. VetMed.*, *32*, 15.
(46) Rice, D. A. et al. (1983) *Vet. Rec.*, *113*, 495.
(47) Kaupinnen, K. (1983) *Acta vet. Scand.*, *24*, 349.
(48) Baker, J. S. et al. (1983) *Comp. cont. Educ.*, *5*, S328.
(49) Grohn, Y. et al. (1983) *J. dairy Sci.*, *66*, 2320.
(50) Kelly, J. M. & Whitaker, D. A. (1984) *Vet. Ann.*, p, 85.
(51) Whitaker, D. A. et al. (1983) *Br. vet. J.*, *139*, 462.
(52) Mills, S. E. et al. (1986) *J. dairy Sci.*, *69*, 362.
(53) Grohn, Y. et al. (1986) *Acta vet Scand.*, *27*, 209.

Fatty infiltration of the liver in cattle (fat cow syndrome, pregnancy toxemia of cattle)

Fatty infiltration of the liver occurs in dairy cattle most commonly within the first 2 weeks after parturition and is associated with periparturient diseases and an increase in the calving to conception interval. In beef cattle it occurs most commonly in late pregnancy when the nutrient intake is decreased in cattle which were previously well fed and in good body condition.

Etiology

The mobilization of excessive quantities of fat from body depôts to the liver, either because of a deprivation of feed in fat beef cattle, more severe in those bearing twins, or because of a sudden demand of energy in the immediate postpartum period in fat lactating dairy cows, is considered to be the cause (1). The disease is an exaggeration of what is a very common occurrence in high-producing dairy cows which are in a state of nutritional energy deficit in early lactation (16). Body fat, especially subcutaneous fat, is mobilized and deposited in many tissues especially liver but also muscle and kidney. Whether or not the cow is actually fat at parturition may not be important in determining the degree of fat mobilization, but the degree of deficiency of energy in early lactation is critical (15).

Epidemiology

Fatty infiltration of the liver is part of a generalized fat mobilization syndrome which occurs in early lactation, particularly in high-yielding dairy cows, as milk production outstrips appetite and body reserves are used to meet the energy deficit (18). The deficit occurs because dietary intake cannot meet the energy requirements for the high yield. Peak yields of milk are reached 4–7 weeks after calving, but the highest levels of voluntary feed intake are not reached until 8–10 weeks after calving. As a result of the energy deficit, the cow mobilizes body reserves for milk production and may lose a large amount of body weight. Most dairy cows develop fatty infiltration of the liver after calving. In about 30% of high-producing cows the fatty infiltration is severe and is associated with reversible but significant effects on liver structure and function.

In North America the introduction of the system of *challenge feeding* of dairy cows appears to have been associated with an increase in the incidence of the disease. The overall effect of the system is to provide excess energy in the diet during late pregnancy or during the dry period generally (5). The diets fed may contain a high percentage of the cereal grains, corn ensilage, or brewer's grains. In this system, dairy cattle are begun on high energy rations a few weeks before parturition. The total daily amount of feed is increased by regular increments to reach a high level at parturition and peak levels to coincide with the peak in the lactation curve several weeks after parturition. This has resulted in some excessively fat cows at the time of parturition when energy demands are high. The disease has also occurred in dairy cows which were fed excessive amounts of high energy rations throughout the dry period. In dairy cattle in problem herds this disease has been associated with an increase in the incidence of parturient hypocalcemia, ketosis and left-sided displacement of the abomasum, all of which are much more difficult to treat successfully because of the fatty liver (11). In a field study the percentage of cattle dying or being culled because of disease was affected by the amount of hepatic triglyceride. The death and cull rates were 15%, 31% and 42% for cattle with mild, moderate, and severe hepatic lipidosis, respectively (16). Cattle have been classified into three groups on the basis of liver fat content determined histologically 1 week after parturition (17). Less than 20% lipid, corresponds to less than 50 mg/g liver by weight, 20–40% lipid, 50–100 mg/g liver, and greater than 40% represents more than 100 mg/g (17). These concentrations correspond to mild, moderate and severe cases of fatty infiltration. Cows with less than 20% lipid in the liver at 1 week after calving are considered normal, and those with more than 20%, are considered to have fatty liver. About 30% of high-yielding dairy cows in the United Kingdom are considered to have fatty liver 1 week after calving. Clinical evidence of hepatic disease may not occur consistently until liver lipid concentrations are in the range of 35–45% or more (29). Outbreaks of the disease have occurred in dairy herds in which up to 25% of all cows were affected with a case fatality rate of 90%. Dairy cows with abnormally long dry periods also have a tendency to become obese and develop the fatty liver syndrome of parturition. The feeding of dairy cows in large groups as in loose housing systems has been associated with an increase in the incidence of the disease.

In dairy cattle there is a relationship between the occurrence of subclinical fatty liver within the first few weeks after parturition and inferior reproductive performance due to a delay in the onset of normal estrus cycles and a reduction in the conception rate which results in an increase in the average days between calving and conception (6). There can be real differences in reproductive performance between cows with mild and moderate fatty livers early after calving (20). Overfeeding in late lactation and during the dry period can result in the fat cow syndrome, which may be associated with an increased incidence of parturient paresis and unresponsive treatment for ketosis in early lactation and inferior reproductive performance (22).

The disease can occur in non-lactating dairy cows by the imposition of a starvation diet in late pregnancy in an attempt to reduce the body weight of cows which were considered to be too fat (23). Changing the diet of pregnant beef cows from silage to straw in an attempt to reduce their body weight and the incidence of dystocia has resulted in outbreaks of the disease (24).

In beef cattle in North America, the disease is seen most commonly in the last 6 weeks of pregnancy in cows which are fat and pregnant with twins. The affected cows are usually well fed until late pregnancy when an unexpected shortage of feed occurs, or the cows are too fat and cannot consume sufficient low energy feed to meet the demands of pregnancy. The disease occurs sporadically: the morbidity is about 1% but the mortality is usually 100%.

The disease has been recognized in pregnant beef cattle in Australia (2) and the United Kingdom (7). It has been more common in first-calf heifers than in older cows and most are in late pregnancy (7–9 months) or have just recently calved. Cows with poor dentition, or those carrying twin calves, are particularly susceptible. Cows exposed to toxic lupins may also develop the disease. In Australia, only beef cattle have been involved in pregnancy toxemia, the fat and the obese being most commonly affected. The circumstances in which the disease has developed are of interest epidemiologically. An enormous expansion of cattle numbers (double in 6 years) took place between 1969 and 1975 in response to an expected demand for beef exports. There was a move to autumn calving (February to April) when feed supplies are likely to be short because of the low summer rainfall. This is particularly true in the southern states in which the main rainfall is in winter with a very hot dry summer. The cows are in good to fat condition because of the lush pastures in the spring and early summer, but by autumn when the calving season approaches the feed supplies may be short and the nutritive value of the pasture may be inadequate. The lack of feed combined with the exploitative atmosphere of the time and the expensive nature of supplementary feeding resulted in an inadequate level of nutrition during late pregnancy. Similarly the control of internal parasitism, especially ostertagiasis, is not intensively practiced. The morbidity is usually from 1 to 3% but may be as high as 10% and the disease is usually fatal.

Pathogenesis

Under normal conditions fat is present in the liver in appreciable amounts at 2 weeks before calving, rises to an average of about 20% at 1 week after calving and declines slowly to the normal level of less than 5% by 26 weeks after calving. However, the levels vary from almost none to 70% among cows 1 week after calving. Fat mobilization begins about 2–3 weeks before calving and is probably induced by a changing hormonal environment prior to calving rather than an energy deficit (31). There is a small increase before calving but a much larger increase at calving.

The heavy demands for energy in the high-producing dairy cow immediately after parturition, or in the pregnant beef cow which may be bearing twins, result in an increased rate of mobilization of fat from body reserves, usually subcutaneous fat, to the blood which transports it to body tissues particularly liver but also muscle and kidney. Any decrease in energy intake caused by a shortage of feed or an inability of the cow to consume an adequate amount of feed during the critical periods of late pregnancy or early lacatation would result in the mobilization of excessive amount of free fatty acids. This results in increased hepatic lipogenesis with accumulation of lipid in enlarged hepatocytes (12), depletion of liver glycogen and inadequate transport of lipoprotein from the liver (3). The serum concentrations of triacylglycerol-rich lipoproteins are reduced in cattle with naturally occurring hepatic lipidosis (25). There is a concurrent loss of body condition and subcutaneous adipose tissue. The degree of mobilization will be dependent on the fatness of the cow and extent of the energy deficit.

Both subcutaneous fat and skeletal muscle mass are decreased after calving and fat cows lose 2·5 times more muscle fiber area than thin cows (31). Thus the loss of body condition is due to total tissue mobilization (protein and fat) rather than fat alone. There appears to be a higher rate of protein mobilization in fat cows than in thin cows. The severity of fatty liver has been arbitrarily classified into severe, moderate and mild based on the amount of triglyceride present in the hepatocytes (17). Fatty infiltration of muscle also occurs and appears to be correlated with the degree of hepatic lipidosis (27) and may be related to the weakness and recumbency seen in severe cases of the fatty liver syndrome. In severe hepatic lipidosis the accumulation of triglyceride in the cytoplasm is accompanied by disturbances in hepatic structure and function which may result in hypoglycemia and ketonemia which are manifested as anorexia and depression and there may be clinical evidence of nervous signs. Some severe cases appear to develop hepatic failure, do not respond to therapy and become weak and recumbent and die. Terminally there is a marked hyperglycemia. The case fatality rate in severe cases may reach 50% or more. A leukopenia has been observed in dairy cows with more than 20% liver fat in the 2nd week after calving (26). This may be related to the increased incidence of postparturient diseases such as mastitis and endometritis observed in cows with subclinical fatty liver. However, this is not necessarily a cause-and-effect relationship.

Cows which are not fat initially do not develop the disease. Pregnant beef cows which are in thin body condition on pasture can become extremely emaciated and eventually recumbent and die of starvation but they do not develop pregnancy toxemia.

The pathogenesis of the relationship between reduced reproductive performance and mild or moderately severe fatty liver dairy cows within the first 2 weeks after calving is unknown (19).

Clinical findings

In dairy cattle, the fat cow syndrome usually occurs within the first few days following parturition and is commonly precipitated by any condition which interferes with their appetite temporarily, such as parturient hypocalcemia, left-sided displacement of the abomasum, indigestion, retained fetal membranes, or dystocia. The affected cow usually does not respond to treatment for some of these conditions and becomes totally anorexic. She may become recumbent and develop a severe form of ketosis, which does not respond to the usual form of therapy. There is marked ketonuria. Affected cows will not eat and gradually become weaker, totally recumbent and die in 7–10 days. Throughout most of the course of the illness, their temperature, heart rate and respirations are within normal ranges. Some cattle exhibit nervous signs consisting of a staring gaze, holding the head high, and muscular tremors of the head and neck. Terminally there is coma and tachycardia (13).

In cattle with moderately severe fatty liver the clinical findings are much less severe and most will recover within several days.

In fat beef cattle shortly before calving, affected cows are aggressive, restless, excited and uncoordinated with a stumbling gait and sometimes have difficulty in rising and they fall easily. The feces are scant and firm and there is tachycardia. When the disease occurs 2 months before calving the cows are depressed for 10–14 days, and do not eat. They become sternally recumbent. The respirations are rapid, there may be an expiratory grunt, the nasal discharge is clear but there may be flaking of the epithelium of the muzzle. The feces are usually scant but terminally there is often a fetid yellow diarrhea. The disease is highly fatal; the course is 10–14 days and terminally there may be coma with cows dying quietly.

Clinical pathology

The changes in the clinical pathology will depend on the severity of the fatty liver, severe cases showing hypoglycemia, ketonemia and ketonuria similar to a severe case of ketosis.

The concentration of serum non-esterified fatty acids is increased, there is an increase in beta-hydroxybutyrate, serum bilirubin and increases in the serum levels of liver enzymes which are released following liver cell injury. In addition there are decreases in cholesterol, albumin, magnesium, and insulin.

In cattle with subclinical fatty liver there may be a leukopenia, neutropenia and lymphopenia (26).

The serum levels of liver enzymes are increased but the values which reliably represent different degrees of fatty infiltration have not been determined (8). Increased serum levels of aspartate aminotransferase are associated with increased total liver lipid but the association is weak (29). However, this enzyme is not exclusively a liver enzyme. It is also present in muscle, kidney and small intestine and any increase may reflect injury to other tissues. The bromosulfophthalein (BSP) clearance test, gamma-glutamyl transpeptidase (GGT) and sorbitol dehydrogenase (SDH) have also been used as liver function tests in cattle with hepatic lipidosis associated with displaced abomasa but are not considered diagnostic (29).

In fatty infiltration of the liver in severely ketotic cows there is a positive correlation between blood ketone body concentrations and the degree of fatty liver (30). However, diurnal variations in the concentrations of plasma beta-hydroxybutyrate make their diagnostic interpretations difficult and unreliable as a diagnostic aid for fatty liver (32).

In experimentally fasted non-lactating dairy cows which developed mild fatty liver the intravenous injection of sodium propionate did not result in a sufficient increase in plasma glucose which suggests a decrease in liver function (36), an observation which may have some potential as a liver function test.

The proposed classification for fatty liver based on liver fat values, while arbitrary, does appear to have a rational basis because cows with moderate or severe fatty infiltration generally have metabolic profile values outside the normal range, whereas cows with mild fatty liver have normal blood chemistry (21). In addition, cows with moderate or severe fatty liver have increased blood concentrations of liver-specific enzymes and ultrastructural evidence of liver damage (34).

Cows with mild fatty liver (less than 20% fat) can be distinguished from cows with moderate fatty liver (more than 20%) using an equation based on the blood concentrations of non-esterified fatty acids, glucose and aspartate aminotransferase (21). The equation is as follows: $Y = -0{\cdot}51 - 0{\cdot}0032$ NEFA (μmol/l + 2·84 glucose (mmol/l) − 0·0528 SGOT (aspartate aminotransferase) (i.u./l). If $Y < 0$, then the cow has moderate fatty liver, if $Y \geqslant 0$ the cow has mild fatty liver.

A liver biopsy can be used to determine the severity of the fatty liver and the concentration of triglyceride. The triglyceride concentration of liver in normal cows ranges from 10 to 15% on a wet weight basis (33). Estimation of the lipid content of bovine liver samples obtained by biopsy may be made by biochemical or histological methods (33). Both methods provide reasonable estimates of liver fat content over a wide range of values. The lipid content of bovine liver is highly correlated with its specific gravity and the submersion of needle biopsy specimens into water and copper sulfate solutions with specific gravities of 1·025 and 1·055 can be used as a test to estimate lipid content (28). For routine clinical diagnosis, three solutions of specific gravities of 1·000, 1·025, and 1·055 can be used. Liver samples which float in all three solutions contain greater than 34% lipid, those that sink in water but float in 1·025 and 1·055 specific gravity solutions are less than 34% but greater than 25% lipid, whereas those that float only in 1.055 specific gravity are less than 25% but greater than 13% lipid. Samples which sink in all three solutions are less than 13%. Some limited evidence indicates that cows with liver lipid concentrations above 34% are severely affected and can be expected to have clinical manifestations of hepatic insufficiency. Those with liver lipid levels between 34 and 25% are moderately affected and might have some clinical evidence of hepatic insufficiency. Those between 25 and 13% are mildly affected, which is the range of most postpartum dairy cows without any evidence of disease. Liver lipid concentrations below 13% are inconsequential (28).

Liver biopsy seems to be the only reliable method of accurately estimating the degree of fatty infiltration of the liver.

Necropsy findings

In severe fatal cases the liver is grossly enlarged, pale yellow, friable and greasy. Mild and moderate cases are usually not fatal unless accompanied by another fatal disease such as peracute mastitis. The degree of fatty infiltration in these is much less obvious. The histological changes include the occurrence of fatty cysts or lipogranulomas, enlarged hepatocytes, compression of hepatic sinusoids, a decreased volume of rough endoplasmic reticulum and evidence of mitochondrial damage (34). The latter two changes are reflected in reduced albumin levels and increased activities of liver enzymes in the blood.

Diagnosis

In dairy cattle the disease must be differentiated from those diseases which occur commonly immediately following parturition. Left-sided displacement of the abomasum results in a secondary ketosis and auscultation and percussion of the left side of the abdomen will usually reveal the characteristic tinkling and metallic sounds. Cows which have had parturient paresis immediately after parturition and do not respond normally to treatment remain recumbent and appear like the downer cow syndrome. However, some of these have pregnancy toxemia in which there is total anorexia, marked ketonuria, which may also be present in the downer cow syndrome, and it may be almost impossible to distinguish between the two diseases. A history of high level grain feeding and the presence of a fat cow will be useful in the differential diagnosis. There is sufficient similarity between the fatty liver syndrome and the *parturition syndrome* to suggest that they are the same disease (10). The latter includes several or all of the following diseases—retained placenta, endometritis, ovarian dysfunction, hypocalcemia, hypomagnesemia, hypoglycemia with ketosis, reduced ruminal activity and mastitis. The result is a chronically sick cow with a much reduced milk production which is more noticeable because the cow is usually a high-producer and the response to intensive and multifaceted treatment is unsatisfactory.

In beef cattle with pregnancy toxemia before parturition, the disease must be differentiated from abomasal impaction, vagus indigestion and chronic peritonitis. These are described elsewhere.

Treatment

The prognosis for severe cases of fatty liver is usually guarded. In general, cows which are totally anorexic for 3 days or more will die; those which continue to eat even a small amount will recover with supportive therapy and nutrition. There is a slight transitory response to parenteral treatment with glucose, calcium and magnesium salts. Glucocorticoids, vitamin B_{12} and cobalt are also used, but the response is unsatisfactory.

Intensive therapy directed at correcting the pathophysiological effects of the ketosis and the fatty liver is required. This means continuous intravenous infusion of glucose electrolyte solution and the intraruminal administration of rumen juice (5–10 litres) from normal cows in an attempt to stimulate the appetite of affected cows. The oral administration of propylene glycol will promote glucose metabolism. The use of insulin (zinc protamine) at 200–300 i.u. subcutaneously twice daily will promote the peripheral utilization of glucose. Affected cattle should be provided with good quality hay and an ample supply of water. Water and balanced electrolytes (10–30 litres) can be administered intraruminally. The use of choline chloride at a dose rate of 25 g every 4 hours, subcutaneously or orally has been recommended for the treatment of severe cases (9). In the mild and moderate cases which are usually subclinical therapy is usually not required. The use of anabolic steroids (Vebenol 300 mg or trenbolone acetate (14) is recommended) provides some improvement but all treatments are less effective the longer their commencement is delayed.

When outbreaks of the disease are encountered in pregnant beef cattle, all remaining cows should be sorted into groups according to body conditions and fed accordingly. Excessively fat cows should be fed the best quality hay which is available with a supplement. Fat cows should be exercised by feeding them on the ground and forcing them to walk.

Control

Because of the large economic losses associated with pregnancy toxemia in cattle, every economic effort must be made to prevent the disease. The principal method of control is to prevent pregnant cattle from becoming fat during the last trimester of pregnancy, particularly during the dry period in dairy cattle. During pregnancy mature cattle should receive sufficient feed to meet the needs for maintenance and pregnancy and the total daily nutrient intake must increase throughout the last trimester to meet the needs of the fetus. However, this increase is usually difficult to control without some cows getting fat and others losing weight. Sorting cows into groups on the basis of size and condition and feeding accordingly is recommended. Metabolic profiles may be used as a means of assessing energy status and correspondingly the likelihood or otherwise of acetonemia or pregnancy toxemia occurring. Both glucose levels are usually used for this purpose, but blood levels of beta-hydroxybutyric acid could also be used.

In dairy cattle, all of the common diseases which occur immediately after parturition must be treated promptly and every effort made to maintain a high energy intake in high-producing cows, particularly those which calved in fat condition. Every effort must be made to maintain their appetite. The use of propylene glycol will promote gluconeogenesis and minimize the mobilization of depôt fat.

Body condition scoring of dairy cows at strategic times can be used to monitor the nutritional status of the herd and minimize the incidence and severity of the fatty liver syndrome (35). The scoring should be done throughout the production cycle as part of a herd health program. Scoring done at calving, at 21–40 days, and 90–110 days postpartum can be used to monitor the nutritional status of the herd. Scoring done at 100–60 days before drying off provides an opportunity for management to make appropriate adjustments in the feeding program so that optimal body condition goals are achieved. The optimum body condition score of a cow at calving which will result in the most economical amount of milk has not yet been determined. On a scale of 5, the suggested optimum score at calving has ranged from 30 to 40 (35). The optimum score will probably depend on the characteristics of the individual herd which include type of cow, type of feedstuffs available, season of the year, environmental temperature and the people doing the actual body condition scoring.

REFERENCES

(1) Morrow, D. A. (1976) *J. dairy Sci.*, *59*, 1625.
(2) Caple, I. W. et al. (1977) *Aust. vet. J.*, *53*, 289.
(3) Reid, I. M. (1973) *Exp. molec. Pathol.*, *18*, 316.
(4) Kelly, J. M. (1977) *Vet. Rec.*, *101*, 499.
(5) Morrow, D. A. (1979) *J. Am. vet. med. Assoc.*, *174*, 161.
(6) Reid, I. M. (1983) *Anim. Reprod. Sci.*, *5*, 275.
(7) Spence, A. B. (1978) *Vet. Rec.*, *102*, 458.
(8) Bogin, E. & Sommer, H. (1978) *Zentralbl. VetMed.*, *25A*, 458.
(9) McCormack, J. (1978) *Vet. Med. SAC*, *73*, 1057.
(10) Sommer, H. (1975) *Vet. Med. Rev.*, *1/2*, 42.
(11) Frank, T. J. et al. (1980) *J. dairy Sci.*, *63*, 1080.
(12) Collins, R. A. & Reid, I. M. (1980) *Res. vet. Sci.*, *28*, 373.
(13) Reid, I. M. et al. (1979) *Vet. Sci. Commun.*, *3*, 231.
(14) Heitzmann, R. J. et al. (1977) *Vet. Rec.*, *100*, 317.
(15) Reid, I. M. (1980) *Vet. Rec.*, *107*, 281.
(16) Gerloff, B. J. et al. (1986) *J. Am. vet. med. Assoc.*, *188*, 845.
(17) Gaal, T. et al. (1983) *Res. vet. Sci.*, *34*, 245.
(18) Reid, I. M. & Roberts, C. J. (1983) *Irish vet. J.*, *37*, 104.
(19) Watson, E. D. (1985) *Br. vet. J.*, *141*, 576.
(20) Reid, I. M. et al. (1983) *J. agric. Sci.*, *101*, 499.
(21) Reid, I. M. et al. (1983) *J. agric. Sci.*, *101*, 473.
(22) Higgins, R. J. & Anderson, W. S. (1983) *Vet. Rec.*, *113*, 461.
(23) Gerloff, B. J. & Herdt, T. J. (1984) *J. Am. vet. med. Assoc.*, *185*, 223.
(24) Doxey, D. L. & Scott, P. R. (1983) *Vet. Rec.*, *113*, 112.
(25) Herdt, T. H. et al. (1983) *Am. J. vet. Res.*, *44*, 293.
(26) Reid, I. M. et al. (1984 *Res. vet. Sci.*, *37*, 63.
(27) Roberts, C. J. et al. (1983) *Vet. Pathol.*, *20*, 23.
(28) Herdt, T. H. et al. (1983) *J. Am. vet. med. Assoc.*, *182*, 953.
(29) Herdt, T. H. & Gerloff, B. J. (1982) *Proc. 12th World Congr. Dis. Cattle, The Netherlands* Vol. 1, pp. 522–525.
(30) Grohn, Y. et al. (1983) *J. dairy Sci.*, *66*, 2320.
(31) Roberts, C. J. (1982) *Proc. 12th World Congr. Dis. Cattle, The Netherlands* Vol. 1, pp. 501–507.
(32) Gaal, T. et al. (1983) *Vet. Rec.*, *113*, 53.
(33) Collins, R. A. et al. (1985) *J. comp. Pathol.*, *95*, 437.
(34) Reid, I. M. & Collins, R. A. (1980) *Invest. cell. Pathol.*, *3*, 237.
(35) Braun, R. K. et al. (1987) *Comp. cont. Educ. pract. Vet.*, *9*, F 62.
(36) Bruss, M. L. et al. (1986) *Am. J. vet. Res.*, *47*, 336.

Hyperlipemia

Hyperlipemia is a metabolic disease of ponies occurring mainly in late pregnancy or early lactation. The serum of affected ponies has a milk-like opalescent character associated with hyperlipidemia. The clinical signs are related to widespread vascular thrombosis and hepatic and renal failure and are manifest principally by somnolence, progressing to hepatic coma, diarrhea, acidosis and vascular disorders. The disease has been reported principally from continental Europe (1–3) and Shetland ponies may be especially susceptible.

Etiology

The disease appears to result from changes secondary to a severe hyperlipidemia but the factors initiating the occurrence of excessive circulating blood lipids are obscure. Hyperlipidemia is a response of some ponies to a period of fasting but the clinical syndrome of hyperlipidemia does not necessarily occur in all hyperlipidemic fasted ponies (4–6). Clinical cases of hyperlipemia frequently have a history of nutritional stress either from a pre-existing or underlying disease or as the result of a falling nutritional plane during a period of high nutrient requirement. The metabolic changes associated with this nutritional stress may result in the severe hyperlipidemia observed. Thus, in Australia, the disease is concentrated in its occurrence during late pregnancy or during lactation. Severe feed stress at this time precipitates the disease (10). The mortality rate is very high, nearly 100%, but with good nursing and encouragement to the patient to eat it can be reduced to 55–60% (5).

Epidemiology

The disease is sporadic in occurrence but certain farms may experience multiple cases. It occurs principally in late pregnant ponies or ponies in early lactation. Cases in barren mares and stallions have been observed but invariably are associated with other underlying disease. In Europe the disease is reported as occurring with greatest frequency in pregnant mares and it most commonly follows, or is associated with, some other underlying disease such as parasitism or sand colic. A high proportion of horses in one study had been recently transported (2).

In Australia, hyperlipemia is more common in lactating pony mares that foal late in the foaling season and are at peak lactation during the period of summer drying off of pasture. The onset is usually 4–8 weeks after foaling. The condition appears more prevalent in older mares of the 'heavy type' but there is little evidence of a familial predisposition.

Pathogenesis

The pathogenesis of the disease is obscure. It appears as a disturbance in fat metabolism occurring secondarily to some underlying disease or spontaneously as a result of nutritional deprivation. There are similarities between the factors that lead to this condition and those that lead to pregnancy toxemia or acetonemia on sheep and cattle. However, blood glucose levels are frequently normal or elevated in hyperlipemia (2) and ketonuria is not a feature. The fact that hyperlipidemia can be produced by fasting normal ponies, but not horses, suggests that a period of nutritional deprivation is central to the initiation of this disease. It is also apparent that the very high levels of serum triglycerides which occur in clinical hyperlipemia are likely to be achieved only if there is a block in removal of the triglycerides from the serum, as well as the unusually high rate of mobilization. Such a metabolic block is known to exist in azotemic horses (11). Ponies do have a marked insensitivity to insulin compared to larger horses and this is thought to exacerbate the effects of stress-induced cortisol release and participate in the massive mobilization of triglycerides in an obese animal (13). A severe hyperlipidemia is associated with widespread lipidosis and extensive vascular thrombosis, and the clinical syndrome is a reflection of these changes with some case to case variation in the severity of individual organ dysfunction.

Clinical findings

The clinical course varies between 3 and 22 days but is generally 6–8 days. The initial signs are depression, weight loss and inappetence. A significant proportion of cases show signs of neuromuscular irritability in the early stages with fine repetitive twitching of muscles of the limb, trunk or neck (muscle fasciculation). Ventral edema unrelated to parturition occurs in approximately 30% of cases. Inappetence progresses to anorexia and the depression progresses to somnolence and hepatic coma. A proportion of cases show compulsive walking or mania terminally. Jaundice is not a feature. Many animals show a willingness to drink but are unable to draw water into the mouth and swallow. Others continually lap at water. The temperature is normal or moderately elevated and heart rate and respiratory rates are increased above the normal. An irreversible metabolic acidosis occurs in the terminal stages. Diarrhea is constant in the terminal stages, the feces are fetid and of a thick porridge consistency. There is a high case fatality except in those cases with an underlying disease that can be successfully treated. Pregnant mares that abort during the clinical course may recover. A method of prognosis based on an estimate of myocardial function has been described (7).

Clinical pathology

Serum and plasma show a milk-like opalescence due to hyperlipidemia. Total lipids may be as high as 4–8 g/dl serum. Plasma triglycerides, part of the total fat fraction, may be increased by 30 times normal levels (12). There is usually a leukocytosis with neutrophilia. Hemoglobin and the packed cell volume are elevated except in those cases where an underlying disease such as parasitism produces anemia. Blood glucose levels are variable and an abnormal glucose tolerance may be present (2). A proportion of cases show hypophosphatemia. Abnormal hepatic and renal function is usually present and may be detected by a prolongation in retention time of bromsulfthalein and an elevated blood urea nitrogen. A marked metabolic acidosis occurs in the terminal stages.

Necropsy findings

Extensive fatty change is present in most internal organs. The most striking is the liver which is enlarged and yellow to orange in color. Liver rupture with intra-abdominal hemorrhage may be present. Fatty change is also prominent in the kidney, skeletal muscle, and adrenal cortex. Histologically widespread vascular thrombosis with nephrosis and generalized skeletal muscle degeneration are evident.

Diagnosis

Hyperlipemia should be considered in any pony with a history of weight loss, inappetence and progressive somnolence, especially in late pregnancy or early lactation. The hyperlipidemia visible in drawn blood is characteristic. Neuromuscular irritability occurs in hypocalcemia, but the onset is rapid and it responds to treatment with calcium salts. Ventral edema occurs prior to foaling in low parity pony mares but is not associated with depression, inappetence and the other signs of hyperlipemia. The toxic hepatopathies of horses are considered elsewhere in this text but can generally be differentiated on history and access.

Treatment

Every effort should be made to ascertain if there is some underlying disease such as parasitism. In these cases recovery may follow successful correction of the underlying problem. In those cases where no infectious initiating factor can be determined, consideration should be given to a nutritional initiating factor. Parenteral administration of glucose may be of value in the initial stages of the disease but the specific treatment of hyperlipemia is unrewarding and the case fatality is high. A regimen consisting of the administration of 30 i.u. insulin parenterally with 100 g glucose orally, and 15 i.u. insulin parenterally with 100 g galactose orally on alternate days has been reported to decrease the fatality rate (8, 9). Supportive treatment and the correction of metabolic acidosis is essential.

Control

An adequate parasite and disease control program should be instituted to cover ponies in late pregnancy and early lactation. Transport of ponies during this period should be avoided. The nutritional requirements during these periods should be met. In problem herds it is possible that periodic blood examination will detect early cases and allow corrective measures to be taken before irreversible changes have occurred.

REVIEW LITERATURE

Jeffcott, L. B. & Field, J. R. (1985) Current concepts of hyperlipemia in horses and ponies. *Vet. Rec.*, *116*, 461–466.

REFERENCES

(1) Schotman, A. J. H. & Wagenaar, G. (1969) *Zentralbl. VetMed.*, *A16*, 1.
(2) Eriksen, L. & Simensen, M. G. (1970) *Nord. VetMed.*, *22*, 273.
(3) Rognerud, B. (1976) *Norsk VetTidsskr.*, *88*, 227.
(4) Baetz, A. & Pearson, J. E. (1972) *Am. J. vet. Res.*, *33*, 1941.
(5) Jeffcott, L. B. & Field, J. R. (1984) *Aust. vet. J.*, *62*, 140.
(6) Wensing, T. H. et al. (1974) *Tijdschr. Diergeneeskd.*, *99*, 855.
(7) Deegen, E. (1972) *Dtsch Tierärztl. Wochenschr.*, *79*, 297.
(8) Wensing, T. H. et al. (1973) *Neth. J. vet. Sci.*, *5*, 145.
(9) Wensing, T. H. et al. (1975) *Clin. chim. Acta*, *58*, 1.
(10) Gay, C. C. et al. (1978) *Aust. vet. J.*, *54*, 459.
(11) Naylor, J. M. et al. (1980) *Am. J. vet. Res.*, *41*, 899.
(12) Bauer, J. E. (1983) *Am. J. vet. Res.*, *44*, 378.
(13) Jeffcott, L. B. & Field, J. R. (1985) *Vet. Rec.*, *116*, 461.

Neonatal hypoglycemia (baby pig disease)

Neonatal hypoglycemia occurs most commonly in piglets in the first few days of life if they do not ingest sufficient milk or are unable to digest milk normally because of an enteropathy. Hypoglycemia also occurs in hypothermic lambs, and occasionally in calves with acute diarrhea.

Etiology

An inadequate intake of milk is always the primary cause of hypoglycemia of piglets. This may be due to failure of the sow's milk supply or to failure of the piglets to nurse. Failure to nurse may be due to such diseases as coliform septicemia, transmissible gastroenteritis, streptococcal infections, myoclonia congenita and hemolytic disease of the newborn (1). Piglets under 4 days of age rapidly develop hypoglycemia under fasting conditions; older pigs do not (8).

In piglets affected with transmissible gastroenteritis there is decreased digestion of lactose, reduced absorption of glucose following the severe and diffuse intestinal villous atrophy and, combined with the low energy reserves of the newborn piglet, severe hypoglycemia can occur (3). Hypoglycemia may occur in newborn calves with acute severe diarrhea and when they are deprived of milk or a source of carbohydrates for more than a few days.

Hypoglycemia occurs in twin or triplet lambs which become hypothermic after 12 hours of age (9).

Epidemiology

Newborn pigs encounter several challenges to their survival during the initial hours of life. One is the inherent problem of glucose homeostasis with the first day of life being the most critical period. Liver glycogen is rapidly depleted postnatally (12–24 hours) for the maintenance of blood glucose. Little insulation against heat loss is provided by the sparse hair coat and the 1–2% total body fat at birth. There is only a small amount of carcass fat and no brown fat and consequently the piglet is dependent almost exclusively on carbohydrate metabolism for subsistence. Therefore, maintenance of the physiologically critical energy metabolite, glucose, depends on the ability of the neonatal pig to compete with its littermates for regular nourishment from its dam.

Neonatal hypoglycemia in piglets occurs primarily during the first 3 days after birth. The disease has been recorded mainly from North America and the United Kingdom. Most affected piglets die if left untreated and the morbidity is usually 30–70% and may be as high as 100% in individual litters. Apart from deaths due to hypoglycemia, many piglets are too weak to avoid the sow and are killed by overlaying. Piglets which fail to ingest sufficient colostrum or milk because of a failure of the sow's milk supply or because of an inability of the piglet to suck normally are the most common primary circumstances. A secondary determinant occurs when piglets affected with an enteritis such as transmissible gastroenteritis are unable to properly digest the lactose in milk and absorb sufficient glucose.

Hypoglycemia occurs in twin and triplet lambs which may be immature or undersized and are subjected to cold exposure and hypothermia (9). About 50% of the total lipid present in the newborn lambs is in the adipose tissue in the form of brown fat which is used by the lambs for non-shivering thermogenesis during the first 24 hours following birth (11). However, the lipid content of newborn lambs can vary from 1·5 to 4·5% of birthweight and small lambs have low levels. Neonatal viability of lambs decreases as birthweight decreases which may be related to their low lipid content in relation to body size (11). Additional factors include mismothering and complete absence of the ewe in lambs only a few days of age.

Hypoglycemia in calves has been recorded as a concurrent disease with diarrhea (5, 14). The hypoglycemia may be secondary to the interference with absorption and digestion caused by the diarrhea. The signs are characteristic but the hypoglycemia does not respond to glucose therapy as quickly, if at all, as in other species (5). However, hypoglycemia in diarrheic calves is not considered to be a significant problem if affected calves receive a supply of milk or milk replacer during the convalescent period.

Pathogenesis

The piglet is born with liver glycogen levels which may be as high as 200 mg/g (wet weight), while muscle glycogen may reach 120 mg/g (wet weight). The blood glucose level at birth is low at 30–60 mg/dl (1·66–3·33 mmol/l) and increases rapidly after feeding on colostrum to 95 mg/dl (5·25 mmol/l) (6). Satisfactory gluconeogenesis does not develop in piglets until the 7th day after birth, and during this period glycogen stores are likely to be rapidly exhausted if the intake of milk is restricted. The blood glucose level is then extremely unstable and dependent entirely upon dietary sources. The 1st week of life is thus the danger period (1). Deprivation of food after this produces only loss of weight and has no effect on blood glucose levels. This particular susceptibility to hypoglycemia in the early postnatal period seems to be characteristic of the pig and may play a major role in causing losses in piglets by contributing to the effects of various infectious and non-infectious agents.

Signs appear first when blood glucose levels fall to

about 50 mg/dl (2·775 mmol/l) although further depression to levels as low as 7 mg/dl (0·388 mmol/l) has been observed. Even in such extreme cases, complete recovery is possible after the administration of glucose (1). The hypoglycemic comatose state induced in piglets by fasting occurs as blood glucose values fall below 40 mg/dl (2·2 mmol/l) (3). Experimental hypoglycemia produced by the injection of insulin causes a clinical syndrome similar to that of the naturally occurring disease.

In piglets with transmissible gastroenteritis the blood glucose levels decreased from a normal of 119 mg/dl (6·6 mmol/l) to 36 mg/dl (2·0 mmol/l) (3). This hypoglycemia coincides with the onset of lethargy followed by a comatose state in a few hours.

Clinical findings

Only piglets less than a week old are affected. Uncertainty in gait is apparent first and the piglet has progressive difficulty in maintaining balance until recumbency becomes permanent. There is shivering, dullness and anorexia, and often a typical weak squeal. A characteristic feature is the subnormal rectal temperature and the cold, clammy skin which also evidences marked pallor and ruffling of the hair. The pallor is related to the failing circulation. The heart rate becomes increasingly feeble and slow and may fall as low as 80/minute. In many cases there are few additional signs but convulsions are recorded as a common occurrence by some observers (1). These vary from aimless movements of the head and forelimbs to severe tetanic convulsions. In the latter there are violent galloping movements, particularly with the hindlegs, opisthotonus and champing of the jaws. Tortuous movements and rigidity of the neck and trunk also occur. Terminally coma develops and death follows 24–36 hours after the onset of signs.

Clinical pathology

Blood glucose levels of less than 50 mg/dl (2·775 mmol/l) in piglets are considered to indicate clinical hypoglycemia. The hypoglycemic comatose state induced in piglets by fasting occurs as blood glucose values fall below 40 mg/dl (2·2 mmol/l) (3). Significant rises in blood non-protein nitrogen and urea nitrogen are often observed but appear to be related to catabolism rather than to renal dysfunction (7).

In calves with acute severe diarrhea the blood glucose may fall to below 40 mg/dl (2·2 mmol/l) in 30–50% of cases (14).

Necropsy findings

There are no visible lesions. Absence of curd in the stomach is good contributory evidence of lack of intake of milk but in many cases it will be obvious that some milk was consumed. Hepatic glycogen levels are usually negligible.

Diagnosis

Unless blood glucose levels are estimated the predominantly nervous signs may lead to an error in diagnosis. However, hypoglycemia and a good response to treatment with glucose may occur when the hypoglycemia is secondary to another disease. A definite diagnosis of neonatal hypoglycemia must depend on elimination of other diseases as primary causes. Viral encephalomyelitis and pseudorabies cause an almost identical clinical picture but are not restricted in occurrence to pigs less than a week old. Bacterial meningoencephalitis including streptococcal septicemia and listeriosis may also affect pigs of this age. Necropsy examination should make definition of viral and bacterial infections a relatively easy task.

Treatment

Piglets with primary hypoglycemia should be given glucose (15 ml of 20% solution) intraperitoneally repeated at 4–6 hours until the animal will suck a foster-dam or drink an artificial diet. Protection from cold is important and an environmental temperature of (27–32°C) (80–90°F) will improve the survival rate of piglets (7). The combined use of oral fluid therapy and the intraperitoneal administration of 5% dextrose at a rate of 25 ml/kg body weight to piglets affected with hypoglycemia associated with transmissible gastroenteritis did not correct the hypoglycemia (4). A newborn piglet weighing 1250 g requires 170 kcal (711 kJ) per day when maintained at 30°C (88°F), 30 ml of a 5% dextrose solution would provide approximately 1·5 g of glucose which would yield only 5·6 kcal (23 kJ) per dose. It would be difficult to provide the energy requirements by parenteral administration of 5% dextrose because the amount of fluid injected per day should not exceed 8% of their body weight (4).

Hypoglycemia and hypothermic lambs can be resuscitated by the intraperitoneal injection of a 20% solution of glucose at a rate of 10 ml/kg body weight followed by rewarming the air at 40°C (104°F) (10).

Control

Avoidance of the causative factors described above constitutes prevention. Piglets should be carefully observed during the 1st week of life for early signs of any disease and treatment instituted promptly. Maintenance of a stable environmental temperature at 32°C (90°F) may delay the onset of the disease, or in marginal circumstances prevent its occurrence.

Lambs require between 180 and 210 ml colostrum/kg body weight during the first 18 hours after birth in order to provide sufficient energy for heat production (12). The administration of colostrum at a rate of 30 ml/kg body weight within a few minutes after birth, directly into the stomach using a catheter and syringe, is recommended to boost the energy supply of the small lamb (11). Ewes which are well fed during late pregnancy produce more colostrum than their lambs need, those with singletons have enough for a second lamb, but in most underfed ewes the lamb requirements for colostrum exceed the ewe's production. Colostrum can be readily obtained by milking those ewes with excess production. The effects of feeding ewe colostrum, cow colostrum, or ewe milk replacer, on plasma glucose in newborn lambs have been compared (13). Both ewe and cow colostrum resulted in a 2-fold increase in plasma glucose within 1–3 hours; the milk replacer caused marked hyperglycemia.

REFERENCES

(1) Goodwin, R. F. W. (1955) *Br. vet. J.*, *111*, 301.
(2) Swiatek, K. R. et al. (1968) *Am. J. Physiol.*, *214*, 400.
(3) Drolet, R. et al. (1984) *Can. J. comp. Med.*, *48*, 282.
(4) Drolet, R. et al. (1985) *Can. J. comp. Med.*, *49*, 357.
(5) Tennant, B. et al. (1968) *Cornell Vet.*, *58*, 136.
(6) Mersmann, H. J. (1974) *J. anim. Sci.*, *38*, 1022.
(7) Morrill, C. C. (1952) *Am. J. vet. Res.*, *13*, 164, 171, 322, 325, 327.
(8) Goodwin, R. F. W. (1957) *Vet. Rec.*, *69*, 1290.
(9) Eales, F. A. et al. (1982) *Vet. Rec.*, *110*, 118.
(10) Eales, F. A. et al. (1982) *Vet. Rec.*, *110*, 121.
(11) Robinson, J. J. (1981) *Livestock Prod. Sci.*, *8*, 273.
(12) Mellow, D. J. & Murray, L. (1986) *Vet. Rec.*, *118*, 351.
(13) Eales, F. A. et al. (1982) *Vet. Rec.*, *111*, 451.
(14) Lewis, L. D. et al. (1975) *Am. J. vet. Rec.*, *36*, 413.
(15) Boyd, R. D. et al. (1981) *J. anim. Sci.*, *53*, 1316.

Postparturient hemoglobinuria

Postparturient hemoglobinuria is a disease of high-producing dairy cows occurring soon after calving and characterized by intravascular hemolysis, hemoglobinuria and anemia.

Etiology

The current hypothesis is that ingested hemolytic agents, some of them identified, for example in rape, some of them not, cause erythrocyte lysis in some circumstances. The particular circumstances in which the erythrocytes of a cow become more sensitive than normal to these hemolysins include hypophosphatemia and hypocupremia, and in New Zealand possibly in selenium deficiency (3). Diets low in phosphorus or unsupplemented with phosphorus are usually associated with the development of the disease. Experimental production of the disease in one cow has been reported after feeding a low phosphorus diet for three pregnancies (1). In this instance other signs of phosphorus deficiency occurred 18 months before hemoglobinuria developed, and the case responded well to supplementary feeding with bone meal. A prolonged hypophosphatemia is thus considered to be a major predisposing cause. For example, in a group of animals in which the disease occurs it is sometimes found that dry cows and yearlings have normal serum inorganic phosphorus levels, milking cows are in the low-normal range, and cows which have calved within the preceding 2 months have low levels. The feeding of cruciferous plants has been associated with the disease (2, 3) but many cases occur unassociated with such diets which creates some uncertainty about their role as a cause. In New Zealand, copper deficiency is considered to be an important etiological factor because copper supplementation reduces the incidence of the disease in herds in marginally copper deficient areas (4). However, no abnormality in copper status is present in most cases of postparturient hemoglobinuria in other countries.

Epidemiology

Although this disease has been observed in many countries its relatively low incidence makes it one of minor importance. The case fatality rate may be as high as 50% but only one or two animals in a herd are affected at a time.

Only adult cows develop the typical hemolytic syndrome, usually in the period 2–4 weeks after calving. Heavy-producing cows in their third to sixth lactations are most commonly affected. The disease does not occur commonly in beef cattle. Phosphorus-deficient soils and drought conditions are thought to be predisposing and the disease is often a problem on particular farms. Cases occur more commonly when the cows graze rape, turnips or other cruciferous plants (2) or when large quantities of beet pulp are fed. These diets are normally low in phosphorus, beet pulp (0·10% dry matter) and turnips (0·22% dry matter). In areas of severe phosphorus deficiency the disease may occur at pasture, but in Europe and North America it is more common during prolonged periods of housing. In New Zealand, in dairy herds with a serious problem with the disease, a high proportion of cows have a Heinz-body anemia without hemoglobinuria (5). Low levels of copper in the blood and liver of cows with the Heinz-body anemia and in the pasture grazed are also observed. The low copper status appears to be related to the application of molybdenum and lime. The ingestion of cold water or exposure to extremely cold weather may precipitate attacks of the disease (6). A similar condition accompanied by hypophosphatemia has been observed in late pregnancy in Egyptian buffalo (7) and in the postparturient period in Indian buffalo (8).

Pathogenesis

There is a constant association with hypophosphatemia and a low dietary intake of phosphorus, and it is presumed that the drain of lactation causes further depletion of phosphorus reserves. The importance of copper and possibly selenium is because of their frequent deficiency in natural foodstuffs. As set out under etiology both are thought to be necessary to provide against orally acquired hemolytic agents (10, 11). The signs observed are those of acute hemolytic anemia and in fatal cases death is due to anemic anoxia.

Clinical findings

Hemoglobinuria, inappetence and weakness develop suddenly and there is a severe depression of the milk yield although, in some less acute cases, the cow continues to eat and milk normally for 24 hours after discoloration of the urine is evident. Dehydration develops quickly, the mucous membranes are pallid, and the cardiac impulse and jugular pulse are much augmented. A moderate temperature rise (40°C, 103·5°F) often occurs. The feces are usually dry and firm. Shortness of breath and tachycardia are evident and jaundice may be apparent in the late stages. Pica may be observed in the other animals in the group. The disease runs an acute course for 3–5 days, the cow becoming weak and staggery and finally recumbent. Gangrene and sloughing of the tip of the tail or the digits has been observed occasionally. Death follows within a few hours. In non-fatal cases convalescence requires about 3 weeks and recovering animals often show pica. Ketosis commonly occurs coincidentally.

In a herd where the disease occurs there may be additional signs of phosphorus deficiency although when the deficiency is marginal the general condition of the herd may be excellent. A similar acute syndrome to that described above, and less severe cases of anemia, may occur sporadically in animals on lush spring pasture.

Clinical pathology

In marginal phosphorus-deficient areas normal non-lactating animals in an affected herd may have serum inorganic phosphorus levels in the normal range. Lactating cows in an affected herd may have moderately low levels of 2–3 mg/dl (0·65–0·97 mmol/l) and affected animals extremely low levels of 0·4–1·5mg/dl (0·13–0·48 mmol/l). Erythrocyte counts and hemoglobin levels are also greatly reduced. Heinz bodies may be present in erythrocytes in the New Zealand disease (9). The urine is dark red-brown to black in color and usually moderately turbid. No red cells are present. A low copper status of the blood and liver of affected cows and the pasture grazed is also recorded (5).

Necropsy findings

The blood is thin and the carcass jaundiced. The liver is swollen, and fatty infiltration and degeneration are evident. Discolored urine is present in the bladder.

Diagnosis

Postparturient hemoglobinuria is characterized by an acute hemolytic anemia in cows calved within the preceding 4 weeks. Other causes of acute hemolytic anemia are not confined to the postcalving period. Laboratory examination is usually necessary to confirm the diagnosis and to eliminate hematuria as a cause of the discoloration of the urine. The differential diagnosis of red urine in cattle is summarized in Table 62.

Treatment

The transfusion of large quantities of whole blood may be the only treatment capable of saving the life of a severely affected animal. The treatment must be given quickly. A delay of 12 hours often seems to lead to an irreversible state. A minimum of 5 liters of blood to a 450 kg cow is recommended. This will usually suffice for up to 48 hours by which time an additional transfusion may be necessary if the cow is weak and the mucous membranes pale. Following successful blood transfusions, fluid therapy is recommended as both supportive therapy and to minimize the danger of hemoglobinuric nephrosis. The administration of phosphorus to acutely ill animals should include the intravenous injection of 60 g of sodium acid phosphate in 300 ml of distilled water and a similar dose subcutaneously, followed by further subcutaneous injections at 12-hour intervals on three occasions and similar daily doses by mouth. Oral dosing with bone meal (120 g twice daily) or dicalcium phosphate or a suitable source of calcium and phosphorus daily for 5 days is recommended followed by inclusion in the ration. Hematinics during convalescence are recommended. Ketosis is a common complication of the disease and additional treatment for it may be required.

Control

An adequate intake of phosphorus according to the requirements for maintenance and milk production should be ensured particularly in early lactation. A decrease in the incidence of the disease is reported after copper supplementation of cattle in a copper-deficient area (4).

REVIEW LITERATURE

MacWilliams, P. S. et al. (1982) Postparturient hemoglobinuria: a review of the literature. *Can. vet. J.*, *23* 309–312.

REFERENCES

(1) Madsen, D. E. & Nielsen, H. M. (1944) *J. Am. vet. med. Assoc.*, *105*, 22.
(2) Tarr, A. (1947) *J. S. Afr. vet. med. Assoc.*, *188*, 167.
(3) Ellison, R. S.et al. (1986) *NZ vet. J.*, *34*, 7.
(4) Smith, B. et al. (1975) *NZ vet. J.*, *23*, 73, 109
(5) Gardner, D. E. et al. (1976) *NZ vet. J.*, *24*, 107.
(6) Penny, R. H. C. (1956) *Vet. Rec.*, *68*, 238.
(7) Awad, F. I. & El-Latif, K. A. (1963) *Vet. Rec.*, 75, 11, 298.
(8) Kurundkar, V. D. et al. (1981) *Ind. J. anim. Sci.*, *51*, 35.
(9) Martinovich, D. & Woodhouse, D. A. (1971) *NZ vet. J.*, *19*, 259.
(10) MacWilliams, P. S. et al. (1982) *Can. vet. J.*, *23*, 309.
(11) Wang, X. L. et al. (1985) *Res. vet. Sci.*, *39*, 373.

Paralytic myoglobinuria (azoturia)

Paralytic myoglobinuria is a disease of horses, occurring during exercise after a period of inactivity on full rations. It is characterized by myoglobinuria and muscular degeneration.

Etiology

The commonly accepted theory is that large stores of glycogen are laid down in muscles during a period of idleness and when exercise is taken the glycogen is rapidly metabolized to lactic acid. If the rate at which lactic acid is produced exceeds the rate at which it can be removed in the bloodstream, accumulation occurs and causes coagulation of the muscles and liberation of myoglobin which escapes in the urine. There are doubts about the general applicability of this hypothesis and many alternatives, including a nutritional deficiency of vitamin E or selenium, have been suggested (13). Most attention is being given to the occurrence of enzymic defects in individual horses, as is suspected in the tying-up syndrome.

Epidemiology

The disease was once of great economic importance in draft horses but is now reduced to sporadic cases occurring particularly in racehorses fed heavily on grain.

In most instances there is a history of a period of complete inactivity for 2 or more days immediately preceding the onset of the disease. An attack is unusual if the period of rest is as brief as 1 day or as long as 2 weeks. Horses taken off track work because of minor injuries or illness are often maintained on full working rations and become affected when taken back to work. Attacks are not uncommon after general anesthesia. Sporadic cases (1) and extensive outbreaks (12, 15) have also been recorded in horses running at pasture and taking no exercise. They have been suggested as resulting from the ingestion of a mycotoxin. A severe outbreak in horses maintained at pasture during the week but ridden at the weekend has been reported (2). A clinically similar disease has been recorded in single cases in cattle 2–8 days after their release onto pasture from winter housing (3). It is dealt with in selenium/vitamin E deficiency (pp. 000, 000). 'Exertional rhabdomyolysis' is also recorded in sheep already receiving selenium supplementation of their diet (11).

Pathogenesis
Coagulation necrosis of muscle fibers causes hard, painful swelling of the large muscle masses. The gluteal muscles are most commonly involved and this is thought to be due to their high content of glycogen. The primary myopathic lesion may cause pressure on the sciatic and other crural nerves and result in a secondary neuropathic degeneration of the rectus femoris and vastus muscles. These latter muscles are said to be the only ones which subsequently atrophy in surviving animals (4). The liberation of myoglobin from the necrotic muscle fibers is followed by the passage of dark red-brown urine. Death is usually due to decubital septicemia or myohemoglobinuric nephrosis and uremia, depending upon the extent of muscle damage. Degeneration of myocardium is sometimes observed and may in some instances be the cause of death.

Clinical findings
Signs develop 15 minutes to 1 hour after the beginning of exercise, which need not be vigorous. There is profuse sweating, stiffness of the gait and reluctance to move. The signs may disappear in a few hours if the horse is given complete rest immediately but the condition usually progresses to recumbency, the horse first assuming a dog-sitting position followed by lateral recumbency.

Severe pain and distress are accompanied by restlessness, struggling and repeated attempts to rise. The respirations are rapid, the pulse small and hard and the temperature may rise to 40·5°C (105°F) in the late stages in severe cases. One limb or all four may be affected but the common finding is involvement of both hindlegs. The quadriceps femoris and gluteal muscles are hard and board-like. The urine is of deep red-brown color and urination may be inhibited. Appetite and water intake are often normal.

Many subacute cases in which signs are mild and myoglobinuria is absent occur in circumstances in which azoturia might be expected to occur. There is lameness, soreness over the rump, crouching, and great restriction of movement of the hindlimbs. If exercise is stopped as soon as lameness occurs the horse may recover in 2–4 days. The prognosis is good if the animal remains standing, recovery occurring in 2–4 days , but recumbency is usually followed by fatal uremia or decubital septicemia.

Clinical pathology
The urine contains myoglobin which can only be differentiated from hemoglobin by spectroscopic examination. There is no discoloration of the serum because the renal threshold for myoglobin is very low. Protein and casts are present in the urine which has a high specific gravity. There is a marked polycythemia. A high proportion of horses with paralytic myoglobinuria have demonstrable ECG abnormalities (5).

In horses the creatinine phosphokinase levels are highest in skeletal and cardiac muscles. SGOT is high in these muscles and liver. Because of its specificity to muscle SCPK levels are the preferred indicator of degree of muscle necrosis (6).

Necropsy findings
Gross and microscopic changes are present, mainly in the large gluteal and quadriceps groups of thigh muscles, and in the iliopsoas and vastus muscles. There is extensive, pale discoloration with a waxy, cooked appearance of the cut surface. Similar degenerative lesions have also been observed in myocardium and muscles of the larynx and diaphragm in some cases (7) but this has not been a general finding. Dark brown urine is present in the bladder and renal medulla shows dark brown streaks.

Diagnosis
Severe cases present no major difficulty in diagnosis. Similar lameness may occur in laminitis but the history is different, there is no discoloration of urine and pain is evident at the coronet. Reddish discoloration of the urine is more commonly due to presence of hemoglobin, and diseases in which hemoglobinuria occurs are not usually accompanied by lameness or local pain. A local maxillary myositis and a generalized polymyositis have also been recorded in horses (8). The former develops slowly and affects only the muscles of the jaw, and the latter is a muscular dystrophy comparable to that caused by vitamin E deficiency. Selenium deficiency does occur in horses but there is no evidence that it plays any part in paralytic myoglobinuria. Iliac thrombosis can be detected on rectal palpation. 'Tying-up', which occurs primarily in light horses, includes a number of conditions, one of which may be mild paralytic myoglobinuria. Exertional rhabdomyolysis is a disease classification with an uncertain cause or group of causes. It is discussed under the heading of myositis/myopathy (in Chapter 13).

Treatment
Further exercise should be avoided and the animal either cared for where it is or taken home by low-level trailer and kept in a box-stall. Every effort should be made to keep the horse standing, and slinging may be advisable in some cases. Narcosis with chloral hydrate or ataractic drugs may be necessary if pain is severe or the horse makes repeated efforts to rise. Corticosteroids, administered intravenously, are recommended. Thiamine hydrochloride is claimed to give favorable results. Intramuscular injections of 0·5 g are usually repeated daily (9, 10). The administration of antihistamines and vitamin E is probably warranted, especially in the early stages of the disease. Ancillary treatment includes the intravenous or oral administration of large quantities of electrolyte solutions to maintain a high rate of urine flow and avoid tubular blockage, catheterization if urination is difficult and the maintenance of soft feces. The urine should be kept alkaline to avoid precipitation of myoglobin in renal tubules. This is usually effected by administering sodium bicarbonate orally or by intravenous injection. It is common practice to administer bicarbonate to combat an expected acidosis. However, the acidosis of the initial attack passes off very quickly and the horse is not

likely to be acidotic at the time of treatment (14). Hot applications to the affected parts may ease the discomfort.

Control

The disease can be avoided by reducing the grain ration to half when the horse is getting no exercise. If there is a chance that the disease may develop exercise should be kept very light initially and increased only gradually.

REVIEW LITERATURE

Arighi, M. et al. (1984) Equine exertional rhabdomyolysis. *Comp. cont. Educ.*, 6, S726–733.

REFERENCES

(1) Pope, D. C. & Heslop, C. H. (1960) *Can. vet. J.*, *1*, 171.
(2) Tritschler, L. A. & Miles, D. (1966) *Vet. Med.*, *61*, 649.
(3) Christl, H. (1971) *Dtsch Tierärztl. Wochenschr.*, *78*, 204.
(4) Merillat, L. A. (1944) *J. Am. vet. med. Assoc.*, *104*, 223.
(5) Maclean, J. (1973) *Aust. vet. J.*, *49*, 41.
(6) Gerber, H. (1969) *Equ. vet. J.*, *1*, 129.
(7) Goto, M. et al. (1953) *Jap. J. vet. Sci.*, *15*, 227.
(8) Alstrom, I. (1948) *Skand. Vet Tidskr.*, *38*, 593.
(9) Bauch, R. E. (1945) *Vet. Med.*, *40*, 169.
(10) Stroup, N. L. (1945) *Vet. Med.*, *40*, 170.
(11) Peet, R. L. et al. (1980) *Aust. vet. J.*, *56*, 155.
(12) Linklater, K. A. (1985) *Vet. Rec.*, *116*, 86.
(13) Harris, P. & Snow, D. H. (1986) *Equ. vet. J.*, *18*, 346.
(14) Koterba, A. & Carlson, G. P. (1982) *J. Am. vet. med. Assoc.*, *180*, 305.
(15) Hosie, B. D. et al. (1986) *Vet. Rec.*, *119*, 444.

Low milk fat syndrome

The secretion of a normal volume of milk but with its milk fat reduced, often to less than 50% of normal, is a significant cause of wastage in high producing cows. It occurs most commonly in cows on low fibre diets, for example, lush, irrigated pasture or grain rations that are ground very finely or fed as pellets (1). It is assumed that a decreased formation of acetate in the rumen is the cause of a depletion of fatty acid precursors and the fall in butterfat.

REFERENCE

(1) van Beukelen, P. et al. (1982) *Bov. Practnr*, *17*, 150.

29

Diseases Caused by Nutritional Deficiencies

INTRODUCTION

THE following criteria are suggested for the assessment of the importance of nutrition in the etiology of a disease state in a single animal or in a group of animals:

- Is there evidence from an examination of the diet that a deficiency of a specific nutrient or nutrients may be occurring?
- Is there evidence from an examination of the animals that a deficiency of the suspected essential nutrient or nutrients could cause the observed disease?
- Does supplementation of the diet with the essential nutrient or nutrients prevent or cure the condition?

The difficulties encountered in satisfying these criteria and making an unequivocal diagnosis of a nutritional deficiency have increased as investigations have progressed into the area of trace elements and vitamins. The amounts of such substances as selenium present in feedstuffs and body tissues are exceedingly small and their estimation difficult and expensive. Because of these difficulties it is becoming more acceptable to describe individual syndromes as 'responsive diseases', i.e. which satisfy only the third of the above criteria. The practice leaves much to be desired but has the advantage that applicable control measures are more readily available.

Evidence of existence of deficiency

General evidence will include either evidence of deficiency in the diet or abnormal absorption, utilization or requirement of the nutrient under consideration. Special evidence may be obtained by chemical or biological examination of the feed.

Diet

The diet for a considerable period prior to the occurrence of the disease must be considered because body stores of most dietary factors may delay the appearance of clinical signs. Specific deficiencies are likely to be associated with particular soil types and in many instances soil and geological maps may predict the probable occurrence of a nutritional disease (1). Diseases of plants may also indicate specific soil deficiencies, e.g. 'reclamation disease' of oats indicates a copper deficiency in the soil. Domination of the pasture by particular plant species may also be important, e.g. subterranean clover selectively absorbs copper, legumes selectively absorb molybdenum and *Astragalus* spp. are selector plants for selenium.

Farming practices may have a marked bearing on the presence or absence of specific nutrients in livestock feed. For example, heavy applications of nitrogen fertilizer can reduce the copper, cobalt, molybdenum and manganese content of the pasture. On the other hand, many applications of lime reduce plant copper, cobalt, zinc and manganese levels but increase the molybdenum content (2). Effects such as these are sufficiently severe to suggest that animals grazing the pasture might suffer trace element deficiency (3). Modern haymaking methods, with their emphasis on the artificial drying of immature forage, tend to conserve vitamin A but may result in a gross deficiency of vitamin D. Soil and pasture improvement by exaggeration of the depletion of nutrients, particularly trace elements, from marginally deficient soil may give rise to overt deficiency disease. Thus local knowledge of farming and feeding practices in a particular area is of primary importance in the diagnosis of nutritional deficiency states.

Abnormal absorption

Even though a diet may contain adequate amounts of a particular nutrient, some other factor, by decreasing the absorption of the nutrient, may reduce the value of the dietary supply. For instance, excess phosphate reduces calcium absorption, excess calcium reduces the absorption of iodine, and absence of bile salts prevents proper absorption of the fat-soluble vitamins. Chronic enteritis reduces the absorption of most dietary essentials. The list of antagonisms that exist between elements grows all the time, most of them being interferences with absorption (4). For example, excess calcium in the diet interferes with the absorption of fluorine, lead, zinc and cadmium, so that it may cause nutritional deficiencies of these elements, but it also reduces their toxic effects when they are present in the diet in excessive amounts.

Abnormal utilization of ingested nutrients
This may also have an effect on the development of conditioned deficiency diseases. For example, molybdenum and sulfate reduce copper storage, vitamin E has a sparing effect on vitamin A and thiamine reduces the dietary requirements of essential fatty acids.

Abnormal requirement
Stimulation of the growth rate of animals by improved nutrition or other practices may increase their requirement of specific nutrients to the point where deficiency disease occurs. There seems to be little doubt that there is a genetic variation in mineral metabolism and it has even been suggested that it may be possible to breed sheep to 'fit' actual deficiency conditions, but the significance of the inherited component of an animal's nutritional requirement is unknown and probably small (2). It should not be overlooked, however, when policies of upgrading livestock in deficient areas are initiated.

Evidence of a deficiency as the cause of the disease

Evidence is usually available from experimental work to indicate the clinical signs and necropsy findings one can expect to be produced by each deficiency. Several modifying factors may confuse the issue. Deficiencies under natural circumstances are unlikely to be single and the clinical and necropsy findings will be complicated by those caused by deficiencies of other factors or by intercurrent infections. In addition most of the syndromes are both variable and insidious in onset and the minimal nature of the necropsy lesions in many nutritional deficiency diseases adds further difficulty to the making of a diagnosis.

Special clinical and laboratory examinations of the animals are valuable aids to diagnosis in many instances. However, the ranges of blood or tissue concentrations of minerals and vitamins, or their biochemical markers, in normal animals and those values which indicate deficiency have not been well established. In other words, the cutoff values above which animals are normal and below which they are abnormal or deficient have not been adequately determined in naturally occurring nutritional deficiencies. Experimentally induced nutritional deficiencies provide an indication of the changes which occur in the concentrations of a particular nutrient marker but variations due to age, genotype, production cycle, length of time on the inadequate diet, previous body stores of the element and other stressors commonly complicate the results and render them difficult to interpret accurately and with repeatability.

In most cases, nutritional deficiencies affect a proportion of the herd or the flock at the same time and the clinicopathological examination should include both normal with clinically affected animals. Comparison of the laboratory results of normal and abnormal animals allows for more accurate and reliable interpretation and the making of a diagnosis.

Evidence based on cure or prevention by correction of the deficiency

The best test of the diagnosis in suspected nutritional deficiency is to observe the effects of specific additions to the ration. Confounding factors are frequently encountered. Spontaneous recoveries may occur and adequate controls are essential. Curative responses may be poor because of an inadequate dose rate or because of advanced tissue damage or the abnormality may have been only a predisposing factor or secondary to a complicating factor which is still present. Another common cause of confusion in therapeutic trials is the impurity of the preparations used, particularly when trace elements are involved. Finally the preparations used may have intrinsic pharmacological activity and produce some amelioration of the disease without a deficiency having been present.

REVIEW LITERATURE

Jacobson, N. L. et al. (1978) Nutrient requirements of domestic animals; *No. 3, Nutrient Requirements of Dairy Cattle, 5th ed.* National Academy of Sciences, Washington, DC.

McDonald, I. W. (1968) The nutrition of grazing ruminants. *Nutr. Abst. Rev.*, *38*, 381.

REFERENCES

(1) Thornton I. et al. (1972) *Vet. Rec.*, 90, 11.
(2) Pope, A. L. (1971) *J. anim. Sci.*, *33*, 332.
(3) Mudd, A. J. (1970) *Br. vet. J.*, *126*, 38.
(4) Pond, W. G. (1975) *Cornell Vet.*, *65*, 441.

DEFICIENCIES OF ENERGY AND PROTEIN

Deficiency of energy

Insufficient quantity or quality of feed is a common nutritional deficiency and practical problem of feeding livestock (1, 2). The term *protein-energy* malnutrition is used to describe a form of incomplete starvation in which energy and protein are present in the diet in suboptimal quantities. Protein and energy deficiencies usually occur concurrently in underfed livestock and often cannot be strictly separated.

A deficiency of energy is the most common nutrient deficiency which limits performance of farm animals. There may be inadequate amounts of feed available or the feed may be of low quality. Supplies of feed may be inadequate because of overgrazing, drought, snow covering or it may be too expensive to be fed to the animals. Available feed may be of such low quality and digestibility that animals cannot consume enough to meet energy requirements. In some cases, forage may contain a high concentration of water which limits total energy intake.

The clinical findings in an energy deficiency will depend on the age of the animal, whether or not it is pregnant or in lactation, the presence of concurrent deficiencies of other nutrients and environmental influences. In general, an insufficient supply of energy in young animals results in retarded growth and delay in the onset of puberty. In mature animals, there is a marked decline in milk production and a shortened lactation. A prolonged energy deficiency in pregnant beef heifers will result in a failure to produce adequate quantities of colostrum at parturition. In mature animals there is also a marked loss of body weight especially during high demands for energy as in late pregnancy and early lactation. There are prolonged periods of anestrus lasting up to several months which has a marked effect on reproductive performance in the herd. Primigravid females are particularly susceptible to protein-energy malnutrition because of growth and maintenance requirements (1). A prolonged deficiency of energy during late gestation may result in undersized, weak neonates with a high mortality rate. A deficiency of energy during prolonged periods of cold weather, especially in pregnant beef cattle, and ewes being wintered on poor quality roughage may result in abomasal impaction. Heat loss from the animal to the environment increases remarkably during cold weather and when ambient temperatures are below the critical temperatures the animal responds by increasing metabolic rate to maintain normal body core temperature. If sufficient feed is available when temperatures are below the lower critical temperature, ruminants will increase their voluntary feed intake to maintain body temperature. If sufficient feed is not available the animal will mobilize energy stored as fat or muscle to maintain body temperature and thus lose body weight. In the case of ruminants and horses if the feed is of poor quality, for example, poor quality roughage, the increased feed intake may result in impaction of the abomasum and forestomachs in cattle and of the large intestine in the horse.

Cold, windy and wet weather will increase the needs for energy and the effects of a deficiency are exaggerated, often resulting in weakness, recumbency and death. A sudden dietary deficiency of energy in fat pregnant beef cattle and ewes can result in starvation ketosis and pregnancy toxemia. Hyperlipemia occurs in fat pregnant or lactating ponies which are on a falling plane of nutrition.

Protein-energy malnutrition occurs in neonatal calves which are fed inferior quality milk replacers which may contain insufficient energy or added non-milk proteins which may be indigestible by the newborn calf. A major portion of the body fat present at birth can be depleted in diarrheic calves which are deprived of milk and fed only fluids and electrolytes for 4–7 days. Feeding only fluids and electrolytes to normal healthy newborn calves for 7 days can result in a significant loss of perirenal and bone marrow fat and depletion of visible omental, mesenteric and subcutaneous fat stores (3). The amount of body fat present in a calf at birth is an important determinant of the length of time an apparently healthy calf can survive in the face of malnutrition. Calves born from dams on an adequate diet usually have sufficient body fat to provide energy for at least 7 days of severe malnutrition. The absence of perirenal fat in a calf at 2–4 days of age suggests inadequate reserves of fat at birth and chronic fetal malnutrition (3).

Deficiency of protein

A deficiency of protein commonly accompanies a deficiency of energy. However, the effects of the protein deficiency, at least in the early stages, are usually not as severe as those of energy. Insufficient protein intake in young animals results in reduced appetite, lowered feed intake, inferior growth rate, lack of muscle development and a prolonged time to reach maturity. In mature animals there is loss of weight and decreased milk production. In both young and mature animals there is a drop in hemoglobin concentration, packed cell volume, total serum protein and serum albumin. In the late stages there is edema associated with the hypoproteinemia. Ruminants do not normally need a dietary supply of essential amino acids, in contrast to swine which need a natural protein supplement in addition to the major portion of total protein supplied by the cereal grains. The amino acid composition of the dietary protein for ruminants is not critical because the ruminal flora synthesize the necessary amino acids from lower quality proteins and non-protein sources of nitrogen.

Diagnosis

The clinical findings of an energy deficiency are similar to those of a protein deficiency and the clinical findings of both resemble many other specific nutrient deficiencies and subclinical disease. Protein-energy malnutrition in beef cattle occurs most commonly in late gestation and is characterized clinically by weakness, clinical recumbency, marked loss of body weight, a normal mental attitude, and a desire to eat (1, 2). Cows with concurrent hypocalcemia will be anorexic. If the condition occurs at the time of parturition there will be an obvious lack of colostrum. Calves of these cows may attempt to vigorously suck their dams, attempt to eat dry feed, drink surface water or urine and bellow continuously. Affected cows and their calves may die within 7–10 days.

Protein-energy malnutrition is less common in dairy cattle because they are usually fed to meet the requirements of maintenance and milk production. Dairy calves fed inferior quality milk replacers during periods of cold weather will lose weight, become inactive, lethargic and may die within 2–4 weeks. Affected calves may maintain their appetites until just before death. Diarrhea may occur concurrently and be confused with acute undifferentiated diarrhea due to the enteropathogenic viruses or cryptosporidiosis. Affected calves recover quickly when fed cow's whole milk.

Protein-energy malnutrition also occurs in sheep and less commonly in goats. Excessive dental attrition is a common cause in grazing sheep which is exacerbated by the excessive ingestion of soil.

The diagnosis will depend on an estimation of the concentration of energy and protein in the feed, or a feed analysis, and comparing the results with the estimated nutrient requirements of the affected animals. In some cases, a sample of feed used several weeks earlier may no longer be available or the daily amount of feed intake may not be known. Marginal deficiencies of energy and protein may be detectable with the aid of a metabolic profile test. Specific treatment of livestock affected with protein-energy malnutrition is usually not undertaken because of the high cost and prolonged recovery period. Oral and parenteral fluid and electrolyte therapy can be given as indicated. The provision of high quality feeds appropriate to the species is recommended.

The prevention of protein-energy malnutrition requires the provision of the nutrient requirements of the animals according to age, stage of pregnancy and production, the environmental temperature and the cost of the feeds. Body-condition scoring of cattle and sheep can be used as a guide to monitor body condition and nutritional status. Regular analysis of feed supplies will assist in the overall nutritional management program. The published nutrient requirements of domestic animals are only guidelines to estimated requirements since they were determined in experimental animals selected for uniform size and other characteristics. Under practical conditions, all of the common factors which affect requirements must be considered.

REVIEW LITERATURE

Oetzel, G. R. & Berger, L. L. (1985) Protein-energy malnutrition in domestic ruminants. Part 1. Predisposing factors and pathophysiology. *Comp. cont. Educ. pract. Vet.*, *7*, S672–S679.

Oetzel, G. R. & Berger, L. L. (1986) Protein-energy malnutrition in domestic ruminants. Part 2. Diagnosis, treatments and prevention. *Comp. cont. Educ. pract. Vet.*, *8*, S16–S21.

REFERENCES

(1) Oetzel, G. R. & Berger, L. L. (1985) *Comp. cont. Educ. pract. Vet.*, *7*, S672.
(2) Oetzel, G. R. & Berger, L. L. (1986) *Comp. cont. Educ. pract. Vet.*, *8*, S16.
(3) Schoonderwoerd, M. et al. (1986) *Can. vet. J.*, 365.

DISEASES CAUSED BY DEFICIENCIES OF MINERAL NUTRIENTS

An enormous literature exists on the subject of mineral nutrient deficiencies in animals and it is not possible to review it all here. However, some general comments should be made. The era of large-scale deficiencies affecting very large numbers of animals and comprising single elements has now largely passed in developed countries. The diagnostic research work has been done and the guidelines for preventive programs have been outlined and put into action in the field, so that the major breakthroughs have already been made, and what remains is in many ways a tidying-up operation after large-scale control campaigns. The loose edges which need to be refined include correcting overzealous application of minerals which can produce toxicoses (7), sorting out the relative importance of the constituent elements in combined deficiencies which are characterized by incomplete response to provision of single elements, and devising means of detecting marginal deficiencies (2).

Despite increasing experimental evidence that anomalies in trace element supply can influence growth, reproductive performance or immunocompetence of livestock, few data exists from which the incidence and economic significance of such problems can reliably be assessed. Most published reports of the more readily recognized trace element-related diseases continue to provide insufficient quantitative information to assess their incidence and true economic impact. Despite these deficiencies in information the FAO/WHO Animal Health yearbooks indicate that, of the countries providing information on animal diseases, 80% report nutritional diseases of moderate or high incidence and trace element deficiencies or toxicities are involved in more than half of those whose causes were identified. In the United Kingdom it has been estimated that despite the activities of its nutritional and veterinary advisory services and extensive policies of ration supplementation, characteristic clinical signs of copper deficiency develop annually in about 0·9% of the cattle population (10). In the light of recently described evidence that copper deficiency can predispose to increased mortality due to infectious diseases in lambs, the economic losses from copper deficiency may be grossly underestimated (9).

In developed countries with highly developed animal industries the emphasis is on disease prevention rather than therapy and elimination or economical control of trace element deficiencies is a matter of education rather than research. However, because copper, cobalt, selenium and iodine deficiencies can affect reproductive performance, appetite, early postnatal growth and immunocompetence on a herd or flock basis, increasing emphasis is being placed on diagnostic methods which will identify a developing risk long before specific clinical manifestations appear. In addition, it is not good enough to merely define the distribution of animal populations with an abnormal trace element status indicated by blood or tissue analysis or to detect a deficiency of the trace element in the diet. The only feasible way of monitoring the preclinical stages of trace element deficiency is the identification of a biochemical indicator which reflects changes in the activity of the enzyme involved or the concentration in tissues of its substrate or products. The demand is growing for techniques which will predict when the likely pathological outcome of such anomalies justifies the introduction of protective measures. For example, recent observations indicate that a high proportion of grazing cattle become hypocupremic if maintained on forage but fail to develop characteristic clinical signs of deficiency and, furthermore, only a small percentage of these animals exhibit any physiological response to the administration of copper. This illustrates the lack of understanding of the variables involved in the development of clinical manifestations of copper deficiency and whether they are induced by a simple dietary deficiency of copper or by specific copper antagonists present in the diet. A relatively new and interesting area of development is the observation of genetic variation in dietary requirements for copper among different breeds of sheep (4) and that sheep can be selected for a high or low concentration of plasma copper which in turn will have profound physiological consequences in the low group. There is now evidence that heredity is involved in the utilization of trace elements by animals. A small amount is necessary but a larger amount may be toxic and there is a need to determine the optimal economic balance.

Thus it is likely that trace element deficiencies are widespread but their incidence and importance are probably underestimated because subclinical forms of deficiency can occur and go unnoticed for prolonged periods.

In developing countries the trace element problem is confounded by the common deficiencies of energy, protein, phosphorus and water which affect postnatal growth and reproductive performance. Undernutrition is commonly accepted as the most important limitation to herbivore livestock production in tropical countries. However, mineral deficiencies or imbalances in soils and forages have long been held responsible for low production and reproduction problems among grazing tropical cattle. Cattle grazing forages in areas which are severely deficient in phosphorus, cobalt or copper are even more limited by lack of these elements than either that of energy or protein.

At least 15 mineral elements are nutritionally essential for ruminants. The macrominerals are calcium, phosphorous, potassium, sodium, chlorine, magnesium and sulfur. The trace elements, or microminerals, are copper, selenium, zinc, cobalt, iron, iodine, manganese and molybdenum.

The trace elements are involved as component parts of many tissues and one or more enzyme activities and their deficiency leads to a wide variety of pathological consequences and metabolic defects (1). These are summarized in Table 84.

The physiological basis of trace element deficiency is very complex (1). Some elements are involved in a single enzyme, some in many more and a lack of one element may affect one or more metabolic processes. Furthermore, there are wide variations in how individual animals respond clinically to lowered blood or tissue levels of a trace element. For example, two animals in a herd or flock with the same copper levels in their blood may be in different bodily condition. The susceptibility to clinical disease may be a function of the stage of physiological development at which they occur, genetic differences within a species and interrelationships with other trace elements. There is now good evidence to show that the amounts of dietary copper adequate for some breeds of sheep were deficient for others, and even toxic to others.

The soil–plant–animal interaction in relation to the incidence of trace element deficiencies in livestock are being examined (5). The soil and its parent materials are the primary sources of trace elements on which soil–plant–animal relationships are built. The natural ranges in concentration of most trace elements in soils are wide and range from deficient soils to those which are potentially toxic. The availability of trace elements to plants is controlled by their total concentration in the soil and their chemical form. Certain species of plants take up more trace elements than do others. The ingestion of soil can have a profound effect on trace element nutrition and metabolism. Geochemical surveys can now

Table 84. Principal pathological and metabolic defects in essential trace element deficiencies (1).

Deficiency	*Pathological consequence*	*Associated metabolic defect*
Copper	Defective melanin production	Tyrosine/DOPA oxidation
	Defective keratinization; hair, wool	—SH oxidation to S—S
	Connective tissue defects	Lysyl oxidase
	Ataxia, myelin aplasia	Cytochrome oxidase
	Growth failure	?
	Anaemia	?
	Uricaemia	Urate oxidase
Cobalt	Anorexia	Methyl malonyl CoA mutase
	Impaired oxidation of propionate	Tetrahydrofolate methyl transferase
	Anaemia	
Selenium	Myopathy; cardiac/skeletal	Peroxide/hydroperoxide destruction
	Liver necrosis	Glutathione peroxidase
	Defective neutrophil function	OH; O_2 generation
Zinc	Anorexia, growth failure	?
	Parakeratosis	Polynucleotide synthesis, transcription, translation?
	Perinatal mortality	
	Thymic involution	
	Defective cell-mediated immunity	
Iodine	Thyroid hyperplasia	Thyroid hormone synthesis
	Reproductive failure	
	Hair, wool loss	
Manganese	Skeletal/cartilage defects	Chondroitin sulfate synthesis
	Reproductive failure	?

assist in the identification of areas in which livestock are exposed to excessive ingestion or deficiencies of trace elements.

The dose–response trial will continue to play a significant role in the delineation of trace element disorders because it is often difficult to determine the role of individual trace elements (6). A deficiency of one trace element may result in clinical disease which may be indistinguishable from a deficiency of more than one trace element. Many of the trace element disorders may produce non-specific as well as specific effects.

The *ad hoc* field observations made by veterinarians who make a diagnosis of a trace element deficiency followed by treatment or dietary changes are subjective and usually lack controls but are nevertheless of value in indicating the magnitude and variability of response that might be expected in future experimental studies. Dose–response trials help to establish a link between a trace element and certain clinical signs; they may identify factors which modify the response to a trace element and, of paramount importance, give an indication of the economic importance of adequate supplementation of the element in the diet.

A dose–response trial can be defined as the application of a test and a control substance to a group, or replicates, of individuals and the measurement of the response to the treatment. The requirements for a reliable dose–response trial include a careful appraisal of the basis for conducting the trial, a suitable form of the test substance for treatment, the careful selection of animals for the test, a reliable biochemical method for monitoring the response to the trace element, a measurable production response, an adequate system for measurement of the variable which may influence the response and a means of measuring the economic impact.

There are major problems in the diagnosis and anticipation of trace element deficiencies in grazing livestock (8). Because of the interplay between the constituents of the diet and the homeostatic mechanisms of the body it is often impossible to predict from dietary composition alone whether a particular nutritional regime will result in clinical disease. The assessment of the absorbable rather than the total concentration of elements in the diet is now considered to be more important in understanding the nutritional basis for the deficiencies (3).

A dietary deficiency does not necessarily lead to clinical disease. Several factors predispose the animal to clinical disease and they include: the age at which the deficiency occurs (for example fetal lambs are highly susceptible to demyelination due to copper deficiency in late fetal life); differences in genotype requirements; discontinuous demands for trace elements because of changes in environment; the challenge of infections, diet and production demands; individual variations in response to the deficiency, the use of alternative pathways by the body in the face of a deficiency; and the size of the functional reserves.

The diagnosis of mineral deficiencies, particularly trace element deficiencies will depend heavily on the interpretation of the biochemical criteria of the trace element status. This is because deficiencies of any one or more of several trace elements can result in nonspecific clinical abnormalities such as loss of weight, growth retardation, anorexia and inferior reproductive performance.

The three important principles which should govern the interpretation of biochemical criteria of trace element status are its relationship with intake, time and function. The relationship between the tissue concentrations of a direct marker and the intake of the element will generally be sigmoid in shape (a dose–response curve). The important point on the curve is the intake at which the requirement of the animal is passed which is the intake of the nutrient which is needed to maintain normal physiological concentrations of the element and or avoid impairment of essential functions. For several markers of trace element status, the position on the x axis at which requirement is passed coincides with the end of the lower plateau of the response in marker concentration. Under these conditions, the marker is an excellent index of sufficiency and body reserves but an insensitive index of a deficiency. If requirement is passed at the beginning of the upper plateau, the marker is a poor index of sufficiency but a good index of deficiency. This principle allows direct markers to be divided into *storage* and *non-storage* types corresponding to the former and latter positions on the x axis. In the second principle, non-storage criteria can be divided into indicators of acute and chronic deficiency and two types of relationships can be distinguished; a rapid early decline in marker concentration followed by a plateau and a slow linear rate of decline. Markers with a slow linear response will be good indices of a chronic deficiency but unreliable indices of acute deficiency because they cannot respond quickly enough. Conversely, the marker with a rapid early decline will be a good index of acute deficiency but an unreliable indicator for chronic deficiency if the low plateau is reached before functions are impaired. Those biochemical criteria which are based on metalloenzyme or metalloprotein concentrations in erythrocytes are of the slow type because the marker is incorporated into the erythrocyte before its release into the bloodstream, and thereafter its half-life is determined by that of the erythrocyte which is 150 days or more. Metalloenzymes or metalloproteins in the plasma which have short half-lives provide markers of the rapid type. The third principle states that a deficiency can be divided into four phases, *depletion*, *deficiency* (marginal), *dysfunction* and *clinical disease* (8).

Depletion is a relative term which describes the failure of the diet to maintain the trace element status of the body and it may continue for weeks or months without observable clinical effects when substantial body reserves exist. When the net requirement for an essential element exceeds the net flow of absorbed element across the intestine then depletion occurs. The body processes may respond by improving intestinal absorption or decreasing endogenous losses. During the depletion phase there is a loss of trace element from any storage sites such as the liver during which time the plasma concentrations of the trace element may remain constant. The liver is a common store for copper, iron, and vitamins A and B_{12}.

If the dietary deficiency persists, eventually there is a

transition from a state of depletion to one of *deficiency* which is marked by biochemical indications that the homeostatic mechanisms are no longer maintaining a constant level of trace elements necessary for normal physiological function. After variable periods of time the concentrations or activities of trace-element containing enzymes will begin to decline leading to the phase of *dysfunction*. There may be a further lag period, the *subclinical phase* before the changes in cellular function are manifested as *clinical disease*. The biochemical criteria can be divided, according to the phase during which they change, into indicators of marginal deficiency and dysfunction. The rate of onset of clinical disease will depend on the intensity of the dietary deficiency, the duration of the deficit and the size of the initial reserve. If reserves are non-existent as with zinc metabolism, the effects may be acute and the separate phases become superimposed. The application of these principles to the interpretation of biochemical criteria of trace element status are presented later in this chapter where applicable under each mineral nutrient.

The definitive etiological diagnosis of a trace element deficiency will depend on the response in growth and health obtained following parenteral treatment or supplementation of the diet. The concurrent measurement of biochemical markers will aid in the interpretation and validation of those markers for future diagnosis. The strategies for anticipating and preventing trace element deficiencies include regular analysis of the feed and soil, which are not highly reliable, and monitoring samples from herds and flocks to prevent animals from entering the zone of marginal trace element deficiencies which precedes the onset of functional deficiency. The decision to intervene can be safely based on the conventional criteria of marginal trace element status.

REVIEW LITERATURE

Hansard, S. L. (1983) Microminerals for ruminant animals. *Nut. Abstr. Rev. Series B*, *53*, 1–24.

Mills, C. F. (1985) Changing perspectives in studies of the trace elements and animal health. In: *Trace Elements in Man and Animals. Proc. 5th Int. Symp.*, (eds) C. F. Mills, I. Bremner & J. K. Chesters. Commonwealth Agricultural Bureaux, pp. 1–10.

New Zealand Ministry of Agriculture and Fisheries (1982) Laboratory diagnosis of trace element deficiency disease. *Proc. Trace Element Workshop, June 1982 Surveillance, NZ*, 9, 24.

Reid, R. L. & Howath, D. J. (1980) Soil chemistry and mineral problems in farm livestock. A review. *Anim. Feed Sci. Technol.*, 5, 95–167.

Suttle, N. F. (1986) Problems in the diagnosis and anticipation of trace element deficiencies in grazing livestock. *Vet. Rec.*, *119*, 148–152.

Suttle, N. F., Gunn, R. G., Allen W. M., Linklater, K. A. & Wiener, G. (1983) *Trace Elements in Animal Production and Veterinary Practice*. Occasional publication No. 7 *Br. Soc. Anim. Prod.*

Underwood, E. J. (1981) *The Mineral Nutrition of Livestock*, 2nd edn. Commonwealth Agricultural Bureaux.

REFERENCES

(1) Mills, C. F. (1983) *Trace Elements in Animal Production and Veterinary Practice*. Occasional Publication, no. 7, British Society of Animal Production, pp. 1–10.

(2) Lewis, G. & Anderson, P. H. (1983) *Trace Elements in Animal Production and Veterinary Practice*. Occasional Publication no. 7, British Society of Animal Production, pp. 11–16.

(3) Suttle, N. F. (1983) *Trace Elements in Animal Production and Veterinary Practice*. Occasional Publication no. 7, British Society of Animal Production, pp. 19–27.

(4) Wiener, G. & Wooliams, J. A. (1983) *Trace Elements in Animal Production and Veterinary Practice*. Occasional Publication no. 7, British Society of Animal Production pp. 27–35.

(5) Thornton, I. (1983) *Trace Elements in Animal Production and Veterinary Practice*. Occasional Publication no. 7, British Society of Animal Production, pp. 39–49.

(6) Phillipo, M. (1983) *Trace Elements in Animal Production and Veterinary Practice*. Occasional Publication no. 7, British Society of Animal Production, pp. 51–61.

(7) Howell, J. Mc C. (1983) *Trace Elements in Animal Production and Veterinary Practice*. Occasional Publication no. 7, British Society of Animal Production, pp. 107–117.

(8) Suttle, N. F. (1986) *Vet. Rec.*, *119*, 148.

(9) Suttle, N. F. (1986) *Vet. Rec.*, *119*, 519.

(10) Mills, C. F. (1985) In: *Trace Elements in Man and Animals. Proc. 5th Int. Symp.*, eds C. F. Mills, I. Bremner, & J. K. Chesters. Commonwealth Agricultural Bureaux, pp. 1–10.

Cobalt deficiency

Etiology

The disease is caused by a deficiency of cobalt in the diet and characterized by anorexia and wasting.

Epidemiology

Cobalt deficiency is known to be of major importance in Australia, New Zealand, the United Kingdom and North America and probably occurs in many other parts of the world. Where the deficiency is extreme, large tracts of land have been found to be unsuitable for the raising of ruminants and in marginal areas suboptimal growth and production may be limiting factors in the husbandry of sheep and cattle.

Cattle and sheep are similarly affected and the signs are identical in both species. Cattle are slightly less susceptible than sheep, and lambs and calves are more seriously affected than adults. Frank deficiency is unlikely to occur in pigs, or in other omnivores or carnivores because vitamin B_{12} is present in meat and other animal tissues, but there are some reports of improved weight gains following supplementation of the ration with cobalt. Horses appear to be unaffected.

Primary cobalt deficiency occurs only on soils which are deficient in cobalt. Such soils do not appear to have any geological similarity, varying from wind-blown shell sands to soils derived from pumice and granite. Japanese soils composed largely of volcanic ash are seriously deficient (15). A survey in New Brunswick, Canada, revealed the average value for grass samples was 0·028 mg/kg and for legume samples, 0·088 mg/kg which justifies supplementation of ruminant diets with cobalt (27). The soils in New Brunswick are naturally acidic and with the heavy annual rainfall of 120 cm the cobalt content of the soil is decreased by leaching. Outbreaks of cobalt deficiency have occurred in cattle grazing on pastures on the granite-derived northern tablelands of New South Wales in Australia (28) and in sheep grazing pasture on soils derived from weathered rhyolite and ignimbrite, the former being inherently low in cobalt (29). Cobalt deficiency is now occurring in areas where it has never before been diagnosed and in seasons of lush spring and summer pasture growth, cobalt deficiency should be suspected as a cause of unthriftiness.

Although soils containing less than 0·25 mg/kg cobalt

are likely to produce pastures containing insufficient cobalt, the relationship between levels of cobalt in soil and pasture is not always constant (1). The factors governing the relationship have not been determined although heavy liming is known to reduce the availability of cobalt in the soil. Manganese appears to have a similar action but the agricultural significance of the relationship is unknown (2).

Pastures containing less than 0·07 and 0·04 mg/kg dry matter lead to the development of clinical signs in sheep and cattle respectively. The daily requirement for sheep at pasture is 0·08 mg/kg dry matter of cobalt; for growing lambs the need is somewhat greater and at pasture levels of less than 0·10 mg/kg dry matter inefficient rates of gain are likely. For growing cattle an intake of 0·04 mg/kg dry matter in the feed is just below requirements levels (4). Variations in the cobalt content of pasture occur with seasonal variations in pasture growth and with drainage conditions. The increased incidence of the disease which has been observed in the spring may be related to domination of the pasture by rapidly growing grasses which have a lower cobalt content than legumes. There is also a great deal of variation between years in the severity of the losses encountered due to variations in the cobalt status of the animals. Forage grown on well-drained soils has a greater cobalt content than that grown on poorly drained soils of the same cobalt status. Plant growth is not visibly affected by a low cobalt content of the soil but the addition of excessive quantities may retard growth.

Although the disease occurs most commonly in ruminants at pasture in severely deficient areas, sporadic cases occur in marginal areas especially after long periods of stable feeding. Bulls, rams and calves are the groups most commonly affected although dairy cows kept under the same conditions may develop a high incidence of ketosis.

Pathogenesis

Cobalt is peculiar as an essential trace element in ruminant nutrition in that it is stored in the body in limited amounts only and not in all tissues. In the adult ruminant its only known function is in the rumen and it must, therefore, be present continuously in the feed.

The effect of cobalt in the rumen is to participate in the production of vitamin B_{12} (cyanocobalamin) and compared to other species the requirement for vitamin B_{12} is very much higher in ruminants. In sheep the requirement is of the order of 11 μg/day and probably 500 μg/day are produced in the rumen, most being lost in the process (5). Animals in the advanced stages of cobalt deficiency are cured by the oral administration of cobalt or by the parenteral administration of vitamin B_{12}. On cobalt-deficient diets the appearance of signs is accompanied by a fall of as much as 90% in the vitamin B_{12} content of the feces, and on oral dosing with cobalt the signs disappear and vitamin B_{12} levels in the feces return to normal. Parenteral administration of cobalt is without appreciable clinical effect although some cobalt does enter the alimentary tract in the bile and leads to the formation of a small amount of cobalamin.

The essential defect in cobalt deficiency in ruminants is an inability to metabolize propionic acid, which is accompanied by a failure of appetite and death from inanition. The efficiency of cobalt in preventing staggers in sheep grazing pasture dominated by *Phalaris tuberosa*, and possibly by canary grass (*Phalaris minor*) or Rhompa grass, a hybrid *Phalaris* spp., is also unexplained. A suggestion that a dietary deficiency of cobalt can lead to the development of polioencephalomalacia (9) appears not to be valid (3). A specific hepatic dysfunction of sheep has been described in New Zealand, Australia (10) and in the United Kingdom (30). It has been called 'white liver disease' because of the grayish color of the liver (10). Clinically, it is manifested by photosensitization when the disease is acute, and anemia and emaciation when the disease is chronic. It seems likely that the disease is a toxic hepatopathy against which adequate levels of dietary cobalt (or thiamin) would be protective.

Clinical findings

No specific signs are characteristic of cobalt deficiency. A gradual decrease in appetite is the only obvious clinical sign. It is accompanied by loss of body weight and final emaciation and weakness, and these are often observed in the presence of abundant green feed. Pica is likely to occur, especially in cattle. There is marked pallor of the mucous membranes and affected animals are easily fatigued. Growth, lactation and wool production are severely retarded and the wool may be tender or broken. Infertility, diarrhea and lacrimation may be observed in the later stages. In sheep severe lacrimation with profuse outpouring of fluid sufficient to mat the wool of the face is one of the most important signs in advanced cases. Signs usually become apparent when animals have been on affected areas for about 6 months and death occurs in 3–12 months after the first appearance of illness, although severe wasting may be precipitated by the stress of parturition or abortion.

Clinical pathology

Estimation of the cobalt or vitamin B_{12} content of the liver, as set down under necropsy findings, is the most valuable diagnostic test available. All tests suffer from the disadvantage that tissue cobalt levels will reflect the cobalt intake for a considerable time prior to the estimation and animals suffering from acute cobalt deficiency may be observed to have normal tissue levels of the element. Estimations of the cobalt content of soils and pasture have limited value because of the seasonal variations which occur.

Cobalt concentrations in the plasma of normal sheep are of the order of 1–3 μg/dl (0·17–0·51 μmol/l) and in deficient animals these are reduced to 0·03–0·41 μmol/l. Clinical signs of cobalt deficiency in sheep are associated with serum vitamin B_{12} levels of less than 0·20 mg/ml and serum vitamin B_{12} levels are used as a laboratory test of cobalt status in animals. Levels of 0·2–0·25 μg/l are indicative of cobalt deficiency. These rise rapidly to 0·5–1·0 μg/l on treatment. The value of serum vitamin B_{12} assay as a diagnostic tool is in some doubt, but correctly interpreted they appear to be worthwhile (14). Radioassay methods for measuring serum and liver vitamin B_{12} in cattle and sheep have now replaced the microbiological assays (31). Serum vitamin B_{12} values greater than 0·2 μg/l are indicative of a normal vitamin B_{12} status in cattle (32). Deprivation of feed from sheep for 24 hours results in a marked increase in serum vitamin B_{12} (31). The serum vitamin B_{12} levels of sheep at pasture are unreliable indicators of liver vitamin B_{12} (31).

Because of some of the difficulties with the interpretation of serum vitamin B_{12} levels, attention has been diverted to other biochemical tests, especially methylmalonic acid (MMA) in plasma and urine as diagnostic and prognostic indicators (34) and formiminoglutamic acid (FIGLU) tests. The determination of MMA has the potential of being able to distinguish between subclinically and clinically affected which serum vitamin B_{12} cannot do (34).

The concentration of formiminoglutamic acid in urine was considered to be a reliable indicator of the cobalt status of lambs. Levels of 0·08–20 μmol/ml in the urine of affected lambs return to zero rapidly after treatment (1).

Methylmalonic acid is ordinarily metabolized in ruminants by a vitamin B_{12} enzyme system. In a cobalt-deficient animal the methylmalonic content of urine is abnormally high and this has some merit as a test for the presence of the deficiency (5, 11). However, recent observations indicate that the concentration of formiminoglutamic acid only increases in the urine of lambs in the later stages of cobalt deficiency when there is weight loss and illthrift (35). Animals with subclinical cobalt deficiency do not produce urinary formiminoglutamic acid at levels which would be useful diagnostically (35). Neither methylmalonic acid nor formiminoglutamic acid is a normal constituent of urine and their presence in urine, without the need for a quantitative measurement, is probably a positive indication of cobalt deficiency (1, 12). An unequivocal result for methylmalonic acid is a concentration of greater than 30 μg/ml for ten animals selected randomly from a flock (6). If the urine is kept for more than 24 hours it should be acidified to avoid degradation of the methylmalonic acid.

Affected animals are anemic, but their hemoglobin and erythrocyte levels are often within the normal range because of an accompanying hemoconcentration. The anemia is normocytic and normochromic. There is also a decrease in cellularity of the bone marrow in cobalt-deficient sheep. It is not repaired by the administration of vitamin B_{12} nor by the parenteral administration of cobalt. Affected animals are also hypoglycemic (less than 60 mg glucose per dl of plasma) and have low serum alkaline phosphatase levels (less than 20 i.u./liter) (4). The response to cobalt administration is matched by a very rapid return to normal of these levels. Unfortunately there are too many other factors which affect their concentration for them to be of much value in diagnostic work.

Necropsy findings

At necropsy, emaciation is extreme. Heavy deposits of hemosiderin in the spleen, and to a less extent in the liver, cause pigmentation of these organs. Biochemical estimations reveal very high iron levels in the liver and spleen and low cobalt levels in the liver. In normal sheep cobalt levels in the liver are usually above 0·20 mg/kg dry matter and in affected sheep are less than 0·07 mg/kg dry matter, 0·05 mg/kg dry matter appearing to be the critical level. Liver cobalt levels in cattle which are fed excessive amounts of cobalt and are thought to be affected by cobalt poisoning can be as high as 69 mg/kg dry matter (26).

Normal levels of vitamin B_{12} in the liver are of the order of 0·3 mg/kg, falling to 0·1 mg/kg in deficient lambs (16). Comparable figures for cattle are: clinical signs occur with liver vitamin B_{12} levels of less than 0·10 mg/kg, and levels of more than 0·3 mg/kg of liver are necessary for optimum growth (17). Normal levels of the vitamin of cattle in New Zealand are 0·70–1·98 mg/kg of liver (18). After oral dosing with cobalt the level of the element in the liver rises but returns to the pretreatment level in 10–30 days.

Diagnosis

The chief difficulty encountered in the field is to differentiate the condition from other causes of 'illthrift' or 'enzootic marasmus'. In young animals, in which this situation is most often encountered, nutritional deficiencies of copper, selenium and vitamin D are possible causes but by far the most important cause is internal parasitism. Lack of total digestible nutrients is the commonest cause of thin animals, but owners are usually aware of the shortage and do not present their animals for diagnosis. However, it does happen, especially with urban people who become farmers and are unaware of the actual needs of animals. So it is best to check the feed supply and also to check whether or not the animals have any teeth. These circumstances are seen so commonly in today's era of hobby farms that a new disease category 'hobby farm malnutrition' is warranted. Careful necropsy or fecal examination will determine the degree of worm infestation but cobalt-deficient animals are more susceptible to parasitism and the presence of a heavy parasite load should not rule out the diagnosis of primary cobalt deficiency (19). It is also common to have parasitic disease and cobalt deficiency occur together in the one animal. It is then necessary to make two diagnoses and conduct two control programs. In sheep special care is needed to differentiate the disease from Johne's disease. The differential diagnosis of anemia has been discussed elsewhere (p. 347).

The response of animals to dietary supplementation with cobalt is generally accepted as a diagnostic test but laboratory analysis of tissues may be necessary to confirm the diagnosis, especially as ruminants with poor appetites due to many causes may show a marked response to dosing with cobalt.

A new approach to defining mineral deficiencies is based on constructing response curves for any specified level of serum vitamin B_{12} that can be used to determine live weight response to supplementation and the probability of obtaining a response (36). The technique closely relates the tissue mineral or biochemical indicator with the degree of production response to treatment. The advantages of this method over the traditional method have been described (36).

Treatment

Affected animals respond satisfactorily to oral dosing with cobalt or the intramuscular injection of vitamin B_{12}. Oral dosing with vitamin B_{12} is effective but much larger doses are required. Oral dosing with cobalt sulfate is usually at the rate of about 1 mg cobalt/day in sheep and can be given in accumulated doses at the end of each week. Intervals of 2 weeks between dosing are inadequate for the best possible response. On the other hand the monthly dosing of lambs with oral doses of 300 mg of cobalt is sufficient to greatly reduce deaths and permit some growth at suboptimal levels (20). The response to dosing is very quick, significant elevation of serum vitamin B_{12} levels being evident within 24 hours. When large doses of cobalt are administered to some sheep, other undosed sheep on the same pasture may find sufficient additional cobalt on the pasture from the feces of their flockmates to meet their needs (21). No exact data are available on dose rates for cattle but ten times the prophylactic rate should be effective. Vitamin B_{12} should be given in 100–300 μg doses for lambs and sheep at weekly intervals (19). Vitamin B_{12} therapy is not likely to be used generally because of the high cost and the comparable effect of oral cobalt administration. However, vitamin B_{12} (hydroxycobalamin) may be a suitable therapeutic agent. One injection of 1 mg provides protection to lambs for 14 weeks, and for weaners protection for up to 40 weeks (13).

Overdosing with cobalt compounds is unlikely but toxic signs of loss of weight, rough hair coat, listlessness, anorexia and muscular incoordination appear in calves at dose rates of about 40–45 mg of elemental cobalt per 50 kg body weight per day. Sheep appear to be much more resistant to the toxic effects of cobalt than are cattle (22). Pigs have tolerated up to 200 mg cobalt/kg of diet. At intakes of 400 and 600 mg/kg there is growth depression, anorexia, stiff legs, incoordination and muscle tremors (8). Supplementation of the diet with methionine, or with additional iron, manganese and zinc alleviate the toxic effects.

Control

The recommended safe level of cobalt in the diet for sheep and cattle is 0·11 mg cobalt kg/dry matter diet (37). If this is not available, supplementation of the diet with cobalt is necessary. Calves reared on cobalt-deficient pastures require cobalt or vitamin B_{12} supplementation prior to weaning (33). Cobalt deficiency in grazing animals can be prevented most easily by the top-dressing of affected pasture with cobalt salts. The amount of top-dressing required will vary with the degree of deficiency. Recommendations include 400–600 g/ha cobalt sulfate annually or 1·2–1·5 kg/ha every 3–4 years. The response to pasture treatment is slow, requiring some weeks to complete. Affected animals should be treated orally or by injection of vitamin B_{12} to obtain a quick, interim response. Supplementation of the diet with 0·1 mg cobalt/day for sheep and 0·3–1·0 mg cobalt/day for cattle should be aimed at and this can be accomplished by inclusion of the cobalt in salt or a mineral mixture. Cobalt can also be supplied to cattle in their drinking water supply (38).

The use of 'heavy pellets' containing 90% cobalt oxide is an alternative means of overcoming the difficulty of maintaining an adequate cobalt intake in a deficient area. The pellet is in the form of a bolus (5 g for sheep, 20 g for cattle) which, when given by mouth, lodges in the reticulum and gives off cobalt continuously in very small but adequate amounts. Reports on their use in sheep and cattle indicate that they are effective (7, 8, 23). Administration of the pellets to lambs and calves less than 2 months old is likely to be ineffective because of failure to retain them in the undeveloped reticulum. The problem of cobalt deficiency in sucking animals can be overcome in part if the dams are treated because of the increased vitamin B_{12} content of their milk (24), but the daily intake of the lambs will still be much below the minimal requirement. In about 5% of animals the pellets do not lodge in the reticulum and approximately 20% are rejected during the year after administration (25). If no response occurs retreatment is advisable. A further possible cause of failure is where pellets become coated with calcareous material, particularly if the drinking water is highly mineralized or if pasture top-dressing is heavy. The effects of pellet coating can be overcome by simultaneous dosing with an abrasive metal pellet. The cost is relatively high and where top-dressing of pastures is practiced addition of cobalt to the fertilizer is the cheaper form of administration. Pellets are preferred in extensive range grazing where top-dressing is impracticable and animals are seen only at infrequent intervals.

Boluses of controlled release glass containing cobalt are available for oral administration to cattle and sheep. The boluses are retained in the forestomachs for up to several months and slowly release cobalt (39).

REVIEW LITERATURE

Robertson, W. W. (1971) *Vet. Rec.*, *89*, 5.

REFERENCES

(1) Russell, A. J. F. (1975) *Vet. Rec.*, *96*, 194.
(2) Pfander, W. H. et al. (1966) *Fedn Proc. Fedn Am. Socs exp. Biol.*, *25*, 431.
(3) Edwin E. E. (1978) *Vet. Rec.*, *101*, 393.
(4) McPherson, A. et al. (1973) *Br. vet. J.*, *129*, 414.
(5) Smith, R. M. & Marston, H. R. (1970) *Br. J. Nutr.*, *24*, 615, 857.
(6) Miller, K. R. & Lorentz, P. P. (1979) *NZ vet. J.*, *27*, 90.
(7) Givens D. I. et al. (1979) *Vet. Rec.*, *104*, 508.
(8) Huck, D. W. & Clawson, A. J. (1976) *J. anim. Sci.*, *43*, 1231.
(9) Macpherson, A. et al. (1977) *Vet. Rec.*, *101*, 231.
(10) Richards, R. B. & Harrison, M. R. (1981) *Aust. vet. J.*, *57*, 565.
(11) Andrews, E. D. & Hogan, K. C. (1972) *NZ vet. J.*, *20*, 33.
(12) Hogan, K. G. et al. (1973) *NZ vet. J.*, *21*, 234.
(13) Hannam, R. J. et al. (1980) *Aust. J. agr. Res.*, *31*, 347.
(14) Sutherland, R. J. (1980) *NZ vet. J.*, *28*, 169.
(15) Kobayashi, Y. et al. (1980) *Jap. agric. Res. Q.*, *14*, 63.
(16) Andrews, E. D. & Hart, L. I. (1962) *NZ J. agric. Res.*, *5*, 403.
(17) Dewey, D. W. et al. (1969) *Aust. J. agric. Res.*, *20*, 1109.
(18) Rammell, C. G. & Poole, W. S. W. (1974) *NZ vet. J.*, *22*, 167.
(19) Andrews, E. D et al. (1970) *NZ J agric. Res.*, *13*, 950.
(20) Andrews, E. D. et al. (1966) *NZ vet. J.*, *14*, 191.
(21) Findlay, C. R. (1972) *Vet. Rec.*, *90*, 468.
(22) Andrews, E. D. (1965) *NZ vet. J.*, *13*, 101.
(23) Skerman, K. D. et al. (1961) *Aust. vet. J.*, *37*, 181.
(24) Skerman, K. D. & O'Halloran, M. W. (1962) *Aust. vet. J.*, *38*, 98.
(25) Millar, K. R. & Andrews, E. D. (1964) *NZ vet. J.*, *12*, 9.
(26) Dickson, J. & Bond, M. P. (1974) *Aust. vet. J.*, *50*, 236.
(27) Nicholson, J. W. G. (1986) *Can. J. anim. Sci.*, *66*, 559.
(28) Duncan, I. F. et al. (1986) *Aust. vet. J.*, *63*, 127.
(29) Clark, R. G. et al. (1985) *NZ vet. J.*, *33*, 218.

(30) McLoughlin, M. F. et al. (1984) *Vet Rec.*, *115*, 325.
(31) Millar, K. R. et al. (1984) *NZ vet. J.*, *32*, 65.
(32) MacPherson, A. (1981) In: *Proc. 4th International Symposium on Trace Element Metabolism in Man and Animals*, (eds) J. McC. Howell, J. M. Cawthorne & C. L. White, Canberra: Aust. Acad. Sciences, p. 58.
(33) Judson, G. J. et al. (1982) *Aust. vet. J.*, *58*, 249.
(34) McMurray, C. H. et al. (1985) In: *Trace Elements in Man and Animals—TEMA 5. Proc. 5th Int. Symp. Trace Elements in Man and Animals* (eds) C. F. Mills, I. Bremner & J. K. Chesters. Commonwealth Agricultural Bureaux, pp. 603–608.
(35) Stebbings, R. St & Lewis, G. (1986) *Br. vet. J.*, *142*, 270.
(36) Clark, R. G. et al. (1985) *NZ vet. J.*, *33*, 1.
(37) Agric. Res. Council (1980) *The Nutrient Requirements of Ruminant Livestock*. Commonwealth Agricultural Bureaux.
(38) MacPherson, A. (1983) *Trace Elements in Animal Production and Veterinary Practice*. British Society of Animal Production Occasional publication no. 7, p. 93.
(39) Allen, W. M. et al. (1985) *Vet. Rec.*, *116*, 175.

Copper deficiency

Copper deficiency occurs primarily in young ruminants resulting in a range of clinical manifestations including unthriftiness, diarrhea, lameness, demyelination of the central nervous system in neonates, anemia in the later stages of deficiency and falling disease. Some minor syndromes occur in the horse and pig.

Etiology

Copper deficiency may be *primary*, when the intake in the diet is inadequate, or *secondary* (conditioned) when the dietary intake is sufficient but the utilization of the copper by tissues is impeded.

Primary copper deficiency

The amount of copper in the diet may be inadequate when the forage is grown on deficient soils or on soils in which the copper is unavailable.

Secondary copper deficiency

There are many disease states in ruminants in which clinical signs are caused by a deficiency of copper in tissues and in which the administration of copper is preventive and curative but in which the copper intake in the diet appears to be adequate. Such secondary copper deficiencies are summarized in Table 85. The conditioning factor is known only in some instances, a dietary excess of molybdenum being most frequently incriminated. Zinc, iron, lead and calcium carbonate are also considered to be conditioning agents and in New Zealand the administration of selenium to sheep on copper-deficient pastures has been shown to increase copper intake by the sheep, and improve the growth rate of lambs. Experimentally, a high zinc maternal diet can result in copper deficiency in neonatal piglets (65). The use of zinc sulfate for the control of facial eczema may cause a depression of plasma copper levels which can be alleviated by the injection of copper glycinate (72). A high molybdenum intake can induce copper deficiency even when the copper content of the pasture is quite high, and a higher copper intake can overcome the effect of the molybdenum. Conversely, supplementation of the diet with molybdenum can be used to counteract the copper intake when its content in the diet is dangerously high. There are species differences in response to high copper and molybdenum intake; sheep are much more susceptible to copper poisoning, cattle to excess molybdenum. Reduction in copper absorption has been produced experimentally in ponies by adding molybdenum to the diet (64).

Dietary inorganic sulfate in combination with molybdenum has a profound effect on the uptake of copper by ruminants. For example, an increase of sulfate concentration in a sheep diet from 0·1 to 0·4% can potentiate a molybdenum content as low as 2 mg/kg (0·02 mmol/kg) to reduce copper intake below normal levels (5). Additional sulfate in the diet also has a depressing effect on the absorption of selenium so that areas of a country which have marginal copper and selenium levels in the soil may produce deficiency syndromes in animals if sulfate is added; this is likely to happen when heavy dressings of superphosphate are applied. Such combined deficiencies are becoming more common. The possibility of interaction between copper and selenium must also be considered because of the reported failure of animals to respond to treatment unless both elements are provided.

Epidemiology

Causes of wastage

Copper deficiency causes diseases of economic importance in many parts of the world and may be sufficient to render large areas of otherwise fertile land unsuitable for grazing by ruminants. Based on serum copper surveys of cattle herds in Britain, copper deficiency constitutes a serious problem in animal agriculture which requires vigilance (66). It is estimated that characteristic clinical signs of copper deficiency develop annually in about 0·9% of the cattle population in the United Kingdom (107). In some surveys the lowest levels of serum copper

Table 85. Secondary copper deficiency states.

Disease	*Country*	*Species affected*	*Copper level in liver*	*Probable conditioning factor*
Swayback	Britain, United States	Sheep	Low	Unknown
Renguerra	Peru	Sheep	Low	Unknown
Teart	Britain	Sheep and cattle	Unknown	Molybdenum
Scouring disease	Holland	Cattle	Unknown	Unknown
Peat scours	New Zealand	Cattle	Low	Molybdenum
Peat scours	Britain	Cattle	Unknown, low level in blood	Unknown
Peat scours	Canada	Cattle	Unknown	Molybdenum
Salt sick	Florida (United States)	Cattle	Unknown	Unknown
'Pine' (unthrifty)	Scotland	Calves	Low	Unknown

were in heifers being reared as heifer replacements (67). Although heavy mortalities occur in affected areas the major loss is due to failure of animals to thrive. Enzootic ataxia may affect up to 90% of a lamb flock in badly affected areas and most of these lambs die of inanition. In falling disease, up to 40% of cattle in affected herds may die.

Age susceptibility

Apart from falling disease which occurs only in adult cattle, young animals are much more susceptible to primary copper deficiency than are adults. Calves on dams fed deficient diets may show signs at 2–3 months of age. As a rule the signs are severe in calves and yearlings, less severe in 2-year-olds and of minor degree in adults. Enzootic ataxia is primarily a disease of sucking lambs whose dams receive insufficient dietary copper. Ewes with a normal copper status take some time to lose their hepatic reserves of copper after transfer to copper-deficient pastures and do not produce affected lambs for the first 6 months. The occurrence of the disease in sucklings, and its failure to appear after weaning, point to the importance of fetal stores of copper and the inadequacy of milk as a source of copper. Milk is always a poor source of copper and when it is the sole source of nourishment the intake of copper will be low. Milk from normal ewes contains 20–60 μg/dl (3·1–9·4 μmol/l) copper, but under conditions of severe copper deficiency this may be reduced to 1–2 μg/dl (0·16–0·31 μmol/l).

Breed susceptibility

There are marked genetic differences in copper metabolism between breeds of sheep. The Welsh Mountain ewe can absorb copper 50% more efficiently than the Scottish blackface (1) and the Texel cross blackface 145% greater than pure blackface lambs (1). It is now apparent that the sheep's susceptibility to or protection from the effects of copper deficiency, and also copper poisoning, is influenced from birth by genetic effects (49). These affect copper status of the lamb at birth, through the maternal environment controlled by the dam's genes and through the effect of the lamb's own genes. Later in life, the animal's own genes become the predominant influence determining its copper status on any given nutritional regime. These genetic differences have been found to have physiological consequences reflected in differences in the incidence of swayback, both between and within breeds, and in effects on growth and possibly on reproduction. The differences observed are due to genetic differences in the efficiency of absorption of dietary copper.

The genetic effects determining the copper status of the lamb are already present *in utero* and the effects appear not to be controlled by the lamb's own genotype but by that of its dam. The maternal effect is still present at weaning at 9 weeks of age but disappears after weaning when the genetic differences are due to the sheep's own genotype.

The existence of genes which determine plasma copper has been shown by the successful continued selection for high and low concentrations in closed lines of a single breed type. Ram selection is made on the basis of plasma copper concentrations at 18 and 24 weeks of age. The proportion of the normal variation in plasma copper that is heritable is 0·3. The high line female sheep retain more copper in the liver than the low line females which is caused by a positive correlation between the concentration of copper in plasma and the efficiency of absorption (110, 111).

The evidence for genetic variation in the copper metabolism of sheep has important physiological consequences. Breeds show wide variation in their susceptibility to swayback; the incidence of swayback may vary from 0 to 40% between breeds within one flock, and the incidence according to breed type is closely related to the differences in the concentration of copper in the liver than in blood. When these high and low female lines are placed on improved and limed pasture, which can induce a severe copper deficiency, soon after birth there are indications of swayback, general dullness, lack of vigor and mortality in the lambs. By 6 weeks of age the mortality rate was higher in the lambs from the low copper line than in those from the high copper line. In addition, at 6 weeks of age, lambs from the low line were 2 kg lighter than those in the high line.

Fetal liver copper

The developing bovine fetus obtains its copper by placental transfer and at birth the liver concentration of copper is high and declines postnatally to adult levels within the first few months. Placental transfer is less efficient in sheep, and lambs are commonly born with low liver reserves which makes the neonatal lambs susceptible to copper deficiency (71). The young mixed-fed animal is able to absorb about 80% of its copper intake, but the efficiency of absorption declines with age as the rumen becomes functional, when only 2–10% of available copper is absorbed (68). Colostrum is rich in copper which allows the newborn with its preferential ability to absorb copper to increase hepatic stores. Later, the copper content of milk declines rapidly so that it is usually insufficient to meet the requirements of the sucking neonate for copper (69). In copper deficient cattle, the accumulation of liver copper in the fetus continues independent of the dam's liver copper until the fetus is about 180 days, then a gradual decline in fetal liver copper occurs (70). The liver copper concentration in fetuses from dams on a copper adequate diet continues to increase and not decline at 180 days of gestation (70).

Seasonal prevalence

Both primary and secondary copper deficiency occur most commonly in spring and summer coinciding with the time at which the copper content of the pasture is lowest.

There are large monthly variations in the serum levels of copper in both beef and dairy cattle. The variations are commonly correlated with the rainfall; the higher the rainfall the lower the copper level (4).

However, in some cases of secondary copper deficiency, the incidence may be highest at other times depending upon the concentration of the conditioning factor in the forage. For example, the molybdenum content may be highest in the autumn when rains stimulate a heavy growth of legumes.

Pasture composition
The absorption (or availability) of copper is influenced by the type of diet, the presence of other substances in the diet such as molybdenum, sulfur and iron, the interaction between the type of diet and the chemical composition of the diet and the genetic constitution of the animals (1). Copper is well absorbed from diets low in fiber such as cereals and brassicas but poorly absorbed from fresh forage. Conservation of grass as hay or silage generally improves its availability. This explains why copper deficiency is a problem of the grazing animal and seen only rarely in housed ruminants receiving diets which are commonly adequate in copper.

Only small increases in the molybdenum and sulfur concentration of grass will cause major reductions in the availability of copper (1). This is especially notable in ruminants grazing improved pastures in which the molybdenum and sulfur concentrations were increased. It is now accepted that the copper content of feedstuffs should be expressed in terms of available copper concentration, using appropriate equations, which will permit the more accurate prediction of clinical disease and can be used for more effective control strategies.

The effect of changes in molybdenum and sulfur concentrations in grass on the availability of copper is changed by conservation; at a given concentration of sulfur, the antagonistic effect of molybdenum is proportionately less in hay than in fresh grass. At a low concentration of molybdenum the effect of sulfur is more marked in silage than in fresh grass. The use of formaldehyde as a silage additive may weaken the copper sulfur antagonism and yield material of high availability (1). Thus, fields of herbage high in molybdenum should be used for conservation when possible and sulfuric acid should not be used as an additive for silage unless accompanied by a copper salt because it significantly raises the sulfur concentration of the silage.

For general purposes it may be assumed that pasture containing less than 3 mg/kg dry matter of copper will produce signs of deficiency in grazing ruminants. Levels of 3–5 mg/kg dry matter can be considered as dangerous and levels greater than 5 mg/kg dry matter (preferably 7–12) can be considered as safe unless complicating factors cause secondary copper deficiency. The extreme complexity of minimum copper requirements, affected as they are by numerous conditioning factors, necessitates examination under each particular set of circumstances. For example, plant molybdenum levels are related directly to the pH reaction of the soil. Grasses grown on strongly acidic molybdenum-rich soils are characterized by low molybdenum values (less than 3 mg/kg), whereas those associated with alkaline molybdenum-poor soils may contain up to 17 mg/kg (12). Thus, it seems likely that conditioned copper deficiency can be related to regionally enhanced levels of plant available rather than soil molybdenum. Heavily limed pastures are often associated with a less than normal copper intake and a low copper status of sheep grazing them. Secondary copper deficiency is also recorded in pigs whose drinking water contains very large amounts of sulfate (22).

The presence of iron salts in the diet can interfere with copper metabolism (3). Ruminants obtain iron from ingested soil and mineral supplements and in areas where hypocuprosis is likely to occur, the risk can be minimized by avoiding the use of mineral supplements of high iron content, minimizing the use of bare winter pasture and avoiding the excessive contamination of silage with soil during harvesting.

Stored feeds
Livestock that are housed, are in a different position to those on pasture. Concentrates and proprietary feeds tend to contain adequate copper. Pasture is less likely to contain sufficient of the mineral, especially in early spring when the grass growth is lush. Silage and haylage may be very deficient in copper. Hay will be more mature and contain more of all minerals, so that animals that are housed for the winter are protected against copper deficiency for a few weeks after they come out onto pasture in the spring. Young growing animals will be first affected. These comments should not be interpreted to mean that housed or feedlot animals cannot be affected by hypocuprosis. They can if the locally produced feed is copper-deficient, or more likely has a high concentration of molybdenum (19). Both are likely to be prevented or less severe if there is some supplementary feeding.

Soil characteristics—copper deficiency
In general there are two types of soil on which copper-deficient plants are produced. Sandy soils, poor in organic matter and heavily weathered, such as occur on the coastal plains of Australia, and in marine and river silts, are likely to be absolutely deficient in copper as well as other trace elements, especially cobalt. The second important group of soils are 'peat' or muck soils reclaimed from swamps, and are soils more commonly associated with copper deficiency in the United States, New Zealand and Europe. Such soils may have an absolute deficiency of copper, but more commonly the deficiency is relative in that the copper is not available and the plants growing on the soils do not contain adequate amounts of the element. The cause of the lack of availability of the copper is uncertain, but is probably the formation of insoluble organic copper complexes. An additional factor is the production of secondary copper deficiency on these soils due to their high content of molybdenum. A summary of the relevant levels of copper in soils and plants is given in Table 86.

Soil characteristics—molybdenum excess
In general terms, pastures containing less than 3 mg/kg dry matter of molybdenum are considered to be safe, but clinical signs may occur at 3–10 mg/kg if the copper intake is low. Pastures containing more than 10 mg/kg of molybdenum are dangerous unless the diet is supplemented with copper. Excess molybdenum may occur in soils up to levels of 10 and even 100 mg/kg. Perhaps more dangerous is the risk that overzealous application of molybdenum to pasture to increase bacterial nitrogen fixation may have similar effects which are likely to be longlasting.

In the United Kingdom, appreciable land is underlain by marine black shales rich in molybdenum which results in a high content of molybdenum in the soil and pastures and a secondary copper deficiency (10, 11)

Table 86. Copper levels of soils and plants in primary and secondary copper deficiency.

Condition	*Area*	*Soil type*	*Soil copper mg/kg*	*Plant copper (mg/kg dry matter)*
Normal	—	—	18–22	11
Primary copper deficiency	West Australia	Various	1–2	3–5
	New Zealand	Sand	0·1–1·6	3
	New Zealand	Peat	—	3
	Holland	Sand	—	<3
Secondary copper deficiency	New Zealand	Peat	5	7
	Britain	Peat	—	7–20
	Britain	Limestone	—	12–27
	Britain	Stiff clay	—	11
	Ireland	Shale deposits, peat marine alluvial soils		
	Holland	Sand	—	>5
	Canada	Burned-over peat	20–60	10–25

which potentially limits livestock performance. Secondary (conditioned) copper deficiency is now recognized in cattle in many parts of Canada. Large areas of west-central Manitoba are underlain by molybdeniferous shale bedrocks and the soils contain up to 20 mg/kg of molybdenum (12). However, in the same geographical location hypocupremia may be associated with a primary deficiency of copper in the forage (9) or a secondary copper deficiency due to molybdenum in the forages (12).

Geographic distribution
The diseases caused by a primary deficiency of copper in ruminants are enzootic ataxia of sheep in Australia, New Zealand and the United States, licking sickness, or *liksucht* of cattle in Holland, and falling disease of cattle in Australia. In pigs, copper deficiency may cause anemia in sucking pigs and on experimental diets an unusual abnormality of the limbs, characterized by lack of rigidity in the joints, has been observed. Adult horses are unaffected, but there have been reports of abnormalities of the limbs and joints of foals reared in copper-deficient areas.

A concurrent deficiency of both copper and cobalt occurs in Australia (coast disease) and Florida, United States (salt sickness) and is characterized by the appearance of clinical signs of both deficiencies. All species of ruminants are affected. The disease is controlled by supplementation of the diet with copper and cobalt as set out under those specific headings.

The diseases caused by secondary copper deficiency, mostly due to high dietary intakes of molybdenum and sulfate, are listed in Table 85. They include syndromes characterized by diarrhea or by unthriftiness. Another syndrome is 'yellow calf', a disease of nursing calves that is widespread on Hawaii's rangeland where copper content of forages ranges from 2·6 to 11·8 mg/kg and the molybdenum from less than 1–39 mg/kg (14). Swayback of lambs in the United Kingdom has been classed as a secondary copper deficiency, but no conditioning factor has been determined. Lead has been suggested in this connection and does appear to reduce blood and liver concentrations of copper, but seems to have little effect on the incidence of swayback in the United Kingdom. Recent work on swayback suggests that the naturally occurring disease is caused by a primary deficiency of copper, but identical lesions are produced experimentally by feeding molybdenum and sulfate to the ewes. There is some evidence that heavy lime dressing of a pasture may predispose to swayback (106). Similar clinical and histopathological changes to those of enzootic ataxia of lambs have been observed in pigs with low levels of copper in their livers. A wasting disease similar to peat scours, and preventable by the administration of copper, and unthriftiness ('pine') of calves, both occur in the United Kingdom, but in both instances the copper and molybdenum intakes are normal. Molybdenum appears to be the conditioning agent in enzootic ataxia in the United States. A dietary excess of molybdenum is known to be the conditioning factor in the diarrheic diseases, peat scours in New Zealand, California and Canada, and 'teart' in Britain.

Pathogenesis—effects on tissues
Copper plays an important role in tissue oxidation by either supplementing cytochrome oxidase systems or entering into their formation. Ceruloplasmin is the copper-containing enzyme through which copper exerts its physiological function. The pathogenesis of most of the lesions of copper deficiency has been explained in terms of faulty tissue oxidation because of failure of these enzyme systems (16). This role is exemplified in the early stages of copper deficiency by the changes in the wool of sheep.

Wool
The straightness and stringiness of this wool is due to inadequate keratinization due probably to imperfect oxidation of free thiol groups. Provision of copper to such sheep is followed by oxidation of these free thiol groups and a return to normal keratinization within a few hours.

Body weight
In the later stages the impairment of tissue oxidation causes interference with intermediary metabolism and loss of condition or failure to grow.

Diarrhea
The role of copper deficiency in causing diarrhea is probably of the same functional order. There are no

histological changes in gut mucosa, although villous atrophy is recorded in severe, experimentally produced cases (20). However, diarrhea is usually only a major clinical finding in secondary copper deficiency associated with molybdenosis.

Anemia
The known importance of copper in the formation of hemoglobin accounts for the anemia that occurs in deficient animals. In view of the heavy hemosiderin deposits in tissues of copper-deficient animals, it is probable that copper is necessary for the reutilization of iron liberated from the normal breakdown of hemoglobin. There is no evidence of excessive hemolysis in copper-deficiency states. Anemia may occur in the later stages of primary copper deficiency, but is not remarkable in the secondary form unless there is a marginal copper deficiency as occurs in peat scours in New Zealand. The unusual relationship in New Zealand between copper deficiency and postparturient hemoglobinuria is unexplained.

Bone
The osteoporosis which occurs in some natural cases of copper deficiency is caused by the depression of osteoblastic activity (21). In experimentally induced primary copper deficiency, the skeleton is osteoporotic and there is a significant increase in osteoblastic activity. There is a marked overgrowth of epiphyseal cartilage especially at costochondral junctions and in metatarsal bones (63). This is accompanied by beading of the ribs and enlargement of the long bones (43). There is also an impairment of collagen formation. When the copper deficiency is secondary to dietary excesses of molybdenum and sulfate, the skeletal lesions are quite different. There is widening of the growth plate and metaphysis, and active osteoblastic activity (17). Copper deficiency has been implicated but not yet adequately substantiated in osteochondrosis of sucking foals (7).

Connective tissue
Copper is a component of the enzyme lysyl oxidase, secreted by the cells involved in the synthesis of the elastin component of connective tissues and has important functions in maintaining the integrity of tissues such as capillary beds, ligaments and tendons (113).

Heart
The myocardial degeneration of falling disease may be a terminal manifestation of anemic anoxia or be due to interference with tissue oxidation. In this disease it is thought that the stress of calving and lactation contribute to the development of heart block and ventricular fibrillation when there has already been considerable decrease in cardiac reserve.

Blood vessels
Experimentally produced copper deficiency has also caused sudden death due to rupture of the heart and great vessels in a high proportion of pigs fed a copper-deficient diet (25). The basic defect is degeneration of the internal elastic laminae. There is no record of a similar, naturally occurring disease. A similar relationship appears to have been established between serum copper levels and fatal rupture of the uterine artery at parturition in aged mares (27).

Pancreas
Lesions of the pancreas may be present in clinically normal cattle with a low blood copper status (73). The lesions consist of an increase in dry matter content and a reduction in the concentrations of protein and copper in wet tissue. The cytochrome oxidase activity and protein: RNA ratio are also reduced. There are defects in acinar basement membranes, splitting and disorganization of acini, cellular atrophy and dissociation, and stromal proliferation.

Nervous tissue
The mechanism by which copper deficiency halts the formation of myelin and causes demyelination in lambs has not yet been established although it appears probable that there is a specific relationship between copper and the maintenance of myelin sheaths. It is evident that defective myelination can commence as early as the midpoint of the fetus's uterine life (23). In experimental animals it has been shown that copper deficiency does interfere with the synthesis of phospholipids. While anoxia is a cause of demyelination, and an anemic anoxia is likely to occur in highly deficient ewes, and anemic ewes do produce a higher proportion of lambs with enzootic ataxia, there is often no anemia in ewes producing lambs with the more common subacute form of the disease. Severely deficient ewes have lambs which are affected at birth and in which myelin formation is likely to have been prevented. The lambs of ewes less severely deficient have normal myelination at birth, and develop demyelination in postnatal life (24).

Reproductive performance
There are conflicting reports on the role of copper deficiency in dairy cows (35). Recent field evidence indicates that the injection of cattle with copper glycinate did not affect the average interval between calving and first observed heat, services per conception or first service conception rate, compared to untreated cows in the same population (28). It appears inadvisable to ascribe poor reproductive performance to subclinical hypocuprosis on the evidence of blood copper analysis alone. Other factors such as management, and energy and protein intake should be examined.

Immune system
Copper deficiency has been implicated in the impaired function of the immune defence system in several species (77). Subclinical copper deficiency in laboratory mice is associated with an increased susceptibility to experimental infections with *Pasteurella hemolytica* (77). The severity of copper depletion needed for immune dysfunction is less than required to induce clinical signs of copper deficiency and endogenous copper may contribute to the regulation of both non-immune and immune inflammatory responses (78). Copper may also have a role in the mechanism of cell-mediated immunity in sheep infected with *Trichostrongylus* spp. (79). There is evidence that low molecular weight complexes have an

anti-inflammatory effect in animal models of inflammation, and it is postulated that the elevation of plasma copper-containing components during inflammatory disease represents a physiological response (80).

Sequence of sign development
In experimental copper deficiency in calves, beginning at 6 weeks of age, subclinical and clinical abnormalities appear after the following intervals: hypocupremia at 15 weeks, growth retardation from 15 to 18 weeks, rough hair coat at 17 weeks, diarrhea at 20 weeks and leg abnormalities at 23 weeks. These signs correlate well with the onset of hypocupremia and are indicative of a severe deficiency (16). Even with these signs of deficiency, the histological abnormalities may be only minor in degree.

In experimental primary copper deficiency begun in calves at 12 weeks of age, clinical signs of the deficiency were not apparent for about 6 months (18). Musculoskeletal abnormalities included a stilted gait, a 'knock-kneed' appearance of the forelimbs, overextension of the flexors, splaying of the hooves and swellings around the metacarpophalangeal and carpometacarpal joints. Changes in hair pigmentation occur after about 5 months and diarrhea between 5 and 7 months. The diarrhea ceased 12 hours after oral administration of a small amount (10 mg) of copper.

Pathogenesis: copper–molybdenum–sulfate relationship
Secondary or conditioned copper deficiency occurs when the dietary intake of copper is considered to be adequate, but absorption and utilization of the copper are inadequate because of the presence of interfering substances in the diet. Molybdenum and sulfate alone or in combination can affect copper metabolism and the mechanisms by which this occurs are now being clarified. This effect also operates in the fetus and interferes with copper storage in the fetal liver. Besides the relationship with molybdenum an interaction between the absorption of copper and selenium has been demonstrated, the administration of selenium to sheep on copper-deficient pastures causing an improvement in copper absorption (36). There is now definitive evidence that decreased resistance to infection is a clinical consequence of naturally occurring copper deficiency in sheep which is amenable to treatment with copper and genetic selection (108). In lambs genetically selected for low and high concentrations of plasma copper the mortality from birth to 24 weeks of age in the high line was half that in the low line. Most of the losses were due to a variety of microbial infections.

Copper absorption
On the basis of a response to copper injections and no response to copper administered orally to sheep on a high molybdenum intake, it is suggested that interference occurs with the absorption of copper from the gut (8).

It is proposed that thiomolybdates form in the rumen from the reaction of dietary molybdenum compounds with sulfides produced from the reduction of dietary sulfur compounds by rumen bacteria. The thiomolybdates reduce the absorption of dietary copper from the intestine and also inhibit a number of copper containing enzymes including ceruloplasmin, cytochrome oxidase, superoxide dismutase and tyrosine oxidase (29).

The toxicity of any particular level of dietary molybdenum is affected by the ratio of the dietary molybdenum to dietary copper. The critical copper : molybdenum ratio in animal feeds is 2 and feeds or pasture with lower ratio may result in conditioned copper deficiency. In some regions of Canada, the copper to molybdenum ratio will vary from 0·1 to 52·7 (30). Higher critical ratios closer to 4·1–5·1 have been recommended for safety (31). The influence of dietary molybdenum on copper metabolism in ponies has been examined experimentally (63).

Copper utilization
This can be affected by sulfate and molybdate by interference with mobilization of copper from the liver, inhibition of copper intake by the tissues and possibly inhibition of copper transport both into and out of the liver, and inhibition of the synthesis of copper-storage complexes and ceruloplasmin (29). The experimental intravenous injection of trithiomolybdate into cattle results in retention or accumulation of copper in plasma by a three-way interaction between trithiomolybdate, albumin and copper (81).

Hepatic storage
When sheep are fed a copper-deficient diet, both molybdate alone and sulfate alone will decrease the levels of copper in plasma, liver and kidney as well as decreasing ceruloplasmic activity. When both molybdate and sulfate are added together in the diet, there is an increased plasma copper which does not result in an increase in ceruloplasmin activity. There is depletion of both stores of copper which occurs via an increased urinary excretion of copper (29). The liver copper status appears to depend on whether the animals are receiving adequate dietary copper. With adequate dietary levels, the liver copper levels are less in the presence of molybdate and sulfate. If the animals are receiving a copper-deficient diet such that copper is being removed from the liver, then the molybdate plus sulfate animals retain more copper in their liver than copper-deficient animals not receiving sulfate plus molybdate. It would appear to support the hypothesis that molybdate and sulfate together impair the movement of copper into or out of the liver, possibly by affecting copper transport. Sulfate alone exerts an effect. An increase in intake reduces hepatic storage of both copper and molybdenum (46).

Tissue utilization
It is known that clinical signs of hypocuprosis (such as steely wool) can occur in sheep on diets containing high levels of molybdenum and sulfate even though blood copper levels are high. This suggests that under these circumstances copper is not utilizable in tissues and the blood copper rises in response to the physiological needs of the tissues for the element. Work with pigs has shown that a copper–molybdenum complex can exist in animals and that in this form the copper is unavailable. This would interfere with hepatic metabolism of copper and the formation of copper–protein complexes such as ceruloplasmin (33).

Summary
The overall effect of these interactions is most simply described in the following terms. Molybdate reacts with sulfides to produce thiomolybdates in the rumen. The subsequent formation of copper–thiomolybdate complexes isolates the copper from being biologically available (8). The thiomolybdates also appear to be effective in tissues in that they reduce the effectiveness of enzymes containing copper (29).

Clinical findings
The general effects of copper deficiency are the same in sheep and cattle, but in addition to these general syndromes there are specific syndromes more or less restricted to species and to areas. What follows is a general description of the disease caused by copper deficiency, in turn followed by the specific syndromes of enzootic ataxia, swayback, falling disease, peat scours, teart and unthriftiness (pine).

COPPER DEFICIENCY SYNDROMES IN CATTLE

Subclinical hypocuprosis: cattle
No clinical signs occur, blood copper levels are marginal or below 57 mg/dl (9·0 mmol/l) and there is a variable response in productivity after supplementation with copper. Some surveys in copper-deficient areas have shown that about 50% of beef herds and 10% of dairy herds within the same area have low blood levels of blood copper associated with low copper intake from natural forages (13, 38). As set out in Chapter 1, the deficiency is likely to be suspected only if production is monitored and found to be supoptimal. One of the earliest indicators could be an increase in the occurrence of no visible estrus cows in a dairy herd. There is an increasing tendency to carry out large-scale geochemical surveys to define areas which are marginally deficient in one or more elements (39).

A perplexing feature of subclinical hypocuprosis is the wide variation in improved growth rate obtained when cattle of the same low copper status are given supplementary copper under field conditions (112).

General syndrome—primary copper deficiency: cattle
Primary copper deficiency causes unthriftiness, loss of milk production and anemia in adult cattle. An increased occurrence of postparturient hemoglobinuria is also recorded (40), but only in New Zealand and is likely to have other etiological complications. The coat color is affected, red and black cattle changing to a bleached, rusty red, and the coat itself becomes rough and staring. Calves grow poorly, sometimes have chronic diarrhea, and there is an increased tendency for bones to fracture, particularly the limb bones including the scapula. In some cases ataxia develops after exercise, there being a sudden loss of control of the hindlimbs with the animal falling or subsiding into a sitting posture. Normal control returns after rest. Itching and hair-licking is also recorded as a manifestation of copper deficiency in cattle (42). Although diarrhea occurs, persistent scouring is not characteristic of primary copper deficiency and its frequent occurrence should arouse suspicion of molybdenosis or helminthiasis. In some affected areas, calves have been observed to develop stiffness and enlargement of the joints and contraction of the flexor tendons causing the affected animals to stand on their toes. These signs may be present at birth or occur before weaning. Paresis and incoordination are not evident.

General syndrome—secondary copper deficiency: cattle
The syndrome caused by secondary copper deficiency include the signs of primary copper deficiency except that anemia occurs less commonly. This is probably due to the relatively better copper status in the secondary state, anemia being largely a terminal sign in primary copper deficiency. For example, anemia occurs in peat scours of cattle in New Zealand, but in this instance the copper intake is marginal. In addition to the other signs, however, there is a general tendency for scouring to occur, particularly in cattle. Because diarrhea is not a major sign in naturally occurring primary copper deficiency it is possible that it is due to the conditioning factor which reduces the availability of copper. For example, the severity of the scouring is roughly proportional to the level of intake of molybdenum. On the other hand diarrhea is a prominent sign in experimental copper deficiency (16).

FALLING DISEASE OF CATTLE

The characteristic behavior in falling disease is for cows in apparently good health to throw up their heads, bellow and fall. Death is instantaneous in most cases, but some fall and struggle feebly on their sides for a few minutes with intermittent bellowing and running movement attempts to rise. Rare cases show signs for up to 24 hours or more. These animals periodically lower their heads and pivot on the front legs. Sudden death usually occurs during one of these episodes.

PEAT SCOURS ('TEART') OF CATTLE AND SHEEP

Persistent diarrhea with the passage of watery, yellow-green to black feces with an inoffensive odor occurs soon after the cattle go on to affected pasture, in some cases within 8–10 days. The feces are released without effort, often without lifting the tail. Severe debilitation results although the appetite remains good. The hair coat is rough and depigmentation is manifested by reddening or gray flecking, especially around the eyes, in black cattle. The degree of abnormality varies a great deal from season to season and year to year and spontaneous recovery is common. Affected animals usually recover in a few days following treatment with copper.

UNTHRIFTINESS (PINE) OF CALVES

The earliest signs are a stiffness of gait and unthriftiness. The epiphyses of the distal ends of the metacarpus and metatarsus may be enlarged and resemble the epiphysitis of rapidly growing calves deficient in calcium and phosphorus or vitamin D (51). The epiphyses are painful on palpation and some calves are severely lame (32, 51). The pasterns are upright and the animals may appear to have contracted flexor tendons. The unthriftiness and emaciation are progressive and death may occur in 4–5 months. Grayness of the hair, especially around the eyes in black cattle, is apparent. Diarrhea may occur in a few cases.

COPPER DEFICIENCY SYNDROMES IN SHEEP

General syndrome—primary copper deficiency: sheep
Abnormalities of the wool are the first observed signs and may be the only sign in areas of marginal copper deficiency. Fine wool becomes limp and glossy and loses its crimp, developing a straight, steely appearance. Black wool shows depigmentation to gray or white, often in bands coinciding with the seasonal occurrence of copper deficiency. The straight, steely defect may occur in similar bands and the staple may break easily. There appear to be some differences between breeds in susceptibility to copper deficiency, Merino sheep appearing to have a higher copper requirement than mutton sheep. The fleece abnormalities of Merino sheep in Australia have not been observed in Romney Marsh sheep in copper-deficient areas in New Zealand, but this may be due in part to the difficulty of detecting abnormality in wool which is normally rather straight and steely. Anemia, scouring, unthriftiness and infertility may occur in conditions of extreme deficiency, but in sheep the characteristic findings are in the lamb, the disease enzootic ataxia being the major manifestation. Retardation of growth, diarrhea, delay to marketing and increased mortality are common clinical findings in lambs genetically selected for low plasma copper and placed on improved and limed upland pastures (109). Osteoporosis with increased tendency of the long bones to fracture has also been recorded under conditions of copper deficiency insufficient to cause enzootic ataxia.

ENZOOTIC ATAXIA AND SWAYBACK IN LAMBS AND GOAT KIDS

These diseases have much in common, but there are differences in epidemiology and some subtle clinical ones.

Swayback is the only authentic manifestation of a primary nutritional deficiency of copper in the United Kingdom (49). There is a suggestion that a predisposition to it is inherited (50). It comes in several forms: a congenital form, cerebrospinal swayback, which occurs only when the copper deficiency is extreme. Affected lambs are born dead or weak and unable to stand and suck. Incoordination and erratic movements are more evident than in enzootic ataxia and the paralysis is spastic in type. Blindness also occurs occasionally. There is softening and cavitation of the cerebral white matter and this probably commences about day 120 of gestation (45). *Progressive (delayed) spinal swayback* begins to develop some weeks after birth with lesions and clinical signs beginning to appear at 3–6 weeks of age.

Postnatal acute fatal swayback may be a third form of the disease which appears to occur only in Wales. It resembles the more usual delayed form, but develops suddenly. There is a sudden onset of recumbency with death occurring 1–2 days later due to acute swelling of the cerebrum.

Enzootic ataxia affects only unweaned lambs. In severe outbreaks the lambs may be affected at birth, but most cases occur in the 1–2 month age group. The severity of the paresis decreases with increasing age at onset. Lambs affected at birth or within the first month usually die within 3–4 days. The disease in older lambs may last for 3–4 weeks and survival is more likely, although surviving lambs always show some ataxia and atrophy of the hindquarters. The first sign to appear in enzootic ataxia is incoordination of the hindlimbs appearing when the lambs are driven. Respiratory and cardiac rates are also greatly accelerated by exertion. As the disease progresses the incoordination becomes more severe and may be apparent after walking only a few yards. There is excessive flexion of joints, knuckling over of the fetlocks, wobbling of the hindquarters and finally falling. The hindlegs are affected first and the lamb may be able to drag itself about in a sitting posture. When the forelegs eventually become involved recumbency persists and the lamb dies of inanition. There is no true paralysis, the lamb being able to kick vigorously even in the recumbent stage. The appetite remains unaffected.

Enzootic ataxia due to copper deficiency has been reported in young goat kids (15, 41). The disease is similar in most respects to the disease in lambs. Kids may be affected at birth or the clinical signs may be delayed until the animals are several weeks of age. Cerebellar hypoplasia is a frequent finding in goats.

COPPER DEFICIENCY SYNDROMES IN OTHER SPECIES

Deer
Enzootic ataxia in red deer is surprisingly different from the disease in lambs in that it develops in young adults well past weaning age and in adults. The clinical signs include ataxia, swaying of the hindquarters, a dog-sitting posture and eventually inability to use the hindlimbs. Spinal cord demyelination and midbrain neuronal degeneration are characteristic (46).

Pigs
The few recorded cases of naturally occurring enzootic ataxia in pigs have been in growing pigs 4–6 months old. Posterior paresis progresses to complete paralysis in 1–3 weeks (76). Dosing with copper salts had no effect on the clinical conditions, but hepatic copper levels were 3–14 mg/kg (0·05–0·22 mmol/kg). Copper deficiency in piglets 5–8 weeks of age has been reported and was characterized clinically by ataxia, posterior paresis, nystagmus, inability to stand, paddling movements of the limbs and death in 3–5 days (75). Pathologically there was demyelination of the spinal cord and degenerative lesions of the elastic fibers of the walls of the aorta and pulmonary arteries (75).

Anemia in young, growing pigs, which responded to treatment with copper, has been observed to occur naturally, and anemia has been produced experimentally in young pigs by the feeding of diets deficient in copper. Low levels of liver copper in pigs in New Zealand which receive milk whey as the main part of their diet may be associated with a greater frequency of illthrift and anemia compared with animals with higher levels of liver copper (74). In experimentally produced cases there are abnormalities of the limbs, with lack of rigidity of joints and excessive flexion of the hocks, leading to the adoption of a sitting posture. The forelegs show varying types and degrees of crookedness. In extreme cases the use of the forelimbs is lost and the animal is recumbent. These abnormalities also respond to treatment with copper. Attempts to produce congenital copper deficiency syndromes in baby pigs have been unsuccessful although hypocuprosis is produced easily enough (47).

The inclusion of copper sulfate, at levels of 125–200 mg/kg of copper, in the diets of pigs 11–90 kg liveweight and fed *ad libitum*, results in slight improvements in growth rate and feed efficiency, but has no significant effect on carcass characteristics (48). The supplemental copper causes a marked increase in liver copper concentration which poses a potential hazard and it is recommended that copper supplementation be limited to starter and grower diets fed to pigs weighing less than 50 kg liveweight (48).

Horses

Adult horses appear to be unaffected by copper deficiency, but there are unconfirmed reports of abnormalities of limbs of foals. Foals in copper-deficient areas have been observed to be unthrifty and slow-growing, with stiffness of the limbs and enlargement of the joints (34). Contraction of the flexor tendons causes the animal to stand on its toes. There is no ataxia or indication of involvement of the central nervous system. Signs may be present at birth or develop before weaning. Recovery occurs slowly after weaning and foals are unthrifty for up to 2 years.

Clinical pathology

The laboratory evaluation of the copper status of farm animals is difficult because the biochemical values are often difficult to interpret and to correlate with the clinical state of the animal. This is particularly true when only an individual animal is being evaluated. The evaluation of the copper status of the herd or flock is usually easier.

Blood samples should be taken at random from at least 10% of clinically affected animals and from 10% of normal animals. Each class of animal according to age groups, diet and production status should also be sampled. Follow-up samples should be taken from the same animals following therapy or the institution of control measures.

For many years the laboratory diagnosis of copper deficiency in cattle and sheep centered on the determination of serum or plasma copper and liver copper. However, experience has indicated that serum and liver copper levels are not consistently reliable as indicators of copper status. Apparently clinically normal animals may have marginal levels of serum copper, or unthrifty animals may have marginal or deficient serum levels of copper. Furthermore, when either the normal animals with the marginal levels of copper or the unthrifty animals with the marginal or deficient levels are treated with copper there may or may not be an improvement in weight gain as might be expected in the former or improvement in clinical condition in the latter.

The development of a deficiency can be divided into four phases: depletion, deficiency (marginal), dysfunction and disease. During the depletion phase there is loss of copper from any storage site such as liver but the plasma concentrations of copper may remain constant. With continued dietary deficiency the concentrations of copper in the blood will decline during the phase of marginal deficiency. However, it may be some time before the concentrations or activities of copper containing enzymes in the tissues begin to decline and it is not until this happens that the phase of dysfunction is reached. There may be a further lag before the changes in cellular function are manifested as clinical signs of disease.

The three principles which govern the interpretation of biochemical criteria of trace element status include: the relationships between the concentration of the marker and the intake of the element; the time the animal is on an adequate diet; and disturbances of tissue function (2). From these principles, the concentrations of liver copper are shown to be insensitive indices of deficiency but good indicators of excess and plasma copper less than 57 μg/dl (9 μmol/l) is a good index of marginal deficiency but values may have to fall to below 19 μg/dl (3 μmol/l) before there is a risk of dysfunction and loss of production in sheep and cattle. *However, these are only guidelines. The range of values and the cutoff levels above which animals are normal or below which they are deficient have not been well established.* There is considerable biological variation dependent on the species, the breed of animal, the length of time over which the depletion has occurred and the presence of intercurrent disease.

Estimations of copper in liver and blood may be of diagnostic value but should be interpreted with caution since clinical signs of copper deficiency may appear before there are significant changes in the levels of copper in the blood and liver. Conversely, the plasma levels of copper may be very low in animals which are otherwise normal and performing well (26, 28).

In general, plasma copper levels between 19 μg/dl and 57 μg/dl (3·0 and 9·0 μmol/l) represent marginal deficiency and levels below 19 μg/dl (3 μmol/l) represent functional deficiency or hypocuprosis. Plasma copper levels of 49·9 μg/dl (7·85 μmol/l) or less are indicative of low liver copper levels. Plasma copper levels above 90·2 μg/dl (14·2 μmol/l) are usually associated with liver levels above 38·1 mg/kg (0·6 mmol/kg) dry matter (53). Of the two estimations, that on liver is the most informative as levels in blood may remain normal for long periods after liver copper levels commence to fall and early signs of copper deficiency appear (54). Levels of copper in adult liver above 200 mg/kg dry matter (3·14 mmol/kg) in sheep and above 100 mg/kg dry matter (1·57 mmol/kg) in cattle are considered to be normal. Levels of less than 80 mg/kg dry matter (1·5 mmol/kg) in sheep and less than 30 mg/kg dry matter (0·5 mmol/kg) in cattle are classed as low. Liver copper levels in fetuses and neonates are usually much higher than in adults, and normal foals have had levels of 219 mg/kg (3·4 mmol/kg) compared to a normal of 31 mg/kg (0·49 mmol/kg) in adults (55). The levels of copper in milk and hair are also lower in deficient than in normal cattle and estimation of the copper content of hair is now acceptable as a diagnostic aid (62). It has the advantage of providing an integrated progressive record of nutritional intake. The levels of copper in bovine hair are more markedly depressed when extra molybdenum is fed.

It is necessary to be especially careful when collecting specimens for copper analysis to avoid contamination by needles, copper distilled water, vial caps, cans for liver specimens and other possible sources of copper. There is an additional problem, that of the effect of intercurrent disease on plasma levels of copper and selenium (44).

The difficulty of interpreting plasma levels of copper led to the estimation of plasma levels of copper–protein complexes especially ceruloplasmin. Ceruloplasmin contains greater than 95% of the circulating copper in normal animals. There is a highly significant correlation between plasma copper levels and plasma ceruloplasmin activity which is a less complicated and more rapid procedure than plasma copper. The regression analyses indicate a strongly positive correlation coefficient of ceruloplasmin with serum of cattle and sheep of 0·83 and 0·92, respectively (37). The correlation between serum ceruloplasmin activity and hepatic copper concentrations in cattle was only 0·35 indicating an unreliable relationship. Normal plasma ceruloplasmin levels in sheep are in the region of 45–100 mg/l. Normal levels of serum ceruloplasmin activity in cattle range from 120 to 200 mg/l. The mean copper and ceruloplasmin levels are higher in plasma than serum (82); the percentage of copper associated with ceruloplasmin is less in serum (55%) than in plasma (66%). Normal plasma ceruloplasmin levels in sheep range from 4.5 to 10 mg/dl. In experimental primary copper deficiency in calves, rapid decreases occur in plasma ceruloplasmin activity at least 80 days before overt clinical signs of deficiency (18).

The measurement of the activity of erythrocyte superoxide dismutase (ESOD), a copper-containing enzyme, is now being evaluated as a procedure for the diagnosis of copper deficiency (56). The activity of this enzyme decreases more slowly than plasma or liver copper in copper-deficient animals and may be more closely correlated with the presence of imminence of hypocuprosis. In marginal deficiency, the ESOD value ranges from 2 to 5 i.u./mg hemoglobin and in functional deficiency the value is below 2 (2).

Because the liver is a storage compartment for copper the concentrations of liver copper indicate the state of depletion rather than deficiency. There is no particular threshold value for liver copper below which the performance and health of livestock are likely to be impaired. A broad range of values may, for example, coincide with the marginally deficient state e.g., 5·1–20·3 mg (0·08 to 0·32 mmol) copper/kg liver dry matter. The concentration of hepatic copper in sheep is uniform and a single biopsy sample should be representative of the whole liver (57). The technique of liver biopsy for assessing the copper status of sheep has been evaluated (58). Frequency of biopsy does not affect copper concentration, the variability between successive samples is small and the biopsy procedure does not reduce body weight or rate of gain. Copper concentrations in the kidney cortex may be of more diagnostic value because concentrations are normally within a narrow range of 12·7–19·0 mg/kg (0·2–0·3 mmol/kg) dry matter. Thus concentrations below 12·7 mg/kg (0·2 mmol/kg) dry matter in the kidney may be a more reliable indicator of dysfunction than liver copper concentration.

The mean hepatic copper concentrations of horses fed diets containing 6·9–15·2 mg copper/kg dry matter were 17·1–21·0 μg/g (0·27–0·33 μmol/g) dry matter tissue (83). The plasma copper concentrations ranged from 3·58 to 4·45 μg/dl (22·8–28·3 μmol/l). There was no simple mathematical relationship between plasma and hepatic copper concentrations. The range of serum copper concentrations in Thoroughbred horses at grass was 63–196 μg/dl (9·91–30·85 mmol/l) and in stabled Thoroughbreds the range was 47–111 μg/dl (7·40–17·47 mmol/l) (84).

Anemia may occur in advanced cases of primary copper deficiency, hemoglobin levels being depressed to 50–80 g/l and erythrocytes to 2–4 × 10^{12}/l. A high proportion of cows in problems herds may have a Heinz-body anemia without evidence of hemoglobinuria and the severity of the anemia will be related to the hypocupremia (52).

The guidelines for the laboratory diagnosis of primary and secondary copper deficiency in cattle and sheep are summarized in Table 87.

Necropsy findings

The characteristic findings in copper deficiency are those of anemia and emaciation. Extensive deposits of hemosiderin can be found in the liver, spleen and kidney in most cases of primary copper deficiency and in the secondary form if the copper status is sufficiently low. In cattle the bones appear normal in spite of the predisposition to fractures but in lambs there may be severe osteoporosis.

In experimental primary copper deficiency in calves there is fibrous thickening of the stratum fibrosum of the synovial capsule surrounding the carpal and tarsal joints. Radiographically there is bone rarefaction and a reduction in the cortical bone index of the humerus, radius, femur, tibia, metacarpus and metatarsus (18). Histologically there is osteoporosis with a decrease in osteoblastic size and number and delayed ossification of calcified cartilage at the epiphysis. There is defective elastogenesis in the ligamentum nuchae attributable to the low monoamine activity. Villous atrophy of the small intestine is severe and may account for the diarrhea.

In naturally occurring secondary copper deficiency in cattle, associated with high dietary molybdenum and sulfate, there is widening of the epiphyseal plate with delayed or impaired provisional calcification in the presence of active osteoblasts (17).

Necropsy examinations should include assay of copper in viscera. The levels of copper in liver are usually low (see Table 87), and in secondary copper deficiency there may be a high level of copper in the kidney and high levels of molybdenum in the liver, kidney and spleen.

The most significant findings in enzootic ataxia is demyelination of cerebellar tracts and the tracts of Lissauer in the spinal cord. In a few extreme cases and in most cases of swayback the demyelination also involves the cerebrum and there is destruction and cavitation of

Table 87. Copper levels in body tissues and fluids in primary and secondary copper deficiency.

Species and tissue	*Normal level*	*Primary copper deficiency*	*Secondary copper deficiency*
Cattle			
Blood plasma (μg/ml) (convert to SI units by multiplying by 15.7 which gives μmol/l).	1·26 ± 0·31	Less than 0·5 and as low as 0·1–0·2	Less than 0·5 and as low as 0·2–0·3
Adult liver (mg/kg dry matter) (convert to SI units by multiplying by 0.0157 which gives mmol/kg)	More than 100 (usually 200)	Less than 20 and as low as 4	Less than 10
Milk (mg/l)	0·05–0·20	0·01–0·02	—
Hair (mg/kg)	6·6–10·4	1·8–3·4	5·5
Sheep			
Blood plasma (μg/ml)	0·7–1·3	0·1–0·2	0·4–0·7
Adult liver (mg/kg dry matter)	More than 200 (usually 350+)	20	15–19

the white matter. There is marked internal hydrocephalus in these cases, the cerebrospinal fluid is increased in quantity and the convolutions of the cerebrum are almost obliterated. Acute cerebral edema with marked brain swelling and cerebellar herniation, reminiscent of polioencephalomalacia, have been observed in lambs with hypocuprosis and the more typical lesions of nervous tissue (59). Although there is no anemia in affected lambs hemosiderosis of the liver and pancreas may be observed.

In falling disease the heart is flabby and pale and on histological examination there is atrophy of the muscle fibers and considerable replacement with fibrous tissue. Venous congestion is marked and the liver and spleen are enlarged and dark. Deposits of hemosiderin are present in the liver, spleen and kidney and there is some glomerular destruction. Congestion of the abomasal and intestinal mucosae is evident.

Diagnosis

Although field diagnosis depends largely on recognition of distinctive signs of copper deficiency and clinical response to treatment with copper, attention is drawn to the need for recognition of a subclinical copper deficiency. For example, a geochemical reconnaissance in a large area in the United Kingdom revealed a low status of soil and animal copper, and a related unthriftiness and infertility. Supplementation with copper improved weight gains and blood copper levels (39). However, there are wide variations in the response to copper supplementation of cattle with the same low copper status (112). In common with supplementation with cobalt, improvement in body weight of copper-deficient animals occurs after supplementation in most cases. Depigmentation of hair and steeliness of wool are probably the most sensitive indicators of deficiency. Laboratory confirmation may be obtained by estimation of the copper content of tissues and body fluids and of the diet. When the copper deficiency appears to be secondary, estimation of the content of molybdenum and inorganic sulfate in the feed, and the molybdenum content of tissues, will aid in determining the etiological significance of these substances.

The radiographic changes in cattle with secondary copper deficiency consist of widened irregular epiphyseal plates with increased bone density in the metaphysis and metaphyseal lipping. These findings are similar to those described for rickets and secondary nutritional hyperparathyroidism in cattle (17). In specific instances such as enzootic ataxia, swayback and falling disease, histological evidence may assist in establishing the diagnosis.

Confusion may arise in differentiating the general syndrome of copper deficiency from that caused by internal parasitism. The general signs of diarrhea, emaciation and anemia are common to both diseases which may also coexist. The response to the addition of copper to the ration is an adequate field test although a fecal examination for helminth eggs, or preferably a total worm count, should always be carried out.

Enzootic ataxia and swayback of lambs are seldom confused with other diseases because of their restricted occurrence in young lambs although cerebellar agenesis and poisoning by pea-vine ensilage cause similar syndromes in this age group. White muscle disease of lambs is characterized by typical lesions of muscular dystrophy.

Peat scours in cattle resembles Johne's disease but usually affects a much larger proportion of a group, with growing animals being more severely affected. Winter dysentery of cattle, salmonellosis, coccidiosis and mucosal disease are acute diseases characterized by diarrhea but are accompanied by other signs and clinicopathological findings which facilitate their identification. Many poisons, particularly arsenic, lead and salt, cause diarrhea in ruminants but there are usually additional diagnostic signs and evidence of access to the poison. Assay of feed and tissues helps to confirm a diagnosis of poisoning. A diagnosis of peat scours is usually made if there is an immediate response to oral dosing with a copper salt.

Falling disease occurs only in adult cattle while enzootic muscular dystrophy affects chiefly young calves. Poisoning by the gidgee tree (*Acacia georgina*) produces a similar syndrome in cattle.

Treatment

The treatment of copper deficiency is relatively simple but if advanced lesions are already present in the nervous system or myocardium complete recovery will not occur. Oral dosing with 4 g of copper sulfate for calves from 2 to 6 months of age and 8–10 g for mature cattle given weekly for 3–5 weeks is recommended for the treatment of primary or secondary copper deficiency. Parenteral injections of copper glycinate may also be used and the dosages are given under control.

The diet of affected animals should also be supplemented with copper. Copper sulfate may be added to the mineral–salt mix at a level of 3–5% of the total mixture. A commonly recommended mixture for cattle is 50% calcium–phosphorus mineral supplement, 45% cobalt–iodized salt and 3–5% copper sulfate. This mixture is offered free of choice or can be added to a complete diet at the rate of 1% of the total diet.

Control

Dietary requirements

The minimum dietary requirement for copper for cattle is 10 mg copper/kg dry matter and 5 mg/kg for sheep (18).

The requirement necessary to prevent hypocupremia and/or clinical copper deficiency will depend on the presence of interfering substances such as molybdenum, sulfur and iron in the diet and possibly the genotype of the animal. Although there is a marked difference between breeds of sheep in their susceptibility to hypocuprosis this would not seem to have an immediate practical application (54). The estimated copper requirement for mature ponies is 3·5 mg/kg (63).

Copper can be supplied to livestock in several different ways as outlined below. The dose rates given are those recommended for the control of primary copper deficiency and these may have to be increased or treatment given more frequently in some instances of secondary copper deficiency. In these circumstances it is often necessary to determine the most satisfactory dosing strategy by a field trial.

Copper sulfate (oral dosing or dietary supplementation)

Oral dosing with copper sulfate (4 g to cattle, 1·5 g to sheep, weekly) is adequate as prophylaxis and will prevent the occurrence of swayback in lambs if the ewes are dosed throughout pregnancy. Lambs can be protected after birth by dosing with 35 mg of copper sulfate every 2 weeks. However, regular oral dosing with copper sulfate is laborious and time-consuming and is no longer widely practiced.

Mineral mixtures of salt licks containing 0·25–0·5% of copper sulfate for sheep and 2% for cattle will supply sufficient copper provided an adequate intake of the mixture is assured. Iron preparations administered orally to pigs to prevent anemia usually contain adequate amounts of copper.

In some deficient areas an effective method of administering copper is by the annual topdressing of pasture with 5–6 kg/ha copper sulfate, although the amount required may vary widely with the soil type and the rainfall. Topdressing may cause copper poisoning if livestock are turned onto pasture while the copper salt is still adherent to the leaves. Treated pasture should be left unstocked for 3 weeks or until the first heavy rain. It is also possible that chronic copper poisoning may result if the copper status of the soil increases sufficiently over a number of years.

Addition of copper salts to drinking water is usually impractical because the solution corrodes metal piping, and maintenance of the correct concentration of copper in large bodies of water is difficult. However, if the need is great, some way around these difficulties can usually be found and a system has been devised for automatic supplementation for short periods via the drinking water (60), and has been effective in controlling copper deficiency in cattle (64).

Removal of sulfates

The removal of sulfates from drinking water by water purification, using a process of reverse osmosis, may have a positive effect on the copper status of beef cows (85). Cows drinking desulfated water had an increased availability of copper compared to those drinking water containing a large concentration of sulfates.

Parenteral injections of copper

To overcome the difficulty of frequent individual dosing or topdressing of pasture, periodic parenteral injection of copper compounds which release copper gradually have given good results. They have the advantage of avoiding fixation of copper by molybdenum in the alimentary tract (105). For the past 20 years the use of injectable preparations of copper has been the method of choice for the prevention of swayback in lambs (91). Copper calcium ethylenediamine tetra-acetate (copper calcium edetate), copper methionate, copper glycinate and copper oxyquinoline sulfonate have been developed and evaluated under field conditions. The criteria used to judge these injections are minimal damage at the site of injections, satisfactory liver storage (90–100%) of the administered dose and a safe margin between therapeutic and toxic doses (91). The dose of copper in any of the compounds for cattle is 400 mg and for sheep 150 mg. Copper calcium edetate has the advantage of giving maximum copper storage very quickly—1 week after injection, and blood levels are elevated within a few hours (60). Because of the rapidity of the absorption, toxic effects can be encountered unless proper dose levels are observed. As well as deaths from serious overdosing, some deaths occur in groups of sheep for unexplained reasons. It is suggested that stress be minimized and simultaneous other therapy be avoided.

Calves are protected at birth and do not need an injection of 50 mg until they are 6 weeks old. One of the other advantages of parenteral administration is the opportunity that it gives for providing copper at exactly the right time, for example, in late pregnancy when the storage demands of the fetus are rapidly followed by the demand of copper excretion in milk. If infertility is a problem in copper-deficient flock an injection just before joining can be helpful in correcting the reproductive efficiency. And an injection just before parturition can give the neonate a good start.

A marked local reaction occurs at the site of injection so that subcutaneous injection is preferable in animals to be used for meat, although to avoid an unsightly blemish breeding animals should receive an intramuscular injection. There may be some danger of precipitating blackleg in cattle on farms where this disease occurs. For sheep a single injection of 45 mg of copper as copper glycinate in midpregnancy is sufficient to prevent swayback in the lambs.

The subcutaneous injection of copper calcium edetate or copper oxyquinoline sulfonate into sheep results in a rapid increase in the concentration of copper in whole blood, serum and urine within the first 24 hours (87). Following the injection of copper methionate, the concentration of copper in blood and serum rises steadily over a period of 10 days and there is no detectable increase in urinary copper. After the injection of all three compounds there is a steady increase in serum ceruloplasmin activity over a period of 10–20 days followed by a slow fall to preinjection activity by 40 days. The lower toxicity of copper injected as methionate compared with that as copper calcium edetate or copper oxyquinoline sulfonate is due to the slower absorption and transport of the copper to the liver and kidney. Death has occurred in sheep following the parenteral administration of diethylamine oxyquinoline sulfonate at recommended doses (104). Affected sheep manifested signs of hepatic encephalopathy and at necropsy there was acute, severe, generalized, centrilobular hepatocellular necrosis (104). The use of copper disodium edetate at recommended doses in calves has also resulted in deaths associated with liver necrosis and clinical signs of hepatic encephalopathy (103).

Injectable copper glycinate is an excellent source of supplementary copper for increasing the concentration of copper in the serum of copper deficient cattle and maintaining grazing cattle in an adequate copper status (86). One dose of copper glycinate will maintain adequate copper levels for about 60–90 days. The recommended dose in beef herds is 120 mg of copper for adult cattle and 60 mg of copper for calves. A supplemental source of copper is required for the calf during the pasture season because milk is a poor source of copper, particularly from copper-deficient cows, and calves do not have the opportunity to increase or maintain body stores of copper while grazing. When the dam is severely hypocupremic in the spring, the calf is also severely hypocupremic or copper-deficient (9). Insufficient copper is secreted into the milk of copper-treated cows. Therefore, where the dam has not received an adequate copper intake during pregnancy, direct treatment of the calf will be required in early life. The copper reserves of newborn calves are increased in fetal liver at the expense of copper stores in the dam's liver which are dependent on the availability of dietary or supplemental copper to the dam. Because of the higher requirements for copper during the last trimester of pregnancy (demands of the fetal liver) a program of copper supplementation should involve the use of copper supplements, throughout the year as required. One dose of copper glycinate is sufficient when cattle are grazing forage which contains no more than 3 mg/kg of molybdenum and 3 g/kg of sulfur. With higher levels of molybdenum and sulfur, repeated injections of copper glycinate are recommended. The injectable copper may be supplemented by the use of copper sulfate in a mineral supplement at a level of 1%. The inclusion of copper sulfate in the mineral supplement may be adequate for cows but the calves may not consume an adequate amount of mineral and injectable copper. The level of supplementation required to prevent a drop in serum copper over the pasture season will depend upon the concentration of dietary molybdenum and sulfur and their effect upon the coefficient of absorption of copper.

Four injectable copper complex compounds have been evaluated as supplementary copper for grazing beef cattle under Canadian conditions (87). Copper edetate at 100 mg of copper, copper glycinate at 120 mg and copper methionate at 120 mg were used and were equally effective in improving copper status of copper-deficient cattle and maintaining them in an adequate copper status for 90 days (88). The copper methionate was least acceptable because of the incidence and severity of reactions at the site of injection.

Death due to poisoning is one of the dangers of parenteral administration because it is difficult to control the rate at which the supplement releases the copper especially if the controlling mechanism is chemical binding. Methods used to control the release include the development of soluble *controlled release glass* containing copper which are implanted subcutaneously (91).

Controlled release glass boluses containing copper are now available for oral administration to sheep and cattle (89). The copper is slowly released, absorbed and stored in the liver. Initial field evaluations indicate that the boluses may not contain sufficient copper to maintain normal levels of copper for a sufficient length of time compared to the use of copper oxide needles (90).

Copper oxide needles

Copper oxide needles or wire particles (fragments of oxidized copper wire up to 8 mm in length and 0·5 mm in diameter) are available for oral dosing (6) and are considered to be one of the most effective and safest methods for the control of copper deficiency in ruminants (91–93). This method of supplementation offers the major advantages of prolonged effectiveness and low cost. A single treatment can be effective for an entire summer or winter season. The needles are retained in the forestomachs and abomasum for up to 100 days or more and the copper is slowly released, absorbed and stored in the liver. The response in liver copper concentrations is dose-dependent. In sheep given doses ranging from 2·5 to 20 g per animal the liver copper concentrations will peak 10 weeks after administration and will thereafter decline in a linear fashion over the next 40 weeks (93). A single dose of 20 g of copper oxide needles to hypocupremic suckler cows was sufficient to maintain adequate copper status for at least 5 months (91). The use of 20 g of copper oxide needles to young cattle weighing 190 kg effectively prevented growth retardation and severe hypocupremia which occurred in an undosed control over a 70-day trial period (94). The currently recommended doses for beef cattle are 5 g for calves, 10 g for yearlings and 20 g for heavier or adult cattle which will give protection for at least 6 months

(95). The use of 50 g of needles in adult cows (55 kg body weight) sustained higher levels of plasma concentrations than the subcutaneous injection of copper glycinate (98) and 100, 200 or 300 g of needles given orally did not cause clinical effects. The administration of a single dose of 2 g cupric oxide needles orally to lambs between 3 and 5 weeks of age is an effective method for the prevention of induced hypocuprosis manifested as illthrift in lambs grazing pastures improved by liming and reseeding (96). The treatment maintained the lambs in normocupremia, provided adequate liver copper reserves, prevented clinical signs of hypocuprosis and produced a liveweight gain advantage. The administration of the needles to ewes in the first half of pregnancy is also effective for the prevention of swayback in their lambs (97). The administration of cupric oxide needles to ewes at parturition is effective in preventing hypocupremia for up to 17 weeks in animals on pasture previously shown to cause a molybdenum–sulfur-induced copper deficiency (100). The treatment of the ewes at parturition also resulted in higher concentrations of copper in the milk in the initial weeks of lactation. However, this increase in milk copper will not be effective in preventing hypocupremia and hypocuprosis in the lambs which can be treated with cupric oxide needles at 6 weeks of age. Because some breeds of sheep may have a propensity to concentrate excess quantities of copper in the liver, it is important to adhere to the recommended dosage (99). Cupric oxide needles at a dose of 4 g per animal have also been used for the prevention of swayback in goats (101).

Genetic selection

It is now possible to manipulate trace element metabolism by genetic selection in farm animals (49). Within a period of 5 years, selection of sheep based on plasma concentration of copper resulted in two divergent sets of progeny, one with a high level of copper status, the other with a low level which resulted in clinical manifestations of copper deficiency in the low level and protection in the high level (102).

General guidelines

Several rules of thumb are worth remembering. An intake of copper equivalent to 10 mg/kg dry matter of the diet will prevent the occurrence of primary copper deficiency in both sheep and cattle; diets containing less than 5 mg/kg dry matter will cause hypocuprosis; diets with copper : molybdenum ratios of less than 5 : 1 are conducive to conditioned (secondary) hypocuprosis; the newborn calf is protected against neonatal hypocuprosis by donations from the dam, but newborn lambs assume the same copper status as the ewe; cattle are more susceptible to copper deficiency than are sheep (61).

REVIEW LITERATURE

Brewer, N. R. (1987) Comparative metabolism of copper. *J. Am. vet. med. Assoc.*, *190*, 654–658.

Hidiroglou, M. (1980) Zinc, copper and manganese deficiencies and the ruminant skeleton: a review. *Can. J. anim. Sci.*, *60*, 579–590.

Hidiroglou, M. & Knipfel, J. E. (1981) Maternal-fetal relationships of copper, manganese and sulfur in ruminants. A review. *J. dairy Sci.*, *64*, 1637–1647.

Mason, J. (1986) Thiomolybdates: mediators of molybdenum toxicity and enzyme inhibitors. *Toxicology*, *42*, 99–109.

National Research Council (1977) Copper. National Academy of Sciences, Washington, DC.

Poole, D. B. R. (1982) Bovine copper deficiency in Ireland—the clinical disease. *Irish vet. J.*, *36*, 169–73.

Suttle, N. F. (1986) Problems in the diagnosis and anticipation of trace element deficiencies in grazing livestock. *Vet. Rec.*, *119*, 148–152.

Suttle, N. F. (1986) Copper deficiency in ruminants, recent developments. *Vet. Rec.*, *119*, 519–522.

Underwood, E. J. (1977) Copper. In: *Trace Elements in Human and Animal Nutrition*, 4th edn. London: Academic Press.

REFERENCES

(1) Suttle, N. F. (1986) *Vet. Rec.*, *119*, 519.
(2) Suttle, N. F. (1986) *Vet. Rec.*, *119*, 148.
(3) Humphries, W. R. et al. (1983) *Br. J. Nutr.*, *49*, 77.
(4) Bain, M. S. et al. (1986) *Vet. Rec.*, *119*, 593.
(5) Goodrich, R. D. & Tillman, A. D. (1966) *J. Nutr.*, *90*, 76.
(6) Whitelaw, A. et al. (1980) *Vet. Rec.*, *107*, 87.
(7) Bridges, C. H. et al. (1984) *J. Am. vet. med. Assoc.*, *185*, 173.
(8) Suttle, N. F. & Field, A. C. (1983) *J. comp. Pathol.*, *93*, 379.
(9) Boila, R. J. et al. (1984) *Can. J. anim. Sci.*, *64*, 919.
(10) Thornton, I. & Webb, J. S. (1975) *Copper in Farming, Symposium of the Copper Development Assoc.*, p. 320.
(11) Poole, D. B. R. (1982) *Irish vet. J.*, *36*, 169.
(12) Boila, R. J. et al. (1984) *Can. J. anim. Sci.*, *64*, 899.
(13) Brockman, R. P. (1977) *Can. vet. J.*, *18*, 168.
(14) Campbell, C. M. et al. (1976) In: *Molybdenum in the Environment.* (eds) W. R. Chappel & K. K. Petersen, vol. 1, pp. 75–84.
(15) Wouda, W. et al. (1986) *Vet. Q.*, *8*, 45.
(16) Suttle, N. F. & Angus, K. W. (1976) *J. comp. Pathol.*, *86*, 595.
(17) Irwin, M. R. et al. (1974) *J. comp. Pathol.*, *84*, 611.
(18) Mills, C. F. et al. (1976) *Br. J. Nutr.*, *35*, 309.
(19) Irwin, M. R. et al. (1976) *J. Am vet. med. Assoc.*, *174*, 590.
(20) Fell, B. F. et al. (1975) *Res. vet. Sci.*, *18*, 274.
(21) Suttle, N. F. et al. (1972) *J. comp. Pathol.*, *82*, 93.
(22) Jericho, K. W. F. et al. (1973) *Can. J. comp. Med.*, *37*, 228.
(23) Smith, R. M. et al, (1977) *J. comp. Pathol.*, *87*, 119.
(24) Lewis, G. et al. (1974) *Vet. Rec.*, *95*, 313.
(25) Waisman, J. et al. (1969) *Lab. Invest.*, *21*, 548.
(26) Suttle, N. F. et al. (1980) *Vet. Rec.*, *106*, 302.
(27) Stowe, H. D. (1968) *J. Nutr.*, *95*, 179.
(28) Whitaker, D. A. (1982) *Br. vet. J.*, *138*, 40.
(29) Mason, J. (1986) *Toxicology*, *42*, 99.
(30) Miltimore, J. E. & Mason, J. L. (1971) *Can. J. anim. Sci.*, *51*, 193.
(31) Alloway, B. J. (1973) *J. agric. Sci., Camb.*, *80*, 521.
(32) Smart, M. E. & Gudmundson, J. (1980) *Calif. Vet.*, *34*, 22.
(33) Marcilese, N. A. et al. (1969) *J. Nutr.*, *99*, 177.
(34) Carbery, J. T. (1978) *NZ vet. J.*, *26*, 279.
(35) Kappel, L. C. et al. (1984) *Am. J. vet. Res.*, *45*, 346.
(36) Thomson, G. G. & Lawson, B. M. (1970) *NZ vet. J.*, *18*, 79.
(37) Blakley, B. R. & Hamilton, D. L. (1985) *Can. J. comp. Med.*, *49*, 405.
(38) Davies, D. G. & Baker, M. H. (1974) *Vet. Rec.*, *94*, 561.
(39) Thornton, I. et al. (1972) *J. agric. Sci., Camb.*, *78*, 157.
(40) Goold, G. J. & Smith, B. (1975) *NZ vet. J.*, *23*, 233.
(41) Cordy, D. R. & Knight, H. D. (1978) *Vet. Pathol.*, *15*, 179.
(42) Deland, M. P. B. et al. (1979) *Aust. vet. J.*, *55*, 493.
(43) Hiridoglou, M. (1980) *Can. J. anim. Sci.*, *60*, 579.
(44) Corrigall, W. et al. (1976) *Vet. Rec.*, *99*, 396.
(45) Done, J. T. (1976) *Adv. vet. Sci.*, *20*, 101.
(46) Ryssen, J. B. & Stielau, W. J. (1980) *S. Afr. J. anim. Sci.*, *10*, 49.
(47) Cancilla, P. A. et al. (1967) *J. Nutr.*, *93*, 438.
(48) Castell, A. G. et al. (1975) *Can. J. anim. Sci.*, *55*, 113.
(49) Wiener, G. & Wooliams, J. A. (1983) In: *Trace Elements in Animal Production and Veterinary Practice.* Occasional publication no. 7, British Society of Animal Production.
(50) Wiener, G. (1971) *J. comp. Pathol.*, *81*, 515.
(51) Smith, B. P. et al. (1975) *J. Am. vet. med. Assoc.*, *166*, 682.
(52) Gardner, D. E. (1976) *NZ vet. J.*, *24*, 117.
(53) Claypool, D. W. et al. (1975) *J. anim. Sci.*, *41*, 911.
(54) Wiener, G. et al. (1976) *J. comp. Pathol.*, *86*, 101.
(55) Egan, D. A. & Murrin, M. P. (1973) *Res. vet. Sci.*, *15*, 147.

(56) Suttle, N. F. & McMurray, C. H. (1983) *Res. Vet. Sci.*, *35*, 47.
(57) Osborn, P. J. et al. (1983) *NZ vet. J.*, *31*, 144.
(58) Donald, G. E. et al. (1984) *Aust. vet. J.*, *61*, 121.
(59) Ishmael, J. et al. (1971) *J. comp. Pathol.*, *81*, 455.
(60) Smith, B. & Moon, G. H. (1976) *NZ vet. J.*, *24*, 132.
(61) Roberts, H. E. (1976) *Vet. Rec.*, *99*, 496.
(62) Kellaway, R. C. et al. (1978) *Res. vet. Sci.*, *22*, 352.
(63) Cymbaluk, N. F. et al. (1981) *J. Nutr.*, *111*, 87 & 96.
(64) Farmer, P. E. et al. (1982) *Vet. Rec.*, *111*, 193.
(65) Hill, G. M. et al. (1983) *J. Nutr.*, *113*, 867.
(66) Leech, A. et al. (1982) *Vet. Rec.*, *111*, 203.
(67) Clegg, F. G. et al. (1983) *Vet. Rec.*, *112*, 34.
(68) Suttle, N. F. (1975) *J. agric. Sci.*, *Camb. 84*, 255.
(69) Smyth, P. J. et al. (1977) *Vet. Sci. Commun.*, *1*, 235.
(70) Smart, M. E. et al. (1983) *Can. J. anim. Sci.*, *63*, 1021.
(71) Hidiroglou, M. & Knipfel, J. E. (1981) *J. dairy Sci.*, *64*, 1637.
(72) Towers, N. R. et al. (1981) *NZ vet. J.*, *29*, 113.
(73) Fell, B. F. et al. (1985) *J. comp. Pathol.*, *95*, 573.
(74) Hodges, R. t. & Fraser, A. J. (1983) *NZ vet. J.*, *31*, 96.
(75) Pletcher, J. M. & Banting, L. F. (1983) *J. S. Afr. vet. Assoc.*, *54*, 43.
(76) Wilson, P. R. et al. (1979) *NZ vet. J.*, *27*, 252.
(77) Jones, D. G. & Suttle, N. F. (1983) *J. comp. Pathol.*, *93*, 143.
(78) Jones, D. G. (1984) *Res. vet. Sci.*, *37*, 205.
(79) Young, W. K. et al. (1985) *Aust. J. exp. Biol. med. Sci.*, *63*, 273.
(80) Sorenson, J. R. J. et al. (1984) *Inorganica Chim. Acta*, *91*, 285.
(81) Mason, J. et al. (1986) *Res. vet. Sci.*, *41*, 108.
(82) Kincaid, R. L. et al. (1986) *Am. J. vet. Res.*, *47*, 1157.
(83) Cymbaluk, N. F. & Christensen, D. A. (1986) *Can. vet. J.*, *27*, 206.
(84) Stubley, D. et al. (1983) *Equ. vet. J.*, *15*, 253.
(85) Smart, M. E. et al. (1986) *Can. J. anim. Sci.*, *66*, 669.
(86) Boila, R. J. et al. (1984) *Can. J. anim. Sci.*, *64*, 675.
(87) Mahmoud, D. M. & Ford, E. J. H. (1983) *J. comp. Pathol.*, *93*, 551.
(88) Boila, R. J. et al. (1984) *Can. J. anim. Sci.*, *64*, 365.
(89) Allen, W. M. et al. (1984) *Vet. Rec.*, *115*, 55.
(90) Gallagher, J. & Cottrill, B. R. (1985) *Vet. Rec.*, *117*, 468.
(91) MacPherson, A. (1983) *Trace Elements in Animal Production and Veterinary Practice*. Occasional publication no. 7, British Society for Animal Production, Edinburgh, p. 93.
(92) Suttle, N. F. (1981) *Vet. Rec.*, *108*, 417.
(93) Judson, G. J. et al. (1982) *Aust. J. agric. Res.*, *33*, 1073.
(94) Whitelaw, A. et al. (1984) *Vet. Rec.*, *115*, 357.
(95) MacPherson, A. (1984) *Vet. Rec.*, *115*, 354.
(96) Whitelaw, A. et al. (1983) *Vet. Rec.*, *112*, 382.
(97) Whitelaw, A. et al. (1982) *Vet. Rec.*, *110*, 522.
(98) Deland, M. P. B. et al. (1986) *Aust. vet. J.*, *63*, 1.
(99) Britt, D. P. & Yeoman, G. H. (1985) *Vet. Res. Commun.*, *9*, 57.
(100) Whitelaw, A. et al. (1983) *Anim. Prod.*, *37*, 441.
(101) Inglis, D. M. et al. (1986) *Vet. Rec.*, *118*, 657.
(102) Wooliams, J. A. et al. (1986) *Anim. Prod.*, *43*, 303.
(103) Bulgin, M. S. et al. (1986) *J. am. vet. med. Assoc.*, *188*, 406.
(104) Mason, R. W. et al. (1984) *Aust. vet. J.*, *61*, 38.
(105) Allen, W. M. & Mallinson, C. B. (1984) *Vet. Rec.*, *114*, 451.
(106) Edwards, W. A. (1980) *Vet. Rec.*, *106*, 494.
(107) Mills, C. F. (1985) In: *Trace Elements in Man and Animals. Proc. 5th Int. Symp*. Commonwealth Agricultural Bureaux, pp. 1–10.
(108) Woolliams, C. et al. (1986) *Anim. Prod.*, *43*, 293.
(109) Wooliams, J. A. et al. (1986) *Anim. Prod.*, *43*, 303.
(110) Wiener, G. et al. (1985) *Anim. Prod.*, *40*, 465.
(111) Wooliams, J. A. et al. (1985) *Anim. Prod.*, *41*, 219.
(112) Phillip, M. (1983) In: *Trace Elements in Animal Production and Veterinary Practice*. Occasional publication no. 7, British Society for Animal Production.
(113) Mills, C. F. (1983) In: *Trace Elements in Animal Production and Veterinary Practice*. Occasional publication no. 7, British Society for Animal Production.

Iodine deficiency

The cardinal sign of iodine deficiency is goiter. The major clinical manifestation is neonatal mortality, with alopecia and visible and palpable enlargement of the thyroid gland occurring in some animals.

Etiology

The iodine deficiency may be primarily due to deficient iodine intake or secondarily conditioned by a high intake of calcium, diets consisting largely of *Brassica* spp. or gross bacterial pollution of feedstuffs or drinking water. A continued intake of a low level of cyanogenetic glucosides, e.g. in white clover, is commonly associated with a high incidence of goitrous offspring. Linamarin, a glucoside in linseed meal, is thought to be the agent producing goiter in newborn lambs from ewes fed the meal during pregnancy. A continued intake of the grass *Cynoden aethiopicus* with low iodine and high cyanogenetic glucoside contents is also recorded as a cause of goiter in lambs (1). Rapeseed and rapeseed meal are also goitrogenic.

Epidemiology

Goiter caused by iodine deficiency occurs in all of the continental land masses. It is not now of major economic importance because of the ease of recognition and correction but if neglected may cause heavy mortalities in newborn animals. The sporadic occurrence of the disease in marginal areas attracts most attention. An epidemiological survey in Germany revealed that up to 10% of cattle and sheep farms and 15% of swine herds were affected with iodine deficiency which were both primary and secondary due to the presence of nitrates, thiocyanates or glucosinates in the diet (21).

The importance of subclinical iodine deficiency, that is deaths in the newborn without goiter, could be much greater than that of the clinical disease. For example, in southern Australia ewes supplemented with iodine by the single injection of iodine in oil, have had less mortality in the lambs, or grown larger lambs or performed the same as controls (8).

Young animals are more likely to bear goitrous offspring than older ones and this may account for the apparent breed susceptibility of Dorset Horn sheep which mate at an earlier age than other breeds.

A simple deficiency of iodine in the diet and drinking water occurs and is related to geographical circumstances. Areas where the soil iodine is not replenished by cyclical accessions of oceanic iodine include large continental land masses and coastal areas where prevailing winds are offshore. In such areas iodine deficiency is most likely to occur where rainfall is heavy and soil iodine is continually depleted by leaching (4). Soil formations rich in calcium or lacking in humus are also likely to be relatively deficient in iodine. The ability of soil to retain iodine under conditions of heavy rainfall is directly related to their humus content and limestone soils are in general low in organic matter. A high dietary intake of calcium also decreases intestinal absorption of iodine and in some areas heavy applications of lime to pasture are followed by the development of goiter in lambs. This factor may also be important in areas where drinking water is heavily mineralized.

Apart from these circumstances, there are a number of situations in which the relationship between iodine intake and the occurrence of goiter is not readily apparent. Goiter may occur on pasture which on analysis contains adequate iodine and is then usually ascribed to a secondary or conditioned iodine deficiency. The conditioning factors which produce secondary iodine deficiency have not been properly determined but there are some circumstances in which secondary iodine deficiency is known to occur. A diet rich in plants of the *Brassica* spp., including cabbages and brussels sprouts, may cause simple goiter and hypothyroidism in rabbits, which is preventable by administered iodine. Hypothyroidism has also been produced in rats by feeding rape seed and in mice by feeding rape seed oil meal. A heavy diet of kale to pregnant ewes causes a high incidence of goiter and hypothyroidism, also preventable by administered iodine in the newborn lambs (6). The goitrogenic substance in these plants is probably a glucosinolate which is capable of producing thiocyanate in the rumen. The thiocyanate content, or potential content, varies between varieties of kale, being much less in rape–kale, which also does not show the two-fold increase in thiocyanate content which other varieties show in autumn (5). Small young leaves contain up to five times as much thiocyanate as large, fully formed leaves. Some of these plants are excellent sources of feed, and in some areas it is probably economic to continue feeding them, provided suitable measures are taken to prevent goiter in the newborn. Although kale also causes mild goiter in weaned lambs this does not appear to reduce their rate of gain.

A diet high in linseed meal (20% of ration) given to pregnant ewes may also result in a high incidence of goitrous lambs, iodine or thyroxine being preventive in these circumstances. Under experimental conditions groundnuts are goitrogenic for rats, the goitrogenic substance being a glycoside–arachidoside. The goitrogenic effect is inhibited by supplementation of the diet with small amounts of iodine. Soybean byproducts are also considered to be goitrogenic. Gross bacterial contamination of drinking water by sewage is a cause of goiter in humans in countries where hygiene is poor. There is a record of a severe outbreak of goitrous calves from cattle running on pasture heavily dressed with crude sewage. Prophylactic dosing of the cows with potassium iodide prevented further cases. Feeding sewage sludge is also linked to the occurrence of goiter.

Goiter in lambs may occur when permanent pasture is plowed up and resown. This may be due to the sudden loss of decomposition and leaching of iodine-binding humus in soils of marginal iodine content. In subsequent years the disease may not appear. There may be some relation between this occurrence of goiter and the known variation in the iodine content of particular plant species especially if new pasture species are sown when the pasture is plowed. The maximum iodine content of some plants is controlled by a strongly inherited factor and is independent of soil type or season. Thus, in the same pasture, perennial rye grass may contain 146 μg iodine per 100 g dry matter and Yorkshire fog grass only 7 μg/100 g dry matter (10). Because goiter has occurred in lambs when the ewes are on a diet containing less than 30 μg iodine per 100 g dry matter the importance of particular plant species becomes apparent. A high incidence of goiter associated with heavy mortality has been observed in the newborn lambs of ewes grazing on pasture dominated by white clover (11) and by subterranean clover and perennial rye-grass (12).

Congenital goiter has been observed in foals born to mares on low iodine intake (14), but also to mares fed an excessive amount of iodine during pregnancy (13).

Pathogenesis

Iodine deficiency results in a decreased production of thyroxine and stimulation of the secretion of thyrotropic hormone by the pituitary gland. This commonly results in hyperplasia of thyroid tissue and a considerable enlargement of the gland. Most cases of goiter of the newborn are of this type. The primary deficiency of thyroxine is responsible for the severe weakness and hair abnormality of the affected animals. Although the defect is described as hairlessness, it is more properly described as a hypoplasia of the hairs, with many very slender hairs present and a concurrent absence and diminution in size of hair follicles (20). A hyperplastic goiter is highly vascular and the gland can be felt to pulsate with the arterial pulse and a loud murmur may be audible over the gland. Colloid goiter is less common in animals and probably represents an involutional stage after primary hyperplasia.

Other factors, particularly the ingestion of low levels of cyanide, probably exert their effects by inhibiting the metabolic activity of the thyroid epithelium and restricting the uptake of iodine. Thiocyanates and sulfocyanates are formed during the process of detoxication of cyanide in the liver and these substances have a pronounced depressing effect on iodine uptake by the thyroid. Some pasture and fodder plants, including white clover, rape and kale are known to have a moderate content of cyanogenetic glucosides. These goitrogenic substances may appear in the milk and provide a toxic hazard to both animals and man. The inherited form in cattle appears to be due to the increased activity of an enzyme which deiodinates iodotyrosines so rapidly that the formation of thyroxine is largely prevented.

Iodine is an essential element for normal fetal brain and physical development in sheep. A severe iodine deficiency in pregnant ewes causes reduction in fetal brain and body weight from 70 days of gestation to parturition (22). There is also evidence of fetal hypothyroidisms, and absence of wool growth and delayed skeletal maturation near parturition.

Clinical findings

Although loss of condition, decreased milk production and weakness might be anticipated these signs are not usually observed in adults. Loss of libido in the bull, failure to express estrus in the cow and a high incidence of aborted, stillborn or weak calves have been suggested as manifestations of hypothyroidism in cattle whereas prolonged gestation is reported in mares, ewes and sows.

A high incidence of stillbirths and weak, newborn animals is the most common manifestation of iodine deficiency. Partial or complete alopecia and palpable enlargement of the thyroid gland are other signs which occur with varying frequency in the different species.

Foals show a normal hair coat and little thyroid enlargement but are very weak at birth. In most cases they are unable to stand without support and many are too weak to suck. Excessive flexion of the lower forelegs and extension of lower parts of the hindlegs has also been observed in affected foals. Defective ossification has also been reported, the manifestation is collapse of the central and third tarsal bones leading to lameness and deformity of the hock (9). Enlargement of the thyroid also occurs commonly in adult horses in affected areas, thoroughbreds and light horses being more susceptible than draft animals.

In cattle the incidence of thyroid enlargement in adults is much lower than in horses and the cardinal manifestations are gross enlargement of the thyroid gland and weakness in newborn calves. If they are assisted to suck for a few days recovery is usual but if they are born on the range during inclement weather many will die. In some instances the thyroid gland is sufficiently large to cause obstruction to respiration. Partial alopecia is a rare accompaniment.

In pigs the major finding is the birth of hairless, stillborn or weak piglets often with myxedema of the skin of the neck. The hairlessness is most marked on the limbs. Most affected piglets die within a few hours of birth. Thyroid enlargement may be present but is never sufficiently great to cause visible swelling in the live pig. Survivors are lethargic, do not grow well, have a waddling gait and leg weaknesses due to weakness of ligaments and joints.

Adult sheep in iodine-deficient areas may show a high incidence of thyroid enlargement but are clinically normal in other respects. Newborn lambs manifest weakness, extensive alopecia and palpable, if not visible, enlargement of the thyroid glands. Goats present a similar clinical picture except that all abnormalities are more severe than in lambs. Goats' kids are goitrous and alopecic. The degree of alopecia varies from complete absence of hair, through very fine hair, to hair which is almost normal.

Animals which survive the initial danger period after birth may recover except for partial persistence of the goiter. The glands may pulsate with the normal arterial pulse and may extend down a greater part of the neck and cause some local edema. Auscultation and palpation of the jugular furrow may reveal the presence of a murmur and thrill, the 'thyroid thrill', due to the increased arterial blood supply of the glands.

Experimental hypothyroidism produced in horses by surgical excision of the gland results in a syndrome of poor growth, cold sensitivity, long, dull hair coat, docility, lethargy, edema of hindlimbs and a coarse thick appearance of the face. The rectal temperature is depressed and blood cholesterol levels are high. Administration of thyroprotein reverses the syndrome (10).

Clinical pathology

Estimations of iodine levels in the blood and milk are reliable indicators of the thyroxine status of the animal. Organic or protein-bound iodine is estimated in serum or plasma and used as an index of circulating thyroid hormone provided access to exogenous iodine in the diet or as treatment is adequately controlled. There may be between-breed differences in blood iodine levels but levels of 2·4–14 μg of protein-bound iodine per 100 ml of plasma appear to be in the normal range. In ewes an iodine concentration in milk of below 8 μg/l indicates a state of iodine deficiency (15).

Levels of thyroxine in the blood have not been much used to measure thyroid gland sufficiency in animals. Work in ewes has shown that normal lambs at birth have twice the serum thyroxine levels of their dams, but goitrous lambs have levels less than those of their dams (7). However, low mean thyroxine levels (50 nmol/l is normal) are not a definitive indication of iodine deficiency because of the variety of factors which affect thyroxine levels. These levels fall rapidly soon after birth and approximate the dam's levels at 5–6 weeks of age (8).

Blood cholesterol levels have been used as an indicator of thyroid function in humans but are not used in the investigation of goiter in animals.

In determining the iodine status of an area iodine levels in soil and pasture should be obtained but the relationship between these levels, and between them and the status of the grazing animal, may be complicated by conditioning factors.

Necropsy findings

Macroscopic thyroid enlargement, alopecia and myxedema may be evident. The weights of thyroid glands have diagnostic value. In full-term normal calves the average fresh weight is 6·5 g, in lambs 2 g is average. The iodine content of the thyroid will also give some indication of the iodine status of the animal. At birth a level of 0·03% of iodine on a fresh weight basis (0·1% on dry weight) can be considered to be the critical level in cattle and sheep. On histological examination of the glands evidence of hyperplasia should be sought. The hair follicles will be found to be hypoplastic. Delayed osseous maturation, manifested by absence of centers of ossification, is also apparent in goitrous newborn lambs (12). Severe dietary iodine deficiency in pregnant ewes results in evidence of retarded fetal brain development, delayed skeletal maturation and absence of wool growth (22).

Diagnosis

Iodine deficiency is easily diagnosed if goiter is present but the occurrence of stillbirths without obvious goiter may be confusing. Abortion due to infectious agents in cattle and sheep must be considered in these circumstances. In stillbirths due to iodine deficiency gestation is usually prolonged beyond the normal period although this may be difficult to determine in animals bred at pasture. Inherited defects of thyroid hormone synthesis are listed under the heading of inherited diseases. Hyperplastic goiter without gland enlargement has been observed in newborn foals in which rupture of the common digital extensor tendons, forelimb contracture and mandibular prognathism also occur (14). The cause of the combination of defects in unknown.

Treatment

Treatment must be undertaken with care as overdosage will cause toxicity, the chief signs in cattle being anorexia and severe pityriasis. Experimental intoxication in lambs causes anorexia, restlessness, hyperthermia and eventually bronchopneumonia (16). In baby pigs signs appear at feed levels of 400 and 800 mg/kg of iodine (as iodate) in the diet (17) and the minimum toxic level must be considered to be less than 400 mg/kg (18). For calves the minimum toxic level is less than 50 mg/kg and even levels of 25 mg/kg were undesirable (19). The recommendations for control can be adapted to the treatment of affected animals.

Control

The recommended dietary intake of iodine for cattle is 0·8–1·0 mg/kg dry matter of feed for lactating and pregnant cows, and 0·1–0·3 mg/kg dry matter of feed for empty cows and calves.

Iodine can be provided as a fertilizer or in salt or a mineral mixture. The loss of iodine from salt blocks may be appreciable and an iodine preparation which is stable but which contains sufficient available iodine is required. Potassium iodate satisfies these requirements and should be provided as 200 mg of potassium iodate per kg of salt. Potassium iodide alone is unsuitable but when mixed with calcium stearate (8% of the stearate in potassium iodide) it is suitable for addition to salt—200 mg/kg of salt.

Individual dosing of pregnant ewes, on two occasions during the 4th and 5th months of pregnancy, with 280 mg potassium iodide or 370 mg potassium iodate has been found to be effective in the prevention of goiter in lambs when the ewes are on a heavy diet of kale (6). For individual animals, weekly application of tincture of iodine (4 ml cattle, 2 ml pig and sheep) to the inside of the flank is also an effective preventive. The iodine can also be administered as an injection in poppy seed oil (containing 40% bound iodine): 1 ml given intramuscularly 7–9 weeks before lambing is sufficient to prevent severe goiter and neonatal mortality in the lambs. Control of goiter can be achieved for up to 2 years (23). The gestation period is also reduced to normal. A similar injection 3–5 weeks before lambing is less efficient.

A device to release iodine slowly into the forestomachs, while still retaining its position there, has given good results in preventing congenital goiter in lambs when fed to ewes during late pregnancy (3).

REFERENCES

(1) Rudert, C. P. & Oliver, J. (1976) *Rhod. J. agric. Res.*, *14*, 67.
(2) Falconer, I. R. (1966) *Biochem. J.*, *100*, 190.
(3) Mason, R. W. & Laby, R. (1978) *Aust. J. exp. Agric. Anim. Husb.*, *18*, 653.
(4) Walton, E. A. & Humphrey, J. D. (1979) *Aust. vet. J.*, *55*, 43.
(5) Paxman, P. J. & Hill, R. (1974) *J. Sci. Food Agric.*, *25*, 323.
(6) Sinclair, D. P. & Andrews, E. D. (1958) *NZ vet. J.*, *6*, 87.
(7) Andrewartha, K. A. et al. (1980) *Aust. vet. J.*, *56*, 18.
(8) Caple, I. W. et al. (1980) *Vict. vet. Proc.*, *38*, 43.
(9) Shaver, J. R. et al. (1979) *J. equ. med. Surg.*, *3*, 269.
(10) Lowe, J. E. et al. (1974) *Cornell Vet.*, *64*, 276.
(11) George, J. M. et al. (1966) *Aust. vet. J.*, *42*, 1.
(12) Setchell, B. P. et al. (1960) *Aust. vet. J.*, *36*, 159.
(13) Baker, H. J. & Lindsey, J. R. (1968) *J. Am. vet. med. Assoc.*, *153*, 1618.
(14) Doige, C. E. & McLaughlin, B. G. (1981) *Can. vet. J.*, *22*, 42 & 130.
(15) Mason, R. W. (1976) *Br. vet. J.*, *132*, 374.
(16) McCauley, E. H. et al. (1973) *Am. J. vet. Res.*, *34*, 65.
(17) Newton, G. L. & Clawson, A. J. (1974) *J. anim. Sci.*, *39*, 879.
(18) Newton, G. L. (1973) *Diss. Abstr. int.*, *33B*, 5591.
(19) Newton, G. L. (1974) *J. anim. Sci.*, *38*, 449.
(20) Itakura, C. et al. (1979) *Am. J. vet. Res.*, *40*, 111.
(21) Korber, R. et al. (1985) *Mh VetMed.*, *40*, 220.
(22) Potter, B. J. et al. (1982) *Neuropathol. appl. Neurobiol.*, *4*, 303.
(23) Statham, M. and Keen, T. B. (1982) *Aust. J. exp. Agric. anim. Husb.*, *22*, 29.

Iron deficiency

A deficiency of iron in the diet causes anemia and failure to thrive. It is most likely to occur in young piglets maintained under artificial conditions.

Etiology

Iron deficiency is usually primary and is most likely to occur in newborn animals whose sole source of iron is the milk of the dam, milk being a poor source of iron. Deposits of iron in the liver of the newborn are insufficient to maintain normal hemopoiesis for more than 2–3 weeks, and are particularly low in piglets.

Epidemiology

More than half the iron in the animal body is found as a constituent of hemoglobin. A relatively small amount is found in myoglobin and in certain enzymes which play a part in oxygen utilization. Iron-deficiency states are not common in farm animals except in the very young confined to a milk diet. Sucking pigs are the only group in which the disease achieves economic importance and in some piggeries the incidence of the disease may be as high as 90%. The losses that occur include those due to mortality, which may be high in untreated pigs, and to failure to thrive. Continued blood loss by hemorrhage in any animal may bring about a subclinical anemia and an associated iron deficiency. Cattle heavily infested with sucking lice may develop serious and even fatal anemia. The chronic form is characterized by a non-regenerative anemia with subnormal levels of serum iron and treatment with iron is necessary for an optimal response. Horses carrying heavy burdens of blood-sucking strongylid worms often have subnormal hemoglobin levels and respond to treatment with iron. Low serum iron concentration and low serum ferritin have been observed in hospitalized young foals (21). On occasions veal calves, and possibly young lambs and kids, may also suffer from an iron deficiency.

Lack of access to the usual sources of iron may occur in veal calves reared intensively in crates on a milk or milk-substitute diet but naturally occurring cases of anemia have not been recorded in these circumstances, and diets containing 25–30 mg soluble iron/kg dietary dry matter are known to provide sufficient hemoglobin for maintenance of health and yet give light-colored meat (1). At levels of less than 19 mg/kg dry matter of feed the situation is likely to be unsatisfactory and supplementation to be needed (2). The objective in veal calf management is to walk the narrow line between the maximum production of white meat and a degree of anemia insufficient to interfere with maximum production. Asymptomatic iron-deficiency anemia also occurs in newborn calves and kids but there is debate as to whether the condition has practical significance (3). In newborn calves which are affected with a normochromic, normocytic and poikilocytic anemia the levels of serum iron are not significantly different from normal calves (22). Clinicopathological anemia, without clinical signs, is most likely to occur when calves are born with low hemoglobin and hematocrit levels, a relatively common occurrence in twins (4). It is possible that suboptimal growth may occur during the period of physiological anemia during early postnatal life. There is some evidence for this in calves in which hemoglobin levels of 11 g/dl at birth fall to about 8 g/dl between the 30th and 70th days and only begin to rise when the calves start to eat roughage. The daily intake of iron from milk is 2–4 mg in calves and their daily requirement during the first 4 months of life is of the order of 50 mg, so that iron supplementation of the diet is advisable if the calves are fed entirely on milk. Even when hay and grain are fed to calves and lambs in addition to milk there is a marked growth response to the administration of iron-dextran preparations at the rate of 5·5 mg/kg body weight (5). The dietary iron requirement for fast-growing lambs is between 40 and 70 mg/kg and growth rate is suboptimal on diets of less than 25 mg/kg iron (6).

The addition of calcium carbonate to the diet of weaned, fattening pigs is known to cause a conditioned iron deficiency and a moderate anemia but this effect is not apparent in mature pigs. Manganese may exert a similar antagonistic effect.

Anemia caused by iron deficiency occurs in those piglets confined in pens with concrete or other impervious floors and where the sole diet is the milk of the sow. The disease is of major importance in rearing units designed to control parasitic infestations, and in cold climates where indoor housing is essential. Access to earthen yards in most cases provides sufficient iron to overcome the deficiency in the sow's milk. On soils with an exceedingly low iron content the typical disease may occur.

Signs may be present at birth but do not usually appear until the piglets are 3–6 weeks old. Considerable variation occurs in the incidence of cases between litters kept under identical conditions. Black pigs are more prone to the disease than white animals. There may be some difference in the age at which piglets begin to eat supplementary creep feed which may provide additional iron but under usual circumstances the amount of solid feed taken is not significant until about 5 weeks of age, by which time the disease may have already developed.

Withholding iron dextran normally given to piglets at 1–3 days of age to prevent anemia results in a neutropenia and a reduction in the response of the piglets to an interferon inducer (23). This may explain the apparent increased susceptibility of anemic piglets to infections. However, this conflicts with reports which indicate that the administration of iron dextran to newborn piglets actually promotes bacterial growth (24). When iron is present in the body in excess of the ability to properly bind it, an increase in the susceptibility to a variety of infections has been shown to occur (25).

Pathogenesis

Piglets at birth have hemoglobin levels of about 9–11 g/dl. A physiological fall to 4–5 g/dl occurs in all pigs, the lowest levels occurring at about the 8th–10th day of life. Levels of iron in the liver at birth are unusually low in this species and cannot be increased appreciably by supplementary feeding of the sow during pregnancy. The intramuscular injection of iron–dextran preparations to sows during late pregnancy does elevate the hemoglobin levels of the piglets during the first few weeks of life but not sufficiently to prevent anemia in them. Piglets with access to iron show a gradual return to normal hemoglobin levels starting at about the 10th day of life, but in pigs denied this access the hemoglobin levels continue to fall. One of the important factors in the high incidence of anemia in piglets is the rapidity with which they grow in early postnatal life. Piglets normally reach four to five times their birth weight at the end of 3 weeks and eight times their birth weight at the end of 8 weeks. The daily requirement of iron during the first few weeks of life is of the order of 15 mg. The average intake in the milk from the sow is about 1 mg/day and the concentration in sow's milk cannot be elevated by feeding additional iron during pregnancy or lactation. Apart from the specific effect on hemoglobin levels, iron-deficient piglets consume less creep feed, and after the first 3 weeks of life make considerably slower weight gains than supplemented piglets. Although specific pathogen-free pigs show a less marked response to the administration of iron than pigs reared in the normal manner, it is obvious that they need supplementary iron to prevent the development of anemia. Iron-deficient piglets appear to be more susceptible to diarrhea at about 2 weeks of age than in piglets which have received iron (26). A marked impairment of gastric secretion of acid and chloride and atrophic gastritis occurs in iron-deprived piglets (26). Villous atrophy of the small intestine (27) and changes in the gastrointestinal flora also occur in iron-deficient piglets which may contribute to the increased susceptibility to diarrhea (28).

Clinical findings

The highest incidence occurs at about 3 weeks of age although the disease can occur in pigs up to 10 weeks of age.

Affected pigs may be well grown and in good condition but the growth rate of anemic pigs is significantly lower than that of normal pigs (10) and food intake is obviously reduced. Diarrhea is very common, but the feces are usually normal in color and the diarrhea further reduces growth rate. Severe dyspnea, lethargy and a marked increase in amplitude of the apex beat occur with exercise. The skin and mucosae are pale and often quite yellow in white pigs, and there may be edema of the head and forequarters giving the animal a fat, puffed-up appearance. A lean, white hairy look is probably more common. Death usually occurs suddenly, or affected animals may survive in a thin, unthrifty condition. A high incidence of infectious diseases, especially enteric infection with *Escherichia coli*, is associated with the anemia and streptococcal pericarditis is a well recognized complication. Under experimental conditions similar signs occur in calves and there is, in addition, an apparent atrophy of the lingual papillae. A high incidence of stillbirths is recorded in the litters of sows suffering from iron-deficiency anemia (8).

Clinical pathology

In normal piglets there is a postnatal fall of hemoglobin levels to about 8 g/dl and sometimes to as low as 4–5 g/dl during the first 10 days of life. In iron-deficient pigs there is secondary fall to 2–4 g/dl during the 3rd week. The hemoglobin level at which clinical signs appear in pigs is about 4 g/dl (5). Erythrocyte counts also fall from a normal of $5-8 \times 10^6$ down to $3-4 \times 10^6$/µl and may be a better index of iron status than hemoglobin levels (10). Iron deficiency anemia in piglets is a microcytic hypochromic anemia. In chronic blood loss anemia in cattle infested with sucking lice there is a non-regenerative anemia and a decrease in serum iron levels. Serum levels of iron considered to be normal in sheep and cattle are 100–200 µg/dl (17·9–35·8 µmol/l). In newborn calves, the levels are 170 µg/dl (30·4 µmol/l) at birth and 67 µg/dl (12·0 µmol/l) at 50 days of age (11). Serum ferritin concentration is an index for monitoring prelatent iron deficiency of calves (29).

Anemia is a matter of great importance to horse owners, and iron has come under intense scrutiny as a potential philosopher's stone to transmute all the dross of poor horses into gold. Without intending to decry the importance of high hemoglobin levels in the racing horse it is necessary to point out that serum iron levels are not the most favored indicator of hematological efficiency. They vary widely between normal horses, and are very labile within the one horse, fluctuating widely, especially after feeding (12).

Necropsy findings

The necropsy appearance is characterized by pallor, thin and watery blood, and moderate anasarca. The heart is always dilated, sometimes extremely so. The cardiac dimension in severely anemic neonatal pigs has been measured and cardiac dilatation and hypertrophy occur consistently (30). The liver in all cases is enlarged, and has a mottled appearance and the grayish yellow color of fatty infiltration. The mucosa of the gastric fundus in cases of the experimentally induced disease is characteristically shallower and less cellular and shows a pronounced decrease in parietal cells (26) and there is a greatly reduced capacity of the stomach to secrete acid.

Diagnosis

Confirmation of the diagnosis will depend upon hemoglobin determinations and curative and preventive trials with administered iron. The possibility that anemia in piglets may be caused by copper deficiency should not be overlooked especially if the response to administered iron is poor. Isoimmunization hemolytic anemia can be differentiated by the presence of jaundice and hemoglobinuria and the disease occurs in much younger pigs. Eperythrozoonosis occurs in pigs of all ages and the protozoan parasites can be detected in the erythrocytes.

Treatment

The recommendations for the prevention of the disease are set out below and can be followed when treating clinically affected animals. Horses with poor racing performance often have suboptimal blood levels of hemoglobin and a blood loss anemia due to parasitism and respond well to treatment with iron. Treatment is usually parenteral and consists of organic iron preparations such as iron-dextran, iron-sorbitol-citric acid complex, iron saccharate or gluconate. These must be given exactly as prescribed by the manufacturer as some are quite irritant, causing large sloughs when injected intramuscularly. The dose rate is 0·5–1 g elemental iron in one injection once each week. When given intravenously or even intramuscularly some horses show idiosyncratic reactions and literally drop dead (13). Vitamin B_{12} (cyanocobalamin) is often used in the same injection at a dose rate of 5000 µg per week in a single dose. Other additives especially folic acid and choline are also used but with little justification. Oral treatment with iron sulfate or gluconate at a dose rate of 2–4 daily for 2 weeks is as effective and much cheaper but lacks the style of the parenteral injection. It has the disadvantage of being unpalatable and is best dispensed in liquid form to be mixed with molasses and poured onto dry feed.

Control

Preventive measures must be directed at the baby pigs because treatment of the sows before or after farrowing is generally ineffective, although some results are obtained if the iron preparations are fed at least 2 weeks before farrowing. Ferric choline citrate appears to have some special merit in this field (14). Allowing the suckers access to pasture or dirt yards, or periodically placing sods in indoor pens, offer adequate protection. Where indoor housing on impervious floors is necessary, iron should be provided at the rate of 15 mg/day until weaning either by oral dosing with iron salts of a commercial grade or by the intramuscular injection of organic iron preparations. These methods are satisfactory but the results are not usually as good as when piglets are raised outdoors. However, indoor housing is practiced in many areas to avoid exposure to parasitic infestation and some bacterial diseases, especially erysipelas. If sods are put into pens care must be taken to ensure that these diseases are not introduced.

The feeding to sows a diet supplemented with 2000 mg iron/kg of diet will satisfactorily prevent iron-deficiency anemia in the piglets (31). The piglets will ingest about 20 g of sows feces per day which will contain sufficient iron and obviate the need for intramuscular injection of iron–dextran (32). The piglets grow and thrive as well as those which receive the iron–dextran.

Oral dosing

Daily dosing with 4 ml of 1·8% solution of ferrous sulfate is adequate. Iron pyrophosphate may also be used (300 mg/day for 7 days). To overcome the necessity for daily dosing, several other methods of administering iron have been recommended. A single oral treatment with iron–dextran (15) or iron–galactan (7) has been recommended, provided an excellent creep feed is available but the method seems unnecessarily expensive. With this oral treatment it is essential that the iron be given within 12 hours of birth because absorption has to occur through the perforate neonatal intestinal mucosa; later administration is not followed by absorption (16). Reduced iron (British Veterinary Codex) can be administered in large doses because it does not cause irritation of the alimentary mucosa. A single dose of 0·5–1 g once weekly is sufficient to prevent anemia. Alternatively, the painting of a solution of ferrous sulfate on the sow's udder has been recommended (450 g ferrous sulfate, 75 g copper sulfate, 450 g sugar, 2 liters water—applied daily) but has the disadvantage of being sticky and of accumulating litter. Pigs raised on steel gratings can derive enough iron from them to avoid the need for other supplementation (16). Excessive oral dosing with soluble iron salts may cause enteritis, diarrhea and some deaths in pigs and high intakes of ferric hydroxide cause diarrhea, loss of weight and low milk production in cattle. The presence of diarrhea in a herd prevents absorption of orally administered iron and treatment by injection is recommended in this circumstance.

Intramuscular injection of iron preparations

Suitable preparations must be used and are usually injected intramuscularly in piglets on one occasion only, between the 3rd and 7th day of life. Iron–dextran, fumarate and glutamate are most commonly used (18, 19). A dose of 200 mg of a rapidly absorbed and readily utilizable form of iron within the first few days of life will result in greater body weights at 4 weeks of age than piglets given only 100 mg (33). Multiple injections give better hemoglobin levels but have not been shown to improve weight gain and thus a second injection at 2–3 weeks of age may not be economical. A total dose of 200 mg is usually recommended as being required to avoid clinically manifest iron deficiency anemia, but in order to avoid any chance of a subclinical deficiency the feed should contain additional iron at the level of 240 mg/kg (8). A new preparation (Heptomer) contains 200 mg/ml of iron permitting a full dose in one injection (9). Contrasting information is that one injection of 100 mg of iron is adequate for baby pigs (17). Acute poisoning and rapid death occurs in piglets given iron–dextran compounds parenterally if the piglets were born from sows which were deficient in vitamin E and selenium during gestation. This is discussed under iron hypersensitivity. In normal piglets the iron–dextran compounds are safe and are usually not toxic even on repeated injection. These preparations are ideal for treatment because of the rapid response which they elicit and the absence of permanent discoloration of tissues after their use if given during the first month of life (20).

Comparable doses of parenteral iron–dextran compounds have been used for the treatment of iron deficiency or iron loss anemias in other species but accurate doses have not been established and the use of these preparations in cattle and horses is expensive. In addition, iron–dextran preparations given intramuscularly to horses may cause death within a few minutes after administration (13). The most inexpensive method of supplying iron is to use ferrous sulfate orally at a dose of 2–4 g daily for 2 weeks to adult cattle and horses with iron-deficiency anemia.

Iron injection of beef calves in the 1st week after birth will result in an increase in packed cell volume (PVC), hemoglobin (Hb), mean corpuscular volume (MCV) and mean corpuscular hemoglobin (MCH) which persists for 12 weeks (34). However, weight gains during the first 18 weeks of life were not affected.

Dietary supplementation

For calves being raised for white veal the diet should contain 25–30 mg actual soluble iron per kg dietary dry matter. The best indicator of the onset of anemia in calves on these vealer diets is loss of appetite. It is a more sensitive indicator than biochemical measurement (1).

REFERENCES

(1) Bremner, I. et al. (1976) *Vet. Rec.*, *99*, 203.
(2) Mollerberg, L. et al. (1975) *Acta vet. Scand.*, *16*, 197.
(3) Kolb, E. (1963) *Adv. vet. Sci.*, *8*, 50.
(4) Tennant, B. et al. (1975) *Cornell Vet.*, *65*, 543.
(5) Carlson, R. H. et al. (1961) *J. Am vet. med. Assoc.*, *139*, 457.
(6) Lawlor, M. J. et al. (1965) *J. anim. Sci.*, *24*, 742.
(7) Webster, W. R. et al. (1978) *Aust. vet. J.*, *54*, 345.
(8) Rudolphi, K. & Pfau, A. (1978) *Blauen Hefte Tierärztl.*, *58*, 383.
(9) Becker, W. & Towlerton, R. (1979) *Tierärztl. Umschau*, *34*, 708.
(10) Hannan, J. (1971) *Vet. Rec.*, *88*, 181.
(11) Mollerberg, L. & Jacobsson, S. O. (1970) *Svensk VetTidskr.*, *22*, 851.
(12) Osbaldistone, G. W. & Griffith, P. R. (1972) *Can. vet. J.*, *13*, 105.
(13) Wagenaar, G. (1975) *Tijdschr. Diergeeneskd.*, *100*, 562.
(14) Smithwick, G. A. et al. (1967) *Am. J. vet. Res.*, *28*, 469.
(15) Blomgren, L. & Lannek, N. (1971) *Nord. VetMed.*, *23*, 529.
(16) Harmon, B. G. et al. (1974) *J. anim. Sci.*, *39*, 699.
(17) Kay, R. M. et al. (1980) *Vet. Rec.*, *106*, 408.
(18) Froysedal, K. & Slagsvold, P. (1976) *Nord. Vet Tidskr.*, *88*, 393.
(19) Thoren-Tolling, K. (1975) *Acta vet. Scand.*, *16*, Suppl. *54*, 121.
(20) Miller, E. R. et al. (1967) *J. Am. vet. med. Assoc.*, *150*, 735.
(21) Smith, J. E. et al. (1986) *J. Am. vet. med. Assoc.*, *188*, 285.
(22) McGillivray, S. R. et al. (1985) *Can. J. comp. Med.*, *49*, 286.
(23) Grainer, J. H. & Guarnieri, J. (1985) *Cornell Vet.*, *75*, 454.
(24) Knight, C. D. et al. (1983) *J. anim. Sci.*, *57*, 387.
(25) Weinberg, E. D. (1984) *Physiol. Rev.*, *64*, 65–102.
(26) Larkin, H. A. & Hannan, J. (1983) *Res. vet. Sci.*, *34*, 11.
(27) Larkin, H. A. & Hannan, J. (1984) *Res. vet. Sci.*, *36*, 199.
(28) Larkin, H. A. & Hannan, J. (1985) *Res. vet. Sci.*, *39*, 5.
(29) Miyata, Y. et al. (1984) *J. dairy Sci.* *67*, 1256.
(30) Lee, J. C. et al. (1983) *Am. J. vet. Res.*, *44*, 1940.
(31) Gleed, P. T. & Sanson, B. F. (1982) *Vet. Rec.*, *111*, 136.
(32) Gleed, P. T. & Sanson, B. F. (1982) *Br. J. Nutr.*, *47*, 113.
(33) Daykin, M. M. et al. (1982) *Vet. Rec.*, *110*, 535.
(34) Reece, W. O. et al. (1984) *Am. J. vet. Res.*, *45*, 2119.

Sodium chloride deficiency

A dietary deficiency of sodium is most likely to occur during lactation, as a consequence of losses of the element in the milk, in rapidly growing young animals fed on low-sodium, cereal-based diets; under very hot environmental conditions where large losses of water and sodium occur in the sweat and where the grass forage and the seeds may be low in sodium; in animals engaged in heavy or intense physical work and in animals grazing pastures on sandy soils heavily fertilized with potash, which depresses forage sodium levels (1).

There is a lack of firm evidence that naturally occurring salt deficiency causes illness in grazing animals but it is also the consensus that it does occur in certain special circumstances. Of these the most commonly cited occurrences are on alpine pastures and heavily fertilized pasture leys. Pasture should contain at least 0·15 g/100 g dry matter and animals begin to show signs after about 1 month on pasture containing 0.1 g/100 g. Under experimental conditions lactating cows give less milk until the chloride deficiency is compensated. After a period of up to 12 months there is considerable deterioration in the animal's health and anorexia, a haggard appearance, lusterless eyes, rough coat and a rapid decline in body weight occur. Heavily producing animals are most severely affected and some of these may collapse and die. The oral administration of sodium chloride is both preventive and rapidly curative. Experimental sodium depletion in horses for up to 27 days has no deleterious effect on general health.

In dairy cattle on a sodium-deficient diet there is a marked polyuria, polydipsia, salt hunger, pica, including licking dirt and each other's coats, drinking urine, loss of appetite and weight, and a fall in milk production (3). There is frequent urination of urine with a lower than normal specific gravity and the urinary concentrations of sodium and chloride are decreased and the potassium increased. The salivary concentration of sodium is markedly decreased, the potassium is increased and the salivary sodium:potassium ratio is decreased. The concentration of serum sodium and chloride are also decreased but the measurement of urinary or salivary sodium concentration is a more sensitive index of sodium intake than plasma sodium concentration (3). Of these it is urinary sodium which is depressed first and is therefore the preferred indicator in cattle (2) and horses (5). It is suggested that the polyuria associated with severe sodium depletion may be an antidiuretic hormone insensitivity due to lack of an effective countercurrent mechanism and hyperaldosteronism (3).

Experimental restriction of chloride in the diet of dairy cows in early lactation results in a depraved appetite, lethargy, reduced feed intake, reduced milk production, scant feces, gradual emaciation and severe hypochloremia and secondary hypokalemic metabolic alkalosis (9). Lethargy, weakness and unsteadiness occur after about 6 weeks on the chloride-deficient diet (7). Bradycardia is also common. The concentration of chloride in cerebrospinal fluid is usually maintained near normal while the serum concentrations decline (8). The experimental induction of a severe total body chloride deficit by the provision of a low-chloride diet and the daily removal of abomasal contents results in similar clinical findings to those described above and lesions of nephrocalcinosis (10).

The diagnosis of salt deficiency is dependent on the clinical findings, analysis of the feed and water supplies, serum levels of sodium and chlorine and determination of the levels of sodium in the saliva, urine and feces of deficient animals (4). The concentration of sodium in saliva is a sensitive indicator of sodium deficiency. In cattle receiving an adequate supply of sodium and chlorine the sodium levels in saliva vary from 140 to 150 mmol/l, in deficient cattle the levels may be as low as 70–100 mmol/l (4). The levels of sodium in the urine are low with a reciprocal rise in potassium (5). The serum sodium levels are less reliable but licking begins when the level falls to 137 mmol/l and signs are intense at 135 mmol/l.

Experimentally induced sodium deficiency in young pigs causes anorexia, reduced water intake and reduced weight gains (6).

The provision of salt in the diet at a level of 0·5% is considered to be fully adequate for all farm animal species. Under practical conditions salt mixes usually contain added iodine and cobalt. In some situations the salt mixes are provided on an *ad libitum* basis rather than adding them to the diet. However, voluntary consumption is not entirely reliable. The daily amount consumed by animals having unrestricted access to salt can be highly variable and often wasteful. Two factors which influence voluntary salt intake include the physical form of the salt and the salt content of the water and feed supplies. Some cattle consume much more loose than block salt, though the lower intakes of block salt may be adequate. Also, animals dependent on high saline water for drinking consume significantly less salt than when drinking non-saline water. Voluntary salt consumption is generally high in cows on low-sodium pastures which are low inherently or as a result of heavy potash fertilization. Lactating gilts may require 0·7% salt in their diets (11) and energy efficiency in feedlot cattle may be improved by feeding high levels (5% of diet) of salt in the diet of finishing steers (12).

REVIEW LITERATURE

Aitken, F. C. (1976) Sodium and potassium in nutrition of mammals. *Commw. Bur. anim. Nutr. techn. Commun.*, 26.

Michell, A. R. (1985) Sodium in health and disease: A comparative review with emphasis on herbivores. *Vet. Rec.*, *116*, 653–657.

REFERENCES

(1) Underwood, E. J. (1981) *The Mineral Nutrition of Livestock*, 2nd edn. Commonwealth Agricultural Bureaux.
(2) Launer, P. & Storm, R. (1979) *Mh VetMed.*, *34*, 364.
(3) Whitlock, R. H. et al. (1975) *Cornell Vet.*, *65*, 512.
(4) Murphy, G. M. & Gartner, R. J. W. (1974) *Aust. vet. J.*, *50*, 280.
(5) Meyer, H. & Ahlswede, L. (1979) *Zentralbl. VetMed.*, *26A*, 212.
(6) Yusken, J. W. & Reber, E. F. (1957) *Trans. Ill. Acad. Sci.*, *50*, 118.
(7) Fettman, M. J. et al. (1984) *J. Am. vet. med. Assoc.*, *185*, 167.
(8) Fettman, M. J. et al. (1984) *Am. J. vet. Res.*, *45*, 403.
(9) Fettman, M. J. et al. (1984) *J. dairy Sci.*, *67*, 2321.
(10) Blackmon, D. M. et al. (1984) *Am. J. vet. Res.*, *45*, 1638.
(11) Friend, D. W. & Wolynetz, M. S. (1981) *Can. J. anim. Sci.*, *61*, 429.
(12) Croom, W. J. et al. (1982) *Can. J. anim. Sci.*, *62*, 217.

Magnesium deficiency

Although a nutritional deficiency of magnesium does play a part in causing lactation tetany in cows and hypomagnesemic tetany of calves, these diseases are dealt with in Chapter 28 on metabolic diseases because in both instances there are complicating factors which may affect the absorption and metabolism of the element.

Magnesium appears to be an essential constituent of rations for recently weaned pigs (1). Experimentally induced deficiency causes weakness of the pasterns, particularly in the forelegs causing backward bowing of the legs, sickled hocks, approximation of the knees and hocks, arching of the back, hyperirritability, muscle tremor, reluctance to stand, continual shifting of weight from limb to limb, and eventually tetany and death. A reduction in growth rate, feed consumption and conversion, and levels of magnesium in the serum also occur.

The requirement of magnesium for pigs weaned at 3–9 weeks of age is 400–500 mg/kg of the total ration.

REFERENCE

(1) Mayo, R. H. et al. (1959) *J. anim. Sci.*, *18*, 264.

Zinc deficiency

Zinc deficiency occurs in pigs, sheep, cattle and goats and causes parakeratosis, alopecia, wool-eating, abnormal hoof growth and lameness and unthriftiness.

Etiology

A zinc deficiency in young growing swine can cause parakeratosis. The cause is not a simple zinc deficiency. The availability of zinc in the diet is adversely affected by the presence of phytic acid, a constituent of plant protein sources such as soybean meal (1). Much of the zinc in plant protein is in the bound form and unavailable to the monogastric animal such as the pig (4). The use of meat meal or meat scraps in the diet will prevent the disease because of the high availability of the zinc. Another unique feature of the etiology of parakeratosis in swine is that an excess of dietary calcium (0·5–1·5%) can favor the development of the disease, and the addition of zinc to such diets at levels much higher (0·02% zinc carbonate or 100 mg/kg zinc) than those normally required by growing swine prevents the occurrence of the disease. The level of copper in the diet may also be of some significance, increasing copper levels decreasing the requirement for zinc (3). A concurrent enteric infection with diarrhea exacerbates the damage done by a zinc deficiency in pigs (8).

It has been suggested that parakeratosis occurs because very rapidly growing pigs outstrip their biosynthesis of essential fatty acids, and when the diet is high in calcium the digestibility of fat in the diet is reduced at the same time. The net effect in rapidly growing pigs could be a relative deficiency of essential fatty acids.

A low level of dietary zinc intake during pregnancy and lactation of gilts can result in skin lesions, stressful parturition and an increased incidence of intrapartum mortality of piglets and deleterious effects on neonatal growth (41).

In ruminants a primary zinc deficiency due to low dietary zinc is rare but does occur (40). Many factors influence the availability of zinc from soils including the degree of compaction of the soil, and the nitrogen and phosphorus concentration. The risk of zinc deficiency increases when soil pH rises above 46·5 and as fertilization with nitrogen and phosphorus increases. Some legumes contain less zinc than grasses grown on the same soil and zinc concentration decreases with aging of the plant. Several factors may deleteriously affect the availability of zinc to ruminants and cause a secondary zinc deficiency. These include the consumption of immature grass which affects digestibility, the feeding of late-cut hay which may be poorly digestible and the presence of excessive dietary sulfur. The contamination of silage with soil at harvesting can also affect the digestibility of zinc (40).

The disease in cattle has been produced experimentally on diets low in zinc (6) and naturally occurring cases have responded to supplementation of the diet with zinc (40). Calves remain healthy on experimental diets containing 40 mg/kg zinc but parakeratosis has occurred in cattle grazing pastures with a zinc content of 20–80 mg/kg (normal 93 mg/kg) and a calcium content of 0·6% (7). There is also an apparently improved response in cattle to zinc administration if copper is given simultaneously (9). Parakeratosis has also been produced experimentally in goats (10) and sheep (12).

Epidemiology

Parakeratosis in swine was first recorded in North America in rapidly growing pigs particularly those fed on diets containing growth promoters. The disease occurs most commonly during the period of rapid growth, after weaning and between 7 and 10 weeks of age. From 20 to 80% of pigs in affected herds may have lesions and the main economic loss is due to a decrease in growth rate. In general, the incidence is greater in pigs fed in dry lot on self-feeders of dry feed than in pigs which have access to some pasture which is preventive and curative.

Naturally occurring cases in cattle, sheep and goats have been recorded. The disease is well recognized in Europe, especially in calves (16). Naturally occurring cases are common in some families of cattle and an inherited increased dietary requirement for zinc is suspected (18). The inherited disease occurs in Friesian and Black Pied cattle and is known as lethal trait A46. Signs of deficiency appear at 4–8 weeks of age and the main defect is an almost complete inability to absorb zinc from the intestine; zinc administration is curative (33).

Outbreaks of the disease have occurred in Sudanese Desert ewes and their lambs fed on a zinc-deficient diet of Rhodes grass containing less than 10 mg/kg of zinc (34). The disease has also been diagnosed in mature sheep and goats and the cause of the deficiency could not be determined (35). A marginal zinc deficiency, characterized by subnormal growth and fertility and low concentration of zinc in serum, but without other clinical signs, can occur in sheep grazing pastures containing less than 10 mg/kg zinc (37).

Pathogenesis

The pathogenesis of zinc deficiency is not well understood. Zinc is a component of the enzyme carbonic anhydrase which is located in the red blood cells and parietal cells of the stomach and is related to the transport of respiratory carbon dioxide and the secretion of hydrochloric acid by the gastric mucosa. Zinc is also associated with RNA function and related to insulin, glucagon and other hormones (20). It also has a role in keratinization, calcification, wound healing and somatic and sexual development. Because it has a critical role in nucleic acid and protein metabolism a deficiency may adversely affect the cell-mediated immune system.

A zinc deficiency results in a decreased feed intake in all species (37) and is probably the reason for the depression of growth rate in growing animals and body weight in mature animals. Failure of keratinization resulting in parakeratosis, and loss and failure of growth of wool and hair and lesions of the coronary bands probably reflect the importance of zinc in protein synthesis. There are lesions of the arteriolar walls of the dermis (19). The bones of zinc-deficient ruminants reveal abnormal mineralization and reduction of zinc concentration in bones (11). Retarded testicular development occurs in ram lambs and complete cessation of spermatogenesis suggests impairment of protein synthesis.

Clinical findings

Pigs

A reduced rate and efficiency of body weight gain is characteristic (13). Circumscribed areas of erythema appear in the skin on the ventral abdomen and inside the thigh. These areas develop into papules 3–5 mm in diameter which are soon covered with scales followed by thick crusts. These crusts are most visible in areas about the limb joints, ears and tail, and are distributed symmetrically in all cases. The crusts develop fissures and cracks, become quite thick (5–7 mm) and easily detached from the skin. They are crumbly and not flaky or scaly. No greasiness is present except in the depths of fissures. Little scratching or rubbing occurs. Diarrhea of moderate degree is common. Secondary subcutaneous abscesses occur frequently but in uncomplicated cases the skin lesions disappear spontaneously in 10–45 days if the ration is corrected.

Ruminants

In the naturally occurring disease in cattle severe cases shows parakeratosis and alopecia affecting about 40% of the skin area. The lesions are most marked on the muzzle, vulva, anus, tail-head, ears, backs of the hindlegs, kneefolds, flank and neck. Most animals are below average condition and are stunted in growth. After treatment with zinc, improvement is apparent in 1 week and complete in 3 weeks. Experimentally produced cases show poor growth, a stiff gait, swelling of the coronets, hocks and knees, soft swelling containing fluid on the anterior aspect of the hind fetlocks, alopecia and wrinkling of the skin of the legs and scrotum and on the neck and head, especially around the nostrils, hemorrhages around the teeth and ulcers on the dental pad (21). The experimental disease in cattle (6) is manifested by parakeratotic skin mainly on the hindlimbs and udder and similar lesions on teats which tend to become eroded during milking. The fetlocks and pasterns are covered with scabby scales. There is exudation first with matting of hair, then drying and cracking. The skin becomes thickened and inelastic. Histologically there is parakeratosis. Clinical signs develop about 2 weeks after calves and lambs go onto a deficient diet so that there is no evidence of storage of zinc in tissues in these animals. In goats, hair growth, testicular size and spermatogenesis are reduced and growth rate is less than normal. Return to a normal diet does not necessarily reverse these signs and the case fatality rate is high (14). There is a marked delay in wound healing (22).

The natural disease in sheep is characterized by loss of wool and the development of thick, wrinkled skin. Wool eating also occurs in sheep and may be one of the earliest signs noticed in lambs after being on a zinc-deficient diet for 4 weeks (35). Induced cases in lambs have exhibited reduced growth rate, salivation, swollen hocks, wrinkled skin and open skin lesions around the hoof and eyes (10–12). The experimental disease in goats is similar to that in lambs.

One of the most striking effects of zinc deficiency in ram lambs is impaired testicular growth and complete cessation of spermatogenesis (23). Diets containing 2·44 mg/kg caused poor growth, impaired testicular growth and cessation of spermatogenesis and other signs of zinc deficiency within 20–24 weeks. A diet containing 17·4 mg/kg of zinc is adequate for growth but a content of 32·4 mg/kg is necessary for normal testicular development and spermatogenesis. On severely deficient experimental diets other clinical signs in young rams are drooling copious amounts of saliva when ruminating, parakeratosis around eyes, on nose, feet and scrotum, shedding of the hooves, dystrophy and shedding of wool which showed severe staining, and development of a pungent odor. In naturally occurring cases in rams the animals stood with their backs arched and feet close together (35).

Infertility in ewes and a dietary deficiency of zinc have not been officially linked but a zinc responsive infertility has been described in ewes. Again attention is drawn to the need for response trials when soil and pasture levels of an element are marginal (24).

Experimentally induced zinc deficiency in goats causes poor growth, low food intake, testicular hypoplasia, rough dull coat with loss of hair, and the accumulation of hard, dry, keratinized skin on the hindlimbs, scrotum, head and neck. On the lower limbs the scabs fissure and crack and produce some exudate. In naturally occurring cases in pygmy goats there was extensive alopecia, a kyphotic stance, extensive areas of parakeratosis, abnormal hoof growth and flaky, painful coronary bands (35).

A marginal zinc deficiency in ewes may be characterized by only a reduction in feed intake and a slightly reduced body weight, and no other external signs of disease (36). This is important because in grazing ruminants the lack of external signs indicates that zinc deficiency could easily pass undetected.

An experimental zinc deficiency in pregnant ewes results in a decrease in the birth weight of the lambs and a reduced concentration of zinc in the tissues of the lambs which are due to the reduced feed intake which is characteristic of zinc deficiency (36, 37). The zinc content of the diet did not significantly influence the ability of the ewes to become pregnant or maintain pregnancy. The combination of pregnancy and zinc deficiency in the ewe leads to highly efficient utilization of ingested zinc and the developing fetus will accumulate about 35% of the total dietary intake of zinc of the ewe during the last trimester of pregnancy (36). The disease is correctable by the supplementary feeding of zinc (13).

Immediately before parturition in cows there is a precipitate fall in plasma zinc concentration which returns to normal slowly after calving. The depression of zinc levels is greater in cows that experience dystocia. This has led to the hypothesis that dystocia in beef heifers may be caused in some circumstances by a nutritional deficiency of zinc and that preparturient supplementation of the diet with zinc may reduce the occurrence of difficult births (2). This phenomenon does not appear to occur in sheep (15).

Clinical pathology
Laboratory examination of skin scrapings yields negative results but skin biopsy will confirm the diagnosis of parakeratosis. Serum zinc levels may have good diagnostic value. Normal levels are 80–120 μg/dl in sheep and cattle. Calves and lambs on deficient diets may have levels as low as 18 μg/dl (3·0 μmol/l). Normal serum zinc levels in sheep are above 78 μg/dl (12 μmol/l) and values below 39 μg/dl (6 μmol/l) or less are considered as evidence of deficiency (37). There is a general relationship between the zinc content of the hair and the level of zinc in the diet (25) but the analysis of hair is not considered to be a sufficiently accurate indicator of an animal's zinc status (26). In the experimental disease in piglets there is a reduction in serum levels of zinc, calcium and alkaline phosphatase (27) and it is suggested that the disease could be detected by measuring the serum alkaline phosphate and serum zinc levels (28). Levels of zinc in the blood are very labile and simple estimations of it alone are likely to be misleading (29). For example, other intercurrent diseases commonly depress serum calcium and copper levels (30); also zinc levels in plasma fall precipitately at parturition in cows (31); they are also depressed by hyperthermal stress (32). After 1 week on a highly deficient diet serum zinc levels fall to about 50% of normal, or pretreatment levels.

Necropsy findings
Necropsy examinations are not usually performed but histological examination of skin biopsy sections reveals a marked increase in thickness of all the elements of the epidermis. Tissue levels of zinc differ between deficient and normal animals but the differences are statistical rather than diagnostic (25).

Diagnosis
Sarcoptic mange may resemble parakeratosis but is accompanied by much itching and rubbing. The parasites may be found in skin scrapings and treatment with appropriate parasiticides relieves the condition. Exudative epidermitis is quite similar in appearance but occurs chiefly in unweaned pigs. The lesions have a greasy character which is quite different from the dry, crumbly lesions of parakeratosis and the mortality rate is higher.

Treatment
In outbreaks of parakeratosis in swine, zinc should be added to diet immediately at the rate of 50 mg/kg (200 mg of zinc sulfate or carbonate per kg of feed). The calcium level of the diet should be maintained at between 0·65 and 0·75%. The injection of zinc at a rate of 2–4 mg/kg body weight daily for 10 days is also effective (17). Zinc oxide suspended in olive oil and given intramuscularly at a dose of 200 mg of zinc for adult sheep and 50 mg of zinc for lambs will result in a clinical cure within 2 months (38). The oral administration of zinc at the rate of 250 mg zinc sulfate daily for 4 weeks resulted in a clinical cure of zinc deficiency in goats in 12–14 weeks (35).

Control
The calcium content of diets for growing pigs should be restricted to 0·5–0·6%. However, rations containing as little as 0·5% calcium and with normal zinc content (30 mg/kg) may produce the disease. Supplementation with zinc (to 50 mg/kg) as sulfate or carbonate has been found to be highly effective as a preventive and there appears to be a wide margin of safety in its use, diets containing 1000 mg/kg added zinc having no apparent toxic effect. The standard recommendation is to add 200 g of zinc carbonate or sulfate to each tonne of feed. Weight gains in affected groups are also appreciably increased by the addition of zinc to the diet. The addition of oils containing unsaturated fatty acids is also an effective preventive. Access to green pasture, reduction in food intake and the deletion of growth stimulants from rations will lessen the incidence of the disease but are not usually practicable.

For cattle the feeding of zinc sulfate (2–4 daily) is recommended as an emergency measure followed by the application of a zinc-containing fertilizer (7). As an alternative to dietary supplementation for ruminants an intraruminal pellet has been demonstrated in sheep (17). It was effective for 7 weeks only and would not be satisfactory for longterm use. The creation of subcutaneous depots of zinc by the injection of zinc oxide or zinc metal dust has been demonstrated. The zinc dust offered a greater delayed effect (15).

REVIEW LITERATURE

Lamand, M. (1984) Zinc deficiency in ruminants. *Irish vet. J.*, *38*, 40–47.

Luecke, R. W. (1984) Domestic animals in the elucidation of zinc's role in nutrition. *Fed. Proc.*, *43*, 2823–2828.

REFERENCES

(1) Luecke, R. W. (1984) *Fed. Proc.*, *43*, 2823.
(2) Dufty, J. H. et al. (1977) *Aust. vet. J.*, *53*, 519.
(3) Ritchie, H. D. et al. (1963) *J. nutr. Soc.*, *24*, 21.
(4) Forbes, R. M. (1984) *Fed. Proc.*, *43*, 2835.
(5) McSporran, K. D. et al. (1977) *Res. vet. Sci.*, *22*, 393.
(6) Schwarz, W. A. & Kirchgessner, M. (1975) *Vet. med. Rev.*, *112*, 19.
(7) Grashuis, J. (1963) *Landbouwk. Tijdschr.*, *75*, 1127.
(8) Whitenack, D. L. et al. (1978) *Am. J. vet. Res.*, *39*, 1447.
(9) Haaranen, S. (1965) *Nord. VetMed.*, *17*, 36.
(10) Miller, W. J. et al. (1964) *J. dairy Sci.*, *47*, 556.
(11) Hiridoglou, M. (1980) *Can. J. anim. Sci.*, *60*, 579.
(12) Mills, C. F. et al. (1967) *Br. J. Nutr.*, *21*, 751.
(13) Smith, M. C. (1981) *J. Am. vet. med. Assoc.*, *178*, 724.
(14) Neathery, M. W. et al. (1972) *J. dairy Sci.*, *56*, 98.
(15) Lamand, M. et al. (1980) *Ann. Rech. Vet.*, *11*, 147.
(16) van Adrichem, P. W. M. et al. (1970) *Tijdschr. Diergeneeskd.*, *95*, 1170.
(17) Masters, D. G. & Moir, R. S. (1980) *Aust. J. exp. Agric. Anim. Husb.*, *20*, 547.
(18) Stober, M. (1971) *Dtsch Tierärztl. Wochenschr.*, *78*, 257.
(19) Hill, E. G. et al. (1957) *Proc. Soc. exp. Biol. Med.*, *95*, 274.
(20) Hansard, S. L. (1983) *Nutr. Abst. Rev.*, *53*, 1.
(21) Ott, E. A. et al. (1965) *J. anim. Sci.*, *24*, 735.
(22) Blackmon, D. M. et al. (1967) *Vet. Med.*, *62*, 265.
(23) Underwood, E. J. (1969) *Aust. J. agric. Res.*, *20*, 889.
(24) Egan, A. R. (1972) *Aust. J. exp. Agric.*, *12*, 131.
(25) Miller, W. J. et al. (1966) *J. dairy Sci.*, *49*, 1446.
(26) Schwarz, W. A. Kirchgessner, M. (1975) *Dtsch Tierärztl. Wochenschr.*, *82*, 141.
(27) Miller, E. R. et al. (1968) *J. Nutr.*, *95*, 278.

(28) Kirchgessner, M. & Schwarz, W. A. (1975) *Zentralbl. VetMed.*, *22A*, 572.
(29) Schwarz, W. A. & Kirchgeessner, M. (1975) *Z. Tierphysiol. tierernähr. Futtermittelk.*, *34*, 289.
(30) Corrigall, W. et al. (1976) *Vet. Rec.*, *99*, 396.
(31) Pryor, W. J. (1976) *NZ vet. J.*, *24*, 57.
(32) Wegner, T. N. et al. (1973) *J. dairy Sci.*, *56*, 748.
(33) Price, J. & Wood, D. A. (1982) *Vet. Rec.*, *110*, 478.
(34) Mahmoud, O. M. et al. (1983) *J. comp. Pathol.*, *93*, 591.
(35) Nelson, D. R. et al. (1984) *J. Am. vet. Med. Assoc.*, *184*, 1480.
(36) Masters, D. G. & Moir, R. J. (1983) *Br. J. Nutr.*, *49*, 365.
(37) Underwood, E. J. (1981) *The Mineral Nutrition of Livestock*, 2nd edn. Commonwealth Agricultural Bureaux.
(38) Mahmoud, O. M. et al. (1985) In: *Proc. 5th Int. Symp. on Trace Elements in Man and Animals*, (eds) C. F. Mills, I. Bremner & J. K. Chesters. Commonwealth Agricultural Bureaux.
(39) McErlean, B. A. (1984) *Irish vet. J.*, *38*, 48.
(40) Lamand, M. (1984) *Irish vet. J.*, *38*, 40.
(41) Kalinowski, J. & Chavez, E. R. (1986) *Can. J. anim. Sci.*, *66*, 201, 217.

Manganese deficiency

Dietary deficiency of manganese is thought to cause infertility and skeletal deformities both congenitally and after birth.

Etiology

A primary deficiency occurs enzootically in some areas because of a geological deficiency in the local rock formations (1, 4). Apart from a primary dietary deficiency of manganese the existence of factors which depress the availability of ingested manganese is suspected. An excess of calcium and/or phosphorus in the diet is known to increase the requirements of manganese in the diet of calves (5), and is considered to reduce the availability of dietary manganese to cattle generally (6).

Epidemiology

Soils containing less than 3 mg/kg of manganese are unlikely to be able to support normal fertility in cattle (6). In areas where manganese-responsive infertility occurs, soils on farms with infertility problems have contained less than 3 mg/kg of manganese, whereas soils on neighboring farms with no infertility problems have had levels of more than 9 mg/kg. A secondary soil deficiency is thought to occur and one of the factors suspected of reducing the availability of manganese in the soil to plants is high alkalinity. Thus heavy liming is associated with manganese-responsive infertility. There are three main soil types on which the disease occurs:

1. Soils low in manganese have low output even when pH is less than 5·5.
2. Sandy soils where availability starts to fall at pH of 6·0.
3. Heavy soils where availability starts to fall at pH of 7·0.

Many other factors are suggested as reducing the availability of soil manganese but the evidence is not conclusive. For example, heavy liming of soils to neutralize sulfur dioxide emissions from a neighboring smelter is thought to have reduced the manganese intake of grazing animals (2).

Herbage on low manganese soils, or on marginal soils where availability is decreased (possibly even soils with normal manganese content), is low in manganese. A number of figures are given for critical levels. It is suggested (6) that pasture containing less than 80 mg/kg of manganese is incapable of supporting normal bovine fertility and that herbage containing less than 50 mg/kg is often associated with infertility and anestrus. The Agricultural Research Council (7) feels that, although definite figures are not available, levels of 40 mg/kg in the diet should be adequate. Other authors state that rations containing less than 20 mg/kg may cause anestrus and reduction in conception rates in cows (8–10) and the production of poor quality semen by bulls (11). Most pasture contains 50–100 mg/kg (12). Skeletal deformities in calves occur when the deficiency is much greater than the above; for example, a diet containing more than 200 mg/kg is considered to be sufficient to prevent them (4).

Rations fed to pigs usually contain more than 20 mg/kg of manganese and deficiency is unlikely unless there is interference with manganese metabolism by other substances.

There are important variations in the manganese content of seeds, an important matter in poultry nutrition (1). Maize and barley have the lowest content. Wheat or oats have three to five times as much, and bran and pollard are the richest natural sources with 10–20 times the content of maize or wheat. Cows' milk is exceptionally low in manganese.

Pathogenesis

Manganese plays an active role in bone matrix formation, and in the synthesis of chondroitin sulfate, responsible for maintaining the rigidity of connective tissue. In magnesium deficiency these are affected deleteriously and skeletal abnormalities result (3).

Clinical findings

In cattle the common syndromes are infertility, calves with congenital limb deformities (4, 10) and calves with manifest poor growth, dry coat and loss of coat color. The deformities include knuckling over at the fetlocks (13), enlarged joints and possibly twisting of the legs (10). The bones of affected lambs are shorter and weaker than normal and there are signs of joint pain, hopping gait and reluctance to move (14). A manganese responsive infertility has been described in ewes (15) and is well known in cattle. In cattle it is manifested by slowness to exhibit estrus, and failure to conceive, often accompanied by subnormal size of one or both ovaries. Subestrus and weak estrus have also been observed.

Some years ago it was proposed that functional infertility occurred in cattle on diets with calcium to phosphorus ratios outside the range of 1 : 2 to 2 : 1 (8). This was not upheld on investigation but may have been correct if high calcium to phosphorus intakes directly reduced manganese (or copper or iodine) availability in diets marginally deficient in one or other of these elements.

In pigs experimental diets low in manganese cause reduction in skeletal growth, muscle weakness, obesity, irregular, diminished or absent estrus, agalactia and resorption of fetuses or the birth of stillborn pigs (16). Leg weakness, bowing of the front legs and shortening of bones also occur (17).

Clinical pathology

The blood of normal cattle contains 18–19 μg/dl (3·3–3·5 μmol/l) of manganese (18) although considerably lower levels are sometimes quoted (10). The livers of normal cattle contain 12 mg/kg (0·21 mmol/kg) of manganese and down to 8 mg/kg (0·15 mmol/kg) in newborn calves (19) which also have a lower content in hair. The manganese content of hair varies with intake. The normal level is about 12 mg/kg (0·21 mmol/kg) and infertility is observed in association with levels of less than 8 mg/kg (0·15 mmol/kg) (19). In normal cows the manganese content of hair falls during pregnancy from normal levels of 12 mg/kg (0·21 mmol/kg) in the first month of pregnancy to 4·5 mg/kg (0·08 mmol/kg) at calving (20). All of these figures require much more critical evaluation than they have had, before they can be used as diagnostic tests.

Although tissue manganese levels in normal animals have been described as being between 2 and 4 mg/kg (0·04 and 0·07 mmol/kg) in most tissue (1) there appears to be more variation between tissues than this (18). However, tissue levels of manganese do not appear to be depressed in deficient animals except for ovaries in which levels of 0·6 mg/kg (0.01 mmol/kg) (3) and 0·85 mg/kg (0·02 mmol/kg) (9) are recorded in contrast to a normal level of 2 mg/kg (0·04 mmol/kg).

There is then no simple, single diagnostic test which permits detection of manganese deficiency in animals. Reproductive functions, male and female, are most sensitive to manganese deficiency and are affected before possible biochemical criteria, e.g. blood and bone alkaline phosphatase, liver arginase levels, are significantly changed. The only certain way of detecting moderate deficiency states is by measuring response to supplementation. Findings which may provide contributory evidence of manganese deficiency are set out below.

Treatment and control

Young cattle have shown a general response in fertility to 2 g $MnSO_4$ daily (3) but the general recommendation is daily supplementation with 4 g manganese sulfate providing 980 mg elemental manganese. This level of feeding is estimated to raise the dietary intake by 75 mg/kg (estimated on a daily intake of 12 kg dry matter by a 450 kg cow). In some herds a full response was obtained only after doubling this rate of feeding (13). Although the feeding of 15 g of manganese sulfate daily is reported to cause no signs of toxicity, manganese is known to interfere with the utilization of cobalt and zinc in ruminants (21). Very large levels of intake to calves can reduce growth rate and hemoglobin levels (22). The recommended procedure is to feed the supplement for 9 weeks commencing 3 weeks before the first service (13).

Excessive supplementation, up to 5000 mg/kg, of the diet with manganese for periods of up to 3 months appeared to cause only a reduction in appetite and weight gain (22).

For pigs the recommended dietary intakes are 24–57 mg manganese per 45 kg body weight (23). Expressed as a proportion of food intake the recommended dietary level is 40 mg/kg in feed (7).

REVIEW LITERATURE

Hiridoglou, M. (1979) Manganese in ruminant nutrition. *Can. J. anim. Sci.*, *59*, 217.

REFERENCES

(1) Underwood, E. J. (1981) *The Mineral Nutrition of Livestock*, 2nd edn. Commonwealth Agricultural Bureaux.
(2) Cowgill, U. M. et al (1980) *Environ. Poll.*, *22*, 259.
(3) Hiridoglou, M. (1980) *Can. J. anim. Sci.*, *60*, 579.
(4) Dyer, I. A. & Rojas, M. A. (1965) *J. Am. vet. med. Assoc.*, *147*, 1393.
(5) Hawkins, G. E. et al. (1955) *J. dairy Sci.*, *38*, 536.
(6) Wilson, J. G. (1966) *Vet. Rec.*, *79*, 562.
(7) Agricultural Research Council (1965) *The Nutrient Requirements of Farm Livestock, No. 2, Ruminants*. Technical Reviews and Summaries. London.
(8) Hignett, S. L. (1956) *Proc. 3rd int. Congr. Anim. Reprod., Cambridge*, 116.
(9) Bentley, O. G. & Phillips, P. H. (1951) *J. dairy Sci.*, *34*, 396.
(10) Rojas, M. A. et al. (1965) *J. anim. Sci.*, *24*, 664.
(11) Lardy, H. A. et al. (1942) *J. anim. Sci.*, *1*, 79.
(12) Thompson, A. (1957) *J. Sci. Food Agric.*, *8*, 72.
(13) Wilson, J. G. (1965) *Vet. Rec.*, *77*, 489.
(14) Lassiter, J. W. & Morton, J. S. (1968) *J. anim. Sci.*, *27*, 776.
(15) Egan, A. R. (1972) *Aust. J. exp. Agric.*, *12*, 131.
(16) Plumlee, M. P. et al. (1956) *J. anim. Sci.*, *15*, 352.
(17) Neher, G. M. et al. (1956) *Am. J. vet. Res.*, *17*, 121.
(18) Sawhney, P. C. & Kehar, N. D. (1961) *Ann. Biochem. exp. Med.*, *21*, 125.
(19) van Koetsveld, E. E. (1958) *Tijdschr. Diergeneeskd.*, *83*, 229.
(20) Ushev, D. (1968) *Vet. Sbir. Sofia*, *65*, 57; in *Vet. Bull.* (1969) *39*, 129.
(21) Pfander, W. H. et al. (1966) *Fedn Proc. Fedn Am. Socs exp. Biol.*, *25*, 431.
(22) Cunningham, G. N. et al. (1966) *J. anim. Sci.*, *25*, 532.
(23) Littlejohn, A. & Lewis, G. (1960) *Vet. Rec.*, *72*, 137.

Potassium deficiency

Naturally occurring dietary deficiency of potassium is thought to be rare. However, calves fed on roughage grown on soils which are deficient in potassium or in which the availability of potassium is reduced may develop a clinical syndrome of poor growth, anemia and diarrhea. Supplementation of the diet with potassium salts appears to be curative. A similar syndrome has been produced experimentally in pigs (1) which manifested poor appetite, emaciation, rough coat, incoordination and marked cardiac impairment as indicated by electrocardiographic examination. The optimum level of potassium in the diet of young growing pigs is about 0·26% and in ruminants 0·5% (i.e. 65 mg/kg body weight) (2). Electrocardiographic changes have also been observed in cattle on potassium-deficient diets and these are probably related to the degeneration of Purkinje fibers of the myocardium which occurs on such diets. Similar changes have been recorded on diets deficient in magnesium or vitamin E.

An intake of potassium above requirement is more likely to occur than a deficiency, and although very large doses of potassium are toxic, ruminants are capable of metabolizing intakes likely to be encountered under natural conditions (3). It seems probable, however, that potassium interferes with the absorption of magnesium and heavy applications of potash fertilizers to grass pastures may contribute to the development of the hypomagnesemia of lactation tetany.

REFERENCES

(1) Cox, J. L. et al. (1966) *J. anim. Sci.*, *25*, 203.
(2) Telle, P. P. et al. (1964) *J. anim. Sci.*, *23*, 59.
(3) Ward, G. M. (1966) *J. dairy Sci.*, *49*, 268.

Selenium and/or vitamin E deficiencies

It is now evident that several diseases of farm animals are caused by or associated with a deficiency of either selenium or vitamin E alone or both, usually in association with important predisposing factors such as dietary unsaturated fatty acids, unaccustomed exercise and rapid growth in young animals.

The diseases which are considered to be caused by a deficiency of selenium and/or vitamin E are summarized in Table 88. We have decided to incorporate all of these diseases under one heading because the available evidence suggests that both selenium and vitamin E are important in the etiology, treatment and control of the major diseases caused by their deficiencies. These diseases are also known as selenium–vitamin E-responsive diseases because, with some exceptions, they can be prevented by adequate supplementation of the diet with both nutrients.

The term 'selenium-responsive disease' has created some confusion relative to the selenium deficiency diseases. In some regions of the world, particularly New Zealand and in parts of Australia and North America, diseases such as illthrift in sheep and cattle and poor reproductive performance respond beneficially to selenium administration and while these usually occur in selenium-deficient regions, these diseases have not necessarily been proved to be due to selenium deficiency. Therefore, it is probable that there are reasonably well-defined selenium deficiency diseases and ill-defined 'selenium-responsive' responses.

Selenium is an essential nutrient for animals, and diseases due to selenium inadequacy in livestock are of world-wide distribution (1). The biochemical role of selenium is as a component of the enzyme glutathione peroxidase (GSH-PX) (2). The activity of the enzyme in erythrocytes is positively related to the blood concentration of selenium in cattle, sheep, horses (60) and swine (11), and is a useful aid for the diagnosis of selenium deficiency and to determine the selenium status of the tissues of these animals. The enzyme from the erythrocytes of both cattle and sheep contains 4 g atoms of selenium per mol of enzyme (15).

Glutathione peroxidase protects cellular membranes and lipid containing organelles from peroxidative damage by inhibition and destruction of endogenous peroxides, acting in conjunction with vitamin E to maintain integrity of these membranes (10). Hydrogen peroxide and lipid peroxides are capable of causing irreversible denaturation of essential cellular proteins which leads to degeneration and necrosis. Glutathione peroxidase catalyzes the breakdown of hydrogen peroxide and certain organic hydroperoxides produced by glutathione during the process of redox cycling. This dependence of GSH-PX activity on the presence of selenium offers an explanation for the interrelationship of selenium, vitamin E and sulfur-containing amino acids in animals. The sulfur-containing amino acids may be precursors of glutathione which in turn acts as a substrate for GSH-PX and maintains sulfhydryl groups in the cell. Selenium is also a component of several other proteins such as selenoprotein of muscle, selenoflagellin, Se-transport proteins, and the bacterial enzymes, formate dehydrogenase and glycin reductase. Selenium also facilitates significant changes in the metabolism of many drugs and xenobiotics. For example, selenium functions to counteract the toxicity of several metals such as arsenic, cadmium, mercury, copper, silver and lead.

The biochemical role of vitamin E is considered to be that of an antioxidant, preventing oxidative damage to sensitive membrane lipids by decreasing hydroperoxide formation (2). Vitamin E has a central role in protection of cellular membranes from lipoperoxidation, especially membranes rich in unsaturated lipids, such as mitochondria, endoplasmic reticulum and plasma membranes (15).

An important interrelationship exists between selenium, vitamin E and the sulfur-containing amino acids in preventing some of the nutritional diseases caused by their deficiency. If vitamin E prevents fatty acid hydroperoxide formation, and the sulfur amino acids (as precursors of GSH-PX) and selenium are involved in peroxide destruction, these nutrients would produce a similar biochemical result, that is, lowering of the concentration of peroxides or peroxide-induced products in the tissues (2). Protection against oxidative damage to susceptible non-membrane proteins by dietary selenium but not by vitamin E might explain why some nutritional diseases respond to selenium but not to vitamin E. On the other hand, certain tissues or subcellular components may not be adequately protected from oxidant damage because they are inherently low in GSH-PX even with adequate dietary selenium. Damage to such tissues would be expected to be aggravated by diets high

Table 88. Diseases considered to be caused by or associated with a deficiency of either selenium or vitamin E or both (including 'selenium-responsive' diseases).

Cattle	*Horse*	*Swine*	*Sheep*
Nutritional (enzootic) muscular dystrophy	Nutritional muscular dystrophy	Mulberry heart disease	Nutritional (enzootic) muscular dystrophy
Retained fetal membranes		Hepatosis dietetica	Illthrift } 'selenium-responsive'
		Exudative diathesis	Reproductive inefficiency } 'selenium-responsive'
		Iron hypersensitivity	Bone marrow abnormalities
		Nutritional muscular dystrophy	
		Anemia	

in unsaturated fatty acids and to respond adequately to vitamin E but not to selenium. The variations in GSH-PX activity between certain tissues such as liver, heart, skeletal and myocardial muscles would explain the variations in the severity of lesions between species.

There are both selenium-dependent glutathione peroxidase and non-selenium-dependent glutathione peroxidase activities in the tissues and blood (102). The non-selenium-dependent enzyme does not contain selenium and does not react with hydrogen peroxide but shows activity toward organic hydroperoxide substrates. The spleen, cardiac muscle, erythrocytes, brain, thymus, adipose tissue and striated muscles of calves contain only the selenium-dependent enzyme. The liver, lungs, adrenal glands, testes, and kidney contain both enzymes. Hepatic tissue contains the highest level of non-selenium-dependent enzyme.

Etiology

The selenium and vitamin E-responsive or deficiency diseases of farm animals are caused by diets which are deficient in selenium and/or vitamin E, with or without the presence of conditioning factors such as an excessive quantity of polyunsaturated fatty acids in the diet. Almost all of the diseases which occur naturally have been reproduced experimentally using diets deficient in selenium and/or vitamin E. Conversely, the lesions can usually be prevented with selenium and vitamin E supplementation (15). In certain instances, as for example in hand-fed dairy calves, the incorporation of excessive quantities of polyunsaturated fatty acids was a major factor in the experimental disease and this led to the conclusion that certain myopathic agents were necessary to produce the lesion, which may no longer be tenable. It appears that the presence of polyunsaturated fatty acids in the diet may cause a conditioned vitamin E deficiency because the vitamin acts as an antioxidant. In the case of naturally occurring muscular dystrophy in calves, lambs and foals on pasture, the myopathic agent, if any, is unknown and selenium is protective. On the other hand, selenium is not protective against the muscular dystrophy associated with the feeding of cod liver oil to calves.

Interactions between selenium and trace minerals may occur (7). Lesions of selenium and vitamin E deficiency can be reproduced experimentally in pigs and ducklings fed excessive quantities of trace mineral elements such as cobalt, silver, tellurium, zinc and vanadium (7). Selenium–vitamin E supplementation can provide protection against cobalt-induced cardiomyopathy (8).

In summary, it would appear that these diseases are associated with diets which are naturally low in selenium because of the selenium deficiency of the soil on which they were grown, combined with a deficiency of vitamin E which may be primary or secondary due to factors which destroy the vitamin. These factors will be discussed under epidemiology and pathogenesis.

Epidemiology

Nutritional muscular dystrophy

This occurs in all farm animal species but is most important in young, rapidly growing calves, lambs and foals, born from dams which have been fed for long periods, usually during the winter months, on diets low in selenium and vitamin E. The disease occurs in pigs usually in association with other more serious diseases, such as mulberry heart disease and hepatosis dietetica. Nutritional muscular dystrophy in calves, lambs and foals has been reported from most countries of the world but is common in the United Kingdom, the United States, Scandinavia, Europe, Canada, Australia and New Zealand. In North America it is common in the northeast and northwest and uncommon on the relatively high selenium soils of the Great Plains, where selenium toxicity has occurred. Soils, and therefore the pastures they carry, vary widely in their selenium content, depending largely on their geological origin. In general, soils derived from rocks of recent origin, e.g., the granitic and pumice sands of New Zealand, are notably deficient in selenium. Soils derived from igneous rocks are likely to be low in selenium. Sedimentary rocks, which are the principal parent material of agricultural soils, are richer in selenium. Forage crops, cereal grains and corn grown in these areas are usually low in selenium content (below 0·1 mg/kg), compared to the concentration in crops (above 0·1 mg/kg) grown in areas where the available soil selenium is much higher and usually adequate (19).

In the United States the states of the Pacific northwest and of the northeastern and southeastern seaboard are generally low in selenium (16). In Canada, western prairie grains generally contain relatively high levels of selenium, whereas in the eastern provinces, soils and feedstuffs usually have low selenium concentrations (21). Most soils in the Atlantic provinces of Canada are acidic and consequently the forages are deficient in selenium. Most forage samples contain less than 0·10 mg/kg of selenium and enzootic nutritional muscular dystrophy is common throughout the region (79).

Surveys in the United Kingdom reveal that the selenium status may be low in sheep and cattle fed locally produced feedstuffs without any mineral supplementation (13, 99). In one survey of 329 farms, the selenium status was low on 47% of the farms, which places a large number of animals at risk (13). There are also differences in the selenium concentrations of different feeds grown in the same area. For example, in some areas it has been estimated that about 75% of cattle fed primarily corn silage or 46% of the cattle fed sedge hay might be considered to be under varying degrees of stress because of inadequate selenium. In contrast, only 20% of the cattle fed primarily grass and legume forage from the same area might be similarly stressed due to an inadequate intake of selenium (22).

There may be wide variations in the serum selenium concentrations and glutathione peroxidase activities in cattle grazing forages of various selenium concentrations within the same geographic area (3). In a certain geographic area some cattle will have adequate levels of serum selenium while others in neighboring farms will have inadequate levels and are at risk of developing selenium-deficiency diseases. Several factors influence the availability of soil selenium to plants. The pH of the soil—alkalinity encourages selenium absorption by plants—and the presence of a high level of sulfur which competes for absorption sites with selenium in both plants and animals are two factors reducing availability. There is also much variation between plants in their ability to absorb selenium; 'selector' and 'converter' plants are listed under the heading of selenium poisoning; legumes take up much less selenium than do grasses. Seasonal conditions also influence the selenium content of pasture, the content being lowest in the spring and when rainfall is heavy. In this way a marginally deficient soil may produce a grossly deficient pasture if it is heavily fertilized with superphosphate, thus increasing its sulfate content, if the rainfall is heavy and the sward is lush and dominated by clover as it is likely to be in the spring months (23).

Primary vitamin E deficiency occurs most commonly when animals are fed on inferior quality hay or straw and on root crops. Cereal grains, green pasture, and well-cured fresh hay contain adequate amounts of the vitamin.

Alpha-tocopherol levels are very high in green grasses and clovers but there are wide variations in the concentrations from one area to another (108). Many factors influence the tocopherol content of pasture and hence the animals' intake. The level of tocopherol in pasture declines by up to 90% as it matures. Levels as low as 0·7 mg/kg have been reported in dry summer pastures grazed by sheep. The alpha-tocopherol content of ryegrass and clover pasture ranges from 22 to 350 and 90 to 210 mg/kg dry matter, respectively. After harvesting and storage, the tocopherol content of pasture and other crops may fall further, sometimes to zero. Preservation of grain with propionic acid does not prevent the decline. Thus the dietary intake of alpha-tocopherol by cattle and sheep may be expected to vary widely and lead to wide variations in tissue levels (108).

The serum tocopherol levels are higher in calves born from cows fed grass silage than in those born from cows fed the same grass as hay (6). Outbreaks of muscular dystrophy with myoglobinuria have been reported, with increasing frequency recently, in yearling cattle fed on high-moisture grain which was treated with propionic acid as a method of inexpensive storage and protection from fungal growth (25). There is a marked drop in the vitamin E content of acid-treated grain, and an increase in the levels of peroxides of fat which is consistent with a loss of naturally occurring antioxidants such as the tocopherols (25) (secondary vitamin E deficiency). The levels of selenium in the feed were below 0·05 mg/kg which is inadequate and emphasizes the interdependence of selenium and vitamin E. The tocopherol content of moist grain (barley and maize) stored for 6 months, with or without propionic acid, falls to extremely low levels compared to conventionally stored grain in which the tocopherol levels usually persist over the same length of time (26). Selenium-deficient barley treated with sodium hydroxide to deplete it of vitamin E can be used to induce muscular dystrophy when fed to yearling cattle (12). Nutritional muscular dystrophy may occur in weaner sheep with low alpha-tocopherol levels in liver with an adequate selenium status (98) which emphasizes the interdependence of the two nutrients.

Those diets which are rich in unsaturated fatty acids such as cod liver oil, other fish oils, fishmeal used as a protein concentrate, lard, linseed oil, soybean and corn oils have all been implicated in the production of muscular dystrophy, particularly in calves fed milk replacers containing some of these ingredients. Experimentally, linolenic acid in a protected-fat form, added to a vitamin E and selenium-deficient diet and fed to calves 6–9 months of age can result in muscular dystrophy (27). Fresh spring grass containing a sufficient concentration of linolenic acid to equal the amount necessary to produce muscular dystrophy in calves may explain the occurrence of the naturally occurring disease in the spring months. The oxidation during rancidification of the oils causes destruction of the vitamin, thus increasing the dietary requirements (a conditioned vitamin E deficiency), and the presence of myopathic agents in the oils may also contribute to the occurrence of the disease. A secondary vitamin E deficiency can be said to occur when muscular dystrophy develops on rations containing vitamin E in amounts ordinarily considered to be adequate, but the disease is prevented by further supplementation with the vitamin. The lack of specificity of vitamin E in the prevention of muscular dystrophy in some circumstances is indicated by its failure, and by the efficiency of selenium, as a preventive agent in lambs on lush legume pasture.

It is generally held that although enzootic muscular dystrophy can result from a dietary deficiency of selenium and/or vitamin E, a precipitating factor, such as myopathic agents in the feed, sudden unaccustomed exercise, prolonged transport, exposure to other dietary or climatic stress or intercurrent disease, may convert an asymptomatic deficiency state to one of frank disease of the musculature.

The myopathic agents concerned in the development of muscular dystrophy in farm animals have not all been identified. Unsaturated fatty acids in fish and vegetable oils appear to be important myopathic agents in many outbreaks of enzootic muscular dystrophy (white muscle disease of calves and stiff-lamb disease). In other circumstances the agent or agents have not been identified although a high content of unsaturated fatty acids in the milk of some dams has been suggested. There is some limited evidence that plants containing cyanogenic glycosides can precipitate outbreaks of nutritional muscular dystrophy in lambs (9).

Nutritional muscular dystrophy occurs principally in young, rapidly growing calves, lambs and foals. Until recently the disease was recognized most commonly in rapidly growing, well-nourished beef calves 2–4 months of age, shortly following unaccustomed exercise. This was commonplace in countries where calves were born and raised indoors until about 6–8 weeks of age when they were turned out onto new pasture in the spring of the year. This is a standard practice in small beef herds in the United Kingdom, Europe and North America. A similar situation applies for ewes which lambed indoors and the lambs were let out to pasture from 1–3 weeks of age. Thus, unaccustomed activity in calves and lambs running and playing following their turnout onto pasture has been considered as an important precipitating factor but is not necessarily a prerequisite for the disease. In lambs, the vigorous exertion associated with running and sucking may account for the peracute form of myocardial dystrophy in young lambs on deficient pastures and from deficient ewes. In older lambs up to 3 months of age, outbreaks of acute myocardial dystrophy and stiff-lamb disease may be associated with the driving of flocks long distances. A similar situation applies for calves which are moved long distances from calving grounds and early spring pastures to lush summer pastures. Experimentally, in lambs, regular exercise had a modifying influence on the development of muscular dystrophy in lambs fed dystrophogenic diets (28). The wandering and bellowing which occurs in beef calves weaned at 6–8 months of age may precipitate outbreaks of subacute muscular dystrophy. Degenerative myopathy of yearling cattle (feedlot cattle, housed yearling bulls and heifer replacements) is now being recognized with increased frequency (30, 37). The disease resembles subacute enzootic muscular dystrophy of calves and in the United Kingdom is often seen when yearlings are turned outdoors in the spring of the year after being housed during the winter and fed a poor quality hay or straw or propionic acid treated grain. Unaccustomed exercise is a common precipitating factor but the disease has occurred in housed yearling bulls with no history of stress or unaccustomed exercise but the diet was deficient in selenium and vitamin E (32). Whether or not congenital nutritional muscular dystrophy occurs in farm animals is not known. Isolated cases are reported by veterinarians but these have not been well documented (35). Certainly the disease can occur in calves and lambs only a few days of age, but these are uncommon.

Nutritional muscular dystrophy in horses occurs most commonly in foals to about 7 months of age (34). The concentration of selenium in the blood of the mares was subnormal, the concentrations of selenium and vitamin E in the feedstuffs were subnormal, the level of unsaturated fatty acids in the feed was high and vitamin E and selenium supplementation prevented the disease. The disease is not well recognized in adult horses, but sporadic cases of dystrophic myodegeneration are recorded in horses from 5 to 10 years of age (33). Some baseline data for selenium and vitamin E concentration in horses from breeding farms is available (20). In horses subjected to exercise there is an increase in erythrocyte malondialdehyde, a product of peroxidation, but selenium supplementation has no beneficial effect (5). There is inconclusive evidence that a selenium–vitamin E deficiency causes nutritional muscular dystrophy in adult horses. There is no evidence that paralytic myoglobinuria and the 'tying-up' syndrome are due to a deficiency of selenium and vitamin E.

In pigs, muscular dystrophy has been produced experimentally on vitamin E and selenium-deficient rations but is usually only a part of the more serious complex of mulberry heart disease and hepatosis dietetica (36).

Mulberry heart disease, hepatosis dietetica, exudative diathesis and muscular dystrophy

These occur naturally in rapidly growing pigs, usually during the postweaning period (3 weeks to 4 months), particularly during the finishing period. The pigs are usually fed on diets which are deficient in both selenium and vitamin E and may contain a high concentration of unsaturated fatty acids (15). The diets commonly associated with this complex in pigs include those which contain mixtures of soybean, high-moisture corn and the cereal grains grown on soils with low levels of selenium (36–38). The feeding of a basal ration of cull peas, low in selenium and vitamin E, to growing pigs resulted in the typical syndrome (39) and low tissue levels of selenium were present in swine with spontaneously occurring hepatosis dietetica (40). However, in naturally occurring cases of mulberry heart disease of swine in Sweden, the tissue levels of selenium were not lower than levels of control pigs with mulberry heart disease, muscular dystrophy and hepatosis dietetica (41). Natural occurrence of the disease complex in swine is not uncommonly associated with diets containing 50% coconut meal, fish-liver oil emulsion, fish scraps with a high content of unsaturated fatty acids, or flaxseed, which produces yellow and brown discoloration of fat preventable by the incorporation of adequate amounts of alpha-tocopherol or a suitable antioxidant. The quality of the dietary fat does not necessarily influence blood vitamin E levels, but the presence of oxidized fat reduces the resistance of the red blood cells against peroxidation (42). The higher requirement for vitamin E by pigs fed oxidized fat may be due to the low vitamin E content in such fat.

Selenium-responsive unthriftiness

This occurs in sheep and cattle, primarily in New Zealand (43, 44) and in some restricted areas of the western states of the United States (18) and to a lesser extent in Australia (45). In New Zealand a condition known as 'illthrift' occurs in lambs at pasture and in beef and dairy cattle of all ages, particularly in the autumn and winter months. The causes of economic loss are inferior growth rate, decreased wool growth, chronic diarrhea in calves, all of which are usually improved following selenium supplementation. Selenium deficiency appears not to be a major factor enhancing susceptibility to facial eczema and rye-grass staggers in sheep (17). Based on some preliminary observations of the selenium content of hair samples of young calves there may be some evidence that higher selenium levels in newborn calves may have some protective effect against morbidity (18). There is some limited evidence that neonatal piglets with high blood levels of glutathione peroxidase activity may be more resistant to infectious diseases or other causes of neonatal mortality and that routine supplementation of newborn piglets with selenium may be beneficial (107).

Reproductive performance

The evidence regarding the effect of selenium and vitamin E deficiency on reproductive performance in sheep is conflicting. Earlier work reported that selenium deficiency was responsible for decreased fertility and/or prolificacy in sheep. In addition, the supplementation of ewes, low or marginal in selenium status, with selenium did not improve reproductive performance (46). Recent experimental work using selenium-deficient diets in ewes was unable to show any adverse effect of selenium depletion on ewe conception rates, embryonic mortality or numbers of lambs born (47).

The possible role of selenium deficiency as a cause of retained fetal membranes and inferior reproductive performance in dairy cattle has been examined and the results are inconsistent. A high incidence (more than 10%) of retained fetal membranes has been associated with marginal levels of plasma selenium compared to herds without a problem. In some cases the incidence could be reduced to below 10% by the injection of pregnant cattle with selenium and vitamin E about 3 weeks prepartum (51). While in other studies similar prepartum injections did not reduce the incidence of retained placenta nor improved reproductive performance (50). A single injection of selenium 3 weeks prepartum can reduce the number of days postpartum required for the uterus to reach minimum size (52) and to reduce the incidence of metritis and cystic ovaries during the early postpartum period (13). The importance of selenium and vitamin E for the maintenance of optimum reproductive performance is not clear. The intramuscular injection of dairy cattle with selenium and vitamin E 3 weeks prepartum did not have any effect on average days to first estrus or first service, average days to conception, services per conception, or number of uterine infusions required (53). Following the treatment of dairy cows with oral selenium pellets there was an improvement in first service conception rate and significantly higher blood levels of glutathione peroxidase (14). The inconsistent results obtained following the use of selenium and vitamin E in pregnant cows may be related to the selenium status of the animals; in some herds the blood levels are marginal and in other the levels are within the normal range. The complex nature of the etiology of retained fetal membranes also requires a well-designed experimental trial to account for all of the possible factors involved.

Resistance to infectious disease

There is evidence that selenium deficiency can affect the function of polymorphonuclear neutrophils which is associated with physiological changes in glutathione peroxidase levels (56). In calves on an experimental selenium-deficient diet the oxygen consumption and the activities of glutathione peroxidase are lower than normal in neutrophils (43). In selenium-deficient goats, the production of leukotriene B_4, a product of neutrophil arachidonic acid lipoxygenation and a potent chemotactic and chemokinetic stimulus for neutrophils is decreased which results in dysfunction of the neutrophils (60). These changes may render selenium-deficient animals more susceptible to infectious disease but there is no available evidence to indicate that naturally occurring selenium and vitamin E deficiencies are associated with an increase in the incidence or severity of infectious diseases. Neutrophils from selenium-deficient animals lose some ability to phagocytose certain organisms but how relevant this observation is in naturally occurring infections is unclear.

There may be a relationship between the prevalence of mastitis in dairy herds and the concentrations of blood selenium (67). In a study of 32 dairy herds, those with low somatic cell counts had significantly higher mean blood glutathione peroxidase and higher whole blood concentrations of selenium than in herds with high somatic cell counts (67). The prevalence of infection due to *Str. agalactiae* and *Staph. aureus* was higher in herds with the high somatic cell counts compared to those with the low somatic cell counts. These observations may indicate that phagocytic function in the mammary gland may be decreased by a marginal selenium deficiency.

Pathogenesis

The available evidence suggests that dietary selenium, sulfur-containing amino acids and vitamin E act synergistically to protect tissues from oxidative damage (1). It is evident that glutathione peroxidase, which depends on dietary selenium, plays a major role in detoxifying lipid peroxides by reducing them to non-toxic hydroxy fatty acids, and vitamin E prevents fatty acid hydroperoxide formation. The presence of high levels of unsaturated fatty acids in the diet increases the requirements for vitamin E and, with an inadequate level of selenium in the diet, tissue oxidation occurs resulting in degeneration and necrosis of cells. Vitamin E protects cellular membranes from lipoperoxidation, especially membranes rich in unsaturated lipids such as mitochondric, endoplasmic reticulum and plasma membranes. Thus it would appear that the presence of unsaturated fatty acids in the diet is not a necessary prerequisite for the disease. Diets low in selenium and/or vitamin E do not provide sufficient protection against the 'physiological' lipoperoxidation which occurs normally at the cellular level.

The relative importance of selenium, vitamin E and sulfur-containing amino acids in providing protection in each of the known diseases caused by their deficiency is not clearly understood. Selenium appears to have a sparing effect on vitamin E and is an efficient prophylactic against enzootic muscular dystrophy of calves and lambs at pasture but does not prevent muscular dystrophy in calves fed on a diet containing cod liver oil. The current understanding of the biochemical function of selenium and its relation to vitamin E and the mechanisms of action of selenium and vitamin E in protection of biological membranes has been reviewed (14).

A simplified integrated concept which explains the pathogenesis of the nutritional muscular dystrophy would be as follows. Diets deficient in selenium and/or vitamin E permit widespread tissue lipoperoxidation leading to hyaline degeneration and calcification of muscle fibers. One of the earliest changes in experimental selenium deficiency in lambs is the abnormal retention of calcium in muscle fibers which are undergoing dystrophy. Selenium supplementation prevents the retention of calcium. Unaccustomed exercise can accelerate the oxidative process and precipitate clinical signs. The muscle degeneration allows the release of enzymes such as lactate dehydrogenase, aldolase and creatine phosphokinase, the last of which is of paramount importance in diagnosis. Degeneration of skeletal muscle is rapidly and successively followed by invasion of phagocytes and regeneration. In myocardial muscle, replacement fibrosis is the rule.

In calves, lambs and foals the major muscles involved are skeletal, myocardial and diaphragmatic. The myocardial and diaphragmatic forms of the disease occur most commonly in young calves, lambs and foals, resulting in acute heart failure, respiratory distress and rapid death, often in spite of treatment. The skeletal form of the disease occurs more commonly in older calves, yearling cattle and older foals and results in weakness and recumbency and is usually less serious and responds to treatment. The biceps femoris muscle is particularly susceptible in calves and muscle biopsy is a reliable diagnostic aid (54).

In foals with muscular dystrophy there is a higher proportion of type IIC fibers and lower proportions of types I and IIA fibers than in healthy foals (31). The type IIC fibers are found in fetal muscle and are undifferentiated and still under development. During the recovery period, fibers of types I, IIA and IIB increase and the proportion of type IIC fibers decreases. A normal fiber type composition is present in most surviving foals 1–2 months after the onset of the disease.

Acute muscular dystrophy results in the liberation of myoglobin into the blood, which results in myoglobinuria. This is more common in horses, older calves and yearling cattle than in young calves which have a lower concentration of myoglobin in their muscles. Hence, the tendency to myoglobinuria will vary depending on the species and age of animal involved.

The specific pathogenesis of the complex of mulberry heart disease, hepatosis dietetica, exudative diathesis and muscular dystrophy of swine has not been fully elucidated. The available evidence from both the naturally occurring and experimentally reproduced disease suggests that vitamin E and selenium are necessary to prevent widespread degeneration and necrosis of tissues, especially liver, heart, skeletal muscle and blood vessels (15). Selenium and vitamin E deficiency in swine results in massive hepatic necrosis (hepatosis dietetica), degenerative myopathy of cardiac and skeletal muscles, edema, microangiopathy and yellowish discoloration of adipose tissue. In addition, in some cases, there is esophagogastric ulceration, but it is still uncertain whether or not this lesion is caused by a selenium and/or vitamin E deficiency. Anemia has also occurred in selenium and vitamin E deficiency in swine and has been attributed to a block in bone marrow maturation, resulting in inadequate erythropoiesis, hemolysis or both (39). However, there is no firm evidence that anemia is a feature of selenium and vitamin E deficiency in swine (81). The entire spectrum of lesions has been reproduced experimentally in swine with natural or purified diets which are deficient in selenium and vitamin E or in which an antagonist was added to inactivate vitamin E or selenium (39, 55). However, in some studies the selenium content of tissues of pigs which died from mulberry heart disease was similar to that of control pigs without the disease (41).

The extensive tissue destruction which occurs in swine explains the sudden death nature of the complex (mulberry heart disease and hepatosis dietetica) and the muscle stiffness which occurs in some feeder pigs and sows of farrowing time with muscular dystrophy. The tissue degeneration is associated with marked increases in serum enzymes related to the tissue involved (36). An indirect correlation between vitamin E intake and peroxide hemolysis in pigs on a deficient diet suggests that lipoperoxidation is the ultimate biochemical defect in swine and that vitamin E and selenium are protective.

The pathogenesis of illthrift in cattle and sheep is unknown. There is no firm evidence that vitamin E and selenium deficiency adversely affects the reproductive function of domestic animals. The pathogenesis of retained fetal membranes due to selenium and vitamin E deficiency in cattle is also not understood.

Nutritional muscular dystrophy

Nutritional muscular dystrophy occurs most commonly in young calves, lambs and foals. The disease is most common in rapidly growing calves 2–4 months of age and younger or older, and sudden unaccustomed exercise often precedes the acute disease by a few days. The disease is now recognized in grain-fed yearling cattle, and often stressors such as being turned outdoors after winter housing, walking long distances, the jostling and movement associated with vaccination and dehorning procedures and the like are precipitating factors. The disease has occurred in steers and bulls 12–18 months of age under feedlot conditions (37). There was laboratory evidence of subclinical myopathy in several animals which was determined after the index case was recognized clinically (37). Outbreaks of severe and fatal muscular dystrophy in heifers at the time of parturition which were previously on a diet deficient in both selenium and vitamin E have been recorded (57). The disease may also occur sporadically in adult horses which are deficient in selenium (33).

There are two major syndromes, an acute form—myocardial dystrophy, which occurs most commonly in young calves and lambs, and occasionally foals—and a subacute form—skeletal muscular dystrophy, which occurs in older calves and yearling cattle. The two forms are not mutually exclusive.

Clinical findings

Acute enzootic muscular dystrophy

Affected animals may die suddenly without premonitory signs, especially after exercise. The excitement associated with the hand-feeding of dairy calves may precipitate peracute death in animals with low levels of blood selenium and glutathione peroxidase (10). In calves under close observation a sudden onset of dullness and severe respiratory distress, accompanied by a frothy or blood-stained nasal discharge, may be observed in some cases. Affected calves, lambs and foals are usually in lateral recumbency and may be unable to sit up in sternal recumbency even when assisted. The heart rate is usually increased up to 150–200/min and often grossly irregular. The temperature is usually normal. The eyesight and mental attitude are normal and affected calves are usually thirsty and can swallow unless the tongue is affected. Affected animals commonly die 6–12 hours after the onset of signs in spite of therapy. Outbreaks of the disease occur in calves and lambs in which up to 15% of susceptible animals may develop the acute form and the case mortality approaches 100%.

Subacute enzootic muscular dystrophy

This is the most common form of the disease in rapidly growing calves, '*white muscle disease*', and in young lambs, '*stiff-lamb disease*'. Affected animals may be found in sternal recumbency and unable to stand but with an obvious desire to stand. In those which are standing the obvious signs are stiffness, trembling of the limbs, weakness and, in most cases, an inability to stand for more than a few minutes. The gait in calves is accompanied by rotating movements of the hocks and in lambs a stiff, goose-stepping gait. Muscle tremor is evident if the animal is forced to stand for more than a few minutes. On palpation the dorsolumbar, gluteal and shoulder muscle masses tend to be bilaterally swollen and firmer than normal. These abnormalities are always symmetrical. Most affected animals retain their appetite and will suck if held up to the dam or eat if hand-fed. Major involvement of the diaphragm and intercostal muscles occurs in many cases and causes dyspnea with labored and abdominal-type respiration. The temperature is usually in the normal range but there may be a transient fever (41°C, 105°F) due presumably to the pyrogenic effects of myoglobinemia and pain. The heart rate may be elevated but there are usually no gross irregularities in the myocardial form. Following treatment, affected animals usually show marked improvement in a few days and within 3–5 days they are able to stand and walk unassisted.

In the more severe and experimentally produced cases, the upper borders of the scapulae protrude above the vertebral column and are widely separated from the chest, the toes are spread, there is relaxation of carpal and metacarpal joints or knuckling at the fetlocks and standing on tip-toe, inability to raise the head, difficulty in swallowing, inability to use the tongue and relaxation of abdominal muscles. Choking may occur when the animals attempt to drink. In 'paralytic myoglobinuria' of yearling cattle, there is usually a history of recent turning out on pasture following winter housing. Clinical signs occur within 1 week and consist of stiffness, recumbency, myoglobinuria, hyperpnea and dyspnea. Severe cases may die within a few days and some are found dead without premonitory signs. In rare cases, lethargy, anorexia, diarrhea and weakness are the first clinical abnormalities recognized followed by recumbency and myoglobinuria (31).

In foals, muscular dystrophy occurs most commonly during the first few months of life and is common in the first week. The usual clinical findings are failure to suck, recumbency, difficulty in rising and unsteadiness and trembling when forced to stand. The temperature is usually normal but commonly there is polypnea and tachycardia. In adult horses with muscular dystrophy, a stiff gait, myoglobinuria, depression, inability to eat, holding the head down low and edema of the head and neck are common (33). The horse may be presented initially with clinical signs of colic.

Muscular dystrophy is not commonly recognized clinically in pigs because it is part of the more serious disease complex of mulberry heart disease and hepatosis dietetica. However, in outbreaks of this complex, sucking piglets, feeder pigs and sows after farrowing will show an uncoordinated, staggering gait suggestive of muscular dystrophy.

Subclinical nutritional muscular dystrophy occurs in apparently normal animals in herds at the time clinical cases are present. The serum levels of creatine phosphokinase levels may be elevated in susceptible animals for several days before the onset of clinical signs and treatment with vitamin E and selenium will return the level of serum enzymes to normal (31). Grossly abnormal electrocardiograms have been observed in some animals and may be of value in diagnosis. In some instances the changes in the ECG are detectable before clinical signs are evident (53).

Clinical pathology

Myopathy

Plasma creatine phosphokinase (CPK) activity is the most commonly used laboratory aid in the diagnosis of muscular dystrophy in calves, lambs and foals. Creatine phosphokinase is highly specific for cardiac and skeletal muscle and is released into the blood following unaccustomed exercise and myodegeneration. In cattle and sheep it has a half-life of 2–4 hours and plasma levels characteristically drop quickly unless there is continued myodegeneration but remain a good guide to the previous occurrence of muscle damage for a period of about 3 days. The normal plasma levels of CPK (i.u./liter) are: sheep 52 ± 10; cattle 26 ± 5; horses 58 ± 6; and pigs 226 ± 43 (59). In cattle and sheep with acute muscular dystrophy the CPK levels will be increased usually above 1000 i.u./liter, commonly increased to 5000–10 000 i.u./liter and not uncommonly even higher. Following turnout of housed cattle onto pasture the CPK levels will increase up to 5000 i.u./liter within a few days (54). The CPK levels will usually return to normal levels within a few days following successful treatment. Persistent high levels suggest that muscle degeneration is still progressive or has occurred within the last 2 days.

The SGOT activity is also an indicator of muscle damage but not as reliable as the CPK because increased SGOT levels may also indicate liver damage. The SGOT activity remains elevated for 3–10 days because of a much longer half-life than CPK. In acute cases of muscular dystrophy levels of 300–900 i.u./liter in calves and 2000–3000 i.u./liter in lambs have been observed. In normal animals of these species, serum levels are usually less than 100 i.u./liter.

The magnitude of the increase in SGOT and CPK is directly proportional to the extent of muscle damage. Both are elevated initially; an elevated SGOT and declining CPK would suggest that muscle degeneration is no longer active. The levels of both enzymes will be increased slightly in animals which have just been turned out and subjected to unaccustomed exercise, horses in training, and in animals with ischemic necrosis of muscle due to recumbency caused by diseases other than muscular dystrophy. However, in acute muscular dystrophy the levels are usually markedly elevated.

Creatine excretion increases markedly and is a useful method of diagnosing the disease and following its progress. The ratio of creatine to creatinine is most informative. Values of less than 0·7 occur in normal lambs, and values over 1 and as high as 5 are found in dystrophic lambs. In calves the normal excretion rate in the urine of 200–300 mg/24 hours may be increased to 1·3 g/24 hours, although in the late stages of the disease when much of the muscle mass has undergone degeneration, the creatine excretion may be lower than normal.

Selenium status

Although information on the critical levels of selenium in soil and plants is accumulating gradually, the estimations are difficult and expensive and most field diagnoses are made on the basis of clinicopathological findings and the response to treatment and control procedures using selenium. The existence of enzootic muscular dystrophy is accepted as presumptive evidence of selenium deficiency which can now be confirmed by analyses of glutathione peroxidase and the concentrations of selenium in soil, feed samples and animal tissues. Tentative critical levels of the element are as follows.

Forages and grains A content of 0·1 mg/kg is considered to be adequate.

Soil Soils containing less than 0·5 mg/kg are likely to yield crops which are inadequate in selenium concentration (16).

Animal tissues, blood and milk The concentration of selenium in various tissues are reliable indicators of the selenium status of the animal. The values fluctuate with the dietary intake of the element (16). Levels of 3·5–5·3 mg/g (67–101 nmol/g) dry matter in the kidney cortex and 0·90–1·75 μg/g (11–22 nmol/g) dry matter in the liver of cattle are indicative of adequate selenium. Levels of 0·6–1·4 μg/g (8–18 nmol/g) in the kidney cortex and 0·07–0·60 μg/g (0·9–8 nmol/g) in the liver represent a deficient state.

There is a positive correlation between the selenium content of feed and the selenium content of the tissues and blood of animals ingesting that feed. Blood and milk levels of selenium are also used as indicators of selenium status in cattle. Dams of affected calves have had levels of 1·7 ng/ml (2·2 nmol/l) (blood) and 4·9 ng/ml (6·2 nmol/l) (milk); their calves have blood levels of 5–8 ng/ml (6·3–10·1 nmol/l). Normal supplemented cows have 19–48 ng/ml (24·1–60·8 nmol/l) in blood and 10–20 ng/ml (12·7–25·3 nmol/l) in milk, and their calves have blood levels of 33–61 ng/ml (41·8–77·2 nmol/l) (61). Mean selenium concentrations in the blood of normal mares have been 26–27 ng/ml (32·9–34·2 nmol/l).

Surveys done in Thoroughbred horses indicate that selenium concentrations in serum range from 39·5 to 18·5 mg/ml (50 to 150 μmol/l) and that there are significant differences between stables (103). Information on the selenium concentrations in a variety of animal tissues, fish, cereal grains and miscellaneous materials is available (104).

Glutathione peroxidase

There is a direct relationship between the glutathione peroxidase (GSH-Px) activity of the blood and the selenium levels of the blood and tissues of cattle, sheep, horses, and pigs (1). The normal selenium status of cattle is represented by whole blood selenium concentration of 100 ng/ml (126·6 nmol/l) and blood GSH-Px activity of approximately 30 mU units/mg hemoglobin (66). There is a high positive relationship (r = 0·87–0·958) between blood GSH-Px activity and blood selenium concentrations in cattle (66). Blood selenium levels less than 50 ng/ml are considered as selenium-deficient, while levels between 50 ng/ml and 100 (126·6) are marginal, and greater than are adequate (1). Comparable whole blood levels of GSH-Px are deficient if less than 30 mU/mg hemoglobin, marginal if 30–60 mU/mg, and adequate if greater than 60 mU/mg hemoglobin (1). There is some evidence of variation in GSH-Px activities between breeds of sheep and levels may also decrease with increasing age (95). It is postulated that low levels in some breeds of sheep may be a reflection of adaptation to low selenium intake because of low levels of selenium in the soil and forages.

The GSH-Px activity is a sensitive indicator of the level of dietary selenium intake and the response to the oral or parenteral administration of selenium (1, 16). Because selenium is incorporated into erythrocyte GSH-Px only during erythropoiesis, an increase in enzyme activity of the blood will not occur for 4–6 weeks following administration of selenium (1). Plasma GSH-Px will rise more quickly and will continue to increase curvilinearly with increasing dietary selenium levels because it is not dependent on incorporation of the selenium into the erythrocytes. The liver and selenium concentration and serum GSH-PX activity may respond to changes in dietary selenium more rapidly than either whole blood selenium or erythrocyte GSH-PX activity (24). The response in GSH-PX activity may depend upon the selenium status of the animals at the time when selenium is administered. Larger increases in the enzyme activity occur in selenium-deficient animals (101). The GSH-PX activity in foals reflects the amount of selenium given to the mare during pregnancy (94, 97).

The GSH-PX activity can be determined rapidly using a spot test which is semiquantitative and can place a group of samples from the same herd or flock into one of three blood selenium categories: deficient, low marginal and marginal adequate (77). A commercial testing kit known as the Ransel Kit is now available (105). The stability of GSH-PX in swine plasma samples has been examined. For absolute measurements, it is suggested that swine plasma GSH-PX activity be measured immediately after separation from the blood cells or be assayed within 24 hours under specified laboratory conditions (106).

Vitamin E status

Vitamin E occurs in nature as a mixture of alpha-tocopherol, beta-tocopherol, gamma-tocopherol, delta-tocopherol and possibly other tocopherols in varying proportions. The compounds vary widely in their biological activity so that chemical determination of total tocopherols is of much less value than biological assay. Tocopherol levels in blood and liver provide good information on the vitamin E status of the animal. However, because of the difficulty of the laboratory assays of tocopherols they are not commonly done and insufficient reliable data are available. Analysis of liver

Table 89. Glutathione peroxidase activity and selenium levels in blood and body tissues of animals deficient in selenium.

Species	*Clinical state or degree of deficiency*	*Erythrocyte glutathione peroxidase (GSH–PX) Activity µmol/min at 37°C/g hemoglobin*	*Serum selenium (µg/ml)*	*Liver selenium (µg/g dry matters)*	*Renal cortex selenium (µg/g dry matter)*
Cattle	Normal or adequate	19.0–36.0	0.080–0.300	0.90–1.75	3.5–5.3
	Marginal	10.0–19.0	0.030–0.070	0.45–0.90	1.4–3.5
	Deficient	0.2–10.0	0.002–0.025	0.07–0.60	0.6–1.4
Sheep	Normal or adequate	60–180	0.080–0.500	0.90–3.50	3.2–10.5
	Marginal	8–30	0.030–0.050	0.52–0.90	2.5–3.9
	Deficient	2–7	0.006–0.030	0.02–0.35	0.2–2.1
Pigs (76)	Adequate	100–200	0.120–0.300	1.40–2.80	5.3–10.2
	Deficient	<50	0.005–0.060	0.10–0.35	1.4–2.7
Horse	Adequate (20, 33)	30–150	0.140–0.250	1.05–3.50	2.5–7.0
	Deficient	8–30	0.008–0.055	0.14–0.70	0.9–4.0

from clinically normal animals on pasture reveal a mean alpha-tocopherol level of 20 mg/kg for cattle and 6 mg/kg for sheep (109). The corresponding ranges were 6·0–53 mg/kg for cattle and 1·8–17 mg/kg in sheep. The critical level below which signs of deficiency may be expected are 5 mg/kg for cattle and 2 mg/kg for sheep. Tocopherol levels in the serum of less than 2 mg/l in cattle and sheep are considered to be critical levels below which deficiency diseases may occur. However, if the diet contains adequate quantities of selenium, but not an excessive quantity of polyunsaturated fatty acids, animals may thrive on low levels of serum tocopherols. In summary, there is insufficient reliable data available on the vitamin E status on animals with muscular dystrophy to be of diagnostic value.

The mean plasma vitamin E levels in stabled Thoroughbred horses in training was 3.34 mg/l (7.7 µmol/l) (110). The serum vitamin E levels in horses with azoturia-tying up syndrome were not lower than control horses which indicates that low vitamin E or selenium is not the cause of the disease (111).

A summary of the glutathione peroxidase activity, tocopherol and selenium levels in blood and body tissues of animals deficient in selenium and/of vitamin E appears in Table 89. Normal values are also tabulated for comparison (100). Both the abnormal and normal values should be considered as guidelines for diagnosis because of the wide variations in levels between groups of animals. The level of dietary selenium may fluctuate considerably which may account for variations in glutathione peroxidase.

Necropsy findings

The microscopic and histological appearance of the muscle lesions is quite constant but their distribution varies widely in different animals. Affected groups of skeletal muscle are always bilaterally symmetrical. In skeletal muscle and the diaphragm there are localized white or graying areas of degeneration with the appearance of fish flesh. These areas may be in streaks, involving a large group of muscle fibers, running through the center of the apparently normal muscle or as a peripheral boundary around a core of normal muscle. In the diaphragm the distribution of dystrophic bundles gives the organ a radially striated appearance. The affected muscle is friable and edematous and may be calcified. Secondary pneumonia often occurs in cases where the muscles of the throat and chest are affected. In cases with myocardial involvement, white areas of degeneration are visible particularly under the endocardium of the left ventricle in calves and both ventricles in lambs. The lesions may extend to involve the interventricular septum and papillary muscles. There may be cardiac hypertrophy and pulmonary congestion and edema, and calcification of lesions has also been observed.

Histologically the muscle lesions are non-inflammatory. Hyaline degeneration is followed by coagulation necrosis. Biochemical analysis of affected muscle will indicate whether degeneration has occurred, as the creatine content of degenerate muscle falls markedly. A degeneration of Purkinje fibers in the myocardium has also been described but is reported also in calves fed diets deficient in potassium or manganese. Yellowish brown discoloration of fat deposits is a feature of the disease in older (2–7 months) but not in younger foals.

Diagnosis

Enzootic muscular dystrophy may be easily confused with other disease, particularly when the myocardial or diaphragmatic involvement is severe. Dyspnea is evident and there may be a high fever so that the disease is often difficult to distinguish from pneumonia. However, severely affected calves are usually recumbent and unable to rise. They appear to be in a state of collapse. If picked up and placed on their feet they may make no effort to bear weight. The heart rate is rapid (150–200/min) and irregularities are common. The disease usually occurs in young calves and lambs in the spring of the year and more than one animal is commonly affected. Differentiation from the infectious diseases which cause septicemia, pneumonia and toxemia is necessary. In acute enzootic muscular dystrophy serum CPK and SGOT levels are markedly elevated and serve as a very reliable diagnostic aid.

Subacute enzootic muscular dystrophy in which skeletal muscle lesions predominate may be readily confused with other forms of paresis and paralysis. The disease is most common in young rapidly growing animals which are on a selenium–vitamin E deficient ration or their dams were on a deficient unsupplemented ration throughout the winter months. The onset is usually sudden and with calves and lambs, many animals may be affected simultaneously or within a few days, particularly following unaccustomed exercise. The major clinical signs are stiffness in walking, recumbency, inability to rise, a normal mental attitude and appetite and no abnormal neurological findings to account for the recumbency. The levels of serum creatine phosphokinase are usually markedly elevated.

The differentiation of the other diseases which cause recumbency, particularly in calves, from subacute muscular dystrophy may be difficult. Other common causes of stiffness or recumbency, paresis and paralysis in calves include: spinal cord compression, polyarthritis, recent treatment with organophosphatic insecticides, tetanus, *Haemophilus* meningoencephalitis, osteodystrophies in older calves 6–8 months of age, traumatic injuries to muscles, bones and joints, and other causes of acute myopathy such as blackleg.

In lambs with 'stiff-lamb' disease there is stiffness and a stilted gait, affected animals prefer recumbency, they are bright and alert and will suck the ewe if assisted. The serum levels of CPK and SGOT are also markedly elevated. Differentiation may be necessary from enzootic ataxia and swayback but in these two diseases stiffness is not a characteristic.

Vitamin E and selenium deficiencies in swine

This group includes mulberry heart disease, hepatosis dietetica, exudative diathesis, muscular dystrophy, iron hypersensitivity in piglets and, perhaps, esophagogastric ulcers. Mulberry heart disease and hepatosis dietetica have received the most attention as vitamin E and selenium deficiencies of swine. Exudative diathesis and muscular dystrophy usually accompany hepatosis dietetica. The cause of esophagogastric ulcers in swine is still uncertain. They often occur in experimental pigs, fed diets which produce vitamin E and selenium deficiencies, but vitamin E and selenium will not necessarily prevent them.

Mulberry heart disease

This is one of the most common forms of selenium and vitamin E deficiency of swine. It occurs most commonly in rapidly growing feeder pigs (60–90 kg) in excellent condition being fed on a high-energy diet low in vitamin E and selenium. The diets most commonly incriminated are soybean, corn and barley. The alpha-tocopherol content of corn is usually low and it is virtually absent from solvent-extracted soybean meal. Both are low in selenium. The use of high-moisture corn may further exacerbate the tocopherol deficiency. The level of polyunsaturated fatty acids in the diet was thought to be an important etiological factor but this is now not considered to be a necessary prerequisite. Outbreaks of the disease may occur in which 25% of susceptible pigs are affected and the case mortality rate is about 90%. The disease has occurred in young piglets (62) and in adult sows.

Hepatosis dietetica and nutritional muscular dystrophy

Hepatosis dietetica appears to be less common than mulberry heart disease but the epidemiological characteristics are similar. It affects young growing pigs up to 3–4 months of age.

Nutritional muscular dystrophy in swine usually occurs in cases of mulberry heart disease and hepatosis dietetica but it has occurred alone in gilts (11–12 months of age) 48 hours after farrowing. The gilts had been fed on a diet of barley and lupin seed which contained only 0.03 mg/kg of selenium (63).

Clinical findings

In mulberry heart disease, affected animals are commonly found dead without premonitory signs. More than one pig may be found dead. When seen alive, animals show severe dyspnea, cyanosis, recumbency and forced walking can cause immediate death. In some outbreaks about 25% of pigs will show a slight inappetence and inactivity and these are probably in the subclinical stages of the disease. The stress of movement, inclement weather or transportation will precipitate further acute deaths. The temperature is usually normal, the heart rate rapid and irregularities may be detectable. The feces are usually normal.

In hepatosis dietetica most pigs are found dead. In occasional cases, before death there will be dyspnea, severe depression, vomiting, staggering, diarrhea and a state of collapse. Some pigs are icteric. Outbreaks also occur similar to the pattern in mulberry heart disease. Muscular dystrophy is almost a consistent necropsy finding in both mulberry heart disease and hepatosis dietetica but is usually not recognized clinically because of the seriousness of the two latter diseases. Clinical muscular dystrophy has been described in gilts at 11 months of age. About 48 hours after farrowing, there was muscular weakness, muscular tremors and shaking. This was followed by collapse, dyspnea and cyanosis. There were no liver or heart lesions. In experimental selenium and vitamin E deficiency in young growing pigs, a subtle stiffness occurs along with a significant increase in the CPK and SGOT values (38).

Clinical pathology

An increase in the activity of several plasma enzymes occurs in selenium and vitamin E deficiencies of swine. The measurement of SGOT, CPK, LDH and ICD can be used to detect the onset of degeneration of skeletal and myocardial muscles and liver. However, these are not commonly used for diagnostic purposes because of the acuteness of the illness. The hematological and biochemical changes in pigs with experimental vitamin E and selenium deficiencies have been described (64). While anemia has been reported to accompany vitamin E deficiency in swine, experimental work has shown that vitamin E is not a limiting factor for normal erythropoiesis in young growing pigs (64). Chronic low grade disseminated intravascular coagulation (DIC) may occur as a terminal event.

The determination of the levels of selenium in feed

supplies, tissues and blood of affected pigs is much more useful as an aid to diagnosis and for guidelines for supplementation of the diet.

The clinicopathologic findings of selenium/vitamin E deficiency in swine are serum selenium values of less than 2·5 ng/ml (3·2 nmol/l), hepatic selenium of less than 0·10 mg/kg (1·3 μmol/kg), plasma alpha-tocopherol values of less than 0·40 μg/ml and hepatic alpha-tocopherol concentrations of less than 0·75 μg/g of tissue (87). In experimentally induced vitamin E selenium deficiency in swine the depletion time may be short and the erythrocytic GSH-PX activity indicator of selenium status because of the slow turnover of erythrocytes; only plasma GSH-PX will accurately reflect short-term selenium status.

There is a close relationship between blood vitamin E and resistance of erythrocytes against lipid peroxidation (65). Red cell resistance against peroxidation is a reliable indicator of the vitamin E status of pigs. The supplementation of the diet of pigs with vitamin E will increase both the serum levels of vitamin E and the resistance of the erythrocytes to lipid peroxidation.

Necropsy findings

In mulberry heart disease the carcass is in good condition. All body cavities contain excessive amounts of fluid and shreds of fibrin. In the peritoneal cavity, the fibrin is often in the form of a lacy net covering all the viscera. The liver is enlarged, mottled and has a characteristic nutmeg appearance on the cut surface. Excessive fluid in the pleural cavities is accompanied by collapse of the ventral parts of the lungs. The lungs are edematous and the interlobular septa are distended with gelatinous material. The pericardial sac is filled with gelatinous fluid interlaced with bands of fibrin. Beneath the epicardium are multiple hemorrhages of various sizes. The hemorrhages often run in a linear fashion in the direction of the muscle fibers. Similar hemorrhages are present under the endocardium and local edema is often present over the face and elsewhere. Marked reddening of the gastric mucosa is also common. Histologically, the characteristic lesion is widespread myocardial congestion, hemorrhage and parenchymal degeneration and there is lysis of cerebral white matter in some cases. There are multiple hyaline microthrombi composed mainly of fibrin in the microcapillaries of the myocardium (80).

In hepatosis dietetica the liver is swollen and has a mottled to mosaic-like appearance throughout its lobes. Histologically there is a distinct lobular distribution of hemorrhage, degeneration and necrosis (68). In muscular dystrophy of swine the most striking lesions are bilateral muscular dystrophy and Zenker's degeneration (63). There is hyalinization, loss of striation and fragmentation of myofibers. In some cases there is selective destruction of type I skeletal muscle fibers (36).

Selenium-responsive unthriftiness in sheep and cattle

In New Zealand, a variety of diseases have become known as selenium-responsive diseases (45), because they respond beneficially to the strategic administration of selenium. These include illthrift in lambs and calves on pasture, ewe infertility, and diarrhea in older calves and lactating ewes. The pathogenesis of these selenium-responsive diseases is not known but it would appear that the selenium deficiency is only marginal. Most investigations into selenium-responsive conditions have related mainly to areas that could be described as selenium-deficient and in which diseases such as white muscle disease of calves and lambs occur (45). The evidence that selenium deficiency in breeding ewes can result in a decline in reproductive performance has not been substantiated experimentally (47). Reproductive performance was not affected in ewes on a selenium depleted diet. A recent report indicated that selenium-responsive infertility in ewes may be present when the whole blood levels of selenium are below 10 ng/ml (12·7 nmol/l) (45).

Selenium-responsive unthriftiness in sheep has received considerable attention in New Zealand where the response to selenium administration has been most dramatic compared to Australia where the syndrome has also been recognized but where the response is much smaller. The oral administration of selenium to lambs in these areas results in greater body weight gains from weaning to 1 year of age compared to lambs which do not receive selenium supplementation (45). The mean fleece weight of selenium-treated lambs is also greater.

The diagnosis of selenium-responsive unthriftiness depends on analyses of the soil, pasture and animal tissues for selenium and response trials to selenium supplementation. A deficiency state might be encountered when the selenium content of the soil is below 0·45 mg/kg, the pasture content below 0·02 mg/kg, the liver content below 21 μg/kg (0·27 μmol/kg) (wet weight) and wool concentrations below 50–60 μg/kg (0·63–0·76 μmol/kg) (44). For the blood in selenium-responsive unthriftiness of sheep the following criteria are suggested (45):

Selenium status	*Mean blood selenium (μg/dl)*
Deficient	<1·0
Doubtful	1·1–1·9
Normal	>2·0

The glutathione peroxidase activity (GSH-Px) is a good index of the selenium status of sheep with a selenium-responsive disease. If measured on a regular basis, it can provide an indication of the selenium status of grazing sheep in individual flocks. Single measurements of GSH-Px activity may fail to detect recent changes in grazing area, differences in pasture species and pasture composition and alterations in the physiological state of the animals.

Retained fetal membranes

Recent evidence indicates that retained fetal membranes in mature dairy cows, when not induced mechanically or by infectious agents, may be due to a selenium and/or vitamin E deficiency (50). Blood selenium levels were lower in cows from herds with a retained fetal membrane problem than in herds with no history of a problem. The injection, 20 days prepartum, of 50 mg of selenium and 680 i.u. of vitamin E effectively reduced the incidence of retained fetal membranes in one series (50), but did not in another series (48). The plasma selenium concentration at parturition ranged from 0·02 to 0·05 ppm in control cows in which there was an incidence of 51% retained membranes and from 0·08 to 0·1 ppm in treated cows in which the incidence was reduced to 9%. A dietary level of 0·1 mg/kg selenium is recommended to minimize the incidence of the problem.

Blood abnormalities

In young cattle from areas where white muscle disease is endemic, and particularly at the end of winter housing, the erythrocytes have an increased susceptibility to hemolysis following exposure to hypotonic saline (69). During clinical and subclinical white muscle disease in calves, there is a significant increase in both the osmotic and the peroxidative hemolysis of the erythrocytes. This defect is thought to be the result of alterations in the integrity of cell membranes of which tocopherols are an essential component (69). Abnormalities of the bone marrow associated with vitamin E deficiency in sheep have been described (70), and abnormal hematological responses have been described in young growing pigs on an experimental selenium and vitamin E-deficient diet (64).

Anemia characterized by a decreased packed cell volume (PCV), decreased hemoglobin concentration and Heinz body formation has been observed in cattle grazing on grass grown on peaty muck soils in the Florida everglades (25). Selenium supplementation corrected the anemia, prevented Heinz body formation, increased the body weight of cows and calves, and elevated blood selenium.

Myleoencephalopathy

Equine degenerative myeloencephalopathy which may have an inherited basis (29) has been associated with a vitamin E deficiency. The vitamin E status is low in some affected horses and supplementation with the vitamin was associated with a marked reduction in the incidence of the disease.

Generalized steatitis

There are reports of steatitis in farm animals and other species associated with vitamin E and/or selenium deficiency (58). Most reported cases in horses have involved nursing or recently weaned foals. Generalized steatitis in the foal has been described as either generalized cachexia due to steatitis alone or as a primary myopathy or myositis with steatitis of secondary importance. The terms used have included steatitis, generalized steatitis, fat necrosis, yellow fat disease, polymyositis and muscular dystrophy. The relationships between steatitis and vitamin E and selenium deficiency in the horse are not clear. In fact, there may be no relationship at all. Many more clinical cases must be examined in detail before a cause-and-effect relationship can be considered.

Treatment

Because of the overlapping functions of selenium and vitamin E, and because it is not always possible to know the relative etiological importance of one nutrient or the other in causing some of the acute conditions already described, it is recommended that a combined mixture of selenium and alpha-tocopherol be used in treatment. Alpha-tocopherol is the most potent form of the tocopherols and is available in a number of pharmaceutical forms which also vary in their biological activity. It has become necessary to express the unitage of vitamin E in terms of international units of biological activity. (1 i.u. ≡ 1 mg synthetic racemic alpha-tocopherol acetate. Natural D-alpha-tocopherol acetate 1 mg ≡ 1 i.u. and natural D-alpha-tocopherol 1 mg ≡ 0·92 i.u.).

For muscular dystrophy in calves, lambs and foals the recommended mixture of intramuscular injection contains 3 mg selenium (as sodium or potassium selenite) and 150 i.u./ml of DL-alpha-tocopherol acetate, and the dose rate for treatment is 2 ml/45 kg body weight. One treatment is usually sufficient. Animals with acute enzootic muscular dystrophy with myocardial involvement will usually not respond to treatment and the case mortality rate is about 90%. However, all in-contact animals in the herd (calves, lambs and foals) should be treated prophylactically with the same dose of selenium and vitamin E. They should be handled carefully during treatment to avoid precipitating acute muscular dystrophy. Animals with subacute skeletal muscular dystrophy will usually begin to show improvement by 3 days following treatment and may be able to stand and walk unassisted within a week.

In outbreaks of mulberry heart disease, hepatosis dietetica and related selenium and vitamin E deficiency diseases in pigs, all clinically affected pigs and all pigs at risk should be treated with individual injections of selenium and vitamin E.

Control

The control and prevention of the major diseases caused by selenium and vitamin E deficiencies can generally be accomplished by the provision of both nutrients to susceptible animals which are fed on deficient rations. The following points are considered to be important:

- While selenium alone is protective against a greater spectrum of diseases than is vitamin E, there are situations in which vitamin E is more protective. However, there is firm evidence that both selenium and vitamin E should be provided in diets which are deficient
- Diseases caused by selenium deficiency can be successfully prevented by the administration of selenium to the dam during pregnancy or directly to the young growing animal. Selenium is transported across the placenta and provides protection for the neonate. Oral supplementation of beef cattle with selenium will provide sufficient to maintain blood levels in the dam and for adequate transfer to the fetus which can sequester selenium when the levels are low in the dam (78). The colostrum of selenium-supplemented cattle also contains an adequate

amount of selenium to prevent severe selenium-deficiency diseases. However, by 7 days after parturition the levels in milk are inadequate to maintain adequate serum levels in calves. The strategic administration of selenium and vitamin E before the expected occurrence of the disease is also a reliable method of preventing the disease (92)

- Besides being an essential nutrient, selenium is also toxic and any treatment and control program must be carefully monitored. Selenium injected into or fed to animals concentrates in liver, skeletal muscle, kidney and other tissues, and withdrawal periods before slaughter must be allowed. There is some concern that selenium may be a carcinogen for man. The only tissues that appear likely to consistently accumulate more than 3–4 mg/kg of selenium are the kidney and liver, and these are very unlikely to constitute more than a very small part of the human diet. There have been no reports of untoward effects of selenium on human health when it has been used at nutritional levels in food-producing animals. The incorporation of selenium into commercially prepared feeds for some classes of cattle and swine has been approved in some countries (82)

  The use of selenium in the diet of lactating dairy cows has caused concern about possible adulteration of milk supplies. However, the addition of selenium to the diets of lactating dairy cows at levels which are protective against the deficiency diseases do not result in levels in the milk which are hazardous for human consumption (49). The feeding of excessive quantities of selenium to dairy cattle would cause toxicity before levels became toxic for man
- The dietary requirement of selenium for both ruminants and non-ruminants is 0·1 mg/kg of the element in the diet. There may be nutritionally important differences in the selenium status between the same feeds grown in different regions and between different feeds within a region (22). Even within a region featuring high selenium concentrations, some feeds may contain levels of selenium below the 0·1 mg/kg minimum requirement for livestock. Thus a selenium analysis of feeds appears necessary in order to supplement livestock appropriately. Some geographical areas are known to be deficient in selenium and the feeds grown in these areas must be supplemented with selenium and vitamin E on a continuous basis
- Avoidance of high sulfate diets is desirable but provision of adequate selenium overcomes the sulfate effect
- The levels of whole blood glutathione peroxidase (GSH-Px) activity is a reliable and useful index for monitoring the selenium status of cattle and sheep, perhaps not as reliable in pigs (87), and not a good indicator in the horse (40)
- The control and prevention of the major diseases caused by selenium and vitamin E deficiencies can be achieved by several different methods which include dietary supplementation in the feed or water supplies, individual parenteral injections or oral administration and pasture topdressing (91). The method used will depend on the circumstances of the farm, the ease of administration, the cost, the labor available, the severity of the deficiency which exists, and whether or not the animals are being dosed regularly for other diseases such as parasitism. The subcutaneous injection of barium selenate, the administration of an intraruminal pellet, and the addition of selenium to the water supply were compared in cattle and each method was effective for periods ranging from 4 to 12 months (91).

Dietary supplementation

The inclusion of selenium and vitamin E in the feed supplies or salt and mineral mixes has been generally successful in preventing the major diseases caused by deficiencies of these two nutrients. Under most conditions, enzootic muscular dystrophy of calves and lambs can be prevented by providing selenium and vitamin E in the diets of the cow or ewe during pregnancy at the rate of 0·1 mg/kg of actual selenium and alpha-tocopherol at the rate of 1 g daily per cow and 75 mg daily per ewe. If possible, the supplementation should be continued during lactation to provide a continuous source of selenium to the calves and lambs. Under some conditions the level of 0·1 mg/kg may be inadequate. In some circumstances the optimal selenium concentration in the feed is considerable higher than 0·1 mg/kg, and levels up to 1·0 mg/kg in the feed result in increases in GSH-Px activity which may be beneficial but the cost-effectiveness has not been determined (85). Pregnant ewes being fed on alfalfa hay may require selenium at a level of up to 0·2 mg/kg to prevent white muscle disease in their lambs (83). Young growing cattle, particularly beef cattle which are likely to receive hay and straw deficient in selenium and those which are fed high-moisture grain, should receive a supplement of selenium at the rate of 0·1 mg/kg and alpha-tocopherol at 150 mg per head per day (32).

Nutritional muscular dystrophy can be prevented in unweaned beef calves and lambs by the inclusion of selenium (14·8 mg/kg) and vitamin E (2700 i.u./kg) in the mineral supplement provided *ad libitum* to the pregnant cows and ewes on a selenium-deficient ration during the latter two-thirds of gestation and for the first month of lactation (71). Under most conditions this will provide selenium at the rate of 0·1 mg/kg in the diet.

The provision of sodium selenite in a salt–mineral mixture to provide 90 mg of selenium/kg salt–mineral mixture on a year-round basis, even under range conditions, increased GSH-Px activity levels into normal ranges in beef cows by 3 months when fed to extremely deficient animals (86). Calves of these cows had increased weaning weights and decreased incidence of infectious diseases but the trial was uncontrolled. The provision of 30 mg selenium/kg salt–mineral mixture was insufficient to raise the GSH-Px activity levels to normal ranges. A level of 25 mg/kg selenium of a salt–mineral mixture provided *ad libitum* for sheep will result in sufficient levels of selenium in the dam's blood and milk to prevent selenium deficiency diseases (84).

Each ewe must consume from 8 to 12 g of the salt mineral mixture per day.

Milk replacers for dairy calves should contain a suitable antioxidant and be supplemented with 300 i.u./kg dry matter of alpha-tocopherol acetate at the rate of 0·1 mg/kg in the dry matter of the milk replacer.

In growing swine, both selenium and vitamin E at 30 i.u./kg of feed are necessary for the prevention of the diseases caused by diets deficient in vitamin E and selenium (87). Injections of selenium and vitamin E may prevent selenium vitamin E deficiency in pigs but repeated injections are required if a severely deficient diet is fed. The supplementation of the diet of the sow will result in an adequate transfer to the piglets (72). Satisfactory protection of the diseases of swine caused by vitamin E selenium deficiency depends on the correct balance between selenium, alpha-tocopherol, polyunsaturated fatty acids in the diet and the presence of a suitable antioxidant to conserve the alpha-tocopherol.

Individual prophylactic injections and oral administration

Prophylactic injections of selenium and vitamin E have been used successfully for prevention particularly in circumstances where the diet cannot be easily supplemented. Following intramuscular injections of sodium selenite into calves, lambs and piglets, the selenium concentration of the tissues, particularly the liver, increases and then declines to reach preinjection levels in 23 days in calves and 14 days in lambs and piglets (73). Animals deficient in selenium are more susceptible to selenium toxicosis than those which are selenium-adequate (73).

The generally recommended dose of selenium is 0·1 mg/kg body weight subcutaneously. The glutathione peroxidase activity will increase to peak levels at about 30 days following the administration of the selenium (88). The subcutaneous administration of selenium at 0·10 or 0·15 mg/kg body weight, as sodium selenate, will increase and maintain the blood selenium and glutathione peroxidase activity in dairy cattle for up to 6 months following injection (89). A single subcutaneous or oral dose of 5 mg of selenium at strategic intervals to prevent or treat selenium deficiency in weaned lambs will increase the selenium residues in the meat, but not at levels which are considered hazardous to the public (90).

A slow-release preparation of barium selenate for subcutaneous injection is now available for use in cattle and sheep. At a dose of 1 mg/kg body weight to pregnant ewes the glutathione peroxidase (GSH-Px) activity is increased and maintained at adequate levels for up to 5 months and there is adequate transfer of selenium to the lambs which provides protection for up to 12 weeks of age which covers the period when lambs are at greatest risk (93). In one study a dose of 1·2 mg selenium/kg body weight provided adequate selenium status for as long as two consecutive lambing seasons (113). A dose of 1 mg selenium/kg body weight (barium selenate) to cattle subcutaneously increased the GSH-Px activity within 4 weeks and was maintained at high levels for up to 5 months (112). The relative safety of barium selenate is due to its slow rate of release from the site of injection. By comparison, when selenium is administered as a soluble salt, such as sodium selenite, acute toxicity may occur at doses of 0·45 mg selenium/kg body weight. Treatment with barium selenate increases the concentration of selenium in blood, liver and muscle and persists for at least 4 months. One disadvantage of barium selenate is that a large residue persists at the site of injection for long periods. The use of sodium selenite also increases tissue and blood concentrations of selenium but they begin to decline by 23 days (112). The bovine liver rapidly removes approximately 40% of injected selenium salts (soluble) from the systemic plasma, binds it to a plasma component and within 1 hour of injection releases it back into circulation (96).

A reduction in the incidence of retained fetal membranes in dairy cattle has been claimed by the injection of 50 mg selenium and 680 mg vitamin E 20 days prepartum (114). However, the results are conflicting (50, 51) and further well-designed clinical trials are necessary to examine the efficacy of vitamin E and selenium as a prophylactic for retained fetal membranes.

For the prevention of enzootic muscular dystrophy, if the danger period in the area is in the first few weeks of life, the selenium can be given to the dam; if it is later, at say 2–3 months of age, it is administered to the lamb or calf. The recommended dose rates of repeated injections at monthly intervals are: 1 mg of selenium to lambs, 5 mg to ewes, 10 mg to calves and 30 mg to adult cattle. The injections are administered about 1 month before the anticipated danger period. In calves on a selenium-deficient pasture a dose of 0·1 mg/kg body weight every 2 months or 0·2 mg/kg body weight every 4 months may be necessary (24). Comparable dose rates of the various compounds in use are: 1 mg selenium is equivalent to 2·2 mg anhydrous sodium selenite, 2·4 mg anhydrous sodium selenate, or 4·7 mg hydrated sodium selenate. These doses may be repeated without danger at monthly intervals. A mixture of selenium and vitamin E can also be used as a preventive at half the dose recommended under the heading of treatment above. It can be administered to the young or to the dam and repeated at 2–4 week intervals.

The parenteral injection of 50 mg of selenium, as sodium selenite, approximately equal to 1 mg selenium/10 kg body weight to dairy cattle 10 days before parturition did not reduce the incidence of the weak calf syndrome which is often attributed to a selenium deficiency (115).

In swine, the injection of selenium at the rate of 0·06 mg/kg body weight into piglets under 1 week of age, repeated at weaning time and into the sow 3 weeks before farrowing will be effective (38). The minimum lethal dose of selenium for piglets is 0·9 mg/kg body weight which provides a reasonably wide range of safety.

Little information is available on the need of horses for selenium but the optimum intake in this species is estimated to be 6 mg/week or 2·4 μg/kg body weight daily. The oral supplementation of 1 mg selenium per day will increase blood selenium concentrations above levels associated with myodegeneration in horses and foals (20). To ensure nutritional adequacy, and to have an adequate safety margin, adult Standardbred horses should receive 600–1800 mg DL-alpha-tocopherol daily in their feed (118). The parenteral administration of vitamin E and selenium to mares in late pregnancy and to their foals beginning at birth will increase blood selenium to adequate levels (20). In selenium-deficient areas or when mares are fed selenium-deficient hay, the prepartum injections of selenium and vitamin E are indicated followed by intermittent injection of the foals, or supplementation of the diet with selenium at 0·1 mg/kg.

Selenium pellets for deposition in the rumen, similar to those used in cobalt deficiency, have produced satisfactory blood levels in sheep for up to 12 months (74). A satisfactory pellet is composed of elemental selenium and finely divided metallic iron. The heavy pellets contain 0·5g of elemental selenium and may last for up to 4 years (83). The technique is efficient but not completely so, due to wide variations between animals in the absorption rate of the selenium. The average delivery of selenium is 1 mg/day and there is no danger of toxicity. In sheep grazing selenium-deficient pastures, the ruminal pellets increase the selenium status and weight gains compared to controls. About 15% of treated sheep reject the pellets within 12 months and in varying degrees the pellets acquire deposits of calcium phosphate. Sheep fed pellets recovered from sheep have low selenium levels which suggest a low release of selenium from pellets which have been in the rumen of other sheep for several months (75). The peak levels of selenium occur 3 months after administration; there is a rapid decline in activity between 5 and 13 months (75).

A selenium pellet containing 10% selenium and 90% iron grit is available for cattle and will maintain plasma selenium and glutathione peroxidase activity above the critical level for up to 2 years (116). When given to beef cows in the last 3 months of pregnancy the selenium levels in milk are higher than in controls, and the selenium status of the calves was sufficient to prevent nutritional muscular dystrophy.

Oral dosing using sodium selenite is sometimes combined with the administration of anthelmintics and vaccinations. The dose rate should approximate 0·044 mg/kg body weight. A routine program in a badly deficient area comprises three doses of 5 mg of selenium (11 mg sodium selenite) each to ewes, one before mating, one at mid-pregnancy and one 3 weeks before lambing, and four doses to the lambs. The first dose to lambs (of 1 mg) is given at docking and the others (2 mg each) at weaning and then at 3-month intervals. The levels of GSH-Px activity may be monitored on a regular basis following the drenching with selenium and provide a good indication of selenium availability and selenium status of grazing sheep.

Pasture topdressing

The application of sodium selenate as a topdressing to pasture is now practiced and permitted in some countries (117). Topdressing at the approved rate of 10 g/ha of selenium is effective for 12 months and has a toxicity margin of safety of about 20 times. Sodium selenate is now used in preference to sodium selenite because only about one-fifth is required to raise the pasture level of selenium to the same concentrations provided by sodium selenite. Topdressing severely deficient pumice soils in New Zealand prevented deficiency for at least 12 months, sheep were protected against white muscle in lambs, and reproduction performance and weight gains were improved. It is recommended that sodium selenate be applied annually to all selenium-deficient soils at the rate of 10 g/ha selenium added to the superphosphate fertilizer or as prills of sodium selenate alone (117). Topdressing is an economical alternative to individual animal dosing particularly in severely deficient areas with a high stocking rate. At the approved rate no adverse effects are anticipated in human or animal health or on the environment.

REVIEW LITERATURE

Barton, C. R. Q. (1977) Degenerative myopathy of yearling cattle: aspects of clinical differential diagnoses. *Vet. Ann.*, *17*, 51.

Dill, S. D. & Rebhun, W. C. (1985) White muscle disease in foals. *Comp. cont. Educ. pract. Vet.*, 7, S627–S632, S634–S635.

Koller, L. D. & Exon, J. H. (1986) The two faces of selenium-deficiency and toxicity are similar in animals and man. *Can. J. vet. Res.*, *50*, 297–306.

National Academy of Sciences (1983) *Selenium in Nutrition*. Washington, DC: National Research Council.

Rammell, C. G. (1983) Vitamin E status of cattle and sheep. 1: A background review. *NZ vet. J.*, *31*, 179–181.

Ullrey, D. E. (1981) Vitamin E for swine. *J. anim. Sci.*, *53*, 1039–1056.

Van Vleet, J. F. (1980) Current knowledge of selenium-vitamin E deficiency in domestic animals. *J. Am. vet. med. Assoc.*, *176*, 321–325.

Van Vleet, J. F. & Ferrara, V. J. (1986) Myocardial diseases of animals. *Am. J. Pathol.*, *126*, 98–178.

Watkinson, J. H. (1983) Prevention of selenium deficiency in grazing animals by annual topdressing of pasture with sodium selenate. *NZ vet. J.*, *31*, 78–85.

REFERENCES

(1) Koller, L. D. & Exon, J. H. (1986) *Can. J. vet. Res.*, *50*, 297.
(2) Rotruck, J. T. et al. (1973) *Science, N. W.*, *179*, 588.
(3) Stevens, J. B. et al. (1985) *Am. J. vet. Res.*, *46*, 1556.
(4) Caple, I. W. et al. (1978) *Aust. vet. J.*, *54*, 57
(5) Brady, P. S. et al. (1978) *J. anim. Sci.*, *47*, 492.
(6) Hidiroglou, M. et al. (1978) *Can. J. comp. Med.*, *42*, 128.
(7) Van Vleet, J. F. et al. (1981) *Am. J. vet. Res.*, *42*, 789.
(8) Van Vleet, J. F. et al. (1977) *Am. J. vet. Res.*, *38*, 991.
(9) Rudert, C. P. & Lewis, A. R. (1978) *Rhod. J. agric. Res.*, *16*, 109.
(10) Cawley, G. D. & Brandley, R. (1978) *Vet. Rec.*, *103*, 239.
(11) Jensen, P. T. et al. (1979) *Acta vet. Scand.*, *20*, 92.
(12) Rice, D. A. & McMurray, C. H. (1986) *Vet. Rec.*, *118*, 173.
(13) Harrison, J. H. et al. (1984) *J. dairy Sci.*, *67*, 123.
(14) McClure, T. J. et al. (1986) *Aust. vet. J.*, *63*, 144.
(15) Van Vleet, J. F. (1980) *J. Am. vet. med. Assoc.*, *176*, 321.
(16) National Academy of Sciences (1983) *Selenium in Nutrition*. Washington, DC National Research Council.
(17) Sissons, C. H. et al. (1982) *NZ vet. J.*, *30*, 9.
(18) Waltner-Toews, D. et al. (1986) *Can. J. vet. Res.*, *50*, 347.
(19) Allaway, W. H. (1973) *Cornell Vet.*, *63*, 151.
(20) Maylin, G. A. et al. (1980) *Cornell Vet.*, *70*, 272.
(21) Arthur, D. (1971) *Can J. anim. Sci.*, *51*, 71.
(22) Miltimore, J. E. et al. (1975) *Can. J. anim. Sci.*, *55*, 101.
(23) Gardiner, M. R. & Gorman, R. C. (1963) *Aust. J. exp. Agric.*, *2*, 261; *3*, 284.
(24) Thompson, K. G. et al. (1980) *Res. vet. Sci.*, *28*, 321.
(25) Morris, J. G. et al. (1984) *Science*, *223*, 491.
(26) Young, L. E. et al. (1972) *J. anim. Sci.*, *35*, 1112.
(27) Michel, R. L. et al. (1972) *J. dairy Sci.*, *55*, 498.
(28) Godwin, K. O. (1972) *Aust. J. exp. Agric. anim. Husb.*, *12*, 473.

(29) Mayhew, I. G. et al. (1987) *J. vet. int. Med.*, *1*, 45.
(30) Barton, C. R. Q. (1977) *Vet. Ann.*, *17*, 51.
(31) Roneus, B. & Essen-Gustavsson, B. (1986) *J. vet. Med.*, *A33*, 1.
(32) Hunter, A. G. & Boyd. J. H. (1977) *Vet. Rec.*, *100*, 103.
(33) Owen, ap R. R. et al. (1977) *J. Am. vet. med. Assoc.*, *171*, 343.
(34) Schougaard. H. et al. (1972) *Nord. VetMed.*, *24*, 67.
(35) Cawley, G. D. & Bradley, R. (1979) *Vet. Rec.*, *105*, 398.
(36) Ruth, G. R. & Van Vleet, J. F. (1974) *Am. J. vet. Res.*, *35*, 237.
(37) Smith, D. L. et al. (1985) *Can. vet. J.*, *26*, 385.
(38) Van Vleet, J. F. et al. (1975) *Am. J. vet. Res.*, *36*, 387.
(39) Piper, R. C. et al. (1975) *Am. J. vet. Res.*, *36*, 373.
(40) Shellow, J. S. et al. (1985) *J. anim. Sci.*, *61*, 590.
(41) Lindberg, P. et al. (1972) *Acta vet. Scand.*, *13*, 238.
(42) Jensen, P. T. et al. (1983) *Acta vet. Scand.*, *24*, 135.
(43) Arthur, J. R. & Boyne, R. (1985) *Life Sci.*, *36*, 1569.
(44) Andrews, E. D. et al. (1976) *NZ vet. J.*, *24*, 111.
(45) Sheppard, A. D. et al. (1984) *NZ vet. J.*, *32*, 91.
(46) Vipond, J. E. (1984) *Vet. Rec.*, *114*, 519.
(47) Mitchell, D. et al. (1975) *Can. J. anim. Sci.*, *55*, 513.
(48) Gwazdauskas, F. C. et al. (1979) *J. dairy Sci.*, *62*, 978.
(49) Fisher, L. J. et al. (1980) *Can. J. anim. Sci.*, *60*, 79.
(50) Ishak, M. A. et al. (1983) *J. dairy Sci.*, *66*, 99.
(51) Eger, S. et al. (1985) *J. dairy Sci.*, *68*, 2119.
(52) Harrison, J. H. et al. (1984) *J. dairy Sci.*, *69*, 1421.
(53) Kappel, L. C. et al. (1984) *Am. J. vet. Res.*, *45*, 691.
(54) Anderson, P. H. et al. (1977) *Br. vet. J.*, *133*, 160.
(55) Van Vleet, J. F. (1976) *Am. J. vet. Res.*, *37*, 1415.
(56) Azing, E. S. et al. (1984) *Am. J. vet. Res.*, *45*, 1715.
(57) Hutchinson, L. J. et al. (1982) *J. Am. vet. med. Assoc.*, *181*, 581.
(58) Foreman, J. H. et al. (1986) *J. Am. vet. med. Assoc.*, *189*, 83.
(59) Boyd, J. W. (1976) *J. comp. Pathol.*, *86*, 23.
(60) Azing, E. S. & Klesius, P. H. (1986) *Am. J. vet. Res.*, *47*, 148, 426.
(61) Jacobson, S. O. et al. (1970) *Acta vet. Scand.*, *11*, 324.
(62) Gudmundson, J. (1976) *Can. vet. J.*, *17*, 45.
(63) Mercy, A. R. et al. (1977) *Proc. 54th ann. Conf. Aust. vet. Assoc.*, 141.
(64) Fontaine, M. et al. (1977) *Can. J. comp. Med.*, *41*, 41, 57 & 64.
(65) Simesen, M. G. et al. (1982) *Acta vet. Scand.*, *23*, 425.
(66) Koller, L. D. et al. (1984) *Can. J. comp. Med.*, *48*, 431.
(67) Erskine, R. J. et al. (1987) *J. Am. vet. med. Assoc.*, *190*, 417
(68) Nafstad, I. & Tollersrud, S. (1970) *Acta vet. Scand.*, *11*, 452.
(69) Kursa, J. & Kroupoua, V. (1976) *Res. vet. Sci.*, *20*, 97.
(70) Kimber, R. J. & Allen, S. A. (1975) *Br. J. Nutr.*, *33*, 357.
(71) Jenkins, K. J. et al. (1974) *Can. J. anim. Sci.*, *54*, 49.
(72) Mahan, D. C. et al. (1977) *J. anim. Sci.*, *45*, 738.
(73) Van Vleet, J. F. (1975) *Am. J. vet Res.*, *36*, 1335.
(74) Paynter, D. I. (1979) *Aust. J. agric. Res.*, *30*, 695.
(75) Wilkins, J. F. & Hamilton, B. A. (1980) *Aust. vet. J.*, *56*, 87.
(76) Wegger, I. et al. (1980) *Livestock Prod. Sci.*, *7*, 175.
(77) Peter, D. W. (1980) *Vet. Rec.*, *107*, 193.
(78) Koller, L. D. et al. (1984) *Am. J. vet. Res.*, *45*, 2507.
(79) Winter, K. A. & Gupta, U. C. (1979) *Can. J. anim. Sci.*, *59*, 107.
(80) Van Vleet, J. F. & Ferrara, V. J. (1977) *Am. J. vet. Res.*, *38*, 2077.
(81) Niyo, Y. et al. (1980) *Am. J. vet. Res.*, *41*, 474.
(82) Van Houweling, C. D. (1979) *J. Am. vet. med. Assoc.*, *175*, 298.
(83) Whanger, P. D. et al. (1978) *J. anim. Sci.*, *47*, 1157.
(84) Overnes, G. et al. (1985) *Acta. vet. Scand.*, *26*, 405.
(85) Moksnes, K. & Norheim, G. (1983) *Acta vet. Scand.*, *24*, 45.
(86) Koller, L. D. et al. (1983) *Cornell Vet.*, *73*, 323.
(87) Van Vleet, J. (1982) *Am. J. vet. Res.*, *43*, 1180.
(88) Allen, W. M. et al. (1978) *Vet. Rec.*, *102*, 222.
(89) Little, W. et al. (1979) *Res. vet. Sci.*, *26*, 193.
(90) Stephenson, J. B. & Grant, A. B. (1979) *NZ vet. J.*, *27*, 232.
(91) MacPherson, A. & Chalmers, J. S. (1984) *Vet. Rec.*, *115*, 544.
(92) McMurray, C. H. & McEldowney, P. K. (1977) *Br. vet. J.*, *133*, 535.
(93) Cawley, G. D. & McPhee, I. (1984) *Vet. Rec.*, *114*, 565.
(94) Roneus, B. (1982) *Nord. VetMed.*, *34*, 350.
(95) Atroshi, F. et al. (1981) *Res. vet. Sci.*, *31*, 269.
(96) Symonds, H. W. et al.(1981) *Br. J. Nutr.*, *45*, 117.
(97) Roneus, & Lindholm, A. (1983) *Nord. VetMed.*, *35*, 337.
(98) Steele, P. et al. (1980) *Aust. vet. J.*, *56*, 529.
(99) Arthur, J. R. et al. (1979) *Vet. Rec.*, *104*, 340.
(100) Puls, R. (1981) *Veterinary Trace Mineral Deficiency and Toxicity Information.* Publication No. 5139 Information Services, Agriculture Canada, Ottawa, pp. 1–101.
(101) Peter, D. W. (1980) *Aust. J. agric. Res.*, *31*, 1005.
(102) Scholy, R. W. et al. (1981) *Am. J. vet. Res.*, *42*, 1724.
(103) Blackmore, D. J. et al. (1982) *Equ. vet. J.*, *14*, 139.
(104) Sheppard, A. D. et al. (1984) *NZ vet. J.*, *32*, 97.
(105) Rice, D. A. & Blanchflower, W. J. (1986) *Vet. Rec.*, *118*, 479.
(106) Zhang, W. R. et al. (1986) *Can. J. vet. Res.*, *50*, 390.
(107) Friendship, R. M. & Wilson, M. R. (1985) *Can. J. comp. Med.*, *49*, 311.
(108) Rammell, C. G. (1983) *NZ vet. J.*, *31*, 179.
(109) Rammell, C. G. & Cuncliffe, B. (1983) *NZ vet. J.*, *31*, 203.
(110) Butler, P. & Blackmore, D. J. (1983) *Vet. Rec.*, *112*, 60.
(111) Roneus, B. & Hakkarainer, J. (1985) *Acta vet. Scand.*, *26*, 425.
(112) Mallinson, C. B. et al. (1985) *Vet. Rec.*, *117*, 405.
(113) Overnes, G. et al. (1985) *Acta vet. Scand.*, *26*, 164.
(114) Julien, W. E. et al. (1976) *J. dairy Sci.*, *59*, 1960.
(115) Rice, D. A. et al. (1986) *Vet. Rec.*, *119*, 571.
(116) Hidiroglou, M. & Proulx, J. (1985) *J. dairy Sci.*, *68*, 57.
(117) Watkinson, J. H. (1983) *NZ vet. J.*, *31*, 78.
(118) Roneus, B. O. et al. (1986) *Equ. vet. J.*, *18*, 50.

Dietary deficiency of phosphorus, calcium and vitamin D and imbalance of the calcium : phosphorus ratio

A dietary deficiency or disturbance in the metabolism of calcium, phosphorus or vitamin D, including imbalance of the calcium : phosphorus ratio, is the principal cause of the osteodystrophies. The interrelation of these various factors is often very difficult to define and because the end result in all these deficiencies is so similar the precise etiological agent is often difficult to determine in any given circumstance.

In an attempt to simplify this situation the diseases in this section have been dealt with in the following order:

Calcium deficiency (*hypocalcicosis*)
(a) *Primary*—an absolute deficiency in the diet.
(b) *Secondary*—when the deficiency is conditioned by some other factor, principally an excess intake of phosphorus.

Phosphorus deficiency (*hypophosphatosis*)
(a) *Primary*—an absolute deficiency in the diet.
(b) *Secondary*—when the deficiency is conditioned by some other factor. Although in general terms an excessive intake of calcium could be such a factor, specific instances of this situation are lacking.

Vitamin D deficiency (*hypovitaminosis D*)
(a) *Primary*—an absolute deficiency in intake of the vitamin.
(b) *Secondary*—when the deficiency is conditioned by other factors of which excess carotene intake is the best known.

In different countries with varying climates, soil types and methods of husbandry, these individual deficiencies are of varying importance. For instance in South Africa, northern Australia and North America the most common of the above deficiencies is that of phosphorus; vitamin D deficiency is uncommon. In Britain, Europe and parts of North America, a deficiency of vitamin D can also be of major importance. Animals are housed indoors for much of the year and they are exposed to little ultraviolet irradiation, and their forage may contain little vitamin D. Under such conditions the absolute and relative amounts of calcium and phosphorus in the diet need to be greater than in other areas if vitamin D deficiency is to be avoided. In New Zealand where much lush pasture and cereal grazing is used for feed, the vitamin D status is reduced not only by poor solar irradiation of the animal and plant sterols, but in addition an antivitamin D factor is present in the diet possibly in the form of carotene.

Now that the gross errors of management with respect to calcium and phosphorus and vitamin D are largely avoided, more interest is devoted to the marginal errors; in these, diagnosis is not nearly so easy and the deficiency can be evident only at particular times of the year (1). The conduct of a response trial in which part of the herd is treated is difficult unless they are hand-fed daily; there are no suitable reticular retention pellets or long-term injections of calcium or phosphorus because the daily requirement is so high. Two methods suggest themselves: analysis of ash content of samples of spongy bone from the tuber coxae (2) and the metabolic profile method (3). The latter program may have some value as a monitoring and diagnostic weapon in the fields of metabolic disease, nutritional deficiency and nutritional excesses.

Absorption and metabolism of calcium and phosphorus

In ruminants, dietary calcium is absorbed by the small intestine according to body needs. Whereas young animals with high growth requirements absorb and retain calcium in direct relation to intake over a wide range of intakes, adult male animals, irrespective of intake, absorb only enough calcium to replace that lost by excretion into urine and intestine, retaining none of it (4). Calcium absorption is increased in adult animals during periods of high demand such as pregnancy and lactation or after a period of calcium deficiency, but a substantial loss of body stores of calcium appears to be necessary before this increase occurs. The dietary factors which influence the efficiency of absorption of calcium include the nature of the diet, the absolute and relative amounts of calcium and phosphorus present in the diet and the presence of interfering substances. Calcium of milk is virtually all available for absorption but calcium of forage-containing diets has an availability of only about 50%. The addition of grain to an all-forage diet markedly improves the availability of the calcium.

Phosphorus is absorbed by young animals from both milk and forage-containing diets with a high availability (80–100%), but the availability is much lower (50–60%) in adult animals. Horses fed diets containing adequate amounts of calcium and phosphorus absorb 50–65% of the calcium and slightly less than 50% of the phosphorus present in a variety of feedstuffs. In grains, 50–65% of the phosphorus is in the phytate form which is utilizable by ruminants but not as efficiently by non-ruminants like the horse and pig. An average availability of 70% has been assumed for phosphorus in early weaning diets for young pigs and a value of 50% in practical cereal-based feeds as supplied to growing pigs, sows and boars.

The metabolism of calcium and phosphorus is influenced by the parathyroid hormone calcitonin and vitamin D. Parathyroid hormone is secreted in response to hypocalcemia and stimulates the conversion of 25-dihydroxycholecalciferol to 1,25-dihydroxycholecalciferol (1,25-DHCC). Parathyroid hormone and 1,25-DHCC together stimulate bone resorption and 1,25-DHCC alone stimulates intestinal absorption of calcium. Calcium enters the blood from bone and intestine and when the serum calcium level increases above normal, parathyroid hormone is inhibited and calcitonin secretion stimulated. The increased calcitonin concentration blocks bone resorption and the decreased parathyroid hormone concentration depresses calcium absorption.

REVIEW LITERATURE

Schryver, H. F. et al. (1974) Calcium and phosphorus in the nutrition of the horse. *Cornell Vet.*, *64*, 493.

REFERENCES

(1) Little, D. A. (1970) *Aust. vet. J.*, *46*, 241.
(2) Priboth, W. & Fritzsche, H. (1969) *Arch. exp. VetMed.*, *23*, 653.
(3) Payne, J. M. et al. (1970) *Vet. Rec.*, *87*, 150.
(4) Braithwaite, G. D. (1976) *J. dairy Res.*, *43*, 501.

Calcium deficiency

Calcium deficiency may be primary or secondary, but in both cases the end result is an osteodystrophy, the specific disease depending largely on the species and age of the animals affected.

Etiology

A primary deficiency due to a lack of calcium in the diet seldom occurs, although a secondary deficiency due to a marginal calcium intake aggravated by a high phosphorus intake is not uncommon. In ponies such a diet depresses intestinal absorption and retention of calcium in the body, and the resorption of calcium from bones is increased (1). The effects of reduced calcium intake and parathyroidectomy are understandably additive in pigs (2) but parathyroid insufficiency seems an unlikely natural phenomenon.

Epidemiology

Calcium deficiency is a sporadic disease which occurs in particular groups of animals rather than in geographically limited areas. Although death does not usually occur there may be considerable loss of function and disabling lesions of bones or joints.

Horses in training, cattle being fitted for shows, and valuable stud sheep are often fed artificial diets containing cereal or grass hays which contain little calcium, and grains which have a high content of phosphorus. The secondary calcium deficiency which occurs in these circumstances is often accompanied by a vitamin D deficiency because of the tendency to keep animals confined indoors. Pigs are often fed heavy concentrate rations with insufficient calcium supplement. Dairy cattle may occasionally be fed similarly imbalanced diets, the effects of which are exaggerated by high milk production. There are no well-established records of calcium deficiency in grazing sheep or cattle but there are records of low calcium intake in feedlots (3) accompanied by clinical osteodystrophy. There is also a well-recognized field occurrence of calcium deficiency in young sheep in southeast Australia (4). Outbreaks can affect many sheep and are usually seen in winter and spring, following exercise or temporary starvation. In most outbreaks the characteristic osteoporosis results from a long-term deprivation of food due to poor pasture growth. Occasional outbreaks occur on green oats used for grazing. The calcium intake in some cases is as low as 3–5 g per week in contrast to the requirement of 3–5 g/day.

In females there is likely to be a cycle of changes in calcium balance, a negative balance occurring in late pregnancy and early lactation and a positive balance in late lactation and early pregnancy and when lactation has ceased. The negative balance in late pregnancy is in spite of a naturally occurring increased absorption of calcium from the intestine at that time, at least in ewes (5).

Osteodystrophia fibrosa is the well-recognized manifestation of calcium deficiency in pigs. A further disease, slipped femoral head in sows, is considered by some to be a form of calcium deficiency because of the way it responds to heavy supplementation of the diet with calcium. Not all observers are convinced of the relationship (6). The more interesting controversy centers on the suggestion that atrophic rhinitis is due to resorption of nasal turbinate bones as part of a general osteodystrophy (7). Recent experimental work has shown that while deviation of the nasal septum occurred in pigs fed diets with varying levels of calcium and phosphorus, the deviation was not related to dietary levels of calcium or phosphorus (8).

Pathogenesis

The main physiological functions of calcium are the formation of bone and milk, participation in the clotting of blood and the maintenance of neuromuscular excitability. In the development of osteodystrophies, dental defects and tetany the role of calcium is well understood but the relation between deficiency of the element and lack of appetite, poor growth, loss of condition, infertility, and reduced milk flow is not readily apparent. The disinclination of the animals to move about and graze and poor dental development may contribute to these effects.

It must be remembered that nutritional factors other than calcium, phosphorus and vitamin D may be important in the production of osteodystrophies which also occur in copper deficiency, fluorosis and chronic lead poisoning. Vitamin A is also essential for the development of bones, particularly those of the cranium.

Clinical findings

The clinical signs, apart from the specific syndromes dealt with below, are less marked in adults than they are in young animals, in which there is decreased rate or cessation of growth and dental maldevelopment. The latter is characterized by deformity of the gums, poor development of the incisors, failure of permanent teeth to erupt for periods of up to 27 months and abnormal wear of the permanent teeth due to defective development of dentine and enamel, occurring principally in sheep (9, 10).

A calcium deficiency may occur in lactating ewes and sucking lambs whose metabolic requirements for calcium are higher than in dry and pregnant sheep. There is a profound fall in serum calcium. Tetany and hyperirritability do not usually accompany hypocalcemia in these circumstances probably because it develops slowly. However, exercise and fasting often precipitate tetanic seizures and parturient paresis in such sheep. This is typical of the disease as it occurs in young sheep in southeast Australia (4). Attention is drawn to the presence of the disease by the occurrence of tetany, convulsions and paresis but the important signs are illthrift and failure to respond to anthelmintics. Serum calcium levels will be as low as 5·6 mg/dl. There is lameness but fractures are not common even though the bones are soft. A simple method for assessing this softness is compression of the frontal bones of the skull with the thumbs. In affected sheep the bones can be felt to fluctuate.

Pigs fed on heavy concentrate rations may develop a hypocalcemic tetany which responds to treatment with calcium salts. Tetany may also occur in young growing cattle in the same circumstances.

Inappetence, stiffness, tendency of bones to fracture, disinclination to stand, difficult parturition, reduced milk flow, loss of condition and reduced fertility (11) are all non-specific signs recorded in adults.

Specific syndromes

Primary calcium deficiency

No specific syndromes are recorded.

Secondary calcium deficiency

Rickets, osteomalacia, osteodystrophia fibrosa of the horse and pig, and degenerative arthropathy of cattle are the common syndromes in which secondary calcium deficiency is one of the specific causative factors. In sheep, rickets is seldom recognized but there are marked dental abnormalities. Rickets has been produced experimentally in lambs by feeding a diet low in calcium (12).

Clinical pathology

Because of the effect of the other factors listed above on body constituents, examination of specimens from living animals may give little indication of the primary cause of the disturbance. For example, hypocalcemia need not indicate a low dietary intake of calcium. Data on serum calcium and phosphorus and plasma phosphatase levels, radiographical examination of bones and balance studies of calcium and phosphorus retention are all of value in determining the presence of osteodystrophic disease, but determination of the initial causative factor will still depend on analysis of feedstuffs and comparison with known standard requirements. The levels of serum calcium may be within the normal range in most cases (15). However, in spite of evidence to the contrary it seems that calcium deficiency is followed, at least in sheep, by a marked fall in serum calcium levels to as low as 3·5 mg/dl (0·87 mmol/l). In an uncomplicated nutritional deficiency of calcium in sheep there is only a slight reduction in the radiopacity of bone in contrast to sheep with a low phosphorus and vitamin D status which show marked osteoporosis (10). The response to dietary supplementation with calcium is also of diagnostic value.

Necropsy findings

Severe osteoporosis and parathyroid hyperplasia are the significant findings. The ash content of the bone is low because the bone is resorbed before it is properly mineralized.

Diagnosis

A diagnosis of calcium deficiency depends upon proof that the diet is, either absolutely or relatively, insufficient in calcium, that the lesions and signs observed are characteristic and that the provision of calcium in the diet alleviates the condition. The diseases which may be confused with calcium deficiency are described under the diagnosis of each of the specific disease entities described below.

The close similarity between the dental defects in severe calcium deficiency of sheep and those occurring in chronic fluorosis may necessitate quantitative estimates of fluorine in the teeth or bone to determine the cause.

Treatment

The response to treatment is rapid and the preparations and doses recommended below are effective as treatment. Parenteral injections of calcium salts are advisable when tetany is present.

Control

The provision of adequate calcium in the diet, the reduction of phosphorus intake where it is excessive, and the provision of adequate vitamin D are the essentials of both treatment and prevention. Some examples of estimated minimum daily requirements for calcium, phosphorus and vitamin D are set out in Table 90. These are estimated minimum requirements and may need to be increased by a safety factor of 10% to allow for variation in individual animal requirements, the biological availability of nutrients in the feedstuffs and the effect which total amount of feed intake has on absolute intake of minerals. For example, the use of a complete swine ration on a restricted basis may require that the concentration of both calcium and phosphorus be increased in order for that ration to deliver the actual total quantity of calcium and phosphorus necessary to meet a particular requirement for growth, pregnancy or lactation. The information in Table 90 is presented merely as a guideline. When investigating a nutritional problem of formulating rations it is recommended that the most recently available publications on the nutrient requirements of domestic animals be consulted.

Ground limestone is most commonly used to supplement the calcium in the ration, but should be prepared from calcite and not from dolomite. Variations in availability of the calcium in this product occur with variations in particle size, a finely ground preparation being superior in this respect. Bone meal and dicalcium phosphate are more expensive and the additional phosphorus may be a disadvantage if the calcium : phosphorus ratio is very wide. Alfalfa, clover and molasses are also good sources of calcium but vary in their content. The optimum calcium to phosphorus ratio is within the range of of 2 : 1 to 1 : 1. In cattle absorption of both elements is better at the 2 : 1 ratio (13). For optimum protection against the development of urolithiasis in sheep a ratio of 2–2·5 calcium to 1 phosphorus is recommended (14).

The dustiness of powdered limestone can be overcome by dampening the feed or adding the powder mixed in molasses. Addition to salt or a mineral mixture is subject to the usual disadvantage that not all animals partake of it readily when it is provided free-choice, but this method of supplementation is often necessary in pastured animals. High-producing dairy cows should receive the mineral mixture in their ration as well as having access to it in boxes or in blocks.

REVIEW LITERATURE

Braithwaite, G. D. & Glascock, R. F. (1976) Metabolism of calcium in sheep. In *Biennial Reviews*, Nat. Inst. Res. Dairying, Shinfield, Reading, UK.

REFERENCES

(1) Schryver, H. F. et al. (1971) *J. Nutr. 101*, 259
(2) Littledike, E. T. et al. (1968) *Am. J. vet. Res.*, *29*, 635.
(3) Curtis, R. A. et al. (1969) *Can. vet. J.*, *10*, 20.
(4) Palmer, N. C. (1969–70) *Vict. vet. Proc.*, *28*, 55.
(5) Braithwaite, G. D. et al (1970) *Br. J. Nutr.*, *24*, 661.
(6) Duthie, I. F. & Lancaster, M. C. (1964) *Vet. Rec.*, *76*, 263.
(7) Brown, W. R. et al (1966) *Cornell Vet.*, *56*, Suppl. 1.
(8) Doige, C. E. et al. (1975) *Can. J. anim. Sci.*, *55*, 147.
(9) Franklin, M. C. (1950) *Cwlth Aust. sci. ind. Res. Org.*, *Bull.*, *252*, 34.
(10) McRoberts, M. R. et al. (1965) *J. agric. Sci.*, *Camb.*, *65*, 1.
(11) Hignett, S. L. (1956) *Proc. 3rd int. Cong. anim. Reprod.*, *Camb.*, 116.
(12) Dutt, B. & Sawhney, P. C. (1965) *Ind. J. vet. Sci.*, *35*, 345.
(13) Manston, R. (1967) *J. agric. Sci.*, *Camb.*, *68*, 263.
(14) Pope, A. L. (1971) *J. anim. Sci.*, *33*, 1332.
(15) Heaney, D. P. et al. (1985) *Can. J. anim. Sci.*, *65*, 163

Phosphorus deficiency

Phosphorus deficiency is usually primary and is characterized by pica, poor growth, infertility and, in the later stages, osteodystrophy.

Etiology

Phosphorus deficiency is usually primary under field conditions but may be exacerbated by a deficiency of vitamin D and possibly by an excess of calcium. Experimentally large doses of vitamin A decrease the absorption of phosphorus in cattle (1), and this may contribute to the development of nutritional osteodystrophies.

Epidemiology

In contrast to calcium deficiency, a dietary deficiency of phosphorus is widespread under natural conditions. It has a distinct geographical distribution depending largely upon the phosphorus content of the parent rock from which the soils of the area are derived, but also upon the influence of other factors, such as excessive calcium, aluminum or iron, which reduce the availability of phosphorus to plants. Large areas of grazing land in many countries are of little value for livestock production without phosphorus supplementation. In New Zealand,

Table 90. Some examples of estimated daily requirements of calcium, phosphorus and vitamin D.

Species, kg body weight and function	*Calcium*	*Phosphorus*	*Vitamin D*
		(g/animal)	
DAIRY CATTLE			
Growing heifers (large breeds)			300 i.u. kg dry matter intake
159	15	12	
300	24	18	
400	26	20	
Growing heifers (small breeds)			
100	9	7	
200	15	11	
300	19	14	
Growing bulls (large breeds)			
300	27	20	
400	30	23	
500	30	23	
Maintenance of mature lactating cows			
400	17	13	
500	20	15	
600	22	17	
Maintenance and pregnancy			
400	23	18	
500	29	22	
600	34	26	
Milk production	Add 2–3 g calcium and 1.7–2.4 g phosphorus to the maintenance requirement for each kg of milk produced		
		(% of ration)	
BEEF CATTLE			
Dry mature pregnant cows	0.16	0.16	300 i.u./kg dry matter intake
Cows nursing calves	0.30	0.25	
Bulls, growth and maintenance	0.26	0.20	
Growing heifers (200 kg live-weight gaining 0.8 kg/day)	0.33	0.26	
Growing steers (200 kg live-weight gaining 0.8 kg/day)	0.36	0.28	
SWINE			
Growing swine (from 10 to 100 kg live-weight)	0.65	0.50	200 i.u./kg ration
Breeding swine (gilts, sows and boars)	0.75	0.50	275 i.u./kg ration
SHEEP			
Ewes			
Maintenance	0.30	0.28	250–300 i.u./kg dry matter intake
Pregnant (early)	0.27	0.25	
Pregnant (late)	0.24	0.23	
Lactating	0.52	0.37	200 i.u./kg dry matter intake
Rams (40–120 kg live-weight)	0.35	0.19	200 i.u./kg dry matter intake
Lambs			
Early weaned (10–30 kg live-weight)	0.40	0.27	
Finishing (30–55 kg live-weight)	0.30	0.20	150 i.u./kg dry matter intake
HORSES			
Mature horses (400–600 kg live-weight)	0.30	0.20	6–8 i.u./kg body weight
Mares (400–600 kg live-weight)			
Last 90 days pregnancy	0.38	0.30	
Peak of lactation	0.50	0.40	
Growing horses (400 kg mature weight)			
3 months old	0.68	0.43	
6 months old	0.68	0.48	
12 months old	0.45	0.30	
Growing horses (500 kg mature weight)			
3 months old	0.69	0.44	
6 months old	0.82	0.51	
12 months old	0.43	0.28	

for example, where fertilization of pasture with superphosphate has been practiced for many years, phosphorus deficiency may still occur in dairy herds because of inadequate maintenance of application over several years (14). There is evidence also that the quality of the superphosphate declined over a period of several years. Soil reserves of phosphorus may also be low because of high phosphate retention soils. Animals in affected areas mature slowly and are inefficient breeders and additional losses due to botulism and defects and injuries of bones may occur. Apart from areas in which frank phosphorus deficiency is seen, it is probable that in many other areas a mild degree of deficiency is a limiting factor in the production of meat, milk and wool.

Heavy leaching by rain and constant removal by cropping contribute to phosphorus deficiency in the soil, and the low phosphorus levels of the plant cover may be further diminished by drought conditions. Pastures deficient in phosphorus are classically also deficient in protein.

Under range conditions milking cows are most commonly affected, but under intensive conditions it is the dry and young stock receiving little supplementation which suffer. The incidence of the disease varies: it is most common in animals at pasture during drought seasons but can also be a serious problem in housed cattle fed on hay only. The dietary requirements of phosphorus are given in Table 91. Cattle which constantly graze pasture in the southern hemisphere appear to require somewhat less phosphorus in their diet (0·20% is probably adequate) than do higher-producing, partly housed livestock (4). The dietary requirements of phosphorus for beef cows weighing 450 kg which have been recommended by the National Research Council may exceed the basic requirements (15). Over a period of several gestations a daily allowance of 12 g of phosphorus/day per animal was adequate for beef cows (15). Cattle given a phosphorus-deficient diet did not develop detectable signs of phosphorus deficiency until they had been on a severely deficient diet for 6 months. Sheep and horses at pasture are much less susceptible to the osteodystrophy of phosphorus deficiency than are cattle and their failure to thrive on phosphorus-deficient pasture is probably due in part to the low protein content of the pasture. In fact there has been no clear demonstration of a naturally occurring phosphorus deficiency in sheep, nor is there any record of infertility in sheep caused by phosphorus deficiency.

Table 91. Approximate levels of phosphorus in soil and pasture (quoted as phosphate radical) at which phosphorus deficiency occurs in cattle.

	Levels at which deficiency does not occur	*Levels at which deficiency occurs*
Soil	0·005%	0·002%
Pasture	0·3%	<0·2%–osteophagia <0·01%–rickets and osteomalacia
Daily intake (cattle)	40–50 g	25 g

All figures are on a dry matter basis and soil phosphate is citrate-soluble.

A primary deficiency can occur in swine kept in confinement. Lactating sows are more commonly affected than growing pigs.

Secondary phosphorus deficiency is of minor importance compared with the primary condition. A deficiency of vitamin D is not necessary for the development of osteodystrophy although with suboptimal phosphate intakes deficiency of this vitamin becomes critical. Excessive intake of calcium does not result in secondary phosphorus deficiency although it may cause a reduction in weight gains, due probably to interference with digestion, and may contribute to the development of phosphorus deficiency when the intake is marginal. The presence of phytic acid in plant tissues, which renders phosphate unavailable to carnivora, is a major consideration in pigs but of only minor importance in herbivora, except that increasing intakes of calcium may reduce the availability of phytate phosphorus even for ruminants. Rock phosphates which contain large amounts of iron and aluminum have been shown to be of no value to sheep as a source of phosphorus (2). A high intake of magnesium, such as that likely to occur when magnesite is fed to prevent lactation tetany, may cause hypophosphatemia if the phosphorus intake of dairy cows is already low (3).

Pathogenesis

Phosphorus is essential for the laying down of adequately mineralized bones and teeth and a deficiency will lead to their abnormal development. Inorganic phosphate, which may be ingested as such or liberated from esters during digestion or in intermediary metabolism, is utilized in the formation of proteins and tissue enzymes and is withdrawn from the plasma inorganic phosphate for this purpose.

Inorganic phosphate also plays an important role in the intermediary metabolism of carbohydrate and of creatine in the chemical reactions occurring in muscle contraction. This may be of importance in those cows which are recumbent after calving and have hypophosphatemia. The loss of phosphorus in the phospholipids of milk due to the onset of profuse lactation may be the crucial factor in the development of postparturient hemoglobinuria. An increased susceptibility to bloat has been postulated as an effect of phosphorus deficiency.

Clinical findings

Primary phosphorus deficiency is common only in cattle. Young animals grow slowly and develop rickets. In adults there is an initial subclinical stage followed by osteomalacia. In cattle of all ages a reduction in voluntary intake of feed is a first effect of phosphorus deficiency and is the basis of most of the general systemic signs. Retarded growth, low milk yield and reduced fertility are the earliest signs of phosphorus deficiency. For example, in severe phosphorus deficiency in range beef cattle the calving percentage has been known to drop from 70% to 20%. Although it is claimed that relative infertility occurs in dairy heifers on daily intakes of less than 40 g of phosphate, the infertility being accompanied by anestrus, subestrus and irregular estrus and delayed sexual maturity (6) this has not been borne out by other experimental work which indicates that fertility is independent of the calcium or phosphorus content or the calcium:phosphorus ratio of the diet in cattle (7). The effects of malnutrition on fertility are likely to be general and the infertility may often be related to lack of total energy intake rather than to specific deficiency (8). The development and wear of teeth are not greatly affected, in contrast with the severe dental abnormalities which occur in a nutritional deficiency of calcium. However, malocclusion may result from poor mineralization and resulting weakness of the mandible.

The experimental production of phosphorus deficiency in beef cows indicates that several months on a deficient diet are necessary before clinical signs develop (15). The clinical signs included general unthriftiness, marked body weight loss, reduced feed consumption, reluctance to move, abnormal stance, bone fractures, and finally impaired reproduction.

In a severely deficient area a characteristic conformation develops and introduced cattle revert to the district type in the next generation. The animals have a leggy appearance with a narrow chest and small girth, the pelvis is small and the bones are fine and break easily. The chest is slab-sided due to weakness of the ribs and the hair coat is rough and staring and lacking in pigment. In areas of severe deficiency the mortality rate may be high due to starvation especially during periods of drought when deficiencies of phosphorus, protein and vitamin A are exaggerated. Osteophagia is common and may be accompanied by a high incidence of botulism. Cows in late pregnancy often become recumbent and although they continue to eat are unable to rise. Such animals present a real problem in drought seasons because many animals in the area may be affected at the same time. Parenteral injections of phosphorus salts are ineffective and the only treatment which may be of benefit is to terminate the pregnancy by the administration of corticosteroids or by cesarean section.

Although sheep and horses in phosphorus-deficient areas do not develop clinically apparent osteodystrophy they are often of poor stature and unthrifty and may develop perverted appetites. An association between low blood phosphorus and infertility in mares has been suggested but the evidence is not conclusive. The principal sign in affected sows is posterior paralysis.

Clinical pathology

Blood levels of phosphorus are not a good indicator of the phosphorus status of an animal because they can remain at normal levels for long periods after cattle have been exposed to a serious deficiency of the element (9). Serum inorganic phosphorus levels are affected by such factors as age of animal, milk yield, stage of pregnancy, season of year, breed, feeding patterns and dietary phosphorus (16). The times of sampling in a herd must be standardized to reduce the effect of diurnal variation in serum concentrations of inorganic phosphorus. Hair does not reflect the status either. However, a marked hypophosphatemia is a good indicator of a severe phosphorus deficiency. The mild to moderate deficiencies, which are the most common ones, are usually accompanied by normal blood levels of phosphorus (10). As a rule clinical signs occur when blood levels have fallen from the normal of 4–5 mg/dl (1·3–1·7 mmol/l) to 1·5–3·5 mg/dl (0·5–1·2 mmol/l) and a response to phosphate supplementation in body weight gain can be anticipated in cattle which have blood inorganic phosphorus levels of less than 4 mg/dl (1·3 mmol/l). Levels may fall as low as 1 mg/dl (1·3 mmol/l) or less in severe clinical cases. Serum levels of calcium are unaffected. Estimation of the mineral content in pasture and drinking water is a valuable aid in diagnosis, but has major difficulty in representing what the animal has actually been taking in. A technique has been devised for determining phosphorus intake of sheep by estimating the phosphorus content of feces (5). A pool of three pellets from each of 30 sheep is used as a sampling technique. There is usually a marked deterioration in the radiopacity of the bones. Attention is drawn to the need to use standard methods of collection because of the effect that technique can have on phosphorus levels in blood. In cattle the recommended procedure is to collect blood from the tail and preserve it in buffered trichloracetic acid (11). However, the bone content of phosphorus is still considered as the most accurate indication of phosphorus status.

Necropsy findings

The necropsy findings are those of the specific diseases, rickets and osteomalacia.

Diagnosis

A diagnosis of phosphorus deficiency depends upon evidence that the diet is lacking in phosphorus, that the lesions and signs are typical of those caused by phosphorus deficiency and can be arrested or reverted by the administration of phosphorus. Differentiation from those diseases which may resemble rickets and osteomalacia is dealt with under those headings (pp.1211 and 1213).

Treatment

The preparations and doses recommended under control can be satisfactorily used for the treatment of affected animals. In cases where the need for phosphorus is urgent, as in postparturient hemoglobinuria and in cases of parturient paresis complicated by hypophosphatemia, the intravenous administration of sodium acid phosphate (30 g in 300 ml distilled water) is recommended.

Control

Under field conditions the difficulty usually encountered is that of providing phosphorus supplements to large groups of cattle running under extensive range conditions. The minimum daily requirement of cattle for phosphorus (as phosphate) is 15 g and 40–50 g is considered optimal.

Bone meal, dicalcium phosphate, disodium phosphate and sodium pyrophosphate may be provided in supplementary feed or by allowing free access to their mixtures with salt or more complicated mineral mixtures. The availability of the phosphorus in feed supplements varies and this needs to be taken into consideration when compounding rations. The relative biological values for young pigs in terms of phosphorus are: dicalcium phosphate or rock phosphate 83%, steamed bone meal 56%, and colloidal clay or soft phosphate 34% (12). It is suggested that in deficient areas adult dry cattle and calves up to 150 kg body weight should receive 225 g bone meal per week, growing stock over 150 kg body weight 350 g per week and lactating cows 1 kg weekly, but experience in particular areas may indicate the need for varying these amounts. The topdressing of pasture with superphosphate is an adequate method of correcting the deficiency and has the advantage of increasing the bulk and protein yield of the pasture but is often impractical under the conditions in which the disease occurs.

The addition of phosphate to drinking water is a much more satisfactory method provided the chemical can be added by an automatic dispenser to water piped into troughs. Adding chemicals to fixed tanks introduces errors in concentration, excessive stimulation of algal growth and precipitation in hard waters. Monosodium dihydrogen phosphate (monosodium orthophosphate) is the favorite additive and is usually added at the rate of 10–20 g/20 liters of water. Superphosphate may be used instead but is not suitable for dispensers, must be added in larger quantities (50 g/20 liters) and may contain excess fluorine. A reasonably effective and practical method favored by Australian dairy farmers is the provision of a supplement referred to as 'super juice'. Plain superphosphate at a rate of 2·5 kg in 40 liters of water is mixed and stirred vigorously in a barrel. When it has settled for a day the 'super juice' is ready for use and is administered by skimming off the supernatant and sprinkling 100–200 ml on the feed of each cow.

The use of phosphate supplements in the diet is not without hazards (13). Phosphoric acid is directly toxic and should not be used, and monosodium phosphate is unpalatable to many animals and the depression of appetite which results may discount the improved feed utilization which it provides.

REFERENCES

(1) Manston, R. (1964) *Br. vet. J.*, *122*, 443.
(2) Reinach, N. & Louw, J. G. (1958) *Onderstepoort J. vet. Res.*, *27*, 611.
(3) McTaggart, H. S. (1959) *Vet. Rec.*, *71*, 709.
(4) Little, D. A. (1979) *Res. vet. Sci.*, *28*, 258.
(5) Belonje, P. C. & van den Berg, A. (1980) *Onderstepoort J. vet. Res.*, *4*, 163 & 169.
(6) Morrow, D. A. (1969) *J. Am. vet. med. Assoc.*, *154*, 761.
(7) Littlejohn, A. I. & Lewis, G. (1960) *Vet. Rec.*, *72*, 1137.
(8) Hart, B. & Mitchell, G. L. (1965) *Aust. vet. J.*, *41*, 305.
(9) Cohen, R. O. H. (1972) *Aust. J. exp. Agric. anim. Husb.*, *13*, 5.
(10) Krook, L. (1968) *Cornell Vet.*, Suppl. 59.
(11) Teleni, E. et al. (1976) *Aust. vet. J.*, *52*, 529.
(12) Morrison, S. H. (1964) *Proc. 101st ann. Mtg Am. vet. Med. Assoc., Chicago*, 41.
(13) McMeiniman, N. D. (1973) *Aust. vet. J.*, *49*, 1590.
(14) Brooks, H. V. et al. (1984) *NZ vet. J.*, *32*, 174.
(15) Call, J. W. et al. (1986) *Am. J. vet. Res.*, *47*, 475.
(16) Forar, F. L. et al. (1982) *J. dairy Sci.*, *65*, 760.

Vitamin D deficiency

Vitamin D deficiency is usually caused by insufficient solar irradiation of animals or their feed and is manifested by poor appetite and growth, and in advanced cases by osteodystrophy.

Etiology

A lack of ultraviolet solar irradiation of the skin, coupled with a deficiency of preformed vitamin D complex in the diet, leads to a deficiency of vitamin D in tissues.

Epidemiology

Although the effects of clinically apparent vitamin D deficiency have been largely eliminated by improved nutrition the subclinical effects have received little attention. For example, retarded growth in young sheep in New Zealand and southern Australia during winter months has been recognized for many years as responding to vitamin D administration.

However, general realization of the importance of this subclinical vitamin D deficiency in limiting productivity of livestock has come only in recent years. This is partly due to the complexity of the relations between calcium, phosphorus and the vitamin and their common association with protein and other deficiencies in the diet. Much work remains to be done before these individual dietary essentials can be assessed in their correct economic perspective.

The lack of ultraviolet irradiation becomes important as distance from the equator increases and the sun's rays are filtered and refracted by an increasing depth of the earth's atmosphere. Cloudy, overcast skies, smokeladen atmospheres and winter months exacerbate the lack of irradiation. The effects of poor irradiation are felt first by animals with dark skin (particularly swine and some breeds of cattle) or heavy coats (particularly sheep), by rapidly growing animals and those that are housed indoors for long periods. The concentration of plasma vitamin D_3 recorded in grazing sheep varies widely throughout the year. During the winter months in the United Kingdom the levels in sheep fall below what is considered optimal, while in the summer months the levels are more than adequate (13). There is a marked difference in vitamin D status between sheep with a long fleece and those which have been recently shorn, especially in periods of maximum sunlight. The higher blood levels of vitamin D in the latter group are probably due to their greater exposure to sunlight. Pigs reared under intensive farming conditions and animals being prepared for shows are small but important susceptible groups.

The importance of dietary sources of preformed vitamin D must not be underestimated. Irradiated plant sterols with antirachitic potency occur in the dead leaves of growing plants. Variation in the vitamin D content of hay can occur with different methods of curing. Exposure to irradiation by sunlight for long periods causes a marked increase in antirachitic potency of the cut fodder whereas modern haymaking technique with its emphasis on rapid curing tends to keep vitamin D levels at a minimum. Grass ensilage also contains very little vitamin D.

Based on a survey of the concentrations of vitamin D in the serum of horses in the United Kingdom the levels may be low (8). In the absence of a dietary supplement containing vitamin D the concentration of 25-OHD_2

and 25-OHD_3 are, respectively, a reflection of the absorption of vitamin D_2 from the diet and of biosynthesis of vitamin D_3.

Information on the vitamin D requirements of housed dairy cattle is incomplete and contradictory. It appears, however, that in some instances natural feedstuffs provide less than adequate amounts of the vitamin for optimum reproductive performance in high-producing cows (2).

The grazing of animals, especially in winter time, on lush green feed including cereal crops, leads to a high incidence of rickets in the young. An antivitamin D factor is suspected because calcium, phosphorus and vitamin D intakes are usually normal, but the condition can be prevented by the administration of calciferol. Carotene, which is present in large quantities in this type of feed, has been shown to have antivitamin D potency but the existence of a further rachitogenic substance seems probable. The rachitogenic potency of this green feed varies widely according to the stage of growth and virtually disappears when flowering commences. Experimental overdosing with vitamin A causes a marked retardation of bone growth in calves. Such overdosing can occur when diets are supplemented with the vitamin and may produce clinical effects (4).

The importance of vitamin D to animals is now well recognized and supplementation of the diet where necessary is usually performed by the livestock owner. Occasional outbreaks of vitamin D deficiency are experienced in intensive systems where animals are housed and in areas where specific local problems are encountered, e.g., rickets in sheep on green cereal pasture in New Zealand.

Pathogenesis

Vitamin D is a complex of substances with antirachitogenic activity. The important components are as follows:

- *Vitamin D_3* (cholecalciferol) is produced from its precursor 7-dehydrocholesterol in mammalian skin and by natural irradiation with ultraviolet light.
- *Vitamin D_2* is present in suncured hay and is produced by ultraviolet irradiation of plant sterols. Calciferol or viosterol is produced commercially by the irradiation of yeast. Ergosterol is the provitamin.
- *Vitamin D_4* and *D_5* occur naturally in the oils of some fish.

Vitamin D produced in the skin or ingested with the diet and absorbed by the small intestine is transported to the liver. In the liver 25-hydroxycholecalciferol is produced which is then transported to the kidney where at least two additional derivatives are formed. One is 1,25-dihydroxycholecalciferol, and the other is 24,25-dihydroxycholecalciferol (DHCC). Under conditions of calcium need or calcium deprivation the form predominantly produced by the kidney is 1,25-DHCC. At the present time it seems likely that 1,25-DHCC is the metabolic form of vitamin D which is most active in eliciting intestinal calcium transport and absorption and is at least the closest known metabolite to the form of vitamin D which functions in bone mineralization. The metabolite also functions in regulating the absorption and metabolism of the phosphate ion, and especially its loss from the kidney. A deficiency of the metabolite may occur in animals with renal disease resulting in decreased absorption of calcium and phosphorus, decreased mineralization of bone and excessive losses of the minerals through the kidney. A deficiency of vitamin D *per se* is governed in its importance by the calcium and phosphorus status of the animal.

Because of the necessity for the conversion of vitamin D to the active metabolites, there is a lag period of 2–4 days following the administration of the vitamin parenterally before a significant effect on calcium and phosphorus absorption can occur. The use of synthetic analogs of the active metabolites such as 1-alpha-hydroxycholecalciferol (an analog of 1,25-dihydroxycholecalciferol) can increase the plasma concentration of calcium and phosphorus within 12 hours following administration (5) and has been recommended for the control of parturient paresis in cattle.

Maternal vitamin D status is important in determining neonatal plasma calcium concentration. There is a significant correlation between maternal and neonatal calf plasma concentrations of 25-OHD_2, 25-OHD_3, 24,25-$(OH)_2D_2$, 24,25-$(OH)_2D_3$ and 25,26-$(OH)_2D_3$. This indicates that the vitamin D metabolite status of the neonate is primarily dependent on the 25-OHD status of the dam (3). The maternal serum concentrations of calcium, phosphorus and magnesium do not determine concentrations of these minerals found in the newborn calf. The ability of the placenta to maintain elevated plasma calcium or phosphorus in the fetus is partially dependent on maternal 1,25-$(OH)_2D$ status. Parenteral cholecalciferol treatment of sows before parturition is an effective method of supplementing neonatal piglets with cholecalciferol via the sow's milk and its metabolite via placenta transport (5).

When the calcium:phosphorus ratio is wider than the optimum (1:1 to 2:1), vitamin D requirements for good calcium and phosphorus retention and bone mineralization are increased. A minor degree of vitamin D deficiency in an environment supplying an imbalance of calcium and phosphorus might well lead to disease, whereas the same degree of vitamin deficiency with a normal calcium and phosphorus intake could go unsuspected. For example, in growing pigs vitamin D supplementation is not essential provided calcium and phosphorus intakes are rigidly controlled but under practical circumstances this may not be possible.

The minor functions of the vitamin include maintenance of efficiency of food utilization and a calorigenic action, the metabolic rate being depressed when the vitamin is deficient. These actions are probably the basis for the reduced growth rate and productivity in vitamin D deficiency.

Clinical findings

The most important effect of lack of vitamin D in farm animals is reduced productivity. A decrease in appetite and efficiency of food utilization cause poor weight gains in growing stock and poor productivity in adults. Reproductive efficiency is also reduced and the overall effect on the animal economy may be severe.

In the late stages lameness, which is most noticeable in the forelegs, is accompanied in young animals by bending of the long bones and enlargement of the joints. This latter stage of clinical rickets may occur simultaneously with cases of osteomalacia in adults. An adequate intake of vitamin D appears to be necessary for the maintenance of fertility in cattle particularly if the phosphorus intake is low. In one study in dairy cattle, the first ovulation after parturition was advanced significantly in vitamin D supplemented cows (2).

Clinical pathology

A pronounced hypophosphatemia occurs in the early stages and is followed some months later by a fall in serum calcium. Plasma alkaline phosphatase levels are usually elevated. The blood picture quickly returns to normal with treatment, often several months before the animal is clinically normal. Typical figures for beef cattle kept indoors are serum calcium 8·7 mg/dl (10·8 normal); 2·2 mmol/l, (2·7 normal), serum inorganic phosphate 4·3 mg/dl (6·3 normal); 1·1 mmol/l, (1·6 normal) and alkaline phosphatase 5·7 units (2·75 normal) (1).

The normal ranges of plasma concentrations of vitamin D and its metabolites in the farm animal species are now available (7) and can be used to monitor the response of the administration of vitamin D parenterally or orally in sheep (9, 10). The serum concentrations of vitamin D in the horse have been determined (8).

Diagnosis

A diagnosis of vitamin D deficiency depends upon evidence of the probable occurrence of the deficiency and response of the animal when vitamin D is provided. Differentiation from clinically similar syndromes is discussed under the specific osteodystrophies.

Treatment

It is usual to administer vitamin D in the dose rates set out under control. Affected animals should also receive adequate calcium and phosphorus in the diet.

Control

The administration of supplementary vitamin D to animals by adding it to the diet or by injection is necessary only when exposure to sunlight or the provision of a natural ration containing adequate amounts of vitamin D is impractical.

A total daily intake of 7–12 i.u./kg body weight is optimal. Sundried hay is a good source but green fodders are generally deficient in vitamin D. Fish liver oils are high in vitamin D but are subject to deterioration on storage particularly with regard to vitamin A. They have the added disadvantage of losing their vitamin A and D content in premixed feed, of destroying vitamin E in these feeds when they become rancid and of seriously reducing the butterfat content of milk. Stable water-soluble vitamin A and D preparations do not suffer from these disadvantages. Irradiated dry yeast is probably the simplest and cheaper method of supplying vitamin D in mixed grain feeds.

Stable water-soluble preparations of vitamin D are now available and are commonly added to the rations of animals which are being fed concentrate rations. The classes of livestock which usually need dietary supplementation include:

- Calves raised indoors on milk replacers
- Pigs raised indoors on grain rations
- Beef cattle receiving poor quality roughage during the winter months
- Cattle raised indoors for prolonged periods and not receiving suncured forage containing adequate levels of vitamin D. These include calves raised as herd replacements, yearling cattle fed concentrate rations, bulls in artificial insemination centers and purebred bulls maintained indoors on farms
- Feedlot lambs fed grain rations during the winter months or under total covered confinement
- Young growing horses raised indoors or outdoors on rations which may not contain adequate concentrations of calcium and phosphorus. This may be a problem in rapidly growing well-muscled horses which are receiving a high level of grain.

Because there is limited storage of vitamin D in the body, compared to the storage of vitamin A, it is recommended that daily dietary supplementation be provided when possible for optimum effect. In situations where dietary supplementation is not possible, the use of single intramuscular injections of vitamin D_2 (calciferol) in oil will protect ruminants for 3–6 months. A dose rate of 11 000 units/kg body weight is recommended and should maintain an adequate vitamin D status for 3–6 months.

In mature non-pregnant sheep weighing about 50 kg a single intramuscular injection at a dose of 6000 i.u./kg body weight produced concentrations of 25-hydroxyvitamin D_3 at adequate levels for 3 months (9). The parenteral administration of vitamin D_3 results in both higher tissue and plasma levels of vitamin D_3 than does oral administration, and intravenous administration produces higher plasma levels than does the intramuscular injection (12). The timing of the injection should be selected so that the vitamin D status of the ewe is adequate at the time of lambing (9). The vitamin D_3 status of lambs can be increased by the parenteral administration of the vitamin to the pregnant ewe (11). Dosing pregnant ewes with 300 000 i.u of vitamin D_3 in a rapidly available form, approximately 2 months before lambing, provides a safe means of increasing the vitamin D status of the ewe and the newborn lambs by preventing seasonally low concentrations of 25-hydroxyvitamin D_3 (14). In adult sheep there is a wide margin of safety between the recommended requirement and the toxic oral dose which provides ample scope for safe supplementation if such is desirable (10). In adult sheep given 20 times the recommended requirements for 16 weeks there was no evidence of pathological calcification (10). Oral dosing with 30–45 units/kg body weight is adequate provided treatment can be given daily. Massive oral doses can also be used to give long-term effects, e.g. a single dose of 2 million units is an effective preventive for 2 months in lambs. Excessive doses may cause toxicity with signs of drowsiness, muscle weakness, fragility of bones and calcification in the walls of blood vessels. The latter finding has been recorded in cattle receiving 10 million units per day and in unthrifty lambs receiving a single dose of 1 million units, although larger doses are tolerated by healthy lambs.

REVIEW LITERATURE

Dobson, R. C. & Ward, G. (1974) Vitamin D physiology and its importance to dairy cattle; a review. *J. dairy Sci.*, *57*, 985.
Horst, R. L. & Reinhardt, T. A. (1983) Vitamin D metabolism in ruminants and its relevance to the periparturient cow. *J. dairy Sci.*, *66*, 661–678.
Wasserman, R. H. (1975) Metabolism, function and clinical aspects of vitamin D. *Cornell Vet.*, *65*, 3.

REFERENCES

(1) Levchenko, V. I. et al. (1979) *Veterinariya, Moscow*, *5*, 57.
(2) Ward, G. et al. (1971) *J. dairy Sci.*, *54*, 204.
(3) Goff, J. P. et al. (1982) *J. Nutr.*, *112*, 1387.
(4) Grey, R. M. et al. (1965) *Pathol. Vet.*, *2*, 446.
(5) Goff, J.P. (1984) *J. Nutr.*, *114*, 163.
(6) Burgisser, H. et al. (1964) *Schweiz. Arch. Tierheilkd.*, *106*, 714.
(7) Horst, R. L. et al. (1981) *Anal. Biochem*, *116*, 189.
(8) Smith, B. S. W. & Wright, H. (1984) *Vet. Rec.*, *115*, 579.
(9) Smith, B. S. W. & Wright, H. (1985) *Res. vet. Sci.*, *39*, 59.
(10) Smith, B. S. W. et al. (1985) *Res. vet. Sci.*, *38*, 317.
(11) Hidiroglou, M. & Knipfel, J. E. (1984) *Can. J. comp. Med.*, *48*, 78.
(12) Hidiroglou, M. et al. (1984) *Can. J. anim. Sci.*, *64*, 697.
(13) Smith, B. S. W. & Wright, H. (1984) *Vet. Rec.*, *115*, 537.
(14) Smith, B. S. W. et al. (1987) *Vet. Rec.*, *120*, 199.

Vitamin D toxicity

Vitamin D toxicity has occurred in cattle (4), horses (3, 5, 6) and swine (1, 2, 7) following the parenteral or oral administration of excessive quantities of the vitamin.

In cattle large parenteral doses of vitamin D_3, 15–17 million i.u., results in prolonged hypercalcemia, hyperphosphatemia and large increases in plasma concentrations of vitamin D_3 and its metabolites (4). Clinical signs of toxicity occur within 2–3 weeks and include marked anorexia, loss of body weight, dyspnea, tachycardia, loud heart sounds, weakness, recumbency, torticollis, fever and a high case fatality rate (4). Pregnant cows 1 month before parturition are more susceptible than non-pregnant cows.

Accidental vitamin D_3 toxicity has occurred in horses fed a grain diet which supplied 12 000–13 000 i.u./kg body weight of vitamin D_3 daily for 30 days (5) equivalent to about 1 million i.u. vitamin D_3/kg of feed. Clinical findings included anorexia, stiffness, loss of body weight, polyuria and polydipsia. There was also evidence of hyposthenuria, aciduria and soft-tissue mineralization and fractures of the ribs (5). Calcification of the endocardium and the walls of large blood vessels are characteristic (6).

Severe toxicity in pigs occurs at a daily oral dose of 50 000–70 000 i.u./kg body weight. Signs include a sudden onset of anorexia, vomiting, diarrhea, dyspnea, apathy, aphonia, emaciation and death (3,5). Clinical signs are commonly observed within 2 days after consumption of the feed containing excessive vitamin D. At necropsy hemorrhagic gastritis and interstitial pneumonia are commonly present (7).

REFERENCES

(1) Hascheck, W. M. et al. (1978) *Cornell Vet.*, *68*, 325.
(2) Sansom, B. F. et al. (1976) *Vet. Rec.*, *99*, 310.
(3) Muyelle, E. et al. (1974) *Zentralbl. VetMed.*, 21A, 638.
(4) Littledike, E. T. & Horst, R. L. (1982) *J. dairy Sci.*, *65*, 749.
(5) Harrington, D. D. & Page, E. H. (1983) *J. Am. vet. med. Assoc.*, *182*, 1358.
(6) Harrington, D. D. (1982) *J. Am. vet. med. Assoc.*, *180*, 867.
(7) Long, G. C. (1984) *J. Am. vet. med. Assoc.*, *184*, 164.

Rickets

Rickets is a disease of young growing animals characterized by defective calcification of growing bone. The essential lesion is a failure of provisional calcification with persistence of hypertrophic cartilage and enlargement of the epiphyses. The poorly mineralized bones are subject to pressure distortions.

Etiology

The etiology of rickets has been discussed under the heading of calcium, phosphorus and vitamin D deficiency. Deficiencies of one or more of these factors may be the cause of rickets in individual situations and the effects of the deficiency are likely to be exacerbated by a rapid growth rate.

An inherited form of rickets has been described in pigs (1). It is indistinguishable from rickets caused by nutritional inadequacy.

Epidemiology

Clinical rickets is not as important economically as the subclinical stages of the various dietary deficiencies which produce it. The provision of diets adequate and properly balanced with respect to calcium and phosphorus, and sufficient exposure to sunlight, are mandatory in good animal husbandry. Rickets is no longer a common disease because these requirements are widely recognized but the incidence can be high in extreme environments including purely exploitative range grazing, intensive feeding in fattening units and heavy dependence on lush grazing, especially in winter months.

Rickets is a disease of young, rapidly growing animals and occurs naturally under the following conditions.

Calves

Primary phosphorus deficiency in phosphorus-deficient range areas, and vitamin D deficiency in calves housed for long periods are the common circumstances (2).

In young rapidly growing cattle raised intensively indoors a combined deficiency of calcium, phosphorus and vitamin D can result in leg weakness characterized by stiffness, reluctance to move and retarded growth. In some cases rupture of the Achilles tendon and spontaneous fracture occur (16). The Achilles tendon may rupture at the insertion of, or proximal to, the calcaneus.

Lambs

Lambs are less susceptible to primary phosphorus deficiency than cattle but rickets does occur under the same conditions (4). Green cereal grazing and to a less extent pasturing on lush rye-grass during winter months may cause a high incidence of rickets in lambs and this is considered to be a secondary vitamin D deficiency.

Pigs
Rickets in young pigs occurs in intensive fattening units where the effects of diet containing excessive phosphate (high cereal diets) are exacerbated by vitamin D and calcium deficiencies (6).

Foals
Rickets is uncommon in foals under natural conditions although it has been produced experimentally (3).

Pathogenesis
Dietary deficiencies of calcium, phosphorus and vitamin D result in defective mineralization of the osteoid and cartilaginous matrix of developing bone. There is persistence and continued growth of hypertrophic epiphyseal cartilage, increasing the width of the epiphyseal plate. Poorly calcified spicules of diaphyseal bone and epiphyseal cartilage yield to normal stresses resulting in bowing of long bones and broadening of the epiphyses with apparent enlargement of the joints. Rapidly growing animals on an otherwise good diet will be first affected because of their higher requirement of the specific nutrients.

Clinical findings
The subclinical effects of the particular deficiency disease will be apparent in the group of animals affected and have been discussed previously. Clinical rickets will be evidenced by a stiffness in the gait, enlargement of the limb joints, especially in the forelegs, and enlargement of the costochondral junctions. The long bones show abnormal curvature, usually forward and outward at the knee in sheep and cattle. Lameness and a tendency to lie down are common. Arching of the back and contraction, often to the point of virtual collapse, of the pelvis occur and there is an increased tendency for bones to fracture.

Eruption of the teeth is delayed and irregular, and the teeth are poorly calcified with pitting, grooving and pigmentation. They are often badly aligned and wear rapidly and unevenly. These dental abnormalities, together with thickening and softness of the jaw bones, may make it impossible for severely affected calves and lambs to close their mouths. As a consequence the tongue protrudes, and there is drooling of saliva and difficulty in feeding. In less severely affected animals dental malocclusion may be a significant occurrence (5). Severe deformity of the chest may result in dyspnea and chronic ruminal tympany. In the final stages the animal shows hypersensitivity and tetany, recumbency and eventually dies of inanition.

Clinical pathology
An elevation of plasma alkaline phosphatase is always evident but serum calcium and phosphorus levels will depend upon the causative factor. If phosphorus or vitamin D deficiencies are the cause the serum phosphorus level will usually be below the normal lower limit of 3 mg/dl. Serum calcium levels will be lowered only in the final stages. In leg weakness of young rapidly growing cattle, the serum concentration of 25-hydroxyvitamin D may be non-detectable and the serum levels of calcium and inorganic phosphorus may be low (16).

Radiographic examination of bones and joints is one of the most valuable aids in the detection of rickets. Rachitic bones have a characteristic lack of density compared to normal bones. The ends of long bones have a 'woolly' or 'motheaten' appearance and have a concave or flat, instead of the normal convex, contour. Surgical removal of a small piece of costochondral junction for histological examination has been used extensively in experimental work and should be applicable in field diagnosis.

Necropsy findings
Apart from general poorness of condition the necropsy findings are restricted to abnormal bones and teeth. The bone shafts are softer and larger in diameter, due in part to the subperiosteal deposition of osteoid tissue. The joints are enlarged and on cutting, the epiphyseal cartilage can be seen to be thicker than usual. Histological examination of the epiphysis is desirable for final diagnosis and in the sheep the best results are obtained from an examination of the distal cartilages of the metacarpal and metatarsal bones (7).

A valuable diagnostic aid is the ratio of ash to organic matter in the bones. Normally the ratio is three parts of ash to two of organic matter but in rachitic bone this may be depressed to 1:2, or 1:3 in extreme cases. A reduction below 45% of the bone weight as ash also suggests osteodystrophy. Because of the difficulty encountered in repeating the results of bone ash determinations, a standardized method has been devised in which the ash content of green bone is determined, using either the metacarpus or metatarsus, and the ash content related to the age of the animal, as expressed by the length of the bone. Although normal standards are available only for pigs (7) the method suggests itself as being highly suitable for all species.

Diagnosis
Rickets occurs in rapidly growing young animals and is characterized by stiffness of the gait and enlargement of the distal physes of the long bones, particularly noticeable on the metacarpus and metatarsus as circumscribed painful swellings. A history of a dietary deficiency of any of calcium, phosphorus or vitamin D will support the clinical diagnosis. Radiographic evidence of widened and irregular physes suggests rickets. Copper deficiency in young cattle under 1 year of age can also result in clinical, radiographic and pathological findings which are similar to rickets. Clinically there is an arched back, severe stiffness of gait, reluctance to move and loss of weight. There are marked swellings of the distal aspects of metacarpus and metatarsus and radiographically there is a widened zone of cartilage and lipping of the medial and lateral areas of the physeal plate (8). Copper concentration in plasma and liver are low and there is usually dietary evidence of copper deficiency.

Epiphysitis occurs in rapidly growing yearling cattle raised and fed intensively under confinement (9). There is severe lameness, swelling of the distal physes, and radiographic and pathological evidence of a necrotizing epiphysitis. The etiology is uncertain but thought to be related to the type of housing.

Congenital and acquired abnormalities of the bony

skeletal system are frequent in newborn and rapidly growing foals. Rickets occurs but only occasionally. 'Epiphysitis' in young foals resembles rickets and is characterized by enlargements and abnormalities of the distal physes of the radius, tibia, third metacarpal and metatarsal bones and the proximal extremity of the proximal phalanx (10). There may or may not be deviation of the limbs caused by uneven growth rates in various growth plates. The suggested causes include improper nutrition, faulty conformation and hoof growth, muscle imbalance, overweight, and compression of the growth plate. Recovery may occur spontaneously or require surgical correction (11).

It is usually difficult to make a definitive diagnosis of rickets in swine. The disease is usually suspected in young rapidly growing swine in which there is stiffness in the gait, walking on tiptoes, enlargements of the distal ends of long bones and dietary evidence of a marginal deficiency of calcium or phosphorus. The radiographic and pathological findings may suggest a rickets-like lesion. Mycoplasmal synovitis and arthritis clinically resemble rickets of pigs. There is a sudden onset of stiffness of gait, habitual recumbency and a decrease in feed consumption, enlargements of the distal aspects of the long bones which may or may not be painful and spontaneous recovery usually occurs in 10–14 days. The locomotor problems in young growing pigs raised in confinement and with limited exercise must be considered in the differential diagnosis (12, 14). In performance testing stations, up to 20% of boars may be affected with leg weakness (15).

In lambs, rickets must be differentiated from chlamydial and erysipelas arthritis which are readily diagnosed at necropsy.

Treatment and control

Recommendations for the treatment of the individual dietary deficiencies have been provided under their respective headings. Lesser deformities recover with suitable treatment but gross deformities usually persist. A general improvement in appetite and condition occurs quickly and is accompanied by a return to normal blood levels of phosphorus and alkaline phosphatase.

REFERENCES

(1) Plonait, H. (1969) *Zentralbl. VetMed.*, *16A*, 271, 289.
(2) Spratling, F. R. et al. (1970) *Br. vet. J.*, *126*, 316.
(3) Groenewald, J. W. (1949) *Rep. 14th int. vet. Cong.*, *3*, 34.
(4) Rossow, N. et al. (1977) *Mh VetMed.*, *32*, 256.
(5) Nisbet, D. I. et al. (1968) *J. comp. Pathol.*, *78*, 73.
(6) Pepper, T. A. et al. (1978) *Vet. Rec.*, *103*, 4.
(7) Pullar, E. M. (1960) *Aust. vet. J.*, *36*, 31.
(8) Smith, B. P. et al. (1975) *J. Am. vet. med. Assoc.*, *166*, 682.
(9) Murphy, P. A. et al. (1975) *Vet. Rec.*, *97*, 445.
(10) Brown, M. P. & MacCallum, F. J. (1976) *Vet. Rec.*, *98*, 443.
(11) Vaughan, L. C. (1976) *Vet. Rec.*, *98*, 165.
(12) Elliot, J. I. & Doige, C. E. (1973) *Can. J. anim. Sci.*, *53*, 211.
(13) Grondalen, T. (1974) *Nord. VetMed.*, *26*, 534.
(14) Hogg, A. et al. (1975) *Am. J. vet. Res.*, *36*, 965.
(15) McPhee, C. P. & Laws, L. (1976) *Aus. vet. J.*, *52*, 123.
(16) Sturen, M. (1985) *Acta vet. Scand.*, *26*, 169.

Osteomalacia

Osteomalacia is a disease of mature animals affecting bones in which endochondral ossification has been completed. The characteristic lesion is osteoporosis and the formation of excessive uncalcified matrix. Lameness and pathological fractures are the common clinical findings.

Etiology

Generally speaking the etiology and occurrence of osteomalacia are the same as for rickets except that the predisposing cause is not the increased requirement of growth but the drain of lactation and pregnancy.

Epidemiology

Osteomalacia occurs under the same conditions and in the same areas as rickets in young animals but is recorded less commonly. Its main occurrence is in cattle in areas seriously deficient in phosphorus (1, 2). It is also recorded in sheep again in association with hypophosphatemia (3). In pastured animals osteomalacia is most common in cattle, and sheep raised in the same area are less severely affected. In feedlot animals excessive phosphorus intake without complementary calcium and vitamin D is likely as a cause, especially if the animals are kept indoors (7). It also occurs in sows which have recently weaned their pigs after a long lactation period (6–8 weeks) while on a diet deficient usually in calcium. A marginal deficiency of both phosphorus and vitamin D will exaggerate the condition.

Pathogenesis

Increased resorption of bone mineral to supply the needs of pregnancy, lactation and endogenous metabolism leads to osteoporosis and weakness and deformity of the bones. Large amounts of uncalcified osteoid are deposited about the diaphyses. Pathological fractures are commonly precipitated by sudden exercise or handling of the animal during transportation.

Clinical findings

In the early stages the signs are those of phosphorus deficiency, including lowered productivity and fertility and loss of condition. Licking and chewing of inanimate objects begins at this stage and may bring their attendant ills of oral, pharyngeal and esophageal obstruction, traumatic reticuloperitonitis, lead poisoning and botulism.

The signs specific to osteomalacia are those of a painful condition of the bones and joints, and include a stiff gait, moderate lameness often shifting from leg to leg, crackling sounds while walking and an arched back. The hindlegs are most severely affected and the hocks may be rotated inwards. The animals are disinclined to move, lie down for long periods, and are unwilling to get up. The colloquial names 'pegleg', 'creeps', 'stiffs', 'cripples' and 'bog-lame' describe the syndrome aptly. The names 'milkleg' and 'milk-lameness' are commonly applied to the condition when it occurs in heavily milking cows. Fractures of bones and separation of tendon attachments occur frequently, often without apparent precipitating stress. In extreme cases deformities of bones occur, and when the pelvis is affected dystocia may result. Finally weakness leads to permanent recumbency and death from starvation.

Affected sows are usually found recumbent and unable to rise from lateral recumbency or from the dog-sitting position. The shaft of one femur or the neck of the femur is commonly fractured. The fracture usually occurs within a few days following weaning of the pigs. The placing of the sow with other adult pigs usually results in some fighting and increased exercise which commonly precipitates the pathological fractures.

Clinical pathology

In general the findings are the same as those for rickets, including increased serum alkaline phosphatase and decreased serum phosphorus levels. Radiographic examination of long bones shows decreased density of bone shadow.

Necropsy findings

Lighter bones with a low ratio of ash to organic matter, and deposits of osteoid, as in rickets, are the characteristic findings. Epiphyseal enlargement is not apparent but severe erosions of articular cartilages have been recorded in cattle in primary phosphorus deficiency (2).

Diagnosis

The occurrence of non-specific lameness with pathological fractures in mature animals should arouse suspicion of osteomalacia. There may be additional evidence of subnormal productivity and reproductive performance and dietary evidence of a recent deficiency of calcium, phosphorus or vitamin D. A similar osteoporotic disease of cattle in Japan has been ascribed to a dietary deficiency of magnesium (4). The cattle are on high concentrate, low roughage diets, have high serum calcium and alkaline phosphatase levels, but a low serum magnesium level. The osteoporosis is observable at slaughter and clinical signs observed are those of intercurrent disease, especially ketosis, milk fever and hypomagnesemia. Reproductive and renal disorders occur concurrently.

In cattle it must be differentiated from chronic fluorosis in mature animals but the typical mottling and pitting of the teeth and the enlargements on the shafts of the long bones are characteristic. In some areas, e.g. northern Australia, where the water supply is obtained from deep subartesian wells, the two diseases may occur concurrently. Analysis of water supplies and foodstuffs for fluorine may be necessary in doubtful cases.

In sows, osteomalacia with or without pathological fractures must be differentiated from spinal cord compression due to a vertebral body abscess and chronic arthritis due to erysipelas.

Treatment and control

Recommendations for the treatment and control of the specific nutritional deficiencies have been described under their respective headings. Some weeks will elapse before improvement occurs and deformities of the bones are likely to be permanent.

REFERENCES

(1) Theiler, A. & Green, H. H. (1932) *Nutr. Abst. Rev.*, *1*, 359.
(2) Barnes, J. E. & Jephcott, B. R. (1955) *Aust. vet. J.*, *31*, 302.
(3) Nisbet, D. I. et al. (1970) *J. comp. Pathol.*, *80*, 535.
(4) Yoshida, S. (1980) *J. Fac. appl. Biol. Sci.*, *19*, 39.

Osteodystrophia fibrosa

Osteodystrophia fibrosa is very similar in its pathogenesis to osteomalacia but differs in that soft, cellular, fibrous tissue is laid down as a result of the weakness of the bones instead of the specialized uncalcified osteoid tissue of osteomalacia. It occurs in horses, goats and swine.

Etiology

A secondary calcium deficiency due to excessive phosphorus feeding is the common cause in horses and probably also in pigs. The disease can be readily produced in horses on diets with a ratio of calcium to phosphorus of 1:2·9 or greater, irrespective of the total calcium intake, and calcium to phosphorus ratios of 1:0·9 to 1:1·4 have been shown to be preventive and curative. With a very low calcium intake of 2–3 g/day and a calcium to phosphorus ratio of 1:13 the disease may occur within 5 months. With a normal calcium intake of 26 g/day and a calcium to phosphorus ratio of 1:5, obvious signs appear in about 1 year but shifting lameness may appear as early as 3 months (1). The disease is reproducible in pigs on similar diets to those described above and also on diets low in both calcium and phosphorus (2). The optimum calcium to phosphorus ratio is 1·2:1·0 and the intake for pigs should be within the range of 0·6–1·2% of the diet.

Epidemiology

Osteodystrophia fibrosa is principally a disease of horses and other Equidae, and to a lesser extent of pigs. It has also occurred in goats (8). Amongst horses, those engaged in heavy city work and in racing are more likely to be affected because of the tendency to maintain these animals on unbalanced diets. The major occurrence is in horses fed a diet high in phosphorus and low in calcium. Such diets include cereal hays combined with heavy grain or bran feeding. Legume hays, because of their high calcium content, are preventive.

The disease may reach enzootic proportions in army horses moved into new territories, whereas local horses, more used to the diet, suffer little. Although horses may be affected at any age after weaning it is the 2–7 year age group which suffer most, probably because they are the group most likely to be exposed to the rations which predispose to the disease.

A novel occurrence has been recorded of an enzootic form of the disease affecting large numbers of horses at pasture (3). The dietary intake of calcium and phosphorus, and their proportions, were normal. The occurrence was thought to be due to the continuous ingestion of oxalate in specific grasses *Cenchrus ciliaris*, *Panicum maximum* var. *trichoglume*, *Setaria anceps*, *Brachiaria mutica* and *Pennisetum clandestinum*.

Pathogenesis

Defective mineralization of bones follows the imbalance of calcium and phosphorus in the diet and a fibrous dysplasia occurs. This may be in response to the weakness of the bones or it may be more precisely a response to hyperparathyroidism stimulated by the excessive intake of phosphorus (1). The weakness of the bones predisposes to fractures and separation of muscular and tendinous attachments. Articular erosions occur commonly and displacement of the bone marrow may cause the development of anemia.

Clinical findings

As in most osteodystrophies the major losses are probably in the early stages before clinical signs appear or on diets where the aberration is marginal. In horses a shifting lameness is characteristic of this stage of the disease and arching of the back may sometimes occur. The horse is lame but only mildly so and in many cases no physical deformity can be found by which the seat of lameness can be localized. Such horses often creak badly in the joints when they walk. These signs probably result from relaxation of tendon and ligaments and appear in different limbs at different times. Articular erosions may contribute to the lameness. In more advanced cases severe injuries, including fracture and visible sprains of tendons, may occur but these are not specific to osteodystrophia fibrosa, although their incidence is higher in affected than in normal horses. Fracture of the lumbar vertebrae while racing has been known to occur in affected horses.

The more classical picture of the disease has largely disappeared because cases are seldom permitted to progress to this advanced stage. Local swelling of the lower and alveolar margins of the mandible is followed by soft, symmetrical enlargement of the facial bones, which may become swollen so that they interfere with respiration. Initially these bony swellings are firm and pyramidal and commence just above and anterior to the facial crests. The lesions are bilaterally symmetrical. Flattening of the ribs may be apparent and fractures and detachment of ligaments occur if the horse is worked. There may be obvious swelling of joints and curvature of long bones. Severe emaciation and anemia occur in the final stages.

In pigs the lesions and signs are similar to those in the horse and in severe cases pigs may be unable to rise and walk, show gross distortion of limbs and enlargement of joints and the face. In less severe cases there is lameness, reluctance to rise, pain on standing, bending of the limb bones but normal facial bones and joints. With suitable treatment the lameness disappears but affected pigs may never attain their full size. The relationship of this disease to atrophic rhinitis is discussed under the latter heading.

Clinical pathology

There are no significant changes in blood chemistry in horses affected with severe osteodystrophia fibrosa. However, the serum calcium level will tend to be lower than normal, the serum inorganic phosphorus higher than normal and the alkaline phosphatase activity higher than normal (8). The levels of alkaline phosphatase which are diagnostic have not been determined (4). Affected horses may be unable to return their serum calcium levels to normal following the infusion of a calcium salt (5). Radiographic examination reveals increased translucency of bones.

Necropsy findings

The entire skeleton shows marked osteoporosis. The hard bone of the mandible, maxilla and nasal bones is replaced by soft fibrous tissue and there is characteristically replacement of red bone marrow with the same fibrous tissue.

Diagnosis

In the early stages diagnosis may be difficult because of the common occurrence of traumatic injuries to horses' legs. A high incidence of lameness in a group of horses warrants examination of the ration and determination of their calcium and phosphorus status. An identical clinical picture has been described in a mare with an adenoma of the parathyroid gland (6). Inherited multiple exostosis has been described in the horse (7).

In pigs, osteodystrophia can be the result of hypovitaminosis A and experimentally as a result of manganese deficiency.

Treatment and control

A ration adequately balanced with regard to calcium and phosphorus (calcium:phosphorus should be in the vicinity of 1:1 and not wider than 1:1·4) is preventive in horses and affected animals can only be treated by correcting the existing imbalance. Even severe lesions may disappear in time with proper treatment. Cereal hay may be supplemented with alfalfa or clover hay, or finely ground limestone (30 g daily) should be fed. Dicalcium phosphate or bone meal are not as efficient because of their additional content of phosphorus.

REFERENCES

(1) Krook, L. & Lowe, J. E. (1964) *Pathol. vet.*, *1*, Suppl. 98.
(2) Storts, R. W. & Koestner, A. (1965) *Am. J. vet. Res.*, *26*, 280.
(3) Walthall, J. C. & McKenzie, R. A. (1976) *Aust. vet. J.*, *52*, 11.
(4) Krook, L. (1968) *Cornell Vet.*, *58*, 59.
(5) Argenzio, R. A. et al. (1974) *J. Nutr.*, *104*, 18.
(6) Bienfet, V. et al. (1964) *Ann. Méd. vét.*, *108*, 252.
(7) Morgan, J. P. et al. (1962) *J. Am. vet. med. Assoc.*, *140*, 1320.
(8) Andrews, A. H. et al. (1983) *Vet. Rec.*, *112*, 404.

'Bowie' or 'bentleg'

This is a disease of lambs of unknown etiology. There is a characteristic lateral curvature of the long bones of the front legs but the lesions differ from those of rickets. It has been observed only on unimproved range pasture in New Zealand (1). The cause is unknown although phosphorus deficiency has been suggested. Improvement of the pasture by topdressing with superphosphate and sowing improved grasses is usually followed by disappearance of the disease. Only sucking lambs are affected and cases occur only in the spring at a time when rickets does not occur. Up to 40% of a group of lambs may be affected without breed differences in incidence. A similar syndrome has been produced by the feeding of wild parsnip (*Trachemene glaucifolia*) and, experimentally, by the feeding of a diet low in both calcium and phosphorus (2).

Some tenderness of the feet and lateral curvature at

the knees may be seen as early as 2–3 weeks of age and marked deformity is present at 6–8 weeks with maximum severity at weaning. The forelimbs are more commonly affected than the hindlimbs. Medial curvature occurs in rare cases. The sides of the feet become badly worn and the lateral aspects of the lower parts of the limbs may be injured and be accompanied by lameness. The lambs grow well at first but by weaning affected lambs are in poor condition because of their inability to move about and feed properly. A rather similar syndrome has been observed in young Saanen bucks but the condition showed more tendency to recover spontaneously (3).

The levels of calcium and inorganic phosphate in serum are normal. At necropsy in spite of the curvature of the limbs there is no undue porosis, and although the epiphyseal cartilages are thickened they are supported by dense bone. There may be excessive synovial fluid in the joints and in the later stages there are articular erosions. Increased deposition of osteoid is not observed.

Supplementation of the diet with phosphorus or improvement of the pasture seems to reduce the incidence of the disease. Dosing with vitamin D or providing mineral mixtures containing all trace elements is ineffective (4).

REFERENCES

(1) Fitch, L. W. N. (1954) *NZ vet. J.*, *2*, 118.
(2) Field, A. C. et al. (1975) *J. agric. Sci., Camb.*, *85*, 435.
(3) Murphy, W. J. B. et al. (1959) *Aust. vet. J.*, *35*, 524.
(4) Cunningham, I. J. (1957) *NZ vet J.*, *5*, 103.

Degenerative joint disease

A degenerative arthropathy occurs in cattle of all breeds but reaches its highest incidence as a sporadic affliction of young beef bulls (1). The disease has been identified as hip dysplasia because of the pre-existing shallow contour of the acetabulum. It is considered to be inherited as a recessive characteristic and exacerbated by rapid weight gain in young animals. The occurrence of the condition in these animals is usually associated with rearing on nurse cows, housing for long periods, provision of a ration high in cereal grains and byproducts (i.e. a high phosphorus:calcium ratio) and possibly with an inherited straight conformation of the hindlegs. Although the disease occurs in all beef breeds there is a strong familial tendency which appears to be directly related to the rate of body weight gain and the straightness of the hindleg. If the potential for rapid weight gain is being realized in animals which are being force fed, the rate of occurrence appears to be dependent on their breeding (2) and animals in the same herd which are allowed to run at pasture under natural conditions are either not affected or are affected at a much later age. Thus, animals in a susceptible herd may show signs as early as 6 months of age if they are heavily hand-fed and raised on dairy cow foster mothers. In the same herd signs do not appear until 1–2 years of age if supplementary feeding is not introduced until weaning, and not until 4 years if there is no significant additional feeding (3).

Clinically there is a more or less gradual onset of lameness in one or both hindlegs. The disease progresses with the lameness becoming more severe over a period of 6–12 months. In some animals there is a marked sudden change for the worse, usually related to violent muscular movements as in breeding or fighting. In badly affected animals the affected limb is virtually useless and on movement distinct crepitus can often be felt and heard over the affected joints. This can be accomplished by rocking the animal from side to side or having it walk while holding the hands over the hip joints. An additional method of examination is to place the hand in the rectum close to the hip joint, whilst the animal is moved. Passive movement of the limb may also elicit crepitus or louder clinking or clicking sounds. Radiographic examination is possible and may provide confirmatory or diagnostic evidence. The hip joints are always most severely affected but in advanced cases there may be moderate involvement of the stifles and minimal lesions in other joints. Affected animals lie down most of the time and are reluctant to rise and to walk. The joints are not swollen, but in advanced cases local atrophy of muscles may be so marked that the joints appear to be enlarged. There is an occurrence of the disease on record in which the lesions were confined mainly to the front fetlocks (4).

At necropsy the most obvious finding is extensive erosion of the articular surfaces, often penetrating to the cancellous bone, and disappearance of the normal contours of the head of the femur or the epiphyses in the stifle joint. The synovial cavity is distended with an increased volume of brownish, turbid fluid, the joint capsule is much thickened and often contains calcified plaques. Multiple, small exostoses are present on the periarticular surfaces. When the stifle is involved the cartilaginous menisci, particularly the medial one, are very much reduced in size and may be completely absent (5). In cattle with severe degenerative changes in the coxofemoral joint, an acetabular osseous bulla may be present at the cranial margin of the obturator foramen (8).

Adequate calcium, phosphorus and vitamin D intake and a correct calcium:phosphorus ratio in the ration should be ensured. Supplementation of the ration with copper at the rate of 15 mg/kg has also been recommended for the control of a similar disease (6).

Degenerative joint disease of cattle is recorded on an enzootic scale in Chile (7) and is thought to be due to gross nutritional deficiency. The hip and tarsal joints are the only ones affected and clinical signs appear when animals are 8–12 months old. There is gross lameness and progressive emaciation. An inherited osteoarthritis is described under that heading. Sporadic cases of degenerative arthropathy, with similar signs and lesions, occur in heavy producing, aged dairy cows, and are thought to be caused by long-continued negative calcium balance. Rare cases also occur in aged beef cows but are thought to be associated with an inherited predisposition (2). In both instances the lesions are commonly restricted to the stifle joints.

REFERENCES

(1) Weaver, A. D. (1978) *Vet. Rec.*, *102*, 54.
(2) Carne, H. R. et al. (1964) *Aust. vet. J.*, *40*, 382.
(3) Palmer, N. C. (1968–69) *Vict. vet. Proc.*, *27*, 68.
(4) Studer, E. & Nelson, J. R. (1971) *Vet. Med. small Anim. Clin.*, *66*, 1007.
(5) Shupe, J. L. (1959) *Lab. Invest.*, *8*, 1190; (1961) *Can. vet. J.*, *2*, 369.
(6) Washburn, L. E. (1946) *J. anim. Sci.*, *5*, 395.
(7) Schulz, L. C. (1964) *Proc. int. Mtg Dis. Cattle, Copenhagen*, 284.
(8) Weaver, A. D. (1982) *Br. vet. J.*, *138*, 123.

DISEASES CAUSED BY DEFICIENCIES OF FAT-SOLUBLE VITAMINS

Vitamin A deficiency (hypovitaminosis A)

A deficiency of vitamin A may be caused by an insufficient supply of the vitamin in the ration or its defective absorption from the alimentary canal. In young animals the manifestations of the deficiency are mainly those of compression of the brain and spinal cord. In adult animals the syndrome produced includes night blindness, corneal keratinization, pityriasis, defects in the hooves, loss of weight, and infertility. Congenital defects are common in the offspring of deficient dams.

Etiology

Vitamin A deficiency occurs either as a primary disease, due to an absolute deficiency of vitamin A or its precursor carotene in the diet, or as a secondary disease in which the dietary supply of the vitamin or its precursor is adequate, but their digestion, absorption or metabolism is interfered with to produce a deficiency at the tissue level.

Epidemiology

Vitamin A deficiency is of major economic importance in groups of animals on pasture or diets deficient in the vitamin or its precursors. Animals at pasture get adequate supplies of the vitamin, except during prolonged droughts, but animals confined indoors and fed on prepared diets may suffer from a severe deficiency if adequate precautions are not taken. For example, a diet of dried sugar beet pulp, concentrates and poor quality hay has produced a syndrome of hypovitaminosis A in confined beef cattle (8).

Primary vitamin A deficiency occurs most commonly because of lack of green feed or failure to add vitamin A supplements to deficient diets. The status of the dam is reflected in that of the fetus only in certain circumstances, in that carotene, as it occurs in green feed, does not pass the placental barrier and a high intake of green pasture before parturition does not increase the hepatic stores of vitamin A in newborn calves, lambs or kids and only to a limited extent in pigs. However, vitamin A in the ester form, as it occurs in fish oils will pass the placental barrier in cows and feeding of these oils, or the parenteral administration of a vitamin A injectable preparation before parturition will cause an increase in stores of the vitamin in fetal livers. Antepartum feeding of carotene and the alcohol form of the vitamin does, however, cause an increase in the vitamin A content of the colostrum. Young animals depend on the dam's milk for their early requirements of the vitamin which is always in higher concentration in the colostrum although it returns to normal levels within a few days of parturition. Pigs which are weaned very early—at 4 weeks—may require special supplementation.

The addition of vitamin A supplements to diets may not always be sufficient to prevent deficiency. Carotene and vitamin A are readily oxidized particularly in the presence of unsaturated fatty acids. Oily preparations are thus less satisfactory than dry or aqueous preparations particularly if the feed is to be stored for any length of time. Pelleting of feed may also cause a serious loss up to 32% of the vitamin A in the original feedstuff.

Heat, light, and mineral mixes are known to increase the rate of destruction of vitamin A supplements in commercial rations. In one study, 47–92% of the vitamin A in several mineral supplements was destroyed after 1 week of exposure to the trace minerals, high relative humidity, sunlight and warm temperatures (20).

Primary vitamin A deficiency occurs in cattle and sheep on dry range country during periods of drought. Clinical vitamin A deficiency does not occur commonly under these conditions because hepatic storage is usually good beforehand and the period of deprivation not sufficiently long for these stores to reach a critically low level (24). Young sheep grazing natural, drought stricken pasture can suffer serious depletion of reserves of the vitamin in 5–8 months but normal growth is maintained for 1 year at which time clinical signs develop. Adult sheep may be on a deficient diet for 18 months before hepatic stores are depleted and the disease becomes evident. Cattle subsist on naturally deficient diets for 5–18 months before clinical signs appear.

Primary vitamin A deficiency is still relatively common in beef cattle which depend on pasture and roughage for the major portion of their diet. Beef calves coming off dry summer pastures at 6–8 months of age are commonly marginally deficient. Beef cattle, particularly pregnant cows, wintered on poor quality roughage commonly need supplementation with vitamin A throughout the winter months to ensure normal development of the fetus and an adequate supply of the vitamin in the colostrum at parturition.

Pigs and poultry housed indoors, and feedlot cattle (20) and sheep may be fed rations low in carotene and vitamin A. Grains, with exception of yellow corn, contain negligible amounts of carotene and cereal hay is often a poor source. Any hay which has been cut late, leached by rain, bleached by sun or stored for long periods loses much of its carotene content. The carotene content of yellow corn also deteriorates markedly with long storage. Moreover, under conditions not yet completely understood, the conversion by ruminants of carotene present in feeds such as silage may be much less complete than was formerly thought. Young pigs on a deficient diet may show signs after several months but as in other animals the length of time required before signs appear is governed to a large extent by the status before depletion commences. As a general rule it can be anticipated that signs will appear in pigs fed deficient rations for 4–5 months, variations from these periods probably being due to variations in the vitamin A status of the animal when the deficient diet is introduced. Congenital defects occur in litters from deficient sows but the incidence is higher in gilts with the first litter than in older sows. It is presumed that the hepatic stores of vitamin A in older sows are not depleted as readily as in young pigs. Adult horses may remain clinically normal for as long as 3 years on a deficient diet.

Secondary vitamin A deficiency may occur in cases of chronic disease of the liver or intestines because much of the conversion of carotene to vitamin A occurs in the intestinal epithelium, and the liver is the main site of storage of the vitamin. Highly chlorinated naphthalenes interfere with the conversion of carotene to vitamin A and animals poisoned with these substances have a very low vitamin A status. The intake of inorganic phosphorus also affects vitamin A storage, low phosphate diets facilitating storage of the vitamin. This may have a sparing effect on vitamin A requirements during drought periods when phosphorus intake is low, and an exacerbating effect in stall-fed cattle on a good grain diet. On the other hand, phosphorus deficiency may lower the efficiency of carotene conversion. Vitamins C and E help to prevent loss of vitamin A in feedstuffs and during digestion. Additional factors which may increase the requirement of vitamin A include high environmental temperatures, a high nitrate content of the feed (1) which reduces the conversion of carotene to vitamin A, and rapid rate of gain. Both a low vitamin A status of the animal and high levels of carotene intake may decrease the biopotency of ingested carotene.

The continued ingestion of mineral oil (liquid paraffin), which may occur when the oil is used as a preventive against bloat in cattle, causes a severe depression of plasma carotene and vitamin A esters and the carotene levels in buffer fat. The vitamin is fat-soluble and is probably absorbed by and excreted in the mineral oil. Deleterious effects on the cattle are unlikely under the conditions in which it is ordinarily used because of the short period for which the oil is administered and the high intake of vitamin A and carotene.

Pathogenesis

Vitamin A is essential for the regeneration of the visual purple necessary for dim-light vision, for normal bone growth and for maintenance of normal epithelial tissues. Deprivation of the vitamin produces effects largely attributable to disturbance of these functions. The same tissues are affected in all species but there is a difference in tissue and organ response in the different species and particular clinical signs may occur at different stages of development of the disease.

Night vision

Ability to see in dim light is reduced because of interference with regeneration of visual purple.

Cerebrospinal fluid pressure

An increase in CSF pressure is one of the first abnormalities to occur in hypovitaminosis A in calves (2). It is a more sensitive indicator than ocular changes and, in the calf, it occurs when the vitamin A intake is about twice that needed to prevent night blindness. The increase in CSF pressure is due to impaired absorption of the CSF due to reduced tissue permeability of the arachnoid villi and thickening of the connective tissue matrix of the cerebral dura mater. The increased CSF pressure is responsible for the syncope and convulsions which occur in calves in the early stages of vitamin A deficiency. The syncope and convulsions may occur spontaneously or be precipitated by excitement and exercise. It is suggested that the CSF pressure is increased in calves with subclinical deficiency and that exercise further increases the CSF pressure to convulsive levels.

Bone growth

Vitamin A is necessary to maintain normal position and activity of osteoblasts and osteoclasts. When deficiency occurs there is no retardation of endochondral bone growth but there is incoordination of bone growth in that shaping, especially the finer molding of bones, does not proceed normally (3). In most locations this has little effect but may cause serious damage to the nervous system. Overcrowding of the cranial cavity occurs with resulting distortion and herniations of the brain and an increase in cerebrospinal fluid pressure up to four to six times normal. The characteristic nervous signs of vitamin A deficiency, including papilledema, incoordination and syncope, follow. Compression, twisting and lengthening of cranial nerves and herniations of the cerebellum into the foramen magnum, causing weakness and ataxia (4), and of the spinal cord into intervertebral foraminae cause damage to nerve roots and localizing signs referable to individual peripheral nerves. Facial paralysis, and blindness due to constriction of the optic nerve (5), are typical examples of this latter phenomenon. The effect of excess vitamin A on bone development by its interference with vitamin D has been discussed elsewhere.

Epithelial tissues

Vitamin A deficiency leads to atrophy of all epithelial cells but the important effects are limited to those types of epithelial tissue which have a secretory as well as a covering function. The secretory cells are without power to divide and develop from undifferentiated basal epithelium. In vitamin A deficiency these secretory cells are gradually replaced by the stratified, keratinizing epithelial cells common to non-secretory epithelial tissues. This replacement of secretory epithelium by keratinized epithelium occurs chiefly in the salivary glands, the urogenital tract (including placenta but not ovaries or renal tubules) and the paraocular glands and teeth (disappearance of odontoblasts from the enamel organ). The secretion of thyroxine is markedly reduced. The mucosa of the stomach is not markedly affected. These changes in epithelium lead to the clinical signs of placental degeneration, xerophthalmia and corneal changes.

Embryological development
Vitamin A appears to be essential for organ formation during growth of the fetus. Multiple congenital defects occur in pigs and rats and congenital hydrocephalus in rabbits on maternal diets deficient in vitamin A. In pigs administration of the vitamin to depleted sows before the 17th day of gestation prevented the development of eye lesions but administration on the 18th day failed to do so (6).

Clinical findings
Generally speaking, similar syndromes occur in all species but because of species differences in tissue and organ response some variations are observed. The major clinical findings are set out below.

Night blindness
Inability to see in dim light is the earliest sign in all species, except in the pig in which it is not evident until plasma vitamin A levels are very low. The inability of affected animals to see obstructions in half light (twilight or moonlit night) is an important diagnostic sign.

Xerophthalmia
True xerophthalmia, with thickening and clouding of the cornea, occurs only in the dog and calf. In other species a thin, serous mucoid discharge from the eyes occurs, followed by corneal keratinization, clouding and sometimes ulceration and photophobia.

Changes in the skin
A rough dry coat with a shaggy appearance and splitting of the bristle tips in pigs is characteristic but excessive keratinization such as occurs in cattle poisoned with chlorinated naphthalenes does not occur under natural conditions of vitamin A deficiency. Heavy deposits of bran-like scales on the skin are seen in affected cattle. Dry, scaly hooves with multiple, vertical cracks are another manifestation of skin changes and are particularly noticeable in horses. A seborrheic dermatitis may also be observed in deficient pigs but is not specific to vitamin A deficiency.

Body weight
Under natural conditions a simple deficiency of vitamin A is unlikely to occur and the emaciation commonly attributed to vitamin A deficiency may be largely due to multiple deficiencies of protein and carbohydrate. Although inappetence, weakness, stunted growth and emaciation occur under experimental conditions of severe deficiency, in field outbreaks severe clinical signs of vitamin A deficiency are often seen in animals in good condition. Experimentally, sheep maintain their body weight under extreme deficiency conditions and with very low plasma vitamin A levels.

Reproductive efficiency
Loss of reproductive function is one of the major causes of loss in vitamin A deficiency. Both the male and female are affected. In the male, libido is retained but degeneration of the germinative epithelium of the seminiferous tubules causes reduction in the number of motile, normal spermatozoa produced. In young rams the testicles may be visibly smaller than normal. In the female, conception is usually not interfered with but placental degeneration leads to abortion and the birth of dead or weak young. Placental retention is common. Although beta-carotene (as distinct from vitamin A) has earned a reputation as an aid to fertility in dairy cows (10) there is a lack of hard data on the subject.

Nervous system
Signs related to damage of the central nervous system include paralysis of skeletal muscles due to damage of peripheral nerve roots, encephalopathy due to increased intracranial pressure, and blindness due to constriction of the optic nerve canal. These defects occur at any age but most commonly in young growing animals and they have been observed in all species except horses.

The paralytic form is ushered in by disturbances of gait due to weakness and incoordination. The hindlegs are usually affected first and the forelimbs at a later stage. In pigs there may be stiffness of the legs initially with a stilted gait or flaccidity with knuckling of the fetlocks and sagging of the hindquarters. Complete limb paralysis occurs terminally. Other manifestations of peripheral nerve injury include facial paralysis and rotation of the head in pigs and calves and curvature of the spinal column.

Encephalopathy, associated with an increase in CSF pressure, is manifested by convulsive seizures which are common in beef calves at 6–8 months, usually following removal from a dry summer pasture at weaning time. Spontaneously or following exercise or handling, affected calves will collapse (syncope) and during recumbency a clonic–tonic convulsion will occur lasting for 10–30 seconds. Death may occur during the convulsion or the animal will survive the convulsion and lie quietly, for several minutes, as if paralyzed, before another convulsion may occur. Affected calves are usually not blind and the menace reflex may be slightly impaired or hyperactive. Some calves are hyperesthetic to touch and sound. During the convulsion there is usually ventroflexion of the head and neck, sometimes opisthotonus and commonly tetanic closure of the eyelids and retraction of the eyeballs. Outbreaks of this form of hypovitaminosis A in calves have occurred and the case fatality rate may reach 25%. The prognosis is usually excellent; treatment will effect a cure in 48 hours but convulsions may continue for up to 48 hours following treatment.

The ocular form of hypovitaminosis A occurs usually in yearling cattle and up to 2–3 years of age (7). These animals have usually been on marginally deficient rations for several months. Night blindness may or may not have been noticed by the owner. The cattle have usually been fed and housed for long periods in familiar surroundings and the clinical signs of night blindness may have been subtle and not noticeable. The first sign of the ocular form of the disease is blindness in both eyes during daylight. Both pupils are widely dilated and fixed and will not respond to light. There is prominent optic disc edema and some loss of the usual brilliant color of the tapetum. Varying degrees of peripapillary retinal detachment, papillary and peripapillary retinal hemorrhages and disruption of the retinal pigment epithelium may also be present (20). The menace reflex is usually totally absent but the palpebral and corneal reflexes are present and the animal is aware of its surroundings and usually eats and drinks unless placed in unfamiliar surroundings. The CSF pressure is usually increased in these but not as high as in the calves described earlier. These cattle may also develop convulsions if forced to walk or if loaded on to a vehicle for transportation. The prognosis for these is unfavorable and treatment is ineffective because of the degeneration of the optic nerves. Some cattle also show exophthalmos and excessive lacrimation.

Congenital defects

These have been observed in rabbits, rats, piglets and calves. In calves the defects are limited to congenital blindness due to optic nerve constriction, and encephalopathy. In piglets complete absence of the eyes (anophthalmos) or small eyes (microphthalmos), incomplete closure of the fetal optic fissure, degenerative changes in the lens and retina, and an abnormal proliferation of mesenchymal tissue in front of and behind the lens (12) are some of the defects encountered. Other congenital defects attributed to vitamin A deficiency in pigs include cleft palate and harelip, accessory ears, malformed hindlegs, subcutaneous cysts, abnormally situated kidneys, cardiac defects, diaphragmatic hernia, aplasia of the genitalia, internal hydrocephalus, herniations of the spinal cord and generalized edema (11). Affected pigs may be stillborn, or weak and unable to stand, or may be quite active. Weak pigs lie on their sides, make slow paddling movements with their legs and squawk plaintively.

Other diseases

Increased susceptibility to infection is often stated to result from vitamin A deficiency. The efficacy of colostrum as a preventive against scours in calves was thought at one time to be due to vitamin A content but the high antibody content of colostrum is now known to be the important factor. A high incidence of otitis media and enteritis has often been reported in conjunction with vitamin A deficiency.

Clinical pathology

Vitamin A levels in the plasma are used extensively in diagnostic and experimental work. Plasma levels of 20 μg/dl are considered to be the minimal concentration for vitamin A adequacy (7, 21). Papilledema is an early sign of vitamin A deficiency which develops before nyctalopia and at plasma levels below 18 μg/dl (22). Normal serum vitamin A concentrations in cattle range from 25 to 60 μg/dl.

The clinical signs may correlate with the serum concentrations of vitamin A (26). In one outbreak, feedlot cattle with serum concentrations between 8·89 and 18·05 μg/dl had only lost body weight, those between 4·87 and 8·88 μg/dl had varying degrees of ataxia and blindness and those below 4·88 μg/dl had convulsions and optic nerve constriction (26). Clinical signs can be expected when the levels fall to 5 μg/dl. For complete safety optimum levels should be 25 μg/dl or above (7). Some information on the plasma retinol values in stabled Thoroughbred horses is available (23). The mean plasma level of retinol in 71 horses 2–3 years of age was 16·5 μg/dl (23).

Plasma carotene levels vary largely with the diet. In cattle levels of 150 μg/dl are optimum and in the absence of supplementary vitamin A in the ration, clinical signs appear when the levels fall to 9 μg/dl. In sheep carotene is present in the blood in only very small amounts even when they are on green pasture.

It is noteworthy that a direct relationship between plasma and hepatic levels of vitamin A need not exist since plasma levels do not commence to fall until the hepatic stores are depleted. A temporary precipitate fall occurs at parturition and in acute infections in most animals. The secretion of large amounts of carotene and vitamin A in the colostrum of cows during the last 3 weeks of pregnancy may greatly reduce the level of vitamin A in the plasma.

Hepatic levels of vitamin A and carotene can be estimated in the living animal from a biopsy specimen. Biopsy techniques have been shown to be safe and relatively easy provided a proper instrument is used. Hepatic levels of vitamin A and carotene should be of the order of 60 and 4·0 μg/g of liver respectively. These levels are commonly as high as 200–800 μg/g. Critical levels at which signs are likely to appear are 2 and 0·5 μg/g for vitamin A and carotene respectively.

Cerebrospinal fluid pressure is also used as a sensitive indicator of low vitamin A status. In calves normal pressures of less than 100 mm of water rise after depletion to more than 200 mm. In pigs normal pressures of 80–145 mm rise to above 200 mm in vitamin A deficiency. An increase in pressure is observed at a blood level of about 7 μg vitamin A per dl plasma in this species. In sheep normal pressures of 55–65 mm rise to 70–150 mm when depletion occurs. In the experimentally induced disease in cattle, there is a marked increase in the number of cornified epithelial cells in a conjunctival smear and distinctive bleaching of the tapetum lucidum as viewed by an ophthalmoscope. These features may have value as diagnostic aids in naturally occurring cases (7).

Necropsy findings

Gross changes at necropsy are not characteristic of vitamin A deficiency. Careful dissection may reveal a decrease in size of the cranial vault and of the vertebrae, and compression and injury of the cranial and spinal nerve roots, especially the optic nerve, may be visible. The lesions caused by secondary bacterial infections including pneumonia and otitis media are also common.

Squamous metaplasia of the interlobular ducts of the parotid salivary gland is considered to be pathognomonic of vitamin A deficiency in pigs, calves and lambs but the change is transient and may have disappeared 2–4 weeks after the intake of vitamin A is increased. The change is most marked and occurs first at the oral end of the main parotid duct (13). Focal necrotic hepatitis occurs in calves but no specific renal lesions are present. The anasarcous lesions which are recorded in vitamin A deficiency in feedlot cattle are associated with vascular damage and degeneration of muscles. Cattle also show hyperkeratinization of the epithelium of the prepuce, reticulum and rumen and a high incidence of pituitary cysts (14).

The abnormalities which occur in congenitally affected pigs have already been described. Generalized edema is present to a marked degree.

Diagnosis

When the characteristic signs or lesions of vitamin A deficiency are observed a deficiency of the vitamin should be suspected if green feed or vitamin A supplements are not being provided. The detection of papilledema and testing for night-blindness are the easiest methods of diagnosing early vitamin A deficiency in ruminants. Incoordination, paralysis and convulsions are the early signs in pigs. Increase in CSF pressure is the earliest measurable change in both pigs and calves. Laboratory confirmation depends upon estimations of vitamin A in plasma and liver, the latter being most satisfactory. Unless the disease has been in existence for a considerable time, response to treatment is rapid. For confirmation at necropsy, histological examination of parotid salivary gland, and assay of vitamin A in the liver are suggested.

The loss of condition, failure to grow and poor reproductive efficiency are general signs which are not limited to vitamin A deficiency. Convulsive seizures as occur in calves, and posterior paralysis as occurs in growing pigs on vitamin-A-deficient diets also resemble the syndromes which occur in many other diseases. Clinically it may be impossible to distinguish between encephalopathy caused by vitamin A deficiency and hypomagnesemic tetany, polioencephalomalacia, enterotoxemia caused by *Cl. perfringens* type D, and acute lead poisoning. Rabies, however, is usually accompanied by a disturbance of consciousness and anesthesia. Sporadic bovine encephalomyelitis is always accompanied by high fever and by serositis. Several other poisonings as listed below are more likely to occur in pigs than in calves and may cause clinical signs similar to those caused by vitamin A deficiency.

In pigs posterior paralysis is a more common observation in vitamin A deficiency than are convulsive episodes. The other diseases which may be confused with vitamin A deficiency in this species include pseudorabies and viral encephalomyelitis. A number of poisonings, including salt, organic arsenic and organic mercury also cause nervous signs. As in calves clinical differentiation is extremely difficult and a careful examination of the local environment and the feeding history is necessary to attempt to limit the diagnostic possibilities.

Congenital defects similar to those caused by vitamin A deficiency may be caused by deficiencies of other essential nutrients, by inheritance or by viral infections in early pregnancy. Final diagnosis often depends upon the necropsy findings although the clinical pathology may be of assistance.

Treatment

Animals which show clinical signs of vitamin A deficiency should be treated immediately with vitamin A at a dose rate equivalent to 10–20 times the daily maintenance requirement. As a rule 440 i.u/kg body weight is the dose rate used. Parenteral injection of an aqueous rather than an oily solution is preferred. The response to treatment in cases of severe, acute deficiency is often rapid and complete but the disease may be irreversible in chronic cases, especially when deficiency has continued over more than one generation. Calves with clinical signs due to increased cerebrospinal fluid will usually return to normal in 48 hours following treatment. Cattle with the ocular form of the deficiency will not respond to treatment and should be slaughtered for salvage.

Daily heavy dosing (about 100 times normal) of calves causes reduced growth rate, lameness, ataxia, paresis, exostoses on the plantar aspect of the third phalanx of the fourth digit of all feet and disappearance of the epiphyseal cartilage (15–17). Persistent heavy dosing in calves causes lameness, retarded horn growth and depressed cerebrospinal fluid pressure. At necropsy, exostoses are present on the proximal metacarpal bones and the frontal bones are thin (18). Very high levels fed to young pigs may cause sudden death through massive internal hemorrhage, and excessive doses during early pregnancy are reputed to result in fetal anomalies. However, feeding vitamin A for prolonged periods at exceptionally high levels is unlikely to produce severe embryotoxic or teratogenic effects in pigs (9).

Control

The minimum daily requirement in all species is 40 i.u. of vitamin A per kg body weight. However, this is only a guideline for the maintenance requirements. In the formulation of practical diets for all species, the daily *allowances* of vitamin A are commonly increased by 50–100% of the daily minimum requirements. During pregnancy, lactation or rapid growth the allowances are usually increased by 50–75% of the requirements. The supplementation of diets to groups of animals is governed

Table 92. Daily dietary allowances of vitamin A.

Animal	*Vitamin A (i.u./kg body weight daily)*
CATTLE	
Growing calves	40
Weaned beef calves at 6–8 months	40
Calves 6 months to yearlings	40
Maintenance and pregnancy	70–80
Maintenance and lactation	80
Feedlot cattle on high energy ration	80
SHEEP	
Growth and early pregnancy and fattening lambs	30–40
Late pregnancy and lactation	70–80
PIGS	
Growing pigs	40–50
Pregnant gilts and sows	40–50
Lactating gilts and sows	70–80
HORSES	
Working horse	20–30
Growing horse	40
Pregnant mare	50
Lactating mare	50

also by their previous intake of the vitamin and its probable level in the diet being fed, and the rate of supplementation can vary from 0 to 110 i.u./kg body weight per day (one i.u. of vitamin A is equivalent in activity to 0·3 μg of retinol; 5–8 μg beta-carotene has the same activity as 1 μg of retinol (25)).

The amounts of the vitamin to be added to the ration of each species to meet the requirements for all purposes should be obtained from published recommended nutrient requirements of domestic animals. Some examples of daily allowances of vitamin A for farm animals are set out in Table 92.

The method of supplementation will vary depending on the class of livestock and the ease with which the vitamin can be given. In swine, the vitamin is incorporated directly into the complete ration usually through the protein supplement. In feedlot and dairy cattle receiving complete feeds, the addition of vitamin A to the diet is simple. In beef cattle which may be fed primarily on carotene-deficient roughage during pregnancy it may not be possible to supplement the diet on a daily basis. However, it may be possible to provide a concentrated dietary source of vitamin A on a regular basis by feeding a protein supplement once weekly. The protein supplement will contain 10–15 times the daily allowance which permits hepatic storage of the vitamin.

An alternative method to dietary supplementation is the intramuscular injection of vitamin A at intervals of 50–60 days at the rate of 3000–6000 i.u./kg body weight. Under most conditions, hepatic storage is good and optimum plasma and hepatic levels of vitamin A are maintained for up to 50–60 days. In pregnant beef cattle the last injection should not be longer than 40–50 days before parturition to ensure adequate levels of vitamin A in the colostrum. Ideally, the last injection should be given 30 days before parturition but this may not be practical under some management conditions. However, it must be emphasized that the most economical method of supplementing vitamin A is in most cases through the feed and when possible should be used. Furthermore the use of injectable mixtures of vitamin A, D and E is not always justifiable. In one study their use in dairy cattle did not improve reproductive performance or herd health (19).

REVIEW LITERATURE

Barnett, K. C. et al. (1970) Ocular changes associated with hypovitaminosis A in cattle. *Br. vet. J.*, *126*, 561.

Clark, L. (1971) Hypervitaminosis A. A review. *Aust. vet. J.*, *47*, 568.

Mitchell, G. E. (1967) Vitamin A nutrition of ruminants. *J. Am. vet. med. Assoc.*, *151*, 430.

Thompson, S. Y. (1975) Role of carotene and vitamin A in animal feeding. *World Rev. Nutr. Diet*, *21*, 224.

REFERENCES

(1) Hoar, D. W. et al. (1968) *J. anim. Sci.*, *27*, 1727.
(2) Thompson, S. Y. (1975) *World Rev. Nutr. Diet.*, *21*, 224.
(3) Davis, T. E. et al. (1970) *Can. vet. J.*, *30*, 90.
(4) Mills, J. H. L. et al. (1967) *Acta vet. Scand.*, *8*, 324.
(5) Hayes, K. C. et al. (1968) *Arch. Ophthal.*, *80*, 777.
(6) Palludan, B. (1964) *Arsberetn. int. Sterilitetsforsk.*, 59.
(7) Eaton, H. D. et al. (1970) *J. dairy Sci.*, *53*, 1775.
(8) Shlosberg, A. et al. (1977) *Refuah Vet.*, *34*, 25.
(9) Wrathall, A. E. et al. (1979) *Zentralbl. VetMed.*, *26A*, 106.
(10) Lotthammer, K. H. (1979) *Feedstuffs*, *51, 16, 37 & 50.*
(11) Palludan, B. (1961) Acta vet. Scand., *2*, 32.
(12) Palludan, B. (1976) *Int. J. Vit. Nutr. Res.*, *46*, 223.
(13) Nielsen, S. W. et al. (1966) *Am. J. vet. Res.*, *27*, 223.
(14) Nielsen, S. W. et al. (1966) *Res. vet. Sci.*, *7*, 143.
(15) Hazzard, D. G. et al. (1964) *J. dairy Sci.*, *47*, 391.
(16) Pryor, W. J. et al. (1969) *Aust. vet. J.*, *45*, 563.
(17) Wolke, R. E. et al. (1968) *Am. J. vet. Res.*, *29*, 1009.
(18) Gallina, A. M. et al. (1970) *Arch. exp. VetMed.*, *24*, 1091.
(19) Hartman, D. A. et al. (1976) *J. dairy Sci.*, *59*, 91.
(20) Divers, T. J. et al. (1986) *J. Am. vet. med. Assoc.*, *189*, 1579.
(21) Chew, B. P. et al. (1984) *J. dairy Sci.*, *67*, 1316.
(22) Thompson, S. Y. (1975) *World Rev. Nutr. Diet*, *21*, 224.
(23) Butler, P. & Blackmore, D. J. (1982) *Vet. Rec.*, *111*, 37.
(24) Molokwu, E. C. I. (1978) *Br. vet. J.*, *134*, 493.
(25) Commonwealth Agricultural Bureaux (1980) *The Nutrient Requirements of Ruminant Livestock*, p. 270.
(26) Booth, A. et al. (1987) *J. Am. vet. med. Assoc.*, *190*, 1305.

Vitamin K deficiency

A primary deficiency of vitamin K is unlikely under natural conditions in domestic animals because of the high content of substances with vitamin K activity in most plants, and the substantial synthesis of these substances by microbial activity in the alimentary canal (1). Sporadic cases may occur when impairment of the flow of bile reduces the digestion and absorption of this fat-soluble vitamin. Experimentally produced vitamin K deficiency in piglets is manifested by hypersensitivity, anemia, anorexia, weakness and a marked increase in prothrombin time (2). The minimum daily requirement for newborn pigs is 5 μg/kg body weight and the minimum curative injection dose is four times this.

A hemorrhagic disease of recently weaned pigs from 6 to 15 weeks of age is considered to be associated with vitamin K deficiency (3–5). Affected pigs fail to grow, become pale, develop large subcutaneous hematomas and exhibit lameness and epistaxis (3). Excessive and fatal hemorrhagia following routine castration may occur in pigs from 30 to 40 days of age but not at 15–20 days of age (4). Subcutaneous massive hemorrhage is more common in pigs at 40–70 days of age. Prothrombin time and activated partial thromboplastin time are prolonged along with decreased levels of vitamin K dependent factors II, VII, IX and X (4). At necropsy, hemorrhages are extensive in the muscles of the hindlimbs, forelimbs, and axillar and mandibular region. Vitamin K, or vitamin K_2 given at a dose of 3 mg/kg body weight intramuscularly as a single dose will restore the blood coagulation defects to normal (5). Vitamin K_3 added to the feed at a rate of 25 mg/kg for 4 days was also effective. The cause of the vitamin K deficiency was considered to be related to the use of antibacterial drugs in the feed but this has not been substantiated.

The most important therapeutic use of vitamin K in domestic animals is in sweet clover poisoning where toxic quantities of coumarin severely depress the prothrombin levels of the blood and interfere with its clotting mechanism. Industrial poisons used in rodent control which contain anticoagulants of the coumarin type, e.g. warfarin, cause fatal hypothrombinemia and vitamin K is an effective antidote. For warfarin-induced anticoagulation in the horse the administration of 300–500 mg of vitamin K_1 subcutaneously every 4–6 hours until the prothrombin time returns to baseline values is recommended (6).

REVIEW LITERATURE

Mount, M. E. & Feldman, B. F. (1982) Vitamin K and its importance. *J. Am. vet. med. Assoc.*, *180*, 1354–1356.

REFERENCES

(1) Kon, S. K. & Porter, J. W. G. (1947) *Nutr. Abst. Rev.*, *17*, 31.
(2) Schendel, H. E. & Johnson, B. C. (1962) *J. Nutr.*, 76, 124.
(3) Newsholme, S. J. et al. (1986) *J. S. Afr. vet. Assoc.*, 56, 101.
(4) Sasaki, Y. et al. (1982) *Jap. J. vet. Sci.*, *44*, 933.
(5) Sasaki, Y. et al. (1985) *Jap. J. vet. Sci.*, *47*, 435.
(6) Byars, T. D. et al. (1986) *Am. J. vet. Res.*, *47*, 2309.
(7) Mount, M. E. & Feldman, B. F. (1982) *J. Am. vet. med. Assoc.*, *180*, 1354.

DISEASES CAUSED BY DEFICIENCIES OF WATER-SOLUBLE VITAMINS

Water-soluble vitamins including vitamin C and the B complex are of little importance in herbivorous animals (except for vitamin B_{12}) because of their synthesis in the alimentary tract of these animals. Thiamin, nicotinic acid, riboflavin, pantothenic acid, pyridoxine, biotin and folic acid are all synthesized by microbial activity, and nicotinic acid and vitamin C are synthesized by other means. The young calf or lamb, in the period before ruminal activity begins, is likely to receive inadequate supplies of these vitamins and deficiency states can be produced experimentally. In the preruminant stage colostrum and milk are good sources of the water-soluble vitamins, ewe's milk being much richer than cow's milk. The production of signs of deficiency of the B vitamins in horses by the feeding of deficient diets has raised some doubts as to the availability of the B vitamins synthesized in the large bowel in this species.

Vitamin C is synthesized by all species and is not an important dietary essential in any of the domestic animals. Synthesis occurs in tissues and although blood levels fall after birth in the newborn calf they begin to rise again at about 3 weeks of age. However, a dermatosis of young calves has been associated with low levels of ascorbic acid in their plasma and responds to a single injection of 3 g of ascorbic acid (6). A heavy dandruff, followed by a waxy crust, alopecia and dermatitis commences on the ears and spreads over the cheeks, down the crest of the neck and over the shoulders. Some deaths have been recorded but spontaneous recovery is more usual.

Thiamin deficiency (hypothiaminosis)

The disease caused by deficiency of thiamin in tissues is characterized chiefly by nervous signs.

Etiology

Thiamin deficiency may be primary, due to deficiency of the vitamin in the diet, or secondary, because of destruction of the vitamin in the diet by thiaminase. A primary deficiency is unlikely under natural conditions because most plants, especially seeds, yeast and milk contain adequate amounts. Thiamin is normally synthesized in adequate quantities in the rumen of cattle and sheep on a well-balanced roughage diet. The degree of synthesis is governed to some extent by the composition of the ration, a sufficiency of readily fermentable carbohydrate causing an increase of synthesis of most vitamins of the B complex, and a high intake in the diet reducing synthesis. The etiology of polioencephalomalacia has been discussed in detail under that heading. Microbial synthesis of thiamin also occurs in the alimentary tract of monogastric animals and in young calves and lambs but not in sufficient quantities to avoid the necessity for a dietary supply, so that deficiency states can be readily induced in these animals with experimental diets. Thiamin in relatively unstable and easily destroyed by cooking.

The coccidiostat amprolium is a thiamin antagonist and others are produced by certain plants, bacteria, fungi and fish.

Epidemiology

Three major occurrences of secondary thiamin deficiency are recorded. The inclusion of excess raw fish in the diet of carnivores leads to destruction of thiamin because of the high content of thiaminase in the fish. In horses the ingestion of excessive quantities of bracken fern (*Pteridium aquilinum*) and horsetail (*Equisetum arvense*) causes nervous signs because of the high concentration of thiaminase in these plants. The disease has been induced in a pig fed bracken rhizomes and the possibility exists of it occurring under natural conditions. It has also been reported in horses fed large quantities of turnips (*Beta vulgaris*) without adequate grain (4). The third important occurrence of thiamin deficiency is in the etiology of polioencephalomalacia and is discussed under that heading.

A thiaminase-induced subclinical thiamin deficiency causing suboptimal growth rate of weaner lambs has been described (28). High levels of thiaminase activity were present in the feces and rumen contents of lambs with poor growth rate compared to normal lambs. *Bacillus thiaminolyticus* was isolated from the feces and ruminal fluids of affected lambs and supplementation of thiaminase-excreting lambs with intramuscular injections of thiamine-hydrochloride was associated with significantly improved growth rate (28).

Pathogenesis

The only known function of thiamin is its activity as a cocarboxylase in the metabolism of fats, carbohydrates and proteins and a deficiency of the vitamin leads to the accumulation of endogenous pyruvates. Although the brain is known to depend largely on carbohydrate as a source of energy, there is no obvious relationship between a deficiency of thiamin and the development of the nervous signs which characterize it. Polioencephalomalacia has been produced experimentally in preruminant lambs on a thiamin-free diet. There are other prodromal indications of deficiency disease. For example, there is a decrease in erythrocyte precursors and in erythrocyte transketolase (13). Additional clinical signs do occur too in the circulatory and alimentary systems but their pathogenesis cannot be clearly related to the known functions of thiamin. Subclinical thiamin deficiency due to thiaminases in the alimentary tract is associated with low erythrocyte transketolase activities and elevated thiamin pyrophosphate effects which may explain the poor growth rate (28).

The efficiency of thiamin in the treatment of paralytic myoglobinuria in horses may be open to doubt but the high carbohydrate diet which precedes the attack, and the accumulation of lactic acid in the affected muscles suggest that its use is justified.

Clinical findings

Bracken fern (Pteridium aquilinum) *and horsetail* (Equisetum arvense) *poisoning in the horse*
Incoordination to the point of falling, and bradycardia due to cardiac irregularity, are the cardinal clinical signs of bracken fern poisoning in the horse and these signs disappear after the parenteral administration of thiamin. Similar clinical effects occur with horsetail. Swaying from side to side occurs first, followed by pronounced incoordination, including crossing of the forelegs and wide action in the hindlegs. When standing the legs are placed well apart, and crouching and arching of the back are evident. Muscle tremor develops and eventually the horse is unable to rise. Clonic convulsions and opisthotonus are the terminal stage. Appetite is good until late in the disease when somnolence prevents eating. Temperatures are normal and the heart rate slow until the terminal period when both rise to above normal levels. Some evidence has also been presented relating the occurrence of hemiplegia of the vocal cords in horses with a below normal thiamin status (3). Neither plant is palatable to horses and poisoning rarely occurs at pasture. The greatest danger is when the immature plants are cut and preserved in meadow hay.

Experimental syndromes
These syndromes have not been observed to occur naturally but are produced readily on experimental rations.

In pigs, inappetence, emaciation and leg weakness, and a fall in body temperature, respiratory rate and heart rate occur. The electrocardiogram is abnormal and congestive heart failure follows. Death occurs in 5 weeks on a severely deficient diet. In calves, weakness, incoordination, convulsions and retraction of the head occur and in some cases anorexia, severe scouring and dehydration. Lambs 1–3 days old placed on a thiamin-deficient diet show signs after 3 weeks. Somnolence, anorexia and loss of condition occur first, followed by tetanic convulsions.

Horses fed amprolium (400–800 mg/kg body weight daily) developed clinical signs of thiamin deficiency after 37–58 days (7). Bradycardia with dropped heart beats, ataxia, muscle fasciculation and periodic hypothermia of hooves, ears and muzzle were the common signs with blindness, diarrhea and loss of body weight occurring inconstantly.

Clinical pathology
Blood pyruvic acid levels in horses are raised from normal levels of 2–3 μg/dl to 6–8 μg/dl. Blood thiamin levels are reduced from normals of 8–10 μg/dl to 2·5–3·0 μg/dl. Electrocardiograms show evidence of myocardial insufficiency. In pigs blood pyruvate levels are elevated and there is a fall in blood transketolase activity. These changes occur very early in the disease (10).

Necropsy findings
No macroscopic lesions occur in thiamin deficiency other than non-specific congestive heart failure in horses. The myocardial lesions are those of interstitial edema and lesions are also present in the liver and intestine.

In the experimental syndrome in pigs there are no degenerative lesions in the nervous system but there is multiple focal necrosis of the atrial myocardium accompanied by macroscopic flabbiness and dilatation without hypertrophy of the heart.

Diagnosis
Diagnosis of secondary thiamin deficiency in horses must be based on the signs of paralysis and known access to bracken fern or horsetail. A similar syndrome may occur with poisoning by *Crotalaria* spp., perennial rye-grass, *Indigophera enneaphylla* and ragwort (*Senecio jacobea*) but is accompanied by hepatic necrosis and fibrosis. The encephalomyelitides are usually accompanied by signs of cerebral involvement, by fever and failure to respond to thiamin therapy.

Treatment
In clinical cases the injection of a solution of the vitamin produces dramatic results (5 mg/kg body weight given every 3 hours). The initial dose is usually given intravenously followed by intramuscular injections for 2–4 days. An oral source of thiamin should be given daily for 10 days and any dietary abnormalities corrected.

Control
The daily requirement of thiamin for monogastric animals is in general 30–60 μg/kg body weight. The addition of yeast, cereals, grains, liver and meat meal to the ration usually provides adequate thiamin.

Riboflavin deficiency (hyporiboflavinosis)

Although riboflavin is essential for cellular oxidative processes in all animals, the occurrence of deficiency under natural conditions is rare in domestic animals because actively growing green plants and animal protein are good sources, and some synthesis by alimentary tract microflora occurs in all species. Synthesis by microbial activity is sufficient for the needs of ruminants but a dietary source is required in these animals in the preruminant stage. Milk is a very good source. Daily requirements for pigs are 60–80 μg/kg body weight and 2–3 g/tonne of feed provides adequate supplementation (26). The trend towards confinement feeding of swine has increased the danger of naturally occurring cases in that species.

On experimental diets the following syndromes have been observed:

In *pigs* slow growth, frequent scouring, rough skin and matting of the hair coat with heavy, sebaceous exudate are characteristic. There is a peculiar crippling of the legs with inability to walk and marked ocular lesions including conjunctivitis, swollen eyelids and cataract. The incidence of stillbirths may be high.

In *calves* anorexia, poor growth, scours, excessive salivation and lacrimation, and alopecia occur. Areas of hyperemia develop at the oral commissures, on the edges of the lips and around the navel. There are no ocular lesions.

Nicotinic acid deficiency (hyponiacinosis)

Nicotinic acid or niacin is essential for normal carbohydrate metabolism. Because of the high content in most natural animal feeds, deficiency states are rare in ordinary circumstances except in pigs fed rations high in corn. Corn has both a low niacin content and a low content of tryptophan, a niacin precursor. A low protein intake exacerbates the effects of the deficiency but a high protein intake is not fully protective.

In ruminants, synthesis within the animal provides an adequate source. Even in young calves signs of deficiency do not occur and because rumen microfloral activity is not yet of any magnitude, extraruminal synthesis appears probable.

The oral supplementation of niacin in the diet of periparturient dairy cows may result in an increase in serum inorganic phosphorus and a decrease in serum potassium, calcium, and sodium concentrations (30). Niacin has been used to study the effects of artificially induced ketonemia and hypoglycemia in cattle (30).

The daily requirements of niacin for mature pigs are 0·1–0·4 mg/kg body weight, but growing pigs appear to require rather more (0·6–1 mg/kg body weight) for optimum growth.

Experimentally induced nicotinic acid deficiency in pigs is characterized by inappetence, severe diarrhea, a dirty yellow skin with a severe scabby dermatitis and alopecia. Posterior paralysis also occurs. At necropsy hemorrhages in the gastric and duodenal walls, congestion and swelling of the small intestinal mucosa and ulcers in the large intestine are characteristic and resemble closely those of necrotic enteritis caused by infection with *Salmonella* spp. Histologically there is severe mucoid degeneration followed by local necrosis in the wall of the cecum and colon. Experimental production of the disease in pigs by the administration of an antimetabolite to nicotinamide causes ataxia or quadriplegia accompanied by distinctive lesions in the gray matter of the cervical and lumbar enlargements of the ventral horn of the spinal cord. The lesions are malacic and occur in the intermediate zone of the gray matter. The identical lesions and clinical picture have been observed in naturally occurring disease (1).

The oral therapeutic dose rate of nicotinic acid in pigs is 100–200 mg; 10–20 g/tonne of feed supplies sufficient nicotinic acid for pigs of all ages. Niacin is low in price and should always be added to swine rations based on corn.

Pyridoxine (vitamin B_6) deficiency (hypopyridoxinosis)

A deficiency of pyridoxine in the diet is not known to occur under natural conditions. Experimental deficiency in pigs is characterized by periodic epileptiform convulsions, and at necropsy by generalized hemosiderosis with a microcytic anemia, hyperplasia of the bone marrow and fatty infiltration of the liver. The daily requirement of pyridoxine in the pig is of the order of 100 μg/kg body weight or 1 mg/kg of solid food (13) although higher levels have been recommended on occasions. Certain strains of chickens have a high requirement for pyridoxine and the same may be true of swine.

Experimentally induced deficiency in calves is characterized by anorexia, poor growth, apathy, dull coat and alopecia. Severe, fatal epileptiform seizures occur in some animals (14). Anemia with poikilocytosis is characteristic of this deficiency in cows and calves.

Pantothenic acid deficiency (hypopantothenosis)

Pantothenic acid is a dietary essential in all species other than ruminants, which synthesize it in the rumen. Deficiency under natural conditions has been recorded mainly in pigs on rations based on corn.

In pigs (15, 16) a decrease in weight gain due to anorexia and inefficient food utilization occurs first. Dermatitis develops with a dark brown exudate collecting about the eyes and there is a patchy alopecia. Diarrhea and incoordination with a spastic, goose-stepping gait are characteristic. At necropsy a severe, sometimes ulcerative, colitis is observed constantly, together with degeneration of myelin.

Calcium pantothenate (500 μg/kg body weight per day) is effective in treatment and prevention (17). As a feed additive 10–12 g/tonne is adequate.

Experimentally induced pantothenic acid deficiency in calves is manifested by rough hair coat, dermatitis under the lower jaw, excessive nasal mucus, anorexia, and reduced growth rate and is eventually fatal. At necropsy there is usually a secondary pneumonia, demyelination in the spinal cord and peripheral nerves, and softening and congestion of the cerebrum (18).

Biotin deficiency (hypobiotinosis)

Biotin has several important biochemical functions. It is a cofactor in several enzyme systems involved in carboxylation and transcarboxylation reactions and consequently has a significant effect on carbohydrate metabolism, fatty acid synthesis, amino acid deamination, purine synthesis and nucleic acid metabolism. Biotin is found in almost all plant and animal materials and, being required in very small quantities, is unlikely to be deficient in diets under natural conditions especially as microbial synthesis occurs in the alimentary tract.

However, the principal source of biotin for the pig is the feed which it receives and feeds vary greatly in their biotin content and in the biological availability of that biotin. The biotin content in basal diets fed to pigs has varied from 29 to 15 μg/kg available biotin and supplementation of these diets has resulted in improvements in litter size (12). Continuous feeding of sulfonamides or antibiotics may induce a deficiency. An antivitamin to biotin (avidin) occurs in egg white, and biotin deficiency can be produced experimentally by feeding large quantities of uncooked egg white (8).

Experimental biotin deficiency has been shown to cause paralysis of the hindlegs in calves (19). In pigs, experimental biotin deficiency is manifested by alopecia, dermatitis and painful cracking of the soles and the walls of the hooves (8, 9). Naturally occurring outbreaks of lameness in gilts and sows associated with lesions of the soles and the walls of the hooves which responded to biotin supplementation have now been well described (8, 9, 11). The severe lameness and long course of convalescence have been responsible for a high rate of culling in breeding animals. Affected animals become progressively lame after being on a biotin-deficient ration for several months. Arching of the back and a haunched stance with the hindlegs positioned forward occurs initially. This posture has been described as a 'kangaroo'-sitting posture. The foot pads become softer and the hoof horn less resilient. The feet are painful and some sows will not stand for breeding. Deep fissures at the wall–sole junction may extend upwards beneath the wall horn, and gaping cracks may separate the toe and heel volar surfaces. The foot pads initially show excessive wear but later longitudinal painful cracks develop. In well-developed cases the foot pads appear enlarged, the cracks are obvious and covered by necrotic debris. The foot pads of the hindfeet are usually more severely affected that those of the forefeet and the lateral digit is more frequently affected. The dewclaws also are affected by cracks and the accumulation of necrotic tissue.

Skin lesions also develop in affected gilts and sows. There is gradual alopecia particularly over the back, the base of the tail and the hindquarters. The hairs are more bristly than normal and break easily. The alopecia is accompanied by a dryness of the skin.

As the lesions of the feet and skin develop there is a marked drop in the serum biotin concentrations which is considered as a sensitive index of biotin deficiency (8). Adequate biotin status may be indicated by serum biotin level (ng/l) > 700; marginal, 600–700; inadequate, 400–600 and deficient below 400 (8). Compression and hardness tests made on external hoof have also been used as an indirect measure of biotin adequacy in pigs (9). The tests indicate that significant improvements in the strength and hardness of pig hoof horn are produced by biotin.

Reproductive performance of sows is also influenced by their biotin status (12, 31). Supplementation of the diet with biotin may increase litter size born, increase the number of pigs weaned, decrease the mean interval in days from weaning to service and improve conception rate. Over a period of four parities, piglet production increased by 1·42 pigs/sow year (12).

The daily requirements of biotin for swine have not been well defined, but certain amounts have been associated with an absence of lameness and improved reproductive performance. Basic diets for gilts contain 35–50 μg/kg, and the addition of 350–500 μg/kg is recommended. This provides a daily intake of 4.0–5.0 mg/sow/day. The response to dietary supplementation may take several months and therefore supplementation should begin at weaning.

The dietary supplementation of horses with 10–30 mg biotin/day for 6–9 months is considered to be effective as an aid in the treatment of weak horn hoof in horses (32). Supplementation of a basal diet, calculated to contain 56 μg/kg available biotin with daily allowances of biotin at 1160 μg/sow/day in pregnancy and 2320 μg/sow/day in lactation produced significant improvements in litter size in second and fourth parity sows (31). It is suggested that the requirement is in excess of 175 μg/kg available biotin diet (12). In a swine herd with a lameness problem, the supplementation of the sow's ration during pregnancy and lactation with daily intakes of biotin of 400 and 800 μg/sow/day respectively and the rations of the weaners and growers to 150 and 250 was effective (11).

Folic acid deficiency (hypofolicosis)

Folic acid (pteroylglutamic acid) is necessary for nucleic acid metabolism and its deficiency in humans leads to the development of pernicious anemia. A dietary source is necessary to all species and an adequate intake is provided by pasture. Although naturally occurring deficiencies have not been diagnosed positively in domestic animals, folic acid has numerous and complex interrelationships with other nutrients and the possibility of a deficiency playing a part in inferior animal performance should not be overlooked. The vitamin has a particular interest for equine nutritionists. Permanently stabled horses and some horses in training may require additional folic acid, preferably on a daily basis by the oral route (2).

Choline deficiency (hypocholinosis)

Choline is a dietary essential for pigs and young calves. Calves fed on a synthetic choline-deficient diet from the second day of life develop an acute syndrome in about 7 days (21). There is marked weakness and inability to get up, labored or rapid breathing and anorexia. Recovery follows treatment with choline. Older calves are not affected. On some rations the addition of choline increases daily gain in feedlot steers, particularly during the early part of the feeding period. In pigs, ataxia, fatty degeneration of the liver and a high mortality rate occur. Enlarged and tender hocks have been observed in feeder pigs. For pigs 1 kg/tonne of food is considered to supply sufficient choline (12).

Congenital splayleg of piglets has been attributed to choline deficiency but adding choline to the ration of the sows does not always prevent the condition (22).

Vitamin B_{12} deficiency (hypocyanocobalaminosis)

Vitamin B_{12} deficiency is unlikely to occur under natural conditions other than because of a primary dietary deficiency of cobalt, which is an important disease in many countries of the world.

Although microbial synthesis of the vitamin occurs in the rumen in the presence of adequate cobalt, and in the intestines of other herbivora such as the horse (23, 24), it is probably a dietary essential in the pig and young calf. Animal protein is a good source. A deficiency syndrome has been produced in young calves on a synthetic ration. Signs include anorexia, cessation of growth, loss of condition and muscular weakness. The daily requirement under these conditions is 20–40 μg of vitamin B_{12} (25). Sows vary in their ability to absorb the vitamin and those with poor absorption ability or on deficient diets show poor reproductive performance (26). For pigs 10–50 mg/tonne of feed is considered to be adequate (12). The vitamin is used empirically in racing dogs and horses to alleviate parasitic and dietetic anemias in these animals at a dose rate of 2 μg/kg body weight. Cyanocobalamin zinc tannate provides effective tissue levels of vitamin B_{12} for 2–4 weeks after one injection (27) and normal and abnormal blood levels have been established for all species (24). It is also used as a feed additive for fattening pigs usually in the form of fish or meat meal or as 'animal protein factor'. It is essential as a supplement if the diet contains no animal protein, and maximum results from the feeding of antibiotics to pigs are obtained only if the intake of vitamin B_{12} is adequate.

REVIEW LITERATURE

Blair, R. & Newsome, F. (1985) Involvement of water soluble vitamins in diseases of swine. *J. anim. Sci.*, *60*, 1508.

REFERENCES

(1) O'Sullivan, B. M. & Blakemore, W. F. (1978) *Vet. Rec.*, *103*, 543.
(2) Roberts, M. D. (1983) *Aust. vet. J.*, *60*, 106.
(3) Cymbaluk, N. F. et al. (1977) *Vet. Rec.*, *101*, 97.
(4) Gratzl, E. (1960) *Wien. Tierärztl. Monatschr.*, *47*, 25.
(5) Halama, A. K. (1979) *Wien. Tierärztl. Monatschr.*, *66*, 370.
(6) Scott, D. W. (1981) *Bov. Pract.*, *2*, 22.
(7) Cymbaluk, N. F. et al. (1978) *Am. J. vet. Res.*, *39*, 255.
(8) Misir, R. et al. (1986) *Can. vet. J.*, *27*, 6.
(9) Webb, N. G. et al. (1984) *Vet. Rec.*, *114*, 185.
(10) Evans, W. C. et al. (1972) *Vet. Rec.*, *90*, 471.
(11) Money, D. F. L. & Laughton, G. L. (1981) *NZ vet. J.*, *29*, 33.
(12) Simmins, P. H. & Brooks, P. H. (1983) *Vet. Rec.*, *112*, 415.
(13) Thornber, E. J. et al. (1981) *Aust. vet. J.*, *57*, 21.
(14) Johnson, B. C. et al. (1950) *J. Nutr.*, *40*, 309.
(15) Maclean, C. W. (1965) *Vet. Rec.*, *77*, 578.
(16) Sharma, G. L. et al. (1952) *Am. J. vet. Res.*, *13*, 298.
(17) Ellis, N. R. (1946) *Nutr. Abst. Res.*, *16*, 1.
(18) Sheppard, A. J. & Johnson, B. C. (1957) *J. Nutr.*, *61*, 195.
(19) Wiese, A. C. et al. (1946) *Proc. Soc. exp. Biol. Med.*, *63*, 521.
(20) Lehrer, W. P. et al. (1952) *J. Nutr.*, *47*, 203.
(21) Johnson, B. C. et al. (1951) *J. Nutr.*, *43*, 37.
(22) Dobson, K. J. (1971) *Aust. vet. J.*, *47*, 587.
(23) Davies, M. E. (1971) *Br. vet. J.*, *1*, 34.
(24) Alexander, F. & Davies, M. E. (1969) *Br. vet. J.*, *125*, 169.
(25) Lassiter, C. A. et al. (1953) *J. dairy Sci.*, *36*, 997.
(26) Frederick, G. L. (1965) *Can. J. anim. Sci.*, *45*, 22.
(27) Thompson, R. E. & Hecht, R. A. (1959) *Am. J. clin. Nutr.*, *7*, 311.
(28) Thomas, K. W. (1986) *Vet. Res. Commun.*, *10*, 125.
(29) Frank, G. R. et al. (1984) *J. anim. Sci.*, *59*, 1567.
(30) Dufua, G. S. et al. (1984) *Am. J. vet. Res.*, *45*, 1835, 1838.
(31) Penny, R. H. C. et al. (1981) *Vet. Rec.*, *109*, 80.
(32) Comben, N. et al. (1984) *Vet. Rec.*, *115*, 642.

30

Diseases Caused by Physical Agents

Environmental pollutants and noise

ALTHOUGH there is now an extensive literature on this subject as it affects man it is not proposed to deal with it here in depth as a veterinary problem. The major chemical pollutants of the environment are cadmium, lead and mercury, but silver, gold, chromium, copper, tin, thallium, antimony and zinc are also listed as having high hazard potential (1). Fluorine and arsenic are also important as pollutants from the veterinary viewpoint. Another important group of compounds is the polychlorinated biphenyls and the polybrominated biphenyls, and the chlorinated hydrocarbons generally. These substances are extensively used in agriculture and in industry. They have a very long half-lives, and although they are not in themselves dangerous, they cause a great deal of trouble if they get into the human food chain and become deposited in fatty tissues. Most of these substances are dealt with individually in Chapters 31 and 32 on poisoning. The significance and alleviation of the problems caused by the pollution of the atmosphere appears to us to be a subject for a textbook on preventive medicine. There remains the subject of air pollution by physical agents, of which smoke and dust are the most significant. In both instances the effects are most noticeable in the lungs after inhalation but ingestion after deposition on fodder can be important also. Dust may be the carrier of pathogenic bacteria or viruses, or antigens which provoke a hypersensitivity reaction, e.g. interstitial pneumonia (8). For definitive work on this form of animal disease it is necessary to use established techniques for measuring the degree of pollution and be aware of the composition of the polluting agent. For example, automobile fumes contain poisons such as carbon monoxide, fumes irritant to lungs and carbon particles capable of soiling animal exteriors (2).

Pollution of the environment by animal feces and urine is now a matter of great importance especially to intensive animal farmers located near population centers (13). Biological degradation of cow pats on pasture or barn debris in a large compost pile is no longer acceptable to environmental protectionists. Nor is pumping of a slurry onto pasture. This introduces health problems such as salmonellosis, colibacillosis, leptospirosis, tuberculosis and brucellosis under which headings the subject is discussed.

One of the important pollutants for housed animals is ammonia from urine. When it is combined with dust it can cause severe inflammation of the respiratory mucosae (10). Shallow wells near animal accommodation are also likely to contain high levels of nitrates derived from urine filtering through surrounding earth. Such water is a potential source of nitrate poisoning especially in pigs. Sulfur dioxide is also an environmental contaminant capable of causing respiratory tract irritation in animals (11). A more esoteric subject is the depletion of the stratospheric ozone layer by the invasion of it with jet aircraft and with the widespread use of chlorofluoromethane propellants from spray cans (12).

Pollution by noise, a matter of increasing importance for veterinarians who police codes of practice for animal welfare and for those who are called upon to act as expert witnesses in cases involving excessive noise and its effects on animals, is also an important subject. An extensive review is available (3).

Some examination has been made of the effects of the sonic bang produced by aircraft (4) but the effects on cattle, sheep, ponies, chickens and wild and laboratory animals appear to be minimal (5–7). Most of the effects reported are shortlived and are due to fear reactions and include injury due to sudden flight, killing of young by mink and rabbits, suffocation in panic-stricken chickens and reduced egg production. Cows appear to be unaffected. Experimentally, loud noises of 90–100 phons applied to horses cause an increase in heart rate (9).

REVIEW LITERATURE

Collins, M. & Algers, B. (1986) Effect of stable dust on farm animals. A review. *Vet. Res. Commun.*, *10*, 415.

Jones, P. W. (1980) Disease hazards associated with slurry disposal. *Br. vet. J.*, *136*, 529.

Kopecky, K. E. (1978) Ozone depletion. Implications for the veterinarian. *J. Am. vet. med. Assoc.*, *173*, 729.

Lillie, R. J. (1970) *Air Pollutants Affecting the Performance of Domestic Animals*. US Dept. Agric., Agricultural Research Service, Agricultural Handbook No. 380.

REFERENCES

(1) Pond, W. G. (1975) *Cornell Vet.*, *65*, 441.

(2) Lillie, R. J. (1970) *Air Pollutants Affecting the Performance of Domestic Animals*. US Dept. of Agriculture, Agricultural Research Service, Agriculture Handbook No. 380.

(3) Ewbank, R. (1977) *Vet. Am.*, *17*, 296.
(4) Boutelier, C. (1967). *Rev. Corps vet. Armée*, *20*, 112.
(5) Brewer, W. F. (1974) *Clin. Toxicol.*, 7, 179.
(6) Espmark, Y. et al. (1974) *Vet. Rec.*, *94*, 106.
(7) Cottereau, P. (1972) *Rev. Méd. vét.*, *123*, 1367.
(8) Collins, M. & Algers, B. (1986) *Vet. Res. Commun.*, *10*, 415.
(9) Sakurai, N. et al. (1967) *Exp. Rep. equ. Hlth Lab. Jap. Racing Assoc., Tokyo*, *4*, 14.
(10) Doig, P. A. & Willoughby, R. A. (1971) *J. Am. vet. med. Assoc.*, *159*, 1353.
(11) Marin, S. W. & Willoughby, R. A. (1971) *J. Am. vet. med. Assoc.*, *159*, 1518.
(12) Kopecky, K. E. (1978) *J. Am. vet. med. Assoc.*, *173*, 729.
(13) Jones, P. W. (1980) *Br. vet. J.*, *136*, 529.

Radiation injury

Animals exposed to radioactive material may suffer radiation injury. They may also serve as reservoirs for radioactive material which could be passed to man in meat, milk and other animal products. This hazard to man is a problem of public health and the following discussion is restricted to the effects of irradiation on the health of animals exposed to it.

Etiology

Radiation injury can be caused in a number of ways including atomic bomb injury and exposure to roentgen rays, but the effects on the tissues are the same, differences occurring only in depth of penetration and degree of injury caused.

The effects of atomic explosions on animals are due to the three major results of such explosions, blast, heat and irradiation. Irradiation is the main cause of animal mortality and studies of its effects have been extensively reviewed (1, 2, 9).

Epidemiology

There is considerable variation in the effects of an atomic explosion depending on the distance from and the time after the blast and whether the explosion occurs in the air or on the ground surface. Animals within the range of immediate irradiation are more severely affected than those exposed only to the 'fallout' of fissionable material on pasture. However, grazing animals are exposed to very great risk because of this fallout. Of the radioactive materials produced by an atomic explosion, a number of radionuclides, including iodine 131, barium 140, strontium 89 and 90, and cesium 137, are likely to enter biological systems. Of these, radioactive iodine, barium and strontium 89 are of limited importance because of their short half-lives. On the other hand, strontium 90 and cesium 137 are produced in very large quantities and have long half-lives and are therefore of greatest biological significance. If sufficient of these radionuclides is ingested and tissue levels of them reach critical points, injury similar to that produced by external irradiation will occur. The effects of exposure of animals to strontium 90 and iodine 131 have been exhaustively reviewed (3).

Pathogenesis

Veterinarians are concerned with the effects of radiation injury to animals at two levels, the somatic dose resulting from acute, direct exposure to irradiation, and the cumulative dose due to the gradual accumulation of radioactivity in tissues resulting from continued exposure to small but toxic levels of radioactive materials.

Somatic doses

With median lethal doses (MLD) (500 roentgen, 'rem' or 'r' units received during a period of 24 hours is an approximate median lethal dose for most domestic animals (4)) 'radiation sickness' develops, manifested by signs of acute irritation of the alimentary tract. With high lethal doses the animal may die at this stage but more commonly progresses to a second stage of apparent normality for a few days.

The third phase commences at the end of the first week due to profound depression of bone marrow activity. Initially there is a lymphopenia followed by a depression of granulocyte and platelet counts. The leukopenia permits invasion by bacteria from the alimentary tract and bacteremia and septicemia develop 1–4 weeks after irradiation. The clotting mechanism and antibody production are impaired and facilitate the invasion. Progressive necrosis of the gut wall without inflammation is characteristic. Thrombocytopenic hemorrhages into the lymphatic system and other tissues lead to the development of a profound anemia.

The activity of germinative epithelium is also profoundly depressed and if the animal survives the early stages listed above, the hair commences to shed, the skin to ulcerate and a gross reduction in fertility occurs. Degenerative changes in the lens of the eye, particularly cataract, may also occur. Very longterm effects of irradiation include a high rate of mutations and a high incidence of tumors, mostly of the hemopoietic system and particularly of the leukemic series.

Chronic exposure

When 'fallout' contaminates pasture there may be sufficient fissionable material on the leaves of the plants to produce the same effects as those which occur with direct irradiation with median lethal doses, except that radiation sickness does not occur. Two indexes are used to measure the chronic effects of low level exposure, the genetic and leukemogenic indexes. The first depends on assessment of the increase in mutation rate in the population and the second on the increase in leukemia rate. Actual doses measured physically at this level are estimated in 'millirems' (one-thousandth of one 'rem' unit). With smaller doses the effects are quite different and depend on the radioactive substances formed, their solubilities and decay periods. Iodine and strontium are of importance when contamination of leaves occurs, but when the effects are due mainly to contamination of the soil and absorption by plants, strontium and cesium are the significant elements. Radioactive iodine causes damage to the thyroid gland and strontium causes destruction of bone tissue, depression of leukocyte and platelet production and a terminal depression of erythropoiesis. Both are excreted in the milk of animals and may cause deleterious effects in humans and animals drinking the milk. The maximum permissible concentration of radioactive substances in milk would be reached at much lower levels of pasture contamination than would be required to cause physical injury to the cattle.

Clinical findings

Acute syndrome

After immediate irradiation with high doses, damage to the alimentary tract occurs and there is a resulting intense, refractory diarrhea. Death occurs in a few days due to dehydration and salt depletion. Local contact of radioactive materials to skin causes changes within a few hours. Observable lesions vary from depilation and slight desquamation to extensive necrosis depending upon the irradiation dose.

Subacute syndrome

Immediately after irradiation with median doses there is an initial phase of 'radiation sickness' characterized by anorexia, vomiting and profound lethargy which lasts from several hours to several days. The second phase is one of apparent normality lasting until 1–4 weeks after irradiation and is followed by a third phase in which most deaths occur. There is fever, knuckling at the fetlocks, swelling of one or more legs and diarrhea developing to melena and dysentery sometimes with tenesmus. Anorexia is complete but there is great thirst. Weakness, recumbency and hyperirritability are present. Respiration is rapid and panting and there is a profuse nasal discharge, sometimes bloodstained. Severe anemia and septicemia occur in the terminal stages, death usually occurring about 20 days after irradiation.

In general if the animal survives this period, there is a long period of convalescence which is accompanied by failure to make normal weight gains, alopecia, sterility and lenticular defects. The sterility may be permanent, or normal fertility may be restored by the end of 8 months in pigs and 2 years in cattle. During the ensuing years, recovered animals may produce mutant offspring. Tumors, especially of the hemopoietic system, and of areas of skin which suffer radiation injury (5) are also likely to occur. Experimental irradiation of pregnant animals causes fetal death and resorption, defects of individual organ and limb development, decreased survival of young born alive and depressed growth rate and fertility of surviving young, the type of abnormality depending upon the stage of pregnancy at which exposure is experienced (6).

These general statements do not apply to cows which survive one median somatic dose. Provided such cows survive for 40 days after irradiation they appear to recover quickly and conceive readily. Congenital anomalies appear to occur only rarely and only in calves which are irradiated in *utero*.

Chronic exposure to gamma and mixed neutron-gamma radiation for several years produced lenticular opacities (7). At levels of irradiation which cause lesions in the human lens similar opacities occur in the lens of cattle, but not pigs or burros.

Clinical pathology

In cattle receiving median somatic doses the total leukocyte count falls precipitately during the first few days after irradiation with the peak of fall at the 15th–25th postirradiation (PI) day. In this species the most sensitive leukocyte is the neutrophil, in contrast to the lymphocyte which is most seriously affected by irradiation in man. Platelet counts begin to decrease from a normal of 500 000/mm^3 on the 7th PI day to 40 000/mm^3 about PI day 21. Erythrocyte counts and hematocrit levels also fall and prothrombin times increase in parallel to the other changes mentioned. The return to preirradiation levels requires about a year for granulocytes and platelets, but from 4 to 5 years for agranulocytes (8).

Necropsy findings

Gastroenteritis, varying from hemorrhagic to ulcerative, is constant, and ulceration of the pharyngeal mucosa and pulmonary edema occur commonly. Hemorrhages into tissues are also characteristic and include all degrees from petechiae and ecchymoses to hematomas and large extravasations. In experimentally produced irradiation sickness a severe fibrinous pneumonia, pleuropneumonia and pericarditis are common. Degenerative lesions are present in all organs (10). Degeneration of bone marrow and lymphoid tissue is evident histologically. Many bacterial colonies are present in ulcerated areas and in parenchymatous organs.

Diagnosis

The subacute syndrome closely resembles poisoning by bracken fern in cattle and by trichloroethylene-extracted soybean meal, but the diagnosis will usually depend upon a knowledge of exposure to irradiation.

Control

The problems of veterinary civil defense in the event of thermonuclear warfare are too extensive to discuss here and the necessary information is provided by most governments.

REVIEW LITERATURE

Garner, R. J. (1969) Radiation and radiation hazards. *Vet. Ann.*, 240.

REFERENCES

(1) Trum, B. F. & Rust, J. H. (1958) *Adv. vet. Sci.*, *4*, 51.
(2) Wilkins, J. H. (1963) *J. R. Army vet. Corps*, *34*, 64.
(3) McClellan, R. D. & Bustad, L. K. (1964) *Ann. NY Acad. Sci.*, *111*, 793.
(4) Wilkins, J. H. (1962) *J. R. Army vet. Corps*, *33*, 74.
(5) Brown, D. G. et al. (1966) *Am. J. vet. Res.*, *27*, 1509.
(6) O'Brien, C. A. et al. (1966) *Am. J. vet. Res.*, *27*, 711.
(7) Brown, D. G. et al. (1972) *Am. J. vet. Res.*, *33*, 309.
(8) Noonan, T. R. et al. (1976) *Radiation Res.*, *66*, 626.
(9) Johansen, U. et al. (1978) *Arch. exp. vet. Med.*, *32*, 537 & *34*, 623.
(10) Koch, F. et al. (1978) *Mh VetMed.*, *35*, 138.

Brisket disease (mountain sickness)

This is a sporadic disease of cattle, and possibly other species, kept at high altitudes. Clinically it is characterized by a syndrome of congestive heart failure.

Etiology

At high altitudes the low density of the atmosphere results in environmental anoxia and this is presumed to be the predisposing cause of brisket disease. The fact that the incidence is greater in introduced than in indigenous cattle suggests that cattle reared at high altitudes may become adapted to the environment. Any additional factor such as myocardial dystrophy, anemia, pulmonary disease, or hypoproteinemia may exacerbate the primary cardiac decompensation and this probably accounts for the sporadic occurrence of the disease in herds kept at high altitudes. The additional effort required to obtain feed on sparse pasture may also be a predisposing cause.

Epidemiology

The disease in cattle is most common in yearlings. Although it occurs in all ages and breeds there is good evidence that susceptibility to altitude disease is inherited (1) and that Friesians are more susceptible than other breeds (2). Horses which are moved up from 300 to 2400 m above sea level show standard increases in pulse and respiratory rates, and hemoglobin and erythrocyte levels. They also lose weight, fatigue easily, become weak and rough-coated, show pain and many suffer from flatulent colic (3). Mules are much less susceptible and appear to be unaffected by altitudes as high as 3200 m (4). Goats, sheep and donkeys are also reputed to be affected in that order of reducing susceptibility. Llamas and alpacas are adapted to hypoxia at high altitudes, in particular by an oxygen dissociation curve in their hemoglobin which increases oxygen uptake (5).

Brisket disease is recorded commonly only in animals which have been maintained for some months at heights of over 1800 m above sea level. At lower altitudes other factors are likely to be involved in causing the myocardial insufficiency (13).

Brisket disease occurs sporadically in high mountainous areas in the United States and South America. The morbidity rate in indigenous cattle seldom exceeds 1%, but may be much higher in newly introduced cattle. Recovery is rare.

Pathogenesis

Anoxic anoxia at high altitudes causes pulmonary vasoconstriction and circulatory embarrassment because the oxygen requirements of tissues exceed the available oxygen supplies. In normal animals and man this is usually compensated by the development of polycythemia, an increase in lung volume, and an increased volume of cardiac output. It has been shown that continued hypoxia can cause sufficient myocardial weakness to interfere with cardiac compensation and thus lead to congestive heart failure. This is most likely to occur if the animal has to walk long distances to get feed. The development of any additional factor, such as pregnancy, pneumonia or anemia, which exacerbates the oxygen deficit will also increase the susceptibility to cardiac decompensation. Animals affected by these diseases can often exist satisfactorily at lower altitudes where their cardiac decomposition is compatible with the environment. That brisket disease can develop in the absence of these diseases has been proved experimentally. The removal of cattle from an altitude of 1100 up to 3000 m has been shown to cause hypertrophy of the right ventricle, an increase in pulmonary arterial pressure from 27 mmHg (3·6 kPa) to from 45 (6·0) to over 100 mmHg (13·3 kPa) and the development of right heart failure (6, 7). Experimental creation of altitude stress has made it possible to demonstrate the exacerbation of pulmonary hypertension which occurs in late pregnancy in susceptible cows (14). One of the significant differences between susceptible and resistant cows was the hyperventilation which occurred in the latter.

Clinical findings

The animal has a dejected appearance, loses condition rapidly, has a rough, lusterless coat, and stands with the elbows abducted. Jugular vein engorgement is followed by the appearance of edema of the brisket, spreading up the neck to the intermandibular space and back along the ventral aspect of the body. Abdominal enlargement due to the development of ascites is accompanied by diarrhea. There is hyperpnea at rest, and dyspnea and weakness on slight exertion. The mucosae may be cyanotic, particularly after exercise, and the lung sounds vary from an increased vesicular murmur, to moist crackles and an absence of breath sounds when pneumonia is present, and to crepitant crackles in the presence of emphysema. Auscultation of the heart reveals tachycardia, increased absolute intensity of the sounds, or a decrease when there is hydropericardium, and an increase in the size of the heart. A hemic murmur may also be present. The appetite is normal until the late stages and the temperature is normal unless secondary pneumonia develops.

Clinical pathology

In affected cattle there is a significant reduction in the packed cell volume coincident with a fall in mean cell volume, and in hemoglobin levels. Hypocalcemia, hyperphosphatemia and hyperkalemia also occur (8).

The effect of altitude on normal horses is of interest. In horses elevation from sea-level to 2200 m causes elevation of heart rate, respiratory rate before and after exercise, ratio of heart to respiratory rate and an increase in red and white cell counts. A stabilization period of 21–28 days is considered necessary before horses perform at their best (9). In sheep and cattle elevations of 1800–3500 m cause rises in hemoglobin (35% in sheep, 9% in cattle) and packed cell volumes (27% in sheep but no change in cattle) and hemoglobin concentration in red cells (8–9% increase in cattle and sheep) (10). Central pulmonary arterial pressures increase significantly immediately after cattle are moved to high altitudes, but the high pressures subside as adaptation develops. Pressures rise from a normal of 22–26 mmHg (2·9–3·5 kPa) up to 37–55 mmHg (4·9–7·3 kPa) depending on whether the calf is susceptible or resistant to the effects of altitude (11). Cattle accustomed to live at high altitudes have much less pulmonary hypertension than introduced cattle (12).

Necropsy findings

There is enlargement of the heart, with marked hypertrophy and dilatation of the right ventricle (8). There is an accompanying severe edema of the pericardial, pleural and peritoneal sacs and subcutaneous tissues. The edema may also involve the wall of the alimentary tract. Minor lesions are present on the heart valves and there may be areas of calcification in the large arteries. Typical congestive changes are evident in the liver—enlargement, rounding of the edges, dilatation of the hepatic veins, and a marked deposition of fibrous tissue around the central veins. In the lungs there is often severe alveolar emphysema, and in some cases bronchitis and pneumonia are also present.

Diagnosis

Congestive heart failure occurs in several diseases of cattle including traumatic pericarditis, lymphomatosis affecting the myocardium, congenital cardiac defects and valvular endocarditis. In these diseases there is cardiac involvement and care is necessary in differentiating the accompanying abnormal heart sounds. The occurrence of congestive heart failure in cattle at high altitudes should arouse suspicion of brisket disease.

Treatment

The cardiac reserve must be maintained and compensation encouraged. Avoidance of excessive exercise by the supplementary feeding of affected animals may cause temporary improvement and individual animals may be helped by the administration of digitalis or related glucosides but the drugs must be given parenterally and the improvement may be only temporary (10). Diuretics to promote fluid loss and antibiotics to combat secondary infection may be indicated in individual cases. Temporary relief can be obtained by housing the animal in a hyperbaric chamber for a brief period (10). Return of affected cattle to lower altitudes results in recovery in many cases.

Control

Control measures are difficult to implement. Restriction of grazing, hand feeding with particular emphasis on a high protein diet, and prompt treatment of cases of pulmonary disease are recommended as worthwhile procedures.

REVIEW LITERATURE

Bisgard, G. E. (1977) Pulmonary hypertension in cattle. *Adv. vet. Sci.*, *21*, 151–172.

REFERENCES

(1) Will, D. H. et al. (1975) *J. appl. Physiol.*, *38*, 491.
(2) Ruiz, A. V. et al. (1973) *Pflügers Arch.*, *34*, 275.
(3) Rao, R. et al. (1973) *J. Remount vet. Corps*, *12*, 11.
(4) Riar, S. S. & Malhotra, M. S. (1974) *J. Remount vet. Corps*, *13*, 25.
(5) Reynafarje, C. et al. (1975) *J. appl. Physiol.*, *38*, 806.
(6) Guilbride, P. D. L. & Sillau, H. (1970) *Span*, *13*, 177.
(7) Wagenwoort, C. A. et al. (1969) *J. comp. Pathol.*, *79*, 517.
(8) Blake, J. T. (1966) *Am. J. vet. Res.*, *26*, 68, 76.
(9) de Aluja, A. S. et al. (1968) *Vet. Rec.*, *82*, 368.
(10) Hansen, R. W. et al. (1984) *Am. Soc. agric. Engin. papers*, no. 4523.
(11) Will, D. H. et al. (1975) *J. appl. Physiol.*, *38*, 495.
(12) Will, D.H. et al. (1975) *Proc. Soc. exp. Biol. med.*, *150*, 564.
(13) Hull, M. W. & Anderson, C. K. (1978) *Cornell Vet.*, *68*, 199.
(14) Moore, L. G. et al. (1979) *J. appl. Physiol., resp. Environ., exercise Physiol.*, *46*, 184.

Lightning stroke and electrocution

Exposure to high-voltage electric currents in the form of lightning stroke or electrocution causes sudden nervous shock with temporary unconsciousness or immediate death. Residual nervous signs may persist after recovery from nervous shock.

Etiology

The three common causes are flashes of linear lightning during thunderstorms, broken overhead electrical transmission wires which usually carry very high voltages, and faulty electrical wiring in cowsheds and barns. In lightning stroke, trees, fences, barns and pools of water may become electrified and it is not unusual for damp ground to act as a conductor for electricity passing along the roots of stricken trees. Animals electrocuted by standing on electrified earth are unlikely to show burn marks on the body. Oak trees are particularly prone to lightning stroke and because of their spreading foliage and extensive root system are common mediators of electrocution deaths in pastured animals. Poplar, elm, walnut, beech, ash and conifer are also highly susceptible (1). Transmission wires are most dangerous when they fall into pools of water, as they are likely to do during the storms which bring the wires down. In such cases the entire pool is electrified and animals passing through it may be killed instantly. In accidents caused by faulty wiring, voltages of 110–220 V are sufficient to kill adult cattle provided they make good contact with the source and the ground (2). Water pumps and milking machines are the common sources of electricity which may electrify water pipes or the milk line through the earth wire or a short circuit. The use of very heavy fuse wire (30–60 A) may cause continuance of the trouble which could be avoided if lower capacity fuses were used.

Epidemiology

The area incidence is never high but on individual farms heavy mortalities may occur when a barn or a group of animals sheltering under a tree is struck. As many as 20 head of cattle may be killed by one lightning flash. Faulty wiring in barns may kill occasional animals and lower production in others.

Most fatalities caused by lightning stroke occur during the summer months when the cattle are at pasture. Deaths due to electrocution in barns may occur at any time.

Pathogenesis

Exposure to high-voltage electrical currents causes severe nervous shock with complete unconsciousness and flaccid paralysis. In some instances focal destruction of nervous tissue occurs and residual signs of damage to the nervous system persist after nervous shock disappears. Death when it occurs is usually due to paralysis of vital medullary centers. Ventricular fibrillation may also occur and contribute to the fatal outcome (1). Superficial burns may be evident at the site of contact with the current or along the path of flow from the point of contact to ground. The burn is produced by heat generated from the resistance of tissues to the passage of the electricity.

Clinical findings

Varying degrees of shock occur. With high voltage currents and good earth contacts such as wet concrete floors, water, and damp earth, the animal may fall dead without a struggle. Singeing and burning are likely to occur because of the severity of the shock. The burns may be localized to the muzzle or feet and be in the form of radial deposits of carbon with or without disruption of tissue, or they may appear as tree-like, branching patterns of singeing running down the trunk and limbs.

In less severe shocks the animal falls unconscious but there is some struggling, followed by a period of unconsciousness varying from several minutes to several hours. When consciousness is regained the animal may rise and be perfectly normal, or show depression, blindness, posterior paralysis, monoplegia and cutaneous hyperesthesia. In some cases there may be more local signs including nystagmus and unilateral paralysis (3, 4). Sloughing of the skin at the sites of burns may occur after a few days. These signs may persist or disappear gradually over a period of 1–2 weeks. In one severe episode of lightning stroke in pigs a large number of animals were affected by posterior paralysis due apparently to fracture of the ileum, ischium and the transverse processes of the lumbar vertebrae (5).

With minor shocks, especially as they occur in barns on low-voltage domestic current, the animal may be knocked down or remain standing. Consciousness is not lost and the clinical picture is one of restlessness and periodic convulsive episodes of short duration. In these episodes the animal may kick violently at the stanchion or the dividing rail. The attacks may be intermittent and occur only when the cattle supply a good ground contact such as standing in the gutter, when they are drinking, or when they are wet. In some cases the shock is so mild that no clear signs are evident but drinking may be interfered with and production lowered drastically (6). Dairy farmers are often unaffected in the same environment because their rubber boots provide effective insulation.

Clinical pathology

Laboratory examinations are of no value in diagnosis.

Necropsy findings

Diagnostic lesions are often minimal (7) but singe marks or damage to the environment, or both, occur in about 90% of lightning deaths.

Rigor mortis develops but passes off quickly. Accumulation of gas in the alimentary tract is rapid and the carcass swells up and decomposes rapidly. Blood may exude from the external orifices and a bloodstained froth from the nostrils. The pupils are usually dilated and the anus relaxed. All viscera are congested and the blood is dark and unclotted. Petechial hemorrhages may occur throughout the body, including the trachea, endocardium, meninges and central nervous system. The superficial lymph nodes, particularly the prescapular and the interior cervical, are often hemorrhagic. Superficial singeing of the hair, burn marks on the feet or muzzle, and internal or subcutaneous extravasations of blood in arboreal patterns also occur. In some cases there are longitudinal fractures of long bones, and in one serious incident involving pigs extensive fractures of the bones in the pelvic area and local hemorrhage have been observed. Fractures of the ribs occurred in other pigs. If electrocution is suspected it is best to ensure that possible sources of electric power are shut off before proceeding with a postmortem examination. Magnetization of metal eartags by lightning strike has been proposed as an aid to diagnosis, but is of no value because most unused tags are already magnetic (8).

Diagnosis

Great care must be taken in accepting an owner's suggestion than an animal has been killed or injured by lightning stroke. Insurance against loss by lightning is commonly carried and the many other causes of sudden death or injury are seldom covered by insurance. To confirm a diagnosis there should be a history of exposure and evidence of sudden injury or death. In the latter case half-chewed food may still be present in the mouth. Burns on the skin, scorching of the grass and tearing of the bark on nearby trees are also accepted as contributory evidence. The possibility of electrocution caused by faulty wiring should be considered when sudden shocks or death occur in animals confined in stanchions. Snakebite, gunshot wound, acute heart failure and trauma of the brain may also result in sudden death without other signs and a careful necropsy examination may be necessary to determine the cause of death. There are very few agents other than electricity which can kill a number of animals within a few minutes. Hydrocyanic acid is the other common cause of such an incident.

Acute septicemias including anthrax and blackleg, and some poisonings including hydrocyanic acid and nitrite, may produce a similar syndrome but are detectable on necropsy or suitable laboratory examination. Unexpected outbreaks of bloat may need to be differentiated from electrocution because of the frequency with which ruminal tympany occurs rapidly after death in the latter.

Treatment

Central nervous system stimulants and artificial respiration should be provided for unconscious animals but in most instances the animals are dead or recovered before treatment can be instituted.

Control

Precautions taken to avoid lightning stroke in animals are largely ineffective, but proper installation of all electric equipment in barns and milking parlors is essential to prevent losses. All motors should be earthed to a special iron spike or pipe driven at least 2·5 m into the ground, preferably in a damp spot. Earthing to water pipes should not be permitted. A rubber connection between the pump of the milking machine and the vacuum line will prevent electrification of the line. Minimum amperage fuses should be used to provide protection in cases of short-circuiting.

REFERENCES

(1) Milis, J. H. L. & Kersting, E. J. (1966) *J. Am. vet. med. Assoc.*, *148*, 647.
(2) Fox, F. H. (1954) *Cornell Vet.*, *44*, 103.

(3) Holgado Rivas, D. E. (1970) *Gac. vet.*, *32*, 124.
(4) Barr, M. (1966) *Vet. Rec.*, *79*, 170.
(5) Best, R. H. (1967) *Can. vet. J.*, *8*, 23.
(6) Salisbury, R. M. & Williams, F. M. (1967) *NZ vet. J.*, *15*, 206.
(7) Ramsey, F. K. & Howard, J. R. (1970) *J. Am. vet. med. Assoc.*, *156*, 1472.
(8) Shannon, D. (1980) *Vet. Rec.*, *107*, 48.

Volcanic eruptions

Active and potentially active volcanic chains exist in several countries in close proximity to significant livestock production areas. However, major volcanic eruptions are rare and there is little documentation of their effects on livestock production and health. The two notable eruptions of recent times, the Mount Hecla eruption in Iceland and the Mount St Helens eruption in Washington, United States, are both recorded as being inconvenient to orderly livestock production, but with minimal effects on animal health, and 7 years after the eruption there is no evidence of a problem in livestock.

Volcanic eruption can result in devastation of land areas from the effects of lateral blast, and pyroclastic, laval and mud flows. Livestock losses which occur in this way can be total, but the affected areas are restricted to the immediate vicinity of the eruption. Significantly greater land areas can be affected by tephra fallout consisting of ash and rock fragments from the volcanic eruption. The size of the sector affected by ash fallout will be determined by the strength and direction of winds at the altitude reached by the ash column at the time of the eruption. In the case of the major Mount St Helens eruption, an area of several thousand square kilometers received ash fallout varying from a light dusting to falls several centimeters in depth, with even heavier falls near to the volcano. Much of this was over agricultural land.

The hazards to livestock during the fallout period appear minimal although in areas where the ash fall is heavy there is virtually total darkness. As a result flocks of sheep and possibly other animals may mill about excessively and some may die of suffocation or misadventure including drowning.

The immediate effect of the fallout is to blanket pastures with ash, and in heavy fallout areas taller succulents may become lodged and unavailable for grazing. Livestock may be forced to graze more robust, but toxic, plant species if stored feeds are not provided and loss from plant poisoning was observed following the Mount St Helens eruption. Hypocalcemia, apparently resulting from food deprivation, was also observed in the immediate post-fallout period and was also recorded following the Mount Hecla eruption (1). In the period immediately following the fallout the investigation and alleviation of livestock ill-health is hampered in badly affected areas by the blocking of roads and the immobilization of automobiles resulting from clogging of air filters and in engine failure and damage.

Potential hazards to livestock health exist in the chemical composition and physical structure of ash. In the fallout from Mount St Helens several potentially toxic heavy metals and trace elements were present, but none in a concentration sufficient to be a hazard to livestock health (4). However, significant livestock mortality resulted from acute fluorine poisoning in association with high fluoride levels in ash and ash-contaminated grasses and water in the period immediately following the Mount Hecla eruption (1). It is therefore advisable to remove livestock from ash-contaminated pastures until this hazard is determined. In most circumstances this will necessitate removal to indoor housing and feeding of stored feed and well water if they are available. During the airborne stage, wind sorting of the dust into particles of varying size, shape and density results in area variation in the composition of the fallout. Consequently, area variations in chemical analysis over the fallout area can occur. However, in the case of the Mount St Helens eruption these were minor. Analyses based on acid-leachable or water-soluble analysis are more relevant to immediate animal health than those reporting total content.

The ash particulate count in air and the respiratory exposure to livestock is highest during the fallout period, but can remain high for long periods following the fallout when ground ash is disturbed by animal movement, winds and normal farming practices. A significant proportion of this material is of small particulate size and is respirable (4). Chemical and/or physical irritation of the respiratory tract, with a significant increase in the prevalence of respiratory disease, might be expected in these circumstances. This did not occur following the Mount St Helens eruption, even in animals with known preexisting respiratory disease, nor was it a reported problem following the eruption of Mount Hecla (1). Signs of irritation such as lacrimation were observed widely, but with no untoward sequelae.

Volcanic ash is composed predominantly of pumiceous volcanic glass and crystalline mineral silicates such as feldspar. These materials have no innate pulmonary toxicity. Volcanic ash may also contain variable amounts of free crystalline silica such as quartz, cristobalite and tridymite which, if present in respirable sized particles for prolonged exposure periods, can induce pulmonary fibrosis. Silicosis is primarily a human health concern, although spontaneous silicosis is recorded in livestock (2). The hazard from the Mount St Helens eruption appears remote. Seven years following the eruption there have been two appreciable effects on livestock health. The first has been a marked increase in the incidence of hypomagnesemia. This has possibly resulted from the reflective nature of the ash layer on the soil reducing soil temperature increase during early grass growth and thus reducing magnesium uptake. Certainly grass magnesium concentrations are low while potassium levels are high. However, there are no preeruption values for comparison. In the semiarid channelled scab lands of central Washington the problem has been particularly severe. Magnesium supplementation via mineral mixes and salt blocks has not been particularly effective and on some ranches it has been necessary to fence off the majority of water sources and to supplement with magnesium salts in the remaining sources to achieve control. The second effect has been an increase in the severity of selenium deficiency. The association between selenium deficiency and recent volcanic origin soils is well recognized. Problems have been corrected by additional and more intensive selenium supplementation.

Animals may ingest considerable quantities of ash from grazing contaminated pastures or from hay subsequently prepared from these areas. There is little field evidence for disturbance of digestive function in livestock following the Mount St Helens eruption and feeding trials of ash to cattle and sheep have shown no clinical or postmortem evidence of untoward effects nor any depression of production except that associated with decreased feed palatability at high ash feed levels (3).

Ash fallout may have a devastating effect on insect life and this may be followed soon afterwards by death from starvation of insectivorous avian species. This may be misinterpreted as evidence for ash toxicity.

REFERENCES

(1) Georgsson, G. & Petursson, G. (1973) *Fluoride Q. Rep.*, 5, 58.
(2) Schwartz, L. et al. (1980) *Proc. 23rd Aspen Lung Conf.*, *Aspen, Colo.*
(3) Preston, R. L. (1981) *Mount St Helens: One Year Later. Proc. Symp. Eastern Wash. Univ.*, May 17–18.
(4) Fruchter, J. S. et al. (1980) *Science*, *209*, 1116.

Bushfire injury

The treatment of burns is by common consent a surgical subject but there are aspects of bushfire or forest fire injury which warrant discussion in a textbook of large animal medicine. For example, when large numbers of animals are affected the most important questions to be decided are whether to treat them, and what to treat them with and, if they are not to be treated, whether they are to be summarily destroyed or salvaged for meat.

Although no written information is readily available about forest fires in softwood forests it is assumed that few would survive the suffocating effects of intense heat and high smoke concentration. The intensity of the heat arises from the fact that the entire forest from leaves to trunks is burned. In hardwood forests, such as eucalyptus forests in Australia, the heat is not so severe because the tops only are destroyed. Underbrush is burned but the tree trunks are only scorched and usually survive to regrow. Depending on the density of the forest and the amount of underbrush there may be many survivors as badly burned animals. The most severe burns are on the lower surfaces and undersurfaces of the body and are caused by burning of the litter on the forest floor. The most serious situation is caused by a grass or prairie fire for the same reason. Many animals will die of suffocation, especially sheep, but the majority survive in various states of burn injury (2).

The problems created by large-scale burnings are three-fold. The first is that national disaster services are usually recruited to deal with the damage to property and welfare problems of human beings. They are often poorly equipped to deal with animal problems and assume authority over their fate in the temporary absence of the owners. The normal reaction of the average person is to judge that burn injuries are much more serious than in fact they are and to shoot burned animals out of hand. The second problem is that the facilities for penning and treating burned animals have usually been destroyed in the fire so that a general feeling of helplessness prevails. Insurance also exerts an influence on the owner's decision on the course to be followed. Most livestock are protected by fire insurance, and there will be no argument with a veterinarian's decision that burned animals should be destroyed for humane reasons. And this is often done unnecessarily if the interest of insurers are to be protected (1, 2). Salvage for slaughter is often difficult to arrange at such short notice for such large numbers, and public sentiment is against the practice. However, delayed salvage must be kept in mind for animals which will have impaired functions because of burns, e.g. ewes with teat injuries, rams with preputial injuries, bulls with scrotal injury and so on.

The parts most affected by burning are the face, especially the eyelids, conjunctivae and lips, the undersurface of the body especially udder, teats and perineum, and the coronets (4). Badly damaged corneas take many weeks to heal but badly swollen lips and eyelids can be almost normal within 48 hours. Marked edema is always a feature of skin burns in animals, but badly burned skin will be dry and ready to slough in a week. The teats of dairy cows may be damaged to the point where they will not be milkable again and wethers and rams may suffer urethral obstruction. In dairy cattle it is heifers that have the worst prognosis with respect to machine milkability. Separation of the coronary band from the hoof is a common occurrence as a result of burning and there may be sufficient weeping at the separation to suggest that the hoof is about to slough, but they seldom do, and hooves that appear quite loose do heal normally. In fires where there is a great deal of smoke, pulmonary congestion is evident at the beginning and may lead to the animal's death during the next 4 days.

The position and posture of the animals may affect the location of burns. Animals which lie down are burnt on the back, not the belly; those that face the fire are burnt on the face. Wool protects and sheep are burnt worst on woolless parts of the body. The length of grass and the type of herbage and scrub present decide what lesions are produced.

Recommended criteria for deciding the fate of sheep burnt by pasture fire depend on the presence of burns to the hooves and legs below the carpal and tarsal joints which cause local swelling and a dry leathery appearance of the skin. Such sheep are likely to be recumbent and immobile and to die. Burns which do not cause swelling of the lower limbs, or to other parts of the body are not likely to be fatal, nor to produce chronic ill-health (3), unless they affect a large part, more than 15–20%, of the body surface. Animals which are unconscious or very distressed, cannot walk, or have severe difficulty in breathing are poor prospects for recovery and are best euthanized forthwith. It may be necessary to monitor sheep for 10 days after a fire before deciding what to do with them. It is necessary at all times to consider the need to avoid inflicting suffering on the animals, but to also consider the farmer's need to retrieve his assets. If the animals are insured against fire it is also highly desirable to keep the insurer advised of developments.

Animals which have been trapped in a burning building are likely to be burned all over and to have tracheitis and laryngitis and pulmonary edema so that they are dyspneic and have a purulent nasal discharge.

The treatment is symptomatic and low in intensity. Cooling astringent lotions containing calamine and an antihistamine are excellent. Ointment is difficult to apply to a sore wet skin. Supportive antibiotic therapy, sometimes accompanied by an analgesic, is usually administered. It may be necessary to apply fly repellent preparations.

REVIEW LITERATURE

Geiser, D. R. et al. (1984) Management of thermal injuries in large animals. *Vet. Clin. N. Am., large Anim. Pract.*, *6(1)*, 91–105.

REFERENCES

(1) French, G. T. et al. (1965–66) *Vict. vet. Proc.*, *24*, 52.
(2) Pierson, R. E. et al. (1969) *Vet. Med.*, *64*, 218.
(3) McAuliffe, R. R. et al. (1980) *Aust. vet. J.*, *56*, 123.
(4) Willson, R. L. (1966) *Aust. vet. J.*, *42*, 101.
(5) Morton, J. M. et al. (1987) *Aust. vet. J.*, *64*, 69.

Wetness

Frequent exposure to wetting, sufficient to keep the skin permanently wet for long periods, is most important in sheep in which it causes fleece rot. In horses it leads to a superficial dermatitis along the dorsum especially over the croup and is known as scald. Frequent immersion of the lower limbs of cattle on irrigated pasture causes dermatitis on the backs of the pasterns leading to mycotic dermatitis. Frequent wetting is also a contributing cause in mycotic dermatitis in all species.

Standing in cold water for a period of more than 3 days causes the immersed parts to become edematous and congested and slough their skin in the form of a cuff around the limb. Recovery is slow and incomplete (1).

REFERENCES

(1) Bracken, F. K. et al. (1986) *Vet. Med.*, *81*, 562, 564, 566.

Fleece rot of sheep

Fleece rot of sheep is a dermatitis caused by prolonged wetting of the skin and resulting in matting of the wool by exudate. A common accompaniment of the disease is discoloration produced by the growth of chromogenic bacteria in the matted wool.

Etiology

Experimentally, continued skin-wetting plus the application of a culture of *Pseudomonas aeruginosa* (1) produces the disease and this is thought to be the main etiological group of factors.

Epidemiology

When rainfall is sufficient to wet sheep to the skin for a week, fleece rot may occur. Young sheep are more susceptible than old, and heritable differences in fleece characters affect the susceptibility of individual sheep.

These characters are probably related to the ease with which the skin can be wetted. The degree of 'grip' and skin wrinkling were found to be unimportant as factors affecting susceptibility. A long fleece dries slowly and for this reason predisposes to the condition. Fleeces with a high wax content are less susceptible probably because of the waterproofing effect of the wax. This view is supported by the observation that disruption of the sebaceous layer on the skin increases its susceptibility to wetting. Changes that occur in the skin and wool wax as a result of wetting subsequently increase the wettability of the skin and wool and their susceptibility to fleece rot (12). Wool with a high suint content is highly susceptible and selection against this character should increase the resistance of a flock (5). Selection against wettability as such is not expected to achieve much gain against the prevalence of fleece rot (12). A dense fleece protects against wetting of the skin but during prolonged periods of wet weather such fleeces do become wet and predispose to fleece rot because of the slowness with which they dry out. Microanatomical identification of susceptible sheep, and susceptible strains of sheep is possible and is based on size and density of primary follicle groups, those with smaller and more dense follicle groups being more susceptible (7). Other characteristics that increase susceptibility to fleece rot include high fiber diameter and irregular fiber diameter (2). These characteristics produce visible differences between fleeces. Resistant sheep have closely packed elliptical wool staples with blocky tips and even crimp. Susceptible fleeces have thin staples of unevenly crimped wool and with a fringe-tipped appearance due to the protrusion of thicker wool fibers above the top of the staple. This fringed appearance is visible along the back and sides.

Discoloration of the fleece may or may not occur depending upon the presence of chromogenic bacteria. The type of discoloration varies with the type of bacteria present. For example, a blue discoloration can be produced by *Pseudomonas indigofera* and a green one by *Ps. aeruginosa* (3).

Fleece rot occurs in sheep only in wet seasons and when the fleece is predisposed to wetting by its physical characters. The disease is common in most parts of Australia during wet years and causes considerable financial loss because of the depreciation in the value of the damaged fleeces. The general health of the sheep is unaffected. A positive relationship has been demonstrated in the United Kingdom between the rainfall 2 years previously and the amount of wool rejected for quality. The high rainfall is thought to encourage the multiplication and distribution of *Dermatophilus congolensis* infection, the cause of mycotic dermatitis (4).

Pathogenesis

Dermatitis develops due to the wetness. It commences in as short a time as 6 hours after the skin is wetted (9). This is followed by the leakage of plasma onto the skin surface from damaged follicles. These discrete 'hot-spots' carry a high protein level and attract blowflies (2). The exudation causes a matting of the wool fibers and provides a suitable medium for the proliferation of chromogenic bacteria. The predominant bacteria is usually

Pseudomonas spp. which inhibits the growth of other bacteria. The odor produced by the bacteria and the serum protein on the skin surface is very attractive to blowflies (6), and most body strikes are due to preexisting fleece rot lesions. To add a further complication *P. aeruginosa* also proliferates in the presence of organophosphorus insecticides and facilitates its biodegradation (11). The skin also shows increasing acanthosis followed by hyperkeratosis (9).

Clinical findings

Lesions occur most commonly over the withers and along the back. The wool over the affected part is always saturated and the tip is more open than over unaffected areas. The wool is leached and dingy and in severe cases can be plucked easily. Coloration of the skin changes from normal pink to purple, and a matted layer appears across the staple. Coloration of the wool by green, brown, orange, pink and blue bands occurs at any level in the staple, often separate from the matted layer.

Clinical pathology and necropsy findings

Autopsy examinations are not carried out and laboratory examination of the living animal is not usually necessary. Culture of the skin lesion to ascertain whether *Pseudomonas aeruginosa* is present might be performed in doubtful cases.

Diagnosis

Fleece rot resembles mycotic dermatitis but there is no scab development and no skin ulceration.

Control

Treatment is unlikely to be of value but some degree of control may be effected by selection of sheep with suitable fleeces and skins for use in susceptible localities. In these same localities shearing before the wet season should facilitate drying of the fleece and lessen susceptibility. Chemical means of drying the living fleece have been shown to reduce wetness, fleece-rot and blowfly strike (8). A mixture of zinc and aluminum oxides with sterols and fatty acids (the mixture identified as B26), applied at the rate of 100–200 ml per sheep as a mist-like simulated rain, caused significant reduction in fleece moisture for 10–12 weeks and this could be extended by further applications. Fleece rot was reduced by 60% and blowfly strike by 75%. A vaccine containing killed *Pseudomonas aeruginosa* has protected against the severe exudative form of fleece rot (10).

REFERENCES

(1) Burrell, D. H. et al. (1982) *Aust. vet. J.*, *59*, 140.
(2) Watts, J. E. & Merritt, G. C. (1981) *Aust. vet. J.*, *57*, 98.
(3) Tonder, E. M. et al. (1976) *J. S. Afr. vet. Assoc.*, *47*, 223.
(4) Smith, L. P. & Austwick, P. K. C. (1975) *Vet. Rec.*, *96*, 246.
(5) Lipson, M. et al. (1982) *Aust. J. exp. Agric.*, *22*, 168.
(6) Merritt, G. C. & Watts, J. E. (1978) *Aust. vet. J.*, *54*, 513 & 517.
(7) Watts, J. E. et al. (1980) *Aust. vet. J.*, *56*, 57.
(8) Hall, C. A. et al. (1980) *Res. vet. Sci.*, *29*, 181 & 186.
(9) Chapman, R. E. et al. (1984) *Anim. Prod. Aust.*, *15*, 290.
(10) Burrell, D. H. (1985) *Aust. vet. J.*, *62*, 55.
(11) Merritt, G. C. et al. (1981) *Aust. vet. J.*, *57*, 531.
(12) Pascoe, L. (1982) *Aust. J. agric. Res.*, *33*, 141.

31

Diseases Caused by Chemical Agents—I

When animals are sick and the cause is not immediately apparent a diagnosis of suspected poisoning is often made. An analyst is faced with a hopeless task if he is provided with this information only. The toxicological examination of tissues and other materials is an expensive and laborious procedure and every effort should be made to provide information on the circumstances which have led to the diagnosis, some suggestion as to the poison or class of poisons suspected; and material for examination should be carefully selected and properly packed for transport.

The conditions which usually arouse suspicion of poisoning are illness in a number of previously healthy animals, affected at the same time, and showing the same signs and necropsy findings. These conditions, of course, may also apply to some infections, metabolic and nutritional deficiency diseases. It is only by acquaintance with the syndromes produced by the common poisons, particularly those likely to occur locally, that this primary differentiation can be made. Poisonous plants often show a geographical limitation in distribution; particular industrial enterprises may create poison hazards in local areas; certain agricultural practices, including the spraying of orchards, the dipping or spraying of cattle for ectoparasites and the use of prepared concentrate feed for pigs and cattle, may also lead to poisoning in groups of animals. So many chemical agents are used in agriculture today that a section of miscellaneous farm chemicals likely to cause poisoning of animals has been included. The appearance of clinical illness soon after feeding, after a change of ration, after medication or spraying, or after change to new pasture is a common history in many outbreaks of disease caused by chemical agents.

The report which accompanies material for toxicological analysis should include a full record of history, clinical signs and necropsy findings and particularly the results of a search of the environment for access to a poison. If the animal has been treated, the drugs that were used and the dates of administration should be given as they may create difficulties for the analyst. The poison or group of poisons suspected should be defined.

Specimens for analysis should include a sample of the suspected source material. Next most important is a specimen of alimentary tract contents, so that ingestion of the material can be proven, and a sample of tissue, usually liver, to prove that absorption of the poison has occurred. Most toxic chemicals are ingested but percutaneous absorption and inhalation must be considered as possible portals of entry. One of the advantages of an examination of alimentary tract contents is that qualitative tests can be carried out and in many cases this determines whether or not further examination of tissues is necessary.

Additional specimens required, other than liver and alimentary tract and contents, vary with the poison and the following list is suggested for the common chemicals:

Arsenic	Kidney, skin and hair
Lead	Kidney, bones and blood
Phosphorus	Kidney and muscle
Mercury	Kidney
Copper	Kidney and blood
Sodium chloride	Alimentary tract and contents only
Fluorine	Bones, teeth and urine
Hydrocyanic acid	Ingesta in a filled and airtight container, blood and muscle
Nitrate and nitrite	Ingesta (plus chloroform or formalin) in an airtight, filled container, blood
Strychnine	Blood, kidney and urine

Careful packing of specimens is necessary to avoid loss of some poisons by escape as gas or conversion by bacterial fermentation, or to prevent contamination. No preservative should be added except in the case of suspected nitrite poisoning. If a preservative is necessary because of distance from the laboratory, packing in dry ice or ethyl alcohol (1 ml/g of tissue) is advisable but in the latter instance a specimen of the alcohol should also be sent. Ingesta and tissues must be kept separate as diffusion is likely to occur between the two. Specimens should be packed in glass or plastic to prevent contamination by lead in soldered joints of cans. Metal tops on jars should also be separated from the tissues by a layer of plastic or other impervious material. A suitable amount of material should be submitted for analysis; 1 kg of ingesta, 1 kg of liver and proportionate amounts of other viscera are suggested to cover all contingencies. A special situation is when plant poisoning is suspected. It is possible to ascertain the identity of the plants eaten recently by a careful examination of the ruminal contents. The freshest, least macerated material is best and whole leaves preferred. An atlas of epidermal plant fragments is available to aid in identification of ingested plant species in agricultural animals (1). Commonly, with plant poisonings, there are perplexing epidemiological features. For example, animals already grazing in the dangerous field are often unaffected and only those recently introduced may be poisoned. Some of the factors which affect susceptibility to plant poisonings are:

- Hungry, ravenous animals are more likely to be affected
- Curious, excited animals are likely to sample the plants they would not otherwise eat
- Young animals are less discerning and are less easily put off
- Plants that are different in texture, e.g. sprayed weeds, lopped foliage, often appear to be attractive
- Pica due to other cause
- Genetic selection of animals towards tolerance of a particular poison, e.g. fluoroacetate.

Poisoning is in most instances accidental although it may occasionally be deliberate. Deliberate or criminal poisoning is often suspected but is rarely proved. If there is a strong suspicion of criminal poisoning, or if litigation appears possible in accidental poisoning, specimens should be collected in duplicate and placed in sealed containers in the presence of witnesses. A complete set of specimens should be available to both plaintiff and defending parties for independent analysis. Also, if litigation appears possible, the veterinarian should make detailed observations of the clinical, pathological and epidemiological findings and record them in detail. The taking of photographs of affected animals and the environmental surroundings is also recommended for future reference and documentation if necessary.

Mineral tolerance of animals

One of the very important aspects of toxicology as it applies to agricultural animals is the determination of levels of dietary constituents which the animals will tolerate for a limited period without impairing their performance and without producing unsafe residues in products destined for the human food chain. There is a great deal of information on this subject and it has been collated and published (2). Table 93 is an adapted summary of the information.

Table 93. Maximum tolerance levels of dietary minerals for domestic animals.

	Cattle	*Sheep*	*Pig*	*Horse*
Arsenic mg/kg				
inorganic	50	50	50	(50)
organic	100	100	100	(100)
Cobalt mg/kg	10	10	10	(10)
Copper mg/kg	100	25	250	800
Fluorine mg/kg				
dairy	40	breeding 60	150	(40)
mature beef	50	finishing 150		
finishing beef	100			
Iodine mg/kg	50	50	400	5
Iron mg/kg	1000	500	3000	(500)
Lead mg/kg	30	30	30	30
Mercury mg/kg	2	2	2	(2)
Molybdenum mg/kg	10	10	20	(5)
Phosphorus %	1	0·6	1·5	1
Selenium mg/kg	(2)	(2)	(2)	(2)
Silicon %	(0·2)	(2)	2	(2)
Sodium chloride %				
lactating	4	9	8	(3)
non-lactating	9			
Sulfur %	(0·4)	(0·4)	no data	no data
Zinc mg/kg	500	300	1000	(500)

Courtesy of National Research Council, USA
(Figures in parentheses are extrapolation from data on other species)

Principles of treatment in cases of poisoning

There are certain principles which apply to all cases of poisoning and they are listed briefly below. The two main principles are the removal of the residual poison from the alimentary tract or skin, and the provision of chemical and physiological antidotes to the poison that has been absorbed.

In farm animals gastric lavage and emetics are of little or no practical value and the removal of residual poison from the alimentary tract depends largely upon the use of adsorbents and purgatives. The only effective adsorbent is activated charcoal. The dose rate is 1–3 g/kg body weight repeated as necessary. It adsorbs chlorinated hydrocarbons, organophosphorus compounds, mycotoxins and plant alkaloids, the common feed additives, antibacterial agents and bacterial toxins. It does not adsorb heavy metals, halogens, nitrite, alcohols, caustics, sodium chloride or chlorate. A purgative is necessary to remove the combined adsorbent and poison; it can be administered simultaneously with the adsorbent (3). The use of irritant purgatives is not advisable when the poison is an irritant and has already caused gastroenteritis, and oily purgatives are preferable in these cases. Saline purgatives are of value in the treatment of non-irritant poisons such as cyanogenetic glucosides. Neutralization of residual poison in the alimentary tract can be effected in some cases. For example, oxidizing agents or tannic acid preparations are effective in precipitating alkaloids; proteins, including milk and eggs, are effective chemical antidotes for poisons that coagulate proteins; lead is precipitated by the addition of sulfates to the alimentary tract contents.

Poison that has already been absorbed can in some instances be inactivated or its excretion facilitated by the provision of chemical antidotes. For instance sodium nitrite and sodium thiosulfate are effective systemic antidotes to hydrocyanic acid, and calcium versenate is an effective antidote against lead.

Treatment of the effects of a poison includes provision of physiological antidotes, for example the injection of a calcium salt in cases of overdosing with magnesium salts, and treatment of the effects of the poison. Ancillary treatment, including the provision of fluids in dehydration due to diarrhea, demulcents in gastroenteritis, sedatives in excitement, stimulants in cases of central nervous system depression, all come under the latter heading.

It is essential when undertaking the treatment of animals for poisoning, especially those which are producing milk or which are destined to become meat in a short time, to take into account the possible unsuitability of the product for human consumption because of the presence of the poison or the antidote (4).

REVIEW LITERATURE

Bailey, E. M. (1979) Management and treatment of toxicosis in cattle. *Bov. Practnr*, *14*, 180.
Buck, W. B. (1969) Laboratory toxicological tests and their interpretation. *J. Am. vet. med. Assoc.*, *155*, 1928.
Edwards, W. C. (1980) Forensic toxicology and the bovine practitioner. *Bov. Practnr*, *18*, 155.
Galitzer, S. & Oehme, F. W. (1979) Emergency procedures for equine toxicosis. *Equ. Practnr*, *1*, 49.

REFERENCES

(1) Howard, G. S. & Samuel, M. J. (1979) *Tech. Bull. US Dept. Agric.*, No. 1582.
(2) National Research Council, Subcommittee on Mineral Toxicity (1980) *Mineral Tolerance of Domestic Animals*. National Academy of Sciences, Washington: National Academy Press.
(3) Buck, W. B. & Bratich, P. M. (1986) *Vet. Med.*, *81*, 73.
(4) Egyed, M. N. & Shlosberg, A. (1984) *Proc. 13th World Cong. Dis. Cattle*, p. 717.

DISEASES CAUSED BY INORGANIC POISONS

Lead poisoning (plumbism)

Lead is one of the commonest causes of poisoning in farm animals, particularly cattle, sheep and horses.

Etiology

The cause of lead poisoning is the accidental ingestion of sources of lead compounds or the ingestion of feed, usually forage, containing lead usually from pollution of the environment.

Epidemiology

Lead is one of the commonest poisonings in farm animals, especially young cattle. Sheep and horses are affected too, but not as commonly. Pigs are not often exposed to lead and appear to be extremently tolerant to it (35). In one diagnostic toxicology laboratory over a period of 15 years, lead poisoning in cattle was one of the most common poisonings diagnosed (52). The disease occurred most commonly in younger cattle with 52% of the cases reported in animals 6 months of age or less (53). Approximately 60% of the cases occurred during the summer months from May to August when the cattle have ready access to lead-containing materials such as crankcase oil and batteries which are being changed in agricultural machinery.

Lead poisoning in cattle is usually the result of the accidental ingestion of a toxic quantity of lead over a short period of time. The natural curiosity, licking habits and lack of oral discrimination of cattle makes any available lead-containing material a potential source of poisoning. Horses, on the other hand, are much more selective than cattle in their eating habits. They usually do not lick old paint cans, lead storage batteries, and peeling paint, nor do they seem to find the taste of used motor oil attractive (2). Several enzootics of lead poisoning in domestic animals have been recorded throughout the world where the source of the metal was contamination of pasture or crops by nearby industrial lead operation (2). Animals eating vegetation in these areas may accumulate amounts of lead sufficient to produce clinical signs of lead poisoning. While the mortality rate may approximate 100%, the overall occurrence rate is still relatively low (1) and it would not appear to be profitable to use the mortality rate in pastured animals as a device to monitor environmental pollution. Horses appear to be more susceptible to lead poisoning from grazing on pastures contaminated with lead than cattle. Young horses are particularly more susceptible than older horses and cattle grazing on the same pasture (3). Sheep are usually affected by eating forage contaminated by environmental sources of lead.

Sources of lead

Lead poisoning occurs most commonly in cattle at pasture, particularly if the pasture is poor and the animals are allowed to forage in unusual places, such as rubbish dumps. Phosphorus deficiency may also be a predisposing cause in that affected animals will chew solid objects as a manifestation of osteophagia. However, cattle on lush pasture may also seek out foreign material to chew. Confined housing of calves with or without overcrowding is often followed by the appearance of pica which may be caused by boredom or by mineral deficiency.

In many countries the incidence of the disease is highest in cattle in the spring (4) of the year, a few days after the animals have been turned out on to pasture. Young cattle, particularly, are curious and amazingly seem to find sources of lead.

The common sources of lead are lead-bearing paints and metallic lead. Discarded paint cans are particularly dangerous but fences, boards and the walls of pens, painted canvas and burlap are also common sources in calves. Painted silos may cause significant contamination of the ensilage.

Metallic lead in the form of car batteries, lead shot, solder or leaded windows has caused mortalities although under experimental conditions sheet lead does not cause toxic effects. Lead sheeting which has been exposed to the weather or subjected to acid corrosion appears to be more damaging, possibly because of the formation of a fine coating of a soluble lead salt. Lead poisoning appears to be a major hazard in the vicinity of oil fields, and engine sump oil may contain over 500 mg lead per 100 ml. Automotive and other mineral oils are very palatable to young beef calves. In one study, used crackcase oil was the most common source of lead poisoning in cattle (7), followed by paint, grease and lead car batteries. Less common but still potent sources of lead are linoleum, roofing felt, putty, automobile oil filters and aluminum paint. Some of the latter paints contain large quantities of lead, others none at all. Only lead-free aluminum paint should be used on fixtures to which animals have access.

The contamination of forage supplies with shotgun lead, pellets used in hunting and shooting exercises can serve as a source of lead for cattle grazing the pasture or consuming haylage or silage made from the contaminated field (55).

Lead parasiticide sprays, particularly those containing lead arsenate, have caused heavy losses in cattle grazing in recently sprayed orchards or vegetable crops. Lead pipes carrying soft water may lead to the ingestion of excess lead. Boiled linseed oil contains lead, and its accidental use as a laxative may result in lead poisoning.

Ruminants are most commonly affected and this may be due in part to the tendency for particulate material to settle in the reticulum and be converted to soluble lead acetate by the action of the acid medium of the forestomachs. In addition cattle in particular seem to be attracted to lead paint.

Environmental pollution with lead

This is a common occurrence in cities and on their edges. For farm animals, significant pollution is more likely to occur near smelters or other industrial enterprises (2, 10), or near major highways where pasture is contaminated by exhaust fumes of automobiles (11). A great deal of attention has been paid in recent years to this form of lead poisoning in ruminants and a good deal of literature, not referred to here, is available on the subject. Much of the poisoning caused is subclinical because of the low level of absorption, and any program intending to use domestic animals as monitors of pollution would need to be based on tissue lead levels. Pasture beside heavily used roads may carry as much as 390 mg/kg of lead, in contrast to 10 mg/kg on lightly used roads (11). The concentration of lead on pasture varies markedly with proximity to the traffic, falling rapidly the greater the distance, and with the time of the year (23). Pastures contaminated by smelters are recorded as carrying 325 mg/kg of lead (equivalent to a daily intake for an animal of 6·4 mg/kg body weight). In some locations near lead smelters, lead poisoning is considered to be a predictable occurrence in horses which are allowed to graze on local pastures. As a result horses are either not raised in these areas or hay is imported from others areas (56). Although ingestion is the principal method of poisoning of animals, inhalation may also be a significant method of entry for cattle grazing close to smelters or highways (28).

Lead as an environmental contaminant is often combined with cadmium which has effects similar to those of lead so that the effects are additive. Experimental poisoning with both elements causes reduced weight gains in calves at dose levels up to 18 mg/kg body weight of each, and clinical signs appear at levels above 18 mg/kg of each (12). Lead is also combined with chromate for industrial purposes. It is not toxic when combined with lead at lead intake levels of 100 mg/kg (13).

There is some concern that toxic levels of lead may occur in the human food chain. Canadian studies of the lead and mercury residues in kidney and liver of slaughter animals have shown that all levels were below the official tolerance level of 2 mg/kg for lead and 0·5 mg/kg for mercury (14). Levels of lead in beef randomly selected from supermarkets in the United States were for muscle 0·46, liver 0·50 and kidney 0·45 mg/kg (wet matter) (15). The upper range of liver levels exceeded the 1 mg/kg guideline which may be cause for concern about the source of the lead. Moderate exposure of people to meat, including liver and kidney, from animals exposed to lead poisoning is thought not to represent a human health hazard (44).

Toxic levels of lead

There is considerable variation between species in their susceptibility to lead, and the chemical composition of the compound containing lead may influence its toxicity. The toxicity also varies with the chemical form of the lead. Lead acetate is very soluble and more toxic than insoluble lead oxide, or solid lead sheeting.

Acute lethal single doses Some figures are available in terms of body weight. For example, for calves acute single lethal doses are 400–600 mg/kg, body weight, for adult cattle 600–800 mg/kg (16) and for goats 400 mg/kg (17), but a warning sign is again sounded about variability of toxicity of different compounds. The acute dose toxicity for horses is less than for ruminants, one horse having survived 1000 mg/kg body weight on two occasions 6 months apart. Pigs are also reputed to be much less susceptible but single lethal dose levels are not recorded.

Less exact figures for acute single lethal doses of lead acetate are for horses 500 g, cattle 50 g, sheep 30 g, calves 0·2–0·4 g/kg body weight. By contrast a single dose of finely ground lead oxide at the rate of 4·8 mg/kg body weight is reported to have killed a cow.

Young animals, for example, milk-fed calves are more susceptible. A daily intake of 2·7 mg/kg body weight of lead can kill calves fed a milk diet in 20 days or less, while 5 mg/kg body weight of lead consistently causes signs of poisoning or death within 7 days (57). The absorption rate of lead is rapid and tissue depositions are high in calves on a milk replacer diet and given lead. In toxicity studies, calves on a milk diet absorb lead much more quickly than calves fed a grain diet (58). The addition of lactose to a grain diet will also increase the absorption of lead (59).

Daily dose levels likely to lead to chronic poisoning These are important because of the impact that contamination of the environment by industrial effluents has had. Daily dose levels likely to lead to chronic plumbism in cattle are 6–7 mg/kg body weight (equivalent to 100–200 mg/kg in the diet) (16). This dose level must be close to the definitive point because dose levels of 100 mg/kg are also recorded as being without effect (19). A dose level of 15 mg/kg body weight produces definite effects of loss of weight gain and normochromic anemia (20). In sheep dose levels of more than 4·5 mg/kg appear to be necessary to produce a toxic effect

(21). Horses appear to be slightly more susceptible to daily administration of lead, 100 mg/kg body weight producing toxic effects in 28 days (17), and a dose rate of 15–30 mg/kg body weight of lead for up to 190 days causing toxicity and some deaths (22), and deaths are recorded on pastures carrying 100–300 mg/kg on foliage. Pigs appear to be more resistant, and daily doses of 33–66 mg/kg are required for periods of up to 14 weeks to produce fatal effects, a more serious end point than for the other dose rates quoted.

Pathogenesis

Irrespective of the chemical form of the ingested lead only a small proportion is absorbed because of the formation in the alimentary tract of insoluble lead complexes which are excreted in the feces. For example, only 1–2% of lead ingested as lead acetate or carbonate is absorbed from the alimentary tract of sheep. Of the lead absorbed, some is excreted in the bile, milk and urine and the blood levels of lead provide a reliable indication of the lead status of the animal. Urine levels may not be as reliable. Deposition in tissues occurs, particularly in the liver and renal cortex and medulla in acute poisoning and in the bones in chronic poisoning. The deposition of lead in the brain is not high compared to other tissues. The deposited lead is gradually liberated from tissues into the bloodstream and excreted via the bile and urine. Consideration must be given to these aspects of lead metabolism when assessing the results of chemical analyses of tissues.

The toxic effects of lead are manifested in three main ways: lead encephalopathy, gastroenteritis, and degeneration of peripheral nerves. In general, acute nervous system involvement occurs following the ingestion of large doses in susceptible animals such as calves, alimentary tract irritation following moderate doses, and peripheral nerve lesions following long-term ingestion of small amounts of lead. The mechanism by which the nervous signs of encephalopathy and the lesions of peripheral nerve degeneration are produced appears to be related to the degenerative changes seen in nervous tissue. In tissues, lead localizes principally in the cytoplasm of capillary endothelial cells and these localizations are later associated with the development of edema. The basic lesion is likely to be vascular with a basic change in transport mechanisms between the blood and brain (25). The pathological effects of lead have been reviewed (26). Gastroenteritis is produced by the caustic action of lead salts on the alimentary mucosa. Ruminal atony occurs in cattle and sheep and causes an initial constipation, later followed in some cases by diarrhea due to gastroenteritis. The rumen protozoa in cattle with acute lead poisoning are commonly absent or inactive. Peripheral nerve degeneration occurs principally in horses.

The lesions, including degeneration of the liver and kidney, vary in their severity with the tissue levels of lead attained. Lead does not remain in tissues for long periods except in bone where it is deposited in an inert form, but from which it can be liberated at a later date in sufficient quantities to cause chronic lead poisoning. This is particularly likely to occur during periods of acidosis.

The blue 'lead-line' at the gum–tooth junction, which is seen in man and the dog, does not commonly occur in ruminants because of failure to form tartar but may be present in the horse. The 'lead-line' is a deposit of lead sulfide formed by the combination of lead with sulfide from the tartar. Lead is transferred across the placental barrier and high liver levels occur in the lambs of ewes fed more than normal amounts of lead. Calves born from cows experimentally poisoned with lead have elevated levels of lead in bone, kidney and liver (27).

The mechanism by which osteoporosis is produced in young lambs affected by chronic lead poisoning has not been explained, nor has the paresis and paralysis of lambs which occur in the same circumstances. The paralysis in the former condition is caused by compression of the spinal cord by collapsed lumbar vertebrae.

Although acute lead poisoning usually develops rapidly there may be a delay of several days after toxic material has been ingested before clinical signs appear.

Anemia is an early manifestation of both acute and chronic lead poisoning but is most common in the chronic form. In chronic lead poisoning the erythrocytes are microcytic and hypochromic and reticulocytosis and basophilic stippling may be observed. However, basophilic stippling is non-specific and probably does not correlate well with levels of lead exposure. The basophilic stippling of erythrocytes is usually an indication of bone marrow response to anemia, although it can occur, rarely, in chronic lead poisoning. It may be related to the effects of lead on pyrimidine nucleotidase activity (60). The anemia in chronic lead poisoning is caused by two basic defects: a shortened erythrocyte lifespan and impairment of heme synthesis. Lead causes increased concentration of protoporphyrin by inhibiting heme synthetase, the enzyme which combines protoporphyrin and iron to form heme. The measurement of free erythrocyte porphyrin is considered to be a sensitive indicator of chronic lead poisoning in calves (61). It also causes inhibition of the enzyme-δ aminolevulinic acid dehydratase (ALA-D), resulting in a failure of utilization of δ-aminolevulinic acid which is excreted in increased quantities in the urine (26).

A number of factors affect the toxicity of a given dose of lead. Age and sex are two such factors and calcium phosphorus and sulfur content of the diet also affect lead assimilation (9), but the effect in field situations is not recorded.

Clinical findings

Cattle

Both acute and subacute syndromes occur in cattle, the former being more common in calves and the latter in adults. In the acute syndrome there is usually a sudden onset of signs and a short course of 12–24 hours so that many animals, especially those at pasture, are found dead without signs having been observed. Affected calves commence to stagger and show muscle tremor, particularly of the head and neck, with champing of the jaws and frothing at the mouth. There is snapping of the eyelids, rolling of the eyes and, in many cases, bellowing. Blindness and cervical, facial and auricular twitching are consistent clinical findings in acute lead poisoning of cattle (7). The animal collapses and intermittent tonic–clonic convulsions develop and may continue until death occurs. Pupillary dilatation, opisthotonus and muscle tremor are marked and persist between the convulsive episodes. There is hyperesthesia to touch and sound and the pulse and respiratory rates are increased. In some cases, particularly in adults, the cow remains standing and shows evidence of blindness and mania, charging into fences, attempting to climb walls and pressing strongly with the head against fixed objects. The general appearance of the animal is one of frenzy and on some occasions they will attack humans but the gait is stiff and jerky and progress is impeded. Death usually occurs during a convulsion and is due to respiratory failure.

In the subacute form the animal remains alive for 3–4 days. There is dullness, complete lack of appetite, blindness and some abnormality of gait including incoordination and staggering, and sometimes circling. The circling is intermittent and not always in the same direction. Muscle tremor and hyperesthesia are present as in the more acutely affected animals. Salivation, grinding of the teeth, and abdominal pain as evidenced by kicking at the belly are other common signs. Alimentary tract dysfunction is one of the most common abnormalities. Ruminal atony is accompanied by constipation in the early stages. Later a fetid diarrhea occurs in most cases. The animal presents a picture of extreme dullness, will not eat or drink, and stands immobile for very long periods. Death frequently occurs by misadventure, the animal walking blindly into a waterhole or being trapped in a fence or between trees. In other circumstances the animal becomes recumbent and dies quietly. In both the acute and subacute forms, the palpebral eye preservation reflex is absent or markedly diminished. This is a useful distinguishing feature from polioencephalomalacia in which this reflex is usually normal. Edema of the optic disc may be present but is not common.

In experimental lead poisoning in young milk-fed calves the latter first become depressed and develop hypoglossal paresis which interferes with sucking. Within the next 12–24 hours the calves become unsteady, develop a trunkal ataxia, exhibit muscular tremors of the head and forelimbs and finally convulsions, opisthotonus and die in respiratory failure during status epilepticus (57).

Sheep

Lead poisoning in sheep is usually manifested by a subacute syndrome similar to that seen in cattle. There is anorexia and an initial constipation followed by the passage of dark, foul-smelling feces. Weakness and ataxia follow, often with evidence of abdominal pain, but there is no excitement, tetany or convulsions. Polyuria occurs when the intake of lead is small but with large amounts there is oliguria.

Although ruminants are supposed to be resistant to chronic lead intoxication, two syndromes of posterior paresis have been described in young lambs in old lead-mining areas and tissue levels of lead are abnormally high in both instances. In both of the paretic syndromes there is impairment of the gait. In one it is caused by osteoporotic changes in the skeleton but in the other there is no suggestion of skeletal changes. In the osteoporotic disease the signs occur only in lambs 3–12 weeks of age and never in adults. There is stiffness of gait, lameness and posterior paralysis. Affected lambs are unthrifty and the bones, including the frontal bones, are very fragile. The paralysis is caused by lesions of the vertebrae, usually affecting one or more of the lumbar bones, and resulting in compression of the spinal cord. In the second form of the disease, gait abnormalities occur in the same lamb age group and are manifested initially by incomplete flexion of the limb joints so that the feet drag while walking. In a later stage the fetlocks are flexed, the extensor muscles paretic, and the lamb soon becomes recumbent. Recovery is common although many lambs die of intercurrent disease.

Chronic ingestion of metallic lead by pregnant sheep can cause abortion and transitory infertility (6).

Goats

Goats show little clinical evidence of fatal experimental poisoning by lead (29). Anorexia and fetid diarrhea are constant, with tenesmus and bloating in some animals.

Horses

Horses are not commonly affected by lead poisoning although chronic plumbism is sometimes seen, usually in the vicinity of lead mines and processing works (30). Some horses die without showing previous clinical illness. Where signs are apparent they are usually distinct and dramatic rather than subtle. In clinical cases inspiratory dyspnea caused by paralysis of the recurrent laryngeal nerve is the commonest syndrome (46). This may be accompanied by pharyngeal paralysis in which recurrent choke and regurgitation of food and water through the nostrils occur. Aspiration pneumonia may result after inhalation of ingesta through the paralyzed larynx. Paralysis of the lips occasionally accompanies the other signs. General muscle weakness and stiffness of the joints occur commonly and the coat is usually harsh and dry. When chronic poisoning with both lead and zinc occurs the signs in zinc poisoning predominate despite high lead levels in liver and kidney (31). In experimental chronic lead poisoning in horses, there is noisy breathing constantly, but no lesions in the pharynx or larynx. Recumbency and convulsions are characteristic signs (22).

When large amounts of lead are ingested by horses a syndrome similar to that of the subacute form in cattle occurs. There is complete anorexia, severe nervous depression, partial paralysis of the limbs followed in most cases by complete paralysis and recumbency. Mild to severe abdominal pain and clonic convulsions may also occur.

Pigs

Early signs include squealing as though in pain, mild diarrhea, grinding of the teeth and salivation. The disease is usually a prolonged one and listlessness, anorexia and loss of weight develop followed by muscle tremor, incoordination, partial or complete blindness, enlargement of the carpal joints and disinclination to stand on the front feet. Convulsive seizures occur in the terminal stages.

Subclinical lead poisoning
Because of the present preoccupation with environmental pollution the effects of the chronic low-level intake of lead have been examined and defined. In cattle at intake levels below those which cause clinical signs there are metabolic changes, and changes in blood characteristics accompanied by a decreased rate of growth (32). One of the fears is that continuous low level consumption by pregnant females will result in teratogenic effects in the newborn. Trials to detect this manifestation in ewes have shown no effect on their lambs (33). No detailed information is available about subclinical mercury and cadmium poisoning in animals, although these poisonings commonly accompany lead in natural circumstances (34).

Clinical pathology
In the living animal which has ingested lead the element can be detected in blood, feces, urine and milk. The estimation of blood levels is generally useful for determining the lead status of the animal and is used most frequently to support or refute a clinical diagnosis of lead poisoning. However, when used alone, blood lead concentrations do not permit evaluation of length of exposure, amount of lead deposition in the body or the effects of lead on physiological systems (5). Blood lead concentrations also fluctuate markedly after administration of lead and consequently the clinical importance of blood lead concentrations is often questionable and a diagnosis based on this single determinant is equivocal. Because of this, other indirect measurements of lead poisoning such as the levels of delta-aminolevulinic acid dehydratase (ALA-D) in blood are being used to supplement blood lead determinations (62). Blood lead concentration also has limited value for assessing the effectiveness of therapy for lead poisoning. Blood level concentrations may change rapidly during chelation therapy, often decreasing by 50% or more within 24 hours after initiation of treatment despite certain body tissues still containing high concentrations of lead. Thus the evaluation of biochemical indicators such as ALA-D may be useful.

Representative values of lead for normal and poisoned animals are summarized in Table 94.

An often successful maneuver when examining a patient for chronic lead poisoning, or for an acute incident which occurred some time before, and when blood and urine levels are low, is to measure the response in blood and urine of the animal to treatment with calcium versanate. The treatment extracts lead from depots in bones and causes a transitory rise in lead levels in body fluids.

Table 94. Lead levels in blood and feces of normal and poisoned animals (16, 36, 47).

Specimen	*Lead levels (ppm)* *Normal*	*Poisoned*
Whole blood (ruminants and horses)	0·05–0·25	More than 0·35 (deaths commence at 1·0)
Whole blood (pigs)	0·05–0·25	1·2
Feces (dry matter) (cattle)	1·5–35	Up to 1000
Pasture		350

Fecal levels of lead represent unabsorbed and excreted lead deriving from the bones, and are of limited value unless considered in conjunction with blood levels because ingested lead may have been in an insoluble form and harmless to the animal. When fecal levels are high it can be assumed that the lead has been ingested in the preceding 2–3 weeks but high blood levels may be maintained for months after ingestion. Thus high blood and low fecal levels indicate that the lead was taken in some weeks previously but high blood and high fecal levels suggest recent ingestion and significant absorption.

Urine levels are variable, rarely high (0·2–0·3 mg/kg), and although elevated urine levels are usually associated with high blood levels this relationship does not necessarily hold.

Because of the frequency with which lead appears in the environment as a pollutant there is often concern for the validity of the normal values for establishment of a diagnosis. In the average city polluted atmosphere it seems that lead intake will be significantly elevated (36). The lead content of hair of cattle and horses, and of the wool of sheep (37), is reported to be raised significantly in poisoned animals but hair is not routinely used in diagnosis of acute poisoning. However, the lead content of hair when cattle are exposed to longterm ingestion as a result of industrial contamination can reach as high as 88 mg/kg (in a clean environment comparable figures are of the order of 0.1 mg/kg) (38). There is likely to be a seasonal variation in deposition and intake of lead. Hair is also a valuable source of information on environmental pollution with cadmium, copper and zinc (39).

Indirect indicators of lead poisoning are also available. For example, the best method of detecting the presence of lead poisoning in its early stages, except in the horse, is the estimation of delta-aminolevulinic acid dehydratase (ALA-D) in the blood (26). At dietary intakes as low as 15 mg/kg of lead in cattle there are detectably lowered levels of ALA-D (19, 20). At the same time, the urinary levels of delta-aminolevulinic acid (ALA) are increased (20); delta-aminolevulinic acid dehydratase is important in the synthesis of heme and is probably the most sensitive enzyme in the heme pathway. Inhibition of the enzyme results in a block in the utilization of delta-ALA, a subsequent decline in heme synthesis and a marked increase in the urinary excretion of delta-ALA (26). In cattle, sheep and pigs affected with chronic lead poisoning the plasma levels of delta-ALA-D are decreased and the urinary levels of delta-ALA are increased before clinical signs are detectable (41). In sheep, erythrocyte delta-ALA-D is recommended as the most sensitive diagnostic test available (24). The disadvantages of the assay for blood delta-ALA-D include age-related variations particularly in calves; the methods used for analysis are not yet uniform and blood must be collected in polystyrene or polyethylene tubes rather than glass tubes and an anticoagulant other than EDTA must be used (5). The levels of erythrocyte delta-ALA-D increase in calves from birth to 10 weeks of age and age-matched controls should be evaluated simultaneously when conducting the test in calves under 6 months of age (62). In cattle under 1 year of age erythrocyte ALA-D values of less than 200 mmol of porphobilinogen (PBG)/ml of RBC/

hour should be suspected of having ingested lead. In this same age range values below 100/mmol would confirm ingestion of lead. In cattle equal to or less than 2 years of age values of RBC ALA-D of less than 100 mmol of PBG/ml of RBC/hour would indicate ingestion of lead (62). Severe inhibition of ALA-D occurs rapidly in calves given 1 mg of lead/kg body weight/day or 5 mg of lead/kg body weight/day. Inhibition of ALA-D will reach approximately 50% of preexposure levels when blood lead concentrations are above 0·5 mg/kg, and if the initial dose of lead increases blood lead concentration above 0·5 mg/kg the ALA-D becomes maximally depressed and remains so with continued exposure. The ALA-D is so sensitive to lead that it remains inhibited even after lead exposure has ceased. Following treatment with a chelating agent the blood lead levels will often decline giving a false indication of a positive treatment effect. If the ALA-D levels do not decrease following therapy it indicates that there is sufficient lead present to continue to depress the enzyme. In summary, the evaluation of ALA-D and blood lead concentrations together can assist in resolving diagnostic situations in which the blood lead concentration is in the questionable range of 0·25–0·35 mg/kg.

The levels of free erythrocyte zinc protoporphyrin increase in lead poisoning and this is indicative of the chronic metabolic effect of lead on the erythroid cells being released from bone marrow into the peripheral circulation (5). A mean value of 21·56 μg coproporphyrin/100 ml of erythrocytes has been determined (42). It may be of some value along with determinations of blood lead and ALA-D.

In chronic lead poisoning, hematological examination may reveal a normocytic, normochronic anemia in some, and although basophilic stippling does not occur often enough to be diagnostic, it is recorded in some experimental poisonings (20, 29). It is recorded as occurring in lead-exposed pigs (35) and a horse (40). In some, poikilocytosis and anicytosis were marked (20). The CSF is approximately normal with slightly elevated leukocyte numbers but no increase in protein or other biochemical components (50).

Necropsy findings

In most acute cases there are no gross lesions at necropsy. In cases of longer standing there may be some degree of abomasitis and enteritis, diffuse congestion of the lungs and degeneration of the liver and kidney. Epicardial hemorrhages are common. Congestion of meningeal and cerebral vessels may also be observed and hemorrhages may be present in the meninges. An increase in cerebrospinal fluid is often recorded but is of minor degree in most cases. In chronic cases gross lesions are recorded in cattle (25). These include cerebrocortical softening, cavitation and yellow discoloration with most severe lesions in the occipital lobes. Histological lesions were most severe at the tips of the gyri. Similar lesions were produced experimentally. Acid-fast inclusion bodies deep in the renal cortex have diagnostic significance (43). Examination of the contents of the reticulum in ruminants for particulate lead matter is essential. Flakes of paint, lumps of red lead or sheet lead usually accumulate in this site. Their absence is not remarkable especially if animals have licked fresh paint but their presence does give weight to the provisional diagnosis.

The submission of alimentary tract contents and tissues for analysis forms an important part of the diagnosis of lead poisoning but results must be interpreted with caution. In cattle 25 mg/kg of lead in wet kidney cortex is diagnostic and is a more reliable tissue for assay than liver which may contain 10–20 mg/kg wet matter. Levels of 4–7 mg/kg of lead have been found in the livers of horses dying of chronic lead poisoning but 25–250 mg/kg are more likely, and 40 mg/kg in the livers of affected pigs. Tissue lead levels in cattle from industrial areas are significantly higher (liver 0·23 mg/kg body weight, kidney 0·42 mg/kg) than in cattle from clear air zones (liver and kidney less than 0·1 mg/kg body weight) (45). Tissues which have been fixed in formalin are useful when they are the only tissues available (63).

Diagnosis

Other nervous diseases of cattle which may require differentiation from lead poisoning are hypovitaminosis A, hypomagnesemic tetany, nervous acetonemia, tetanus, poisoning due to arsenic, mercury or *Claviceps paspali*, brain abscess, cerebral edema and hemorrhage, and the encephalitides and encephalomalacias. The differential diagnosis of brain dysfunction and lead poisoning in cattle is summarized in Table 95.

In all cases much importance must be attached to the possibility of access to lead and the environmental circumstances which may arouse suspicion of other poisonings or errors in management. Estimation of the lead content of blood and feces should be carried out at the earliest opportunity and tissues from necropsy specimens submitted for analysis.

The chronic forms of lead poisoning in lambs require to be differentiated from other forms of posterior paralysis, particularly enzootic ataxia. Polyarthritis due to bacterial infection and enzootic muscular dystrophy may cause lameness and paresis similar in many ways to the paralysis of these forms of lead poisoning, but may be distinguished clinically by careful examination of the joints and skeletal muscles.

Treatment

Acute lead poisoning of cattle is almost always fatal because of the nature of the material ingested and the susceptibility of members of this species. Sedation by intravenous injection of anesthetic doses of pentobarbital sodium in calves and chloral hydrate in adults temporarily relieves the convulsions. Rumenotomy is often attempted but is seldom satisfactory because of the difficulty of removing particulate material from the recesses of the reticular mucosa. Oral dosing with small amounts of magnesium sulfate is often recommended on the grounds that soluble lead salts will be precipitated as the insoluble sulfate. The method is limited in value because the lead is often present in large quantities and in the form of particles which are only slowly dissolved.

Calcium versenate (calcium disodium ethylenedia-

Table 95. Differential diagnosis of diseases of cattle with clinical findings referable to brain dysfunction.

Disease	*Epidemiology*	*Clinical findings*	*Clinical pathology and pathology*	*Response to treatment*
Lead poisoning	All ages. Calves and cows on pasture with access to dumps. Case mortality rate high	*Acute in calves*: *blindness*, 'chewing gum' champing of jaws, convulsions, charging, rapid death. *Subacute in adults: blindness*, stupor, head-pressing, grinding teeth, rumen static, protozoa dead	Blood and tissues for lead. Malacia in brain microscopically	Will respond favorably to treatment in early stages if not too severe but most cases do not return to normal
Polioencephalomalacia	Grain-fed rapidly growing feedlot cattle. Occasionally on pasture. Rare over 2 years. Outbreaks occur	Sudden onset, blindness, twitching of head and ears, head-pressing, opisthotonus, nystagmus, strabismus, rumen clinically normal, CSF pressure increased	Blood biochemistry (see text). Brain for histopathology	Responds to thiamin in early stages
Hypovitaminosis A	Calves 6–8 months of age off dry pasture (CSF form). Young bulls and steers fed deficient ration for several months (ocular form)	*CSF form*: sudden onset; syncope and convulsions followed by recovery, eyesight usually normal, pupils normal. Nyctalopia. CSF pressure increased *Ocular form*: complete blindness, pupils dilated and fixed, marked disk edema. Syncope and convulsions will occur too. Preceded by nyctalopia	Plasma and liver vitamin A. Optic nerve constriction. Squamous cell metaplasia of parotid ducts	*CSF form*: recover in 48 hours following treatment *Ocular form*: will not recover because of optic nerve degeneration
Haemophilus meningoencephalitis (thromboembolic meningoencephalitis)	Feedlot cattle (8–12 months), outbreaks, preceded by respiratory disease in group. High mortality if not treated early	Found down, ataxic, not usually blind, fundic lesions, irritation signs uncommon, weakness and paresis common, synovitis, laryngitis, pleuritis, *fever common*. May die in 8–10 hours	Neutrophilia. CSF contains neutrophils. Typical gross lesions in brain	Respond favorably to antibiotics if treated early. Later, mortality high
Listeria meningoencephalitis	Sporadic. Fed silage. Yearlings and adults	Unilateral facial paralysis, deviation of head and neck, mild fever, endophthalmitis, may be recumbent	CSF for cells. Brain for histopathology	Gradual recovery may occur with early treatment. Residual signs in survivors common
Nervous signs with coccidiosis (see text)	In 20% of young cattle affected with dysentery due to coccidiosis. Mortality high	Tonic–clonic convulsions, normal eyesight, sometimes hyperesthetic, normal temperature, dysentery, may live for 2–4 days	Feces for oocysts. Not all have oocysts. Disease may not be coccidiosis	Unfavorable response to treatment. Most die
Rabies	Cattle exposed to wildlife, one or more affected, all ages, incubation 3 weeks to few months	Quiet and dull (dumb form) or excitable and easily annoyed (furious form). Bellowing, yawning, drooling saliva, eyesight normal, tenesmus, ascending paralysis beginning with *anesthesia over tail head*, progressive course, die in 4–6 days, *usually no gross muscular tremors or convulsions*, mild fever early	Hemogram normal. Brain for laboratory diagnosis	Nil
Pseudorabies	Not common except when pigs run together with and bite cattle	Intense, local pruritus, excitement, bellowing, convulsions, paralysis, death 2–3 days	Tissues for injection into rabbit.	Nil

Table 95 (cont.)

Disease	*Epidemiology*	*Clinical findings*	*Clinical pathology and pathology*	*Response to treatment*
Hypomagnesemic tetany (lactation tetany)	Lactating dairy cows on lush pasture, late pregnant beef cows, cold, windy weather in spring. May be precipitated by long transportation or deprivation of feed and water. Outbreaks occur. Seen in yearlings too. Case mortality can be high	*Acute*: sudden onset of irritability, hyperesthesia; convulsions, recumbency, loud heart sounds, tachycardia, polypnea *Subacute*: gradual onset (2–4 days), hyperirritable, difficult to handle, stilted gait, falling, stumbling, sudden movement may precipitate convulsion	Serum magnesium levels low	Responds to magnesium sulfate early
Nervous acetonemia	2–6 weeks postpartum. High-producing cow. Single animal	Sudden onset, bizarre mental behavior, chewing, licking bellowing, hyperesthesia, sweating	Ketonuria, hypoglycemia	Responds to glucose parenterally and/or propylene glycol orally
Bovine Bonkers (Bovine hysteria)	Mature cattle and calves consuming ammoniated feeds (lucerne hay, bromegrass hay, fescue hay, wheat hay, maize stalks or silage). May also occur when animals have access to molasses–urea–protein blocks. Toxic agent may be substituted imidazole formed by combination of soluble carbohydrates and ammonia. Usually occurs when high quality forage treated with ammonia at rate of more than 3% dry matter by weight. Can occur in calves nursing cows fed ammoniated feedstuffs	Periodic episodes of hyperexcitability, bellowing, running, charging, circling, convulsions, weaving, episodes last 30 sec and may recurr every 5–10 min. Some die. Most recover following removal of feed	Information not available	Recover spontaneously following removal of feed source
Hepatic encephalopathy (i.e. ragwort poisoning)	Cattle with access to plants containing pyrrolizidine alkaloids. Many cattle may be affected	Loss of body weight, gradual onset of aggressive behavior, ataxia, muscular tremors, recumbency, convulsions, tenesmus and bellowing	Hyperbilirubinemia, decreased excretion of BSP, liver lesions	No treatment
Brain abscess	Sporadic, young cattle (6 months to 2 years of age) may have history of previous infections	Localizing signs, rotation or deviation head and neck, loss of equilibrium, circling, mild fever, may be blind in one eye, nystagmus one eye	Neutrophilia, neutrophils in CSF	Unfavorable response to therapy
Enterotoxemia due to *Clostridium perfringens* type D	Calves 2–4 months of age sucking high producing cows grazing on lush pasture. Outbreaks	*Peracute*: found dead *Acute*: bellowing, mania, convulsions, blindness, death in 1–2 hours *Subacute*: dull, depressed, blind	Hyperglycemia (150–200 mg/dl), glycosuria marked. Smear intestinal contents. Recover toxin (mouse protection tests)	Hyperimmune serum. Most die. Vaccination effective.
Whole milk hypomagnesemic tetany of calves	Calves 2–4 months of age on whole milk. Also in calves on milk replacers, concentrates and hay and occasionally in nursing calves on pasture	Sudden alertness, hyperesthesia, head-shaking, opisthotonus, muscular tremors, frothing at mouth, convulsions, heart rate 200–250/minute, die or recover from convulsion	Serum magnesium levels usually below 0·8 mg/dl	Magnesium sulfate intravenously gives good response, must follow up daily because of previous depletion of bone reserves

Table 95 (cont.)

Disease	*Epidemiology*	*Clinical findings*	*Clinical pathology and pathology*	*Response to treatment*
Sporadic bovine encephalomyelitis (Buss disease)	Young calves and yearlings, occasionally adults	Depression, ocular and nasal discharge, high fever, weakness, knuckling, stumbling, falling recumbency and opisthotonus, dyspnea, pleuritis	Leukopenia, neutropenia and lymphopenia. Serology for diagnosis	Responds to tetracyclines when treated early
Traumatic injury to brain	Not common. Single animal. May have history of trauma	Sudden loss of consciousness, dilated and fixed pupils, reflexes absent or sluggish. Die in few hours or improve up to certain point and remain static with residual deficits for several days	Cerebral edema, hemorrhage. Examine CSF	Nil
Mercury poisoning	Not common. Access to source of mercury	Incoordination, blindness, headpressing, muscular tremors, prolonged recumbency	Mercury in feces and urine and tissues. Histological changes in brain	Usually not treated

NB Congenital and acquired defects of newborn calves are not included. Diseases are not included in which significant signs of brain dysfunction occur but in which the main clinical abnormality relates to some other system. Some of these are arsenic poisoning (severe diarrhea), organophosphate poisoning (severe dyspnea, pupillary constriction), bovine malignant catarrh (mucosal erosions, severe diarrhea), severe anoxic anemia, e.g., any acute pneumonia, terminal bloat. One exception included in this table is the nervous form of coccidiosis.

mine tetra-acetate) has been used successfully in cases of lead poisoning produced experimentally in calves and in natural cases in cattle. A 12·5% solution should be used for intravenous injection but solutions of this strength given subcutaneously cause local pain and a more dilute solution (1–2% in 5% dextrose) is recommended. The optimum treatment is infusion intravenously by continuous drip to deliver 110–220 mg/kg over 12 hours or two rapid intravenous injections 6 hours apart and each of 110 mg/kg.

Calcium versanate removes lead directly from bone sensitive sites in bone and not from parenchymatous organs because cell membranes form a barrier to the therapeutic removal of intracellular lead. The lead is removed from soft tissues by equilibration with bone. The process takes time and thus necessitates multiple treatment. Thus it is recommended that calcium versanate be given on alternate days to allow redistribution of lead from soft tissues to available bone sites (47, 64). An increase in the heart and respiratory rates and the development of muscle tremors during injection indicates a toxic reaction but can be avoided by slow administration. Recovery may take 5–15 days and parenteral or stomach tube alimentation may be required. Blindness may persist for several days after general recovery and may continue indefinitely. Dramatic improvement has also been reported in cases of chronic lead poisoning in horses after the use of calcium versanate.

A recent development has been the observation that the subcutaneous administration of thiamin hydrochloride reduces the deposition of lead in most tissues especially liver, kidney and brain of experimentally poisoned calves (65). Thiamin also decreased the deposition of lead in both the central and peripheral nervous systems. Thiamin hydrochloride was given at the rate of 2 mg/kg body weight subcutaneously daily. The lead concentrations in liver, kidney, and blood from thiamin-treated calves remained below the levels considered diagnostic, while the lead concentrations in the same tissues from calves dosed only with lead were within those considered diagnostic of lead poisoning. However, the levels of erythrocyte delta-aminolevulinic acid dehydratase (ALA-D) activity were decreased by 70% from pretreatment levels which indicated that thiamin had no protective effect on the ability of lead to inhibit the enzyme. But thiamin appeared to decrease tissue accumulation of lead.

Control

Animals should be prevented from having access to lead paint. If the interior of barns or pens are to be painted care should be taken to avoid the use of a lead-bearing paint. Chewing of foreign objects by cattle and sheep may be minimized by appropriate feeding practices. Practical antidotes to poisoning by environmental pollution have yet to be defined. However, the daily feeding of sodium sulfate to lambs appears to have been effective (48) and the addition of a high level of calcium in the diet also appears to be preventive in pigs (49). When pasture contamination has occurred it is recommended that livestock be removed, forage cut and removed and stubble burned (18).

REVIEW LITERATURE

Aronson, A. L. (1978) Outbreaks of plumbism in animals associated with industrial lead operations. In: *Toxicity of Heavy Metals in the Environment*, Pt. 1, ed. F. W. Oehme, pp. 173–177. New York: Marcel Dekker.

Neathery, M. W. & Miller, W. J. (1975) Metabolism and toxicity of cadmium, mercury and lead in animals. A review. *J. dairy Sci.*, *58*, 1767.

Osweiler, G. D. et al. (1978) Epidemiology of lead poisoning in animals In: *Toxicity of Heavy Metals in the Environment*, Pt. 1, ed. F. W. Oehme, pp. 143–171. New York: Marcel Dekker.

REFERENCES

(1) Priester, W. A. & Hayes, H. M. (1974) *J. Am. vet. med. Assoc.*, *35*, 567.
(2) Aronson, A. L. (1972) *Am. J. vet. Res.*, *33*, 627.
(3) Schmidt, N. et al. (1971) *Arch. envir. Hlth*, *23*, 185.
(4) Blakeley, B. R. & Brockman, R. P. (1976) *Can. vet. J.*, *17*, 16.
(5) Bratton, G. R. & Zumdzki, J. (1984) *Vet. hum. Toxicol.*, *26*, 387.
(6) Sharma, R. M. & Buck, W. B. (1976) *Vet. Toxicol.*, *18*, 186.
(7) Osweiler, G. D. et al. (1973) *Clin. Toxicol.*, *6*, 367.
(8) Osweiler, G. D. & Ruhr, L. P. (1978) *Am. J. vet. med. Assoc.*, *172*, 498.
(9) Quarterman, J. et al. (1977) *J. comp. Pathol.*, *87*, 405.
(10) Hapke, H. G. & Abel, J. (1978) *Tierärztl. Wochenschr.*, *85*, 288.
(11) Kopp, C. (1974) *Tierärztl. Umschau*, *29*, 496, 500, 565, 568.
(12) Lynch, G. P. et al. (1976) *J. anim. Sci.*, *42*, 410.
(13) Dinius, D. A. et al. (1973) *J. anim. Sci.*, *37*, 169.
(14) Prior, M. G. (1976) *Can. J. comp. Med.*, *40*, 9.
(15) Edwards, W. C. et al. (1976) *Vet. Toxicol.*, *18*, 70.
(16) Buck, W. B. (1975) *J. Am. vet. med. Assoc.*, *166*, 222.
(17) Dollahite, J. W. et al. (1975) *SW Vet.*, *28*, 40.
(18) Edwards, W. C. & Clay, B. R. (1977) *Vet. hum. Toxicol.*, *19*, 247.
(19) Hapke, H. J. & Prigge, E. (1973) *Berl. Münch. Tierärztl. Wochenschr.*, *86*, 410.
(20) Kelliher, D. J. et al. (1973) *Irish J. agric. Res.*, *12*, 61.
(21) Carson, T. L. et al. (1973) *Clin. Toxicol.*, *6*, 389.
(22) Dollahite, J. W. et al. (1978) *Am. J. vet. Res.*, *39*, 961.
(23) Arfert, H. & Harlos, H. (1977) *Zeitschr. Ges. Hyg.*, *23*, 455.
(24) Roltov, C. E. et al. (1978) *Aust. vet. J.*, *54*, 394.
(25) Wells, G. A. H. et al. (1976) *Neuropathol. appl. Neurobiol.*, *2*, 175.
(26) Goyer, R. A. & Rhyne, B. C. (1973) *Int. Rev. exp. Pathol.*, *12*, 1.
(27) Wright, F. C. et al. (1976) *Bull. envir. Contam. Toxicol.*, *16*, 156.
(28) Ward, N. I. et al. (1978) *Bull. envir. Contam. Toxicol.*, *20*, 44.
(29) Davis, J. W. et al. (1976) *Cornell Vet.*, *66*, 490.
(30) Knight, H. D. & Burau, R. G. (1973) *J. Am. vet. med. Assoc.*, *162*, 781.
(31) Willoughby, R. A. et al. (1972) *Vet. Rec.*, *91*, 382.
(32) Lynch, G. P. et al. (1976) *J. dairy Sci.*, *59*, 1490.
(33) McLain, R. M. & Becker, B. A. (1975) *Toxicol. appl. Pharmacol.*, *31*, 72.
(34) Neathery, M. W. & Miller, W. J. (1975) *J. dairy Sci.*, *58*, 1767.
(35) Lassen, E. D. & Buck, W. B. (1979) *Am. J. vet. Res.*, *40*, 1359.
(36) Willoughby, R. A. & Brown, G. (1971) *Can. vet. J.*, *12*, 165.
(37) Ward, N. I. & Brooks, R. R. (1979) *Bull. envir. Contam. Toxicol.*, *21*, 403.
(38) Sterner, W. (1972) *Arch. Lebensmittelhyg.*, *23*, 209.
(39) Dorn, C. R. et al. (1974) *Bull. envir. Contam. Toxicol.*, *12*, 626.
(40) Wilson, G. L. et al. (1979) *J. equ. med. Surg.*, *3*, 386.
(41) Fassberder, C. P. (1976) *Zentralbl. VetMed.*, *23A*, 283.
(42) Rhur, L. P. (1984) *Vet. hum. Toxicol.*, *26*, 105.
(43) Thomson, R. G. (1972) *Can. vet. J.*, *13*, 88.
(44) Sharma, R. P. & Street, J. C. (1980) *J. Am. vet. med. Assoc.*, *177*, 149.
(45) Grahwit, G. (1972) *Arch. Lebensmittelhyg.*, *23*, 213.
(46) Voros, K. et al. (1980) *Magy Allatorv. Lap.*, *35*, 253.
(47) Hammond, P. B. & Sorenson, D. K. (1957) *J. Am. vet. med. Assoc.*, *130*, 23.
(48) Morrison, J. N. et al. (1975) *Proc. Nutr. Soc.*, *34*, 77A.
(49) Hsu, F. S. et al. (1975) *J. Nutr.*, *105*, 112.
(50) Clausen, H. H. et al. (1980) *Münch. Tierärztl. Wochenschr.*, *93*, 437.
(51) Bratton, G. R. et al. (1981) *Toxicol. appl. Pharmacol.*, *59*, 164.
(52) Blakley, B. R. (1984) *Can. vet. J.*, *25*, 17.
(53) Blakley, B. R. (1984) *Vet. hum. Toxicol.*, *26*, 505.
(54) Clausen, B. et al. (1981) *Nord. VetMed.*, *33*, 65.
(55) Frape, D. L. & Pringle, J. D. (1984) *Vet. Rec.*, *114*, 615.
(56) Burrows, G. E. & Borchard, R. E. (1982) *Am. J. vet. Res.*, *43*, 2129.
(57) Zmudzki, J. et al. (1983) *Bull. envir. Contam. Toxicol.*, *30*, 4345.
(58) Zmudzki, J. et al. (1984) *Toxicol. appl. Pharmacol.*, *76*, 490.
(59) Zmudzki, J. et al. (1986) *Bull. envir. Contam. Toxicol.*, *36*, 356.
(60) George, J. W. & Duncan, J. R. (1982) *Am. J. vet. Res.*, *43*, 17.
(61) George, J. W. & Duncan, J. R. (1981) *Am. J. vet. Res.*, *42*, 1630.
(62) Bratton, G. R. et al. (1986) *Am. J. vet. Res.*, *47*, 2068.
(63) Bratton, G. R. et al. (1985) *Vet. hum. Toxicol.*, *27*, 7.
(64) Kowalczyk, D. F. (1984) *J. Am. vet. med. Assoc.*, *184*, 858.
(65) Bratton, G. R. et al. (1981) *Toxicol. appl. Pharmacol.*, *59*, 164.

Arsenic poisoning

Etiology

Arsenic poisoning usually occurs after ingestion of the toxic substance but percutaneous absorption can occur especially if the skin is abraded or hyperemic and percutaneous toxic dose is much lower than (probably one-tenth of) the oral toxic dose. The toxicity of arsenic compounds varies widely with their solubility and particle size. Soluble salts are highly poisonous; arsenic trioxide and sodium arsenate are much less soluble and thus less toxic than sodium arsenite. Organic arsenicals are quite rapidly absorbed but liberate their arsenic slowly.

Toxic doses vary with the animal species (1). The toxic doses (mg/kg body weight) of sodium arsenite are: horse 6·5, cattle 7·5, sheep 11 and pig 2. Toxic doses of arsenic trioxide are 7·5–11 mg/kg body weight for pigs and 33–55 mg/kg body weight for horses, cattle and sheep.

Epidemiology

Arsenic is one of the more common causes of poisoning in livestock but the incidence varies widely with farm practices and industrial undertakings which cause exposure to the poison. The morbidity rate is variable but the mortality rate usually approximates 100% except for poisoning by organic compounds in which recovery is more usual.

In cases of poisoning the commonest source of arsenic is in fluids used for dipping and spraying of animals to control ectoparasites. Animals may swallow the solution while in the dip or in the draining yards after dipping. Animals that are not allowed to drain completely may contaminate the pasture, and faulty disposal of drainage from yards and dips may contaminate the environment. Opened containers of dipping solutions or powders may provide a source for accidental contamination of feed or for mistaken application to the skin (20). An appreciable amount of arsenic is absorbed through the skin after dipping in sodium arsenite solution in both cattle and sheep. The absorption is increased if the animals are dipped when hot, if the fleece is long, if they are crowded too tightly in draining yards or driven too soon after dipping. However, in most outbreaks of poisoning some ingestion appears to occur and supplements the cutaneous absorption. There is some danger in dipping rams at mating time when erythema of the skin of the thighs and scrotum is present. Dipping immediately after shearing is also a predisposing cause and jetting at high pressure or with excessively strong solutions may also cause increased absorption. Most arsenical dipping and jetting solutions contain sodium arsenite.

Arsenical weed killers including sodium arsenite, arsenic pentoxide and monosodium acid methanearsonate sprays used to kill potato haulms prior to mechanical harvesting and containing sodium or potassium arsenite, and insecticidal sprays used in orchards, particularly lead arsenate, are less common causes of poisoning (1). Pasture may also be contaminated by use of calcium arsenate for the treatment of Colorado beetle grubs (16). In most instances poisoning occurs when animals accidentally gain access to recently sprayed areas although drifting of windblown spray may result in accidental contamination of pasture. Grass clippings from lawn areas treated with arsenical herbicides 6 months earlier have been shown to carry 15 000 mg/kg arsenic (2). Ash from timber treated with arsenicals may be toxic for several months. With lead arsenate the major effects are usually ascribed to the effects of the lead but this does not always appear to be so. In several outbreaks of lead arsenate poisoning in cattle the clinical signs were primarily those of arsenic poisoning and the concentration of arsenic in tissues was greater than that of lead (3). Insect baits often contain Paris green (cupric acetoarsenite) mixed with bran and when these are laid over large areas of land in an attempt to control grasshopper plagues they constitute a major hazard to livestock. Arsenical preparations used as wood preservatives may cause poisoning when used in wooden calf pens. One of the less obvious sources of arsenic poisoning is the licking of ashes from burned timber fence posts which have been treated with arsenic (17). Cattle in particular have a predilection for ash. Arsenic is indestructible and adds a salty taste to contaminated materials.

Some metal-bearing ore deposits including iron, gold and copper ores (18) contain large quantities of arsenic which may be carried off in the fumes from smelters and contaminate surrounding pastures and drinking water supplies. Arsenic found in lake weed (including water hyacinths) in New Zealand is thought to be of geothermal origin. When fed continuously to sheep to provide a daily intake of 200 mg/kg of arsenic no apparent disease was produced (4).

Arsenic is still used therapeutically and overdosing may occur. Inorganic preparations are little used now although lead arsenate still has some devotees as an anthelmintic. At 88 mg/kg body weight a cumulative toxicity occurs after 7 doses at monthly intervals in sheep (5). Organic arsenicals, particularly arsanilic acid and sodium arsanilate, are used both as feed additives and in the control and treatment of vibrionic dysentery in animals, and as antidotes to selenium poisoning. Phenylarsonic acid is also used, but has a different toxicity mechanism from the arsanilates (19). Overdosage can accidentally occur when the administration is carried on for too long or when there is an error in mixing a batch of feed. In one outbreak in pigs the feed contained 450–650 mg/kg of arsenic. In another outbreak long-term feeding of feed containing 375 mg/kg of arsanilic acid caused poisoning (7). Experimentally the disease is reproduced by feeding feed containing 611 mg/kg or more. The toxicity of feed containing arsanilic acid depends to a certain extent on the intake of drinking water but moderate water restriction does not make normal dose rates dangerous (9). Experimentally arsanilic acid at concentrations of 0·25% produces clinical signs in pigs and levels of 0·2–0·4% cause deaths in lambs. The feeding of the growth promotant 3-nitro-4-hydroxyphenylarsonic acid at five times the recommended dose rate causes severe toxic signs in pigs (8).

Another organic arsenical compound used in the control of swine dysentery is 3-nitro-4-hydroxyphenyl arsonic acid in pigs (8, 21). The clinical signs caused by poisoning with this substance are quite different from those caused by arsanilic acid and occur only with exercise. There is a sudden onset of muscle tremor, incoordination and agitation, some pigs putting their nose to the ground for support. Screaming is a feature in some. When the pigs lie down all the signs disappear, but they recur if the pig gets up. Recovery is usual if the compound is withdrawn and there are no gross lesions at necropsy.

Arsenic is, for the most part, excreted rapidly after absorption, chiefly in the urine. After the ingestion of non-toxic amounts by the cow there is no detectable excretion in the milk. When much larger doses are taken arsenic may be excreted in the milk, as well as urine and feces, but the concentration is quite low (1). The principal interest with arsenic and its possible entry into the human food chain is the contamination of tissues when pigs are fed arsanilic acid. The biological half-life of arsenic taken this way is 4·2 days in liver, 5·7 days in kidney and 15 days in muscle. In pigs fed arsanilic acid at 200 mg/kg in the feed the level of arsenic in muscle is still more than the admissible level of 0·1 mg/kg 18 days after withdrawal (6). The usual recommendation is to withdraw arsanilic acid 5–7 days before slaughter (9). This is adequate at normal dose levels.

Pathogenesis

Arsenic is a general tissue poison and exerts its toxic effect by combining with and inactivating the sulfhydryl groups in tissue enzymes. Trivalent arsenicals are most toxic because of their greater affinity for these sulfhydryl groupings. The efficiency of sulfur-containing compounds including BAL (dimercaptopropranol) as antidotes depends on the ability of these compounds to compete with sulfur-containing compounds of enzyme systems for the available arsenic. Although all tissues are affected, deposition and toxic effects are greatest in those tissues which are rich in these oxidation systems. Thus alimentary tract wall, liver, kidney, spleen and lung are most susceptible. When these organs are affected there is a general depression of metabolic activity. The alimentary tract lesion is the one which produces the most obvious clinical signs. The primary effect in this site is extensive damage to capillaries causing increased permeability and exudation of serum into tissue spaces. The mucosa is lifted from the underlying muscle coat and is shed with the resulting loss of large quantities of fluid from the body. A direct local effect of arsenic on alimentary tract mucosa is not likely to be important as indicated by the observation that the parenteral injection of arsenic produces lesions in the gut wall which are identical with those caused by the ingestion of arsenic. Moreover arsenic does not precipitate protein and does not thereby limit its own absorption, and there is a considerable timelag after ingestion, whereas corrosive substances produce lesions immediately.

When arsenic is absorbed from the skin it may cause local necrosis without systemic signs if the peripheral circulation is poor or the concentration of arsenic is excessively high, but if the cutaneous circulation is good the arsenic is quickly carried away and causes a systemic disease without skin necrosis. The chronic toxicity of arsenic at low levels of intake is due to its accumulation in particular organs especially the liver, kidney and alimentary tract wall. The epidermis, spleen and lung also have a special affinity for arsenic. Organic arsenicals appear to have a particular affinity for nervous tissue and cause only nervous signs, the characteristic sign of blindness being caused by atrophy of the optic nerve (10).

Clinical findings

In acute arsenic poisoning caused by the ingestion of large amounts of inorganic arsenic there is a severe gastroenteritis. Clinical signs do not appear until some time after the arsenic has been ingested, the time varying with the fullness of the stomach at the time of ingestion. There may be a delay of 20–50 hours in ruminants. Distress develops suddenly, the animal showing severe abdominal pain, restlessness, groaning, an increased respiratory rate, salivation, grinding of the teeth and vomiting, even in cattle. There is usually complete ruminal atony but a fluid and fetid diarrhea develops especially in the late stages. The heart rate is greatly increased and the pulse small in amplitude. Many animals, especially cattle and sheep, show little except depression and prostration and die before signs of enteritis develop. There may be a fluid sound in the abdomen if the animal is shaken. Death occurs 3–4 hours after commencement of the illness and is usually preceded by clonic convulsions and diarrhea. Additional signs in horses include marked congestion of the mucosae and a very sudden onset of severe colic which passes off in a few hours in horses which survive. Severe diarrhea may be followed by a period of complete stasis of the alimentary tract with diarrhea recurring just before death.

In less severe cases the course may extend over 2–7 days. The emphasis clinically is still on gastroenteritis manifested by vomiting in occasional animals, diarrhea and sometimes dysentery, complete anorexia, absence of gut sounds, severe thirst and dehydration, and evidence of peripheral circulatory failure as indicated by a rapid heart rate and a rapid small pulse. Abdominal pain is evident and affected animals are stiff and reluctant to move. Nervous signs including muscle tremor and incoordination, and clonic convulsions occur quite commonly and terminally there is always coma.

In chronic cases the most commonly observed abnormalities are unthriftiness, poor growth, a dry, staring coat which is easily shed, and loss of vigor and spirit. The appetite is capricious, and unexplained bouts of indigestion occur. Reddening of the conjunctiva and visible mucosae is common and there may be edema of the eyelids and conjunctivitis. Erythema of the buccal mucosa may be accompanied by ulceration which may extend to the muzzle. The milk yield in dairy cattle is seriously reduced and abortions and stillbirths may occur. When local skin lesions are the only manifestation there is an initial hyperemia followed by necrosis and sloughing of the skin. The lesions are indolent and extremely slow to heal.

In chronic poisoning in swine and lambs resulting from overdosing with arsanilic acid the clinical signs are restricted to the nervous system. In one outbreak clinical signs of incoordination and blindness did not appear until 7 days after the contaminated diet was first fed. Consciousness, body temperature and appetite were unaffected. The signs became gradually more severe over a period of 4 days but disappeared within a few days after the feed was changed. Some pigs remained permanently blind. In the experimental disease the clinical signs are tremor of the head, incoordination, blindness, ataxia and paresis. Naturally occurring and experimental cases of arsanilic acid poisoning in pigs caused by feeding a ration containing 8000 mg/kg of arsanilic acid recovered completely provided the ration was withdrawn as soon as signs appeared (11). Rations containing 1000 mg/kg and fed to pigs over longer periods caused similar signs which did not disappear when the medication was stopped (12).

Clinical pathology

Arsenic can be detected in the urine, feces and milk for periods of up to about 10 days beginning shortly after the toxic material is ingested. The rate of excretion is faster with organic compounds than with inorganic arsenic and urine levels may be back to normal in 5 days (14). The most satisfactory material for laboratory examination from a living animal is a large volume (about 1 liter) of urine in which arsenic levels may be as high as 16 mg/kg (1). Levels in milk are low. Normal levels of up to 0·25 mg/kg in cows' milk may be elevated to 0·34–0·47 mg/kg in cases of acute poisoning and to 0·8–1·5 mg/kg in the milk of normal cows which graze arsenic-contaminated pasture for long periods. Deposition in the hair occurs and the arsenic persists there until the hair is shed making possible the detection of prior arsenic ingestion in the absence of arsenic from the blood and feces. The hair of animals not exposed to arsenic should contain less than 0·5 mg/kg but that of normal animals may contain as much as 5–10 mg/kg. Estimations of the amount of arsenic present in suspected materials should be carried out, but if there is delay in sampling of herbage after a contaminating incident has occurred, the concentration of soluble compounds may be greatly decreased by leaching.

Arsanilic acid has specific clinicopathological effects when fed to pigs. There is an increase in blood urea nitrogen, alkaline phosphatase and gamma-glutamyl transpeptidase, all being increased (9).

Necropsy findings

In acute and subacute cases there is pronounced hyperemia and patchy submucosal hemorrhage in the stomach, duodenum and cecum. In ruminants the forestomachs are unaffected but typical lesions are present in the abomasum. The gut contents are very fluid, and contain much mucus and shreds of mucosa. Profuse subendocardial hemorrhages are common and ulceration of gallbladder mucosa is often observed in sheep. Macroscopic lesions may be minimal in cases which die after a very short course. Histologically there are severe degenerative lesions in the liver, kidney, myocardium and adrenal glands. Severe intravascular hemolysis has been observed in sheep. In chronic cases the gastroenteritis is not severe but there may be ulceration of the mucosa. Fatty degeneration of the liver and kidneys is characteristic.

The liver is the best source of arsenic and levels of over 10–15 mg/kg wet matter of arsenic trioxide in kidney or liver are considered to be diagnostic of arsenic poisoning. However, it is probable that many animals die of arsenic poisoning when their hepatic levels are much lower than this. Maximum concentrations of arsenic in tissues occur about 8 hours after ingestion and animals which survive for 2–3 days may have levels as low as 3 mg/kg; and conversely normal animals which are dipped routinely in arsenical dips may have hepatic levels of the element as high as 8 mg/kg. The concentration in ingesta varies widely but is reported to average about 36 mg/kg (13).

Animals poisoned with organic arsenicals show no significant gross pathological changes although a distended urinary bladder has been noted as a frequent occurrence in pigs. Histologically degeneration of the optic nerves and tracts and peripheral nerves is apparent. The animals maintain tissue levels of arsenic for longer periods and although the levels fall rapidly during the first 7 days after feeding of the arsenic ceases, normal levels are not reached until a further 7 days. Levels of about 6 mg/kg arsenic trioxide on a fresh, wet-matter basis indicate poisonous levels of intake. A part of the lower alimentary tract including contents, and in chronic cases hair, should also be submitted for analysis. Because the stomach and intestinal wall appear to attain maximum concentrations of arsenic most rapidly after poisoning, the use of these tissues for quantitative assay has been recommended. Levels of 1–3 mg/kg are obtained in cattle dying from arsenic poisoning after percutaneous ingestion and levels of over 10 mg/kg in cattle which ingest arsenical dip. In cases of poisoning with phenyl arsonic acid where there has been exposure to the compound for 2–3 weeks (19), demyelination can be detected in peripheral nerves sectioned longitudinally.

Diagnosis

Arsenic poisoning presents a clinical syndrome of gastroenteritis with minor signs of nervous system involvement. This combination is not common in other diseases. Lead poisoning has some similarity but the emphasis is on nervous system signs with gastroenteritis an inconstant accompaniment. Bovine malignant catarrh develops in somewhat the same manner especially in the alimentary tract form but there are diagnostic lesions in the eyes and buccal mucosa. Mucosal disease is also characterized by erosions in the buccal and nasal mucosae. Of the bacterial enteritides salmonellosis is often confused with arsenic poisoning especially when the disease is seen in the later stages and the fever has subsided. There are several miscellaneous poisonous plants which cause nervous signs and gastroenteritis.

Chronic inorganic arsenical poisoning causes a syndrome not unlike that caused by inanition and internal parasitism and suspicion will probably only be aroused when a mining or smelting undertaking is in the vicinity.

The nervous syndrome in pigs poisoned by organic arsenicals may be confused with organic mercury poisoning, salt poisoning and the encephalitides but the mildness of the signs, the lack of effect on appetite and the absence of fever rather set it apart from the others.

Treatment

In acute cases treatment is of little value because of the large amounts ingested and the delay between ingestion and the appearance of illness. Nevertheless since affected animals are not suitable for human consumption treatment is usually undertaken. Residual arsenic in the gut should be removed by the administration of an oil demulcent. Dehydration is usually severe and drastic purgatives should be avoided. Several products are used in an attempt to precipitate arsenic in the gut lumen. Ferric hydrate is most commonly used but has little apparent effect on the course of the disease.

Compounds containing sulfur are theoretically the best antidotes and of these sodium thiosulfate is practicable and of some value. The compound is almost completely non-toxic and can be given in large amounts and without accurate measurement. Intravenous injection is desirable as an initial treatment using 15–30 g of the salt in 100–200 ml of water and this should be followed by oral dosing of 30–60 g at 6 hour intervals. Treatment should be continued until recovery occurs which may require 3–4 days. BAL (2:3-dimercaptopropranol) is an efficient antidote for poisoning by organic arsenicals but is often disappointing in cases of poisoning by inorganic salts. Dosing at 4 hourly intervals is necessary and the oily injections cause some local pain. Although BAL has a general beneficial effect and is recommended as a treatment the drug is quite toxic itself and in the doses required may cause deaths in sheep. It also causes a reaction at the injection site sometimes serious enough to warrant the animal's destruction (16). A comparison of these treatments in experimentally poisoned cattle showed little benefit from sodium thiosulfate administration and most effect with a combination of BAL and thioetic acid (15).

Severe dehydration occurs and supportive treatment must include the provision of ample fluids preferably by parenteral injection. An adequate supply of drinking water containing electrolytes should be provided and the animals should be disturbed as little as possible and provided with shelter from the sun. Astringent preparations given by mouth may help to reduce the loss of body fluids.

After the treatment of pigs with arsanilic acid the arsenic content of their livers may exceed 1 mg/kg, the statutory level of arsenic in food for human consumption. At least 10 days should be permitted between ceasing to feed the arsanilate and slaughter to avoid poisoning of humans.

Control

Arsenical preparations must be handled and stored with care and contamination of feed and pasture avoided.

Therapeutic preparations containing arsenic should be labeled 'Poison' and strict instructions given on dosage and particularly the length of time for which administration should continue. Farmers are sometimes inclined to overdose in the hope of expediting recovery and to continue treatment for long periods when the response to treatment is poor rather than call for further assistance. Animals to be dipped in arsenical solutions should be allowed to cool off before dipping, to drain properly afterwards and to dry before being driven. They should be watered before dipping to prevent them drinking the dip. Many mortalities have occurred when instructions for mixing dip solutions are not closely followed. Dipping solutions containing more arsenic than is safe usually occur when tanks which have lost water by evaporation are reconstituted by guesswork. The maximum safe concentration of arsenic trioxide in a dip for cattle is 0·20% (14).

REFERENCES

(1) Morgan, S. E. et al. (1984) *Vet. Med. SAC*, *79*, 1525.
(2) Buck, W. B. (1973) *Vet. Toxicol.*, *15*, 25.
(3) McParland, P. J. et al. (1971) *Vet. Rec.*, *89*, 450.
(4) Lancaster, R. J. et al. (1971) *NZ vet. J.*, *19*, 141.
(5) Bennett, D. G. & Schwarz, T. E. (1971) *Am. J. vet. Res.*, *32*, 727.
(6) Suren, K. & Kreuzer, W. (1979) *Schlacht. Vermarkt.*, *49*, 203.
(7) Menges, R. W. et al. (1970) *Vet. Med. small. Anim. Clin.*, *65*, 565.
(8) Rice, D. A. et al. (1985) *Res. vet. Sci.*, *39*, 47.
(9) Ferslew, K. E. & Edds, G. T. (1979) *Am. J. vet. Res.*, *40*, 1365.
(10) Witzel, D. A. et al. (1976) *Am. J. vet. Res.*, *37*, 521.
(11) Keenan, D. M. (1973) *Aust. vet. J.*, *49*, 229.
(12) Ledet, A. E. et al. (1973) *Clin. Toxicol.*, *6*, 439.
(13) Hatch, R. C. & Funnell, H. S. (1968) *Can. vet. J.*, *10*, 117.
(14) Littlejohn, A. & Virlas, D. (1980) *Br. vet. J.*, *136*, 190.
(15) Hatch, R. C. et al. (1978) *Am. J. vet. Res.*, *39*, 1411.
(16) Deckert, W. et al. (1983) *Mh VetMed.*, *38*, 650.
(17) Thatcher, C. D. et al. (1985) *J. Am. vet. med. Assoc.*, *187*, 179.
(18) Bergeland, M. E. et al. (1977) *Proc. 19th ann. Mtg Am. Assoc. vet. Lab. Diagnost.*, pp. 311–316.
(19) Ledet, A. E. & Buck, W. B. (1978) In: *Toxicology of Heavy Metals*, Pt. 1, (ed.) F. W. Oehme. New York: Marcel Dekker.
(20) Robertson, I. D. et al. (1984) *Aust. vet. J.*, *61*, 366.
(21) Gilbert, F. R. et al. (1981) *Vet. Rec.*, *109*, 158.

Selenium poisoning

Selenium poisoning occurs in specific areas where the selenium content of the soil is high. Acute cases show mainly signs of nervous system involvement with blindness and head-pressing. Chronic cases are manifested by emaciation, lameness and loss of hair.

Etiology

The effective selenium is contained in the top 60–90 cm of the soil profile, selenium at lower levels than this not being within reach of most plants. Selenium poisoning may occur on soils containing very little selenium—as low as 0·01 mg/kg (1)—but some soils may contain as much as 1200 mg/kg. Most pasture plants seldom contain selenium in excess of 100 but several species, the so-called converter or indicator plants, take up the element in such large quantities that selenium levels may reach as high as 10 000 mg/kg (2). Such plants constitute a serious hazard in areas where the selenium content of the soil is high. *Astragalus* and *Oxytropis* spp. are two of the common converter plants in North America. *Artemisia canescens* (fourwinged salt bush) is also a selenium converter (24) and has caused poisoning. *Morinda reticulata*, *Neptunia amplexicaulis* and *Acacia cana* have been shown to be converter plants in Australia (1, 3). These plants have the advantage that they tend to grow preferentially on selenium-rich soils and are thus 'indicator' plants. They are in general unpalatable because of a strong odor. They are discussed in relation to other *Astragalus* sp. plants under that heading.

Selenium may also contaminate pasture by aerial deposition of material from industrial enterprises. Fly ash from soft coal has been shown to cause increased selenium levels in tissues from sheep fed the material (1).

Because of the number of factors which affect the toxicity of selenium there is much discrepancy between toxic doses quoted by different workers and the following information is subject to this limitation. There are many case reports of unexpected illness and mortality in animals dosed with selenium preparations and it is apparent that not all of the factors affecting selenium toxicity are known (5). Factors known to affect the toxicity of selenium compounds are the cobalt and protein status of the animal, deficiencies of either causing increased susceptibility, the length and rate of the ingestion period and the animal species, cattle being more tolerant than sheep. Organic selenium compounds, especially those occurring naturally in plants, are generally considered to be much more toxic than inorganic compounds but this difference may not be apparent in ruminants because of alterations in ingested compounds produced by digestive processes in the rumen. There is a difference of opinion as to whether the selenite or the selenate salts are more toxic but both are more damaging than selenium dioxide (4).

Selenium in feeds should not exceed 5 mg/kg dry matter if danger is to be avoided and feeding on pasture containing 25 mg/kg dry matter for several weeks can be expected to cause chronic selenium poisoning. Pasture may contain as much as 2000–6000 mg/kg of selenium and causes the acute form of the disease when fed for a few days. Daily intakes of 0·25 mg/kg body weight are toxic for sheep and cattle and feed containing 44 mg/kg selenium for horses and 11 mg/kg for pigs causes poisoning (4), the daily intake of a diet containing 2 mg/kg of selenium can be marginally toxic for sheep (8). Toxic single oral doses (as mg/kg body weight) are 2·2 for horses and sheep, 9 for cattle and 15 for pigs. An oral dose of 10–15 mg of selenium has been known to kill lambs (5). It is now common practice to combine a selenium compound with an anthelmintic drench or injection and, if the mixture is incorrectly prepared, poisoning may occur (20, 21). Feeding pigs on a concentrate ration containing 84 mg/kg of selenium caused an outbreak of poisoning in pigs (19). A less toxic mixture was fed for 6 weeks before signs appeared (22).

Because of the present popularity of selenium in the treatment of enzootic muscular dystrophy it has become necessary to determine toxic levels of selenium compounds administered by injection. In general the ratio between toxic and therapeutic doses is 50–100:1 and dosing accidents should not be common (4). The subcutaneous injection of selenium, as sodium selenite, causes poisoning in sheep at doses of 0·8 mg/kg body weight and doses of 1·6 mg/kg are lethal (9). A single injection of 5 mg of selenium may kill some lambs (5) and the toxic level for single injections in lambs has been reported as 455 μg/kg body weight (11). Lethal doses by injections are 1·2 mg/kg body weight for cattle (4) and between 1 and 2 mg/kg in pigs (6). In ponies relatively large doses, e.g. 6–8 mg/kg body weight seem necessary to cause fatality (7).

Epidemiology

Selenium poisoning occurs in restricted areas in North America where the soils are derived from particular rock formations containing a high content of selenium. It has also been recorded in Ireland, Israel, Canada and Australia and is suspected of contributing to the development of 'geeldikkop' and toxemic jaundice in South Africa. Losses are caused by failure of animals to thrive on pasture grown on seleniferous soils and some deaths occur.

Selenium poisoning occurs chiefly when animals feed on plants grown on seleniferous soils which may be restricted to small, very distinct areas. The incidence of the disease is highest when selector plants are growing in the pasture. A low rainfall predisposes to selenium poisoning because soluble, available selenium compounds are not leached out of the topsoil and lack of competing forage may force animals to eat large quantities of indicator plants. If the use of selenium in the prevention of enzootic muscular dystrophy becomes widespread induced selenium poisoning may increase in incidence. An acute syndrome occurs rarely if animals are forced to eat large amounts of highly toxic converter plants. More commonly, animals are affected by one of the two chronic forms—blind staggers and alkali disease.

Pathogenesis

Selenium occurs in plants in analogs of the sulfur-containing amino acids, and the probable mechanism of intoxication is by interference with enzyme systems which contain these amino acids. Arsenic and antimony exert their toxic effects in the same way and both of these elements reduce the toxicity of selenium compounds. Selenium reduces the sulfur and protein content of sheep's liver and high protein diets have a protective effect against selenium poisoning. Selenium is deposited in greatest concentration in the liver, kidney and hair. It has a marked dystrophic effect on skeletal musculature and causes a marked rise in SGOT levels after subcutaneous administration.

It has not been possible to reproduce the chronic natural disease by the experimental administration of small amounts of selenium and it may be that a toxic action of the converter plant itself may contribute to the disease which is seen in the field. In the experimentally produced disease there is a gradual accumulation of selenium in tissues followed by the sudden onset of the acute form of the disease in which sheep die with dyspnea and pulmonary edema caused by acute heart failure. Poisoning in pigs caused by a single injection similarly causes acute heart failure (25).

Clinical findings

In acute selenium poisoning there is severe respiratory distress, watery diarrhea, fever, tachycardia, abnormal posture and gait, prostration and death after a short illness. Mildly affected pigs show posterior ataxia, walking on tiptoe, sternal recumbency but able to rise, tremor and vomiting in some. More severe cases are in lateral recumbency (19).

One chronic form of the disease is known as 'blind staggers', because affected animals are blind, stumble, and wander aimlessly and often in circles, and show head-pressing. The appetite may be depraved and abdominal pain is evidenced. The terminal stage is one of paralysis with death due to respiratory failure. Essentially the same picture is produced by the experimental oral dosing of sheep with sodium selenite but dilatation of the pupils and cyanosis are also present (14). The experimental disease in pigs is characterized by vomiting, diarrhea, lethargy, dyspnea and coma. Terminally there is ataxia, head-pressing, recumbency and convulsions (15).

Chronic poisoning (alkali disease) is manifested by dullness, emaciation, rough coat, lack of vitality, stiffness and lameness. In cattle, horses, and mules the hair at the base of the tail and switch is lost and in pigs and horses there may be general alopecia. There are hoof abnormalities including swelling of the coronary band, and deformity or separation and sloughing of the hooves in all species. Lameness is severe. Congenital hoof deformities may occur in newborn animals whose dams have received diets containing an excess of selenium. Feeding pigs on rations containing 20–27 mg/kg causes paralysis due to poliomyelomalacia and necrosis of the coronary band (22, 23). Marginal levels of intake of selenium (10 mg/kg) are reported to lower the conception rate and increase neonatal mortality in pigs. This syndrome is not recorded in sheep.

Clinical pathology

Selenium can be detected in the urine, milk and hair of affected animals but critical data are not available. Clinical illness is evident at blood levels of 3 mg/kg and at urine levels of more than 4 mg/kg of selenium. Critical levels of selenium in hair include the following:

- Less than 5·0 mg/kg suggests that chronic selenosis is unlikely
- From 5·0 to 10·0 mg/kg suggests that borderline problems will occur
- More than 10 mg/kg is diagnostic of chronic selenosis (12).

A moderate anemia occurs in acute and chronic poisoning and a depression of hemoglobin levels to about 7 g/dl is one of the early indications of selenium poisoning.

Necropsy findings

In cases of acute selenium poisoning there is congestion and necrosis of the liver, congestion of the renal medulla, epicardial petechiation, impaction of the rumen, and hyperemia and necrosis, sometimes with ulceration, in the abomasum and small intestine. The hooves are not involved but there may be erosion of the articular surfaces, particularly of the tibia. In acute poisoning of cattle with a massive accidental overdose of a selenium preparation there was histological evidence of extensive damage in liver, lungs and myocardium (16). Gross overdosage in sheep by overdrenching with sodium selenite has caused hydrothorax and pulmonary edema (17).

In animals suffering from chronic selenium poisoning there is atrophy and dilatation of the heart, cirrhosis and atrophy of the liver, glomerulonephritis, mild gastroenteritis and erosion of articular surfaces (7). Deformities of the feet are usually apparent as described under clinical findings. In experimentally induced cases in sheep the significant lesions are degeneration and necrosis in the myocardium, and edema and interstitial petechiation in the lungs (13, 18). In pigs symmetrical spinal poliomalacia is recorded in chronic poisoning (23).

In chronic selenosis in sheep hepatic levels of selenium are about 20–30 mg/kg and levels in wool are in the range of 0·6–2·3 mg/kg. In horses hair levels of more than 5 mg/kg are recorded (10).

Diagnosis

The diagnosis of selenium poisoning rests largely on the recognition of the typical syndromes in animals in areas where the soil content of selenium is high. The acute form of the disease resembles subacute lead poisoning, encephalopathy due to liver insufficiency and many encephalitides and encephalomalacias. Chronic cases bear some resemblance to hypovitaminosis A.

Treatment

A number of substances have been tried in the treatment of selenium poisoning, including potassium iodide, ascorbic acid and beet pectin but without apparent effect. BAL is contraindicated (2).

Control

Protection against the toxic effects of selenium in amounts up to 10 mg/kg in the diet has been obtained by the inclusion in the ration fed to pigs of 0·01–0·02% of arsanilic acid or 0·005% of 3-nitro-4-hydroxyphenyl arsonic acid. In cattle 0·01% arsanilic acid in the ration or 550 mg/day to grazing steers gives only slight protection. The addition of linseed oil to the ration improves the efficiency of this protection. A high protein diet also has a general protective effect. Pretreatment with copper is also known to be an effective preventive measure in all species (7). The mechanism of this protection is unknown. Single oral doses of 20–40 mg/kg of copper given 24 hours beforehand protected ponies.

REFERENCES

(1) Knott, S. G. & McCray, C.W.R. (1959) *Aust. vet. J.*, *35*, 161.
(2) Hart, J. R. & Muth, O.H. (1972) *Clin. Toxicol.*, *5.*, 175.
(3) McCray, C. W. R. & Hurwood, I. S. (1964) *Queensland J. agric. Sci.*, *20*, 475.
(4) Muth, O. H. & Binns, W. (1964) *Ann. NY Acad. Sci.*, *111*, 583.
(5) Gabbedy, B. J. (1970) *Aust. vet. J.*, *46*, 223.
(6) MacDonald, D. W. et al. (1981) *Can. vet. J.*, *22*, 279.
(7) Stowe, H. D. (1980) *Am. J. vet. Res.*, *41*, 1925.
(8) Pope, A. L. (1971) *J. anim. Sci.*, *33*, 1332.
(9) Caravaggi, C. & Clark, F. L. (1969) *Aust. vet. J.*, *45*, 383.
(10) Crinion, R. A. P. & O'Connor, J. P. (1978) *Irish vet. J.*, *32*, 81.
(11) Caravaggi, C. et al. (1970) *Res. vet. Sci.*, *11*, 146.
(12) James, L. F. et al. (1981) *J. Am. vet. med. Assoc.*, *178*, 146.
(13) Glenn, M. W. et al. (1964) *Am. J. vet. Res.*, *23*, 1479, 1486.
(14) Morrow, D. A. (1968) *J. Am. vet. med. Assoc.*, *152*, 1625.
(15) Herigstad, R. R. et al. (1973) *Am. J. vet. Res.*, *34*, 1227.
(16) Shortridge, E. H. et al. (1971) *NZ vet. J.*, *19*, 47.
(17) Lambourne, D. A. & Mason, R. W. (1969) *Aust. vet. J.*, *45*, 208.
(18) Gabbedy, B. J. & Dickson, J. (1969) *Aust. vet. J.*, *45*, 470.
(19) Hill, J. (1985) *Aust. vet. J.*, *62*, 207.
(20) Hopper, S. A. (1985) *Vet. Rec.*, *116*, 569.
(21) Anderson, P. H. et al. (1985) *Vet. Rec.*, *116*, 647.
(22) Casteel, S. W. et al. (1985) *J. Am. vet. med. Assoc.*, *186*, 1084.
(23) Harrison, L. H. et al. (1983) *Vet. Pathol.*, *20*, 265.
(24) James, L. F. et al. (1982) *J. Am. vet. med. Assoc.*, *180*, 1478.

Phosphorus poisoning

Phosphorus poisoning is characterized by severe inflammation of the alimentary mucosa and acute necrosis of the liver. Gastroenteritis and acute hepatic insufficiency are the clinical syndromes produced.

Etiology

Phosphorus is rarely used as a rodent poison nowadays and this comprises the only likely source of phosphorus for animals. Toxic effects are most likely to occur when the phosphorus is finely divided and mixed with oils or fats which facilitate its absorption.

Epidemiology

Phosphorus poisoning is rare in farm animals because of lack of exposure. Small animals are rather more exposed to rat baits containing white phosphorus and amongst farm animals most cases are likely to occur in swine.

Rat or rabbit baits containing lumps of white phosphorus may be left about in barns or at pasture and be ingested accidentally by farm livestock. Phosphorus used for military purposes may cause extensive contamination of pasture.

Pathogenesis

Phosphorus has a local caustic action and on ingestion causes severe irritation of the alimentary mucosa with signs of gastroenteritis appearing within an hour or two. Some phosphorus may be absorbed and cause acute hepatic necrosis but signs do not appear for several days.

Clinical findings

Violent gastroenteritis occurs with severe diarrhea, acute abdominal pain, salivation and intense thirst. Pigs vomit violently and the vomitus is described as being luminous and having a garlic odor. The animal often dies of acute shock during this stage. If it survives this initial period of illness signs of hepatic and renal insufficiency appear 4–10 days later. There is jaundice, weakness and anorexia, oliguria and hematuria. Death may occur in coma or be accompanied by convulsions.

Clinical pathology

Phosphorus can be detected in the vomitus and feces of affected animals.

Necropsy findings

Macroscopically there is congestion and hemorrhagic inflammation of the alimentary mucosa, enlargement of the liver with hemorrhage and yellowish pallor of lobules. Histologically there is acute hepatic necrosis and nephrosis. For analytic purposes liver, kidney and muscle should be supplied as well as a portion of the alimentary canal and its contents. The latter is most important as tissues are often negative for phosphorus. No preservative of any kind should be added to the specimens.

Diagnosis

Clinically phosphorus poisoning is characterized by acute gastroenteritis and differentiation from other causes requires evidence of access to the poison and the detection of large amounts of it in the alimentary tract.

Treatment

An emetic or purgative should be given immediately. Copper sulfate (1% solution) given orally is an effective emetic in small animals and tends to reduce the solubility of the particles of phosphate by covering them with a coating of insoluble copper phosphide. In small animals 15 g of the solution is given by mouth every 10 minutes until vomiting occurs and presumably this form of therapy could be instituted in the other species. A hydragogue cathartic is preferred for purgation, oils facilitating absorption of the phosphorus. Supportive treatment includes the administration of astringents to allay the gastroenteritis and parenteral electrolyte solutions to relieve the dehydration.

Mercury poisoning

Poisoning by mercury causes inflammation of the alimentary mucosa and damage to the kidneys. It is manifested clinically by gastroenteritis and terminally by signs of uremia.

Etiology

The toxicity of mercury compounds depends on their solubility and the susceptibility of the animals. Cattle are highly susceptible. Mercuric chloride and mercury biniodide are highly poisonous, the toxic dose for horses and cattle being about 8 g and for sheep 4 g. Mercury is a cumulative poison because of its slow excretion from the intestines and kidney. Organic mercury taken regularly in the diet at a level of 1 mg/kg causes chronic poisoning in pigs (1). A level of 6 mg/kg has been recorded as causing deaths in pigs within 5 days (2).

Epidemiology

Mercury poisoning is becoming increasingly common in farm animals, principally because of accidental feeding of grain treated with organic mercurial compounds used as antifungal agents. In some cases the grain is processed into pellets and concentrate mixtures.

Accidental administration of medicines containing mercury, licking of skin dressings and absorption from liberally applied skin dressings (3) may cause sporadic cases. The continued administration of a strong mercuric ointment to horses has been shown to cause poisoning by inhalation of mercury vapor by cattle in the same stable (4).

Seed grain which has been treated with antifungal preparations containing organic mercury compounds has been one of the commonest sources of outbreaks of mercury poisoning in farm animals. Because of the availability of other fungicidal agents it is currently common to limit the use of mercuric agents by legislation. It may also be practicable to limit the use of compounds so that only those excreted rapidly by animals, the phenylmercury compounds, are used and those retained in animal tissues, the ethyl and methyl compounds, are prohibited. The commonest agent used is Ceresan which contains 5·25% methoxyethylmercury silicate or 1·75% mercury. Methylmercury dicyandiamide is another common poisonous agent (1, 5). It and ethylmercuric chloride are toxic when fed to pigs at the rate of 0·19–0·76 mg of mercury per kg body weight per day for 60–90 days (6). Other measures of the toxicity of methylmercury dicyandiamide include the observation that feeding to pigs at the rate of 2·5 mg/kg body weight causes no apparent illness. Also feeding at dose levels of 5–15 mg/kg body weight caused illness, while levels of 20 mg/kg body weight caused some deaths. A delay of 3 weeks between dosing and illness was characteristic (5). The sensitivity to mercury poisoning varies between the species, toxicosis occurring in cattle on an average daily intake of 10 mg/kg body weight per day of mercury as organic mercury, while toxic effects were only obtained in sheep with intakes of 17·4 mg/kg body weight per day (7). In horses, feeding inorganic mercury at the rate of 0·4 mg/kg body weight produced only mild signs of poisoning (10), and feeding methylmercury chloride (10 g over 10 weeks) caused serious illness including exudative dermatitis, renal insufficiency and degenerative neuropathy (11).

The seed is usually not harmful if it comprises only 10% of the ration and must be fed in large amounts for long periods before clinical illness occurs (9). A single feeding even of large amounts of grain is thought to be incapable of causing mercury poisoning in ruminants but a fatal case has been reported in a horse.

A matter of vital interest in chronic poisoning by organic mercurials is the use of the meat from such animals for human consumption. There is one record of a family being poisoned in this way (10). The question of excretion of mercury into milk also arises but very little appears to be so excreted and the real risk of drinking poisonous milk appears to be very small (11).

Pathogenesis

Inorganic mercury compounds cause coagulation of the alimentary mucosa and this caustic action results in the rapid development of gastroenteritis. Animals that survive the alimentary tract disorder may show signs of systemic effects from absorbed mercury. This effect is largely one of damage to peripheral capillaries especially those at the sites where mercury is excreted, in the kidney, colon and mouth. Systemic involvement leads to the development of nephrosis, colitis and stomatitis. Organic mercurials in small doses liberate their mercury slowly into tissues and cause degenerative changes in brain and peripheral nerves (12, 13) and in kidney. In some cases of phenylmercuric acetate poisoning there are extensive subcutaneous hemorrhages and a bleeding tendency and the animals die suddenly (19). With larger doses there is stasis of the alimentary tract and with doses of 0·23 g/kg body weight there is general collapse (14). Toxic and lethal doses will vary with the compound used. The primary lesion in chronic organic mercurial poisoning is a segmental demyelination of peripheral nerves (8). There are no effects on reproduction or unborn offspring (4).

Clinical findings

In very severe cases where large amounts of inorganic mercury are ingested there is an acute gastroenteritis with vomiting of bloodstained material and severe diarrhea. Death occurs within a few hours due to shock and dehydration. In less acute cases salivation, a fetid breath and anorexia accompany the gastroenteritis and the animal survives for several days. There is oliguria, an increase in heart and respiratory rates and in some cases posterior paralysis. Convulsions occur in the final stages.

The common form of the disease is chronic mercurialism where small amounts of mercury are ingested over long periods. There is depression, anorexia, emaciation, and a stiff stilted gait which may progress to paresis. Alopecia, scabby lesions around the anus and vulva, pruritus, petechiation and tenderness of the gums and shedding of the teeth are accompanied by chronic diarrhea. Nervous signs are present and include weakness, incoordination and convulsions (14, 15).

Poisoning of pigs by organic mercurial compounds causes blindness, staggering, continuous walking and inability to eat although the appetite appears to be good. Cattle poisoned in this way evidence a staggery gait, standing on tiptoe and paresis. The animals lie down most of the time but appear normal in other respects, often eating well. Clinical signs may not develop until 30 days after feeding is commenced. Cattle poisoned experimentally show marked nervous signs including incoordination, head-pressing, muscle tremor with twitching of the eyelids, tetanus-like spasms on stimulation, excessive salivation, recumbency and inability to eat or drink. These are followed by tonic–clonic convulsions with opisthotonus (14).

Clinical pathology

Mercury can be detected in the feces and urine of affected animals and in the toxic source material. Among the earliest and most accurate indicators of nephrotoxicity due to mercury intoxication are the urinary concentrations of alkaline phosphatase and gamma-glutamyl transpeptidase (16).

Necropsy findings

In acute cases there is severe gastroenteritis with edema, hyperemia and petechiation of the alimentary mucosa. The liver and kidneys are swollen and the lungs are congested and show multiple hemorrhages. There may be an accompanying catarrhal stomatitis. Histologically there are degenerative changes in the renal tubules. In chronic mercurialism caused by organic mercury compounds there are also degenerative changes in nerve cells in the cortex of cerebrum, brain stem and spinal cord. The lesions include neuronal necrosis, neuronophagia, cortical vacuolation and gliosis (17). Mercury reaches its greatest concentration in kidney and this tissue should be submitted for assay. Levels of 100 mg/kg may be present in the kidney of animals poisoned with inorganic mercury (15). With chronic organic mercurial poisoning in swine levels of mercury up to 2000 mg/kg may be present in the kidney (18).

Diagnosis

Acute mercury poisoning is rare but should be suspected in animals which are exposed to inorganic mercury compounds and which show signs of gastroenteritis and nephritis. The occurrence of nervous signs results in a syndrome similar to that of poisoning by lead or arsenic. Pigs poisoned by organic mercury compounds manifest a syndrome similar to that caused by poisoning with organic arsenic preparations.

Treatment

In acute cases large amounts of coagulable protein such as eggs should be given by mouth immediately, followed by mild purgatives to facilitate removal from the gut before digestion and absorption occur. Treatment with sodium thiosulfate as described in arsenic poisoning is recommended. BAL has the same limitations here as in arsenic poisoning and delay in treatment of any sort is likely to be fatal. If the case can be treated early an injection of BAL (6·5 mg/kg body weight) should be given every 4 hours. Supportive treatment includes astringents given orally to control the gastroenteritis and fluids given parenterally to correct the dehydration.

Control

Seed grains dusted with mercury compounds should not be fed to animals but the practice is reasonably safe if only small amounts are used.

REFERENCES

(1) Kahrs, R. F. (1968) *Cornell Vet.*, *58*, 67.
(2) Loosmore, R. M. et al. (1967) *Vet. Rec.*, *81*, 268.
(3) Irving, F. & Butler, D. G. (1975) *Can. vet. J.*, *16*, 260.
(4) Chang, C. W. et al. (1977) *J. anim. Sci.*, *45*, 279.
(5) Piper, R. C. et al. (1971) *Am. J. vet. Res.*, *32*, 263.
(6) Tryphonas, L. & Nielsen, N. O. (1973) *Am. J. vet. Res.*, *34*, 379.
(7) Palmer, J. S. et al. (1973) *Clin. Toxicol.*, *6*, 425.
(8) Charlton, K. M. (1974) *Can. J. comp. Med.*, *38*, 75.
(9) Palmer, J. S. (1963) *J. Am. vet. med. Assoc.*, *143*, 1385.
(10) Roberts, M. C. & Seawright, A. A. (1978) *Vet. hum. Toxicol.*, *20*, 410.
(11) Seawright, A. A. et al. (1978) *Vet. hum. Toxicol.*, *20*, 6.
(12) Miyakawa, T. et al. (1971) *Acta Neuropathol.*, *17*, 6, 80.
(13) Tryphonas, L. (1971) *Diss. Abst. int.*, *31B*, 4423.
(14) Herigstad, R. R. et al. (1972) *J. Am. vet. med. Assoc.*, *160*, 173.
(15) Reinders, J. S. (1972) *Neth. J. vet. Sci.*, *4*, 79.
(16) Robinson, M. & Trafford, J. (1977) *J. comp. Pathol.*, *87*, 275.
(17) Davies, T. S. et al. (1976) *Cornell Vet.*, *66*, 32.
(18) Alekseeva, A. A. (1969) *Veterinariya, Moscow*, *5*, 58.
(19) Boyd, J. H. (1985) *Vet. Rec.*, *116*, 443.

Fluorine poisoning

Fluorosis is a chronic disease caused by the continued ingestion of small but toxic amounts of fluorine in the diet or drinking water, and is characterized by mottling and excessive wear of developing teeth and osteoporosis. Acute fluorine poisoning usually occurs as a result of the inhalation of fluorine-containing gases or accidental administration of large amounts of fluoride and is manifested by gastroenteritis.

Etiology

The toxic effects of fluorine depend on the amount ingested, the solubility and availability of the fluorine compound, and the age of the animal. The intake may be expressed as parts per million (ppm) in drinking water or feed, or as mg/kg body weight. The most satisfactory measure is the concentration in the total dry matter consumed.

Levels in excess of 100 ppm of dry ration consumed are likely to cause disease in cattle, sheep and pigs when the fluorine is contained in rock phosphate or cryolite. At this or lower levels minor teeth lesions may occur but not to such a degree that they will affect the animal's wellbeing during an ordinary commercial lifespan. If the fluorine is in the form of calcium fluoride much higher intakes are innocuous. Sodium fluorosilicate is also relatively non-toxic, intakes of 400 mg to 2 g/kg body weight being necessary for fatal effects (2). On the other hand sodium fluoride is approximately twice as toxic and a general level of 50 mg/kg of dry ration should not be exceeded. In experimentally induced fluorosis in cattle mottling of the tooth enamel occurs at intakes of 27 mg/kg but there is no pitting until levels of 49 mg/kg are fed, bony lesions are slight at intakes of 27 mg/kg, moderate at 49 mg/kg and marked at 93 mg/kg, and milk production in dairy cows is supposed not to be affected by intakes of 50 mg/kg of fluorine in the diet until about the fourth lactation (3). A more recent view, especially relative to high-producing cows with high food intakes and calcium loss, is that the existing tolerance level for dairy cows of 40 mg/kg is too high and will lead to serious loss of production and some dental fluorosis (31).

Contamination from industrial plants is a complex problem because of variation in the form of the contaminating compound. Two of the common effluent substances are hydrofluoric acid and silicon tetrafluoride, both of which are highly toxic. Grass can absorb and retain gaseous fluoride from the ambient air, and the extent to which this happens can now be determined based on its content of fluoride and the nature of the compound (21). Hay contamination by these effluents is as toxic as sodium fluoride and dental lesions occur in 100% of young ruminants on an intake of 14–16 mg/kg dry matter of these substances. Severe cases occur on pastures containing more than 25 mg/kg dry matter and similar lesions develop much more rapidly in cattle grazing on pasture containing 98 mg/kg dry matter. Fluoracetamide is also known to be a toxic factory effluent.

The available data for drinking water suggest that although minor teeth lesions occur at 5 mg/kg of fluorine it is not until levels of 10 mg/kg are exceeded that excessive tooth wear occurs and the nutrition of the animal is impaired. More serious systemic effects do not occur until the water contains 30 mg/kg. It seems highly unlikely that the fluoridation of water supplies to prevent human tooth decay would have any deleterious effect on animal health.

In terms of body weight daily intakes of 0·5–1·7 mg/kg body weight of fluorine as sodium fluoride produce dental lesions in growing animals without affecting general wellbeing. Intakes equal to twice these amounts are consumed by adult animals without ill-effect. In heifers a continuous intake of 1·5 mg/kg body weight per day was sufficient to cause severe dental fluorosis without affecting growth rate or reproductive function. However, extensive osteofluorosis and periods of severe lameness occurred (6). An intake of 1 mg/kg body weight is the maximum safe limit for ruminants. An intake of 2 mg/kg body weight produces clinical signs after continued ingestion. The fluorine content of the bones of newborn calves depends on the dam's intake of fluorine in the last 3–4 months of pregnancy and not on her own bone composition. An uptake of up to 9 mg fluorine/kg body weight per day by the dam was not dangerous to the calf (7). In pigs an intake of 1 mg/kg body weight added fluorine for long periods has no deleterious effect and has no apparent beneficial effect on the formation of bone (8).

Epidemiology

Fluorine intoxication has been observed in most countries, usually in association with specific natural or industrial hazards. In Europe and Great Britain losses are greatest on summer grazing of pastures contaminated by industrial fumes, including dust from factories converting rock phosphate to superphosphate. Ingestion of superphosphate itself has been incriminated as a cause of fluorosis but a supernatant liquid of a suspension of the fertilizer will contain no fluorine. Iceland is extensively affected by contamination from volcanic ash. Drinking water from deep wells, industrial contamination of pasture and the feeding of fluorine-bearing phosphatic supplements are the common causes in North America. Deep wells also are an important source in Australia and South America. In Africa the important cause is the feeding of phosphatic rock supplements. Some wood preservatives may contain large quantities of fluoride which may cause acute poisoning in some circumstances (11).

Death losses are rare and restricted largely to acute poisoning, the major losses taking the form of unthriftiness caused by chronic fluorosis. Although it is possible for animal tissues to contain amounts of fluorine in excess of permissible amounts this is not usually so in chronic fluorosis. The fluorine content of milk in these circumstances is below that permitted in fluoridated drinking water (1 mg/l) (12).

Fluorine occurs naturally in rock, particularly in association with phosphate, and these rocks, the soils derived from them and surface water leaching through the soils, may contain toxic quantities of fluorine. In such areas the soil content of fluorine may be as high as 2000—4000 mg/kg even up to 12 000 mg/kg (9) and the levels in water up to 8·7 mg/kg. Levels of fluorine likely to be toxic to animals are not usually encountered in natural circumstances, interference by man being necessary in most instances to increase fluorine ingestion above the critical level.

Plants, with few exceptions, do not absorb appreciable quantities of fluorine. Major outbreaks of intoxication occur as the result of the ingestion of pasture contaminated with fluorine, and drinking water and mineral supplements which contain excessive amounts of fluorine. General undernutrition exacerbates the effects of ingested fluorine.

Most recorded occurrences of fluorosis are in cattle, but sheep and goats (9) are also affected and the pathogenesis in these species is as for cattle.

Pasture contamination

Topdressing of pasture with phosphatic limestone is a common cause of fluorosis. Most phospatic limestones, particularly those from North Africa, are rich in fluorine (0·9–1·4%). Non-phosphatic limestones contain insignificant amounts. Contamination of pasture by smoke, vapor or dust from industrial plants is also common, and such pasture may contain 20–50 mg/kg of fluorine. Factories producing aluminum by the electrolytic process, iron and steel with fluorine-containing fluxes, superphosphate, glazed bricks, copper, glass and enamels are likely to be potent sources and may cause toxic levels of contamination as far as 14 km downwind from the factory. Dust from factories manufacturing superphosphate from rock phosphate may contain as much as 3·3% fluorine (15). Industrial plants engaged in the calcining of ironstone have also been incriminated as sources of fluorine. Dust and gases from volcanic eruptions may cause acute fatal fluorine intoxication in the period immediately after the eruption, and contamination of pasture may be sufficient to cause subsequent chronic intoxication in animals eating the herbage, although the fluorine content of the contaminated materials falls very rapidly if rainfall occurs. Iceland is particularly afflicted with fluorine intoxication deriving from this source.

Supplementary feeding of phosphates

The common occurrence of phosphorus deficiency in animals has led to the search for cheap phosphatic materials suitable for animal feeding. Rock phosphates are commonly used and many deposits contain dangerous amounts of fluorine (3–4%) (17). It is quite possible to reduce the fluorine content of the mineral, but the cost of doing so encourages the use of marginally safe material (21).

Drinking water

Although surface drinking water varies considerably in its fluorine content the major occurrence of fluorine intoxication is from water obtained from deep wells or artesian bores. Chronic intoxication has occurred in sheep drinking bore water containing 12–19 mg/kg and in cattle drinking deep well water containing 16 mg/kg fluorine. Reported occurrences of fluoride poisoning in cattle at intakes of 1·5–4·0 mg/kg fluorine and with metacarpal fluorine levels of 4000 mg/kg must be open to some doubt with respect to etiology (17).

Pathogenesis

Fluorine is a general tissue poison; its exact mode of action does not appear to have been closely examined. When large amounts of soluble inorganic fluorine compounds are ingested there is immediate gastrointestinal irritation due to the formation of hydrofluoric acid in the acid medium of the stomach. Nervous signs including tetany and hyperesthesia may follow as a result of the fixation of serum calcium to form physiologically inactive calcium fluoride in the blood plasma. Blood clotting is inhibited for the same reason. Death occurs quickly. Organic fluorides, including sodium fluoracetate, also known as 1080, and fluoracetamide cause sudden death by poisoning the enzyme aconitase, leading to the accumulation of diagnostically significant levels of citrate in tissues and permanent damage to myocardium.

Chronic intoxication due to the ingestion of small amounts of inorganic fluorides over long periods of time is more common in animals. An initial effect is a marked reduction in the activity of ruminal infusoria, a reduction in food intake, and a decreased production of fatty acids (18). The level of fluorine intake is critical and intakes of 150 mg/kg or less have no effect on food intake of cattle. Levels of 150–200 mg/kg have a depressing effect on milk production. At 200 mg/kg the intake of grain is reduced (5). These effects are matched by an accompanying hypothyroidism and anemia (6). The more widely known and clinically diagnostic effect is the detoxication process which takes the form of deposition of fluorine in association with phosphate in the teeth and bones. Deposition in bone occurs throughout life but in teeth only in the formative stages. In bones the degree of deposition varies being greatest on the periosteal surface of the long bones where exostoses commonly develop. Thus lesions in teeth occur only if the intake is high before the teeth have erupted but bone lesions occur at any stage. When the tissue levels of fluorine are moderate, characteristic lesions due to hypoplasia of the enamel appear in the teeth. At higher levels the storage capacity of these organs is exceeded and blood and urine levels rise. General signs of toxicity thus appear in tissues at the same time as bone lesions develop. The bone lesions of osteomalacia, osteoporosis and exostosis formation are caused by excessive mobilization of calcium and phosphorus to compensate for their increased urinary excretion in conjunction with fluorine. The other tissues particularly prone to fluorine intoxication and in which degenerative changes occur are bone marrow, kidney, liver, adrenal glands, heart muscle and central nervous system. A severe anemia may occur as a result of toxic depression of bone marrow activity although this is not a constant sign. The facility of storage in bone explains the long latent period which occurs in animals subjected to chronic intoxication. There has been controversy about whether fluorine passes the placental barrier in significant amounts. It does because cases of neonatal dental fluorosis have now been identified in cattle (32). Thus temporary teeth may be affected. Fluorine does not occur in significant quantities in the milk or colostrum of poisoned cows.

After storage has occurred in bones a decrease in the intake of fluorine leads to lowering of blood levels and mobilization from bones and teeth commences. This is of importance when interpreting urine and blood levels of the element.

Clinical findings

Acute intoxication

Gastroenteritis occurs with complete anorexia, vomiting

and diarrhea in pigs and dogs, and ruminal stasis with constipation or diarrhea in ruminants. Affected animals are dyspneic. Vomiting acts as a protective mechanism and toxic doses in pigs may be eliminated in this way without the development of other signs. Nervous signs are characteristic and include muscle tremor and weakness, a startled expression, pupillary dilatation, hyperesthesia and constant chewing. Tetany and collapse follow and death usually occurs within a few hours.

Chronic intoxication—fluorosis

Lesions of the teeth and bones are characteristic of chronic fluorine intoxication and the signs are largely referable to these lesions. Teeth changes are the earliest and most diagnostic sign but may not produce clinical effects until other signs have developed. Consequently they are often missed until other clinical findings suggest that the teeth be examined. Because of the distinct clinical separation between animals with dental lesions and those which have in addition signs of lameness and general ill-health it is customary to refer to two forms of the disease—dental fluorosis and osteofluorosis.

Osteofluorosis In this disease lameness and unthriftiness are the signs usually observed first by farmers. These occur in animals of any age. There is lameness and stiffness with a painful gait, most marked in the loins, hip joints and hindlegs. The occurrence of hip lameness on a herd scale in cattle is thought to be diagnostic of fluorosis (19). Pain is evinced on pressure over limb bones and particularly over the bulbs of the heels. The bones may be palpably and visibly enlarged. This is most readily observed in the mandible, sternum, metacarpal and metatarsal bones and the phalanges, all of which are increased in thickness. This overall thickness may be subsequently replaced by well-defined exostoses. The bones are subject to easy fracture. These well-defined lesions occur only in advanced cases and are often accompanied by extensive tooth lesions in young animals. In addition to the generalized lameness there are cases which show a sudden onset of very severe lameness, usually in a forelimb, caused by transverse fracture of the third phalanx.

Dental fluorosis Temporary teeth of animals poisoned while *in utero* and permanent teeth exposed to intoxication before eruption will be affected. The earliest and mildest sign is mottling with the appearance of pigmented (very light yellow, green, brown or black) spots or bands arranged horizontally across the teeth. Occasional vertical bands may be seen where pigment is deposited along enamel fissures. Mottling and staining occur on incisors and cheek teeth and are not evident when the affected tooth erupts and in fact may not appear until some months later. If the period of exposure to intoxication has been limited only some of the teeth may be affected but the defects will always be bilateral. Mottling may not progress any further but if the intoxication has been sufficiently severe defective calcification of the enamel leads to accelerated attrition or erosion of the teeth, usually in the same teeth as the mottling. The mottled areas become pits and the teeth are brittle and break and wear easily and unevenly. Patterns of accelerated attrition are dependent upon the chronological occurrence of the intoxication and the eruption time of the teeth. Uneven and rapid wear of the cheek teeth makes proper mastication impossible. Infection of the dental alveoli and shedding of teeth commonly follow. The painful condition of the teeth and the inability to prehend and masticate seriously reduce the food intake and cause poor growth in the young and unthriftiness and acetonemia in adults. Affected cattle may lap cold drinking water to avoid the discomfort occasioned by normal drinking. Eruption of the teeth may be abnormal, resulting in irregular alignment. A standard for the classification of fluorosis has been proposed based on the degree of mottling, pitting and rate of wear of the teeth (10). The additional clinically apparent abnormalities include delayed eruption of permanent incisor teeth, necrosis of alveolar bone resulting in recession of bone and gingiva, oblique eruption of permanent teeth, hypoplasia of teeth, wide spaces between teeth and rapid development of any dental lesions (16).

Fluorosis generally

Reproduction, milk yield and wool growth are not usually considered to be adversely affected except indirectly by the reduced food intake. However, there is a record of a significant increase in postcalving anestrus in cows receiving a diet containing 8–12 mg/kg fluorine for a year with further declines in fertility with further exposure. Other signs of fluorine intoxication were not observed (22). Additional signs including diarrhea in cattle and sheep and polydipsia and polyuria in pigs are recorded in the naturally occurring disease but cannot be considered as constant or pathognomonic.

In animals that are housed for part of the year and grazed on pasture contaminated by factory effluent during the summer there may be considerable clinical improvement during the winter and an annual recrudescence of signs when the animals are at pasture.

Horses with chronic fluorosis have a similar clinical picture to that of ruminants (23). There is lameness, dental lesions including excessive molar abrasion, and hyperostotic lesions of the metatarsus, metacarpus, mandible and ribs.

Clinical pathology

Laboratory examination of specimens from living animals can be of value in diagnosis. Normal cattle have blood levels of up to 0·2 mg fluorine per mg/dl of blood and 2–6 mg/kg in urine. Cattle on fluorine intakes sufficient to cause intoxication may have blood levels of 0·6 mg/dl, and urine levels of 16–68 mg/kg although blood levels are often normal. Such high levels may not be an indication of high intakes immediately preceding the examination as heavy deposits in bones may cause abnormally high blood and urine fluorine levels for some months after the intake has been reduced to normal. Urine levels should be corrected to a specific gravity of 1·040. Serum calcium and phosphorus levels are usually normal and there is a significant correlation between the amount of fluoride fed and the concentration of alkaline phosphatase in the serum. The increase in phosphatase activity is probably related to the abnormal formation of bone. The increased SAP activity may be three to seven times the normal level (4).

Significant changes can be detected by radiographic examination of bones containing more than 4000 mg/kg of fluorine. These changes include increased density or abnormal porosity, periosteal feathering and thickening, increased trabeculation, thickening of the compact bone and narrowing of the marrow cavity. Spontaneous rib fractures show incomplete union. Good data are available for fluorine concentrations in rib bones and estimations of fluorine content in biopsy samples of ribs have been used in the clinicopathological study of the disease (3). Samples of tail bone and the spongiosa of the tuber coxae have also been used for these purposes.

Organic fluorides are difficult to assay in excretions and tissues, and even in contaminated feed sources. In affected animals indirect measurement based on tissue concentrations of citrate may be necessary. An additional suggested procedure is the administration of an aqueous extract of suspected poisoned tissues or feed material to guinea-pigs and the measurement of tissue levels of citrate in them (24).

Necropsy findings

Severe gastroenteritis is present in acute poisoning. In fluorosis the bones have a chalky, white appearance, are brittle and have either local or disseminated exostoses particularly along the diaphyses (25). Intra-articular structures are not primarily affected although there may be some spurring and bridging of the joints. Histologically there is atrophy of spongiosa, defective and irregular calcification of newly formed osseous tissue and active periosteal bone formation. Hypoplasia of the enamel and dentine are consistent physical and histological defects in the teeth of affected young animals (30). Degenerative changes in kidney, liver, heart muscle, adrenal glands and central nervous system have been reported in severe cases. Degeneration of bone marrow and aplastic anemia also occur.

Chemical examination of necropsy specimens is of considerable assistance in diagnosis. The fluorine content of bones is greatly increased. Levels of up to 1200 mg/kg are observed in normal animals but may be increased up to 3000 mg/kg in animals exposed to fluorine and showing only mottling of the teeth. Animals showing severe clinical signs have levels greater than 4000 mg/kg of bone on a dry, fat-free basis and after prolonged heavy feeding levels may be as high as 1·04% (26). Care must be taken in selecting samples of bone because of the great variation in the concentration of fluorine which occurs between different bones. Good data are available for comparison between metacarpal, metatarsal, rib, pelvic and mandibular bones (3). Mandibles usually show the greatest concentrations and in the long bones the distal and proximal quarters are more sensitive indicators than the center half (1). There is also a greater concentration in periosteal than in endosteal bone, and there is also great variation between the various structures of the tooth. The highest concentration is in the cementum (13).

The concentration of fluorine is greater in cancellous than in compact bone. Soft tissues are unreliable as a criterion for fluorosis because of their low levels of fluorine. In bone and teeth, ash levels of 0·01–0·15% fluorine are found in normal animals. Levels up to 1.5% fluorine indicate excessive intake but are not usually accompanied by anatomical changes. Where clinical signs of intoxication appear there is usually up to 2% fluorine in bone ash and 1% in teeth ash.

Diagnosis

Most confusion in the diagnosis of fluorine intoxication in the past has been in differentiating the disease from dietary deficiencies of phosphorus, calcium and vitamin D. The dental lesions of fluorosis are characteristic and the bone lesions are unlike those which occur in any of the deficiency diseases. Final diagnosis must depend upon fluorine assay of food and water, of blood and urine of affected animals, and bones and teeth at necropsy.

Treatment

The treatment of animals suffering from chronic fluorine intoxication, apart from removing them from the source of fluorine, is largely impractical. Acute cases require gastrointestinal sedatives, treatment to neutralize residual fluorine in the alimentary tract and calcium salts intravenously. Aluminum salts should be effective as neutralizers of the hydrofluoric acid produced in the stomach and because of their insolubility they are unlikely to have any deleterious effects even when given in large quantities. Doses of 30 g of aluminum sulfate daily have been used in the prevention of chronic fluorosis and relatively larger doses may be useful in treatment. The calcium salts given intravenously to replace the precipitated calcium should be given to effect, using the disappearance of tetany and hyperesthesia as a guide. This treatment will probably have to be repeated. The parenteral administration of glucose solutions is recommended at the same time because of the interference by fluorine with glucose metabolism. Irrespective of treatment used, no improvement in dental or osseous lesions can be anticipated but amelioration of the other clinical signs may occur.

Control

Phosphatic feed supplements should contain not more than 0·2% for milking or breeding cattle or 0·3% for slaughter cattle (20), of fluorine, and should not comprise more than 2% of the grain ration if the fluorine content is of this order. In spite of this recommendation the feeding of rock phosphate containing 1–1·5% fluorine to cattle for long periods has been recommended and appears to have no major deleterious effects on health in certain circumstances (27). Some deposits of rock phosphate have much higher contents of fluorine than others and commercial defluorination makes these toxic deposits safe for animal feeding. Bone meal in some areas may contain excessive quantities of fluorine and should be checked for its fluorine content. Access to superphosphate made from rock phosphate with a high fluorine content should be avoided. Water from deep wells and artesian bores should be assayed for fluorine content before use. Where levels are marginal careful husbandry including the watering of young, growing stock on fluorine-free supplies, and permitting only adults to be watered on the dangerous supplies, and rotating the animals between safe and dangerous waters at 3 month intervals may make it possible to utilize land areas otherwise unsuitable for stock raising. In some areas dairy herds may have to be maintained by the purchase of replacements rather than by the rearing of young stock. In areas where longterm ingestion of fluorine is likely to occur the aim should be to provide a diet of less than 50 mg/kg of the total diet of dairy cows.

Adequate calcium and phosphorus intakes should be ensured as these facilitate maximum bone storage of fluorine. Aluminum salts are the only substances used in an attempt to reduce the toxic effects of fluorine. They are relatively ineffective, reducing the accumulation of fluorine in bone by only 20–30%, and are thus referred to as 'alleviators'. The sulfate and phosphate have been used but all the salts are unpalatable and can only be administered daily to animals being hand-fed relatively large amounts of concentrates. It is presumed that highly insoluble aluminum fluoride is formed in the alimentary canal. An extensive field trial of aluminum as an alleviator has not justified its use as a practicable control measure. Best results are obtained by improvement in nutrition of the animals and better grassland management (28). If effective control measures are introduced it will be some years before the affected teeth have erupted and become visible and the cows culled or otherwise disposed of.

The fluorine content of drinking water can be considerably reduced (from 10 to 0·95 mg/kg) by adding freshly slaked lime to the water, 500–1000 mg/kg should be added and the water allowed to settle for 6 days. The method requires the use of large storage tanks (29).

Legislation to control fluoride emission from factories is now general but the usual limitation of not more than 1 $\mu g/m^3$ does not completely avoid danger and serious losses can still occur at these emission levels (14). Tolerances for pasture contamination also appear to be incompletely protective.

REVIEW LITERATURE

Ammerman, C. B. et al. (1980) Symposium on fluoride toxicosis in cattle. *J. anim. Sci.*, *51*, 744 et seq.
Krook, L. & Maylin, G. A. (1979) Industrial fluoride pollution. *Cornell Vet.*, *69*, Suppl. 8, 69 pp.
Wheeler, S. M. & Fell, L. R. (1983) Fluorides in cattle nutrition. *Nutr. Abst. Rev.*, *53*, 741–766.

REFERENCES

(1) Ammerman, C. B. et al. (1964) *J. anim. Sci.*, *23*, 409.
(2) Egyed, M. & Rosner, M. (1969) *Refuah Vet.*, *25*, 6.
(3) Shupe, J. L. et al. (1964) *Ann. NY Acad. Sci.*, *111*, 618.
(4) Miller, G. W. et al. (1977) *Fluoride*, *10*, 67.
(5) Suttie, J. W. & Kostad, D. L. (1977) *J. dairy Sci.*, *60*, 1568.
(6) Hillman, D. et al. (1979) *J. dairy Sci.*, *62*, 416.
(7) Rosenberger, G. & Grunder, H. D. (1967) *Berl. Münch. Tierärztl. Wochenschr.*, *80*, 41.
(8) Spencer, G. R. et al. (1971) *Am. J. vet. Res.*, *32*, 1751.
(9) Kessabi, M. et al. (1986) *Maghreb Vet.*, *2* (Suppl), 51.
(10) National Academy of Sciences (1974) *Effects of Fluorides in Animals*, Committee on Animal Nutrition, Subcommittee on fluorosis, Washington, DC, p. 23.
(11) Padberg, W. (1972) *Tierärztl. Umschau*, *27*, 428.
(12) Oelschlager, W. et al. (1972) *Zentralbl. VetMed.*, *19A*, 743.
(13) Shearer, T. R. et al. (1978) *Am. J. vet. Res.*, *39*, 1392.
(14) Crissman, J. W. et al. (1980) *Cornell Vet.*, *70*, 183.
(15) Zumpt, I. (1975) *J. S. Afr. vet. med. Assoc.*, *46*, 61.
(16) Krook, L. et al. (1983) *Cornell Vet.*, *73*, 340.
(17) Obel, A. L. & Erne, K. (1971) *Acta vet. Scand.*, *12*, 164.
(18) Leeman, W. & Stahel, O. (1972) *Fluoride*, *5*, 200.
(19) Griffith-Jones, W. (1977) *Vet. Rec.*, *100*, 84.
(20) Shupe, J. L. (1980) *J. anim. Sci.*, *51*, 746.
(21) Bunce, H. W. F. (1985) *J. dairy Sci.*, *68*, 1706.
(22) van Rensburg, S. W. J. & de Vos, W. H. (1966) *Onderstepoort J. vet. Res.*, *33*, 185.
(23) Shupe, J. L. & Olson, A. E.(1971) *J. Am. vet. med. Assoc.*, *158*, 167.
(24) Egyed, M. N. & Shlosberg, A. (1973) *Refuah Vet.*, *30*, 112.
(25) Lasarov, E. et al. (1972) *Wien. Tierärztl. Monatschr.*, *59*, 258.
(26) Mortensen, F. N. et al. (1964) *J. dairy Sci.*, *47*, 186.
(27) Snook, L. C. (1962) *Aust. vet. J.*, *38*, 42.
(28) Burns, K. N. & Allcroft, R. (1967) *4th int. mtg World. Assoc. Buiatrics, Zurich, 1966*, p. 22.
(29) Mariakulandai, A. & Venkatamariah, M. A. (1955) *Ind. J. vet. Sci.*, *25*, 183.
(30) Shearer, T. R. et al. (1978) *Am. J. vet. Res.*, *39*, 597.
(31) Eckerlin, R. H. et al. (1986) *Cornell Vet.*, *76*, 403.
(32) Maylin, G. A. et al. (1987) *Cornell Vet.*, *77*, 84.

Molybdenum poisoning

Molybdenum poisoning causes a secondary hypocuprosis and is manifested clinically by persistent diarrhea and depigmentation of the hair.

Etiology

Soil molybdenum levels in problem areas vary between 10 and 100 mg/kg. Illness may occur on pasture producing forage containing 3–10 mg/kg. Although levels of less than 3 mg/kg are usually considered to be safe, signs of toxicity may occur at levels as low as 1 mg/kg if the sulfate intake is high and the copper status low. Forage containing 10 mg/kg must be considered dangerous at all times and with aerial contamination levels of 10–200 mg/kg may be encountered. A daily intake of 120–250 mg has proved to be toxic for cattle although the toxic dose varies widely with the intake of sulfate, copper and possible other factors. Such intakes can be provided by industrial fallouts of 5–40 ng/m^3 of air or 2 mg/m^2/month on pasture (10).

Molybdenum in the drinking water may not be as toxic as the same amount in fresh forages. For calves, the minimum toxic concentration in drinking water is between 10 and 50 mg/kg when dietary copper and sulfur intake in the diet is normal (5).

Epidemiology

Molybdenum poisoning is being recorded with increased frequency as the search for it is intensified. The disease is not highly fatal but severe stunting and loss of production occur. Sheep and cattle are clinically affected in field outbreaks of the disease and signs are most marked in young growing animals. Cattle are much more susceptible than sheep. The concentration of molybdenum in forage varies with the season, being highest in the spring and autumn, and with the plant species, legumes, particularly alsike clover, taking up molybdenum in much greater quantities than grasses (1). On the basis of apparent increases in the digestibility of cellulose and improvement in weight gains in lambs fed added molybdenum it has been suggested that the element is an essential one for ruminants.

The major occurrence of molybdenum poisoning is on pasture growing on molybdenum-rich soils usually derived from particular geological formations. Such soils are those of the 'teart' pastures of Somerset (United Kingdom), the United States and Canada. In the United Kingdom, marine black shales may be rich in molybdenum and be potentially limiting to livestock performance for this reason (2). In addition, excess molybdenum intake with or without a marginal deficiency of copper causes peat scours of cattle in New Zealand, Canada, Ireland and Australia. The use of molybdenum in fertilizer mixtures to increase nitrogen fixation by legumes may lead to excessive amounts of molybdenum in soils.

Aerial contamination of pastures by fumes from aluminum and steel alloy factories and oil refineries using molybdenum is also recorded (1, 3). In these conditions simple contamination of the herbage may occur without an increase in soil molybdenum.

Pathogenesis

An extended discussion of the role of molybdenum in copper metabolism is provided in the section on secondary deficiency. Excess molybdenum intake interferes with the hepatic storage of copper and produces a state of copper deficiency. This situation is exacerbated by a high intake of sulfur or a low intake of copper. The syndrome of molybdenum intoxication resembles that of copper deficiency and treatment and prevention by the administration of copper is effective. However, some of the signs of molybdenum poisoning, particularly diarrhea, are not characteristic of copper deficiency and may represent a specific toxic effect of molybdenum (4). One such specific toxic effect is that of causing the development of exostoses and hemorrhages about the long bones, and separation of the great trochanters of the femur in some sheep fed molybdenum experimentally (6). The lesions appear to be due to defects in connective tissue at muscle insertion points, and to defects in the epiphyseal growth plates. The experimental feeding of molybdenum produces a syndrome identical with that seen in the naturally occurring disease in cattle but liver and plasma levels of copper may not be depressed as is usual in naturally occurring cases (4). Experimental feeding of a large dose, up to 40 g, of molybdenum may cause only transient diarrhea. Most of the molybdenum is rapidly absorbed and excreted, 90% in the first week.

Clinical findings

Persistent scouring commences within 8–10 days of the animals having access to affected pasture. Emaciation and a dry, staring coat develop and there is profound depression of milk production. Depigmentation of black hair causes a red or gray tinge to appear. This may be particularly noticeable around the eyes, giving a bespectacled appearance. Intense craving for copper supplement has been noted. Young cattle (3 months to 2½ years) show in addition abnormalities of locomotion including marked stiffness of the legs and back, difficulty in rising and great reluctance to move. The gait is suggestive of laminitis but the feet appear normal. The lameness may be due to the periosteal lesions described above. The appetite remains good (3).

Clinical pathology

Blood copper levels are reduced from the normal of 15 μmol/l to 2·5 μmol/l. Seasonal variations occur depending on the intake of molybdenum. Blood molybdenum levels in normal animals are of the order of 0·05 mg/kg and rise to about 0·10 mg/kg when excess molybdenum is ingested. Levels as high as 0·70 and 1·4 mg/kg have been recorded in cattle and horses grazing on pasture contaminated by smelter fumes (7). On very large intakes of molybdenum cattle which are clinically normal may have molybdenum levels of 1000 mg/kg in feces, 45 mg/kg in urine, 10 mg/kg in blood and 1 mg/kg in milk (8).

Necropsy findings

There are no gross or histological findings which characterize the disease, enteritis being conspicuously absent. The carcass is emaciated and dehydrated and there may be anemia if there is an accompanying copper deficiency. Tissue copper levels will be below normal.

Diagnosis

The most effective method of confirming the diagnosis is to treat affected animals orally with copper sulfate (2 g daily or 5 g weekly for adult cattle and 1·5 g for adult sheep). The diarrhea ceases in 2–3 days and improvement in the other signs is rapid.

The persistence of the diarrhea without other clinical signs, particularly in young cattle and sheep, may suggest internal parasitism and examination of feces for worm eggs is necessary for differentiation. Johne's disease affects only adults and usually only one animal in a herd shows clinical signs at any one time. The acute enteridites including salmonellosis, winter dysentery and virus diarrhea are acute diseases and are accompanied by other diagnostic signs.

Treatment and control

In problem areas the administration of copper to large numbers of animals presents a number of problems. The methods available and their respective advantages are discussed under copper deficiency, but in general terms molybdenum toxicity can be controlled by increasing the copper content of the diet by 5 mg/kg (9).

REFERENCES

(1) Verweij, J. H. P. (1971) *Tijdschr. Diergeneeskd.*, *96*, 1508.
(2) Thomson, L. et al. (1972) *J. Sci. Food Agric.*, *23*, 879.
(3) Gardner, A. W. & Hall-Patch, P. K. (1968) *Vet. Rec.*, *82*, 86.
(4) Cook, G. A. et al. (1966) *J. anim. Sci.*, *25*, 96.
(5) Kinkaid, R. L. (1980) *J. dairy Sci.*, *63*, 608.
(6) Pitt, M. et al. (1980) *J. comp. Pathol.*, *90*, 567.
(7) Hallgren, W. et al. (1954) *Nord. VetMed.*, *6*, 469.
(8) Tolgyesi, G. & Abd Elmothy, I. (1967) *Magy Allatorv. Lap.*, *22*, 123.
(9) Pope, A. L. (1971) *J. anim. Sci.*, *33*, 1332.
(10) Alary, J. et al. (1981) *Sci. total Envir.*, *19*, 111.

Copper poisoning

Copper poisoning is a complex problem because of the many factors which influence the metabolism of copper. Both acute and chronic copper poisoning occur under field conditions and although acute poisoning is relatively straightforward those diseases which are grouped under the general heading of chronic copper poisoning are difficult to define. Acute copper poisoning usually occurs because of the accidental administration of large quantities of soluble copper salts, but chronic copper poisoning is mainly a disease which occurs in certain areas where the soil is naturally rich in copper. The toxicity of the plants growing on these soils is governed not only by the absolute amount of copper in the soil but also by the interaction of a number of factors including the amount of molybdenum and probably of sulfate present in the diet and the presence or absence of specific plants and the level of protein in the diet. In fact either copper deficiency or copper poisoning can occur on soils with apparently normal copper levels, the syndrome depending on the particular conditioning factors present. There is also a competitive relationship between copper and zinc in the internal metabolism of ruminants. The 'toxemic jaundice' group of diseases result from the complex interactions of these factors. For convenience copper poisoning is dealt with here as primary and secondary copper poisoning. *Primary copper poisoning* includes acute copper poisoning caused by the accidental ingestion of large amounts of copper salts at one time, and chronic poisoning caused by the continued ingestion of small amounts over a long period. *Secondary copper poisoning* includes *phytogenous chronic copper poisoning*, in which relatively small amounts of copper are ingested but excessive retention occurs because of the presence of specific plants which cause no apparent liver damage, and *hepatogenous chronic copper poisoning* in which excessive retention of copper is caused by the ingestion of specific plants which cause liver damage. One of the plants which commonly contributes to hepatogenous chronic copper poisoning is *Heliotropum europaeum* which is also capable of causing uncomplicated toxipathic hepatitis without abnormality of copper metabolism. The toxemic jaundice group of diseases includes all of these forms of secondary copper poisoning and toxipathic hepatitis caused by *Heliotropum europaeum*.

PRIMARY COPPER POISONING

Etiology

Sheep are much more susceptible than adult cattle and single doses of 20–110 mg of copper per kg body weight produce acute copper poisoning in sheep and young calves. Sheep are peculiar in the way in which copper is handled metabolically. Increased absorption is not easily achieved but abnormally high excretion is more difficult still, so that there is the general tendency for copper to accumulate in the body of the sheep. In cattle a dose rate of 220–880 mg/kg body weight is necessary to cause death. Chronic copper poisoning occurs in sheep and calves with daily intakes of 3·5 mg of copper/kg body weight (3). Pasture containing 15–20 mg/kg dry matter of copper causes chronic copper poisoning in sheep but there are few records of cattle being affected by chronic copper poisoning while at pasture. Pelleted feeds containing 50 mg/kg and mineral mixtures containing 1400 mg/kg have caused fatalities in sheep and accidental feeding of 2 kg daily of a pig-meal containing 250 mg/kg of copper to a heifer for 4 months has also been fatal. In lambs a concentrate ration containing 27 mg/kg fed for 16 weeks caused mortality (4). Poisoning is recorded of housed sheep by copper ions shed by a copper water pipe supplying troughs (34). Copper is presently being used as a feed additive in pig rations and may result in poisoning of pigs especially when the mixing of the ration is faulty (30). Concentrate feeds containing 20 mg/kg are dangerous for artificially fed lambs indoors and if the molybdenum content of the feed is very low, levels of 8–11 mg/kg can produce toxicity (5). This is a real and frequent problem in housed experimental sheep on pelleted feeds. Ponies fed copper experimentally appear to be very resistant to poisoning, daily intakes of 791 mg/kg of copper leading to tissue concentrations of over 4000 mg/kg in liver produced no signs of illness (6). Horses housed in yards made of treated pine timber reputedly died of copper poisoning after gnawing the timber. The tissues contained high enough levels to support the diagnosis (36). Arsenic poisoning is also recorded from this source. The status of goats generally is uncertain, but Nubian goats appear to be more resistant than sheep (10).

Copper by injection is being increasingly used to prevent copper deficiency in grazing ruminants when other cheaper methods are not applicable. The paste preparations, usually copper glycinate, appear to be non-toxic but the soluble preparations, e.g. copper edetate, when given at abnormally high levels (twice recommended dose levels), can cause heavy mortalities in sheep (8) and calves. Copper as copper methionate is not toxic at the rate of 6 mg/kg of copper, but as copper calcium ethylene diamine tetra-acetate (EDTA) deaths occur within 48 hours of injection of 3–4 mg/kg (22). Copper as the diethylamine oxyquinoline sulfonate has also caused deaths in sheep after ingestion of recommended dose rates (39). This variable toxicity may be due to the speed with which copper is absorbed into the bloodstream. The absorption is fast and the blood levels high with copper calcium edetate and copper oxyquinoline sulfonate but not with copper methionate (31). Similar toxicity is recorded with copper disodium edetate administered at recommended dose levels. Deaths commenced 24 hours later and were due to massive liver necrosis (35). Clinical signs are not recorded, but postmortem findings included hepatic centrilobular necrosis, nephrosis, pleural and peritoneal effusions. The illness lasts 2–7 days.

Epidemiology

Sporadic outbreaks of primary copper poisoning occur in many circumstances. In both acute and chronic cases the mortality rate approximates 100%.

Most cases of acute poisoning are caused by the accidental administration of large quantities of soluble copper salts, by contamination of plants with fungicidal sprays containing copper, by overdosage with copper-containing parasiticide drenches, by contamination of drinking water when snail eradication programs are in progress, by too liberal ingestion of mineral mixtures containing copper and when animals are grazed on pasture soon after it has been topdressed with a copper salt to correct a copper deficiency. In this circumstance the copper salt remains on the leaves and the pasture should not be grazed for at least 3 weeks or until heavy rain falls. Chronic poisoning may occur on soils rich in copper, or when pasture is contaminated by smelter fumes or by drippings from overhead power cables made of copper but corroded by the constituents of industrially polluted area, by the feeding of seed grain which has been treated with antifungal agents containing copper and by the inclusion of excessive amounts of copper in licks and mineral mixtures. Prophylactic injections of copper salts into animals are commonly used, and care needs to be taken with the more soluble, aqueous preparations that excessive doses are avoided. The amount recommended is usually related to body weight of the animals and farmers may fail to read the instructions or accurately estimate the body weight.

Copper has achieved some prominence as a feed additive for pigs and is normally fed at levels of 125–250 mg/kg of copper in the total ration. However, pigs will eat feed containing as much as 1000 mg/kg of copper and poisoning accidents in this species can easily occur especially if the feed is improperly mixed (23). In diets, concentrations of copper greater than 250 mg/kg are toxic (11) and those greater than 500 mg/kg can cause deaths, but high levels of protein in, or supplementation of the diet with zinc and iron exert some protective effect. If copper-supplemented rations are to be fed, great care should be taken to ensure that the recommended level is adhered to, mixing is adequate and that none of the supplemented diet is fed to sheep. The latter are more susceptible to copper poisoning than are pigs with cattle occupying an intermediate position (3). The application of pig feces as slurry to pasture has caused concern that pollution of the pasture plants and soil with copper may occur if the pigs have been fed high copper rations. It seems unlikely that this will occur unless ruminants graze the pasture soon after the slurry is applied and the plants are physically contaminated, or if very large amounts are applied over long periods. However, there is one record of a mortality in sheep fed hay from a pasture treated with copper-rich pig slurry (14). The hay contained 42 mg/kg of copper. Ewes on pasture dressed with chicken litter from a house in which chickens had been supplemented with copper in their diet also developed chronic copper poisoning (2). Dried poultry waste in the diet of lambs has similarly caused chronic copper poisoning (13).

Pathogenesis

Soluble copper salts in high concentrations are protein coagulants. The ingestion of large quantities causes intense irritation of the alimentary mucosa and profound shock. Severe intravascular hemolysis occurs if the animal survives long enough. When excessive amounts of copper are injected the response is rapid and animals begin to die the next day and with a peak of mortality about the third day after dosing. Early deaths appear to be due to severe hepatic insufficiency and later deaths to renal failure due to tubular necrosis (7, 10, 35). There appear to be no renal lesions in sheep affected with chronic copper poisoning unless a hemolytic crisis occurs in which case there is a hemoglobinuric nephrosis.

The frequent ingestion of small amounts produces no ill-effects while copper accumulates in the liver. When maximum hepatic levels are reached, after periods of exposure often as long as 6 months, the copper is released into the bloodstream, the animal dying of acute intravascular hemolysis. Thus there is really no such thing as 'chronic' copper intoxication; syndromes so called are fatal as acute hemolytic crises. One of the dangers of cumulative copper poisoning is that animals show normal health until the hemolytic crisis when they become acutely ill and die very quickly. Death is ascribed to acute anemia and hemoglobinuric nephrosis. Two other abnormalities have been observed during and after the hemolytic crisis. One is the occurrence of methemoglobinemia; the other is the presence of degenerative lesions in the white matter of the brain (16). The accumulated copper can lead to the occurrence of an hemolytic crisis after ingestion of copper has ceased, and recurrent attacks can therefore occur in sheep that survive the attacks (17). There are a number of explanations for the development of hemolysis. The most attractive is that the erythrocytes in affected sheep become immunogenic as a result of the copper accumulation. It is suggested that this immunogenicity leads to the development of an autoantibody and the final result of an autoimmune hemolytic anemia (21).

The liberation of the hepatic copper is incompletely understood. Various stresses including a fall in plane of nutrition, traveling and lactation, are considered to precipitate the liberation. Complex mechanisms relating to disorders of cell membranes, a marked change in hemoglobin composition, including the development of methemoglobinemia and an increase in the oxidative status of the sheep are described as occurring during the critical stages (18). During the prehemolytic stage of several weeks before the crisis there is hepatic necrosis and an elevation of levels of liver specific enzymes. A much more serious necrosis of liver occurs at the time of the hemolytic crisis. Sheep on a selenium-deficient diet and with low blood levels of glutathione peroxidase are more susceptible to chronic copper poisoning (7). Some sheep are also conditioned by inheritance to have low blood glutathione levels in spite of a normal dietary intake of selenium. They also have low glutathione peroxidase blood levels and may be more susceptible for this reason. A particular susceptibility to copper poisoning has been reported in the Orkney breed of sheep (9). Finnish Landrace are also reported to be less susceptible than Scottish Blackface sheep (12).

There is also a difference between breeds in their capacity to reduce copper absorption in response to the administration of zinc, Texels being much more responsive than Friesians (3). Sheep of the North Ronaldsay breed are also known to be highly susceptible (8). These sheep normally subsist on seaweed which has a very low content of copper and molybdenum. When the sheep are fed on terrestial herbage containing normal levels of copper and molybdenum and high levels of zinc they develop copper poisoning (37).

Clinical findings

Acute intoxication

Severe gastroenteritis occurs accompanied by abdominal

pain and severe diarrhea and vomiting in some species. The feces and vomitus contain much mucus and have a characteristic green to blue color. Vomiting occurs in the pig and dog and intense thirst is apparent. Severe shock with a fall in body temperature and an increase in heart rate is followed by collapse and death usually within 24 hours. If the animal survives for a longer period dysentery and jaundice become apparent (19).

Acute poisoning caused by the injection of copper salts is manifested only by anorexia, depression and dehydration. In calves that survive the illness for 3 days or more massive ascites and hydrothorax and hydropericardium are apparent and hemoglobinuria and massive hemorrhages also occur. Lambs similarly poisoned and with similar postmortem lesions died within 24 hours of injection (1).

Chronic intoxication

In ruminants anorexia, thirst, hemoglobinuria, pallor and jaundice appear suddenly. There is no disturbance of alimentary tract function. Depression is profound and the animal usually dies 24–48 hours after the appearance of signs. The signs in toxemic jaundice are identical with these. In pigs signs of illness are uncommon, most pigs being found dead without premonitory signs, although dullness, anorexia, poor weight gain, melena, weakness, pallor, hyperesthesia and muscle tremor may be observed occasionally (3, 23).

Subclinical disease

Lambs receiving a high experimental intake of copper have shown a slight weight-gain loss on an intake of 27 μg/g dry matter of copper in the diet and a marked loss of weight-gain on an intake of 41 μg/g. No clinical illness was apparent (20).

Clinical pathology

Levels of copper in the blood and liver are markedly increased in chronic copper poisoning. In acute intoxications several days are required after ingestion before these levels rise appreciably. Fecal examination may show large amounts (8000–10 000 mg/kg) of copper. Liver biopsy is a satisfactory diagnostic technique and serves a most useful purpose in the detection of chronic copper poisoning as blood levels do not rise appreciably until the hemolytic crisis occurs just before death. Because of the greater concentration of copper in the caudate lobe as compared to other parts of the liver an autopsy specimen is to be preferred (21). Blood levels of copper during the hemolytic crisis are usually of the order of 78–114 μmol/l, compared to about 15·7 μmol/l in normal animals. Normal liver levels of less than 5·5 mmol/kg dry matter rise to above 15·7 mmol/kg in the latter stages of chronic copper poisoning in sheep, to 95 mmol/kg in pigs, and to 30 mmol/kg in calves. In sheep, liver values greater than 7·85 mmol/kg and kidney values of greater than 1·25–1·57 mmol/kg dry matter are diagnostic (5). After a massive single dose it is important to include kidney among specimens submitted for copper assay because levels may be high (more than 25 mg/kg dry matter) while liver copper levels have not yet risen (24).

The packed cell volume of the blood decreases sharply, from 40 down to 10% in 48 hours, during an acute hemolytic episode. Methemoglobinemia may be present and the urine should be checked for hemoglobin.

Serum enzyme activity is greatly increased just before the hemolytic episode, and there is a significant reduction in the rate of bromosulfalein clearance during this period in sheep (25) and in calves poisoned experimentally. In sheep the SGOT levels may rise as high as 880 SF units per ml up to 6 weeks before obvious clinical signs appear (27), and the rest is regarded as a suitable monitor of copper poisoning in this species (28).

Necropsy findings

In acute copper poisoning severe gastroenteritis is evident with erosion and ulceration particularly in the abomasum. Rupture of the abomasum may occur. If intravascular hemolysis has occurred the lesions characteristic of chronic intoxication may also be present. In calves poisoned by injected solutions of copper salts there is extensive centrilobular necrosis, massive fluid accumulations in body cavities and extensive renal tubular necrosis (10).

In chronic copper poisoning a swollen, yellow liver, a friable spleen with soft pulp, swollen kidneys of a dark gunmetal color, jaundice and hemoglobinuria are characteristic findings. Casts are present in the renal tubules and hemosiderin deposits in the liver and spleen. In both instances the analysis of tissues and alimentary tract contents is essential for confirmation of the diagnosis. Details of the critical copper levels of tissues are provided under clinical pathology. Although the lesions described above do occur in some outbreaks of the disease in pigs, they are not as pronounced as in ruminants and they are often accompanied by severe hemorrhage into the stomach, from ulcers in the pars esophagea, or large intestine (12).

Diagnosis

Histological examination of liver tissue is necessary to determine whether or not liver damage is present. The history and the examination of feedstuffs and pastures are valuable aids in determining the cause. Acute hemolytic diseases which may be mistaken for chronic copper poisoning include leptospirosis, postparturient hemoglobinuria, bacillary hemoglobinuria, rape poisoning and some cases of acute pasteurellosis. The bacterial infections are usually accompanied by fever and toxemia but rape poisoning and postparturient hemoglobinuria can only be diagnosed tentatively by an examination of the environment and consideration of the history. Acute copper poisoning can usually be differentiated from acute gastroenteritis caused by other agents by the blue green color of the ingesta.

Treatment

In acute cases gastrointestinal sedatives and symptomatic treatment for shock are recommended. Dimercaprol intravenously increases copper excretion but there are no reports of its clinical use. Penicillamine is effective, but is too expensive for general field use (15). There could be a rational use for it in valuable animals because it exerts its effects by inducing cupruresis and thus facilitates reduction of tissue levels (28). Calcium EDTA and DMPS (a mercaptan) should theoretically be effective, but has not been of value under experimental conditions (15). Daily oral treatment of affected lambs with 100 mg ammonium molybdate and 1 g anhydrous sodium sulfate significantly reduced the copper content of tissues (28) and appears to prevent deaths in lambs known to have toxic amounts of copper. The mode of action is by increasing the fecal excretion of copper (28). Under experimental conditions ammonium thiomolybdate injected intravenously has an ameliorating effect on copper poisoning by reducing the capacity of circulating copper to enter erythrocytes and cause their lysis (33). Injection of the compound (three to six times intravenously at 2–3-day intervals at a dose rate of 168 mg/100 kg body weight in saline) had a very good effect and the treatment is recommended for field use (38).

Control

When chronic intoxication is occurring or appears probable the provision of additional molybdenum in the diet as described under the control of phytogenous chronic copper poisoning (see below) should be effective as a preventive. Ferrous sulfide is effective but difficulty is usually encountered in getting the animals to eat it. In pigs and sheep the administration of iron and zinc reduces the risk of copper poisoning on diets supplemented by this element (29) and a diet high in calcium encourages the development of copper poisoning, probably by creating a secondary zinc deficiency (12). None of these agents appears to have been used to control copper poisoning in field situations.

SECONDARY COPPER POISONING ('TOXEMIC JAUNDICE' COMPLEX)

Phytogenous chronic copper poisoning

This occurs in sheep grazing pasture containing normal amounts of copper. Although the copper intake may be low, liver copper levels are high and a hemolytic crisis typical of chronic copper poisoning occurs. The occurrence of this form of the disease is related to the domination of the pasture by subterranean clover (*Trifolium subterraneum*) which may contain lower than normal quantities of copper (15–20 mg/kg). British breeds of sheep and their crosses with merinos are most susceptible.

Control of copper poisoning of this type is aided by encouragement of grass growth in pastures. Outbreaks can also be avoided if sheep are prevented from grazing lush, clover-dominant pastures in the autumn. Avoidance of stress, particularly malnutrition, is also important in the prevention of outbreaks. The daily administration of molybdenum in the feed (7 mg/kg molybdenum) has been shown to greatly reduce the uptake of copper by lambs on diets of high copper content (26) and this has been used as a practical preventive measure. Molybdenized superphosphate (70 g/ha molybdenum mg/kg) is valuable to increase the molybdenum content of the pasture and reduce the retention of copper. Molybdenized licks or mineral mixtures (86 kg salt, 63 kg finely ground gypsum, 0·45 kg sodium molybdate) can be used alternatively. When an outbreak occurs the administration of ammonium molybdate (50–100 mg/head/day) together with sodium sulfate (0·3–1·0 g/head/day) has stopped further deaths in sheep within 3 days. Solutions of the above salts may be sprayed onto hay and administration should be continued for several weeks. Addition of copper sulfate to drinking water by a mechanical proportioner that adds 2–3 mg/l of drinking water of copper has been an effective measure (32). A number of other methods have been used with satisfactory results (5) but daily drenching of lambs for 3–13 weeks does not appeal as a practical procedure and administration in salt-lick and pellets is unsatisfactory.

Hepatogenous chronic copper poisoning

This form of the disease occurs most commonly following the ingestion of sufficient quantities of the plant *Heliotropum europaeum*, over a period of 2–5 months, to produce morphological and biochemical changes in liver cells without major impairment of liver function. Other plants containing hepatotoxic alkaloids (*Senecio* spp. and *Echium plantagineum*) (38) also cause this syndrome. After ingestion of these plants the liver cells have an increased affinity for copper and abnormally high amounts accumulate in the liver with an increased risk of a hemolytic crisis. Sheep grazed on *H. europaeum* and then on subterranean clover are particularly prone to this form of the disease. Control depends upon preventing the ingestion of hepatotoxic plants and restricting copper retention by the methods described above.

Poisoning by Heliotropum europaeum

Heliotrope contains hepatotoxic alkaloids and continued ingestion of the plant causes liver damage. If a high copper storage occurs, hepatogenous chronic copper poisoning may develop. On the other hand if the sheep's copper status remains normal liver damage proceeds until the animal suffers from a simple toxipathic hepatitis. The effects of the plant are cumulative and grazing for one season may cause little apparent harm but further grazing in the subsequent year may cause heavy mortality. Control must aim at eradication of the plant.

REVIEW LITERATURE

Bath, G. F. (1979) Enzootic icterus. A form of chronic copper poisoning. *J. S. Afr. vet. Assoc.*, *50*, 3.

Buck, W. B. (1978) Copper/molybdenum toxicity in animals. In: *Toxicity of Heavy Metals in the Environment*, (ed.) F. W. Oehme. New York: Marcel Dekker.

Mason, J. (1986) Thiomolybdates: mediators of molybdenum toxicity and enzyme inhibitors. *Toxicology*, *42*, 99.

Soli, N. E. (1980) Chronic copper poisoning in sheep. *Nord. VetMed.*, *32*, 75.

REFERENCES

(1) Gardiner, B. (1978) *Vet. Rec.*, *103*, 408.
(2) Miller, S. & Nelson, H. A. (1978) *J. Am. vet. med. Assoc.*, *173*, 1587.
(3) Schee, W. van der et al. (1983) *Vet. Q.* 5, 171, in *Tijdschr. Diergeneeskd.*, *108*, 20.
(4) Tait, R. et al. (1971) *Can. vet. J.*, *12*, 73.
(5) Pope, A. L. (1971) *J. anim. Sci.*, *33*, 1332.
(6) Smith, J. D. et al. (1975) *J. anim. Sci.*, *41*, 1645.
(7) Andrewartha, K. A. (1978) *Vict. vet. Pract.*, *36*, 42.
(8) Britt, D. P. & Yeoman, G. H. (1985) *Vet. Res. Commun.*, *9*, 57.
(9) Wiener, G. et al. (1977) *Vet. Rec.*, *101*, 424.
(10) Adam, S. E. I. et al. (1977) *J. comp. Pathol.*, *87*, 623.

(11) De Goey, L. W. et al. (1971) *J. anim. Sci.*, *33*, 52.
(12) Suttle, N. F. (1977) *Anim. Feed Sci. Tech.*, *2*, 235.
(13) Suttle, N. F. et al. (1978) *Anim. Prod.*, *26*, 39.
(14) Feenstra, P. & van Ulsen, F. W. (1973) *Tijdschr. Diergeneeskd.*, *98*, 632.
(15) Soli, N. E. et al. (1978) *Acta vet. Scand.*, *19*, 422.
(16) Howell, J. McC. et al. (1974) *Acta neuropathol.*, *29*, 9.
(17) Gopinath, C. & Howell, J. McC. (1975) *Res. vet. Sci.*, *19*, 35.
(18) Thompson, R. H. & Todd, J. R. (1976) *Res. vet. Sci.*, *20*, 257.
(19) Cabadaj, R. & Gdovin, T. (1970) *Vet. Med. Praha*, *15*, 21.
(20) Hill, R. & Williams, H. L. (1965) *Vet. Rec.*, *77*, 1043.
(21) Wilhelmsen, C. L. (1979) *Cornell Vet.*, *69*, 225.
(22) Mahmoud, O. H. & Ford, E. J. H. (1981) *Vet. Rec.*, *108*, 114.
(23) Hatch, R. C. et al. (1979) *J. Am. vet. med. Assoc.*, *174*, 616.
(24) Sharman, J. R. (1969) *NZ vet. J.*, *17*, 67.
(25) Ishmael, J. et al. (1971) *Res. vet. Sci.*, *13*, 22.
(26) Harker, D. B. (1976) *Vet. Rec.*, *99*, 78.
(27) McPherson, A. & Hemingway, R. G. (1969) *Br. vet. J.*, *125*, 213.
(28) Hidiroglou, M. et al. (1984) *Can. vet. J.*, *25*, 377.
(29) Bremner, I. et al. (1976) *Br. J. Nutr.*, *36*, 551.
(30) Higgins, R. J. (1981) *Vet. Rec.*, *109*, 134.
(31) Mahmoud, O. M. & Ford, E. J. H. (1983) *J. comp. Pathol.*, *93*, 551.
(32) Farmer, P. E. et al. (1982) *Vet. Rec.*, *111*, 193.
(33) Gooneratne, S. R. et al. (1981) *Br. J. Nutr.*, *46*, 457.
(34) Clegg, M. S. et al. (1986) *Agripractice*, *7(1)*, 19.
(35) Bulgin, M. S. et al. (1986) *J. Am. vet. med. Assoc.*, *188*, 406.
(36) Dewes, H. F. & Lowe, M.D. (1985) *NZ vet. J.*, *33*, 159.
(37) Maclachlan, G. K. & Johnston, W. S. (1982) *Vet. Rec.*, *111*, 299.
(38) Seaman, J. T. (1985) *Aust. vet. J.*, *62*, 247.
(39) Mason, R. W. et al. (1984) *Aust. vet. J.*, *61*, 38.

Sodium chloride poisoning

The ingestion of excessive quantities of sodium chloride causes inflammation of the alimentary tract with the production of gastroenteritis and diarrhea. The toxic effect produced when the salt intake is not excessive but the water intake is restricted is one of cerebral edema with a clinical picture characterized mainly by nervous signs.

Etiology

Feed and water containing excessive quantities of salt are usually unpalatable to animals but in certain circumstances listed below excessive quantities of salt are taken, especially in saline drinking waters. The problem of the degree of salinity of drinking water which is compatible with health in animals has received a great deal of attention, but specific details are difficult to provide because of the variation in the salts which occur in natural saline waters. Many of them contain appreciable amounts of fluorine and magnesium which exert a much greater effect on alimentary mucosa than does sodium. Variation also occurs in the relative proportions of the acid radicals, particularly sulfates, carbonates and chlorides. In Australia the two principal artesian basins provide waters of quite different composition. One which is classified as a 'chloride' water is safe for livestock up to a 1% concentration of total salts; at 1·3% concentration there is reduction in lambing percentage in ewes and weight gain in lambs and some increase in mortality rate. The other is classed as a 'bicarbonate' water, containing 0·5% total salts, and has no apparent effect other than a reduction in lambing percentage (1).

Sheep, beef cattle and dry dairy cattle appear to be less susceptible than dairy cows in milk, which are in turn less susceptible than horses. Heavy milking cows, especially those in the early stages of lactation, are highly susceptible to salt poisoning because of their unstable fluid and electrolyte status. Environmental temperatures have an effect on toxicity, signs occurring in the summer on water containing levels of salt which appear to be non-toxic in the winter time. Australian recommendations (2) are that the maximum concentration for sodium chloride or total salts in drinking water should not exceed 1·3% for sheep, 1% for cattle and 0·9% for horses. South African recommendations (3) are considerably lower than these and it is suggested that a concentration of 0·5% total salts in drinking water is excessive for stock. Canadian data (4) recommended much lower levels than the above but there does not appear to be any proof that such low levels of total and individual salts are necessary to avoid poisoning of livestock. Apart from overt signs of toxicity which occur when too much salt is taken it is apparent that lower levels of intake can suppress growth. Also, the use of drinking water containing 0·25% salt significantly reduces the milk yield of high-producing dairy cows (11). In cattle signs of toxicity occur in heifers drinking water containing 1·75% sodium chloride, the animals only maintain weight at a level of 1·5% and show suboptimal weight gains when the water contains 1·25% sodium chloride. Saline waters often contain a mixture of salts and those containing high levels of fluorine may be quite toxic. Water containing 0·2–0·5% magnesium chloride may cause reduced appetite and occasional diarrhea in sheep, especially if the sodium chloride content is also high, but water containing similar quantities of sodium sulfate does not have any harmful effect.

Toxic doses quoted for acute sodium chloride poisoning are for pigs, horses and cattle 2·2 g/kg body weight and for sheep 6 g/kg. The toxicity of salt is significantly influenced by the age and body weight of the subject. For example, dose rates which kill pigs of 6·5–10 kg body weight have little effect on pigs of 16–20 kg (5).

In the circumstances where animals are fed prepared feeds containing the standard recommendation of 2% salt, disease does not occur unless the supply of drinking water is temporarily restricted. It is probable that the physiological disturbance in this instance is one of water intoxication rather than salt poisoning in the absolute sense. High salt intakes are extensively used in sheep to restrict food intake during drought periods and in the control of urolithiasis in feeder wethers but salt poisoning does not occur if there is free access to water. Rations containing up to 13% of sodium chloride have been fed to ewes for long periods without apparent ill effects although diets containing 10–20% and water containing 1·5–2% sodium chloride do reduce food consumption (6). This may be of value when attempting to reduce feed intake but can be a disadvantage when sheep are watered on saline artesian water.

Epidemiology

Salt poisoning is of major importance in some areas where animals are kept under range conditions and have to depend on saline water supplies for drinking purposes. Many animals may be clinically affected and the mortality rate may be high. In animals kept under intensive conditions salt poisoning occurs only sporadically but most affected animals die and heavy losses may occur in groups of pigs.

In animals at pasture salt poisoning can occur in a number of circumstances. A sudden change from fresh water to saline water may cause poisoning, especially if the animals are thirsty when first allowed access to the saline water. Water accumulating in salt troughs during drought periods may also cause poisoning. Animals previously deprived of salt may eat excessive amounts if they are suddenly allowed access to unlimited quantities.

In animals kept in barns and small yards salt poisoning (10) may occur if prepared feeds contain too much salt, if the salt is provided only at long intervals, and when trough space is limited and animals tend to gorge on swill or concentrate. Swill fed to pigs may contain excessive amounts of salt when it contains dough residues from bakeries, brine from butchers' shops, salt whey from cheese factories or salted fish waste. Excessive administration of sodium sulfate to pigs as a treatment for gut edema also produces the disease if the water intake is restricted (7). Another rather special occurrence of salt poisoning is via environmental pollution by oil wells. Cattle are attracted to oil residues because of their salty flavor and may ingest toxic amounts (8).

One of the major occurrences in all species is when animals are being fed a high-normal salt intake but the water supply is temporarily restricted (16, 17). Poisoning occurs when they are again allowed access to unlimited water. Pigs brought into new pens where drinking water is supplied in automatic drinking cups may not be accustomed to their use and be deprived of water for several days until they learn to operate the cups. Feeder lambs and cattle may also be deprived of water when their troughs are frozen over. This form of salt poisoning is recorded most commonly in pigs 8–12 weeks of age but does occur in lambs and calves. A similar occurrence has been recorded in wild life in the northern United States. The source of salt was material deposited on road surfaces to reduce the hazards of ice.

A severe eosinophilic dermatitis has been observed at meat inspection in pigs transported in trucks which were salted to prevent slipping. The pigs were killed 48 hours after transport. The condition was reproduced experimentally by rubbing salt in the skin (9).

Pathogenesis

When excessive amounts of salt are ingested gastroenteritis occurs because of the irritating effects of the high concentrations of salt. Dehydration results and is exacerbated by the increased osmotic pressure of the alimentary tract contents. Some salt is absorbed and may cause involvement of the central nervous system as in chronic poisoning. Poisoning which occurs in these circumstances is described as acute poisoning in contradistinction to the chronic form in which sodium ions accumulate in tissues gradually.

In chronic poisoning where the defect is one of decreased water but normal salt intake there is an accumulation of sodium ions in tissues, including the brain, over a period of several days. When water is made available in unlimited quantities there is a sudden migration of water to the tissues to establish the normal salt–water equilibrium. In the brain this causes acute cerebral edema and the appearance of signs referable to a sudden rise in intracranial pressure (13). The response is the same in all species but in pigs there is, in addition, an accumulation of eosinophils in nervous tissue and the meninges and before the cause of the disease was established it was known as eosinophilic meningoencephalitis. The sodium ion is the one that accumulates in the tissues, identical syndromes being produced by the feeding of sodium propionate or sodium sulfate (7). It has also been observed that the feeding of soluble substances such as urea, which are excreted unchanged by the kidney, may cause anhydremia and an increase in the sodium ion concentration in brain tissue and the development of encephalomalacia.

This form of salt poisoning is chronic only in the sense that the sodium ion accumulates gradually. The clinical syndrome is acute in much the same way as the syndrome is acute in chronic copper poisoning. There is an apparent relationship between this form of salt poisoning and polioencephalomalacia in all species. Many outbreaks of this latter disease occur in circumstances which suggest chronic salt poisoning. It is dealt with in detail under the heading of polioencephalomalacia. Sheep become adapted to a continuous high salt intake (up to 1·3% sodium chloride in the drinking water) by significant changes in numbers of microflora in the rumen but this is not usually accompanied by any change in total metabolic activity (12). The same levels of intake are reported to cause some mortality, chronic diarrhea and reduction in fertility, weight gain and wool growth (1).

Clinical findings

Acute salt poisoning in cattle

With very large doses the clinical signs are largely those of an alimentary tract disturbance. There is vomiting, diarrhea with mucus in the feces, abdominal pain and anorexia. The more common syndrome, which accompanies poisoning by the size of dose usually encountered, is one of numerous signs including opisthotonus, nystagmus, tremor, blindness, paresis and knuckling at the fetlocks. There may be a nasal discharge and polyuria occurs constantly. A period of recumbency with convulsions follows and affected animals die within 24 hours of the appearance of clinical signs. Sheep show similar signs (16). In swine the syndrome suggests less alimentary tract involvement, the signs being largely referable to the nervous system (10). There is great weakness, and prostration, muscle tremor, clonic convulsions, coma and death after a course of about 48 hours.

Chronic salt poisoning

In pigs this is ushered in by the appearance of constipation, thirst and pruritus 2–4 days after exposure commences. A characteristic nervous syndrome follows within 12–24 hours. Initially there is apparent blindness and deafness, the pig remaining oblivious to normal stimuli and wandering about aimlessly, bumping into objects and pressing with the head. There may be circling or pivoting on one front leg. Recovery may occur at this stage or epileptiform convulsions may appear. These convulsive episodes recur at remarkably constant time intervals, usually 7 minutes, and commence with tremor of the snout and neck. Clonic contractions of the neck muscles may result in the jerky development of opisthotonus until the head is almost vertical and the pig walks backwards and assumes a sitting posture. This may be followed by a complete clonic convulsion with the pig laterally recumbent. During the convulsion there is champing of the jaws, salivation and respiratory distress. Death may occur due to respiratory failure or the pig relaxes into a state of coma for a few moments, revives and wanders about aimlessly until the next episode occurs. The pulse and temperature are normal except in convulsive pigs when both may be elevated. The course is variable and death may occur in a few hours or not for 3–4 days after the first appearance of illness.

A syndrome which is often described as chronic salt poisoning occurs in cattle and sheep on saline drinking water. There is a depression of appetite, loss of body weight, dehydration, depression of body temperature, weakness and occasional diarrhea. If affected cattle are forced to take exercise they may collapse and have tetanic convulsions. In dairy cattle acetonemia may occur in these circumstances.

Clinical pathology

In pigs serum sodium levels are elevated appreciably above normal levels (135–145 mmol/l), to about 180–190 mmol/l during the severe stage of chronic sodium salt poisoning (13). Also polydipsia is recorded at blood serum levels of sodium chloride of 900 mg/dl, typical signs of salt poisoning at 1300 mg/dl, and death when levels exceeded 1500 mg/dl (5). An eosinopenia is also evident during this stage and a return to normal levels usually indicates recovery. In cattle the same changes occur but there is no eosinopenia. Samples of feed and drinking water should be collected for salt assay.

Necropsy findings

In acute salt poisoning of cattle there is marked congestion of the mucosae of the omasum and abomasum. The feces are fluid and in some cases sufficiently dark in color to suggest that they contain blood. Animals which have survived for several days show edema of the skeletal muscles and hydropericardium. The blood appears to be thinner than normal. Gastroenteritis may be evident in some pigs poisoned with large doses of salt but in chronic poisoning there are no gross lesions. Histologically the lesions of chronic poisoning in the pig are quite diagnostic. There is acute cerebral edema and meningoencephalitis accompanied by an invasion by eosinophils of the meninges and perivascular spaces around the blood vessels of the brain. In pigs that survive the acute stages there may be residual polioencephalomalacia especially of the cerebral cortex. Chemical estimation of the amount of sodium and chloride in tissues, especially brain, may be of diagnostic value. Levels exceeding 150 mg/dl of sodium in the brain and liver, and of chlorides in excess of 180 mg in the brain, 70 mg in muscle and 250 mg/dl in the liver are considered to indicate salt poisoning (14). Comparison of levels in serum and CSF is worthwhile. In salt poisoning the sodium content is significantly higher in CSF than serum (15).

Diagnosis

The appearance of typical signs in pigs which have been just moved to new quarters or subjected to change of ration during the preceding week, or which have not had access to water at all times, immediately suggests sodium salt poisoning. Other diseases of the nervous system in feeder pigs may resemble salt poisoning. If convulsions occur the temperature in pigs poisoned with salt may be sufficiently high to suggest encephalitis. Pseudorabies is restricted in its occurrence to young sucking pigs, viral encephalomyelitis occurs in pigs of all ages, but in both the syndrome may be very similar to that of salt poisoning. Polioencephalomalacia in pigs and ruminants is almost identical with chronic salt poisoning and occurs in many instances under the same set of circumstances. Gut edema occurs in rapidly growing pigs in the same age group as chronic salt poisoning. There are some differences in the clinical syndromes as they occur in the field, particularly the periodicity of the convulsive episodes in salt poisoning and the altered squeal in gut edema, but in many instances it will be impossible to decide on the diagnosis without reference to the history of salt and water intake. Mulberry heart disease may be accompanied by nervous signs similar to those of salt poisoning but the disease is usually restricted to older pigs and deaths occur quite suddenly.

Gastroenteritis caused by excessive ingestion of saline drinking water has few diagnostic features and the diagnosis depends upon detection of the salinity of the water. A recent change in the source of drinking water is often a part of the history. Laboratory analysis of feed and water is necessary for confirmation.

Treatment

In both acute and chronic salt poisoning the toxic feed or water must be removed immediately. Initially access to fresh water should be restricted to small amounts at frequent intervals as unlimited access to water may result in a sudden increase in the number of animals affected. In advanced cases animals may be unable to drink and water may have to be administered by stomach tube.

Symptomatic treatment includes alimentary tract sedatives when gastroenteritis is present and the provision of isotonic fluids when dehydration has occurred. When there is evidence of cerebral edema it may be necessary to administer a sedative and cerebral decompression may be attempted by the use of diuretics or hypertonic solutions injected parenterally.

Control

Drinking water for all classes of livestock should not contain more than 0·5% sodium chloride or total salts although sheep and beef cattle can survive on water containing as much as 1·7% sodium chloride or total salts. Waters containing a high concentration of fluoride or magnesium are particularly dangerous to livestock. Both salt and water should be freely available at all times. Diets fed to pigs should not contain more than 1% salt. The way in which whey is fed to pigs—with minimum water intake—makes prevention difficult unless the whey can be kept free of salt at the cheese factory.

REFERENCES

(1) Pierce, A. W. (1968) *Aust. J. agric. Res.*, *19*, 577, 589.
(2) Pierce, A. W. (1963) *Aust. J. agric. Res.*, *14*, 815.
(3) Steyn, D. G. & Reinach, N. (1939) *Onderstepoort J. vet. Sci.*, *12*, 167.
(4) Ballantyne, E. E. (1957) *Can. J. comp. Med.*, *21*, 254.
(5) Adamesteanu, I. et al. (1972) *Bull. Soc. Sci. vet. Med. comp. Lyon*, *74*, 265.
(6) Wilson, A. D. (1966) *Aust. J. agric. Res.*, *17*, 503.
(7) Dow, C. et al. (1963) *Vet. Rec.*, *75*, 1052.
(8) Monlux, A. W. et al. (1971) *J. Am. vet. med. Assoc.*, *158*, 1379.
(9) Anderson, P. & Petaja, E. (1968) *Nord. VetMed.*, *20*, 706.
(10) Sandals, W. C. D. (1978) *Can. vet. J.*, *19*, 136.
(11) Jaster, E. H. et al. (1979) *J. dairy Sci.*, *61*, 66.
(12) Potter, B. J. et al. (1972) *Br. J. Nutr.*, *27*, 75.
(13) Smith, D. L. T. (1957) *Am. J. vet. Res.*, *18*, 825.
(14) Bohosiewicz, M. (1962) *Veterinariya, Moscow*, *11*, 3.
(15) Osweiler, G. D. & Hurd, J. W. (1974) *J. Am. vet. med. Assoc.*, *165*, 165.
(16) Scarratt, W. K. et al. (1985) *J. Am. vet. med. Assoc.*, *186*, 977.
(17) Pearson, E. G. & Kallfelz, F. A. (1982) *Cornell Vet.*, *72*, 142.

Zinc poisoning

Poisoning by zinc compounds occurs only rarely and the syndrome reported is poorly defined.

Etiology

Soluble zinc salts causing poisoning in animals usually originate from galvanized ironware used as piping or drinking utensils. Toxic doses are not well defined but drinking water containing 6–8 mg/kg of zinc has caused constipation in cattle (1), and 200 g of zinc as lactate fed over a period of 2 months as a 0·1% solution has caused arthritis in pigs (2). Zinc chromate used as a paste in joining electrical cables has caused poisoning in calves (3); the acute toxicity appears to be due to the chromic oxide content of the paste but chronic intoxication may be caused by the accumulation of zinc. Experimental zinc poisoning in sheep and cattle caused reduced weight gains and feed efficiency when zinc was fed at the rate of 1 g/kg body weight. At 1·5–1·7 g/kg body weight there was reduced feed consumption in both species and depraved appetite in cattle (5). The accidental inclusion of zinc oxide in a prepared feed for dairy cows led to the ingestion by some of 150 g daily resulting in serious illness in many cattle and death in 7% of them (6). Zinc dust may be an industrial hazard, but dose rates up to 45 mg/kg body weight have no effect on cattle. At dose rates of 50 mg/kg anemia occurs, and deaths occur at daily dose rates of 110 mg/kg body weight (7). Zinc sulfate is now a popular prophylactic and treatment for poisoning by fungi, especially *Pithomyces chartarum*. It is also a favored part of the treatment of ovine foot rot and is used orally in the treatment of lupinosis. It is reasonable to expect poisoning due to accidental access to or to accidental dosing with prepared solutions; sheep may also voluntarily drink the footbath solution (17). It is apparent that daily doses of 50–100 mg zinc/kg body weight in these circumstances can cause severe abomasal lesions and pancreatic damage and cause death in sheep, provided the material is administered with a drenching gun. The same dose administered by ruminal intubation is non-toxic (12). It seems likely that the zinc triggers a closure of the reticular groove resulting in its immediate deposition in the abomasum. Oral dosing with large doses of zinc oxide to provide protection for 3–18 days can also cause hypocalcemia and a syndrome comparable to milk fever (14).

Epidemiology

Zinc may be released from galvanized surfaces when subjected to electrolysis as occurs when galvanized and copper pipes are joined. Cattle may be poisoned by fumes from a nearby galvanizing factory (8). Zinc, often associated with cadmium, is a common pollutant from industrial plants handling a variety of ores (1). The pasture may contain more than 500 mg/kg of zinc (15). Zinc-based paints, with a 50–55% zinc content, are a common source of poisoning when cattle lick freshly painted ironwork. An outbreak of poisoning has been recorded in pigs fed buttermilk from a dairy factory. The buttermilk was piped to the pigpens each day through a long galvanized iron pipe. The buttermilk lay in pools in the pipe after each batch was run through, souring occurred and the lactic acid produced caused the formation of zinc lactate which was passed to the pigs in the next batch of buttermilk. The concentration of zinc in the milk (0·066%) was slightly higher than the minimum toxic strength (0·05%). The addition of zinc to pig rations as a preventive against parakeratosis is unlikely to cause poisoning because of the low toxicity of the element and the unpalatability of rations containing excessive amounts. The maximum amount tolerated by pigs is 0·1% zinc (as zinc carbonate) in the diet. Levels greater than this cause decreased food intake, arthritis, hemorrhages in the axillae, gastritis and enteritis. Death may occur within 21 days (4). Zinc fed experimentally to foals causes pharyngeal and laryngeal paralysis, stiffness and lameness resulting from swelling of the epiphyses of long bones (9). Zinc has been added to calf-grower rations for no specific reason of dietary deficiency and serious poisoning incidents have occurred as a result (20).

Interbreed differences between sheep in their susceptibility to zinc poisoning has been proposed but not demonstrated (18).

Pathogenesis

The pathogenesis of zinc poisoning has not been determined, but it is likely that the arthritic lesions observed will be due to faulty calcium absorption.

Clinical findings

Pigs fed buttermilk containing zinc show anorexia, unthriftiness, rough coat, subcutaneous hematomas (24), stiffness and lameness. There is progressive weakness with enlargement of the joints, particularly the shoulder joint. Chronic poisoning in horses causes a non-specific, degenerative arthritis (1, 10) especially at the distal end of the tibia. The lesion is accompanied by an effusion into the joint capsule and the obvious enlargement of the hock joint (13). There may also be a generalized osteoporosis, lameness, and illthrift (5). Dairy cattle drinking contaminated water show chronic constipation and a fall in milk yield. Experimental dosing with large quantities of soluble zinc salts causes diarrhea, dysentery, or subcutaneous edema, jaundice, posterior weakness and death. A natural outbreak in cattle caused scouring and drastic reduction in milk yield. Severely affected cattle, poisoned by licking zinc paint, show additional signs including somnolence, paresis and a light green-colored diarrhea.

Clinical pathology

After experimental feeding high levels of zinc are detectable in tissues, especially liver, pancreas and kidney, and serum and liver levels of copper are reduced. Serum zinc levels in affected cattle may be as high as 500 μg/ml, in contrast with the usual levels of about 140 μg/ml in normal cattle (8). Fecal levels of zinc are likely to be elevated from an average of 220 mg/kg in normal animals to 8740 mg/kg in affected ones.

Necropsy findings

Severe, acute poisoning in sheep is accompanied by abomasitis and duodenitis the mucosa of which will be green in color (16) and a severe, later fibrosing pancreatitis. Acute poisoning in cattle has been accompanied by generalized pulmonary emphysema, pale flabby myocardium, hemorrhages in kidney and severe hepatic degeneration (6). In chronic poisoning there are lesions in all organs but the most consistent ones are in the pancreas, and it is essential that it be examined when zinc is the object of the search (11).

In chronic zinc poisoning in pigs there is a nonspecific, degenerative arthritis affecting particularly the head of the humerus, the articular cartilage being separated from the underlying bone which has undergone extensive osteoporotic changes. There may be some renal damage. In more severe poisoning there is gastritis, enteritis, arthritis, hemorrhages under the skin, in the ventricles of the brain and in lymph nodes and spleen (4). There are similar lesions, and nephrosclerosis in foals (1). Ingesta, liver, kidney, spleen and bone should be submitted for analysis. The zinc content of liver in normal animals is high (30–150 mg/kg wet matter in calves) and may reach levels of 400–600 mg/kg wet matter after continued ingestion of zinc chromate paste without being accompanied by signs of zinc poisoning. In acute poisoning by zinc oxide in cattle levels of 2000 mg/kg dry matter in liver and 300–700 mg/kg dry matter in kidney may be achieved; tissue copper levels in these animals may be reduced to 10–20 mg/kg (6).

Diagnosis

Arthritis caused by zinc poisoning in pigs must be differentiated from rickets and erysipelas. Chronic constipation as a herd problem in cattle is most unusual and zinc poisoning should be considered as a possible cause when it occurs.

Treatment

Special treatments have not been recommended and removal of the source of zinc and symptomatic treatment are suggested as the only measures available.

Control

Galvanized utensils and piping should be rinsed after each use in carrying milk. The addition of extra amounts of calcium to the diet of pigs is capable of preventing the toxic effects of zinc if the calcium supplementation is heavy and the zinc intake is not too high.

REFERENCES

(1) Gunson, D. E. et al. (1982) *J. Am. vet. med. Assoc.*, *180*, 295.
(2) Grimmett, R. E. R. et al. (1939) *NZJ Agric.*, *59*, 140.
(3) Harrison, D. L. & Staples, E. L. J. (1955) *NZ vet. J.*, *3*, 63.
(4) Palmer, J. S. (1963) *J. Am. vet. med. Assoc.*, *143*, 994.
(5) Eamens, J. G. et al. (1984) *Aust. vet. J.*, *61*, 205.
(6) Allen, G. S. (1968) *Vet. Rec.*, *83*, 8.
(7) Rosenberger, G. & Grunder, H. D. (1976) *Proc. 20th World vet. Congr.*, *3*, 2059.
(8) Wentink, G. H. et al. (1985) *Vet. Q.*, *7*, 153.
(9) Willoughby, R. A. et al. (1972) *Can. J. comp. Med.*, *36*, 348.
(10) Kronemann, J. & Goedegebuirne, S. A. (1980) *Tijdschr. Diergeenskd.*, *105*, 1049.
(11) Allen, J. G. et al. (1983) *J. comp. Pathol.*, *93*, 363.
(12) Smith, B. L. et al. (1979) *NZ J. exp. Agr.*, *7*, 107.
(13) Messer, N. T. (1981) *J. Am. vet. med. Assoc.*, *178*, 294.
(14) Smith, B. L. et al. (1984) *NZ vet. J.*, *32*, 48.
(15) Hoskam, E. G. et al. (1982) *Tijdschr. Diergeneeskd.*, *107*, 672.
(16) Allen, J. G. (1986) *Aust. vet. J.*, *63*, 93.
(17) Dargatz, D. A. et al. (1986) *Agripractice*, *7*, 30.
(18) Ellis, T. M. et al. (1984) *Aust. vet. J.*, *61*, 296.
(19) Pritchard, G. C. et al. (1985) *Vet. Rec.*, *117*, 545.
(20) Graham, T. W. et al. (1987) *J. Am. vet. med. Assoc.*, *190*, 668.

Sulfur poisoning

Elemental sulfur (flowers of sulfur) is often fed to livestock as a tonic and to control external parasites. It is also used in feedlots to restrict the consumption of feed by lambs and thus reduce the incidence of enterotoxemia. In small doses the substance is relatively nontoxic but excessive doses can cause fatal gastroenteritis and dehydration (1). Most deaths occur because of inadvertent overdosing. The feeding of 85–450 g per head to cattle has been fatal (2), as has 45 g of sulfur in feed pellets to ewes (3), and the minimum lethal dose of a sulfur-protein concentrate for sheep is estimated to be 10 g/kg body weight. Continuous feeding of sulfur at the rate of 7 g per day can be fatal to adult sheep (3). Accidental feeding of flowers of sulfur to adult horses at a dose level of 0·2–0·4 kg per horse has caused poisoning (4). It is possible that sulfur is most toxic when fed in a ration containing a high level of protein. Sodium metabisulfite and sulfur dioxide gas are used in the preparation of ensilage but at the levels used are unlikely to have toxic effects in animals eating the ensilage. Hydrogen sulfide gas is often present in gases emanating from oil and natural gas wells, in cesspools and in wells but animals are not likely to be exposed to concentrations of the gas which are sufficiently high to cause illness, although a slatted floor system of manure disposal, if functioning imperfectly, might present problems.

Clinically the syndrome is characterized by dullness, abdominal pain, muscle twitching, black diarrhea and a strong odor of hydrogen sulfide on the breath. Dehydration is severe and the animals soon become recumbent and dyspneic, develop convulsions and die in a coma.

At necropsy the lungs are congested and edematous, the liver is pale, the kidneys congested and black in color and there is severe gastroenteritis with peritoneal effusion. Petechial hemorrhages have been observed to occur extensively in all organs and in musculature (3).

One of the early blows in the battle over pollution of animal environments has been struck in an examination of the effects of constant exposure of pigs to an atmosphere containing 35 mg/kg of sulfur dioxide for 1–6 weeks. Increased salivation was apparent and was accompanied by clinical and histological evidence of irritation of the conjunctiva and respiratory mucosa (5, 6).

REFERENCES

(1) Julian, R. J. & Harrison, K. B. (1975) *Can. vet. J.*, *16*,28.
(2) McFarlane, D. F. (1952) *Vet. Rec.*, *64*, 345.
(3) White, J. B. (1964) *Vet. Rec.*, *76*, 278.
(4) Corke, M. J. (1981) *Vet. Rec.*, *109*, 212.
(5) Lawson, G. H. F. & McAllister, J. V. S. (1966) *Vet. Rec.*, *79*, 274.
(6) Martin, S. W. & Willoughby, R. A. (1971) *J. Am. vet. med. Assoc.*, *159*, 1518.

Poisoning by organic iron compounds

Heavy fatalities have occurred in young piglets soon after the injection of organic iron compounds used to prevent anemia. Death is due to acute iron poisoning (1). Within an hour or two of injection sudden deaths occur, sometimes accompanied by vomiting and diarrhea. At necropsy examination there is severe myodegeneration (2) of skeletal but not cardiac muscle. The progeny of vitamin E deficient sows are most susceptible (3) and the most toxic compounds are those which contain a high proportion of their iron in ionic, and therefore readily absorbable form. In the absence of vitamin E the muscle cell membranes are damaged and extensive biochemical changes results. One of these is a great increase in extracellular potassium levels causing cardiac arrest and sudden death (1). Pigs at 2 days of age are much more susceptible to the toxic effects of these iron compounds than are 8-day-old pigs, apparently because of the older pigs' better renal functional ability to excrete iron. Another possible reason for this age difference in combating iron toxicity is the greater mobilization of calcium by older pigs in response to iron administration. This mobilization, or calciphylaxis, can be great enough to result in deposition of calcium in damaged tissues or cause death. This effect appears to be precipitated by simultaneous or immediately preceding (within 24 hours) injection of vitamin D_3 (4) but the injection is not essential to it. Much of the administered iron is taken up by the reticuloendothelial system, and it has been suggested that blockage of the system with the iron preparation has removed the buffering action of the system against absorbed toxins whether they are bacterial or inorganic (5).

There is an additional possible damaging effect of iron injection in young pigs, the development of asymmetric hindquarters (1, 6). In this condition there is asymmetry but the muscles are normal in composition and appear to have asymmetric blood supplies. Deaths have also occurred in horses within a few minutes of intramuscular injection of iron compounds. Other horses have shown severe shock but recovered. Death when it occurs appears to be due to acute heart failure (7).

REFERENCES

(1) Patterson, D. S. P. & Allen, W. M. (1972) *Br. vet. J.*, *128*, 101.
(2) Arpi, T. & Tollerz, G. (1965) *Acta vet. Scand.*, *6*, 360.
(3) Tollerz, G. & Lannek, N. (1964) *Nature, Lond.*, *201*, 846.
(4) Penn, G. B. (1970) *Vet. Rec.*, *86*, 718.
(5) Lindvall, S. et al. (1972) *Acta vet. Scand.*, *13*, 206.
(6) Hoorens, J. & Oyaert, W. (1970) *Vlaams Diergeneeskd. Tijdschr.*, *39*, 246.
(7) Lannek, N. & Persson, S. (1972) *Svensk VetTidn.*, *24*, 341.

Iodine poisoning

Poisoning with iodine is not regarded as a likely cause of illness in animals because the toxic dose is so great. Doses of 10 mg/kg body weight daily are required to produce fatal illness in calves (1). In cattle and sheep lacrimation, anorexia, hyperthermia, nasal discharge, hypersalivation and coughing due to bronchopneumonia result from moderate poisoning. Severe cases may die of bronchopneumonia, and exophthalmos occurs in some cases. Heavy dusting of the hair coat with large-sized dandruff scales, accompanied by hair loss and dryness of the coat are also common. Squamous metaplasia of tracheal and parotid duct epithelium is also recorded and serum vitamin A levels are also reduced. Serum iodine levels are raised from the normal level of 5–10 μg/100 ml up to 20–130 μg/ml (7).

Toxicity has also occurred at much lower levels of intake (e.g., 160 mg/day per cow) and appears to be a practical risk when cows or calves are fed organic iodides such as ethylene diamine dihydroiodide constantly as a prophylactic against footrot (2, 8, 9). The toxic effects include a serious increased susceptibility to calf pneumonia, and to abortion in pregnant cows.

Iodism is not recorded often in horses. It is characterized by alopecia and heavy dandruff (6). There appears to be a special occurrence of goiter in foals when the foal and the dam are fed an excessive amount of iodine (5). Intakes of 35–40 mg iodine/day to a mare can cause the development of goiter in her foal. Daily intakes of iodine as high as 432 mg have been achieved with mares fed kelp as a nutritional supplement and congenital goiter may also occur in the foals of these mares (3).

REVIEW LITERATURE

Stowe, C. M. (1981) Iodine, iodides and iodism. *J. Am. vet. med. Assoc.*, *179*, 334–335.

REFERENCES

(1) Mongkoewidjojo, S. et al. (1980) *Am. J. vet. Res.*, *41*, 1057.
(2) Hillman, D. & Curtis, A. R. (1980) *J. dairy Sci.*, *63*, 55.
(3) Baker, H. J. & Lindsey, J. R. (1968) *J. Am. vet. med. Assoc.*, *153*, 1618.
(4) Olson, W. G. et al. (1984) *J. Am. vet. med. Assoc.*, *184*, 179.
(5) Conway, D. A. & Cosgrove, J. S. (1980) *Irish vet. J.*, *34*, 29.
(6) Fadok, V. A. (1983) *J. Am. vet. Med. Assoc.*, *183*, 1104.
(7) Stowe, C. M. (1981) *J. Am. vet. med. Assoc.*, *179*, 334.

(8) Andersson, L. & Tornquist, M. (1983) *Vet. Rec.*, *113*, 215.
(9) Morrow, D. A. & Edwards, L. (1981) *Bov. Practnr*, p. 114.

Cadmium poisoning

Cadmium salts have little currency as anthelmintics, but there is a mention of cadmium poisoning under that heading. There is, however, a good deal of interest in the element with respect to its occurrence as an environmental pollutant and its likelihood of entering the human food chain. Naturally occurring cases of poisoning by cadmium salts are rare in animals, most cases resulting from accidental administrations of farm chemicals. For example, in an outbreak of poisoning in ponies characterized by colic, disorientation and ataxia, it was thought that the consumption of paint containing cadmium was the cause (2). Sewage and sewage sludge may have higher than desirable levels of cadmium but have not been shown to cause poisoning when used as pasture topdressing or as feed (1). Conversely cattle are seen to be an effective screen or filter between the high content of cadmium in the diet and the human consumer of the meat (11).

Chronic experimental dosing of calves at the daily rate of 18 mg/kg body weight, combined with a similar dose of lead, produced clinical evidence of poisoning (3). In sheep, levels of 60 μg/g of feed for 137 days are needed to cause illness (4). For young pigs, levels in the feed of 50 mg/kg for 6 weeks proved toxic and reduced growth rate. A significant anemia results (5) and this is preventable by high doses (800–1000 μg) of iron as a single injection (6).

Chronic poisoning in cattle causes inappetence, weakness, loss of weight, poor hoof keratinization, dry brittle horns, matting of the hair, keratosis and peeling of the skin. At necropsy there is hyperkeratosis of forestomach epithelium and degenerative changes in most organs (7). Experimental poisoning of sheep causes anemia, nephropathy and bone demineralization at a dose rate of 2·5 mg/kg body weight/day (8). A cadmium-containing fungicide is also toxic causing abortion, congenital defects and stillbirths when fed to pregnant cows and ewes (9). The cutaneous effect of cadmium poisoning resembles that produced by a dietary deficiency of zinc, and the effect of the cadmium can be partly offset by the administration of zinc (10).

The chances of cadmium accumulating in lean meat are not very great because the levels of ingestion required to produce significant levels are so high that they would cause observable clinical illness. However, kidney and liver do accumulate cadmium much more readily (12).

REFERENCES

(1) Osuna, O. et al. (1981) *Am. J. vet. Res.*, *42*, 1542.
(2) Sass, B. et al. (1972) *Vet. Med. SAC*, *67*, 745.
(3) Lynch, G. P. et al. (1976) *J. anim. Sci.*, *42*, 410.
(4) Doyle, J. J. (1974) *Diss. Abstr. Int.*, *35B*, 611.
(5) Cousins, R. J. et al. (1973) *J. Nutr.*, *103*, 964.
(6) Pond, W. G. et al. (1973) *J. anim. Sci.*, *36*, 1122.
(7) Rotkiewiez, T. et al. (1979) *Med. Weterynaryjna*, *25*, 486.
(8) Glaser, U. et al. (1978) *Zentralbl. VetMed.*, *25A*, 685 & 821.
(9) Wright, F. C. et al. (1977) *J. agric. Food Chem.*, *25*, 293.
(10) Powell, G. W. et al. (1964) *J. Nutr.*, *84*, 205.
(11) Ligget, A. D. et al. (1985) *J. Am. vet. med. Assoc.*, *187*, 72.
(12) Sharma, R. P. & Street, J. C. (1980) *J. Am. vet. med. Assoc.*, *177*, 149.

Chromium poisoning

Use of a protein concentrate prepared from tannery waste is not recommended because of the material's high chromium content. Trivalent chromium salts given orally to pigs at the rate of 0·5–1·5 and at 3 mg/kg body weight produced transient diarrhea. With the higher dosage there was also tremor, dyspnea and anorexia (1).

REFERENCES

(1) Vishnyakov, S. I. et al. (1985) *Veterinariya, Moscow*, *5*, 69.

Vanadium poisoning

Experimental (1) and natural (2) poisoning of adult cattle and calves are recorded. These include diarrhea, sometimes dysentery, oliguria, difficulty in standing and incoordination. Field cases are only likely to be encountered when industrial contamination of pasture occurs.

REFERENCES

(1) Platonow, N. & Abbey, H. K. (1968) *Vet. Rec.*, *82*, 292.
(2) Milhaud, G. & Bouye, H. (1977) *Rec. med. Vet.*, *153*, 369.

Bromide poisoning

Accidental access to sodium bromide by goats has resulted in a syndrome of somnolence, lateral recumbency, drooping of the ears, eyelids and tail and dribbling of urine. At biochemical examination the high level of bromide in the blood gave a spuriously high level of serum chloride (1).

REFERENCES

(1) Liggett, A.D. et al. (1985) *J. Am. vet. med. Assoc.*, *187*, 72.

Cobalt poisoning

Overdosing with cobalt compounds is unlikely but toxic signs of loss of weight, rough hair coat, listlessness, anorexia and muscular incoordination appear in calves at dose rates of about 40–55 mg of elemental cobalt per 50 kg body weight per day. Sheep appear to be much more resistant to the toxic effects of cobalt than are cattle (1) and can withstand continued daily intake of 15 mg/kg body weight of cobalt without apparent effect (2). Pigs have tolerated up to 200 mg cobalt/kg of diet. At intakes of 400 and 600 mg/kg there is growth depression, anorexia, stiffness of the legs, incoordination and muscle tremors (3). Supplementation of the diet with methionine, or with additional iron, manganese and zinc alleviate the toxic effects.

REFERENCES

(1) Andrews, E.D. (1965) *NZ vet. J.*, *13*, 101.
(2) Corrier, D.E. et al. (1986) *Vet. hum. Toxicol.*, *28*, 216.
(3) Huck, D.W. & Clawson, A.J. (1976) *J. anim. Sci.*, *43*, 1231.

32

Diseases Caused by Chemical Agents—II

DISEASES CAUSED BY ORGANIC POISONS

Hydrocyanic acid poisoning

ACUTE poisoning by hydrocyanic acid causes a histotoxic anoxia with a syndrome of dyspnea, tremor, convulsions and sudden death. Chronic poisoning may lead to the development of goiter in newborn animals.

Etiology

Most outbreaks of hydrocyanic acid poisoning are caused by the ingestion of plants which contain cyanogenetic glucosides. In this form the acid is nontoxic but it may be liberated from the organic complex by the action of an enzyme which may also be present in the same or other plant, or by the activity of rumen microorganisms. Horses and pigs are much less susceptible to the glucosides because the acidity of the stomach in monogastric animals helps to destroy the enzyme. Sheep are much more resistant than cattle, apparently because of differences between enzyme systems in the forestomachs of the two animals.

Many plants contain cyanogenetic glucosides and it is not proposed to list them all here. Many of them are weeds including native couch (*Brachyachne convergens*). Bermuda and blue couch grasses, arrowgrass (*Triglochin* sp.), tall mannagrass (*Glyceria maxima* sp.) (4, 15), chokecherry, native fuchsia (*Eremophila maculata*) and particularly plants of the flax family. Saskatoon serviceberry (*Amelanchier alnifolia*) foliage is also cyanogenetic and when the animal's diet contains 75% of this plant severe toxicity can be expected (7). Cyanide poisoning of goats has resulted from the ingestion of foliage of the sugargum tree (*Eucalyptus cladocalyx*) (13). Reed sweet grass (*Poa aquatica*) can contain 1·52 mg hydrocyanic acid (HCN) per g dry material and is thought to have caused heavy mortalities in hungry traveling stock (1). Some garden plants, including the cherry laurel tree (*Prunus laurocerasus*), flowering quince (*Chaenomeles* spp.), *Nandina domestica*, *Photinia* spp. (syn. Christmas berry) (16) and the common crab-apple (*Malus sylvestris*) (14) are potent sources, but their content of cyanogenetic glucosides varies widely between seasons and between different parts of the plant (17). Of greatest importance are a number of common pasture and cultivated plants. Johnson grass (*Sorghum halepense*), Sudan grass (*S. sudanense*) and sorghum (*S. vulgare*) are used extensively in some countries for forage and may cause heavy mortalities in particular circumstances. Sugar cane contains a cyanogenetic glucoside from which hydrocyanic acid can be released. Release occurs through the action of an enzyme in algarrobo pods (*Prosopsis glandulosa*) when the two are fed together (2). Linseed in the form of cake or meal may also be highly toxic if eaten in large quantities. Some clovers, particularly white clover (*Trifolium repens*) (6) and members of the *Brassica* genus may also contain significant amounts of cyanogenetic glucosides, but poisoning by cyanide is not recorded on clovers, probably because of their high content of sulfur.

Drying, haymaking and physical factors such as chilling and freezing may appear to reduce the toxicity of cyanogenetic material because of the destruction of the enzyme beta-glucosidase, but the plant material remains as potentially toxic as previously, requiring only to encounter the enzyme in the rumen to become fully poisonous.

A number of specific glucosides have been isolated and include linamarin from linseed and flax, lotaustralin from white clover, dhurrin from sorghum, lotusin from *Lotus arabicus* and amygdalin from bitter almonds. The glucosides are byproducts of plant metabolism and their concentration in the different plant species is variable depending upon climatic and other conditions which influence plant growth.

The minimum lethal dose of hydrocyanic acid is about 2 mg/kg body weight for cattle and sheep when taken in the form of a glucoside. The minimum lethal dose (MLD) of lotaustralin for sheep approximates 4 mg/kg body weight (3). Plant material containing more than 20 mg of hydrocyanic acid per 100 g (200 ppm) is likely to cause toxic effects and highly poisonous samples may contain as much as 6000 ppm. The toxic doses quoted must be accepted with some reservation as the toxicity of a particular specimen varies with a number of factors including the concentration of the hydrolyzing enzyme in the plant, the preceding diet of the animals and particularly the speed with which the material is eaten.

Epidemiology

Hydrocyanic acid poisoning occurs in most countries because of the common occurrence of plants which contain toxic quantities of cyanides. When the disease occurs most affected animals die and although the overall economic effects are not great, the losses may be heavy on individual farms.

Poisoning is most likely to occur when the cyanide content of the material is high and it is eaten quickly. The glucoside content is highest when plants grow rapidly after a previous period of retardation. This is most likely to occur when autumn rains cause rapid growth after stunting during a summer drought, or when a crop is eaten back by livestock or grasshoppers, or following the application of herbicides. Wilted, frost-bitten and young plants are also likely to be more poisonous than normal, mature plants. A high soil concentration of nitrogen is one of the principal precursors of a high hydrocyanic acid content of plants, and a low phosphorus status is similarly conducive (12). The greatest danger exists when animals which are hungry are allowed access to heavy concentrations of the poisonous plants. Traveling or recently introduced animals may not be accustomed to local plants and thus may be poisoned on pastures that indigenous stock graze with impunity. There is evidence that animals become accustomed to the poison and can tolerate increasing doses with experience (3). Cattle or sheep may break out of dry, summer pastures into fields of immature sorghum or Sudan grass and gorge themselves. In these circumstances, heavy mortalities are likely to occur within an hour, sometimes within about 15 minutes. Toxic forage made into ensilage loses much of its cyanide content and on exposure to air may give off large quantities of free hydrocyanic acid.

Deaths due to the ingestion of excessive linseed meal or cake occur under the same circumstances. Sheep fed large quantities of linseed meal at the end of a period of starvation have died of hydrocyanic acid poisoning. Calves fed on milk replacer containing linseed which has been soaked but not boiled may also ingest lethal amounts of cyanogenetic linamarin. Occasional cases of hydrocyanic acid poisoning occur when animals are exposed to chemicals used for fumigation or the fertilizer, calcium cyanamide.

Pathogenesis

Acute cyanide intoxication causes a histotoxic anoxia, and a resultant tissue asphyxia, by paralysis of tissue enzyme systems. Oxygen exchange is suspended and oxygen is retained in the blood, giving it a characteristic bright red color. If the course is prolonged the blood may be dark red due to inhibition of respiration and restriction of oxygen intake. Because of the severity of the anoxia the major manifestation of cyanide poisoning is that of cerebral anoxia with muscle tremor and convulsions, and dyspnea. Cyanogenetic glucosides may be of importance as contributory causes of bloat in ruminants.

Doses which do not produce clinical effects appear to be well tolerated and the tolerance appears to increase with experience. Cyanides ingested in small amounts, however, are known to be goitrogenic and may be important in the production of clinical goiter in lambs on marginal intakes of iodine. Pregnant ewes grazing on star grass (*Cynodon plectostachyus*) develop goiter due partly to a low iodine intake and partly due to the large amounts of thyrotoxic cyanides in the grass.

Hydrocyanic acid is normally detoxicated by its conversion to thiocyanate in the liver through the action of a specific enzyme system. After the administration of hydrocyanic acid to sheep the thiocyanate content of the liver may rise from 2·3–17·6 mg/dl. Bovine liver also contains this enzyme system but thiocyanate levels do not rise after the administration of hydrocyanic acid in clover, suggesting that there may be more effective excretion or an alternative method of detoxication in cattle.

Clinical findings

In its common form hydrocyanic acid poisoning is always acute and affected animals rarely survive for more than 1–2 hours. In the most acute cases animals become affected within 10–15 minutes of eating toxic material and die within 2–3 minutes of first showing signs. The onset of signs may be delayed if the ingested material is relatively indigestible, such as crabapples (14). These include dyspnea, anxiety, restlessness, moaning, recumbency and terminal clonic convulsions with opisthotonus. The mucosae are bright red in color. In the more common, less acute cases the animals show depression, staggering, gross muscle tremor and dyspnea. There may be hyperesthesia and lacrimation. The muscle tremor is evident first in the head and neck but soon spreads to involve the rest of the body; the animal becomes weak and goes down. The pulse is small, weak and rapid. There is dilatation of the pupils, nystagmus and cyanosis in the terminal stages, usually accompanied by clonic convulsions and in some cases by vomiting and aspiration of ingesta into the lungs. Vomition is not a typical sign in cyanide poisoning and, when it does occur, it may be the result of bloating in the recumbent animal and during the final convulsions. The course in these cases may be as long as 1–2 hours.

Ataxia and urinary incontinence are recorded in cattle grazing wilted grain sorghum. The disease appears not to be related to cyanide poisoning and is listed under the heading of poisoning by sorghum.

Clinical pathology

The suspected plant material or ruminal contents may be tested for the presence of hydrocyanic acid (8, 9). The rumen sample, or shredded plant material, is placed in a test tube containing a little water and a few drops of chloroform and heated very gently in the presence of sodium picrate paper. A rapid change in the color of the reagent paper from yellow to red indicates the presence of free hydrocyanic acid. Once started the color change occurs rapidly although it may require

5–10 minutes of gentle warming before the change commences. The tube should be corked while being warmed and the paper hung from the top without touching the test material. Reagent papers are easily prepared by mixing 0·5 g picric acid, 5 g sodium carbonate in 100 ml water. Filter paper is dipped in the reagent and allowed to dry in a dark place. The reagent is stable for at least 6 months if kept in a cool place but the papers deteriorate if kept for more than a week. Ruminal contents may also be tested by placing a drop of ruminal fluid on a test paper. A red discoloration is a positive reaction. The test is designed to detect free hydrocyanic acid and may not be positive even when cyanides are present if the gas is not liberated. Samples of suspected plant material sent to a laboratory for analysis should be immersed in a 1–3% solution of mercuric chloride.

Necropsy findings

In very acute cases the blood may be bright red in color but in most field cases it is dark red due to anoxemia. The blood clots slowly, the musculature is dark and there is congestion and hemorrhage in the trachea and lungs. Patchy congestion and petechiation may be evident in the abomasum and small intestines. Subepicardial and subendocardial hemorrhages occur constantly. A smell of 'bitter almonds' in the rumen is described as typical of hydrocyanic acid poisoning. It may occur with some plants but is not apparent with others. Specimens submitted for laboratory examination should include rumen contents, liver and muscle. Much hydrocyanic acid may be lost from specimens during transit and they should be immersed in a 1–3% solution of mercuric chloride or despatched in a very tightly stoppered bottle. Muscle is least likely to lose its hydrocyanic acid and is the preferred tissue if the delay between death and necropsy has been long. To be satisfactory, liver samples must be taken within 4 hours of death and muscle tissue within 20 hours. A level of hydrocyanic acid of 0·63 μg/ml in muscle justifies a diagnosis of poisoning (9).

Diagnosis

The development of an acute anoxic syndrome in ruminants pasturing on plants, or being fed on feeds, known to be cyanogenetic usually suggests the occurrence of hydrocyanic acid poisoning. Acute pulmonary edema and emphysema may resemble it clinically but it is less acute and auscultation of the lungs usually indicates the presence of fluid and emphysema. Nitrite poisoning produces an almost identical syndrome but the blood is dark and tends to be coffee-colored. A similar syndrome may also occur in poisoning by algae. Occasional cases of anaphylaxis in cattle, particularly young calves, are manifested by acute dyspnea but there are usually additional signs of an allergic reaction including bloat and sometimes urticaria or angioneurotic edema, and, if the case is sufficiently severe, there is a profuse discharge of bloodstained froth from the nose. Cases occur only sporadically whereas hydrocyanic acid poisoning is likely to affect a number of animals at one time.

Treatment

The standard treatment for many years has been the intravenous injection of a mixture of sodium nitrite and sodium thiosulfate, and field experience with it has been very good. However, it is now apparent that the results in cattle poisoned experimentally can be improved by using just sodium thiosulfate, but in a much heavier dose (660 mg/kg body weight compared to the previous level of 66 mg/kg). This can be combined with either sodium nitrite (22 mg/kg body weight) or 1·5 mg/kg body weight aminopropriophenone (5) or cobaltous chloride (10·6 mg/kg body weight), but these products appear unlikely to improve the efficacy of the sodium thiosulfate alone. Sodium thiosulfate has very low toxicity and treatment with that product alone would avoid the potential for toxicity inherent in the use of nitrites intravenously. This position could be very dangerous if a combined cyanide and nitrite poisoning was encountered. The other antidote recently identified in experimental studies is *p*-aminopropriophenone which has been used alone (1–1·5 mg/kg body weight) or together with sodium thiosulfate. It is less effective than sodium thiosulfate when the dose level of cyanide is high (11).

It seems probable that the heavy sodium thiosulfate dose will supersede the traditional nitrite–thiosulfate (5 g sodium nitrite, 15 g sodium thiosulfate in 200 ml water for cattle; 1 g sodium nitrite, 3 g sodium thiosulfate in 50 ml water for sheep). Treatment may have to be repeated because of further liberation of hydrocyanic acid. The sodium nitrite produces methemoglobin which combines with the hydrocyanic acid to produce cyanmethemoglobin which is not toxic. The acid is released gradually from this compound and is taken up by the thiosulfate to form thiocyanate which is also nontoxic and which is readily excreted. There is an upper limit of safe methemoglobinemia beyond which anemic anoxia occurs and doses of nitrite greater than those recommended may exacerbate the tissue anoxia.

In all cases sodium thiosulfate should be given orally or intraruminally to fix the free hydrocyanic acid in the rumen. Doses of 30 g are used in cattle and are repeated at hourly intervals. Animals that have been exposed showing no clinical signs may be treated similarly.

The interesting laboratory observation that cobalt has a marked antagonistic effect against cyanide, which is enhanced by combination with thiosulfate or nitrite (10), is still unexplained, but it is now an alternative treatment as set out above.

Non-specific treatment including respiratory stimulants and artificial respiration are unlikely to have any effect on the course of the disease.

Control

Hungry cattle and sheep should not be allowed access to toxic plants, especially cultivated *Sorghum* spp. when they are immature, wilted, frostbitten or growing rapidly after a stage of retarded growth. Plants of the sorghum family should be in flower before they are grazed or chopped to be fed green. If there is doubt as to the toxicity of a field of these plants a sample may be tested by the method described under clinical pathology. Linseed meal should be fed in small quantities without soaking and gruel containing linseed should be thoroughly boiled to drive off any free hydrocyanic acid.

REVIEW LITERATURE

Burrows, G. E. (1981) Cyanide intoxication in sheep: therapeutics. *Vet. hum. Toxicol.*, *23*, 22.

REFERENCES

(1) Sharman, J. R. (1967) *NZ vet. J.*, *15*, 19.
(2) Seifert, H. S. H. & Beller, K. A. (1969) *Berl. Munch. Tierärztl. Wochenschr.*, *82*, 88.
(3) Coop, I. E. & Blakeley, R. L. (1950) *NZ J. Sci. Technol.* (A), *31*, 44.
(4) Puls, R. et al. (1978) *Can. vet. J.*, *19*, 264.
(5) Burrows, G. E. & Way, J. L. (1979) *Am J. vet. Res.*, *40*, 613.
(6) Gurnsey, M. P. et al. (1977) *NZ vet. J.*, *25*, 128.
(7) Majak, W. et al. (1980) *Can vet. J.*, *21*, 74.
(8) Bergsten, M. L. (1964) *Vet. Med.*, *59*, 720.
(9) Terblanche, M. et al. (1964) *J. S. Afr. vet. med. Assoc.*, *35*, 503, 199.
(10) Isom, G & Way, J. L. (1973) *Toxicol. appl. Pharmacol.*, *24*, 449.
(11) Burrows, G. E. (1981) *Vet. hum. Toxicol.*, *23*, 22.
(12) Kriedman, P. E. (1964) *Aust. J. exp. Agric.*, *4*, 15.
(13) Webber, J. J. et al. (1985) *Aust. vet. J.*, *62*, 28.
(14) Shaw, J. M. (1986) *Vet. Rec.*, *119*, 242.
(15) Barton, N. J. et al. (1983) *Aust. vet. J.*, *60*, 220.
(16) Burrows, G. E. & Tyrl, R. J. (1983) *Bov. Practnr*, *18*, 188.
(17) Majak, W. et al. (1981) *Can. J. anim. Sci.*, *61*, 681.

Nitrate and nitrite poisoning

Nitrates and nitrites are closely linked as causes of poisoning. Nitrates may cause gastroenteritis when ingested in large quantities but their chief importance is as a source of nitrite which may be formed before or after ingestion of the nitrate. The nitrites cause a syndrome of respiratory distress because of the formation of methemoglobin which results in anemic anoxia.

Etiology

The toxic principle as it occurs in growing plants is always nitrate, usually as potassium nitrate, and may be ingested as such in sufficient quantities to cause gastroenteritis. The nitrate may be reduced to nitrite in the plant before ingestion. This occurs in oaten hay in the stack, particularly if it is wet and hot, or if the hay is overheated in the sun (30) or damp for some time before feeding. The gentle cooking of mangels may also convert nitrate to nitrite and cause poisoning of pigs. There is considerable variation between species in their susceptibility to nitrite poisoning, pigs being most susceptible followed by cattle, sheep and horses in that order. The susceptibility of cattle relative to sheep is due either to their ability to convert nitrate to nitrite in the rumen or because of the known greater ability of sheep to convert nitrite to ammonia. Pigs are highly susceptible to nitrite poisoning but are affected only if they ingest it preformed.

Cattle reduce nitrate to nitrite in the rumen and their capacity to do this is enhanced by continued feeding of nitrate. The enhanced capacity, due to changes in microbial activity, is transferred naturally to nearby animals not receiving additional nitrate (35). Cases of nitrate poisoning that occur in sheep are caused either by the ingestion of preformed nitrite or by ruminal conditions which favor reduction of nitrate. A diet rich in readily fermentable carbohydrate reduces nitrite production in the rumen of the sheep (1). Also nitrite poisoning occurs in sheep fed an inadequate ration after dosing with nitrite at a level which is innocuous to sheep fed on a good ration. There is often a delay of a few days in the appearance of signs of poisoning after sheep go onto toxic forage. It seems likely that ruminal flora need to adapt to the changed nutrients (2). The degree of methemoglobinemia also varies with the quality of the diet.

The common sources of nitrate for farm animals include cereal crops, certain specific plants and water from deep wells. Oat hay may contain 3–7% nitrate. Immature green oats, barley, wheat and rye hay, and Sudan grass, corn or sorghum fodder may contain toxic amounts. Very heavy growths of ryegrass in pastures have been incriminated in New Zealand (3) and Australia (22). Freshly pulled mangels may also contain high concentrations. Turnip tops may contain 8% nitrate, and sugar beet tops and rape have caused nitrite poisoning. Of the specific plants variegated thistle (*Silybum marianum*), redroot (*Amaranthus reflexus*), winged thistle (*Carduus tenuiflorus*), *Astragalus* and *Oxytropis* spp. and mintweed (*Salvia reflexa*) are well known as causes of nitrite poisoning and these plants have caused heavy losses in cattle. Linseed grass (*Urochloa panicoides*) is less well known, but equally poisonous (4). It may contain as much as 5·5% of nitrate in its stems, a level much in excess of that tolerated by cattle. Outbreaks of nitrite poisoning have occurred in sheep grazing heavy swards of capeweed (*Arctotheca calendula*), a normally safe plant, after a prolonged drought. In such circumstances some normally safe plants with a capacity for fast growth may become dangerous. It is presumed that high levels of nitrate accumulate in the soil during the drought and are absorbed in large amounts when the drought ends. Plants that accumulate more than 1·5% by dry matter of nitrate are potentially toxic although poisoning is more likely to occur when the feeding pattern is green chop fed indoors than when animals graze the material. For animals at pasture probably 2% dry matter as nitrate is safe (21, 29). Levels of potassium nitrate in plants may be as high as 20% of dry matter (7) and 3% is not uncommon in recognized forage plants such as sorghum (8) and sudax (32) and heavy mortality has occurred on them. There is one recorded incident of what appeared to be a facilitation of development of nitrite poisoning in cattle by the feeding of monensin (13). Deep wells filled by seepage from highly fertile soils may contain levels as high as 1700–3000 ppm of nitrate and water of condensation in barns may trap ammonia and eventually contain 8000–10 000 ppm of nitrate. Composition lining board in animal barns may become highly impregnated with nitrite and cause poisoning if chewed (5).

Toxic doses are hard to compute because of variation in susceptibility, and in production of nitrite from nitrate. The lethal dose of sodium nitrite for pigs is 88 mg/kg body weight. Doses of 48–77 mg/kg cause moderate to severe but not fatal methemoglobinemia. Potassium nitrate in doses of 4–7 g/kg body weight causes fatal gastritis in pigs and the lethal dose of potassium or sodium nitrite is about 20 mg/kg (10). Measured as nitrate nitrogen the LD_{50} for pigs is 19–21 mg/kg body weight (11). At dose levels of 12–19 mg clinical signs occur but the pigs recover (12). In cattle the minimum lethal dose of nitrite is 88–110 mg/kg body weight or about 0·6 g of potassium nitrate per kg body weight. In sheep the lethal dose of nitrite is 40–50 mg/kg body weight. Daily doses of about 0·15 g potassium nitrate have caused abortion in cattle after 3–13 doses but continued low-level dosing does not appear to affect sheep. Drinking water containing 1000 ppm of nitrate nitrogen causes appreciable methemoglobin formation in sheep but has no obvious clinical effect. Plants to be safe for feeding should contain less than 1·5% potassium nitrate on a dry matter basis. Less than 0·6% of the total diet is recommended. Cattle can eat sufficient quantities of toxic plants to cause death in 1 hour.

Epidemiology

Nitrate and nitrite poisoning are being diagnosed with increasing frequency as heavy fertilization with nitrogenous compounds becomes more widespread. While there is no doubt that the dangers have increased it is also evident that 'nitrate poisoning' is enjoying a vogue and that many cases so reported, particularly of chronic toxicity, rest on inadequate evidence.

Cereals and root crops are likely to contain high concentrations when heavily fertilized with nitrogenous manures and when growth is rapid during hot, humid weather. Heavy dressings of crude sewage are credited with increasing the nitrate content of pasture to a point where nitrite poisoning occurs (6). Ensiled material usually contains less nitrate than the fresh crop, because normal silage fermentation destroys nitrate, but juices draining from silos containing high-nitrate materials may be toxic. On the other hand, hay made from nitrate-rich material contains almost as much as when it was made, unless some of it is converted to nitrite by overheating and the activities of molds. Heavily fertilized grass made into grass cubes may contain as much as 0·71% nitrate (dry matter) and cause nitrite poisoning (15). Corn stalks in fields previously damaged by drought may be dangerous. Cereal hay, especially oat hay, grown under these conditions and cut when sappy, may develop a high concentration of nitrite when the stacked material develops some heat. Dry oat hay which is damp for some time before it is eaten is also likely to contain a high concentration of nitrite. The nitrite is present chiefly in the leafy part of the hay. Weeds and sugar beet tops may contain toxic quantities of nitrate after spraying with the herbicide 2,4-D because of changes produced in the metabolism of the plants. Pigs are most likely to be poisoned when fed on cooked mangels which have not been thoroughly boiled, on whey to which potassium nitrate has been added in the cheese-making process, or on swill containing salt-brine from butchers' shops, or made with well water containing a high concentration of nitrate. Water containing 2300 ppm of nitrate and less than 10 ppm of nitrite when mixed into a swill, stored in tins and then cooked has resulted in the production of a mixture containing 1200–1400 ppm of nitrite. Well waters containing 200–500 ppm of potassium nitrate equivalent may also cause poisoning in cattle and sheep, the nitrate being reduced to nitrite in the rumen. Open surface storage tanks collecting rain runoff from roofs may also contain toxic amounts of nitrite in the plant debris which collects at the bottom (17).

Accidental poisoning with nitrates occurs sporadically when sodium or potassium nitrate is used in mistake for sodium chloride or magnesium sulfate, or when ammonium nitrate solution is used instead of whey. In such an outbreak the water contained 3000 mg/l for 3 days (the maximum tolerance is for 1320 mg/l) and caused death by nitrite poisoning (18). Ingestion of ammonium nitrate in granular form appears not to kill by nitrite poisoning but possibly by ammonia or nitrate poisoning (33, 34). Poorly fed animals are more susceptible to nitrite poisoning than those on good diets and this probably influences the susceptibility of introduced and traveling cattle to this form of poisoning, although lack of acquaintance with the plants, and possibly adaptation, may also affect their susceptibility. Prior exposure to nitrate reduces susceptibility under experimental conditions but the practical significance of the observation is uncertain. The most important factor influencing susceptibility appears to be the rate of ingestion of the nitrate-bearing plant (20).

Pathogenesis

Nitrates have a direct caustic action on alimentary mucosa and the ingestion of sufficiently large quantities causes gastroenteritis. Absorption of nitrites causes methemoglobinemia and the development of an anemic anoxia. Nitrites are also vasodilators which may contribute to the development of tissue anoxia by causing peripheral circulatory failure, but this effect appears to be of little significance compared to that of methemoglobin formation. When nitrite is ingested preformed the effects may be very rapid but when conversion of nitrate to nitrite occurs in the rumen there is a delay of some hours before clinical illness occurs. In cattle and sheep the maximum methemoglobinemia occurs about 5 hours after ingestion of nitrate (9). In pigs it is 90–150 minutes (11).

Death does not occur until a certain level of methemoglobinemia is attained. In farm animals lethal levels in cattle are about 9 g methemoglobin per 100 ml blood (15); in pigs when 76–88% of hemoglobin has been altered to methemoglobin deaths occur (11).

In cattle, abortion and a greatly increased requirement of vitamin A have been believed to result from the long-term ingestion of nitrite. Both have been discredited (25) and prolonged ingestion of sublethal amounts of nitrite is not known to have any significant effect on productivity (12). However, abortion is commonly recorded as a sequel to an acute outbreak of poisoning.

Clinical findings

In animals poisoned by nitrate there is salivation, abdominal pain, diarrhea and vomiting even in ruminants. The more typical syndrome is that caused by the anoxia of nitrite poisoning. Dyspnea, with a gasping, rapid respiration is the predominant sign. Muscle tremor, weakness, staggering gait, severe cyanosis followed by blanching of the mucosae, a rapid, small, weak pulse, and a normal or subnormal temperature are other typical signs. The affected animals go down and there are terminal clonic convulsions. Frequent urination and abortion are other recorded signs, and in some outbreaks in cattle the principal problem is abortion a few days after exposure.

Clinical signs are delayed for about 6 hours after the ingestion of nitrate, the time necessary for conversion of the nitrate to nitrite and for the nitrite to be absorbed and to form methemoglobin. Death usually occurs within 12–24 hours of ingestion of the toxic plant, although in acute poisoning the duration of illness may be even shorter and clinical signs may not be observed.

In one report acute cardiac and circulatory failure without other observed clinical signs was much the most common syndrome in cattle (26).

Clinical pathology

Nitrite poisoning is difficult to diagnose unless blood samples are collected during life and its content of nitrite estimated, usually by the diphenylamine test. Contributory information is provided by blood levels of methemoglobin. Methemoglobinemia may be detected by examination of the blood in a reversion spectrometer but it is not diagnostic of nitrite poisoning and results are not dependable unless the blood has been collected for less than an hour or two. Methemoglobin levels of 9 g/dl of blood are lethal in cattle; levels of 1·65–2·97 g/dl are recorded in association with obvious clinical signs (7) compared to normal levels of 0·12–0·2 g/dl. Lower blood levels are toxic in animals with chronic hepatitis (31). An alternative method is the diphenylamine blue test (13) which is very sensitive to the presence of nitrite but not entirely specific. A satisfactory test can be conducted on a thick air-dried blood smear. Laboratory tests are available for the rough estimation of the nitrite or nitrate content of fodder but they are not sufficiently simple for field use nor accurate enough for critical assay. A modified diphenylamine reagent provides a qualitative test suitable for field use (27). The test solution (0·5 diphenylamine, 20 ml distilled water and concentrated sulfuric acid to make up to 100 ml) is placed on the tissues of the inside of the stem (to avoid contact with possible iron contamination on the outside surface). An intense blue color within 10 seconds indicates a concentration of greater than 1% of nitrate (8). The test is also suitable for use with plant material. Roots and stems usually contain more nitrate than leaves, and a total plant content of 6000–10 000 ppm dry matter of nitrate is considered to be potentially toxic (19). The diphenylamine test does have disadvantages and can give inaccurate results. To avoid these errors it is recommended that the blood be diluted with phosphate buffer (1 part in 20). It is also worthwhile submitting a sample of urine as nitrite appears to pass unchanged into the urine (28).

Necropsy findings

In nitrate poisoning there is gastroenteritis. In nitrite poisoning the blood is dark red to coffee-brown in color and clots poorly. Petechial hemorrhages may be present in the heart muscle and trachea and there is general vascular congestion and a variable degree of congestion in the rumen and abomasum. Specimens for laboratory examination should include blood for methemoglobin estimation, ingesta and suspected plants or water, with added chloroform or formalin to prevent conversion of nitrates by bacterial fermentation. If the animals have been dead for some time, chemical analysis should be attempted on the aqueous humor of the eye and the cerebrospinal fluid. All of these specimens are submitted to the diphenylamine test. Postmortem specimens must be collected within 1–2 hours of death to be of any value.

Diagnosis

The acute dyspnea, short course and nervous signs of tremor and convulsions resemble the signs of hydrocyanic acid poisoning but in acute cases the blood is dark red to brown in color in contradistinction to the bright red color of the blood in the latter poisoning. Caution should be exercised in interpreting this sign, as a dark red appearance of the blood occurs commonly in the later stages of both poisonings. The source of the toxic material is also different. Analysis of tissues, ingesta and suspected material may be necessary to confirm the diagnosis, although the rapid response to treatment with methylene blue is a good criterion for field use. Acute pulmonary edema and emphysema and anaphylaxis must also be considered in the differential diagnosis.

Treatment

Methylene blue is the specific treatment. The standard dose rate is traditionally 1–2 mg/kg body weight, injected intravenously as a 1% solution. This dose rate should be retained for use in pigs and horses, but in ruminants it has been shown that high dose rates of methylene blue do not cause methemoglobinemia in sheep and cattle, and a higher dose rate of 20 mg/kg body weight has been recommended for treatment in these animals (23) but the standard dose rate appears to be adequate (9). Treatment may have to be repeated when large amounts of toxic material have been ingested. The half-life of methylene blue in tissues is about 2 hours, and a repetition of treatment is recommended as necessary at intervals of 6–8 hours (14). Methylene blue in large amounts causes methemoglobinemia, hence its use in cyanide poisoning, but in small amounts causes rapid reconversion of methemoglobin to hemoglobin.

Control

Ruminants likely to be exposed to nitrites or nitrates should receive adequate carbohydrate in their diet and travelling or hungry animals should not be allowed access to dangerous plants. Poisonous well water can be made safe by boiling. Haylage or silage suspected of dangerous levels of nitrate should be allowed to aerate overnight before feeding. If feed known to contain toxic quantities of nitrate has to be fed, supplementation of the diet of sheep and cattle with chlortetracycline (30 mg/kg of feed) is partially effective for a period of about 2 weeks in suppressing the reduction of nitrate to nitrite (24). For safety it is recommended that cows not be fed on feed containing more than 1% nitrate when at pasture, and slightly less when zero grazing (16).

REVIEW LITERATURE

Clay, R. R. et al. (1976) Toxic nitrate accumulation in the sorghums. *Bov. Practnr*, *11*, 28.
Deeb, B. S. & Sloan, K. W. (1975) Nitrates, nitrites and health. *Bull. Ill Agric. exp. Stn*, *750*, 521.

REFERENCES

(1) Miyazaki, A. & Kawashima, R. (1976) *Jap. J. zootech. Sci.*, *47*, 158.
(2) Nakamura, Y. et al. (1976) *Jap. J. zootech. Sci.*, *47*, 63.
(3) O'Hara, P. J. & Fraser, A. J. (1975) *NZ vet. J.*, *23*, 45.
(4) Hill, B. D. & Blaney, B. J. (1980) *Aust. vet, J.*, *56*, 256.
(5) McParland, P. J. et al. (1980) *Vet. Rec.*, *106*, 201.
(6) Jones, T. O. & Jones, D. R. (1977) *Vet. Rec.*, *101*, 266.
(7) Nakamura, R et al. (1972) *Jap. J. zootech. Sci.*, *43*, 286.
(8) Clay R. R. et al. (1976) *Bov. Practnr*, *11*, 28.
(9) van Dijk, S. et al. (1983) *Vet. Rec.*, *112*, 272.
(10) London, W. T. et al. (1967) *J. Am. vet. med. Assoc.*, *150*, 398.
(11) Curtin, R. M. & London, W. T. (1967) *Proc. US live Stk sanit Assoc., Buffalo*, 339.
(12) London, W. T. et al. (1967) *J. Am. vet. med. Assoc.*, *150*, 398.
(13) Malone, P. (1978) *Vet. Rec.*, *103*, 477.
(14) Anon. (1980) *J. Am. vet. med. Assoc.*, *177*, 82.
(15) Purcell, D. A. et al. (1971) *Res. vet. Sci.*, *12*, 598.
(16) Wiesner, E. et al. (1979) *Vet. Med.*, *34*, 487.
(17) Counter, D. E. et al. (1975) *Vet. Rec.*, *96*, 412.
(18) Egyed, M. N. et al. (1980) *Refuah Vet.*, *37*, 101.
(19) Edwards, W. C. & McCoy, C. P. (1980) *Vet. Med. SAC*, *75*, 457.
(20) Crawford, R. F. et al. (1966) *Cornell Vet.*, *56*, 3.
(21) Geurink, J. H. et al. (1982) *Neth. J. agric. Sci.*, *30*, 105.
(22) Nicholls, T. J. & Miles, E. J. (1980) *Aust. vet. J.*, *56*, 95.
(23) Burrows, G. E. & Way, J. C. (1975) *Proc. ann. US anim. Hlth Assoc.*, *79*, 266.
(24) Emerick, R. J. & Embry, L. B. (1961) *J. anim. Sci.*, *20*, 844.
(25) Dodd, D. C. (1967) *Proc US live Stk sanit. Assoc., Buffalo*, 581.
(26) Johanssen, U. & Kuhnert, M. (1969) *Arch. exp. VetMed.*, *23*, 375.
(27) Householder, G. T. et al. (1966) *J. Am. vet. med. Assoc.*, *148*, 662.
(28) Watts, H. et al. (1969) *Aust. vet. J.*, *45*, 492.
(29) Haraszti, E. et al. (1983) *Magy. allatorv. Lap.*, *38*, 495.
(30) Prasad, B. et al. (1983) *Ind. J. vet. Med.*, *3*, 69.
(31) Prasad, B. et al. (1985) *Ind. J. vet. med.*, *5*, 27.
(32) Carrigan, M. J. & Gardner, I. A. (1982) *Aust. vet. J.*, *59*, 155.
(33) Jones, T. O. (1982) *Vet. Rec.*, *111*, 211.
(34) Horner, R. F. (1982) *Vet. Rec.*, *110*, 472.
(35) Cheng, K. J. et al. (1985) *Can. J. anim. Sci.*, *65*, 647.

Oxalate poisoning

The ingestion of excess oxalate causes some gastrointestinal irritation but the major effect is that of precipitation of blood calcium and the production of a hypocalcemic syndrome of muscular weakness and paralysis. Continued ingestion of small amounts of oxalate may lead to renal damage or to the development of urinary calculi and in horses to the development of nutritional secondary hyperparathyroidism.

Etiology

Plants usually contain oxalate in the form of the potassium salt, and this is much less toxic than if it is given experimentally as the pure salt. High concentrations are present in halogeton (*Halogeton glomeratus*), pigweed (*Amaranthus retroflexus*), fat hen (*Chenopodium album*), soursob (*Oxalis cernua*, *O. pescaprae*), *Bassia hyssopifolia* (2), greasewood (*Sarcobatus vermiculatus*), dock and orchard sorrell (*Rumex acetosella*), *R. venosus* (15), *Isotropis* sp., *Anagallis* sp., *Portulacca oleracea*, *Salsola bali*, *Trianthema portulacastrum* and *Threlkeldia proceriflora*, and in the leaves of cultivated rhubarb, mangels and sugar beet, especially when the plants are in the green leafy stage. Young fresh plants may contain as much as 17% potassium oxalate whilst old, dry plants rarely contain more than 1% (3). On the other hand *Halogeton*, probably the most important of the above plants, becomes more toxic as the growing season advances and is most dangerous when frosted and dried. The plant may contain as much as 16·6% of soluble oxalate (4). Grasses rarely contain significant amounts of oxalate but *Setaria sphacelata* has been shown to contain up to 7% oxalate and cause poisoning in cattle and horses (6). This plant was specially introduced into Australia because of its ability to grow well in tropical conditions. It now dominates large areas of pasture. Toxicity caused by the grass is also recorded in Costa Rica (1). Other grasses which have the same effect are *Brachiaria* spp., *Cenchus ciliaris*, *Digitaria decumbens* and *Panicum* spp. Ingestion of these grasses by horses leads to them being in serious negative calcium and phosphorus balance (17). Cattle metabolize soluble oxalates in the rumen and are not at such a disadvantage as horses, although they may still be in slight negative calcium balance (18). There is a high incidence of a milk fever-like condition in dairy cattle grazing the grass *Setaria* spp. The trees, *Terminalia oblongata and Quercus* sp., also carry heavy concentrations of oxalate. Some fungi are capable of producing significant amounts of oxalate and their presence on moldy feedstuffs may contribute to the occurrence of poisoning (8, 14).

Large quantities of a toxic plant must be ingested to cause poisoning because not all the oxalate is absorbed and much is broken down in the alimentary tract. Up to 450 g of sodium oxalate given by mouth is required to produce fatal effects in horses, and 6 g/day of anhydrous oxalic acid is required to produce toxic effects in sheep. Cattle can eat as much as 685 g of oxalic acid without harmful effect and buffalo are similarly tolerant of the poison (9). The natural disease does not appear to have been recorded in pigs, but renal damage has been produced in this species by experimental administration of oxalate (13).

Oxalate is normally metabolized in the rumen and the continued ingestion of oxalate in small quantities by sheep results in increased ability to decompose the oxalate to the point where relatively large quantities (up to 75 g daily by sheep) can be ingested without toxic effects. This may explain the relative susceptibility of sheep and cattle when they are grazed for the first time on pasture containing the toxic plants, although it seems likely that other factors in the rumen will also affect the amount of oxalate rendered insoluble as calcium oxalate or digested to bicarbonate. Of these the level of calcium in the diet and the activities of bacteria in the rumen are considered to be important. It is the microbial population of the ruminal flora which is responsible for the intraruminal degradation of the oxalate and requires 3–4 days to adapt to the occurrence of oxalate in the diet (10).

Epidemiology
Plants containing oxalates in dangerous quantities grow principally in specific areas. Heavy mortalities may occur in groups of animals which are not accustomed to grazing the toxic pasture.

The disease occurs principally in sheep which are more likely to be grazed on the kind of pasture in which the toxic plants commonly occur. Pasture is at its most dangerous stage when there is a rapid growth of lush plants in a warm autumn after a dry summer. Traveling and recently introduced animals are more likely to be affected than indigenous animals and as a group pregnant and lactating animals are probably more susceptible than others. Clinical signs may appear within 2–4 hours of eating an oxalate-containing plant. There is an increased susceptibility if the animals are hungry and consume large amounts of the plants. Salt hunger has been suggested as a predisposing factor in the etiology of oxalate poisoning.

Cattle fed large amounts of *Oxalis cernua* containing high concentrations of oxalates, 85% of it water-soluble, have been able to metabolize it without harmful effect. Calves drinking the milk from these cows exclusively are reputed to develop diarrhea (3). However, oxalate poisoning and death have been observed in cattle eating *Setaria sphacelata*, a pasture grass grown in tropical areas (5). Poisoning has also occurred in hungry cattle having access to *Halogeton glomeratus* (5) and *Rumex venosus* containing up to 13·9% of oxalate (16). The plants are not very palatable, but hungry and inexperienced cattle can succumb.

Pathogenesis
Broadly speaking, three syndromes occur, depending on the amount of oxalate ingested. With large quantities the major effect is the absorption of free oxalate and precipitation of blood calcium as calcium oxalate to produce a *hypocalcemia*. Immobilization of calcium in the alimentary tract may contribute significantly in the development of this hypocalcemia. The resulting syndrome in sheep is indistinguishable from that caused by hypocalcemia at parturition or on starving.

Continuous ingestion of soluble oxalates causes *nephrosis* due to precipitation of oxalate crystals in the lumen of the renal tubules. Up to 25% of sheep may be affected in some flocks. Such damage is likely to be cumulative if the sheep are periodically exposed to oxalate-bearing plants. At intermediate levels of oxalate intake there is marked damage to vascular tissues especially in alimentary tract and lungs (7). Invasion of the *chemical rumenitis* that results may lead to an irreversible fungal or bacterial rumenitis or hepatitis. A possible fourth pathogenetic pattern is the apparent relationship between continuous oxalate ingestion and the enzootic development of nutritional secondary hyperparathyroidism in horses in Australia, described under that disease. It is assumed that this results from precipitation of dietary calcium in the gut and reduction of its absorption (16). Also, it is possible that the disease is due partly to a concurrent dietary deficiency of calcium (12). Nephrosclerosis has also been recorded separately as a result of chronic ingestion of oxalate by horses (8, 11).

Continued low level dosing in sheep may cause ruminal dysfunction due to changes in pH of its contents and interference with cellulose digestion. The importance of oxalate ingestion over long periods in the production of urinary calculi is discussed elsewhere.

Clinical findings
In acute poisoning in sheep the clinical signs include paresis, muscle tremor, staggering and final recumbency and death in coma. The heart rate is rapid, ruminal movements are decreased, and the pupils dilated. There may be slight bloating, frequent getting up and lying down, eventually recumbency, frequent attempts to urinate, frothy blood-tinged nasal discharge and occasionally red-brown urine. In sheep, chronic cases with renal damage show poor appetite, failure to grow, poor bodily condition, ascites and a significant anemia (14).

Oxalate poisoning in horses caused by eating *Setaria sphacelata* in pasture dominated by the grass is manifested by osteodystrophia fibrosa (6). Within 4 months of going onto the pasture, affected animals show a stiff, stilted gait, most evident at gaits faster than walking. The horses resent having to trot or canter. There is bilateral swelling of the maxilla around the molar teeth and the mandibles, and the swellings are hard and bony. The horses are unthrifty in spite of an ample supply of feed.

Clinical pathology
Suspected plants should be assayed for oxalate content. Estimation of the level of calcium in serum is of debatable value as the levels of total calcium may be normal, the clinical illness being caused by depression of the ionizable fraction of the calcium. Albuminuria and sometimes hematuria may be observed in the nephrotic syndrome, the packed cell volume may be as low as 15–20%, the blood urea nitrogen (BUN) is of the order of 85 mg/dl (30·3 mmol/l). The proteinuria which occurs is almost diagnostic of the disease in sheep grazing *Oxalis* spp. A biopsy of the thickened bone of chronically affected horses shows lesions typical of osteodystrophia fibrosa.

Necropsy findings
There are no gross findings at necropsy which are characteristic of oxalate poisoning although there may be deposition of crystals in the renal tubules and pelvis and even in the ureters and urethra. In experimental poisoning in the horse and sheep, severe gastroenteritis and dehydration have been observed. Vesicular inflammation and necrosis of the epithelium of the esophagus and rumenoreticulum occurs in cattle poisoned by ammonium oxalate in the grass, *Setaria sphacelata* (7).

Diagnosis
The hypocalcemic syndrome is characteristic and oxalate poisoning must be differentiated from parturient paresis, hypocalcemia due to starvation or forced exercise, and lactation tetany. Environmental conditions and the presence of known toxic plants give some indication of the cause. Acute indigestion due to overeating on grain may cause a similar syndrome but a history of free access to grain or concentrate is usually available in such cases.

Treatment
The parenteral injection of solutions of calcium salts is a specific treatment. Calcium borogluconate as a 25% solution given intravenously or subcutaneously in doses of 300–500 ml in cattle and 50–100 ml in sheep usually effects recovery. Ancillary treatment should include the provision of ample fluids to decrease precipitation of oxalate crystal in the urinary tract.

Control
Hungry sheep and cattle should not be allowed to feed on large quantities of the toxic plants. The water intake of sheep also affects the oxalate intake. Halogeton poisoning is more likely to occur when sheep are watered and then allowed to graze (15). Alternative sources of food should be provided for animals grazing pasture dominated by one of the oxalate-bearing plants. Prophylactic feeding of dicalcium phosphate is effective, other calcium salts and bone meal being ineffective and adequate salt should be made available. Horses on oxalate-containing grass pasture can be protected against nutritional secondary hyperparathyroidism by feeding them 1 kg of a mixture of 1 part calcium carbonate and 2 parts dicalcium phosphate, in 1·5 kg molasses each week (19).

REFERENCES

(1) Kiatoko, M. et al. (1978) *J. dairy Sci.*, *61*, 324.
(2) James, L. F. et al. (1976) *J. Range Mgmt*, *29*, 284.
(3) Lai, P. & Cosseddu, A. M. (1967) *Arch. vet. Ital.*, *18*, 171.
(4) James, L. F. & Butcher, J. E. (1972) *J. anim. Sci.*, *35*, 1233.
(5) Lincoln, S. D. & Black, B. (1980) *J. Am. vet. med. Assoc.*, *176*, 717.
(6) Groenendyk, S. & Seawright, A. A. (1974) *Aust. vet. J.*, *50*, 131.
(7) James, M. P. et al. (1971) *Aust. vet. J.*, *47*, 9.
(8) Andrews, E. J. (1971) *J. Am. vet. med. Assoc.*, *159*, 49.
(9) Sudarshan, S. et al. (1977) *Ind. J. anim. Sci.*, *47*, 323.
(10) Allison, M. J. et al. (1977) *J. anim. Sci.*, *45*, 1173.
(11) Webb, R. F. & Knight, P. R. (1977) *Aust. vet. J.*, *53*, 554.
(12) Swartzman, J. A. et al. (1978) *Am. J. vet. Res.*, *39*, 1621.
(13) Wilson, G. D. A. & Harvey, D. G. (1977) *Br. vet. J.*, *133*, 318.
(14) Linklater, K. A. & Angus, K. W. (1979) *Vet. Rec.*, *104*, 429.
(15) James, L. F. et al. (1970) *J. Range Mgmt*, 23, 123.
(16) Dickie, C. W. et al. (1978) *J. Am. vet. med. Assoc.*, *173*, 73.
(17) Blaney, B. J. et al. (1981) *J. agric. Sci., Camb.*, 97, 69, 507, 581, 639.
(18) Blaney, B. J. et al. (1982) *J. agric. Sci., Camb.*, *99*, 533.
(19) McKenzie, R. A. et al. (1981) *Aust. vet. J.*, *57*, 554.

Strychnine poisoning

Strychnine poisoning is an uncommon occurrence in farm animals and is usually caused by accidental overdosing with strychnine preparations, or accidental access to grain treated with strychnine and to be used for rodent control (1). Cattle are particularly susceptible to parenteral administration (30–60 mg of strychnine hydrochloride may be fatal) but less susceptible to oral administration because of destruction of the drug in the rumen. Lethal doses by parenteral injection are 200–250 mg in horses, 300–400 mg in cattle and 15–50 mg in pigs.

In strychnine poisoning there is greatly increased reflex excitability and, after an initial period of muscle stiffness and tremor, tetanic convulsions occur. These can be provoked by the application of minor external stimuli. In these convulsive episodes there is extension of the limbs, opisthotonus and protrusion of the eyeballs. Respiratory arrest may lead to death from respiratory paralysis. The seizures may last for 3–4 minutes and are followed by periods of partial relaxation which become progressively shorter as the disease develops.

Strychnine is rapidly excreted and detoxicated and sedation of the animal with barbiturate anesthetics or chloral hydrate for a sufficiently long period may result in recovery. Tannic acid preparations administered orally precipitate the alkaloid in the alimentary tract and interfere with further absorption.

REFERENCES

(1) Lilley, C. W. (1985) *Equ. Pract.*, 7(2), 7.

DISEASES CAUSED BY FARM CHEMICALS

Poisoning of animals by agricultural chemicals has become a major growth sector in farm animal medicine. This is because of the multiplicity of the products used, and the difficulty of determining generic composition from trade names, or the even greater difficulty of remembering the exact chemical formula of complicated organic compounds. It is possible to come to a diagnosis by observing clinical signs and necropsy lesions if one of the more common compounds has been used, but in many other instances it is not possible, and even hazardous to do so. It is necessary in the case of any suspected poisoning to enquire in great detail into the history of exposure of the affected animals to any noxious materials. Having identified possible exposure it is then necessary to define exactly the compound used and then consult a suitable information source, usually the manufacturer, about toxicity problems.

Although poisoning of animals is the prime concern of veterinarians when dealing with agricultural chemicals, there is now a further area of involvement, the contamination of animal products intended for human consumption. Part of the responsibility is to adequately warn owners of the dangers when dispensing drugs which are looked upon as contaminants in human food, for example, penicillin. The other way in which veterinarians become involved is in the detection of sources of contamination when public health authorities advise that rules concerning food purity have been violated. In some countries these contamination problems have now been designated as animal 'diseases' to bring them within legislative control by government veterinarians.

The subject has now become so large that it forms a complete new literature. It is not possible to review all the known toxic compounds in a few pages and only the more common substances are dealt with here. The reader is referred to the more exhaustive treatises below for detailed descriptions.

REVIEW LITERATURE

O'Brien, J. J. (1970) Toxicological aspects of some modern anthelmintics. *Aust. vet. J.*, *46*, 297.
Palmer, J. & Radeleff, R. D. (1964) *Ann. NY Acad. Sci.*, *111*, 729.
Radeleff, R. D. (1970) *Veterinary Toxicology*, 2nd ed. Philadelphia: Lea & Febiger.
Scott, W. N. (1964) *Vet. Rec.*, 76, 964.

Anthelmintics

CARBON TETRACHLORIDE POISONING

Etiology
Deaths following dosing with carbon tetrachloride may occur within 24 hours and result from anesthetic depression and severe pulmonary edema, or may occur 3–7 days later resulting from renal and hepatic insufficiency. Carbon tetrachloride is sometimes accidentally administered in excessive quantities but deaths more commonly occur when sheep are given standard doses or cattle are dosed by mouth, instead of by injection.

Epidemiology
The standard dose of 2 ml per sheep to kill adult *F. hepatica* or 1 ml/10 kg body weight to obtain efficiency against immature forms has been widely used but in some circumstances these doses can be highly toxic. Doses as low as 0·5 ml/10 kg body weight cause liver damage in calves and clinical effects are apparent at 1 ml/10 kg body weight in goats. Damage to the liver by plant (1, 2) or chemical poisons or the ingestion of oxalate-rich plants (3) predisposes to carbon tetrachloride poisoning. Cold stress in shorn sheep also increases susceptibility (4).

Accidental administration of the dose directly into the respiratory tract or inhalation of vapor due to faulty placement of the dose may cause immediate collapse. Outbreaks of death in sheep given the standard dose are recorded when sheep are held without food for long periods, when they are put onto lush pasture after treatment (5), or when they are treated concurrently with a hepatotoxic anthelmintic. Lactating ewes may be more susceptible than dry sheep.

Pathogenesis
Inhalation of carbon tetrachloride causes an immediate and acute depression of the central nervous system and peripheral and circulatory collapse. Diffuse pulmonary edema occurs and sheep that survive show hepatic and renal damage (4). Ingestion of toxic doses causes delayed deaths occurring 3–4 days later. Deaths are associated with almost complete liver (6) and kidney failure but damage to the renal tubules appears to be the critical lesion (7). It has been suggested that carbon tetrachloride is metabolized to a toxic compound and that factors that increase hepatic microsomal activity also increase the toxicity of carbon tetrachloride. Thus lush pastures will increase activity while poorly fed sheep should be more resistant (8). Dieldrin and phenobarbitone have the same effect on the mitochondria and significantly increase the toxicity of CC14 (6).

Clinical findings
With gross overdosing or after inhalation there is an immediate onset of staggering, falling, progressive narcosis, collapse, convulsions, and death due to respiratory failure. Animals that survive this stage or, as in the most common form of carbon tetrachloride poisoning, in which animals absorb insufficient to produce narcosis, additional signs may be manifested in 3–4 days. These comprise anorexia, depression, muscle weakness, diarrhea and jaundice. After a further 2–3 days affected sheep go down and mild to moderate clonic convulsions may occur, but death is always preceded by a period of coma. Those that survive are emaciated and weak, and are prone to develop photosensitization or shed their wool. They are very susceptible to environmental stresses, particularly inclement weather, and isolated deaths may occur for several months.

Clinical pathology
In the first 3 days after dosing liver dysfunction is suggested by a pronounced elevation of SGOT levels and renal dysfunction by an elevation of blood urea levels. After 4 days from dosing the SGOT levels return to normal but blood urea levels remain high (9). A complete spectrum of responses by hepatic enzymes (13) and other biochemical responses (14) to carbon tetrachloride poisoning have been recorded. The BSP test is highly positive and gamma-glutamyl transferase levels are increased.

Necropsy findings
Animals dying after inhalation of the drug show marked pulmonary, hepatic and renal damage. Those dying of massive oral overdosing may show abomasitis and inflammation of the duodenum in addition to the hepatic and renal lesions observed in animals which die after the ingestion of small doses. In the latter animals there is acute hepatitis with swelling, pallor and mottling of the liver. The lobules are more obvious than usual and histologically there is centrilobular necrosis in animals which die within 3 days of dosing and fatty degeneration in sheep dying more than 4 days afterwards (10). The renal lesions comprise extensive degeneration and necrosis of the tubular epithelium on histological examination.

Diagnosis
The history of deaths commencing in sheep 3–4 days after drenching with carbon tetrachloride usually suggests the diagnosis. When poisoning from inhalation is suspected pulmonary lesions should be sought. Acute hepatitis affecting a number of sheep may occur in animals grazing on perennial rye-grass or following access to some poison plants including ragwort, *Crotalaria* spp., and heliotrope.

Treatment
In inhalation poisoning, artificial respiration and respiratory center stimulants are indicated. There is no specific treatment for the hepatitis but supportive treat-

ment should include the parenteral administration of calcium solutions and the provision of readily digestible carbohydrate. In valuable and seriously affected animals the latter are probably best provided by the repeated parenteral injection of glucose and protein hydrolysate solutions. In the experimentally produced disease in cows the intravenous administration of 100 mg/kg body weight of 2-mercaptopropionyl-glycine daily for several days appeared to have a beneficial effect (4).

Control

Carbon tetrachloride should not be used if sheep are stressed by cold or lack of feed, or if they have been grazing hepatotoxic plants. It should never be given simultaneously with anthelmintics that damage the liver. Sheep should be drenched into the pharynx when standing naturally so that the dose can be swallowed immediately (11). An observation of potential importance is that carbon bisulfide given orally significantly reduces the toxicity of carbon tetrachloride, suggesting that its inclusion in commercial drenches may reduce toxicity (12).

REFERENCES

(1) Setchell, B. P. et al. (1964) *Aust. vet. J.*, *40*, 30.
(2) Hunt, E. R. (1972) *Aust. vet. J.*, *48*, 57.
(3) Setchelll, B. P. (1962) *Aust. vet. J.*, *38*, 487.
(4) Gallagher, C. H. (1964) *Aust. vet. J.*, *40*, 229.
(5) Kondos, A. C. & McClymont, G. L. (1965) *Aust. vet. J.*, *41*, 349.
(6) Abdelsalam, E. B. et al. (1982) *Zentralbl. VetMed.*, *29*, 142.
(7) Setchell, B. P. (1961) *Aust. J. agric. Res.*, *12*, 944.
(8) Fowler, J. S. L. (1971) *Br. vet. J.*, *127*, 304.
(9) Setchell, B. P. (1962) *Aust. vet. J.*, *38*, 580.
(10) Gallagher, C. H. (1963) *Aust. vet. J.*, *39*, 49.
(11) Jones, B. E. V. & Shah, M. (1982) *Nord. VetMed.*, *34*, 25.
(12) Seawright, A. A. et al. (1973) *Res. vet. Sci.*, *15*, 158.
(13) Alemu, P. et al. (1977) *J. comp. Pathol.*, *41*, 420.
(14) Kawamura, S. et al. (1985) *J. Jap. vet. med. Assoc.*, *38*, 375.

PHENOTHIAZINE POISONING

Several modes of poisoning are recorded and only the more common ones are discussed.

Keratitis has been recorded most commonly in calves and to a lesser extent in pigs and goats. In most cases the disease results from a heavy dose of phenothiazine, but it is also recorded in calves receiving phenothiazine daily in a dietary premix calculated to keep them free from intestinal nematodes. The phenothiazine was presented as a 1·25% mixture with a protein supplement fed at the rate of 170 g/day in ensilage, free choice. Phenothiazine is absorbed from the rumen as the sulfoxide, conjugated in the liver and excreted in the urine. Cattle are unable to detoxify all the sulfoxide and some escapes into the circulation and can enter the aqueous humor of the eye, causing photosensitization (1). Other photodynamic agents are produced which cannot enter the eye, but they, with the sulfoxide, cause photosensitization of light-colored parts of the body. Lacrimation commences 12–36 hours following treatment and is followed by the development of a white opacity on the lateral or dorsal aspects of the cornea, depending on which is exposed to sunlight. There is marked blepharospasm and photophobia. Most animals recover within a few days, particularly if kept inside or in a shaded paddock. If the animals continue to be exposed a severe conjunctivitis with keratitis may result. Phenothiazine should not be used in white pigs, not only because more efficient compounds are now available, but because of the generalized photosensitization that may occur.

In sheep gradually deprived of water over 12–14 days, the administration of normal doses of phenothiazine can cause fatal renal papillary necrosis. Similar lesions can be produced in cattle but only with higher than normal doses (2).

REFERENCES

(1) Arundel, J. H. (1962) *Aust. vet. J.*, *38*, 307.
(2) Salisbury, R. M. et al. (1969) *NZ vet. J.*, *17*, 187, 227.

Poisoning caused by miscellaneous anthelmintics

TETRACHLORETHYLENE POISONING

Tetrachlorethylene rarely produces toxic effects in cattle or sheep. The signs are similar to those of carbon tetrachloride poisoning and in calves incoordination may be evident for an hour or two after dosing. Treatment is not usually necessary.

HEXACHLOROETHANE POISONING

Hexachloroethane is preferred to carbon tetrachloride for the treatment of fascioliasis in cattle but it is not completely without danger. Emaciated animals may show narcosis and recumbency after administration of the standard dose (15 g per 6 months of age up to a maximum of 60 g) and such animals should be given half this dose on two occasions at 48-hour intervals.

Occasional animals show an idiosyncrasy to the drug, the reaction taking the form of ataxia, dullness, anorexia and sometimes abdominal pain, diarrhea and dysentery. In severe cases the signs are identical with those of parturient paresis. Outbreaks of poisoning also occur in certain areas under certain dietary conditions and possibly when the liver damage caused by fluke infestation is severe. High protein diets, rape and kale are reported to predispose to toxicity. Parturient or heavily lactating cows may also show increased susceptibility. Animals that die show acute abomasitis and enteritis, with edema of the abomasal mucosa, and hepatic centrilobular necrosis. Deaths are rare in cattle (1 in 20 000 treated), and in sheep (1 in 40 000) but non-fatal illness is not uncommon.

Hexachloroethane poisoning in sheep may occur at a dose level of 0·4 g/kg body weight and the clinical signs include narcosis, staggering and falling. There is muscle tremor, a weak pulse and shallow respiration. In cattle and sheep there is a rapid response to treatment with calcium borogluconate as used in parturient paresis.

HEXACHLOROPHENE

At high dose rates (25–50 mg/kg body weight) hexachlorophene causes atrophy of seminiferous epithelium of the testis of the young adult ram (1). Repeated dosing causes periportal fatty changes in liver.

RAFOXANIDE

Rafoxanide is capable of poisoning sheep (2). The obvious result is blindness caused by degeneration of optic nerve tracts and other optic pathways in the brain.

NICOTINE POISONING

Nicotine poisoning seldom occurs in animals except in lambs and calves where nicotine sulfate is still incorporated in some vermifuges. Doses of 0·2–0·3 g nicotine sulfate have been toxic for lambs weighing 14–20 kg. Animals in poor condition are more susceptible than well-nourished animals. Animals are affected within a few minutes of dosing and show dyspnea with rapid shallow respirations, muscle tremor and weakness, recumbency and clonic convulsions. Death is due to respiratory failure. At necropsy there may be abomasitis and inflammation of the duodenum, and animals that survive the depression of the respiratory center may show abdominal pain, salivation and diarrhea.

Treatment should include artificial respiration and the administration of respiratory center stimulants. Oral dosing with tannic acid preparations will precipitate the alkaloid and retard further absorption.

TOLUENE

Toluene has wide applicability as an anthelmintic but its use may be followed by toxic effects. It causes severe irritation of mucous membranes and has a depressant effect on the central nervous system. Repeated exposure causes depression of bone marrow activity and anemia. With overdosing vomiting and slight purgation may occur, and in young animals incoordination and muscle tremor may appear transiently soon after treatment.

CADMIUM SALTS

Cadmium oxide and cadmium anthranilate used to be used extensively for the treatment of ascariasis in swine. However, these compounds are quite toxic and can be administered only once because of their marked tendency to accumulate in tissues. In acute poisoning, gastroenteritis with vomition is the most obvious sign of toxicity but deaths due to uremia may occur some days later. These compounds are no longer in general use.

PIPERAZINE

Piperazine compounds are relatively non-toxic but poisoning can occur in horses on normal or excessive doses. Signs follow a delay of 12–24 hours and include incoordination, pupillary dilatation, hyperesthesia, tremor, somnolence and either swaying while at rest or lateral recumbency. Recovery follows in 48–72 hours without treatment (8).

THIABENDAZOLE (2-(4′-THIAZOLYL)-BENZIMIDAZOLE)

At an oral dose rate of 800 mg/kg body weight in sheep transient signs of salivation, anorexia and depression appear. There are similar signs at larger dose rates and death is likely at a dose rate of 1200 mg/kg body weight (9). Toxic nephrosis is the cause of death and is reflected in the clinical and pathological findings of hypokalemia, hypoproteinemia and uremia (5). An unusual occurrence, due possibly to direct entry of the chemical into the abomasum, resulted in steers which received eight times the standard dose. They became acutely ill within an hour of dosing; clinical signs included aggression, incoordination and collapse (6).

LEVAMIZOLE (1–2, 3, 5, 6-TETRAHYDRO-6-PHENYLIMIDAZO (2, 1-*b*) THIAZOLE)

When first introduced as tetramisole, the compound consisted of equal parts of the levo and dextro isomers. The anthelmintic activity was confined to the levo isomer while both were equally toxic, and the margin between the therapeutic and toxic dose rates in tetramisole was low. All commercial material now consists of the levo isomer. Following treatment at standard doses some cattle, and more rarely sheep, show signs of lip-licking, increased salivation, head-shaking, skin tremors and excitability. The excitability is more marked in calves; when released they tend to raise their tails and run around the paddock. Coughing may commence within 15–20 minutes, but this is due to the death and expulsion of lung worms and stops in 24 hours (3). With higher doses the signs are more pronounced, defecation is frequent and hyperesthesia in the form of a continuous twitching of the skin may be seen (3). Double doses in goats produce mild depression and ptosis, while higher doses produce, in addition, head-shaking, twitching of facial muscles, grinding of teeth, salivation, tail-twitching, increased micturition and straining (4). Accidental injection of swine caused vomiting, salivation, ataxia, recumbency and a high mortality within a few minutes of injection (18).

PARBENDAZOLE (METHYL 5-BUTYL-2-BENZIMIDAZOLE CARBAMATE), CAMBENDAZOLE (ISOPROPYL 2-(4-THIAZOLYL)-5-BENZIMIDAZOLE CARBAMATE) AND ALBENDAZOLE (METHYL (5-(PROPYL THIO)-1H-BENZIMIDAZOLE-2YL) CARBAMATE)

The teratogenic effects of parbendazole (10) and cambendazole (11) have been identified and these compounds are specifically contraindicated in pregnant animals especially during the first third of pregnancy and at dose rates higher than normal. The safety margin is small and their use at any dose level is not recommended in these females. The defects include rotational and flexing deformities of the limbs, overflexion of the carpal joints, abnormalities of posture and gait, vertebral fusion and asymmetric cranial ossification (19). Cerebral hypoplasia and hydrocephalus have also been reported (2). Albendazole at four times the standard dose also produces some abnormalities if given early in pregnancy (12), but dosing at 75% of these levels to cows during the 5th to 33rd week of pregnancy had no deleterious effects on the fetuses (17). Deaths are also recorded in calves which received high dose rates of cambendazole combined with concentrate feeding (7).

FENBENDAZOLE (METHYL 5-(PHENYLTHIO)-2-BENZIMIDAZOLE CARBAMATE)

The use of fenbendazole and the flukicide, bromsalans, to cattle either simultaneously or within a few days of each other may be accompanied by deaths. As fenbendazole and the other tertiary benzimidazoles, oxfendazole and albendazole, are extremely valuable in removing dormant *O. ostertagi* larvae, it is suggested that fascol (bromsalans) should not be used where this is an important problem or that 2 weeks should elapse between treatments.

IVERMECTIN

The intravenous injection into horses of a cattle formulation of ivermectin, contrary to the recommended usage, may cause immediate collapse with coma and periodic nystagmus (16). Treatment intravenously with flumethasone and flunixin meglumine was followed by recovery at 9 hours and normal muscular coordination at 3 days. Intramuscular injection is attended by a variety of untoward sequels (20). These include ventral midline edema caused possibly by a reaction to dead microfilariae, edema of limbs, edema of eyelids, fever, dyspnea, disorientation, colic and sudden death. Transient swelling at the injection site is common.

HYGROMYCIN B

This aminoglycoside antibiotic is given to pigs at 13·2 g/453 kg feed to control *A. suum*, *Oesophagostomum* spp. and *T. suis*. The recommended regime is to place it in the ration for 8 weeks and then feed non-medicated feed for the next 8 weeks. This alternation of medicated and non-medicated feed should continue until the pigs are 55 kg. The product is also used in sows in the periparturient period. Continual use of that dose rate causes cortical cataracts (14) and the correct alternating treatment for extended periods may also result in cataracts in some sows (15).

ORGANOPHOSPHATIC ANTHELMINTICS

These are dealt with in the next section on insecticides. Industrial organophosphates and organophosphatic defoliants are dealt with in the section on miscellaneous farm chemicals.

TETRACHLORODIFLUORETHANE (FREON-112)

Tetrachlorodifluorethane is an effective anthelmintic against mature liver flukes but some samples of the product are highly toxic to sheep and cattle and its use in treatment is not recommended. The degree of toxicity appears to depend on the concentration of the asymmetric isomer of the compound in the sample. Fatal poisoning, including marked prolongation of the blood clotting time, widespread hemorrhages, kidney, liver and myocardial damage, venous congestion and anasarca, occur at recommended therapeutic levels for cattle (200 mg/kg body weight) and at levels of 1000 mg/kg body weight for sheep (13).

REFERENCES

(1) Thorpe, E. (1969) *J. comp. Pathol.*, *79*, 167.
(2) Prozesky, L. & Joubert, J. P. L. (1981) *J. S. Afr. vet. Assoc.*, *52*, 75.
(3) Forsythe, B. A. (1966) *J. S. Afr. vet. Assoc.*, *37*, 403.
(4) Smith, J. P. & Bell, R. R. (1971) *Am. J. vet. Res.*, *32*, 871.
(5) Clark, R. G. & Lewis, K. H. C. (1977) *NZ vet. J.*, *25*, 187.
(6) Hennessy, P. R. & Pritchard, R. K. (1979) *Aust. vet. J.*, *55*, 298.
(7) Main, D. C. & Vass, D. E. (1980) *Aust. vet. J.*, *56*, 273.
(8) McNeil, P. H. & Smyth, G. B. (1978) *J. equ. med. Surg.*, *2*, 321.
(9) Bell, R. R. (1964) *Ann. NY Acad. Sci.*, *111*, 662.
(10) Saunders, L. Z. et al. (1981) *Onderstepoort J. vet. Res.*, *48*, 159.
(11) Dalatour, P. et al. (1975) *Bull Soc. Sci. vet. Med. comp. Lyon*, *77*, 197.
(12) Johns, D. J. & Philip, J. R. (1977) *Proc. 8th int. Wld Assoc. Adv. vet. Parasit Conf., Sydney*.
(13) Gallagher, C. H. (1965) *Aust. vet. J.*, *41*, 167.
(14) Cargill, C. F. et al. (1983) *Aust. vet. J.*, *60*, 312.
(15) Norton, J. J. (1980) *Aust. vet. J.*, *56*, 403.
(16) Burrough, S. (1986) *NZ vet. J.*, *34*, 137.
(17) Wetzel, H. (1985) *Zentralbl. VetMed.*, *32*, 375.
(18) Cook, W. O. et al. (1985) *Vet. hum. Toxicol.*, *27*, 388.
(19) Drudge, J. H. et al. (1983) *Am. J. vet. Res.*, *44*, 110.
(20) Karns, P. A. & Luther, D. G. (1984) *J. Am. vet. med. Assoc.*, *185*, 782.

Insecticides

CHLORINATED HYDROCARBONS

This group includes DDT, benzene hexachloride (and its pure gamma isomer—lindane), aldrin, dieldrin, chlordane, toxaphene, methoxychlor, DDD, isodrin, endrin and heptachlor. The toxic effects produced by the members of this group include increased excitability and irritability followed by muscle tremor, weakness and paralysis and terminal convulsions in severe cases. Salivation and teeth grinding occur in large animals and vomiting in pigs. Complete anorexia occurs constantly. Most of the substances accumulate in the fat depots, may be excreted in the milk in dangerous amounts, and may be concentrated still further in butter and cream. Fat depots are a potential source of danger in that sudden mobilization of the fat may result in liberation of the compound into the bloodstream and the appearance of signs of toxicity. This information is of incidental value when a diagnosis of chlorinated hydrocarbon poisoning is required. The removal of a fat biopsy from the fat pad near the cow's tail offers a satisfactory means of providing samples for tissue analysis (3).

To produce systemic signs these insecticides must enter the bloodstream and ingestion, inhalation, aspiration and percutaneous absorption are all possible portals of entry. Dipping is the most hazardous method of application because entry may occur through all portals. Spraying is safer, percutaneous absorption and inhalation being the only portals of entry. Small particle size of the compound and concentration of animals in confined spaces while spraying increase the possibility of poisoning. Although oily preparations are not usually used for animal treatment they may be used inadvertently and in this form are readily absorbed through the skin. Concentrations used for spraying barns are usually much higher than those used for animals. Of the usual spray preparations simple solutions are most dangerous followed by emulsions and least of all suspensions of wettable powder. Dusting is safest and is preferred to other methods. Preparations for use on plants are often fast-breaking emulsions, that is they are relatively unstable and come out of suspension quickly when they contact the plant. If these preparations are used in animal dips the first few animals through the dip can be heavily contaminated and suffer acute, lethal toxic effects. Although the treatment of pastures to control their insect pests is usually, with an occasional notable exception, safe to animals grazing the treated pasture or hay made from it, contamination of animal products occurs often. This contamination can be avoided by incorporating the insecticide into superphosphate granules ('prills') instead of applying it as sprays or dusts. The use of chlorinated hydrocarbons to protect stored seeds provides a hazard to animals if they are fed on the treated seed. The speed of onset of illness after exposure varies from a few minutes to a few hours, varying with the portal of entry and the compound and its formulation, but it is never very long.

The compounds vary in their ability to pass the skin barrier. Benzene hexachloride, aldrin, dieldrin and chlordane are readily absorbed. Species susceptibility to skin absorption also varies widely. Very young animals of any species are more susceptible than adults and lactating and emaciated animals also show increased susceptibility. General toxicity data for the more common compounds are given in Table 96. Methoxychlor is less toxic than DDT, and isodrin and endrin are more toxic than aldrin and dieldrin.

When these compounds were first used in dips, skin and foot infections occurred frequently because of contamination of the dip in the absence of a bactericidal agent. Cases of otitis media occurred for the same reason but more rarely.

At necropsy there are no specific lesions and specimens of hair, if the portal is percutaneous, and of the ingesta, if oral intake is probable, should be sent to the laboratory for assay. If possible the specimens should be deep frozen and the suspected compound should be nominated as assay procedures are long and involved.

DDT AND METHOXYCHLOR

DDT and methoxychlor cause initial stimulation of the central nervous system followed by terminal depression and death due to respiratory failure. Chronic poisoning causes liver damage, and a fall in blood sugar and liver glycogen levels and elevation of blood lactate and potassium.

At necropsy there are no lesions in the nervous system but in chronic cases there is focal centrilobular necrosis in the liver. Treatment comprises sedation with pentobarbital sodium, intravenous injections of glucose and calcium and the administration of a non-oily purgative. Residual DDT should be removed from the coat.

BENZENE HEXACHLORIDE, LINDANE, CHLORDANE, TOXAPHENE, DIELDRIN, ENDRIN, ALDRIN AND HEPTACHLOR

Poisoning with these compounds has been recorded in horses (11) and in dogs, lambs, calves and steers (2). Clinical signs resemble those of DDT poisoning but to a more extreme degree. Muscle tremors are not evident but there is excitement with grinding of the teeth, dyspnea, tetany, snapping of the eyelids and frequent micturition. Movements are frenzied and include walking backwards, climbing walls, violent somersaults and aimless jumping. In steers salivation, incoordination and muscle tremor are recorded. In pigs poisoned by tox-

Table 96. Toxic oral doses and maximum concentrations of insecticides (1).

Compound	*Method of application*	*Calves to 2 weeks*	*Cattle*	*Sheep*	*Pig*	*Goat*	*Horse*
DDT	Oral single dose (mg/kg body weight)	—	450	200	200	200	200
	Maximum safe spray (%)			In general above 5%			
Benzene hexachloride	Oral single dose (mg/kg body weight)	—	1000	1000	1000	1000	1000
Lindane	Oral single dose (mg/kg body weight)	5	25	25	—	—	—
	Maximum safe spray (%)	0·025	0·1	1·0	1·0	—	0·5
Aldrin	Oral single dose (mg/kg body weight)	2·5–5·0	10–25	>10	—	—	—
	Oral daily dose (mg/kg body weight)	—	2–5	2–5	—	—	—
Dieldrin	Oral single dose (mg/kg body weight)	5–10	10–25	<25	25–50	—	<25
	Maximum safe spray (%)	0·1–0·25	1–2	0·2–0·3 (lambs)	4·0	4·0	100
Toxaphene	Oral single dose (mg/kg body weight)	5.0	—	25	—	50	—
	Maximum safe spray (%)	0·5	2·0	1·5	4·0	—	—
Chlordane and heptachlor	Oral single dose (mg/kg body weight)	25	—	100	—	—	—
	Maximum safe spray (%)	0·5	2–3	2–3 (1·0 lambs)	—	—	—

aphene head-pressing, ataxia, depression, lethargy and diarrhea are listed as signs. So are paddling convulsions at short intervals, with persistent recumbency in some (4). The clinical signs are not inconsistent with those of salt poisoning, but the characteristic lesions of eosinophilic meningoencephalitis are missing (11). Recovery may occur but with smaller animals paralysis follows and finally collapse and death ensue. Repeated doses of pentobarbital sodium are recommended until signs disappear. Similar clinical effects are produced by poisoning with chlordane, toxaphene, dieldrin, aldrin and heptachlor. In one outbreak in lambs in which undiluted aldrin was applied to oral lesions of contagious ecthyma 105 of 107 lambs died. Deaths began soon after application of the aldrin and 45% of the lambs were dead within 36 hours. Although histological changes were evident in the brain, they were mild and probably reversible. The significant lesions appeared to be an acute toxic hepatitis and an acute tubular nephritis (4). An outbreak of dieldrin poisoning in shedded sheep continued over a period of over a year because of repeated contamination from the shed (15). Long-term, low-level dosing of goats with aldrin produces severe nephrosis (8). An outbreak of benzene hexachloride (Gammexane) poisoning has been observed in horses which ate contaminated bran. Grasshopper baits containing toxaphene and chlordane have caused poisoning in cattle which ate large quantities of the bait.

Heptachlor is used extensively in agriculture to control soil pests. It is incorporated in the soil before the crop of potatoes or maize is sown. Subsequent grazing of the same field may result in contamination of the cattle. This may continue for long periods and affected paddocks are not suitable for animal pasturing (6). It has caused hyperesthesia and tetanic convulsions in horses (14, 16). Endrin is a particularly toxic pesticide which causes hyperesthesia, convulsions, hypersalivation, teeth grinding and mania in pigs (13).

All of these compounds are soluble in fat and accumulate in body stores of it. They are also excreted in significant amounts in milk and enter the human food chain at this point. They also represent a threat to sucklings. However, the degree of contamination in fetuses and suckling animals is much less than in their dams (5).

The chlorinated hydrocarbons have come under so much criticism that they are not often used directly on animals nowadays so that outbreaks of clinical illness caused by them are much less common than they were. However, the compounds are still widely used in agriculture, principally on growing plants to control insect pests, and on stored seed grain to control fungi. If the plants or grain are fed to animals they can cause problems of tissue residues, or if they are fed in sufficient quantities they can cause clinical illness (7). These insecticides may also contaminate soil and persist there for many years (17). Rooting animals such as pigs are particularly susceptible to this source of poisoning. These compounds are also sometimes fed accidentally in lieu of feed additives (8). They are then usually fed in large amounts and cause acute poisoning. With the more usual chronic poisoning the end-result is the contamination of animal tissues at levels which are not acceptable by modern health standards. These contaminations become the subject of veterinary investigations, and are susceptible to standard techniques of epidemiological examination. If the source is determined the only practicable procedure is to deny animals access to it.

Treatment

Treatment to reduce the contamination of tissues is unsuccessful, and in most cases the time required for the contamination to subside naturally is long, of the order of 3–6 months but varying between specific compounds. For example cows fed DDT prepartum have required an average of 189 days from parturition for the level in the milk fat to decline to 125 ppm (9). Contamination in other species and with other chlorinated hydrocarbon compounds also tends to be persistent. After the source of contamination is removed it is recommended that cows be drenched with up to 2 kg of activated charcoal and that 1 kg be incorporated in their feed daily for 2 weeks. Sodium phenobarbitone has been shown to increase the excretion rate of chlorinated hydrocarbons significantly when fed to dairy cows at the rate of 5 g per day for up to a month. Charcoal and phenobarbitone has a similar effect on contaminated swine (10). Mineral oil by mouth is recommended as a means of removing chlorinated hydrocarbons from the alimentary tract; small amounts are given at short intervals (12).

REVIEW LITERATURE

Harrison, D. L. (1971) Veterinary aspects of insecticides: organochlorines. *NZ vet. J.*, 19, 227.

World Health Organization (1973) Safe use of pesticides. Twentieth report of the WHO Expert Committee on Insecticides. *WHO tech. Rep. Ser.*, *513*, 54.

REFERENCES

(1) Mount, M. E. et al. (1980) *J. Am. vet. med. Assoc.*, *177*. 445.
(2) Alsupp, T. N. & Wharton, M. H. (1967) *Vet. Rec.*, *80*, 583.
(3) Weinland, K. M. & Henderson, B. M. (1977) *J. Am. vet. med. Assoc.*, *170*, 1095.
(4) DiPietro, J. A. & Haliburton, J. C. (1979) *J. Am. vet. med. Assoc.*, *175*, 452.
(5) Czoukwu, M. & Sleight, S. D. (1972) *J. Am. vet. med. Assoc.*, *160*, 1641.
(6) Harradine, I. R. & McDougall, K. W. (1986) *Aust. vet. J.*, *63*, 419.
(7) Neumann, G. (1973) *Mh Vet. Med.*, *28*, 50.
(8) Singh, K. K. et al. (1985) *Zentrall. VetMed.*, *32*, 437.
(9) Miller, D. D. (1967) *J. dairy Sci.*, *50*, 1444.
(10) Dobson, R. C. et al. (1971) *Bull. envir. Contam. Toxicol.*, *6*, 189.
(11) Nazario, W. et al. (1980) *Biologico*, *46*, 191.
(12) Rozman, K. et al. (1984) *Bull envir. Contam. Toxicol.*, *32*, 27.
(13) Reid, G. G. et al. (1982) *Aust. vet. J.*, *59*, 160.
(14) Dickson, J. et al. (1983) *Aust. vet. J.*, *60*, 311.
(15) Walker, R. I. et al. (1982) *Aust. Adv. vet. Sci.*, p. 215.
(16) Dickson, J. et al. (1984) *Aust. vet. J.*, *61*, 331.
(17) Casteel, S. W. & Carson, T. L. (1985) *Vet. Med.*, *80*(3), 93.

Organophosphorous compounds and carbamates

Organophosphorous compounds and carbamates inactivate cholinesterase and produce a syndrome of salivation, diarrhea, and muscle stiffness indicative of stimulation of the parasympathetic nervous system. Some compounds cause a delayed neurotoxicity.

Etiology

Organophosphorous compounds and carbamates act in essentially the same way, both therapeutically and toxicologically. A large number of compounds are included in the group and there is a great deal of variation in their toxicity for animals. Those used for the direct treatment of animals have been selected for their low toxicity. A large amount of information has become available on the relative toxicities of the many compounds which are now commercially available. It is not possible to provide extended details here and the information does not lend itself to summarization.

Epidemiology

The introduction of these compounds into animal therapeutics as treatments for nematode, botfly, sheep nasal botfly and warble-fly infestations and as insecticidal sprays on plants and soil (e.g. fonofos as a pasture spray) (22) has increased their importance as possible causes of poisoning, and as causes of pollution of milk, meat and eggs. They also have a role in the poisoning of the native birdlife (20). They are now one of the most important causes of poisoning of agricultural animals.

Substances in this OP group are included in the instruments of modern biological warfare as 'nerve gases'. Their use in war would be expected to have effects similar to those described here. The famous 'Utah sheep kill' phenomenon is thought to have been due to an accidental release of an OP from a defense forces proving ground (1).

A number of factors including age, breed, sex, diet and species affect the toxicity of these compounds (26). For example, young animals are usually much more susceptible than adults but with some compounds the reverse is the case. Brahman and Brahman-cross cattle appear to be more susceptible to some compounds than other cattle (2) and there is a suggestion of a higher than normal susceptibility of Dorset Down sheep (3). Restriction of water intake renders animals more susceptible to the toxic effects especially after oral treatment with these compounds to control warble-fly infestations. The toxicity of some compounds appears to increase with storage. Chlorpyrifos is more toxic for male animals with high tissue levels of testosterone and is not recommended for use in bulls over 8 months of age (24).

Accidental exposure may occur when animals are allowed to graze in recently sprayed areas, particularly orchards where the most toxic compounds are frequently used. Accidental contamination of pasture may occur when spray used on cereal crops and in orchards is carried by wind on to pasture fields. Lucerne cubes made from plants which had been sprayed with organophosphate compounds produced signs of poisoning in dairy cattle. There was probably an uneven distribution of the insecticide on the feed (9). Failure to prevent cattle going onto freshly sprayed pasture, use of old insecticide buckets and contamination of water supplies are potent sources of poisoning (10).

Many accidents occur as a result of improper use of sprays, either because of too high a concentration of the insecticide or, more commonly, because of the application to animals of products containing oily bases and designed specifically for spraying on walls and other inanimate objects. In the race for supremacy with anthelmintics a number of compounds have been released which are not safe in all circumstances. The reasons for outbreaks of toxicity with these compounds are often not understood but in most cases the recommended dose rate has been exceeded. On the other hand with proper care these compounds can be safe. In Australia it has been reported that in $17{\cdot}5 \times 10^6$ cattle dippings there were 563 deaths—an incidence of 0·033% (4), while in the United Kingdom the incidence of deaths following the use of organophosphorous compounds as warblefly dressings was 1 in 93 000 animals treated (14).

Pathogenesis

Organophosphorous compounds are highly toxic and are readily absorbed by ingestion, inhalation and by percutaneous and perconjunctival absorption. There are two forms of toxicity, cholinesterase inactivation and an organophosphorus-induced, delayed neurotoxicity.

The *inactivation of cholinesterase* by these organophosphorous compounds causes an increase in acetylcholine in tissues and increased activity of the parasympathetic nervous system and of the postganglionic cholinergic nerves of the sympathetic nervous system. The toxic effects thus reproduce the muscarinic and nicotinic responses of acetylcholine administration. The muscarinic effects are the visceral responses of increased peristalsis, salivation, bronchial constriction, increased mucous secretion by bronchiolar glands, pupillary constriction and sweating. The nicotinic effects are the skeletal muscle responses of twitching, tremor and tetany initially followed by weakness and flaccid paralysis. There is a difference in the relative muscarinic and nicotinic responses between species, the visceral effects being more marked in ruminants and the muscular effects more evident in pigs in which posterior paralysis is the common manifestation (5). Effects additional to those quoted include terminal effects on the nervous system, particularly drowsiness, convulsions and coma.

Some organophosphorous compounds cause only temporary interference with cholinesterase and do not cause any permanent effects in recovered animals but with some compounds, especially coumaphos and Ronnel, the recovery period may be quite long, up to 3 months in the case of Ronnel, because of slow excretion of the compound. Also the fluid diarrhea which is a transient sign in moderate intoxication in foals may be expanded to a severe gastroenteritis with heavier dose rates.

Organophosphorous-induced delayed neurotoxicity is manifested by distal axonopathy commencing 1 or 2 weeks after the poisoning incident. There is a dieback of neurones causing regional flaccid paralysis, especially in long neurones (16). Typical examples of this effect are congenital defects in young carried by poisoned pregnant females, bilateral hemiplegia of the larynx in horses, and possibly the paralytic ileus caused by chlorpyrifos. The most severe effects in this category are caused by industrial organophosphorous compounds and are discussed under that heading. Haloxon has this neurotoxic effect in that it causes only a slight depression in cholinesterase levels, but a neurotoxic response in the form of hindleg ataxia has been reported in a proportion of sheep (15) and pigs (5) that are dosed. The susceptibility of sheep is determined by their ability to metabolize this class of organophosphorous compounds and this is genetically controlled (15).

An unexpected side-effect of the use of organophosphorous anthelmintics in the horse is their effect in potentiating the action of succinylcholine chloride for up to 1 month after the administration of the organophosphorous compound (6). The administration of the relaxant to a sensitized horse can be followed by persistent apnea and death. There are a number of other interactions with drugs which may themselves have toxic effects, but there are no clearcut generalizations about these effects and the manufacturer's instructions must be followed explicitly.

Clinical findings

Cattle

In cattle the premonitory signs in acute cases, and the only signs in mild cases, are salivation, dyspnea, diarrhea and muscle stiffness with staggering. It is the dyspnea which is most obvious and it may be heard from some distance away because a number of animals are usually affected and the breathing is accompanied by grunting (18). In the acute cases additional signs include protrusion of the tongue, constriction of the pupils with resulting impairment of vision, muscle tremor commencing in the head and neck and spreading over the body, bloat, collapse, and death without convulsions or severe respiratory distress. In sheep the signs are similar and include also abdominal pain.

Chlorpyrifos should not be applied to adult dairy cattle nor to any mature bulls because of its toxicity for them. When it is used it does not have a clinical effect until 4–7, sometimes as many as 22, days later. The signs include anorexia, depression, recumbency, a distended abdomen, ruminal stasis and diarrhea, and fluid-splashing sounds on succussion of the right flank. There are no intestinal sounds due to paralytic ileus, and severe dehydration may cause death (21).

Pigs

In pigs visceral effects are less pronounced and salivation, muscle tremor, nystagmus and recumbency are characteristic. In some instances, the syndrome is an indefinite one with muscle weakness and drowsiness the only apparent signs. Respiratory distress and diarrhea do not occur. There is a record of a series of outbreaks of posterior paralysis after dosing of pigs with an organophosphorous anthelmintic (5). Clinical signs vary in severity from knuckling in the hindlegs to complete flaccid paralysis. The hindlegs may be dragged behind while the pigs walk on the front legs. These signs are recorded as not having occurred until 3 weeks after dosing. Affected pigs were bright and alert and ate well. There were constant degenerative lesions in the spinal cord. The picture closely resembles that recorded in poisoning caused by industrial organophosphorous compounds and dealt with under that heading.

Sheep

A similar outbreak has been recorded in sheep after the administration of a recommended dose rate of the same anthelmintic (7), and after the oral administration of an insecticide (13). Also, clinical signs did not appear until 5–90 days after dosing. The signs were ataxia and posterior paralysis, and there were striking degenerative lesions in the spinal cord.

Horses

In horses signs of toxicity include abdominal pain and grossly increased intestinal sounds, a very fluid diarrhea, muscle tremor, ataxia, circling, weakness and dyspnea. Increased salivation occurs rarely (8). Acute bilateral laryngeal paralysis has been recorded in foals after dosing with an organophosphatic anthelmintic (23). It is described under laryngeal hemiplegia (p. 386).

Congenital defects in the offspring of dams treated with organophosphorous compounds during midpregnancy have been suggested as an effect–cause relationship many times. It is now reported as a natural and experimental effect of dosing with organophosphorous compounds in pregnant sows (11). Ataxia and tremor are observed clinically, and cerebellar and spinal cord hypoplasia at necropsy. Teratogenicity may be a characteristic of only some organophosphorous compounds, e.g. trichlorphon is teratogenic, dichlorvos is not (17).

Illness may occur within minutes of inhalation or ingestion of solutions of the more toxic compounds and deaths may commence 2–5 minutes later. With less toxic compounds in solid form signs may not appear for some hours and deaths may be delayed for 12–24 hours.

Clinical pathology

The estimation of cholinesterase in body tissues and fluids is the most satisfactory method of diagnosing this poisoning, but it is essential that proper methods and standards of normality be used (8). The degree of depression of blood cholinesterase levels varies with the dose rate and the toxicity of the compound used but the duration of the toxic effect will also play a large part in the duration of the depression. For example, cholinesterase levels in cattle poisoned with terbufos, an agricultural insecticide, did not commence to rise towards normal until 30 days and were not normal for 150 days after the poisoning incident (14).

A potentially useful clinicopathological tool for the detection of exposure to organophosphorous compounds is the estimation of *O,O*-diethyl phosphorothionate (DETP) in urine; its concentration rises sharply after exposure (25).

Suspected food material can be assayed for its content of organophosphorous compounds but assay of animal tissues or fluids is virtually valueless and may be misleading.

Necropsy findings

There are no gross or histological lesions at necropsy, but tissue specimens should be collected for toxicological analysis. Material sent for laboratory analysis for cholinesterase should be refrigerated but not deep frozen.

Diagnosis

Dyspnea, salivation and muscle stiffness and constriction of the pupils after exposure to organophosphorous insecticides suggest intoxication with these compounds. Occasional animals may show a similar syndrome when affected by anaphylaxis, and groups of cattle affected by fog fever may show a sudden onset of dyspnea but pulmonary edema is obvious on auscultation, and salivation and muscle stiffness are absent. In pigs the signs are less diagnostic and may suggest arsenic, rotenone, salt or mercury poisoning, or avitaminosis A. In pigs the recovery rate is good and all pigs may recover if the intake has been low and access is stopped. With the other poisons listed above, death is much more common and residual defects including blindness and paralysis occur in a proportion of the survivors. The history of exposure to the various poisons or of nutritional deficiency may give the clue to the diagnosis but it is usually necessary to depend on assay of the food material for confirmation. It should be remembered that reactions following organophosphorous treatment for grubs may be due either to the drug or to the damaged grub, and treatment with atropine would be contraindicated in the latter.

Treatment

Atropine in large (about double the normal) doses is the rational and approved treatment (19). Recommended doses are 0·25 mg/kg body weight in cattle and 1 mg/kg body weight in sheep. In very sick animals about one third of this dose should be given very slowly intravenously in a dilute (2%) solution and the remainder by intramuscular injection (11). Injections may have to be repeated at 4–5 hourly intervals as signs return, and continued over a period of 24–48 hours. Cows that have received very large doses of the poison may or may not respond to treatment (18).

A group of compounds known as oximes have some efficiency in treatment. The oxime trimedoxime bromide is superior to 2-pyridine aldoxime methiodide (2-PAM) and diacetylmonoxime (DAM). Recommended dose rates for 2-pyridine aldoxime methiodide are 50–100 mg/kg body weight given intravenously and for trimedoxime bromide 10–20 mg/kg body weight (12). These dose rates can also be used for subcutaneous and intraperitoneal injection. Administration by any route is as a 10% solution in normal saline. In horses 2-pyridine aldoxime methiodide at doses of 20 mg/kg body weight has given good results. Combination of an oxime and atropine is recommended (13). Treatment with pyridine aldoxime methiodide may need to be repeated for up to 10 days to counteract slower acting compounds such as coumaphos (12). Atropine appears to have low efficiency in sheep. This is not a serious drawback as sheep are much less susceptible than cattle to larger doses of atropine.

Animals that have been dipped or sprayed should be washed with water to which soap, soda or a detergent is added to remove residual organophosphorous material.

Control

Most outbreaks occur after accidental access to compounds and this cannot always be avoided. Animals to be treated orally with organophosphorous insecticides should be permitted ample fresh drinking water beforehand. Chlorpyrifos is restricted to use in beef cattle and then not in calves less than 12 weeks old nor in bulls over 8 months of age (1).

REVIEW LITERATURE

Abdelsalam, E. B. (1987) Factors affecting the toxicity of organophosphorous compounds in animals. *Vet. Bull.*, *57*, 441–448.

Barrett, D. S., Oehme, F. W. & Kruckenberg, S. M. (1985) A review of organophosphorous ester-induced delayed neurotoxicity. *Vet. hum. Toxicol.*, *27*, 22–37.

Maddy, K. T. & Riddle, L. C. (1977) Pesticide poisonings in domestic animals. *Mod. Vet. Pract.*, *58*, 3.

REFERENCES

(1) Van Kampen, K. R. et al. (1969) *J. Am. vet. med. Assoc.*, *154*, 623.
(2) Randell, W. F. & Bradley, R. E. (1980) *Am. J. vet. Res.*, *41*, 1423.
(3) Smith, I. D. (1970) *Vet. Rec.*, *86*, 284.
(4) Boermans, H. J. et al. (1985) *Can. vet. J.*, *26*, 350.
(5) Stubbings, D. P. et al. (1976) *Vet. Rec.*, *99*, 127.
(6) Himes, J. A. et al. (1967) *J. Am vet. med. Assoc.*, *151*, 54.
(7) Williams, J. F. & Dade, A. W. (1976) *J. Am. vet. med. Assoc.*, *169*, 1307.
(8) Abdelsalam, E. B. & Ford, E. J. H. (1983) *Zentralbl. VetMed.*, *32*, 518.
(9) Egyed, M. N. et al. (1978) *Refuah Vet.*, *35*, 4.
(10) Maddy, K. T. et al. (1977) *Calif. vet.*, *31*, 9.
(11) Pope, A. M. et al. (1986) *J. Am vet. med. Assoc.*, *189*, 781.
(12) Younger, R. L. & Wright, F. C. (1971) *J. Am. vet. med. Assoc.*, *32*, 1053.
(13) El-Sebae, A. H. et al. (1979) *J. env. Sci. Hlth*, *14B*, 247.
(14) Andrews, A. H. (1981) *Vet. Rec.*, *109*, 171.
(15) Baker, N. F. et al. (1980) *Am. J. vet. Res.*, *41*, 1857.
(16) Wilson, R. D. et al. (1982) *Am. J. vet. Res.*, *43*, 222.
(17) Wrathall, A. E. et al. (1980) *Zentralbl. VetMed.*, *27A*, 662.
(18) Boermans, H. J. et al. (1984) *Can. vet. J.*, *25*, 335.
(19) Lekeux, P. et al. (1986) *Res. vet. Sci.*, *40*, 318.
(20) Henny, C. J. et al. (1985) *J. Wildl. Mgt*, *49*, 648.
(21) Lein, D. H. et al. (1982) *Cornell Vet.*, *72*, Suppl. 9, pp. 1–58.
(22) Kurtz, D. A. & Hutchinson, L. (1982) *Am. J. vet. Res.*, *43*, 1672.
(23) Rose, R. J. et al. (1981) *Equ. vet. J.*, *13*, 171.
(24) Haas, P. J. et al. (1983) *Am. J. vet. Res.*, *44*, 879.
(25) Mount, M. E. (1984) *Am. J. vet. Res.*, *45*, 817.
(26) Abdelsalam, E. B. (1987) *Vet. Bull.*, *57*, 441.

Rotenone

Rotenone is relatively non-toxic when taken orally but toxic effects have been observed in pigs fed a ration containing 2·5% of rotenone. In this instance, assay of ingesta at necropsy revealed the presence of 2130 ppm of rotenone. Clinically there was salivation, muscle tremor, vomiting, ascending paralysis accompanied by incoordination, followed by paralysis of all four limbs. Respiratory depression and coma preceded death which occurred in all of the ten pigs exposed (1).

REFERENCE

(1) Oliver, W. T. & Roe, C. K. (1957) *J. Am. vet. med. Assoc.*, *130*, 410.

Amitraz

This formamidine compound is widely used against ticks affecting cattle and sheep and against mange mites in a variety of species. It is prohibited from use in horses but when it is used accidentally it causes a syndrome characterized by somnolence, incoordination, depression, reduction of intestinal sounds and impaction of the large intestine may occur within 12–24 hours. Concentration of the dipping fluid, environmental temperature and the condition of the skin may influence absorption and the susceptibility of the animal. There is one record of poisoning in horses that had been previously sprayed without ill-effects. It was thought that the amitraz in the spray had broken down during storage of a prepared mix and was more toxic (2). Residual amitraz should be removed from affected animals by hosing with cold water and the animal should be treated with large volumes of lubricant by stomach tube at intervals of 12–24 hours. Oral fluids containing electrolytes should be given by stomach tube to counter dehydration and intravenous fluids may be necessary (1).

REFERENCES

(1) Roberts, M. C. and Seawright, A. A. (1979) *Aust. vet. J.*, *85*, 553.
(2) Auer, D. E. et al. (1984) *Aust. vet. J.*, *61*, 257.

Herbicides

Herbicides vary widely in their composition and also in their toxicity. Arsenicals are still widely used because of their long-term effects and the arsenic poisoning of animals which results is discussed elsewhere. Sodium chlorate is also toxic in its own right. Poisoning by the organic herbicides, including the dinitro compounds, the chlorphenoxy compounds (2, 4-D and 2, 4, 5-T) and the dipyridyl compounds (paraquat, diquat), is rare unless the animals are exposed to the concentrated chemical in its undiluted form. One of the recently recognized hazards has been the contamination of these relatively safe compounds by highly toxic ones as a result of faults in the manufacturing process. An example is the dioxins which have been found to be significant contaminants of the 2, 4, 5-T chemical. An additional problem is that some herbicides, e.g. glyphosate, make pasture that is sprayed with them more palatable, thus creating their own toxicity hazard (19).

DINITROPHENOL COMPOUNDS

Dinitrophenols find considerable use in agriculture because of their versatility as herbicides and fungicides. Animals can be poisoned accidentally by inhalation, ingestion or percutaneous absorption of these compounds which have the effect of increasing the basal metabolic rate. Poisoning is manifested by an acute onset of restlessness, sweating, deep, rapid respiration, fever and collapse. The unmetabolized chemicals cause dyspnea and hyperthermia. In ruminants but not in non-ruminants the metabolites of these compounds cause methemaglobinemia, hypoproteinemia and hemolysis. Death may occur 24–48 hours later.

Dinitrophenol (DNP) and dinitro-orthocresol (DNOC) are the commonest members of this group. In all species doses of 25–50 mg/kg body weight are usually toxic but much smaller doses produce toxicity when environmental temperatures are high. There is no accumulation of the drug within the body.

HORMONE WEED KILLERS

2, 4-D, Silvex, MCPA and 2, 4, 5-T are reputed to be non-toxic in the concentrations used on crops and pasture but dosing with 300–1000 mg/kg as a single dose, causes deaths in 50% of cattle. They have also been linked with the high prevalence of small intestinal carcinomas in sheep; the relationship is suggestive only. The picolinic acid herbicides, piclorum and clopyralid have also been suspected of the same relationship (7). The organic weedkiller Barban is toxic at doses of 25 mg/kg for cattle, 10 mg/kg body weight for sheep (4). A fatal accident is recorded in a cow receiving a dose between 150 and 188 mg/kg body weight of 2, 4-D orally. A toxic non-fatal dose to another cow was between 105 and 132 mg/kg body weight (5). Reversible toxic effects are produced with single doses of 2, 4-D in calves with doses of 200 mg/kg and in pigs with 100 mg/kg (6). Repeated administration of 50 mg/kg is toxic to pigs. In adult cows the signs of poisoning include recumbency, ruminal stasis, salivation and rapid heart rate. In calves the clinical signs are dysphagia, tympanites, anorexia and muscular weakness; in pigs there is in addition incoordination, vomiting and transient diarrhea. In very long-term experiments with pigs (500 ppm in the diet for 12 months) moderate degenerative changes in kidney and liver were produced. 2, 4-D may cause poisoning indirectly by its effect on the metabolism of weeds and sugar beets, resulting in a significant increase in the nitrate content of the leaves. A commonly used mixture of 2, 4-D, 2, 4, 5-T and a brushwood killer, monosodium methyl arsenate, is very toxic by mouth or after application to the skin; the chief clinical signs are anorexia, diarrhea, loss of weight and death in most cases. Repeated dosing of sheep with Silvex causes death after dosing for about 30 days at dose rates of 150 mg/kg body weight. Single doses of 250 mg/kg body weight of other compounds used as herbicides (carbamate, triazine, propionanilide and diallylacetamide) are fatal to sheep. Repeated smaller doses of carbamate A caused marked alopecia. Acute poisoning with any of these compounds is unlikely unless large amounts are ingested accidentally (8). Paraquat causes fibrosing pneumonitis in pigs but this does not develop in sheep or cattle with doses large enough to be fatal (9). Poisoning with this substance is unlikely to occur unless it is administered accidentally or maliciously. A dose rate of 100 mg/kg body weight is uniformly fatal in pigs with signs of vomiting, diarrhea and dyspnea (10). Accidental poisoning of sheep due to contamination of pasture by diquat has caused widespread illness manifested principally by diarrhea and a significant mortality (11). In cattle accidental poisoning with diquat has caused fatal abomasitis and enteritis, hepatic and myocardial degeneration and pulmonary emphysema (12). The herbicide triallate causes severe illness and some deaths with single oral doses of 300 mg/kg body weight to sheep and 800 mg/kg to pigs. Salivation, bradycardia, vomiting, muscular weakness, dyspnea, tremor and convulsions are followed by death in 2–3 days (12, 13). The organic herbicide is also toxic when given in small amounts continuously (14). The triazine herbicides atrazine and prometone appear to be non-toxic at natural levels of ingestion (15). Accidental poisoning of sheep with atrazine causes paralysis, exophthalmos, grinding of the teeth, diarrhea, dyspnea and tachycardia (2). Accidental poisoning of cattle causes slobbering, tenesmus, stiff gait, weakness (23). Experimental dosing of heifers with large doses of atrazine causes fatal poisoning, but animals treated with activated charcoal survive (21). Simazine and aminonitrazole in combination have caused death in sheep and horses allowed access to pasture which had been sprayed with the mixture (16). In sheep the signs were staggering, inappetence and depression. In horses colic was the important feature. Triclopyr, a selective postemergence herbicide, is toxic to horses at five times the estimated maximum intake from herbage. It causes digestive and respiratory signs, ataxia, stiff gait, sometimes tremor (22).

SODIUM CHLORATE

This substance is still widely used as a weed killer and constitutes a potential hazard to grazing stock. Animals seldom ingest sufficient sprayed plant material to produce clinical illness and the principal danger is from accidental dosing or permitting salt-hungry cattle to have access to the chemical.

The lethal oral dose is 2–2·5 g/kg body weight for sheep, 0·5 g/kg for cattle and 3·5 g/kg for dogs. Irritation of the alimentary tract causes diarrhea and deep, black erosions of the abomasal and duodenal mucosae. Hemoglobinuria, anemia and methemoglobinemia result and somnolence and dyspnea are characteristic. At necropsy the blood, muscles and viscera are very dark (20). No specific treatment is available. Sodium thiosulfate and methylene blue appear to have little effect on the course of the disease but copious blood transfusions have been recommended.

DELRAD

Delrad is an algaecide used to control the growth of algae on ponds and other water reservoirs. Cattle and sheep are unharmed by the ingestion of water containing 100 ppm of the compound. Dose rates of 250 g/kg body weight in adult cattle, 150 mg/kg in calves and 500 mg/kg sheep cause toxic effects.

DEFOLIANTS

Substances used to remove the leaves from plants used for harvesting seed may represent a toxic hazard if the residual stalks are fed to livestock. Monochloroacetate (SMCA) is commonly used for this purpose and although it is unlikely to cause poisoning unless very large quantities of the stalks are fed, animals which gain access to recently sprayed fields may be seriously affected. Toxic signs in cattle include diarrhea, colic, muscular tremor, stiff gait, ataxia and dyspnea (17). Terminally there may be convulsions, hyperexcitability and aggressiveness. The course is short, most animals dying within a few hours. Sheep have also been killed by this compound. An organophosphorous compound, tributyl phosphorotrithioite, used as a defoliant for cotton plants, produces typical signs of organophosphorous poisoning (18). *Thidiazuron*, a cotton defoliant, appears not to be toxic for animals, but may enter the human food chain, at least via goat's milk and chicken eggs (3).

REVIEW LITERATURE

McIntosh, I. G. (1967) Herbicides and their toxicity to livestock. *NZ vet. J.*, *15*, 70.

Osweiler, G. D. (1979) Diagnosis and management of bovine chemical toxicoses. *Bov. Practnr*, *14*, 155.

REFERENCES

(1) Froslie, A. (1974) *Acta vet. Scand.*, Suppl. *49*, 61.
(2) Simon, P. & Kharalampier, P. (1984) *Vet. Sbirka*, *82*, 43.
(3) Benezet, H. J. et al. (1978) *J. agric. Food Chem.*, *26*, 622.
(4) Palmer, J. S. (1972) *J. Am. vet. med. Assoc.*, *160*, 338.
(5) McLennan, M. W. (1974) *Aust. vet. J.*, *50*, 578.
(6) Bjorklund, N. E. & Erne, K. (1966) *Acta vet. Scand.*, *7*, 364.
(7) Ross, A. D. (1986) *Aust. adv. vet. Sci.*, 152.
(8) Palmer, J. S. (1964) *J. Am. vet. med. Assoc.*, *145*, 787, 917.
(9) Smalley, H. E. & Radeleff, R. D. (1970) *Toxicol. appl. Pharmacol.*, *17*, 305.
(10) Rogers, P. A. M. et al. (1973) *Vet. Rec.*, *93*, 144.
(11) Schulz, O. et al. (1976) *Mh VetMed.*, *31*, 647.
(12) Jopek, Z. et al. (1980) *Medycyna wet.*, *36*, 479.
(13) Verkovskii, A. P. (1972) *Veterinariya, Moscow*, *6*, 97.
(14) Palmer, J.S. et al. (1972) *Am. J. vet. Res.*, *33*, 543.
(15) Johnson, A. E. et al. (1972) *Am. J. vet. Res.*, *33*, 1433.
(16) Egyed, M. N. & Shlosberg, A. (1977) *Vet. hum. Toxicol.*, *19*, 83.
(17) Quick, M. P. et al. (1983) *Vet. Rec.*, *113*, 155.
(18) Palmer, J. S. & Schlinke, J. C. (1973) *J. Am. vet. med. Assoc.*, *163*, 1172.
(19) Kisseberth, W. C. et al. (1986) *Am. J. vet. Res.*, *47*, 696.
(20) Ganiere, J. P. et al. (1981) *Rev. med. Vet.*, *132*, 127, 131.
(21) Kobel, W. et al. (1985) *Vet. hum. Toxicol.*, *27*, 185.
(22) Osweiler, G. D. (1984) *Proc. Ann. Mtg Am. Assoc. vet. Lab. Diagnost.*, *26*, 193.
(23) Jowett, L. H. et al. (1986) *Vet. hum. Toxicol.*, *28*, 539.

FUNGICIDES

Zinc ethylene dithiocarbonate (Zineb) may cause thyroid hyperplasia and degeneration of myocardium and skeletal muscle (1). See also the poisons listed under the heading of seed dressings.

REFERENCE

(1) Guarda, F. et al. (1985) *Wien. Tierarztl. Monatsschr.*, *72*, 161.

Rodenticides

The commonly used rodenticides are sodium fluoroacetate, alphanaphthyltiourea (ANTU), warfarin (3-acetonylbenzyl)-4-hydroxycoumarin) and zinc phosphide. They are all toxic to domestic animals and may cause deaths when ingested accidentally.

SODIUM FLUOROACETATE

Fluoroacetate occurs naturally in some plants, and in the form of 1080 is used as a rodenticide in agriculture. Its mode of action is by inhibition of the enzyme aconitase, thus blocking the intracellular energy cycle. The operative chemical compound is fluorocitrate, to which fluoroacetate must be converted before exerting a toxic effect. A search for substances which interfere with this conversion has as yet not provided an effective antidote. (7).

Two actions are manifest, myocardial depression with ventricular fibrillation, and stimulation of the central nervous system producing convulsions. In sheep the predominant effect with acute poisoning is on myocardium; in dogs it is the nervous system. In herbivora there is sudden death, the animals being found dead without evidence of a struggle, or there are tetanic convulsions and acute heart failure with the animals showing weakness and dyspnea accompanied by cardiac arrhythmia, a weak pulse and electrocardiographic evidence of ventricular fibrillation. In sheep with subacute poisoning the signs are similar but are not apparent when the animal is at rest. When they are disturbed the nervous signs of tremor and convulsions appear but disappear when the sheep lies down (8).

Pigs manifest the nervous form of the disease, including hyperexcitability and violent tetanic convulsions. In all cases there is a period of delay of up to 2 hours after ingestion before signs appear. A dose rate of 0·3 mg/kg body weight seems to have been established as a toxic dose level for domestic species and 0·4 mg/kg is lethal for sheep and cattle (3). Sublethal doses may be cumulative if given at sufficiently short intervals. The fluoroacetate ion is present in sufficient quantities in the leaves of the gidgee tree and the plant *Gastrolobium grandiflorum* to cause poisoning of livestock. Poisoning by these plants is discussed under their headings. The use of 1080 (fluoroacetate) as a bait poses something of a hazard for grazing farm animals because it is usually spread out across fields with cereals, carrots or bread which are attractive to ruminants.

ALPHANAPHTYLTHIOUREA (ANTU)

Horses, pigs, calves and dogs are susceptible as well as rats. Tolerance develops after the ingestion of sublethal doses. Death occurs within 24–48 hours after ingestion due to marked pleural effusion, pulmonary edema, and to a less extent pericardial effusion. The toxic dose rate is of the order of 20–40 mg/kg body weight in a single dose.

'VALOR' (N-3-PYRIDYL METHYL N^1-P-NITROPHENYL UREA)

Poisoning of horses with this rodenticide is reported, but the product has been withdrawn from sale because of the risk to humans. Clinical signs in horses included dehydration, abdominal pain, hindlimb weakness, inappetence and a fishy smell, especially of urine (1). In the event of poisoning immediate emptying of the stomach is recommended. Nicotinamide is the complete antidote, but to be effective it must be given within 1 hour of ingestion of the poison (6).

WARFARIN

Warfarin and its related compounds, pindone and diphacinone, exert their effects by inhibiting the blood clotting mechanism. The action is the same as that of coumarin in moldy sweet clover in that it inhibits the thrombin to prothrombin complex and prevents clotting of the blood. All of these products are used by incorporating them into baits and they are in widespread use because they cause no poison shyness.

Although most deaths occur because of misuse by farmers, contamination of feedstuffs at the milling plant is not unknown and may cause death when the history of warfarin use is negative. Calves and poultry are not usually affected, most outbreaks being recorded in pigs, cats and dogs (4). Single doses, unless massive, are unlikely to cause poisoning but repeated ingestion for some days may do so. Daily doses of 0·2–0·5 mg/kg body weight are fatal to pigs in 6–12 days. In cattle dose rates of up to 200 mg/kg daily for 5 days cause 50% mortality. At a dose rate of 0·25 mg/kg for 10 days prothrombin times are depressed 20% and at 0·1–0·3 mg/kg abortions occur (5). Sudden massive hemorrhage into body cavities or brain may cause sudden death, or death may occur slowly with accompanying lameness due to hemorrhage into subcutaneous tissues. Massive or multiple hemorrhages are characteristic at necropsy. Vitamin K is the antidote and blood transfusions are also indicated in treatment. Horses are not commonly affected, but warfarin poisoning has been produced experimentally in ponies (2). The intravenous injection of a single dose of 50–75 mg/kg body weight of vitamin K_1 is suggested as an effective antidote. The prothrombin time is returned to normal in 12–24 hours after this treatment and persists at this level for as long as 96 hours.

Another derivative of warfarin, coumatetralyl, has been introduced to overcome the problem of resistance to warfarin which has developed in some rodent populations. It has about the same level of toxicity as warfarin but the signs produced are rather more specific. In pigs it causes lameness, swelling of the legs and hemorrhage. Vitamin K is an effective antidote. It is rather more hazardous for domestic animals than the original warfarin because it can be used in a concentrated form by laying it across rodent tracks; the rodents lick it from their paws. Brodifacoum is also a dicoumarol derivative being used for rodent control. It is recommended that it be not used where food-producing animals could have access to it because of fear of contaminating their meat (9). It is potent and acts over a long period. It is detectable in liver up to 128 days after intake.

RED SQUILLS

Poisoning by red squills seldom occurs because the material is extremely unpalatable and when eaten is usually vomited (5). In all species large doses (100–500 mg/kg body weight) must be administered to produce toxic effects. Young calves are most susceptible and goats least. Experimental poisoning causes convulsions, gastritis and bradycardia.

ZINC PHOSPHIDE

Zinc phosphide is also unpalatable to domestic animals (4), and requires an acid stomach to release its toxic phosgene gas. It is not therefore a likely poison for ruminants, but could be a hazard for pigs and horses. Experimental poisoning with doses of about 40 mg/kg body weight causes death in most species. A general toxemia with depression of appetite, dullness and some increase in respiratory rate occurs but there are no diagnostic signs. Necropsy lesions include congestion and hemorrhages in all organs, fatty degeneration of the liver and inflammation in the small intestine. Chemical assay is necessary to establish a diagnosis.

REFERENCES

(1) Russell, S. H. et al. (1978) *J. Am. vet. med. Assoc.*, *172*, 270.
(2) Scott, E. A. et al. (1978) *Am. J. vet. Res.*, *39*, 1888.
(3) Robison, W. H. (1970) *J. Wildlife Mgmt*, *34*, 647.
(4) Ashworth, B. (1973) *Vet. Rec.*, *93*, 50.
(5) Pugh, D. M. (1968) *Br. J. Pharmacol. Chemotherap.* *33*, 210P.
(6) Peoples, S. A. & Maddy, K. T. (1979) *Vet. hum. Toxicol.*, *21*, 266.
(7) Buck, W. B. (1978) *Vet. Med. SAC*, *73*, 810.
(8) Schultz, A. et al. (1982) *Onderstepoort J. vet. Res.*, *49*, 237.
(9) Laas, F. J. et al. (1985) *NZ J. agric. Res.*, *28*, 357.

Molluscicides

METALDEHYDE

Metaldehyde is in common use as a molluscicide in domestic gardens and because it is usually dispensed in a bran base and is toxic to animals it represents a poisoning hazard to farm livestock. Clinical signs include incoordination, hyperesthesia, muscle tremor, salivation, dyspnea, diarrhea, partial blindness, unconsciousness, cyanosis and death due to respiratory failure. All the signs are exacerbated by excitement or activity, and a mortality rate of 3% may be expected. Hyperthermia with temperatures up to 43·5°C (110°F) have been observed in sheep (1). Outbreaks of poisoning have been observed in cattle, horses and sheep, and experimental cases have been produced in a donkey and a goat (2).

In cattle a dose rate as low as 0·2 g/kg body weight in adults, and less in calves, can be lethal (3). The only effective treatment is likely to be rumenotomy, supplemented by sedation. In horses a dose rate of 0·1 g/kg body weight has been lethal (4). Signs are similar to those in cattle, plus heavy perspiration, hypersalivation and muscle fasciculation, and death in 3–5 hours. A tranquilizer, sedative or muscle relaxant is usually given. In horses, mineral oil by stomach tube is recommended to delay further absorption of the metaldehyde (5).

REFERENCES

(1) Simmons, J. R. & Scott, W. A. (1974) *Vet. Rec.*, *95*, 211.
(2) Egyed, M. N. & Brisk, Y. L. (1966) *Vet. Rec.*, *78*, 753.
(3) Stubbings, P. D. et al. (1976) *Vet. Rec.*, *98*, 356.
(4) Harris, W. F. (1975) *Mod. vet. Pract.*, *56*, 336.
(5) Miller, R. M. (1972) *Vet. Med. small Anim. Clin.*, *67*, 1141.

METHIOCARB

This is a carbamate molluscicide which has anticholinesterase and nicotinic and muscarinic activities. Poisoning of sheep causes depression, hypersalivation, diarrhea, dyspnea, aimless wandering and ataxia. Death is due to pulmonary edema (1, 3). A poisoned horse showed sweating, dribbling, muscle tremor, hypersalivation and finally recumbency and death due to pulmonary edema (2). The compound is usually in pellet form and dyed blue so that affected animals can be detected by the blue staining of their mouths. Atropine is an effective antidote but may be required to be repeated if the amount of bait taken is large.

REFERENCES

(1) Giles, C. J. et al. (1984) *Vet. Rec.*, *114*, 642.
(2) Edwards, H. G. (1986) *Vet. Rec.*, *119*, 556.
(3) Ogilvie, T. W. B. (1986) *Vet. Rec.*, *119*, 407.

Wood preservatives

Phenolic compounds

Lumber used in the construction of barns, stables, pens and yards is often treated with wood preservatives, chiefly pentachlorophenol, dinitro-orthophenols, dinitro-orthocresols (DNOC), dinitrophenol, and coal tar creosote, or mixtures of these, and animals which have access to freshly treated material or the neat preservative may be poisoned. A high mortality may be encountered in newborn pigs and there may be a greater than normal incidence of stillbirths when sows are farrowed in treated crates. Weaned pigs may show depression, skin irritation and occasionally death. The toxic cresols may be imbibed orally or absorbed percutaneously and contact with freshly treated wood may cause local cutaneous necrosis (1). Coal tar sealers for concrete floors may cause similar phenolic poisoning (4). Acute fatal doses in all species are in the range of 120–140 mg/kg body weight for pentachlorophenol and chronic fatal doses range from 30 to 50 mg/kg body weight. Fatal doses for coal tar creosote are 4–6 g/kg body weight as a single dose and 0·5 g/kg body weight daily (2). Creosote, applied as a treatment for ringworm, has shown marked toxic effects in cattle (3).

Besides the known toxic effects of these chemicals there has been a great deal of interest in possible subclinical intoxications in animals housed in barns made of treated lumber. There is a lack of definitive evidence on the subject (5) but calves fed pentachlorophenol daily for 6 weeks showed no toxic signs at a daily dose rate of 1 mg/kg body weight. At 10 mg/kg body weight there was anorexia and loss of body weight. The necropsy lesions were equivocal (6).

Copper–chrome–arsenate

Softwood preserved against rot by the application of a patented mixture containing copper, chromate and arsenic, has become very popular for use in yards and buildings used by livestock. The materials have been carefully tested to ensure that there is virtually no risk of poisoning. It is recorded that animals would need to eat at least 28 g of the treated wood daily for a month before a chronic poisoning occurred (7). Horses that have the chewing habit could eat more than that and could theoretically become poisoned.

REFERENCES

(1) Schipper, I. A. et al. (1964) *N. Dak. Farm. Res.*, *23*, 4.
(2) Harrison, D. L. (1959) *NZ vet. J.*, *7*, 89, 94.
(3) Blandford, T. B. et al. (1968) *Vet. Rec.*, *82*, 323.

(4) Hunneman, W. A. (1979) *Tijdschr. Diergeenskd.*, *104*, 322.
(5) Osweiler, G. D. et al. (1984) *Am. J. vet. Res.*, *45*, 244.
(6) Hughes, B. J. et. al. (1985) *J. anim. Sci.*, *61*, 1587.
(7) Bick, J. (1975) *Vet. Rec.*, *96*, 187.

Seed dressings

There is an increasing number of poisoning incidents caused by livestock gaining access to seed which has been dressed in some way. Some of the more common ones are listed below, but each is dealt with under the heading of the toxic agent.

- Grain treated with *arsenic* used to poison birds
- Grain treated with highly toxic *organophosphorous* substances used to make baits for market garden pests
- Bran mixed with *metaldehyde* as a bait for snails
- Grain to be used as seed which has been treated with a *mercurial* fungistatic agent.

Additional poisonous substances are bird repellants, grain fumigants and fungistatic agents.

Bird repellants
Baits of corn or wheat are mixed with various substances and spread over areas to protect them from damage by bird droppings or to avoid damage to aircraft. One of these bird repellants, 4-aminopyridine, has caused poisoning in horses which ate grain treated with it. Clinical signs include signs of fright, profuse sweating, severe convulsions, fluttering of the third eyelid and death 2 hours after the onset of signs and 6–8 hours after ingesting the material (1). In cattle the signs of poisoning include anorexia, frequent passage of small amounts of feces, and tenesmus with some animals also showing tremor, ataxia, erratic behavior, especially walking backwards, and some sudden deaths (5).

Grain fumigants
There is an increasing number of disease incidents, usually in cattle, in which grain treated by a fumigant to control weevils, is fed out to animals. One such substance is dibromoethane which has caused mortality in sheep to which it was fed (2). The principal damage caused is in the lungs which show pulmonary edema, septal fibrosis and alveolar epithelialization. Pleural effusion may also be present. Death occurs 48–120 hours after exposure to the poison. Methyl bromide, described under soil fumigants, is also used for stored grain.

Fungistatic agents
Hexachlorobenzene (HCB) is widely known because of its indestructibility and capacity to pass from grain through cattle and into humans. Legislation against chlorinated hydrocarbons being found in the human food chain is very harsh and hexachlorobenzene is a prime target for public health veterinarians. Its specific toxicity is not high, although experimental poisoning has been carried out with pigs (3, 4). At large doses, hepatic injury is produced.

REFERENCES

(1) Ray, A. C. et al. (1978) *Am. J. vet. Res.*, *39*, 329.
(2) Badman, R. T. (1979) *Aust. Adv. vet. Sci.*, p.54.
(3) Tonkelaar, E. M. et al. (1978) *Toxicol. appl. Pharmacol.*, *43*, 137.
(4) Hansen, L. G. et al. (1979) *Toxicol. appl. Pharmacol.*, *51*, 1.
(5) Nicholson, S. S. & Prejean, C. J. (1981) *J. Am. vet. med. Assoc.*, *178*, 1277.

Additives in feeds

Many substances including antibiotics, fungistatics, vermicides, estrogens, arsenicals, urea, iodinated casein and copper salts are added to prepared feed mixes to improve food utilization and hasten growth and fattening. Many of these substances may be toxic if improperly used. The toxic effects of arsanilic acid are described under arsenic poisoning (p. 1250). Copper sulfate has recently been introduced as an additive to rations for pigs and feeding of the treated material for long periods to cattle has caused chronic copper poisoning.

IODINATED CASEIN

Iodinated casein has been used as a feed additive to increase milk production in dairy cows but its use is not without risk, particularly in hot weather. The feeding of 20 g per day for 6 weeks has caused illness in dairy cows, although the milk yield is significantly increased in the early stages. Clinical signs of toxicity include abnormality of cardiac rhythm, high respiratory rate, nervousness, digestive disorders and scouring.

ESTROGENIC SUBSTANCES

Improvement in fattening and weight gains occurs when estrogenic substances are fed to growing animals or injected in a repository form. Toxicity occurs with overdosage and has been observed in animals grazing particular pasture plants including lucerne, subterranean clover, red clover and ladino clover, and in some cases mixed pasture and green forage crops in which the estrogen-rich plants have not been identified. The estrogenic activity of individual plant species is discussed under each of them. Small quantities of estrogens are also present in rye-grasses during the spring. White clover does not usually contain detectable amounts but plants heavily infested with fungi may contain significant amounts (5). Estrogens may also be present in large amounts in moldy corn and produce toxic effects when fed to pigs. An outbreak of poisoning in pigs has been recorded in which the source was probably hexestrol implants in capon necks fed to the pigs. Cattle treated orally or by subcutaneous implants with estrogenic substances pass significant amounts in the feces, especially when the substance is fed and there is one record of abortions in heifers fed on ensilage contaminated by the manure of steers fed hexestrol. In all these circumstances the clinical findings and necropsy lesions are referable to the urogenital system.

Standard recommendations are for the feeding of 510 mg of stilbestrol daily to fattening cattle of 180–270 kg body weight. The feeding of up to 20 mg/day to cattle has no visible effect on the reproductive tract. Larger doses of stilbestrol to cattle may cause prolapse of the rectum and vagina with relaxation of the pelvic ligaments, elevation of the tail-head and susceptibility to fracture of the pelvic bones and dislocation of the hip.

Nymphomaniac behavior in such animals invites skeletal injury.

Heavy mortalities have occurred in feeder lambs after the use of 12 mg implants of estrogens. Prolapse of the rectum, vagina and uterus occurred together with urethral obstruction. In another outbreak 20% of 300 feedlot wethers died within 35 days of implantation with pellets containing 30 mg of stilbestrol whereas none of 150 control wethers was affected. In these outbreaks the calculi consisted largely of desquamated epithelial and pus cells which formed a nidus for the deposition of mineral, the desquamation probably being stimulated by the estrogen. The possibility also exists that partial urethral obstruction caused by the estrogen facilitated complete obstruction by the calculi.

The daily feeding of 0·75 mg/kg body weight of stilbestrol has also caused poisoning in pigs; clinical signs included straining, prolapse of the rectum, incontinence of urine, anuria and death. At necropsy there was inflammation and necrosis of the rectal wall, enlargement of the kidneys, thickening of the ureters and distension of the bladder, and gross enlargement of the prostate and seminal vesicles.

A number of specific pasture plants may contain large amounts of estrogenic substances but increased estrogenic activity has also been observed in mixed pasture. This activity may be apparent only at certain times and is often restricted to particular fields. Clinically the effects are those of sterility, some abortions, swelling of the udder and vulva in pregnant animals and in virgin heifers, and endometritis with a slimy, purulent vaginal discharge in some animals. Estrus cycles are irregular. In milking cows there is depression of the milk yield, reduction in appetite and an increase in the cell count of the milk.

UREA

Urea has been introduced as a feed additive for ruminants to provide a cheap protein substitute. It is also used as a fertilizer on crop and pasture fields, and accidental access to the powder or liquid form of the compound can cause severe mortalities (2, 9). Poisoning occurs when cattle or sheep accidentally gain access to large quantities of urea, or are fed large quantities when they are unaccustomed to it, or when feeds are improperly mixed. Some care is required in bringing the animals on to urea gradually and an adequate proportion of carbohydrate must be included in the ration. The toxic effects are due to the sudden production of large quantities of ammonia and signs occur within 20–30 minutes of feeding. Absorption of the ammonia in the forestomachs results in the very rapid onset of signs (3). The severity of signs is related to blood ammonia levels and not to levels of ammonia in the rumen. The rapidity with which the ammonia is released in the rumen may be increased if soybean meal is being fed—soya beans contain urease which facilitates the breakdown of urea to ammonia. Other ammonia-rich materials are by products of industrial products and are attractive as sources of nitrogen for lot feeding of ruminants. Some of these have been tested and can in general be expected to perform in the same way as urea. One of them, diureido isobutane (DUIB) has been determined to have this effect (4).

Toxic dose levels vary, but in cattle which have been starved beforehand dose levels up to 0·33 g/kg body weight cause increases in blood levels of ammonia and dose levels of 0·44 g/kg body weight produce signs of poisoning within 10 minutes of dosing (11) and dose rates of 1–1·5 g/kg body weight cause death. Animals unaccustomed to urea may show clinical illness when fed 20 g/50 kg body weight, but by gradually increasing the quantity fed this amount can be tolerated. This tolerance is lost rapidly and animals which receive no urea for 3 days are again susceptible. Tolerance is also reduced by starvation and by a low protein diet. Sheep can eat 6% of their total ration as urea provided it is well mixed with roughage and fed throughout the day, preferably by spraying the urea mixed with molasses onto the roughage. Much more urea is tolerated if given to sheep in molasses (18 g), than if given as a drench (8 g) and prior feeding on lucerne further increases the tolerance and fasting for 24 hours reduces it. A dose rate of 1 g/kg body weight to sheep appears to be non-toxic but 2 g/kg is quickly fatal (53). In general, urea should not constitute more than 3% of the concentrate ration of ruminants. Horses appear to be tolerant to relatively large doses of urea but the disease has been produced experimentally in ponies by administering 450 g by stomach tube. The clinical picture is similar to that in cattle, being largely related to the central nervous system (12). There is a sharp increase in blood ammonia levels after ingestion of the urea and it is assumed that hydrolysis of the urea occurs in the cecum. Pigs are quite unaffected by very large doses of urea (29) unless they are deprived of water or have developed a cecal flora which produces urease.

Clinical signs of toxicity in cattle include severe abdominal pain, muscle tremor, incoordination, weakness, dyspnea, bloat, and violent struggling and bellowing. The course is short and death occurs about 4 hours after ingestion. The death rate in affected animals is high. There are no characteristic lesions at necropsy, but most cases show generalized congestion and hemorrhages and pulmonary edema. Death is thought to result from respiratory arrest due to ammonia intoxication (1). Clinical signs of toxicity appear in cattle when blood ammonia nitrogen concentrations reach 0·7–0·8 mg/100 ml (14). In sheep deaths occur at levels of ammonia nitrogen of 33 μg/ml of blood (15). The ruminal contents are alkaline when tested with litmus paper (pH elevated from 6·94 to 7·90) and ruminal ammonia levels rise from 6 to 50 mg/100 ml (14). Clinical signs in sheep are identical with those in cattle (14).

Treatment is unlikely to be effective but the oral administration of a weak acid such as vinegar (0·5–1 liter to a sheep, 4 liters to a cow) may reduce the amount of ammonia absorbed. The administration of 5% acetic acid is recommended as an antidote but it must be administered as soon as the first clinical signs appear and repeated dosings may be necessary as clinical signs tend to recur about 30 minutes after treatment (11). The only really effective treatment is prompt and efficient emptying of the rumen, either via a large bore tube or by rumenotomy (16). Encephalomalacia has been produced in pigs by feeding a ration containing 15% urea (38). The clinical picture and histopathological findings were similar to those of salt poisoning except that no eosinophilic aggregations were present in the cerebral lesions.

PROPYLENE GLYCOL

Propylene glycol is an unlikely poison but it is used extensively in veterinary practice and can cause poisoning if it is accidentally administered to horses. Dose rates of 3 liters to horses of 500 kg by stomach tube can cause severe ataxia, depression and a fetid odor of the feces. Much larger doses (8 liters) can be fatal. Moderate to severe inflammation of the lining of the gut and edema of the brain are noticeable at necropsy examination (18).

DRIED POULTRY WASTES

Feeding dried poultry wastes to ruminants provides them with a source of nitrogen, and gets rid of the chicken farmer's disposal problem. There are problems, dealt with elsewhere, when the chickens are fed on diets supplemented with copper. High levels of phosphorus are also found in the waste. In addition, a problem arises of hepatic necrosis, hypoalbuminemia and ascites in lambs fed large amounts of poultry waste from hen batteries. This problem is not observed with broiler waste, but renal damage does ensue. There is also a great deal of variation in toxicity between different groups of chickens (7). Botulism can also be a serious problem with chicken wastes.

CHEMICALLY TREATED NATURAL FEEDS

Formalin treated grain
This is a special diet fed to dairy cows to produce dairy products containing an increased proportion of polyunsaturated fats for special human diets. Fats in the grain are protected against hydrogenation in the rumen by coating the grains with formalin. If the formalin and the grain are not properly mixed, the free formalin left as a residue causes rumenitis and severe diarrhea.

Caustic treated grain
Grain treated with caustic to improve its digestibility is recorded as causing focal interstitial nephritis, rumenitis and abomasal ulceration in feedlot steers. The lesions were detected at slaughter and may have little clinical effect if the feeding is of short duration (8).

Ammoniated forage
Anhydrous ammonia is added to hay to improve its digestibility and nitrogen content. If the forage is high quality and has a high carbohydrate content it may undergo chemical change, possibly with the formation of a substituted imidazole, which causes hysteria in the cattle eating it (6). The clinical signs include hyperexcitability, circling and convulsions. Tremor, commencing at the head, and opisthotonus were obvious early signs. Between convulsions affected sheep walk in circles and have a stiff gait. Calves sucking cows fed ammoniated hay may also be affected by this same syndrome (46).

NEWSPRINT

Newsprint is being fed commercially to ruminants as an alternative roughage. Toxicological hazards of the material have been examined (10). In sheep fed colored magazines for 6 months and comprising 23% of their ration, there was a significant deposition of lead in tissues, an increase in enzyme activity in liver, but there were no clinical signs and no histopathological lesions (10).

PYREXIA—PRURITUS—HEMORRHAGIC SYNDROME OF DAIRY COWS (POSSIBLE 'SYLADE' POISONING)

Very large numbers of cows are fed on ensilage made with the assistance of 'Sylade', a combination of formalin and sulfuric acid, and there are only a few records of the 'pruritus–pyrexia–hemorrhage' syndrome in dairy cattle. So the suggestion that the disease is caused by 'Sylade', if it is correct, must include the intervention of other physical characteristics or substances in the environment (28). The disease was recorded in the United Kingdom first in 1977, but there have been a number of serious outbreaks since then (30–32).

Clinical signs of the disease include pruritus, hair loss, papular dermatitis, variable appetite with roughage being taken, fever up to 40·5°C (104·5°F), petechiation on conjunctiva and visible mucosae. The dermatitis is widespread, exudative, initially papular, and itching. It occurs principally on the head, neck, perineum and udder. There is an accompanying fever (40–41·5°C; 104–106·7°F). Pruritus is variable in degree, but is often so marked that rubbing causes the affected skin to become raw and bleeding. The dermatitis subsides but the fever persists, and over a period of 4–7 weeks the animal becomes so unthrifty that it is usually sent for slaughter. The morbidity rate is usually 10%, but may be as high as 100%. Seriously affected animals die (32). A similar but more severe syndrome occurs in which there is petechiation in all tissues especially subserosally (33, 34). In these cases there are multiple hemorrhages in all mucosae and free blood at the anus and other orifices.

Necropsy examination shows petechiation in all organs and tissues, although they are absent altogether in some cases. Histological findings include low-grade, longstanding interstitial nephritis and very little else of significance. Hematology, blood chemistry and serum enzymes are similarly normal. Antibody reactivity to some components of ruminal contents may be elevated, but not apparently significantly.

The cause is still undetermined, but the epidemiology of a variable number of cows being affected simultaneously in a number of herds in the same locality suggests that a chemical intoxicant is the cause. Diureidoesobutane (DUIB) poisoning (35) and poisoning by the hairy vetch (*Vicia villosa*) (36) have been suggested, but silage made with the adjuvant 'Sylade' appears to be the most likely prospect at the moment (30). However, none of the proposed agents can account epidemiologically for the territorial distribution of cases. Because most cases occur in cows which are eating prepared feeds, a feed contaminant or mycotoxin are the principal possibilities.

SEWAGE SLUDGE

Urban sewage sludge is used as top-dressing for pasture and may cause spread of infectious disease as well as goiter. Sewage sludge may also be fed directly to animals, but may lead to chronic poisoning by lead and cadmium (13).

MONENSIN, LASOLOCID AND SALINOMYCIN POISONING

Monensin is an ionophore antibiotic, a monovalent cationic substance, used in agriculture principally as a coccidiostat in poultry and as a growth stimulant in cattle. Lasolocid is a chemically and pharmacologically similar compound, it is a divalent cationic substance, and is dealt with in the same way as monensin (25). Another monovalent ionophore antibiotic similar to monensin is salinomycin used a a growth promotant and coccidiostat in pigs. It has similar chemical and pathological properties to monensin and lasolocid but is even more toxic for horses (50). Monensin has minor additional uses in the treatment of acetonemia, lactic acidosis, bloat and atypical interstitial pneumonia. It has a reasonable safety margin but is very poisonous if used carelessly. Its use in horses at any time is prohibited because of its toxicity for that species. Lasolocid is a chemically and pharmacologically very similar compound and is dealt with in exactly the same way as monensin (25). The recommended doses of monensin vary depending on the age and size of the livestock and the purpose for which it is administered and the manufacturer's recommendations should be adhered to strictly. Approximate levels, orally and usually in the feed, are: cattle, 50–200 mg per head per day, 16·5–33 ppm; sheep 5–10 ppm in feed (44).

The poisonous properties of the agent are well known and poisoning is usually accidental due to failure to dilute a concentrate, poor mixing or because of wrong identification of containers. Also some liquid preparations settle out and need to be constantly mixed before and during mixing with a batch of feed.

For monensin, dosage levels at which clinical signs of poisoning can be expected to occur are: cattle 10, sheep 4, pig 7·5 and horse 1 mg/kg body weight. Deaths in cattle are likely to commence at intakes of 100 mg/kg body weight and in horses at 2–3 mg/kg. Toxic feed concentrations are for pigs 200–220 mg/kg of feed. Comparative LD_{50} in mg/kg body weight are: cattle 50–80, horse 2–3, sheep 12, pig 16–50 and goat 24 (20). It is common for cattle to be poisoned with more than ten times the recommended dose (17, 26, 49). The LD_{50} for salinomycin for the horse is 0·6 mg/kg body weight (50).

The principal pathogenesis of monensin poisoning is damage to muscles. In cattle the cardiac muscle is most severely affected, in sheep the skeletal muscle is most seriously affected. In cattle, signs commence with feed refusal followed by tremor, weakness, tachycardia and ruminal atony, and animals may die at this stage from acute heart failure. Those that survive for a day or two develop congestive heart failure manifested by brisket edema, engorgement of the jugular veins, ascites, fluid feces, dyspnea and tachycardia (45). Clinical pathology tests show increases in serum levels of creatinine phosphokinase and aspartate aminotransferase and there may be myoglobinuria. At necropsy there is myocardiopathy, pulmonary edema, and enlargement of the liver and heart, hydropericardium, hydrothorax and ascites (52).

In sheep (41, 43, 51) the syndrome commences with feed refusal followed by muscle weakness, a stilted gait and recumbency. Myoglobinuria may be evident. The postmortem changes include necrosis in both skeletal and cardiac muscles but there are no signs of heart failure. Chronic cases show atrophy of the muscles of the hindquarters and a stiff gait. Neonatal lambs less than a month old show only gastrointestinal hemorrhage. Pretreatment with vitamin E–selenium reduces the effects of the poisoning without completely preventing it (40).

Poisoning of pigs causes anorexia, ataxia, paresis, myoglobinuria and cyanosis, diarrhea, tympany and puritis. Death follows in about 6 hours (20, 42). Clinical and clinicopathological changes are the same as in cattle. As in ruminants, pretreatment using vitamin E–selenium reduces some of the effects of the poisoning without completely preventing it (20).

Horses are very susceptible to poisoning by these antibiotics and great care is needed to ensure that feed contaminated by them and used for cattle is not left around for horses to eat. In horses, cardiac and skeletal muscle are affected but it is the myocardium that creates the prominent syndrome. Some horses are just found dead having suffered an acute heart attack. In most cases there is respiratory distress, diarrhea, mucosal congestion, sweating, sometimes myoglobinuria, cardiac irregularity and tachycardia (50–60 per minute) (21–23). The course of the disease is short and affected horses may not show much clinical evidence of heart failure. Clinicopathological findings include increases in serum creatinine phosphokinase, lactate dehydrogenase and aspartate aminotransferase levels (22). Horses that survive develop a poor performance syndrome or congestive heart failure up to several months later (27). Necropsy lesions in acute cases include pulmonary congestion, hepatic swelling and in some cases include pulmonary petechiation. Chronic cases show marked cardiac myopathy with obvious fibrosis. Some feeds fed to horses have contained as much as 125–250 g/tonne of feed (22, 23) and their stomach contents have contained 50–100 ppm (22).

Besides these major involvements of monensin and lasolocid there are a number of less well-known ones. There is a risk that cattle fed on a nitrogen-rich diet will be likely to suffer an outbreak of nitrite poisoning if they are also fed monensin (17, 24). There is also a shift of ruminal flora to one which is a more efficient converter of nitrate to nitrite. Another undesirable outcome may be a fall in butterfat because of shift from acetate to proprionate production in the rumen (19).

There is no effective treatment and only supportive procedures are recommended. Activated charcoal or mineral oil have been standard treatments aimed at removing the residue of the poison from the alimentary tract. They are of no value if the poison has already been absorbed; recovery is unlikely once the myocardium is affected.

Monensin–tiamulin poisoning in pigs

The mycotoxicity of monensin for pigs is enhanced by the simultaneous administration of the two antibiotics. Both of the substances are used as coccidiostats and it is not unusual for farmers to combine them. However, both agents use the same detoxication pathways in the liver with tiamulin having the priority. Monensin accumulates to the point of being toxic (24). The clinical syndrome consists of anorexia and weight loss and at necropsy there are lesions of myonecrosis in the tongue, diaphragm and limbs (39). A similar toxicological situation arises in pigs with simultaneous dosing with tiamulin and salinomycin (48).

PLURONICS POISONING

These substances are administered to adult cattle in their feed as a prevention against bloat. They are unpalatable and unlikely to be consumed in dangerous amounts unless they are well masked in feed. When they are fed accidentally to calves in their milk they cause dyspnea, ruminal tympany, bellowing, protrusion of the tongue, nystagmus, opisthotonus, recumbency and convulsions. Death after 24 hours is the usual outcome (47).

REVIEW LITERATURE

Hanson, L. J. et al. (1981) Toxic effects of lasolocid in horses. *Am. J. vet. Res.*, *42*, 456.

Langston, V. C. et al. (1985) Toxicity and therapeutics of monensin; a review. *Vet. Med.*, *80*, 75–84.

REFERENCES

(1) Itabisahi, T. (1977) *Natl Inst. Hlth Q.*, *17*, 115, 128, 130 & 151.
(2) Salam Abdullah, A. et al. (1986) *Vet. Rec.*, *119*, 407.
(3) Davidovich, A. et al. (1977) *J. anim. Sci.*, *45*, 551.
(4) Mullen, P. A. (1978) *Res. vet. Sci.*, *24*, 8.
(5) Wong, E. et al. (1971) *NZ J. agric. Res.*, *14*, 639.
(6) Johns, J. T. et al. (1984) *J. Am. vet. med. Assoc.*, *185*, 215.
(7) Suttle, N. F. et al. (1981) *J. comp. Pathol.*, *91*, 545.
(8) Nelson, J. R. (1980) *Vet. Rec.*, *107*, 139.
(9) Morris, J. G. & Payne, E. (1970) *J. agric. Sci.*, *Camb.*, *74*, 259.
(10) Helfron, C. L. et al. (1979) *Cornell Vet.*, *69*, 356.
(11) Word, J. D. et al. (1969) *J. anim Sci.*, *29*, 786.
(12) Hintz, H. F. et al. (1970) *J. Am. vet. med. Assoc.*, *157*, 693.
(13) Edds, G. T. et al. (1978) *Proc. 82nd Mtg US anim. Hlth Assoc.*, p. 207.
(14) Bargai, U. (1980) *Refuah Vet. 37*, 150.
(15) Kirkpatrick, W. C. et al. (1973) *Am. J. vet. Res.*, *34*, 587.
(16) Davidovich, A. et al. (1977) *J. anim. Sci.*, *44*, 702.
(17) Janzen, E. D. et al. (1981) *Can. vet. J.*, *22*, 92.
(18) Myers, V. S. & Usenik, E. A. (1969) *J. Am. vet. med. Assoc.*, *155*, 1841.
(19) Rogers, P. A. M. & Hope-Cawdery, M. J. (1980) *Vet. Rec.*, *106*, 311.
(20) van Vleet, J. F. et al. (1983) *Am. J. vet. Res.*, *44*, 1460, 1469.
(21) Ordidge, R. M. et al. (1979) *Vet. Rec.*, *104*, 375.
(22) Nuytten, J. L. et al. (1981) *Vlaams Diergeneeskd. Tijdschr.*, *50*, 242.
(23) Gerhards, H. et al. (1986) *Dtsch Tierärztl. Wochenschr.*, *93*, 323.
(24) Pott, J. M. & Skov, B. (1981) *Vet. Rec.*, *109*, 545.
(25) Galitzer, S. J. et al. (1982) *Vet. hum. Toxicol.*, *24*, 406.
(26) Sauvageau, R. et al. (1984) *Med. Vet. Quebec*, *14*, 170.
(27) Muylle, E. et al. (1981) *Equ. vet. J.*, *13*, 107.
(28) Holden, A. R. (1980) *Vet. Rec.*, *106*, 413.
(29) Button, C. et al. (1982) *J. S. Afr. vet. Assoc.*, *53*, 67.
(30) Thomas, G. W. (1979) *Vet. Rec. (In Practice)*, *1 (6)*, 16.
(31) Turner, S. J. et al. (1978) *Vet. Rec.*, *102*, 488.
(32) Matthews, J. G. (1978) *Vet. Rec.*, *103*, 408.
(33) Ducroz, G. & Ducroz, J. (1979) *Bull. Mens Soc. vet. Prat. France*, *63*, 709.
(34) Matthews, J. G. & Shreeve, B. J. (1978) *Vet. Rec.*, *103*, 408.
(35) Breuckink, H. J. et al. (1978) *Vet. Rec.*, *103*, 221.
(36) Panciera, R. J. et al. (1966) *J. Am. vet. med. Assoc.*, *148*, 804.
(37) Mollenhauer, H. H. et al. (1981) *Am. J. vet. Res.*, *42*, 35.
(38) Done, J. T. et al. (1959) *Vet. Rec.*, *71*, 92.
(39) Umemura, T. et al. (1985) *Vet. Pathol.*, *22*, 409.
(40) van Vleet, J. F. et al. (1985) *Am. J. vet. Res.*, *46*, 2221.
(41) Nation, P. N. et al. (1982) *Can. vet. J.*, *23*, 323.
(42) Frantova, E. et al. (1986) *Veterinarstvi*, *36*, 270.
(43) Newsholme, S. J. et al. (1983) *J. S. Afr. vet. Assoc.*, *54*, 29.
(44) Langston, V. C. et al. (1985) *Vet. Med.*, *80 (10)*, 75.
(45) Galitzer, S. J. et al. (1986) *J. anim. Sci.*, *62*, 1308.
(46) Weiss, W. P. et al. (1986) *J. anim. Sci.*, *63*, 525.
(47) Teague, W. R. (1986) *NZ vet. J.*, *34*, 104.
(48) Miller, D. J. S. et al. (1986) *Vet. Rec.*, *118*, 73.
(49) Gear, R. J. & Robinson, W. F. (1985) *Aust. vet. J.*, *62*, 130.
(50) Amstel, S. R. van & Guthrie, A. J. (1985) *Proc. 31st Ann. Conv. AAEP*, 373.
(51) Bourque, J. G. et al. (1986) *Can. vet. J.*, *27*, 397.
(52) Galitzer, S. J. et al. (1986) *Am. J. vet. Res.*, *47*, 2624.
(53) McLennan, M. W. (1987) *Aust. vet. J.*, *64*, 26.

Miscellaneous farm chemicals

POLYBROMINATED BIPHENYLS

Mixtures of polybrominated biphenyls find a great deal of use in industry, particularly as flame retardants. They are not especially poisonous, nor are they a greater risk to farm animals because of degree of exposure, than many other industrial chemicals. But they happen to have found their way into the cattle food chain in one much discussed incident in the United States (1, 2). The use of secondhand oil in back rubbers for cattle and pigs has also produced a serious poisoning incident because the oil contained high levels of polychlorinated biphenyls (PCB) (10). A naturally occurring incident due to contamination of ensilage by paint off the silo wall caused pollution of dairy products (14). Experimental dosing with 67 mg/kg body weight daily for long periods caused poisoning but levels of 9.65 mg/kg body weight were not toxic. Clinical signs of illness are anorexia, diarrhea, lacrimation, salivation, emaciation, dehydration, depression and abortion. These signs are accompanied by postmortem findings of mucoid enteritis, degenerative renal lesions, hyperkeratosis in the glands and epithelium of the eyelids. Similar signs plus extensive cutaneous hyperkeratosis were reported in naturally occurring cases (3). The principal lesion in experimental cases in cattle is renal. Large doses (e.g., 25 g daily) are required (6). Experimental poisoning in pigs caused no ill-effects in sows, but high concentrations of polybrominated biphenyls (PBB) developed in the sow's milk with death of some nursing pigs resulting (11).

Apart from the illness caused by the very large dose levels to which some animals were exposed, there were far greater losses of animals destroyed because they had become contaminated by the compounds in what has been described as the worst agricultural contamination disaster in US history (9). Much of this destruction of animals was carried out because of fear of adverse effects on humans who ate the meat, milk or eggs of the contaminated animals. Exhaustive examination of areas in which animals were exposed failed to find any evidence of illness in them after exposure to low levels of the toxins (8). Similar results were obtained after examination of people in the area (4). PCBs pass the placenta and are found in fetuses but appear to cause no health problems in the offspring (12, 13).

The excretion of these compounds occurs principally in feces and urine but as much as 25% of ingested substance may be present in the milk. Also these compounds are lipotrophic and accumulate in fat depots (5), especially in the liver. Attempts to hasten excretion have not produced a satisfactory method (7).

REFERENCES

(1) Moorhead, P. D. et al. (1977) *J. Am. vet. med. Assoc.*, *170*, 307.
(2) Mercer, H. D. et al. (1976) *J. Am. vet. med. Assoc.*, *168*, 762.
(3) Jackson, T. F. & Halbert, F. L. (1974) *J. Am vet. med. Assoc.*, *165*, 437.
(4) Dunckel, A. E. (1975) *J. Am. vet. med. Assoc.*, *167*, 838.
(5) Fries, G. F. (1978) *J. Am. vet. med. Assoc.*, *173*, 1479.
(6) Durst, H. I. et al. (1978) *J. dairy Sci.*, *61*, 197.
(7) Cook. R. M. et al. (1978) *J. dairy Sci.*, *61*, 414.
(8) Fries, G. F. et al. (1983) *J. dairy Sci.*, *66*, 1303.
(9) Sterner, E. F. (1978) *Bov. Practnr*, *13*, 111.
(10) Robens, J. & Anthony, H. D. (1980) *J. Am. vet. med. Assoc.*, *177*, 613.
(11) Werner, P. R. & Sleight, S. D. (1981) *Am. J. vet. Res.*, *42*, 183.
(12) Perry, T. W. et al. (1984) *J. dairy Sci.*, *67*, 224.
(13) Willett, L. B. et al. (1982) *J. dairy Sci.*, *65*, 81.
(14) Sorensen, N. D. (1982) *Dansk Vet Tidsskr.* *65*, 462.

POLYCHLORINATED BIPHENYLS

These substances have a number of industrial uses and are common environmental contaminants. They are lipophilic so that they accumulate in body fat, and have low rates of biotransformation and excretion so that they persist in animal tissues for long periods (1, 2). Although deleterious effects of the compounds in animal tissues are not often recorded, their presence in animal tissues is likely to cause rejection of meat from the human food chain. Recorded damage refers to unidentified reproductive inefficiency (1, 3) and reduction in efficiency of food conversion (4) and possibly hepatic hypertrophy and gastric erosion, but in the same species a positive growth stimulating effect has also been recorded (5). Experimental poisoning of gnotobiotic pigs has caused diarrhea, erythema of the nose and anus, distension of the abdomen, growth retardation and, at doses of more than 25 mg/kg body weight, coma and death. The disease is more severe than in conventional piglets (6). A naturally occurring case of poisoning is recorded in rhesus monkeys. Weight loss, alopecia and diarrhea were prominent and at necropsy the obvious lesion was hypertrophy of the glandular stomach and the colon (7).

REFERENCES

(1) Platonow, N. S. & Geissinger, H. D. (1973) *Vet. Rec.*, *93*, 287.
(2) Furr, A. K. et al. (1974) *J. Agric. Food Chem.*, *22*, 954.
(3) Hansen, L. G. et al. (1975) *Am. J. vet. Res.*, *36*, 23.
(4) Hansen, L. G. et al. (1976) *Am. J. vet. Res.*, *37*, 1021.
(5) Matthews, H. B. & Dedrick, R. (1984) *Ann. Rev. Pharmacol. Toxicol.*, *24*, 85.
(6) Miniats, O. P. et al. (1978) *Can. J. comp. Med.*, *42*, 192.
(7) Altman, N. H. et al. (1979) *Lab. anim. Sci.*, *29*, 661 & 666.

SOIL FUMIGANT: METHYL BROMIDE

Soil fumigants used to prepare fields for planting may cause toxicity hazards in animals grazing them or in feed harvested from them. Methyl bromide has caused poisoning in horses, cattle and goats when used in this way (1). Clinical signs in horses include ataxia, stumbling and somnolence to produce a drunken behavior. Cattle and goats showed similar signs.

REFERENCE

(1) Knight, H. D. & Costner, G. C. (1977) *J. Am. vet. med. Assoc.*, *171*, 446.

FORMALIN

Formalin is used to preserve colostrum for calf feeding, and in the preparation of formalin-treated grain (p. 1300). Milk containing too much formalin causes severe gastroenteritis and some deaths in calves that drink it. The clinical signs include salivation, abdominal pain, diarrhea and recumbency (1).

REFERENCE

(1) Egyed, M. N. et al. (1981) *Refuah Vet.*, *33*, 31.

OIL AND PETROLEUM PRODUCT POISONING

Crude oil or petroleum distillates, including diesel oil, lamp oil, kerosene and gasoline are all poisonous to animals. Cattle will drink all of them and appear to have a positive liking for some products, especially used sump oil and liquid paraffin (mineral oil). Gasoline up to the level of 3 ppm in the drinking water does not appear to depress water intake or to interfere with growth performance of pigs (8). Crude oil coming directly from wells is usually repellent to animals, but they can consume lethal quantities of it if they are salt-deficient and salt-hungry: a characteristic of crude oil is that it is usually mixed with salty water which represents a problem in disposal and is often left lying in ponds and pits nearby (1). Therefore, access to oilfield installations where overflow oil has accumulated, and to storage dumps where these products are accessible in open dumps, may lead to outbreaks of poisoning. When highly chlorinated naphthalenes were used as lubricants, access to oil dumps could lead to hyperkeratosis. On farms access to tractor fuel (paraffin, diesolene, kerosene) is most likely (2). Kerosene has an unwarranted reputation as a therapeutic agent for bloat and constipation, but it is unlikely to be given in amounts sufficient to cause more than slight illness, unless it is given repeatedly.

The toxicity of the various products varies. In general those with the highest content of volatile and inflammable components, especially naphtha and petrol (gasoline) fractions, are the most toxic. Of natural crude oils those with the highest content of sulfur ('sour crude') are most unpalatable and most toxic. With commercial gasoline and oily lubricants the additives used, especially lead, may also contribute significantly to the poisoning (3). Most crude oils are extracted from their subterranean locations combined with saline water, and are temporarily stored in installations where lead paint is available so that salt and lead poisoning commonly occur with oil poisoning and may be confused with it. Other toxic agents of all kinds can be encountered when reject sludge oil is available to animals. For example, a serious outbreak of fatal poisoning has been recorded in horses working out on a riding school which has been sprayed with sludge oil containing tetrachlorodibenzodioxin (4). Colic, hematuria, alopecia, dermatitis, emaciation, edema, laminitis and conjunctivitis were among the signs and diseases observed.

Most records of naturally occurring cases are of cattle (10) being poisoned, but sheep (5) and goats (9) can also be affected. Accurate dose levels are difficult to determine in field outbreaks. In experimental trials crude oil at the rate of 37 ml/kg body weight in a single dose or 123 ml/kg in five divided daily doses were poisonous to cattle. Kerosene at 20 ml/kg body weight as a single dose and 62 ml/kg body weight in five equal daily doses was poisonous (6). Tractor paraffin (kerosene) at a single dose rate of 13 ml/kg body weight caused severe illness and at 21 ml/kg was fatal to cattle (2).

In naturally occurring cases the clinical signs are not accurately recorded. When large volumes of crude oil are consumed (1, 7) there are signs of toxemia and incoordination, regurgitation (vomiting) may or may not occur, and death occurs quickly. Bloating is inconstant. In the terminal stages the pupils are dilated, the heart and respiratory rates are increased and the temperature elevated. The animals smell of oil, and oil is often present on the skin around the mouth and anus, and in the feces. The feces vary from constipation to diarrhea. Recovered animals often do poorly after the incident. The oil persists in the alimentary tract for very long periods and may be found in the cud and feces, and at postmortem as long as 16 days after ingestion (2). In naturally occurring cases in goats dullness, pneumonia and nervous signs are prominent (9).

In experimentally produced cases the early signs which occurred soon after dosing included incoordination, shivering, head-shaking and mental confusion. Within 24 hours anorexia, vomiting and moderate to severe bloating occurred (6). The early signs are thought to be due to regurgitation of the oil, aspiration of it to cause aspiration pneumonia, and absorption of the volatile components through the pulmonary mucosa. The later signs are thought to be caused by the direct effect of the oil on the alimentary tract. Animals that survive the acute toxic syndrome eat poorly, lose weight and die at variable periods from 16 to 36 days later. Oil appears at the anus on about the 8th day after administration. It may also appear in the nasal discharge, reaching there via the lungs. The vomitus always contains the oil. The feces are usually oily, often soft to semifluid, and frequently black if the oil taken has been crude oil. With kerosene the feces are often dry and firm in the later stages and the regurgitus may be in the form of gelatin-like cuds, smelling strongly of kerosene.

There are no specific clinicopathological findings but hypoglycemia, acetonemia and transient hypomagnesemia are all recorded.

At necropsy examination the important lesion in poisoning with crude oil or kerosene is aspiration pneumonia. It is recorded constantly in naturally occurring and experimentally produced cases. How it develops is not sure but it is thought to be the result of vomiting and aspiration from the alimentary tract of already swallowed oil. There is thought to be a relationship between the ability of the oil to cause bloat and vomiting, and therefore aspiration, and its overall toxicity (6). Oil is always still present in the alimentary tract and there may be thickening and inflammation of the alimentary mucosa. Degenerative changes in liver and kidney are recorded in some cases (2).

No particular form of treatment has been recommended but if the animal has survived the initial acute phase the replacement of the ruminal contents with material from a normal rumen suggests itself as a rational treatment.

REFERENCES

(1) Monlux, A. W. et al. (1971) *J. Am. vet. med. Assoc.*, *158*, 1379.
(2) Parker, W. H. (1951) *Vet. Rec.*, *63*, 430.
(3) Winkler, J. K. & Gibbons, W. J. (1973) *Mod. vet. Pract.*, *54*, 45.
(4) Carter, C. D. et al. (1975) *Science, NY*, *188*, 738.
(5) Ranger, S. F. (1976) *Vet. Rec.*, *99*, 508.
(6) Rowe, L. D. et al. (1973) *J. Am. vet. med. Assoc.*, *162*, 61.
(7) McConnell, W. C. (1957) *Vet. Med.*, *52*, 159.
(8) Mitchell, L. H. et al. (1978) *Can. vet. J.*, *19*, 10.
(9) Toofanian, F. et al. (1979) *Trop. anim. Hlth Prod.*, *11*, 98.
(10) Meadows, D. L. & Walter-Toews, D. (1979) *Vet. Med. SAC*, *75*, 545.

TIN POISONING

Dibutyl tin dilaurate is a coccidiostat fed to chickens in their feed. Errors in mixing may lead to cattle receiving toxic amounts in concentrates or pellets (1, 2). Calves usually die acutely with signs of tremors, convulsions, weakness and diarrhea. Older animals usually suffer a chronic illness characterized by persistent diarrhea, severe weight loss, inappetence, polyuria and depression. The syndrome is reminiscent of arsenic poisoning. Affected animals may not be suitable for human consumption because of the high content of tin in their tissues.

REFERENCES

(1) Mayer, E. et al. (1978) *Refuah Vet.*, *35*, 83.
(2) Shlosberg, A. & Egyed, M. N. (1979) *Vet. hum. Toxicol.*, *21*, 1.

SODIUM FLUOROSILICATE

Sodium fluorosilicate is a white, odorless and tasteless powder used as a poison in baits for crickets, grasshoppers and the like. Because of the way it is prepared in pellets in a bran base it is attractive to all animal species and the disease is recorded in cattle, sheep and horses. The disease is likely to occur unless care is taken to retrieve unused baits after a baiting program. In sheep mild illness occurs after doses of 25–50 mg/kg body weight and death after 200 mg/kg.

Clinical signs include drowsiness, anorexia, constipation, ruminal stasis, abdominal pain and diarrhea. Bradycardia is recorded in horses and grinding of the teeth in sheep (1).

REFERENCE

(1) Egyed, M. N. & Shlosberg, A. (1975) *Fluoride*, *8*, 134.

POISONING BY HIGHLY CHLORINATED NAPHTHALENES

The local application or ingestion of highly chlorinated naphthalenes to cattle produces a disease characterized by thickening and scaliness of the skin, due to hyperkeratosis, emaciation and eventual death (1). The toxic compounds interfere with the conversion of carotene to vitamin A and, in effect, cause hypovitaminosis A. The naphthalenes were extensively used in industry as lubricants, insulants and wood-preserving agents. Recognition of their toxicity has resulted in their exclusion from the farm environment and virtual elimination of the disease. Occasional outbreaks are still recorded (2, 3). When poisoning results from accidental emission from industrial plants there are additional signs due to ocular, nasal and tracheobronchial irritation. Infertility and abortion also occur (3).

REFERENCES

(1) Olson, C. (1968) *Adv. vet. Sci.*, *13*, 101.
(2) Bohosiewicz, M. & Houska, M. (1973) *Med. wet.*, *29*, 610.
(3) Fleckinger, R. et al. (1976) *Bull. Acad. vet., France*, *49*, 459.

COAL TAR PITCH POISONING

Pigs may be exposed to coal tar pitch and its toxic cresols when housed in pens with tarred walls or floors, or when they have access to 'clay pigeons' used as targets by gun clubs (1). Bitumen and asphalt appear to be non-toxic. Affected pigs nibble the tarred material in pens or ingest fragments of the 'clay pigeons' at pasture. Young pigs 6–20 weeks of age are most commonly affected and the incidence in this group may be as high as 20%. Clinically there may be an acute illness or the disease may run a chronic course of some weeks. In the acute illness there are non-specific signs of inappetence, rough coat, tucked-up abdomen, weakness and depression. The chronic illness is characterized by anorexia, depression, weakness, anemia and jaundice, and pigs affected subclinically may manifest only a reduction in growth rate of up to 20–30% (2). A severe reduction in hemoglobin concentration and erythrocyte count is detectable on examination of the blood. Vitamin A storage is also reduced.

At necropsy there may be jaundice, ascites and anemia but the characteristic finding is a red and yellow mottling of the hepatic surfaces. On histological examination there is severe centrilobular necrosis of the liver and the necrotic zones are suffused with blood (3, 4). Cresols can be detected in the ingesta and liver of affected pigs.

REFERENCES

(1) Graham, R. et al. (1940) *J. Am. vet. med. Assoc.*, *96*, 135.
(2) Maclean, C. W. (1969) *Vet. Rec.*, *84*, 594.
(3) Libke, K. G. & Davis, J. W. (1967) *J. Am. vet. med. Assoc.*, *151*, 426.
(4) Davis, J. W. & Libke, K. G. (1968) *J. Am. vet. med. Assoc.*, *152*, 382.

METHYL ALCOHOL

Accidental ingestion of methyl alcohol by cattle has caused vomiting, recumbency and death. A high concentration of methyl alcohol was present in the ruminal contents. Methyl alcohol is used as an antifreeze in gasoline engines for pumps working continuously on oilfields in cold regions. Accidental access to the pump enclosure may result in a poisoning incident (1).

REFERENCE

(1) Rousseaux, C. R. (1982) *Can. vet. J.*, *23*, 252.

ETHYLENE GLYCOL

Accidental poisoning with antifreeze mixture containing ethylene glycol may occur in swine (1) and calves (2). The pathogenesis of the disease is dependent upon the development of an oxalate nephrosis. In *pigs* this is manifested by ascites, hydrothorax and hydropericardium, depression, weakness and posterior paralysis. In *cattle* there is dyspnea, incoordination, paraparesis, recumbency and death. There is accompanying uremia and hypocalcemia. Calcium oxalate crystals are present in large numbers in the kidney and brain and there is a fatal nephrosis (2). The toxic dose rates determined experimentally for cattle are 5–10 ml/kg body weight in adults and 2 ml/kg in non-ruminant calves (2).

REFERENCES

(1) Osweiler, G. D. et al. (1972) *J. Am. vet. med. Assoc.*, *160*, 746.
(2) Crowell, W. A. et al. (1979) *Cornell Vet.*, *69*, 272.

POISONING BY INDUSTRIAL ORGANOPHOSPHATES

Organophosphatic compounds are used industrially, as well as for anthelmintics and insecticides. Their principal uses are as fire-resistant hydraulic fluids, as lubricants and as coolants. A number of compounds including tri-*o*-tolyl phosphate (1), tri-*o*-cresyl phosphate (TOCP) (2) and triaryl phosphates (TAP) (3) have come to veterinary notice as causes of poisoning in animals. Triaryl phosphates contain a number of isomers as well as TOCP, e.g. *m*-cresol, *p*-cresol, *o*-cresol, all of them more poisonous than TOCP (5). They have also caused serious outbreaks of poisoning in humans when they accidentally contaminate food. Poisoning may occur by ingestion or cutaneous absorption. Clinical signs do not occur until several weeks after contact and comprise irreversible neurological signs of knuckling, leg weakness and posterior paralysis. Characteristic lesions are present in the spinal cord and peripheral nerves (4). The lesions are characteristic of the neurotoxicosis discussed under insecticides.

REFERENCES

(1) Kruckenberg, S. M. et al. (1973) *Am. J. vet. Res.*, *34*, 403.
(2) Julian, R. J. & Galt, D. E. (1966) *J. Am. vet. med. Assoc.*, *168*, 248.
(3) Sanders, D. E. et al. (1985) *Cornell Vet.*, *75*, 493.
(4) Soliman, S. A. et al. (1983) *Toxicol. appl. Pharmacol.*, *69*, 417.
(5) Sugden, E. A. (1981) *Can. vet. J.*, *22*, 211.

SUPERPHOSPHATE

This customary form of applying phosphorus-rich fertilizers to the soil is available to animals on most farms in many countries with phosphorus-deficient soils. The product is not highly palatable but sheep will eat it when it is in pill form; it resembles grain in texture and particle size. The fertilizer is also used to prepare 'superjuice' which is administered to cows as a phosphorus supplement. Overdosing will cause poisoning, due largely to the fluorine present; the phosphate seems unlikely to play more than a contributory role (1).

The LD_{50} of superphosphate for sheep is 100–300 mg/kg body weight. Clinical signs of poisoning include anorexia, thirst, diarrhea, weakness and ataxia. Death follows in about 48 hours (2) and is due to uremia caused by tubular nephrosis, possibly the result of fluorine poisoning (1).

REFERENCES

(1) O'Hara, P. J. et al. (1982) *NZ vet. J.*, *30*, 199.
(2) O'Hara, P. J. & Cordes, D. O. (1982) *NZ vet. J.*, *30*, 153.

MANURE GAS POISONING

Confinement housing of cattle and swine has resulted in the concentrated production of manure and its storage for varying periods of time in large holding pits, usually under slatted floors (1, 2). Oxygen from the air is excluded from manure stored within a confinement unit and under such conditions, anaerobic bacteria degrade the organic and inorganic constituents of manure yielding hydrogen sulfide, ammonia, methane and carbon dioxide as major gases. When diluted with water to facilitate handling, liquid manure in storage separates by gravity. The solid wastes form a sediment, the lightweight particles float to the top leaving a middle layer which is relatively fluid. Thorough remixing is necessary before pits are emptied to prevent the fluid fraction from flowing out and the solids remaining. The remixing or agitation results in the release of large quantities of toxic gases from the slurry. The exposure of man or cattle and swine to high concentrations of manure gases, particularly hydrogen sulfide, can be rapidly fatal. Exposure and inhalation of hydrogen sulfide in concentrations above 700 ppm may be rapidly fatal in man. Peracute deaths usually occur in cattle and swine which are lying directly over slatted floors over manure storage pits which are being agitated and emptied in barns which are usually inadequately ventilated. Necropsy of cattle which have died from acute hydrogen sulfide poisoning reveals pulmonary edema, extensive hemorrhage in muscles and viscera and bilaterally symmetrical cerebral edema and necrosis (7).

There is insufficient information available on the effects on livestock of sublethal concentrations of hydrogen sulfide over varying lenghts of time. Chronic exposure to low levels of hydrogen sulfide is thought to be associated with reduced performance in cattle and swine. However, it is often difficult to differentiate from other causes of suboptimal performance. Two diseases of the limbs, a necrosis of the outer claw, and a local cellulitis with fever are also ascribed to manure gas poisoning (6), but seem more likely to arise because of trauma from a rough floor surface.

High concentration of ammonia (100–200 ppm) will cause conjunctivitis, sneezing and coughing for a few days but pigs will commonly acclimatize after which no effects may be detectable. An increased incidence of pneumonia and reduced daily weight gains in pigs are associated with exposure to a combination of ammonia at levels of 50–100 ppm and the presence of atmospheric dust in barns (3).

The production of hydrogen sulfide in manure can be inhibited by aeration using air as the oxidizing agent or the use of chemical oxidizing agents (4). The use of ferrous salts virtually eliminates hydrogen sulfide evolution (5).

Adequate ventilation with all doors and windows wide open during remixing and agitation of the slurry will reduce the concentration of hydrogen sulfide to nontoxic levels. Animals and personnel should not enter closed barns when the pits are being emptied.

REFERENCES

(1) Nordstrom, G. A. & McQuitty, J. B. (1976) *Manure Gases in the Environment. A Literature Review (with Particular Reference to Cattle Housing)*. Dept. of Agricultural Engineering, Faculty of Agriculture & Forestry, Univ. of Alberta, Edmonton, Canada.
(2) Barber, E. M. & McQuitty, J. B. (1971) *Hydrogen Sulfide Evaluation from Anaerobic Swine Manure*. Dept. of Agricultural Engineering, Faculty of Agriculture & Forestry, Univ. of Alberta, Edmonton, Canada.
(3) Doig, R. A. & Willoughby, R. A. (1971) *J. Am. vet. med. Assoc.*, *159*, 1353.
(4) Barber, E. M. & Mcquitty, J. B. (1975) *Can. agric. Engin.*, *17*, 90.
(5) Barber, E. M. & McQuitty, J. B. (1977) *Can. agric. Engin.*, *19*, 15.
(6) Simensen, E. & Grandahl, J. (1977) *Norsk VetTidsskr.*, *89*, 541.
(7) Dahme, E. et al. (1983) *Dtsch Tierärztl. Wochenschr.*, *90*, 316.

POISONING BY ALGAE

Many green or blue-green algae (water bloom), including *Microcystis* spp. (syn. *Anacystis cyanea*), *Anabaena circinalis* (1), *A. spiroides* (5), *Aphanizomenin*, *Gloeatrichia*, *Coelosphaerium* and *Oscillatoria* sp. (8) and *Nodularia spemengioma* (2), contain toxic substances but outbreaks of poisoning in farm animals are uncommon, occurring chiefly on lakes when the algae are concentrated by onshore winds so that large quantities may be ingested by animals while drinking, and on dams, ponds and waterholes which may be completely covered. Smaller animals who drink near the edge of the lake get more toxin because it is concentrated in the superficial layers at the edge (3). The disease has been recorded in the United States, Canada, Norway, South Africa, Australia and New Zealand and affects all animals and birds. In New South Wales the algae occur seasonally in most dams in the area but deaths do not necessarily occur, especially if animals are able to avoid large concentrations. Heavy growth occurs in the late summer to autumn period. Factors which increase the chances of animals being poisoned include high water temperature, especially sunny weather when the water is very shallow, high electrolyte concentration as a result of massive water loss by evaporation, and a high concentration of other nutrients such as nitrogen, caused by animals defecating and urinating in the water. All of these factors promote algal growth and increase the concentration of toxic materials in the water. In small waterholes, dams and dugouts the surface water is often completely covered with a very thick coat of gelatinous algae, and animals are unable to drink without ingesting some of it. The period of toxicity of a water supply is often very brief, and if there is suspicion of it water samples for examination need to be collected at the earliest opportunity. Laboratory examination for the presence of high concentrations of known toxic algae is required. Not many laboratories are equipped to carry out the examination, and a negative result should be treated with caution, especially as there may be as yet unidentified algae species. The toxins in a variety of algae species appear to be the same or similar.

The toxic effects of algae vary widely depending on the strains of algae present, the types of bacteria growing in association with the algae, the conditions of growth, accumulation and decomposition and the amounts of toxic material consumed. Two distinct forms of toxicity occur, a fast death and a slow death. *Microcystis* spp. is the most common algae and the most toxic, and is unusual in that it secretes an exotoxin. Previously, it was thought bacteria associated with the algae produced substances capable of causing gastroenteritis and hepatitis—the slow-death factor (7). However, it has been demonstrated that the experimental administration of large doses of toxin from *Microcystis aeruginosa* to sheep (4), causes sudden death and the repeated administration of the same toxin in small doses causes toxipathic hepatopathy (9)—the slow-death syndrome. The fast-death factor secreted by *Anabaena flos-aquae* has also been shown to cause a postsynaptic neuromuscular blockade and death by respiratory arrest (6). Clinical signs may become apparent within 30 minutes after exposure. In acute cases the affected animals show muscle tremor, stupor, staggering, recumbency, and in some cases hyperesthesia to touch so that slight stimulation provokes a convulsion with opisthotonus. Abdominal pain, diarrhea and dyspnea are additional signs. After experimental dosing death may occur within a few minutes of the first appearance of clinical signs but in field cases the course may be prolonged for several hours. Necropsy lesions which occur in animals that die suddenly include massive hepatic necrosis, generalized petechiation, plasma transudates in body cavities and congestion of most viscera (4).

In the chronic form of the disease there is severe liver damage accompanied by jaundice and photosensitization in cattle and sheep. Severe gastroenteritis with intestinal hemorrhage has also been observed in some outbreaks. The photosensitization is caused by the presence of a photodynamic pigment, phyocyan, the excretion of which is retarded by the liver damage.

The intravenous injection of a mixture of sodium nitrite and sodium thiosulfate as recommended for cyanide poisoning is credited with curative properties. Excessive growth of algae is favored by the presence of large quantities of organic matter in the water and by hot weather. Algal growth can be controlled by the use of copper sulfate or other algaecides such as Delrad.

REFERENCES

(1) McBarron, E. J. et al. (1975) *Aust. vet. J.*, *51*, 587.
(2) Main, D. C. et al. (1977) *Aust. vet. J.*, *53*, 578.
(3) Hammer, C. T. (1968) *Can. vet. J.*, *9*, 221.
(4) Jackson, A. R. B. et al. (1984) *Vet. Pathol.*, *21*, 102.
(5) Simon, J. et al. (1983) *J. Am. vet. med. Assoc.*, *182*, 413.
(6) Codd, G. A. (1983) *Vet. Rec.*, *113*, 223.
(7) Flint, E. A. (1966) *NZ vet. J.*, *14*, 181.
(8) Berg, K. & Soli, N. E. (1985) *Nord. VetMed.*, *26*, 363.
(9) Elleman, T. C. et al. (1978) *Aust. J. biol. Sci.*, *31*, 209.

POISONING BY FUNGI (MYCOTOXICOSIS)

The importance of fungi as poisonous agents has been appreciated for many years but it is only recently that the scope and magnitude of the losses that they cause have become apparent. Partly this has come about because of the greater accuracy of definition of other diseases with which mycotoxicoses have been confused. There has also been a significant improvement in the investigational effort used to identify fungi. One of the problems that remains is the experimental production of these diseases. In the absence of evidence produced by such experiments the relationship between the fungi and specific cases of naturally occurring disease must continue to remain speculative.

One of the problems confronting the experimental toxicologist is that the cultivation of fungi in large quantities is difficult and it seems that on many occasions the fungi become poisonous because of their conditions of growth, especially the composition of the substrate on which they are growing. In general fungi require warm, moist conditions to prosper but they are also individually very demanding with respect to their environmental requirements for optimum growth, so that fungal overgrowth is likely to occur suddenly and dramatically when their critical needs are satisfied. It is not possible to predict when this will happen by simply sniffing the wind; instrumental measurement is essential. It is usually simpler to monitor the yield of spores obtained from a given area or volume of the substrate. However, there is a need to know the growth requirements of each fungus if any attempt is to be made to restrain its growth in agricultural materials (1).

Another current problem in mycotoxicology is that of providing authoritative evidence when litigation arises out of a suspected poisoning incident. There is a great lack of laboratory tests for identification of the actual toxins in feed. Even if the fungi can be demonstrated this is only circumstantial evidence that the toxins are there also.

Molds grow on any stored feeds, the highest incidence being on feeds with high moisture content. Thus a common fungal poisoning is on moldy corn or maize, which is a high moisture grain and difficult to harvest or store at the correct stage of maturity and moisture content. A degree of spoilage must be expected in corn grain with a moisture content in excess of 20%. The frequent occurrence of fungal growth on stored feeds ensures that mycotoxicoses occur more commonly in housed animals and in those confined to zero grazing in dry lots.

Molds also grow on standing plants, especially seed heads. Examples are ergots on rye and paspalum, and *Phomopsis* sp. on lupins. Growth on green foliage is much less likely, but herbivores can ingest toxic amounts of soil fungi, e.g. *Penicillium* sp., and fungi which grow on plant litter, e.g. *Pithomyces chartarum* is a fungus which does this. An increasing number of poisonings previously thought to be due to plants are turning out to be mycotoxic. A recent example is myrotheciotoxicosis on kikuyu grass.

Many of the molds on feeds are non-toxic, many are toxic only at certain times and many have an as yet undetermined status. Many syndromes generally considered to be caused by fungal toxins, e.g. the hemorrhagic diathesis which occurs on feeding moldy lespedeza hay (2), corn grain (3), hay, chaff and bedding, have no recognized specific mycotoxic origin. On the other hand, there are some well-identified organ specificities. These include aflatoxin affecting the liver, ochratoxin and citrinin causing renal disease, ergotamine and zearalenone affecting uterus, and tremorgens affecting the nervous system. There is also the relatively unexplored area of subclinical disease in which animals exposed to moldy feeds suffer a reduction in productivity without showing overt clinical signs (8).

Much of the research work on mycotoxicoses relates to the effects of poisoning by pure cultures or even by their separated toxins. In practice, many poisonings arise as a result of multiple infections in the feed being fed; for example, sorghum stems infected with *Aspergillus flavus, A. ochraceus, A. niger, Penicillium citrinum, Curvularia lunta, Botryodiplodia theobromae* contained the toxins aflatoxin, citrinin, ochratoxin and penicillic acid (9). Such combinations of poisonings make for great difficulty in clinical and pathological recognition (4).

The important and immediate problem is the prevention of mycotoxicoses. Suggested techniques include careful surveillance of all stored feeds for evidence of fungal infestation. Feed that is dusty or showing obvious, usually patchy, discoloration should be examined with a strong magnifying glass. This should be sufficient to identify spores and hyphae. Infested or suspicious feeds should be discarded or diluted to at the most 10% with undamaged feeds, and preferably fed to a sample, pilot group of animals. Lactating, pregnant and growing animals are most likely to be seriously affected and these are best avoided.

The principal part of the losses caused by mycotoxins has probably not yet been revealed. Only the acute and common chronic syndromes are known, and these are the only ones dealt with here. They are summarized in Table 97. The subclinical diseases and most of the chronic ones await definition and represent a major task. One of the major fields of investigation in mycotoxicoses which has yet to be explored is the development of techniques and protocols for effectively, but cheaply, monitoring the contamination of feedstuffs used by animals and man. Much attention is now being directed to this phase of mycotoxicology, because of the known carcinogenicity of some fungal toxins (5). Most methods of examination of feedstuffs made to determine the presence of mycotoxins are chromatographic analyses. Mycological techniques and methods of using animals to measure toxicity have also been described (6, 7).

An additional cause for concern in animal mycotoxicoses is the possibility that the toxins will 'carry over' into the milk or other animal products used as human food (2). This fear applies to all toxins, but is understandably greater with carcinogens. With the possible exception of aflatoxin in cows' milk, there is no identified occurrence of such human mycotoxicoses. Experimental administration of toxin T_2 in large doses has resulted in detectable toxin in cows' milk, but at levels not considered to be dangerous for man (3).

Because of the rate of occurrence of contamination of feedstuffs by mycotoxins, and because of the enormous industry involved in the handling and processing of grain, the problem of monitoring food for these toxins is very complex. Part of the surveillance strategy must include knowing the grains industry and where in the processing opportunities for mold growth occur (5). One other aspect of the problem is the possibility of treating poisonous grain commercially so as to render it non-toxic. The treatment of grain containing aflatoxin with ammonia shows promise.

The invasion of tissues by fungi is dealt with in Chapter 24.

REVIEW LITERATURE

Harwig, J. & Munro, I. C. (1975) Mycotoxins of possible importance in diseases of Canadian farm animals. *Can. vet. J.*, *16*, 125.

Lynch, G. P. (1972) Mycotoxicosis in feedstuffs and their effects on dairy cattle. *J. dairy Sci.*, *5*, 1243.

Morehouse, L. G. (1979) Mycotoxicosis of the bovine. *Bov. Practnr*, *14*, 175.

Pier, A. C. (1981) Mycotoxins and animal health. *Adv. vet. Sci.*, *25*, 185–243.

Shreeve, B. J. & Patterson, D. S. P. (1975) Investigation of suspected causes of mycotoxicoses in farm animals in Britain. *Vet. Rec.*, *97*, 275 & 279.

USA Nat. Res. Ccl. (1979) Interactions of mycotoxins in animal production. *Proc. of a Symposium, July 13, 1978, Michigan State Univ., Natl Acad. Sci., Washington, DC.*

Wyllie, T. D. & Morehouse, L. G. (1977) *Mycotoxicoses of Domestic and Laboratory Animals, Poultry and Aquatic Invertebrates and Vertebrates*, vol. 2. New York: Marcel Dekker.

REFERENCES

(1) Lillehoj, E. B. (1973) *J. Am. vet. med. Assoc.*, *163*, 1281.
(2) Shreeve, B. J. et al. (1979) *Food Cosmetic Toxicol.*, *17*, 151.
(3) Robinson, T. S. et al. (1979) *J. dairy Sci.*, *62*, 637.
(4) Tapia, M. O. & Seawright, A. A. (1985) *Aust. vet. J.*, *62*, 33.
(5) Wessel, J. R. & Stoloff, L. (1973) *J. Am. vet. med. Assoc.*, *163*, 1284.
(6) Shreeve, B. J. & Patterson, D. S. P. (1975) *Vet. Rec.*, *97*, 275.
(7) Prior, M. G. (1976) *Can. J. comp. Med.*, *40*, 75.
(8) Marrassis, W. F. O. & Smalley, E. B. (1972) *Onderstepoort J. vet. Res.*, *39*, 1.
(9) Manickam, A. et al. (1985) *Ind. vet. J.*, *62*, 711.

Table 97. Common mycotoxicoses in farm animals.

Disease	*Clinical syndrome*	*Pathogenesis*	*Animal species affected*	*Causative fungus*	*Causative toxin*	*Substrate*
Aflatoxicosis	Drop in milk production, jaundice, nervous signs of blindness, circling, falling, convulsions	Hepatotoxicosis, also carcinogenic, teratogenic and immune suppressant	Cattle, pigs	*Aspergillus flavus*	Aflatoxin	Stored grain, ground nuts
Facial eczema	Photosensitization	Hepatotoxicosis (cholangiohepatitis)	Sheep, occasionally cattle	*Pithomyces chartarum*	Sporidesmin	Pasture litter
Rubratoxin poisoning	Hepatotoxicosis and hemorrhages	Hepatotoxicosis and hemorrhagic diatheses	Cattle	*Penicillium rubrum* and *P. purpurogenum*	Not identified	Stored feeds
Lupinosis	Drop in milk production, jaundice, nervous signs of hepatopathy	Hepatotoxicosis	Cattle, sheep, pigs	*Phomopsis leptostromiformis*	Not identified	Standing mature lupins
Moldy corn disease	Necrotic lesions and hemorrhages skin, mouth intestines, liver, kidneys. In pigs vomition and food refusal	Hemorrhage and necrosis of epithelium	Cattle	*Fusarium tricinctum* and other *Fusarium* spp.	T_2 toxin (tricothecenes)	Stored grain usually corn (maize)
Stachybotry-toxicosis	Thrombocytopenic purpura stomatitis, hemorrhagic enteritis, death	Bone marrow depression, immuno-suppression	Horses, cattle	*Stachybotrys alternans*	Satratoxins B and H	Hay, straw
Myrotheciotoxicosis	Hemorrhages in gut especially abomasum; hepatitis, pulmonary congestion	General tissue damage	Calves, sheep	*Myrothecium roridum* etc.	Not identified	Standing grasses, clovers and stored feeds
Slaframine toxicosis	Excessive salivation, lacrimation, bloat, urination, defecation	Not known	Cattle	*Rhizoctonia leguminicola*	Slaframine, swainsonine	Red clover hay
Mycotic nephropathy or ochratoxicosis	Polydipsia, polyuria, enlarged kidneys	Nephrosis	Pig	*Penicillium virodicatum (Aspergillus ochraceus)*	Ochratoxin A and citrinin and viomellen	Stored feeds
Interstitial pneumonia	Respiratory distress	Lesions similar to atypical interstitial pneumonia	Cattle	*Fusarium solani*	Ipomeanols	Sweet potatoes
Ergotism (reproductive disease)	Reduced fertility, agalactica	Uterine tonicity changes	Pig, sheep	*Claviceps purpurea*	Ergot alkaloids	Rye and other stored grains. Standing rye-grass pasture
Fusaritoxicosis (1).	Enlarged mammae, vulva, prepuce, splayleg piglets. Infertility (anestrus), neonatal deaths	Estrogenic disease	Pig (possibly cattle, sheep)	*Fusarium graminareum (F. roseum)*	Zearalenone (or F_2 toxin)	Maize or barley grain

Table 97. (Cont.)

Disease	*Clinical syndrome*	*Pathogenesis*	*Animal species affected*	*Causative fungus*	*Causative toxin*	*Substrate*
Fusaritoxicosis (2)	No syndrome	Leukopenia	Sheep	*Fusarium* spp.	T_2 toxin	Grain
Fusaritoxicosis (3)	Congenital skin defect	Teratogenic	Pig	*Fusarium* spp.	T_2 toxin	Grain
Fusaritoxicosis (4)	Food refusal	Not known	Pig	*Fusarium moniliforme*	*Deoxynivalenol*	Grain
Tremorgen intoxication	Tremor, ataxia, muscular rigidity, convulsions	Functional muscle tremor	Cattle, sheep, pigs	*Acremonium lolii*	Lolitrems ABC and D	Stored feeds or while grazing on *Lolium perenne*
Leukoencephalo-malacia	Tremor, ataxia, circling, depressed consciousness, recumbency, death	Encephalopathy—brain abscess (possibly hepatitis)	Horse and donkey	*Fusarium moniliforme*	Not identified	Maize corn
Ergotism (nervous form)	Convulsions	Vascular spasm nervous system	Sheep	*Claviceps purpurea*	Ergot alkaloids	Rye and other grains, rye-grass
Paspalum ergot poisoning	Cerebellar ataxia; recovery on removal from pasture	Functional nervous disability	Cattle, sheep, horse	*Claviceps paspali*	Not identified	Standing paspalum or water-couch or dallas grass
Ergotism (skin form)	Skin gangrene ear tips, tail tip, coronet	Peripheral vascular spasm	Cattle	*Claviceps purpurea*	Ergot alkaloids	Rye and other grains, rye-grass
Fescue foot	Skin gangrene feet	Peripheral vascular spasm	Cattle	*Epichloe typhina* or *Acremonium coenophialum* (syn. *Sphacelia typhina*)	Ioline	Standing tall fescue grass or hay, or seed
Diplodiosis	Lacrimation, salivation, tremor, ataxia, paralysis	Not known	Cattle, sheep, goats, horses	*Diplodia maydis*	Unidentified neurotoxin	Prolonged growth on maize

POISONING BY *FUSARIUM* SPP.

Fusarium spp. fungi produce a variety of toxins which are capable of producing a great variety of diseases. The principal ones are dealt with below. The toxins include an estrogenic substance, zearalenone (syn. F_2), toxin T_2, diacetoxyscirpenol (syn. DAS) (the latter two are both trichothecenes), deoxynivalenol (syn. vomitoxin), and ipomeanols capable of causing acute interstitial pneumonia of cattle. The T_2 toxin is a cause of leukopenia and thymic involution and of reduced blood coagulability (25).

Vulvovaginitis of swine (estrogenism, zearalenone poisoning)

Fusarium roseum (***F. graminearum, Gibberella zea***) growing on moldy maize or barley grain produces estrogenic substances, especially one identified as F_2, or zearalenone (1). *F. **culmorum*** growing on oat herbage also produces much zearolenone but not when growing on perennial rye grass (9, 34). Ingestion of the infected grain causes a number of syndromes. The severest one occurs in pigs and is identified as vulvovaginitis (3), but the main presenting sign may be infertility including absence of estrus (4), high levels of stillbirth, neonatal mortality and reduced litter size (6). Small fetal size, fetal malformations, pseudopregnancy and constant estrus are also recorded (9). The newborn piglets may have splayleg and hindlimb paresis. In cattle, the effect is largely on conception rate and the rate of services per conception may rise but the overall effect is very small (3). Estrogenic disturbances are also suspected in sheep (8). Abortion is suspected to result and mild vulvovaginitis and hypertrophy of the uterus are recorded (8). The T_2 toxin given experimentally to pigs causes small litters, repeat breeders (16) and abortion (21).

The classical clinical picture in vulvovaginitis includes tumefaction of the vulva, enlargement of mammary glands and increased size and weight of uterus (3). The syndrome is indistinguishable from that produced by long-term overdosing with diethyl stilbestrol. Signs appear 3–6 days after feeding of the moldy grain commences and disappears soon after the feeding stops. The basic lesion is an engorgement of the genital mucosa. Pigs of all ages including sucklings may be affected but the worst are gilts 6–7 months old. The vulva is swollen to three to four times normal size and the lips are edematous and congested. These abnormalities extend only as far as the external urethral opening but on autopsy examination the ovaries and uterine horns can be observed to be enlarged (10). There may be a thin catarrhal exudate from the vulva and moderate enlargement of the mammary glands. Prolapse of the vagina occurs commonly (up to 30% of affected pigs) and prolapse of the rectum in some (5–10%). In males there may be enlargement of the prepuce and enlargement of erythema of the rudimentary teats and mammary glands. Symmetrical enlargement of the mammary glands is recorded in prepubertal dairy heifers feeding on fungus-infected corn (19). Experimental feeding of zearalenone to boars had some depressing effect subsequently on libido but all structural parameters, such as testicular size, were unaffected (30).

All female pigs exposed to the moldy feed are likely to be clinically affected, and the mortality rate is high due to the secondary development of cystitis, uremia, and septicemia. At high doses the zearalenone is passed through the milk of sows in sufficient dose rates to produce clinical signs of vulvar enlargement in the sucking pigs (5). At other dose rates neither effect has been produced (7). Young swine will refuse rations containing the toxin. Experimental feeding of zearalenone to lactating cows and ewes does result in minor contamination of their milk sufficient to produce hyperestrogenism in a lamb sucking a poisoned ewe (17). In small pigs it causes degenerative changes in seminiferous tissue (20).

Leukoencephalomalacia in horses and other neurotoxic syndromes

The commonest clinical entity in this group is leukoencephalomalacia, a febrile, non-infectious disease of horses and donkeys (23) caused by the ingestion of moldy corn grain. The significant fungus is *Fusarium moniliforme* (syn. *F. verticilloides*) and the disease has been produced experimentally by dosing with cultures of the fungus (12). It seems likely that the same fungus can cause hepatosis and leukoencephalomalacia, and that the outcome may depend on the size of the dose, and the frequency of dosing with toxin, the more acute syndrome being the hepatic one. The fungus is commonly found growing on moldy corn grain that has been affected by rain while on the stalk or which has been stored wet. The disease also occurs in horses fed commercial, including pelleted, feeds (27); some large-scale outbreaks are reported (11). No specific toxin has been isolated.

Clinically the disease is manifested by muscle tremor and weakness, staggering, circling, inability to swallow, and marked depression of consciousness. Jaundice may occur in some cases. Death occurs after a course of 48–72 hours. At necropsy there are macroscopic areas of softening accompanied by hemorrhages in the white matter of the cerebral hemisphere.

This fungus has also caused deaths due to pulmonary edema when fed to sheep, and nephrosis and hepatosis when fed to pigs (28).

Alimentary tract syndromes: vomiting, mucosal lesions

F. roseum produces toxins associated with emesis and refusal of feed (13) and toxins lethal to pigs (14) as well as estrogenic substances. *F. culmorum* also causes inappetence, scouring, ataxia and a fall in milk yield when fed to cattle. *F. sporotrichiella* can cause hemorrhagic enteritis and death in 24 hours, or up to 5 days later in less severe cases. The toxin which produces this syndrome is deoxynivalenol, but other agents may also be involved (2).

However, the most important disease in this group is the one caused by *F. tricinctum*, a fungus common on ear corn. It produces a potent toxin (diacetoxyscirpenol) which causes necrotic lesions and hemorrhages in the skin, mouth, intestine, liver and kidneys (18). In pigs the experimental disease is manifested by hemorrhagic bowel lesions, but the toxin also produces a syndrome including emesis, lethargy, hunger, frequent defecation of normal stools and posterior paresis (16). The clinical syndrome includes mucosal hemorrhages and erosions, intermittent salivation, and depression. The stomatitis is characteristic and needs to be differentiated from similar lesions caused by viruses. Continued exposure to the fungus can cause heavy mortalities in cattle (18). The potent T_2 toxin produced by the fungus may cause generalized hemorrhages, but experimental administration of the purified toxin parenterally produces a quite different range of signs including emesis, posterior paresis, lethargy, hunger and frequent defecation of normal stools (21). Other experimental evidence is that the oral administration of the T_2 toxin or cultures containing it to piglets and calves causes no hemorrhagic disease (15). Field evidence of the relationship between the ingestion of the fungus and the appearance of hemorrhagic disease is strong, but the identity of the specific toxic agent may be in doubt.

Necropsy findings are limited to engorgement of the genitalia, and vaginal prolapse and its complications. Assay of the feed for estrogenic activity by feeding it to laboratory animals may be attempted. A high incidence of rectal and vaginal prolapse is also recorded in pigs fed stilbestrol as a feed additive. Outbreaks of rectal prolapse, without vaginal prolapse, occur in swine with diarrheic diseases.

Complete recovery follows when the feeding of the affected grain is stopped and no treatment other than surgical repair of the prolapsed organs is attempted.

Congenital defect T_2 toxin has been cited as the probable cause of congenital skin defects about the head and tarsus of pigs (33).

Immunosuppression T_2 toxin is known to produce immunosuppression when fed to laboratory animals but no identified disease is recorded in farm animals as being caused by it. Experimental feeding to sheep causes leukopenia and lymphopenia, and atrophy of lymph nodes and spleen (29) but the immunosuppression is minor (31).

Food refusal The fungus *Fusarium moniliforme* causes this syndrome in cattle (24). It is also recorded with zearalenone and with deoxynivalenol poisoning (26) in pigs although the latter appears not to affect cattle (32) or lambs (36). Feed consumption in pigs is reduced by 15–17% (34) and vomiting occurs if sufficient vomitoxin is eaten (35).

Respiratory tract disease

Isolates of *Fusarium solani* have been reported to cause a disease identical to atypical interstitial pneumonia of cattle and is discussed under that heading.

REFERENCES

(1) Nelson, G. H. et al. (1973) *J. Am. vet. med. Assoc.*, *163*, 1276.
(2) Forsyth, D. M. (1977) *Appl. exp. Microbiol.*, *34*, 547.
(3) Weaver, G. A. et al. (1986) *Am. J. vet. Res.*, *47*, 1395, 1826.
(4) Long, G. G. & Diekman, M. A. (1986) *Am. J. vet. Res.*, *47*, 184.
(5) Palyusik, M. et al. (1979) *Magy. Allatorv. Lap.*, *34*, 836.
(6) Sharma, V. D. et al. (1974) *J. anim. Sci.*, *38*, 598.
(7) Shreeve, B. J. et al. (1978) *Br. vet. J.*, *134*, 421.
(8) Vanyi, A. et al. (1973) *Magy. Allatorv. Lap.*, *28*, 303.
(9) Gallagher, R. T. (1985) *NZ vet. J.*, *33*, 37.
(10) Blaney, B. J. et al. (1984) *Aust. vet. J.*, *61*, 24.
(11) Guo, Y. X. & Li, J. Y. (1983) *Chin. J. vet. Med.*, *9*, 14.
(12) Marasas, W. F. O. et al. (1976) *Onderstepoort J. vet. Res.*, *43*, 113.
(13) Vesonder, R. F. et al. (1976) *Appl. envir. Microbiol*, *31*, 280.
(14) Pathre, S. V. et al. (1976) *J. agric. Food Chem.*, *24*, 97.
(15) Patterson, D. P. S. et al. (1979) *Vet. Rec.*, *105*, 252.
(16) Weaver, G. A. et al. (1981) *Res. vet. Sci.*, *31*, 131.
(17) Hagler, W. M. et al. (1980) *Acta vet. Acad. Sci., Hung.*, *21*, 348.
(18) Smalley, E. B. (1973) *J. Am. vet. med. Assoc.*, *163*, 1278.
(19) Bloomquist, C. et al. (1982) *J. Am. vet. med. Assoc.*, *180*, 164.
(20) Vanyi, A. & Szeky, A. (1980) *Magy. Allatorv. Lap.*, *35*, 242.
(21) Weaver, G. A. et al. (1978) *Can. vet. J.*, *19*, 72.
(22) Weaver, G. A. et al. (1980) *Can. vet. J.*, *21*, 210.
(23) Halliburton, J. C. et al. (1979) *Vet. hum. Toxicol.*, *21*, 348.
(24) Beasley, V. R. et al. (1982) *Vet. Rec.*, *111*, 393.
(25) Gentry, P. A. & Cooper, M. L. (1983) *Am. J. vet. Res.*, *44*, 741.
(26) Cote, L. M. et al. (1984) *J. Am. vet. med. Assoc.*, *184*, 189.
(27) Wilson, T. M. et al. (1985) *Vet. Med.*, *80 (11)* 63, 66, 68.
(28) Kriek, N. D. J. et al. (1981) *Onderstepoort J. vet. Res.*, *48*, 129.
(29) Friend, S. C. E. et al. (1983) *Can. J. comp. Med.*, *47*, 291.
(30) Berger, T. et al. (1981) *J. anim. Sci.*, *53*, 1449.
(31) Friend, S. C. E. et al. (1983) *Can. J. comp. Med.*, *20*, 737.
(32) Trenholm, H. L. et al. (1985) *J. dairy Sci.*, *68*, 1000.
(33) Barnikol, H. et al. (1985) *Tierärztl. Umschau.*, *40*, 658.
(34) Friend, D. W. et al. (1984) *Can. J. anim. Sci.*, *64*, 733.
(35) Moore, C. J. et al. (1985) *Aust. vet. J.*, *62*, 60.
(36) Harvey, R. B. et al. (1986) *Am. J. vet. Res.*, *47*, 1630.

Poisoning caused by *Claviceps purpurea* (ergot of rye) (ergotism)

Poisoning caused by the ingestion of large quantities of the naturally occurring ergots of *Claviceps purpurea* is manifested by derangement of the central nervous system, constriction of arterioles and damage to capillary endothelium. Two distinct syndromes occur, one in which there is gangrene of the extremities and the other characterized by signs of central nervous system stimulation.

Etiology

Claviceps purpurea is a fungus which under natural conditions infests cereal rye and less commonly other cereals, including maize, rye-grasses, tall fescue grass, timothy, cocksfoot, Yorkshire fog, crested dogstail and tall oat grasses and bulrush millet. Tall fescue also has a specific fungus as well. It is harvested commercially for the manufacture of pharmaceutical ergot preparations. Ingestion of large quantities of seedheads infested with the fungus causes ergotism in cattle, sheep, pigs, horses, dogs and birds. The ergots contain a number of alkaloids and amines with pharmacological activity and these vary in concentration with the maturity of the ergot. There is some evidence that corn smut may have pharmacological activity similar to that of *Cl. purpurea*. An unidentified ergot (*Claviceps* spp.) on Bermuda or couch grass (*Cynodon dactylon*) may be related to the tremor syndrome which occurs occasionally in cattle grazing this grass (1).

Epidemiology

Ergot of rye is widespread in its distribution but it is seldom that sufficient is ingested in its toxic stage to cause poisoning. Poisoning is most likely to occur in warm, wet seasons which are conducive to the growth of the fungus.

Ergotism occurs commonly only in cattle and usually in stall-fed animals feeding on heavily contaminated grain over a considerable period of time. Other species are not usually exposed to the infested grain. Ergot-infested pasture may cause the disease (2). Cows may show early signs of lameness in as short a period as 10 days after going onto an infested pasture, but most animals do not become affected until 2–4 weeks after exposure.

Pathogenesis

The alkaloids of ergot, particularly ergotamine, cause central nervous system stimulation with the production of convulsions when taken in large amounts, and arteriolar spasm and capillary endothelial damage with restriction of the circulation and gangrene of the extremities when small amounts are taken over long periods. Chronic ergotism is much more common in animals because of the circumstances in which the disease occurs. In spite of the known abortifacient action of *Cl. purpurea*, abortion does not usually occur in poisoned animals.

The experimental feeding of ergots (1–2% of ration) caused severe reduction in feed intake and growth rate in young pigs without producing overt signs of ergotism (3, 4).

Clinical findings

There are two well-known syndromes: chronic ergotism, characterized by gangrene of the extremities, and the acute form characterized by neurotoxicity. There is a third form, recently identified (17) characterized by hyperthermia.

Chronic ergotism

The extremities, particularly the lower part of the hindlimbs, the tail and ears are affected. There are reddening, swelling, coldness, loss of hair or wool, and lack of sensation of the parts initially, followed by the development of a blue-black color, dryness of the skin and its separation from normal tissues. The gangrene usually affects all local tissues and after the lapse of some days the affected part becomes obviously separated and may eventually slough. The lesions are not painful but some lameness is evident even in the early stages and the animal may remain recumbent most of the time. Severe diarrhea is often an accompanying sign. Although the gangrenous form of the disease is most common in cattle acute poisoning with nervous signs has been recorded (5).

Long-term low-level feeding of ergot to fattening beef cattle can result in reduced feed intake and weight gain, increased water intake and urination, failure to shed winter coat and increased susceptibility to heat stress (6).

In sheep under experimental conditions there is no gangrene of the limbs but ulceration and necrosis occur on the tongue, and the mucosae of the pharynx, rumen, abomasum and small intestine.

In pigs the chronic syndrome is manifested by lack of udder development and agalactia in sows and the birth of small pigs which suffer a heavy neonatal mortality. Some of the piglets survive and subsequently suffer gangrene of the ear edges and tail tip (7). In pigs the chronic feeding of *Cl. purpurea* may not disturb existing pregnancies (8), but premature births, mummified fetuses and low litter size are recorded (9). Levels up to 0.2% in the diet appear to be safe (18). Feeding of ergot reduces the chance of the fetuses surviving, so that relative infertility occurs, and feeding pregnant ewes on ergotized grain is not recommended (10). A specific ergot, *Claviceps fusiformis*, which grows on bulrush millet (*Pennisetum typhoides*), is known to be a cause of agalactia in sows in Zimbabwe (11).

Acute ergotism

Convulsive episodes are the major manifestations of this form of the disease but may be preceded by signs of nervous depression (12). These signs, which may be transient, include drowsiness, staggering and a tendency to fall. There may be intermittent blindness and deafness and the skin may also show alternating periods of increased and decreased sensitivity. In mild cases these may be the only signs observed but in severe cases they are followed by convulsions which are usually generalized but may be restricted to one limb or other part of the body. The generalized convulsions are epileptiform in type, are followed by temporary paralysis and coma, and appear to cause pain, the animals crying out during the period of muscular activity.

Apparent recovery may occur between convulsions but there is usually cardiac irregularity, and diarrhea and vomiting occur in some species. The appetite is often good, although some animals show pharyngeal paralysis and eating may precipitate a convulsion. The course of the disease is very irregular, some animals dying during the first convulsions and others only after several days. Some animals persist in a state of chronic ill-health for several months. Gangrene of the extremities may occur in this form of the disease.

In spite of the rarity of abortion occurring as a result of ergot poisoning there is one report of a brief exposure to a heavily ergotized pasture causing abortion in late pregnant cows (15).

Hyperthermia form

There is hyperthermia with temperatures of 41–42°C (105–107°F), dyspnea, and hypersalivation (17). Milk production and growth rate are depressed and morbidity is about 100%. The syndrome is more severe in hot weather when affected ?nimals seek water or shade.

Clinical pathology

Samples of fungus-infested material may be submitted for assay or test feeding.

Necropsy findings

In cattle gangrene of the extremities is the principal gross lesion. There may be evidence of congestion, arteriolar spasm and capillary endothelial degeneration in the vicinity of the gross lesions and in the central nervous system. Ulceration and necrosis of the oral, pharyngeal, ruminal and intestinal mucosae are recorded in sheep.

Diagnosis

Gangrene of the extremities may occur after trauma or exposure to extreme cold or possibly, in calves, following infection with *Salmonella* spp. (13). It is also recorded in buffalo fed on rice straw and suspected to be due to poisoning by the fungi *Fusarium equiseti* and *Aspergillus tereus* which contaminated the straw (14). The nervous signs of the acute form, which is rare in farm animals, are not diagnostic and may be confused with those of many other diseases in which convulsions occur. A number of poisonous fungi produce similar nervous signs as does poisoning with nematode larvae which infest the seedheads of some grasses. The galls produced by the larvae are not unlike the sclerotia of ergot but are much harder in consistency. The best known occurrence is with Wimmera rye-grass infested with the nematode *Anguina* spp. (16). The disease is described under the heading of Wimmera rye-grass.

Treatment

Treatment is not usually attempted although vasodilator drugs may have some beneficial effect. The infested grain should be withdrawn from the ration immediately.

Control

Heavily ergotized grain or pasture fields containing ergotized grasses should not be used for animal feeding. Pasture fields may be grazed if the seedheads are mowed with the mower blade set high. Feed should not contain more than 0.1% of ergot-infested heads. Ergot infested feed should not be fed to pregnant sows.

REVIEW LITERATURE

Burfening, P. J. (1973) Ergotism. *J. Am vet. med. Assoc.*, **163**, 1288.

REFERENCES

(1) Porter, K. J. et al. (1974) *J. agric. Food Chem.*, *22*, 838.
(2) Woods, A. J. et al. (1966) *Vet. Rec.*, *78*, 742.
(3) Friend, D. W. & Maclntyre, T.M. (1970) *Can. J. comp. Med.*, *34*, 198.
(4) Whittemore, C. T. et al. (1977) *Res. vet. Sci.*, *22*, 146.
(5) Dillon, B. E. (1955) *J. Am. vet. med. Assoc.*, *126*, 136.
(6) Dinnusson, W. E. et al. (1971) *N. Dak. Fm Res.*, *29*, 20.
(7) Anderson, J. F. & Werdin, R. E. C. (1977) *J. Am. vet. med. Assoc.*, *170*, 1089.
(8) Bailey, J. et al. (1973) *Br. vet. J.*, *129*, 127.
(9) Barnikol, H. et al. (1982) *Tierärztl. Umschau*, *37*, 524.
(10) Burfening, P. J. (1975) *Theriogenology*, *3*, 193.
(11) Loveless, A. R. (1967) *Trans. Br. mycol. Soc.*, *50*, 18.

(12) Gutlhon, J. (1955) *Rev. Pathol. gen.*, *55*, 1467.
(13) O'Connor, P. J. et al. (1972) *Vet. Rec.*, *91*, 459.
(14) Kwatra, M. S. (1980) *Ind. J. anim. Hlth.*, *19*, 67.
(15) Appleyard, W. T. (1986) *Vet. Rec.*, *118*, 48.
(16) Gwynn, R. & Hadlow, A. J. (1971) *Aust. vet. J.*, *47*, 408.
(17) Burgess, L. W. et al. (1986) *Proc. nutr. Soc. Aust.*, *11*, 120.
(18) Dignean, M. A. et al. (1986) *J. vet. Med.*, *36*, 757.

Poisoning caused by *Claviceps paspali* (ergot of paspalum or dallas grass)

Claviceps paspali is an ergot which parasitizes paspalum or dallas grass (*Paspalum dilatatum*), *Argentine bahia grass* (*Paspalum notatum*) *and water-couch grass* (*P. distichum*). The degree of infestation of pastures varies widely with climatic conditions, being heaviest after wet, humid summers. Outbreaks of the disease occur in winter when animals at pasture graze the seedheads because of a shortage of other feed. The ergots are most toxic when they are passing from the sticky 'honeydew' (sphacelial) stage to the hard, black (sclerotical) stage. The 'honeydew' stage itself is comparatively non-toxic (5). Illness can occur when mature ergots are eaten but the disease is not so severe. Cattle are most commonly affected but sheep and horses are less susceptible (1). A very similar syndrome is produced by *Claviceps cinerea* (2). The husk of the seeds of *Paspalum scrobiculatum*, when fed to buffalo calves, causes severe tremors without other signs of ergotism (3). The toxin has not been positively identified, but it is chemically related to the tremorgen of *Penicillium cyclopium*, and is not related to the ergot alkaloids (5). The neurological effect of the *Penicillium* sp. and *Claviceps paspali* ergots is almost identical.

The clinical signs are all manifestations of nervous system derangement. There is hypersensitivity to noise or movement but not to touch. Muscle tremor is at first only noticeable on exercise but is later continuous, even at rest, and is sufficiently severe to cause shaking of the limbs and trunk and nodding of the head. Involuntary movements may prevent grazing. There is a severe ataxia with gross incoordination of movement, sideways progression and frequent falling into unusual postures. Animals which fall paddle violently in attempts to rise. After a period of rest they can usually rise unassisted.

The appetite is always unaffected but there may be scouring, salivation and some loss of condition. Abortion does not occur. Some deaths are caused by misadventure but recovery occurs quickly in most cases if the animals are removed from affected pastures. At necropsy there are no gross changes, except for some increase in cerebrospinal fluid volume, and histological examinations are negative. No treatment is necessary but livestock should be removed from the affected pasture, which may, however, be used by permitting only intermittent grazing or after mowing and raking of the seedheads (4).

REFERENCES

(1) Ehret, W. J. et al. (1968) *J. S. Afr. vet. med. Assoc.*, *39*, 103.
(2) Dollahite, J. W. (1963) *SWest. Vet.*, *16*, 295.
(3) Gupta, I. & Bhide, N. K. (1967) *Indian vet. J.*, *44*, 787.
(4) Cysewski, S. J. (1973) *J. Am. vet. med. Assoc.*, *163*, 1291.
(5) Mantle, P. G. et al. (1977) *Res. vet. Sci.*, *24*, 49.

Poisoning caused by *Pithomyces chartarum* (*Sporidesmium bakeri*) (facial eczema)

Facial eczema is a disease characterized by hepatitis and photosensitization in sheep and cattle, caused by the ingestion of a fungus which grows on dead and damaged plant material in pasture.

Etiology

Facial eczema is caused by a hepatotoxic agent—sporidesmin—present in the fungus *Pithomyces chartarum (Sporidesmium bakeri)* which infests dead plant material on pastures. Sporidesmin has been isolated and identified as a resinous substance. The environmental factors which encourage the growth of the fungus and the production of sporidesmin have been accurately determined. Although the disease is commonly associated with rye-grass pastures, the causative fungus is capable of growing on all kinds of dead leaf material. Facial eczema has been observed in sheep fed on cereal hay which was heavily infested with *P. chartarum* (1). In South Africa it is thought that the ingestion of *Tribulus terrestris* enhances the toxicity of *Pithomyces chartarum* (6).

Of the farm animals only sheep and cattle are affected.

Epidemiology

The disease has been recorded most commonly in New Zealand and occurs to a limited extent also in Europe, Australia and South Africa. The incidence varies widely depending on climatic conditions; in some years the disease does not occur, in others the morbidity rate in affected flocks of sheep may be 70–80% and 5–50% of these may die (2). Of the survivors many are unthrifty and make less than normal weight gains. In cattle the morbidity rate is much lower and rarely exceeds 50%. In spite of the obvious weight loss caused by the nonfatal form of the disease, there is no appreciable effect on the palatability of the carcass meat (1).

Facial eczema occurs extensively only when pasture is short and contains recently killed plant material in abundance, and under climatic conditions of warm, humid weather, which favor a heavy infestation with the fungus. This is most likely to be a problem in autumn when the summer has been hot and dry, the pasture well eaten back and good rains fall when the ground is still warm. In such circumstances the grass and the fungus grow rapidly. This is a different set of conditions to those which favor the appearance of rye-grass staggers, the other disease occurring on this type of pasture, and the two diseases are not usually seen together.

Pathogenesis

Sporidesmin causes acute toxipathic hepatitis and biliary obstruction and a resulting severe hepatic insufficiency manifested by loss of condition, obstructive jaundice and photosensitization. Sporidesmin administered by mouth is excreted unchanged in high concentrations in urine and bile, especially the latter where it reached 100 times the concentration in serum. The resulting inflammation of the bile ducts and progressive obliterative cholangiolitis slow down the rate of bile flow to negligible levels over a period of about 14 days (7). The photodynamic agent is phylloerythrin, a normal metabolic product of chlorophyll, which is retained in tissues because of failure of its excretion through the damaged liver and bile ducts. The frequent observation that only part of the liver is involved is probably explained by the deposition of toxin in particular parts of the liver, due to portal streaming, on its first passage through hepatic sinusoids: the toxin which reaches the general circulation is probably destroyed.

Clinical findings

In cattle and sheep the disease starts suddenly with the appearance of lethargy, dullness, anorexia, jaundice and photosensitive dermatitis. The skin lesion and jaundice are both variable in occurrence and sheep may die without either having been observed. Many animals die during this acute stage but some survive and pass into a state of chronic ill-health manifested by poor bodily condition and a susceptibility to minor environmental stresses. Many others show no clinical signs but have significant changes in serum enzyme systems indicative of an acute hepatic injury, and measurable reductions in reproductive efficiency and lamb weights (14). Occasional animals develop encephalopathy manifested by dullness, depression, progressing to tremor and lateral recumbency. Wider spread spongy vacuolation of brain tissue is observable histologically (15). A moderate fall in the plane of nutrition, parasitic infestation and pregnancy may cause further mortalities, and photosensitive dermatitis may recur if the animals are fed on lush green pasture. Cattle are not as commonly affected by the chronic form of the disease as are sheep but dermatitis of the teats may lead to the development of mastitis. Details of the clinical findings in photosensitive dermatitis are given under the heading of photosensitization.

Clinical pathology

Tests of hepatic function especially the bromosulfalein clearance test, should be of value in determining the presence of liver damage. In the very early stages serum enzyme estimations should also be of value. Serum gamma-glutamyl transferase levels are regarded as the best indicator of hepatic damage in cattle and continue high for at least several months after an attack of facial eczema (10).

Necropsy findings

In the acute stages of facial eczema there is jaundice and a swollen, mottled liver with thickened bile-duct walls. In the chronic phase there is extensive hepatic fibrosis, the liver is tough and contracted and the left lobe is almost completely atrophic. Areas of regeneration are usually apparent macroscopically. Histologically there is perilobular fibrosis with obliteration of the bile ducts and pressure atrophy of hepatic cells. The changes are much more marked in the left lobe.

Diagnosis

Facial eczema must be differentiated from those other diseases in which photosensitization and hepatitis occur. It bears a marked resemblance to a disease of cattle of the southern United States believed to be caused by the ingestion of dead forage on which a fungus (*Periconia* spp.) is growing.

Treatment

General, supportive treatment for hepatitis and photosensitization, as outlined under those headings, and the administration of antibiotics and antihistamines to control secondary infection and shock may be applicable in animals of sufficient economic value. The provision of drinking water containing 6 g zinc sulfate per 100 liters for 28 days is claimed to hasten recovery of affected cattle (9).

Control

One of the major difficulties in the control of the disease is that of predicting the occurrence of an outbreak. Meteorological observation can be of value but the counting of spores by a mobile spore catcher is now routinely used in danger areas.

In bad seasons the incidence of facial eczema can be reduced by alternating grazing between native and improved pastures or by reducing the intake of the fungus in any other way. Because of the proclivity of the fungus for dead grass two acceptable management procedures for prevention are summer irrigation and hard grazing, both of which reduce the amount of foliar substrate available for fungal growth. Avoidance of sandy soils in bad seasons is also advisable because of the greater tendency for grass death on this kind of soil. Allowing pasture to flower, the sward to grow long, the pasture to be damaged by diseases and pests, and frequent mowing, encourages facial eczema (10).

In a comparison of fungicides used to control the growth of *P. chartarum* Carbendazim was best (at 0·15 and at 0·30 kg/ha of active ingredient) while Benomyl and thiophanate methyl was effective only at 0·30 kg/ha (11). The original methods of applying fungistatic agents to pasture included thiabendazole or Benlate sprayed on at the rate of 272 g/ha in January. The growth of *P. chartarum* was controlled (13) and the development of facial eczema prevented.

The daily oral administration of zinc (30 mg/kg zinc body weight/day) to lactating dairy cows (4) has been shown to reduce the toxic effects of sporidesmin. The zinc salt can be administered by drench as a slurry of zinc oxide (5), by spraying zinc oxide onto pasture, and adding zinc sulfate to the drinking water (12).

Vaccination against sporidesmin has so far been unsuccessful in protecting sheep against facial eczema (3). Resistance to sporidesmin as reflected in the degree of liver damage created is strongly inherited, so much so that a severe field challenge does not overpower the resistance mechanism (8).

REVIEW LITERATURE

Richard, J. L. (1973) Mycotoxin photosensitivity. *J. Am. vet. med. Assoc.*, *163*, 1298.

Smith, B. L. & O'Hara, P. J. (1978) Bovine photosensitization in New Zealand. *NZ vet. J.*, *26*, 2.

REFERENCES

(1) Kirton, A. H. et al. (1979). *NZ J. agric. Res.*, *22*, 399.

(2) Clare, N. T. (1952) *Photosensitization in Diseases of Domestic Animals.* Farnham Royal, England: Commonwealth Agriculture Bureaux.

(3) Fairclough, R. J. et al. (1984) *NZ vet. J.*, *32*, 101.
(4) Smith, B. L. et al. (1978). *NZ vet. J.*, *26*, 314.
(5) Wright, D. E. et al. (1978) *NZ J. agric. Res.*, *21*, 215.
(6) Kellerman, T. S. et al. (1980) *Onderstepoort J. vet. Res.*, *47*, 231.
(7) Mortimer, P. H. & Stanbridge, T. A. (1969) *J. comp. Pathol.*, *79*, 267.
(8) Campbell, A. G. et al. (1981) *Proc. NZ Soc. anim. Prod.*, *41*, 273.
(9) Rickard, B. F. (1975) *NZ vet. J.*, *23*, 41.
(10) Towers, N. R. & Stratton, G. C. (1978) *NZ vet. J.*, *26*, 109.
(11) Wallace, E. G. R. (1976) *NZ J. exp. Agric.*, *4*, 243.
(12) Smith, B. L. & Towers, N. R. (1985) Plant toxicology. *Proc of an Australian USA Seminar*, 1984.
(13) McKenzie, E. H. C. (1971) *NZ J. agric. Res.*, *14*, 379.
(14) Smeaton, D. C. et al. (1985) *Proc. NZ Soc. anim. Prod.*, *45*, 133.
(15) Thompson, K. G. et al. (1979) *NZ vet. J.*, *27*, 221.

Poisoning by *Aspergillus* spp.

Much the most important disease caused by the ingestion of this fungus is aflatoxicosis caused by the aflatoxins, but other important toxins produced by them are ochratoxin and patulin, a lactone and sterigmatocystin.

AFLATOXICOSIS

A restricted number of strains of *Aspergillus* spp. (especially *A. flavus* and *A. parasiticus*) produce a series of hepatotoxins, the aflatoxins, of which aflatoxin B_1 is the most important. The first observed and most common source of the toxin was groundnuts infested by *A. flavus* but peanut hay carrying some nuts-in-shells (15), green chop sorghum (25), moldy bread (21), cotton seed meal, sorghum grain and corn can also be sources. The fungus grows on stored feeds when temperature and humidity are high. It is not destroyed by milling and can continue to produce aflatoxin again. Aflatoxins are also produced by other fungi, notably *Penicillium puberulum*. All animal species are susceptible. A carcinogen, aflatoxin M_1, has also been identified (5). *A. clavatus* has produced similar effects to *A. flavus* in cattle (6).

The aflatoxins are not related to the pyrrolizidine alkaloids but produce almost identical effects in that they produce severe hepatic insufficiency. They are bifuranocoumarin derivatives related to warfarin. At certain dose rates and in some species, e.g. trout, aflatoxin B_1 can also be a powerful carcinogen. There is some experimental evidence pointing towards the carcinogenic effects of aflatoxin in pigs (7). Aflatoxin B_1 has been isolated and its toxic properties accurately calibrated. At a dose rate of 4 mg/kg to wethers, death occurs at 15–18 hours due to acute hepatic insufficiency; at dose rates of 2 mg/kg there is increased respiratory rate, a rise in temperature of 1·5°C (34°F) and diarrhea with blood and mucus; at a dose rate of 0·23 mg/kg there is anorexia and diarrhea (8). Similar dose relationships have been established for calves and for pigs.

Cattle

In cattle the clinical signs include blindness, walking in circles, frequent falling, ear-twitching, teeth grinding, diarrhea, severe tenesmus and anal prolapse. Terminally there are convulsions, and abortion is common (12). Affected animals usually die within 48 hours, calves in the 3–6 months group being most susceptible. Aflatoxicosis is also reputed to interfere with clotting of the blood in cattle leading to the development of hematomas (3). Amounts of toxin insufficient to cause overt disease in cows may be sufficient to reduce food intake, weight gains, and milk production (13). Diarrhea may also occur.

The toxin is passed in the milk and this may cause aflatoxicosis in the sucklings and there is the possibility that the disease may be caused in humans drinking the milk. Typical hepatic lesions have been observed in newborn calves, and are thought to result from passage of the toxin through the placenta (17).

The concentration of aflatoxin in cow's milk may be as high as 0·33 µg/l (1) and may continue to be as high for 3–4 days after ingestion (4). A great deal of aflatoxin taken in in the feed by cattle is physically bound to ruminal contents and as little as 2–5% reaches the intestine (9). Levels of aflatoxin B in excess of 100 µg/kg of feed are considered to be poisonous for cattle. Since the advent of reliable and accurate methods of assaying aflatoxin in feeds there has been a notable tendency for feed to be less contaminated. Supplementation of the diet with zinc has not been effective in preventing aflatoxicosis in calves (18).

Pigs

In pigs the period between when the toxin is ingested and when signs appear is thought to be quite long, at least 6 weeks, and varies with the toxicity of the batch of feed (14). The mortality rate is often 20% (2), but may be as high as 40%. Feeder pigs are more susceptible than adults. In pigs there is no clearly defined clinical syndrome, and diagnosis depends on the detection of aflatoxin in the feed and blood serum, and the characteristic gross and histopathological findings in the liver. A pronounced lower enterocolitis, with diarrhea and dysentery is common, but not constant. Abortion is a commonly reported sequel but there is doubt about the relationship (4). Also described in pigs after feeding on *A. flavus* is a syndrome of depression, fever, reduced liver function and marked elevation of SGOT and OCT levels (16). At necropsy there is icterus, ascites, swelling of the liver, and mesenteric edema. Selenium, in the form of glutathione peroxidase, reduces the toxic effects of aflatoxin B_1 on the liver cells of pigs, but this appears not to have been developed into a practical application (11).

Horses

Aflatoxicosis in horses is recorded, but is unusual probably because horses are not likely to be fed damaged feeds. No clinical signs are reported, but illness lasted 5 days after a prodromal period of anorexia lasting 3–4 days which began a few days after access to contaminated feeds. Necropsy lesions included encephalomalacia, hepatitis and hepatic fibrosis, bile duct hyperplasia, hemorrhagic enteritis and myocardial degeneration. The experimental disease (26, 28) is characterized by depression, inappetence, tremor and prostration with death following in 2–6 weeks.

OTHER SYNDROMES CAUSED BY *ASPERGILLUS* SPP.

Aspergillus fumigatus administered to sheep may cause erosive lesions on the buccal mucosa, and renal cortical necrosis (19). Ochratoxin A is a very potent renal toxin produced by *A. ochraceus*, also thought to cause fetal death and resorption and thus cause abortion (20). It is also produced by other fungi, especially *Penicillium viridicatum* and it is dealt with under that heading. Hyperkeratosis of the skin of the cheeks and neck, and erosive lesions of the buccal mucosa are attributed to *A. clavatus* and *A. chevalieri* (22). *A. clavatus* has also been shown to cause hypersensitivity, incoordination, stiff gait, severe generalized tremor, opisthotonus, paresis, paralysis and constipation in cattle. At postmortem examination there is neuronal degeneration and necrosis in the midbrain, medulla oblongata and spinal cord (23, 24). *A. terreus* is confirmed as the cause of gangrene of the extremities in cattle. The fungus grows on tall fescue grass (*Festuca arundinacea*) and the toxic principle has been extracted from hay and used to produce the lesions (25, 26). *Aspergillus fumigatus* in moldy corn silage produces tremorgens and toxins capable of causing enteritis (3).

Also isolated from *A. flavus* is cyclopiazonic acid which causes weakness, anorexia, loss of body weight and diarrhea in pigs. Postmortem lesions include gastric ulceration and hemorrhages throughout the alimentary tract (10). *A. oryzae* administration to newborn foals as a digestive inoculant to promote fast development of digestion is suspected of producing mycotoxins and causing acute hepatic insufficiency including encephalopathy (27).

REVIEW LITERATURE

Edds, G. T. & Osuna, O. (1976) *Aflatoxicosis. Proc. 80th ann. Mtg US anim. Hlth Assoc.*, pp. 434–458.

Newberne, P. M. (1973) Chronic aflatoxicosis. *J. Am. vet. med. Assoc.*, *163*, 1262, 1269, 1284.

REFERENCES

(1) Patterson, D. S. P. et al. (1980) *Food Cosm. Toxicol.*, *18*, 35.
(2) Hayes, A. W. et al. (1978) *J. Am. vet. med. Assoc.*, *172*, 1295.
(3) Cole, R. J. et al. (1977) *J. agric. Food Chem.*, *25*, 826.
(4) Piscak, A. et al. (1978) *Vet. Med.*, *23*, 219.
(5) Stoloff, L. et al. (1971) *Food cosmet. Toxicol.*, *9*, 839.
(6) Abadjieff, W. et al. (1966) *Mh VetMed.*, *21*, 452.
(7) Shalkop, W. T. & Ambrecht, B. H. (1974) *Am. J. vet. Res.*, *35*, 623.
(8) Armbrecht, B. H. et al. (1970) *Nature, Lond.*, *225*, 1062.
(9) Engel, G. & Hagemeister, H. (1978) *Milchwissenschaft*, *33*, 21.
(10) Lomax, L. G. et al. (1984) *Vet. Pathol.*, *21*, 418.
(11) Davila, J. C. et al. (1983) *Am. J. vet. Res.*, *44*, 1877.
(12) Ray, A. C. et al. (1986) *J. Am. vet. med. Assoc.*, *188*, 1187.
(13) Duthie, I. F. et al. (1966) *Vet. Rec.*, *79*, 621.
(14) Loosmore, R. M. & Harding, J. D. J. (1961) *Vet. Rec.*, *73*, 1362.
(15) McKenzie, R. A. et al. (1981) *Aust. vet. J.*, *57*, 284.
(16) Cyzewski, S. J. et al. (1968) *Am J. vet. Res.*, *29*, 1577, 1591.
(17) Adamesteanu, I. et al. (1973) *Dtsch Tierarztl. Wochenschr.*, *81*, 141.
(18) Neathery, M. W. et al. (1980) *J. dairy Sci.*, *63*, 789.
(19) Thornton, R. H. et al. (1968) *NZ J. agric. Res.*, *11*, 1.
(20) Munro, I. C. et al. (1973) *J. Am. vet. med. Assoc.*, *163*, 1269.
(21) Ketterer, P. J. et al. (1982) *Aust. vet. J.*, *59*, 113.
(22) Wogan, G. N. (1969) *Foodborne Infections and Intoxications*. New York: Academic Press.
(23) Kellerman, T. S. et al. (1984) *Onderstepoort J. vet. Res.*, *57*, 271.
(24) Jiang, C. S. et al. (1982) *Acta vet. Zoot. Sinica*, *13*, 247.
(25) Edwards, A. J. et al. (1982) *Vet. hum. Toxicol*, *24*, 94.
(26) Cysewski, S. J. et al. (1982) *Toxicol. appl. Pharmacol.*, *65*, 354.
(27) Swerczek, T. W. & Crowe, M. W. (1983) *Calif. Vet.*, *37*, (7), 23.
(28) Bortell, R. et al. (1983) *Am. J. vet. Res.*, *44*, 2111.

Myrotheciotoxicosis

Myrothecium spp. are fungi isolatable from growing ryegrass and white clover plants and from stored roughages.

Experimental oral dosing of cultured fungus to calves and sheep caused death in 24 hours with hemorrhages in the alimentary tract, especially the abomasum, hepatitis, and pulmonary congestion and edema. With smaller doses the same signs and lesions were produced but the course was 7–10 days before death. Very small doses for 30 days caused weight loss and growth retardation in lambs without histological lesions (1).

The principal toxic species are *M. roridum* and *M. verrucaria* and their toxins have been identified (2). There is a strong resemblance between this disease and the so-called kikuyu grass poisoning.

REFERENCES

(1) di Menna, M. E. & Mortimer, P. H. (1971) *NZ vet. J.*, *19*, 246.
(2) Mortimer, P. H. et al. (1971) *Res. vet. Sci.*, *12*, 508.

Stachybotrytoxicosis

Forage molded by *Stachybotrys alternans* produces the disease known as stachybotrytoxicosis, a favorite subject in Russian literature (1). Toxins isolated are the macrocyclic tricothecenes, the satratoxins G and H (2). Horses, cattle, sheep and pigs may be affected and the disease is characterized by fever, ruminal atony, diarrhea, necrotic ulceration of the mucosae and skin, hemorrhages into tissue and agranulocytosis (2–4). The important lesion appears to be depression of leukocyte formation which produces a disease not unlike that caused by bracken poisoning in cattle (5). Hemorrhages are visible in the mucosae, there is also a hemorrhagic enteritis and, in sheep, *Pasteurella haemolytica* can often be isolated from tissues (3). The infection is thought to occur as a result of the immunosuppression caused by the toxins. In horses there is also a subacute or acute myositis (6). The disease resembles alimentary toxic aleukia, caused by the ingestion of toxin from *Fusarium poae* and *F. sporotrichoides* in man.

REFERENCES

(1) Spesiwzewa, N. A. (1963) *Proc. 17th Wld vet. Congr. Hanover*, *1*, 305.
(2) Harrach, B. et al. (1983) *Appl. envir. Microbiol.*, *45*, 1419.
(3) Hajtos, I. et al. (1983) *Acta vet. Hung.*, *31*, 181.
(4) Szabo, I. & Szeky, A. (1970) *Magy. Allatorv. Lap.*, *25*, 633.
(5) Danko, G. (1976) *Magy. Allatorv. Lap.*, *31*, 226.
(6) Servantie, J. et al. (1985) *Rev. med. Vet.*, *136*, 687.

Poisoning by *Rhizoctonia leguminicola*

Profuse salivation is a characteristic sign produced by the ingestion or experimental dosing (2) of the fungus *Rhizoctonia leguminicola* in cattle, goats and horses. Excessive lacrimation, frequent urination, bloat, anorexia and diarrhea also occur. The salivation is at its peak at 5–6 hours after ingestion and disappears at about 24 hours.

The fungus infests standing alfalfa or red clover plants (1) and clover hay (4), especially red clover hay. Infested plants carry bronze to black spots or rings and the hay is usually dusty and discolored by black patches on the stems and leaves. Clinical signs usually subside within several days of substituting normal hay. Atropine may be used to control the salivation (3). The toxic principle is an alkaloid metabolite of the fungus—slaframine. Swainsonine, the phytotoxin found in *Swainsona* and *Astralagus* spp. has also been isolated (5).

REFERENCES

(1) Sockett, D. C. et al. (1982) *J. Am. vet. med. Assoc.*, *181*, 606.
(2) Isawa, K. et al. (1971) *Bull. Natl. Inst. Anim. Ind.*, Summaries *24*, 10.
(3) Crump, M. H. (1973) *J. Am vet. med. Assoc.*, *163*, 1300.
(4) Hagler, W. M. & Behlow, R. F. (1981) *Appl. envir. Microbiol.*, *42*, 1067.
(5) Broquist, H. P. et al. (1984) *Appl. envir. Microbiol.*, *48*, 386.

Poisoning by *Penicillium* spp.

Fungi of the *Penicillium* family produce a number of important toxins as set out below.

OCHRATOXIN A: NEPHROSIS

Ochratoxin is produced by many fungi, but particularly by *Penicillium viridicatum* (1). The most significant result produced by this intoxication is nephrosis. This occurs naturally and in experimental animals (16). The natural disease has been widespread in Denmark for many years (3). This fungus also produces viomellein, another nephrotoxic mycotoxin (4). The principal lesion is a degenerative change of the renal tubules and there is a consequential impairment of tubular function (14). The toxin does not appear to cross the porcine placental barrier and fetal pigs are not affected (15). Although ochratoxin is the principal cause of the renal lesion, another toxin, citrinin, also present in the fungus, enhances the lesion (2). It resembles Balkan nephropathy, a naturally occurring disease of man.

Clinically the disease is characterized by diarrhea, polyuria and polydipsia. Postmortem findings include dehydration, enteritis, generalized edema, renal enlargement and fibrosis, and necrosis of renal tubular epithelium (5). The fungus grows on stored barley or corn grain, and nephrosis results when the grain is fed. The species most often involved is pigs (6). Experiments with cattle indicate that they are likely to be affected only at very high dose rates, but goats are rather more susceptible (3). There is some evidence that chickens and horses can also be affected (12). The ochratoxin has been detected as a 'carryover' in pigs and poultry meats and has some significance for persons eating contaminated pig meats (18). Affected pigs placed on an ochratoxin-free diet are decontaminated in about 1 month (11).

TREMORGENS: 'STAGGERS'

Small repeated doses of *P. cyclopium* cultures to sheep cause a disease identical with rye-grass staggers (7). *P. palitans* has been shown to produce ataxia and convulsions in cattle (8). A tremorgen penitrem A has been isolated from *P. puberulum* and *P. crustosum* (20), and a more potent one, verrucologen, from *P. crustosum* and *P. simplicissimum* (21). Penitrem A closely resembles the tremorgen produced by *Claviceps paspali*. It produces tremor, ataxia, muscular rigidity and convulsive episodes in calves (9). The tremor is very fine, and increases with excitement. It increases until calves sway rhythmically, standing with their legs wide apart and stiff. The gait is stiff and ataxic and the calves fall often. The worst affected calves are laterally recumbent, with tetanic convulsions, opisthotonus and severe tremor. Nystagmus and profuse salivation occur sometimes (10). Other soil penicillia produce tremorgens. *P. piscarium* produces verrucologen and fumitremorgen B. *P. estinogenum* also produces verrucologen. *P. nigricans* yields penitrem A (16). *P. jantinellum* and *P. cyclopium* also produce penitrem A. The list is still growing (18).

The disease 'rye-grass staggers' is now known to be caused by the endophyte *Acremonium lolii* but it is possible that some outbreaks of incoordination in sheep and other species may be contributed to or even caused by other tremorgens such as those produced by *Penicillium* spp. The disease is discussed in detail in the section on poisonous grasses. A subsidiary effect of tremorgenic fungi is a depression of testosterone production in rams and bulls (17). To confirm a diagnosis that fungal intoxication is the cause of cases of staggers depends on the isolation of tremorgenic fungi from the feces of affected animals. The fungal elements survive passage through the ruminant gut and can be cultured from the feces (18).

P. rubrum causes frothing at the mouth, champing of the jaws, jaundice, cutaneous erythema, and collapse in goats and pigs (1). In horses the clinical signs of intoxication include incoordination, chronic spasm, jaundice, diarrhea, abdominal pain and vomiting. These fungi are soil-borne and could be accidentally ingested by cattle and sheep while grazing.

RUBRATOXINS: HEPATOTOXINS, HEMORRHAGIC DISEASE

Penicillium rubrum and *P. pururogenum* produce rubratoxins suspected of causing hepatic and hemorrhagic diseases (1), and rubratoxin administered experimentally to calves has produced mild hepatitis (13).

OTHER DISEASES ASCRIBED TO POISONING BY *PENICILLIUM* SPP.

P. roqueforti is suspected of causing bovine abortion and placental retention (14). It grows on moldy mixed grains and ensilage. A subacute illness without any diagnostic signs killed lambs in which the critical lesion was oxaluric nephrosis. This was thought to have been due to contamination of the feed by an oxalate-producing fungus, *Penicillium* sp. (19).

REVIEW LITERATURE

Edds. G. T. & Osuna, O. (1976) *Proc. 80th ann. Mtg US Anim. Hlth Assoc.*, pp. 34–458.

Krogh. P. (1976) Mycotoxic nephropathy. *Adv. vet. Sci.*, *20*, 147.

REFERENCES

(1) Wilson, B. J. & Harbison, R. D. (1973) *J. Am. vet. med. Assoc.*, *163*, 1274.
(2) Krogh, P. (1978) *Acta Pathol. Microbiol. Scand.*, Suppl. 269A, 28.
(3) Ribelin, W. E. et al. (1978) *Can. J. comp. Med.*, *42*, 172.
(4) Krogh, P. et al. (1984) *Dansk Vet Tidsskr.*, *67*, 123.
(5) Zimmerman, J. L. et al. (1979) *Vet. Pathol.*, *16*, 583.
(6) Carlton, W. W. et al. (1973) *J. Am. vet. med. Assoc.*, *163*, 1295.
(7) Gallagher, R. T. et al. (1977); *NZ J. agric. Res.*, *20*, 431.
(8) Krogh, P. & Elling, F. (1977) *Vet. Sci. Commun.*, 1, 51.
(9) Cyzewski, S. J. et al. (1975) *Am. J. vet. Res.*, *36*, 53.
(10) Cyzewski, S. J. (1973) *J. Am. vet. med. Assoc.*, *163*, 1291.
(11) Elling, F. (1979) *Dansk Vet Tidsskr.*, *62*, 14.
(12) Krogh, P. (1976) *Adv. vet. Sci.*, *20*, 147.
(13) Pier, A. C. et al. (1976) *Proc. 80th ann. Mtg U.S. Anim. Hlth Assoc.*, p. 130.
(14) Krogh, P. et al. (1979) *Vet. Pathol.*, *16*, 466.
(15) Shreeve, B. J. et al. (1977) *Br. vet. J.*, *133*, 412.
(16) Mantle, P. G. et al. (1978) *Vet. Rec.*, *103*, 403.
(17) Peterson, A. J. et al. (1978) *Res. vet. Sci.*, *25*, 266.
(18) di Menna, M. E. & Mantle, P. G. (1980) *Res. vet. Sci.*, *24*, 347.
(19) Linklater, K. A. & Angus, K. W. (1979) *Vet. Rec.*, *104*, 129.
(20) Dorner, J. W. et al. (1984) *J. agric. Food Chem.*, *32*, 411.
(21) Peterson, D. W. et al. (1982) *Res. vet. Sci.*, *33*, 183.

Poisoning caused by other miscellaneous fungi

A number of aberrations of reproductive function in animals are caused by fungal intoxications. The production of estrogenic substances by *Fusarium* spp. fungi has been described above. White clover does not normally contain estrogens but when heavily infested with fungi it may contain significant amounts (1). Barley smut fungus (*Ustilago hordei*) is thought to be toxic to farm animals; feeding it to experimental animals has caused infertility and stillbirths (2). The wheat smut fungus *Tilletia tritici* should not be included in rations for pigs at more than 5% of infested grain in the ration because it is thought to cause glomerulonephritis and failure to gain weight in pigs (3). In southeastern Australia a common infertility–abortion–mummified fetus syndrome has been ascribed to an onion-like weed, *Romulea rosea*. There is now a suspicion that the disease may be due to a toxin produced by a fungus, *Helminthosporium biseptatum*, growing on the weed (4). *H. ravenelli* growing on esparto grass is credited with producing a syndrome of excitement, dyspnea, tachycardia, hypersalivation, tremor, jaundice and some deaths in Argentinian cattle (19).

A fungus, *Periconia* sp., which grows on forage in the field is also suspected of causing hepatic damage and photosensitization in cattle in the southern United States (5): there is a close resemblance in clinical signs and circumstances of occurrence to facial eczema and myrotheciotoxicosis.

Ngaione, a hepatotoxic ketone, is found in sweet potato tubers infested with black rot due to one of the fungi *Ceratostomella fimbriata* (6) or *Ceratocystis* spp. (20). Three other toxins have been isolated from sweet potatoes infested by fungi, especially *Fusarium javanicum*, which caused serious mortality when fed to beef cattle (7). The toxins were present in tubers with only minor blemishes. One of the toxins produces pulmonary edema and respiratory distress, another is a specific hepatotoxin; renal lesions are also produced. The respiratory form of the disease has been produced experimentally by feeding sweet potatoes and the mold (8).

Drechslera campanulata (syn. *Helminthosporium* spp.) occurs as brown-red spots on the leaves of cereal oat plants and causes diarrhea, milk yield reduction and death in some cows. Similar syndromes are caused in sheep and goats except that photosensitivity is also apparent in goats (21). At necropsy there is ulceration of the forestomach mucosae.

Phomopsis leptostromiformis and *P. rossiana* are accepted as being the cause of so-called 'lupinosis' of cattle and sheep (9, 10). Typical hepatic injury is produced experimentally by feeding sheep on pure cultures of the fungus. In the early stages of the hepatitis serum enzyme tests are the best aids to diagnosis. The gamma-glutamyl transpeptide test is preferred in the early subacute stages, and glutamate oxalate transminase when the disease is more severe. In the late stages of the disease liver function tests are preferred (15). The disease has been reproduced experimentally in pigs (9). It is dealt with in more detail under the heading of lupin poisoning (page 1337).

Nervous signs predominate in the toxic effects ascribed to the ingestion of *Trichothecium roseum* (11). Sterigmatocystin is a fungal toxin capable of causing hepatic carcinoma. It has been isolated from *Bipolaris* spp. (12) and *Aspergillus nidulans* (13) growing on groundnuts.

Dendrochium toxicum is reported to produce a great variety of disorders when fed to pigs (14). A hemorrhagic diathesis, a thrombocytopenia, leukocytosis and necrotic, ulcerative and degenerative lesions in viscera are only some of the effects.

Diplodia maydis causes diplodiosis, a neuromycotoxicosis when fed to cattle, sheep, goats and horses. The disease is characterized by lacrimation, salivation, tremor, ataxia, paresis and paralysis. The fungus grows on maize and develops its toxin only after a prolonged (more than 6 weeks) period of growth. This may explain frequent reports that the fungus is not poisonous (17). The same applies to cultured fungus used to produce the disease experimentally; it must be a culture which is at least 8 weeks old (18). Affected animals recover if feeding of the infected grain is stopped. The infection is a serious disease of the maize crop.

Acremonium lolii is generally accepted as the cause of rye-grass staggers under which heading it is discussed.

Acremonium coenophialum (syn. *Epichloe typhina*) is accepted as the cause of fescue foot discussed under the heading of tall fescue grass poisoning.

REFERENCES

(1) Wong, E. et al. (1971) *NZ J. agric. Res.*, *14*, 633.
(2) Ibragimov, Kh. Z. & Khabiev, M. S. (1970) *Veterinariya, Moscow*, *8*, 77.
(3) Muller, E. (1977) *Dtsch Tierärztl. Wochenschr.*, *84*, 143.
(4) Fisher, E. E. & Finnie, E. P. (1967) *Nature, Lond.*, *215*, 1276.
(5) Kidder, R. W. et al. (1961) *Bull. Fla agric. Exp. Stn.*, *630*, 21.
(6) Denz, F. A. & Hanger, W. G. (1961) *J. Pathol. Bacteriol.*, *81*, 91.
(7) Wilson, B. J. et al. (1970) *Nature, Lond.*, *227*, 521.
(8) Peckham, J. et al. (1972) *J. Am. vet. med. Assoc.*, *160*, 2, 169.
(9) Rensburg, I. J. B. et al. (1975) *J. S. Afr. vet. med. Assoc.*, *46*, 197.
(10) Gardiner, M. R. & Petterson, D. S. (1972) *J. comp. Pathol.*, *82*, 5.
(11) Richard, J. L. et al. (1969) *Mycopathol. Mycol. appl.*, *38*, 313.
(12) Purchase, I. F. H. & van der Watt, J. J. (1969) *Food Cosmet. Toxicol.*, 7, 135.
(13) Holzapfel et al. (1966) *S. Afr. med. J.*, *40*, 1100.
(14) Stepushin, E. A. & Chernov, K. S. (1969) *Veterinariya, Moscow*, 7, 60, 62.
(15) Malherbe, W. D. et al. (1977) *Onderstepoort J. vet. Res.*, *44*, 29.
(16) Kellerman, T. S. et al. (1985) *Onderstepoort J. vet. Res.*, *52*, 35.
(17) Blaney, B. J. et al. (1981) *Aust. vet. J.*, *57*, 196.
(18) Rabie, C. J. et al. (1985) *Food Chem. Toxicol.* *23*, 349.
(19) Vallejo, L. C. et al. (1981) *Gaceta Vet.*, *43*, 638.
(20) Liu, C. I. (1982) *J. Chin. Soc. vet. Sci.*, *8*, 155.
(21) Schneider, D. J. et al. (1985) *Onderstepoort J. vet. Res.*, *52*, 93.

Mushroom and toadstool poisoning

Reports of poisoning caused by mushrooms and toadstools in animals are rare. *Amanita verna* has been shown to cause fatal poisoning in cattle (1) but large quantities must be eaten before toxic effects occur. Severe pain at defecation and matting of the perianal regions with feces is caused by vesicular and necrotic eruption about the anus and vulva (1, 2). At necropsy there is severe inflammation of the alimentary mucosa.

A large cauliflower-like toadstool (*Ramaria* sp.) is credited with causing death in cattle (3). Clinical signs include salivation, mucosal erosions, ocular lesions, abortion and anorexia. Similar signs plus loosening of the hair and hooves and nervous signs have been observed in sheep and cattle and attributed to consumption of fungi of genus *Clavaria* (4).

The mushroom *Cortinarius speciocissimus* has caused deaths in sheep in Norway with renal tubular necrosis and terminal uremia (2).

REFERENCES

(1) Piercy, P. L. et al. (1944) *J. Am. vet. med. Assoc.*, *105*, 206.
(2) Overas, J. et al. (1979) *Acta vet. Scand.*, *20*, 157.
(3) Paschoal, J. P. et al. (1983) *Biolojico*, *49*, 15.
(4) de Freitas, J. et al. (1967) *Proc. 5th panam. Congr. vet. med. Zootechnol.* (*Caracas 1966*), *2*, 818.

DISEASES CAUSED BY POISONOUS PLANTS

Ferns

BRACKEN FERN (*PTERIDIUM AQUILINA*) POISONING

Bracken fern poisoning in horses and pigs causes a conditioned thiamin deficiency and has been described under that heading (page 1224). In ruminants the defect is one of depression of bone marrow activity with pancytopenia expressed primarily as ecchymotic hemorrhages and often followed by bacterial invasion of tissues. There is also a relationship between bracken and the disease enzootic hematuria which is discussed under that heading. Tumors of the alimentary tract including benign adenomatous polyps in the small intestine of rat, neoplasms in mice, and carcinomas of the intestine in sheep and cattle have also been attributed to the ingestion of bracken for long periods.

Etiology

The toxic factor in bracken fern which causes poisoning in ruminants has not been identified. Thiaminase or toxopyrimidine administered to cattle do not produce the disease and thiamin, vitamin B_1 and folic acid do not prevent the occurrence of the disease (1). Most field outbreaks of the disease occur in cattle but it can be produced in sheep by feeding bracken fern over a much longer period and natural outbreaks have been recorded (2). Large amounts of bracken fern must be eaten before poisoning occurs but the toxicity of the plant varies with the stage of growth, younger plants being more toxic. The underground stems (rhizomes) of the fern also contain the toxic principle, in approximately five times the concentration of that found in the fronds, and have been used to produce the disease experimentally in cattle (3). Cattle allowed access to recently ploughed fields of bracken eat the rhizomes avidly and may suffer heavy mortalities. A norsequiterpene glucoside of the illudane type and *p*-hydroxystyrene glucosides, known as ptaquiloside or PT, has been extracted from the fern and used to produce hematuria and neoplasia in experimental animals (11).

Epidemiology

Bracken fern poisoning occurs in most countries as a sporadic disease. The disease is highly fatal in cattle. Although the losses due to the disease are usually small because of the high intake of the fern required to produce illness, heavy mortalities have been observed in some outbreaks. Sheep are less commonly affected by this form of bracken poisoning but it has been produced experimentally (18).

Animals do not eat bracken fern readily but samples of meadow hay may contain toxic amounts and animals at pasture may eat large quantities especially when young, green fronds appear after drought or burning off or when other forage is sparse. Bracken used as bedding may also be ingested in dangerous amounts by animals with a poor nutritive status. The toxin is excreted in the milk in significant quantity (4), and may cause neoplasia in offspring drinking it.

Pathogenesis

Bracken fern poisoning in ruminants is caused by the depression of bone marrow activity, an increased capillary fragility, prolonged bleeding time and defective clot retraction but with normal clotting and prothrombin times. The clotting defect in calves appears to be due to the formation of heparinoid substances and the presence of toxic amines in the blood (5).

In the bone marrow there is depression of granulopoiesis and thrombopoiesis. The myeloid cells are particularly affected leading to a severe reduction in blood platelets and granular leukocytes. The erythrocyte series in bone marrow is affected but only in the terminal stages. It has been suggested that hemorrhage into the alimentary mucosa or submucosa occurs as the result of the thrombocytopenia and ulcers develop at these hemorrhage sites. Bacterial invasion follows and the resulting bacteremia may cause infarction in the liver if small vessels are blocked by clumps of bacteria, or the organisms may be carried into the systemic circulation and cause infarction in other organs including the kidneys, lungs and heart.

The capillary fragility, intestinal ulceration and laryngeal edema which occur in some cases are thought to be due to damage to tissue mast cells and the liberation of histamine (6). The carcinogenicity of bracken has been extensively investigated and synoptically described (15).

Clinical findings

Pancytopenic disease of cattle

Signs characteristic of bracken fern poisoning may not appear in cattle until there has been access to bracken for from 2 to 8 weeks. Initially there is loss of condition and dryness and slackness of the skin. Clinical signs occur suddenly and include high fever (40·5–43°C, 105–109°F), dysentery or melena, bleeding from the nose, eyes and vagina, and drooling of saliva. Nasolabial ulcers and hematuria may be observed. Petechial and ecchymotic hemorrhages may be visible under mucosae and skin and in the anterior chamber of the eye. An increase in respiratory and heart rates occurs at this stage. Death usually follows in 1–3 days.

Cattle may continue to become ill for up to 6 weeks after being taken off the bracken fern. Calves 2–4 months of age show essentially the same clinical and necropsy picture as adult animals except that marked bradycardia and death from heart failure are common, and a laryngitic form, with marked dyspnea due to laryngeal edema, is not uncommon. Although only a few animals in a group are affected most of those showing clinical signs die.

Sheep are not commonly affected by this form of bracken poisoning but it has been produced experimentally (18).

'Bright-blindness' in sheep

A syndrome known as 'bright-blindness' in sheep has been observed to occur on pastures heavily infested with bracken and the disease has been produced experimentally in sheep fed bracken nuts (8). There are no indications of inheritance having any effect on the occurrence of the disease. Affected sheep are blind, the pupils are dilated and show a poor light reflex and on ophthalmoscopic examination there is retinal degeneration. This degeneration may be observable in many more sheep than those clinically blind. Affected sheep are always more than 18 months old. The number of sheep affected is increasing and there is concern that the cause should be positively identified. An association between blindness and leukopenia (a hallmark of bracken poisoning) has been established but little else.

A *carcinogenic action* has also been ascribed to bracken because of the high incidence of malignant adenocarcinoma in the ileum of sheep and rats on experimental diets high in bracken (1, 10). A very high prevalence of neoplasms, especially of the alimentary tract, and including the jaws and liver, is recorded in sheep grazing pasture heavily infested with bracken (14). Dairy cattle on farms infested with bracken are reported to have a high prevalence of carcinoma of the intestine and tumors of the urinary bladder (13). Cancer of the alimentary tract generally with lesions on the lateral dorsum of the tongue, the soft palate and oropharynx, esophagus, esophageal groove and the rumen is also common in upland Scotland and northern England (16). The epidemiological evidence suggests that papillomas caused by the papilloma virus are transformed into carcinomas by the carcinogenic effect of an environmental agent, probably bracken. The simultaneous production of bladder and intestinal neoplasms is recorded in mice on diets of bracken for long periods (1) and in rats fed milk from cows fed on bracken (12). Many of the signs and lesions of *enzootic hematuria* have been produced by the prolonged feeding of bracken (7) but the role of bracken in the etiology of this disease is unknown.

Clinical pathology

Estimations of the occurrence of platelets in blood smears appear to be the most valuable laboratory test in diagnosis and prognosis of the disease. Platelet counts fall gradually from normals of about 500 000/μl to about 40 000/μl just before death. Total leukocyte levels fall gradually at first and then precipitously to about 1000/μl in the terminal stages. Polymorphonuclear leukocytes are the most profoundly depressed and often none are visible in a smear. Hematological changes may not be sufficiently marked to enable prophylactic treatment to be undertaken in clinically normal animals.

Bone marrow biopsy is valuable as an indication of the status of the platelet and granulocyte series. Increase in capillary fragility is detectable and defective clot retraction is also a feature of this disease. A fall in erythrocyte count and hemoglobin content may be detectable in the late stages. Depression of erythropoiesis is more marked in sheep than in cattle. Urine examination may reveal the presence of erythrocytes and many epithelial cells.

Necropsy findings

Death is due to the combined effects of multiple internal hemorrhages and bacteremia. Multiple hemorrhages, varying in size from petechiae to large extravasations occur in all tissues. In some organs, particularly the alimentary tract, necrosis and sloughing occur over the hemorrhages. Areas of edema are also common in the gut wall. The bone marrow is paler than normal. Multiple small, pale or red areas representing infarcts and areas of necrosis are present in the liver, kidney and lungs.

Diagnosis

Bracken fern poisoning may be readily confused with many of the acute septicemias of cattle, including anthrax, blackleg, septicemic pasteurellosis and leptospirosis, but bacteriological findings are negative for these specific infections except for the occasional occurrence of a pasteurella septicemia. Hemorrhages are not a common finding in babesiosis and anaplasmosis and the causative protozoa can usually be demonstrated. Exposure to a high intake of bracken fern is usually sufficient reason for a presumptive diagnosis of poisoning when the characteristic lesions are present.

Several other poisonings including sweet clover and some molds produce similar lesions and signs to those caused by bracken fern but there is no fever or leukopenia. Trichloroethylene-extracted soybean meal causes aplasia of bone marrow and produces a syndrome indistinguishable on clinical, hematological and necropsy grounds from that produced by bracken fern. Granulocytopenic disease of calves is a similar disease.

Treatment

DL-Batyl alcohol, a known bone-marrow stimulant, has been recommended as a treatment but has not always been successful (17). It should be combined with an antibiotic; 1 g of the alcohol is injected intravenously or subcutaneously daily for 4–5 days. Treatment is not likely to be successful in advanced cases when the leukocyte count is below 2000/μl and the platelet count is less than 50 000–100 000/μl because of the effects of secondary bacterial invasion and hemorrhage.

Additional supportive treatment may include blood transfusions in those animals in which serious depression of erythrocyte and leukocyte counts have occurred. The transfusions should be large and 4·5 liters is considered to be a minimum dose in adult cattle.

Control

Fields containing large quantities of bracken fern should not be harvested for hay, and animals forced to graze affected areas should be supplied with a supplementary diet when the pasture is short.

REFERENCES

(1) Pamukcu, A. M. et al. (1977) *Vet. Fakultesi Dergesi*, *24*, 28.
(2) Parker, W. H. & McCrea, C. T. (1965) *Vet. Rec.*, *77*, 861.
(3) Evans, W. C. et al. (1961) *Vet. Rec.*, *73*, 852.
(4) Evans, I. A. et al. (1972) *Nature, Lond.*, *237*, 107.
(5) Yamane, O. (1975) *Jap. J. vet. Sci.*, *37*, 335, 341, 577.
(6) Ishii, K. et al. (1974) *J. Fac. Agric. Tottori Univ.*, *9*, 27.
(7) Pamukcu, A. M. et al. (1976) *Vet. Pathol.*, *13*, 110.
(8) Watson, W. A. et al. (1972) *Br. vet. J.*, *128*, 457.
(9) Mason, J. et al. (1973) *Exp. Eye Res.*, *15*, 51.
(10) Evans, I. A. & Mason, J. (1965) *Nature, Lond.*, *208*, 913.
(11) Hirono, I. et al. (1984) *Vet. Rec.*, *115*, 375.
(12) Pamukcu, A. M. et al. (1978) *Cancer Res.*, *38*, 1556.
(13) Jarrett, W. F. H. (1980) *Br. med. Bull.*, *36*, 79.
(14) McCrea, C. T. & Head, K. W. (1978) *Br. vet. J.*, *134*, 154.
(15) Evans, I. A. (1979) *Res. vet. Sci.*, *26*, 339.
(16) Jarrett, W. F. H. et al. (1978) *Nature, Lond.*, *274* (5668), 215.
(17) Dalton, R. G. (1964) *Vet. Rec.*, 76, 411.
(18) Sunderman, F. M. (1987) *Aust. vet. J.*, *64*, 25.

Poisoning caused by miscellaneous ferns

HORSETAIL (*EQUISETUM SPP.*)

This plant contains thiaminase and causes a syndrome of thiamin deficiency in horses which is described under that heading.

BURRAWANG PALM (*MACROZAMIA SPP.*)

The leaves of plants of this species cause incoordination of the hindquarters when eaten. Many members of the family are toxic, particularly the young shoots of *Macrozamia spiralis*, *Zamia integrifolia* and *Z. media*, and *Cycas* and *Bowenia* spp. (1). Initial signs include frequent dribbling of urine, holding the tail to one side, and walking sideways because of a tendency of the hindquarters to fall to one side, due to increased tone in the opposite hindleg. There is an uncontrolled extension and flexion of the hindlimbs, the hindquarters tending to sag or sway when moving. In the early stages overextension of the lower joints gives rise to a 'goose-stepping gait', and this is followed in the later stages by flexion of the fetlocks and walking on the anterior aspect of the foot. The gait worsens with exercise and the animal either falls or drags itself along on its forelegs with the hindlegs trailing behind. The falling is *en bloc*, so that the animal crashes to the ground heavily, or in farmers' terms, with a wamp, hence the colloquial name of 'the wamps'. Some recovery occurs if ingestion ceases but is never complete. The experimental feeding of leaves of *Bowenia serrulata* and *Macrozamia lucida* to cattle produced degenerative lesions in the nerve fibers of the fasciculus gracilis and dorsal spinocerebellar pathways. Similar lesions are found in natural cases (2). Eosinophilic, spheroid masses, thought to be axonal swellings caused by axonal dystrophy, have also been observed in the central nervous system of affected cattle. They occur in all parts of the spinal cord and in the cuneate nucleus of the medulla. Degeneration of spinal ganglia is also sometimes seen (3). Cattle and sheep are affected and cattle may show some addiction to the plant particularly when other forage is not available.

Acute hepatic necrosis is also caused in sheep by the ingestion of fresh leaves of *Macrozamia reidlei*. The toxicity of the leaves is readily destroyed by drying (7).

The seeds of *Macrozamia* spp. contain a toxic alkaloid, macrozamin, which has caused gastroenteritis and jaundice in sheep. Experimental feeding with the nuts has caused hepatic cirrhosis, proliferative gastroenteritis, myocarditis, pancreatitis, pneumonitis and arteriosclerosis in pigs, cattle, horses (5) and sheep (6). The seeds of the South African cycad *Encephelartos lavatus* also contain a macrozamin known to be a potent hepatoxin and, in rats, a carcinogen (10). *Cycas* spp. contain the toxic glucoside cycasin which is capable of causing liver damage and demyelination of spinal cord tracts (11).

GRASS TREE (*XANTHORRHOEA HASTILE* syn. *X. RESINOSA*)

Ingestion of the flower spikes of this plant causes poisoning in cattle and there is some evidence that a dietary deficiency of phosphorus predisposes to the disease. In some cases the appearance of clinical signs may be delayed for 2 or 3 weeks after consumption of the plant has ceased. Incoordination is the cardinal sign, the affected animal lurching to one side while walking and swinging laterally or spinning around, often falling heavily. The hindlegs are most seriously affected and there is lateral flexion of the spine and incontinence of urine. Even severely affected animals recover if fed and watered and prevented from eating the plant. An unusual incidental finding in poisoning by *X. minor* is a red discoloration of urine caused by resins in the plant (4).

ROCKFERNS

Cheilanthes tenuifolia and *Notholoena distans* cause a slow stumbling gait and severe depression of consciousness in sheep in Australia. Affected sheep appear to be blind.

MALE FERN

Dryopteris borreri and *D. flix-mas* are thought to poison cattle causing a profound drowsiness, a tendency to stand in water, blindness and low mortality rate. Recovery is common, but some animals remain blind. Perineuronal and perivascular edema are detectable at necropsy (8, 9).

REFERENCES

(1) Hall, W. T. K. & McGavin, M. D. (1968) *Pathol. vet.*, *5*, 26.
(2) Mason, M. M. & Whiting, M. G. (1968) *Cornell Vet.*, *58*, 541.
(3) Hooper, P. T. et al. (1974) *Aust. vet. J.*, *50*, 146.
(4) Harrison, M. A. et al. (1978) *Aust. vet. J.*, *54*, 40.
(5) Gardiner, M. R. (1970) *Aust. J. agric. Res.*, *21*, 519.
(6) Healey, P. J. (1968) *Clin. chim. Acta*, *22*, 603.
(7) Gabbedy, B. J. et al. (1975) *Aust. vet. J.*, *51*, 303.
(8) Edgar, J. T. & Thin, I. M. (1978) *Vet. Rec.*, *82*, 33.
(9) Macleod, N. S. M. et al. (1978) *Vet. Rec.*, *102*, 239.
(10) Tustin, R. C. (1983) *J. S. Afr. vet. Assoc.*, *54*, 33 & 38.
(11) Shimizu, T. et al. (1986) *Jap. J. vet. Sci.*, *48*, 1291.

Fodder crops

Many crops grown to provide feed for livestock may cause poisoning in some circumstances.

RAPE (*BRASSICA NAPUS*) OR CANOLA POISONING (ALSO KALE OR COLE (*BRASSICA OLERACEA*), CHOU MOELLIER, TURNIPS AND SWEDES)

Plants of all the *Brassica* species cause several syndromes including hemolytic anemia, blindness, pulmonary emphysema, and digestive disturbances which may occur separately or in combination.

Etiology

The acute pulmonary emphysema syndrome observed in cattle grazing on rape is probably acute interstitial pneumonia. The blindness syndrome has been determined to be a mild form of polioencephalomalacia. Chief interest in poisoning by plants of the *Brassica* family is the hemolytic anemia which is the commonest form of poisoning. The anemia-producing agent in kale, and presumably in other plants, is dimethyl disulfide, produced by ruminal bacteria from naturally occurring substance S-methyl cysteine sulfoxide (SMCO) (1). The SMCO content of kale and other forage brassicas varies, increasing as the plant matures. The toxic dose of SMCO is 15 g/100 kg body weight daily to produce severe, fatal anemia. Intakes of 10 g/100 kg body weight cause a subacute low-grade anemia. Particular note should be taken of the occurrence of SMCO in cabbages, swedes and stubble turnips. The level may be insufficiently high to cause anemia, but may cause failure to gain weight satisfactorily, or clinically evident ill-thrift (8). SMCO is a rare amino acid occurring only in these plants and onions, hence onion-induced anemia.

Although there is probably no etiological relationship it is not uncommon for the hemolytic disease to occur in the presence of hypophosphorosis, and therefore at the same time as postparturient hemoglobinuria. The pulmonary emphysema associated with grazing on rape and allied plants also occurs at the same time of year on other types of pasture and there is probably no direct causal relationship between them and the disease. Some outbreaks have been observed to be caused by atypical interstitial pneumonia.

The seeds and leaves of these plants may contain significant quantities of cyanogenetic substances and this may be related to their capacity to produce goiter in lambs and occasional outbreaks of bloat in cattle. Nitrate and nitrite poisoning have also been recorded on kale feeding. Rape seed meal has also been shown to cause goiter in pigs when fed in the proportion of 10–20% of the diet.

The thyroid enlargement is not preventable by dietary iodine. No toxic effects have been observed in ruminants, and chickens appear to be the principal target species (7). The goitrogenic effects of rapeseed meal, which are not necessarily matched by low thyroxin outputs, appear to be related to the meal's content of glucosinolate, from which goitrogens are released in the gut.

Epidemiology

Rape and kale poisoning are well known where these plants are grown for fodder and in some areas they are no longer used because of their dangerous propensities. The overall prevalence of poisoning is probably not great but on individual farms the number affected is usually significant, and the mortality rate is high.

Only ruminants are affected by poisoning with kale and other fodder brassicas, and the hemolytic effect is produced only when the diet consists largely of the plants. The characteristic anemic disease which they produce only develops when the animals are on the feed for at least 1 and usually 3 weeks. The plants are more toxic as they mature and when secondary growth begins; the flowers and seeds are particularly poisonous (1). The toxicity of the plants varies from year to year, and on rape grazing most outbreaks occur in wet years when early frosts occur and the leaves assume a purple color. The toxicity of kale also varies significantly between varieties of the plant (2) but the important factors in most outbreaks are the maturity of the crop and the amount eaten (3). The toxic principle in kale is destroyed in heat-dried or ensiled material but is still present in frozen (4) and dried (5) material. Rape and kale anemia are also thought to be more common when the phosphorus status of animals is low and possibly also during spells of colder weather (6).

Pathogenesis

The effect of the toxic agent, dimethyl disulfide, is to precipitate hemoglobin molecules in the erythrocytes to form the Heinz–Ehrlich bodies which are characteristic of the disease. These are extruded from the red cells and removed from the circulation by the spleen. The resulting hemolytic anemia affects all classes of animals but its effects are most serious in heavily pregnant and recently parturient females (6). The observed tendency for cycles of spontaneous improvement followed by recrudescence of the anemia (9) may be related to variations in the cellular content of reduced glutathione which prevents the formation of Heinz–Ehrlich bodies. There appears to be some chance that some families of animals are inherently deficient in glutathione and therefore predisposed to this disease (8). The goiter produced in some incidents is the result of poisoning with glucosinolates which are goitrogenic because of their capacity to produce thiocyanates. The subject is dealt with in the section on goiter caused by iodine deficiency (page 1274).

Clinical findings

Bloat, goiter, nitrate and nitrite poisonings are discussed separately under those headings. In the anemia syndrome, the onset in severe cases may be so sudden that no signs are observed before the animal collapses and dies. If clinical illness is apparent hemoglobinuria is observed first and is soon followed by weakness and dejection. Pallor of the mucosae, moderate jaundice, tachycardia and a slight increase in respiratory rate and depth are also observed. Diarrhea occurs commonly and, although body temperatures are usually normal to low, there may be fever up to 40·5°C (105°F). Death is common unless effective treatment is provided and surviving animals require a long period of convalescence. A normal hematological status may not be regained for up to 6 weeks. In an affected herd it is common to find a number of animals which are not seriously ill but which have a subclinical anemia.

'Rape blindness'

This is manifested by the sudden appearance of blindness in cattle and sheep grazing on rape. More severe nervous signs including head-pressing and mania have been observed in steers. The eyes are normal on ophthalmoscopic examination, the pupils show some response to light and may or may not be dilated. Complete recovery usually occurs but may take several weeks.

Pulmonary emphysema

This has been observed only in cattle. Affected animals show severe dyspnea, with stertorous rapid respiration, mouth breathing and subcutaneous emphysema. The temperature may or may not be elevated. Affected animals may survive but often remain chronically affected and do poorly.

Digestive disturbances

These disturbances in steers on rape are usually accompanied by anorexia, the passage of small amounts of feces, absence of ruminal sounds and the presence of a solid, doughy mass in the rumen. Only a small quantity of sticky, black material is present on rectal examination.

Clinical pathology

In the hemolytic anemia syndrome the erythrocyte count, hemoglobin level, hematocrit and leukocyte levels are reduced and Heinz–Ehrlich bodies are present in up to 100% of erythrocytes. They are significantly increased in numbers before anemia appears (10). The anemia is macrocytic and the hemoglobin level falls from 110 g/l to 6 g or less. Hemoglobin is present in the urine. There is often a concurrent hypophosphatemia. The dimethyl disulfide content of the blood, which will be high at the time of occurrence of the poisoning, can be measured chromatographically (4).

Necropsy findings

In the hemolytic syndrome there is pallor, jaundice, hemoglobinuria, thin, watery blood, dark coloration of the kidney, and accentuation of the lobular appearance of the liver. Histologically there is moderate hepatic necrosis in the liver. In the emphysema syndrome there is emphysema and edema, sometimes accompanied by the hepatic lesions of the anemic syndrome, and the accumulation of dark-colored ingesta and patchy congestion of the alimentary mucosa which characterize the digestive form of the disease.

Diagnosis

The occurrence of the disease when cattle or sheep are grazing on plants of the *Brassica* spp. suggests the presumptive diagnosis. There are many other causes of hemolytic anemia including postparturient hemoglobinuria, which is limited to cows which have calved recently, leptospirosis, bacillary hemoglobinuria, anaplasmosis, and babesiosis all of which are accompanied by fever and toxemia. Chronic copper poisoning can only be proved by estimation of blood and liver copper levels.

Acute pulmonary edema and emphysema occur in 'fog fever' and other allergies. 'Rape blindness' has some clinical signs in common with poisoning by lead, *Senecio* spp. and other hepatotoxic plants as well as rabies and other encephalitides.

Treatment

In severe cases of anemia immediate blood transfusion is necessary if the animal is to be saved. Ancillary treatment includes the use of hematinic preparations and the provision of a highly nutritious diet. 'Rape blindness' and pulmonary emphysema respond poorly to treatment but antihistamines are recommended and in violent cases sedatives may be of value. The treatment of acute pulmonary edema and emphysema is discussed in detail under acute interstitial pneumonia (page 1426). In the digestive form it is usual to treat the animal with mild rumenatorics over a period of 7–10 days but the response is poor.

Control

The provision of ample hay either daily before the animals are pastured on the rape, or as a stack in the rape field, or allowing access to a field of rough grass, are recommended to reduce the consumption of rape. Rape showing purple discoloration should be regarded with suspicion and only limited grazing permitted until doubts as to its safety are satisfied. Cattle and sheep grazing on these plants should be kept under close observation so that affected animals can be treated in the early stages of the disease. An adequate phosphorus intake is particularly necessary when ruminants are grazed on plants of this species. If feeding is stopped the hemoglobin levels return to normal in about 3 weeks. Even if feeding is continued there is a strong tendency for a spontaneous recovery and further similar cycles, to occur. Some varieties of kale have lower concentrations of SMCO, the hemolytic agent, and a genetic approach to preventing the disease might be worth examining.

REVIEW LITERATURE

Smith, R. H. (1980) Kale poisoning. The *Brassica* anemia factor. *Vet. Rec.*, *107*, 12.

REFERENCES

(1) Smith, R. H. (1977) *Vet. Ann.*, *17*, 28.
(2) Greenhalgh, J. F. D. et al. (1970) *Res. vet. Sci.*, *11*, 232.
(3) Greenhalgh, J. F. D. et al. (1972) *Res. vet. Sci.*, *13*, 15.
(4) Earl, C. R. A. et al. (1983) *J. Sci. Food Agric.*, *34*, 23.
(5) Pelletier, G. & Martin, L. H. (1973) *Can. J. anim. Sci.*, *53*, 229.
(6) Clegg, F. G. (1967) *4th int. Mtg World Assoc. Buiatrics, Zurich, 1966*, p. 11.
(7) Hill, R. (1979) *Br. vet. J.*, *135*, 3.
(8) Smith, R. H. (1980) *Vet. Rec.*, *107*, 12.
(9) Tucker, E. M. (1969) *Br. vet. J.*, *125*, 472.
(10) Grant, C. A. et al. (1968) *Acta vet. Scand.*, *9*, 126, 141.

Miscellaneous fodder crops

SORGHUM (*SORGHUM VULGARE*), JOHNSON GRASS (*S. HALEPENSE*), SUDAN GRASS (*S. SUDANENSE*) AND THEIR HYBRIDS, AND COMMON FLAX (*LINUM USITATISSIMUM*)

The sorghums are commonly used to provide green fodder, ensilage, or grain. Flax is grown commercially for fiber and linseed oil and meal. The plants may contain high concentrations of cyanogenetic glucosides, especially when growing rapidly after a period of retarded growth, and cause heavy mortalities due to cyanide poisoning. The nitrate content of the plants may be sufficiently high to cause nitrite poisoning in cattle.

In recent years a syndrome characterized by cystitis, urinary incontinence, loss of hair due to scalding and ataxia, which is most marked in the hindlegs when the horse is backed or turned, has been reported as occurring in horses grazing sudan or hybrid sudan grass pastures in southwestern United States (1). A similar syndrome has been reported in cattle and sheep grazing grain sorghum in Australia (3). Degeneration of white matter was observed in the spinal cord. The occurrence of poisoning incidents appeared to be related to stunting of the crop by lack of rain, or by attacks of grasshoppers.

Fetal deformities are also recorded in horses (2) and cattle (8) after ingestion of the plant and death in adult horses is usually due to pyelonephritis (3). Only the growing plant produces this effect and the factors responsible are unknown. Focal axonal degeneration and demyelination are present in lumbar and sacral parts of the spinal cord (1). The fetal deformities comprise fixation of all joints causing dystocia (2, 8).

TRITICALE

This is a hybrid between wheat and rice used mainly for grain production. If it is harvested green as a crop and made into hay the dried awns are prohibitively irritating to the pharynx and mouth of cattle and horses. The clinical signs that result in about a week include, in horses, cough, mucoid nasal discharge, foul breath, hypersalivation, quidding and loss of body weight. Some horses develop submandibular edema and there are severe ulcerations in the mouth with many awns embedded in the ulcers. The ulcers are very painful, up to 5 cm in diameter at the labial gingival junction, the lingual frenulum, the base of the lingual dorsum, soft palate and the sides of the tongue (7).

SUGAR BEETS, MANGELS AND FODDER BEETS (*BETA VULGARIS*)

These roots are in common use as feeds for animals but they may cause toxic effects in some circumstances. When frozen they may cause indigestion and when fed in excessive amounts mangels, sugar and fodder beet may cause acute rumen impaction with lactic acidemia in cattle. The latter disease is not identical with that caused by overeating on grain because dehydration is not always present and deaths occur irrespective of the degree of hemoconcentration. Hypocalcemia and hypermagnesemia also occur. The recommended maximum intake of fodder beet is 30 kg daily for adult cattle and 3 kg for sheep. Recently lifted or partly cooked mangel roots may cause nitrite poisoning. The tops of the growing plants may contain large amounts of oxalates and may cause oxalate poisoning and in some circumstances blindness and hemolytic anemia similar to the diseases caused by ingestion of plants of the *Brassica* spp. Beet pulp is a highly regarded and expensive feed but if it is the sole article of diet, or almost entirely so (4), it can cause encephalopathy with blindness, keratoconjunctivitis and degeneration of the optic nerve. Vitamin A deficiency is thought to be the basis for the disease.

POTATO (*SOLANUM TUBEROSUM*)

Potatoes are toxic if they are green and sprouted and the toxic alkaloid solanin is concentrated in the sprouts and green skin. Pigs are most commonly affected but all species are susceptible. Potatoes must constitute more than 50% of the diet before toxicity occurs. Clinical signs appear several days after feeding commences. In pigs there is dullness, copious diarrhea, anorexia and a subnormal temperature, and coma in the terminal stages. The mortality rate in groups of affected pigs may be high. In horses the signs include depression and prostration but usually there are no signs of alimentary tract irritation. In cattle a dermatitis, manifested by vesicles and scabs, appears on the legs. At necropsy in all species there is a moderate hyperemia of the alimentary mucosa.

Treatment should include central nervous system stimulants and alimentary tract astringents. Recovery follows when the potatoes are omitted from the diet of pigs. Sprouted or diseased potatoes can be fed safely if they are boiled and the amount fed restricted to less than 25% of the diet.

Fatal diarrhea is recorded in a horse that ate rotten ungreened potatoes (6).

ONION (*ALLIUM* SP.)

Cultivated and wild onions are capable of causing Heinz body anemia when eaten in large quantities by horses and cattle (5). Poisoning is unlikely to occur at pasture, most incidents being recorded when penned animals are fed large amounts of cull onions. Cattle are most susceptible, and sheep and goats least susceptible. The toxic agent is a disulfide, *n*-propyldisulfide, as described in rape poisoning. The clinical picture is one of hemolytic anemia, characterized by hemoglobinuria, mucosal pallor, and jaundice.

CORNSTALK POISONING

Cornstalk poisoning is an all-inclusive term which may include nitrite poisoning, bloat or various fungal intoxications but not all of the reported outbreaks can be so classified.

Poisoning is reported in cattle fed on corn plants which are stunted by drought conditions or early frosts. Although the incidence is usually low, the morbidity rate may reach 50% in affected herds and the mortality rate approximates 100%. Clinical signs usually commence 7–10 days after the cattle are turned on to the stalk field and include dullness, recumbency and muscle tremor affecting the ears, thorax and abdomen. If the animal is forced to rise the gait is weak and staggery. The pulse, temperature and respiration are normal but there is atony of the rumen, complete closure of the iris, so that the animal is unable to see, and dribbling of urine. Clonic convulsions may precede death. At necropsy petechial hemorrhages are present under most serous surfaces and striped zones of hemorrhage are present in the mucosa of the terminal portion of the large bowel. The liver and kidneys are swollen. No effective treatment has been found, although dextrose solutions administered intravenously may cause temporary improvement.

CEREAL CROP POISONING

Grazing of cereal crops when in the young growing stages often results in a condition allied to lactation tetany and known colloquially as 'wheat poisoning'. Heavily fertilized crops may contain sufficient nitrate to cause nitrite poisoning in cattle but clinical illness does not usually occur unless the crop is made into hay and undergoes heating or wetting. Stunted mature crops are sometimes grazed when they are too short to harvest. The crops may contain sufficient grain to cause acute rumen impaction.

BUCKWHEAT (*FAGOPYRUM SAGITTATUM, F. ESCULENTUM*)

Buckwheat is grown for its seeds and they and the vegetation contain a photodynamic substance, fagopyrum, which may cause photosensitive dermatitis in all species of the animals.

PEA VINE ENSILAGE

Pea vines salvaged from pea-canning factories are made into ensilage, usually in stacks, and when fed out to ewes in the winter have produced a nervous disorder in 90% of the young lambs. Silage which has turned black rather than the normal dark green is most frequently involved. The lambs are normal at birth but signs appear at 1–3 days of age. While standing the lambs show tetany and either walk backwards or run forwards with the head lowered and back depressed. After a period of activity they become recumbent, limp and unable to stand but after a few minutes can get up and appear normal. The nervous syndrome reappears with exercise or excitement. Normal growth occurs if the lambs are confined. Dietary supplementation with added minerals and vitamins does not prevent the condition. At necropsy there is degeneration of Purkinje cells in the cerebellar cortex and vacuolar degeneration of cerebral neurones.

REFERENCES

(1) Adams, L. G. et al. (1969) *J. Am. vet. med. Assoc.*, *155*, 518.
(2) Prichard, J. T. & Voss, J. L. (1967) *J. Am. vet. med. Assoc.*, *150*, 871.
(3) McKenzie, R. A. & McMicking, L. I. (1977) *Aust. vet. J.*, *53*, 496.
(4) Alibasoglu, M. et al. (1973) *Vet. Fak. Derg. Ankara Univ.*, *20*, 239.
(5) Verhoeff, J. et al. (1985) *Vet. Rec.*, *117*, 497.
(6) Owen, R. R. (1985) *Vet. Rec.*, *117*, 246.
(7) McCosker, J. E. et al. (1983) *Aust. vet. J.*, *60*, 259.
(8) Seaman, J. T. et al. (1981) *Aust. vet. J.*, *54*, 351.

Miscellaneous plant byproducts used as feed

TOBACCO

Stalks of the tobacco plant (*Nicotiana tabacum*) have a teratogenic effect when fed to pregnant sows at 10–48 days of pregnancy (1). The defect produced is arthrogryposis affecting limb and intervertebral joints. *Nicotiana glauca* (wild tree tobacco), containing anabasine, produces similar congenital defects when fed to cows during the period of days 40–75 of pregnancy (3). The most sensitive period is that of days 43–55 (3). There are no abnormalities of the nervous system (14). Woody material has a low concentration of the teratogen, but leaves and bark contain much more (7). *Nicotiana glauca* also causes cleft palate in pigs (3). In ewes *N. glauca* causes hypersalivation, ataxia, recumbency and death, and lambs *in utero* at the time develop flexed limb joints, rotation of limb bones, lordosis and cleft palate (11).

TRICHLOROETHYLENE-EXTRACTED SOYBEAN MEAL

Soybean meal prepared by the trichloroethylene extraction of soybeans contains an unidentified toxic substance which causes aplastic anemia, leukopenia and damage to vascular endothelium. The disease has been known for many years but is now of historic interest only, other methods of extracting soybean oil having been introduced. The disease produced has a striking resemblance to radiation sickness and the ruminant form of bracken poisoning. All farm animal species other than pigs are susceptible.

LINSEED CAKE

Linseed cake is a common constituent of animal feeds. In certain circumstances it may cause toxic effects because of its high content of cyanide present in the form of the glucoside linamarin. Hydrocyanic acid poisoning may occur when large quantities of the cake are fed to hungry sheep, or calves are fed on cake which has been soaked. A high incidence of goiter in newborn lambs may result when large quantities are fed to ewes during late pregnancy. The cake can be detoxicated by soaking and then boiling for 10 minutes to eliminate the hydrocyanic acid.

COTTONSEED CAKE

Gossypol, a poisonous phenolic substance present in variable amounts in cottonseed cake, causes damage to the myocardium and liver parenchyma and significant changes in the electrocardiographs of treated pigs (2). Most recorded outbreaks of gossypol poisoning refer to pigs. Sheep are susceptible if the toxin is injected but appear to be unaffected when it is fed. Calves consuming 800–1000 g cottonseed meal/day died of heart failure (13). Illness and mortality have also been produced by feeding gossypol to adult dairy cows (4). Clinical signs do not appear until animals have been fed on rations containing cottonseed cake for 1–3 months. Anorexia, dyspnea and weakness are the characteristic signs and death occurs after an illness of several days. Hematuria is also recorded (13).

Cottonseed cake may be fed with safety to pigs provided it constitutes less than 10% of the ration, or in large quantities if the material is detoxified. Cooking of the cake or the addition of 1% calcium hydroxide or 0·1% ferrous sulfate to it are efficient methods of detoxification. In experimental trials the addition of iron in equal proportions to gossypol up to 600 mg/kg of the ration will protect pigs. At necropsy there is generalized edema due to congestive heart failure, and histologically there is degeneration of the myocardium and skeletal musculature. Centrilobular necrosis in the liver is also a characteristic lesion.

Many of the outbreaks of disease ascribed to the feeding of cottonseed cake have probably been due to deficiencies of essential nutrients, especially vitamin A.

RAPESEED MEAL

Rapeseed meal is goitrogenic for pigs when fed in quantities of 10–20% of the total diet. One incident is recorded in which 34–80% of pigs in a 10 000 pig fattening unit had enlarged thyroid glands when the diet contained 3–10% of rapeseed meal. The clinical signs were limited to inefficient weight gain. Treatment with iodine was corrective (5). The goiterogenic substance is goitrin, a thioglucoside (6), and a degradation product of the plant's glucosinolates, produced in the rumen by its bacteria (15). The content of glucosinolate in the seed varies with species of rape used. *Brassica napus* seed is much more goitrogenic than *B. campestris*. Including the rapeseed in ensilage does not reduce its goiter-generating capacity (12). Toxicity has also occurred when the rapeseed used to make the cake comes to be contaminated by other toxic seeds, e.g. crotonyl isosulfocyanate, which causes a severe hemorrhagic gastroenteritis.

Poisoning also occurs when large quantities of the seeds of cruciferous plants, especially if they have been stored for long periods, are fed to cattle. The high concentration of glucosinolates leads to a toxic level of isothiocyanates, which are damaging to tissues, and goitrin (16). The clinical syndrome is one of abdominal pain but without diarrhea. A necropsy there is edema in the subepithelial tissue of the rumen and separation of the ruminal epithelium from the muscle layer.

BREWERS' GRAIN

Wet brewers' grain may develop high concentrations of lactic acid especially when kept in a heap rather than being spread out. If large amounts are fed, especially to cows on heavy grain rations, lactic acid poisoning, similar to that caused by overeating on grain, may result. Important clinical signs include ataxia, dehydration, sinking of the eyes, and sticky, foul-smelling feces. Treatment by the oral administration of sodium bicarbonate is recommended (8). Brewer's grain may also contain residual ethanol and cause poisoning of cattle and deaths due to acute heart failure (17).

HERRING MEAL

Certain batches of herring meal have been reported as causing widespread poisoning of ruminants in Norway (9). The toxic principle is thought to be dimethylnitrosamine (10) and the essential lesion is liver necrosis. Clinical signs appear after feeding the meal for 2–3 weeks and include depression, loss of appetite and milk yield and ruminal atony, sometimes progressing to complete anorexia, ataxia of the hindlimbs and abdominal pain with marked contractions of the abdominal muscles. There is a characteristic unpleasant odor on the breath and milk. Convulsions are observed occasionally but more often severe cases develop a 'dummy' syndrome followed by coma and death. The bromosulfalein clearance test appears to be of diagnostic value in both cattle and sheep.

REFERENCES

(1) Crowe, M. W. (1978) In: *Effects of Poisonous Plants on Livestock*, ed. R. F. Keeler et al., p. 419. New York: Academic Press, Inc.
(2) Albrecht, J. E. et al. (1968) *J. anim. Sci.*, *27*, 976.
(3) Keeler, R. F. & Crowe, M. W. (1983) *Clin. Toxicol.*, *20*, 47.
(4) Lindsey, T. O. et al. (1980) *J. dairy Sci.*, *63*, 562.
(5) Seidel, H. et al. (1977) *Mh VetMed.*, *32*, 693.
(6) Marangoes, A. & Hill, R. (1975) *Vet. Rec.*, *96*, 377.
(7) Keeler, R. F. et al. (1981) *Cornell Vet.*, *71*, 47.
(8) Owens, E. L. (1959) *NZ vet. J.*, *7*, 43.
(9) Hansen, M. A. (1964) *Nord. VetMed.*, *16*, 323.
(10) Sakshaug, J. et al. (1965) *Nature, Lond.*, *206*, 1261.
(11) Keeler, R. F. & Crowe, M. W. (1984) *Cornell Vet.*, *74*, 50.
(12) Schone, F. et al. (1986) *Arch. exp. Vet. Med.*, *40*, 507.
(13) Osgad-Klopfer, U. & Adler, H. (1986) *Israel J. vet. Med.*, *42*, 16.
(14) Keeler, R. F. et al. (1981) *Am. J. vet. Res.*, *42*, 1231.
(15) Bell, J. M. (1984) *J. anim. Sci.*, *58*, 996.
(16) Mason, R. W. & Lucas, P. (1983) *Aust. vet. J.*, *60*, 272.
(17) Hibbs, C. M. et al. (1986) *Proc. 14th World Cong. Dis. Cattle*, *2*, 733.

Grasses

POISONING CAUSED BY CANARY GRASSES (*PHALARIS SPP.*) (PHALARIS STAGGERS)

The ingestion of *Phalaris* spp. grasses causes two distinct syndromes: sudden death and incoordination in sheep, and incoordination in cattle. The oral administration of cobalt prevents the nervous form of the disease.

Etiology

Toowoomba canary grass (*Phalaris aquatica* syn. *P. tuberosa*) is known to cause this disease and it is possible that canary grass (*P. minor*) and a hybrid species, rhompa grass, can also cause it. *P. arundinacea* is assumed to cause the staggers and acute death syndromes. As in *P. aquatica* poisoning there is a slate-gray discoloration of the brain stem and diencephalon (1). Provision of cobalt appears to stimulate the proliferation in the rumen of microorganisms which are capable of destroying the causative agent. Sheep affected with phalaris staggers do not usually show any signs of cobalt deficiency.

Epidemiology

The disease has been recorded in many parts of Australia and in New Zealand, and South Africa where these grasses are in common use as pasture plants. Up to 30% of a flock may be affected.

The disease occurs only when the *P. aquatica* dominates the pasture or is preferentially grazed, and toxicity is greatest when the plants are young and growing rapidly especially after a break in a dry season. On lightly stocked pastures the acute syndrome, with signs appearing within 4 hours but usually between 12 and 72 hours after going on to the pasture, is most likely to occur. Hungry animals are understandably most commonly affected. Deaths are most common in the early morning or in foggy or cloudy weather. The nervous form of the disease occurs in similar circumstances but in sheep which have protracted or repeated exposure (2). In this case clinical signs appear 2–3 weeks after sheep are put on to pasture showing new growth, usually in the autumn or early winter. Both forms may occur in the one flock of sheep. Sheep of all ages are affected and mild cases may occur among cattle. The acute form of the disease is also recorded in cattle on irrigated *Phalaris* spp. pasture in hot humid weather (3).

Pathogenesis

Three tryptamine alkaloids, structurally similar to serotonin, are present in the grass under certain conditions and are thought to be the causative toxins (4). The alkaloids are capable of interfering with the functions of serotonin, a chemical transmitter in the autonomic nervous system with functions analogous to those of acetylcholine. As such the alkaloids are capable of causing both neurological signs and the cardiac abnormalities of tachycardia and ventricular block. The nervous disturbance appears to be functional initially but anatomical changes may occur in advanced cases.

The relevant tryptamine alkaloids vary significantly in their toxicity so that plants in a pasture can vary greatly in the danger they present (5). Other factors which affect the concentration of tryptamines, and hence the toxicity of the grass, are high environmental temperature and growing in shade (6). There are still further details that need to be known before the causes of the disease are completely understood. Under some circumstances plants which have a low content of the causative tryptamine alkaloids precipitate the syndrome (8).

Clinical findings

The 'sudden death' or cardiac syndrome is manifested by sudden collapse, especially when excited, a short period of respiratory distress with cyanosis, and then death or rapid recovery. During the stage of collapse there is arrhythmic tachycardia followed by ventricular fibrillation and cardiac arrest. Consciousness is retained.

In the initial stages of the nervous form of the disease in sheep signs appear only when the animals are disturbed. Hyperexcitability and generalized muscle tremor, including nodding of the head, occur first. On moving, the limb movements are stiff and there is inability to bend the hocks causing dragging of the hindfeet. Incoordination and swaying of the hindquarters follow. In the most severe cases tetanic convulsions occur with lateral recumbency, paddling movements of the legs, and irregular involuntary movements of the eyeballs. There is rapid respiration and irregular tachycardia. The sheep may die at this stage but if left undisturbed it may recover from the convulsion and walk away apparently unaffected. If the sheep are left on the pasture the condition worsens in individual cases, the animal becoming recumbent and manifesting repeated clonic convulsions until death occurs.

There is a great deal of variation from day to day in the number of sheep which show signs and in the severity of the signs observed. Even after sheep are removed from the pasture the clinical state may deteriorate and, although some appear to recover, clinical signs can usually be elicited by forcing them to exercise. Deaths are reported to continue for 1 week after removal of sheep from toxic pasture and clinical signs of the nervous form of the disease may persist for as long as 2 months. The extraordinary situation is recorded where new cases continued to occur for as long as 12 weeks after sheep were moved onto pasture which contained no *Phalaris* spp.

In cattle the signs may be restricted to stiffness of the hocks and dragging of the hind toes but severe cases similar to the common syndrome in sheep also occur. Additional signs observed in cattle include an extraordinary incoordination of the tongue and lips in prehension so that the hungry animal trying desperately to eat can only prehend a few stalks of grass at a time. The movements are quite strong, but the tongue stabs and darts and lacks the sinuous curling movements normally present. There may also be an inability to put the muzzle to the ground so that prehension can only be effected from a raised manger or hayrack.

Clinical pathology

Laboratory tests on antemortem material are of no value in diagnosis.

Necropsy findings

Exhaustive histological examinations have not been carried out and gross lesions are absent. Degeneration of spinal cord tracts and of the ventral portion of the cerebellum has been observed in the nervous form of the disease but is not a consistent finding (2). Abnormal greenish pigmentation of tissues occurs in the renal medulla and the brain stem and midbrain.

In the 'sudden death' or cardiac syndrome sheep are usually found dead on their sides with their heads strongly dorsiflexed and legs rigidly extended. Some sheep have bloodstained nasal discharges and many have been frothing at the mouth (7). Abdominal visceral congestion, epicardial and duodenal hemorrhages are present and indicate acute heart failure.

Diagnosis

The association between the disease and the plants should suggest the diagnosis. The appearance of signs only on exercise is significant, suggesting a functional rather than a physical lesion. Poisoning caused by *Claviceps paspali*, perennial ryegrass, marshmallow, stagger weed and other plants produces a very similar syndrome and the diagnosis must depend on the identification of the toxic plant.

Treatment

Flocks of affected sheep should be removed immediately from the toxic pasture.

Control

No preventive measures are available against the acute form of the disease but the nervous form can be prevented by the oral administration of cobalt.

Affected pastures may be grazed if sheep are dosed with cobalt (at least 28 mg per week) at intervals of not more than a week, or if alternative grazing is provided in rotation. Dosing at too long intervals or with inadequate amounts may account for some failures in prevention. The parenteral administration of cobalt or vitamin B_{12} is not effective. The additional cobalt can be provided by drenching the sheep individually or spreading it on the pasture mixed with fertilizer as described under cobalt deficiency.

REFERENCES

(1) Simpson, B. H. et al. (1969) *NZ vet. J.*, *17*, 240.
(2) Gallagher, C. H. et al. (1966) *Aust. vet. J.*, *42*, 279.
(3) Kerr, D. R. (1972) *Aust. vet. J.*, *48*, 421.
(4) Gallagher, C. H. et al. (1964) *Nature, Lond.*, *204*, 542.
(5) Rendig, V. V. et al. (1970) *Crop Sci.*, *10*, 682.
(6) Moore, R. M. et al. (1967) *Aust. J. biol. Sci.*, *20*, 1131.
(7) Gallagher, C. H. et al. (1967) *Aust. vet. J.*, *43*495.
(8) Kennedy, D. J. et al. (1986) *Aust. vet. J.*, *63*, 88.

POISONING CAUSED BY PERENNIAL RYE-GRASS (*LOLIUM PERENNE*) (RYE-GRASS STAGGERS, MIGRAM)

Two distinct syndromes occur in animals on rye-grass dominant pastures, one of liver damage and photosensitization, and one of incoordination. The former is caused by a fungus growing on the rye-grass and is dealt with under the heading of poisoning caused by *Pithomyces chartarum*.

Etiology

Knowledge about the cause of rye-grass staggers has changed dramatically during the past decade. It is now known to be caused by tremorgenic mycotoxins produced by the endophytic fungus *Acremonium lolii* (13). The mycotoxins are intensely fluorescent complex indoles called lolitrems (10). Lolitrem B is the abundant one and lolitrems A, C and D are present in only small quantities. The endophytes grow in the plant tissues and are also present in the seeds. Different cultivars of perennial rye-grass vary in their degree of contamination by the endophyte, some, such as Nui and Ruanui carry only 30% infection whereas Yatsyn and Droughtmaster are 100% infected. *A. lolii* produces another metabolite peramine that is repellent to insect pests especially the devastating Argentine stem weevil (3, 7). *A. lolii* also has an ameliorating effect on the growth of the plants that it infests causing increases in dry matter production of 30–40% (12). This may be due to the deterrent effect on insect pests.

Epidemiology

Rye-grass staggers occurs chiefly in New Zealand but also to a limited extent in Australia and Great Britain. The incidence is extremely variable depending on climatic conditions. Rye-grass staggers affects a variable number of animals (5–75%) but causes few, if any, deaths. Sheep, cattle, horses and wapiti deer (4) are all affected.

Rye-grass staggers occurs most commonly in the autumn but when the grass is dry and short and making only a small amount of slow growth. A sudden fall of rain and rapid growth of the grass is followed by disappearance of the disease. For this reason facial eczema and rye-grass staggers do not occur together in the same flocks at the same time. Lolitrems A and B are present in high concentrations in the seeds of *L. perenne* and feeding the seed to sheep causes rye-grass staggers syndromes (11). Rye-grass staggers has also occurred in horses fed on the cleanings of perennial rye-grass seed; heavier cleanings containing more seed were more toxic than the husk-rich cleanings (6).

Pathogenesis

Because of the transient nature of the disease, the nervous signs in rye-grass staggers are presumed to be caused by a functional derangement of nervous tissue. The disease produced experimentally by the administration to sheep of material containing the tremorgenic mycotoxin penitrem A is very similar to naturally occurring rye-grass staggers (4). Fine tremor, manifested as muscle fasciculations, is followed by coarse tremor causing movement of the head and body. The tremor is enhanced by movement. There is incoordination with a bounding gait, and abnormality of postural reflexes leading to lateral recumbency, or sternal recumbency with the hindlegs stretched out behind. Eating and drinking are unaffected. There are no diagnostic lesions except in prolonged cases and the disease is likely to be a reversible biochemical toxicosis (4).

Bulls grazing toxic rye-grass pastures have lower than normal blood levels of testosterone (8) and sheep make lower weight gains than normal (9).

Clinical findings

In sheep the disease occurs commonly in animals in very good bodily condition. In mild cases signs are observed only on driving, the limbs being moved without flexion of the joints, so that the gait is bounding. In severe cases the animal is unable to make any movement without the legs becoming extended and abducted causing it to fall. Tetanic convulsions follow. If the sheep are left undisturbed they appear to recover, get up and move off, only to repeat the performance within a few yards. In extreme cases the sheep are permanently prostrate.

In cattle the syndrome is similar to that which occurs in sheep. There is some nodding of the head at rest and occasionally head tremor, but the convulsions are more severe and flexion of the limbs is more marked than extension.

In horses there is tremor, hypersensitivity, and a reeling, drunken gait which may proceed to posterior paralysis. Recovery occurs in a few days when the animals are moved to new pasture. Horses and cattle affected mildly are unable to move quickly because of limb and trunk stiffness and a tendency to fall. Turning is achieved only with difficulty. The signs are not apparent when the animals are grazing, occurring only when they are disturbed.

Clinical pathology

There are no tests available which aid in the diagnosis of rye-grass staggers. Heinz-body anemia is common in cattle grazing rye-grass but its significance in relation to rye-grass staggers is unknown.

Necropsy findings

The necropsy findings in rye-grass staggers include macroscopic pallor of skeletal muscles and focal areas of hyaline necrosis on histological examination. Degenerative lesions of Purkinje cell neurones are described in longstanding cases (5).

Diagnosis

Rye-grass staggers resembles many other functional diseases of the nervous system especially those caused by poisonous plants. Nervous syndromes caused by *Claviceps paspali*, *Phalaris aquatica* and rough-bearded grass (*Echinopogon ovatus*) are very similar to rye-grass staggers.

Treatment

Livestock should be immediately removed from affected pasture but no treatment is required since spontaneous recovery is rapid.

Control

Sheep and cattle should not be allowed to graze potentially toxic pasture for more than 2–3 hours a day unless it is more than 30 cm high. Supplementation of the diet with vitamin E, vitamin A and minerals has had no effect on the incidence of the disease.

REFERENCES

(1) Gallagher, R. T. (1981) *NZ vet. J.*, *29*, 189.
(2) White, E. P. et al. (1980) *NZ vet. J.*, *28*, 123.
(3) Prestidge, R. A. et al. (1985) *NZ agric. Res.*, *28*, 87.
(4) Mackintosh, C. G. (1982) *NZ vet. J.*, *30*, 106.
(5) Mason, R. W. (1968) *Aust. vet. J.*, *44*, 428.
(6) Munday, B. L. et al. (1985) *Aust. vet. J.*, *62*, 207.
(7) Rowan, D. D. & Graynor, D. L. (1986) *J. chem. Ecol.*, *12*, 647.
(8) Peterson, A. J. et al. (1984) *NZ vet. J.*, *32*, 36.
(9) Fletcher, L. R. & Barrell, G. K. (1984) *NZ vet. J.*, *32*, 139.
(10) Gallagher, R. T. et al. (1981) *NZ Vet. J.*, *29*, 189.
(11) Gallagher, R. T. et al. (1982) *NZ Vet. J.*, *30*, 183.
(12) Latch, G. C. M. et al. (1985) *NZ J. agric. Res.*, *28*, 165.
(13) Fletcher, L. R. & Harvey, I. C. (1981) *NZ vet. J.*, *29*, 185.

Poisoning caused by miscellaneous grasses

WIMMERA RYE-GRASS (*LOLIUM RIGIDUM*)

Nematode larvae which infest the seedheads of Wimmera rye-grass (*Lolium rigidum*) and chewing fescue (*Festuca rubra commutata*) resemble the sclerotia of ergot but are much harder. Sheep and cattle grazing infested grass, provided the nematode (*Anguina lolii*) is accompanied by the appropriate bacteria (*Corynebacterium* sp.), are poisoned, with the development of a characteristic clinical picture. The original view was that the poisoning was caused by toxins in galls produced by the nematode larvae, but it is now known that the poison is a glycolipid corynetoxin which originates from galls containing a yellow-pigmented *Corynebacterium* sp. (2). It is capable of causing cerebral vascular lesions in experimental animals (6). The technique of assaying the toxicity of a suspected stand of pasture has been described (19). A similar tunicamycin has been isolated from water-damaged wheat which when fed to pigs caused clinical signs and deaths similar to those caused by corynetoxin (32).

The disease has become a very important cause of death losses on farms in western Australia and is also recorded in South Africa (1). Pasture improvement based on annually alternating crop–pasture rotations seem to predispose to the disease, with the worst outbreaks occurring after the end of a cropping year. This can be avoided by burning the pasture in the autumn. It is introduced onto farms by the introduction of infested grass seed or agricultural implements contaminated with it. The standing grass becomes toxic as soon as the seed head appears, and loses the toxicity as soon as heavy rain falls. Hay made from infested grass remains poisonous for 5–6 years. Sheep are not commonly affected, probably because of their more selective grazing habits (4).

The clinical signs include tremor, nystagmus, opisthotonus and ataxia, convulsions, and a high mortality rate. Multiple hemorrhages and abortion also occur. The nervous signs are precipitated by driving. During recumbency there may be other nervous signs including neck ventroflexion, opisthotonus, head nodding, extension of limbs, tetanic and clonic convulsions and, in sheep, posterior extension of the hindlimbs. Some sheep can get up and move about between such episodes, but the gait is either stiff, swaying or jumping. Such animals soon go down again and death occurs in up to 24 hours. Additional signs include nystagmus, dyspnea, frothing at the mouth and tachycardia. The diagnostic lesion is perivascular edema, particularly in cerebellar meninges, in animals with appropriate nervous signs which have had access to wimmera rye parasitized by the nematode (18). Other lesions include significant liver damage, and hemorrhages in most tissues (5). Further cases occur for up to 10 days after affected animals are removed from the pasture (3). Attempts at controlling the development of the nematodes have been unsuccessful (30) and there are no practicable means of controlling the disease. A high recovery rate has been demonstrated after the treatment of experimentally affected sheep. The treatment was with chlordiazepoxide (20 mg/kg body weight), a tranquilizer (20). Injections of magnesium sulfate have given temporary relief in the early stages but have no significant effect on the outcome of the disease (5).

MILLET AND PANIC GRASSES (*PANICUM SPP.*)

Panicum effusum, *P. miliaceum* and possibly *P. decompositum* (native millet), *P. coloratum* (Kleingrass) (21), and other *Panicum* spp. (cereal millet) contain hepatotoxic substances which cause liver damage and photosensitization in sheep. Photosensitive dermatitis is the major manifestation but it may be accompanied by jaundice and other signs of liver insufficiency in severe cases giving rise to the colloquial name of 'yellow bighead'. The plants are most toxic when young and growing rapidly.

TALL FESCUE GRASS (*FESTUCA ARUNDINACEA*)

There are two major diseases caused by this grass, fescue summer toxicosis and fescue foot, and these and the minor syndromes listed below may or may not be related etiologically (10).

Fescue summer toxicosis

Fescue summer toxicosis or summer slump is an unaccountable poor production syndrome manifested by a fall in milk production or a failure to grow adequately in fat cattle, both in the presence of what looks like an optimum amount of nutritious pasture. The same poor weight gain is experienced by steers fed on fescue seed (16). In cattle grazing at pasture the depressing effect on production is made worse by environmental temperatures above 31°C (87°F) (23). Affected cattle show hyperthermia with temperatures as high as 40·5°C (104·5°F) dyspnea, hypersalivation, inappetence, and rough coat and they may seek out water in which to stand (9, 24). The syndrome is related to the presence of loline mycotoxins and the fungus *Epichloe typhina*. *Acremonium coenophialum* (syn. *Sphacelia typhina*), a very similar fungus, has also been identified as the cause (22, 28). The lowered milk yield is accompanied by low blood levels of prolactin. These levels can be significantly increased by the administration of metoclopramide, a dopamine antagonist (31). There is a great deal of variation in the toxicity of different varieties of the grass; KY-31 is most toxic, Kenhy, Mo-96 and Kenmont are intermediate and Fawn is least toxic. The disease has also been observed in animals fed on hay made from affected pastures and the active principle has been extracted from the hay (11).

Control of the disease can be effected by growing endophyte-resistant varieties, by rotating cattle through fescue and other grass and clover varieties. Treatment of parental plants with the fungicide benomyl produced seed and resulting pasture with the reduced infection rate and lower toxicity for cattle grazing it (17). Oral administration of thiabendazole just before the cattle go onto the toxic pasture prevents the onset of signs. The recommended regimen is a dose rate of 5 g/45·5 kg body weight repeated every 7 days (12).

Epidemic hyperthermia An increasing number of incidents have been reported in cattle in which hypersalivation is the most obvious presenting sign. This is accompanied by hyperthermia. The prevalence in the herd is virtually 100%. One of the known causes is tall fescue poisoning. Another is poisoning with *Claviceps purpurea*.

Fescue foot

Fescue foot also occurs in cattle which are grazing pasture dominated by tall fescue, usually within 10–14 days of being turned onto the pasture. Cattle permanently pastured on the field do not appear to be affected and horses appear to be able to graze it with impunity. The lesions and clinical signs include severe lameness followed 2 or more weeks later by gangrene and sloughing of the extremities especially the digits and to a less extent the tail. There is a close similarity to the disease caused by the ingestion of *Claviceps purpurea* and ergot may be present on fescue (*Festuca octoflora*) so that the specific cause of gangrene of the extremities of goats may not be capable of decision (29). The incidence in a herd may be as high as 10%. The lesions are thought to be caused by vasoconstrictive agents in the mycotoxins but no specific toxin has been identified. In freezing temperatures frostbite may be a complicating factor. New cases may continue to appear for up to 1 week after removal from the affected pasture. The grass heads are commonly infested by *Claviceps purpurea* but the disease occurs in its absence and the toxic principle is distinct from ergot.

Miscellaneous diseases

Mares grazing on tall fescue pasture may suffer from agalactia after foaling (15). There is no adverse effect on the udder which is normal in subsequent lactations. A high incidence of rectally palpable fat necrosis is recorded in cattle grazing fescue that has been heavily fertilized with nitrogen (14).

BERMUDA OR COUCH GRASS (*CYNODON DACTYLON*) AND BLUE COUCH GRASS (*CYNODON INCOMPLETUS*)

Both of these grasses have been known, in some circumstances, to cause hydrocyanic acid poisoning. A disease of cattle characterized chiefly by nervous signs has also been attributed to the consumption of Bermuda grass but may be caused by the *Claviceps* sp. fungus which commonly infests the grass. The disease has also been reproduced experimentally in goats (26). Bermuda grass is a common pasture grass and is eaten readily and without danger under most conditions.

ROUGH-BEARDED GRASS (*ECHINOPOGON OVATUS*)

Ingestion of this grass when it is in the early, flowering stages causes incoordination and convulsions in lambs and calves. Affected animals nod their heads continuously while standing still. The limbs are stiff, the animals bounding rather than running. On exercise they go down and have clonic convulsions during which they bawl with pain. The respiration rate is rapid and there is marked sweating and hypersensitivity. Recovery occurs if the animals are moved from the pasture for a few days.

KIKUYU GRASS (*PENNISETUM CLANDESTINUM*)

Kikuyu grass is very extensively grown as a pasture plant in many countries and it is only recently that there have been reports of poisoning from it. The reports come from New Zealand and southern Australia and at first the poisoning was attributed to lactic acid indigestion, but the more recent suggestion is that it is a poisoning caused by the fungi *Myrothecium verrucaria* spp. and *Phoma herbarum* growing on the grass (14), an unlikely cause in some outbreaks (7).

The disease occurs in sheep and cattle in late summer and autumn (7, 15). There is depression, salivation, abdominal pain, ruminal tympany and stasis, paralysis of the tongue and pharynx, sham drinking, fine muscle tremor, incoordination, recumbency, diarrhea, cyanosis of mucosae and dehydration. In the forestomachs there is distension, mucosal reddening and extensive necrosis in the rumen and abomasum (8). Epidemiologically the disease occurs concurrently with circumstances conducive to fungal growth, including warmth, moisture, and litter under the grass, often due to the depredations of heavy infestations with army caterpillars (*Pseudoletia separata*).

YELLOW BRISTLE GRASS (*SETARIA LUTESCENS*)

This grass carries heavy bristles (13) which cause mechanical stomatitis in cattle and horses. Affected horses are slow eaters, refuse to eat hay and show excess salivation. There are proliferative and ulcerative lesions at the gumtooth margins and at the mucocutaneous junction of the lips. Individual lesions are up to 25 mm diameter. There are obvious plant fibers in the lesions. After careful cleaning up, the lesions heal slowly over about 3 weeks.

Setaria sphacelata is an Australian grass which contains sufficient oxalate to cause oxalate poisoning under which heading the disease is described.

YELLOW OAT GRASS (*TRICETUM FLAVESCENS*)

Enzootic calcinosis caused by this grass is discussed under the heading of poisoning by *Solanum malacoxylon* (page 1343).

REVIEW LITERATURE

Bryson, R. W. (1982) Kikuyu poisoning and the army worm. *J. S. Afr. vet. Assoc.*, *53*, 161–165.

Hemken, R. W. et al. (1984) Toxic factors in tall fescue. *J. anim. Sci.*, *58*, 1011–1016

REFERENCES

(1) Schneider, J. (1981) *Onderstepoort J. vet. Res.*, *48*, 251.
(2) Vogel, P. et al. (1981) *Aust. J. exp. Biol.*, *59*, 455.
(3) Richards, I. S. (1982) *Aust. vet. J.*, *58*, 115.
(4) Martinovitch, D. S. & Smith, B. (1972) *NZ vet. J.*, *20*, 169.
(5) Berry, P. H. et al. (1982) *Res. vet. Sci.*, *32*, 148.
(6) Finnie, J. W. & Mukherjee, T. M. (1986) *J. comp. Pathol.*, *96*, 205.
(7) Newsholme, S. J. et al. (1983) *Onderstepoort J. vet. Res.*, *50*, 157.
(8) Heerden, J. van der, et al. (1978) *J. S. Afr. vet. Assoc.*, *49*, 27.
(9) Hemken, R. W. et al. (1979) *J. anim. Sci.*, *49*, 641.
(10) Hammond, A. D. et al. (1982) *Bov. Practnr*, *17*, 137.
(11) Williams, M. et al. (1975) *Am. J. vet. Res.*, *36*, 1353.
(12) Farnell, D. R. et al. (1975) *J. envir. Quality*, *4*, 120.
(13) Linnabary, R. D. et al. (1986) *J. equ. vet. Sci.*, *6*, 20.
(14) Stuedemann, J. A. et al. (1985) *Am. J. vet. Res.*, *46*, 1990.
(15) Heimann, E. D. et al. (1981) *Proc. 7th Equ. Nutr. Physiol. Symp.*, p. 62.
(16) Jackson, J. A. et al. (1984) *J. anim. Sci.*, *58*, 1057.
(17) Jackson, J. A. et al. (1981) *J. dairy Sci.*, *64* (Suppl), p. 152.
(18) Berry, P. H. et al. (1980) *Aust. vet. J.*, *56*, 402.
(19) Stynes, B. A. et al. (1979) *Aust. J. agric. Res.*, *30*, 201.
(20) Norris, R. T. et al. (1981) *Aust. vet. J.*, *57*, 302.
(21) Muchiri, D. J. et al. (1980) *J. Am. vet. med. Assoc.*, *177*, 353.
(22) Lyons, P. C. et al. (1986) *Science USA*, *232*, 487.
(23) Hemken, R. W. et al. (1981) *J. anim. Sci.*, *52*, 710.
(24) Brookbanks, E. D. et al. (1985) *NZ vet. J.*, *33*, 57.
(25) Davis, C. B. et al. (1983) *Vet. hum. Toxicol.*, *25*, 408.
(26) Strain, G. M. et al. (1982) *Am. J. vet. Res. 43*, 158.
(27) Cornell, C. N. et al. (1982) *J. anim. Sci.*, *55*, 180.
(28) Jackson, J. A. et al. (1984) *J. dairy Sci.*, *67*, 104.
(29) Hibbs, C. M & Wolf, N. (1982) *Mod. vet. Pract.*, *63*, 126.
(30) McKay, A. C. et al. (1982) *Aust. J. agric. Res.*, *34*, 403.
(31) Kitzman, J. V. et al. (1986) *Mississippi vet. J.*, Fall, p. 13.
(32) Bourke, C. A. (1987) *Aust. vet. J.*, *64*, 127.

Pasture and cultivated legumes

SWEET CLOVER POISONING

Sweet clover poisoning is caused by the ingestion of moldy sweet clover hay or silage which contains dicoumarol. It is characterized by extensive hemorrhages into tissues and severe blood loss after injury or surgery.

Etiology

Coumarol is a normal constituent of sweet clover (*Melilotus alba*) and is converted to dicoumarol (dicoumarin or bishydroxycoumarin) through the action of molds. Not all moldy sweet clover hay or silage contains dicoumarol and the degree of spoilage is no indication of the toxicity of the hay sample. Varieties of sweet clover differ in their content of coumarol and thus in their potential toxicity. For example, the Cumino variety has a low, and the Arctic variety a high, coumarol content (1). The disease can occur in all species but is most common in cattle. Sheep are less susceptible, clinicopathological evidence of toxicity occurring on diets containing 10 mg/kg of dicoumarol. However, significant changes in clotting time do not occur on diets containing less than 20–30 mg/kg. Similar changes commence to occur in lambs and calves when the dietary intake of dicoumarol rises to above 2 mg/kg body weight (1). *Melilotus indica* (Hexham Scent or King Island Melilot) also contains a dicoumarol-like substance and hay containing the plant can be highly toxic (2).

Sweet vernal grass (*Anthoxanthum odoratum*) may also contain dicoumarol, and when fed to cattle may cause a hemorrhagic syndrome similar to that caused by moldy sweet clover (12).

Epidemiology

The disease is recorded most commonly in North America where sweet clover is grown fairly extensively as a fodder crop. Sweet clover is a popular high yielding legume forage. It is drought-resistant and is valuable in soil improvement, silage, hay and pasture production and a prized crop for the honey producer. It is the most saline-tolerant of the legumes and is particularly useful on saline 'white alkali' soils where cereals and other crops cannot grow (10). The occurrence of the disease has brought the plant into some disfavor and the disease incidence has been greatly reduced for this reason. Severe losses may occur when affected animals are dehorned or castrated.

It is difficult to make sweet clover hay without the development of mold because of the succulent nature of the plant, and the heaviness of the stems and the degree of spoilage is directly related to the moisture content of the cut material. Grazing the crop is not dangerous but the presence of dicoumarol in moldy sweet clover ensilage has been reported (3). Sweet clover is an excellent silage crop because of its high forage yield and it is usually harvested as silage rather than hay. The dicoumarol concentrations in sweet clover hay bales, hay stacks or silage may vary widely (11). The concentrations are highest in small bales; round bales contain more than hay stacks, and the levels are low in sweet clover silage (11). Properly cured silage contains low levels because of the anaerobic conditions which exist in silage; dicoumarol-producing fungi require oxygen. The levels of dicoumarol are highest in the outer parts of hay bales, presumably because they are exposed to moisture. There is no difference in the dicoumarol levels between crimped and non-crimped hay (11).

The toxic level of dicoumarol in moldy sweet clover feed samples is approximately 20 mg/kg of feed (14). Hay containing 10–20 mg/kg dicoumarol can be fed safely for at least 100 days; 30 mg/kg caused illness after 4 months of feeding and 60–70 mg/kg caused illness after only 17–23 days (14). Clinical signs may appear without apparent precipitating cause but trauma and surgery are often followed by deaths from hemorrhage. Migrating warble larvae are also suspected of precipitating fatal hemorrhages (4). Newborn calves may die of the disease during the first few days of life when their dams have been fed affected hay without the dams being clinically affected (5). There is a record of the occurrence of the disease in a horse (9).

In affected herds the morbidity rate is about 12% with a case fatality rate of 65% (13). Aborted fetuses and calves less than 2 weeks of age may be affected most often in some herds. The disease occurs most commonly in western Canada during the winter months from January to April when stored feed is fed to cattle. In beef cattle, large or small hay bales are most commonly implicated, while in dairy cattle silage may be the primary source of moldy sweet clover.

Pathogenesis

Dicoumarol interferes with the synthesis of vitamin K-dependent coagulation factors VII, IX, X and prothrombin. Inadequate synthesis of these factors results in impaired fibrin stabilization of platelet plugs and affected animals are subjected to internal and external hemorrhage and anemia. The degree of hypoprothrombinemia is directly related to the amount and duration of dicoumarol ingestion. Large extravasations of blood into tissues may provide signs of disease because the pressure exerted on internal organs. Large hemorrhages in the pelvic cavity and broad ligament of postpartum cows often delay uteral involution and shedding of fetal membranes.

Clinical findings

Extensive hemorrhages into subcutaneous tissues, intermuscular planes and under serous surfaces cause pain and discomfort. The hemorrhages may be visible and palpable but are not painful or hot and do not crepitate. They may cause stiffness and disinclination to move. There are no signs of toxemia, the affected animal continues to eat well and the temperature, respiration and heart rate are normal until the terminal stages. Accidental and surgical wounds cause severe bleeding but hemorrhages in the mucosae and from the orifices seldom occur except for nosebleed in an occasional animal. Newborn calves may become weak from internal or external hemorrhages within a few hours of birth.

When the loss of whole blood is severe signs of hemorrhagic anemia appear. The animal is weak, the mucosae pallid, the heart rate increases, and the absolute intensity of the heart sounds increases markedly.

Clinical pathology

Severe anemia with markedly increased clotting and prothrombin times are characteristic of the disease. Extension of prothrombin times occurs before there is any increase in clotting time and the former is therefore a useful prognostic test.

Coagulation assays for sweet clover poisoning are as follows.

Bleeding time

This test lacks precision in animals and unless grossly prolonged must be rigidly controlled to be meaningful. It would also be difficult to do this test on several animals in a herd.

Whole blood clotting time

The Lee-White method is preferred and is conducted as follows:

- Obtain at least 3 ml of blood in a plastic syringe by careful venepuncture
- Place 1 ml of blood in each of three 10 × 75 mm tubes
- After 2 minutes, one of the three tubes is gently tipped at 1 minute intervals until the blood is clotted
- Next tip another tube in the same manner
- The elapsed time between appearance of blood in the syringe and clotting in the second tube is the clotting time
- Most cattle should clot between 3 and 12 minutes.

The capillary tube method is less precise than the Lee-White method. A skin puncture is made and after wiping away the first drop a large plain capillary tube is filled with blood. The tube is broken every 30 seconds until a strand of fibrin is detected. Bovine blood should clot within 15 minutes.

Prothrombin time

The prothrombin time is the preferred test when sweet clover toxicity is suspected because impaired coagulation can be detected prior to clinical evidence of hemorrhage. The test should be performed by a laboratory whose technologists are familiar with the procedure. Before obtaining samples the laboratory should be contacted to ensure proper scheduling of the tests and use of the correct anticoagulant.

The prothrombin time measures the time required for fibrin clot formation in recalcified fresh citrated plasma after addition of tissue thromboplastin *in vitro*. If the samples cannot be presented in the laboratory within 30 minutes the plasma should be removed and frozen.

The prothrombin time in normal cattle is less than 15 seconds although some variation may occur between laboratories. It is prolonged in sweet clover poisoning because coumarins interfere with synthesis of the vitamin K-dependent coagulation factors within hepatocytes. These factors are prothrombin, and factors VII and X which result in a long prothrombin time.

Dicoumarol analysis

Representative samples of suspected feed should be submitted for analysis of the content of dicoumarol.

The analysis for dicoumarol is complex and often it is difficult to detect any dicoumarol in a sample of forage being consumed by cattle clinically affected with the disease. Two obvious reasons for this are failure to take a representative feed sample, or the inability of the assay to detect the presence of dicoumarol. Samples should be taken from at least two bales of the suspected hay (11).

The quantitative determinations of dicoumarol levels in blood and tissues of affected animals especially aborted fetuses and newborn calves in which there may have been inadequate opportunity for clinical examination are now possible (13) but normal and toxic ranges must yet be determined.

Necropsy findings

The common lesions include: subcutaneous hemorrhages and large hematomata in areas where normal activity produces mild contusion such as the flanks, carpal and tarsal joints and the side of the body where the animal exerts pressure while lying down; hemorrhages of the peritoneal surface of the rumen; massive retroperitoneal hemorrhage around the kidneys; and absence of hemorrhages in the lungs, kidneys, pancreas and adrenals. The carcass is pale and there is no intravascular hemolysis, jaundice, hemoglobinuria or hemosiderosis.

Diagnosis

A similar syndrome has been recorded after poisoning by some molds which occur on feeds. Extensive subcutaneous extravasatons of blood and serum also occur in purpura hemorrhagica but this disease is uncommon except in the horse and rarely affects more than one animal in a group. The clotting and prothrombin times are not abnormal, the defect being one of vascular damage. Other extensive subcutaneous swellings such as those caused by angioneurotic edema are not usually accompanied by an anemia. There is some similarity between sweet clover poisoning and poisoning by bracken fern and trichloroethylene-extracted soybean meal.

Treatment

Feeding of the suspected hay or silage should be stopped immediately. New cases may continue for up to about 6 days after the first case is recognized, presumably because of the persistent effect of the ingested dicoumarol. Animals with clinical evidence of severe hemorrhage should be given a whole blood transfusion at the rate of 10 ml/kg body weight. This will usually return the prothrombin time to normal within several hours.

Vitamin K_1 (naturally occurring vitamin K) is an effective antidote for sweet clover poisoning (6, 15). A single dose of vitamin K_1 at a rate of 1·1–3·3 mg/kg body weight intramuscularly is effective in restoring the prothrombin times to within normal range within 24 hours in cattle which have been fed moldy sweet clover hay containing 90 mg/kg of dicoumarol (15).

Vitamin K_3 (synthetic vitamin K), menadione sodium bisulfite, in either the injectable or oral form, is available for both treatment and prevention, but is not as effective as vitamin K_1.

Vitamin K_3 is metabolized within 30–40 minutes when given intravenously compared with several days for vitamin K_1. At the present time the vitamin K_3 sterile injection is used by veterinarians for the treatment of sweet clover poisoning in cattle, but no clinical or pharmacokinetic studies have been done in cattle to substantiate its use. The currently available vitamin K_3 is intended for use in dogs, cats and horses as an aid in the treatment of hypoprothrombinemia related to injury or destruction of the biliary tract and intestinal disorders interfering with normal alimentary absorption and hepatic injury. Dosage rates have not been determined for cattle, but 2–11 mg/kg body weight given intravenously, intramuscularly or subcutaneously every 10–12 hours has been recommended for dogs, cats and horses. In cattle, experimentally given a measured amount of dicoumarol daily, the oral administration of a large dose of vitamin K_3 (5000 mg to steers weighing an average of 373 kg) reduced the prothrombin time markedly within 24 hours, followed by a rebound increase for 2 days and then a gradual return to normal in 6–8 days (8). However, the dicoumarol administration was also stopped on the same day of the vitamin K administration and the prothrombin times in dicoumarol-fed animals which did not receive vitamin K also returned to normal within 1 week after cessation of the dicoumarol. This illustrates the beneficial effect of withdrawing the toxic feed and the persistent effect of ingested dicoumarol which may last several days. This necessitates that oral vitamin K_3 be repeated daily for several days until recovery is apparent. The oral form of vitamin K_3 is available in powder form and daily doses are dispensed and administered in gelatin capsules.

The use of the oral form of vitamin K as a supplement in feed of cattle consuming moldy sweet clover has been considered. Vitamin K_3 fed at a level of 500–1000 mg/day to cattle (373 kg body weight) consuming 500–1000 mg of dicoumarol daily provided some moderate control of prothrombin times compared to cattle receiving only dicoumarol (8). However, the levels of dicoumarol consumed by cattle ingesting moldy sweet clover are probably highly variable from day to day and the beneficial effect of a uniform daily dose of vitamin K may be unreliable. Large daily doses of 10 g per animal (500 kg body weight) may be protective, but clinical trials are necessary before such a recommendation can be substantiated.

Control

Sweet clover forage must be carefully prepared, and not fed if it is damaged or spoiled during curing. Moldy portions of hay or silage should be discarded and representative samples of suspected feed should be submitted for analysis of dicoumarol content.

If the disease is suspected, discontinue the feed immediately. After 3 weeks, the sweet clover forage may be fed alone, but preferably mixed with another type of unspoiled roughage at the rate of one part sweet clover to three parts unspoiled feed. This may be continued for 2 weeks after which time the sweet clover should be discontinued completely for 1 week. The removal of suspected feed for about 1 week is considered sufficient time to allow the prothrombin times to return to normal. Following 1 week off, the feed may be fed for 2 weeks, followed again by 1 week off. If a problem still persists, a 1 week on, 1 week off feeding regime should be followed.

Suspected feed should not be fed for at least 3 weeks before surgery such as castration or dehorning. Pregnant cows should not receive sweet clover during the last 3 weeks of pregnancy.

REVIEW LITERATURE

Friedman, P. A. (1984) Vitamin K dependent proteins. *New Engl. J. Med.*, *310*, 1458–1460.

REFERENCES

(1) Williams, G. F. (1965) *J. dairy Sci.*, *48*, 1135.
(2) Wignall, W. N. et al. (1961) *Aust. vet. J.*, *37*, 456.
(3) White, W. J. et al. (1954) *Can. J. agric. Sci.*, *34*, 601.
(4) Meads, E. B. et al. (1964) *Can. vet. J.*, *5*, 65.
(5) Fraser, C. M. & Nelson, J. H. (1959) *J. Am. vet. med. Assoc.*, *135*, 283.
(6) Radostits, O. M. et al. (1980) *Can. vet. J.*, *21*, 155.
(7) Linton, J. H. (1963) *Can. J. anim. Sci.*, *43*, 344, 353; *44*, 76.
(8) Goplen, B. P. (1980) *Can. vet. J.*, *21*, 149.
(9) McDonald, G. K. (1980) *Can. vet. J.*, *21*, 250.
(10) Goplen, B. P. (1980) *Can. vet. J.*, *21*, 149.
(11) Benson, M. E. et al. (1981) *Am. J. vet. Res.*, *42*, 2014.
(12) Pritchard, D. G. et al. (1983) *Vet. Rec.*, *113*, 78.
(13) Blakley, B. R. (1985) *Can. vet. J.*, *26*, 357.
(14) Casper, H. H. et al. (1983) *Proc. Ann. Mtg Am. Assoc. vet. Lab. Diag.*, *25*, 41.
(15) Alstad, A. D. et al. (1985) *J. Am. vet. med. Assoc.*, *187*, 729.

Poisoning caused by miscellaneous legumes

SUBTERRANEAN CLOVER (*TRIFOLIUM SUBTERRANEUM*)

A special form of infertility has been observed in sheep grazing pasture dominated by subterranean clover. The infertility is caused by the high content of estrogenic substances in the leaves of the plant. Of the isoflavones or phytoestrogens which occur it is formononetin which is the most active biologically and the risk of a pasture can be determined by its chemical assay. The various strains of the clover vary greatly in their estrogenic activity. Thus Dinninup, Dwalganup and Yarloop are very active while Clare, Mt Barker, Bacchus Marsh, Daliak, Northam A and Woogenellup are poorly active and Geraldton occupies an intermediate position (1). Pastures containing the first three varieties cannot be considered as safe if they comprise more than 30% of the pasture. A number of environmental factors affect the concentration of the important isoflavones in the pasture. They are much higher when the soil is deficient in phosphorus. In the search for other factors affecting estrogenic potency it has been observed that clover leaves that are entirely red or have red margins have a much higher content of estrogenic isoflavones than green leaves (3). It is assumed that the leaf redness is due to a viral infection.

One of the difficulties encountered in research work on phytoestrogens in ruminants has been the different results obtained by chemical analysis, by laboratory biological assay and by assay in ruminants in long-term grazing experiments. Ruminants are now known to develop ruminal detoxication mechanisms against some phytoestrogens and not others.

Plants which have matured in the field and set seed have no estrogenic potency, but the making of potent fodder into hay causes little depression of estrogen content. Clover ensilage can contain high levels of estrogens and the ensiling process is considered to increase the estrogenic effect of clover 3–5 fold (7). The clover is most potent estrogenically in the spring, and sheep eating a lot of the plant at this time can become temporarily infertile, but are normally fertile again by the usual breeding season in the autumn. However, ingestion of the plant in several successive years causes 'permanent clover disease'—infertility from which ewes do not recover. The disease is important only in sheep. Cattle are generally considered to be unaffected but the subject is still a controversial one with the weight of evidence against cattle being affected. Horses appear to be able to graze the toxic pasture without ill-effects.

The most commonly observed abnormality is a failure to conceive even with multiple matings, and the flock breeding status worsens progressively, with the lambing percentage falling from a normal 80% down to 30%. Under these conditions sheep farming becomes unprofitable and large areas of country have been made unsuitable for sheep raising by this disease. Although there are records of temporary infertility in sheep which were grazing subterranean clover pastures in most cases the infertility is permanent and affected sheep moved to other pastures do not recover. The demonstration and duration of estrus may be normal, or it may be depressed (5), and the defect is one of sperm transport (11) due to changes in the composition of cervical mucus, and the structure of cervical glands. The change is to a more watery mucus and this is the basis of a test in affected sheep in which the watery mucus is more readily absorbed by a cottonwool plug inserted in the vagina. The increased weight of the plug is a positive test. At necropsy there is severe cystic degeneration of the endometrium. Similar clinical and histopathological changes have been produced by the daily injection of 0·03 mg of diethylstilbestrol per ewe for a period of 6 months. There is also a long-term change in the cervix with an increased incidence of cervicitis and a histologically observable transformation to a uterine-like appearance. In ewes on a long-term intake of toxic pasture there are additional external signs of elevation of the tailhead and partial fusing of the vulvar labia and clitoridal hypertrophy (10).

In affected flocks there may also be a high incidence of maternal dystocia due to uterine inertia, or failure of the cervix or vagina to dilate (8). Affected ewes show little evidence of impending parturition and many full-term fetuses are born dead. Because of the similarity between this form of the disease and the disease 'ringwomb' in ewes in the United Kingdom it has been suggested that the latter may be caused by an excessive intake of phytoestrogens (14). The mortality rate in lambs may be as high as 40%, and 15–20% of ewes may die of metritis and toxemia. Uterine prolapse may also occur in unbred and virgin ewes and in mature ewes some months after lambing. The incidence of prolapse is usually 1–2% but may be as high as 12%. There is marked udder development and copious milk secretion in the ewes. Wethers may also secrete milk, and metaplasia of the prostate and bulbourethral glands is evident. These can be detected at an early stage of development by digital rectal palpation. Continuing hyperplasia and cystic dilatation of these glands causes their prolapse in a subanal position, followed by rapid weight loss and fatal rupture of the bladder. Rams usually show no clinical abnormality and their fertility is not impaired. However, there is one record of lactation in rams grazing subterranean clover-dominated pasture, without apparent effect on fertility.

It is possible that a good deal of the infertility seen in ewes on improved clover pasture may be caused by its high estrogen content, in spite of the absence of the more dramatic evidence of hyperestrogenism described above. Because of the necessity to utilize this pasture a great deal more needs to be known about the seasonal occurrence of the estrogenic substances and the management of sheep grazing the pasture so that the effects of the disease can be minimized. One of the major difficulties in field investigations has been the absence of a suitable method of estrogen assay. Increase in the length of the teats of wethers has been used as a method (17).

The syndrome seen in cattle is manifested clinically by anestrus and by swelling of the vulva and lactation in maiden heifers.

Another syndrome caused by subterranean clover and unrelated to the infertility syndrome is that of obstructive urolithiasis in sheep, discussed under that heading. This disease occurs in outbreaks in spring in merino wethers grazing estrogenic strains of the clover. As the isoflavone concentrations in the plants rise the daily excretion of phenols and acid-precipitable material in the urine increases, and so does the occurrence of obstruction by the characteristic soft yellow calculi containing benzocoumarins (18).

Prevention of clover disease can only be achieved by proper management of sheep and pasture to avoid ingestion of excessive amounts of estrogens. Vaccination with a phytoestrogen–immunogenic protein conjugate has produced good levels of antibodies but has not been successful in preventing the problem (12).

WHITE CLOVER (*TRIFOLIUM REPENS*)

This clover is in widespread use as a pasture plant and although it may contain significant amounts of hydrocyanic acid, acute poisoning due to this substance does not occur in pastures dominated by the clover. However, the high cyanide content may contribute to a high incidence of bloat, and of goiter in lambs. The plant, in contradistinction to Ladino clover, does not have a high content of estrogens. However, when heavily infested with fungi it can contain significant amounts (19). It is believed that the production of estrogens is a byproduct of the plant's mechanism of resistance to the fungal infection.

LADINO CLOVER (*TRIFOLIUM REPENS*)

Ladino clover, a large-growing variety of white clover, may contain large quantities of a highly active estrogen (coumestrol), and when it dominates a pasture and is grazed when the pasture is lush it may cause cornification of vaginal epithelium and functional infertility in ewes.

RED CLOVER (*TRIFOLIUM PRATENSE*)

Three estrogenic compounds have been isolated from red clover and where this plant dominates the pasture a clinical syndrome similar to that caused by subterranean clover may be observed. Ewes grazing on red clover pasture, especially a toxic cultivar of the plant, may have their conception rate at the first mating cycle reduced from 75% to as low as 25% (35). One of the features of the infertility which occurs in ewes is its reversibility, ewes which have grazed estrogenic red clover pasture for 21–33 days returning to normal fertility 3 weeks or more after being removed from the pasture (21). However, permanent sterility due to cystic hyperplasia of the endometrium can result from prolonged exposure. Cows can ingest large amounts of estrogens (over 40 g/day/cow) in red clover without showing any reduction in reproductive efficiency (37).

LUPINS (*LUPINUS ANGUSTIFOLIUS* AND *L. VARIUS*)

Lupins are grown extensively to provide protein-rich feed in winter months. The green plants are usually safe to feed, but the dried mature plants can be toxic in several ways:

- A nervous syndrome caused by alkaloids in the seeds. The toxicity varies between varieties of lupins and within the variety in different years, depending on the climate
- An hepatic syndrome—lupinosis—caused by fungi (e.g., *Phomopsis leptostromiformis* and *P. rossiana* (23)) growing on the plant. The degree of infestation determines the crop's toxicity
- A congenital series of deformities in calves—the 'crooked calf syndrome'
- Intermittent photosensitization due to previous hepatic injury
- Myopathy
- Pregnancy toxemia/ketosis in fresh cows
- Possibly precipitation of an acute episode of copper poisoning (25, 26).

In the *nervous* form of the disease convulsive episodes occur in which there is staggering, falling, clonic convulsions, dyspnea and frothing at the mouth, the signs often appearing only with exercise. There is no liver damage and the mortality rate varies from very low to as high as 50%.

Lupinosis is the commoner of the two syndromes. It is characterized clinically by anorexia, depression, loss of body weight and jaundice. Photosensitization is not uncommon. Death may occur within a few days of first illness or be delayed for months, affected animals standing immobile for long periods or wandering aimlessly, often dying from misadventure. Recovery may occur if animals in the early stages of the disease are taken off the dangerous pasture but severely affected animals usually die. At necropsy there is jaundice and the liver is mottled, friable and bright yellow in color in acute cases, and small and fibrotic in chronic cases. Spongy transformation of the brain has been recorded in naturally occurring cases and has also been produced experimentally (16). Affected sheep also have a higher hepatic concentration of copper and selenium and a lower concentration of zinc, due to necrosis of liver cells (22). This affinity for copper may lead to the development of a complicating chronic copper poisoning in affected sheep. It is evident that many cases of illness in the pregnant and recently calved cows that have been diagnosed as lupinosis are cases of pregnancy toxemia or fat cow syndrome.

Cattle and especially sheep are most commonly affected, probably because of their greater exposure. Most occurrences are animals which graze lupin stubble in which there is dry foliage, seed pods and seeds. The disease occurs also in sheep fed only on the seeds (36), and has also occurred in pigs fed ground lupin seeds (27). Poisoning of horses occurs, but rarely (28). The disease is common in Europe, Australia, New Zealand and South Africa.

Factors which increase the chances of poisoning caused by fungal infestation of the mature plants include the following: summer rain is conducive, but not essential; toxic lupins remain poisonous for several months; the provision of alternative feed, and the presence of other plants, including weeds, in a crop may reduce its toxicity. Similarly, if good quantities of lupin seed are available either still on the standing plant or spilled onto the ground there is less chance of poisoning. The mature stalks are the most poisonous so that a heavy stocking rate which encourages the ingestion of all parts of the plants increases its prevalence. Stubble from which lupin seeds have been harvested is the most common source of fungal poisoning on this plant. The stems of the plant are most toxic and some varieties are much more susceptible to fungal infections than others (13).

Prevention of the disease is assisted by restricting grazing on mature, standing, dry plants during warm, humid weather which favors fungal growth, by avoiding copper supplementation near danger periods and by encouraging the administration of cobalt. Hay made from lupins appears to be free of toxicity and this may be a useful technique in the prevention of the disease (9). Fungistatic agents, such as Benomyl, are also sprayed onto lupins to reduce fungal growth but no specific recommendations have been made (30). Additional protection may be gained by the oral administration of zinc which has been shown to reduce the severity of liver damage caused by lupins/fungal poisoning, but commercial application of this knowledge is not yet possible, partly because of the toxicity of the administered zinc (20). It is advisable to be wary at all times when grazing mature lupin crops. If they are used the crops should be inspected regularly for evidence of fungal infection. If this does occur livestock should be permitted to have access for short periods only, and alternate and supplementary feed should be available (32).

The *crooked calf syndrome* occurs principally in the western United States and the consumption of lupins, especially *Lupinus sericeus*, is thought to be the cause. An alkaloid, anagyrine, is thought to be the specific cause (31). It has been identified in 14 species of lupins, and a grazing program designed to avoid access to the plants during the susceptible period of pregnancy (days 40–70 in cows) is recommended. Toxic plant concentrations are those above 1·44 g/kg dry matter of anagyrine (6). In some cases the alkaloid may be contained in an aphis, *Aphis craccivova*, infesting the plant (33). It seems likely that there is a similarity of action to the effects produced by aminoacetonitrile, a lathyrogen, or an extract of *Lupinus caudatus*, both of which produce fetuses with excessive flexure, malpositioning, malalignment and rotation of limbs. (31). Hemimelia in lambs may be due to grazing on Australian Blue lupin stubble (sand plain lupin, *Lupinus consentinii*) (41, 42).

Calves with the crooked calf syndrome show arthrogryposis or torticollis and scoliosis or both, and occasionally cleft palate. The dam is most susceptible between the 40th and 70th day of gestation. Affected calves bear a marked similarity to those reported under the heading of manganese deficiency. The possibility of a lupin-associated *myopathy* being caused by lupins has been raised because the prevalence of enzootic muscular dystrophy appears to be much higher on lupin than on other pasture (16). Lupins are low in selenium and vitamin E content, and classical white muscle disease may also occur. Histological and biochemical examination of affected calves discount myopathy as the primary lesion (43).

Pregnancy toxemia/ketosis in cows recently calved also appears to be more common if the cows are grazing lupins because the stresses of early lactation, probable nutritional stress, are worsened by hepatic insufficiency (2).

Reducing the toxicity of lupin stubbles has been achieved by spraying them with 4–8% of sodium hydroxide solution and leaving them ungrazed for 3 weeks (2). The treatment also increased the digestibility of the material in the stubble. There is a good reduction in the incidence of lupinosis with this treatment but when the feed is heavily infested animals may still die.

LUCERNE OR ALFALFA (*MEDICAGO SATIVA*)

Lucerne may, in certain circumstances, such as water damage, produce photosensitization in all animal species due probably to the transient occurrence of a photodynamic agent. It has also a high bloat-producing potential and may contain sufficient estrogens to cause infertility. This appears to be due to a depression in ovulation rate of the ewes. The lambing rate may be as low as 38% (29).

BURR TREFOIL (*MEDICAGO DENTICULATUM*)

Natural pastures may be dominated by this plant especially in the spring when luxuriant growth occurs. Large amounts of the plant may be eaten by all animal species and photosensitization may result. Skin lesions disappear quickly when animals are taken of the pasture and there is no liver damage or permanent after-effects. The photosensitive dermatitis was thought at one time to be due to the aphids which commonly infest the plant in very large numbers. Aphids do contain large amounts of a photodynamic agent and may be important in some outbreaks of the disease. Medics, particularly annual varieties, may also contain significant amounts of estrogens. *Medicago littoralis* and *M. truncatula* are the most active varieties and the most potent portions of the plants are the mature leaves of dry pasture (34).

ALSIKE CLOVER (*TRIFOLIUM HYBRIDUM*)

Alsike clover causes photosensitization in all animals but whether this is due to the presence of a photodynamic agent in the plant or to liver damage and accumulation of phylloerythrin is not clear. In horses alsike clover poisoning is associated with signs of liver disease including jaundice, dullness, staggering and blindness and gross enlargement of the liver.

Alsike clover is a converter plant for molybdenum and, in areas where the molybdenum content of the soil is above normal, grazing on the clover may contribute to the development of clinical molybdenosis in animals.

KALEY-PEA OR WILD WINTER PEA (*LATHYRUS HIRSUTUS*)

This plant is often sown with grasses to provide early spring grazing. In late spring, signs of toxicity may occur in cattle grazing mature plants bearing seed pods. Pain in the feet is the most evident sign, affected animals being lame, sitting with the feet under the body and showing a marked disinclination to rise.

HAIRY VETCH (*VICIA VILLOSA*)

This is a weedy legume which causes poisoning in cattle manifested by dermatitis commencing on the tailhead, udder and neck and then spreading to other parts of the body. There is alopecia, formation of a yellow-brown crust and pruritus (38). Conjunctivitis and eyelid edema occur in some. Rarely there is hypersalivation, nasal discharge, and in advanced cases diarrhea and dysentery (39). The mortality rate averages 50% and at postmortem examination there are multiple extensive eosinophilic cellular infiltrations in many organs. A similar disease is recorded in cattle grazing a *V. villosa* hybrid with *V. dasycarpa* (40) and a similar disease is recorded in cattle grazing an actively growing sward of *V. dasycarpa* (15). A number of other less well-known syndromes are caused by *Vicia villosa* and other vetches. They include cyanide poisoning, photosensitization, a bellowing–ataxia–convulsions syndrome and one of subcutaneous swellings, alopecia, cyanosis, purulent nasal discharge, coughing, dyspnea and a low mortality rate (40).

REVIEW LITERATURE

Bickoff, E. M. (1968) *Oestrogenic Constituents of Forage Plants*, Commonwealth Agricultural Bureaux Review Series, No. 1.

Gardiner, M. R. (1967) Lupinosis. *Adv. vet. Sci.*, *11*, 85.

Keeler, R. F. (1984) Teratogens in plants. *J. anim. Sci.*, *58*, 1029–1030.

REFERENCES

(1) Rossiter, R. C. (1970) *Aust. vet. J.*, *46*, 141.
(2) Allen, J. G. et al (1986) *Aust. vet. J.*, *63*, 350.
(3) Thain, R. I. & Robinson, E. C. (1968) *Aust. J. Sci.*, *31*, 121.
(4) Adams, N. R. (1986) *Aust. vet. J.*, *63*, 279.
(5) Adams, N. R. (1979) *Aust. vet. J.*, *55*, 481.
(6) Davis, A. M. & Stout, D. M. (1986) *J. Range Mtg.*, *39*, 29.
(7) Ludewig, C. (1973) *Mh VetMed.*, *28*, 853.
(8) Adams, N. R & Nairu, M. E. (1983) *Aust. vet. J.*, *60*, 124.
(9) Allen, J. G. et al. (1979) *Aust. vet. J.*, *55*, 38.
(10) Adams, N. R. (1979) *Aust. vet. J.*, *55*, 22.
(11) Lightfoot, R. J. et al. (1974) *Aust. J. biol. Sci.*, *27*, 409.
(12) Cox, R. I. (1984) Plant toxicology symposium. *Proc. Brisbane, Australia*, pp. 98–108.
(13) Arnold, G. W. et al. (1978) *Austr. J. exp. Agric.*, *18*, 92.
(14) Ward, W. R. (1975) *Vet. Ann.*, *15*, 75.
(15) Peet, R. L. & Gardner, J. J. (1986) *Aust. vet. J.*, *63*, 381.
(16) Allen, J. G. & Nottle, F. K. (1979) *Vet. Rec.*, *104*, 31.
(17) Braden, A. W. H. et al. (1964) *Aust. J. agric. Res.*, *15*, 142.
(18) Parr, W. H. et al. (1970) *Aust. J. agric. Res.*, *32*, 933.

(19) Wong, E. et al. (1971) *NZ J. agric. Res.*, *14*, 633.
(20) Allen, J. G. & Masters, H. G. (1980) *Aust. vet. J.*, *56*, 168.
(21) Morley, F. H. W. et al. (1966) *Aust. vet. J.*, *42*, 204.
(22) Allen, J. G. et al. (1979) *Vet. Rec.*, *105*, 434.
(23) Allen, J. G. et al. (1983) *Aust. vet. J.*, *60*, 206.
(24) Allen, J. G. (1981) *Aust. vet J.*, *57*, 212.
(25) Gardiner, M. R. (1966) *J. comp. Pathol.*, *76*, 107.
(26) Gardiner, M. R. (1967) *Aust. vet J.*, *43*, 243.
(27) Marczewski, H. (1955) *Med. vet. Varsovie*, *211*, 738.
(28) Gardiner, M. R. & Seddon, H.D. (1966) *Aust. vet. J.*, *42*, 242.
(29) Scales, G. H. et al. (1977) *Proc. NZ Soc. Anim. Prod.*, *37*, 149 & 152.
(30) Wood, P. McR. et al. (1975) *Aust. vet. J.*, *51*, 381.
(31) Keeler, R. F. (1976) *J. Toxicol. envir. Hlth*, *1*, 887.
(32) Croker, K. P. et al. (1979) *Aust. J. agric. Res.*, *30*, 551 & 929.
(33) Mohamed, F. H. A. et al. (1977) *Bull. anim. Hlth Prod. in Africa*, *25*, 184.
(34) Francis, C. M. & Millington, A. J. (1965) *Aust. J agric. Res.*, *16*, 927.
(35) Kelly, R. W. et al. (1980) *NZ J. exp. Agric.*, *8*, 87.
(36) Allen, J. G. et al. (1983) *Aust. vet. J.*, *60*, 206.
(37) Petterson, H. et al. (1984) *Svensk VetTidn.*, *36*, 677.
(38) Kerr, L. A. & Edwards, W. C. (1982) *Vet. Med. SAC*, *77*, 257.
(39) Panciera, R. J. et al. (1978) *J. Am. vet. med. Assoc.*, *148*, 804.
(40) Burroughs, G. W. et al. (1983) *J. S. Afr. vet. Assoc.*, *54*, 75.
(41) Hawkins, C. D. et al. (1983) *Aust. vet. J.*, *60*, 23.
(42) Allen, J. G. et al. (1983) *Aust. vet. J.*, *60*, 283.
(43) Abbott, L. C. et al. (1986) *Vet. Pathol.*, *23*, 734.

Weeds

WEEDS CONTAINING HEPATOTOXINS

All the following plants contain hepatotoxic substances and cause a syndrome of hepatic insufficiency plus photosensitization and, in many instances, marked signs of central nervous system derangement.

Crotalaria	*Crotalaria* spp.
Ragwort or tansy ragwort	*Senecio jacobaea* (1)
Common fireweed	*Senecio lautus* (32)
Other ragworts	*S. tweedii*, *S. burchelli* (8)
Threadleaf groundsel	*S. douglasii* (46)
Tarweed	*Amsinckia intermedia*
Caltrops or puncture vine	*Tribulus terrestris*
Lantana	*Lantana camara*
Heliotrope	*Heliotropum europaeum*
	H. ovalifolium (47), *H. amplexicaule* (54)
Sacahuiste	*Nolina texana*
Horsebrush	*Tetradymia glabrata* (or *canescens*) (2)
Hound's tongue	*Cynoglossum officinale* (38)
Paterson's curse or salvation jane	*Echium plantagineum* (*E. lycopsis*)
Ganskweed	*Lasiospermum bipinnatum* (3)
	Asaemia axillaris (4)
	Indigofera spicata
	Brachyglottis reponda
Zamia	*Cycas* spp.
	Ipomoea carnea
	Lippia spp.
Bog asphodel	*Narthecium ossifragum* (5)
Summer cypress	*Kochia scoparia*, *K. sedifolia*, *K. brevifolia* (49, 52)
	Acanthospermum hispidum (14)
	Capparis tomentosa (17)
	Pteronia pallens (35)
	Athanasia trifurcata (45)

Etiology

Toxic substances are present in all of the above plants, and in all parts of these plants. *Senecio* spp. contain an alkaloid, retrorsine; heliotrope contains two alkaloids, lasiocarpine and heliotrine, and monocrotaline, fulvine and crispatine are present in *Crotalaria* spp. They are all pyrrolizidine alkaloids. They survive for long periods without change in hay but are degraded in ensilage but not to the point where the silage can be considered to be safe for cattle (43). Lantana contains a hepatotoxic substance lantadene A, a terpene compound (6). Other toxic principles are present in *Crotalaria* spp. and cause erosion of the esophageal and gastric mucosae of horses. Affected animals are unable to swallow and may die of starvation. The concentration of pyrrolizidines varies widely between seasons in the same part of the plant and all parts of the plant need to be examined if the content of alkaloids is being assayed.

It is important to know how much of the plant or its toxic alkaloid represents a toxic or lethal dose. There is little definite information except that experimental feeding of ragwort has established that cattle can tolerate up to 1·5% of their body weight during a 15-day period, but that 2% during a 20-day period is lethal (7), but sheep and goats can withstand a diet of 2–3% of the plant (41). The toxic dose of *Senecio brasiliensis* for cattle is 2–4% of body weight for the acute illness (42). Seeds of *Crotalaria retusa* at a rate of 0·1% of the ration are highly fatal, 0·5% reduces feed intake, but levels of 0·1% are safe and should not be exceeded (11).

Epidemiology

Disease caused by the ingestion of these plants occurs in many countries. Ragwort and tarweed poisoning have been recorded most commonly in the United States as a cause of 'walking disease' in horses and cattle. Ragwort causes 'Winton disease' of horses and cattle in New Zealand and, with *Crotalaria* spp. causes 'dunsiekte' of horses in South Africa. *Crotalaria retusa* and *C. crispata* are causes of the disease known as 'walkabout' or 'Kimberley horse disease' in northern Australia, and *C. sagittalis* is suspected as the cause of hepatic fibrosis of horses which occurs commonly in the southeastern United States. *Crotalaria saltiana* causes mortalities in cattle in the Sudan (36). *Crotalaria macronata* has been shown to be poisonous for sheep. Experimental feeding of the leaves of the plant causes sudden death with pulmonary lesions the only prominent finding at necropsy. *Crotalaria spectabilis* was introduced into the southern United States many years ago to act as a soil-binder and improver. It now grows uncontrolled in the area. If the seeds are harvested along with the intended grain harvest the contaminated grain represents a stock hazard. Pigs have been poisoned this way.

Heliotrope causes severe losses in sheep in Australia and is commonly associated with 'toxemic jaundice' in this species causing hepatitis and playing a part in the development of hepatogenous chronic copper poisoning (39). Provided the heliotrope is in a sufficient concentration in the pasture, young cattle can also be affected but the disease is much less common in cattle than in sheep and goats are relatively insusceptible. The disease occurs mostly when livestock graze the standing plant but mortalities have occurred in calves housed indoors and bedded on straw containing the plant which the calves ate (40). Caltrops poisoning is common in South Africa and lantana poisoning in Australia, the Indian subcontinent, Florida, the United States and Mexico. *Echinum plantagineum* poisoning has occurred in sheep, horses, cattle and pigs, in Australia. The monogastric animals are more susceptible, ruminants metabolizing some of the pyrrolizidine alkaloids, principally echimidine, in the rumen (12). Sheep are more resistant to pyrrolizidine alkaloids than cattle; the mechanism of the resistance is not understood but is related in some way to ruminal activity (53). Poisoning by *Myoporum* spp. is reported in Australia and New Zealand. Ganskweed poisoning is reported in South Africa (13). Lantana is a very pungent plant and not very palatable, but in times of famine cattle may eat it in large quantities (15). *Bos taurus* cattle are more susceptible to poisoning by this plant than *Bos indicus* cattle (48). *Tetradymia* sp. is poisonous in its own right, but there is a synergistic interaction with sagebrush (*Artemisia nova*) which makes the plant much more poisonous (16). *Capparis tomentosa*, recorded in the Sudan, causes degenerative lesions in spinal cord and kidney, as well as liver (17). The morbidity rate with all plants is often high and the majority of affected animals die.

Crotalaria spp. have some value as soil-improvers and have been introduced to some areas for this purpose but usually become a pest. These weeds are for the most part not readily eaten by animals, except heliotrope which is not unpalatable, but when other feed is short they may be consumed in quantities sufficient to cause toxic effects. Outbreaks have occurred in animals feeding on silage, hay and pelleted feeds contaminated by *Senecio jacobaea*, and wheat screenings contaminated by the seeds of *Amsinckia intermedia*. Although sheep which eat these plants, especially *Heliotropum europaeum* and *S. jacobaea*, suffer a chronic hepathopathy they are much less susceptible than cattle. Pigs have been poisoned experimentally with *S. jacobaea*, the chief clinical signs being dyspnea and fever.

Narthecium ossifragum causes a disease of sheep in Norway called alveld which is reproducible by the oral administration of saponins from the plant (37). *Kochia scoparia* also contains an antithiamin and may cause polioencephalomalacia (50).

Pathogenesis

The pyrrolizidine alkaloids of *Senecio* and *Crotalaria* spp. have a primary toxic effect on liver parenchyma causing a megalocytosis, and secondarily on centrilobular and hepatic veins causing proliferation of the endothelium and occlusion of the vessels. This venoocclusive effect is characteristic of these alkaloids and does not appear to occur in sheep poisoned by *Heliotropum* spp. Clinical signs do not occur until there is sufficient liver damage to impair its function. Thus, the development of lesions occurs gradually but the onset of clinical signs is usually quite sudden and often some time after the animals have stopped ingesting the toxic material. The relationship between disease of the liver and the nervous signs which are a major manifestation in these diseases is difficult to explain. It is suggested that the hepatic damage interferes with the animal's ability to synthesize urea with a resulting ammonia intoxication of the central nervous system and the elevated levels of ammonia in the blood (and glutamine in the CSF) are directly related to the occurrence of spongy degeneration of the brain of sheep (19). It is known that some pyrrolizidine alkaloids have severe toxic effects on lung (20) and *S. quadridentatis*, which has this effect, is listed elsewhere. Although some pyrrolizidine alkaloid absorbed by cows is secreted into their milk, the amount and composition of it does not give cause for immediate alarm, but goats secrete enough ingested pyrrolizidine alkaloids in their milk to cause liver disease in rats drinking the milk (22). Experimentally induced poisoning by *S. vulgaris* in horses showed a gradual loss of hepatic function as demonstrated by clinicopathological tests. At necropsy the liver damage varied from a hemorrhagic centrilobular necrosis to a fibrotic occlusive lesion in horses that lived longer. Focal myocardial necrosis and edema of the intestinal wall were also evident (34).

In poisoning by *Tribulus terrestris* there is a concurrent hepatic and renal dysfunction and a low-grade intravascular hemolysis and a degenerative disease of the spinal cord of sheep (Coonabarabran disease) is reported elsewhere. A subclinical intoxication by selenium is also thought to contribute to the disease (23). One of the difficulties with this poisoning is the high level of confusion between it and geeldikkop and enzootic icterus. The latest view is that geeldikkop is caused by the simultaneous ingestion of *T. terrestris* and sporidesmin, each of the agents supplementing the toxic effects of the other (21, 29).

Lantana poisoning causes hepatic insufficiency and renal tubular lesions, neither of which are specific (4). The triterpene acids lantadene A and lantadene B are the toxic agents which cause damage to bile canaliculi, gallbladder paralysis and intrahepatic cholestasis. Jaundice, photosensitization and ruminal stasis result (25). One of the principal objectives of treatment must be to prevent further absorption of the toxins from the rumen. In all of these poisonings it is recognized that there is much variation in the toxicity of the plants and it has been shown that the pyrrolizidine content is highest in the preflower (early bud) stage (24).

Clinical findings

Disturbances of consciousness, muscle weakness, jaundice and, to a less degree, photosensitization are the major clinical abnormalities in these diseases.

Cattle

In severe cases of poisoning by *S. jacobaea* in cattle there is dullness with occasional periods of excitability and frenzy, severe diarrhea with straining, staggering and partial blindness. Abdominal pain may be evident and the straining may be sufficiently severe to cause rectal prolapse. Rectal prolapse is recorded as being the most important presenting sign in some outbreaks of the disease (26). The staggering gait is most noticeable in the hindlegs and the feet are dragged rather than lifted. Walking in circles may also occur. The excitability may be extreme, with animals charging moving objects. Jaundice may be present but pallor of the mucosae is more usual. Most acute cases die within a few days but occasional animals linger on for several weeks. In less severe cases of poisoning by *Senecio* spp. there is little or no excitability, and jaundice and photosensitization are more common.

Horses

In horses poisoned by *Senecio* spp. (51) there is profound dullness and depression, the animal standing with the head held down and often ceasing to eat halfway through a mouthful. There is muscle tremor, particularly of the head and neck, frequent yawning and difficulty in swallowing, sometimes to the point where food and water are regurgitated through the nose or aspirated into the lungs. Blindness is apparent and the horse may walk compulsively in circles, or in a straight line for long distances, bumping into objects, becoming wedged in inaccessible situations and being unable to back out, falling into streams and often walking into houses and outbuildings. Head-pressing is common and there may be sudden attacks of frenzy with violent, uncontrollable galloping. Most affected horses die after a period of illness varying from a week to several months.

Pigs

Crotalaria poisoning in pigs is manifested by signs of pneumonia and renal insufficiency. The disease is chronic and progressive, and most affected pigs die (27).

The clinical picture in poisonings caused by other hepatotoxic plants is in general the same as those described above for poisoning by *Senecio* spp. *Lantana* spp. have secondary toxic effects on kidneys causing a terminal nephrotoxicosis, nephrosis and uremia and on alimentary tract smooth muscle causing chronic constipation (28).

Clinical pathology

Liver function tests, liver biopsies and serum transaminase activity have been used to try to predict the outcome of the disease in individual animals. The bromosulfalein test is laborious, but it has been suggested as a practical means of assessing hepatic efficiency of sheep flocks exposed to poisoning with pyrrolizidine alkaloids. Flocks which demonstrate significant hepatic damage are withdrawn from further exposure to the responsible plant (18). As a means of predicting early hepatic damage in cattle having access to ragwort, gamma-glutamyl transpeptidase and glutamate dehydrogenase estimations on serum are recommended (30). For assessment of the degree of damage in chronic cases with a view to deciding which animals should be discarded a bromosulfalein clearance test and a liver biopsy give the best information (44). A rapid simple laboratory method for assessing the hepatotoxicity of a plant sample is available (9).

Necropsy findings

A necropsy picture of progressive destruction of liver cells and replacement fibrosis is common to poisonings by this group of plants.

In acute cases of poisoning there may be inflammation of the abomasum with acute hepatic degeneration and petechial hemorrhages scattered through the subcutaneous tissue and viscera. In more chronic cases there is fibrosis and shrinkage of the liver, ascites, anasarca and inconstantly, jaundice and photosensitization. A renal lesion is also characteristic, and pulmonary epithelialization occurs in some cases. Spongy degeneration of the brain, as referred to above, will not necessarily be a characteristic lesion, but should be of some assistance in diagnosis. It is well-defined histologically and chemically (31).

Diagnosis

This group of plants produces a syndrome which is similar in many ways to primary disease of the nervous system, particularly the encephalomyelitides. In the horse the disease may be mistaken for infectious equine encephalomyelitis except that fever is not present and there may be signs of liver dysfunction. Leukoencephalomalacia caused by eating moldy corn is also similar and may be accompanied by jaundice. Nigropallidal encephalomalacia caused by ingestion of yellow star thistle is another similar disease but affects only the nervous system.

In cattle rabies, lead and coal tar pitch poisoning, herring meal poisoning, and poisoning by other plants may resemble poisoning by these hepatotoxic plants and again the differentiation depends on diagnosis of the presence of primary liver disease and recognition of the toxic plant. In sheep the difficulties in diagnosis are similar except that photosensitization is a frequent sign in these diseases and they must be differentiated from the other causes of photosensitive dermatitis.

Treatment

Treatment is of uncertain value but the provision of a high intake of carbohydrate by forced oral intravenous feeding may help to tide the animal over the period of severe liver dysfunction. Activated charcoal (500 g for sheep, 2–2·5 kg for cattle) by mouth is an effective treatment but should be supported by treatment for dehydration and photosensitization (24).

Control

These plants are toxic at all times and their eradication from grazing areas is the only satisfactory method of controlling the disease. If *Crotalaria* spp. are to be used as soil-improvers *C. giant striata* is preferred to other species because of its lower toxicity. A high carbohydrate diet may aid in preventing the disease in horses and the feeding of molasses and sugar is recommended as a prophylactic measure. With some of these plants significant damage occurs only after prolonged grazing. Thus it is possible, for example with *H. europaeum*, to utilize the plants as fodder provided sheep are grazed on them for only one season. Sheep are relatively resistant to *Senecio* spp. and stocking infested pastures with sheep is suggested as a control measure (33). As a long-term project the selection of pyrrolizidine-resistant sheep is a logical solution to the problem of poisoning by these plants. However, it is unlikely to be any more practicable than the simultaneous feeding of iodoform which significantly delays the onset of poisoning by heliotrope (10).

REVIEW LITERATURE

Adams, S. E. I. (1974) Hepatoxic activity of plant poisons and mycotoxins in domestic animals. *Vet. Bull.*, *44*, 767.

REFERENCES

(1) Johnson, A. E. (1974) *Am. J. vet. Res.*, *35*, 1583.
(2) Pearson, E. G. (1977) *Mod. vet. Pract.*, *58*, 421.
(3) Fair, A. E. et al. (1970) *J. S. Afr. vet. med Assoc.*, *41*, 231.
(4) Coetzer, J. A. W. & Bergh, T. (1983) *Onderstepoort J. vet. Res.*, *50*, 55.
(5) Lakesvela, B. & Dishington, I. W. (1983) *Vet. Rec.*, *112*, 375.
(6) Seawright, A. A. & Allen, J. G. (1972) *Aust. vet. J.*, *48*, 323.
(7) Johnson, A. E. (1978) *Am. J. vet. Res.*, *39*, 1542.
(8) Carrillo, B. J. et al. (1976) *Rev. Med. Vet., Argentina*, *57*, 205, 209, & 213.
(9) Molyneux, R. J. et al. (1979) *J. agric. Food Chem.*, *27*, 494.
(10) Lanigan, G. W. et al. (1978) *Aust. J. agric. Res.*, *29*, 1281.
(11) Ross, A. J. (1977) *J. agric. Sci.*, *89*, 101.
(12) Peterson, J. E. (1984) *Proc. Aust. USA Symposium on Poison Plants, Brisbane*, p. 191.
(13) Thornton, D. J. (1977) *J. S. Afr. vet. Assoc.*, *48*, 210
(14) Bakhita, Ali & Adam, S. E. I. (1978) *J. comp. Pathol.*, *88*, 553.
(15) Yadava, J. N. S. & Verma, N. S. (1978) *Ind. vet. med. J.*, *2*, 1.
(16) Johnson, A. E. (1978) In: *Effects of Poisonous Plants on Livestock*, eds R. F. Keeler et al. New York: Academic Press.
(17) Ahmed, O. M. M. et al. (1981) *Vet. hum. Toxicol.*, *23*, 403.
(18) Lanigan, G. W. & Peterson, J. E. (1979) *Aust. vet. J.*, *55*, 220.
(19) Hooper, P. T. et al. (1974) *Res. vet. Sci.*, *16*, 216.
(20) McLean, E. K. (1970) *Pharmacol. Rev.*, *22*, 429.
(21) Glastonbury, J. R. W. & Boal, G. K. (1985) *Aust. vet. J.*, *62*, 62.
(22) Goeger, D. E. et al. (1982) *Am. J. vet. Res.*, *43*, 1631.
(23) Brown, J. M. M. (1968) *Onderstepoort J. vet. Res.*, *35*, 319.
(24) Johnson, A. E. et al. (1985) *J. Agr. Food Chem.*, *33*, 50.
(25) Pass, M. A. (1986) *Aust. vet. J.*, *63*, 169.
(26) Wiltjer, J. C. & Walker, C. E. S. (1974) *Aust. vet. J.*, *50*, 579.
(27) Hooper, P. T. & Scanlan, W. A. (1977) *Aust. vet J.*, *53*, 109.
(28) Seawright, A. A. (1963) *Aust. vet. J.*, *39*, 340.
(29) Kellerman, T. S. et al. (1980) *Onderstepoort J. vet. Res.*, *47*, 231.
(30) Craig, A. M. (1980) *Am. Assoc. vet. Lab. Diagnosis., Proc. 21st ann. Mtg.*, p. 161.
(31) Hooper, P. T. (1975) *Acta neuropathol.*, *31*, 325, 335.
(32) Walker, K. H. & Kirkland, P. D. (1981) *Aust. vet. J.*, *57*, 1.
(33) Muth, O. H. (1968) *J. Am. vet. med. Assoc.*, *153*, 310.
(34) Qualls, C. W. (1980) *Diss. Abst. Inter.*, *41B*, 2080.
(35) Prozesky, L. et al. (1986) *Onderstepoort J. vet. Res.*, *53*, 9.
(36) Bassi, M. E. S. & Adam, S. E. I. (1981) *J. comp. Pathol.*, *91*, 261.
(37) Abdelkader, S. V. et al. (1984) *Acta. vet. Scand.*, *25*, 76.
(38) Knight, A. P. et al. (1984) *J. Am. vet. med. Assoc.*, *185*, 647.
(39) Seaman, J. T. (1985) *Aust. vet. J.*, *62*, 247.
(40) Harper, D. A. W. et al. (1985) *Aust. vet. J.*, *62*, 382.
(41) Cheeke, P. R. (1984) *Can. J. anim. Sci.*, *64*, (Suppl.) 201.
(42) Tokarnia, C. H. & Dobereiner, J. (1984) *Pesquisa, vet. Brasileira*, *4*, 39.
(43) Candrian, U. et al. (1984) *J. agric. Food Chem.*, *32*, 935.
(44) Klopfer, U. et al. (1981) *Refuah Vet.*, *38*, 88.
(45) Kellerman, T. S. et al. (1983) *Onderstepoort J. vet. Res.*, *50*, 45.
(46) Johnson, A. E. & Molyneux, R. J. (1984) *Am. J. vet. Res.*, *45*, 26.
(47) Damir, H. A. et al. (1982) *Br. vet. J.*, *138*, 463.
(48) Frisch, J. E. et al. (1984) *J. agric. Sci. UK*, *102*, 191.
(49) Sprowls, R. W. (1981) *Vet. lab. Diagnost.*, *24*, 397.
(50) Dickie, C. W. & James, L. F. (1983) *J. Am. vet. med. Assoc.*, *183*, 765.
(51) Giles, C. J. (1983) *Equ. vet. J.*, *15*, 248.
(52) Thilsted, J. et al (1986) *Proc. 14th World Cong. Dis. Cattle*, *2*, 738.
(53) Craig, A. M. et al. (1986) *Israel J. vet. Med.*, *42*, 376.
(54) Ketterer, P. J. (1987) *Aust. vet. J.*, *64*, 114.

Poisoning by *Astragalus* sp.

There are a very large number of species of *Astragalus* (used here to include the genus *Oxytropis*) many of them poisonous, many of them not. Although many of them provide excellent forage, the two genera *Astragalus* and *Oxytropis* spp., contain many plants which are severely destructive. They are all leguminous herbs, most of them perennials. They have the capacity to dominate a pasture, especially the desert range in the spring in the United States. Animals appear to become addicted to them. Toxicity occurs in four ways:

- As selenium converter plants
- Poisonings by 'nitro compounds'
- 'Loco'—a form of madness
- Congenital defects and abortion.

An important characteristic of this poisoning is that the toxin can be secreted in the milk of cows eating the plant (9).

Astragalus *spp. as selenium converter plants*
On seleniferous soils the effective converters (e.g., *A. bisulcatus, A. pattersonii, A. praelongus, A. pectinatus* and *A. racemosus*) accumulate selenium to a much higher level (up to several thousand mg/kg) than in other plants on the same soil. These plants also grow preferentially on soils high in selenium and have some value as indicators of possible toxicity. Their other advantage is that they are, for the most part, unpalatable due to their unpleasant odor. The clinical syndromes produced by selenium poisoning are described under that heading. Because these plants also cause clinical signs referable to the 'nitro compounds' it is thought that they contain toxic compounds as well as accumulating selenium (15).

Poisoning by 'nitrocompounds'
Some species, e.g. *A. emoryanus, A. tetrapterus, A. pterocarpus, A. viser* var. *serotinus, A. m.* var. *oblongifolus, A. hyperphylus* and *A. canadensis*, contain aliphatic nitrocompounds, notably miserotoxin, which is metabolized in the rumen to highly toxic compounds such as 3-nitro l-propanolol and 3-nitro-proprionic acid. These compounds have two toxic effects: liberation of nitrite (1) which causes methemoglobin on absorption (see under nitrite poisoning; and an undetermined compound which produces a group of apparently unrelated effects. Cattle and sheep are both affected, but cattle are the more susceptible. Poisoning may be acute with severe respiratory distress including dyspnea, cyanosis, general weakness, staggery gait and wobbly hindlegs with death in as short a time as 3 hours, but usually as long as 24 hours. Chronic poisoning is also manifested by nervous signs, especially incoordination in the hindlegs which may develop into almost complete paralysis, temporary blindness, drooling of saliva and very loud respiratory stertor. The latter is a more prominent sign in sheep, the former more prominent in cattle. The mortality rate in both forms of the disease is very high. Necropsy lesions are minimal except for some pulmonary emphysema and pneumonia, and increased volume of cerebrospinal fluid. Histopathological lesions include pulmonary alveolar emphysema, bronchiolar constriction, interlobular edema and fibrosis, and in the nervous

system degenerative changes in the spinal cord and peripheral nerves, especially the sciatic nerve. The course of the chronic disease may be as long as several months. A similar syndrome and postmortem picture are recorded in horses poisoned by *O. kansuensis* (17).

'Loco' or locoweed poisoning
Species which have this effect are *A. lentiginosus, A. mollissimus, A. wootonii, A. thurberi, A. northoxys, Oxytropis sericea, O. lambertii, O. soximontana*. The toxic principle in these plants is unknown, but ingestion of the plant by cattle or horses over long periods (at least 2 weeks, up to 8 weeks) causes the development of bizarre nervous signs. These include staggery gait, a staring look from the eyes, extreme nervousness including hypersensitivity to stimuli, and hyperexcitability, making them difficult to handle and impossible to work or ride, isolation from other animals and difficulty in eating and drinking. In time, the animal's coat becomes dry and staring, the animals become thin, then emaciated and die. Removal from the plant is followed by disappearance of signs, but these are visible subsequently if the animal is physically stressed. The disease is essentially irreversible, but there is some evidence of regression with time in both maternal and fetal tissues (2). At necropsy, the diagnostic lesion is extensive vacuolation of tissues, especially the kidney and brain (3). These lesions have been observed in tissues as widely separated as the brain of affected horses (4) and the fetuses of ewes fed on the plant (5).

Abortion and congenital deformity
Abortions in ewes grazing *Astragalus* sp. may be as prevalent as 100%, and they also occur in cows. It is thought to be due to interference by the cytoplasmic vacuolation of chorionic epithelial cells with the transfer of nutrients across the placenta (6). Skeletal malformations occur in the newborn of both sheep and cattle (7), the commonest deformities including lateral rotation of the forelimbs, contracted flexor tendons, flexure and hypermobility of the hock joints and flexure of the carpus. Similar deformities have occurred in foals produced by mares which consumed *A. mollisimus* (14). The deformities either recovered spontaneously or were susceptible to surgical treatment. There were also abortions in the same band of mares.

Miscellaneous other problems
There appears to be an increased prevalence of minor infections in poisoned animals, and there are some indications that *Astragalus* spp. may reduce cell-mediated immune responses (10). A relationship has been demonstrated between the consumption of *Oxytropis sericea* and the occurrence of right-sided congestive heart failure in cattle grazing high-altitude pasture. The disease is clinically similar to altitude sickness (16).

Pathogenesis
There is a similarity between the pathogenesis and lesions of poisoning by *Astragalus* sp. and that caused by *Swainsona* sp. (8), and swainsonine, an alkaloid present in *Swainsona* sp. and some of its derivatives occur in *Astragalus* and *Oxytropis* spp. (11). This alkaloid is now considered to be the principal toxin in the development of locoweed poisoning (13). There is also a similarity in the histopathological lesions caused by *Astragalus* spp. in pigs and those caused by selenium accumulators and selenium poisoning (12). The cytoplasmic vacuoles observed in both species appear to be the result of continued enlargement by lysosomes and the development of acquired, rather than congenital as in mannosidosis, lysosomal storage disease. There is similarity also to the abortifacient and teratological effects of *Lathyrus* and *Vicia* spp. and to the teratological effects of lupins.

REVIEW LITERATURE

James, L. F. et al. (1981) Syndromes of *Astragalus* sp. poisoning in livestock. *J. Am. vet. med. Assoc.*, *178*, 146.

REFERENCES

(1) Williams, M. C. et al. (1979) *Am. J. vet. Res.*, *40*, 403.
(2) Hartley, W. J. & James, L. F. (1975) *Am. J. vet. Res.*, *36*, 825.
(3) van Kampen, K. R. & James, L. F. (1970) *Pathol. Vet.*, *7*, 503.
(4) Harries, W. N. et al. (1972) *Can. vet. J.*, *13*, 141.
(5) Hartley, W. J. & James, L. F. (1973) *Am. J. vet. Res.*, *34*, 209.
(6) Balls, L. D. & James, L. F. (1973) *J. Am. vet. med. Assoc.*, *162*, 291.
(7) James, L. F. et al. (1969) *Am. J. vet. Res.*, *30*, 337.
(8) James, L. F. et al. (1970) *Pathol. Vet.*, *7*, 116.
(9) James, L. F. & Hartley, W. J. (1977) *Am. J. vet. Res.*, *38*, 1263.
(10) Sharma, R. P. et al. (1984) *Am. J. vet. Res.*, *45*, 2090.
(11) Molyneux, R. J. et al. (1984) *Proc. Aust. US Symposium on Poison Plants, Brisbane*, p. 266.
(12) Hartley, W. J. et al. (1984) *Proc. Aust. US Symposium on Poison Plants, Brisbane*, p. 141.
(13) Tulsiani, D. R. P. et al. (1984) *Arch. Biochem. Biophys.*, *232*, 76.
(14) McIllwraith, C. W. & James, L. F. (1982) *J. Am. vet. med. Assoc.*, *181*, 225.
(15) James, L. F. et al. (1983) *Vet. hum. Toxicol.*, *25*, 86.
(16) James, L. F. et al. (1986) *J. Am. vet. med. Assoc.*, *189*, 1549.
(17) Chang, S. et al. (1981) *Acta. vet. Zootechnol. Sinica*, *12*, 145.

Poisoning by *Solanum malacoxylon* (Enteque seco, Manchester wasting disease, naalehu)

Manchester wasting disease occurs in cattle in Jamaica, and similar diseases are recorded as 'Enteque seco' in Argentina, 'Espichamento' in Brazil and 'naalehu' in Hawaii. In Brazil only cattle are affected; in Argentina sheep and possibly horses are also affected. In Europe horses are affected after feeding on *Trisetum flavescens* (9). Pigs appear to be quite resistant (2) and modification of the active principle by ruminants in the rumen to produce the toxic effect is postulated (11). Clinically there is progressive wasting and stiffness of the joints with reluctance to rise or lie down. The stiffness is most severe in the forelegs and the animal stands for long periods with stiff legs and an arched back, the thorax fixed and distended. Heart murmurs are audible and severe distress develops with exercise. Cattle aged 15 months and over may be affected. Regression of the disease occurs when affected animals are hand-fed or are moved to a 'clean' area.

At necropsy the carcass is emaciated and shows anasarca and ascites. Calcification of small blood vessels, patchy edema and pale discoloration of skeletal musculature are evident. Calcification of the coronary arteries, endocardium and aorta occurs commonly and may extend into the large arteries. Calcification is also present in the pleura and in the emphysematous parenchyma of the lung and, in varying degrees, in most other viscera. Degenerative arthritis occurs in the limb joints, and calcification of tendons and ligaments is also present (3).

The cause of the disease has been identified in South America as the ingestion of the weed *Solanum malacoxylon*. Blood levels of calcium and phosphorus are 20–25% above normal. The disease has been produced experimentally and the mode of action of *S. malacoxylon* determined to be a dramatic increase in calcium absorption from the diet. It has in fact a mode of action similar to that of 1,25-dihydroxycholecalciferol, the active principle of vitamin D_3 (7), and the available evidence is consistent with the view that the leaves of *S. malacoxylon* are a potent source of this active metabolite of vitamin D (6). Similar views are also held about *Tricetum flavescens* (10).

A very similar disease has been described in Europe in recent years under the name of 'enzootic calcinosis' (8). On affected farms many animals become affected at about 3 years of age and introduced animals are affected about 1½ years after introduction to the alpine pastures on which the disease occurs. The disease is chronic and may take several years to run its course, and is worst when the animals are at pasture. There is chronic wasting, reluctance to walk, constant shifting of weight from foot to foot. Calcification of vessels is palpable, especially on rectal examination. Serum calcium (up to 3·4 mmol/l) and phosphorus (up to 4 mmol/l) levels are elevated and radiological examination of soft tissues suggests itself as a diagnostic aid. At necropsy examination the calcification of endocardium, vessels generally, lungs and tendons is very evident in advanced cases. It occurs principally on alpine pastures and consumption of a grass, *Tricetum flavescens* or yellow (golden) oatgrass, is the cause (9–11). The plant is common in these alpine pasture. It is most toxic when young, and silage, but not hay, exerts a calcinogenic effect (12). The diet has to include a large proportion (50% or more) of the plant over a long period (5–6 months) before all sheep are affected (1). Heating reduces the toxic effect of *T. flavescens* only slightly, but significantly depresses the toxicity of *S. malacoxylon* (4). It is possible by careful management of the pasture to significantly reduce the occurrence of the disease (13).

Enzootic calcinosis has now been tentatively identified in many countries including Papua-New Guinea, where the causative plant is *S. torvum* (5), Israel, India and South Africa, but a positive diagnosis and accurate identification of the cause are usually not made. *Cestrum diurnum*, which is described elsewhere, produces an almost identical disease in the southern United States.

REFERENCES

(1) Simon, U. et al. (1978) *Dtsch Tieräztl. Wochenschr.*, *85*, 363.
(2) Done, S. H. et al. (1976) *Res. vet. Sci.*, *20*, 217.
(3) Dobereiner, J. et al. (1971) *Pequisa Agropecuaria Brasileira. Ser. Vet.*, *6*, 91.
(4) Ullrich, W. (1979) *Berl. Münch. Tierärztl. Wochenschr.*, *92*, 220.
(5) Morris, K. M. L. et al. (1979) *Res. vet. Sci.*, *27*, 264.
(6) Collins, W. T. et al. (1977) *Am. J. Pathol.*, *87*, 603.
(7) Peterlik, M. et al. (1976) *Biochem. Biophys. Res. Comm.*, *70*, 797.
(8) Dirksen, G. et al. (1970) *Dtsch Tierärztl. Wochenschr.*, *77*, 321.
(9) Kohler, H. (1981) *Zentralbl. VetMed.*, *28*, 187.
(10) Peterlik, M. et al. (1977) *Dtsch Tierärztl. Wochenschr.*, *84*, 253.
(11) Ruckson, B. F. et al. (1978) *Vet. Rec.*, *103*, 153.
(12) Kohler, H. et al. (1978) *Zentralbl. VetMed.*, *25A*, 617.
(13) Libiseller, R. et al. (1978) *Zentralbl. VetMed.*, *25A*, 1 & *26A*, 290.

Miscellaneous poison weeds

Many weeds which occur in cultivation and pasture land are thought to be poisonous in certain circumstances and it is impossible to include them all here. Many countries publish bulletins dealing with the common poison plants of the area and a list of these is provided at the end of this section. In the following list an attempt has been made to group the plants according to the disease syndromes that they produce.

WEEDS WHICH CAUSE PRINCIPALLY NERVOUS SIGNS

Darling pea (Swainsona *spp.*)
This species includes *S. galegifolia*, *S. canescens*, *S. greyana*, *S. luteola*, *S. procumbens*, *S. swainsonoides*. A native of Australia, this plant causes nervous signs including stiffness of the limbs, incoordination and muscle tremor. Unusual postures, particularly a 'stargazing' attitude, are adopted. Terminally, sheep, which are the species most commonly affected, are unable to rise and may die of starvation. Loss of condition is a common and sometimes the only sign. The course is long, sometimes several months long, but death usually follows several weeks after the onset of nervous signs. Addiction to the pea is common. Necropsy findings are restricted to microscopic lesions of vacuolation of cytoplasm in neurones throughout the central nervous system. Vacuolations in cells occur in other organs also. Their presence in circulating lymphocytes may have diagnostic value (2). The plant contains swainsonine, an indolizidine alkaloid, which is an inhibitor of alpha-mannosidase. Ingestion of this toxin causes the lysosomal accumulation of mannoside and the development of a lysosomal storage disease similar to genetically initiated mannosidosis (3). Identical lesions and clinical signs are produced by *S. canescens* (4). The disease is very similar to that caused by *Astragalus* spp. (see above) and swainsonine has been isolated from plants of that genus and from the fungus *Rhizoctonia leguminicola*. Poisoning with Darling pea has also been recorded in cattle in which there are neurological signs similar to those which occur in sheep but in addition there is emaciation and a poor breeding performance (5). The disease is also recorded in horses (6). The lesions are identical with those described in cattle and sheep. Loss of condition, hyperesthesia and excitability are the important clinical signs. There may be abnormality of gait and balance. Ventroflexion of the head, rearing over backwards when stimulated, and defective visions are other observed signs. The resemblance in horses to poisoning with *Indigofera dominii (enneaphylla)* is close, and differentiation needs to be based on identification of botanical specimens and the presence of vacuolated lymphocytes in the leukon of animals affected by *Swainsona* sp. poisoning (4).

Affected animals will recover if removed from access to the plant while they are still in the early stages of the disease. Chronic cases are usually irreversible.

Trachyandra *spp.*
The plants *T. laxa* and *T. divaricata* cause paralysis, with decreased withdrawal reflexes, in ewes and horses (120). The histopathological lesions are those of a lysosomal storage disease (73) and include prominent neuronal pigmentation in the brain and spinal cord (81). The pigment is a lipofuscin.

Romulea *spp., e.g.* Romulea bulbocodium
These cause poisoning in sheep if they dominate pasture so that sheep can eat very little else (7, 8). The two principal manifestations are incoordination and a very low conception rate, down to as low as 20%. If affected sheep are driven they develop incoordination and fall down but are able to walk again within a few minutes. Affected sheep can be detected because they walk with heads elevated above those of other sheep. After 3 or 4 weeks of periodic paralysis the sheep passes into a final stage of recumbency. The many fetal deaths which occur may be the sole explanation for the low birth rate. The plant also causes the development of phytobezoars in cattle which is dealt with elsewhere. The plant grows prolifically in southern Australia and, because of its ability to survive droughts, it comes to dominate pastures in dry autumns in some areas. It is also host to fungal infections which may be as important to the relevant diseases as the plant itself. All the diseases have a strict seasonal and geographical distribution which corresponds with the growth characteristics of the plant. The development of intestinal obstructions, as distinct from the formation of the phytobezoars, probably depends on additional factors such as physical activity and softness of the manure.

Matricaria *spp.*
M. nigellifolia causes cattle to become clumsy and docile and to head-push against fixed objects. There is a histopathologically recognized encephalopathy. The disease is called pushing disease, or snootsiekte. Sheep are resistant to the unidentified toxin in the plant (82).

Redleg, pigweed, red amaranth, Prince of Wales' feather (Amaranthus retroflexus *or* reflexus) *and lambsquarters, fat hen* (Chenopodium album)
Consumption of these weeds, commonly found in pig yards, by feeder pigs unaccustomed to them has been related to a syndrome characterized by trembling, incoordination of the hindquarters, coma and a high mortality (9). A consistent finding on postmortem examination is perirenal edema. There are also degenerative changes in the brain and kidneys (10). In cattle tubular nephrosis causes terminal uremia. *C. album* also contains large amounts of oxalate and may produce hypocalcemia (12). *A. retroflexus* is also often high in oxalate.

Narthecium asiaticum
Cattle grazed on this lily-like plant develop acute renal tubular necrosis, fluid in body cavities, anasarca, oliguria, anorexia, elevation of BUN levels and glycosuria and proteinuria. There is a high mortality rate (86).

Jimson weed, false castor oil plant (Datura stramonium)
This plant contains a nephrotoxin and ingestion of it causes a dry mouth, dilated pupils, tachycardia, partial blindness, polyuria, convulsions, coma and death. In cattle ruminal atony limits the intake (107). The seeds fed to horses in a contaminated meal have caused a similar syndrome (69). The toxic principles on the plant are atropine, hyoscine and hyoscyamine. Poisoning by the plant is unlikely in cattle because of the high toxic dose rate and because the plant is very unpalatable. It is also reported to cause arthrogryposis in piglets when fed to pregnant sows (55).

Larkspur
Tall and small larkspur (*Delphinium* spp.) are both toxic. Experimentally tall larkspur administered to cattle produces muscle tremor, ataxia, recumbency and death from respiratory paralysis (36). Cattle are more susceptible than sheep. The toxic principle is methyllycaconitine which acts as a postsynaptic cholinergic blocker in cattle. Physostigmine appears to be an effective antidote (108).

Sneezeweed (Helenium autumnale)
This is a common weed of wet pastures in eastern North America. Sheep, cattle and horses may be affected, the flowering heads being the most toxic part of the plant. Clinical signs of toxicity include hypersensitivity, incoordination, dyspnea and tachycardia. *Smallhead sneezeweed (H. microcephalum)* contains a toxic lactone helenalin (23). Clinical signs in sheep include salivation, nasal discharge, bloat, severe abdominal pain and diarrhea.

Hemlock water dropwort (Oenanthe cracata)
The roots of this plant contain a poisonous substance which causes severe convulsions similar to those of acute lead poisoning in cattle. Most affected animals die and at necropsy there is hyperemia of the oral and ruminal mucosae and a celery-like odor in the rumen.

Perennial broomweed (Gutierrezia microcephala)
This plant is most toxic when growing rapidly on sandy soils. In the United States it is known to cause acute illness and rapid death, but more commonly it is associated with abortion or the birth of premature, weak calves and retention of the placenta.

Tribulus terrestris
This causes liver damage and the clinical syndrome of jaundice, photosensitization and mental depression and is discussed under that heading. From epidemiological observations it appears to also be the cause of a posterior paralysis of sheep in Australia called also Coonabarabran disease (85). Only adults are affected and only when they graze pure stands of the plant for long periods. The disease is characterized by the slow development of an irreversible asymmetrical weakness of the hindlimbs. *T. micrococcus* (yellow vine) causes a transient ataxia in sheep after prolonged ingestion. Death may result from inanition (102). A related plant species *Kallstroemia* spp. (e.g. *K. parviflora* or watery caltrop; *K. hirsutissima*, hairy caltrop) causes a similar knuckling of the rear

fetlocks followed by recumbency and convulsions in some (103).

Birdsville indigo (Indigophera dominii *or* I. enneaphylla)
Birdsville indigo causes poisoning in horses in desert areas of Australia. All ages and classes of horses are affected and most cases occur in spring and summer with variation in incidence from year to year. The plant is equally poisonous when dry or green, although most cases occur in the spring when the plant is succulent. Animals need to graze the plant for about 10 days before signs appear.

The clinical syndrome, known locally as 'Birdsville disease', is ushered in by inappetence, segregation and somnolence, the animal often standing out in the open in the hot sun when unaffected horses have sought the shade. There is marked incoordination, the front legs being lifted and extended in an exaggerated manner. The hocks are not flexed, causing the fronts of the hind hooves to be dragged on the ground. The head is held in an unnaturally high position and the tail is held out stiffly. There is difficulty in changing direction and incoordination increases as the horse moves. The horse commences to sway and at the canter there is complete disorientation of the hindlegs so that the animal moves its limbs frantically but stays in the one spot with the legs becoming gradually abducted until it sits down and rolls over. Rapid emaciation and labored respiration are commonly seen in acute cases. Terminally there is recumbency with intermittent tetanic convulsions which may last for up to 15 minutes and during which death usually occurs.

A chronic syndrome may develop in some animals subsequent to an acute attack. Affected animals can move about but there is incoordination and dragging of the hindfeet with wearing of the toe, and inspiratory dyspnea may also occur. Detailed necropsy findings have not been recorded but liver changes have been suggested. Supplementation of the diet with arginine-rich protein feeds prevents development of the disease (24). Peanut meal (0·5–1 kg/day) and gelatin provide readily available and cheap sources of arginine. *E. dominii* contains two toxic alkaloids, indospicine, an analog of arginine, and canavanine.

Water hemlock (Cicuta *spp., e.g.* C. douglasii *and* C. maculata)
Many water hemlocks are poisonous. They occur in most countries of the northern hemisphere and have caused losses, particularly in cattle. Initially there is frothing at the mouth and uneasiness followed by tetanic convulsions during which the animal bellows as though in pain. Diarrhea may occur and there may be bloating and spasmodic contractions of the diaphragm. The course is extremely short and death may occur within a few minutes (105).

Poison hemlock (Conium maculatum)
This plant is not as poisonous as *Cicuta* spp. The standing plant may be eaten (90) and severe outbreaks have been recorded in cattle fed on hay containing up to 60% of the plant (45). Clinical signs include trembling, ataxia, coma, and death in respiratory failure. Gastroenteritis with dysentery may occur, and hypersalivation, frequent regurgitation resembling vomiting, and frequent urination and ruminal stasis are also recorded. In pigs the signs include ataxia, tremor, lacrimation, mydriasis, tachycardia, dyspnea and fever. Vision also appears to be impaired (117). Congenital defects of limbs, nervous system and cleft palate of piglets have been related to the consumption of poison hemlock by their sows (26). Experimentally, congenital defects have been produced in calves, but not in lambs or foals (25). The principal defects were arthrogryposis and spinal curvature, coniceine is the teratogen in cleft palate in pigs (77).

Fadogia monticola and four other plants (*Pachystigma* and *Pavetta* spp.) occur in southern Africa and after a period of eating the plant lasting 4–8 weeks sudden death occurs. The causative lesion is myocarditis. The disease is called gousiekte or quick disease.

Rubber vine (Cryptostegia grandiflora)
This poisonous vine causes sudden death in cattle and sheep in north Queensland. After experimental ingestion of the plant sudden death occurs after short periods of vigorous exercise.

Ascelapias labriformis and *A. eriocarpa* are toxic milkweeds which can cause death at the time of eating the plant (28).

Albizia tanganyicensis
The disease occurs naturally in cattle and has been produced experimentally in sheep. Hyperthermia, hypersensitivity, tetanic convulsions and dyspnea are the important clinical signs and at necropsy petechiation in many tissues, pulmonary edema, degenerative changes in myocardium and other organs and in some cases in the brain (29).

Iceland poppy (Papaver nudicaule)
This elegant member of many winter gardens is blamed for causing ataxia and muscle tremor in horses (30) and other species. To their credit is the apparent restriction of their toxicity to the postflowering stage.

White snakeroot (Eupatorium rugosum)
A toxic alcohol, tremetol, is present in this plant which is common in North America. The alcohol is excreted in the milk of cattle which ingest the plant and may cause clinical illness and even death in humans drinking the milk. Severe muscle tremor is characteristic of the disease and is accompanied by salivation, nasal discharge, vomiting and dyspnea. The animal becomes progressively weaker and is finally unable to stand, lapsing into a coma before death. In horses there is heavy sweating, regurgitation of food through the nostrils and the passage of dark, hard feces (74). Depression and hindlimb ataxia may also be present and there may be congestive right heart failure with electrocardiographic abnormalities and extensive mycardial damage (84).

Yellow star thistle (Centaurea solstitialis) *and Russian knapweed* (C. repens)
The disease nigropallidal encephalomalacia of horses is caused by the continued ingestion of large quantities of yellow star thistle and has been recorded in the United States, South America (20), and Australia (34). There is

a sudden onset with difficulty in eating and drinking, varying from complete inability to less obvious defects such as difficulty in prehension, in moving feed back to the molars or in swallowing. A fixed facial expression is common, the mouth being held half-open or the lips drawn into a straight line. Wrinkling of the skin of the lips and muzzle and protrusion of the tongue are present in many cases. Tongue and lip movements are often awkward and persistent chewing movement without food in the mouth, and rhythmic protrusion of the tongue occur. Yawning and somnolence are evident but the horse is easily aroused. Some horses show aimless, slow walking and, in the early stages, transient circling. The gait is not grossly abnormal, a slight stiffness at the walk being the only abnormality except for weakness in the terminal stages. Signs fluctuate in severity for 2–3 days and then remain static until the animal dies or is destroyed.

No major liver lesions are present at necropsy but areas of necrosis or softening are visible macroscopically in the brain, in the globus pallidus and substantia nigra. The lesions are bilateral in most cases. The disease occurs in summer and late autumn in horses on weedy pasture and experimental feeding with thistle plants produces the disease. The plant does not appear to be toxic to ruminants, rodents or monkeys, and is thought to contain an antimetabolite which is specific to the horse (35). Sheep do well on a sole diet of the plant.

Gomphrena celosiodes

Ingestion of this weed causes extensive outbreaks of incoordination in horses in northern Australia. When moving the hindquarters sway and the toes are dragged. The horse is dull, eats little and stands with the feet bunched well underneath the body. If the disease progresses the horse stands with the legs spread wide apart. When movement is attempted the head is pushed forward and the limbs moved uncertainly, and the animal may rear backwards or collapse forward and fall heavily. Completely incoordinated movements are made in attempts to rise. Recovery occurs if ingestion of the plant ceases.

Marshmallow (Malva parviflora), *staggerweed* (Stachys arvencies)

In Australia these plants cause abnormalities of gait in sheep. Signs do not appear until the sheep have grazed affected pasture for some weeks. Exercise provokes the abnormal gait which commences with muscle tremor, weakness and incoordination in the hindlimbs and frequent urination. If the animals are forced to move they go down with extension of the limbs but without convulsions. After a short rest they get up and walk normally again. Removal from the affected pasture usually results in recovery within 3–4 days.

Urginea *sp.*

Urginea sanguinea (syn. *Urginea burkei*) contains a bufadienolide cardiac glycoside, transvaalin, which causes dyspnea, tachycardia, cardiac irregularity, ruminal atony, diarrhea, and posterior paresis (110).

Cotyledon *spp.*

Plants of *Cotyledon*, *Crassula* and *Andromischus* spp. cause cotyledonosis or krimpsiekte characterized by spasmodic contractions especially of the muscles of the neck. The toxic principle is a group of bufadeniolides which are cardiac glycosides (79). The disease in goats is manifested by prostration, weakness, tachycardia and pupillary constriction (80).

Kalanchoe *spp.* (*syn.* Bryophyllum *spp.*)

These herbaceous plants cause scouring, sometimes with tenesmus, plus dyspnea, incoordination, dribbling of urine, lacrimation, lethargy and immobility and cardiac irregularity in calves (70, 101). The toxic agents are bufadienolides which are potent cardiac glucosides and they cause mild to severe multifocal cardiomyopathy in sheep. In Africa, the syndrome is called krimpsiekte. A similar disease with a similar pathogenesis is caused by *Tycelodon* spp. (71). Treatment with atropine and propanolol is effective.

Moraea polystachya

This lily-like plant contains toxic glycosides which cause cardiac irregularities, tachycardia and dyspnea. Activated charcoal is an effective treatment but needs to be repeated. The minimum effective dose of charcoal is 2 g/kg body weight (72).

Baccharis *spp.*

Baccharis spp. including *B. pteronioides* (syn. *B. ramulosa*), *B. glomeruliflora*, *B. halimifolia* cause tremor, stiff gait and convulsions and some deaths in cattle and sheep. *B. coridifolia* is thought to derive its toxicity from a symbiotic relationship with the fungus *Myrothecium* spp. (98).

Ipomoea *spp.*

Ipomoea muelleri is a straggling prostrate vine which contains hallucinogenic compounds of the lysergic acid type and causes poisoning of sheep, and probably cattle, in Australia. Clinical signs include ataxia, posterior weakness, rapid fatigue accompanied by dyspnea, loss of weight and death after a long period of illness. There are no significant lesions at necropsy.

Ipomoea carnea causes nervous signs referable to hepatic necrosis in calves, sheep and goats. Clinically there is weakness, tremor and paralysis (38).

Sarcostemma viminale, Sarcostemma australe *and* Euphorbia mauritanica

Sarcostemma viminale and *Euphorbia mauritanica* in Africa (39) and *S. australe* produce marked nervous signs in sheep, including hypersensitivity, stiffness, incoordination, recumbency, tremor and convulsions. There is also hyperglycemia and a postmortem picture resembling that of *Clostridium perfringens* (type D) poisoning.

Cocklebururs (Xanthium *spp.*)

These annual weeds, especially *X. strumarium* (Noogoora burr, small burdock) and *X. orientale* cause anorexia, prostration, dyspnea, depression, clonic convulsions, opisthotonus and death in sheep, cattle and pigs. The plants, the seeds and the sprouted seeds are all poisonous but the spiny burr seeds are most toxic (75, 106).

Helichrysum *spp.*

H. argyrosphaerum causes blindness and paresis, and

spongy degeneration of the brain in sheep and cattle in South Africa (41), and *H. blandowskianum* (woolly daisy) has caused death and similar brain lesions in cattle in Australia (42).

Tansy mustard (Descurainia pinnata)
This is a poisonous plant affecting all species in the southern United States. Clinical signs are depression, impaired vision, paresis of the tongue and muscles of mastication and swallowing; spasmodic contractions of neck muscles causing head bobbing occur in some animals (43).

Blind grass, candyup poison (Stypandra imbricata)
This causes incoordination and posterior weakness. Blindness is characteristic and is accompanied by dilatation and immobility of the pupil. There is axonal degeneration of optic nerve fibers and the photoreceptor cells of the retina (11). Only the young green shoots are poisonous.

Jessamine (Gelsemium sempervirens)
This is a perennial evergreen vine that causes hypothermia, mydriasis, recumbency and convulsions (116).

WEEDS WHICH CAUSE GASTROENTERITIS AND NERVOUS SIGNS

A very large number of plants cause gastroenteritis manifested by salivation, grinding of the teeth, abdominal pain, vomiting and diarrhea, usually accompanied by muscle tremor, incoordination and convulsions. There are some differences between the syndromes caused by individual plant species but for brevity the common plants are listed below. For greater detail the reader is referred to the extensive reference list at the end of the section.

Spurges	*Euphorbia* spp.
Castor oil bean	*Ricinus communis*
Black nightshade	*Solanum nigrum*
Silver-leafed nightshade	*S. elaeagnifolium*
	Tephrosia apollinea (109).
Cape tulip	*Homeria collina*
Natal yellow tulip	*Homeria glauca*
Cockleburr	*Xanthium orientale*
Death camas	*Zygadenus gramineus*
Timber milk vetch	*Astragalus* spp.
Monkshood	*Aconitum* spp.
Pokeweed	*Phytolacca americana*
	P. dodecandra
Cockles	*Agrostemma* spp. and *Saponaria* spp.
Buttercup	*Caltha palustris* and *Ranunculus* spp.
Dutchman's breeches	*Dicentra cucularia*
Squirrel corn	*D. canadensis*
Indian tobacco	*Lobelia inflata*
Dogbane	*Apocymum* spp.
Laurel	*Kalmia* spp.
Whorled milkweed	*Asclepias verticillata*
Short-crown milkweed	*A. brachystephana* (48)
Meadow saffron	*Colchicum autumnale* (49)
Alfombrilla	*Drymaria arenarioides* (27)
Pingue (Colorado rubber weed)	*Hymenoxis richardsonii*

WEEDS CAUSING MISCELLANEOUS CLINICAL SIGNS

Privet (Ligustrum vulgare)
An unidentified toxin present in the leaves and berries of this hedge plant causes gastroenteritis manifested by diarrhea, vomiting, colic and ataxia (116).

Castor oil plant (Ricinus communis)
The seeds contain a potent toxin, ricin, which causes hepatitis and severe diarrhea.

Bur buttercup (Ceratocephalus testiculatus)
This has caused heavy mortality in sheep at a dose rate of about 10 g green plant/kg body weight (112). Clinical signs include diarrhea, dyspnea and fever in some. At necropsy there is edema of the serosal surface of the ruminoreticulum. The plant's toxicity is thought to be due to its content of the toxic alkaloid ranunculin.

Aristolochia *spp.*
Aristolochia spp. contain an alkaloid aristolochine which appears to be the toxic principle in this plant. In goats *A. bracteata* causes diarrhea, dyspnea, alopecia and hindlimb weakness (104).

Sesbania *spp.*
Sesbania spp., including *S. punicea*, *S. cannabina*, contain saponins and cause diarrhea and food refusal in cattle. There is some confusion in their nomenclature and they are also called *Daubentonia* spp. and *Glottidium* spp.

Citrullus *spp.*
These vines contain bitter irritant substances that cause diarrhea in ruminants, e.g. *C. colocynthis* (syn. *Colocynthis vulgaris*) (115).

Jute (Corchorus olitorius)
The seeds of the jute plant may contaminate other grain and poison pigs causing diarrhea, vomiting and inappetence (78).

Gnidia latifolia
Gnidia latifolia at dose rates of 1–2 kg/body weight causes acute poisoning of cattle manifested by abdominal pain, inappetence, ocular and nasal discharge and diarrhea in some. Chronic poisoning causes loss of condition, anorexia, anasarca, alopecia and leukopenia (95).

Crofton weed (Eupatorium adenophorum (*syn.* glandulosum) *and* E. riparium)
Poisoning by these plants causes pulmonary consolidation of horses. Clinically there is coughing, cyanosis and respiratory distress on exercise. Access to the plant for some months is necessary before the disease develops. Pulmonary fibrosis is the principal lesion (33). The disease is recorded in Hawaii and Australia. *E. riparium* (mist flower) produces similar lesions (88).

Perilla frutescens (purple mint plant) contains toxins similar to ipomeanols produced by the mold *Periconia* sp. on sweet potatoes, and like them produces acute bovine pulmonary emphysema (32).

Crown beard (Verbesina encelioides)
Verbesina encelioides (crown beard) contains glycosides which cause hydrothorax and pulmonary edema in cattle

and sheep, manifested clinically by frothing of the mouth, dyspnea, tongue protrusion and bloat. *Wedelia asperrima* and *Galega officinalis* (goat's rue) (91, 92) have the same pathological and clinical effects.

Cotton fireweed (Senecio quadridentatus)
This has been shown to cause severe respiratory distress and death in cattle in western Australia (50). At autopsy there are changes in the lungs similar to those in atypical interstitial pneumonia, and also hepatic damage.

Halogeton (Halogeton glomeratus), *greasewood* (Sarcobatus vermiculatus), *docks and sorrels* (Rumex *spp.*), *soursob* (Oxalis cernua), Portulacca oleracea, Salsola kali, Trianthema portulacastrum *and* Threlkeldia proceriflora
The leaves of these plants may contain sufficient oxalate to cause oxalate poisoning, which is described under that heading.

Variegated thistle (Silybum marianum), *mintweed* (Salvia reflexa)
Both plants are known to cause nitrite poisoning in ruminants when the plants are lush and growing rapidly but on many occasions cattle can eat them in large quantities without ill-effects.

Seaside or marsh arrowgrass (Triglochin maritima)
These plants cause cyanide poisoning in parts of North America.

St John's wort or Klamath weed (Hypericum perforatum), H. triquetrifolium (31), *lecheguilla* (Agave lecheguilla), *lady's thumb* (Polygonum *spp.*), *bishop's weed* (Ammi majus), *spring parsley* (Cymopterus watsonii (37, 40)), Thamnosma texana (*Dutchman's breeches*)
These plants contain photodynamic agents (hypericin in St John's wort) which cause photosensitive dermatitis when ingested by animals. Sheep and cattle are most commonly exposed. All parts of the plant are toxic when eaten in large quantities. They are not very palatable and most outbreaks occur when the plants are in the young stage and dominate the pasture. Clinical signs may appear within a few days of stock going on to affected fields and usually disappear within 1–2 weeks after removal from the fields. Experimental production of poisoning with *H. perforatum* has shown that the plant contains a primary photodynamic agent (1). There is no evidence of liver damage or loss of hepatic function. *Ammi majus* (18) has the particular characteristic of being photosensitizing by contact, without the need for ingestion, and causes serious lesions in humans.

Thamnosma texana (Dutchman's breeches, blister-weed) contains primary photodynamic agents in the form of linear furocoumarins (psoralens) and is also capable of causing photosensitization by contact but in animals does so by ingestion (89, 97).

Heracleum mantegazzianum (giant hogweed) also contains compounds related to furocoumarin and has caused severe stomatitis in a goat (94).

Skunk cabbage, western hellebore, false hellebore or wild corn (Veratrum californicum)
This plant is unusual among poisonous plants in that its ingestion by ewes on the 14th to 30th day of pregnancy causes severe congenital cyclopean deformities of the head, absence or displacement of the pituitary gland with prolonged gestation, and giantism in their lambs. Similar cyclopean lesions have been produced experimentally in calves and kids (51). Many other defects have been produced experimentally in lambs. Some of them are cleft palate, harelip, syndactyly, various leg deformities, and supernumerary claws. Tracheal stenosis in neonatal lambs resulted from feeding the plant to ewes pregnant for 28–33 days (96). Fetal death and resorption occurs when the plant is fed in the 19th–29th day period of pregnancy. The plant grows naturally in alpine pastures in the United States and contains a number of toxic amines, some of which have been shown to produce the relevant defects if fed to ewes on the 14th day of pregnancy (53). The specific teratogen in this plant is cyclopamine (19). The plant is also toxic for adult sheep causing salivation, purgation, diuresis, vomiting, weakness, cardiac irregularity, dyspnea, cyanosis and terminal convulsions (54).

Salsola tuberculata *var.* tomentosa
This plant has caused prolonged gestation if it was fed to pregnant ewes during the last 50 days of pregnancy (55). There are no signs of toxicosis in the ewes. Affected lambs show atrophy of the pituitary, adrenal and thymus glands. Gestation is prolonged to as long as 213 days, and the fetuses are so large that assistance is essential during parturition. The pelts of karakul sheep are rendered economically worthless by the excessive growth of curly locks. A similar prolongation of pregnancy is recorded in Scottish ewes but the cause was not identified (118).

Wild coffee, coffee senna (Cassia occidentalis) *and* Karwinskia humboldtiana (Corutilin)
These have all attracted attention because of their capacity to cause degenerative lesions in skeletal muscle. In both plants the mature fruits contain the most toxin. Reports of outbreaks of poisoning by these plants come chiefly from Texas, United States. Empirical treatment with selenium and vitamin E had been used but is not recommended because either preparation, especially vitamin E, enhances the poisonous effect of the plant (59). An axonal dystrophy has been observed in the cerebellum and spinal cord and the lesions have a close correlation with clinical signs (60). The clinical picture of coyotillo poisoning (58) in goats includes increased alertness, hypersensitivity, tremor and disturbances of gait such as stiff, stilted movements, hypermetria and terminal recumbency. Patellar and gastrocnemius reflexes disappear. These clinical findings suggest decreased function of peripheral nerves and cerebellum (61).

In coffee senna poisoning (56, 57) the early signs are anorexia and diarrhea and these are followed in horses (15) and goats (52) by hyperpnea, tachycardia, ataxia, staggering and recumbency. At autopsy there is a fatal cardiomyopathy. The muscle lesion is accompanied by marked elevations of SGOT and CPK levels (62). Pigs have been poisoned by *Cassia occidentalis* seeds which contaminated a prepared ration (76).

Ixiolaena brevicompta is also suspected of causing mortality in sheep due to skeletal muscle dystrophy. Cardiac myopathy and nephrosis, hepatosis and degeneration of the central nervous system also occur (17).

Geigeria ornativa
This plant and others of the same genus cause vomition of ruminal contents and stiffness and paralysis of limbs. The causative lesion is a degeneration of muscle fibers (63).

Solanum esuriale
This plant was thought at one time to be the cause of 'humpy back' in sheep in Australia. This appears now not to be so (119). On forced exercise affected sheep show gait abnormalities of stiffness of hindlimbs with shortness of steps. This is followed by an inability to keep walking and the adoption of a peculiar humpbacked stance. The disease occurs only in summer after heavy rainfall. At necropsy there is degeneration of spinal cord tracts.

All *Solanum* sp. plants (64) should be considered as poisonous, but there is little firm evidence about the toxicity of most of them. *Solanum malacoxylon* is dealt with elsewhere (page 1343) and has special characteristics. For most of the members of the genus toxicity takes the form of gastrointestinal irritation plus dysfunction, by way of paralysis, of the nervous system. *S. dimidiatum* in the United States causes a 'crazy cow syndrome' of staggering and incoordination with a selective loss of Purkinje cells from the cerebellum (16). A similar syndrome is caused by *S. kwebense* in South Africa (14), and one by *S. fastigiatum* var. *fastigiatum* in Brazil (83). The latter appears to be an acquired gangliosidosis. It is characterized by cytoplasmic membranous bodies in the Purkinje cells and a syndrome of falling, opisthotonous, nystagmus and extension of the neck and thoracic limbs. The cattle act normally until frightened or disturbed when the signs appear. In mild cases the cattle adopt a straddle-legged posture and their movements are hypermetric. After an attack of several to 60 seconds, the animal returns to normal. Affected animals do not recover but do not die unless by misadventure. The animals can be provoked to have an attack by raising their heads. There are probably other plants, e.g. *S. fastigiatum* var. *acicularium* and *S. bonariensis* that cause this disease which is called *lurubeba*.

Trachymene *spp. ('bentleg')*
'Bentleg' (see also p.1216) is a disease of sheep recorded for many years in eastern Australia. Clinically the disease is characterized by abnormal curvature of the long bones and angulation of the joint cartilages. The lesion appears to result from irregular retardation of growth of epiphyseal plates, thought to be due to the ingestion of plants of *Trachymene* spp. (65). Up to 25% of a flock may be affected and, although some lambs are affected at birth, others are normal until much later.

Desert rice flower, flaxweed, wild flax, mustard weed, broom bush (Pimelea trichostachya, P. simplex, P. altior, P. continual) *and* P. neo-angelica (113)
The disease caused in cattle by this plant has been known in Queensland for many years under the name of 'St George disease', but the cause has only recently been identified. The findings are edema under the jaw and down the brisket, intermittent diarrhea and death. The causative substance in the plant causes constriction of pulmonary venules, pulmonary venous hypertension and right heart failure (66). Inhalation of the powdered plant causes the pulmonary lesion only, ingestion causes the congestive heart failure/pulmonary lesions plus diarrhea. The usual field picture is that cattle graze looking for feed between old dry flaxweed plants and inhale it so that the pulmonary cardiac form is the common one and the commonest occurrence is in summer. There is also a severe anemia shown to be due to a significant hemodilution. Experimentally it has been possible to produce two forms of the disease, the subacute with diarrhea, weakness and anemia as the predominant signs, and the chronic form characterized by circulatory failure as evidenced by anasarca, hydrothorax and cardiac dilatation (46). The toxin is simplexin, an irritant, diterpenoid daphnane ester (114).

The disease is recorded only in cattle. Sheep are resistant under experimental conditions. Fatal necrotic gastroenteritis is produced by feeding *Pimelea* spp. to horses but it is unlikely that they would eat the plant in natural circumstances.

Whiteheads (Sphenosciadium capitellatum)
This alpine pasture plant has caused disease in horses and cattle. It acts in a manner similar to an anaphylactic reaction with pulmonary edema and photosensitization.

Mercurialis *spp.*
Dog's mercury (*M. perennis*) causes gastritis and hemolytic anemia in sheep. *M. annua* has also caused mortality in sheep (67) and calves (22). The pathogenesis of the disease is hemolytic anemia.

Allium validum
Also called wild onion, this causes hemoglobinuria, and a severe hemolytic crisis in sheep and horses (47).

Isotropis *spp.*
These are plants confined in their distribution to Australia. They cause serious kidney damage and fatal uremia in cattle and sheep. *I. forrestii*, and *I. cuneifolia* cause renal tubular necrosis and acute primary renal failure (100). *Anagallis arvensis* also causes mortality in sheep because of its nephrotoxicity (21).

Bitterweed (Hymenoxys odorata), *khaki weed, cape khaki weed* (Inula graveolens) *foxglove* (Digitalis purpurea)
Hymenoxys odorata causes poisoning in sheep in southwestern United States. There is anorexia, salivation, vomiting and lethargy, and at autopsy there is severe pulmonary congestion and hemorrhage. Hemorrhages are also present in most other tissues. Subacute poisoning characterized by congestion and mucosal erosion of the forestomachs and abomasum has also been produced experimentally. The toxicity of the plant can be reduced by supplementing the diet of sheep with sodium sulfate and/or additional protein (13) and the identified toxin is hymenoxon, a sesquiterpene lactone (68).

Inula graveolens is recorded as a cause of fatal gastroenteritis in sheep, the result of penetration of the intestinal mucosa by the bristles of this plant (11). Foxglove is not very palatable, but some livestock can develop a taste for it and die of acute heart failure (44).

Giant fennel (Ferula communis)
Ferula communis causes poisoning manifested by a hemorrhagic tendency. The prothrombin time is prolonged with intakes of 2·5–5·0 g/kg body weight/day in lambs. Vitamin K_1 is an effective antidote (93). The anticoagulant principle has not been identified.

Sweet vernal (Anthoxanthum odorata)
Hay made from this plant contains dicoumarol and causes prolongation of the prothrombin time and a serious hemorrhagic disease which is often fatal. Vitamin K_1 is a satisfactory antidote (111).

Narrowleaf sumpweed (Iva angustifolia)
This causes abortion in cattle (99).

REVIEW LITERATURE

Bailey, E. M. (1979) Major poisonous plant problems in cattle. *Bov. Pract.*, *14*, 169.

Campbell, J. B. et al. (1956) *Poisonous Plants of the Canadian Prairies*. Canada Dept. Agric., Pub. 900, Ottawa, Canada.

Connor, H. E. (1951) *The Poisonous Plants of New Zealand*. Dept. Sci. Ind. Res., Bull. 99, Wellington, NZ.

Everist, S. L. (1972) *Poisonous Plants of Australia*. Sydney: Angus & Robertson.

Keeler, R. F. et al. (1978) Effects of poisonous plants on livestock. *Proc. Joint US.-Australian Symposium, Utah*, 1977.

Kingsbury, J. M. (1958) Plants poisonous to livestock. *J. dairy Sci.*, *41*, 875.

McBarron, E. J. (1978) *Poisonous Plants of Western NSW*, Dept. Agric., NSW, Sydney, Australia.

Nwude, N. & Parsons, L. E. (1977) Nigerian plants that may cause poisoning in livestock. *Vet. Bull.*, *47*, 811.

Ministry of Agriculture, Food and Fisheries (1979) *British Poisonous Plants*, Ed. 2. London: HMSO.

REFERENCES

(1) Araya, O. S. & Ford, E. J. (1981) *J. comp. Pathol.*, *91*, 135.
(2) Huxtable, C. R. et al. (1982) *Acta Neuropathol.*, *58*, 27.
(3) Huxtable, C. R. & Dorling, P. R. (1982) *Aust. vet. J.*, *59*, 50.
(4) Locke, K. B. et al. (1980) *Aust. vet. J.* *56*, 379.
(5) Hartley, W. J. & Gibson, A. J. F. (1971) *Aust. vet. J.*, *47*, 301.
(6) O'Sullivan, B. M. & Goodwin, J. A. (1977) *Aust. vet. J.*, *53*, 446.
(7) Gorrie, C. J. R. (1962) *Aust. vet. J.*, *38*, 138.
(8) Everist, S. L. (1972) *Poisonous Plants of Australia*, pp. 264–266. Sydney: Angus & Robertson.
(9) Sturart, B. P. et al. (1975) *J. Am. vet. med. Assoc.*, *167*, 949.
(10) Osweiler, G. D. et al. (1969) *Am. J. vet. Res.*, *30*, 557.
(11) Schneider, D. J. & Plessis, J. L. du (1980) *J. S. Afr. vet. Assoc.*, *51*, 159.
(12) Herweijer, C. H. & Den Houter, L. F. (1971) *Neth. J. vet. Sci.*, *4*, 52.
(13) Bridges, G. W. et al. (1980) *Vet. hum. Toxicol.*, *22*, 87.
(14) James, L. F. et al. (1980) *Am. J. vet. Res.*, *41*, 377.
(15) Martin, B. W. et al. (1981) *Vet. hum. Toxicol.*, *23*, 416.
(16) Menzies, J. S. et al. (1979) *SW vet.*, 32, 45.
(17) Walker, K. H. et al. (1980) *Aust. vet. J.*, *56*, 64.
(18) Egyed, M. N. et al. (1974) *Refuah Vet.*, *31*, 128.
(19) Keeler, R. F. (1978) *Lipids*, *13*, 708.
(20) Perdomo, E. & Freitas, A. de (1978) *Veterinaria, Montevideo, Uruquay*, *14*, 137.
(21) Rothwell, J. T. & Marshall, D. J. (1986) *Aust. vet. J.*, *63*, 316.
(22) Sendil, C. (1978) *Vet. Fac. Dergisi*, *25*, 480.
(23) Witzel, D. A. et al. (1976) *Am. J. vet. Res.*, *37*, 859.
(24) Hooper, P. I. et al. (1971) *Aust. vet. J.*, *47*, 326.
(25) Keeler, R. F. (1980) *Cornell Vet.*, *70*, 19.
(26) Dyson, D. A. & Wrathall, A. E. (1977) *Vet. Rec.*, *100*, 241.
(27) Williams, M. C. (1978) *J. Range Mgmt*, *31*, 182.
(28) Benson, J. M. et al. (1978) In: *Effects of Poisonous Plants on Livestock*, eds R. F. Keeler et al., p. 273. London: Academic Press.
(29) Basson, P. A. et al. (1970) *J. S. Afr. vet. med. Assoc.*, *41*, 117.
(30) de Malmanche, I. (1970) *NZ vet. J.*, *18*, 96.
(31) Bale, S. (1978) *Refuah Vet.*, *35*, 36.
(32) Kerr, L. A. et al. (1986) *Vet. hum. Toxicol.*, *28*, 412.
(33) O'Sullivan, B. M. (1985) *Aust. vet. J.*, *62*, 30.
(34) Gard, G. P. et al. (1973) *Aust. vet. J.*, *49*, 107.
(35) Mettler, F. A. & Stern, G. M. (1963) *J. Neuropathol.*, *22*, 164.
(36) Olsen, J. D. (1978) *J. Am. vet. med. Assoc.*, *173*, 762.
(37) Dollahite, J. W. et al. (1978) *Am. J. vet. Res.*, *39*, 193.
(38) Adam, S. E. I. et al. (1973) *J. comp. Pathol.*, *83*, 531.
(39) Terblanche, M. et al. (1966) *J. S. Afr. vet. med. Assoc.*, *37*, 3, 311, 317.
(40) Witzel, D. A. et al. (1978) *Am. J. vet. Res.*, *39*, 319.
(41) Basson, P. A. et al. (1975) *Onderstepoort J. vet. Res.*, *42*, 135.
(42) McAuliffe, P. R. & White, W. E. (1976) *Aust. vet. J.*, *52*, 366.
(43) Staley, E. (1976) *Bovi. Practnr*, *11*, 36.
(44) Corrigall, W. et al. (1978) *Vet. Res.*, *102*, 119.
(45) Kubilk, M. et al. (1980) *Veterinarstri*, *30*, 157.
(46) Kelly, W. R. (1975) *Aust. vet. J.*, *51*, 233, 504 & 325.
(47) Pierce, K. R. et al. (1972) *J. Am. vet. med. Assoc.*, *160*, 323.
(48) Rowe, L. D. et al. (1970) *SW. Vet.*, *23*, 219.
(49) Tribunskii, M. P. (1970) *Veterinariya, Moscow*, *6*, 71.
(50) Dickson, J. & Hill, R. (1977) *Proc. 54th ann. Congr. Aust. vet. Assoc.*, 92.
(51) Binns, W. et al. (1972) *Clin. Toxicol.*, *5*, 245.
(52) Suliman, H. B. & Shommein, A. M. (1986) *Vet. hum. Toxicol.*, *28*, 6.
(53) Keeler, R. F. (1973) *Proc. Soc. exp. Biol. Med.*, *142*, 1287.
(54) Binns, W. et al. (1964) *Ann. NY Acad. Sci.*, *111*, 571.
(55) Joubert, J. F. et al. (1972) *Onderstepoort J. vet. Res.*, *39*, 59.
(56) Henson, J. B. & Dollahite, J. W. (1966) *Am. J. vet. Res.*, *27*, 947.
(57) Mercer, H. D. et al. (1967) *J. Am. vet. med. Assoc.*, *151*, 735.
(58) Dewan, M. L. et al. (1965) *Am. J. Pathol.*, *46*, 215.
(59) O'Hara, P. J et al. (1970) *Am. J. vet. Res.*, *31*, 2151.
(60) Charlton, K. M. et al. (1970) *Pathol. vet.*, *7*, 385, 408, 420, 435.
(61) Charlton, K. M. et al. (1971) *Am. J. vet. Res.*, *32*, 1381.
(62) O'Hara, P. J. & Pierce, K. R. (1974) *Vet. Pathol.*, *11*, 97.
(63) Pienaar, J. G. et al. (1973) *Onderstepoort J. vet. Res.*, *40*, 127.
(64) O'Sullivan, B. M. (1976) *Aust. vet. J.*, *52*, 414.
(65) Clark, L. et al. (1975) *Aust. vet. J.*, *51*, 4.
(66) Kelly, W. R. & Bick, I. R. C. (1976) *Res. vet. Sci.*, *20*, 311.
(67) Landau, M. et al. (1973) *Refuah Vet.*, *30*, 131.
(68) Roberts, A. J. & Camp, B. J. (1984) *Vet. hum. Toxicol.*, *26*, 1.
(69) Williams, S. & Scott, P. (1984) *NZ vet. J.*, *32*, 47.
(70) Anderson, L. A. P. et al. (1983) *Onderstepoort J. vet. Res.*, *50*, 295.
(71) Anderson, L. A. P. et al. (1983) *Onderstepoort J. vet. Res.*, *50*, 301.
(72) Joubert, J. P. J. & Schultz, R. A. (1982) *J. S. Afr. vet. Assoc.*, *52*, 249, 265.
(73) Newsholme, S. J. et al. (1985) *Onderstepoort J. vet. Res.*, *52*, 87.
(74) Olson, C. T. et al. (1984) *J. Am. vet. med. Assoc.*, *185*, 1001.
(75) Martin, T. et al. (1986) *J. Am. vet. med. Assoc.*, *189*, 562.
(76) Colvin, B. M. et al. (1986) *J. Am. vet. med. Assoc.*, *189*, 423.
(77) Panter, K. E. et al. (1985) *Am. J. vet. Res.*, *46*, 1368.
(78) Johnson, S. J. & Toleman, M. A. (1982) *Aust. vet. J.*, *58*, 264.
(79) Anderson, L. A. P. et al. (1984) *Onderstepoort J. vet. Res.*, *52*, 21.
(80) Tustin, R. C. et al. (1984) *J. S. Afr. vet. Assoc.*, *55*, 181
(81) Grant, R. C. et al. (1985) *Onderstepoort J. vet. Res.*, *52*, 255.
(82) Newsholme, S. J. et al. (1984) *Onderstepoort J. vet. Res.*, *51*, 119, & 277.
(83) Riet-Correa, F. et al. (1983) *Cornell Vet.*, *73*, 240.
(84) Smetzer, D. L. et al. (1983) *Equ. Pract.*, *5*, 26.
(85) Bourke, C. A. (1984) *Aust. vet. J.*, *61*, 360.

(86) Suzuki, K. et al. (1985) *Cornell Vet.*, *75*, 348.
(87) Main, D. C. et al. (1981) *Aust. vet. J.*, *57*, 132.
(88) Gibson, J. A. & O'Sullivan, B. M. (1984) *Aust. vet. J.*, *61*, 271.
(89) Oertli, E. H. et al. (1983) *Am. J. vet. Res.*, *44*, 1126.
(90) Hannam, D. A. R. (1985) *Vet. Rec.*, *116*, 322.
(91) Keeler, R. F. et al. (1986) *Vet. hum. Toxicol.*, *28*, 309.
(92) Puyt, J. D. & Faliu, L. (1984) *Proc. 13th World Cong. Dis. Cattle*, *2*, 670.
(93) Shlosberg, A. & Egyed, M. N. (1985) *Zentralbl. VetMed.*, *A32*, 778.
(94) Andrews, A. H. et al. (1985) *Vet. Rec.*, *116*, 205.
(95) Mugera, G. M. et al. (1982) *Bull Anim. Hlth Prod. Africa*, *30*, 251.
(96) Keeler, R. F. et al. (1986) *Vet. Med.*, *81*, 449.
(97) Oertli, E. H. et al. (1984) *Phytochemistry*, *23*, 439.
(98) Habermehl, G. (1985) *Veterinaria Argentina*, *2*, 330, 332.
(99) Murphy, M. J. et al. (1984) *Proc. Ann. Mtg Am. Assoc. Vet. Lab Diagnost.*, *26*, 161.
(100) Cooper, T. B. et al. (1986) *Aust. vet. J.*, *63*, 178.
(101) McKenzie, R. A. & Dimster, P. J. (1986) *Aust. vet. J.*, *63*, 222.
(102) Bourke, C. A. & MacFarlane, J. A. (1985) *Aust. vet. J.*, *62*, 282.
(103) Dollahite, J. W. (1975) *SW Vet.*, *28*, 135.
(104) Barakat, S. E. M. et al. (1983) *Vet. Pathol.*, *20*, 611.
(105) Dijkstra, R. G. & Falkera, R. (1981) *Tijdschr. Diergeneeskd.*, *106*, 1037.
(106) Oelkers, S. (1982) *Bov. Pract.*, *3*, 11.
(107) Nelson, P. D. et al. (1982) *Vet. hum. Toxicol.*, *24*, 321.
(108) Nation, P. N. et al. (1982) *Can. vet. J.*, *23*, 264.
(109) Suliman, H. B. et al. (1982) *J. comp. Pathol.*, *92*, 309.
(110) Joubert, J. P. J. & Schultz, R. A. (1982) *J. S. Afr. vet. Assoc.*, *53*, 25.
(111) Pritchard, D. G. et al. (1983) *Vet. Rec.*, *113*, 78.
(112) Olsen, J. D. et al. (1983) *J. Am. vet. med. Assoc.*, *183*, 538.
(113) Storie, G. J. et al. (1986) *Aust. vet. J.*, *63*, 235.
(114) Seawright, A. A. (1984) *Vet. hum. Toxicol.*, 26, 208.
(115) Elawad, A. A. et al. (1984) *Vet. hum. Toxicol.*, *26*, 481.
(116) Burrows, G. E. & Tyrl, R. J. (1983) *Bov. Practnr*, *18*, 188.
(117) Widmer, W. R. (1984) *Vet. Med.*, *79*, 405.
(118) Barlow, R. M. et al. (1985) *Vet. Rec.*, *117*, 124.
(119) Dunster, P. J. & McKenzie, R. A. (1987) *Aust. vet. J.*, *64*, 119.
(120) Huxtable, C. R. et al. (1987) *Aust. vet. J.*, *64*, 105.

Trees and shrubs

Oak (Quercus *spp.*)
Young oak (*O. robur* syn. *O. pedunculata*, European oak) leaves and acorns or windfall acorns (26) are sometimes browsed by animals and cause no illness when they form only a small part of the diet but if little else is eaten they may cause polyuria, ventral edema, abdominal pain and constipation followed by the passage of feces containing mucus and blood. Blood urea nitrogen (BUN) levels are elevated and the specific gravity of the urine is low and there is proteinuria (26). At necropsy there are alimentary tract lesions including edema of the gastrointestinal wall and mesentery (60) and a characteristic nephrosis (1). The alimentary tract lesions are ulcerations consistent with the presence of uremia. The toxic principle has not been accurately identified, but is likely to be one or more breakdown products of tannin, such as gallic acid or pyrogallol (42). All species of animals are affected, losses in sheep and cattle being reported most commonly, with occasional cases occurring in horses (52). Goats are thought to be capable of surviving much greater intakes of tannin than cattle because of greater concentrations of tannase enzymes in their ruminal mucosae (30). Experimental administration of tannic acids to goats has produced anemia, but there is no record of the natural occurrence of the disease. Extensive areas of oak-brush range in the United States can be utilized for cattle grazing but require careful management if losses are to be avoided. All parts of the sand shin oak (*Quercus havardi*), a low shrub common in southwest United States, are toxic to cattle causing emaciation, edema and constipation. The toxic agent is a tannin. Other species of oak e.g. *O. marilandica* (blackjack oak) and *O. garryanna* (63), are also toxic and cause signs similar to those listed above. Calcium hydroxide (15% of the ration) is an effective antidote under experimental conditions.

Red maple (Acer rubrum)
The ingestion by horses of the wilted leaves of lopped maple tree branches is thought to be a significant contributor to a syndrome including acute hemolytic anemia and methemoglobinemia in northeast United States (41, 45). The principal clinical signs were weakness, pallor, hemoglobinemia, jaundice and brown discoloration of mucosae. Horses which had methemoglobinemia died; those without it survived. The disease was reproduced experimentally (59).

Blackeyes, horse chestnut (Aesculus *spp.*)
All of the known species of this tree must be considered to be poisonous. The nuts and young growth are most poisonous. Incoordination, tremor and hyperexcitability occur in poisoned animals of all species. Convulsions and some deaths are also recorded in calves (2).

Laburnum (Cytisus laburnum) *and broom* (Cytisus scoparius)
Cytisine, a toxic alkaloid, is present in both laburnum and broom trees, particularly the flowers and seeds. Ingestion results in excitement, incoordination, convulsions and death due to asphyxia.

Cherry laurel (Prunus laurocerasus), *choke cherry* (Prunus demissa)
A cyanogenetic glucoside, amygdalin, is present in the leaves of the cherry laurel tree, and hydrocyanic acid poisoning may result if large quantities of the leaves are eaten. The leaves of choke cherry also cause hydrocyanic acid poisoning.

Mountain laurel (Kalmia *spp.*)
Leaves of this plant are not ordinarily palatable but poisoning of ruminants can occur when other feed is scarce. Clinical signs in cattle included hyperexcitability, incoordination and paralysis. The toxic principle is andromedotoxin as in rhododendron.

Rhododendron (Andromeda *spp.*)
A toxic glucoside, andromeditoxin (syn. acetylandromedol) present in the leaves of rhododendron, causes anorexia, repeated swallowing or eructation, excessive salivation, abdominal pain, weakness, staggering and collapse. Vomiting is common even in ruminants. Other signs are tachycardia, cardiac irregularities, tremor and dyspnea (53). Death follows after several days of illness. The Japanese pieris (*Pieris japonica*) also contains andromedotoxin and can cause poisoning (38) including mummification of fetuses (39).

Oleander (Nerium oleander)
This decorative shrub is very poisonous and there are many records of deaths due to feeding prunings to animals, usually cattle, or when animals break into gardens. In goats, salivation, vomiting, tremor, uneasiness, mydriasis, frequent defecation and urination, bradycardia or tachycardia, arrhythmia, excitement and convulsions occur (6). Death is sudden and due to ventricular fibrillation. Treatment is not usually possible but atropine is recommended (6).

Palo santo tree (Bulnesia sarmientii)
The seed pods and foliage contain a toxic saponin which causes convulsions, licking of forelimbs, geophagia, chewing movements, ruminal atony, bradycardia and frequent urination and defecation (54).

Cestrum (Cestrum aurantiacum *and* C. laevigatum, C. parqui)
This hedge and windbreak bush causes mortality in goats and cattle (7). It causes a hemorrhagic gastroenteritis and degenerative lesions in the liver, kidney and brain. *C. parqui* (57) causes primarily liver damage and may cause nervous signs as well as diarrhea.

Wild jessamine (Cestrum diurnum)
Ingestion of the leaves of *C. diurnum* has been implicated as the cause of chronic debilitating disease of horses and cattle in Florida, United States (8). The disease is characterized by wasting, lameness, hypercalcemia, osteoporosis and generalized tissue calcinosis especially of vessels, tendons and ligaments. The plant contains a substance with actions similar to those of biologically active vitamin D_3 (1,25-dihydrocholecalciferol). Similar lesions have been produced experimentally in lambs (23) and in pigs by feeding 3% of the ration as *C. diurnum* leaves (9). The disease is identical with that caused by *Solanum malocoxylon* and is dealt with under that heading (page 1343).

Chinese tallow tree (Sapium sebiferum)
This ornamental tree causes gastroenteritis in cattle.

Box tree (Buxus sempervirens)
The foliage causes ataxia, severe diarrhea and other nervous signs, e.g. inability to swallow, in cattle (50).

Ficus *spp.*
Several species of figs are thought to be poisonous but there are few reports. *F. tsiela* leaves cause cerebral edema and hepatic and renal necrosis in cattle. The clinical syndrome includes hypersalivation, tremor, nystagmus and convulsions (49).

Cassia spp.
Several species of this bush, e.g. *C. italica* (46) cause severe gastroenteritis. The clinical syndrome includes diarrhea, dyspnea, ataxia and anemia. Necropsy lesions include hemorrhagic enteritis and pulmonary emphysema.

Yew (Taxus baccata)
All parts of the yew tree contain a highly poisonous alkaloid, taxine, which has a strong depressive effect on the heart. Commonly there is sudden death without obvious clinical signs. Signs, if they appear, include dyspnea, muscle tremor, weakness and collapse. The Japanese yew tree (*Taxus cuspitata*) is as toxic as *T. baccata* and is a more common decorative tree. Clinical signs of toxicity are depression, tremor, ataxia, bradycardia, hypothermia and weakness (62). Sudden death is recorded in horses and cattle which have eaten the plant (12). Removal of the ruminal contents of goats via a rumenotomy has been followed by recovery (47). There are no significant findings at necropsy (11).

Yellowwood tree (Terminalia oblongata)
The leaves of this tree may be eaten when other food is scarce and cause some losses in cattle and sheep in northeast Australia. In an acute form of the disease there is a sudden onset of profuse diarrhea, dullness, anorexia, dyspnea and dryness of the muzzle. Marked edema of the jowl, neck and brisket occurs constantly. At necropsy there is ascites, anasarca and a toxic nephrosis. A more chronic syndrome is manifested by scouring, emaciation, photophobia, a purulent ocular discharge, keratitis and blindness. There may be incontinence of urine with frequent straining and continuous dribbling. At necropsy the bladder wall is thickened and the bladder much enlarged. Renal tubular damage is also present. Bromosulfalein clearance tests indicate that there is also a serious depression of liver function present (13). The mortality rate is 100%, most deaths occurring after an illness of less than 6 weeks (14).

Ironwood tree (Erythrophloeum chlorostachys)
This is a common tree in Australia and the leaves contain a highly toxic alkaloid, erythrophleine. All animal species seem to be affected, clinical signs including anorexia, a staring expression, partial blindness, contraction of abdominal muscles, increased heart sounds, mucosal pallor, and terminal dyspnea (14). *E. guineense* has also been shown to be toxic; force-feeding of the leaves to sheep can cause death within a few hours or after several days. Increased heart sounds, tremor and ataxia, and dysentery are included in the syndrome produced (32).

Gidgee or gidyea tree (Acacia georgina)
In northern Australia poisoning by this tree has caused heavy mortalities in sheep and cattle and seriously reduced the productivity of large areas of grazing land (14). The toxic principle has been identified as the fluoroacetate ion which is present in the leaves and seed pods, particularly the latter. The toxicity of the plant varies and in some areas may be eaten with no apparent ill-effects. Clinically there is a sudden onset of tachycardia with heart rates up to 300/min, dyspnea, cyanosis, convulsions and death within a few minutes to several hours. Cardiac irregularity, moderate bloat and frequent micturition are also observed in some cases. Signs commonly appear when affected animals are driven. At necropsy there is congestion of the alimentary mucosa, flabbiness of the myocardium and multiple subendocardial and subepicardial hemorrhages. There may be edema and congestion of the lungs. The plants *Gastrolobium*

grandiflorum and *Oxylobium* sp. also cause poisoning because of their content of monofluoroacetic acid. Similar to other organic fluorides, fluoroacetate is known to exert its effect by poisoning the enzyme aconitase leading to the accumulation of significant amounts of citrate in tissues and to irreversible cardiac damage (17).

Australian herbivorous mammals have evolved a high level of genetic tolerance to this toxin and this has been used as a genetic marker to trace the evolutionary history of some of the continent's indigenous marsupials (34).

Dichapetalum *spp.*

Dichapetalum spp., e.g. *D. cymosum* (Gibflaar), *D. ruhlandii* (35), *D. barteri* (33), are poisonous shrubs common in Africa but also in the tropics generally. The fresh green leaves contain fluoroacetate, and ingestion of them by any animal species causes clinical illness about 12 hours later (18). There is staggering, restlessness, frequent urination, tachycardia, an imperceptible pulse and almost continuous recumbency. Death is the common outcome and may occur a few minutes to several days after the illness begins. Degenerative changes in the myocardium are accompanied by lesions of acute heart failure. Acetamide 2 g/kg given experimentally soon after the ingestion of *Dichapetatum* spp. appears to have helped animals against the poison (64).

Ngaio tree (Myoporum laetum, M. deserti (*19*), *and* M. serratum)

The leaves of these trees contain ngaione, a hepatoxic ketone which causes jaundice, photosensitization and death in all animal species that ingest them. Poisoning is recorded in Australia, China, Japan and New Zealand. *Myoporum tetrandrum*, the common Australian boobialla tree, is also poisonous, containing hepatotoxic substances. The principal agent is dehydrongaione (36). Mortality in cattle due to poisoning by *M.* affinity *insulare* is also associated with acute hepatic injury (61).

Yellow pine tree (Pinus ponderosa), Pinus radiata *and* Pinus cubensis

The pine needles of all of these trees are credited with producing abortion in cattle, and a phytoestrogen has been detectable in the leaves of the tree (65). Poisoning is most likely to occur when cattle graze amongst the trees and have access to the wilted foliage on lopped or broken branches (10). Feeding trials with the needles of *P. cubensis* appear to show conclusively that the leaves are abortifacient for cattle (3). Early abortions have also been procured by feeding *P. ponderosa* to cows (21). Ewes are unaffected (22). A contrary view based on work with mice is that these abortions are in fact caused by a concomitant infection with *Listeria monocytogenes* (4). The feeding of pine needle extracts to mice does cause fetal resorptions in them (43).

Cupressus macrocarpa

Abortion and cerebral leukomalacia of the aborted fetus are both ascribed to ingestion of the foliage of this tree (24). Attempts at induction of premature birth in ewes have been unsuccessful (28).

Stinkwood (Zieria arborescens)

This tall shrub or small tree occurs in areas of over 75 cm annual rainfall in Tasmania and eastern Australia. Cattle eat it when other food is scarce. The natural disease is reproducible by feeding 15–30 kg of the herbage during a period of 2–4 weeks. The clinical signs appear as tachypnea up to 80/minute, grunting, extension of the head, mouth breathing, abdominal respiration and a nasal discharge. In bad cases the temperature and pulse are elevated. Death occurs after an illness of 1–21 days; some cases survive. At necropsy examination there is massive pulmonary edema and emphysema (29). The disease resembles closely atypical interstitial pneumonia as it occurs in western United States. It has been produced experimentally in rabbits.

Supple jack (Ventilago viminalis)

This tree is a palatable and valuable fodder tree but if it is used as the major part of the diet of sheep for about 3 weeks (an unlikely field occurrence) toxicity appears. The principal signs are hypersensitivity to external stimuli, resulting in repeated tetanic convulsions. Autopsy findings include abomasal ulceration and hepatic and renal degenerative lesions (31).

Black walnut (Juglans nigra)

Shavings from black walnut timber have produced edema of the lower legs, and laminitis in horses stabled on them (14, 16). A toxic compound, juglone, present in the tree produces similar signs inconsistently.

Leucaena leucocephala

This leguminous browse shrub causes the disease known as 'jumbey' (Bahamas), 'lamtoro' (Indonesia) or 'koa haole' (Hawaii). The tree is used extensively as fodder in many tropical countries, but it contains a toxic amino acid mimosine, some varieties containing more than others. Because of its ease of cultivation, high yield and high content of protein, it is as valuable as lucerne/alfalfa. Its use is likely to increase (5). Mimosine occurs in all parts of the plant, but is at its highest concentration in the leaves of growing tips. Cattle and goats in Hawaii eat very large amounts of the plant without ill-effect. This is explained as being the result of adaptation of ruminal microflora which then degrade the mimosine (44).

The degree of degradation can be varied by changing the diet, being much greater on a concentrate diet than on a roughage one (58). The degradation is in two stages, from mimosine to 3-hydroxy-4(IH)-pyridone (3, 4 DHP) which is a potent goitrogen. The 3, 4 DHP is then degraded to innocuous metabolites. The ability to degrade 3, 4 DHP is present in animal rumens only in some countries, e.g. Hawaii and Indonesia. A transfer of rumen contents from Hawaiian to Australian cattle has been carried out as a preventive veterinary procedure (56). Acceptable daily intakes of mimosine (48) are 0·18 g/kg body weight for cattle, 0·14 g/kg body weight for sheep and 0·18 g/kg body weight for goats.

There is a great deal of variation in the effects of poisoning with *Leucaena leucocephala* depending on the variety of the tree, the amount of other fodder available, and the selection of the feed by the animal. Horses, sheep and cattle are commonly affected. Goats are reported not to be, but in fact are (5). Alopecia (depilation) is the common and important effect of poisoning with mimosine, but nervous signs are also constant. Other recorded but inconstant effects are cataract, gingival atrophy, lingual epithelial ulceration, goiter, infertility and low birth weight (51). In experimental animals hepatic injury is one of the most marked effects (20), but this is not recorded in domestic animals.

Horses show loss of hair, especially the mane and tail, and around the hocks and knees. Ring formation in the hooves and emaciation also occur. In cattle and sheep, shedding of hair or wool occurs soon (7–14 days) after the first exposure to the plant or when very large amounts are fed. The alopecia is not necessarily general but is symmetrical. Experimental feeding of large amounts of the plant to steers has caused hair loss especially on the tail, pizzle and escutcheon. If ruminants are introduced to the plant gradually the ruminal microflora develops the capacity of metabolizing mimosine so that poisoning is not a problem. In addition to alopecia which occurs acutely, cattle which are fed on the plant for long periods develop other chronic syndromes including incoordination, temporary blindness and hyperactivity to the point of severely interfering with normal handling procedures (25).

The secondary phase of poisoning caused by the formation of DHP is recorded in some countries but not others. It is characterized by enlarged thyroid glands, poor breeding performance and goitrous, weak calves recorded in experimental feeding to cattle in some countries but not in others. All of these toxic effects are quickly reversible by removing animals from access to the plants so that animals do not usually die of the poisoning. However, in pen feeding trials where large amounts are fed, listlessness, poor appetite, poor weight gains, increased DHP secretion in urine and decreased serum T_3 levels are observed and the severity of the abnormality is proportional to the dose of mimosine given (37). The goitrogenic effect is limited to ruminants and is not responsive to iodine administration. Mimosine is converted into a potent goitrogen in the rumen (27).

In pigs, the feeding of diets containing up to 15% of dried *L. leucocephala* to pregnant gilts causes a high proportion of fetuses to be resorbed and some to have limb deformities. Feeding 1% ferrous sulfate in the diet reduces these effects, and supplementation of the diet of ruminants with iron, copper and zinc is also claimed to reduce the toxic effects.

Mimosine is under examination as a defleecing agent for sheep and although there are problems of toxicity (15), the method has promise. Much of the recent information on toxic doses and blood levels, which has clarified the field observations of the disease, is the result of work on this possible commercial application of mimosine.

REVIEW LITERATURE

Burrows, G. E. & Tyrl, R. J. (1983) Ornamental plants potentially hazardous to cattle. *Bov. Practnr*, *18*, 188–194.

Knight, A. P. (1987) Poisonous plants. *Comp. cont. Educ.*, 9, F26.

REFERENCES

(1) Strober, M. et al. (1976) *Bov. Practnr*, *11*, 38.
(2) Magnusson, R. A. et al. (1983) *Bov. Practnr*, *18*, 195.
(3) Hernandez, J. et al. (1979) *Ciencia Tec. agric. vet. (Cuba)*, *1*, 55.
(4) Adams, C. J. et al. (1979) *Infect. Immunol.*, *25*, 117.
(5) Jones, R. J. (1979) *Anim. Rev.*, *31*, 13.
(6) Mahin, L. et al. (1984) *Vet. hum. Toxicol.*, *26*, 303.
(7) Mugera, G. M. & Nderito, P. (1968) *Bull. epizoot. Dis., Afr.*, *16*, 501.
(8) Krook, L. et al. (1975) *Cornell Vet.*, *65*, 26, 557.
(9) Kasali, O. B. et al. (1977) *Cornell Vet.*, *67*, 190.
(10) Knowles, R. L. & Dewes, H. F. (1980) *NZ vet. J.*, *28*, 103.
(11) Thomson, G. W. & Barker, I. K. (1978) *Can. vet. J. 19*, 320.
(12) Karns, P. A. (1983) *Equ. Pract.*, *5 (1)*, 12.
(13) Hunt, S. E. & McCosker, P. J. (1968) *Am. J. vet. clin. Pathol.*, *2*, 161.
(14) True, R. G. & Lowe, J. E. (1980) *Am. J. vet. Res.*, *41*, 944.
(15) Reis, P. J. (1978) *Aust. J. agric. Res.*, *39*, 1043 & 1065.
(16) Ralston, S. L. & Rich, V. A. (1983) *J. Am. vet. med. Assoc.*, *183*, 1095.
(17) Allcroft, R. et al. (1969) *Vet. Rec.*, *84*, 403.
(18) Vickery, B. & Vickery, M. L. (1973) *Vet. Bull.*, *43*, 537.
(19) Allen, J. G. & Seawright, A. A. (1973) *Res. vet. Sci.*, *15*, 167.
(20) Lee, J. S. (1979) *Kor. J. vet. Res.*, *19*, 85 & 127.
(21) Stevenson, A. H. et al. (1972) *Cornell Vet.*, *62*, 519.
(22) McCall, J. W. & James, L. F. (1976) *J. Am. vet. med. Assoc.*, *169*, 1301.
(23) Simpson, C. F. & Bruss, M. L. (1979) *Calcified Tissue Int.*, *29*, 245.
(24) Mason, R. W. (1974) *Aust. vet. J.*, *50*, 419.
(25) Falvey, L. (1976) *Aust. vet. J.*, *52*, 243.
(26) Holliman, A. (1985) *Vet. Rec.*, *116*, 546.
(27) Hegarty, M. P. et al. (1976) *Aust. vet. J.*, *52*, 489.
(28) Mason, R. W. (1984) *Aust. vet. J.*, *61*, 192.
(29) Munday, B. L. (1968) *Aust. vet. J.*, *44*, 501.
(30) Begovic, S. (1978) *Veterinaria, Yugoslavia*, No. 4, 443, 445 & 459x.
(31) Pryor, W. J. et al. (1972) *Aust. vet. J.*, *48*, 339.
(32) Nwude, N. & Chimene, C. N. (1980) *Res. vet. Sci.*, *28*, 112.
(33) Nwude, N. et al. (1977) *Toxicology*, *7*, 23.
(34) Oliver, A. J. et al. (1979) *Aust. J. Zool.*, *27*, 363.
(35) Kamau, J. A. et al. (1978) *Ind. vet. J. 55*, 626.
(36) Allen, J. G. et al. (1978) *Aust. vet. J.*, *54*, 287.
(37) Jones, R. J. & Hegarty, M. P. (1984) *Aust. J. agric. Res.*, *35*, 317.
(38) Smith, M. C. (1978) *J. Am. vet. med. Assoc.*, *173*, 78.
(39) Smith, M. C. (1979) *Cornell Vet.*, *69*, 85.
(40) Sloss, V. & Brady, J. W. (1983) *Aust. vet. J.*, *60*, 223.
(41) Tennant, B. et al. (1981) *J. Am. vet. med. Assoc.*, *179*, 143.
(42) Sandusky, G. E. et al. (1977) *J. Am. vet. med. Assoc.*, *171*, 627.
(43) Kubik, M. & Jackson, L. L. (1981) *Cornell Vet.*, *71*, 34.
(44) Jones, R. T. (1981) *Aust. vet. J.*, *57*, 55.
(45) Divers, T. J. et al. (1982) *J. Am. vet. med. Assoc.*, *180*, 300.
(46) Galal, M. et al. (1985) *Acta vet. Yugoslavia*, *35*, 163.
(47) Casteel, S. W. & Cook, W. O. (1985) *Mod. vet. Pract.*, *66*, 875.
(48) Szyszka, M. & Meulen, U. (1984) *Dtsch Tierärztl. Wochenschr.*, *91*, 260.
(49) Rajan, A. et al. (1986) *Ind. vet. J.*, *63*, 184.
(50) Camy, G. et al. (1986) *Point Vet.*, *18*, 203.
(51) Holmes, J. H. G. et al. (1981) *Aust. vet. J.*, *57*, 257.
(52) Warren, C. G. B. & Vaughan, S. M. (1985) *Vet. Rec.*, *116*, 82.
(53) Higgins, R. J. et al. (1985) *Vet. Rec.*, *116*, 294.
(54) Williams, M. C. et al. (1984) *Vet. Rec.*, *115*, 646.
(55) Hill, B. D. et al. (1985) *Aust. vet. J.*, *62*, 107.
(56) Jones, R. J. & Megarrity, R. G. (1986) *Aust. vet. J.*, *63*, 259.
(57) McLennan, M. W. & Kelley, W. R. (1984) *Aust. vet. J.*, *61*, 289.
(58) Kudo, H. et al. (1984) *Can. J. anim. Sci.*, *64*, 937.
(59) George, L. W. et al. (1982) *Vet. Pathol.*, *19*, 521.
(60) Anderson, G. A. et al. (1983) *J. Am. vet. med. Assoc.*, *182*, 1105.
(61) Jerrett, I. V. & Chinnock, R. J. (1983) *Aust. vet. J.*, *60*, 183.
(62) Kerr, L. A. & Edwards, W. C. (1981) *Vet. Med.*, *76*, 1339.
(63) Kasari, T. R. et al. (1980) *Comp. cont. Educ.*, *8*, F17.
(64) Egyed, M. N. & Schultz, R. A. (1986) *Onderstepoort J. vet. Res.*, *53*, 231.
(65) Wagner, W. D. & Jackson, L. L. (1983) *Theriogenology*, *19*, 507.

DISEASES CAUSED BY ANIMAL AND INSECT BITES AND TOXINS

Snakebite

The bites of venomous snakes may cause serious effects in farm animals, but mortalities are rare. Nervous signs occur and there may or may not be local swelling depending on the type of snake.

Etiology

At least four toxic actions can result from snake venoms and different snakes have varying combinations of toxins in their venoms. The toxins include necrotizing and coagulant fractions as well as neurotoxic and hemolytic fractions. Although there is often insufficient toxin injection to cause death in large animals a serious secondary bacterial infection may be set up in the local swelling and cause the subsequent death of the animal.

Epidemiology

The incidence of snakebite is controlled by the geographical distribution of the snakes and their numbers. Asia, India, Africa, Central and South America, Australia and the southern United States are areas in which snake populations are large. In general the morbidity rate in farm animals is not high although a mortality rate of 20% has been recorded in a small group of bitten animals (1).

Most snakebite accidents occur during the summer months and bites are mainly about the head because of the inquisitive behavior of the bitten animal. Pigs are not highly susceptible but not, as generally believed, because of their extensive subcutaneous fat depots (2). Sheep may be bitten on the udder but their long wool coat is generally effective as a protective mechanism on other parts of the body. Large animals tend to be resistant because of their large size and the large dose rate required to cause death. However, horses appear to be much more susceptible to venom than any other species.

Pathogenesis

The effects of snakebite (envenomation) depend upon the size and species of the snake, the size of the bitten animal and the location of the bite, particularly with reference to the thickness of the hair coat and the quantity of subcutaneous fat. As a general rule the venom is injected by fangs which leave a bite mark comprising a row of small punctures with two large punctures outside them. An exception is the coral snake which must chew to inoculate the venom. The bites may be visible on hairless and unpigmented skin but can only be seen on reflection of the skin at necropsy in many instances. Non-poisonous snakes may bite animals but the bite mark is in the form of two rows of small punctures.

The toxins in venom include *neurotoxins*, causing flaccid paralysis, pupillary dilatation and paralytic respiratory failure, *cytolisins* which cause tissue necrosis, including platelets, leading to intravascular coagulation, *hemolysins*, *coagulant* or *thrombase*, *anticoagulants* leading to a hemorrhagic tendency (10) and *myotoxins* causing muscle necrosis and myoglobinuria. The overall effect of a bite by a snake depends on the mix of specific venoms in the dose delivered and the actual dose which depends on the size of the snake and the period since the snake last bit. Examples of the effects of specific snake envenomations are as follows. Tiger snake venom contains neurotoxins and coagulants. Death adder venoms contain only neurotoxin, brown snake has coagulant and some neurotoxin. Rattlesnake venom causes necrosis of arterioles and arteriolar thrombus formation (12).

Clinical findings

Bites by adder-type snakes cause a local swelling which develops very rapidly and causes severe pain, usually sufficient to produce signs of excitement and anxiety. Bites about the head may be followed by swellings of sufficient size to cause dyspnea. If sufficient neurotoxin has been injected a secondary stage of excitement occurs and is followed by marked dilatation of the pupils, salivation, hyperesthesia, tetany, depression, recumbency and terminal paralysis. In small animals, death may occur due to asphyxia during convulsions in the excitement stage of the disease. In animals that recover there is usually local sloughing at the site of the swelling (3).

Bites by cobra-type snakes cause local swelling in animals that survive the effects of the neurotoxin. These commonly develop local swellings due to bacterial infection 3–4 days later. The major effects after bites of cobra-type snakes are excitement with convulsions, and death due to asphyxia. The signs appear quickly and death occurs usually within 1–10 hours in dogs and in up to 48 hours in horses. In calves the effects of the neurotoxin are manifested by marked pupillary dilatation, excitement, incoordination and later paralysis (4).

Clinical signs in horses bitten by tiger snakes (*Notechis scutatus*) in Australia (5) include pronounced pupillary dilatation without pupillary response to light but the menace reflex is present and the animal can see. Muscle tremor is most obvious in the standing patient and the horse is very fidgety and wants to lie down. The tremor disappears when the animal lies down, but it will not stay down and insists on rising and wandering about in a compulsive way.

Clinical signs in foals bitten by brown snakes (*Demansia textilis*) in Australia are similar to those caused by tiger snake envenomation (6). There is drowsiness, drooping of eyelids and lips, partial tongue paralysis, muscle tremor and weakness, leading to recumbency; pupillary dilatation occurs in some. The respiration becomes labored and abdominal. Sweating, inability to suck, swallow or whinny, occur late in the course. Adults also show inability to swallow, with salivation and accumulation of food in the mouth.

Rattlesnake bite in calves causes restlessness, teeth-grinding, vomiting, hypersalivation, dyspnea, ataxia and convulsions (13).

Clinical pathology

An ELISA for identification of venom in blood, urine or other body tissue or fluid is available. It is highly accurate, suitable for field or office use, immediate but expensive. It is limited to the snake species for which reagents are available (14).

Necropsy findings

Local swellings at the site of the bite are due to exudation of serous fluid which is often deeply bloodstained. Fang marks are usually visible on the undersurface of the reflected skin.

Diagnosis

In acute cases death has usually occurred by the time the animal is seen. If the actual bite is observed the diagnosis is made on the history. Bacterial infection of bite wounds may be confused with blackleg, anthrax or non-specific phlegmonous infections.

Treatment

Recommended local treatment for animals still includes the application of a tourniquet above the bite to restrict the circulation and the application of suction if possible. The tourniquet should be released for a few minutes at 20 minute intervals. If the bite area is incised the incision should reach the site of deposition of the venom but does not require to be more than 0·5 cm in depth. If it can be carried out quickly after the bite has occurred, excision of the part is recommended for the bites of snakes which cause a serious local reaction (7). In human medicine this treatment has been replaced: a firm pressure bandage is applied over the bite to keep the venom in the site and allow systemic administration of antivenin.

Systemic treatment should include antivenin, antibiotics and antitoxin (8). Antivenin containing antibodies against the venoms of all the snakes in the area can usually be obtained locally, often in highly purified form. It is expensive to use but highly effective. Speed is essential and the intravenous route is preferred. A portion of the antivenin should be injected locally around the bite. The dose rate varies widely with the size of the animal, one unit often being sufficient for animals weighing 70 kg or more, but smaller animals of 9–18 kg body weight require about 5 units. A broad-spectrum antibiotic should also be administered to control the local infection at the site of the bite. The occurrence of clostridial infections after snakebite suggests the administration of antitoxins against tetanus and gas gangrene. Supportive fluid treatment may be advisable when shock is severe and the administration of a sedative may be necessary to control pain and excitement.

Many other treatments have been used in snakebite including particularly ACTH, cortisone and antihistamines. These drugs have been found to be valuable as a protection against possible anaphylaxis after treatment with antivenin but in cases where local tissue damage is evident they are without value and in many cases exert deleterious effects (9). Adrenalin or epinephrine have little or no value and calcium salts do not significantly reduce mortality. The application of chemicals to the incised bite area is also of no value and may exacerbate tissue damage. Attention has been drawn to the need to appreciate the mode of action of one's local snakes before attempting a general program of treatment — what may be effective in one country may very well be lethal in another (7).

REVIEW LITERATURE

Clarke, E. G. C. & Clarke, M. L. (1969) Snakes and snakebite. *Vet. Ann.*, *10*, 27.

Garnet, J. R. (1968) *Venomous Australian Animals Dangerous to Man.* Melbourne: Commonwealth Serum Laboratories.

Prescott, C. W. (1984) The snake venom intoxications. *Aust. vet. Practnr*, *14*, 53–63.

REFERENCES

(1) Parrish, H. M. & Scatterday, J. E. (1957) *Vet. Med.*, *52*, 135.
(2) Araujo, P. et al. (1963) *Archos Inst. biol. S Paulo*, *30*, 43, 49.
(3) Swanson, T. D. (1976) *Proc. 22nd ann. Conf. Am. Assoc. equ. Practnrs*, p. 267.
(4) Couttie, P. M. (1969) *Aust. vet. J.*, *45*, 384.
(5) Fitzgerald, W. E. (1975) *Aust. vet. J.*, *51*, 37.
(6) Pascoe, R. R. (1975) *J. S. Afr. vet. med. Assoc.*, *46*, 129.
(7) Liefman, C. E. (1970) *Aust. vet. J.*, *46*, 182.
(8) Horak, I. G. (1964) *J. S. Afr. vet. med. Assoc.*, *35*, 343.
(9) Parish, H. M. et al. (1957) *J. Am. vet. med. Assoc.*, *130*, 548.
(10) Crawford, A. M. & Mills, N. J. (1985) *Aust. vet. J.*, *62*, 185.
(11) Akhtari, A. et al. (1984) *Ind. J. vet. Med.*, *4*, 19.
(12) Saliba, A. M. et al. (1983) *Dtsch Tierärztl. Wochenschr.*, *90*, 513.
(13) Akhtari, A. et al. (1983) *Ind. J. vet. Med.*, *3*, 21.
(14) Prescott, C. W. (1984) *Aust. vet. Practnr*, *14*, 53.

Bee stings

Multiple stings by bees may cause severe local swelling in animals. Pain may result in pronounced excitement and in severe cases in horses there may be diarrhea, hemoglobinuria, jaundice, tachycardia and prostration. Animals attacked about the head may show dyspnea because of severe local swelling. In rare cases the attack may be fatal (1). Treatment includes the local application of a weak solution of ammonia or sodium bicarbonate, nervous system stimulants if prostration is severe and tracheotomy if asphyxia threatens.

REFERENCE

(1) Wirth, D. (1943) *Wien. Tierärztl. Monatsschr.*, *30*, 129.

Ant bites

Bites from the aggressive fire ant (*Solenopsis invicta*) can cause focal necrotic ulcers of the cornea and conjunctiva of newborn calves (1). Weak calves are most likely to be injured.

REFERENCE

(1) Joyce, J. R. (1983) *Vet. Med.*, *78*, 1109.

Tick paralysis

Infestations with a variety of species of ticks (see Table 79) cause paralysis of animals (1, 2). Dogs are most commonly affected but losses can occur in lambs, calves, goats and foals and even children (3). *Ixodes holocyclus* have been shown to paralyse calves of 25–50 kg body weight. Between four and ten adult female ticks are required to produce this effect and paralysis occurs 6–13 days after infestation occurs (4). The ticks under natural conditions parasitize wild fauna, and infestations of other species occur accidentally. The disease is limited in its distribution by the ecology of the ticks and the natural host fauna. The paralysis which is characteristic of the disease is caused by a toxin secreted by the salivary glands of female ticks and which is present in much greater concentration in the glands of adults than in other stages. The severity of the paralysis is independent of the number of ticks involved; susceptible animals may be seriously affected by a few ticks. The toxin of *Dermacentor andersoni* interferes with liberation or synthesis of acetylcholine at the motor end-plates of muscle fibers (5). The disturbance is functional and paralysis of the peripheral neurones is the basic cause (6). Continuous secretion of toxin by the ticks is necessary to produce paralysis, recovery occurring rapidly as soon as the ticks are removed.

Clinically there is an ascending, flaccid paralysis commencing with incoordination of the hindlegs, followed by paralysis of the forelimbs and chest muscles. The respiration is grossly abnormal because of its diaphragmatic form; there is a double expiratory effort and the rate is slow but deep. All limb reflexes are absent, the pupils dilate widely and death is due to respiratory paralysis. In dogs there are additional signs including vomiting, absence of voice and secondary aspiration pneumonia. Death, due to respiratory failure, may occur in 1–2 days but the course is usually 4–5 days. The mortality rate may be as high as 50% in dogs but is usually much lower in farm animals. Since tick-borne diseases, such as tularemia, often coexist with tick paralysis, this possibility should always be considered in arriving at a diagnosis (7).

Hyperimmune serum is used in the treatment of dogs but in farm animals removal of the ticks in the early stages is usually followed by rapid recovery. Control necessitates eradication of the ticks or host fauna. The use of appropriate insecticides is an effective preventive.

REFERENCES

(1) Clumies-Ross, I. (1935) *Counc. sci. ind. Res. J., Aust.*, *8*, 8.
(2) Neitz, W. O. (1963) *Rep. 2nd meet. FAO/OIE Panel Tick-borne Dis., Cairo 1962*, p. 24.
(3) Bootes, B. W. (1962) *Aust. vet. J.*, *38*, 68.
(4) Doube, B. M. et al. (1977) *Aust. vet. J.*, *53*, 39.
(5) Emmons, P. & McLennan, H. (1959) *Nature, Lond.*, *183*, 474.
(6) Abbott, K. H. (1943) *Proc. Mayo Clin.*, *18*, 39, 59.
(7) Jellison, W. et al. (1965) *Proc. US live Stk sanit. Assoc.*, 60.

Cantharides poisoning (blister beetle poisoning)

Poisoning of horses by the consumption of the blister beetle (*Epicauta vittata*) has been recorded in the southern United States (1, 2). The beetle, which contains cantharidin, is found in lucerne hay. Administration of 1 g of ground beetles by stomach tube is fatal to a pony. Cattle are not affected.

Signs include irritation in the mouth, frequent urination, colic and occasionally synchronous diaphragmatic flutter. Clinicopathologically there may be hematuria, hemoconcentration and a neutrophilic leukocytosis, but these lesions are not diagnostic and the presence of beetles in the feed should be established (4). An analytical method for detection of cantharidin in field specimens is available (3). The amount found in the different species varies greatly (4).

REFERENCES

(1) Shawley, R. V. & Rolf, L. L. (1984) *Am. J. vet. Res.*, *45*, 2261.
(2) Schoeb, T. R. & Panciera, R. J. (1978) *J. Am. vet. med. Assoc.*, *173*, 75.
(3) Ray, A. C. et al. (1980) *Am. J. vet. Res.*, *41*, 932.
(4) Capinera, J. L. et al. (1985) *J. econ. Entomol.*, 78, 1052.

Sawfly larvae

The larvae of the sawfly (*Lophyrotoma interrupta*) accumulate in large piles under their host eucalyptus trees where they are eaten by cattle. They contain an octapeptide, lophyratomin, which causes renal and hepatic damage and a clinical syndrome including depression, mania, coma and death in a few days. Polyuria occurs in some (1).

REFERENCE

(1) Dadswell, L. P. et al. (1985) *Aust. vet. J.*, *62*, 94.

33

Diseases Caused by Allergy

Alloimmune hemolytic anemia of the newborn (neonatal isoerythrolysis, isoimmune hemolytic anemia of the newborn)

THIS is a hemolytic disease of newborn animals caused by an incompatible blood group reaction between the serum antibodies of the mother and the erythrocytes of the newborn.

Etiology

In horses and mules the disease is caused by the natural occurrence of inherited blood groups. The foal inherits erythrocyte antigens from the sire and these pass through the placenta into the dam's circulation. If the antigens are not also part of the dam's normal complement, antibodies are produced in the dam's circulation against the foal's erythrocytes. The antibodies are usually produced in large quantities by the 8th–10th month of pregnancy but do not affect the fetus because they are unable to pass the placental barrier. Thus, no reaction occurs until the foal is born and ingests colostrum which contains the antibodies in high concentration. Experimental immunization of mares against donkey erythrocytes has resulted in the birth of affected mule foals, suggesting that placental transmission of antibodies can occur (1).

Not all incompatible pregnancies result in sensitization of the mare. It has been suggested that abnormality of the placenta, such as fetomaternal hemorrhage, permits passage of the fetal red cell antigen into the mare's circulation in some instances only. Vaccination of mares against equine viral rhinopneumonitis using fetal tissue vaccines has been considered as a possible cause of the disease. A rise in hemagglutination titer does occur after such vaccination but in most cases there are no clinical effects in the foals, probably because of the disappearance of the antibodies by foaling time. If vaccination is carried out twice during pregnancy the clinical syndrome may occur and the danger is greatest when the mares are vaccinated during the last 3 months of pregnancy. The disease has been produced experimentally in adult horses by the injection of ovine antihorse serum (2), and in calves by the injection of sire erythrocytes into the dams (3).

Although the disease is recorded as occurring spontaneously in pigs (5) the main occurrence is manmade and is related to repeated vaccination against hog cholera, using the crystal violet vaccine. The vaccine contains erythrocytes, and isoantibodies to the cells are produced in the sows and transmitted to the piglets in the colostrum. This may cause isoagglutination if the piglets have blood groups to which the sow has become sensitized. The disease is much more common in the litters produced by mating Large White boars with Essex or Wessex sows than in litters produced by Large White sows, and the variation is thought to be due to a differential inheritance of erythrocyte antigens (6). In pigs the high antibody titers may persist for several years causing losses in successive litters, or recede rapidly with no piglets affected at subsequent farrowings (7).

The natural occurrence of the disease has been related to the immunization of the sow against the boar's erythrocyte antigens via the fetus at parturition (9). If the breeding were repeated a significant antibody level could develop. A feature of naturally occurring neonatal erythrolysis is that it rarely if ever occurs in primiparous females because the induced antibody is not sufficiently high to induce the disease until later pregnancies. However, first pregnancy offspring are often affected by manmade erythrolysis after vaccination (10).

The disease has also occurred in calves whose dams had been vaccinated against babesiosis (11) or anaplasmosis (12) using a vaccine containing bovine blood. The calves had inherited blood group antigens from the sire that were not present in the dam's blood. As a result of vaccination the dam had developed lytic antibodies against the same sire antigens, and the presence of these antibodies in the colostrum provided the mechanism for the acute hemolytic anemia in the calves. Attempts to produce the disease experimentally in lambs have been unsuccessful (13).

Epidemiology

The disease in horses occurs in most parts of the world. Both horse and mule foals are affected. In one area in France an incidence of 10% in mule foals was recorded, apparently due to sensitization of mares to donkey red cells. In England a very low incidence, about 0·2%, seems likely. In the United States in a group of 65 Thoroughbred mares observed over a 4-year period, nine affected foals were born to four mares. There is no record of the occurrence of the disease in Shetland ponies even though the distribution of blood group genes in them suggests that they should be the most affected breed (10).

The incidence of the disease in pigs after hog cholera vaccination did assume some importance in Britain, and it also occurred in the United States, where there has been a marked increase in the disease in calves following vaccination of their dams against anaplasmosis (10).

Pathogenesis

At parturition the antibody is concentrated in the dam's colostrum and soon after ingestion it is absorbed into the suckling's circulation. The interaction between the antibody and the red cells of the newborn is followed by intravascular hemolysis with resultant anemia, hemoglobinuria and jaundice. Permeability of the intestine of the newborn foal to antibody disappears at about 36 hours and hourly milking of the mare rapidly reduces the antibody content of the colostrum. The duration of the alimentary permeability in piglets has not been determined. In the experimental disease in horses (2) anemia developed soon after the injection of the antihorse serum, there was a pronounced leukopenia, albuminuria, and hemoglobinuria which persisted for up to 3 days. The same sorts of reaction occurred in the experimental disease of calves (3). There were in addition high levels of fibrinogen degradation products indicating that disseminated intravascular coagulation (DIC) had occurred and contributed to the deaths of calves.

The cause of death is usually the acute anemia, although neonatal hypoglycemia may also play a part in piglets with only moderate anemia. It has been pointed out that many cases in pigs may be subclinical and be unobserved (7).

Clinical findings

In the mare, pregnancy and parturition are uneventful and the foal is normal for some hours after birth. Signs appear only if colostrum is taken, and vary a great deal in severity.

Horses

Peracute cases develop within 8–36 hours of birth, show severe hemoglobinuria and pallor but little jaundice. The first observed abnormality may be complete collapse. The mortality rate is high. In *acute cases* signs do not develop until 2–4 days after birth and jaundice is marked, with only moderate pallor and hemoglobinuria. *Subacute cases* may not show signs until 4–5 days after birth. Jaundice is marked, there is no hemoglobinuria and only mild pallor of mucosae. Many subacute cases recover.

General signs include lassitude, weakness and disinclination to suck and the foal lies down in sternal recumbency for long periods and yawns frequently. There is no febrile reaction but the heart rate is increased up to 120/min. The cardiac impulse is readily palpable over a wide area and may be visible. Cardiac sounds are increased in amplitude and the area of auscultation is increased. The sounds have a metallic quality and a systolic thrill is audible over the left base of the heart and posteriorly. The arterial pulse has a very small amplitude and there is a well-marked positive jugular pulse in severe cases. Respiration is normal until severe anemia develops when hyperpnea, dyspnea (respiratory rate up to 80/min) and yawning are observed. Peripheral edema does not occur and there are no signs of involvement of the central nervous system. Constipation may occur late in the syndrome.

Pigs

Piglets show essentially the same syndrome, being normal at birth but developing jaundice at 24 hours, and weakness at 48 hours with most affected pigs dying by the 5th day. Peracute cases occur and piglets may die within 12 hours of birth, showing acute anemia but no jaundice or hemoglobinuria. A proportion of subclinical cases also occurs in which hemolysis can be detected only by hematological examination.

Cattle

In calves clinical signs develop within 24–48 hours after birth and the calves die during the first week of life (12). Surviving calves are returned to normal health in 2–3 weeks. Peracute cases die within 24 hours, and at necropsy examination are characterized by pulmonary edema and splenomegaly.

Clinical pathology

There is acute anemia; erythrocyte counts, packed cell volumes and hemoglobin levels are low and although the blood cells appear normal there is greatly increased erythrocyte fragility and sedimentation rate. In piglets, the erythrocyte count may be as low as 1 million/μl and the hemoglobin level below 2 g/dl. Leukocyte counts are normal and immune isoantibodies to the red cells of the foal or piglet and the sire are present in the dam's serum, colostrum and milk.

Clinicopathological tests are used in two definitive ways to determine that the hemolytic disease is in fact an autoimmune hemolysis, and to predict its occurrence. The same tests are used, but the protocols differ. Those for prediction are set out under the heading of control. For diagnosis it is necessary to determine that the foal's erythrocytes are sensitive to the mare's serum.

The antigenic determinants involved in erythrolysis are the same as those which characterize blood groups, so that blood group typing tests provide the basic clinical pathology of the disease. The vital test is the direct sensitization test between the mare's serum and the foal's erythrocytes, and this test is considered to be the most reliable in diagnosis (14). The same test is of course applicable to all species. It has been found that careful drying of a few drops of blood from affected piglets on a glass slide shows marked erythrocyte agglutination. The slide is rocked gently to wash the cells in the plasma. A positive result is indicated by the appearance of the erythrocytes in clumps rather than as a homogeneous smear on the drying slide (15). This test is based on the agglutinating part of the antigen–antibody reaction. It has been pointed out that the lytic aspect of the reaction provides a more sensitive and dependable test (10, 16), and hemolytic tests are available for use in foals (18).

There is some prognostic significance in determining which of the blood group antigens are present and responsible for the hemolysis in individual horses (8). The *Aa* antigen produces very potent antibodies and therefore acute, severe cases. *Qa* are less potent and give rise to milder cases developing at about 24 hours. *R* or *S* antigens are less potent still with milder cases developing even later.

Necropsy findings

In affected foals, marked pallor is evident but jaundice is slight in peracute cases. No gross change is observable in the liver but the spleen is greatly enlarged, and is almost black in color due to the accumulation of lysed and lysing erythrocytes. In less severe cases jaundice is marked but pallor is only moderate in degree. Bacteriological examination is negative and histopathological changes are not marked. In piglets hemoglobinuria is an important sign, and jaundice or portwine coloration of tissues occur constantly (15). The presence of blood-stained peritoneal fluid and an enlarged spleen is also typical of the disease in piglets.

Diagnosis

There are no diseases of the newborn which present the same clinical picture as that of isoimmune hemolytic anemia. Physiological icterus of the newborn may occur occasionally but rarely causes clinical illness. However, many cases of foal septicemia are erroneously diagnosed as isoerythrolysis. Unless there is jaundice or hemoglobinuria a sleepy foal is much more likely to be affected by septicemia. An isoimmune hemorrhagic anemia has been recorded in newborn pigs, but gross hemorrhages were evident at necropsy and the age incidence was 5–14 days (17).

Treatment

The treatment is time-consuming and complicated so that a positive diagnosis should be made first. Then there is the need for clinical evaluation to determine whether the case is severe enough for intensive treatment. A severely affected foal 15 hours after birth needs intensive heroic treatment if it is to survive. A mildly affected, badly jaundiced foal at 3–4 days may need only gently supportive treatment. The aims of treatment are to repair the anemia and prevent damage from anemic anoxia and hemoglobinuric nephrosis. A transfusion of compatible blood causes a marked and rapid improvement. Because of the possibility of transfusion reactions in horses compatibility tests should be performed (14). If the necessity for rapid action makes this impossible any donor other than the dam may be used. It is also possible to select a donor by testing the donor's blood against the dam's serum. The blood of the dam, or other animal in which incompatibility appears probable, may be used after separating the cells, washing them free of plasma and resuspending them in saline or preferably donor plasma. The procedure has obvious practical limitations. A decision on when to give a transfusion must be made in the light of the circumstances. In general terms a packed cell volume of 15% and a red blood cell count of less than $3 \times 10^6/\mu l$ is a good rule-of-thumb decision point (4).

Whole blood may be stored for 5 days at 4°C (30°F) before use but hemolysis is likely if resuspended blood is stored. The intravenous injection of 500–600 ml of blood into the saphenous vein is recommended. The transfusion should be repeated in 12–24 hours but phlebitis, thrombosis and embolism are likely to occur after multiple venepunctures. The transfusion should take 30 minutes as overdosage or too rapid injection may cause circulatory embarrassment. Exchange transfusions overcome this danger and a highly efficient method has been devised (14). However, a general anesthetic is required and unless expert anesthetic advice is available the technique is best avoided. The alternative is a straight transfusion from a compatible donor or of washed cells, preferably concentrated by centrifugation. Both methods give excellent results (8). Four liters of whole blood and 500 ml of blood concentrated by sedimentation is recommended as a suitable dose.

In cases occurring in the first 3 days of life, the foal should be placed on a foster mother or on reconstituted cow's milk. After 48 hours it is safe to permit sucking of the mare. If the fluid intake is low 200–400 ml of normal saline containing 4% glucose and 3% sodium bicarbonate, should be administered to foals by stomach tube twice daily.

In pigs the prevention of sucking for periods of up to 24 hours does not prevent the disease. In piglets the safest procedure is to remove them from the sow, feed them artificially for 48 hours and then return them to the sow. Frozen bovine colostrum collected as soon as possible after calving is a satisfactory substitute for sow colostrum but is improved by the addition of pig serum. When transfusion is necessary the intraperitoneal is a practical and safe route (19). In both species it is also advisable to use penicillin or other antibiotics to prevent secondary infection if colostrum is not provided.

Control

In horses the theoretically correct method is to test the mare's serum against the sire's cells during the last 2 weeks of pregnancy. A positive agglutination reaction will suggest fostering or hand-rearing the foal. If the test can be repeated on several occasions at 2-week intervals a rapid rise in titer of the mare's serum suggests the probability of an incompatible mating. Precolostrum can be used instead of the mare's serum. The more practical procedure is to test the mare's serum against antigens (red cells) from horses with known blood groups, one of each. A sensitized mare will react with one of these and the titer will rise rapidly in late pregnancy (8). These measures are only likely to be taken in mares known or suspected to have had a jaundiced foal previously. After birth the foal's erythrocytes may be submitted to an agglutination test with the mare's serum. If the test is positive (at titers of 1:32 or above), in either case, the foal should be muzzled for 48 hours and fed cow's milk and lime water (2:1) or colostrum from a non-sensitized dam. Many veterinary practices now have access to colostrum banks maintained by breeding farms. Addition of vitamins A and C to the milk improves its nutritive value. Suckling is permitted for 5 minutes at the end of this time and if after 12 hours there is no apparent reaction the foal is put back on the dam. Hourly milking of the dam in the meantime will reduce the hemagglutination titer of the milk from 1:64 to less than 1:2.

The frequent occurrence of the disease after the use of crystal violet vaccine against hog cholera in the litters of Essex and Wessex sows gave rise to the suggestion that vaccine for use in these breeds should be prepared from homologous blood rather than from blood of another breed (6). Blood samples from sows and cows which are to be used for examination for the presence of antibodies can be taken at any time during pregnancy instead of the last few weeks, because the antibody titer is not dependent on the presence of the fetus. Avoidance of vaccines based on whole blood or cellular parts of blood is recommended, and if they have to be used it should be as far away as possible from parturition and should be restricted to one injection and one booster (1).

REVIEW LITERATURE

Becht, J. L. (1986) Neonatal isoerythrolysis in the foal. Part 1. Background, blood group antigens and pathogenesis. *Comp. cont. Educ. 5*, S591–S596.

Clarke, C. A. et al. (1978) Symposium. Hemolytic disease of the newborn foal. *J. Roy. Soc. Med.*, *71*, 574.

Morris, D. D. (1986) Immunologic diseases of foals. *Comp. cont. Educ.*, *8*, S139–S150.

Scott, A. M. & Jeffcot, L. B. (1978) Haemolytic disease of the newborn foal. *Vet. Rec.*, *103*, 71.

Stormont, C. (1975) Neonatal isoerythrolysis in domestic animals: A comparative review. *Adv. vet. Sci.*, *19*, 23.

REFERENCES

(1) Searl, R. C. (1980) *Vet. Med. SAC*, *75*, 101.
(2) Sonoda, M. & Mari, K. (1976) *Exp. Rèp. equ. Hlth Lab., Tokyo*, *13*, 50.
(3) Dimmock, C. K. et al. (1977) *Res. vet. Sci.*, *20*, 244.
(4) Lui, I. K. M. (1980) *J. Am. vet. med. Assoc.*, *176*, 1247.
(5) Nansen, P. et. al. (1970) *Nord. VetMed.*, *22*, 1.
(6) Goodwin, R. F. W. & Saison, R. (1956) *J. comp. Pathol.*, *66*, 163.
(7) Goodwin, R. F. W. (1957) *Vet. Rec.*, *69*, 1290.
(8) Scott, A. M. & Jeffcott, L. B. (1978) *Vet. Rec.*, *103*, 71.
(9) Linklater, K. A. (1968) *Vet. Rec.*, *83*, 203.
(10) Stormont, C. (1975) *Adv. vet. Sci.*, *19*, 23.
(11) Dowsett, K. F. et al. (1978) *Aust. vet. J.*, *54*, 65.
(12) Dennis, R. A. et al. (1970) *J. Am. vet. med. Assoc.*, *156*, 1861.
(13) Tucker, E. M. (1961) *Nature, Lond.*, *189*, 847.
(14) Becht, J. L. et al. (1983) *Cornell Vet.*, *73*, 380.
(15) Goodwin, R. F. W. (1957) *Vet. Rec.*, *69*, 505.
(16) Sonoda, M. et al. (1972) *Expl. Rep. equ. Hlth Lab.*, *9*, 103.
(17) Stormorken, H. et al. (1963) *Nature, Lond.*, *198*, 1116.
(18) Becht, J. L. & Page, E. H. (1980) *Proc. ann. Conv. Am. Assoc. equ. Pract.*, *25*, 247.
(19) Edwards, B. L. (1965) *Vet. Rec.*, *77*, 268.

Purpura hemorrhagica

This is an acute, non-contagious disease, occurring chiefly in the horse, and characterized by extensive, edematous and hemorrhagic swellings in subcutaneous tissues, accompanied by haemorrhages in the mucosae and viscera.

Etiology

The cause of the disease is uncertain. Its common association with streptococcal infection of the upper respiratory tract has led to the suggestion that it is caused by an allergic reaction to streptococcal protein. However, in some instances there is no history of prior occurrence of streptococcal infection. Anaphylactoid purpura is similar in that it occurs commonly after streptococcal infection. It is very rare in animals, but well known in man (7).

Epidemiology

Purpura hemorrhagica is most common in horses although it has been recorded in pigs and is observed occasionally in cattle. In the horse it occurs only sporadically and usually as a sequel to upper respiratory infections. It achieves its highest incidence in large groups of horses used for military purposes, or during and after shipment. Most affected animals die of the disease.

Most commonly the disease occurs as a sequel to strangles in horses, or in association with infectious equine arteritis or infectious equine rhinopneumonitis. Only a small proportion of horses become affected but the incidence is highest when extensive outbreaks of strangles occur, possibly because of reinfection with streptococci of horses already sensitized by previous infection.

Pathogenesis

Damage to capillary walls with extravasation of plasma and blood into the tissues is the basis of the disease process (3). The disease appears to be immune complex-mediated because immune complexes are found in the serum of horses with post-strangles purpura. The immune complexes contain IgA and *S. equi*-specific antigens (10). In anaphylactoid purpura there is basically a vasculitis also, but instead of large extravasations of blood there are patches of hemorrhage and necrosis of the intestinal wall. A case is reported in a horse in which there was an associated membranoproliferative and mesangioproliferative glomerulonephritis (9).

Clinical findings

Extensive subcutaneous, edematous swellings are the characteristic sign of the disease. They occur most commonly about the face and muzzle, but are often present on other parts of the body and are not necessarily symmetrical in distribution. The swellings may appear suddenly or develop gradually over several days. They are cold and painless and pit on pressure and merge gradually in normal tissue without a definite line of demarcation between. There is no discontinuity of the skin although it may be tightly distended and even ooze serum. Swellings about the head may cause pressure on the pharynx and dyspnea and difficulty in swallowing. Extensive edema of the limbs, with a sharply defined upper margin, may occur but typical, discrete swellings do not develop below the knees or hocks.

Submucous hemorrhages occur in the nasal cavities and mouth, and petechiae may be present under the conjunctiva. Hemorrhage and edema of the gut wall may cause severe, fatal colic but in most cases there is no diarrhea or constipation. In anaphylactoid purpura recorded in a horse the principal clinical sign was colic. The temperature is normal or slightly elevated but the heart rate is frequently raised (90–100/min) probably because of loss of plasma or blood. The course of the disease is usually 1–2 weeks and many animals die at the end of this time from blood loss and secondary bacterial infections. Relapses occur commonly during convalescence.

Clinical pathology
In severe cases there is a fall in the erythrocyte count and hemoglobin level, a marked neutrophilia but no marked depression of platelet counts. A leukocytosis occurs in less severe cases. There is no defect in the clotting mechanism. There may be oligocythemia or polycythemia depending upon the degree of loss of the plasma or whole blood. The urine is normal although there may be oliguria.

Necropsy findings
Petechial hemorrhages are present generally throughout the body. The subcutaneous swellings contain plasma which may be bloodstained, or whole blood and plasma, and blood may be present in the body cavities. The intestines, lungs and spleen may be congested and there may be edematous thickening of the intestinal wall.

Diagnosis

Horses
In horses purpura hemorrhagica may be mistaken for idiopathic thrombocytopenic purpura which is readily distinguishable by its low platelet count. In other species it is thought to be immune-mediated. It is characterized by a bleeding tendency, mucosal hemorrhages and large bullous hematomas. Corticosteroid therapy for 7–10 days is effective in most cases but may need to be repeated (5, 8). Purpura hemorrhagica may also be mistaken for congestive heart failure but in the latter the edema is of the dependent parts only and hemorrhages are not present in the mucosae. Angioneurotic edema is accompanied by large subcutaneous swellings but again there are no hemorrhages and the lesions disappear quickly after treatment. There is also some resemblance between purpura hemorrhagica and infectious equine arteritis and, to a less extent, infectious equine rhinopneumonitis, but both of these diseases spread rapidly to other horses while purpura hemorrhagica affects only occasional animals and the edema in the viral diseases is restricted to the limbs. Petechial hemorrhages of the mucosae and anemia also occur in infectious equine anemia but this disease is characterized by a regional distribution, a chronic recurrent course, jaundice, and restriction of edema to dependent parts. Dourine is a venereal disease, and although edematous swellings occur they originate in the external genitalia. 'Blue nose' is a photosensitization which occurs in the United Kingdom in horses on spring grass. Purplish coloration of the unpigmented skin around the muzzle, and urticarial swellings in other parts of the body, may create a resemblance to purpura hemorrhagica (6).

Pigs
In pigs a thrombocytopenic purpura occurs in the newborn. Bleeding commences at 5 days of age and continues for more than 7 days (1–3). There are antibodies against the piglet's thrombocytes in the dam's serum.

Cattle
In cattle hemorrhagic septicemia, poisoning by bracken fern and sweet clover, fungal intoxications such as stachybotrytoxicosis, and some other septicemias are more likely causes of a hemorrhagic syndrome than is purpura hemorrhagica. A hemorrhagic disease which is similar in many respects to purpura hemorrhagica affects Charolais cattle in France (4).

Treatment
Many treatments have been tried, including blood transfusions, antihistamine drugs, and formalin and calcium administered parenterally, but with very poor results in most cases and the prognosis should be very grave. Blood transfusions give the greatest chance of recovery and are usually supported by full and continuous doses of corticosteroids. At least 4 liters of blood should be given every 48 hours. Calcium gluconate (100–200 ml of a 7.5% solution), or calcium lactate (600 ml of a 10% solution) given intravenously daily have also been found useful. Adrenaline (10 ml of 1:1000) given daily as a subcutaneous injection may have some value. If corticosteroids will temporarily control the disease they should be given continuously for periods of about 2 weeks and then discontinued to determine whether signs return. A total course of 3 months may be necessary before the sensitivity finally abates.

Control
The control and prevention of upper respiratory tract infections in horses should lead to a reduction in the incidence of purpura hemorrhagica.

REFERENCES

(1) Stormorken, H. et al. (1963) *Nature, Lond.*, *198*, 1116.
(2) Nordstoga, K. (1965) *Pathol. vet.*, *2*, 601.
(3) Saunders, C. N. et al. (1966) *Vet. Rec.*, *79*, 549.
(4) Cottereau, P. (1965) *Encycl. vet. period.*, *22* , 33.
(5) Larson, V. L. et al. (1983) *J. Am. vet. med. Assoc.*, *183*, 328.
(6) Greatorex, J. C. (1969) *Equ. vet. J.*, *1*, 157.
(7) Gunson, D. E. & Rooney, J. R. (1977) *Vet. Pathol.*, *14*, 325.
(8) Byars, T. D. & Greene, C. E. (1982) *J. Am. vet. med. Assoc.*, *180*, 1422.
(9) Roberts, M. C. & Kelly, W. R. (1982) *Vet. Rec.*, *110*, 144.
(10) Galan, J. E. & Timoney, J. F. (1985) *J. Immunol.*, *135*, 3134.

Laminitis

Laminitis is a disease of all species, particularly the horse, characterized by damage to the sensitive laminae of the hooves. Clinically it is manifested by severe lameness with heat and pain around the coronets.

Etiology
Laminitis is thought to be caused by an intoxication, in horses usually related to bacterial toxins after an alimentary tract disturbance, usually overeating on grain, or related to a local infection such as metritis, or retention of the placenta in the mare. The disease has been produced experimentally in the horse by the administration of a gruel made of starch and wood flour. It has been produced in cattle by the injection of histamine (22). It has also been produced experimentally in lambs by the intraruminal injection of lactic acid. However,

the predisposing and precipitating causes in cattle are less well identified.

Epidemiology

Laminitis occurs only sporadically but a number of cases may occur at one time in a group of animals in special circumstances. It is of most importance in horses and cattle on heavy concentrate feed and has attracted particular attention in young cattle (4½–6 months of age) being fattened on heavy grain diets—the 'barley beef' calves—in the United Kingdom and Japan (24). Amongst horses, ponies are much more susceptible, up to four times as many cases occurring in them as in other horses. However, sex and age exert very little influence, although the castrated male is less susceptible than the entire male, and the middle age group of 4–10 years is the most susceptible group (4). Death is unusual, but the severe lameness may cause a great deal of inconvenience and affected horses may develop permanent deformities of the feet.

Laminitis is most common in horses which engorge moderately on grain feed; it seldom occurs in those which eat sufficient to cause acute dilatation of the stomach, or death due to lactic acidosis and cardiovascular collapse (28). There seems to be a predisposition to laminitis in individual animals. Mares which retain the placenta are often affected. Fat ponies running at pasture and getting little exercise commonly develop the chronic form of the disease. The pasture is most contributory if it is lush, and there is correspondingly a peak of cases in spring and autumn. Concussion of excessive weight-bearing in one or more legs, e.g. when a horse is very lame in the contralateral one, or paws persistently, can be followed by laminitis. This is usually defined as traumatic laminitis, as distinct from the more common form, which is designated as 'metabolic laminitis'. Horses standing for periods of several days during transport may develop the acute form.

In ruminants, the disease is uncommon but is being reported with increasing frequency. Cattle and lambs introduced too quickly to heavy grain rations in feedlots may be affected and occasionally individual dairy cows which overeat develop the disease. Beef cattle being prepared for shows are often grossly overfed on high grain rations and become affected with a chronic form of the disease which markedly affects their gait and may cause permanent foot deformity. This is a serious matter to owners of show cattle because they have difficulty in regulating the food intake to achieve fatness and yet avoid laminitis. As in horses there appears to be a variation in susceptibility between individual animals, one or two animals in a group kept under identical conditions often developing the disease.

In cattle the disease is also reported to occur after metritis, retained placenta, mastitis and mammary edema but the incidence is not usually very high. It is not uncommon, however, to come upon herds of cattle which appear to be having a special problem with laminitis. The heifers are usually worst affected (24) and the disease usually develops soon after calving, with more than 50% of cases occurring in the period 30 days before and 30 days after calving (21). It seems to be associated with a high incidence of metritis. There may be a relationship between being introduced to the herd, with the frequent harassment by bossy cows, when heavily pregnant and when the surface of the yards is rough. It is possible that the disease, or rather a susceptibility to it, is inherited, especially as it occurs more frequently in Guernseys and in Jerseys. For example, a specific laminitis, conditioned by the inheritance of an autosomal recessive gene, is recorded in Jersey heifers (23).

Housing may be important including standing in slurry or having to twist and turn in narrow passageways and races. Trauma to the feet is also thought to be important in an unexpectedly high prevalence of related postmortem lesions observed in African cattle (30). The disease has been produced experimentally in postcalving cows by feeding a high starch, low-fiber diet. The resulting high incidence of laminitis was accomplished by a significantly increased prevalence of sole ulcers (32).

Laminitis has been recorded in pigs but the disease is difficult to diagnose in this species and many cases secondary to other diseases, e.g. postparturient fever, may be missed. The disease is also recorded in this species when pigs are fed very heavy concentrate diets.

Pathogenesis

Until recently, it was considered that laminitis was caused by engorgement of the vascular bed in the structures of the foot and that histamine was the causative mechanism of the engorgement. There is a good deal of evidence on the subject, most of it negative, and the hypothesis has little currency (26). The present hypothesis is that the vascular engorgement is caused by other toxic substances, especially lactic acid, produced in the gut by fermentation of excessive carbohydrate, and bacterial endotoxins released by bacteria destroyed in the same process and absorbed through a mucosa also damaged by the abnormal circumstances in the gut. This damage to the cecal mucosa has been quantified in experimental grain overload in horses and has been assessed as substantial (3). Cecal fluid lactate and bacterial endotoxin levels have been shown to increase after grain engorgement and prior to the development of laminitis (6). There are also significant rises in blood levels of endotoxins, e.g. from a normal of less than 0·1 ng/l of plasma to as high as 80 ng/l in horses later affected with laminitis (34). Appropriate changes in cecal flora also occur (6).

An important suggested corollary to this hypothesis is that the changes which occur in the foot are only part of a general vascular change in which peripheral resistance to blood flow is increased by the causative agent, and this results in a significant increase in arterial blood pressure (12). However, the absence of demonstrably increased peripheral vascular resistance to blood flow in grain engorgement produced experimentally in horses (13) casts some doubt on this proposal. It is supported by evidence derived from angiographic techniques which indicate that there is vasoconstriction of the terminal vessels and a reduction in blood flow in the foot with laminitis (9).

A second hypothesis is that the vascular changes in laminitis are secondary, and that the primary defect is one of epidermal horn formation resulting in the weakening of the bond between horn and sensitive laminae (10). In this hypothesis the presence of additional blood within the hoof is the result of the traumatic separation of the two structures. There is good correlation between the occurrence of laminitis-inducing diseases such as acute intestinal disease, septicemia and abnormalities of the pulmonary and secondary epidermal laminae (11).

On the evidence available it seems more probable that the disease is primarily vascular, with the vascular response being caused by bacterial toxins when the initiating cause is for example metritis or digestive upset, or being part of a general vascular response to shock after such events as abdominal crises. The effective vascular mechanism is thought to be a diversion of blood supply from the laminar corium because of the operation of arteriovenous shunts which are characteristic of the anatomy of the area. The deprivation of blood to the corium results in a deficient supply of nutrients to it, especially methionine, cysteine and cystine, so that incomplete keratin is produced and the onchygenic bridge between the laminar epithelium and the horn breaks down. The hoof then separates from the digital cushion and the third phalanx, blood pools in distended vessels which result, and serum exudes into the potential space created. The toe, which is freed from its attachment most, moves most, and it angles down towards the sole causing the characteristic, and diagnostic, rotation of the pedal bone. The sole is pushed downwards or 'dropped', and the point of the toe of the third phalanx may actually penetrate the sole. This rotation of the third phalanx is most likely to occur in overweight, middle-aged females with laminitis in all four feet, and subsequent to a primary disease such as metritis or grain overload (7).

Two further hindrances to the development of a coherent hypothesis on pathogenesis are the observations that disseminated intravascular coagulopathy develops just before the lameness of laminitis appears (19), and that anti-inflammatory corticosteroids are capable of inducing laminitis (27). Another observed phenomenon, which has not been explained, is the significantly lower sensitivity to insulin of laminitic ponies than that of other ponies. Ponies generally are less sensitive to insulin than other types but there may be some relationship between this physiological characteristic and the known susceptibility of ponies to laminitis (2).

The experimental production of laminitis in horses has made a significant contribution to an understanding of the pathogenesis of the disease. It has made possible the careful mapping of the physiological and pathological responses to the laminitis-inducing insults although the occurrence of some of the reported effects is disputed.

Clinical findings

Horses

Laminitis may develop as an acute disease and be followed by recovery or persistence of a chronic state, or it may develop in a mild form from the beginning. In *acute cases* there is severe pain in all four feet, but especially the front feet; in occasional cases only the hindfeet are affected. In 36% of one series of cases the lesion was unilateral (15). The clinical signs are all manifestations of pain and include an expression of great anxiety, muscle shivering, sweating, a marked increase in heart rate to as high as 75/min, rapid, shallow respiration and a moderate elevation of temperature. The posture is characteristic, all four feet being placed forward of their normal position, the head held low and the back arched. There is usually a great deal of difficulty in getting the animal to move and when it does so the gait is shuffling and stumbling and the animal evidences great pain when the foot is put to the ground. The act of lying down is accomplished only with difficulty, often after a number of preliminary attempts. There is also difficulty in getting the animals to rise and some horses may be recumbent for long periods. It is not unusual for horses to lie flat on their sides. The diagnostic sign in laminitis is pain on palpation around the coronet, light palpation causing a marked pain reaction. In bad cases there may be an exudation of serum at the coronet.

In the chronic stages of the disease there is separation of the wall from the sensitive laminae and a consequent dropping of the sole. The hoof wall spreads and develops marked horizontal ridges, and the slope of the anterior surface of the wall becomes accentuated and concave. Eventually the lameness may disappear but the animal is clumsy, goes lame easily with exercise and may suffer repeated, mild attacks of laminitis. In occasional cases the separation of the wall from the laminae is acute and the hoof is shed.

Cattle and sheep

Here the clinical picture is similar to but less marked than that observed in the horse. In calves 4–6 months of age and in heifers an acute syndrome similar to that seen in the horse has been described. Affected animals lie down much of the time, and are reluctant to rise. When they attempt to rise they remain kneeling for long periods. Their standing posture is with all four feet bunched together and the back is arched, they shift their weight from foot to foot frequently and they walk with a shuffling painful gait. The feet are painful when squeezed and later become flattened and enlarged and look as though slippers are being worn. There is severe ventral rotation of the third phalanx. In adult cows some cases have acute signs, others show only local lesions (21). These include sole ulcers and patchy changes in the horn including softening, waxy yellow discoloration, and red-brown patches suggestive of previous hemorrhage. The cow is chronically lame (29). A long-term study of the effects of an acute attack of laminitis on the subsequent performance of the horn has been conducted in cattle (16) and has shown that the solar horn of affected animals was thinner and more soft and waxy than that of normal animals. Also previously affected animals were much more susceptible to injury to the sole.

Pigs

In sows the clinical signs are similar and include arching of the back, bunching of the feet, awkwardness of movement, increased pulsation in the digital arteries and pain when pressure is applied to the feet (8).

Clinical pathology

The important clinicopathological findings in acute laminitis include an elevation of arterial blood pressure which occurs at about 48 hours after the dietary insult. There is a synchronous and significant increase in heart rate, and a precipitate fall in central venous blood pressure; there is also a rise in temperature and total leukocyte count, and a rise in packed cell volume and total protein concentration (17). Hyponatremia, hypochloremia and marked hypovolemia are part of the acute laminitis syndrome in horses but not in ponies (14). The same findings are characteristic of experimental grain engorgement, and are indications of hemoconcentration (31). A significant alteration in platelet function is recorded by many observers. Initially there is an increase in platelet aggregation and subsequently a hypocoagulability and sharp decline in blood platelet numbers, and these are related to the severity of clinical signs of laminitis (5). Disseminated intravascular coagulopathy is thought to be involved in the pathogenesis of laminitis in either a primary or secondary role (19). The systolic arterial blood pressure is now an essential diagnostic ingredient in a case of laminitis (12); it will be elevated from a normal of 120 mmHg to as high as 150 mmHg (1).

Blood histamine levels and eosinophil counts may be raised but are often within the normal range and other hematological findings are normal. Radiological examination is an essential part of the diagnosis of laminitis, especially chronic laminitis in the horse. The downward tilting of the toe of the third phalanx and the ventral displacement of the whole phalanx are characteristic. The degree of rotation of the phalanx can be used as a basis for prognosis in terms of returning to sports action. Horses with a pedal rotation of more than 11·5° will not return to sports. Horses with rotation less than 5·5° have good prospects for complete recovery (1). Angiographic delineation of the vascular changes in the affected horse's feet is described (12). In cattle there are rarefaction of the pedal bone, particularly the toe, and the development of osteophytes at the heel and on the pyramidal process (18).

Necropsy findings

The disease is not usually fatal but if a necropsy examination is carried out on an acute case the stomach contents usually contain excessive amounts of grain, have a pasty, mealy consistency and an odor suggestive of putrefaction of protein. Retained placenta and metritis may be present in postparturient laminitis in mares. No other gross findings are visible although there may be perceptible engorgement of the vessels of the sensitive laminae of the digital cushion. Histological examination reveals disappearance of some of the keratogenic structures of the inner zone of cornification in the epidermal laminae. This is followed by vascular engorgement, edema and some necrosis of laminar tissues. These changes have been accurately defined in terms of time after the insult by serial postmortem examinations carried out on experimental cases (17). In subacute and chronic laminitis there are obvious gross changes in the shape of the foot. Histological findings in the feet of cows affected by laminitis are similar to those in horses (8).

Diagnosis

Laminitis is easily missed unless a typical history is available. The animal's distress, immobility and increased pulse and respiration always suggest severe pain but it is only when the posture and gait and pain in the feet are taken into consideration that it is possible to localize the lesion. Cases of laminitis in horses have been mistaken for tetanus, azoturia, rupture of the stomach or bladder, or colic, but in none of these diseases is the pain localized in the feet and there are other differentiating signs. In cattle and lambs recumbency after overeating is usual and the presence of laminitis may be difficult to detect. A clinically similar condition in young Hereford bulls appears to be genetic in origin. There is epiphysitis at the distal metacarpus and first phalanx and calcium deposits in the testes and kidneys (20).

Treatment

The treatment of acute laminitis is reasonably effective but the critical factor is the time elapsed between when the disease commences and when treatment is initiated. Any delay beyond 24 hours could be fatal, and cases which have been untreated for 48 hours are unlikely to have a favorable outcome, unless it is a spontaneous one. Even if treatment is begun within a few hours of onset the outcome cannot be guaranteed because it is the severity of the damage in the hoof which is critical. In summary, laminitis must always be dealt with as an emergency. The treatment program generally used includes phenylbutazone, mineral oil and methionine, and feeding techniques which reduce the sodium intake.

In the past, antihistamine drugs have been recommended in the treatment of acute cases and appeared to have a good effect if given parenterally early. Corticosteroids have been widely used, but they are now omitted from treatment programs because of fears that they might exacerbate the condition. Phenylbutazone is now generally used because of its vascular effects, and because of its analgesic properties. If a corticosteroid is used it should not be used beyond the second day because of the possibility of further reducing the protein status of the hoof horn (21). Excellent recoveries are reported after the treatment of acute and chronic cases with methionine. The treatment is based on the known requirement for methionine in the chondroitin complex of collagen (22). There is some rationale for the treatment but it seems more appropriate as a supportive than as a principal treatment. The recommended oral dose rate is 10 g/day for 3 days followed by 5 g/day for 10 days (11). Ancillary treatment should include an analgesic in severe cases, cold packs to the feet (either ice packs or standing the horse in mud or a water bath), and a mild purgative to hasten elimination of the toxic ingesta. The latter is a required treatment when toxic ingesta needs to be evacuated quickly, and is recommended in all cases. Mineral oil by stomach tube is the standard product used. Every effort should also be made to eliminate other sources of bacterial toxins, such as infection in the uterus. If the animal will walk, forced exercise for short periods at frequent intervals is recommended in order to increase movement of blood through the foot. This could be improved further by locally anesthetizing the volar nerves in the affected leg. This remains as one of the important features in promoting recovery—gentle exercise to cause alternate expansion and contraction of the digital cushion by exerting and releasing pressure on it by the hoof during walking. The intravenous administration of butazolidine is the most effective means of relieving the pain so that the animal can walk. If pedal rotation has already occurred the horse will be reluctant to walk and should not be encouraged to do so. To facilitate the reduction of blood pressure, salt should be removed from the diet and be replaced by 30 g/day potassium chloride. Experimental administration of isoxuprine (1·8 mg/kg intravenously every 12 hours) is thought to improve the affected horse's chance of recovery (33).

Additional non-specific treatments which have been used include venesection either from the jugular vein or from the sole of the foot, and autogenous blood therapy. In the latter 50 ml of whole blood collected from the jugular vein is injected immediately in a deep intramuscular site. Excellent results are claimed for the procedure in both horses (25), and cattle, but it is not recommended. The administration of diuretics is rational to reduce the circulating blood volume, and antibiotics are used by most to avoid secondary microbial invasion under the hoof. Spontaneous recovery from the acute disease does occur, often very rapidly and after an illness of only 24 hours. The acute disease in intensively fed calves does not appear to respond to any of these recommended treatments.

Medical treatment of chronic cases is seldom satisfactory and surgical procedures are recommended. Reduction of weight by a high quality protein, low-calorie diet may be advisable, along with butazolidine when pain persists. Animals affected for more than 7 days are unlikely to make a complete recovery.

Control

The disease is not readily subject to control because of its sporadic nature. Heavily fed or fat horses should be given some exercise when not working; if possible horses in transit should be removed from the transport vehicle, given light exercise and rested for several hours at the end of each day; retained placenta in mares should be completely removed and early metritis treated promptly. Heavy carbohydrate feeding should be avoided. The best policy is to use high quality roughage only and to supplement this with an absolute minimum of grain. Horse owners in general use far more feed than is necessary to maintain growth and performance capability. Protein intake should be assured by the use of legume hay. Cattle and lambs which are brought into feedlots should be gradually introduced to grain feeds and a higher forage : grain ratio provided in the feed. Exercise should be provided around calving time. Housing errors need to be corrected. Vaccination with a Gram-negative bacterin–endotoxoid combination vaccine has provided some protection against laminitis induced by grain overload (18).

REVIEW LITERATURE

Colles, C. M. & Jeffcott, C. D. (1977) Laminitis in the horse. *Vet. Rec.*, *100*, 262.

Edwards, G. B. (1982) Acute and subacute laminitis in cattle. *Vet. Ann.*, *22*, 99–106.

Garner, H. E. (1980) Update on equine laminitis. *Vet. Clin. N. Am., large Anim. Pract.*, *2(1)*, 25–32.

REFERENCES

(1) Stick, J. A. et al. (1982) *J. Am. vet. med. Assoc.*, *180*, 251.
(2) Coffman, J. R. & Colles, C. M. (1983) *Can. J. comp. Med.*, *47*, 347.
(3) Krueger, A. S. et al. (1986) *Am. J. vet. Res.*, *47*, 1804.
(4) Dorn, C. R. et al. (1975) *Cornell Vet.* *65*, 57.
(5) Bell, T. et al. (1979) *Fed. Proc.*, *38*, 1411.
(6) Garner, H. E. et al. (1978) *Equ. vet. J.*, *10*, 249.
(7) Baxter, G. M. (1986) *J. Am. vet. med. Assoc.*, *189*, 326.
(8) Andersson, L. & Bergman, A. (1980) *Acta vet. Scand.*, *21*, 559.
(9) Hood, D. M. et al. (1978) *J. equ. med. Surg.*, *2*, 439.
(10) Obel, N. (1948) *Coll. Pap. vet. Inst., Stockholm*, 63.
(11) Roberts, E. D. et al. (1980) *Vet. Pathol.*, *17*, 656.
(12) Garner, H. E. et al. (1975) *J. Am. vet. med. Assoc.*, *166*, 56, 58.
(13) Robinson, N. E. et al. (1977) *Vet. Rec.*, *100*, 427.
(14) Clarke, L. L. et al. (1982) *Am. J. vet. Res.*, *43*, 1551.
(15) Kameya, T. (1973) *Rep. equ. Hlth Lab.*, *10*, 19.
(16) Maclean, C. W. (1971) *Vet. Rec.*, *89*, 34.
(17) Garner, H. E. et al. (1974) *Proc. 20th ann. Cont. Am. Assoc. equ. Practnrs*, 61.
(18) Garner, H. E. et al. (1985) *Proc. 31st AAEP Ann. Conv.*, p. 525.
(19) Hood, D. M. et al. (1979) *J. equ. med. Surg.*, *3*, 355.
(20) Brown, C. J. et al. (1967) *J. anim. Sci.*, *26*, 201, 206.
(21) Slone, D. E. et al. (1981) *Proc. 27th Ann. Conv. AAEP*, p. 469.
(22) Takahashi, K. & Young, B. A. (1981) *Jap. J. vet. Sci.*, *43*, 261, 375.
(23) Edwards, G. N. (1972) *7th Int. Mtg on Dis. Cattle, London*, pp. 663–668.
(24) Bazeley, K. & Pinsent, P. J. N. (1984) *Vet. Rec.*, *115*, 619.
(25) Siemens, J. W. (1979) *Equ. Pract.*, *1*, 8.
(26) Robinson, N. E. & Scott, J. B. (1981) *Am. J. vet. Res.*, *42*, 205.
(27) Eyre, P. et al. (1979) *Am. J. vet. Res.*, *40*, 135.
(28) Garner, H. E. et al. (1977) *J. anim. Sci.*, *45*, 1037.
(29) Greenough, P. R. (1985) *Bov. Practnr*, *20*, 144.
(30) Mgassa, M. N. et al. (1984) *Vet. Rec.*, *115*, 413.
(31) Moore, J. N. et al. (1981) *Equ. vet. J.*, *13*, 240.
(32) Livesey, C. T. (1985) *Proc. 1984/85 British Cattle vet. Assoc.*, p. 161.
(33) Kirker-Head, C. A. et al. (1986) *J. equ. vet. Sci.*, *6*, 293.
(34) Sprouse, R. F. et al. (1987) *Equ. vet. J.*, *19*, 25.

Allergic dermatitis (Queensland itch, sweet itch)

This is an intensely itchy dermatitis of horses caused by hypersensitivity to insect bites.

Etiology

Hypersensitivity to the bites of sandflies and other insects is the cause. *Culicoides brevitarsus* is the cause in Australia (1), *C. pulicaris* in the United Kingdom and Europe (7), and *C. obsoletus* in Canada (8). *Stomoxys calcitrans* has been identified as a causative insect in Japan (2). *C. pulicaris* has a predilection for landing at the mane and tail of horses where the lesion is most commonly seen (3). Occasional cases in areas where sandflies do not exist suggest that other allergens may cause the disease.

Epidemiology

The disease is quite common in Australia, particularly in hot, humid coastal areas and similar conditions are recorded in Japan, Israel, Hong Kong, North America, the Philippines, India and France. A clinically identical disease occurs in ponies in the United Kingdom during the summer months. It is identified as 'sweet itch' (4) and up to 3% of ponies are reported to be affected. Only a proportion of horses in a group will be affected. Deaths do not occur but badly affected horses may be of little use as working animals because of the intense pruritus.

Most cases occur during the hot humid months of summer and disappear during cooler weather. Only horses are affected and characteristic lesions have been observed in animals of all ages. Lesions disappear when the horses have been stabled for several weeks or are moved to an unaffected area.

Pathogenesis

Local accumulations of eosinophils and a general eosinophilia, together with a significant, seasonal increase in blood histamine levels occur and are suggestive of hypersensitivity (5).

Clinical findings

Lesions are usually confined to the butt of the tail, rump, along the back, withers, crest, poll and ears. In severe cases the lesions may extend down the sides of the body and neck and on to the face and legs. Itching is intense, especially at night, and the horse scratches against any fixed object for hours at a time. In the early stages slight, discrete papules, with the hair standing erect, are observed. Constant scratching may cause severe inflammatory lesions and loss of hair. Scaliness and loss of hair on the ears and tail-butt may be the only lesions in mildly affected horses.

The general condition of the horse is unaffected except for some loss of condition due to interference with grazing.

Clinical pathology

Affected animals have significantly elevated blood eosinophil and platelet counts. In early lesions, before trauma masks the true picture, edema, capillary engorgement and eosinophil infiltration can be observed in a biopsy specimen. Immediate sensitivity reactions can be elicited by the intradermal injection of extracts of *Culicoides* and *Stomoxys* spp.

Diagnosis

The intense scratching, the dorsal distribution of the dermatitis and the seasonal occurrence of the disease in association with biting insects are characteristic of this form of dermatitis.

A very similar disease occurs in cattle in Japan. It is thought to be due to an allergy to the bite of an external parasite (6).

Treatment

Local and parenteral application of antihistamine drugs may have some transient value. Longacting corticosteroids can give relief for about 4 weeks.

Control

Prevention of the disease necessitates protection against sandfly bites by stabling in insect-proof quarters. Continuous spraying of the horses with insecticides or repellents may be of some value.

REVIEW LITERATURE

Baker, K. P. (1978) The rational approach to the management of sweet itch. *Vet. Ann.*, *18*, 163.

REFERENCES

(1) Quinn, P. J. & Baker, K. P. (1983) *Equ. Vet. J.* *15*, 266.
(2) Hasselholt, M. & Agger, N. (1977) *Dansk. VetTidskr.*, *60*, 715.
(3) Mellor, P.S. & McCaig, J. (1974) *Vet. Rec.*, *95*, 411.
(4) McCaig, J. (1975) *Vet. Ann.*, *15*, 204.
(5) Riek, R. F. (1955) *Aust. J. agric. Res.*, *6*, 161.
(6) Arisawa, M. (1971) *Bull. Nippon vet. zootech. College*, *19*, 46.
(7) Anderson, L. & Bergman, A. (1980) *Acta Vet. Scand.*, *21*, 559.
(8) Kleider, N. & Lees, M. J. (1984) *Can. vet. J.*, *25*, 26.

Milk allergy

Signs of allergy, principally urticaria, are often manifested by cows during periods of milk retention (1, 2). Most of these occur as the cow is being dried off. Cattle of the Channel Island breeds are most susceptible and the disease is likely to recur in the same cow at subsequent drying off periods; it is almost certainly inherited as a familial trait.

The important clinical signs relate to the skin. There is urticaria which may be visible only on the eyelids or be distributed generally. Local or general erection of the hair may also be seen. A marked muscle tremor, respiratory distress, frequent coughing, restlessness to the point of kicking at the abdomen and violent licking of themselves and even maniacal charging with bellowing may occur. Other cows may show dullness, recumbency, shuffling gait, ataxia and later inability to rise. The temperature and pulse rates are usually normal or slightly elevated but the respiratory rate may be as high as 100/minute.

Diagnosis of milk allergy can be made by the intradermal injection of an extract of the cow's own milk. A positive reaction occurs with milk diluted as much as 1 in 10 000 and the edematous thickening is present within minutes of the injection. Other clinicopathological observations include the development of eosinopenia, neutrophilia and hyperphosphatemia during an attack.

Spontaneous recovery is the rule but antihistamines are effective, especially if administered early and repeated at short intervals for 24 hours. Prevention is usually a matter of avoiding milk retention in susceptible cows, but in many cases it is preferable to cull them.

REFERENCES

(1) Campbell, S. G. (1970) *Cornell Vet.*, *60*, 684.
(2) Campbell, S. G. (1971) *Allergy. clin. Immunol.*, *48*, 230.

Enzootic nasal granuloma of cattle (bovine atopic rhinitis)

Of the three known clinical types of chronic nasal obstruction in cattle two have been identified etiologically. One recorded in beef cattle appears to be caused by a fungus, *Rhinosporidium* sp. Another is caused by the parasite *Schistosoma nasalis*. The third type, enzootic nasal granuloma, occurs commonly in southern Australia (1). An extensive survey of dairying areas showed that 22% of cattle had lesions, and that the prevalence was greater in areas where the average annual rainfall was over 70 cm, than where it was less than 70 cm; the prevalence varied between 4% and 48%; Jerseys were more commonly affected than Friesians. In New Zealand 40% of farms and 36% of culled cattle are reported to be affected whereas only 3·6% of young beef cattle showed lesions (2). The disease has been identified as an allergic rhinitis and has been produced experimentally (5). Specific antigens have not been identified as the cause but cows with nasal granuloma are much more sensitive to a number of common allergens in the environment than are unaffected cows (5). Additional possible causes include infestation of the nasal cavities with pasture mites (*Tyrophagus palmarum*) (7). An allied condition has been described in the United States as maduromycosis (8, 10) and an enzootic nasal adenocarcinoma occurring in sheep has been recorded (9). In maduromycosis there are nasal granulomas plus multiple granulomatous lesions of the skin of the ears, tail, vulva and thigh (6). The granulomas contain many eosinophils and fungal elements identified provisionally as *Helminthosporium* sp.

Enzootic nasal granuloma occurs sporadically in some herds but may reach an incidence of 30%. In an area as many as 75% of herds may have the disease. Animals aged between 6 months and 4 years are most commonly affected and the chronic disease may or may not be preceded by an attack of acute rhinitis. Most cases commence in the autumn months. It is apparent that nasal granuloma develops as a continuous and progressive response to acute episodes of hypersensitivity. This accords with the gradual development of the stertorous respiration (10).

Acute cases are characterized by a sudden onset of ocular and nasal discharge and swelling of the nasal mucosa causing difficult, noisy breathing. Affected animals shake their heads and snort and rub their noses in hedges. As a result they commonly block their nostrils with twigs. This form of the disease is commonest in cattle of the Channel Island breeds and their crossbreeds. The nasal discharge in these breeds is usually yellow to orange in color.

Established cases of enzootic nasal granuloma have lesions, consisting of granulomatous nodules 1–4 mm in diameter and height, in both nostrils. The lesions extend from just inside the nostril posteriorly for 5–8 cm. They may be few in number or packed closely together. Their texture is firm and the mucosa over them appears to be normal. They have a characteristic histopathology and contain large numbers of eosinophils and mast cells (3). A mucopurulent discharge occurs in many animals. The predominant clinical sign is respiratory stertor and dyspnea caused by obstruction to the air flow. The severity of these signs may fluctuate but in general they progress slowly over several months and then remain static. Although the respiratory distress may be sufficiently severe to cause a loss of condition and marked reduction in milk yield, affected animals do not die. A good proportion of them have to be culled as uneconomic units.

The clinical picture in *mycotic nasal granuloma* is superficially similar with respect to noisy breathing, respiratory distress and nasal discharge. However, the visible and palpable lesions in the anterior part of the nasal cavities are polyps up to 5 cm in diameter which occur singly or in confluent masses. Their cut surfaces are yellow to green and they are sometimes ulcerated (4). Histologically the lesions are eosinophilic granulomas containing fungal spores and sometimes hyphae. Fungi (*Drechslera rostrata*) have been isolated from the lesions.

REFERENCES

(1) Hore, D. E. et al. (1973) *Aust. vet. J.*, *49*, 330.
(2) Gallagher, P. (1972) *NZ vet. J.*, *20*, 40.
(3) Carbonell, P. L. (1979) *Vet. Pathol.*, *16*, 60.
(4) McKenzie, R. A. & Connole, M. D. (1977) *Aust. vet J.*, *53*, 268.
(5) Pemberton, D. H. et al. (1977) *Aust. vet. J.*, *53*, 201.
(6) Patton, C. S. (1977) *Cornell Vet.*, *67*, 236.
(7) James, M. P. et al. (1975) *NZ vet. J.*, *23*, 63.
(8) Roberts, E. D. et al. (1963) *J. Am. vet. med. Assoc.*, *142*, 42.
(9) Duncan, J. R. et al. (1967) *J. Am. vet. med. Assoc.*, *151*, 732.
(10) Pemberton, D. H. & White, W. E. (1974) *Aust. vet. J.*, *50*, 85.

34

Diseases Caused by the Inheritance of Undesirable Characters

THERE are two principal problems for the field veterinarian in the area of inherited diseases; the first is to be able to diagnose that a disease is or is not inherited, and it is just as important to be able to prove the latter as it is to prove the former; the second is to be able to select the heterozygotes for a particular disease so that some attempt can be made to reduce the gene frequency for it or, more rarely, to eradicate it.

The importance of inherited disease

In recent times inherited diseases have assumed a position of greater importance because of intensive inbreeding systems introduced to hasten the multiplication of desirable characteristics. If there is added to this the even greater intensification of inbreeding which attends the introduction of a few foundation members of exotic breeds which are then mated and remated within a small group, the multiplication frequency of undesirable genes can be very rapid. This is the 'founder' effect which is capable of still further enhancement by modern breeding techniques, especially superovulation and ovum transplantation (7).

Another important and emerging aspect of inherited disease is the importance of inheritance in predisposing animals to the occurrence of disease caused by other agents, e.g. susceptibility to bloat, to mastitis, to ovarian malfunction. The lethal and seriously inconvenient defects conditioned by inheritance and listed in the following pages are numerically and financially important, especially to the individual farmer, but they may be overshadowed by the effect of inheritance on these much more widespread chronic diseases. A particular facet of this relationship which is of even greater importance is the interaction between inheritance and infection. Enzootic bovine leukosis and scrapie are the classical examples of diseases in which genetic selection is likely to be able to eliminate an infectious disease.

Some other diseases not listed in this chapter are ones which are sometimes inherited, sometimes caused by other factors. Thus, goiter may be inherited, but is more commonly the result of a nutritional deficiency of iodine. Laminitis in cattle may be inherited, but is more commonly of the 'traumatic' or 'metabolic' variety. Other diseases in this category are porcine congenital tremor, porcine stress syndrome, asymmetric hindquarters and splayleg, both of swine, pityriasis rosea, also of pigs, inherited and nutritional forms of cardiomyopathy in cattle and hydrocephalus in all species.

The diagnosis of inherited disease in farm animals

It is not easy to define the point during the examination of a series of cases of disease, which are sufficiently similar to suggest that they have the same cause, at which it becomes evident that the cause may be hereditary. Any case of disease may be inherited but the possibility is often dismissed early in the investigation for one reason or other. Set out below are the features of a disease which attract attention to the possibility of inheritance as a cause.

The nature of the disease

Conditioning of the function or structure of the body by genes can be exerted in several ways. Usually it is structural, so that a congenital deformity results. Less commonly it is functional, as in inherited porphyria. It can also be abiotrophic, in which premature degeneration or a structural lesion which is not congenital develop. These are readily understandable modes of inheritance of disease. Less simple modes include those in which susceptibility to relatively mild pathogens is greater than normal; thus the Arabian foal may die of pneumonia caused by an adenovirus, but the real cause of death is the immunodeficiency which the foal has inherited. In the same way animals may inherit susceptibility to bloat and to mastitis, and to a nutritional deficiency, e.g. to zinc deficiency in inherited parakeratosis of calves.

Although the common modes of inheritance of disease are readily recognizable it is also apparent that the clinical picture in many inherited diseases can be exactly simulated by environmental influences. Thus goiter may be inherited or the result of a nutritional deficiency of iodine; immunosuppression can be due to combined immunodeficiency inherited in Arab ponies, or be the result of failure to ingest colostrum.

It is therefore unsafe to diagnose inheritance as the cause of the disease *because* the defect, structural or functional, is known to be inherited. If this evidence can be supported by a laboratory indicator such as cytogenetic marker, a specific biochemical reaction, or a specific pathological lesion such as an overfilled lysosome, the diagnosis can be more certain. But the laboratory tests are usually stimulated by the specific epidemiological behavior of the disease which suggests inheritance as the basic disorder.

Epidemiology of inherited disease

The following features are suggested to be good pointers to the probability of inheritance playing a part in causing a disease, assuming that inheritance is conditioned by single recessive genes.

- A gradual increase in the number of cases over a period of years (assuming the same sire and dams are retained)
- The sudden appearance of a new disease accompanies the introduction of a new sire
- Evenness of spread through a season, within a mating group, provided the females are a homogeneous lot genetically. A sudden burst of cases without evidence of genetic influence is a common finding in environmentally induced defects
- Repeat of a mating to a group should produce the same result mathematically
- A numerical level of occurrence appropriate to the probable gene frequency in the group. Thus a sire mated to his daughters, produced by a group of cows with a negative gene frequency, should produce 12·5% of defective calves. A bull mated to his half-sisters should produce 25% of affected calves. The problems with inherited disease so often arise on stud farms, or in new or small breeds, where most of the population is related to each other, that a fictitious relationship between inheritance and the occurrence of the disease can often be established
- Purebred animals are the most commonly affected because their genetic base is much more standardized, often stereotyped. However, crossbreds can be involved, but the chance is less great. The role of studs in maintaining the prevalence of inherited disease depends to an extent on the selection pressure which is exerted in them to foster the development of some characteristics. The selection pressure may be consciously directed at the fault, for example, the policy of selecting short-legged, straight-hocked Hereford cattle has subconsciously selected bulls for achondroplastic dwarfism
- Notorious breeds, and even families, arise because of intense inbreeding and consequent increase in gene frequencies of good and bad traits
- Identicality of the defect is a characteristic of inherited disease. Although there may be variation in the severity of the lesion, the same lesions should be present in all cases. There is greater variability in environmentally acquired defects.

DIAGNOSTIC PROCEDURES AND THEIR PROBLEMS

Retrospective epidemiological data

An important procedure in the diagnosis of inherited disease is to get epidemiological evidence retrospectively about the environment at the time that the noxious influence was applied. It is routine, for example, in the examination of a congenital defect to attempt to determine whether a toxin, a nutritional deficiency or a viral infection could have exerted its influence during the first third of pregnancy, the period of organogenesis. In diseases in which incomplete development of the cellular components of an organ occurs, for example amyelination in the central nervous system, the period of influence is later and longer. This question is discussed in some detail in the section on neonatal disease and congenital defects in Chapter 3.

Mode of inheritance

Most inherited defects are conditioned by recessive genes and the numerical rate of occurrence in the offspring is identifiable and predictable in a naturally occurring population and in test matings. Difficulties occur when recessive genes exert incomplete penetrance and when partially dominant genes are encountered. The numerical distributions are not then predictable although they can be highly standardized for a particular defect.

Other modes of inheritance other than single autosomal recessive characters need consideration. Lethal dominants which occur by mutation are self-destructing. Sublethal dominants are rare but will affect large numbers, usually 50% of the population mated to the mutants, and are therefore quickly recognizable and easily removed. Sex-linked or sex-limiting dominants or recessives express themselves by limitation to one sex. Incomplete dominants provide three phenotypes, the two homozygotes at the extremes, and the heterozygote between in terms of expressing the inherited characteristic.

Test-mating

A provisional diagnosis of inheritance of a defect is usually made on the basis of similarity to prerecorded defects, and on epidemiological information as set out above. To confirm the diagnosis it is necessary to predict that such and such a mating program will produce such and such cases of the disease, in fact to carry out a test-mating.

The principal difficulty in field work is to convince farmers that they should conduct test matings to determine whether their own bull carries a flawed inheritance. Most are not prepared to do this but dispose of the bull forthwith. If artificial insemination is being used the situation is different; the artificial insemination center has usually invested a great deal of money in the bull, but on the other hand it is not ethical for the center to maintain a defective bull. A relatively simple method is to subsidize farmers to breed the daughters back to the sire in the expectation of a 12·5% crop of defective calves if the character is inherited as a simple recessive and the bull is heterozygous and the cows all negative. The technique has been used to estimate the heritability of spastic paresis in Friesians (1) producing the startling conclusion that the anomaly had very low heritability, if any. The enormous problem which can arise in artificial insemination systems is well recognized and most artificial insemination organizations monitor offspring in search of defects. The multiplication of desirable qualities by artificial insemination from one sire is now further multiplied by ova transfers from one cow. In such circumstances undesirable inherited characters can become widespread very quickly. The New Zealand Dairy Board has successfully maintained surveillance over artificial insemination centers under their control for many years (2).

The disinclination of farmers to conduct test-matings is largely economic, and there is certain to be an interference with production efficiency and with longevity by the test-mating program. It will also take time to bring suspect, non-pregnant females to the suspected sire and then view the resulting offspring; 2 years is a minimum period before a result can be obtained.

Diagnosis of heterozygotes based on biochemical data

Blood typing or enzyme estimations for the detection of enzymopathies such as glycogenosis are used to detect heterozygotes. Interpretation of the assays is not always easy nor accurate, but provided adequate data is available on values for homozygous animals good use can be made of these techniques. Interpretation is facilitated if there is information available on the subject's relatives.

The control of inherited disease

The policy of control of inherited disease by individual farmers is often shortsighted in that diseases which are inherited can be ignored and their prevalence even enhanced by positive selection pressure. Breed societies are more likely to press for a culling program and there are excellent records of performance in this respect. Artificial insemination services have the best control over farmers and over breeding programs and one of their major advantages in animal management is the eradication, or at least limitation, of inherited disease. This is not to say that breed societies or even individual farmers cannot do an excellent job. A practical demonstration of what can be achieved is contained in the record of eradication of 'bulldog' calves from the Guernsey breed (3). Satisfactory evidence of freedom from the character was the birth of normal calves sired by the bull from ten known carrier cows, or from 20 daughters of known carrier cows.

Another example of cooperative enthusiasm is the test-mating herd set up by breeders of Galloway cattle to provide an opportunity for farmers to detect heterozygotes of tibial hemimelia away from their own farms (5). Suspect animals are mated with known heterozygotes in the test herd. To help reduce the long delays in identification of affected calves a procedure has been adopted of terminating pregnancy at 90 days by the administration of prostaglandin. The technique has great merit because two fetuses can be obtained in 1 year from the one cow. It is subject to the need for the defect under examination to be detectable at such an early fetal age.

Other means of shortening the period required to obtain a positive answer include procuring multiple births by superovulation and embryo transfer and by terminating pregnancy by cesarean operation (6, 8).

The major difficulty in a control program for an inherited disease is the recognition of the clinically normal heterozygote. Test-matings are a theoretically suitable, but in most cases impractical, means. There is therefore a constant search for indirect tests including examination for chromosomal abnormalities, evidence of biochemical aberrations, and radiologically identifiable defects. When such tests are available they are included in the details of the defect concerned. Only the more common inherited defects are described here and for greater detail more comprehensive works are set out under review literature.

The problems of control of inherited disease are largely economical and it is necessary to be philosophically inclined when attempting to convince farmers to commence an eradication program. Consider the difficulties in his way:

- The generation interval is long and he must wait a long time for the result of a test-mating or to see the effects of a control program
- Births are mostly single and it takes many births to make up enough data to be statistically significant
- Most agricultural animals have a relatively short reproductive life and produce relatively few offspring from which to extrapolate a genetic hypothesis.
- Experimental herds or flocks are almost impossible to maintain because of high costs. There is a similar difficulty in assembling herds of known or suspected genetic inadequacy
- Inbreeding which is likely to highlight the presence of an inherited defect is really very little used so that gene frequencies for defects in commercial herds are likely to be very low.

In spite of these difficulties there can be handsome profits. An economic assessment of genetic screening programs to select heterozygous carriers of inherited diseases of cattle shows that a 300–400% return on the investment is likely over a 20-year period and over an infinite time-span. This assumes that the gene prevalence is of the order of 10% (4).

REVIEW LITERATURE

Foley, C. W. et al. (1979) *Abnormalities of Companion Animals. Analysis of Heritability of Abnormalities of the Horse. Pt. IV*. Ames, Iowa: Iowa State Univ. Press.

Hutt, F. B. (1964) *Animal Genetics*. New York: Ronald Press.

Jolly, R. D. & Healey, P. J. (1986) Screening for carriers of genetic diseases by biochemical means. *Vet. Rec.*, *119*, 264.

Jolly, R. D. et al. (1981) Screening for genetic disease: principles and practice. *Adv. vet. Sci.*, *25*, 245–276.

Leipold, H. W. et al. (1978) Genetics and diseases of cattle. *Proc. 11th ann. Conv. Amer. Assoc. Bov. Pract.*, pp. 18–31.

Preister, W. A. et al. (1970) Congenital defects in domesticated animals; general consideration. *Am. J. vet. Res.*, *31*, 1871.

REFERENCES

(1) Dawson, P. L. L. (1975) *Vet. Rec.*, *97*, 432.
(2) Jolly, R. D. & Leipold, H. W. (1973) *NZ vet. J.*, *21*, 147.
(3) Jones, W. A. (1961) *Vet. Rec.*, *73*, 937.
(4) Jolly, R. D. & Townley, R. J. (1980) *NZ vet. J.*, *28*, 3.
(5) Pollock, D. L. et al. (1979) *Vet. Rec.*, *104*, 258.
(6) Johnson, J. L. et al. (1980) *J. Am. vet. med. Assoc.*, *176*, 549.
(7) Jolly, R. D. (1977) *NZ vet. J.*, *25*, 109.
(8) Leipold, H. W. & Peeples, J. G. (1981) *J. Am. vet. med. Assoc.*, *179*, 69.

DISEASES CHARACTERIZED BY CHROMOSOMAL ANOMALIES

It is only a few years since the first application of cytogenetic study to animals revealed the first chromosomal abnormality associated with the presence of an inherited disease. Even in man the science is not yet well developed so that in all species there are relatively few diseases which have been identified by this means. In animals these diseases have been reviewed (1, 2). The proportion of affected animals in the population is very low as indicated by a survey of 743 bulls in artificial insemination centers in the United States (3). Many inherited diseases characterized by congenital defects have been examined for the presence of chromosomal abnormality, but with very little success.

Chromosomal analysis techniques are based on tissue culture using leukocytes collected in a highly aseptic manner. The blood is placed in tissue culture medium containing a stimulant to cell division. After brief incubation, cell division is arrested by the addition of a cytotoxic agent and the cells then swollen osmotically by treatment with a hypotonic solution, then fixed and dried onto slides and then stained. Microscopic examination of dividing cells allows the total number of chromosomes in each cell to be counted, the sex chromosomes and abnormal chromosomes identified. The individual chromosomes are cut out from photographic prints, paired and stuck onto cards constructing the identifying document—the *karyotype*. The number of cells subjected to chromosomal analysis in each case is usually 10–20 but 50 is recommended for satisfactory accuracy. The technique is described in detail (2, 24) and the interpretation is described in the several races of cattle (23).

Freemartinism in calves

In normal calves the chromosomal identification of females is 60 XX (60 chromosomes, both X chromosomes) and of males is 60 XY (the Y being smaller and not readily paired with its opposite X chromosome). In freemartins (phenotypically a female, but carrying also male cells) there is a mixture of mostly 60 XX chromosomes to a cell, and a small proportion of 60 XY cells. A large number of cells needs to be analysed if only the freemartin calf is available because the proportion of abnormal cells present may be as low as 2%. It is, however, possible to make a diagnosis on the examination of 10–20 cells provided the male twin is also analysed; the female may have very few XY chromosomes but the male will have a very high proportion of XX chromosomes. The technique is much more accurate than blood group analysis, or clinical observations of a short vagina, enlarged clitoris and the presence of a vulval tuft of hair.

The freemartin is the classical example of the chimera in cytogenetics. They are the individuals which contain two or more cell types which originated in separate individuals. The only way in which chimera can develop is via the fusion of circulations or zygotes *in utero*. Sex chromosome chimerism is also reported in goats, sheep and pigs, and although the male partners of female twins are usually anatomically normal they often have reduced fertility (2). Bulls born co-twin with freemartin females may also be chimeric and have low reproductive efficiency (18). Special cytogenetic techniques are also available which facilitate the diagnosis of freemartinism in a female calf of a male–female twinning (31, 32).

Chromosomal translocations in cattle

When two chromosomes which have previously been broken have fused to form a morphologically distinct chromosome this is known as a translocation. It is further identified by the chromosomal series involved. Thus a 1/29 translocation represents a fusion between a chromosome of each of the pairs numbered 1 and 29. *Translocation 1/29* has been identified in many breeds of cattle and has been associated with reduced fertility due to early death of embryos produced by fertilization of affected gametes or fertilization of normal gametes by spermatozoa carrying the *1/29* translocation. There is no abnormality of serving behavior or semen quality (19). The translocation has been shown to be inherited in Swedish Red and White, Charolais and Red Poll breeds (1) and in the wild British White cattle (4). The frequency of affected animals in a breed may vary between 1 and 20%. *Translocations 2/4* and *13/21* have also been identified in bulls, the latter seeming to be widespread in Simmental cattle. Neither has been linked with a disease but it is becoming accepted practice not to use such animals for artificial insemination, and in some countries to refuse their importation. *Translocation 27/29* is suspected of being associated with reduced fertility in Guernsey cattle (5). Other translocations recorded for bulls engaged in the artificial insemination industry have been listed (6). These and other abnormalities of chromosomal structure were detected in an examination of a large number of infertile dairy heifers (27).

Other chromosomal abnormalities

Cattle

Bulls with an extra X chromosome have been identified (22) and are characterized by testicular hypoplasia. They usually have a 61XXY chromosome complement which has been likened to human Klinefelter's syndrome (25). Anestrus heifers with ovarian inactivity may have an additional X chromosome (2n=61XXX) i.e. an X-trisomy karyotype (30). A bull with an XX/XY chimerism and arrested spermogenesis has also been identified (28).

A numerical anomaly of an additional chromosome has been related to the development of achondroplastic dwarfism in calves but a number of other reported searches for chromosomal abnormality in that disease have been negative (8).

Horses
A number of mares with chromosomal abnormalities have been identified. All have had abnormalities of ovaries or estrus and were infertile (16, 20, 21). It has been suggested that it could be a common cause of infertility in mares (21). A cryptorchid (bilateral) Belgian stallion has been identified as possibly having a female karyotype (10).

There are several reports of chromosomal abnormalities in equine intersexes. Some intersexes have had a mosaiac of 63, X/64, XY or 65, X/66, Y, but others have no trace of a male chromosome and have a 2n=64, XX configuration (29). A male pseudohermaphrodite Arabian horse with mixoploidy has been described (14). There was an enlarged clitoris which had an urethral process opening on its dorsal aspect. The vulva consisted of only a small fossa and on laparotomy there were small gonads in each internal inguinal ring. The genetic sex of the animal was considered to be 63XO?/64XX/65XXY.

Two other equine intersexes, one a Welsh pony, and one a Standardbred, with karyotypes of 64 XX/64 XY and 63SO/64XY have also been described (9).

Sheep
A chromosomal translocation has been associated with infertility in Romney sheep (11). Rams with normal testicles and libido, but with XXY karyotypes (i.e., Klinefelter syndrome) are also recorded (26). An extensive investigation of sheep with a Robertsonian translocation manifested as multiple centric fusions has shown that these sheep are no different in their fertility rate or prevalence of congenital defects from other sheep (7, 13).

Pigs
A chromosomal translocation has been related to congenital abnormalities in pigs (12), to infertility (17) and to infertility due to embryonic mortality.

REVIEW LITERATURE

Bruere, A. N. (1980) Application of cytogenetics to domestic animals. *Vet. Ann.*, *20*, 29.

Gustavsson, I. (1979) Symposium. Cytogenetics of farm animals. The 1/29 Robertsonian translocation. *J. dairy Sci.* *52*, 825.

Halnan, C. R. E. (1985) Equine cytogenetics: role in equine veterinary practice. *Vet. Rec.*, *17*, 173.

Long, S. (1980) Veterinary cytogenesis. *Vet. Ann.* *20*, 24.

REFERENCES

(1) Harvey, M. J. A. (1976) *Vet. Rec.*, *98*, 479.
(2) McFeely, R. A. (1976) *Vet. Ann.*, *16*, 39.
(3) Fechheimer, N. S. (1973) *Vet. Rec.*, *93*, 535.
(4) Eldridge, F. E. (1977) *Vet. Rec.*, *97*, 71.
(5) Bongso, A. & Basrur, P. K. (1976) *Cornell Vet.*, *66*, 476.
(6) Pollock, D. L. (1974) *Vet. Rec.*, *95*, 266.
(7) Bruere, A. N. & Ellis, P. M. (1979) *J. Reprod. Fertil.*, *57*, 363.
(8) Weaver, A. D. (1975) *Vet. Ann.*, *15*, 7.
(9) Dunn, H. O. et al. (1981) *Cornell Vet.*, *71*, 123.
(10) Dunn, H. O. et al. (1974) *Cornell Vet.*, *64*, 265.
(11) Long, S. E. (1978) *Vet. Rec.*, *102*, 399.
(12) Hans-Melander, E. & Melander, Y. (1970) *Hereditas*, *69*, 101.
(13) Moraes, J. C. et al. (1981) *Vet. Rec.*, *107*, 489.
(14) Fretz, P. B. & Hare, W. C. D. (1976) *Equ. vet. J.*, *8*, 130.
(16) Eilts, B. E. et al. (1983) *J. Am. vet. med. Assoc.*, *182*, 1120.
(17) Potter, W. L. et al. (1980) *Aust. vet. J.*, *56*, 133.
(18) Dunn, H. O. et al. (1979) *J. Reprod. Fertil.*, *57*, 21.
(19) Logue, D. N. & Harvey, M. J. A. (1978) *J. Reprod. Fertil.*, *54*, 159.
(20) Blue, M. G. et al. (1978) *NZ vet. J.*, *26*, 137.
(21) Bruere, A. N. et al. (1978) *NZ vet. J.*, *26*, 145.
(22) Logue, D. N. et al. (1979) *Vet. Rec.*, *104*, 500.
(23) Potter, W. L. et al. (1979) *Aust. vet. J.*, *55*, 560.
(24) Gustavsson, I. (1980) *Adv. vet. Sci.*, *24*, 245.
(25) Dunn, H. O. et al. (1980) *Cornell Vet.*, *70*, 137.
(26) Bruere, A. N. & Kilgour, R. (1974) *Vet. Rec.*, *95*, 437.
(27) Swartz, H. A. & Vogt, D. W. (1983) *J. Hered.*, *74*, 320.
(28) Bongso, T. A. et al. (1981) *Cornell Vet.*, *71*, 376.
(29) Haynes, S. E. (1984) *Aust. Adv. vet. Sci.*, p. 70.
(30) Buoen, L. C. et al. (1981) *J. Am. vet. med. Assoc.*, *179*, 810.
(31) Shanker, V. & Bhalio, S. (1983) *Vet. Rec.*, *113*, 17, & *112*, 230.
(32) Balakrishnan, C. R. et al. (1981) *Vet. Rec.*, *109*, 162.

INHERITED METABOLIC DEFECTS

Inherited congenital porphyria and protoporphyria

There are congenital defects of porphyrin metabolism in cattle and swine characterized by excessive excretion of porphyrins in urine and feces and deposition of porphyrins in tissues, especially bones and teeth. Photosensitization occurs in affected cattle.

Etiology
The commoner of these two diseases, congenital porphyria, is similar to erythropoietic or Gunther's porphyria of man. Erythropoietic protoporphyria is similar to the same disease in man. The protoporphyria is a similar disease to, but milder than, the porphyria. It occurs in cattle and is thought to be inherited (2).

Most cases of porphyria in cattle are due to the inheritance of a single recessive factor, heterozygotes being clinically normal (1). Although there is no strict sex linkage in the mode of inheritance, the incidence is higher in females than in males. In pigs the pattern of inheritance is uncertain but may be due to one or more dominant genes. Porphyria in man is of three types and must be differentiated from the porphyrinuria which occurs in liver insufficiency and which is the result of deficient conversion rather than excess production of porphyrins. Cattle and pigs are the only domestic species in which congenital porphyria has been recorded.

Epidemiology
The disease occurs rarely and as yet is of little economic importance. It has been recorded in Shorthorn, Hol-

stein, Black and White Danish (1), Jamaica Red and Black cattle and Ayrshires (4). Affected cattle suffer from incapacitating photosensitization when exposed to sunlight and must be kept indoors. In countries where sunlight hours are limited the disease may go unnoticed. The disease is also recorded in pigs, which appear to suffer little harm (2).

Pathogenesis

The porphyrins are natural pigments but in these diseases they are present in larger than normal concentrations in the blood, urine and feces. In porphyria the metabolic defect is probably one of abnormal synthesis of heme due to enzymatic insufficiency at the stage of conversion of pyrrol groups to series 3 porphyrins. Excess series 1 porphyrins are produced as a result and there is flooding of the tissues with these coloring and photosensitizing substances. Thus this disease is one of overproduction of physiologically inactive porphyrins. Photosensitivity occurs in cattle because the high tissue levels of porphyrins sensitize the skin to light. In protoporphyria there is deficient activity of the enzyme ferrochalase, resulting in excessive protoporphyrin synthesis with high levels appearing in the erythrocytes and feces.

Clinical findings

The passage of amber to portwine colored urine, a pink to brown discoloration of the teeth and bones, and severe photosensitization are characteristic of porphyria in cattle. Additional signs include pallor of the mucosae and retardation of growth. The health of affected pigs is usually normal and photosensitivity does not occur but the disease can be recognized by the red-brown discoloration of the bones and teeth which is present even in the newborn. In *protoporphyria* the only abnormality is photosensitive dermatitis.

Clinical pathology

In *porphyria* the urine is amber to portwine in color when voided due to the high content of porphyrins. The urine of affected cattle with inherited congenital porphyria may contain 500–1000 μg/dl of uroporphyrins and 356–1530 μg/dl of coproporphyrins (4). The urine of normal cattle contains 1·84 μg/dl of coproporphyrins and no significant quantity of uroporphyrins. The color darkens to brown on exposure to light. Spectroscopic examination is necessary to identify the pigment as porphyrin. Erythrocyte survival time is reduced considerably. A macrocytic, normochromic anemia occurs and its severity appears to be related to the level of uroporphyrins in the erythrocytes (5, 6), and there is evidence of a hemolytic anemia. Cattle with the highest erythrocyte uroporphyrin levels are also the most sensitive to sunlight (7).

Necropsy findings

In *porphyric* animals the teeth and bones are stained brown or reddish purple, the pigment occurring chiefly in the dentine in teeth and often in concentric layers in the bones. Affected bones and teeth show a red fluorescence under illumination with ultraviolet light. The histological findings are unique to this disease (3).

Diagnosis

Classical porphyria must be differentiated from photosensitization due to other causes and symptomatic porphyrinuria caused by liver insufficiency. Affected cattle and pigs can be detected at birth by the discoloration of the teeth. Breeding trials are necessary to detect heterozygous, normal carrier animals. Protoporphyria must be differentiated from the other causes of photosensitization.

Treatment

Non-specific treatment for photosensitization may be necessary. Affected cattle should be reared indoors.

Control

Elimination of affected carrier animals from the breeding program is the only measure available. Periodic examination of the urine and feces for excessive quantities of coproporphyrin is carried out on bulls used for artificial insemination in breeds in which the disease occurs (1).

REFERENCES

(1) Jorgensen, S. K. (1961) *Br. vet. J.*, *117*, 61.
(2) Ruth, G. R. et al. (1979) *Proc. Am. Assoc. Vet. lab. Diagnost. 21*, 91.
(3) Scott, D. W. et al. (1979) *Cornell Vet.*, *69*, 145.
(4) Haydon, M. (1975) *Can. vet. J.*, *16*, 118.
(5) Kaneko, J. J. & Mille, R. (1970) *Cornell Vet.*, *60*, 52.
(6) Kaneko, J. J. et al. (1971) *Am. J. vet. Res.*, *32*, 1981.
(7) Wass, W. M. & Hoyt, H. H. (1965) *Am. J. vet. Res.*, *26*, 654, 659.

Familial polycythemia

This inherited defect has been observed only in Jersey cattle. Attention is drawn to the presence of the disease by early calfhood deaths and a clinical syndrome including congestion of mucosae, dyspnea and poor growth. Hematologically there is marked elevation of erythrocyte count, hemoglobin concentration and packed cell volume (1, 2). The disease appears to be a primary polycythemia inherited as a simple autosomal recessive.

REFERENCES

(1) Tennant, B. et al. (1969) *Cornell Vet.*, *49*, 594.
(2) Kaneko, J. J. et al. (1968) *Am. J. vet. Res.*, *29*, 949.

Congenital methemoglobinemia

The disease is rarely recorded and its heritability is unproven. The one series of cases recorded in horses was familial (1). Clinically there is decreased exercise tolerance, pale mucosae, and a hemic heart murmur. There is a hemolytic anemia and decreased levels of erythrocyte glutathione reductase and glutathione, and high levels of methemoglobin.

REFERENCE

(1) Dixon, P. M. et al. (1977) *Equ. vet. J.*, *9*, 198.

UMP synthase deficiency

This is a partial deficiency of an enzyme which is involved in the conversion of orotate to uridine-5′ monophosphate (UMP) as a step in the synthesis of pyrimidine nucleotides. It occurs in heterozygotes for a condition which is likely to be lethal in the homozygous state (1). It is characterized by the secretion of high levels of orotate in the milk but is clinically benign. Heterozygous animals have a partial deficiency of UMP synthase but have no individual or herd abnormalities (2).

REFERENCES

(1) Robinson, J. L. (1984) *J. Hered.*, *75*, 277.
(2) Shanks, R. D. et al. (1987) *J. anim. Sci.*, *64*, 695.

Inherited goiter

This disease is recorded in Merino sheep (1, 2), Afrikander cattle (3, 6, 7), crossbred Saanen dwarf goats (5), Boer goats (8) and possibly polled Dorset sheep (4) and appears to be inherited as a recessive character. The essential defect is in the synthesis of abnormal thyroid hormone leading to increased production of thyrotropic factor in the pituitary gland, causing in turn a hyperplasia of the thyroid gland. In Afrikander cattle the defect stems from an abnormality of the basic RNA (3). Clinically in sheep there is a high level of mortality, enlargement of the thyroid above the normal 2·8 g, but varying greatly up to 222 g, and the appearance of 'lustrous' or 'silky' wool in the fleeces of some lambs. Other defects which occurred concurrently were edema and floppiness of ears, enlargement of, and outward or inward bowing of, the front legs at the knees, and dorsoventral flattening of the nasal area. The thyroglobulin deficiency in the neonatal lamb may result in defective fetal lung development and the appearance of a neonatal respiratory distress syndrome; there is dyspnea at birth (10). The clinical picture in goats is the same as for lambs. It includes retardation of growth, sluggish behavior, rough, sparse haircoat, which worsens as the goats get older, and a thick scaly skin (5). In Afrikander cattle most of the losses are from stillbirths or from early neonatal deaths (11). Some are caused by tracheal compression from the enlarged gland. It is the calves with the largest glands that have the greatest mortality. In these cattle there may be a concurrent inherited gray coat colour, a defect in a red breed (9).

REFERENCES

(1) Rac, R. et al. (1968) *Res. vet. Sci.*, *9*, 209.
(2) Mayo, G. M. E. & Mulhearn, C. J. (1969) *Aust. J. agric. Res.*, *20*, 533.
(3) Tassi, V. P. N. et al. (1984) *J. Biol. Chem.* *259*, 10507.
(4) Davis, G. B. et al. (1979) *NZ vet. J.*, *27*, 126.
(5) Rijnberk, A. et al. (1977) *Br. vet. J.*, *133*, 495.
(6) Pammenter, M. et al. (1979) *Endocrinology*, *104*, 1853.
(7) Vijlder, J. J. Mde. et al. (1978) *Endocrinology*, *102*, 1214.
(8) van Jaarsveld, P. et al. (1971) *J. S. Afr. vet. med. Assoc.*, *42*, 295.
(9) Schulz, K. C. A. & Groenewald, J. W. (1983) *J. S. Afr. vet. med. Assoc.*, *54*, 147.
(10) Jones, B. R. et al. (1986) *NZ vet. J.*, *34*, 145.
(11) Ricketts, M. H. et al. (1985) *J. Hered.*, *76*, 12.

Inherited combined immunodeficiency (CID) in foals of Arabian breeding

This is an inherited disease of young foals characterized by lymphopenia, lack of immunoglobulin synthesis, absence of cell-moderated immunity, thymic hypoplasia and a marked reduction in the numbers of splenic and lymph node lymphocytes. Affected foals are highly susceptible to secondary infections which usually cause death by 3 months of age.

Etiology

The immunodeficiency is inherited as an autosomal recessive defect (3). Affected foals are susceptible to infections of all kinds, but mostly of the respiratory tract (13). Adenoviral pneumonia is the most common complication, but infections with bacteria and *Pneumocystis carinii* also occur. The foals are particularly susceptible to *Listeria monocytogenes*, but the infection is recorded only rarely (12). *Cryptosporidium* sp. has also been recorded in a number of foals with diarrhea (2) which is also a common complication.

Epidemiology

In one survey of Arabian foals in the United States the prevalence rate of affected foals was 2·3% of 257 foals of Arabian breeding, and 25·7% of the parents of affected foals were estimated to be carriers of the genetic defect. The disease occurs in purebred and part-Arabian horses. It has also occurred in an Appaloosa foal which had an Arab stallion in the fifth past generation of its mother's pedigree (1). Affected foals usually appear normal at birth but are highly susceptible to infections from 2 to 65 days after birth and usually die from one or more infections by 3 months of age. The sires and dams of affected foals are clinically normal and have normal lymphocyte counts and serum immunoglobulin levels.

Pathogenesis

Affected foals are born with a combined immunodeficiency associated with a deficiency in both B-lymphocytes (which produce immunoglobulins) and T-lymphocytes (which provide cellular immunity). There is a marked lymphopenia and failure of immunoglobulin (IgM) synthesis (5) and absence of delayed hypersensitivity of skin responses (6). Foals which receive immunoglobulins from the dam's colostrum derive passive immunity and may survive for as long as 4 months. Foals which do not receive colostrum die much earlier. Adenoviral pneumonia is considered to be the most common secondary complication probably because adenovirus infection is so widespread in the horse population. Affected foals also die from hepatitis, enteritis and infection of other organs without pulmonary involvement. An extensive literature has grown up which deals with the comparative medical aspects of this disease, which is an excellent animal model of the similar disease in humans, but this has not been included here.

Clinical findings

Affected foals usually become ill from 10 to 35 days of age. Commonly there is a history suggesting a mild disease of the respiratory tract, especially the appearance of a bilateral nasal discharge which often becomes sufficiently thick to interfere with sucking. The foal is unthrifty, lethargic, tires easily but still nurses and eats solid feed. A deep dry cough and a serous to mucopurulent ocular and nasal discharge are common when pneumonia is present. There is moderate fever (39·5°C, 103°F) and an increase in the heart and respiratory rates. The depth of respirations is increased and a double expiratory effort is common. On auscultation loud bronchial tones and moist and dry crackles are common over the anterior ventral aspects of both lungs. A chronic diarrhea is present in some foals, and alopecia and dermatitis, commonly associated with an infection by *Dermatophilus congolensis*, also occur. An important clinical feature is that affected foals do not respond favorably to treatment with antimicrobial agents. The course of the illness will vary from a few days to a few weeks and probably depends on the degree of immunodeficiency and the nature of the infection. Most affected foals become progressively worse over a period of 2–4 weeks, and death by 3 months of age is the usual outcome.

Clinical pathology

Lymphopenia is a constant finding with counts often less than 1000/μl and there is a concurrent hypogammaglobulinemia. There is no IgM in precolostral serum of the foal. Following ingestion of colostrum, all subclasses of immunoglobulin will be present but in affected foals the level of IgM will steadily decrease weekly until at about 36 days no levels are detectable because of lack of synthesis (6). The determination of immunoglobulin subclasses is considered essential for a definitive diagnosis and practical methods are described (9). The determination of serum gammaglobulin levels of all valuable foals at 24 hours of age may assist in differentiating foals with failure to achieve passive transfer of immunoglobulin, due to lack of colostrum or failure to absorb gammaglobulins, from foals with CID. Additional tests include enumeration of B-lymphocyte and T-lymphocyte responses to phytolectin stimulation (9) and other tests of lymphocytic immunological function (4).

Necropsy findings

The lymph nodes are small and splenic follicles are not visible. A viral interstitial pneumonia and a secondary bacterial bronchopneumonia are common. The thymus gland is usually hypoplastic. Histologically the lymph nodes and spleen are depleted of lymphocytes and germinal centers are absent. In some foals there are foci of necrosis of the intestinal epithelium but with minimal infiltration of inflammatory cells. Inclusion bodies of adenovirus may be present in the cells of several different body systems. In Australian foals *Corynebacterium* (*Rhodococcus*) *equi* can be commonly isolated from pulmonary abscesses. Additional histological findings include a severe adenoviral pancreatitis and adenitis of the salivary glands.

Diagnosis

The chronic pneumonia secondary to CID in foals may resemble the septicemia and pneumonia of foals, caused by *Corynebacterium* (*Rhodococcus*) *equi*. The two diseases may be indistinguishable clinically in older foals (6–8 weeks of age) but the lymphopenia is characteristic of CID. The failure of passive transfer of immunoglobulins may terminate in a disease identical with CID except that the lymphocyte count should be normal.

It has become apparent that there is a series of immunological defects in foals. The identified ones are set out in Table 98. Foals with these and probably other unidentified deficits are very susceptible to a variety of infectious diseases and are usually chronically ill, most often with respiratory infections. However, because they have partial protection, they survive and their lifespan is much longer than that of foals with CID, usually over a year and often 18 months. Hematologically the animal is normal unless an infection is in process, but electrophoretic examination usually reveals a marked deficit of betaglobulins. Further tests are needed to identify the exact deficiency (10). A radioimmunodiffusion assay is used to quantitate serum immunoglobulins —IgA and IgM levels are usually at negligible levels, but IgG levels are discernible although diminished. An intradermal test by injection of phytohemagglutinin determines T-lymphocyte status—a normal response is migration of mononuclear cells. The overall effects of hypoimmune states are discussed under that heading in Chapter 2.

Additionally, an isoimmune neonatal leukopenia has been reported as a cause of immune deficiency in foals (7); antibodies to the sire's lymphocytes were detectable in mares' sera. Extensive surveys of the immune status of foals has uncovered the information that about 20% of newborn foals are immunologically deficient, mostly because of ineffective transfer of antibodies from colostrum (8). The differential clinical and laboratory diagnosis of the immunodeficiency states in newborn foals is summarized in Table 98.

Treatment and control

There is no satisfactory treatment for CID in foals. Hyperimmune serum, whole blood transfusions and broad-spectrum antibiotics are all used without more than a temporary response. Immunotherapy using a transplant of bone marrow, and a fetal thymus transplant has been attempted without success (11). Corticosteroids are contraindicated. Selection against carrier dams and sires of the genetic defect is the only rational control program. Affected foals may be kept alive by twice-weekly injections of hyperimmune serum and a constant antibiotic cover (13).

REVIEW LITERATURE

Campbell, T. M. & Studdert, M. J. (1983) Reconstitution of primary, severe, combined immunodeficiency in man and horse. *Comp. Immun. Microbiol. infect. Dis.*, *6*, 101–114.

Perryman, L. E. (1979) Primary and secondary immune deficiencies of domestic animals. *Adv. vet. Sci.*, *23*, 23.

Splitter, G. A. et al. (1980) Combined immunodeficiency of horses. A review. *Develop. comp. Immunol.*, *4*, 21.

Studdert, M. J. (1978) Primary, severe combined immunodeficiency diseases of Arabian foals. *Aust. vet. J.*, *54*, 411.

REFERENCES

(1) Perryman, L. E. et al. (1984) *Vet. Pathol.*, *21*, 547.
(2) Gibson, J. A. et al. (1983) *Aust. vet. J.*, *60*, 378.

Table 98. Differential diagnosis of immunodeficiency states in newborn foals (8).

Immunodeficiency state	*Breed*	*Lymphocyte count*	*B-lymphocyte numbers*	*T-lymphocyte function*	*IgM*	*Immunoglobulin concentrations IgG, IgA, IgG (T)*
Combined immunodeficiency	Arabian and part-Arabian	Low, below 1000/µl	Low or none	Impaired	None at birth and after 4–6 weeks	Incapable of synthesis. Concentrations prior to 3 months depend on colostral transfer
Agammaglobulinemia	Thoroughbred and Standardbred	Normal	None	Normal	None	Incapable of synthesis. Concentrations prior to 3 months depend on colostral transfer
Hypogammaglobulinemia from failure in transfer of colostral antibody	All	Normal	Normal	Normal	Normal	Capable of synthesis. Concentrations low until 2–3 months of age
Selective IgM deficiency	Arabs and Quarterhorses	Normal	Normal	Normal	Low or absent	Capable of synthesis. Concentrations normal by 3 months of age, concentrations prior to 3 months depend on colostral transfer of antibody
Transient hypogammaglobulinemia	Arabian	Normal	Normal	Impaired	Normal	IgG (T) is low at birth but reaches normal levels later

(3) Perryman, L. E. & Torbeck, R. L. (1980) *J. Am. vet. med. Assoc.*, *176*, 1250.
(4) Lew, A. M. et al. (1980) *Am. J. vet. Res.*, *41*, 1161.
(5) Perryman, L. E. et al. (1977) *J. Am. vet. med. Assoc.*, *170*, 212.
(6) McGuire, T. C. et al. (1974) *J. Am. vet. med. Assoc.*, *164*, 70.
(7) Lendl, W. et al. (1980) *Berl., Münch. Tierärztl. Wochenschr.*, *93*, 141.
(8) Perryman, L. E. & McGuire, T. C. (1980) *J. Am vet. med. Assoc.*, *176*, 1374.
(9) Buening, G. M. et al. (1977) *J. Am. vet. med. Assoc.*, *171*, 455.
(10) Deem, D. A. et al. (1979) *J. Am. vet. med. Assoc.*, *175*, 469.
(11) Campbell, T. M. et al. (1983) *Equ. vet. J.*, *15*, 233.
(12) Clarke, E. G. et al. (1978) *J. Am. vet. med. Assoc.*, *172*, 363.
(13) Perryman, L. E. et al. (1978) *Am. J. vet. Res.*, *39*, 1043.

Chediak–Higashi syndrome

This inherited disease occurs in man, in mink and in Hereford Japanese Black, and possibly other breeds of cattle. Affected animals are incomplete albinos and have a defect in immune defense mechanisms so that they often die of septicemia. The defect has been identified as one of insufficient bactericidal activity within abnormal leukocytes (1). It is readily diagnosed by the detection of anomalous enlarged cytoplasmic granules in neutrophils, lymphocytes, monocytes, and eosinophils (2). The granules are swollen lysosymes, and the disease is a lysosomal storage disease (3). There is also a defect in blood clotting, and this has been identified as a metabolic defect within structurally abnormal platelets (4–6). The platelets have a storage pool deficiency of dense granules and produce much less serotonin, ATP and ADP than normal platelets (7). The platelets also fail to aggregate normally in response to the presence of collagen (4). Clinically affected animals have poor growth, reduced pigmentation of skin and hair, anemia, enlarged edematous lymph nodes and a predilection for bacteremia and septicemia (2). Their average lifespan is 12·4 months. There are ocular abnormalities and fundic hypopigmentation (5). The disease is conditioned by a factor inherited as a single autosomal recessive.

REFERENCES

(1) Renshaw, H. W. et al. (1974) *Infect. Immunol.*, *10*, 928.
(2) Padgett, G. A. (1968) *Adv. vet. Sci.*, *12*, 240.
(3) Jolly, R. D. & Blakemore, W. F. (1973) *Vet. Rec.*, *92*, 391.
(4) Bell, T. G. et al. (1976) *Blood*, *48*, 175.
(5) Collier, L. L. et al. (1979) *J. Am. vet. med. Assoc.*, *175*, 587.
(6) Prieur, D. J. et al. (1976) *Lab. Invest.*, *35*, 197.
(7) Meyers, K. M. et al. (1981) *Am. J. Physiol.*, *237*, R239.

Pseudoalbinism and lethal whites

True albino horses rarely if ever occur in nature, but white horses with pigmented eyes do. They are more accurately called pseudoalbinos. There are a number of forms of pseudoalbinism in domestic animals. There is a non-lethal form in cattle (1) and a lethal dominant in horses (2) in which 25% of conceptions produced by mating dominant white horses die *in utero* in early gestation. The only pigment in the affected foals is in the eyes (5).

The disease in cattle occurs in Angus, Brown Swiss, Holstein and Hereford cattle (6). The Angus cattle have a brown coat and two-tone irises with an outer pale brown ring and an inner blue one. There appears to be no defect in digestion or metabolism (1). Hereford incomplete albinos have the Chediak–Higashi syndrome. The other breeds do not appear to have defects other than in pigmentation and the defect in Angus is probably more accurately called 'oculocutaneous hypopigmentation' (7). They do have one problem; they are photophobic and prefer to be out of the sun.

A recessive lethal white can also be produced by mating two Overo paint horses (an Overo is a horse with a coat color pattern where white is continuous over the body, but there is pigmented hair in a patch stretching from the ears to the tail). Affected foals develop colic soon after birth, fail to pass meconium and die at 2–4 days of age. At necropsy there is an irreparable atresia or contraction of the colon associated with a congenital absence of myoenteric ganglia in the terminal portion of the ileum and the cecum and colon. The colon is patent but unable to dilate (3).

A complete albinism in Icelandic sheep is manifested by white skin color, pink eyes, and impaired vision in bright light. It is an autosomal recessive (4).

REFERENCES

(1) Strasia, C. A. et al. (1983) *Bov. Practnr*, *18*, 147.
(2) Umemura, T. et al. (1983) *Jap. J. vet. Sci.*, *45*, 241.
(3) Hultgren, B. D. et al. (1982) *J. Am. vet. med. Assoc.*, *180*, 289.
(4) Adalsteinsson, S. (1977) *J. Hered.*, *68*, 347.
(5) Jones, W. E. (1979) *J. equ. med. Surg.*, *3*, 54.
(6) Ojo, S. A. et al. (1982) *Bov. Practnr*, *17*, 115.
(7) Cole, D. et al. (1984) *Bov. Practnr*, *19*, 92.

INHERITED DEFECTS OF THE ALIMENTARY TRACT

Inherited harelip

Harelip in cattle often has a distinct familial tendency but little work appears to have been done on the mode of inheritance (1). An apparently inherited harelip combined with poor growth and accompanying cryptorchidism is recorded in Holstein Friesian cattle (3). Bilateral cleavage of the lip which also involves the maxilla is recorded in Texel sheep as being conditioned by a single recessive autosomal gene (2).

REFERENCES

(1) Wheat. J. D. (1960) *J. Hered.*, *51*, 99.
(2) Hoekstra, P. & Wensvoort, P. (1976) *Tijdschr. Diergeneeskd.*, *101*, 71.
(3) Reike, H. (1979) *Dtsch Tierärztl. Wochenschr.*, *86*, 108.

Inherited rectovaginal constriction of Jersey cattle

The defect is inherited and is manifested as stenosis of the rectum in either sex and stenosis of the vaginal vestibule in females. It is regulated by an autosomal recessive gene. Affected cows are difficult to inseminate and have difficulty in calving. Their udders are small and hard and productivity is low (1). The condition is due to the presence of bands of non-elastic fibrous bands (2, 3). Edema of the udder is also a common complication (4).

REFERENCES

(1) Leipold, H. W. & Saperstein, G. (1975) *J. Am. vet. med. Assoc.*, *166*, 231.
(2) McGhee, C. C. & Leipold, H. W. (1982) *Cornell Vet.*, *72*, 427.
(3) Troyer, D. & Leipold, H. W. (1985) *Zentralbl. VetMed.*, *A32*, 752.
(4) Leipold, H. W. et al. (1981) *Bov. Practnr*, *16*, 76 & *18*, 13.

Inherited atresia of alimentary tract segments

Atresia ani occurs quite commonly in pigs, sheep and to a less extent in cattle. Affected animals may survive for up to 8 days but develop marked abdominal distension. Surgical repair is possible in some cases but in others a large segment of rectum is missing and creation of a colonic fistula in the inguinal region is necessary. The condition is thought to be inherited in pigs and calves: the evidence is less clear in sheep (1).

Inherited atresia coli, with complete closure of the ascending colon at the pelvic flexure, has been recorded in Percheron horses (3). A clinically similar defect in Overo horses, described in the section on pseudoalbinism, is in fact an aganglionosis. Death occurs during the first few days of life. The defect appears to be inherited as a simple recessive character.

Inherited atresia ilei has been recorded in Swedish Highland cattle (4). Affected calves manifest marked abdominal distension causing fetal dystocia. The distension is caused by accumulation of intestinal contents. Inheritance of a single recessive gene conditions the occurrence of the defect in some species and breeds but the prevalence may be higher than would be expected with that form of inheritance, especially in Jersey cattle with atresia coli (2).

REFERENCES

(1) Dennis, S. M. & Leipold, H. W. (1972) *Vet. Rec.*, *91*, 219.
(2) Willer, S. et al. (1984) *Mh VetMed.*, *39*, 473.
(3) Hutt, F. B. (1946) *Cornell Vet.*, *36*, 180.
(4) Nihleen, B. & Eriksson, K. (1958) *Nord. VetMed.*, *10*, 113.

Smooth tongue (epitheliogenesis imperfecta linguae bovis)

A defect of Holstein-Friesian and Brown Swiss cattle, this condition is inherited as an autosomal recessive factor (1, 2). The filiform papillae on the tongue are small, there is hypersalivation and poor haircoat and the calves do not fare well. The heterozygote is normal.

REFERENCES

(1) Weisman-Hamerman, Z. M. (1970) *Proefschr. Vet. Fak. Rijksuniv. Utrecht*, 135.
(2) Huston, K. et al. (1968) *J. Hered.*, *59*, 65.

INHERITED DEFECTS OF THE CIRCULATORY SYSTEM

Inherited cardiomyopathy

There are three types recorded.

Type 1

Sudden death of Poll Hereford calves up to 3 months of age may be due to inherited cardiomyopathy (1). The calves are often identifiable before death by their very rapid growth rate, short curly coat and rather protuberant eyes. Death is usually precipitated by stress or exercise and is characterized by dyspnea, the passage of bloody froth from the nose and a course of a few minutes to a few hours. Less acute cases have a syndrome of congestive heart failure for several days before death. Life expectancy is less than 6 months. At necropsy there is an obvious patchiness of the myocardium, reminiscent of a bad case of white muscle disease. The disease appears to be conditioned by a single autosomal recessive gene (1).

Type 2

A second form of inherited cardiomyopathy is recorded in Japanese Black cattle (2). Death is preceded by a brief period (a few minutes to a few hours) of agonizing dyspnea in calves about 30 up to 120 days of age. At necropsy there is edema, ascites, hydrothorax and marked dilatation of the left ventricle. This is matched by acute myocardial necrosis. A new autosomal recessive gene is credited with initiating the disease.

Type 3

Type 3 is a dilated or congestive cardiomyopathy in young-adult cattle and has been reported in Holstein-Friesian cattle in Japan and Canada (3) and in Simmental-Red Holstein crossbred cattle and Black Spotted Friesian cattle in Switzerland (4). Similar family lines in the Holstein breed have been identified in affected cattle in all three countries and it has been suggested that there is an inherited predisposition to cardiomyopathy in the Holstein breed (3). The disease occurs in cattle from 1½–6 years of age with the peak prevalence in 3 and 4-year-old cattle. The stress of pregnancy and lactation may precipitate clinical disease and the majority of cases occur in late pregnancy or early lactation. The onset is sudden and the majority of cases manifest with signs of congestive right heart failure. Edema of the submandibular area, brisket, ventral abdomen and udder is prominent and there is venous engorgement, hepatomegaly, pleural and pericardial effusion and ascites. Muffling of the heart sounds, tachycardia and a gallop rhythm are evident on auscultation of the heart. Postmortem examination shows congestive heart failure and histological findings compatible with congestive cardiomyopathy. There can be a high incidence in certain herds possibly associated with some unrecognised environmental precipitating factor but probably due to a high coefficient of inbreeding (3).

REFERENCES

(1) Morrow, C. J. & McOrist, S. (1985) *Vet. Rec.*, *117*, 312.
(2) Watanabe, S. et al. (1979) *J. Hered.*, *70*, 255.
(3) Baird, J. et al. (1986) *Proc. 14th World Cong. Dis. Cattle, Dublin*, *1*, 89.
(4) Martig, J. & Tschudi, P. (1985) *Dtsch Tierärztl. Wochenschr.*, *92*, 363.

Inherited lymphatic obstruction of Ayrshire calves

This defect has been recorded in Ayrshire calves in New Zealand (1), Scotland (2), Australia (3), the United States (4) and Finland (5). Males are more often affected than females; it has been suggested that some affected females may not be detected. The defect appears to be inherited as a single, autosomal recessive character.

The outstanding clinical feature is edema, the degree varying from slight to severe, severe cases causing dystocia to the point where embryotomy or cesarean section is necessary. Some mortality occurs among the dams. Many calves are dead at birth and those born alive may be reared but the edema persists. Before parturition the cow may show evidence of hydrops amnii and have difficulty in rising. In calves the edema may be generalised or, more commonly, be localised to the head, neck, ears, legs and tail. Drooping of the ears caused by increased weight is characteristic and accessory lobes are commonly situated behind and at the base of the ears.

The edema is caused by a developmental abnormality of the lymphatic system. The lymph nodes are small and contain cystic dilatations and the lymphatic vessels are enlarged, tortuous and dilated. Edema of the subcutaneous tissues and body cavities varies in degree; the skin is usually thickened and there is edema of the stomach wall. A cyst has been described in the pituitary gland of one animal (4). The liver is usually small. A similar condition is observed in newborn pigs born to sows vaccinated with attenuated hog cholera virus during the first 30 days of pregnancy.

REFERENCES

(1) Hancock, J. (1950) *Proc. 10th ann. Conf. NZ Soc. Anim. Prod.*, p. 91.
(2) Donald, H. P. et al. (1952) *Br. vet. J.*, *108*, 227.
(3) Morris, B. et al. (1954) *Aust. J. exp. Biol. med. Sci.*, *32*, 265.
(4) Herrick, E. H. & Eldridge, F. E. (1955) *J. dairy Sci.*, *38*, 440.
(5) Korkman, N. (1940) *Nord. JordbrForsk.*, *22*, 225.

Ventricular septal defect

There is one report of the occurrence of ventricular septal defect in Hereford cattle in such a way as to suggest that the condition is inherited (1).

REFERENCE

(1) Belling, T. H. (1962) *Vet. Med.* 57, 965.

Inherited aortic aneurysm

An inherited defect of the abdominal aorta, resulting in a high mortality from intra-abdominal hemorrhage, has been observed in cattle in Holland (1). The breed of cattle is not recorded.

REFERENCE

(1) Schuiringa-Sybesma, A. M. (1961) *Tijdschr. Diergeneeskd.*, *86*, 1192.

INHERITED DEFECTS OF THE NERVOUS SYSTEM

Inherited idiopathic epilepsy of cattle

Idiopathic epilepsy has been reported as an inherited condition in Brown Swiss cattle (1) and appears to be inherited as a dominant character. Typical epileptiform convulsions occur especially when the animals become excited or are exercised. Attacks do not usually commence until the calves are several months old and disappear entirely between the ages of 1 and 2 years.

REFERENCE

(1) Atkeson, F. W. et al. (1944) *J. Hered.*, *35*, 45.

Doddler calves

An inherited congenital defect in Hereford cattle produced by intensive breeding of half-sibs (1). It is no longer recorded. It was characterized by continuous clonic convulsions, nystagmus and pupillary dilatation. Stimulation by touch or sound exacerbated the convulsions.

REFERENCE

(1) High, J. W. et al. (1958) *J. Hered.*, *49*, 250.

Mannosidosis (neuronopathy and pseudolipidosis)

Mannosidosis is the best known of the inherited lysosomal storage diseases in agricultural animals. These are diseases in which there is a genetically determined deficiency of a specific lysosomal hydrolase enzyme. As a result of the deficiency, metabolic substrates accumulate in the lysosomes. The lysosomes themselves are concerned with the hydrolysis of polymetric material which enters the vacuolar system and converting it to monomeric units such as amino acids, monosaccharides and nucleotides which can be dealt with by the better known metabolic processes. There are other lysosomal storage diseases caused by poisonings and these are dealt with elsewhere. The best known ones are caused by poisoning with *Swainsona* sp., *Astragalus* sp., *Oxytropis* sp., and *Phalaris* sp. (the chronic form of that disease).

Alpha-mannosidosis is a lysosomal storage disease in which a deficiency of the enzyme alpha-mannosidase results in the accumulation of a metabolite rich in mannose and glucosamine in secondary lysosomes in neurones, macrophages and reticuloendothelial cells of lymph nodes causing apparent vacuolations in them. Similar vacuoles are found in exocrine cells in pancreas, abomasum, and lacrimal and salivary glands (3). Storage appears to be cumulative in the fetus, but after birth stored material is lost from the kidney into the urine via desquamated tubular epithelium. On the other hand, postnatal storage continues in the brain, pancreas and lymph nodes (9). The disease occurs in Angus, Murray Grey (5) and Galloway (8) cattle, is inherited as a simple recessive, and is recorded as occurring in the United States (9), Australia and New Zealand. Clinically it is characterized by ataxia, fine lateral head tremor, slow vertical nodding of the head, intention tremor, an aggressive tendency, failure to thrive and death or the necessity of euthanasia before reaching 1 year of age. These signs appear at 1–15 months of age and worsen over a period of 3–4 months. The first sign observed is a swaying of the hindquarters especially after exercise or with excitement. The stance becomes widebased and the gait jerky, stilted and high stepping, with slight overflexion of the hindquarters so that the animal appears to be squatting as it moves.

The nervous signs are exacerbated by excitement, diarrhea is common, the calves are usually stunted and unthrifty. They are also aggressive and attempt to charge but are usually impeded by their incoordination. Many calves die after having shown general ill-thrift and with minimal nervous signs. Death may occur due to paralysis and starvation, or to misadventure and some appear to die during a 'fit' following a period of excitement. Many others are euthanized because of persistent recumbency. The nervous syndrome of mannosidosis is well known but there is in addition the probability that the disease also causes neonatal mortality in calves disadvantaged by it (6); an alpha-mannosidosis is recorded in Galloway cattle (10) and is manifested by stillbirth, moderate hydrocephalus, enlargement of the liver and kidneys and arthrogryposis. A very similar disease has been recorded in Aberdeen Angus crossbred calves in South Africa (1).

Normal heterozygotes carrying genes for mannosidosis are identifiable because of their reduced tissue or plasma levels of alpha-mannosidase. The mannosidase test for beta-mannosidase in goats is specific and does not cross-react with alpha-mannosidase (5).

In New Zealand a control program for control of the disease in cattle is in hand in which heterozygotes are identifiable for the most part on their plasma mannosidase levels. Those animals which are equivocal are identified by reference to their parents, or to a more sensitive test on blood neutrophils (2). An Australian program is based on the granulocyte test because of the inaccuracy of the plasma mannosidase test (4). A program of screening cattle in herds which produce bulls for sale to commercial herds should stop the spread of the disease very quickly because the number of heterozygous females in the population will be irrelevant to the continuation of the disease in the absence of affected sires. A similar program is mooted for goats (7).

Beta-mannosidosis occurs in goats; it is recorded in Anglo-Nubian goats (9), is present at birth and characterized clinically by tetraplegia, tremor and nystagmus. Additional signs include clinical deafness, bilateral Horner's syndrome, carpal contractures, pastern joint hyperextension, thickened skin and a dome-shaped skull (11).

REVIEW LITERATURE

Baker, H. J. et al. (1979) The gangliosidoses. *Vet. Pathol.*, *16*, 635.
Jolly, R. D. & Hartley, W. J. (1977) Storage diseases of domestic animals. *Aust. vet. J.*, *53*, 1.

Jolly, R. D. (1975) Mannosidosis of Angus cattle. A prototype control programme for some genetic diseases. *Adv. vet. Sci.*, *19*, 1.

REFERENCES

(1) Coetze, J. A. W. & Louw, T. A. T. (1979) *Onderstepoort J. vet. Res.*, *45*, 245.
(2) Jolly, R. D. (1978) *NZ vet. J.*, *26*, 194.
(3) Jolly, R. D. & Thompson, K. G. (1977) *J. Pathol.*, *121*, 59.
(4) Healy, P. J. et al. (1983) *Aust. vet. J.*, *60*, 135.
(5) Dunstan, R. W. et al. (1983) *Am. J. vet. Res.*, *44*, 685.
(6) Jolly, R. D. & Thompson, K. G. (1976) *NZ vet. J.*, *24*, 184.
(7) Sewell, C. A. & Healy, P. J. (1985) *Aust. vet. J.*, *62*, 286.
(8) Hart, K. G. & Healey, P. J. (1980) *Aust. vet. J.*, *56*, 255.
(9) Shapiro, J. L. et al. (1985) *Can. vet. J.*, *26*, 155.
(10) Emberry, D. H. & Jerrett, I. V. (1985) *Vet. Pathol.*, *22*, 548.
(11) Kumar, K. et al. (1986) *Vet. Rec.*, *118*, 325.

Other lysosomal storage diseases of the central nervous system

Gangliosidoses

There are at least five types of gangliosidosis known to occur in man and animals. Two have so far been identified in agricultural animals:

GM1 gangliosidosis is an inherited lysosomal storage disease recorded in Friesian cattle (1) in which the activity of an enzyme beta-galactosidase in nervous tissue is greatly reduced. As a result there is an accumulation of the ganglioside (GM1) in the tissue. Clinical signs of progressive neuromotor dysfunction and a reduction in growth rate appear at about 3 months of age. The growth rate is reduced, the animal is in poor condition, blind and has a staring coat. The neuromotor signs include lack of response to external stimuli, sluggish mastication and swallowing, hindquarter sway while walking, a wide stance, a tendency to fall, reluctance to move, stiff high-stepping gait, aimless walking, headpressing and convulsions (1). Abnormal ECG tracings are common (2). The blindness results from lesions in the retina and the optic nerve. Ophthalmoscopic examination of the retina is recommended as an aid to diagnosis (7). A positive diagnosis is made on the grounds of intraneuronal lipid storage plus reduced beta-galactosidase activity plus identification of the stored lipid (1). In the live animal enzyme assays are carried out on leukocytes. The enzymatic defect is also detectable in liver, skin and leukocytes (3).

GM2 gangliosidosis has been identified in Yorkshire pigs and also causes decreased growth rate, incoordination appearing after 3 months of age, gray-white spots in the retina and dark blue granules in neutrophils, and azurophilic granules in lymphocytes. A serum enzyme assay is a suitable method of detecting 'carrier' heterozygous pigs. The test is based on the amount of *N*-acetyl-beta-D-hexosaminidase in tissues (10). It is also present in Suffolk sheep (15).

Ceroid lipofuscinosis is a disease of South Hampshire sheep, resembling neuronal ceroid lipofuscinosis of man, and has been recorded in New Zealand. The clinical findings include blindness. The necropsy lesion is atrophy of the cerebral cortex with eosinophilic granulation of neurons and macrophages in the central nervous system (3) followed by progressive retinal atrophy. There is a progressive storage of lipopigment in nervous tissue especially retinal photoreceptors (5). The mechanism of the accumulation is not understood but the disease is not a lipidosis nor does the lipopigment arise from the abnormal peroxidation of lipids; it may result from an inherited defect of liposomal protein catabolism (16). The disease provides a good animal model for discussing the similar disease (Batten's disease) of humans (12). It also occurs in Devon cattle (4).

Bovine generalised glycogenosis is a glycogen storage disease of Corriedale sheep (6), Shorthorn (5) and Brahman (13) beef cattle which resembles Pompe's disease in man. Clinical signs include poor growth, muscle weakness, incoordination of gait and difficulty in rising. The animals become permanently recumbent. The disease is identified as a lysosomal storage disease with lesions present in skeletal and cardiac muscle, and central nervous tissue. During the course of the disease there is progressive muscular damage, and acute degeneration of muscle fibers in the terminal stage (9). Affected Brahman calves die at 8–9 months of age (13) and British breed cattle at over one year (5). Only histopathological lesions are evident and include extensive vacuolation and accumulations of granular material in affected tissues. Amongst the biochemical lesions are greatly diminished alpha-glucosidase activity in liver and muscle, and a correspondingly high level of glycogen. Animals in affected herds are divisible into normal heterozygotes and homozygotes on the basis of alpha-1, 4-glucosidase activity in lymphocytes (8) or in muscle, especially semitendinosus muscle (14).

Globoid cell leukodystrophy has been identified in polled Dorset sheep in Australia (11). Incoordination in the hindlimbs progressed until the animals were tetraplegic. Only histological changes were evident at necropsy. These included myelin destruction and the accumulation of characteristic globoid cells in nervous tissue. There was greatly decreased galactocerebrosidase activity in affected tissue.

REFERENCES

(1) Donnelly, W. J. C. & Sheahan, B. J. (1981) *Irish vet. J.*, *35*, 45.
(2) Howell, J. Mc C. et al. (1981) *J. Pathol.*, *134*, 266.
(3) Donnelly, W. J. C. et al. (1977) *Vet. Rec.*, *100*, 318.
(4) Cook, R. W. (1984) *Univ. of Sydney Postgrad. Comm. Proc. No. 68*, p. 461.
(5) Armstrong, D. & Jolly, R. (1986) *Vet. Res. Commun.*, *10*, 79.
(6) Richards, R. B. et al. (1977) *Neuropathol. appl. Neurobiol.*, *3*, 45.
(7) Sheahan, B. J. et al. (1978) *Acta Neuropathol.*, *41*, 91.
(8) Cook, R. D. et al. (1978) *J. Neuropathol. exp. Neurol.*, *37*, 603.
(9) Edwards, J. R. & Richards, R. B. (1979) *Br. vet. J.*, *135*, 338.
(10) Kosanke, S. D. et al. (1978) *Vet. Pathol.*, *15*, 685 & *16*, 6.
(11) Pritchard, D. H. et al. (1980) *Vet. Pathol.*, *17*, 399.
(12) Mayhew, I. G. et al. (1985) *Neuropathol. appl. Neurobiol.*, *11*, 273.
(13) O'Sullivan, B. M. et al. (1981) *Aust. vet. J.*, *57*, 227.
(14) Howell, J. M. et al (1984) *Neuropathol. appl. Neurobiol.*, *10*, 255, 379.
(15) Ahern-Rindell, A. et al. (1985) *Fed. Proc.*, *44*, 744.
(16) Palmer, D. N. et al. (1986) *J. Biol. Chem.*, *261*, 1773.

Inherited congenital hydrocephalus

Congenital hydrocephalus without abnormality of the frontal bones occurs sporadically but is also known to be an inherited defect in Holstein and Hereford and possibly in Ayrshire (1) and Charolais (2) cattle. Two specific inherited entities have been described (2). In one there is obstruction to drainage of the cerebrospinal fluid from the lateral ventricles which become distended with fluid and may cause bulging of the forehead, often sufficient to cause fetal dystocia. Hereford calves with this defect have partial occlusion of the supraorbital foramen, a domed skull and poorly developed teeth, and at necropsy the cerebellum is found to be small and there may be microphthalmia and skeletal muscle myopathy (2). They are usually born a few days prematurely, are small in size and unable to stand or suck. In some cows the amniotic fluid is increased in volume. Another form of inherited hydrocephalus due to malformation of the cranium and with no enlargement of the cranium has also been observed in Hereford cattle (2–4). The ventricular dilatation is not marked, and microphthalmia and cerebellar hypoplasia are not features. Affected calves may be alive at birth, are blind and unable to stand. Some bawl continuously and some are dumb. They do not usually survive for more than a few days. At necropsy there is internal hydrocephalus of the lateral ventricles with marked thinning of the overlying cerebrum. Other lesions include constriction of the optic nerve, detachment of the retina, cataract, coagulation of the vitreous humor, and a progressive muscular dystrophy (4). The condition is inherited as a recessive character. Internal hydrocephalus inherited in combination with multiple eye defects in White Shorthorns is dealt with elsewhere, as are non-inherited forms of the disease.

Congenital hydrocephalus in Yorkshire and European pigs (5) has been recorded. The abnormality varies from a small protrusion of dura (meningocele) to an extensive brain hernia in which the cerebral hemispheres protrude through the frontal suture, apparently forced there by increased fluid pressure in the lateral and third ventricles. The condition is thought to be inherited in a recessive manner, but exacerbated in its manifestation by a coexisting hypovitaminosis A. An outbreak of congenital meningoencephalocele in Landrace pigs is recorded in circumstances suggesting that it was inherited (6).

REFERENCES

(1) Barlow, R. M. & Donald, L. B. (1963) *J. comp. Pathol.*, *73*, 410
(2) Greene, H. J. (1974) *Cornell Vet.*, *64*, 596.
(3) Baker, M. L. et al. (1961) *J. Hered.*, *52*, 135.
(4) Urman, H. K. & Grace, O. D. (1964) *Cornell Vet.*, *54*, 229.
(5) Meyer, H. & Trautwein, G. (1966) *Pathol. vet.*, *3*, 529, 543.
(6) Wijeratne, W. V. S. et al. (1974) *Vet. Rec.*, *95*, 81.

Inherited cranium bifidum of pigs

The disease occurs in a number of breeds, but has been shown to be inherited only in Poland China pigs and their crossbreds (1). There is a deficit in the cranial bones such that the defect would more properly be called cranioschisis. Meningoceles or encephaloceles may result. The pigs are not viable. Genetic experiments have shown the inheritance to be of a recessive character with varying penetrance.

REFERENCE

(1) Stewart, R. W. et al. (1972) *Vet. Med. small Anim. Clin.*, *67*, 677.

Inherited congenital cerebellar defects

Several inherited cerebellar defects occur congenitally in calves, lambs and foals. Lesions of the cerebellum may or may not be obvious. They all need to be differentiated from similar defects known to be caused by viral infections such as swine fever, bovine mucosal disease/virus diarrhea and bluetongue in early pregnancy.

Cerebellar hypoplasia of cattle

This occurs in Herefords, Guernseys, Holsteins (1), Shorthorns (3) and Ayrshires and appears to be conditioned by a factor inherited in a recessive manner. Most calves are obviously affected at birth. While lying down there is no marked abnormality although a moderate lateral tremor of the neck occurs, causing a gentle side-to-side swaying of the head. Severely affected calves are blind, have widely dilated pupils and their pupils do not react to light. Such calves are unable to stand, even when assisted, because of flaccidity of limb muscles. When less severely affected animals attempt to rise the head is thrown back excessively and the limb movements are exaggerated in force and range and are grossly incoordinated, and many calves are unable to rise without assistance. If they are placed on their feet the calves adopt a straddle-legged stance with the feet wide apart and the legs and neck extended excessively. On attempting to move, limb movements are incoordinated and the calf falls, sometimes backwards because of overextension of the forelimbs. Affected animals drink well but have great difficulty in getting to the teat or pail, attempts usually being wide of the mark. There are no defects of consciousness and no convulsions. Tremor may be evident while standing and postrotational nystagmus after rapid lateral head movements may occur. Sight and hearing are unimpaired and, although complete recovery does not occur, the calf may be able to compensate sufficiently to enable it to be reared to a vealing weight.

At necropsy the most severe defect comprises complete absence of the cerebellum, hypoplasia of the olivary nuclei, the pons and optic nerves and partial or complete absence of the occipital cortex. Less severe defects include a reduction in size of the cerebellum and absence of some neuronal elements in a cerebellum of normal size.

Inherited cerebellar ataxia in horses

The disease is recorded principally in Arabs (5, 6) but occurs also in the Australian pony, which was developed from the Arab, and in the Gotland breed from Sweden (7). A similar clinical syndrome occurs in the Oldenberg breed but the pathological picture is quite different.

The disease may be present at birth but is often not observed until the foal is 6–9 months old. The characteristic signs are vertical head-nodding (some cases show horizontal head tremors), especially when excited, and ataxia which is most noticeable at a fast gait. It may not be evident while the foal is walking. Very badly affected foals are unable to stand or suckle at birth, less severe ones are normal until about 4 months of age when head-nodding becomes obvious. The degree of ataxia varies from inability to stand to slight incoordination. A 'goosestepping' gait which slams the front feet into the ground occurs in some. All foals can see but there is an absence of the menace reflex in many. Nystagmus is not recorded as occurring in this disease.

Necropsy findings are limited to histopathological lesions in the cerebellum (5). These include widespread loss of Purkinje cells and the presence of a gliosis. There are no degenerative lesions in the spinal cord. In the similar disease in Oldenberg horses the cerebellum is often reduced in size. The disease is an abiotrophy, a premature aging of tissues.

Although the disease is dealt with generally as an inherited one there is no firm evidence to substantiate this view, and there are sporadic, non-inherited cases in other breeds (11).

Cerebellar atrophy of lambs (daft lamb disease)

This has been recorded in many breeds in Britain and in Corriedales in Canada. Affected lambs are normal at birth but are unable to walk properly. At 3 days of age it is obvious that there is severe incoordination of limb movement, opisthotonus, tremor, and a straddle-legged stance. At necropsy the cerebellum may be of normal size but on histological examination there is gross atrophy of cerebellar neurons. The disease appears to be conditioned by a recessive gene but not as a simple homozygous recessive. A clinically similar disease has been observed in Border Leicester lambs (4, 10). There is no histopathological lesion in the cerebellum, but there are significant lesions in the cervical muscles and the nerve supply to them. The disease is inherited, most likely as an autosomal recessive trait (8).

Inherited ataxia of calves

This is a true cerebellar ataxia inherited as a recessive character in Jerseys, Shorthorns and Holsteins. Clinically the condition resembles cerebellar hypoplasia except that signs may not occur until the calves are a few days to several weeks old. At necropsy the cerebellum is normal in size but histologically aplasia of neurons is evident in the cerebellum and also in the thalamus and cerebral cortex. An inherited condition, manifested by cerebellar ataxia which did not develop until calves were 6 weeks to 5 months old, has also been recorded but the cerebellum was small and macroscopically abnormal. Conspicuous degeneration of cerebellar Purkinje cells was evident on histological examination.

Cerebellar abiotrophy

A fourth disease in this group is described as cerebellar abiotrophy of Holstein calves (9) and of Merino sheep in Australia (12). In the calves ataxia appears for the first time when they are 3–8 months old. The calves are not blind but they often fail to exhibit a menace reflex. The onset of clinical signs is sudden but progression is slow or inapparent. Some become recumbent. Those that remain standing have a spastic, dysmetric ataxia. All are strong and have good appetites. Abiotrophy, or premature aging, is evident only microscopically and consists of degeneration of cerebellar neurons. The disease appears to be inherited.

The disease in sheep does not appear until about 3 years of age. There is incoordination and dysmetria so that the gait is awkward and disorganized and there is frequent falling. There are also a reduced menace response, an apprehensive manner and a wide-based stance in the hindlimbs. At necropsy there is diffuse cerebellar degeneration and severe loss of Purkinje cells.

A congenital progressive cerebellar abiotrophy is also reported in piglets of the offspring of Saddleback sows and an unrelated Large White boar. The disorder behaves epidemiologically like an inherited disease conditioned by a simple autosomal recessive trait (13). Clinical signs included dysmetria, ataxia and tremor at standing but not at rest. There was gradual adjustment so that the piglets could walk and stand at 5 weeks of age but by 15 weeks they were no longer able to do so. Affected pigs also had a coarse matted hair coat caused by a disproportionate number of coarse to fine hairs. Histopathological lesions were confined to the cerebellum where there was a significant loss of Purkinje cells.

Familial convulsions and ataxia in cattle

A neurological disease is recorded as being inherited in Aberdeen Angus cattle and their crossbreds (1). In young calves there are intermittent attacks of convulsions, and in older animals these are replaced by a residual ataxia. The first signs appear within a few hours of birth, up to several months later there are single or multiple tetanic convulsions lasting for 3–12 hours. As these episodes disappear a spastic goose-stepping gait becomes apparent in the forelegs and there is difficulty placing the hindlegs. The characteristic necropsy lesion is a very selective cerebellar cortical degeneration. The epidemiology of the disease is consistent with the operation of an autosomal dominant gene with incomplete penetrance, but there is sufficient other evidence to suggest that other causative agents should still be considered (1). A similar syndrome and lesion have been recorded in a Charolais calf, and inheritance was suggested as the cause (2).

Inherited congenital spasms of cattle

This condition has been recorded only in Jersey cattle and appears to be conditioned by a factor inherited in a recessive manner. Affected calves show intermittent, vertical tremor of the head and neck and there is a similar tremor of all four legs which prevents walking and interferes with standing. Although the calves are normal in all other respects they usually die within the first few weeks of life. No histological examinations have been reported but a cerebellar lesion seems probable. A similar condition, described as being inherited as a single recessive character, has been described in horses in Europe.

REFERENCES

(1) Barlow, R. M. (1981) *Vet. Pathol.*, *18*, 151.
(2) Cho, D. Y. & Leipold, H. W. (1978) *Vet. Pathol.*, *15*, 264.
(3) O'Sullivan, B. M. & McPhee, C. P. (1975) *Aust. vet. J.*, *51*, 469.
(4) Bradley, R. & Terlecki, S. (1977) *J. Pathol.*, *123*, 225.
(5) Palmer, A. C. et al. (1973) *Vet. Rec.*, *93*, 62.
(6) Baird, J. D. & Mackenzie, C. D. (1974) *Aust. vet. J.*, *50*, 25.

(7) Bjorck, G. et al. (1973) *Zentralbl. VetMed.*, *20A*, 341.
(8) Terlecki, S. et al. (1978) *Br. vet. J.*, *134*, 299.
(9) White, M. E. et al. (1975) *Cornell Vet.*, *65*, 476.
(10) Bradley, R. (1978) *J. Pathol.*, *125*, 205.
(11) Beech, J. (1976) *Proc. 22nd ann. Conv. Am. Assoc. equ. Pract.*, p.77.
(12) Harper, P. A. W. et al. (1986) *Aust. vet. J.*, *63*, 18.
(13) Kidd, A. R. M. et al. (1986) *Br. vet. J.*, *142*, 275.

Inherited spastic paresis of cattle (Elso-heel)

This disease occurs in the Holstein, Aberdeen Angus, Red Danish, Ayrshire, Beef Shorthorn (1), Poll Hereford (9), Murray Grey and several Dutch and German breeds of cattle and probably in many others. It has been observed in an Ayrshire X Beef Shorthorn crossbred steer (2). The disease occurs principally in calves with signs appearing from several weeks to 6 months or more after birth. Occasional cases are reported as developing in adult European cattle and there is one report of the occurrence of the disease in adult Indian cattle (3).

It has been held for a long time that the disease is inherited, and the principal argument has centered on the mode of inheritance. Attempts to determine this have shown that the rate of occurrence in planned test matings is so low that, if inheritance is involved, it can only be the inheritance of a susceptibility to the disease. It is firmly believed that a bull suspected of producing affected calves should not necessarily be withdrawn from a breeding program (10). There is also a disquieting observation of a mild, non-suppurative encephalitis in some calves (11).

It is suggested that different time appearances represent a single disease entity with varying expressivity, the late forms being affected by cumulative environmental factors (4). In both diseases there is excessive tone of the gastrocnemius muscle and straightness of the hock, usually more marked in one hindleg. If only one leg is affected it may be thrust out behind while the calf is walking and advanced with a restricted, swinging motion often without touching the ground. There is no resistance to passive flexion of the limb. The gastrocnemius and perforatus muscles are rigid and in a state of spastic contraction. There is a characteristic elevation of the tail. The lameness becomes progressively worse and affected animals spend much time lying down. Much body weight is lost and the animal is usually destroyed between 1 and 2 years of age. Minor lesions described as regressive changes in the neurons of the red nucleus, in the reticular substance and the lateral vestibular nucleus (5) are of doubtful significance (1), as are the observed reduction in inorganic phosphate and ascorbic acid levels in the blood and cerebrospinal fluid of affected calves (6). A lower CSF concentration than normal of a central neurotransmitter, dopamine, could also be an effect rather than a cause (7). There are demonstrable lesions on radiological examination of the tarsus but exhaustive examinations of muscles and tendons fail to reveal histological abnormalities (8). The absence of any structural lesion and the variation in intensity of the abnormality suggests that it is a functional one. The hypersensitivity of the myotic reflex which has been observed (13) could be such a defect.

In Europe affected animals are kept for breeding purposes, especially if they are double-muscled. They are kept for this reason and because of the efficacy of the curative surgical operation (9, 12) and in view of the high incidence of double muscling in such calves. In the Holstein breed, and several German breeds, bulls which sire affected calves have been observed to have very straight hocks and to suffer from various forms of stifle and hock lameness early in life.

REFERENCES

(1) Leipold, H. W. et al. (1967) *J. Am. vet. med. Assoc.*, *151*, 598.
(2) Love, J. & Weaver, A. D. (1963) *Vet. Rec.*, *75*, 394.
(3) Gadgil, B. A. et al. (1970) *Vet. Rec.*, *86*, 694.
(4) van Huffel, X. et al. (1986) *Vlaams Diergeneeskd. Tijdsch.*, *55*, 21.
(5) Chomiak, M. & Szteyn, S. (1970) *Schweiz. Arch. Tierheilk*, *112*, 397.
(6) Bijleveld, K. & Binkhorst, G. J. (1973) *Tiidschr. Diergeneeskd.*, *98*, 803.
(7) de Ley, G. & de Moor, A. (1975) *Am. J. vet. Res.*, *36*, 227.
(8) de Ley, G. & de Moor, A. (1976) *Zentralbl. VetMed.*, *23A*, 89.
(9) Browning, G. F. et al. (1986) *Aust. vet. J.*, *63*, 367.
(10) Dawson, P. L. L. (1975) *Vet. Rec.*, *97*, 432.
(11) Baird, J. D. et al. (1974) *Aust. vet. J.*, *50*, 239.
(12) Osinga, A. & de Boer, G. (1973) *Tijdschr. Diergeneeskd.*, *98*, 795.
(13) de Ley, G. & de Moor, A. (1980) *Vet. Sci. Commun.*, *3*, 289.

Inherited periodic spasticity of cattle

This disease has been observed in Holstein and Guernsey cattle and usually does not appear until the animals are adults (1). It is a particular problem in mature bulls maintained in artificial insemination centers. In the early stages the signs are apparent only on rising, the hindlegs being stretched out behind and the back depressed. Marked tremor of the hindquarters may be noted. Initially the attacks persist only for a few seconds but are of longer duration as the disease progresses and may eventually last for up to 30 minutes. Movement is usually impossible during the attacks. The tetanic episodes fluctuate in their severity from time to time but there is never any abnormality of consciousness. Lesions of the vertebrae have been recorded but no lesions have been found in the nervous system. The disease is familial and the mode of inheritance appears to be by inheritance of a single recessive factor with incomplete penetrance (2).

Administration of the spinal cord depressant, mephenesin (3–4 g/100 kg/body weight given orally in three divided doses and repeated for 2–3 days) controls the more severe signs. A single course of treatment may be effective for some weeks.

REFERENCES

(1) Roberts, S. J. (1965) *Cornell Vet.*, *55*, 637.
(2) Sponenberg, D. P. et al. (1985) *Vet. Med.*, *80(8)*, 92.

Inherited neonatal spasticity

The defect is recorded in Jersey and Hereford cattle (1). Affected calves are normal at birth but develop signs 2–5 days later. The signs commence with incoordination and bulging of the eyes and a tendency to deviation of the neck causing the head to be held on one side.

Subsequently the calves are unable to stand and on stimulation develop a tetanic convulsion in which the neck, trunk and limbs are rigidly extended and show marked tremor. Each convulsion is of several minutes duration. Affected calves may survive for as long as a month if nursed carefully. There are no gross or histological lesions at necropsy. Inheritance of the defect is conditioned by a single, recessive character.

REFERENCE

(1) Gregory, K. E. et al. (1962) *J. Hered.*, *53*, 130.

Inherited maple syrup urine disease

Calves affected with this disease are normal at birth and develop signs only at 1–3 days of age. It is inherited as an autosomal recessive and occurs principally in Poll Hereford and Hereford cattle but probably occurs also in Angus, Jersey and Australian Illawarra Shorthorn calves (1, 2). The disease is characterized by dullness, recumbency, tremor, tetanic spasms and opisthotonus. When held in a standing position some calves have tetanic paralysis, others have flaccid paralysis. The disease is caused by an accumulation of branched chain amino acids including valine, leucine and isoleucine presumably due to an absence of branched chain ketoacid decarboxylase. The urine smells of burnt sugar. At necropsy there is a characteristic severe status spongiosus of the central nervous system similar to that found in comparable hereditary aminoacidurias in humans.

REFERENCE

(1) Harper, P. A. W. et al. (1986) *Vet. Rec.*, *119*, 62.
(2) Baird, J. D. et al. (1987) *Can. Vet. J.*, *28*, 505.

Inherited congenital myoclonus (hereditary neuraxial edema)

This congenital defect of the nervous system has been reported only in polled Hereford cattle (1, 2) or their crossbreds (3) and appears to be transmitted by inheritance in an autosomal recessive pattern (7). At birth affected calves are unable to sit up or rise and are very sensitive to external stimuli, manifested by extreme extensor spasm, including fixation of thoracic muscles and apnea, especially if lifted and held upright. The intellect of the calves seems unaffected, vision is normal, they drink well and can be reared but at great cost in time. Intercurrent disease is common and calves usually die of pneumonia or enteritis before they are a month old.

All affected calves have subluxations of the hip joints or epiphyseal fractures of the femoral head caused by muscle spasms in the fetus. Their gestation length is shorter than that of normal calves by 9 days (7).

There are no microscopic lesions or biochemical defects in the central nervous system (8). The disease needs to be differentiated from two other congenital, presumed hereditary diseases of newborn Herefords, maple syrup urine disease and 'congenital brain edema', in which spongy degeneration of the CNS is accompanied by severe edema of the gray and white matter (5). These two diseases are assumed to represent those cases of congenital disease, originally bracketed with inherited congenital myoclonus, but in which there was vacuolation of nervous tissue in the central nervous system (4, 6).

REFERENCES

(1) Cordy, D. R. et al. (1969) *Pathol. vet.*, *6*, 487.
(2) Blood, D. C. & Gay, C. C. (1971) *Aust. vet. J.*, *47*, 520.
(3) Davis, G. B. et al. (1975) *NZ vet. J.*, *23*, 181.
(4) Weaver, A. D. (1974) *Dtsch Tierätzl. Wochenschr.*, *81*, 572.
(5) Jolly, R. D. (1974) *J. Pathol.*, *114*, 199.
(6) Cho, D. Y. & Leipold, H. W. (1978) *Pathol. Res. Pract.*, *163*, 158.
(7) Healy, P. J. & Harper, P. A. W. (1984) *Aust. Adv. vet. Sci.*, p. 34.
(8) Harper, P. A. W. et al. (1986) *Vet. Rec.*, *119*, 59.

Inherited citrullinemia

The clinical disease manifested by depression, recumbency, opisthotonus and convulsions, begins in the first week of life in Holstein–Friesian calves in Australia (1). The calves are normal at birth. Other signs include compulsive walking, blindness, head-pressing, tremor and hyperthermia. The calf dies 6–12 hours after the onset of illness. Blood citrulline levels are of the order of 40–1200 times normal. Arginosuccinate synthetase deficiency is the likely cause.

REFERENCE

(1) Harper, P. A. W. et al. (1986) *Aust. vet. J.*, *63*, 378.

Shaker calf syndrome

This is an inherited, degenerative disorder of horned Hereford calves (1). Newborn calves show severe tremor, difficulty in rising, spastic gait and aphonia. Terminally there is spastic paraplegia. Histologically there are accumulations of neurofilaments within neurons.

REFERENCE

(1) Rousseaux, C. G. et al. (1985) *Vet. Pathol.*, *22*, 104.

Inherited congenital posterior paralysis

Two inherited forms of congenital posterior paralysis are recorded in cattle (1). In Norwegian Red Poll cattle posterior paralysis is apparent in affected calves at birth. Opisthotonus and muscle tremor are also present. No histological lesions have been found. The disease is conditioned by an inherited recessive factor. In red Danish and Bulgarian Red (2) cattle a similar condition occurs but there is spastic extension of the legs, particularly the hindlegs, and tendon reflexes are exaggerated. Histological examination has revealed degenerative changes in mid-brain motor nuclei. Both defects are lethal because of prolonged recumbency.

An inherited posterior paralysis has been recorded in several breeds of swine in Europe (1). Affected pigs are able to move their hindlegs but are unable to stand on them. They are normal in other respects. Degeneration of neurons is evident in cerebral cortex, mid-brain, cerebellum, medulla and spinal cord. The disease is conditioned by the inheritance of a recessive character. An inherited progressive ataxia is also recorded in Yorkshire pigs (3).

REFERENCES

(1) Innes, J. R. M. & Sunders, L. Z. (1957) *Adv. vet. Sci.*, *3*, 35.
(2) Guerov, K. et al. (1973) *Rev. Med. Vet.*, *124*, 1139.
(3) Rimaila-Parnanen, E. (1982) *Hereditas*, *97*, 305.

Inherited congenital myotonia of goats

This disease has been observed in goats and possibly in a horse (1) and because of its great similarity to Thomsen's disease (myotonia congenita) of humans, affected goats have been used in experimental studies to determine the nature of the disease in man. There is no apparent defect of the nervous system and the condition is thought to be due to abnormality of the muscle fibers. The specific defect is thought to be one of cell membranes and because, in affected animals, the erythrocytes are less susceptible than normal to hemolysis, it is suggested that the membrane abnormality may be generalized (4). Affected animals run when startled but quickly develop extreme rigidity of all four limbs and are unable to move. Relaxation occurs in a few seconds and the animal can then move again. Signs are not usually present until some time after birth and may vary from day to day for no apparent reason (2). They tend to diminish immediately before and after parturition. When water is withheld from affected goats for 2–3 days clinical signs disappear but reappear when drinking is permitted (3). The disease is inherited but the mode of inheritance is unknown.

REFERENCES

(1) Steinberg, S. & Botelho, S. (1962) *Science, NY*, *137*, 979.
(2) Bryant, S. H. et al. (1968) *Am. J. vet. Res.*, *29*, 2371.
(3) Hegyeli, A. & Szent-Gyorgi, A. (1961) *Science, NY*, *133*, 1011.
(4) Atkinson, J. B. et al. (1980) *Proc. Soc. exp. Biol. Med.*, *163*, 69.

Inherited congenital tremor of pigs

Congenital tremor of pigs has a multiple etiology and some of the causes are not yet identified. For this reason the disease as a whole is dealt with in Chapter 35. The inherited diseases are noted here. There are two of them, congenital tremor type A-IV of British Saddleback pigs, and congenital tremor type A-III, a sex-linked inherited form of cerebrospinal hypomyelinogenesis of Landrace pigs. The A-IV disease is characterized by the presence of poorly myelinated axons in all parts of the central nervous system. The specific defect in A-IV is one of fatty acid metabolism (1). The structural abnormalities in the A-III disease have been identified (2); splayleg is a common accompaniment (3).

Both diseases are characterized by muscle tremor, incoordination, difficulty in standing, and some squealing. The A-III disease occurs only in males. Both are inherited as recessive characters.

REFERENCES

(1) Patterson, D. S. P. et al. (1973) *J. Neurochem.*, *21*, 397.
(2) Blakemore, W. F. et al. (1974) *Res. vet. Sci.*, *17*, 174.
(3) Miry, C. et al. (1983) *Dtsch Tierärztl. Wochenschr.*, *90*, 358.

Bovine progressive ataxia

This well-recognized disease is in Charolais cattle. The first onset of signs is at about 12 months of age when the gait is seen to be stiff and stumbling, especially in the hindlegs. The ataxia progresses over a period of 1–2 years. Affected animals tend to be down a lot and have difficulty in rising and posturing for urination. Urination is abnormal being a squirting but continuous flow which soils the tail. Some affected animals nod their heads from side to side when excited (1, 2). Both males and females are affected (3). Characteristic necropsy lesions are confined to the central nervous system and are histopathological. The white matter of the cerebellum and internal capsule contains multiple foci of oligodendroglial dysplasia (4). The somatic lymph nodes contain nodules of hyperplastic lymphoid follicles, some catarrh of the medullae of the nodes and an accumulation of eosinophils.

There is a similar progressive spinal myelinopathy in Murray Grey cattle which is possibly genetic in origin (5). There are degenerative lesions in spinal cord, midbrain and cerebellum.

REFERENCES

(1) Palmer, A. C. et al. (1972) *Vet. Rec.*, *91*, 592.
(2) Palmer, A. C. & Blakemore, W. F. (1975) *Bov. Practnr*, *8*, 84.
(3) Ogden, A. L. et al. (1974) *Vet. Rec.*, *94*, 555.
(4) Cordy, D. R. (1986) *Vet. Pathol.*, *23*, 78.
(5) Richards, R. B. & Edwards, J. R. (1986) *Vet. Pathol.*, *23*, 35.

Weaver syndrome in Brown Swiss (bovine progressive degenerative myeloencephalopathy)

The defect is inherited in Brown Swiss. It appears first in calves when they are 6–8 months old and is manifested by hindlimb ataxia followed by recumbency (1, 2). Histopathologically there are abnormalities of the synaptic junctions in the cerebral cortex (3).

REFERENCES

(1) Hansen, K. M. (1984) *Dansk Veterinaertidssk.*, *67*, 425.
(2) Stuart, L. K. & Leipold, H. W. (1983) *Bov. Practnr*, *18*, 129 & 133.
(3) Aitchison, C. S. et al. (1985) *Am. J. vet. Res.*, *46*, 1773.

Exophthalmos with strabismus of cattle

This disease has been recorded in Shorthorn (1) and Jersey cattle. In the former it is not manifested until the first pregnancy or lactation but in the latter may appear at 6–12 months of age. Defective vision is the first sign and is followed by severe protrusion and anteromedial deviation of both eyeballs. The defects may get worse over a long period. It appears to be inherited in a recessive manner, with relative absence of neurons in the abducens nerve (2).

REFERENCES

(1) Holmes, J. R. & Young, G. B. (1957) *Vet. Rec.*, *69*, 148.
(2) Schultz-Hanke, W. et al. (1979) *Dtsch Tierärztl. Wochenschr.*, *86*, 185.

Familial undulatory nystagmus

This is an inherited defect of Finnish Ayrshire cattle characterized by a tremor-like, synchronous movement of the eyeballs (1). The tremor has small amplitude (1–2 mm) and fast (200/minute) rate and is usually vertical. It is present at all times, there is no sign of impaired vision, and the eye reflexes are normal. The condition is a blemish rather than a disease because there is no functional deficiency.

REFERENCE

(1) Nurmio, P. et al. (1982) *Nord. VetMed.*, *34*, 130.

INHERITED DEFECTS OF THE MUSCULOSKELETAL SYSTEM

Inherited osteoarthritis of cattle

There are strong indications from field evidence that both degenerative arthropathy, in which the hip joint is principally involved (1), and degenerative osteoarthritis affecting particularly the stifle joint, are inherited in cattle. In both diseases other factors, particularly nutritional deficiency and the stress of lactation, exert an important influence on the appearance of the clinical disease and in degenerative arthropathy there is no clear evidence that it is in fact inherited. On the other hand there is good evidence that osteoarthritis can be inherited, at least in Holstein-Friesian and in Jersey cattle (2).

In inherited degenerative osteoarthritis in which the stifle joints are most severely affected there is usually a gradual onset of lameness in both hindlegs in aged animals of both sexes. Occasionally only one leg appears to be involved. Progression of the disease proceeds over a period of 1–2 years and is evidenced by failure to flex the limb resulting in the foot not being lifted high from the ground. Crepitation in the stifle joint can be heard and felt, the muscles of the limb atrophy and the joints are enlarged. Movement is slow, the hindlegs at rest are placed further forward than normal, the stifles are abducted and the feet held together. Joint fluid can be aspirated and is clear and straw-colored. Appetite and milk yield remain normal until the late stages, except in cattle running at pasture.

At necropsy there is severe osteoarthritis involving particularly the stifle, with extensive erosion of the articular cartilages, great increase in synovial fluid and the development of many osteophytes around the edges of the articular surfaces. Less severe changes are evident in other joints. It is suggested that the disease is conditioned by the inheritance of a single autosomal recessive character.

An inherited defective development of the acetabulum occurs in Dole horses. There is no clinical evidence of the disease at birth but osteoarthritis of the joint and disruption of the round ligament develop subsequently (3).

REFERENCES

(1) Carnahan, D. L. (1968) *J. Am. vet. med. Assoc.*, *158*, 1150.
(2) Kendrick, J. W. & Sittmann, K. (1966) *J. Am. vet. med. Assoc.*, *149*, 17.
(3) Sokoloff, L. (1960) *Adv. vet. Sci.*, 6.

Inherited arachnomelia of cattle

This suspected inherited disease of Simmental, Brown Swiss and other European (2) breeds of cattle is manifested by excessively long, thin, distal extremities which give the calves a spidery look, hence arachnomelia. The bones are very fragile, there is curvature of the spine, foreshortening of the mandible, and associated cardiac and vascular defects. It is thought to be inherited as a simple recessive (1). A similar disease of sheep, known as spider disease, is listed under that name. There is no evidence that it is inherited but it is most common in Suffolks.

REFERENCES

(1) Rieck, G. W. & Schade. W. (1975) *Dtsch Tierärztl. Wochenschr.*, *84*, 342.
(2) Brem, G. et al. (1984) *Berl. Munch. Tierärztl. Wochenschr.*, 97, 393.

Inherited multiple ankylosis of cattle

Multiple ankylosis affecting all limb joints has been recorded as an inherited congenital defect in Holstein calves (1). The abdomen of the dam shows marked enlargement at the 6th–7th month of pregnancy and this may occasion some respiratory distress. Excessive fetal fluids are present and insertion of the hand per rectum is impeded by the distended uterus. Abortion during the last month of pregnancy is a common occurrence. Affected fetuses have a very short neck, ankylosed intervertebral joints and varying degrees of ankylosis of all limb joints. The limbs are fixed in flexion and there is some curvature of the spine. Fetal dystocia always occurs and embryotomy or cesarean section is necessary to deliver the calf.

Ankylosis of limb joints combined with cleft palate occurs occasionally in Charolais cattle and is suspected of being inherited (2). Ankylosis of the coffin joint, developing at several weeks of age, has been reported in Simmental calves. The etiology of the condition is not clear (3).

REFERENCES

(1) Murray, M. D. (1951) *Aust. vet. J.*, *27*, 73, 76.
(2) Lauvergne, J. J. & Blin, P. C. (1967) *Ann. Zootechnol.*, *16*, 291.
(3) Martig, J. et al. (1972) *Vet. Rec.*, *91*, 307.

Inherited arthrogryposis (inherited multiple tendon contracture)

Inherited fixation of limb joints present at birth is recorded in many breeds of cattle especially in the Charolais (1) and Piedmont (2) breeds. There are many other environmental causes (3) of which the best known is Akabane virus infection of early pregnancy and discussed under that heading.

This disease has been recorded in Shorthorn calves and is thought to be inherited as a single recessive character. It resembles closely the non-inherited disease of calves, arthrogryposis. The limbs of affected calves are fixed in flexion or extension and cause dystocia due to abnormal positioning and lack of flexibility. There is no involvement of joint surfaces and the joints can be freed by cutting the surrounding tendons or muscles. There is atrophy of limb muscles and those calves which are born alive are unable to stand and usually die or are destroyed within a few days. Clinically similar defects have been observed to be inherited amongst Dole cattle in Norway.

A defect similar in some respects to the above syndrome has been recorded in cattle (13) and appears to be inherited in a dominant manner. The front legs are straight and rigid down to the fetlock which is permanently flexed. The hindlegs are sickle-shaped but the joints are freely movable in all directions. The teeth are soft, fleshy and easy to bend. There is no defect of bones or joints other than marked softness and the presence of excess cartilage at the epiphyses. There is abnormal ossification of the cartilage. The calves are of normal size, do not cause dystocia and although they are unable to stand because of the excessive flexibility of the limbs, they can suck. Hypostatic pneumonia usually develops and causes death of the calf.

In the inherited disease it is common to have other defects associated with the articular rigidity (3). Probably the commonest is the cleft palate seen in the Charolais breed (4) which is known in France as the syndrome of arthrogryposis and palatoschisis (SAP) (5, 6). It is inherited as a simple recessive with low penetrance in pure French Charolais in France and high penetrance in 7/8 Charolais cattle in Canada (5). In the Canadian studies the frequency of carriers appears to be high in Charolais and hybrid-Charolais population. The gene is usually carried by heterozygous animals with one normal and one deleterious gene. However, some animals are able to survive with a double recessive genotype. Among pure-bred Charolais cattle, a high percentage of homozygous individuals show slight to no visible effect of the gene. Among cross-bred Charolais cattle, the homozygous condition is almost always markedly expressed and lethal (11). Arthrogryposis carrier dams show improved fertility and longevity which may be advantageous in a breeding program (7). Because of the low rate of prevalence in France, attempted eradication does not appear to be economical (5).

In this syndrome all limbs are usually affected but the front limbs more than the hindlimbs, and the more distal joints more rigidly fixed than proximal ones. The muscles of affected limbs are atrophic and pale in color. Histological changes in the spinal cord suggest that the muscle atrophy is neurogenic (8). In affected calves the gestation period may be longer than normal by an average of 2 weeks.

There is one record of a Charolais calf with arthrogryposis and cleft palate which also had a 1/29 translocation in its karyotype but this was thought not to be related to the deformity (9). In Simmentals a combined set of defects includes arthrogryposis, underdevelopment of the mandible, curvature of the spine and defects of the heart and main vessels (10).

Suspected inherited arthrogryposis without cleft palate is often associated with the limbs in a 'wraparound' position around the body (4). Inherited arthrogryposis has also been recorded in pigs and sheep (4) and in Merino and Corriedale sheep (15). The defect in Norwegian Landrace pigs is thought to be inherited as a simple recessive (16). The Corriedale defect is associated with other lesions including brachygnathia inferior, hydranencephaly and thoracic scoliosis. Contracture of appendicular joints also occurs congenitally in calves and foals but often appears not to be inherited (12). An inherited form of the disease does occur in horses of the Norwegian Fjord breed (14). The arthrogryposis affects the hindlegs and there are accompanying defects of polydactyly (13), palatoschisis and brachygnathia in some. Most foals are unable to stand and the defect must be considered to be a lethal one.

REVIEW LITERATURE

Lauvergne, J. J. & Faucon, A. (1976) The syndrome of arthrogryposis and palatoschisis (SAP) in Charolais cattle, an annotated bibliography: 1967–1975. *Ann. genet. Sel. Anim.*, *8*, 51.

Nawrot, P. et al. (1980) Arthrogryposis; an inherited defect in newborn calves. *Aust. vet. J.*, *56*, 359.

REFERENCES

(1) Cole, A. E. (1976) *Proc. 53rd ann. Conf. Aust. vet. Assoc.*, Melbourne, 116–118.
(2) Pancani, I. et al. (1976) *Atti. Soc. ital. Butatria*, 7, 241.
(3) Greene, H. J. et al. (1973) *Am. J. vet. Res.*, *34*, 887.
(4) Swatland, H. J. (1974) *Vet. Bull.*, *44*, 179.
(5) Lauvergne, J. J. & Faucon, A (1976) *Ann. génet. Sel. Anim.*, *8*, 51.
(6) Lauvergne, J. J. (1975) *Ann. génet. Sel. Anim.*, 7, 321.
(7) Goonewardene, L. A. & Berg, R. T. (1976) *Ann. génet. Sel. Anim.*, *8*, 493.
(8) Leipold, H. W. et al. (1974) *Vet. Med.*, *68*, 1140, 1142, 1146.
(9) Logue, D. N. et al. (1977) *Vet. Rec.*, *100*, 509.
(10) Rieck, G. W. & Schade, W. (1975) *Dtsch Tierärztl. Wochenschr.*, *82*, 342.
(11) Hanset, R. et al. (1978) *Ann. Med. Vet.*, *122*, 591.
(12) Rooney, J. R. (1966) *Cornell Vet.*, *56*, 172.
(13) Johnston, W. G. & Young, G. B. (1958) *Vet. Rec.*, *70*, 1219.
(14) Nes, N. et al. (1982) *Nord. VetMed.*, *34*, 425.
(15) Whittington, R. J. et al. (1985) *Aust. Adv. vet. Sci.*, p. 122.
(16) Lomo, O. M. (1985) *Acta vet. Scand.*, *26*, 419.

Inherited splayed digits

Recorded only in Jersey cattle (1), this defect appears to be conditioned by an inherited gene, probably a monogenic autosomal recessive. Lameness becomes apparent at 2–4 months of age, the toes becoming increasingly widely spread and the toes themselves misshapen. Affected animals lie down increasingly and become disinclined to stand and to stay standing. Walking and standing are painful, especially on the front feet so that some animals tend to graze and walk on their knees. The apparent abnormality is a defect of the muscles and ligaments holding the phalanges together.

REFERENCE

(1) Mead, S. W. et al. (1949) *Genetics*, *40*, 151.

Inherited patellar subluxation

Unilateral or bilateral subluxation occurs as an inherited defect in *Bos indicus* cattle and in water buffalo (*Bubalus bubalis*) (1). There is periodic lameness with the affected limb held in rigid extension; the patella is displaced medially. If the animal shakes the limb the patella may go back into its normal position and the problem is relieved.

REFERENCE

(1) Sharma, K. B. et al. (1984) *Ind. vet. J.*, *61*, 689.

Inherited hypermobility of joints

The inherited disease is recorded only in Jersey cattle (1). It has assumed great importance because of the great popularity of a sire which carried the gene. There is abnormal flexure and extension of all joints but especially the hock, stifle, hip, knee, elbow and shoulder joints. The muscles are much atrophied and the joints look very enlarged as a result. It is impossible for the calves to stand but they are bright, alert and eat well. The limbs are so flexible that they can be bent into extraordinary positions, and almost tied in knots. A drawer sign, a displacement of the articular surfaces laterally produced by manual pressure, can be elicited easily and with a displacement of up to 2 cm. There are no detectable lesions in the nervous or musculoskeletal systems. Although the disease is known to be inherited as a simple autosomal recessive, it has also been seen in circumstances which preclude inheritance being the cause.

REFERENCE

(1) Lamb, R. C. et al. (1976) *J. Hered.*, *67*, 241.

Bovine osteogenesis imperfecta

This disease is recorded as being inherited in Holstein-Friesian cattle (1). It is transmitted as an autosomal dominant trait. Calves are clinically abnormal at birth with the main presenting signs being bright pink teeth and slackness of the flexor tendons on all four feet. The calves become progressively worse to the point where they cannot walk. The full list of abnormalities in this syndrome includes smaller than normal body size at birth and a dome-shaped cranial vault, and fragility of bones, manifested by multiple fractures occurring during birth. The defect is one of connective tissue cells so that there is a faulty production of collagen and intercellular cement. Radiological examination demonstrates growth-arrest lines and multiple fractures in the long bones, and thin dentine and enamel layers on the teeth which are pink because of the exposed condition of the enlarged pulp. The excessive mobility of the joints results from the small bulk of the ligaments and tendons. A syndrome of simple bone fragility occurs in Charolais cattle and is called osteogenesis imperfecta (2).

REFERENCES

(1) Denholm, L. J. & Cole, W. G. (1983) *Aust. vet. J.*, *60*, 9.
(2) Jensen, P. J. et al. (1976) *Nord. VetMed.*, *28*, 304.
(3) Straube, E. et al. (1978) *Vict. vet. Proc.*, *36*, 50.

Ovine osteogenesis imperfecta

Affected lambs are of normal size at birth but, although bright and alert, are unable to stand. The main feature of the condition is bone fragility with multiple fractures particularly of the limbs and ribs. The bones are of normal length and thickness and, in contrast to a similar disease in cats, the thyroid appears normal. The essential change appears to be a defect in the formation of bone matrix. Affected lambs may show a temporary response to calcium therapy. A genetic etiology appears certain although the mode of inheritance is not clear (1). A similar hereditary disease is recorded in Charolais cattle (2).

REFERENCES

(1) Holmes, J. R. et al. (1964) *Vet. Rec.*, *76*, 980.
(2) Jensen, P. T. et al. (1976) *Nord. VetMed.*, *28*, 304.

Multiple defects of limbs

'Mole' calves of the Danish Black and White breed are characterized by shortened and malformed limbs especially the extremities which are sometimes missing altogether (1). There is also hydrocephalus, hypoplasia of the mandible and absence of part of the face. The body is edematous. Many are aborted during the latter part of pregnancy. The condition is conditioned by a single recessive gene.

REFERENCE

(1) Hansen, K. M. (1974) *Hereditas*, *78*, 315.

Inherited reduced phalanges

This defect has been recorded in cattle and appears to be inherited as a single recessive character. The limbs are normal down to the metacarpal and metatarsal bones, which are shorter than usual, but the first two phalanges are missing and the normal hooves and third phalanges are connected to the rest of the limb by soft tissues only. The calves are unable to stand but can crawl about on their knees and hocks.

Bilateral absence of the patella, and shortening or

absence of the tibia, accompanied by hydrocephalus, meningoceles, ventral abdominal hernia, and cryptorchidism comprise the syndrome known as *tibial hemimelia*. It is inherited in the Galloway breed of cattle (1). An autosomal recessive mode of inheritance is assumed (7). A concerted program of eradicating the defect has been undertaken (6), based on test-matings and examination for defects of 90-day fetuses obtained by terminating pregnancy with prostaglandin.

An even more serious defect, in which the mandible and all the bones below the humerus and stifle were vestigial or absent has been reported in British (2), French (3) and German (4) Friesians. It appears to be conditioned by the inheritance of a single recessive gene. Similar 'amputates' have been shown not to be inherited (5).

REFERENCES

(1) Ojo, S. A. et al. (1974) *J. Am. vet. med. Assoc.*, *165*, 548.
(2) Bishop, M. W. H. & Cembrowicz, H. J. (1964) *Vet. Rec.*, *76*, 1049.
(3) Lauvergne, J. J. & Cu, Q. P. (1963) *Ann. Zootechnol.*, *12*, 181.
(4) Rieck, G. W. & Bähr, H (1967) *Tierärztl. Wochenschr.*, *74*, 356.
(5) Harbutt, P. R. et al. (1965) *Aust. vet. J.*, *41*, 173.
(6) Pollock, D. L. et al. (1979) *Vet. Rec.*, *104*, 258.
(7) Leipold, H. W. et al. (1978) *Zeitschr. Tierzucht. Zuchtungsbiol.*, *94*, 291.

Inherited defects of claws

Extra claws (polydactylism) (4) and fusion of the claws (syndactylism) are known hereditary defects of cattle, the former in the Normandy breed (2) and the latter in Holsteins (3), Angus, Hereford and Chianina (4). Dactylomegaly (enlarged dew claws), often associated with syndactyly or deviation of the adjacent major digit and creating a clubfooted appearance, may be inherited in Shorthorn cattle (1). In most cases they cause no more than inconvenience but an association of syndactyly with susceptibility to hyperthermia is recorded (5). Some animals subjected to high environmental temperatures die of hyperthermia.

There is good field evidence that *corkscrew claw* or *curled toe* is an inherited defect in cattle (6), especially in beef breeds, but also in Holstein-Friesians (7). It is almost always the lateral claw which is affected, and in some breeds is more common in the hindfeet, in others it is more common in the front feet. In the affected digit the third phalanx is much smaller than normal and is narrower and longer. The soft tissue and the horn are correspondingly deformed so that the horn grows much longer and narrower and tends to curl over the sole so that the cow walks on the wall of the hoof. The claw also curls over the front of the other digit of the limb. There are often cracks in the front of the claw, originating at the coronet and causing serious lameness. All affected animals suffer gait abnormalities as they get older and heavier. Much of this is due to distortion and wear of the articular surfaces in the companion claw which has to carry much more weight than is usual. Marked changes in the affected digit are detectable by anteroposterior radiography (8).

REFERENCES

(1) Hawkins, C. D. & Grandage, J. (1983) *Aust. vet. J.*, *60*, 55.
(2) Lauvergne, J. J. (1962) *Ann. Zootechnol.*, *11*, 151.
(3) Hart-Elcock, L. et al. (1987) *Vet. Pathol.*, *24*, 140.
(4) Ojo, S. A. et al. (1975) *J. Am. vet. med. Assoc.*, *166*, 607.
(5) Leipold, H. W. et al. (1974) *J. dairy Sci.*, *57*, 1401.
(6) McCormack, J. (1977) *Auburn Vet.*, *34*, 24.
(7) Glicken, A. & Kendrick, J. W. (1977) *J. Hered.*, *68*, 386.
(8) Edwards, G. B. (1987) *Vet. Ann.*, *27*, 81.

Inherited multiple exostosis

Multiple exostosis affecting both cortical and medullary bone of the limbs and ribs has been described in Quarterhorses and Thoroughbreds in the United States. The lesions are visible externally but cause little apparent inconvenience (1, 2). It is inherited as a single dominant autosomal gene (3).

REFERENCES

(1) Morgan, J. P. et al. (1962) *J. Am. vet. med. Assoc.*, *140*, 1320.
(2) Shupe, J. L. (1970) *Mod. vet. Pract.*, *51*, 34.
(3) Gardner, E. J. et al. (1975) *J. Hered.*, *66*, 318.

Inherited thick forelegs of pigs (inherited congenital hyperostosis)

This defect is thought to be caused by the inheritance of a simple recessive character (1). Affected piglets show obvious lesions at birth and although many of them die or are destroyed immediately a proportion of them may survive. The forelegs are markedly enlarged below the elbows and the skin is tense and may be discolored. There is difficulty in standing and moving about and starvation and crushing contribute to the mortality rate. There is extensive edema of the subcutaneous tissues, thickening of the bones and roughness of the periosteum (2). It is thought that the primary lesion is a separation of the periosteum from the bone (3).

REFERENCES

(1) Kaye, M. M. (1962) *Can. J. comp. Med.*, *26*, 218.
(2) Gibson, J. A. & Rogers, R. J. (1980) *Aust. vet. J.*, *56*, 254.
(3) Doizé, B. & Martineau, G. P. (1984) *Can. J. comp. Med.*, *48*, 414.

Inherited rickets in pigs

The disease is indistinguishable from rickets due to nutritional inadequacy. The pigs are healthy at birth. Subsequently there is hypocalcemia, hyperphosphatemia and increased serum alkaline phosphatase. The defect is failure of active transport of calcium through the wall of the small intestine (1).

REFERENCE

(1) Plonait, H. (1969) *Zentralbl. VetMed.*, *16A*, 271, 289.

Inherited dwarfism

Most inherited food animal dwarfs are chondrodysplastic; they occur commonly only in cattle and are of two kinds, snorter dwarfs and Dexter bulldog calves.

Snorter dwarfs

These are short-legged with short, wide heads and protruding lower jaws. The mandibular teeth may protrude 2–4 cm beyond the dental pad, preventing effective grazing and necessitating handfeeding if the animal is to survive. There is protrusion of the forehead and distortion of the maxillae, and obstruction of the respiratory passages results in stertorous respiration and dyspnea. The tip of the tongue usually protrudes from the mouth and the eyes bulge. There is some variation between affected animals in their appearance at birth. In most cases the defects are as described above but they become more exaggerated as the calf grows. In addition abdominal enlargement and persistent bloat develop. The head is disproportionately large. The calves fail to grow normally and are about half the weight of normal calves of the same age.

The predominant form of the condition appears to be inherited as a simple recessive character although the relationship of the 'comprest' types to the total syndrome is more complex (1). Heterozygotes vary widely in conformation but some of them show minor defects which may be attractive to cattle breeders who are seeking a chunkier, short-legged type of animal. For this reason, unconscious selection towards the heterozygote has undoubtedly occurred, resulting in widespread dissemination of the character. Herefords and Aberdeen Angus are the breeds most commonly affected but similar dwarfs occur also in Holstein and Shorthorn cattle, and typical dwarf animals have been produced by mating heterozygous Aberdeen Angus and Herefords. A similar inherited defect occurs in Danish Landrace pigs (3). Besides the shortness of limbs there is also a looseness of attachment of limbs and abnormal mobility of joints.

The detection of the heterozygous carrier animals is of first importance and many tests have been proposed to effect this differentiation. Careful examination of the head using a special 'profilometer' has been widely used. Radiographic examination of the lumbar vertebrae during the first 10 days of life may reveal compression of the vertebrae, disappearance of the concavity in the ventral surface of the vertebral body and bending forward of the lumbar transverse processes in affected animals (2). It is claimed that carrier, heterozygous animals have these defects in less, but recognizable, degree. Premature closure of the spheno-occipital synchondrosis is characteristic of dwarfism. Closure is reported to occur at 5½ months compared to 24–36 months in normals and can be detected by radiographic examination (3). Other characteristics of dwarf calves which are detectable by radiographic examination are the presence of two intracranial projections and shortening of the shafts of the long bones of the limbs (4).

Physiological tests have also been used. Because of a possible relationship between the disease and hypothyroidism, tests of thyroid function have been carried out and dwarf calves may have significantly lower plasma cholesterol levels than normal calves. Tests of pituitary and adrenal cortical function have also been studied. It is reported that after an injection of insulin the blood sugar level falls to a greater degree and returns to normal more slowly in dwarf animals and that there is a much smaller leukocytic response. Heterozygotes react in an intermediate manner but the variation in degree of abnormality in this group makes the test impractical as a means of selecting them. Serum protein, calcium, phosphorus and magnesium levels are within the normal limits in affected calves. 'Snorter' dwarf calves have been shown to excrete glycosaminoglycans at levels 30 times greater than those in the urine of normal calves, suggesting an enzymatic error of metabolism similar to the mucopolysaccharidoses of humans (5). However, this biochemical peculiarity is not necessarily common to all achondroplastic dwarfs. There is a significant difference between the cerebrospinal fluid pressure in normal and dwarf animals, but the estimation of cerebrospinal fluid pressure is not a feasible method of differentiating between carrier and non-carrier animals. There is no conclusive evidence of association between dwarfism and chromosomal abnormalities (6) but there is one record of dwarfism associated with a chromosomal defect (7). Affected calves also showed marked involution of the pituitary gland.

The margin of error in all indirect tests is too great for general acceptance and the testing of animals with unknown genetic constitution by mating them with known carriers is still the most efficient method of detecting dwarf genes. This has the obvious disadvantage of requiring the maintenance of a carrier herd but is thought to be worthwhile by some breeders of valuable cattle.

Whether or not a fetus is affected by inherited dwarfism can be determined at the 125th day of pregnancy. Multiple ovulations, artificial insemination and early cesareans make it possible to progeny-test a suspect bull very quickly (10).

Inherited congenital achondroplasia with hydrocephalus (bulldog calves)

First recorded in Dexter cattle this inherited defect has since been observed in a variety of forms in other breeds, including Jerseys, Guernseys and Holsteins. Affected calves are often aborted but some reach full term and cause fetal dystocia because of the extreme hydrocephalus (12). The forehead bulges tremendously over a foreshortened face with a depressed, short nose. The tongue protrudes, the palate is cleft or absent, the neck is short and thick and the limbs are shortened. Accompanying defects are fetal anasarca and hydrops amnii in the dam (13). An apparently identical syndrome has been recorded in fallow deer in the United Kingdom (15).

The defect is primarily a chondrodystrophy rather than an achondroplasia and the nasal bones and maxillae do not grow. Hydrocephalus develops because of the deformed cranium. In most breeds the condition is inherited as a simple recessive character but a dominant form has occurred in Jerseys (14). The heterozygous form in Dexters is easily recognized by the shortness of the limbs. The heterozygote in other breeds is normal in appearance.

Miscellaneous dwarfs

Other types of dwarfs have been described (3) and include 'comprest' and 'compact' cattle in Herefords and Shorthorns and various other forms of proportionate dwarfs. For example, in Charolais, miniature calves which are exact replicas of normal calves, but which weigh only 5–16 kg at birth and which are born 2 or more weeks prematurely, have been recorded (9). Most are dead at birth or die soon after so that the condition is effectively lethal. Proportional dwarfs occur also in Simmentals (11).

Other forms of chondrodystrophy, including 'bulldog calves' and one which causes fatal nasal obstruction in the German Black Spotted breed of cattle have also been recorded. In the latter there are multiple deformities of limb bones and the condition appears to be inherited due to the influence of a single recessive gene (5).

Dwarf lambs occur sporadically. The best known is the mutant Ancon which has appeared and disappeared three times, with one incidence in New Zealand and one in the United Kingdom (8). The defect is chondrodysplasia and the lambs are not viable.

REFERENCES

(1) Gregory, P. W. et al. (1964) *Growth*, *28*, 191.
(2) Emmerson, M. A. & Hazel, L. N. (1956) *J. Am. vet. med. Assoc.*, *128*, 381.
(3) Jensen, P. T. et al. (1984) *Nord. VetMed.*, *36*, 32.
(4) Tyler, W. S. et al. (1961) *Am. J. vet. Res.*, *22*, 693.
(5) Hurst, R. E. et al. (1975) *J. comp. Pathol.*, *85*, 481.
(6) Weaver, A. D. (1975) *Vet. Ann.*, *15*, 7.
(7) Gluhovischi, N. et al. (1972) *Vet. Med. Rev.*, *2*, 107.
(8) Duffell, S. J. et al. (1985) *Vet. Rec.*, *117*, 571.
(9) Gregory, K. E. & Spahr, S. L. (1979) *J. Hered.*, *70*, 217.
(10) Jones, J. & Jolly, R. D. (1982) *NZ vet. J.*, *30*, 185.
(11) Pirchner, F. & Kaiser, E. (1986) *Wein. Tierärztl. Monatsschr.*, *73*, 173.
(12) Jones, W. A. (1961) *Vet. Rec.*, *73*, 937.
(13) Weaver, A. D. (1975) *Vet. Ann.*, *15*, 7.
(14) Innes, J. R. M. & Saunders, L. Z. (1957) *Adv. vet. Sci.*, *3*, 35.
(15) Baker, J. R. et al. (1979) *Vet. Rec.*, *104*, 450.

Inherited displaced molar teeth

Inherited as a simple recessive character this defect usually results in the death of affected calves within the first week of life. The six premolars of the lower jaw are impacted or erupted in abnormal positions, often at grotesque angles. The mandible is shorter and narrower than normal. There is no abnormality of the incisors or upper jaw (1).

REFERENCE

(1) Heizer, E. E. & Hervey, M. C. (1937) *J. Hered.*, *28*, 123.

Inherited progressive muscular dystrophy

This is a primary skeletal muscle disease with a strong probability of having a genetic mode of transmission (1). It is recorded in Merino flocks in Australia and is characterized by a gradually progressive failure to flex the joints of the hindlimbs commencing at 3–4 weeks of age. Eventually the limbs are rigid at all times and running becomes an impossibility. The forelimbs and the head and neck are normal. Affected sheep are easily detected when they are 1 year old and will have mobility problems by the time they are 2–3 years old. At necropsy there are pale areas in skeletal muscle, and sometimes the muscles of the diaphragm in sheep which have a tendency to bloat.

REFERENCE

(1) Richards, R. B. et al. (1986) *Aust. vet. J.*, *63*, 396.

Inherited mandibular prognathism

Defective apposition of upper and lower incisors, or lower incisors and dental pad in ruminants, may result in inefficient grazing and malnutrition. This is of most importance in ruminants and there is good evidence that abnormal length of the mandible is inherited. Among British breeds the defect is more common in beef than in dairy breeds. In Herefords (2) and Angus (1) the inheritance is thought to be conditioned by a single recessive gene. Underdevelopment of the mandible has also been recorded in Dairy Shorthorn, Jersey, Holstein, Ayrshire and Simmental (5) cattle, with the defect so severe in some cases that the animals are unable to suck (3). Inheritance of the defect is probably conditioned by a recessive gene, although one study in Jerseys suggests that the defect can occur without being conditioned by inheritance (4). A less severe degree of mandibular underdevelopment has been recorded in Merino and Rambouillet sheep and designated as brachygnathia. The mode of inheritance is suggested to be by the interaction of several pairs of genes. Mandibular prognathism occurs as a part of other more general defects including achondroplastic dwarfism and inherited displaced molar teeth.

REFERENCES

(1) Heidari, M. et al. (1985) *Am. J. vet. Res.*, *46*, 708.
(2) Gregory, K. E. et al. (1962) *J. Hered.*, *53*, 168.
(3) Grant, H. T. (1956) *J. Hered.*, *47*, 165.
(4) Moller, K. & James, J. P. (1975) *NZ vet. J.*, *23*, 175.
(5) Stur, I. et al. (1978) *Wien. Tierärztl. Monatsschr.*, *65*, 200.

Inherited agnathia

Partial or complete absence of the mandibles with ventral displacement of the ears is common in sheep and is categorized as a lethal recessive because the sheep may not safely graze (1).

REFERENCE

(1) Dennis S. M. & Leipold, H. W. (1979) *Vet. Bull.*, *49*, 708.

Inherited craniofacial deformity

The defect is incompatible with life. It is reported in Border Leicester lambs and is characterized by a variable degree of nasomaxillary hypoplasia often associated with incomplete cerebral development with less pronounced sulci and gyri than normal (1). It appears to be inherited in a simple autosomal recessive mode. A similar lethal defect is recorded in Angus cattle (as brachygnathica superior) in association with generalized degenerative joint disease (2).

REFERENCES

(1) Morrow, C. J. & Roth I. J. (1985) *Aust. Adv. vet. Sci.*, p. 124.
(2) Jayo, M. et al. (1987) *Vet. Pathol.*, *24*, 148.

Congenital osteopetrosis

This inherited defect is recorded in Aberdeen Angus calves which are stillborn and undersized. The major manifestations are shortening of the mandible with protrusion of the tongue, impaction of the lower molars, a patent fontanelle, and the characteristic lesion of shortness of the long bones and absence of a marrow cavity in them (1–3). The absence of the marrow cavity, caused by defective remodeling of the bone, gives it a homogeneous shaft leading to the colloquial name of 'marble bone'. Radiographic examination makes antemortem diagnosis simple. It is considered to be an autosomal recessive trait (5). It is reported also in foals but there is doubt about its genetic origin in that species (4).

REFERENCES

(1) Leipold, H. W. et al. (1986) *Bov. Practnr*, *21*, 96.
(2) Greene, H. J. (1974) *J. Am. vet. med. Assoc.*, *164*, 389.
(3) Ojo, S. A. et al. (1975) *J. Am. vet. med. Assoc.*, *166*, 781.
(4) Nation, P. N. & Clavono, C. G. (1986) *Can. vet. J.*, *27*, 74.
(5) Young, U. M. et al. (1985) *Fed. Proc.*, *44*, 475.

Inherited probatocephaly (sheepshead)

This defect is inherited in Limousin cattle (1). The cranial bones are deformed so that the head resembles that of a sheep. The accompanying defects in heart, buccal cavity, tongue and abomasum increase the chances of an early death.

REFERENCE

(1) Blin, P. C. & Lauvergne, J. J. (1967) *Ann. Zootechnol.*, *16*, 65.

Inherited umbilical and scrotal hernias, cryptorchidism and hermaphroditism

Umbilical hernias in cattle and scrotal hernias and cryptorchidism in pigs have been considered to be inherited defects for many years. Umbilical hernias of Holstein cattle has been shown to occur because of the influence of either one or more pairs of autosomal recessive factors of rather low frequency (1). It is unlikely that the responsible genes are sex-linked, in spite of the apparent greater incidence in females. Umbilical hernias in Holstein-Friesian cattle can also be conditioned by a dominant character with incomplete penetrance, or be due to environmental factors (2). Scrotal hernias of pigs have also been shown to be inherited and evidence suggesting the inheritance of cryptorchidism in swine, sheep (6), horses and Hereford cattle (3) and hermaphroditism in swine (4) has also been presented. Cryptorchidism in horses appears to be inherited with a polygenic pattern of transmission (7). Hernias of various types are seen in lambs but their etiology is uncertain (5).

REFERENCES

(1) Gilman, J. P. W. & Stringham, E. W. (1953) *J. Hered.*, *44*, 113.
(2) Angus, K. & Young, G. B. (1972) *Vet. Rec.*, *90*, 245.
(3) Wheat, J. D. (1961) *J. Hered.*, *52*, 244.
(4) Pond, W. G. et al. (1961) *Cornell Vet.*, *51*, 394.
(5) Dennis, S. M. & Leipold, H. W. (1968) *J. Am. vet. med. Assoc.*, *152*, 999.
(6) Claxton, J. H. & Yeates, N. T. M. (1972) *J. Hered.*, *63*, 141.
(7) Leipold, H. W. et al. (1985) *Proc. 31st ann. Mtg AAEP*, 579.

Inherited taillessness and tail deformity

Complete absence of the tail or deformity of the appendage occur relatively commonly as a congenital defect and is thought to be inherited in Holstein cattle and in Landrace and Large White pigs. It is often seen in combination with other deformities of the hindquarters such as atresia ani and urogenital tract abnormalities (1).

REFERENCE

(1) Greene, H. J. et al. (1973) *Giessener Beitr. Erbpathol. Zuchthyg.*, 5, 158.

Myofiber hyperplasia (double muscling, doppellender, culard)

This is an inherited condition, characterized by an increased bulk of skeletal muscles due to the presence of a greater than normal number of muscle fibers, and is well known in many breeds of cattle but appears to be most common in the Charolais, Belgian blue, Piedmont and South Devon breeds (1). The condition is recorded only rarely in sheep (2) and not at all in pigs. Pietrain pigs exhibit many of the characteristics of double-muscled cattle, including large muscle mass and susceptibility to stress. Severely affected animals show a marked increase in muscle mass most readily observed in the hindquarters, loin and shoulder, an increase in the muscle/bone ratio and a decrease in body fat (3). Since these changes are in the direction of the current demand for lean, meaty carcasses, there is interest, especially in Europe, in the exploitation of this anomaly for meat production (4).

Affected calves demonstrate above-average weight gains during the first year of life if well fed and managed, although mature size is somewhat reduced. Well-marked grooves along the intramuscular septa in the hindquarters are a distinguishing feature as is an apparent forward positioning of the tail head. The skin tends to be thinner than normal. These features vary widely in their expression. The muscle mass appears to be normal, and to be characterized by a disproportionate number of glycolytic, anaerobic fibers (5).

The condition often gives rise to dystocia, possibly due to increased gestation length, and affected females are said to be less fertile than normal. Macroglossia, prognathism and a tendency toward muscular dystrophy and rickets have been observed in affected calves. Blood lactate is increased as is susceptibility to stress (6). These findings are interpreted as indicators of cell membrane fragility which is also manifested by fragility of the erythrocytes (8). There is also a very high incidence of Elso-heel in affected cattle and this interferes greatly with their economic value. Other associated defects are brachygnathia, deviation of the incisor arch and hypertrophy of the tongue (7). The mode of inheritance has not been established but heterozygotes usually show some degree of hypertrophy.

REVIEW LITERATURE

Bradley, R. (1978) Double muscling of cattle. *Vet. Ann.*, *18*, 51.

REFERENCES

(1) Swatland, H. J. (1974) *Vet. Bull.*, *44*, 179.
(2) Dennis, S. M. (1972) *Cornell Vet.*, *62*, 263.
(3) Butterfield, R. M. (1966) *Aust. vet. J.*, *42*, 37.
(4) Lauvergne, J. J. et al. (1963) *Ann. Zootechnol.*, *12*, 133.
(5) Ashmore, C. R. (1974) *Growth*, *38*, 501.
(6) Holmes, J. H. G. et al. (1972) *J. anim Sci.*, *35*, 1011.
(7) Hanset, R. & Michaux, C. (1978) *Ann. MedVet.*, *122*, 649.
(8) King, A. W. & Basrur, P. K. (1979) *Acta vet. Scand.*, *20*, 245.

Pietrain creeper pigs

A progressive muscular weakness found in stress-susceptible Pietrain pigs (1). The syndrome commences with muscle tremor at 2–4 weeks of age leading to complete recumbency by 12 weeks of age. At this stage the pigs move with a creeping gait with the limbs flexed. There are no neuropathological lesions but there are myopathic changes especially in the forelimbs.

REFERENCE

(1) Bradley, R. & Wells, G. A. H. (1980) In: *Animal Models of Neurological Disease*, (eds) Rose, F. C. & Behan, P. O. London: Pitman Medical Ltd, pp. 36–44.

Quarterhorse episodic tremor

The disease occurs in certain families of the Quarterhorse breed and is characterized by brief (10–15 minute) episodes of generalized muscle tremor and stiffness. Between attacks the horse may be normal or have a continuous localized tremor, e.g., in the flank. The tremor episodes are unrelated to exercise but are marked by a significant elevation of serum potassium, increased myotonic discharge as measured by an EMG and a response to treatment with hydrochlorothiazide (1).

REFERENCE

(1) Steiss, J. E. & Naylor, J. M. (1986) *Can. vet. J.*, *27*, 332.

Porcine stress syndrome (PSS)

Three closely related stress syndromes occur in pigs. The *porcine stress syndrome* is characterized by acute death induced by stressors such as transport, high ambient temperature, exercise and fighting, which results in progressive dyspnea, hyperthermia, disseminate vasoconstriction and the rapid onset of rigor mortis. *Pale, soft and exudative pork* (PSE) occurs post mortem in some pigs slaughtered by conventional methods. *Malignant hyperthermia* (MH) is a drug-induced stress syndrome characterized by muscle rigidity and hyperthermia occurring in susceptible pigs following the use of halothane or the muscle-relaxant suxamethonium (1–3). *Back muscle necrosis* of pigs is a special manifestation of the porcine stress syndrome (4).

Etiology

There is considerable evidence that susceptibility to the syndrome complex is inherited as a single recessive gene with a high penetrance (6–8). The recessive gene is now commonly known as the *halothane gene* because pigs with the homozygous genotype can be identified with the halothane test which results in malignant hyperthermia (5). The halothane gene is located within a group of blood type genes on the same chromosome which allows identification of affected pigs by blood typing (8–10).

Stress-susceptible pigs have a biochemical lesion which precipitates the rapid onset of anaerobic glycolysis and loss of control of skeletal muscle metabolism in response to stress and anoxia.

Epidemiology

The porcine stress syndrome occurs worldwide, but there is considerable breed and area variation in its prevalence. In some European countries this syndrome has increased in prevalence over recent years to the point where it is now a major problem in pig production. This has resulted from the inadvertent selection for this syndrome in genetic improvement programs and it underlies the problems of selection based purely on performance and production characteristics.

The syndrome probably occurs in all breeds of pigs, but it has high incidence in pigs selected for heavy muscling and stress-susceptible pigs are leaner and more meaty (5). It is especially prevalent in the Pietrain and Poland China breeds and also in some European strains of Landrace where a score for muscling as well as growth rate, food conversion and back fat has been included in the selection index.

Susceptibility to the syndrome is inherited and the biochemical events leading to PSE, transport death or malignant hyperthermia may be triggered by several external influences or stressors in the living animal. The most important precipitating factors are transportation at high environmental temperatures and humidity, exhaustive exercise, and under experimental conditions, the more specific reaction towards the anesthetic halothane (10). Experimentally, psychological mechanisms can precipitate the PSS (11). The effects of mixing, transportation and duration of lairage can have profound effects on carcass characteristics of susceptible pigs (12). Death during transportation and PSE are associated with fear, defensive or aggressive reactions in unfamiliar social environments or conflict with other strange pigs or man.

The prevalence of the syndrome in the swine population can be determined by the use of screening tests applied on the farm or when pigs enter swine performance test stations. The halothane test and the creatine-kinase (C-K) test are useful for this purpose (15). Surveys in the United Kingdom indicate that the prevalence in the British Landrace varies from 0 to 23% of herds with an average of 11% (13). In general, in the

United Kingdom, there is no indication for the introduction of tests to identify affected animals (16). In European breeds the prevalence varies from 0 to 88% with up to 100% in the Pietrain breed (13). None is present in the Large White breed although one isolated report describes malignant hyperthermia in a single Large White pig (3). The prevalence of halothane susceptibility is low in the Danish Landrace breed in Denmark (14). Based on the halothane test, 1·5% of young boars entering a Record of Performance Test Station in Canada were positive reactors (41). The reactors originated from 7·5% of 107 herds. The halothane-succinylcholine test was a more sensitive test because 18% of the same pigs were identified as reactors. There is a correlation between halothane susceptibility and carcass traits. Halothane-positive animals usually score higher for visual conformation of the loin and ham than pigs which are halothane-negative (17). The progeny of reactor boars are also more susceptible than the progeny of non-reactors (17). The major limitation of the halothane test is that it identifies only those pigs which are stress-susceptible to the syndrome. The test does not detect the heterozygote.

The economic losses associated with the syndrome are due to mortality from transport death, and inferior meat quality due to pale, soft, exudative pork. PSE carcasses yield less bacon and the drip loss from fresh PSE meat is more than doubled compared to normal carcasses (42).

Landrace pigs can be divided into those which are sensitive to halothane and develop pale, soft, exudative pork *post mortem*, those which are resistant to halothane but develop pale, soft, exudative pork, and those resistant to halothane and pale, soft, exudative pork (the normal pig) (18, 19). Muscle from pigs susceptible to malignant hyperthermia and pale, soft, exudative pork has significantly higher glucose-6-phosphate levels and lower phosphocreatine under thiopentone anesthesia than muscle from pigs susceptible to PSE and normal pigs (19). Altered muscle fiber type is not the primary basis of the disease complex (43).

Pathogenesis

Stress-susceptible pigs cannot tolerate stress and lose control of skeletal muscle metabolism. The stress may be from external influences such as transportation, fear and excitement or halothane anesthesia. The biochemical defect is considered to be in intracellular calcium homeostasis. There is excessive catecholamine release and the sudden onset of anaerobic glycolysis of skeletal muscle, excessive production of lactate and excessive heat production which, in conjunction with peripheral vasoconstriction, leads to hyperthermia. Following exertional or thermal stress, susceptible pigs undergo more extensive physiological change than do resistant pigs (44).

Depending upon the nature, severity and duration of the stress, the syndrome may manifest in different ways. The porcine stress syndrome causes rapid death following severe stress, the pale, soft and exudative pork is seen after slaughter which may have been preceded by mild stressors during lairage, and the malignant hyperthermia is drug-induced.

Malignant hyperthermia is the drug-induced often fatal stress syndrome which occurs in susceptible pigs within 3 minutes following the inhalation of a mixture of halothane and oxygen (5). Susceptible pigs develop limb rigidity and a hyperthermia which are not easily reversed and may result in death. The current hypothesis for the pathogenesis is an increased rate of intracellular ATP hydrolysis leading to a progressive failure of ATP dependent Ca^{2+} accumulation by sarcoplasmic reticulum and/or the mitochondria with a rise in myoplasmic concentration of Ca^{2+} and consequent contraction of muscle (23). The mitochondria from predominantly red muscle fibers have a greater calcium-binding capacity than those from predominantly white muscle fiber areas (45). There is extreme rigidity of skeletal muscles, hyperthermia, tachycardia, cardiac arrhythmia, an increase in oxygen consumption, lactate formation and high-energy phosphate hydrolysis in muscle, respiratory and metabolic acidosis and a rise in the creatine-kinase activity and concentration of potassium, lactate, glucose, free fatty acids and catecholamines in blood. There is a large release of glucose and potassium from the liver which contributes to the hyperglycemia and hyperkalemia (21). There is a marked alpha-adrenergic stimulation which is responsible for the heat production in malignant hyperthermia susceptible pigs (22). The lactic acidemia is severe due to the overproduction of lactate peripherally and failure of normal lactate uptake. The syndrome can also be induced using methoxyflurane, isoflurane and enflurane (20). There are no histochemical differences between muscles of susceptible and normal swine (24).

Clinical findings

Porcine stress syndrome (transport death)

Death during or following transport to market may also be significant and is more prevalent when overcrowding occurs and during the hot summer period. If seen alive, affected pigs initially show a rapid tremor of the tail, general stiffness associated with increased muscular rigidity, and dyspnea to the extent of mouthbreathing. The body temperature becomes markedly elevated, often beyond the limits of the clinical thermometer, and there are irregularly shaped areas of skin blanching and erythema. At this stage the affected pig is frequently attacked by other pigs within the group. The pig collapses and dies shortly afterwards and the total time course of the syndrome is generally of the order of 4–6 minutes.

Malignant hyperthermia

Malignant hyperthermia is also a manifestation of the porcine stress syndrome. It may be induced in stress-susceptible pigs by anesthesia with potent volatile anesthetics such as halothane or by the administration of succinylcholine. It is characterized by the development during anesthesia of increased muscle metabolism with muscular rigidity, lactic acidosis and a marked increase in basal metabolic rate, increased oxygen consumption, carbon dioxide production and severe hyperthermia and tachycardia, tachyarrhythmia and death (5). Once fully developed the syndrome is irreversible. The syndrome poses a hazard in swine anesthesia which can be averted by prior medication with dantrolene (27) and has received considerable study as a model for an analogous syndrome in man. It has also been used as a method for determining stress-susceptibility for genetic selection programs.

Pale, soft and exudative pork (PSE)
Stress-susceptible pigs frequently show inferior quality meat after slaughter with pale, soft, exudative characteristics. This is related to excessive postmortem glycolysis with lactic acid production and a rapid fall in muscle pH with depigmentation and reduced water binding as a consequence (10). In affected muscle, rigor mortis occurs rapidly after slaughter, but then decreases so that affected carcasses have been 'set' and postmortem drip is excessive. Affected pork has a pH of less than 6 and generally a temperature of 41°C (104°F) or greater 45 minutes after slaughter, as opposed to the normal pH above 6 and temperature less than 40°C (106°F). Affected meat has inferior taste, cooking and processing qualities and does not accept curing as readily. The occurrence of this syndrome is considerably influenced by the stress of transport and handling prior to and during slaughter and this aspect of the syndrome is of major economic importance. The occurrence of dark firm meat in slaughter pigs subjected to prolonged transport with fasting may be a related condition.

Back muscle necrosis
Acute necrosis of the longissimus dorsi has been reported in German Landrace pigs and other breeds (4, 28). The acute syndrome lasts approximately 2 weeks and is characterized by swelling and pain over the back muscles with arching or lateral flexion of the spine and reluctance to move. Following this the swelling and pain subside, but there is atrophy of the affected muscle and development of a prominent spinal ridge. Some regeneration may occur after several months. Acute cases may die. The syndrome occurs in young adults weighing from 75 to 100 kg. The mild form may be undetectable except for pigs lying down near the feed trough. In the severe form, affected pigs may assume the dog-sitting position with a hunched-up back (28).

Clinical pathology
There are several testing methods which are available for predicting susceptibility and these have been reviewed (8, 10, 14–16).

Halothane test
The halothane test is highly reliable for the identification of pigs which are homozygous for the single recessive gene responsible for susceptibility to the PSS (5). However, the halothane test detects the worst clinical outcomes, does not identify the heterozygote and will not identify all the pigs which will develop PSE. Stress-susceptible pigs are sensitive to halothane at 8 weeks of age and if the anesthetic challenge is removed immediately after obvious signs of limb rigidity develop and before the development of fulminant hyperthermia, the mortality from the procedure is negligible. Pigs that remain unreactive for a challenge period of 5 minutes are considered normal. This test has been found to be of good predictive value for the occurrence of PSE. However, there may be breed variations as mentioned above.

Halothane concentration markedly affects the outcome of halothane testing and either higher halothane concentrations or longer exposure might be required to identify positive reactors in a heterogeneous population (46). The ionophore A23187, a lipophilic carboxylic antibiotic which binds and transports divalent cations across both natural and artificial membrane bilayers allows clear differentiation between the muscles of normal and pathological animals and may be a useful adjunct to the halothane test (48).

Blood creatine-kinase levels
The blood creatine-kinase (CK) levels are higher in stress-susceptible pigs and were originally considered to be useful for the identification of susceptible pigs (29). Pigs are subjected to a standard exertion test and blood samples are taken 8–24 hours later and analyzed for creatine kinase. The original work indicated a good correlation between the creatine-kinase levels and the halothane test (29). There is also an increase in the serum enzyme levels in pigs as they are transported from the farm to the abattoir (31). However, not all pigs which develop PSE have increased serum levels of creatine kinase (19). The initial test was modified so that blood could be collected as drops on a filter paper and sent to a laboratory for identification by a bioluminescent technique (40). A recent evaluation of a commercial creatine kinase screening test using the method of bioluminescence compared with the halothane challenge test on young boars entering a Record of Performance Test Station revealed that it was an inadequate indicator of susceptibility to the PSS or MH (30). In a different study the creatine-kinase levels of piglets 8–10 weeks of age predicted halothane-induced stress syndrome with an accuracy of 87–91% (47).

Blood-typing
Blood-typing is also used as a method for the identification of susceptible pigs (8, 10, 32). On one of the chromosomes of the pig, a region with four known loci has been identified. These loci contain the genes responsible for variants of the enzymes 6-phosphogluconate dehydrogenase and phosphoferose isomerase (PHI). The *H*-blood group system is determined by one of the loci and halothane sensitivity is also determined by genes at a locus in this region. This region is of special interest because a close connection has been found between this and important carcass traits such as the PSE condition. Thus, blood grouping may be used to detect halothane-sensitive pigs as well as heterozygote carriers (14).

Pale, soft and exudative pork
This is evaluated by a meat quality index which combines meat color, pH at 24 hours *post mortem* and water-binding capacity (14). Susceptible lines can be identified by carcass inspection and the results applied to sibling or progeny selection. A recent approach is the measurement of mitochondrial calcium efflux. Mitochondria isolated from longissimus dorsi muscle exhibit a rate of Ca^{2+} efflux twice that of normal pigs (38). Most of the

tests readily predict the worst examples of the syndrome, but are not sufficiently precise to be able to identify tendencies towards it, which restricts their value in breeding programs.

Erythrocyte osmotic fragility
Erythrocyte osmotic fragility may be correlated with malignant hyperthermia and is being examined as a possible aid in the determination of susceptibility to the defect (49).

Necropsy findings
In the porcine stress syndrome rigor mortis is present following death and carcass putrefaction occurs more rapidly than normal. On postmortem examination the viscera are congested and there is usually an increase in pericardial fluid and the presence of pulmonary congestion and edema. The muscles, especially the gluteus medius, biceps femoris and longissimus dorsi, are pale and putty-like in consistency. This may be evident following death, but is maximally developed within 2 hours (25). The lesions are similar to those seen in experimental restraint stress (26). Histologically, there is myocardial and skeletal muscle degeneration (33).

In back muscle necrosis the acute lesions are restricted to the multifidi and longissimus dorsi muscles which are pale, soft and exudative. Histologically, there are floccular and hyaline changes and transverse banding. In chronic cases there is phagocytosis, mineralization and regeneration of muscle cells together with fibrosis.

Diagnosis
The acute nature of the porcine stress syndrome and its relation to stress serve to differentiate it from most other syndromes producing death in pigs. Hypocalcemic tetany resulting from severe vitamin D deficiency can produce a similar clinical syndrome that is also initiated by excitement as may pyridoxine deficiency. Both are rare and restricted generally to home-mixed diets. Porcine viral encephalomyelitis may also result in a similar clinical syndrome in postweaned pigs. Pathological and biochemical examinations differentiate all three conditions from the porcine stress syndrome. Similarly, the myopathy associated with vitamin E/selenium deficiency has distinguishing pathological characteristics from this syndrome (26).

Treatment
Treatment of the acute syndromes is usually not undertaken. Several drugs are available for the protection of pigs against drug-induced malignant hyperthermia. A combination of acepromazine and droperidol will delay the onset or prevent the occurrence of halothane-induced malignant hyperthermia (35). Dantrolene is also effective for treatment and prevention (27, 36). The therapeutic dose recommended for swine is 7·5 mg/kg body weight (36). Carazolol is effective for the prevention of transport death when given 3–8 hours before transportation and improves meat quality compared to untreated susceptible animals (37, 50). Acute back necrosis has been treated successfully with isopyrin and phenylbutazone (28).

Control
The control of this syndrome relies on the reduction of the severity of stress imposed on pigs and genetic selection against the disease. Control through reduction of stress is not easily applied because frequently the syndrome is induced by routine minor procedures within the piggery. The incidence of transport deaths or the necessity for immediate slaughter salvage of severely stressed pigs on arrival at the abattoir and the occurrence of pale, soft, exudative meat characteristics are a significant economic problem in some countries and can be reduced by prior treatment of pigs with 40–80 mg of azaperone. The necessity to climb an upper deck in the transport has been found to pose a significant stress for the causation of these problems, and the use of single-deck transports or mechanical lifts for multiple deck transports, and the shipment of pigs in containers has resulted in a decreased incidence, as has the provision of spacious, well-ventilated transport vehicles and spray-cooling of pigs on arrival at the holding pens (39). Pigs should not be slaughtered directly after arrival at the abattoir but should be rested for at least 1–2 hours if they have been stressed only by transportation (51). In cases of severe physical exertion even more time should be allowed for recovery. Where possible transport distance should be kept to a minimum and transport should be avoided on excessively hot days.

The ultimate control of the syndrome will be achieved by genetic selection against it. The various testing methods described under clinical pathology are used to identify pigs with the halothane gene. The tests can be applied to breeding stock entering swine performance test stations or on a herd basis.

REVIEW LITERATURE

Aldrete, J. A. & Britt, B. A. (Eds) (1978) *Second International Symposium on Malignant Hyperthermia*. New York: Grune & Stratton.

Jorgensen, P. F. & Hyldgaard-Jensen, J. (1981) Blood parameters and meat quality. *Pigs News Info.*, *2*, 9–15.

Lucke, J. N. (1981) Halothane anaesthesia as a method of identifying stress-susceptible pigs. *Vet. Ann.*, *21*, 140–143.

Mitchell, G. & Heffron, J. J. A. (1982) Porcine stress syndrome. *Adv. food Res.*, *28*, 167–230.

McGloughlin, P. (1980) Genetic aspects of pig meat quality. *Pig News Info.*, *1*, 5–9.

McLoughlin, J. V. (1977) Malignant hyperthermia in the pig: etiology, therapy and implications. *Vet. Sci. Commun.*, *1*, 153–160.

Webb, A. J. (1981) Role of the halothane test in pig improvement. *Pig News Info.*, *2*, 17–23.

Wegger, I., Hyldgaard-Jensen, J. & Moustgaard, J. (Eds) (1979) *Proceedings of the Symposium on Muscle Function and Porcine Meat Quality. Acta Agric. scand.*, *Suppl. 21*, 516 pp.

REFERENCES

(1) Bergmann, V. (1979) *Mh VetMed.*, *34*, 21.
(2) McLoughlin, J. V. (1977) *Vet. Sci. Commun.*, *1*, 153.
(3) Meredith, M. J. & Williams, L. A. (1980) *Br. vet. J.*, *136*, 195.
(4) Bradley, R. et al. (1979) *Vet. Rec.*, *104*, 183.
(5) Webb, A. J. (1981) *Pig News Info.*, *2*, 17.
(6) Eikelenboom, G. et al. (1979) *Proc. 30th ann. Mtg European Assoc. anim. Prod., Harrogate*, Paper MP 2.3.
(7) Smith, C. & Bampton, P. (1977) *Genet. Res.*, *29*, 287.
(8) McGloughlin, P. (1980) *Pig News Info.*, *1*, 5.
(9) Andersen, E. (1979) *Nord. VetMed.*, *31*, 443.
(10) Jorgensen, P. F. & Hyldgaard-Jensen, J. (1981) *Pig News Info.*, *2*, 9.

(11) Johansson, G. & Jonsson, L. (1979) *Acta agric. Scand., Suppl. 21*, 322.
(12) Moss, B. W. (1980) *J. Sci. food Agric.*, *31*, 308.
(13) Webb, A. J. (1980) *Anim. Prod.*, *31*, 101.
(14) Jensen, P. & Andersen, E. (1980) *Livestock Prod. Sci.*, *7*, 325.
(15) Schworer, D. et al. (1980) *Livestock Prod. Sci.*, *7*, 337.
(16) Allen, W. M. et al. (1980) *Livestock Prod. Sci.*, *7*, 305.
(17) Eikelenboom, G. et al. (1980) *Livestock Prod. Sci.*, *7*, 283.
(18) Mitchell, G. & Heffron, J. J. A. (1980) *Br. vet. J.*, *136*, 500.
(19) Mitchell, G. & Heffron, J. J. A. (1981) *Br. vet. J.*, *137*, 374.
(20) McGrath, C. J. et al. (1981) *Am. J. vet. Res.*, *42*, 604.
(21) Hall, G. M. et al. (1980) *Br. J. Anaesth.*, *52*, 11.
(22) Hall, G. M. et al. (1977) *Br. J. Anaesth.*, *49*, 855.
(23) Ahern, C. P. et al. (1980) *J. comp. Pathol.*, *90*, 177.
(24) Gallant, E. M. (1980) *Am. J. vet. Res.*, *41*, 1069.
(25) Tapel, D. G. et al. (1968) *Mod. vet. Pract.*, *49*, 40.
(26) Johansson, G. & Jonsson, L. (1977) *J. comp. Pathol.*, *87*, 67.
(27) White, M. D. et al. (1983) *Biochem. J.*, *212*, 399.
(28) Erhard, G. & Elmar, G. (1979) *Tierärztl. Umschau*, *34*, 626.
(29) Thoren-Tolling, K. (1979) *Acta vet. Scand.*, *20*, 309.
(30) McDonell, W. N. et al. (1986) *Can. J. vet. Res.*, *50*, 494.
(31) Moss, B. W. & McMurray, C. H. (1979) *Res. vet. Sci.*, *26*, 1.
(32) Andersen, E. (1980) *Livestock Prod. Sci.*, *7*, 155.
(33) Johannsen, U. & Menger, S. (1980) *Arch. exp. VetMed.*, *34*, 797.
(34) Bickhardt, K. et al. (1977) *Vet. Sci. Commun.*, *1*, 225.
(35) McGrath, C. J. et al. (1981) *Am. J. vet. Res.*, *42*, 195.
(36) O'Brien, P. J. & Forsyth, G. W. (1983) *Can. vet. J.*, *24*, 200.
(37) Gregory, N. G. & Wilkins, L. J. (1982) *Vet. Res. Commun.*, *5*, 277.
(38) Cheah, K. S. & Cheah, A. M. (1979) *Experientia*, *35*, 1001.
(39) Allen, W. M. & Herbert, C. N. (1974) *Vet. Rec.*, *94*, 212.
(40) Addis, P. B. et al. (1976) *Proc. 4th Int. Congr. Pig Vet. Soc.*, 7.
(41) Seeler, D. C. et al. (1983) *Can. J. comp. Med.*, *47*, 284.
(42) Smith, W. C. & Lesser, D. (1982) *Anim. Prod.*, *34*, 291.
(43) Heffron, J. J. A. et al. (1982) *Br. vet. J.*, *138*, 45.
(44) D'Allaire, S. & DeRoth, L. (1986) *Can. J. vet. Res.*, *50*, 78.
(45) Somers, C. J. & McLoughlin, J. V. (1982) *J. comp. Pathol.*, *92*, 191.
(46) McGrath, C. J. et al. (1984) *Am. J. vet. Res.*, *45*, 1734.
(47) Mabry, J. W. et al. (1983) *J. Hered.*, *74*, 23.
(48) Reiss, G. et al. (1986) *Can. J. Physiol. Pharmacol.* *64*, 248.
(49) O'Brien, P. J. et al. (1985) *Am. J. vet. Res.*, *46*, 1451.
(50) Schmidt, W. & Worner, B. (1981) *Prakt. Tierärztl.*, *62*, 279.
(51) Kallweit, E. (1982) In: *Transport of Animal Intended for Breeding, Production and Slaughter*, (ed.) R. Moss. The Hague, Netherlands: Martinus Nijhoff, pp. 75–84.

INHERITED DEFECTS OF THE SKIN

Inherited symmetrical alopecia

This is an inherited skin defect of cattle in which animals born with a normal hair coat lose hair from areas distributed symmetrically over the body. It has been observed in Holstein cattle (1) as a rare disease but its appearance among valuable pure-bred cattle has economic importance. It appears to be inherited as a single autosomal recessive character.

Affected animals are born with a normal hair coat but progressive loss of hair commences at 6 weeks to 6 months of age. The alopecia is symmetrical and commences on the head, neck, back and hindquarters, and progresses to the root of the tail, down the legs and over the forelimbs. The affected skin areas become completely bald. Pigmented and unpigmented skin is equally affected; there is no irritation and the animals are normal in other respects. Failure of hair fibers to develop in apparently normal follicles can be detected by skin biopsy.

The disease is similar to congenital hypotrichosis which is, however, present at birth or very soon afterwards.

REFERENCE

(1) Holmes, J. R. & Young, G. B. (1954) *Vet. Rec.*, *66*, 704.

Inherited congenital hypotrichosis

In this congenital disease there is partial or complete absence of the hair coat with or without other defects of development. The disease is inherited in pigs and is associated with low birth weights, weakness and high mortality (1). It has also been reported in poll Dorset sheep (2). There are six known forms of congenital hypotrichosis in cattle (3). One form, recorded in North America in Guernsey cattle (4), is usually viable provided the calves are sheltered. They grow normally but are unable to withstand exposure to cold weather or hot sun. In most instances hair is completely absent from most of the body at birth but eyelashes and tactile hair are present about the feet and head. Occasionally hair may be present in varying amounts at birth but is lost soon afterwards. There is no defect of horn or hoof growth. The skin is normal but has a shiny, tanned appearance and on section no hair follicles are present in the skin. The condition is inherited as a single, recessive character. A similar form of hypotrichosis has been observed in Jersey cattle. A non-viable form of complete hypotrichosis occurs in British Friesian cattle (5). In this form there is an abnormally small and hypofunctional thyroid and the calves die shortly after birth. The third form of the disease is hypotrichosis with anodontia. The calves are born hairless and without teeth (3). Inheritance of the defect is conditioned by a sex-linked recessive gene.

In Holsteins a sex-linked semidominant gene causes development of a streaked hairlessness in which irregular narrow streaks of hypotrichosis occur. The defect is present only in females (6). A partial hypotrichosis has also been observed in Hereford cattle (7). At birth there is a fine coat of short, curly hair which later is added to by the appearance of some very coarse, wiry hair. The calves survive but do not grow well. The character is inherited as a simple recessive. A similar disease in Poll Herefords has the same short curly coat and a deficiency of hair in the switch, and over the poll, brisket, neck and legs in some cattle. Some have a much lighter hair coat color. Histologically there is a characteristic accumulation of large tricohyalin granules in the hair follicles (8). Hypotrichosis also occurs in adenohypophyseal hypoplasia in Guernseys and Jerseys.

REFERENCES

(1) Meyer, H. & Drommer, W. (1968) *Dtsch Tierärztl. Wochenschr.*, *75*, 13.
(2) Dolling, C. H. S. & Brooker, M. G. (1966) *J. Hered.*, *57*, 86.
(3) Hutt, F. B. (1963) *J. Hered.*, *54*, 186.

(4) Becker, R. B. (1963) *J. Hered.*, *54*, 3.
(5) Shand, A. & Young, G. B. (1964) *Vet. Rec.*, 76, 907.
(6) Eldridge, F. W. & Atkeson, F. W. (1953) *J. Hered.*, *44*, 265.
(7) Young, J. G. (1953) *Aust. vet. J.*, *29*, 298.
(8) Olson, T. A. et al. (1985) *Bov. Practnr*, *20*, 4.

Baldy calves

This is an inherited defect of calves characterized by alopecia, skin lesions, loss of bodily condition and failure of horns to grow.

The disease has so far been observed only in heifers of the Holstein breed. The calves are normal at birth but at 1–2 months of age begin to lose condition in spite of good appetites, and develop stiffness of the joints and abnormalities of the skin. These include patches of scaly, thickened and folded skin especially over the neck and shoulders, and hairless, scaly and often raw areas in the axillae and flanks and over the knees, hocks and elbow joints. There is usually alopecia about the base of the ears and eyes. The tips of the ears are curled medially. The horns fail to develop and there is persistent slobbering although there are no mouth lesions. Gross overgrowth of the hooves and stiffness of joints cause a shuffling, restricted gait. Severe emaciation leads to destruction at about 6 months of age. The similarity of this condition to inherited parakeratosis, described below, and to experimental zinc deficiency suggests an error in zinc metabolism. There is no record of this having been investigated.

There is a definite familial incidence and inheritance is of the autosomal recessive type (1).

Another disease has been described in this breed which has much in common with 'baldy calves' and inherited parakeratosis of calves (2). The hooves are not affected as they are in 'baldy calves' and there are ulcerative lesions in the mouth, esophagus and forestomachs.

REFERENCES

(1) Ackerman, L. (1983) *Mod. vet. Pract.*, *64*, 807.
(2) McPherson, E. A et al. (1964) *Nord, VetMed.*, *16*, Suppl. 1, 533.

Inherited parakeratosis of calves (lethal trait A46, adema disease)

This defect is recorded in Black Pied Danish cattle (1) but probably occurs in a number of European breeds of cattle (2, 3), including Friesian-type cattle. It is inherited as an autosomal recessive character (4). Calves are normal at birth and signs appear at 4–8 weeks of age; untreated animals die at about 4 months of age. There is exanthema and loss of hair, especially on the legs, parakeratosis in the form of scales or thick crusts around the mouth and eyes, under the jaw, and on the neck and legs and a very poor growth rate. At necropsy the characteristic lesion is hypoplasia of the thymus. A report that animals affected by the disease have chromosomal aberrations has been denied (7).

There is a significant response to oral treatment with zinc (0·5 g zinc oxide/day) and an apparently complete recovery can be achieved in a few weeks if treatment is continued. The disease reappears if treatment is stopped. The dose rate needs to be increased as body weight increases (5). It is thought that the disease is an inherited excessive requirement for zinc and that the thymic hypoplasia is due to the dietary deficiency. Absorption studies with radioactive zinc have shown that there is impaired absorption of the element (6).

REFERENCES

(1) Brummerstedt, F. et al. (1971) *Acta Pathol. Microbiol. scand.*, *79A*, 686.
(2) Stober, M. (1971) *Dtsch Tierärztl. Wochenschr.*, *78*, 265.
(3) Trautwein, G. (1971) *Dtsch Tierärztl. Wochenschr.*, *78*, 265.
(4) Andersen, E. et al. (1974) *Nord. VetMed.*, *26*, 275, 279.
(5) Stober, M. et al. (1974) *Zentralbl. VetMed.*, *20*, 165.
(6) Flagstad, T. (1976) *Nord. VetMed.*, *28*, 160 and *29*, 96.
(7) Bosma, A. & Kroneman, J. (1979) *Tijdschr. Diergeneenskd.*, *104*, 121.

Inherited congenital absence of the skin

Classical epitheliogenesis imperfecta

This is characterized by absence of mucous membrane, or more commonly, absence of skin over an area of the body surface has been recorded at birth in pigs (1), calves (2) and foals (3). There is complete absence of all layers of the skin in patches of varying size and distribution. In *cattle* the defect is usually on the lower parts of the limbs and sometimes on the muzzle and extending onto the buccal mucosa. The disease is best known in Holstein-Friesians, but is also recorded in Japanese Black (9), Shorthorn and Angus cattle (7). In *pigs* the skinless areas are seen on the flanks, sides, back and other parts of the body. The defect is usually incompatible with life and most affected animals die within a few days. Inheritance of the defect in cattle is conditioned by a single recessive gene.

Familial acantholysis

This is recorded in Angus calves (4) and is suspected of being inherited. The basic defect is one of defective collagen bridges in the basal and prickle layers of the epidermis so that skin is shed at carpal and metacarpophalangeal joints and coronet, and there is separation of horn at the coronet.

Epidermolysis bullosa

This is a congenital disease of Suffolk and South Dorset Down sheep (5) and Simmental (10) and Brangus calves (8). It is characterized by the formation of epidermal bullae in the mouth and on exposed areas of skin leading to shedding of the covering surface and separation of the horn from the coronet. Simmental calves grow poorly, have hypotrichosis and suffer repeated breaks in the skin. The disease in Brangus calves is very similar to familial acantholysis in Angus cattle.

Red-foot disease of sheep

This is similar to both of the above diseases. It is recorded only in Scottish Blackface sheep (6). The lesions are not present at birth but become apparent at 2–4 days of age when there is sloughing of skin of the limbs, the accessory digits, the ear pinna and the external areas, and of the epidermal layers of the cornea and buccal mucosa especially the dorsum of the tongue. There is also an absence of head horn and a separation of hoof horn from the coronet. Pieces of horn become completely detached exposing the red corium below, hence 'red-foot'. The cutaneous and mucosal lesions often commence as blood-filled or fluid-filled blisters. The corneal lesions are similarly the result of sloughing of epidermal layers. Although the cause is unknown there are indications that it is inherited.

REFERENCES

(1) Sailer, J. (1955) *Tierärztl. Umschau*, *10*, 215.
(2) Dyrendahl, S. (1956) *Nord. VetMed.*, *8*, 953.
(3) Butz, H. & Meyer, H. (1957) *Dtsch Tierärztl. Wochenschr.*, *64*, 555.
(4) Jolly, R. D. et al. (1973) *Vet. Pathol.*, *10*, 473.
(5) Alley, M. R. et al. (1974) *NZ vet. J.*, *22*, 55.
(6) McTaggart, H. S. et al. (1974) *Vet. Rec.*, *94*, 153.
(7) Jayasekara, M. U. & Leipold, H. W. (1979) *Zentralbl. VetMed.*, *26A*, 497.
(8) Thompson, K. G. et al. (1985) *Vet. Pathol.*, *22*, 283.
(9) Hamana, K. (1986) *Proc. 14th World Cong. Dis. Cattle, Dublin*, *1*, 81.
(10) Bassett, H. (1986) *Proc. 14th World Cong. Dis. Cattle, Dublin*, *1*, 75.

Inherited photosensitization

An inherited photosensitization has been observed in Southdown sheep in New Zealand and the United States (1).

The lambs are normal at birth but severe, persistent photosensitization develops at 5–7 weeks, that is, as soon as they commence to eat a chlorophyll-containing diet. Blindness is apparent. Death follows in 2–3 weeks if the lambs are left without shelter.

Liver insufficiency is present but the liver is histologically normal. Phylloerythrin and bilirubin excretion by the liver is impeded and the accumulation of phylloerythrin in the bloodstream causes the photosensitization. There is also a significant deficiency in renal function (2). The disease is conditioned by a single recessive gene. Symptomatic treatment of photosensitization and confining the animals indoors may enable the lambs to fatten to market weight. The persistent hyperbilirubinemia is accompanied by an inability of the kidneys of these sheep to concentrate urine and the ultimate death of the sheep from renal insufficiency (4).

A similar photosensitivity is inherited in Corriedales (3).

REFERENCES

(1) Cornelius, C. E. & Gronwall, R. R. (1968) *Am. J. vet. Res.*, *29*, 291.
(2) McGavin, M. D. et al. (1972) *Vet. Pathol.*, *9*, 142.
(3) Gronwall, R. R. (1970) *Am. J. vet. Res.*, *31*, 213.
(4) Filippich, L. J. et al. (1977) *Res. vet. Sci.*, *23*, 204.

Inherited congenital ichthyosis (fish-scale diseases)

Congenital ichthyosis is a disease characterized by alopecia and the presence of plates of horny epidermis covering the entire skin surface. It has been recorded only in Holstein (1) and Norwegian Red Poll and probably in Brown Swiss calves among the domestic animals, although it occurs also in man.

The newborn calf appears to be either partly or completely hairless and the skin is covered with thick, horny scales separated by fissures which follow the wrinkle lines of the skin. These may penetrate deeply and become ulcerated. There are plenty of normal hair follicles and normal hairs but these are lost in the areas covered by the growth of scales (2). A skin biopsy section will show a thick, tightly adherent layer of keratinized cells. The disease is incurable and although it may be compatible with life most affected animals are disposed of for esthetic reasons. The defect has been shown to be hereditary and to result from the influence of a single recessive gene.

REFERENCES

(1) Julian, R. J. (1960) *Vet. Med.*, *55*, 35.
(2) Barber, J. R. & Ward, W. R. (1985) *Br. vet. J.*, *141*, 1.

Inherited dermatitis vegetans of pigs

This disease appears to be conditioned by the inheritance of a recessive, semilethal factor (1). Affected pigs may show defects at birth but in most instances lesions appear after birth and up to 3 weeks of age. The lesions occur at the coronets and on the skin. Those on the coronets consist of erythema and edema with a thickened, brittle, uneven hoof wall. Lesions on the belly and inner surface of the thigh commence as areas of erythema and become wart-like and covered with gray-brown crusts. Many affected pigs die but some appear to recover completely. Many of the deaths appear to be due to the giant-cell pneumonitis which is an essential part of the disease. The pathology of the disease indicates that it is the result of a genetic defect which selectively affects mesodermal tissue (2). It is known to have originated in the Danish Landrace breed (3).

REFERENCES

(1) Flatla, J. L. et al. (1961) *Zentralbl. VetMed.*, *8*, 25.
(2) Jericho, K. W. F. (1974) *Res. vet. Sci.*, *16*, 176.
(3) Done, J. T. et al. (1967) *Vet. Rec.*, *80*, 292.

Dermatosparaxia (hyperelastosis cutis)

This is an extraordinary fragility of skin and connective tissue in general, with or without edema. It is probably inherited as a recessive character (1). It occurs in cattle (2) and horses (5) has been recorded in the United States (2), in Norwegian lambs (3), in Finnish sheep (8), and a mild form is seen in Merino sheep (7). The latter is inherited as a simple autosomal recessive. The skin is hyperelastic, as are the articular ligaments, and marked cutaneous fragility, delayed healing of skin wounds and the development of papyraceous scars are also characteristic. Pieces of skin may be ripped off when affected sheep are being handled. The defect appears to be related to a defect in collagen metabolism (4), probably a deficiency in aminopropeptidase activity.

The *Ehlers–Danlos syndrome* of cattle, recorded in Charolais and Simmental (6) is also characterized by extreme fragility of skin and laxness of joints in newborn calves. There is a defect in collagen synthesis, and histopathological findings include fragmentation and disorganization of collagen fibers.

REFERENCES

(1) Hanset, R. & Lapiere, C. M. (1974) *J. Hered.*, *65*, 356.
(2) Stober, M. et al. (1982) *Prakt. Tierärztl.*, *63*, 139.
(3) Fjolstad, M. & Helle, O. (1974) *J. Pathol.*, *112*, 183.
(4) Wick, G. et al.(1978) *Lab. Invest.*, *39*, 151.
(5) Lerner, D. J. & McCracken, M. D. (1978) *J. equ. med. Surg.*, *2*, 350.
(6) Jayasekara, M. U. et al. (1979) *Zeitschr. Tierzucht. Zuchtungsbiol.*, 96, 100.
(7) Ramshaw, J. A. M. et al. (1983) *Aust. vet. J.*, *60*, 149.
(8) Atroshi, F. et al. (1983) *Zentralbl. VetMed.*, *A30*, 233.

MISCELLANEOUS INHERITED DEFECTS

Inherited eye defects

Iridiremia (total or partial absence of iris), microphakia (smallness of the lens), ectopia lentis and cataract have been reported to occur together in Jersey calves. The mode of inheritance of the characters is as a simple recessive (1). The calves are almost completely blind but are normal in other respects and can be reared satisfactorily if they are hand-fed. Although the condition has been recorded only in Jerseys, similar defects, possibly inherited, have also been seen in Holsteins and Shorthorns.

An inherited, congenital opacity of the cornea occurs in Holstein cattle. The cornea is a cloudy blue color at birth and both eyes are equally affected. Although the sight of affected animals is restricted they are not completely blind, and there are no other abnormalities of the orbit or the eyelids. Histologically there is edema and disruption of the corneal lamellae (2). Brown Swiss cattle are affected by an inherited congenital blindness with a cloudy shrunken lens as the cause (3). Japanese Black cattle also suffer from an inherited blindness caused by defects in the pupil, retina and optic disc (4).

Although the vision appears unaffected a large number of congenital defects of the eye have been observed in cattle, including Herefords, affected by partial albinism (5). The defects include iridal heterochromia, tapetal fibrosum and colobomas. Congenital blindness is also seen in cattle with white coat color, especially Shorthorns (6). The lesions are multiple including retinal detachment, cataract, microphthalmia, persistent pupillary membrane and vitreous hemorrhage. Internal hydrocephalus is present in some, and hypoplasia of optic nerves also occurs. The inheritance is a simple autosomal recessive mode of inheritance (10). Bilateral cataract has been observed to be an inherited defect in Romney sheep. It is inherited as an autosomal dominant and can be eradicated easily by culling (7).

Complete absence of the iris in both eyes is also recorded as an inherited defect in Belgian horses (8). Affected foals develop secondary cataract at about 2 months of age. Total absence of the retina in foals has also been recorded as being inherited in a recessive manner (9).

Microphthalmia is reported to be an inherited defect in Texel sheep, but the incidence is low (11).

REFERENCES

(1) Saunders, L. Z. & Fincher, M. G. (1951) *Cornell Vet.*, *41*, 351.
(2) Deas, D. W. (1959) *Vet. Rec.*, *71*, 619.
(3) Geyer, H. et al. (1974) *Schweiz. Arch. Tierheilkd.*, *116*, 147.
(4) Fujimura, T. et al. (1972) *J. Jap. vet. med. Assoc.*, *25*, 288.
(5) Gelatt, K. N. et al.(1969) *Am. J. vet. Res.*, *30*, 1313.
(6) Greene, H. J. & Leipold, H. W. (1974) *Cornell Vet.*, *64*, 367.
(7) Brooks, H. V. et al. (1982) *NZ vet. J.*, *30*, 113.
(8) Erikson, K. (1955) *Nord. VetMed.*, *7*, 773.
(9) Koch, P. (1952) *Rep. 2nd int. Congr. Physiol. Pathol. Anim. Reprod. artif. Insem.*, *2*, 110.
(10) Green, H. J. et al. (1978) *Irish vet. J.*, *32*, 65.
(11) Wagenaar, G. (1980) *Tijdschr. Diergeneeskd.*, *105*, 275.

Inherited typical colobomata

These inherited congenital defects of eyes have assumed a more prominent position than they used to have because of their high level occurrence in Charolais cattle (1). The lesions are present at birth and do not progress beyond that stage. They affect vision very little, if at all. However, because they are defects they should be named in certificates of health but they are not usually considered as being a reason for disqualification from breeding programs. In Charolais cattle the inheritance of the defect is via an autosomal dominant gene with complete penetrance in males and partial (52%) penetrance in females (2). The prevalence may be as high as 6% and in most cases both eyes are affected (3).

The defect is one of incomplete closure of one of the ocular structures at or near the line of the embryonic choroidal fissure. Failure of the fissure to close represents the beginnings of a coloboma. The retina, choroid and sclera are usually all involved.

REFERENCES

(1) Barnett, K. C. & Ogden, A. L. (1972) *Vet. Rec.*, *91*, 592.
(2) Falco, M. & Barnett, K. C. (1978) *Vet. Rec.*, *102*, 102.
(3) Walker, K. H. et al. (1977) *Aust. vet. Practnr*, *7*, 25.

Inherited entropion

Entropion is inherited in sheep and this is known to occur in a number of breeds including Oxfords, Hampshires and Suffolks (1). Affected lambs are not observed until about 3 weeks of age when attention is drawn to the eyelids by the apparent conjunctivitis. A temporary blindness results but even without treatment there is a marked improvement in the eyelids and the lambs do not appear to suffer any permanent harm.

REFERENCE

(1) Taylor, M. & Catchpole, J. (1986) *Vet. Rec.*, *118*, 361.

Inherited ocular dermoids

These are recorded as genetically transmitted in Hereford cattle (1). They occur as multiple small masses of dystopic skin complete with hair on the conjunctiva of both eyes of affected cattle. They can be anywhere on the cornea, on the third eyelid or the eyelid and may completely replace the cornea and there may be a resulting marked dysplasia of the internal ocular structures.

REFERENCE

(1) Barkyoumb, S. D. & Leipold, H. W. (1984) *Vet. Pathol.*, *21*, 316.

Inherited prolonged gestation

Prolonged gestation occurs in cattle and sheep in several forms and is usually, although not always, inherited. The two recorded forms of the disease are prolonged gestation with fetal giantism and prolonged gestation with deformed fetuses of normal or small size. The latter form is accompanied by adenohypophyseal hypoplasia. Other sporadic cases occur originating apparently from absent or developmentally abnormal adrenal and pituitary glands (3).

Prolonged gestation with fetal giantism
This disease is recorded in Holstein, Ayrshire and Swedish cattle and in Karakul sheep (1). The cause of the disease in the sheep is unknown. A similar condition of prolonged gestation with fetal giantism in sheep has been found to be caused by the ingestion of *Veratrum californicum* or the shrub *Salsola tuberculata* (2). The disease in cattle is familial in most instances, but cases resulting from poisoning with *Veratrum album* are also recorded (9).

The usual clinical picture in this form of the disease is prolongation of pregnancy for periods of from 3 weeks to 3 months. The cows may show marked abdominal distension but in most cases the abdomens are smaller than one would expect. Parturition, when it commences, is without preparation in that udder enlargement, relaxation of the pelvic ligaments and loosening and swelling of the vulva do not occur. There is also poor relaxation of the cervix and a deficiency of cervical mucus. Dystocia is usual and cesarean section is usually advisable in Holstein cattle but the Ayrshire calves have all been reported as having been born without assistance. The calves are very large (48–80 kg body weight) and show other evidence of post-term growth, with a luxuriant hair coat and large, well-erupted teeth which are loose in their alveoli, but the birth weight is not directly related to the length of the gestation period. At birth the calves exhibit a labored respiration with diaphragmatic movements more evident than movements of the chest wall. They invariably die within a few hours in a hypoglycemic coma. At necropsy there is adenohypophyseal hypoplasia and hypoplasia of the adrenal cortex. The progesterone level in the peripheral blood of cows bearing affected calves does not fall before term as it does in normal cows.

Prolonged gestation with adenohypophyseal hypoplasia
This form of the disease has been observed in Guernsey and Jersey cattle, and in one Ayrshire cow (5). It differs from the previous form in that the fetuses are dead on delivery, show gross deformity of the head and are smaller than the normal calves of these breeds born at term. In Guernseys the defect has been shown to be inherited as a single recessive character and it is probable that the same is true in Jerseys. The gestation period varies widely with a mean of 401 days.

Clinical examination of the dams carrying defective calves suggests that no development of the calf or placenta occurs after the seventh month of pregnancy. Death of the fetus occurs and is followed in 1–2 weeks by parturition unaccompanied by relaxation of the pelvic ligaments or vulva or by external signs of labor. The calf can usually be removed by forced traction because of its small size. Mammary gland enlargement does not occur until after parturition.

The calves are small and suffer varying degrees of hypotrichosis. There is hydrocephalus and in some cases distension of the gut and abdomen due to atresia of the jejunum. The bones are immature and the limbs are short. Abnormalities of the face include cyclopian eyes, microphthalmia, absence of the maxilla and the presence of only one nostril. At necropsy there is partial or complete aplasia of the adenohypophysis. The neural stalk is present and extends to below the diaphragm sellae. Brain abnormalities vary from fusion of the cerebral hemispheres to moderate hydrocephalus. The other endocrine glands are also small and hypoplastic.

The disease has been produced experimentally in ewes by severe ablation of the pituitary gland, or destruction of the hypothalamus, or section of the pituitary stalk in the fetus (6) and by adrenalectomy of the lamb (7) or kid (4). Infusion of ACTH into ewes with prolonged gestation due to pituitary damage produces parturition but not if the ewes have been adrenalectomized beforehand.

A third form of prolonged gestation, which occurs in Hereford cattle and is thought to be inherited, is accompanied by arthrogryposis, scoliosis, torticollis, kyphosis and cleft palate (8).

Other forms of non-inherited prolonged gestation are recognized in sheep and caused by the poisonous plants *Salsola tuberculata*, *Veratrum californicum* and possibly *Lysichiton americanus* (10).

REVIEW LITERATURE

Holm, L. W. (1967) *Adv. vet. Sci.*, *11*, 159, 206.

REFERENCES

(1) De Lange, M. (1962) *Proc. 4th int. Congr. Anim. Reprod., The Hague*, 1961 *3*, 590.
(2) Basson, P. A. et al. (1969) *Onderstepoort J. vet. Res.*, *36*, 59.
(3) Frerking, H. & Benten, K. van (1977) *Dtsch Tierärztl. Wochenschr.*, *84*, 239.
(4) Rawlings, N. C. & Ward, W. R. (1978) *J. Reprod. Fertil.*, *52*, 249.
(5) Lindberg, L. A. et al. (1980) *Nord. VetMed.*, *32*, 400.
(6) Liggins, G. C. et al. (1966) *J. Reprod. Fertil.*, *12*, 419.
(7) Drost, M. & Holm, L. W. (1968) *J. Endocrinol.*, *40*, 293.
(8) Shupe, J. J. et al. (1967) *J. Hered.*, *58*, 311.
(9) Hosokawa, K. (1978) *Theriogenology*, *10*, 147.
(10) Barlow, R. M. et al. (1985) *Vet. Rec.*, *117*, 124.

'Barker' syndrome in pigs

A possibly inherited disease of pigs recorded only once (1) is characterized by severe respiratory distress, including the emission of a barking sound and high mortality and short course, most being dead at 12–24 hours after birth. Affected piglets have a rolypoly appearance, show severe respiratory distress and 'bark' repeatedly. Some show aimless wandering and apparent blindness. The skin is very thin and papery and the bristles appear as a very fine hair. At necropsy examination there were significant changes in lungs and the thyroid was small.

REFERENCE

(1) Gibson, E. A. et al. (1976) *Vet. Rec.*, *98*, 476.

35

Specific Diseases of Uncertain Etiology

INTRODUCTION

It was anticipated that, with time, this chapter would shrink in succeeding editions and eventually disappear. As the causes of individual diseases are demonstrated they are removed to other chapters but in the past newly identified diseases have been added at approximately the same rate so that the net effect on the chapter has been negligible. The process could have been hastened by moving diseases when the consensus of opinion, short of proof, was that the cause had been identified. We have thought it preferable to leave those diseases here, together with those in which the combination of causes is complex—thus 'weaner illthrift' and acute diarrhea of horses.

DISEASES CHARACTERIZED BY SYSTEMIC INVOLVEMENT

Unthriftiness in weaner sheep (weaner illthrift)

Loss of weight at weaning and failure to make satisfactory weights subsequently, in spite of the presence of ample feed and when adult sheep are faring well, has been a problem in sheep for many years (1). The problem has seemed to be most severe in the southern hemisphere but this may be because sheep are so prevalent there. It may also be due partly to the predominance of Merino and Merino-type sheep; the disease is most common in these breeds which have their own particular timorous nature which makes weaning and the need to shift for themselves more traumatic than in most other breeds. This trait is particularly noticeable if there is overcrowding on pasture. Other management factors likely to lead to unthriftiness are multibirth lambs, small ewes, ewes with little milk and lambs born late in the season (2).

Apart from the need for more gentle and considerate handling of the young at weaning in order to ensure a smooth transition, a number of less abstract measures are often practiced. Examination of the teeth to ensure that there is no excessive attrition of the teeth, or even breaking of the incisors if the sheep are being fed roots, is an essential preliminary step in any investigation of an illthrift problem. Supplementation of the diet to replace deficient items is most common and of the deficiencies the most likely one in many environments is protein, especially at the end of a dry summer. Diagnosis by response to cobalt, selenium, perhaps copper or vitamin D, the latter in areas far from the equator, is often used in situations where deficiencies of these trace elements or vitamins are suspect (3). Clinical or subclinical infestations with nematodes are also common occurrences at this time in the sheep's life before immunity is properly developed and infections with coccidia, cryptosporidia, or *Eperythrozoon ovis* are probably significant causes of illthrift (3).

Examination of the above-mentioned possible causes is time-absorbing and costly and, if there is a residuum of unsolved cases, they are likely to remain undiagnosed. An additional factor which might be taken into consideration is the villous atrophy seen in ruminal epithelium in young sheep grazing on pasture composed of a pure stand of one pasture plant species, especially perennial rye-grass (4,5). The change in the epithelium is similar to that which occurs in sheep fed heat-treated pellets. It has been pointed out (3) that this lesion, with its attendant malabsorption, can arise by virtue of trauma by coccidia or nematodes which are no longer in evidence at the time of postmortem examination or response trial.

There is also the possibility that infections with coronaviruses may cause the same villous atrophy. In all of these cases the malabsorption which results may be manifested by weight loss, but also by chronic diarrhea. Both of these clinical signs are also characteristic of grossly inadequate diets, especially when there is excessive fiber and inadequate protein. In that circumstance the ruminal contents will be undigested.

In bad years there may be many deaths; in any circumstance there is a gross delay in maturation so that maiden lambing may be delayed to as late as 3 years of age (5). The economic effects can be disastrous.

REFERENCES

(1) Pulsford M. R. et al. (1966) *Aust. vet. J.*, *42*, 165, 169, 388.
(2) Findlay, G. R. & Heath, G. B. S. (1969) *Vet. Rec.*, *85*, 547.
(3) Pout, D. D. & Harbutt, P. (1968) *Vet. Rec.*, *83*, 373.
(4) Lancashire, J. A. & Keogh, R. G. (1966) *NZ J. agric. Res.*, *9*, 916.
(5) McLoughlin, J. W. (1967) *Vict. vet. Proc.*, *25*, 60.

Weak calf syndrome

A disease of newborn calves called the 'weak calf syndrome' was first recognized in Montana in 1964. The morbidity rate varied from 5 to 15% and the case mortality rate was often as high as 80%. The disease or a similar condition has been reported frequently from the northwestern United States and is considered a major economic loss in cattle herds (1, 2).

The etiology has not been determined (2). Some bacteria and viruses have been isolated from affected calves, but a causal relationship has not yet been shown (3, 4). Similar calves have occurred experimentally after intra-amnionic exposure to an adenovirus (6). The serum immunoglobulin concentrations in the precolostral serum of affected calves have been normal, suggesting that infections are not occurring during the stage of gestation when the fetus is immunologically competent (5). Fetal hypoxemia due to a prolonged parturition may also be a cause which is presented in Chapter 3 on diseases of the newborn.

The epidemiological observations which have been made include:

- Cows that have delivered an affected calf rarely have another affected calf
- First-calf heifers or recently introduced herd replacements more commonly give birth to calves which are affected at birth or soon after
- Rapid changes in weather or very inclement weather are usually associated with an outbreak of the disease
- Transfusion of blood from a cow which has had an affected calf has increased the survival rate of affected calves (2).

Affected calves are usually found in sternal recumbency, depressed, reluctant to stand unassisted, reluctant to walk, and not interested in sucking. While standing, their backs are arched and from a distance they appear stiff and are obviously gaunt. Diarrhea may be present but is usually not profuse and watery. The muzzle may be reddened and crusty. The joints may be slightly swollen and painful to touch. The temperature, heart rate and respirations are usually within the normal range.

At necropsy the prominent lesions are marked edema and the hemorrhages of the subcutaneous tissues over the carpal and tarsal joints and extending distally down the limbs. The synovial fluid may be blood-tinged and contain fibrinous deposits. Erosions or ulceration of the gastrointestinal tract, petechial hemorrhage of internal organs, involution of the thymus gland and hemorrhages in skeletal muscle have also been described (1, 2).

Nothing specific for the treatment and control of the disease can be recommended because the etiology is not known (2).

REFERENCES

(1) Card, C. S. et al. (1974) *Proc. 77th ann. Mtg US Anim. Hlth Assoc.*, *77*, 67.
(2) Stauber, E. H. (1976) *J. Am. vet. med. Assoc.*, *168*, 223.
(3) McClurkin, A. W. & Coria, M. F. (1975) *J. Am. vet. med. Assoc.*, *167*, 139.
(4) Cutlip, R. C. & McClurkin, A. W. (1975) *Am. J. vet. Res.*, *36*, 1095.
(5) Ivanoff, R. M. & Renshaw, H. W. (1975) *Am. J. vet. Res.*, *36*, 1131.
(6) Stauber, E. & Card, C. S. (1978) *Can. J. comp. med.*, *42*, 466.

Watery mouth of lambs

A condition of lambs mostly 24–48 hours, up to 72 hours, old characterized by excessive mucoid saliva around and hanging from the mouth, depression to the point of coma, anorexia and in the late stages, abdominal distension and recumbency. Some lambs have hypothermia but the average temperature is normal. A small proportion have diarrhea. The mortality rate is about 40% most dying 6–24 hours after the first signs of illness. Biochemical examination reveals hypoglycemia in the final stages and a hypogammaglobulinemia in some. Most of the young lambs are ram lambs that have been castrated by the use of an elastic band and the resulting pain may have dissuaded them from feeding.

The cause of watery mouth is undecided and there is some doubt as to its separate identity as a disease. Many cases with similar signs do occur in lambs and calves with toxipathic colibacillosis. Factors that appear to increase the probability of the disease occurring are: rubber ring castration at a very young age (down to 3 days) (1), inclement weather, twins or triplets, ewes in poor condition, the incidence is much less in lambs given prophylactic oral antibiotics at birth (2) and inadequate intake of colostrum. It seems likely that this is a multifactorial disease in which hypersalivation results from one of several primary causes such as alimentary tract distention due to paralytic ileus. Abomasal distention and slow emptying time result from the inclusion of colostrum in the diet and the application of rubber castration rings (3).

REVIEW LITERATURE

Eales, F. A. (1987) Watery mouth. *In Practice*, *9(1)*, 12.

REFERENCES

(1) Collins, R. O. et al. (1985) *Br. vet. J.*, *141*, 135.
(2) Eales, F. A. et al. (1986) *Vet. Rec.*, *119*, 543.
(3) Eales, F. A. et al. (1985) *Vet. Rec.*, *117*, 332.

Cold cow syndrome

A herd disease problem reported from the United Kingdom in cows freshly turned out onto lush pasture with a high (27–43%) soluble carbohydrate content (1). There is a high morbidity (up to 80%) and a large number of outbreaks in an area. The syndrome includes hypothermia, dullness, inappetence, agalactia and profuse diarrhea. Affected cows feel cold to the touch. Some have perineal edema, some collapse. The herd milk yield falls disastrously but there is a quick return to normal if the cows are moved to a different field. The problem may occur on the same pasture each year and recur if the cows are returned to the same pasture. There is no obvious clinicopathological abnormality.

REFERENCE

(1) Veterinary information service (1984) *Vet. Rec.*, *114*, 603.

Thin sow syndrome

The 'thin sow syndrome' must be classified as a problem rather than as a disease because of its probable multiple etiology. Admittedly it has been recorded much more in recent years (1) but it is by no means new. At one time it was possible to evade the problem but in today's cost-conscious and waste-conscious agriculture, the thin-sow syndrome needs to be admitted, quantified and examined. Its effects on fertility and overall farm productivity can be formidable (2).

Affected sows lose more than the usual amount of weight during pregnancy and after farrowing, the latter being more noticeable. No abnormalities are evident on clinical examination but the sow fails to regain weight after weaning and the most critical period for weight loss is the first 2 weeks after weaning. Affected sows have a poor appetite but often show pica and excessive water intake and are anemic. The most important characteristic of the disease is the failure to respond to treatment and culling is usually advisable.

In some instances the problem is parasitic and accompanied by high egg counts and a significant population of *Oesophagostomum* spp. and *Hyostrongylus rubidus* and this group is discussed under those headings. In others the problems appear to arise because of errors in management which are likely to be exaggerated and multiplied on farms where intensive management is practiced. The most common errors are cold or drafty housing, low-level feeding to avoid obesity and low fertility, wet bedding and lack of drinking water. Modern-day rapid remating of sows and very early weaning increase the chances of metabolic breakdown, especially if nutrition is inadequate. The latter is most likely when sows are run in large groups with different stages of pregnancy present and where timid sows are likely to be bullied out of their fair share of food. When breeds are mixed it is often the Landrace, Saddleback and their crossbreds which are the most timid and most likely to become affected (2). Individual stalls give an opportunity for individual feeding and tend to avoid this problem. A satisfactory level of feed intake must be maintained during lactation because most affected sows fail to respond to improved nutrition after weaning.

REFERENCES

(1) Maclean, C. W. (1968) *Vet. Rec.*, *83*, 308.
(2) Maclean, C. W. (1969) *Vet. Rec.*, *85*, 675.

Postvaccinal hepatitis of horses

The disease has been recorded chiefly as a sequel to infectious encephalomyelitis, occurring 1–3 months after an outbreak of this disease. Outbreaks have occurred in the United Kingdom (1), Nigeria (2) and China (6) where infectious equine encephalomyelitis (IEE) does not occur. Although the hepatitis is thought to be related to the use of serum and vaccine used in the control of infectious equine encephalomyelitis, cases have occurred in horses which do not appear to have received any biological preparation in the period of several months prior to the development of the disease. This form of hepatitis bears some resemblance to infectious hepatitis of man and its possible method of spread on hypodermic needles further heightens the resemblance. However, attempts to transmit the disease have been unsuccessful and it is thought that a hepatotoxic agent may be present in any equine serum or tissue extract used as vaccine. Occurrence of the disease in horses is recorded after vaccination against abortion due to *Salmonella abortisequi* in mares (6), infectious equine encephalomyelitis, African horse sickness, anthrax, enterotoxemia, tetanus (tetanus antitoxin) (3) and influenza (1).

Clinically the disease is characterized by intense icterus, cessation of alimentary tract movement and oliguria, absence or rare occurrence of fever, and severe nervous signs including stupor and mania.

There may be a straddle-legged posture with continuous head-pressing, violent, uncontrolled movement and walking in circles. Hemoglobinuria occurs terminally in some cases. Most affected animals die within 12–48 hours. Some animals recover and without apparent after-effects while others manifest imbecility and an intractable disposition. The mortality rate varies between 40 and 60%. Clinicopathological aids in diagnosis depend on serum liver enzyme tests, the sorbitol dehydrogenase and serum glutamic oxalacetate transferase tests being preferred (3).

At necropsy the most significant changes are seen in the liver which, although normal in size, is light or greenish in color and soft and friable in texture (4, 5). Degenerative changes may also be seen in the kidneys. There is hyperemia or submucosal hemorrhage of the small intestine, and petechial and ecchymotic hemorrhages are present under the serous membranes and in the musculature. Icterus is present throughout the carcass.

Treatment with antibiotics, glucose and electrolyte solutions and B-complex vitamins may be of some value (4).

REFERENCES

(1) Thomsett, L. R. (1971) *Equ. vet. J.*, *3*, 15.
(2) Oduye, O. O. et al. (1974) *J. Nigerian vet. med. Assoc.*, *3*, 86.
(3) Rose, J. A. et al. (1974) *Proc. 20th ann. Conf. Am. Assoc. equ. Practnrs, Las Vegas, 1974*, 175.
(4) Hjerpe, C. A. (1964) *J. Am. vet. med. Assoc.*, *144*, 734.
(5) Panciera, R. J. (1969) *J. Am. vet. med. Assoc.*, *155*, 408.
(6) China, Zootechnic & Veterinary Division (1983) *Chin. J. vet. Med.*, *9*, 10.

Granulocytopenic disease of calves

A fairly widespread disease of recent origin, granulocytopenic disease of calves is commonly ascribed to poisoning with furazolidone. The calves are always being reared on milk-replacer and sometimes, but not always, receiving prophylactic antibiotics (1–3). Affected calves show fever, and increased salivation and nasal discharge, and there are hemorrhages and necrotic lesions in the mouth and lower alimentary tract. The disease is characterized by decreased myelopoiesis in bone marrow, neutropenia and thrombocytopenia. The course varies from 2 to 5 days, and the mortality rate is high, apparently from bacterial invasion. *Fusobacterium necrophorum* is reported in one case (5). Pneumonia, peritonitis and enteritis are common accompaniments.

The disease has been related to longterm feeding of furazolidone (2 mg/kg body weight daily) and the disease can be reproduced by this means. At higher dose rates (20–30 mg/kg body weight) nervous signs, including convulsions, and death follow within a few days (4). These clinical, pathological and hematological findings resemble those of radiation sickness.

REFERENCES

(1) Gay, C. C. et al. (1974) *Aust. vet. J.*, *50*, 126.
(2) Hayashi, T. (1976) *Jap. J. vet. Sci.*, *38*, 225
(3) Hoffman, W. et al. (1977) *Dtsch Tierärztl. Wochenschr.*, *84*, 1.
(4) Buck, W. B. (1975) *J. Am. vet. Assoc.*, *166*, 222.
(5) Nimmo-Wilkie, J. & Radostits, O. M. (1981) *Can. vet. J.*, *22*, 166.

Sweating sickness (tick toxicosis)

This is an acute non-infectious disease of calves caused by the bites of the tick *Hyalomma* spp. and characterized by fever, salivation, lacrimation, hyperemia of mucosae, epistaxis and extensive and severe dermatitis.

Etiology

The cause has not been identified, but it behaves as though it were an epitheliotropic toxin produced by the salivary glands of the tick *Hyalomma truncatum*.

Epidemiology

Attempts to transmit the disease between animals by mediate or immediate contact and by injections of tissue or blood are unsuccessful. The disease occurs in Central, East and South Africa, Sri Lanka and probably southern India. Only calves 2–6 months of age are affected as a rule but rare cases occur in adults. Sheep, pigs and goats are susceptible, although the disease does not naturally occur in them, and the disease has been produced experimentally in dogs. Sweating sickness occurs at all times of the year but is most prevalent during the wet season when ticks are more plentiful. The morbidity rate varies with the size of the tick population but is usually 10–30%. The case fatality rate is up to 30%.

Pathogenesis

The clinical signs begin 4–7 days after the ticks attach, probably 3 days in experimental infestations. The effects are dose-specific; if the ticks are removed very early there is no clinical response and the animal remains susceptible; with a longer exposure before the ticks are removed the animal becomes immune but shows no clinical signs. With longer exposure of more than 5 days the subject develops the full-blown clinical disease and may die. If it recovers it has a solid and durable immunity.

Clinical findings

There is a sudden onset of fever up to 41°C (106°F), anorexia, hyperemia of the mucosae and hyperesthesia. The animal is lethargic, depressed, dehydrated and has a serous then mucopurulent oculonasal discharge, an arched back and a rough coat. There is an extensive, moist dermatitis commencing in the axilla, groin, perineum and at the base of the ears which extends to cover the entire body in bad cases. The hair is matted together by exudate and moisture collects in the form of beads on the surface. The eyelids may be stuck together. Subsequently patches of the skin and hair are rubbed off or can be pulled off to leave raw, red areas of subcutaneous tissue exposed. The tips of the ears and tail may slough. Affected calves seek shade and their skin is very sensitive to touch. Later it becomes dry and hard, and cracks develop. Secondary bacterial infection and infestation with blowflies or screwworm larvae are common sequelae. The oral mucosa is hyperemic at first and then becomes necrotic with the formation of ulcers and diphtheritic membranes. The calf salivates profusely, cannot eat or drink and becomes emaciated and rapidly dehydrated. There are similar mucosal lesions in the vagina and nasal cavities, the latter causing dyspnea. The severity of the mucosal lesions appears to vary with different 'strains' of the toxin (3). There may be abdominal pain and diarrhea in some calves. The course may be as short as 2 days but is usually 4 or 5 days. In recovered animals the skin may heal and the hair regrow but there may be permanent, patchy alopecia and the calves may remain stunted and unthrifty.

Clinical pathology

There is a severe neutropenia and eosinopenia and a degenerative left shift. Alpha-globulin and beta-globulin levels are raised. Urinalysis indicates the existence of nephrosis but serum creatinine levels are normal (2). Dermatological examination fails to reveal the presence of any of the usual infectious causes of dermatitis.

Necropsy findings

The lesions are essentially those seen clinically plus evidence of severe toxemia, dehydration, emaciation and hyperemia of all internal organs. The necrosis of the oral epithelium extends into the esophagus and may reach the forestomachs.

Diagnosis

The combination of extensive dermatitis and mucosal necrosis is unusual. Mucosal disease and bovine malignant catarrh may bear some resemblance and there could be difficulty in differentiation in areas where the tick *Hyalomma truncatum* occurs.

Treatment
There is no specific treatment which should be directed at relieving the severity of the dermatitis and mucosal loss. Non-steroidal anti-inflammatory drugs (NSAIDs) and broad-spectrum antibiotic cover is a logical regimen. Hyperimmune serum, produced in sheep and cattle by infesting them with *Hyalomma truncatum* at 6 week intervals for two to five occasions, is an effective treatment in pigs, sheep and to a less extent calves (1).

Control
Control is limited to control of the causative tick. No vaccine is available.

REVIEW LITERATURE

Bwangamoi, O. (1979) In *Diseases of Cattle in Tropical Africa*, (ed.) Mugera, G. M. Kenya Literature Bureau, Nairobi, p. 405.

REFERENCES

(1) Oberem, P. T. et al. (1985) *Onderstepoort J. vet. Res.*, *52*, 283.
(2) Amstel van, S. R. (1984) *Proc. 13th Wld Cong. Dis. Cattle*, *1*, 520.
(3) Bezuidenhout, J. D. & Oberem, P. T. (1984) *Proc. 13th Wld Cong. Dis. Cattle*, *1*, 515.

DISEASES CHARACTERIZED BY ALIMENTARY TRACT INVOLVEMENT

Grass sickness of horses

Grass sickness is a non-infectious disease of horses of unknown etiology. It is characterized clinically by alimentary stasis, emaciation and severe mental depression. Degenerative lesions are detectable on histological examination of the sympathetic ganglia.

Etiology
The cause is unknown. Viral infection has been suggested because of the nature of the lesions in the sympathetic ganglia but the disease has not been transmitted. Cases do tend to occur close together and if an infectious agent is involved an incubation period of about 7 days is suggested (1). Intoxification has also been suggested as a cause because most cases occur in horses at pasture, and on particular farms. Also the lesions characteristic of the disease have been reproduced by the injection of blood from an affected horse (2). Intoxication caused by *Clostridium perfringens* type D was suggested but vaccination with an anaculture of the organism, while producing antibodies, did not prevent the disease (3). An association between the disease and intoxification with *Clostridium perfringens* A toxin has also been suggested (6), but is not a favored candidate (11, 12).

Epidemiology
Grass sickness is not common and appears to be restricted in occurrence to Scotland and Northern England and to Sweden. Most affected horses die or are destroyed because of weakness and emaciation. Horses are the only species affected and all breeds and age groups, other than sucking foals, are susceptible, but the incidence is highest in the 3–6 years age group. The disease is also recorded in two zoo animals, a zebra and a Przewalski horse, and a donkey (3).

Most cases develop while horses are at pasture but sporadic cases occur in stabled animals (4), and horses receiving supplementary feed are not susceptible to the disease. Cases occur throughout the year but the highest incidence is in the summer months. In Scotland the occurrence of the disease is dependent on rain and on an increasing environmental temperature (5) with a high point of prevalence in May and a peak incidence in horses 3 years of age, but the disease is common in horses of 2–7 years of age. The disease is most likely to occur on farms where the disease has occurred previously, and horses which have been on the farm for less than 2 months are more likely to develop the disease than those which have been there longer.

Pathogenesis
The early hypothesis of sympatheticotonia has not been refuted and the clinical picture is, apart from the absence of pupillary dilatation, one of increased sympathetic tone. The alimentary signs are those of paralytic ileus due to functional stasis. The lesions in the sympathetic ganglia bear out the suggestion that the sympathetic nervous system is the site of the important defect. However, one might expect that the degenerative nature of the lesions would cause a decrease in sympathetic tone, rather than the observed sympathetic dominance. Whether or not identical lesions occur in normal horses is debatable. However, there seems to be no doubt that the disease is caused by a primary axonal lesion, probably caused by neurotoxin, and resulting in the accumulation of noradrenaline nerve fibers (8, 9).

Peristalsis ceases, the contents of the large intestine become dehydrated, the digestive tract becomes distended with decomposing ingesta and gas, and rupture is the usual termination (1).

Clinical findings
Acute, subacute and chronic cases occur. In all cases, there is lethargy and difficulty in swallowing, resulting in drooling of saliva and trickling of ingesta from the nose. The pulse rate is increased to 80–90/min. Bowel movements cease, peristaltic sounds are absent and there may be tympanites. Abnormal discomfort may suggest the presence of subacute impaction of the large intestine. On rectal examination, the feces are hard, dry pellets covered with sticky mucus. Urination is frequent and may be accompanied by tenesmus. Affected horses may wander about in a restless manner and a fine muscle tremor occurs constantly, especially in the upper forelimb. Periodic attacks of patchy sweating occur commonly.

The course of the disease varies. Acute cases die in 1–5 days and may or may not show signs of colic. In subacute cases, the course is usually 2–3 weeks and, during this time, the animal loses much condition and becomes extremely gaunt. The skeletal muscles appear to be stretched tight and are very hard to the touch. Chronic cases may appear to recover but are incapable of hard work. Rupture of the stomach causes sudden death in some.

Clinical pathology
All hematological and biochemical examinations on affected horses have failed to show any significant abnormalities. There is a radiological discernible defect in esophageal motility in horses with grass sickness (7).

Necropsy findings
In cases of short duration, the stomach and small intestines are distended with an excess of fluid and gas, and the colon contains small, hard, black pellets of manure. The spleen is always enlarged. In chronic cases, the alimentary tract is empty and of very small caliber. Histologically there is extensive degeneration of neurones in the sympathetic ganglia without evidence of inflammation (10) and neuronal necrosis in the central nervous system; the lesions are present in oculomotor, facial, lateral vestibular, hypoglossal and vagal nuclei (4).

Diagnosis
Grass sickness is strictly limited in its geographical distribution. Early acute cases may resemble subacute impaction of the colon except for difficult swallowing and the accumulation of fluid in the alimentary tract. Failure of cases of grass sickness to respond to treatment for colonic impaction may serve as a further aid in diagnosis. A disease of horses described in Colombia as 'grass sickness' and which bears some resemblance to the disease described in this section, has significant clinical and pathological differences from it. For example, the Colombian disease is always acute, lasting about 3 days, and the mortality rate is only 70–80%.

Treatment
All attempts at treatment have been without effect. Decompression of the stomach by drainage and the administration of large quantities of isotonic solutions parenterally prolong the life of affected animals but do not influence the final outcome of the disease (7).

Control
Successful measures have not been satisfactorily established and no recommendations can be made.

REFERENCES

(1) Limont, A. G. (1971) *Vet. Rec.*, *88*, 98.
(2) Gilmour, J. S. (1973) *Vet. Rec.*, *92*, 565.
(3) Ashton, D. G. et al. (1977) *Vet. Rec.*, *100*, 406.
(4) Gilmour, J. S. (1973) *Res. vet. Sci.*, *15*, 197.
(5) Gilmour, J. S. & Jolly, G. M. (1974) *Vet. Rec.*, *95*, 77.
(6) Ochoa, R. & Velandia, S. (1978) *Vet. Rec.*, *95*, 77.
(7) Greet, T. R. M. & Whitwell, K. E. (1986) *Equ. vet. J.*, *18*, 294.
(8) Bishop, A. E. et al. (1984) *Experientia*, *40*, 801.
(9) Gilmour, J. S. & Mould, D. L. (1977) *Res. vet. Sci.*, *22*, 1.
(10) Hodson, N. P. et al. (1984) *J. Pathol.*, *142*, A21.
(11) Anon (1981) *Equ. vet. J.*, *13*, 1.
(12) Gilmour, J. S. et al. (1981) *Equ. vet. J.*, *13*, 56.

Acute diarrheas of horses

A great deal of attention is now focused on acute diarrhea in horses. The interest derives largely from the high case fatality rate and very short course of the disease and the uncertainty about the cause or causes. The two common causes are salmonellosis and colitis-X and these are dealt with in detail under these specific headings. Some uncertainty still exists with regard to the diagnosis of salmonellosis. In typical cases there is a preclinical leukopenia and fever, a severe foul-smelling diarrhea containing mucus, blood and some epithelial shreds, and a high fecal leukocyte count (23) and at necropsy a severe hemorrhagic enteritis affecting the entire length of the intestine and large numbers of salmonellae can be isolated on primary culture of intestinal contents and mesenteric lymph nodes. In many less typical cases the final diagnosis of salmonellosis may be made but laboratory findings are not characteristic. Salmonellae can be isolated in only small numbers after careful culture of mesenteric lymph nodes which is the kind of result one would expect in a 'carrier' animal. In areas where it occurs Potomac horse fever would be a prime suspect in cases of equine acute diarrhea. A coronavirus has also been isolated from such cases but an etiological relationship was not established (24). *Polymorphella ampulla*, a commensal organism in normal circumstances, may assume a secondary pathogenic role in the presence of other enteritides (25).

Because of the recognized association between the imposition of stress on an animal and the development of these diarrheas it is not unreasonable to suggest that salmonellosis could be the superimposed disease. In the cases which occur after the administration of tetracyclines it is also possible that the intestinal flora is radically altered as a result of this treatment and this allows the overgrowth of salmonellae, lying dormant until now, or of *E. coli* with resulting toxin production leading either to salmonellosis or colitis-X (1, 2).

ANTIBIOTIC-INDUCED DIARRHEA

There are a number of records of acute diarrhea occurring after dosing with tetracyclines (2–4), and debilitated horses may die within 24 hours because of the severity of the dehydration which results. In most of the recorded cases there has been prior stress, often an infection, requiring administration of the antibiotic (5). The dose rate of tetracycline used may be very high but the disease also occurs at normal doses of the order of 1–2 mg/kg body weight given parenterally (6).

The onset is sudden, usually 3–4 days after the antibiotic is administered, and the course is short, sometimes as short as 24 hours, but mostly 4–15 days. The mortality rate is high. At necropsy there is edema of the wall of the large bowel wall with an attendant typhlitis and colitis reminiscent of colitis-X. The probability is that most cases of post-tetracycline scours would be classified as colitis-X. Chronic equine diarrhea can be initiated by dosing with antibiotics and is the more common outcome.

A similar syndrome is recorded after the feeding of tylosin at the rate of 0·88 g per Thoroughbred colt or filly on one or two occasions, 1–2 days apart. There was profuse diarrhea 1–2 days later. The same medicated feed caused chronic diarrhea in adult horses (20). Lincomycin, trimethoprim-sulfonamide, massive doses of penicillin, and erythromycin have all been associated with attacks of acute colitis in horses (21). An outbreak of fatal acute diarrhea was caused by horses eating grain containing 50 g/tonne of lincomycin (22).

COLITIS-X

This disease of horses has come to public attention only during recent times and although it is known to occur in the United States (7), Canada, the West Indies and Australia, there are few written reports on which to base an accurate description. Because of its highly fatal nature, most affected horses dying within 24 hours of first illness, and because it sometimes occurs as an 'outbreak' with a number of horses in a group (up to 20%) becoming affected within a space of 1–2 weeks, this disease is of major economic importance. Most cases occur in adult horses but affected animals may be in the range of 1–10 years. The cause is unknown and no treatment appears to have any effect on the course of the disease. Cases may occur sporadically or as 'outbreaks' but no infectious agent has been isolated nor are the lesions suggestive of viral, bacterial or other infection. Two causes have been suggested, endotoxemia due to a bacterial toxin (8), and exhaustion shock (9). *E. coli* endotoxin, infused rapidly intravenously into ponies, produces a similar clinical and pathological picture (10). Although the histories of many cases of colitis-X suggest that the animals were subjected to stress, including transport, deprivation of food or water, disease or abdominal surgery for the treatment of colic, prior to the development of the disease, many horses are affected without such a history. On the other hand the lesions seen do suggest that spontaneous exhaustion shock is the cause of death.

Clinically there is a very sudden onset of enteritis, or occasionally intestinal distention with gas, and death in 3–24 hours (11). The horse suddenly becomes depressed, shows muddy, discolored mucosae, a very fast (100/min) small amplitude pulse, patchy sweating, moderate dyspnea and abdominal pain. In the early stages the temperature may rise to 39·5°C (103°F) but soon falls to become subnormal terminally, and the skin feels cold and clammy almost from the first signs of illness. The horse becomes very weak and is inclined to collapse where it stands, lie over on its side and die quietly a few minutes later. The pupils are dilated. Profuse diarrhea may or may not occur, animals surviving for less than 3–4 hours tending to have normal feces even on rectal examination. There is a complete absence of intestinal sounds. Dehydration is evident in animals which survive for longer periods. On hematological examination elevation of the blood urea nitrogen (BUN) (over 60 mg/dl) and hemoconcentration are evident; the packed cell volume may be as high as 70%. A marked acidosis develops and there may be a leukopenia. There is a severe hypokalemia, serum potassium levels may be as low as 1·5 mmol/l down from a normal of 2·5–3·7 mmol/l, and the oral administration of potassium is recommended as part of the treatment, the potassium content of erythrocytes being used as a guide to the effectiveness of the treatment (19).

There are extensive lesions at necropsy examination (10), the most dramatic being in the large intestine, especially the cecum and ventral colon. These include hyperemia, extensive petechiation, and edema of the gut wall in the early stages, and later an intense, greenish black, hemorrhagic necrosis. The contents are fluid, often foamy and foul-smelling and may be bloodstained. Lesions in the small intestine are minimal (12).

From clinical and necropsy examinations it is possible to confuse the disease with enteritis due to salmonella infection, to treatment with tetracyclines, or to arsenic poisoning. Before death, difficulty may be encountered in distinguishing between colitis-X and acute intestinal obstruction, or thromboembolic colic caused by occlusion of the cecocolic arteries by *Strongylus vulgaris* larvae.

EQUINE INTESTINAL CLOSTRIDIOSIS

This is a rare acute highly fatal diarrhea in horses associated with large numbers of *Clostridium perfringens* type A in the intestinal tract (13, 16). The disease is characterized clinically by a sudden onset of depression, a profus, watery, foul-smelling diarrhea, circulatory failure and death within 24 hours (17). Hyperemia, edema and hemorrhages of the cecum and colon are characteristic and degenerative lesions of the liver and myocardium are common. The lesions are attributed to abnormally high numbers of *Clostridium perfringens* type A in the intestinal tract but the cause of the colonization and excessive proliferation of the organism is unknown. The feeding of a diet rich in protein with a relatively low content of cellulose in combination with stress is being considered as a triggering mechanism. Equine intestinal clostridiosis is very similar to colitis-X. It has been produced experimentally by dosing horses with a culture of the organism (13) and by injecting *Cl. perfringens* type A toxin intravenously (18). Clinicopathological findings included hypoglycemia and leukopenia.

Treatment of acute equine diarrhea

If a horse with acute diarrhea is to survive it must have massive parenteral fluid therapy and very large doses of corticosteroids; the oral administration of fluids containing electrolytes is likely to exacerbate the condition (14). The methods to be used in correcting the errors of fluid and electrolyte status, and of acid–base balance are presented elsewhere under that heading. It is possible to make generalizations about the nature and the volume of the treatments to be administered, based on the duration of the diarrhea and on whether or not a foal is being suckled. However, the departures from these general rules are so frequent and so potentially dangerous that decisions about optimal fluid therapy should be based on the patient's blood gas and electrolyte status (26).

The use of antimicrobials in acute diarrheas of the horse is controversial. If the case is one of salmonellosis it is considered by some to be essential to treat it with antibiotics; by others it is thought to be contraindicated because it is likely to damage the existing intestinal flora. It is probably best to follow the middle path and restrict treatment to parenteral routes, and use broad-spectrum products such as ampicillin, chloramphenicol or potentiated sulfonamides. It is generally agreed that treatment of salmonellosis with an antibiotic (intravenous chloramphenicol, 20–30 mg/kg body weight every 6–8 hours) is highly recommended provided it can be administered *very* early. What constitutes early is the crux of the matter. In our experience a very careful clinical surveillance needs to be maintained, and the onset of diarrhea with a temperature of 38·5°C (101°F) or more should be an indication for immediate treatment with the chosen antibacterial agent. If the animal has had diarrhea for 24 hours before treatment is administered a good response would not be anticipated, and antibiotics should be withheld. The surveillance should include hematological examination because in animals affected by salmonellosis there is a preclinical precipitate fall in total leukocyte count and an elevation of temperature. This sort of surveillance is profitable, and probably necessary, in a hospital environment where the stress of surgery could be expected to lead to clinical salmonellosis in a previously symptomless salmonella 'carrier'. A similar circumstance would be in a group of horses in which one or more cases of salmonellosis had already occurred.

Additional supportive therapy is restricted largely to the use of a corticosteroid. This needs to be given early and in a large dose. Dexamethasone at a dose rate of 250 mg intravenously, and repeated at 8 hour intervals is recommended (15). Oral treatment with astringent mixtures including kaolin, chalk and catechu are used but with minimal expectations.

REVIEW LITERATURE

O'Brien, K. (1985) Differential diagnosis of diarrhea in adult horses. *In Practice*, 7 (2), 52 to 60.

Whitlock, R. H. (1986) Colitis: differential diagnosis and treatment. *Equ. vet. J.*, *18*, 278–283.

REFERENCES

(1) Argenzio, R. A. (1975) *Cornell Vet.*, *65*, 303.
(2) White, G. & Prior, S. D. (1982) *Vet. Rec.*, *111*, 316.
(3) Cook, W. R. (1973) *Vet. Rec.*, *93*, 15.
(4) Baker, J. A. & Leyland, A. (1973) *Vet. Rec.*, *93*, 583.
(5) Manahan, E. F. (1970) *Aust. vet. J.*, *46*, 231.
(6) Baker, J. R. (1975) *Vet. Ann.*, *15*, 178.
(7) Teigland, M. B. (1960) *Proc. 6th ann. Mtg Am. Assoc. equ. Practnrs*, 81.
(8) Carroll, E. J. et al. (1965) *J. Am. vet. med. Assoc.*, *146*, 1300.
(9) Rooney J. R. et al. (1966) *Cornell Vet.*, *56*, 220.
(10) Burrows, G. E. & Cannon, J. (1970) *Am. J. vet. Res.*, *31*, 1967.
(11) Pickrell, J. W. (1968) *Mod. vet. Pract.*, *49*, 63.
(12) Hudson, R. S. (1968) *Auburn Vet.*, *24*, 92.
(13) Wierup, M. (1977) *Acta vet. Scand.*, Suppl. 62, 1.
(14) Merritt, A. M. (1975) *J. S. Afr. vet. med. Assoc.*, *46*, 89.
(15) Olson, N. E. (1966) *J. Am. vet. med. Assoc.*, *48*, 418.
(16) Ackermann, W. & Kleine, B. (1978) *Berl. Münch. Tierärztl. Wochenschr.*, *91*, 141.
(17) Bojorquez, N. L. (1979) *Rev. latinoam. Microbiol.*, *21*, 61.
(18) Ochoa, R. & Kern, S. R. (1980) *Vet. Pathol.*, *17*, 738.
(19) Muylle, E. et al. (1984) *Equ. vet. J.*, *16*, 450.
(20) Suzuki, T. et al. (1986) *J. Jap. vet. med. Assoc.*, *39*, 13.
(21) Whitlock, R. H. (1984) *J. Am. vet. med. Assoc.*, *185*, 1210.
(22) Raisbeck, M. F. et al. (1981) *J. Am. vet. med. Assoc.*, *179*, 362.
(23) Morris, D. D. et al. (1983) *Cornell Vet.*, *73*, 265.
(24) Huang, J. C. M. et al. (1983) *Vet. Rec.*, *113*, 262.
(25) Gregory, M. W. et al. (1986) *J. comp. Pathol.*, **96**, 109.
(26) Wilson, E. A. & Green, R. A. (1986) *J. equ. vet. Sci.*, 6, 321.

Chronic undifferentiated diarrhea of horses

This is a group of diseases with almost identical clinical signs of chronic diarrhea, long course, moderate appetite and gradual weight loss. Most cases are irreversible after a short period and most affected animals are destroyed.

Etiology

A group of diseases has been identified as causes of chronic diarrhea and on physical clinical examination they are not readily separable. Of the causes of chronic diarrhea, massive strongyle larval migration is most commonly recorded (1), followed by granulomatous enteritis, which may itself be a manifestation of tissue strongylosis (2), and primary hepatic insufficiency. Less common causes include avian tuberculosis, lymphosarcoma (3), gastric carcinoma, and chronic infections with *Corynebacterium* (*Rhodococcus*) *equi* or *Strongylus* spp. Less common still are the multifactorial cases with a number of significant causative agents present in the one animal, e.g. ulcerative colitis, salmonellosis and histoplasmosis (4). There is still an unidentifiable residuum, which may in some series be as many as two-thirds of the cases. Of these idiopathic cases about one-half have a history of preceding stress such as illness or exposure, severe exertion, or treatment with large doses of tetracycline. In some cases the prior illness has been treated with antibiotics including penicillin and streptomycin or a combination of both. This has led to the commonly held view that antibiotics which are excreted via the bile, and thus reach the intestine, frequently cause colitis. Terramycin has the worst reputation in this regard (15).

One of the earlier suggested causes, *Trichomonas fecalis* (or *T. equi*) (5) is no longer considered to have any significance. It is true that in a minority of cases the flora on wet fecal smear is dominated by these protozoa, but this is now regarded as a result of the altered physical and chemical composition of the intestinal content rather than a cause of it (6–8). The accepted association in other species and foals between rotavirus and coronavirus and diarrhea suggests the possibility of this association in adult horses. Such a virus infection would not be expected to produce the extreme chronicity characteristic of many cases of chronic diarrhea in adult horses.

The strong suggestion remains that many cases are parasitic in origin because of the common occurrence of colitis and vasculitis, but there is the disconcerting occurrence of the same lesions in clinically normal horses which tends to refute the hypothesis. It may be a matter of measuring the lesions and relating cause and effect in a quantitative way. It would seem to be simpler to compare the incidence of the disease in groups of horses in which strongylosis was, or was not, eliminated. There is a recurring clinical suspicion that foals can be congenitally deficient in intestinal disaccharidase,

Table 99. Causes of chronic diarrhea in horses.

Identified cause	*Percentage of all causes* US data (9)	Australian data (6)
Strongyle larval migration	43	10
Stress induced	nil	35
Granulomatous enteritis	11	nil
Edema small intestinal wall	11	nil
Chronic liver disease	7	10
Chronic *Corynebacterium* (*Rhodococcus*) *equi* infection	4	nil
Salmonellosis	4	nil
Neoplasia (gastric carcinoma, intestinal lymphosarcoma)	4	3
Tetracycline-induced	nil	3
No cause identified	18	39
Total number	28	31

at least temporarily, and that this can be a cause of diarrhea.

It is probable that there are many causes and that their relative importance varies between locations. To give some idea of the etiological complexities of the disease a comparison of causes is set down in Table 99.

Epidemiology

Several series of cases have been published recently (6, 9, 10, 18) and the disease has attracted increasing interest over the past 15 years. Although it appears so, it is not possible to say whether the prevalence has increased. The occurrence is sporadic, with only single cases occurring in a group. In-contact horses are not affected. The case fatality rate is about 35%. Most of the fatal cases are horses which eventually have to be destroyed. For an individual horse owner, the loss can be heavy if, as is usual, a great deal of time and money is devoted to treating the horse. There appears to be no age-related, sex-related, or breed-related variation in incidence, but a majority of cases are reported to commence in the colder half of the year (6). Most affected horses, like most unaffected horses, are aged 2–5 years. In these cases which appear to result from previous stress or illness there is an interval of 3–12 days between stress and signs.

Pathogenesis

No lesion other than those recorded as specific to parasitic gastroenteritis, lymphosarcoma, or carcinoma is identifiable. The myoneural plexuses are normal. The disease appears to be functional in many cases and may be due to malabsorption caused by a primary biochemical lesion in the mucosa of the small intestine. There may (20) or may not (17) be protein loss into the intestine, perhaps related to the age and severity of the lesion. Hypoalbuminemia does occur, but may be caused by factors other than a protein-losing enteropathy. In a search for a pathogenetic mechanism, an investigation has been conducted of the volatile fatty acid concentration in the colonic contents, but with no definite results (14). However, the colonic contents of affected horses have a greatly different fermentative capacity to those of normal horses, reinforcing the hypothesis that the disease is essentially one of abnormal colonic digestion and absorption (19).

Clinical findings

The characteristic finding is chronic diarrhea. The feces vary in consistency from thick porridge, through undigested fibers in liquid, to liquid without fiber. The consistency of the feces in an individual horse may vary widely from one day to the next. The duration of the diarrhea may be as long as a year and a half but most cases are terminated by death, euthanasia or recovery in 5–8 weeks.

The onset of diarrhea is sudden and there is severe weight loss initially followed by a long period of relative stability, or at most gradual weight loss. There is an accompanying anemia but no fever and no apparent toxemia, the horses for the most part remaining bright and alert and maintaining their appetite. The feces remain porridge-like. For no apparent reason there are intermittent periods of several days duration during which there is depression, inappetence and a more watery diarrhea. Biochemical tests of absorption and digestion are limited in their applicability for the reason that a period of enforced starvation is usually followed by an episode of severe diarrhea.

Clinical pathology

An examination of feces for helminth eggs should be undertaken. An investigation should also be undertaken for the oocysts of *Eimeria leuckarti*. It is also a common practice to examine a wet smear, taken directly from the horse to avoid death of the protozoa which do not survive cooling, storage or transport. Large numbers of motile protozoa are found in these smears in a few cases but have no apparent significance. The use of a glucose or xylose (11) absorption test or a corn starch digestion/absorption test (6) is warranted to determine whether there is a specific malabsorption of carbohydrates. Of these tests the D(+)xylose absorption test is most recommended (9). A protein-losing enteropathy is not usually present but a total protein estimation, and an albumin-globulin separation, should be carried out to detect if it is (23). A mild to moderate hypoalbuminemia should suggest the presence of liver disease or granulomatous enteritis. Conversely an increase in serum beta-globulin is indicative of prepatent strongylosis. To check for the presence of eosinophilia a differential leukocyte count should be carried out on blood, and on peritoneal fluid obtained by paracentesis. A bromosulfalein clearance test to detect reduced hepatic function is recommended because of the surprisingly frequent occurrence in horses of a non-specific hepatopathy, although most such cases have constipation rather than diarrhea.

Culture of feces is recommended because the rare cases of chronic salmonellosis, enteritis due to *Corynebacterium* (*Rhodococcus*) *equi*, and *Mycobacterium avium* need to be detected. The latter is more likely to be detected by examination of a rectal mucosal biopsy for acid-fast organisms. Although *Salmonella* sp. are occasionally incriminated in a search for a cause, they are not often detectable in a fecal swab from the living horse. Biopsy of the intestinal wall is helpful in determining the presence of enteritis but because it requires general anesthesia and laparotomy, it is not usually used.

Necropsy findings

There are no identifying gross necropsy findings. Bacteriological examination occasionally detects salmonellae in mesenteric lymph nodes but their etiological significance is doubtful. Histopathological examination may reveal the presence of enteritis in the large intestine, and occasionally in the small intestine. The tissue reaction may be primarily eosinophilic or basophilic (12). The colitis varies in severity but is strongly reminiscent of parasitic colitis, and there are also vascular lesions in the blood vessels of the colon in most cases. The findings in the specific causes, e.g. lymphosarcoma, gastric carcinoma, granulomatous enteritis, are characteristic of those diseases.

Diagnosis

There may be difficulty in defining undifferentiated chronic diarrhea in horses. It is suggested that the criteria should include the presence of diarrhea for a period of more than 1 week, stability of clinical signs other than the gradual decline of body weight, and lack of response to standard treatment.

The existence of large numbers of migrating strongyle larvae is usually treated by the administration of large doses (500 mg/kg body weight) of thiabendazole, sometimes on 2 successive days. Recovery is usually accepted as establishing the causal relationship. More difficult to interpret is the frequent temporary remission of diarrhea for several days. This could be due to the destruction of larvae in blood vessels, but continuation of the signs because irreversible damage has been done to the intestinal vasculature by the larvae. Although little significance can be attached to the nature of the feces it is our experience that in strongylosis the feces are cow-like in consistency, in the other diseases they are profuse and watery. The presence of a verminous aneurysm may provide contributory evidence of strongylosis, but the frequency with which these are detected in pastured horses, even when they are clinically normal, detracts from their significance. A marked eosinophilia is more noteworthy and is regarded as being diagnostic of strongyle larval migration. The consistency of its presence is doubtful, and one of the great needs in strongylosis control is a laboratory test to detect the presence of larvae in tissues, a test comparable to the plasma pepsinogen test in ostertagiasis in cattle.

In specific locations Potomac horse fever (equine intestinal ehrlichiosis) must now be considered in the differential diagnosis. Laboratory tests are essential for this task.

The diagnosis of chronic hepatic insufficiency is dealt with elsewhere and there is no special characteristic of it in horses. Squamous cell carcinoma of the stomach is not usually accompanied by diarrhea and lymphosarcoma is a more likely neoplastic cause of chronic diarrhea in horses (3). Its detection depends on the presence of lymphocytes with mitotic figures in the peritoneal fluid, and possibly by physically palpable mesenteric lymph nodes.

Treatment

The only treatment which appears to have a curative effect on a significant number of cases is ten times the normal dose of thiabendazole orally (i.e. 500 mg/kg body weight). Some authors (9) recommend that the dose be repeated on successive days.

Many other treatments have been recorded but none is recommended. They are listed below but there is little information about the results obtained. Spontaneous recovery does occur, particularly in young horses, and this, and the often lengthy duration (6–12 months) of the illness, make it difficult to decide accurately the value of the treatment. On the basis that many cases are due to an immunodeficiency, affected horses have been treated with equine immunoglobulins. Parenteral treatment has not been effective but excellent results are recorded after the oral administration of normal horse serum (1 liter daily for 3 days by stomach tube) (13). In spite of inability to isolate a virus, or to produce significant titers of antibody in experimental horses, the administration of serum from these horses in large quantities by mouth has been claimed to be a successful treatment (16).

Symptomatic relief can be obtained by the oral administration of tincture of opium (30–80 ml twice daily for 2 days then once daily). Overdosing may result in the development of impaction colic and a number of horses show severe disorientation, compulsive walking and intractability, characteristic of opium toxicity. Diarrhea returns unabated within 24 hours of ceasing treatment. Corticosteroids in standard doses consistently stop the diarrhea but only transiently. Other treatments which have a similar temporary effect when applied over a 3–5 day period are penicillin, streptomycin, sulfonamides, salazopyrine, sodium arsanilate, iodochlorhydroxyquin (Vioform, Enterovioform) and metronidazole (1·5–2·5 g daily for 5 days), all given orally. Parenterally administered drugs to which the same comments apply are sulfadimidine, streptomycin, neomycin, chloramphenicol, ampicillin, a combination of trimethoprim and sulfadiazine, antihistamines and intravenous macrodex (a high molecular weight dextran in 6% solution). Phenoxybenzamine is used extensively and gives many temporary improvements and some complete recoveries. The dose rate is 2 mg/kg body weight given intravenously in two or three divided doses at 24 hour intervals (1, 21). Two other related antidiarrheals, iodochlorhydroxyquinoline (clioquinol) and chlorhydroxyquinoline (Halquinol) bring temporary relief to the diarrhea (22). Vioform (Enterovioform) is among the most effective drugs but still has only a temporary effect. The recommended treatment regimen consists of Vioform 15 g daily until the feces are firm, then reduce the dose by 1 g daily until the dose is 2 g and maintain this level for a further 7 days. The treatment is exhausting to both the horse and the veterinarian because it lasts 4–5 weeks.

A frequently used but invariably unsuccessful treatment is to attempt to repopulate the bowel with normal flora (5) on the assumption that defloration is the basis of the disease. Daily infusions by stomach tube for 3 days with 12 liters of an infusion of feces or intestinal contents from a normal horse are recommended. To avoid destruction of the administered protozoa as they pass through the stomach, and the small intestine, 100 g of sodium bicarbonate are added to the infusion but without apparent advantage. A few cases have recovered after intestinal biopsy, during which a similar infusion was introduced directly into the cecum. Administration of an infusion by enema is unsuccessful.

Supportive therapy must include fluids and electrolytes. At most times the provision of electrolytes in the drinking water is sufficient to maintain body electrolyte levels. However, during severe bouts of diarrhea it may be necessary to provide them by parenteral infusion. Horses which become very lethargic after long periods of diarrhea, may be severely depleted of plasma sodium and may require an intensive course of parenteral sodium administration.

REVIEW LITERATURE

Roberts, M. C. (1985) Malabsorption syndromes in the horse. *Comp. cont. Educ.*, *7*, S637–S646.

REFERENCES

(1) Hunt, J. M. & Gerring, E. L. (1985) *Equ. vet. J.*, *17*, 399.
(2) Blackwell, N. J. (1973) *Vet. Rec.*, *93*, 401.
(3) Crawley, G. R. (1985) *Vet. Med.*, *80*, 66.
(4) Goetz, T. E. & Coffman, J. R. (1984) *Equ. vet. J.*, *16*, 439.
(5) Laufenstein-Duff, H. (1969) *J. Am. vet. med. Assoc.*, *155*, 1835.
(6) Gay, C. C. & Blood, D. C. (1976) *Proc. 53rd ann. Conf. Aust. vet. Assoc., Melbourne*, 130.
(7) Damron, G. W. (1976) *Am. J. vet. Res.*, *37*, 25.
(8) Manahan, F. F. (1970) *Aust. vet. J.*, *46*, 231.
(9) Merritt, A. M. et al. (1975) *J. S. Afr. vet. Assoc.*, *46*, 73, 89.
(10) Lundvall, R. L. & Romberg, P. F. (1960) *J. Am. vet. med. Assoc.*, *137*, 481.
(11) Roberts, M. C. (1974) *Equ. vet. J.*, *6*, 28.
(12) Pass, D. A. et al. (1984) *Vet. Pathol.*, *21*, 362.
(13) Targowski, S. P. (1976) *Am. J. vet. Res.*, *37*, 29.
(14) Merritt, A. M. & Smith, D. A. (1980) *Am. J. vet. Res.*, *41*, 928.
(15) Owen, R. A. P. (1980) *Vet. Rec.*, *107*, 94.
(16) Gustafson, D. P. & Page, E. H. (1977) *Proc. 22nd ann. conv. Am. Assoc. equ. Practnrs*, p. 167.
(17) Merritt, A. M. et al. (1977) *Am. J. vet. Res.*, *38*, 1769.
(18) Nielsen, K. & Vibe-Petersen, G. (1979) *Nord. VetMed.*, *31*, 376.
(19) Minder, H. P. et al. (1980) *Am. J. vet. Res.*, *41*, 564.
(20) Dietz, H. H. & Nielsen, K. (1980) *Nord. VetMed.*, *32*, 369.
(21) Hood, D. M. et al. (1982) *J. Am. vet. med. Assoc.*, *180*, 758.
(22) O'Brien, J. K. (1981) *Vet. Rec.*, *109*, 60.
(23) Platt, H. (1986) *J. comp. Pathol.*, *96*, 671.

Granulomatous enteritis of horses

The disease is reported in horses of all ages after 1 year. It is characterized by persistent weight loss, and some of the horses have chronic diarrhea and edema associated with hypoproteinemia (4). There is malabsorption of carbohydrate and lipid and in some cases gastrointestinal loss of protein (3). Clinicopathological findings include hypoalbuminemia and decreased phagocytic activity of mesothelial cells collected in the peritoneal fluid by paracentesis. Grossly the intestinal wall is thickened uniformly especially in the jejunum and ileum. Histologically the principal lesion is in the lamina propria of the small intestine. It is infiltrated through most of its length by lymphocytes and histiocytes. There is granuloma formation under the muscularis mucosa and partial villous atrophy (1, 3–5). Minor lesions may be present in the stomach and colon. In most cases the cause is not identified but cyathastome infestation is present in some (6). No acid-fast organisms are present (7).

The lymph nodes are enlarged and also contain granulomatous nodules. When there are local thickenings and enlarged lymph nodes these can be readily palpated by rectal examination.

The serum albumin level is of the order of 0·8 g/dl and is accompanied by subcutaneous edema. It appears to be due to a protein-losing enteropathy. Mild colic sometimes occurs intermittently. The lesions can be identified by laparotomy through the right flank in the standing horse (2). Xylose absorption tests are informative but may be positive or negative depending on whether there is diffuse involvement of the small intestine.

REFERENCES

(1) Cimprich, R. E. (1974) *Vet. Pathol.*, *11*, 535.
(2) Merritt, A. M. et al. (1976) *J. Am. vet. med. Assoc.*, *169*, 603.
(3) Meuten, D. J. et al. (1978) *J. Am. vet. med. Assoc.*, *172*, 326.
(4) Roberts, M. C. & Kelly, W. R. (1980) *Aust. vet. J.*, *56*, 230.
(5) Bester, R. C. & Coetzer, J. A. W. (1978) *J. S. Afr. vet. Assoc.*, *49*, 351.
(6) Jasko, D. J. & Roth, L. (1984) *J. Am. vet. med. Assoc.*, *185*, 553.
(7) Sweeney, R. W. et al. (1986) *J. Am. vet. med. Assoc.*, *188*, 1192.

Chronic eosinophilic gastroenteritis of horses

This sporadic disease of young, adult horses is characterized by soft, formless feces or diarrhea, malabsorption and loss of body weight and by the presence of eosinophilic infiltrates in a chronic inflammatory reaction affecting the esophagus, stomach, small and large intestines and mesenteric lymph nodes (1). The cause has not been identified but the lesion suggests a continuing hypersensitivity reaction to an ingested allergen.

REFERENCE

(1) Pass, D. A. & Bolton, J. R. (1982) *Vet. Pathol.*, *19*, 486.

Porcine proliferative enteritis complex (intestinal adenomatosis, necrotic enteritis, regional enteritis, proliferative hemorrhagic enteropathy of swine)

The porcine proliferative enteritis complex affects pigs from weaning age to feeder pigs and young gilts, sows and boars and is characterized clinically by diarrhea, loss of body weight and inappetence in recently weaned pigs, and sudden death in feeder pigs, young gilts and boars. Pathologically the lesions are characterized by proliferation of immature crypt epithelial cells, elongation of crypts, loss of villi and inflammation of the lamina propria of primarily the ileum, but the jejunum, cecum and colon may be involved. The essential lesions are proliferative and there seems to be an etiological and pathological relationship between porcine intestinal adenomatosis, necrotic enteritis, regional enteritis and hemorrhagic enteropathy of swine.

Etiology

The etiology is uncertain but *Campylobacter sputorum* subsp. *mucosalis* and *Campylobacter hyointestinalis* can be isolated from the intestines of pigs with lesions of proliferative ileitis (1–3). Proliferative hemorrhagic enteropathies are frequently associated with the presence of a proliferative enteropathy; however, attempts to transmit the hemorrhagic syndrome have failed (15). It has been more difficult to recover the organism from cases of proliferative hemorrhagic enteropathy than from cases of porcine intestinal adenomatosis. The organism can usually be recovered in large numbers from the affected mucosa of adenomatosis cases. On the other hand, the organism may not be present or present only in small numbers in the mucosa of pigs dying of proliferative hemorrhagic enteropathy (4). It has been suggested that proliferative hemorrhagic enteropathy is a particular manifestation of porcine intestinal adenomatosis in which intestinal hemorrhage is a feature (4). The difficulty in recovering the organism may be related to the observation that large amounts of IgA are present in affected intestinal tissues of pigs with proliferative hemorrhagic enteropathy (4) despite the visible presence of large numbers of bacteria.

The strains of *Campylobacter sputorum* subsp. *mucosalis* isolated in the United Kingdom and Australia are biochemically identical and there is a strong crossreaction between the strains isolated in both countries from proliferative hemorrhagic enteropathy in pigs in Australia and porcine intestinal adenomatosis in pigs in the United Kingdom (5).

Epidemiology

Porcine proliferative enteritis occurs in recently weaned pigs and is characterized by a sudden onset of loss of condition and weight and inappetence. Subclinical porcine intestinal adenomatosis may be the cause of suboptimal weight loss in growing pigs (21). There is some evidence to suggest that the porcine intestinal adenomatosis complex may be associated with malabsorption of dietary proteins (25). A cumulative sum technique reveals that about 2·5% of all pigs in a closed herd may be affected with porcine intestinal adenomatosis which can be detected only by necropsy of randomly selected pigs (21). Sera collected from healthy pigs at slaughter reveal a large percentage of animals with high titers to *C. sputorum* subsp. *mucosalis* (31). Serological surveys of swine sera indicate that the majority of pigs have agglutinating antibodies to both species of *Campylobacter* and that newborn pigs obtain colostral titers (14).

There is a positive correlation between the presence of *Campylobacter hyointestinalis* and/or *Campylobacter sputorum* subsp. *mucosalis* and lesions of proliferative enteritis (16). It is unusual to recover *C. sputorum* subsp. *mucosalis* in any numbers from the alimentary tract of pigs other than those affected with proliferative enteritis or one of the related diseases. However, it is present in the oral cavity of some pigs in herds in which the disease is occurring (19). This suggests that the organism may be spread through contact in the saliva. *C. sputorum* subsp. *mucosalis* cannot be recovered from histologically normal areas of the intestine of pigs with lesions of porcine intestinal adenomatosis which yield the organism (17). Experimentally the organism spreads from inoculated piglets to uninoculated piglets within 24–48 hours after infection (17). The organism can be isolated from mouth swabs of experimentally infected pigs for several weeks (19). The weaned pigs are resistant to experimental infection unless pretreated with benzetimide to reduce gastrointestinal peristalsis (18).

Campylobacter hyointestinalis can also be isolated from pigs with lesions of proliferative enteritis (3) and in association with other enteropathogens of pigs (20). It can be distinguished from other *Campylobacter* spp. (24).

Proliferative hemorrhagic enteropathy is one form of the proliferative enteritis complex and has been reported from the United Kingdom (7), Europe (9), Australia (6), Asia and the United States (10), but appears to occur in most countries. It is especially common in hysterectomy-derived or specific pathogen free (SPF) herds and has a higher prevalence in the hot summer period. In some countries its prevalence is increasing and it is emerging as a major syndrome in SPF herds. The disease can occur in all ages of postweaned pigs, but it has a high incidence in young replacement gilts and boars at 6–9 months of age and in pigs approximately 4–8 weeks after weaning. The high incidence in replacement gilts may be due to suppression of the disease by low-level feeding of antibacterial agents during the growing period (6), but frequently the syndrome appears first in gilts and some time later in the growing pigs. In gilts the outbreak is explosive, but generally shortlived with morbidity of up to 50% of the group occurring within a 2–3 week period. Mortality is generally no greater than 6%. In large herds with continual addition to the replacement gilt herd and in herds where the disease occurs in grower pigs outbreaks may be more prolonged. The disease in growers generally has equivalent morbidity and mortality rates, but is more severe in that runting of surviving and contemporary pigs may occur.

The disease in all ages is frequently associated with the concurrent occurrence of porcine intestinal adenomatosis, but it is unknown whether the hemorrhagic syndrome results from some insult to the intestine which also predisposes to a proliferative enteropathy and invasion by *Campylobacter* spp., or whether it is simply an acute manifestation of this disease. The related syndromes of necrotic enteritis and regional ileitis can be found in apparently healthy pigs examined at slaughter (7).

Pathogenesis

The pathogenesis is not well understood. In porcine intestinal adenomatosis there is proliferation of the epithelial cells of the mucosa of the ileum and the development of an adenomatous epithelium which is deficient in enzymes normally found in mature absorptive cells (8). The affected epithelial cells contain the bacteria free in the cytoplasm. It is suggested that the proliferative lesion of porcine intestinal adenomatosis is the primary lesion of the four enteropathies.

Experimental inoculation of neonatal piglets with *Campylobacter sputorum* subsp. *mucosalis* results in infection of the intestinal mucosa, but adenomatous changes do not occur (17). The oral inoculation of gnotobiotic piglets with *C. sputorum* subsp. *mucosalis* results in colonization of the intestine for several weeks but did not induce adenomatosis (17). The oral inoculation of specific-pathogen free (SPF) pigs (26) or cesarean-derived colostrum-deprived piglets (27) with a crude inoculum from intestinal mucosa or cultures of *Campylobacter sputorum* subsp. *mucosalis* resulted in lesions of proliferative enteritis. The necessity for a crude inoculum of homogenized intestinal mucosa suggests that other agents, or more than one species of *Campylobacter*, are involved in the etiology and pathogenesis of porcine intestinal adenomatosis. The oral inoculation of gnotobiotic pigs with broth cultures of both *C. sputorum* subsp. *mucosalis* and *C. hyointestinalis* resulted in colonization of the intestine but did not induce proliferative enteritis (28). It has not been possible to reproduce porcine intestinal adenomatosis with pure cultures of either *C. sputorum* subsp. *mucosalis* or *C. hyointestinalis* (30).

The proliferative lesion may result in suboptimal performance in otherwise normal pigs or unthriftiness, or be manifested as acute intestinal hemorrhage during the recovery stages of intestinal adenomatosis.

Clinical findings

Porcine intestinal adenomatosis occurs in pigs weaned 4–6 weeks previously and is characterized by a sudden onset of loss of condition and weight and inappetence. Affected pigs are afebrile and diarrhea occurs, but is unremarkable. Often it is a chronic, non-specific, intermittent diarrhea in pigs from 7 to 16 weeks of age (2). Most cases recover spontaneously within 6 weeks of the onset of signs. When inflammation and necrosis have resulted in necrotic enteritis and regional ileitis, diarrhea and severe weight loss occur followed by death, often by ileal perforation in the case of regional ileitis.

Proliferative hemorrhagic enteropathy occurs in young gilts and boars and is manifested primarily by sudden death associated with the presence of large amounts of blood in loose feces. Others within the group may show skin pallor and hemorrhagic feces with fibrin casts but otherwise appear clinically normal. In some pigs there is continual blood loss and death occurs within 48 hours of the onset of hemorrhage but in the majority the hemorrhage is transient. Fever is not a feature and the majority of pigs suffer only a minor setback for a 2 week period. A small percentage develop chronic illthrift.

In grower pigs the disease is economically more severe. As in gilts acute death with marked skin pallor and without premonitory signs can occur but survivors show illthrift and as the outbreak progresses contemporary pigs may show a chronic syndrome of illthrift with the periodic passage of bloody feces.

Necropsy findings

In pigs with porcine intestinal adenomatosis the prominent lesions are in the terminal ileum and anterior portion of the large intestine. Grossly there is thickening of the mucosa and submucosa of the terminal ileum and histologically the lesion consists of immature proliferating epithelial cells (benign adenoma). The organism is visible intracellularly and can be recovered in large numbers. *C. sputorum* subsp. *mucosalis* can be recovered in large numbers from adenomatous tissue, in lower numbers from luminal contents, and is absent or present in only low numbers in non-adenomatous mucosa of affected pigs. A microagglutination test can be used to distinguish between the different species of *Campylobacter* (14). An indirect fluorescent antibody test can be used to detect *C. sputorum* subsp. *mucosalis* and *C. hyointestinalis* in sections of ileal mucosa (16). In necrotic enteritis the thickened mucosa is yellow-gray due to the coagulation necrosis of the adenomatous mucosa. In regional ileitis (called hosepipe gut) the distal ileum is rigid due to thickening of the intestinal wall caused by muscular hypertrophy and granulation tissue formation.

In proliferative hemorrhagic enteropathy there is marked pallor and often a marble-white appearance to the carcass. The characteristic findings are in the intestine. In contrast to porcine intestinal adenomatosis in which there is an absence of an inflammatory response, in proliferative hemorrhagic enteropathy there is evidence of an acute inflammatory response. There is massive hemorrhage into the intestinal lumen with free blood and frequently the presence of fibrinous casts (29). The mucosa and submucosa are thickened and the lumen may contain a solid cast consisting of a large blood clot contoured to the mucosal folds. In some cases there is a fibrinous membrane covering and adhering to the mucosa. The hemorrhage extends from a variable level of the small intestine, but usually from the ileum throughout the large intestine. Although the intestinal wall may be hemorrhagic there may be no obvious points of hemorrhage. Histologically, there is evidence of vascular congestion, fibrin thrombi, increased permeability of blood vessels and necrosis of intestinal mucosa. The lesion resembles an acute bacterial infection and type I hypersensitivity reaction. Extensive accumulations of eosinophils are visible throughout the mucosa. The organisms can be seen in proliferating immature cells which line greatly elongated crypts that are devoid of villi. The organism is difficult to recover from cases of proliferative hemorrhagic enteropathy.

Diagnosis

The characteristic clinical findings of porcine intestinal adenomatosis are inappetence, loss of weight and mild diarrhea in recently weaned pigs. This must be differentiated from postweaning coliform gastroenteritis which is much more severe clinically and rapid deaths occur. The postweaning drop in average daily gain (*postweaning check*) occurs within several days after weaning and recovery occurs within several days following consumption of a normal daily intake of feed.

Proliferative hemorrhagic enteropathy occurs in feeder pigs, young gilts and boars and is characterized by sudden death and extreme pallor of the skin. It must be differentiated from fatal hemorrhagic esophagogastric ulceration, acute swine dysentery and intestinal hemorrhage syndrome.

Esophagogastric ulcer occurs in all ages of pigs but especially in growers and the necropsy finding of ulceration in the non-glandular portion of the stomach at the esophageal entrance along with hemorrhage into the stomach with passage into the intestines provides easy differentiation. Acute death with intestinal hemorrhage occurs occasionally in swine dysentery. It is more common in adults affected with the disease and at the onset of an outbreak, skin pallor is not as marked and the hemorrhage is restricted to the large intestine and is associated with the characteristic lesions of swine dysentery in this area. Contemporary pigs show clinical and necropsy findings typical for this disease and the diagnosis can be confirmed with laboratory studies.

The intestinal hemorrhage syndrome is more difficult to differentiate from the proliferative hemorrhagic enteropathy. It occurs most commonly in 3–6-month-old pigs that are well-nourished and many but not all outbreaks have been associated with whey feeding (11, 12). Typically, it is associated with abdominal distention and evidence of abdominal pain preceding death and the presence of marked intestinal tympany on postmortem examination. In many cases, hemorrhage in the intestine appears to result from torsion which occludes the mesenteric veins. It occurs in all areas of the intestine except the proximal duodenum and stomach which have separate drainage. Due to intestinal distention the torsion may be easily missed but it is best determined by the abnormal cranial direction of the blind end of the cecum and palpation of the mesentery. This distribution of hemorrhage may occur without the occurrence of torsion and the etiology in these cases is unknown.

Other diseases such as infectious necrotic enteritis associated with *Clostridium perfringens* type C may cause hemorrhage into the intestine but they are easily differentiated on clinical, epidemiological and laboratory findings (13).

Treatment and control

Treatment of individually affected pigs is not usually undertaken. Recovery is prolonged. There are varying reports of the efficacy of individual antibiotics in the control of the disease which might reflect its possible varied etiology. In one outbreak, furazolidine (200 mg/kg) in the feed apparently prevented the disease but other antibiotics proved of little value in control (32). In outbreaks associated with proliferative enteropathy and *Campylobacter sputorum* subsp. *mucosalis* the disease has been controlled with tylosin (200 mg/kg feed) or a combination of penicillin and chlortetracycline at 50 and 100 mg/kg of feed respectively (6)

Porcine intestinal adenomatosis can usually be controlled in newly introduced pigs by allowing them to mingle with infected recovered pigs followed by the use of medicated feed (22). This allows the development of immunity. Vaccines have been ineffective (23).

REVIEW LITERATURE

Roberts, L. (1985) Porcine intestinal adenomatosis. In: *Campylobacter*, ed. K. P. Lander. Commission of European Communities, pp. 109–121.

Yates, W. D. G., Clark, E. G., Osborne, A. D., Erweani, C. C., Radostits, O. M. & Theede, A. (1979) Proliferative hemorrhagic enteropathy in swine: an outbreak and review of the literature. *Can. vet. J.*, *20*, 261–268.

REFERENCES

(1) Lomax, L. G. & Glock, R. D. (1982) *Am. J. vet. Res.*, *43*, 1608.
(2) Wilson, T. M. et al. (1986) *Can. J. vet. Res.*, *50*, 217.
(3) Gebhart, C. J. et al. (1983) *Am. J. vet. Res.*, *44*, 361.
(4) Lawson, G. H. K. et al. (1979) *Res. vet. Sci.*, *27*, 46.
(5) Love, D. N. et al. (1977) *Vet. Rec.*, *101*, 407.
(6) Love, R. J. & Love, D. N. (1977) *Vet. Rec.*, *100*, 473.
(7) Rowland, A. C. & Hutchings, D. A. (1978) *Vet. Rec.*, *103*, 338.
(8) Rowland, A. C. et al. (1978) *Res. vet. Sci.*, *24*, 191.
(9) Meyer, P. et al. (1974) *Tijdschr. Diergeneenskd.*, *99*, 664.
(10) Kurtz, H. J. (1976) *Proc. 4th int. Congr. Pig Vet. Soc.*, N 6.
(11) O'Hara, P. J. (1972) *Vet. Rec.*, *91*, 517.
(12) Todd, J. N. et al. (1977) *Vet. Rec.*, *100*, 11.
(13) Penny, R. H. C. (1975) *Vet. Ann.*, *15*, 115.
(14) Chang, K. et al. (1985) *Am. J. vet. Res.*, *45*, 1373.
(15) Rowlands, A. C. & Rowntree, P. G. M. (1972) *Vet. Rec.*, *91*, 235.
(16) Chang, K. et al. (1984) *Am. J. vet. Res.*, *45*, 703.
(17) McCartney, E. et al. (1984) *Res. vet. Sci.*, *36*, 290.
(18) Roberts, L. et al. (1980) *Res. vet. Sci.*, *28*, 148.
(19) Roberts, L. (1981) *Vet. Rec.*, *109*, 17.
(20) Lambert, M. et al. (1984) *Vet. Rec.*, *115*, 128.
(21) Roberts, L. et al. (1979) *Vet. Rec.*, *104*, 366.
(22) Love, R. J. et al. (1977) *Vet. Rec.*, *100*, 65.
(23) Lawson, G. H. K. et al. (1980) *Vet. Rec.*, *107*, 424.
(24) Gebhart, C. J. et al. (1985) *J. clin. Microbiol.*, *21*, 715.
(25) Rowan, T. G. & Lawrence, T. L. J. (1982) *Vet. Rec.*, *110*, 306.
(26) Lomax, L. G. et al. (1982) *Am. J. vet. Res.*, *43*, 1615.
(27) Lomax, L. G. et al. (1982) *Am. J. vet. Res.*, *43*, 1622.
(28) Boosinger, T. R. et al. (1985) *Am. J. vet. Res.*, *46*, 2152.
(29) Love, D. N. & Love, R. J. (1979) *Vet. Pathol.*, *16*, 41.
(30) Roberts, L. (1985) In: *Campylobacter*, ed. K. P. Lander. Commission of European Communities, pp. 109–121.
(31) Lawson, G. H. K. et al. (1982) *Res. vet. Sci.*, *32*, 89.
(32) Chu, R. M. & Hong, C. B. (1973) *Vet. Rec.*, *93*, 562.

Esophagogastric ulceration of swine

Esophagogastric ulceration of swine has become a disease of major proportions during recent years. Examination of pigs' stomachs at abattoirs in various countries has shown that a high proportion of pigs may have ulcers or potential or healed ulcers. The incidence generally varies between 2 and 25% of stomachs examined (4) and the varying incidence between countries may reflect differences in feeding or husbandry methods. The incidence of clinical disease is not very high but the mortality rate is so great that individual farmers may suffer significant losses.

The cause of the disease has not been fully determined but largely by inference from the suspected causes of gastric ulcer in other species many agents, including rough feed and conversely the absence of sufficient fiber in the ration, high concentrations of irritant mineral mixtures improperly mixed with the grain ration, hyperacidity due to stress, and erosion of the mucosa by keratolytic fungi encouraged by a high sugar content of the diet, have been advanced as etiological agents (6). The physical form of the ration in terms of its fiber content and particle size appears of paramount importance in the induction of esophagogastric ulceration. There is now considerable evidence that cereal particle size is a major cause of gastric abnormalities. Finely ground barley (1, 5) or wheat (3) are associated with a marked increase in gastric abnormalities compared to the use of coarsely ground grains. The size of particles in feed is significant whatever feed is used, even straw; coarsely ground barley straw at 5–10% of the ration gives almost complete protection (14). On the other hand, pelleting of feed seems to increase the number of ulcers occurring (15). Oat hulls in the diet are also highly effective, 25% coarsely ground oats in a corn ration being protective (16). The physical texture can influence pepsin and acid secretion, and the fluidity of the stomach contents induced by ulcerogenic diets may destroy the normal pH gradient within the stomach. This allows greater pepsin and acid contact to the esophagogastric area (5).

The occurrence is limited to penned pigs and particularly to those receiving a heavy grain diet and growing rapidly, although the disease also occurs in pigs being fed large quantities of whey (10). On grain rations there is a much higher incidence on diets containing a higher proportion of corn (maize) than other grains (11). The tendency is greater still if the corn is finely ground (12) or is gelatinized or expanded (13). Esophagogastric ulcers in some pigs may be associated with *Ascaris suis* infection (7), but in other studies there is no significant association between the parasite and ulcers (8).

Of the suspected causes there is good evidence, from the administration of histamine and reserpine, that gastric hyperacidity is an important factor (9). This is probably related to the effects of psychological stress, including noise, excessive disturbing and overcrowding of pigs, which is known to be a significant contributor to the development of gastric ulcer in pigs (17). It is probably safe to assume that a dietary factor and a management factor (psychological stress) are capable, either singly or together, of causing the disease (17, 19). However, in some controlled trials the incidence of ulcers was higher in pigs fed *ad libitum* than in pigs fed a restricted diet and which had to compete for feeder space (2). The daily administration of prednisone to pigs will result in hemorrhages in the fundus of the stomach (23).

Plasma gastrin and plasma pepsinogen levels are the same in normal pigs as in those with epithelial hyperplasia or ulceration of the pars esophagia (18). If ulcers of this region arise from hypersecretion of gastric acid, some factor other than gastrin appears to be involved.

Esophagogastric ulceration is most common in pigs of 45–90 kg body weight but the disease may also occur in significant proportions in pigs after weaning and in adult sows and boars. All breeds are affected. A high heritability for esophagogastric ulcer has been determined and it appears related to selection for fast growth rate and low back fat (20).

The clinical signs are dependent on the severity of the ulcers. The majority of pigs with esophagogastric ulcers may show no evidence of the disease and growth rate and feed intake appear unaffected. However, the effect of ulceration on production does not appear to be well documented. Some observations suggest that there is no effect of ulceration on growth rate (3) while others indicate that the presence of esophagogastric ulcers resulted in a marked decrease in growth rate and an increase in the length of time required to reach market weight (24). Affected pigs also ate slowly and regurgitated frequently.

The erosion of a blood vessel within the ulcer will result in acute to subacute gastric hemorrhage. These cases are usually sporadic causing deaths of individuals within a group, with cases occurring over a period of several weeks. Clinical signs are often not observed, affected pigs being found dead from acute hemorrhage into the stomach.

A few subacute cases survive for 12–18 hours with signs of marked pallor, weakness, anorexia and black pasty feces changing to mucus-covered pellets in small amounts. The weakness may be sufficient to cause recumbency. Animals that survive are often unthrifty, usually due to anemia from chronic blood loss with a few cases affected by chronic peritonitis. When the disease is occurring careful observation may detect early cases. Suggestive signs are a darkening of the feces and the development of pallor.

At necropsy the ulcers are confined to the esophageal region of the stomach. They may be acute or chronic with the latter often showing signs of recent exacerbation, and fresh blood may be found in the stomach and intestines. Early lesions in clinically unaffected animals include hyperkeratinization of the mucosa and epithelial denudation without actual ulceration. Affected stomachs consistently have more fluid contents than unaffected ones (21). Evidence of bile staining in some affected stomachs has led to the suggestion that duodenal regurgitation of bile into the stomach may cause ulceration (22).

The occurrence of sudden death with a carcass that shows extreme pallor and a marble-white skin should immediately suggest the possibility of esophagogastric ulcer. The disease must be differentiated at necropsy from proliferative hemorrhagic enteropathy. Acute swine dysentery may also be manifested occasionally by sudden death with significant hemorrhage into the large intestine. Esophagogastric ulceration may also be a feature in pigs poisoned with pyrrolizidine alkaloid containing seeds but hepatic and renal damage are also evident.

Supplementation of the diet with vitamin E (18 mg/kg of feed), with or without selenium, has given mixed results as a prophylactic in field cases (25). Supplementation of the diet with antibiotics, copper sulfate, vitamins A and E, antihistamines or tranquilizers failed to prevent ulceration in pigs fed rations high in corn (26).

The incorporation of sodium polyacrylate at 0·1–0·5% in the diet will effectively control esophagogastric ulceration and also increase weight gain and feed conversion (27). Polyacrylate is an ideal compound because it is non-toxic and does not accumulate in body tissues.

Some control of the disease can usually be achieved by increasing the fiber content of the ration to 7% by the addition of coarsely ground oat hulls or barley straw in conjunction with the feeding of a more coarsely ground ration. Supplemental vitamin E is added to a level of 30 mg/kg feed. Where applicable a reduction of the amount of corn in the ration and the feeding of meal rather than pellets may also be of value. The reduction of psychologically stressful situations, with attention to stocking rates and environmental stress, may be of value. The genetic predisposition of pigs to esophagogastric ulceration requires further investigation as a possible longterm method of control.

REVIEW LITERATURE

Kowalczyk, T. (1969) Etiologic factors of gastric ulcers in swine. *Am. J. vet. Res.*, *30*, 393.

Lawrence, T. L. J. (1972) A review of some effects on health and performance of variations in the physical form of the diet of the growing pig. *Vet. Rec.*, *91*, 67, 84, 108.

O'Brien, J. J. (1969) Gastric ulceration in the pig. *Vet. Bull.*, *39*, 75.

REFERENCES

(1) Lawrence, T. L. et al. (1980) *Anim. Prod.*, *31*, 93.
(2) Blackshaw, J. K. et al. (1980) *Aust. vet. J.*, *56*, 384.
(3) Dobson, K. J. et al. (1979) *Aust. vet. J.*, *54*, 601.
(4) Penny, R. H. C. & Hill, F. W. G. (1973) *Vet. Ann.*, *14*, 55.
(5) Simorsson, A. & Bjorklund, N. E. (1978) *Swed. J. agric. Res.*, *8*, 97.
(6) Kadel, W. L. et al. (1969) *Am. J. vet. Res.*, *30*, 401.
(7) Qureski, S. R. et al. (1978) *Vet. Pathol.*, *15*, 353.
(8) Hani, H. & Indermuhle, N. A. (1979) *Vet. Pathol.*, *16*, 617.
(9) Kokue, E. I. et al. (1978) *J. vet. Pharmacol. Therap.*, *1*, 217.
(10) O'Brien, J. J. (1968) *Vet. Rec.*, *83*, 245.
(11) Reese, N. E. et al. (1966) *J. anim. Sci.*, *25*, 14, 21.
(12) Bjorklund, N. E. et al. (1970) *Proc. 11th nordic vet. Congr. Bergen, 1970*, 274.
(13) Mason, D. W. et al. (1968) *J. anim. Sci.*, *27*, 1006.
(14) Baustad, B. & Nafstad, I. (1969) *Pathol. vet.*, *6*, 546.
(15) Chamberlain, C. C. et al. (1967) *J. anim. Sci.*, *26*, 72, 214, 1054.
(16) Maxwell, C. V. (1970) *Diss. Abstr. int.*, *31B*, 777.
(17) Kowalczyk, T. et al. (1971) *Vet. med. small Anim. Clin.*, *66*, 1185.
(18) Bunn, C. M. et al. (1981) *Res. vet. Sci.*, *30*, 376.
(19) Reese, N. A. et al. (1963) *J. anim. Sci.*, *22*, 1129.
(20) Grondalen, T. & Vangen, O. (1974) *Nord. VetMed.*, *26*, 40.
(21) Muggenburg, B. A. et al. (1964) *Am. J. vet. Res.*, *25*, 1354.
(22) Reed, J. H. & Kidder, D. E. (1970) *Res. vet. Sci.*, *11*, 438.
(23) Zamora, C. S. et al. (1980) *Am. J. vet. Res.*, *41*, 885.
(24) Blackshaw, J. K. & Kelly, W. R. (1980) *Vet. Rec.*, *106*, 52.
(25) Dobson, K. J. (1967) *Aust. vet. J.*, *43*, 219.
(26) Nuwer, A. J. et al. (1965) *J. anim. Sci.*, *24*, 113.
(27) Yamaguchi, M. et al. (1981) *Am. J. vet. Res.*, *42*, 960.

DISEASES CHARACTERIZED BY RESPIRATORY TRACT INVOLVEMENT

Atrophic rhinitis (turbinate atrophy of swine)

Atrophic rhinitis is a disease affecting primarily young pigs but causing anatomical lesions which may persist for life. The disease is characterized clinically by an initial episode of acute rhinitis followed by chronic atrophy of the turbinate bones and deformity of the face.

Etiology

Several different causes have been proposed and examined in the last 30 years. There is now substantial experimental evidence that infection of the nasal cavities initially with *Bordetella bronchiseptica* followed by toxigenic strains of *Pasteurella multocida* results in progressive turbinate atrophy which is similar to the naturally occurring disease (1). The proposal that the disease was a manifestation of a deficiency or imbalance of calcium and phosphorus has now been discounted (1). There is no evidence that the disease has an inherited basis. Other non-infectious causes have been suggested, but it is generally agreed that they predispose to the disease or contribute to its severity. These include inadequacies in housing, ventilation and general nutritional status.

Epidemiology

Atrophic rhinitis occurs worldwide in areas where swine are reared under intensive conditions. The incidence of clinical disease varies from 5 to 30%, and its incidence or the presence of gross lesions depends on the method of detection. Abattoir surveys of the snouts of slaughtered pigs indicate that the incidence of gross lesions ranges from 14 to 50% (2). However, the incidence of gross lesions in abattoir surveys will reflect the source of the pigs; the incidence may be low in pigs from herds which have attempted to control the disease and high in some commercial herds with no control program. In pigs slaughtered from pig testing stations the incidence of lesions may be uniform over a long period (2). The published data on the incidence of gross lesions is also variable because of the lack of a uniform method of evaluating and quantifying the lesions. However, major improvements in the development of uniform and repeatable methods of evaluating lesions have occurred in recent years.

Infection of the nasal cavities of pigs with *Bordetella bronchiseptica* is widespread. The infection is present in almost every swine herd and the prevalence of infection in pigs in commercial herds will vary from 25 to 50%. Serological surveys of individual herds reveal that up to 90% of the pigs are positive, which indicates that there is no reliable relationship between the frequency of isolation of the organism and the percentage of animals with antibody (3). The incidence is just as high in specific pathogen free (SPF) herds as in non-SPF herds (3). *Bordetella bronchiseptica* readily colonizes the ciliated mucosa of the respiratory tract of swine. Direct contact and droplet infection are presumed to be the most likely methods of transmission. The reservoir of infection is probably the infected sow, and litters of piglets become infected at an early age; thus the carrier sow is an important source of the organism for newborn piglets. The infection is usually introduced into a herd by the purchase of infected pigs. Spread between piglets is probably enhanced after weaning when mixing of litters occurs and 70–80% of a large weaned group become infected. Infection persists for up to several weeks and months followed by a gradual reduction in the intensity and rate of infection. In herds where *B. bronchiseptica* is the initiating agent, up to 90% of pigs from 4 to 10 weeks of age will have nasal infection, but this infection rate falls to approximately 15% by 12 months of age and the proportion of carrier pigs within the breeding herd decreases with increasing age of sow (5). The prevalence of infection is also much higher during the period from October to March than at other times of the year, and the prevalence of serologically positive animals is highest from July to December.

The age at which piglets first become infected with *B. bronchiseptica* has an important effect on the development of lesions. The most severe lesions occur in non-immune animals infected during the first week of life. Animals infected at 4 weeks of age develop less severe lesions, while those infected at 10 weeks do not develop significant lesions.

The level of immunity in the young pigs will influence the level of infection and the incidence of clinical disease. Colostral immunity from sows serologically positive to *B. bronchiseptica* is transferred to piglets and provides protection for 2–5 weeks. Clinical disease does not occur in piglets with high levels of passive antibody (6). Older pigs from 10 to 12 weeks of age may become infected, but are less likely to develop severe turbinate atrophy and may develop inapparent infection and become carriers (7). Vaccination of the sow before parturition to increase colostral immunity or vaccination of the young pig will increase the rate of clearance of the organism from the nasal cavity and reduce the incidence of clinical disease. In chronically affected herds a level of immunity develops with increasing age of the breeding herd.

The epidemiology of toxigenic strains of *Past. multocida* as a causative agent of atrophic rhinitis is not as well understood. The organism colonizes the tonsils of clinically normal pigs. In contrast to *B. bronchiseptica* which is ubiquitous in swine herds the toxigenic isolates of *Past. multocida* appear to be restricted to herds affected with progressive atrophic rhinitis (1, 4). The organism is invariably present in herds with progressive atrophic rhinitis, but may also be present in about 5% of the pigs in a herd with no clinical history of atrophic rhinitis. The main source of toxigenic isolates of *Past. multocida* for young pigs appears to be the pharyngeal tissues of the breeding stock. About 10–15% of sows in farrowing houses may be infected with toxigenic isolates and piglets became infected within a week after birth. In contrast to *B. bronchiseptica*, infection of piglets at 12–16 weeks of age with toxigenic *Past. multocida* will still result in varying degrees of severity of lesions.

The prevalence of infection of toxigenic *Past. multocida*, serotype D, is higher in herds with clinical disease (48). The organism can be present in 50–80% of weaned pigs in a herd with clinical disease in the finishing pigs.

While *B. bronchiseptica* is eliminated from the respiratory tract of most infected pigs leaving only a few infected at slaughter, *Past. multocida* often persists.

For many years it was accepted as dogma that atrophic rhinitis was an important cause of economic loss in swine herds because of apparent decreased growth rate, less than optimal feed efficiency, and was a major predisposing factor in enzootic swine pneumonia. However, recent field studies have failed to show that the disease has an effect on growth rate in fattening pigs or that there is a cause and effect relationship between atrophic rhinitis and pneumonia (8, 9). The presence of pneumonia in pigs from a test station reduced mean daily weight gains by 33% for each 10% of affected lung, but atrophic rhinitis did not affect daily gain and there was no association between the development of atrophic rhinitis and the development of pneumonia (9). Pigs vaccinated against *B. bronchiseptica* had turbinate atrophy scores or mean daily gains no different from those in unvaccinated pigs. In another study there was a low positive correlation between the herd mean turbinate atrophy score and the herd mean percentage pneumonia score (10). A recent report from Illinois indicates that the prevalence of clinical atrophic rhinitis in farrow-to-finish herds ranged from 0 to 20% and in pigs from those herds examined at the abattoir the incidence of turbinate lesions ranged from 5 to 92% (11). In some of the herds the mean daily weight gain was 15–18% higher than in herds where pigs had severe turbinate lesions. In an Australian report there was no correlation between the severity of atrophic rhinitis and growth rate or back fat thickness (12).

The virulence characteristics of *B. bronchiseptica* and the toxigenic isolates of *Past. multocida* are now considered to be important epidemiological determinants of atrophic rhinitis. The virulence of *B. bronchiseptica* is dependent on the ability to produce heavy, persistent colonization in the nasal cavity and the production of a heat-labile toxin (13). Only certain porcine phase 1 cultures possess both properties. However, even the most virulent of 10 isolates of *B. bronchiseptica* did not cause progressive turbinate atrophy or significant snout deformation in experimental infections (14). The severe lesions of atrophic rhinitis cannot be attributed to this organism alone. Experimental inoculation of SPF or gnotobiotic pigs with the organism results in a non-progressive moderately severe turbinate atrophy 2–4 weeks after infection followed frequently by regeneration of the turbinates. These virulence characteristics of *B. bronchiseptica* are consistent with the observations that in herds where the organism is common it can provoke sneezing and coughing but no evidence of clinical turbinate atrophy. The examination of the turbinates within 2 weeks after the sneezing will reveal some mild lesions but no lesions will be evident when the pigs are examined at slaughter (19). Both organisms are required to produce lesions similar to the naturally occurring progressive disease.

Toxigenic isolates of *Past. multocida* can colonize the nasal cavity, elaborate several toxins and produce progressive lesions of the turbinate bones and snout. There is some evidence that the presence of *B. bronchiseptica* can enhance the colonization of *Past. multocida*, particularly the toxigenic type-D strains isolated from pigs. Severe turbinate damage and shortening of the snout can be reproduced in SPF and gnotobiotic pigs by combined infection with *B. bronchiseptica* and certain strains of *Past. multocida* (16, 17). Following experimental infection both organisms may persist in the nasal cavities for up to 64 days. The cell envelope proteins and lipopolysaccharides of *Past. multocida* strains associated with atrophic rhinitis have been characterized and compared (18). At least three protein patterns and six lipopolysaccharide patterns can be distinguished, which can be used to predict the pathogenic character of some of the strains. This will obviate the need to use the guinea-pig skin test to distinguish strains associated with atrophic rhinitis and those which are not.

The effects of housing, population density and adequacy of ventilation on the prevalence of infection of *B.*

bronchiseptica and toxigenic isolates of *Past. multocida*, and on the incidence and severity of atrophic rhinitis have not been examined in detail. Undocumented field observations suggest that the disease is more common and severe when pigs are confined, overcrowded, and housed in poorly ventilated unsanitary barns, all of which promotes the spread of infection. There is no effect of high levels of ammonia on the severity of turbinate atrophy (15). Management factors such as confinement farrowing and the use of continual throughput farrowing houses and weaner houses are also considered as important epidemiological determinants.

Pathogenesis

Following infection of the nasal cavity, *B. bronchiseptica* becomes closely associated with the ciliated epithelium of the respiratory tract. The organism produces a heat-labile toxin which results in a non-progressive, moderately severe turbinate atrophy which is apparent within 2 to 4 weeks after infection, followed frequently by regeneration of the turbinates. There is hyperplasia and metaplasia of the nasal epithelium, fibrous in the lamina propria, and resorption and replacement fibrosis of the osseous core. Experimental infection with *B. bronchiseptica* alone does not result in severe persistent turbinate atrophy or twisting or shortening of the snout.

Infection and colonization of the nasal cavities with the toxigenic strains of *Past. multocida* results in the elaboration of a toxin which cause progressive turbinate atrophy. The toxin is thermolabile, dermonecrotic and has been named as the *atrophic rhinitis* toxin (48). The inoculation of a toxin from a toxigenic strain of type D *Past. multocida* into the nasal cavities of gnotobiotic pigs results in severe bilateral atrophy of the turbinates (23). Atrophy of the ventral conchae can be produced experimentally with pathogenic *B. bronchiseptica* in piglets at 6 weeks of age and with toxigenic *Past. multocida* strains in piglets as old as 16 weeks of age (48). The toxin enhances osteoclastic resorption and impairs osteoblastic synthesis of the turbinate osseous core and irreversible changes can occur within a few days. The epithelium and the submucosa undergo secondary atrophy and the turbinates may disappear almost completely within 10–14 days (20, 21). These lesions can persist until the animal is 90 kg body weight. The turbinate atrophy is not accompanied by an inflammatory reaction. The effect of the *Past. multocida* toxin is restricted to the nasal cavity which is supported by the intriguing observation that the parenteral injection of the toxin into gnotobiotic piglets results in turbinate lesions and shortening and twisting of the snout (22). The culture filtrate of a non-atrophic rhinitis pathogenic *Past. multocida* will not cause lesions after intramuscular injection. The disappearance of the turbinates and the involvement of the bones of the face lead to deformity of the facial bones with the appearance of dishing and bulging of the face and, if the lesion is unilateral, to lateral deviation of the snout. The effect on growth rate, if any, may be due to the chronic irritation and interference with prehension.

Clinical findings

The clinical findings of atrophic rhinitis depend on the stage of the lesions. In acute cases in piglets 3–9 weeks of age irritation of the nasal mucosa causes sneezing, some coughing, small amounts of serous or mucopurulent nasal discharge and transient unilateral or bilateral epistaxis. The frequency of sneezing may be a measure of the incidence and severity of the disease. In piglets, born from sows vaccinated with *B. bronchiseptica* and *Past. multocida* vaccine before farrowing, followed by two vaccinations within 3 weeks of age, the frequency of sneezing at 3–9 weeks of age was much less than in piglets given only *B. bronchiseptica* vaccine (32). There may be rubbing of the nose against objects or on the ground. A watery ocular discharge usually accompanies this and may result in the appearance of dried streaks of dirt below the medial canthus of the eyes. There may be a decrease in growth rate. In infection with *B. bronchiseptica* these clinical signs will disappear spontaneously in a few weeks when the pigs will appear normal. In severe cases, respiratory obstruction may increase to the point of dyspnea and cyanosis, and sucking pigs may have great difficulty in nursing. The nasal secretions become thicker and nasal bleeding may also occur. In the more chronic stages, inspissated material may be expelled during paroxysms of sneezing. During this chronic stage, there is often pronounced deformity of the face due to arrested development of the bones, especially the turbinates, and the accumulation of necrotic material in the nasal cavities. The nasal bones and premaxillae turn upwards and interfere with approximation of the incisor and, to a less extent, the molar teeth. There are varying degrees of brachygnathia superior and protrusion of the lower incisor teeth. Prehension and mastication become difficult with a resulting loss of body condition. Facial distortion in the final stages takes the form of severe 'dishing' of the face with wrinkling of the overlying skin. If the condition is unilateral, the upper jaw may be twisted to one side. These visible facial deformities develop most commonly in pigs 8–10 weeks old within 3–4 weeks after infection, but they may occur in younger pigs.

The most serious effects of the advanced disease are depression of growth rate and unthriftiness. The appetite may be unaffected but much feed is lost by spillage and feed efficiency may be reduced in some instances.

Clinical pathology

It is important to be able to detect infected animals in a herd, especially the carrier animal. Nasal swabs are used to detect the bacteria and to determine their drug sensitivity. The collection of the nasal swabs must be done carefully and require special transport medium to ensure a high recovery rate. A sampling technique and a special culture medium to facilitate the isolation and recognition of *B. bronchiseptica* are described (24). The external nares are cleaned with alcohol and a cotton-tipped flexible wire pushed into the nasal cavity (of each side in turn) until it reaches a point midway between the nostril and the level of the medial canthus of the eye. On removal, the cotton tip is cut off into 0·5 ml of an ice-cold sterile transport medium comprising phosphate-buffered saline (PBS, pH 7·3) with fetal calf serum (5% v/v). The samples are then placed on special media preferably within 4 hours (24). Normally the organism grows well on conventional culture media, especially when younger pigs are sampled. However, in the carrier pig the organism may be sparse and the selective medium is recommended (24).

The nasal culturing procedure has been used as an aid in the control of atrophic rhinitis caused by *B. bronchiseptica*. A series of three nasal swabs from each animal is considered to be about 77% efficient in detecting infected animals for possible culling and elimination from the herd (26).

Agglutination tests and ELISA test are available for the detection of pigs infected with *B. bronchiseptica* especially carrier animals (27). Serology is of value in the assessment of the response of pigs vaccinated with the *B. bronchiseptica* vaccines (40). There are currently no reliable serological tests for *Past. multocida*.

Pasteurella multocida grow readily in the laboratory but are difficult to isolate from nasal swabs because they are frequently overgrown by commensal flora. Selective laboratory media containing antimicrobial agents have been developed to promote the isolation of *Past. multocida* from nasal swabs (41). The most sensitive method for recovering them is by passage of the material through mice.

A cell culture assay for using embryonic bovine lung cell cultures is available and is a sensitive *in vitro* test for the differentiation of toxigenic from non-toxigenic isolates of *Past. multocida* (25). This test can replace the lethal tests in mice or the dermonecrotic tests in guineapigs.

Some aids to the clinical diagnosis have been examined, but are not highly accurate. Radiography of the nose is not reliable in detecting the severity of turbinate atrophy (31).

Necropsy findings

The typical lesions of atrophic rhinitis are restricted to the nasal cavities though concurrent diseases, especially virus pneumonia of pigs, may produce lesions elsewhere. In the early stages, there is acute inflammation, sometimes with the accumulation of pus but, in the later stages, there is evidence only of atrophy of the mucosa, and decalcification and atrophy of the turbinate and ethmoid bones, which may have completely disappeared in severe cases. The inflammatory and atrophic processes may extend to involve the facial sinuses. There is no evidence of interference with the vascular supply to the affected bones. The changes in the nasal cavities are most readily seen if the head is split in the sagittal plane but for accurate diagnosis the degree of turbinate symmetry, volume and atrophy and medial septum deviation should be assessed by inspection of a vertical cross-section of the skull made at the level of the second premolar tooth.

The clinical diagnosis is confirmed and the severity of the lesions is assessed by the postmortem examination of a cross-section of the snout. The snout must be sectioned at the level of the second premolar tooth because the size of the turbinate bone reduces anteriorly and may give a false positive result if the section is taken too far forward. Quantitation of the severity of the lesions has been of value for monitoring the incidence and severity of the disease in a herd. Several systems for grading the severity of lesions of the snout have been used. Most of them have used a subjective visual scoring system in which snouts are grade 0 (complete normality) to 5 (complete conchal atrophy).

The standards for each grade are as follows (2):

Grade 0 No deviation from absolute normality, with nasal septum straight and turbinates symmetrical and filling nasal cavities.
Grade 1 Slight irregularity, asymmetry or distortion of the nasal structures without atrophy.
Grade 2 Marked distortion of nasal structure but without marked atrophy.
Grade 3 Definite atrophy of the turbinates with or without distortion.
Grade 4 More severe atrophy with severe atrophy of one or more turbinates.
Grade 5 Very severe atrophy in which all turbinates have virtually disappeared.

Such a discontinuous grading system does not provide a direct quantitative relationship. Regular examination of the snouts from heads of pigs sent to slaughter can be used to assess the level of turbinate atrophy in the herd. Morphometric methods, using either point counting or semiautomated planimetry applied to photographic or impression prints of sections of the snout to measure the extent of conchal atrophy on a continuous scale as a morphometric index, are now available. Cross-sections of the snout are photographed or used to make impression prints which are then measured (28). A morphometric index is determined, which is the ratio of free space to total cross-sectional area of the nasal cavity. The system correlates well with the visual grading system of 0–5 but is labor-intensive and relatively expensive. Descriptions of the methods for making snout impressions are available (29, 30).

A major limitation of the grading system is that turbinate atrophy occurs as a continuous spectrum and it is difficult to decide, for example, if a pig with a grade 3 lesion represents the more severe manifestation of *B. bronchiseptica* infection, which may not progress further, or an early manifestation of infection with toxigenic *Past. multocida*, which could develop into a severe herd problem.

Diagnosis

The occurrence of sneezing in the early stages and of facial deformity in the later stages are characteristic of this disease. Inclusion body rhinitis due to a cytomegalovirus is a common infection in young piglets in which there is sneezing and conjunctivitis. However, by itself it does not progress to produce turbinate atrophy and facial distortion. Under good hygienic conditions the course of the disease is about 2 weeks and the economic effects are minimal. In the early acute stages, atrophic rhinitis may be mistaken for swine influenza which, however, usually occurs as an outbreak affecting older pigs and is accompanied by a severe systemic reaction without subsequent involvement of facial bones. Necrotic rhinitis is manifested by external lesions affecting the face, and virus pneumonia of pigs is characterized by coughing rather than sneezing. The inherited prognathic jaw of some breeds of pigs has been mistaken for the chronic stage of atrophic rhinitis and protrusion of the lower jaw is quite common in adult intensively housed pigs and has been attributed to behavioral problems of pushing the snout against fixed equipment such as bars and nipple drinkers.

Treatment

Treatment early in the course of the disease will reduce the severity of its effects, but it is of little value in chronically affected pigs, and due to persistent poor growth rate and high food conversion these pigs are best culled at an early age. Tylosin at 20 mg/kg body weight, oxytetracycline at 20 mg/kg body weight or trimethoprim-sulfadoxine (40 mg/200 mg/ml) at 0·1 ml/kg body weight may be given parenterally or the creep feed may be medicated with sulfamethazine and/or tylosin at 200 and 100 mg/kg of feed respectively (36). Parenteral injections need to be repeated every 3–7 days for at least three injections and feed medication should be given for 3–5 weeks. The problem with early creep medication is in obtaining adequate intakes of the antibacterial. This is seldom achieved before 2 weeks of age and parenteral antibiotics may be required if significant infection occurs before this stage.

The parenteral administration of antimicrobial agents to individual piglets at 3–7 day intervals beginning at 3 days of age for a total of three to five injections per piglet has been recommended for the treatment and control of atrophic rhinitis (45, 47). However, in a large herd such a treatment regimen would be a major task and until a cost-benefit analysis indicates a beneficial effect over other methods we cannot recommend such a practice.

The treatment of experimental *B. bronchiseptica* infection in young pigs has been successful with the use of trimethoprim-sulfadiazine in the drinking water at levels of 13·3 and 77·6 μg/ml respectively, for 3 weeks (50). This method would remove the necessity to inject pigs repeatedly.

Control

The methods which have been recommended and used for the control of atrophic rhinitis were based largely on the premise that *B. bronchiseptica* was the major etiological agent. The methods of control were aimed at eradication of the organism from the herd or decreasing the prevalence of infection in the herd, and presumably clinical disease, by strategic mass medication of the feed with antimicrobials, or by vaccination of the pregnant sow and/or the piglets in order to increase the level of specific immunity against *B. bronchiseptica*. However, it is now accepted that *B. bronchiseptica* does not cause progressive atrophic rhinitis and therefore control programs aimed solely at elimination or control of this organism will be ineffective. Effective control will likely depend on developing methods of eliminating or controlling the prevalence of toxigenic isolates of *Past. multocida* which do cause progressive atrophic rhinitis if they can become established in the nasal cavity (20). Previous infection of the nasal cavity with *B. bronchiseptica* can enhance the establishment of toxigenic *Past. multocida* and result in progressive atrophic rhinitis.

While there is considerable information available on the ecology of *B. bronchiseptica* and the methods by which it might be eliminated or controlled in a herd, there is little documented information available on methods which can be used for control of the toxigenic isolates of *Past. multocida* associated with atrophic rhinitis. The control methods outlined here are guidelines and are based on the traditional methods used for control by infection due to *B. bronchiseptica*.

Control of atrophic rhinitis can be attempted in at least four ways: total eradication; reduction of infection pressure; mass medication with antimicrobials to reduce the severity and adverse effects of infection; and vaccination. Regardless of the method employed any effective control program must have a system for monitoring the incidence of clinical disease in the herd and the incidence and severity of turbinate lesions of the pigs sent to slaughter (51). Accurate and reliable methods for monitoring clinical disease are not available but the incidence of acute rhinitis and facial deformities could be recorded regularly. At slaughter, snouts can be examined for lesions of turbinate atrophy and assessing a mean snout score for each group of pigs slaughtered.

Eradication

Total eradication can only be achieved with confidence by complete depopulation for a 4 week period and repopulation with primary or purchased specific pathogen free (SPF) stock. This approach has the added advantage of also eliminating enzootic pneumonia which may be a significant contributing factor to the economic importance of this disease. However, this method of control is extremely costly and the economic importance of the disease would need to be carefully evaluated in relation to this cost before this method was instituted. Other techniques of obtaining pigs free of atrophic rhinitis, such as the isolated farrowing of older and presumed non-carrier sows with subsequent clinical and postmortem examinations of a proportion of the litters, have had a significant failure rate in the field and are not recommended. Eradication by repopulation with cesarean-derived stock may be essential in breeding nucleus herds where a high generation turnover results in a low herd sow age and a low herd level of immunity. The breakdown rate of herds established by this method can be significant presumably because the initiating organisms are not solely confined to pigs.

A pilot control scheme was initiated in Britain in which a herd had to meet the following conditions:

- It must be inspected by a veterinarian every 6 months over a period of 2 years over which time there must be no clinical evidence of atrophic rhinitis
- The herd owner must certify that atrophic rhinitis has not been suspected over the same time period
- Cross-sections of snouts taken from at least 30% of marketed pigs must be examined regularly by a veterinarian, and over a 2 year probationary period the average 6 monthly snout score must not exceed 0·5
- There must be no vaccination or treatment for atrophic rhinitis

- New breeding stock can be introduced only from other qualified herds or herds derived by hysterectomy, artificial insemination or embryo transfer techniques.

Over a 5 year period 45 herds qualified at some stage, and 34 were still qualified at the end of 5 years (33).

Reduction of infection
Reduction of infection pressure can be attempted. Infection of piglets occurs primarily either from carrier sows or from other infected piglets in the immediate environment and severe atrophic rhinitis generally results from infection of piglets under 3 weeks of age. If these factors can be minimized the incidence and severity of the disease can be reduced. The level of infection with *B. bronchiseptica* and other respiratory pathogens decreases with age, and in herds where high genetic turnover is not of primary concern, the simple expedient of allowing the average age of the sow herd to increase may significantly increase herd resistance and decrease infection pressure. In small herds the farrowing of older sows and the rearing of their litters until weaning in areas separate from young sows and their litters may also effectively reduce the incidence of the disease.

The detection and elimination from the herd of affected and carrier animals can also be attempted. Clinical examination with especial attention to snout deformity and malposition of the incisor teeth with brachygnathia superior and wrinkling of the skin of the snout will detect a proportion of affected animals but snout radiography is required for the detection of turbinate changes. The technique and interpretation of snout radiography is presented elsewhere (31). However, it would appear impractical for most circumstances. In herds where *B. bronchiseptica* is the initiating pathogen, control has been achieved by elimination of carriers detected from nasal cultures. Usually this procedure is preceded by a period of feed medication of the breeding herd with sulfamethazine at 450–1000 mg/kg of feed for a period of 4–6 weeks in order to reduce the incidence of carriers. Deep nasal swabs are taken at 3 week intervals taking care to avoid contamination and attempting to swab the medium septum. Positive carriers are eliminated from the herds as soon as convenient and sows are considered non-carriers when three consecutive swabs prove negative. By the use of this technique a significant reduction and even virtual elimination of atrophic rhinitis has been achieved in herds where *B. bronchiseptica* is the significant etiological agent (26).

Since severe lesions depend upon infection of the piglet under 3 weeks of age every attempt should be made to minimize the severity of the challenge to young piglets. It is a common observation that the effects of atrophic rhinitis are minimal under good systems of management and adequate ventilation, non-dusty conditions and good hygiene. The use of continual throughput farrowing houses and weaner houses allows a buildup of infection with the presence of actively infected pigs that can provide a high infection pressure on piglets born into or introduced into these areas. The use of all-in/all-out systems of management in these areas is recommended and young piglets should be kept in a separate area from older pigs.

Mass medication
The prophylactic use of antimicrobials is frequently used to reduce the incidence of the disease within the herd. These are used both within the breeding herd to reduce the prevalence of carriers, and in young suckling and weaner pigs to reduce the severity of the infection. The medication is begun about 2 weeks before farrowing, continued throughout lactation and incorporated in the creep feed for the sucking pigs and the starter feeds for the weaned pigs. In this way there is continuous medication of the sow and the piglets during the most susceptible period. For the breeding herd, sulfamethazine at levels of 450–1000 mg/kg feed, with the higher levels being given to dry sows on restricted feeding, has been recommended (7). Sulfonamide resistance has proved a problem in some countries (39) but beneficial results may still be achieved with these levels (7). It is recommended that medication be continued for a 4–6 week period (7). Carbadox at a level of 55 ppm in combination with sulfamethazine at 110 ppm is reported to be effective in clearing experimentally induced *B. bronchiseptica* infection, and when used alone improved growth rate and feed efficiency in pigs with naturally occurring atrophic rhinitis (35). In the starter period, carbadox fed alone or in combination with sulfamethazine improved average daily gain in piglets from herds with naturally occurring atrophic rhinitis (37). Use of the medication, however, did not result in a reduction of mean nasal lesion scores due to atrophic rhinitis. Sulfamethazine at 110 mg/kg of feed is more effective than sulfathiazole at the same concentration for the control of experimentally induced atrophic rhinitis due to *B. bronchiseptica* (38). Sulfamethazine may also be incorporated in creep rations and the use of tetracyclines (200 mg/kg), tylosin (50–100 mg/kg), chloramphenicol (200–400 mg/kg) and penicillin (200 mg/kg) have also been suggested (36).

The concept of medicated early weaning is recommended to obtain pigs free from pathogens, including *B. bronchiseptica*, which are endemic in the herd of origin (34). The sows are fed medicated feed from 5 days before and after weaning and the piglets are dosed from birth to 10 days of age.

Vaccination
There has been considerable interest in the development of vaccines for the control and prevention of atrophic rhinitis due to *B. bronchiseptica* (40). Inactivated vaccines have been used to vaccinate the pregnant sow 4–6 weeks before farrowing, and in some cases, followed by vaccination of the piglets at 7 and 28 days of age. In general, the use of the vaccine in pregnant sows in herds where the disease has been endemic has reduced the incidence of clinical atrophic rhinitis. However, the results from one study to another have been highly variable. Vaccination of the pregnant sow does result in an increase in colostral antibody titer which does improve the clearance rate of *B. bronchiseptica* in the piglets. However, it has been difficult to evaluate the efficacy of

the *B. bronchiseptica* used alone because the turbinate atrophy caused by infection of piglets with *B. bronchiseptica* experimentally or naturally heals and regenerates completely when they are reared to about 70–90 kg body weight in good housing conditions.

Vaccination of pregnant gilts with a *B. bronchiseptica* vaccine at mid-pregnancy and again 3 weeks before farrowing provided some protection against experimentally induced atrophic rhinitis using *B. bronchiseptica* followed by *Past. multocida* (19). The nasal lesions in piglets born from vaccinated sows were significantly reduced but complete protection was not achieved. The mean daily weight gains were reduced in pigs with severe atrophic rhinitis. The use of a vaccine containing crude toxin of *Past. multocida* in pregnant gilts provided significant protection against the experimental disease in SPF piglets (42). The use of a vaccine containing antigens from both *B. bronchiseptica* and *Past. multocida* also provided protection and the weight gains in vaccinated piglets were superior to those in unvaccinated piglets (43). Experimentally, piglets born from sows vaccinated with *Past. multocida* are protected from a challenge with atrophic rhinitis toxin (49). This indicates that artificial immunization for atrophic rhinitis should be possible.

Experimental infection and vaccination of pregnant minimum-disease sows with *B. bronchiseptica* resulted in much higher agglutinins in serum and colostrum than in sows only vaccinated or control animals and the piglets were provided with protection against experimental disease (44).

There is conflicting evidence about the efficacy of vaccinating piglets with a *B. bronchiseptica* vaccine (40). The original reports indicated significant protection when the piglets were vaccinated at 7 and 28 days of age (45). However, in colostrum-fed piglets, from vaccinated or experimentally infected sows, the presence of passive antibody interferes with their ability to respond actively to parenteral vaccination at 7 and 28 days of age (44). Current evidence indicates that additional vaccination of piglets from vaccinated sows results in no benefits over those obtainable from vaccination of the sow alone.

In the light of the possible effect of nutrition on the disease it would be unwise to neglect the calcium and phosphorus status of the diet, especially in pregnant and lactating sows and in young pigs. The recommended levels of intake are 1·2% calcium and 1% phosphorus in the ration. The high intake of calcium necessitates the intake of more zinc than is usually recommended. A level of 100 mg/kg of total diet is suggested as adequate. It is also recommended that attention be given to the control of any infectious disease, particularly enteric disease, which might limit the assimilation of minerals in the diet.

REVIEW LITERATURE

Giles, C. J. & Smith, I. M. (1983) Vaccination of pigs with *Bordetella bronchiseptica*. *Vet. Bull.*, *53*, 327–338.

Pedersen, K. B. & Nielsen, N. C. (1983) Atrophic rhinitis in pigs. A seminar in the CEC Programme of Coordination of Research on Animal Pathology held in Copenhagen, May 25–26, 1983, pp. 205.

Rutter, J. M. (1985) Atrophic rhinitis in swine. *Adv. vet. Sci. comp. Med.*, *29*, 239–279.

REFERENCES

(1) Rutter, J. M. (1985) *Adv. vet. Sci. comp. Med.*, *29*, 239.
(2) Jackson, G. H. et al. (1982) *Br. vet. J.*, *138*, 480.
(3) Shashidhar, B. Y. et al. (1983) *Am. J. vet. Res.*, *44*, 1123.
(4) Rutter, J. M. et al. (1984) *Vet. Rec.*, *115*, 615.
(5) Jenkins, E. M. et al. (1977) *Am. J. vet. Res.*, *38*, 2071.
(6) Rutter, J. M. (1981) *Vet. Rec.*, *108*, 451.
(7) Farrington, D. O. & Switzer, W. P. (1979) *Am. J. vet. Res.*, *40*, 1347.
(8) Straw, B. E. et al. (1983) *J. Am. vet. med. Assoc.*, *182*, 607.
(9) Straw, B. E. et al. (1984) *J. Am. vet. med. Assoc.*, *185*, 1544.
(10) Morrison, R. B. et al. (1986) *Can. vet. J.*, *26*, 95.
(11) Backstrom, L. et al. (1985) *J. Am. vet. med. Assoc.*, *187*, 712.
(12) Love, R. J. et al. (1985) *Aust. vet. J.*, *62*, 377.
(13) Collings, L. A. & Rutter, J. M. (1985) *J. med. Microbiol.*, *19*, 247.
(14) Rutter, J. M. et al. (1982) *J. med. Microbiol.*, *15*, 105.
(15) Drummond, J. C. et al. (1981) *Am. J. vet. Res.*, *42*, 963.
(16) Rutter, J. M. (1983) *Res. vet. Sci.*, *34*, 287.
(17) Rutter, J. M. & Rojas, X. (1982) *Vet. Rec.*, *110*, 531.
(18) Lugtenberg, B. et al. (1984) *Infect. Immun.*, *46*, 48.
(19) Pedersen, K. B. & Barford, K. (1981) *Nord. VetMed.*, *33*, 513.
(20) Pedersen, K. B. & Elling, F. (1984) *J. comp. Pathol.*, *94*, 203.
(21) Elling, F. & Pedersen, K. B. (1985) *Vet. Pathol.*, *22*, 469.
(22) Rutter, J. M. & MacKenzie, A. (1984) *Vet. Rec.*, *114*, 89.
(23) Dominck, M. A. & Rimler, R. B. (1986) *Am. J. vet. Rec.*, *47*, 1532.
(24) Smith, I. M. & Baskeville, A. J. (1979) *Res. vet. Sci.*, *27*, 187.
(25) Rutter, J. M. & Luther, P. D. (1984) *Vet. Rec.*, *114*, 393.
(26) Farrington, D. O. & Switzer, W. P. (1977) *J. Am. vet. med. Assoc.*, *170*, 34.
(27) Venier, L. et al. (1984) *Am. J. vet. Res.*, *45*, 2634.
(28) Done, J. T. et al. (1984) *Vet. Rec.*, *114*, 33.
(29) Done, J. T. et al. (1984) *Br. vet. J.*, *140*, 418.
(30) Lund, L. J. & Beckett, P. (1983) *Vet. Rec.*, *113*, 473.
(31) Webbon, P. M. (1978) *Br. vet. J.*, *134*, 193.
(32) Douglas, R. G. A. & Ripley, P. H. (1984) *Vet. Rec.*, *114*, 321.
(33) Goodwin, R. F. W. & Whittlestone, P. (1983) *Vet. Rec.*, *113*, 411.
(34) Alexander, T. J. L. et al. (1980) *Vet. Rec.*, *106*, 114.
(35) Farrington, D. O. & Shively, J. E. (1979) *J. Am. vet. med. Assoc.*, *174*, 597.
(36) Done, J. T. (1977) *Vet. Ann.*, *17*, 96.
(37) Wheelhouse, R. K. et al. (1984) *Can. J. anim. Sci.*, *64*, 951.
(38) Kobland, J. D. et al. (1984) *Am. J. vet. Res.*, *45*, 720.
(39) Hodges, R. T. & Young, G. W. (1984) *NZ vet. J.*, *32*, 111.
(40) Giles, C. J. & Smith, I. M. (1983) *Vet. Bull.*, *53*, 327.
(41) Smith, I. M. & Baskerville, A. J. (1983) *Br. vet. J.*, *139*, 476.
(42) Pedersen, K. B. & Barfod, K. (1982) *Nord. VetMed.*, *34*, 293.
(43) Barfod, K. & Pedersen, K. B. (1984) *Nord. VetMed.*, *36*, 337.
(44) Smith, I. M. et al. (1982) *Vet. Rec.*, *110*, 488.
(45) Goodnow, R. W. et al. (1979) *Am. J. vet. Res.*, *40*, 58.
(46) deJong, M. F. (1983) In: *Atrophic Rhinitis in Pigs*, eds K. B. Pedersen and N. C. Nielsen. Commission of European Communities, pp. 165–176.
(47) Gois, M. et al. (1983) *Am. J. vet. med. Assoc.*, *183*, 445.
(48) deJong, M. F. & Akkermans, J. P. W. M. (1986) *Vet. Q.*, *8*, 204.
(49) deJong, M. F. et al. (1986) *Vet. Q.*, *8*, 215.
(50) Giles, C. J. et al. (1981) *Vet. Rec.*, *108*, 136.
(51) Done, J. T. (1983) In: *Atrophic Rhinitis in Swine*, eds K. B. Pedersen and N. C. Nielsen. Commission of the European Communities, pp. 193–198.

Interstitial pneumonia of cattle

Interstitial pneumonia of cattle has been known for many years under many different terms including atypical interstitial pneumonia, acute pulmonary emphysema and edema, bovine pulmonary emphysema, 'panters', 'lungers', bovine asthma, pneumoconiosis and 'fog fever'.

Diffuse or patchy damage to alveolar septa is the essential feature of interstitial pneumonia which may be acute or chronic and can be caused by many forms of pulmonary injury. There is an obvious lack of lesions of the small airways which differentiates interstitial pneumonia from bronchopneumonia. Traditionally it was thought that interstitial pneumonias were characterized by chronic inflammation in which there is a predominantly proliferative response involving the alveolar walls and supporting stroma. However, acute diffuse damage of the alveolar walls accompanied by an early intra-alveolar exudative phase, which can be followed by proliferation of type 2 alveolar epithelial cells and fibroblasts, is now commonly recognized. The recognition that interstitial pneumonia can have an acute exudative phase was the reason for the designation of acute interstitial pneumonia in cattle as 'atypical' interstitial pneumonia (4). It is apparent that the use of the word 'atypical' has created confusion in the interpretation and diagnosis of lesions and in the conveying of information (1). Thus we have decided to abandon the use of the term *atypical interstitial pneumonia* in favor of interstitial pneumonia and to specify where possible, clinically, epidemiologically and pathologically the various forms of interstitial pulmonary disease in cattle.

The diseases in which interstitial pneumonia is the essential lesion are listed in Table 100. Pulmonary congestion and edema, alveolar exudation, hyaline membrane formation, interstitial emphysema and alveolar epithelial cell hyperplasia and fibrosis of the supporting stroma without lesions of the smaller airways are the characteristic lesions, with their presence and extent varying according to the stage of the disease process. The term atypical interstitial pneumonia as originally proposed (4) was useful in describing the above diseases clinically and it set them apart from the common acute infectious diseases of the respiratory tract of cattle. Clinically, they are atypical with regard to most clinical signs, especially those related to bacterial pneumonias. Some are acute, like fog fever, while others are chronic as in 'bovine farmer's lung'. There is usually acute or chronic respiratory distress and a relative absence of toxemia; most are progressive and non-responsive to treatment; the pathology consists of varying degrees of pulmonary emphysema, edema, hyaline membrane formation and alveolar epithelial cell and interstitial tissue hyperplasia. While there are obvious clinical, and particularly epidemiological, differences between the various diseases, there are fewer differences between the pathological findings which tend to merge from one to another.

Table 100. Diseases of the lungs of cattle in which the essential lesion is interstitial pneumonia.

A. *Diseases of uncertain etiology*
   1. Acute bovine pulmonary emphysema and edema (ABPEE) also known as 'fog fever', in cattle moved from dry to lush pasture (may be due to D, L-tryptophan). Usually occurs in outbreak form (2)
   2. Diffuse fibrosing alveolitis. Chronic disease which occurs sporadically in mature cows (1)
   3. Sporadic cases of acute interstitial pneumonia of young cattle (6–18 months of age)

B. *Hypersensitivity diseases*
   1. Extrinsic allergic alveolitis (bovine farmer's lung). Epidemiologically associated with moldy feeds in housed cattle. May be sudden in onset in individual animals or develop insidiously as a chronic disease in several cows (3)
   2. Milk allergy. Occurs sporadically and is sudden in onset (1)

C. *Plant poisoning*
   1. *Ipomoea batatas* (sweet potatoes infested with the mold *Fusarium solani*) (23)
   2. *Zieria arborescens* (stinkwood)
   3. *Perilla frutescens* (purple mint) (24)
   4. *Brassica* spp.

D. *Parasitic diseases*
   1. *Dictyocaulus viviparus* (6) (including the hypersensitivity aspect)
   2. *Ascaris suum (12)*

E. *Exposure to irritant gases and fumes*
   1. Nitrogen dioxide (13)
   2. Zinc oxide (16)

F. *Endotoxic or metabolic*
   Shock lung due to endotoxemia such as in peracute coliform mastitis

Etiology

The precise etiology cannot usually be determined.

Acute bovine pulmonary emphysema and edema (ABPEE) or fog fever

This is acute interstitial pneumonia and has also been described as acute respiratory distress syndrome of cattle. Several causes have been suggested based on epidemiological findings but invariably the cause cannot be determined. The cause in adult cattle which have been moved from a dry to a lush pasture in the autumn season is considered to be the ingestion of a toxic level of D, L-tryptophan in the forage. The experimental oral administration of toxic amounts of D, L-tryptophan to cattle causes clinical and pathological findings similar, if not identical, to those of the naturally occurring disease (5, 6). D, L-tryptophan is converted in the rumen to 3-methylindole which, when given orally or intravenously, also produces the characteristic lesions in cattle and goats (7). It is thought that the 3-methylindole exerts a direct effect upon cells and cell membranes of bronchioles and alveolar walls, perhaps as a result of strong lipophilic properties (7). Specific forages have not been implicated, but affected cattle have often been consuming alfalfa, kale, rape, turnip tops, rapidly growing pasture grass, and several other feeds (9). In one study, however, pasture levels of trypotophan were not higher in those associated with the disease compared to normal pastures (10). In some naturally occurring cases of fog fever in beef cows changed from a dry summer range to a lush green pasture, there was a marked increase in the ruminal levels of 3-methylindole (39) while in other cases the levels were not abnormal (40). Failure to detect abnormally high levels in the rumen and plasma of naturally occurring cases may be related to the rapid metabolism and elimination of 3-methylindole. The levels of tryptophan in lush pasture are considered to be sufficient to yield toxic doses of 3-methylindole. A 450 kg cow eating grass at an equivalent dry weight intake of 3·5% of body weight per day with a tryptophan concentration of 0·3% of dry weight would ingest 0·11 g tryptophan/kg body weight/day. The total amount ingested over a 3 day period would approximate the single oral dose of 0·35 g/kg body weight needed to reproduce the disease experimentally (6).

In the experimental disease, the typical clinical signs of respiratory disease appear within 24–36 hours after the oral administration of L-tryptophan to adult cattle, and within 4 days 50% of the dosed cows will die (7). The predominant pulmonary lesions include edema, interstitial emphysema, hyaline membranes, and hyperplasia of alveolar lining cells (7). The L-tryptophan is converted to indolacetic acid which is decarboxylated to 3-methylindole which is absorbed and metabolized by a mixed function oxidase system in the lung to produce pneumotoxicity (7). The lesions have also been produced in cattle, sheep and goats following oral or intravenous administration of 3-methylindole (7). Calves may be more resistant to experimental toxicity with 3-methylindole than adults which supports the observation that the naturally occurring disease is uncommon in calves grazing the same pasture in which adults are affected (41). Indole, a ruminal metabolite of L-tryptophan, when given experimentally does not cause acute pulmonary edema and emphysema in cattle, but high doses can result in hemoglobinuric nephrosis (42).

Diffuse fibrosing alveolitis

This is a chronic interstitial pneumonia of cattle which occurs sporadically and is suspected of being caused by repeated subclinical incidents of ABPEE or from recovered cases of the disease (1). Experimentally, repeated oral doses of 3-methylindole can result in diffuse pulmonary fibrosis and alveolitis in cattle (11).

Parasitic infestation

For many years it was thought that massive infestation of the lungs by large numbers of lungworm larvae in a lungworm-sensitized animal could cause an allergic reaction resulting in the development of acute bovine pulmonary emphysema. The possibility of such a hypersensitivity as a cause of fog fever cannot be totally ignored but at the present time there is no evidence to support such a theory (2). Such a hypersensitivity can happen when the level of larval infestation of pasture is extremely high but it is not involved in the great majority of cases. In most cases of naturally occurring fog fever there is no laboratory evidence of lungworms in the lungs or feces of affected and in-contact animals. Reinfection of cattle with lungworm will occur 2–3 weeks following introduction to an infected pasture and cause acute respiratory distress which is indistinguishable clinically from fog fever. The migration of abnormal parasites, particularly *Ascaris suum*, has been observed to cause an acute interstitial pneumonia in cattle which were allowed access to areas previously occupied by swine (12).

Inhalation of irritant gases

The experimental inhalation of nitrogen dioxide gas is capable of causing acute interstitial pneumonia in cattle and severe alveolar edema and emphysema in pigs (13) but it seems unlikely that animals of either species would be exposed naturally to a significant concentration of the gas for a sufficiently long period to produce such lesions. However, one report suggests that silo-fillers' disease has occurred in cattle (14).

Pigs which survived experimental exposure to silo gas do not have the lesions seen in silo-fillers' disease in man, and experimental exposure of cattle to nitrogen dioxide gas produces lesions which do not occur in naturally occurring fog fever (15). Acute pulmonary emphysema and deaths have occurred in cattle exposed to zinc oxide fumes produced by the welding of galvanized metal in an enclosed barn housing cattle (16).

Hypersensitivity to molds

The ingestion or inhalation of molds has been suspected as a cause of the disease in cattle. Earlier work suggested that the disease was associated with hypersensitivity to moldy hay based on the presence of serum precipitins of the thermophilic antigens of *Thermopolyspora polyspora* (17), *Micropolyspora faeni* (18) and *Thermoactinomyces vulgaris* (18). These serum precipitins have been present in cattle affected with extrinsic allergic alveolitis or bovine farmers' lung (3).

While these serum precipitins were frequently found in cattle exposed to moldy hay, they were absent from the serum of cases of ABPEE in grazing cattle (19). In Switzerland a high incidence of precipitin against *Micropolyspora faeni* (60%) and moldy hay antigen (80%) was demonstrated in exposed but apparently healthy cattle from an area where 'allergic pneumonia' is common. Many animals lost their precipitins during the pasture season and regained them during winter housing (20).

An outbreak of acute respiratory disease in cattle has been described in Canada in which 90% of the adults in a dairy herd developed acute bovine allergic pneumonitis about 15 hours after the introduction of severely moldy hay (8). The results of the serological investigation and provocative challenge indicated a hypersensitivity pneumonitis due to allergens of *Micropolyspora faeni*. A hypersensitivity pneumonitis has been produced experimentally in calves by exposure to aerosols of *Micropolyspora faeni* with or without prior sensitization by subcutaneous injection of the antigen (8).

One relationship which is thought to be of importance in Canada is the occurrence of the disease in cattle standing near the hay chute from which hay and bedding are thrown down from the storage area to the barn floor. It is not uncommon to have a selective distribution of the disease so that only animals which stand near the chute, and are thus more exposed to the inhalation of the dust, become affected. Similarly, feedlot cattle which are fed too finely ground mixed feed are commonly exposed to dusty feed particles and this may explain certain outbreaks.

The high incidence of ABPEE in the autumn when many legumes and other pasture plants are in flower, and the common occurrence at this time of allergic rhinitis in cattle, suggest that the inhalation of pollen may cause an allergic response of the alveolar epithelium. However, many outbreaks of the disease have occurred in cattle solely on grass pasture with no flowers and intradermal tests of sensitivity to many pasture plants and to the ruminal contents of affected animals have been negative and blood histamine levels are within the normal range (22).

Plant poisoning
In North America the ingestion of sweet potatoes infested with the mold *Fusarium solani* has been incriminated as a cause of acute interstitial pneumonia in cattle (23). Growth of the mold on the potatoes produces the toxins ipomeamarone and ipomeamaronol, and a lung edema factor. The latter is a collective term for a group of substances capable of causing death associated with severe edema and a proliferative alveolitis of the lungs of laboratory animals. It produces a respiratory syndrome which is clinically and pathologically indistinguishable from ABPEE.

A weed, *Perilla frutescens*, is considered to be a cause of the disease in cattle in the United States and wherever the plant is found (24). High morbidity and high case fatality rates are characteristic and the plant contains a perilla ketone which can be used to produce the disease experimentally (24).

Viral and/or bacterial infections
The possibility that viral and/or bacterial infections of the lung may cause a acute interstitial pneumonia cannot be excluded. Many veterinarians have experienced cases of what they thought clinically was pneumonic pasteurellosis, particularly in yearling cattle, which failed to respond to the usual successful therapy and which died unexpectedly in 2–4 days with lesions similar to or indistinguishable from those of acute interstitial pneumonia (37). One syndrome occurs in young cattle between 6 and 24 months of age which have been recently introduced into a feedlot. There is a sudden onset of what appears clinically to be pneumonic pasteurellosis which responds initially to antibiotic therapy. However, 2–4 days later the animal develops acute respiratory distress and dies in a few days. At necropsy there are lesions of acute interstitial pneumonia. In the second syndrome, young calves from 3 to 6 months of age appear to develop the disease a few weeks following recovery from enzootic pneumonia. Some of these resemble the disease seen in housed feedlot cattle in the United Kingdom (25). In the interstitial pneumonias caused by the bovine respiratory viruses there is a bronchiolitis in addition to the alveolitis and these should be termed bronchiointerstitial pneumonias (21). The bovine respiratory syncytial virus is considered to be an important cause of outbreaks of acute interstitial pneumonia in beef calves 2–4 weeks after weaning. The clinical and pathological manifestations of the pulmonary response in experimentally induced anaphylaxis and naturally occurring ABPEE in cattle on pasture in the autumn are different which suggests that an acute anaphylaxis is not the mechanism (26).

Other less likely causes of ABPEE have been suggested, including a nutritional deficiency of phosphorus and *Clostridium perfringens* intoxication, but these lack support.

Epidemiology
Acute pulmonary emphysema and edema or fog fever, occurs almost exclusively in adult cows and bulls usually 4–10 days after being moved abruptly from a dry or overgrazed summer pasture to a lush autumn pasture. The new pasture may or may not have been grazed during that summer and the species of grass or plants does not seem to make a difference, but usually there is some lush regrowth of grass, legume or other palatable plants. Merely changing pasture fields in the autumn has precipitated the disease. In the mountainous areas of North America the disease occurs commonly in cattle brought down from high altitude grasslands to the cultivated and perhaps irrigated lush pastures (9, 27).

ABPEE usually occurs in outbreaks, the morbidity ranging from 10% in some herds up to 50% and higher in others with a case fatality ranging from 25 to 50%. It is not unusual to observe a mild form of the disease in about one-third of the adults at risk but only 10% of those at risk may be severely affected. Often, a number of cows are found dead without premonitory signs; many others are severely ill and die within 24 hours and the owner believes that the entire herd will die because of the sudden onset and the large number of animals which are affected at once. Calves and young growing cattle up to 1 year of age grazing the same pasture are usually unaffected.

A retrospective analysis and random sample survey of cattle ranches in northern California revealed that the type of forage management has a significant effect on the occurrence of the disease (34). The greatest occurrence of the disease was in herds where the cattle were moved from summer ranges to second-growth hay fields or to irrigated pastures or from one irrigated field to another. The adult morbidity rate was 2.6% and the case fatality rate about 55% (34). The disease did not occur on ranches with limited or no movement of cattle from summer ranges to lush autumn pastures.

Placing cattle on rape or kale forage fields, or in fields where turnips have been pulled and the cattle allowed access to the tops, may have the same effect. The disease has also occurred commonly in western Canada when cattle have been placed in a stubble field following harvesting of any of the cereal crops. Veterinarians have noted that the timespan over which the disease occurs during the autumn months is only 2–4 weeks and that, following the first frost in the fall, the incidence of the disease declines rapidly. The disease has also occurred in the same herd on the same pasture in successive years.

ABPEE in adult cattle in autumn have been recorded from Canada (4) and the United States (9), Great Britain (27) Holland and New Zealand (30). The disease is rare in Australia. The chronic form of the disease in housed cattle appears to be the predominant form of the disease in Switzerland, but the acute form in cattle which have been changed from a dry to lush pasture is now reported (31). The disease has been recognized in France for many years as *aftermath disease* or *aftermath emphysema*, especially in the Normandy region (36). Some reports have suggested a breed incidence, Herefords being more commonly affected than the Jersey, Holstein, Shorthorn and Angus breeds, but there are few exact epidemiological data to support the observation. One report suggested that the chronic type in housed cattle was more common in the Channel Island breeds (4).

Acute interstitial pneumonia has been recorded in sheep and there was extensive alveolar epithelialization (32). In Norway, an acute respiratory distress syndrome has occurred in lambs moved from mountain pastures onto lush aftermath pasture (29). The lesions were those of acute interstitial pneumonia and alveolar epithelial hypersensitivity to molds in the grass is being explored (35, 44). The experimental oral administration of 3-methylindole to lambs will result in acute dyspnea and lesions similar to those which occur in cattle and adult sheep following dosing with 3-methylindole (48). However, the lesions in experimental lambs are different from those which occur in lambs affected with the naturally occurring disease (48).

The other types of interstitial pneumonia occur sporadically and may affect only a single animal or several over a period of time. There is not necessarily a seasonal incidence except in areas where cattle are housed and fed dusty and moldy hay during the winter months. The disease has occurred in feedlot cattle in open feedlots (28) and in young cattle fed on fattening rations indoors (25). Acute interstitial pneumonia occurs in weaned beef calves about 4 weeks after weaning (38). The interstitial pneumonia which may be the result of anaphylaxis also occurs sporadically and therefore not in outbreaks.

Pathogenesis

Because of the number and variety of circumstances in which acute or chronic interstitial pneumonia occurs, it is difficult to suggest a basic underlying cause, or to explain the mechanisms for the development of the lesions and the variations which occur from one circumstance to another. Our interpretation is that the reaction which occurs is a non-specific but fundamental reaction of the pulmonary parenchyma to a wide variety of insults which may be ingested, inhaled or produced endogenously. The fundamental reaction of the pulmonary parenchyma to sublethal injury is a combination of congestion, edema and an outpouring of protein-rich fluid into the alveolus, hyaline membrane formation, alveolar and interstitial emphysema which is secondary, and proliferation of alveolar septal cells and fibrosis of the interstitial spaces. Unlike the bacterial pneumonias, the emphasis is on edema and proliferation rather than on necrosis as in the bacterial pneumonias. Because mild cases of ABPEE may recover completely, it is suggested that the lesion can be reversible.

Considerable effort has been expended to experimentally induce ABPEE similar to the naturally occurring disease, by the oral administration of D, L-tryptophan or one of its metabolites, 3-methylindole, to cattle, sheep and goats (7). The L-isomer of tryptophan is metabolized by ruminal microorganisms to indolacetic acid which is then converted to 3-methylindole. The conversion of L-tryptophan to 3-methylindole is maximal at a ruminal pH near neutrality (51). Under field conditions, when cattle are abruptly changed from a relatively dry pasture to a lush green pasture, this change is associated with an increase in ruminal ammonia, a decrease in ruminal pH, and a decrease in ruminal buffering capacity (6). The 3-methylindole is absorbed from the rumen and metabolized by a mixed-function oxidase system to an active intermediate which has pneumotoxic properties. Pulmonary edema is the first morphological change seen in ruminants given 3-methylindole, and the severity and extent of this lesion is probably the single most important factor which determines the severity of the clinical response and the likelihood of survival. The edema is preceded by degeneration, necrosis and exfoliation of type 1 alveolar septal cells. During this acute phase, the most dramatic features of the lesion are flooding of the alveoli with serofibrinous exudate, and congestion and edema of alveolar walls. There is also hyaline membrane formation. Varying degrees of severity of interstitial emphysema develop. This interstitial emphysema may spread within the lymphatics to the mediastinum and into the subcutaneous tissues over the withers. It may even spread over the entire dorsum of the back and, occasionally, over the entire body including the legs. If the acute phase is severe enough there is marked respiratory distress and rapid death from hypoxemia.

If the animal survives the acute phase, proliferation of alveolar type 2 cells marks the beginning of the shift from the exudative to the proliferative stages of pneumonia. There is alveolar epithelialization and interstitial fibrosis, the latter being progressive and irreversible. The central features of chronic interstitial pneumonia are intra-alveolar accumulation of mononuclear cells, proliferation and persistence of alveolar type 2 cells, and interstitial thickening by accumulation of lymphoid cells and fibrous tissue. Diffuse fibrosing alveolitis is a form of chronic interstitial pneumonia of uncertain etiology, but possibly the chronic form of ABPEE. Repeated oral administration of 3-methylindole in cattle provides a good experimental model for diffuse pulmonary fibrosis (11).

The effects of 3-methylindole on pulmonary function and gas exchange have been examined in cattle, goats and horses. In cattle there is impairment of sympathetic pulmonary vasconstriction (33), and changes in intra-acinar pulmonary arteries which may be related to a sudden elevation in arterial and venous pressures in the pulmonary system (49). There are large increases in respiratory rate, minute viscous work, $P\text{aco}_2$ and large decreases in tidal volume dynamic lung compliance, and $P\text{ao}_2$. All of these are compatible with the severe pulmonary edema and alveolar injury (50). In goats there is a pronounced decrease in lung compliance, a moderate increase in airway resistance, a concomitant hypoxemia, a progressive decrease in tidal volume and alveolar ventilation and an increase in the dead space-to-tidal volume ratio (52). These changes are characteristic of a restrictive type of respiratory tract disease in goats in which pulmonary edema and the pulmonary function changes are similar to those of adult respiratory distress syndrome in man. In the horse, 3-methylindole causes decreased dynamic compliance and increased functional residual capacity and minimal volume, all of which are compatible with small airway obstruction produced by necrotizing bronchiolitis (53). Phenobarbital, an inducer of cytochrome P_{450}, increases the clearance of 3-methylindole from plasma and therefore the severity of the lesions in ponies (54).

Clinical findings

Acute bovine pulmonary emphysema and edema

This disease, also known as 'fog fever', is usually obvious because of its characteristic clinical presentation.

The onset is sudden. Within 4–10 days after adult cattle have been turned onto a new pasture, they may be found dead without any premonitory signs. Many cattle show labored breathing, often with an expiratory grunt, open-mouthed breathing, frothing at the mouth, and anxiety. Severely affected cattle to not graze, stand apart from the herd and are reluctant to walk. If forced to move they may fall down and die within a few minutes. Often, removal of the affected herd from the pasture will result in an increased number of deaths. Moderately affected cattle will continue to graze but their respirations are increased above normal. Coughing is infrequent regardless of the severity. The temperature is normal to slightly elevated (38·5–39·5°C, 102–103°F) but may be up to 41–42°C (106–108°F) during very warm weather. There is a similar variation in the heart rate (80–120/min) and those with a rate of more than 120/min are usually in the terminal stages of the disease. Bloat and ruminal atony are common in severe cases. Subcutaneous emphysema is common over the withers and extending down to the axillae and ventral aspects of the thorax. The nostrils are flared and the nasal discharge is normal. Diarrhea is not uncommon but is mild and transient.

Loud, clear bronchial tones audible over the ventral aspects of the lung, indicating consolidation without bronchial involvement, are the characteristic findings on auscultation in the early stages of the acute disease. There may be a relative absence of breath sounds over the dorsal parts of the lung if involvement is severe, but in animals which live for several days the loud friction rubs and dry crackling sounds characteristic of interstitial emphysema are signs of diagnostic significance. Most severely affected cases will die within 2 days of onset but less severe cases will live for several days and then die with diffuse pulmonary involvement. Those which survive longer than 1 week will often have chronic emphysema and remain unhealthy. Of those moderately affected cattle which recover in a few days, some will develop congestive heart failure a few months later, due to chronic interstitial pneumonia. Calves running with their adult dams will usually not be affected.

Other interstitial pneumonias

These diseases usually occur sporadically, but several animals may be affected over a period of time. There may or may not be a history of a change of feed or the feeding of moldy or dusty feed. In many cases, a few days elapse after the appearance of signs before the owner is sufficiently concerned to call a veterinarian. Commonly, the owner has treated the animal with an antibiotic for what he thought was a bacterial pneumonia, with little or no response. There is dyspnea, increased respiratory effort sometimes with a grunt, frequently deep coughing, a fall in milk production, an absence of toxemia, a variable temperature (38·5–40°C, 102–104°F) and a variable appetite. On auscultation there are loud bronchial tones over the ventral aspects of the lungs and dry crackling sounds over both dorsal and ventral aspects. The presence of moist crackling sounds suggests secondary bacterial bronchopneumonia; subcutaneous emphysema is uncommon in these and most will become progressively worse. Yearling cattle with acute interstitial pneumonia which may be viral in origin will become much worse and die in a few days in spite of therapy. Mature cattle affected with bovine farmers' lung will survive in an unthrifty state with the chronic disease for several weeks and even months. The major clinical features of all these are obvious respiratory disease, lack of toxemia, poor response to treatment, progressive worsening, and abnormal lung sounds distributed over the entire lung fields.

Clinical pathology

In this disease there are no clinicopathological findings which have any diagnostic significance, although bacteriological examination of a nasal swab may indicate the cause of the secondary bronchopneumonia. Examination of feces and herbage for lungworm larvae should also be carried out. The observed high levels of 'farmers' lung hay' antibodies in serum are not of much value diagnostically because of the similar levels found in many clinically normal cows (3) and many cases of classical fog fever have negative serum precipitin levels (19).

Necropsy findings

In ABPEE, the lungs are enlarged and firm and do not collapse on cutting. In the early stages of acute cases they contain much fluid which is more viscid than usual edema fluid. The pleura is pale and opaque and appears to be thickened. In peracute cases, the entire lungs are homogeneously affected in this way. Such cases usually have edema of the larynx. In the more common acute case, the lung has a marbled appearance. Adjacent lobes may be affected with any one of four abnormalities. Areas of normal, pink lung are restricted to the dorsal part of the caudal lobes. There are areas of pale tissue indicative of alveolar emphysema, areas of a dark pink color affected by early alveolar exudation, yellow areas in which the alveoli are filled with coagulated protein-rich fluid, and dark red areas where epithelialization has occurred. The latter two lesions are firm on palpation and resemble thymus or pancreas. They are more common in the ventral parts of the cranial lobes. In chronic cases, as a sequel to the acute form described above, the obvious differences in the age of the lesions suggests that the disease progresses in steps by the periodic involvement of fresh areas of tissue. In all cases there is usually a frothy exudate, sometimes containing flecks of pus, in the bronchi and trachea, and the mucosa of these passages is markedly hyperemic.

Histologically, the characteristic findings are an absence of inflammation, except in the case of secondary bacterial invasion, and the presence of an eosinophilic, protein-rich fluid which coagulates in the alveoli, or may subsequently be compressed into a hyaline membrane. This is more apparent in acute cases and, if animals live for a few days, there is evidence of epithelialization of the alveolar walls. In longstanding cases, there is extensive epithelialization and fibrosis.

The pathology of bovine farmers' lung (3) and diffuse fibrosing alveolitis (1) has been described and consists of variations of the lesions of chronic interstitial pneumonia.

Bacteriological examination of the lungs is often negative, although in cases of long standing in which secondary bacterial pneumonia has developed *Pasteurella multocida*, *Past. haemolytica*, *Streptococcus* spp., and *Corynebacterium* (*Rhodococcus*) *pyogenes* may be found. A careful search should be made for nematode larvae.

Diagnosis

The differential diagnosis of bovine respiratory disease is summarized in Table 53, p. 000.

The diagnosis of acute bovine pulmonary emphysema and edema is usually obvious when presented with an outbreak of acute respiratory disease in adult cattle which have recently been moved onto a new pasture. The onset is sudden, many cattle are found dead and many dyspneic. The disease may resemble pneumonic pasteurellosis if the cattle were moved recently but there are usually fever, toxemia, mucopurulent nasal discharge, less dyspnea, and young cattle are more commonly affected. Organophosphatic insecticide poisoning may resemble the pasture form of pulmonary emphysema because of the dyspnea but additionally there is pupillary constriction, mucoid diarrhea, muscular tremor and stiffness of the limbs, and no abnormal lung sounds. An outbreak of nitrate poisoning may occur in cows moved into a new pasture with high levels of nitrate. Many cows are affected quickly, they are weak, stagger, gasp, fall down and die rapidly. The chocolate brown coloration of the mucous membranes, the lack of abnormal lung sounds, and the response to treatment are more common in nitrate poisoning.

All of the other types of acute interstitial pneumonia in cattle not associated with a change of pasture in the autumn are difficult to diagnose clinically and pathologically, especially when they occur in a single animal. Their epidemiological characteristics summarized in Table 53 will often offer some clues.

The chronic and subacute types of interstitial pneumonia are difficult to differentiate from each other and from other pneumonias of cattle. Bovine farmers' lung or extrinsic allergic alveolitis occurs in housed cattle exposed to dusty or moldy feeds for a prolonged period and is characterized by a history of chronic coughing, weight loss, poor milk production, occasionally green-colored nasal discharge, and dry crackles over most aspects of the lungs (3). Not infrequently, acute cases occur and die within a week after the onset of signs. Reinfection or primary infections with lungworm may occur in cattle at grass in the autumn months and result in subacute or acute disease which may resemble bovine farmers' lung clinically but not epidemiologically and necropsy will provide the diagnosis of both types of lungworm pneumonia. The acute interstitial pneumonia occurring in recently weaned beef calves or feedlot cattle is characterized by the sudden onset of acute respiratory distress, absence of toxemia, lack of abnormal nasal discharge, and a poor response to treatment with antibiotics. It can be difficult to differentiate clinically from acute viral interstitial pneumonia or pneumonic pasteurellosis. However, in acute interstitial pneumonia there is marked dyspnea and the abnormal lung sounds are usually distributed over the entire lung fields.

Enzootic pneumonia of calves may resemble acute or chronic interstitial pneumonia but it is almost entirely restricted to housed calves less than 6 months of age and they respond to treatment gradually over a few days. The pneumonia caused by aberrant migration of *Ascaris suis* larvae may be indistinguishable from acute interstitial pneumonia, but a history of previous occupation of the area by pigs may provide the clue to the diagnosis which can only be confirmed on histological examination of tissues. It is impossible to differentiate clinically between verminous pneumonia and some of the acute interstitial pneumonias seen in yearling cattle except by identification of the larvae in the feces or tissues of affected animals.

Treatment

The treatment of fog fever in cattle is empirical and symptomatic because the etiology is poorly understood. The lesion is probably irreversible in severe cases and treatment is therefore unlikely to be effective. When outbreaks of the disease occur on pasture the first reaction is usually to remove the entire herd from the pasture to avoid the development of new cases. Many veterinarians have observed that almost all new cases in an outbreak will usually occur by the 4th day after the onset of the outbreak and that removal from the pasture will not necessarily prevent new cases. Conversely, leaving the herd on pasture will not usually result in additional cases. Severely affected cattle should be removed from the pasture with extreme care and very slowly and only if necessary to move them to shelter from sun or to load them for shipment to slaughter. Immediate slaughter for salvage may be indicated in severe cases. Mild or moderately affected cases will commonly recover spontaneously without any treatment if left alone and this fact has not been given due consideration when the use of certain drugs has provided remarkable results.

Several different drugs have been advocated and used routinely for the treatment of ABPEE in cattle. None of them has been properly evaluated and it is difficult to make definitive recommendations. Corticosteroids have been used routinely in an attempt to reduce the development and the effects of the alveolar edema but their efficacy has been difficult to evaluate. The use of dexamethazone, 1 mg/5–10 kg body weight intramuscularly, may be beneficial in severe cases. Combinations of adrenaline and antihistamines are also used routinely but must be repeated every hour because of their short pharmacological action. Atropine is also used at a rate of 1 g/450 kg body weight intramuscularly, with variable results. Because of its bronchodilatory effect it may provide some relief from the dyspnea temporarily but probably has no effect on the basic lesion. Diuretics have been recommended for the pulmonary edema but have not been investigated in the field. Treatment with antihistamines provided no observable clinical improvements.

Drugs which act as antagonists to postulated mediators of bovine anaphylaxis or hypersensitivity such as acetylsalicylic acid, mepyramine maleate, sodium meclofenamate and dexomethazone are ineffective against the effects of experimental administration of 3-methylindole (45).

The treatment of the chronic interstitial pneumonias is also unsatisfactory because the lesion is progressive and irreversible. Treatment with a course of antibiotics and corticosteroids for several days is recommended but there is no evidence to support the beneficial claims.

Control

There are no known reliable methods for the prevention of ABPEE in pastured cattle. If lush autumn pasture contains toxic levels of the substance that causes the acute disease it would seem rational to control the introduction of cattle to the new pasture. This can be done by controlling the total grazing time during the first 10 days: allow the cattle to graze for 2 hours on the first day, increasing by increments of 1 hour per day, and leave them on full time at the end of 10–12 days. Such a management procedure is laborious, requires supplementation with other feeds and daily removal of cattle from the pasture, and may not be practical depending on the size and terrain of the pasture and the holding yards which are available.

A possible approach to the field problem would be the use of inhibitors which prevent the conversion of tryptophan in forage to 3-methylindole. The experimental tryptophan-induced acute bovine pulmonary edema and emphysema can be prevented by the simultaneous oral administration of chlortetracycline or polyether antibiotics such as monensin (43). The daily oral administration of 2·5 g of chlortetracycline beginning 1 day before and for 4 days following administration of a toxin of L-tryptophan will prevent clinical signs (46). The daily oral administration of monensin at the rate of 200 mg/head/day beginning one day before and for 7 days after an abrupt change from a poor quality hay diet to a lush pasture reduced the formation of 3-methylindole during the 7 days of treatment, but the effect of the drug was diminished on day 10, 3 days after its withdrawal (6). Because the effects of monensin on ruminal 3-methylindole are diminished within 48 hours after withdrawal of the drug, effective prevention of acute pulmonary edema and emphysema may require continuous administration of monensin for the critical period of approximately 10 days after the mature animals are exposed to the lush pasture (47). The daily feeding of monensin in either an energy or protein supplement will effectively reduce ruminal 3-methylindole formation in pasture-fed cattle (56). Lasalocid at a dose of 200 mg per head once daily in ground grain for 12 days reduced the conversion of tryptophan to 3-methylindole and prevented pulmonary edema (55). The daily administration of inhibitors during the critical period immediately before and after the cattle are turned onto the lush pasture may be a practical problem.

The control of non-pasture cases of interstitial pneumonia will depend on the suspected cause and removal of it from the environment of the animals. Every attempt must be made to control the concentration of dust and moldy foods to which cattle are exposed. Feed supplies must be harvested, handled, and stored with attention to minimizing dust and molds. In the preparation of mixed ground feed for cattle, the fineness of grind must be controlled to avoid dusty feed particles which may be inhaled. If dusty feeds must be used they should be wetted to assist in dust control.

The control of lungworm is essential in endemic areas where the disease occurs. This may necessitate careful monitoring and regular treatment to reduce the level of infestation on pasture.

In countries where cattle are housed, especially during the winter months, the provision of adequate ventilation is necessary to minimize aerosol viral infection which may cause acute interstitial pneumonia. Because of the creation of dust, the grinding and mixing of dry feeds like hay, straw and grains should not be done in the same enclosed area in which cattle are housed.

REVIEW LITERATURE

Breeze, R. G. & Carlson, J. R. (1982) Chemical-induced lung injury in domestic animals. *Adv. vet. Sci. comp. Med.*, *26*, 201–231.

Dungworth, D. L. (1982) Interstitial pulmonary disease. *Adv. vet. Sci. comp. Med.*, *26*, 173–200.

Wilkie, B. N. (1982) Allergic respiratory disease. *Adv. vet. Sci. comp. Med.*, *26*, 233–265.

REFERENCES

(1) Selman, I. E. & Wiseman, A. (1983) *Irish vet. J.*, *37*, 28.
(2) Selman, I. E. & Wiseman, A. (1983) *Irish vet. J.*,*37*, 54.
(3) Wiseman, A. et al. (1983) *Irish vet. J.*, *38*, 22.
(4) Blood, D. C. (1962) *Can. vet. J.*, *3*, 40.
(5) Schiefer, B. et al. (1974) *Vet. Pathol.*, *11*, 327.
(6) Carlson, J. R. et al. (1983) *Am. J. vet. Res.*, *44*, 118.
(7) Breeze, R. G. & Carlson, J. R. (1982) *Adv. vet. Sci. comp. Med.*, *26*, 207.
(8) Wilkie, B. N. (1982) *Adv. vet. Sci. comp. Med.*, *26*, 233.
(9) Blake, J. T. & Thomas, D. W. (1971) *J. Am vet. med. Assoc.*, *158*, 2047.
(10) MacKenzie, A. et al. (1975) *Res. vet. Sci.*, *19*, 227.
(11) Logan, A. et al. (1982) *Res. Vet. Sci.*, *34*
(12) McLennan, M. W. (1974) *Aust. vet. J.*, *50*, 266.
(13) Giddens, W. E. et al. (1970) *Am. J. vet. Res.*, *31*, 1779.
(14) Brightwell, A. H. (1972) *Can. vet. J.*, *13*, 224.
(15) Cutlip, R. C. (1966) *Pathol. Vet.*, *3*, 474.
(16) Hilderman, E. & Taylor, P. A. (1974) *Can. vet. J.*, *15*, 173.
(17) Jenkins, P. A. & Pepys, J. (1965) *Vet. Rec.*, *77*, 464.
(18) Lacey, J. (1968) *J. gen. Microbiol.*, *51*, 173.
(19) Pirie, H. M. et al. (1971) *Res. vet. Sci.*, *12*, 586.
(20) Nicolet, J. et al. (1972) *Infect. Immun.*, *6*, 38.
(21) Dungworth, D. L. (1982) *Adv. vet. Sci. comp. Med.*, *26*, 173.
(22) Moulton, J. E. (1961) *J. Am. vet. med. Assoc.*, *139*, 669.
(23) Doster, A. R. et al. (1978) *Vet. Pathol.*, *15*, 367.
(24) Kerr, L. A. et al. (1986) *Vet. hum. Toxicol.*, *28*, 412.
(25) Omar, A. R. & Kinch, D. A. (1966) *Vet. Rec.*, *78*, 766.
(26) Ladiges, W. C. et al. (1974) *Am. J. vet. Res.*, *35*, 389.
(27) Selman, I. E. et al. (1974) *Vet. Rec.*, *95*, 139.
(28) Jensen, R. et al. (1976) *J. Am. vet. med. Assoc.*, *169*, 507.
(29) Ulvund, M. J. & Gronstol, H. (1984) *Nord. VetMed.*, *36*, 88.
(30) Bennell, D. G. (1966) *NZ vet. J.*, *14*, 73.
(31) Eigenmann, U. J. E. et al. (1979) *Schweiz. Arch. Tierheilkd.*, *121*, 49.
(32) Pascoe, R. R. & McGavin, M. D. (1969) *Vet. Rec.*, *85*, 376.
(33) Perry, M. S. et al. (1985) *Am. J. vet. Res.*, *46*, 905.
(34) Heron, B. R. & Suther, D. E. (1979) *Bov. Pract.*, *14*, 2.
(35) Ulvund, M. J. et al. (1984) *Nord. VetMed.*, *36*, 98.
(36) Espinasse, J. & Savey, M. (1979) *Vet. Rec.*, *104*, 397.
(37) Curtis, R. A. et al. (1979) *Can. vet. J.*, *20*, 141.
(38) Hibbs, C. M. et al. (1981) *Mod. vet. Pract.*, *62*, 381.
(39) Hammond, A. C. et al. (1979) *Am. J. vet. Res.*, *40*, 1398.
(40) Mackenzie, A. et al. (1977) *Res. vet. Sci.*, *23*, 47.
(41) Cornelius, L. M. et al. (1979) *Am. J. vet. Res.*, *40*, 571.
(42) Hammond, A. C. et al. (1980) *Vet. Rec.*, *107*, 344.

(43) Hammond, A. C. et al. & Carlson, J. R. (1980) *J. anim. Sci.*, *51*, 207.
(43) Hammond, A. C. & Carlson, J. R. (1980) *J. anim. Sci.*, *51*, 207.
(44) Ulvund, M. J. & Gronstol, H. (1984) *Nord. VetMed.*, *36*, 170.
(45) Hammond, A. C. et al. (1979) *Bov. Pract.*, *14*, 9 & 12.
(46) Hammond, A. C. et al. (1978) *Am. J. vet. Res.*, *39*, 1404.
(47) Hammond, A. C. et al. (1982) *Am. J. vet. Res.*, *43*, 753.
(48) Ulvund, D. M. J. (1984) *Nord. VetMed.*, *36*, 253.
(49) Atwal, O. S. & Persofsky, M. S. (1984) *Am. J. Pathol.*, *114*, 472.
(50) Lekeux, P. et al. (1985) *Am. J. vet. Res.*, *46*, 1629.
(51) Hammond, A. C. et al. (1984) *Am. J. vet. Res.*, *45*, 2247.
(52) Mesina, J. E. Jr et al. (1984) *Am. J. vet. Res.*, *45*, 1526.
(53) Derksen, F. J. et al. (1982) *Am. J. vet. Res.*, *43*, 603.
(54) Tark, A. M. & Thomas, D. E. (1986) *Am. J. vet. Res.*, *47*, 901.
(55) Nocerini, M. R. et al. (1985) *J. anim. Sci.*, *60*, 232.
(56) Potchoiba, M. J. et al. (1984) *Am. J. vet. Res.*, *45*, 1389.

Chronic obstructive pulmonary disease of horses (COPD)

Chronic obstructive pulmonary disease (COPD) in the horse is characterized clinically by decreased work performance, chronic coughing, abnormal lung sounds and varying degrees of pulmonary and cardiac dysfunction. Pathologically, there are varying degrees of bronchitis, bronchiolitis and pulmonary emphysema. The disease was formerly known as 'heaves', pulmonary emphysema or 'broken wind'.

Etiology

The cause of the disease is uncertain, but clinical and epidemiological evidence suggests that chronic bronchiolitis which is present in affected horses is due to a hypersensitivity reaction to the allergens found in barn dust and moldy and dusty feeds (1). *Micropolyspora faeni* and *Aspergillus fumigatus* are recognized as common causes of respiratory hypersensitivity in horses affected with chronic obstructive pulmonary disease (2, 5). The hypersensitivity reactions are determined by an intradermal test or by inhalation challenge with the suspected antigen.

The serum precipitins to *Micropolyspora faeni* and *Aspergillus fumigatus* occur more frequently in horses with chronic obstructive pulmonary disease than in normal horses. Some horses without detectable precipitins will respond clinically to inhalation challenge with these antigens (3). The chymotrypsin-like enzymes of *M. faeni* and *A. fumigatus* do not play a major role in the precipitation of clinical signs of COPD (26). Horses with 'haysickness' in Iceland have serum precipitins to *M. faeni* similar to 'farmer's lung' in man (31).

There is some epidemiological evidence that chronic obstructive pulmonary disease may occur as a sequel to viral infection of the upper respiratory tract of horses. However, sufficient microbiological evidence to support the relationship is not yet available. High levels of hemagglutination inhibiting activity against influenza A equine 1 in mucus samples of horse with COPD may indicate a role for the virus in the disease (27). Similarly, elastase-producing bacteria have been isolated from some horses with the disease but the significance of their presence is unknown (28).

The possible genetic predisposition to this disease has been examined and there is no evidence to indicate an inherited basis (1). The major antiproteases in equine serum have been identified and characterized (4) and there is no evidence that the alpha-1-antitrypsin inhibitor plays a role in chronic obstructive pulmonary disease in the horse as it does in man.

Because 3-methylindole is a potent pneumotoxicant which is formed in the gastrointestinal tract and appears to be important in the pathogenesis of acute interstitial pneumonia in cattle, it has been suggested that it may be the agent responsible for forage-related COPD in horses which are pastured year round (29). The oral and intravenous administration of 3-methylindole, at a rate of 0·1 or 0·03 mg/kg body weight, to horses results in a severe and sometimes fatal pulmonary disease characterized by bronchiolitis (30). These observations raise the possibility that other air pollutants and dietary factors may cause chronic airway inflammation. In horses, the toxicity of 3-methylindole correlates with its saturable dose-dependent pharmacokinetics which precludes the possibility that 3-methylindole is pneumotoxic when exposure is at or below saturation level dose (29). Thus horses could consume small amounts of 3-methylindole or its precursors over long periods without any observed pulmonary dysfunction. However, if horses ingest slightly larger doses of 3-methylindole or indole precursors from grasses of rapid-growing pastures, acute toxicosis can result when the nearly saturated mechanisms for non-toxic elimination become saturated (29). However, to date there is no evidence that 3-methylindole plays a major role in naturally occurring COPD.

Epidemiology

The disease occurs most commonly in horses over 5 years of age and sporadic cases may occur as early as 4 months of age. In some countries in Europe the disease is a major cause of premature loss among the horse population. The disease is most common where horses are housed for long periods and are exposed to dusty or moldy feeds (6). Ponies with a history of COPD go into clinical remission when pastured, and develop an acute exacerbation of the disease due to airway hyperactivity when housed in a barn where dusty feed is used (37). As a result of the constant air pollution in barns, the air inhaled always contains potentially irritating materials. Inadequate ventilation of horse barns increases the chance of a horse becoming affected. The sex, body weight and season of the year when epidemic coughing begins, have no influence on the occurrence of the disease (6). The incidence may be highest in ponies because they are exposed to poor quality dusty feed and bedding more often than other classes of horses (6).

Pathogenesis

The most important lesion is considered to be bronchiolitis of the small airways and the clinical findings can be attributed to this lesion. Bronchospasm may also play a role in the pathogenesis. In most mammals, intrapulmonary airways are supplied throughout their length by parasympathetic bronchoconstrictor and sympathetic bronchodilator nerves. The distribution of nerves has not been established in horses, but in some species vagally induced bronchoconstriction results from stimulation of laryngeal and tracheal irritant receptors, by physical agents such as dust, chemical mediators of the immune response, and possibly by cold and turbulent air.

The net effect of the bronchiolitis or bronchospasm is a decrease in dynamic compliance and a reduction of expiratory flow rates because of the obstruction. The interference of normal airflow is the result of bronchoconstriction, thickening of the airway epithelium, excess mucus production with inflammatory cell infiltration and ineffective mucociliary clearance mechanism. The horse fails to passively exhale the previously inspired volume in the time available. Consequently, the functional residual capacity of the lung increases and if the obstruction is severe enough a forced expiratory effort may be necessary (11). Although forced expiration occurs, it may provide no effective increase in expiratory flows because of dynamic compression of the intrathoracic airways occurring when intrapleural pressure becomes greater than atmospheric pressure (7). In horses with bronchiolitis, resistance of small airways increases and airway compression may be occurring in the majority of the airways, so that forced expiratory flow may not exceed passive flow at functional residual capacity.

Because small airways contribute only a small fraction of total airway resistance, their obstruction may not increase the work of breathing, but does cause uneven distribution of ventilation, and this may be accentuated as respiratory frequency increases. This causes hypoxemia (reduced partial pressure of arterial oxygen Pa_{O_2}) (7, 32) but has little effect on arterial CO_2 tension (Pa_{CO_2}). During exercise there is a decrease in Pa_{O_2} which may be due to a greater release of oxygen from the capillary blood to supply the oxygen needs of the tissues. During the gallop of the horse with COPD there is a marked hypoxemia (Pa_{O_2} about 50 mmHg) which is compensated for by a greater release of oxygen from capillary blood to tissues and an increase in heart rate and cardiac output (32). Pulmonary hypertension also occurs secondary to the systemic arterial hypoxemia but there is a low prevalence and degree of right heart failure (cor pulmonale) probably because of the reversibility of the pulmonary hypertension associated with the disease (8).

Maldistribution of ventilation and perfusion is thus probably the major factor in the genesis of the hypoxemia. The mean percentage alveolar dead space in horses with COPD is about three times greater than that of normal horses (33). The mean percentage venous admixture of COPD horses is also more than three times that of normal horses which indicates that a larger proportion of alveoli are hypoventilated compared to normal horses (34). Uneven distribution of ventilation and hypoxemia during exercise may occur in horses failing to perform following viral diseases, but showing no clinical signs at rest.

The poor collateral ventilation in the horse may be sufficient to prevent atelectasis, but insufficient to improve gas exchange following airway obstruction. In the exercising horse with small airway obstruction a decrease in the alveolar pressure in the obstructed segment may increase capillary transmural pressure sufficiently to result in rupture and hemorrhage into the lung. In this way, airway obstruction may be a cause of intrapulmonary hemorrhage in race horses (11).

The net effect of chronic obstructive pulmonary disease in the horse is arterial hypoxemia, pulmonary arterial hypertension, an increase in the maximum change in intrapleural pressure, a decrease in compliance, decreased work performance and an increase in the expiratory effort. The chronic cough and the abnormal lung sounds are due to the bronchiolitis.

The bronchiolitis may result in functional alveolar emphysema or structural emphysema, depending on the duration and severity of the inciting agent. In functional alveolar emphysema, which is reversible, there is excessive dilatation of the alveoli and minimal rupture. This is the situation in the early stages of chronic obstructive pulmonary disease and in the acute form of equine asthma occurring on pasture. As the lesion becomes more severe, irreversible structural emphysema develops with rupture of alveoli and the development of centrilobular, panlobular and bullous emphysema. Whether there is simple overdistension of alveoli, or whether their walls are also ruptured, is very important in prognosis and treatment. There is no reliable method of differentiating clinically between functional and structural emphysema, although a corticosteroid or atropine test may be a guide if an immediate answer is required in an advanced case.

In horses with functional emphysema, the bronchiolitis will presumably heal and full recovery can occur. However, relapses may occur. In the case of structural emphysema, full recovery does not occur and the degree of respiratory insufficiency will depend on the extent of the lesion.

Clinical findings

The disease occurs most commonly in adult horses from 6 to 10 years of age. The usual history is that the horse has been stabled for several weeks or months and has a chronic cough. The animal may have had an infectious respiratory disease 1 or 2 months previously, recovered from the acute illness but began coughing recently. In affected animals, heaves can be precipitated by exposure to hay in a barn, but disease remission occurs in most of them when pastured and removed from hay. There may be a history of reduced exercise tolerance in some horses, but this is not a major feature initially.

On clinical examination, the horse is usually bright and alert, the temperature is normal and the appetite is usually normal. Coughing is common and may consist of a single cough every few seconds or there may be a paroxysm of coughing. The cough can also be elicited by digital massage of the larynx and proximal part of the trachea. The cough becomes more pronounced and wheezing with exercise. It also occurs more frequently when the horse is exposed to cold air, physical activity, excitement, and when placed in a dusty environment, or if dusty feed is offered.

An intermittent, bilateral nasal discharge is a common sign in affected horses. It may consist of serous fluid, mucus, mucopus, or blood, or a combination of these. In some cases sputum may be actually coughed out. Bilateral bloodstained nasal discharge is very suggestive of hemorrhage into the lungs after vigorous exercise.

When the blood originates in the nasal cavities or guttural pouch it is present even at rest, and is not stimulated by exercise. Race horses with early chronic obstructive pulmonary disease may develop exercise-induced pulmonary hemorrhages, the so-called 'bleeder', and exhibit epistaxis. A hunter or showjumping horse may also develop epistaxis or discharge bloodstained mucus following exercise, but for hemorrhage to be precipitated by a degree of exercise less vigorous than racing, more advanced disease must be present (9).

The resting respiratory rate is increased from a normal of 12/min up to 24–36/min. There is also an increase in the depth of respiration. The expiratory phase of respiration is prolonged and expiratory effort is clinically obvious. In advanced cases the expirations which are normally biphasic become exaggerated. During expiration there is normal collapse of the rib cage followed by a clearly visible contraction of the abdominal muscles of the flank. In longstanding cases this results in the so-called 'heave-line' which is a trough which follows along the costal arch. In advanced cases the nostrils may be visibly dilated during inspiration and the force of the expiratory effort causes the anus to protrude.

In the resting horse with COPD the heart rate is commonly within the normal range or only slightly increased. In advanced cases pulmonary arterial hypertension may result in an increase in the heart rate up to 50–60/min. In horses with chronic obstructive pulmonary disease the heart rate is significantly higher during exercise than in clinically healthy horses (16).

Auscultation of the lungs in the early stages of the disease may reveal only a slight increase in the amplitude of normal breath sounds. Abnormal lung sounds become audible as the disease progresses. Wheezing and crackling sounds occur at the end of inspiration and the end of expiration. These abnormal sounds are audible over most of the lung but are usually easiest to detect over the upper one-half of both lung fields. The abnormal sounds may be barely audible in the resting horse but they can be accentuated by 10–15 minutes exercise on a lunge line. Also, the placement of a plastic bag over the horse's nostrils for 1 minute will cause the horse to hyperventilate and abnormal sounds then become more clearly audible. Because of the wide range of interpretation of lung sounds between different clinicians it is perhaps best to recognize the presence of the abnormal lung sounds rather than identify them specifically as wheezing or crepitant sounds. It is assumed that the origin of the abnormal lung sounds is primarily from the bronchiolitis. However, because detailed correlation between the sounds heard and the pathological findings are not available, the most that can be concluded is the presence of abnormal lung sounds in a horse with the other common clinical findings of chronic obstructive pulmonary disease (12). Certainly, in the early stages the severity of the pulmonary lesion cannot be reliably assessed by auscultation.

Percussion of the thorax may reveal an increase in the area of resonance by as much as one to two intercostal spaces caudally. However, the area of resonance delineated by percussion is too labile and ill-defined to be of diagnostic value (9). Routine clinical methods for accurate measurement of exercise tolerance are not available.

The course of the disease is dependent on the removal or continual presence of the precipitating cause. If the cause is removed in the early stages, complete recovery can occur. The degree of improvement will depend on how much emphysema is functional and how much is structural. In the continual presence of the precipitating cause relapses occur commonly or the disease becomes progressive and affected horses become severely incapacitated. With conscientious management and adequate housing, breeding animals and hunters or showjumpers can remain useful for many years. The prognosis for racehorses with exercise-induced epistaxis is less hopeful because even a small degree of persistent emphysema is a serious handicap for a racehorse (9).

Most horses even with advanced chronic obstructive pulmonary disease do not die from the disease, but are usually euthanitized because of severe incapacitation.

Clinical pathology and special examinations

There are no significant changes in the hemogram or serum biochemistry of affected horses. The $Pa{O_2}$ is below normal and the $Pa{CO_2}$ is increased.

The mean values and standard deviations for blood gas and acid–base status in 20 horses with COPD were as follows: $Pa{O_2}$ = 60·8 ± 9·1 mmHg; $Pa{CO_2}$ = 42·3 ± 7·13 mmHg; and arterial pH = 7·369 ± 0·052 (32). The values for Thoroughbred horses in training were: $Pa{O_2}$ = 77·4 ± 4·3 mmHg; $Pa{CO_2}$ = 40·9 ± 5·8 mmHg and arterial pH = 7·358 ± 0·051. The $Pa{O_2}$, $Pa{CO_2}$ and arterial pH were significantly correlated to the respiratory rate in horses with COPD.

Pulmonary function tests in horses are now available but are not used routinely because of the laboratory equipment and technology required (13, 14). However, there is considerable variation in the results of the tests for healthy and diseased horses because of the many different types of equipment used and the lack of standard description of the horse with COPD (13). Affected horses have an increased respiratory and expiratory flow rate, a decreased dynamic compliance, increased pulmonary resistance and prolongation of the nitrogen washout. Most of these changes can be normalized temporarily by an intravenous injection of atropine sulfate at a rate of 0·02 mg/kg bodyweight or clenbuterol at 0·8 μg/kg bodyweight. Any of these will provide clinical relief to horses with COPD within 10–20 minutes after treatment. Histamine given by an aerosol or intravenously to normal horses or those with COPD has been recorded (14, 35). Horses with COPD are much more sensitive to histamine given intravenously, as determined by a change in breathing mechanics, than are horses with no respiratory disease (36).

Precipitins against fungi have been identified in the serum of affected horses (3) and allergic skin tests and antigen inhalation tests have also been used (2). A crude natural inhalation challenge can be done by exposing suspected horses to moldy hay or straw for 12–24 hours. Sensitive horses develop a distinct worsening of clinical signs within 8–12 hours. Cytological examination of tracheobronchial aspirates or bronchoalveolar lavage samples of horses with COPD reveal excessive mucus and a predominance of neutrophils (38, 39). In ponies with recurrent airway obstruction, acute exacerbation of the disease initiated by barn exposure results in a marked increase in the numbers of neutrophils in the bronchoalveolar lavage sample and the neutrophil numbers return to normal when the ponies are pastured (39).

Cytological examination of transtracheal washings can aid in the differential diagnoses from infectious diseases of the lung. The presence of eosinophils in the tracheal fluid sample suggests an allergic cause. However, their absence does not preclude allergy as a cause. Endoscopic examination of the upper respiratory tract can aid in the detection of horses with evidence of pulmonary hemorrhage secondary to this disease. Also, in the horse with advanced bronchitis, an excess of mucus may be seen in the pharynx, larynx or upper trachea (9). Radiography of the thorax may be useful in differentiating chronic obstructive pulmonary disease from other diseases of the lungs of horses.

Necropsy findings

Horses with bronchiolitis and functional emphysema do not die from the lung lesion. If they die from other causes the lungs may appear normal. Grossly and microscopically there is diffuse bronchiolitis and alveolar emphysema. The major lesions are restricted to lungs and heart. The lesions in the lungs are primarily in the small airways, those which are less than 2 mm in diameter. There is chronic bronchiolitis marked by diffuse epithelial hyperplasia plugs of mucus in the lumina of the small airways, peribronchiolar fibrosis and cellular infiltration by lymphocytes, plasma cells and mast cells (23). Alveolar emphysema or acinar overinflation is present usually without destructive changes in the interalveolar septa. Eosinophil infiltration of the bronchiolar walls and lumina, peribronchiolar and perivascular connective tissue and of the interlobular and interalveolar septa also occur. Destructive emphysema may occur but is uncommon. Right ventricular hypertrophy also occurs in advanced cases but cor pulmonale does not usually develop. In horses with advanced chronic obstructive pulmonary disease the lungs are enlarged, puffy, do not collapse, are pale in color and subpleural bullous emphysema is present. Microscopically there is panlobular and centrilobular emphysema, atrophy and loss of smaller airways. The alveolar walls are disrupted and the airspaces confluent. The pulmonary and bronchial arterial networks are reduced in size. The bronchioles are infiltrated with chronic inflammatory cells. The bronchiolar lesions of emphysema differ from those seen in isolated cases of equine bronchiolitis which is distinguished chiefly by the presence of dense, inflammatory reaction without apparent destruction or atrophy (15).

Diagnosis

The important clinical features of chronic obstructive pulmonary disease in the horse include the following:

- Mature horse 6–10 years of age
- History of prolonged confinement and exposure to a dusty environment
- Remission of clinical signs if the horse is placed on pasture
- Exacerbation of the disease if a suspected case is housed in a barn with access to dusty feed
- Chronic coughing for several days or weeks
- Reduced exercise performance
- Dyspnea in an otherwise normal horse
- Wheezing and crepitant lung sounds
- An obvious expiratory effort following exercise
- Lack of toxemia.

The disease must be differentiated from acute pneumonia in which there is toxemia, fever, coughing and increased bronchial tones on auscultation. A transtracheal wash will reveal the presence of an exudate. A concurrent pleuritis will result in a pleural effusion and muffling of lung sounds and a fluid line. Thoracentesis will reveal the presence of an exudate.

Acute equine asthma is similar to chronic obstructive pulmonary disease but occurs with an acute onset in pastured horses. Presumably, bronchospasm occurs as a result of exposure to an allergen on pasture. There is a sudden onset of acute dyspnea and respiratory distress which responds dramatically to a combination of corticosteroids and antihistamines.

Lungworm pneumonia in the horse is uncommon, but usually occurs in young animals and is characterized clinically by coughing and dyspnea with forced expiration. Knowledge of the occurrence of disease in the area is important; examination of the feces for larvae is necessary and treatment with anthelmintics is beneficial.

Pleurisy in the horse is characterized by varying degrees of toxemia, inappetence to anorexia, an increase in respiratory rate, a muffling or absence of lung sounds over the ventral one-half or two-thirds of both lung fields, a fluid line on percussion and ventral body edema. Thoracentesis will reveal the presence of pleural fluid.

Pulmonary or mediastinal neoplasms will cause progressive weight loss, reduced exercise performance, dyspnea, hydrothorax, areas of absence of lung sounds and dullness on percussion. Examination of pleural fluid may assist in the diagnosis if neoplastic cells have exfoliated.

'Farmer's lung' in the horse is characterized by chronic pulmonary disease due to progressive alveolar epithelial hyperplasia and fibrosis of the lungs. The presence of serum precipitins to *Micropolyspora faeni* and *Aspergillus fumigatus* in affected horses suggests a type III allergic reaction causing alveolar cell proliferation. The disease is clinically similar to chronic obstructive pulmonary disease but is progressive and unresponsive to treatment.

Acute viral infection of the upper respiratory tract of horses may result in animals which continue to cough and have reduced exercise tolerance for 2–3 weeks following recovery from the acute illness. Wheezing and crepitant sounds of the lungs may be audible and differentiation from bronchiolitis associated with chronic obstructive pulmonary disease is difficult. With good management and adequate housing recovery is usual.

The presence of reversible uncomplicated bronchiolitis (functional alveolar emphysema) may be determined by the use of bronchodilators which are presented under treatment. The beneficial response to corticosteroids is also indirect evidence of the presence of the early stages of disease in which bronchiolitis is the major lesion.

Treatment and control

The best treatment for early cases is the provision of fresh air (9). The effects of environmental control on pulmonary function of horses affected with COPD have been examined (9). A controlled environment in which affected horses were bedded on shredded paper and fed a complete cubed diet resulted in remission of the clinical signs of COPD in from 4 to 24 days. There were significant changes in several pulmonary function parameters such as the maximum change in intrathoracic pressure, tidal volume, minute volume and $Pa{O_2}$(9). The pulmonary function values returned to those found in normal horses which indicates that the respiratory function changes which occur in COPD are reversible. It also indicates that destructive emphysema is not a major feature of the disease. Thus environmental control is of major importance therapeutically. Ideally, the horse should be kept permanently in the open air, if not actually on pasture. A partly covered and well-protected outside yard is also suitable. During the winter months blankets may be necessary for horses kept outdoors. For horses which must be housed, the loose box should not be less than 3 × 3·6 m and even larger boxes 5·4 × 5·4 m are recommended for large Thoroughbred horses. The box should be well ventilated with eight to ten air changes per hour. Every effort must be made to ensure that stable dust is kept to a minimum. All dust should be removed from roof rafters, windowsills, ledges and feed boxes. In order of preference, peat, woodchippings or sawdust should be used for bedding, instead of straw. If hay is fed it should be of the best quality and must be thoroughly wetted with water prior to feeding. The feeding of hay as wet chaff at ground level will encourage the horse to keep its head down for long periods which facilitates the drainage of bronchial exudate. The two major advantages of pasture are the lowering of the head to graze and the breathing of fresh air. An alternative to hay is to feed a complete pelleted ration which contains molasses to minimize dust which may occur if the pellets break. Advanced cases of pulmonary emphysema in the horse are unlikely to recover but with proper care and feeding as outlined above they can be maintained as breeding animals for months and even years. The prognosis is quite good for a pleasure horse, but for a racehorse the disease is usually sufficient to make it a respiratory invalid, and if it 'bleeds' it may drop dead at the track or be disqualified from racing.

Many drugs including corticosteroids, antihistamines, expectorants, inhalants, bronchodilators and antibiotics have been used for the treatment of chronic obstructive pulmonary disease in the horse. The rationale for the use of some of these drugs is not documented. Regardless of which ones are used the precipitating causes in the environment must be removed. Dexamethasone (esterified) is used at a dose of 25 mg per animal intramuscularly every 2nd day for up to 2 weeks and may give remarkable results (12). Presumably the corticosteroids are effective because of their anti-inflammatory effect on the bronchiolitis.

Bronchodilator drugs can be used as an aid in the clinical diagnosis and temporary treatment of chronic obstructive pulmonary disease. Isoprenaline is a sympathomimetic drug which stimulates both beta-1 (or cardiac) receptors and beta-2 (or smooth muscle) receptors causing cardiac stimulation and bronchial muscle relaxation. Terbutaline is a sympathomimetic drug which exhibits action selectively for beta-2 receptors, thereby causing bronchodilation with little or no cardiac stimulation (10). Atropine is a parasympatholytic drug. Administration of these three bronchodilators by inhalation or atropine intravenously at a rate of 0·02 mg/kg body weight will result in a marked decrease in intrathoracic pressure, a decrease in respiratory rate, an initial decrease followed by an increase in arterial oxygen partial pressure and clinical improvement. The wheezing sounds audible over the lung will also be markedly reduced. Clinical improvement persists for 1–2 hours following isoprenaline and atropine and for 2–6 hours following terbutaline treatment. The atropine also results in mydriasis which may persist for 12–24 hours. Within 10–20 minutes after the intravenous administration of atropine and isoprenaline inhalation the heart rate will increase by twice the normal rate in normal horses and those affected with chronic obstructive pulmonary disease. Because terbutaline is a highly selective adrenoreceptor drug which causes bronchial dilatation lasting from 2 to 6 hours it may prove to be of value in the symptomatic treatment of this disease in the horse particularly if oral preparations become available and are effective (10).

Clenbuterol hydrochloride is also a beta-2-sympathomimetic for use as a bronchodilator in horses with COPD (22, 42). Clenbuterol has no untoward effects on the circulatory system of exercising horses (41). It also exerts an antiallergenic effect by stabilizing mast cells, increasing mucociliary clearance and demonstrates a bronchosecretolytic effect (22). Preliminary reports indicate that clenbuterol is effective in providing temporary relief when given by the parenteral or the oral routes.

It would appear that the combination of an effective longacting bronchodilator combined with the provision of fresh air and the removal of the precipitating cause is a rational approach to therapy.

Bromohexine, a mucinolytic agent given at the rate of 15–20 g/day in the field for 10 days and sometimes for up to 45 days has resulted in marked improvement in horses with suspected chronic obstructive pulmonary disease (17). The use of mucinolytic drugs and bronchodilators is discussed in a review (24). Antibiotics are used in the treatment of this disease in the horse, but there is only limited clinical evidence of their value (20). Procaine penicillin at a dose rate of 25 000 i.u./kg body weight intramuscularly daily for 2 weeks is recommended (20). Sulfamethazine or tetracycline has also been recommended. There is no effective treatment for the pulmonary hemorrhage associated with chronic obstructive pulmonary disease in horses.

There is no evidence that furosemide has any significant effect on pulmonary arterial pressures of normal horses or those with chronic obstructive pulmonary disease and it is thus unlikely that the drug would prevent pulmonary hemorrhage (18). In one study approximately

44% of horses had evidence of pulmonary hemorrhage following a race and there was no evidence that furosemide was beneficial (19). Experimentally, sodium cromoglycate, an inhibitor of histamine release, given by inhalation, will protect horses which are sensitive to *Micropolyspora faeni* against challenge from the antigen for a period of several days (21). This may be further support for hypersensitivity to fungi as a cause of COPD in the horse.

REVIEW LITERATURE

Deegen, E. & Beadle, R. E. (1985) (eds) *Lung Function and Respiratory Diseases in the Horse. International Symposium in Hannover, Germany, June 27–29, 1985.* Hippiatrika Verlagsgesellschaft mbH Calw.

Genetzky, R. M. (1985) Chronic obstructive pulmonary disease in horses. Part 1. *Comp. cont. Educ. pract. Vet.*, 7, S407–S414.

Littlejohn, A. (1979) Chronic obstructive pulmonary disease in horses. *Vet. Bull.*, *49*, 907–917.

McPherson, E. A. & Thomson, J. R. (1983) Chronic obstructive pulmonary disease in the horse. 1. Nature of the disease. *Equ. vet. J.*, *15*, 203–206.

Robinson, N. E. & Sorenson, P. R. (1978) Pathophysiology of airway obstruction in horses: a review. *J. Am. vet. med. Assoc.*, *172*, 299–303.

Robinson, N. E. (Ed.) (1979) In: *Symposium on Equine Respiratory Disease. Vet. Clin. N. Am. large Anim. Pract. 1.*

Thomson, J. R. & McPherson, E. A. (1983) Chronic pulmonary disease. 2. Therapy. *Equ. vet. J.*, *15*, 207–210.

REFERENCES

(1) Littlejohn, A. (1979) *Vet. Bull.*, *49*, 907.
(2) McPherson, E. A. et al. (1979) *Equ. vet. J.*, *11*, 159.
(3) Lawson, G. H. G. et al. (1979) *Equ. vet. J.*, *11*, 172.
(4) Matthews, A. G. (1979) *Equ. vet. J.*, *11*, 177.
(5) Halliwell, R. E. W. et al. (1979) *J. Am. vet. med. Assoc.*, *174*.
(6) McPherson, E. A. et al. (1979) *Equ. vet. J.*, *11*, 167.
(7) McPherson, E. A. et al. (1978) *Equ. vet. J.*, *10*, 47.
(8) Dixon, P. M. et al. (1982) *Equ. vet. J.*, *14*, 80.
(9) Thomson, J. R. & McPherson, E. A. (1984) *Equ. vet. J.*, *16*, 35.
(10) Murphy, J. R. et al. (1980) *Equ. vet. J.*, *12*, 10.
(11) Robinson, N. E. & Sorenson, P. R. (1978) *J. Am. vet. med. Assoc.*, *172*, 299.
(12) Gerber, H. (1973) *Equ. vet. J.*, *5*, 26.
(13) Stadler, P. & Deegen, E. (1986) *Equ. vet. J.*, *18*, 171.
(14) Mirbahar, K. B. et al. (1985) *Can. J. comp. Med.*, *49*, 211.
(15) McLaughlin, R. F. & Edwards, D. W. (1966) *Am. Rev. resp. Dis.*, *93*, 22.
(16) Littlejohn A. et al. (1977) *Equ. vet. J.*, *9*, 75.
(17) Pearce, H. G. et al. (1978) *NZ vet. J.*, *26*, 28.
(18) Dixon, P. M. (1980) *Equ. vet. J.*, *12*, 28.
(19) Pascoe, J. R. et al. (1981) *Am. J. vet. Res.*, *42*, 703.
(20) Larson, V. L. (1980) *J. Am. vet. Assoc.*, *176*, 1091.
(21) Murphy, J. R. et al. (1979) *Vet. Immun. Immunopathol.*, *1*, 89.
(22) Genetzky, R. M. & Loparco, F. V. (1985) *J. equ. vet. Sci.*, *5*, 320.
(23) Breeze, R. G. (1979) In: *Symposium on Equine Respiratory Diseases. Vet. Clin. N. Am. large Anim. Pract.*, *1*, 219–230.
(24) Littlejohn, A. (1980) *Onderstepoort J. vet. Res.*, *47*, 159, 187, and 193.
(25) Littlejohn, A. & Bowles, F. (1981) *Onderstepoort J. vet. Res.*, *48*, 37.
(26) Thomson, J. R. et al. (1983) *Vet. Immunol. Immunopathol.*, *4*, 387.
(27) Thorsen, J. et al. (1983) *Can. J. comp. Med.*, *47*, 332.
(28) Grunig, G. et al. (1986) *Equ. vet. J.*, *18*, 396.
(29) Thomas, D. E. et al. (1985) *Am. J. vet. Res.*, *46*, 1619.
(30) Breeze, R. G. et al. (1984) *Equ. vet. J.*, *16*, 108.
(31) Asmundson, T. et al. (1983) *Equ. vet. J.*, *15*, 229.
(32) Littlejohn, A. & Bowles, F. (1981) *Onderstepoort J. vet. Res.*, *48*, 37, 239.
(33) Littlejohn, A. & Bowles, F. (1982) *Onderstepoort J. vet. Res.*, *49*, 71.
(34) Littlejohn, A. et al. (1982) *Onderstepoort J. vet. Res.*, *49*, 211.
(35) Derksen, F. J. et al. (1985) *Am. J. vet. Res.*, *46*, 774.
(36) Klein, H. J. & Deegen, E. (1986) *Am. J. vet. Res.*, *46*, 1796.
(37) Derksen, F. J. et al. (1985) *J. appl. Physiol.*, *58*, 584.
(38) Nuytten, J. et al. (1983) *Zentralbl. VetMed. A30*, 114.
(39) Derksen, F. J. et al. (1985) *Am. Rev. resp. Dis.*, *132*, 1066.
(40) McPherson, E. A. & Thomson, J. R. (1983) *Equ. vet. J.*, *15*, 203.
(41) Rose, R. J. et al. (1983) *Res. vet. Sci.*, *35*, 301.
(42) Thomas, J. R. & McPherson, E. A. (1983) *Equ. vet. J.*, *15*, 207.

DISEASES CHARACTERIZED BY URINARY TRACT INVOLVEMENT

Enzootic hematuria

Enzootic hematuria is a chronic, non-infectious disease of cattle characterized by the development of hemangiomatous lesions of the wall of the urinary bladder and clinically by intermittent hematuria and death due to anemia.

Etiology

The specific cause is still undecided but the great bulk of evidence points to chronic poisoning with bracken as the principal cause. There is also strong support for the interaction of bracken fern and papilloma virus in the etiology (11). A high incidence has been observed where bracken fern is growing (1) and the disease has been reproduced by the experimental feeding of bracken, either green or dried or as hay (3). On the other hand cases are seen in cattle which have no access to bracken. Many other plants have been incriminated from time to time but their etiological significance remains unproved. Research workers have gone to extraordinary lengths to establish the presence of carcinogens in bracken fern (4). Neoplasms histologically indistinguishable from natural lesions of enzootic hematuria have been produced experimentally by feeding cattle on fresh bracken from an area where enzootic hematuria was common (5). A high incidence of vesicular carcinomas, similar to the bladder lesions of enzootic hematuria in cattle, has been recorded in sheep grazing bracken for 18 months (6). Rats fed bracken develop a high frequency of urinary bladder carcinoma and this is greatly increased by the supplementation of the diet by thiamin (7). Multiple intestinal tumors also developed and tumors have been observed affecting the upper digestive tract of cattle in field cases in Brazil (8). The disease is also recorded in cattle grazing pasture containing rock or mulga ferns (*Cheilantes sieberi*) in Australia (2).

Attempts at transmission by the oral administration or infusion into the bladder of urine and bladder tissue. extracts have not been successful. It is generally agreed that some irritant substance is present in the urine of affected animals although its nature has not been determined. A similar lesion has been produced experimentally by the submucosal injection into the bladder of a suspension of bovine cutaneous papilloma (9), but repeated vaccination with partly inactivated papilloma virus does not prevent the development of lesions (10). Many other possible causes have been considered but evidence is lacking to incriminate any particular agent. Cows affected with the disease excrete large quantities of tryptophan metabolites in their urine and one tryptophan metabolite, 3-hydroxy-L-kyneurenine, is a known bladder carcinogen. It is possible that abnormal metabolism of tryptophan could occur in cattle in specific dietary circumstances (12). The disease is sometimes associated with a high content of molybdenum in pasture and its incidence appears to be reduced by heavy applications of gypsum.

Epidemiology

Enzootic hematuria occurs as an area problem on all continents. The overall incidence is not great but the disease may cause heavy losses in affected areas. It is usually fatal. Cattle over 1 year of age are most commonly affected and the disease has also been recorded in water buffalo.

The disease is confined mainly to poor, neglected or recently opened up land and tends to disappear as soil fertility and land management improves. It is not closely associated with a particular soil type although it is recorded most commonly on lighter soils.

Pathogenesis

The mode of development of the lesions is unknown. Hemorrhage from the hemangiomata in the bladder wall occurs intermittently and results in varying degrees of blood loss. Deaths are due to hemorrhagic anemia.

Clinical findings

Acute cases are manifested by the passage of large quantities of blood, often as clots, in the urine. Acute hemorrhagic anemia develops and the animal becomes weak and recumbent and may die after an illness lasting 1–2 weeks. Subacute cases are characterized by intermittent, mild clinical hematuria or persistent subclinical hematuria. In these cases there is a gradual loss of condition over several months and eventually clinical evidence of anemia. On rectal examination acute cases may show nothing but subacute cases usually evidence marked thickening of the bladder wall. Secondary bacterial infection of the bladder may lead to the development of cystitis and pyelonephritis.

Clinical pathology

In the absence of gross hematuria, a urine sample should be centrifuged and the deposit examined for erythrocytes. Repeated examinations may be necessary. Non-specific anemia and leukopenia are detectable by hematological examination.

Necropsy findings

Hemorrhages in the bladder mucosa are typical of the disease. In the later stages, there are raised pedunculated tumors which are friable and bleed easily and these are accompanied by fibrotic thickening with scarring and distortion of the bladder wall. The tumors probably arise from transitional epithelium and often show evidence of malignancy, metastasis to regional lymph nodes and lungs having been observed. In uncomplicated cases, the remainder of the urinary tract is usually unaffected although lesions have been observed in ureters and the renal pelvis. The severity of the hemorrhage is not necessarily related to the extent of the lesions and animals may bleed to death when only minor lesions are present.

Diagnosis

It is necessary to determine by microscopic examination that the redness of the urine is due to the presence of erythrocytes and not to the presence of free hemoglobin. Other causes of hematuria in cattle are few. Cystitis and pyelonephritis are usually accompanied by fever, frequent urination and the presence of pus and debris in the urine. Bacteriological examination of the urine will reveal the presence of infection.

Treatment

Blood transfusion is necessary in acute cases and hematinic mixture should be provided in chronic cases. Little can be done to cause regression of the bladder lesions and affected animals are best disposed of.

Control

A general improvement in nutrition is often followed by a decrease in the number of animals affected. A specific recommendation is to apply gypsum (225–335 kg/ha) to the pasture as a fertilizer, a measure which is reputed to delay the onset of the disease.

REFERENCES

(1) Smith, B. L. & Beatson, N. S. (1970) *NZ vet. J.*, *18*, 115.
(2) McKenzie, R. (1978) *Aust. vet. J.*, *54*, 61.
(3) Pamukcu, A. M. & Bryan, G. T. (1976) *Firat Univ. vet. Fakult. Dergisi*, *3*, 27.
(4) Pamukcu, A. M. et al. (1971) *Cancer Res.*, *30*, 902.
(5) Pamukcu, A. M. et al. (1976) *Vet. Pathol.*, *13*, 110.
(6) Harbutt, P. R. & Leaver, D. D. (1969) *Aust. vet. J.*, *45*, 473.
(7) Pamukcu, A. M. et al. (1970) *Cancer Res.*, *30*, 2671.
(8) Tokarnia, C. H. et al. (1969) *Pesquisa agropec. bras.*, *4*, 209.
(9) Olson, C. et al. (1959) *Am. J. Pathol.*, *35*, 672.
(10) Pamukcu, A. M. et al. (1967) *Cancer Res.*, *27*, 2197.
(11) Hopkins, N. C. G. (1986) *Vet. Rec.*, *118*, 715.
(12) Pamukcu, A. M. (1963) *Ann. NY Acad. Sci.*, *108*, 938.

DISEASES CHARACTERIZED BY NERVOUS SYSTEM INVOLVEMENT

Polioencephalomalacia (cerebrocortical necrosis) of ruminants

Polioencephalomalacia occurs sporadically in young cattle and sheep, and is characterized clinically by sudden onset of blindness, head-pressing, opisthotonus and convulsions, a rapid response following thiamine therapy in the early stages and pathologically by acute cerebral edema and laminar necrosis of the cerebral cortex.

Etiology

The cause of the disease is not completely understood although there appears to be sufficient evidence available that a thiamin inadequacy is associated with the disease (1). The evidence for this includes:

- Affected animals respond to the parenteral administration of thiamin if given within a few hours after the onset of clinical signs
- Affected animals have biochemical findings consistent with thiamin diphosphate (TDP) inadequacy
- The clinical signs and pathological lesions can be reproduced in sheep and cattle by the administration of large daily doses of pyrimidine containing structural analogs of thiamin, principally amprolium, given orally or intraperitoneally (2).

While there has been general agreement that thiamin inadequacy is associated with the cause of the disease, the possible mechanisms by which this occurs are uncertain (1). Thiamin inadequacy in ruminants could theoretically occur in any of the following situations:

- There may be inadequate net microbial synthesis of thiamin in the rumen which may occur in concentrate-fed animals receiving inadequate roughage (3), impaired absorption and/or phosphorylation of thiamin, the presence of a thiamin inhibitor in the tissues of the host, lack of sufficient or appropriate apoenzyme or coenzyme–apoenzyme binding for thiamin dependent systems, increased metabolic demands for thiamin in the absence of increased supply, and increased rate of excretion of thiamin resulting in its net loss from the body
- Thiamin can be destroyed by thiaminases of which significant amounts can be found in the rumen contents and feces of cattle and sheep affected with naturally occurring polioencephalomalacia (7, 25).

There is now considerable evidence that the major cause of polioencephalomalacia in cattle and sheep is a progressive severe state of thiamin deficiency caused by the destruction of thiamin by bacterial thiaminases in the rumen and intestines (7, 45). Certain species of bacteria which provide thiaminases have been found in the rumen and intestines of animals with polioencephalomalacia. *Bacillus thiaminolyticus* and *Clostridium sporogenes* produce thiaminase type I and *Bacillus aneurinolyticus* produces thiaminase type II (7). While there is good circumstantial evidence that the thiaminases from these bacteria are the real source of thiaminases associated with the disease, it is not entirely certain. The experimental oral inoculation of large numbers of thiaminase type I producing *Clostridium sporogenes* into lambs did not result in the disease (43). The properties of thiaminases associated with cerebrocortical necrosis have been examined (42).

Certain species of fungi from moldy feed are thiaminase producers but the evidence that they destroy thiamin and are associated with polioencephalomalacia is contradictory and uncertain (10).

High levels of thiaminase type I are present in the rhizomes of bracken fern (*Pteridium aquilinum*) and horsetail (*Equisetum arvense*). The feeding of the bracken fern rhizomes (*Pteridium esculentum*) to sheep will cause acute thiamin deficiency and lesions similar to those of polioencephalomalacia (13) but neither of these plants is normally involved in the natural disease. The disease has occurred in sheep grazing the Nardoo fern, *Marsilea drummordi*, in flood-prone or low-lying wet areas in Australia. The fern contains a high level of thiaminase type I activity (26).

The experimental disease can be produced in young lambs fed a thiamine-free milk diet and it may unnecessary to postulate that thiamin analogs produced in the rumen are essential components of the etiology (11).

Cobalt deficiency in sheep has been incriminated as a possible contributing cause of polioencephalomalacia (14).

In Cuba molasses toxicity occurs in cattle fed on a liquid molasses–urea feeding system with limited forage (7). The clinical and necropsy findings are identical to polioencephalomalacia. However, molasses toxicity is not thiamin responsive and can be reversed by feeding forage. It has been suggested that a deficiency in the ruminal production of propionic acid must be an important causative factor.

Epidemiology

The disease has been reported from most parts of the world and occurs primarily in cattle and sheep and has been reported in goats, antelope and whitetail deer (37, 38). A similar disease has been recorded in pigs (15). It is most common in cattle and sheep which are being fed concentrate rations under intensified conditions such as in cattle and lamb feedlots. It usually occurs in well-nourished thrifty cattle 6–18 months of age (peak incidence 9–12 months of age) which have been in the feedlot for several weeks. Similarly, feedlot lambs are usually affected only after being on feed for several weeks (3). In Cuba, the disease occurs in feedlot cattle which are fed primarily on molasses with a minimal quantity of roughage, and can be reproduced in cattle fed a molasses–urea and roughage diet by gradual removal of the roughage without the use of thiamin analogs (33). The disease has occurred in pastured cattle usually 5–10 days after change from a poor to a good pasture. The disease may occur in range cattle grazing on dry, short, grama grass pasture (35). There is circumstantial evidence that *Kochia scorpia* (summer cypress or Mexican fireweed) may be associated with disease in range cattle (36). A high concentrate of sulfates in the diet of cattle has also been associated with episodes of the disease in 6-to-18 month old cattle. Inorganic sulfate salts in the form of gypsum were added to the rations in order to control total daily intake of the diet (8). The disease occurs only rarely in adult cattle which may be a reflection of the greater quantities of roughage they usually consume.

In some outbreaks there is a history of deprivation of feed and water for 24–28 hours, because of either a managerial error or frozen water supplies. In other cases, a rapid change in diet appears to precipitate an outbreak. Some outbreaks are associated with a temporary deprivation of water for 24–36 hours, followed by sudden access to water and an excessive supply of salt, a situation analogous to salt poisoning in pigs, but these require more documentation to ensure that they indeed are not salt poisoning (37). In sheep flocks, a drastic change in management, such as occurs at shearing time, will precipitate outbreaks in which only the yearlings are affected. Changing the diet of sheep from hay to corn silage resulted in a decrease in thiamin concentrations in ruminal fluid to about 25% of control values on hay (4). The cause of the drop in thiamin concentrations is unknown.

Accurate morbidity and mortality data are not available, but outbreaks can occur suddenly in which up to 25% of groups of feeder cattle may be affected, with case mortality rates from 25 to 50%. Mortality rates are higher in young cattle (6–9 months) than in the older age group (12–18 months) and mortality increases if treatment with thiamin is delayed for more than a few hours after the onset of signs. In feedlot lambs, it has been suggested that approximately 19% of all deaths are due to polioencephalomalacia (3).

The disease may affect goats from 2 months to 3 years of age and is commonly associated with milk-replacer diets in kids or concentrate feeding in older goats (31).

In a survey of cattle under farm conditions, using transketolase activity as a measurement of thiamin status, it has been shown that up to 23% of cattle under 2 years of age and 5% over 2 years may be in a thiamin-low state (16). A survey of newly weaned beef calves on a hay diet are not subject to a thiamin deficiency (6). A low and variable proportion of young cattle on barley-based feedlot diets (1·7%) had some evidence of thiamin deficiency based on a thiamin pyrophosphate activity effect in excess of 15% (6). The supplementation of the diet of feedlot steers on an all-concentrate barley-based diet with 1·9 mg thiamin per kg of diet resulted in an increase in average daily gain and final carcass weights, which indicated that some animals were marginally deficient in thiamin and decreased production in cattle fed all-concentrate diets is possibly due to thiamin inadequacies (40). However, thiamin supplementation of cattle on all-concentrate diets does not consistently result in improved animal performance (44).

The factors which promote the colonization and growth of thiaminase-producing bacteria in the rumen are unknown. Attempts to establish the organism in the rumen of healthy calves or lambs has been unsuccessful (9). Thiaminases have also been found in the rumen contents and feces of normal animals which may suggest the existence of a subclinical state of thiamin deficiency (12, 46). Poor growth of unweaned and weaned lambs can be associated with a thiaminase-induced subclinical thiamin deficiency (46). Weekly testing of young lambs over a period of 10 weeks revealed that 90% of unthrifty lambs were excreting high levels of thiaminase in their feces, low levels of thiaminase activity were present in 20% of clinically normal animals, and there were significant differences in the mean erythrocyte transketolase activity of the unthrifty animals excreting thiaminase compared to the thiaminase-free normal animals (46). Field and laboratory investigations have supported an association between inferior growth rate of weaner sheep in Australia and a thiaminase-induced thiamin deficiency (47). The parenteral or oral administration of thiamin to normal calves raised under farm conditions resulted in a marked reduction in the percentage thiamin pyrophosphate effect which is an indirect measurement of thiamin inadequacy (12).

Pathogenesis

Current evidence is that high levels of thiaminases are formed in the rumen which destroy thiamin that is naturally synthesized in the rumen (1, 7). The circumstances in the diet or in the rumen which allow for the development of high levels of thiaminases are unknown but may be related to the nature of the ruminal microflora in young cattle and sheep fed concentrate rations which results in the development of ruminal acidosis (17, 45). These rations may also allow for the development and growth of thiaminase-producing bacteria which, combined with a smaller net synthesis of thiamin in the rumens of concentrate-fed ruminants, could explain the higher incidence in feedlot animals. Experimentally the disease has been produced in lambs by continuous intraruminal infusion of a highly fermentable diet (18). Animals changed very rapidly to high concentrate rations develop increased ruminal thiaminase levels (19). The possibility that intraruminal thiaminases may also create thiamin analogs capable of acting as thiamin antimetabolites and accentuating the disease has been studied but the results are inconclusive (5). The presence of naturally occurring second substrates (cosubstrates) in the rumen could produce, by the thiaminase type I reaction, a potent thiamin antimetabolite capable of accentuating the condition. *In vitro* studies have shown that thiaminase only caused rapid destruction of thiamin when a second substrate was added, and a large number of drugs commonly used as anthelmintics or tranquilizers may be active as second substrates (45). Many compounds found in the rumen of cattle are potential cosubstrates (22).

Amprolium has been used extensively to produce the lesions in the brains of cattle and sheep that are indistinguishable from the naturally occurring disease (1). However, since amprolium has been found in the brain tissue, the experimental disease should perhaps be known as 'amprolium poisoning encephalopathy' (2, 23). The administration of other antagonists such as oxythiamin and pyrithiamin does not produce the disease (2). This suggests that polioencephalomalacia is a particular form of thiamin deficiency in which the supply of thiamin is reduced by the action of intraruminal thiaminase. Thus, the thiamin status of the animal will be dependent on dietary thiamin intake, thiamin synthesis, the presence of thiaminase in the rumen and the effects of possible antimetabolites. Subclinical states of thiamin deficiency probably exist in apparently normal cattle and sheep being fed diets which are conducive to the disease (46). This suggests that in outbreaks of the disease the unaffected animals of the group should be considered as potential new cases and perhaps treated prophylactically.

Thiamin is an essential component of several enzymes involved in intermediary metabolism and a state of deficiency results in increased blood concentration of pyruvate, a reduction in the lactate to pyruvate ratio and depression of erythrocyte transketolase. These abnormalities affect carbohydrate metabolism in general, but in view of the specific requirements of the cerebral cortex for oxidative metabolism of glucose, it is possible that a thiamin inadequacy could have a direct metabolic effect on neurones (1). The brain of the calf has a greater dependence on the pentose pathway for glucose metabolism, in which pathway the transketolase enzyme is a rate-limiting enzyme (17). Ultrastructural examination of the brain of sheep with the natural disease reveals that the first change which occurs is an edema of the intracellular compartment, principally involving the astrocytes and satellite cells (24). This is followed by neuronal degeneration which is considered secondary. It has been suggested that the edema may be due to a reduction in ATP production following a defect of carbohydrate metabolism in the astrocyte (39). There are three basic lesions which are not uniform: compact necrosis, edema necrosis, and edema alone (39). This may suggest that a uniform etiology such as thiamin deficiency cannot be fully supported.

Acute cerebral edema and laminar necrosis occur and the clinical signs are usually referable to increased intracranial pressure from the edema, and the widespread focal necrosis. Recovery can occur with early treatment which suggests that the lesions are reversible up to a certain point.

Clinical findings

In acute cases there is a sudden onset of blindness, muscle tremor, particularly of the head, champing of the jaws and frothy salivation, and headpressing, and the animal is particularly difficult to handle. Initially, the irritation signs may occur in episodes, and convulsions may occur, but within several hours the irritation signs may be continuous. The animal usually then becomes recumbent, there is marked opisthotonus, nystagmus, clonic-tonic convulsions, particularly when the animal is stimulated, and tetany of the forelimbs is common. The temperature is usually normal but elevated if there has been excessive muscular activity. The heart rate may be normal, subnormal or increased and is probably not a reliable diagnostic aid.

The frequency of the rumen movements remains normal for a few days, which is an important differential feature from lead poisoning in which the rumen is invariably static.

The menace reflex is always absent in the acute stage and its slow return to normal following treatment is a valuable aid in prognosis. The palpebral eye-preservation reflex is usually normal. The pupils are usually of normal size and responsive to light. In severe cases the pupils may be constricted. Dorsal strabismus due to stretching of the trochlear nerve is seen commonly. Nystagmus is common and may be vertical or horizontal. Optic disc edema is present in some cases but is not a constant finding.

Calves 6–9 months of age may die in 24–48 hours, while older cattle up to 18 months of age may survive for several days. Recovery is more common in the older age group.

In less severe cases, affected animals are usually blind, show head-pressing and remain standing for several hours or a few days. In an outbreak of the disease, some cattle will be recumbent with the severe form, others will remain standing with obvious blindness, while others are anorexic, mildly depressed and have only partial impairment of eyesight. These latter cases will usually return to normal. Some survivors are permanently blind but may begin to eat and drink if provided with assistance.

Sheep usually begin to wander aimlessly, sometimes in circles, or stand motionless and are blind, but within a few hours become recumbent with opisthotonus, extension of the limbs, hyperesthesia, nystagmus and periodic tonic-clonic convulsions. Hoggets affected at shearing time may show blindness and head-pressing but, if fed and watered, usually recover within a few days. Occasional animals show unilateral localizing signs, including circling and spasmodic deviation of the head. In goats, early signs may include excitability and elevation of the head. Blindness, extreme opisthotonus and severe extensor rigidity and nystagmus are common.

There are some preliminary reports from Australia of unthriftiness in unweaned and weaned lambs being associated with thiamin deficiency due to the presence of thiaminases in the alimentary tract (46, 47). In affected flocks the incidence of illthrift in lambs is much higher than the usual incidence and other causes of unthriftiness were ruled out. Affected lambs lose weight, may have chronic diarrhea and become emaciated and die from starvation. In some flocks, clinical signs of polioencephalomalacia may occur in a small percentage of animals. The disease occurs most commonly in early July which is the coldest part of the year in Australia for lambs which are born in May and June (47). In affected lambs the fecal thiaminase levels are high and the blood transketolase level activity is increased above normal. Treatment of affected lambs with thiamin resulted in an increase in growth rate (46).

Clinical pathology

The biochemical changes occurring in cattle and sheep with the disease have not been well-defined diagnostically based thoroughly investigated naturally occurring clinical cases. However, some estimates are available including the changes which occur in experimental disease. Interpretation of the values may also be unreliable if the animals have been treated prior to death. The erythrocyte transketolase activity is decreased and the thiamin pyrophosphate (TPP) effect is increased (25, 27). The erythrocyte transketolase activities in normal sheep will range from 40 to 60 i.u./ml red blood cells (47). A TPP effect of 30–50% is commonly found in normal healthy cattle and sheep (20, 47) and an increase to above 70–80% occurs in animals with polioencephalomalacia (20, 47). The thiamin concentrations of blood of animals with polioencephalomalacia have varied widely and may be difficult to interpret because of the possibility of thiamin analogs inducing deficiency even when blood thiamin levels are normal. However, this would not apply when blood thiamin levels are below normal. A normal reference of 15·1–45·2 μg/dl (50–150 nmol/l) for pastured animals has been suggested and levels below 15·1 μg/dl (50 nmol/l) are significant (29). Levels as low as 1·8–3·6 μg/dl (6–12 nmol/l) have been found in suspected cases of polioencephalomalacia. The thiamin concentrations of liver, heart and brain of cattle and sheep with polioencephalomalacia are decreased (25, 27). The levels of blood pyruvate and lactate are also increased and thiamin pyrophosphate-dependent enzymes such as pyruvate kinase are decreased (7). The thiaminase activity of the feces is increased (46, 47).

The procedure for obtaining blood and tissue samples from suspected cases is shown in Table 101 (25).

The hemogram is usually normal; the total and differential leukocyte counts may indicate a mild stress reaction, a finding which may be useful in differentiation from encephalopathies due to bacterial infections.

The cerebrospinal fluid pressure is usually increased from a normal range of 120–160 mm saline to levels of 200–350 mm. The level of protein in the cerebrospinal fluid may be normal to slightly or extremely elevated. A range from 15 to 540 mg/dl with a mean value of 90 mg/dl in affected cattle is recorded (41). There may also be a slight to severe pleocytosis in the cerebrospinal fluid in which monocytes or phagocytes predominate.

Necropsy findings

Diffuse cerebral edema with compression and yellow discoloration of the dorsal cortical gyri is evident and the cerebellum is pushed back into the foramen magnum with distortion of its posterior aspect. In recovered animals, there is macroscopic decortication about the motor area and over the occipital lobes. The lesion can be identified grossly using ultraviolet illumination which results in a fluorescence that indicates necrosis of brain and engulfment of necrotic tissue by lipophages (21, 28). In general, there is a good correlation between the presence of characteristic fluorescence and the biochemical changes in cases of polioencephalomalacia (21). A small percentage of false negatives may occur (28). Histologically the lesions are widespread but most common in the cerebral cortex. There is bilateral laminar necrosis and necrosis of deeper cerebral areas. The necrosis is most prominent in the dorsal occipital and parietal cortex, but bilateral areas of necrosis are also seen less frequently in the thalamus, lateral geniculate bodies, basal ganglia and mesencephalic nuclei (30). Lesions of the cerebellum are also present (32). The severity and distribution of the lesions probably depend on the interrelationships between clinical severity, age of affected animal and length of illness before death. Subnormal levels of thiamin are detectable in the liver and brain (25, 27) of calves with the natural disease and low levels are also found in the experimental disease (2). In the molasses-induced disease in Cuba, the tissue thiamin levels were within the normal range (33).

Table 101. Procedure for obtaining blood and tissue samples.

Tissue	*Treatment*	*Storage and shipment*
Blood (heparinized, about 10 ml)	Centrifuge at 3000 *g* for 10 minutes; discard plasma	Freeze packed cells at −20°C (−6°F); send frozen
Liver (about 10 g)	Place in small carton and freeze	Send frozen
Heart (about 10 g)	Sample of left ventricle	Send frozen
Brain (about 10 g)	Section longitudinally. Place half in carton and freeze; place other half in buffered formalin	Send at ambient temperature
Ruminal contents	Take six separate samples from different areas of rumen	Send frozen
Feces	Separate samples from each animal	Store and send frozen

Diagnosis

Polioencephalomalacia in cattle occurs primarily in young growing animals 6–9 months of age on concentrate rations and is characterized clinically by a sudden onset of blindness, muscular tremors of the head and neck, head-pressing, nystagmus and opisthotonus. The clinical findings of polioencephalomalacia in cattle closely resemble lead poisoning and hypovitaminosis A, and may resemble *Haemophilus* meningoencephalitis. The differential clinical diagnosis for cattle is given in Table 95.

In unvaccinated sheep, especially feedlot lambs, enterotoxemia (pulpy kidney) due to *Cl. perfringens* type D causes almost identical clinical findings and occurs under the same management conditions as polioencephalomalacia. However, enterotoxemia in lambs usually occurs within several days after being placed on a grain ration, whereas polioencephalomalacia occurs after several weeks of grain feeding. Glycosuria occurs in pulpy kidney disease and may assist the diagnosis but a necropsy is usually more informative. Focal symmetrical encephalomalacia also resembles polioencephalomalacia but is sporadic, usually involves only a few animals and will not respond to treatment.

In goats the disease must be differentiated from caprine leukoencephalomyelitis, listeriosis, enterotoxemia, pregnancy toxemia, lead poisoning and meningoencephalitis.

None of the biochemical tests described under clinical pathology is practicable under usual practice conditions. The clinician must usually make the diagnosis on the basis of clinical findings and the readily available simple tests which rule out other diseases that resemble polioencephalomalacia. A careful consideration of the epidemiological history will often assist in arriving at the diagnosis.

Treatment

The treatment of choice is thiamin hydrochloride at 10 mg/kg body weight given intravenously initially and followed by similar doses every 3 hours for a total of five treatments. When treatment is given within a few hours of the onset of signs, a beneficial response within 1–6 hours is common and complete clinical recovery can occur in 24 hours. Goats and sheep will commonly respond within 1–2 hours. For those which take longer to recover, the eyesight and mental awareness will gradually improve in a few days and the animal will usually begin to eat and drink by the 3rd day after treatment. Rumen transplants of rumen juice from roughage-fed cattle are often indicated to improve appetite and rumen function in those which are responding slowly. In affected sheep, following treatment with thiamin the blood transketolase activity begins to return to normal in 2–4 hours and is considered normal 24 hours after treatment (48). Some cattle improve to a subnormal level within a few days and fail to continue to improve. These are usually affected with diffuse cortical and subcortical necrosis and will usually not improve further in spite of continued treatment. Those which return to a clinically normal state will usually do so by 48 hours or sooner after initial treatment. Those which are still clinically subnormal and anorexic by the end of the 3rd day will usually remain at that level and should be slaughtered for salvage.

Treatment is relatively ineffective in advanced cases, but unless an accurate history is available on the length of the illness, it is usually difficult to predict the outcome until 6–12 hours following treatment. Therefore, it is usual practice to treat most affected cases with thiamin at least twice and monitor the response. If there is no beneficial response in 6–8 hours, emergency slaughter for salvage should be considered.

Hypertonic solutions (mannitol, urea) have been used for the treatment of cerebral edema in the dog and may be indicated in polioencephalomalacia. Mannitol and urea, each given intravenously at a dose of 1·5 g/kg body weight, effectively reduced cerebrospinal fluid pressure for 1·5 hours in the dog (34). A larger dose of mannitol (4·5 g/kg body weight) reduces pressure for 3 hours. In severe cases of polioencephalomalacia in which diffuse cerebral edema may be present, the use of mannitol may be indicated. However, because of the short duration of effect and the impracticability of administering mannitol every few hours and the potential hazard of causing severe dehydration, the use of corticosteroids to maintain the reduction in cerebrospinal fluid pressure is indicated. Dexamethasone at a rate of 1 mg/5–10 kg body weight is recommended. While the use of hypertonic solutions and corticosteroids for the treatment of the cerebral edema is rational, their efficacy has not been sufficiently evaluated and only cautious reliance should be placed on their value. The reduction of the cerebral edema with these drugs will at best provide only a temporary clinical improvement unless thiamin is also used to correct the biochemical defect which exists and which is the cause of the edema and the widespread necrosis. The use of the hypertonic solutions will cause diuresis which may lead to dehydration and fluid therapy may be indicated. Also, the high costs associated with hypertonic solutions and corticosteroids at the dose rates suggested above may be prohibitive.

The oral administration of thiamin or thiamin derivatives is now considered necessary for the treatment of cattle and sheep affected with polioencephalomalacia caused by the presence of thiaminases in the alimentary tract (22). Thiamin hydrochloride at a rate of 1 g for goats and lambs and 5 g for calves, in a drench, is recommended. However, because the action of thiaminase type I on thiamin may result in the production of thiamin analogs which may act as inhibitors of thiamin metabolism, the use of thiamin derivatives which are resistant to thiaminases, lipid soluble and absorbed from the intestine are being explored as therapeutic and prophylactic agents (7). Thiamin propyldisulfide can depress the thiaminase activities in the ruminal fluid of sheep with polioencephalomalacia within 2 hours after oral administration (22). The blood pyruvate levels and transketolase activities are also restored to normal and treated animals recovered clinically (22).

In outbreaks of the disease, the in-contact unaffected animals which have been on the same diet as the affected animals are probably on the brink of acute clinical disease. The diet should be changed to one containing at least 50% roughage or 1·5 kg of roughage per 100 kg body weight. Thiamin may be added to the ration at the rate of 50 mg/kg of feed for 2–3 weeks as a preventive against clinical disease, followed by a level of 20–30 mg/kg of feed (cattle and sheep) if the animals remain on a diet that may predispose them to the disease.

Control

Because the present state of knowledge indicates that polioencephalomalacia is a conditioned thiamin inadequacy, it would appear that a rational approach to control is to supplement the rations of concentrate-fed cattle and sheep with thiamin on a continuous basis. The daily requirements for protection have not been recommended (35). This level may not be protective in all situations and response trials may be necessary to determine protective levels for different situations. A level of 20–30 mg/kg of feed may be necessary for protection. Most natural feedstuffs for ruminants contain thiamin at the rate of about 2 mg/kg of dry feed which when combined with the thiamin synthesized in the rumen will meet animals' requirements. However, the presence of thiaminases in the rumen will necessitate dietary supplementation with thiamin, but the optimal amounts that will provide protection under practical conditions is uncertain.

The intramuscular injection of 500 mg thiamin three times weekly into 6-month-old calves raised under practical farm conditions will steadily reduce the percentage thiamin pyrophosphate effect to zero in about 6 weeks (12). The daily oral administration of 100 mg thiamin to young calves fed initially on milk substitutes and then on concentrates and hay results in a decrease in percentage pyrophosphate effect (12).

For animals which are fed diets associated with thiamin inadequacy, it is recommended that thiamin be added to the diet at the rate of 5–10 mg/kg of dry feed (35). Cattle and sheep on concentrate-fed rations must also receive supplements containing all necessary vitamins and minerals, especially cobalt, a deficiency of which may be associated with some outbreaks of the disease.

The minimum amount of roughage which should be fed to feedlot cattle and sheep in order to prevent the disease and still maintain them on high levels of concentrates is unknown. A level of 1·5 kg of roughage per 100 kg body weight has been recommended but this may not be economical for the feedlot whose profits are dependent on rapid growth in grain-fed cattle. Supplementation of the diet with thiamin appears to be the only alternative.

The prevention of the disease in sheep which are being moved long distances or gathered together for shearing and other management practices will depend on ensuring an ample supply of roughage and water and avoiding drastic changes in management.

REVIEW LITERATURE

Edwin, E. E. & Jackman, R. (1982) Ruminant thiamine requirements in perspective. *Vet. Res. Commun.*, *5*, 236–250.
Jackman, R. (1985) The diagnosis of CCN (cerebrocortical necrosis) and thiamine deficiency in ruminants. *Vet. Ann.*, *25*, 71–77.
Markson, L. M. (1980) Cerebrocortical necrosis: an encephalopathy of ruminants. *Vet. Ann.*, *20*, 180–188.
Rammel, C. G. & Hill, J. H. (1986) A review of thiamine deficiency and its diagnosis, especially in ruminants. *NZ. vet. J.*, *34*, 202–204.

REFERENCES

(1) Loew, F. M. (1975) *Wld Rev. Nutr. Diet.*, *20*, 168.
(2) Markson, L.M. (1980) *Vet. Ann.*, *20*, 180.
(3) Pierson, R.E. & Jensen, R. (1975) *J. Am. vet. med. Assoc.*, *166*, 557.
(4) Candau, M & Massengo, J. (1982) *Ann. Rech. vet.*, *13*, 329.
(5) Edwin, E. E. et al. (1982) *Br. vet. J.*, *138*, 337.
(6) Grigat, G. A. & Mathison, G. W. (1983) *Can. J. anim. Sci.*, *63*, 715.
(7) Edwin, E. E. & Jackman, R. (1982) *Vet. Res. Commun.*, *5*, 237.
(8) Raisbeck, M. F. (1982) *J. Am. vet. med. Assoc.*, *180*, 1303.
(9) Boyd, J. W. & Walton, J. R. (1977) *J. comp. Pathol.*, *87*, 581.
(10) Loew, F. M. et al.(1972) *Vet. Rec.*, *90*, 657.
(11) Thornber, E. J. et al. (1980) *J. Neurochem.*, *35*, 713.
(12) Edwin, E. E. et al. (1976) *J. agric. Sci., Camb.*, *87*, 679.
(13) Bakher, H. J. et al. (1980) *Vet . Rec.*, *107*, 464.
(14) MacPherson, A. et al. (1977) *Vet. Rec.*, *101*, 231.
(15) Newman, W. F. et al (1969) *Vet. Rec.*, *84*, 577.
(16) von Rehm, W. F. et al. (1971) *Berl. Munch. Tierärztl. Wochenschr.*, *4*, 64.
(17) Loew, F. M. (1975) *J. Am. vet. med. Assoc.*, *166*, 219.
(18) Lusby, K. S. & Brent, B. E. (1972) *J. anim. Sci.*, *35*, 270.
(19) Sapienza, D. A. & Brent, B. E. (1974) *J. anim. Sci.*, *39*, 251.
(20) Bogin, E. et al. (1985) *Zentralbl. VetMed. A32*, 135.
(21) Jackman, R. & Edwin, E. E. (1983) *Vet. Rec.*, *112*, 548.
(22) Thomas, K. W. (1986) *J. vet. Pharmacol. Therap.*, *9*, 402.
(23) Morgan, K. T. (1974) *J. Pathol.*, *122*, 229.
(24) Askaa, J. & Moller, T. (1978) *Nord. VetMed.*, *30*, 126.
(25) Edwin, E. E. et al. (1979) *Vet. Rec.*, *104*, 4.
(26) Pritchard, D. & Eggleston, G. W. (1977) *Aust. vet. J.*, *54*, 204.
(27) Jackman, R (1985) *Vet. Ann.*, *25*, 71.
(28) Markson, L. M. & Wells, G. A. H. (1982) *Vet. Rec.*, *111*, 338.
(29) Rammell, C. G. & Hill, J. H. (1986) *NZ vet. J.*, *34*, 202.
(30) Little, P. B. & Sorenson, D.K. (1969) *J. Am. vet. med. Assoc.*, *155*, 1892.
(31) Smith, M. C. (1979) *J. Am. vet med. Assoc.*, *174*, 1329.
(32) Pill, A. H. (1967) *Vet. Res.*, *81*, 178.
(33) Mella, C. M. et al. (1976) *Can. J. comp. Med.*, *40*, 105.
(34) Zintzen, H. (1973) *Ubers. Tierarnahr.*, *1*, 273.
(35) Dickie, C. W. & Berryman, J. R. (1979) *J. Am. vet. med. Assoc.*, *175*, 463.
(36) Padovan, D. (1980) *Cornell Vet.*, *70*, 153.
(37) Wobeser, G. & Runge, W. (1979) *Can. vet. J.*, *20*, 323.
(38) Robertson, D. M. et al. (1968) *Am J. Pathol.*, *52*, 1081.
(39) Bestetti, G. & Frankhauser, R (1979) *Schweiz. Arch. Tierheilkd.*, *121*, 467.
(40) Grigat, G. A. & Mathison, G. W. (1982) *Can. J. anim. Sci.*, *62*, 807.
(41) Eigenmann, U. J. E. et al. (1980) *Wein. Tierheilkd. Monatsschr.*, 67, 273.
(42) Edwin, E. E. et al. (1982) *J. agric. Sci.*, *99*, 271.
(43) Cushnie, G. H. et al. (1979) *Vet. Rec.*, *105*, 480.
(44) Grigat, G. A. & Mathison, G. W. (1983) *Can. J. anim. Sci.*, *63*, 117.
(45) Brent, B. E. & Bartley, E. E. (1984) *J. anim. Sci.*, *59*, 813.
(46) Thomas, K. W. (1986) *Vet. Res. Commun.*, *10*, 125.
(47) McDonald, J. W. (1982) *Aust. vet. J.*, *58*, 213.
(48) Roberts, G. W. & Boyd, J. W. (1974) *J. comp. Pathol.*, *84*, 365.

Neonatal maladjustment syndrome of foals (barkers and wanderers in Thoroughbred foals)

This series of abnormalities appears to occur only in Britain (1) and only in Thoroughbred horses. Cases occur after easy parturitions and may reach an incidence of 1–2%. It seems probable that only foals which are assisted at birth are affected and it has been suggested that too early severance of the cord may deprive the foal of large quantities of blood in the placental vascular bed and precipitate the disease. By the same token, oxygen deprivation due to any cause is likely to cause the disease and it has been classified as a pulmonary dysfunction (2). A very similar syndrome has been described in hunter foals and is ascribed to hypoglycemia because of rapid response to oral administration of colostrum (3). A similar hypoxic disease occurs in human infants and has been produced experimentally in laboratory animals. In calves hypoxic encephalomalacia is well identified as a sequel to prolonged parturition. One case is recorded in a foal born without assistance and with late placental separation from the foal, but at postmortem examination there was extensive pulmonary consolidation (4).

Clinically there are three stages of the disease, affected foals in each stage being known as 'barkers', 'dummies' or 'wanderers'. Foals that show the 'barkers' syndrome pass through the other stages during recovery but some may begin as 'dummies' or 'wanderers' and these progress to recovery. In the first stage, about 50% die but, in the other stages, improvement or recovery is the rule. The disease always commences during the first day of life, sometimes as early as 10–30 minutes after birth, but usually after an hour or two.

The barking stage may be ushered in by prodromal signs of weakness, aimless movements and blindness. The characteristic signs in this stage are a barking sound emitted during severe clonic convulsions in which the foal paddles wildly, champs the jaws, shows clonic contractions of the head and neck and often bruises itself extensively about the head by banging it on the floor. Nystagmus is also present and sweating may be profuse. A period of coma follows such a convulsive episode but the foal can be aroused and subsequent, less severe convulsions may occur. The foal is unable to stand or suck and is blind. Affected foals may die during this stage or remain in a coma for hours or days and then pass into the 'dummy' stage. The rectal temperature may be as high as 40·6°C (105°F) during convulsions and as low as 32·2°C (90°F) when in a coma. Normally, the foal's heart rate during the first day of life is about 120/min. In foals affected with neonatal maladjustment syndrome, it will be over 150 during periods of active convulsion, and during coma about 80/min.

The 'dummy' and 'wandering' stages are manifested by blindness and failure to respond to most external stimuli. The sucking reflex is absent, the foal shows no fear and there is no excitement or abnormal movement. The foal can walk and wanders about aimlessly, bumping into fixed objects. Most such foals go on to recover completely in 3–10 days. Much of the success or failure of treatment of these cases depends on the accuracy of assessment of the foal's status. This includes a complete clinical examination, radiological examination of the chest, a complete hemogram and blood gas analysis. Blood gas anomalies are characteristic. There is a decreased P_{O_2} (< 45 mmHg) and an increased P_{CO_2} (> 50 mmHg) but there is no alkalosis (8).

At necropsy, there is extensive consolidation of the upper parts of both lungs, ischemic necrosis of the cerebral cortex and local hemorrhage in the brain. In less affected foals the lesions are restricted to hemorrhage, brain swelling and edema. These lesions appear likely to be the result of circulatory disturbances occurring at the time of parturition (5, 6).

Differentiation from the following diseases as set out in Table 59 is necessary: the foal septicemias, especially *Escherichia coli* and *Actinobacillus equuli*, retention of meconium, rupture of the bladder, and isoimmune hemolytic anemia.

In the acute stage, sedation is necessary to prevent excessive injury and, in the chronic stage, the foal must be fed by nasal tube, preferably four to five times a day, until it can learn to drink from a dish or suck from the mare. The amount of milk (mare's or reconstituted dried milk) fed should be 80 ml/kg body weight per day in ten divided feeds; the fluid intake should be at least 4–5 liters per day and the milk should be at 38°C (100°F). The foal must be kept warm during the comatose stage and should be in an environment of 28–32°C (82–89·5°F). If hypoxia is likely, oxygen administration through a nasal catheter at a flow rate of 10 liters per minute is recommended (7).

A degree of sophistication is now available in the treatment of these foals (9). It is based primarily on ventilatory support of assisted, controlled respiration and intermittent mandatory ventilation and the provision of oxygen at just the right rate to avoid hypoxia.

REVIEW LITERATURE

Clabough, D. L. & Martens, R. J. (1985) Equine neonatal maladjustment syndrome. *Comp. cont. Educ. pract. vet.*, 7, S497–S505.

Sonea, I. (1985) Respiratory distress syndrome in neonatal foals. *Comp. cont. Educ.*, 7, S462–S470.

REFERENCES

(1) Mahaffey, L. W. & Rossdale, P. D. (1957) *Vet. Rec.*, *69*, 1277.
(2) Rossdale, P. D. (1969) *Res. vet. Sci.*, *10*, 279.
(3) Smith, G. A. (1968) *Vet. Rec.*, *83*, 588.
(4) Baird, J. D. (1973) *Aust. vet. J.*, *49*, 530.
(5) Palmer, A. C. & Rossdale, P. D. (1976) *Res. vet. Sci.*, *20*, 267.
(6) Johnson, P. & Rossdale, P. D. (1976) *J. Reprod. Fertil*, Suppl. *23*, 695.
(7) Rossdale P. D. (1972) *Vet. Rec.*, *91*, 581.
(8) Kosch, P. C. et al. (1984) *Equ. vet. J.*, *16*, 312.
(9 [illegible] 1984) *Equ. vet. J.*, *16*, 319.

Shaker foal syndrome

This naturally occurring syndrome can be produced experimentally by the intravenous injection of *Clostridium botulinum* type A toxin. There is difficulty in assuming that the disease is a form of botulism in that there is a very strict limitation in the age group affected—3–8 weeks of age. The disease occurs sporadically in the United States (1) and the United Kingdom (2) where it has been known for many years. It occurs rarely and never more than one or two cases per farm in a year. Either sex and both Standardbreds and Thoroughbreds are affected.

Clinically there is a sudden onset of severe muscular weakness and prostration, with the foal going down and being unable to rise. If it is held up there is a gross muscle tremor which is not evident when the foal is lying down. Prostrate foals are bright and alert and respond to pinching. They go through periods of rising, followed by onset of the tremor and recumbency and complete prostration.

During this latter period there is a complete cessation of peristalsis and dilatation of the pupils with a sluggish response to light. The temperature varies from being slightly elevated to slightly depressed. Death occurs about 72 hours after the onset of signs and is due to respiratory failure.

There is no significant clinicopathological change although extreme acidosis has been recorded terminally. At necropsy examination the colon is tightly contracted and contains small amounts of dry, hard fecal material. The liver is enlarged and unevenly mottled. The pericardial sac contains excessive clear yellow fluid with fibrin flakes. There are no lesions in the nervous system. There are some similarities to grass sickness. As discussed under the heading of botulism, there has been a proposal that the disease is toxicoinfectious botulism in which the botulinus bacteria are located in tissues.

An heroic treatment schedule of 2 mg neostigmine every 2 hours (plus mineral oil, steroids, antibiotics and tube feeding) for 4–7 days is recorded as curing both of the two cases thus treated (1).

REFERENCES

(1) Rooney, J. E. & Prickett, M. E. (1967) *Mod. vet. Pract.*, 48, 44.
(2) Rossdale, P. D. & Mullen, P. A. (1969) *Vet. Rec.*, *85*, 702.

Equine narcolepsy/cataplexy

Affected horses, mostly Shetland ponies (1), suffer recurrent episodes of uncontrollable sleep. It is difficult to differentiate this from cataplexy, in which the patient loses all control of voluntary muscles during the episode, so that the animal falls to the ground. Respiration continues and there are no involuntary movements, but consciousness appears to be lost. The duration of the fit is several minutes, after which the horse is completely normal. It is sometimes possible to precipitate an attack by feeding or handling. A forceful blow may terminate an attack.

REFERENCE

(1) De Lahunta, A. (1978) *Cornell Vet.*, *68*, 122.

Congenital tremor syndromes of piglets

This group of at least four etiologically distinct congenital diseases of the nervous system have a similar clinical and pathological identity (1, 2). In particular they all have congenital tremor (myoclonia congenita) and these rhythmic tremors are most evident while the piglet is standing, are reduced when it lies down, and disappear when it is asleep. It is therefore not an encephalitis but an increased sensitivity of the spinal cord reflexes.

Although the tremor is present at birth it may not be observed until the piglets are 2 or 3 days old and beginning to move about actively. The tremor varies from a very rapid twitch affecting only the head to a slow tremor causing the pig to 'dance'; there may be such a severe tremor that the body and head tremble violently and rock from side to side. There is no muscular weakness and the piglets get up and scamper about, but there may be ataxia and dysmetria so that the gait may be badly affected. Mildly affected piglets are not greatly incapacitated and can survive and eventually recover in 2–8 weeks; the tremor fades gradually, and near the end of the course it may be evident only during exercise. Badly affected piglets may be unable to get to the teat to suck and may die of starvation. Many are fatally crushed or trampled by the sow.

For convenience, entities within the syndrome have been classified as type A, in which there are types AI, AII, AIII and AIV for which the causes are known (7). Type AV occurs naturally in Scandinavia and has been experimentally produced following dosing of pregnant sows between 45 and 75 days of gestation with trichlorfon (6). Type B is a form of congenital tremor not yet adequately characterized and is of unknown etiology (9, 11).

The four identified causes include transplacental infection of the fetus with the swine fever virus, similar transplacental infection with an unidentified virus, and two inherited forms, one a sex-linked recessive and the other an autosomal recessive (2). In litters affected by swine fever virus usually about 40% of the litter are affected. The characteristic lesions are cerebellar hypoplasia and cerebrospinal dysmyelinogenesis (5). When the disease caused by the unidentified viral infection of the fetus first appears in a piggery all litters are affected. Most pigs in each litter have the disease, but after a period of several months the disease disappears, apparently because of herd immunity. The principal sign as in the swine fever induced disease is myoclonia, and most piglets recover. Spinal dysmyelinogenesis is the characteristic lesion. The inherited sex-linked disease occurs in the progeny of Landrace or Landrace-cross sows. Up to 11% of Landrace piglets may be affected compared to only 0·3–0·8% in the Yorkshire, Hampshire and Duroc breeds (10). The mode of transmission is via a monogenic sex-linked recessive character, and half of all male pigs born are affected. Histologically there is cerebrospinal myelinogenesis. Most affected pigs die. The fourth disease conditioned by the inheritance of a single autosomal recessive character occurs in Wessex Saddleback pigs, in about 25% of the progeny, and is fatal in most of them. Cerebrospinal dysmyelinogenesis is the characteristic lesion.

A fifth disease is recorded in the United Kingdom and Sweden as being similar to the swine fever-induced disease in that there is cerebellar hypoplasia.

The differentiation of these diseases is now possible on the basis of histopathological and neurochemical findings (2) and relating these to the epidemiological data (1). In piglets born from sows inoculated with the Weybridge congenital tremor strain of the swine fever virus in early pregnancy, the severity of the clinical signs was related to the degree of spinal myelin deficiency (7). Semiautomated planimetry can be used to determine the cross-sectional areas of spinal gray and white matter of affected piglets (8). The spinal cord cross-sectional area is significantly reduced in piglets affected with type AI congenital tremor (8). The reduction is similar to type AII (9). The neurochemical findings relate to the presence of particular fatty acid profiles in the cholesterolesters in the lipids of the spinal cord.

Control of the disease depends on its cause. If it is inherited the recommended procedure is to keep none of the affected recovered pigs for breeding. If the cause is one of the maternal infections of early pregnancy it is recommended practice to deliberately expose empty females to affected piglets so that they become immunized before pregnancy. Failure to identify the cause may necessitate adopting both procedures.

The disease appears to have assumed much greater prevalence and importance recently. As many as 15% of litters born in a piggery may be affected, and of these 72% of the piglets may be affected and the case fatality rate amongst these may be as high as 50% (3). The specific cause of the increased prevalence has not been identified but it is possibly the unidentified virus referred to above. There is also the possibility that the observed concurrent increase in prevalence between congenital tremor and splayleg of piglets may indicate that splayleg is also caused by the same virus (4).

REVIEW LITERATURE

Done, J. T. (1976) The congenital tremor syndrome in pigs. *Vet. Ann.*, *16*, 98.

Faulkes, J. A. (1974) Myelin and demyelination in domestic animals. *Vet. Bull.*, *44* 441.

REFERENCES

(1) Done, J. T. (1976) *Vet. Ann.*, *16*, 98.
(2) Patterson, D. S. P. & Done, J. T. (1977) *Br. vet. J.*, *133*, 111.
(3) Hamori, D. et al. (1976) *Magy. Allatorv. Lap.*, *31*, 119.
(4) Gustafson, D. P. & Kanitz, C. L. (1974) *Proc. ann. Mtg US Anim. Hlth Assoc.*, *78*, 338.
(5) Vannier, P. et al. (1981) *Am. J. vet. Res.*, *42*, 135.
(6) Bolske, G. et al. (1978) *Nord. VetMed.*, *30*, 534.
(7) Bradley, R. et al. (1983) *J. comp. Pathol.*, *93*, 43.
(8) Done, J. T. et al. (1984) *Zentralbl. VetMed.*, *31*, 81.
(9) Done, J. T. et al. (1986) *Br. vet. J.*, *142*, 145.
(10) Lindstrom, K. & Lundeheim, N. (1986) *Nord. Vet Med.*, *38*, 22.
(11) Miry, C. et al. (1984) *Vlaams Diergeneeskd. Tijdschr.*, *53*, 31, 38.

Hypomyelinogenesis congenita

This congenital disease has been recorded in lambs in the United Kingdom (1, 2) and Canada (3) and in calves in the United States (4). It occurs extensively in Australia. Congenital hypomyelinogenesis is also a common finding in some forms of congenital tremor of piglets discussed in the previous section.

The disease recorded in lambs is manifested by severe muscle tremors affecting the whole body and head. The tremor disappears when the lambs are asleep. The gait is erratic and incoordinated and the lambs tend to hop or jump with the hindlegs, but they follow the ewe, and suck and grow well. Defecation, urination and the voice are unaffected. Many lambs recover spontaneously but severely affected lambs may die of starvation within the first few days of life, or nervous signs, including intermittent head-shaking and mild, coarse muscle tremor with ataxia of the hindlegs, may persist for as long as 5 months. These lambs appear normal at rest and grow normally if carefully nursed but appear to be more susceptible than usual to intercurrent disease. The disease has occurred in outbreak form with an incidence as high as 13% (5).

There is a great deal of similarity between hypomyelinogenesis congenita and 'hairy shaker' or 'border' disease of lambs (6). Although these diseases are known to be transmissible (7, 8) and to be reproducible by the injection of mucosal disease virus into pregnant ewes (9), the possibility remains that congenital hypomyelinogenesis can also be caused by other as yet unidentified pathogens. Hence, we continue to maintain its description in two places, under mucosal disease, and amongst the diseases whose causes are not fully known. The histopathological lesion is an absence of myelin but without any defect of the nerve fiber.

Affected calves are well formed, alert and have normal eyes but are unable to stand or achieve normal postures from birth. Persistent general tremor is evident at all times, is more pronounced on stimulation and may be accompanied by brief periods of spastic rigidity and moderate opisthotonus and occasionally nystagmus. At necropsy there is a marked deficiency of myelin particularly in the cerebellum and brainstem. Although the cause of the disease has not been determined, an inherited factor does not appear to be responsible (4). Epidemiological evidence suggests strongly that it is a viral infection contracted in the middle third of pregnancy which causes no apparent ill-effect in the dam. The usual pattern is for a high proportion of the first calves to be born in a calving season to be affected over a period of about a month and for subsequent calves to be unaffected.

REFERENCES

(1) Markson, L. M. et al. (1959) *Vet. Rec.*, *71*, 269.
(2) Hughes, L. E. et al. (1959) *Vet. Rec.*, *71*, 313.
(3) Darcel, C. LeQ. et al. (1961) *Can. J. comp. Med.*, *25*, 132.
(4) Young, S. (1962) *Cornell Vet.*, *52*, 84.
(5) Barr, M. (1964) *Vet. Rec.*, *76*, 815.
(6) Barlow, R. M. & Dickinson, A. G. (1965) *Res. vet. Sci.*, *6*, 230.
(7) Shaw, J. G. et al. (1967) *Vet. Rec.*, *81*, 115.
(8) Dickinson, A. G. & Barlow, R. M. (1967) *Vet. Rec.*, *81*, 114.
(9) Acland, H. M. et al. (1972) *Aust. vet. J.*, *48*, 70.

Enzootic incoordination ('wobbles', foal ataxia, equine sensory ataxia)

Enzootic incoordination is a group of diseases of young horses affecting the cervical spinal cord and characterized clinically by chronic incoordination. This is the only clinical syndrome presented and there are many other diseases characterized by transience of the incoordination or by additional other signs.

Etiology

Earlier confusion about the cause of incoordination of young horses has been greatly improved by an analysis of case material into morphological entities, some with known causes, some without (10). The principal group is equine degenerative myeloencephalopathy in which the cause is not identified (7). Another important group comprises those diseases caused by injury to the cord. These may be static, due to simple narrowing of the vertebral column, as in osteochondrosis and osteoporosis, or dynamic due to vertebral instability resulting in intermittent compression when the neck is flexed in an exaggerated manner (13). The stenotic myelopathy is believed to be the result of a combination of fast growth rate (or large size) and overnutrition. Inflammatory lesions caused most commonly by protozoal coccidial infection identified as *Sarcocystis* sp. (12), are also a large group.

The part played by nutritional deficiency or inheritance in causing any of these diseases has not been determined. There is an overall tendency for 'wobbles' to be inherited (1), but the relationship could be as distant as the relationship between genetics and growth rate. The excessive mobility between the vertebrae which probably results in pressure being exerted on the spinal cord may be nutritional in origin and be exerted through disease of the intervertebral discs and ligaments and articular surfaces (2).

Epidemiology

Details of incidence are not available but the disease occurs sporadically in most countries, and is of importance in that affected horses are useless for further work, and the disease is irreversible.

Most cases are first observed in sucklings and yearlings but clinical signs may appear for the first time in horses up to 2 years of age. Often the horses affected in a group are those in best condition.

The disease occurs in young Thoroughbreds, trotting and saddle horses but no association has been noted between the occurrence of the disease and any management or nutritional factor. Males are most commonly affected, and overall the incidence is very low.

Pathogenesis

The basis of each of the diseases in the group is a symmetric, focal, cervical myelopathy which may be the result of pressure from outside the cord (*cervical vertebral stenotic myelopathy*) or be an intrinsic degenerative lesion (*equine degenerative myeloencephalopathy*) or an inflammatory one (*equine protozoal meningoencephalitis*). The incoordination which is characteristic of these diseases always takes the form of symmetric ataxia and tetraparesis.

When the disease is the result of pressure in the cervical spinal cord there is secondary ascending and descending nerve fiber degeneration.

Continued contusion of the cervical spinal cord is accepted as the basic lesion, the contusion occurring by overflexion of the neck and momentary dorsal displacement of the vertebral body, or because of fleeting protrusion of the capsule of the lateral spinal joint into the spinal canal (2). It is suggested that the occurrence of the abnormality is related to the length of neck, longer necked horses being more susceptible because of greater bending and retroflexing force (5). Serious exacerbations occur from time to time, often associated with falls or other violent movements. The clinical picture then is one of gradual deterioration in coordination of movement, which may go undetected in horses which are not under restraint, until the more serious errors occur.

The specific degenerative lesion of this disease, due to pressure from subluxation of vertebral bodies, may be primarily due to venous occlusion (6). The abnormalities observed are more readily explained as both motor and sensory rather than a purely sensory ataxia (6, 7).

Clinical findings

Although a history of sudden onset is sometimes obtained it is usually found that in these cases there were mild signs previously and that a fall, violent activity or casting have precipitated a more severe disturbance. In most cases the onset is insidious, the first signs being a slight incoordination of leg movements. This may be apparent in mild cases only when the horse is being ridden. Neck movements are restricted and pain may be elicited on sudden movement of, or pressure over, the cervical vertebrae but there is no cutaneous hypersensitivity in the usual sense.

The defect of gait is difficult to describe. There may be insufficient or excessive flexion or extension or excessive abduction. There is usually a degree of weakness. While moving, there is clumsiness when the horse is turned sharply, and pulling up sharply at a fast gait causes knuckling over at the fetlocks. During walking there may be lurching and swaying, particularly of the hindquarters, and the horse often has difficulty maintaining a normal posture for urination and grazing. The forelimbs may be more seriously involved than the hindlimbs and one of a pair may be more affected than the other. The signs are most marked when walking and often disappear at the trot. There is some difference of opinion about the effect of blindfolding on the gait (6, 7) but the consensus is that it has no effect. Dragging of the toes, often intermittently, is an early sign in many cases and there may be difficulty in getting up after the horse has rolled or been cast.

A useful aid could be the 'slap test' for laryngeal adductory function (3). With an endoscope in place so that the vocal cords can be observed the horse is slapped just behind the withers on the saddle place. A positive response is a flickering adductory withdrawal of the contralateral arytenoid cartilage. Failure of the cartilage to respond indicates the presence of spinal cord inefficiency, inefficiency of the innervation of the larynx and, if the horse is excited, inhibition by higher brain centers.

After the initial appearance of signs, there may be progression of the disease for several weeks, followed by a long period during which the signs remain static. Recovery does not occur but death is unusual unless the animal has a severe accident.

Clinical pathology

No laboratory examinations have diagnostic value. Blood levels of calcium and phosphorus are within normal limits. Radiographic examination offers some assistance in differentiation. It is possible to predict the occurrence of contusion to the cord by observing abnormal flexibility of the intervertebral joints (11).

Necropsy findings

In 30–50% of cases, there are projections of vertebrae or intervertebral discs into the spinal canal and some evidence of compression of the cord (4). Areas of malacia are present in the spinal cord and there is symmetrical degeneration of ascending and descending spinal cord tracts. Inflammation of the articular processes of both thoracic and cervical vertebrae may be present with involvement of the spinal nerves. Severe inflammation of peripheral nerves may also be present in early cases. Slight atrophy of cervical muscles is sometimes evident. There is histological evidence of stretching and tearing of the ligamentum flavum and joint capsule at affected joints especially C6 or C7 (15).

Diagnosis

Traumatic injury to the spinal cord causes a sudden onset of paralysis often followed by gradual improvement. Pressure on the spinal cord due to space occupying lesions in the vertebral canal may cause almost identical signs (6). Spinal meningitis or myelitis usually develops slowly; meningitis is accompanied by rigidity and hyperesthesia of the neck and myelitis by some signs of encephalitis. Incoordination during moderate exercise is a prominent sign in iliac thrombosis but usually only one leg is affected and there are circulatory signs on palpation of the affected limb. In tropical countries, cerebrospinal nematodiasis is a more common cause of an almost identical syndrome. A fatal, inherited ataxia of foals in the Oldenburg breed is much more severe and develops to the stage of recumbency and finally complete paralysis. A spinal ataxia in zebras (8) characterized by degeneration of spinal cord tracts without the malacic lesions of 'wobbler' disease, has clinical similarities to wobbles. So does disseminated necrotizing myeloencephalitis caused by the rhinopneumonitis virus (9). But both diseases are progressive and euthanasia is necessary.

Treatment

The surgical treatment of focal compression of the spinal cord is now undertaken in selected cases (14).

Control

Because of the possible inherited nature of the disease, a corrective breeding program may be advisable.

REVIEW LITERATURE

Beech, J. (1976) Cervical cord compression and wobbles in horses. *Proc. 22nd ann. Conv. Am. Assoc. equ. Pract.*, p. 79.

De Lahunta, A. (1978) Diagnosis of equine neurologic problems. *Cornell Vet.*, *88*, 122.
Whitwell, K. E. (1980) Cause of ataxia in horses. *Vet. Rec. in Practice*, *2*(4), 17.

REFERENCES

(1) Falco, M. J. et al. (1976) *Equ. vet. F.*, *8*, 165.
(2) Dahme, E. & Schebitz, H. (1970) *Zentralbl. VetMed.*, *17A*, 120.
(3) Greet, T. R. C. et al. (1980) *Equ. vet. J.*, *12*, 127.
(4) Pohlenz, J. & Schulz, L. C. (1966) *Dtsch Tierärztl. Wochenschr.*, *73*, 533.
(5) Rooney, J. R. (1972) *Mod. vet. Pract.*, *53*, 42.
(6) Fraser, H. & Palmer, A. C. (1967) *Vet. Rec.*, *80*, 338.
(7) Mayhew, I. G. et al. (1977) *Am. J. vet. med. Assoc.*, *170*, 195.
(8) Montali, R. J. et al. (1974) *Vet. Pathol.*, *11*, 68.
(9) Little, P. B. & Thorsen, J. (1976) *Vet. Pathol.*, *13*, 161.
(10) Mayhew, I. G. et al. (1978) *Cornell Vet.*, *68*, Suppl. 6, pp. 1–207.
(11) Bohm, D. & Hekeler, W. G. (1980) *Berl. Münch. Tierärztl.* Wochenschr., *93*, 181.
(12) Simpson, C. F. & Mayhew, I. G. (1980) *J. Protozool*, *27*, 228.
(13) Nixon, A. J. et al. (1982) *Proc. 28th Ann. Conv. Am. Assoc. equ. Pract.* *28*, 253.
(14) Wagner, P. C. et al (1981) *Comp. cont. Educ.*, *3*, S192.
(15) Power, B. E. et al (1986) *Vet. Pathol.*, *23*, 392.

Stringhalt

Stringhalt is an involuntary, exaggerated flexion of the hock during progression. It may affect one or both hindlimbs. Classical stringhalt occurs sporadically and is irreversible without surgical intervention. A clinically identical disease, Australian stringhalt, occurs in outbreaks and most horses recover without treatment (1). It has been recorded in Australia, New Zealand and California. In the most severe cases the horse is unable to rise without assistance. In the mildest form the abnormal movement is only elicited when the horse begins to move, or is backed or turned. The average case is manifested by a flexion of the hock violent enough for the horse to kick itself in the abdomen. The hoof is held in this position for a moment and then stamped hard on the ground. If both legs are affected progress is very slow and difficult. The horse's general health is unaffected although it may be difficult for it to graze. There is a selective wasting of the muscles of the thigh. Some cases have other nervous signs such as stiffness of the forelimbs.

It is generally conceded that Australian outbreaks are caused by eating flatweed or catsear (*Hypochaeris radicata*); but good evidence of its role is lacking. Pathological findings are restricted to a peripheral neuropathy in the tibial, superficial peroneal and medial plantar nerves (2).

REVIEW LITERATURE

Cahill, J. I. et al. (1985) A review and some observations on stringhalt. *NZ vet. J.*, *33*, 101–104.

REFERENCES

(1) Pemberton, D. H. & Caple, I. W. (1980) *Vet. Ann.*, *20*, 167.
(2) Friend, S. C. E. & Jeffcott, L. B. (1985) *Aust. Adv. vet. Sci.*, p.60.

DISEASES CHARACTERIZED BY INVOLVEMENT OF THE MUSCULOSKELETAL SYSTEM

Sporadic lymphangitis (bigleg, weed)

This is a non-contagious disease of horses characterized by acute fever, lymphangitis and severe swelling of one or both hindlegs. The disease commences abruptly with fever (40·5–41°C, 105–106°F), shivering and a rapid pulse rate and respiration. Pain is severe and the horse is usually quite distressed. There is severe pain on palpation of the affected leg and lameness may be so severe that the horse may refuse to put its foot to the ground. The limb is swollen and hot, the swelling commencing at the top of the leg and extending down to the coronet. There is cording of the lymphatics on the medial aspect of the leg and palpable enlargement of the lymph nodes. Anorexia, thirst and patchy sweating may also be in evidence and constipation is usual. The acute stage lasts for 2–3 days but the swelling persists for 7–10 days. Occasionally abscesses develop in the lymph nodes and vessels. There is a tendency for the disease to recur and cause chronic fibrotic thickening of the lower part of the limb.

Sporadic lymphangitis usually occurs in horses fed highly nutritious rations with restricted exercise for a number of days. It is usually associated with superficial wounds and ulcers on the lower parts of the limbs, and the disease is thought to develop as a lymphadenitis of the deep inguinal nodes as a result of these wounds. The affected lymph nodes obstruct lymphatic and venous drainage and, because of lack of stimulation of these by exercise, lymphangitis develops, causing lymphatic obstruction, edema and, in some cases, cellulitis (1).

Affected horses require energetic treatment. Penicillin or other antibiotic should be administered parenterally to control the infection. A sedative to ease the pain, and vigorous hot fomentation and massage of the leg to remove the edema fluid are also advised. The administration of a laxative and a diuretic has long been a standard practice. Hot fomentations, with upward massage of the limb, should be applied frequently and the leg bandaged tightly in the intervals. The efficiency with which this part of the treatment is carried out would determine largely the speed of recovery. Exercise should be encouraged as soon as the horse can put its foot to the ground.

Prevention of the disease necessitates prompt and careful treatment of all wounds of the lower limbs. Provision of daily exercise, restriction of the diet during prolonged rest periods and dry standing in the stable also help to prevent the disease.

REFERENCE

(1) Tufvesson, G. (1952) *Nord. VetMed.*, *4*, 529, 729, 817, 1046.

Asymmetric hindquarter syndrome of pigs

This condition has been reported from continental Europe (1, 2) and the United Kingdom (3). The syndrome is manifest by variable asymmetry of the hindquarters which is generally evident during the early grower period and obvious by 80 kg live-weight stage. Several breeds have been found affected but the problem is generally restricted to certain herds and to certain families within these herds, suggesting that a genetic liability exists for this condition (3). Both sexes may be involved and the condition may involve either hindlimb. Despite a marked reduction in muscle mass there is no detectable abnormality in gait. The cause is unknown although it appears to result from suboptimal muscle growth rather than degenerative loss (4). Perineural fibrosis and myopathy have been observed in some cases but have not been found consistently (1, 3, 4).

REFERENCES

(1) Bickhardt, K. et al. (1967) *Dtsch Tierärztl. Wochenschr.*, *74*, 324.
(2) Hoorens, J. & Oyaert, W. (1970) *Vlaams Diergeneeskd. Tijdschr.*, *39*, 246.
(3) Done, J. T. et al. (1975) *Vet. Rec.*, *96*, 482.
(4) Swatland, H. J. & Cassens, R. G. (1972) *J. anim. Sci.*, *35*, 336.

Splayleg syndrome in newborn pigs (spraddle leg, myofibrillar hypoplasia)

This syndrome occurs in newborn piglets in most countries and is characterized by a temporary inability to stand with the hindlimbs (1).

The etiology of the disease is not known, but based on epidemiological evidence it is thought to be multifactorial (1). The overall prevalence of the disease in the United Kingdom is 0·4% and the morbidity in affected herds varies from 2 to 27%. The case fatality rate is approximately 50% and is due to crushing, chilling and starvation because affected piglets are not able to move around normally. The disease is more common in the Welsh Landrace and Large White breeds of swine; Landrace pigs may be especially susceptible. This suggests a genetic basis, but test-matings, with the exception of a few, have not been successful in reproducing the disease (1, 2). On most farms the disease affects both male and female piglets. In a recent retrospective analysis of the incidence of the disease in a swine herd over a period of 5 years, the overall frequency was 1.74 times more in males than females and the birth weight of splayleg piglets tended to be subnormal (3). The current hypothesis is that the disease is caused by an interaction of genetic and non-genetic factors—a polygenic mode or expression of many genes. The environmental factors which have been associated with some outbreaks include slippery floors, a dietary choline deficiency and the ingestion of *Fusarium* toxin by pregnant sows. Choline deficiency is unlikely to be a factor (4) and none of the other factors have been substantiated as etiological factors or epidemiological determinants (1).

Recent evidence indicates that splayleg may represent a congenital form of glucocorticoid myopathy resulting from stress and hormonal imbalance of pregnant sows (10–12). Myofibrillar hypoplasia can be induced experimentally in piglets by treatment of the sows in the late pregnancy with dexamethasone (10, 12).

The pathogenesis of the disease is known. Detailed microscopic examination of the muscles of the limbs of affected pigs have revealed evidence of myofibrillar hypoplasia. However, because myofibrillar hypoplasia can also be found in normal unaffected littermates (1) it has been difficult to explain the pathogenesis of the muscular weakness. However, in addition to myofibrillar hypoplasia, in splayleg pigs there is a higher content of sarcoplasmic RNA, reflected ultrastructurally by the presence of numerous ribosomes. The extramyofibrillar space was also filled with glycogen in splayleg pigs. In myofibrillar hypoplasia induced experimentally by the administration of glucocorticoids to the pregnant sow, none of the pigs had splayleg but the extramyofibrillar space contained little glycogen (10). In the latter there were also many glycogen-filled phagosomes and residual bodies which indicate a difference in the metabolism of glycogen in the first 2 or 3 days after birth. Quantitative image analysis of skeletal muscle revealed that the arrangement of the myofibrils within the fascicles of affected and unaffected pigs was different (5).

Some studies have indicated that there are both quantitative (hypoplastic-type) and qualitative (dystrophic-type) insufficiencies in affected pigs and that these changes represent a temporary perinatal developmental disturbance. This could explain the muscular weakness and the recovery which occurs (6, 7).

The clinical signs are usually obvious in 2–3 hours after birth when the litter should be up and walking around the creep area. Affected piglets are unable to stand and their hindlimbs are splayed sideways or forwards and the animals are resting in sternal recumbency. Sometimes the forelimbs are also splayed. Most severely affected piglets are unable to move, less severely affected animals are able to move slightly. As a result, the piglets are likely to be crushed or have difficulty gaining access to their source of nourishment. Affected piglets are normal in other respects and have a normal appetite and will suck the sow if placed near a teat. If they are able to suck or if fed artificially for 2–4 days recovery will occur within 1 week in about 50% of cases. The ambulatory capacity of affected pigs can be improved, and mortality reduced, by taping or loosely tying together the hindlimbs for a period of up to 1 week. The method of loose-tying of the hindlimbs consists of a figure-of-eight bandage (2·5 cm wide adhesive tape) being fixed around the metatarsal bones, leaving a space between the legs of up to 7 cm depending on the size of the piglet. The legs should be tied together within a few hours after the syndrome is obvious; a delay of several hours will decrease the prognosis. The provision of a non-slip floor surface such as a carpet or sack may also be helpful.

Whether or not to cull the boar depends on the pedigree value of the animal, the incidence of the disease and the probability that the boar is responsible. There is no evidence that the disease is monogenic. However, the incidence is highest in the Landrace breed which suggests a hereditary predisposition. In deciding whether to use a suspected carrier animal, there is a need to distinguish between different situations. The consequences of disease are felt differently at the different levels of organization of the pig industry. A boar of high merit for performance traits may be more economical to retain as breeding stock even though some progeny are affected with the disease than a less superior boar whose progeny are unaffected. If stress of the pregnant sow is a factor, control of the disease may be dependent upon the selection of stress-resistant boars and sows (12).

REVIEW LITERATURE

Ward, P. S. (1978) The splayleg syndrome in newborn pigs: a review. Part I, *Vet. Bull.*, *48*, 279–295. Part II, *Vet. Bull.*, *48*, 381–399.

REFERENCES

(1) Ward, P. S. (1978) *Vet. Bull.*, *48*, 279 & 381.
(2) Law, T. (1971) *J. Hered.*, *62*, 250.
(3) Vogt, D. W. et al. (1984) *Am. J. vet. Res.*, *45*, 2408.
(4) Tucek, S. et al. (1985) *Zentralbl. VetMed.*, *A32*, 1.
(5) Cox, C. S. et al. (1979) *Br. vet J.*, *135*, 370.
(6) Bergmann, V. (1976) *Mh VetMed.*, *31*, 129.
(7) Bergmann, V (1976) *Arch. exp. Vet. Med.*, *30*, 239.
(10) Ducatelle, R. et al. (1986) *J. comp. Pathol.*, *96*, 433.
(11) Jirmanova, I. (1983) *Vet. Res. Commun.*, *6*, 91.
(12) Jirmanova, I. & Lojda, L. (1985) *Zentralbl. VetMed.*, *A32*, 445.

Leg weakness in pigs (osteochondrosis and arthrosis, epiphyseolysis)

Locomotor disability is a significant cause of loss and mandatory culling in pig herds. Infectious arthritis, especially that associated with *Erysipelothrix insidiosa*, is an important cause but syndromes associated with non-infectious arthropathy and osteopathy have become of increasing importance with intensification of rearing and performance selection of pigs.

The etiology and factors underlying these syndromes are poorly defined, partly because of the difficulty of definitive clinical examination of affected pigs and the frequent lack of apparent significant pathological changes in necropsy examination of mild cases.

The clinical syndrome has been given the name of leg weakness and varies in severity from locomotor abnormality that results from conformation and leg defects such as narrow lumbar area and board hips, hyperflexion of the carpus, bowing of the forelimbs and 'knock knees', hyperextension of the phalanges, lateral angulation of the foot and sickle hocks to more severe lameness and, in the extreme, inability to rise and paresis (1–3).

In growing animals, the superficial layer of joint cartilage is articular cartilage, and the deeper layer is epiphyseal cartilage which undergoes endochondral ossification as the animal matures. The articular cartilage persists in the mature animal while the epiphyseal cartilage becomes a layer of calcified cartilage and underlying subchondral bone. The cartilage of the physis is known as the growth plate and is involved in metaphyseal growth. Osteochondrosis is a generalized disease in which there are focal areas of failure of endochondral ossification in the physeal (metaphyseal growth) and epiphyseal growth cartilages. In osteochondrosis the primary abnormality is an increased thickness of the joint cartilages combined with degenerative changes which result in infoldings and erosion of articular cartilages. Defects of the growth plates (physes) result in short deformed bones. Pathologically, severe clinical cases are characterized by osteochondrosis and secondary degenerative joint disease especially involving the medial aspects of the larger joints, epiphyseolysis and lumbar intervertebral disc degeneration and spondylosis (4–6). Osteochondrosis has been used to encompass lesions involving the physes and the articular epiphyseal complexes. However, because of morphologic changes that have been observed in growing pigs, dyschondroplasia is now the preferred term to be used generically and then qualified by the location and nature of the morphological description since the causes may be different (20).

It has been postulated that osteochondrosis is the underlying defect in this syndrome (7). Osteochondrosis, defective endochondral ossification in the deep layers of cartilage, has been found to occur commonly in growing pigs at predilection sites of the medial condyle of the humerus and femur, the epiphyseal plates of the distal ulna and the femoral head and the intervertebral joints (5, 7). It may heal spontaneously or it may progress to osteochondritis dessicans and osteoarthrosis. Its progression in either direction is influenced by local loading (3) and by joint stability which depends upon joint shape and muscle and ligamentous support. The age-related changes and osteochondrosis in the articular and epiphyseal cartilage have been described (13). The cartilage increases with age up to 5 weeks and then begins to decrease in thickness. Deleterious influences such as defects in conformation, heavy muscling with skeletal immaturity, muscular weakness resulting from myofibrillar hypoplasia, myopathies or lack of exercise, inadequate flooring or even simple trauma may adversely affect this progression and lead to severe skeletal change (8). Porcine synovial fluid contains both hyaluronic acid and chondroitin sulfate and the chondroitin sulfate-to-hyaluronic acid ratio is not influenced by relatively advanced stages of osteochondrosis (17).

The cause of the primary osteochondrosis is not known. The occurrence of osteochondrosis is significantly associated with rapid early growth (4), but it does not appear related to protein, vitamins A and D or calcium and phosphorus imbalance in the ration. It is possible that it is related to an effect of increased growth hormone (4). Rapid growth, especially during the early period, was thought to have a significant influence on the occurrence of this syndrome and there is also some breed variation in susceptibility (3). However, in some feeding trials of pigs from weaning to slaughter weight there was no direct effect of rapid growth rate on the incidence and severity of osteochondrosis (16).

The problem occurs in both male and female pigs and a prevalence of 20–30% or even higher is not unusual. It is a particular problem in gilt and boar testing stations where it may necessitate slaughter of affected animals before the testing period is complete. The lesions develop most commonly in growing pigs, particularly boars, raised in confinement, from 20 to 30 weeks of age

(6, 9). The effect of the quality of floor has been examined and there is no clear evidence that hardness of floor contributes to an increased frequency of lesions (9). However, the incidence and severity of joint lesions may be related to the duration of confinement in pigs confined individually (10). Exercise will prevent abnormalities such as bow legs, flexion of the carpus and sickle-legs from impairing the mobility of boars, but does not influence the severity of joint lesion (11). Experimentally, feed restriction appears to have no effect on the incidence of lesions in growing pigs (12). The peak period of clinical manifestation is from the late grower stage until 18 months of age although the effect of osteoarthrosis may carry through to the adult period. The milder syndromes of poor movement and lameness associated with defects in leg conformation in the grower stage are not necessarily associated with bone or joint lesions and may regress spontaneously or improve if affected pigs are placed on pasture (10). However, severe lameness at this age, and that which occurs in replacement stock and young adults is frequently associated with severe bone and joint lesions which may be irreversible (4).

Well-established lesions typical of osteochondrosis associated with the physes can be found in young pigs between 25 and 30 days of age (20). The earliest change associated with a dyschondroplasia of the physis is a focus of persistent hypertrophied chondrocytes which do progress but heal (20). Lesions associated with physes and articular epiphyseal complexes develop continuously and regress as pigs grow older (21).

There is no evidence that vascular damage is a factor in the pathogenesis of the lesions (19).

Because foci of dyschondroplastic lesions are associated with physes of pigs between birth and the stage of rapid growth they could be regarded as part of the usual growth patterns in contemporary commercial swine (18). However, clinical signs of dyschondroplasias, or degenerative joint disease secondary to dyschondroplasias, usually do not appear until pigs are almost 6 months of age (18).

The clinical syndrome is largely one of locomotor disorder and it usually involves the hindlimbs. Mild cases show stiffness, especially immediately after a period of lying down and lameness. Slowness to rise and a tendency to walk with short steps on tiptoes frequently in association with a marked inward curve of hindlimb motion during forward progression and side-to-side motion of the buttocks is frequently seen. More severely affected pigs sit on their hindquarters and show marked reluctance to rise. They carry one or both hindlimbs more forward under the body and walk with a short goose-stepping giant. Wasting is not a feature except in severely affected animals and the locomotor disorder may be minor unless exacerbated by physical exertion. However, the syndrome is of particular importance in breeding animals as it may interfere with successful mating. Boars may show initial interest in mounting but subsequently slide off the sow or dummy before mating is complete presumably due to the pain of the limb lesions. In Europe this problem has been called *impotentia coeundi*. There may be no meaningful association between visual scores for physical soundness in the live animal and the degree of joint damage (10). Some pigs with severe lesions are not lame and conversely other pigs are severely lame with minor lesions. Epiphyseolysis of the femoral head produces severe unilateral lameness and if bilateral is usually manifest by marked reluctance to rise and severe locomotor disability. Initial signs are frequently deceptively mild and follow physical exertion such as mating, transport, farrowing or fighting but they progress to severe lameness over a 7–10-day period. Epiphyseolysis of the tuber ischii may also occur following physical exertion but is more common in second or third parity sows (15) and is manifest by 'paralysis' with the hindlimbs in forward extension under the body of the sow.

Because of the pain and muscle contraction, it is frequently difficult to determine the site and severity of the lesion by simple clinical examination, and palpation following general anesthesia or radiography may be required for proper clinical assessment. While the lesions of the physes and articular epiphyseal complexes are detectable in pigs under 14 days of age they are not detectable radiographically in live animals until the pigs are over 100 days of age (21). Only 21% of the lesions associated with the physes and 22% of the lesions associated with the articular epiphyseal complexes were detectable in radiographs of bones of live pigs (21).

The histological, radiological and angiomicrographical findings of dyschondroplasias of growth cartilages in crossbred commercial pigs at 1 and 15 days of age have been described (18). The ultrastructural characteristics of normal epiphyseal cartilage of the articular epiphyseal cartilage complex in growing swine has been examined and found to be different from the articular cartilage and the cartilage of the physis (22).

The syndrome must be differentiated from other conditions which produce lameness and paralysis in growing and young adult pigs and include infectious arthritis, laminitis, traumatic foot lesions, foot lesions produced by biotin deficiency and footrot, osteodystrophy resulting from calcium, phosphorus and vitamin D imbalance in rations, vitamin A deficiency and viral poliomyelitis (14).

There is no effective treatment. Early cases may respond to corticosteroids or phenylbutazone in conjunction with being placed outside on pasture or housing individually inside on deep straw litter. Short-term control measures of restricted feeding of potential breeding stock with adequate exercise and care of feet and flooring underfoot have been suggested (2). Longterm control measures include the genetic selection of pigs with good conformation that can withstand highlevel feeding with little exercise (3, 6).

REVIEW LITERATURE

Bradley, R. & Wells, G. A. H. (1978) Developmental muscle disorders in the pig. *Vet. Ann.*, *18*, 144–157.

Grondalen, T. (1974) Osteochondrosis, arthrosis and leg weakness in pigs. *Nord. VetMed.*, *26*, 534.

Nakano, T., Aherne, F. X. & Thompson, J. R. (1981) Leg weakness and osteochondrosis in pigs. *Pig News Info.*, *2*, 29–34.

REFERENCES

(1) Vaughan, L. C. (1971) *Vet. Rec.*, *89*, 81.
(2) McPhee, C. P. & Laws, L. (1976) *Aust. vet. J.*, *52*, 123.
(3) Grondalen, T. (1974) *Acta vet. Scand.*, *555*, 574.
(4) Nakano, T. et al. (1981) *Pig News Info.*, *2*, 29.
(5) Doige, C. E. (1980) *Can. J. comp. Med.*, *44*, 382.
(6) Nakano, T. et al. (1979) *Can. J. comp. Med.*, *59*, 167.
(7) Reilard, S. (1978) *Acta Radiol.*, *Suppl. 358*, 23.
(8) Grondalen, T. (1974) *Acta vet. Scand.*, *15*, 1, 26, 43, 53, 61.
(9) Perrin, W. R. et al. (1978) *Can. J. anim. Sci.*, *58*, 129.
(10) Fredeen, H. T. & Sather, A. P. (1978) *Can. J. anim. Sci.58*, 759.
(11) Perrin, W. R. & Bowland, J. P. (1977) *Can. J. anim. Sci.*, *57*, 245.
(12) Nakano, T. et al. (1979) *Can. J. anim. Sci.*, *59*, 491.
(13) Bhatnagar, R. et al. (1981) *Can. J. comp. Med.*, *45*, 188.
(14) Penny, R. H. C. (1979) *Pig vet. Soc. Proc.*, *4*, 85.
(15) Penny, R. H. C. (1972) *Vet. Ann.*, *13*, 31.
(16) Nakano, T. et al. (1984) *Can. J. anim. Sci.*, *64*, 139.
(17) Nakano, T. et al. (1984) *Can. J. comp. Med.*, *48*, 434.
(18) Hill, M. A. et al. (1985) *Vet. Rec.*, *116*, 40.
(19) Hill, M. A. et al. (1985) *Res. vet. Sci.*, *38*, 151.
(20) Hill, M. A. et al. (1984) *Am. J. vet. Res.*, *45*, 903.
(21) Hill, M. A. et al. (1984) *Am. J. vet. Res.*, *45*, 917.
(22) Carlson, C. S. et al. (1985) *Am. J. vet. Res.*, *46*, 306.

Hyena disease

This disease of cattle has been recorded only in recent years (1). It is characterized by a slow growth rate and marked dissimilarity in growth and development between the forequarters and the hindquarters, the latter being comparatively underdeveloped. This gives the animal the classical contours of the hyena and this resemblance is heightened by a crest of thick, stiff bristles along the back in the midline. An aggressive attitude also develops. Affected calves are normal at birth and only develop the abnormality at 5–6 months of age. There is no apparent abnormality of sex hormones (2). The femur and tibia are shorter in affected than in normal animals (3). There are accompanying difficulties of locomotion with a tendency to fall sideways, and to frequently adopt a position of lateral recumbency. German Simmental, Charolais, Black Pied, German Holstein-Friesian, and German Red Pied cattle have been involved. Genetic analysis appears to indicate that the disease is inherited as a simple recessive with incomplete penetrance (4) but this is obviously not so in some herds. The lesion is a chondrodystrophy affecting particularly the long bones and the lumbar vertebrae (5).

REFERENCES

(1) Espinasse, J. & Parodi, A. (1976) *1ere Congr. int. mal. bétail (Paris, 1976)*, *2*, 519.
(2) Thibier, M. et al. (1978) *Br. vet. J.*, *134*, 462.
(3) Klee, W. & Lengfelder, K. (1979) *Tierärztl. Umschau*, *34*, 663.
(4) Herzog, A. et al. (1986) *Dtsch. Tierärztl. Wochenschr.*, *93*, 309.
(5) Parodi, A. L. et al. (1985) *Rec. med. Vet.*, *161*, 419.

'Tying-up' syndrome of horses

The all-embracing terms 'tying-up' or 'set-fast' are used to denote horses which become stiff and sore in their limbs, showing cramped and slow movement without actual lameness. They include also horses which stumble a little when walking and have a general appearance of rigidity, stiffness and gauntness of the abdomen after exercise, a real problem for racehorse trainers. In many cases the problem is one of muscle soreness due to a sudden change from a soft to a hard track, or overwork, especially in horses coming back into work after a rest. It may be due to a trainer demanding too much too soon. If such factors can be eliminated, and a decision reached that the horse's reaction is abnormal, the following possible causes should be considered (2).

Myopathy (polymyositis)
Most of the following entities are poorly defined, this being no exception. It is characterized by muscle soreness, often to the point where the horse literally will not move, a sudden onset after brisk exercise, and greatly elevated levels of serum enzymes including glutamic oxalate transaminase (SGOT), aldolase and creatine phosphokinase (CPK). Needle biopsy of gluteus muscle in affected horses shows hyaline degeneration, a low content of glycogen, adenosine triphosphate and creatinine phosphate, and a high content of lactate and glucose, suggesting a local hypoxia (3). It is identical to azoturia except that there is no myoglobinuria, and there is no immediately preceding history of an enforced rest on a full grain ration. There are distinct clinical and epidemiological differences from the enzootic equine myositides of Scandinavia and New Zealand which are described elsewhere; the principal difference is the tendency for this disease to be a characteristic of a particular horse which is inclined to have successive or intermittently repeated attacks (4). These make it an impossible training proposition and of doubtful suitability for other equine occupations. They are understandably significant sources of client dissatisfaction for veterinarians.

The onset of an attack may occur while the horse is being ridden; within a few strides it falters, goes gingerly and then stops. If it can be persuaded to move it does so with reluctance and with short shuffling steps. The pulse rate and temperature are elevated and the horse is obviously in pain. The muscles are not palpably abnormal. Lesser attacks are usually evident when the horse has cooled off after work; the signs are the same but less marked. SGOT levels are often as high as 4000 SF units, normal horses rarely go above 600 (occasionally to 1000) SF units after exercise (5). SGOT is a fairly non-specific enzyme although it is largely influenced by skeletal muscle status. Serum creatine phosphokinase and aspartate aminotransferase levels in serum are the best indicators, the former peaking 4–8 hours after exercise, the latter at 24–48 hours (10). They are sensitive and reliable indicators of muscle cell damage, rather than specifically skeletal muscle. Aldolase is fairly specific for muscle injury but lactic dehydrogenase is too non-specific (6). Susceptible horses often have suspiciously high serum enzyme levels at rest. Serum and urine myoglobin levels are directly related to the severity of the lesions and clinical signs (1).

An abnormality of mitochondria has been observed in a horse which was predisposed to the disease (12). The muscle stiffness passes off in 1–3 days depending on the severity of the attack. The serum enzymes subside irregularly, CPK levels being back to normal at 4–6 days but SGOT levels take 4–5 weeks to return to normal (7). There is still a large percentage of cases of 'tying-up' (it may be as many as 25%) in which there are no detectable changes in muscle enzymes. As set out in Chapter 2 under the heading of physical exercise, there is an increasing body of information on the biochemical effects of exercise and this should be referred to when assessing a case of 'tying-up' so that the appropriate examinations can be carried out.

The development of biochemical and biophysical profiles in racing horses are an urgent need for the investigation of performance potentials. Such examinations could also be added to routine physical examinations for soundness, and be carried out on horses which are under offer to sell, or horses coming back into training. They should also be included in a standard protocol for examination of those horses submitted for clinical examination and diagnosis as being 'thin horses' or 'horses performing below potential'.

With little justification, horses suffering from 'tying-up' myositis are treated with a combination of selenium and vitamin E. Spontaneous recovery occurs without treatment.

Grain or oat sickness

The existence of this entity depends on observations that individual horses on heavy grain diets develop a 'tying-up' syndrome which can be alleviated by reducing the grain intake or by administering 30–60 g magnesium sulfate daily in the feed (2). The characteristic stiffness and restriction of movement are most noticeable 1–2 hours after exercise.

Verminous arteritis/iliac thrombosis

This is a well-known disease. The development of weakness and incoordination during fast work, the obvious pain, lack of sweating, diminution of pulse amplitude in the internal iliac arteries on rectal examination and the volar digital arteries, and lack of warmth in the skin of the affected limb are the diagnostic features. There may be an abnormality of gait while walking and failure of the superficial veins to distend normally.

Spondylopathy

The early stages or mild forms of enzootic incoordination due to repeated contusion of the cervical spinal cord may resemble 'tying-up' and is described elsewhere. There are in addition other poorly defined syndromes caused by damage to the spinal cord and pressure to or irritation of dorsal spinal nerve roots (2). Causes of such pressure include vertebral dislocation, fracture or osteoarthritis, or abscess or hematoma. The stiffness and pain which result can be relieved by anti-inflammatory and painkilling agents.

Neuritis of the cauda equina

This is characterized by paralysis of the tail, loss of tone of the anal sphincter, distention of the rectal ampulla, paralysis of the bladder and cutaneous anesthesia of the tail, perineum and caudal upper parts of the hindlegs as reflected by an absence of anal and cutaneous reflexes. The animal has difficulty urinating and defecating and there is an associated weakness and incoordination of gait in the hindlimbs (8). It has been suggested that the lesion may have an etiological relationship to the 'wind-sucking' that occurs in some horses (2). There is a non-suppurative inflammation of nerve trunks of the cauda equina (9) and there may be concurrent cranial nerve neuropathies of one or more cranial nerves. Lesions of the cauda equina can be diagnosed using an ELISA test based on proteins derived from bovine or equine myelin as an antigen (13).

Degenerative arthritis

Mild cases of osteodystrophia fibrosa still occur but knowledge of the disease has resulted in its virtual elimination by dietary management. A number of cases of degenerative arthritis still occur (2). They represent a problem dealt with in surgical textbooks, and are mentioned here only as additions to the list of diagnostic possibilities.

REFERENCES

(1) Watanabe, H. et al. (1978) *Exp. Rep. equ. Hlth Lab. (Japan)*, *15*, 79.
(2) Steel, J. D. (1969) *Aust. vet. J.*, *45*, 162.
(3) Lindholm, A. et al. (1974) *Acta vet. Scand.*, *15*, 325.
(4) Wagner, P. C. et al. (1977) *J. equ. med. Surg.*, *1*, 282.
(5) Hansen, M. A. (1970) *Nord. VetMed.*, *22*, 617.
(6) Gerber, H. (1969) *Equ. vet. J.*, *1*, 129.
(7) Lindholm, A. (1972) *Svensk VetTidn.*, *24*, 871.
(8) Rousseaux, C. G. et al. (1984) *Can. vet. J.*, *25*, 214.
(9) Scarratt, W. K. & Jortner, B. S. (1985) *Comp. cont. Educ.*, 7, S197.
(10) McEwen, S. A. & Hulland, T. J. (1986) *Vet. Pathol.*, *23*, 400.
(11) Edington, N. et al. (1984) *Res. vet. Sci.*, *37*, 252.
(12) van den Hoven, R. et al. (1986) *Equ. vet. J.*, *18*, 418.
(13) Fordyce, P. S. et al. (1987) *Equ. vet. J.*, *19*, 55.

'Acorn' calves

A non-inherited condition has been described in the United States and Australia (1) which bears some resemblance to inherited dwarfism. The disease occurs on poor range country and is thought to be due to a maternal nutritional deficiency during the middle trimester of pregnancy. The specific dietary factors involved have not been determined although supplementary feeding during pregnancy eliminates the condition. Osseous development of the head is abnormal with either a shortened or long, narrow head. Shortening of the shafts of the long bones of the limbs is accompanied by bending of the joints, and calves nurse and stand with difficulty. Incoordination, arching of the back and a tendency to bloat, which may cause death, also occur. The dentition is normal. Muscle spasticity, wry neck, circling, falling backwards and goose-stepping occur rarely. Most of the calves are born alive and, in badly affected herds, as many as 15% of calves may be affected. The condition derives its name from the common occurrence of acorns in the diet of affected herds, although the acorns are not thought to have any etiological significance.

REFERENCE

(1) Barry, M. R. & Murphy, W. J. B. (1964) *Aust. vet. J.*, *40*, 195.

Spider lamb syndrome

A congenital osteopathy is recorded in Suffolk and Hampshire lambs (1, 2) in which the limbs are thin, disproportionately long and have abnormal positions of the bones about the joints causing abnormalities of posture. There is also less muscle than normal. In severe cases the deformities are obvious at birth and may be lethal. In less severe cases the deformities do not become apparent until the lambs are several weeks old. Spinal deformities, especially kyphoscoliosis, are observed in some sheep. The cause is unknown but inheritance seems probable.

REFERENCES

(1) Vanek, J. A. et al. (1986) *Vet. Med.*, *81*, 663.
(2) Rook, J. S. et al. (1986) *Comp. cont. Educ.*, *8*, S402.

Slipped capital femoral epiphysis in calves

This condition occurs in newborn calves of the well-muscled, rapidly growing European breeds such as the Charolais, Maine-Anjou and Simmental. It is characterized by varying degrees of lameness, palpable crepitus over the greater trochanter on passive manipulation of the affected limb, muscle atrophy in longstanding cases, and prolonged recumbency. Some calves carry the affected limb or drag the foot, whereas others tolerate slight weight-bearing during standing or walking. Most calves are lame at birth or within a few days after birth. About 75% of cases are associated with a dystocia and forced traction delivery (1). Radiographically, there are varying degrees of displacement of the femoral neck from the head. In chronic cases there is partial resorption of the femoral head. Excision arthroplasty has been attempted with some encouraging results.

The disease must be differentiated from perinatal femoral nerve degeneration and neurogenic atrophy of the quadriceps femoris muscle which also occurs most commonly in the same breeds of cattle. The right hindleg is most commonly affected and affected calves are unable to bear weight on the leg, and there is obvious neurogenic atrophy of the quadriceps muscle (2). There is no known effective treatment.

REFERENCES

(1) Hamilton, G. F. et al. (1978) *J. Am. vet. med. Assoc.*, *172*. 1318.
(2) Tryphonas, L. et al. (1974). *J. Am. vet. med. Assoc.*, *164*, 801.

DISEASES CHARACTERIZED BY INVOLVEMENT OF THE SKIN

Pityriasis rosea

This skin disease of pigs resembles ringworm closely but skin scrapings do not reveal the presence of fungal hyphae or spores, and cultures for fungal growth are usually negative. Treatment with standard preparations used for ringworm is usually ineffective although spontaneous recovery may occur.

The disease occurs in sucking pigs (1) and young pigs in the 10–14-weeks age group. Up to 50% of each litter may be affected and in large groups of feeder pigs there may be only individual pigs or the majority of the group with lesions. The disease is usually innocuous although digestive disturbances, particularly anorexia and, to a lesser extent, diarrhea and vomiting may accompany the appearance of lesions and affected pigs lose some body weight. There is no fever.

Lesions occur most commonly on the ventral abdomen but may spread to the rest of the body. They commence as small, red nodules which enlarge to flat plaques and become covered with thin, dry, brown scales. The lesions appear to enlarge centrifugally leaving a center of normal appearance surrounded by a narrow zone of elevated, erythematous skin covered by typical scales. Individual lesions are generally circular except that they often coalesce to produce a large, irregular lesion. There is little irritation and the skin lesions, although obvious, are superficial. There is no loss of bristles.

The cause is unknown although there is strong evidence of familial susceptibility, either through inheritance or by vertical transmission of an infectious agent (2, 3). Transmission experiments have been unsuccessful and the disease has been observed in SPF pigs produced by cesarean section (4). By analogy with a similar condition affecting man, it may be a viral infection. Treatment appears to be completely ineffective but in general consists of the local application of a salve containing 5% salicylic or iodized mineral oil. Affected pigs should be isolated from the group. Spontaneous recovery occurs in 6–8 weeks in most instances.

REFERENCES

(1) Thomson, R. (1960) *Can. vet. J.*, *1*, 449.
(2) Wellman, G. (1963) *Berl. Münch. Tierärztl. Wochenschr.*, 107.
(3) Corcoran, C. J. (1964) *Vet. Rec.*, *76*, 1407.
(4) McDermid, K. A. (1964) *Can. vet. J.*, *5*, 95.

Anhidrosis (non-sweating syndrome, puff disease, dry coat)

Anhidrosis is a disease characterized by absence of sweating, occurring mainly in horses, and less commonly in cattle.

Etiology

The disease is basically a failure in adaptation to a hot climate. Work done in horses suggests that although blockage of sweat gland ducts occurs this is a secondary lesion and that the basic disturbance is one of insensitivity of sweat glands to adrenaline, the sweat glands having been conditioned by persistent high blood adrenaline levels caused by exposure to consistently high environmental temperatures (2). In cattle the capacity of animals reared in temperate climates to adapt themselves to tropical conditions appears to be quite strongly inherited. This may or may not be the case in horses.

Epidemiology

The disease occurs most commonly in horses in countries with hot, humid climates including India, Indonesia, Sri Lanka, Burma, Malaysia, Australia, Puerto Rico, Trinidad, and the Gulf of Mexico coast in the United States (7). It is most severe in hot summer months, if seasons occur in the area. Males and females are equally affected. Indigenous horses may be affected and the prevalence in them may be as high as in imported horses but there is more concern because of their greater capital value. The major problem is in racehorses imported into tropical areas from temperate climates. A similar condition has been described in cattle (1). The indigenous animals, particularly zebus and their crosses, are unaffected and stock imported for breeding purposes present the major difficulty. High-producing dairy cows are more susceptible than other types. Affected animals rarely die of the disease but are seriously incapacitated and may have to be returned to cooler climates if they are to function efficiently.

Pathogenesis

The failure of the sweating mechanism results in reduction of heat loss from the body and a rise in body temperature, particularly on exercise. Respiration is stimulated by the need for heat dissipation by other routes and the resulting dyspnea may be so severe that the animal is unable to function efficiently.

Clinical findings

In the early stages in horses, excessive sweating and dyspnea after exercise are observed. The skin area over which sweating can be observed is gradually reduced over a period of weeks until sweating can be observed only under the mane. In addition, the skin becomes dry and scurfy and loses its elasticity, and there may be alopecia, especially of the face. Dyspnea may become extreme, and the animals continually seek the shade. The animals become thin, and exercise tolerance declines to the point where any sort of work is impossible. Death from heart failure may occur if exercise is forced. High body temperatures are observed after exercise, sometimes reaching 41·5–42°C (107–108°F) and persist for long periods. At this stage, the disease is analogous to heat stroke. If animals are returned to cool climates, the condition gradually disappears.

Clinical pathology

Blood chloride levels are low and blood adrenaline levels are high but these observations are unlikely to be used in clinical diagnosis. Normal horses respond to an intradermal injection of adrenaline by sweating at the site of the injection of a dilute solution, e.g., one in a million. Badly affected horses do not sweat in response to an injection and moderately affected horses respond only to more concentrated solutions, e.g., one in a thousand (3). Skin biopsies reviewed under electron microscopy show atrophy of the sweat glands and other abnormalities indicative of progressive secretory failure (6).

Necropsy findings

There are no characteristic lesions at necropsy.

Treatment and control

Treatment is empirical because of the doubtful etiology of the disease. An adequate salt intake should be maintained, and in severe cases intravenous injections of physiological saline are recommended. The ration should contain adequate green feed. The feeding of iodinated casein (containing 0·72% 1-thyroxin) is claimed to cure the disease in horses when given in daily doses of 10–15 g for 4–8 days and good results are reported after the use of thyroid gland extract (50 g daily for 20 days) (4). The daily administration orally of 1000–3000 units of vitamin E is also reported to be effective (5). Removal of affected animals to cooler climates is often necessary, although air conditioning of stables and maintenance of horses in higher country where they can be returned after a day's racing may enable susceptible horses to be kept locally (1).

REVIEW LITERATURE

Warner, A. & Mayhew, I. G. (1983) Equine anhidrosis: a review of pathophysiologic mechanisms. *Vet. res. Commun.*, 6, 249–264.

REFERENCES

(1) Stewart, C. M. (1956) *Irish vet. J.*, *10*, 189, 208.
(2) Evans, C. L. (1966) *Br. vet. J.*, *122*, 117.
(3) Currie, A. K. & Seager, S. W. J. (1976) *Proc. 22nd ann. Conv. AAEP*, p. 249.
(4) Correa, J. E. & Calderin, G. G. (1966) *J. Am. vet. med. Assoc.* *149*, 1556.
(5) Marsh, J. H. (1961) *Vet. Rec.*, *73*, 1124.
(6) Jenkinson, D. M. et al. (1985) *Equ. vet. J.*, *17*, 287.
(7) Warner, D. E. & Mayhew, I. G. (1982) *J. Am. vet. med. Assoc.*, *180*, 627.

'Cancer eye' (squamous cell carcinoma of eye)

This is a common neoplasm of the eyelids and the eyeball of cattle and is best known by its colloquial name of 'cancer eye'. The initial lesion may be on the eyelid or any structure in the conjunctival sac, except the avascular cornea or pigmented eyelid. They can encroach on these tissues from others nearby, carrying a blood supply with them.

The lesions develop through three stages. The first two, a plaque and then a papilloma, are non-malignant and have high regression rates. The third stage is the squamous cell carcinoma which does not regress. The carcinomas develop most commonly on the third eyelid or the corneal limbus. They grow rapidly and are actively invasive often metastasizing to the local lymph nodes. Primary lesions of the lids are most likely to metastasize to these nodes.

The etiology is not well understood but is obviously multifactorial. The carcinoma is probably a papilloma-associated tumor because papilloma virus can be found in the precursor lesions and papillomavirus DNA in the carcinomas (20). Bovine herpesvirus-5 has also been suggested as a causative agent because of its presence in bovine ocular lesions (18). Heredity plays some part and Hereford cattle are more commonly affected than other beef breeds and Ayrshires appear to be the most susceptible dairy breed (1). But the relative importance of heredity, lack of pigment in the eye structures, sunlight and viruses is still uncertain (8). Nutritional status also seems to affect the rate of occurrence of the disease. Animals do not appear to develop resistance to the cancer; only two of 35 cows with the disease had measurable antibodies in their sera (2). It is one of the characteristics of this disease that the carcinomas appear to produce immunosuppressive substances. Removal of tumor mass reduces blood levels of these immunosuppressive substances (20). An occurrence rate of 14% is recorded in cattle on a high-level feed intake while the rate was 1·5% in cattle on low-level feed intake.

Because of the strong correlation between absence of pigmentation of the eyelids and the occurrence of the disease, and because of the high heritability of this pigmentation in Hereford cattle it is suggested that a breeding program aimed at increasing the degree of pigmentation of eyelids could quickly reduce the incidence of the disease in this breed (1). A positive approach to the problem would be to crossbreed susceptible *Bos taurus* cattle with *Bos indicus* cattle which always have pigmented eyelids and have much less eye cancer (3). In Ayrshires there is a corresponding predilection for squamous cell carcinomata of the vulva, but the neoplasm does not occur on both sites in the one cow. However, selection on the basis of the occurrence of lesions results in only limited reduction in incidence. Treatment of early bovine cases by excision, especially by cryosurgery (6), is often successful and treatment by the use of radioactive implants has also aroused favorable comment. Radical surgery, including removal of the local lymph nodes and parts of the salivary gland, may be desirable in some bovine cases (15). It is often combined with immunotherapy, for example, with BCG vaccination.

Other treatments which have received favorable comment, but need to be evaluated in the light of the known natural recovery rate of the benign precursor lesions, are electrothermal hyperthermia (13) and non-specific immunotherapy, usually with BCG vaccine injected systemically or into the lesion (7). That there is a significant immune body response at the normal tissue–corneal interface has been demonstrated (4), but whether this plays any part in the rejection of the tumors is not known. One controlled trial in cattle showed that intralesional injection of BCG vaccine can interrupt neoplastic progression and prevent malignant disease (16). In horses treatment is largely surgical but all of the above techniques have been used. So has local irradiation therapy with ^{90}Sr or ^{222}Rn (17).

A favorable response to a single injection of a saline phenol extract of fresh tumor tissue has been reported, and a well-controlled trial has reported a high rate of regression of tumors after vaccination (11) with a higher recovery rate after the use of 200 mg of lyophilized tumor extract as compared to an injection of 100 mg. The injection may need to be repeated (11).

Some tumors show enhancement of growth after vaccination, especially if it is repeated (10). The vaccine does not need to be autologous, and only one injection is required. A freeze-dried preparation of tumor antigen has been used successfully. In general, the use of a vaccine seems likely to provide a satisfactory method for controlling an esthetically distressing and financially important disease.

One of the difficulties encountered in the field is the clinical differentiation of benign precursor lesions from the malignant carcinomas and failure to do so may account for the high rates of spontaneous regression recorded, especially in Hereford cattle (12), where a spontaneous recovery rate of 88% is recorded. To avoid this inaccuracy, exfoliative cytology by the examination of smears of lesions is helpful. Combined with a clinical assessment this is the recommended method of confirming the diagnosis (5).

In countries and in herds where ocular carcinoma is common, it is not unusual to encounter lesions on the labia of the vulva especially if there are patches of unpigmented skin (19).

REVIEW LITERATURE

Spradbrow, P. B. (1984) Cancer eye. Treatment and prevention. *Univ. Syd. Postgrad. Comm. vet. Sci. Proc. Refr. Course No. 68*, p. 171.

Spradbrow, P. B. & Hoffman, D. (1980) Bovine ocular squamous cell carcinoma. *Vet. Bull.*, *50*, 449.

REFERENCES

(1) Hunermund, G. (1973) *Berl. Münch. Tierärztl. Wochenschr.*, *86*, 414.
(2) Dennis, M. W. et al. (1985) *Am. J. vet. Res.*, *46*, 1975.
(3) Nishimura, H. & Frisch, J. E. (1977) *J. exp. Agric. Anim. Husb.*, *17*, 709.
(4) Hamir, A. N. J. etal. (1980) *J. comp. Pathol.*, *90*, 535.
(5) Hoffman, D. et al. (1978) *J. comp. Pathol.*, *88*, 497.
(6) Ferris, H. E. & Frauenfelder, F. T. (1976) *J. Am. vet. med. Assoc.*, *168*, 213.
(7) Kleinschuster, S. J. et al. (1977) *J. Natl Cancer Inst.*, *58*, 1807.
(8) Russell, W. C. et al. (1976) *J. anim. Sci.*, *43*, 1156.
(9) Spradbrow, P. B. (1986) *Aust. Adv. vet. Sci.*, p. 51.
(10) Fivaz, B. H. (1978) *Rhod. vet. J.*, *9*, 24.
(11) Hoffman, D. et al. (1981) *Aust. vet. J.*, *57*, 159.
(12) Taylor, R. L. & Hanks, M. A. (1972) *Vet. Med. small Anim. Clin.*, *67*, 669.
(13) Grier, R. L. et al. (1980) *J. Am. vet. med. Assoc.*, 177, 55.
(14) Heeney, J. L. & Valli, V. E. O. (1985) *Can. J. comp. Med.*, *49*, 21.
(15) Klein, W. R. et al. (1984) *Vet. Surg.*, *13*, 236.
(16) Kleinschuster, S. J. et al. (1983) *J. Natl Cancer Inst.*, *70*, 771.
(17) Frauenfelder, H. C. et al. (1982) *J. Am. vet. med. Assoc.*, 307 & 310.
(18) Anson, M. A. et al. (1982) *Can. J. comp. Med.*, *46*, 334.
(19) Omara-Opeyne, A. L. et al. (1984) *Kenya Vet.*, *8*, 5.

'Cockle'

This is a disease of the skin of sheep recorded only in New Zealand (1). Lesions commence on the neck and shoulders and may extend over the entire pelt. The lesions are worst in unshorn sheep; they are inflammatory nodules, possibly allergic in origin but their response to diazinon suggests that the primary cause is parasitic. Diazinon (0·04%) applied as shower dip, tip spray or plunge dip protected sheep for 6 months, and cured affected sheep within 3 weeks. Treated sheep made a significantly greater weight gain than untreated sheep (2, 3).

REFERENCES

(1) Dempsey, M. et al. (1972) *NZ J. agric. Res.*, *15*, 741.
(2) Dempsey, M. et al. (1974) *NZ J. agric. Res.*, *17*, 423.
(3) Dempsey, M. et al. (1975) *NZ J. exp. Agric.*, *3*, 305.

Wool slip

This is a condition in which housed ewes lose part of their fleece and develop bald patches over a large area of the rear half of the back (1). There is no systemic disease; the skin is normal and the wool regrows immediately. The sheep are shorn in winter and the lesions begin to develop 2–3 weeks later. All breeds are equally susceptible; up to 40% of a flock may be affected. The wool loss occurs because of a premature and synchronized shedding of wool fibers and not a pathological process which damages the wool fiber. The current explanation for the wool shedding is that blood corticosteroid levels rise after the stress of shearing and are maintained for a long period because of the trauma of being housed and shorn and kept in the cold. Prevention is aimed at lessening these traumas and arranging for them to be kept together and not spread out in time.

REFERENCE

(1) Morgan, K. L. et al. (1986) *Vet. Rec.*, *119*, 621.

Conversion Tables

CONVERSION FACTORS FOR OLD AND SI UNITS

	Old units	Multiplication factors: Old units to SI units	Multiplication factors: SI units to old units	SI units
RBC	$\times 10^6/mm^3$	10^6	10^{-6}	$\times 10^{12}/l$
PCV	%	0·01	100	l/l
Hb	g/dl	None	None	g/dl
MCV	μ^3	None	None	fl
MCH	$\mu\mu g$	None	None	pg
MCHC	%	None	None	g/dl
WBC	$\times 10^3/mm^3$	10^6	10^{-6}	$\times 10^9/l$
Platelets	$\times 10^3/mm^3$	10^6	10^{-6}	$\times 10^9/l$
Total serum protein	g/dl	10	0·1	g/l
Albumin	g/dl	10	0·1	g/l
Bicarbonate	mEq/l	None	None	mmol/l
Bilirubin	mg/dl	17·1	0·0585	μmol/l
Calcium	mg/dl	0·25	4·008	mmol/l
Chloride	mEq/l	None	None	mmol/l
Cholesterol	mg/dl	0·0259	38·7	mmol/l
Copper	μg/dl	0·157	6·35	μmol/l
Cortisol	μg/dl	27·6	0·0362	nmol/l
Creatinine	mg/dl	88·4	0·0113	μmol/l
Globulin	g/dl	10	0·1	g/l
Glucose	mg/dl	0·0555	18·02	mmol/l
Inorganic phosphate	mg/dl	0·323	3·10	mmol/l
Iron	μg/dl	0·179	5·59	μmol/l
Lead	μg/dl	0·0483	20·7	μmol/l
Magnesium	mg/dl	0·411	2·43	mmol/l
Molybdenum	μg/dl	0·104	9·6	μmol/l
Potassium	mEq/l	None	None	mmol/l
Selenium	μg/dl	0·126	7·9	μmol/l
Sodium	mEq/l	None	None	mmol/l
Triglyceride	mg/dl	0·0113	88·5	mmol/l
Urea	mg/dl	0·166	6·01	mmol/l
Zinc	μg/dl	0·152	6·54	μmol/l

CONVERSIONS

To convert grams per 100 ml into grains per US fluid ounce, multiply by 4·564.
To convert grams per 100 ml into grains per Imperial fluid ounce, multiply by 4·385.
To convert grams into ounces avoirdupois, multiply by 10 and divide by 283.
To convert liters into US pints, multiply by 2·114.
To convert liters into Imperial pints, multiply by 88 and divide by 50.
To convert kilos into pounds, multiply by 1000 and divide by 454.

MASS

Metric

1 kilogram (kg) = 15 432 grains
or 35·274 ounces
or 2·2046 pounds
1 gram (g) = 15·432 grains
1 milligram (mg) = 0·015432 grain

US/Imperial

1 ton (2240 lb) = 1016 kilograms
1 hundredweight (112 lb) (cwt) = 50·80 kilograms
1 stone (14 lb) (st) = 6·35 kilograms
1 pound (avoirdupois) (lb) = 453·59 grams
1 ounce (avoirdupois) (oz) = 28·35 grams
1 grain (gr) = 64·799 milligrams

CAPACITY

Metric

1 liter (l) = 2·114 US pints = 1·7598 Imperial pints
1 milliliter (ml) = 16·23 US minims = 16·894 Imperial minims

US Liquid

1 gallon (128 fl oz) (gal) = 3·785 liters
1 pint (pt) = 473·17 milliliters
1 fluid ounce (fl oz) = 29·573 milliliters
1 fluid dram (fl dr) = 3·696 milliliters
1 minim (min) = 0·061610 milliliters

Imperial

1 gallon (160 fl oz) (gal) = 4·546 liters
1 pint (pt) = 568·25 milliliters
1 fluid ounce (fl oz) = 28·412 milliliters
1 fluid drachm (fl dr) = 3·5515 milliliters
1 minim (min) = 0·059192 milliliters

LENGTH

Metric

1 kilometer (km) = 0·621 miles
1 meter (m) = 39·370 inches
1 decimeter (dm) = 3·9370 inches
1 centimeter (cm) = 0·39370 inch
1 millimeter (mm) = 0·039370 inch
1 micrometer (μm) = 0·000039370 inch

US/Imperial

1 miles = 1·609 kilometers
1 yard = 0·914 meters
1 foot = 30·48 centimeters
1 inch = 2·54 centimeters
or 25·40 millimeters

TEMPERATURE

Celsius (Centigrade)	*Fahrenheit*
110°	230°
100	212
95	203
90	194
85	185
80	176
75	167
70	158
65	149
60	140
55	131
50	122
45	113
44	111·2
43	109·4
42	107·6
41	105·8
40·5	104·9
40	104·0
39·5	103·1
39	102·2
38·5	101·3

Celsius (Centigrade)	*Fahrenheit*
38°	100·4°
37·5	99·5
37	98·6
36·5	97·7
36	96·8
35·5	95·9
35	95·0
34	93·2
33	91·4
32	89·6
31	87·8
30	86
25	77
20	68
15	59
10	50
+5	41
0	32
−5	23
−10	14
−15	+5
−20	−4

To convert Fahrenheit into Celsius, subtract 32, multiply the remainder by 5, and divide the result by 9.
To convert Celsius into Fahrenheit, multiply by 9, divide by 5, and add 32.

Normal Laboratory Values

Normal values of laboratory data are offered as a guide and the reader must be aware that values may vary depending on the sex, age and geographical habitat of the animal and on the laboratory. These tables are normal values used at the Western College of Veterinary Medicine, University of Saskatchewan, and have been compiled from the clinical laboratory, Department of Pathology; from O.W. Schalm, N.C. Jain and E.J. Carroll (1975) *Veterinary Hematology*, 3rd ed. Philadelphia: Lea & Febiger; and from J.J. Kaneko (1980) *Clinical Biochemistry of Domestic Animals*, 3rd ed. New York: Academic Press. Courtesy G.P. Seancy, Department of Veterinary Pathology, University of Saskatchewan.

HEMATOLOGY

	Ox	*Sheep*	*Goat*	*Swine*	*Horse*
Hemoglobin (g/dl)	8·0–15·0	9·0–15·0	8·0–12·0	10·0–16·0	11·0–19·0
PCV (%)	24·0–46·0	27·0–45·0	22–38·0	32·0–50·0	32·0–53·0
RBC ($\times 10^6/\mu l$)	5·0–10·0	9·0–15·0	8·0–18·0	5·0–8·0	6·8–12·9
MCV (fl)	40·0–60·0	28·0–40·0	16·0–25·0	50·0–68·0	37·0–58·5
MCH (pg)	11·0–17·0	8·0–12·0	5·2–8·0	17·0–21·0	12·3–19·7
MCHC (g/dl)	30·0–36·0	31·0–34·0	30·0–36·0	30·0–34·0	31·0–38·6
Thrombocytes ($\times 10^5/\mu l$)	1·0–8·0	2·5–7·5	3·0–6·0	3·2–5·2	1·0–3·5
WBC ($/\mu l$)	4000–12 000	4000–12 000	4000–13 000	11 000–22 000	5400–14 300
Neutrophils (mature) ($/\mu l$)	600–4000	700–6000	1200–7200	3080–10 450	2260–8580
Neutrophils (bands) ($/\mu l$)	0–120	Rare	Rare	0–880	0–100
Lymphocytes ($/\mu l$)	2500–7500	2000–9000	2000–9000	4290–13 640	1500–7700
Monocytes ($/\mu l$)	25–840	0–750	0–550	200–2200	0–1000
Eosinophils ($/\mu l$)	0–2400	0–1000	0–650	55–2420	0–1000
Basophils ($/\mu l$)	0–200	0–300	0–120	0–440	0–290
Plasma proteins (g/dl)	6·6–7·8	6·0–7·5	6·0–7·5	6·0–8·0	5·8–8·7
Fibrinogen (mg/dl)	300–700	100–500	100–400	100–500	100–400

International System of Units (SI)

	Ox	*Sheep*	*Goat*	*Swine*	*Horse*
Hemoglobin (g/l)	80–150	90–150	80–120	100–160	110–190
PCV (l/l)	0·24–0·46	0·27–0·45	0·22–0·38	0·32–0·50	0·32–0·53
RBC ($\times 10^{12}/l$)	5·0–10·0	9·0–15·0	8·0–18·0	5·0–8·0	6·8–12·9
MCV (fl)	40–60	28–40	16·0–25·0	50–68	37–58
MCH (pg)	11–17	8–12	5·2–8·0	17–21	12–20
MCHC (g/l)	300–360	310–340	300–360	300–340	310–386
Thrombocytes ($\times 10^9/l$)	100–800	250–750	300–600	320–520	100–350
WBC ($\times 10^9/l$)	4·0–12·0	4·0–12·0	4·0–13·0	11·0–22·0	5·4–14·0
Neutrophils (mature) ($\times 10^9/l$)	0·6–4·0	0·7–6·0	1·2–7·2	3·0–10·0	2·3–8·5
Neutrophils (bands) ($\times 10^9/l$)	0–0·1	Rare	Rare	0–0·8	0–0·1
Lymphocytes ($\times 10^9/l$)	2·0–7·0	2·0–9·0	2·0–9·0	4·2–13·6	1·5–7·7
Monocytes ($\times 10^9/l$)	0–0·8	0–0·8	0–0·55	0·2–2·2	0–1·0
Eosinophils ($\times 10^9/l$)	0–2·0	0–1·0	0–0·65	0·5–2·4	0–1·0
Basophils ($\times 10^9/l$)	0–0·2	0–0·3	0–0·12	0–0·4	0–2·9
Plasma proteins (g/l)	66–78	60–75	60–75	60–80	58–87
Fibrinogen (g/l)	3–7	1–5	1–4	1–5	1–4

CHEMISTRY

	Ox	*Sheep*	*Swine*	*Horse*
Sodium (mEq/l)	132–152	145–160	140–150	132–150
Potassium (mEq/l)	3·9–5·8	4·8–5·9	4·7–7·1	3·0–5·0
Chloride (mEq/l)	95–110	98–110	100–105	98–110
P_{CO_2} (mmHg)	34–45	38		38–46
pH	7·35–7·50	7·32–7·50		7·32–7·55
HCO_3^- (mmol/l)	20–30	21–28	18–27	23–32
Anion gap (mEq/l)	14–26	12–24	10–25	10–25
Calcium (mg/dl)	8·0–10·5	11·5–13·0	11·0–11·3	11·2–13·8
Phosphorus (mg/dl)	4·0–7·0	4·0–7·0	4·0–11·0	3·1–5·6
Magnesium (mg/dl)	1·2–3·5	1·9–2·5	1·9–3·9	1·8–2·5
Iron ($\mu g/dl$)	57–162	166–222	73–140	91–199

Urea (mg/dl)	6·0–27	8·0–20	8·0–24	10–20
Creatinine (mg/dl)	1·0–2·7	1·2–1·9	1·0–2·7	1·2–1·9
Glucose (mg/dl)	35–55	30–65	65–95	60–100
Cholesterol (mg/dl)	39–177	40–58	117–119	46–177
Total bilirubin (mg/dl)	0–1·9	0–0·4	0–0·2	0·2–6·0
Direct bilirubin (mg/dl)	0–0·4	0–0·3		0–0·4
Alkaline phosphatase (iu/l)	35–350	68–387		95–233
AST (SGOT) (iu/l)	60–150	260–350	25–57	200–400
Creatine phosphokinase (CPK) (iu/dl)	65	65	65	65
SDH (iu/l)	0–15			0–15
γ-Glutamyltransferase (iu/l)	0–31	0–70	0–25	0–25
Total protein (g/dl)	5·7–8·1	6·0–7·9	3·5–6·0	6·0–7·7
Albumin (g/dl)	2·1–3·6	2·4–3·0	1·9–2·4	2·9–3·8
α_1-Globulin (g/dl)	0·7–1·2	3·0–6·0	1·0–1·3	0·7–1·3
α_2-Globulin (g/dl)		3·0–6·0		0·7–1·3
β-Globulin (g/dl)	0·6–1·2	1·1–2·6	0·8–1·1	0·4–1·2
γ-Globulin (g/dl)	1·6–3·2	0·9–3·3	0·3–0·7	0·9–1·5

International System of Units (SI)

	Ox	*Sheep*	*Swine*	*Horse*
Sodium (mmol/l)	132–152	145–160	140–150	132–150
Potassium (mmol/l)	3·9–5·8	4·8–5·9	4·7–7·1	3·0–5·0
Chloride (mmol/l)	95–110	98–110	100–105	98–110
$P\text{CO}_2$ (mmHg)	34–45	38		38–46
pH	7·35–7·50	7·32–7·50		7·32–7·55
HCO_3^- (mmol/l)	20–30	21–28	18–27	23–32
Calcium (mmol/l)	2·00–2·62	2·86–3·24	2·74–2·82	2·80–3·44
Phosphorus (mmol/l)	1·30–2·25	1·30–2·25	1·30–3·55	1·00–1·80
Magnesium (mmol/l)	0·50–1·44	0·78–1·02	0·78–1·60	0·74–1·02
Iron (μmol/l)	10–29	30–40	13–25	16–36
Urea (mmol/l)	2·0–9·5	3·0–7·0	3·0–8·5	3·5–7·0
Creatinine (μmol/l)	90–240	110–170	90–240	110–170
Glucose (mmol/l)	1·9–3·1	1·7–3·6	3·6–5·3	3·3–5·6
Cholesterol (mmol/l)	1·00–4·60	1·05–1·50	3·05–3·10	1·20–4·60
Total bilirubin (μmol/l)	0–32	0–6	0–4	4–102
Direct bilirubin (μmol/l)	0–6	0–6		0–6
Alkaline phosphatase (u/l)	35–350	68–387		95–233
AST (SGOT) (u/l)	60–150	260–350	25–57	200–400
Creatine kinase (CK) (u/l)	65	65	65	65
SDH (u/l)	0–15			0–15
γ-Glutamyltransferase (u/l)	0–31	0–70	0–25	0–25
Total protein (g/l)	57–81	60–79	35–60	60–77
Albumin (g/l)	21–36	24–30	19–24	29–38
α_1-Globulin (g/l)	7–12	3–6	10–13	7–13
α_2-Globulin (g/l)		3–6		7–13
β-Globulin (g/l)	6–12	11–26	8–11	4–12
γ-Globulin (g/l)	16–32	9–33	3–7	9–15

Index

Page numbers in **bold** type indicate principal references, those in *italic* type refer to tables

I

M

Q

R

T

U

V